VASCULAR SURGERY

VASCULAR SURGERY

FIFTH EDITION

ROBERT B. RUTHERFORD, M.D., F.A.C.S., F.R.C.S. (Glasg.)

Emeritus Professor of Surgery

University of Colorado School of Medicine

Denver, Colorado

W.B. SAUNDERS COMPANY
A Division of Harcourt Brace & Company
Philadelphia   London   Sydney   Toronto

W.B. SAUNDERS COMPANY
A Division of Harcourt Brace & Company

The Curtis Center
Independence Square West
Philadelphia, Pennsylvania 19106

Library of Congress Cataloging-in-Publication Data

Vascular surgery [edited by] Robert B. Rutherford. —5th ed.

p.   cm.

Includes bibliographical references and index.

ISBN 0–7216–8078–X (set)

1. Blood-vessels—Surgery.   I. Rutherford, Robert B.

[DNLM: 1. Vascular Surgical Procedures.   WG 170 V3311 2000]
RD598.5.V37 2000

617.4'13—dc21

DNLM/DLC   98–52324

ISBN 0-7216-8078-X
Vol. 1 ISBN 0-7216-8100-X
Vol. 2 ISBN 0-7216-8101-8

VASCULAR SURGERY

Last digit is the print number: 9   8   7   6   5   4   3   2   1

To my wife Kay, who has sacrificed more than anyone, in lost time and patience strained, as I happily labored through all these editions.

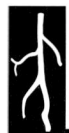 # EDITORS

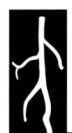

CONTRIBUTORS

ALI F. ABURAHMA, M.D.
Professor, Department of Surgery, West Virginia University School of Medicine and Robert C. Byrd Health Sciences Center. Chief, Vascular Section, and Medical Director, Vascular Laboratory, Charleston Area Medical Center, Charleston, West Virginia.
Causalgia and Post-traumatic Pain Syndromes

C. ALAN ANDERSON, M.D.
Assistant Professor of Neurology and Emergency Medicine, University of Colorado School of Medicine, Denver, Colorado.
Diagnosis, Evaluation, and Medical Management of Patients with Ischemic Cerebrovascular Disease

ENRICO ASCHER, M.D.
Professor of Surgery, State University of New York Health Science Center at Brooklyn. Director, Division of Vascular Surgery, Maimonides Medical Center, Brooklyn, New York.
Secondary Arterial Reconstructions in the Lower Extremity

J. DENNIS BAKER, M.D.
Professor of Surgery, University of California, UCLA School of Medicine. Chief, Vascular Surgery Section, West Los Angeles Veterans Affairs Medical Center, Los Angeles, California.
The Vascular Laboratory

WILLIAM H. BAKER, M.D., F.A.C.S.
Professor of Surgery, Loyola University Stritch School of Medicine. Chief, Division of Vascular Surgery, Loyola University Medical Center, Maywood, Illinois.
Arteriovenous Fistulae of the Aorta and Its Major Branches

JEFFREY L. BALLARD, M.D., F.A.C.S.
Associate Professor of Surgery, Loma Linda University School of Medicine. Program Director, Vascular Surgery Residency, and Medical Director, Noninvasive Vascular Laboratory, Loma Linda University Medical Center, Loma Linda, California.
Cervicothoracic Vascular Injuries

DENNIS F. BANDYK, M.D.
Professor of Surgery and Director, Division of Vascular Surgery, University of South Florida College of Medicine, Tampa, Florida.
Infection in Prosthetic Vascular Grafts

RICHARD A. BAUM, M.D.
Assistant Professor of Radiology, University of Pennsylvania School of Medicine, Philadelphia, Pennsylvania.
Magnetic Resonance Imaging and Angiography

B. TIMOTHY BAXTER, M.D.
Professor of Surgery, University of Nebraska College of Medicine. Chief of Vascular Surgery, Omaha Veterans Affairs Hospital, Omaha, Nebraska.
Arterial Aneurysms: Etiologic Considerations

MICHAEL BELKIN, M.D.
Associate Professor of Surgery, Harvard Medical School. Program Director in General Surgery, Brigham and Women's Hospital, Boston, Massachusetts.
Infrainguinal Bypass

MARSHALL E. BENJAMIN, M.D.
Vascular Fellow, Division of Surgical Sciences, Department of General Surgery, Wake Forest University School of Medicine, Winston-Salem, North Carolina.
Techniques of Operative Management

THOMAS M. BERGAMINI, M.D.
Associate Professor of Surgery, University of Louisville School of Medicine. Chief, Section of Vascular Surgery, Veterans Administration Medical Center, Louisville, Kentucky.
Long-Term Venous Access

JOHN J. BERGAN, M.D., F.A.C.S.
Professor of Surgery, University of California, San Diego, School of Medicine, San Diego; Loma Linda University School of Medicine, Loma Linda, California; and U.S. United Health Service, Bethesda, Maryland. Attending Surgeon, Scripps Memorial Hospital, La Jolla, California.
Adventitial Cystic Disease of the Popliteal Artery; Varicose Veins: Treatment by Surgery and Sclerotherapy

RAMON BERGUER, M.D., Ph.D.
Professor of Surgery, Wayne State University School of Medicine. Chief, Section of Vascular Surgery, Harper Hospital, Detroit, Michigan.
Vertebrobasilar Ischemia: Indications, Techniques, and Results of Surgical Repair

SCOTT S. BERMAN
Associate Professor of Biomedical Engineering and Associate Professor of Clinical Surgery, University of Arizona College of Medicine. Section Head, Vascular Surgery, Carondelet St. Mary's Hospital. Medical Director, Vascular Program, Tucson Heart Hospital, Tucson, Arizona.
Patient Evaluation and Preparation for Amputation

VICTOR M. BERNHARD, M.D.
Visiting Scholar, Department of Surgery, Section of Vascular Surgery, University of Chicago, Chicago, Illinois.
Profundaplasty

MICHAEL J. BLOCH, M.D.
Instructor, Department of Medicine, Division of Hypertension, Cornell University Medical College. Assistant Attending Physician, Department of Medicine, New York Presbyterian Hospital, New York, New York.
Renal Artery Imaging: Alternatives to Angiography

FRED BONGARD, M.D.
Professor of Surgery, University of California, Los Angeles, UCLA School of Medicine, Los Angeles. Chief, Division of Trauma and Critical Care, Department of Surgery, Harbor–UCLA Medical Center, Torrance, California.
Thoracic and Abdominal Vascular Trauma

THOMAS C. BOWER, M.D.
Associate Professor of Surgery, Mayo Graduate School of Medicine. Program Director, Vascular Surgery Fellowship Program, Mayo Clinic and Mayo Foundation, Rochester, Minnesota.
Diagnosis and Management of Tumors of the Inferior Vena Cava

DAVID C. BREWSTER, M.D.
Clinical Professor of Surgery, Harvard Medical School. Attending Surgeon, Division of Vascular Surgery, Massachusetts General Hospital, Boston, Massachusetts.
Prosthetic Grafts; Direct Reconstruction for Aortoiliac Occlusive Disease

JOHN G. CALAITGES, M.D.
Clinical Instructor in Surgery, University of Missouri–Columbia School of Medicine. Vascular Resident, University of Missouri–Columbia Hospitals and Clinics, Columbia, Missouri.
Principles of Hemostasis; Antithrombotic Therapy

KEITH D. CALLIGARO, M.D.
Associate Clinical Professor of Surgery, University of Pennsylvania School of Medicine. Chief, Section of Vascular Surgery, Pennsylvania Hospital, Philadelphia, Pennsylvania.
Renal Artery Aneurysms and Arteriovenous Fistulae

RICHARD P. CAMBRIA, M.D.
Associate Professor of Surgery Harvard Medical School. Visiting Surgeon, Massachusetts General Hospital, Boston, Massachusetts.
Thoracoabdominal Aortic Aneurysms

ROBERT A. CAMBRIA, M.D., F.A.C.S.
Associate Professor of Surgery, Medical College of Wisconsin, Milwaukee, Wisconsin.
Iatrogenic Complications of Arterial and Venous Catheterizations

MICHAEL T. CAPS, M.D., M.P.H.
Assistant Professor of Surgery, University of Washington School of Medicine, Seattle, Washington.
The Epidemiology of Vascular Trauma

JEFFREY P. CARPENTER, M.D.
Associate Professor of Surgery, University of Pennsylvania School of Medicine, Philadelphia, Pennsylvania.
Magnetic Resonance Imaging and Angiography

KENNETH J. CHERRY, JR., M.D.
Professor of Surgery, Mayo Medical School. Chair, Division of Vascular Surgery, Mayo Clinic, Rochester, Minnesota.
Arteriosclerotic Occlusive Disease of Brachiocephalic Arteries

JAE-SUNG CHO, M.D.
Senior Staff Surgeon, Henry Ford Hospital, Division of Vascular Surgery, Detroit, Michigan.
Surgical Treatment of Chronic Deep Venous Obstruction

G. PATRICK CLAGETT, M.D.
Jan and Bob Pickens Professor of Medical Science; Chairman, Division of Vascular Surgery, and Director, Center for Vascular Disease, University of Texas Southwestern Medical Center at Dallas. Chief of Vascular Surgery and Attending Staff, Zale Lipshy University Hospital and Parkland Memorial Hospital. Attending Staff, Vascular General Surgery, and Consulting Member, Department of Surgery, Children's Medical Center, Dallas, Texas.
Upper Extremity Aneurysms

ELIZABETH T. CLARK, M.D.
Chief, Section of Vascular Surgery, Catholic Health Partners, Chicago, Illinois.
Anastomotic and Other Pseudoaneurysms

ALEXANDER W. CLOWES, M.D.
Professor of Surgery, University of Washington School of Medicine. Attending Surgeon, University of Washington Medical Center, Seattle, Washington.
Pathologic Intimal Hyperplasia as a Response to Vascular Injury and Reconstruction

JON R. COHEN, M.D.
Professor of Surgery, Albert Einstein College of Medicine of Yeshiva University, Bronx, New York. Chairman, Department of Surgery, and Chief of Vascular Surgery, Long Island Jewish Medical Center, New Hyde Park, New York.
Ruptured Abdominal Aortic Aneurysms

ANTHONY J. COMEROTA, M.D., F.A.C.S.
Professor of Surgery, Department of Surgery, Temple University School of Medicine. Chief of Vascular Surgery, Temple University Hospital, Philadelphia, Pennsylvania.
Clinical and Diagnostic Evaluation of Deep Venous Thrombosis

DANIEL P. CONNELLY, M.D.
Assistant Professor of Surgery, Uniformed Services University of the Health Sciences, Bethesda, Maryland. Chairman, Department of Surgery, Overland Park Regional Medical Center, Overland Park, Kansas.
The Arterial Autograft

JOHN P. COOKE, M.D., Ph.D.
Associate Professor, Division of Cardiovascular Medicine, Stanford University School of Medicine, Stanford, California.
Atherogenesis and the Medical Management of Atherosclerosis

MICHAEL A. COOPER, M.D.
Assistant Clinical Professor, University of Colorado School of Medicine. Attending Physician, Rose Medical Center, Denver, Colorado.
Neurogenic Thoracic Outlet Syndrome

ENRIQUE CRIADO, M.D., F.A.C.S.
Associate Professor of Surgery, University of North Carolina at Chapel Hill, Chapel Hill, North Carolina. Head, Vascular Surgery Unit, Fundación Hospital de Alcorców, Madrid, Spain.
Physiologic Assessment of the Venous System

JACK L. CRONENWETT, M.D.
Professor of Surgery and Chief, Section of Vascular Surgery, Dartmouth Medical School, Hanover, New Hampshire, and Dartmouth-Hitchcock Medical Center, Lebanon, New Hampshire.
Overview, Section XII; Abdominal Aortic and Iliac Aneurysms

MICHAEL D. DAKE, M.D.
Associate Professor of Radiology and Medicine (Pulmonary), Stanford University School of Medicine. Chief, Cardiovascular and Interventional Radiology, Stanford University Hospital and UC San Francisco–Stanford Health Care, Stanford, California.
Radiographic Evaluation and Treatment of Renovascular Disease; Endovascular Treatment of Chronic Occlusions of Large Veins

HERBERT DARDIK, M.D.
Clinical Professor of Surgery, Mount Sinai School of Medicine of the City University of New York. Chief of Vascular Surgery, Englewood Hospital and Medical Center, Englewood, New Jersey.
Biologic Grafts for Lower Limb Revascularization

RICHARD H. DEAN, M.D.
Interim Vice-President for Health Affairs, Wake Forest University School of Medicine, Winston-Salem, North Carolina.
Atherosclerotic Renovascular Disease: Evaluation and Management of Ischemic Nephropathy; Techniques of Operative Management

JONATHAN S. DEITCH, M.D.
Vascular Fellow, Wake Forest University School of Medicine, Winston-Salem, North Carolina.
Renal Complications

RALPH G. DePALMA, M.D., F.A.C.S.
Professor of Surgery, Vice Chair Department of Surgery, and Associate Dean, University of Nevada School of Medicine. Chief of Surgery, Veterans Affairs Medical Center, Reno, Nevada.
Vasculogenic Impotence; Superficial Thrombophlebitis: Diagnosis and Management

LARRY-STUART DEUTSCH, M.D., C.M. F.R.C.P.(C.)
Professor and Chief-of-Service, University of California, Irvine, College of Medicine, Irvine. Chief-of-Service, Vascular and Interventional Radiology, UC Irvine Medical Center, Orange, California.
Anatomy and Angiographic Diagnosis of Extracranial and Intracranial Vascular Disease

JOHN A. DORMANDY, D.Sc., F.R.C.S.
Professor of Vascular Sciences, St. Georges Hospital Medical School. Consultant Vascular Surgeon, Department of Vascular Surgery, St. George's Hospital, London, England.
Circulation-Enhancing Drugs

MATTHEW J. DOUGHERTY, M.D.
Assistant Clinical Professor of Surgery, University of Pennsylvania School of Medicine; Section of Vascular Surgery, Pennsylvania Hospital, Philadelphia, Pennsylvania.
Renal Artery Aneurysms and Arteriovenous Fistulae

JOSEPH R. DURHAM, M.D., R.V.T.
Chairman, Department of Surgery, Oak Forest Hospital of Cook County, Oak Forest, Illinois.
Lower Extremity Amputation Levels: Indications, Determining the Appropriate Level, Technique, and Prognosis

JAMES M. EDWARDS, M.D.
Associate Professor of Surgery, Oregon Health Sciences University School of Medicine, Portland, Oregon.
Upper Extremity Ischemia: Approach to Diagnosis; Occlusive and Vasospastic Diseases Involving Distal Upper Extremity Arteries—Raynaud's Syndrome

BO EKLOF, M.D., Ph.D.
Clinical Professor of Surgery, John A. Burns School of Medicine, University of Hawaii. Vascular Surgeon, Straub Clinic and Hospital, Honolulu, Hawaii.
Interventional Treatments for Iliofemoral Venous Thrombosis

ERROL E. ERLANDSON, M.D.
Clinical Associate Professor of Surgery, University of Michigan Medical School. Director, Noninvasive Vascular Laboratory, St. Joseph Mercy Hospital, Ann Arbor, Michigan.
Upper Extremity Revascularization

CALVIN B. ERNST, M.D.
Professor of Surgery, MCP Hahnemann University School of Medicine. Chief, Division of Vascular Surgery, MCP Hahnemann University Hospital, Philadelphia, Pennsylvania.
Aortoenteric Fistulae; Infected Aneurysms; Colon Ischemia Following Aortic Reconstruction

MICHAEL M. FAROOQ, M.D.
Assistant Professor of Surgery, University of California, Los Angeles, UCLA School of Medicine. Attending Vascular Surgeon, UCLA Medical Center, UCLA Olive View Medical Center, West Los Angeles Veterans Affairs Medical Center, Los Angeles.
Peritoneal Dialysis

RISHAD M. FARUQI, M.B.B.S., F.R.C.S.(Eng.), F.R.C.S.(Ed.)
Clinical Instructor of Surgery, Division of Vascular Surgery, University of California, San Francisco School of Medicine, San Francisco, California.
The Arterial Autograft

CARLOS M. FERRARIO, M.D.
Professor, Wake Forest University School of Medicine. Director, Hypertension and Vascular Disease Center, North Carolina Baptist Hospitals, Inc., Winston-Salem, North Carolina.
Pathophysiology, Functional Studies, and Medical Therapy of Renovascular Hypertension

MARK F. FILLINGER, M.D.
Assistant Professor of Surgery, Dartmouth Medical School, Hanover, New Hampshire, and Dartmouth-Hitchcock Medical Center, Lebanon, New Hampshire.
Computed Tomography and Three-Dimensional Reconstruction in Evaluation of Vascular Disease

DANIEL F. FISHER, JR., M.D., F.A.C.S.
Associate Professor, Department of Surgery, University of Tennessee, Chattanooga, College of Medicine. Chief of Surgery, Erlanger Medical Center, Chattanooga, Tennessee.
Complications of Amputation

D. PRESTON FLANIGAN, M.D.
Clinical Professor of Surgery, University of California, Irvine, College of Medicine, and UC Irvine Medical Center, Orange, California.
Postoperative Sexual Dysfunction After Aortoiliac Revascularization

RICHARD J. FOWL, M.D.
Associate Professor of Surgery, Mayo Medical School. Vascular Surgeon, Mayo Clinic, Scottsdale, Arizona.
Popliteal Artery Entrapment

JULIE A. FREISCHLAG, M.D.
Professor of Surgery, University of California at Los Angeles, UCLA School of Medicine. Chief of Vascular Surgery, The Gondo Vascular Center, Los Angeles, California.
Hemodialysis Access; Peritoneal Dialysis

GAIL L. GAMBLE, M.D.
Assistant Professor, Mayo Medical School. Co-Director, Lymphedema Center, and Consultant, Department of Physical Medicine and Rehabilitation, Mayo Clinic, Rochester, Minnesota.
Nonoperative Management of Chronic Lymphedema

HUGH A. GELABERT, M.D.
Associate Professor, Division of Vascular Surgery, University of California, UCLA School of Medicine, Los Angeles, California.
Hemodialysis Access

BRUCE L. GEWERTZ, M.D., F.A.C.S.
Dallas B. Phemister Professor and Chairman, Department of Surgery, The University of Chicago Pritzker School of Medicine, Chicago, Illinois.
Anastomotic and Other Pseudoaneurysms; Acute Occlusive Events Involving the Renal Vessels

JOSEPH M. GIORDANO, M.D.
Professor of Surgery, George Washington University School of Medicine. Chairman, Department of Surgery, George Washington University Medical Center, Washington, DC.
Embryology of the Vascular System; Takayasu's Disease: Nonspecific Aortoarteritis

SEYMOUR GLAGOV, M.D.
Professor of Pathology, Medicine, and Surgery, University of Chicago Pritzker School of Medicine, Chicago, Illinois.
Artery Wall Pathology in Atherosclerosis

BOBBY S. GLICKMAN, M.D.
Resident in General Surgery, University of Nebraska Medical Center, Omaha, Nebraska.
Arterial Aneurysms: Etiologic Considerations

PETER GLOVICZKI, M.D.
Professor of Surgery, Mayo Medical School. Vice Chair, Division Vascular Surgery, Mayo Clinic and Foundation, Rochester, Minnesota. Staff Surgeon, Saint Mary's Hospital of Rochester and Rochester Methodist Hospital, Rochester, Minnesota.
Principles of Venography; Lymphatic Complications of Vascular Surgery; Venous Disease: An Overview; Management of Perforator Vein Incompetence; Surgical Treatment of Chronic Deep Venous Obstruction; Surgical Treatment of Superior Vena Cava Syndrome; Lymphedema: An Overview; Clinical Diagnosis and Evaluation of Lymphedema; Nonoperative Management of Chronic Lymphedema; Lymphatic Reconstructions

JERRY GOLDSTONE, M.D.
Professor of Surgery, University of California, San Francisco, School of Medicine. Chief, Vascular Surgery, San Francisco General Hospital, San Francisco, California.
Aneurysms of the Extracranial Carotid Artery

MICHAEL J. V. GORDON, M.D., F.A.C.S.
Associate Professor and Director, Hand Surgery, University of Colorado School of Medicine; University Hospital, Veterans Administration Medical Center, The Children's Hospital, Denver Health Medical Center, Denver, Colorado.
Upper Extremity Amputation

FRANK A. GOTTSCHALK, M.D., F.R.C.S.Ed., F.C.S.(S.A.)Orth.
Professor, Orthopaedic Surgery, University of Texas Southwestern Medical Center at Dallas Southwestern Medical School. Orthopaedic Consultant, Zale Lipshy University Hospital, Parkland Memorial Hospital, and University of Texas Southwestern Medical Center, Dallas, Texas.
Complications of Amputation

LINDA M. GRAHAM, M.D.
Professor of Surgery, University of Michigan Medical Center. Chief of Vascular Surgery at Department of Veterans Affairs Medical Center, Ann Arbor, Michigan.
Femoral and Popliteal Aneurysms

ROY K. GREENBERG, M.D.
Instructor in Surgery, The University of Rochester School of Medicine and Dentistry, Rochester, New York.
Arterial Thromboembolism

LAZAR J. GREENFIELD, M.D.
Frederick A. Coller Distinguished Professor and Chairman, Department of Surgery, The University of Michigan Medical School. Surgeon-in-Chief, University of Michigan Hospitals, Ann Arbor, Michigan.
Caval Interruption Procedures

NAVYASH GUPTA, M.D.
Fellow, Vascular Surgery, The University of Chicago Hospitals, Chicago, Illinois.
Acute Occlusive Events Involving the Renal Vessels

JOHN W. HALLETT, JR., M.D., F.A.C.S.
Professor of Surgery, Associate Dean for Faculty Affairs, Mayo Medical School. Attending Physician, Mayo Clinic. Rochester, Minnesota.
Iatrogenic Complications of Arterial and Venous Catheterizations

SHARON L. HAMMOND, M.D.
Vascular Surgeon, Rose Medical Center, and Chairman, President Health Center, Denver, Colorado.
Neurogenic Thoracic Outlet Syndrome

KIMBERLEY J. HANSEN, M.D.
Professor of Surgery, Division of Surgical Sciences, Department of General Surgery, Wake Forest University School of Medicine.
Renal Complications; Renovascular Disease: An Overview; Atherosclerotic Renovascular Disease: Evaluation and Management of Ischemic Nephropathy; Techniques of Operative Management

JOHN P. HARRIS, M.S., F.R.A.C.S., F.R.C.S., F.A.C.S., D.D.U.
Professor of Vascular Surgery, University of Sydney. Chairman, Division of Surgery, Royal Prince Alfred Hospital, Sydney, Australia.
Upper Extremity Sympathectomy

DOMINIC F. HEFFEL, M.D.
Resident, Division of General Surgery, University of California, Los Angeles, UCLA School of Medicine, Los Angeles, California.
Excisional Operations for Chronic Lymphedema

W. SCOTT HELTON, M.D.
Professor of Surgery, University of Illinois College of Medicine, Chicago, Illinois.
Operative Therapy for Portal Hypertension

NORMAN R. HERTZER, M.D.
Staff Vascular Surgeon, Department of Vascular Surgery, The Cleveland Clinic Foundation, Cleveland, Ohio.
Postoperative Management and Complications Following Carotid Endarterectomy

WILLIAM R. HIATT, M.D.
Professor of Medicine, University of Colorado School of Medicine and University of Colorado Health Sciences Center. Executive Director, Colorado Prevention Center, Denver, Colorado.
Atherogenesis and the Medical Management of Atherosclerosis

JOHN R. HOCH, M.D.
Assistant Professor of Surgery, University of Wisconsin Medical School. Chief, Section of Vascular Surgery, William S. Middleton Veteran Affairs Medical Center, Madison, Wisconsin.
Long-Term Venous Access

KIM J. HODGSON, M.D.
Professor and Chief of Peripheral Vascular Surgery, Southern Illinois University School of Medicine. Attending Surgeon, Memorial Medical Center and St. John's Hospital, Springfield, Illinois.
Principles of Arteriography; Fundamental Techniques in Endovascular Surgery

GARY S. HOFFMAN, M.D.
Chairman, Department of Rheumatic and Immunologic Diseases, Cleveland Clinic Foundation, Cleveland, Ohio.
Takayasu's Disease: Nonspecific Aortoarteritis

DOUGLAS B. HOOD, M.D.
Assistant Professor of Surgery, University of Southern California School of Medicine; USC University Hospital, Los Angeles, California.
Vascular Injuries of the Extremities

RICHARD L. HUGHES, M.D.
Associate Professor of Neurology, University of Colorado School of Medicine. Chief, Neurology, Denver Health Medical Center, Denver, Colorado.
Diagnosis, Evaluation, and Medical Management of Patients with Ischemic Cerebrovascular Disease

RUSSELL D. HULL, M.B.B.S., M.Sc.
Professor of Medicine, University of Calgary Faculty of Medicine. Foothills Hospital, Calgary, Alberta, Canada.
Prevention and Medical Treatment of Acute Deep Venous Thrombosis

SCOTT N. HURLBERT, M.D.
Clinical Vascular Fellow, Southern Illinois University School of Medicine, Springfield, Illinois.
Subclavian-Axillary Vein Thrombosis

KARL A. ILLIG, M.D.
Assistant Professor of Surgery, University of Rochester School of Medicine and Dentistry. Associate Attending Physician, Strong Memorial Hospital and Rochester General Hospital, Rochester, New York.
Perioperative Hemorrhage

GLENN R. JACOBOWITZ, M.D.
Assistant Professor of Clinical Surgery, Division of Vascular Surgery, New York University School of Medicine, New York, New York.
Peripheral Arteriovenous Fistulae

DENNIS M. JENSEN, M.D.
Professor of Medicine, University of California, Los Angeles, UCLA School of Medicine. Staff Physician, Division of Digestive Diseases, UCLA Center for the Health Sciences, West Los Angeles Veterans Affairs Medical Center, and CURE: Digestive Disease Research Center, Los Angeles, California.
Initial Management of Upper Gastrointestinal Hemorrhage in Patients with Portal Hypertension

KAJ H. JOHANSEN, M.D., Ph.D.
Professor of Surgery, University of Washington School of Medicine. Director, Surgical Education, Providence Medical Center, Seattle, Washington.
Compartment Syndrome: Pathophysiology, Recognition, and Management; Portal Hypertension: An Overview; Operative Therapy for Portal Hypertension

GEORGE JOHNSON, JR., M.D.
Emeritus Professor of Surgery, University of North Carolina at Chapel Hill, Chapel Hill, North Carolina.
Superficial Thrombophlebitis: Diagnosis and Management

K. WAYNE JOHNSTON, M.D., F.R.C.S.(C.)
Professor of Surgery and Chair, Division of Vascular Surgery, University of Toronto Faculty of Medicine, Toronto, Ontario, Canada.
Overview, Section VII; Ischemic Neuropathy; Upper Extremity Ischemia: Overview

DARRELL N. JONES, Ph.D.
Research Associate in Vascular Surgery, University of Colorado Health Sciences Center. Associate Director, Vascular Diagnostic Laboratory, University Hospital, Denver, Colorado.
Integrated Assessment of Results: Standardized Reporting of Outcomes and the Computerized Vascular Registry

JOHN W. JOYCE, M.D.
Professor of Medicine, Emeritus, Mayo Medical School, Rochester, Minnesota.
Uncommon Arteriopathies

VIKRAM S. KASHYAP, M.D.
Fellow in Vascular Surgery, University of California, Los Angeles, UCLA School of Medicine, Los Angeles, California.
Principles of Thrombolytic Therapy

JEFFREY L. KAUFMAN, M.D.
Associate Professor of Surgery, Tufts University School of Medicine. Vascular Surgeon, Department of Surgery, Baystate Medical Center, Springfield, Massachusetts.
Atheroembolism and Microthromboembolic Syndromes (Blue Toe Syndrome and Disseminated Atheroembolism)

ANDRIS KAZMERS, M.D., M.S.P.H.
Associate Professor of Surgery, Wayne State University School of Medicine. Medical Director, Vascular Surgery Laboratory, Harper Hospital, Detroit, Michigan.
Intestinal Ischemia Caused by Venous Thrombosis

RICHARD F. KEMPCZINSKI, M.D.
Emeritus Professor of Surgery, University of Cincinnati College of Medicine, Cincinnati, Ohio.
Vascular Conduits: An Overview; The Chronically Ischemic Leg: An Overview; Popliteal Artery Entrapment; Vasculogenic Impotence

K. CRAIG KENT, M.D.
Professor, Department of Surgery, Division of Vascular Surgery, Cornell University Medical College. Attending Physician, Department of Surgery, New York Presbyterian Hospital, New York, New York.
Renal Artery Imaging: Alternatives to Angiography

ROBERT K. KERLAN, JR., M.D.
Clinical Professor of Radiology, University of California, San Francisco, School of Medicine. Interventional Radiologist, Chief, Interventional Radiology, Mount Zion Medical Center of UC–San Francisco, San Francisco, California.
Percutaneous Interventions in Portal Hypertension

LAWRENCE L. KETCH, M.D., F.A.C.S., F.A.A.P.
Associate Professor and Chief, Plastic and Reconstructive Surgery, University of Colorado School of Medicine. Chief, Pediatric Plastic Surgery, The Children's Hospital, Denver, Colorado.
Upper Extremity Amputation

EDOUARD KIEFFER, M.D.
Professor of Vascular Surgery, Pitre-Salpetriere University. Chief, Department of Vascular Surgery, Pitre-Salpetriere University Hospital, Paris, France.
Arterial Complications of Thoracic Outlet Compression; Dissection of the Descending Thoracic Aorta

ROBERT L. KISTNER, M.D.
Clinical Professor of Surgery, University of Hawaii, John A. Burns School of Medicine. Department of Vascular Surgery, Straub Clinic and Hospital, Honolulu, Hawaii.
A Practical Approach to the Diagnosis and Classification of Chronic Venous Disease

STEVEN J. KNIGHT, R.V.T.
Instructor in Surgery, University of Vermont College of Medicine. Technical Director, Vascular Diagnostic Laboratory, Fletcher Allen Health Care, Inc., Burlington, Vermont.
The Role of Noninvasive Studies in the Diagnosis and Management of Cerebrovascular Disease

THOMAS O. G. KOVACS, M.D.
Associate Professor of Medicine, Division of Digestive Diseases, University of California, Los Angeles, UCLA School of Medicine. Director, Cure Clinical Trials Unit, West Los Angeles Veterans Affairs Medical Center, Los Angeles, California.
Initial Management of Upper Gastrointestinal Hemorrhage in Patients with Portal Hypertension

WILLIAM C. KRUPSKI, M.D.
Professor of Surgery, University of Colorado School of Medicine. Chief, Vascular Surgery, University of Colorado Health Sciences Center, Denver, Colorado.
Cardiac Complications and Screening; Thromboendarterectomy for Lower Extremity Arterial Occlusive Disease; Overview, Section XII; Abdominal Aortic and Iliac Aneurysms; Indications, Surgical Technique, and Results for Repair of Extracranial Occlusive Lesions; Uncommon Disorders Affecting the Carotid Arteries; Overview of Extremity Amputations, Section XXI

JEANNE M. LABERGE, M.D.
Associate Professor of Radiology, University of California, San Francisco, School of Medicine. Interventional Radiologist, The Medical Center at UC San Francisco, San Francisco, California.
Percutaneous Interventions in Portal Hypertension

LEWIS J. LEVIEN, M.B., B.Ch., Ph.D., F.C.S.(S.A.)
Honorary Lecturer, Department of Surgery, University of the Witwatersrand. Vascular Surgeon, Milpark Hospital, Johannesburg, South Africa.
Advential Cystic Disease of the Popliteal Artery

PAVEL J. LEVY, M.D.
Assistant Professor, Wake Forest University School of Medicine. Attending Physician, North Carolina Baptist Hospitals, Inc., Winston-Salem, North Carolina.
Pathophysiology, Functional Studies, and Medical Therapy of Renovascular Hypertension

ROBERT P. LIDDELL, M.S.
Royal College of Surgeons and Beaumont Hospital, Dublin, Ireland.
Endovascular Treatment of Chronic Occlusions of Large Veins

ROBERT C. LOWELL, M.D., F.A.C.S., R.V.T.
Vascular Surgeon, The Longstreet Clinic, Gainesville, Georgia.
Lymphatic Complications of Vascular Surgery

JAMES M. MALONE, M.D., F.A.C.S.
Clinical Professor of Surgery, University of Arizona College of Medicine, Tucson, Arizona, and Mayo Graduate School of Medicine, Rochester, Minnesota.
Revascularization Versus Amputation

M. ASHRAF MANSOUR, M.D., F.A.C.S.
Assistant Professor of Surgery, Loyola University Stritch School of Medicine. Attending Vascular Surgeon, Director of Residency Training and Education, Loyola University Medical Center, Maywood, Illinois.
Arteriovenous Fistulae of the Aorta and Its Major Branches

ELNA M. MASUDA, M.D.
Assistant Professor of Surgery, University of Hawaii John A. Burns School of Medicine. Vascular Surgeon and Director of Vascular Laboratory, Straub Clinic and Hospital, Honolulu, Hawaii.
A Practical Approach to the Diagnosis and Classification of Chronic Venous Disease

JAMES MAY, M.D., M.S., F.R.A.C.S., F.A.C.S.
Bosch Professor of Surgery, University of Sydney. Vascular Surgeon, Royal Prince Alfred Hospital, Sydney, Australia.
Endovascular Grafts; Upper Extremity Sympathectomy; Endovascular Treatment of Aortic Aneurysms

KENNETH E. McINTYRE, JR., M.D.
Professor of Surgery, Division of Vascular Surgery, University of Texas Southwestern Medical Center at Dallas Southwestern Medical School. Chief, Vascular Surgery, St. Paul Medical Center, Dallas, Texas.
Patient Evaluation and Preparation for Amputation

W. BURLEY McINTYRE, M.D.
Vascular Surgeon, Everett Clinic, Everett, Washington.
Cervicothoracic Vascular Injuries

MICHAEL A. McKUSICK, M.D.
Assistant Professor of Radiology, Mayo Graduate School of Medicine. Vascular and Interventional Radiologist, Mayo Clinic, Rochester, Minnesota.
Principles of Venography

ROBERT H. MEIER, III, M.D.
Director, Amputee Services of Colorado, Sunspectrum Outpatient Rehabilitation, Thornton, Colorado.
Rehabilitation of the Person with an Amputation

MARK H. MEISSNER, M.D.
Assistant Professor, Department of Surgery, University of Washington School of Medicine; Department of Vascular Surgery, Harborview Medical Center, Seattle, Washington.
Venous Duplex Scanning; Pathophysiology and Natural History of Acute Deep Venous Thrombosis

LOUIS M. MESSINA, M.D.
Professor of Surgery and Chief, Division of Vascular Surgery, University of California, San Francisco, School of Medicine. Attending Surgeon, UC San Francisco–Stanford Hospital, San Francisco, California.
Endarterectomy; Renal Artery Fibrodysplasia and Renovascular Hypertension

MARK MEWISSEN, M.D.
Clinical Associate Professor of Radiology, Medical College of Wisconsin. Interventional Radiologist, Wisconsin Heart and Vascular Clinics, Milwaukee, Wisconsin.
Interventional Treatments for Iliofemoral Venous Thrombosis

TIMOTHY A. MILLER, M.D., F.A.C.S.
Professor of Plastic and Reconstructive Surgery, University of California, Los Angeles, UCLA School of Medicine. Chief, Plastic and Reconstructive Surgery, West Los Angeles Veterans Administration Hospital, Los Angeles, California.
Excisional Operations for Chronic Lymphedema

MARC E. MITCHELL, M.D.
Assistant Professor of Surgery, Division of Vascular Surgery, University of Pennsylvania School of Medicine, Philadelphia, Pennsylvania.
Basic Considerations of the Arterial Wall in Health and Disease

GREGORY L. MONETA, M.D.
Professor of Surgery, Oregon Health Sciences University School of Medicine, Staff Surgeon, Veterans Affairs Medical Center, Portland, Oregon.
Natural History and Nonoperative Treatment of Chronic Lower Extremity Ischemia; Diagnosis of Intestinal Ischemia; Treatment of Acute Intestinal Ischemia Caused by Arterial Occlusions; Treatment of Chronic Visceral Ischemia; Pathophysiology of Chronic Venous Insufficiency; Nonoperative Treatment of Chronic Venous Insufficiency

WESLEY S. MOORE, M.D.
Professor of Surgery, University of California, Los Angeles, UCLA School of Medicine. Vascular Surgeon, UCLA Center for the Health Sciences, Los Angeles, California.
Fundamental Considerations in Cerebrovascular Disease; Indications, Surgical Technique, and Results for Repair of Extracranial Occlusive Lesions

MARK R. NEHLER, M.D.
Assistant Professor of Surgery, University of Colorado School of Medicine and University of Colorado Health Sciences Center, Denver, Colorado.
Cardiac Complications and Screening; Pathophysiology of Chronic Venous Insufficiency

AUDRA A. NOEL, M.D.
Division of Vascular Surgery, Mayo Clinic and Foundation, Rochester, Minnesota.
Lymphatic Reconstructions

SEAN P. O'BRIEN, M.D.
Vascular Surgery Fellow, MCP Hahnemann University Hospitals, Philadelphia, Pennsylvania.
Aortoenteric Fistulae

JEFFREY W. OLIN, D.O.
Chairman, Department of Vascular Medicine, Cleveland Clinic Foundation, Cleveland, Ohio.
Thromboangiitis Obliterans (Buerger's Disease)

KENNETH OURIEL, M.D.
Professor of Surgery, Ohio State University College of Medicine, Columbus. Chairman, Department of Vascular Surgery, The Cleveland Clinic Foundation, Cleveland, Ohio.
Perioperative Hemorrhage; Acute Limb Ischemia; Arterial Thromboembolism

MARC A. PASSMAN, M.D.
Fellow, Division of Vascular Surgery, Department of Surgery, University of North Carolina at Chapel Hill School of Medicine, Chapel Hill, North Carolina.
Physiologic Assessment of the Venous System

GRAHAM F. PINEO, M.D.
Professor of Medicine, University of Calgary Faculty of Medicine; Foothills Hospital, Calgary, Alberta, Canada.
Prevention and Medical Treatment of Acute Deep Venous Thrombosis

JOHN M. PORTER, M.D.
Professor of Surgery (Head), Oregon Health Sciences University School of Medicine, Portland, Oregon.
Natural History and Nonoperative Treatment of Chronic Lower Extremity Ischemia; Upper Extremity Ischemia: Approach to Diagnosis; Occlusive and Vasospastic Diseases Involving Distal Upper Extremity Arteries—Raynaud's Syndrome; Treatment of Acute Intestinal Ischemia Caused by Arterial Occlusions; Treatment of Chronic Visceral Ischemia; Pathophysiology of Chronic Venous Insufficiency; Nonoperative Treatment of Chronic Venous Insufficiency

WILLIAM J. QUIÑONES-BALDRICH, M.D.
Professor of Surgery, University of California, Los Angeles, UCLA School of Medicine. Vascular Surgeon, UCLA Center for the Health Sciences, Los Angeles, California.
Principles of Thrombolytic Therapy; Indications, Surgical Technique, and Results for Repair of Extracranial Occlusive Lesions

RICARDO T. QUINTOS II, M.D.
Clinical Research Fellow, Montefiore Medical Center, New York, New York.
Techniques for Thromboembolectomy of Native Arteries and Bypass Grafts; Secondary Arterial Reconstructions in the Lower Extremity

SESHADRI RAJU, M.D.
Emeritus Professor of Surgery, University of Mississippi School of Medicine. Honorary Surgeon, University Hospital, Jackson, Mississippi.
Surgical Treatment of Deep Venous Valvular Incompetence

DANIEL J. REDDY, M.D.
Head, Division of Vascular Surgery, Program Director, Vascular Fellowship, Henry Ford Hospital, Detroit, Michigan.
Infected Aneurysms

JASON P. REHM, M.D.
Resident in General Surgery, University of Nebraska Medical Center, Omaha, Nebraska.
Arterial Aneurysms: Etiologic Considerations

JEFFREY M. RHODES, M.D.
Clinical Fellow, Division of Vascular Surgery, Mayo Clinic, Rochester, Minnesota.
Management of Perforator Vein Incompetence

MICHAEL A. RICCI, M.D.
Associate Professor of Surgery, University of Vermont College of Medicine. Director, Vascular Diagnostic Laboratory, Fletcher Allen Health Care, Inc., Burlington, Vermont.
The Role of Noninvasive Studies in the Diagnosis and Management of Cerebrovascular Disease

LAYTON F. RIKKERS, M.D.
A.R. Curreri Professor and Chairman, University of Wisconsin Medical School, Madison, Wisconsin.
Operative Therapy for Portal Hypertension

THOMAS S. RILES, M.D.
Professor of Surgery and Director, Division of Vascular Surgery, New York University School of Medicine. Attending Physician, Tisch Hospital and Bellevue Hospital, New York, New York.
Overview, Section XIII; Peripheral Arteriovenous Fistulae; Congenital Vascular Malformations

STEVEN P. RIVERS, M.D.
Associate Professor of Surgery, Albert Einstein College of Medicine of Yeshiva University, Bronx, New York. Division of Vascular Surgery, Montefiore Medical Center, New York, New York.
Nonocclusive Mesenteric Ischemia

THOM W. ROOKE, M.D.
Associate Professor, Mayo Graduate School of Medicine. Head, Section of Vascular Medicine, Mayo Clinic, Rochester, Minnesota.
Uncommon Arteriopathies; Nonoperative Management of Chronic Lymphedema

ROBERT J. ROSEN, M.D.
Associate Professor of Radiology, New York University School of Medicine. Director of Vascular and Interventional Radiology, New York University Medical Center, New York, New York.
Peripheral Arteriovenous Fistulae; Congenital Vascular Malformations

CARLO RUOTOLO, M.D.
Assistant Professor of Surgery, Pitre-Salpetriere University. Staff Surgeon, Department of Vascular Surgery, Pitre-Salpetriere Hospital, Paris, France.
Arterial Complications of Thoracic Outlet Compression

ROBERT B. RUTHERFORD, M.D., F.A.C.S., F.R.C.S.(Glasg.)
Emeritus Professor of Surgery, University of Colorado School of Medicine, Denver, Colorado.
Initial Patient Evaluation: The Vascular Consultation; Evaluation and Selection of Patients for Vascular Interventions; Integrated Assessment of Results: Standardized Reporting of Outcomes and the Computerized Vascular Registry; Basic Vascular Surgical Techniques; Causalgia and Post-traumatic Pain Syndromes; Extra-anatomic Bypass; Endovascular Interventions in the Management of Chronic Lower Extremity Ischemia; Lumbar Sympathectomy: Indications and Technique; Subclavian-Axillary Vein Thrombosis; Abdominal Aortic and Iliac Aneurysms; Diagnostic Evaluation of Arteriovenous Fistulae; Extracranial Fibromuscular Arterial Dysplasia; Interventional Treatments for Iliofemoral Venous Thrombosis

DAVID SACKS, M.D.
Head, Interventional Radiology, The Reading Hospital and Medical Center, West Reading, Pennsylvania.
Angiography and Percutaneous Vascular Interventions: Complications and Quality Improvement

LUIS A. SANCHEZ, M.D.
Associate Professor of Surgery, Albert Einstein College of Medicine of Yeshiva University, Bronx, New York. Chief of Vascular Surgery, Jack D. Weiler Hospital, New York, New York.
Secondary Arterial Reconstructions in the Lower Extremity

RICHARD J. SANDERS, M.D.
Clinical Professor of Surgery, University of Colorado School of Medicine and Health Sciences Center. Attending Surgeon, Rose Medical Center, Denver, Colorado.
Neurogenic Thoracic Outlet Syndrome

ALVIN H. SCHMAIER, M.D.
Professor, Hematology and Oncology Division, Department of Internal Medicine and Pathology, University of Michigan Medical School. Director, Coagulation Laboratory, University of Michigan Medical Center, Ann Arbor, Michigan.
Vascular Thrombosis Due to Hypercoagulable States

PETER A. SCHNEIDER, M.D.
Clinical Assistant Professor of Surgery, University of Hawaii John A. Burns School of Medicine. Vascular and Endovascular Surgeon, Hawaii Permanente Medical Group, Honolulu, Hawaii.
Endovascular Interventions in the Management of Chronic Lower Extremity Ischemia; Extracranial Fibromuscular Arterial Dysplasia

LEWIS B. SCHWARTZ, M.D.
Assistant Professor of Surgery, University of Chicago Pritzker School of Medicine, Chicago, Illinois.
Anastomotic and Other Pseudoaneurysms

GARY R. SEABROOK, M.D.
Associate Professor, Division of Vascular Surgery, Medical College of Wisconsin, Milwaukee, Wisconsin.
Management of Foot Lesions in the Diabetic Patient

CHARLES J. SHANLEY, M.D.
Assistant Professor of Surgery, University of Michigan Medical School, Ann Arbor, Michigan.
Pulmonary Complications in Vascular Surgery

CYNTHIA K. SHORTELL, M.D.
Assistant Professor of Surgery, University of Rochester School of Medicine and Dentistry. Attending Surgeon, Strong Memorial Hospital and Rochester General Hospital, Rochester, New York.
Perioperative Hemorrhage

ANTON N. SIDAWY, M.D.
Professor of Surgery, George Washington University School of Medicine and Health Sciences and Georgetown University School of Medicine. Chief, Surgical Services, Veterans Affairs Medical Center, Washington, DC.
Basic Considerations of the Arterial Wall in Health and Disease

DONALD SILVER, M.D.
Emeritus Professor of Surgery, University of Missouri–Columbia School of Medicine, Columbia, Missouri.
Principles of Hemostasis; Antithrombotic Therapy; Diagnosis of Intestinal Ischemia

SUZANNE M. SLONIM, M.D.
Assistant Professor of Radiology, Stanford University School of Medicine, Stanford, California. Chief, Cardiovascular and Interventional Radiology, Palo Alto Veterans Administration Medical Center, Palo Alto, California.
Radiographic Evaluation and Treatment of Renovascular Disease

RICHARD K. SPENCE, M.D., F.A.C.S.
Director of Surgical Education, Baptist Health System, Birmingham, Alabama.
Blood Loss and Transfusion in Vascular Surgery

JAMES C. STANLEY, M.D.
Professor of Surgery, University of Michigan Medical School. Head, Section of Vascular Surgery, University Hospital, Ann Arbor, Michigan.
Splanchnic Artery Aneurysms; Arterial Fibrodysplasia; Renal Artery Fibrodysplasia and Renovascular Hypertension

ANTHONY STANSON, M.D.
Associate Professor of Radiology, Mayo Medical School. Consultant, Department of Diagnostic Radiology, Mayo Clinic and Mayo Foundation, Rochester, Minnesota.
Diagnosis and Management of Tumors of the Inferior Vena Cava

RONALD J. STONEY, M.D.
Professor of Surgery, Division of Vascular Surgery, University of California, San Francisco, School of Medicine, San Francisco, California.
Endarterectomy; The Arterial Autograft

D. EUGENE STRANDNESS, JR., M.D.
Professor, Department of Surgery, University of Washington School of Medicine, Seattle, Washington.
Pathophysiology and Natural History of Acute Deep Venous Thrombosis

DAVID S. SUMNER, M.D.
Distinguished Professor of Surgery Emeritus, Southern Illinois University School of Medicine, Springfield, Illinois.
Essential Hemodynamic Principles; Physiologic Assessment of Peripheral Arterial Occlusive Disease; Evaluation of Acute and Chronic Ischemia of the Upper Extremity; Hemodynamics and Pathophysiology of Arteriovenous Fistulae; Diagnostic Evaluation of Arteriovenous Fistulae

GENE Y. SUNG, M.D.
Assistant Professor, Neurology, University of Colorado School of Medicine. Director, Neurocritical Care and Stroke, University of Colorado Health Sciences Center, Denver, Colorado.
Diagnosis, Evaluation, and Medical Management of Patients with Ischemic Cerebrovascular Disease

SCOTT W. TABER, M.D.
Assistant Professor of Surgery, University of Louisville School of Medicine, Department of Surgery, Louisville, Kentucky.
Long-Term Venous Access

LLOYD M. TAYLOR, JR., M.D.
Professor of Surgery, Oregon Health Sciences University School of Medicine, Portland, Oregon.
Natural History and Nonoperative Treatment of Chronic Lower Extremity Ischemia; Upper Extremity Ischemia: Approach to Diagnosis; Treatment of Acute Intestinal Ischemia Caused by Arterial Occlusions; Treatment of Chronic Visceral Ischemia

JONATHAN B. TOWNE, M.D.
Professor and Chairman, Division of Vascular Surgery, Medical College of Wisconsin, Milwaukee, Wisconsin.
The Autogenous Vein; Profundaplasty; Management of Foot Lesions in the Diabetic Patient

J. JEAN E. TURLEY, M.D., F.R.C.S.(P.)
Associate Professor, Department of Medicine, University of Toronto Faculty of Medicine. Attending Physician, St. Michael's Hospital, Toronto, Ontario, Canada.
Ischemic Neuropathy

WILLIAM W. TURNER, JR., M.D.
James D. Hardy Professor and Chairman, Department of Surgery, The University of Mississippi School of Medicine, Jackson, Mississippi.
Acute Vascular Insufficiency Due to Drug Injection

R. JAMES VALENTINE, M.D.
Associate Professor, University of Texas Southwestern Medical Center at Dallas Southwestern Medical School. Attending Surgeon, Parkland Memorial Hospital, Zale Lipshy University Hospital, Veterans Affairs Medical Center, Dallas, Texas.
Anatomy of Commonly Exposed Arteries; Acute Vascular Insufficiency Due to Drug Injection

FRANK J. VEITH, M.D.
Professor of Surgery, Albert Einstein College of Medicine of Yeshiva University, Bronx, New York. Chief, Vascular Surgical Services, Montefiore Medical Center, New York, New York.
Techniques for Thromboembolectomy of Native Arteries and Bypass Grafts; Secondary Arterial Reconstructions in the Lower Extremity; Nonocclusive Mesenteric Ischemia

OMAIDA C. VELÁZQUEZ, M.D.
Instructor in Surgery, University of Pennsylvania School of Medicine, Philadelphia, Pennsylvania.
Magnetic Resonance Imaging and Angiography

TERRI J. VRTISKA, M.D.
Department of Diagnostic Radiology, Mayo Clinic and Foundation, Rochester, Minnesota.
Surgical Treatment of Superior Vena Cava Syndrome

HEINZ W. WAHNER, M.D., F.A.C.P.
Professor Emeritus of Radiology, Mayo Clinic, Rochester, Minnesota.
Clinical Diagnosis and Evaluation of Lymphedema

THOMAS W. WAKEFIELD, M.D.
Professor, Section of Vascular Surgery Department of Surgery, University of Michigan Medical School. Director, Noninvasive Diagnostic Vascular Unit, University of Michigan Medical Center. Staff Surgeon, Ann Arbor Veterans Administration Medical Center, Ann Arbor, Michigan.
Arterial Fibrodysplasia; Vascular Thrombosis Due to Hypercoagulable States

DANIEL B. WALSH, M.D.
Professor of Surgery, Dartmouth Medical School, Hanover, New Hampshire. Vice Chair, Department of Surgery, Dartmouth-Hitchcock Medical Center, Lebanon, New Hampshire.
Technical Adequacy and Graft Thrombosis

JAMES C. WATSON, JR., M.S., M.D.
Clinical Instructor, University of Washington School of Medicine; Advanced Surgical Associates, PLLC; Northwest Hospital and Providence Medical Center, Seattle, Washington.
Compartment Syndrome: Pathophysiology, Recognition, and Management

FRED A. WEAVER, M.D., F.A.C.S.
Associate Professor of Surgery, University of Southern California School of Medicine. Chief, Division of Vascular Surgery, USC University Hospital, Los Angeles, California.
Vascular Injuries of the Extremities

ERIC S. WEINSTEIN, M.D.
Assistant Clinical Professor, University of Colorado School of Medicine, Denver. Attending Physician, Swedish Medical Center, Englewood, Colorado; and Rose Medical Center and Porter Medical Center, Denver, Colorado.
Thromboendoarterectomy for Lower Extremity Arterial Occlusive Disease; Neurogenic Thoracic Outlet Syndrome

KURT WENGERTER, M.D.
Director of the Vascular Laboratory, Englewood Hospital and Medical Center, Englewood, New Jersey.
Biologic Grafts for Lower Limb Revascularization

GEOFFREY H. WHITE, M.D., F.R.A.C.S.
Clinical Associate Professor, University of Sydney. Vascular Surgeon, Department of Vascular Surgery, Royal Prince Alfred Hospital, Sydney, Australia.
Endovascular Grafts; Endovascular Treatment of Aortic Aneurysms

JOHN V. WHITE, M.D.
Chairman, Department of Surgery, Lutheran General Hospital, Park Ridge, Illinois.
Integrated Assessment of Results: Standardized Reporting of Outcomes and the Computerized Vascular Registry

THOMAS A. WHITEHILL, M.D.
Associate Professor of Surgery, University of Colorado School of Medicine. Chief of Vascular Surgery, Veterans Administration Medical Center, Denver, Colorado.
Uncommon Disorders Affecting the Carotid Arteries

WALTER M. WHITEHOUSE, JR., M.D.
Clinical Associate Professor of Surgery, University of Michigan Medical School. Chairman, Department of Surgery, St. Joseph Mercy Hospital, Ann Arbor, Michigan.
Upper Extremity Revascularization

ANTHONY D. WHITTEMORE, M.D.
Professor of Surgery, Harvard Medical School. Chief of Vascular Surgery, Brigham and Women's Hospital, Boston, Massachusetts.
Infrainguinal Bypass

KENT WILLIAMSON, M.D.
Surgery Resident, Oregon Health Sciences University School of Medicine, Portland, Oregon.
Upper Extremity Ischemia: Approach to Diagnosis

GARY G. WIND, M.D.
Professor of Surgery, Uniformed Services University of the Health Sciences. Staff Surgeon, National Naval Medical Center, Bethesda, Maryland.
Anatomy of Commonly Exposed Arteries

CHARLES L. WITTE, M.D.
Professor of Surgery, University of Arizona College of Medicine, Tucson, Arizona.
Circulatory Dynamics and Physiology of the Lymphatic System

MARLYS H. WITTE, M.D.
Professor of Surgery and Director, Medical Student Research Program, University of Arizona College of Medicine, Tucson, Arizona.
Circulatory Dynamics and Pathophysiology of the Lymphatic System

JAMES S. T. YAO, M.D., Ph.D.
Magerstadt Professor of Surgery, Northwestern University Medical School. Acting Chair, Department of Surgery, Northwestern Memorial Hospital, Chicago, Illinois.
Occupational Vascular Problems

ALBERT E. YELLIN, M.D., F.A.C.S.
Professor of Surgery, University of Southern California School of Medicine. Associate Chief of Staff, Medical Director of Surgical Services, Los Angeles County–University of Southern California Medical Center, Los Angeles, California.
Vascular Injuries of the Extremities

CHRISTOPHER K. ZARINS, M.D.
Chidester Professor of Surgery, Stanford University School of Medicine. Chief of Vascular Surgery, Stanford University Medical Center, Stanford, California.
Artery Wall Pathology in Atherosclerosis

GERALD B. ZELENOCK, M.D.
Professor of Surgery, Section of Vascular Surgery, University of Michigan Medical School; Attending Staff, Section of Vascular Surgery, University Hospital, and Vascular Surgery Service, Veterans Administration Hospital, Ann Arbor, Michigan.
Pulmonary Complications in Vascular Surgery; Splanchnic Artery Aneurysms

R. EUGENE ZIERLER, M.D.
Professor of Surgery, Department of Surgery, Division of Vascular Surgery, University of Washington School of Medicine. Attending Staff, University of Washington Medical Center, Seattle, Washington.
Physiologic Assessment of Peripheral Arterial Occlusive Disease

ROBERT M. ZWOLAK, M.D., Ph.D.
Associate Professor, Dartmouth Medical School, Hanover, New Hampshire. Director, Noninvasive Vascular Laboratory, Mary Hitchcock Memorial Hospital, Lebanon, New Hampshire.
Arterial Duplex Scanning

PREFACE

The fifth edition of *Vascular Surgery* comes at the millennium, a time when everyone tends to reflect on changes occurring over the past century, the past 25 years, or at least the past decade. I will spare the reader this and will focus primarily on the changes that have occurred in the practice of vascular surgery since the fourth edition and their impact on the current edition.

The inevitable trend of more vascular surgery being done by fewer but better-trained surgeons, who are more committed to this field as their primary or sole activity, has continued. This is just as well, for it offsets other negative trends. The pressure from superimposed cost-containment measures has resulted not only in more conservative indications for intervention, which is mostly appropriate, but also in far less compensation per procedure, which is not. Vascular surgery, dealing as it does primarily with an elderly population (e.g., Medicare participants) has never been compensated on the same scale as some other surgical specialties with which it has been targeted. Endovascular procedures, on the other hand, have not suffered the same fate, even though their relative costs have climbed because of the new technology involved (e.g., better imaging equipment, special devices, catheters and introducers, and other improvements). While the overall number of traditional (i.e., open) vascular surgical procedures might have declined, from the inroads made by managed care and endovascular procedures, this has been offset, for the most part, in the majority of vascular surgery practices by the dwindling numbers of part-time or "occasional" vascular surgeons, the aging of the population, and the increasing degree to which vascular surgeons in North America and Europe have acquired the necessary skills with which to perform endovascular interventions themselves or in collaboration with interventional radiologists. This latter trend was given a boost by the advent of endografts that, at the outset at least, *required* involvement by vascular surgeons but that also honed their skills at manipulations under fluoroscopic monitoring to the point where balloon dilations and stenting and other simpler procedures were reasonably within reach.

This change is reflected in this new edition in an expanded coverage of *endovascular procedures* and *alternative imaging options* in addition to angiography, topics written principally by surgeons. New chapters are devoted to the various types of endovascular grafts, to the endovascular treatment of abdominal aortic aneurysms (AAAs), to the complications of angiography and of endovascular interventions, and to endovascular interventions for lower extremity occlusive disease. Endovascular treatments are also presented in other chapters dealing with the management of variceal hemorrhage, renovascular disease, acute deep venous thrombosis, and chronic large vein obstruction.

Despite the inroads made by imaging-based radiologists into the field of noninvasive vascular diagnosis, vascular surgeons have managed to keep a firm control on duplex scanning by showing the way in extending and standardizing its clinical applications (e.g., as the sole preoperative imaging method for most cases of carotid endarterectomy and in selected cases of lower extremity revascularization). Vascular surgeons have also demonstrated the continued value of certain of the indirect physiologic tests, which are less expensive than duplex scans but foreign to most radiologists. Nevertheless, in this edition separate chapters describe peripheral arterial and venous duplex scanning, and the application in the diagnosis of mesenteric and renal disease has been given expanded coverage.

Other trends that had just surfaced during the writing of the last edition have continued. Thrombolytic therapy has continued to flourish and has become an integral part of the management of acute arterial thromboses, even though several randomized trials have had difficulty in showing advantages, in overall results, over surgery. These disappointing trial results are partly due to a higher than expected (but "real life?") failure to gain access and achieve lysis (i.e., initial technical failure) and to flaws in protocol design, particularly the linking of thrombolysis with the ultimate treatment of the underlying lesion by percutaneous transluminal angioplasty (PTA), even when surgery would have been more effective. Post hoc analysis has helped to identify the settings in which catheter-directed thrombolysis is likely to be of benefit and demonstrated the clear need for careful case selection. Two chapters address these issues, and another one fully discusses the use of catheter-directed thrombolysis in deep venous thrombosis.

Angioaccess, particularly for hemodialysis, continues to play a major role in the practice of many vascular surgeons, and new techniques that improve the opportunity to create autogenous fistulae and enhance the patency of prosthetic shunts have been introduced. Periodic surveillance of surgical and endovascular revascularizations has become a standard of care, even though appropriate reimbursement for these efforts has lagged shamefully behind. The criteria for identifying critical restenoses and the most cost-effective monitoring intervals need to be better defined, but reasonable options have been identified. The advantages and limitations of PTA and stenting for renal artery stenosis have become better recognized, and its relative role vis à vis surgical revascularization has been better delineated. However, the preferred techniques for renal revascularization have clearly shifted away from a clear dominance by aortorenal vein bypass to relatively more endarterectomies, prosthetic grafts, and extra-anatomic bypasses, each used selectively in certain settings.

Carotid endarterectomy has survived its challenge from

randomized prospective trials versus the best medical therapy and, despite the incurable negativity of some neurologists, has come out stronger than ever. Rather than stand pat, however, we have seen a sweeping trend toward the use of duplex scanning instead of arteriography as the preoperative imaging method in the majority of patients, same-day admission for surgery, selective avoidance of monitoring in intensive care units, and discharging a sizable portion of patients from the hospital on the day after surgery. Although these measures have been instigated by competitive pressures related to increased managed care, they have not reduced the safety of carotid endarterectomy—which, if anything, has continued to improve while becoming less costly. This is just as well, for carotid endarterectomy must meet the new challenge of carotid stenting. Critical appraisal of the initial and current results of stenting, particularly in regard to some deceiving reporting practices, suggests that it should not constitute a major threat to modern-day carotid endarterectomy, but the pressures of continued open use by enthusiasts, industry-driven uncontrolled "trials," and its potential attractiveness to patients, have finally prompted proper randomized trials, even though the matter of clinical equipoise is still being debated. The recent announcement that the CAVITAS trial has shown "no significant difference" ensures that its details will be hotly debated and puts more pressure on the CREST trial. I predict that, in the absence of unforeseen major technologic innovations, carotid stenting will still end up having limited applications (e.g., in technical or operative high-risk patients, such as postendarterectomy restenoses and in the patient with a hostile neck from previous cancer surgery or irradiation).

Although not a major part of the practice of most vascular surgeons, operations for the complications of portal hypertension and for congenital vascular malformations have continued to decline. Operations for mesenteric insufficiency and for upper and lower extremity occlusive disease have not declined, except for aortoiliac occlusive disease. Even there, however, when long-term, lesion-specific stratified data become available, particularly for the more extensive lesions that are being treated percutaneously since the advent of stents, and the impact of reintervention is included in outcome assessment, the pendulum can be expected to swing back.

The management of venous disease has made great strides, the major exception being in direct reconstructive surgery for chronic venous *valvular* insufficiency (as opposed to obstructive disease); even here, however, the selective use and results have been more clearly defined, suggesting that it would be better limited to primary cases rather than postphlebitic cases.

The advances in the management of venous disease are reflected in this book in an expanded section, "Management of Venous Diseases." A new section, "Basic Principles in Vascular Disease," includes chapters on embryology of the vascular system, anatomy of commonly exposed arteries, and vascular biology of the arterial wall in health and disease. The acutely ischemic limb and vascular trauma are now covered in separate sections, the latter with two new chapters.

Considering these and many other changes not detailed here, the fifth edition of *Vascular Surgery* has again undergone major revision. The number of chapters totals 166 instead of 153, but there are more new chapters than the numerical difference would suggest. Some chapters have actually been consolidated, so that almost 20 chapters are topically new. In addition, 87 chapters have been written by new authors or a new primary author. Many other primary authors have enlisted new coauthors in bringing about major revisions. Thus, more than two thirds of the chapters are new or have been extensively revised, and the remainder have been appropriately updated. Even those chapters dealing with slowly changing subjects (e.g., lymphedema and amputation, hemodynamic principles, basic vascular surgery techniques, endarterectomy technique, ischemic neuropathy, and the hemodynamics and pathophysiology of arteriovenous fistulae) have not remained the same.

I owe my deep appreciation to the associate and assistant editors who have shared the hard work of putting together yet another comprehensive and thoroughly updated edition. With each new edition, we resist the temptation to cut back or at least to hold it to the same size, for knowledge in this field is increasing and we believe that there should be one text in this field that endeavors to be almost encyclopedic, one in which the reader can expect almost every aspect to be covered. As this textbook is not meant to be read from cover to cover, there is deliberate repetition in addition to thorough cross-referencing.

The associate and assistant editors join me in thanking each and every author and coauthor of the many chapters. Writing chapters is usually a thankless job, with no reward other than being recognized for one's expertise and the satisfaction of contributing to updating and perpetuating a textbook that has become, by these efforts and the efforts of past contributors, a valuable resource in one's chosen field.

Needless to say, I have benefited the most from all these efforts, being given undue credit for the work of so many others. It is my hope that they all will share my pride in a job well done and that their unselfish efforts will continue to sustain *Vascular Surgery* in the role into which it has grown—that of vascular surgery's main textbook—and that they will see it as a legacy worth perpetuating with future editions, long after I cease to wheedle yet one more chapter from them and then cajole them to produce it on time.

ROBERT B. RUTHERFORD

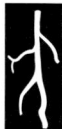CONTENTS

S E C T I O N V

S E C T I O N VI

S E C T I O N VII

S E C T I O N   X I

NEUROVASCULAR CONDITIONS INVOLVING THE UPPER EXTREMITY   1111
Edited by K. Wayne Johnston, M.D., F.R.C.S.(C.)

S E C T I O N   X I I

ARTERIAL ANEURYSMS   1241
Edited by Jack L. Cronenwett, M.D.

S E C T I O N   X I I I

ARTERIOVENOUS COMMUNICATIONS AND CONGENITAL VASCULAR MALFORMATIONS   1398
Edited by Thomas S. Riles, M.D.

S E C T I O N   X V I I I

S E C T I O N   X I X

Plate XXIV

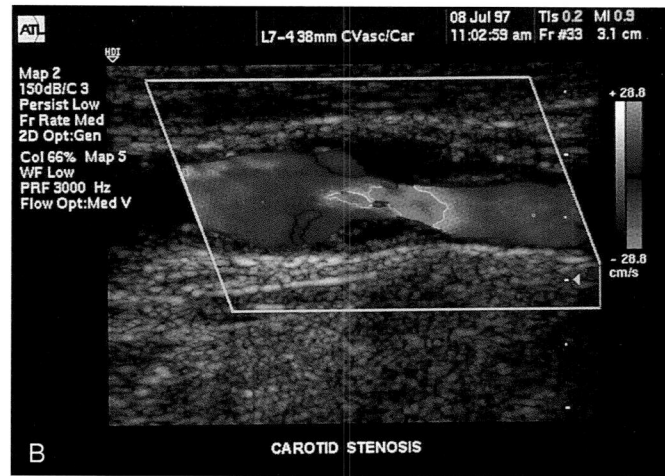

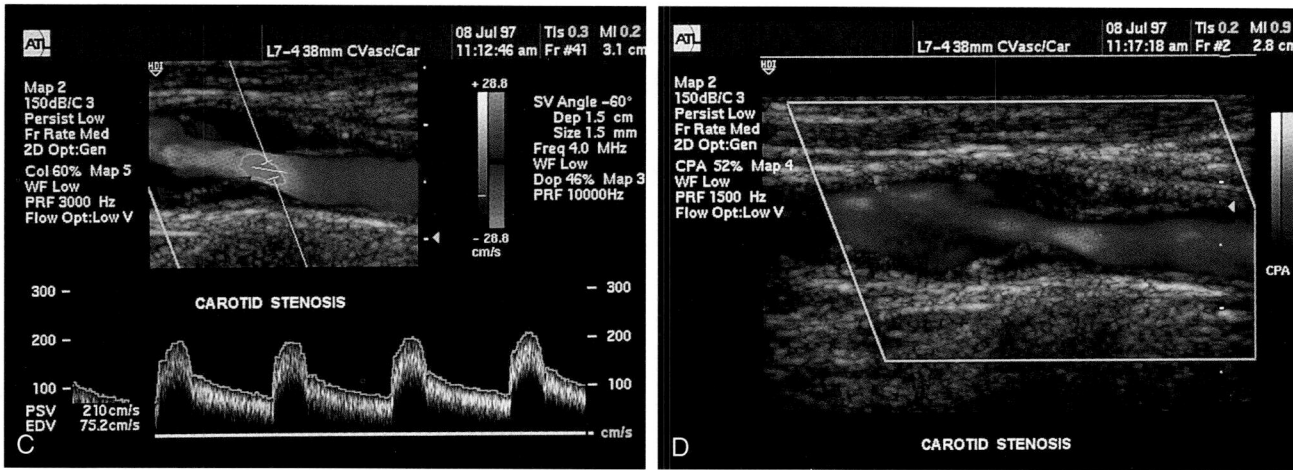

FIGURE 129–18. Ultrasound examination of the carotid artery. *B,* Color flow Doppler image. *C,* Doppler flow velocity measurements used to grade the approximate severity of the stenosis. *D,* Power Doppler image of the same stenosis. (Courtesy of ATL—Advanced Technology Laboratories, Bothell, Wash.)

Plate XXV

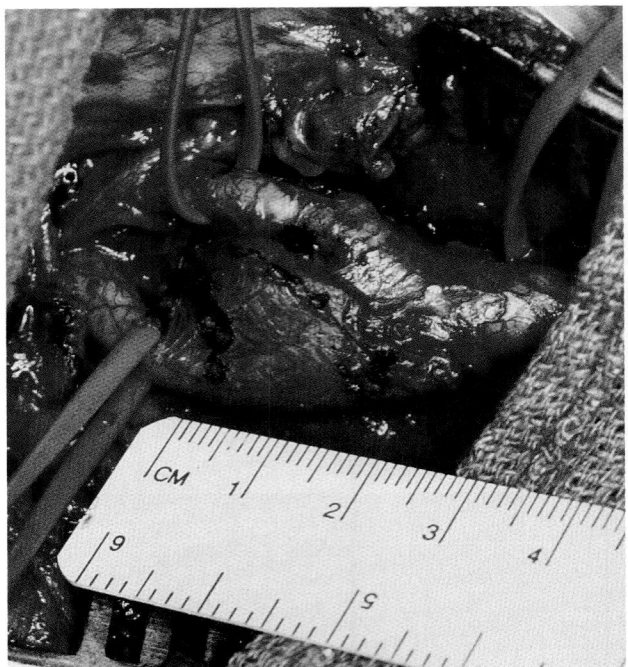

FIGURE 135–7. Operative photograph taken during resection of a small carotid body tumor. Vessel loops encircle the common (*right*), external (*left upper*), and internal (*left lower*) carotid arteries.

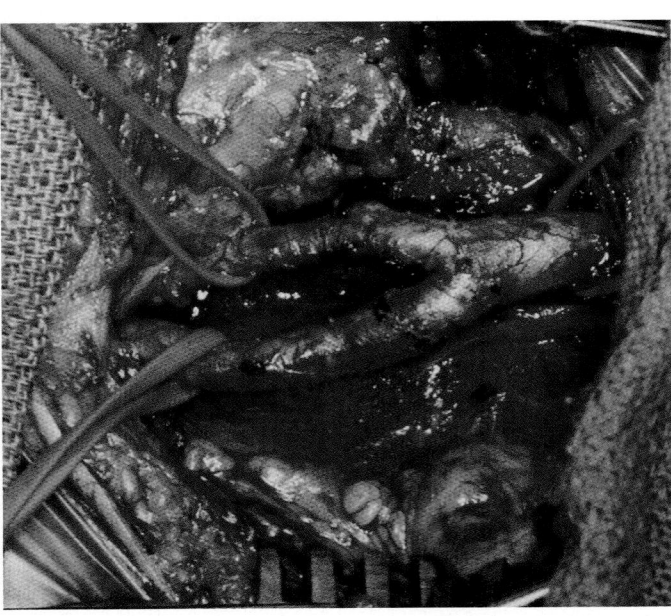

FIGURE 135–12. Postoperative photograph taken after resection of the carotid body tumor shown in Figure 135–7. The adventitia of the carotid arteries is intact; the external carotid artery is preserved.

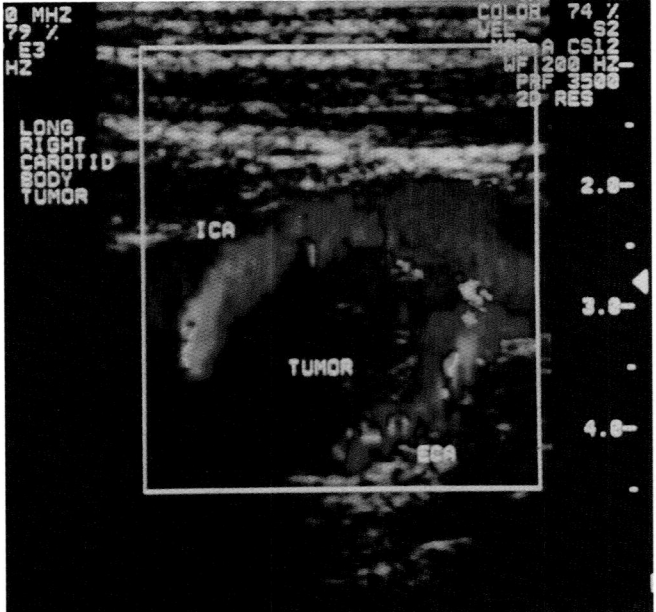

FIGURE 135–8. Characteristic duplex color flow image of a carotid body tumor. The internal and external carotid branches are splayed by the tumor mass. The tumor may exhibit a very active mixed-signal pattern representing the extensive vascularity of the tumor.

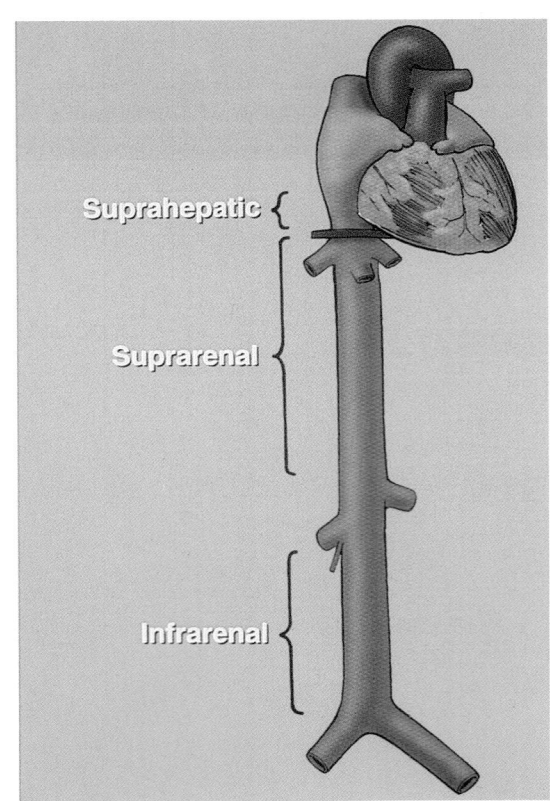

FIGURE 152–1. Segments of the inferior vena cava.

Plate XXVI

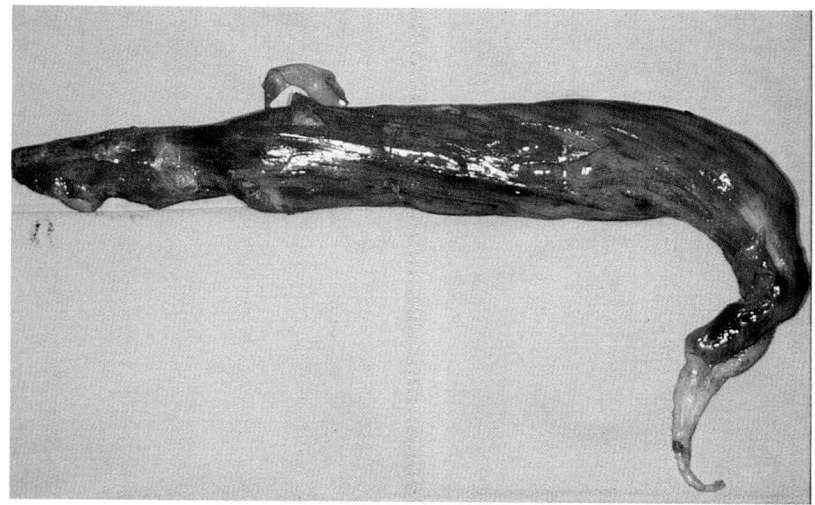

FIGURE 152–5. Intracaval tumor thrombus. Pathologic specimen revealed endometrial stromal cell sarcoma.

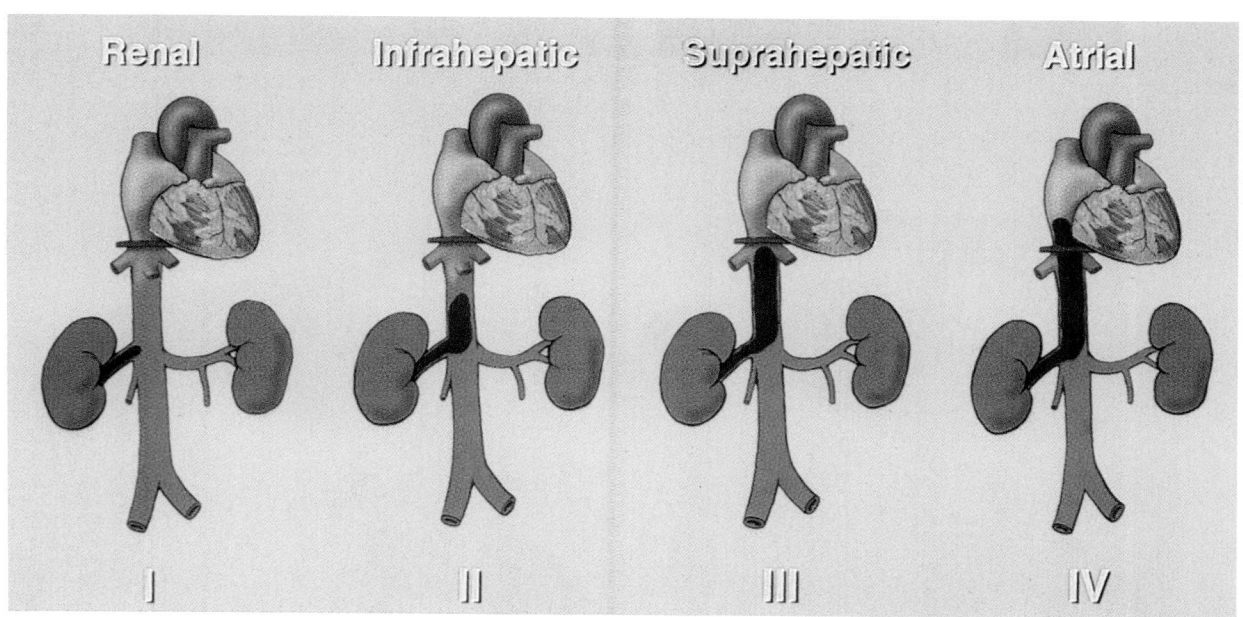

FIGURE 152–6. Classification of level of inferior vena caval thrombus associated with renal cell carcinoma.

Plate XXVII

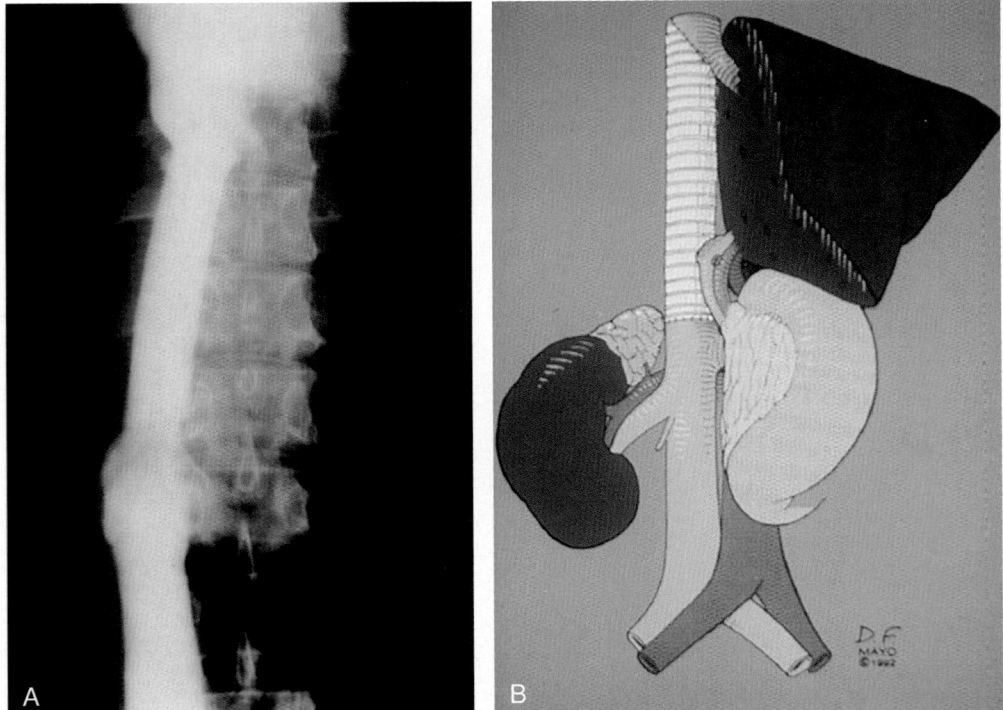

FIGURE 152–8. Postoperative cavograms and accompanying diagrams demonstrating patency of expanded polytetrafluoroethylene grafts used to replace the retrohepatic vena cava after liver resection (*A* and *B*). (From Bower TC, Nagorney DM, Toomey BJ, et al: Vena cava replacement for malignant disease: Is there a role? Ann Vasc Surg 7: 51–62, 1993, with permission).

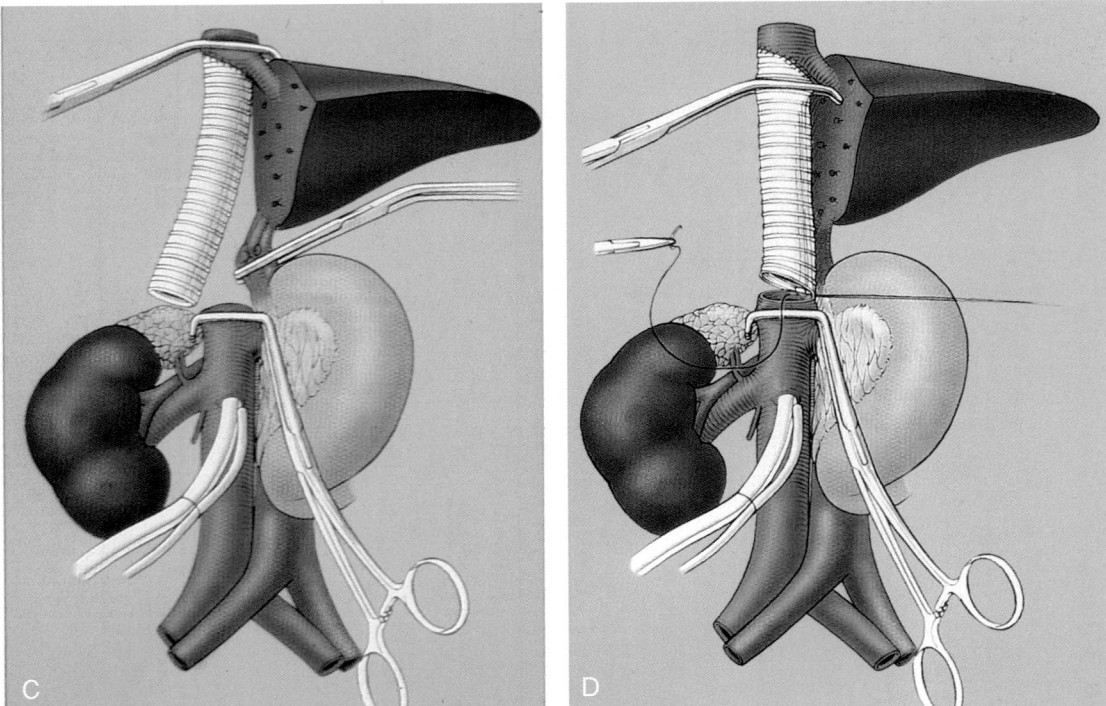

FIGURE 152–9. Operative technique for replacement of the retrohepatic inferior vena cava (IVC) in conjunction with major liver resection. *C,* The upper caval anastomosis is performed first. *D,* The suprahepatic caval clamp is then placed across the graft after acid metabolites have been flushed from the liver. The lower caval anastomosis is completed.

S E C T I O N   X I

NEUROVASCULAR CONDITIONS INVOLVING THE UPPER EXTREMITY

K. WAYNE JOHNSTON, M.D., F.R.C.S.(C.)

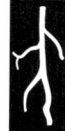

C H A P T E R   7 8

Upper Extremity Ischemia

Overview

K. Wayne Johnston, M.D., F.R.C.S.(C.)

Symptomatic vascular diseases involving the upper extremity are quite rare in comparison to those involving the lower extremity; however, when present, such diseases may be very disabling because they affect the hand function and may carry a poor prognosis because they may be a manifestation of a systemic disorder. In lower extremity arterial occlusive disease, intermittent claudication is the most common associated symptom; in the upper extremity, coldness and color changes of the digits are more common than complaints of tiredness, claudication, or ulceration and gangrene. These differences in the upper extremity symptoms are related to the more frequent distal distribution of the arterial disease and the excellent collateral supply around the shoulder and elbow.

Diagnosis of the anatomic location of the upper extremity arterial occlusive disease is often straightforward and is based on the following:

1. Careful vascular examination, including blood pressure measurements, pulse palpation, Allen's test, and thoracic outlet maneuvers.
2. Noninvasive tests to detect obstruction of large arteries (segmental blood pressure measurements, Doppler recordings, or duplex Doppler studies) and small arteries (digital blood pressure measurements, Doppler recordings, or plethysmographic recordings).
3. Angiography.

Establishing the etiologic diagnosis is often difficult, however, unless there are digital or general manifestations of a systemic disease.

The following topics relevant to upper extremity vascular disease have been covered earlier: Takayasu's disease (see Chapter 21), Buerger's disease (see Chapter 20), vasculitis (see Chapter 25), causalgia (see Chapter 63), cold injury, and proximal arterial injuries (see Chapter 60). The chap-

ters in this section describe the neurovascular diseases of the upper extremity and summarize the most important aspects of the pathogenesis, diagnosis, and management of these diseases. The subchapter by Taylor and colleagues following this overview summarizes the general approach to the diagnosis of upper extremity ischemia.

DIAGNOSIS OF ACUTE AND CHRONIC ISCHEMIA (see Chapter 79)

The assessment of the ischemic upper extremity by clinical evaluation, noninvasive assessment, and arteriography aims to determine (1) the anatomic site of the arterial disease, (2) the severity of the ischemia, and (3) the etiology. The diagnostic approach depends on the results of a comprehensive history taking and a careful physical examination because it can usually reveal the site of obstruction and may suggest the possible cause (see the subchapter "Approach to Diagnosis" by Taylor and coworkers).

This chapter describes the tests used in the further evaluation of arterial disease involving the arch vessels and the subclavian arteries and includes segmental blood pressure measurements; Doppler recordings, duplex scanning, or both; and arteriography. Significant thoracic outlet arterial compression can be detected by palpation of the radial pulse and auscultation for bruits in the infraclavicular area during the various thoracic outlet maneuvers or by noninvasively recording changes in radial artery flow with a Doppler flowmeter or changes in digital flow with a photoplethysmograph.

Acute or chronic obstruction of the axillary, brachial, and forearm arteries can usually be evaluated by clinical examination, segmental blood pressure measurement, Doppler recordings, and sometimes arteriography.

Digital artery involvement may be a result of primary vasospasm, presenting as episodic vasospasm on exposure to cold or emotional stimuli, or it may be due to fixed arterial obstruction (Table 78–1), presenting as similar cold intolerance or more advanced ischemic sequelae. A cold

TABLE 78–1. CAUSES OF UPPER EXTREMITY ISCHEMIA

Arterial Vasospasm

Small Artery (see Chapter 79)
   Idiopathic vasospastic Raynaud's syndrome
   Vibrating tool use (see Chapter 84)
   Vinyl chloride exposure
   Beta adrenergic blocker treatment
Large Artery
   Ergot-containing medications
   Claviceps purpurea–contaminated grain

Arterial Obstruction

Small Artery (see Chapter 79)
   Connective tissue disease
      Scleroderma
      Rheumatoid arthritis
      Mixed connective tissue disease
      Systemic lupus erythematosus
   Myeloproliferative disease
      Thrombocytosis
      Polycythemia
      Leukemia
      Myeloid metaplasia
   Buerger's disease (see Chapter 20)
   Hypersensitivity angiitis
   Cold injury
   Henoch-Schönlein purpura
   Cytotoxic drugs
Large Artery
   Atherosclerosis (see Chapter 18)
   Thoracic outlet syndrome (compression by cervical rib, first rib, or clavicle) (see Chapters 80, 81, and 92)
   Arteritis
      Giant cell (see Chapter 25)
      Takayasu (see Chapter 21)
   Fibromuscular disease (see Chapter 25)

Hypercoagulable states (see Chapter 46)
   Heparin antibodies
   Deficiencies
      Antithrombin III
      Protein C
      Protein S
   Antiphospholipid syndrome
   Malignancy
   Increased blood viscosity
   Macroglobulinemia
   Cryoglobulinemia
   Myeloma

Proximal Large Artery Sources of Embolism to Distal Small Arteries

Ulcerated or stenotic atherosclerotic plaques
   Aortic arch
   Innominate artery
   Subclavian artery
Aneurysms (see Chapters 22 and 92)
   Innominate artery
   Subclavian artery
   Axillary or brachial artery
   Ulnar artery
Thoracic outlet syndrome (see Chapters 83 and 84)
   Compression or stenosis of the subclavian artery with or without post-stenotic aneurysm

---

tolerance test can verify the symptoms but does little to establish the anatomic or etiologic diagnosis. Noninvasive tests distinguish between primary vasospasm and fixed arterial obstruction. The most useful modalities are digital pressure measurements, Doppler recordings, and digital plethysmographic waveform recordings. Arteriography is necessary if the results of the clinical and noninvasive tests are equivocal.

ATHEROSCLEROTIC OCCLUSIVE DISEASE OF THE BRACHIOCEPHALIC ARTERIES (see Chapter 80)

Arterial occlusive disease of the brachiocephalic and aortic arch vessels may be due to atherosclerosis, inflammatory arteritis, or trauma. Chapter 80 describes atherosclerotic occlusive disease; Chapter 21, Takayasu's disease; Chapter 25, arteritis; and Chapter 60, trauma.

Because of the abundant collateral blood supply, lesions of the brachiocephalic vessels are usually asymptomatic, but some patients present with arm claudication or cerebral symptoms resulting from changes in perfusion. Less commonly, if the lesions ulcerate, they may become symptomatic because of platelet or atheromatous embolization to the upper extremities or the brain.

In general, patients complaining of arm claudication or symptoms of cerebral hypoperfusion can be treated conservatively unless their quality of life is adversely affected. In contrast, if the symptoms are the result of emboli to either the arm or the brain, surgical repair is required. When appropriate, extrathoracic operations provide satisfactory long-term results and have a low operative mortality; however, direct repair can be also accomplished with low risk. Many surgeons prefer extrathoracic procedures to intrathoracic endarterectomy or bypass procedures except for the management of complex occlusive disease of two or more major vessels.

The options for repairing an innominate lesion include (1) endarterectomy, (2) aortoinnominate (or carotid or subclavian) bypass through a median sternotomy, and (3) axilloaxillary bypass. A left subclavian lesion can be repaired by carotid-subclavian bypass or subclavian-carotid reimplantation. On the right side, subclavian endarterectomy and carotid-subclavian bypass are possible alternatives. Common carotid occlusion can be repaired by endarterectomy on the right side, but subclavian-carotid bypass is usually a simpler operation. Multiple lesions of the arch vessels are bypassed from the aortic arch.

UPPER EXTREMITY REVASCULARIZATION (see Chapter 81)

In this chapter, we describe the surgical treatment of occlusive disease affecting the axillary, brachial, radial, and ulnar arteries. The most common problems involving these vessels include emboli, trauma, and iatrogenic injury.

In general, except for occlusion of one of the two forearm arteries, acute arterial occlusions should be repaired in order to minimize the risk of late symptoms. The decision to repair a chronic arterial occlusion is based on the presence of disabling forearm and hand claudication with minimal exercise or the presence of severe ischemic sequelae.

Brachial artery thrombosis following cardiac catheterization is often associated with only minor symptoms during the acute stage because of the extensive collateral circulation around the elbow; however, late symptoms are present in up to 45% of patients. Furthermore, because repair is usually straightforward and requires thrombectomy or local resection and anastomosis, early repair is advised.

Thrombosis following transaxillary angiography should be treated promptly, and the hematoma in the axillary sheath should be decompressed before neurologic sequelae develop.

The ischemic consequences of radial artery thrombosis following cannulation for blood pressure monitoring can be minimized if the palmar arch is confirmed to be patent by means of the Allen test. In rare cases of acute ischemia, thrombectomy of the radial artery and the palmar arch may be successful.

Embolic occlusion of the axillary or the brachial artery can usually be treated by embolectomy through the brachial artery at the supracondylar level.

Penetrating traumatic injuries are approached directly. Injuries to the proximal axillary artery can usually be approached through an incision in the deltopectoral groove; however, it may be necessary to control the subclavian artery through a supraclavicular incision or by removal of the middle third of the clavicle to optimize exposure.

Chronic upper extremity arterial occlusions are repaired by saphenous vein bypass grafting if the patient's symptoms are disabling.

OCCLUSIVE AND VASOSPASTIC DISEASES INVOLVING DISTAL UPPER EXTREMITY ARTERIES: RAYNAUD'S SYNDROME (see Chapter 82)

The clinical manifestations of diseases of the distal small arteries of the upper extremity span the spectrum from episodic vasospasm on exposure to cold or emotional stimuli to digital ulceration and gangrene. Episodic spasm of the small arteries and arterioles may affect 20% to 30% of certain patient populations. It results from increased force of vasoconstriction owing to altered sensitivity of the adrenergic receptors in smooth muscle cells, and it may be an early manifestation of diseases that cause fixed arterial obstruction. Ulceration or gangrene is invariably the consequence of fixed organic arterial occlusions, most commonly arteritis associated with autoimmune diseases (scleroderma or a CREST variant, mixed connective tissue disease, rheumatoid arthritis, systemic lupus erythematosus (SLE), Sjögren's syndrome, or unclassified connective tissue disease) or arteriosclerosis. Early in the course of connective tissue diseases, the patient's arteries may exhibit excessive vasospasm; later, diffuse small artery obstruction is present as the consequence of vasculitis and subsequent inflammatory thrombosis.

The clinical picture of cold-induced or emotion-induced episodic digital ischemia is best referred to as *Raynaud's syndrome* because the original classification into Raynaud's disease and Raynaud's phenomenon is difficult and has not proved to be of prognostic significance.

The diagnosis of Raynaud's syndrome is made by a clinical history of episodic digital ischemia, usually associated with color changes (pallor, cyanosis, and the rubor of hyperemia). The proximal arteries are evaluated by measuring systolic blood pressures at three levels and recording Doppler waveforms from the brachial, radial, ulnar, and digital arteries. Obstructive diseases of the small arteries may be detected and are invariably present if there is ulceration, but they are most accurately assessed by digital plethysmography with waveform analysis, digital blood pressure measurements, the occlusive digital hypothermic challenge test, magnification arteriography, or a combination.

Associated diseases causing fixed arterial obstruction are identified on the basis of history, physical examination, and baseline laboratory investigations, including complete blood count, erythrocyte sedimentation rate, chemistry profile, urinalysis, rheumatoid factor, and antinuclear antibody. In selected patients, more detailed investigations may be necessary to detect autoimmune diseases. Because the symptoms associated with Raynaud's syndrome may precede the detection of associated diseases by many months or years, careful follow-up with repeated investigation is justified.

In addition to avoidance of cigarette smoking and cold exposure, the vasospastic symptoms are most often treated with calcium channel blocking agents (nifedipine). Other methods of treatment, including intra-arterial reserpine, infusion of prostaglandins, plasmapheresis, and cervical sympathectomy, are not recommended because symptomatic recurrence almost invariably follows the initial period of improvement. Digital ulcers usually respond to conservative therapy, including soaks, débridement, antibiotics, and length-conserving digital amputation. Specific treatment of the collagen vascular disease may be possible.

NEUROGENIC THORACIC OUTLET SYNDROME (see Chapter 83)

Thoracic outlet syndromes are due to compression of the brachial plexus, the subclavian artery, or the subclavian vein as these structures pass through the thoracic outlet. The anatomic abnormalities are generally congenital in origin and include skeletal abnormalities that can be seen on x-ray studies (e.g., a cervical rib, an elongated transverse process of C7, callus formation from a fractured first rib or clavicle, or hypoplastic first rib) and, more often, soft tissue abnormalities (e.g., fibromuscular bands or scalene muscle anomalies). In patients with an anatomic defect, thoracic outlet syndrome may develop as the result of postural abnormalities, musculoskeletal injury, or a spasm secondary to injury.

Controversy surrounds the etiology and treatment of the symptoms of brachial plexus irritation caused by mechanical abnormalities of the thoracic outlet. Presenting complaints may include pain, paresthesias, and weakness, which are usually exacerbated by the overhead posture. Autonomic disturbances, including coldness and skin color changes, are due to sympathetic nerve irritation because they accompany the roots of the brachial plexus.

The differential diagnosis includes musculoskeletal disorders of the neck and shoulder and nerve root compression (cervical root, ulnar nerve, or carpal tunnel). Diagnosis is made on the basis of a careful clinical examination. Note that Adson's test is not reliable in the diagnosis of neurogenic thoracic outlet. Ancillary studies, including electromyography and nerve conduction tests, are used primarily to exclude other causes of patient complaints.

Conservative measures are usually tried first, and surgical decompression is reserved for patients with disabling complaints. Of the possible alternative operative approaches (supraclavicular, transaxillary, infraclavicular, and parascapular), the approach selected depends on which anatomic structure is considered to be the most important cause of compression (congenital or acquired abnormalities of the scalene muscle, cervical rib, an abnormal transverse process of a cervical vertebra, the first rib, congenital or acquired fibromuscular bands, and others) (see Chapter 83).

Although osseous abnormalities are not a common cause of compression, any such abnormality should be removed. Even though the first rib is not the usual cause, first rib resection is effective because the scalene muscles are also divided and other congenital bands are removed. Some surgeons recommend a supraclavicular approach and total removal of the scalene muscles with brachial plexus neurolysis and excision of congenital and acquired fibromuscular bands.

ARTERIAL COMPLICATIONS OF THORACIC OUTLET COMPRESSION (see Chapter 84)

Although less common than neurologic complications, arterial complications of thoracic outlet syndrome may have serious sequelae. Most often, the compression is due to a congenital bony abnormality (a complete cervical rib or an incomplete rib associated with a fibrous band, an elongated transverse process of C7, a congenital anomaly of the first thoracic rib, or malunion or hypertrophic callus following fracture of the clavicle or first rib); rarely is the compression associated with a fibrous band. The compression produces

subclavian artery stenosis, which is followed in time by post-stenotic dilatation, aneurysm formation, or the development of an intimal lesion. Complications include subclavian artery thrombosis, embolization of mural thrombi, and embolization of platelet aggregates.

Most often, patients complain of symptoms of Raynaud's syndrome that are the result of microembolization to digital arteries or of reduced forearm blood flow due to progressive occlusion of large arteries. A large embolus may produce acute ischemic symptoms and must be distinguished from emboli of cardiac origin.

Although clinical findings of a cervical rib, subclavian aneurysm, or supraclavicular bruit or a history of a fractured clavicle or first rib may lead to the correct diagnosis, most often the diagnosis is established by a combination of cervical and upper thoracic spine x-ray studies, noninvasive tests, and arteriography, which demonstrates abnormalities of the subclavian artery (displacement, stenosis, post-stenotic dilatation, aneurysm, an irregular wall, or filling defects).

Because the thoracic outlet must be decompressed and the artery repaired, the optimal surgical exposure is usually the supraclavicular approach. Surgical repair is considered in three steps:

1. The thoracic outlet decompression usually involves complete removal of a cervical rib and its accompanying muscular or fibrous tissue or clavicular resection if malunion, hypertrophic callus, or both are present after a fracture. Simultaneous removal of the first rib is recommended by some surgeons.

2. Arterial reconstruction is necessary if mural thrombus or an aneurysm is present. The treatment of mild post-stenotic dilatation is controversial; some surgeons believe that this lesion will regress after removal of the compression, whereas others believe that arterial repair is necessary.

3. Distal embolic occlusions are difficult to manage, but the ischemic sequelae may decrease in severity after cervical sympathectomy. Proximal embolic occlusions can be managed conservatively if the collateral blood supply is adequate; however, if significant ischemic symptoms are present, sympathectomy, embolectomy, or bypass grafting should be considered. The prognosis depends on the extent of distal embolization.

SUBCLAVIAN–AXILLARY VEIN THROMBOSIS (see Chapter 85)

Axillary–subclavian vein thrombosis may be due to local trauma from a central venous catheter, a pacemaker lead, a diagnostic catheter, or a dialysis catheter. Patients often have localized thrombosis with good collateralization and few symptoms. If the patient is asymptomatic and the thrombus is discovered coincidentally, no specific treatment is necessary. If edema or enlarging collaterals suggest propagation of the thrombus, anticoagulation, infusion of fibrinolytic agents directly into the thrombus through the partially withdrawn indwelling catheter, or both may be of benefit.

Primary (effort) thrombosis may be multifactorial in origin and may result from reduced flow through the subclavian vein as a result of:

1. Intrinsic venous abnormalities (a congenital web or a valve in the subclavian vein at the border of the first rib that may become thickened by repetitive compression).

2. Venous damage due to extrinsic compression (by the subclavius muscle and tendon, the costoclavicular ligament, or the anterior scalene muscle; by callus from a fractured clavicle or first rib; or by congenital fibromuscular bands) that is aggravated by performing repetitive tasks or heavy work with the arm in the elevated position.

3. Coagulation abnormalities (a less likely cause).

Thus, patients frequently have a history of recent physical exertion or trauma, and they often have an abrupt onset of swelling and venous engorgement and visible shoulder collaterals. Duplex Doppler ultrasonography or venography is diagnostic.

If the diagnosis is delayed, a conservative approach (heparin, elevation, and long-term oral anticoagulants) is justified to reduce the risk of pulmonary embolism and the late incidence of symptoms. However, because many patients have persistent symptoms, especially with vigorous upper extremity activity, an aggressive approach to the management of early disease, which consists of clot removal followed by correction of the predisposing factors, is recommended. Although there is no universal agreement on the optimal method of treatment, catheter-directed local fibrinolytic therapy is recommended, followed by the administration of heparin and warfarin. Subsequent balloon angioplasty of residual vein stenosis with or without stenting can be considered but long-term results are not satisfactory. Thoracic outlet decompression (division of a prominent subclavius muscle, the costoclavicular ligament, congenital fibromuscular bands, or the anterior scalene muscle) is preferred.

UPPER EXTREMITY SYMPATHECTOMY (see Chapter 86)

Although performed less frequently than in the past, upper extremity sympathectomy is still indicated in the treatment of selected patients with hyperhidrosis, ischemia, and post-traumatic pain syndromes.

If excessive debilitating sweating of the hands and axillae is not secondary to a systemic disorder such as hyperthyroidism and does not respond to atropine-like drugs or topical antiperspirant medication, sympathectomy is indicated. It usually results in complete relief of symptoms.

The role of sympathectomy in upper extremity ischemic syndromes is controversial. Patients with Raynaud's syndrome that is not associated with digital artery occlusion usually have a transient benefit, perhaps because many later prove to have a collagen vascular disease. Although Porter and Edwards (see Chapter 86) describe their experience, which indicates that most patients with severe digital ischemia can be treated conservatively, the observations by Harris and colleagues (see Chapter 86) suggest that sympathectomy can relieve pain, improve digital perfusion, and decrease the need for amputation.

Although most patients with a post-traumatic pain syndrome (sympathectomy dystrophy) respond to conservative therapy, those without evidence of atrophic changes may show improvement after sympathectomy.

The surgeon can denervate the upper extremity by cutting the sympathetic trunk below the third thoracic ganglion and severing the rami communicantes of the second and third thoracic ganglia. It is unnecessary to excise any portion of the stellate ganglion or to divide the rami to the first thoracic ganglion. To denervate the axilla, the surgeon divides the sympathetic chain below the fourth thoracic ganglion and its associated rami.

Of the alternative surgical approaches, the endoscopic, supraclavicular, and axillary transthoracic approaches are the most popular. Complications after supraclavicular sympathectomy may include Horner's syndrome, lymphatic interruption, and incisional pain. Respiratory complications are the most frequent when a transthoracic approach is used, but a winged scapula can occur from injury to the long thoracic nerve to the serratus anterior. After either procedure, postsympathectomy neuralgia and compensatory hyperhidrosis may occur. The choice between the two operations is made by balancing these relative risks in the hands of the individual surgeon.

After more experience has been obtained with transthoracic endoscopic sympathectomy, this less invasive procedure may gain widespread acceptance.

OCCUPATIONAL VASCULAR PROBLEMS (see Chapter 87)

Arterial and venous injuries occur in the work environment as a result of excessive physical force to the shoulder or hand. Vibration-induced *white finger syndrome* is due to vasospasm and segmental occlusion of digital arteries caused by the prolonged use of vibrating tools (e.g., pneumatic drills, chainsaws). In the early stages, the worker presents with numbness and tingling, but later attacks of cold-induced Raynaud's syndrome predominate. Prevention is important; treatment of established cases by a change of job or the use of a calcium channel blocker may be effective.

The *hypothenar hammer syndrome* is caused by injury to the ulnar artery in its vulnerable subcutaneous position in the area of the hypothenar eminence owing to the repetitive injury to the palm of the hand. The symptoms of Raynaud's syndrome are due to ulnar and digital arterial spasm, ulnar artery thrombosis, or digital artery occlusion secondary to emboli from an ulnar artery aneurysm. Treatment is often supportive, but it may be possible to resect an ulnar artery aneurysm.

Exposure to polyvinylchloride may result in occupational *acro-osteolysis*. Patients present with symptoms of Raynaud's syndrome, owing to multiple digital arterial occlusions; tapering of the tips of the fingers similar to that observed in scleroderma, resulting from resorption of the distal phalangeal tufts; or clubbing secondary to hypervascularity adjacent to the areas of bony resorption.

High-voltage (>1000 V) electrical injuries are associated with widespread tissue damage, but arterial necrosis, thrombosis, stenosis, and aneurysm formation may be observed at any site between the point of entrance and the point of exit during early or late follow-up.

Athletes may experience hand ischemia owing to the arterial damage that results from repeated local trauma associated with such sports as handball, baseball, and karate; thoracic outlet syndrome may result if shoulder movement is overextended, as in baseball pitchers and swimmers performing the butterfly stroke.

Approach to Diagnosis

Lloyd M. Taylor, Jr., M.D.,
Kent Williamson, M.D.,
James M. Edwards, M.D.,
and John M. Porter, M.D.

Vascular surgeons treat large numbers of patients with lower extremity ischemia caused by atherosclerosis with monotonously consistent patterns of symptoms and with well-established diagnostic methods leading to localization of the responsible lesions. In contrast, symptomatic upper extremity ischemia most often is not caused by atherosclerosis. Regardless of etiology, the pathophysiology and, importantly, the prognosis of upper extremity ischemia differ considerably from those of lower extremity ischemia caused by atherosclerosis. To complicate matters further, vasospasm is a normal component of the vasculature of the upper extremity, and misunderstanding how the normal and the abnormal kinds of vasospasm interact in the production of upper extremity ischemic symptoms can lead to confusion in diagnosis.

This chapter describes an approach to diagnosis of upper extremity ischemia that has proved useful at Oregon Health Sciences University. In 1971, the senior author (J.M.P) instituted a long-term clinical research center to which patients with upper extremity ischemia could be referred.[1] In the 28 years since, this project has enrolled over 1600 new patients with symptomatic upper extremity ischemia, allowing refinement of diagnostic methods based upon a large and varied experience. The subjects discussed include (1) the pathophysiology of upper extremity ischemic symptoms, (2) the specific diagnostic steps that allow clinicians to classify the type of arterial disease producing the symptoms, and (3) the specific etiologic factors within each type. For details on the many various causes of upper extremity ischemia, see the other chapters in Section XI and the references listed in Table 78–1 (see "Overview" earlier).

PATHOPHYSIOLOGY

Two pathophysiologic features distinguish ischemia occurring in the upper extremities from the more familiar type occurring in the lower extremities: (1) vasospasm plays a prominent role in the nature of the symptoms that occur, and (2) the available collateral supply in the upper extremities vastly exceeds those in the lower extremities. A knowledge of the role of normal and abnormal vasospasm leads to an understanding of the nature of upper extremity ischemic symptoms, and a knowledge of the role of the abundant collaterals leads to an understanding of the natural history and prognosis of upper extremity ischemia.[2]

Normal Upper Extremity Vasospasm

The hands, like the head, face, and neck, are very involved in regulating heat loss or gain for the whole body. This means that resting blood flow is large, there are many functional arteriovenous shunts, and flow to the hands and fingers varies greatly in response to ambient and body temperature and in response to emotional states. Placing the entire body or the hands in cold results in a marked reduction in hand and finger blood flow owing to spasm of palmar and digital arteries. A similar response may accompany strong emotions.

Abnormal Upper Extremity Vasospasm (Raynaud's Syndrome)

Although it is normal for hand and finger blood flow to decrease in response to cold or emotions, spastic closure of digital arteries resulting in cessation of digital artery flow is abnormal. When this occurs, the stereotypical symptoms produced are known as Raynaud's syndrome. With cessation of digital artery flow, *pallor* occurs. With relaxation of the vasospasm, the first returning arterial blood is rapidly desaturated, producing *cyanosis*. Postischemic hyperemia rapidly replaces cyanosis with *rubor*. Many Raynaud's attacks do not include all three classic color changes, either because they do not occur or because they are sufficiently transient to not be recognized by the patient. Episodes of Raynaud's syndrome vary in duration from a few minutes to, at most, an hour. Raynaud's syndrome resulting from abnormal vasospasm always resolves spontaneously, in response to external warming, or to cessation of the precipitating emotional stress.

Digital artery closure producing Raynaud's syndrome symptoms can occur through two distinctly different mechanisms. In *vasospastic Raynaud's syndrome*, patients with normally patent digital arteries suffer intermittent complete arterial closure as a result of an abnormally forceful vasospastic response to cold (Fig. 78–1). In *obstructive Raynaud's syndrome*, digital arteries that have reduced intraluminal pressure caused by fixed arterial occlusive disease suffer intermittent complete arterial closure as a result of the normal vasospastic response to cold, which is not eliminated by the underlying arterial disease.[3]

Relationship of Raynaud's Syndrome to the Spectrum of Upper Extremity Ischemia

Nearly all patients with symptomatic upper extremity ischemia complain of Raynaud's syndrome. Skin color changes may not be the only symptoms present, but it is rare to have other symptoms, such as exercise-induced muscle pain, ischemic pain at rest, and ischemic ulceration without also having Raynaud's syndrome. The distinctive nature of the Raynaud's symptoms and the fact that the prominent

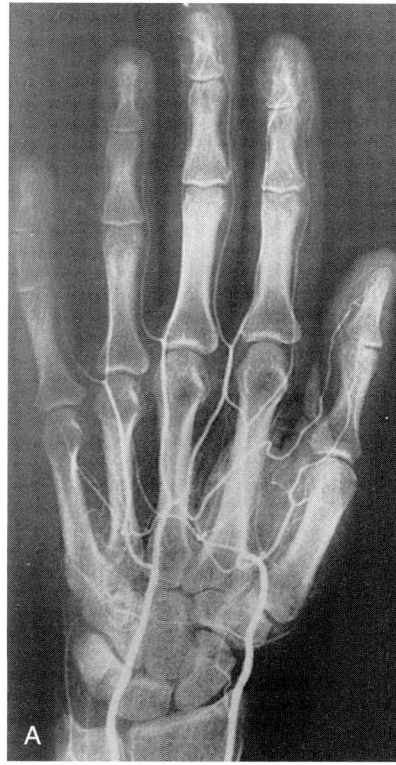
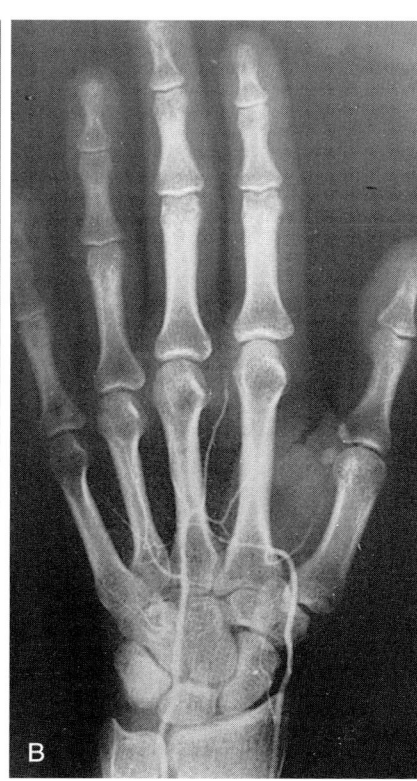

FIGURE 78–1. Magnification hand angiogram showing abnormal cold-induced vasospasm in a patient with idiopathic Raynaud's syndrome. *A,* Normal arterial anatomy with hand at room temperature. *B,* Complete spastic obstruction of digital arteries after immersion of the hand in ice water.

skin color changes are quite visible to patients and to observers among friends and family mean that the Raynaud's symptoms may well be the most prominent. Understanding how these stereotypical symptoms can result from myriad causes is central to an orderly diagnosis of upper extremity ischemia.[4]

Role of Collateral Vessels in Upper Extremity Ischemia

The collateral supply in the upper extremity is more extensive than that in the lower extremity. The familiar progression of severe ischemia from localized distal gangrene to more extensive changes ultimately resulting in limb loss, which occurs with regular frequency in the lower extremities, is vanishingly rare in the upper extremities. The need for limb amputation for ischemia is also extraordinarily rare in the upper extremities. The extensive collateral network means that patients with advanced occlusive disease may be asymptomatic until further progression of disease finally results in occlusion of vital collaterals and symptoms. Such symptoms may be erroneously interpreted as an indication of an acute disease process, when in fact the opposite is true. The abundance of collateral supply in the upper extremity is the most important reason why classification of upper extremity ischemia into acute and chronic causes is not clinically very relevant.

INITIAL APPROACH TO DIAGNOSIS

Experience indicates that it is convenient and clinically relevant to classify the various disorders producing upper extremity ischemia according to (1) whether the affected

vessels are large arteries (proximal to the wrist) or small arteries (distal to the wrist) and (2) whether the symptoms result from vasospasm or from arterial obstruction. In a few patients, upper extremity ischemic symptoms occur when embolism from proximal large arterial sources results in obstruction of distal small arteries.[5] Although these events are rare, the potential for surgical correction of the proximal large artery source of embolism means that any approach to diagnosis must include methods to identify this clinically important group. The diverse disorders that produce upper extremity ischemic symptoms are listed in Table 78–1 according to this classification. It is nearly always possible to determine whether large or small arteries are involved and whether the involvement is vasospastic or obstructive. If obstructive, obstruction is differentiated from intrinsic embolic disease by history, physical examination, appropriate vascular laboratory testing and, when indicated, by arteriography.

History

We can differentiate vasospasm from arterial obstruction by understanding a basic fact: *Symptoms caused by vasospasm are intermittent, and the involved extremity is asymptomatic and normal in appearance and to examination between attacks; thus, constant symptomatic ischemia is always caused by arterial obstruction,* although the severity may wax and wane as normal vasospasm induced by cold occurs. The single exception occurs when abnormal vasospasm is caused by toxins or medications, as is the case with ergotism.[6] Consequently, *all symptoms of severe upper extremity ischemia, including ischemic rest pain, fixed cyanosis, ischemic ulceration, and gangrene, are caused by fixed arterial obstruction, not by vasospasm.* Again, an exception is recognized in the case of ergotism.

We can distinguish between large and small artery involvement by history by recognizing the extent of the symptomatic involvement. Exercise-induced pain in upper extremity muscle groups is obviously related to large artery obstruction. Symptoms confined to the hands and fingers may result from either large or small artery obstruction or from embolic occlusion of small arteries from large artery sources.

Embolization of distal small arteries from proximal large artery sources should be suspected whenever symptoms are unilateral. Although further testing may reveal that the involvement is in fact bilateral, unilateral symptoms from abnormal vasospasm alone or from diffuse small artery disease is rare.

The history should include specific questions to elicit causes of environmental or occupational exposure known to be related to upper extremity arterial disease, such as ergot exposure, vibrating tool use, vinyl chloride exposure, and use of the hands as a hammer (e.g., as with carpenters and mechanics). Diabetes or symptoms of atherosclerotic disease at other sites, smoking history, and any history of connective tissue or hematologic disorders should also be specifically considered.[7]

Physical Examination

Palpation of axillary, brachial, radial, and ulnar pulses and inspection of the hands and fingers for ischemic lesions are the basic steps in initial physical examination. Normal pulses to the level of the wrist with ischemic lesions on the hands establishes the presence of small artery obstruction. An embolic source should be suspected if the findings are unilateral. Cervical ribs and aneurysmal dilation of the subclavian and axillary arteries should be specifically evaluated by palpation.

Just as with the history, the presence of ischemic lesions establishes that the patient's condition is the result of arterial obstructive disease, not abnormal vasospasm. Because of the excellent collateral supply of the upper extremity, it is possible for a large amount of arterial obstruction to exist in the presence of normal pulses and normal arterial pressures. For this reason, vascular laboratory testing for both abnormal vasospasm and arterial obstruction is an important extension of the physical examination.[8]

Vascular Laboratory Examination

Bilateral arm segmental pressures and Doppler analogue waveforms allow detection of hemodynamically significant large artery obstruction. Photoplethysmographic waveforms obtained from the fingertips, combined with digital artery blood pressures using the photoplethysmograph as a detector and finger cuffs, is the most accurate test for detecting obstruction of palmar and digital arteries. When results are abnormal, the digital pressure and waveform testing are quite specific for arterial obstruction.[9] These tests, however, are not ideally sensitive. This is because each finger has two digital arteries, and it is possible for one to be obstructed completely while patency of the other maintains normal finger blood pressure. Similarly, because the finger cuffs are applied at the level of the proximal phalanx, it is possible for considerable distal digital occlusive disease to exist and for the detected finger blood pressure to remain normal.

Abnormal vasospasm is detected by digital hypothermic challenge testing with the machine designed by Nielsen and Lassen.[10] Details of this testing including criteria for normal and abnormal and accuracy are in Chapter 79.

Embolization of distal small arteries from proximal large artery sources is suggested by vascular laboratory findings of abnormal finger pressures and waveforms in the symptomatic hand with normal findings in the contralateral hand. Involvement of only a few digits in the symptomatic hand is even more suggestive of emboli. In contrast, if only one hand is symptomatic but the digital artery and waveform testing shows bilateral involvement, intrinsic small artery obstructive disease is the most likely explanation.[11]

Radiographic Examination

For patients with large artery obstructions and for those with suspected embolic occlusion of distal small arteries, chest radiographs are recommended to detect bony abnormalities of the thoracic outlet (cervical rib, abnormal first rib). For patients with intrinsic small artery obstructive disease, hand radiographs are necessary to detect the soft tissue calcifications characteristic of scleroderma and mixed connective tissue disease.[7]

Arteriography

Detailed arteriography of upper extremity vessels from the aortic arch to the fingers should be performed in patients with symptomatic large artery obstruction and in all patients with suspected embolic occlusion of distal small arteries from proximal large artery sources. We do not perform arteriograms in patients with history, physical examination, or vascular laboratory testing compatible with abnormal vasospasm (*idiopathic vasospastic Raynaud's syndrome*). Arteriograms are also not required in patients with noninvasive findings showing diffuse bilateral small artery obstructive disease and laboratory evidence clearly diagnostic of connective tissue disease, defined hematologic disorder, or other known cause of small artery disease, as listed in Table 78–1.

In our practice, arteriograms are performed in patients with severe symptoms and probable small artery disease in whom a diagnosis of cause cannot be made based on laboratory testing (see next section) because the arteriographic appearance of the abnormalities may be diagnostic (i.e., fibromuscular disease) and because proximal large artery source of distal embolic occlusions may be difficult or impossible to detect without arteriography (Fig. 78–2).

Upper extremity arteriography, including adequate views of palmar and digital arteries, can be quite difficult to perform.[12] Normal vasospasm may mimic arterial obstruction of both large and small arteries. Magnification views, hand warming, and administration of multiple pharmacologic agents may be necessary to produce images of diagnostic quality. Digital images, particularly on older machines, may not have high enough resolution to see digital emboli; conventional "cut-film" images are superior.

Most upper extremity arteriograms should be bilateral

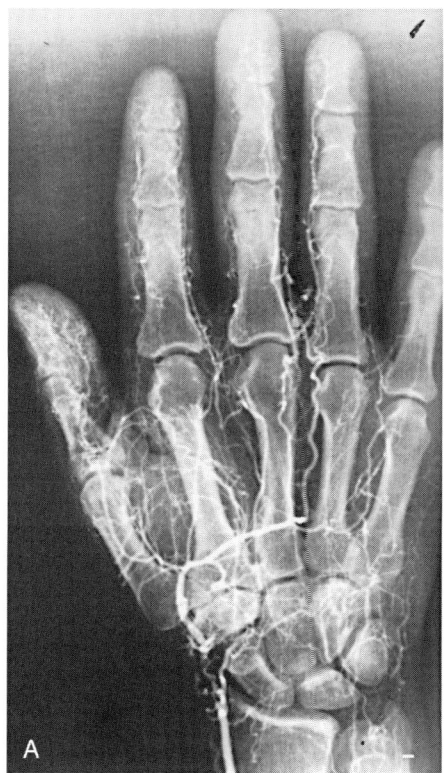 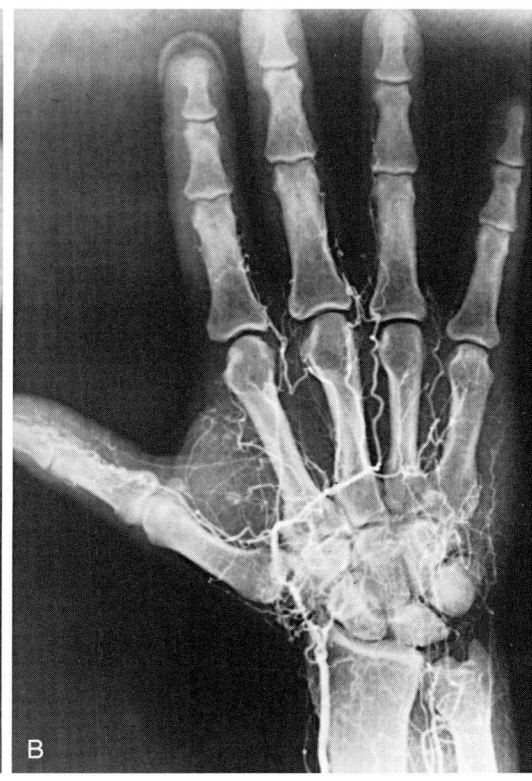

FIGURE 78–2. Small artery obstruction. *A,* Multiple palmar and digital artery occlusions in a patient with scleroderma. *B,* Appearance of arteriogram after ice water immersion. Normal cold-induced vasospasm still occurs in the presence of the extensive arterial disease.

even if only one extremity is symptomatic, because it is the bilateral nature of diffuse small artery obstructive disease that allows differentiation from diffuse small artery obstructions produced by embolism from proximal sources, which should nearly always be unilateral. This is especially important when proximal atherosclerotic lesions are suspected as the source of distal emboli. Bilateral small artery obstructions may identify the atherosclerosis as being merely coexistent with the independent diffuse small artery disease, instead of being its cause, as would be the case if the small artery obstructions were unilateral.

Echocardiography

Rarely, patients are encountered with unilateral ischemic symptoms from palmar and digital artery occlusions in whom arteriography fails to reveal a proximal embolic source. Some of these patients have embolism of athero-thrombotic material from ulcerated atherosclerotic plaques in the aortic arch, near the origin of the innominate or left subclavian arteries that cannot be detected by arteriography. Transesophageal echocardiography has proved capable of demonstrating such lesions, including the adherent thrombus, with greater sensitivity than can be obtained with arteriographic visualization.[13, 14]

LABORATORY DIAGNOSIS OF SPECIFIC DISORDERS

Small Artery Vasospasm

Abnormally forceful vasospasm in small arteries distal to the wrist most frequently results from idiopathic Raynaud's

syndrome, a condition that affects as many as 25% of young women in cool damp climates (see Fig. 78–1).[15] Idiopathic Raynaud's syndrome is by far the most frequent cause of hand ischemia of any type. The laboratory tests which are routinely obtained in patients with small artery vasospasm are listed in Table 78–2. Screening tests for hematologic disorders (complete blood count with platelets) and for connective tissue disease (erythrocyte sedimentation rate, antinuclear antibody, rheumatoid factor) are indicated because Raynaud's syndrome may be the initial symptomatic manifestation of these diseases, symptoms that may precede other manifestations by years.[1] Although connective tissue disease and hematologic disorders produce arterial obstruction, vascular laboratory testing may be insufficiently sensitive to detect the obstructions in patients with minimal disease. Abnormal small artery vasospasm can also result from use of vibrating tools and from occupational exposure to vinyl chloride or therapeutic use of beta-adrenergic blocking agents.[16, 17]

Large Artery Vasospasm

Significant vasospasm of large arteries proximal to the wrist is only seen in ergot toxicity.[6] In modern practice, the source of ergot is nearly always from medication intended to treat migraine or uterine bleeding, although occasional outbreaks of ergotism from grain, contaminated by the fungus *Claviceps purpurea,* continue to occur.

Small Artery Obstructive Disease

Small arteries distal to the wrist are most frequently obstructed by lesions resulting from connective tissue disease

TABLE 78–2. LABORATORY TESTING IN PATIENTS WITH
UPPER EXTREMITY ISCHEMIA

Small Artery Vasospasm

 Complete blood count with platelet count
 Urinalysis
 Multichemistry screen
 Erythrocyte sedimentation rate
 Antinuclear antibody
 Rheumatoid factor

Large Artery Vasospasm

 No tests; caused only by ergotism

Small Artery Obstruction

 Same tests as for small artery vasospasm plus the following, as
   indicated:
  Serum protein electrophoresis
  Total hemolytic complement
  Hep-2 antinuclear antibody
  Extractable nuclear antigen
  Anti-native DNA antibody
  Cold agglutinins
  Complement (C3, C4)
  Protein C
  Protein S
  Antithrombin III
  Anticardiolipin antibody
  Lupus anticoagulant
  Heparin-associated antibodies
  Factor V Leiden
  Prothrombin gene mutation

Large Artery Obstruction

 Same tests as for small artery vasospasm
 Appropriate evaluation for atherosclerosis when indicated
  Lipid panel
  Blood glucose
  Hypercoagulability testing

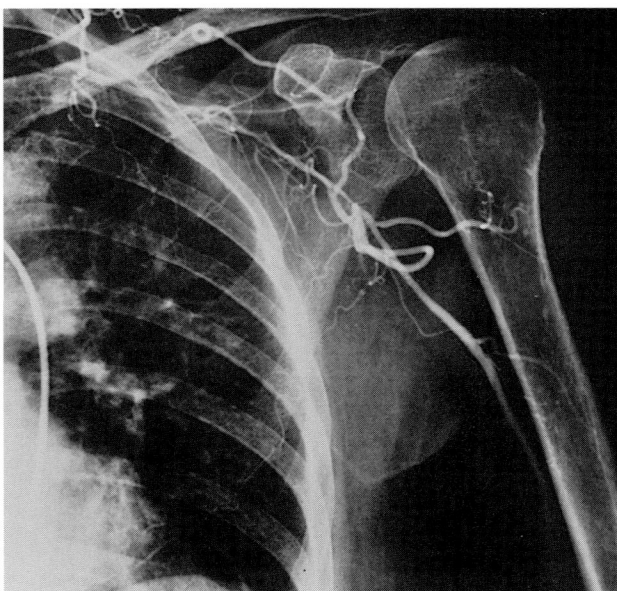

FIGURE 78–3. Large artery obstruction. Typical long tapered stenosis of the axillary artery in a patient with exercise-induced arm muscle pain and Raynaud's syndrome. The patient has giant cell arteritis.

or arteritis or by myeloproliferative disorders or hypercoagulable states, the most frequent types of which are listed in Table 78–1 (see Fig. 78–2). Buerger's disease and malignancy are also relatively frequent causes. Laboratory evaluation required in such patients may be extensive and should be guided by the other features of history and physical examination and the findings of the initial screening laboratory examination. Extensive bilateral small artery obstruction in the absence of any laboratory features of connective tissue disease, hypercoagulable states, hematologic abnormality, or other identified cause has been called *hypersensitivity angiitis*, based on the presumption that it has an immune origin and the fact that such patients almost always suffer a discrete symptomatic episode followed by gradual improvement through collateral vessel formation without recurrence.

Large Artery Obstructive Disease

Atherosclerosis and arterial compression by bony abnormalities of the thoracic outlet (cervical rib, abnormal first rib or clavicle) are the most frequent causes of large artery obstruction (Fig. 78–3). Emboli from cardiac sources, Takayasu's or giant cell arteritis, and fibromuscular disease are more rare. Basic laboratory screening, as listed in Table 78–2, is indicated because of the frequent coexistence of underlying atherosclerosis with connective tissue disease or

hematologic and myeloproliferative disorders or hypercoagulable states.

Large Artery Diseases That May Produce Embolization in the Absence of Proximal Arterial Obstruction

Ulcerated atherosclerotic plaques, subclavian artery aneurysms, and ulnar artery aneurysms that are vulnerable to

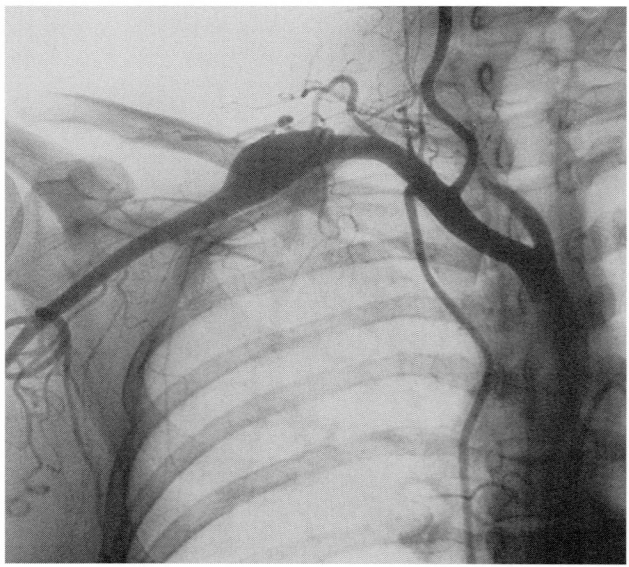

FIGURE 78–4. Proximal large artery source of emboli. Subclavian aneurysm associated with a cervical rib in a patient who presented with unilateral finger ischemia. (From Porter JM, Taylor LM, Friedman EI: Indications for cervical and first rib excisions. In Greenhalgh R [ed]: Indications in Vascular Surgery. Philadelphia, WB Saunders, 1988, pp 101–116.)

occupational trauma may all serve as sources for emboli that occlude distal palmar and digital arteries (Fig. 78–4) These lessons may not produce hemodynamically significant stenosis of the involved proximal arteries, leading to the mistaken impression that the symptoms are the result of intrinsic small artery occlusive disease. Clinicians must maintain a high level of suspicion leading to arteriography to make certain that such lesions are not overlooked. It is important to remember that idiopathic vasospastic Raynaud's syndrome affects as many as 25% of persons in cool climates. Unilateral severe symptoms of ischemia with contralateral mild Raynaud's syndrome symptoms should not be regarded as evidence of systemic bilateral disease, since this condition may simply result from the coincidence of the very common idiopathic Raynaud's syndrome with a far more serious source of arterial embolism.

SUMMARY

In our experience, the most frequent errors in diagnosing the source of upper extremity ischemic symptoms have been those resulting from (1) attribution of symptoms of severe ischemia to vasospasm, (2) failure to recognize that acute symptoms of upper extremity ischemia are most frequently the result of a long period of asymptomatic progression of a chronic disease process, and (3) inability to recognize that unilateral small artery obstruction frequently results from a proximal large artery source of emboli. Essential to avoiding such errors is understanding the pathophysiology of upper extremity ischemia, including the role of normal and abnormal vasospasm, and why Raynaud's syndrome symptoms occur in nearly all patients with upper extremity ischemia, regardless of cause. The abundant collateral supply of the upper extremities explains why extensive occlusive disease can remain asymptomatic until far advanced changes are present. Recognizing that all causes of intrinsic small artery obstruction are systemic diseases should eliminate the failure to search for an embolic source when only unilateral involvement is present.

The approach to diagnosis (Fig. 78–5), which consists of initial classification into vasospastic versus obstructive and large artery versus small artery involvement, followed by detailed evaluation to determine the actual diagnosis within each category, has proved serviceable to the authors during a large experience with more than a thousand patients referred for nearly 30 years.

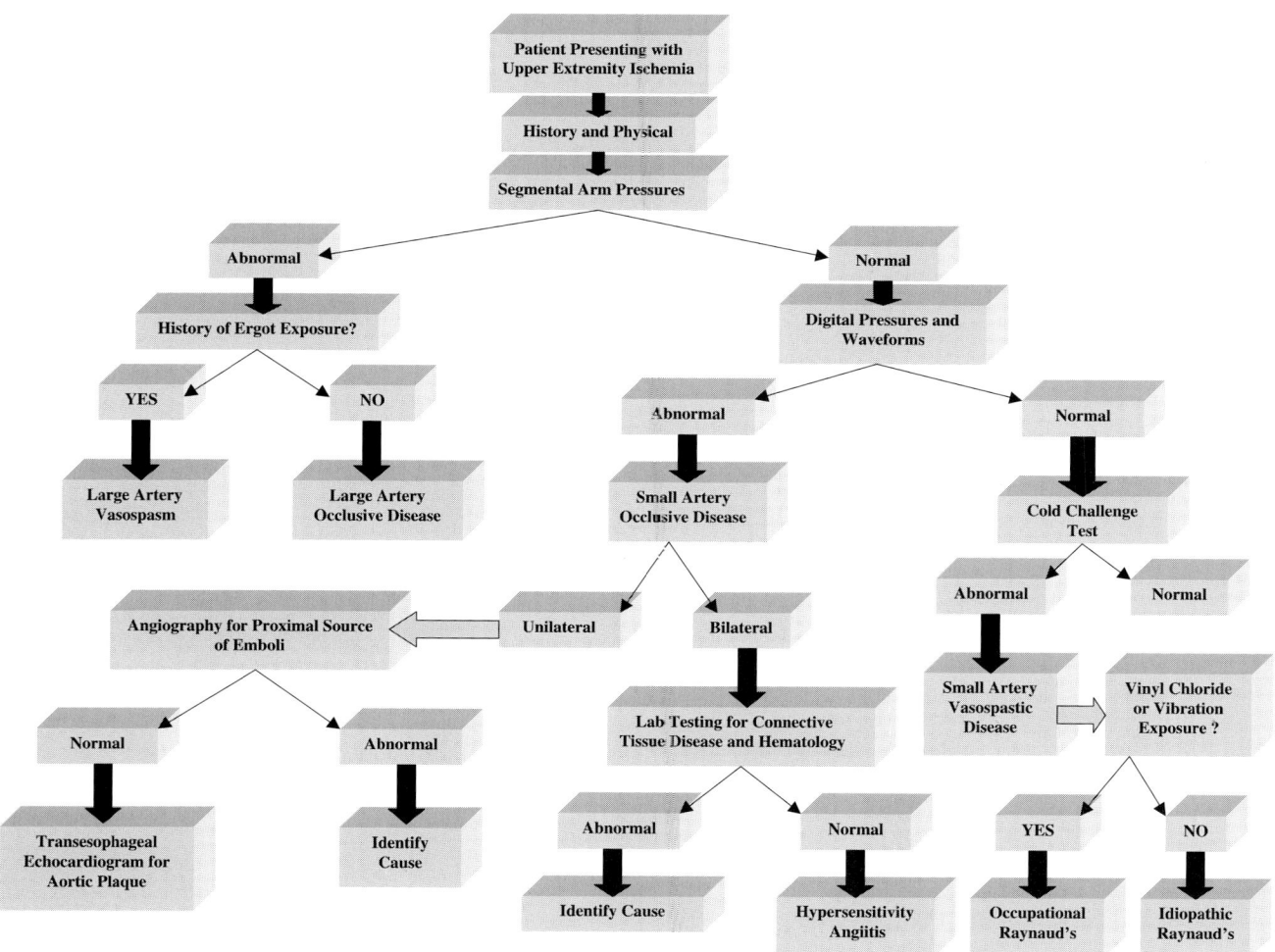

FIGURE 78–5. Schematic approach to diagnosis of upper extremity ischemia.

REFERENCES

1. Landry GJ, Edwards JM, McLafferty RB, et al: Long-term outcome of Raynaud's syndrome in a prospectively analyzed patient cohort. J Vasc Surg 23:76–86, 1996.
2. Porter JM, Bardana EJ, Baur CM, et al: The clinical significance of Raynaud's syndrome. Surgery 80:756, 1976.
3. Porter, JM, Snider RL, Bardana EJ, et al: The diagnosis and treatment of Raynaud's phenomenon. Surgery 77:11, 1975.
4. Spittell JA Jr: Raynaud's phenomenon and allied vasospastic conditions. In Juergens JL, Spittell JA Jr, Fairbairn JF (eds): Allen-Barker-Hines Peripheral Vascular Disease, 5th ed. Philadelphia, WB Saunders, 1980, p 555.
5. McNamara MF, Takali HS, Yao JST, Bergan JJ: A systemic approach to severe hand ischemia. Surgery 83:1, 1978.
6. Merhoff CG, Porter JM: Ergot intoxication: Historical review and description of unusual clinical manifestations. Ann Surg 180:773–779, 1974.
7. Edwards JM, Taylor LM Jr, Porter JM: Small Artery Disease of the Upper Extremity. In Machleder HI (ed): Vascular Disorders of the Upper Extremity, 2nd ed. Mount Kisco, NY, Futura Press, 1989, p 103.
8. Dale WA, Lewis MR: Management of ischemia of the hand and fingers. Surgery 67:62, 1970.
9. Holmgren K, Baur GM, Porter JM: The role of digital photoplethysmography in the evaluation of Raynaud's syndrome. Bruit 5:19, 1981.
10. Nielsen SL, Lassen NA: Measurement of digital blood pressure after local cooling. J Appl Physiol 43:907–910, 1977.
11. Mills JL, Friedman EI, Taylor LM Jr, Porter JM: Upper extremity disease caused by small artery disease. Ann Surg 205:521–528, 1987.
12. Rosch J, Porter JM, Gralino B: Cryodynamic hand angiography in the diagnosis and management of Raynaud's syndrome. Circulation 55:807–810, 1977.
13. Weinberger J, Azhar S, Danisi F, et al: A new noninvasive technique for imaging atherosclerotic plaque in the aortic arch of stroke patients by transcutaneous real-time B-mode ultrasonography: An initial report. Stroke 29:673–676, 1998.
14. Laperche T, Laurian C, Roudaut R, Steg PG: Mobile thromboses of the aortic arch without aortic debris: A transesophageal echocardiographic finding associated with unexplained arterial embolism: The Filiale Echocardiographie de la Societe Francaise de Cardiologie. Circulation 96:288–294, 1977.
15. Olsen N, Nielsen SL: Prevalence of primary Raynaud's phenomenon in young females. Scand J Clin Lab Invest 37:761, 1978.
16. Chatterjee DS, Petrie A, Taylor W: Prevalence of vibration-induced white finger in flourspar mines in Weardale. Br J Indust Med 35:208, 1978.
17. Taylor W, Pelmear PL: Raynaud's phenomenon of occupational origin: An epidemiological survey. Acta Chir Scand (Suppl) 465:27, 1976.
18. Porter JM, Taylor LM, Friedman EI: Indications for cervical and first rib excisions. In Greenhalgh R (ed): Indications in Vascular Surgery. Philadelphia, WB Saunders, 1988, pp 101–116.

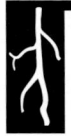

CHAPTER 79
Evaluation of Acute and Chronic Ischemia of the Upper Extremity

David S. Sumner, M.D.

The evaluation of ischemic disorders of the upper extremity often challenges the diagnostic ability of even the most experienced clinician.[27, 65, 82] Not only are there multiple causes, but many of the disease processes are poorly understood. Ischemia may be constant or intermittent; may be a manifestation of a fixed arterial obstruction, vasospasm, or both; and may reflect involvement of large proximal arteries, small distal arteries, or the microvasculature. Although much can be learned from the history and physical examination findings, simple noninvasive tests contribute important diagnostic information that can prove useful in selecting further investigative modalities, such as arteriography, blood tests, or nerve blocks.[9, 10, 50, 96] They provide an accurate assessment of the severity of the circulatory impairment, locate the site or sites of obstruction, differentiate between obstruction and vasospasm, and may also suggest a cause.

Finally, noninvasive tests help to define the natural history of the disease process and lend objectivity to the evaluation of the results of medical and surgical treatment.

PATHOPHYSIOLOGY

Some knowledge of the pathophysiology of upper extremity ischemic syndromes is necessary in order to understand the results of noninvasive testing. As in the lower extremities, the system responsible for delivering blood to the tissues of the arms and hands consists of (1) inflow arteries (innominate and subclavian); (2) intrinsic arteries (axillary, brachial, antecubital, radial, ulnar, palmar, and digital); and (3) arterioles, which terminate in sphincters that control flow into the capillaries. The collateral circulation around the shoulder, axilla, and elbow is particularly well developed; also, within the forearm, hand, and fingers, the radial and ulnar arteries, the deep and superficial palmar arches, and the paired proper digital arteries provide parallel systems in which either one of the pair can usually sustain circulation independent of the other. Arteriovenous anastomoses, which are situated proximal to the capillary bed and which divert blood away from the capillaries, are more frequent than in the lower extremities and are especially numerous in the tips of the fingers. They are also found in the volar surfaces of the fingers and hands but are essentially absent in the forearm.

Fixed Arterial Obstruction

The term *fixed* is used to designate obstructions that are due to well-defined anatomic changes involving the wall or lumen of the artery. A host of disparate entities can produce fixed obstruction of the upper extremity arteries, including atherosclerosis; thrombosis; emboli; dissection; toxins; autoimmune disorders (connective tissue diseases), Buerger's disease (thromboangiitis obliterans); and vibratory, blunt, and penetrating trauma. As discussed in Chapter 7, lesions seldom produce recognizable hemodynamic changes unless the cross-sectional area of the arterial lumen is diminished by more than 75%. Disturbances of pressure and flow are less severe when the process is localized and when collaterals are well developed. Impairment is more severe when the disease is extensive or multisegmental, when entrance or exit of collaterals is blocked, or when terminal arteries or those without efficient collateral beds are involved. Lesions that are asymptomatic under normal resting conditions may become symptomatic during exercise or when stimuli that produce vasospasm are superimposed.

Chronic stenoses or occlusions isolated to the subclavian, axillary, or brachial arteries are usually well tolerated because of the abundant collateral circulation. Although peripheral blood pressures are reduced, blood flow at rest remains normal. Exercise, however, may produce claudication. In the forearm, hand, and fingers, chronic (and even some acute) occlusions limited to either one of the paired arteries may cause few or no hemodynamic changes. Lesions in these areas are often completely asymptomatic. Multiple occlusions, on the other hand, may be so extensive or so critically located that they overwhelm the compensatory mechanisms, resulting in ischemia. Chronic obstruction of an end artery (such as the common digital) or of both proper digital arteries frequently causes ischemia of the involved finger.

As a rule, acute occlusions, especially those involving unpaired or terminal arteries, prove to be more devastating. Owing to the instantaneous nature of the obstruction, blood flow distal to the site of trauma or an embolic occlusion must be maintained by preexisting collaterals, which may not be adequate to sustain tissue viability. Moreover, emboli tend to lodge at bifurcations, where they obstruct both the main arterial channel and the collateral input. Consequently, peripheral arterial pressure is usually severely reduced and may not be measurable.

Intermittent Obstruction

The two major causes of intermittent episodes of arm or hand ischemia are (1) extrinsic compression of the large inflow arteries and (2) vasospasm of the digital arteries. Although the two sometimes occur together, their clinical manifestations and pathophysiology are radically different. Both may also occur in conjunction with fixed arterial obstruction.

Extrinsic Compression

The structures responsible for extrinsic arterial compression include bones, muscles, tendons, and ligaments. In the upper extremity, compression is most likely to occur at the thoracic outlet, where the subclavian artery must traverse a narrow triangular opening bounded by the first rib, the scalenus anticus and medius muscles, and their associated ligaments. Compression may also occur around the pectoralis minor muscle. In these areas, obstruction is related to the position of the arm. Unless emboli arising from a poststenotic dilatation of the subclavian artery have lodged in the more peripheral arteries of the arm, hemodynamic changes are evident only while the artery is actually being compressed.

Vasospasm

The peripheral arterioles of the upper extremity, especially those in the fingertips, are normally quite sensitive to sympathetic or alpha-adrenergic stimuli. Emotional factors, pain, respiratory reflexes, local cold exposure, and total body cooling all cause arteriolar constriction. Release of arteriolar constriction by local or total body heating, administration of sympatholytic agents or vasodilating drugs, or surgical or pharmacologic sympathectomy ordinarily causes a great increase in blood flow. Much of this increase is due to the opening of arteriovenous shunts, which are abundant in the fingertips. Flow through the capillaries is less affected. Fingertip blood flow is therefore quite variable, ranging from 1.0 ml/100 ml/min to as much as 150 ml/100 ml/min in normal individuals.[66]

Ischemia caused by vasospasm is much more common in the upper extremities than in the lower extremities. The episodic color changes in the fingers and toes of patients with cold sensitivity are known as *Raynaud's phenomenon*, for the French physician who initially described the condition in 1862. Classically, in response to cold exposure, the fingers initially become pallid, then cyanotic, and finally red, as the vasospasm subsides. Variations are common, and many patients never experience the typical triphasic color changes. The causes of Raynaud's phenomenon are multifactorial and, despite intensive investigation, remain incompletely understood. Although many classifications have been proposed, none is entirely satisfactory.

For the purpose of discussing the hemodynamics of vasospastic disease, this chapter employs the term *secondary Raynaud's phenomenon* to designate conditions in which a fixed anatomic obstruction has been identified (or is strongly suspected) and the term *primary Raynaud's disease* to identify conditions in which the cause remains obscure.[3, 6, 44, 93]

Secondary Raynaud's Phenomenon

Arteriolar constriction is usually tolerated well, but when it is superimposed on a substrate of fixed arterial obstruction, the previously adequately perfused fingers may become ischemic (Fig. 79–1).[36, 67, 93] This is the mechanism principally responsible for the appearance of Raynaud's phenomenon in patients with autoimmune diseases (e.g., scleroderma), Buerger's disease, or traumatic arteritis. Although the fingers typically display hemodynamic alter-

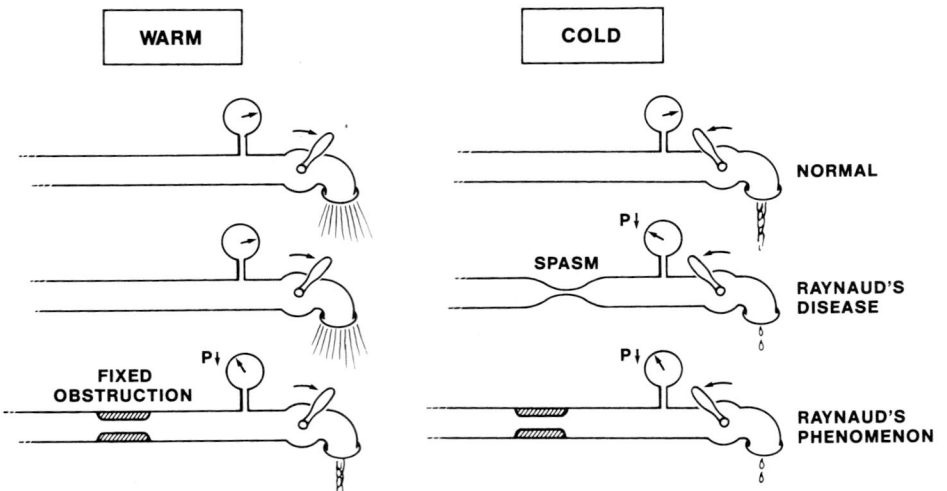

FIGURE 79–1. Effect of cold exposure on normal fingers, fingers with primary Raynaud's disease, and fingers with Raynaud's phenomenon secondary to fixed arterial obstruction. Faucets represent arteriolar sphincters. When the handle is turned to the right, the arterioles are dilated; when it is turned to the left, the arterioles are constricted. Gauges represent digital arterial pressure, with increasing pressure indicated by clockwise rotation of the hand. Digital blood flow is represented by the output of the faucets.

ations even when they are warm, the changes become more marked with cold exposure.

Primary Raynaud's Disease

Although the digital arteries in patients with this form of episodic ischemia may be histologically normal, they are hypersensitive to cold and to alpha-adrenergic stimuli.[16, 24, 29, 45, 55, 57] Unlike the digital arteries of normal individuals, which are relatively unresponsive to cold, those of patients with primary Raynaud's disease display a remarkable ability to constrict, with complete closure occurring when the skin temperature falls below a threshold level.[92] This, together with cold-induced arteriolar constriction, produces profound but temporary digital ischemia (see Fig. 79–1).[52, 77, 89] Even when the hands are warm, enhanced sympathetic activity is evident. Although the digital arterial pressure is normal, blood flow in the fingers is moderately reduced.[77, 85] Whereas the arterioles are sensitive both to local and to remote cold exposure, the digital arteries respond almost exclusively to local cold.[77]

Comment: Admittedly, this classification into secondary Raynaud's phenomenon and primary Raynaud's disease is arbitrary. Not infrequently, patients in one category show responses consistent with the other. For example, digital artery vasospasm may occur in patients with histologic features of autoimmune disease; in addition, autoimmune phenomena may contribute to the hypersensitivity of the anatomically normal digital arteries in patients with primary Raynaud's disease.[82] There may well be a continuum of pathophysiologic features that extends from one class to the other. This notion is supported by the observation that patients who initially appear to have the more benign primary Raynaud's disease are eventually diagnosed as having scleroderma or some other autoimmune problem. Nonetheless, for the purposes of the initial hemodynamic evaluation, the author has found the classification to be quite useful.

Yet, the dichotomous classification proposed by Edwards and Porter has considerable merit because it makes no assumptions about the presence or absence of a currently diagnosable associated disease in patients who have no demonstrable organic obstruction of the digital or palmar arteries.[26] Patients who have normal digital blood pressures between attacks are said to have *vasospastic Raynaud's syndrome*. Patients whose resting digital blood pressure is reduced and who, by definition, have an associated disease are said to have *obstructive Raynaud's syndrome*.

NONINVASIVE STUDIES

Noninvasive studies are designed to answer the following questions:

1. Is there fixed arterial obstruction? If so, what is its location and how severe is the hemodynamic impairment?
2. Is there intermittent obstruction related to arm position?
3. Is there cold-induced vasospasm?
4. Do the arterioles retain the ability to dilate?
5. Is sympathetic activity present?

Answers to the first three questions help to determine the cause of the patient's complaints, and answers to the last two aid in selecting therapy.

Segmental Pressure Measurements

The examination of any patient with complaints suggestive of upper extremity ischemia should begin with the measurement of segmental arterial pressures. Techniques for noninvasive pressure measurements are described in Chapter 10. Pneumatic cuffs are placed around the brachial area, the upper forearm, and the wrist; each cuff in turn is inflated above the systolic pressure and then slowly deflated while the return of flow, signifying the pressure at each level, is detected by a Doppler probe placed over the radial or ulnar artery or the palmar arch. In the absence of an arterial signal, the return of flow can be monitored plethysmographically.

At each of the three anatomic levels, the pressure in one arm is compared with that in the other.[97] Normally, the difference in pressure between the two arms at any given

TABLE 79–1. PRESSURE DATA: NORMAL ARMS*

	MEAN ± SD	RANGE
Difference (mmHg): Higher Pressure Minus Lower Pressure		
Brachial	5.4 ± 4.6	0–16
Forearm	7.6 ± 4.6	2–16
Wrist	7.2 ± 6.1	0–22
Index: Lower Pressure Divided by Higher Pressure		
Brachial	0.96 ± 0.03	0.88–1.00
Forearm	0.93 ± 0.04	0.85–0.98
Wrist	0.94 ± 0.05	0.83–1.00

Data from Sumner DS, Lambeth A, Russell JB: Diagnosis of upper extremity obstructive and vasospastic syndromes by Doppler ultrasound, plethysmography, and temperature profiles. In Puel P, Boccalon H, Enjalbert A (eds): Hemodynamics of the Limbs 1. Toulouse, France, GEPESC, 1979, pp 365–373.
*Pressures in one arm compared with those in the other arm at the same level. SD = standard deviation.

site seldom exceeds 15 to 20 mmHg and is usually considerably less (~5 to 8 mmHg) (Table 79–1). Indices obtained by dividing the lower of the two pressures by the higher average about 0.95 and are rarely less than 0.85 (see Table 79–1). Pressure gradients between adjacent levels of the same arm are usually less than 15 mmHg, with a mean in the range of 5 to 7 mmHg (Table 79–2). Because the relationship between cuff width and arm diameter varies between levels, and perhaps because peripheral augmentation of systolic pressure may occur, the gradients are occasionally reversed, with pressures at the more distal sites exceeding those measured farther up the arm. Indices obtained by dividing the pressure at the forearm or wrist by the ipsilateral brachial pressure fluctuate around 1.0 and almost always exceed 0.85 (see Table 79–2).

A reduction in the brachial pressure indicates occlusive disease of the ipsilateral innominate, subclavian, axillary, or upper brachial artery.[32, 105] In a series of patients with lesions in one or more of these arteries, our group observed that the brachial pressures in the involved arms were 20 to 124 mmHg less than those in the control arms, with a mean difference of 50 ± 33 mmHg.[97] The average ipsilateral-contralateral pressure index was 0.65 ± 0.15, with a range of 0.38 to 0.81. Because bilateral subclavian artery obstruction is not uncommon, both brachial pressures may be reduced. Bilateral disease is suggested by the presence of bruits over both subclavian arteries and may be confirmed by the detection of abnormal Doppler signals from the subclavian arteries. In such cases, the ankle pressure

TABLE 79–2. PRESSURE DATA: NORMAL ARMS*

	GRADIENT (mmHg)	
Brachial-forearm	5.0 ± 4.8	−6 to +15
Forearm-wrist	6.6 ± 4.6	−19 to +14
	INDEX	
Forearm-brachial	0.97 ± 0.06	0.87 to 1.06
Wrist-brachial	0.99 ± 0.06	0.89 to 1.15

Data from Sumner DS, Lambeth A, Russell JB: Diagnosis of upper extremity obstructive and vasospastic syndromes by Doppler ultrasound, plethysmography, and temperature profiles. In Puel P, Boccalon H, Enjalbert A (eds): Hemodynamics of the Limbs 1. Toulouse, France, GEPESC, 1979, pp 365–373.
*Pressures at different levels in the same arm.

can be used as a reference value, provided there is no evidence of arterial obstruction in the lower limbs.

An abnormally large pressure gradient between any two adjacent levels in the arm implies significant obstructive disease of the arteries in the intervening segment.[7] As with similar studies in the leg, segmental pressure measurements lack sensitivity and specificity (see Chapter 10). Gradients, for example, may be reduced when the ipsilateral brachial pressure is also low. Our group measured gradients of 42 ± 30 mmHg in a series of arms with occlusions of the distal brachial, antecubital, radial, and ulnar arteries.[97] The range, however, was large (12 to 114 mmHg). Forearm-brachial and wrist-brachial indices in these patients ranged from 0.37 to 0.86, with a mean of 0.68 ± 0.16. A marked difference between the pressure measured at the wrist with the Doppler probe over the radial artery and that obtained with the probe over the ulnar artery indicates which of these two vessels is more severely diseased.

Finger Pressure Measurements

The technique for measuring systolic blood pressures in the fingers is analogous to that employed in the arms (see Chapter 10).[23, 33, 35, 74] To avoid vasoconstriction, one should perform all measurements in a warm (~25°C), draft-free room. The patient should be relaxed, and efforts should be made to allay apprehension. A pneumatic cuff with a width of at least 1.2 times the diameter of the finger is wrapped around the proximal phalanx. A Doppler probe applied to a volar digital artery at the distal interphalangeal joint may be used to detect the return of blood flow as the cuff is deflated. Alternatively, a mercury strain-gauge or a photoplethysmograph placed over the distal phalanx can be used. The values obtained with the cuff at the proximal phalangeal level reflect pressures in the common and proximal proper digital arteries. When it is necessary to record pressures at the middle phalangeal level, the cuff may be moved to this position. By wrapping the cuff around both the distal phalanx and a photoplethysmographic sensor, one can even obtain reasonably accurate pressure measurements at the fingertip. Hirai and colleagues have devised a bladder-free cuff specifically for this purpose.[38]

Nielsen and colleagues, using a 2.4-cm cuff, found that finger pressures exceeded brachial pressures by 9 ± 7 mmHg in subjects 17 to 31 years of age.[74] The range was from 3 mmHg lower to 21 mmHg higher. In normal older subjects (43 to 57 years of age), the average pressure difference was approximately zero, with a standard deviation of ± 7 mmHg. Using a somewhat larger cuff (3.8 cm), Downs and associates observed that simultaneously measured pressures in corresponding fingers of both hands differed by only 3.5 ± 3.2 mmHg.[23] Only 3% had a difference greater than 9 mmHg. In their study, finger pressures averaged 9.5 ± 6.8 mmHg less than wrist pressures, which in turn were 9.6 ± 7.0 mmHg lower than those at the brachial level. They considered a pressure difference exceeding 15 mmHg between corresponding fingers, a wrist-digital gradient of greater than 30 mmHg, and an absolute finger pressure of less than 70 mmHg abnormal. Hirai, whose results were similar to those of Nielsen and colleagues, considers any arm-finger pressure gradient that exceeds 19 mmHg in subjects younger than age 50 or 25 mmHg in older subjects to be abnormal.[35]

In a series of normal subjects, our group found the mean finger–ipsilateral brachial index to be 0.97 ± 0.09. Values ranged from 0.78 to 1.27 (Fig. 79–2).[97] Finger–ipsilateral brachial indices in patients thought to have primary Raynaud's disease on the basis of clinical criteria and laboratory test findings were similar to those of normal persons (mean, 0.96 ± 0.11; range, 0.60 to 1.23). When, however, there was evidence of proximal digital or palmar arterial obstruction in limbs with no inflow disease, the finger–ipsilateral brachial indices were markedly decreased, averaging 0.56 ± 0.27 and ranging from 0 to 0.95 (see Fig. 79–2). Low pressures were found in the fingers of both hands in 57% of the patients. Only one finger was affected in 17% of the hands, two fingers were affected in 11%, three or four were affected in 39%, and all five were affected in 33%. As shown in Figure 79–3, finger pressures accurately predict arteriographic findings.

According to one report of finger pressures in patients with connective tissue disease, mean digital pressure indices were 0.62 in patients with rheumatoid arthritis, 0.53 in patients with systemic lupus erythematosus (SLE), and 0.38 in patients with scleroderma.[90] Indices of zero were observed only in patients with scleroderma.

Interpretation

Pressures in all fingers are reduced in proportion to any reduction in the ipsilateral brachial, forearm, or wrist pressure. When the disease is confined to the arm arteries and the palmar or digital arteries are spared, pressures in all fingers are approximately equal and the wrist-finger gradi-

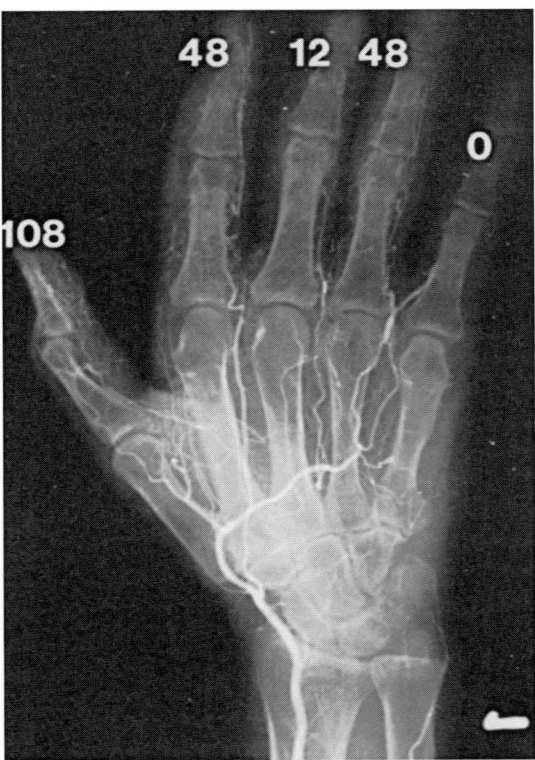

FIGURE 79–3. Digital artery pressures from the proximal phalanges of a 49-year-old man with an ischemic ulcer on the tip of the middle finger. The ipsilateral brachial pressure was 108 mmHg. The arteriogram shows major obstruction of the proper digital arteries to all fingers except the thumb, which has a normal pressure. Pressures in all the other fingers are markedly reduced.

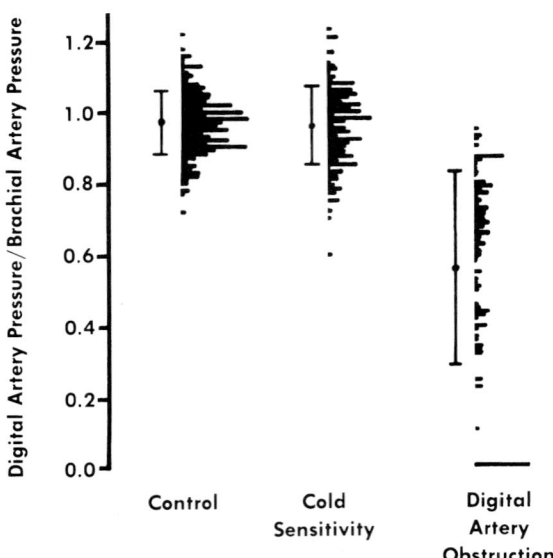

FIGURE 79–2. Finger pressure indices (mean ± 1 standard deviation). Data for cold sensitivity are derived from patients with primary Raynaud's disease. Those in the digital artery obstruction category are from patients who may or may not have secondary Raynaud's phenomenon. (From Sumner DS, Lambeth A, Russell JB: Diagnosis of upper extremity obstructive and vasospastic syndromes by Doppler ultrasound, plethysmography, and temperature profiles. *In* Puel P, Boccalon H, Enjalbert A [eds]: Hemodynamics of the Limbs 1. Toulouse, France, GEPESC, 1979, pp 365–373.)

ents are within normal limits. When the pressure in one or more fingers is distinctly lower than that in the others, however, obstruction of the palmar or digital arteries must also be present.

When arm pressures are normal at all levels, a reduction in finger pressure indicates disease in the palmar or digital arteries. If pressures in all fingers are equally decreased, the lesion must involve the palmar arch or the terminal portions of both the radial and the ulnar arteries. A reduction in pressure limited to the fingers on one side of the hand suggests that the palmar arch is incomplete or occluded at some point. Isolated obstruction of a common digital artery is implied when the pressure reduction is confined to a single finger and pressures in adjacent fingers remain normal.

Occlusion of only one of the paired proper digital arteries may have no perceptible effect on finger pressure.[23, 35] Not infrequently, the disease process is confined to arteries in the middle or distal phalanx, in which case the pressure measured at the base of the finger is likely to be normal.[23] In such cases, pressures representing the true perfusion potential can be obtained by moving the cuff to the middle or the terminal phalanx.[35, 38, 59]

Doppler Flow Studies

The contour of the blood flow signal in the upper extremity is similar to that in the leg. Normally, the velocity rises rapidly to a peak in early systole. It then falls abruptly to the baseline value, frequently reversing in early diastole (Fig. 79–4). In late diastole, a final, low-level forward flow phase may be present. This gives rise to the typical biphasic or triphasic audible signal that is easily recognized by the experienced observer. Beyond or distal to an obstruction or a high-grade stenosis, the signals become attenuated and have a slower upslope, a more rounded peak, and a downslope that continues throughout diastole. Flow reversal no longer occurs (see Fig. 79–4). Audible signals have a low frequency and are monophasic. When the probe is placed over or just distal to a stenosis, noisy, high-frequency signals are obtained, reflecting the presence of distrubed high-velocity flow. No signals are obtained over a totally occluded artery.

An examination of the subclavian, axillary, brachial, radial, and proper digital arteries often identifies the exact location of the obstruction.[5, 105] In most cases, the audible signal suffices; recordings are seldom required.

Because of the extensive collateral network in the forearm and hand, signals obtained from the radial and ulnar arteries at the wrist may sound normal, even though one of the pair may be occluded proximally. Clues to the true condition of either one of the two arteries can be obtained by observing the direction of flow and the effect of compression of the other major artery. For example, if flow in the radial artery at the wrist is reversed or if compression of the ulnar artery obliterates the signal, it is evident that an obstruction of the proximal radial artery is present. We can ascertain the patency of the distal radial and ulnar arteries and the palmar arch by noting the effect of sequential compression of the radial and ulnar arteries on the mid-palmar signal.[71] Normally, there should be no interruption of flow when either one of the arteries is compressed. When both arteries are compressed simultaneously, flow in the palm should disappear or be markedly decreased, unless a well-developed interosseous arterial communication exists. Flow should resume with release of the compression,

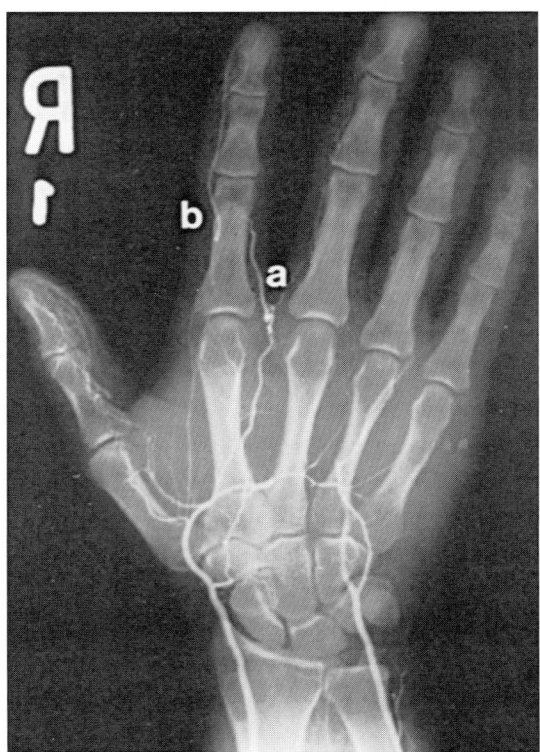

FIGURE 79–5. Arteriogram showing a crossover collateral from the proximal ulnar proper digital artery (a) to the distal radial proper digital artery (b) at the level of the proximal phalanx of the index finger. Compression of the ulnar digital artery at the base of the finger obliterated the Doppler signal heard on the radial side at the level of the middle phalanx.

provided that the artery being compressed was patent and communicated with the palmar arch. This test is easy to interpret, can be performed rapidly, and is more objective and more informative than the classic Allen's test. With the probe placed over a digital artery, similar compression maneuvers can be used to determine the primary source of the blood supply to any one of the fingers.

The hands must be warm when the digital arteries are being studied in order to avoid vasoconstriction, which may lead to a false-positive interpretation.[5] A complete examination requires interrogation of the volar proper digital arteries on both sides of each finger at the proximal and distal interphalangeal joints. Signals from each finger should be compared with those obtained from other fingers on both hands. It is not unusual to detect a signal at the distal interphalangeal joint in the absence of a signal at the proximal interphalangeal joint or at the base of the finger.[5, 97] In this event, compression of the proximal digital artery on the other side of the finger often obliterates the signal, thus confirming the existence of a crossover collateral derived from the contralateral artery (Fig. 79–5). Examination of the signal over the volar surface of the fingertip is also often informative. A loud signal in this area signifies good perfusion and is typical of the hyperemic phase of primary Raynaud's disease. Poor or absent signals imply vasospasm or fixed arterial obstruction.

A complete Doppler survey of the upper extermities is time-consuming and need not be performed in most cases. The history and physical examination findings, coupled

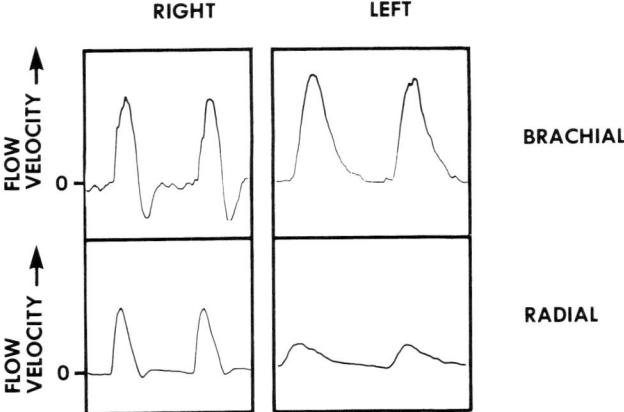

FIGURE 79–4. Analog recordings of Doppler flow signals from the right and left brachial and radial arteries of an 89-year-old woman with occlusion of the left subclavian artery. Brachial pressure: right, 164 mmHg; left, 101 mmHg. Wrist pressure: right, 154 mmHg; left, 77 mmHg. (From Sumner DS: Vascular laboratory diagnosis and assessment of upper extremity vascular disorders. In Machleder HI [ed]: Vascular Disorders of the Upper Extremity, 2nd ed. Mount Kisco, NY, Futura Publishing Company, 1989, pp 9–57.)

with pressure data, usually permit the examiner to focus on a particular artery. For example, extensive digital artery surveys are required only when digital pressure study results are normal and do not coincide with the clinical assessment.

Duplex and Color Flow Scanning

As in all other areas of the peripheral circulation, duplex scanning has had a significant effect on the evaluation of upper extremity arterial disease.[43, 49, 80, 101] Unlike other noninvasive methods, duplex scanning provides precise anatomic information, locates stenotic or occlusive lesions and evaluates their extent and severity, identifies collateral pathways, and defines the patency of arteries distal to an occlusion. Arteriographic verification is infrequently required. In addition, arteriovenous malformations and aneurysms of the upper extremity arteries are easily recognized and differentiated from other masses.[47, 73] Now that these sophisticated and versatile instruments are widely available and technologists have become skilled in their operation, duplex scanning is rapidly replacing many of the more cumbersome and less specific noninvasive tests, especially when the information required is largely anatomic.

Although conventional duplex instruments are satisfactory, color flow mapping facilitates scanning by making vessels easier to locate and to follow longitudinally. All major arteries of the arm, forearm, wrist, and hand are readily identified, and even those of the digits can be studied. Absence of color in an artery clearly visualized by B-mode imaging is diagnostic of total occlusion, and a color shift from red to white (or to yellow or green in some instruments) identifies stenotic sites, where flow velocities are increased. This feature reduces the need for serial Doppler investigation of flow patterns.

The subclavian artery is less easily visualized than the other major arteries of the upper extermity, owing to its origin in the thorax and to the "blind spot," where it passes under the clavicle. Lesions in these areas can be detected and their severity evaluated, albeit indirectly, by examining Doppler flow patterns in accessible portions of the subclavian artery above or below the clavicle.

Because of their small size, finger arteries are the most challenging of the upper extremity vessels to study.[101] Encouraging results, however, have been reported by Langholz and coworkers.[54] In their study, color duplex scans of 450 digital arteries in 45 hands of 41 symptomatic patients were compared to conventional hand arteriograms. Of 160 occluded arteries, 138 (86%) were correctly identified by color duplex scanning. Of 290 arteriographically patent arteries, 270 (93%) were correctly identified. The positive predictive value of the color duplex interpretations was 87%, and the negative predictive value was 93%. In terms of the whole hand, 39 (95%) of the diagnoses were accurate. Most false-positive results were due to incomplete visualization of the entire length of the digital arteries. False-negative studies were attributed to segmental occlusions that were overlooked by the ultrasound scan and to mistaking collateral vessels for the native artery.

Plethysmographic Studies

Volume pulses can be recorded from the tips of the fingers with a variety of plethysmographs. For most clinical stud-

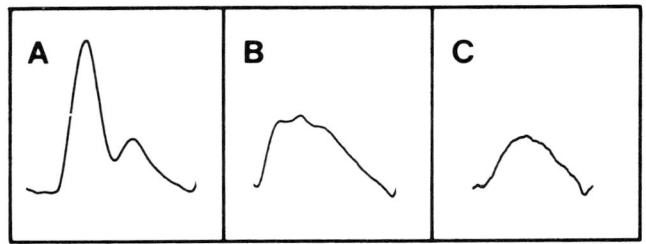

FIGURE 79–6. Plethysmographic pulse contours. A, Normal. B, Peaked. C, Obstructed. (A–C, From Sumner DS: Noninvasive assessment of upper extremity ischemia. In Bergan JJ, Yao JST [eds]: Evaluation and Treatment of Upper and Lower Extremity Circulatory Disorders. Orlando, Fla, Grune & Stratton, 1984, pp 75–95.)

ies, the photoplethysmograph is entirely satisfactory and is somewhat easier to use than the mercury strain-gauge. Quantification, however, requires a strain-gauge.[95] Although venous occlusion plethysmography can be used to measure digit volume flow, these measurements are cumbersome and are reserved for research purposes.[22, 29, 77, 86] For diagnostic evaluations, recording the pulse volume and contour is sufficient.

Pulse Contour

The normal fingertip pulse has a rapid upslope, a sharp systolic peak, and a downslope that bows toward the baseline. A dicrotic notch or wave is usually present on the downslope (Fig. 79–6A). The pulse recorded distal to a hemodynamically significant stenosis or occlusion has a delayed upslope, a rounded peak, and a downslope that bows away from the baseline (Fig. 79–6C). No dicrotic wave is present on the downslope. An intermediate form, characterized by a rapid ascending limb, an anacrotic notch or an abrupt bend terminating in a systolic peak, and a dicrotic notch high on the downslope, has been called a *peaked pulse* (Fig. 79–6B).[98] Another variant resembles the normal pulse but has a dicrotic notch high on the downslope just after the systolic peak.[78, 99]

Initial studies should be conducted with the fingers warm to eliminate the effects of vasoconstriction. Not only must the room temperature be warm, but it may also be necessary to warm the hands by immersing them in warm water. Although mild vasoconstriction merely decreases the pulse amplitude, more severe vasoconstriction may alter the contour of the pulse or result in its disappearance.[34]

Absence of a fingertip pulse or an obstructed pulse recorded under conditions conducive to vasodilatation suggests fixed arterial obstruction somewhere in the vascular pathway supplying the terminal phalanx.[81] The obstruction may be confined to the digital arteries or the palmar arch, or it may involve the forearm, brachial, axillary, or subclavian arteries. Multilevel disease may be present. Obstructions limited to one of the paired digital arteries or one of the forearm arteries may not produce an obstructed pulse if collateral channels are well developed. This finding, of course, is not unexpected; to affect the contour of the plethysmographic pulse adversely, a stenosis must be hemodynamically significant and all vessels feeding the fingertip must be involved. As a rule, plethysmographic pulses tend to be less sensitive than pressure measurements to the presence of disease. Normal pulses, on the other hand, are highly specific for the absence of fixed arterial disease.

Owing to the lack of sensitivity, some patients with secondary Raynaud's phenomenon may have relatively normal pulse contours in one or more fingers and, occasionally in all.[106] Thus, the negative predictive value of a normal pulse may not be great, particularly if the population has a high prevalence of obstructive disease. Nonetheless, in the author's experience, the finding of a normal pulse in all fingers of both hands in a patient complaining of cold sensitivity is highly suggestive of primary Raynaud's disease.

Although the significance of peaked pulses remains uncertain, they have been observed frequently in patients with autoimmune (collagen) disorders who do not have major arterial obstruction proximal to the terminal phalanges.[2, 42, 93, 98] They may also be present in a significant number of patients thought, on the the basis of other criteria, to have primary Raynaud's disease. Ohgi and associates showed that normal pulses can be converted to peaked pulses by both direct and indirect exposure to cold, even in subjects with no history of cold sensitivity.[78] Peaked pulses, therefore, at least in some cases appear to be associated with vasospasm of the digital arteries and arterioles.[2]

Additional diagnostic information can be obtained if one observes the effects of cold exposure and spontaneous rewarming on the amplitude of the finger pulse.[40] Cooling of normal fingers to 20°C or below markedly reduces the pulse amplitude, which, on rewarming, rapidly and steadily returns to pre-exposure levels. Similarly, in patients with secondary Raynaud's phenomenon, exposure to cold causes the pulse either to disappear or to become barely detectable; recovery to pre-exposure levels is gradual and takes longer than in normal subjects. Reflecting the critical closure phenomenon that characterizes the vasospastic response in patients with primary Raynaud's disease, plethysmographic pulses in patients with this condition disappear entirely on cold exposure and remain undetectable until the finger temperature rises above 24° to 26°C; a normal waveform then suddenly reappears. Other investigators have found this test to be more useful for assessing vasospasm in the foot than in the hand.[25, 46]

McLafferty and coworkers have proposed a "plethysmographic digital obstruction index" for evaluating patients with hand ischemia.[64] For each finger, a score of 8 points is assigned if the digital waveform is normal, 4 points if the upstroke time is greater than 0.2 seconds and the dicrotic notch is lost, 2 points if minimal waveform activity is detected, and 0 points if there is no digital waveform. The scores of all five fingers of each hand are added, and the result is divided by 40 (a perfectly normal score). The investigators observed that the plethysmographic index corresponded well with a similar index based on arteriography and that it was significantly greater in hands with moderate ischemia (0.75 ± 0.15) than in hands with severe ischemia (0.51 ± 0.20). An index less than 0.65 in patients with connective tissue disorders predicted digital ulceration with sensitivity of 77%, specificity of 100%, a positive predictive value of 100%, and a negative predictive value of 73%. These observations led the authors to conclude that digital photoplethysmography is the test of choice for evaluating patients with hand ischemia. Arteriography is required only for ruling out a source of emboli and for investigating patients who have no evidence of systemic illness that would explain the hand ischemia.

Responses to Sympathetic Stimuli

In normal limbs, both the amplitude of the digital pulse and the volume of the fingertip vary with respiration. Respiratory waves are superimposed on larger, but less frequent, alpha-, beta-, and gamma-waves.[15, 41, 93] For these responses to occur, the sympathetic innervation must be intact. Absence of these waves is therefore abnormal, suggesting lack of sympathetic activity. One can also monitor sympathetic activity by recording the response of the pulse amplitude and fingertip volume to a deep breath, performing mental arithmetic, or placing ice on the chest or forehead (Fig. 79–7, *left*).[14, 21, 45, 97] Normally, these maneuvers cause significant vasoconstriction. Reduction of the pulse amplitude reflects a comparable decrease in digital blood flow, and a reduction in fingertip volume reflects both a decrease in arterial inflow and constriction of the terminal arteries and veins. A diminished response or none

FIGURE 79–7. Effect of sympathetic stimuli on digit volume and digital pulse amplitude in a patient with primary Raynaud's disease and in a patient with scleroderma. Recordings in the right-hand panels were made at a higher sensitivity than those in the left. The patient with scleroderma shows little or no response. (From Sumner DS, Lambeth A, Russell JB: Diagnosis of upper extremity obstructive and vasospastic syndromes by Doppler ultrasound, plethysmography, and temperature profiles. *In* Puel P, Boccalon H, Enjalbert A [eds]: Hemodynamics of the Limbs 1. Toulouse, France, GEPESC, 1979, pp 365–373.)

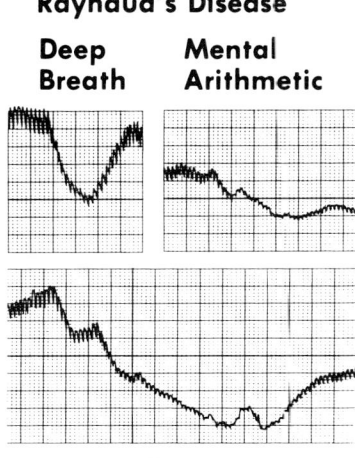
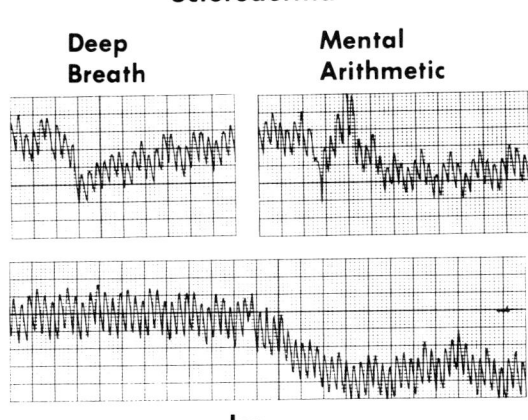

(commonly seen in patients with collagen diseases) indicates impaired sympathetic activity (see Fig. 79–7, *right*). Sympathectomy is unlikely to be effective in limbs that display little evidence of sympathetic activity. To record the larger, slower changes in fingertip volume, it is necessary to employ direct current (DC) coupling; the more rapid changes in digital pulse amplitude are more conveniently recorded with an alternating current (AC)–coupled plethysmograph.[95]

Reactive Hyperemia

The capacity of the digital arterioles to dilate can be determined by monitoring the response of the pulse amplitude to a short period of ischemia (reactive hyperemia test).[95] A pneumatic cuff is placed around the arm, inflated for 5 minutes to a suprasystolic pressure, and then rapidly deflated. In normal limbs and in limbs with purely vasospastic disease, the finger pulse returns promptly and its amplitude increases rapidly (within 30 seconds) to double that of the control pulse (Fig. 79–8).[97] In contrast, when the peripheral arterioles have dilated maximally to compensate for increased proximal resistance imposed by a fixed arterial lesion, little or no increase in pulse amplitude is observed. A similarly poor response is also frequently observed in the limbs of patients whose microvasculature has been stiffened by autoimmune disease.[97] Although sympathectomized limbs may continue to display reactive hyperemia, lack of vasodilatation after a period of ischemia is usually associated with a similarly poor response to a surgical sympathectomy or to administration of vasodilator drugs.

Vasodilatation can also be induced by warming the patient with an electric blanket, by oral administration of alcohol, or by immersing the hands in warm water.

Laser Doppler Examination

Although laser Doppler recordings do not permit quantitative measurement of blood flow, the output is related to

changes in microcirculatory flow. Results are expressed in millivolts or in arbitrary units.

Direct and indirect cooling cause more profound reductions in fingertip laser Doppler flux in patients with Raynaud's syndrome than in subjects without cold senstivity.[4, 50, 53] Recovery to baseline levels is also delayed. The increase in laser Doppler flux in response to a reactive hyperemia test is similar in fingers of patients with primary Raynaud's disease to that in normal subjects and is much larger than that observed in fingers of patients with fixed digital arterial obstruction.[103] Observations, therefore, are similar to those obtained with plethysmographic methods.

Attempts to correlate digital flux parameters with capillary microscopic findings have met with some success, suggesting a role for laser Doppler in predicting which patients who have what appears to be primary Raynaud's disease will eventually be found to have scleroderma.[12] Others have found that because of overlapping flux values, the laser Doppler is less discriminating than capillary microscopy for this purpose.[56] Recordings of laser Doppler flux have proved useful as an adjunct to physiologic studies of Raynaud's disease and as an objective method of documenting the efficacy of drug therapy.[31, 86]

Cold Tolerance Tests

Although the testimony of a reliable patient may be sufficient to establish the diagnosis of cold sensitivity, there are cases—especially those involving industrial injury or workers compensation—when a more objective method is desirable. Moreover, an accurate assessment of the results of therapy requires objective documentation. All investigators who have attempted to reproduce the typical triphasic changes in the laboratory are aware of how frustrating such efforts may be.

The simple cold tolerance test described by Porter and associates has, in the author's experience, proved to be reasonably reliable.[83] Thermistors are taped to the fingertips, and pre-exposure temperatures are noted. The hands are immersed in ice water for 20 seconds and then removed and dried; post-exposure temperatures are monitored for 20 minutes or until temperatures return to pre-exposure levels. Because the relationship between skin temperature and digit blood flow is so markedly curvilinear, temperature measurements do not accurately reflect blood flow.[77] Recovery times after cold exposure are, however, roughly comparable, signifying the end of vasoconstriction.

Under the same environmental conditions, fingertip temperatures in normal subjects tend to be several degrees higher than those in patients with cold sensitivity (Fig. 79–9). Immersion in ice water cools the fingertips of both groups to similar levels; however, within 10 minutes after exposure, most normal fingers recover to pre-exposure temperatures, whereas relatively few cold-sensitive fingers do.[97] Recovery in cold-sensitive fingers is often delayed 20 minutes or more.[25]

In the author's laboratory, this test was 87% sensitive and 79% specific for detecting or ruling out cold-induced vasospasm (when, after a 20-second cold exposure, a 10-minute recovery time was used to divide normal from abnormal responses).[97] Using a modification of their original protocol (in which cold exposure was limited to 5 to

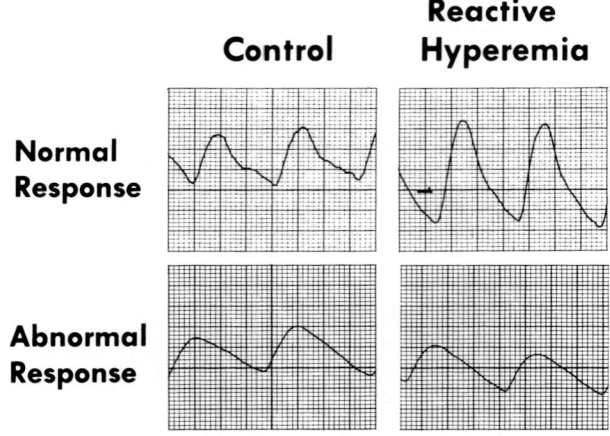

Control   **Reactive Hyperemia**

Normal Response

Abnormal Response

FIGURE 79–8. Normal and abnormal reactive hyperemia responses in a patient with primary Raynaud's disease (*upper panels*) and a patient with scleroderma (*lower panels*). Both patients had normal digital pressures at the level of the proximal phalanges. (From Sumner DS, Lambeth A, Russell JB: Diagnosis of upper extremity obstructive and vasospastic syndromes by Doppler ultrasound, plethysmography, and temperature profiles. *In* Puel P, Boccalon H, Enjalbert A [eds]: Hemodynamics of the Limbs 1. Toulouse, France, GEPESC, 1979, pp 365–373.)

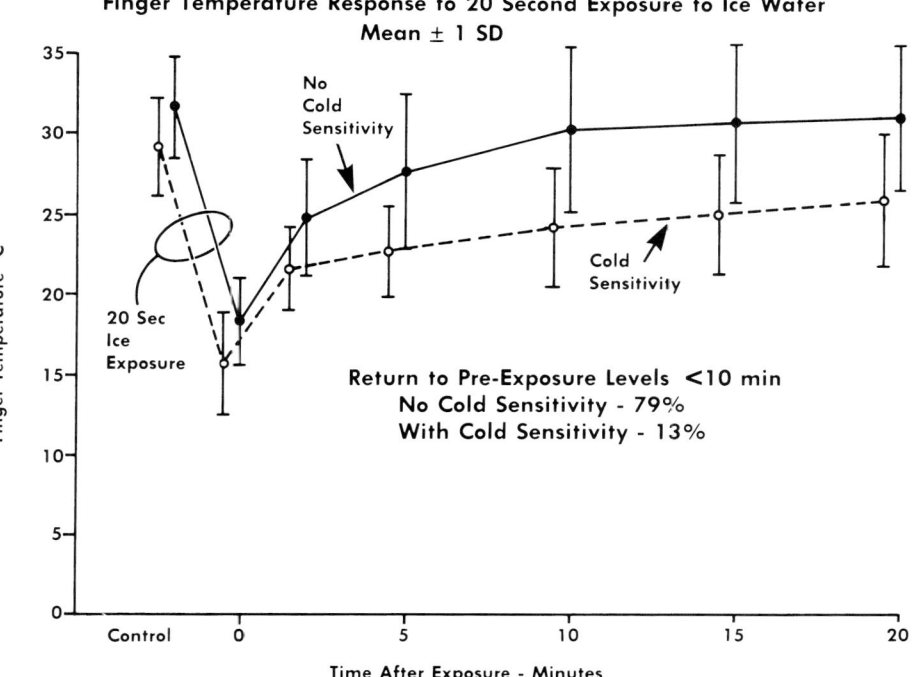

FIGURE 79–9. Fingertip temperatures before, during, and after 20-second immersion of the hands in ice water. (From Sumner DS, Lambeth A, Russell JB: Diagnosis of upper extremity obstructive and vasospastic syndromes by Doppler ultrasound, plethysmography, and temperature profiles. *In* Puel P, Boccalon H, Enjalbert A [eds]: Hemodynamics of the Limbs 1. Toulouse, France, GEPESC, 1979, pp 365–373.)

10 seconds and a 5-minute recovery time was taken as the upper limit of normal), Edwards and Porter reported specificity of 95% but disappointingly low sensitivity of 50% to 60%.[25]

Nielsen and Lassen have devised a more elegant test that measures the decrease in digital blood pressure as the finger is cooled.[39, 52, 75] A cuff with a double inlet, placed around the middle phalanx, is used first to cool the finger and the underlying arteries to the desired temperature and then to measure blood pressure at that level. To ensure rapid and complete cooling, the finger is made ischemic by inflating a cuff placed around the proximal phalanx to suprasystolic pressure while a cooling solution is circulated through the more distal cuff. When the desired temperature has been attained, the distal cuff is inflated, the proximal occluding cuff is deflated, and finger pressure is measured by noting the return of blood flow with a mercury strain-gauge or photoplethysmograph placed around the fingertip as the distal cuff is gradually deflated. The process is repeated at progressively lower temperatures until 10°C is reached. (Newer instruments use the same cuff for producing ischemia, cooling the finger, and measuring pressure. Two fingers may be examined simultaneously; one, which is not cooled, serves as the reference finger.)

Whereas the digital artery pressure in normal subjects decreases only $16 \pm 3\%$ at a skin temperature of 10°C, the pressure in patients with primary Raynaud's disease falls rapidly with decreasing temperature and then precipitously to undetectable levels as a "trigger point" is reached. The trigger point at which zero pressures are reached varies from 10° to 20°C, depending on the individual patient, but it is reproducible in any given patient. In a study reported by Alexander and colleagues, the Nielsen test had sensitivity of 100%, specificity of 79%, positive predictive value of 95%, and negative predictive value of 100% for identifying

the presence or absence of digital artery vasospasm in patients with primary Raynaud's disease and secondary Raynaud's phenomenon.[2] According to Carter and associates, the test is most sensitive during total body cooling and is more accurate in patients with secondary Raynaud's phenomenon than in patients with primary disease.[16] Corbin and coworkers also noted low sensitivity in patients with primary Raynaud's disease.[17]

Using a modification of Nielsen's method, Maricq and associates found that digital-brachial pressure ratios in patients with scleroderma approached zero at a finger temperature of 10° to 15°C.[62] Mean ratios in patients with primary Raynaud's disease were significantly higher (30%), and both were much lower than ratios in normal patients (75% to 80%) and in patients with cold sensitivity that did meet the clinical criteria for Raynaud's phenomenon (60% to 70%). From these observations, they concluded that Nielsen's test may be helpful for differentiating between primary Raynaud's disease and Raynaud's phenomenon associated with scleroderma.

Unfortunately, Nielsen's test is time-consuming, requires special equipment not available in most vascular laboratories, and is somewhat artificial in that ischemia is necessary to ensure local cooling.[16] In fact, the lower pressure measured in the cooled finger may be in part the result of prolonged digital artery contraction or delayed relaxation caused by the combined effects of suprasystolic cuff pressure and increased stiffness of the cooled digital artery. For this reason, the measurements are more appropriately termed *apparent systolic pressures*.[16]

Another, and perhaps more physiologic, method of studying the effect of cold on finger pressures is to make the measurements while the entire hand is immersed in a water bath at progressively lower temperatures (Fig. 79–10).[77] Arterial occlusion is not used. In normal fingers,

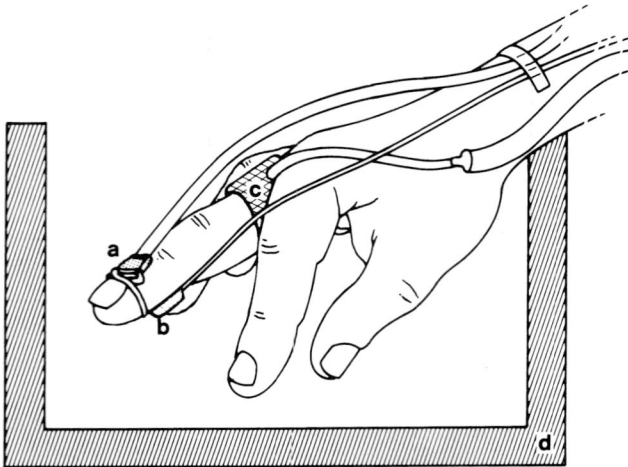

FIGURE 79–10. Apparatus for measuring skin temperature, finger blood flow, and finger pressure during local cold exposure. The apparatus consists of a mercury-in-Silastic strain-gauge (a), an insulated thermistor probe (b), a digital blood pressure cuff (c), and an insulated water bath (d). (From Ohgi S, Moore DJ, Miles RD, et al: The effect of cold on circulation in normal and cold-sensitive fingers. Bruit 9:9, 1985.)

there is little change in pressure at 10°C, but in cold-sensitive fingers, blood pressure drops precipitously, reaching zero in about half the subjects. In a study by DiGiacomo and associates, finger pressures in patients with primary Raynaud's disease averaged 105 ± 24 mmHg in 40°C water and 13 ± 38 mmHg in 10°C water.[22]

Naidu and associates have described a more direct test for detecting digital artery spasm.[72] Their method uses a 20-MHz ultrasonic probe to measure the diameters of finger arteries at room temperature (25°C) and then again after the hand has been immersed in cold water (10°C) for 5 minutes. At room temperature, the average diameter of normal arteries (1.18 ± 0.17 mm) was only slightly greater than that of cold-sensitive arteries (1.06 ± 0.26 mm). After cold exposure, the diameters of normal arteries decreased by only $8.7 \pm 11.5\%$, to 1.07 ± 0.15 mm, whereas those of cold-sensitive arteries decreased by $92.4 \pm 16.4\%$, to 0.09 ± 0.21 mm. When a cold-induced decrease in diameter of 45% was used as a cut-off point, vasospastic arteries were identified with sensitivity of 97% and normal arteries with specificity of 100%. Although this method is of interest to clinical scientists investigating cold sensitivity, it is too technically demanding to be used routinely to evaluate patients with Raynaud's phenomenon.

Capillary Microscopy

Capillary loops can be observed in the nailfold with a microscope adjusted to magnify 20 to 40 times. If photographs are not required, a standard ophthalmoscope set at the highest magnification (+40) may suffice. To facilitate visualization, a drop of immersion oil is placed on the skin. Normally, the loops are uniformly distributed and are similar in size and morphology. Findings associated with connective tissue diseases include enlarged, dilated, distorted loops with dropout of adjacent capillaries and areas of avascularity. Megacapillaries are not usually seen in patients with rheumatoid arthritis, systemic lupus erythema-

tosus, or polymyositis but are found in 90% to 100% of patients with scleroderma.[13, 60] According to a recent report, megacapillaries were observed in 86% of patients with dermatomyositis, 73% of patients with *CREST syndrome* (calcinosis cutis, Raynaud's phenomenon, esophageal dysfunction, sclerodactyly, telangiectasia) and 55% of patients with mixed connective tissue disease.[13]

Abnormal nailfold capillaries may be the first indication that patients with the clinical diagnosis of primary Raynaud's disease will eventually be found to have an underlying connective tissue disease. Priollet and associates noted abnormal nailfold capillary patterns in 13 of 14 patients originally classified as having primary Raynaud's disease who were later determined to have scleroderma or another connective tissue disease.[84] Similarly, in a prospective study of patients who had Raynaud's phenomenon without an associated illness, Fitzgerald and associates found abnormal results on capillary microscopy to be the variable most strongly associated with subsequent development of a connective tissue disease.[28] The odds ratio was 27:1. Thus, capillary microscopy provides important prognostic information and may be the best noninvasive method for confirming the presence of an underlying connective tissue disease.

APPLICATION OF NONINVASIVE TESTS

A careful history and physical examination often suggest a diagnosis or at least eliminate a number of disease categories. This information enables the examiner to select the noninvasive tests that are apt to be most productive. In most cases, only a few tests are required. The diagnostic approach should be modified according to the suspected site of obstruction, the duration of symptoms, the presence or absence of cold sensitivity or vasospasm, and the constant or intermittent character of the complaints. Simple algorithms, such as those in Figure 79–11, serve as rough guidelines for the efficient use of noninvasive diagnostic tests.[96]

Obstruction of Arm and Forearm Arteries

When symptoms suggest ischemia of the arm or forearm, the diagnosis of obstruction involving the subclavian, axillary, brachial, radial, or ulnar arteries is usually easily established by measuring and comparing the segmental pressures in both arms. Pressure levels also serve to define the severity of the circulatory impairment. A rapid survey with a Doppler flow detector often localizes the obstruction to one or more of these arteries and may indicate the approximate site of obstruction. More precise definition of the problems can be obtained with a duplex scanner or with a real-time, color-coded Doppler flow-mapping device. Unless intermittent obstruction or hand involvement is suspected, additional noninvasive tests are not required (see Fig. 79–11).

Acute Obstruction

Acute ischemia of the arm may be caused by emboli originating from the heart or ipsilateral subclavian artery or by

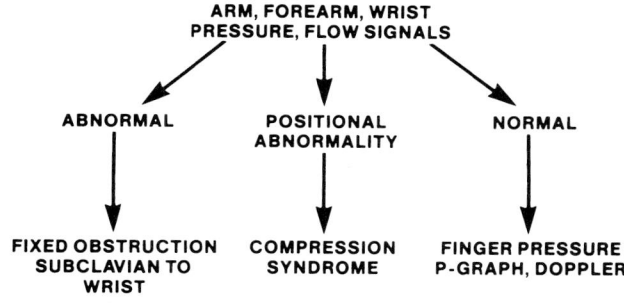

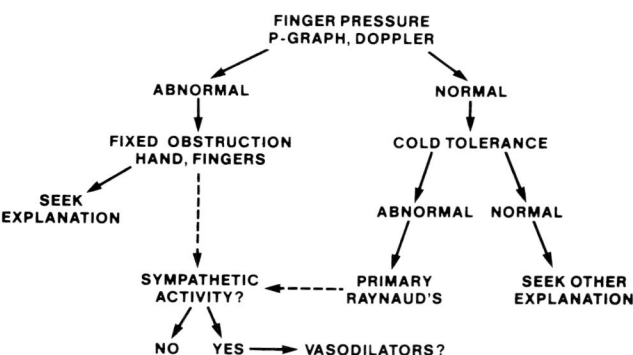

FIGURE 79–11. Approach to noninvasive diagnosis of upper extremity ischemia. P-graph = plethysmograph. (From Sumner DS: Noninvasive assessment of upper extremity and hand ischemia. J Vasc Surg 3:560, 1986.)

penetrating, blunt, or iatrogenic trauma. When symptoms are compatible with an embolus, especially in patients with atrial fibrillation or a recent myocardial infarction, noninvasive tests will confirm the diagnosis and help the surgeon to choose the appropriate incision. Duplex scanning is especially helpful for locating the obstruction. Preoperative arteriography is seldom necessary, but intraoperative arteriography should be employed to confirm the patency of the distal vessels after the embolus has been extracted.

Although a decreased pressure or an abnormal Doppler signal distal to the site of penetrating trauma establishes the diagnosis of arterial injury, normal distal pressure does not necessarily rule out the diagnosis. In all cases of external bleeding or extensive hematoma formation, an arterial injury must be excluded (or identified) by duplex scanning, arteriography, or surgical exploration.

Arterial obstruction caused by blunt trauma, fractured bones, joint dislocations (especially at the elbow), or prolonged extrinsic pressure (e.g., crutch injuries) can be recognized by a reduction in arterial pressure distal to the site of the injury. It must be emphasized that the presence of an audible Doppler signal or even a palpable pulse does not exclude an injury, because collateral development may continue to supply some blood flow to the peripheral tissues. Careful pressure measurements are necessary to avoid overlooking a potentially disastrous injury. A duplex scan should be obtained whenever there is any question. Depending on the clinical presentation, the nature of the

trauma, and the certainty of the noninvasive diagnosis, arteriography may or may not be required.

Cardiac catheterization, diagnostic venous or arterial puncture, and radial artery pressure monitoring still occasionally cause iatrogenic injuries.[7, 47, 58] Many of these mishaps may initially be attributed to spasm. True vasospasm, however, usually causes relatively little reduction in distal arterial pressure even though the radial or ulnar pulses may be difficult to palpate. A distinct reduction in pressure implies mechanical obstruction. If the pressure is only moderately reduced, it is safe to delay further investigation for a few hours. In the event that vasospasm was indeed the culprit, the pressure will have returned to normal levels. Some transient obstructions attributed to vasospasm are in reality due to thrombi that undergo lysis or fragmentation, the fragments then being dispersed to "silent" areas of the forearm or hand.

Although prompt operative intervention is the recommended approach in most cases of acute obstruction of the arteries of the upper extremity, it is possible to temporize when the patient's condition makes immediate surgery hazardous or otherwise inadvisable and the noninvasive findings are compatible with continued viability of the arm and hand. As long as distal pressures exceed 40 mmHg, digital plethysmographic pulses are present, and Doppler signals can be detected in the hand and fingers, the potential for tissue survival is good. Because the condition can deteriorate at any time, these parameters must be monitored frequently until it is certain that the limb is out of danger.

Chronic Obstruction

Although atherosclerosis is infrequently responsible for obstruction of the axillary, brachial, or forearm arteries, it is a common cause of proximal subclavian artery obstruction. Beyond the origin of the subclavian artery, retained emboli and neglected trauma are other etiologic factors to be considered. Rarely, giant cell arteritis or Takayasu's disease may affect the subclavian or brachial arteries. Thromboangiitis obliterans (*Buerger's disease*), another rare condition, tends to involve the distal arteries of the forearm, sparing those in the more proximal parts of the extremity. Segmental pressure measurements will establish the diagnosis, determine the severity of the circulatory compromise, and usually provide some clue to the site of obstruction. More information regarding the location of the obstructive process can be obtained with the Doppler flow detector or with duplex scanning. Digital plethysmography and finger pressure measurements are necessary only when involvement of the hand arteries is also suspected. Arteriography is required only when operative intervention is being considered.

As with similar diseases of the lower extremity, the decision to intervene surgically should be based primarily on symptoms and on the degree to which the patient is incapacitated; however, regardless of the symptoms, finding a distal pressure within the ischemic range (<40 mmHg) provides a strong impetus.

Intermittent Claudication

An occasional patient with symptoms compatible with arm claudication may have essentially normal segmental pressures at rest. In such cases, a distinct drop in arm pressure after exercise of sufficient intensity to duplicate the symptoms provides confirmation of the diagnosis.[32, 105] Comparing the effect of reactive hyperemia on the blood pressure in both arms is another technique for demonstrating subtle degrees of arterial obstruction. If the pressure drop in the symptomatic arm is significantly greater (≥20 mmHg) than that in the asymptomatic arm, arterial obstruction is the likely explanation for the patient's complaints. Most patients, however, tolerate chronic upper extremity arterial obstruction quite well, especially when the lesion is confined to the proximal subclavian artery. In fact, pressure differentials between the arms that exceed 20 mmHg are frequently observed in completely asymptomatic patients.

Subclavian Steal

Although a normal brachial artery pressure essentially eliminates the diagnosis of subclavian steal, a decreased pressure does not establish the diagnosis because the obstruction responsible for the pressure drop may be distal to the origin of the vertebral artery. If a normal Doppler signal is obtained from the axillary artery or the infraclavicular subclavian artery, the obstruction responsible for the pressure drop must lie farther distally in the arm, thus ruling out the diagnosis of subclavian steal. Finding an abnormal Doppler signal in the supraclavicular subclavian artery increases the likelihood that subclavian steal is present. To confirm the diagnosis, reversed flow must be demonstrated in the vertebral artery. This is best accomplished with duplex scanning or with arteriography.[11, 18, 70]

Intermittent Obstruction

The first rib, the scalene muscles, the pectoralis minor muscle, and associated ligaments may cause intermittent compression of the subclavian and axillary arteries. When the arm is subjected to the various thoracic outlet maneuvers, a reduction in the arterial cross section of 75% or more can be detected noninvasively by monitoring changes in the radial artery flow pattern, the brachial blood pressure, and the digital plethysmographic pulse (Fig. 79–12).[30, 105] Because compression of a lesser degree goes undetected and because pressure on the brachial plexus is responsible for most of the arm symptoms, negative test findings do not exclude the diagnosis of thoracic outlet syndrome. However, positive test results do not confirm the diagnosis, because some degree of arterial compression is often present during these maneuvers, even in normal subjects. In the author's opinion, noninvasive tests add little to a carefully performed physical examination during which the radial pulses are palpated and the infraclavicular area is auscultated for bruits as the arm is manipulated. Objective tests are valuable, however, for detecting emboli originating from post-stenotic subclavian dilatation that obstruct arteries farther distally in the arm or hand.

Repeated trauma to the vessels of the shoulder girdle resulting from strenuous athletic activities, such as pitching a baseball or passing a football, may also cause local thrombosis and emboli to the distal arm arteries. Because highly motivated athletes tend to minimize their symptoms or attribute them to muscle strain, the diagnosis may be overlooked. Noninvasive tests provide an easy way of making the diagnosis and avoiding a result that may prove disastrous to their careers.[63]

Obstruction of Hand and Finger Arteries

Conditions responsible for obstruction of the arteries of the hand and fingers include emboli, vibratory trauma (in chain saw or jackhammer operators), repetitive percussive trauma (hypothenar hammer syndrome, baseball catching), frostbite, autoimmune diseases (scleroderma or rheumatoid arthritis), Buerger's disease, intra-arterial drug administration, and exposure to various toxins. Patients with end-stage renal disease may have heavily calcified obstructed digital arteries. Atherosclerotic involvement does occur but is relatively rare. In many cases, the cause remains unclear despite extensive investigation. Fixed obstruction of the arteries of the hand or fingers may be entirely asymptomatic; may be symptomatic only during cold exposure (secondary Raynaud's phenomenon); or may cause continued pain, fingertip ulcers, or gangrene.

Noninvasive detection of arterial obstruction is usually

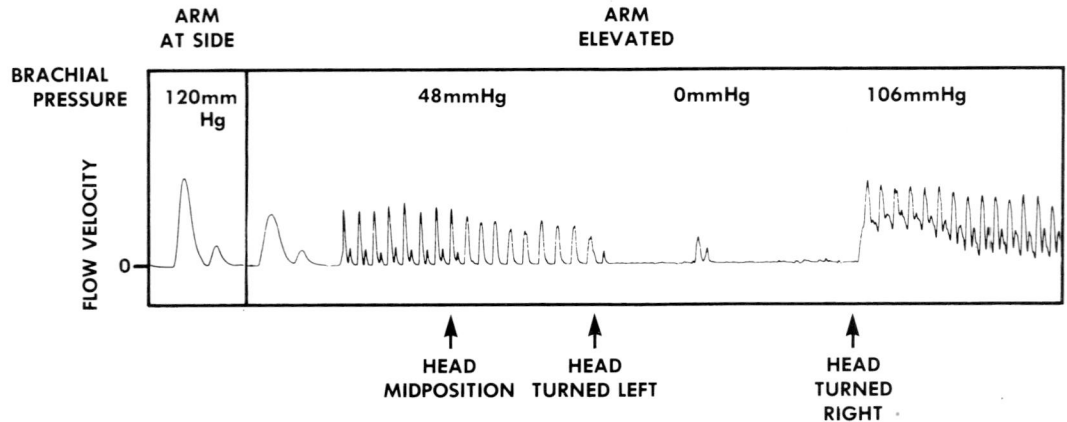

FIGURE 79–12. Doppler flow signals from the right radial artery of a 34-year-old man with thoracic outlet syndrome. Signals decrease with arm elevation and disappear when the head is turned to the left. Hyperemia appears when the head is turned to the right. The brachial blood pressure shows similar changes. (From Sumner DS: Vascular laboratory diagnosis and assessment of upper extremity vascular disorders. *In* Machleder HI [ed]: Vascular Disorders of the Upper Extremity, 2nd ed. Mount Kisco, NY, Futura Publishing Company, 1989, pp 9–57.)

not difficult.[8] Even when symptoms are confined to the hand or fingers, the first step is to ascertain whether disease is present in the more proximal arteries (see Fig. 79–11). If lesions are demonstrated in the subclavian, brachial, or forearm arteries, it is likely that any additional obstructions in the hand are part of the same pathologic process. When the proximal examination is normal, the next step is to determine whether the hand symptoms are indeed due to arterial obstruction or whether they represent an exclusively vasospastic process (see Fig. 79–11). This distinction is important because vasospasm generally has a benign prognosis, whereas that of arterial obstruction is more ominous.

The patency of the palmar arch should be investigated in all cases, and the relative contributions of the radial, ulnar, and interosseous arteries should be determined. Blood pressure at the proximal phalangeal level should be measured in all 10 fingers, especially when symptoms are bilateral.[35, 97] If measurements are restricted to the symptomatic finger or fingers, more generalized involvement may be overlooked. Similarly, digital pulse waveforms should be recorded from the tips of all fingers. When proximal finger pressures are normal, this step is particularly important to avoid missing disease of the intervening arteries. Measurement of pressure at the middle or distal phalangeal level may be revealing in fingers with normal proximal digital pressures and abnormal plethysmographic pulses. Because extensive Doppler surveys and duplex scanning of the digital arteries are time-consuming and may not be rewarding, these tests ordinarily need not be performed on all fingers; however, selective studies of individual fingers may be informative. As emphasized earlier, to prevent vasospasm and arteriolar constriction, studies designed to detect fixed arterial obstruction should be undertaken only when the hands are warm.

The distribution of the lesions identified by noninvasive testing may suggest a cause. An incomplete palmar arch may represent a common congenital variant, in which case the digital pressures and plethysmographic waveforms in all fingers will be normal, or it may be due to any of a host of pathologic entities, including trauma, atherosclerosis, emboli, and collagen diseases. If pressures are decreased and pulses are abnormal in the fourth and fifth fingers and the patient gives a history of repetitive percussive trauma to the palm of the hand, the hypothenar hammer syndrome is a strong possibility.[1, 8, 51, 65] In this event, compression of the radial artery at the wrist obliterates Doppler signals and reduces pressures in the involved fingers, whereas compression of the ulnar artery has no effect.[37]

Patients often present with symptoms and signs confined to one finger. Noninvasive tests, however, may disclose widespread subclinical lesions in both hands, confirming the presence of a generalized process such as scleroderma or another autoimmune disease. At some point, more fingers will inevitably become symptomatic.[106] If the obstructions are diffuse but are confined to one hand, a traumatic or embolic cause should be considered. Possible causes include use of a jackhammer or chain saw or an unrecognized proximal lesion that is a source of emboli. When, after all fingers have been carefully studied, the obstruction appears to be localized to a single finger, it is reasonable to postulate that isolated trauma or a single small embolus

might be responsible. Nonetheless, the clinician should never discount the possibility that the disease process is generalized and that other lesions may eventually appear.

Abnormalities of the plethysmographic pulses may be the only objective evidence of arterial disease. When all other study results are negative, obstructive or peaked pulses imply disease localized to the terminal vasculature. Autoimmune diseases can present in this fashion.[20, 98]

Arteriography is necessary only when an occult embolic focus is suspected or in the relatively rare situation when microsurgical arterial reconstruction is contemplated. Revascularization may be feasible when noninvasive tests reveal patent digital arteries lying distal to an occluded palmar arch (as in the hypothenar hammer syndrome). Doppler surveys and duplex scanning are especially useful for mapping out the extent of arterial involvement. When hand ischemia is due to diffuse arterial involvement, extensive blood tests are required to identify the cause (see Chapter 82).

Although unrelenting pain, digital ulceration, and gangrene suggest severe ischemia, in other, less obvious situations, objective methods may be necessary to define the degree of circulatory impairment. During the acute phase of the disease, digital pressures may lie in the ischemic range and plethysmographic pulses may be absent. Over a period of a few days or weeks, digital pressures often rise and plethysmographic pulses become more nearly normal. Not infrequently, improvement in the circulation of one finger parallels deterioration in the circulation of another. Once the dynamic phase of the disease runs its course, noninvasive findings may remain remarkably stable for long periods. For this reason, the surgeon should avoid precipitous action and adopt a wait-and-see attitude. Because the natural history of digital arterial disease is ordinarily one of fluctuating degrees of ischemia, the clinician must be cautious in attributing improvement to vasodilating drugs, surgical sympathectomy, or other therapeutic measures.[68]

Vasospasm: Intermittent Digital Ischemia

Episodic ischemia of the fingers in response to cold exposure or emotional stimuli (Raynaud's phenomenon) is a frequent complaint of patients referred for vascular evaluation. Estimates of the prevalence of this condition in the general population vary widely, from less than 1.0% to as much as 20%. Of 1752 randomly selected subjects from South Carolina, 10% complained of cold sensitivity.[61] About 5% reported color changes and 3% sought medical attention. Although the apparent prevalence may be considerably higher in regions of the world where the climate is colder and damper, it may reflect more frequent exposure to the triggering stimulus rather than a difference in the prevalence of the underlying disorder.

An attempt to classify the patient's disease process is made in order to formulate a treatment plan and to offer a short-term prognosis. If, in addition to cold sensitivity, the patient has symptoms or signs of fixed arterial obstruction (e.g., trophic skin changes, ulcers, severe pain), or if results of noninvasive tests are positive for arterial obstruction, the process is classified as secondary Raynaud's phenomenon (see Fig. 79–11).[36, 97] In most of these patients, cold sensitivity is overshadowed by other complaints. One or both hands may be symptomatic, but digital involvement is seldom symmetric.

If digital pressures, pulses, and Doppler study results are normal when the hands are warm, a diagnosis of primary Raynaud's disease or vasospastic Raynaud's syndrome can be made, provided that the existence of cold sensitivity can be documented by history, direct observation, or cold tolerance tests (see Fig. 79–11).[36, 98, 100] Patients with primary Raynaud's disease are usually young, and the majority are female. Although these patients may complain of discomfort during the attacks, severe pain is rare. Symptoms are bilateral and symmetric, and there are no skin changes. Responses to sympathetic stimuli are active, and reactive hyperemia studies demonstrate a normal capacity for vasodilatation.[97] In the author's experience, blood test results in all patients with this constellation of symptoms, signs, and normal noninvasive findings have consistently been normal.

Between these two extremes is a group of patients whose history and physical examination findings are consistent with primary Raynaud's disease but whose noninvasive test results suggest an underlying disorder.[6, 20, 98, 106] In some or all of the fingers, digital artery pressures may be moderately decreased and plethysmographic pulses may be peaked or have a high dicrotic notch. The Doppler survey may reveal isolated abnormalities. Laboratory tests may disclose abnormalities in the sedimentation rate, antinuclear antibody (ANA) titers, or serum immunoelectrophoretic patterns; however, in the majority of these patients the results are normal. Although it is likely that some of these patients will ultimately be shown to have scleroderma or another connective tissue disease, currently available data are insufficient to substantiate this prediction.

Among the criteria proposed in the early 1930s by Allen and Brown for primary Raynaud's disease was the stipulation that episodic cold sensitivity must be present for 2 years without the appearance of any associated disease.[3] Subsequently, many investigations have shown that this period is too short and that Raynaud's syndrome may be present for as long as 30 years before an associated disease becomes apparent. Indeed, there seems to be no clearly defined upper limit.

Although it is impossible to predict which patients will ultimately have a connective tissue disease, the likelihood that such diseases will become manifest during follow-up appears to be related to the initial clinical and laboratory findings. If the cumulative results of those articles published after 1980 are extracted from Edwards and Porter's literature review, only 12 of 408 patients (2.9%) classified on the basis of serologic and clinical evaluations as having primary Raynaud's disease developed a connective tissue disease over a follow-up period averaging 3.7 years.[26] In contrast, 60 of 184 patients (32.6%) with one or more clinical or serologic abnormalities but without all the necessary criteria for a definitive diagnosis of connective tissue disease as set forth by the American Rheumatism Association[94] developed a connective tissue disease over an average follow-up period of 4.0 years. The term *suspected secondary Raynaud's phenomenon* has been proposed to differentiate this high-risk group from the group without evident abnormalities.[48, 84]

Among the clinical features that suggest the diagnosis of connective tissue disease in patients with Raynaud's syndrome are sclerodactyly, digital pitting scars, puffy fingers, telangiectasias, pulmonary fibrosis, and esophageal motility problems. Although elevated ANA titers often correlate with the subsequent appearance of an associated disease, positive ANA findings have been reported in 12% of otherwise normal women who manifested no connective tissue disease over a period of 5 years.[26, 104] Perhaps the test with the greatest prognostic value is capillary microscopy.[28, 44, 84] It seems reasonable to speculate that many, if not most, patients classified as having suspected secondary Raynaud's phenomenon will also demonstrate some changes in digital pulse waveforms, Doppler signals, or digital pressures.

THERAPY

When lesions involve the subclavian, axillary, brachial, radial, or ulnar arteries, vascular reconstruction is usually possible. With microvascular techniques, reconstruction of the small arteries of the hand is often feasible.[1, 73, 91] Emboli and thrombi can be treated surgically or with thrombolytic drugs. As discussed previously, noninvasive tests are helpful in identifying the lesions that compromise the circulation sufficiently to require direct therapy. After treatment, these tests are valuable not only for assessing the degree of immediate physiologic improvement but also for following the results longitudinally (Table 79–3).[63, 73] Restoration of flow to completely or partially severed arms, hands, and fingers is now being performed routinely in many centers. Although continued viability of the severed part confirms the patency of the vascular anastomoses, noninvasive measurement of digital pulses, blood flow, and digital pressures provides objective data concerning the adequacy of the blood supply. The author's group showed that perfusion of tissues that survive reimplantation is usually within normal limits but is often lower than that in normal tissues of the same person (Fig. 79–13).[59]

Many patients, however, have lesions that are situated too far distally or are too extensive to be amenable to vascular reconstruction, among them autoimmune and

TABLE 79–3. PRESSURE DATA (mmHg) BEFORE AND AFTER REVASCULARIZATION IN PATIENTS WITH BRACHIAL, RADIAL, AND ULNAR ARTERY OBSTRUCTION

SITE OF OBSTRUCTION	BRACHIAL ARTERY Before	BRACHIAL ARTERY After*	RADIAL (FOREARM) ARTERY Before	RADIAL (FOREARM) ARTERY After†	ULNAR, PALMAR ARCH ARTERY Before	ULNAR, PALMAR ARCH ARTERY After‡
Brachial	100	110	90	100	132	130
Forearm	88	102	70	104	—	—
Wrist	86	94	—	—	—	—
Finger (1)	0	106	22	98	126	128
(2)	46	100	25	82	130	136
(3)	30	102	—	—	130	128
(4)	55	87	—	—	100	124
(5)	25	103	—	—	60	118

*Proximal brachial–antecubital bypass graft.
†Distal brachial–distal radial bypass graft.
‡Distal ulnar–common digital bypass graft.

FINGER BLOOD PRESSURE
(mean ± SEM)

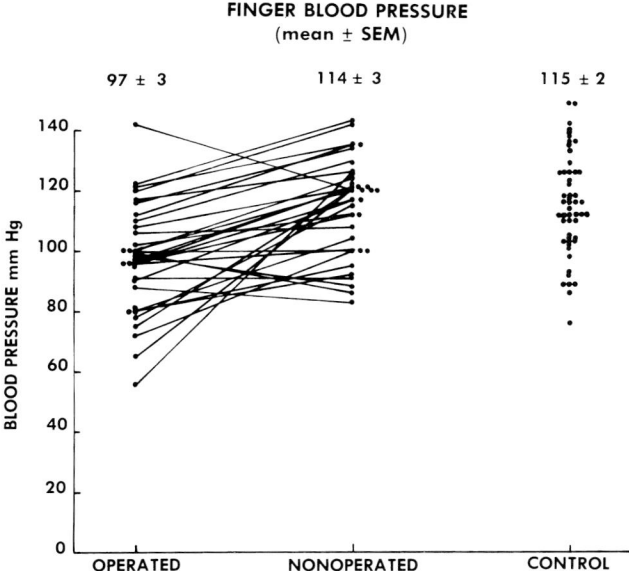

FIGURE 79–13. Blood pressures in the distal phalanges of 32 replanted fingers (operated) compared with those of the comparable fingers of the other hand (nonoperated). Control pressures are from 52 normal fingers. (From Manke DA, Sumner DS, Van Beek AL, et al: Hemodynamic studies of digital and extremity replants or revascularizations. Surgery 88:445, 1980.)

connective tissue diseases, vibratory trauma, frostbite, Buerger's disease, and a host of other problems. To increase blood flow, the physician may turn to vasodilating drugs, calcium channel blockers, prostaglandins, hemorrheologic agents, fish oil supplements, or surgical sympathectomy.[22, 68, 79, 86–88, 102] All of these methods have been reported to be successful by some investigators and unsuccessful by others, but few controlled studies have been performed. Given sufficient time, the circulation of most ischemic fingers improves spontaneously, although the improvement may be temporary and may be concurrent with decreasing circulation to another finger.[68] Noninvasive tests, therefore, provide an objective method of assessing the effect of a specific therapy and of documenting the natural history of the disease.[22, 31, 68, 69, 76, 79, 87] Although alleviation of symptoms is the principal goal, subjective evaluations are notoriously unreliable.

Vasodilating drugs and sympathectomy are likely to be beneficial only when the terminal vasculature is capable of vasodilatation. Noninvasive tests designed to evaluate sympathetic activity should be performed when these forms of therapy are contemplated (see Fig. 79–11). If, in response to a reactive hyperemia test, the digital pulse volume does not increase appreciably, it is doubtful that these measures will be successful (see Fig. 79–8). Even when reactive hyperemia develops, sympathectomy or sympatholytic drugs would not be expected to increase blood flow in the absence of a positive response to a deep-breath test (see Fig. 79–7). Before the patient is subjected to sympathectomy, plethysmographic pulses should be monitored, both before and after sympathetic block, to confirm that vasodilatation is possible.

Patients with primary Raynaud's disease almost invariably demonstrate reactive hyperemia and an active response to

taking a deep breath (see Figs. 79–7 and 79–8). Although sympathectomy usually increases blood flow (at least temporarily), it is seldom if ever indicated in these patients, because their symptoms are rarely severe and the disease does not jeopardize tissue survival. Vasodilators may, however, be helpful. Unfortunately, sympathectomy and sympatholytic drugs are least efficacious in patients with secondary Raynaud's phenomenon who most need increased perfusion, because the arterioles are often maximally dilated to compensate for a proximal obstruction and the compliance of the terminal vessels is impaired by the disease process that is producing the ischemia.[68] A few drugs—particularly calcium channel blockers—do seem to afford some relief, but noninvasive tests show little objective evidence of increased perfusion.[19, 68, 69, 79, 86–88]

SUMMARY

Evaluation of acute or chronic ischemia of the upper extremity is facilitated by selective use of simple noninvasive methods available in most vascular laboratories. They detect arterial obstruction, help locate the site or sites of obstruction, assess the severity of the circulatory impairment, and distinguish between primarily obstructive and vasospastic disease. Although noninvasive tests do not establish a cause, they clarify the need for further laboratory tests or arteriography. Finally, they provide an objective method of evaluating the results of therapeutic intervention and a way of defining the natural history of the disease.

REFERENCES

1. Abshire J, Fruscha JD, Jones TR, Schellack JV: Demonstration of hypothenar hammer syndrome by duplex ultrasound. J Vasc Technol 16:39, 1992.
2. Alexander S, Cummings C, Figg-Hoblyn L, et at: Usefulness of digital peaked pulse for diagnosis of Raynaud's syndrome. J Vasc Technol 12:71, 1988.
3. Allen E, Brown G: Raynaud's disease: A critical review of minimal requisites for diagnosis. Am J Med Sci 183:187, 1932.
4. Allen JA, Devlin MA, McGrann S, et al: An objective test for the diagnosis and grading of vasospasm in patients with Raynaud's syndrome. Clin Sci 82:529, 1992.
5. Balas P, Katsogiannis A, Katsiotis P, et al: Comparative study of evaluation of digital arterial circulation by Doppler ultrasonic tracing and hand arteriography. J Cardiovasc Surg 21:455, 1980.
6. Balas P, Tripolitis AJ, Kaklamanis P, et al: Raynaud's phenomenon: Primary and secondary causes. Arch Surg 114:1174, 1979.
7. Barnes RW, Peterson JL, Krugmire RB, et al: Complications of brachial artery catheterization: Prospective evaluation with the Doppler velocity detector. Chest 66:363, 1974.
8. Bartel P, Blackburn D, Peterson L, et al: The value of non-invasive tests in occupational trauma of the hands and fingers. Bruit 8:15, 1984.
9. Baxter BT, Blackburn D, Payne K, et al: Noninvasive evaluation of the upper extremity. Surg Clin North Am 70:87, 1990.
10. Berger AC, Kleinert JM: Noninvasive vascular studies: A comparison with arteriography and surgical findings in the upper extremity. J Hand Surg 17A:206, 1992.
11. Berguer R, Higgins R, Nelson R: Noninvasive diagnosis of reversal of vertebral-artery blood flow. N Engl J Med 302:1349, 1980.
12. Binaghi F, Cannas F, Mathieu A, et al: Correlations among capillaroscopic abnormalities, digital flow and immunologic findings in patients with isolated Raynaud's phenomenon. Can laser Doppler

flowmetry help identify a secondary Raynaud phenomenon? Int Angiol 11:186, 1992.

13. Blockmans D, Beyens G, Verhaeghe R: Predictive value of nailfold capillaroscopy in the diagnosis of connective tissue diseases. Clin Rheumatol 15:148, 1996.

14. Browse NL, Hardwick PJ: The deep breath–venoconstriction reflex. Clin Sci 37:125, 1969.

15. Burch GE: Digital Plethysmography. New York, Grune & Stratton, 1954.

16. Carter SA, Dean E, Kroeger EA: Apparent finger systolic pressures during cooling in patients with Raynaud's syndrome. Circulation 77:988, 1988.

17. Corbin DOC, Wood DA, Housley E: An evaluation of finger systolic pressure response to local cooling in the diagnosis of primary Raynaud's phenomenon. Clin Physiol 5:383, 1985.

18. Corson JD, Menzoian JO, LoGerfo FW: Reversal of vertebral artery blood flow demonstrated by Doppler untrasound. Arch Surg 112:715, 1977.

19. Creager MA, Pariser KM, Winston EM, et al: Nifedipine-induced fingertip vasodilation in patients with Raynaud's phenomenon. Am Heart J 108:370, 1984.

20. Dabich L, Bookstein JJ, Zweifler A, et al: Digital arteries in patients with scleroderma: Arteriographic and plethysmographic study. Arch Intern Med 130:708, 1972.

21. Delius W, Kellerova E: Reactions of arterial and venous vessels in the human forearm and hand to deep breath or mental strain. Clin Sci 40:271, 1971.

22. DiGiacomo RA, Kremer JM, Shah DM: Fish-oil dietary supplementation in patients with Raynaud's phenomenon: A double-blind, controlled, prospective study. Am J Med 86:158, 1989.

23. Downs AR, Gaskell P, Morrow I, et al: Assessment of arterial obstruction in vessels supplying the fingers by measurement of local blood pressures and the skin temperature response test: Correlation with angiographic evidence. Surgery 77:530, 1975.

24. Edwards JM, Phinney ES, Taylor LM, et al: α_2-Adrenergic receptor levels in obstructive and spastic Raynaud's syndrome. J Vasc Surg 5:38, 1987.

25. Edwards JM, Porter JM: Diagnosis of upper extremity vasospastic disease. In Ernst CB, Stanley JC (eds): Current Therapy in Vascular Surgery, 2nd ed. Philadelphia, BC Decker, 1991, pp 186–190.

26. Edwards JM, Porter JM: Long-term outcome of Raynaud's syndrome. In Yao JST, Pearce WH (eds): Long-term Results in Vascular Surgery. Norwalk, Conn, Appleton & Lange, 1993, pp 345–352.

27. Erlandson EE, Forrest ME, Shields JJ, et al: Discriminant arteriographic criteria in the management of forearm and hand ischemia. Surgery 90:1025, 1981.

28. Fitzgerald O, O'Connor GT, Spencer-Green G: Prospective study of the evolution of Raynaud's phenomenon. Am J Med 84:718, 1988.

29. Freedman RR, Mayes MD, Sabharwal SC: Induction of vasospastic attacks despite digital nerve blood in Raynaud's disease and phenomenon. Circulation 80:859, 1989.

30. Gelabert HA, Machleder HI: Diagnosis and management of arterial compression at the thoracic outlet. Ann Vasc Surg 11:359, 1997.

31. Graafsma SJ, Wollersheim H, Droste HT, et al: Adrenoceptors on blood cells from patients with primary Raynaud's phenomenon. Clin Sci 80:325, 1991.

32. Gross WS, Flanigan P, Kraft RO, et al: Chronic upper extremity arterial insufficiency. Arch Surg 113:419, 1978.

33. Gundersen J: Segmental measurements of systolic blood pressure in the extremities including the thumb and the great toe. Acta Chir Scand 426(Suppl):1, 1972.

34. Hertzman AB, Roth LW: The reactions of the digital artery and minute pad arteries to local cold. Am J Physiol 136:680, 1942.

35. Hirai M: Arterial insufficiency of the hand evaluated by digital blood pressure and arteriographic findings. Circulation 58:902, 1978.

36. Hirai M: Cold sensitivity of the hand in arterial occlusive disease. Surgery 85:140, 1979.

37. Hirai M: Digital blood pressure and arteriographic findings under selective compression of the radial and ulnar arteries. Angiology 31:21, 1980.

38. Hirai M, Ohta T, Shionoya S: Development of a bladder-free cuff for measuring the blood pressure of the fingers and toes. Circulation 61:704, 1980.

39. Hoare M, Miles C, Girvan R, et al: The effect of local cooling on digital systolic pressure in patients with Raynaud's syndrome. Br J Surg 69(Suppl):527, 1982.

40. Holmgren K, Bauer GM, Porter JM: Vascular laboratory evaluation of Raynaud's syndrome. Bruit 5:19, 1981.

41. Honda N: The periodicity in volume fluctuations and blood flow in the human finger. Angiology 21:442, 1970.

42. Huff SE: Observations on peripheral circulation in various dermatoses. Arch Dermatol 71:575, 1955.

43. Hutchison DT: Color duplex imaging: Applications to upper extremity and microvascular surgery. Hand Clin 9:47, 1993.

44. Jacobs MJHM, Breslau PJ, Slaaf DW, et al: Nomenclature of Raynaud's phenomenon: A capillary microscopic and hemorrheologic study. Surgery 101:136, 1987.

45. Jamieson GG, Ludbrook J, Wilson A: Cold hypersensitivity in Raynaud's phenomenon. Circulation 44:254, 1971.

46. Janoff KA, Phinney ES, Porter JM: Lumbar sympathectomy for lower extremity vasospasm. Am J Surg 150:147, 1985.

47. Jones CE, Anderson FA Jr, Cardullo PA: Duplex ultrasound evaluation of radial artery diameter and hemodynamics before and after placement of a radial artery cannula. J Vasc Technol 15:181, 1991.

48. Kallenberg CGM, Pastoor GW, Wouda AA, et al: Antinuclear antibodies in patients with Raynaud's phenomenon: Clinical significance of anticentromere antibodies. Ann Rheum Dis 41:382, 1982.

49. Koman LA, Bond MG, Carter RE, et al: Evaluation of upper extremity vasculature with high resolution ultrasound. J Hand Surg 10:249, 1985.

50. Koman LA, Smith BP, Smith TL: Stress testing in the evaluation of upper-extremity perfusion. Hand Clin 9:59, 1993.

51. Koman LA, Urbaniak JR: Ulnar artery insufficiency: A guide to treatment. J Hand Surg 6:16, 1981.

52. Krähenbühl B, Nielsen SL, Lassen NA: Closure of digital arteries in high vascular tone states as demonstrated by measurement of systolic blood pressure in the fingers. Scand J Clin Lab Invest 37:71, 1977.

53. Kristensen JK, Engelhart M, Nielsen T: Laser-Doppler measurement of digital blood flow regulation in normals and in patients with Raynaud's phenomenon. Acta Derm Venereol (Stockh) 63:43, 1983.

54. Langholz J, Ladleif M, Blank B, et al: Colour coded duplex sonography in ischemic finger artery disease: A comparison with hand arteriography. Vasa 26:85, 1997.

55. Lewis T: Experiments relating to the peripheral mechanism involved in spasmodic arrest of circulation in fingers: A variety of Raynaud's disease. Heart 15:7, 1929.

56. Lütolf O, Chen D, Zehnder TT, et al: Influence of local finger cooling on laser Doppler flux and nailfold capillary blood flow velocity in normal subjects and in patients with Raynaud's phenomenon. Mircrovasc Res 46:374, 1993.

57. Lynn RB, Steiner RE, Van Wyk FAK: Arteriographic appearances of the digital arteries of the hands in Raynaud's disease. Lancet 1:471, 1955.

58. Machleder HI, Sweeney JP, Barker WF: Pulseless arm after brachial artery catheterization. Lancet 1:407, 1972.

59. Manke DA, Sumner DS, Van Beek AL, et al: Hemodynamic studies of digital and extremity replants or revascularizations. Surgery 88:445, 1980.

60. Maricq HR, Spencer-Green G, LeRoy EC: Skin capillary abnormalities as indicators of organ involvement in scleroderma (systemic sclerosis), Raynaud's syndrome and dermatomyositis. Am J Med 61:862, 1976.

61. Maricq HR, Weinrich MC, Keil JE, et al: Prevalence of Raynaud phenomenon in the general population: A preliminary study by questionnaire. J Chron Dis 39:423, 1986.

62. Maricq HR, Weinrich MC, Valter I, et al: Digital vascular responses to cooling in subjects with cold sensitivity, primary Raynaud's phenomenon, or scleroderma spectrum disorders. J Rheumatol 23:2068, 1996.

63. McCarthy WJ, Yao JST, Schafer MF, et al: Upper extremity arterial injury in athletes. J Vasc Surg 9:317, 1989.

64. McLafferty RB, Edwards JM, Taylor LM Jr, et al: Diagnosis and long-term clinical outcome in patients diagnosed with hand ischemia. J Vasc Surg 22:361, 1995.

65. McNamara MF, Takaki HS, Yao JST, et al: A systematic approach to severe hand ischemia. Surgery 83:1, 1978.

66. Mead J, Schoenfeld RC: Character of blood flow in the vasodilated fingers. J Appl Physiol 2:680, 1950.

67. Mendlowitz M, Naftchi N: The digital circulation in Raynaud's disease. Am J Cardiol 4:580, 1959.

68. Mills JL, Friedman EI, Taylor LM Jr, et al: Upper extremity ischemia caused by small artery disease. Ann Surg 206:521, 1987.

69. Mohrland JS, Porter JM, Kahaleh MB, et al: A multiclinic, placebo-controlled, double-blind study of prostaglandin E1 in Raynaud's syndrome. Ann Rheum Dis 44:754, 1985.
70. Mozersky DJ, Barnes RW, Sumner DS, et al: Hemodynamics of innominate artery occlusion. Ann Surg 178:123, 1973.
71. Mozersky DJ, Buckley CJ, Hagood Co Jr, et al: Ultrasonic evaluation of the palmer circulation: A useful adjunct to radial artery cannulation, Am J Surg 126:810, 1973.
72. Naidu S, Baskerville PA, Goss DE, et al: Raynaud's phenomenon and cold stress testing: A new approach. Eur J Vasc Surg 8:567, 1994.
73. Nehler MR, Dalman RL, Harris EJ, et al: Upper extremity arterial bypass distal to the wrist. J Vasc Surg 16:633, 1992.
74. Nielsen PE, Bell G, Lassen NA: The measurement of digital systolic blood pressure by strain gauge technique. Scand J Clin Lab Invest 29:371, 1972.
75. Nielsen SL, Lassen NA: Measurement of digital blood pressure after local cooling. J Appl Physiol 43:907, 1977.
76. Nobin BA, Nielsen SL, Eklov B, et al: Reserpine treatment of Raynaud's disease. Ann Surg 87:12, 1978.
77. Ohgi S, Moore DJ, Miles RD, et al: The effect of cold on circulation in normal and cold-sensitive fingers. Bruit 9:9, 1985.
78. Ohgi S, Moore DJ, Miles RD, et al: Physiology of the peaked finger pulse in normal and cold-sensitive subjects. J Vasc Surg 3:516, 1986.
79. Pardy BJ, Hoare MC, Eastcott HHG, et al: Prostaglandin E1 in severe Raynaud's phenomenon. Surgery 92:953, 1982.
80. Payne MP, Blackburn DR, Peterson LK, et al: B-Mode imaging of the hand and upper extremity. Bruit 10:168, 1986.
81. Peller JS, Gabor GT, Porter JM, et al: Angiographic findings in mixed connective tissue disease: Correlation with fingernail capillary photomicroscopy and digital photoplethysmography findigs. Arthritis Rheum 28:768, 1985.
82. Porter JM, Rivers SP, Anderson CJ, et al: Evaluation and management of patients with Raynaud's syndrome. Am J Surg 142:183, 1981.
83. Porter JM, Snider RL, Bardana EJ, et al: The diagnosis and treatment of Raynaud's phenomenon. Surgery 77:11, 1975.
84. Priollet P, Vayssairat M, Housset E: How to classify Raynaud's phenomenon: Long-term follow-up study of 73 cases. Am J Med 83:494, 1987.
85. Pyykkö I, Kolari P, Fäkkilä M, et al: Finger peripheral resistance during local cold provocation in vasospastic disease. Scand J Work Environ Health 12:395, 1986.
86. Rademaker M, Cooke ED, Almond NE, et al: Comparison of intravenous infusions of iloprost and oral nifedipine in treatment of Raynaud's phenomenon in patients with systemic sclerosis: A double blind randomized study. Br Med J 298:561, 1989.
87. Roald OK, Seem E: Treatment of Raynaud's phenomenon with ketanserin in patients with connective tissue disorders. Br Med J 289:577, 1984.
88. Rodeheffer RJ, Rommer JA, Wigley F, et al: Controlled double-blind trial of nifedipine in the treatment of Raynaud's phenomenon. N Engl J Med 308:880, 1983.
89. Rösch J, Porter JM, Gralino BJ: Cryodynamic hand angiography in the diagnosis and management of Raynaud's syndrome. Circulation 55:807, 1977.
90. Salem ME-S, El-Girby AH, El-Moneim NAA, et al: Value of finger arterial blood pressure in diagnosis of vascular changes in some connective tissue diseases. Angiology 44:183, 1993.
91. Silcott GR, Polich VL: Palmar arch arterial reconstruction for the salvage of ischemic fingers. Am J Surg 142:219, 1981.
92. Singh S, de Trafford JC, Baskerville PA, et al: Digital artery calibre measurement: A new technique of assessing Raynaud's phenomenon. Eur J Vasc Surg 5:199, 1991.
93. Strandness DE Jr, Sumner DS: Raynaud's disease and Raynaud's phenomenon. In Hemodynamics for Surgeons. New York, Grune & Stratton, 1975, pp 543–581.
94. Subcommittee for Scleroderma Criteria of the American Rheumatism Association Diagnostic and Therapeutic Criteria Committee: Preliminary criteria for the classification of systemic sclerosis (scleroderma). Arthritis Rheum 23:581, 1980.
95. Sumner DS: Mercury strain-gauge plethysmography. In Bernstein EF (ed): Noninvasive Diagnostic Techniques in Vascular Disease, 3rd ed. St. Louis, CV Mosby, 1985, pp 133–150.
96. Sumner DS: Noninvasive assessment of upper extremity and hand ischemia. J Vasc Surg 3:560, 1986.
97. Sumner DS, Lambeth A, Russell JB: Diagnosis of upper extremity obstructive and vasospastic syndromes by Doppler ultrasound, plethysmography, and temperature profiles. In Puel P, Boccalon H, Enjalbert A (eds): Hemodynamics of the Limbs 1. Toulouse, France, GEPESC, 1979, pp 365–373.
98. Sumner DS, Strandness DE Jr: An abnormal finger pulse associated with cold sensitivity. Ann Surg 175:294, 1972.
99. Thulesius O: Methods for the evaluation of peripheral vascular function in the upper extremities. Acta Chir Scand 465(Suppl):53, 1975.
100. Tordoir JHM, Haeck LB, Winterkamp H, et al: Multifinger photoplethysmography and digital blood pressure measurement in patients with Raynaud's phenomenon of the hand. J Vasc Surg 3:456, 1986.
101. Trager S, Pignatoro M, Anderson J, et al: Color flow Doppler: Imaging the upper extremity. J Hand Surg 18A:621, 1993.
102. Welling RE, Cranley JJ, Krause RJ, et al: Obliterative arterial disease of the upper extremity. Arch Surg 116:1593, 1981.
103. Wollersheim H, Reyenga J, Thien TH: Postocclusive reactive hyperemia of fingertips, monitored by laser Doppler velocimetry in the diagnosis of Raynaud's phenomenon. Microvasc Res 38:286, 1989.
104. Yadin O, Sarov B, Naggan L, et al: Natural autoantibodies in the serum of healthy women—A five-year follow-up. Clin Exp Immunol 75:402, 1989.
105. Yao JST, Gourmos C, Pathanasiou K, et al: A method for assessing ischemia of the hands and fingers. Surg Gynecol Obstet 135:373, 1972.
106. Zweifler AJ, Trinkaus P: Occlusive digital artery disease in patients with Raynaud's phenomenon. Am J Med 77:995, 1984.

Arteriosclerotic Occlusive Disease of Brachiocephalic Arteries

Kenneth J. Cherry, Jr., M.D.

ETIOLOGY AND INCIDENCE

Atherosclerotic lesions of the innominate, common carotid, and subclavian arteries requiring reconstruction occur much less frequently than those encountered at the carotid bifurcations. The Joint Study of Arterial Occlusion reported that only 17% of lesions demonstrated on arteriography involved the innominate artery and the proximal subclavian arteries.[1] Wylie and Effeney[2] reported that of the 1961 operations at the University of California, San Francisco (UCSF), for carotid bifurcation, vertebral artery, or great vessel disease, only 7.5% were performed for innominate, common carotid, or subclavian artery lesions. The relative rarity of these lesions has meant that their natural history is unknown and that data concerning operations to correct brachiocephalic stenoses and occlusions, especially of the innominate and common carotid arteries, have come from retrospective studies at larger referral centers.[3–10, 74, 75] Recently, the two largest series to date, one from France and one from the United States, have added substantially to our knowledge of the mortality and morbidity of these operations and of the long-term fate of the reconstructions and of the patients undergoing operation.[74, 75]

Innominate artery and other brachiocephalic occlusive lesions occur in a relatively younger age group, with mean or median ages ranging from 50 through 61 years.[3–10, 74, 75] Men predominate slightly. In most of the reports from the United States, women make up 45% to 49% of the patients,[3–5, 7, 10] and in five series they represent a majority.[6, 8, 9, 75] Berguer and colleagues[75] reported that 57% of their 98 patients were female. In distinction to that trend in the United States, Kieffer and coworkers[74] in their series of 148 patients undergoing innominate artery reconstruction reported only 18% were women.

Atherosclerosis is the predominant cause in North America, with Takayasu's arteritis a distant second. The patients with Takayasu's arteritis are more often female and younger. Radiation-induced atherosclerosis obliterans accounts for a smaller fraction of the cases seen, but these patients may prove difficult to treat, especially in the long term.[11, 12, 76] Patients with atherosclerosis may present with either occlusive or atheroembolic symptoms. The symptoms in patients with arteritis are nearly always occlusive, although atheroembolism may occur in patients with combined arteritis and atherosclerosis.[76]

Smoking has been identified as a risk factor in 78% to 100% of patients with brachiocephalic arterial occlusive disease.[4, 7–10, 75] Concomitant coronary artery disease has been identified in 26% to 65% of these patients.[4, 7–10, 74, 75] Four of the larger series of aortic arch reconstructions report coronary disease in approximately 45% of patients, including Berguer's series of 98 patients. Kieffer and colleagues identified concomitant coronary disease in 26% of their patients.[4, 7, 8, 75]

A HISTORY

Savory,[13] in 1856, described a female patient with signs and symptoms referable to multiple occlusive lesions of the brachocephalic vessels. In 1875, Broadbent, reporting on "non-pulsating radial arteries" detailed a male patient with chronic occlusive lesions of the innominate and left subclavian arteries, which were subjected to postmortem examination.[14] In 1908, Takayasu described the ophthalmologic findings in a patient with the disease now bearing his name.[15] In 1926, Harbitz and Raeder reported a case of arteritis in a non-Asian woman.[16] In 1944, Martorell and Fabre described what was called for a time the "Martorell syndrome" in a patient with occlusive disease of all great vessels.[17] In 1951, an article by Shimizu and Sano ("Pulseless Disease") was published and excited new interest.[18] A year later, Caccamise and Whitman described the first patient with arteritis in the United States and again used the term pulseless disease.[19] Ross and McKusick analyzed 100 cases of "aortic arch syndrome" from the literature in 1953.[20] In 1957, Kalmansohn and Kalmansohn reviewed 90 cases from the literature.[21] In 1960, Contorni described a radiologic subclavian steal for the first time.[22]

On September 20, 1950, Murray of Toronto performed a retrograde endarterectomy of the common carotid arteries, presumably through supraclavicular or cervical incisions, for a patient with syphilitic arteritis presenting with occlusion of all his great vessels.[20] The symptoms recurred, and on August 10, 1953, Bahnson and colleagues in Baltimore performed an ascending aorta–innominate artery bypass on this same patient using a pediatric aortic homograft; the patient was known to have done well for 5 years.[20, 23] Davis and coauthors reported the first thromboendarterectomy of the innominate artery through a right anterior thoracotomy, on March 20, 1954.[24] The operation successfully restored flow to the right carotid artery but not to the right upper extremity. The patient was known to have relief of neurologic symptoms for at least a year.

In 1956, Lyons and Galbraith of Alabama reported four subclavian-carotid artery bypass grafts performed for disease of the carotid bifurcation.[25] DeBakey and colleagues reported the first prosthetic aortic-origin grafting in 1958.[26] That same article reported the first left subclavian artery endarterectomy, performed through combined thoracotomy and supraclavicular incisions. Wylie performed the first of his remarkable series of innominate artery endarterectomies in 1960.[3] By 1961, the Houston group had also reported subclavian-carotid artery bypass grafting.[27]

In 1964, Parrott of Minneapolis described subclavian artery transposition in two patients for disease of the right subclavian artery.[28] In 1965, Javid and coworkers reported a series of 44 patients undergoing a combination of innominate endarterectomy and aortic-origin grafting to the carotid, subclavian, and innominate arteries.[29] Diethrich and associates analyzed the Houston group's experience with 125 cases of carotid-subclavian artery bypass grafts in 1967,[30] thereby popularizing that operation. In the report from 1961, DeBakey and colleagues mentioned but did not detail 49 subclavian, 23 innominate, and 22 common carotid artery operations.[27] That experience was detailed in 1969 by Crawford and colleagues.[31]

Axillary-axillary artery grafting was first reported for treatment of innominate or subclavian artery lesions in 1971 by Meyers and coworkers from the Marshfield Clinic.[32] That same year, femoral-axillary artery bypass grafting was also reported as a method to avoid direct reconstruction of the great vessels.[33]

Interest in direct reconstruction of the brachiocephalic vessels waned in all but a few centers during the 1970s, in large part because of the mortality and morbidity associated with the early reconstructions.[31, 34] However, more recent cumulative experience reported by various centers around the world[3–10, 74–76] detailing acceptable morbidity and mortality rates for direct reconstruction, coupled with the suspect patency and unappealing placement of extra-anatomic grafts crossing the neck or anterior chest, has revived interest in direct repair of these lesions.

INNOMINATE ARTERY

Innominate artery lesions are uncommon. Wylie and Effeney found them to represent only 1.7% of the 1961 operations performed at UCSF for occlusive lesions of the brachiocephalic vessels, vertebral arteries, and carotid bifurcations over 20 years.[2] Innominate artery lesions may be asymptomatic. In the past, asymptomatic lesions rarely underwent repair. More recently, however, Kieffer and colleagues reported 22% of their 148 patients were operated on for asymptomatic lesions.[74] Berguer and coauthors reported that 13% of their 98 patients were asymptomatic.[75] Symptomatic patients may present with (1) ischemia of the right upper extremity, (2) symptoms of the anterior (carotid artery) or posterior (vertebral artery) circulations, (or 3) combined upper extremity and neurologic symptoms.

The percentage of patients presenting with neurologic symptoms range from 5% to 90%.[10, 74–76] In our Mayo Clinic series, 76.9% of patients had neurologic symptoms.[9] Of those symptoms, 50% were referable to the anterior cerebral circulation alone, 40% to the vertebrobasilar distribution, and 10% to both. Of the 10 patients with anterior

cerebral circulation symptoms, six had right amaurosis fugax, and four had right hemispheric transient ischemic attacks; none presented with stroke. In the 1991 Texas Heart Institute series, 77.8% of patients had neurologic symptoms.[10] In the more recent series from Kieffer and colleagues, 64% of the patients had neurologic symptoms[74] and Berguer's group reported 83%.[75]

Upper extremity symptoms have been reported in a range from 5% to 63.3% of patients.[3, 6, 7, 9, 10, 74] In the Mayo Clinic series, 53.8% of patients had symptoms of the right upper extremity, with five of the 14 having microembolization and nine having claudication.[9] By and large, those patients with claudication had tightly stenotic lesions, whereas patients with microembolization had ulcerative but less stenotic lesions. In contrast, only 14.8% of the patients in the Houston series had arm ischemia.[10] Kieffer's group reported an identical rate of 14%, and the group from Detroit reported a 5% instance of upper extremity symptoms.[74, 77] Combined upper extremity and neurologic symptoms occurred in 38.5% of the Mayo Clinic patients[9] and in 32% of the Texas Heart Institute patients.[10] In a more recent group of 49 patients seen during the 1990s at the Mayo Clinic, 42.8% of patients had neurologic symptoms, 38.8% had upper extremity symptoms, and 18.4% had combined symptoms.[76]

In the past, few operations had been reported for asymptomatic lesions. Generally, these are performed concomitantly in patients requiring coronary artery bypass or prophylactically in patients needing renal artery or infrarenal aortic reconstruction. A few patients with multiple, albeit asymptomatic, extracranial lesions have also undergone innominate artery reconstruction in this setting. More recently, however, Kieffer's group reported that 22% of the patients were asymptomatic; in Berguer's series, 13% were asymptomatic.[74, 75] Berguer's group concluded, however, that asymptomatic patients should not be offered transsternal repairs because of the relative high morbidity and mortality. None of their asymptomatic patients in this series died; one sustained a stroke.

The diagnosis may be aided by duplex scanning of the carotid and subclavian arteries or waveform analysis of the upper extremity circulation. The bases of diagnosis, however, remain physical examination and aortic arch arteriography. Physical examination should include palpation and auscultation of the proximal as well as mid-cervical carotid artery pulses, and the superficial temporal, subclavian, brachial, radial and ulnar artery pulses. Proximal carotid and subclavian artery bruits or thrills should suggest innominate artery or other great vessel stenotic lesions. Absent proximal cervical or subclavian pulses are evidence of occlusive lesions. Allen's test or its variations may reveal digital artery occlusions. Blood pressure comparison in both upper extremities is mandatory. If bilateral upper extremity occlusive disease is evident, comparison with blood pressure in the lower extremities should be performed. The presence of bluish, painful discolorations in the fingertips, subungual splinter hemorrhages, or livedo reticularis may indicate innominate artery or subclavian artery atheroembolic lesions. Unilaterality of symptoms may help to differentiate atherosclerosis of the innominate or subclavian artery from systemic causes of upper extremity ischemia.

Arch aortography with runoff views of the carotid, sub-clavian, and vertebral artery circulations is the *sine que non* of diagnosis. Aortography is necessary to confirm the diagnosis, to localize the lesions, to determine the etiologic mechanism, and to plan the operation. Magnetic resonance angiography (MRA) with gadolinium enhancement may supplant conventional angiography in the future as computer programming and techniques improve.[78]

Most patients undergoing innominate artery reconstruction have multiple supra-aortic lesions. This fact is very important when one is planning the operation, assessing risks, and interpreting operative results. In the Mayo Clinic series, 73% had multiple arch lesions and another 11.5% had concomitant vertebral artery or carotid bifurcation lesions.[9] Of the patients treated at the Texas Heart Institute, 61% had concomitant arch or bifurcation lesions.[10] Berguer and colleagues reported multiple vessel involvement in 84% of patients, and the group from Wayne State reported that 63% of their patients had multiple supra-aortic lesions.[74, 78] If direct reconstruction is anticipated, the aortogram provides essential information concerning the possibility of less invasive cervical or extrathoracic reconstruction, the feasibility of endarterectomy or bypass grafting and allows planning for reconstruction of multiple arch vessels and concomitant carotid endarterectomy.

Stenotic lesions of the innominate artery requiring reconstruction may be approached directly via arch reconstruction or indirectly via extra-anatomic methods, such as sub-clavian-subclavian artery bypass, axillary-axillary artery bypass, or contralateral carotid-carotid or carotid-subclavian artery bypass. These extra-anatomic methods came into vogue as a means of reducing the high morbidity and mortality encountered in the early experience with direct reconstruction and were initially proposed by the surgeons doing these early direct operations.[31] However, the extra-anatomic operations they espoused, namely carotid-subclavian artery and subclavian-carotid artery bypass grafts, have endured and were proposed for a subset of great vessel lesions, not for all great vessel lesions. Nonetheless, over the past two decades median sternotomy has proved to be a safe procedure with low inherent morbidity and mortality.

Brewster and associates reported a 50% failure rate for axillary-axillary artery grafts.[7] Criado, in his review of the English language literature on extrathoracic operations, found axillary-axillary artery grafts to have the worst patency and recommended against their use.[35] Nonetheless, selected series have reported excellent results with these bypass grafts.[36–39]

All of the 112 patients in these four reports were treated for subclavian artery disease; none underwent surgery for occlusive disease of the innominate artery. One group has reported less morbidity and increased patency with axillary-axillary artery grafts than with carotid-subclavian artery grafts for symptomatic subclavian artery disease.[40] The University of North Carolina group reported their experience with extra-anatomic grafting in 44 patients with great vessel disease; only three of their patients underwent operation for innominate artery disease.[79]

The routes of extra-anatomic bypasses performed for innominate artery disease crossing the trachea or sternum make these tunnels prone to skin erosion and infection. Further, the routes complicate tracheostomy, coronary ar-

tery bypass grafting (CABG), or subsequent arch reconstructions should any of these become necessary (Fig. 80–1). The presence of grafts crossing the sternum, on which patients may well be dependent for cerebral blood flow, in such situations complicates and alters repair. As approximately 45% of patients with brachiocephalic occlusive disease may be expected to have associated coronary artery disease,[4, 7, 8] and because they are relatively young patients, this is a practical and valid concern. Furthermore, 5.2% of patients undergoing brachiocephalic revascularization in the best of hands may be expected to need a subsequent arch reconstruction.[41]

In addition, direct reconstruction is favored in most patients for other reasons. The retrograde origins of extra-anatomic bypass grafts are, at least theoretically, less appealing than prograde reconstructions. Atheroembolic lesions require direct repair rather than extra-anatomic reconstruction if the atheroembolic source is to be removed from the circulation. Finally, multiple great vessel occlusive lesions are better treated by direct arch reconstruction because the aorta offers an excellent source of inflow and diseased arch vessels do not.

Poor patency may be expected from even more complicated and involved attempts at avoiding direct repair, such as femoral-axillary artery bypass grafts.[33]

Direct reconstruction may be accomplished by aortic-origin grafting or by innominate artery endarterectomy (Fig. 80–2). Each method has its proponents, and each gives excellent results and is equally effective in properly selected patients. We found no difference in early reconstructive failures for bypass and endarterectomy.[9] Similarly, no significant differences were reported in the patients from the Massachusetts General Hospital and the Texas Heart Institute.[7, 10] Reul and coworkers reported four late failures, all graft related except for one carotid bifurcation endarterectomy.[10] The Mayo Clinic series found no difference in late symptomatic recurrences for patients undergoing direct repair by either grafting or endarterectomy.[9] It appears, from the literature, that most centers favor direct bypass grafting as a technically less demanding operation that is

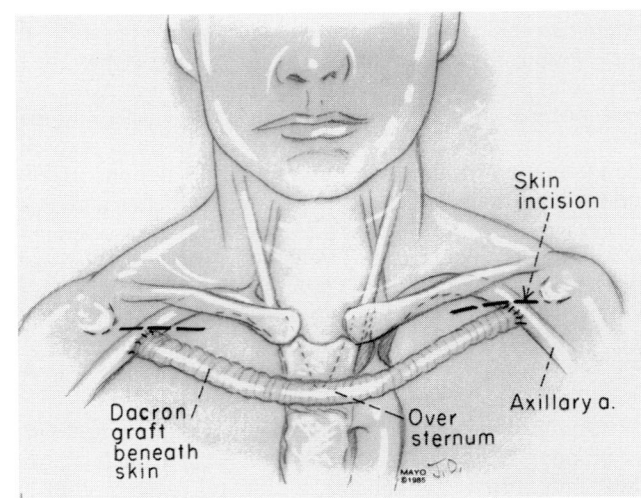

FIGURE 80–1. Schematic drawing of an axillary-axillary graft demonstrating its position overlying the sternum. (By permission of the Mayo Foundation.)

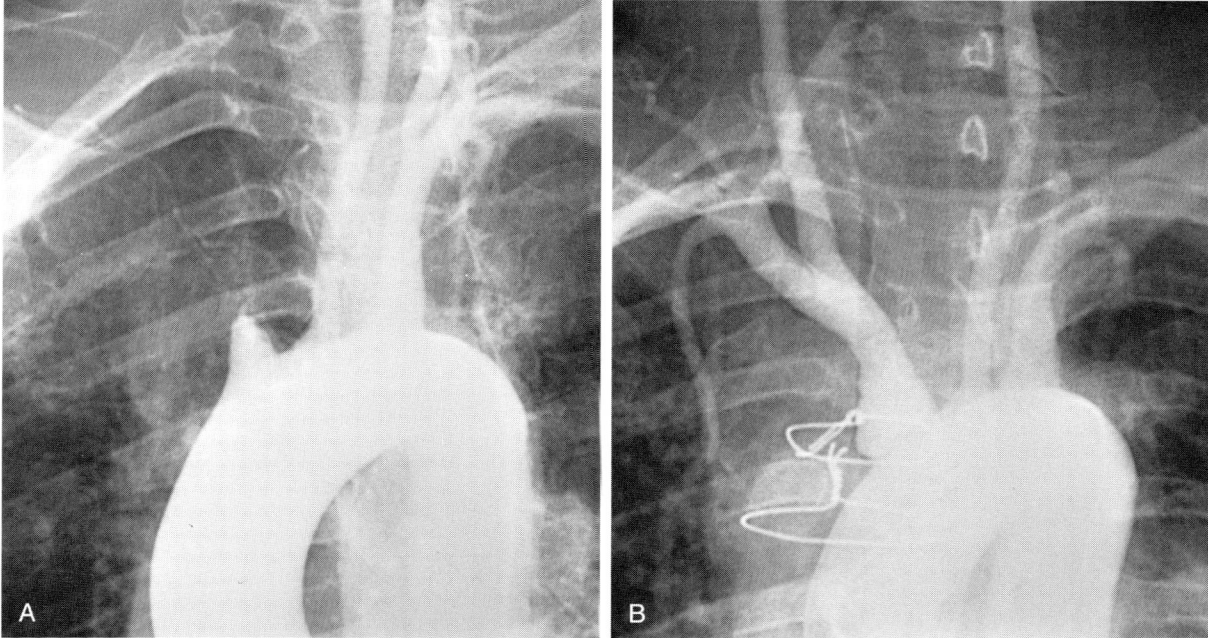

FIGURE 80–2. *A,* Preoperative arteriogram of innominate artery occlusion and global ischemia in a 47-year-old woman. *B,* Postoperative arteriogram of the same patient following innominate artery endarterectomy.

applicable to all good-risk patients,[5, 7] whereas innominate artery endarterectomy is somewhat limited in its applicability, being suitable only for patients with atherosclerotic lesions whose anatomy and extent of disease permit.

Direct bypass grafting is preferred for patients with Takayasu's arteritis (Fig. 80–3) or radiation injury or with recurrent innominate disease. The inflammatory arteritides, by nature of their panmural involvement, are generally not suitable for endarterectomy. Multiple arch lesions are probably more easily handled by bypass than endarterectomy. The extent of the atherosclerotic process and the patient's anatomy may mitigate against endarterectomy of the innominate artery. Carlson and coauthors identified atherosclerosis involving the aortic arch at the base of the innominate artery as a contraindication to innominate artery endarterectomy.[3] Atherosclerosis and calcification in this location precludes safe, hemostatic clamping of the base of the innominate artery without undue risk of intimal disruption, dissection, or embolization. Aortic dissection with innominate artery reconstruction has been reported, albeit with bypass rather than endarterectomy.[8] The San Francisco group also identified the close proximity of the origin of the left common carotid artery to that of the innominate artery as a contraindication, as clamping of the latter would not be possible without also decreasing blood flow to the left hemisphere.[3] A common brachiocephalic trunk, would, therefore, require grafting.

Crawford and colleagues thought that proximal innominate artery lesions, in contrast to distal lesions, were better treated by direct bypass grafting.[5] The surgeons with the largest current experience in the world, Kieffer and Berguer, have used the bypass technique almost exclusively in the last few years.[74, 75] The group from San Francisco has continued to use endarterectomy successfully.

Aortic-origin grafting to the innominate, subclavian, or common carotid artery presents the vascular surgeon with several choices. Simple grafting to the distal innominate artery may be accomplished by means of an 8- or 10-mm polyester (Dacron) graft. Woven grafts are usually used in this location, although collagen-coated knitted grafts may prove preferable in the coming years. If multiple arteries are to be bypassed, two methods of reconstruction are advocated. Compression of the graft by mediastinal contents and the reapproximated sternum has been long recognized as a mechanism of graft failure, venous compression, and even of death by tracheal compression.[5]

Crawford and colleagues proposed the use of single limb grafts with necessary side arms added as an efficient method of reducing bulk in the mediastinum while reconstructing multiple great vessels (Fig. 80–4).[34] Our group agrees, having had at least one failure secondary to the use of a bifurcated graft[9] (see Fig. 80–3). Surgeons from the Texas Heart Institute, however, use bifurcated grafts with excellent results.[10] One noticeable difference that may account for their success is their utilization of a long segment of graft trunk as opposed to the use of a short segment (Fig. 80–5). The use of a short trunk is common practice in infrarenal aortic operations, but it may not be preferred in this setting. The longer trunk probably reduces jet stream turbulence at the divergence of the limbs.

The two methods—bifurcated grafts and single limb grafts with added side arms—are probably equivalent in terms of hemodynamics. The use of the longer trunk places the second limb in approximately the position that an added side arm would take. The method of single graft limbs with added side arms probably does reduce mediastinal bulk more readily than does the use of bifurcated grafts. Other measures that can be performed to reduce the volume of the mediastinal contents include (1) resection of the diseased innominate artery following bypass and (2)

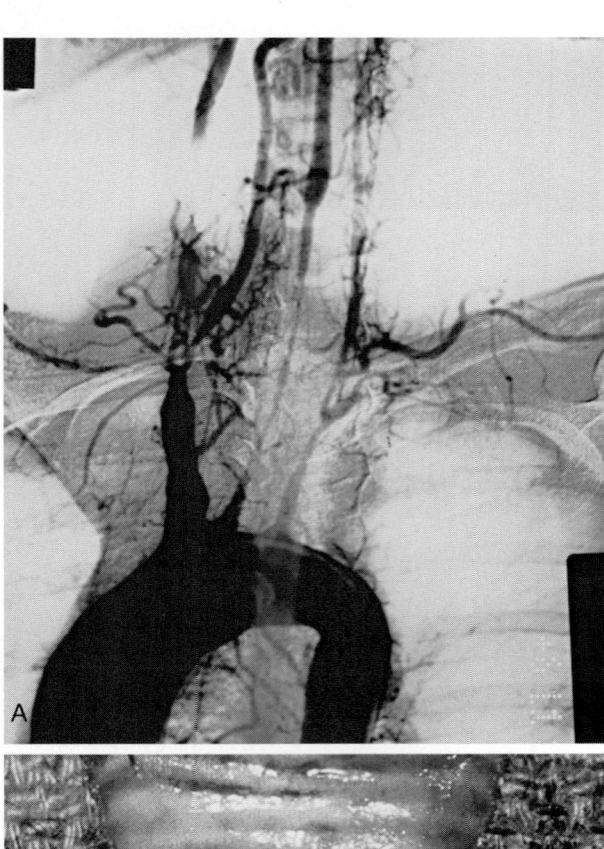

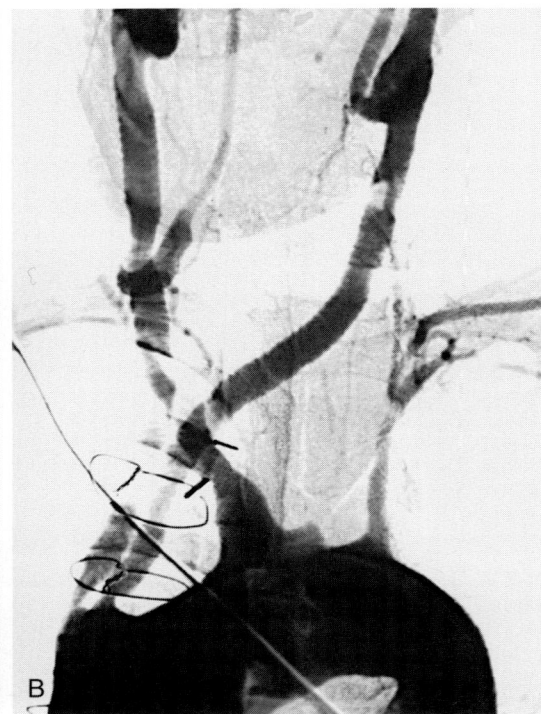

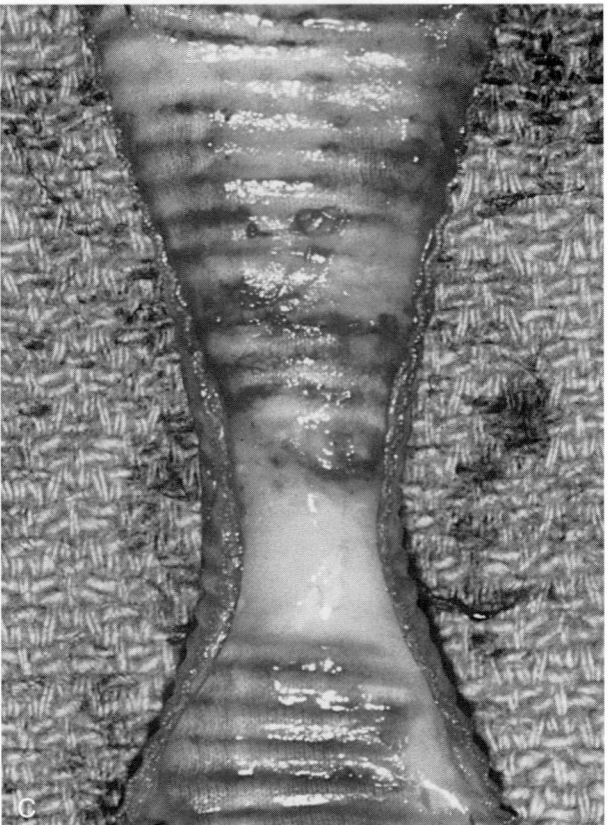

FIGURE 80–3. *A,* Arteriogram of Takayasu's arteritis in a 19-year-old woman who presented with global cerebral ischemia and bilateral upper extremity claudication. *B,* Arteriogram 16 months postoperatively, demonstrating stenoses at origins of the limbs of the bifurcated graft. The claudication was relieved even though the subclavian arteries were not directly reconstructed. (From Cherry KJ Jr, McCollough JL, Hallet J Jr, et al: Technical principles of direct innominate artery revascularization: A comparison of endarterectomy and bypass grafts. J Vasc Surg 9:718, 1989.) *C,* Photograph of resected graft limb demonstrating fibrous stenosis.

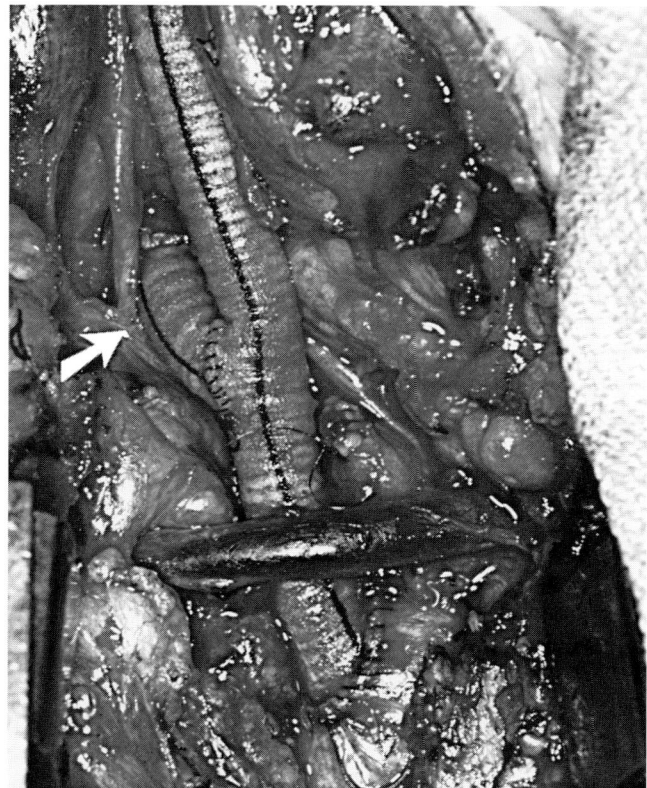

FIGURE 80–4. Photograph of anastomosis of added graft limb to single limb graft originating from the ascending aorta with a clamp placed proximally (arrow).

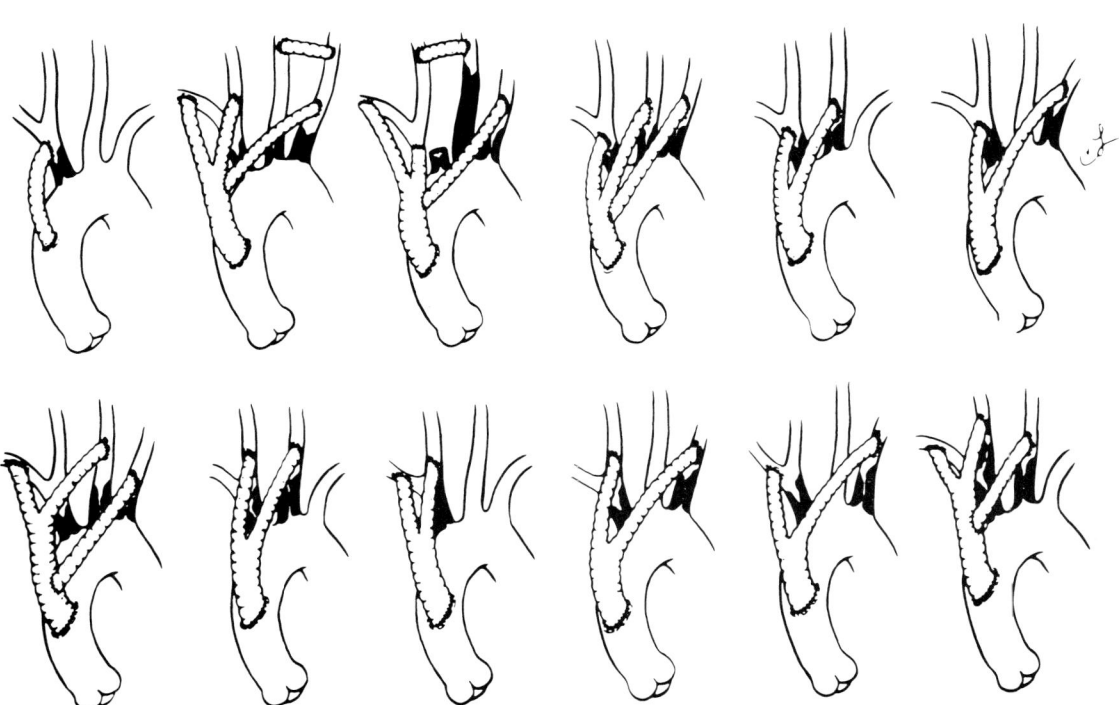

FIGURE 80–5. Schematic drawings demonstrating the Texas Heart Institute method of innominate artery and multiple brachiocephalic artery reconstructions. Note the length of the graft trunk and the reconstruction of all diseased vessels. (From Reul GJ, Jacobs MJ, Gregoric ID, et al: Innominate artery occlusive disease: Surgical approach and long-term results. J Vasc Surg 14:405–412, 1991.)

TABLE 80–1. INNOMINATE ARTERY RECONSTRUCTIONS

INSTITUTION	NO. OF PATIENTS	PERIOPERATIVE TRANSIENT ISCHEMIC ATTACK OR STROKE (%)	MORTALITY (%)	RELIEF OF SYMPTOMS (%)	PROBABILITY OF FREEDOM FROM STROKE (%)	PRIMARY GRAFT PATENCY (%)	SURVIVAL (%)
University of California, San Francisco, 1977	37	2.9	6.0	94			
Cleveland Clinic, 1982	34	0.0	14.7	82			
Baylor, 1983	43	5.5	4.7	94			
University of Michigan, 1985	17	5.9	0	100			
Massachusetts General Hospital, 1985*	29	6.9	3.4	88			
Ohio State University, St. Anthony, 1988	26	7.6	7.6	96			
Mayo Clinic, 1989	26	0.0	3.8	96			
Texas Heart Institute, 1991*	*38	2.7	0	92			
Pitié-Salpêtrière University Hospital, 1995	148	5.4	5.4		88.8 (5 yr); 80.4 (10 yr)	98.4 (5 yr); 96.3 (10 yr)	77.5 (5 yr); 51.9 (10 yr)
Wayne State University, 1998	98	8.0	8.0		87.0 (5 yr); 81.0 (10 yr)	94.0 (5 yr); 88.0 (10 yr)	73.0 (5 yr); 52.0 (10 yr)

Adapted from Cherry KJ Jr, McCullough JL, Hallet JW Jr, Pairolero P: Technical principles of direct innominate artery revascularization: A comparison of endarterectomy and bypass grafts. J Vasc Surg 9:718–724, 1989.
*Intrathoracic approach.

division and ligation of the left brachiocephalic vein. In our experience, this latter maneuver has been safe, with only transient left upper extremity swelling, and it is used selectively at the Mayo Clinic. Kieffer's group uses that technique[42]; however, one of their 148 patients died from hemorrhage from the oversewn venous stump. Permanent left upper extremity swelling has been noted by others.[43, 75] Alternatively, the vein is mobilized by division and ligation of its tributaries and the graft placed behind it. In either circumstance, monitoring lines should not be placed from the left neck or the left upper extremity as the vein is either divided or mobilized extensively.

Another decision to be made at the time of grafting is the extent of reconstruction in patients with multiple lesions. There are two schools of thought. The first, best expressed by the surgeons from the Texas Heart Institute, is to "bypass all diseased vessels."[10] This approach results in placement of multiple grafts (see Fig. 80–5) and has provided excellent results in their hands. Our philosophy has been to reconstruct symptomatic lesions and those lesions needing repair by virtue of their anatomy, such as a left common carotid artery arising from a common brachiocephalic trunk or a stenotic but asymptomatic left common carotid artery. It is the concomitant left subclavian artery lesion that is the point of difference. Adherents of either philosophy would repair concomitant asymptomatic lesions of the left common carotid artery and synchronous carotid bifurcation lesions. In our experience, restoration of flow to the carotid arteries without subclavian reconstruction has resulted in relief of upper extremity claudication even in the most severe cases (see Fig. 80–3). Subsequent left carotid-subclavian artery bypass may be an easier operation than ascending aortic–left subclavian artery grafting, as the left subclavian artery lies far posterior in the mediastinum.

Both approaches work, however, and the choice remains the prerogative of the surgeon. Like Kieffer and Berguer's teams, we employ a selective approach to the diseased left subclavian artery.[74, 75] If both subclavian arteries are occluded, at least one should be reconstructed to allow accurate assessment of blood pressure.

Results of innominate artery reconstructions are very good to excellent, with early relief of symptoms in 95% of patients,[3–10] and long-term relief in 87% to 90% of patients (Table 80–1).[3–10] The best long-term data at present come from Paris and from Detroit. Kieffer and coauthors reported that the probability of freedom from an ipsilateral neurologic event was 92.7% at 5 years and 84.0% at 10 years. The probability of freedom from an ipsilateral stroke was 98.6% at both 5 and 10 years. Primary patency in that series was 98.4% at 5 years and 96.3% at 10 years.[74] In the series from Detroit, stroke-free survival was 87% in 5 years and 81% at 10 years. Primary patency rates at 5 and 10 years were 94% and 88%. Five- and 10-year survival of the patients in both series was remarkably similar (see Table 80–1).[74, 75]

Perioperative stroke ranges from 0 to 8%; mortality ranges from 0 to 14.7%.[3–10, 74, 75] Kieffer and colleagues reported 5.4% mortality and an identical perioperative stroke or TIA rate. Berguer and colleagues reported a combined stroke and death rate of 16%, being equally divided between stroke and death. These latter figures from such excellent centers are disturbing. It is my opinion that these numbers reflect the severity and extent of the disease in their referral populations, with at least two thirds having multiple supra-aortic arterial lesions and a large number having had previous strokes and undergone failed reconstructions. Patients at highest risk for supra-aortic reconstruction (i.e., those with multiple arterial involvement and extensive occlusive processes) are generally not candidates for either extra-thoracic reconstructions or balloon angioplasty and stenting because of the widespread nature of their atherosclerosis. It is the severity of disease rather than the sternotomy itself that contributes to the relatively high mortality and morbidity.

These deaths underscore the necessity to evaluate the status of the coronary circulation and cardiac function in these patients. Concomitant coronary artery bypass grafting has been performed successfully[5, 8, 44] and is probably preferable to staged operations with the necessity of repeated sternotomy. Recently, Takach and colleagues from the Texas Heart Institute have reported a series of 31 patients so treated with a perioperative mortality of only 3.2% and an identical stroke rate. These are obviously exceptional results.[80] Kieffer and associates routinely obtain coronary angiography in these patients.[74] Patients at Wayne State and at the Mayo Clinic undergo functional assessment of cardiac status and selective coronary angiography.[76, 77]

The current and foreseeable debate in repairing lesions of the great vessels is direct repair versus interventional angioplasty and stenting. I believe that for isolated short segment lesions, interventional techniques may prove to be an acceptable option for patients. Most probably, patients with multiple great vessel lesions will need operative repair, either alone or in conjunction with interventional techniques.

Operative Technique

General anesthesia in employed for all the operations described in this chapter. Assessment of the need to shunt blood to the distal carotid artery circulation may be made by any method the surgeon usually employs for carotid artery endarterectomy. Fortunately, these more proximal brachiocephalic lesions seldom require shunting. Placement of arterial lines for blood pressure monitoring in patients with multiple arch lesions requires close communication between the surgeon and the anesthesiologist.

Innominate Artery Endarterectomy

The patient is placed supine on the operating table with the arms at the side. The patient's back is elevated on rolls placed vertically between the scapulae, and the head is supported in an extended position and turned to the left. The neck, chest, and upper abdomen are prepared and draped into the operative field. The surgeon makes a midline incision, dividing the entire sternum and extending a short distance into the right neck along the anterior border of the sternocleidomastoid muscle (Fig. 80–6A). If necessary, the sternal attachments of this muscle are divided. The surgeon mobilizes the thymus and pericardial fat, exposing the left innominate or brachiocephalic vein, which is then either mobilized by division and ligation of its tributaries or divided primarily (Fig. 80–6B). The ascending

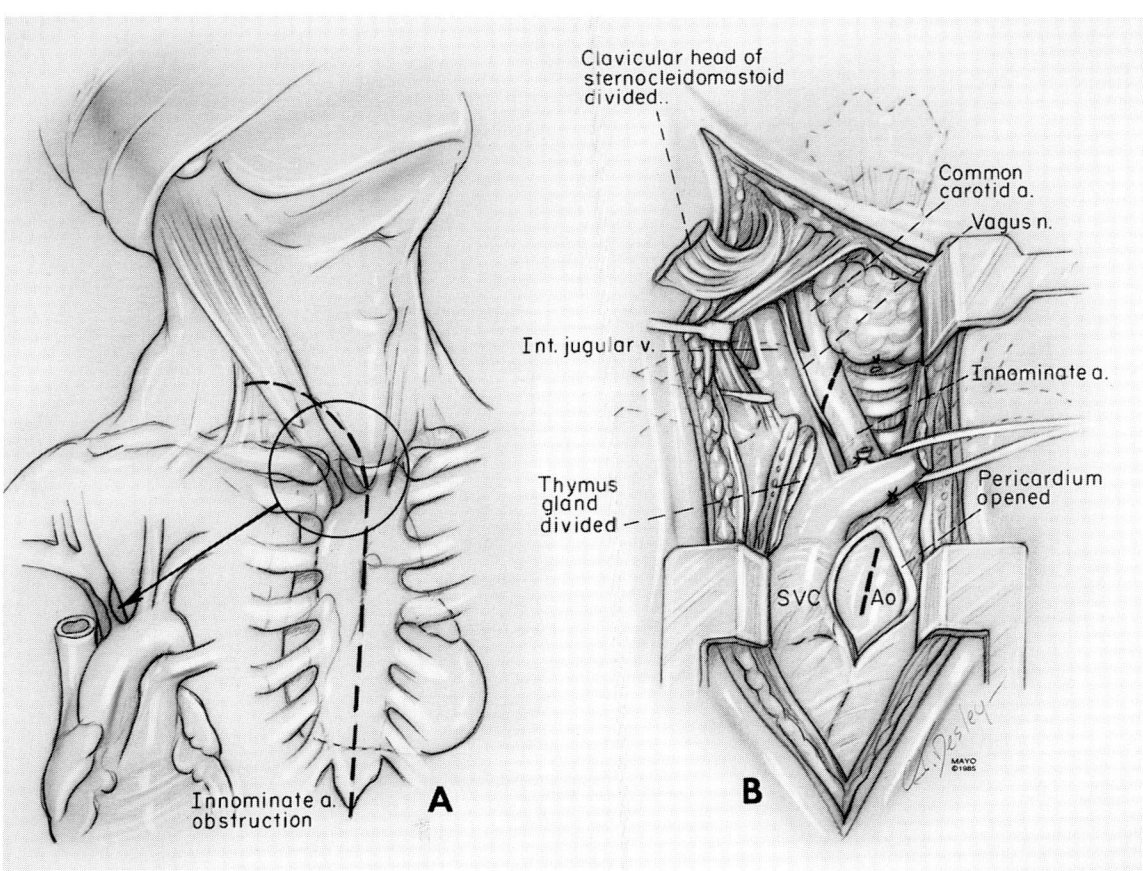

FIGURE 80–6. *A,* Schematic drawing of full median sternotomy with extension into the right neck. *B,* Schematic drawing of the sites of anastomosis for aorta–innominate artery grafting. The vein may be mobilized or divided. The intrapericardial ascending aorta is usually free of atherosclerotic disease. (By permission of Mayo Foundation.)

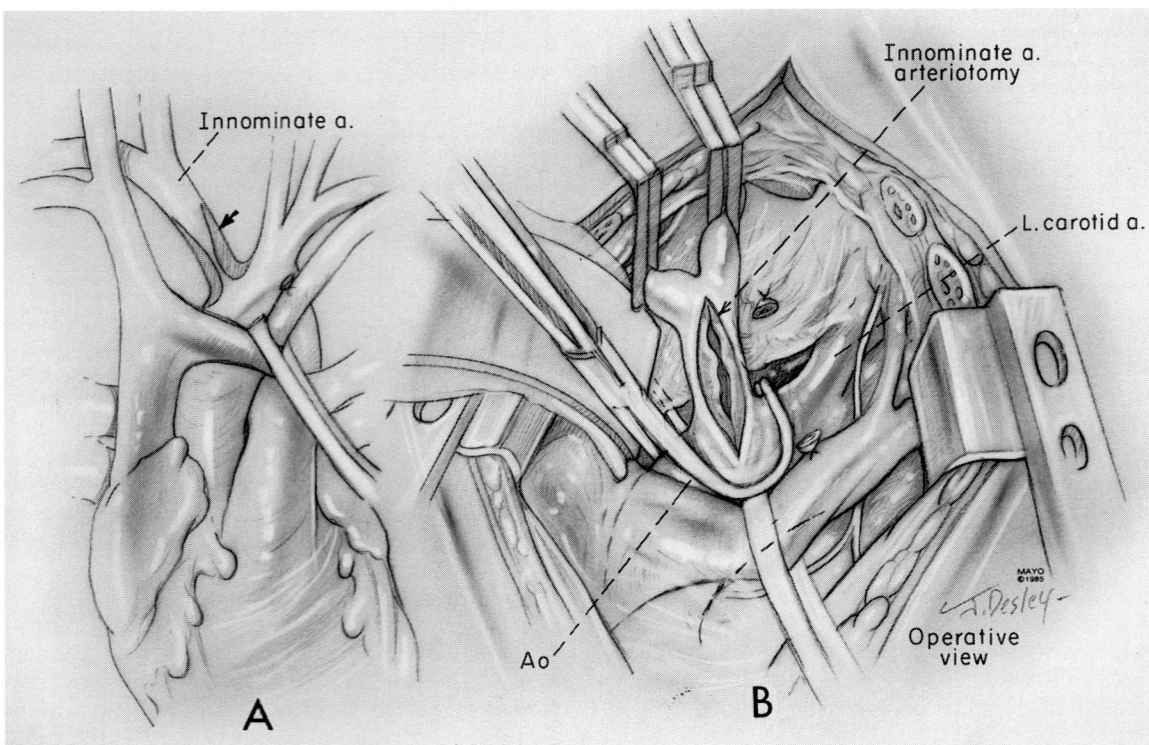

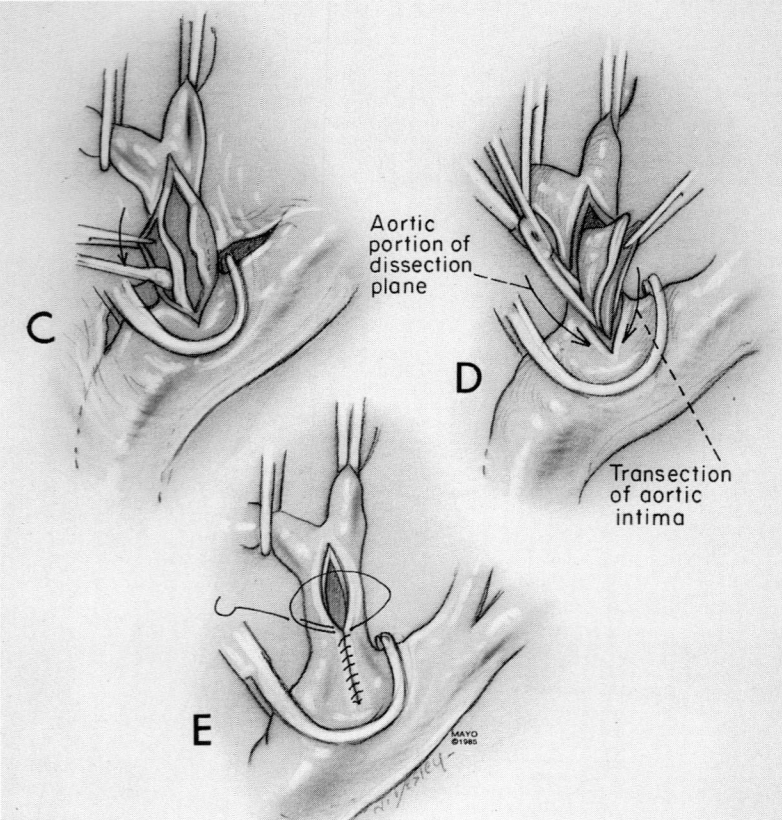

FIGURE 80–7. Schematic drawings of innominate artery endarterectomy. *A,* Endarterectomy is suitable for patients with a soft aorta at the base of the innominate artery and flow through the left common carotid artery unimpaired by clamping. *B,* Schematic demonstrating application of clamps and extension of incision onto the aortic arch. *C,* Schematic showing the initiation of the endarterectomy. *D,* The precise division of the innominate plaque. *E,* Closure with polypropylene sutures. (*A–E,* By permission of the Mayo Foundation.)

aortic arch proximal to the innominate artery and the origins of the innominate and left common carotid arteries are dissected free. The aorta at the base of the innominate artery is inspected, and the distance between the innominate artery and the left common carotid artery is ascertained. If the aorta is normal at the base of the innominate artery and if the origin of the left common carotid artery is sufficiently distant (1.5 to 2 cm) from the innominate artery, endarterectomy is feasible.

The innominate artery is mobilized past the origins of the right common carotid and subclavian arteries. If the disease continues distal to the innominate artery, the atherosclerotic plaque usually extends unto the subclavian rather than the common carotid artery. The vagus and recurrent laryngeal nerves are identified and preserved. If more distal dissection of the subclavian artery is necessary, the phrenic nerve must be identified and also preserved.

The patient is given systemically heparin therapy. First, control of the subclavian and common carotid arteries is obtained to prevent distal atheroembolization. The origin of the innominate artery is then clamped with a narrow, deep partial occlusion clamp, such as the Wylie J-clamp (Pilling). Satisfactory flow into the left common carotid artery should be ascertained by pulse examination.

A vertical innominate arteriotomy is made. If necessary, the arteriotomy is extended into the right subclavian artery or, more rarely, into the right common carotid artery. Proximally, the incision is carried down unto the aorta (Fig. 80–7). If the proximal innominate artery is free of disease, the endarterectomy plane is started just distal to the origin of the innominate artery. It is developed circumferentially at this point, and the specimen is divided. With an arterial elevator, the diseased intima and the inner media are dissected free. The plaque usually has a nice tapered endpoint. If necessary, tacking sutures of fine polypropylene may be used distally. If disease is present at the origin of the innominate artery, it is removed by judicious use of the arterial elevator and fine sharply pointed scissors. Tacking sutures may be necessary or preferred on the aortic intima at the distal, or carotid artery side, of the endarterectomy.

The operative site is inspected for any remnants of the atherosclerotic debris and thoroughly rinsed. If the artery is small, it may be patched with a woven Dacron graft with running 5-0 or 6-0 polypropylene suture. In my experience, most arteries may be closed primarily using these same fine polypropylene (Prolene) sutures. Like the subclavian artery, the innominate artery is fragile, and braided sutures should not be used.

Just before the closure is completed, the proximal clamp is partially opened and reapproximated. Back-bleeding is allowed from the subclavian artery and, finally, from the common carotid artery. After the arteriotomy is closed, the subclavian artery clamp is removed and hemostasis is evaluated. If the closure is hemostatic, flow is restored first to the right subclavian artery and then the right common carotid artery.

Protamine sulfate may be given at this point. Mediastinal and chest tubes are placed, and the wound closed in standard manner with wire reapproximation of the sternum.

Aorta–Innominate Artery Bypass Graft

Positioning of the patient and the incision is the same as described earlier. A more extensive exposure of the as-

cending aorta proximal to the innominate artery is necessary. The pericardium may be entered, and the intrapericardial ascending aorta is dissected free (see Fig. 80–6B). The aorta is usually free of atherosclerosis in this location. A partial occlusion clamp, such as the Cooley Curved Multi-Purpose clamp (V. Mueller) is placed as far laterally on the ascending aorta as possible. At this point, administration of heparin is not necessary.

A vertical aortotomy is made, and the aortic wall is separated with guy sutures of polypropylene. Classically woven Dacron grafts of 8 or 10 mm are chosen for this bypass. The graft is widely spatulated and fashioned to fit the aortotomy. For the anastomosis, running 3-0 or 4-0 polypropylene or Dacron suture is used. After satisfactory hemostasis is achieved, a clamp is placed across the graft and the aortic clamp is removed. The patient is now systemically heparinized. Control of the right subclavian and common carotid arteries, and last of the innominate artery, is obtained to prevent distal embolization.

The innominate artery is divided distally. If necessary, the distal artery is spatulated for anastomosis. If the disease process extends into the subclavian artery, the surgeon must address this appropriately. The distal anastomosis is performed in an end-to-end manner with running 4-0 or 5-0 polypropylene sutures. Appropriate antegrade and retrograde bleeding are allowed, and the anastomosis is completed. Flow is restored, first to the subclavian and then to the common carotid artery (Fig. 80–8).

As much of the innominate artery as feasible is excised to help decompress the mediastinum. The stump is oversewn with horizontal and over-and-over polypropylene suture. The remainder of the operation is conducted in a fashion identical to that of innominate artery endarterectomy.

Ascending Aorta–Carotid Artery and Aorta–Subclavian Artery Bypass

As previously mentioned, bifurcated grafts or single limb grafts with side arms attached may be used. If the left common carotid artery is to be reconstructed at the same time as the innominate artery, a Dacron graft may be sutured to the left lateral wall of the innominate artery graft as a side arm. This step is performed after the proximal anastomosis has been completed. It is done in the upper mediastinum, and a running permanent suture is used. To determine the most advantageous location for this graft, the surgeon may relax the sternal retractor be relaxed to allow the grafts and the mediastinal contents to assume their more nearly permanent positions. Side arms to the subclavian artery, most usually to the right subclavian artery, are performed in the same manner.

If it is necessary to expose the carotid bifurcations, the exposures are performed through standard vertical incisions. On the right side, the sternal incision may simply be continued; on the left side, a separate cervical incision is usually performed.

If the distal anastomosis is to the carotid bifurcations, it is generally performed in an end-to-side manner as with an angioplasty. Proximal ties on the common carotid artery or end-to-end anastomosis may sometimes be necessary, especially those cases involving distal embolization. If nec-

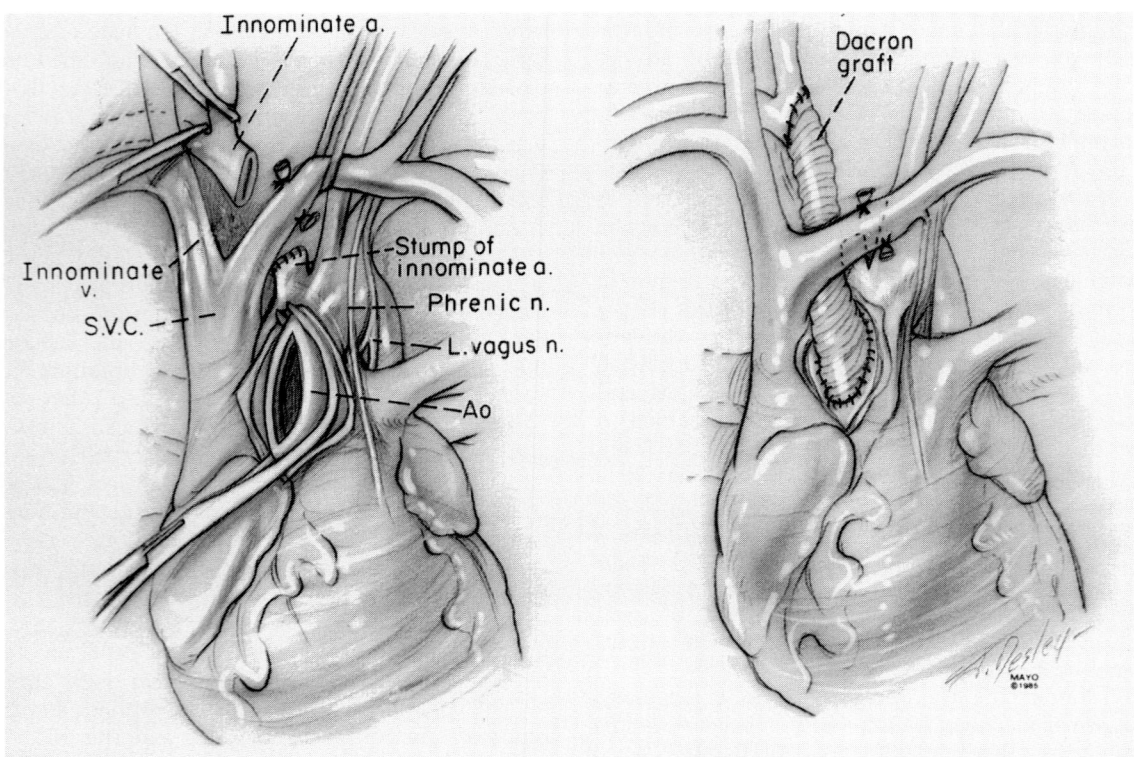

FIGURE 80–8. Schematic drawing demonstrating aortotomy and division of the innominate artery. If the left brachiocephalic vein is mobilized, the graft is placed behind it. The innominate artery is resected following bypass. (By permission of Mayo Foundation.)

essary, endarterectomy of the carotid bifurcation is performed in standard manner.

The mediastinal wound is closed in a fashion identical to that of innominate artery endarterectomy. The closure of the cervical wounds is performed in standard manner.

COMMON CAROTID ARTERY

Occlusive lesions of the common carotid arteries necessitating repair are encountered less frequently than those of the carotid bifurcations. Toole reported only 1% of patients with "carotid artery syndrome" had common carotid artery occlusions and that the right side was involved much less frequently than the left.[45] Riles and coauthors stated that 2% of patients with symptomatic carotid artery disease would be found to have occlusions of the common carotid artery.[46] Wylie and Effeney, in their review of surgery of the aortic arch branches, found only 32 of 1961 patients with great vessel, carotid bifurcation, or vertebral artery disease to have common carotid artery lesions (1.5%).[2] Lesions of the right common carotid artery are seen only rarely in the absence of innominate artery lesions and far less frequently than those of the left common carotid artery. Atherosclerosis, Takayasu's arteritis, and (less infrequently) radiation-induced atherosclerosis are the causes.

Most of the reports dealing with common carotid artery disease focus on occlusions rather than stenoses,[46–48] although stenoses as well as occlusions may give rise to symptoms. A more thorough understanding of the natural history of common carotid artery lesions and the best

methods of their repair has been hindered by the relative rarity of common carotid artery lesions, especially those requiring operation, and a lack of long-term evaluation. Further hampering the acquisition of precise knowledge of these lesions and their treatment has been the grouping of these patients with patients undergoing either reconstruction for subclavian artery lesions or arch reconstruction for multiple lesions.

Physical examination may reveal reduced carotid artery pulses or the presence of a proximal bruit distinct from a bifurcation bruit. No pulse would be palpable with common carotid artery occlusion. Oculoplethysmography may demonstrate hemodynamic significance, and duplex scanning may be expected to demonstrate proximal flow disturbances even if the lesion cannot be visualized. Patients suspected of having strokes should undergo computed tomography (CT) of the head, and the timing of operation should be based accordingly. Arch aortography with four-vessel runoff should be obtained in all patients to localize disease, to determine the etiology, to facilitate planning of operation, and to determine the presence of synchronous extracranial vessel lesions.

Occlusions of the common carotid artery may originate at either end of the artery, ostial stenosis may progress to occlusion with prograde thrombosis, or bifurcation disease may advance to occlusion with retrograde thrombosis. Asymptomatic patients with common carotid artery occlusions, as distinct from stenoses, are usually observed. Symptomatic patients (whether symptoms are primary, recurrent, or persistent) with common carotid artery occlusions merit careful evaluation, because conventional arteriography may fail to demonstrate patent external and internal carotid arteries, either of which is a suitable recipient vessel for such patients. If arteriography does not demonstrate patent internal or external carotid arteries, CT Doppler examination, magnetic resonance angiography (MRA) or another method should be employed to ascertain patency of these bifurcation vessels.

Riles and colleagues used rapid-sequence CT with good results.[46] Podore and associates reported their early experience with directional Doppler investigations to determine internal carotid artery patency.[47] Keller and coworkers combined Doppler examinations and sequential CT scans to evaluate external carotid and internal carotid artery patency.[48] MRA is proving useful in this setting, and as this modality improves, it may become the test of choice. At the Mayo Clinic, we now rely heavily on duplex scanning of the carotid bifurcation in these situations.

Common carotid artery lesions may give rise to symptoms because of reductions in flow, thrombosis, or embolization. The indications for operation are the same as those for bifurcation disease: amaurosis fugax, transient ischemic attack, and stroke. If tandem lesions of both the common carotid artery and the carotid bifurcation exist, it is difficult, if not impossible, to determine which stenosis is the source of the presenting problems. Both lesions, as a consequence, require repair to ensure high flow rates and removal of both potential sources of symptoms (Fig. 80–9). Isolated, asymptomatic, highly stenotic lesions of the common ca-

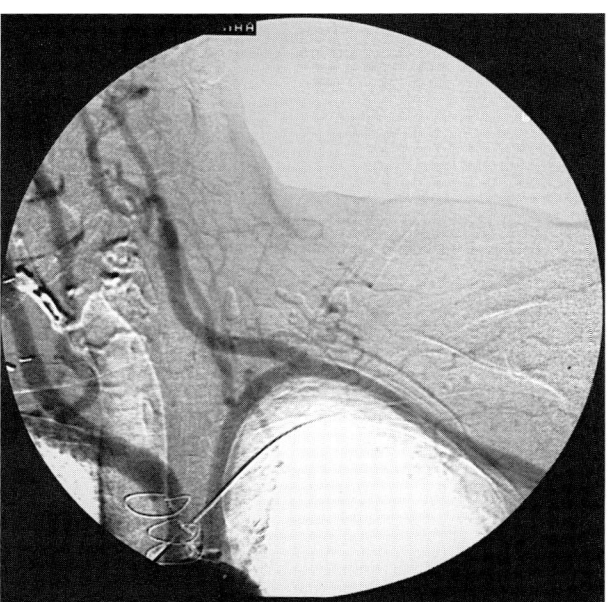

FIGURE 80–10. Postoperative digital subtraction angiogram demonstrating a patent left common carotid artery transposition in a 66-year-old woman. The procedure was performed for a stenosis of the proximal artery and a reversible ischemic neurologic deficit. The left vertebral artery arises from the aortic arch.

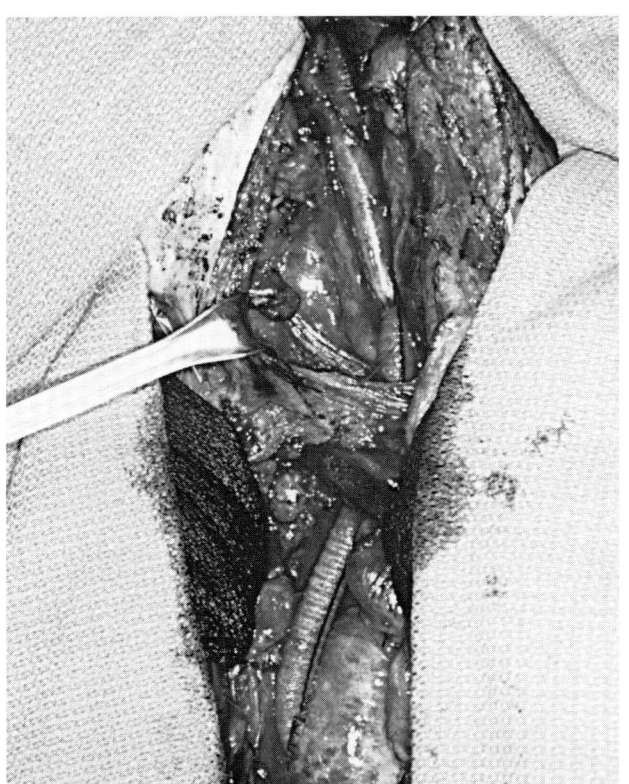

FIGURE 80–9. Intraoperative photograph of aorta–left common carotid artery graft and left carotid bifurcation endarterectomy performed for a 68-year-old man 6 weeks after a left hemispheric stroke. Both the origin of the left common carotid artery and the left carotid bifurcation had 90% stenoses, and the left subclavian artery was occluded.

rotid artery have been repaired, since it is assumed that they have the same propensity to give rise to symptoms as asymptomatic bifurcation lesions. The data for that assumption are admittedly lacking, since the natural history of these lesions is unknown.

If the ipsilateral subclavian artery is patent, a reconstruction based on that artery is the easiest, safest, and best method of reconstruction. These lesions are usually treated by subclavian-carotid artery bypass or, less commonly, by transposition of the distal common carotid artery unto the subclavian artery. Such repairs are feasible, of course, only if the ipsilateral subclavian artery is a good donor vessel.

If the common carotid artery distal to a stenosis is healthy and if the ipsilateral subclavian artery widely patent, a transposition of the distal common carotid unto the subclavian artery is easily performed and attractive. Its only drawback is the necessity of more proximal dissection of the common carotid artery than would be required if bypass were performed. Wylie and Effeney[2] and Ehrenfeld and colleagues[49] described transposition of the carotid artery unto the subclavian artery with good results. The number of patients, of course, was small. We have had similar results in the few patients for whom this has been performed (Fig. 80–10). Stenotic disease extending the length of the common carotid artery or occlusions with thrombosis mitigate against transposition. Law and coauthors, in their review of both carotid-subclavian and subclavian-carotid artery reconstructions, reported five carotid artery transpositions and 32 subclavian-carotid artery bypasses. Patency for the transpositions at 5 years was 100%.[81]

Subclavian-carotid artery bypass grafting is the most commonly performed reconstructive operation for common carotid artery disease. Fry and associates reported 20 patients treated over 12 years.[50] They analyzed their patients separately and did not group them with patients having carotid-subclavian artery grafts or repair of multiple arch lesions. Results were excellent, with no strokes and one death. Four patients underwent concomitant ipsilateral bifurcation endarterectomy. Saphenous vein was used in 15 patients, and prosthetic grafts were used in the other five. In follow-up ranging to 55 months, all grafts were patent and only one patient had cerebrovascular symptoms, which were of the posterior circulation.

Unlike the experience with carotid-subclavian artery grafts,[51] the use of saphenous vein in this series of subclavian-carotid artery bypass grafts provided the same long-term patency as that of prosthetic grafts. Of interest, the majority of patients in this series had right common carotid artery lesions. All the grafts in this series were to the level of the carotid bifurcation or beyond. Five of the 20 patients had external carotid artery outflow only. None of the grafts were placed horizontally to the common carotid artery at the same level as the subclavian artery. The vertical orientation[50] and the decreased resistance of the cerebral vasculature[52] were proposed as possible reasons for better results with vein in this setting than with vein in carotid-subclavian artery bypass grafting. Synn and associates, from the University of Iowa, found vein for these bypasses far superior to prosthetics in their review of 14 patients.[82]

Salam and colleagues reported a 10-year experience with 31 reconstructions for proximal common carotid lesions.[83] Of these patients, 26 underwent subclavian-carotid artery bypass grafting and five underwent carotid-carotid artery bypass grafting. In this series, there were no strokes or deaths. The 3-year patency was 90%.

If the ipsilateral subclavian artery is also involved in the atherosclerotic process, aortic-origin grafting (see Fig. 80–9) or contralateral carotid-carotid artery grafting (Fig. 80–11) is necessary. Berguer and Gonzalez reported very good results in 16 patients undergoing carotid-carotid artery bypass grafting via the retropharyngeal route.[77] There were no deaths, one stroke, and one graft occlusion in this group of patients. Primary patency was 94%, and 5-year survival was 87.5%. In contradistinction, Law and others reported a 5-year survival of patients with proximal carotid disease of 62.7%.[81]

Common carotid artery lesions in association with multiple other arch lesions are best treated by direct arch reconstruction in good-risk patients.[5, 6, 8–10]

Concomitant ipsilateral bifurcation lesions are repaired at the same time for the reasons given earlier. Usually, the distal anastomosis is to the endarterectomy site.

Operative Technique

Subclavian-Carotid Artery Bypass Graft

The patient is placed supine on the operating table, with a roll placed vertically between the scapulae to elevate the shoulders. The neck is extended as much as feasible, and the head turned away from the side of the lesion.

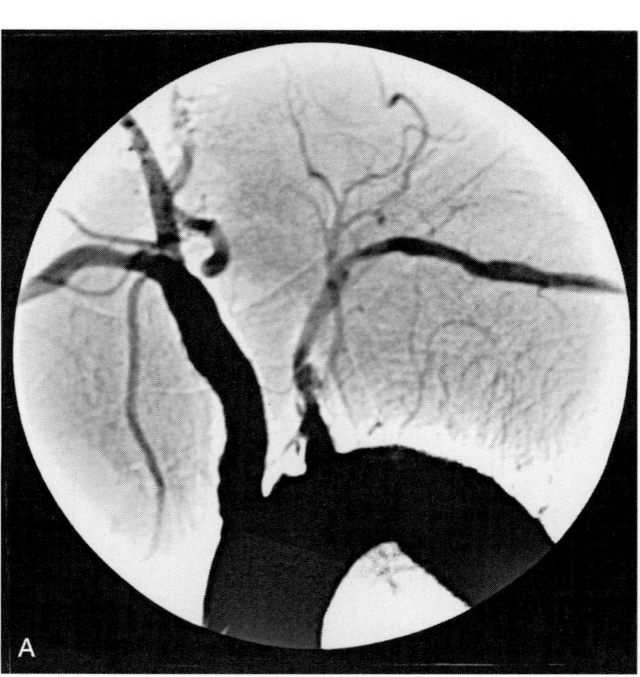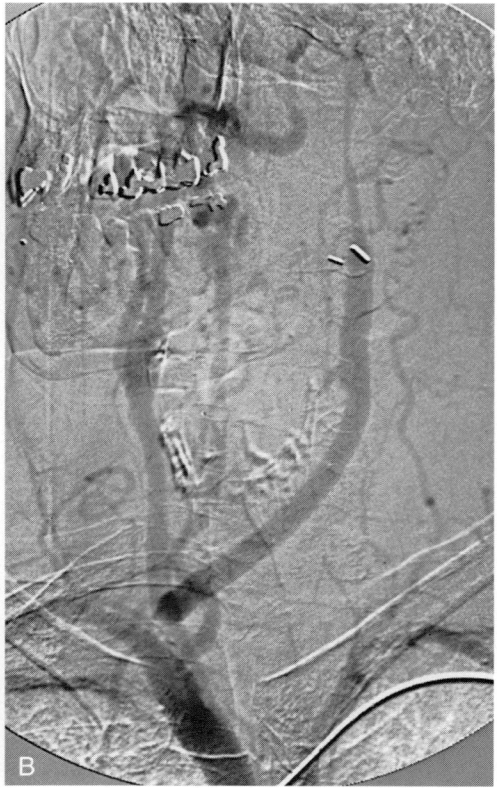

FIGURE 80–11. *A,* Arteriogram with left amaurosis fugax in a 67-year-old woman. Note the occluded left common carotid artery and the markedly diseased left subclavian artery. *B,* Postoperative digital subtraction arteriogram following carotid-carotid artery bypass graft and left carotid endarterectomy. Arterial outflow is through the internal carotid artery. The patient's symptoms were relieved.

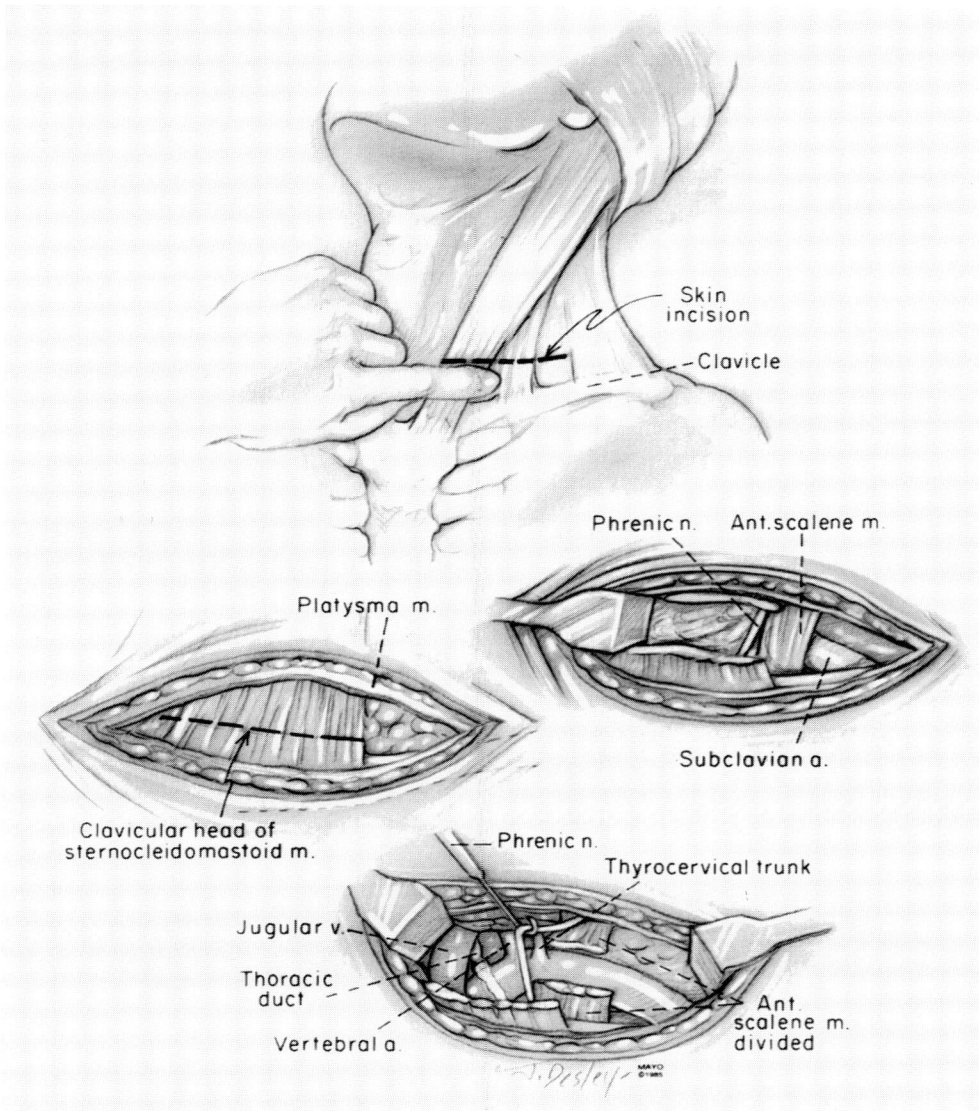

FIGURE 80–12. Schematic drawings demonstrating a left supraclavicular incision and exposure of the subclavian artery. (By permission of Mayo Foundation.)

A supraclavicular incision 2 to 3 cm above and parallel to the clavicle is made with its medial extent overlying the clavicular head of the sternocleidomastoid muscle. After the platysma is incised, the clavicular head of the sterno-cleidomastoid muscle may be transected if necessary. The scalene fat pad is mobilized by clamping, division and ligation, and reflected superiorly. The thoracic duct or right lymphatic duct may be sought at this time and formally ligated. Because the subclavian veins lie more inferiorly than the arteries, the surgeon may elect not to ligate but simply to avoid avulsion injuries by careful dissection.

The anterior scalene muscle is identified with the phrenic nerve coursing medially along its anterior surface. The nerve is identified and protected, and the muscle is transected. Some surgeons elect not to transect this muscle but to retract it. The subclavian artery is identified just posterior to the muscle (Fig. 80–12). Adequate length is mobilized to allow proximal and distal control. Its branches may

be divided and ligated to facilitate mobilization with the exception of the vertebral artery, which must be preserved, and the internal mammary artery, which should be preserved, if at all possible, for subsequent coronary artery revascularization.

If the anastomosis is to be made to the common carotid artery at the same level, that artery may be exposed through the same incision. Medial retraction allows dissection. The jugular vein and the vagus nerve are identified and protected. In most instances, a tunnel is made posterior to the jugular vein. The positions of the vagus and phrenic nerve may depend on the patient's anatomy and should be noted as such in the operative report. If the distal anastomosis is to be made to the carotid bifurcation, that area is exposed through a vertical incision and the bifurcation dissected free in standard manner. The tunnel is made posterior to the jugular vein and the sternocleido-mastoid muscle.

The patient is given systemic heparin therapy. Control of the subclavian artery is obtained, and a vertical arteriotomy is made at the dome of the artery. Usually, a 7- or 8-mm knitted Dacron graft, preclotted, is employed. Expanded polytetrafluoroethylene (PTFE) or venous autografts may also be used. The anastomosis is performed end-to-side to the artery with running 4-0 or 5-0 polypropylene sutures. The subclavian artery is fragile, and braided permanent sutures are not as desirable as monofilament sutures.

After appropriate flushing, the anastomosis is completed and a clamp is placed across the origin of the graft. Flow is restored to the extremity. The graft is brought through the tunnel, and control of the carotid artery is obtained. If the anastomosis is to the common carotid artery at the same level, the arteriotomy is made in the lateral wall. The arteriotomy should not be too long, because the graft will be joining the carotid at a right angle. Otherwise, the anastomosis would be elongated and flattened. If the distal anastomosis is to the carotid bifurcation or either of its two branches, the incision is made in the usual location. It may be combined with carotid endarterectomy if indicated (Fig. 80–13). The wound is closed in standard manner. The platysma is reapproximated with polyglactin (Vicryl) sutures, and the skin is reapproximated with subcuticular or horizontal mattress nylon sutures.

Transposition of the Common Carotid Artery

Positioning of the patient, incision, and exposure are as described earlier. The common carotid artery is dissected free into the mediastinum until adequate length is obtained. After systemic heparinization, the *distal* clamp is placed on the carotid first to prevent clamp injury to the proximal lesion and embolization. The *proximal* clamp is then applied and the artery divided. The proximal stump is oversewn with horizontal and over-and-over polypropylene sutures. Control is obtained at the subclavian artery, and a vertical arteriotomy is made at its apex. The carotid artery is cut to length and sutured end-to-side to the subclavian artery with running 4-0 or 5-0 polypropylene sutures. Again, the surgeon should take care that the arteriotomy not be too long in order to avoid narrowing of this anastomosis. The wound is closed as described earlier (Fig. 80–14A).

SUBCLAVIAN ARTERY

Lesions of the subclavian artery requiring arterial reconstruction are relatively uncommon, but they are encountered more frequently than lesions of the innominate and common carotid arteries. Wylie and Effeney found that they represented 4.3% of the 1961 operative cases they reviewed of carotid bifurcation, vertebral artery, and great vessel reconstructions.[2] Crawford and coauthors reported 80 subclavian artery repairs in their review of 142 great vessel reconstructions.[5] The left subclavian artery is more often atherosclerotic than the right and is involved in approximately 70% of symptomatic cases.

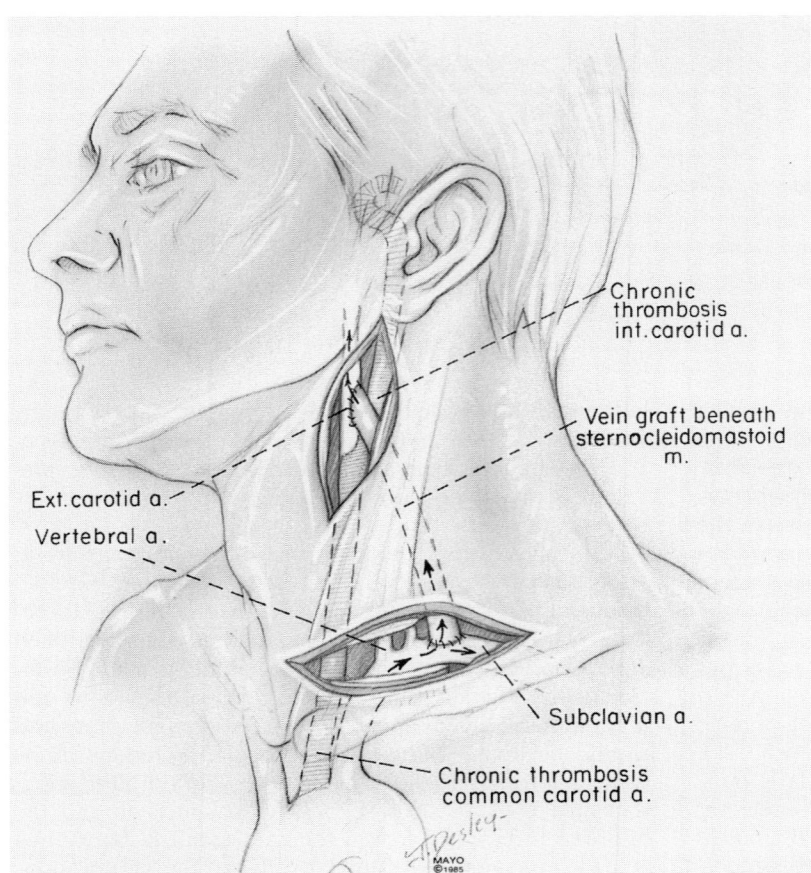

FIGURE 80–13. Schematic drawing of a left subclavian-carotid artery bypass. In this instance, outflow is through the external carotid artery. (By permission of Mayo Foundation.)

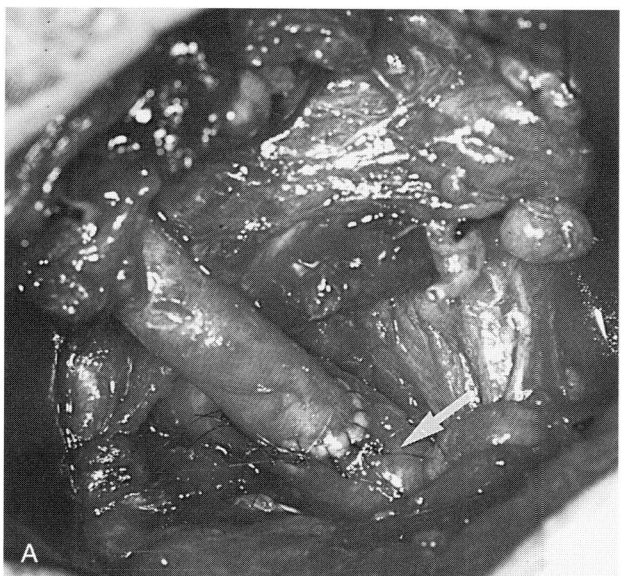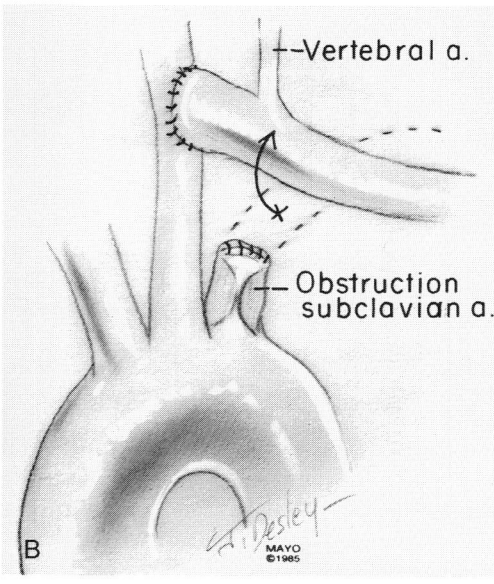

FIGURE 80–14. A, Transposition of the left common carotid artery. (The interposition polyester [Dacron] graft [arrow] pictured here is seldom necessary if the proximal common carotid artery is mobilized sufficiently.) B, Left subclavian artery transposition. (By permission of Mayo Foundation.)

Patients with isolated occlusive lesions of the subclavian artery are usually asymptomatic because of the rich arterial collateral supply of the head, neck, and shoulder. These lesions may give rise to ischemia of either the upper extremity or the posterior cerebral circulation. The mechanism of symptom formation may be hemodynamic or atheroembolic. The latter is especially notable with upper extremity ischemia.

In 1960, Contorni described a radiographic *subclavian steal* (i.e., reversal of flow in the ipsilateral vertebral artery distal to a proximal lesion) in an asymptomatic patient for the first time.[22] The term "subclavian steal" was coined the following year.[53] The so-called subclavian steal syndrome seems to occur when use of the upper extremity increases demand for blood and "steals" it from the cerebral circulation through the ipsilateral vertebral artery distal to the proximal subclavian (or rarely innominate) artery lesion. Despite its simplistic anatomic appeal, however, the existence of such a clinical syndrome—in distinction to radiographic or duplex findings—has been seriously questioned by vascular surgeons,[5, 49] especially in the absence of concomitant extracranial arterial occlusive disease. Reversal of vertebral artery flow, as documented by arteriography or duplex scanning, usually represents a normal pattern of collateral response to a proximal subclavian artery lesion and is not itself an indication for operation. Webster and coworkers, however, with exercise of the upper extremities in six patients having proximal subclavian artery disease and concomitant lesions, demonstrated decreased regional blood flow, thereby giving validity to the concept of a clinical steal.[84]

Symptomatic subclavian artery lesions are associated with concomitant lesions of the contralateral vertebral artery or one or both carotid arteries in 35% to 85% of patients.[1, 5, 54, 55] The Joint Study of Extracranial Arterial Occlusion found that 80% of patients with cerebral steal had concomitant lesions.[1] Walker and associates found 72%

of their 157 patients to have such concomitant lesions.[55] Further, they were unable to correlate symptoms with the presence or absence of reversed flow in the ipsilateral vertebral artery.

In general, it is probable that subclavian artery lesions cause vertebrobasilar insufficiency by virtue of decreases in regional blood flow, thrombosis, or embolization, and that a majority are associated with synchronous lesions of the great vessels, vertebral arteries, or carotid bifurcations.

The indications for operative reconstruction of subclavian artery lesions are classically those of vertebrobasilar insufficiency and upper extremity ischemia. In addition, myocardial ischemia is seen in patients with left internal mammary artery coronary grafts and proximal left subclavian artery disease. Vertebrobasilar insufficiency, discussed more fully elsewhere, may present with multiple and diverse symptoms that are often obscure; these include visual disturbances, often bilateral, vertigo, ataxia, syncope, dysphasia, dysarthria, sensory deficits of the face, and motor and sensory deficits of the extremities.

Symptomatic occlusive disease of the upper extremities, which includes muscle fatigue, or "claudication," ischemic rest pain, ulcers, digital necrosis, or atheroembolization, is much less common than that of the lower extremities, accounting for approximately 5% of patients with limb ischemia.[56–58]

The etiology of upper extremity ischemia is diverse, in contrast to that of lower extremity ischemia, which is most often atherosclerotic in origin. Vasospastic disorders, thoracic outlet syndrome with arterial involvement, arteritis, autoimmune diseases, trauma, and cardiac-source embolization in addition to atherosclerosis, may all produce ischemia of the upper extremity. Those etiologic factors and their management are discussed elsewhere.

In addition to the presence of synchronous lesions of the supra-aortic vessels as a contributing cause of ischemia, atheroembolization from proximal subclavian artery ulcerative lesions is noteworthy (Fig. 80–15). Ischemia of the upper extremity is much more likely than that of the lower extremity to manifest itself by microembolization. Rapp and colleagues found that 47% of their 17 patients with symptomatic proximal subclavian or innominate artery disease had evidence of microembolization.[59] Atheroembolization from a proximal subclavian artery lesion was the most frequent cause of upper extremity ischemia in that series.[59] Similarly, Kadwa and Robbs found 13 patients with atheroembolization and two with cardiac-source embolization in their review of 35 patients with gangrenous fingers presenting over 7 years.[58] Atheroemboli may rise from highly stenotic lesions or from those which are ulcerated but not hemodynamically significant. In the latter situation, radial and ulnar pulses may be readily palpable and blood pressure in the upper extremities may be equal. Palpable pulses may mislead physicians and may prompt a search for systemic disorders, thereby delaying diagnosis. In more advanced cases that have gone undiagnosed or untreated, radial and ulnar pulses may be absent as the digital and palmar arteries have occluded with atheroembolic debris. This low-flow state results in occlusion of the named forearm vessels. That this is a potentially limb-threatening problem is borne out by the study from San Francisco, wherein four major limb amputations were reported following atheroembolization to the upper extremity.[59]

The salient features of the history and physical are the same as those for the innominate artery. CT scans of the head should be obtained for patients thought to have had a stroke. The localization of infarction may help to determine the source of injury (i.e., carotid or vertebrobasilar artery origin). Aortic arch aortography with four-vessel views is necessary in all patients. Runoff views of the arteries of the involved extremity may be necessary to localize embolic occlusions. Selective catheters should not be placed in the subclavian artery before a film of the artery's origin is obtained first, because nonhemodynamically significant but ulcerative lesions may be missed.

The diagnosis of a subclavian artery occlusive lesion as the source of symptoms for upper extremity ischemia is usually evident following arteriography. The etiologic association between a subclavian artery lesion and vertebrobasilar symptoms may be less clear, especially in the presence of synchronous carotid or vertebral artery lesions. Patients presenting with vertebrobasilar symptoms in the presence of both significant subclavian artery and carotid bifucation disease are usually offered carotid artery endarterectomy as a first operation or in combination with ipsilateral carotid-subclavian artery bypass. Synchronous lesions may adversely affect the results of operation. We found that morbidity for carotid-subclavian artery bypass (i.e., stroke) increased when the procedure was performed in the presence of significant concomitant bifurcation disease.[54] Crawford and coworkers noted an increased rate of stroke in the presence of multiple lesions.[5]

Nonetheless, the operative management of subclavian artery lesions causing vertebrobasilar symptoms, upper extremity ischemia, and myocardial ischemia, is technically the same. Patients with myocardial ischemia should not undergo subclavian transposition. Adjunctive measures, such as shunting of the carotid artery, Fogarty embolectomy, and cervical sympathectomy, depend on the particular situation at hand. In some cases, especially involving the right subclavian artery, localized endarterectomy of the subclavian artery may be a viable option. The left subclavian artery is involved far more often than the right, however, and usually subclavian artery endarterectomy cannot suffice.

If the ipsilateral common carotid artery is healthy, a reconstruction based on that vessel is the preferred method of revascularization. Carotid-subclavian artery bypass using prosthetic material has been the most commonly performed operation. The report of Diethrich and colleagues on 125 patients in 1967 brought that extra-anatomic reconstruction into the forefront.[30] Synthetic grafts, most usually of Dacron, almost uniformly have better patency rates than saphenous vein when used in carotid-subclavian artery bypass.[51, 60]

Law and colleagues have reported that PTFE grafts had a patency of 95%, followed by Dacron grafts at 84% and saphenous vein grafts at 65%. These figures were not statistically significant.[81] It is thought the size mismatch of the vein and the arteries and the axial forces generated by movement in the neck and shoulder regions contribute to the decreased patency rates of venous grafts in this location.

Carotid-subclavian artery bypass grafts yield excellent results with low morbidity and mortality rates. Vitti and coworkers reported their experience with 124 patients over 22 years. Operative mortality was 0.8%, and the stroke rate was 0%. Primary patency was 95% at both 5 and 10 years. Survival at 5 years was 83%.[85] Crawford and colleagues reported no deaths and a 1.3% stroke rate for 80 patients having subclavian artery reconstruction.[5] Perler and Williams reported no operative mortality in their 31 patients (three of whom underwent transposition). There were no early graft thromboses, although three grafts become oc-

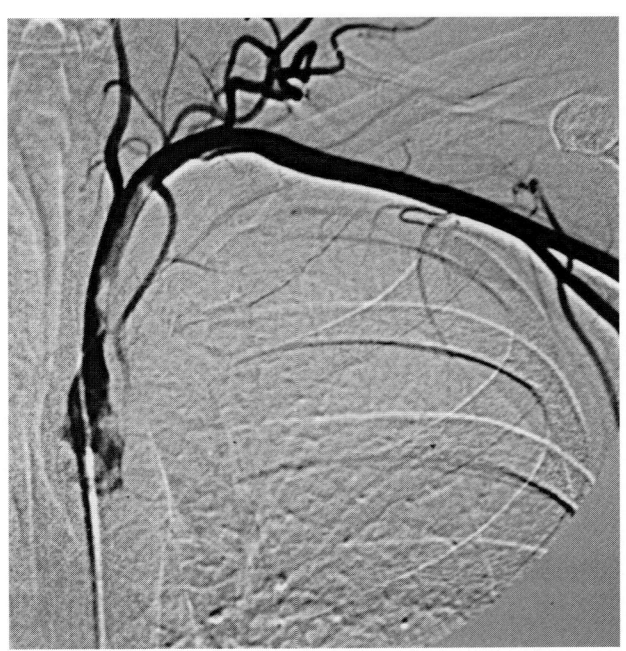

FIGURE 80–15. Arteriogram of an atheroembolization to the left upper extremity and rest pain in a 50-year-old woman. A proximal left subclavian artery lesion and a tailing thrombus are visible. Embolic lesions were demonstrated distally.

cluded during follow-up. Long-term patency (including that in the transposition patients) was 92% at 5 years and 83% at 8 years. There was one stroke in this series.[6] Kretschmer and coauthors reported no deaths and one stroke for 19 patients undergoing carotid-subclavian artery bypass grafting.[62] At our institution, there were no deaths in 40 patients but there were two strokes.[54]

A peculiar mechanism of stroke in these patients is thrombosis of the synthetic graft in the early postoperative period, with protrusion of the thrombus into the common carotid artery and distal embolization into the cerebral circulation. The Houston group reported such a case,[5] and we noted one at the Mayo Clinic.[54] For that reason, we believe that thrombosis of carotid-subclavian artery grafts should be aggressively managed with a full anticoagulation regimen while the patient is being prepared for reoperation or as treatment if reoperation is not planned.

Parrott first reported transposition of the subclavian artery unto the common carotid artery in 1964.[28] Interest in that operation grew because of the series from Germany by Sandmann and associates.[63] Subclavian artery transposition avoids the use of prosthetics in these relatively young patients and, of course, obviates the need for a second anastomosis. This procedure does require more proximal dissection of the subclavian artery, but that requirement would appear to be its only drawback. It is necessary to dissect the artery proximal to the vertebral and internal mammary arteries so that prograde flow into these two important branches may be maintained (Fig. 80–16). The contraindications to transposition are proximal origin of the vertebral artery, the extension of the atherosclerotic process well beyond the origin of the vertebral artery, and the presence of a left internal mammary artery graft to the coronary arteries.

Transposition appears to be superior even to bypass,

both in operative mortality and morbidity and in long-term patency. Schardey and colleagues, in their review of 108 patients undergoing subclavian artery transposition, reported two transient ischemic attacks but no strokes; actuarial patency at 70 months was 100%.[86]

Several retrospective reviews indicate less morbidity and improved patency.[62–65] van der Vliet and colleagues, in a comparison of transposition and bypass grafting, found no difference in morbidity and mortality. Patency of transposition was 100% at 2, 5, and 10 years in distinction to bypass grafting with patency rates of 75%, 62%, and 52% at those time periods, respectively.[87] Similar improved patency was also reported by Law and coworkers from the University of California, Los Angeles (UCLA).[81] Sandmann and others reported 1.4% mortality and 95% late patency for 72 patients undergoing transposition.[63] Sterpetti and associates compared carotid-subclavian artery bypass and subclavian artery transposition in 46 patients with a mean follow-up of 46.9 months.[64] Seven-year actuarial patency was 100% for transpositions and 85% for bypass. Dacron, PTFE, and vein were all used. Dacron grafts demonstrated better patency rates than either PTFE or vein grafts.

Kretschmer and colleagues in Vienna, analyzing 52 patients, found 33 transpositions to have 100% patency, whereas there were five occlusions in the 19 patients undergoing bypass.[62] Ziomek and colleagues, at UCLA, found transposition to have better actuarial patency (100%) than prosthetic grafts (94.1%) or vein grafts (58.3%), although only five transpositions were included in this group of 36 patients.[51] Weimann and coauthors noted no occlusions in their 38 transpositions.[65]

The risk of perioperative stroke may be lower with subclavian artery transposition. Perler and Williams reported a 3.6% stroke rate for 28 patients undergoing bypass.[61] Kretschmer and coworkers documented a 5.3% stroke rate

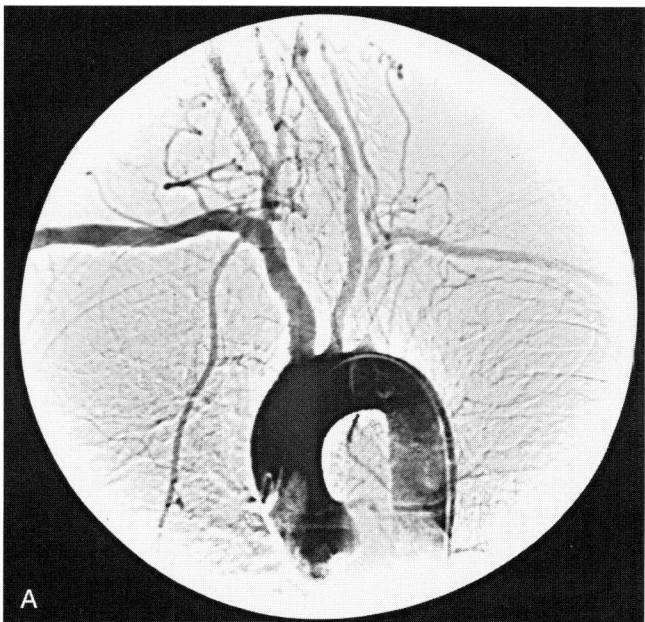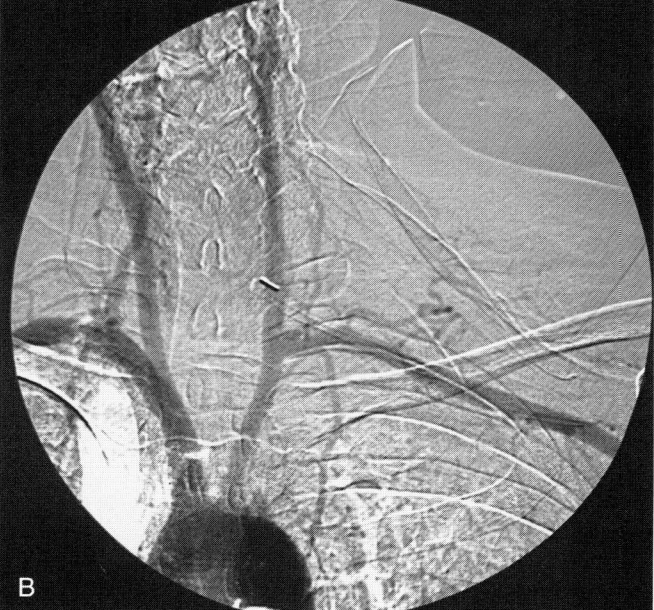

FIGURE 80–16. *A,* Arteriogram of incapacitating left upper extremity "claudication" in a 59-year-old woman. Left subclavian artery occlusion and reconstitution via retrograde flow through the vertebral artery are demonstrated. *B,* Postoperative digital subtraction angiogram demonstrating patent subclavian artery transposition with prograde flow through the vertebral artery and the internal mammary artery.

for their 19 bypass patients and 0% for their 32 transposition patients.[62] Sandmann and others reported no strokes in their 72 patients undergoing transposition.[63] Sterpetti and colleagues reported more neurologic complications with their bypass patients than with those undergoing transposition, but each of the patients having neurologic problems underwent concomitant carotid endarterectomy.[64] The mechanism of synthetic graft thrombosis and distal embolization may account for the difference in the stroke rates for the two operations.

These operations, especially subclavian artery transposition, involve a small supraclavicular incision, a very low morbidity and mortality, short hospital stay, and excellent long-term patency. They remain the gold standards for treatment of these lesions.

Operative Technique

Carotid-Subclavian Artery Bypass Graft

The patient is placed supine on the operating room table with a vertical roll between the scapulae to elevate the shoulders. The neck is extended, and the head is turned away from the side of the lesion.

A supraclavicular incision parallel to the clavicle and 2 to 3 cm above it with its medial extent overlying the clavicular head of the sternocleidomastoid muscle is made. The clavicular head is completely or partially incised. The scalene fat pad is mobilized by division and ligation and reflected superiorly. The thoracic duct may be formally ligated or carefully avoided. The phrenic nerve is identified anterior to the scalene muscle and protected. The anterior scalene muscle is transected, and the subclavian artery is located posteriorly, identified (see Fig. 80–12), and dissected free. Its branches may be divided and ligated to facilitate mobilization. The vertebral and internal mammary arteries should be preserved. Through the same incision, the common carotid artery is dissected free. The vagus nerve is identified and protected. A tunnel is made, usually posterior to the jugular vein. The position of the vagus and phrenic nerve relative to the tunnel may depend on the patient's anatomy and should be stated as such in the operative note.

A 7- or 8-mm prosthetic graft, either knitted Dacron or PTFE, is chosen (Dacron may provide better patency than PTFE).[64] Systemic heparinization therapy is administered. Control of the common carotid artery is obtained, and a lateral arteriotomy is made. The graft originates at a right angle, and care must be taken that the arteriotomy not be too long, lest the anastomosis be elongated and narrowed. The anastomosis is performed with running 4-0 or 5-0 polypropylene or Dacron sutures. After appropriate forward and backward bleeding is allowed, a clamp is placed across the proximal graft and flow restored to the carotid circulation. Shunting is rarely necessary. The graft is brought through the tunnel, and control of the subclavian artery is obtained. A vertical arteriotomy is made at the dome of the artery. The graft is fashioned to fit and sutured end-to-side

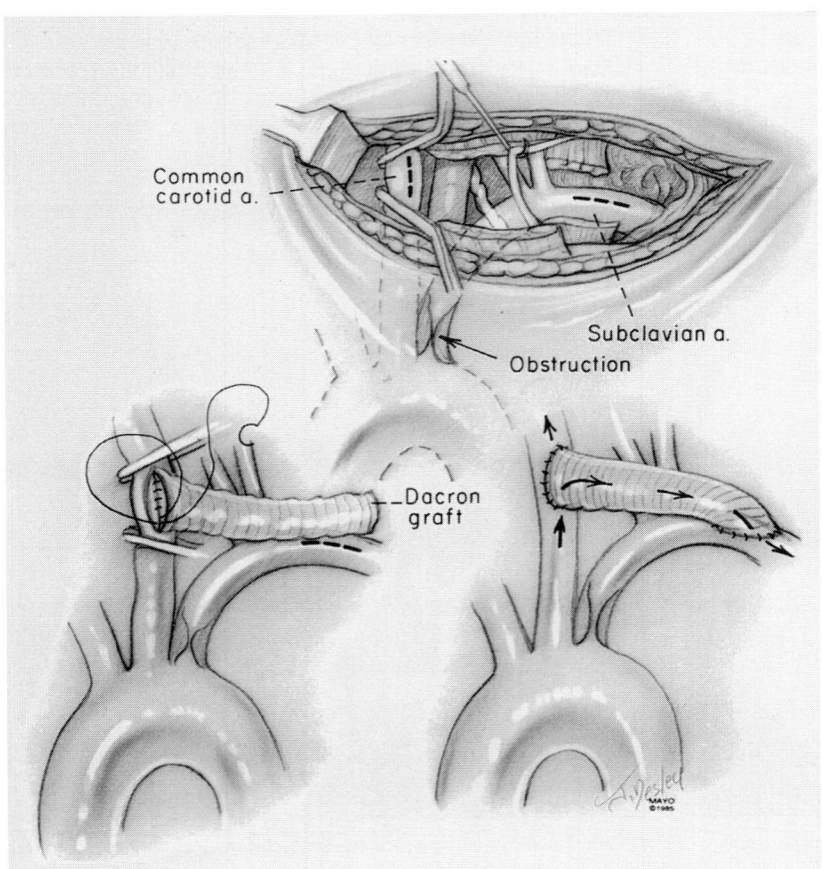

Common carotid a.

Subclavian a.
Obstruction

Dacron graft

FIGURE 80–17. Schematic drawings demonstrating left carotid-subclavian artery bypass graft. (By permission of Mayo Foundation.)

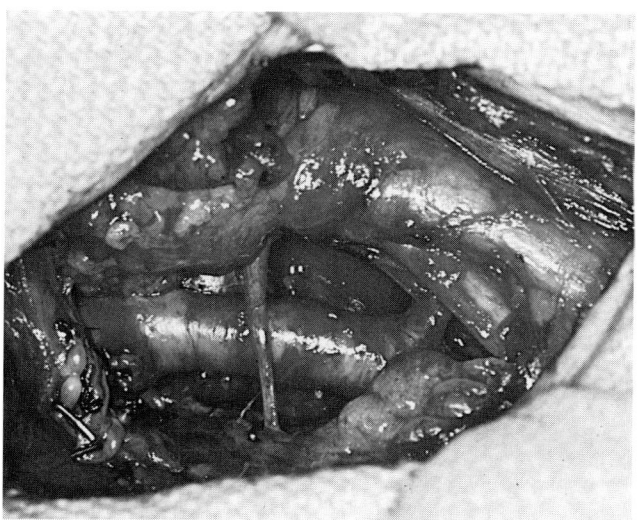

FIGURE 80–18. Intraoperative photograph demonstrating left subclavian artery transposition. The subclavian artery is posterior to the jugular vein and phrenic nerve and anterior to the vagus nerve in this patient. The vertebral artery and the internal mammary artery are obscured by the jugular vein.

with running 4-0 or 5-0 polypropylene suture. Braided suture should probably not be used on the subclavian artery.

Appropriate flushing is allowed and flow instituted to the subclavian artery circulation (Fig. 80–17). If necessary, a tie should be placed about the subclavian artery proximal to the vertebral artery. This is especially vital if the presenting problem is one of atheroembolization and if the lesion is not hemodynamically significant. The platysma is closed with polyglactin sutures, and the skin is closed with subcuticular polyglactin sutures.

Transposition of the Subclavian Artery

Positioning of the patient, incision, and exposure are essentially the same as in the operation just described. The subclavian artery must be dissected and mobilized more extensively into the mediastinum and proximal to the origins of the vertebral and internal mammary arteries. Branches other than these may be divided and ligated, as necessary, to facilitate exposure and mobilization. Systemic heparinization therapy is given. Control of the distal subclavian, vertebral, and internal mammary arteries and then of the proximal subclavian artery is obtained to avoid embolization from the lesion into the distal circulation. The subclavian artery is divided, and the proximal stump is oversewn with horizontal and over-and-over polypropylene sutures. The artery is then brought into approximation with the carotid artery, usually posterior to the jugular vein (Fig. 80–18; see Fig. 80–14B). The phrenic nerve lies anterior to the artery in this operation. Control of the carotid artery is obtained, and a lateral arteriotomy is made. Because the subclavian arises at a right angle to the carotid artery, the arteriotomy must not be too long to avoid narrowing of the anastomosis. After the anastomosis is performed with running 4-0 or 5-0 polypropylene sutures and after appropriate flushing, flow is restored or instituted to the subclavian, internal mammary, vertebral, and carotid arteries. The

remaining portion of the case is then conducted in a fashion identical to that of the carotid-subclavian artery bypass.

PERCUTANEOUS TRANSLUMINAL BALLOON ANGIOPLASTY

Percutaneous transluminal balloon angioplasty (PTA) of the great vessels, especially of the subclavian artery, is being performed with increasing frequency. Early reports emanated from Europe,[66–71] but centers in the United States are performing these procedures with increasing frequency.[72, 88–95] Patients with Takayasu's arteritis as well as patients with atherosclerotic lesions have undergone PTA.[72, 73] These reports chronicle high early success rates and moderate mid-range success. Reports continue to be uncontrolled, anecdotal, and without long-term follow-up.[72, 88–95] Direct comparisons to surgical controls have been lacking.

Kachel and colleagues of Erfurt, Germany, reported 105 patients undergoing PTA of the internal carotid, external carotid, common carotid, vertebral, subclavian, and innominate arteries.[68] Fifty-one occlusions or stenoses of the subclavian artery were dilated. In contrast, in this series there were three stenoses of the innominate artery and two of the common carotid artery. The authors reported "no major complications"; however, a postprocedure transient ischemic attack and a carotid thrombosis necessitating operation occurred, both of which were termed "minor." In their summation of the literature, these authors classified puncture site hematomas, thrombosis of the subclavian artery, thromboembolism to the fingers, and transient ischemic attacks as minor complications.

These same authors found that only one of seven occluded subclavian vessels was successfully opened.[68] Forty-four stenotic subclavian vessels were dilated "successfully," with two late restenoses. The authors recommended dilation of the arch aortic vessels when there was "smooth delineation of the stenoses with no indication of ulceration, heavy calcification or thrombotic deposits." Further, they felt that ulcerated stenoses of the carotid arteries were contraindications to PTA, as were occlusions of all brachiocephalic vessels. Other authors have not agreed with these contraindications. In their report on subclavian and axillary artery PTA, Romanowski and colleagues stated that they had no problems performing dilation in patients with evidence of microembolization.[71] Despite that statement, they report that one patient with multiple occlusive episodes distal to the angioplasty site eventually underwent limb amputation and another patient who lost a previously present radial pulse. They reported 84.2% early success and a 68% long-term success rate.

Düber and colleagues in Mainz, Germany, reported long-term patency of the subclavian artery following PTA to be less than 50%.[70] Farina and colleagues retrospectively compared patients undergoing PTA in Rome with patients having subclavian artery reconstructions in Omaha.[67] The groups were dissimilar in other respects, and 18 subclavian reconstructions were excluded from analysis. Actuarial patency was 87% for operation and 54% for subclavian artery PTA.

More recently, Martinez's group at the Arizona Heart

Institute reported 17 patients undergoing treatment for occlusion of the subclavian arteries. There was a 94% procedural success rate and an 81% cumulative patency rate at 6 months.[93]

Kumar and colleagues, reporting on 27 consecutive patients undergoing subclavian artery stenting, provided no long-term data and wrote that "the incidence of lesion recurrence remains for follow-up studies."[88]

The presence of concomitant aortic arch and carotid bifurcation lesions and associated coronary disease would be expected to influence patient outcome for brachiocephalic vessel PTA, just as they do for operative reconstructions.[3–5, 9, 54] The early and long-term results of PTA for each of the various arch lesions should be carefully assessed in terms of the patient's general health, specific risk factors, and concomitant associated aortic arch and bifurcation lesions. To allow meaningful comparison with reports from the surgical literature, the symptoms prompting PTA must be clearly set forth. Complications such as transient ischemic attacks, occluded arteries, and digital embolization must be considered major. Occlusive lesions should be differentiated from atheroembolic ones. "Claudication" should be differentiated from rest ischemia and tissue loss.

Careful patient selection, with categorization of risk factors and associated atherosclerotic lesions, precise identification of presenting symptoms, close follow-up, and careful analysis are necessary to determine the proper place of these procedures in the treatment of patients with atherosclerotic lesions of the brachiocephalic vessels. Angioplasty with or without stenting is probably an appropriate option for patients with localized disease of the great vessels, most often without concomitant lesions. One must exercise care, however, in considering PTA as the treatment of choice. Both carotid-subclavian artery bypass grafting and, most especially, subclavian artery transposition, with carefully analyzed and excellent results both in short-term and long-term follow-up (up to 10 years), and with low mortality and morbidity and short hospital stay, remain the standards that balloon angioplasty and stenting must meet or exceed.

It is probable that in the future, complex supra-aortic cases with multiple lesions will be addressed not only by surgery and angioplasty singly but also by combinations of the two. These techniques are certainly theoretically attractive in high-risk patients for whom sternotomy is less than an appealing alternative.

REFERENCES

1. Fields WS, Lemak NA: Joint study of extracranial arterial occlusion: VII. Subclavian steal—a review of 168 cases. JAMA 222:1139–1143, 1972.
2. Wylie EJ, Effeney DJ: Surgery of the aortic arch branches and vertebral arteries. Surg Clin North Am 59:669–680, 1979.
3. Carlson RE, Ehrenfeld WK, Stoney RJ, Wylie EJ: Innominate artery endarterectomy: A 16-year history. Arch Surg 112:1389–1393, 1977.
4. Vogt DP, Hertzer NR, O'Hara PJ, Beven EG: Brachiocephalic arterial reconstruction. Ann Surg 196:541–552, 1982.
5. Crawford ES, Stowe CL, Powers RW Jr: Occlusion of the innominate, common carotid, and subclavian arteries: Long-term results of surgical treatment. Surgery 94:781–791, 1983.
6. Zelenock GB, Cronenwett JL, Graham LM, et al: Brachiocephalic arterial occlusions and stenoses: Manifestations and management of complex lesions. Arch Surg 120:370–376, 1985.
7. Brewster DC, Moncure AC, Darling RC, et al: Innominate artery lesions: Problems encountered and lessons learned. J Vasc Surg 2:99–112, 1985.
8. Evans WE, Williams TE, Hayes JP: Aortobrachiocephalic reconstruction. Am J Surg 156:100–102, 1988.
9. Cherry KJ Jr, McCullough JL, Hallett JW Jr, Pairolero P: Technical principles of direct innominate artery revascularization: A comparison of endarterectomy and bypass grafts. J Vasc Surg 9:718–724, 1989.
10. Reul GJ, Jacobs MJHM, Gregoric ID, et al: Innominate artery occlusive disease: Surgical approach and long-term results. J Vasc Surg 14:405–412, 1991.
11. McCready RA, Hyde GL, Bivins BA, et al: Radiation-induced arterial injuries. Surgery 93:306–312, 1983.
12. Levinson SA, Close MB, Ehrenfeld WK, Stoney RJ: Carotid artery occlusive disease following external cervical irradiation. Arch Surg 107:395–397, 1973.
13. Savory WS: Case of a young woman in whom the main arteries of both upper extremities, and of the left side of the neck, were throughout completely obliterated. Med Chir Trans 39:205, 1856.
14. Broadbent WH: Absence of pulsation in both radial arteries, the vessels being full of blood. In Trans of the Clin Soc of London, London, Spottiswoode and Co, 8:165–169, 1875.
15. Takayasu M: Case of queer changes in central blood vessels of retina. Acta Soc Ophthalmol Jpn 12:554, 1908.
16. Harbitz F, Raeder JG: Ansigts- og orienatrofi foraarsaget av symmetrisk karotisaffektion. Norsk mag. Laegevidensk 87:529, 1926.
17. Martorell F, Fabre J: El sindrome de obliteration de los trancos supraaorticos. Med Clin 2:26, 1944.
18. Shimizu K, Sano K: Pulseless disease. J Neurol Clin Neurol 145:1095, 1951.
19. Caccamise WC, Whitman JF: Pulseless disease. Am Heart J 44:629, 1952.
20. Ross RS, McKusick VA: Progress in internal medicine: Aortic arch syndromes—diminished or absent pulses in arteries arising from arch of aorta. Arch Intern Med 92:701–740, 1953.
21. Kalmansohn RB, Kalmansohn RW: Thrombotic obliteration of branches of aortic arch. Circulation 15:237, 1957.
22. Contorni L: Il circolo collaterale vertebro-vertebrale nella obliterazione dell'arteria succlavia alla sua origine. Minerva Chir 15:268–271, 1960.
23. Bahnson HT, Spencer FC, Quattlebaum JK Jr: Surgical treatment of occlusive disease of the carotid artery. Ann Surg 149:711–720, 1959.
24. Davis JB, Grove WJ, Julian OC: Thrombic occlusion of the branches of the aortic arch, Martorell's syndrome: Report of a case treated surgically. Ann Surg 144:124–126, 1956.
25. Lyons C, Galbraith G: Surgical treatment of atherosclerotic occlusion of the internal carotid artery. Ann Surg 146:487–494, 1957.
26. DeBakey ME, Morris GC Jr, Jordan GL Jr, Cooley DA: Segmental thrombo-obliterative disease of branches of aortic arch. JAMA 166:998–1003, 1958.
27. DeBakey ME, Crawford ES, Morris GC, Cooley DA: Surgical considerations of occlusive disease of the innominate, carotid, subclavian, and vertebral arteries. Ann Surg 154:698–725, 1961.
28. Parrott JC: The subclavian steal syndrome. Arch Surg 88:661–665, 1964.
29. Javid H, Julian O, Dye WS, Hunter JA: Management of cerebral arterial insufficiency caused by reversal of flow. Arch Surg 90:634–643, 1965.
30. Diethrich EB, Garrett HE, Ameriso J, et al: Occlusive disease of the common carotid and subclavian arteries treated by carotid-subclavian bypass: Analysis of 125 cases. Am J Surg 114:800, 1967.
31. Crawford ES, De Bakey ME, Morris GC, Howell JF: Surgical treatment of occlusion of the innominate, common carotid, and subclavian arteries: A 10-year experience. Surgery 65:17–31, 1969.
32. Myers WO, Lawton BR, Sautter RD: Axillo-axillary bypass graft. JAMA 217:826, 1971.
33. Sproul G: Femoral-axillary bypass for cerebral vascular insufficiency. Arch Surg 103:746–747, 1971.
34. Crawford ES, De Bakey ME, Morris GC Jr, Cooley DA: Thrombo-obliterative disease of the great vessels arising from the aortic arch. J Thorac Cardiol Surg 43:38–53, 1962.
35. Criado FJ: Extrathoracic management of aortic arch syndrome. Br J Surg (Suppl) 69:45–51, 1982.
36. Posner MP, Riles TS, Ramirez AA, et al: Axilloaxillary bypass for

symptomatic stenosis of the subclavian artery. Am J Surg 145:644–646, 1983.

37. Schanzer H, Chung-Loy H, Kotok M, et al: Evaluation of axillo-axillary bypass for the treatment of subclavian or innominate artery occlusive disease. J Card Surg 28:258–261, 1987.

38. Rosenthal D, Ellison RG Jr, Clark MD, et al: Axilloaxillary bypass: Is it worthwhile? J Card Surg 29:191–194, 1988.

39. Weiner RI, Deterling RA Jr, Sentissi J, O'Donnell TF Jr: Subclavian artery insufficiency: Treatment with axilloaxillary bypass. Arch Surg 122:876–880, 1987.

40. Mingoli A, Feldhaus RJ, Farina C, et al: Comparative results of carotid-subclavian bypass and axillo-axillary bypass in patients with symptomatic subclavian disease. Eur J Vasc Surg 6:26–30, 1992.

41. Kieffer E, Petitjean C, Bahnini A: In Bergan JJ, Yao JST (eds): Reoperative Arterial Surgery: Surgery of Failed Brachiocephalic Reconstructions. Orlando, Fla, Grune & Stratton, 1986, pp 581–607.

42. Kieffer E: Personal communication, 1988.

43. Berguer R: Personal communication, 1988.

44. Selle JG, Cook JW, Elliott CM, et al: Simultaneous revascularization for complex brachiocephalic and coronary artery disease. Surgery 90:91–101, 1981.

45. Toole JF: Syndromes of the carotid artery and its branches. In Toole JF (ed): Cerebrovascular Disorders, 3rd ed. New York, Raven Press, 1984, pp 60–61.

46. Riles TS, Imparato AM, Posner MP, Eikelboom BC: Common carotid occlusion: Assessment of the distal vessels. Ann Surg 199:363–366, 1984.

47. Podore PC, Rob CG, DeWeese JA, Green RM: Chronic common carotid occlusion. Stroke 12:98–100, 1981.

48. Keller HM, Valavanis A, Imhof HG, Turina M: Patency of external and internal carotid artery in the presence of an occluded common carotid artery: Noninvasive evaluation with combined cerebrovascular Doppler examination and sequential computer tomography. Stroke 15:149–157, 1984.

49. Ehrenfeld WK, Chapman RD, Wylie EJ: Management of occlusive lesions of the branches of the aortic arch. Am J Surg 118:236–243, 1969.

50. Fry WR, Martin JD, Clagett P, Fry WJ: Extrathoracic carotid reconstruction: The subclavian-carotid artery bypass. J Vasc Surg 15:83–89, 1992.

51. Ziomek S, Quiñones-Baldrich WJ, Busuttil RW, et al: The superiority of synthetic arterial grafts over autologous veins in carotid-subclavian bypass. J Vasc Surg 3:140–145, 1986.

52. Fry WR, Martin JD, Clagett P, Fry WJ: Extrathoracic carotid reconstruction: The subclavian-carotid artery bypass. Discussion (Rutherford). J Vasc Surg 15:83–89, 1992.

53. Fisher CM: A new vascular syndrome—"the subclavian steal." N Engl J Med 265:912–913, 1961.

54. Hallett JW, Knight CD Jr, Hollier LH, Cherry KJ Jr, Pairolero PC: Early and late results of carotid-subclavian grafts: A 26-year review (unpublished).

55. Walker PM, Paley D, Harris KA, et al: What determines the symptoms associated with subclavian artery occlusive disease? J Vasc Surg 2:154–157, 1985.

56. Whitehouse WM, Zelenock GB, Wakefield TW, et al: Arterial bypass grafts for upper extremity ischemia. In Symposium: Surgical treatment of upper extremity ischemia. 3:569–573, 1986.

57. McCarthy WJ, Flinn WR, Yao JST, et al: Result of bypass grafting for upper limb ischemia. J Vasc Surg 3:741–746, 1986.

58. Kadwa AM, Robbs JV: Gangrenous fingers: The tip of the iceberg. J R Coll Surg Edinb 35:71–74, 1990.

59. Rapp JH, Reilly LM, Goldstone J, et al: Ischemia of the upper extremity: Significance of proximal arterial disease. Am J Surg 152:122–126, 1986.

60. Wylie EJ: Personal communication, 1980.

61. Perler BA, Williams GM: Carotid-subclavian bypass: A decade of experience. J Vasc Surg 12:716–723, 1990.

62. Kretschmer G, Teleky B, Marosi L, et al: Obliterations of the proximal subclavian artery: To bypass or to anatomose? J Cardiol Surg 32:334–339, 1991.

63. Sandmann W, Kniemeyer HW, Jaeschock R, et al: The role of subclavian-carotid transposition in surgery for supra-aortic occlusive disease. J Vasc Surg 5:53–58, 1987.

64. Sterpetti AV, Schultz RD, Farina C, Feldhaus RJ: Subclavian artery revascularization: A comparison between carotid-subclavian artery bypass and subclavian-carotid transposition. Surgery 106:624–632, 1989.

65. Weimann S, Willeit H, Flora G: Direct subclavian-carotid anastomosis for the subclavian steal syndrome. Eur J Vasc Surg 1:305–310, 1987.

66. Jaschke W, Menges HW, Ockert D, et al: PTA of the subclavian and innominate artery: Short- and long-term results. Ann Radiol (Paris) 32:29–33, 1989.

67. Farina C, Mingoli A, Schultz RD, et al: Percutaneous transluminal angioplasty versus surgery for subclavian artery occlusive disease. Am J Surg 158:511–514, 1989.

68. Kachel R, Basche St, Heerklotz I, et al: Percutaneous transluminal angioplasty (PTA) of supra-aortic arteries especially the internal carotid artery. AJNR Am J Neuroradiol 33:191–194, 1991.

69. Nicholson AA, Kennan NM, Sheridan WG, Ruttley MS: Percutaneous transluminal angioplasty of the subclavian artery. Ann R Coll Surg Engl 73:46–52, 1991.

70. Düber C, Klose JK, Kopp H, Schmiedt W: Percutaneous transluminal angioplasty for occlusion of the subclavian artery: Short- and long-term results. Cardiovasc Intervent Radiol 15:205–210, 1992.

71. Romanowski CAJ, Fairlie NC, Procter AE, Cumberland DC: Percutaneous transluminal angioplasty of the subclavian and axillary arteries: Initial results and long term follow-up. Clin Radiol 46:104–107, 1992.

72. Staller BJ, Maleki M: Percutaneous transluminal angioplasty for innominate artery stenosis and total occlusion of subclavian artery in Takayasu's type artiritis. Cathet Cardiovasc Diagn 16:91–94, 1989.

73. Kumar S, Mandalam KR, Rao VRK, et al: Percutaneous transluminal angioplasty in nonspecific aortoarteritis (Takayasu's disease): Experience of 16 cases. Cardiovasc Intervent Radiol 12:321–325, 1990.

74. Kieffer E, Sabatier J, Koskas, et al: Atherosclerotic innominate artery occlusive disease: Early and long-term results of surgical reconstruction. J Vasc Surg 2:326–37, 1995.

75. Berguer R, Morasch MD, Kline RA: Transthoracic repair of innominate and common carotid artery disease: Immediate and long-term outcome for 100 consecutive surgical reconstructions. J Vasc Surg 27:34–32, 1998.

76. Rhodes J, Cherry KJ Jr, Clark RC, et al: Arch reconstruction of the great vessels: Risk factors of early and late complications. Submitted.

77. Berguer R, Gonzalez JA: Revascularization by the retropharyngeal route for extensive disease of the extracranial arteries. J Vasc Surg 19:217–225, 1994.

78. Carpenter JP, Holand GA, Golden MA, et al: Magnetic resonance angiography of the aortic arch. J Vasc Surg 25:145–151, 1997.

79. Owens LV, Tinsley EA Jr, Criado E: Extrathoracic reconstruction of arterial occlusive disease involving the supra-aortic trunks. J Vasc Surg 22:217–222, 1995.

80. Takach TJ, Reul GJ Jr, Cooley DA, et al: Concomitant occlusive disease of the coronary arteries and great vessels. Ann Thorac Surg 65:79–84, 1998.

81. Law MM, Colburn MD, Moore WS, et al: Carotid-subclavian bypass for brachiocephalic occlusive disease: Choice of conduit and long-term follow-up. Stroke 26:1565–1571, 1995.

82. Synn AY, Chalmers RTA, Sharp WJ, et al: Is there a conduit of preference for a bypass between the carotid and subclavian arteries? Am J Surg 166:157–162, 1993.

83. Salam TA, Smith RB, Lumsden AB: Extrathoracic bypass procedures for proximal common carotid artery lesions. Am J Surg 166:163–166, 1993.

84. Webster MW, Downs L, Yonas H, et al: The effect of arm exercise on regional cerebral blood flow in the subclavian steal syndrome. Am J Surg 168:91–93, 1994.

85. Vitti MJ, Thompson BW, Read RC, et al: Carotid-subclavian bypass: A twenty-two-year experience. J Vasc Surg 20:411–418, 1994.

86. Schardey HM, Meyer G, Rau HG, et al: Subclavian-carotid transposition: An analysis of a clinical series and a review of the literature. Eur J Vasc Endovasc Surg 12:431–436, 1996.

87. van der Vliet JA, Palamba HW, Scharn DM, et al: Arterial reconstruction for subclavian obstructive disease: A comparison of extrathoracic procedures. Eur J Vasc Endovasc Surg 9:454–458, 1995.

88. Kumar K, Dorros G, Bates MC, et al: Primary stent deployment in occlusive subclavian artery disease. Cathet Cardiovasc Diagn 34:281–285, 1995.

89. Harris NJ, Cameron I, Beard JD, et al: Percutaneous stenting of proximal subclavian artery occlusion. Eur J Vasc Endovasc Surg 9:479–480, 1995.

90. Robbin ML, Lockhart ME, Weber TM, et al: Carotid artery stents: Early and intermediate follow-up with Doppler US. Radiology 205:749–756, 1997.

91. Watura R, Halpin SFS, Ruttley MS: Percutaneous transluminal angioplasty of an innominate artery occlusion. Cardiovasc Intervent Radiol 18:396–398, 1995.

92. Vozzi CR, Rodriguez AO, Paolantonio D, et al: Extracranial carotid angioplasty and stenting. Tex Heart Inst J 24:167–172, 1997.

93. Martinez R, Rodriguez-Lopez J, Torruella L, et al: Stenting for occlusion of the subclavian arteries. Tex Heart Inst J 24:23–237, 1997.

94. Lyon RD, Shonnard KM, McCarter DL, et al: Supra-aortic arterial stenoses: Management with Palmaz balloon-expandable intraluminal stents. J Vasc Interv Radiol 7:825–835, 1996.

95. Queral LA, Criado FJ: Endovascular treatment of aortic arch occlusive disease. Semin Vasc Surg 9:156–163, 1996.

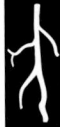

CHAPTER 81
Upper Extremity Revascularization

Walter M. Whitehouse, Jr., M.D.,
and Errol E. Erlandson, M.D.

Occlusive arterial disease resulting in symptomatic upper extremity ischemia occurs much less frequently than ischemia affecting the lower extremities. Arterial reconstructions involving the upper extremity represent only 4% of peripheral arterial procedures performed in contemporary practice. Diseases causing upper extremity ischemia are similar to those affecting the lower limbs; however, significant differences exist in the incidence, symptomatology, complications, and severity of associated disability. Some differences relate to the anatomic and functional variations between the upper and the lower extremities. The collateral circulation of the upper extremity is superior to that of the lower extremity. The upper extremity muscle mass is smaller and is ordinarily subjected to less work. Additionally, the functional importance of the hand in activities of daily living and employment is of major concern to affected patients.

Direct surgical treatment of upper extremity arterial insufficiency was first reported in 1956.[23] Improvement in arteriography and refinement of vascular surgical techniques since then have contributed to the evolution of surgical treatment of the ischemic upper extremity. In this chapter, discussion is limited to diseases affecting the axillary, brachial, radial, and ulnar arteries that may be treated successfully by direct revascularization. Brachiocephalic occlusive disease is described in Chapter 80; diseases affecting the more distal vasculature are discussed in Chapter 82.

ANATOMY

The major blood supply for the upper extremity comes from the subclavian artery.[53, 83] As this vessel passes over the first rib, it becomes the axillary artery, which extends to the lower border of the teres major muscle. Throughout its 15-cm course, the axillary artery gives off six branches of major significance, including the highest thoracic, thoracoacromial, lateral thoracic, subscapular, and anterior and posterior circumflex humeral arteries. All but the first may serve as major collateral vessels around the shoulder girdle. The brachial artery extends from the lower border of the teres major muscle to its bifurcation, which is adjacent to the head of the radius. It is single in approximately 80% of cases. An additional superficial brachial artery occurs in the remaining 20% of cases. It begins at the upper brachial level and descends through the arm superficial to the median nerve. The superficial brachial artery constitutes a high radial or ulnar artery in 10% to 15% and 2% to 3% of cases, respectively. The deep brachial artery, which is the largest branch of the brachial artery, usually originates just below the level of the teres major muscle. Other important branches include the superior and inferior ulnar collateral arteries.

The radial and ulnar arteries are the terminal branches of the brachial artery, with the interosseous artery originating from the ulnar artery. The ulnar recurrent, radial recurrent, and interosseous recurrent arteries anastomose with the collateral arteries of the brachial artery to form a rich collateral bed around the elbow. The superficial palmar arch, the major source of blood flow to the digits, is primarily derived from the ulnar artery. The radial artery supplies the smaller deep palmar arch and dorsal arches of the hand. Superficial and deep palmar arch anatomy is quite variable and has been well described on the basis of both anatomic dissection and analysis of hand arteriograms.[19, 39] An incomplete palmar arch without significant retrograde collateral circulation, such that the hand is perfused primarily by the radial artery, has been reported in 1.6% of patients.[4] Other studies have demonstrated a higher incidence of radial artery dominance.[19, 39, 49]

The abundance of collateral supply at both the shoulder

and the elbow levels is responsible for the low incidence of symptomatic ischemia associated with segmental arterial occlusion at these levels. Except for occlusion of a digital vessel, chronic single-artery occlusion rarely results in severe distal ischemia with tissue loss. Gangrene results from ligation of the axillary artery in approximately 10% to 15% of cases and after brachial artery ligation distal to the deep brachial origin in 3% to 4% of cases.[45]

CLINICAL MANIFESTATIONS

Patients with acute arterial insufficiency of the upper extremity present with the same dramatic signs and symptoms seen with acute arterial insufficiency of the lower extremity, including pulselessness, pallor, pain, paresthesia, and paralysis. Chronic arterial insufficiency of the upper extremity is more subtle. Disabling exertional forearm and hand discomfort is a common manifestation of chronic ischemia and is reported to be the most common indication for surgical treatment in one series.[30] Such discomfort may occur with minimal exercise, such as shaving or combing hair, whereas discomfort associated with less severe ischemia occurs only with prolonged repetitive activity. The degree of disability is directly related to the severity of ischemia and whether the dominant hand is involved. Rest pain and gangrene may be less common manifestations, although one review reported these to be the most frequent indications for surgical treatment.[50] Tissue loss implies the presence of severe distal arterial obstruction, usually involving the palmar arch or digital vessels, but it may also occur with multisegment disease.

ETIOLOGY, DIAGNOSIS, AND TREATMENT

Acute and chronic upper extremity ischemia amenable to direct revascularization results from a multitude of causes. As discussed in the following text, these include:

1. Iatrogenic injury (cannulation of the axillary, brachial, and radial arteries for a cardiac or peripheral arteriographic study or blood pressure monitoring).
2. Emboli.
3. Non-iatrogenic trauma.

Atherosclerosis, a major cause of occlusive disease of the innominate and subclavian arteries, rarely involves the more distal vasculature to such a degree that clinically significant ischemia results. Other disease entities, such as thromboangiitis obliterans and collagen vascular diseases, are important causes of hand ischemia but are seldom successfully treated by direct revascularization. Severe forearm and hand occlusive disease seen in patients with end-stage renal failure (ESRF) has been successfully treated with arterial bypass distal to the wrist.[22, 61] Giant cell arteritis may involve the axillobrachial arterial segment but ordinarily responds to medical therapy.[69] Radiation arteritis may rarely require bypass.[13, 48]

Iatrogenic Injury

Cardiac Catheterization via the Brachial Artery

Brachial arteriotomy for cardiac catheterization is the most common iatrogenic cause of upper extremity ischemia (Fig. 81–1).[1, 8, 11, 14, 24, 41, 46, 47, 57, 58, 62, 64, 66, 68, 72, 79] The incidence of thrombotic complications from this procedure varies, ranging from 0.3%[70] to 28%.[11] The incidence reported in most large contemporary experiences ranges from 0.9% to 4%.[46, 47, 52, 62] This is significantly higher than the 0.4% incidence of thrombotic complications reported with the transfemoral Judkins technique.[24] The transfemoral approach is currently the preferred method of arterial access for cardiac catheterization and coronary angioplasty in most institutions. As a result, the frequency of this form of brachial artery injury has declined. Because of the extensive collateral circulation surrounding the site of brachial arteriotomy, patients may remain asymptomatic despite brachial artery occlusion. Thus, the true incidence of this complication may exceed that reported.

Brachial artery injuries may account for both acute and chronic symptoms. Thrombosis of a long segment of the artery may jeopardize collateral flow and result in acute symptomatology requiring immediate surgical intervention. On the other hand, occlusion of a short segment may not produce significant acute ischemia, and symptoms of

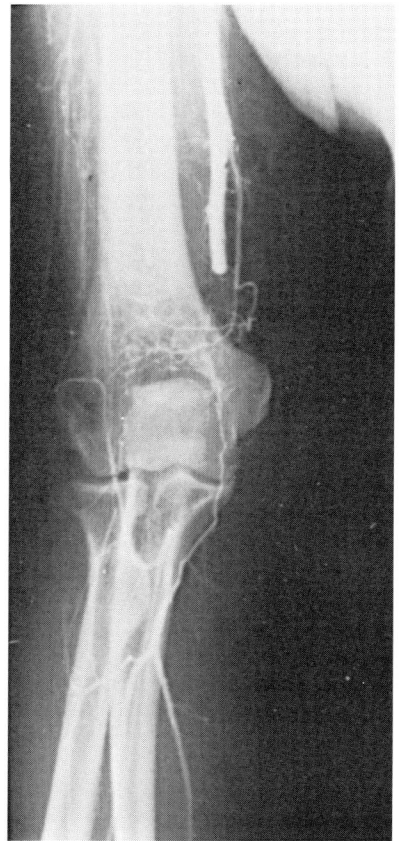

FIGURE 81–1. Acute brachial artery thrombosis following cardiac catheterization. (From Whitehouse WM Jr: Direct revascularization for forearm and hand ischemia. In Bergan JJ, Yao JST [eds]: Evaluation and Treatment of Upper and Lower Extremity Circulatory Disorders. Orlando, Fla, Grune & Stratton, 1984, pp 231–248.)

chronic ischemia may become apparent only after discharge, when upper extremity exercise becomes more vigorous. Because the right brachial artery is ordinarily used for these studies, most patients with significant ischemia are rendered symptomatic in their dominant hand.

Certain factors that predispose to brachial artery thrombosis after cardiac catheterization have been recognized. The method of arteriotomy closure is of importance; pursestring or longitudinal closure may be associated with a higher incidence of complications than a more precise transverse closure. Other factors include

- Multiple catheter changes
- Duration of catheterization
- Presence of brachial artery atherosclerosis
- Female gender
- Experience of the cardiologist
- Lack of anticoagulation during the procedure

The diagnosis of brachial artery thrombosis is ordinarily apparent with reduction in or complete absence of the radial pulse on physical examination. This finding may be accompanied by symptoms of hand ischemia. Assessment of the axillary and proximal brachial artery pulses and measurement of the perfusion pressure of the arm and forearm can aid in the localization of the obstructing lesion.[6] Most lesions are limited to the arteriotomy site; however, proximal axillary or subclavian dissections may result from difficult catheterizations (Fig. 81–2). Although this rarely occurs, failure to recognize this leison promptly may result in recurrent thrombosis after a local brachial procedure has been performed. If a proximal dissection is suspected because of a reduction in arm perfusion pressure or abnormal proximal Doppler waveforms, preoperative arteriography is essential. Radiographic examination should include an arch aortogram followed by selective subclavian injection. The importance of a complete arteriographic study cannot be overemphasized.[26] Major surgical misadventures leading to amputation may be avoided by early diagnosis and treatment of such proximal lesions.

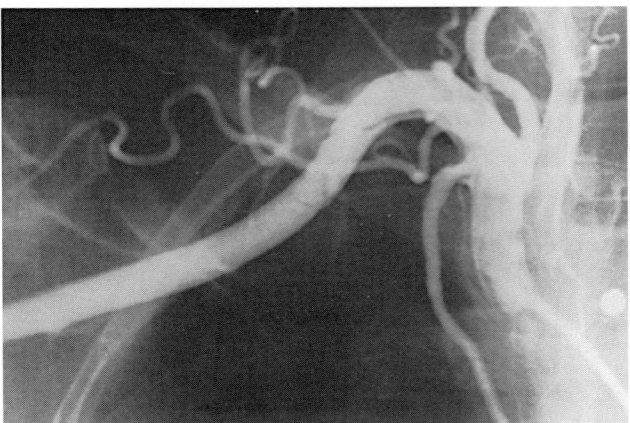

FIGURE 81–2. Intimal dissection of the subclavian artery following cardiac catheterization. This lesion would have gone undetected with a more distal selective injection of contrast. (From Whitehouse WM Jr: Direct revascularization for forearm and hand ischemia. *In* Bergan JJ, Yao JST [eds]: Evaluation and Treatment of Upper and Lower Extremity Circulatory Disorders. Orlando, Fla, Grune & Stratton, 1984, pp 231–248.)

Management of Acute Ischemia

Operative repair is indicated in the presence of acute symptoms of forearm and hand ischemia. Management of the asymptomatic patient has been controversial in the past. Some authors have suggested conservative treatment in patients with forearm pressures exceeding 60 mmHg. However, as many as 45% of patients who are initially asymptomatic despite brachial artery occlusion will have late symptoms,[57] and half of these patients will require late arterial reconstruction. Early surgical therapy usually called for only thrombectomy or local resection, whereas procedures performed later require more complex bypass procedures. Further, the brachial and radial arteries may be needed for repeated cardiac catheterization or blood pressure monitoring at a later date. Thus, an aggressive approach or re-exploration for all occlusions in the absence of significant contraindications to operation is recommended.

Brachial artery exploration may be performed with the patient under local anesthesia either in the cardiac catheterization laboratory or in the operating room. The latter location is usually preferable because of better instrumentation, lighting, and assistance. Preoperative heparinization (150 U/kg) is advisable to limit thrombus propagation. The previously made transverse antecubital incision is extended medially and laterally because the initial exposure is almost always inadequate for proper repair. If further exposure is required, the incision may be extended proximally along the bicipital groove and distally at the lateral extent of the transverse incision. Sufficient mobilization of the brachial artery is gained proximal and distal to the arteriotomy. Care is taken to protect the median nerve during this dissection. After the suture line is opened, the surgeon performs proximal and distal thrombectomy using a 3 French (Fr.) balloon catheter. If adequate inflow cannot be established, a proximal intimal flap must be suspected. In this case, transfemoral aortography is required to define the proximal pathology.

After thrombectomy, the vessel is débrided and then closed transversely with 6-0 monofilament suture. Interrupted suture technique facilitates a precise closure. Alternatively, if the vessel is significantly damaged, segmental resection with primary spatulated end-to-end anastomosis may be required. The technique should include anterior spatulation of the distal artery to ensure direct visualization of the intima at the time of suture placement. If a long segment is damaged, reversed saphenous vein interposition grafting may be necessary.

If preoperative arteriography had demonstrated a proximal intimal dissection, a more complex reconstruction is necessary, using a reversed saphenous vein or prosthetic conduit to bypass the diseased segment. Depending on the location of the arterial injury, a carotid-axillary, carotid-brachial, or axillary-brachial bypass may be necessary. Although prosthetic conduits function well for short, proximal bypasses, saphenous vein is preferable for longer, more distal reconstructions. Such procedures are best performed before brachial artery repair.

Surgical results appear to justify an aggressive approach to postcatheterization brachial artery thrombosis. Thrombectomy alone may be feasible in 34% to 90% of cases, with resection and reanastomosis or vein interposition grafting required in the other 10% to 66%.[41, 46, 47, 52] Early occlusion occurs in approximately 5% of cases; however, even if re-exploration is required, as many as 99% of patients have been reported to leave the hospital with patent reconstructions.[46, 47, 52] The use of short-term postoperative heparinization has been reported to reduce the incidence of early occlusion.[47]

Management of Chronic Ischemia

Symptomatic chronic arterial insufficiency may develop if acute occlusions following cardiac catheterization are not repaired. As many as 45% of such patients may become symptomatic, and 50% of these patients may experience symptoms severe enough to require vascular reconstruction.[57] Generally, symptoms are limited to exercise intolerance, although rest pain may occur. When exercise intolerance significantly limits the patient's lifestyle, surgical intervention should be considered. Rest pain and tissue loss are absolute indications for surgical treatment.

Evaluation of the chronically ischemic upper extremity must include noninvasive laboratory assessment and arteriography if surgical treatment is planned.[6] Exercise studies may occasionally assist the clinician in determining the severity of ischemia. In addition to delimiting the obstructed segment, arteriography demonstrates distal runoff, which is important in planning an optimal procedure. Complete arteriographic studies should include arch aortography in addition to selective views of the entire extremity, including the hand.[26]

Surgical treatment of chronic lesions requires bypassing of the occluded arterial segment. Autogenous saphenous vein is the conduit of choice.[29, 30, 50, 84] Upper extremity veins may be used as alternatives in the absence of an adequate saphenous vein. The use of in situ cephalic vein grafting has been reported.[18, 31] No large clinical series have reported the late results of the use of prosthetic conduits in this position. Prosthetic material should be used only in rare instances when an adequate autogenous vein is not available. The proximal end-to-side anastomosis is created just proximal to the site of occlusion, and the distal end-to-side anastomosis is created distal to the occlusion, usually just proximal to the bifurcation of the brachial artery. This may include an angioplasty of the bifurcation with the hood of the graft. Direct anastomosis to either the radial or the ulnar artery will occasionally be required (Fig. 81–3). Rarely, the interosseous artery may be the only forearm vessel that is patent; anastomosis to this vessel or its anterior or posterior branch is required.

The importance of the interosseous artery in this setting has been emphasized.[50] Completion arteriography is recommended for distal reconstructions. These upper extremity arterial bypass procedures are associated with 2- to 5-year patency rates generally ranging from 60% to 90%.[12, 30, 37, 50, 59, 74, 80, 82] Early failure is usually associated with limited outflow. Late failures are more common when the distal anastomosis is below the brachial bifurcation.[50, 59]

Transaxillary Arteriography

Percutaneous transaxillary arteriographic studies account for additional cases of upper extremity ischemia. Axillary artery thrombosis is reported to occur in 0.8% of patients studied.[35] This is five times the rate associated with trans-

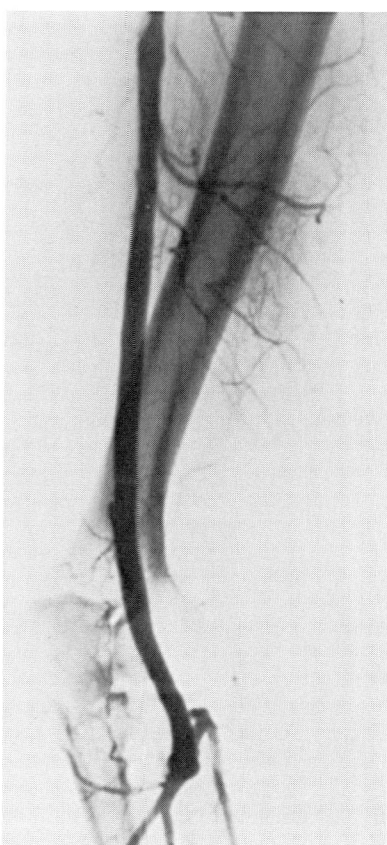

FIGURE 81–3. Reversed saphenous vein brachial-ulnar bypass in a patient with chronic hand ischemia secondary to cardiac catheterization (postoperative arteriogram).

femoral studies but less than that associated with brachial cutdown techniques used for cardiac catheterization. Such axillary artery occlusions are likely to render the patient acutely symptomatic; as a result, the diagnosis is usually obvious. Noninvasive arterial studies are used for confirmation, and arteriography is seldom required.

Surgical treatment is generally indicated when the diagnosis is made. Immediate heparinization is recommended. A longitudinal incision is made over the upper bicipital groove and extended proximally. Arterial control is obtained proximal and distal to the injury. A transverse arteriotomy is made at the puncture site, and proximal and distal thrombectomy is performed with a 3 Fr. balloon catheter. This usually suffices, and the arteriotomy is closed transversely. Occasionally, resection with primary anastomosis or vein interposition grafting is necessary.

Morbidity is more often the consequence of neurologic complications from an axillary sheath hematoma than the result of the vascular injury itself. Many radiologists now prefer to perform percutaneous cannulation of the mid-brachial artery distal to the deep brachial origin rather than cannulation of the axillary artery in order to lessen the potential ischemic and neurologic sequelae of such injuries.

Radial Artery Cannulation

Cannulation of the radial artery is a rare iatrogenic cause of upper extremity ischemia.[4, 7, 27, 43] This technique is frequently used for continuous blood pressure monitoring and arterial blood sampling, both intraoperatively and in critical care units. Recently, percutaneous radial artery cannulation techniques for coronary arteriography, angioplasty, and stent placement have been developed. These techniques are potentially more traumatic than placement of arterial lines for blood pressure monitoring.[78] Demonstration of a patent palmar arch by the Allen test[2] is a prerequisite for radial artery cannulation. More precise assessment may be performed by a Doppler probe to map out the palmar arch and digital arteries, with and without ulnar and radial artery compression.[36, 40, 60] Direct digital pressure measurement with and without radial artery compression may represent a more objective screening test, however.[81]

Radial artery thrombosis occurs in as many as 40% of cases of radial artery cannulation.[7] Factors recognized to predispose to thrombosis include a prolonged period of cannulation, spasm secondary to repeated arterial puncture, diminished systemic perfusion pressure, large catheter size, underlying arterial disease, and sustained local pressure to arrest hemorrhage from the catheter site at the time of removal.[4] Authors have estimated the incidence of severe ischemic complications as a result of radial artery cannulation to be only 0.3% to 0.5% in patients at risk.[60] This complication rate may be significantly higher if underlying palmar arch disease is unrecognized. After the appearance of severe ischemia, tissue loss may occur in as many as 80% of patients.

Severe hand ischemia secondary to radial artery cannulation is significantly more difficult to treat by revascularization compared with the more proximal axillary or brachial artery lesions. Propagation of thrombus into the palmar arch may complicate attempted revascularization. Nonetheless, in view of the high incidence of tissue loss, an aggressive surgical approach is justified when significant ischemic changes are apparent. Arteriography may be helpful in specific instances but is generally not beneficial.

Exposure of the vessel is obtained through a longitudinal incision at the level of cannulation. Proximal and distal thrombectomy is performed carefully with 2 Fr. and 3 Fr. balloon thrombectomy catheters. The use of 2 Fr. catheters may enable the surgeon to maximize distal thrombectomy within the palmar arch. If significant arterial damage is noted at the site of cannulation, segmental resection and primary spatulated end-to-end anastomosis may be required. Optical magnification and the use of interrupted 7-0 monofilament sutures facilitate the creation of a precise anastomosis. Results of this rare procedure are not well documented in the literature. A successful outcome is unlikely if thrombosis of arch and digital arteries is present.

The administration of intra-arterial thrombolytic agents for the treatment of palmar arch and digital thrombus has been used in the past.[42] The combination of catheter thrombectomy and intraoperative intra-arterial lytic therapy has been reported, particularly in the lower extremity.[20, 63, 65, 67] Although both streptokinase and urokinase have been used for this purpose, urokinase appears to be the agent of choice. Slow intra-arterial bolus infusion with up to 150,000 units of urokinase has been successful in lysing residual thrombus inaccessible to balloon catheters. The application of this technique in the upper extremity has been extremely limited. In combination with the use of vasodilators, intra-arterial thrombolytic therapy has been used in the treatment of acute thrombosis of the distal arteries following inadvertent arterial injections by drug abusers.

Placement of Chemotherapeutic Infusion Catheters

Percutaneous transbrachial or axillary placement of long-term chemotherapy infusion catheters is an additional, although infrequent, cause of upper extremity ischemia. The exact incidence of such complications is not well defined, but as many as 24% of patients undergoing such treatment may be affected.[17] The use of implantable infusion pumps and a trend away from hepatic chemotherapy infusion altogether should reduce the number of these complications. Nonetheless, when upper extremity ischemia is recognized, the catheter should be removed and the patient given heparin. Unless significant resolution of ischemia is noted, local exploration with thrombectomy, with or without segmental resection and primary reanastomosis, is appropriate.

Results are variable and poorly documented. Duration of catheterization is an important factor influencing outcome.

Emboli

Embolic arterial occlusion is an additional cause of upper extremity ischemia.[3, 5, 27, 38, 44, 73] Emboli involving the upper extremity arterial tree are uncommon and represent 15% to 32% of all peripheral emboli.[32] A cardiac origin is reported in approximately 90% of cases. Rheumatic heart disease, less common today than in the past, has been replaced by arteriosclerotic heart disease and myocardial infarction as the most common underlying cardiac disease responsible for the embolic event. Atrial fibrillation is present in approximately 80% of these patients.

The brachial artery is the most frequently involved upper extremity vessel; it is the site of the embolus in approximately 60% of patients. The three characteristic locations of lodgment include (1) the upper third of the arm just proximal to the origin of the deep brachial artery, (2) the mid-arm at the origin of the superior ulnar collateral artery, and (3) the brachial bifurcation. The axillary (23%) and subclavian (12%) arteries are less frequently involved.[32] The radial and ulnar arteries are rarely the sites of cardiac embolic occlusion but are more frequently involved with emboli of arterial origin. Such embolic sources include proximal atherosclerotic plaques, aneurysms of the subclavian or axillary artery, and complications of thoracic outlet syndrome.

Although the onset of ischemic symptoms secondary to embolic arterial occlusion may be dramatic, symptoms may also develop slowly over a matter of hours. The level of occlusion is ordinarily detectable by physical examination. The site of disappearance of the axillary or brachial pulse is usually easily assessed by palpation. Doppler studies may also be of assistance in localizing the level of occlusion and assessing the degree of peripheral ischemia. Preoperative arteriography is particularly useful in ruling out a proximal arterial embolic source and is indicated if a cardiac source is not evident.

Embolectomy is indicated in all but the moribund patient. Without treatment, morbidity and mortality may be significant.[32] Prompt systemic heparinization therapy is important not only to limit the propagation of thrombus but also to prevent recurrent embolism. Standard techniques using balloon embolectomy catheters are employed.

Exposure for axillary embolectomy may be obtained through a longitudinal incision in the upper third of the arm over the bicipital groove. This approach may be of particular value with embolic involvement at the level of the deep brachial artery. An alternative approach involves exposure of the brachial artery in the antecubital fossa, with antegrade embolectomy being performed from that location. This is the procedure of choice for mid-brachial and distal brachial lesions. The embolectomy technique should include transverse arteriotomy with interrupted closure. Occasionally, exposure of the brachial artery to its bifurcation is necessary in order to pass catheters selectively down the radial and ulnar arteries. In certain cases with distal thrombus propagation, palmar arch thrombectomy including 2 Fr. thrombectomy catheters may be required through incisions in the radial and ulnar arteries at the wrist. A transverse arteriotomy is used.

After the thrombectomy, the surgeon completes closure using interrupted 7-0 monofilament sutures. Optical magnification facilitates this closure. After embolectomy, fasciotomy is rarely necessary. Intraoperative arteriography should be used if there is any question about the adequacy of distal thrombectomy. The intraoperative use of thrombolytic agents may be efficacious in this setting, as previously described.

Operative mortality rates range from 0 to 19% in this group of patients. Generally, mortality results from associated cardiac disease. Limb salvage rates range from 81% to 100%[3, 5, 32, 38, 55] Gangrene may occur in up to 37% of patients treated conservatively without embolectomy.[32] In certain carefully selected cases, thrombolytic therapy may play an important role in the nonoperative management of upper extremity embolism.

Non-iatrogenic Trauma

Non-iatrogenic injury of the axillary, brachial, radial and ulnar arteries is an important cause of upper extremity ischemia.[10, 15, 28, 44, 55, 66, 72, 75, 77] These injuries are not infrequently encountered by a vascular surgeon associated with a busy trauma service. In civilian experience, the incidence of axillary artery injury is reported to range from 5% to 9%[25, 66] the incidence of brachial artery injury is approximately 30%,[25, 66] and injuries of the radial and ulnar arteries make up 7% to 20%[9, 25, 34, 66, 75] of all arterial injuries. Some series suggest that injuries of the radial and ulnar arteries are more common, but they are rarely of clinical significance if only one vessel is involved. When both vessels are injured, hand viability may be threatened.

Axillary artery injuries range from intimal damage resulting from blunt shoulder girdle trauma and shoulder dislocation to complete transection from a high-velocity missile. Findings associated with axillary artery injury range from an ischemic upper extremity without other significant clinical findings to a rapidly expanding axillary hematoma or hemorrhage from a penetrating axillary wound. Because of the proximity of the brachial plexus and the axillary artery and veins, the incidence of concomitant neurologic and venous injuries is high; brachial plexus injury in the presence of normal vascular examination findings should raise the possibility of a subclinical arterial injury.

The diagnosis is obvious in the presence of frank distal ischemia or hemorrhage; however, palpable distal pulses do not preclude proximal arterial injury and are present in up to 30% of patients.[9, 71, 75, 77] Arteriography is the most precise diagnostic modality, but in the face of frank ischemia and an obvious site of injury, it may only postpone necessary expeditious surgical treatments. Arteriography is of particular importance in ruling out subclinical vascular injury in the face of brachial plexus injury without obvious arterial damage, and if there is a possibility of intrathoracic arterial injury, it is mandatory.

Surgical treatment is indicated whenever axillary arterial injury is identified. The choice of incision depends on the location of the injury. Proximal lesions are best approached through an incision over the deltopectoral groove, whereas distal lesions are approached through a more lateral incision. Occasionally, proximal subclavian artery control through a supraclavicular incision may be necessary before distal exposure. Resection of the middle third of the clavicle may optimize exposure in selected cases. The pectoralis minor and major tendons may be transected if necessary for adequate exposure of more distal lesions. Although expeditious control of hemorrhage is necessary, hasty arterial clamping should be avoided because of the proximity of the brachial plexus. Digital pressure on the vessel as it exits under the clavicle usually provides hemostasis until the vessel can be carefully dissected free of surrounding soft tissue. Only then, under direct vision, should clamps be carefully applied. The ends of the vessel are débrided, and contused vessel segments are resected. After thrombectomy with a balloon catheter, a primary end-to-end spatulated anastomosis is usually sufficient. A reversed vein interposition graft may be required to replace excised segments. Forearm fasciotomy may be required when prolonged ischemia has occurred.

The results of surgical repair of axillary artery injuries should be excellent. The vessel is of satisfactory caliber and sufficiently mobile. Surgical failures are ordinarily due to preventable errors such as inadequate vessel débridement or incomplete distal thrombectomy. Amputation rates range from 0 to 10%.[9, 25, 66] Although gangrene does not occur frequently following ligation, this is not the preferred approach. In fact, when this approach might be most applicable, namely with significant adjacent soft tissue destruction, a higher incidence of gangrene is likely because of collateral vessel destruction. Associated residual neurologic damage is of major importance because it is a greater factor in long-term disability than the consequences of arterial insufficiency.[33, 54, 75, 76]

Most brachial artery injuries are caused by low-velocity missiles or lacerations from glass or knives,[2, 55] but fractures, particularly a supracondylar fracture of the humerus, or dislocations of the humerus and elbow are also causes (Fig. 81–4). Blunt injury of the brachial artery is unusual. Associated injuries include median nerve damage, bone fracture, and venous injury.

Brachial artery injuries are usually obvious, and the diag-

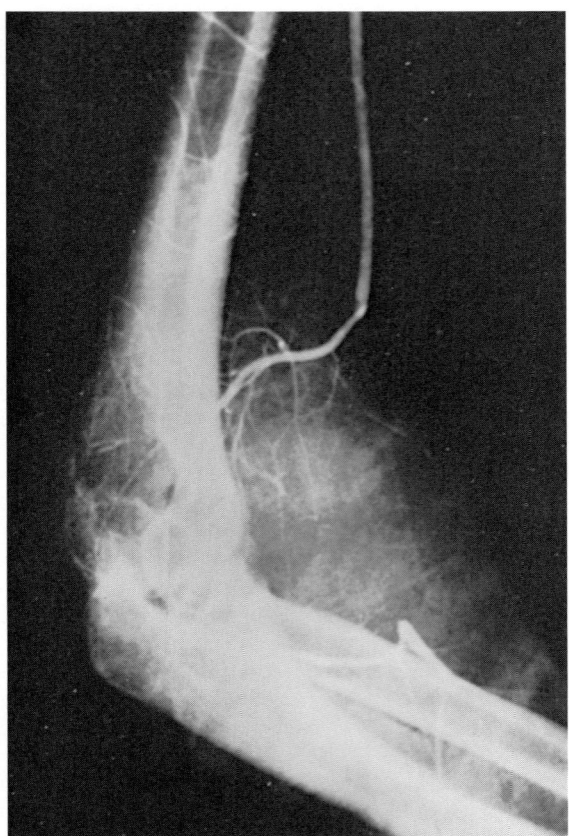

FIGURE 81–4. Brachial artery thrombosis secondary to a fracture-dislocation of the elbow. (From Whitehouse WM Jr: Direct revascularization for forearm and hand ischemia. *In* Bergan JJ, Yao JST [eds]: Evaluation and Treatment of Upper and Lower Extremity Circulatory Disorders. Orlando, Fla, Grune & Stratton, 1984, pp 231–248.)

nosis can be made on the basis of physical examination. Doppler studies are used to document the degree of distal ischemia. Arteriography may be appropriate when the diagnosis is unclear and may be of particular assistance in dealing with blunt trauma.

Surgery is generally indicated for all brachial artery injuries. Sufficient surgical exposure is afforded with an incision along the bicipital groove. If necessary, this can be extended transversely across the antecubital fossa and then farther distally. The surgeon must take care to avoid injury to the median nerve during exposure. Lateral repair is seldom appropriate. Because this vessel lacks many major branches, adequate length of the vessel can usually be mobilized and primary spatulated end-to-end anastomoses can be performed. If interposition grafting is necessary, autogenous saphenous vein is the conduit of choice. Amputation rates range from 0 to 2.5%.[9, 10, 25, 66, 75]

Radial and ulnar artery injuries are frequently deemphasized in reports dealing with vascular trauma. This is due, in part, to the fact that ligation of one of these vessels is ordinarily of no clinical significance. When the vessels are considered in clinical reports, such injuries represent up to 20% of vascular injuries and up to 67% of upper extremity arterial injuries.[75] Lacerations and transections from sharp objects are most frequently reported. Contusion with resulting intimal flaps and thrombosis from blunt trauma

may also occur. The diagnosis can usually be established on the basis of physical examination and Doppler studies. Arteriography may be useful in certain select clinical settings but is seldom used.

Surgical treatment is indicated in the presence of significant hand ischemia. Hemorrhage, if present, can ordinarily be controlled with pressure over the vessel proximal to or at the site of injury. Exposure of the proximal radial and ulnar arteries can be accomplished through the same Z-shaped incision in the antecubital fossa used for exposure of the distal brachial artery. Distal exposure is best afforded by longitudinal incisions overlying the vessels. When only one vessel is injured and collateral flow is satisfactory, ligation is appropriate. When both vessels are injured, however, repair of at least one artery is required. Generally, the ulnar artery is largest and should be repaired if possible. Small defects may also be repaired. Small defects may be repaired with resection and primary end-to-end anastomoses using interrupted 6-0 or 7-0 monofilament sutures. If interposition grafting is required, the distal saphenous vein or cephalic vein serves as a satisfactory conduit. Thrombectomy using 2 Fr. and 3 Fr. catheters should be performed before repair to remove any residual thrombus. Optical magnification facilitates such repairs.

Chronic ischemia of the hand and forearm may occur as a late sequela of traumatic injuries of the axillary, brachial, radial, and ulnar arteries. Surgical treatment is indicated when ischemia causes severe exercise intolerance, tissue loss, or rest pain. The standard surgical approach to these problems includes preoperative arteriography and bypass procedures using saphenous vein, as previously described. In the absence of distal arterial disease, results from such reconstructions are satisfactory.[30, 50] Early failures are associated with limited outflow; late failures are uncommon.

A subset of patients with chronic hand ischemia related to repetitive trauma deserve specific comment. The *hypothenar hammer syndrome* is associated with repetitive trauma over the distal ulnar artery resulting in either arterial thrombosis or aneurysmal degeneration with distal embolization.[21, 51] Recent reports have described direct revascularization with reversed vein bypasses extending beyond the wrist in these cases. One report includes use of this technique in patients with chronic radial and ulnar arterial occlusive disease associated with ESRF. Excellent patency rates have been documented in a limited number of reports.[16, 44, 56, 61]

REFERENCES

 1. Armstrong PW, Parker JO: The complications of brachial arteriotomy. J Thorac Cardiovasc Surg 61:424, 1973.
 2. Ashbell TS, Keinert HE, Kutz JE: Vascular injuries about the elbow. Clin Orthop 50:107, 1967.
 3. Baird RJ, Lajos TZ: Emboli to the arm. Ann Surg 160:905, 1964.
 4. Baker RJ, Chunprapaph B, Nyhus IM: Severe ischemia of the hand following radial artery catheterization. Surgery 80:449, 1976.
 5. Banis JC, Rich N, Whelan TJ: Ischemia of the upper extremity due to noncardiac emboli. Am J Surg 134:131, 1977.
 6. Baxter BT, Blackburn D, Payne K, et al: Noninvasive evaluation of the upper extremity. Surg Clin North Am 70:87, 1990.
 7. Bedford RF, Wollman H: Complications of percutaneous radial-artery cannulation. Anesthesiology 38:228, 1973.

8. Bergqvist D, Ericsson BF, Konrad P, Bergentz SE: Arterial surgery of the upper extremity. World J Surg 7:786, 1983.
9. Bole PV, Purdy RT, Munda RT, et al: Civilian arterial injuries. Ann Surg 183:13, 1976.
10. Borman KR, Snyder WH, Weigelt JA: Civilian arterial trauma of the upper extremity: An 11 year experience in 267 patients. Am J Surg 148:796, 1984.
11. Brener BJ, Couch NP: Peripheral arterial complications of left heart catheterization and their management. Am J Surg 125:521, 1973.
12. Brunkwall J, Berqvist D, Bergentz SE: Long-term results of arterial reconstruction of the upper extremity. Eur J Vasc Surg 8:47, 1994.
13. Butler MJ, Lane RHS, Webster JHH: Irradiation injury to large arteries. Br J Surg 67:341, 1980.
14. Campion BC, Frye RL, Pluth JR, et al: Arterial complications of retrograde brachial arterial catheterization. Mayo Clin Proc 46:589, 1971.
15. Cheek RC, Pope JC, Smith HF, et al: Diagnosis and management of major vascular injuries: A review of 200 operative cases. Am Surg 41:755, 1975.
16. Clark ET, Mass DP, Bassiouny HS, et al: True aneurysmal disease in the hand and upper extremity. Ann Vasc Surg 5:276, 1991.
17. Clouse ME, Ahmed R, Ryan RB, et al: Complications of long term transbrachial hepatic arterial infusion chemotherapy. Am J Roentgenol 129:797, 1977.
18. Cohen ES, Holtzman RB, Johnson GW: Axillobrachial artery bypass grafting with in situ cephalic vein for axillary artery occlusion: A case report. J Vasc Surg 10:683, 1989.
19. Coleman SS, Ansun BJ: Arterial patterns of the hand based upon a study of 650 specimens. Surg Gynecol Obstet 113:409, 1961.
20. Comerota AJ, White JV, Grosh JD: Intraoperative intra-arterial thrombolytic therapy for salvage of limbs in patients with distal arterial thrombosis. Surg Gynecol Obstet 169:283, 1989.
21. Conn J, Bergan JJ and Bell JL: Hypothenar hammer syndrome. Surgery 68:1122, 1970.
22. Dalman RL, Nehler MR, Harris EJ, et al: Upper extremity arterial bypass distal to the wrist. J Vasc Surg 16:633, 1992.
23. Davis JB, Grove WJ, Julian OC: Thrombotic occlusion of the aortic arch, Martorell's syndrome: Report of a case treated surgically. Ann Surg 144:124, 1956.
24. Davis K, Kennedy JW, Kemp HG Jr: Complications of coronary arteriography from the collaborative study of coronary artery surgery. Circulation 59:1105, 1979.
25. Drapanas T, Hewitt RL, Weichert RF, et al: Civilian vascular injuries: A critical appraisal of three decades of management. Ann Surg 172:351, 1970.
26. Erlandson EE, Forrest ME, Shields JJ, et al: Discriminant arteriographic criteria in the management of forearm and hand ischemia. Surgery 90:1025, 1981.
27. Evans PJD, Kerr JH: Arterial occlusion after cannulation. Br Med J 3:197, 1975.
28. Fitridge RA, Miller RS, Faris I: Upper extremity arterial injuries: experience at the Royal Adelaide Hospital, 1969 to 1991. J Vasc Surg 20:941, 1994.
29. Garret HE, Morris GC, Howell JE, et al: Revascularization of upper extremity with autogenous vein bypass graft. Arch Surg 91:751, 1965.
30. Gross WS, Flanigan DP, Kraft RO, et al: Chronic upper extremity arterial insufficiency. Arch Surg 113:419, 1978.
31. Guzman-Stein G, Schubert W, Najarian DW, et al: Composite in situ vein bypass for upper extremity revascularization. Plast Reconstr Surg 83:533, 1989.
32. Haimovic H: Cardiogenic embolism of the upper extremity. J Cardiovasc Surg 23:209, 1982.
33. Hardin WD, O'Connell RC, Adinolfi MF, et al: Traumatic arterial injuries of the upper extremity: Determinants of disability. Am J Surg 150:266, 1985.
34. Hardy JD, Raju S, Neely WA, et al: Aortic and other arterial injuries. Ann Surg 181:640, 1975.
35. Hessel SJ, Adams DF, Abrams HL: Complications of angiography. Radiology 138:273, 1981.
36. Hirai M: Arterial insufficiency of the hand evaluated by digital blood pressure and arteriographic findings. Circulation 58:902, 1978.
37. Holleman JH, Hardy JD, Williamson JW, et al: Arterial surgery for arm ischemia: A survey of 136 patients. Ann Surg 191:727, 1980.
38. James EC, Khuri NT, Fedde CW, et al: Upper limb ischemia resulting from arterial thromboembolism. Am J Surg 137:739, 1979.
39. Javenski BK: Angiography of the Upper Extremity. The Hague, Martinus Nijhoff, 1982.
40. Kamienski RW, Barnes RW: Critique of the Allen test for continuity of the palmar arch assessed by Doppler ultrasound. Surg Gynecol Obstet 142:861, 1976.
41. Karmody AM, Zaman SN, Mirza RA, et al: The surgical management of catheter injuries of the brachial artery. J Thorac Cardiovasc Surg 73:149, 1977.
42. Kartchner MM, Wilcox WC: Thrombolysis of palmar and digital arterial thrombosis by intraarterial thrombolysin. J Hand Surg 1:67, 1976.
43. Katz AM, Birnbaum M, Moylan J, et al: Gangrene of the hand and forearm: A complication of radial artery cannulation. Crit Care Med 2:270, 1974.
44. Katz SG, Kohl RD: Direct revascularization for the treatment of forearm and hand ischemia. Am J Surg 165:312, 1993.
45. Key E: Embolectomy of the vessels of the extremities. Br J Surg 24:350, 1936.
46. Kitzmiller JW, Hertzer NR, Beven EG: Routine surgical management of brachial artery occlusion after cardiac catheterization. Arch Surg 117:1066, 1982.
47. Kline RM, Hertzer NR, Beven EG, et al: Surgical treatment of brachial artery injuries after cardiac catheterization. J Vasc Surg 12:20, 1990.
48. Kretschmer G, Niederle B, Polterauer P, et al: Irradiation-induced changes in the subclavian and axillary arteries after radiotherapy for carcinoma of the breast. Surgery 99:658, 1986.
49. Little JM, Zylstra PL, West J, et al: Circulatory patterns in the normal hand. Br J Surg 60:652, 1973.
50. McCarthy WJ, Flinn WR, Yao JST, et al: Result of bypass grafting for upper limb ischemia. J Vasc Surg 3:741, 1986.
51. McCarthy WJ, Yao JST, Schafer MF, et al: Upper extremity arterial injury in athletes. J Vasc Surg 9:317, 1989.
52. McCollum CH, Mavor E: Brachial artery injury after cardiac catheterization. J Vasc Surg 4:355, 1986.
53. McCormack LJ, Cauldwell EW, Anson BJ: Brachial and antebrachial arterial patterns: A study of 750 extremities. Surg Gynecol Obstet 96:44, 1953.
54. McCready RA, Procter CD, Hyde GL: Subclavian-axillary vascular trauma. J Vasc Surg 3:24, 1986.
55. McCroskey BL, Moore EE, Pearce WH, et al: Traumatic injuries of the brachial artery. Am J Surg 156:553, 1988.
56. Mehlhoff TL, Wood MB: Ulnar artery thrombosis and the role of interposition vein grafting: patency with microsurgical technique. J Hand Surg 16A:274, 1991.
57. Menzoian JO, Corson JD, Bush HL, et al: Management of the upper extremity with absent pulses after cardiac catheterization. Am J Surg 135:484, 1978.
58. Menzoian JO, Doyle JE, Cantelmo NL, et al: A comprehensive approach to extremity vascular trauma. Arch Surg 120:801, 1985.
59. Mesh CL, McCarthy WJ, Pearce WH, et al: Upper extremity bypass grafting: a 15 year experience. Arch Surg 128:795, 1993.
60. Mozersky DJ, Buckley CJ, Hagood CO, et al: Ultrasonic evaluation of the palmar circulation. Am J Surg 126:812, 1973.
61. Nehler MR, Dalman RL, Harris EJ, et al: Upper extremity arterial bypass distal to the wrist. J Vasc Surg 16:633, 1992.
62. Nicholas GG, DeMuth WE Jr: Long-term results of brachial thrombectomy following cardiac catheterization. Ann Surg 183:436, 1976.
63. Norem RF, Short DH, Kerstein MD: Role of intraoperative fibrinolytic therapy in acute arterial occlusion. Surg Gynecol Obstet 167:87, 1988.
64. Page CP, Hagood CO, Kemmerer WT: Management of post-catheterization brachial artery thrombosis. Surgery 72:619, 1972.
65. Parent FN, Bernhard VM, Pabst TS, et al: Fibrinolytic treatment of residual thrombus after catheter embolectomy for severe lower limb ischemia. J Vasc Surg 9:153, 1989.
66. Perry MO, Thal ER, Shires GT: Management of arterial injuries. Ann Surg 173:403, 1971.
67. Quiñones-Baldrich WJ, Zierler RE, Hiatt JC: Intraoperative fibrinolytic therapy: An adjunct to catheter thromboembolectomy. J Vasc Surg 2:319, 1985.
68. Rich NM, Hobson RW, Fedde CW: Vascular trauma secondary to diagnostic and therapeutic procedures. Am J Surg 128:715, 1974.
69. Rivers SP, Baur GM, Inahara T, et al: Arm ischemia secondary to giant cell arteritis. Am J Surg 143:554, 1982.
70. Ross RS: Arterial complications. Circulation 37(Suppl III):39, 1968.

71. Rutherford RB: Diagnostic evaluation of extremity vascular injuries. Surg Clin North Am 68:683, 1988.
72. Sachatello GR, Ernst CB, Griffen WO Jr: The acutely ischemic upper extremity: Selective management. Surgery 76:1002, 1974.
73. Savelyev VS, Zatevakhin JJ, Stepano NV: Artery embolism of the upper limbs. Surgery 81:367, 1977.
74. Schmidt FE, Hewitt RL: Severe upper limb ischemia. Arch Surg 115:1188, 1980.
75. Sitzman JV, Ernst CB: Management of arm arterial injuries. Surgery 96:895, 1984.
76. Smith RF, Szilagyi DE, Elliott JP Jr: Fracture of long bones with arterial injury due to blunt trauma. Arch Surg 99:315, 1969.
77. Smith RF, Elliott JP, Hageman JH, et al: Acute penetrating arterial injuries of the neck and limbs. Arch surg 109:198, 1974.
78. Spaulding C, Lefevre T, Thebault B, et al: Left radial artery approach for coronary angiography: results of a prospective study. Cathet Cardiovasc Diagn 39:365, 1996.
79. Tuzzeo S, Saad SA, Hastings OM, et al: Management of brachial artery injuries. Surg Gynecol Obstet 146:21, 1978.
80. Welling RE, Cranley JJ, Krause RJ, et al: Obliterative arterial diesease of the upper extremity. Arch Surg 116:1593, 1981.
81. Wolk SW, Moores HK, Lampman RM, et al: The use of preoperative noninvasive vascular studies for the evaluation of radial artery conduits for coronary bypass grafting. Vasc Surg 32:249, 1998.
82. Wood PB: Vein graft bypass in axillary and brachial artery occlusions causing claudication. Br J Surg 60:29, 1973.
83. Woodburne RT: Essentials of Human Anatomy. New York, Oxford University Press, 1983, pp. 91–92.
84. Yao JST, Pearce WH: Reconstructive surgery for chronic upper extremity ischemia. Semin Vasc Surg 3:258, 1990.

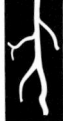

C H A P T E R   8 2

Occlusive and Vasospastic Diseases Involving Distal Upper Extremity Arteries—Raynaud's Syndrome

John M. Porter, M.D., and James M. Edwards, M.D.

Many disparate disease processes may affect the distal small arteries of the upper extremities. Their clinical manifestations range from episodic digital vasospasm to severe hand ischemia with rest pain and gangrene. Although fixed arterial occlusions are present in the distal extremity arteries of patients with digital ulceration and gangrene, patients with episodic digital vasospasm frequently have no identifiable morphologic arterial abnormalities. These patients experience excessive digital artery vasospasm in response to cold provocation or emotional stimulation and are completely normal between attacks. Digital vasospasm and digital arterial occlusion clearly are not mutually exclusive. Many patients with digital ischemia have elements of both arterial obstruction and vasospasm. Additionally, during long-term follow-up, a number of patients with episodic digital vasospasm subsequently develop diffuse palmar and digital arterial occlusions in conjunction with one or more associated diseases. Thus, it appears clear that episodic digital vasospasm and ischemic digital ulceration are components of a continuous clinical spectrum of disease entities that may affect the distal small arteries of the upper extremities.

This chapter reviews the clinical presentation, pathophysiology, diagnosis, and treatment of spastic and obstructive upper extremity small artery diseases. The Division of Vascular Surgery at the Oregon Health Sciences University is conducting an ongoing prospective clinical study of upper extremity small artery diseases. To date, more than 1100 patients have been enrolled, two thirds of whom have been fully analyzed. The contents of this chapter are, in large part, derived from the authors' experience with this patient population.

RAYNAUD'S SYNDROME

Raynaud's syndrome (RS) is a clinical condition characterized by episodic attacks of vasospasm caused by closure of the small arteries and arterioles of the most distal parts of the extremities in response to cold or emotional stress. The fingers and hands are most often affected, although in certain patients, the toes and feet are involved. Classically, the episodes of vasospasm consist of an intense pallor of the distal extremities followed in sequence by cyanosis and rubor on rewarming. Generally, the attacks are over within 30 to 60 minutes, although many patients describe attacks induced by cold exposure that persist until they enter a warm area. Most patients do not experience the complete triple-color response but instead note only pallor or cyanosis during attacks. The authors have encountered a number of patients who complain of cold hands without color changes and who demonstrate abnormal digital arteriographic and blood flow changes that are indistinguishable from those in patients with classic triple-color Raynaud's attacks. Thus, it is questionable whether any color change should be a criterion for diagnosis.

Historical Background

The first description of a group of patients with finger ischemia presumably caused by digital artery vasospasm was published by Maurice Raynaud in 1862.[112] He reported on 25 patients with varying degrees of episodic digital pallor and cyanosis, frequently associated with localized finger gangrene. Raynaud proposed that the observed changes were caused by vasospasm produced by sympathetic overactivity; that is, in most of his patients wrist pulses were palpable, but in some of them large artery patency was documented at autopsy. It is now known that vasospasm alone is insufficient to produce gangrene, and it appears likely that most, if not all, of Raynaud's original patients had far advanced, unrecognized, fixed small artery occlusive disease in addition to episodic vasospasm.

Raynaud's vasospastic hypothesis was challenged by Hutchinson at the turn of the century.[57] He recognized that digital gangrene, like episodic digital ischemia, may be associated with many conditions, such as arteriosclerosis, scleroderma, and heart failure. Hutchinson suggested that the term Raynaud's phenomenon be applied to episodic digital vasoconstriction and that this clinical sign is common to diseases of diverse causes.

The clinical approach to RS was substantially influenced by a publication of Allen and Brown's in 1932.[6] They clearly recognized that the Raynaud's event, namely episodic digital artery vasoconstriction, may occur with a variety of associated disorders, particularly digital artery occlusive diseases. They proposed dividing the syndrome into Raynaud's disease, which was benign, idiopathic, and not associated with systemic disease, and Raynaud's phenomenon, which had a similar symptom complex but occurred in association with various systemic diseases. They presented rigid diagnostic criteria that supposedly allowed individual cases to be categorized as either Raynaud's phenomenon or idiopathic Raynaud's disease.

Ever since 1932, attempts to distinguish Raynaud's disease from Raynaud's phenomenon have dominated the medical literature on this topic. This approach has done little to further understanding of this syndrome, because many authors have varied the diagnostic criteria without changing the terminology. Additionally, this conceptual framework retarded recognition of changing clinical patterns in a given patient.

Since Allen and Brown's article appeared, many investigators have examined the natural history and clinical significance of RS. Lewis and Pickering reported that most of their patients had a benign clinical course.[75] This position was challenged in 1957 by Gifford and Hines, who first described associated disorders in certain patients that developed long after the onset of typical RS.[38] Several years later, deTakats and Fowler accurately noted that a long period of clinical observation is often required before an associated disease can be recognized and that methods available to earlier investigators for identification of these diseases were unsophisticated by present standards.[24] These deficiencies undoubtedly led to the erroneous conclusion, published in the older literature, that RS without any associated disease was more common than it actually was. The striking frequency of associated disease has been confirmed in reports from the authors' service, which, as noted, is conducting an ongoing prospective clinical investigation of small artery and vasospastic diseases.[11, 102–105, 113–115, 142]

The information obtained from their investigations has led the authors to abandon the older terminology of Raynaud's disease and phenomenon, which often implied more than was actually understood about the patient's condition. The authors prefer to use the term Raynaud's syndrome to define cold-induced or emotionally induced episodic digital ischemia. Available evidence clearly shows that patients with RS are not easily separated into a benign "disease" group and a virulent "phenomenon" group, as suggested by Allen and Brown. The increasing sophistication of clinical, radiologic, and immunologic diagnostic techniques is making possible the unequivocal diagnosis of autoimmune and other associated diseases in many patients with mild symptoms whose condition undoubtedly would have been categorized as Raynaud's disease by the Allen and Brown criteria.[102–104]

Epidemiology

Surprisingly little information is available on the incidence of RS in the general population. Lewis and Pickering questioned 122 individuals selected at random and found that 25% of the males and 30% of the females had a history of Raynaud's attacks.[75] Taylor and Pelmear, as part of a study on vibration-induced RS, questioned 254 working men without vibration exposure and found a 5.3% incidence of RS.[135] Olsen and Nielsen questioned a group of apparently healthy women between ages 21 and 50 years in Copenhagen and found that 22% reported symptoms of RS.[95] Heslop and associates found a 17.6% incidence of RS in females and an 8.3% incidence in males who were seen in a stratified random sample of patients selected from a general practice in Hampshire, England. Only about half had sought medical attention for digital ischemia.[50]

Maricq and colleagues conducted a population-based survey in South Carolina to attempt to determine the incidence of RS in the general population.[78] They found an incidence of RS of 5.1% in females and 3.5% in males. Leppert and coworkers sent questionnaires to a random sample of 3000 women in Sweden and found an incidence of RS of 15.6% in the 2705 patients who responded.[73] Silman and associates found an incidence of RS of 19% in females and 11% in males who responded to their questionnaire.[124] The authors questioned 150 individuals selected at random in their institution and found that 30% described symptoms suggestive of RS.[102–104]

Combining all these studies yields an incidence of RS of 11.8% (13.5% in females and 6.7% in males). It appears that a large number of patients who live in cool, damp climates such as those in Denmark, England, and the state of Oregon have mild but definite cold sensitivity, whereas only a small percentage of this group seek treatment for it. Holling stated that cool climates should increase both the frequency and the severity of RS in the population.[55] This intuitive reasoning, however, remains unsupported by conclusive data.

Between 70% and 90% of all reported patients with RS are women. The reason is not known. Random population surveys have revealed that RS affects 20% to 30% of the population in certain geographic areas. It must be remembered that the literature on RS has reported only on patients with vasospastic symptoms severe and persistent enough to prompt them to seek medical treatment. It is unclear whether conclusions derived from these more severely symptomatic patients can be applied accurately to "less symptomatic" patients who do not seek treatment. This seems especially unlikely in the important epidemiologic areas of frequency and type of associated diseases.

Of considerable interest are several population groups in whom RS appears to be a complication of their occupation.[94, 134] The best-studied groups are those whose work requires frequent use of vibrating equipment such as chain saws and pneumatic drills. A number of studies have shown that more than 50% of persons routinely employed in such activities ultimately experience RS.[14, 135]

The exact mechanism of RS in these patients is not understood. Laboratory studies have shown that a vibration frequency of about 125 Hz places severe shear stresses on the arteries of the hands and fingers.[119] Limited pathologic studies have shown increasing subintimal fibrosis after prolonged exposure to vibrating instruments. One study described the angiographic pattern of "vibration white finger" as one of widespread palmar and digital arterial obstruction.[59] Available data suggest that the incidence of RS in chain saw operators has decreased significantly since the introduction of the antivibration chain saw in the early 1980s.

The relationship of chronic industrial cold exposure to RS has great potential importance. One report indicated that 50% of workers in a food-processing industry who were exposed to alternately hot and cold temperatures noted some degree of RS.[77] Control workers for both the vibration and the cold food-processing study groups showed an approximate 5% incidence of RS.[3, 12] Future clarification of the precise relationship between RS and specific employment and working conditions is required and will have great potential medicolegal significance.[65]

Pathophysiology

A classic triphasic Raynaud's attack begins with profound blanching of the digits, and occasionally the proximal part of the hand, in response to cold exposure or emotional stress. The mechanism is complete closure of the palmar and digital arteries, and possibly of the arterioles, which results in the cessation of capillary perfusion. The blanching may be accompanied by a feeling of relative numbness or paresthesias, and both generally persist as long as the exposure does.

Attacks may end spontaneously or when the patient enters a warm environment. The capillaries, and probably the venules, reflexively dilate secondary to regional hypoxia, possibly influenced by an accumulation of the local by-products of anaerobic metabolism. Eventually, slight relaxation of arterial spasm occurs that permits a trickle of blood to enter the dilated capillary bed, where it rapidly desaturates, producing cyanosis. Subsequently, the digits may become ruborous, reflecting reactive hyperemia after transient digital ischemia[101] as more blood flows into the dilated capillaries. The attack terminates with relaxation of the arterial spasm and the return of baseline arterial inflow and capillary perfusion.

The search for the mechanism responsible for the vasoconstriction of a Raynaud's attack has occupied investigators for more than a century. The suggestion of Raynaud that abnormal nervous system function caused the attacks was substantively disproved by the methodical evaluations of Lewis in the 1920s and 1930s.[74, 75] Lewis repeatedly observed that autonomic and somatic nerve blocks with local anesthesia did not prevent the Raynaud's attacks. He therefore proposed that a "local vascular fault" was responsible for the observed vascular wall hyperresponsiveness to cold, exclusive of sympathetic innervation.

Blood flow in an artery ceases when the constrictive force in the arterial wall exceeds the intraluminal distending pressure, the so-called critical closing pressure. Lewis showed that complete digital artery closure occurs during a Raynaud's attack,[74] and the measured digital artery pressure is actually in the range of 5 mmHg.[53] Abundant clinical observations suggest that the critical arterial closing pressure required to produce a Raynaud's attack may be achieved by two distinct pathophysiologic mechanisms, which the authors have termed *obstructive* and *vasospastic*,[21, 104, 150] although a number of patients appear to manifest elements of both mechanisms. This finding further reinforces the assertion that vasospastic and obstructive RS represent a continuum of disease, rather than two separate entities.

Obstructive RS occurs in the presence of fixed organic obstruction of the palmar or digital arteries, with resultant decreased intraluminal distending pressure. In the face of a normal vasoconstrictive response to cold or emotional stimuli, complete digital artery closure occurs and blood flow ceases, thus producing an attack. These small artery obstructions may be caused by a variety of disorders; two of the most common ones are arteriosclerosis and chronic arteritis associated with autoimmune connective tissue disease.[22] The systolic brachial-finger pressure gradient in normal persons is 10 to 15 mmHg. A brachial-finger gradient of more than 15 mmHg, an absolute finger blood pressure less than 70 mmHg, or a difference of more than 15 mmHg between any two fingers indicates significant palmar or digital artery obstruction.[26]

The relationship between arterial occlusive disease and cold sensitivity is a quantitative one. Hirai studied a group of patients who were found to have palmar and digital artery obstruction on plethysmography and digital blood pressure measurements.[53] He found that mild digital artery obstruction was not associated with RS. The production of an obstructive Raynaud's attack required arterial occlusive disease severe enough to produce a significant reduction in resting digital artery pressure, a condition that occurred only with obstruction of both arteries in a single digit. When this degree of occlusive disease was present, a Raynaud's attack was always observed during cooling. A corollary of this observation is the prediction that anyone with palmar or digital artery obstruction capable of causing a significant decrease in digital artery pressure should experience RS. Analysis of the more than 1100 patients undergoing investigation at the authors' center confirms this hypothesis.

In contrast to the relatively straightforward and quantitative relationship between digital artery occlusive disease and RS, the pathophysiology of *vasospastic RS* remains incompletely understood. Patients with vasospastic RS do not have significant palmar or digital artery obstruction and have normal digital artery pressures at room temperature. Plethysmographic and angiographic studies in affected patients demonstrate complete digital artery closure after cold provocation, despite previously normal finger systolic blood pressure and the absence of significant arterial obstruction.[70, 95, 117]

Krahenbuhl and associates examined a group of patients with vasospastic RS by measuring digital artery blood pressure changes induced by external finger cooling.[70] The patients showed a moderate decline in digital artery pressure until a critical temperature of approximately 28°C was reached, at which point total digital artery closure suddenly occurred, and the finger blood pressure abruptly dropped to unmeasurable levels (Fig. 82–1).

The cause of this increased force of arterial vasoconstriction, the "local vascular fault" of Lewis, is not known. Evidence of enhanced adrenergic neuroeffector activity has been suggested by successful clinical use of sympathetic blocking agents, and experimentally by radioisotope clearance studies.

Coffman and Cohen performed detailed studies of finger blood flow before and after cooling in a group of controls and patients with RS.[19, 21] Normal fingers subjected to hypothermia showed a decrease in arteriovenous shunt flow without alterations in nutrient capillary flow. In patients with RS, however, both shunt flow and capillary nutritive flow were reduced at room temperature and after cooling. Pretreatment with the sympathetic blocking agent reserpine significantly increased capillary flow in patients with RS, both at room temperature and after cooling. These findings suggest that enhanced adrenergic neuroeffector activity may contribute to RS.

A local fault that results in intermittent vasospasm is suggested by several observations. The persistence or recurrence of vasospastic symptoms that often follows a sympathectomy may be explained by an unaltered defect in the vessel wall that responds to circulating catecholamines, possibly in association with receptor denervation hypersensitivity. Additionally, vasospastic events are known to occur in isolated and seemingly unrelated vessels, producing such disparate clinical phenomena as variant angina, classic migraine, abdominal migraine, and RS. Indeed, RS has been observed five times more often in patients with variant angina than in a control group.[84]

Alteration of the alpha-adrenergic receptors in vascular smooth muscle, possibly related to repeated exposure to cool temperatures, has also been implicated in the pathophysiology of vasospastic RS.[60] Experimental studies have provided evidence to support this theory.

Keenan and Porter found significantly higher levels of alpha$_2$-adrenergic receptors in circulating platelets of patients with vasospastic RS than in either patients with obstructive RS or normal controls.[66] This observation was subsequently confirmed, and a subset of patients with subnormal alpha$_2$-adrenergic receptor levels was identified.[28] When serum from patients with vasospastic RS was incubated with platelets from controls, an absolute decrease occurred in the measured alpha$_2$-adrenoreceptor levels of the control platelets that was not observed after a control incubation. This observation suggested receptor modulation as a mechanism of increased cellular receptor synthesis.

Although the relationship between receptor levels in platelet membranes, which contain a pure population of alpha$_2$-adrenergic receptors, and vascular smooth muscle remains to be quantitated in humans, extrapolation from other experimental and clinical models supports a direct correlation. The existence of an altered receptor population may prove to be the fundamental abnormality through which any one of a number of factors, such as neurogenic activity, immune system mediators, or elevated serotonin level, may produce vasospasm. This may also help to explain the observation that sympathetic nerve transection with resultant adrenoreceptor hypersensitivity is not as effective as adrenergic receptor blockade in relieving vasospastic symptoms.

Many other factors have been considered in the pathophysiology of vasospastic RS. Alterations in blood viscosity,[42, 137] abnormal serum proteins,[41, 137] elevated serotonin levels,[46] and altered shear stress[90, 119] have all been demonstrated in certain patients with RS. More recently, abnormalities in vasoactive peptides such as calcitonin gene–related peptide and endothelin have been described in patients with RS.[13, 32, 121, 141, 149] Although certain of these factors may occasionally play a significant role in the pathogenesis of symptomatic cold-induced vasospasm, they are uncommon, inconsistently observed, and unlikely to be major factors in a majority of patients.[11, 45, 66, 104]

Clinical Presentation

RS consists of episodic digital coldness associated with pallor or cyanosis brought on by cold exposure or emotional stimuli. Mild pain, paresthesias, and numbness are frequent complaints, but severe pain is rare. RS may coexist with persistent or chronic digital ischemia. Persistent digital cyanosis or painful digital ischemic ulceration may infrequently dominate the clinical picture and be the presenting complaint in patients with a history of long-standing, stable RS.[104] Conversely, previously asymptomatic patients may present with digital ischemia of abrupt onset and then manifest chronic RS after the initial ischemic symptoms

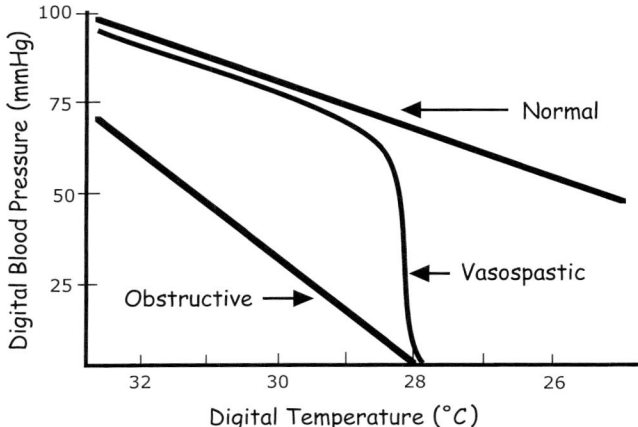

FIGURE 82–1. Alterations in digital artery blood pressure with a decrease in temperature.

resolve.[9, 86, 131] It is important to note that digital ulceration is never caused by vasospasm alone. Ischemic digital ulceration always implies widespread palmar and digital artery obstruction.

Clinical and Laboratory Evaluation

The only absolute requirement for the diagnosis of RS is a history of cold-induced or emotionally induced episodic digital ischemia, usually manifested by color changes. Diagnostic studies should therefore be directed toward precise quantification of the degree of ischemia and identification of associated disorders. History taking is the most important initial diagnostic modality, and findings substantially direct the course and extent of subsequent investigations. A history of arthralgia, dysphagia, xerostomia, or xerophthalmia suggests a connective tissue disorder. Symptoms related to large-vessel arterial occlusive disease, trauma, or a history of malignancy should be sought, because all these disorders may be associated with digital ischemia.

A complete medication profile is essential. The physical examination findings are frequently unremarkable; however, specific attention should be directed to the quality of the peripheral pulses, the presence of digital ulcerations, evidence of previous tissue loss, and joint changes. The skin should be evaluated for telangiectasias or rashes, or thinning and tightening suggestive of scleroderma; the latter is most easily seen in the face and hands.

The extent of laboratory testing depends on the initial clinical suspicions. The minimal evaluation for all patients suspected of having RS includes a complete blood count, determination of the erythrocyte sedimentation rate, a chemistry profile, and urinalysis. A serum rheumatoid factor assay and a screening antinuclear antibody (ANA) titer are useful enough to warrant inclusion in a baseline evaluation. The ANA test is most sensitive when performed on two different substrates.[7] These tests are most helpful in detecting rheumatoid arthritis, systemic lupus erythematosus, mixed connective tissue disease, and scleroderma. Additional laboratory testing should be pursued in selected patients when the results of the screening tests so indicate (Table 82–1).

Vascular Laboratory and Arteriographic Evaluation

The objective vascular laboratory documentation of RS, although not essential for diagnosis in most patients, has

TABLE 82–1. LABORATORY EVALUATION OF RAYNAUD'S SYNDROME

ROUTINE BASELINE TESTS	ADJUNCTIVE TESTS FOR SELECTED PATIENTS
Complete blood count	Serum protein electrophoresis
Erythrocyte sedimentation rate	Extractable nuclear antibody
Chemistry profile	Anti–native DNA antibody
Urinalysis	Antinuclear antibody
Rheumatoid factor	Cryoglobulins
Antinuclear antibody	Complement levels
	Hepatitis B screen
	Anticentromere antibody

DNA = deoxyribonucleic acid.

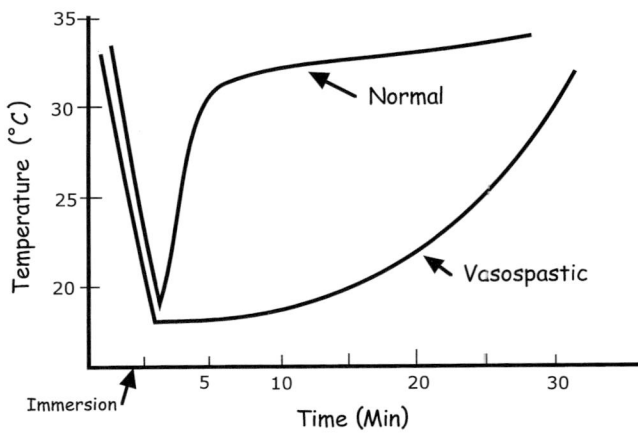

FIGURE 82–2. Digital temperature recovery after ice water exposure. The different curves for the normal and the vasospastic digit are indicated.

great value in certain situations. It is especially useful in evaluating "symptomatic patients" who do not manifest typical color changes, certain patients with medicolegal claims, and for objectively quantitating the results of treatment.

The simplest vascular laboratory test for RS is the hand *ice water immersion test* with determination of fingertip temperatures with a thermistor probe. The patient's hand is immersed in ice water for 30 seconds. The hand is then dried, and fingertip pulp temperatures are measured every 5 minutes for 45 minutes or until the temperature returns to the preimmersion level. The test requires body warming, so that the preimmersion digital temperature is above 30°C. The digital temperature of normal persons returns to normal in 10 minutes or less, whereas in patients with RS it takes much longer. This test appears to be quite specific for RS, but, unfortunately, appears to have low sensitivity.[105] Ice water immersion is also poorly tolerated by patients. A representative temperature recovery curve appears in Figure 82–2.

Sumner and Strandness described a distinctive peaked appearance of the *digital photoplethysmographic waveform* observed in 78% of patients with cold sensitivity and RS.[128] This waveform was found in only 3% of asymptomatic individuals. A detailed assessment of plethysmographic peaked digital pulse waveforms in the diagnosis of RS indicated that presence of the peaked pulse was 66% sensitive and 100% specific and had an overall accuracy rate of 70% in the objective diagnosis of RS.[4]

The *occlusive digital hypothermic challenge test* described by Nielsen and Lassen is the most sensitive and specific test currently available for the diagnosis of RS.[91] Patients are examined at a room temperature of 21°C. A double-inlet cuff for local cooling is placed over the proximal phalanx of the test finger (most often the right second digit). Baseline digital artery pressures are measured in the reference and test fingers with a mercury-in-rubber strain-gauge placed distal to the occlusive finger cuff. Next, the test finger is subjected to 5 minutes of ischemic hypothermic perfusion. After tourniquet release following cooling, the digital blood pressure recovery is recorded. Results are expressed as the percentage of decrease in the cool finger systolic pressure on reperfusion, as compared with pressure in the reference finger. A decrease in digital blood pressure of 20% or more is considered positive for RS. In the authors' vascular laboratory, this test is 100% sensitive and 80% specific, with an accuracy of 97% in the diagnosis of RS.[4, 34]

Several other diagnostic tests have been used to detect RS, although none appears to equal the digital hypothermic challenge test. The tests included thermal entrainment,[71] digital thermography,[15] venous occlusion plethysmography, digital artery caliber measurement,[125] and other methods of digital blood flow measurement.[21, 148]

Digital plethysmography with waveform analysis and *digital blood pressure determination* provide an accurate assessment of the status of the digital arterial circulation.[4, 56] The information obtained with these noninvasive examinations is essential to differentiating between vasospastic and obstructive RS in a given patient and is frequently important in detecting associated disease. Examples of a normal, peaked pulse, and an abnormal digital photoplethysmographic tracing are seen in Figure 82–3.

Early in their experience, the authors used *hand arteriography* extensively to establish the diagnosis of RS. Magnification hand arteriograms were obtained before and after ice water exposure and before and 24 hours after intra-arterial administration of reserpine. An example of a film sequence is shown in Figure 82–4. A typical pattern of total abolition of cold-induced vasospasm by adrenoreceptor-blocking drugs was recognized, and it proved to be a reliable diagnostic test. The early arteriograms were of considerable importance in establishing the role of adrenoreceptor function in the pathophysiology of RS. Today, hand arteriography has been almost entirely replaced by vascular laboratory tests, especially Nielsen's test and digital plethysmography, in the diagnosis of RS.

The authors recommend upper extremity arteriography only for suspected large artery disease proximal to the palmar arch. This may be suggested by the absence of pulses on examination or by unilateral development of digital ischemia.

Treatment

The goal of treatment for RS is palliation because no cure is available. It is important for physicians to understand that the course of RS in most patients is generally benign. The natural history is one of symptomatic periods interspersed with periods of improvement, or even complete remission. Inexorable progression to severe finger ischemia or gangrene is rare and exclusively associated with an underlying obstructive arterial disease. The majority of patients with vasospastic RS have only mild to moderate symptoms and respond satisfactorily to avoidance of cold and tobacco. Use of oral contraceptives,[27] beta-adrenergic blockers,[31, 79] and ergotamine preparations[43, 49, 83, 85] is not recommended, because each of these agents has been reported to exacerbate RS symptoms and equally effective alternatives are generally available. Patients occasionally require pharmacologic intervention during the winter; such treatment is also indicated for those with severe symptoms.

Objective evaluation of the efficacy of drug treatment of RS is impossible because no vascular laboratory test accurately quantitates a drug's effect on the digital circulation. Until such a test is developed, assessment of drug response will be anecdotal and greatly hampered by such uncontrolled variables as environmental temperature, amount of environmental cold exposure, and the patient's emotional state. The efficacy assessments of all the drugs described in this section are anecdotal and are subject to all the inherent disadvantages of this method of drug evaluation.

Sympatholytic agents have been the mainstay of drug therapy for RS.[1, 2, 18, 20, 81, 138, 146] Patients with vasospastic RS generally respond much more favorably than those with obstructive RS. The effectiveness of medical treatment is limited not only by severe arterial obstructive disease but also by frequent side effects of drug treatment.[97]

Oral reserpine was one of the first drugs to be evaluated for treatment of RS,[37, 92, 99] and daily doses of 0.25 mg to as much as 1.0 mg have been used clinically.[69] Other orally administered sympathetic blockers in clinical use that have produced modest benefits include guanethidine,[113] methyldopa,[140] isoxsuprine,[145] phenoxybenzamine,[113, 131] and prazosin.[143] The large doses required when any of these agents is used alone frequently produce intolerable side effects. Low-dose combination regimens can sometimes reduce the frequency and severity of side effects; one such combination, 10 mg of guanethidine and 1 to 2 mg of prazosin per day, has appeared to be beneficial in the treatment of RS in these authors' experience.[106] There are few reported prospective, randomized, double-blind trials of any of these agents in the treatment of RS, and all reports of drug treatment of RS have relied on anecdotal end-points.

Sympathetic blockers have generally been replaced by calcium channel blockers in the treatment of symptomatic RS.[63] Nifedipine, given either as 30 mg orally at bedtime in a sustained-release formulation or as 10 mg orally three times a day, is currently the authors' first-line drug.[40, 89, 103] The sustained-release formulation appears to be tolerated better. Some patients who do not tolerate the standard formulation can take the sustained-release formulation without side effects. Controlled prospective trials have shown improvement in the vasospastic symptoms of patients with RS.[40, 116, 126] Diltiazem, another calcium channel blocker, may be equally effective. The addition of the alpha-adrenergic blocker prazosin may produce further improvement in patients who respond incompletely to a calcium channel blocker alone. Pentoxifylline, 400 mg three times per day, is a hemorheologic agent that appears to be of benefit in some patients, but controlled trials are lacking. The angiotensin-converting enzyme inhibitors captopril, 25 mg one to three times a day, and losartan, 12.5 to 50 mg one to three times a day, may also be of some benefit.[97, 139]

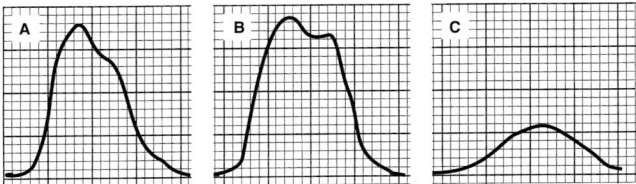

FIGURE 82–3. Photoplethysmographic digital artery waveforms objectively document arterial occlusive disease and diminish the need for angiography. *A,* Normal tracing. *B,* Tracing from a patient with vasospastic Raynaud's syndrome demonstrating a peaked pulse. *C,* Tracing from a patient with obstructive Raynaud's syndrome.

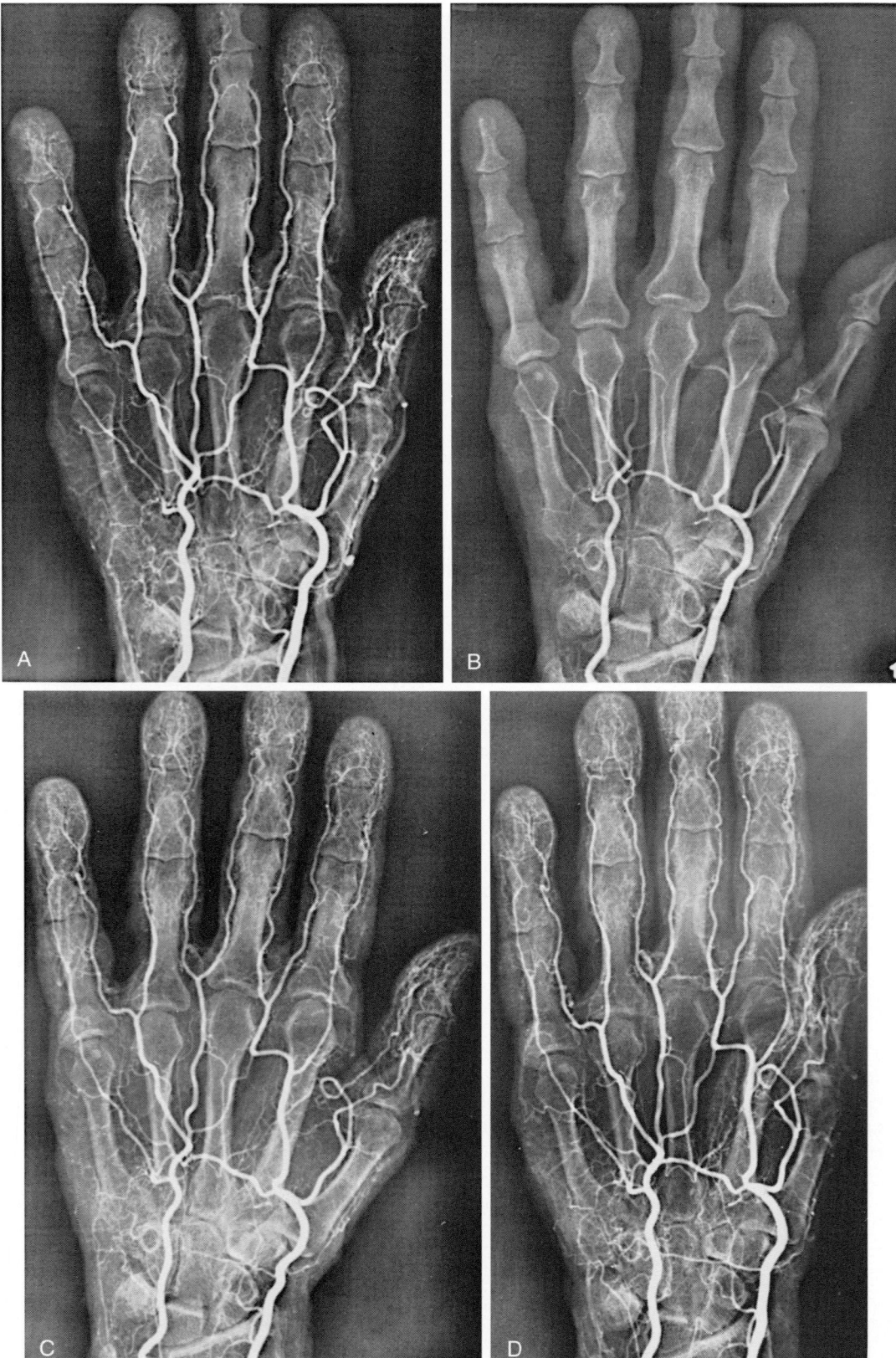

FIGURE 82–4. *A,* Hand arteriogram of a patient with Raynaud's syndrome before exposure to ice water. *B,* After ice water exposure, prominent resting vasospasm and a marked vasospastic response to cold are present. *C* and *D,* Arteriograms obtained 48 hours after intra-arterial injection of reserpine and before and after ice water exposure. Resting vasospasm has been completely eliminated, and there is a marked decrease in the vasospastic response to cold.

The beneficial effect of *intra-arterial reserpine* on RS was first reported by Abboud and associates in 1967.[1] Other investigators have confirmed the abilities of intra-arterial reserpine[2, 81, 108, 138] and tolazoline[101, 104] to improve certain difficult cases, including those with digital ulcers. The effect is generally short-lived, however, lasting from a few hours to a few weeks. Additionally, repeated intra-arterial drug injections are hazardous and present a cumulative risk of arterial damage. An example of the effect of reserpine on cold-induced vasospasm is shown in Figure 82–4.

Bier-block reserpine, with injection of the medication intravenously into the "extravasated" extremity under tourniquet control, has been reported to be safe and appears to be at least as effective as intra-arterial administration.[133] Unfortunately, parenteral reserpine is no longer available in the United States.

The difficulty of treating patients with RS who have associated digital ulceration has prompted investigations of less conventional modalities. Infusion of prostaglandin E (PGE), and prostaglandin I$_2$ (prostacyclin), both potent vasodilators and inhibitors of platelet aggregation,[129] has been studied by Clifford and associates[16, 17] and Pardy and associates,[98] with encouraging initial anecdotal results. Interestingly, a subsequent randomized, double-blind study of prostaglandin E in patients with RS without digital ulceration showed no benefit.[88] A study of an oral prostacyclin analogue demonstrated subjective, but not objective, improvement.[141]

Jarrett and coworkers used the fibrinolytic stimulating agent stanozolol in patients with RS, again with promising results.[61] This treatment, however, was selected because of high fibrinogen levels in a number of patients. High fibrinogen levels have seldom been observed by the authors or other investigators. Therefore, this experimental treatment is not expected to be generally applicable. Likewise, plasmapheresis has been used with satisfactory results in certain patients, supposedly on the basis of defibrination. Plasmapheresis may also affect lysis of established fibrin deposits, induced alterations of platelet function, or reduction of circulating immune complexes.[25, 96, 130] These treatments may be of great benefit to individual patients when unusual factors such as abnormal serum proteins or viscosity play dominant roles. However, they appear to be of little or no benefit in the majority of patients, who do not manifest these specific abnormalities.

Cervicothoracic sympathectomy has been performed frequently in past decades to treat both vasospastic RS and ischemic digital ulceration associated with small-artery occlusive disease.[23, 69, 76] The reported rates of response to sympathectomy vary much in different surgical series; generally, however, symptomatic recurrence has followed an initial period of improvement.[39, 44, 62] Whether this failure of long-term benefit is due to incomplete sympathectomy, regeneration of sympathetic nerves, or catecholamine hypersensitivity after denervation is unclear. Periarterial or local digital sympathectomy has been suggested as an alternative method of sympathectomy associated with fewer recurrences.[33] Local digital artery sympathectomy, performed by stripping the adventitia from distal digital arteries and by dividing the terminal sympathetic nerve branches using microscopic assistance, has been described in the treatment of finger ischemia.[30] These reports are anecdotal, and controlled clinical trials have not been conducted to compare this mode of therapy with others. In addition, distal microsurgical sympathectomy, like the proximal cervicothoracic procedure, does not address the underlying arterial obstructive disease of patients with ischemic digital ulceration and has no effect on the fundamental local vascular deficit of patients with spastic RS. At present, the authors do not recommend or perform upper extremity sympathectomy for RS.

ASSOCIATED DISEASES

RS has been associated with a bewildering variety of clinical conditions (Table 82–2), which at first glance appear to have little relation to each other.[11] In the past, this array of disparate associated conditions significantly confounded the understanding of RS. It now appears clear that the associated conditions should be viewed as related to either vasospastic or obstructive RS. A majority of the conditions listed have an element of distal upper extremity small artery obstruction.

The type and severity of associated diseases that are encountered reflect, in significant part, local referral patterns. In the early years of their study,[105] when only the more severely symptomatic patients from the community were referred, the authors found an associated autoimmune disease in 80% of all patients with RS. As awareness of their continued interest in the condition spread, patients with milder symptoms of shorter duration were also referred. Accordingly, the incidence of associated connective

TABLE 82–2. DISORDERS REPORTED IN ASSOCIATION WITH RAYNAUD'S SYNDROME

Autoimmune connective tissue diseases	Obstructive arterial diseases
Dermatomyositis	Atherosclerosis
Henoch-Schönlein purpura	Buerger's disease
Hepatitis B antigen–induced vasculitis	Peripheral embolization
Mixed connective tissue disease	Atherosclerosis
Polyarteritis nodosa	Thoracic outlet syndrome
Polymyositis	Environmental conditions
Reiter's syndrome	Repetitive trauma
Rheumatoid arthritis	Vibration injury
Scleroderma-CREST syndrome	Cold injury
Sjögren's syndrome	Drug-induced (without arteritis)
Systemic lupus erythematosus	Ergots
Undifferentiated connective tissue disease	Beta-blocking drugs
Hypersensitivity angiitis (rapid-onset vascular occlusion)	Cytotoxic agents
Myeloproliferative disorders	Oral contraceptives
Leukemia	Miscellaneous disorders
Myeloid metaplasia	Chronic renal failure
Polycythemia rubra vera	Drug-induced vasculitis
Thrombocytosis	Vinyl chloride disease
Circulating globulins	Neurologic disorders
Cold agglutinins	Central
Cryoglobulinemia	Peripheral
Malignancy	Polyneuropathy
Macroglobulinemia	Neurofibromatosis
Multiple myeloma	Endocrine disorders
	Hematologic disorders
	Disseminated intravascular coagulation

CREST = calcinosis cutis, Raynaud's phenomenon, esophageal dysfunction, sclerodactyly, telangiectasia.

tissue disease in their patients dropped to approximately 30% and has been stable at this level in more recent years.

In the authors' experience and that reported from other referral centers, approximately 40% of patients with RS have the idiopathic variety caused by vasospasm alone and no evidence of associated small artery obstructive disease.[102–105] RS, however, may be the first symptom of an otherwise silent systemic illness. Therefore, careful long-term follow-up is prudent for all such patients, because the initial symptoms of Raynaud's attacks may antedate, by months or even years, the development of a detectable associated disease.[103] The prognosis for vasospastic RS is benign; in most patients, it is a nuisance condition only that carries no risk of subsequent tissue loss.

In 60% of patients with RS, an underlying disorder associated with palmar and digital artery occlusive disease can be diagnosed using the evaluation plan outlined earlier. The associated diseases found in the authors' most recently tabulated series of 631 patients with RS are shown in Table 82–3. In our experience and that of other referral centers,[102–105, 150] autoimmune connective tissue disorders are the most frequently diagnosed associated conditions, accounting for about 50% of associated diseases.

One third of patients with RS and connective tissue disease have scleroderma or a CREST (calcinosis cutis, Raynaud's phenomenon, esophageal dysfunction, sclerodactyly, telangiectasia) variant; the remainder suffer from one or more autoimmune diseases—mixed connective tissue disease, rheumatoid arthritis, systemic lupus erythemato-

sus, and Sjögren's syndrome, among many. A significant percentage of patients present with abnormal serologic study results and evidence of end-organ involvement but with no pattern associated with a classically defined syndrome; their conditions are classified as undifferentiated connective tissue disease. Other patients have signs and symptoms of more than one clinical syndrome and are categorized as having overlap syndromes.

The common pathophysiologic mechanism of RS in patients with connective tissue disorders is presumed to be patchy or transmural necrotizing vasculitis, possibly secondary to an antigen–antibody or autoantibody reaction.[11, 23] Subsequent inflammatory thrombosis results in areas of fibrous obliteration of multiple digital and palmar arteries. Once diffuse small artery obstruction is present, even a normal vasospastic response to cold induces a Raynaud's attack. Thus, most patients with RS and autoimmune disease appear to have obstructive RS. Early in the course of autoimmune disease, however, patients may manifest spastic RS before widespread small artery obstruction develops. It is estimated that RS is present in more than 80% of patients with scleroderma or mixed connective tissue disease, in 25% of those with rheumatoid arthritis, and in 20% of those with systemic lupus erythematosus.[25, 102, 127] Interestingly, there is currently no explanation for the predilection of autoimmune arteritis to affect the distal upper extremity arteries.

For a patient who presents for evaluation of RS and does not have a connective tissue disease at the time of initial presentation, the risk of subsequently developing a connective tissue disorder appears to depend principally on the presence or absence of other findings suggestive of connective tissue disease, such as positive antinuclear antibody titer, sclerodactyly, or abnormal nailfold capillary microscopy findings. The published reports of which the authors are aware are listed in Table 82–4. Combining these results gives an average risk of developing connective tissue disease of 6% at 3.3 years when there are no signs or symptoms at initial presentation and of 42% at 4 years when there is at least one sign of a connective tissue disease.

Many other obstructive arterial diseases may be associated with RS, including atherosclerosis and Buerger's disease (thromboangiitis obliterans). Upper extremity involvement is frequently reported in Buerger's disease; some 20% to 50% of these patients have associated obstructive RS.[5, 52, 55, 87] Distal embolization resulting in multiple palmar and digital arterial occlusions may result from a proximal innominate or subclavian artery lesion or, rarely, from arterial complications of thoracic outlet syndrome.[58, 107, 120] Various myeloproliferative disorders, including leukemia,[109, 118] myeloid metaplasia, thrombocytosis, and polycythemia rubra vera, may be associated with digital artery obstruction and RS.[93] Pathologic increases in any of the formed elements of the blood may lead to hyperviscosity and cellular sludging, and subsequently to small artery thrombosis.[42, 51] Hyperviscosity caused by circulating serum proteins has been described in numerous conditions and may result in digital ischemia in certain patients with multiple myeloma, cryoglobulinemia,[40] or an epithelial cell–derived malignancy.[48, 93, 132]

The occupational causes of RS are discussed in the section on epidemiology. Chronic vibration injury may cause

TABLE 82–3. ASSOCIATED DISORDERS IN 1137 PATIENTS WITH RAYNAUD'S SYNDROME (OREGON HEALTH SCIENCES UNIVERSITY CLINICAL RESEARCH CENTER, 1970–1987)

DISORDER	NO. OF CASES (%)
Idiopathic (pure vasospasm with no associated disease)	356 (31.3)
CTD	391 (34.4)
Scleroderma, CREST	131
Undifferentiated CTD	36
Mixed CTD	31
Rheumatoid arthritis	20
Systemic lupus erythematosus	30
Sjögren's syndrome	25
Positive ANA/ENA	108
Unknown CTD	10
Other diseases	389 (34.2)
Hypersensitivity angiitis (rapid-onset vascular occlusion)	27
Hematologic disorders	58
Malignancy (solid tumors)	15
Atherosclerosis obliterans	55
Buerger's disease	32
Frostbite	34
Vibration injury	37
Trauma	51
Hypothyroidism	20
Carpal tunnel syndrome	41
Hypothyroidism	18
Multiple sclerosis	2
	1137 (100)

CTD = connective tissue disease; CREST = calcinosis cutis, Raynaud's phenomenon, esophageal dysfunction, sclerodactyly, telangiectasia; ANA = antinuclear antibody; ENA = extractable nuclear antibody.

TABLE 82–4. RISK OF CONNECTIVE TISSUE DISEASE IN PATIENTS WITH RAYNAUD'S SYNDROME WITH NO OR 1 + SIGNS OF SUCH A DISEASE

AUTHOR	FOLLOW-UP (yr)	NO SIGN OF CTD		1+ SIGN OF CTD	
		N	% Progression	N	% Progression
Blain et al, 1951[10]	5+	100	25	—	—
Gifford and Hines, 1957[38]	2+	280	4.6	—	—
Harper et al, 1982[47]	2	37	2.7	17	35.3
Gerbracht et al, 1985[36]	3.7	75	2.7	12	16.7
Sheiner and Small, 1987[122]	3.5	78	0	19	15.8
Priollet et al, 1987[111]	4.7	49	0	24	58.3
Fitzgerald et al, 1988[29]	2.7	33	9	25	32
Kallenberg et al, 1988[64]	6	29	3.4	35	25.7
Wollersheim et al, 1989[147]	3.5	51	7.8	20	65
Gentric et al, 1990[35]	4	16	6.3	9	11
Weiner et al, 1991[144]	4	40	0	23	17.4

*CTD, connective tissue disease.

digital artery obstruction after long exposure.[59] The cause of the syndrome in patients exposed to vibration for only a short time may reflect smooth muscle alterations induced by vibratory shear stresses.[8, 119] With longer exposure, arterial obstruction appears to predominate. A Raynaud's-type syndrome, with associated swelling and pain on cold exposure, frequently follows frostbite injuries.[80]

Drug-induced RS appears to be principally vasospastic, as exemplified by effects of ergot and the beta-blockers.[31] The mechanism of action of cytotoxic[136] and anovulatory[27] drugs in RS is unclear. The precise cause of RS in patients with one or more of the associated diseases listed under the miscellaneous category in Table 82–2 is likewise unclear.

Of special interest has been a group of patients who present with endocrine abnormalities[11] and RS. The associated endocrine conditions seen to date in the authors' patient group include hypothyroidism, Graves' disease, Addison's disease, Cushing's disease, and hypofunctioning pituitary tumors. The temporal association of these conditions with the onset of RS in certain patients has suggested a causal relationship, although to date no pathophysiologic mechanism has been explained.

ISCHEMIC DIGITAL ULCERATION AND GANGRENE

Ischemic digital ulceration occurs infrequently. In the course of evaluating more than 1100 patients with RS since 1970, the authors have encountered more than 100 patients with finger gangrene caused by small artery occlusive disease.[72, 82, 86, 100] The underlying diagnoses established in these patients are listed in Table 82–5. Digital ulceration never results from vasospasm alone; it invariably signals an underlying disease associated with digital artery obstruction. In the authors' experience, the four most common associated diseases are connective tissue disorders, hypersensitivity angiitis, atherosclerosis, and Buerger's disease. More than half of patients with ischemic digital ulceration have connective tissue disease, and half of *them* suffer from scleroderma or the CREST variant.

Hypersensitivity angiitis is an interesting condition characterized by the sudden onset of pain and digital cyanosis

with rapid progression to ulceration and finger gangrene[9] in a previously asymptomatic patient. Twenty-seven patients in the authors' series presented in this manner. All had documented fixed digital artery obstruction as demonstrated by plethysmography, angiography, or both, and in all patients, serologic test findings for autoimmune disease were intially negative. In five patients, serologic abnormalities developed during long-term follow-up and led to the diagnosis of an associated autoimmune condition. In 22 patients, however, all serologic test results remained consistently negative. Ischemic digital lesions healed with conservative treatment in all these patients, and no recurrences were noted on follow-up that extended up to 15 years. This syndrome has been termed *hypersensitivity angiitis with rapid-onset vascular occlusion.* The authors acknowledge that use of this term is speculative, and this condition does not manifest the florid necrotizing panarteritis or systemic symptoms associated with the traditional hypersensitivity angiitides. The clinical picture of sudden-onset digital ischemia without systemic toxicity, with relatively rapid resolution, and with lack of recurrence is consistent with an immune vasculitis with distribution limited to the digital and palmar arteries.

All patients with digital ischemia undergo routine upper extremity three-cuff vascular laboratory evaluation and recording of Doppler waveforms from the brachial, radial, ulnar, and digital arteries. Hand arteriography is performed selectively. When a patient has normal pulses to the wrist,

TABLE 82–5. UNDERLYING DIAGNOSIS ESTABLISHED IN 100 PATIENTS WITH ISCHEMIC FINGER ULCERATION SECONDARY TO SMALL ARTERY OCCLUSIVE DISEASE

DIAGNOSIS	NO. OF PATIENTS
Connective tissue disease	54
Hypersensitivity angiitis (ROVO)	22
Thromboangiitis obliterans (Buerger's disease)	9
Atherosclerosis obliterans	9
Malignancy	4
Combined atherosclerosis and connective tissue disorder	2
TOTAL	100

ROVO = rapid-onset vascular occlusion.

obstructive waveforms in all 10 fingers, and serologic abnormalities typical of autoimmune disease, arteriography is unlikely to show more than the palmar and digital artery obstructive disease documented by the noninvasive tests. The authors currently recommend arteriography only for patients with absent or diminished arm pulses, unilateral finger ischemia, or both. An example of hand arteriography showing marked arterial obstruction in a patient with finger ulceration is shown in Figure 82–5.

Treatment

Healing rates of 80% to 85% for ischemic digital ulcers have been reported after a variety of unconventional therapies, including sympathectomy and vasodilator drug infusion.[23, 68, 76] In the authors' series of 100 consecutive patients with ischemic finger ulceration and gangrene associated with small artery disease, a conservative treatment regimen without sympathectomy was used.[86] This simple regimen consisted of gentle soap-and-water scrubs, débridement of necrotic tissue, fingernail removal to facilitate drainage from areas of underlying infection, administration of culture-specific antibiotics, and delayed, length-conserving digital amputation débridement, as required. With this approach, complete healing without recurrence was achieved in 88% of patients. This outcome apparently

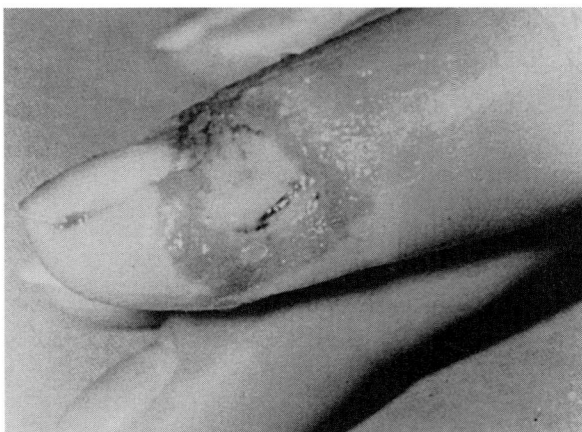

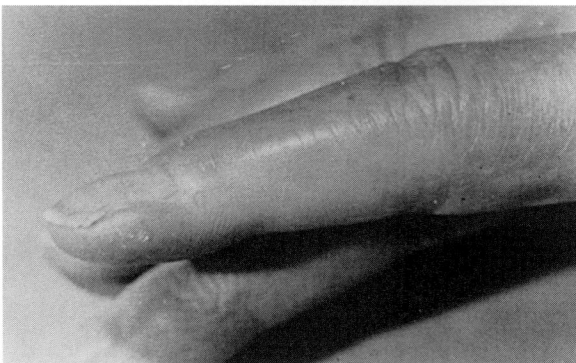

FIGURE 82–6. *Top* and *bottom,* Ischemic digital ulcer in a patient with scleroderma. Total healing was achieved using the conservative treatment regimen outlined.

reflects the natural history of the condition itself; certainly, it is not a specific response to this therapy. A representative photograph of a painful ischemic digital ulcer in a patient with digital artery obstruction is shown in Figure 82–6. Total healing was achieved in 4 weeks after conservative therapy. In the authors' experience, all recurrent digital ulcers have occured in patients with connective tissue disease, most often scleroderma. The authors find no evidence that cervicothoracic or periarterial digital sympathectomy or unconventional drug therapy is of any benefit, and we do not use them to treat ischemic finger ulcerations.

Microsurgical arterial reconstruction of palmar and digital arteries has been reported in a few patients,[123] but the diffuse pattern of involvement in most patients limits the application of this technique to an insignificant minority. Arteriovenous reversal at the wrist has also been reported in a small number of patients, but the reported results, and the authors' experience, do not warrant widespread use of this procedure.[67]

SUMMARY

RS consists of episodic digital pallor or cyanosis with associated numbness induced by cold or emotional stimuli. The condition affects, to some degree, 20% to 30% of persons in cool, damp climates, and a significant majority of affected persons are female. Available evidence suggests

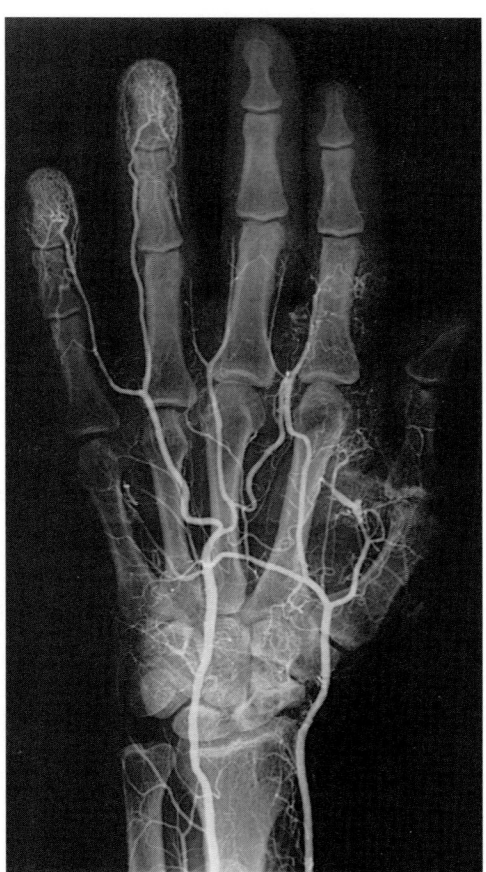

FIGURE 82–5. Hand arteriogram of a 44-year-old man with Buerger's disease, an ischemic digital ulcer, and Raynaud's syndrome. The widespread arterial obstruction is obvious. Compare this pattern with the vasoconstrictive pattern after cold exposure in Figure 82–4B.

that Raynaud's attacks may be produced by two distinct pathophysiologic mechanisms. In certain patients, the digital arteries appear normal, and episodic vasospasm is induced by abnormally forceful muscle contractions of the digital artery. Other patients have significant palmar and digital artery obstructive disease with diminished arterial pressure in the fingers. For them, a presumably normal cold-induced arterial contraction is sufficient to induce an attack. The treatment of RS is entirely symptomatic because no curative therapy is available. Approximately 90% of patients are adequately treated by cold and tobacco avoidance, and no drug therapy is necessary. For the remainder, the best results have been obtained with calcium channel blockers, specifically nifedipine, although drug treatment results in symptomatic improvement in only about 50% of patients and is frequently associated with significant side effects. There is currently no evidence that regional surgical sympathectomy has any long-term benefit for patients with RS.

A small number of patients develop severe finger ischemia, including ischemic finger ulceration, with or without RS. These patients all have severe palmar and digital artery obstructive disease caused by various associated processes. In the authors' experience, the most frequent ones are the arteritis of autoimmune connective tissue disease, hypersensitivity arteritis, arteriosclerosis, and Buerger's disease. The treatment of these patients has been conservative: local cleansing, antibiotics, and limited débridement, as required. There is no convincing evidence that sympathectomy or vasodilator drug therapy is of benefit in the treatment of digital ischemia.

REFERENCES

1. Abboud FM, Eckstein JW, Lawrence MS: Preliminary observations on the use of intra-arterial reserpine in Raynaud's phenomenon. Circulation 35:11, 1967.
2. Acevedo A, Reginato AJ, Schnell AM: Effect of intra-arterial reserpine in patients suffering from Raynaud's phenomenon. J Cardiovasc Surg 19:77, 1978.
3. Adams T, Smith RE: Effect of chronic cold exposure on finger temperature responses. J Appl Physiol 17:317, 1962.
4. Alexander S, Cummings C, Figg-Hoblyn L, et al: Usefulness of digital peaked pulse for diagnosis of Raynaud's syndrome. J Vasc Tech 12:71, 1988.
5. Allen EV, Brown GE: Thrombo-angiitis obliterans: A clinical study of 200 cases. Ann Intern Med 1:535, 1928.
6. Allen EV, Brown GE: Raynaud's disease: A critical review of minimal requisites for diagnosis. Am J Med Sci 1983:187, 1932.
7. Anderson CJ, Bardana EJ, Porter JM, et al: Anticentromere and antinuclear antibodies in Raynaud's syndrome. Clin Res 28:76A, 1980.
8. Azuma T, Onhashi T, Salsaguchi M: An approach to the pathogenesis of "white finger" induced by vibratory stimulation: Acute but sustained changes in vascular responsiveness of canine hindlimb to noradrenaline. Cardiovasc Res 14:725, 1980.
9. Baur GM, Porter JM, Bardana EJ, et al: Rapid onset of hand ischemia of unknown etiology: Clinical evaluation and follow-up of ten patients. Ann Surg 186:184, 1977.
10. Blain A III, Coller FA, Carver GB: Raynaud's disease: A study of criteria for prognosis. Surgery 29:387, 1951.
11. Blunt RJ, Porter JM: Raynaud's syndrome. Semin Arthritis Rheum 11:282, 1981.
12. Buchanan JL, Cranley JJ Jr, Linton RR: Observations on the direct effect of cold on blood vessels in the human extremity and its relation to peripheral vascular disease. Surgery 31:62, 1952.
13. Bunker CB, Terenghi G, Springall DR, et al: Deficiency of calcitonin gene–related peptide in Raynaud's phenomenon. Lancet 336:1530, 1990.
14. Chatterjee DS, Petrie A, Taylor W: Prevalence of vibration-induced white finger in fluorspar mines in Weardale. Br J Ind Med 35:208, 1978.
15. Chucker R, Fowler RC, Molomiza T, et al: Induced temperature gradients in Raynaud's disease measured by thermography. Angiology 22:580, 1971.
16. Clifford PC, Martin MFR, Dieppe PA, et al: Prostaglandin E$_1$ infusion for small vessel arterial ischemia. J Cardiovasc Surg 24:503, 1983.
17. Clifford PC, Martin MFR, Sheddon EJ, et al: Treatment of vasospastic disease with prostaglandin E$_1$. Br Med J 2:1031, 1980.
18. Coffman JD: Effect of vasodilator drugs in vasoconstricted normal subjects. J Clin Pharmacol 8:302, 1968.
19. Coffman JD: Total and nutritional blood flow in the finger. Clin Sci 42:243, 1979.
20. Coffman JD: Vasodilator drugs in peripheral vascular disease. N Engl J Med 300:713, 1979.
21. Coffman JD, Cohen AS: Total and capillary fingertip blood flow in Raynaud's phenomenon. N Engl J Med 285:259, 1971.
22. Cupps TR, Fauci AS: The Vasculitides. Philadelphia, WB Saunders, 1981, pp 116–118.
23. Dale WA: Occlusive arterial lesions of the wrist and hand. J Tenn Med Assoc 57:402, 1964.
24. deTakats G, Fowler EF: Raynaud's phenomenon. JAMA 179:99, 1962.
25. Dodds AJ, O'Reilly MJG, Yates CJP, et al: Hemorrheological response to plasma exchange in Raynaud's syndrome. Br Med J 2:1186, 1979.
26. Downs AR, Gaskell P, Morrow I, et al: Assessment of arterial obstruction in vessels supplying the fingers by measurement of local blood pressures and the skin temperature response test—Correlation with angiographic evidence. Surgery 77:530, 1975.
27. Eastcott HHG: Raynaud's disease and the oral contraceptive pill. Br Med J 2:447, 1976.
28. Edwards JM, Phinney ES, Taylor LM Jr, et al: Alpha-2 adrenergic receptor levels in obstructive and spastic Raynaud's syndrome. J Vasc Surg 5:38, 1987.
29. Fitzgerald O, Hess EV, O'Connor GT, Spencer-Green G: Prospective study of the evolution of Raynaud's phenomenon. Am J Med 84:718, 1988.
30. Flatt AE: Digital artery sympathectomy. J Hand Surg 5:550, 1980.
31. Frolich ED, Tarayi RC, Dutson MP: Peripheral arterial insufficiency as a complication of beta-adrenergic blocking therapy. JAMA 208:2471, 1969.
32. Fyhrquist F, Saijonmaa O, Metsarinne K, et al: Raised plasma endothelin-1 concentration following cold pressor test. Biochem Biophys Res Commun 169:217, 1990.
33. el-Gammal TA, Blair WF: Digital periarterial sympathectomy for ischaemic digital pain and ulcers. Hand Surg 16:382, 1991.
34. Gates KN, Tyburczy JA, Zupan T, et al: The non-invasive quantification of digital vasospasm. Bruit 8:34, 1984.
35. Gentric A, Blaschek MA, Le Noach JF, et al: Serological arguments for classifying Raynaud's phenomenon as idiopathic. J Rheumatol 17:1177, 1990.
36. Gerbracht DD, Steen VD, Ziegler GL, et al: Evolution of primary Raynaud's phenomenon (Raynaud's disease) to connective tissue disease. Arthritis Rheum 28:87, 1985.
37. Gifford RW Jr: Reserpine and Raynaud's phenomenon (Editorial). N Engl J Med 285:290, 1971.
38. Gifford RW Jr, Hines EA Jr: Raynaud's disease among women and girls. Circulation 16:1012, 1957.
39. Gifford RW Jr, Hines EA Jr, Craig WM: Sympathectomy for Raynaud's phenomenon: Follow-up study of 70 women with Raynaud's disease and 54 women with secondary Raynaud's phenomenon. Circulation 17:5, 1958.
40. Gjorup T, Kelbaek H, Hartling OJ, et al: Controlled double-blind trial of the clinical effect of nifedipine in the treatment of idiopathic Raynaud's phenomenon. Am Heart J 111:742, 1986.
41. Gorevic PD: Mixed cryoglobulinemia: Clinical aspects and long-term follow-up of 40 patients. Am J Med 69:287, 1980.
42. Goyle KG, Dormandy JA: Abnormal blood viscosity in Raynaud's phenomenon. Lancet 1:1317, 1976.
43. Graham MR: Methysergide for prevention of headache: Experience in five hundred patients over three years. N Engl J Med 270:67, 1964.

44. Hall KV, Hillestad LK: Raynaud's phenomenon treated with sympathectomy: A follow-up study of 28 patients. Angiology 11:186, 1960.
45. Halperin JL, Coffman JD: Pathophysiology of Raynaud's disease. Arch Intern Med 139:89, 1979.
46. Halpern A, Kuhn PH, Shaftel HE, et al: Raynaud's phenomenon and serotonin. Angiology 11:151, 1960.
47. Harper FE, Maricq HR, Turner RE, et al: A prospective study of Raynaud phenomenon and early connective tissue disease: A five-year report. Am J Med 72:883, 1982.
48. Hawley PR, Johnston AW, Rankin JT: Association between digital ischemia and malignant disease. Br Med J 3:208, 1967.
49. Henry LG, Blockwood JS, Cowley JE, et al: Ergotism. Arch Surg 110:929, 1975.
50. Heslop J, Coggon D, Acheson ED: The prevalence of intermittent digital ischaemia (Raynaud's phenomenon) in a general practice. J R Coll Gen Pract 33:85, 1983.
51. Hild DH, Myers TJ: Hyperviscosity in chronic granulocytic leukemia. Cancer 46:1418, 1980.
52. Hill GL, Moelino J, Tumewee F, et al: The Buerger syndrome in Java: A description of the clinical syndrome and some aspects of the aetiology. Br J Surg 60:606, 1973.
53. Hirai M: Cold sensitivity of the hand in arterial occlusive disease. Surgery 85:140, 1979.
54. Hirai M, Shinoya S: Arterial obstruction of the upper limb in Buerger's disease: Its incidence and primary lesion. Br J Surg 60:124, 1979.
55. Holling HE: Digital ischemia. In Peripheral Vascular Disease: Diagnosis and Management. Philadelphia, JB Lippincott, 1972, p 137.
56. Holmgren K, Baur GM, Porter JM: The role of digital photoplethysmography in the evaluation of Raynaud's syndrome. Bruit 5:19, 1981.
57. Hutchinson J: Raynaud's phenomena. Med Press Circ 123:403, 1901.
58. James EC, Khun NT, Fedde CW: Upper limb ischemia resulting from arterial thromboembolism. Am J Surg 137:739, 1979.
59. James PB, Galloway RW: Arteriography of the hand in men exposed to vibration. In Taylor W, Pelmear PL (eds): Vibration White Finger in Industry. London, Academic Press, 1975, p 31.
60. Jamieson GG, Ludbrook J, Wilson A: Cold hypersensitivity in Raynaud's phenomenon. Circulation 44:254, 1971.
61. Jarrett PEM, Morland M, Browse NL: Treatment of Raynaud's phenomenon by fibrinolytic enhancement. Br Med J 2:523, 1978.
62. Johnston ENM, Summerly R, Birnstingly M: Prognosis in Raynaud's phenomenon after sympathectomy. Br Med J 1:962, 1965.
63. Kahan A, Weber S, Amor B, et al: Nifedipine and Raynaud's phenomenon. Ann Intern Med 94:546, 1981.
64. Kallenberg CG, Wouda AA, Hoet MH, van Venrooij WJ: Development of connective tissue disease in patients presenting with Raynaud's phenomenon: A six-year follow-up with emphasis on the predictive value of antinuclear antibodies as detected by immunoblotting. Ann Rheum Dis 47:634, 1988.
65. Kaminski M, Bourgine M, Zins M, et al: Risk factors for Raynaud's phenomenon among workers in poultry slaughterhouses and canning factories. Int J Epidemiol 26:371, 1997.
66. Keenan EJ, Porter JM: Alpha-2 adrenergic receptors in platelets from patients with Raynaud's syndrome. Surgery 94:204, 1983.
67. King TA, Marks J, Berrettoni BA, Seitz WH: Arteriovenous reversal for limb salvage in unreconstructible upper extremity arterial occlusive disease. J Vasc Surg 17:924, 1993.
68. Kirtley JA, Riddell DH, Stoney WS, et al: Cervicothoracic sympathectomy in neurovascular abnormalities of the upper extremities. Experience in 76 patients with 104 sympathectomies. Ann Surg 165:869, 1967.
69. Kontos HA, Wasserman AJ: Effect of reserpine in Raynaud's phenomenon. Circulation 39:259, 1969.
70. Krahenbuhl B, Nielsen SL, Lassen NA: Closure of digital arteries in high vascular tone states as demonstrated by measurement of systolic blood pressure in the finger. Scand J Clin Lab Invest 37:71, 1977.
71. Lafferty K, deTrafford JC, Roberts VC, et al: Raynaud's phenomenon and thermal entrainment: An objective test. Br Med J 286:290, 1983.
72. Landry GJ, Edwards JM, McLafferty RB, et al: Long-term outcome of Raynaud's syndrome in a prospectively analyzed patient cohort. J Vasc Surg 23:76, 1996.
73. Leppert J, Aberg H, Ringqvist I, Sorensson S: Raynaud's phenomenon in a female population: Prevalence and association with other conditions. Angiology 38:871, 1987.
74. Lewis T: Experiments relating to the peripheral mechanism involved in spastic arrest of the circulation in the fingers, a variety of Raynaud's disease. Heart 15:7, 1929.
75. Lewis T, Pickering GW: Observations upon maladies in which the blood supply to digits ceases intermittently or permanently and upon bilateral gangrene of digits: Observations relevant to so-called Raynaud's disease. Clin Sci 1:327, 1933.
76. Machleder HI, Wheeler E, Barber WF: Treatment of upper extremity ischemia by cervico-dorsal sympathectomy. Vasc Surg 13:399, 1979.
77. Mackiewisz A, Piskorz A: Raynaud's phenomenon following long-term repeated action of great differences of temperature. J Cardiovasc Surg 18:151, 1977.
78. Maricq HR, Weinrich MC, Keil JE, LeRoy EC: Prevalence of Raynaud phenomenon in the general population. J Chron Dis 39:423, 1986.
79. Marshall AJ, Roberts CJC, Barritt DW: Raynaud's phenomenon as a side effect of beta-blockers in hypertension. Br Med J 1:1498, 1976.
80. Martinez A, Golding M, Sawyer P: The specific arterial lesion in mild and severe frostbite: Effect of sympathectomy. J Cardiovasc Surg 35:495, 1965.
81. McFadyen IJ, Housley E, MacPherson AIS: Intra-arterial reserpine administration in Raynaud's syndrome. Arch Intern Med 132:526, 1973.
82. McLafferty RB, Edwards JM, Taylor LM Jr, Porter JM: Diagnosis and long-term clinical outcome in patients presenting with hand ischemia. J Vasc Surg 22:361, 1995.
83. Merhoff CG, Porter JM: Ergot intoxication: Historical review and description of unusual clinical manifestations. Ann Surg 180:773, 1974.
84. Miller D, Waters DD, Warnica W, et al: Is variant angina the coronary manifestation of a generalized vasospastic disorder? N Engl J Med 304:763, 1981.
85. Miller-Schweinitzer E: Responsiveness of isolated canine cerebral and peripheral arteries to ergotamine. Arch Pharmacol 292:113, 1976.
86. Mills JL, Friedman EI, Taylor LM Jr, et al: Upper extremity ischemia caused by small artery disease. Ann Surg 154:123, 1987.
87. Mills JL, Taylor LM Jr, Porter JM: Buerger's disease in the modern era. Am J Surg 154:123, 1987.
88. Mohrland JS, Porter JM, Smith EA, et al: A multiclinic, placebo-controlled, double-blind study of prostaglandin E₁ in Raynaud's syndrome. Ann Rheum Dis 44:754, 1985.
89. Murdoch D, Brogden RN: Sustained release nifedipine formulations. Drugs 41:737, 1991.
90. Nerem RM: Vibration-induced arterial shear stress: The relationship to Raynaud's phenomenon of occupational origin. Arch Environ Health 26:105, 1973.
91. Nielsen SL, Lassen NA: Measurement of digital blood pressure after local cooling. J Appl Physiol 43:907, 1977.
92. Nobin BA, Nielsen SL, Eklov D, et al: Reserpine treatment of Raynaud's disease. Ann Surg 187:12, 1978.
93. O'Donnell JR, Keaveny TV, O'Connell LG: Digital arteritis as a presenting feature of malignant disease. Ir J Med Sci 149:326, 1980.
94. Okada A, Yamashita T, Nagano C, et al: Studies on the diagnosis and pathogenesis of Raynaud's phenomenon of occupational origin. Br J Ind Med 28:353, 1971.
95. Olsen N, Nielsen SL: Prevalence of primary Raynaud phenomena in young females. Scand J Clin Lab Invest 37:761, 1978.
96. O'Reilly MJG, Talops G, Robert VC, et al: Controlled trial of plasma exchange in treatment of Raynaud's syndrome. Br Med J 1:1113, 1979.
97. Pancera P, Sansone S, Secchi S, et al: The effects of thromboxane A₂ inhibition (picotamide) and angiotensin II receptor blockade (losartan) in primary Raynaud's phenomenon. J Int Med 242:373, 1997.
98. Pardy BJ, Lewis JD, Eastcott HHG: Preliminary experience with prostaglandins E₁ and I₂ in peripheral vascular disease. Surgery 88:826, 1980.
99. Peacock JH: The treatment of primary Raynaud's disease of the upper limb. Lancet 2:65, 1960.
100. Porter JM: Upper extremity digital gangrene caused by small artery occlusion. In Machleder HI (ed): Vascular Disorders of the Upper Extremity. Mt. Kisco, NY, Futura Publishing, 1983, p 107.
101. Porter JM: Raynaud's syndrome. In Sabiston DC Jr (ed): Textbook of Surgery, 13th ed. Philadelphia, WB Saunders, 1986, p 1925.
102. Porter JM, Bardana EJ Jr, Baur GM, et al: The clinical significance of Raynaud's syndrome. Surgery 80:756, 1976.
103. Porter JM, Friedman EI, Mills JL Jr: Raynaud's syndrome: Current concepts and treatment. Med Trib Ther 29:23, 1988.

104. Porter JM, Rivers SP, Anderson CJ, et al: Evaluation and management of patients with Raynaud's syndrome. Am J Surg 142:183, 1981.

105. Porter JM, Snider RL, Bardana EJ, et al: The diagnosis and treatment of Raynaud's phenomenon. Surgery 77:11, 1975.

106. Porter JM, Taylor LM Jr: Limb ischemia caused by small artery disease. World J Surg 7:326, 1983.

107. Porter JM, Taylor LM Jr, Friedman EI: Indications for cervical and first rib excisions. In Greenhalgh RM (ed): Indications in Vascular Surgery. Orlando, Fla, Grune & Stratton, 1987, pp 101–118.

108. Porter JM, Wesche D, Rosch J, et al: Intra-arterial sympathetic blockade in the treatment of clinical frostbite. Am J Surg 132:625, 1976.

109. Powell KR: Raynaud's phenomenon preceding acute lymphocytic leukemia. J Pediatr 82:539, 1973.

110. Prandoni AG, Moser M: Clinical appraisal of intra-arterial Priscoline therapy in the management of peripheral arterial diseases. Circulation 9:73, 1954.

111. Priollet P, Vayssairat M, Housset E: How to classify Raynaud's phenomenon: Long-term follow-up study of 73 cases. Am J Med 83:494, 1987.

112. Raynaud M: On local asphyxia and symmetrical gangrene of the extremities. In Selected Monographs. London, New Sydenham Society, 1888.

113. Rivers SP, Porter JM: Clinical approach to Raynaud's syndrome. Vasc Diagn Ther 4:15, 1983.

114. Rivers SP, Porter JM: Management of Raynaud's syndrome. In Bergan JJ (ed): Clinical Surgery International. New York, Churchill Livingstone, 1984, p 185.

115. Rivers SP, Porter JM: Raynaud's syndrome and upper extremity small artery occlusive disease. In Wilson SE, Veith FJ, Hobson RW, et al (eds): Vascular Surgery: Principles and Practice. New York, McGraw-Hill, 1987, p 696.

116. Rodeheffer RJ, Rommer JA, Wigley F, et al: Controlled double-blind trial of nifedipine in the treatment of Raynaud's phenomenon. N Engl J Med 308:880, 1983.

117. Rosch J, Porter JM, Gralino BJ: Cryodynamic hand angiography in the diagnosis and management of Raynaud's syndrome. Circulation 55:807, 1977.

118. Rudolph RI: Vasculitis associated with hairy-cell leukemia. Arch Dermatol 116:1077, 1980.

119. Schmid-Schonbein H: Critical closing pressure or yield shear stress as the cause of disturbed peripheral circulation? Acta Chir Scand 465(Suppl): 10, 1976.

120. Schmidt FE, Hewitt RL: Severe upper limb ischemia. Arch Surg 115:1188, 1980.

121. Shawket S, Dickerson C, Hazelman B, Brown MJ: Prolonged effect of CGRP in Raynaud's patients: A double-blind randomised comparison with prostacyclin. Br J Clin Pharmacol 32:209, 1991.

122. Sheiner NM, Small P: Isolated Raynaud's phenomenon: A benign disorder. Ann Allergy 58:114, 1987.

123. Silcott GR, Polich VL: Palmar arch arterial reconstruction for the salvage of ischemic fingers. Am J Surg 142:219, 1981.

124. Silman A, Holligan S, Brennan P, Maddison P: Prevalence of symptoms of Raynaud's phenomenon in general practice. Br Med J 301:590, 1990.

125. Singh S, de Trafford JC, Baskerville PA, Roberts VC: Digital artery calibre measurement—A new technique of assessing Raynaud's phenomenon. Eur J Vasc Surg 5:199, 1991.

126. Smith CD, McKendry RJR: Controlled trial of nifedipine in the treatment of Raynaud's phenomenon. Lancet 2:1299, 1982.

127. Strandness DE Jr: Episodic digital ischemia. In Peripheral Arterial Disease: A Physiologic Approach. Boston, Little, Brown, 1969, p 265.

128. Sumner DS, Strandness DE Jr: An abnormal finger pulse associated with cold sensitivity. Ann Surg 175:294, 1972.

129. Szczeklik A, Cryglewski RJ, Nizankowski R, et al: Prostacyclin therapy in peripheral arterial disease. Thromb Res 19:191, 1980.

130. Talpos G, White JM, Horrocks M, et al: Plasmapheresis in Raynaud's disease. Lancet 1:416, 1978.

131. Taylor LM Jr, Baur GM, Porter JM: Finger gangrene caused by small artery occlusive disease. Ann Surg 193:453, 1981.

132. Taylor LM Jr, Hauty MG, Edwards JM, et al: Digital ischemia as a manifestation of malignancy. Ann Surg 206:62, 1987.

133. Taylor LM Jr, Rivers SP, Keller F, et al: Treatment of digital ischemia with intravenous Bier block reserpine. Surg Gynecol Obstet 154:39, 1982.

134. Taylor W, Pelmear PL: Vibration White Finger in Industry. London, Academic Press, 1975.

135. Taylor W, Pelmear PL: Raynaud's phenomenon of occupational origin: An epidemiologic survey. Acta Chir Scand 465(Suppl):27, 1976.

136. Teutsch C, Lipton A, Harvey A: Raynaud's phenomenon as a side effect of chemotherapy with vinblastine and bleomycin for testicular carcinoma. Cancer Treat Rep 61:925, 1977.

137. Tietjen GW, Chien S, Leroy C, et al: Blood viscosity, plasma proteins, and Raynaud's syndrome. Arch Surg 110:1343, 1975.

138. Tindall JP, Whalen RE, Burton EE Jr: Medical uses of intra-arterial injections of reserpine: Treatment of Raynaud's syndrome and of some vascular insufficiencies of the lower extremities. Arch Dermatol 110:233, 1974.

139. Trubestein G, Wigger E, Trubestein R, et al: Treatment of Raynaud's syndrome with captopril. Detsch Med Wochenschr 109:857, 1984.

140. Varadi DP, Lawrence AM: Suppression of Raynaud's phenomenon by methyldopa. Arch Intern Med 124:13, 1969.

141. Vayssairat M: Controlled multicenter double blind trial of an oral analog of prostacyclin in the treatment of primary Raynaud's phenomenon: French Microcirculation Society Multicentre Group for the Study of Vascular Acrosyndromes. J Rheumatol 23:1917, 1996.

142. Velayos EE, Robinson H, Porciuncula FU, et al: Clinical correlation analysis of 137 patients with Raynaud's phenomenon. Am J Med Sci 262:347, 1971.

143. Waldo R: Prazosin relieves Raynaud's vasospasm. JAMA 241:1037, 1979.

144. Weiner ES, Hildebrandt S, Senecal JL, et al: Prognostic significance of anticentromere antibodies and anti-topoisomerase I antibodies in Raynaud's disease. A prospective study. Arthritis Rheum 34:68, 1991.

145. Wesseling H, denHeeten A, Wouda AA: Sublingual and oral isoxsuprine in patients with Raynaud's phenomenon. Eur J Clin Pharmacol 20:329, 1981.

146. Willerson JT, Thompson RH, Hookman P, et al: Reserpine in Raynaud's disease and phenomenon: Short-term responses to intra-arterial injection. Ann Intern Med 72:17, 1970.

147. Wollersheim H, Thien T, Hoet MH, Van Venrooy WJ: The diagnostic value of several immunological tests for anti-nuclear antibody in predicting the development of connective tissue disease in patients presenting with Raynaud's phenomenon. Eur J Clin Invest 19:535, 1989.

148. Yao JST, Gourmos C, Papathanasiou K, et al: A method for assessing ischemia of hands and fingers. Surg Gynecol Obstet 135:373, 1972.

149. Zamora MR, O'Brien RF, Rutherford RB, Weil JV: Serum endothelin-1 concentrations and cold provocation in primary Raynaud's phenomenon. Lancet 336:1144, 1990.

150. Zweifler AJ, Trinkaus P: Occlusive digital artery disease in patients with Raynaud's phenomenon. Am J Med 77:995, 1984.

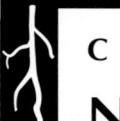

C H A P T E R   8 3

Neurogenic Thoracic Outlet Syndrome

Richard J. Sanders, M.D., Michael A. Cooper, M.D.,
Sharon L. Hammond, M.D., and Eric S. Weinstein, M.D.

CLASSIFICATION AND INCIDENCE

Thoracic outlet syndrome (TOS) is defined as upper extremity symptoms due to compression of the neurovascular bundle in the thoracic outlet area. The neurovascular bundle consists of three elements: nerves, artery, and vein. Each of these structures can be compressed separately and distinct symptom complexes are thus produced, each one different from the others. Therefore when using the term TOS, one should specify neurogenic, venous, or arterial TOS.

Neurogenic TOS is the most common form, constituting more than 95% of cases. Venous TOS makes up 2% to 3%, and arterial TOS about 1%. The symptoms, physical findings, and treatment of each form are different; thus, they are addressed in three separate chapters in this book.

HISTORY

Over the past 100 years, our understanding of TOS has changed considerably. What started out as an arterial disorder attributed to cervical ribs has been found to be a neurologic condition usually due to neck trauma.

The first description of TOS was published early in the 19th century, before the introduction of the term. In 1821, Sir Astley Cooper noted that subclavian artery thrombosis was due to compression by a cervical rib.[6] In the 19th century, this compression became known as cervical rib syndrome. In 1861, Coote performed the first cervical rib resection for the condition[7]; however, it was not until 1895, and the introduction of radiography, that recognition of this condition became generally available and case reporting became significant. By 1916, more than 100 cases of the syndrome had been recorded.[25]

After 1900, focus changed from the cervical rib as the cause of symptoms to other structures in the thoracic outlet area, such as the anterior and middle scalene muscles, first rib, and congenital bands. In patients without cervical ribs, first rib resection[2, 26, 50, 51] and division of congenital bands[17] proved effective.

In his classic article of 1947, Adson described performing division of the anterior scalene muscle rather than cervical rib resection in patients with cervical ribs. This major change in approach was an effort to avoid the frequent nerve complications that accompanied cervical rib resection. The article also describes "Adson's sign," obliteration of the radial pulse and hand paresthesia produced by rotating the head to the ipsilateral side and inspiring.[1]

By 1935, more symptomatic patients without cervical ribs were being recognized and treated with anterior scalenectomy; the term scalenus anticus syndrome became popular; and the relationship of trauma was noted.[27, 29] In 1923, middle scalenectomy was suggested,[50] and in 1943 compression between the clavicle and first rib, the costoclavicular syndrome, was described.[8] By 1956, so many causes of neurovascular compression in the thoracic outlet area had been recognized that there was a need for a single label that could encompass them all. The term thoracic outlet syndrome was introduced and rapidly accepted.[31, 32] In 1962, attention was refocused on first rib resection through a posterior approach,[5] but a few years later, the easier transaxillary and infraclavicular approaches were introduced.[13, 34] In the 1980s, it was realized that the results of first rib resection were no better than those of anterior and middle scalenectomy, and some surgeons have since returned to scalenectomy without rib resection for TOS. More recently, microscopic evidence of scalene muscle fibrosis in TOS patients gave support to the concept that the site of the lesion was in the scalene muscles, not the first rib.[23, 44]

ANATOMY

Three Spaces

The three main spaces in the thoracic outlet area are the scalene triangle, the costoclavicular space, and the pectoralis minor space (Fig. 83–1). The scalene triangle is the most common site of nerve compression. Its contents are the brachial plexus and subclavian artery. The space does not include the subclavian vein, which lies anterior to the anterior scalene muscle and posterior to the costoclavicular ligament. The costoclavicular space is traversed by all three structures: artery, vein, and nerve. The pectoralis minor space is outside the thoracic outlet area and is seldom involved in TOS.

Nerves

The brachial plexus is the central structure in the thoracic outlet area. It is derived from spinal nerves C5 to T1, and in the thoracic outlet area the five nerve roots combine to form three trunks: C5 and C6 fuse into the upper trunk; C8 and T1 join to form the lower trunk; and C7 continues as the middle trunk. It is compression of these nerves that produces the symptoms of neurogenic TOS.

Two other nerves in this area are of surgical importance. The phrenic nerve lies on the surface of the anterior scalene

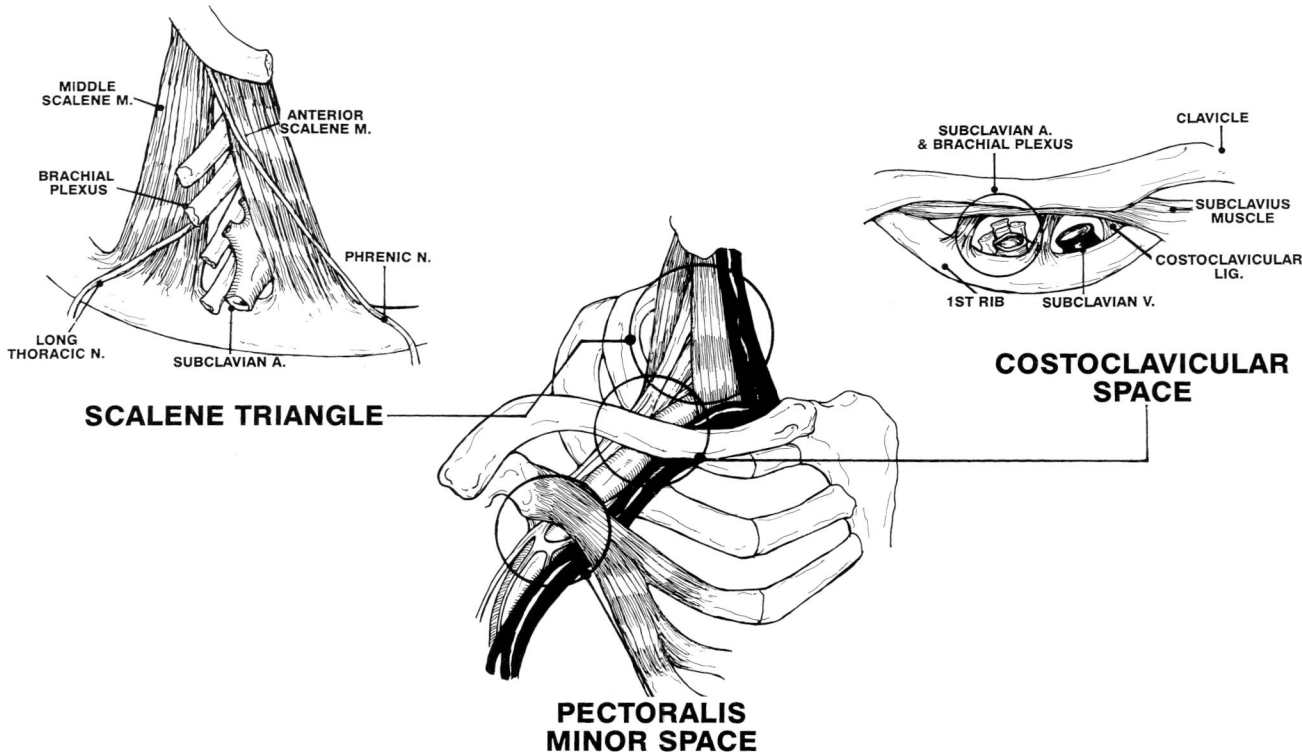

FIGURE 83–1. Anatomy of the thoracic outlet area demonstrating the three main spaces. (From Sanders RJ, Haug CE: Thoracic Outlet Syndrome: A Common Sequela of Neck Injuries. Philadelphia, JB Lippincott, 1991, p 34.)

muscle. It arises primarily from C4 and usually receives branches from C3 and C5. Thirteen per cent of people have a double phrenic nerve.[45] As the phrenic descends, 84% of the time it crosses from the lateral to the medial side of the anterior scalene muscle. It has the distinction of being the only nerve in the body that does not pass from medial to lateral. In 16% of patients, the phrenic nerve remains on the lateral side of the anterior scalene muscle.[45]

The *long thoracic nerve* arises primarily from C6 and usually gets branches from C5 and C7. It runs through the belly of the middle scalene muscle, where its three branches of origin are usually seen separately before they fuse to form a single nerve. The positions of the long thoracic nerve branches are variable. Most pass directly through the belly of the middle scalene muscle; others travel next to their nerve root for several inches before joining other branches.

Cervical and Rudimentary First Ribs

Cervical ribs lie in the midst of the middle scalene muscle. Their incidence in the normal population is 0.45% to 1.5%.[9, 49] For no apparent reason, 68% of all cervical ribs and 70% of all TOS conditions affect women. Cervical ribs are bilateral 63% to 80% of the time.[1]

Rudimentary first ribs are not as well known as cervical ribs, and, unless radiographs are carefully reviewed, rudimentary first ribs can be erroneously labeled cervical ribs. Their incidence averages 0.34%. Unlike cervical ribs, rudimentary first ribs occur equally among men and women.[38]

These ribs tend to lie higher in the neck than the normal first rib, and they often insert into the second rib rather than the sternum. The junction of the rudimentary first rib and second rib is frequently under the clavicle, where it can narrow the costoclavicular space, compress the subclavian artery, and produce arterial aneurysms or thrombosis.

Scalene Muscle Anomalies and Variations

Variations in the scalene muscle anatomy have been identified both in the normal population and in TOS patients. They are too common to be labeled anomalies and are more properly regarded as anatomic variations. Their role in producing symptoms is not clear. We postulate that scalene muscle anatomy most likely is a predisposing factor for nerve compression in the space through which the brachial plexus travels, making it easier for neck trauma to produce symptoms. Some of the more common variations are listed as follows:

1. The anterior scalene muscle frequently splits around C5 and C6.

2. A scalene minimus muscle is present 55% of the time.[15] It originates from the transverse processes of the lower cervical vertebrae, often runs with the anterior scalene muscle in front of C7, C8, and sometimes T1, and posterior to the subclavian artery, and inserts either on the first rib or into Sibson's fascia on top of the pleura.

3. Interdigitating fibers are common between the anterior and middle scalene muscles. These fibers run between the nerves of the brachial plexus.

4. The width of the space between the two scalene

muscles, where they insert on the first rib, varies from 0.3 to 2.0 cm.[24]

5. The anterolateral edge of the middle scalene muscle often has a fibrous band that presses against the lower trunk of the brachial plexus. Middle scalene muscle abnormalities have been observed in 58% of TOS patients.[52]

Congenital Bands and Ligaments

Fibrous bands and ligamentous structures are observed in many places in the thoracic outlet area. They can be simple fibrous thickenings in one of the scalene muscles or discrete bands not attached to muscles. Several separate bands have been identified and numbered, and they are quite common in normal healthy persons as well as patients with TOS. The first study of these bands in control subjects[35] noted an incidence of 37%. A more recent study[14] found the incidence to be 63%. In our opinion, the role of these bands in producing symptoms is similar to that of anatomic muscle variations: they are predisposing factors rather than primary causes.

HISTOPATHOLOGY

Microscopic studies of scalene muscles from patients with neurogenic TOS reveal two consistent findings:

1. Type 1 fiber predominance of 78% (normal is 49% to 56%), with atrophy and pleomorphism of type 2 fibers.
2. Increased endomesial fibrosis, averaging 36% in TOS patients as compared with only 14% in control subjects (Fig. 83–2).[23, 44]

These findings are significant because they are the first objective microscopic changes observed in TOS. It is postulated that they result from muscle injury and are consistent with the high incidence of neck trauma associated with TOS.

ETIOLOGY

The cause of arterial TOS is usually a cervical or rudimentary first rib. Primary venous TOS is generally due to the costoclavicular ligament and subclavius muscle compressing the subclavian vein. In contrast, neurogenic TOS is caused by a combination of (1) predisposing anatomic factors that narrow the thoracic outlet area and (2) neck trauma.

Predisposing Anatomic Factors

Cervical ribs are the best known of the predisposing factors. Most cervical ribs are asymptomatic. In one study, only 12% of 303 patients with cervical ribs had significant symptoms.[21] However, cervical ribs are a predisposing factor in neurogenic TOS in 4.5% of our patients. The incidence may be even higher in other studies, a significant observation because even 4.5% is several times the incidence of cervical ribs in the normal population.

Other predisposing factors for neurogenic TOS include rudimentary first ribs, congenital narrowing of the scalene triangle (Fig. 83–3), variations and anomalies of the anterior and middle scalene muscles, congenital bands, narrowing of the costoclavicular space between the first rib and clavicle, sagging shoulders, and even heavy breasts. The level at which nerves emerge from the scalene triangle may be a significant factor in the development of neurogenic TOS. One study showed that in 83% of patients operated on for TOS, the nerves emerged high, in the narrow part of the scalene triangle. In cadaver controls,[45] the site of emergence of the nerves was high in only 40%. These anatomic factors have been present since birth but usually cause no symptoms until some neck trauma occurs.

Neck Trauma

Neck trauma is the most common predisposing factor for neurogenic TOS with an incidence of close to 80%. The

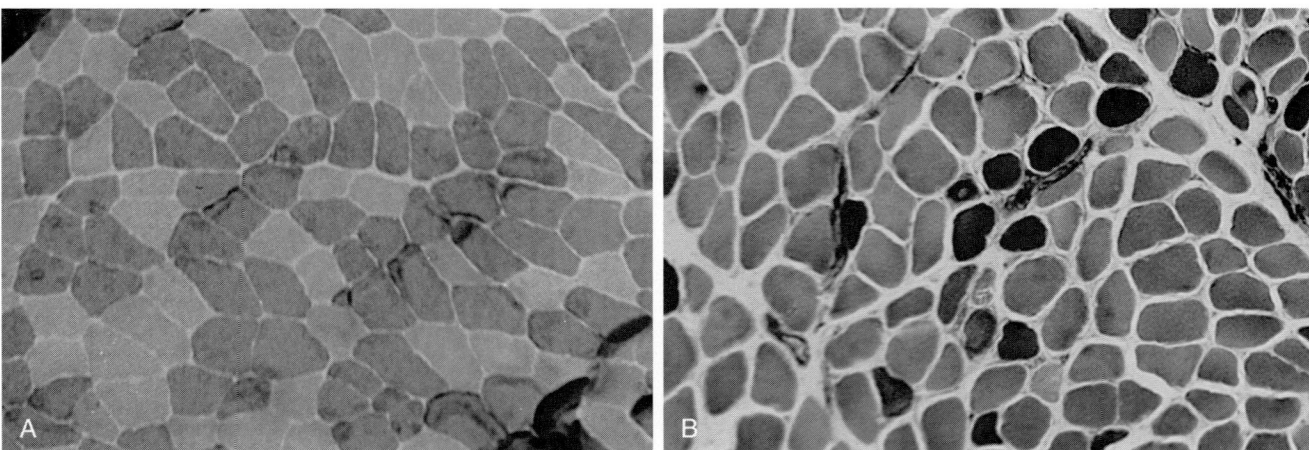

FIGURE 83–2. Scalene muscle histology. *A,* Control patient. *B,* Patient with thoracic outlet syndrome (TOS). Note the increase in connective tissue around each muscle fiber in the TOS patient. Note also the equal distribution of light and dark staining fibers (type 1 and type 2 fibers, respectively) in the control patient in contrast to the reduction in number and pleomorphism of the dark staining type 2 fibers. (From Sanders RJ, Jackson CGR, Banchero J, Pearce WH: Scalene muscle abnormalities in traumatic thoracic outlet syndrome. Am J Surg 159:231–236, 1990.)

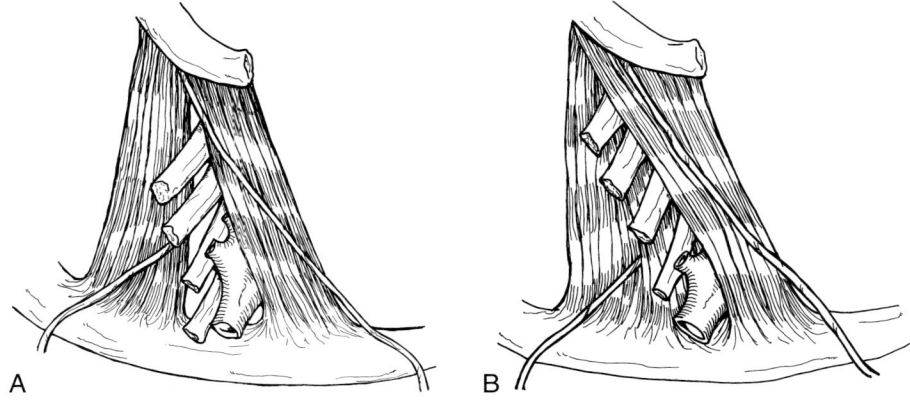

FIGURE 83–3. Variations in the scalene triangle. *A*, The usual relations found in most cadavers. The triangle is wider and the nerves emerge lower in the triangle than in most patients with thoracic outlet syndrome. *B*, A narrow triangle in which the nerves emerge high and are touching the muscles as they emerge. (From Sanders RJ, Roos DB: The surgical anatomy of the scalene triangle. Contemp Surg 35:11–16, 1989.)

two most common mechanisms of neck injury are automobile accidents, which result in hyperextension neck injuries, and repetitive stress injuries. Repetitive stress injuries may be sustained in occupations that require repetitive neck hyperextension and sudden neck stretching. Examples include keyboard jobs such as secretary and data entry clerk; cashier and shelf stocker; and assembly line work. Most of these tasks involve use of the arms and hands, but it is the repetitive movements and frequent jerking of the neck that lead to the scalene muscle injury.

PATHOPHYSIOLOGY

Most patients with neurogenic TOS report a history of a neck trauma. In patients who had acute injuries, neck pain usually appears within a few days; shoulder, chest wall, and arm pain, along with hand paresthesia and occipital headaches, develops in the next few days to weeks. Histologic studies reveal a loss of fast-twitch (type 2) muscle fibers and the development of endomesial fibrosis. In patients with repetitive stress injuries, development of symptoms is more gradual but follows a similar pattern.

It may be possible to explain these clinical observations in TOS with a single theory. Hyperextension neck injuries stretch the scalene muscles, causing hemorrhage and swelling in the muscle. This may lead to spasm and tightness that produce neck pain. Since the muscles arise from the transverse processes of the cervical spine, the muscle spasm may cause referred pain up the back of the neck to the occiput and lead to development of occipital headaches.

Because the nerves of the plexus are intimately involved with the scalene muscle bundles, the swollen, scarred, or spastic muscle fibers irritate the nerves, resulting in extremity pain and paresthesia. The distribution of the arm and hand symptoms depends on which nerves of the plexus are irritated.

Support for this theory includes the beneficial effects of the scalene muscle anesthetic block, the histologic changes observed in the scalene muscles of patients with TOS, and the long-term clinical improvement in two thirds of the patients who receive scalenectomy without first rib resection. When symptoms have been present for a number of years and (in the absence of pending litigation) the inciting trauma may have been forgotten, detailed questioning by the examiner is sometimes required to elicit information on the initial event.

SYMPTOMS

Demographics

Most patients with TOS are in the 20- to 45-year-old group; 70% are women. Patients in their teens as well as septuagenarians have been seen who have TOS, but it is rare at the extremes of life.

Paresthesia

The symptoms of neurogenic TOS are the same as those of nerve compression elsewhere in the body: pain, paresthesia, and weakness. Although ulnar nerve involvement is regarded as typical of TOS, our review of symptoms in several hundred patients revealed that compression of *all* nerves of the brachial plexus was the most common pattern. Next most common was ulnar nerve distribution (lower plexus), and least common was median nerve (upper plexus) involvement.[39]

Pain

Pain in the shoulder, arm, and forearm is a hallmark of neurogenic TOS. The location of the pain depends on which portion of the brachial plexus is compressed. It may follow the specific patterns of upper or lower plexus involvement, but often the picture is mixed. Pain in the neck is usually the result of scalene muscle injury and is associated with tenderness over the scalene muscles.

Headaches

Occipital headaches, which can radiate forward, are a common complaint, noted in 74% of TOS cases.[39] They probably reflect referred pain from the tight scalene muscles arising from the transverse processes of the cervical spine. In contrast, frontal headaches are not due to TOS.

Paraspinal Muscle Pain

Symptoms of pain over the trapezius and rhomboid muscles and around the scapula are common complaints with

TOS, although they usually are not due to brachial plexus compression. Such symptoms probably arise from fibromyalgia produced by the same trauma that caused the TOS or in some cases are due to dorsal scapular nerve compression by the middle scalene muscle.

Weakness

Weakness of the arm and hand is common in patients with TOS, who may complain of difficulty grasping and holding objects.

Vascular Symptoms

Two groups of symptoms are attributable to vascular disease. Claudication, ischemic ulcers, and gangrenous fingertips are indicative of arterial thrombosis and emboli. Cold hands, color changes, and mild swelling can also be symptoms of arterial occlusive disease, but most often they manifest increased sympathetic activity. Sympathetic nerve fibers accompany the lower roots of the brachial plexus, a fact that explains why symptoms of increased sympathetic activity are usually the result of nerve, not arterial, compression. Therefore, when coldness and color changes occur without other arterial symptoms, they usually are due to neurogenic, rather than arterial, TOS.

PHYSICAL EXAMINATION

Physical findings are easier to interpret in patients with unilateral symptoms; however, even with bilateral disease, positive physical findings are usually reliable.

Examination for Thoracic Outlet Syndrome

Positive findings of TOS on physical examination include weak grip strength, as measured by dynamometry; supraclavicular tenderness over the scalene muscles of the involved side; Tinel's sign over the brachial plexus in the supraclavicular area; and radiating pain or paresthesia in the ipsilateral upper extremity in response to pressure over the scalene muscles. Rotating the head, and tilting the head, away from the involved side often produces radiating pain or paresthesia in the contralateral extremity. Abducting the arms to 90 degrees in external rotation (the 90-degree abduction and external rotation [AER], or "stick-em-up," position) reproduces the symptoms in the involved extremity. Reduced sensation to light touch is often demonstrable in the involved fingers in unilateral TOS.

Adson's Sign

Loss of the radial pulse in dynamic positions, such as Adson's maneuver or 90-degree AER, is frequently said to be an important physical finding and often is used to establish or eliminate the diagnosis of neurogenic TOS. This observation is not reliable. Adson's "infallible sign," described in 1947, has been refuted by numerous investigators since 1945. Studies of normal subjects have revealed that 13% to 53% may be able to obliterate their pulses

with such a maneuver. This compares to an average of 31% of persons with TOS who have positive vascular findings.[11, 40]

Other Conditions

Physical examination should include observations of other areas for findings that often accompany TOS:

1. Tenderness over the biceps or rotator cuff tendons suggests tendinitis.
2. Inability to abduct the arm to 180 degrees suggests acromioclavicular joint impingement syndrome.
3. Tenderness over trapezius or rhomboid muscles indicates fibromyalgia.
4. Head tilting that elicits pain or paresthesia in the ipsilateral arm or hand suggests cervical disc disease.
5. Tenderness over the vertebrae may signify cervical and dorsal spine strain.
6. Paresthesia or pain on vertex compression is a sign of cervical disc herniation.
7. Tinel's and Phelan's signs in the wrist may indicate carpal tunnel syndrome.
8. Tenderness over the elbows often means epicondylitis.
9. Tinel's sign over the ulnar nerve at the elbow suggests cuboid tunnel syndrome.
10. Tenderness and Tinel's sign over the pronator and radial tunnels of the forearms may denote nerve compression in these areas.
11. Tenderness over the pectoral muscles suggests pectoralis minor compression.

Atrophy

Atrophy of intrinsic hand muscles innervated by the ulnar nerve is seldom seen with TOS but does occur in a few patients. Atrophy is due to constant pressure on the ulnar nerve, usually from a cervical rib or cervical band. In most cases of TOS, nerve compression is mild. It is strong enough to cause irritation that produces pain and paresthesia but not strong enough to elicit neurophysiologic diagnostic changes and muscle atrophy.

DIAGNOSTIC TESTS

Scalene Muscle Block

Injection of 4 ml of 1% lidocaine into the belly of the anterior scalene muscle was first described in 1939 as a diagnostic test for TOS.[10] A positive response is improvement in physical findings: less pain on neck rotation, head tilt, and 180-degree abduction of the arms; less tenderness over biceps and rotator cuff tendons; and delayed and less intense hand and arm symptoms on positioning the arms in 90 degrees of AER.

In the injection, the needle is directed into the tender area over the anterior scalene muscle and cephalad, beginning just above the clavicle (Fig. 83–4). Aiming the needle straight in can puncture the pleura and produce pneumothorax. Aspirating before injecting is important, lest the

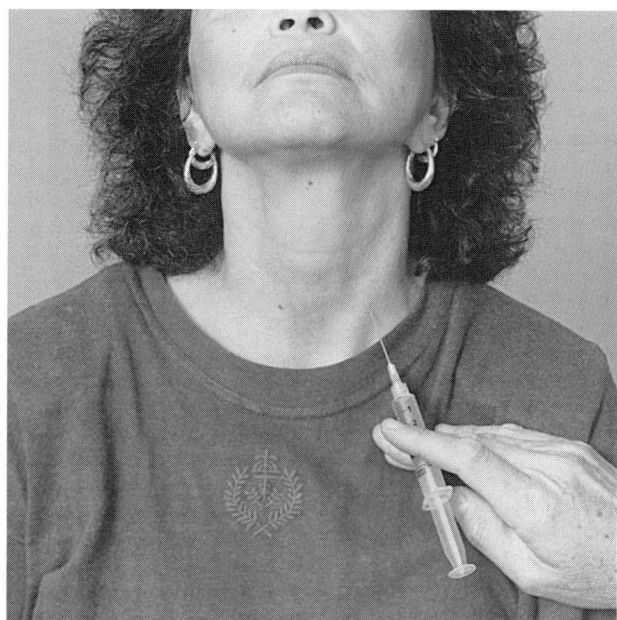

FIGURE 83–4. Scalene muscle block. A No. 22 needle is inserted 2 cm above the clavicle and about 3 cm lateral to the midline, selecting a point directly over the area of scalene tenderness. Four ml of 1% lidocaine is injected into the anterior scalene muscle, constantly moving the needle throughout the injection. (From Sanders RJ, Haug CE: Thoracic Outlet Syndrome: A Common Sequela of Neck Injuries. Philadelphia, JB Lippincott, 1991, p 92.)

jugular vein or an arterial branch be entered. When this misadventure occurs, the needle is withdrawn a few millimeters and redirected. With this technique, in our experience with more than 3000 injections, there have been three cases of pneumothorax and no complications from bleeding.

A good block is indicated by loss of tenderness over the "injected" scalene muscle. If tenderness persists, the block is repeated, and, then, if tenderness still persists, the block is abandoned and no conclusions are drawn. A good response to the scalene muscle block has a 94% correlation with a good early response to surgical decompression of the thoracic outlet area.[41] When there is a poor response to the block, surgery is approached more cautiously and performed only when other clinical criteria are strong.

Neurophysiologic Testing

Although neurogenic TOS is a neurologic condition, it seldom is severe enough to cause neurophysiologic changes, and, when it does produce changes, they are usually nonspecific. Electromyography (EMG) is primarily a measure of motor, not sensory, nerve function. Since in most cases of TOS sensory function is principally involved, EMG findings are usually normal. F-wave responses, nerve conduction velocity (NCV), and somatosensory evoked potentials (SSEP) all measure the responses to various forms of nerve stimulation. When results are positive, they are usually nonspecific. While some reports have favored NCV[54] and SSEP,[22] other investigators have refuted these findings.[16, 55, 56]

Fewer than 1% of patients with TOS have muscle atro-

phy of the intrinsic hand muscles innervated by the ulnar nerve. In patients with atrophy, there is no standard electrophysiologic finding; such findings will evolve with the severity of the syndrome. In those few cases when electrophysiologic changes are present, the first abnormality is observed in the F wave, then in sensory potentials, and finally on EMG. Nerve conduction patterns are the last to change.[30] Unfortunately, once the condition has produced muscle atrophy, surgical correction cannot restore muscle tone; it can only relieve pain and paresthesia. In summary, neurophysiologic studies cannot rule out a diagnosis of neurogenic TOS, and only in patients with muscle atrophy can they confirm one.

Angiography and Vascular Laboratory Studies

Arteriography and venography are indicated to investigate suspected arterial or venous TOS. They are not indicated and have no diagnostic value in neurogenic TOS. The same is true for vascular laboratory studies. Obliteration of the radial pulse can be confirmed by positional studies with a pulse-volume recorder, but it is merely an expensive way to document observations that can be made by palpating the radial pulse in the same elevated positions. Obliteration of the radial pulse by dynamic positioning occurs with about the same frequency in asymptomatic persons and in patients with TOS. Thus, these studies cannot be relied upon to either confirm or rule out neurogenic TOS.

Radiography

Cervical spine films can detect cervical and abnormal first ribs. They may also reveal cervical spine disease, which must be distinguished from TOS.

Cross-Sectional Imaging

Magnetic resonance imaging (MRI) and computed tomography (CT) are helpful in diagnosing herniated cervical discs and spinal stenosis. Neither modality, however, help establish a diagnosis of TOS.

ASSOCIATED AND DIFFERENTIAL DIAGNOSES

Because TOS is often caused by trauma, it is not unusual for TOS to coexist with other conditions. Therefore, in considering the differential diagnosis, one must also think of associated diagnoses. These are some of the conditions to keep in mind:

1. *Shoulder tendinitis or acromioclavicular impingement syndrome.* This finding is suggested by reduced shoulder range of motion and tenderness over the biceps and rotator cuff tendons. Shoulder radiography and MRI are helpful here.

2. *Carpal tunnel and Guyen's tunnel syndromes.* Tinel's and Phelan's signs at the wrist are an indication for neurophysiologic studies to confirm these diagnoses.

3. *Cuboid tunnel syndrome, or ulnar nerve entrapment at*

the elbow. Tenderness and Tinel's sign over the medial epicondyle may indicate epicondylitis; positive neurophysiologic tests confirm nerve entrapment.

4. *Epicondylitis.* The finding can occur at either the medial or the lateral epicondyle. The diagnostic sign is tenderness over the epicondyle.

5. *Pronator and radial tunnel syndromes.* Tenderness and Tinel's sign over these tunnels suggest nerve entrapment of the median and radial nerves, respectively, in the forearm. Neurophysiologic testing confirms these diagnoses.

6. *Fibromyalgia of the trapezius muscles* is commonly associated with TOS and is revealed by pain and tenderness over these muscles.

7. *Cervical spine strain.* This finding is commonly seen with whiplash injuries and is a clinical diagnosis, without positive objective findings, much like TOS. Neck stiffness and reduced range of motion should raise suspicion of this diagnosis.

8. *Cervical disc disease, arthritis, and spinal stenosis.* Symptoms may be improved rather than aggravated by arm elevation (as in TOS). Head tilting causes symptoms in the ipsilateral extremity, whereas in TOS, head tilting elicits symptoms in the contralateral side; and vertex compression reproduces the arm symptoms. The examiner should think of this when symptoms are limited to the thumb and index finger. These conditions are recognized by neck radiography, cross-sectional imaging, and sometimes myelography.

9. *Brachial plexus stretch injury.* This finding is uncommon but is suggested by a history of arm stretching; it can be difficult to diagnose. Neurophysiologic testing is used for diagnosis, but when the condition is mild, even these findings may be normal.

MAKING THE DIAGNOSIS

Most patients with neurogenic TOS exhibit only subjective physical findings on which a diagnosis can be based. Objective findings—cervical ribs, hand atrophy, specific abnormalities on electrophysiological testing, and obliterated pulses in dynamic positions—are present in only a small percentage of cases. It is the absence of these objective findings that leads some concerned physicians to question the diagnosis of TOS. It must be stressed, however, that the presence of these objective findings *alone* cannot establish a diagnosis. The diagnosis of neurogenic TOS can be made only when objective findings are supported by subjective symptoms and physical findings.

In the more than 35 years since first rib resection was reintroduced to treat neurogenic TOS,[52] increased awareness has developed of the many soft tissue abnormalities found in TOS patients that defy preoperative objective testing.[18] Many published studies of the symptoms, signs, therapies, and complications of this condition have provided clinicians with a good database from which a balanced approach to diagnosis has evolved.

TOS should not be regarded as simply a diagnosis of exclusion. Most affected persons exhibit a recognizable pattern of history, symptoms, and physical findings. Conditions that do not fit this pattern should be labeled neurogenic TOS only with caution.

The diagnosis of neurogenic TOS is a clinical one. The typical history is as follows: After a motor vehicle accident or some other type of hyperextension neck injury, symptoms of neck and shoulder pain develop within a few days. Occipital headaches, arm pain, hand paresthesia, and weakness occur within the first few days to weeks. Elevating the arm, to do such things as drive a car or comb one's hair, aggravates the symptoms.

Physical findings present in almost all patients include scalene muscle tenderness, Tinel's sign and positive pressure test over the brachial plexus, and reproduction of the patient's symptoms with the arms in the 90-degree AER position. Other conditions that produce symptoms similar to those of TOS must be investigated to see if they are associated with, or should be distinguished from, TOS.

All of these historical features and physical findings may not be present in every patient, but the absence of hand paresthesia or a history of some type of neck trauma should make the examiner hesitate to make this diagnosis. Although neurogenic TOS does exist without them, both are present in the large majority of patients with TOS. Repetitive stress at work can be a subtle form of neck trauma.

TREATMENT

Conservative Treatment
Stretching, Physical Therapy, and Medication

Therapy for TOS should always begin with nonoperative modalities. The therapy we have found most effective is a home exercise program of (1) neck stretching, (2) abdominal breathing, and (3) posture exercises. Theoretically, abdominal breathing and correct posture help to relax the neck muscles, which are accessory muscles of respiration. After instruction from a physical therapist, the patient performs the stretches at least twice a day at home, taking care to perform each stretch slowly, to hold it for at least 15 seconds, and to do no more than three repetitions at any session. Therapies we have found ineffective include shoulder shrugs, lifting light weights, and neck traction. In fact, strengthening exercises, theraband stretching, and exercising against resistance have made many patients worse.

Drugs should be prescribed for pain relief, muscle relaxation, sleep, and depression. Ergonomic evaluation of work stations may help to minimize aggravating the symptoms. Other important recommendations that all patients should receive include avoiding heavy lifting, repetitive movements, and working with the arms above shoulder level. In some cases, work tasks or occupation may require modification or change. Pain clinics and biofeedback are other modalities that can be offered for pain relief. Finally, all associated conditions should be recognized and treated.

Conservative treatment should be continued until symptoms have "plateaued" for a few months. If the intensity of symptoms has been reduced enough so that the patient can learn to live with them, conservative therapy, particularly neck stretching, should be continued indefinitely.

Results

The majority of patients managed conservatively improve significantly. In one study of patients who had symptoms for an average of 38 months, 25 of 42 improved, 10 had no change, and seven were worse.[28]

Surgical Treatment

Indications

The indications for surgical decompression of the thoracic outlet area include failure of conservative therapy after a minimum of several months; completion of treatment of all associated conditions; and symptoms that are disabling for work, recreation, or activities of daily living. In our practice, we seldom operate on any patient who has had symptoms for less than a year, and many patients have had symptoms for more than 2 years.

Choice of Operation

The goal of surgery is to decompress the brachial plexus, which is accomplished by removing one or more sides of the scalene triangle. Transaxillary first rib resection is probably the most common operation currently performed for neurogenic TOS, but other operations performed through a supraclavicular approach are just as effective and may carry fewer risks and complications. These procedures include anterior and middle scalenectomy, which may be performed alone or with supraclavicular first rib resection. The various operations are described next.

Total Anterior and Middle Scalenectomy

Following general anesthesia and intratracheal intubation, all muscle relaxants are stopped so that the patient is not paralyzed. This is important because it permits the arm or diaphragm to contract if the surgeon pinches or irritates motor nerves. The patient is placed in semi-Fowler's position with the back and neck elevated about 20 degrees from the horizontal. The head is tilted slightly toward the operated side to relax the brachial plexus and then rotated slightly to the opposite side. Often, the wrists are placed on top of the abdomen, overlapped, and gently strapped together to aid shoulder elevation. A folded bath towel is placed beneath the shoulder to elevate the clavicle. A small rolled towel is placed beneath the dorsal spine to extend the spine (Fig. 83–5A).

A 6- to 8-cm supraclavicular transverse incision is made 2 to 3 cm above the clavicle, beginning 1 cm lateral to the midline. The platysma is divided, and the external jugular vein is preserved (Fig. 83–5B). Skin flaps are elevated 4 to 5 cm cephalad and to the clavicle caudad. A Gelpi retractor spreads the skin flaps vertically. The lateral edge of the sternocleidomastoid is freed from the clavicle cephalad as high as possible; division of the clavicular head is unnecessary. The scalene fat pad is divided vertically, at least 1 cm away from the internal jugular vein to avoid the lymphatics that lie next to the vein (Fig. 83–5C). The omohyoid muscle is divided, and a 2- to 3-cm segment is resected to avoid postoperative adherence of the ends of this muscle. A self-retaining miniframe retractor (Omni-Tract Surgical, Minnesota Scientific, Minneapolis) is positioned (Fig. 83–6A).

When present, the transverse cervical artery is ligated and divided. All other bleeding is controlled with a bipolar cautery device. The phrenic nerve is identified on the surface of the anterior scalene muscle and carefully mobilized by dividing connective tissue 2 mm on either side of the nerve without touching the nerve. The phrenic can now be pushed away gently as needed. Placing identifying sutures around the nerve is unnecessary, and they can cause damage if accidentally pulled. During dissection, if the phrenic nerve is in the way, it can be gently elevated with a vessel loop held manually. Double phrenic nerves are always sought, and both branches are preserved when found.

The medial and lateral edges of the anterior scalene muscle are freed, and the muscle divided at its insertion on the first rib (Fig. 83–5D). The lowest muscle fibers lie on the pleura and must be divided carefully to avoid entering it. The muscle is elevated and dissected off the subclavian artery; adhesions to the brachial plexus and interdigitating fibers with the middle scalene muscle are divided; and the muscle is passed below the phrenic nerve and regrasped above it. The muscle origins are divided near the transverse processes (which are not seen but can be felt), and the anterior scalene is removed (Fig. 83–5E).

Brachial plexus neurolysis is performed next on the anterior surface of the plexus. All remaining muscle fibers, bands, and connective tissue over C5 to C7 are excised. The space between C7 and the subclavian artery is dissected free (Fig. 83–5F). It is here that scalene minimus muscle and congenital bands are often found lying over the C8 and T1 nerve roots. All tissue is excised. The transverse scapular artery, frequently encountered arising from the subclavian artery, is ligated flush with the subclavian artery. Its distal end is ligated lateral and posterior to the plexus.

Middle scalenectomy is begun by mobilizing C5 and gently elevating it. The surface of the middle scalene muscle is inspected, and branches of origin of the long thoracic nerve are identified. This often requires gently dissecting the middle scalene fibers to find the branches of origin from C5, C6, and sometimes C7. The dorsal scapular nerve is often seen near the C5 branch. The nerves are kept in view as the lateral half of the middle scalene is divided cephalad at the level of the long thoracic nerve crossing (Fig. 83–5G). The lower end is divided at its first rib insertion. The medial half of the middle scalene is removed next by dividing it on the first rib and again at its origin from the transverse processes. Use of a pediatric oral sucker tip to gently retract the plexus aids in middle scalenectomy. When present, a cervical rib lies in the midst of the middle scalene and is removed with a rongeur as it is encountered (Fig. 83–5H). Neurolysis of the posterior surfaces of the five nerve roots is the final step.

Thus, anterior and middle scalenectomy is completed. The lung is expanded, and any opening in the pleura is noted. A small, round (10 French) suction drain is positioned behind the plexus, and, if the pleura was opened, the end is placed inside the pleura and the lung expanded. The drain exits through the fat pad and out the lateral corner of the wound. The drain is maintained on bulb suction until all drainage stops, usually in 24 to 48 hours. A drain is routinely used, because bloody drainage averages 50 to 75 ml in almost all cases, even when the wound is totally dry at closing. The scalene fat pad is reapproximated in its normal position without attempts to wrap the plexus in fat. We have found that the fat does not prevent postop-

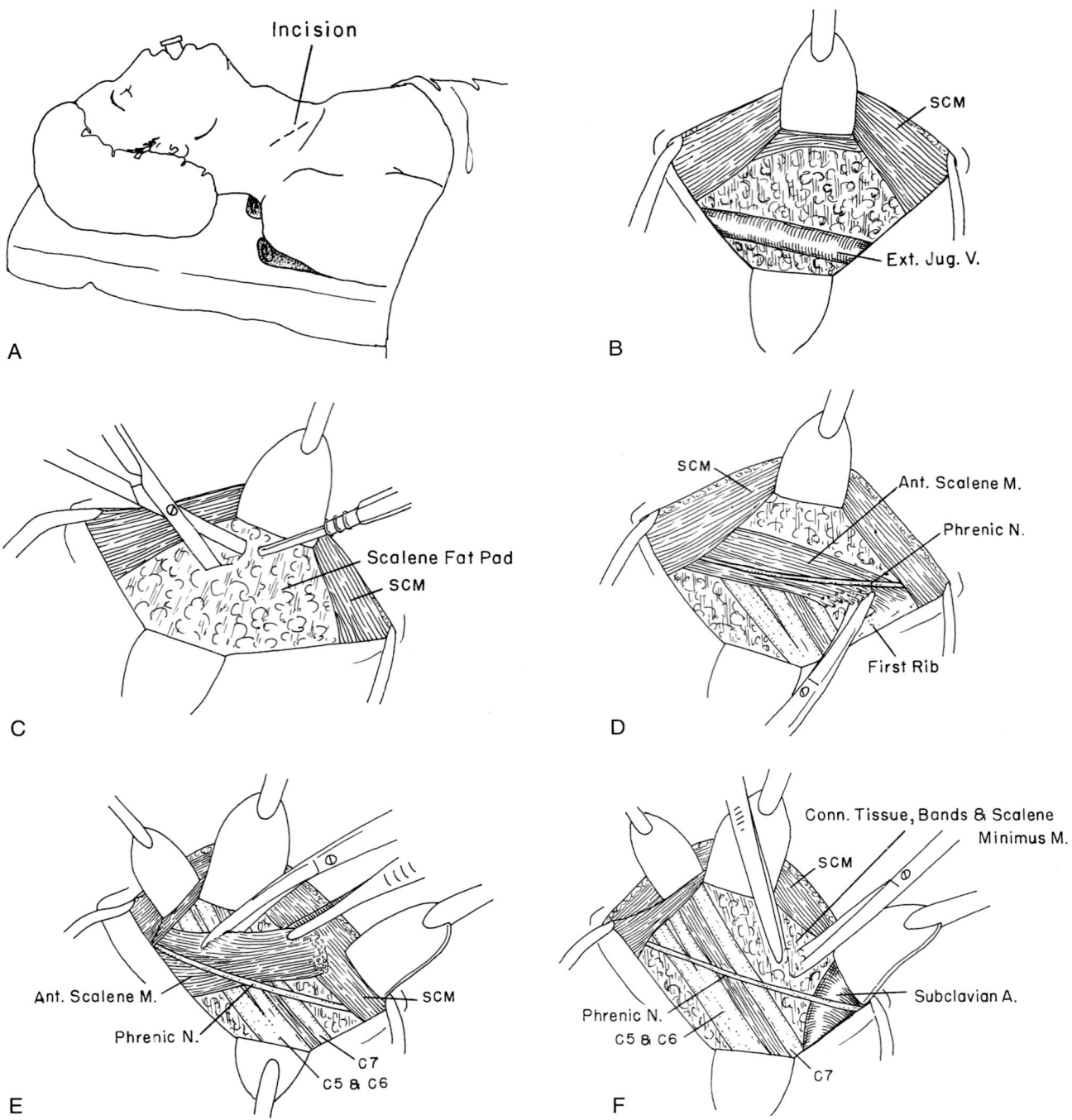

FIGURE 83–5. *A–D,* Technique of supraclavicular scalenectomy. *A,* The patient is positioned with the back of the table elevated about 15 to 20 degrees. A small towel is beneath the upper dorsal spine, and a bath towel is beneath the shoulder. The incision is 5 to 6 cm long and two fingerbreadths above the clavicle. *B,* The lateral edge of sternocleidomastoid muscle (SCM) is mobilized and retracted medially. The external jugular vein is usually preserved. *C,* The scalene fat pad is divided in its mid-portion with a cautery, with the surgeon taking care to lift the fat above the muscle to avoid cautery injury to the phrenic nerve. *D,* The anterior scalene muscle (ASM) is divided at its first rib insertion.

E–H, Technique continued. *E,* The divided end of ASM has been freed from adhesions to the subclavian artery and brachial plexus, passed below the phrenic nerve, and regrasped. The ASM origin is being divided close to the transverse processes. *F,* The space between C7 and the subclavian artery is cleaned of scalene minimus muscle (present about 50% of time), connective tissue, and ligaments. This exposes C8 and T1 nerve roots.

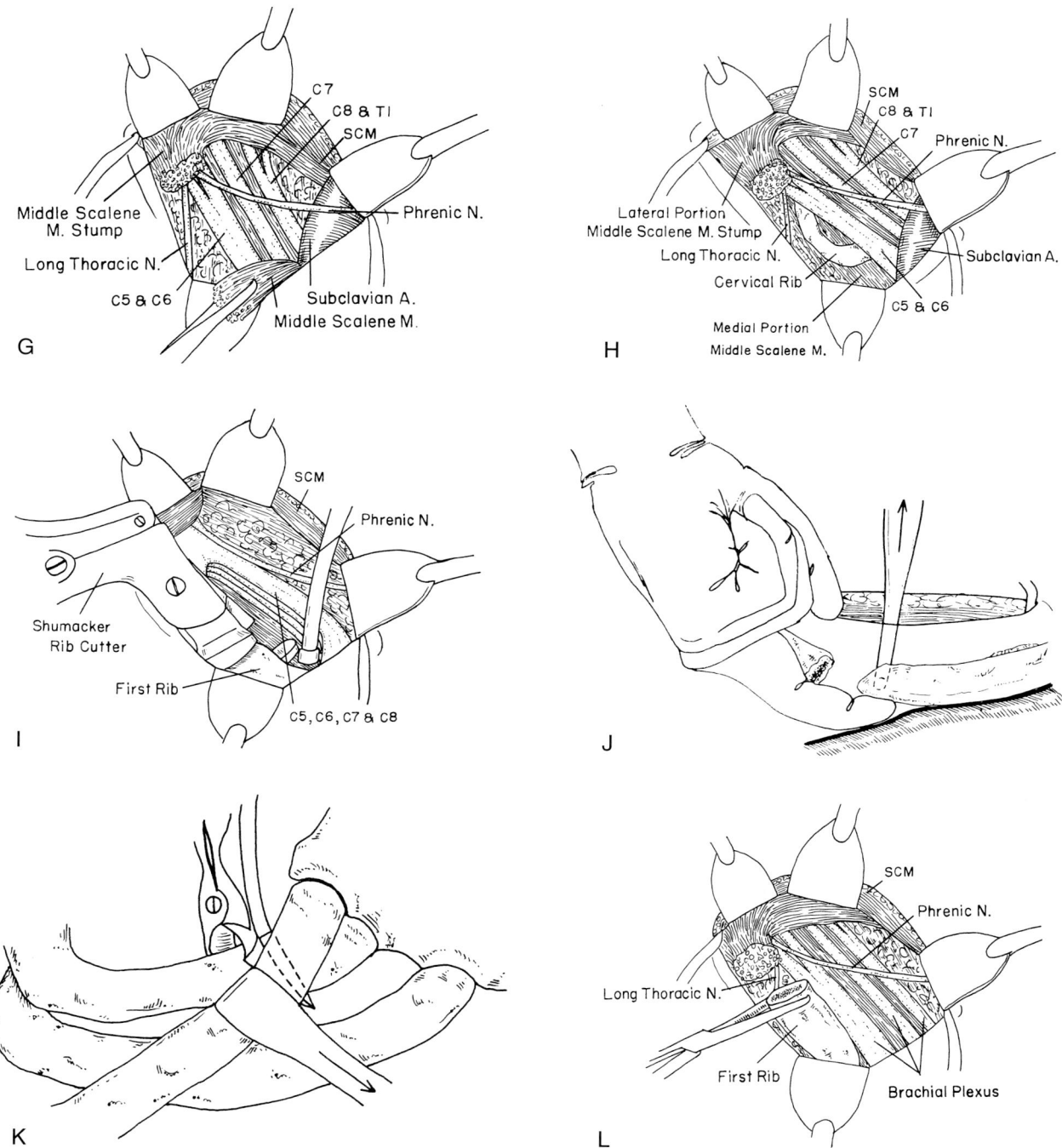

FIGURE 83–5 *Continued G,* The middle scalene muscle (MSM) is exposed lateral to the brachial plexus and the long thoracic nerve (LTN), identified exiting through the muscle. The cephalic end of the lateral portion of MSM is divided above the LTN and again at its first rib insertion. *H,* When present, a cervical rib lies in the midst of the MSM.

I–L, Technique of supraclavicular first rib resection. *I,* After dividing remaining MSM fibers and freeing lateral and medial first rib edges with an Overholt first rib elevator, the surgeon uses a Shumacker rib cutter or Raney rongeur to divide the neck of the first rib near the transverse process. *J,* The divided rib end is lifted with an elevator as finger dissection frees the pleura from the rib. *K,* The anterior rib end is divided below the clavicle by a special infraclavicular first rib cutter (Pilling) after first freeing subclavian artery and pleura from the rib. *L,* The now freed rib is extracted from behind the plexus.

(A–L, Modified from Sanders RJ, Raymer S: The supraclavicular approach to scalenectomy and first rib resection: Description of technique. J Vasc Surg 5:751–756, 1985.)

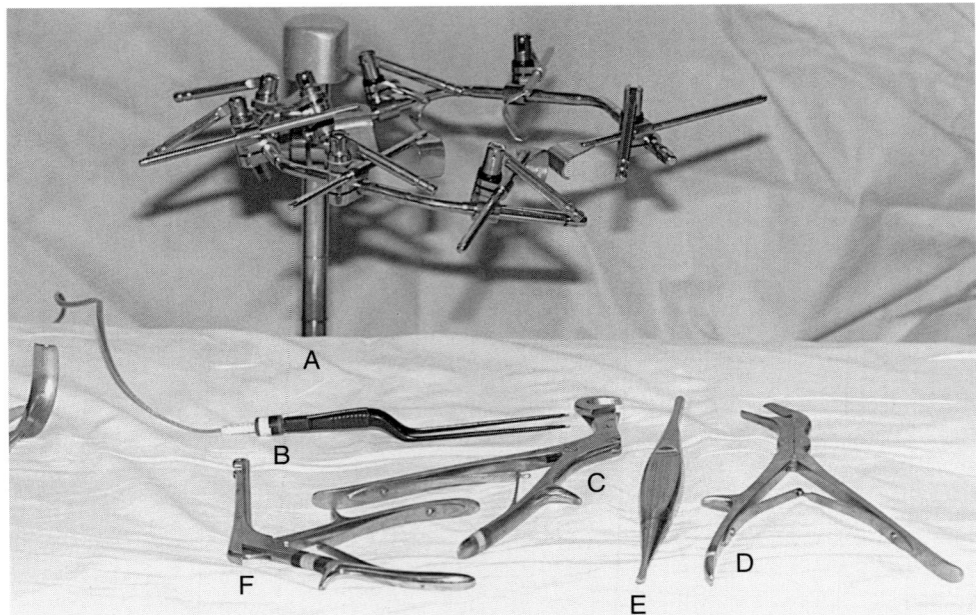

FIGURE 83–6. Instruments used in supraclavicular scalenectomy and first rib resection. *A,* Omni-Tract self-retaining retractor. *B,* Bipolar bovie. *C,* Shumacker rib cutter. *D,* Infraclavicular rib cutter (Pilling). *E,* Overholt No. 1 periosteal elevator. *F,* Raney rongeur. (From Sanders RJ, Cooper MA, Hammond SL, Weinstein ES: Supraclavicular and infraclavicular approach to subclavian artery and vein compression. *In* Yao JST, Pearce WH (eds): Techniques in Vascular and Endovascular Surgery. Stamford, Conn, Appleton & Lange, 1997, p 519.)

erative scarring. The wound is then closed subcutaneously and subcuticularly.

Supraclavicular First Rib Resection

Anterior and middle scalenectomy must precede supraclavicular first rib resection. Once the middle scalene has been resected, the posterior end of the first rib is exposed. Its medial and lateral edges are freed with an Overholt No. 1 first rib elevator (Fig. 83–6E). The neck of the rib is divided with a Shumacker rib cutter (Fig. 83–5I and 6C) or with multiple bites of a Raney (Fig. 83–6F) or Kerrison rongeur. The end of the rib is elevated with the first rib elevator, and, by finger dissection, the pleura is pushed away from the rib by simply rubbing a finger against the rib (Fig. 83–5J). Remaining intercostal muscles are also divided by finger dissection. The anterior end of the rib is then freed to below the clavicle using finger dissection above and below the rib. A special infraclavicular first rib cutter (Fig. 83–6D) (Pilling) is positioned around the rib, as far caudad as possible, and divides the anterior end of the rib with a single bite (Fig. 83–5K).

The rib is removed with a Kocher clamp from behind the plexus (Fig. 83–5L). The posterior rib stump is shortened with rongeurs to the transverse process. The anterior stump is about 2 cm from the costal junction, which is rarely a problem as the subclavian artery and plexus are usually more than 1 cm from the stump. After first rib resection, the scalene fat pad and wound are closed with drainage as described above.

Key Points: Scalenectomy and Rib Resection

1. When performing middle scalenectomy and when excising the first rib, the nerves of the plexus must be relaxed to avoid traction injuries. Relaxing is accomplished by flexing the neck toward the operative side, elevating the head, and elevating the ipsilateral shoulder. Although the patient is initially positioned thus, the head may move during the procedure, and adjustments are made through-

out the operation to permit gentle retraction of the plexus when needed.

2. A bipolar cautery device is invaluable to control bleeding and avoid nerve injury.

3. The self-retaining Omni-Tract mini-retractor provides better and safer exposure than we were ever able to achieve with hand-held retractors.

Combined Supraclavicular and Infraclavicular Rib Resection

In some cases it may be desirable to remove the anterior 2 cm of first rib, which cannot be reached via the supraclavicular approach. Indications for this include combined neurogenic and venous TOS. Exposure is achieved either by adding another infraclavicular incision or by stretching the lower skin flap a few centimeters below the clavicle. The latter technique involves making the initial supraclavicular skin incision only 1 cm above the clavicle and dissecting the lower skin flap 5 to 6 cm caudad. The pectoralis major muscle is split in the direction of its fibers, and the intercostal muscles are divided with an Overholt No. 1 rib elevator. A finger is passed through the upper incision and positioned beneath the first rib to guide the elevator and protect the pleura. The rib is transected with a Raney or Kerrison rongeur at the sternal junction.[33] The costoclavicular ligament must be divided carefully to avoid the nearby subclavian vein.

A look at the chest film helps to determine when this technique should be used. If the anterior end of the first rib descends farther than 1 cm below the clavicle, it is fairly easy to transect the rib there. On the other hand, if the rib lies completely behind the clavicle, exposure is poor. Subclavian vein injury is a risk, and the vein can be difficult to repair.

Removing the anterior 2 cm of the first rib is not necessary in most patients. When a residual segment remains here, there is the potential for subclavian vein adherence and intermittent venous obstruction. Since we have observed this complication in only 1% of our patients, we do not include this measure as a routine part of the procedure.

Cervical Rib Resection

Cervical ribs always lie in the midst of the middle scalene muscle. They are excised through the approach used for anterior and middle scalenectomy. The rib is encountered as middle scalene fibers are excised. The rib is mobilized with elevators and excised piecemeal with rongeurs. Complete cervical ribs with joints that fix them to the first rib are hard to separate from the first rib. Frequently, the first rib must be excised with the cervical rib to adequately remove this cervical–first rib joint. On the other hand, when the cervical rib is incomplete and only a band connects it to the first rib, we often leave the first rib in place provided it is broad and lies low in the field.

Transaxillary First Rib Resection

The patient is placed in a lateral thoracotomy position. The arm is elevated to expose the axilla, and the arm is prepared into the operative field. An assistant or a special arm holder (Dr. Robert Sessions, Marietta, Ga.) supports the arm in an abducted, elevated position throughout the procedure. Even with the mechanical arm holder, we usually find it

necessary for an assistant to manually elevate the arm farther during portions of the operation.

An 8- to 11-cm curvilinear incision is made in the axilla 1 cm below the hairline (Fig. 83–7A). The incision is deepened to the chest wall. The latissimus dorsi muscle lies at the posterior edge of the wound. Freeing the anterior edge of this muscle for 4 to 5 cm improves exposure. Once the chest wall is identified, blunt dissection proceeds over the ribs until the first rib is identified. The second intercostal brachial cutaneous nerve is often seen in the middle of the field, and when possible it is preserved. If in the dissection the nerve is stretched, however, postoperative causalgia develops in the arm. To avoid this complication, the nerve should be divided when it appears to be under severe tension. Preoperatively, the patient is told that numbness under the arm is a common sequela of this procedure and is a less serious complication than burning pain.

Dissection proceeds over the serratus anterior muscle and under the pectoral muscles. Retraction of the pectoral muscles is done with a long, thin vaginal retractor (Simon-Haney) which is positioned over the second rib.

Finding the first rib can be difficult, because frequently the second rib lies high enough to obscure the first rib. When it does, the surgeon must try to push the second rib

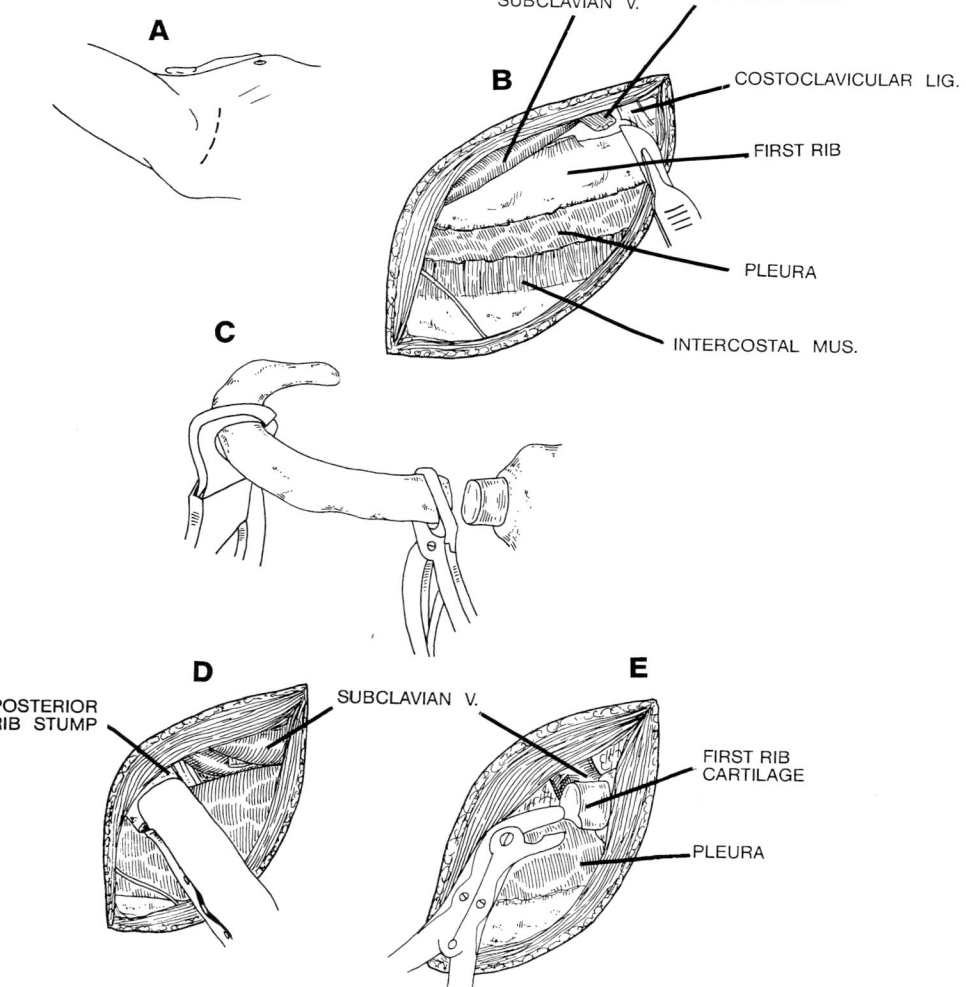

FIGURE 83–7. Technique of transaxillary first rib resection. *A,* An incision (8 to 11 cm) is made 1 cm below the axillary hairline. *B,* After the intercostal, anterior, and middle scalene muscles are divided, the subclavius muscle and costoclavicular ligament are divided. *C,* The anterior end of the rib has been divided and held with a clamp as the posterior end is divided. *D,* The posterior rib stump is shortened as close to the transverse process as is safe. C8 and T1 nerve roots should be visualized and protected at this point. *E,* The anterior rib end is resected to the costal cartilage. (From Sanders RJ, Haug CE: Management of subclavian vein obstruction. *In* Bergan JJ, Kistner RL [eds]: Atlas of Venous Surgery. Philadelphia, WB Saunders, 1992, p 265.)

downward and work over it. When exposure is particularly difficult, some surgeons have even resected portions of the second rib to gain exposure (Dr. David Roos, personal communication). Once identified, the first rib is freed by dividing 2 to 3 cm of intercostal muscle below it. An Overholt No.1 periosteal elevator (Fig. 83–6E) is passed below the rib to free it from the pleura. The right-angle end of the elevator is passed around the medial edge of the rib, and the elevator is moved anteriorly and posteriorly to divide as many of the intercostal muscle fibers as possible. The subclavius muscle and costoclavicular ligament are divided (Fig. 83–7B).

The middle scalene muscle is divided on top of the rib, keeping the scissors against the rib at all times to avoid injuring the long thoracic nerve. Rib resection is now performed by dividing the posterior end with either a right-angle bone cutter (Roos rib cutter, Pilling) or straight bone shears. The anterior end of the rib is then divided near the costochondral junction (Fig. 83–7C). The anterior scalene muscle is now divided as far cephalad as possible by pulling down on the divided first rib segment. The stumps of the rib are shortened with rongeurs, posteriorly to as close to the transverse process as is safe (Fig. 83–7D) and anteriorly to the costal cartilage (Fig. 83–7E). The wound is closed around a suction drain, as described above.[37] When the pleura has been entered, the drain is left inside the pleura and the lung is fully expanded before closing.

Infraclavicular First Rib Resection

Infraclavicular first rib resection can be used for neurogenic TOS, but it is used principally in cases of venous TOS when venolysis and possible endovenectomy or grafting of the subclavian vein is contemplated, as it provides excellent exposure of both the axillary and the subclavian veins. The patient is positioned supine, and a 12- to 15-cm transverse incision is made 2 to 3 cm below the clavicle. The pectoralis major muscle is split between its sternal and clavicular heads. The lower edge of the first rib near the costal margin is found just below the pectoralis muscle. In some cases, the first rib–cartilage junction lies directly behind the clavicle, which makes exposure of the first rib difficult. Elevating the ipsilateral shoulder several centimeters aids exposure.

The intercostal muscle below the anterior portion of the first rib is divided up to the costochondral junction. The intercostal muscle is then divided under the lateral portion of the rib. After identifying the subclavian vein, the anterior scalene muscle is sectioned as far from the first rib insertion as possible. The middle scalene muscle is next divided on top of the rib, staying close to the rib to avoid the long thoracic nerve. Additional exposure is obtained by elevating the shoulder, which raises the clavicle. The remaining posterior fibers of the intercostal muscle are divided.

Rib resection begins by dividing the anterior end of the rib at the costal margin. The subclavian vein lies near the inner margin of the rib and must not be injured. The center of the rib is next divided with a rib cutter that can fit into the narrow space, and the anterior half of the rib is removed. The posterior half is removed piecemeal with rongeurs, as far posteriorly as is safe. Special rongeurs (Urschel from Pilling, and Lexsell) are helpful for this.

In cases of venous TOS, venolysis of the subclavian vein

is easily performed at this stage of the operation. The wound is closed with drainage, as for scalenectomy.

In some patients, the anterior end of the rib lies directly behind the clavicle and the space is too tight to permit safe exposure of the costoclavicular ligament and the subclavian vein. On one occasion, we abandoned this approach and performed the operation through the axilla, as described earlier.

Postoperative Management

An upright chest film is obtained in the recovery room to check for pneumothorax. Small air collections are common when the pleura has been opened, but they require no treatment. A pneumothorax larger than 20% to 30% is tapped with a plastic needle in the second anterior interspace. A chest tube is rarely needed because there is rarely a continuous air leak.

A transcutaneous nerve stimulator (TNS) unit is attached to the patient in the recovery room to reduce pain. It may be used for a few days to several weeks. Postoperative neck stretching and wall-climbing exercises are begun on the first postoperative day and continued daily at home. Most patients leave the hospital on the first or second postoperative day. Return to work on light duty jobs is possible in 2 to 4 weeks; to heavier jobs in 6 to 8 weeks.

Selection of Approach

Indications for the Supraclavicular Approach

As of 1998, transaxillary first rib resection was the most popular approach; however, anterior and middle scalenectomy, with or without supraclavicular first rib resection, was gaining popularity. We have used both approaches in large numbers of cases. We prefer the supraclavicular approach for these reasons:

1. Since the results of scalenectomy and transaxillary first rib resection are similar, it appears that first rib resection is effective not because the rib has been removed, but because the anterior and middle scalene muscles have been divided. In essence, a scalenotomy has been performed.

2. Proponents of the transaxillary approach recognize that, in patients with upper and lower plexus involvement, anterior scalenectomy must be added through a supraclavicular incision to avoid failure or recurrence. If the supraclavicular incision is being used for this, it is easier and faster to do the whole operation through this approach and avoid a second incision.

3. The supraclavicular approach permits good exposure of all scalene muscle variations and anomalies, all congenital ligaments and bands, and cervical ribs. The posterior end of the first rib is more easily exposed and resected through the neck than through the axilla.[3]

4. The supraclavicular route provides better exposure than the transaxillary route and reduces the chances of injuring major vessels and nerves. While nerve and major vessel injuries can occur with either approach, they are easier to avoid through the supraclavicular route. Should vessel injury occur, it is usually easier to repair through this route as well. In the early 20th century, supraclavicular scalenotomy and rib resection had a greater than 30%

incidence of brachial plexus injury.[1] Since then, the incidence has been reduced to less than 1%, because of better retraction, the bipolar cautery, better instruments (see Fig. 83–6), and more experience.

Indications for the Transaxillary Approach

The transaxillary route provides better exposure of the anterior end of the first rib than the supraclavicular route. This is important in venous TOS when it is necessary to remove the entire anterior end of the rib and free the subclavian vein. The transaxillary route is also best for first rib resection in patients who have recurrent symptoms after scalenectomy. Except for these two indications, we have stopped using the transaxillary route in favor of the supraclavicular one.

SURGICAL COMPLICATIONS

Nerve Injuries

Nerve injuries are the most serious complications. In the transaxillary approach, excessive arm traction can cause *brachial plexus* neurapraxia. In removing the posterior rib stump, the T1 nerve root may be cut or stretched. With the supraclavicular approach, brachial plexus injury is most likely to occur from excessive traction on the nerves during exposure of the middle scalene muscle and the posterior end of the first rib. In large series, the incidence of permanent brachial plexus injury is less than 1% with each approach.[3, 36, 46]

Long thoracic nerve injury occurs because this nerve courses through the middle scalene muscle. It then descends over the first rib to reach the serratus anterior muscle. When excising the middle scalene, the branches that will compromise the nerve should be identified before dividing the muscle.

Phrenic nerve injury occurs with both transaxillary and supraclavicular approaches. The nerve can lie in the medial corner of the transaxillary wound and, although it is not identified, it may inadvertently be retracted. The resultant palsy is usually temporary.

During supraclavicular exposure, the phrenic nerve lies on top of the anterior scalene muscle in the middle of the field. It must be gently pushed aside or lifted with a vessel loop to avoid traction injury. Even with careful technique, the incidence of temporary phrenic paresis is 4% to 12%[3, 20, 36, 42] In these patients, postoperative chest fluoroscopy reveals a fixed diaphragm with paradoxical movements. Though the condition usually resolves, it may take a few days or as long as 24 months. The incidence of permanent phrenic injury is about 1%. Postoperative phrenic nerve weakness, as evidenced fluoroscopically by a sluggish diaphragm on the first postoperative day, occurs in more than 10% of all patients. The diaphragm usually returns to normal within a month.

Horner's syndrome has occasionally been seen in supraclavicular operations. Although the cervical sympathetic chain is not identified in this approach, it may be injured by a retractor or cautery, since it can lie on the medial wall of the field. Should this occur and a drooping eyelid result, it can be corrected by shortening the levator muscle of the eyelid. Electric cautery is the cause of some nerve injuries. Using bipolar cautery reduces this risk.

Bleeding

Bleeding can occur from injury to the subclavian artery or vein. Initially, most vessel defects are small, and when they lie in deep or hidden areas, it is worth first trying to control the bleeding with an absorbable gelatin sponge (Gelfoam) soaked in thrombin. Arterial injury in the axillary approach can be difficult to control, because exposure is very deep and limited. Control of the artery may be obtained by making a supraclavicular incision and clamping the artery proximally. Vessel repair may then proceed from either the upper or the lower incision.

Subclavian vein bleeding is more common than arterial bleeding. When it occurs through the axilla, the bleeding is tamponaded with a peanut sponge while the anterior part of the rib is excised. This is necessary because the rib prevents placement of a needle holder to repair the vein. Once the rib has been excised, the hole in the vein can usually be repaired.

Subclavian vein bleeding in the supraclavicular approach is usually caused by tearing a small vein that empties into the subclavian vein. If Gelfoam and thrombin fail, and if control of the bleeding cannot be obtained from above the clavicle, the bleeding is tamponaded and an infraclavicular incision made to control the vein from below. The incidence of major bleeding from one of these vessels is less than 1%.

Lymph Leakage

Lymph leak occurs on the left side from injury to the thoracic duct. On the right side, it is rare. Lymph pooling in the surgical field is an indication to immediately stop the dissection, identify the leak, and control it with sutures or clips. By doing this when the leak is first seen, the repaired area can be observed for additional leaks as the operation proceeds. The incidence of lymph leaks requiring reoperation is less than 1%.

RESULTS OF SURGERY

There are no standard criteria for evaluating the results of surgery. Some authors define success as relief of all symptoms; others define it as relief of most major symptoms; still others let patient satisfaction be the determinant; and finally there are those who do not define their criteria. This disparity may explain why success rates over 1 year vary from 43%[18] to 78%.[12] In general, a good result from surgery means improvement, not total cure. Most patients with good results have fewer, less intense, and less frequent symptoms, but they seldom have none. Depending on their occupation, some patients must modify or change their jobs to avoid recurrent symptoms. Patients most likely to require job modification are those who do repetitive activities, work on assembly lines, do heavy laboring, or work with their arms above shoulder level.

Our success rates are about the same for transaxillary first rib resection, anterior and middle scalenectomy, and combined scalenectomy and rib resection (Fig. 83–8). The 5-year success rate, *success* being defined as enough symptomatic improvement to feel that the surgery was worthwhile, is 68% using life table methods. The results can be several percentage points higher by using short to long ranges of follow-up.[43] Reliable statistics require a minimum of 12 months' follow-up.

The most significant variable in success rate is the cause of TOS. After automobile accidents, good improvement occurs in 80% of cases and fair improvement in another 10%. In contrast, after occupational repetitive stress injuries, the "good success" rate is 65% and the fair rate 16%. Review of our most recent results suggests that combining scalenectomy with first rib resection gave 15% better results than scalenectomy alone.[48] Others have noted just the opposite results, scalenectomy alone giving better results than adding rib resection.[3] These differences have not yet reached statistical significance.

Patients with cervical ribs do not have a better success rate than patients without cervical ribs; the rates are the same. Patients with hand atrophy and typical neurophysiologic changes of ulnar neuropathy actually have poorer success rates than those who have no objective findings.[12]

RECURRENT AND PERSISTENT THORACIC OUTLET SYNDROME

About 10% of patients fail to improve after surgery. Persistence of symptoms could mean an incomplete operation, but it is more likely to reflect a missed diagnosis, which occurs more often in "repetitive stress patients" who have compartment compression in multiple areas. For these patients, decompression of the thoracic outlet area does little to relieve symptoms that arise from compression in other sites. The term *double crush syndrome* describes compression in more than one site.[53] In some patients, surgical decompression in one area is all that is needed, and other areas can be left alone. On the other hand, some patients need decompression of both areas to relieve symptoms.

Recurrence of symptoms after initial improvement occurs in 15% to 20% of patients, most often during the first 18

months after operation. Initial treatment is conservative and includes a search for other diagnoses. Failure to respond to conservative treatment and *disabling* symptoms are the indications for reoperation. The choice of procedures depends on what operation was performed originally. Scalenectomy is preferred for recurrence after transaxillary first rib resection. Transaxillary first rib resection is offered for recurrence after initial scalenectomy.

When the patient has already had both scalenectomy and first rib resection, the only operation that can be offered is brachial plexus neurolysis through a supraclavicular approach, through the axilla, or using both exposures. Our first preference is the supraclavicular route. The rate of long-term improvement after operations for recurrence is 40% to 50%.[4, 47] For this reason, reoperations should be offered with caution, and only as a last resort. The incidence of nerve complications is higher after reoperations than after primary operations.

Intermittent subclavian vein obstruction has occurred as a late complication, several months or more postoperatively, in 1% of the patients undergoing supraclavicular first rib resection. The cause is adherence of the vein to the anterior rib stump, which could not be excised through the supraclavicular approach owing to inadequate exposure of this part of the rib. Diagnosis is confirmed by dynamic venography. Treatment is transaxillary resection of the anterior segment of the first rib with venolysis.

SUMMARY

Several myths regarding neurogenic TOS should be corrected. These include the following:

1. *Adson's test* is no longer regarded as reliable for either confirming or ruling out neurogenic TOS. Many asymptomatic people have abnormal responses; most patients with TOS have negative test results.

2. An abnormal *first rib* is *not* the usual cause of neurogenic TOS. Because first rib resection is a common treatment for TOS, many people erroneously attribute TOS to the first rib. The lesion is in the scalene muscles, not the rib. First rib resection is effective because the scalene mus-

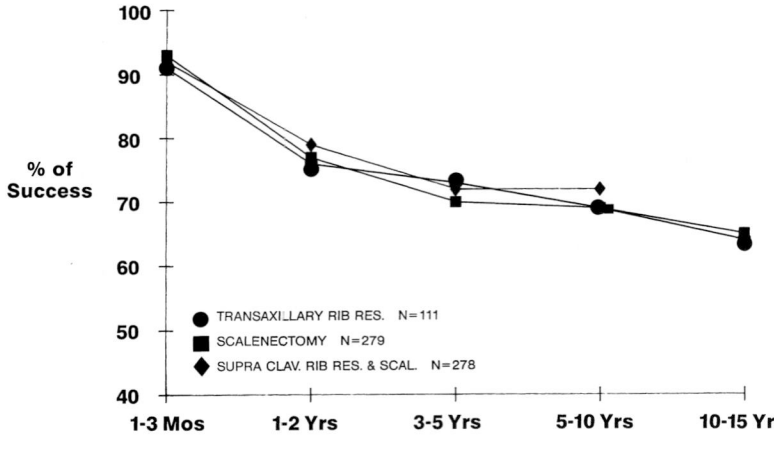

Primary Success Rate

% of Success

TRANSAXILLARY RIB RES.   N=111
SCALENECTOMY   N=279
SUPRA CLAV. RIB RES. & SCAL.   N=278

1-3 Mos   1-2 Yrs   3-5 Yrs   5-10 Yrs   10-15 Yrs

FIGURE 83–8. Results of three primary operations for thoracic outlet syndrome. N = number of operations. (From Sanders RJ, Haug CE: Thoracic Outlet Syndrome: A Common Sequela of Neck Injuries. Philadelphia, JB Lippincott, 1991, p 182.)

cles must be divided to remove the rib. Improvement is probably achieved because the scalene muscles have been released rather than because the rib is removed.

3. *Coldness and color changes* in the hand seldom indicate arterial involvement in TOS. These symptoms are due to sympathetic nerve irritation. The sympathetic nerves accompany the lower nerve roots of the brachial plexus, and, when the plexus is compressed or irritated, the sympathetic fibers are also stimulated and produce coldness and color changes.

4. *TOS surgery* usually is not curative. Seldom does surgery give complete relief of all symptoms. Good results mean improvement of most symptoms, but only occasionally are all symptoms totally relieved.

5. *TOS surgery* seldom makes patients worse. Although serious and disabling complications have occurred from TOS surgery, in experienced hands, the incidence is less than 1%.

6. *Normal electromyographic, nerve conduction velocity, and somatosensory evoked potential* findings are common in patients with neurogenic TOS and cannot be used to rule out TOS. On the other hand, positive study results are usually nonspecific and cannot be used to confirm TOS. However, there is an exception to this. In less than 1% of TOS patients, there is atrophy of the small hand muscles and neuroelectrophysiologic studies reveal changes of ulnar neuropathy.

7. *Patients with objective findings* such as cervical ribs, abnormal neurophysiologic studies, and hand atrophy do not have better surgical success rates than patients who have no objective findings.

REFERENCES

1. Adson AW: Surgical treatment for symptoms produced by cervical ribs and the scalenus anticus muscle. Surg Gynecol Obstet 85:687–700, 1947.
2. Bramwell E: Lesion of the first dorsal nerve root. Rev Neurol Psychiatry 1:236–239, 1903.
3. Cheng SWK, Reilly LM, Nelken NA, et al: Neurogenic thoracic outlet decompression: Rationale for sparing the first rib. Cardiovasc Surg 3:617–623, 1995.
4. Cheng SWK, Stoney RJ: Supraclavicular reoperation for neurogenic thoracic outlet syndrome. J Vasc Surg 19:565–572, 1994.
5. Clagett OT: Presidential address: Research and prosearch. J Thorac Cardiovasc Surg 44:153–166, 1962.
6. Cooper A: On exostosis. *In* Cooper, Cooper, Travers (eds): Surgical Essays, 3rd ed. London, 1821, p 128.
7. Coote H: Exostosis of the left transverse process of the seventh cervical vertebra, surrounded by blood vessels and nerves: successful removal. Lancet 1:360–361, 1861.
8. Falconer MA, Weddell G: Costoclavicular compression of the subclavian artery and vein. Lancet 2:539–543, 1943.
9. Felson B: A review of 30,000 normal chest roentgenograms. *In* Felson B (ed): Chest Roentgenology. Philadelphia, WB Saunders, 1973, p 494.
10. Gage M: Scalenus anticus syndrome: A diagnostic and confirmatory test. Surgery 5:599–601, 1939.
11. Gergoudis R, Barnes RW: Thoracic outlet arterial compression: Prevalence in normal persons. Angiology 31:538–541, 1980.
12. Green RM, McNamara MS, Ouriel K: Long-term follow-up after thoracic outlet decompression: An analysis of factors determining outcome. J Vasc Surg 14:739–746, 1991.
13. Gol A, Patrick DW, McNeel DP: Relief of costoclavicular syndrome by infraclavicular removal of first rib. J Neurosurg 28:81–84, 1968.
14. Juvonen T, Satta J, Laitala P, et al: Anomalies at the thoracic outlet are frequent in the general population. Am J Surg 170:33–37, 1995.
15. Kirgis HD, Reed AF: Significant anatomic relations in the syndrome of the scalene muscles. Ann Surg 127:1182–1201, 1948.
16. Komanetsky RM, Novak CB, Mackinnon SE, et al: Somatosensory evoked potentials fail to diagnose thoracic outlet syndrome. J Hand Surg 21:662–666, 1996.
17. Law AA: Adventitious ligaments simulating cervical ribs. Ann Surg 72:497–499, 1920.
18. Lindgren KA, Oksala I: Long-term outcome of surgery for thoracic outlet syndrome. Am J Surg 169:358–360, 1995.
19. Liu JE, Tahmoush AJ, Roos DB, Schwartzman RJ: Shoulder-arm pain from cervical bands and scalene muscle anomalies. J Neurol Sci 128:175–180, 1995.
20. Loh CS, Wu AVO, Stevenson IM: Surgical decompression for thoracic outlet syndrome. J R Coll Surg Edinb 34:66–68, 1989.
21. Love JG: The scalenus anticus syndrome with and without cervical rib. Proc Mayo Clin 20:65–70, 1945.
22. Machleder HJ, Moll F, Nuwer M, Jordan S: Somatosensory evoked potentials in the assessment of thoracic outlet compression syndrome. J Vasc Surg 6:177–184, 1987.
23. Machleder HI, Moll F, Verity A: The anterior scalene muscle in thoracic outlet compression syndrome: Histochemical and morphometric studies. Arch Surg 121:1141–1144, 1986.
24. Makhoul RG, Machleder HI: Developmental anomalies at the thoracic outlet: An analysis of 200 consecutive cases. J Vasc Surg 16:534–545, 1992.
25. Murphy JB: Cervical rib excision: Collective review on surgery of cervical rib. Clin John B Murphy 5:227–240, 1916.
26. Murphy T: Brachial neuritis caused by pressure of first rib. Aust Med J 15:582–585, 1910.
27. Naffziger HC, Grant WT: Neuritis of the brachial plexus mechanical in origin: The scalenus origin. Surg Gynecol Obstet 67:722–729, 1938.
28. Novak CB, Collins ED, Mackinnon SE: Outcome following conservative management of thoracic outlet syndrome. J Hand Surg 20A:542–548, 1995.
29. Ochsner A, Gage M, Debakey M: Scalenus anticus (Naffziger) syndrome. Am J Surg 28:669–695, 1935.
30. Paradiso PS, Giannini C, Cioni F, et al: Diagnosis of thoracic outlet syndrome: Relative value of electrophysiological studies. Acta Neurol Scand 90:179–185, 1994.
31. Peet RM, Hendriksen JD, Anderson TP, Martin GM: Thoracic outlet syndrome: Evaluation of a theraputic exercise program. Proc Mayo Clin 31:281–287, 1956.
32. Rob CG, Standeven A: Arterial occlusion complicating thoracic outlet compression syndrome. Br Med J 2: 709–712, 1958.
33. Robicsek F, Eastman D: "Above-under" exposure of the first rib: A modified approach for the treatment of thoracic outlet syndrome. Ann Vasc Surg 11:304–306, 1997.
34. Roos DB, Owens JC: Thoracic outlet syndrome. Arch Surg 93:71–74, 1966.
35. Roos DB: New concepts of thoracic outlet syndrome that explain etiology, symptoms, diagnosis, and treatment. Vasc Surg 13:313–321, 1979.
36. Roos DB: The place for scalenectomy and first rib resection in thoracic outlet syndrome. Surgery 92:1077–1085, 1982.
37. Roos DB: Technique of transaxillary decompression for thoracic outlet syndrome. *In* Yao JST, Pearce WH (eds): Techniques in Vascular and Endovascular Surgery. Stamford, Conn, Appleton & Lange, 1997, pp 531–538.
38. Sanders RJ, Haug CE: Thoracic Outlet Syndrome: A Common Sequela of Neck Injuries. Philadelphia, JB Lippincott, 1991, p 41.
39. Sanders RJ, Haug CE: Thoracic Outlet Syndrome: A Common Sequela of Neck Injuries. Philadelphia, JB Lippincott, 1991, p 75.
40. Sanders RJ, Haug CE: Thoracic Outlet Syndrome: A Common Sequela of Neck Injuries. Philadelphia, JB Lippincott, 1991, pp 77–80.
41. Sanders RJ, Haug CE: Thoracic Outlet Syndrome: A Common Sequela of Neck Injuries. Philadelphia, JB Lippincott, 1991, p 93.
42. Sanders RJ, Haug CE: Thoracic Outlet Syndrome: A Common Sequela of Neck Injuries. Philadelphia, JB Lippincott, 1991, p 165.
43. Sanders RJ, Haug CE: Thoracic Outlet Syndrome: A Common Sequela of Neck Injuries. Philadelphia, JB Lippincott, 1991, p 183.
44. Sanders RJ, Jackson CGR, Banchero N, Pearce WH: Scalene muscle abnormalities in traumatic thoracic outlet syndrome. Am J Surg 159:231–236, 1990.
45. Sanders RJ, Roos DB: The surgical anatomy of the scalene triangle. Contemp Surg 35:11–16, 1989.

46. Sanders RJ, Pearce WH: The treatment of thoracic outlet syndrome: A comparison of different operations. J Vasc Surg 10:626–634, 1989.
47. Sanders RJ, Haug C, Pearce WH: Recurrent thoracic outlet syndrome. J Vasc Surg 12:390–400, 1990.
48. Sanders RJ: Results of treatment for TOS. Semin Thorac Cardiovasc Surg 8:221–228, 1996.
49. Southam AH, Bythell WJ: Cervical ribs in children. Br Med J 2:844–855, 1924.
50. Stiles H: Torticollis-congenital elevation of the scapula—cervical ribs. In Jones R, Lovett R (eds): Orthopedic Surgery, 2nd ed. New York, William Wood & Co, 1923.
51. Stopford JS, Telford ED: Compression of the lower trunk of the branchial plexus by a first dorsal rib: With a note on the surgical treatment. Br J Surg 7:168–177, 1919.
52. Thomas GI, Jones TW, Stavney LS, et al: The middle scalene muscle and its contribution to the TOS. Am J Surg 145:589–592, 1983.
53. Upton ARM, McComas AJ: The double crush in nerve-entrapment syndromes. Lancet 2:359–362, 1973.
54. Urschel HC, Razzuk MA: Management of the thoracic outlet syndrome. N Engl J Med 286:1140–1143, 1972.
55. Veilleux M, Stevens JC, Campbell JK: Somatosensory evoked potentials: Lack of value for diagnosis of thoracic outlet syndrome. Muscle Nerve 11:571–575, 1988.
56. Wilbourn AJ: Evidence for conduction delay in thoracic outlet syndrome is challenged. N Engl J Med 310:1052–1053, 1984.

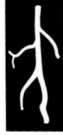

CHAPTER 84
Arterial Complications of Thoracic Outlet Compression

Edouard Kieffer, M.D., and Carlo Ruotolo, M.D.

Arterial complications of thoracic outlet compression have serious prognostic implications, although they are present in fewer than 5% of operations performed for thoracic outlet syndrome (TOS). Long-standing compression of the subclavian artery (SA) may lead to major arterial lesions with post-stenotic dilatation, aneurysmal dilatation, and thromboembolic complications which may in turn impair the function and even jeopardize the viability of the affected upper limb.[1-3, 26, 27] This chapter reviews the anatomic, clinical, and surgical aspects of these complications.

ANATOMIC LESIONS

Arterial complications of TOS are almost always secondary to significant, permanent, and long-standing compression—usually a congenital bony abnormality. There is usually a long delay before arterial lesions develop and symptoms appear. The mean age of patients who have arterial complications is at least 10 years older than that of patients who have neurologic or venous symptoms from TOS. Although the compression may involve any of the three consecutive sites of the thoracic outlet, it affects primarily the costoscalene passage and, less frequently, the costoclavicular passage. Compression of the subclavian artery occurs in the anteroposterior direction in the former case and cephalad to caudad in the latter. To the authors' knowledge, no case of arterial complication due to compression in the retropectoral passage has ever been reported. The following text describes the causes of compression and pathologic arterial findings.

Elements of Compression

Congenital bony abnormalities are the most common cause. *Cervical ribs* are present in most patients with arterial complications of TOS. The arterial consequences of both complete and incomplete cervical ribs have been emphasized by several investigators.[4-6] *Complete* long cervical ribs are articulated or fused to a tubercle on the upper aspect of the first thoracic rib, just behind the distal insertion of the anterior scalene muscle. When the anterior end of the cervical rib is large and spatulate, the resulting arterial compression may be accentuated. *Incomplete* short cervical ribs do not reach the first thoracic rib, although they are commonly associated with a fibrous band that follows the same trajectory as a complete cervical rib. Incomplete cervical ribs, when symptomatic, usually cause nerve compression, whereas complete cervical ribs appear to be the main cause of arterial compression and complications. These complications may also develop as a result of an incomplete cervical rib or an elongated transverse process of the seventh cervical vertebra (C7), but this configuration occurs much less frequently.[7, 8] In both situations, the bony abnormality is usually extended by a fibrous band inserted on the first thoracic rib just behind the tubercle of the anterior scalene muscle.

Congenital abnormalities of the *first thoracic rib* are less common than those of the cervical ribs, but, when present, they seem to be an even more frequent cause of arterial complications than cervical ribs.[9] The most common abnormality is agenesis of the anterior part of the first rib. The posterior part of the rib may articulate with or fuse to the second rib in the same manner that a complete cervical rib articulates with a normal first thoracic rib. In other cases, the anterior end of the partially agenetic first rib may be free and pulled upward by the anterior scalene muscle that inserts on it. Synostosis of the first two ribs,[6] bifidity,[10] and an abnormal tubercle of the first rib[11] are less common findings.

Isolated *congenital bands* as well as hypertrophic anterior scalene muscles have been described in a small number of patients with arterial complications of TOS, although they are responsible mainly for neurologic symptoms.[11–14] *Acquired bony abnormalities* affecting mainly the clavicle, and, less frequently, the first thoracic rib, are even less common.[15] Malunion of a fractured clavicle is more likely to cause arterial problems than is a hypertrophic callus. Anecdotal cases of hypertrophic callus or exostosis of the first thoracic rib, have also been reported, as have cases of sequelae of osteomyelitis of the clavicle.

Whatever its cause, location, and mechanism, arterial compression is usually intermittent at onset. Later, it becomes permanent as a result of various physiologic, pathologic, or traumatic factors. The most important of these is physiologic drooping of the shoulder girdle, which usually takes place during the third decade of life, especially in women.[5, 11] Whiplash cervical injuries sometimes also percipitate arterial compression by causing trauma and subsequent fibrosis of the scalene muscles.

Arterial Lesions

The initial consequence of tight, long-standing compression of the subclavian artery in the costoscalene or costoclavicular passage of the thoracic outlet is *localized stenosis*. Even after many years, this lesion is probably entirely reversible by surgical decompression; however, with the passage of time and the repetitive mechanical trauma caused by shoulder motion, the arterial wall becomes thick and fibrotic and inflammatory changes of the adventitia fix the artery to the surrounding structures. In most cases, post-stenotic dilatation develops, which is a characteristic complication of arterial compression in the thoracic outlet. The most common mechanism of this dilatation, at least with compression in the costoscalene passage, is *post-stenotic turbulence*,[5] which is secondary not only to the presence of a tight stenosis but also to angulation in the frontal plane. Indeed, the bony abnormality usually pushes the artery upward in the lower cervical region, leading to its acute angulation before it reaches the axillary region. The resulting vibrations or abnormal wall shear stress affect the fragile arterial wall, distending and rupturing components of the media and giving rise to a circumferential dilatation of the artery.[16, 17]

Early post-stenotic dilatation is reversible if the underlying cause can be removed; however, with time, the lesion becomes irreversible because of permanent changes to the arterial wall. Localized jet lesions may be present in very tight stenoses and account for the rare occurrence of saccular aneurysms. Similarly, repeated trauma from the moving clavicle may be responsible for a localized lesion of the upper aspect of the subclavian artery when compression takes place in the costoclavicular passage.

These arterial lesions have several consequences, of which thromboembolic complications are the most common and potentially the most dangerous (Fig. 84–1). An intimal lesion may occur either at the site of compression and stenosis of the subclavian artery (Fig. 84–2) or in the post-stenotic dilatation, often at the site of impact of the post-stenotic jet (Fig. 84–3). When distal pulses are normal, distal microembolization of platelet aggregates formed on this intimal lesion is now commonly considered to be the usual mechanism of Raynaud's syndrome and of digital necrosis as a complication of TOS. These microemboli are especially common in the thumb and index finger, probably as a result of the straightforward pathway through the radial artery in contrast to that through the ulnar artery. The formation of a mural thrombus is even more ominous.[18]

Although mechanical factors are usually predominant, they may be accelerated by hematologic or hormonal disturbances, including those induced by contraceptive pills.[1, 8] Ischemic consequences of the resulting macroembolization vary with the site and extent of the distal occlusion. An isolated proximal embolus often has less serious consequences than a more distal one, owing to the greater possibilities for collateral circulation. If the subclavian artery abnormality is not corrected early, emboli will occur repeatedly, with progressive obliteration of the distal arterial bed and aggravation of the ischemia. In some cases, effective treatment may be impossible and major irreversible ischemia follows.

Thrombotic occlusion of the subclavian artery is rare, but when it does occur, initially it usually remains limited to the subclavian and axillary arteries and good collateral circulation develops. In these cases, distal inchemia is usually mild, even absent. When it occurs after many episodes of distal embolization, ischemia is usually severe and may even be irreversible because of difficulties in clearing the distal arterial bed. Retrograde embolization in the cerebral arteries, although rare, is a serious potential complication.[19, 20]

CLINICAL SYMPTOMS

Diagnosis is rarely made at an early stage, before thromboembolic complications appear. Three clinical situations may result in an early diagnosis:

1. A pulsatile supraclavicular mass that reveals an asymptomatic subclavian aneurysm.[21]
2. Isolated neurologic symptoms associated with a cervical rib or any bony abnormality of the thoracic outlet, a situation that, in the authors' opinion, warrants arteriography or ultrasonography.
3. An incidental finding in an arteriogram obtained to investigate a symptomatic lesion of the opposite upper extremity.

In many cases, the disease remains undetected until thromboembolic complications develop. The most frequent early symptoms are a result of embolic occlusions of the digital arteries or the palmar arch. Raynaud's syndrome or its equivalents, including episodic pallor, cyanosis, or both; paresthesias; coldness; pain; and cold sensitivity of the hands and digits are common at this stage of the disease. They must be recognized as vascular symptoms and their

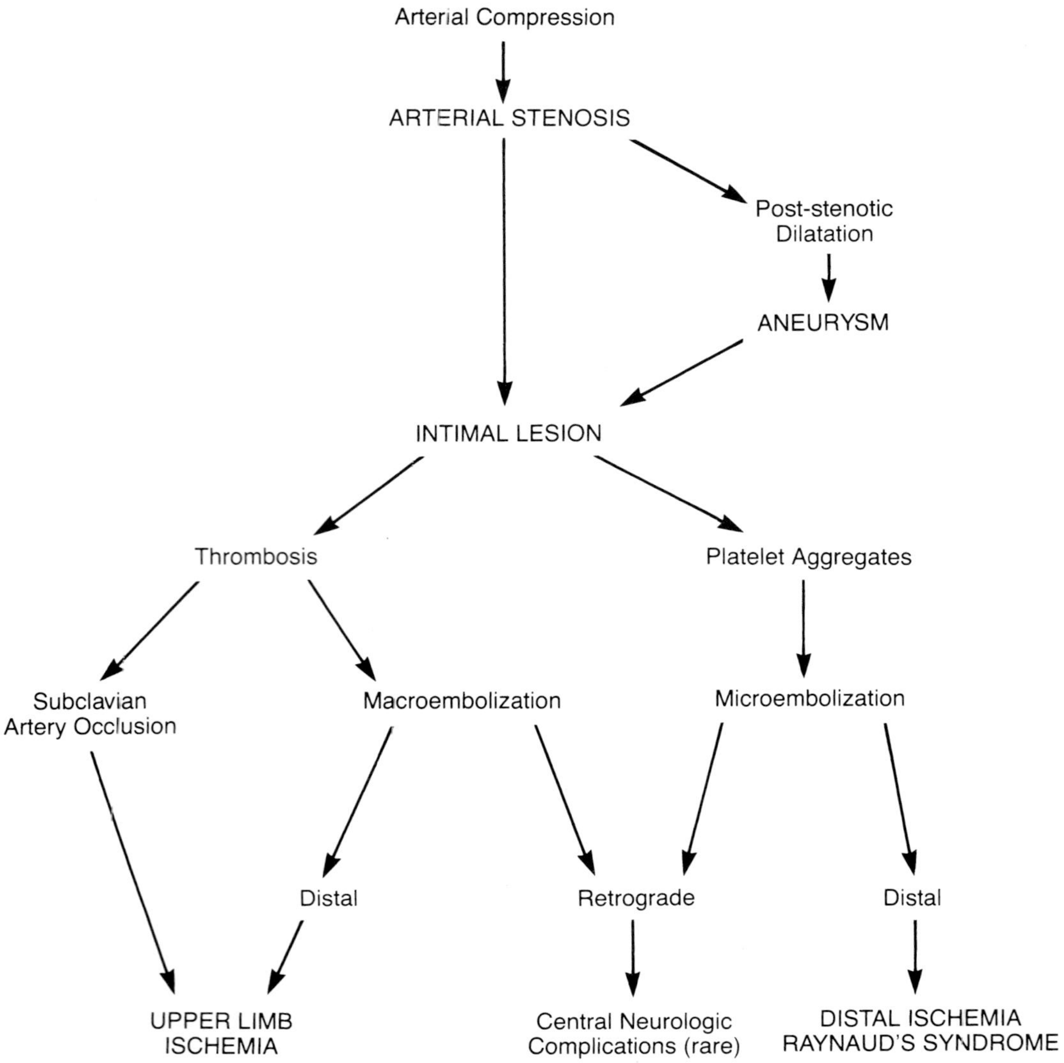

Arterial Compression

↓

ARTERIAL STENOSIS

→ Post-stenotic
Dilatation

↓

ANEURYSM

INTIMAL LESION

Thrombosis   Platelet Aggregates

Subclavian
Artery Occlusion   Macroembolization   Microembolization

Distal   Retrograde   Distal

UPPER LIMB
ISCHEMIA   Central Neurologic   DISTAL ISCHEMIA
                  Complications (rare)   RAYNAUD'S SYNDROME

FIGURE 84–1. Pathophysiology of arterial complications of thoracic outlet syndrome.

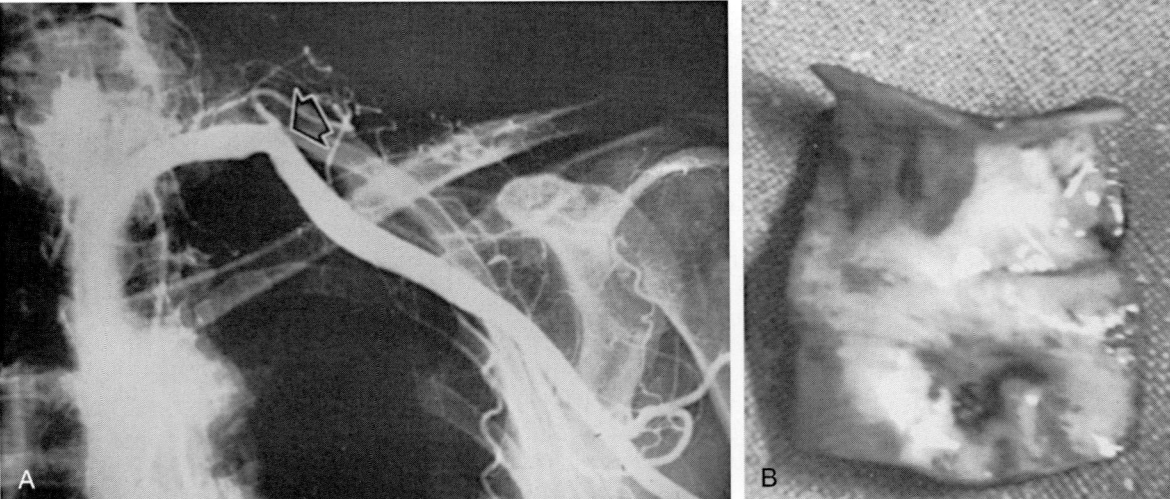

FIGURE 84–2. Preoperative arteriogram (A) and operative specimen (B) of a patient with unilateral Raynaud's syndrome and an ulcerated plaque at the point of compression of the subclavian artery by a cervical rib (*open arrow* in A).

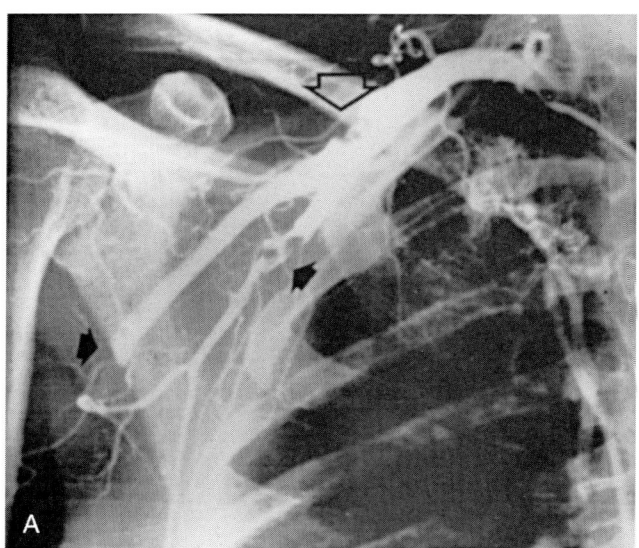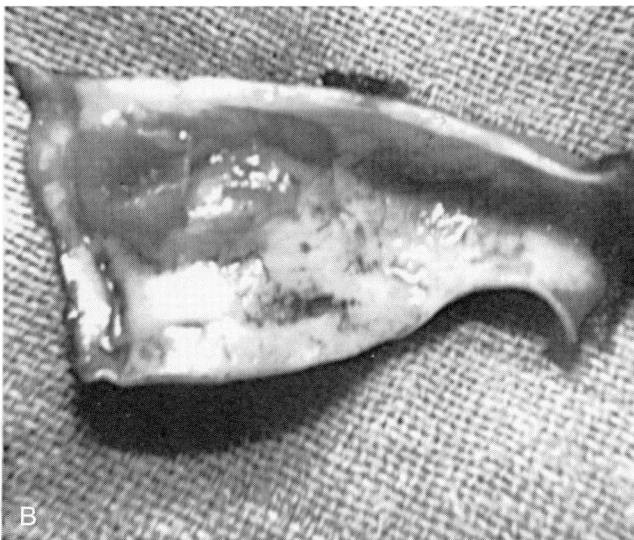

FIGURE 84–3. Preoperative arteriogram (A) and operative specimen (B) of a patient with acute embolic ischemia of the arm (*black arrows* in A) caused by post-stenotic dilatation with mural thrombus of the subclavian-axillary artery (*open arrow* in A) secondary to an anomalous first thoracic rib.

source properly managed before further showers of microemboli or a larger embolus produces ischemic lesions of the fingertips, or even frank gangrene of part or all of one or more digits.[22]

In the presence of such distal vascular findings, the following findings favor the diagnosis of arterioarterial embolism[6, 11]:

- Late age of onset
- Predominant distribution in the radial artery of the hands and digits
- Absence of another cause, such as collagen vascular disease, occupational arterial trauma, or Buerger's disease
- A strictly unilateral condition, clearly indicating their secondary origin

Although digital gangrene is diagnostic of arterial occlusion, Raynaud's syndrome or its equivalents may offer special clinical difficulties. Even if TOS is recognized, these symptoms may have been wrongly attributed to sympathetic irritation because of nerve compression[6]; as a result, the arterial complications may be overlooked. Another diagnostic difficulty may arise from the coincidence of a cervical rib and Raynaud's syndrome of a different cause because both entities are sometimes encountered in one patient.

Microembolization may last months or even years before major embolic complications occur. Acute ischemia due to proximal embolism is the most frequent complication. A proximal artery is the source of 25% to 50% of all upper extremity emboli[23]; of these, complications of TOS are the most common. This source must be suspected in the presence of any proximal embolus in the upper extremity, especially when no cardiac source is found. A major error would be to proceed with standard isolated embolectomy alone.[5, 13, 14, 24]

This first episode of embolization usually has a favorable outcome, even without surgical treatment. The resulting ischemia may become subacute or chronic or may even disappear completely owing to the development of collateral circulation; however, sooner or later, embolization recurs if the cause has not been eradicated through proper management. In these cases, ischemia becomes severe, it does not regress spontaneously, and surgical management becomes extremely difficult because of multiple emboli of different "ages" located at various levels in the limb. The outcome may be unfavorable in more advanced cases, and major amputations are sometimes necessary. Subacute or chronic ischemia is usually produced by a proximal segmental occlusion with good collateral circulation. In a few cases, usually with isolated subclavian artery occlusion, ischemia does not develop, and it may be difficult to establish the differential diagnosis of chronic occlusions because of trauma, cardiogenic embolism, or even Takayasu's arteritis.

In rare cases, arterial damage secondary to TOS may be associated with retrograde cerebral embolization, particularly during exercise that requires atypical positioning of the arm.[29]

DIAGNOSTIC METHODS

History

Diagnosis is usually straightforward if the possibility of a TOS is considered when the clinician treats a patient who has an ischemic upper extremity. A clinical history of a fractured clavicle or first rib, and late complications of hypertrophic callus, malunion, or both, may suggest the diagnosis. More frequently, a cervical rib may have been visualized earlier on a chest film. Symptoms secondary to associated nerve compression are present in only one third of cases.

Physical Examination

The diagnosis may be established by physical examination. A pulsatile mass in the supraclavicular area is often palpable

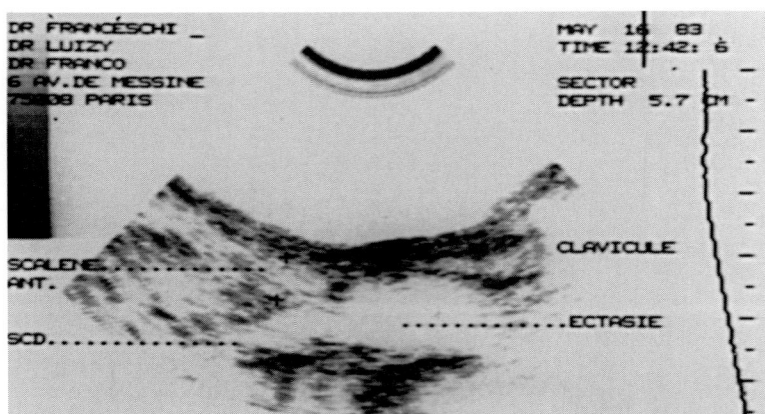

FIGURE 84–4. Ultrasonogram of a case of post-stenotic aneurysm of the subclavian artery.

but does not usually correspond to the subclavian artery aneurysm itself. A more precise examination usually shows that the palpable lesion reflects the bony abnormality pushing the artery upward; the arterial dilatation is slightly more distal, behind the clavicle. A bruit may be heard over the subclavian artery, occasionally only with the upper extremity in extreme positions. Such positions may also diminish or even abolish the distal pulses. Although these findings have some value in these clinical circumstances, they are not specific, because they are often present in normal persons.

Radiography

Anteroposterior and oblique cervical spine and upper thoracic radiographs are most important because a bony abnormality is nearly always present. As mentioned, the most frequent one is a cervical rib, usually long, complete, and fused or articulated to the first rib. Agenesis of the anterior part of the first thoracic rib is less common; still rarer are other congenital abnormalities of the first rib and acquired abnormalities of the clavicle or first rib. The absence of a bony abnormality, however, does not rule out the diagnosis of arterial complications of TOS. In a few cases, only muscular or fibrous elements of compression have been present.

Noninvasive Techniques

Noninvasive techniques have been used to investigate these patients. Doppler examination may be useful in describing and quantifying postural changes in the arterial circulation of the upper extremity. It may also localize the arterial occlusion and assess the collateral circulation. B-mode ultrasonography is useful for establishing the diagnosis of post-stenotic dilatation (Fig. 84–4) and mural thrombus.

Arteriography

The arteriogram should visualize the entire upper extremity, from the aortic arch to the digital arteries. The usual technique is catheterization through the femoral artery and selective injection in the proximal subclavian artery. Arteriographic diagnosis of arterial complications of TOS is not always easy.[24] Subtraction techniques are useful. A fusiform

aneurysm is usually evident, especially one distal to a permanent arterial stenosis (Fig. 84–5). An irregular lining or filling defect strongly suggests mural thrombus (see Fig. 84–3).

Arteriographic findings are seldom entirely normal, but some features may be difficult to recognize. Mural thrombus may obliterate part of the aneurysmal sac. In symptomatic patients, even the smallest post-stenotic dilatation is a strong clue to the diagnosis, and in these patients, mural thrombus is often found at operation or may be demonstrated on ultrasonography. Subclavian stenosis is not always evident on the anteroposterior view because compression in the costoscalene passage occurs in the same plane. Dynamic views help to determine the exact site of compression.

Arteriography is also helpful in demonstrating distal arterial occlusions and the development of the collateral circulation. In the presence of Raynaud's syndrome or distal gangrene secondary to occlusive disease of the digital arteries, magnification films, including those obtained after intra-arterial injection of a vasodilator, may help to distinguish between local lesions and emboli.[25]

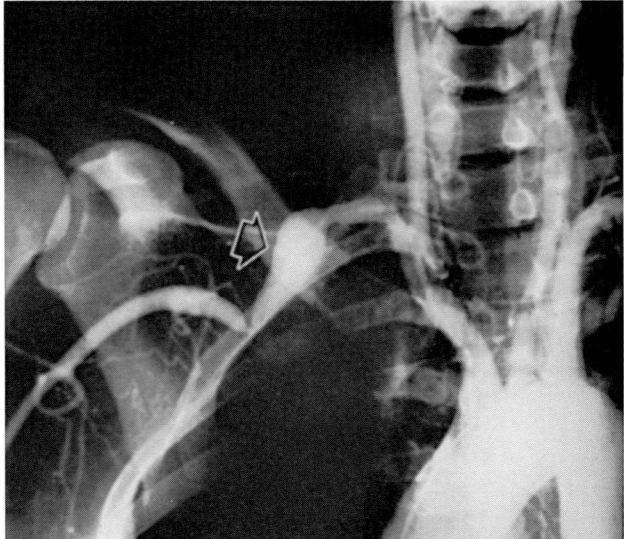

FIGURE 84–5. Post-stenotic aneurysm of the subclavian-axillary artery (open arrow) in an asymptomatic patient with a cervical rib.

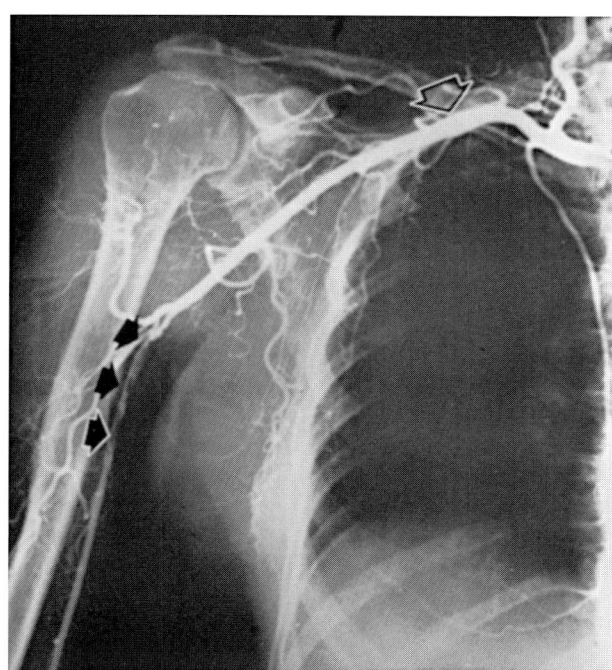

FIGURE 84–6. Minimal post-stenotic dilatation of the subclavian-axillary artery *(open arrow)* in a patient with brachial emboli *(black arrows)* and a cervical rib; mural thrombus of the subclavian-axillary artery was found at operation.

Computed Tomography

Helical computed tomography (CT) may be useful for demonstrating the arterial abnormality, including thrombus in the post-stenotic dilatation or aneurysm and the associated bone abnormality.[30]

Surgical Exploration

In a small number of patients who have cervical ribs or other bony abnormalities and symptoms of thromboembolic disease of the upper extremity, the subclavian artery may appear grossly normal or only slightly dilated on arteriography (Fig. 84–6). In these rare cases, the authors strongly advocate surgical exploration as an integral part of the diagnostic evaluation. Intraoperative arterial palpation is unreliable and may be dangerous because it risks mobilizing the thrombus, resulting in further distal embolization. The authors believe that an exploratory longitudinal arteriotomy is best in these cases. This seemingly aggressive approach is the only way to rule out a small intimal lesion, which must be treated if recurrent emboli are to be avoided.[6, 7, 10, 11] If the arterial intima appears normal, it is simple to close the artery with a continuous suture, tailoring it to correct the post-stenotic dilatation.

SURGICAL MANAGEMENT

The treatment of arterial complications of TOS is surgery. It must often be performed on an emergency or semi-emergency basis, not only in the presence of acute or subacute ischemia of the upper extremity but also every time a mural thrombus has been recognized, because severe embolic complications are unpredictable and may rapidly become difficult to manage.[7] The three anatomic components of the disease process must be treated simultaneously:

• Arterial compression
• Subclavian-axillary arterial lesions
• Distal emboli (less consistently)

Approach

An ideal surgical approach allows simultaneous thoracic outlet decompression, treatment of the subclavian-axillary arterial lesions, and upper dorsal sympathectomy if indicated. The whole upper extremity should be accessible to the surgeon to allow for distal embolectomy when necessary.

The *transaxillary approach* is largely used for isolated rib resection in the presence of neurologic symptoms. An associated upper dorsal sympathectomy may be easily added; however, this approach does not offer satisfactory exposure of the subclavian-axillary artery and is therefore contraindicated for the management of arterial complications. The same objections apply to the *anterolateral thoracic approach*. In addition, a thoracic incision is an unwarranted surgical maneuver, even in young or middle-aged patients.

The *transclavicular approach* allows wide exposure of the supraclavicular and axillary regions. One of two techniques may be used. Although temporary transection of the mid-part of the clavicle, followed by osteosynthesis, seems logical, it may lead to orthopedic complications such as malunion or hypertrophic callus of the clavicle, with or without infection.[8] Resection of the mid-part or the medial two thirds of the clavicle is simpler and has a low incidence of cosmetic and functional impairment[1, 11]; however, because the same surgical procedures can be performed without dividing the clavicle using a supraclavicular approach, the only indications for clavicular resection are the rare cases of arterial complications from malunion or hypertrophic callus of the clavicle.

The *supraclavicular approach* offers complete exposure of the subclavian artery, a cervical rib, and muscular or fibrous bands.[11] With this approach, resection of the normal first rib is safe, provided that the subclavian artery and the brachial plexus are entirely dissected and that the entire upper extremity is prepared and draped so that it may be raised when resection of the anterior part of the rib is undertaken. Complete resection of the posterior part of the first rib can be achieved, and it is a straightforward way to detect and treat any associated muscular or fibrous abnormality. Difficulties may arise when arterial lesions extend to the axillary artery. In these cases, additional exposure is obtained through a deltopectoral or infraclavicular incision, leaving the clavicle undisturbed.[2, 3, 7]

Thoracic Outlet Decompression

Complete resection of a cervical rib or an abnormal first rib is, obviously, necessary. It seems logical to add routine resection of the normal first rib, as in the more common neurologic forms of TOS. Clavicular resection should be performed when malunion or hypertrophic callus complicates a fractured clavicle. In any case, resection of the bony abnormality must be accompanied by removal of any abnormal muscular or fibrous element. Scalenectomy seems definitely preferable to scalenotomy, because the scalene muscles may reattach themselves to the bed of the resected cervical or first rib and cause recurrent arterial or nerve compression.

Proximal Arterial Reconstruction

Arterial reconstruction is necessary in the presence of an arterial aneurysm or mural thrombosis, with or without distal thromboembolic complications. However, mild post-stenotic dilatation without clinical or radiologic evidence of mural thrombus deserves discussion. Many surgeons still consider this entity an indication for conservative management because it is expected to regress after isolated arterial decompression.[4, 8, 21] The authors believe that it is not always a benign condition and that it dictates, at least, surgical exploration. Intimal arterial disease or mural thrombus is difficult to rule out unless exploratory arteriotomy is performed. Very few cases of actual regression of the dilatation after isolated arterial decompression have been reported. Severe arterial complications have been reported after conservative procedures.[10] Although the initial arterial lesions have not always been described precisely, these cases constitute a strong argument in favor of arterial reconstruction in the presence of a seemingly benign post-stenotic dilatation.

Surgical techniques must be tailored to the arterial lesions. Resection is necessary in the presence of a subclavian-axillary aneurysm. Excessive arterial length is usually obtained after resection of the cervical and first thoracic ribs; this allows end-to-end anastomosis in most cases.[2, 3] With a lengthy arterial dilatation, a short segment of graft may have to be interposed to bridge the arterial defect. The preferred graft material is autogenous saphenous vein. When this material is unavailable, the authors favor an arterial autograft[24] rather than a polyester (Dacron) or polytetrafluoroethylene graft.

A mild fusiform post-stenotic dilatation should be opened longitudinally along its entire length and closed with a continuous tailoring suture after an intimal lesion has been ruled out or treated by either intimectomy or limited segmental resection. Although this technique appears easy and appealing, it is sometimes difficult to perform. The use of an internal temporary stent may be necessary for a suitable aneurysmorrhaphy. Proximal or distal transection of the artery may also be useful for arterial lesions that extend behind the clavicle. This measure affords visualization of the entire diseased artery through the supraclavicular or infraclavicular incision. After the aneurysmorrhaphy has been performed, the artery is placed in its normal position and an end-to-end anastomosis is created. Limited arterial resection may be added if the artery is too long.

In rare cases, an isolated intimal fibrous plaque without any associated arterial dilatation may be treated by intimectomy, with or without patch angioplasty closure of the artery. At present, the role of endovascular stents or stent-grafts in managing subclavian artery post-stenotic dilatations or aneurysms is not known.[31]

Management of Distal Embolic Occlusions

Distal embolic occlusions often introduce major surgical difficulties. They are usually multiple and diffuse, with emboli of different ages. Some occlusions are recent and easily cleared by thromboembolectomy; others are older, adherent to the arterial wall, and inaccessible to direct or indirect embolectomy. In such cases, unsuccessful surgical attempts at disobliteration may result in extensive thrombosis. In the presence of a seemingly old and well-compensated distal embolic occlusion, direct surgical treatment is to be avoided.[2, 3] In most such cases, upper dorsal sympathectomy is probably all that is required.

If the distal arterial occlusion involves the large arteries, is apparently of recent onset, and results in severe distal ischemia, an attempt at direct revascularization is appropriate. It may be possible to perform an embolectomy by introducing a Fogarty balloon catheter through the distal subclavian artery at the site of proximal reconstruction. Distal passage of the catheter through the entire upper extremity is often difficult or impossible. Selective catheterization of the radial and ulnar arteries may also be difficult, and a separate approach to the brachial artery bifurcation is usually necessary. Intraoperative arteriography is advisable in most cases, and urokinase infusion can be considered although its role has not been established.

For persistent occlusion of the forearm or hand arteries, a direct approach is required to the radial artery, ulnar artery, or both, at the wrist. The surgeon performs selective embolectomy of the palmar arches using a No. 2 Fogarty balloon catheter. Closure of the arteriotomy is accomplished under loupe magnification. For a chronic brachial occlusion that is complicated by a proximal recent embolus, it may be sufficient to revascularize the deep brachial artery,[10] which plays the same physiologic collateral role in the upper extremity as the deep femoral artery does in the lower extremity, provided that the periarticular arterial network of the elbow is patent.

In subacute cases, and perhaps chronic cases, catheter-directed fibrinolytic therapy can be considered in an attempt to open the distal arterial bed. Although experience is limited, this new therapeutic modality may provide appropriate salvage or permit a more straightforward reconstruction.

If an embolectomy is impossible, ineffective, or incomplete, a distal bypass using autogenous vein may be performed in an attempt to revascularize one of the forearm arteries, usually the interosseous one (Fig. 84–7).

Difficulty in clearing the distal arterial bed accounts for the incomplete revascularization of the forearm and hand in the most advanced cases. Major amputations are still reported, often after multiple surgical attempts to revascularize the upper extremity.[1, 11, 24] Distal amputations are mentioned in most large series, and some patients, although they have a viable upper limb, may experience a disabling ischemic sequela such as Raynaud's syndrome, Volkmann's contracture, claudication, or fatigability of the forearm. These results are in sharp contrast to those obtained in the absence of distal embolization, when clinical and anatomic results are consistently good if the initial surgical management has been appropriate.[2, 3, 21]

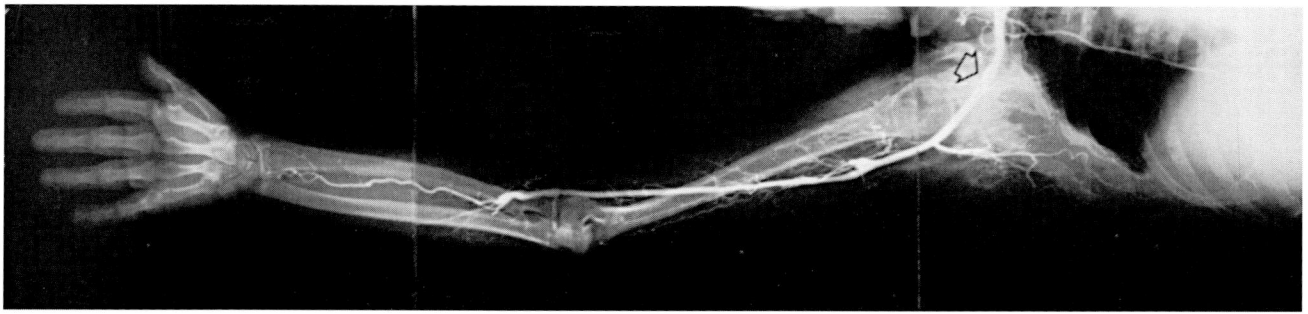

FIGURE 84–7. Postoperative arteriogram 4 years after bony decompression of thoracic outlet, resection and anastomosis of a subclavian aneurysm *(open arrow)*, embolectomy of the axillary and proximal brachial artery, upper dorsal sympathectomy, and brachial artery–interosseous artery saphenous vein bypass.

REFERENCES

1. Judy KL, Heymann RL: Vascular complications of thoracic outlet syndrome. Am J Surg 123:521, 1972.
2. Kieffer E, Jue-Denis P, Benhamou M, et al: Complications artérielles du syndrome de la traversée thoraco-brachiale: Traitement chirurgical de 38 cas. Chirurgie 109:714, 1983.
3. Cormier JM, Amrane M, Ward A, et al: Arterial complications of the thoracic outlet syndrome: Fifty-five operative cases. J Vasc Surg 9:778, 1989.
4. Blank RH, Connar RG: Arterial complications associated with thoracic outlet syndrome. Ann Thorac Surg 17:315, 1974.
5. Short DW: The subclavian artery in 16 patients with complete cervical ribs. J Cardiovasc Surg 16:135, 1975.
6. Swinton NW Jr, Hall RJ, Baugh JH, et al: Unilateral Raynaud's phenomenon caused by cervical–first rib anomalies. Am J Med 48:404, 1970.
7. Martin J, Gaspard DJ, Johnston PW, et al: Vascular manifestations of the thoracic outlet syndrome: A surgical urgency. Arch Surg 111:779, 1976.
8. Mercier C, Houel F, David G, et al: Les complications vasculaires des syndromes de la traversée thoraco-brachiale. Chirurgie 107:433, 1981.
9. Dumeige F, Andre J, Vargas R, et al: Les complications vasculaires des anomalies de la première côte. Chirurgie 112:584, 1986.
10. Banis JC Jr, Rich N, Whelan TJ Jr: Ischemia of the upper extremity due to noncardiac emboli. Am J Surg 134:131, 1977.
11. Bouhoutsos J, Morris T, Martin P: Unilateral Raynaud's phenomenon in the hand and its significance. Surgery 82:547, 1977.
12. Roos DB: Congenital anomalies associated with thoracic outlet syndrome. Am J Surg 132:771, 1976.
13. Dorazio RA, Ezzet F: Arterial complications of the thoracic outlet syndrome. Am J Surg 138:246, 1979.
14. Simon H, Gryska PF, Carlson DH: The thoracic outlet syndrome as a cause of aneurysm formation, thrombosis, and embolization. South Med J 70:282, 1977.
15. Melliere D, Escourrou J, Becquemin JP, et al: Ischémies aigues des membres: Complications tardives de cals hypertrophiques et de pseudarthroses. J Chir (Paris) 118:641, 1981.
16. Roach MR: Changes in arterial distensibility as a cause of poststenotic dilatation. Am J Cardiol 12:802, 1963.
17. Ojha M, Johnson KW, Cobbold RSC: Evidence of a possible link between poststenotic dilation and wall shear stress. J Vasc Surg 11:127, 1990.
18. Gunning AJ, Pickering GW, Robb-Smith AHT, et al: Mural thrombosis of the subclavian artery and subsequent embolism in cervical rib. Q J Med 129:133, 1964.
19. Al-Hassen HK, Sattar MA, Eklof B: Embolic brain infarction: A rare complication of thoracic outlet syndrome: A report of two cases. J Cardiovasc Surg 29:322, 1988.
20. De Villiers JC: A brachiocephalic vascular syndrome associated with cervical rib. Br Med J 2:140, 1966.
21. Pairolero PC, Walls JT, Payne WS, et al: Subclavian axillary artery aneurysms. Surgery 90:757, 1981.
22. Vayssairat M, Fiessinger JN, Housset E: Les nécroses digitales du membre supérieur: 86 cas. Nouv Presse Med 6:931, 1977.
23. Sachatello CR, Ernst CB, Griffen WO Jr: The acutely ischemic upper extremity: Selective managment. Surgery 76:1002, 1974.
24. Etheredge S, Wilbur R, Stoney RJ: Thoracic outlet syndrome. Am J Surg 138:175, 1979.
25. Maiman MH, Bookstein JJ, Bernstein EF: Digital ischemia: Angiographic differentiation of embolism from arterial disease. Am J Roentgenol 137:1183, 1981.
26. Nehler MR, Taylor LMJ, Moneta GL, Porter JM: Upper extremity ischemia from subclavian artery aneurysm caused by bony abnormalities of the thoracic outlet. Arch Surg 132:527, 1997.
27. Desai Y, Robbs JV: Arterial complications of the thoracic outlet syndrome. Eur J Vasc Endovasc Surg 10:362, 1995.
28. Gelabert HA, Machleder HI: Diagnosis and management of arterial compression at the thoracic outlet. Ann Vasc Surg 11:359, 1997.
29. Bearn P, Patel J, O'Flynn WR: Cervical ribs: A cause of distal and cerebral embolism. Postgrad Med J 69:65, 1993.
30. Matsumura JS, Rilling WS, Pearce WH, et al: Helical computed tomography of the normal thoracic outlet. J Vasc Surg 26:776, 1997.
31. Szeimies U, Kueffer G, Stoeckelhuber B, Steckmeier B: Successful exclusion of subclavian aneurysms with covered nitinol stents. Cardiovasc Intervent Radiol 21:246, 1998.

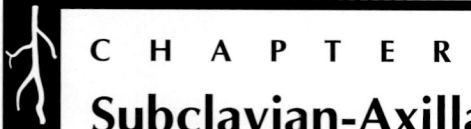

CHAPTER 8 5
Subclavian-Axillary Vein Thrombosis

Scott N. Hurlbert, M.D., and
Robert B. Rutherford, M.D.

HISTORICAL PERSPECTIVE

James Paget[91] described the clinical symptoms of subclavian-axillary vein thrombosis in 1875. He called the syndrome of acute swelling and pain of the upper extremity "gouty phlebitis" and attributed it to vasospasm. In 1884, von Schroetter[122] postulated that a thrombosis of the subclavian and axillary veins caused these symptoms. The term "Paget-Schroetter syndrome" first appeared in 1949 in Hughes'[62] comprehensive review of the world's literature. At that time, subclavian-axillary vein thrombosis was relatively rare, as Hughes found only 320 cases of the disease.

By the 1960s, it had been established that primary subclavian-axillary vein thromboses were seen after exertion of the affected upper extremity, and the term "effort thrombosis" came into use. In the early 1970s, a steady shift in the predominant cause began as more cases of subclavian-axillary vein thrombosis were encountered in patients with indwelling central venous catheters. Aubaniac[8] had described the first use of a subclavian vein catheter in 1952. These central venous lines were used for fluid resuscitation and placed via a cutdown. In 1968, Dudrick and coworkers[38] described the first percutaneous placement of a subclavian vein catheter for total parenteral nutrition. Reports of catheter-associated subclavian-axillary vein thrombosis started appearing in the literature soon after the initial descriptions of placement of these catheters.[29, 114] An autopsy study by McDonough and Altemeier,[84] in 1971, confirmed the association.

The use of central venous catheters experienced rapid growth after 1973 with the introduction of a silicone-rubber (Silastic) catheter, which was more flexible and easier to handle than before.[23] Currently, the subclavian vein is cannulated for a variety of reasons, including nutrition, cardiac monitoring, hemodialysis, chemotherapy, resuscitation, and pacemakers. As the indications for central venous access have increased, so has the incidence of catheter related subclavian-axillary vein thrombosis.

Subclavian-axillary vein thrombosis is a multifactorial disease. The treatment and prognosis depend on the specific cause. Subclavian-axillary vein thromboses can be divided into two major groups: primary and secondary. The *primary* (effort-induced) form implies that no direct cause is obvious on initial evaluation. Often an anatomic defect in the thoracic inlet becomes apparent through repetitive compressive venous trauma or after a period of strenuous use or prolonged positioning that precipitates thrombosis. Thus, although such a mechanism is presumed, Paget-Schroetter syndrome is still considered synonymous with "primary" subclavian-axillary vein thrombosis.

Secondary subclavian-axillary vein thrombosis is a result of multiple etiologic factors exerting their effects through one or more of *Virchow's triad*: stasis, endothelial injury, and hypercoagulability. These conditions all promote thrombosis and include malignancy, heart failure, infection, trauma, polycythemia, drug abuse, estrogens, mediastinal tumors, thrombocytosis, and central venous catheters, although in most series central venous catheters dominate this category.

INCIDENCE

Upper extremity deep venous thrombosis (DVT) occurs in 1% to 4% of all DVTs.[5, 11, 29, 56, 59, 76, 94] As mentioned, the advent of percutaneous techniques and flexible, easily handled catheters brought about a large increase in the number of central venous cannulations and a subsequent rise in the number of catheter-related thromboses. Table 85–1 documents the relative change in incidence between primary and catheter-associated subclavian-axillary vein thrombosis.

Primary subclavian-axillary vein thrombosis is reported to make up about 25% of all upper extremity DVTs, catheter-associated subclavian-axillary vein thrombosis constitutes 40%, and other forms of secondary subclavian-axillary vein thrombosis make up the rest of the upper extremity DVTs. Because primary and secondary subclavian-axillary vein thromboses have different etiologic patterns and treatment considerations, they are considered separately here.

PRIMARY SUBCLAVIAN-AXILLARY VEIN THROMBOSIS

Etiology

The underlying cause of primary subclavian-axillary vein thrombosis is universally accepted as being related to compression of the subclavian vein at the thoracic inlet (Fig. 85–1). This compression, presumably, leads to stasis of blood flow and subsequent thrombosis. Earlier work by Adams and DeWeese[4] demonstrated compression of the subclavian vein in the costoclavicular space with hyperabduction of the arm, hyperextension of the neck, or downward and backward movement of the shoulder *in normal patients* without thrombosis of the subclavian vein.

Anatomic abnormalities or occasionally congenital defects are thought to increase the susceptibility to positional

TABLE 85–1. RELATIVE INCIDENCE OF PRIMARY SUBCLAVIAN-AXILLARY VEIN THROMBOSIS VERSUS CATHETER-ASSOCIATED THROMBOSIS

AUTHOR	YEAR	PRIMARY THROMBOSIS (%)	CATHETER-ASSOCIATED THROMBOSIS (%)
Hughes[62]	1949	84	0
Coon and Willis[29]	1966	28	10
Tilney et al[114]	1970	41	17
Campbell et al[25]	1977	44	36
Painter and Karpf[92]	1984	47	29
Donayre et al[35]	1986	24	24
Horattas et al[59]	1988	18	39
Lindblad et al[76]	1988	40	22
Kerr et al[68]	1990	6	69
Hill and Berry[56]	1990	45	33
AbuRahma et al[1]			
First 5 yr of study	1991	28	17
Second 5 yr of study	1991	29	47
Hingorani et al[57]	1997	21	65

compression of the vein and can be incriminated in most patients with subclavian-axillary vein thrombosis by venographic studies and direct observation at operation. Some of the more common anatomic anomalies are abnormalities of the anterior scalene, subclavius, pectoralis minor, and scalenus minimus muscles.[1, 3, 4, 33, 34, 72, 86, 106, 107, 110, 115] Bony abnormalities of the clavicle and ribs have also been observed.[33, 72, 106, 115, 119] Other authors have found congenital bands,[55, 119] an aberrant phrenic nerve,[62, 107, 114] or an abnormal costocoracoid ligament[9, 33, 36, 107] at the time of thoracic outlet decompression.

Unfortunately, no study has been able to determine the relative involvement of these anatomic defects in the development of subclavian-axillary vein thrombosis. It is unknown how many patients with these abnormalities will have a clinically significant upper extremity thrombosis, but in the studies that specifically looked for anatomic defects, 92% of patients had some anatomic abnormality at surgery.[34, 71, 115] Venographic studies evaluating the contralateral arm in patients with subclavian-axillary vein thrombosis have found venous compression in 56% to 80% of these limbs.[11, 72, 81, 82] Notably, the incidence of bilateral thrombosis is only 2% to 15%.[33, 46, 72, 81, 82, 112, 119]

In addition to the acute compressive event, repetitive compressive trauma to the vein may cause microscopic tears to the intima.[1, 9, 69, 112] Aziz and colleagues[9] hypothesized that fibrosis and thickening of the vein wall and intimal proliferation developed after repetitive minor injuries to the vein with arm motion. The subsequent narrowing of the vein was thought to eventually result in thrombosis.

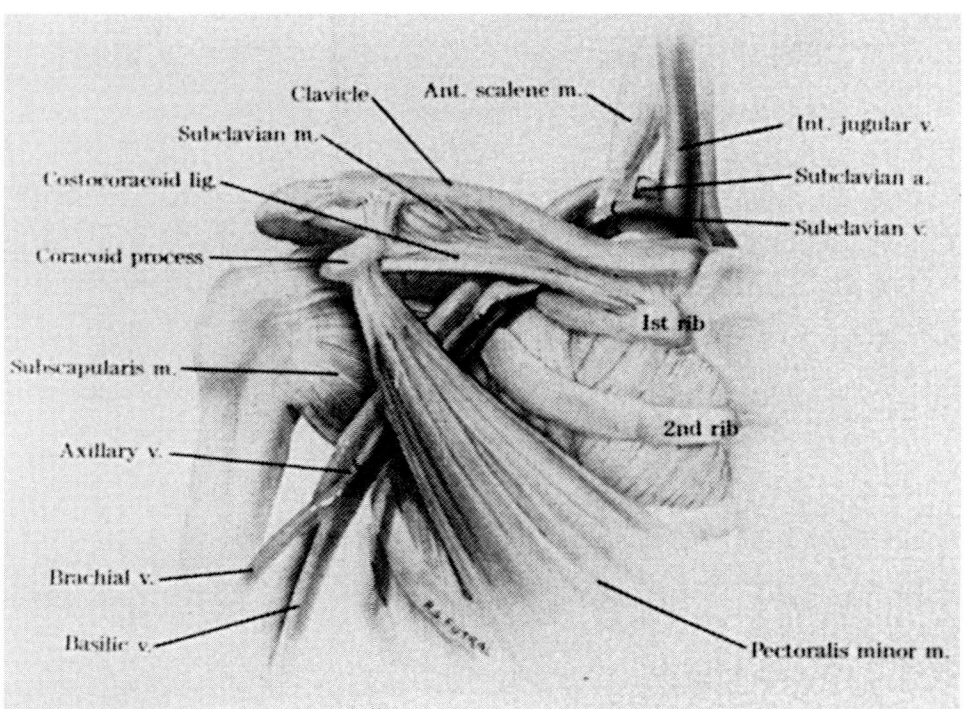

FIGURE 85–1. Anatomy of the thoracic outlet.

This observation was made after chronic fibrous changes, both externally and internally, were noted in the subclavian veins of a series of patients undergoing direct surgical thrombectomy and venolysis. Whether these changes were the cause of the eventual thrombosis or the result of subclinical thrombotic build-up before the final event is not known.

Some authors have suggested that the stress of exercise causes a temporary hypercoagulability.[1, 9, 69] In their study, Sundqvist and coworkers[110] found a decrease in fibrinolytic activity within the subclavian vein in almost half of the 53 patients with subclavian-axillary vein thrombosis. Unfortunately, many of these patients were taking exogenous estrogens, had an underlying cancer, or had other causes of secondary subclavian-axillary vein thrombosis. It is not clear what percentage of the group had pure primary subclavian-axillary vein thrombosis. Whether a systemic or local coagulation defect is present in patients with subclavian-axillary vein thrombosis is not clear. It may play a role in certain patients, such as women taking oral contraceptives, but of Virchow's triad, endothelial injury and flow disturbances predominate.

Clinical Presentation

Most patients with primary subclavian-axillary vein thrombosis are young males. One review of the literature revealed a 2:1 predilection of males over females, with an average age of 31 years.[63] Of the patients, 75% report an antecedent event of strenuous or repetitive activity before onset of symptoms.[1, 3, 5, 25, 29, 72, 82, 114] The dominant extremity is involved in 60% to 80% of cases.[1, 25, 72, 82, 112] There have been variable reports of the association between subclavian-axillary vein thrombosis and arterial or neurogenic thoracic outlet syndrome. The presence of subclavian-axillary vein thrombosis in patients with neurogenic thoracic outlet syndrome is low, (only 4% to 10% of patients).[25, 45, 46, 109] This is not surprising, when one considers that the vein and nerves are at opposite ends of the thoracic outlet. With this in mind, it is surprising that most patients with primary subclavian-axillary vein thrombosis report symptoms of either arterial or neurogenic thoracic outlet syndrome.[46, 72, 81, 112, 115, 119]

The hallmark of subclavian-axillary vein thrombosis is swelling of the involved extremity. Virtually every patient will present with some degree of upper extremity swelling. The edema usually involves the entire arm and hand and is characteristically nonpitting. In time, a variable percentage of patients will have obvious venous engorgement of the superficial collateral veins over the upper arm, base of the neck, and anterior chest. Most patients eventually also complain of pain in the affected extremity. The pain is described as "aching," "stabbing," or a feeling of "tightness" referred to the arm or axilla[3] and usually worsens with exertion. Some patients may have discoloration or cyanosis of the arm, usually mild, and a few have a palpable cord.

The pathophysiology underlying the clinical characteristics of subclavian-axillary vein thrombosis is venous hypertension. The intensity of signs and symptoms is directly related to the length of the occlusion and the amount of activity of the involved extremity.

After recovery from the acute event, most active patients have residual symptoms. Before the advent of surgical or thrombolytic therapy, 80% of patients with primary subclavian-axillary vein thrombosis had persistent symptoms.[3, 5, 35, 69, 112, 114] This likely reflects an above-average activity level with an ongoing need for active use of the involved extremity. Unlike lower extremity DVT symptoms, symptoms in the upper extremity are related to residual obstruction rather than reflux. Most patients complain of pain and swelling that are made worse by dependency and active use of the involved extremity. The increased arterial blood flow to the exercising upper extremity cannot be met by a proportional increase in venous outflow through the limited collateral vessels without significant venous hypertension. Swelling, pain, and even venous claudication result. The incidence of disabling symptoms is high.

In their series of primary subclavian-axillary vein thrombosis patients, Swinton and coauthors[112] found that only 9% had no symptoms, 52% of patients had symptoms but were able to work, and 39% were completely disabled. Tilney and colleagues[114] reported that 55% of patients in their series were unable to work, 18% were working but symptomatic, and 27% had no symptoms. In the Swinton study,[112] the use or nonuse of extended oral anticoagulation after thrombosis made no difference in the degree of disability. Other authors have found a decrease in symptoms with the use of oral anticoagulation agents.[3] In a more recent study, Donayre and associates[35] reported a 78% incidence of persistent symptoms in patients taking warfarin (Coumadin).

In contrast to lower extremity DVT, stasis dermatitis and ulceration are almost never seen in subclavian-axillary vein thrombosis.[5, 35, 69] Venous reflux, which contributes to stasis dermatitis and venous ulceration in the lower extremity, is not a factor in the upper extremity, and the contribution of gravity to increased hydrostatic pressure is much lower.

Pulmonary embolism has been variously reported as occurring from 0% to 28.5% in patients with subclavian-axillary vein thrombosis.[3, 5, 25, 35, 54, 60, 112, 114, 116] As the methods of detecting pulmonary embolism have improved, the incidence has increased. Hughes[62] reported pulmonary embolism in only three of 302 patients in his review. Monreal and coauthors[89] prospectively examined, with ventilation-perfusion scanning, 30 consecutive patients who had upper extremity DVT. They discovered that 15% of patients had evidence of pulmonary emboli. Of these patients, only one was symptomatic. Overall, the symptomatic pulmonary embolism rate is about 12%.[63]

Most studies that reported pulmonary embolism have grouped primary and secondary subclavian-axillary vein thrombosis together. It is difficult to determine whether one form of subclavian-axillary vein thrombosis has a higher rate of pulmonary embolism, but when we compare the rates in studies reporting only primary or secondary subclavian-axillary vein thrombosis, there is not much difference in the incidence.[3, 35, 76, 89, 99, 102, 112] In a retrospective study, Hingorani and colleagues[57] found no difference in the rate of pulmonary embolism between primary or secondary subclavian-axillary vein thrombosis. Their overall incidence was 7%. Regardless of the underlying cause, pulmonary embolism can be a significant complication of subclavian-axillary vein thrombosis. Only the relatively small clot burden reduces its usual clinical impact.

Venous gangrene is an extremely rare complication of upper extremity DVT. It is estimated that upper extremity phlegmasia cerulea dolens constitutes 2% to 5% of all phlegmasia cases.[66] Only 15 cases of upper extremity phlegmasia were reported before 1993.[26] All of these cases were secondary to an underlying hypercoagulable state or malignancy. This same report did document a single patient with venous gangrene secondary to a spontaneous upper extremity DVT. Their extensive evaluation revealed no underlying cause of the thrombosis.[26] To date, there have been no reports of phlegmasia arising from effort-induced subclavian-axillary vein thrombosis.

Diagnosis

The diagnosis of primary subclavian-axillary vein thrombosis is based on the clinical presentation of upper extremity swelling, venous engorgement, and pain of relatively sudden onset. Eighty-five per cent of patients eventually have symptoms within the first 24 hours of the precipitating event.[5, 69, 112] Patients with small occlusions and ample collateral vessels may not have many symptoms. This fact, or the lack of a clear precipitating event, can cause delays in making the diagnosis.

Once subclavian-axillary vein thrombosis is thought to be present, diagnostic studies are indicated to confirm the diagnosis and to determine the extent of the thrombus. Some of the comments that follow apply to both primary and secondary subclavian-axillary vein thrombosis.

Older noninvasive diagnostic modalities, such as continuous-wave Doppler examination and impedance plethysmography, have largely been supplanted by duplex ultrasonography, which has been used extensively in the diagnosis of upper extremity DVT. Compared with venography, duplex scanning has excellent specificity.[51, 70] Although Haire and coworkers[51] found no false-positive results in their prospective series comparing duplex with venography, sensitivity of duplex scanning was only 44% in their study. In this experience, duplex scanning tended to miss occlusions in the vein under the medial one third of the clavicle owing to shadowing and to miss nonocclusive thrombi. In a later study, Koksoy and colleagues[70] found that duplex scanning had a sensitivity of 94% and a specificity of 96% compared with venography. Advances in ultrasound technology (e.g., color flow scan) and adjunctive use of indirect criteria for proximal occlusion (distended, incompressible vein with continuous flow and poor augmentation by compressive maneuvers) may improve sensitivity.

Other noninvasive diagnostic modalities have been used to evaluate subclavian-axillary vein thrombosis. Magnetic resonance angiography (MRA) is specific for complete occlusions of the subclavian and axillary veins, but it has poor sensitivity, especially for nonocclusive thrombi.[51] MRA may also miss short segment occlusions.[41] Other disadvantages include the expense of the study and the production of artefacts by indwelling catheters. Unlike duplex, MRA cannot easily be made portable, and a specialized setting is necessary. Radionuclide venography is useful in detecting the presence of thrombus, but it provides minimal information about the surrounding structures; nuclear medicine studies do not precisely define the extent of the clot either.[41] Computed tomography (CT) has also been used to detect

subclavian-axillary vein thrombosis. Unfortunately, comparison studies with venography are insufficient to determine its specificity and sensitivity. Because of its cost, relative accuracy, and ease of performance, venous duplex ultrasonography remains the screening tool of choice.

Venography is still the "gold standard" in evaluating subclavian-axillary vein thrombosis, and it is required if intervention is contemplated. Performing upper extremity venography can be challenging. Often edema within the arm makes it difficult to locate a suitable vein without ultrasound guidance. The basilic vein is the preferred site for venous access. A more peripheral vein can be used if anticubital veins are not accessible. Digital subtraction methods have allowed for more accurate images from these distal cannulation sites, and they also decrease the amount of contrast material needed to obtain the images.[97] The cephalic vein is not used because it joins directly with the subclavian vein and venography through this vein may miss an axillary vein thrombosis.

Positioning of the patient is very important in upper extremity venography. The patient's arm must be abducted at least 30 degrees. The pectoralis major muscle may compress the axillary vein if the arm is at the patient's side and may mimic a complete occlusion.[68] A positive venogram can show various degrees of occlusion or stenosis of the subclavian-axillary vein (Fig. 85–2). It also shows the presence and extent of the collateral circulation. The extent of the collateral circulation can help determine the chronicity of the occlusion as well as the hemodynamic significance of the occlusion or stenosis.

Patients with a normal venogram with the arm in the neutral position may still have intermittent compression of the subclavian vein.[4] (Fig. 85–3). Patients with symptoms without an occluding thrombus or patients with normal venograms after clot removal by thrombolysis or thrombec-

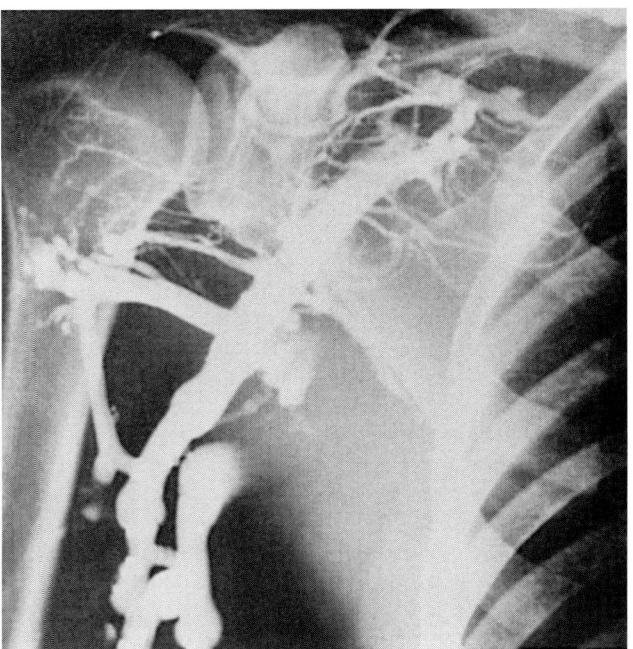

FIGURE 85–2. Venogram of acute primary subclavian-axillary vein thrombosis.

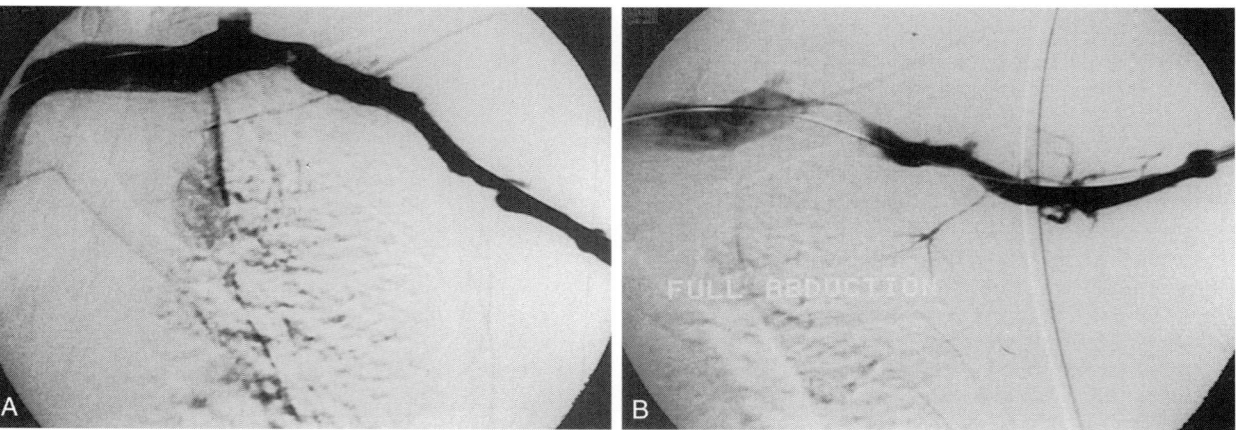

FIGURE 85-3. *A,* Post-thrombolysis venogram with the arm to the side. *B,* Post-thrombolysis venogram with the arm in full abduction.

tomy should undergo provocative maneuvers under fluoroscopy to demonstrate the compression. These maneuvers recreate the most likely positions for compressing the subclavian vein. The abduction and externally rotated (AER) position is commonly recommended, but holding the arm overhead or pulling it down by the side, as if carrying a weight, may also demonstrate extrinsic compression. If one maneuver fails to show compression, others should be tried.

Contrast venography is not without pitfalls. False-positive results are possible from inadequate positioning of the patient or by the inflow of nonopacified blood, as in the confluence of the internal jugular vein and the subclavian vein. The contrast material itself can even precipitate venous thrombosis.[97] Injection of contrast media into the subcutaneous tissues can cause blistering and tissue necrosis. Intravenous contrast media can also induce an anaphylactic reaction or nephrotoxicity. Upper extremity venography is an invasive study with potential complications and is not suitable as a screening test. Even if subclavian-axillary vein thrombosis is suspected and noninvasive findings are negative, a venogram may not be warranted if conservative therapy is planned. Venography is indicated when surgical or endovascular intervention is contemplated.

Treatment

Historically, the treatment of primary subclavian-axillary vein thrombosis relied on rest and elevation of the affected extremity along with systemic anticoagulation therapy. The incidence of long-term morbidity associated with conservative therapy is high.[1, 5, 35, 112, 114] Many of the patients are young and active and are severely limited by their symptoms. Early attempts to treat this disorder with cervical sympathectomy, surgical venolysis, excision of a venous segment, perivenous and periarterial sympathectomies, and even thrombectomy were largely unsuccessful.[62] It was not until investigators realized that the underlying etiology of primary subclavian-axillary vein thrombosis stemmed from venous compression in the thoracic outlet that more effective therapy was developed. It ultimately became accepted that successful treatment of primary subclavian-axillary vein thrombosis required restoration of luminal patency and removal of any extrinsic compression. As will be seen,

with the advent of thrombolytic therapy routinely monitored by venography, residual intrinsic stenoses have been seen with increasing frequency, and when these are significant, treatment is required.

Thrombectomy

Initially, subclavian vein patency was restored by operative thrombectomy. Short-term results were good in small series, but rethrombosis was not uncommon[72] unless thoracic outlet decompression followed. DeWeese and Adams and their colleagues[3, 34] reported a series of six patients who underwent operative thrombectomy along with thoracic outlet decompression via a first rib resection. There were no symptomatic limbs after 0 to 12 years of follow-up. Although the numbers were small, these authors established the effectiveness of this combined therapy.[3, 34]

Operative thrombectomy is attractive because vein recanalization and thoracic outlet decompression can be accomplished in the same setting. Aziz and coworkers[9] noted similar results in their series of four patients treated with combined thrombectomy and first rib resection. Although largely supplanted by thrombolysis (see later), this therapy has proved effective enough that it should be considered in any healthy, low-risk patient with indications for intervention and a contraindication to, or failure of, thrombolytic therapy.

Thrombolytic Therapy

With the advent of thrombolytic therapy, attempts were made to restore patency of the subclavian and axillary veins. Modern thrombolytic techniques generally produce less morbid than operative thrombectomy does, but they too carry poor long-term outcomes if not combined with thoracic outlet decompression. In an early paper, Zimmermann and coauthors[128] gave systemic urokinase to 13 primary patients with subclavian-axillary vein thrombosis. More than half of these patients were still symptomatic after treatment and had residual stenoses, as demonstrated by venography. Subsequent studies of systemic thrombolysis without thoracic outlet decompression have substantiated this finding.[1, 73, 105, 106, 109, 113, 127]

There has been a shift away from the systemic thrombolytic therapy administration to catheter-directed administration. Catheter-directed techniques allow for immediate venographic evaluation of the progress of thrombolysis and provide a means of assessing extrinsic compression with positional phlebography after thrombolysis. When the catheter is placed directly into the clot, the thrombus is exposed to a higher concentration of lytic agent and less time is needed to dissolve the clot. Although local administration also limits the complications associated with a systemic lytic effect, the method of delivery has no effect on the amount of residual stenosis after thrombolysis.[7, 14, 37, 103] In a study by Sheeran and others[103] nine patients underwent catheter-directed thrombolysis with urokinase but did not receive thoracic outlet decompression; 36% of patients had residual lesions, and 55% had symptomatic limbs. Recanalization of the vein without decompression of the thoracic outlet is not adequate for treatment of primary subclavian-axillary vein thrombosis.

The observation that thrombolysis alone was insufficient in treating primary subclavian-axillary vein thrombosis prompted investigators to combine this therapy with thoracic outlet decompression. Kunkel and Machleder[72] reported the first major series of this combined multimodality approach. In their initial 18 patients, 92% returned to work after catheter-directed thrombolysis and first rib resection. In a follow-up to this series, Machleder[82] reported that 86% of 36 patients were asymptomatic after combined therapy. Since the earlier studies, the literature has confirmed the superiority of initial thrombolysis followed by first rib resection in the treatment of primary subclavian-axillary vein thrombosis[6, 16, 58, 83, 85–87, 103, 109, 115, 119]; this is now accepted as the preferred approach (Fig. 85–4). The procedure for first rib resection is described in Chapter 83.

Interval Between Clot Removal and Thoracic Outlet Decompression

One issue raised by multimodal therapy is the appropriate time interval between the initial thrombolysis and the thoracic outlet decompression. In Machleder's first study,[81] it was recommended that the patient receive oral anticoagulation agents and that 3 months elapse from thrombolysis to surgery. This interval was to allow for healing of the endothelium and to avoid thrombosis of the vein at the time of surgery. The delay also provided time to evaluate the need for surgery after return of full use of the arm.[72] The disadvantages to waiting so long are that:

1. There is a definite risk of rethrombosis.
2. The majority of patients who are active cannot return to work or other desired activities for a prolonged period.
3. A second admission is necessary.

Rethrombosis rates in the literature range from 6% to 18%.[6, 58, 85] Molina[86, 87] has advocated immediate first rib resection after thrombolysis to prevent chronic fibrous narrowing of the vein and to decrease the formation of collateral vessels, which may adversely affect the patency of a subsequent stent or operative angioplasty. He reported no episodes of rethrombosis in eight patients who presented with acute, first time subclavian-axillary vein thrombosis.[86] Urschel and Razzuk[119] performed thoracic outlet decompression 4 hours after ceasing lytic therapy in 35 patients and noted no rethromboses or excessive bleeding.

The issue is still unresolved, but since Machleder's first report, his recommended time interval between therapies has decreased. Most authors now wait a month before first rib resection, and treatment outcomes have not been adversely affected.[6, 58, 85, 103] Recently others[27, 74] have successfully tested a policy of treating the acute thrombosis and relieving the thoracic outlet during the same admission, thereby reducing patient "down" time and overall management costs. Lee and colleagues[74] performed thoracic outlet decompression in 11 patients within 4 days of thrombolysis in four, venolysis in seven, patch angioplasty in three, and bypass in two, with good results in nine of 11. Chang and coauthors[27] performed thoracic outlet decompression followed by venography with stenting as needed, all within 24 hours of thrombolysis, with uniformly good results.

The ideal waiting period has yet to be determined; however, while it seems reasonable to wait 3 or 4 weeks from

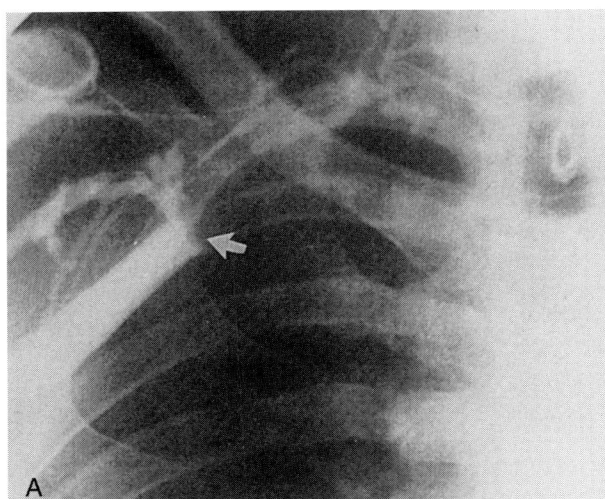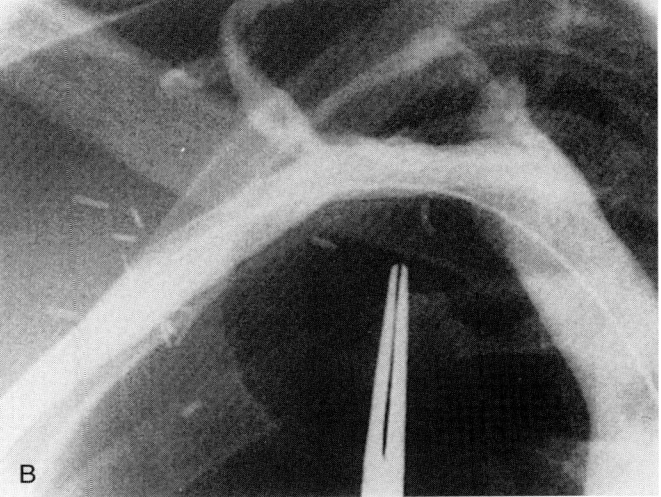

FIGURE 85–4. *A*, Venogram of acute primary subclavian-axillary vein thrombosis prior to therapy. *Arrow* shows site of occlusion. *B*, Venogram following successful thrombolysis and first rib resection. (From Molina JE: Need for emergency treatment in subclavian vein effort thrombosis. J Am Coll Surg 181:414–420, 1995.)

thrombolysis to first rib resection to allow for endothelial healing and decrease the risk of rethrombosis, if attempts to shorten this interval and avoid readmission can be confirmed to do so without penalty, this will likely become common practice.

Other Treatment Scenarios

The preceding recommendations apply to the expected scenario, which ideally consists of (1) catheter-directed lytic therapy with complete lysis, (2) demonstration of extrinsic compression by positional venography, and (3) thoracic outlet decompression after an appropriate interval. Although no report has studied their relative frequency, it is becoming apparent that other scenarios (incomplete lysis, residual intrinsic narrowing) are common enough to deserve greater consideration.

A small group of patients has no residual lesions after thrombolysis, and extrinsic compression cannot be demonstrated by positional phlebography. One explanation is that the appropriate position was not properly mimicked during venography. The other possibility is that the thrombosis may have been caused by conditions specific to the precipitating event, not to repetitive trauma to the vein from aberrant thoracic inlet structures. In such cases, a trial of conservative therapy (i.e., 3 months of anticoagulation therapy and avoidance of vigorous arm use or extremes of position rather than empirical first rib resection) is considered appropriate.[98] If the patient has recurrent symptoms or thrombosis, reevaluation is indicated. There are no data on the long-term outcome with this approach, but many authors do not perform thoracic outlet decompression if the positional venogram results are negative.[1, 2, 6, 46, 56, 72, 82, 85]

After successful thrombolysis, a patient may still have an intrinsic stenosis within the vein (Fig. 85–5). This scenario is more common than initially realized and is more common with treatment delays. These lesions may be treated operatively with venolysis, with or without vein patch angioplasty, or percutaneously with balloon angioplasty, with or without a stent. Operative venolysis, with vein patch angioplasty as needed, has the advantage of combining correction of the venous stenosis with thoracic outlet decompression. Molina[87] treated nine patients with residual

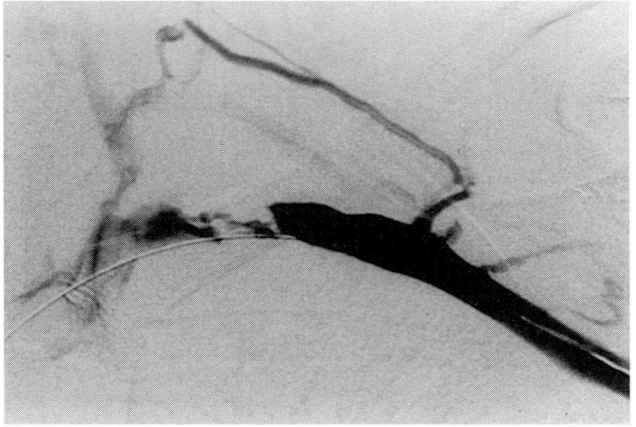

FIGURE 85–5. Venogram following thrombolysis but with a residual intrinsic stenosis.

stenoses by operative vein patch angioplasty and first rib resection. Only one patient had a persistent stenosis, which was successfully treated with balloon angioplasty and stenting. Molina now utilizes an extension of the infraclavicular incision used for thoracic outlet decompression, which involves a limited transverse sternotomy and allows adequate exposure of the subclavian-innominate junction to deal with a stenosis there without the need for claviculectomy.[88] Sanders and Cooper[101] have rongeured bone at the junction of the sternum and clavicular head to obtain additional exposure.

Role of Balloon Angioplasty and Stenting

More emphasis has been placed on percutaneous balloon angioplasty, with or without stenting. This approach does not obviate the need for surgery, because thoracic outlet decompression is still needed (see later), but it can make the surgical procedure less complicated and produce less morbidity. In primary subclavian-axillary vein thrombosis, balloon angioplasty is not generally successful without thoracic outlet decompression.

Glanz and coworkers[44] performed balloon angioplasty in 19 primary subclavian-axillary vein thrombosis patients with persistent stenoses after thrombolysis. The initial success rate was 76% with a 1-year primary patency of 35% and a 2-year patency rate of only 6%. None of these patients underwent thoracic outlet decompression. Machleder[82] reported immediate rethrombosis in seven of 12 balloon angioplasties performed before first rib resection. In nine patients who had thoracic outlet decompression before angioplasty, seven underwent successful dilation of their venous stenoses. Two patients had lesions that could not be crossed with a guide wire.

Other authors have confirmed the high rate of rethrombosis or restenosis in venous stenoses dilated without thoracic outlet decompression.[6, 14, 16, 103] This is not only because balloon angioplasty does nothing to address the underlying problem of extrinsic compression seen in effort thrombosis, for even after thoracic outlet decompression, some patients have stenoses resistant to balloon dilation. Venous stenoses are composed of large amounts of collagen and elastin and may not fracture and remodel like atherosclerotic lesions.[111] Instead, these lesions tend to spring back to their original shape after dilation.

Various types of stents have been used to counteract this intrinsic elastic recoil (Fig. 85–6). If the underlying pathophysiology has not been addressed, primarily stenting venous stenoses (i.e., without thoracic outlet decompression) leads to poor outcomes because of stent deformation or fracture, which has occurred with both balloon-expanded (Palmaz) stents[17] and self-expanding (Wallstent) stents.[85] After problems were reported with the Palmaz stent, it was recognized that once deployed, these stents, having no recoil properties, would be permanently deformed after external compression in the thoracic outlet.[17] It was then thought that self-expanding stents, because they have an inherent memory and resume their shape after external compression, should fare better in this location.[17, 28, 52, 85] However, Meier and associates[85] placed self-expanding Wallstents in four patients without prior first rib resection. Two of these stents fractured (Fig. 85–7), and

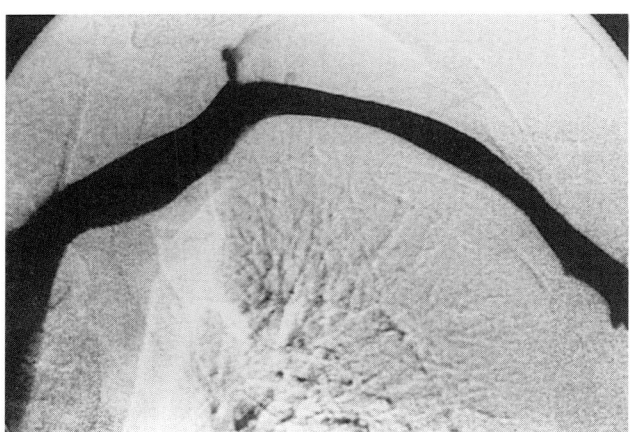

FIGURE 85–6. Venogram following percutaneous transluminal angioplasty and stenting of the subclavian vein with a Wallstent.

the other two stents thrombosed. Four different patients underwent stent placement and thoracic outlet decompression with an acceptable clinical outcome. For this reason, most now suggest that the decision to use a stent to deal with a residual intrinsic stenosis requires a commitment to also perform a thoracic outlet decompression.

The proper timing and sequence of balloon angioplasty and/or stenting is still not defined. Most authors perform thoracic outlet decompression during the same admission if the lesion is stented at the time of its discovery after thrombolysis. In contrast, Chang and colleagues[27] perform a first rib resection immediately after thrombolysis, then bring the patient back to the angiography suite for venography and stenting as necessary (80%). They achieved 100% patency with a mean follow-up of 19.5 months. Even after first rib resection, the subclavian vein may still be subjected to intermittent compression,[52] and a self-expandable stent is thus preferable in this setting.

The main unresolved question in the use of balloon angioplasty and/or stenting in the treatment of primary subclavian-axillary vein thrombosis is the long-term patency rate. Most studies show few numbers and short follow-up, and there are no direct comparisons of endovascu-

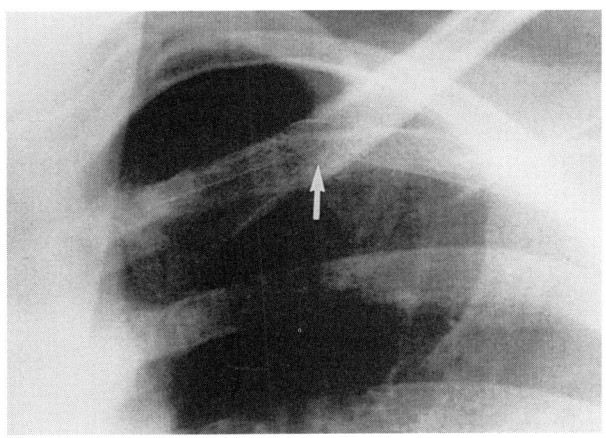

FIGURE 85–7. Fractured Wallstent (*arrow*) in the subclavian vein.

lar and surgical therapies. The relative rarity of primary subclavian-axillary vein thrombosis makes such direct comparisons unlikely. In the hemodialysis literature, percutaneous balloon angioplasty of the upper extremity arm veins has a primary patency of 30% to 60% at 6 months and 10% to 40% at 1 year.[13, 43, 47, 80, 100, 118] The use of stents does not improve patency rates unless the balloon angioplasty was initially unsuccessful.[12, 49, 71, 104, 117, 123]

In the hemodialysis population, balloon angioplasty seems to be more successful in the subclavian and axillary veins than in the peripheral veins. Because the disease process that causes venous stenoses in these patients is more chronic than primary subclavian-axillary vein thrombosis, the patency rates with balloon angioplasty may not be comparable. Until more data are published, the question of surgical versus endovascular treatment of venous stenoses in primary subclavian-axillary vein thrombosis remains unresolved. If stenting proves durable, it will likely continue to be used preferentially along with simple thoracic outlet decompression. If not, venolysis, combined with thoracic outlet decompression through an extended incision,[88, 101] will become popular again. These lesions, if treated early, tend to be more extrinsic, with adventitial scarring and contraction, and therefore are amenable to venolysis without patch angioplasty.

Residual Thrombotic Occlusion After Thrombolysis

In some patients, there is residual occlusion of the subclavian vein following thrombolysis. Success of thrombolytic therapy is a function of the time from thrombosis to the initiation of treatment. Zimmermann and coauthors[128] found residual lesions in 100% of patients given systemic urokinase if therapy was initiated more than 10 days from the onset of thrombosis. Wilson and associates,[127] using systemic streptokinase, had noted a marked increase in the incidence of incomplete thrombolysis if the clot was more than 7 days old. Adelman and colleagues[6] found that catheter-directed thrombolysis was not as successful if the thrombus was more than 8 days old.

For primary subclavian-axillary vein thrombosis, the age of the thrombus that can be successfully lysed varies with opinion, but according to the available data, beyond 10 to 14 days the chances of success diminish markedly. The treatment approach to residual occlusions depends on the length of the occlusion and the presence and severity of symptoms. Patients are more likely to be asymptomatic or to have mild symptoms if the occlusions are short. Most of these patients should be treated conservatively with anticoagulation and elevation, and time should be allowed to determine whether disabling symptoms develop. Patients with persistent disabling symptoms warrant further treatment. For occlusions less than 2 cm in length, Molina[87] advocates first rib resection and operative thrombectomy with vein patch angioplasty. In 19 patients treated this way, all procedures were immediately successful. Four patients eventually required balloon angioplasty for recurrent stenosis.

Sanders and Cooper[101] also had success with this approach when the lesion was short. Longer occlusions do

TABLE 85–2. RESULTS OF SHORT UPPER EXTREMITY VENOUS BYPASS FOR SUBCLAVIAN-AXILLARY VEIN OCCLUSION

AUTHOR	YEAR	NO. OF PATIENTS	TYPE OF BYPASS	PATENCY (%)	FOLLOW-UP
Inahara[65]	1968	1	GSV axillojugular bypass	100	11 mo
Rabinowitz and Goldfarb[96]	1971	2	GSV axillojugular bypass	100	4 mo
Hashmonai et al[55]	1976	1	Cephalic vein crossover	100	5.5 mo
Hansen et al[53]	1985	1	Internal jugular vein turndown	100	1 yr
Currier et al[31]	1986	6	PTFE axillojugular bypass	50	1–3 yr
Malcynski et al[83]	1993	2	Internal jugular vein turndown	100	5 yr
Molina[87]	1995	4	GSV axillojugular bypass	50	4 yr
Sanders and Cooper[101]	1995	5	Internal jugular vein turndown	100	2–4 yr
Sanders and Cooper[101]	1995	1	PTFE axillojugular bypass	100	9 mo

GSV = greater saphenous vein, PTFE = polytetrafluoroethylene.

not respond as well to this approach. Molina[87] reported success in only 37% of patients with lesions longer than 2 cm. Longer occlusions require venous bypass. The experience with *short venous bypass* for upper extremity venous occlusions is favorable but largely anecdotal (Table 85–2). If the patient has the proper anatomy, (i.e., a short occlusion extending not much distal to the entrance of the cephalic vein), internal jugular vein transposition or turndown is a good option. Malcynski[83] and Sanders and Cooper[101] documented excellent results with this procedure.

The paradox is that patients with subclavian vein occlusions short enough so that the internal jugular vein reaches the patent part of the subclavian vein are not as likely to have severe symptoms. Whether or not the cephalic vein, a major collateral pathway, is patent may be a factor in the severity of symptoms. Polytetrafluoroethylene and greater saphenous vein bypasses have shown mixed results, but generally the longer the bypass, particularly with the use of a prosthetic conduit, the worse the outcome.[31, 65, 85, 95, 101] Cephalic vein crossover grafts have also been described.[55]

In constructing these bypasses, most authors recommend placing an arteriovenous fistula distal to the bypass for 6 weeks to 3 months.[31, 53, 55, 83, 85, 95, 101] With longer or prosthetic bypasses, closure of a well-tolerated arteriovenous fistula is not advised. Patients with no accessible patent major veins proximally or with only distal, below-elbow veins patent (i.e., those who are generally most symptomatic), unfortunately cannot be candidates for any bypass.

In general, venous bypasses should be reserved for patients who have severe disabling symptoms and the appropriate anatomy.

In view of the limited options for patients with long, chronic occlusions, prompt and aggressive management along with intervention is recommended for primary subclavian-axillary vein thrombosis in active, healthy patients who have an ongoing need for active use of the involved extremity. Figure 85–8 provides a treatment algorithm.

SECONDARY SUBCLAVIAN-AXILLARY VEIN THROMBOSIS

Secondary subclavian-axillary vein thrombosis can be caused by a variety of factors. Where possible, the treatment is directed at the underlying cause as well as the occlusion itself. Many patients have one or more risk factors for DVT. However, the common denominator in most patients with secondary subclavian-axillary vein thrombosis is a central venous catheter. It is a relatively rare patient who has severe congestive heart failure, sepsis, an underlying malignancy, or other systemic risk factors for thrombosis without a concurrent central venous line. Because of the widespread and increasing use of these catheters and the related increase in upper extremity DVT, this part of the chapter focuses primarily on catheter-related thrombosis.

TABLE 85–3. CATHETER-ASSOCIATED THROMBOSIS: PROSPECTIVE TRIALS

AUTHOR	YEAR	NO. OF LINES	THROMBOSIS (%)	SYMPTOMATIC (%)	STUDY
Warden et al[125]	1973	139	46	5	Autopsy
Ryan et al[99]	1974	34	24	0	Autopsy
Stoney et al[108]	1976	203	31	16	Venography
Brismar et al[20]	1981	60	8	0	Venography
Burt et al[24]	1981	21	33	29	Venography
Valerio et al[120]	1981	18	33	17	Venography
Brismar et al[21]	1982	53	36	0	Venography
Bozzetti et al[19]	1983	52	29	0	Venography
Pottecher et al[93]	1984	52	38	15	Autopsy/venography
Wanscher et al[124]	1988	69	23	13	Autopsy/venography
Bern et al[15]	1990	40	38	67	Venography
Horne et al[60]	1995	80	39	13	Venography
Koksoy et al[70]	1995	44	41	50	Venography

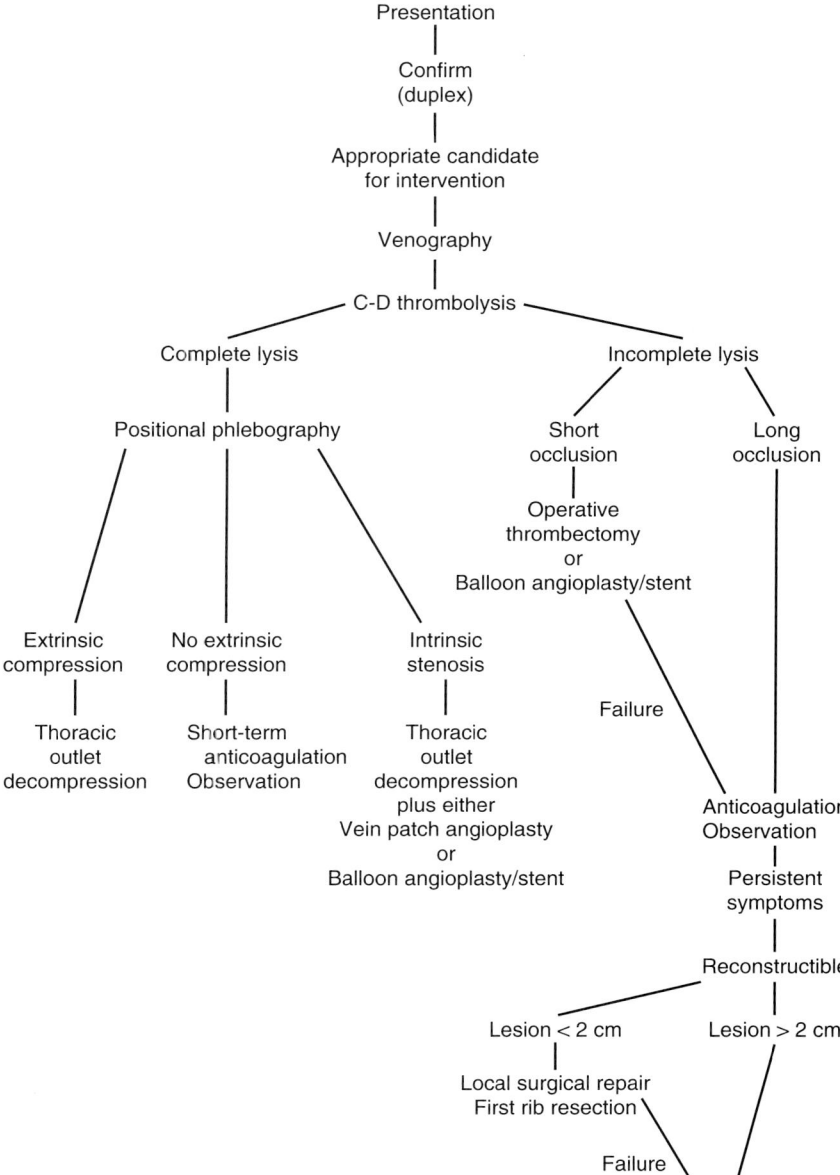

FIGURE 85–8. Algorithm for the treatment of primary subclavian-axillary vein thrombosis. C-D = catheter-directed.

Incidence

The overall incidence of catheter-associated thrombosis has been difficult to determine. The literature has not shown consistency in the degree of aggressiveness or in the methods of detecting the presence of subclavian-axillary vein thrombosis. Estimates of the overall incidence range from 3% to 70% of all central lines placed.[79] Part of the difficulty with catheter-related thrombosis is that a majority of patients are asymptomatic. It is also a blessing, because, as discussed later, durable revascularization is often not achievable. Table 85–3 shows the incidence of catheter-associated thrombosis detected by venography or autopsy in prospective trials. Overall, approximately one third of patients with central lines eventually have DVT, but only 10% to 15% of these are symptomatic.

Etiology

Virchow's triad (stasis, hypercoagulability, and intimal trauma) plays a major role in secondary subclavian-axillary vein thrombosis. From the time a central venous catheter is placed, there is ongoing injury to the vein. The method of insertion, composition, size, and duration of use of the catheter are all important in the development of a thrombus. Difficulty in gaining percutaneous access to a central vein increases the risk of thrombosis.[59, 66, 121] When central venous catheters were first developed, they were composed of relatively inflexible polyvinyl chloride and polyethylene. Newer catheters, composed of Silastic and polyurethane are softer and more flexible and cause less injury to the venous intima. A reduced rate of thrombosis has been found with less rigid catheters.[10, 59, 75, 78, 90, 126] Larger-diameter catheters (e.g., sheath introducers and catheters used for hemodialysis) are also relatively inflexible and result in a higher incidence of subclavian vein thrombosis.[60, 78] Besides intimal injury, larger catheters may also cause stasis within the vein owing to their size in relation to the diameter of the blood vessel.

The risk of thrombosis development is also related to how long the catheter remains in a vein. Many studies have documented an increased rate of thrombosis the longer a line is in place.[10, 48, 59, 121, 126]

Another well-studied risk factor is the *type of fluid* infused through the catheter. Parenteral nutrition and many cancer chemotherapeutic agents are directly toxic to vascular endothelium because of hyperosmolarity and extremes of pH.[39, 42, 59, 75, 126] *Drug incompatibility* may also contribute to venous trauma.[77] Other risk factors related to the catheter include left-sided cannulation,[48] placement of the tip of the catheter in veins other than the superior vena cava,[18, 48, 67] and the presence of bilateral catheters.[50]

Besides local trauma from the catheter, many patients have systemic factors that contribute to thrombosis. The presence of malignancy is probably the best-studied risk factor for thrombosis. The hypercoagulable state associated with malignancy has been well documented.[56, 79] Patients with solid tumors seem to be at higher risk for thrombosis than those with hematologic malignancies.[77, 96, 126] Other disease processes, such as inflammatory bowel disease, sepsis, and obesity, may also be associated with hypercoagulability.[79]

Stasis also plays a role in the development of secondary subclavian-axillary vein thrombosis. Many critically ill patients require central venous access for nutritional support and hemodynamic monitoring. Congestive heart failure, hypotension, dehydration, and prolonged bed rest can all lead to stasis in the venous system.[56, 79]

One final issue in the etiology of catheter-associated thrombosis is the presence of a *fibrin sheath,* which invariably forms around an indwelling catheter. Venographic and autopsy studies have documented the presence of a fibrin sheath in almost all patients whose catheters have been in place for at least 1 week.[10, 20, 32, 61, 77, 126] The fibrin sheath is a result of the catheter surface's being exposed to circulating platelets. To date, there is no evidence to suggest that the fibrin sheath contributes to the formation of an occlusive thrombus.[10, 32, 79, 126]

Clinical Presentation

The clinical presentation of catheter-associated thrombosis may be subtle. The onset of thrombosis is usually slower than in primary subclavian-axillary vein thrombosis, and the affected segment is shorter. This may allow time for adequate collateral vessels to form. Also, many of the patients with long-term indwelling catheters are critically ill or have other debilitating illnesses that limit the use of their upper extremity. Such patients may be asymptomatic mainly because they are unable to use their arms enough to produce symptoms. These reasons may account for the low incidence of clinically evident thrombosis.[35, 56, 76, 79] Symptomatic patients present similarly to those with primary subclavian-axillary vein thrombosis. Most patients have edema of the affected extremity, with some experiencing pain over the vein and in the arm, and distended veins around the shoulder girdle.[10, 35, 50, 57, 76] In a large epidemiologic study, the incidence of pain, distended veins, erythema, and acrocyanosis was lower in catheter-associated thrombosis than in primary subclavian-axillary vein thrombosis.[76]

The natural history of catheter-associated thrombosis is usually indolent. Donayre and colleagues[35] found that of 10 limbs that initially presented with symptomatic thrombosis, with none symptomatic in long-term follow-up. Most patients who are symptomatic initially become asymptomatic without further treatment other than removal of the catheter.[50] The isolated nature of these thromboses and the extensive venous collaterals of the shoulder girdle limit the long-term sequelae of catheter-associated thrombosis. As mentioned, pulmonary embolus is not uncommon, even in secondary subclavian-axillary vein thrombosis. In a prospective study, Monreal and colleagues[90] examined 79 patients, who all had indwelling central venous catheters, with ventilation-perfusion scans. Of these patients, 16% had evidence of pulmonary embolism; of these patients, however, only 31% were symptomatic. Although many patients with subclavian-axillary vein thromboses are clinically asymptomatic, there is still a risk of pulmonary embolism. Venous gangrene is a rare complication of catheter-related thrombosis and is usually a preterminal event.[26, 66]

Treatment

The treatment of catheter-associated thrombosis depends primarily on the patient's symptoms and the need for further central venous access. Because there are no controlled studies on treatment, therapy guidelines are based on observational reports. In symptomatic patients who no longer need lines, catheter removal is adequate treatment for the thrombosis itself.[22, 35, 50] Patients remain asymptomatic even without oral anticoagulation therapy,[79] but short-term anticoagulation is usually indicated to prevent clot extension, recurrence, or pulmonary embolus. If the patient still requires central venous access and if the catheter is functioning, anticoagulation agents are given until the catheter is no longer needed.[22, 48] The thrombus may even resolve without removal of the catheter.[79]

Symptomatic patients should be placed on an anticoagulation regimen, and the catheters should be removed. Symptoms usually resolve after a couple of days of heparin therapy.[22, 35, 50, 75] If the need for central venous access persists, anticoagulation is indicated and should be continued until the catheter can be removed.[48] Even with the catheter still in place, most symptoms resolve with anticoagulation.[22, 35, 48, 50, 75, 79]

Because the course of catheter-associated thrombosis is usually benign, thrombolytic therapy has only a limited role. The direct instillation of thrombolytic agents into a catheter has been successful, at least temporarily, in reopening thrombosed catheters.[22] This procedure can be done expeditiously on an outpatient basis. Thrombolytic therapy has also been employed to salvage catheters in completely occluded veins.

Beygui and colleagues[16] successfully lysed six of six veins with catheter-related thrombosis. Seigel and coworkers[102] treated 38 secondary subclavian-axillary vein thrombosis patients with catheter-directed thrombolysis and were able to salvage catheter access in 87%. Because these patients required 1 to 5 days of thrombolytic therapy to lyse the clot and since this study was uncontrolled, it is unknown how many patients could have had access restored with transcatheter infusion of lytic agents and anticoagulation with less morbidity and cost. Until more data are forthcoming, it seems reasonable to institute thrombolytic therapy only for significantly symptomatic patients when conventional therapy fails or when the patient has an extended need for catheter access and is in danger of running out of available venous sites.

The roles of angioplasty and stenting in catheter-associated thrombosis are not well defined. As stated earlier, the patency rates after angioplasty and stenting of subclavian and axillary venous stenoses in hemodialysis patients are low. Many of the stenoses in these patients are secondary to indwelling catheters. In the Seigel report,[102] only 64% of patients with residual stenoses after thrombolysis had angioplasty that was successful right away. There was no long-term follow-up. Again, until more data are available, these therapies should be reserved for when preservation of venous access is critical.

With the increasing recognition of catheter-associated thrombosis, prevention of thrombus formation has been emphasized. Fabri's group[40] administered 3000 units of heparin per liter of total parenteral nutrition in 24 patients with central venous catheters. There was a significant decrease in the incidence of subclavian-axillary vein thrombosis compared with the control group. Other authors have confirmed that the addition of heparin to total parenteral nutrition formula decreases the incidence of catheter-associated thrombosis.[21, 64] Chemoprophylaxis has also been studied in cancer patients.

Bern and coworkers[15] randomized 82 patients with long-term central venous catheters for cancer chemotherapy to receive 1 mg/day of Coumadin or none. At the end of 90 days, there was a significantly lower incidence of thrombosis in the patients taking Coumadin. There were no adverse bleeding complications in the group receiving oral anticoagulation. For high-risk cancer patients, it may be advantageous to administer low-dose Coumadin to prevent catheter-associated thrombosis.

REFERENCES

1. AbuRahma AF, Sadler D, Stuart P, et al: Conventional versus thrombolytic therapy in spontaneous (effort) axillary-subclavian vein thrombosis. Am J Surg 161:459–465, 1991.
2. AbuRahma AF, Short YS, White JF, et al: Treatment alternatives for axillary-subclavian thrombosis: Long-term follow-up. Cardiovasc Surg 4:783–787, 1996.
3. Adams JT, DeWeese JA: "Effort" thrombosis of the axillary and subclavian veins. J Trauma 11:923–930, 1971.
4. Adams JT, DeWeese JA, Mahoney EB, et al: Intermittent subclavian vein obstruction without thrombosis. Surgery 63:147–165, 1968.
5. Adams JT, McEvoy RK, DeWeese JA: Primary deep venous thrombosis of upper extremity. Arch Surg 91:29–42, 1965.
6. Adelman MA, Stone DH, Riles TS, et al: A multidisciplinary approach to the treatment of Paget-Schroetter syndrome. Ann Vasc Surg 11:149–154, 1997.
7. Appleby DH, Heller MS: Low-dose streptokinase therapy for subclavian vein thrombosis. South Med J 77:536–537, 1984.
8. Aubaniac R: L'injection intraveineuse sousclaviculaire: Avantage et technique. Presse Med 60:1456, 1952.
9. Aziz S, Straehley CJ, Whelan TJ: Effort-related axillosubclavian vein thrombosis. Am J Surg 152:57–61, 1986.
10. Balestreri L, DeCicco M, Matovic M, et al: Central venous catheter-related thrombosis in clinically asymptomatic oncologic patients: A phlebographic study. Eur J Radiol 20:108–111, 1995.
11. Barker NW, Nygaard KK, Watters W, et al: Statistical study of postoperative venous thrombosis and pulmonary embolism: Location of thrombosis. Relation of thrombosis and embolism. Proc Mayo Clin 16:33–37, 1941.
12. Beathard GA: Gianturco self-expanding stent in the treatment of stenosis in dialysis access grafts. Kidney Int 43:872–877, 1993.
13. Beathard GA: Percutaneous transvenous angioplasty in the treatment of vascular access stenosis. Kidney Int 42:1390–1397, 1992.
14. Becker GJ, Holden RW, Rabe FE, et al: Local thrombolytic therapy for subclavian and axillary vein thrombosis. Radiology 149:419–423, 1983.
15. Bern MM, Lokich JJ, Wallach SR, et al: Very low doses of warfarin can prevent thrombosis in central venous catheters. Ann Intern Med 112:423–428, 1990.
16. Beygui RE, Olcott C, Dalman RL: Subclavian vein thrombosis: Outcome analysis based on etiology and modality of treatment. Ann Vasc Surg 11:247–255, 1997.
17. Bjarnason H, Hunter DW, Crain MR, et al: Collapse of a Palmaz stent in the subclavian vein. AJR Am J Roentgenol 160:1123–1124, 1993.
18. Bottino J, McCreadie KB, Groschel DHM, et al: Long-term intravenous therapy with peripherally inserted silicone elastomer central venous catheters in patients with malignant diseases. Cancer 43:1937–1943, 1979.
19. Bozzetti F, Scarpa D, Terno G, et al: Subclavian vein thrombosis due to indwelling catheters: A prospective study on 52 patients. J Parenter Enteral Nutr 7:560–562, 1983.
20. Brismar B, Hardstedt C, Jacobson S: Diagnosis of thrombosis by catheter phlebography after prolonged central venous catheterization. Ann Surg 194:779–783, 1981.
21. Brismar B, Hardstedt C, Jacobson S, et al: Reduction of catheter-associated thrombosis in parenteral nutrition by intravenous heparin therapy. Arch Surg 117:1196–1199, 1982.
22. Brothers TE, Von Moll LK, Niederhuber JE, et al: Experience with subcutaneous infusion ports in three hundred patients. Surg Gynecol Obstet 166:295–301, 1988.
23. Broviac JW, Cole JJ, Scribner BH: A silicone rubber atrial catheter for prolonged parenteral alimentation. Surg Gynecol Obstet 136:603–606, 1973.
24. Burt ME, Dunnick MR, Krudy AG, et al: Prospective evaluation of subclavian vein thrombosis during total parenteral nutrition by contrast venography. Clin Res 29:264A, 1981.
25. Campbell CB, Chandler JG, Tegtmeyer CJ, et al: Axillary, subclavian, and brachiocephalic vein obstruction. Surgery 82:816–826, 1977.
26. Chandrasekar R, Nott DM, Enabi L, et al: Upper limb venous gangrene, a lethal condition. Eur J Vasc Surg 7:475–477, 1993.
27. Chang BB, Kreienberg PB, Darling RC III, et al: One stage definitive therapy for Paget-Schroetter syndrome: A multidisciplinary approach. Presented at the 44th Annual Meeting of the North American chapter of the International Society for Cardiovascular Surgery, Chicago, June 1996.
28. Cohen GS, Braunstein L, Ball DS, et al: Effort thrombosis: effective treatment with vascular stent after unrelieved venous stenosis following a surgical release procedure. Cardiovasc Intervent Radiol 19:37–39, 1996.
29. Coon WW, Willis PW: Thrombosis of axillary and subclavian veins. Arch Surg 94:657–663, 1967.
30. Crowell DL: Effort thrombosis of the subclavian and axillary veins: Review of the literature and case report with two-year follow-up with venography. Ann Intern Med 52:1337–1343, 1960.
31. Currier CB, Widder S, Ali A, et al: Surgical management of subclavian and axillary vein thrombosis in patients with a functioning arteriovenous fistula. Surgery 104:561–567, 1988.
32. Damascelli B, Patelli G, Frigerio L, et al: Placement of long-term central venous catheters in outpatients. AJR Am J Roentgenol 168:1235–1239, 1997.
33. Daskalakis E, Bouhoutsos J: Subclavian and axillary vein compression of musculoskeletal origin. Br J Surg 67:573–576, 1980.
34. DeWeese JA, Adams JT, Gaiser DL: Subclavian venous thrombectomy. Circulation 42(Suppl):158–163, 1970.

35. Donayre CE, White GH, Mehringer SM, et al: Pathogenesis determines late morbidity of axillosubclavian vein thrombosis. Am J Surg 152:179–184, 1986.
36. Drapanas T, Curran WL: Thrombectomy in the treatment of "effort" thrombosis of the axillary and subclavian veins. J Trauma 6:107–119, 1966.
37. Druy EM, Trout HH, Giordano JM, et al: Lytic therapy in the treatment of axillary and subclavian vein thrombosis. J Vasc Surg 2:821–827, 1985.
38. Dudrick JJ, Wilmore DW, Vans HM, et al: Long-term total parenteral nutrition with growth, development, and positive nitrogen balance. Surgery 64:134–142, 1968.
39. Fabri PJ, Mirtallo JM, Ebhert ML, et al: Clinical effect of nonthrombotic total nutrition catheters. J Parenter Enteral Nutr 8:705–707, 1984.
40. Fabri PJ, Mirtallo JM, Rubert RL, et al: Incidence and prevention of thrombosis of the subclavian vein during parenteral nutrition. Surg Gynecol Obstet 155:238–240, 1982.
41. Fielding JR, Nagel JS, Pomeroy O: Upper extremity DVT: Correlation of MR and nuclear medicine flow imaging. Clin Imaging 21:260–263, 1997.
42. Fonkalsrud EW: The effect of pH in glucose infusions on development of thrombophlebitis. J Surg Res 8:539, 1968.
43. Glanz S, Gordon DH, Butt KMH, et al: The role of percutaneous angioplasty in the management of chronic hemodialysis fistulas. Ann Surg 206:777–781, 1987.
44. Glanz S, Gordon DH, Lipkowitz GS, et al: Axillary and subclavian vein stenosis: Percutaneous angioplasty. Radiology 168:371–373, 1988.
45. Glass BA: The relationship of axillary venous thrombosis to the thoracic outlet compression syndrome. Ann Thorac Surg 19:613–621, 1975.
46. Gloviczki P, Kazmier FS, Hollier LH: Axillary-subclavian venous occlusion: The morbidity of a non-lethal disease. J Vasc Surg 4:333–337, 1986.
47. Gmelin E, Winterhoff R, Rinast E: Insufficient hemodialysis access fistulas: Late results of treatment with percutaneous balloon angioplasty. Radiology 171:657–660, 1989.
48. Gould JR, Carloss HW, Skinner WL: Groshong catheter-associated subclavian venous thrombosis. Am J Med 95:419–423, 1993.
49. Gray RJ, Horton KM, Dolmatch BL, et al: Use of Wallstents for hemodialysis access-related venous stenosis and occlusions untreatable with balloon angioplasty. Radiology 195:479–484, 1995.
50. Haire WD, Lieberman RP, Edney J, et al: Hickman catheter-induced thoracic vein thrombosis. Cancer 66:900–908, 1990.
51. Haire WD, Lynch TG, Lund GB, et al: Limitations of magnetic resonance imaging and ultrasound-directed (duplex) scanning in the diagnosis of subclavian vein thrombosis. J Vasc Surg 13:391–397, 1991.
52. Hall LD, Murray JD, Boswell GE: Venous stent placement as an adjunct to the staged, multimodal treatment of Paget-Schroetter syndrome. J Vasc Interv Radiol 6:565–570, 1995.
53. Hansen B, Feins RS, Detmer DE: Simple extra-anatomic jugular vein bypass for subclavian vein thrombosis. J Vasc Surg 2:921–923, 1985.
54. Harley DP, White RA, Nelson RJ, et al: Pulmonary embolism secondary to venous thrombosis of the arm. Am J Surg 147:221–224, 1984.
55. Hashmonai M, Schramek A, Farbstein J: Cephalic vein cross-over bypass for subclavian vein thrombosis: A case report. Surgery 80:563–564, 1976.
56. Hill SL, Berry RE: Subclavian vein thrombosis: A continuing challenge. Surgery 108:1–9, 1990.
57. Hingorani A, Ascher E, Lorenson E, et al: Upper extremity deep venous thrombosis and its impact on morbidity and mortality rates in a hospital-base population. J Vasc Surg 26:853–860, 1997.
58. Hood DB, Kuehne J, Yellin AE, et al: Vascular complications of thoracic outlet syndrome. Am Surg 10:913–917, 1997.
59. Horattas MC, Wright DJ, Fenton AH, et al: Changing concepts of deep venous thrombosis of the upper extremity: Report of a series and review of the literature. Surgery 104:561–567, 1988.
60. Horne MK, May DJ, Alexander HR, et al: Venographic surveillance of tunneled venous access devices in adult oncology patients. Ann Surg Oncol 2:174–178, 1995.
61. Hoshal VC, Ause RG, Hoskins PA, et al: Fibrin sleeve formation on indwelling central venous catheters. Arch Surg 102:353–358, 1971.
62. Hughes ESR: Venous obstruction in the upper extremity. Int Abstr Surg 88:89–127, 1949.
63. Hurlbert SN, Rutherford RB: Primary subclavian-axillary vein thrombosis. Ann Vasc Surg 9:217–223, 1995.
64. Imperial J, Bistrian BR, Bothe Jr A, et al: Limitation of central vein thrombosis in total parenteral nutrition by continuous infusion of low-dose heparin. J Am Coll Nutr 2:63–73, 1982.
65. Inahara T: Surgical treatment of "effort" thrombosis of the axillary and subclavian veins. Am Surg 34:479–483, 1968.
66. Kammen BF, Soulen MC: Phlegmasia cerulea dolens of the upper extremity. J Vasc Interv Radiol 6:283–286, 1995.
67. Kearns RJ, Coleman S, Wehner JG: Complications of long arm-catheters: A randomized trial of central vs. peripheral tip location. J Parenter Enteral Nutr 20:20–24, 1996.
68. Kerr TM, Lutter KS, Moeller DM, et al: Upper extremity venous thrombosis diagnosed by duplex scanning. Am J Surg 160:202–206, 1990.
69. Kleinsasser LJ: "Effort" thrombosis of the axillary and subclavian veins. Arch Surg 59:258–274, 1949.
70. Koksoy C, Kuzu A, Kutlay J, et al: The diagnostic value of colour Doppler ultrasound in central venous catheter related thrombosis. Clin Radiol 50:687–689, 1995.
71. Kovalik EC, Newman GE, Suhocki P, et al: Correction of central venous stenoses: Use of angioplasty and vascular Wallstents. Kidney Int 45:1177–1181, 1994.
72. Kunkel JM, Machleder HI: Treatment of Paget-Schroetter syndrome. Arch Surg 124:1153–1158, 1989.
73. Landercasper J, Gall W, Fischer M, et al: Thrombolytic therapy of axillary-subclavian venous thrombosis. Arch Surg 122:1072–1075, 1987.
74. Lee MC, Belkin M, Mannick JA, et al: Early operative intervention following thrombolytic therapy for primary subclavian vein thrombosis: An effective treatment approach. J Vasc Surg (in press).
75. Lindblad B: Thromboembolic complications and central venous catheters. Lancet 2:936, 1982.
76. Lindblad B, Tengborn L, Bergqvist D: Deep vein thrombosis of the axillary-subclavian veins. Eur J Vasc Surg 2:161–165, 1988.
77. Lokich JJ, Becker B: Subclavian vein thrombosis in patients treated with infusion chemotherapy for advanced malignancy. Cancer 52:1586–1589, 1983.
78. Lokich JJ, Bothe Jr A, Benotte P, et al: Complications and management of implanted venous access catheters. J Clin Oncol 3:710–717, 1985.
79. Lowell JA, Bothe Jr A: Central venous catheter related thrombosis. Surg Oncol Clin North Am 4:479–492, 1995.
80. Lumsden AB, MacDonald MJ, Kikeri DK, et al: Hemodialysis access graft stenosis: Percutaneous transluminal angioplasty. J Surg Res 68:181–185, 1997.
81. Machleder HI: Upper extremity venous thrombosis. Semin Vasc Surg 3:219–226, 1990.
82. Machleder HI: Evaluation of a new treatment strategy for Paget-Schroetter syndrome: Spontaneous thrombosis of the axillary-subclavian vein. J Vasc Surg 17:305–317, 1993.
83. Malcynski J, O'Donnell TF, Mackey WC, et al: Long-term results of treatment for axillary subclavian vein thrombosis. Can J Surg 4:365–371, 1993.
84. McDonough JJ, Altemeier WA: Subclavian venous thrombosis secondary to indwelling catheters. Surg Gynecol Obstet 133:397–400, 1971.
85. Meier GH, Pollak JS, Rosenblatt M, et al: Initial experience with venous stents in exertional axillary-subclavian vein thrombosis. J Vasc Surg 24:974–983, 1996.
86. Molina JE: Surgery for effort thrombosis of the subclavian vein. J Thorac Cardiovasc Surg 103:341–346, 1992.
87. Molina JE: Need for emergency treatment in subclavian vein effort thrombosis. J Am Coll Surg 181:414–420, 1995.
88. Molina JE: A new surgical approach to the innominate and subclavian vein. J Vasc Surg (in press).
89. Monreal M, Lafoz E, Ruiz J, et al: Upper-extremity deep venous thrombosis and pulmonary embolism. Chest 99:280–283, 1991.
90. Monreal M, Raventos A, Lerma R, et al: Pulmonary embolism in patients with upper extremity DVT associated with venous central lines—a prospective study. Thromb Haemostasis 72:548–550, 1994.
91. Paget J: Clinical lectures and essays. London, Longmens Green and Co, 1875.
92. Painter TD, Karpf M: Deep venous thrombosis of the upper extremity: Five years' experience at a university hospital. Angiology 35:743–749, 1984.

93. Pottecher T, Forrler M, Picardat P, et al: Thrombogenicity of central venous catheters: Prospective study of polyethylene, silicone, and polyurethane catheters with phlebography or post-mortem examination. Eur J Anaesthesiol 1:361–365, 1984.

94. Prescott SM, Tikoff G: Deep venous thrombosis of the upper extremity: A reappraisal. Circulation 59:350–355, 1979.

95. Ray S, Stacey R, Imrie M, et al: A review of 560 Hickman catheter insertions. Anaesthesia 51:981–985, 1996.

96. Rabinowitz R, Goldfarb D: Surgical treatment of axillosubclavian venous thrombosis: A case report. Surgery 70:703–706, 1971.

97. Rose SC: Venography. In Rutherford RB (ed): Vascular Surgery, 4th ed. Philadelphia, WB Saunders, 1995, p 1764.

98. Rutherford RB, Hurlbert SN: Primary subclavian-axillary vein thrombosis: Consensus and commentary. Cardiovasc Surg 4:420–423, 1996.

99. Ryan JA, Abel RM, Abbott WM, et al: Catheter complications in total parenteral nutrition: A prospective study of 200 consecutive patients. N Engl J Med 290:757–761, 1974.

100. Saeed M, Newman GE, McCann RL, et al: Stenosis in dialysis fistulas: Treatment with percutaneous angioplasty. Radiology 164:693–697, 1987.

101. Sanders RJ, Cooper MA: Surgical management of subclavian vein obstruction, including six cases of subclavian vein bypass. Surgery 118:856–863, 1995.

102. Seigel EL, Jew AC, Delcore R, et al: Thrombolytic therapy for catheter-related thrombosis. Am J Surg 166:716–719, 1993.

103. Sheeran SR, Hallisey MJ, Murphy TP, et al: Local thrombolytic therapy as part of a multidisciplinary approach to acute axillosubclavian vein thrombosis (Paget-Schroetter syndrome). J Vasc Interv Radiol 8:253–260, 1997.

104. Shoenfeld R, Hermans A, Novick A, et al: Stenting of proximal venous obstruction to maintain hemodialysis access. J Vasc Surg 19:532–539, 1994.

105. Smith-Behn J, Althar R, Katz W: Primary thrombosis of the axillary/subclavian vein. South Med J 79:1176–1178, 1986.

106. Steed DL, Teodori MF, Peitzman AB, et al: Streptokinase in the treatment of subclavian vein thrombosis. J Vasc Surg 4:28–32, 1986.

107. Stevenson IM, Parry EW: Radiological study of the aetiological factors in venous obstruction of the upper limb. J Cardiovasc Surg 16:581–585, 1975.

108. Stoney WS, Addlestone RB, Alford WC, et al: The incidence of venous thrombosis following long-term transvenous pacing. Ann Thorac Surg 22:166–170, 1976.

109. Strange-Vognsen HH, Hauch O, Andersen J, et al: Resection of the first rib, following deep arm vein thrombolysis in patients with thoracic outlet syndrome. J Cardiovasc Surg 30:430–433, 1989.

110. Sundqvist SB, Hedner U, Kullenberg HKE, et al: Deep venous thrombosis of the arm: A study of coagulation and fibrinolysis. Br Med J 283:265–267, 1981.

111. Swedberg SH, Brown BG, Sigley R, et al: Intimal fibromuscular hyperplasia at the venous anastamosis of PTFE grafts in hemodialysis patients. Circulation 80:1726–1736, 1989.

112. Swinton NW, Edgett JW, Hall RJ: Primary subclavian-axillary vein thrombosis. Circulation 38:737–745, 1968.

113. Taylor LM, McAllister WR, Dennis DL, et al: Thrombolytic therapy followed by first rib resection for spontaneous ("effort") subclavian vein thrombosis. Am J Surg 149:644–647, 1985.

114. Tilney NL, Griffiths HJG, Edwards EA: Natural history of major venous thrombosis of the upper extremity. Arch Surg 101:792–796, 1970.

115. Thompson RW, Schneider PA, Nelken NA, et al: Circumferential venolysis and paraclavicular thoracic outlet decompression for "effort thrombosis" of the subclavian vein. J Vasc Surg 16:723–732, 1992.

116. Torosian MH, Meranze S, Mullen JL, et al: Central venous access with occlusive superior central venous thrombosis. Ann Surg 203:30–33, 1986.

117. Trerotola SO, Fair GH, Davidson D, et al: Comparison of Gianturco Z-stents and Wallstents in a hemodialysis access graft animal model. J Vasc Interv Radiol 6:387–396, 1995.

118. Turmel-Rodrigues L, Pengloan J, Blanchier D, et al: Insufficient dialysis shunts: Improved long-term patency rates with close hemodynamic monitoring, repeated percutaneous balloon angioplasty, and stent placement. Radiology 187:273–278, 1993.

119. Urschel HC, Razzuk MA: Improved management of the Paget-Schroetter syndrome secondary to thoracic outlet compression. Ann Thorac Surg 52:1217–1221, 1991.

120. Valerio D, Hussey JK, Smith FW: Central vein thrombosis associated with intravenous feeding. J Parenter Enteral Nutr 5:240–242, 1981.

121. Vanherweghem JL, Yassine T, Goldman M, et al: Subclavian vein thrombosis: A frequent complication of subclavian vein cannulation for hemodialysis. Clin Nephrol 26:235–238, 1986.

122. Von Schroetter L: Erkrankungen der gefasse. In Nathnagel Handbuch der Pathologie und Therapie. Vienna, Holder, 1884.

123. Vorwerk D, Guenther RW, Mann H, et al: Venous stenosis and occlusion in hemodialysis shunts: Follow-up results of stent placement in 65 patients. Radiology 195:140–146, 1995.

124. Wanscher M, Prifelt JJ, Smith-Sivertsen C, et al: Thrombosis caused by polyurethane double-lumen subclavian superior vena cava catheter and hemodialysis. Crit Care Med 16:624–628, 1988.

125. Warden GD, Wilmore DW, Pruitt BA: Central venous thrombosis: A hazard of medical progress. J Trauma 13:620–625, 1973.

126. Williams EC: Catheter-related thrombosis. Clin Cardiol 13 (Suppl IV):IV–34–IV–36, 1990.

127. Wilson JJ, Zahn CA, Newman H: Fibrinolytic therapy for idiopathic subclavian-axillary vein thrombosis. Am J Surg 159:208–211, 1990.

128. Zimmermann R, Morl H, Harenberg J, et al: Urokinase therapy of subclavian-axillary vein thrombosis. Klin Wochenschr 59:851–856, 1981.

CHAPTER 86

Upper Extremity Sympathectomy

John P. Harris, M.S., F.R.A.C.S., F.R.C.S., F.A.C.S., D.D.U., and James May, M.D., M.S., F.R.A.C.S., F.A.C.S.

Thoracic sympathectomy was once commonly performed for conditions as diverse as hypertension, bronchial asthma, angina pectoris, hyperthyroidism, and even the crises of tertiary syphilis.[70] In the absence of effective medical and surgical alternatives, the operation was one of the few options available to surgeons for ischemic disorders of the upper extremity. As a result of more effective medical therapy,[5] chemical sympathetic blockade,[38] and percutaneous techniques[87] to disrupt the sympathetic nerve supply to the upper extremity, open surgical sympathectomy fell into disuse, having limited indications. This was particularly true for pain syndromes and digital ischemia associated with Raynaud's syndrome, since there was little objective evidence to support the efficacy of surgical sympathectomy.[22, 44] The notable exception was hyperhidrosis, for which excellent results could be expected from sympathectomy, although relatively few of the younger patients generally affected were willing to accept the morbidity of open surgical sympathectomy.[1]

Endoscopic thoracic sympathectomy had been used for many years, but the technique did not gain widespread popularity until the 1980s as part of a general upsurge of interest in endoscopic surgery when endoscopic skills and improved instrumentation became generally available.[16] Endoscopic thoracic sympathectomy has clearly emerged as the preferred surgical option for hyperhidrosis. Several large series have confirmed excellent results, safety, and good patient acceptance.[18, 24] Given this favorable experience, the indications for endoscopic thoracic sympathectomy are likely to broaden with reevaluation of sympathectomy for management of upper extremity ischemic and pain syndromes.[64] By 1993, Drott and colleagues[18] had little doubt that open surgical techniques were being relegated to history by the widespread acceptance of endoscopic sympathectomy. However, open surgical upper extremity sympathectomy can be performed in conjunction with thoracic outlet surgery[80] or when endoscopic sympathectomy is contraindicated by dense pleural adhesions or other thoracic lesions.

HISTORY

Sympathetic control of the circulation was described by Bernard and Brown-Sequard in 1852. By 1889, Gaskell and Langley had mapped the anatomy of the autonomic nervous system. Alexander is credited as being the first surgeon to operate on the sympathetic nervous system: he performed cervical sympathectomy for epilepsy in 1889. Leriche, in 1913, described periarterial sympathectomy to increase blood flow to the extremities. Other surgeons, including Jonnesco, Brunning, Gask, and Royle, advocated more proximal upper extremity sympathetic interruption by excision of the stellate ganglion. The history of and past controversy over the exact anatomy, open surgical approach, and indications for upper extremity sympathectomy were reviewed by Welch and Geary.[84]

In 1910, Jacobaeus introduced thoracoscopy as a diagnostic tool, and 32 years later Hughes performed the first thoracoscopic removal of sympathetic ganglia. In 1954, Kux described experience with more than 1400 sympathetic and vagal thoracoscopic procedures. Despite this early success, general acceptance of the method outside Europe was delayed almost 30 years longer (Table 86–1).[16, 18]

The conflicting aims of achieving complete sympathectomy and avoiding the disability of Horner's syndrome (contracted pupil, drooping eyelid, and facial anhidrosis, which occurs when the stellate ganglion is completely excised, have resulted in argument over the extent of sympathectomy, the amount of stellate ganglion to be resected, and the best way to do the procedure.[56, 68, 84]

ANATOMIC CONSIDERATIONS

Anatomy of the Thoracic Sympathetic Chain

The autonomic nervous system has sympathetic and parasympathetic components and controls visceral functions. In the upper extremity, the sympathetic nervous system controls vasomotor activity, piloerection, and sweating. Preganglionic fibers supplying the upper limb are derived from cells in the intermediolateral column of the gray matter of the spinal cord between its second and ninth segments. They pass through the anterior nerve root of the spinal cord into the spinal nerve, then separate to pass into the corresponding ganglia of the paravertebral sympathetic chain that are located on either side of the vertebral column. After entering the ganglia, fibers can take a variable course, forming a synapse with the postganglionic neuron at the same level, passing up or down the sympathetic chain to form synapses in other ganglia, or passing along the chain to exit via a gray communicating ramus to ultimately form synapses with outlying sympathetic ganglia.[71] The majority of the preganglionic outflow to the sweat

TABLE 86–1. HISTORY OF OPEN SURGICAL AND ENDOSCOPIC THORACIC SYMPATHECTOMY

YEAR	AUTHOR	EVENT
	Role of the Sympathetic Nerves in Control of the Circulation	
1852	Bernard and Brown-Sequard	Sympathetic control of the circulation
1889	Gaskell and Langley	Anatomy of the autonomic nervous system
1913	Leriche	Described periarterial sympathectomy
1914	Kramer and Todd	Demonstrated that sympathetic fibers reach periphery via peripheral nerves
	Early Surgical Experience	
1889	Alexander	First surgeon to perform cervical sympathectomy in a patient with epilepsy
1896	Jaboulay and Jonnesco	Sympathectomy tried for exophthalmos
1899	Abadie	Sympathectomy tried for glaucoma
1902	Pappalado	Sympathectomy tried for trigeminal neuralgia
1905	Ball	Sympathectomy tried for optic nerve atrophy
1917	Kotzareff	Sympathectomy tried for external carotid angioma
1920	Kotzareff	Successful excision of cervical ganglia for facial hyperhidrosis
1921	Jonnesco	Stellectomy for angina pectoris
	Evolution of Indications for and Methods of Thoracic Sympathectomy	
1927	Kuntz	Aberrant nerve described bypassing T2–3 ganglia
1935	Telford	Supraclavicular approach
1936	Smithwick	Posterior exposure of the sympathetic chain
1944	Goetz and Marr	Anterior or transaxillary transthoracic approach
1954	Atkins	Transaxillary approach
1956	Palumbo	Anterior transthoracic exposure
1965	Lougheed	Anterior cervical approach
1969	Cloward	Anterior midline approach for bilateral cervical sympathectomy
1971	Roos	Extrapleural approach after transaxillary resection of the first rib
	Percutaneous and Endoscopic Methods	
1927	White	Alcohol injection to destroy sympathetic ganglia
1990	Adler	Phenol injection guided by computed tomography
1984	Wilkinson	Radiofrequency destruction
1988	Chuang	Percutaneous, stereotactic thermocoagulation
1910	Jacobaeus	First thoracoscopy
1942	Hughes	First thoracoscopic removal of sympathetic ganglia
1944	Goetz and Marr	Induced pneumothorax to check patient tolerance
1954	Kux	Published experience with more than 1400 endoscopic sympathectomies and vagotomies, but no widespread acceptance
1980s		Emergence of endoscopic surgery, including thoracoscopic sympathectomy
1990s		Large series of endoscopic sympathectomy for hyperhidrosis

Data from Drott C: Eur J Surg Suppl 572:5–7, 1994; Drott C, et al: Arch Surg 128(2):237–241, 1993; Welch E, et al: J Vasc Surg 1:202, 1984.

glands in the upper extremity arise from the T2 spinal segment. Most vasoconstrictor fibers supplying the arteries of the upper extremity emerge from the spinal cord in the ventral roots of T2 and T3. The surgeon can denervate these arteries by cutting the sympathetic trunk below the third thoracic ganglion and severing the rami communicantes of the second and third thoracic ganglia. The sympathetic nerve supply to the eccrine glands in the upper extremity may be similarly interrupted. It is necessary to divide the trunk below the fourth thoracic ganglion and to divide its associated rami if the eccrine glands of the axilla are to be completely denervated. To produce sympathetic denervation of the upper extremity, it is not necessary to excise any portion of the stellate ganglion or to divide the rami to the first thoracic ganglion.[71, 84]

Kuntz[40] described an intrathoracic nerve passing from the second intercostal nerve to the T1 nerve root. Sympathetic fibers may pass from the spinal cord to the lower brachial plexus along this nerve, bypassing the sympathetic chain, particularly the T2 ganglion (Fig. 86–1). This anomaly occurs in about 10% of the population, and if it is overlooked, sympathectomy will be incomplete.[72] Van der Kloot and coworkers,[83] by microscopic dissection of 18 resected sympathectomy specimens, found several other anatomic variations. They noted that the neuroanatomy of the T1 and T2 ganglia is incompletely described and, because of these anatomic variations, questioned whether complete interruption of all sympathetic fibers to the arm can be accomplished by thoracic sympathectomy.

Sympathetic innervation of the digital arteries has been described by Morgan and colleagues.[62] Sympathetic nerve twigs pass from the digital nerves to the digital arteries. Sympathectomy can be performed in the hand by denervating the digital arteries using microsurgical techniques.[34]

Endoscopic Surgical Anatomy

Various endoscopic landmarks have been suggested to guide the surgeon in determining the exact level of ganglia on the sympathetic chain.[11] The T2 ganglion lies between the second and third ribs.[48] The second rib is the easier to identify, since apical pleural fat protects the stellate ganglion and conceals the neck of the first rib. The first rib can,

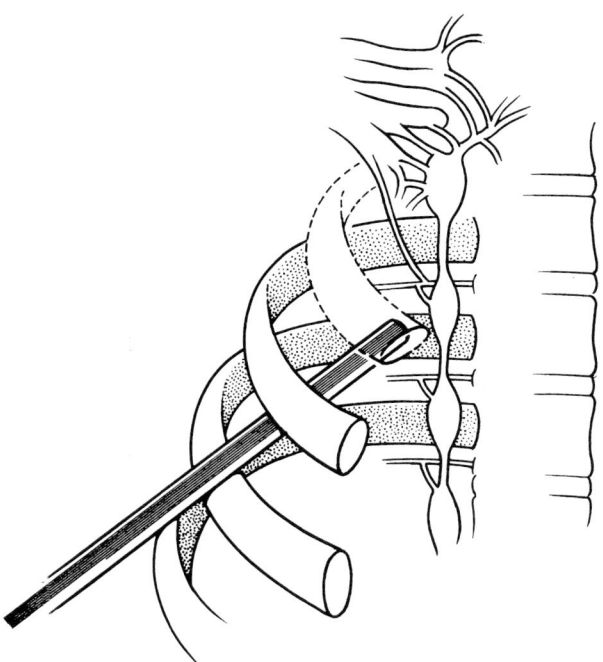

FIGURE 86–1. The right paravertebral sympathetic chain is shown with a thoracoscope introduced through an intercostal space. The nerve of Kuntz bypasses the T2 ganglion and goes directly from the spinal nerve to the T1 nerve root. This anomaly and the sympathetic chain are seen most clearly crossing the second rib because the first rib and stellate ganglion are covered by the apical fat pad.

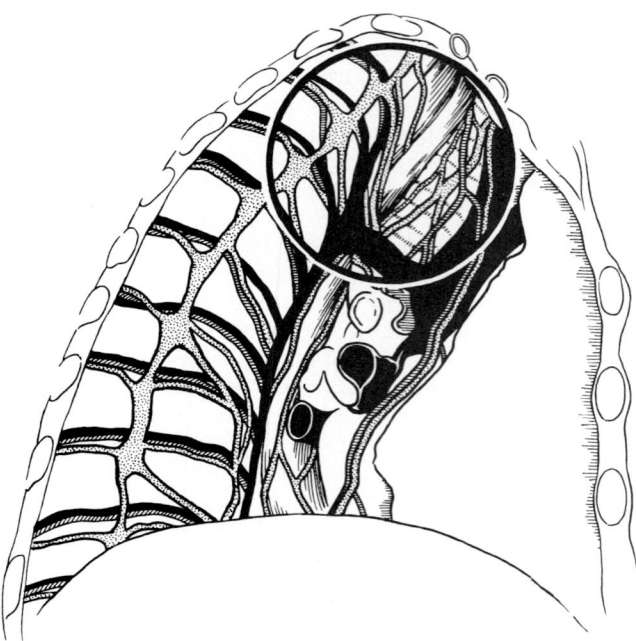

FIGURE 86–2. A view of the right pleural cavity showing the relationship between the sympathetic chain and tributaries of the azygos vein. The first rib is usually covered by a fat pad, whereas the neck of the second rib is more easily identified. The usual field of view through the thoracoscope is indicated by the *circle*.

however, be identified by palpating with an endoscopic probe and by noting the level where the subclavian artery leaves the thoracic cavity. The thoracic sympathetic chain is seen most easily where it crosses the neck of the second rib (see Fig. 86–1).

METHODS OF THORACIC SYMPATHECTOMY

Endoscopic thoracic sympathectomy is now performed far more often than open surgical sympathectomy.[10] Nevertheless, traditional open operations occasionally have a place when endoscopic surgery is not feasible or is preferred by the operating surgeon[89] or when sympathectomy is performed in conjunction with another surgical procedure, for example transaxillary first rib resection.[80] Pleural adhesions are only a relative contraindication to thoracoscopic sympathectomy since in most cases they can be dealt with endoscopically, provided the surgeon is familiar with the anatomy and is well trained in the procedure.[49] The preoperative chest plain film may be normal despite dense pleural adhesions, but it is helpful in alerting the surgeon to potential problems such as apical lung lesions or anomalies of venous drainage.[75]

Endoscopic Sympathectomy: Surgical Technique

As laparoscopic surgical instrumentation is adapted for thoracic endoscopic sympathectomy, similar results have been reported to those of open operation. It is probable

that the best results will be achieved with the endoscopic method as surgeons can handle larger case loads and benefit from the better lighting and magnification afforded by endoscopic instrumentation. Although a double-lumen endobronchial tube can be used to control ventilation to each lung separately during endoscopic surgery,[26] the operation can safely be performed with a single-lumen tube.[88]

A 5-mm thoracoscope with high-intensity light guide, high-resolution video display, and at least one additional operating port enables precise dissection and excision of the thoracic sympathetic chain. The azygos vein and tributaries are at risk on the right, whereas the aortic arch and left subclavian artery may impede visualization of the thoracic sympathetic chain in the left pleural cavity (Figs. 86–2 and 86–3). Our preferred technique is to position the patient supine on the operating table with the arms abducted 90 degrees (Fig. 86–4). The head of the table can be elevated to allow the lung to fall away from the apex of the thoracic cavity, improving exposure.

Although it is possible to perform endoscopic sympathectomy with a modified urologic resectoscope through a single port,[23] we prefer two ports for more precise dissection. A very acceptable cosmetic result is achieved when one of the stab incisions is placed in the inframammary fold (see Fig. 86–4). The overlying pleura is opened, and the sympathetic chain is divided below the stellate ganglion. Simple division of the chain on the neck of the second rib is all that is required to produce a dry hand for almost all patients with hyperhidrosis. A segment of thoracic sympathetic chain from T2 to the T4 ganglion can be excised if histologic confirmation is necessary or if the operation is intended to include the axillary sympathetic supply (Fig. 86–5). This excision is around the T4 level,

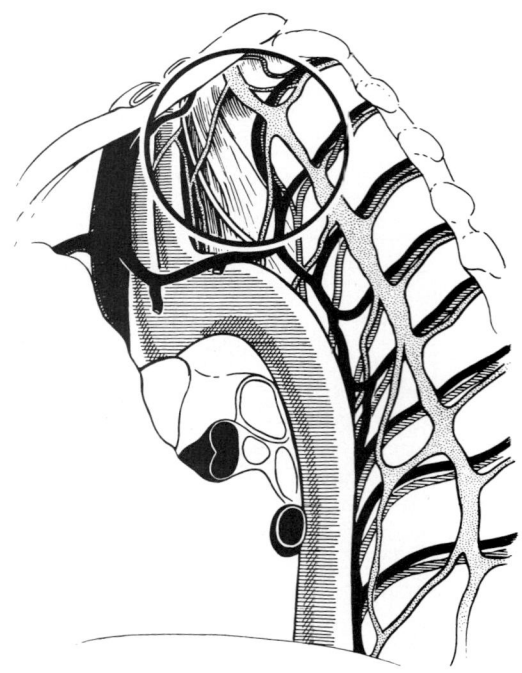

FIGURE 86–3. A view of the left thoracic cavity. The aortic arch is the most prominent structure seen in the left pleural cavity. Care must be taken not to place the electrocautery anywhere near the subclavian artery. The endoscopic view is indicated by the *circle*.

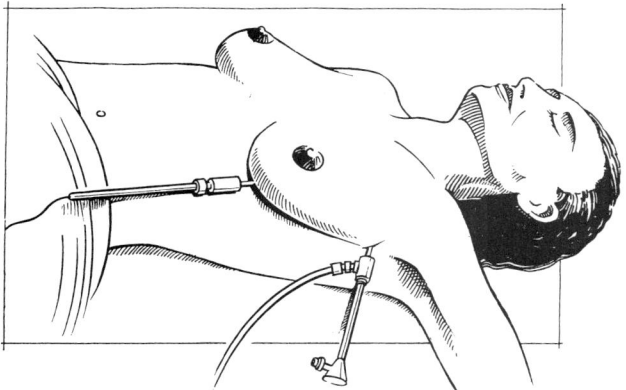

FIGURE 86–4. Bilateral endoscopic sympathectomy can be performed with the patient in the supine position with the arms abducted at 90 degrees to facilitate access. A pleasing cosmetic result is achieved if one of the operating ports is placed in the inframammary fold as shown.

but the relationship is not as constant as that between T2 and the sympathetic supply to the hand. After hemostasis has been verified, lung expansion can be observed on the video display before the camera is removed so that a chest drain is rarely needed.

Bilateral thoracic sympathectomy can safely be performed with a single session of anesthesia or staged, depending on the patient's fitness for surgery and surgical preference. Simultaneous bilateral endoscopic sympathectomy overcomes a problem associated with open operation. About 20% of patients, having undergone successful unilateral open sympathectomy, would not agree to have the same operation on the other side because of the postoperative pain of the initial operation.[77] Postoperative pain can be significantly decreased by interpleural bupivacaine[46] and infusion of a local anesthetic agent into the stab wounds. An erect chest radiograph is taken during recovery to check for any residual pneumothorax. A hospital stay of only 1 or 2 days is typical, and the patient is spared the morbidity associated with thoracotomy.[61]

Open Thoracic Sympathectomy: Surgical Technique

The transaxillary, supraclavicular, and extrapleural approaches are the most frequently used open operations,

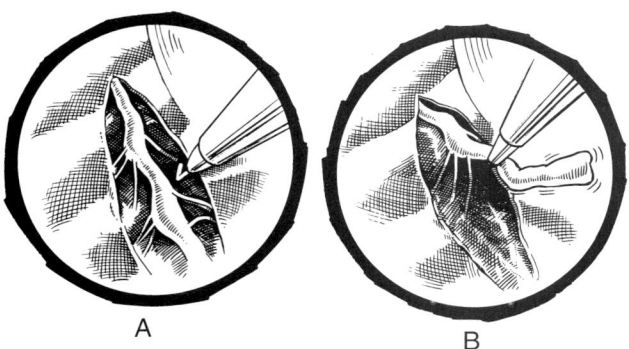

FIGURE 86–5. *A*, Endoscopic view of the thoracic sympathetic chain after the pleura has been incised *B*, Precise dissection of the sympathetic rami is facilitated by the magnified view.

although the posterior thoracic approach still has its advocates,[20] especially among neurosurgeons.[30]

Supraclavicular Sympathectomy

Supraclavicular sympathectomy is performed through a short incision above the medial one third of the clavicle with the patient in the supine position. The clavicular head of the sternocleidomastoid is divided. The phrenic nerve runs down from the lateral to the medial border of the scalenus anterior muscle deep to the investing fascia. The nerve is mobilized, and then the scalenus anterior muscle is divided. The subclavian artery is exposed and retracted without division of any of its branches. The pleura may be opened inadvertently if scalenus pleuralis muscle, which lies over the dome of the lung in more than 35% of persons,[58] is not divided before an attempt is made to depress the apical pleura. It is possible to spare the stellate ganglion, although the incidence of Horner's syndrome as a complication of the supraclavicular approach to the T2 and T3 ganglia is significant.[1]

Axillary Transthoracic Sympathectomy

An advantage of transthoracic transaxillary sympathectomy is that the sympathetic chain can be excised below the stellate ganglion more readily than with the supraclavicular approach.[56] The patient is placed in the lateral position, and the arm is supported to prevent traction on the brachial plexus. Collapse and re-expansion of the lung can be controlled with a double-lumen endotracheal tube, but this is not essential because the lung can be retracted provided the patient is ventilated manually and is not on a ventilator. A transverse incision is made beneath the hair-bearing area of the axilla. The intercostobrachial nerve should be identified and preserved, but some numbness in this nerve's distribution is common postoperatively. The thorax is entered through the second intercostal space.[51] Winging of the scapula can occur if the long thoracic nerve, which supplies the serratus anterior, is injured. This nerve is particularly at risk when the intercostal opening is extended posteriorly. A small rib retractor is inserted and opened slowly to avoid rib fracture. Improved operative illumination can be provided by passing a flexible, cold light source through a stab incision in the fourth intercostal space in the mid-axillary line.[59] An underwater seal drain is conveniently brought out through the track left after the light source has been removed.

The sympathetic chain is identified and its level determined by counting down from the first rib at the apex of the thoracic cavity. After incision of the pleura, the sympathetic chain can be encircled with a polymeric silicone (Silastic) loop if retraction is required to identify and divide the rami. This should be done gently, lest excessive traction on the sympathetic chain result in Horner's syndrome. The extent of the sympathectomy is determined by the indication for surgery.[56] After reinflation of the lung is ensured, the chest is closed and the drain removed within 24 hours of surgery. Chest films are taken to ensure that there is no intrathoracic collection of fluid or residual pneumothorax. Although Campbell and associates[8] considered it safe to perform bilateral axillary sympathectomy using the same anesthetic, most surgeons preferred staged unilateral operations, particularly for older patients, to minimize the risk of pulmonary complications.[60]

Extrapleural Sympathectomy After Resection of the First Rib

Sympathectomy has also been incorporated into surgery for thoracic outlet syndrome, particularly for associated sympathetically mediated pain syndromes.[80] An extrapleural approach,[72] which can be performed after excision of the first rib, has these advantages: there is less postoperative pain because rib retraction is unnecessary, and the operating surgeon is able to determine beyond doubt the exact level of the sympathetic chain and identify and protect the T1 nerve root, which carries the motor fibers to the small muscles of the hand. These advantages notwithstanding, the approach is technically demanding, and the supraclavicular and axillary transthoracic approaches were considered safer options for surgeons unfamiliar with first rib resection for thoracic outlet syndrome.[74]

Endoscopic instrumentation can facilitate conventional thoracic outlet surgery. The magnification and lighting can provide excellent video display of the operative field to guide the surgeon and the assistant during open transaxillary first rib resection combined with dorsal sympathectomy.[79]

Comparative Studies of Open and Endoscopic Sympathectomy

Before thoracoscopic sympathectomy was accepted as the operation of choice, most surgeons chose either supraclavicular or axillary transthoracic sympathectomy (depending on personal preference, since few studies had compared the two procedures). May and Harris[58] found no significant difference in length of hospital stay. Respiratory complications were more common after transaxillary sympathectomy but usually responded promptly to treatment. Horner's syndrome and post-sympathetic neuralgia occurred more frequently after supraclavicular sympathectomy, but there were fewer respiratory problems.[60] Although postoperative pain is more severe after transaxillary sympathectomy, this approach was recommended because it affords easier access to the sympathetic chain for wide excision, it avoids Horner's syndrome, and it has a good cosmetic result.[58]

Morbidity associated with both supraclavicular and transaxillary sympathectomy relates to difficulty of access, risk of injury to major vessels and nerves, and wound pain. These problems are largely avoided with endoscopic thoracic sympathectomy; there is excellent visualization of the sympathetic chain without the morbidity of a neck wound or thoracotomy.[7]

In a comparative study of the short-term results of open supraclavicular sympathectomy and thoracoscopic resection of the T2 to T4 ganglia in two randomly selected groups of 12 patients with palmar hyperhidrosis, Hashmonai and coworkers[27] achieved dry hands in all patients but found that anesthesia time was prolonged and patients in the thoracoscopic group were less satisfied 1 week after surgery. Based on this small trial, they concluded that the supraclavicular sympathectomy did not take longer and

was no more difficult than thoracoscopic sympathectomy, might be associated with less morbidity, and produced greater subjective satisfaction.[27] The same group later reported 106 thoracoscopic sympathectomies in 53 patients with palmar hyperhidrosis.[39] All limbs were completely dry at the end of the procedure and at a mean follow-up time of 19.5 months; 88.5% of patients expressed subjective satisfaction with the procedure. From this experience, they concurred that thoracoscopic sympathectomy was preferred over supraclavicular sympathectomy for severe palmar hyperhidrosis.[39]

Similarly, Yilmaz and colleagues[89] recommended endoscopic sympathectomy in preference to transaxillary sympathectomy. Their efficacies were identical, but there was less postoperative pain, a shorter hospital stay, and more rapid recovery after thoracoscopic sympathectomy.[89] Only minimal changes in pulmonary function, secondary to a temporary small decrease in lung volume and a minor but permanent decrease in forced expiratory flow, have been observed after thoracoscopic sympathectomy.[67] In contrast, more significant respiratory changes were observed after supraclavicular and transaxillary sympathectomy.[60] Partial beta-blocker–like activity has also been observed after T2 to T3 thoracic sympathectomy that resulted in a decrease in heart rate at rest and during rigorous exercise. The long-term consequences are not known.[65]

OBJECTIVE ASSESSMENT OF THE RESULTS OF SYMPATHECTOMY

The diagnosis of hyperhidrosis can usually be made on clinical grounds, so that methods for detecting sympathetic denervation, although well established, have not found widespread clinical application. Most are complex to perform, relatively imprecise, and time-consuming, so that their use is mainly restricted to research settings.[12]

Satchell and associates[73] overcame most of the problems inherent in these tests by finger sudometry, which provided a sensitive measure of sudomotor drive to the fingers. After the patient inserts a finger through a rubber diaphragm into a chamber, continuous measuring of sweat produced by a finger allows the effect of stimuli on sweat output to be quantified in "real time." Such a test can confirm sympathetic-driven sweating in patients with hyperhidrosis and can postoperatively determine whether sympathectomy is complete. This type of test is not yet available for clinical practice, but such a test is needed in the diagnostic workup of patients being considered for sympathectomy, particularly when reoperation is being considered.[37] Measurement of sympathetic skin responses is a simple, electrophysiologic method of assessing sympathetic nerve function and may prove a useful investigational tool.[45] Intraoperative monitoring of palmar skin temperature by infrared thermography has been used to locate the appropriate sympathetic segment and to confirm successful sympathectomy.[13]

INDICATIONS AND RESULTS FOR SPECIFIC CONDITIONS

In modern surgical practice, the most common indication for upper extremity sympathectomy is hyperhidrosis.[15,22]

Less common indications include upper limb ischemia,[64] cold injury,[53] post-traumatic pain syndromes,[22] and unusual cardiac conditions[17] (including the long QT-interval syndrome when it is refractory to medical therapy).[20]

The management of upper extremity ischemic disease is dealt with in Chapters 81 and 82 and of post-traumatic pain syndromes in Chapter 63. The initial and long-term results of sympathectomy for upper extremity ischemic and post-traumatic pain syndromes are not as good as those for hyperhidrosis.[22] Although some investigators have abandoned upper extremity sympathectomy for digital ischemia,[44] others believe that it can help selected patients.[22] Gordon and coworkers,[22] in a review of the role of sympathectomy in current surgical practice, concluded that any benefit for Raynaud's phenomenon affecting the hands was short-lived and had no effect on the prognosis of the disease. Nevertheless, the demonstrated safety and high patient acceptance of endoscopic sympathectomy are such that Nicholson and associates[64] asserted that the indications for surgical thoracic sympathectomy could be extended to more cases of Raynaud's syndrome.

The decision to proceed to surgical sympathectomy still depends on clinical judgment, because a good response to temporary stellate ganglion blockade is only a limited predictor of the outcome of upper extremity sympathectomy.[82] In marked contrast to the debate over the place of upper extremity sympathectomy in these conditions, it is generally agreed that a predictably good outcome will follow upper extremity sympathectomy for hyperhidrosis.

Essential Hyperhidrosis

Hyperhidrosis is sweating in excess of that required for normal thermoregulation. Primary, or essential, hyperhidrosis occurs in the absence of any known structural abnormality of the eccrine glands, sympathetic nerves, or ganglia. Rarely, hyperhidrosis is secondary to systemic disorders, which include hyperthyroidism and pheochromocytoma. A good account of the differential diagnosis and nonoperative management of hyperhidrosis was given by Fitzpatrick.[21]

Most affected patients are young and otherwise healthy. The condition occurs in both sexes. Some authors have observed a familial tendency,[2] although others dispute this.[25] Unusual sweating typically begins in childhood or adolescence. It is usually episodic and is precipitated by thermal, gustatory, or emotional stimuli specific to the individual patient (Table 86–2). Although sweating may be exacerbated by hot weather, climate is not a major causal factor. The mechanism is unclear, but these stimuli produce hyperactivity of the sudomotor drive.[2] Sweating tends to be symmetric and is usually absent during sleep. In severe cases, sweat can drip from the hands, making handling papers impossible and shaking hands a social embarrassment. Moist skin can result in chronic dermatitis and fungal infections.

The clinical picture is usually so clear-cut that extensive investigation is not required.[2, 85] Patients who are mildly affected may obtain sufficient symptomatic relief from a topical antiperspirant and atropine-like drugs.[25] With severe hyperhidrosis, these measures are not sufficient, and surgical sympathectomy is indicated. It is desirable, how-

TABLE 86–2. RELATIVE FREQUENCY OF TRIGGER STIMULI FOR HYPERHIDROSIS OBSERVED IN 270 PATIENTS

TRIGGER	NO.	%
Emotional	119	44.1
Heat	12	4.4
Physical exercise	4	1.5
Gustatory	3	1.1
Others	18	6.7
None	114	42.2
TOTAL	270	100

From Herbst F, Plas EG, Fugger R, Fritsch A: Endoscopic thoracic sympathectomy for primary hyperhidrosis of the upper limbs: A critical analysis and long-term results of 480 operations. Ann Surg 220(1):86–90, 1994.

ever, to allow patients with essential hyperhidrosis to try all conservative measures before concluding that sympathectomy is the only cure. Extensive sympathetic denervation of the upper and lower extremities for hyperhidrosis should be avoided, because orthostatic hypotension has been observed.[47] In rare instances, eccrine glands may be congenitally absent in some areas of the body. For patients thus affected, compensatory localized sweating is the only means of cutaneous thermoregulation and sympathectomy is therefore inappropriate.

Open Thoracic Sympathectomy: Results

After upper extremity sympathectomy, relief of hyperhidrosis can be expected, regardless of the method of sympathectomy. Patients so treated are significantly younger than those who have sympathectomy for other indications.

Adar and colleagues failed to achieve a dry hand in only seven (3.6%) of 198 sympathectomies in 100 patients suffering from hyperhidrosis.[2] When frozen section histologic examination was used to confirm excision of the sympathetic chain, they had no failures. Ninety-one patients who had a good initial result were followed for an average of 18 months; 38 had completely dry hands, and 53 had some return of sweating, but in no case did the hyperhidrosis recur. These good results were confirmed in a later review of 475 patients who underwent simultaneous bilateral supraclavicular T2 and T3 sympathectomies for palmar hyperhidrosis, although there was a 5.3% incidence of recurrent hand sweating.[1]

Greenhalgh and coworkers reported similarly good results in a smaller group of patients, some of whom were followed up as long as 10 years.[25] Mild gustatory sweating was common in the experience of Adar and colleagues, as was some form of compensatory perspiration.[2] Occasionally, patients have residual sweating in part of the axillae. The affected area can be delineated by starch-iodine testing and excised if symptoms are sufficiently troublesome.[25] Temporary sweating of the palms may occur on the third or fourth day after sympathectomy for hyperhidrosis. Greenhalgh's group noted that temporary sweating was frequent following supraclavicular sympathectomy for hyperhidrosis.[25] It is important to be aware of this phenomenon; otherwise the surgeon could be misled into believing that he or she has done an incomplete operation. Awareness of this phenomenon is important if metallic clips have been used for hemostasis, because clips indicating the upper limit of resection usually appear much lower than the superior border of the second rib on postoperative chest films.

May and Harris[58] placed metallic clips at the superior border of the second rib, just lateral to the sympathetic chain, in patients treated with thoracotomy for lung disease through a large incision through which the second rib could be identified with complete confidence. In postoperative radiographs, clips consistently appeared to be below the second rib, despite having been placed at its upper border.

Endoscopic Sympathectomy: Results

The early results of endoscopic or percutaneous upper extremity sympathectomy have been confirmed in larger series as endoscopic sympathectomy has evolved to be the preferred method for surgical control of hyperhidrosis.[18, 24] Percutaneous sympathectomy has been performed as an outpatient procedure.[87]

Malone and associates found that the endoscopic technique could readily be learned.[55] Although endoscopic sympathectomy predictably produces a dry hand in patients with hyperhidrosis, achieving a dry axilla is less certain. Kux[41] reported complete relief of hand sweating in 63 patients after endoscopic sympathectomy, but 19% of them still had some sweating in the axilla. Similarly, in a series of 100 consecutive patients, Noppen and colleagues[66] found that palmar hyperhidrosis was cured in 98% but axillary sweating improved in only 62%. Of interest, 65% had some relief of associated plantar sweating,[66] an observation confirmed by others.[32] The benefit from sympathectomy is lasting in adults[29] and children,[28] although recurrences occasionally take place.

Herbst and associates[29] had an 83.7% response to a questionnaire sent to 323 patients in whom 480 sympathectomies had been performed (mean follow-up period 14.6 years). There were no postoperative deaths and no major complications that required further surgery. Surgical success was achieved in 98.1%, and 95.5% were satisfied initially. Permanent side effects included compensatory sweating in 67.4%, gustatory sweating in 50.7%, and Horner's syndrome in 2.5%. Patient satisfaction declined over time, however, although hand sweating recurred in only 1.5%. Compensatory and gustatory sweating were the reasons most frequently given for dissatisfaction. Individuals whose operation was for axillary hyperhidrosis without palmar involvement were significantly less satisfied.[29]

Kao and coworkers[35] surveyed 9988 patients in 17 hospitals in Taiwan treated for hyperhidrosis by endoscopic sympathectomy over a 5-year period. Although the surgical and anesthetic techniques varied, overall clinical results were excellent and no deaths were reported. Benefit was also achieved in patients with craniofacial hyperhidrosis. Complications such as pneumothorax, hemothorax (0.3%), and Horner's syndrome (0.1%) were rare. The most common late problem was compensatory hyperhidrosis, which was usually tolerated after it was explained. The authors concluded that endoscopic T2 sympathectomy gave effective long-term relief to adults and children affected by essential hyperhidrosis.[35] Patients benefit from early hospital discharge and are spared the morbidity associated with thoracotomy.[61]

Although electrocautery is the usual method used to divide the sympathetic chain, other modalities have been tried. In an experimental study of endoscopic thoracic sympathectomy that compared techniques for sympathetic ablation, Massad and associates found that the excimer laser and the carbon dioxide laser produced discrete lesions and minimal damage to surrounding structures, as compared with radiofrequency-generated thermocoagulation and the neodymium:yttrium-aluminum-garnet (Nd : YAG) laser.[57]

Compensatory Sweating and the Extent of Sympathectomy

Compensatory sweating is the commonest long-term complaint subsequent to upper extremity sympathectomy for hyperhidrosis.[29] Most patients tolerate this, provided they have been informed before surgery. The reported incidence and severity of compensatory hyperhidrosis are generally proportional to the extent of the sympathectomy. Herbst and associates[29] found an incidence of 67.4% for this permanent side effect after T1 to T4 sympathectomy.

Hehir's group,[28] in a small pediatric series using a more limited T2 sympathectomy, reported a 17% incidence of compensatory hyperhidrosis. O'Riordain and coworkers[68] also proposed more localized sympathectomy, noting that axillary sweating is rarely a significant postoperative problem and concluding that extensive sympathectomy to include axillary denervation is unnecessary and should be avoided to minimize compensatory hyperhidrosis.

Although no clinical trial data confirm a direct relationship between compensatory sweating and the extent of sympathectomy, it is appropriate to warn patients of this common postoperative problem[42] and to limit sympathetic transection to the interganglionic trunk or T2 ganglia when treating palmar hyperhidrosis (Fig. 86–6).[7]

Hand and Digital Ischemia
(see Chapters 81 and 82)

Although the place of sympathectomy in upper extremity ischemic syndromes is controversial,[6, 44] upper extremity sympathectomy can help selected patients with upper extremity ischemia, and several broad recommendations can be supported. Only short-term benefit has been associated with upper extremity sympathectomy for Raynaud's syndrome not associated with digital artery occlusion.[4, 6, 84] Symptoms usually recur within 2 to 3 years after surgery. Vasospastic changes in the hands may precede, by many years, clinical manifestations of collagen vascular disease.[9] Van de Wal and coworkers followed up 25 patients thought to have primary Raynaud's disease.[82] Collagen vascular disease was eventually discovered in 20%. Upper extremity sympathectomy for Raynaud's syndrome associated with collagen vascular disease, particularly scleroderma, does not retard the progression of hand ischemia.[33]

Major upper extremity amputation for ischemia is rarely required,[86] although digital ischemia severe enough to warrant local amputation is relatively common. Detailed hand angiography can complement other investigations in detecting underlying reasons for upper extremity ischemia

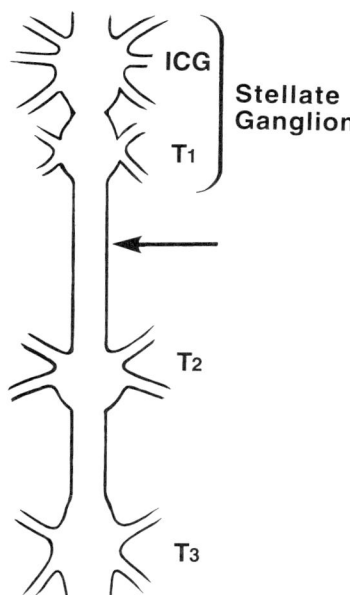

FIGURE 86–6. Transection of the interganglionic trunk *(arrow)* or T2 ganglion gives a predictably dry hand for patients with palmar hyperhidrosis (see text). ICG = inferior cervical ganglion.

and in determining whether arterial reconstruction is feasible.[90] Sympathectomy may be a useful adjunct to proximal arterial reconstruction, but this has not been established. Most patients with digital ischemia are helped by topical and systemic vasodilators and by stellate ganglion blockade.[78] Some surgeons have abandoned upper extremity sympathectomy for digital ischemia[44]; however, others have found that sympathectomy relieves pain, improves digital perfusion, and decreases the need for amputation.[58, 81] The best results are achieved in patients with digital arterial occlusion in the absence of Raynaud's syndrome.[82] Birnstingl found that the prognosis after sympathectomy for digital ischemia was better in males than in females.[6] These observations are supported by van de Wal and coworkers in a long-term study of 57 patients who had 72 thoracic sympathectomies for upper extremity ischemia.[82]

Although there is little good objective evidence to support the efficacy of surgical sympathectomy,[22] some surgeons have had favorable results, and Nicholson and colleagues[64] encouraged reevaluation of the place of sympathectomy in the management of upper extremity ischemia.

Based on these considerations, it seems reasonable to recommend upper extremity sympathectomy for those few patients whose obliterative arterial disease threatens the viability of the hands or digits when the site and extent of the arterial occlusions make reconstructive arterial surgery impossible. Their ultimate prognosis depends on the underlying cause of the upper extremity ischemia.[43]

Post-traumatic Pain Syndromes
(see Chapter 63)

Complex regional pain syndrome has been suggested as a term to replace *reflex sympathetic dystrophy* and *causalgia*.[63]

The diagnosis is based on the presence after a noxious event of regional pain and sensory changes and findings such as abnormal skin color, temperature change, abnormal sudomotor activity, or edema in excess of what would be expected from the inciting event.[76] This syndrome may include somatic and sympathetically maintained pain. A multidisciplinary approach is advocated to determine and specifically treat any associated nerve lesion and to discourage uncontrolled sympathetic blocks.[54] Upper extremity sympathectomy, therefore, has an increasingly limited role in the management of these conditions. The best results of sympathectomy were achived when a diagnosis of sympathetically associated pain was made early, before physical changes occurred.[52]

Kleinert and colleagues reported on a large series of 506 patients who had what they classified as post-traumatic sympathetic dystrophy.[36] Only 23 of them underwent sympathectomy; 19 experienced permanent improvement, and there were four failures in patients with fixed pain patterns and established trophic changes.

Horowitz, stressing the importance of early recognition and reviewing the legal ramifications, studied 11 patients in a civilian practice, all of whose symptoms were thought to be iatrogenic.[31] Two of these patients had had earlier surgery for thoracic outlet syndrome.

On the basis of these considerations, upper extremity sympathectomy will be indicated for few patients with complex regional pain syndrome.[14] Most will get sufficient symptomatic relief from physical therapy, analgesia, and judicious use of nerve blocks. Sympathectomy offers the most benefit when sympathetic pain is clearly differentiated from somatic pain, before trophic changes become established.[14]

COMPLICATIONS

Open Sympathectomy

Complications observed after supraclavicular and transaxillary sympathectomy are summarized in Table 86–3. Numb-

TABLE 86–3. COMPLICATIONS AFTER 80 OPEN UPPER EXTREMITY SYMPATHECTOMIES

Supraclavicular Approach (no. = 29)	
Postsympathectomy neuralgia	3
Pleural effusion	1
Atelectasis	1
Chylous fistula	2
Lymphocele	1
Wound hematoma	1
TOTAL	9
Axillary Approach (no. = 51)	
Empyema	1
Winged scapula	2
Pneumonia	2
Atelectasis	3
Pneumothorax	2
TOTAL	10

From May J, Harris J: In Bergan J, Yao J (eds): Evaluation and Treatment of Upper and Lower Extremity Circulatory Disorders. Orlando, Fla, Grune & Stratton, 1984, p 159.

ness may occur in the distribution of the intercostobrachial nerve after axillary sympathectomy and to a lesser extent in the distribution of the supraclavicular nerve after supraclavicular sympathectomy. Sensory deficit in these areas is rarely reported spontaneously by the patient. Severe postsympathetic neuralgia[69] can be a devastating complication; debilitating pain develops in the upper arm approximately 2 weeks after operation. Major drug and alcohol dependence can develop unless symptoms, which last from 2 to 12 months, can be relieved with repeated brachial plexus nerve blocks and transcutaneous nerve stimulation.[58] Lymphatic complications are observed only after supraclavicular sympathectomy, particularly on the left side, where the thoracic duct may be injured, resulting in a lymph fistula.

The majority of complications observed after axillary transthoracic sympathectomy relate to the thoracotomy and include incomplete expansion of the lung, pulmonary infection, and recurrent pneumothorax, among others.[89] Horner's syndrome is rare, and it is usually temporary if the sympathetic chain is divided below the stellate ganglion. The complication of winged scapula is disfiguring, particularly in young females. It is a preventable complication, and every effort should be made to identify and protect the long thoracic nerve to the serratus anterior muscle. Temporary sweating of the palms may occur on the third or fourth day after sympathectomy for hyperhidrosis.[25] This phenomenon is probably due to a period of transmitter release from degenerating sympathetic postganglionic nerve endings, a phenomenon well documented in animal experiments.[3]

Endoscopic Sympathectomy

Complications of endoscopic sympathectomy are uncommon. Drott and colleagues[19] reported no deaths or life-threatening complications in a series of 850 patients treated by bilateral endoscopic sympathectomy for hyperhidrosis. Nine patients (1%) in this series required intercostal drainage because of pneumothorax or hemothorax. Treatment failure occurred in 18 cases (2%), and symptoms recurred in 18 cases (2%). Satisfactory results were reported in 98% of patients with a median follow up of 31 months.[19] Similar excellent results have been achieved by others with few serious complications. Chen and coworkers[10] undertook a retrospective review by questionnaire of 180 patients with palmar hyperhidrosis, 98% of whom reported successful treatment. No patient required a chest tube for pneumothorax, and no case of Horner's syndrome was recorded; however, 70% were troubled by compensatory sweating.

More serious complications have been encountered, particularly after left thoracic sympathectomy. Chylothorax has occurred after thoracic sympathectomy.[10] Of more concern, Lin and colleagues[50] reported a 0.28% incidence of intraoperative cardiac arrest. This occurred when the left T2–3 sympathetic trunk was transected by the thoracoscopic method (in two in a series of 719 patients). The two patients recovered completely after cardiopulmonary resuscitation.

SUMMARY

Patients with essential hyperhidrosis can expect an excellent result from upper extremity sympathectomy, the com-

monest indication for this operation. Sympathectomy may benefit patients with upper extremity ischemia or complex regional pain syndromes, but the outcome is less predictable.

Of the many options for open operation, the transaxillary transthoracic approach was preferred for its superior exposure, wider sympathetic excision capability, good cosmetic result, and avoidance of Horner's syndrome. When lung disease is present and when the root of the neck must be explored, supraclavicular sympathectomy is indicated. Extrapleural sympathectomy can be combined with first rib resection during thoracic outlet surgery.

Endoscopic sympathectomy has otherwise replaced open operation as the method of choice for upper extremity sympathectomy, particularly for hyperhidrosis. Compensatory sweating is a common late complaint, but the risk may be decreased by limiting the extent of sympathectomy.

REFERENCES

 1. Adar R: Surgical treatment of palmar hyperhidrosis before thoracoscopy: Experience with 475 patients. Eur J Surg Suppl 592:9–11, 1994.
 2. Adar R, Kurchin A, Zweig A, et al: Palmar hyperhidrosis and its surgical treatment: A report of 100 cases. Ann Surg 186, 1977.
 3. Asking B, Svartholm E: Degeneration activity: A transient effect following sympathectomy for hyperhidrosis. Eur J Surg Suppl 572:41–42, 1994.
 4. Baddeley R: The place of upper dorsal sympathectomy in the treatment of primary Raynaud's disease. Br J Surg 52:426, 1965.
 5. Belch JJ, Ho M: Pharmacotherapy of Raynaud's phenomenon. Drugs 52(5): 682–695, 1996.
 6. Birnstingl M: Results of sympathectomy in digital artery disease. Br Med J 2:601, 1967.
 7. Bonjer HJ, Hamming JF, du Bois N, van Urk H: Advantages of limited thoracoscopic sympathectomy. Surg Endosc 10(7):721–723, 1996.
 8. Campbell W, Cooper M, Sponsel W, et al: Transaxillary sympathectomy: Is a one stage bilateral procedure safe? Br J Surg 69(Suppl): S29, 1982.
 9. Cerinic MM, Generini S, Pignone A: New approaches to the treatment of Raynaud's phenomenon. Curr Opin Rheumatol 9(6): 544–556, 1997.
10. Chen HJ, Shih DY, Fung ST: Transthoracic endoscopic sympathectomy in the treatment of palmar hyperhidrosis. Arch Surg 129(6):630–633, 1994.
11. Chiou TS, Liao KK: Orientation landmarks of endoscopic transaxillary T-2 sympathectomy for palmar hyperhidrosis. J Neurosurg 85(2):310–315, 1996.
12. Chu EC, Chu NS: Patterns of sympathetic skin response in palmar hyperhidrosis. Clin Autonom Res 7(1):1–4, 1997.
13. Chuang TY, Yen YS, Chiu JW, et al: Intraoperative monitoring of skin temperature changes of hands before, during, and after endoscopic thoracic sympathectomy: Using infrared thermograph and thermometer for measurement. Arch Phys Med Rehabil 78(1):85-88, 1997.
14. Cooney WP: Somatic versus sympathetic mediated chronic limb pain: Experience and treatment options. Hand Clin 13(3):355–361, 1997.
15. Daniel TM: Thoracoscopic sympathectomy. Chest Surg Clin North Am 6(1):69–83, 1996.
16. Drott C: The history of cervicothoracic sympathectomy. Eur J Surg Suppl 572:5–7, 1994.
17. Drott C, Claes G, Gothberg G, Paszkowski P: Cardiac effects of endoscopic electrocautery of the upper thoracic sympathetic chain. Eur J Surg Suppl 572:65–70, 1994.
18. Drott C, Gothberg G, Claes G: Endoscopic procedures of the upper-thoracic sympathetic chain: A review. Arch Surg 128(2):237–241, 1993.
19. Drott C, Gothberg G, Claes G: Endoscopic transthoracic sympathectomy: An efficient and safe method for the treatment of hyperhidrosis. J Am Acad Dermatol 33(1):78–81, 1995.

20. Epstein AE, Rosner MJ, Hageman GR, et al: Posterior left thoracic cardiac sympathectomy by surgical division of the sympathetic chain: An alternative approach to treatment of the long QT syndrome. Pacing Clin Electrophysiol 19(7):1095–1104, 1996.
21. Fitzpatrick T: Dermatology in General Medicine, 4th ed. New York, McGraw-Hill, 1993.
22. Gordon A, Zechmeister K, Collin J: The role of sympathectomy in current surgical practice. Eur Vasc Surg 8(2): 129–137, 1994.
23. Gothberg G, Claes G, Drott C: Electrocautery of the upper thoracic sympathetic chain: A simplified technique. Br J Surg 80(7):862, 1993.
24. Gothberg G, Drott C, Claes G: Thoracoscopic sympathectomy for hyperhidrosis—surgical technique, complications and side effects. Eur J Surg Suppl 572:51–53, 1994.
25. Greenhalgh R, Rosengarten D, Martin P: Role of sympathectomy for hyperhidrosis. Br Med J 1:332, 1971.
26. Hartrey R, Poskitt KR, Heather BP, Durkin MA: Anaesthetic implications for transthoracic endoscopic sympathectomy. Eur J Surg Suppl 572:33–36, 1994.
27. Hashmonai M, Kopelman D, Schein M: Thoracoscopic versus open supraclavicular upper dorsal sympathectomy: A prospective randomised trial. Eur J Surg Suppl 572:13–16, 1994.
28. Hehir DJ, Brady MP: Long-term results of limited thoracic sympathectomy for palmar hyperhidrosis. J Pediatr Surg 28(7):909–911, 1993.
29. Herbst F, Plas EG, Fugger R, Fritsch A: Endoscopic thoracic sympathectomy for primary hyperhidrosis of the upper limbs: A critical analysis and long-term results of 480 operations. Ann Surg 220(1):86–90, 1994.
30. Herz DA, Looman JE, Ford RD, et al: Second thoracic sympathetic ganglionectomy in sympathetically maintained pain. J Pain Symptom Manage 8(7):483–491, 1993.
31. Horowitz S: Iatrogenic causalgia: Classification, clinical findings, and legal ramifications. Arch Neurol 41:821, 1984.
32. Hsu CP, Chen CY, Lin CT, et al: Video-assisted thoracoscopic T2 sympathectomy for hyperhidrosis palmaris. J Am Coll Surg 179(1):59–64, 1994.
33. Johnson E, Summerlym RMB: Prognosis in Raynaud's phenomenon after sympathectomy. Br Med J 1:962, 1965.
34. Jones N: Ischemia of the hand in systemic disease: The potential role of microsurgical revascularization and digital sympathectomy. Clin Plast Surg 16:547, 1989.
35. Kao MC, Lin JY, Chen YL, et al: Minimally invasive surgery: Video endoscopic thoracic sympathectomy for palmar hyperhidrosis. Ann Acad Med Singapore 25(5):673–678, 1996.
36. Kleinert H, Cole N, Wayne L, et al: Post-traumatic sympathetic dystrophy. Orthop Clin North Am 4:917, 1973.
37. Kloot van der, Rhede van EJ, Jorning PJ: Resympathectomy of the upper extremity. Br J Surg 77:1043, 1990.
38. Kobayashi K, Omote K, Homma E, et al: Sympathetic ganglion blockade for the management of hyperhidrosis. J Dermatol 21(8):575–581, 1994.
39. Kopelman D, Hashmonai M, Ehrenreich M, et al: Upper dorsal thoracoscopic sympathectomy for palmar hyperhidrosis: Improved intermediate-term results. Vasc Surg 24(2):194–199, 1996.
40. Kuntz A: Distribution of the sympathetic rami to the brachial plexus. Arch Surg 15:871–877, 1927.
41. Kux M: Thoracic endoscopic sympathectomy in palmar and axillary hyperhidrosis. Arch Surg 113:264, 1978.
42. Lai YT, Yang LH, Chio CC, Chen HH: Complications in patients with palmar hyperhidrosis treated with transthoracic endoscopic sympathectomy. Neurosurgery 41(1):110–115, 1997.
43. Landry GJ, Edwards JM, McLafferty RB, et al: Long-term outcome of Raynaud's syndrome in a prospectively analyzed patient cohort. J Vasc Surg 23(1):76–85, 1996.
44. Landry GJ, Edwards JM, Porter JM: Current management of Raynaud's syndrome. Adv Surg 30:333–347, 1996.
45. Lefaucheur JP, Fitoussi M, Becquemin JP: Abolition of sympathetic skin responses following endoscopic thoracic sympathectomy. Muscle Nerve 19(5):581–586, 1996.
46. Lieou FJ, Lee SC, Ho ST, Wang JJ: Interpleural bupivacaine for pain relief after transthoracic endoscopic sympathectomy for primary hyperhidrosis. Acta Anaesthesiol Sin 34(1):21–25, 1996.
47. Lieshout van der J, Wieling W, Wesseling K, et al: Orthostatic hypotension caused by sympathectomies performed for hyperhidrosis. Neth J Med 36:53, 1990.
48. Lin C: A new method of thoracoscopic sympathectomy in hyperhidrosis palmaris. Surg Endosc 4:224, 1990.
49. Lin CC, Mo LR: Experience in thoracoscopic sympathectomy for hyperhidrosis with concomitant pleural adhesion. Surg Laparosc Endosc 6(4):258–261, 1996.
50. Lin CC, Mo LR, Hwang MH: Intraoperative cardiac arrest: A rare complication of T2, 3 sympathectomy for treatment of hyperhidrosis palmaris. Two case reports. Eur J Surg (Suppl) 572:43–54, 1994.
51. Little J: Transaxillary transpleural thoracic sympathectomy. In Malt R (ed): Surgical Techniques Illustrated. Vol 2. Boston, Little, Brown, 1977, p 15.
52. Lopez RF: Reflex sympathetic dystrophy: Timely diagnosis and treatment can prevent severe contractures. Postgrad Med 101(4):185–190, 1997.
53. Lowell RC, Gloviczki P, Cherry KJ Jr, et al: Cervicothoracic sympathectomy for Raynaud's syndrome. Int Angiol 12(2): 168–172, 1993.
54. Mackin GA: Medical and pharmacologic management of upper extremity neuropathic pain syndromes. J Hand Ther 10(2):96–109, 1997.
55. Malone P, Cameron A, Rennie J: Endoscopic thoracic sympathectomy in the treatment of upper limb hyperhidrosis. Ann R Coll Surg Engl 68:93, 1986.
56. Mares AJ, Steiner Z, Cohen Z, et al: Transaxillary upper thoracic sympathectomy for primary palmar hyperhidrosis in children and adolescents. J Pediatr Surg 29(3):382–386, 1994.
57. Massad M, LoCicero J, Matano J, et al: Endoscopic thoracic sympathectomy: Evaluation of pulsatile laser, non-pulsatile laser, and radiofrequency-generated thermocoagulation. Lasers Surg Med 11:8–25, 1991.
58. May J, Harris J: Upper extremity sympathectomy: A comparison of the supraclavicular and axillary approaches. In Bergan J, Yao J (eds): Evaluation and Treament of Upper and Lower Extremity Circulatory Disorders. Orlando, Fla, Grune & Stratton, 1984, p 159.
59. McCaughan BC, May J: Illumination and access for transaxillary thoracic sympathectomy. Surg Gynecol Obstet 156:507, 1983.
60. Molho M, Shemesh E, Gordon D, et al: Pulmonary functional abnormalities after upper dorsal sympathectomy: A comparison between supraclavicular and transaxillary approaches. Chest 77:651, 1980.
61. Moran K, Brady M: Surgical management of primary hyperhidrosis. Br J Surg 78:279, 1991.
62. Morgan R, Riesman N, Wiligis E: Anatomic localization of sympathetic nerves in the hand. J Hand Surg 8:283, 1982.
63. Muizelaar JP, Kleyer M, Hertogs IA, DeLange DC: Complex regional pain syndrome (reflex sympathetic dystrophy and causalgia): Management with the calcium channel blocker nifedipine and/or the alpha-sympathetic blocker phenoxybenzamine in 59 patients. Clin Neurol Neurosurg 99(1):26–30, 1997.
64. Nicholson ML, Dennis MJ, Hopkinson BR: Endoscopic transthoracic sympathectomy: Successful in hyperhidrosis but can the indications be extended? Ann Coll Surg Engl 76(5):311–314, 1994.
65. Noppen M, Dendale P, Hagers Y, et al: Changes in cardiocirculatory autonomic function after thoracoscopic upper dorsal sympathicolysis for essential hyperhidrosis. J Autonom Nerv Syst 60(3):115–120, 1996.
66. Noppen M, Herregodts P, D'Haese J, et al: A simplified T2–T3, thoracoscopic sympathicolysis technique for the treatment of essential hyperhidrosis: Short-term results in 100 patients. J Laparoendosc Surg 6(3):151–159, 1996.
67. Noppen M, Vincken W: Thoracoscopic sympathicolysis for essential hyperhidrosis: Effects on pulmonary function. Eur Respir J 9(8):1660–1664, 1996.
68. O'Riordain D, Maher M, Waldron DJ, et al: Limiting the anatomic extent of upper thoracic sympathectomy for primary palmar hyperhidrosis. Surg Gynecol Obstet 176(2):151–154, 1993.
69. Raskin N, Levinson S, Hoffman P, et al: Postsympathectomy neuralgia amelioration with diphenylhydantoin and carbamazepine. Am J Surg 128:75, 1974.
70. Ravitch M: A Century of Surgery. Philadelphia, JB Lippincott, 1982.
71. Riolo J, Gumucio CA, Young AE, Young VL: Surgical management of palmar hyperhidrosis. South Med J 83(10):1138–1143, 1990.
72. Roos D: Transaxillary extrapleural thoracic sympathectomy. In Bergan J, Yao J (eds): Operative Techniques in Vascular Surgery. New York, Grune & Stratton, 1980, p 115.
73. Satchell P, Ware S, Barron J, Tuck R: Finger sudorometry and the sudomotor drive. J Neurosci Methods 53:217–223, 1994.
74. Scher L, Veith F, Samson R, et al: Vascular complications of thoracic outlet syndrome. J Vasc Surg 3:565, 1986.

75. Sieunarine K, May J, White GH, Harris JP: Anomalous azygous vein: A potential danger during endoscopic thoracic sympathectomy. Aust N Z J Surg 67(8):578–579, 1997.
76. Stanton-Hicks M, Janig W, Hassenbusch S, et al: Reflex sympathetic dystrophy: Changing concepts and taxonomy. Pain 63(1): 127–133, 1995.
77. Sternberg A, Brickman S, Kott I, et al: Transaxillary thoracic sympathectomy for primary hyperhidrosis of the upper limbs. World J Surg 6:458, 1982.
78. Taylor L, Baur G, Porter J: Finger gangrene caused by small artery occlusive disease. Ann Surg 193:453, 1981.
79. Urschel HC Jr: Dorsal sympathectomy and management of thoracic outlet syndrome with VATS. Ann Thorac Surg 56(3):717–720, 1993.
80. Urschel HC Jr: The transaxillary approach for treatment of thoracic outlet syndromes. Semin Thorac Cardiovasc Surg 8(2):214–220, 1996.
81. van Damme H, De Leval L, Creemers E, Limet R: Thrombangiitis obliterans (Buerger's disease): Still a limb-threatening disease. Acta Chir Belg 97(5):229–236, 1997.
82. van de Wal HJCM, Skotnicki SH, Wijn PFF, Lacquet LK: Thoracic sympathectomy as a therapy for upper extremity ischemia: A long-term follow-up study. Thorac Cardiovasc Surg 33(3):181–187, 1985.
83. van der Kloot E, Drukker J, Lemmens HAJ, Greep JM: The high thoracic sympathetic nerve system—its anatomic variability. J Surg Res 40:112–119, 1986.
84. Welch E, Geary J: Current status of thoracic dorsal sympathectomy. J Vasc Surg 1:202, 1986.
85. White JW: Treatment of primary hyperhidrosis. Mayo Clin Proc 61(12): 951–956, 1986.
86. Whitehouse W, Zelenock G, Wakefield T, et al: Arterial bypass grafts for upper extremity ischemia. J Vasc Surg 3:569, 1986.
87. Wilkinson HA: Percutaneous radiofrequency upper thoracic sympathectomy. Neurosurgery 38(4):715–725, 1996.
88. Wong RY, Fung ST, Jawan B, et al: Use of a single lumen endotracheal tube and continuous CO_2 insufflation in transthoracic endoscopic sympathectomy. Acta Anaesthesiol Sin 33(1):21–26, 1995.
89. Yilmaz EN, Dur AH, Cuesta MA, Rauwerda JA: Endoscopic versus transaxillary thoracic sympathectomy for primary axillary and palmar hyperhidrosis and/or facial blushing: 5-year-expereince. Eur J Cardiothorac Surg 10(3):168–172, 1996.
90. Zelenock G, Cronenwett J, Graham L, et al: Brachiocephalic arterial occlusions and stenoses: Manifestations and managemnt of complex lesions. Arch Surg 120:370, 1985.

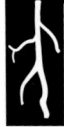

CHAPTER   8 7
Occupational Vascular Problems

James S. T. Yao, M.D., Ph.D.

Occupational and work associations with pain in the shoulders, arms, and hands have been recognized for almost 300 years.[1] Occupational injuries include those caused by work accidents and those caused by cumulative trauma due to the performance of repetitive motions. Injuries in the latter category result from small but additive amounts of tissue damage sustained from repetitive tasks; they are known collectively as *cumulative trauma disorders*. According to data released by the United States Bureau of Labor Statistics, cumulative trauma disorders account for more than 50% of all occupational illnesses in the country today.[2] Although most of these injuries affect the musculoskeletal system, injuries to arteries and veins also occur.[3] These injuries occur because of excessive or exaggerated job-related physical activity involving the shoulder or hands. Arterial occupational trauma includes vibration-induced white finger, hypothenar hammer syndrome, electrical burns, acro-osteolysis, and athletic injuries.

VIBRATION-INDUCED WHITE FINGER

The term *vibration-induced white finger* was favored by the Industrial Injuries Advisory Council in 1970 to describe symptoms somewhat similar to those of Raynaud's disease that, however, were caused by exposure to vibration.[4] Other investigators have used the term *Raynaud's phenomenon of occupational origin* or *traumatic vasospastic disease*. Regardless of the designation, the common and presenting symptoms are those of Raynaud's phenomenon secondary to prolonged use of vibrating mechanical tools.

In the very early stages, vibration injury may be manifested as slight tingling and numbness. Later, the tips of one or more fingers exposed to vibration suffer attacks of blanching, usually precipitated by cold. With continued exposure to vibration, the affected area increases in size and the blanching extends to the entire finger exposed to vibration. Attacks of white finger typically last about 1 hour and terminate with reactive hyperemia (red flush), and often considerable pain. Prolonged exposure to vibration may induce a blue-black cyanosis in the affected fingers. Only about 1% of cases progress to ulceration or gangrene.[5] It is well known that hand-held tools (such as pneumatic hammers and drills, grinders, and chain saws) are associated with vibration-induced white finger. Such injury potential is not restricted to a few types of tools but is present in a variety of situations in which workers' hands are subjected to significant vibration exposure.[4] Table 87–1 lists the types of tools that commonly cause vibration-induced white finger.

The first cases of this type of injury are usually considered to be those reported in Rome in 1911 by Loriga.[6] Blanching and numbness of the hands after using pneu-

TABLE 87–1. TOOLS ASSOCIATED WITH VIBRATION-INDUCED WHITE FINGER

Pneumatic tools
   Riveting
   Caulking
   Drilling
   Clinching and flanging
Rotary bur tools
Pneumatic hammers
Chain saws
Grinders
   Pedestal
   Hand-held
Chipping hammers
Concrete vibrothickener
Concrete-leveling vibrotables

matic drills was noted by Cottingham in 1918,[7] and subsequent reports by Taylor and Pelmear[8] and Ashe and associates[9] firmly established vibration-induced white finger as a discrete clinical entity associated with hand ischemia. According to Taylor and Pelmear,[8] the severity of the disease can be divided into five categories (Table 87–2); this classification has been accepted as a standard by workers in this field. This classification is particularly useful in determining workers' compensation.

The exact mechanism of injury is unknown. Repetitive trauma from the vibration of the tool is obviously the main cause of the problem. Both the frequency of the vibration and the intensity of the trauma it produces affect the extent of damage to the endothelium.[10] Local platelet adhesion appears to be an important factor in arterial occlusion. It has been shown that sympathetic hyperactivity, in combination with local factors such as vibration-induced hyper-responsiveness of the digital vessels to cold, may be responsible for finger-blanching attacks.[11]

Diagnosis is made from a history of using vibrating tools and from the classic Raynaud's symptoms. For a vasospastic condition, the most promising single objective test is cold provocation and recording of the recovery time of digital temperature. Digital artery occlusion is best detected by recording the systolic pressure of the affected fingers with the transcutaneous Doppler ultrasound technique,[12, 13] although more recently the B-mode scanning technique has been adopted.[14] In advanced disease, arteriographic examination is helpful. Barker and Hines first documented arterial occlusion by brachial arteriography in a group of workers who complained of hand blanching and attacks of numbness.[15] Others have reported on the use of arteriography in investigating this injury.[16–18]

Arteriographic changes in vibration tool injury are largely confined to the hands. Multiple segmental occlusions of the digits and sometimes a corkscrew configuration are seen.[18] The extent of digital artery occlusion depends on the duration of exposure to the vibratory insult. In advanced cases, occlusion of digital arteries is common. Of 80 workers (chippers) with vibration-induced white finger investigated at the Blood Flow Laboratory at Northwestern University, 25 (28%) exhibited significant reduction in systolic pressure in one or more digits.[19] In six of the 25 workers, arteriography demonstrated occlusion of digital arteries (Fig. 87–1). Incompleteness of the palmar arch was seen not only in the symptomatic hand but also in the contralateral, asymptomatic one. Seventy-three of 80 workers (91%) had symptoms of Raynaud's phenomenon. Ab-

TABLE 87–2. STAGES OF VIBRATION-INDUCED WHITE FINGER

STAGE	CONDITION OF DIGITS	WORK AND SOCIAL INTERFERENCE
0	Vibration exposure but no signs or symptoms	No complaints
0_T	Intermittent tingling	No interference with activities
0_N	Intermittent numbness	No interference with activities
1	Blanching of one or more fingertips, with or without tingling and numbness	No interference with activities
2	Blanching of one or more fingers with numbness, usually in winter	Slight interference with home and social activities; no interference with work
3	Extensive blanching; frequent episodes in summer and winter	Definite interference at work, at home, and with social activities; restriction of hobbies
4	Same as Stage 3: extensive blanching; most fingers involved; frequent episodes in summer and winter	Same as Stage 3, but occupation changed to avoid further vibration exposure because of the severity of signs and symptoms

Updated from Taylor W, Pelmear PL (eds): Vibration White Finger in Industry. New York, Academic Press, 1975.

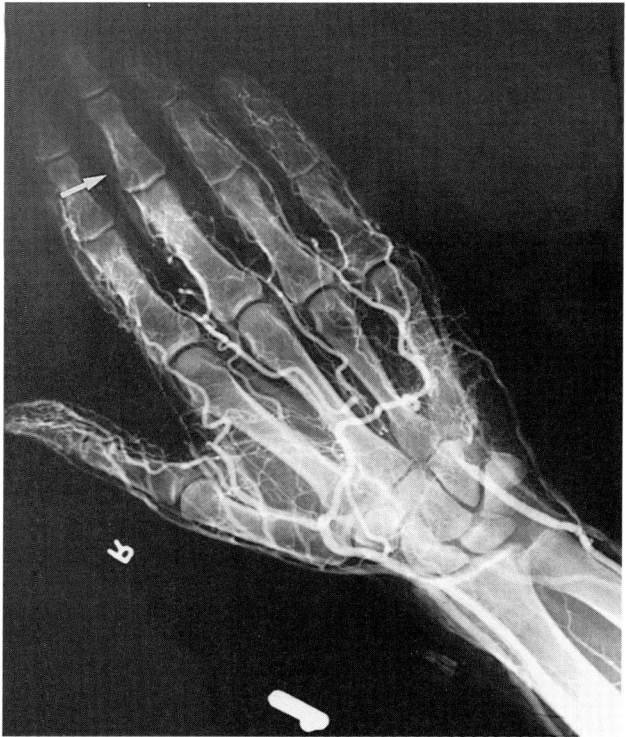

FIGURE 87–1. Arteriogram of the hand in a vibratory tool worker. There is occlusion of the digital arteries (*arrow*).

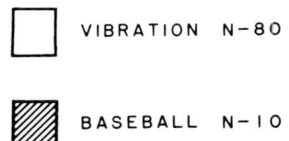

VIBRATION N-80

BASEBALL N-IO

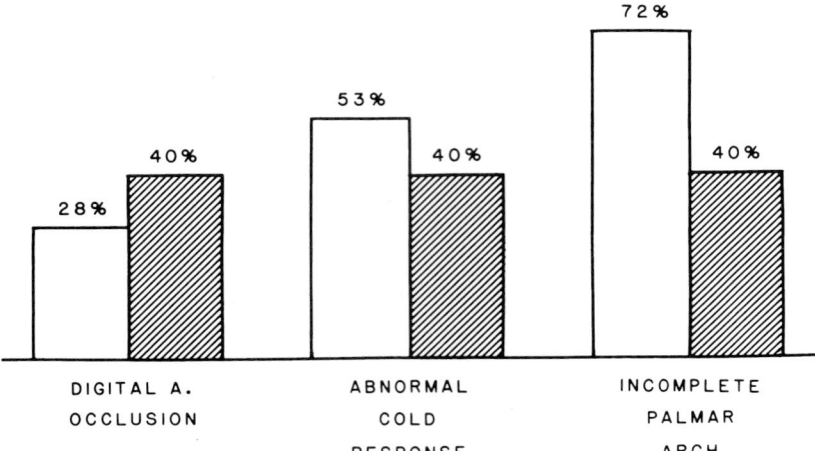

FIGURE 87–2. Incidence of abnormal cold response, digital artery occlusion, and incomplete palmar arch by Doppler examination in vibratory tool workers and baseball players. (From Bartel P, Blackburn D, Peterson L, et al: The value of non-invasive tests in occupational trauma of the hands and fingers. Bruit 8:15, 1984.)

normal cold response was observed in 53% of them (Fig. 87–2).

Treatment of vibration-induced white finger consists of symptomatic relief of Raynaud's symptoms. Surgical treatment such as cervical sympathectomy or digital sympathectomy is rarely indicated or needed. The most important step is to discontinue use of vibrating tools by changing jobs or rotating on and off that particular task. In most instances, prevention is more effective than cure. Factory standards should conform to those suggested by the American Conference of Governmental Industrial Hygienists in 1984,[20] and perhaps more operations should be automated to eliminate human exposure to vibratory insults. In advanced cases, a calcium channel blocker such as nifedipine (30 to 80 mg daily) may be useful. Calcium antagonists inhibit the response of arterial smooth muscle to noradrenaline and have been reported to be effective.[21] Intravenous infusion of a prostanoid (prostaglandin E_1, prostacyclin, or iloprost) is usually reserved for patients with digital gangrene.[22]

HYPOTHENAR HAMMER SYNDROME

The predisposing factor in the development of hypothenar hammer syndrome is repetitive use of the palm of the hand in activity that involves pushing, pounding, or twisting. The anatomic site of the ulnar artery in the area of the hypothenar eminence makes it vulnerable. The terminal branches of the ulnar artery (deep palmar branch and superficial arch) arise in a groove called Guyon's tunnel, which is bounded medially by the pisiform and the hook of the hamate and dorsally by the transverse carpal ligament. Over a distance of 2 cm, the ulnar artery lies quite "superficially" in the palm, being covered only by skin,

subcutaneous tissue, and the palmaris brevis muscle (Fig. 87–3). When this area is repeatedly traumatized, ulnar or digital arterial spasm, aneurysms, occlusion, or a combination of these lesions can result. Embolization from an aneurysm may cause multiple digital artery occlusions distally. The type of arterial abnormality observed often depends on the nature of the vessel damage.

Thus, intimal damage often results in thrombotic occlusion, whereas injury to media causes palmar aneurysms (Fig. 87–4).[23] This type of occupational injury has been called the *hypothenar hammer syndrome.*[24] In 1934, Von Rosen provided the first descriptive report of this condition,[25] but only recently has it been recognized as an occupational disease.[26] Table 87–3 lists the types of workers who developed this syndrome in reported series.[27] Among 79 workers who habitually used their hands as a hammer, Little and Ferguson found that 11 (14%) showed evidence of ulnar artery occlusion in one or both hands. [28]

TABLE 87–3. OCCUPATIONS OF 33 PATIENTS WITH HYPOTHENAR HAMMER SYNDROME

Mechanic/automobile repair	15
Lathe operator	3
Fitter and turner	2
Tire braider	2
Carpenter	2
Engineer	2
Machinist	2
Painter	1
Butcher	1
Gardener	1
Tool and die worker	1
Bus conductor	1

Modified from Pineda CJ, Weisman MH, Bookstein JJ, et al: Hypothenar hammer syndrome: Form of reversible Raynaud's phenomenon. Am J Med 79:561, 1985. With permission of Excerpta Medica, Inc.

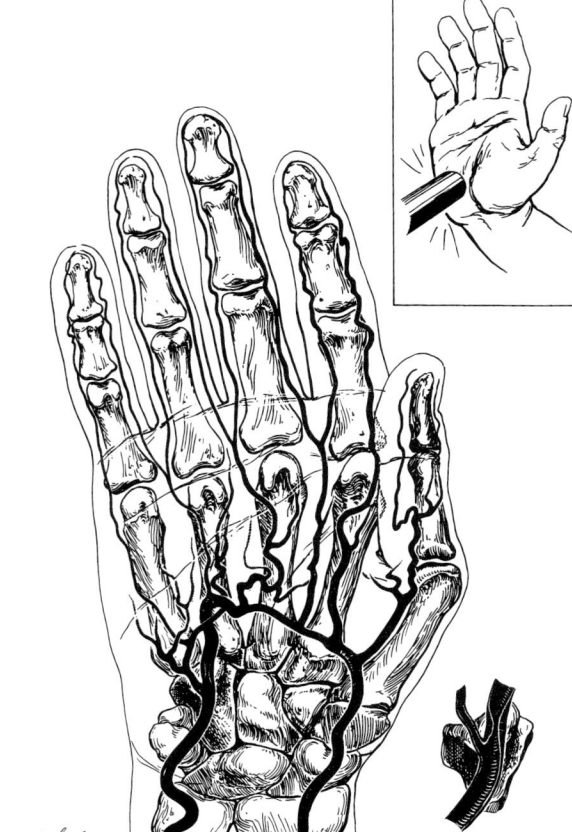

FIGURE 87–3. Mechanism of ulnar artery injury in a patient with hypothenar hammer syndrome. The terminal branch of the ulnar artery is vulnerable to injury because of its close proximity to the hamate bone (inset).

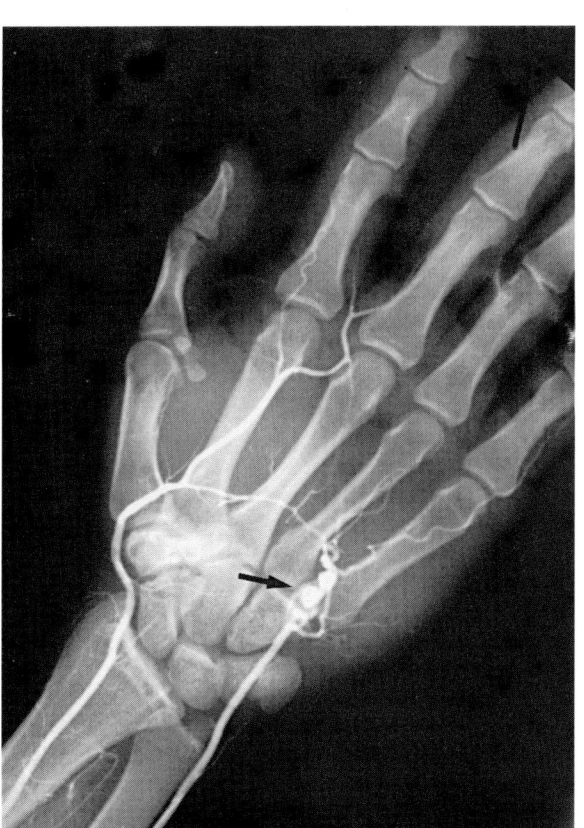

FIGURE 87–4. Arteriogram of the hand in a carpenter. Note the aneurysm of the ulnar artery (arrow) because of repetitive trauma from using the hand as a hammer.

Clinically, the patient reports symptoms of Raynaud's phenomenon, namely numbness, paresthesias, stiffness, coldness, and blanching of one or more digits of the dominant hand. In the series of patients described by Conn and colleagues, the ring finger was most often involved.[24] The traditional triphasic color changes (white-blue-red) and thumb involvement are uncommon.[27] Physical examination may disclose a prominent callus over the hypothenar eminence, coldness or mottling of the involved fingertip, and atrophic ulceration. A positive Allen's test result, which indicates ulnar artery occlusion, is common. Occasionally, an aneurysm is observed as a pulsatile mass in the palm.

The diagnosis is made from a history of trauma and the presenting symptoms and can be confirmed by a noninvasive test. B-mode scanning is particularly useful in detecting ulnar aneurysms. Arteriography is helpful in both diagnosis of hypothenar hammer syndrome and treatment planning. Arteriographic examination defines the type of vascular lesion (spasm, aneurysm, occlusion), demonstrates its site and extent, and demonstrates the presence of significant collateral vessels. Not infrequently, these patients have an incomplete superficial palmar arch, even in the asymptomatic hand.

Treatment of ulnar artery occlusion is often supportive, and surgical intervention is seldom needed or possible. Urokinase infusion may be beneficial if ischemic symptoms occur within 2 weeks. Occasionally, an ulnar aneurysm is uncovered by urokinase infusion. Aneurysms of the ulnar artery should be resected to eliminate the source of emboli and can be treated by resection with end-to-end anastomosis or by an interposed vein graft. Satisfactory long-term results have been reported with this approach by Vayssairat and coworkers.[29]

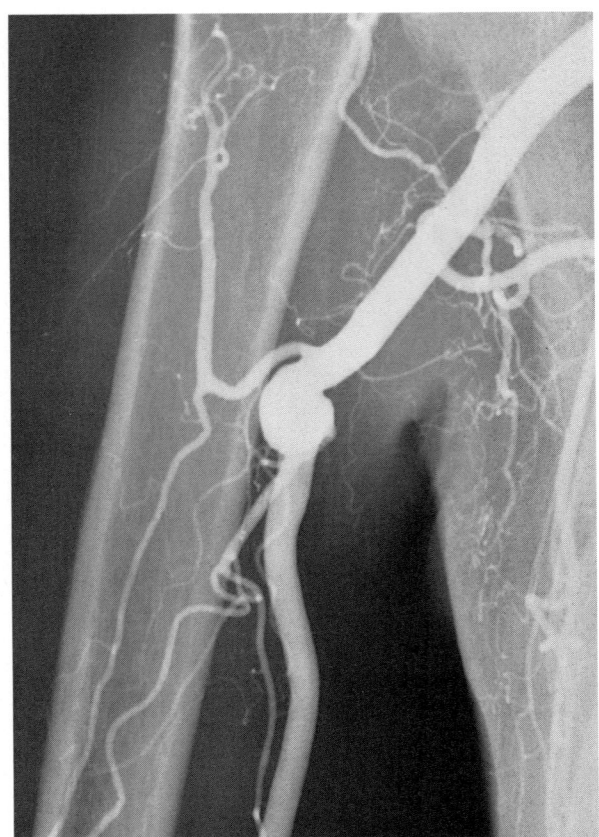

FIGURE 87–5. Aneurysm of the brachial artery in an electrician who had suffered a high-voltage electrical burn 9 months previously.

OCCUPATIONAL ACRO-OSTEOLYSIS

Occupational acro-osteolysis was first described by Wilson and colleagues in workers exposed to polyvinylchloride.[30] Many of them present with ischemic symptoms in the hand. Interestingly, resorption of the distal phalangeal tufts develops, similar to that seen with scleroderma. Once again, the dominant presenting symptoms are of Raynaud's phenomenon. Few reports of angiography in this syndrome have been published to document damage to the digital arteries.[31–33] The findings include multiple arterial stenoses and occlusions of the digital arteries along with nonspecific hypervascularity adjacent to the areas of bony resorption. The reason for the hypervascularity is not clear, but it may be related to stasis of contrast medium in digital pulp arteries secondary to shortening and retraction of the fingers. Some of these digits were clubbed, a finding that has also been associated with hypervascularity in the fingertips.

ELECTRICAL BURNS

Electrical burns inflict tissue destruction in relation to the voltage applied. Currents of less than 1000 V cause injuries limited to the immediate underlying skin and soft tissues. High voltage (>1000 V) usually causes extensive damage

as the current travels from the point of entrance to the point of exit. No tissue is immune to the devastating effects of high-voltage injury, and arterial injury may occur. The upper extremity, especially the hand, is more often involved than other parts of the body because of its grasping function. The arterial injury is often manifested by arterial necrosis with thrombus or bleeding, occasionally producing gangrenous digits.

Bookstein described the angiographic changes in the upper extremity after electrical injury.[31] The findings include extensive occlusion of the ulnar and digital arteries and thrombosis of the radial artery. Arterial spasm may also be present. Later on, damage of the media may cause aneurysm formation. Figure 87–5 shows a brachial artery aneurysm in a patient who had suffered electrical burns 9 months earlier. Treatment depends on the associated soft tissue and bone injuries. Major artery occlusion documented by arteriography requires bypass grafting, and good results have been reported.[34]

ATHLETIC INJURIES

Athletes, particularly professionals who engage in strenuous or exaggerated hand or shoulder activity, may develop hand or upper extremity ischemia as a result of arterial injury. Hand ischemia is often manifested by Raynaud's phenomenon, symptoms of sudden arterial occlusion, or embolization to digits. Two types of arterial injuries are common: hand ischemia and thoracic outlet compression of the subclavian-axillary artery. The exact incidences are unknown; however, vascular injury has been reported in professional or competitive players of baseball, karate, volleyball, handball, Frisbee, and lacrosse and in weightlifters and butterfly swimmers.[19, 27, 35-38]

Hand Ischemia

Repetitive trauma is the principal cause of hand ischemia, and injuries to the digital arteries can occur in hypothenar hammer syndrome or with sudden occlusion of the radial or ulnar arteries. Nearly all hand activity involved in any sport can cause blunt force injury to the arteries. Hand ischemia, however, is more common in handball players, baseball catchers, and practitioners of karate. Figure 87–6 illustrates an occlusion of the palmar arch in a Frisbee player; ischemia of all fingers occurred suddenly after he caught the Frisbee. It has been suggested that handball players with more than 200 hours of accumulated playing time are at greater risk for symptomatic alterations in perfusion.[39, 40]

Professional baseball players, particularly catchers, are likely to develop chronic hand ischemia. Many catchers have symptoms of Raynaud's phenomenon, especially in the off season, when they engage in outdoor activity in cool autumn or winter weather. Lowrey reported decreased digital perfusion to the index finger of the glove hand in

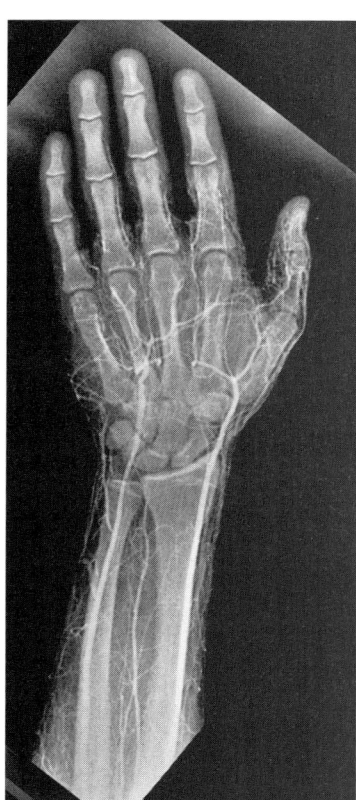

FIGURE 87–6. Occlusion of the palmar arch in a Frisbee player. Because of the injury, there is poor filling of the contrast media in the second, third, fourth, and fifth fingers.

13 of 22 baseball catchers examined by Doppler flow detector and Allen's test.[41] Of 10 professional catchers studied in the author's laboratory, 40% had evidence of digital artery occlusion (see Fig. 87–2).[19] Considering the speed of the baseball and the impact of the force on the hands, perhaps arterial injury in professional baseball catchers occurs more often than would be expected. Another form of hand ischemia occasionally observed in baseball pitchers is compression of the digital artery by Cleland's ligament.

Treating hand ischemia depends on the mode of presentation. With acute injury, a conservative approach using dextran 40 infusion and pain control is in order. Surgical intervention is rarely needed. Once again, preventing injury is important and can be accomplished by the use of gloves with padding and other protective devices.[41]

Thoracic Outlet Compression

Athletes who engage in overextended shoulder motion, such as baseball pitchers, butterfly swimmers, weightlifters, and oarsmen, are potential candidates for thoracic outlet compression. Injuries to the subclavian artery or vein have been reported in these athletes. In professional baseball pitchers, the injury is most likely due to the violent throwing motion. The act of pitching has five phases: (1) windup, (2) cocking, (3) acceleration, (4) release and deceleration, and (5) follow-through. Most injuries occur during the acceleration and deceleration phases.[42] It has been estimated that the fast ball creates 600 inch-pounds of forward momentum at release of the ball. It is thus understandable that soft tissue injury may occur because of the force absorbed by the shoulder and the elbow.[43]

Symptoms are more common in pitchers whose throwing motion is overhand rather than sidearm. Symptoms are pain in the region of the elbow associated with easy fatigue and loss of pitch velocity after several innings. Raynaud's phenomenon has also been observed in these pitchers. Diagnosis is often difficult, and a complete evaluation by an orthopedic surgeon to rule out musculoskeletal abnormalities is mandatory. Duplex scanning and transcutaneous Doppler flow detection with the athlete in pitching position help to detect compression of the subclavian or axillary artery. Finally, definitive diagnosis is established by arteriography with positional exposure (Figs. 87–7 and 87–8).

Arterial injury in the pitching arm affects the subclavian artery,[36] the axillary artery,[35] and the posterior humeral circumflex artery.[44] Compression to the subclavian or axillary artery is often due to hypertrophy of the anterior scalene or the pectoralis minor muscle. In 1964, Tullos, Cooley, and colleagues were the first to report an axillary artery thrombus secondary to pectoralis minor compression in a major league pitcher.[35] In 1978, Strukel and Garrick reported on three competitive baseball pitchers who suffered from thoracic outlet compression.[45] Until Fields' report on athletic injury in the thoracic outlet, the injury had received little attention.[46] The report by Fields and associates on a major league pitcher who suffered a catastrophic stroke resulting from subclavian artery thrombosis is of great interest.[36]

The main trunk of the subclavian-axillary artery is not the only vessel subjected to compression. Cahill and Palmer described the quadrilateral space syndrome—compression

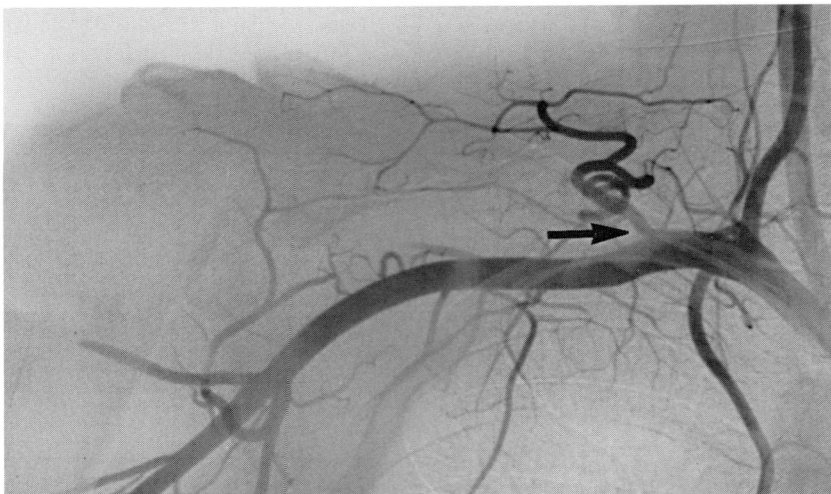

FIGURE 87–7. Arteriogram of the right subclavian artery *(arrow)* in a professional baseball pitcher. No injury is seen when the arm is placed in neutral position.

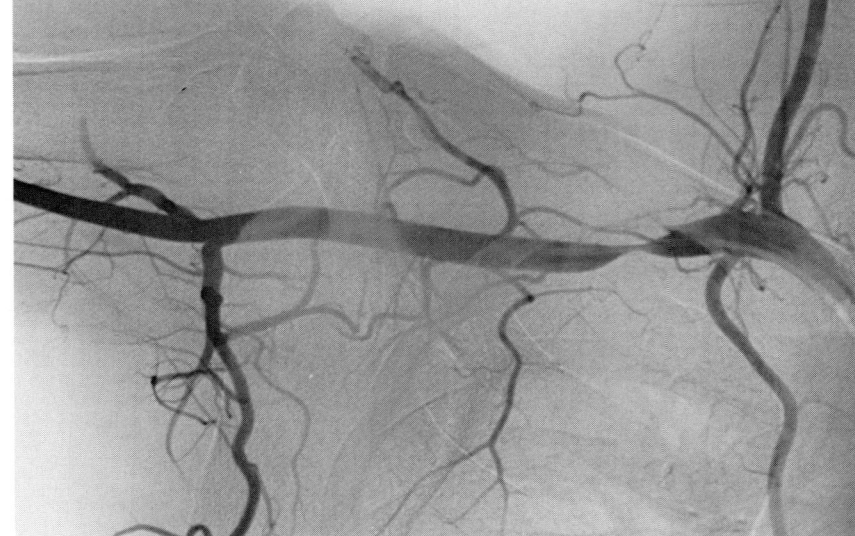

FIGURE 87–8. In the same patient shown in Figure 87–7, there is compression of the subclavian artery when the arm is placed in the pitching position (hyperabduction).

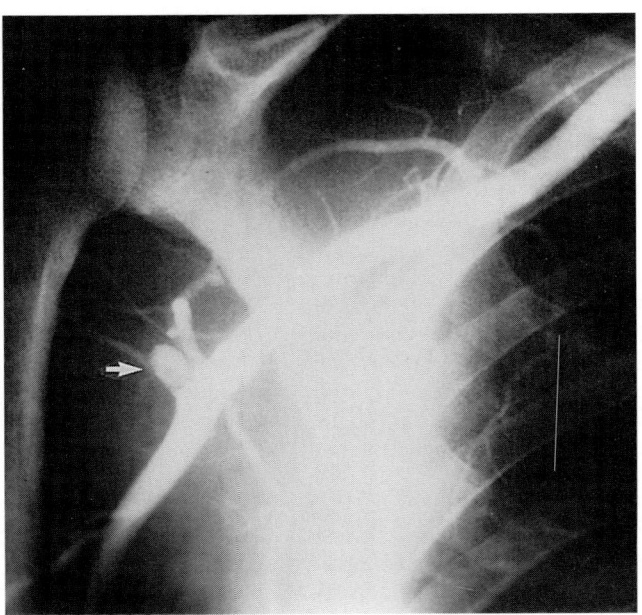

FIGURE 87–9. Artery of a major league baseball pitcher. Note the emboli of the posterior circumflex artery *(arrow)*. (From Yao JST, Upper extremity ischemia in athletes. Semin Vasc Surg 11:1–10, 1998.)

of the posterior humeral circumflex artery or nerve—in the quadrilateral space of 18 patients.[44] It is now recognized that aneurysm formation in the (anterior or posterior) circumflex artery due to repetitive athletic activities is responsible for severe hand ischemia due to embolization.[47] Such injury has been observed in baseball pitchers and volleyball players (Fig. 87–9).[48–50] The circumflex artery is not the only one affected; aneurysm formation in the subscapular artery has also been reported.[51]

The head of the humerus can cause compression to the axillary artery. As a result of repetitive compression, damage to the axillary artery that causes a thromboembolic phenomenon has been reported in baseball pitchers.[48, 49, 52]

In addition to arterial injury, thrombosis of the subclavian-axillary vein, so-called effort thrombosis, has been reported in baseball pitchers,[53] weightlifters,[54] and competitive swimmers.[55]

Treatment depends on the extent of injury. Compression only is best treated by division of the offending muscle and tendon. Occlusion of a major artery requires bypass grafting together with decompression of the thoracic outlet. Aneurysm of the circumflex artery or thrombosis in the axillary artery is best treated by the transaxillary approach with resection of the aneurysm and/or vein grafting if indicated.[52] Venous thrombosis is best treated with heparin and standard anticoagulation therapy. Injury requires cessation of athletic activity and carefully planned rehabilitation. To return a professional athlete to full activity, close consultation with a trainer or sports medicine specialist is necessary.

REFERENCES

1. Buckle PW: Fortnightly review: Work factors and upper limb disorders. BMJ 315:1360–1363, 1997.
2. Bureau of Labor Statistics Reports on Survey of Occupational Injuries and Illness in 1977–1989. Washington, DC, Bureau of Labor Statistics, U.S. Department of Labor, 1990.
3. Rempel DM, Harrison RJ, Barnhart S: Work-related cumulative trauma disorders of the upper extremity. JAMA 267:838, 1992.
4. Griffin MJ: Vibration injuries of the hand and arm: Their occurrence and the evolution of standards and limits. London, Her Majesty's Stationery Office, 1980.
5. Yodaiken RE, Jones E, Kunicki R: The Raynaud phenomenon of occupational origin. In Altura BM, Davis E (eds): Advances in Microcirculation. Vol 12. Basel, Karger, 1985, pp 6–33.
6. Loriga G: Ill lavoro con i martelli pneumatic boll. Ispett Lavoro 2:35, 1911.
7. Cottingham CE: Effects of use of air hammer on hands of Indiana stone cutters. U.S. Bureau of Labor Statistics 19:125, 1918.
8. Taylor W, Pelmear PL (eds): Vibration White Finger in Industry. New York, Academic Press, 1975.
9. Ashe WF, Cook WT, Old JW: Raynaud's phenomenon of occupational origin. Arch Environ Health 5:63, 1962.
10. Newem RM: Vibration-induced arterial shear stress: The relationship to Raynaud's phenomenon of occupational origin. Arch Environ Health 26:105, 1973.
11. Bovenzi M: Some pathophysiological aspects of vibration-induced white finger. Eur J Appl Physiol 55:381, 1986.
12. Pearce WH, Yao JST, Bergan JJ: Noninvasive vascular diagnostic testing. In Ravitch MM (ed): Current Problems in Surgery. Vol 20. Chicago, Year Book Medical Publishers, 1983.
13. Sumner DS: Vascular laboratory diagnosis and assessment of upper extremity vascular disorders. In Machleder HI (ed): Vascular Disorders of the Upper Extremity. Mt. Kisco, NY, Futura Publishing Company, 1983, pp 1–47.
14. Payne KM, Blackburn DR, Peterson LK, et al: B-Mode imaging of the arteries of the hand and upper extremity. Bruit 10:168, 1986.
15. Barker NW, Hines EA Jr: Arterial occlusion in the hands and fingers associated with repeated occupational trauma. Mayo Clin Proc 19:345, 1944.
16. Shatz IJ: Occlusive arterial disease in the hand due to occupational trauma. N Engl J Med 268:281, 1963.
17. Ashe WF, Williams N: Occupational Raynaud's: II. Further studies of this disorder in uranium mine workers. Arch Environ Health 9:425, 1964.
18. Wegelius U: Angiography of the hand: Clinical and postmortem investigations. Acta Radiol Suppl (Stockh) 315:1, 1972.
19. Bartel P, Blackburn D, Peterson L, et al: The value of noninvasive tests in occupational trauma of the hands and fingers. Bruit 8:15, 1984.
20. Threshold limit values approved by ACGIH for hand-arm vibration. Noise Reg Reporter 11:3, 1984.
21. Kahan A, Amor B, Menkes CJ: Nifedipine and allied substances in the treatment of Raynaud's phenomenon. In Altura BM, Davis E (eds): Advances in Microcirculation. Vol 12. Basel, Karger, 1985, pp 95–104.
22. Chetter IC, Kent PJ, Kester RC: The hand arm vibration syndrome: A review. Cardiovasc Surg 6 (1):1–9, 1998.
23. Kleinert HE, Burget GC, Morgan JA, et al: Aneurysms of the hand. Arch Surg 106:554, 1973.
24. Conn J, Bergan JJ, Bell JL: Hypothenar hammer syndrome: Post-traumatic digital ischemia. Surgery 68:1122, 1970.
25. Von Rosen S: Ein Fall von Thrombose in der Arteria ulnaris nach Einwirkung von stumpfer Gewalt. Acta Chir Scand 73:500, 1934.
26. Short DW: Occupational aneurysm of the palmar arch. Lancet 2:217, 1948.
27. Pineda CJ, Weisman MH, Bookstein JJ, et al: Hypothenar hammer syndrome: Form of reversible Raynaud's phenomenon. Am J Med 79:561, 1985.
28. Little JM, Ferguson DA: The incidence of the hypothenar hammer syndrome. Arch Surg 105:684, 1972.
29. Vayssairat M, Debure C, Cormier J, et al: Hypothenar hammer syndrome: Seventeen cases with long-term follow-up. J Vasc Surg 5:838, 1987.
30. Wilson R, McCormick W, Tattum C, et al: Occupational acro-osteolysis. JAMA 201:577, 1967.
31. Bookstein JJ: Arteriography. In Poznanski AK (ed): The Hand in Radiologic Diagnosis with Gamuts and Pattern Profiles, 2nd ed. Vol 1. Philadelphia, WB Saunders, 1984, pp 97–112.
32. Veltman G: Raynaud's syndrome in vinylchloride disease. In Heidrich H (ed): Raynaud's Phenomenon. Berlin, TM-Verlag, 1979, pp 211–216.
33. Falappa P, Magnavita N, Bergamaschi A, et al: Angiographic study of digital arteries in workers exposed to vinyl chloride. Br J Ind Med 39:169, 1982.
34. Wang X, Roberts BB, Zapata-Sirvent RL, et al: Early vascular grafting to prevent upper extremity necrosis after electrical burns: Commentary on indications for surgery. Burns 11:359, 1985.
35. Tullos HS, Erwin WD, Woods GW, et al: Unusual lesions of the pitching arm. Clin Orthop 88:169, 1972.
36. Fields WS, Lemak NA, Ben-Menachem Y: Thoracic outlet syndrome: Review and reference to stroke in a major league pitcher. Am J Neuroradiol 7:73, 1986.
37. Green DP: True and false traumatic aneurysms in the hand: Report of two cases and review of the literature. J Bone Joint Surg 55A:120, 1973.
38. Ho PK, Dellon AL, Wilgis EFS: True aneurysms of the hand resulting from athletic injury: Report of two cases. Am J Sports Med 13:136, 1985.
39. Buckhout BC, Warner MA: Digital perfusion of handball players: Effects of repeated ball impact on structures of the hand. Am J Sports Med 8:206, 1980.
40. McCue FC III, Miller GA: Soft-tissue injuries to the hand. In Pettrone FA (ed): Upper Extremity Injuries in Athletes. St. Louis, CV Mosby, 1986, pp 85–94.
41. Lowrey CW: Digital vessel trauma from repetitive impacts in baseball catchers. J Hand Surg 1:236, 1976.
42. McLeod WD: The pitching mechanism. In Zarins B, Andrews JR, Carson WG Jr (eds): Injuries to the Throwing Arm. Philadelphia, WB Saunders, 1985, pp 22–29.
43. San J, Andrews JR: Proper pitching techniques. In Zarins B, Andrews JR, Carson WG Jr (eds): Injuries to the Throwing Arm. Philadelphia, WB Saunders, 1985, pp 34–36.
44. Cahill B, Palmer R: Quadrilateral space syndrome. J Hand Surg 8:65, 1983.

45. Strukel RJ, Garrick JG: Thoracic outlet compression in athletes: A report of four cases. Am J Sports Med 6:35, 1978.
46. Fields WS: Neurovascular syndromes of the neck and shoulders. Semin Neurol 1:301, 1981.
47. Nijhuis HHAM, Muller-Wiefel H: Occlusion of the brachial artery by thrombus dislodged from a traumatic aneurysm of the anterior humeral circumflex artery. J Vasc Surg 13:408, 1991.
48. McCarthy WJ, Yao JST, Schafer MF, et al: Upper extremity arterial injury in athletes. J Vasc Surg 9:317, 1989.
49. Rohrer MJ, Cardullo PA, Pappas AM, et al: Axillary artery compression and thrombosis in throwing athletes. J Vasc Surg 11:761, 1990.
50. Reekers JA, den Hartog BMG, Kuyper CF, et al: Traumatic aneurysm of the posterior circumflex humeral artery: A volleyball player's disease? J Vasc Interv Radiol 4:405–408, 1993.
51. Kee ST, Dake MD, Wolfe-Johnson B, et al: Ischemia of the throwing hand in major league baseball pitchers: Embolic occlusion from aneurysms of axillary artery branches. J Vasc Interv Radiol 6:979–982, 1995.
52. Durham JR, Yao JST, Pearce WH, et al: Arterial injuries in the thoracic outlet syndrome. J Vasc Surg 21:57–70, 1995.
53. Dale WA: Thoracic outlet compression syndrome. *In* Dale WA (ed): Management of Vascular Surgical Problems. New York, McGraw-Hill, 1985, pp 562–587.
54. Baker CL, Thornberry R: Neurovascular syndromes. *In* Zarins B, Andrews JR, Carson WG Jr (eds): Injuries to the Throwing Arm. Philadelphia, WB Saunders, 1985, pp 176–188.
55. Vogel CM, Jensen JE: "Effort" thrombosis of the subclavian vein in a competitive swimmer. Am J Sports Med 13:269, 1985.

SECTION XII

ARTERIAL ANEURYSMS

JACK L. CRONENWETT, M.D.

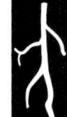

CHAPTER 88

Overview

Jack L. Cronenwett, M.D., and William C. Krupski, M.D.

The term aneurysm is derived from the Greek word *aneurysma*, meaning "a widening." By current reporting standards, an aneurysm is defined as a permanent localized dilation of artery having at least a 50% increase in diameter compared with the expected normal diameter.[25] Arterial dilation less than 50% above normal is termed *ectasia*. Unfortunately, normal arterial diameter is dependent on age, gender, body size, and other factors. Thus, by practical convention, an aneurysm is defined as a localized dilation at least 50% larger than an adjacent normal portion of the same artery.[25] If there is no adjacent normal artery segment, this definition must rely on an estimate of the expected normal diameter (Table 88–1). Diffuse arterial enlargement involving several arterial segments with an increase in diameter greater than 50% above normal is termed *arteriomegaly*. This is distinct from "multiple" aneurysms, which are separated by normal diameter arterial segments, although arteriomegaly is often associated with multiple aneurysms.

HISTORICAL PERSPECTIVE

Arterial aneurysms have been recognized since ancient times. One of the earliest texts known, the Ebers Papyrus (2000 B.C.), contains a description of traumatic aneurysms of the peripheral arteries.[30] Galen (131–200) defined an aneurysm as a localized pulsatile swelling that disappeared on pressure and wrote, "if an aneurysm be wounded, the blood is spouted out with so much violence that it can scarcely be arrested."[16] The first elective operation for treatment of an aneurysm was reported by Antyllus in the 2nd century. He recommended ligating the artery above and below the aneurysm and then incising the sac and evacuating its contents.[31] This recommendation for aneurysm repair remained the basis of direct arterial operations for the next 1500 years; few operations have withstood the test of time so well. In the 7th century, details of operative repair of an arterial aneurysm were recounted by Aetius of Amida

in his book *De Vasorum Dilatatione* ("On the Dilation of the Vessels"), now in the Vatican Library. Like Antyllus, Aetius recognized the difference between true degenerative aneurysms and traumatic false aneurysms. He wrote[22]:

> An aneurysm located in the bend of the elbow is treated thus. First we carefully trace the artery leading to it, from armpit to elbow, along the inside of the upper arm. Then we make an incision on the inside of the arm, three or four finger-breadths below the armpit, where the artery is felt most easily. We gradually expose the bloodvessel and, when it can be lifted free with a hook, we tie it off with two firm ligatures and divide it between them. We fill the wound with incense and lint dressing, then apply a bandage. Next we open the aneurysm itself and no longer need fear bleeding. We remove the blood clots present, and seek the artery which brought the blood. Once found, it is lifted free with the hook, and tied as before. By again filling the wound with incense, we stimulate good suppuration.

Modern surgeons will recognize the failure to obtain distal control in these instructions. Moreover, Aetius, like others of his time, believed Galen's teachings that no wound heals properly without the formation of pus, brought about by the application of dried herbs (incense).

In medieval times, brachial artery aneurysms were frequent iatrogenic complications of blood letting during attempted puncture of the median cubital vein. Ambrose Paré (1510–1590), who contributed so much to the principles of proper wound care, applied his observations to aneurysm operations. He vividly described the death of a patient whose brachial artery aneurysm had been treated by application of a caustic, contrary to Paré's advice, resulting in a torrential fatal hemorrhage.[24] Paré's prestigious contemporary, Andreas Vesalius, wrote one of the first descriptions of an abdominal aortic aneurysm.[30] In 1590, Peter Lowe (1550–1612), personal physician to King James VI in Scotland and founder of the medical and surgical faculty at Glasgow, reported that one of the highest ranking officers in the Spanish Regiment presented with a peripheral arterial aneurysm. Whereas Lowe prescribed apothecary remedies against its growth, a second physician consulted a barber,

TABLE 88–1. REPORTED DIAMETER OF NORMAL ADULT ARTERIES

ARTERY	DIAMETER (cm)	GENDER
Aorta, thoracic		
Root	3.50–3.72	F
	3.63–3.91	M
Ascending	2.86	F, M
Descending, mid	2.45–2.64	F
	2.39–2.98	M
At diaphragm	2.40–2.44	F
	2.43–2.69	M
Aorta, abdominal		
Supraceliac	2.10–2.31	F
	2.50–2.72	M
Suprarenal	1.86–1.88	F
	1.98–2.27	M
Infrarenal	1.19–2.16	F
	1.41–2.39	M
Celiac	0.53	F, M
Superior mesenteric	0.63	F, M
Iliac		
Common	0.97–1.02	F
	1.17–1.23	M
Internal	0.54	F, M
Common femoral	0.78–0.85	F
	0.78–1.12	M
Popliteal	0.9	M
Posterior tibial	0.3	M
Carotid		
Common	0.77	F
	0.63–0.84	M
Bulb	0.92	F
	0.99	M
Internal	0.49	F
	0.55	M
Brachial	0.39	F
	0.42–0.44	M

From Johnston KW, Rutherford RB, Tilson MD, et al: Suggested standards for reporting on arterial aneurysms. J Vasc Surg 13:452, 1991.
F = female; M = male.

who opened the swelling with a lance and "blood spewed out so violently that the Captain died some hours later."[22]

Almost a century later, Richard Wiseman (1625–1686), known as "the father of English surgery," described an aneurysm in the arm of a cooper from Maidenhead.[22] During operative exposure of the aneurysm, it ruptured. Wiseman instructed an assistant to place his thumb over the hole. According to the detailed report, onlookers were eager to see the patient bleed to death. Instead, Wiseman inserted an instrument beneath the artery and ligated it, whereupon the assistant removed his finger and the bleeding subsided.

John Hunter (1728–1793) performed perhaps the most famous operation for an arterial aneurysm.[22] Hunter had observed that the blood supply to the horns of deer changed under different conditions. A rich blood supply was present when the crest was full, but the blood vessels decreased in number and size when the horns shed. Hunter inferred that reserve vessels, now termed collaterals, might develop in humans if obstruction occurred in their arteries. In the autumn of 1785, a beer delivery man was admitted to St. George's Hospital with a pulsatile mass in the popliteal fossa, possibly secondary to repetitive trauma against

the coachman's seat while driving on rough streets. He complained of leg pain on walking and rested frequently, presumably owing to arterial occlusion distal to the aneurysm. Standard treatment at that time entailed above-knee amputation, as strongly advocated by another renowned London surgeon, Percival Pott (1714–1788).[33] Hunter's experiments with deer, however, suggested that collateral vessels must have formed around the obstruction or the leg would have developed gangrene. Thus, he incised above the knee at a location now known as *Hunter's canal* and tied four ligatures around the artery. Four sutures were used to avoid sawing through the vessel. After a bout of local infection, the patient survived and was discharged. Later, Hunter performed four similar operations and three were successful; the fourth patient died 26 days postoperatively.

Astley Paston Cooper (1768–1841) was John Hunter's most acclaimed disciple. In contrast to Hunter's irascible, sullen, and unsophisticated behavior, Cooper was handsome, charming, and well mannered. Although he is best remembered for his contributions to inguinal hernia repair and female breast anatomy, his most celebrated operation was performed for a leaking iliac artery aneurysm in 1817.[9] Before the operation, he visited the autopsy room and practiced every detail of the procedure on a cadaver. His attempt to ligate the abdominal aorta seemed initially successful, but the patient died suddenly after 40 hours. Cooper[9] also reported the first documented case of a spontaneous aortoenteric fistula caused by aneurysmal disease and cautioned that patients who present with one aneurysm should be evaluated for the coexistence of others, advice that is equally applicable today.[9]

The 18th century can be characterized as the era of arterial ligation for treatment of aneurysms, with surgeons such as Anel, Brasdor, and Wardrop defending the merits of different sites of ligation in relation to the aneurysm. Interestingly, arterial ligation, accompanied by extra-anatomic bypass, was resurrected in the 1970s by the group at Albany, N.Y., for treatment of abdominal aortic aneurysms in high-risk patients. Unfortunately, many individuals so treated suffered outcomes similar to that of Cooper's patient.[7]

In 1804, Antonio Scarpa (1752–1832) wrote a definitive treatise on the forms and diagnosis of arterial aneurysms. About this time several ingenious treatments were introduced. Giovanni Monteggia (1762–1815) unwisely attempted to cure an aneurysm by injecting a sclerosant into it, which predictably failed because of rapid blood flow. Attempts to thrombose aneurysms by passing an electric current between needles stuck into the vessel were begun in 1832 and were still going on in the 1930s. Charles Hewitt Moore (1821–1870), at Middlesex Hospital in London, introduced obliteration of aneurysms by inserting steel wires in 1864, once using 26 yards of the material.[22] One of the most prominent Americans known to have aneurysmal disease in the 19th century was Kit Carson, who died of a ruptured abdominal aortic aneurysm in rural Colorado in 1868[1]; Albert Einstein also died of this entity.[8] Unlike Kit Carson, Einstein had been treated for his disorder by means of wrapping the aneurysm in cellophane, a technique introduced by Rea[34] in 1948.

A better method of treatment of peripheral aneurysms

had been developed in 1888 by the legendary New Orleans surgeon, Rudolph Matas (1860–1957). His technique of endoaneurysmorrhaphy involved clamping above and below the aneurysm, opening it, ligating branches from within, and buttressing the wall with imbricated sutures. By 1906, he had performed 22 obliterative operations and seven restorative operations (preserving the arterial lumen) with no recurrences. Matas[29] performed the first successful proximal ligation of an aortic aneurysm in 1923, some 106 years after Astley Cooper's innovative operation. Matas' endoaneurysmorrhaphy presaged the current prevailing method of "internal" or intrasaccular reconstruction conceived by Oscar Creech and Michael DeBakey.[12]

Another notable achievement at the beginning of the 20th century is attributed to José Goyanes of Madrid.[21] In 1906, Goyanes excluded a popliteal aneurysm by proximal and distal ligation; in addition, he mobilized the adjacent popliteal vein and used it as an in situ interposition graft between the proximal femoral artery and the distal popliteal artery by means of end-to-end anastomoses. Unfortunately, this important contribution, which had a good outcome, remained largely ignored until many years later.

Modern techniques of aneurysm repair were made possible by Alexis Carrel (1873–1948), who demonstrated in animals that a segment of aorta could be replaced with a piece from another artery or vein and who successfully anastomosed blood vessels. Carrel won the Nobel Prize for this work in 1912. However, it was not until March 29, 1951, that his countryman Charles DuBost performed the first successful replacement of an aneurysm with a freeze-dried homograft.[15] He was inspired by a similar operation for an occluded abdominal aorta by Jacques Oudot[32] in 1950. The second and third aortic aneurysm repairs in which patients survived were both performed on October 25, 1952, one by Ormand Julian's group[26] in Chicago and the other by Russel Brock and associates[5] in London. DeBakey and Cooley[13] in Houston soon reported survival of five of six patients operated on for replacement of abdominal aortic aneurysms. In a series of 17 aortic aneurysm operations, Bahnson[2] from Johns Hopkins described the first successful repair of a ruptured aortic aneurysm. In 1953, Voorhees and colleagues[36] introduced a major innovation by substituting Vinyon-N cloth for the unreliable homograft. The modern era of aneurysm repair had truly begun.

The first successful repair of a thoracoabdominal aortic aneurysm was reported by Sam Etheredge and associates[17] in 1955. E. Stanley Crawford[10] became the authority on this formidable procedure beginning with his 1974 report delineating good results with 28 consecutive operations for thoracoabdominal aortic aneurysms. Crawford's contributions to the repair of complex aortic aneurysms were extraordinary and have greatly reduced the risk of surgery. Throughout the late 1950s and early 1960s, aortic aneurysm repair became a common and safe surgical procedure throughout the world.

CLASSIFICATION

Aneurysms are typically classified according to their (1) location, (2) size, (3) shape, and (4) etiology (Table 88–2).

TABLE 88–2. ANEURYSM CLASSIFICATION BY ETIOLOGY

TYPE	EXAMPLE
Congenital	Idiopathic
	Tuberous sclerosis
	Turner's syndrome
	Menkes' syndrome
Connective tissue disorder	Marfan's syndrome
	Ehlers-Danlos syndrome
	Cystic medial necrosis
	Berry (cerebral)
Degenerative	Nonspecific (atherosclerotic)
	Fibromuscular dysplasia
Infectious	Bacterial
	Fungal
	Syphilis
Inflammatory—arteritis	Takayasu's disease
	Behçet's disease
	Kawasaki disease
	Polyarteritis nodosa
	Giant cell arteritis
	Systemic lupus erythematosus
	Periarterial (e.g., pancreatitis)
Post-dissection	Idiopathic
	Cystic medial necrosis
	Trauma
Post-stenotic	Thoracic outlet syndrome
	Coarctation
Pseudoaneurysm	Trauma
	Anastomotic disruption
Miscellaneous	Pregnancy-associated
	Inflammatory abdominal aortic

By definition, aneurysms represent a dilation of all layers of the arterial wall. Confusion exists concerning the definition of false aneurysms (*pseudoaneurysms*) because these have often been described as an aneurysm that does not involve all layers of the arterial wall. In reality, false aneurysms are just that; they are not arterial aneurysms. Rather, they represent contained hematomas that result from localized arterial trauma and simply have the appearance of an arterial aneurysm on examination (Fig. 88–1). In fact, these pseudoaneurysms do not contain any of the layers of the arterial wall; they represent a disruption of the arterial wall with extravasation of blood that is contained by surrounding layers of connective tissue. If the fibrotic reaction around such hematomas is chronic, it can become very well organized and may have an aneurysmal appearance when exposed at surgery.

Historically, pseudoaneurysms most frequently resulted from penetrating trauma. Nowadays, they more frequently result from iatrogenic injury during arterial catheterization or arterial-graft anastomotic disruption. Pseudoaneurysms are discussed in detail in Chapter 48.

The shape of an aneurysm is commonly described as saccular versus fusiform (spindle-shaped), although these represent a continuum rather than discrete entities. In general, saccular or eccentric aneurysms are believed to have a higher risk of rupture (see Chapter 89).[37] Aneurysm size is described by diameter and length, with diameter being the important risk factor for rupture.

The etiology is the most clinically relevant classification system because it directly influences not only natural history but also treatment. Although the specific cause of some aneurysms is well known (see Table 88–2), most

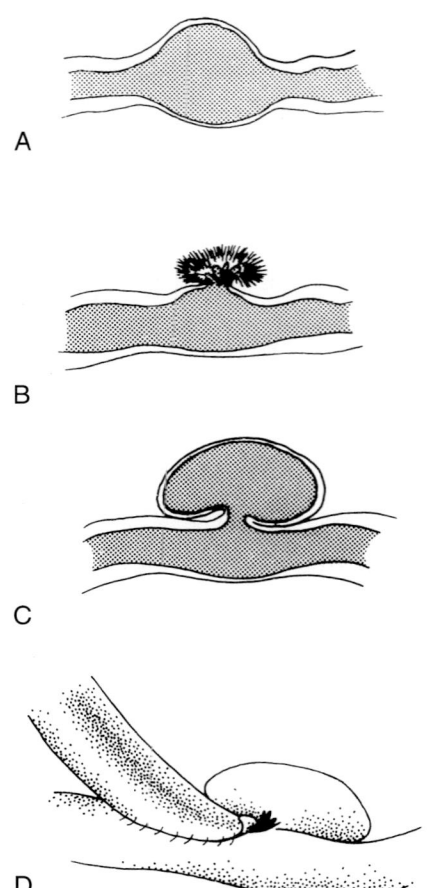

FIGURE 88–1. *A*, "True" aneurysms represent expansion of all layers of the artery wall. *B–D*, "False" aneurysms (pseudoaneurysms) are locally contained hematomas that result from arterial injury (*B* and *C*) or artery-graft disruption (*D*) and are contained by surrounding tissue rather than the arterial wall.

aneurysms are nonspecific in etiology. Such aneurysms were formerly termed "atherosclerotic" because they are universally associated with atherosclerotic changes in the arteries of elderly patients. However, it now appears that the etiology of these degenerative aneurysms is much more complex (see Chapter 22). Hence, for lack of a better descriptor, they are termed *nonspecific* or *degenerative* and make up the majority of all aneurysms. Congenital aneurysms and those associated with arteritis and connective tissue abnormalities are rare. Infected aneurysms are more common. Aneurysms that result from wall weakness after arterial dissection represent the most common specific cause.

Considerable confusion also exists concerning the term *dissecting aneurysm*. As discussed in Chapter 93, arterial dissection is a distinct pathologic entity that does not necessarily result in aneurysm formation. However, chronic arterial dissections are frequently associated with aneurysmal degeneration, leading to the confusion in terminology.

ANEURYSM LOCATION

The most common site for nonspecific aneurysms is the infrarenal abdominal aorta. In a large autopsy series of patients with aortoiliac aneurysms, the relative frequency was abdominal aorta alone, 65%; thoracic aorta alone, 19%; abdominal aorta plus iliac, 13%; thoracoabdominal, 2%; and isolated iliac, 1%.[6] Population-based studies estimate the incidence of clinically apparent abdominal aortic aneurysms to be 21 per 100,000 person-years,[3] compared with 6 per 100,000 person-years for thoracic aortic aneurysms.[4] Whereas nearly all the abdominal aortic aneurysms are nonspecific in etiology, thoracic aortic aneurysms are much more diverse in etiology, with approximately 50% resulting from aortic dissection.[4] Abdominal aortic aneurysms also cause the largest number of deaths from aneurysm rupture. In a Swedish study with a high autopsy rate, ruptured abdominal aortic aneurysms caused 0.6% of all annual deaths in men, a rate of 648 per 100,000 deaths.[35] This was seven times higher than deaths caused by ruptured thoracic aneurysms and twice as common as deaths from aortic dissection. In women, the mortality rate from ruptured abdominal aortic aneurysms was only 285 per 100,000 deaths, which was three times higher than deaths caused by ruptured thoracic aneurysms but less common than deaths from aortic dissection, which is relatively more common in women (343 per 100,000 deaths in this study).[35]

Non-aortic aneurysms are much less common. The incidence of abdominal aortic aneurysms in hospitalized patients in the United States is approximately 50 per 100,000,[19] compared with only 3 per 100,000 for iliac aneurysms and 4 per 100,000 for femoropopliteal aneurysms.[27] Popliteal aneurysms account for 70% of all peripheral aneurysms, whereas carotid aneurysms make up less than 4%.[18, 38] Visceral and renal artery aneurysms are rare. The common femoral artery is the most common site for pseudoaneurysms because arterial grafts commonly begin or end there, and it is the preferred entry site for radiologic and interventional procedures. The femoral artery is also the most common location of infected aneurysms because of the frequency of vascular intervention there and because it is a preferred location for intravenous drug abuse.

CLINICAL PRESENTATION

The clinical presentation of aneurysms depends on the type, size, location, and confounding factors in the patient, such as connective tissue disorders, hypertension, and intravenous drug abuse. In general, aneurysms can rupture, thrombose, embolize contained thrombus; can cause symptoms from local compression of adjacent structures; or can be detected in an asymptomatic state. Occasionally, systemic signs (such as sepsis) may be the first manifestation. The relative frequency of these presentations varies significantly among different aneurysm types and locations. Among nonspecific aneurysms, those involving the aorta, iliac and visceral arteries are most prone to rupture; femoral, popliteal, renal, and brachiocephalic aneurysms are more likely to thrombose or embolize. Aneurysms of specific etiology, including congenital, infectious, dissecting, and those associated with arteritis are usually complicated by rupture. Details of the clinical presentation of different aneurysms are discussed later. Because renal and carotid artery aneurysms are treated with methods similar to those used for other disorders of these arteries, they are discussed separately in Chapters 125 and 134.

ARTERIOMEGALY AND MULTIPLE ANEURYSMS

Arteriomegaly was originally described by Leriche[28] as diffuse ectasia of the aorta and iliofemoral arteries without discrete aneurysm formation, which he termed "dolicho-meaga-artere." In nearly 6000 patients who underwent aortofemoral arteriography, Hollier and coworkers[23] identified arteriomegaly in 5%, of whom one third also had discrete aneurysms in at least three different arterial segments. All of these patients with arteriomegaly and multiple aneurysms were men, approximately 5 years younger than the average-aged patient with a solitary aneurysm. Arteriomegaly associated with femoral and popliteal aneurysms appeared to increase the risk of thrombosis in this segment. Surgical reconstruction varied according to the exact location of aneurysms but generally included intervening ectatic segments.

Although the term arteriomegaly is generally applied to the infrarenal aortoiliofemoral-popliteal segments, the more proximal aorta is often involved with diffuse aneurysmal changes. In a review of more than 1500 patients treated for aortic aneurysms in a specialized referral practice, Crawford and Cohen[11] found that 13% had multiple aneurysms. Most of these patients (72%) presented with multiple aneurysms synchronoulsy, whereas others (28%) later developed metachronous aneurysms. The cause of most aneurysms was nonspecific (62%), followed by dissection (23%) and other specific causes (e.g., Marfan's syndrome). The most common location of the primary aneurysm was the abdominal aorta (63%), followed by the thoracoabdominal aorta (14%), descending aorta (13%), aortic arch (5%), and ascending aorta (5%). The most common pattern for multiple aneurysms was an infrarenal aortic aneurysm associated with a discrete descending thoracic aortic aneurysm. Whereas 12% of patients with abdominal aneurysms had thoracic aneurysms, 68% of those with thoracic aneurysms had other aneurysms.

In a 1990 review of multiple aortic aneurysms, Gloviczki and colleagues[20] reported similar findings, although multiple aneurysms were found in only 3.4% of all patients with aortic aneurysms, of whom 75% were men. These studies indicate the need for evaluation of the entire aorta in patients with a known aortic aneurysm. This is especially true for patients with a thoracic aortic aneurysm because of the high likelihood of finding an abdominal aortic aneurysm. Thus, patients who present with thoracic or thoracoabdominal aneurysms should have an initial imaging study of the infrarenal aorta, with subsequent follow-up dictated by patient age and other risk factors. Conversely, for a patient with an abdominal aortic aneurysm, initial computed tomography (CT) scanning to exclude a thoracic aneurysm is appropriate if the chest radiography suggests an aneurysm, if there is evidence of dissection or suprarenal aneurysmal involvement, or if the patient is young at presentation, when multiple aneurysms are more likely.[20]

In addition to multiple aortic aneurysms, patients with abdominal aortic aneurysms have a proclivity for lower extremity aneurysms. In a review of nearly 1500 patients with nonspecific aortoiliac aneurysms, 3.5% had other aneurysms, of which 3% were femoral or popliteal and 0.5% were visceral.[14] All of these patients with aortoiliac and other aneurysms were men. The likelihood of detecting an abdominal aortic aneurysm was very high in men with peripheral aneurysms—92% for those with a common femoral artery aneurysm and 64% for those with a popliteal aneurysm. Although other reviews have found somewhat lower probabilities for this association, it is generally agreed that at least one third of patients with femoral or popliteal aneurysms have an associated abdominal aortic aneurysm (see Chapter 94). This emphasizes the necessity for abdominal aortic imaging to exclude an aneurysm in such patients. Although it is likely that other aneurysms (renal, visceral, or carotid) are more likely in patients with aortic aneurysms, these are so rare that screening is generally not recommended. Details concerning the specific aneurysms discussed in this overview are presented in subsequent chapters.

REFERENCES

1. Abernathy CM, Baumgartner R, Butler HG, et al: The management of ruptured abdominal aortic aneurysms in rural Colorado: With a historical note on Kit Carson's death. JAMA 256:587, 1986.
2. Bahnson HT: Considerations in the excision of aortic aneurysms. Ann Surg 97:257, 1953.
3. Bickerstaff LK, Hollier LH, Van Peenen HJ, et al: Abdominal aortic aneurysms: The changing natural history. J Vasc Surg 1:6, 1984.
4. Bickerstaff LK, Pairolero PC, Hollier LH, et al: Thoracic aortic aneurysms: A population-based study. Surgery 92:1103, 1982.
5. Brock RC, Rob CG, Forty F: Reconstructive arterial surgery. Proc R Soc Med 46:115, 1953.
6. Brunkwall J, Hauksson H, Bengtsson H, et al: Solitary aneurysms of the iliac arterial system: An estimate of their frequency of occurrence. J Vasc Surg 10:381, 1989.
7. Cho SI, Johnson WC, Bush HL, et al: Lethal complications associated with nonresective treatment of abdominal aortic aneurysms. Arch Surg 117:1214, 1982.
8. Cohen JR, Graver LM: The ruptured abdominal aortic aneurysm of Albert Einstein. Surg Gynecol Obstet 170:455, 1990.
9. Cooper AP: Lectures on the Principles and Practice of Surgery, 2nd ed. London, FC Westley, 1830.
10. Crawford ES: Thoraco-abdominal and abdominal aortic aneurysms involving renal, superior mesenteric and celiac arteries. Ann Surg 179:763, 1974.
11. Crawford ES, Cohen ES: Aortic aneurysm: A multifocal disease: Presidential address. Arch Surg 117:1393, 1982.
12. Creech O Jr: Endoaneurysmorrhaphy and treatment of aortic aneurysm. Ann Surg 164:935, 1966.
13. DeBakey ME, Cooley DA: Surgical treatment of aneurysm of abdominal aorta by resection of continuity with homograft. Surg Gynecol Obstet 97:257, 1953.
14. Dent TL, Lindenauer SM, Ernst CB, et al: Multiple arteriosclerotic arterial aneurysms. Arch Surg 105:338, 1972.
15. DuBost C, Allary M, Deconomos N: Resection of an aneurysm of the abdominal aorta: Reestablishment of the continuity by a preserved human arterial graft, with a result after five months. Arch Surg 64:405, 1952.
16. Erichsen J: Observations on Aneurism, London, C&J Allard, 1844.
17. Etheredge SN, Yee J, Smith JV, et al: Successful resection of a large aneurysm of the upper abdominal aorta and replacement with homograft. Surgery 38:1071, 1955.
18. Gaylis H: Popliteal arterial aneurysms: A review and analysis of fifty-five cases. S Afr Med J 48:75, 1974.

19. Gillum RF: Epidemiology of aortic aneurysm in the United States. J Clin Epidemiol 48:1289, 1995.
20. Gloviczki P, Pairolero P, Welch T, et al: Multiple aortic aneurysms: The results of surgical management. J Vasc Surg 11:19, 1990.
21. Goyanes J: The Arteries: Part I. Austin, TX, Silvergirl, 1988.
22. Haeger K: The Illustrated History of Surgery. New York, Bell Publishing, 1988.
23. Hollier LH, Stanson AW, Gloviczki P, et al: Arteriomegaly: Classification and morbid implications of diffuse aneurysmal disease. Surgery 93:700, 1983.
24. Johnson T: The Works of That Famous Chirurgeon Ambrose Paré. London, Coates & Dugard, 1649.
25. Johnston KW, Rutherford RB, Tilson MD, et al: Suggested standards for reporting on arterial aneurysms. J Vasc Surg 13:452, 1991.
26. Julian OC, Grove WJ, Dye WS, et al: Direct surgery of atherosclerosis: Resection of abdominal aorta with homologous aortic graft replacement. Ann Surg 138:387, 1953.
27. Lawrence PF, Lorenzo-Rivero S, Lyon JL: The incidence of iliac, femoral and popliteal artery aneurysms in hospitalized patients. J Vasc Surg 22:409, 1995.
28. Leriche R: Dolicho et mega-artere dolicho et mega-veine. Presse Med 51:554, 1943.
29. Matas R: Ligation of the abdominal aorta. Ann Surg 81:457, 1925.
30. Osler W: Aneurysm of the abdominal aorta. Lancet 2:1089, 1905.
31. Osler W: Remarks on arterio-venous aneurysm. Lancet 2:949, 1915.
32. Oudot J: La greffe vasculaire dans les thromboses du carrefour aortique. Presse Med 59:234, 1951.
33. Pott P: Remarks on the Necessity and Propriety of the Operation of Amputation in Certain Cases. London, J Johnson, 1779.
34. Rea CE: The surgical treatment of aneurysm of the abdominal aorta. Minn Med 31:153, 1948.
35. Svensjo S, Bengtsson H, Bergqvist D: Thoracic and thoracoabdominal aortic aneurysm and dissection: An investigation based on autopsy. Br J Surg 83:68, 1996.
36. Voorhees A, Jaretzki A, Blakemore AH: The use of tubes constructed from Vinyon "N" cloth in bridging arterial defects. Am Surg 135:332, 1952.
37. Vorp DA, Raghavan ML, Webster MW: Mechanical wall stress in abdominal aortic aneurysm: Influence of diameter and asymmetry. J Vasc Surg 27:632, 1998.
38. Welling RE, Taha JA, Goel T, et al: Extracranial carotid artery aneurysms. Surgery 93:319, 1983.

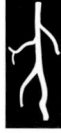

C H A P T E R   8 9
Abdominal Aortic and Iliac Aneurysms

Jack L. Cronenwett, M.D., William C. Krupski, M.D., and Robert B. Rutherford, M.D.

HISTORY

Since the first description of abdominal aortic aneurysms (AAAs) by the 16th century anatomist Vesalius,[166] the history of this disease has reflected the remarkable progress of vascular surgery. Before the development of modern surgical techniques, successful management was rare. Initial attempts at ligation of the aorta failed. In 1923, Matas performed the first successful aortic ligation in a patient with an AAA.[185] Others attempted to induce thrombosis of AAAs by inserting intraluminal wires.[224] In 1948, Rea wrapped reactive cellophane around the neck and over the anterolateral surfaces of an aneurysm to induce a fibrotic reaction and thereby limit expansion.[229] In 1949, Nissen used this technique to treat the symptomatic AAA of Albert Einstein, who survived 6 years before succumbing to eventual rupture.[59] Durable and successful management of AAAs, however, was not achieved until recection and graft replacement was first performed in 1951. Although Dubost and coworkers published the first account of successful replacement of an AAA,[85] a case subsequently reported by Schaffer and Hardin[242] actually preceded that of Dubost and coworkers. The current standard procedure, endoaneurysmorrhaphy with intraluminal graft placement, was popularized by Creech,[67] DeBakey, and their colleagues.

AAAs are the most common type of true aneurysm and have a high propensity to rupture, which makes them a significant health care problem. In the United States, ruptured AAAs are the 15th leading cause of death overall and the 10th leading cause of death in men over age 55 years.[258] In 1991, AAAs caused more than 8500 hospital deaths in the United States,[108] which is an underestimate of their true number because 30% to 50% of all patients with ruptured AAAs die before they reach a hospital.[21] In addition, 30% to 40% of patients with ruptured AAAs die after hospitalization but without operation.[21] When combined with an operative mortality rate of 40% to 50%,[93] these data indicate an overall mortality rate of 80% to 90% for AAA rupture.[21, 144] Unfortunately, this high mortality rate has not changed over the past 20 years despite improvements in operative technique and perioperative management that have reduced elective surgical mortality to less than 5% in most cases.

The effectiveness of elective AAA repair means that most deaths from AAAs are theoretically preventable. In fact, elective AAA repair is one of the most frequent vascular surgery procedures, with a relatively constant rate of 40,000 operations performed annually in the United States during the past 10 years.[108] Despite the frequency of the elective repair, however, death from AAA rupture has remained relatively constant because many AAAs are undetected or untreated. In a review of ruptured AAAs that were easily palpable, more than 50% were either not detected or not referred for treatment despite recent medical examination.[60]

Unfortunately, ruptured aneurysms also impose a substantial financial burden on overall health care costs. One report estimated that $50 million and 2000 lives could have been saved if AAAs had been repaired before they ruptured.[210] Another study showed that emergency operations for AAAs resulted in a mean financial loss to the hospital of $24,655 per patient.[33] For all of these reasons, AAAs remain a central focus for vascular surgeons and a common health care problem for all physicians.

Nearly all AAAs involve the infrarenal aorta, but only about 5% of those being surgically repaired also involve the suprarenal aorta.[203] By definition, suprarenal AAAs extend above the renal arteries so that they require reimplantation of at least one renal artery during AAA repair. The term *juxtarenal* is used to describe AAAs that do not involve the renal arteries, but, because of proximity, require clamping above the renal arteries to complete the proximal aortic anastomosis. Although 25% of AAAs also involve the iliac arteries,[203] isolated iliac artery aneurysms are rare (<1%).[41] Aneurysms of the suprarenal aorta are extremely rare unless they have an associated thoracic or infrarenal component. Concomitant thoracic aneurysms have been found in as many as 12% of patients with AAAs, but this is a high estimate based on a selected referral practice.[61] Peripheral aneurysms of the femoral or popliteal artery are present in approximately 3.5% of patients with AAAs.[79] As aneurysmal dilation of the aorta occurs, elongation also results, leading to a tortuous configuration of the aneurysmal aorta and iliac arteries.

Aneurysms are defined as a focal dilation at least 50% larger than the expected normal arterial diameter.[137] Thus, a practical working definition of an AAA is a transverse diameter of at least 3 cm and for a common iliac aneurysm a transverse diameter of at least 1.8 cm. As shown by Pearce and coworkers, normal aortic diameter gradually decreases from the thorax (28 mm in men) to the infrarenal location (20 mm in men).[215] At all levels, normal aortic diameter is approximately 2 mm larger in men than in women and increases with age and increased body surface area.[215] In a recent large ultrasound screening study, Lederle and coworkers found that increasing age, male gender, African American race, and increasing height, weight, body mass index, and body surface area were all independently associated with increased infrarenal aortic diameter but that the effects of these variables were small.[162] Because the average normal infrarenal aortic diameter was 2.0 cm for these patients, Lederle and associates recommended using a 3.0 cm definition for an infrarenal AAA without the need to consider a more complicated definition based on factors such as gender or body surface area. Although such definitions are useful for large patient groups, in clinical practice with individual patients it is more common to define an aneurysm based on 50% or more enlargement compared with the diameter of the adjacent, nonaneurysmal artery diameter.[137] This is particularly true for patients with unusually small arteries in whom even a 2.5 cm local dilation of the infrarenal aorta might be aneurysmal if the adjacent aorta is only 1.5 cm in diameter.

Most AAAs are spindle shaped, beginning below the renal arteries and ending at the aortic bifurcation. However, considerable variation exists, with saccular aneurysms and other eccentric geometry being quite common. Computer modeling of AAA wall stress suggests that asymmetry may significantly influence rupture risk.[294] It appears that 10% to 20% of AAAs have focal outpouchings or "blebs" that may also increae the risk of rupture.[97, 132] As AAAs enlarge, thrombus is laminated along the aneurysm wall, often preserving a relatively normal arterial lumen despite considerable aneurysmal dilation (Fig. 89–1).

PATHOGENESIS

AAAs represent a degenerative process that has often been attributed to atherosclerosis because of the elderly age of affected patients and the universal atherosclerotic changes found in AAAs. An atherosclerotic cause of AAAs fails to explain the alternative development of occlusive rather than aneurysmal changes in the aorta of similar patients, however, which implies a more complex cause. Thus, rather than being termed *atherosclerotic*, AAAs are more accurately referred to as *degenerative* or nonspecific in etiology. Extensive research is being conducted to better understand the etiology of aneurysms, which is discussed in detail in Chapter 22 and in several recent reviews.[114, 212, 284, 286, 289, 299] Issues particularly relevant to aneurysms of the abdominal aorta are briefly considered here.

The aortic wall contains not only vascular smooth muscle cells but also the important matrix proteins elastin and collagen, which are arranged in organized, concentric layers to withstand arterial pressure.[120] In the normal aorta there is a gradual but marked reduction in the number of medial elastin layers from the proximal thoracic aorta (60 to 80 layers) to the infrarneal aorta (28 to 32 layers), accompanied by medial thinning and intimal thickening in the more distal aorta.[120, 304] Associated with this structural change is a reduction in both collagen and elastin content from the proximal to distal aorta, as reported by Halloran and colleagues.[120] These investigators also found a marked 58%

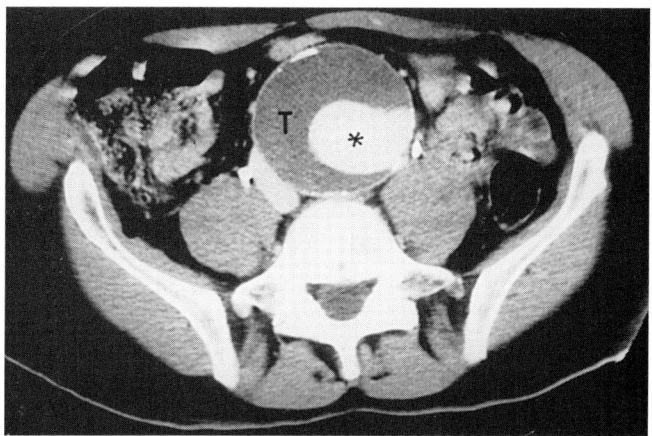

FIGURE 89–1. CT scan of an abdominal aortic aneurysm showing contrast-filled lumen (*asterisk*) surrounded by thrombus (T) within the aneurysm sac.

decrease in elastin content between the suprarenal and the infrarenal aorta and noted that this was the only location within the aorta where the proportion of elastin decreases relative to collagen. Because elastin fragmentation and degeneration are observed histologically in aneurysm walls, these observations help to explain the predilection for aneurysm formation in the infrarenal aorta.[114, 299] Elastin is the principal load-bearing element in the aorta that resists aneurysm formation, while collagen acts as a strong "safety net" to prevent rupture after an aneurysm occurs.[83]

Of note, elastin is not synthesized in the adult aorta but has a half-life of 40 to 70 years, accounting for its reduction with age and for the occurrence of AAAs primarily in elderly patients.[253] In addition to reduced elastin content in the infrarenal aorta, increased susceptibility to aneurysm formation has been attributed to hemodynamic, structural, and autoimmune factors unique to this location. Reflected waves from the aortic bifurcation increase pulsatility and wall tension in the distal, less-compliant atherosclerotic aorta.[193] Increased prevalence of AAAs many years after above-knee amputation has been attributed to increased aortic pulsatility due to increased peripheral resistance,[293] although this relationship was not found in another study.[176] Absence of vasa vasorum in the infrarenal aorta has been suggested to reduce nutrient supply and to potentiate degeneration.[212] In 1998, Tilson found that immunoreactive protein is more conspicuously expressed in the abdominal than in the thoracic aorta, which may also explain the increased frequency of aneurysms in this location, and proposed an autoimmune mechanism for aneurysm formation.[285]

Degradation of proteolytic aortic media in aneurysmal disease implies an increase in proteolytic enzymes relative to their inhibitors. Numerous reports have documented increased expression and activity of matrix metalloproteinases (MMPs) in the wall of aortic aneurysms.[114, 187, 212, 299] Pearce and associates found threefold higher activity of MMP-9 (the primary elastolytic enzyme) in 5- to 7-cm diameter AAAs compared with smaller than 5-cm AAAs, consistent with the increased expansion rates observed for larger AAAs. Other MMPs, as well as serine proteinases such as plasmin, and neutrophil elastase have been found in higher concentrations in AAAs than in normal aortic tissue, while their inhibitors appear unchanged, leading to a net increase in matrix-degrading activity in AAAs.[114] Animal studies have shown that elastase infusion recruits an inflammatory reaction that results in aneurysm formation, which can be prevented by inhibiting inflammatory cell recruitment or by blocking MMP activity with an inhibitor such as doxycycline.[6, 31, 218, 234] These studies emphasize the importance of proteinase activity in the development of AAAs and the likely inflammatory source of stimulation of these enzymes.

Histologic studies of AAAs demonstrate not only fragmentation of elastin fibers and decreased elastin content but also a chronic adventitial and medial inflammatory infiltrate that is different from aortic occlusive disease in which the inflammatory reaction is found primarily in the intimal plaque.[289] This transmural inflammatory response in AAAs appears central to their development, but what causes the response is not clearly understood. The finding of *Chlamydia pneumoniae* in the wall of AAAs suggests that infection with this common pathogen could be a stimulus.[139, 217] Characteristics of this infiltrate, however, including the presence of B-lymphocytes, plasma cells, and large amounts of immunoglobulin (including Russell's bodies), suggest an autoimmune component.[37, 286, 299]

Tilson and associates[286] and Juvonen and associates[116] identified a 40-kD matrix protein that is immunoreactive with immunoglobulin G isolated from the aneurysm wall. This putative autoantigen appears to be a collagen-associated microfibril that Tilson's group found to be most conspicuous in the abdominal aorta and termed *aortic aneurysm antigenic protein* (AAAP-40).[285] Microfibrillar integrity is known to be important for preventing aneurysms because defective fibrillin in Marfan's syndrome leads to aneurysm formation.[82] Interestingly, AAAP-40 shares amino acid sequence homologies with both *Treponema pallidum* and cytomegalovirus, microorganisms associated with aneurysmal disease.[207] This raises the possibility that aneurysms in these infections might result from an immune response against the pathogen that also attacks a similar self-protein in the aneurysm wall, a concept known as *molecular mimicry*.[207]

Numerous studies have noted familial clustering of AAAs in 15% to 25% of patients undergoing AAA repair.[76, 135, 291, 295] Although there is disagreement about the mode of inheritance, the most recent studies by Majumder and colleagues[180] and Verloes and coworkers[291] suggest a single dominant gene with low penetrance that increases with age. A potential genetic basis for the autoimmune manifestations of AAAs was reported in an interesting study by Tilson and coworkers,[286] who identified potential susceptibility alleles for AAAs involving the DRB1 major histocompatibility locus. The alleles they have identified occur rarely in North American blacks but were found in all five black patients with AAAs who were studied.[286] Importantly, these DRB1 alleles were found in 75% to 100% of white patients with AAAs, depending on the degree of similarity required. This research points to a specific DRB1 genetic basis for AAA development, which could lead to genetic testing for susceptibility. The DRB1 major histocompatibility locus has also been recently identified as a likely genetic basis for inflammatory AAAs.[228] Although other candidate genes have been identified in a very small proportion of patients with familial AAAs, these recent findings concerning the DRB1 locus appear to have more widespread implications.

Degenerative aneurysms account for more than 90% of all infrarenal AAAs; less frequent causes include infection, cystic medial necrosis, arteritis, trauma, inherited connective tissue disorders, and pseudoaneurysm from anastomotic disruption. Aortic aneurysms are rare in children and are of diverse etiology,[240] infection from umbilical artery catheters being the most common cause.[265]

EPIDEMIOLOGY

AAAs are generally a disease of elderly white males. AAAs increase steadily in frequency after age 50 years, are 5 times more common in men than in women, and are 3.5 times more common in white than in African American men.[142, 157] The reported incidence, or likelihood of developing an AAA, varies from 3 to 117 per 100,000 person-years.[300] More accurate incidence estimates for asymptomatic AAAs in a community are not possible because sequential screening surveys of the same population have not been conducted. In men, AAAs begin to occur at about age 50 years and reach a peak incidence near age 80 years.[189] In women, AAA onset is delayed, beginning around age 60 years, with incidence continuing to rise thereafter (Fig. 89–2).[189] Overall, the age-adjusted incidence is fourfold to sixfold higher in men than in women for both asymptomatic and ruptured AAAs.

A significant increase in the incidence of asymptomatic AAAs has been noted during the 1990s,[189, 300] in part because of increased case finding due to more frequent use of ultrasonography and other abdominal imaging modalities. In addition to increased case finding, however, there appears to have been a real increase in the incidence of aortic aneurysmal disease. This is supported by the finding of a 2.4% per year increase in the age-adjusted incidence of death from AAA rupture from 1952 to 1988[300] because this statistic is less influenced by more frequent abdominal imaging. A 1995 analysis of hospital deaths in the United States indicates that AAA rupture rates stabilized from 1979 to 1990, with 4 deaths per 100,000 in white males.[108] The reported incidence of ruptured AAA varies from 1 to 21 per 100,000 person-years.[300]

For patients over age 50 years, the incidence of AAA rupture is much higher because the risk of rupture increases dramatically with age (see Fig. 89–2).[21] A recent population-based study by Chosky and coworkers of ruptured AAAs in patients in England noted an incidence of 76 per 100,000 person-years for men and 11 per 100,000 person-years for women over 50 years of age, giving a male:female ratio of 4.8:1.[57] The median age at rupture was 76 years for men and 81 years for women. The median AAA size at rupture was 8 cm, but 4.5% of the ruptured AAAs were less than 5 cm in diameter (measured at autopsy or during operation). The overall mortality rate from rupture was 78%, and three fourths of these deaths occurred

outside the hospital. Interestingly, most deaths from ruptured AAAs, like those from coronary artery disease, occur in winter months.[53]

Prevalence estimates for asymptomatic AAAs are more accurate than incidence estimates now that large ultrasound screening surveys have been performed. Ultrasound screening and autopsy series indicate that the prevalence of AAAs (≥ 3 cm) is 3% to 10% for patients over 50 years of age in the western world.[300] In a 1997 Veterans Administration screening study of more than 73,000 patients aged 50 to 79 years, the prevalence of AAAs at least 3 cm was 4.6%; for those at least 4 cm, the prevalence was 1.4%.[161] Prevalence of AAAs in a given population depends on risk factors that are associated with AAAs, including older age, male gender, white race, positive family history, smoking, hypertension, hypercholesterolemia, peripheral vascular occlusive disease, and coronary artery disease.[3] Although these risk factors are associated with increased AAA prevalence, they may not be independent predictors and may be markers rather than causes of AAA disease. Of these risk factors, however, age, gender, and smoking have the largest impact on AAA prevalence.[165, 300]

In the 1997 Veterans Administration study, smoking was the risk factor most strongly associated with AAA.[161] The relative risk of an AAA of 4 cm or larger was 5.6 fold higher in smokers than in nonsmokers, and the risk increased significantly with the number of years of smoking. The excess prevalence associated with smoking accounts for 78% of all AAAs that were at least 4 cm in this study. Other relatively important risk factors that increased AAA prevalence in this study were male gender (4.5-fold risk), white race (two-fold risk), and positive family history (two-fold risk), while diabetes had a decreased risk (0.5-fold risk). Less important independent risk factors for increased AAA prevalence were increased age, height, coronary artery disease, any atherosclerosis, high cholesterol level, and hypertension. There is less agreement that hypertension increases AAA prevalence, although it does increase rupture risk in patients with established AAAs (see later). A recent population-based study found that atherosclerosis increased the prevalence of AAAs, that smoking was an independent risk factor (relative risk, 2.6-fold), but that diastolic hypertension did not increase AAA prevalence.[165] Among smokers, however, AAA prevalence is increased not only by the number of cigarettes smoked and increasing depth of inhalation but also by elevated mean arterial or diastolic blood pressure.[103] The estimated impacts of various risk factors on AAA prevalence are listed in Table 89–1.

Familial clustering of patients with AAAs is well described in the literature. Of patients undergoing AAA repair, 15% to 25% have a first-degree relative with a clinically apparent AAA compared with only 2% to 3% of age-matched control patients without AAAs.[76, 135, 291, 295] Conversely, and more clinically relevant, approximately 7% of siblings of patients with AAAs have a clinically apparent AAA.[223] This prevalence increases if ultrasound screening of relatives is performed. Webster and coworkers demonstrated that ultrasound screening of siblings of a patient with an AAA yielded AAAs of 3 cm or greater in 25% of the male and 7% of the female siblings older than age 55 years.[295] The likelihood that relatives have AAAs increases if the proband (patient with the AAA) is a woman. Thus,

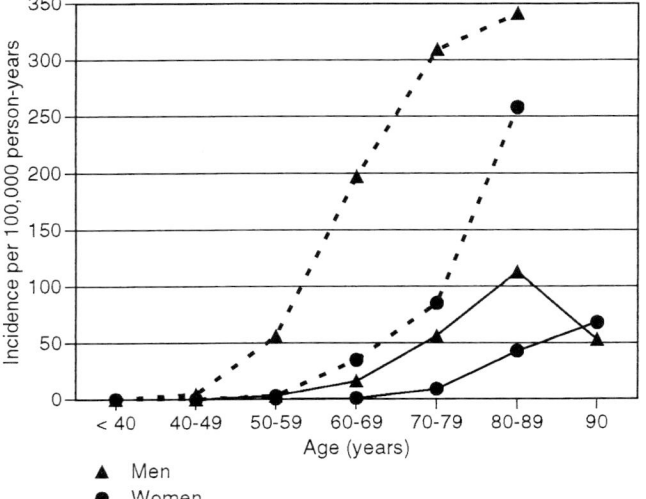

FIGURE 89–2. Incidence of clinically apparent[27] and ruptured abdominal aortic aneurysms (AAAs)[21] from population-based studies. *Dashed lines* = incidence of all AAAs; *solid lines* = incidence of ruptured AAAs.

TABLE 89–1. INDEPENDENT RISK FACTORS FOR DETECTING AN UNKNOWN ABDOMINAL AORTIC ANEURYSM 4 CM IN DIAMETER OR LESS DURING ULTRASOUND SCREENING

RISK FACTOR	ODDS RATIO*	95% CI
Increased Risk		
Smoking history	5.6	4.2–7.3
Family history of AAA	2.0	1.6–2.4
Older age (per 7-year interval)	1.7	1.5–1.8
Coronary artery disease	1.6	1.4–1.8
High cholesterol level	1.5	1.3–1.8
COPD	1.3	1.1–1.5
Height (per 7-cm interval)	1.2	1.1–1.3
Decreased Risk		
Abdominal imaging within 5 years	0.8	0.7–0.9
Deep vein thrombosis	0.7	0.5–0.9
Diabetes mellitus	0.5	0.4–0.7
Black race	0.5	0.4–0.7
Female gender	0.2	0.1–0.7

From Lederle FA, Johnson GR, Wilson SE, et al: Prevalence and associations of abdominal aortic aneurysm detected through screening: Aneurysm Detection and Management (ADAM) Veterans Affairs Cooperative Study Group. Ann Intern Med 126(6): 441, 1997.
*Odds ratio indicates relative risk compared to patients without that risk factor.
CI = confidence interval; COPD = chronic obstructive pulmonary disease.

if the proband is male, 7% of parents or siblings have a clinically apparent AAA, but, if the proband is female, 12% of these relatives have an AAA.[223] It is estimated that first-degree relatives of a patient with an AAA have a 12-fold increased risk for aneurysm development.[135] Brothers of a patient with an AAA have an 18-fold increased risk for AAA development, highest in the 50- to 60-year-old range and decreasing thereafter.[291] Analyses of patients with familial aneurysms indicate that, on average, these patients are 5 to 7 years younger and are more frequently women than those without familial aneurysms.[76, 291] In the surgical series of Darling and associates of patients undergoing AAA repair, women accounted for 35% of patients with a positive family history of AAAs but for only 14% of patients without familial AAAs.[76] Thus, although AAAs in women are much less common than in men, women with AAAs are more likely to have affected relatives.

CLINICAL PRESENTATION AND DIAGNOSIS

Physical Examination

Most AAAs are asymptomatic, which leads to difficulty in their detection. Occasionally, patients may describe a "pulse" in their abdomen or may actually palpate a pulsatile mass. Although most clinically significant AAAs are potentially palpable during routine physical examination, the sensitivity of this technique depends on the AAA size, the obesity of the patient, the skill of the examiner, and the focus of the examination.[163] Although a focused physical examination detected 50% of 3.5- to 6-cm diameter AAAs, these had all been missed on a recent, nonfocused examination.[163] Conversely, AAAs may be falsely suspected in thin patients with a prominent, but normal-sized aorta or in

patients with a mass overlying the aorta that transmits a prominent pulse. Patients with hypertension, a wide pulse pressure, or a tortuous aorta can also have a prominent aortic pulsation that may be mistaken for an AAA. In fact, the positive predictive value of physical examination for identifying AAAs larger than 3.5 cm diameter is only 15%.[19] The accuracy of physical examination for measuring size of a known AAA is also poor, usually resulting in an overestimate of size due to intervening intestine and abdominal wall fat. Because of these factors, most AAAs are detected by incidental abdominal imaging studies done for other reasons.

In a review of 243 patients who underwent elective AAA repair, Chervu and associates found that 38% were initially detected by physical examination, whereas 62% were detected by incidental radiologic studies even though 43% of these were palpable on subsequent examination.[56] Importantly, 23% of these clinically significant AAAs were not palpable even when the diagnosis was known, and, in obese patients, fully two thirds were not palpable. This emphasizes the potential role for ultrasound screening in high-risk patients, as discussed later.

Imaging

Several imaging modalities confirm the diagnosis of AAA. Abdominal B-mode ultrasonography is the least expensive, least invasive, and most frequently used examination, particularly for initial confirmation of a suspected AAA or for follow-up of small AAAs. Diameter measurements using ultrasound have an interobserver variability of less than 5 mm in 84% of studies and are more accurate in the anteroposterior than the lateral dimension.[134] Visualization of the suprarenal aorta and iliac arteries may be obscured by bowel gas and be difficult to achieve in obese patients. Furthermore, ultrasonography cannot accurately determine the presence of rupture[255] and often cannot accurately determine the upper extent of an AAA.[214]

Computed tomography (CT) scanning is more expensive than ultrasonography and involves radiation and intravenous contrast exposure, but it provides somewhat more accurate diameter measurement, with 91% of studies showing an interobserver variability of less than 5 mm.[134] Accuracy can be increased with standardized techniques, calipers, and magnification.[164] More importantly, CT scanning precisely defines the proximal and distal extent of an AAA, more accurately images the iliac arteries, and provides other important information for operative planning (see later). It is particularly useful for excluding AAA rupture in a stable but symptomatic patient, for defining the proximal extent of an AAA, and for detecting other unsuspected pathology, such as an inflammatory aneurysm. Both ultrasonography and CT scanning can overestimate AAA diameter if an oblique rather than a perpendicular section is obtained in a tortuous aneurysm. The oblique angle results in an elliptical rather than a circular cross section, and the larger diameter of the ellipse overestimates the true AAA diameter, as discussed in Chapter 14. Compared with CT scanning, ultrasonography appears to underestimate the diameter of AAAs systematically by 2 to 4 mm in the anteroposterior direction.[134, 164, 283] Spiral CT scanning is a new, more rapid method of CT scanning that provides excellent resolution of even visceral aortic branches when thin "slices" are obtained. Refinements of spiral CT scanning include three-dimensional reconstruction, which provides more user-friendly images and facilitates accurate measurement for endovascular graft sizing (see Chapter 14).

Magnetic resonance imaging (MRI) is comparable in accuracy to CT scanning for AAA measurement and evaluation and avoids radiation exposure (see Chapter 15). However, this technique is more expensive, less readily available, and less well tolerated by claustrophobic patients than CT scanning. MRI is particularly valuable when intravenous contrast is contraindicated, such as in patients with renal failure. Improvements in the spatial resolution of spiral CT scanning, combined with its more rapid, less expensive technique, however, have largely relegated MRI to a secondary role in the evaluation of AAAs. Magnetic resonance angiography (MRA) may be valuable in the preoperative evaluation of AAAs when information about occlusive disease in adjacent arteries is required (see later). Arteriography is not an accurate technique with which to confirm the diagnosis of AAA or to measure diameter accurately because thrombus within an AAA usually diminishes the size of the contrast-filled lumen. Rather, arteriography is used in the preoperative evaluation of some patients with AAAs to define pathology in adjacent arteries that might impact the AAA repair (see Preoperative Assessment, later).

Diagnosis of Rupture

Most AAAs that become symptomatic do so because of rupture or acute expansion. Patients with a ruptured AAA experience abrupt onset of abdominal or back pain that can radiate into the flank or groin. Most ruptured AAAs are palpable, if not prevented by obesity or abdominal distention, and are usually tender. When rupture occurs, extravasation of blood takes place through the disrupted aortic wall. The extents of hemorrhage and cardiovascular compensation then determine the severity of hypotension and shock associated with rupture. This, in turn, usually depends on the specific location of rupture, which in 20% occurs anteriorly into the peritoneal cavity.[75] In that location little tamponade can be expected so that massive hemorrhage ensues. Fortunately, 80% of ruptures occur posteriorly into the retroperitoneal space where the hematoma is usually initially contained, increasing the possibility of survival.

Most patients with ruptured AAAs present with at least transient hypotension, which develops into frank shock over a period of hours. Occasionally, rupture is so effectively contained within the retroperitoneum that symptoms can persist for days or even weeks without hypotension. These patients with chronic "contained rupture" can be difficult to diagnose because their symptoms often mimic an acute inflammatory condition. Although the classic presentation of a ruptured AAA includes abdominal or back pain, hypotension, and a pulsatile abdominal mass, all three findings are seen in only 26% of patients with proven AAA rupture.[183] Temporary loss of consciousness is a potentially important symptom of ruptured AAA because it occurs in combination with pain in 50% of patients and as the only initial symptom in 17% of patients with AAA

rupture.[21] Ruptured AAAs are discussed in detail in Chapter 91.

Early diagnosis of patients with ruptured AAAs who do not have hypotension or other signs of bleeding can be difficult, particularly in obese patients if an AAA is not palpable. Accordingly, a high index of suspicion for ruptured AAA must exist in patients who present with back or abdominal pain, especially if they are older males in whom the prevalence is higher. If an AAA is not palpable, such patients should have an abdominal imaging study to exclude an AAA unless the abdomen is so thin that physical examination is completely reliable. If such patients have a palpable or known AAA, CT scanning is useful to diagnose or exclude rupture and may provide useful information concerning alternative diagnoses. The accuracy of CT scanning for determining AAA rupture in this setting is approximately 90%.[153, 251] In a review of stable but symptomatic patients with a suspected ruptured AAA, CT scanning demonstrated aneurysm rupture in 30%, a nonruptured AAA in 50%, and other pathologic causes to explain the symptoms in 20% of patients.[153] This is valuable information because patients with symptomatic but nonruptured aneurysms (termed *acutely expanding*) have a substantially higher operative mortality rate than that associated with the elective AAA repair (average, 23%[144]).[272] This higher rate likely results from a combination of factors, including suboptimal preoperative evaluation and management of co-morbid disease, as well as fatigue or inexperience of the emergency surgical and anesthesia teams. Because acute expansion is considered an immediate precursor of rupture, however, such patients must undergo expeditious AAA repair. Therefore, in-hospital evaluation and preoperative preparation of patients with symptomatic but nonruptured AAAs are recommended to reduce perioperative morbidity and mortality but allow emergent operation should rupture occur.[272]

Other Symptoms

Much less frequently, AAAs may present with symptoms unrelated to rupture. Rarely, large AAAs cause symptoms from local compression, such as early satiety, nausea, or vomiting from duodenal compression; urinary symptoms due to hydronephrosis from ureteral compression; or venous thrombosis from iliocaval venous compression. Posterior erosion of AAAs into adjacent vertebrae can lead to back pain. Even without bony involvement, AAAs can cause chronic back pain or abdominal pain that is vague and ill defined. Acute ischemic symptoms can result from the distal embolization of thrombotic debris contained within an AAA. This appears to be more common in smaller AAAs, especially if the intraluminal thrombus is irregular or fissured.[17] Acute thrombosis of an AAA occurs rarely, but causes catastrophic ischemia comparable with any acute aortic occlusion. Embolism is much more common than acute AAA thrombosis, but both combined occur in less than 2% to 5% of patients with AAAs.[17] Nonetheless, an aortic aneurysm source for distal emboli must always be considered, especially in patients without overt atherosclerotic occlusive disease. Such symptoms are nearly always in indication for AAA repair.

Although AAAs are primarily a disease of the elderly, they can present in patients younger than 50 years of age.

As reported by Muluk and coworkers, these AAAs are more often symptomatic and on average are 1 cm larger at presentation than in older patients.[196] This may relate to fewer incidental abdominal imaging studies performed in younger patients such that AAAs escape detection until they are larger or symptomatic. Younger patients tend to have more proximally located AAAs, with 46% being juxtarenal or higher compared with 18% at this level in older patients. Smoking is nearly universal in young patients with AAAs, whereas only 23% have a defined cause, such as Marfan's syndrome.[196]

Screening

Because asymptomatic AAAs are often not discovered until they rupture, the potential benefit of ultrasound screening programs has been suggested. Although not yet popular in the United States, a number of such programs have been introduced in other countries.[22, 171, 192, 249] Two recent population-based studies investigated the impact of such a screening program on subsequent AAA rupture rate. In 1995, Scott and colleagues reported a study of nearly 16,000 men and women aged 65 to 80 years in which prevalence of AAAs of at least a 30-cm diameter was 4.0% overall (7.6% in men, 1.3% in women).[250] Patients with small AAAs were subsequently followed up with ultrasound size measurements and offered elective AAA repair if a 6-cm-diameter threshold was reached or if expansion of at least 1 cm per year of symptoms developed. The incidence of rupture was reduced by 55% in men who participated in this screening program compared with age-matched randomized controls. Women in both the screened and control groups had low rupture risk. In a similar study in 1997 of men over age 50 years who were offered ultrasound screening (plus appropriate follow-up and AAA repair when indicated), the subsequent incidence of AAA rupture was 2.8 per 10,000 person-years compared with 6.7 per 10,000 person-years in the control, unscreened group.[300] These studies indicate that ultrasound screening for AAAs in men over 50 years of age can reduce AAA rupture rate by more than 50% when accompanied by appropriate follow-up and timely elective repair.

Other studies have suggested the value of identifying high-risk groups for AAA screening. In addition to male gender and advanced age, smoking history increases the positive yield of a screening program.[301] As noted earlier, the recent Veterans Administration screening study found that smoking increased the risk for detecting AAAs of 4 cm or more by nearly sixfold.[161] In a study of ultrasound screening for AAAs in patients undergoing lower extremity noninvasive arterial examination, Wolf and coworkers found AAAs of at least 4 cm in 9% of male smokers over age 65 years compared with 3% in the entire population.[302] Nonetheless, the cost-effectiveness of screening programs to detect asymptomatic AAAs continues to be debated. In part, this relates to inadequate knowledge concerning the natural history of the mostly small AAAs that are identified by such screening. Formal cost-effectiveness studies have suggested that ultrasound screening for AAAs is cost-effective, however, if performed once in patients with a reasonably high prevalence of AAA, such as male patients over 60 years of age who are smokers or who have other risk factors associated with increased AAA prevalence.[101, 260] Such recommendations appear appropriate and are likely to be the only successful method to reduce mortality from AAA rupture.

RISK OF RUPTURE

Estimates of AAA rupture risk are imprecise because large numbers of patients with AAAs have not been followed up without intervention. Studies conducted before the widespread application of surgical repair documented the likelihood of large AAAs to rupture, although many of these AAAs were not only large, but also symptomatic.[95, 243] Contemporary reports have necessarily focused on the natural history of small AAAs because larger ones are nearly always repaired when detected. Unfortunately, there are still insufficient data to develop an accurate prediction rule for AAA rupture in individual patients, which makes surgical decision making difficult. However, knowledge of available natural history data can assist these decisions, as discussed here.

Risk Factors for Rupture

From a hemodynamic perspective, AAA rupture occurs when the forces within an AAA exceed the wall's bursting strength. Laplace's law indicates that the wall tension of an ideal cylinder is directly proportional to its radius and intraluminal pressure and inversely proportional to wall thickness. Real AAAs are not ideal cylinders and have wall thicknesses of variable strength. Theoretically, however, Laplace's formula predicts that larger AAA diameter and hypertension should increase wall tension and thus rupture risk. Decreasing wall thickness (or strength), while difficult to measure clinically, should also theoretically increase the probability of rupture.

The paramount importance of diameter in determining AAA rupture risk is universally accepted, based initially on a pivotal study reported by Szilagyi and colleagues in 1966.[277] These authors compared the outcomes of patients with large (>6 cm by physical examination) and small (<6 cm) AAAs who were managed nonoperatively even though at least half were considered fit for surgery in that era. During follow-up, 43% of the larger AAAs ruptured compared with only 20% of the small AAAs, although the actual size at the time of rupture is unknown. This difference in rupture rate contributed to a 5-year survival rate of only 6% for patients with large AAAs compared with 48% for patients with small AAAs. These results were confirmed with 51% for AAAs of more than 6 cm in patients managed nonoperatively.[100] Because the imaging techniques used now were not available in the 1960s to measure these aneurysms accurately, it is likely that diameter was overestimated by physical examination such that the "large" 6-cm AAAs in these studies were closer to 5 cm by today's standards. Nonetheless, the influence of size on AAA rupture risk was firmly established and has provided a sound basis for recommending elective repair for large AAAs especially because both these studies demonstrated a marked improvement in survival after operative repair.[100, 277]

Autopsy studies have also demonstrated that larger AAAs are more prone to rupture. In an influential study in 1977, Darling and colleagues analyzed 473 consecutive patients who had an AAA at autopsy, of which 25% had ruptured.[75] Probability of rupture increased with diameter: less than 4 cm, 10%; 4 to 7 cm, 25%; 7 to 10 cm, 46%; more than 10 cm, 61%. These results were later confirmed by Sterpetti and coworkers in an autopsy series of 297 patients with AAAs in which the rate of rupture was 5% for AAAs of 5 cm or less diameter; 39% for 5- to 7-cm AAAs; and 65% for 7 cm or more diameter AAAs.[263] Although these autopsy studies have clearly shown the impact of relative AAA size on rupture rate, absolute diameter measurements at autopsy likely underestimate actual size because the aorta is no longer pressurized. After rupture, size measurement is even more difficult because the AAA is not intact. Furthermore, autopsy series are biased toward patients with larger AAAs that rupture and more likely lead to autopsy than smaller AAAs in asymptomatic patients who die of other causes. Thus, the rupture rates assigned to specific aneurysm diameters by autopsy studies almost certainly overestimate true rupture risk.

Estimates of Rupture Risk

Despite the inability to relate rupture risk with size precisely, there is widespread agreement that rupture risk primarily depends on AAA diameter and increases substantially for very large AAAs. There appears to be a transition point between a diameter of 5 and 6 cm below which rupture risk is quite low and above which rupture risk is quite high.[198] A recent survey of members of the Society for Vascular Surgery yielded median estimates for annual rupture risk of 20% per year for a 6.5-cm diameter AAA and 30% per year for a 7.5-cm diameter AAA, but there was large variability in these responses, reflecting the lack of precise data.[160] However, because more than 90% of vascular surgeons agreed that the annual rupture risk of a 6-cm or larger AAA is at least 10% per year, elective repair is recommended for nearly all patients with large AAAs unless the predicted operative mortality rate is extremely high. Thus, a precise definition of rupture risk for large AAAs is only relevant for patients with high operative risk or poor life expectancy. For this reason, current attention is focused on the natural history of small AAAs (4 to 6 cm diameter) whose lower rupture risk makes decision making more difficult even for patients with low operative risk.

Rupture Risk of Small Abdominal Aortic Aneurysms

A large number of contemporary series have examined the outcomes of patients with small, asymptomatic AAAs. In most of these series "selective management" was practiced in which patients were followed up with periodic AAA size measurement until the AAA reached a threshold size for elective repair or rapid AAA expansion or symptoms developed. Four prospective series of selective management of 378 patients with small AAAs yielded remarkably similar results.[26, 72, 172, 266] In these studies, elective repair was generally recommended at a threshold diameter of 5 cm for good risk patients and 6 cm for higher risk patients or for rapid

expansion (>1 cm per year) or AAA symptoms. After an average follow-up of 31 months, 38% of patients met these criteria and underwent elective AAA repair, while 6% required emergent surgery for rupture or acute expansion. Death from other causes occurred in 29%, and 27% were alive with their AAA at final follow-up.[69] These results provide an estimate of the anticipated outcome of selective management of patients with small AAAs. It appears that few experience AAA rupture during careful follow-up but that a large proportion require elective repair.

A population-based study by Brown and coworkers from Kingston, Ontario, Canada, confirmed this conclusion in a group of 492 patients with AAAs less than 5 cm diameter who entered a prospective measurement program of ultrasonography or CT scanning every 6 months.[39, 40] Of these patients, 41% underwent elective repair during the 2.5-year mean follow-up period because their AAA reached the 5-cm threshold size (32%), expanded by more than 0.5 cm in 6 months (5%), or for other reasons (4%). Aneurysm size and patient age at entry significantly affected the subsequent likelihood of elective repair. Of patients 70 years or older, with AAAs less than 4 cm at entry, only 26% underwent elective repair during follow-up compared with 72% of patients younger than 70 with AAAs of at least 4 cm. While rupture did not occur in AAAs less than 5 cm diameter, six AAAs ruptured at 5.0 to 5.6 cm in diameter in patients who did not undergo elective repair at the 5-cm threshold. Because AAAs in the 4.5- to 4.9-cm diameter range expanded rapidly (0.7 cm per year), the authors recommended a threshold size of 4.5 cm for elective repair in good risk patients to avoid the possibility of exceeding the 5-cm threshold when rupture was observed.[40]

It is difficult to derive accurate estimates of rupture risk for small aneurysms from so-called natural history studies because most of these are actually reports of selective management in which 30% to 40% of patients with small AAAs underwent elective repair during follow-up, thus eliminating the possibility of rupture.[69] Within any size range, AAAs selected for elective repair are usually ones with more rapid expansion or vague symptoms in which rupture risk is highest. Accordingly, when rupture risk is calculated from such studies, it is systematically underestimated. Cronenwett and colleagues reported the outcomes of 67 patients with 4- to 6-cm diameter AAAs, only 3% of whom underwent elective repair during the 3-year follow-up.[71] In this series, the annual rupture rate was 6% per year, causing a 5% annual mortality rate from AAA rupture. Most AAAs expanded during follow-up to a larger size before rupture, however, so that the rupture rate for AAAs that remained less than 5 cm in diameter was only 3% per year.[144]

Different results from similar studies illustrate the difficulty in accurately defining the rupture risk of small AAAs given current data. After a population-based study in Minnesota, Nevitt and colleagues reported the outcome of 176 patients initially selected for nonoperative management and noted no rupture during 5 years of follow-up for AAAs less than 5 cm in diameter, but a 5% annual rupture risk for AAAs larger than 5 cm at initial presentation.[198] In a later analysis of the same patients, these authors examined rupture risk as a function of the most recent ultrasound diameter measurement rather than AAA size at entry.[231] They estimated annual rupture risk to be zero for AAAs less than 4 cm, 1% per year for AAAs 4.0 to 4.9 cm, but 11% per year for AAAs 5.0 to 5.9 cm. These conclusions likely underestimate rupture risk, however, because 45% of AAAs underwent elective repair during follow-up, presumably those at greatest risk for rupture within any size category.[231]

In another study of 114 patients with small AAAs initially selected for nonoperative management, Limet and coworkers observed rupture in 12% during a 2-year follow-up period despite elective repair because of rapid expansion in 38%.[169] This yielded an annual rupture rate of zero for AAAs less than 4 cm in diameter, 5.4% per year for AAAs 4 to 5 cm, and 16% per year for AAAs more than 5 cm in diameter. Because this was a referral-based study, it probably overestimated rupture risk of the entire population, but may accurately portray the group of patients referred for surgical consultation. In another referral-based study of 300 patients with AAAs initially managed nonoperatively, however, the observed annual rupture risk over 4 years' follow-up was only 0.25% per year for AAAs less than 4 cm, 0.5% per year for AAAs 4 to 4.9 cm, and 4.3% per year for AAAs more than 5 cm in diameter, even though only 8% of patients underwent elective repair.[118] These differences in the estimated rupture risk of small AAAs undoubtedly reflect subtle differences in the populations analyzed and indicate the current error range in these estimates.

Other Variables

The simple observation that not all AAAs rupture at a specific diameter indicates that other patient-specific and aneurysm-specific variables also influence rupture. Variations in AAA wall thickness and strength affect rupture risk, but, at present, these cannot be measured and thus do not have current clinical relevance. Two groups of investigators used multivariate analysis to examine the predictive value of various clinical parameters on AAA rupture risk. In a group of patients with small AAAs, some of which ruptured during follow-up, Cronenwett and associates determined that larger initial AAA diameter, hypertension, and chronic obstructive pulmonary disease (COPD) were independent predictors of rupture.[71] After comparing patients with ruptured and intact AAAs at autopsy, Sterpetti and coworkers also concluded that larger initial AAA size, hypertension, and bronchiectasis were independently associated with AAA rupture.[263] Patients with ruptured AAAs had significantly larger aneurysms (8.0 versus 5.1 cm), more frequently had hypertension (54% versus 28%), and more frequently had both emphysema (67% versus 42%) and bronchiectasis (29% versus 15%).

In a review of 75 patients with AAAs managed nonoperatively, Foster and associates noted that death from rupture occurred in 72% of patients with diastolic hypertension, but in only 30% of the entire group.[100] Among 156 patients with AAAs managed nonoperatively, Szilagyi and colleagues found that hypertension (>150 per 100 mmHg) was present in 67% of patients who experienced rupture but in only 23% of those without rupture.[275] Thus, in addition to AAA size, these reports strongly implicate both hypertension and COPD as important risk factors for AAA rupture. The explanation for a causative role of hypertension is

straightforward, based on Laplace's law. An explanation for the association of COPD with rupture is less straightforward, but may relate to a systemic imbalance in proteinase activity affecting both pulmonary and aortic connective tissues.[70]

Smoking also appears to be an important risk factor associated with AAA rupture, although a potential interaction with COPD cannot be excluded. A large study of male civil servants in England found that the relative risk of death from AAA rupture increased 4.6-fold for cigarette smokers, 2.4-fold for cigar smokers, and 14.6-fold for smokers of hand-rolled cigarettes.[270] It was not possible in this large epidemiologic study, however, to separate the potential confounding influence of COPD, and the two studies noted earlier specifically identified COPD, but not smoking, as predictive of rupture.[71, 263] Nonetheless, from a clinical prospective, the nearly fivefold increase in AAA rupture risk observed in cigarette smokers cannot be overlooked when counseling patients.

Although a positive family history of AAA is known to increase the prevalence of AAAs in other first-degree relatives (FDRs), it also appears that familial AAAs have a higher rupture risk. Darling and coworkers reported that the frequency of ruptured AAAs increased with the number of FDRs who have AAAs: 15% with two FDRs, 29% with three FDRs, and 36% with four or more FDRs.[76] Women with familial aneurysms were more likely (30%) to present with rupture than men with familial AAAs (17%). Verloes and associates found that the rupture rate was 32% in patients with familial versus 9% in patients with sporadic aneurysms and that familial AAAs ruptured 10 years earlier (65 versus 75 years of age).[291] These observations suggest that patients with a strong family history of AAA may have an individually higher risk of rupture, especially if they are female. However, these studies did not consider other potentially confounding factors, such as AAA size, that might have been different in the familial group. Thus, further epidemiologic research is required to determine whether a positive family history is an independent risk factor for AAA rupture in addition to a risk factor for increased AAA prevalence.

In addition to absolute AAA diameter, many surgeons believe that the ratio of the aneurysm diameter to the adjacent normal aorta is important in determining rupture risk. Thus, a 4-cm AAA in a small woman with a 1.5-cm diameter native aorta would be considered at greater rupture risk than a comparable 4-cm AAA in a large man with a native aortic diameter of 2.5 cm. The validity of this concept, however, has not been proven. Ouriel and colleagues have suggested that a relative comparison between aortic diameter and the diameter of the third lumbar vertebra may increase the accuracy for predicting rupture risk by adjusting for differences in body size.[205] The improvement in prediction potential appears minimal, however, when compared with absolute AAA diameter.

Clinical opinion also holds that eccentric saccular aneurysms represent greater rupture risk than more diffuse, cylindrical aneurysms. One analysis based on computer modeling found that wall stress is substantially increased by an asymmetric bulge in AAAs.[294] The influence of asymmetry was as important as diameter over the clinically relevant range tested. This raises the possibility that estimates of AAA rupture risk might be improved with biomechanical modeling of individual AAAs. In addition to a large bulge over the entire AAA, localized outpouchings or "blebs," ranging from 5 to 30 mm, can be observed on AAAs intraoperatively or on CT scans.[132] These areas of focal wall weakness demonstrate marked thinning of the tunica media elastin and have been suggested to increase rupture risk, although this is not firmly established.[97] The effect of intraluminal thrombus on rupture risk is also debated. One study has reported a thinner thrombus in AAAs that ruptured,[152] and thrombus has been suggested to reduce aneurysm wall tension.[195] The practical impact of these variables on AAA rupture risk requires further study.

Although rapid AAA expansion is presumed to increase rupture risk, it is difficult to separate this effect from the influence of expansion rate on absolute diameter, which alone could increase rupture risk. Two studies have reported that expansion rate was larger in ruptured than in intact AAAs, but these ruptured AAAs were also larger.[169, 244] Other studies have found that absolute AAA diameter, rather than expansion rate, predicted rupture.[71, 198] Thus, although not proven, rapid AAA expansion is generally regarded as a risk factor for rupture and is often used as a criterion for elective repair of small AAAs. Corroborative evidence for this assumption was recently reported in which not only initial diameter but also, more importantly, subsequent expansion rate were independent predictors of rupture of thoracoabdominal aneurysms.[173]

Conclusion

In summary, AAA rupture risk requires more precise definition. Currently available data suggest the following estimates for rupture risk as a function of diameter: AAAs less than 4 cm, 0% per year; 4 to 5 cm, 0.5% to 5% per year; 5 to 6 cm, 3% to 15% per year; 6 to 7 cm, 10% to 20% per year; 7 to 8 cm, 20% to 40% per year; more than 8 cm, 30% to 50% per year. For a given sized AAA, hypertension and COPD appear to be independent risk factors for rupture. Smoking is also a risk factor, although potential interactions between COPD and smoking require clarification. Family history and rapid expansion are probably risk factors for rupture; the influences of shape, thrombus content, and diameter ratio are less certain.

EXPANSION RATE

Estimating the expected AAA expansion rate is important to predict the likely time when a given AAA will reach threshold diameter for elective repair. Numerous studies have established that aneurysms expand more rapidly as they increase in size.[24, 72, 117, 125, 169] Expansion rate is most accurately represented as an exponential rather than a linear function of initial AAA size. Limet and coworkers calculated the median expansion rate of small AAAs to be $e^{0.106t}$, where t = years.[169] For a 1-year time interval, this formula predicts an 11% increase in diameter per year, nearly identical to the 10% per year calculation reported by Cronenwett and colleagues.[72] At least two other studies have confirmed this estimate of approximately 10% per year for

clinically relevant AAAs in the size range of 4 to 6 cm in diameter.[23, 125] Screening studies that have identified very small AAAs suggest that expansion rate may be less than 10% per year for AAAs smaller than 4 cm.[117]

Although average AAA expansion rate can be estimated for a large population, it is important to realize that individual AAAs behave in a more erratic fashion. Periods of rapid expansion may be interspersed with periods of slower expansion.[55, 266] Episodes of sudden, rapid expansion do not appear predictable.[266] Chang and associates found that, in addition to large initial AAA diameter, rapid expansion is independently associated with advanced age, smoking, severe cardiac disease, and stroke.[55] The influence of smoking has been confirmed by others.[179] In addition to these factors, hypertension and pulse pressure have been identified as independent predictors of more rapid expansion rate.[72, 244] Finally, Krupski and coworkers[150] and Wolf and coworkers[303] have shown that increased thrombus content within an AAA and the extent of the aneurysm wall in contact with thrombus are associated with more rapid expansion.

Clinical studies have suggested that beta-blockade, particularly with propranolol, may decrease the rate of AAA expansion. In a small group of patients with AAAs, Leach and coworkers noted that only 8% of patients treated with beta-blockers had rapid expansion (greater than the mean rate) compared with 53% of other patients.[159] Similarly, Gadowski and coworkers noted rapid expansion in only 19% of patients with small AAAs treated with beta-blockers compared with 60% of other patients.[105] In a recent multivariate analysis of patients with small AAAs, Englund and associates found that beta-blockade treatment had an independent effect to reduce AAA expansion rate.[91] Possible mechanisms for this effect include a reduction in heart rate, blood pressure, or cardiac contractility or a possible direct effect on the aortic wall. Based on animal models, propranolol was initially thought to stabilize collagen cross-linking, but later studies showed that this does not occur.[38, 194] Propranolol blocks circulating tissue plasminogen activator, and it may decrease expansion rate by reducing plasmin-mediated MMP activation.[246] Although not yet tested prospectively in a clinical trial, these results provide a reasonable basis, if no contraindications exist, to prescribe propranolol for patients with small AAAs managed medically.

ELECTIVE OPERATIVE RISK

Modern series from vascular centers of excellence report operative mortality rates of less than 5% for elective AAA repair.[138, 145] Population-based studies demonstrate somewhat higher mortality rates, such as 6.8% in male and 10.6% in female patients from Michigan from 1980 to 1990.[142] As expected, considerable variation occurs among individual patients and depends on specific operative risk factors.

In a meta-analysis, Steyerberg and colleagues identified seven prognostic factors that were independently predictive of operative mortality after elective AAA repair and calculated the relative risks for these factors (Table 89–2).[267] The

TABLE 89–2. INDEPENDENT RISK FACTORS FOR OPERATIVE MORTALITY AFTER ELECTIVE ABDOMINAL AORTIC ANEURYSM REPAIR

RISK FACTOR	ODDS RATIO*	95% CI
Creatinine > 1.8 mg/dl	3.3	1.5–7.5
Congestive heart failure	2.3	1.1–5.2
ECG ischemia	2.2	1.0–5.1
Pulmonary dysfunction	1.9	1.0–3.8
Older age (per decade)	1.5	1.2–1.8
Female gender	1.5	0.7–3.0

From Steyerberg EW, Kievit J, Alexander de Mol Van Otterloo JC, et al: Perioperative mortality of elective abdominal aortic aneurysm surgery: A clinical prediction rule based on literature and individual patient data. Arch Intern Med 155:1998, 1995.
*Odds ratio indicates relative risk compared to patients without that risk factor.
CI = confidence interval; ECG = electrocardiographic.

most important risk factors for increased operative mortality were renal dysfunction (creatinine level > 1.8 mg/dl), congestive heart failure (cardiogenic pulmonary edema, jugular vein distention, or the presence of a gallop rhythm), and ischemic changes on resting electrocardiogram (ECG) (ST depression > 2 mm). Age had a limited effect on mortality when corrected for the highly associated co-morbidities of cardiac, renal, and pulmonary dysfunction (mortality increased 1.5-fold per decade). This explains the excellent results reported in multiple series in which selected octogenarians who underwent elective AAA repair had mortality rates comparable with those of younger patients.[146]

Based on their own analysis, Steyerberg and associates developed a clinical prediction rule to estimate the operative mortality risk for individual patients undergoing elective AAA repair (Table 89–3).[267] This scoring system takes into account the seven independent risk factors plus the average overall elective mortality rate from a specific medical center. To demonstrate the impact of the risk factors listed earlier on a hypothetical patient, the predicted operative mortality rate for a 70-year-old man in a medical center with an average operative mortality rate of 5% could range from 2% if no risk factors were present to over 40% if cardiac, renal, and pulmonary co-morbidities were all present. Obviously, this would have a substantial impact on the decision to perform elective AAA repair.

A similar Bayesian model for perioperative cardiac risk assessment in vascular patients was reported by L'Italien and coworkers, who demonstrated the added predictive value of dipyridamole-thallium studies in patients with intermediate risk for cardiac death.[154] This study also demonstrated the protective effect of coronary artery bypass surgery within the previous 5 years, which reduced the risk of myocardial infarction or death following AAA repair by 2.2-fold. Although this type of statistical modeling cannot substitute for experienced clinical judgment, it helps to identify high-risk patients who might benefit from further evaluation, risk factor reduction, or medical management if AAA rupture risk is not high.

Medical center–specific mortality rate is an important consideration because results vary between centers and individual surgeons, independent of patient-specific risk factors. In part, this variation is due to volume and experience because low-volume hospitals and surgeons have demonstrably worse outcomes for AAA repair than higher-volume centers. In New York State in 1985 to 1987, age-adjusted and severity-adjusted operative mortality rate was 9% for elective AAA repair among surgeons who performed five or fewer procedures per year compared with only 4% for surgeons who performed more than 26 procedures per year.[290] Similarly, for hospitals where fewer than five procedures per year were performed, the operative mortality rate was 12% versus only 5% in hospitals where more than 38 procedures were performed per year. These results are significant because the average number of AAA repairs per surgeon was only 3.6 per year and per hospital, 10.2 per year. Thus, more than half of the procedures were performed by surgeons in hospitals with demonstrably worse results. In Norway, the operative mortality rate following elective AAA repair was 2.7-fold higher in hospitals performing fewer than 10 procedures per year and 2.6-fold lower in hospitals where more than 100 major vascular procedures were performed per year.[5] Similar observations in large series have been made by others.[142, 145]

SURGICAL DECISION MAKING

For patients with symptomatic AAAs, operative repair is usually appropriate because of the high mortality rate associated with rupture or thrombosis and the high likelihood of limb loss associated with peripheral embolism. Occa-

TABLE 89–3. PREDICTING OPERATIVE MORTALITY AFTER ELECTIVE ABDOMINAL AORTIC ANEURYSM (AAA) REPAIR

1. *Surgeon-specific average operative mortality*

Mortality (%):	3	4	5	6	8	12	
Score:	−5	−2	0	+2	+5	+10	_____

2. *Individual patient risk factors*

Age (years):	60	70	80	
Score:	−4	0	+4	_____

Gender:	Female	Male	
Score:	+4	0	_____

Cardiac co-morbidity:	MI	CHF	ECG ischemia	
Score:	+3	+8	−8	_____

Renal co-morbidity:	Creatinine > 1.8 mg/dl	
Score:	+12	_____

Pulmonary co-morbidity:	COPD, dyspnea	
Score:	+7	_____

3. *Estimated individual surgical mortality* TOTAL SCORE: _____

Total score:	−5	0	5	10	15	20	25	30	35	40
Mortality (%):	1	2	3	5	8	12	19	28	39	51

Based on total score from sum of scores for each risk factor (2), including surgeon-specific average mortality for elective AAA repair (1), estimate patient specific mortality from the table, line (3).

From Steyerberg EW, Kievit J, Alexander de Mol Van Otterloo JC, et al: Perioperative mortality of elective abdominal aortic aneurysm surgery: A clinical prediction rule based on literature and individual patient data. Arch Intern Med 155:1998, 1995.
MI = myocardial infarction; CHF = congestive heart failure; COPD = chronic obstructive pulmonary disease; ECG = electrocardiographic.

sionally, very-high-risk patients, or those with a short life expectancy, may choose to forego emergency repair of symptomatic AAAs, but, in general, surgical decision making for symptomatic AAAs is straightforward. For patients with asymptomatic AAAs, however, surgical decision making is often difficult. Repair of these aneurysms represents a prophylactic intervention designed to avoid rupture and to prolong life. Thus, appropriate decision making requires an accurate estimate of AAA rupture risk versus elective operative risk.

These factors must be considered in the context of an individual patient's life expectancy. On a population basis, age is the best predictor of life expectancy, which in the United States is approximately 18 years for a 60-year-old man, decreasing to 5 years for an 85-year-old man.[68] Obviously, however, for an individual patient, many other factors that influence life expectancy must also be considered, including both coexisting medical problems and family history of longevity. After successful AAA repair, long-term survival is reduced for patients with coronary artery disease, renal insufficiency, hypertension, and peripheral atherosclerosis.[68] With consideration of these factors in the context of patient age, it is possible to make reasonably accurate predictions of life expectancy to compare with rupture risk and operative mortality, as discussed later.

Because of the complexity of interaction among variables that influence AAA management, formal decision-analysis models have been constructed to aid in risk comparisons.[144, 190] It is reassuring that such models confirm the central importance of three key variables that have long been accepted by clinicians: elective operative risk, AAA rupture risk, and life expectancy. These models demonstrate that for a 70-year-old man with average life expectancy and average elective operative mortality (5%), AAA repair will improve life expectancy if annual AAA rupture risk exceeds

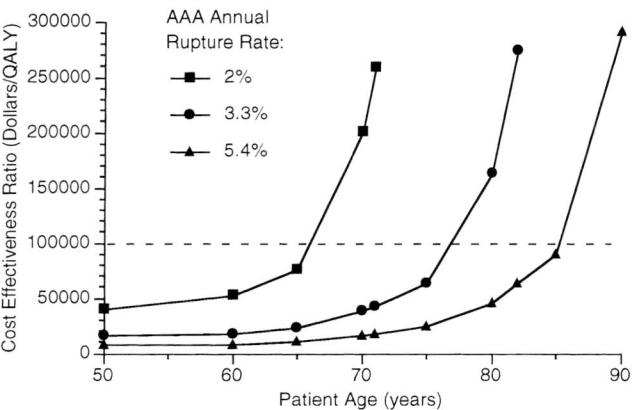

FIGURE 89–4. Cost-effectiveness of elective abdominal aortic aneurysm (AAA) repair as a function of age, at three different rupture risks, assuming an operative mortality of 5%.[143] Cost increases exponentially with age such that elective repair is not cost-effective above age 75 years for an AAA with a 3.3% annual rupture risk (~4.5 to 5 cm in diameter). (From Katz DA, Cronenwett JL: The cost-effectiveness of early surgery versus watchful waiting in the management of small abdominal aortic aneurysms. J Vasc Surg 19:980, 1994.)

1.5% per year.[144] For younger patients, the "threshold" AAA diameter (and rupture risk) that justifies elective repair is lower while for older patients the threshold diameter for elective repair increases as shown in Figure 89–3.

Of the three key factors that influence AAA decision-making, elective operative risk is most accurately estimated, followed by life expectancy and then rupture risk, which is most difficult to estimate accurately for individual AAAs. Thus, decision-analysis models are more helpful for guiding policy decisions concerning large populations than for individual patient decision making. However, such models help to focus attention on the most relevant variables for decision making and provide a framework with which to evaluate individual patients.

In addition to evaluating life expectancy, decision-analysis techniques can be used to evaluate cost-effectiveness, allowing a comparison of the value of AAA repair with other health care measures.[143] Although some physicians object to applying cost considerations to individual patients, decisions concerning scarce resource allocation, such as limiting preoperative cardiac testing or limiting intensive care postoperatively, are common. Furthermore, such analyses point out the impact of key variables on the cost-effectiveness of a procedure, such as the impact of age on the cost-effectiveness of elective AAA repair (Fig. 89–4).

Although there is no universal definition of "cost-effectiveness," it is generally agreed that an incremental cost-effectiveness ratio of less than $20,000 per quality adjusted life year (QALY) saved is very cost-effective, while an incremental cost of more than $100,000 per QALY is not cost-effective. Intermediate costs from $20,000 to $100,000 per QALY may be cost-effective and depend on societal values for the specific health care measure. As shown in Figure 89–4, the incremental cost of initial AAA repair compared with selective management and subsequent repair increases exponentially with age. Thus, for an AAA with a rupture risk of 3% per year (~4.5 to 5 cm in diameter), AAA repair is quite cost-effective for patients below age 70 to 75 years,

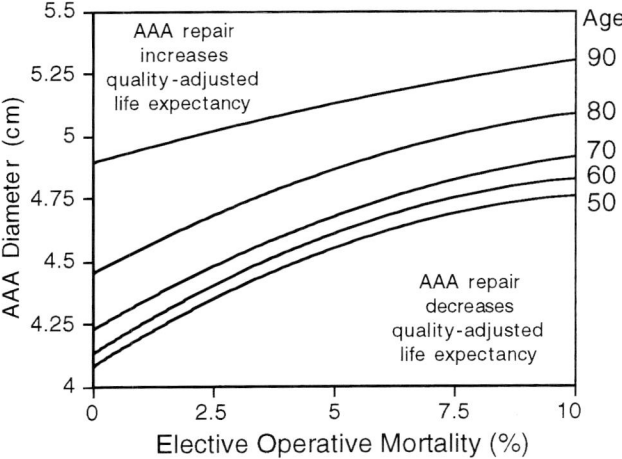

FIGURE 89–3. Impact of abdominal aortic aneurysm (AAA) diameter (rupture risk) and elective operative risk on optimal decision making for small AAAs based on decision analysis. For a 70-year-old man with a 5% elective operative risk, repair of AAAs larger than 4.7 cm optimizes life expectancy. At older ages or increased operative risk, this threshold diameter increases. At younger age or lower operative risk, the optimal threshold diameter for elective repair decreases, as shown. Based on decision analysis with average rupture risk = 1% for 4 to 4.9 cm in diameter and 11% for 5 to 5.9 cm in diameter (see Reed[231]), assuming a 10% per year expansion rate (see Cronenwett et al[72]).

but above this age the cost rises rapidly. Thus, for an 85-year-old man, AAA rupture risk needs to exceed approximately 5% per year (~6 cm in diameter) for elective repair to be "cost-effective." As discussed previously, age is only a surrogate for life expectancy in this model and must be carefully individualized. Furthermore, precise rupture risk is difficult to determine and may be influenced by factors other than diameter alone.

Based on the above discussion it is obvious that appropriate selection of patients for AAA repair is a complex process that is critically dependent on clinical judgment and on a patient's approach to current versus future risk taking. In general, patients with AAAs less than 4 cm in diameter should be followed by ultrasound size measurement at 6-month intervals and offered repair only if the aneurysm expands. Patients with AAAs of 4 to 5 cm in diameter may benefit from elective repair if they are young, have low risk, and have good life expectancy such that eventual repair is almost certain if a 5-cm diameter threshold is used. Depending on preference, these patients may be offered elective repair or ultrasound follow-up, assuming that a low perioperative risk can be ensured. Most patients with AAAs will not benefit from elective repair until the aneurysm is 5 cm in diameter, however, unless they have other risk factors for rupture (such as hypertension or COPD), because most aneurysms occur in older patients, with higher operative risk and reduced life expectancy. For higher-risk patients or very old patients, the optimal threshold for elective AAA repair may be as large as 6 to 7 cm in diameter. Thus, it is impossible to establish a precise or generic diameter criterion for elective AAA repair that applies to all patients. Careful, individual decision making is required to achieve optimal outcome.

PREOPERATIVE ASSESSMENT

Patient Evaluation

A careful history, thorough physical examination, and basic laboratory data are the most important factors for estimating perioperative risk and subsequent life expectancy. These factors may not only influence the decision to perform elective AAA repair but may also focus preoperative management to reduce modifiable risk. Because coronary artery disease is the largest single cause of early and late mortality after AAA repair,[237] it is discussed in detail in Chapter 40 and summarized briefly later.

The first issue to consider in preoperative evaluation, however, is whether a patient's current quality of life is sufficient in his or her opinion to justify a surgical procedure to potentially prolong life. In some debilitated elderly patients or those with mental deterioration this decision is difficult and must be made in conjunction with the extended family. Once this decision is made, attention must be directed to identifying risk factors that would increase operative risk or decrease otherwise expected survival such that prophylactic repair might not be warranted. Assessment of activity level, stamina, and stability of health is important in this regard and can be translated into metabolic equivalents to help assess both cardiac and pulmonary risks.[88] Because COPD is an independent predictor of oper-

ative mortality,[136] it should be assessed by pulmonary function studies or room air arterial blood gas measurement in patients who have suspected pulmonary disease. In some cases, preoperative treatment with bronchodilators and pulmonary toilet can reduce operative risk. In more extreme cases, pulmonary risk may substantially reduce life expectancy, and, in these cases, formal pulmonary consultation may be helpful to estimate survival. Serum creatinine level is one of the most important predictors of operative mortality[136] and must be assessed. The impact of other diseases, such as malignancy, on expected survival should also be carefully considered. It is well established that patients with AAAs have a high prevalence of coronary artery disease (CAD). By performing routine preoperative coronary arteriography at the Cleveland Clinic, Hertzer and colleagues established that only 6% of patients with AAAs had normal arteries; 29% had mild to moderate CAD; 29% had advanced compensated CAD; 31% had severe correctable CAD; and 5% had severe uncorrectable CAD.[123] Furthermore, Hertzer and colleagues established that clinical prediction of the severity of CAD was imperfect because 18% of patients without clinically apparent CAD had severe correctable CAD on arteriography compared with 44% of patients whose CAD was clinically apparent. This pivotal study led to intense efforts to identify risk factors and algorithms that more accurately predict the presence of severe CAD to justify its correction before AAA repair or to avoid AAA repair.

A number of clinical parameters, such as angina, history of myocardial infarction, Q-wave on ECG, ventricular arrhythmia, congestive heart failure, diabetes, and increasing age have been reported to increase the risk of postoperative cardiac events.[89, 305] Various combinations of these risk factors have been used to generate prediction algorithms for perioperative cardiac morbidity.[88, 208] These algorithms usually identify low-risk, high-risk, and intermediate-risk patients. For high-risk patients, such as those with unstable angina, more sophisticated cardiac evaluation is required, while low-risk patients may undergo elective AAA repair without further testing. For intermediate-risk patients, who comprise the vast majority with AAAs, decision making is more difficult and may be facilitated by additional cardiac testing.[89]

Radionuclide stress scanning (either exercise-induced or dipyridamole-induced), or stress echocardiography (dolbutamine-induced), is most frequently used for this purpose and has a high negative predictive value; that is, patients with a normal stress response have a very low probability of perioperative myocardial complications.[73, 156] For patients with abnormal stress response, however, the positive predictive value of these tests is low because many such patients can safely undergo elective AAA repair. Although many initial studies demonstrated a high predictive value for dipyridamole-thallium scanning in patients undergoing AAA repair,[30, 167, 168] later studies have not found that routine screening is cost-effective.[42, 74, 247] In fact, it appears that increasing age and clinical indicators of CAD are better predictors of adverse cardiac outcome after AAA repair.[8] This has led to considerable debate about the appropriateness of extensive cardiac evaluation and potential treatment of patients before elective AAA repair.

If significant CAD or other cardiac risk such as valvular

disease or congestive heart failure is identified preoperatively in a patient with an AAA, three options are possible: (1) delay or avoid AAA repair, (2) perform AAA repair with more intensive cardiac monitoring and management, or (3) reduce cardiac risk before AAA surgery with coronary artery bypass graft, coronary angioplasty, or stenting. Option 1 is most applicable to patients with small, low-risk AAAs or to elderly patients in whom the added benefit of AAA repair is marginal. Proponents of option 2 cite the low mortality of AAA repair without preoperative cardiac surgery and the added mortality from cardiac intervention that must be considered.[280] In contrast, proponents of option 3 point out the need to ensure long-term survival in order to gain the benefit of AAA repair and the survival benefit of coronary artery bypass graft in appropriately selected patients.[122, 126] Because no randomized trial has been conducted to address the benefit of prophylactic coronary revascularization before elective AAA repair, this question remains an issue for individualized decision making based on local outcomes.

With improved techniques for perioperative management of AAA patients, however, such as the routine use of perioperative beta-blockade, there is a trend toward less extensive preoperative cardiac evaluation. In this regard, the American Heart Association has developed consensus recommendations regarding the preoperative cardiac evaluation of patients with peripheral vascular disease.[88] The impact of cardiac risk assessment is particularly relevant for AAA repair (or any prophylactic operation) because it can change the decision of whether to repair a given risk aneurysm. For patients without clinically apparent heart disease, sophisticated cardiac testing has little impact on decision making for large, high-risk AAAs but is more relevant for lower-risk, small AAAs for which operative mortality must be especially low to justify elective repair.[247] For the rare patient with unstable CAD and a very large (or symptomatic) AAA, coronary revascularization combined with AAA repair may be indicated.[124, 238]

Alternatively, perioperative intra-aortic balloon counterpulsation has been used successfully in high-risk cardiac patients who required AAA repair.[128] In these cases, the intra-aortic balloon can be introduced via the femoral artery and advanced through the graft after completing the proximal aortic anastomosis. The distal aortic or iliac anastomosis is then constructed with the device in place, maintaining hemostasis with a Rummel's tourniquet around the proximal graft. These techniques are seldom required, however, because elective AAA repair is not likely to prolong life in patients with such severe cardiac disease unless this can be corrected. Lower-risk endovascular AAA repair appears particularly well suited for such patients (see Chapter 90).

Aneurysm Evaluation

Most surgeons recommend a preoperative imaging study with CT scanning, MRI or MRA, or arteriography. Contrast-enhanced CT scanning appears to be the most useful study for preoperative AAA evaluation with regard to information obtained, invasiveness, and cost. This is particularly true for spiral CT scanning, with thin "slices" in the region of interest. This allows not only accurate size measurements but also accurate definition of the relationship of an AAA

to visceral and renal arteries. Iliac artery aneurysms are easily detected by CT scanning, and even occlusive disease of intra-abdominal vessels is often apparent. Furthermore, CT scanning aids in the identification of venous anomalies, such as a retroaortic left renal vein or a duplicated vena cava, or renal abnormalities, such as horseshoe or pelvic kidney, which would influence operative techniques and approach.

CT scanning is thus the technique of choice for identifying suspected inflammatory aneurysms and may reveal unsuspected abdominal pathology, such as associated malignancy or gallbladder disease. Furthermore, for juxtarenal or suprarenal aneurysms, CT scanning can define the most appropriate location for suprarenal cross-clamping, based on the detailed relationship of the visceral arteries, and can identify potentially associated aortic wall calcification (see Chapter 14).

MRI is comparable to CT scanning in terms of AAA measurement accuracy and other preoperative planning issues. It avoids intravenous contrast, which may represent an advantage over CT scanning for selected patients. Because it is more expensive and time-consuming, however, MRI is not as widely utilized as CT scanning. When MRA is included with MRI, however, it can significantly increase the value when arteriography would otherwise be required. In medical centers with surgeons who have sufficient experience using this technique, MRA has been demonstrated to be accurate for determining the presence of occlusive disease in intra-abdominal arteries (see Chapter 15).

Historically, arteriography was usually used for preoperative evaluation of AAAs and adjacent arteries. Unfortunately, it has substantially more risk than the other imaging techniques due to its invasive nature, is associated with both contrast and radiation exposure, and is very expensive. This has led to more reliance on CT scanning for routine preoperative AAA evaluation, especially because CT scanning can detect associated pathologic problems that cannot be detected with arteriography. Thus, arteriography is now reserved for the preoperative evaluation of AAAs in patients who have suspected disease of adjacent arteries and detailed evaluation of the arterial lumen will affect the conduct of the AAA repair.[51] Usually these are patients with associated renal or mesenteric disease, iliofemoral occlusive disease, or anomalies such as horseshoe or pelvic kidney. The development of endovascular AAA repair has renewed the need for arteriography for precise preoperative device measurement, but even for this indication three-dimensional CT scanning appears to have comparable value (see Chapter 14).

MEDICAL MANAGEMENT

For patients with low-risk AAAs (small diameter without other risk factors for rupture) being followed with periodic size measurements, attempts should be made to reduce both expansion rate and rupture risk. Thus, smoking cessation is critical, and hypertension should be aggressively controlled. Although not definitively proven, there is increasing evidence to support treatment with propranolol if contraindications (e.g., bronchospastic conditions, congestive heart failure) are not present.[91, 105, 159] Because the optimal dose of propranolol has not been established in clinical trials, a schedule of 40 mg twice daily seems reasonable if tolerated. For patients with small AAAs and hypertension, propranolol is an ideal component of the antihypertensive regimen.

Because diameter measurement by CT scanning is more accurate than by ultrasound, it has been suggested that AAAs should be followed by CT rather than ultrasound size measurements. Because ultrasonography is much less expensive and less invasive, however, most physicians continue to use this technique. Comparing sequential ultrasound scans should provide increased accuracy in terms of relative change if current and previous images are actually compared. The question remains whether CT scanning should be used as the final determinant for recommending repair of "borderline"-sized AAAs. Because most patients undergo a CT scan for preoperative planning, however, this is usually a moot point. It can also be argued that the accuracy of ultrasonograpy is as precise as our present knowledge of AAA rupture risk based on size. Nonetheless, because ultrasound appears to underestimate AAA diameter systematically by 2 to 4 mm compared with CT scanning,[134, 164, 283] it seems reasonable to recommend a CT size measurement for AAAs followed by ultrasound examination if the AAAs approach the threshold for elective repair.

SURGICAL TREATMENT

Since about 1960, AAAs have been repaired with the technique of endoaneurysmorrhaphy with intraluminal graft placement, as described by Creech.[67] This procedure is described later (see Transperitoneal Approach). The development of this technique was based in part on the failure of previous "nonresective" operations, including aneurysm ligation, wrapping, and attempts at inducing aneurysm thrombosis, that yielded uniformly dismal results. AAA thrombosis by iliac ligation combined with axillobifemoral bypass enjoyed a brief resurgence in popularity for very-high-risk patients but had a high complication rate, including late aneurysm rupture, and an operative mortality rate comparable with conventional repair in similar patients.[127, 133, 141, 177, 248] Thus, this technique was similarly abandoned.

As an alternative to standard, open AAA repair, Shah and colleagues proposed exclusion of an AAA with bypass to reduce operative blood loss.[252] This technique is also described later (see Retroperitoneal Approach). A promising technique for AAA repair using an endovascular approach was devised by Parodi and coworkers in 1991.[209] This method involves the transfemoral placement of a prosthetic graft that incorporates some type of stent-like attachment device. Because this less-invasive technique has the potential to reduce morbidity and mortality, it has received considerable attention and is described in detail in Chapter 90.

In another attempt to reduce the invasiveness of AAA repair, the use of laparoscopy was suggested to assist AAA repair. Laparoscopic techniques were used to dissect the aneurysm neck and iliac arteries followed by a standard endoaneurysmorrhaphy through a minilaparotomy. Kline and associates reported their results in 20 patients to demonstrate the feasibility of this approach, but a clear benefit has not been shown because the intraoperative, intensive care unit, and total hospital duration appear comparable with those of conventional AAA repair.[148] Further experience with this technique may identify a subgroup of patients for whom a laparoscopic-assisted AAA repair is advantageous.

Perioperative Management

Preoperative intravenous antibiotics (usually a cephalosporin) are administered to reduce the risk of prosthetic graft infection.[140] Ample intravenous access, intra-arterial pressure recording, and Foley catheter monitoring of urine output are routine. For patients with associated cardiac disease, pulmonary artery catheters are frequently used to guide volume replacement and vasodilator or inotrope therapy both intraoperatively and in the early postoperative period. Mixed venous oxygen tension measurements, available with these catheters, can provide an additional estimate of global circulatory function. Transesophageal echocardiography can be useful in selected patients to monitor ventricular volume and cardiac wall motion abnormalities and to guide fluid administration and the use of vasoactive drugs. Despite the frequent use of pulmonary artery catheters during AAA surgery, studies examining their efficacy have been unable to easily demonstrate added value.[20, 308] These studies, however, have usually excluded very-high-risk patients, who are most likely to benefit from such monitoring. Because these techniques are not without risk, selective use is probably more appropriate than routine application.

Because the blood lost during AAA repair often requires replacement, intraoperative autotransfusion as well as preoperative autologous blood donation have become popular, primarily to avoid the infection risk associated with allogeneic transfusion. Studies of the cost-effectiveness of such procedures, however, question their routine use.[28, 113, 131] Autologous blood donation is less important for elderly patients in whom life expectancy is shorter than the usual time for development of transfusion-associated viral illness. Because the allogeneic blood pool has become safer and the transfusion requirement for elective AAA repair lower, autologous blood donation does not appear to be cost-effective for elderly cardiovascular patients.[28] Intraoperative autotransfusion during AAA repair is widely used because of its documented safety.[204] Systems that use cell separation and return only red blood cells cause fewer coagulation disturbances than systems that return whole blood.[11] Because of the fixed costs associated with autotransfusion equipment, however, studies have shown that this technique is not cost-effective unless an approximately 1000 ml blood loss occurs.[113, 131] Because it is usually difficult to predict the volume of blood loss during AAA repair, most surgeons employ autotransfusion in case blood loss becomes extensive. An intermediate solution is to employ only the reservoir component of an autotransfusion system and process the collected blood (using the more expensive components of these systems) only if blood loss is sufficient to justify this.[131] Optimizing oxygen delivery to patients with reduced cardiac output by maintaining an adequate hematocrit appears beneficial for patients undergoing AAA repair. One study has shown that a postoperative hematocrit less than 28% was associated with significant cardiac morbidity in vascular surgery patients.[197]

Maintenance of normal body temperature during aortic surgery is important to prevent coagulopathy, allow extubation, and maintain normal metabolic function. In a review of patients undergoing elective AAA repair, Bush and associates noted significantly more organ dysfunction (53% versus 29%) and higher mortality (12% versus 1.5%) in hypothermic patients (temperature < 34.5°C) than in normothermic patients.[45] The only predictor of intraoperative hypothermia was female gender, and prolonged hypothermia was related to initial hypothermia, indicating the difficulty in rewarming cold patients. A recent randomized trial found significantly reduced cardiac morbidity (1.4% versus 6.3%) in patients who were normothermic (36.7°C) versus hypothermic (35.4°C) intraoperatively.[102] To prevent hypothermia, a recirculating warm forced-air blanket should be placed in contact with the patient and intravenous fluids, including any blood returned from an autotransfusion device, should be warmed before administration.

Anesthesia

Most patients undergo general anesthesia for AAA repair. The use of supplemental continuous epidural anesthesia, begun immediately preoperatively and continued for postoperative pain control, is increasing.[184] This technique allows a lighter level of general anesthesia to be maintained while pain is controlled through the epidural blockade. Additional benefits may include a reduction in the sympathetic-catecholamine stress response, which might decrease cardiac complications. One randomized trial comparing general anesthesia with combined general-epidural anesthesia demonstrated decreased rates of deaths, cardiac events, infection, and overall complications.[306] However, these benefits were not observed in another randomized trial,[10] suggesting that the details of perioperative management and patient selection may determine the impact of epidural anesthesia. Furthermore, it is possible that the major benefit of epidural anesthesia accrues in the postoperative period rather than intraoperatively.[227] Although concern has been raised about possible complications of epidural hematoma in patients whose blood is anticoagulated, this has proven to be extremely rare when the epidural catheter is inserted before and removed after anticoagulation.[9]

Preoperative beta-adrenergic blockade is an important adjunct to reduce left ventricular work by decreasing heart rate, blood pressure, and cardiac contractility. This blockade decreases myocardial oxygen demand to reduce or prevent ischemia. Pasternack and coworkers demonstrated that patients who underwent vascular surgery and received metoprolol immediately before operation had significantly lower heart rate and less intraoperative myocardial ischemia than untreated controls.[211] A recent randomized, placebo-controlled trial assessed the effect of atenolol (given intravenously immediately before and after surgery and orally during that hospitalization) in patients at risk for CAD who underwent noncardiac surgery.[181] A significant reduction in mortality extending 2 years after discharge was observed in the atenolol-treated patients (3% versus 14% 1-year mortality) due to a reduction in death from cardiac causes. This

simple and low-risk adjunctive treatment is applicable to most patients undergoing AAA repair unless contraindications of congestive heart failure, third-degree heart block, and bronchospasm are present.

Choice of Incision

AAA repair can be accomplished through an anterior transperitoneal incision (midline or transverse) or through a retroperitoneal approach (left or right side). Midline, transperitoneal incisions can be performed rapidly and provide wide access to the abdomen, but may be associated with more pulmonary complications due to postoperative splinting from upper abdominal pain. Transverse abdominal incisions, just above or below the umbilicus, require more time to open and close, but may be associated with fewer pulmonary complications and late incisional hernias. Retroperitoneal incisions, from the lateral rectus margin extending into the tenth or eleventh intercostal space, afford good exposure of both the infrarenal and suprarenal aorta, but limit exposure of the contralateral renal and iliac arteries. In addition, this exposure does not allow access to intra-abdominal organs unless the peritoneum is purposely opened so that associated abdominal disease can remain undetected.

The left retroperitoneal approach is used more often than the right approach for exposure of the upper abdominal aorta because the spleen is easier to mobilize and retract than the liver. The right retroperitoneal approach is used when specific abdominal problems, such as a stoma, preclude the left-sided approach.[54] In recent years, the left retroperitoneal approach has become more popular due to suggestions that pulmonary morbidity, ileus, and intravenous fluid requirements are decreased postoperatively. Randomized trials have resulted in different conclusions about the potential advantages of retroperitoneal over transabdominal incisions, however. Sicard and associates reported more prolonged ileus, small bowel obstruction, and overall complications after transabdominal than retroperitoneal aortic surgery, although pulmonary complications were similar.[256] Cambria and coworkers found no differences in these incisions in terms of pulmonary complications, fluid or blood requirements, or other postoperative complications except slightly prolonged return to oral intake after the transperitoneal approach.[49]

In the most recent randomized trial, Sieunarine and coworkers found no difference in operating time, cross-clamp time, blood loss, fluid requirement, analgesia requirement, gastrointestinal function, intensive care unit stay, or hospital stay for transperitoneal versus retroperitoneal approaches for aortic surgery.[257] In long-term follow-up, however, there were significantly more wound problems (hernias, bulging, and pain) in the retroperitoneal group. These results suggest that, in most cases, the choice of incision for AAA repair is a matter of personal preference.

Both the transperitoneal and retroperitoneal approaches, however, have advantages in certain patients. Relative indications for retroperitoneal exposure include a "hostile" abdomen due to multiple previous transperitoneal operations, an abdominal wall stoma, a horseshoe kidney, an inflammatory aneurysm, or anticipated need for suprarenal endarterectomy or anastomosis. Relative indications for a transperitoneal approach include a ruptured AAA, coexistent intra-abdominal pathologic problems, uncertain diagnosis, left-sided vena cava, large bilateral iliac aneurysms, or need for access to both renal arteries. Exposure of sufficient normal aorta proximal to a juxtarenal AAA may be difficult via a transperitoneal approach. Ligation and division of the left renal vein is an alternative, but can lead to renal dysfunction.[2, 48, 136] Left retroperitoneal exposure, with displacement of the left kidney anteriorly, avoids this problem and facilitates suprarenal exposure.[254] Need for concomitant renal or mesenteric revascularization may dictate specific operative approaches. The left retroperitoneal approach is optimal for left renal, celiac, and superior mesenteric artery (SMA) revascularization, as well as transaortic endarterectomy of these vessels. Bypass grafting (and endarterectomy) of the right renal artery is more easily accomplished by a transperitoneal exposure (or a right retroperitoneal approach if other visceral arteries need not be exposed). Because of the advantages of each approach in the situations described, it is advisable for surgeons to become proficient with both techniques.

Transperitoneal Approach

After the abdomen is entered through a transperitoneal incision, it is thoroughly explored to exclude other pathology and to assess the extent of the aneurysm. The transverse colon is then retracted superiorly, and the ligament of Treitz is divided to allow retraction of the small bowel to the right. Exposure is greatly facilitated with a fixed, self-retaining retractor. A longitudinal incision is made in the peritoneum just to the left of the base of the small bowel mesentery to expose the aneurysm. This incision extends from the inferior border of the pancreas proximally to the level of normal iliac arteries distally. Care must be taken to avoid the ureters, especially if exposure includes the iliac bifurcation where the ureters normally cross. Autonomic nerves to the pelvis course anterior to the proximal left common iliac artery and should be retracted with associated retroperitoneal tissue rather than incised to prevent sexual dysfunction in men. The left renal vein should be identified and retracted superiorly, if necessary, to fully expose the neck of the aneurysm. The surgeon must take care not to avulse renal vein tributaries, particularly a descending lumbar vein, frequently encountered to the left of the aorta, which must be divided before the left renal vein is mobile enough to allow upward retraction.

Rarely, proximal exposure cannot be obtained without division of the left renal vein. In such cases, this should be done at its junction with the vena cava to maintain patency of collateral drainage via adrenal and gonadal branches. In most cases, reanastomosis is not required, but can be performed if proximal renal vein engorgement suggests inadequate collateral drainage.

After adequate aortoiliac exposure is obtained, the normal aorta and iliac arteries are dissected sufficiently to place a vascular clamp proximal and distal to the aneurysm. Regardless of the proximal extent of an infrarenal AAA, it is desirable to construct the proximal aortic anastomosis near the renal arteries to avoid subsequent aneurysmal degeneration of residual infrarenal aorta. When an AAA approaches or involves the renal arteries, it can be safer to apply the cross-clamp proximal to the celiac artery rather than between the renal arteries and the SMA.

Green and coworkers demonstrated much higher operative mortality (32% versus 3%) and renal failure requiring dialysis (23% versus 3%) after infrarenal AAA repair when clamping was performed between the SMA and renal arteries versus proximal to the celiac artery.[115] They attributed this to the greater likelihood of dislodging atherosclerotic debris in the pararenal aorta as opposed to the supraceliac aorta, which is usually less diseased. Complications resulted from atheroembolization to the kidneys, legs, and intestine or from injury to the aorta or renal arteries.

Others have also noted the relative safety of clamping the supraceliac aorta, which can easily be accessed by dividing the gastrohepatic ligament and the diaphragmatic crus.[32] Aortic clamping between the renal arteries and the SMA is also safe, however, when performed in properly selected patients without extensive plaque in this region.[201] Occasionally, it is possible to obtain distal control of an AAA on the aorta, but usually aneurysmal changes or calcification in this location make iliac clamping preferred. A disease-free area of proximal aorta and iliac arteries should be identified for clamping to minimize the possibility of clamp injury or embolization of arterial debris. Some iliac arteries may be so diffusely calcified that clamping without injury is impossible. In such cases, internal occlusion with a balloon catheter or extension of the graft to the femoral arteries is required. In most cases, it is unnecessary to encircle the aorta and iliac arteries completely because vascular clamps can be placed in the anteroposterior direction, leaving the back wall undissected. This minimizes the likelihood of injury to both lumbar and iliac veins. Sometimes posterior arterial plaque necessitates placement of a vascular clamp transversely on either the aorta or iliac arteries, which then require careful posterior dissection precisely on the plane of the artery to avoid venous injury.

AAA repair can be accomplished with a straight ("tube") graft in 40% to 50% of patients without extension onto the iliac arteries.[138, 203] Although concern has been raised about the potential for future aneurysm development in the iliac arteries after tube graft repair of AAAs, late follow-up has shown that this is not clinically significant if the iliac arteries were not aneurysmal at the time of AAA repair.[225] Extension to the iliac arteries with a bifurcated graft for AAA repair is necessary in the remaining 50% to 60% of patients due to aneurysmal involvement of the iliac arteries or to severe calcification of the aortic bifurcation. Extension of the graft to the femoral level is indicated for severe concomitant iliac occlusive disease or rarely because of technical difficulties associated with a deep pelvic anastomosis. Iliac anastomoses are preferred, however, due to decreased infection and pseudoaneurysm complications compared with femoral anastomoses.

Prosthetic grafts available for AAA repair include knitted polyester (Dacron), knitted Dacron impregnated with collagen or gelatin to decrease porosity, woven Dacron, and polytetrafluoroethylene (PTFE). These and other graft choices are discussed in detail in Chapter 37. There is no clear evidence that any of these graft types provides superior outcome. In a prospective randomized comparison of PTFE and Dacron, long-term patency was equivalent, but PTFE had a higher incidence of early graft failure and graft sepsis.[222] In contrast, in a smaller trial with shorter follow-up, PTFE was found to be superior.[175] Most surgeons prefer an impervious graft to avoid the need for preclotting and thus select impregnated knitted Dacron, PTFE, or woven Dacron.[220] This not only saves time and more reliably prevents bleeding through the graft, but also allows graft selection to be delayed until the aneurysm is opened so that a graft diameter corresponding to the inner diameter of the normal proximal aorta can be selected. It also allows delayed selection of a straight versus bifurcated graft that may not always be obvious before the aneurysm is open and the distal aorta can be carefully inspected.

Most surgeons use heparin anticoagulation during aortic cross-clamping to reduce lower extremity thrombotic complications. Heparin dosage varies from 50 to 150 units/kg based on personal preference. Activated clotting time (ACT) measurement is useful to determine the need for supplemental heparin in prolonged cases and the appropriate dose of protamine sulfate to reverse anticoagulation after declamping.[178]

The sequence for applying proximal and distal vascular clamps is selected to apply the initial clamp in the area of least atherosclerotic disease in order to reduce the risk of distal embolization. The aneurysm is opened longitudinally along its anterior surface, away from the inferior mesenteric artery (IMA) in case this requires later reimplantation. The proximal aorta is then incised horizontally at the level selected for proximal anastomosis (Fig. 89–5). To avoid potential injury to posterior veins, this incision does not

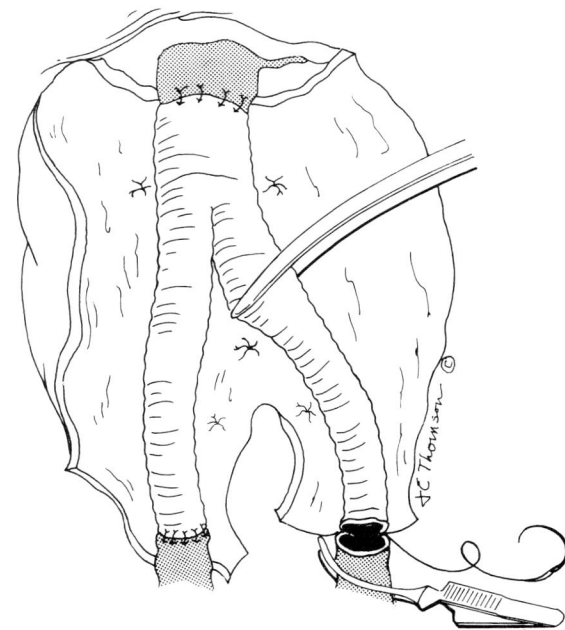

FIGURE 89–6. Completing the iliac anastomosis of an abdominal aortic aneurysm repair. Lumbar artery orifices have been suture ligated. Flow has already been established through the right graft limb.

need to extend through the back wall of the aorta, although some surgeons prefer complete transection for better exposure. Intraluminal thrombotic material and atherosclerotic debris are extracted from the aneurysm, which usually discloses several back-bleeding lumbar artery orifices that require suture ligation. If the IMA is patent, it should be controlled temporarily with a small vascular clamp (see Fig. 89–5) so that its need for reimplantation can be assessed after the revascularization is completed. IMA revascularization may be advised if the hypogastric arteries are diseased or if one requires ligation for technical reasons.

Once hemostasis within the opened aneurysm sac has been achieved, the proximal anastomosis is performed. There is often a distinct ring at the aneurysm neck that defines the appropriate level for this anastomosis. Most surgeons use a polypropylene suture, taking large aortic "bites" and incorporating a double thickness of posterior aortic wall for added strength. If the aortic wall is friable, pledgets of PTFE (Teflon) or Dacron can be incorporated into the suture line. After the proximal anastomosis is completed, the graft is clamped and the proximal aortic clamp is released briefly to check for and correct any suture line bleeding. If the distal anastomosis is to the aorta, a similar technique is used just above its bifurcation, with sutures from within the lumen that encompass both iliac artery orifices within the suture line. If iliac artery aneurysms exist, these are incised anteriorly so that the limbs of a bifurcated graft can be sutured to the normal iliac artery beyond these aneurysms (Fig. 89–6). Often this requires graft extension to the common iliac bifurcation, including the orifices of both the internal and external iliac arteries within the distal anastomosis. In rare instances, aneurysmal involvement of the distal common iliac artery may preclude anastomosis to both the internal and external iliac artery orifices because these are widely separated. In

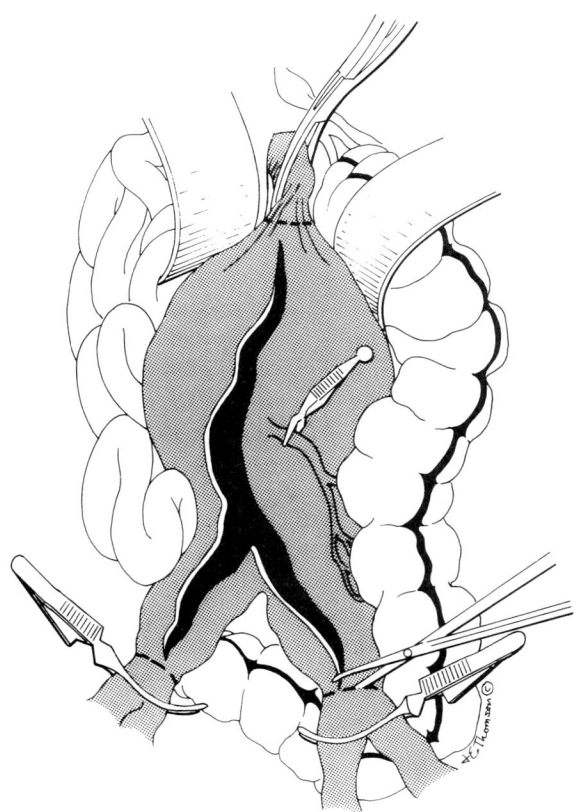

FIGURE 89–5. Transabdominal aortic aneurysm exposure, vascular clamps in place, incising the aneurysm.

such cases, an external iliac artery anastomosis can be constructed, but care must be taken to preserve adequate pelvic blood flow, which may mean direct revascularization of at least one internal iliac artery.

The need for internal iliac revascularization is usually assessed by the extent of back-bleeding, as discussed later (see Isolated Iliac Aneurysms). For large aneurysms of the left iliac artery, medial reflection of the sigmoid mesocolon facilitates a retroperitoneal approach to the distal common iliac artery and prevents unnecessary dissection of autonomic nerves crossing the proximal left common iliac artery. Before the distal anastomoses are completed, arterial clamps are carefully removed and vigorous irrigation is used to flush out any thrombus or debris.

When the first iliac (or distal aortic) anastomosis is completed, flow into that extremity should be restored, releasing the clamp slowly to minimize "declamping" hypotension. Declamping shock is rare if adequate intravenous fluid replacement has been administered. However, sudden restoration of blood flow into a dilated distal vascular bed and the associated venous return of vasoactive substances that have accumulated in the ischemic limbs usually cause some hypotension. Declamping should therefore be gradual and carefully coordinated with the anesthesia team because additional volume administration can be required. In some cases, the clamp must be intermittently reapplied to allow adequate volume resuscitation and prevent hypotension.

After restoration of lower extremity and pelvic blood flow, the IMA and sigmoid colon are inspected. The IMA can be ligated with a transfixing suture applied to its internal orifice if it is small and not associated with known SMA occlusive disease, if it has good back-flow on release of its vascular clamp, if the sigmoid color and arterial pulsations are good, and if at least one internal iliac artery is patent. In questionable cases, Doppler signals from the sigmoid colon or an assessment of IMA stump pressure[94] may be necessary to determine the need for IMA reimplantation (see Chapter 113). In the rare circumstances when sigmoid colon perfusion appears marginal, a circular cuff

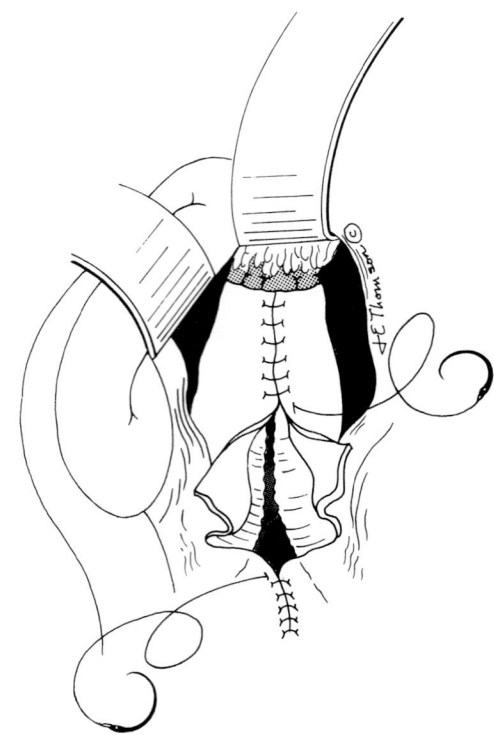

FIGURE 89–8. Closing the aneurysm sac and retroperitoneum between the graft and duodenum.

of the aortic wall around the IMA orifice is excised (Carrel patch) and anastomosed to the left side of the graft (Fig. 89–7).

Next, the adequacy of lower extremity blood flow is determined by visual inspection of the feet, palpation of distal pulses, or more sophisticated Doppler or pulse volume recording. If reduced blood flow is detected, intraoperative arteriography can differentiate thrombosis or embolism from peripheral vasoconstriction, which is relatively common if the procedure is prolonged and the patient is cold. Embolism or thrombosis requires prompt surgical correction, while vasoconstriction requires correction of any volume deficit and rewarming.

After adequate intestinal and lower extremity circulation is ensured, heparin effect is reversed with protamine sulfate if sufficient heparin has been given to justify reversal and hemostasis is achieved. The aneurysm wall and retroperitoneum are then closed over the graft to provide a tissue barrier between the prosthesis and the adjacent intestine (Fig. 89–8). The aortic prosthesis and upper anastomosis must be isolated from the overlying duodenum during closure; if necessary, a pedicle of greater omentum can be interposed to achieve this purpose. The small bowel should be inspected carefully and replaced in its normal position before abdominal closure.

Retroperitoneal Approach

Proper patient positioning is essential to achieve optimal exposure with the retroperitoneal approach. For most infrarenal AAAs, a left retroperitoneal incision centered on the 11th or 12th rib is employed. The patient's left shoulder

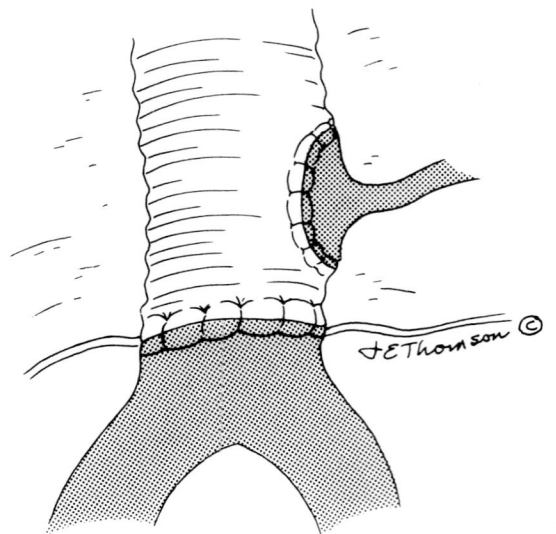

FIGURE 89–7. Reimplanting the inferior mesenteric artery with Carrel patch technique after aneurysm repair with tube graft.

is elevated at a 45- to 60-degree angle relative to the table while the pelvis is positioned relatively flat. The table is flexed, with the break positioned at a level midway between the iliac crest and the costal margin (Fig. 89–9). An air-evacuating "bean bag" is helpful to maintain proper positioning.

Beginning at the lateral border of the left rectus muscle midway between the pubis and umbilicus, the skin incision is carried superiorly and then curved laterally up to the tip of the 11th or 12th rib. If extensive exposure of the right iliac artery is required, the incision can be extended infero-laterally into the right lower quadrant, or a separate right lower quadrant retroperitoneal incision can be used. The underlying lateral abdominal wall muscles are divided, exposing the underlying peritoneum and the anterior edge of the properitoneal fat layer at the lateral aspect of this exposure. Dissection in the retroperitoneal plane is then developed, either anterior or posterior to the left kidney, until the aorta is encountered.

For infrarenal aneurysm exposure, it is often sufficient to proceed anteriorly and leave the left kidney in its normal position. For juxtarenal or suprarenal aneurysms that require more cephalad exposure, the kidney is mobilized anteriorly to approach the aorta from behind the left renal artery (Fig. 89–10). If the need for higher exposure is anticipated, the incision should be directed more cephalad over the ninth or 10th rib and the shoulders positioned as near perpendicular to the table as possible. In this case,

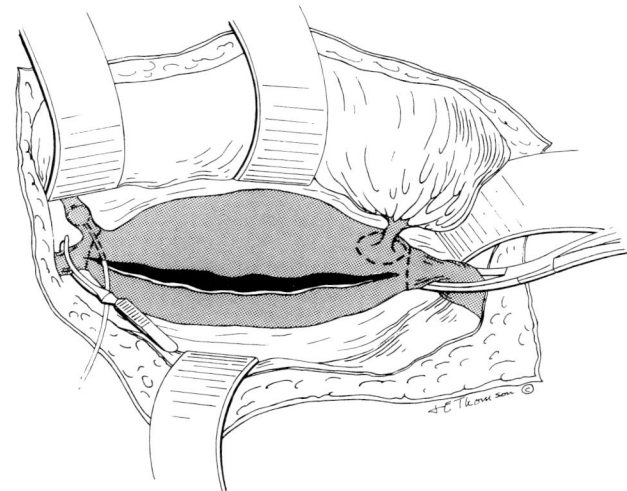

FIGURE 89–10. Retroperitoneal aortic exposure with left kidney retracted anteriorly for repair of a suprarenal abdominal aortic aneurysm. The left renal artery is to be reimplanted as a Carrel patch. The right iliac artery is controlled with a balloon catheter.

more table flexion is required to open the space between the pelvis and ribs, and the trunk is twisted so that the angle between the pelvis and the table is about 30 degrees.

When the aorta is approached from behind the left renal artery, it is necessary to divide a large lumbar branch of the left renal vein to mobilize the kidney and renal vein anteriorly. The ureter must be identified and retracted medially with the kidney, with care taken to separate it from the iliac bifurcation distally. Medial mobilization of the peritoneal contents exposes the IMA, which usually is divided for more complete exposure of the aortic bifurcation and right renal artery, depending on the size of the AAA. Exposure is greatly facilitated by using a fixed, self-retaining retractor. If necessary, exposure of the right iliac artery and right renal artery is easier after the AAA is opened and decompressed. Right iliac artery control is often best accomplished with a balloon occlusion catheter after entering the aneurysm (see Fig. 89–10).

After adequate exposure is achieved, repair of the AAA is usually carried out as described for the transperitoneal approach. The retroperitoneal technique does not normally afford an opportunity to inspect colonic and intestinal viability, but the peritoneum can be opened to accomplish this if any concern exists.

As an alternative to open AAA repair with in-lying graft replacement, it is possible to exclude and bypass an AAA without opening the sac.[252] The potential advantage of this technique is avoidance of blood loss associated with back-bleeding lumbar arteries during conventional open repair. A potential disadvantage is possible continued expansion and rupture of an excluded AAA if thrombosis does not occur. Shah and associates reported the outcome of 280 AAAs treated by exclusion and bypass with the retroperitoneal approach.[252] Operative mortality was 4%, morbidity was 6%, blood loss was minimal, and only two patients with anticoagulation required further treatment for aneurysm sac expansion and rupture during long-term follow-up.

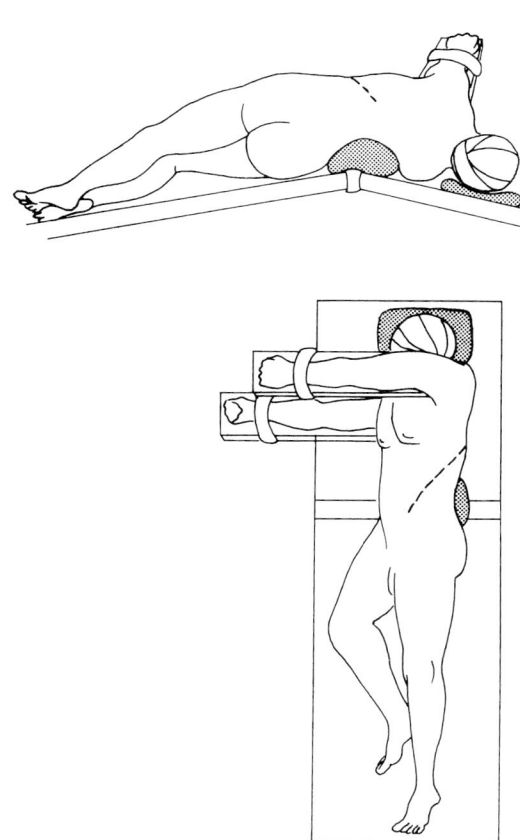

FIGURE 89–9. Positioning and the skin incision for the retroperitoneal approach to abdominal aortic aneurysm repair.

In a randomized trial that compared open endoaneurysmorrhaphy versus exclusion and bypass, Paty and associates found lower postoperative complications (10% versus 24%), lower blood loss (700 versus 1000 ml), and shorter hospital stay in the exclusion-bypass group than the open group.[213] Only 4% of excluded and bypassed AAAs failed to thrombose, and none ruptured during 10 months' follow-up. Despite the reported advantages of this technique compared with open AAA repair, the exclusion-bypass procedure has not achieved widespread usage and these study results have not been duplicated in other medical centers.

Associated Arterial Disease

Indications for concomitant mesenteric or renal artery revascularization during elective AAA repair are comparable with those for isolated disease in these arteries. Occasionally, patients with asymptomatic, high-grade stenoses of these arteries will warrant "prophylactic" concomitant reconstruction if the patient is at low operative risk and the AAA repair proceeds uneventfully. Although the natural history of asymptomatic mesenteric artery stenosis is not well characterized, it appears that patients with critical disease of all three mesenteric arteries are at sufficiently high risk for future complications of mesenteric ischemia that concomitant revascularization is justified.[282]

Progression of renal artery stenosis has been better documented,[287, 309] but the ultimate clinical impact of such progression appears minimal in nonhypertensive patients with normal renal function.[77] The adjacency of the renal arteries to the operative field for AAA repair has led some to recommend prophylactic repair of critical, but asymptomatic, renal artery stenoses.[50] Although this may be appropriate for younger, good-risk patients, it adds morbidity and mortality to the AAA repair, leading others to recommend the combined procedure only for standard indications of hypertension or ischemic nephropathy.[25]

COMPLICATIONS OF AAA REPAIR

Despite major improvements in the outcome of elective AAA repair, major complications occur and must be correctly managed or avoided to maintain the low mortality necessary to justify prophylactic AAA repair. Myocardial infarction is the leading single-organ cause of both early and late mortality in patients undergoing AAA repair[136] and must be carefully assessed and managed to reduce mortality. In a recent review of patients undergoing elective AAA repair, however, Huber and coworkers found that multisystem organ failure (MSOF) caused more deaths (57%) than cardiac events (25%).[131] Visceral organ dysfunction was the most common cause of MSOF, followed by postoperative pneumonia. Most patients with MSOF, however, had associated cardiac dysfunction, which may have aggravated visceral ischemic injury.

Several factors may be responsible for the emergence of MSOF as a more prominent cause of death after elective AAA repair. First, with modern techniques of intensive care, it is uncommon for patients to die with single-system failure (even cardiac) after AAA repair. Second, strict atten-

tion to cardiac risk in these patients may have reduced the relative impact of cardiac complications. Finally, older patients with more associated visceral and renal artery disease underwent AAA repair in this series and had the highest likelihood of MSOF postoperatively. The relative frequencies of single-system complications after elective AAA repair are listed in Table 89–4.

Cardiac Complications

Most cardiac ischemic events occur within the first 2 days after surgery during which time intensive care monitoring is appropriate for high-risk patients. To prevent myocardial ischemia postoperatively, surgeons can maximize myocardial function with adequate preload, control oxygen consumption by the reduced heart rate and blood pressure product, ensure adequate oxygenation, and establish effective analgesia. Patients with cardiac dysfunction have a greater risk of myocardial infarction when the postoperative hematocrit is less than 28% even though this level is well tolerated by normal individuals.[197] Postoperative epidural analgesia, in addition to providing excellent pain control, may reduce myocardial complications by decreasing the catecholamine stress response.[306]

Hemorrhage

Intraoperative or postoperative hemorrhage usually results from difficulties with the proximal aortic anastomosis or from iatrogenic venous injury. Proximal suture line bleeding, particularly when posterior, can be difficult to control, especially if the proximal anastomosis is juxtarenal. In this event, temporary supraceliac aortic compression facilitates anastomotic repair without excessive additional blood loss. Interrupted pledgeted sutures can be helpful if the aortic wall is friable. Venous bleeding usually results from injury to the iliac or left renal veins during initial exposure. Often the distal aortic aneurysm or common iliac aneurysm is densely adherent to the associated iliac vein, making cir-

TABLE 89–4. EARLY (30 DAY) COMPLICATIONS AFTER ELECTIVE ABDOMINAL AORTIC ANEURYSM REPAIR AS ESTIMATED FROM SOME SURGICAL SERIES

COMPLICATION	FREQUENCY (%)
Death	<5
All cardiac	15
Myocardial infarction	2–8
All pulmonary	8–12
Pneumonia	5
Renal insufficiency	5–12
Dialysis dependent	1–6
Deep vein thrombosis	8
Bleeding	2–5
Ureteral injury	<1
Stroke	1
Leg ischemia	1–4
Colon ischemia	1
Spinal cord ischemia	<1
Wound infection	<5
Graft infection	<1
Graft thrombosis	<1

Data from AbuRahma,[1] Diehl,[81] Johnston,[136, 138] Olsen,[203] and Richardson.[236]

cumferential arterial dissection hazardous. In such cases, vascular clamps can usually be applied successfully without complete dissection of the posterior wall of the iliac artery, or vascular control can be obtained with balloon occlusion catheters.

A posterior left renal vein or a large lumbar vein may pose similar hazards during the proximal dissection. If undetected by preoperative CT scanning, such anomalies pose a high risk for venous injury. Careful suture repair of venous injuries is required and is occasionally facilitated by temporary division of the overlying artery. Diffuse bleeding after substantial intraoperative blood loss is usually due to exhausted coagulation factors and platelets, combined with hypothermia. Aggressive rewarming with platelet and coagulation factor replacement is required to overcome this complication.

Hemodynamic Complications

Aortic clamping (especially supraceliac) results in a sudden increase in cardiac afterload, evidenced by hypertension, which can precipitate myocardial ischemia. Gradual clamp application, carefully coordinated with anesthetic and vasoactive drug administration, is required to avoid this problem. In contrast, sudden aortic declamping is often associated with significant hypotension. This is due to a combination of reduced cardiac afterload, "washout" of potassium, acidic metabolites, and myocardial depressant factors from reperfusion of ischemic legs with a preload reduction due to increased venous capacitance in the legs. Gradual declamping combined with adequate fluid and blood replacement is critical to avoid this complication. Careful intraoperative monitoring, including pulmonary capillary wedge pressure recording and transesophageal echocardiography, may facilitate fluid, anesthetic, and vasoactive drug administration in patients at known cardiac risk.

Iatrogenic Injuries

Injury to an adjacent organ is possible during AAA repair. Ureteral injury is rare during elective surgery unless the course of the ureter has been distorted by a large AAA, fibrosis, or inflammation. If injury occurs, it should be repaired immediately. A double-J stent is inserted through the injury site to traverse the ureter from the renal pelvis to the urinary bladder. The ureter is then closed with fine, interrupted absorbable sutures. Omentum can be mobilized on a vascular pedicle and wrapped around the site of injury. After copious irrigation, repair of the aneurysm can proceed, assuming the urine is not infected.

After repair, early postoperative CT imaging is advised to detect possible urinoma formation. This is unlikely to occur if the stent is working properly, but, if present, percutaneous closed drainage should be instituted with CT or ultrasound guidance. If ureteral injury is unrecognized, hydronephrosis or urinoma may develop, requiring re-exploration and more complex repair. Careful identification of the ureter, especially during pelvic dissection, successfully prevents this complication. Splenic injury due to excessive retraction may result in hemorrhage that should be controlled by splenectomy because late hemorrhage is poorly

tolerated if attempted splenic repair fails. Inadvertent enterotomy before graft placement should prompt termination of the procedure with subsequent elective AAA repair in order to avoid graft infection.

Pancreatitis is an unusual complication of AAA repair that has been attributed to a retractor injury at the base of the transverse mesocolon. It should be suspected as a cause for prolonged postoperative ileus, particularly when proximal aortic exposure has been difficult.

Renal Failure

Although once common after infrarenal AAA repair, renal failure is now rare owing to adequate volume replacement and maintenance of normal cardiac output and renal blood flow. Precautions are still required, however, to reduce the risk of this complication. Because of the renal toxicity of intravenous contrast media, it is prudent to delay AAA repair after arteriography or contrast-enhanced CT scanning to be certain that renal dysfunction has not been induced. A more likely cause of renal failure after infrarenal AAA repair is embolization of aortic atheromatous debris into the renal arteries during proximal aortic cross-clamping. Preoperative CT scanning may reveal pararenal atheromatous debris or thrombus, which should prompt temporary supraceliac cross-clamping until the infrarenal aorta is open. At this point, such material can be removed and the clamp moved to the normal infrarenal location. During such manipulation the renal arteries should be temporarily clamped and the orifices carefully irrigated before blood flow is restored.

Because preoperative renal insufficiency is the best predictor of postoperative renal failure,[136, 191] special precautions are appropriate for patients with indications of renal insufficiency. There is some evidence to support a beneficial effect of intravenous mannitol when given before aortic cross-clamping (~25 gm).[191] Although some have advocated maintenance of higher urine volume with furosemide, the efficacy of this approach has not been proven and may hinder the assessment of fluid balance by artificially increasing urine output. Because renal failure is more likely in patients who require prolonged suprarenal clamping,[136] special measures such as renal cooling are recommended, as discussed later.

Gastrointestinal Complications

Some degree of bowel dysfunction occurs after any major abdominal procedure. The paralytic ileus that occurs after evisceration and dissection of the base of the mesentery during transperitoneal AAA repair, however, often lasts longer than that occurring after other procedures. Dysmotility may be exacerbated by premature discontinuation of gastric decompression. Consequently, one must use caution when reinstituting oral feeding postoperatively. Anorexia, periodic constipation, and diarrhea are commonly seen in the first few weeks after aneurysm surgery.

Sigmoid colon ischemia following AAA repair is a rare but devastating complication that occurs after approximately 1% of elective AAA repairs.[15, 174] This may result from embolization into, or ligation of, the IMA or internal iliac arteries. Although the IMA is often chronically occluded, ligation too far from the aneurysm wall can obliterate important SMA collaterals. Fortunately, the abundance of collateral flow to the sigmoid colon usually prevents ischemia. Complicated distal iliac artery anastomoses may inadvertently obliterate the internal iliac orifice, however, while dislodgment of aneurysmal debris during dissection or clamping may cause embolism. Sigmoid ischemia is three to four times more likely following ruptured AAA repair, presumably due to the associated hypotension and shock added to the usual risk of this complication.[15, 297]

Careful inspection of the sigmoid colon after graft placement is important and may be facilitated by Doppler insonation of the bowel wall and mesentery. Preoperatively patent IMAs should be carefully inspected for back-bleeding after the aortic reconstruction and ligated only when back-bleeding is pulsatile and colon viability is ensured. In questionable circumstances, IMA reimplantation or direct internal iliac revascularization is indicated.[92] Preoperative arteriographic indicators of risk for sigmoid ischemia include (1) a stenotic or occluded SMA, (2) a large patent IMA with ascending collateral flow, and (3) occlusion of both internal iliac arteries. Postoperatively, colon ischemia should be suspected in the presence of early diarrhea usually containing blood, left lower quadrant abdominal pain, unexplained fever or leukocytosis, or excessive intravenous fluid requirement. These indications should prompt immediate flexible sigmoidoscopy or colonoscopy. In most cases, patchy, partial-thickness mucosal necrosis and sloughing are detected and often resolve with antibiotic therapy and bowel rest. In more severe cases of transmural infarction, however, early re-exploration is indicated to avoid the high mortality rate associated with delayed treatment of this complication. Treatment requires sigmoid resection and colostomy, rarely combined with aortic graft excision followed by extra-anatomic bypass if substantial graft contamination has occurred. This complication is discussed in detail in Chapter 113.

Distal Embolization

Lower extremity ischemia may occur after AAA repair, usually from embolization of aneurysmal debris that occurs during aneurysm mobilization or aortoiliac clamping. Usually such emboli are small (termed *microemboli*), not amenable to surgical removal, and result in transient, patchy areas of dusky skin or "blue toes." This can result in persistent pain or skin loss, occasionally necessitating amputation. Some investigators have recommended treatment with low-molecular-weight dextran or even sympathectomy for such microembolic lesions, but their management is largely expectant. Occasionally, larger emboli or distal intimal flaps, particularly in diseased iliac arteries, may require operative intervention. For this reason, the legs should be carefully inspected intraoperatively for ischemia after AAA repair while the incision is still open and arterial access can be easily obtained if necessary.

Paraplegia

Paraplegia, due to spinal cord ischemia, is rare following infrarenal AAA repair. It can result when important spinal artery collateral flow via the internal iliac arteries or an abnormally low origin of the accessory spinal artery (arterial magna radicularis or artery of Adamkiewicz) is obliterated or embolized during AAA repair.[276] Because the accessory spinal artery normally originates from the descending thoracic or upper abdominal aorta, this complication is much more common after thoracoabdominal aneurysm repair. Recent reports have emphasized the importance of preserving normal internal iliac artery perfusion of important spinal artery collateral vessels to avoid paraplegia.[111, 219] Occlusive disease of the spinal collateral arteries, combined with severe hypotension, may also result in paraplegia, accounting for the higher frequency of this complication during ruptured AAA repair.[276] Interestingly, paraplegia has been reported as the presenting symptom of infrarenal AAAs, suggesting that important spinal artery collateral blood flow originating from the distal aorta can be occluded by mural thrombus within the aneurysm or actual aneurysm thrombosis.[188]

Impaired Sexual Function

Impotence or retrograde ejaculation may result after AAA repair due to injury of autonomic nerves during para-aortic dissection.[80] The incidence of this complication is difficult to determine due to the multiple causes of impotence in the age group usually affected by AAAs and to frequent underreporting. Careful preservation of nerves, particularly as they course along the left side of the infrarenal aorta and around the IMA and cross the proximal left common iliac artery, has been shown to substantially reduce this complication, which can otherwise occur in up to 25% of patients.[99, 296] Other possible causes of postoperative impotence include reduction in pelvic blood flow due to internal iliac occlusion or embolization.

Venous Thromboembolism

Pulmonary embolism and deep vein thrombosis are less common after AAA repair than after other abdominal operations, perhaps due to intraoperative anticoagulation. Unrecognized deep vein thrombosis, however, can occur in up to 18% of untreated patients.[202] Therefore, perioperative prophylaxis with intermittent pneumatic compression stockings and subcutaneous heparin is appropriate for high-risk patients.

Late Complications

Late complications after successful AAA or iliac aneurysm repair are infrequent.[68] In a recent population-based study, only 7% of patients experienced such complications within 5 years after AAA repair.[119] Anastomotic disruption, usually due to arterial degeneration, can result in a pseudoaneurysm (a hematoma locally contained by surrounding connective tissue). After 3-year follow-up, the incidence of anastomotic pseudoaneurysm was only 0.2% for aortic anastomoses, 1.2% for iliac anastomoses, and 3% for femoral anastomoses.[278] Aortic pseudoaneurysms appear to increase progressively with time, however, and for young patients who survive many years after AAA repair, follow-up imaging studies may be appropriate to detect late asymptomatic pseudoaneurysms.

One study reported an incidence of aortic pseudoaneurysms of only 1% after 8 years but 20% after 15 years.[90] After their population-based study, Hallett and colleagues reported a 4% likelihood of anastomotic pseudoaneurysm after 10 years.[119] These results suggest a potential benefit of CT scan surveillance at 5-year intervals after AAA repair in the subgroup of generally younger patients who survive this long. When identified, aortic and iliac pseudoaneurysms warrant repair because of the high likelihood of mortality if rupture occurs.[288] Pseudoaneurysms are discussed in detail in Chapter 48.

Graft infection after AAA repair is also rare unless a femoral anastomosis is required.[43] For aortoiliac grafts, the likelihood of infection is 0.5%, usually presenting 3 to 4 years after implantation.[98] Early presentation is possible and more likely if a femoral anastomosis is present.[279] The development of a secondary aortoenteric fistula after AAA repair is also unusual (0.9%), but much more frequent than a primary aortoenteric fistula associated with an AAA.[44] Aortoenteric fistulae usually develop approximately 5 years after AAA repair, nearly always involve the duodenum at the proximal suture line and usually present with gastrointestinal hemorrhage. Less commonly, aortoenteric fistulae may involve the central portion of the graft and lead to infection rather than to hemorrhage. The combined likelihood of graft infection and graft-enteric fistula appears to be 5% after 10 years.[119] Aortic graft infection and aortoenteric fistula usually require graft resection and extra-anatomic bypass. Both of these complications have a high associated mortality rate and are discussed in Chapters 47 and 49.

Thrombosis of an aortoiliac graft after AAA repair is unusual unless extensive iliac occlusive disease coexists, which can lead to early graft thrombosis if unrecognized. Hallett and coworkers estimated the likelihood of graft thrombosis to be only 3% after 10 years.[119] In long-term follow-up after AAA repair, approximately 5% of patients will develop complications due to other aneurysms at a mean interval of 5 years postoperatively.[46] These are usually true aneurysms of the thoracic or more proximal abdominal aorta and occasionally the iliac arteries. If these secondary aneurysms rupture, fewer than 5% of patients survive.[221] Thus, it is important to detect these aneurysms before rupture occurs. Hypertension significantly increases the risk of secondary aneurysm development[221] and suggests that initial screening and subsequent follow-up imaging should be performed for other aneurysms in hypertensive patients with AAAs. If a tortuous, possibly dilated thoracic aorta is seen on chest radiographs, screening and follow-up imaging should also be performed. In total, fewer than 10% of patients will experience late complications of AAA repair during their lifetime. Most of these are severe, however, and often fatal.[68]

LONG-TERM SURVIVAL

As noted previously, the early (30-day) mortality rate after elective AAA repair in properly selected patients is 5% or less, whereas the early mortality rate after ruptured AAA repair averages 54% (not including patients who died of rupture before repair).[144] The 5-year survival rate after successful AAA repair in series during the 1980s and 1990s is approximately 70%, with a 10-year survival rate of 40%.[64, 126, 149, 203, 259, 292] Survival rates after successful elective and ruptured AAA operations are comparable if the patient survives the initial 30 days.[268] Overall, survival after AAA repair is reduced compared with an age-matched and sex-matched population because of greater associated comorbidity in patients with aneurysms.[126]

Not surprisingly, systemic complications of atherosclerosis cause most late deaths after AAA repair in the predominately elderly, male population. The cause of late deaths after AAA repair are cardiac disease (44%), cancer (15%), rupture of another aneurysm (11%), stroke (9%), and pulmonary disease (6%).[64, 121, 126] When cardiac causes, aneurysmal disease, and stroke are combined, vascular complications account for two thirds of the late deaths following AAA repair. When outcome is stratified according to these risk factors, the 5-year survival rate improves to 84% in patients without heart disease, which is substantially better than the 54% survival rate observed in patients with known heart disease.[64] Hypertension also reduces 5-year survival rate after AAA repair (from 84% to 59%).[64] In patients without hypertension or heart disease, late survival rate after AAA repair is identical to that of normal, age-matched controls.[126]

Multivariate analyses indicate that uncorrected coronary artery disease is the most significant variable associated with late mortality after AAA repair but that age, renal dysfunction, and peripheral occlusive disease also contribute.[203, 232] An analysis of coronary artery bypass graft performed in preparation for AAA repair indicates that improved long-term survival is likely in patients under age 70 years with severe coronary artery disease but that older patients do not benefit from this aggressive approach.[232] A recent prospective, multicenter study identified not only age and cardiac, carotid, and renal diseases as independent predictors of late mortality after elective AAA repair, but also aneurysm extent, as judged by size, suprarenal extension, and external iliac involvement, which has not been previously reported.[149]

SPECIAL CONSIDERATIONS

Suprarenal Aneurysms

By definition, AAAs that extend above at least one renal artery but end below the diaphragm are termed *suprarenal* and constitute approximately 5% of aortic aneurysms within the abdomen. If these aneurysms extend above the celiac artery, and thus above the crus of the diaphragm, they are classified as *thoracoabdominal aneurysms* (discussed in Chapter 92). CT or MRI is required to define the proximal extent of an AAA and is especially important for discerning the detailed anatomy of a suprarenal aneurysm. Arteriography usually detects suprarenal extension (although it may underestimate this due to intraluminal thrombus) but is more useful to delineate associated renal or mesenteric occlusive disease. It is rare for an AAA to be isolated to the suprarenal segment unless an infrarenal AAA has been previously repaired.

The natural history of suprarenal AAAs is even less well defined than that of infrarenal AAAs because suprarenal AAAs are less frequently encountered. Without other data, the rupture risk of suprarenal AAAs should be considered comparable with that of infrarenal AAAs for comparably sized aneurysms.[63] Surgical risk is higher, however, owing to the necessity for renal and mesenteric artery revascularization and to potential ischemic injury during suprarenal cross-clamping.[4, 201] Thus, most surgeons use a threshold size for elective repair of a suprarenal AAA that is approximately 1 cm larger than would be used for an infrarenal AAA in the same patient. Surgical treatment of ruptured suprarenal AAAs is even more complicated and is associated with nearly 100% mortality.

Suprarenal AAAs are best approached surgically with a left retroperitoneal incision, which can be extended into the chest if more proximal exposure is required. If an unsuspected suprarenal aneurysm is discovered during transperitoneal exposure, medial visceral rotation (reflecting the left colon, spleen, pancreas, and stomach medially to gain proximal retroperitoneal exposure) can be used.[233] Optimal placement of the aortic cross-clamp in these cases depends on the proximal extent of the AAA, the proximity of the renal arteries to the SMA, and associated aortic atherosclerosis and calcified plaque.[201] If the AAA does not extend above the renal arteries and sufficient length of undiseased aorta exists above the AAA but below the SMA, clamping in this location avoids visceral ischemia. Often the aorta is less diseased above the celiac artery, however, in which case clamping in this location is safer and well tolerated despite the associated temporary visceral ischemia.[115] This must be individualized and can be facilitated by preoperative CT scanning, especially with three-dimensional reconstruction to visualize the location of calcified plaque in relation to visceral and renal orifices (see Chapter 14). In many cases, the proximal aortic anastomosis for a low suprarenal AAA can be constructed on an angle that allows incorporation of the right renal artery orifice and calls for only reimplantation of the left renal artery as an onlay patch.

If a suprarenal AAA extends to involve the SMA and celiac arteries, repair is accomplished with the inclusion technique popularized by Crawford and associates in which the orifices of the mesenteric and renal arteries are attached to the bypass graft as a patch.[65] Usually the celiac, SMA, and right renal arteries can be incorporated as one large patch, with the left renal artery reimplanted separately. The proximal aortic anastomosis for a suprarenal (but not thoracoabdominal) aneurysm can often incorporate the visceral and right renal artery origins with a beveled technique that excludes the entire aneurysm except for the small portion of the wall where these arteries originate. Ischemic injury to the liver, intestines and kidneys is unlikely if proximal aortic clamp time can be kept below 30 minutes.

After the visceral and renal arteries are revascularized, the aortic clamp is moved onto the graft, distal to these vessels, before the distal aortic or iliac anastomosis is completed. Intraoperative cooling by iced saline perfusion of the renal or mesenteric arteries is useful if more than 30 minutes of ischemia is anticipated, which is usually the case for the left renal artery when it must be reimplanted separately.[4]

Significantly greater hemodynamic changes occur with aortic clamping and declamping above the celiac artery, necessitating careful coordination of anesthesia, fluid administration, and vasoactive drug use. Long-term outcome after successful repair is comparable with that for infrarenal AAAs, although the operative mortality rate is higher on average (4% to 10%).[4, 201, 226] Compared with infrarenal AAA repair, increased postoperative renal failure is more likely after suprarenal aneurysm repair.[32] Although many of these issues are discussed in more detail for thoracoabdominal aneurysms in Chapter 92, they also apply to the management of suprarenal aneurysms that are entirely within the abdomen.

Inflammatory Abdominal Aortic Aneurysms

Inflammatory AAAs are a distinct clinical entity characterized by marked thickening of the aneurysm wall, especially in the anterior and lateral aspects, with extensive perianeurysmal and retroperitoneal fibrosis and dense adhesions to adjacent abdominal organs.[66, 216, 264] The thickened aneurysm wall consists of an intense fibrotic, inflammatory response in the adventitial and periadventitial layers with a lymphocytic (primarily T-cell) and monocytic infiltrate.[228] Although these changes suggest an immune mechanism, the exact cause is unclear. Because mild chronic inflammation is often present in the walls of typical degenerative aneurysms, it has been suggested that inflammatory aneurysms simply reflect an accentuation of this reaction.[228] The inflammatory process may be a response to the aneurysm rather than a cause because AAA repair is accompanied by resolution of the inflammation and fibrosis in more than half the patients.[262] This process may also be related to more diffuse retroperitoneal fibrosis, but is unique because of its predominance in the aneurysm wall. Inflammatory changes of this magnitude occur in approximately 5% of infrarenal AAAs.[228, 264]

Patients with inflammatory AAAs nearly always complain of abdominal or back pain, which frequently leads to urgent exploration for suspected AAA rupture. Patients may also present with a febrile illness, elevated sedimentation rate, and systemic symptoms (including weight loss) that confuse the diagnosis. Patients with inflammatory aneurysms are more likely to have a positive family history of AAAs and are more likely to be current smokers.[199] Inflammatory AAAs usually present 5 to 10 years sooner than noninflammatory aneurysms and on average are 1 cm larger. Most studies have found that the diagnosis of inflammatory AAA can be accurately made by CT scanning, which reveals a "halo" of soft tissue around the anterior AAA that is enhanced by intravenous contrast (Fig. 89–11). One study, however, questions the accuracy of CT scanning and suggests that MRI is more accurate, demonstrating characteristic arrays of concentric alternating layers of high and low signal intensity on T1-weighted images.[281] Preoperative recognition of an inflammatory aneurysm may facilitate management with a retroperitoneal approach to avoid the most thickened and inflamed portion of the anterior wall.

Although the dense fibrotic reaction around inflammatory AAAs might suggest protection from rupture, this is not the case, probably because rupture may occur through the less thickened posterior wall. Thus, current indications

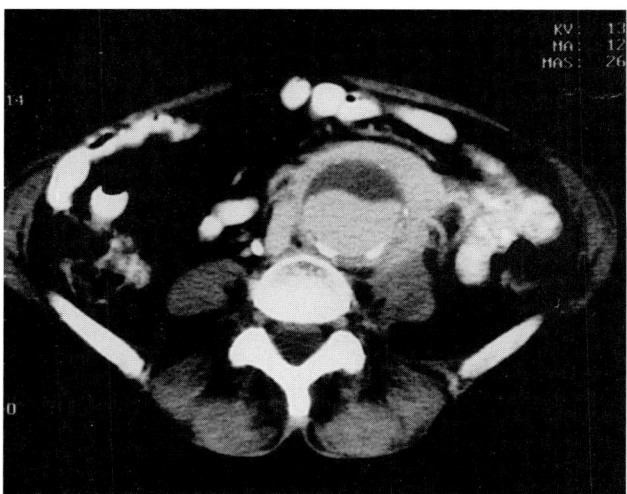

FIGURE 89–11. CT scan of an inflammatory aneurysm showing contrast-enhanced, thickened aortic wall along anterolateral aspects of the abdominal aortic aneurysm.

for repair of inflammatory AAAs are identical to those for noninflammatory aneurysms. When approached transabdominally, the fibrosis around these aneurysms has a characteristic shiny, pearly gray appearance and extends to involve the duodenum in more than 90% of cases, the vena cava and left renal vein in more than 50%, and the ureters in more than 25%.[228] To avoid injuring these structures during operative repair, supraceliac control, direct AAA incision without duodenal dissection, and endoaneurysmal repair (analogous to a ruptured AAA) are recommended if a transperitoneal approach is used. The left retroperitoneal approach avoids anterior fibrosis and thus reduces the risk to adjacent structures and is recommended when inflammatory AAAs are recognized preoperatively.

Complications associated with injury to adjacent structures should be minimal if these techniques are used. Preoperative ureteral stenting can facilitate the identification of ureters and also treats hydronephrosis if present. Two reports suggest that ureters may remain entrapped in one third of patients, but fewer than 5% require dialysis.[199, 262] Thus, prophylactic ureterolysis is generally not recommended because injury is common. Rather, ureteral obstruction can be managed with a stent placed preoperatively and left in place until the inflammation resolves after AAA repair. In a comparative study of patients treated with ureterolysis versus temporary stent decompression, no difference in renal function was noted.[170]

If associated retroperitoneal fibrosis does not resolve and the ureter remains obstructed, steroid therapy can be used successfully,[269] and later surgical decompression or drainage can be undertaken if necessary. Results of inflammatory AAA repair indicate that elective operative mortality is similar to that of noninflammatory aneurysms, with a somewhat greater risk of operative complications.[155, 199, 264] Steroid treatment of inflammatory AAAs has been reported to reduce the fibrotic reaction and AAA wall thickness.[13] The benefit of reducing aneurysm wall thickness is controversial, however, because reduced strength might precipitate rupture, which has been reported during steroid treatment.[13] Thus, appropriately sized or symptomatic inflammatory AAAs should be repaired surgically, whereas steroid treatment might be useful for postsurgical treatment of associated retroperitoneal fibrosis, especially if ureteral compression persists.

Infected Abdominal Aortic Aneurysms

An infected AAA can result from degenerative changes caused by the primary infection of a previously normal aorta or as a secondary infection of an already established aneurysm.[96, 112, 230] If sufficiently severe, primary aortic infection can lead to aortic degeneration, localized wall disruption, and aneurysm formation, usually in a localized, asymmetric fashion. The source of aneurysm infection can be septic embolization from a distant site, bacteremia, or contiguous spread from local infection. Fortunately, primary aortoiliac infection leading to aneurysm formation is rare, accounting for fewer than 1% of aneurysms in this location. Before the era of antibiotics, systemic syphilis and septic emboli from bacterial endocarditis were common causes of AAAs. Although any bacterial or fungal infection can lead to an infected aneurysm, the most common pathogens are *Salmonella* species and *Staphylococcus aureus*.

Clinically significant secondary infection of an already established AAA is also rare. However, inapparent infection, more appropriately described as *bacterial colonization* is frequent because up to 37% of AAAs produce positive intraoperative cultures.[98] In these cases, the most frequent organisms cultured are consistent with normal skin flora (coagulase-negative *Staphylococcus*, *Corynebacterium*, and *Streptococcus faecalis*). The significance of this bacterial colonization appears minimal because the finding of a positive intraoperative culture has not increased the rate of subsequent prosthetic graft infection. Bacterial colonization must be differentiated from more severe infections that often result from contiguous spread of an established infection and lead to marked inflammatory changes of the AAA wall, or even purulence.

Because infected AAAs are rare and the symptoms are nonspecific, diagnosis can be delayed or unsuspected until surgery. Abdominal pain, fever, bacteremia, and a pulsatile abdominal mass should suggest an infected AAA, but these findings may not all be present, and the AAA may be small enough to escape detection. For this reason, an infected AAA should be considered in the differential diagnosis of fever of unknown origin, particularly if *Salmonella* is cultured from the blood of a patient older than 50 years of age.

In the absence of systemic signs of infection, a localized, noncalcified, asymmetric AAA in an otherwise normal-appearing aorta should suggest a primary infected AAA. Traditionally, the treatment for an infected infrarenal AAA has been aortic excision with proximal and distal closure, débridement of surrounding infected tissue, and extra-anatomic (axillobifemoral) bypass.[230] Complications of proximal aortic stump "blowout" after this procedure have led some to recommend in situ graft replacement after débridement of all infected tissue. Experience suggests that aortic excision with extra-anatomic bypass is optimal for patients with overtly purulent infections, especially those caused by *Salmonella, Pseudomonas,* or other gram-negative organisms.

In situ replacement is more applicable to less purulent

infections, especially from gram-positive organisms or infections involving the suprarenal aorta where visceral reconstruction requires in situ replacement. Infected iliac aneurysms are more easily treated by local excision and femorofemoral bypass because the risk of aortic blowout is not present. Experimental evidence suggests that PTFE grafts may be more resistant to infection than Dacron, although this has not been proven clinically.[307] Aortic replacement with autogenous tissue should resist infection more than prosthetic replacement, but size mismatch with peripheral veins is unsatisfactory. Good results have been described with larger, deep veins harvested from the leg for aortoiliac replacement in infected circumstances.[58] Similarly, aortic homografts have been used effectively in this setting.[147] Fortunately, infected AAAs are rare so that most experience with aortic replacement for infection arises from previously placed infected aortofemoral prosthetic grafts. Concomitant antibiotic treatment is important for these patients, with the duration sometimes extended indefinitely for more virulent organisms.[112] Infected aneurysms are discussed in detail in Chapter 97.

Primary Aortocaval Fistulae

Rarely, large AAAs may erode into the adjacent vena cava or proximal left iliac vein leading to a direct aortovenous (AV) fistula.[35, 107] Usually such patients experience symptoms of pain associated with AAA rupture, but sometimes a chronic, stable AV fistula may result.[130] Sudden AAA rupture into the vena cava may also be associated with more typical retroperitoneal hemorrhage, in which case the aortocaval fistula may not be recognized until emergent surgery is performed. The extent of hemodynamic compromise due to the aortocaval fistula depends on its size. A typical machinery bruit is present in more than half the cases, while venous hypertension leads to leg swelling in one third.[106] Renal vein hypertension may lead to microscopic or gross hematuria.[239] Acute congestive heart failure results in 25% of patients when the fistula is large or if baseline cardiac function is poor.[107] In the rare case of a stable, chronic aortocaval fistula, sustained increased venous pressure can result in lower extremity swelling, venous thrombosis, perineal and hemorrhoidal varices, scrotal edema, and hematuria.[241] In these cases, an abdominal bruit and high-output congestive heart failure may aid an otherwise confusing diagnosis that is best confirmed by arteriography.

Surgical treatment of an aortocaval fistula consists of conventional repair of the AAA, with closure of the fistula from within the aneurysm. Dissection of the vena cava or iliac vein away from the aneurysm is extremely hazardous. Control of the vena cava adjacent to the fistula with direct pressure from within the aneurysm allows the fistula to be closed without excessive bleeding or air embolization. Mortality from an aortocaval fistula remains high (30%).[107] This condition is discussed in detail in Chapter 101.

Primary Aortoenteric Fistulae

It is possible for an AAA to erode into adjacent intestine, usually the fourth portion of the duodenum.[47, 274, 298] This very rare but dramatic complication is usually associated with large AAAs. Much more common is the "secondary" aortoenteric fistula that arises as a late anastomotic complication of a prosthetic aortic graft (see Chapter 49). Initially, gastrointestinal (GI) bleeding may be limited, leading to melena or anemia. Eventually, and often abruptly, severe hemorrhage leads to hematemesis and shock. Classically, patients with aortoenteric fistulae present with a small "herald" hemorrhage due to bowel mucosal bleeding before sudden brisk hemorrhage and collapse.

A primary aortoduodenal fistula should be suspected in a patient with GI hemorrhage, abdominal pain, and a pulsatile abdominal mass. Due to the rarity of this complication, however, it is much more frequent for patients with AAAs to develop upper GI hemorrhage from the more common causes of peptic ulcer disease, gastritis, or even esophageal varices. Accordingly, the first diagnostic step in these patients should be upper GI endoscopy, which often localizes the source of bleeding. An aortoenteric fistula should be suspected when no obvious source of bleeding is found. Rarely, a mucosal defect may be seen in the third or fourth portion of the duodenum. Because severe hemorrhage can occur suddenly, evaluation must proceed rapidly in a patient with a known or suspected AAA and GI hemorrhage. A CT scan can confirm the diagnosis of AAA, but will not usually demonstrate local inflammatory changes diagnostic of an aortoduodenal fistula. Similarly, arteriography is usually not beneficial unless it localizes an alternative source of GI hemorrhage.

Often, the diagnosis of primary aortoduodenal fistula cannot be definitively established. Thus, when other more common sources of GI bleeding have been excluded, exploratory laparotomy is indicated because of the universal mortality of an untreated aortoduodenal fistula. Closure of the duodenum, aortic ligation with aneurysm exclusion, and extra-anatomic bypass are usually required, although in situ AAA repair has been successfully accomplished if contamination is minimal. This problem is discussed in detail in Chapter 49.

Associated Developmental Anomalies

Renal developmental anomalies may complicate AAA repair.[62] Multiple renal arteries are relatively frequent (15% to 30%), whereas pelvic kidney, horseshoe kidney, and multiple ureters are quite rare.[16] These anomalies may be detected by preoperative arteriography, spiral CT scanning, or MRA. Accessory renal arteries can also be found during careful dissection of the aorta, usually arising more anteriorly than the normal lateral renal artery orifices. Those that are sufficiently large to supply distinct areas of renal parenchyma should be reimplanted onto the aortic graft if they arise from the AAA. This is facilitated by excising a surrounding collar (Carrel patch) of associated aortic wall along with the orifice.

Pelvic kidneys usually have a single renal artery, but their origin may be displaced to the distal aorta or even iliac arteries and thus require reimplantation. Distal origins of a renal artery require special consideration to avoid prolonged ischemic injury when the more proximal aorta is clamped. This may be accomplished by perfusing the renal artery with cold saline or with blood via a shunt from the aortic graft after the proximal aortic anastomosis is constructed.[245]

Horseshoe kidneys pose more technical difficulties both because they limit access to the distal aorta and because they are usually supplied by multiple renal arteries arising from the aorta, the AAA itself, or the iliac arteries.[261] The isthmus of the horseshoe kidney should not be divided unless it is extremely thin and atrophic. Rather, the aortic graft usually can be tunneled beneath the kidney if the aorta is approached anteriorly. Care must be taken, however, to revascularize the major, multiple arteries by reimplantation and cold perfusion for renal preservation during temporary ischemia.[129] Preoperative arteriography facilitates identification of these branches, but careful intraoperative dissection and inspection are required to avoid injury. A retroperitoneal approach offers significant advantages because the graft can be easily placed behind the horseshoe kidney and the renal arteries reimplanted similar to the inclusion technique used for suprarenal aneurysms.

Major venous anomalies, although rare, can also pose technical difficulties during AAA repair. Failure to recognize these anomalies can lead to venous injury and significant hemorrhage. A retroaortic left renal vein (2% to 3% incidence) and a circumaortic anterior and posterior left renal vein (7% incidence) are the most common anomalies encountered.[7, 18, 110] These should be suspected if the left renal vein is not encountered anteriorly during the proximal aortic dissection or if it appears small.[34] Preoperative CT scanning discloses these anomalies, as well as less frequently encountered left-sided or duplicated inferior vena cava.[12] Except in cases of situs inversus, a left-sided vena cava usually crosses anteriorly to the right side of the aorta at the level of the renal veins.[86] If this is not the case, the right renal vein crosses the aorta to join the left-sided vena cava. These venous anomalies complicate aortic exposure and must be approached with care. Duplicated veins may often be ligated to facilitate exposure, but the details of venous anatomy must be fully appreciated to avoid inadvertent ligation of a nonduplicated system.

Associated Abdominal Disease

Frequently an AAA is detected during the evaluation of another disease process such as prostate cancer, lumbar disc disease, cholelithiasis, or even colon or renal cancer. If such an AAA warrants surgical repair, a decision must be made concerning the prioritization of treatment of the two disease processes. The general guidelines are to treat the most life-threatening process first and to avoid simultaneous operations that increase the risk of prosthetic graft infection. Usually the AAA takes priority, such as in patients with lumbar disc disease or prostate cancer, when the other procedure can be secondarily staged without increased risk. More difficult decisions arise with cholelithiasis and abdominal malignancies for which simultaneous surgical treatment is attractive but may increase the risk of prosthetic graft contamination. This is especially true for colon operations so that AAA repair and colon resection should be staged except in extraordinary circumstances. The larger the AAA, the more likely that it should be treated first. Alternatively, colon cancers that are obstructing, and potentially liable to perforate or to cause total obstruction (particularly those on the left side), should usually be treated before AAA repair.[200]

In contrast, nephrectomy for renal malignancy does not appear to increase the risk of prosthetic graft infection and can usually be performed during the same operation as AAA repair.[14, 109] The same consideration would apply to other "clean" procedures such as oophorectomy if required in patients undergoing AAA repair. When performed, such additional procedures should be done after the AAA is repaired and the retroperitoneal closure is complete, provided that the patient's condition remains stable. Although there have been anecdotal reports of AAA rupture after unrelated abdominal surgery,[273] a cause-effect relationship has not been proven.[87] Thus, this should not affect decision making for patients with large AAAs who require urgent surgical treatment of an unrelated problem. For patients with very large AAAs, repair should be offered soon after the preceding operation, optimally during the same hospitalization.

There is controversy concerning the advisability of cholecystectomy at the time of AAA repair. Because positive bile culture specimens may be present in up to 33% of cases,[271] many surgeons have avoided concomitant cholecystectomy for asymptomatic cholelithiasis due to the fear of prosthetic graft infection. This complication has been reported,[206] but concomitant cholecystectomy has been performed in many patients during AAA repair without an apparent increase in graft infection.[206, 271] The incidence of graft infection is sufficiently low in general and the onset so delayed, however, that these optimistic results must be viewed cautiously. The likelihood of acute cholecystitis after AAA repair is also very low, even if cholelithiasis is present.[104] As many as half of these patients, however, will develop symptoms that require cholecystectomy during the next 5 years.[271] For this reason, adjunctive cholecystectomy has been recommended by some when cholelithiasis is present during AAA repair.[206, 271]

If performed, cholecystectomy should follow AAA repair and careful closure of the retroperitoneum to minimize the possibility of graft contamination. The possible advantages of this combined procedure have been reduced somewhat by laparoscopic techniques, which allow later cholecystectomy with very low morbidity. In general, when an unsuspected intra-abdominal problem is discovered during AAA repair, the AAA reconstruction should proceed and the other (probably asymptomatic) condition treated secondarily if concomitant treatment would lead to an increased risk of prosthetic graft infection. Rarely, an unexpected intra-abdominal process such as widespread metastatic disease or abscess would warrant abandoning the planned AAA repair.

ISOLATED ILIAC ARTERY ANEURYSMS

Isolated iliac aneurysms, without an associated AAA, are rare (Fig. 89–12). A population-based study estimates their prevalence to be 0.03% based on autopsy findings.[41] Of all aortoiliac aneurysms, only 0.6% were isolated to the iliac arteries.[41] Based on hospital admissions in the United States, the incidence of known, isolated iliac aneurysms in

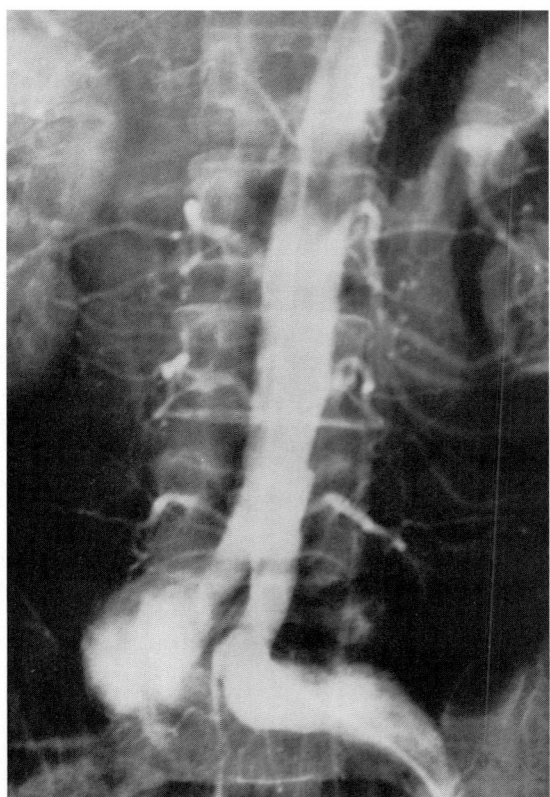

FIGURE 89–12. Arteriogram of an isolated common iliac aneurysm associated with a normal-caliber aorta (confirmed by CT scan).

men aged 65 to 75 years is 70 per 100,000 years, while in women the incidence is only 2 per 100,000 years, emphasizing the predominance of these aneurysms in men.[158] Like AAAs, isolated iliac artery aneurysms increase in frequency with age and are rare before age 60 years. Their deep location in the pelvis makes detection by physical examination nearly impossible, although large iliac aneurysms are sometimes discovered by rectal examination.

Because of the increased performance of abdominal imaging studies for other reasons, more small iliac aneurysms are now being detected. The common iliac artery is most frequently involved (70% to 90%), followed by the internal iliac artery (10% to 30%), with the external iliac usually spared, for reasons not understood.[186, 235] There is a clear male predominance (male:female ratios of 5–16:1), with most patients being 65 to 75 years old in surgical series.[151, 186, 235] Approximately 50% are bilateral.[151] Although iliac artery aneurysms are usually asymptomatic until rupture, they may present with unique signs due to local compression of adjacent pelvic structures. Ureteral obstruction, hematuria, iliac vein thrombosis, large bowel obstruction, and lower extremity neurologic deficit may be present, but are much more frequently caused by other entities, often confusing the initial diagnosis of an iliac aneurysm.

Before the widespread use of CT and MRI, most isolated iliac aneurysms presented with rupture, with a resulting high mortality rate. The natural history of small iliac aneurysms is not well defined, however, because iliac aneurysms are uncommon and have usually not been followed with sequential imaging. In most surgical series, the average size of these aneurysms is 4 to 5 cm, while the average size of ruptured iliac aneurysms has been estimated to be 6 cm.[29] During follow-up of iliac aneurysms, reported rates of rupture have ranged from 10% to 70% after 5 years.[36, 235] Furthermore, follow-up of large iliac aneurysms from 4 to 12 cm diameter indicates that there is not a clear relationship between rupture and size in this range.[36] Mortality from rupture is high, from 25% to 57%, whereas mortality from elective repair is less than 5%.[151, 186, 235] Thus, despite the vagaries concerning natural history, most surgeons recommend elective repair of isolated iliac aneurysms at a threshold diameter of approximately 3 cm in good-risk patients. However, all of the issues concerning decision making for patients with AAAs apply here, primarily a comparison of rupture risk versus operative risk.

Iliac aneurysms can be approached through a lower abdominal retroperitoneal incision, but when they are bilateral or potentially requiring aortic repair, a transabdominal approach is more versatile. Unilateral common iliac aneurysms can be repaired with a simple interposition graft, but bilateral aneurysms are more easily treated with aortoiliac reconstruction. If preclinical aneurysmal changes are present in the infrarenal aorta, even though this is not excessively enlarged, aortoiliac reconstruction should be employed to prevent later aneurysmal degeneration of the aorta. Proximal ligation of an internal iliac aneurysm without distal ligation or endoaneurysmorrhaphy may lead to persistent aneurysm expansion and rupture.[78] Therefore, internal iliac artery aneurysms should either be repaired with an interposition graft or, more often, be excluded by distal ligation, with endoaneurysmal ligation of branches because these are usually large, deep, and difficult to reconstruct.

When internal iliac aneurysms are bilateral, or the contralateral artery is occluded, pelvic blood flow must be carefully assessed. In these cases, one internal iliac artery may require direct revascularization. Although back-pressure recording from the distal internal iliac artery is possible, the adequacy of pelvic circulation is usually assessed by clinical grading of back-bleeding, as well as visual and Doppler assessment of the sigmoid colon blood flow after temporary iliac clamping. Rare complications of iliac aneurysm rupture into adjacent rectum, bladder or small intestine may require ligation with reconstruction outside the surgical field if contamination is significant.

Endovascular repair of isolated iliac aneurysms with a supported graft (or a covered stent) is possible if a sufficient length of normal iliac artery exists above and below the aneurysm to allow graft sealing. In some cases this would necessitate occluding the internal iliac artery, so that adequate contralateral pelvic blood flow would need to be ensured. Early experience with endovascular repair of isolated iliac aneurysms is disappointing, with an early and late adverse event rate of 27% in the largest published series.[52] This is a rapidly developing technique, however, and improved results can be expected with increased experience and more refined devices. Although follow-up is short, more encouraging results have been published in recent, small series.[84, 182]

REFERENCES

1. AbuRahma AF, Robinson PA, Boland JP, et al: Elective resection of 332 abdominal aortic aneurysms in a southern West Virginia community during a recent 5-year period. Surgery 109:244, 1991.

2. AbuRahma AF, Robinson PA, Boland JP, et al: The risk of ligation of the left renal vein in resection of the abdominal aortic aneurysm. Surg Gynecol Obstet 173:33, 1991.
3. Alcorn HG, Wolfson SK Jr, Sutton-Tyrrell K, et al: Risk factors for abdominal aortic aneurysms in older adults enrolled in the cardiovascular health study. Arterioscler Thromb Vasc Biol 16:963, 1996.
4. Allen BT, Anderson CB, Rubin BG, et al: Preservation of renal function in juxtarenal and suprarenal abdominal aortic aneurysm repair. J Vasc Surg 17:948, 1993.
5. Amundsen S, Skjaerven R, Trippestad A, et al: Abdominal aortic aneurysms: Is there an association between surgical volume, surgical experience, hospital type and operative mortality? Acta Chir Scand 156:323, 1990.
6. Anidjar S, Dobrin PB, Eichorst M, et al: Correlation of inflammatory infiltrate with the enlargement of experimental aortic aneurysms. J Vasc Surg 16(2):139, 1992.
7. Baldridge ED Jr, Canos AJ: Venous anomalies encountered in aorto-iliac surgery. Arch Surg 122:1184, 1987.
8. Baron JF, Mundler O, Bertrand M, et al: Dipyridamole-thallium scintigraphy and gated radionuclide angiography to assess cardiac risk before abdominal aortic surgery. N Engl J Med 330:663, 1994.
9. Baron HC, LaRaja RD, Rossi G, et al: Continuous epidural analgesia in the heparinized vascular surgical patient: A retrospective review of 912 patients. J Vasc Surg 6(2):144, 1987.
10. Baron JF, Bertrand M, Barre E, et al: Combined epidural and general anesthesia versus general anesthesia for abdominal aortic surgery. Anesthesiology 75:611, 1991.
11. Bartels C, Bechtel JV, Winkler C, et al: Intraoperative autotransfusion in aortic surgery: Comparison of whole blood autotransfusion versus cell separation. J Vasc Surg 24:102, 1996.
12. Bartle EJ, Pearce WH, Sun JH, et al: Infrarenal venous anomalies and aortic surgery. J Vasc Surg 6:590, 1987.
13. Baskerville PA, Blakeney CG, Young AE, et al: The diagnosis and treatment of peri-aortic fibrosis ('inflammatory' aneurysms). Br J Surg 70(6):381, 1983.
14. Baskin LS, McClure RD, Rapp JH, et al: Simultaneous resection of renal cell carcinoma and abdominal aortic aneurysm. Ann Vasc Surg 5:363, 1991.
15. Bast TJ, van der Biezen JJ, Scherpenisse J, et al: Ischaemic disease of the colon and rectum after surgery for abdominal aortic aneurysm: A prospective study of the incidence and risk. Eur J Vasc Surg 4:253, 1990.
16. Bauer S, Perlmutter A, Retik A: Anomalies of the upper urinary tract. In Walsh P, Retik A, Stamey T, et al (eds): Campbell's Urology, 6th ed. Philadelphia, WB Saunders, 1992, p 1357.
17. Baxter BT, McGee GS, Flinn WR, et al: Distal embolization as a presenting symptom of aortic aneurysms. Am J Surg 160(2):197, 1990.
18. Beckman CF, Abrams HL: Circumaortic venous ring: Incidence and significance. Am J Radiol 132:561, 1979.
19. Beede SD, Ballard DJ, James EM, et al: Positive predictive value of clinical suspicion of abdominal aortic aneurysm: Implications for efficient use of abdominal ultrasonography. Arch Intern Med 150(3):549, 1990.
20. Bender JS, Smith-Meek MA, Jones CE: Routine pulmonary artery catheterization does not reduce morbidity and mortality of elective vascular surgery: Results of a prospective, randomized trial. Ann Surg 225(3):229, 1997.
21. Bengtsson H, Bergqvist D: Ruptured abdominal aortic aneurysm: A population-based study. J Vasc Surg 18:74, 1993.
22. Bengtsson H, Bergqvist D, Ekberg O, et al: A population based screening of abdominal aortic aneurysms (AAA). Eur J Vasc Surg 5:53, 1991.
23. Bengtsson H, Ekberg O, Aspelin P, et al: Ultrasound screening of the abdominal aorta in patients with intermittent claudication. Eur J Vasc Surg 3:497, 1989.
24. Bengtsson H, Nilsson P, Bergqvist D: Natural history of abdominal aortic aneurysm detected by screening. Br J Surg 80(6):718, 1993.
25. Benjamin ME, Hansen KJ, Craven TE, et al: Combined aortic and renal artery surgery: A contemporary experience. Ann Surg 223(5):555, 1996.
26. Bernstein EF, Chan EL: Abdominal aortic aneurysms in high risk patients: Outcome of selective management based on size and expansion rate. Ann Surg 200:255, 1984.
27. Bickerstaff LK, Hollier LH, Van Peenen HJ, et al: Abdominal aortic aneurysms: The changing natural history. J Vasc Surg 1:6, 1984.
28. Birkmeyer JD, AuBuchon JP, Littenberg B, et al: Cost-effectiveness of preoperative autologous donation in coronary artery bypass grafting. Ann Thorac Surg 57(1):161, 1994.
29. Bolin T, Lund K, Skau T: Isolated aneurysms of the iliac artery: What are the chances of rupture? Eur J Vasc Surg 2(4):214, 1988.
30. Boucher CA, Grewster DC, Darling RC, et al: Determination of cardiac risk by dipyridamole-thallium imaging before peripheral vascular surgery. N Engl J Med 312:389, 1985.
31. Boyle JR, McDermott E, Crowther M, et al: Doxycycline inhibits elastin degradation and reduces metalloproteinase activity in a model of aneurysmal disease. J Vasc Surg 27(2):354, 1998.
32. Breckwoldt WL, Mackey WC, Belkin M, et al: The effect of suprarenal cross-clamping on abdominal aortic aneurysm repair. Arch Surg 127:520, 1992.
33. Breckwoldt WL, Mackey WC, O'Donnell T Jr: The economic implications of high-risk abdominal aortic aneurysm. J Vasc Surg 13:798, 1991.
34. Brener BJ, Darling C, Frederick PL, et al: Major venous anomalies complicating abdominal aortic surgery. Arch Surg 108:160, 1974.
35. Brewster DC, Cambria RP, Moncure AC, et al: Aortocaval and iliac arteriovenous fistulas: Recognition and treatment. J Vasc Surg 13:253, 1991.
36. Brin BJ, Busuttil RW: Isolated hypogastric artery aneurysms. Arch Surg 117:1329, 1982.
37. Brophy CM, Reilly JM, Smith GJ, et al: The role of inflammation in nonspecific abdominal aortic aneurysm disease. Ann Vasc Surg 5(3):229, 1991.
38. Brophy CM, Tilson JE, Tilson MD: Propranolol stimulates the cross-linking of matrix components in skin from the aneurysm-prone blotchy mouse. J Surg Res 46(4):330, 1989.
39. Brown PM, Pattenden R, Gutelius JR: The selective management of small abdominal aortic aneurysms: The Kingston study. J Vasc Surg 15:21, 1992.
40. Brown PM, Pattenden R, Vernooy C, et al: Selective management of abdominal aortic aneurysms in a prospective measurement program. J Vasc Surg 23:213, 1996.
41. Brunkwall J, Hauksson H, Bengtsson H, et al: Solitary aneurysms of the iliac arterial system: An estimate of their frequency of occurrence. J Vasc Surg 10:381, 1989.
42. Bry JDL, Belkin M, O'Donnell TF Jr, et al: An assessment of the positive predictive value and cost-effectiveness of dipyridamole myocardial scintigraphy in patients undergoing vascular surgery. J Vasc Surg 19:112, 1994.
43. Bunt TJ: Synthetic vascular graft infections. I. Graft infections. Surgery 93(6):733, 1983.
44. Bunt TJ: Synthetic vascular graft infections. II. Graft-enteric erosions and graft-enteric fistulas. Surgery 94(1):1, 1983.
45. Bush HL Jr, Hydo LJ, Fischer E, et al: Hypothermia during elective abdominal aortic aneurysm repair: The high price of avoidable morbidity. J Vasc Surg 21:392, 1995.
46. Calcagno D, Hallett J Jr, Ballard DJ, et al: Late iliac artery aneurysms and occlusive disease after aortic tube grafts for abdominal aortic aneurysm repair. A 35-year experience. Ann Surg 214:733, 1991.
47. Calligaro KD, Bergen WS, Savarese RP, et al: Primary aortoduodenal fistula due to septic aortitis. J Cardiovasc Surg 33:192, 1992.
48. Calligaro KD, Savarese RP, McCombs PR, et al: Division of the left renal vein during aortic surgery. Am J Surg 160:192, 1990.
49. Cambria RP, Brewster DC, Abbott WM, et al: Transperitoneal versus retroperitoneal approach for aortic reconstruction: A randomized prospective study. J Vasc Surg 11:314, 1990.
50. Cambria RP, Brewster DC, L'Italien G, et al: Simultaneous aortic and renal artery reconstruction: Evolution of an eighteen-year experience. J Vasc Surg 21(6):916, 1995.
51. Campbell JJ, Bell DD, Gaspar MR: Selective use of arteriography in the assessment of aortic aneurysm repair. Ann Vasc Surg 4:419, 1990.
52. Cardon JM, et al: Endovascular repair of iliac artery aneurysm with Endoprosystem I: A multicentric French study. J Cardiovasc Surg (Torino) 37:45, 1996.
53. Castleden WM, Mercer JC: Abdominal aortic aneurysms in Western Australia: Descriptive epidemiology and patterns of rupture. Br J Surg 72:109, 1985.
54. Chang BB, Paty PS, Shah DM, et al: The right retroperitoneal approach for abdominal aortic surgery. Am J Surg 158(2):156, 1989.

55. Chang JB, Stein TA, Liu JP, et al: Risk factors associated with rapid growth of small abdominal aortic aneurysms. Surgery 121:117, 1997.

56. Chervu A, Clagett GP, Valentine RJ, et al: Role of physical examination in detection of abdominal aortic aneurysms. Surgery 117:454, 1995.

57. Chosky SA, Wilmink ABM, Quick CRG: Ruptured abdominal aortic aneurysm in the Huntingdon district: A 10-year experience. Br J Surg 84(Suppl 1):44, 1997.

58. Clagett GP, Bowers BL, Lopez-Viego MA, et al: Creation of a neo-aortoiliac system from lower extremity deep and superficial veins. Ann Surg 218:239, 1993.

59. Cohen JR, Graver LM: The ruptured abdominal aortic aneurysm of Albert Einstein. Surg Obstet Gynecol 170:455, 1990.

60. Craig SR, Wilson RG, Walker AJ, et al: Abdominal aortic aneurysm: Still missing the message. Br J Surg 80:450, 1993.

61. Crawford ES, Cohen ES: Aortic aneurysm: A multifocal disease. Presidential address. Arch Surg 117(11):1393, 1982.

62. Crawford ES, Coselli JS, Safi HJ, et al: The impact of renal fusion and ectopia on aortic surgery. J Vasc Surg 8:375, 1988.

63. Crawford ES, Hess KR, Cohen ES, et al: Ruptured aneurysm of the descending thoracic and thoracoabdominal aorta: Analysis according to size and treatment. Ann Surg 213:417, 1991.

64. Crawford ES, Saleh SA, Babb JW, et al: Infrarenal abdominal aortic aneurysm: Factors influencing survival after operation performed over a 25-year period. Ann Surg 193(6):699, 1981.

65. Crawford ES, Snyder DM, Cho GC, et al: Progress in treatment of thoracoabdominal and abdominal aortic aneurysms involving celiac, superior mesenteric, and renal arteries. Ann Surg 188(3):404, 1978.

66. Crawford JL, Stowe CL, Safi HJ, et al: Inflammatory aneurysms of the aorta. J Vasc Surg 2:113, 1985.

67. Creech O Jr: Endo-aneurysmorrhaphy and treatment of aortic aneurysm. Ann Surg 164:935, 1966.

68. Cronenwett JL: Factors influencing the long-term results of aortic aneurysm surgery. In Yao J, Pearce W (eds): Vascular Surgery: Long Term Results. East Norwalk, Conn., Appleton & Lange, 1993. p 171.

69. Cronenwett JL, Katz DA: When should infrarenal abdominal aortic aneurysms be repaired: What are the critical risk factors and dimensions? In Veith FJ (ed): Current Critical Problems in Vascular Surgery. Vol 5. St. Louis, Quality Medical Publishing, 1993, p 256.

70. Cronenwett JL: Factors increasing the rupture risk of small aortic aneurysms. In Veith FJ (ed): Current Critical Problems in Vascular Surgery. Vol 3. St. Louis, Quality Medical Publishing, 1991. p 234.

71. Cronenwett JL, Murphy TF, Zelenock GB, et al: Actuarial analysis of variables associated with rupture of small abdominal aortic aneurysms. Surgery 98(3):472, 1985.

72. Cronenwett JL, Sargent SK, Wall MH, et al: Variables that affect the expansion rate and outcome of small abdominal aortic aneurysms. J Vasc Surg 11:260, 1990.

73. Cutler BS, Hendel RC, Leppo JA: Dipyridamole-thallium scintigraphy predicts perioperative and long-term survival after major vascular surgery. J Vasc Surg 15:972, 1992.

74. D'Angelo AJ, Puppala D, Farber A, et al: Is preoperative cardiac evaluation for abdominal aortic aneurysm repair necessary? J Vasc Surg 25(1):152, 1997.

75. Darling RC, Messina CR, Brewster DC, et al: Autopsy study of unoperated abdominal aortic aneurysms: The case for early resection. Circulation 56(3 Suppl):II 161, 1977.

76. Darling RC III, Brewster DC, Darling RC, et al: Are familial abdominal aortic aneurysms different? J Vasc Surg 10(1):39, 1989.

77. Dean RH, Benjamin ME, Hansen KJ: Surgical management of renovascular hypertension. Curr Probl Surg 34(3):209, 1997.

78. Deb B, Benjamin M, Comerota AJ: Delayed rupture of an internal iliac artery aneurysm following proximal ligation for abdominal aortic aneurysm repair. Ann Vasc Surg 6:537, 1992.

79. Dent TL, Lindenauer SM, Ernst CB, et al: Multiple arteriosclerotic arterial aneurysms. Arch Surg 105(2):338, 1972.

80. DePalma R, Levine SB, Feldman S: Preservation of erectile function after aortoiliac reconstruction. Arch Surg 113:958, 1978.

81. Diehl JT, Cali RF, Hertzer NR, et al: Complications of abdominal aortic reconstruction: An analysis of perioperative risk factors in 557 patients. Ann Surg 197:49, 1983.

82. Dietz HC, Cutting GR, Pyeritz RE, et al: Marfan syndrome caused by a recurrent de novo missense mutation in the fibrillin gene. Nature 352(6333):337, 1991.

83. Dobrin PB, Mrkvicka R: Failure of elastin or collagen as possible critical connective tissue alterations underlying aneurysmal dilatation. Cardiovasc Surg 2(4):484, 1994.

84. Dorros G, Cohn JM, Jaff MR: Percutaneous endovascular stent-graft repair of iliac artery aneurysms. J Endovasc Surg 4:370, 1997.

85. Dubost C, Allary M, Oeconomos N: Resection of an aneurysm of the abdominal aorta: Reestablishment of the continuity by a preserved arterial graft, with result after five months. Arch Surg 64:405, 1952.

86. Dupont JR: Isolated left-sided vena cava and abdominal aortic aneurysm. Arch Surg 102:211, 1971.

87. Durham SJ, Steed DL, Moosa HH, et al: Probability of rupture of an abdominal aortic aneurysm after an unrelated operative procedure: A prospective study. J Vasc Surg 13:248, 1991.

88. Eagle KA, Brundage BH, Chaitman BR, et al: Guidelines for perioperative cardiovascular evaluation for noncardiac surgery. Report of the American College of Cardiology/American Heart Association Task Force on Practice Guidelines (Committee on Perioperative Cardiovascular Evaluation for Noncardiac Surgery). J Am Coll Cardiol 27(4):910, 1996.

89. Eagle KA, Coley CM, Newell JB, et al: Combining clinical and thallium data optimizes preoperative assessment of cardiac risk before major vascular surgery. Ann Intern Med 110:859, 1989.

90. Edwards JM, Teefey SA, Zierler RE, et al: Intraabdominal paraanastomotic aneurysms after aortic bypass grafting. J Vasc Surg 15:344, 1992.

91. Englund R, Hudson P, Hanel K, et al: Expansion rates of small abdominal aortic aneurysms. Aust NZ J Surg 58:21, 1998.

92. Ernst CB: Prevention of intestinal ischemia following abdominal aortic reconstruction. Surgery 93:102, 1983.

93. Ernst CB: Abdominal aortic aneurysm. N Engl J Med 328(16):1167, 1993.

94. Ernst CB, Hagihara PF, Daugherty ME, et al: Inferior mesenteric artery stump pressure: A reliable index for safe IMA ligation during abdominal aneurysmectomy. Ann Surg 187:641, 1978.

95. Estes E: Abdominal aortic aneurysm: A study of one hundred and two cases. Circulation 2:258, 1950.

96. Ewart JM, Burke ML, Bunt TJ: Spontaneous abdominal aortic infections: Essentials of diagnosis and management. Am Surg 1983:37, 1983.

97. Faggioli GL, Stella A, Gargiulo M, et al: Morphology of small aneurysms: Definition and impact on risk of rupture. Am J Surg 168:131, 1994.

98. Farkas J, Fichelle J, Laurian C, et al: Long-term followup of positive cultures in 500 abdominal aortic aneurysms. Arch Surg 128:284, 1993.

99. Flanigan DP, et al: Elimination of iatrogenic impotence and improvement of sexual function after aortoiliac revascularization. Arch Surg 117:544, 1982.

100. Foster JH, Bolasny BL, Gobbel WG, et al: Comparative study of elective resection and expectant treatment of abdominal aortic aneurysm. Surg Gynecol Obstet 129:1, 1969.

101. Frame PS, Fryback DG, Patterson C: Screening for abdominal aortic aneurysm in men ages 60 to 80 years. A cost-effectiveness analysis. Ann Intern Med 119:411, 1993.

102. Frank SM, Fleisher LA, Breslow MJ, et al: Perioperative maintenance of normothermia reduces the incidence of morbid cardiac events. A randomized clinical trial. JAMA 277(14):1127, 1997.

103. Franks PJ, Edwards RJ, Greenlaugh RM, et al: Risk factors for abdominal aortic aneurysms in smokers. Eur J Vasc Endovasc Surg 11:487, 1996.

104. Fry RE, Fry WJ: Cholelithiasis and aortic reconstruction: The problem of simultaneous therapy. J Vasc Surg 4:345, 1986.

105. Gadowski GR, Pilcher DB, Ricci MA: Abdominal aortic aneurysm expansion rate: Effect of size and beta-adrenergic blockade. J Vasc Surg 19:727, 1994.

106. Ghilardi G, Scorza R, Bortolani E, et al: Rupture of abdominal aortic aneurysms into the major abdominal veins. J Cardiovasc Surg 34:39, 1993.

107. Gilling-Smith GL, Mansfield AO: Spontaneous abdominal arteriovenous fistulae: Report of eight cases and review of the literature. Br J Surg 78:421, 1991.

108. Gillum RF: Epidemiology of aortic aneurysm in the United States. J Clin Epidemiol 48:1289, 1995.

109. Ginsberg DA, Modrall JG, Esrig D, et al: Concurrent abdominal

aortic aneurysm and urologic neoplasm: An argument for simultaneous intervention. Ann Vasc Surg 9(5):428, 1995.

110. Giordano JM, Trout HH: Anomalies of the inferior vena cava. J Vasc Surg 3:924, 1986.

111. Gloviczki P, Cross SA, Stanson AW, et al: Ischemic injury to the spinal cord or lumbosacral plexus after aorto-iliac reconstruction. Am J Surg 162(2):131, 1991.

112. Gomes MN, Choyke PL, Wallace RB: Infected aortic aneurysms. A changing entity. Ann Surg 15:435, 1992.

113. Goodnough LT, Monk TG, Sicard G, et al: Intraoperative salvage in patients undergoing elective abdominal aortic aneurysm repair: An analysis of cost and benefit. J Vasc Surg 24:213, 1996.

114. Grange JJ, Davis V, Baxter BT: Pathogenesis of abdominal aortic aneurysm: An update and look toward the future. Cardiovasc Surg 5(3):256, 1997.

115. Green RM, Ricotta JJ, Ouriel K, et al: Results of supraceliac aortic clamping in the difficult elective resection of infrarenal abdominal aortic aneurysm. J Vasc Surg 9:125, 1989.

116. Gregory AK, Yin NX, Capella J, et al: Features of autoimmunity in the abdominal aortic aneurysm. Arch Surg 131(1):85, 1996.

117. Grimshaw GM, Thompson JM: The abdominal aorta: A statistical definition and strategy for monitoring change. Eur J Endovasc Surg 10:95, 1995.

118. Guirguis EM, Barber GG: The natural history of abdominal aortic aneurysms. Am J Surg 162:481, 1991.

119. Hallett JW Jr, Marshall DM, Petterson TM, et al: Graft-related complications after abdominal aortic aneurysm repair: Reassurance from a 36-year population-based experience. J Vasc Surg 25:277, 1997.

120. Halloran BG, Davis VA, McManus BM, et al: Localization of aortic disease is associated with intrinsic differences in aortic structure. J Surg Res 59(1):17, 1995.

121. Hertzer NR: Fatal myocardial infarction following abdominal aortic aneurysm resection. Ann Surg 192:667, 1980.

122. Hertzer NR, Young JR, Beven EG, et al: Late results of coronary bypass in patients with infrarenal aortic aneurysms. Ann Surg 205:360, 1987.

123. Hertzer NR, Young JR, Kramer RJ, et al: Routine coronary angiography prior to elective aortic reconstruction. Arch Surg 114:1336, 1979.

124. Hinkamp TJ, Pifarre R, Bakhos M, et al: Combined myocardial revascularization and abdominal aortic aneurysm repair. Ann Thorac Surg 51:470, 1991.

125. Hirose Y, Hamada S, Takamiya M: Predicting the growth of aortic aneurysms: A comparison of linear vs exponential models. Angiology 46:413, 1995.

126. Hollier LH, Plate G, O'Brien PC, et al: Late survival after abdominal aortic aneurysm repair: Influence of coronary artery disease. J Vasc Surg 1:290, 1984.

127. Hollier LH, Reigel MM, Kazmier FJ, et al: Conventional repair of abdominal aortic aneurysm in the high-risk patient: A plea for abandonment of nonresective treatment. J Vasc Surg 3:712, 1986.

128. Hollier LH, Spittell JA, Puga FJ: Intra-aortic balloon counterpulsation as adjunct to aneurysmectomy in high-risk patients. Mayo Clin Proc 56:565, 1981.

129. Hollis HW, Rutherford RB: Abdominal aortic aneurysms associated with horseshoe or ectopic kidneys. Techniques of renal preservation. Semin Vasc Surg 1:148, 1988.

130. Houben PF, Bollen EC, Nuyens CM: "Asymptomatic" ruptured aneurysm: A report of two cases of aortocaval fistula presenting with cardiac failure. Eur J Vasc Surg 7:352, 1993.

131. Huber TS. et al: Intraoperative autologous transfusion during elective infrarenal aortic reconstruction: A decision analysis model. J Vasc Surg 25:984, 1997.

132. Hunter GC, Smyth SH, Aguirre ML, et al: Incidence and histologic characteristics of blebs in patients with abdominal aortic aneurysm. J Vasc Surg 24:93, 1996.

133. Inahara T, Geary GL, Mukherjee D, et al: The contrary position to the nonresective treatment for abdominal aortic aneurysm. J Vasc Surg 2:42, 1985.

134. Jaakkola P, Hippelainen M, Farin P, et al: Interobserver variability in measuring the dimensions of the abdominal aorta: Comparison of ultrasound and computed tomography. Eur J Vasc Endovasc Surg 12:230, 1996.

135. Johansen K, Koepsell T: Familial tendency for abdominal aortic aneurysms. JAMA 256:1934, 1986.

136. Johnston KW: Multicenter prospective study of nonruptured abdominal aortic aneurysm. Part II. Variables predicting morbidity and mortality. J Vasc Surg 9(3):437, 1989.

137. Johnston KW, Rutherford RB, Tilson MD, et al: Suggested standards for reporting on arterial aneurysms. Subcommittee on Reporting Standards for Arterial Aneurysms, Ad Hoc Committee on Reporting Standards, Society for Vascular Surgery and North American Chapter, International Society for Cardiovascular Surgery. J Vasc Surg 13(3):452, 1991.

138. Johnston KW, Scobie TK: Multicenter prospective study of nonruptured abdominal aortic aneurysms I. Population and operative management. J Vasc Surg 7:69, 1988.

139. Juvonen J, Juvonen T, Laurila A, et al: Demonstration of Chlamydia pneumoniae in the walls of abdominal aortic aneurysms. J Vasc Surg 25(3):499, 1997.

140. Kaiser AB, Clayson KR, Mulherin JL Jr, et al: Antibiotic prophylaxis in vascular surgery. Ann Surg 188(3):283, 1978.

141. Karmody AM, Leather RP, Goldman M, et al: The current position of non-resective treatment for abdominal aortic aneurysm. Surgery 94:591, 1983.

142. Katz DJ, Stanley JC, et al: Operative mortality rates for intact and ruptured abdominal aortic aneurysms in Michigan: An eleven-year statewide experience. J Vasc Surg 19:804, 1994.

143. Katz DA, Cronenwett JL: The cost-effectiveness of early surgery versus watchful waiting in the management of small abdominal aortic aneurysms. J Vasc Surg 19(6):980, 1994.

144. Katz DA, Littenberg B, Cronenwett JL: Management of small abdominal aortic aneurysms. Early surgery vs watchful waiting. JAMA 268(19):2678, 1992.

145. Kazmers A, et al: Abdominal aortic aneurysm repair in Veterans Affairs medical centers. J Vasc Surg 23:191, 1996.

146. Kazmers A, Perkins AJ, Jacobs LA: Outcomes after abdominal aortic aneurysm repair in those > or =80 years of age: Recent Veterans Affairs experience. Ann Vasc Surg 12(2):106, 1998.

147. Kieffer E, Bahnini A, Koskas F, et al: In situ allograft replacement of infected infrarenal aortic prosthetic grafts: Results in forty-three patients. J Vasc Surg 17:349, 1993.

148. Kline RG, D'Angelo AJ, Chen MH, et al: Laparoscopically assisted abdominal aortic aneurysm repair: First 20 cases. J Vasc Surg 27(1):81, 1998.

149. Koskas F, Kieffer E: Long-term survival after elective repair of infrarenal abdominal aortic aneurysm: Results of a prospective multicentric study. Association for Academic Research in Vascular Surgery (AURC). Ann Vasc Surg 11:473, 1997.

150. Krupski WC, Bass A, Thurston DW, et al: Utility of computed tomography for surveillance of small abdominal aortic aneurysms. Arch Surg 125:1345, 1990.

151. Krupski WC, Selzman CH, Floridia R, et al: Contemporary management of isolated iliac aneurysms. J Vasc Surg 28:1, 1998.

152. Kushihashi T, Munechika H, Matsui S, et al: [CT of abdominal aortic aneurysms—aneurysmal size and thickness of intra-aneurysmal thrombus as risk factors of rupture.] Nippon Igaku Hoshasen Gakkai Zasshi 51(3):219, 1991.

153. Kvilekval KHV, Best IM, Mason RA, et al: The value of computed tomography in the management of symptomatic abdominal aortic aneurysms. J Vasc Surg 12:28, 1990.

154. L'Italien GJ, Paul SD, Hendel RC, et al: Development and validation of a Bayesian model for perioperative cardiac risk assessment in a cohort of 1,081 vascular surgical candidates. J Am Coll Cardiol 27:779, 1996.

155. Lacquet JP, Lacroix H, Nevelsteen A, et al: Inflammatory abdominal aortic aneurysms. A retrospective study of 110 cases. Acta Chir Belg 97:286, 1997.

156. Lalka SG, Sawada SG, Dalsing MC, et al: Dobutamine stress echocardiography as a predictor of cardiac events associated with aortic surgery. J Vasc Surg 15:831, 1992.

157. LaMorte WW, Scott TE, et al: Racial differences in the incidence of femoral bypass and abdominal aortic aneurysmectomy in Massachusetts: Relationship to cardiovascular risk factors. J Vasc Surg 21:422, 1995.

158. Lawrence PF, Lorenzo-Rivero S, Lyon JL: The incidence of iliac, femoral and popliteal artery aneurysms in hospitalized patients. J Vasc Surg 22:409, 1995.

159. Leach SD, Toole AL, Stern H, et al: Effect of beta-adrenergic blockade on the growth rate of abdominal aortic aneurysms. Arch Surg 123:606, 1988.

160. Lederle FA: Risk of rupture of large abdominal aortic aneurysms: Disagreement among vascular surgeons. Arch Intern Med 156(9): 1007, 1996.
161. Lederle FA, Johnson GR, Wilson SE, et al: Prevalence and associations of abdominal aortic aneurysm detected through screening: Aneurysm Detection and Management (ADAM) Veterans Affairs Cooperative Study Group. Ann Intern Med 126(6):441, 1997.
162. Lederle FA, Johnson GR, Wilson SE, et al: Relationship of age, gender, race and body size to infrarenal aortic diameter. J Vasc Surg 26:595, 1997.
163. Lederle FA, Walker JM, Reinke DB: Selective screening for abdominal aortic aneurysms with physical examination and ultrasound. Arch Intern Med 148(8):1753, 1988.
164. Lederle FA, Wilson SE, Johnson GR, et al: Variability in measurement of abdominal aortic aneurysms. J Vasc Surg 21:945, 1995.
165. Lee AJ, Fowkes FGR, Carson MN, et al: Smoking, atherosclerosis and risk of abdominal aortic aneurysm. Eur Heart J 18:671, 1997.
166. Leonardo R: History of Surgery. New York, Froben Press, 1943.
167. Lette J, Waters D, Lassonde J, et al: Multivariate clinical models and quantitative dipyridamole-thallium imaging to predict cardiac morbidity and death after vascular reconstruction. J Vasc Surg 14:160, 1991.
168. Levinson JR, Boucher CA, Coley CM, et al: Usefulness of semiquantitative analysis of dipyridamole-thallium-201 redistribution for improving risk stratification before vascular surgery. Am J Cardiol 66:406, 1990.
169. Limet R, Sakalihassan N, Albert A: Determination of the expansion rate and incidence of rupture of abdominal aortic aneurysms. J Vasc Surg 14:540, 1991.
170. Lindblad B, Almgren B, Bergqvist D, et al: Abdominal aortic aneurysm with perianeurysmal fibrosis: Experience from 11 Swedish vascular centers. J Vasc Surg 13(2):231, 1991.
171. Lindholt JS, Henneberg EW, Fasting H, et al: Mass or high-risk screening for abdominal aortic aneurysm. Br J Surg 84:40, 1997.
172. Littooy FN, Steffan G, Greisler HP, et al: Use of sequential B-mode ultrasonography to manage abdominal aortic aneurysms. Arch Surg 124:419, 1989.
173. Lobato A, Puech-Leao P: Predictive factors for rupture of thoracoabdominal aortic aneurysm. J Vasc Surg 27:446, 1998.
174. Longo WE, Lee TC, Barnett MG, et al: Ischemic colitis complicating abdominal aortic aneurysm surgery in the U.S. veteran. J Surg Res 60:351, 1996.
175. Lord RSA, Nash PA, Raj PT, et al: Prospective randomized trial of polytetrafluoroethylene and Dacron aortic prosthesis. I. Perioperative results. Ann Vasc Surg 3:248, 1988.
176. Lorenz M, Panitz K, Grosse-Furtner C, et al: Lower-limb amputation, prevalence of abdominal aortic aneurysm and atherosclerotic risk factors. Br J Surg 81(6):839, 1994.
177. Lynch K, Kohler T, Johansen K: Nonresective therapy for aortic aneurysm: Results of a survey. J Vasc Surg 4:469, 1986.
178. Mabry CD, Thompson BW, Read RC: Activated clotting time (ACT) monitoring of intraoperative heparinization in peripheral vascular surgery. Am J Surg 138(6):894, 1979.
179. MacSweeney ST, Ellis M, Worrell PC, et al: Smoking and growth rate of small abdominal aortic aneurysms. Lancet 344(8923):651, 1994.
180. Majumder PP, St. Jean PL, Ferrell RE, et al: On the inheritance of abdominal aortic aneurysm. Am J Hum Genet 48(1):164, 1991.
181. Mangano DT, Layug EL, Wallace A, et al: Effect of atenolol on mortality and cardiovascular morbidity after noncardiac surgery: Multicenter Study of Perioperative Ischemia Research Group. N Engl J Med 335(23):1713, 1996.
182. Marin ML, Veith FJ, Lyon RT, et al: Transfemoral endovascular repair of iliac artery aneurysms. Am J Surg 170:179, 1995.
183. Marston WA, Ahlquist R, Johnson G, et al: Misdiagnosis of ruptured abdominal aortic aneurysm. J Vasc Surg 16:17, 1992.
184. Mason RA, Newton GB, Cassel W, et al: Combined epidural and general anesthesia in aortic surgery. J Cardiovasc Surg (Torino) 31(4):442, 1990.
185. Matas R: Ligation of the abdominal aorta: Report of the ultimate result, one year, five months and nine days after the ligation of the abdominal aorta for aneurysm of the bifurcation. Ann Surg 81:457, 1925.
186. McCready RA, Pairolero PC, Gilmore JC, et al: Isolated iliac artery aneurysms. Surgery 93:688, 1983.
187. McMillan WD, Tamarina NA, Cipollone M, et al: Size matters: The relationship between MMP-9 expression and aortic diameter. Circulation 96(7):2228, 1997.
188. Meagher AP, Lord RS, Graham AR, et al: Acute aortic occlusion presenting with lower limb paralysis. J Cardiovasc Surg (Torino) 32(5):643, 1991.
189. Melton LJ, Bickerstaff LK, Hollier LH, et al: Changing incidence of abdominal aortic aneurysms: A population-based study. Am J Epidemiol 120:379, 1984.
190. Michaels JA: The management of small abdominal aortic aneurysms: A computer simulation using Monte Carlo methods. Eur J Vasc Surg 6:551, 1992.
191. Miller DC, Meyers BD: Pathophysiology and prevention of acute renal failure associated with thoracoabdominal or abdominal aortic surgery. J Vasc Surg 5:518, 1987.
192. Morris GE, Hubbard CS, Quick CRG: An abdominal aortic aneurysm screening programme for all males over the age of 50 years. Eur J Vasc Surg 8:156, 1994.
193. Moulder PV: Physiology and biomechanics of aneurysms. In Kerstein MD, Moulder PV, Webb WR (eds): Aneurysms. Baltimore, Williams & Wilkins, 1983, p 19.
194. Moursi MM, Beebe HG, Messina LM, et al: Inhibition of aortic aneurysm development in blotchy mice by beta adrenergic blockade independent of altered lysyl oxidase activity. J Vasc Surg 21(5):792, 1995.
195. Mower WR, Quinones WJ, Gambhir SS: Effect of intraluminal thrombus on abdominal aortic aneurysm wall stress. J Vasc Surg 26(4):602, 1997.
196. Muluk SC, Gertler JP, Brewster DC, et al: Presentation and patterns of aortic aneurysms in young patients. J Vasc Surg 20:880, 1994.
197. Nenhaus HP, Javid H: The distinct syndrome of spontaneous aortic-caval fistula. Am J Med 44:464, 1968.
198. Nevitt MP, Ballard DJ, Hallett JW: Prognosis of abdominal aortic aneurysms: A population based study. N Engl J Med 321:1009, 1989.
199. Nitecki SS, et al: Inflammatory abdominal aortic aneurysms: A case-control study. J Vasc Surg 23:860, 1996.
200. Nora JD, et al: Concomitant abdominal aortic aneurysm and colorectal carcinoma: Priority of resection. J Vasc Surg 9:630, 1989.
201. Nypaver TJ, Shepard A, Reddy DJ, et al: Repair of pararenal abdominal aortic aneurysms: An analysis of operative management. Arch Surg 128:803, 1993.
202. Olin JW, Graor RA, O'Hara P, et al: The incidence of deep venous thrombosis in patients undergoing abdominal aortic aneurysm resection. J Vasc Surg 18:1037, 1993.
203. Olsen PS, Schroeder T, Agerskov K, et al: Surgery for abdominal aortic aneurysms: A survey of 656 patients. J Cardiovasc Surg (Torino) 32(5):636, 1991.
204. Ouriel K, Shortell CK, Green RM, et al: Intraoperative autotransfusion in aortic surgery. J Vasc Surg 18:16, 1993.
205. Ouriel K, Green RM, Donayre C, et al: An evaluation of new methods of expressing aortic aneurysm size: Relationship to rupture. J Vasc Surg 15:12, 1992.
206. Ouriel K, Ricotta JJ, Adams JT, et al: Management of cholelithiasis in patients with abdominal aortic aneurysms. Ann Surg 198:717, 1983.
207. Ozsvath KJ, Hirose H, Xia S, et al: Molecular mimicry in human aortic aneurysmal diseases. Ann NY Acad Sci 800:288, 1996.
208. Palda VA, Detsky AS: Guidelines for assessing and managing the perioperative risk from coronary artery disease associated with major noncardiac surgery: American College of Physicians. Ann Intern Med 127(4):309, 1997.
209. Parodi JC, Palmaz JC, Barone HD: Transfemoral intraluminal graft implantation for abdominal aortic aneurysms. Ann Vasc Surg 5:491, 1991.
210. Pasch AR, Ricotta JJ, May AG, et al: Abdominal aortic aneurysm: The case for elective resection. Circulation 70(Suppl I):I, 1984.
211. Pasternack PF, Grossi EA, Baumann FG, et al: Beta blockade to decrease silent myocardial ischemia during peripheral vascular surgery. Am J Surg 158:113, 1989.
212. Patel MI, Hardman DT, Fisher CM, et al: Current views on the pathogenesis of abdominal aortic aneurysms. J Am Coll Surg 181(4):371, 1995.
213. Paty PS, Darling RC III, Chang BB, et al: A prospective randomized study comparing exclusion technique and endoaneurysmorrhaphy for treatment of infrarenal aortic aneurysm. J Vasc Surg 25:442, 1997.

214. Pavone P, Di Cesare E, Di Renzi P, et al: Abdominal aortic aneurysm evaluation: Comparison of US, CT, MRI, and angiography. Magn Reson Imaging 8:199, 1990.
215. Pearce WH, Slaughter MS, LeMaire S, et al: Aortic diameter as a function of age, gender, and body surface area. Surgery 114:691, 1993.
216. Fennell RC, Hollier LH, Lie JT, et al: Inflammatory abdominal aortic aneurysms: A thirty-year review. J Vasc Surg 2:859, 1985.
217. Petersen E, Boman J, Persson K, et al: *Chlamydia pneumoniae* in human abdominal aortic aneurysms. Eur J Vasc Endovasc Surg 15(2):138, 1998.
218. Petrinec D, Liao S, Holmes DR, et al: Doxycycline inhibition of aneurysmal degeneration in an elastase-induced rat model of abdominal aortic aneurysm: Preservation of aortic elastin associated with suppressed production of 92 kD gelatinase. J Vasc Surg 23(2):336, 1996.
219. Picone AL, Green RM, Ricotta JR, et al: Spinal cord ischemia following operations on the abdominal aorta. J Vasc Surg 3:94, 1986.
220. Piotrowski JJ, McCroskey BL, Rutherford RB: Selection of grafts currently available for repair of abdominal aortic aneurysms. Surg Clin North Am 69:827, 1989.
221. Plate G, Hollier LA, O'Brien PO, et al: Recurrent aneurysms and late vascular complications following repair of abdominal aortic aneurysms. Arch Surg 120:590, 1985.
222. Polterauer P, Prager M, Holzenbein T, et al: Dacron versus polytetrafluoroethylene for Y-aortic bifurcation grafts: A six-year prospective, randomized trial. Surgery 111:626, 1992.
223. Powell JT, Greenhalgh RM: Multifactorial inheritance of abdominal aortic aneurysm. Eur J Vasc Surg 1:29, 1987.
224. Power DA: The palliative treatment of aneurysms by "wiring" with Colt's apparatus. Br J Surg 9:27, 1921.
225. Provan JL, Fialkov J, Ameli FM, et al: Is tube repair of aortic aneurysm followed by aneurysmal change in the common iliac arteries? Can J Surg 33(5):394, 1990.
226. Qvarfordt PG, Stoney RJ, Reilly LM, et al: Management of pararenal aneurysms of the abdominal aorta. J Vasc Surg 3:84, 1986.
227. Raggi R, Dardik H, Mauro AL: Continuous epidural anesthesia and postoperative epidural narcotics in vascular surgery. Am J Surg 154(2):192, 1987.
228. Rasmussen TE, Hallett JW Jr: Inflammatory aortic aneurysms: A clinical review with new perspectives in pathogenesis. Ann Surg 225:155, 1997.
229. Rea CE: The surgical treatment of aneurysm of the abdominal aorta. Minn Med 31:153, 1948.
230. Reddy DJ, Shepard AD, Evans JR, et al: Management of infected aortoiliac aneurysms. Arch Surg 126:873, 1991.
231. Reed WL, Hallett JW Jr, Damiano MA, et al: Learning from the last ultrasound. A population-based study of patients with abdominal aortic aneurysm. Arch Intern Med 157:2064, 1997.
232. Reigel MM, Hollier LH, Kazmier FJ, et al: Late survival in abdominal aortic aneurysm patients: The role of selective myocardial revascularization on the basis of clinical symptoms. J Vasc Surg 5:222, 1987.
233. Reilly LM, Ramos TK, Murray SP, et al: Optimal exposure of the proximal abdominal aorta: A critical appraisal of transabdominal medial visceral rotation. J Vasc Surg 19(3):375, 1994.
234. Ricci MA, Strindberg G, Slaiby JM, et al: Anti-CD 18 monoclonal antibody slows experimental aortic aneurysm expansion. J Vasc Surg 23(2):301, 1996.
235. Richardson JW, Greenfield LJ: Natural history and management of iliac aneurysms. J Vasc Surg 8:165, 1988.
236. Richardson JD, Main KA: Repair of abdominal aortic aneurysms. A statewide experience. Arch Surg 126:614, 1991.
237. Roger VL, Ballard DJ, Hallett JW, et al: Influence of coronary artery disease on morbidity and mortality after abdominal aortic aneurysmectomy: A population-based study 1971–1987. J Am Coll Cardiol 14:1245, 1989.
238. Ruby ST, Whittemore AD, Couch NP, et al: Coronary artery disease in patients requiring abdominal aortic aneurysm repair. Selective use of a combined operation. Ann Surg 201:758, 1985.
239. Salo JA, Verkkala KA, Ala-Kulju KV, et al: Hematuria is an indication of rupture of an abdominal aortic aneurysm into the vena cava. J Vasc Surg 12:41, 1990.
240. Sarkar R, Coran AG, Cilley RE, et al: Arterial aneurysms in children: Clinicopathologic classification. J Vasc Surg 13(1):47, 1991.
241. Saxon SR, Glover WM, Youkey JR: Aortocaval fistula and contained

rupture of an abdominal aortic aneurysm presenting with pelvic venous congestion. Ann Vasc Surg 4:381, 1990.
242. Schaffer PW, Hardin CW: The use of temporary and polyethylene shunts to permit occlusion, resection and frozen homologous artery graft replacement of vital vessel segments. Surgery 31:186, 1952.
243. Schatz IJ, Fairbairn JF, Jugens JL: Abdominal aortic aneurysms: A reappraisal. Circulation 26:200, 1962.
244. Schewe CK, Schweikart HP, Hammel G, et al: Influence of selective management on the prognosis and the risk of rupture of abdominal aortic aneurysms. Clin Invest 72(8):585, 1994.
245. Schneider JR, Cronenwett JL: Temporary perfusion of a congenital pelvic kidney during abdominal aortic aneurysm repair. J Vasc Surg 17(3):613, 1993.
246. Schneiderman J, Adar R, Engelberg I, et al: Medical control of abdominal aortic aneurysm expansion rate. J Vasc Surg 24(2):297, 1996.
247. Schueppert MT, Kresowik TF, Corry DC, et al: Selection of patients for cardiac evaluation before peripheral vascular operations. J Vasc Surg 23:802, 1996.
248. Schwartz RA, Nichols WK, Silver D: Is thrombosis of the infrarenal abdominal aortic aneurysm an acceptable alternative? J Vasc Surg 3(3):448, 1986.
249. Scott RA, Ashton HA, Kay DN: Abdominal aortic aneurysm in 4237 screened patients: Prevalence, development and management over 6 years. Br J Surg 78:1122, 1991.
250. Scott RAP, Wilson NM, Ashton HA, et al: Influence of screening on the incidence of ruptured abdominal aortic aneurysm: 5-year results of a randomized controlled study. Br J Surg 82:1066, 1995.
251. Seeger JM, Kieffer RW: Preoperative CT in symptomatic abdominal aortic aneurysms: Accuracy and efficacy. Am Surg 52:87, 1986.
252. Shah DM, Chang BB, Paty PS, et al: Treatment of abdominal aortic aneurysm by exclusion and bypass: An analysis of outcome. J Vasc Surg 13:15, 1991.
253. Shah PK: Inflammation, metalloproteinases, and increased proteolysis: An emerging pathophysiological paradigm in aortic aneurysm. Circulation 96:2115, 1997.
254. Shepard AD, Tollefson DF, Reddy DJ, et al: Left flank retroperitoneal exposure: A technical aid to complex aortic reconstruction. J Vasc Surg 14(3):283, 1991.
255. Shuman WP, Hastrup WJ, Kohler TR, et al: Suspected leaking abdominal aortic aneurysm: Use of sonography in the emergency room. Radiology 168(1):117, 1988.
256. Sicard GA, Reilly JM, Rubin BG, et al: Transabdominal versus retroperitoneal incision for abdominal aortic surgery: Report of a prospective randomized trial. J Vasc Surg 21:174, 1995.
257. Sieunarine K, Lawrence-Brown MM, Goodman MA, et al: Comparison of transperitoneal and retroperitoneal approaches for infrarenal aortic surgery: Early and late results. Cardiovasc Surg 5:71, 1997.
258. Silverberg E, Boring CC, Squires TS: Cancer statistics, 1990. Cancer 40:9, 1990.
259. Soreide O, Lillestol J, Christensen O, et al: Abdominal aortic aneurysms: Survival analysis of four hundred thirty-four patients. Surgery 91(2):188, 1982.
260. St Leger AS, Spencely M, McCollum CN, et al: Screening for abdominal aortic aneurysm: A computer assisted cost-utility analysis. Eur J Vasc Endovasc Surg 11:183, 1996.
261. Starr DS, Foster WJ, Morris GC Jr: Resection of abdominal aortic aneurysm in the presence of horseshoe kidney. Surgery 89:387, 1981.
262. Stella A, Gargiulo M, Faggioli GL, et al: Postoperative course of inflammatory abdominal aortic aneurysms. Ann Vasc Surg 7:229, 1993.
263. Sterpetti AV, Cavallaro A, Cavallari N, et al: Factors influencing the rupture of abdominal aortic aneurysm. Surg Obstet Gynecol 173:175, 1991.
264. Sterpetti AV, Hunter WJ, Feldhaus RJ, et al: Inflammatory aneurysms of the abdominal aorta: Incidence, pathologic, and etiologic considerations. J Vasc Surg 9:643, 1989.
265. Sterpetti AV, Hunter WJ, Schultz RD: Congenital abdominal aortic aneurysms in the young: Case report and review of the literature. J Vasc Surg 7:763, 1988.
266. Sterpetti AV, Schultz RD, Feldhaus RJ, et al: Factors influencing enlargement rate of small abdominal aortic aneurysms. J Surg Res 43:211, 1987.
267. Steyerberg EW, Kievit J, Alexander de Mol Van Otterloo JC, et al:

Perioperative mortality of elective abdominal aortic aneurysm surgery: A clinical prediction rule based on literature and individual patient data. Arch Intern Med 155:1998, 1995.

268. Stonebridge PA, Callam MJ, Bradbury AW, et al: Comparison of long-term survival after successful repair of ruptured and non-ruptured abdominal aortic aneurysm. Br J Surg 80(5):585, 1993.
269. Stotter AT, Grigg MJ, Mansfield AO: The response of peri-aneurysmal fibrosis—the "inflammatory" aneurysm—to surgery and steroid therapy. Eur J Vasc Surg 4(2):201, 1990.
270. Strachan DP: Predictors of death from aortic aneurysm among middle-aged men: The Whitehall study. Br J Surg 78:401, 1991.
271. String ST: Cholelithiasis and aortic reconstruction. J Vasc Surg 1:664, 1984.
272. Sullivan CA, Rohrer MJ, Cutler BS: Clinical management of the symptomatic but unruptured abdominal aortic aneurysm. J Vasc Surg 11:799, 1990.
273. Swanson RJ, Littooy FN, Hunt TK, et al: Laparotomy as a precipitating factor in the rupture of intra-abdominal aneurysms. Arch Surg 115:299, 1980.
274. Sweeney MS, Gadacz TR: Primary aortoduodenal fistula: Manifestation, diagnosis, and treatment. Surgery 96:492, 1984.
275. Szilagyi DE, Elliott JP, Smith RF, et al: Clinical fate of the patient with asymptomatic aortic aneurysm and unfit for surgical treatment. Arch Surg 104:600, 1972.
276. Szilagyi DE, Hageman JH, Smith RF, et al: Spinal cord damage in surgery of the abdominal aorta. Surgery 83:38, 1978.
277. Szilagyi DE, Smith RF, DeRusso FJ, et al: Contribution of abdominal aortic aneurysmectomy to prolongation of life. Ann Surg 164:678, 1966.
278. Szilagyi DE, Smith RF, Elliott JP, et al: Anastomotic aneurysms after vascular reconstruction: Problems of incidence, etiology, and treatment. Surgery 78:800, 1975.
279. Szilagyi DE, Smith RF, Elliott JP, et al: Infection in arterial reconstruction with synthetic grafts. Ann Surg 176(3):321, 1972.
280. Taylor L Jr, Yeager RA, Moneta GL, et al: The incidence of perioperative myocardial infarction in general vascular surgery. J Vasc Surg 15:52, 1991.
281. Tennant WG, et al: Radiologic investigation of abdominal aortic aneurysm disease: Comparison of three modalities in staging and the detection of inflammatory change. J Vasc Surg 17:703, 1993.
282. Thomas J, Blake K, Pierce G, et al: The clinical course of asymptomatic mesenteric arterial stenosis. J Vasc Surg 27:840, 1998.
283. Thomas PR, Shaw JC, Ashton HA, et al: Accuracy of ultrasound in a screening programme for abdominal aortic aneurysms. J Med Screen 1(1):3, 1994.
284. Thompson RW: Basic science of abdominal aortic aneurysms: Emerging therapeutic strategies for an unresolved clinical problem. Curr Opin Cardiol 11(5):504, 1996.
285. Tilson MD: Personal communication, 1998.
286. Tilson MD, Ozsvath KJ, Hirose H, et al: A genetic basis for autoimmune manifestations in the abdominal aortic aneurysm resides in the MHC class II locus DR-beta-1. Ann NY Acad Sci 800:208, 1996.
287. Tollefson DF, Ernst CB: Natural history of atherosclerotic renal artery stenosis associated with aortic disease. J Vasc Surg 14(3):327, 1991.
288. Treiman RL, Hartunian SL, Cossman DV, et al: Late results of small untreated abdominal aortic aneurysms. Ann Vasc Surg 5:359, 1991.

289. van der Vliet JA, Boll AP: Abdominal aortic aneurysm. Lancet 349(9055):863, 1997.
290. Veith FJ, Goldsmith J, Leather RP, et al: The need for quality assurance in vascular surgery. J Vasc Surg 13:523, 1991.
291. Verloes A, Sakalihasan N, Koulischer L, et al: Aneurysms of the abdominal aorta: Familial and genetic aspects in three hundred thirteen pedigrees. J Vasc Surg 21(4):646, 1995.
292. Vohra R, Reid D, Groome J, et al: Long-term survival in patients undergoing resection of abdominal aortic aneurysm. Ann Vasc Surg 4(5):460, 1990.
293. Vollmar JF, Paes E, Pauschinger P, et al: Aortic aneurysms as late sequelae of above-knee amputation. Lancet 2(8667):834, 1989.
294. Vorp DA, Raghavan ML, Webster MW: Mechanical wall stress in abdominal aortic aneurysm: Influence of diameter and asymmetry. J Vasc Surg 27:632, 1998.
295. Webster MW, Ferrell RE, St. Jean PI, et al: Ultrasound screening of first-degree relatives of patients with an abdominal aortic aneurysm. J Vasc Surg 13:9, 1991.
296. Weinstein MH, Machleder HI: Sexual function after aortoiliac surgery. Ann Surg 181:787, 1975.
297. Welling RE, Roedersheimer LR, Arbaugh JJ, et al: Ischemic colitis following repair of ruptured abdominal aortic aneurysm. Arch Surg 120:1368, 1985.
298. Wheeler WE, Hanks J, Raman VK: Primary aortoenteric fistulas. Am Surg 58:53, 1992.
299. Wills A, Thompson MM, Crowther M, et al: Pathogenesis of abdominal aortic aneurysms—cellular and biochemical mechanisms. Eur J Vasc Endovasc Surg 12(4):391, 1996.
300. Wilmink ABM, Hubbard CS, Quick CRG: The influence of screening for asymptomatic abdominal aortic aneurysms in men over the age of 50 on the incidence of ruptured abdominal aneurysms in the Huntington district. Br J Surg 84(Suppl 1):11, 1997.
301. Wilmink ABM, Quick CRG: Epidemiology and potential for prevention of abdominal aortic aneurysm. Br J Surg 85:155, 1998.
302. Wolf YG, Otis SM, Schwend RB, et al: Screening for abdominal aortic aneurysms during lower extremity arterial evaluation in the vascular laboratory. J Vasc Surg 22:417, 1995.
303. Wolf YG, Thomas WS, Brennan FJ, et al: Computed tomography scanning findings associated with rapid expansion of abdominal aortic aneurysms. J Vasc Surg 20:529, 1994.
304. Wolinsky H, Glagov S: Comparison of abdominal and thoracic aortic medial structure in mammals: Deviation of man from the usual pattern. Circ Res 25(6):677, 1969.
305. Wong T, Detsky AS: Preoperative cardiac risk assessment for patients having peripheral vascular surgery. Ann Intern Med 116:743, 1992.
306. Yeager MP, Glass DD, Neff RK, et al: Epidural anethesia and analgesia in high-risk surgical patients. Anesthesiology 66:729, 1987.
307. Zdanowski Z, Ribbe E, Schalen C: Bacterial adherence to synthetic vascular prostheses and influence of human plasma: An in vitro study. Eur J Vasc Surg 7:277, 1993.
308. Ziegler DW, Wright JG, Choban PS, et al: A prospective randomized trial of preoperative "optimization" of cardiac function in patients undergoing elective peripheral vascular surgery. Surgery 122(3):584, 1997.
309. Zierler RE, Bergelin RO, Davidson RC, et al: A prospective study of disease progression in patients with atherosclerotic renal artery stenosis. Am J Hypertens 9(11):1055, 1996.

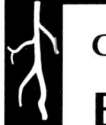

C H A P T E R   9 0

Endovascular Treatment of Aortic Aneurysms

James May, M.D., M.S., F.R.A.C.S., F.A.C.S., and
Geoffrey H. White, M.D., F.R.A.C.S.

This chapter concentrates on the endovascular treatment of abdominal aortic aneurysms (AAAs) and the endovascular treatment of aneurysms of the descending thoracic aorta. The endovascular method of treating AAAs has attracted much interest since the first report of its feasibility in 1991.[1] The conventional method of AAA repair by open operation, however, produces excellent long-term results, and this is the standard by which the endovascular technique will be judged.

Endovascular aneurysm repair involves the transluminal placement of a graft within the aneurysm that completely excludes the sac from the general circulation. The graft is anchored in place by a balloon-expandable or self-expanding metal frame that supports all or part of the graft and provides a watertight seal proximal and distal to the dilated segment of the artery. Because it avoids the need for laparotomy, cross-clamping of the aorta, and the obligatory blood loss associated with opening the aneurysm sac, the technique has much to recommend it. It has the potential to reduce the morbidity and mortality associated with conventional open AAA repair and extend the scope of repair to those patients with severe medical co-morbidities who were previously denied treatment.

Despite the advantages, there are two major areas of concern with the endovascular method. One is the unknown long-term outcome and, specifically, whether the deployment of an endograft in the proximal neck of the AAA will arrest the natural history of progressive aneurysm degeneration in that segment of the aorta. Similarly, the durability of the prosthesis in the long term is unknown, with structural failure already having been reported in two types of device.[2, 3]

The second area of concern is for those complications that are specific to endovascular repair. Manipulation of endovascular devices within an aneurysm has resulted in massive microembolization that has proved to be fatal.[4] Despite improvements in technology and increasing experience, endoleak, a phenomenon unique to endovascular repair, remains a problem in up to 20% of patients.[5, 6] The term *endoleak* refers to incomplete exclusion of the aneurysm sac where a leakage remains within the confines of the vessel but external to the endovascular graft. Aneurysms with this clinical course usually continue to expand and may go on to rupture.

There are reports of historic comparison[7] and concurrent comparison[8] of the two methods in attempts to determine the place of endovascular repair of aortic aneurysms relative to open repair. No prospective randomized trials have been published.

HISTORICAL BACKGROUND

Endovascular treatment of aortic aneurysms is not new. As early as 1684, Moore is said to have attempted thrombosis of an aneurysm by introducing 75 feet of intraluminal wire into it.[9] Before antibiotics were used, most aneurysms were syphilitic in origin and saccular in morphology. This made them more amenable to treatment by wiring than the fusiform variety seen today. Corradi in 1879 modified the process by passing an electric current along an insulated wire.[10] Power described a device, credited to his house surgeon, Colt, that delivered a self-expanding wire umbrella into the aneurysm via a trocar.[11] The method encouraged thrombosis and had limited success. As late as 1938, Blakemore and King were reporting electrothermic coagulation of aortic aneurysms.[12] The technique was largely abandoned after graft replacement of aneurysms was developed.

INDICATIONS FOR TREATMENT

The indications for elective repair of an AAA include asymptomatic aneurysms more than 5 cm in diameter and all symptomatic and ruptured aneurysms, provided that coexisting medical conditions do not preclude operation.[13] It was in the high-risk patients who were unfit for conventional open repair that endovascular repair was first used in the management of aortic aneurysms. Although many high-risk patients were thus able to be treated, there were important implications if the endovascular technique failed and required conversion to open repair in patients denied conventional surgery due to medical co-morbidities. The mortality in patients with this clinical course proved to be very high.[14] With improvements in technology and increasing experience, however, the incidence of conversion from endovascular to open operation is falling.[15] High-risk patients may therefore continue to be considered for endovascular repair provided that the size of the aneurysm justifies intervention and the patient understands the increased risk.

A diameter of 6 cm is an approximate guide to the point at which the risk of rupture begins to exceed the risk of endovascular repair in a high-risk patient. High-risk patients have been defined by the Endovascular Graft Committee[16] as "patients with large, threatening aneurysms whose operative risk is excessive, for example, in excess of three to four times normal, on the basis of heart, lung, or liver disease or previous abdominal scarring or infection." This is clearly important when outcomes are compared and patients are informed of the relative risks.

Now that the feasibility and relative safety of endovascular repair have been established, the procedure can be offered to patients who are good risk and considered fit for conventional open repair. It is important, however, that these patients understand that the long-term outcome of these procedures is unknown and that concurrent comparison of endovascular and open repair of AAAs demonstrates a significantly higher failure rate for the endovascular method after mid-term follow-up of several years.[8]

At this stage in the evolution of the endovascular method of repair, ruptured aneurysms are best avoided. Because the technique necessitates careful imaging, measurement and sizing, there are logistic problems in the acute situation. Despite the problems, Yusuf and coworkers have achieved success in a small group of hemodynamically stable patients with ruptured aneurysms.[17]

Selective screening of older patients to identify those who would be suitable for endovascular repair, even with an AAA less than 4 cm, has been suggested. Until the long-term outcome is known, however, this approach is premature.

CRITERIA FOR ENDOVASCULAR TREATMENT

Not all aneurysms are anatomically suitable for endovascular repair. The major determinants of suitability are the size and the morphologic features of the proximal neck of the aneurysm. A collar of normal aorta between the renal arteries and the aneurysm of 15 mm or greater and a diameter of 28 mm or less are required for currently available devices. The presence of heavy circumferential calcification, mural thrombus, or an inverted funnel-shaped collar are contraindications to the endovascular method.

Tortuosity is also an important determinant of suitability for endovascular repair. Because aneurysms expand longitudinally as well as transversely, the increase in size longitudinally may be accommodated by angulation in the neck, the

aneurysm itself, the iliac arteries, or any combination of the three. The angles have been defined by the Ad Hoc Committee of the Joint Societies of Vascular Surgery and North American Chapter of the International Society for Cardiovascular Surgery (SVS/ISCVS) for uniform reporting standards for endovascular abdominal aortic aneurysm repair (Fig. 90–1).[18] The recommended maximum angulation in the neck is 120 degrees (180 degrees representing a straight course without angulation), and in the iliac arteries it is 90 degrees.[19] Angulation in the aneurysm is less critical.

The natural history of AAAs involves not only expansion and resulting tortuosity but also extension of aneurysmal degeneration into the adjacent arteries. This may cause a number of different morphologic combinations, which have been classified as grades I through IV (Fig. 90–2).[18] Each type has implications for endovascular repair. Grade I, for example, is suitable for a tube endograft, whereas grades III and IV are unsuitable for any endograft due to the absence of a proximal neck. Grades IIA and IIB are suitable for treatment with either an aortouni-iliac or bifurcated endograft.

Because the endovascular method of aneurysm repair requires isolation of the aneurysm sac from the circulation, the presence of large patent collateral channels such as the inferior mesenteric artery and the internal iliac arteries communicating with the aortic or iliac sac is a relative contraindication. However, these may be occluded by coil embolization preoperatively and need not necessarily preclude the use of the endovascular method.

PREOPERATIVE IMAGING

Preoperative imaging is very important because patient selection and sizing of the endograft depend on it. Contrast-enhanced spiral computed tomography (CT) is the preferred initial method of investigation. The scans are rapidly acquired, which allows uniform vascular enhancement at peak intensity with similar or lower contrast load compared with conventional CT. The contrast allows thrombus to be distinguished from flowing blood and enables the proximal neck to be assessed for suitability for endovascular repair. The dimensions of the proximal neck can be accurately determined and the presence of calcification or mural thrombus noted. The size of the iliac arteries

Grade I: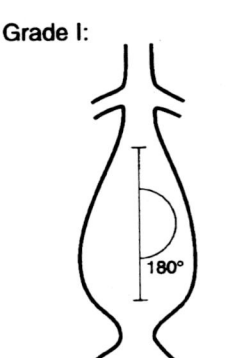

Grade II: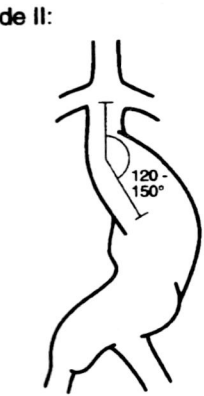

Grade III: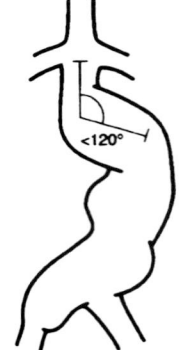

FIGURE 90–1. Angulation of the proximal neck of the aneurysm as defined by the Ad Hoc Committee for Uniform Reporting Standards. (From Ahn SS, Rutherford RB, Johnston KW, et al: Reporting standards for infrarenal endovascular abdominal aortic aneurysm repair. J Vasc Surg 25:405–410, 1997.)

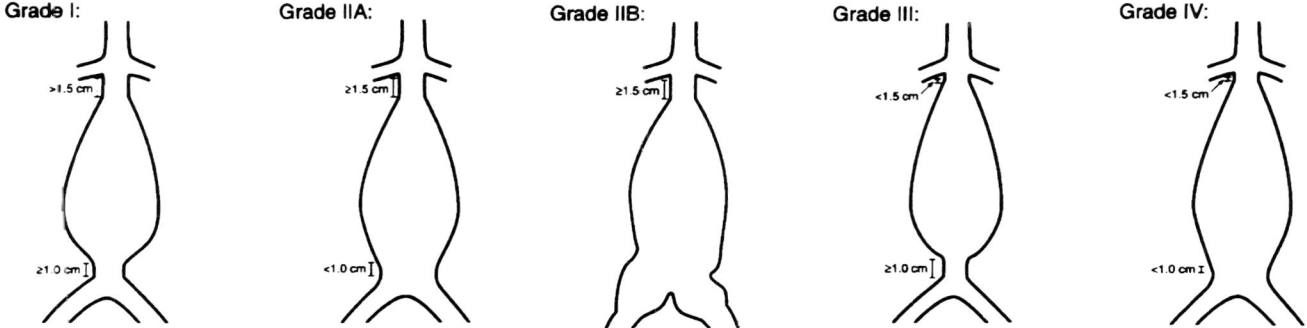

FIGURE 90–2. Morphologic classification of abdominal aortic aneurysms (Ad Hoc Committee for Uniform Reporting Standards). (From Ahn SS, Rutherford RB, Johnston KW, et al: Reporting standards for infrarenal endovascular abdominal aortic aneurysm repair. J Vasc Surg 25:405–410, 1997.)

and the presence of aneurysm disease and calcification can also be noted.

Software packages are available that plot the axial line of the aorta and aneurysm and enable cuts to be made at right angles to that line. This enables more accurate measurements of the diameter of the aorta and the distance from the renal arteries to the aortic and iliac bifurcations to be made. (See Chapter 14 for details.)

Although the anatomy of the iliac arteries and accessory renal arteries can be demonstrated by spiral CT, in most medical centers aortography is performed when the patient has been found to be suitable for endovascular repair by CT. The aortogram should be performed with a calibrated catheter to allow accurate measurements to be made without the magnification that occurs with external calibration. Anteroposterior and lateral views are required to demonstrate tortuosity in the neck of the aneurysm and the iliac arteries. Because the aortogram demonstrates the lumen of the aorta and CT demonstrates the arterial wall in addition to the lumen, the diameter of the neck of the aneurysm is usually greater when measured by CT than by angiography.

ENDOVASCULAR PROSTHESES

The early endovascular prostheses comprised tubular or tapered fabric grafts anchored in place by balloon-expandable or self-expanding stents at each end. Hooks or barbs were incorporated in the stents to minimize migration of the device. Initially, the configuration of the endografts was tubular. To increase the number of patients who were suitable for endovascular repair, endovascular aortoiliac and aortofemoral tapered grafts were combined with extravascular femorofemoral crossover grafts to revascularize the contralateral limb and interruption of the contralateral common iliac artery to exclude the aneurysm sac (Fig. 90–3). One-piece bifurcated prostheses were developed that required the contralateral limb to be pulled across the aortic bifurcation to the contralateral side by a crossover wire. Both iliac limbs were anchored by metal stents.

The limitations of these devices became apparent, and a second generation of prostheses was developed. In these, the fabric was supported throughout by a metallic frame to prevent kinking and to add column strength. The modular method was used to deploy bifurcated grafts, with compo-

nent parts being delivered from both groins. The French (Fr.) size of the delivery system's internal diameter was reduced from 24 to 21 and the flexibility increased. There are now four commercially available prostheses commonly used throughout the world (Fig. 90–4). A review of endovascular prostheses may be found in Chapter 38.

TECHNIQUE OF ENDOVASCULAR REPAIR

Endovascular repair is best performed in the operating room under general or regional anesthesia. The patient should be draped for open repair in the event of failed endovascular repair or occurence of complications needing open operation. A radiolucent operating table, preferably of carbon fiber and with a C-arm to provide cine loop angiography with the capability of digital subtraction and frame-by-frame replay, is required. The patient is positioned so that the C-arm can be placed beneath the abdomen and lower chest without obstruction from the table. A radiopaque ruler is placed beneath the patient as a reference point during deployment.

The common femoral artery in the ipsilateral groin is exposed and the patient given heparin. A preprocedure aortogram is performed with a power injector, and a calibrated pigtail catheter is placed with the holes immediately above the renal arteries. The positions of the renal arteries, aortic bifurcation, and iliac bifurcation are noted relative to the ruler. The position of one of the digits on the ruler is identified on the image intensifier screen by a piece of tape. This enables the image intensifier to be moved inferiorly to monitor the introduction of the prosthesis and returned to the same position without introducing errors of parallax. A straight angiographic catheter is introduced percutaneously over a guide wire into the contralateral femoral artery.

An extra-stiff guide wire is introduced through the pigtail catheter as far as the descending thoracic aorta and the catheter is removed. A transverse arteriotomy is made in the ipsilateral common femoral artery in such a way that the guide wire is situated within the arteriotomy. The catheter and prosthesis within it are introduced over the extra-stiff guide wire after checking the orientation of the device under the image intensifier. The catheter is advanced under radiographic control until the superior end of the prosthesis

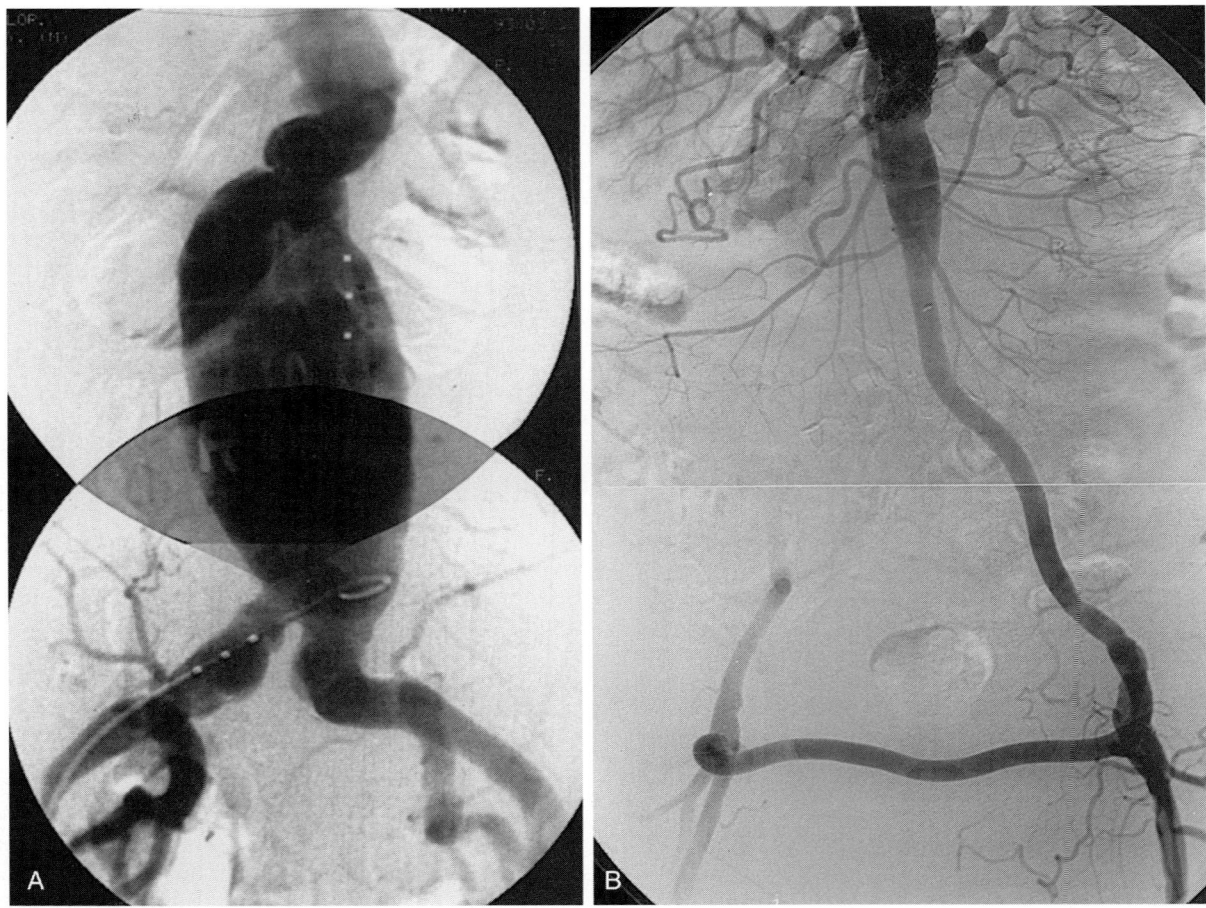

FIGURE 90–3. *A*, Aortogram demonstrating 6.5 cm abdominal aortic aneurysm with common iliac artery ectasia. *B*, Postoperative aortogram performed on patient from Figure 90–3*A* 2 years after endoluminal repair using an aortofemoral endograft. The right common iliac artery has been occluded by a detachable balloon, and the right limb has been revascularized by a femorofemoral crossover graft. (From May J, White GH, Yu W, et al: Repair of abdominal aortic aneurysms by the endoluminal method: Outcome in the first 100 patients. Med J Aust 165:549–551, 1996.)

is immediately below the renal arteries. The image intensifier is moved superiorly to place the superior end of the prosthesis (and therefore the renal arteries) in the center of the field. The straight angiographic catheter is withdrawn to the point where contrast injected through it will accurately locate the exact position of the renal arteries. These last maneuvers eliminate parallax and avoid errors caused by the catheter straightening an angled aorta and moving the renal arteries to a different level.

After it is ascertained that the systolic blood pressure is less than 100 mmHg, the trunk and ipsilateral limb of the bifurcated prosthesis are deployed under radiographic control. A detailed description of technique of deployment for individual prostheses is beyond the scope of this chapter and is discussed in general here. After ipsilateral limb deployment, attention is directed to passing a guide wire from the contralateral femoral artery through the stump of the prosthesis. This can usually be achieved from below with an angled guiding catheter. If difficulty is experienced, the guide wire may be passed from the ipsilateral groin through the ipsilateral limb of the prosthesis and, again with the aid of a guiding catheter, inferiorly through the contralateral stump into the aneurysm sac. From here it may be retrieved by a snare passed from the contralateral groin.

An approach from the left brachial artery may also be used if the two previous methods fail. A guide wire is passed from the left brachial artery and directed down the descending thoracic aorta by either a guiding catheter or a balloon catheter, which can be inflated in the aorta and carried distally by blood flow to reach the aneurysm sac via the contralateral stump. The brachial approach is also very useful in cases of extreme tortuosity in the iliac arteries. After retrieval of the brachial guide wire in the aneurysm sac by snare, tension can be applied from the brachial and femoral ends. This results in considerable straightening of the iliac arteries (Fig. 90–5), allowing passage of the catheter.

After cannulation of the contralateral stump, the contralateral limb, within its catheter, is delivered under radiographic control to a position within and overlapping the contralateral stump (see Fig. 90–4). This position is identified by clearly visible radiopaque markers on the stump and endograft limb (see Fig 90–9*B*, later). The limb is now deployed, again under radiographic control. The pigtail catheter is reintroduced, and a postprocedure digital subtraction aortogram is performed. The cine loop is examined several times for the presence of extravasation of contrast, which suggests an endoleak. Flow of contrast through the iliac arteries is also examined for any kinking or twisting.

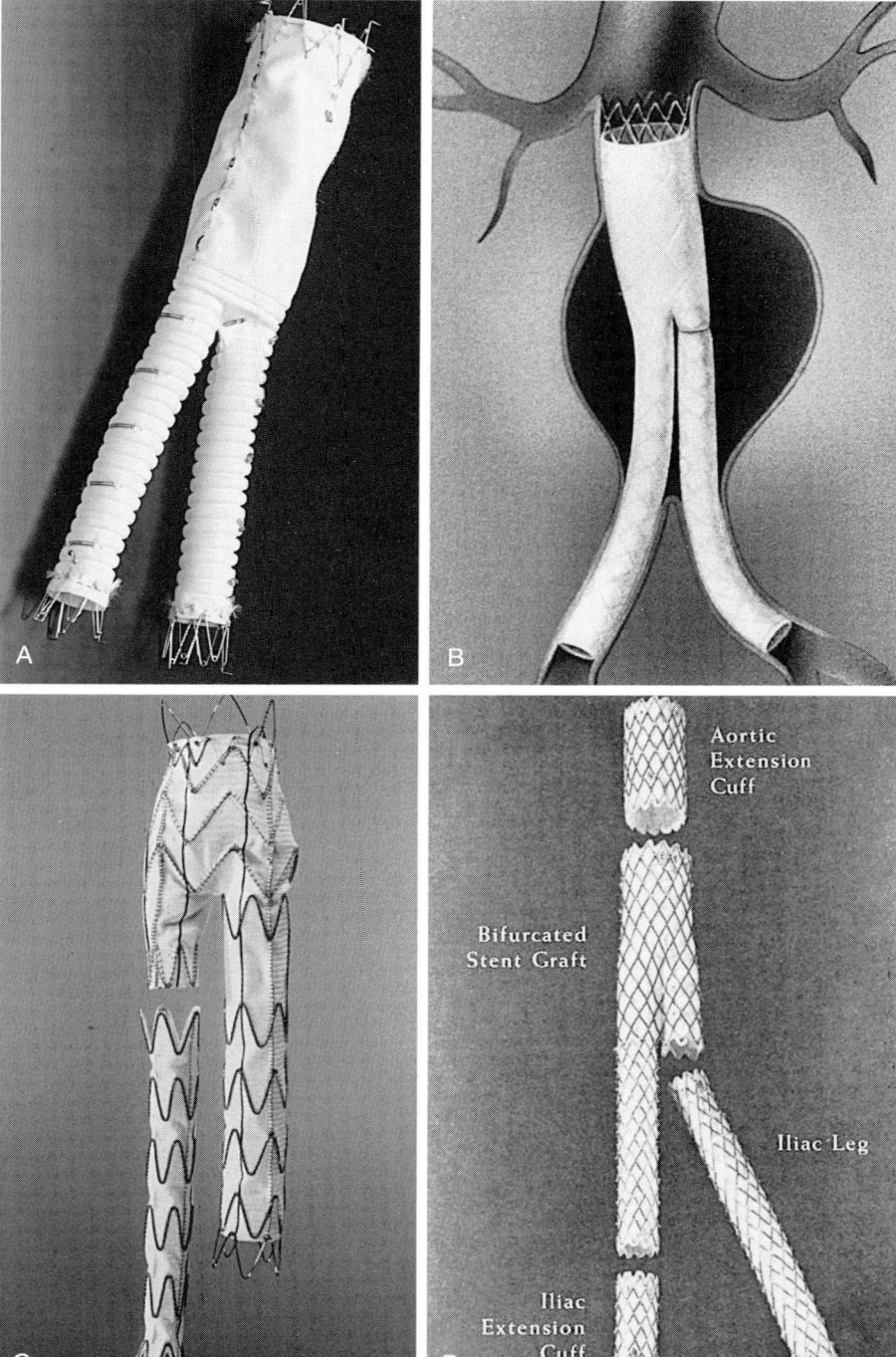

FIGURE 90–4. Endovascular techniques. A, One-piece bifurcated endograft. B, Boston Scientific modular bifurcated endograft. C, World Medical modular bifurcated endograft. D, Medtronic modular bifurcated endograft.

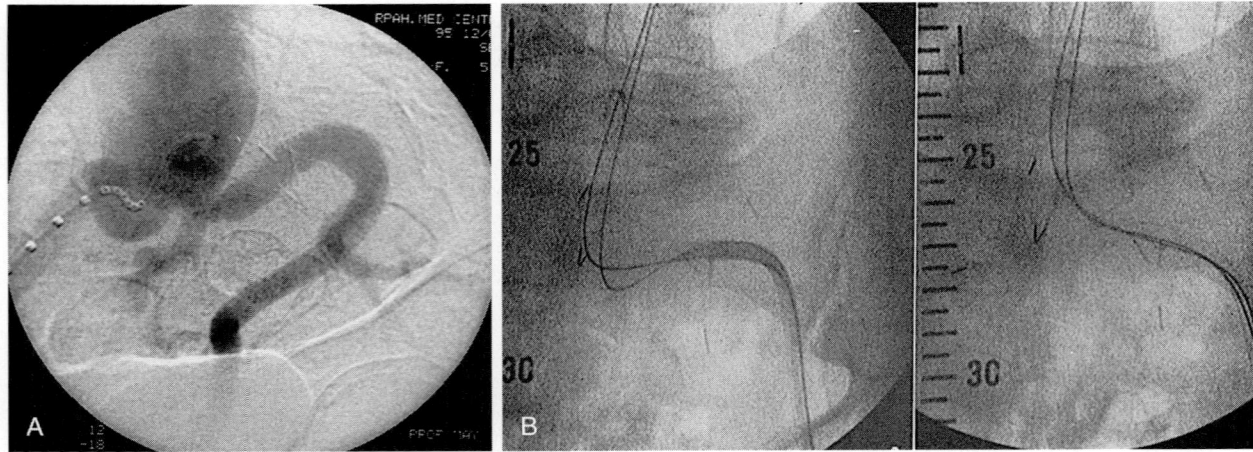

FIGURE 90–5. *A,* Aortogram demonstrating abdominal aortic aneurysm (7 cm diameter) and extreme tortuosity of the left common iliac artery. *B,* Guide wires traversing the aorta and left iliac arteries in the patient from Figure 90–5A *(left panel).* Appearance following traction on the brachial and femoral ends of the through-and-through guide wire. Note disappearance of the acute angle between the aneurysm and the left common iliac artery.

FOLLOW-UP AFTER ENDOVASCULAR REPAIR

Because the long-term outcome of endovascular repair is unknown, careful and prolonged follow-up is required. Physical examination and contrast-enhanced CT within 1 week of operation and at 6, 12, and 18 months after operation and annually thereafter are recommended. Color-coded duplex ultrasonography has also been used successfully, but its accuracy is very operator-dependent. It does, however, have the advantages of demonstrating blood flow within the sac, not requiring contrast, and being less costly than CT.

CHANGES IN MORPHOLOGY AFTER ENDOVASCULAR REPAIR

After successful endoluminal repair of an AAA, the sac undergoes a reduction in size as measured by maximum transverse diameter[20-22] and volume.[23] Conversely, the sac increases in size in the presence of an endoleak. Persistent untreated endoleak may lead to rupture of the aneurysm.[20]

Most investigators have reported an increase in diameter of the proximal neck of the aneurysm after endoluminal repair.[20, 22] This increase is about 10% and is thought to be due to deliberate oversizing of the prostheses to ensure secure anchoring and watertight seal with the aorta. The increased diameter is related in time and magnitude to the deployment and degree of oversizing of the prostheses. Of significance, neither Parodi[27] nor the authors have noted progressive dilatation of the proximal neck in patients who have undergone endoluminal AAA repair more than 4 years previously. This is in contrast to the findings of those who have studied the segment of aorta between the renal arteries and the superior end of the prosthetic graft after conventional open repair of AAA.[28] Here dilatation, often of considerable degree, has been noted. Further long-term follow-up studies are required to confirm this divergence in outcomes of the two methods of treatment.

Although the reduced size of the aneurysm after endoluminal repair is a welcome sign, and indeed an important criterion of success, it can also lead to problems. Because the reduction in size occurs not only transversely but also longitudinally, it can lead to kinking and dislocation of component parts of a modular prosthesis within the aneurysm sac (see Complications later).

PATHOLOGY OF HEALING AFTER ENDOLUMINAL REPAIR

Information on the pathology of healing after endoluminal aneurysm repair has come from autopsy reports of patients who died of unrelated illness.[29, 30] The human response to the placement of an endoluminal graft in an AAA is essentially an acellular one at the level of the proximal neck and a thrombotic one within the isolated aneurysm sac. There is some infiltration of host cells into the interstices of the fabric of the endograft adjacent to the intima of the neck of the aneurysm, but it is minimal. The fabric of the graft is covered on its interior surface by a thin pseudointima. This is usually complete at the superior end of the prosthesis, but coverage is patchy in the inferior portion. This minimal cellular response to the radial force of an endograft deployed in the proximal neck of an aneurysm is in marked contrast to the hypercellular response that accompanies balloon dilatation and stent placement in the treatment of occlusive arterial disease.

The practical implication of these findings is that the degree of incorporation of the endograft in the treatment of aneurysm disease is insufficient to maintain the integrity of the junction of the native aorta and the endograft. The anchoring of the endograft and the seal that isolates the aneurysm sac is permanently dependent on the radial force applied by the endograft. This is not surprising when one considers that the integrity of the anastomoses between aorta and graft in open aneurysm repair is permanently dependent on the nonabsorbable nature of the suture material.

COMPLICATIONS

Complications have been divided into *remote* or *systemic* and *local* or *vascular* by the Ad Hoc Committee of the Joint Societies of Vascular Surgery and North American Chapter of the International Society for Cardiovascular Surgery for uniform reporting standards. The *remote/systemic* complications after endoluminal AAA repair do not vary greatly from those following open aneurysm repair and are not covered further here. The *local/vascular* complications, however, are important, as many of them are specific to the endoluminal method of aneurysm repair. A complete list of these complications is given in Table 90–1, the more important of which are considered in detail next.

Injuries to Arteries of Access

It is not surprising that the passage of comparatively large-bore catheters, containing endografts, through tortuous and diseased iliac arteries may result in rupture. It is important to recognize that such rupture may become apparent not only during the introduction of the catheter but also following withdrawal of the catheter. After the catheter is introduced and the artery damaged, the onset of bleeding is delayed by the tamponading effect of the catheter. Although second-generation prostheses are capable of being introduced through iliac arteries with a considerable degree of tortuosity, the presence of heavy circumferential calcification increases the risk of rupturing the artery considerably.

Suprarenal arteries are also vulnerable to injury when the brachial route is used to complement access of the AAA. The seemingly harmless passage of a guide wire from the brachial artery down the descending thoracic aorta may result in substantial intraperitoneal bleeding if it passes inadvertently and unnoticed into the superior mesenteric artery and ruptures one of the terminal branches of this artery.

Embolization

Manipulation of endovascular devices within the sac of an AAA has resulted in widespread microembolization and

TABLE 90–1. LOCAL AND VASCULAR COMPLICATIONS AFTER ENDOLUMINAL REPAIR

Injury to arteries of access
    Iliac
    Suprarenal

Embolization
    Microembolization, renal failure
    Distal embolization, ischemia

Endoleak
    Type 1 (graft-related)
    Type 2 (collateral channels)

Postimplant syndrome

Graft limb thrombosis

Groin wound complications

Conversion to open repair: current indications
    Aortic rupture
    Endograft migration obstructing iliac outflow
    Persistent endoleak after unsuccessful secondary endoluminal repair
    Endograft infection

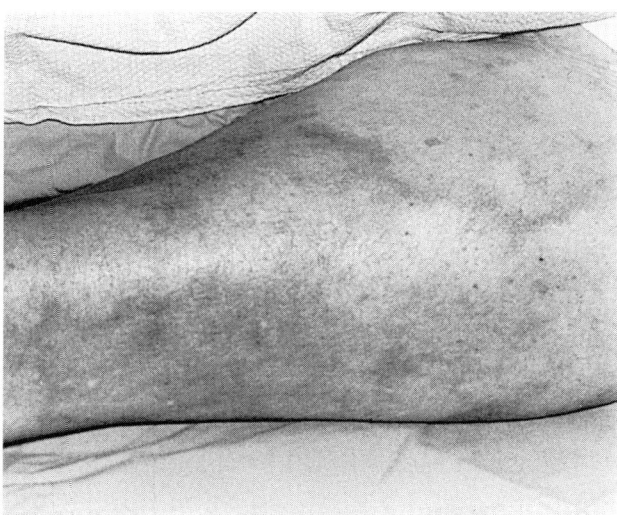

FIGURE 90–6. Skin changes in the left thigh following distal embolization in a patient with mural thrombus in the proximal neck of an abdominal aortic aneurysm treated by endoluminal repair.

death from renal failure.[4] Every effort should be made to reduce the catheter introduction process to one pass in which the prosthesis is delivered to the level of the renal arteries. The movement of all component parts of the catheter from this point should be in the direction of withdrawal, not advancement, to minimize the risk of thrombus dislodgment.

Distal embolization resulting in ischemia is also a recognized complication (Fig. 90–6). In the authors' experience, this has been limited to patients in whom an endograft has been deployed in the presence of mural thrombus in the proximal neck of the aneurysm. It is recommended therefore to avoid the endoluminal method in patients with this finding or to clamp both common femoral arteries during deployment if a decision is made to take a calculated risk in poor-risk patients with mural neck thrombus.

Endoleak

Endoleak is a condition associated with endoluminal vascular grafts, defined by the persistence of blood flow outside the lumen of the endoluminal graft but within an aneurysm sac or adjacent vascular segment being treated by the graft. Endoleak is due to incomplete sealing or exclusion of the aneurysm sac or vessel segment as evidenced by imaging studies such as contrast-enhanced CT, ultrasonography, and angiography.[5]

Classification

A clear distinction should be made between endoleak related to the graft device itself and endoleak associated with flow from collateral arterial branches as classified by the following system[31]:

- *Type 1 endoleak (graft-related endoleak).* Type 1 occurs when a persistent channel of blood flow develops owing to inadequate or ineffective seal at the graft ends (or between segments of overlapping graft segments). It can usually be determined whether the endoleak is at the proximal, mid-graft, or distal graft aspect, and these qualifiers should be used. Endograft at the mid-graft region may be due to leakage through a defect in the graft fabric or may be between segments of a modular multisegment graft (Fig. 90–7).

• *Type 2 endoleak (non–graft-related endoleak).* Type 2 occurs when there is persistent collateral blood flow into the aneurysm sac flowing retrogradely from patent lumbar arteries, the inferior mesenteric artery, the intercostal arteries (in thoracic aneurysms), or other collateral vessels. In this situation, there is usually a complete seal around the graft attachment zones so that the complication is not related directly to the graft itself.

Endoleak may also be classified according to the time of occurrence:

• *Primary endoleak.* A primary endoleak is present from the time of the implantation procedure or from the initial diagnosis during the 30-day perioperative period.
• *Secondary (late) endoleak.* This endoleak occurs as a late event after a successful endoluminal graft implantation procedure. No endoleak is present at the time of implantation or during the perioperative period.
• *Recurrent endoleak.* This endoleak can seal spontaneously and then recur.

Incidence and Natural History

The incidence of endoleak has been variously reported to be 44% by Moore and Rutherford,[32] 27% by Marin and

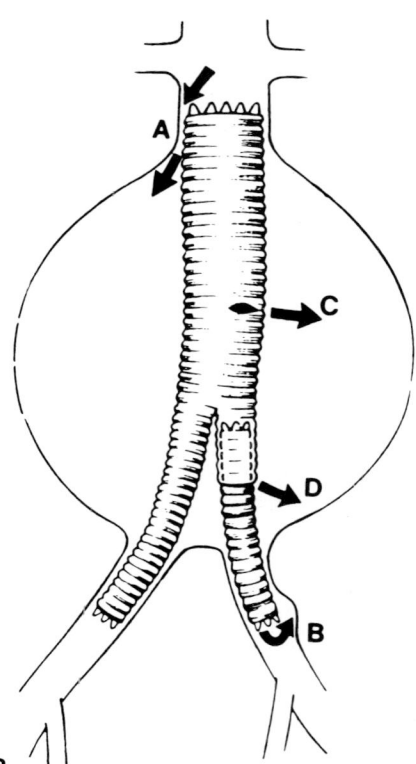

FIGURE 90–7. Sites of endoleak classified as type 1 or graft-related endoleak. (From White GH, Yu W, May J, et al: Endoleak as a complication of endoluminal grafting of abdominal aortic aneurysms: Classification, incidence, diagnosis, and management. J Endovasc Surg 4:152–168, 1997.)

coworkers,[33] and 10% or less by Blum and coworkers,[34] Parodi,[4] and May and coworkers.[35] Untreated, an endoleak leads to continued expansion of the AAA.[20–22] The endoleak may seal spontaneously by thrombosis. This occurred in over half the cases of endoleak reported by Moore and Rutherford, resulting in a permanent endoleak rate of 21%.[32] Spontaneous sealing of the endoleak is accompanied by reduction in the diameter of the AAA (Fig. 90–8). Conversely, the diameter of the AAA increases when a secondary endoleak develops in a previously isolated AAA after successful endoluminal repair.

Bernhard, after reviewing an extensive series of patients with EVT (EndoVascular Technologies, Menlo Park, Calif.) grafts, reported that type 2 endoleaks were more likely to seal spontaneously than type 1 leaks.[36] It has also been suggested that type 2 endoleaks may be less likely to rupture. This supposition may be dangerous, however, because the Albany group[37] has reported rupture of an AAA due to collateral channels in patients treated by ligation and bypass. Untreated endoleak (type 1) resulting in AAA rupture has been reported on three occasions.[24–26]

Management

Endoleaks may be managed by (1) observation, (2) a further endovascular procedure comprising either a supplementary endoluminal repair or embolization, (3) surgical band ligature of the aneurysm neck, and (4) conversion to open repair of the aneurysm.

Observation

Because some endoleaks seal spontaneously, the majority of vascular surgeons are prepared to observe endoleaks despite the knowledge that aneurysm rupture may occur in patients with this clinical course. Although there is no proof that spontaneous sealing of an endoleak by thrombosis removes systemic arterial pressure from the aneurysm sac, there is presumptive evidence that this is so in the form of reduction in the diameter of aneurysms in this situation. The duration of observation varies according to the size of the aneurysm. Patient safety would dictate that aneurysms in excess of 6 cm in diameter should not be observed longer than 3 months. It should also be noted that spontaneous seals do not necessarily continue indefinitely. It has been our experience that recurrent endoleak may follow spontaneous seal.

Further Endovascular Procedures

Type 1 endoleaks may be treated by secondary endoluminal repair with a cuff endograft for a proximal endoleak, an extension endograft for a distal iliac endoleak, and an intersegmental endograft for distraction of component parts of a modular graft (Fig. 90–9). A distal endoleak from a tube endograft may be treated by either a cuff endograft or conversion to an endoluminal aortoiliac graft with crossover graft and interruption of the contralateral common iliac artery or conversion to an endoluminal bifurcated graft. Coil embolization has also been used in the treatment of type 1 endoleaks. The place of this maneuver, in the authors' opinion, however, remains to be established.

Type 2 endoleaks arising from the lumbar arteries may be treated by coil embolization with selective catheterization of branches of the superior gluteal artery (Fig. 90–10). Type

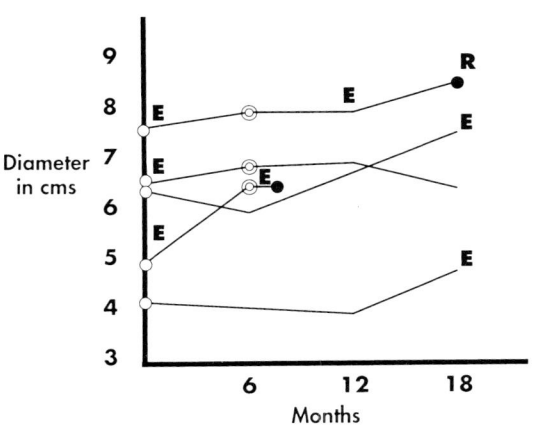

FIGURE 90–8. Relationship of abdominal aortic aneurysm diameter and the presence of endoleak in five patients following endoluminal repair. (From May J, White GH, Yu W, et al: A prospective study of anatomicopathological changes in abdominal aortic aneurysms following endoluminal repair. Is the aneurysmal process reversed? Eur J Vasc Endovasc Surg 12:11–17, 1996.)

2 endoleak resulting from retrograde flow into the inferior mesenteric artery has also been treated by embolization with selective catheterization of the middle colic artery via the superior mesenteric artery.[38]

Surgical Band Ligature of the Aortic Aneurysm Neck

Surgical band ligature has been used by the Nottingham group[17] and involves open exposure and placement of an external ligature to achieve a seal around the proximal graft attachment device. Although it necessitates laparotomy, this approach is clearly less disturbing hemodynamically than conversion to open repair in high-risk patients.

Conversion to Open Repair

Conversion to open repair may be indicated when supplementary endoluminal repair is not possible or has failed.

Post-implant Syndrome

Post-implant syndrome is characterized by back pain and fever but absence of leukocytosis or other evidence of infection. It follows implantation directly, lasts up to 7 days, and is usually associated with thrombosis within the aneurysm sac. The cause is unknown, and the incidence may be as high as 50%. Despite some early reports of an associated coagulopathy, the course of post-implant syndrome is generally considered to be benign; indeed, some hold it to be a favorable sign signifying thrombosis of the aneurysm sac and successful endoluminal repair.

Graft Limb Thrombosis
Due to Dissection During Introduction of the Catheter

The passage of catheters containing prostheses through the common femoral and iliac arteries may result in dissection. If suspected, the complication may be diagnosed by withdrawing the catheter and replacing it with an 8 Fr. introducing sheath, thus allowing an angiogram to be performed through the side port. Although it may be technically possible to correct the dissection by endovascular means, we recommend placing a polyester (Dacron) graft from the common iliac bifurcation to the common femoral artery via an extraperitoneal approach. This allows simultaneous revascularization of the affected limb and ensures access to the common iliac artery for delivery of the prosthesis into the aneurysm.

Due to Kinking Within the Iliac Arteries

First-generation endografts with unsupported fabric were prone to thrombosis of the limbs of the graft due to kinking and twisting within the native iliac arteries. Even with later prostheses in which the fabric is supported by a metallic frame, the problem persists. Postprocedure on-table angiography in one plane is no guarantee that kinking has not occurred. Plain x-ray studies in anteroposterior and lateral planes in the immediate postoperative period are recommended to identify a problem in the metal frame before thrombosis occurs and while correction may be carried out by endovascular rather than open means.

Due to Kinking Within the Aneurysm Sac

Successful endoluminal repair results in reduction in the size of the aneurysm sac in both length and transverse diameter. This may lead to kinking of the previously straight limbs of an endoluminal graft, with progression to thrombosis. Such kinking may also encourage or result in dislocation of the limbs of endograft from the native iliac arteries or the contralateral limb from the contralateral stump of the endograft (see Fig. 90–9). Fortunately, kinks in the iliac arteries and within the aneurysm sac are amenable to endovascular correction, thus avoiding open operation.

Conversion to Open Repair

Conversion to open repair may be required under the following circumstances[15]:

1. Aortic rupture during endoluminal repair or subsequently during observation of an endoleak awaiting spontaneous thrombosis.

2. After migration of an endograft into a position that obstructs the outflow of blood into the iliac arteries.

3. In the presence of a persistent endoleak where supplementary attempts at endoluminal repair have been unsuccessful.

4. In the presence of an infected endograft.

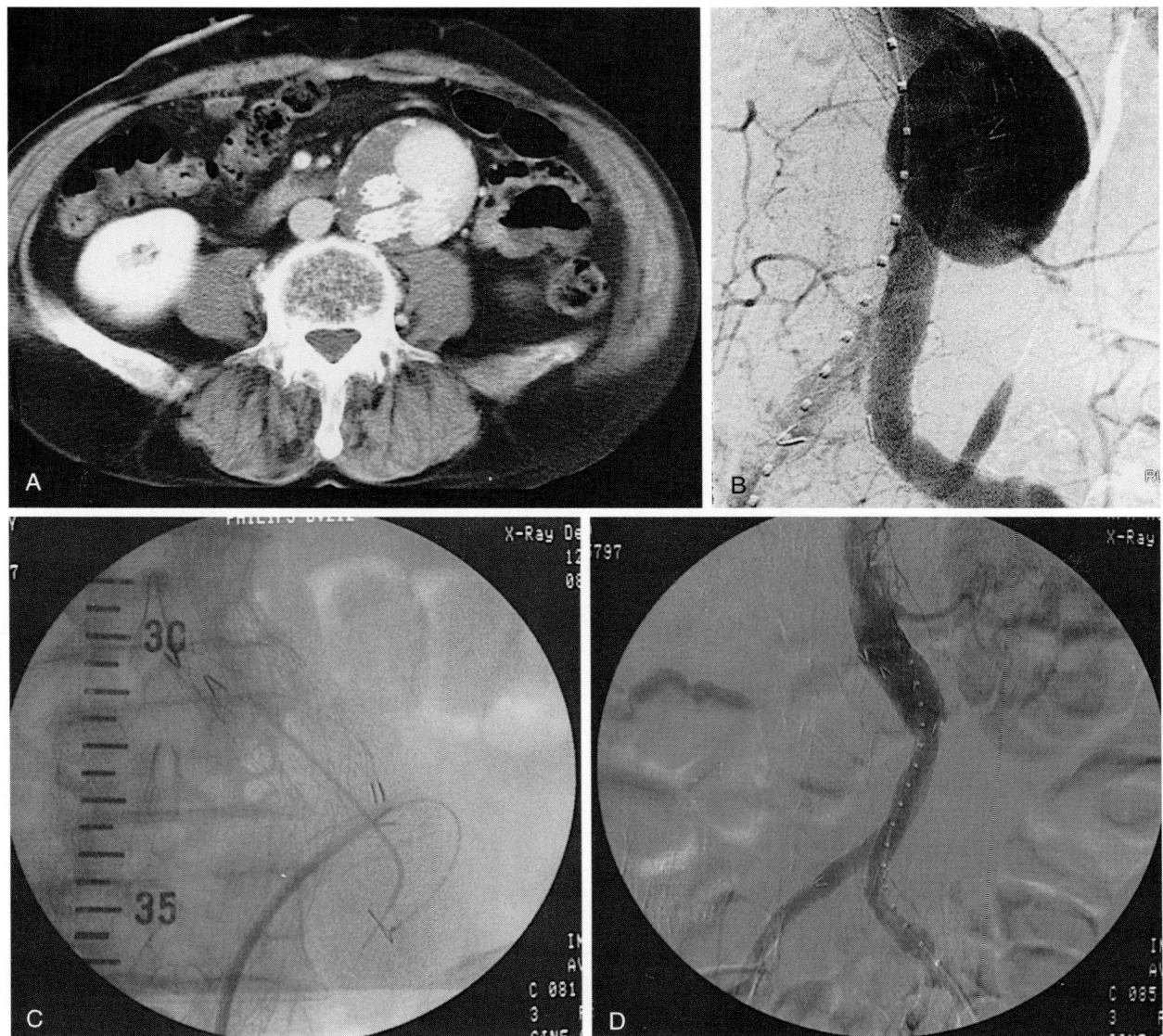

FIGURE 90–9. *A,* Contrast CT scan demonstrating an endoleak 1 year after endoluminal repair of an abdominal aortic aneurysm with a bifurcated endograft. The right limb of the endograft is circular in cross section, indicating vertical disposition. The left limb is lying transversely. *B,* On the table, preprocedure aortogram of the patient in Figure 90–9A. A large circular endoleak due to dislocation of the left (contralateral) limb of the endograft is shown. Note the V-shaped radiopaque markers on the dislocated limb and the two vertical radiopaque markers on the contralateral stump. *C,* Hard copy from image intensifier demonstrating a guide wire that has been passed from the left brachial artery into the endograft and out through the contralateral stump into the aneurysm sac. A snare has been passed superiorly through the dislocated contralateral limb to pull the brachial guide wire down to the femoral artery in the left groin. *D,* Postprocedure aortogram following deployment of an intrasegmental endograft to reunite the contralateral stump and contralateral limb. Note the absence of endoleak and restoration of flow through the left limb of the endograft. (From May J, White GH: Endovascular leak. *In* Whittemore A [ed]: Advances in Vascular Surgery. Vol 6. St. Louis, Mosby–Year Book, 1998, pp 65–79.)

RESULTS

The primary success rate for endoluminal repair of AAAs has been variously reported within the range of 75% to 90%. These reported results are summarized in Table 90–2 together with complication rates and 30-day mortality rates. It should be reemphasized that rapid changes have been made from first-generation to second-generation devices over the past 6 years. These changes need to be taken into account when interpreting the data.

The only study to date that has attempted a concurrent comparison of endoluminal versus open repair of AAA demonstrated that the endoluminal method is safe.[8] Despite having 44% high-risk patients, the endoluminal group had the same perioperative mortality (5.6%) as the open group. Kaplan-Meier curves for survival after endoluminal and open repair of 303 patients treated concurrently showed no significant difference when analyzed by log rank test (Fig. 90–11). Demonstration of this acceptable survival probability of 83% at 5 years in the endoluminal group is important, considering the cost of endoluminal prostheses. It would be difficult to justify this expense in a group of patients whose life expectancy was approximately 12 to 18 months.

Graft failure rate was significantly higher in the endoluminal group than in the open group. The success probability at 3 years was 70% (Fig. 90–12). The higher failure rate,

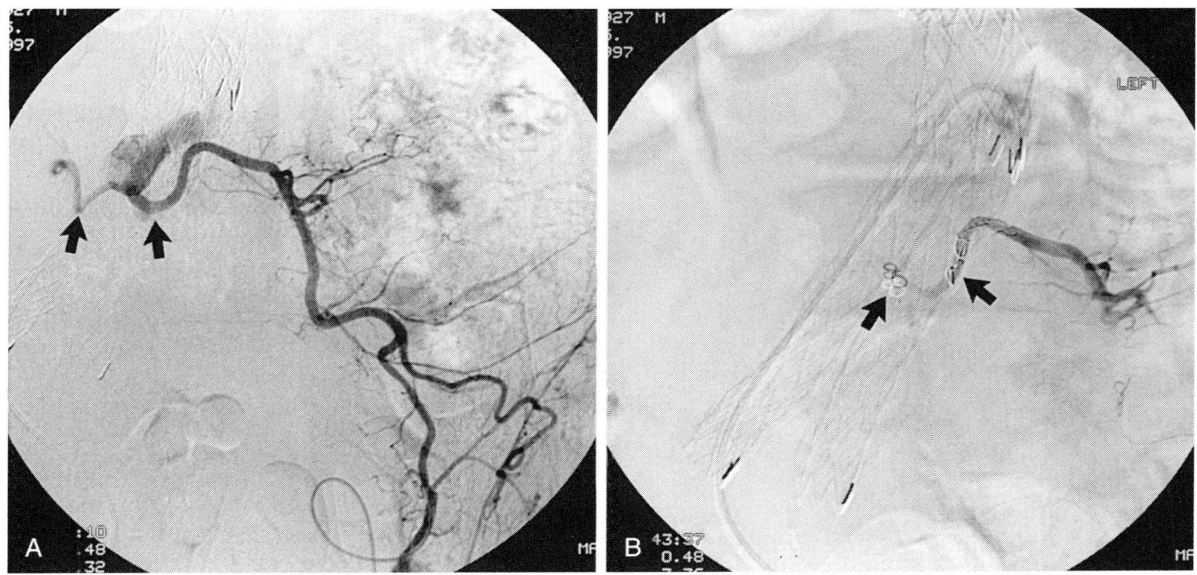

FIGURE 90–10. *A,* Angiogram demonstrating selective catheterization of left lumbar artery (*right arrow*) and filling the right lumbar artery (*left arrow*). Between the two lumbar arteries contrast can be seen to be entering the aneurysm sac, constituting a type 2 endoleak. *B,* Angiogram following successful coil embolization of both lumbar arteries with no evidence of endoleak. (From May J, White JH: Endovascular leak. *In* Whittemore A [ed]: Advances in Vascular Surgery, Vol 6. St. Louis, Mosby–Year Book, 1998, pp 65–79.)

TABLE 90–2. REPORTED RESULTS OF ENDOLUMINAL REPAIR OF ABDOMINAL AORTIC ANEURYSMS

SERIES	DEVICE	NO.	PRIMARY TECHNICAL SUCCESS*	SUCCESS AFTER ADDITIONAL ENDOLUMINAL PROCEDURE	CONVERT TO OPEN REPAIR	PERSISTING ENDOLEAK OR OTHER LATE FAILURE	OTHER POSTOPERATIVE COMPLICATIONS	30-DAY MORTALITY (OVERALL IN-HOSPITAL DEATHS)
Blum[34]	Aortoaortic	21	18 (86%)	21 (100%)	0			
	Aortobi-iliac (Vanguard/ Passager)	133	116 (87%)	128 (3) (96%)†	3	9 (6%)	15 (10%)	1 (1%)
Parodi[4, 25]	Aortoaortic	51	81 (74%)	93 (2) (86%)†	4	16 (15%)	8 (7%)	5 (4%)
	Aortouni-iliac	46						
	Aortobi-iliac (Parodi Device)	12						
Chuter[42]	Aortobi-iliac (Chuter-Gianturco)	54	43 (80%)	NS	3	14 (30%)	NS	3 (5%)
Moore[32]	Aortoaortic (EVT)	46	22 (48%)	32 (9) (70%)†	7	7 (32%)	27 complications (rate not stated)	0
Balm[2]	Aortoaortic (EVT)	31	24 (77%)	27 (3) (87%)†	1	3 (10%)	34 complications in 23 patients	1 (3%)
Yusuf[17]	Aortouni-iliac (Ivancev-Malmo)	30	25 (83%)	25 (83%)	5	3 (10%)	6 (20%)	2 (3) (7/10%)
Lawrence-Brown[43]	Aortobi-iliac (Perth device)	21	17 (81%)	NS	0	7 (33%)	11 (52%)	1 (4%)
White[26]	Aortoaortic	36	29 (81%)	32 (1) (89%)†	2	6		
	Aortouni-iliac	20	19 (95%)	19 (95%)	1	0 (17%)	33%	3 (4%)
	Aortobi-iliac (White-Yu GAD)	20	15 (75%)	15 (75%)	5	0		
May[35, 44]	Aortoaortic	54	106 (88%)	NS	15	NS	15%	6 (4%)
	Aortouni-iliac	26						
	Aortobi-iliac (GAD and others)	41						
Marin[33]	All types (EVT and Parodi)	18	16 (90%)	NS	NS	0	8 (42%)	5 (28%)
Thompson[45]	Aortouni-iliac (Leicester device)	25	20 (80%)	NS	5	NS	6 (24%)	2 (8%)

*Primary success refers to primary technical success rate as defined in the Reporting Standards of the Society for Vascular Surgery/International Society for Cardiovascular Surgery; updated from Ahn SS, Rutherford RB, Johnston KW, et al: Reporting standards for infrarenal endovascular abdominal aortic aneurysm repair. J Vasc Surg 25:405–410, 1997 (see Balm R, et al: Eur J Endovasc Surg 11:214–220, 1996).
†These totals include cases in which spontaneous thrombosis of endoleaks occurred (numbers in parentheses) within 6 months of surgery (primary clinical success²).
NS, Not specified; GAD = graft attachment device; EVT = EndoVascular Technologies, Menlo Park, Calif.

Survival

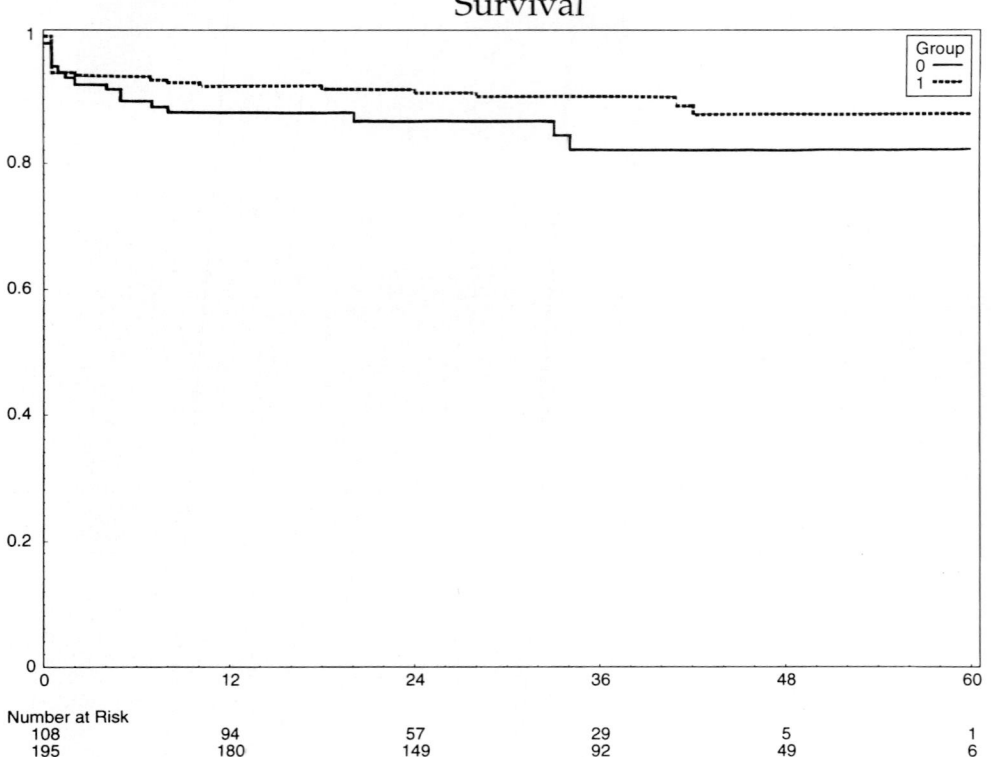

Number at Risk

| 108 | 94 | 57 | 29 | 5 | 1 |
| 195 | 180 | 149 | 92 | 49 | 6 |

FIGURE 90–11. Kaplan-Meier curves for survival following endoluminal and open repair in 303 patients with abdominal aortic aneurysms treated concurrently. (From May J, White GH, Yu W, et al: Concurrent comparison of endoluminal versus open repair in the treatment of abdominal aortic aneurysms: Analysis of 303 patients by life table method. J Vasc Surg 27:213–222, 1998.)

Graft Failure

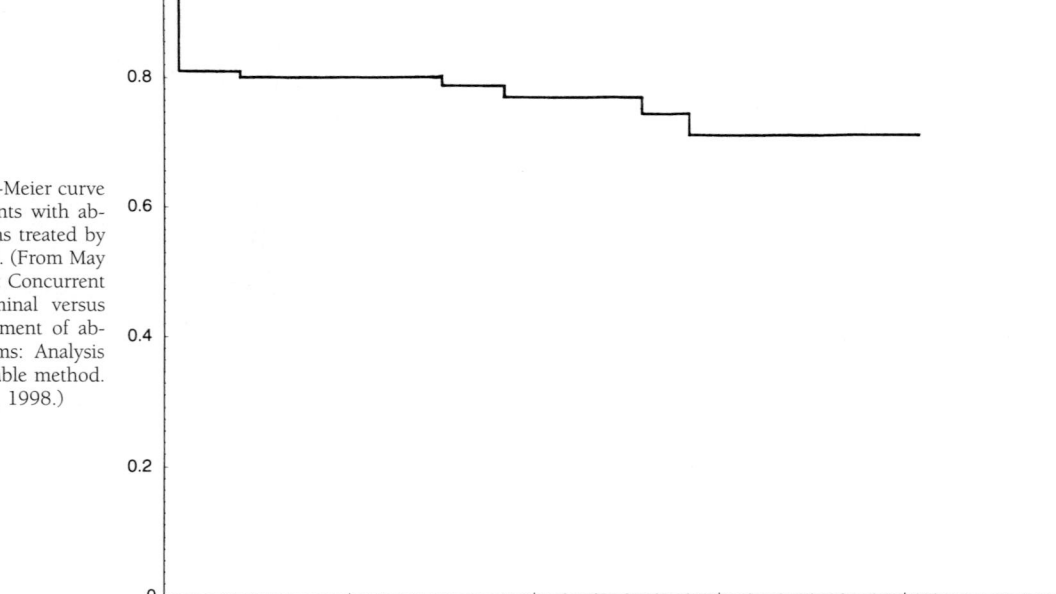

Number at Risk

| 108 | 78 | 41 | 18 | 1 | 0 |

FIGURE 90–12. Kaplan-Meier curve for graft failure in patients with abdominal aortic aneurysms treated by the endoluminal method. (From May J, White GH, Yu W, et al: Concurrent comparison of endoluminal versus open repair in the treatment of abdominal aortic aneurysms: Analysis of 303 patients by life table method. J Vasc Surg 27:213–222, 1998.)

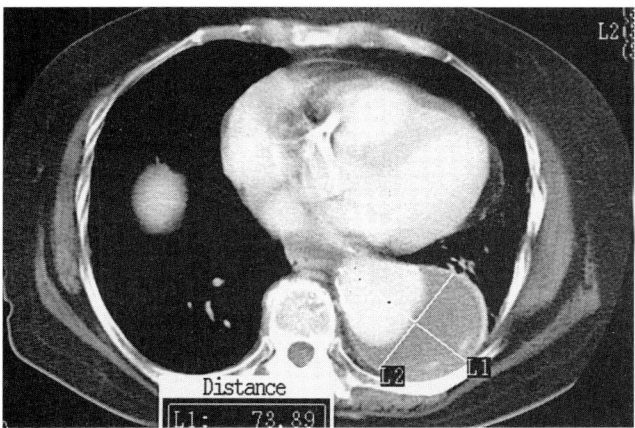

FIGURE 90–13. Contrast CT demonstrating a 7.4-cm-diameter aneurysm in the descending thoracic aorta.

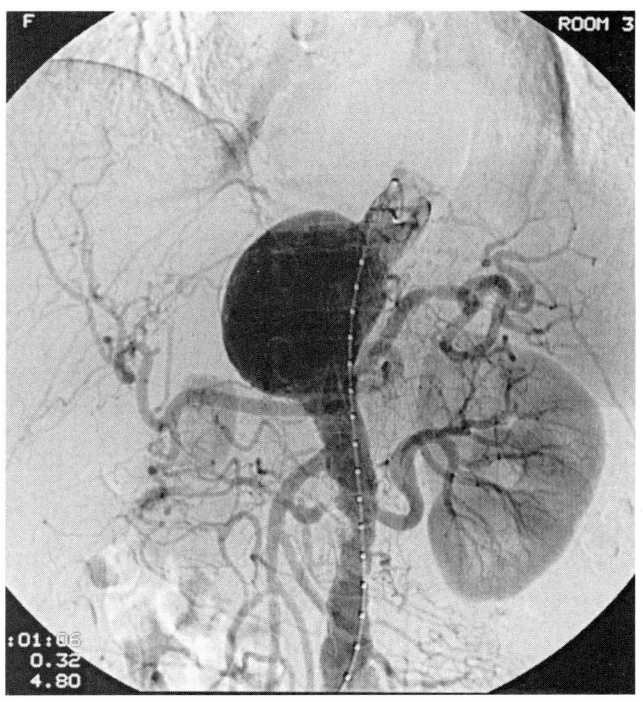

FIGURE 90–15. Preoperative aortogram demonstrating a thoracoabdominal aneurysm from which the celiac trunk is arising.

however, was compensated for by a decrease in blood loss at operation, need for intensive care, and length of hospital stay.

ANEURYSMS OF DESCENDING THORACIC AORTA

On theoretical grounds, there is much to recommend the endoluminal method for treatment of aneurysms of the descending thoracic aorta. To begin with, there are no natural barriers such as the renal arteries and aortic bifurcation that exist in the abdominal aorta. The problems of deployment of endografts in the descending thoracic aorta are limited to availability of a prosthesis of sufficiently large diameter to match the aorta adjacent to the aneurysm, the difficulty of accurate graft placement in a large, high-flow artery, and the risk of paraplegia.

There are sound reasons, however, why the risk of para-

plegia should be less when the endoluminal method rather than the open method is used. The patient is more likely to be hemodynamically stable during endoluminal repair and thus avoid spinal cord ischemia due to low flow in the intercostal arteries during periods of hypotension. The short period of interference with flow in the thoracic aorta during endoluminal graft deployment virtually guarantees good perfusion of the important intercostal arteries distal to the aneurysm without the complexity and complications of using a shunt. The seminal work of Dake and associates[39] in the clinical setting supports the theoretical advantages

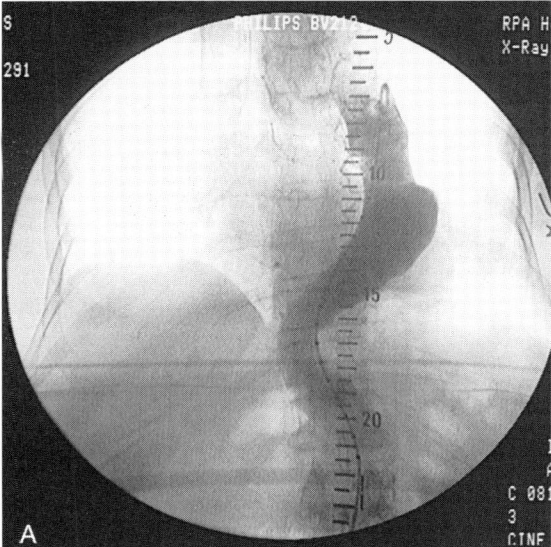

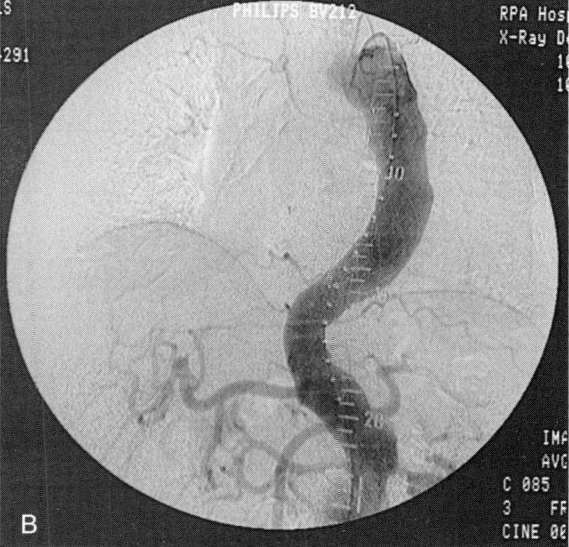

FIGURE 90–14. *A,* On the table, a preprocedure aortogram of the patient in Figure 90–13. *B,* On the table, a postprocedure aortogram following deployment of a 10-cm endoluminal graft. Note exclusion of the aneurysm sac from the circulation.

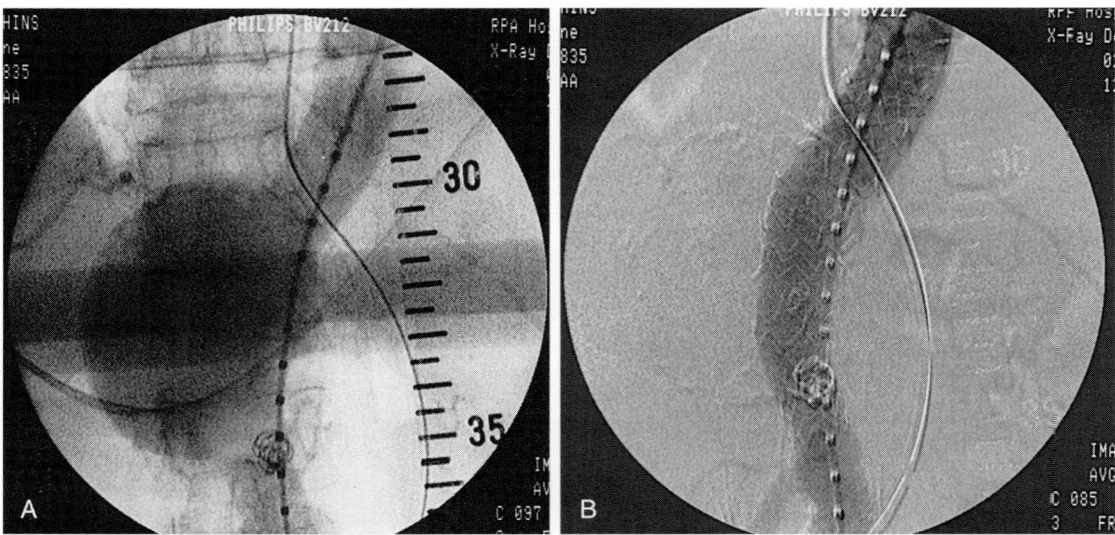

FIGURE 90–16. *A*, On the table, a preprocedure aortogram demonstrating the thoracoabdominal aortic aneurysm in Figure 90–15. Note the embolization coils opposite the 35-cm marker. These have blocked flow in the celiac artery. *B*, On the table, a postprocedure aortogram following deployment of an 11-cm endograft. The aneurysm sac has been excluded from the circulation, and there is no retrograde filling of the aneurysm sac via the celiac artery.

referred to earlier. Paraplegia was limited to four of 121 patients undergoing endoluminal repair of aneurysms of the descending thoracic aorta. Interestingly, all four patients had previously undergone open repair of AAAs.[40]

As with AAA endoluminal repair, further careful long-term follow-up is required to ensure that mechanical device failure is not a limiting factor. Advances in technology seem certain to provide prostheses of adequate diameter for the thoracic aorta, and Dorros and Cohn[41] have developed a novel method of deliberately producing a temporary period of cardiac asystole using intravenous adenosine to assist with accurate deployment of the prosthesis.

Two examples of endoluminal repair for aneurysms of the descending thoracic aorta are included to demonstrate the utility of the method in this site. The first is a frail 80-year-old woman with a 7.4-cm aneurysm in the lower descending thoracic aorta (Fig. 90–13). She was unfit for open repair and referred for consideration of endoluminal repair. This procedure was performed with a 10-cm long endograft after she gave informed consent regarding the risk of paraplegia (Fig. 90–14). Even though the aneurysm was situated in a site where spinal cord ischemia may have been expected, the patient made an uneventful recovery, with postoperative contrast CT confirming exclusion of the aneurysm sac from the circulation.

The second patient, who had a 6-cm thoracoabdominal aortic aneurysm, was also an unsuitable candidate for open repair. The aneurysm was situated in the distal descending thoracic aorta and proximal abdominal aorta with the celiac artery arising from the aneurysm sac (Fig. 90–15). Sufficient normal aorta was present proximal to the aneurysm and between the celiac and superior mesenteric artery to enable the endoluminal method of repair to be used. Coil embolization of the celiac artery was undertaken to avoid the development of an endoleak resulting from retrograde flow in the celiac artery supported by collateral channels. Successful endoluminal repair was undertaken without complication (Fig. 90–16).

REFERENCES

1. Parodi JC, Palmaz JC, Barone HD: Transfemoral intraluminal graft implantation for abdominal aortic aneurysm. Ann Vasc Surg 5:491–499, 1991.
2. Balm R, Eikelboom BC, May J, et al: Early experience with transfemoral endovascular aneurysm management (TEAM) in the treatment of aortic aneurysms. Eur J Vasc Endovasc Surg 11:214–220, 1996.
3. Schunn CD, Heilberger P, Krauss M, et al: Aortic aneurysm size and graft behaviour after endovascular stent-grafting—two years of clinical experience and follow-up. Paper presented to the 23rd World Congress of the International Society for Cardiovascular Surgery, London, September 21–26, 1997.
4. Parodi JC: Endovascular repair of abdominal aortic aneurysms and other arterial lesions. J Vasc Surg 21:549–555. 1995.
5. White GH, Yu W, May J, et al: Endoleak as a complication of endoluminal grafting of abdominal aortic aneurysms: Classification, incidence, diagnosis, and management. J Endovasc Surg 4:152–168, 1997.
6. May J, White GH: Endovascular leak. *In* Whittemore A (ed): Advances in Vascular Surgery. Vol 6. St. Louis, Mosby–Year Book 1998, pp 65–79.
7. White GH, May J, McGahan T, et al: Historical control comparison of outcome for matched groups of patients undergoing endoluminal versus open repair of abdominal aortic aneurysms. J Vasc Surg 2:201–212, 1996.
8. May J, White GH, Yu W, et al: Concurrent comparison of endoluminal versus open repair in the treatment of abdominal aortic aneurysms: Analysis of 303 patients by life table method. J Vasc Surg 27:213–222, 1998.
9. Keen WW: Surgery: Its Principles and Practice. Philadelphia, WB Saunders, 1921, pp 216–349.
10. Wiley FB: Clio Chirurgica: The Arteries Part 1. Austin, Tex, Silvergirl, Inc, 1998.
11. Power D: The palliative treatment of aneurysms by "wiring" with Colt's apparatus. Br J Surg 9:27, 1921.
12. Blakemore AH, King BG: Electrothermic coagulation of aortic aneurysms. JAMA 111:1821, 1938.
13. Ernst CB: Abdominal aortic aneurysm. N Engl J Med 328:1167–1172, 1993.
14. May J, White GH, Yu W, et al: Conversion from endoluminal to open repair of abdominal aortic aneurysms: A hazardous procedure. Eur J Vasc Endovasc Surg 14:4–11, 1997.
15. May J, White GH, Yu W, et al: Endovascular grafting for abdominal

aortic aneurysms: Changing incidence and indications for conversion to open operation. Cardiovasc Surg 6:194–197, 1998.

16. Veith FJ, Abbott WM, Yao JST, et al: Guidelines for development and use of transluminally placed endovascular prosthetic grafts in the arterial system. J Vasc Surg 21:670–685, 1995.

17. Yusuf SW, Whitaker SC, Chuter TA, et al: Early results of endovascular aortic aneurysm surgery with aortouniiliac graft, contralateral iliac occlusion and femoro-femoral bypass. J Vasc Surg 25:165–172, 1997.

18. Ahn SS, Rutherford RB, Johnston KW, et al: Reporting standards for infrarenal endovascular abdominal aortic aneurysm repair. J Vasc Surg 25:405–410, 1997.

19. May J, White GH: Basic data underlying clinical decision making: Endovascular treatment of infrarenal abdominal aortic aneurysms. Ann Vasc Surg 12:4:391–395, 1998.

20. May J, White GH, Yu W, et al: A prospective study of anatomico-pathological changes in abdominal aortic aneurysms following endoluminal repair: Is the aneurysmal process reversed? Eur J Vasc Endovasc Surg 12:11–17, 1996.

21. Matsumara JS, Pearce WH, McCarthy WJ, Yao JST, for the EVT Investigators: Reduction in aortic aneurysm size: Early results after endovascular graft placement. J Vasc Surg 25:113–123, 1997.

22. Malina M, Invacev K, Chuter TAM, et al: Changing aneurysmal morphology after endovascular grafting: Relation to leakage or persistent perfusion. J Endovasc Surg 4:23–30, 1997.

23. Broeders IAMJ, Blankensteijn JD, Gvakharia A, et al: The efficacy of transfemoral endovascular aneurysm management: A study on size changes of the abdominal aorta during mid-term follow-up. Eur J Vasc Endovasc Surg 14:84–90, 1997.

24. Lumsden AB, Allen RC, Chaikof EL, et al: Delayed rupture of aortic aneurysms following endovascular stent grafting. Am J Surg 170:174–178, 1995.

25. Parodi JC, Barone A, Piraino R, Schonholz C: Endovascular treatment of abdominal aortic aneurysms: Lessons learned. J Endovasc Surg 4:102–110, 1997.

26. White GH, Yu W, May J, et al: Three-year experience with the White-Yu endovascular GAD graft for transluminal repair of aortic and iliac aneurysms. J Endovasc Surg 4:124–136, 1997.

27. Parodi JC: Personal communication.

28. Baker DM, Hund R, Yusuf W, et al: (Abstract). Dilatation of proximal neck following open aneurysm repair. Int Angiol 14:158, 1995.

29. McGahan TJ, Berry GA, McGahan SL, et al: Results of autopsy 7 months after successful endoluminal treatment of an infrarenal abdominal aortic aneurysm. J Endovasc Surg 348–355, 1995.

30. May J, White GH, Yu W, et al: Pathology of healing and changes in morphology of abdominal aortic aneurysms treated by endoluminal prostheses. In Chuter TAM, Donayre CE, White RA (eds): Endolumi-

nal Vascular Prostheses, 2nd ed. Armonk, NY, Futura Publishing Co, 1998 (in press).

31. White GH, May J, Waugh RC, Yu W: Type I and type II endoleak: A more useful classification for reporting results of endoluminal repair of AAA (Letter). J Endovasc Surg 5:189–191, 1998.

32. Moore WS, Rutherford RB, for the EVT Investigators: Transfemoral endovascular repair of abdominal aortic aneurysm: Results of the North American EVT phase 1 trial. J Vasc Surg 23:543–553, 1996.

33. Marin ML, Veith FJ, Cynamon J, et al: Initial experience with transluminally placed endovascular grafts for the treatment of complex vascular lesions. Ann Surg 222:449–469, 1995.

34. Blum U, Voshage G, Lammer J, et al: Endoluminal stent-grafts for infrarenal abdominal aortic aneurysms. N Engl J Med 336:13–20, 1997.

35. May J, White GH, Yu W, et al: Repair of abdominal aortic aneurysms by the endoluminal method: Outcome in the first 100 patients. Med J Aust 165:549–551, 1996.

36. Bernhard V: Personal communication, 1998.

37. Lloyd WE, Darling RC, Chang BB, et al: The fate of the excluded abdominal aortic aneurysm sac: Long-term follow-up of 852 patients. Poster presentation of the Society for Vascular Surgery/International Society for Cardiovascular Surgery (SVS/ISCVS) meeting, New Orleans, 1997.

38. Schie G, Sieunarine K, Holt M, et al: Successful embolization of persistent endoleak from a patent inferior mesenteric artery. J Endovasc Surg 4:312–315, 1997.

39. Dake MD, Miller DC, Semba CP, et al: Transluminal placement of endovascular stent grafts for the treatment of descending thoracic aortic aneurysms. N Engl J Med 331:1729–1734, 1994.

40. Kee S: Stanford experience of endoluminal repair of thoracic aneurysms. Presented at Critical Issues in Endovascular Surgery, Nottingham, U.K., January 22–23, 1998.

41. Dorros G, Cohn JM: Adenosine-induced transient cardiac asystole enhances precise deployment of stent-grafts in the thoracic or abdominal aorta. J Endovasc Surg 3:270–272, 1996.

42. Chuter TAM, Chuter-Gianturco: Bifurcated stent grafts for abdominal aortic aneurysm exclusion. In Hopkinson B, Yusuf W, Whitaker S, Veith F (eds): Endovascular Surgery for Aortic Aneurysms. London, WB Saunders, 1997, pp 88–103.

43. Lawrence-Brown MM, Hartley D, MacSweeney ST, et al: The Perth endoluminal graft system—development and early experience. Cardiovasc Surg 4:706–712, 1996.

44. May J, White GH, Yu W: Endoluminal repair of abdominal aortic aneurysms: Strengths and weaknesses of various prostheses observed in a 4–5 year experience. J Endovasc Surg 4:147–151, 1997.

45. Thompson MM, Sayers RD, Nasim A, et al: Aortomonoiliac endovascular grafting: Difficult solutions to difficult aneurysms. J Endovasc Surg 4:174–181, 1997.

Ruptured Abdominal Aortic Aneurysms

Jon R. Cohen, MD

With major advances in surgical expertise and anesthesia over the past 20 years, the mortality for elective repair of abdominal aortic aneurysm (AAA) has gradually decreased to approximately 4%. However, the mortality for ruptured aneurysms has not changed significantly and continues to be 40% to 70%. In fact, the true mortality for ruptured aneurysms is much closer to 80% to 90% if deaths occurring before patients reach the hospital are included. With the increasing age of the population, the incidence of AAAs is also increasing to between 25 and 30 per 100,000 patients and now accounts for approximately one in every 200 deaths in the general population. Ruptured AAAs now rank 15th among all causes of death for men in the United States. The prevalence of AAAs as well as the proportion of elderly patients with AAAs appears to be increasing. As a result, the number of ruptured AAAs continues to increase.[1, 2] Some of the more famous people who have died of a ruptured AAA include Albert Einstein (1955), Charles De Gaulle (1972), and the singer Conway Twitty (1996).

ETIOLOGY OF RUPTURE

The pathophysiologic event that causes an AAA to rupture is unknown. There is, however, a distinct relationship between aneurysm size and rupture. In 1950, Estes[3] reported a classic study on the relationship between aneurysm rupture and size. In this series, the rupture rate was 20% within the first year and 40% to 50% within the first 5 years after diagnosis of large aneurysms. As the aneurysm increases in size the rupture rate increases at an exponential rate such that at 5 to 6 cm the rate rapidly increases. Aneurysm rupture risk is discussed in detail in Chapter 89.

There is some scientific evidence that an increase in circulating proteases that results from other pathologic conditions may increase aneurysm rupture. Analysis of the abdominal aortic wall in patients with ruptured AAAs indicates that there is a significant increase in aortic wall proteolytic activity compared with patients undergoing elective AAA repair (Fig 91–1).[4] A frequent clinical cause of an increase in circulating proteases is elective operations. Surgery causes a release of proteolytic enzymes from circulating white blood cells into the plasma in the normal postoperative period. This may be the reason why stable aneurysms sometimes rupture after surgical procedures unrelated to the AAA, such as after coronary artery bypass surgery.

DIAGNOSIS

A high index of suspicion is critical to early diagnosis and, in many cases, survival of patients with a ruptured AAA. Interestingly, fewer than 15% of patients are known to have an AAA prior to rupture. Unfortunately, the mean time from onset of symptoms (pain) to presentation in an emergency department is usually long; in one study, it was 37 hours.[5] Any patient over age 50 years without a history of trauma who is hypotensive or who suffers a cardiac arrest without a history suggestive of a cardiac etiology may have a ruptured AAA. Lower back, flank, or groin pain that is unremitting in nature should immediately suggest the possibility of a ruptured AAA. A careful history is very important because abdominal pain alone without back pain is unusual and frequently reflects another pathologic process. Aortic dissection must be considered in the differential diagnosis with high back pain, hypotension, and no prior history of an AAA.

Physical examination in patients with ruptured AAAs usually reveals a pulsatile abdominal mass if the systolic blood pressure is above 90 mmHg unless the patient is obese. Often patients with rupture have tender aneurysms, but this is not a reliable sign in the diagnosis of rupture. The presence and quality of all distal pulses must be documented because intraoperative decisions may depend on the pulse examination before surgery. Common symptoms and findings of ruptured AAA at admission are listed in Table 91–1. The examination of popliteal pulses is also important because 15% of patients with AAA have popliteal artery aneurysms.

The three most common diagnostic studies available for the diagnosis of a ruptured AAA are computed tomography (CT) scan, abdominal ultrasonography, and a lateral abdominal radiograph. The CT scan is the most accurate but may cause a significant delay if the scanner is not located near the emergency department (Fig. 91–2). There continues to be some debate about the role of CT scanning in patients with suspected AAA rupture. Patients with a known AAA who present with pain and hypotension should be taken immediately to the operating room for emergent repair.[7] Patients with an obvious pulsatile mass, hypotension, and pain should also undergo immediate, emergent surgery. The most important role of the CT scan is to detect the presence of an aneurysm, if not otherwise known, and to determine whether an AAA has ruptured in a hemodynamically stable patient if this is not clinically apparent. Some emergency departments have the availabil-

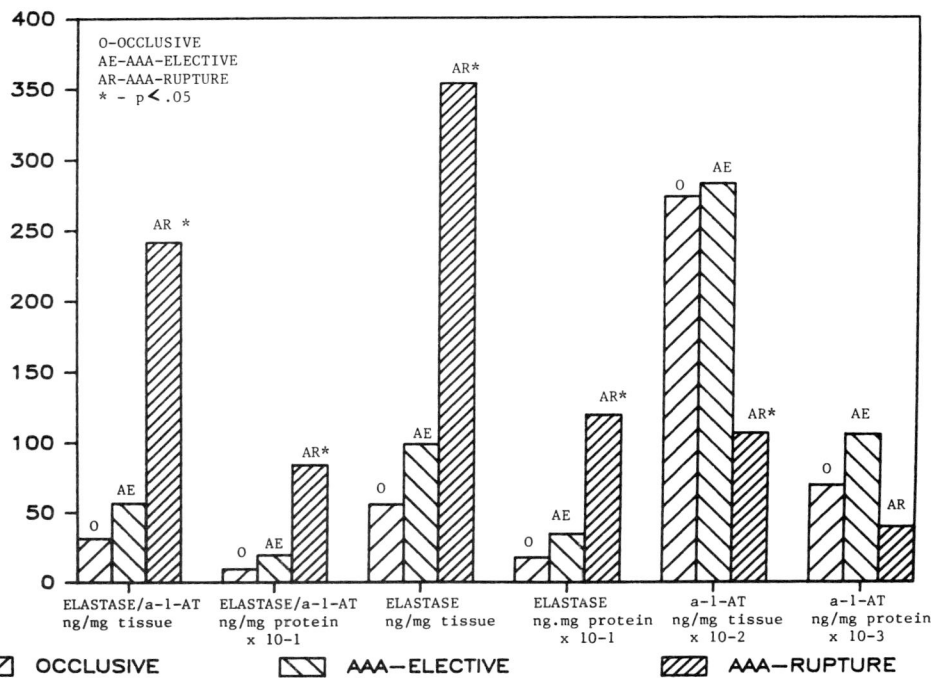

FIGURE 91–1 Elastase and elastase/alpha$_1$-antitrypsin (AT) were significantly higher and alpha$_1$-antitrypsin significantly lower in patients with a ruptured abdominal aortic aneurysm (AAA) compared with patients who underwent an elective procedure for AAA or had occlusive aortic disease. O = occlusive; AE-AAA = elective; AR-AAA = rupture. *Asterisk* represents P <.05. (Modified from Cohen JR, Mandell C, Margolis I, et al: Altered aortic protease and antiprotease activity in patients with ruptured abdominal aortic aneurysms. Surg Gynecol Obstet 164: 355–358, 1987.

ity of immediate ultrasound technology that can rapidly determine the presence of an AAA; unfortunately, it cannot reliably distinguish between a rupture and a nonruptured AAA. A cross-table lateral x-ray study of the abdomen sometimes reveals a calcified aneurysmal aortic wall, which also can aid in diagnosis of the AAA but contributes little to the diagnosis of rupture.

In one study, 65 patients with suspected ruptured AAAs who were hemodynamically stable underwent CT.[8] The average duration of the examination was 63 minutes, and no episodes of hypotension occurred in that group. Of the CT scans showing rupture, only one of 17 AAAs was not actually ruptured, for a specificity of 94%. In patients with rupture, CT provided useful additional information, including the presence of left-sided inferior vena cava, inflammatory aneurysm, thoracic aneurysm, and lung cancer. Among patients in this study who had aneurysms and

abdominal symptoms but did not have rupture, other intra-abdominal pathologic features were often identified to explain the symptoms. Thus, in this study, the use of CT scanning in patients with ruptured aortic aneurysms who were hemodynamically stable was helpful for evaluation of rupture, and did not adversely affect patient outcome. Beneficial information was gained from CT scan that was helpful for preoperative and intraoperative management in some of the cases.[8]

In a more recent study of 74 patients with a diagnosis of possible AAA rupture who underwent a CT scan, the sensitivity for detecting rupture was only 79% and the specificity was 77%. In this study, CT scanning actually had little additional diagnostic value when compared with the clinical impression of an experienced vascular surgeon.[7]

TABLE 91–1. SYMPTOMS AND FINDINGS AT ADMISSION IN 81 PATIENTS WITH RUPTURED ABDOMINAL AORTIC ANEURYSM

Symptoms	
Pain	96.3%
Abdominal	58.0%
Back	70.4%
Fainting	29.6%
Vomiting	22.2%
Findings	
Mass	91.3%
Tenderness	77.5%
Blood pressure <80 mmHg	41.7%
Hematocrit <38%	42.2%
White blood cell count >10,000/μL	79.4%
Abdominal aortic aneurysm seen on abdominal x-ray film	74.4%

From Donaldson MC, Rosenberg JM, Bucknam CA: Factors affecting survival after ruptured abdominal aortic aneurysm. J Vasc Surg 2:564–570, 1985.

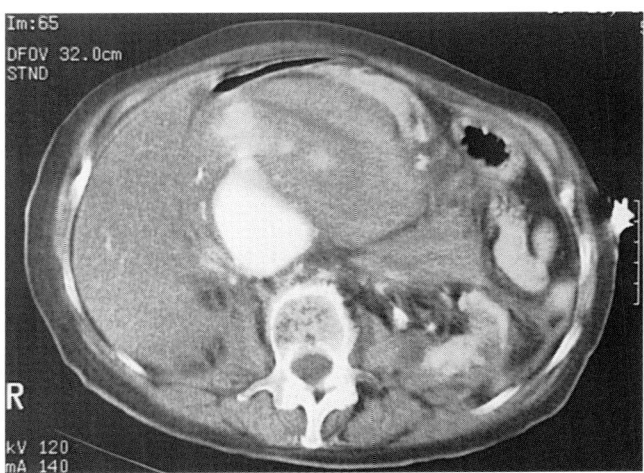

FIGURE 91–2 Ruptured abdominal aortic aneurysm with large retroperitoneal hematoma.

In some stable patients with questionable AAA rupture, expeditious CT scanning is helpful and may avoid unnecessary emergent procedures if rupture is not present (see Chapter 89).

RESUSCITATION AND PREPARATION FOR SURGERY

In the past 10 years, a debate has ensued about whether vigorous resuscitation of patients with suspected ruptured AAA is appropriate. Many suggest that, as in the treatment of any trauma victim, bleeding from a ruptured AAA is best managed by the rapid infusion of intravenous fluids, followed by immediate surgery for control of the hemorrhage. An alternative opinion has now emerged, namely that fluid resuscitation may promote further bleeding by increasing the blood pressure and causing a temporarily sealed rupture site in the aorta to reopen and bleed.

Crawford[9] suggested that the optimal strategy is to use blood for resuscitation until the time of surgery and that the systolic blood pressure should be maintained at approximately 50 to 70 mmHg until the aorta is crossed-clamped. Aortic clamping in his series was usually performed at the diaphragm while blood and fresh frozen plasma were given to maintain blood pressure and coagulation. Crawford argued that saline resuscitation increased the risk of hemodilution and coagulopathy, making the operation more technically difficult. Lawrie and associates[10] also reported a low mortality for ruptured aneurysms and attributed this low mortality to early diagnosis, immediate transfer to the operating room, and little, if any, infusion of fluids to avoid increased blood pressure. These views regarding fluid resuscitation have been supported by other evidence in the trauma literature in which the mortality for severe life-threatening hemorrhage has not been improved by preoperative administration of large amounts of fluids[11] and, in fact, has been worsened in certain circumstances.[12, 13]

The case for more aggressive fluid resuscitation argues that in many studies of patients with ruptured AAAs, the incidence of multisystem organ failure correlates directly with the duration of preoperative hypotension and shock. Organ hypoperfusion resulting in renal failure, ischemic colitis, and respiratory distress syndrome is almost universally lethal. Data from retrospective studies in which fluid resuscitation was restricted failed to support a benefit of this strategy. In fact, several studies of more aggressive, early fluid resuscitation have reported low mortality for ruptured AAAs, similar to Crawford's reported 26% mortality.[16] In contrast, Johanssen and coworkers reported a high mortality of 78% in 186 patients in a retrospective study of ruptured aneurysms despite optimal management in the field; this included prehospital aggressive fluid resuscitation, rapid transportation to a designated trauma center, immediate emergency department evaluation, and aneurysm repair by a vascular specialist.[14] The high mortality seen in this series, however, likely reflects the fact that nearly all patients survived long enough to undergo surgery, compared with other studies in which many of the highest-risk patients died of rupture before surgery.

There have been no prospective studies evaluating different fluid replacement regimens in treating ruptured aneurysms; furthermore, there are no clear data to indicate that either increased resuscitation or more rapid transit without resuscitation has made any difference in survival, which, unfortunately, has not changed much since the 1980s. Most surgeons would agree that transport to the nearest surgical facility with the capability to treat AAA rupture in association with a moderate infusion of intravenous fluids to maintain the systolic blood pressure above 90 mmHg is appropriate.

One of the most important factors that predicts outcome of ruptured AAA is initial blood pressure on admission to the emergency department, independent of the resuscitative effort. The expertise of the surgeon repairing the ruptured AAA is also important, as is any inadvertent intraoperative injury, such as inferior vena caval or renal vein injury, which is almost uniformly fatal. There are no specific preoperative co-morbid medical conditions that have accurately predicted mortality. An analysis of the most common co-morbid conditions reveals that there is no difference between survivors and nonsurvivors (Table 91–2)

Patients with known or strongly suspected AAA rupture should be brought to the operating room with at least two large-bore intravenous catheters and 6 units of blood available. Patients are usually prepared and draped before induction of anesthesia, because hypotension often worsens on induction. If time permits, a Foley catheter and introducer for a pulmonary artery catheter should be placed in addition to an arterial line. Only when the surgeon is ready to make the incision should the patient be anesthetized. Any of the maneuvers discussed previously, including the arterial line, central venous pressure line, or Foley catheter, should not be so uncomfortable to the patient as to raise the blood pressure and cause further bleeding of a stable rupture. Other helpful adjuncts include a nasopharyngeal temperature probe, rapid-infusion devices, a warming blanket, blood warmers, and a humidifier. The anesthesiologist should be aware of the most common coexisting diseases, particularly that 50% of patients have associated coronary artery disease (Table 91–3).

OPERATIVE TECHNIQUE

The first successful repair of a ruptured AAA was by Cooley and DeBakey in 1954.[18] Rupture into the retroperitoneal

TABLE 91–2. ASSOCIATION OF PREOPERATIVE RISK FACTORS WITH THE OUTCOME OF RUPTURED ABDOMINAL AORTIC ANEURYSMS

CO-MORBID CONDITIONS	ALIVE	DEAD	p
Diabetes mellitus	13%	3%	0.084
Chronic obstructive lung disease	21%	26%	0.254
Chronic renal failure or insufficiency	16%	26%	0.186
Coronary artery disease	50%	47%	0.871
Hypertension	34%	41%	0.313
Congestive heart failure	3%	2%	0.638
Smoking	45%	36%	0.266
Total patients (n)	38	58	

From Halpern VJ, Kline RG, D'Angelo AJ, Cohen JR: Factors that affect the survival rate of patients with ruptured abdominal aortic aneurysms. J Vasc Surg 26:939–948, 1997.

TABLE 91–3. PREVALENCE OF COEXISTING DISEASE IN PATIENTS WITH RUPTURED ABDOMINAL AORTIC ANEURYSMS

Coronary artery disease or cardiac failure	50%
Preexisting hypertension	30–50%
Obstructive airway disease	30–40%
Chronic renal disease	5%
Cerebrovascular disease	6%

From Brimacombe J, Berry A: A review of anaesthesia for ruptured abdominal aortic aneurysm with special emphasis on preclamping fluid resuscitation. Anaesth Intensive Care 21:311–323, 1993.

space occurs in 88% of cases, and free rupture into the intraperitoneal cavity occurs in 12%. Occasionally, rupture occurs into the duodenum or the inferior vena cava.

The most important surgical concept is proximal control of the aorta above the ruptured segment. More than 98% of ruptures occur below the renal arteries. It has been our policy to approach these patients in a very systematic fashion. First, exploration is accomplished through a long mid-line incision. A quick examination of the retroperitoneum should disclose whether rupture exists and the extent of hematoma in the area of the aortic neck below the renal arteries. If the surgeon can comfortably approach the aorta at the infrarenal level, the aorta should be clamped at this level. In the presence of a large amount of blood or continued hemorrhage, proximal control of the aorta at the level of the diaphragm should be obtained through the gastrohepatic ligament. The aorta just below the diaphragm is exposed, and an aortic clamp is put in place. In the severely hypotensive patient, this clamp is applied immediately. In the more stable patient, this clamp is put in place but not clamped unless hemorrhage is encountered during isolation of the infrarenal aneurysm neck. The plan minimizes suprarenal clamp time. In many cases, because of a large retroperitoneal hematoma, it is easier to clamp the aorta at the diaphragm, to proceed to open the infrarenal AAA, and to identify the neck by dissection from within the aorta.

Once the aorta is identified below the renal arteries, the aorta is clamped at this level and the proximal clamp at the diaphragm is released. The combination of long clamp times above the renal arteries plus hypotension frequently results in renal failure, which is usually fatal.

Other methods have been used for control of the proximal aorta, including compression at the diaphragm or placement of aortic balloon catheters or large Foley catheters via puncture of the aneurysm. However, it has been our experience that direct control of the suprarenal aorta at the diaphragm is most reliable. Identification of the iliac arteries in the retroperitoneal hematoma can also be difficult if these are not sufficiently calcified to facilitate easy palpation. Often, control of iliac back-bleeding with balloon occlusion catheters after the AAA is open is most expeditious and potentially avoids hazardous dissection around iliac veins that are obscured by hematoma. In most cases, a tube graft repair of the ruptured AAA can be accomplished.

It is our policy not to give heparin for ruptured AAA repair. Patients should be given antibiotics immediately prior to or during the operative procedure. Iatrogenic injury occurs in 10% of cases to such structures as the left renal

vein, renal artery, iliac veins, vena cava, superior mesenteric vein and artery, spleen, and duodenum. Unfortunately, these iatrogenic injuries are almost universally fatal because of increased bleeding, prolonged surgery, and direct, adverse effects of the injury.[6]

VARIABLES ASSOCIATED WITH MORTALITY AND SURVIVAL

Considerable analysis has been done to identify specific factors that might accurately predict outcome in patients with ruptured AAAs (Table 91–4).[19–31] Mortality in most series is associated with one or more of these 10 factors.[6]

TABLE 91–4. RISK FACTORS ASSOCIATED WITH MORTALITY FOLLOWING RUPTURED ABDOMINAL AORTIC ANEURYSM REPAIR

	MORTALITY RATE (%)
Age (yr)	
<70	58
70–80	62
>80	58
Admission systolic blood pressure (mmHg)	
<90	84
>90	46
Preoperative creatinine	
<1.5	44
1.5–1.9	50
>2	86
Loss of consciousness	
Present	77
Absent	52
Preoperative hemoglobin (g/dl)	
<9	77
9–10	78
11–12	48
>13	37
Intraoperative average SBP (mmHg)	
<90	77
>90	29
Operative blood loss (L)	
<4	45
4–7	54
>7	77
Unknown	90
Operative urine output (ml)	
<200	85
200–800	54
>800	54
Unknown	74
Blood transfused (units)	
<5	38
5–10	59
>10	77
Temperature at procedure completion	
<91° F	91
91°–96° F	52
>96° F	33

From Halpern VJ, Kline RG, D'Angelo AJ, Cohen JR: Factors that affect the survival rate of patients with ruptured abdominal aortic aneurysms. J Vasc Surg 26:939–948, 1997.

TABLE 91–5. RISK FACTORS ASSOCIATED WITH DEATH FOLLOWING RUPTURED ABDOMINAL AORTIC ANEURYSM REPAIR BY UNIVARIATE ANALYSIS

RISK FACTOR	p VALUE	ODDS RATIO
Age >70 yr	0.5	—
Age >80 yr	0.53	—
ECG changes	0.33	—
Loss of consciousness	0.014	3.0
Preoperative		
Hemoglobin <10 g/dl	0.01	3.8
Hemoglobin <9 g/dl	0.19	—
Creatinine >1.5 mg/dl	0.06	0.4
Creatinine >1.9 mg/dl	0.09	—
Creatinine >2 mg/dl	0.04	7.1
Systolic blood pressure <90 mmHg	0.0002	6.1
Intraoperative		
Systolic blood pressure <90 mmHg	<0.0001	8.2
Operative		
Urine output <200 ml	0.037	0.21
Temperature <93°F	0.017	0.32
Estimated blood loss >6L	0.04	0.347
Transfusion >7 units PRBC	0.013	2.822

From Halpern VJ, Kline RG, D'Angelo AJ, Cohen JR: Factors that affect the survival rate of patients with ruptured abdominal aortic aneurysms. J Vasc Surg 26:939–948, 1997.
ECG = electrocardiogram; PRBC = packed red blood cell.

TABLE 91–7. MORTALITY AFTER RUPTURED ABDOMINAL AORTIC ANEURYSM REPAIR

AGE (yr)	MORTALITY (%)
0–59	42
60–69	81
70–79	74
>79	38

From Cohen JR, Birnbaum E, Kassan M, Wise L: Experience in managing 70 patients with ruptured abdominal aortic aneurysms. N Y State J Med 91:97–100, 1991.

treatment. Attempts to classify institutions as community or university or tertiary centers and to correlate this with patient survival, however, have been unsuccessful.[33–35] In contrast, several studies have indicated that the degree of specialization of the surgeon (i.e., vascular surgeon versus general surgeon) may have a role in determining survival after a ruptured AAA.[36] In one study, patient survival after repair by vascular surgeons was significantly higher than after repair by general surgeons.[37] This may have related to a higher volume of cases by vascular surgeons than general surgeons because outcome is related to case volume.[33]

COMPLICATIONS

Major postoperative complications after ruptured AAA repair are common and occur in 50% to 70% of patients. Respiratory failure requiring mechanical ventilation for more than 3 days is most frequent, renal failure is second, and sepsis is the third most common complication (Table 91–8). Many of the complications reflect multisystem organ failure that occurs as a result of severe hypoperfusion at the time of rupture. Many of these complications are almost uniformly fatal after ruptured AAA repair, including myocardial infarction, renal failure, and ischemic colitis. Renal failure occurs as a result of hypoperfusion caused by hypotension, prolonged suprarenal clamp times, or a combination of both. The only reliable way of preventing renal failure is by maintaining renal perfusion, which may be impossible given the hypotension often associated with AAA rupture. Acute tubular necrosis is the most common cause of renal failure following AAA rupture and is treated

In a series of patients with a ruptured AAA, we reported the relative risk of factors associated with mortality by univariate analysis (Table 91–5). By multivariate analysis, three factors were identified to predict death: initial hemoglobin below 10 gm/dl, loss of consciousness, and a creatinine above 1.5 mg/dl. Mortality increased significantly as the number of these three factors increased (Table 91–6). In fact, the presence of all three of these factors was associated with death at a rate of 100%. Increased age has been suggested to be significant in predicting death from ruptured AAA; in most studies, however, there is not a clear correlation between age and mortality.[32] In fact, some studies indicate that patients who have survived to old age may have less coronary artery disease and do just as well as their younger counterparts after ruptured AAA repair (Table 91–7).

Attempts have been made to identify the specific type of medical facility that might be best for the management of ruptured AAAs in an effort to promote regionalization in

TABLE 91–6. MORTALITY RATE AFTER RUPTURED ABDOMINAL AORTIC ANEURYSM REPAIR: EFFECT OF SIGNIFICANT RISK FACTORS (MULTIVARIATE ANALYSIS)

RISK FACTOR	ALL PATIENTS	ADMISSION SYSTOLIC BLOOD PRESSURE	
		<90 mmHg	>90 mmHg
LOC present	77% (n = 34)	83% (n = 23)	64% (n = 11)
Creatinine >1.5 mg/dl	64% (n = 31)	82% (n = 12)	58% (n = 19)
Hemoglobin <10 g/dl	68% (n = 19)	82% (n = 11)	58% (n = 8)
Hemoglobin <10 + creatinine >1.5	50% (n = 4)	50% (n = 2)	50% (n = 2)
Hemoglobin <10 + LOC	100% (n = 5)	100% (n = 5)	0% (n = 0)
Creatinine >1.5 + LOC	50% (n = 6)	67% (n = 3)	100% (n = 3)
LOC + creatinine >1.5 + hemoglobin <10	80% (n = 5)	67% (n = 3)	100% (n = 2)

From Halpern VJ, Kline RG, D'Angelo AJ, Cohen JR: Factors that affect the survival rate of patients with ruptured abdominal aortic aneurysms. J Vasc Surg 26:939–948, 1997.
LOC = loss of consciousness.

expectantly with postoperative dialysis until such time as renal function may return. This may occur as late as 3 weeks postoperatively.

Ischemic colitis is very common after ruptured AAAs, also as a result of hypoperfusion from the initial event. Any patient who has a bowel movement within 24 hours after repair of a ruptured AAA should have a sigmoidoscopic examination of the colon to confirm or exclude colonic ischemia. In addition, patients requiring excessive fluid resuscitation and ongoing lactic acidosis should undergo sigmoidoscopic examination because this may be the only sign of colon ischemia. Severe colonic ischemia requires emergent colectomy, which is required in 50% of those patients with ischemic colitis after ruptured AAAs, and is associated with a mortality of approximately 50%.[39]

Other common complications of ruptured AAA repair include prolonged respiratory failure often requiring tracheostomy, sepsis, myocardial infarction, congestive heart failure, bleeding, stroke, lower extremity ischemia, paraplegia, and paraparesis. All of these complications are associated with high mortality rates.[40]

SURVIVAL AND QUALITY OF LIFE SURVIVAL

Patients with ruptured AAAs do not survive without operative repair. In one study of nonoperated ruptured AAAs, following the onset of symptoms, 80% of patients survived 6 hours; 50%, 24 hours; 30%, 6 days; and 10%, 6 weeks.[46] Survival beyond 3 months is uncommon. In patients who survive operation, quality-of-life surveys indicate no difference in lifestyle, degree of independence, or productivity following repair of ruptured AAAs compared with elective AAA repair. Survivors have an excellent long-term prognosis and a good to very good quality of life; 80% of patients have reported a good quality of life, and 77% of patients with ruptured AAAs function independently or with minimal help following successful repair.[41, 42] Long-term survival does not differ significantly after successful repair of ruptured compared with nonruptured AAA. Coronary artery disease is responsible for 38% of late deaths and is the most frequent cause of death after ruptured AAA repair.[44–46]

TABLE 91–8. POSTOPERATIVE COMPLICATIONS AFTER RUPTURED ABDOMINAL AORTIC ANEURYSM REPAIR

COMPLICATION	FREQUENCY (%)	MORTALITY (%)
Respiratory failure	48	34
Tracheostomy	14	44
Renal failure	29	76
Sepsis	24	45
Myocardial infarction or congestive heart failure	24	66
Bleeding	17	90
Stroke	6	50
Ischemic colitis	5	67
Lower extremity ischemia	3	17
Paraplegia or paraparesis	2	50

Modified from Gloviczki P, Pairolero PC, Mucha P Jr, et al: Ruptured abdominal aortic aneurysms: Repair should not be denied. J Vasc Surg 15:851–859, 1992.

TABLE 91–9. LATE CAUSES OF DEATH FOR PATIENTS SURVIVING AT LEAST 3 MONTHS AFTER ELECTIVE REPAIR VERSUS REPAIR OF RUPTURED ABDOMINAL AORTIC ANEURYSMS

LATE DEATH CAUSE	ELECTIVE (%)	RUPTURED (%)
Coronary artery disease	41	38
Other cardiac related	4	6
Lung cancer	11	14
Other malignancy	9	5
Rupture of thoracic aortic aneurysm	5	8
Cerebrovascular disorders	13	10
Gastrointestinal disease	2	1
Renal failure	2	1
Respiratory failure	5	6
Pulmonary embolism	2	0
Graft-enteric fistula	2	2
Graft thrombosis	1	0
Graft infection	1	0
Other	2	9
TOTAL	100%	100%

From Soisalon-Soininen S, Salo JA, Takkunen O, Mattila S: Comparison of long-term survival after repair of ruptured and non-ruptured abdominal aortic aneurysm. Vasa 24:42–48, 1995.

Other causes of late death are listed in Table 91–9. There is no significant difference in the cause of late deaths for patients with ruptured aneurysms and patients with elective AAA repair.

REFERENCES

1. Department of Health and Human Services, Office of Health Research, Statistics and Technology: Detailed Diagnosis and Surgical Procedures for Patients Discharged from Short Stay Hospitals. Hyattsville, Md., National Center for Health Statistics, 1982, p 30.
2. Graves EJ: Detailed Diagnosis and Procedures, National Hospital Discharge Survey: National Center for Health Statistics. Vital Health Stat 100:72, 1989.
3. Estes JE: Abdominal aortic aneurysms: A study of one hundred and two cases. Circulation 2:258, 1950.
4. Cohen JR, Mandell C, Margolis I, et al: Altered aortic protease and antiprotease activity in patients with ruptured abdominal aortic aneurysms. Surg Gynecol Obstet 164:355–358, 1982.
5. Farooq MM, Freischlag JA, Seabrook GR, et al: Effect of the duration of symptoms, transport time, and length of emergency room stay in morbidity and mortality in patients with ruptured abdominal aortic aneurysm. Surgery 119:9–14, 1996.
6. Donaldson MC, Rosenberg JM, Bucknam CA: Factors affecting survival after ruptured abdominal aortic aneurysm. J Vasc Surg 2:564–570, 1985.
7. Adam DJ, Bradbury AW, Stuart WP, et al: The value of computed tomography in the assessment of suspected ruptured abdominal aortic aneurysm. J Vasc Surg 27:431–437, 1998.
8. Kvilekval KHV, Best IM, Mason RA, et al: The value of computed tomography in the management of symptomatic abdominal aortic aneurysms. J Vasc Surg 12:28–33, 1990.
9. Crawford ES: Ruptured abdominal aortic aneurysm: An editorial. J Vasc Surg 13:348–350, 1991.
10. Lawrie GM, Morris GC, Crawford ES, et al: Improved results of operation for ruptured abdominal aortic aneurysms. Surgery 85:483–488, 1979.
11. Martin RR, Bickell WH, Pepe PE, et al: Prospective evaluation of preoperative fluid resuscitation in hypotensive patients with penetrating truncal injury: A preliminary report. J Trauma 33:354–362, 1992.
12. Bickell WH, Wall MJ Jr, Pepe PE, et al: Immediate versus delayed fluid resuscitation for hypotensive patients with penetrating torso injuries. N Engl J Med 331:1105–1109, 1994.

13. Bickell WH, Bruttig SP, Millnamow GA, et al: The detrimental effects of intravenous crystalloid after aortotomy in swine. Surgery 110:529–536, 1991.
14. Johansen K, Kohler T, Nicholls S, et al: Ruptured abdominal aortic aneurysm: The Harborview experience. J Vasc Surg 13:240–247, 1991.
15. Halpern VJ, Kline RG, D'Angelo AT, et al: Factors that affect the survival rate of patients with ruptured abdominal aortic aneurysms. J Vasc Surg 26:939–948, 1997.
16. Martin RS, Edwards WH, Jenkins JM, et al: Ruptured abdominal aortic aneurysm: A 25-year experience and analysis of recent cases. Am Surg 54:539–543, 1988.
17. Brimacombe J, Berry A: A review of anaesthesia for ruptured abdominal aortic aneurysm with special emphasis on preclamping fluid resuscitation. Anaesth Intensive Care 21:311–323, 1993.
18. DeBakey ME, Crawford ES, Cooley DA, et al: Aneurysm of abdominal aorta analysis of results of graft replacement therapy one to eleven years after operation. Ann Surg 160:622, 1964.
19. Harris LM, Faggioli GL, Fiedler R, et al: Ruptured abdominal aortic aneurysms: Factors affecting mortality rates. J Vasc Surg 14:812–820, 1991.
20. Katz DJ, Stanley JC, Zelenock GB: Operative mortality rates for intact and ruptured abdominal aortic aneurysms in Michigan: An eleven-year statewide experience. J Vasc Surg 19:804–817, 1994.
21. Marty-Anè CH, Alric P, Picot MC, et al: Ruptured abdominal aortic aneurysm: Influence of intraoperative management on surgical outcome. J Vasc Surg 22:780–786, 1995.
22. Maynard ND, Taylor PR, Mason RC, et al: Gastric intramucosal pH predicts outcome after surgery for ruptured abdominal aortic aneurysm. Eur J Vasc Endovasc Surg 11:201–206, 1996.
23. Bradbury AW, Bachoo P, Milne AA, et al: Platelet count and the outcome of operation for ruptured abdominal aortic aneurysm. J Vasc Surg 21:484–491, 1995.
24. Wakefield TW, Whitehouse WM Jr, Wu SC, et al: Abdominal aortic aneurysm rupture: Statistical analysis of factors affecting outcome of surgical treatment. Surgery 91:586–596, 1982.
25. AbuRahma AF, Woodruff BA, Lucente FC, et al: Factors affecting survival of patients with ruptured abdominal aortic aneurysm in a West Virginia community. Surg Gynecol Obstet 172:377–382, 1991.
26. Murphy JL, Barber GG, McPhail NV, et al: Factors affecting survival after rupture of abdominal aortic aneurysm: Effect of size on management and outcome. Can J Surg 33:201–205, 1990.
27. Soreide O, Lillestol J, Christensen O, et al: Abdominal aortic aneurysms: Survival analysis of four hundred thirty-four patients. Surgery 91:188–193, 1982.
28. Hardman DTA, Fisher CM, Patel MI, et al: Ruptured abdominal aortic aneurysms: Who should be offered surgery? J Vasc Surg 23:123–129, 1996.
29. Bauer EP, Redaelli C, von Segesser LK, et al: Ruptured abdominal aortic aneurysms: Predictors for early complications and death. Surgery 114:31–35, 1993.
30. Johnston KW, Canadian Society for Vascular Surgery Aneurysm Study Group: Ruptured abdominal aortic aneurysm: Six-year follow-up results of a multicenter prospective study. J Vasc Surg 19:888–900, 1994.
31. Chen JC, Hildebrand HD, Salvian AJ, et al: Predictors of death in nonruptured and ruptured abdominal aortic aneurysms. J Vasc Surg 24:614–623, 1996.
32. Aune S, Amundsen SR, Evjensvold J, et al: The influence of age on operative mortality and long-term relative survival following emergency abdominal aortic aneurysm operations. Eur J Vasc Endovasc Surg 10:338–341, 1995.
33. Jenkins AM, Ruckley CV, Nolan B: Ruptured abdominal aortic aneurysm. Br J Surg 73:394–398, 1986.
34. Burke PM Jr, Sannella NA: Ruptured abdominal aortic aneurysm: A community experience. Cardiovasc Surg 1:239–242, 1993.
35. Katz SG, Kohl RD: Ruptured abdominal aortic aneurysm: A community experience. Arch Surg 129:284–290, 1994.
36. Rutledge R, Oller DW, Meyer AA, et al: A statewide, population-based, time-series analysis of the outcome of ruptured abdominal aortic aneurysm. Ann Surg 223:492–505, 1996.
37. Ouriel K, Geary K, Green RM, et al: Factors determining survival after ruptured abdominal aortic aneurysm: The hospital, the surgeon, and the patient. J Vasc Surg 11:493–496, 1990.
38. Cohen JR, Birnbaum E, Kassan M, et al: Experience in managing 70 patients with ruptured abdominal aortic aneurysms. NY State J Med 91:97–100, 1991.
39. Levison JA, Halpern VJ, Kline RG, et al: Perioperative predictors of colonic ischemia following ruptured abdominal aortic aneurysm. Presented at the Society for Vascular Surgery, June 1998. J Vasc Surg 29(1):40–45, 1999.
40. Panneton JM, Lassonde J, Laurendeau F: Ruptured abdominal aortic aneurysm: Impact of comorbidity and postoperative complications on outcome. Ann Vasc Surg 9:535–54l, 1995.
41. Rohrer MJ, Cutler BS, Wheeler HB: Long-term survival and quality of life following ruptured abdominal aortic aneurysm. Arch Surg 123:1213–1217, 1988.
42. Magee TR, Scott DJ, Dunkley A, et al: Quality of life following surgery for abdominal aortic aneurysm. Br J Surg 79:1014–1016, 1992.
43. Soisalon-Soininen S, Salo JA, Takkunen O, et al: Comparison of long-term survival after repair of ruptured and non-ruptured abdominal aortic aneurysm. Vasa 24:42–48, 1995.
44. Poulias GE, Doundoulakis N, Skoutas B, et al: Abdominal aneurysmectomy and determinants of improved results and late survival: Surgical considerations in 672 operations and 1–15 year follow-up. J Cardiovasc Surg (Torino) 35:115–121, 1994.
45. Hollier LH, Plate G, O'Brien PC, et al: Late survival after abdominal aortic aneurysm repair: Influence of coronary artery disease. J Vasc Surg 1:290–299, 1984.
46. Vohra R, Reid D, Groome J, et al: Long-term survival in patients undergoing resection of abdominal aortic aneurysm. Ann Vasc Surg 4:460–465, 1990.
47. Gloviczki P, Pairolero PC, Mucha P Jr, et al: Ruptured abdominal aortic aneurysms: Repair should not be denied. J Vasc Surg 15:851–859, 1992.

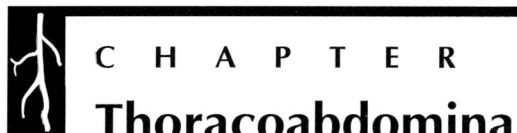

C H A P T E R   9 2

Thoracoabdominal Aortic Aneurysms

Richard P. Cambria, M.D.

OVERVIEW

Aneurysms that simultaneously involve the thoracic and abdominal aorta or those aneurysms including the visceral aortic segment are referred to as thoracoabdominal aortic aneurysms (TAAs). Such aneurysms are uncommon when compared with isolated infrarenal aneurysms (abdominal aortic aneurysms [AAAs]), composing no more than 2% to 5% of the total spectrum of degenerative aortic aneurysms. Patients with a TAA represent one point on a spectrum of disease continuity involving various segments of the aorta. For example, most studies examining natural history data for thoracic aortic aneurysms indicate that between 20% and 30% of these patients will also be found to have aneurysms of the abdominal aorta.[8, 90, 119] In a large Mayo Clinic series encompassing nearly 6000 aortic resections for aneurysm disease, 2% of patients undergoing AAA repair versus 18% of patients with a TAA underwent repairs for multiple aneurysms.[65] Crawford and Cohen[40] noted in a series of 1500 patients treated for AAA that some 12.5% harbored aneurysms in other aortic segments.

Aside from the obvious more proximal extent of aorta involved, TAAs can also be distinguished from the more routine AAAs because of varying causes and demographic profiles. Although most TAAs are degenerative in nature and occur in association with hypertension, smoking, and frequently evidence of vascular disease in other territories, up to 20% of TAAs in most series are the sequelae of chronic aortic dissection.[3, 13, 30, 108, 122] Furthermore, the male:female ratio of TAAs in our patients is 1:1, whereas our experience with patients with AAAs is consistent with the 5 to 6:1 male:female ratio frequently reported in the literature. Others have noted the tendency for aneurysm disease in females to more often involve proximal aortic segments.[8, 74, 98]

Because graft replacement of TAAs implies at least temporary interruption of splanchnic, renal, and potentially spinal cord blood flow, operative management of these lesions may be complicated by ischemic damage in these vascular beds, thereby increasing the overall scope and potential morbidity of the operation. Accordingly, acceptable surgical results with TAA have been achieved in most environments only over the past decade. Successful management of abdominal aneurysms involving the visceral aortic segment was first performed by Etheredge in 1955.[52] Thereafter, DeBakey and associates[46] reported using a polyester (Dacron) graft replacement and a multiple side-arm technique for reconstruction of the visceral vessels.

The modern era in the successful surgical management of TAAs began with the pioneering work of E. Stanley Crawford of Houston. In a series of publications that laid the foundation for the widespread successful management of TAAs, Crawford and colleagues described a simplified operative approach to these lesions using the inclusion technique, wherein visceral and intercostal vessels were reconstructed from within the aneurysm by directly anastomosing openings in the main Dacron graft to the aortic origin of these vessels (see Fig. 92–4).[34] Despite various surgical and adjunctive strategies applied in different centers to minimize overall operative morbidity, the state of the art in contemporary management of these patients still entails a 5% to 10% risk of perioperative mortality or morbidity in the form of renal, respiratory, and spinal cord ischemic complications.[3, 13, 30, 64, 72, 108]

ETIOLOGY AND EXTENT

Most TAAs are degenerative in nature and indistinguishable on either gross or microscopic pathology from the more typically encountered AAA. Genetic predisposition is likely an important etiologic factor in some patients with familial aneurysm. Although there is debate about whether aneurysmal disease is a sequela of atherosclerosis or a primary connective tissue weakness, the terms "atherosclerotic" and "degenerative" are used interchangeably.

About 20% of TAAs are the sequelae of chronic aortic dissection. Available information indicates that a minimum of 25% of patients who sustain spontaneous aortic dissection will eventually have chronic aneurysmal dilatation of the outer wall of the false lumen and be at risk for death from late aneurysm rupture.[47, 95, 113] This is further confused by the fact that at least some patients who sustain spontaneous aortic dissection will do so in aortas with preexistent aneurysmal dilatation.[12] Patients with Marfan's syndrome may have true cystic medial necrosis, a rare pathology, predisposing such patients to aneurysm formation and aortic dissection. The majority of patients with Marfan's syndrome who undergo surgical treatment for TAAs harbor aneurysms caused by chronic dissection.

Our data are consistent with published reviews on the distribution of the various causes of TAA; namely, some 80% are degenerative; 15% to 20% are the sequelae of chronic dissection, including the 5% of patients who harbor Marfan's syndrome); 2% are related to infection; and 1% to 2% are the sequelae of previous aortitis.[13, 97] Patients with aneurysms secondary to chronic dissection are significantly younger than their counterparts with degenerative aneurysms, but their aneurysms tend to be more extensive. Aneurysms secondary to the sequelae of giant cell arteritis

1303

are typically seen in women and can result from either Takayasu's disease or the nonspecific variety of giant cell aortitis. In addition, in some patients there may be no known prior diagnosis of aortitis or other associated collagen vascular diseases. Such aneurysms can be either focal or diffuse along the thoracoabdominal aorta and are frequently associated with other known sequelae of inflammatory aortitis (namely, visceral aneurysm) and renal artery occlusive disease.

TAAs secondary to an infectious process present challenging management issues because the dual goals of eradication of sepsis and arterial reconstruction typically demand an in situ type of reconstruction, that is, placement of a prosthetic graft in a contaminated field. The term *mycotic aneurysm* continues to be applied to these lesions, although it more precisely relates to the aneurysms secondary to embolization from an infected cardiac vegetation. In contemporary practice, the pathogenesis of infected TAAs is usually hematogenous seeding of atherosclerotic plaque, the development of focal aortitis with dissolution of the aortic wall, and the formation of a false aneurysm. All such aneurysms are, in fact, contained ruptures of false aneurysms.

TAAs are classified according to the scheme originally devised by Crawford.[37] In the most basic terms, this scheme considers whether the lesion is primarily a caudal extension of a descending thoracic aneurysm or a cephalad extension of a total abdominal aneurysm (Fig. 92–1). This classification is clinically useful because it has direct implications for both the technical conduct of operations and the incidence of operative complications, in particular, ischemic spinal cord injury. There is considerable variation in the spectrum and overall scope of operation required to deal with lesions within the classification of TAA.

In contemporary practice, the management of a *type IV* aneurysm should be accomplished with an overall morbidity and mortality very similar to the management of routine AAAs[114]; however, the same cannot be said for the more extensive *type I* and *type II* lesions. The designation *type II* aneurysm is reserved for patients in whom the entire descending thoracic aorta is involved. Repair of these aneurysms typically requires a clamp placed directly at or even proximal to the left subclavian artery. Some authors consider any aneurysm wherein more than half of the descending thoracic aorta is involved to be a type II lesion. Furthermore, the aneurysm should be classified according to the extent of aorta resected during a single procedure. For example, it is commonplace to resect a type I aneurysm down to a prior infrarenal aneurysm repair. Such lesions should be classified as a type I rather than a type II aneurysm.

Considerable variation is reported in the literature with respect to the distribution of TAAs. Although this reflects, to a degree, referral biases, the issue of precision in aneurysm classification, as discussed previously, likely also accounts for some of the variability. Table 92–1 displays data from representative contemporary series with respect to the relative distribution of TAA extent. Although the degree of variability is evident, some 50% to 60% of treated aneurysms fall into the more extensive type I and type II categories.

Virtually all major clinical series emphasize a significant incidence of prior aortic resections. In our experience, this is seen in one third of patients presenting for TAA resection. The most common pattern is the patient who has undergone a prior infrarenal AAA repair (60% of total prior resections). Virtually every pattern can be seen, however, including prior proximal thoracic aortic grafts or earlier TAA resections in which part of the visceral aortic segment was encompassed in the original operation.[29, 32]

The classification scheme outlined in Figure 92–1 does not consider the patient with incontinuity aneurysm of parts or all of the ascending aorta and aortic arch. Whereas synchronous proximal aneurysm is noted in 6% to 13% of degenerative TAA patients, contiguous arch aneurysm is rare, typically occurring only in patients with a previous DeBakey type I aortic dissection, especially those with Marfan's syndrome.[97] Patients with incontinuity arch and TAA

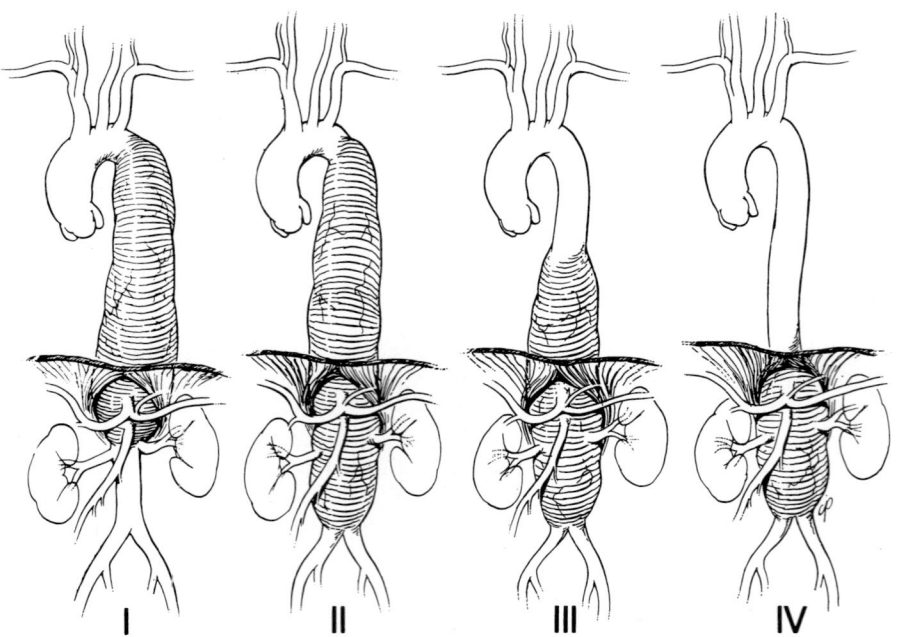

FIGURE 92–1. Crawford classification of thoracoabdominal aortic aneurysm extent (I–IV).

I   II   III   IV

TABLE 92–1. ANEURYSM EXTENT (CRAWFORD CLASSIFICATION) AMONG MAJOR CLINICAL SERIES OF PATIENTS TREATED FOR THORACOABDOMINAL ANEURYSMS

ARTICLE	YEAR	NO. OF PATIENTS	TYPE I (%)	TYPE II (%)	TYPE III (%)	TYPE IV (%)
Grabitz et al[66]	1996	232	29	35	25	10
Safi et al[104]	1998	343	32	34	11	23
Coselli et al[31]	1999	1220	35	30	16	18
Acher et al[3]	1998	176	19	37	16	26
Cambria et al[13]*	1997	210	32	21	28	19
Svensson[122]	1993	1509	25	29	23	23
Total/mean (range)		3690	29 (19–35)	30 (15–37)	21 (11–34)	20 (10–26)

*Updated.

aneurysm usually require complex, staged procedures.[70] Because patients with degenerative TAA or prior distal dissections most often have an aneurysm "neck" in the region of the aortic isthmus, TAA resection is usually (and more safely) staged from the treatment of ascending or arch aneurysms, the separate management of which is not further considered in this chapter.

NATURAL HISTORY

Irrespective of etiology, the expected natural history of TAAs is progressive enlargement and eventual rupture. Because TAAs are uncommon compared with infrarenal AAAs, few natural history studies are available. Furthermore, natural history studies of degenerative TAA are confused by the inclusion of patients with acute aortic dissection, many of whom die in the acute phase of the disease.[8, 74] Natural history data are essential to the clinician in balancing the risk of aneurysm rupture with that of surgical morbidity. Size threshold criteria for recommending operation in patients with TAA are not clearly defined compared with those for patients with infrarenal AAA. This is further complicated by the fact that the typical degenerative TAA is not uniform in size and may present the surgeon with the dilemma as to the wisdom of extending the resection to encompass often modestly dilated aortic segments.

Natural history data gleaned from university referral center populations are inherently biased. Accordingly, population-based studies, although few in number, are frequently cited. Bickerstaff and colleagues[8] from the Mayo Clinic reported an incidence of 5.9 thoracic aortic aneurysms per 100,000 person-years over a 30-year period in Rochester, Minn. These investigators found that rupture occurred in 74% of their patients and was nearly always fatal. Actuarial 5-year survival for their patients was a mere 13%. If patients with aortic dissection were eliminated, the prognosis of degenerative thoracic aortic aneurysm in the first 3 years after diagnosis was considerably worse compared with a prior Mayo Clinic study of unoperated AAAs.[51]

Similar data with respect to the incidence of concomitant AAA (25%), the higher risk of rupture for aortic dissection, and a substantial risk of rupture for thoracic aortic aneurysm were reported by McNamara and Pressler.[90] This study is valuable because no patients were operated upon and the 3-year survival rate of patients with degenerative tho-

racic aortic aneurysm was only 35%. Almost half of the deaths were related to aneurysm rupture.

Johansson and coworkers[74] reported on the incidence of ruptured thoracic aortic aneurysm in two separate time intervals (1989 and 1980). The incidence of patients presenting for treatment for ruptured thoracic aortic aneurysm was 5 per 100,000 patient-years, and the incidence was stable over the decade examined. Rupture was nearly uniformly fatal, and approximately half of all ruptures occurred in the ascending aorta. There was an equal sex distribution with respect to ruptured thoracic aortic aneurysm, but the data are clearly complicated by the inclusion of acute proximal aortic dissections.

Although natural history data from referral center populations are biased, such studies remain valuable because the practicalities of triage for operative or conservative therapy are among the variables considered. Crawford and DeNatale[36] reported on nearly 100 patients referred for, but subsequently denied, surgical treatment for TAA, usually related to advanced age or associated co-morbid conditions. Survival at 2 years was only 24%, and half of all deaths were related to aneurysm rupture. Data on aneurysm diameter were not available from this study, but chronic obstructive pulmonary disease (COPD), interestingly, was noted in 80% of the subgroup whose operation was deferred because of associated co-morbid conditions. Not surprisingly, the comparative 2-year survival (70%) in these authors' comparative series of surgically treated patients was far superior to the observed survival in the nonoperated cohort.[36]

Data with respect to size criteria for recommending operation were inferred from another report from Crawford's group. In a series of 117 patients treated for ruptured thoracic aneurysms or TAAs, Crawford and coworkers[35] noted that 80% of all ruptures occurred in aneurysms smaller than 10 cm, dispelling the previously held myth that only exceedingly large thoracic aneurysms ruptured. Rupture occurred in smaller aneurysms when acute dissection was the pathologic feature, and indeed, 13% of all ruptures occurred at a site where the aneurysm was less than 6 cm in diameter. Rupture occurred with equal frequency in the chest and abdominal cavities, and 60% of all TAA ruptures occurred in cases in which the abdominal component was less than 8 cm in diameter. Because rupture was observed in some 10% of patients with aneurysms smaller than 6 cm in diameter, the authors recommended elective operation for TAA when a 5 cm diameter threshold was exceeded.

Some reports provide insight into the expected natural history and rupture risk in patients referred for consideration of TAA resection. Cambria and colleagues,[15] reporting on 57 patients with TAAs initially managed nonoperatively (mean follow-up, 37 months), found that rupture occurred in 14% of patients, accounting for 24% of all deaths. Variables weakly ($p = .06$) associated with aneurysm rupture included a history of COPD and chronic renal failure. The mean size of the ruptured TAAs in their series was 5.8 cm, and no aneurysm less than 5 cm ruptured. Median expansion rate was only 0.2 cm per year for the entire cohort but was significantly accelerated in patients with a history of COPD. The risk of rupture in their patients must be considered a minimum estimate because 25% of the original cohort subsequently underwent repair of TAA during the study interval. This report is consistent with other data indicating that COPD, in particular, and likely chronic renal failure are additional factors (in addition to absolute aneurysm diameter) that increase the risk of aneurysm expansion and rupture.[85, 98]

Juvonen and coworkers,[75] using detailed computer-generated representations of the thoracoabdominal aorta, reported on 114 patients managed without surgery and followed with sequential computed tomography (CT) scans over a mean interval of 28 months. Although only 10% of their patients had a true TAA extent of the aneurysm, the data are valuable because these authors maintained a relatively conservative threshold of 7 cm in recommending elective operation for thoracic aortic aneurysms and TAAs. Aneurysm rupture occurred in a sobering 23% of their patients, and another 20% met previously defined or clinically compelling indications for operation. Relatively modest mean diameter values (5.8 cm for the thoracic component and 4.5 cm for the abdominal component) were observed in patients whose aneurysm ruptured. Not surprisingly, however, mean diameters in both the thoracic and abdominal aorta were significantly larger in patients with rupture than in those without. Expansion rates in the abdominal component of TAA were significantly higher in the patients who experienced rupture.[75]

Reproduced in Table 92–2 are the results of these authors' multivariate analysis of risk factors associated with aneurysm rupture. Although the association of aneurysm rupture with increasing diameter of either the thoracic or

TABLE 92–2. RISK FACTORS FOR RUPTURE OF DESCENDING THORACIC AND THORACOABDOMINAL ANEURYSMS: MULTIVARIATE ANALYSIS

RISK FACTOR	p VALUE	RELATIVE RISK
Age	0.02	2.6†
Pain*	0.04	2.3
Chronic obstructive pulmonary disease	0.004	3.6
Descending aortic diameter	0.003	1.9‡
Abdominal aortic diameter	0.05	1.50§

From Juvonen T, Ergin MA, Galla JD, et al: Prospective study of the natural history of thoracic aortic aneurysm. Ann Thorac Surg 63:1533–1545, 1997.

*Considers the presence of even uncharacteristic pain.

†Relative risk increases by a factor of 2.6 for each decade of age.

‡Relative risk increases by a factor of 1.9 for each cm of descending aortic diameter.

§Relative risk increases by a factor of 1.5 for each cm of abdominal aortic diameter.

the abdominal component is expected, the striking association of COPD with aneurysm rupture fits with the observations made by the Mayo Clinic investigators and in previous reports of variables associated with rupture risk for infrarenal aneurysm.[41] These authors also observed that pain possibly related to the aneurysm was a variable associated with aneurysm rupture, findings reported by others.[98] This suggests that the chronic back pain syndrome not uncommonly related by patients with TAAs (see later) should be considered in formulating a recommendation for operation in these patients.

Although incomplete (and likely to remain so because of ethical considerations), reasonable natural history data for TAAs are now available and are consistent with extrapolations from the more completely documented AAA studies. As with AAA studies, there is adequate information to indicate that increasing aneurysm diameter, the presence of COPD, and possibly female sex, advanced age, and the presence of renal insufficiency increase the risk of TAA rupture.[15, 85] The mean expansion rate of TAAs is less than 5 mm/year when all patients under observation are considered, but larger TAAs (>5.5 cm) expand at a more rapid rate.

Several investigators have correlated increased rates of expansion with TAA rupture.[60, 83, 85] Inferences made from the previously noted studies indicate that the risk of TAA rupture is negligible in aneurysms smaller than 5 cm, is likely no higher than the risk of surgical morbidity in the range of 5 to 6 cm in diameter, and increases substantially at aneurysm diameters larger than 6 cm. Perko and associates[98] found that risk of rupture increased fivefold when the 6-cm diameter threshold was exceeded. The rupture risk of greater than 20% reported by Juvonen and coworkers[75] when operation was recommended for aneurysms 7 cm and larger indicates that this size threshold is excessively conservative with respect to recommendation for operation in most patients.

These observations have led us to the general recommendation of 6 cm as an appropriate size threshold for surgical intervention for degenerative types I to III TAAs after an appropriate consideration of age and other co-morbid conditions. Since type IV TAA is a total abdominal aneurysm, a 5-cm threshold for operation is maintained. In TAAs secondary to chronic dissection, particularly in patients with Marfan's syndrome, a size threshold of 5 cm is maintained, because most natural history studies have demonstrated a tendency for TAAs secondary to dissection to rupture at smaller sizes.

CLINICAL PRESENTATION, ASSOCIATED DISEASES, AND DIAGNOSIS

Although presentation in totally asymptomatic fashion is common, as is detection of a TAA during radiographic investigations carried out for other causes, symptoms referable to the TAA are often seen. In addition to sudden development of severe pain that may be associated with aneurysm expansion, rupture, or acute dissection, large TAA may produce symptoms of back, epigastric, or flank pain presumably related to local compressive phenomena.

The usual dismissal of such complaints if they are chronic is inappropriate in patients with TAAs. Frequently reported symptoms include back pain localized to the left lower hemithorax or typical mid-back and epigastric pain if the aneurysm is largest in the region of the aortic hiatus. When the aneurysm erodes into the thoracolumbar spine or chest wall, complaints of chest and back pain can be prominent and may be present for even weeks or months. In severe cases, such complaints are often related to a chronic state of contained aneurysm rupture (Fig. 92–2).

Depending on the topography of the aneurysm, other symptoms may be referable to a variety of compression or erosion phenomena. Possible but uncommon symptomatic manifestations of TAAs include (1) new onset of hoarseness related to left recurrent laryngeal nerve palsy; (2) compression or erosion of the tracheobronchial tree or pulmonary parenchyma producing cough, hemoptysis, or dyspnea; and (3) dysphasia lusoria.[27] As with AAAs, distal embolization of atheromatous debris can be observed but has constituted a rare indication for operation in our experience.

Perhaps related to reluctance to recommend operation in asymptomatic patients because of the threat of surgical morbidity, up to 40% of patients with TAAs eventually have symptoms.[13, 122] This explains the higher incidence of patients treated for ruptured TAA when compared with AAA operations. Our results are consistent with those available from a review of the literature indicating that about 25% of patients with TAAs will be treated in urgent or emergent circumstances, with approximately half of these treated for frank rupture.[3, 13, 31, 104, 122]

Associated vascular diseases and co-morbid conditions are commonplace in patients presenting for treatment of TAA. Synchronous aneurysms typically involving the ascending aorta or arch have been observed in some 10% of patients at the time of treatment of TAA. A familial aneurysm history was noted in 7.5% of our patients. Earlier operation for aortic aneurysmal disease is seen in one third of patients. As noted previously, the most common of these is a previous infrarenal aneurysm repair.

Coselli and colleagues[29] detailed their experience in 123 patients undergoing TAA resection after a prior infrarenal AAA repair. These patients were likely to present with symptoms at a mean interval of 8.2 ± 5.4 years after the initial AAA repair. Although many of these represent de novo development of a second aneurysm, an initial repair of only the infrarenal aorta in a patient with more diffuse aneurysmal disease creates the necessity for a second, more definitive procedure. The presence of a previous infrarenal or more proximal thoracic aortic graft does not unduly complicate the subsequent TAA repair. Coselli and coworkers[32] in another study have indicated that operation after a prior aortic graft produces results similar to those seen with de novo TAA resection, although a prior proximal graft appears to increase the risk of spinal cord ischemia.

Because most patients seen for consideration of TAA resection are those with degenerative aneurysm, demographic and clinical features typical of a patient population with diffuse atherosclerosis are the rule. Patients treated for degenerative aneurysms average 70 years of age and usually have a history of hypertension. Cigarette smoking and significant COPD are frequently encountered. Pulmonary function studies have been routinely performed prior to operation, and 25% of patients will have significant COPD, as manifested by an FEV_1 of less than 50% predicted. Cerebrovascular disease, prior stroke, and symptomatic manifestations of lower extremity arterial occlusive disease occur in 15% of patients. Associated visceral and renovascular occlusive disease occurs to some degree in 30% of patients. Such lesions, of course, have direct implications for the technical conduct of the operation and the incidence and significance of chronic renal insufficiency.

Coselli and colleagues[31] reported the incidence and implications of associated visceral and renal artery occlusive disease in more than 1000 TAA operations. Some degree of mesenteric or renovascular occlusive disease occurred in 30% of patients. These patients were more likely to be older and to have some degree of compromised renal function. Their overall incidence of complications after operation, in particular renal failure, was significantly increased

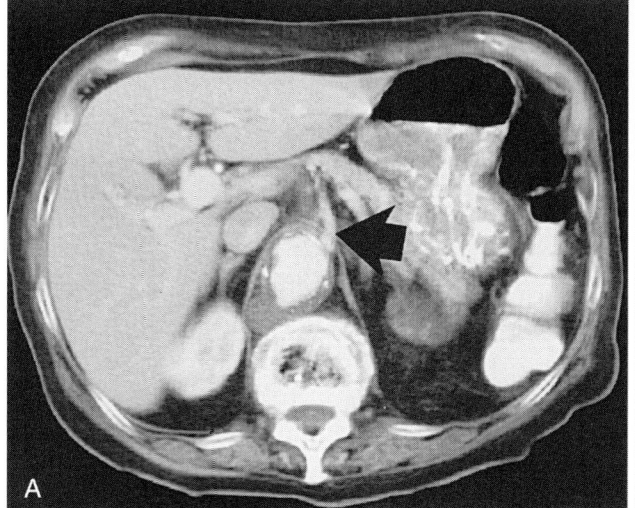
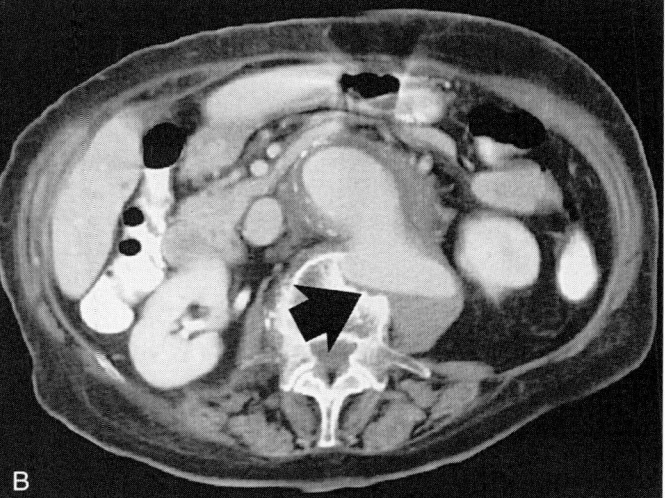

FIGURE 92–2. Type III thoracoabdominal aortic aneurysm associated with months of severe back pain. The aneurysm (A) is of modest size at the level of the celiac axis (arrow) but produced dramatic vertebral body erosion (B, arrow) in the juxtarenal aorta associated with chronic contained rupture.

when compared with patients without visceral artery occlusive disease.

In our experience, 15% of patients will have significant renal insufficiency, as manifested by a preoperative serum creatinine of at least 1.8 mg/dl.[13] The coexistence of renovascular disease and some degree of renal insufficiency is both commonplace in patients with TAAs and has important implications for accurate assessment of perioperative risk and long-term preservation of renal function. With the exception of type I TAAs, which frequently terminate just proximal to the renal artery level, types II, III, and IV TAAs imply aneurysmal degeneration of the entire visceral aortic segment. Such aneurysmal involvement of this region of the aorta is frequently accompanied by occlusive lesions of the mesenteric or renal arteries or total ostial occlusion of one or more of these vessels. Accordingly, some patients with renal insufficiency will have the potential for retrieval or salvage of renal function with renal artery reconstruction during TAA repair.

We believe that extreme levels of preoperative azotemia (serum creatinine > 2.5 cm/dl) constitute a relative contraindication to elective operation unless preoperative studies indicate some potential for salvage or retrieval of renal function with renal artery reconstruction. In many series, the presence of an abnormal preoperative serum creatinine level is at least a univariate correlate of perioperative mortality.[3, 13, 33, 64, 111, 122] Accordingly, assessment of renal function and associated renovascular disease becomes an important component of preoperative patient evaluation and surgical decision making.

An accurate assessment of associated co-morbid conditions is mandatory to guide appropriate decision making with respect to recommending operation. We believe that all patients should undergo dipyridamole thallium scanning or the equivalent thereof to evaluate perioperative myocardial ischemic potential. In patients with a history or symptoms suggestive of heart failure, left ventricular function should be assessed. Although patients with significant impairments of pulmonary reserve can usually be detected on a historical basis alone, we routinely obtain preoperative pulmonary function studies. Advanced age is an important component only because it is accompanied by overall fragility and impaired functional status. We routinely hospitalize patients for at least 12 hours prior to surgery for intravenous fluid hydration, intravenous dopamine infusions if any degree of renal insufficiency is present, and a mechanical and antibiotic bowel preparation. The latter is based on evidence indicating that bacterial translocation during the course of supraceliac clamping may contribute to disorders of blood coagulation during the operation.[20]

DIAGNOSIS

Accurate and complete radiographic evaluation is essential for precise operative planning. Based on a review of preoperative studies, there should be no equivocation in the surgeon's mind as to the proximal and distal extent of aortic resection. In contemporary practice, a dynamic, fine-cut, contrast-enhanced computed tomography (CT) scan with or without helical reconstruction provides the surgeon with the following:

1. The location for proximal aortic cross-clamping and anastomosis.
2. A qualitative assessment of the aorta in the region of the proximal cross-clamp.
3. The assessment of at least patency if not orificial stenosis of the visceral vessels.
4. The topography of the renal artery origins in relation to aneurysm contour, in addition to kidney size and adequacy of perfusion.
5. The distal extent of the resection, including major aneurysmal disease of the iliac vessels.

Traditionally, complete contrast arteriography was also used to evaluate patients treated in elective settings, and this remains helpful for evaluation of the aortic arch (in types I and II aneurysm) and for the assessment of intercostal and visceral and renal artery patency. Surgeons who utilize retrograde transfemoral aortic perfusion are well served with a pelvic arteriogram to exclude significant iliac occlusive disease. All iodinated contrast diagnostic studies, whether CT scans or catheter arteriography, are performed well in advance of actual surgery. Irrespective of the patient's baseline level of renal function, interruption of renal blood flow, which is an obligatory component of operation, should be avoided within days of intravenous contrast administration. In type I and II TAAs, a CT scan without helical reconstruction may be inadequate for the delineation of distal arch anatomy.

The aortic arch and the adequacy of a proximal aneurysm neck in the distal portion of the transverse arch or the proximal descending thoracic aorta can be more thoroughly evaluated with either angiography or magnetic resonance imaging (MRI) scan (Fig. 92–3). In addition, our own experience with magnetic resonance angiography (MRA) for evaluation of renal and visceral artery stenosis has been favorable, such that it can be readily substituted for contrast arteriography with respect to evaluation of the visceral vessels.[99] We prefer to avoid contrast studies in patients with any degree of renal insufficiency and to avoid intravascular catheter manipulation in patients with excessive atherosclerotic debris in the visceral aortic segment. In such patients, an adequate preoperative evaluation can be obtained with a combination of a non-contrast CT scan and an MRI or MRA.

Because the surgeon has the ability to directly interrogate the origins of the visceral and renal vessels during the conduct of operation, preoperative arteriography for the evaluation of visceral and renovascular disease is not absolutely necessary. In our practice, contrast arteriography is most useful in providing some assessment of the number and locations of patent intercostal arteries. Whereas decisions about intercostal vessels are ultimately made intraoperatively, knowledge of multiple patent intercostal arteries in the critical aortic segment (T9 to L1) can prepare the surgeon for the potential reconstruction of these vessels. Although we prefer to use preoperative contrast arteriography selectively, the presence of chronic dissection and the complexities thereof mandate complete arteriography in these patients.

As in contemporary practice with respect to acute presentations of patients with abdominal aneurysms, the CT scan is the initial diagnostic test of choice in patients

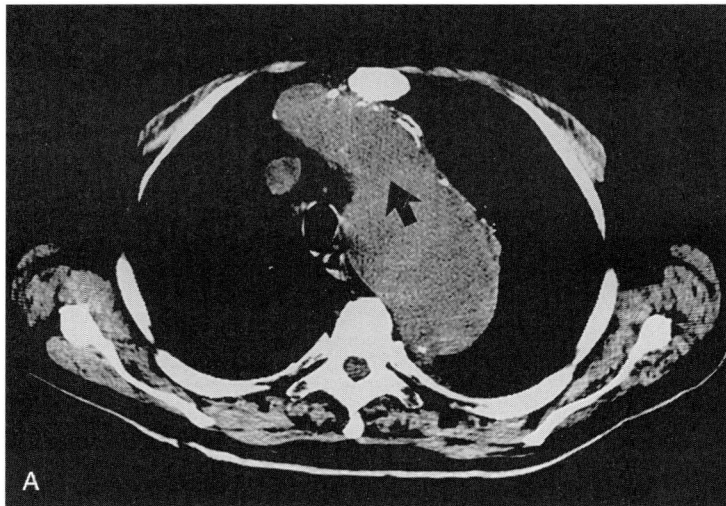

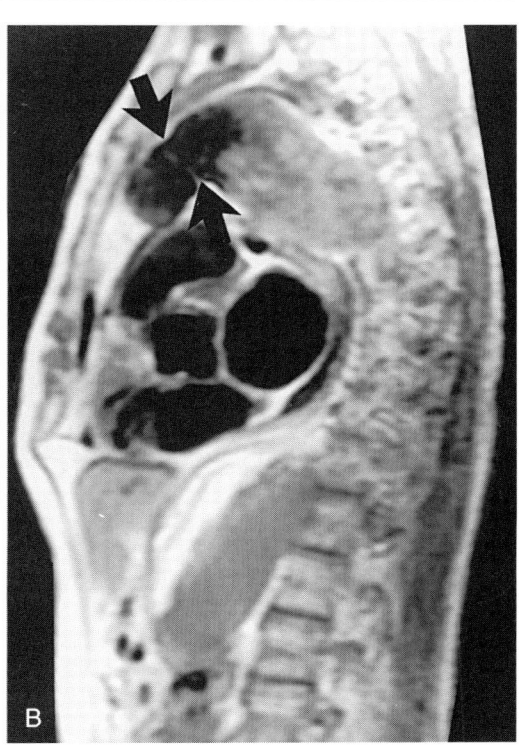

FIGURE 92–3. Determination of aortic arch anatomy in a patient with a type II aneurysm and renal insufficiency, which made contrast arteriography undesirable. *A*, The CT scan suggests that an ectatic aortic arch may be contiguous *(arrow)* with the aneurysmal proximal descending thoracic aorta. *B*, Coronal section of the MRI scan demonstrates adequate aneurysm "neck" *(arrows)* in the region of the aortic isthmus.

presenting with acute pain or whenever the possibility of TAA rupture is entertained. If rupture is documented, no further studies are indicated and prompt operation is carried out. If rupture is not found, contrast administration is carried out to more completely delineate the pathology and evaluate the possibility of other acute presentations, such as acute dissection, dissecting intramural hematoma, and penetrating aortic ulcer.

PRINCIPLES OF TREATMENT

Graft replacement by a direct surgical approach is the only effective treatment for TAAs. Endovascular graft placement, which has been applied to lesions isolated to the descending thoracic aorta,[43] is not applicable to TAAs because of the inability to reconstruct intercostal or visceral vessels with this technique. Nonoperative therapy may be selected initially in very elderly patients, those with modest-sized aneurysms (see previously), and those in whom associated co-morbid conditions make the short-term risk of surgery prohibitive or limit the life expectancy to a degree that surgical treatment is not rational. Patients selected for nonoperative therapy should be treated aggressively with beta-blockade, hypertension control, and cessation of cigarette smoking.[59] Our experience is that most patients with aneurysms 6 cm in diameter or larger are fit to undergo operation after cardiopulmonary profiling and a current assessment of renal function.

There is a consensus that the inclusion technique described by Crawford and associates is the preferred operative technique for repair of TAAs (Fig. 92–4). This method was the principal component of a general approach to the operative management of TAAs advocated by Crawford, which also included an emphasis on operative expediency and simplicity, without the use of external shunts or by-passes,[38] minimal cross-clamp times, minimal dissection on the anterior aspect of the aorta, and avoidance of systemic anticoagulation because of its potential contribution to intraoperative bleeding complications.

We have continued to apply these general principles of operation with certain modifications. In contemporary practice, several schemes of operative management are utilized (Fig. 92–5; see Fig. 92–4). The two general approaches involve a "clamp and sew" technique, often supplemented by adjuncts to minimize the principal complications, versus the use of distal aortic perfusion usually combined with a sequential clamping technique. The rationale for distal aortic perfusion is the reduction of ischemic times to the intercostal, visceral, and renal vessels because these vascular beds are perfused during creation of the proximal anastomosis. For this reason, distal perfusion has been favored for repair of isolated thoracic aneurysms.[130]

Distal aortic perfusion can be provided in either passive fashion with an indwelling Gott shunt wherein inflow is taken from the proximal aorta, the left subclavian artery, or the left ventricular apex, and distal perfusion provided either to the aorta below the aneurysm or via a retrograde transfemoral approach.[49] There are sufficient technical and anatomic complications associated with providing inflow for the Gott shunt, however, that some surgeons have adopted the use of an initial right axillary to femoral bypass graft to provide passive distal aortic perfusion.[25] However, partial left heart bypass techniques have been sufficiently refined that most authors who report distal aortic perfusion use active distal perfusion with atrial-femoral bypass utilizing the Bio-Medicus pump. This centripetal, motorized

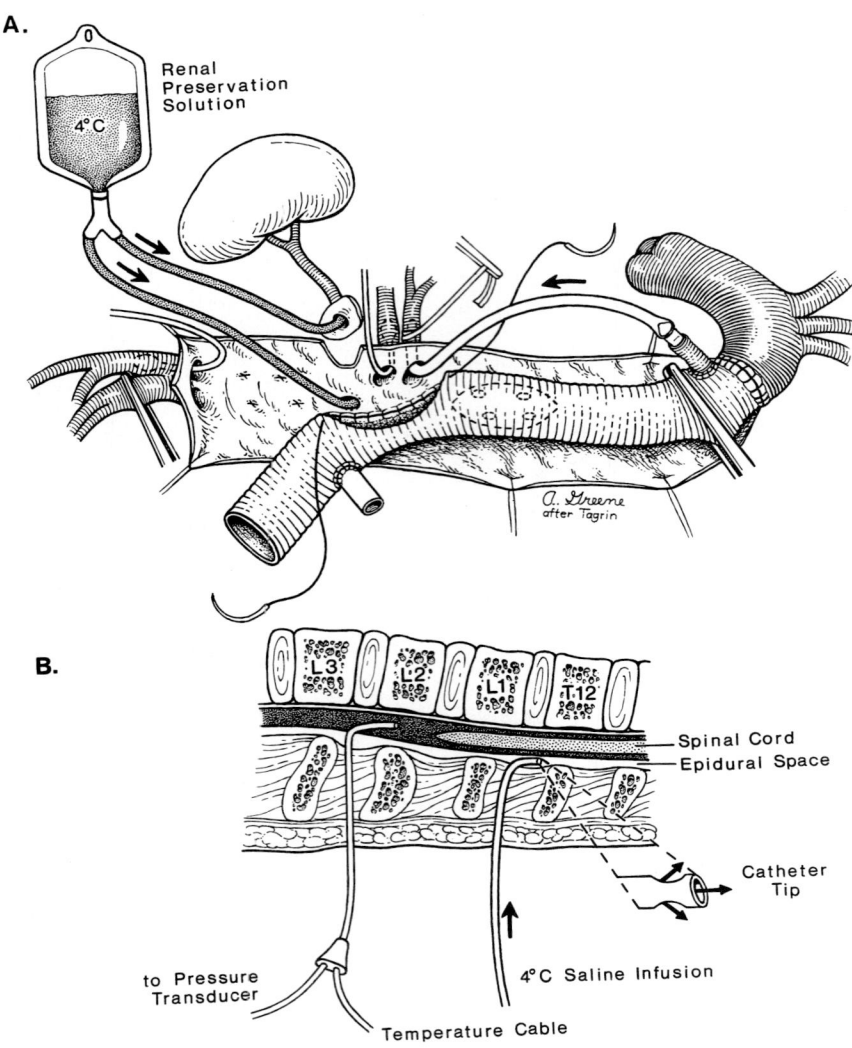

A.

Renal Preservation Solution

4°C

a. Greene
after Tagrin

B.

L3 L2 L1 T-12

Spinal Cord
Epidural Space

Catheter Tip

to Pressure Transducer

Temperature Cable

4°C Saline Infusion

FIGURE 92–4. Operative approach for repair of type II thoracoabdominal aortic aneurysm with a clamp and sew technique supplemental with regional hypothermic adjuncts for renal and spinal cord protection.[13] *A,* The entire aneurysm sac is continuously exposed after proximal cross-clamp application. After completion of the proximal anastomosis, pulsatile arterial perfusion is established into the mesenteric circulation via in-line mesenteric shunting into either the celiac axis (as depicted) or the superior mesenteric artery. Thereafter, critical intercostal vessels are reconstructed (*dotted line*), and a single inclusion button anastomosis for reconstruction of celiac, superior mesenteric, and right renal arteries is possible in most cases. The left renal artery is reconstructed with a side-arm graft. *B,* Regional spinal cord hypothermic protection is achieved via epidural cooling. A 4°C epidural saline infusion is begun in anticipation of cross-clamping. Cerebrospinal fluid temperature and pressure are monitored simultaneously with a separate intrathecal catheter. See text for details.

pump is elegant in its simplicity and, when used with heparinized impregnated tubing, can be placed without the need for systemic heparin.[26] Most surgeons, however, prefer at least low-dose heparin if atrial-femoral bypass is utilized. Partial left heart bypass using a femoral vein to femoral artery technique becomes more complicated because of the necessity to add an in-line oxygenator. Our principal criticism of the atrial-femoral bypass technique with sequential clamping is that it only saves the cross-clamp time required to complete the proximal aortic anastomosis, which in our experience, has been a minimum of the overall clamp time.

After the proximal aortic anastomosis, reconstruction of critical intercostal vessels and the visceral aortic segment must then proceed with distal perfusion during this stage of the operation, providing only retrograde pelvic perfusion and, at least in theory, some additional spinal cord circulation via the lateral sacral branches of the hypogastric vessels. This objection can be overcome by the use of a variety of "octopus" visceral perfusion catheter arrangements (see Fig. 92–5). The drawback is that multiple catheters in the surgical field interfere with surgical exposure. The pressure-flow relationships of multiple small catheters may be diffi-

cult to overcome. At least one study demonstrated a paradoxical detrimental effect of renal function using multiple selective visceral perfusion catheters.[106]

Whereas some have been aggressive about the application of distal perfusion methods for all TAAs,[105, 112] others advocate this use only in the more extensive type I and type II aneurysms, and still others utilize atrial-femoral bypass and distal aortic perfusion selectively in accordance with individual patient anatomy.[28, 30] Our current posture is in agreement with the highly selective use of atrial-femoral bypass. Because its principal advantage is during the performance of the proximal aortic reconstruction, we utilize this method only in circumstances in which the proximal reconstruction is likely to be complex, in particular in patients with chronic aortic dissection. Comparable results have been achieved in contemporary practice using both clamp and sew and distal perfusion techniques.[3, 12, 28, 88, 112] In addition, atrial-femoral bypass provides easily adjustable mechanical unloading of the left ventricle, which may be desirable in patients with antecedent aortic valvular dysfunction or significant degrees of left ventricular dysfunction.

Our general approach to the technical conduct of opera-

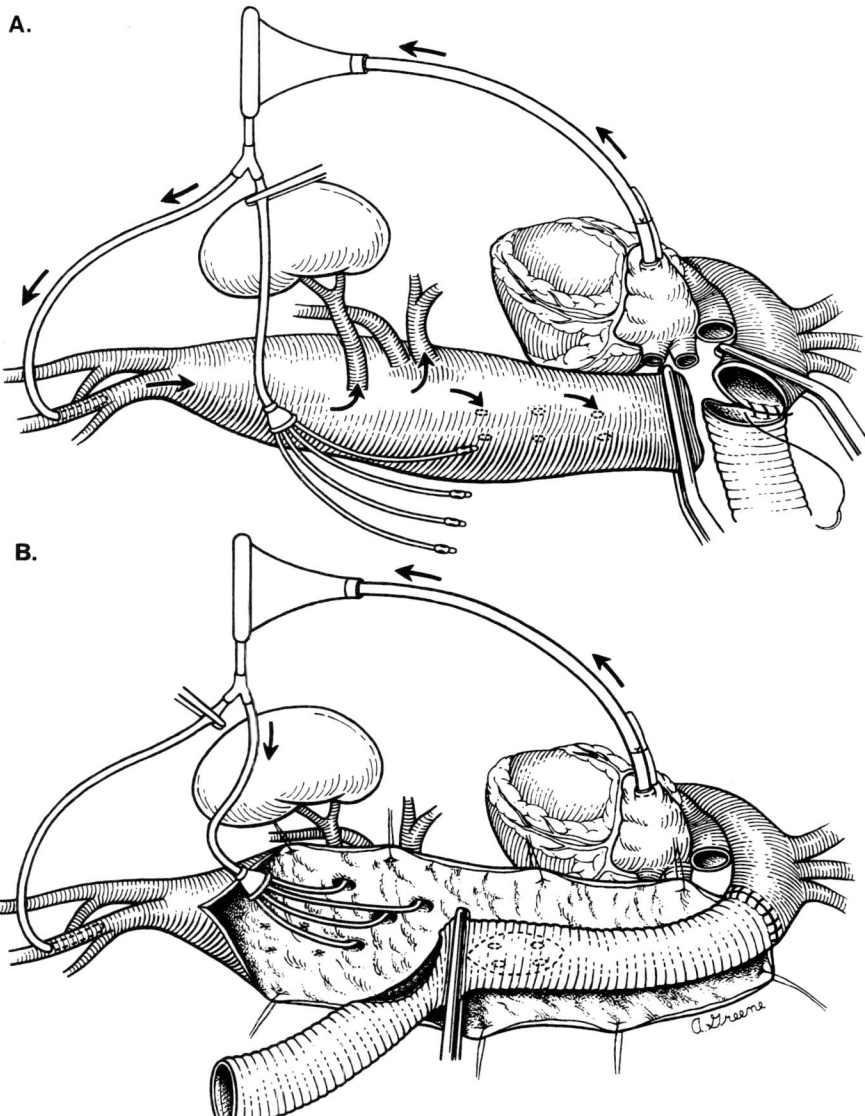

FIGURE 92–5. Repair of type II thoracoabdominal aortic aneurysm with distal aortic perfusion via atriofemoral bypass and sequential clamping technique. *A,* Two clamps are applied proximally, and distal, retrograde, transfemoral perfusion is provided to visceral, renal, and intercostal arteries during construction of the proximal aortic anastomosis. *B,* Thereafter, the aneurysm sac is opened and visceral-renal perfusion can be provided with multiple catheter "octopus" arrangement while intercostal (*dotted line*) and visceral-renal artery reconstruction proceeds.

tion for TAA emphasizes the principles of operative expediency and simplicity without the use of external bypasses and avoiding systemic hypothermia and heparin. As shown in Figure 92–4, we use a clamp and sew technique with specific regional hypothermic adjuncts for spinal cord and renal protection. We have developed and applied a technique for the provision of regional hypothermic protection to that segment of the spinal cord typically at risk for ischemic injury during TAA repair.[17, 45] The system uses an iced saline epidural infusion that provides for moderate (25 to 27°C) hypothermia to the spinal cord during the critical period when the aorta is cross-clamped. Direct instillation of renal preservation fluid (4°C lactated Ringer's solution with 25 gm/L of mannitol and 1 gm/L methylprednisolone) into the renal artery ostia is performed after the aorta is opened. Initially, 250 ml of this solution is instilled into each renal artery ostium, followed by a continuous drip of the same solution begun through 6 French (Fr.) perfusion balloon-tipped catheters. Experience has shown that such

an infusion results in a rapid decline of renal parenchymal temperature to 15°C after the bolus infusion. During the continuous infusion, renal core temperatures remain in the 25°C level as monitored by direct temperature probes in the renal cortex.

The final adjunct in our overall approach involves in-line mesenteric shunting. A 10-mm Dacron side-arm graft is sewn to the main aortic graft so as to be located just beyond the region of the proximal anastomosis (see Fig. 92–4). A 20 to 24 Fr. arterial perfusion cannula is attached to the side-arm graft, and immediately after performance of the proximal anastomosis, prograde pulsatile perfusion can be established into either the celiac axis or superior mesenteric artery to minimize visceral ischemic time and its potential contribution to coagulopathic bleeding. In our experience, pulsatile arterial perfusion can thus be reestablished to the mesenteric circulation within 25 minutes of initial aortic cross-clamp placement.[18] This system can be modified by using a bifurcation graft and placing a separate cannula into the left renal artery origin in patients at particular risk for perioperative renal failure.

Finally, the concept of hypothermic protection for spinal cord and visceral organs can be extended to the extreme by the use of a complete cardiopulmonary bypass technique, profound hypothermia, and circulatory arrest. Although this method has been utilized as a routine operative approach for patients with extensive TAA in at least one center,[79] Most surgeons specifically avoid this technique because of the potential for bleeding and pulmonary complications. Whereas this technique is essential for the repair of complex lesions of the ascending aorta or aortic arch, its use is only recommended for TAA repair in those circumstances in which proximal control and clamping of the aorta is either hazardous or not technically possible.[103]

ANESTHETIC MANAGEMENT

Successful conduct of a TAA operation requires close coordination between the surgeon and anesthesiologist. An 8 Fr. introducer is placed in an upper extremity or neck vein for volume replacement in conjunction with a high-flow fluid warming device. An arterial catheter is placed in an upper extremity after confirming equal blood pressures. If aortic clamping is to be proximal to the left subclavian artery then the right radial artery is used. A thoracic epidural catheter is placed at the T10 level, and a cerebrospinal fluid (CSF) drainage catheter is placed in the lower lumbar area and connected to a pressure transducer. A multilumen thermistor pulmonary artery catheter is placed via the internal jugular vein to monitor cardiac function. The additional lumina of the catheter are used for administering vasoactive drugs. Electrocardiogram (ECG) monitoring includes a precordial V_5 lead.

Prior to the induction of anesthesia, 2% lidocaine with epinephrine is injected into the epidural catheter to ensure its function. Anesthesia is induced with increments of barbiturates, narcotics, and a muscle relaxant and is maintained with nitrous oxide, an inhalation agent, and further narcotics. The epidural is supplemented with lidocaine as indicated by the need for more anesthesia. Muscle relaxation is provided with cisatracurium so that reversal can easily be achieved at the end of the procedure. An upper body warming blanket is used to maintain core temperature as we specifically avoid systemic hypothermia.

A double-lumen endotracheal tube is placed to provide lung isolation in types I, II, and III TAA. A right-sided tube is used with type I and II TAA operations when surgical dissection may impinge on the mediastinum around the carina. Evidence of hypoxemia during one-lung anesthesia may require increasing FiO_2, the addition of positive end-expiratory pressure (PEEP) to the dependent lung, and inflation of oxygen into the collapsed lung. Systemic heparin is rarely used. Packed red blood cells and fresh frozen plasma are started early as the primary fluid replacement; platelets are administered when the visceral or distal aortic anastomoses are completed. Autotransfusion is used to retrieve shed blood and generally accounts for half the red blood cell volume returned to the patient.

In preparation for aortic cross-clamping, mannitol (25 gm) or furosemide is administered to promote diuresis. Patients with renal insufficiency are maintained on dopamine infusions. Before clamping, 20 ml of CSF is removed. The epidural anesthetic agent is often reinforced to aid in lowering the blood pressure prior to aortic clamping. Operative cases involving a very difficult proximal aortic reconstruction or significant renal dysfunction preoperatively may benefit from partial left heart bypass and distal aortic perfusion. Aortic cross-clamping proceeds slowly. Sequential clamping of the left iliac and visceral vessels prior to proximal aortic clamping facilitates blood pressure manipulation with vasodilator agents. The more proximal the TAA, the lower the blood pressure is maintained during the cross-clamp time.

Controversy exists about the use of vasodilators, particularly sodium nitroprusside, as part of the management of proximal hypertension associated with aortic cross-clamping. Nitroprusside has been shown, in animal models, to reduce distal aortic perfusion pressure to the spinal cord. If the spinal cord is relying on distal perfusion during cross-clamping, then reducing this pressure could increase the risk of ischemia to the cord.[19, 115, 117] These data, like those related to CSF drainage to improve distal cord perfusion, are of uncertain importance in patients.[77] Because it provides rapid and easily reversible manipulation of arterial pressure, we continue to use sodium nitroprusside as the principal afterload-reducing agent. CSF is removed to maintain preclamp baseline CSF pressures. An infusion of sodium bicarbonate is given prior to visceral vessel unclamping unless an in-line mesenteric shunt has been used (see Fig. 92–4). Further administration of lidocaine through the epidural catheter is not employed so that a neurologic examination of the lower extremities can be done at the end of the procedure.

Aortic declamping is associated with significant hemodynamic alterations during two stages—visceral reperfusion and distal aortic reperfusion. Temporary use of vasopressors may be required during this time. Emergence from anesthesia usually requires therapy for hypertension. All patients are evaluated for lower extremity neurologic function on the operating table, and the double-lumen endotracheal tube is changed to a single-lumen tube. In the intensive care unit (ICU), the blood pressure is usually maintained in the upper levels of normal and hypotension is aggressively treated. The CSF catheter is transduced and maintained at pressures below 10 mmHg for 24 to 28 hours after the operation. The epidural catheter is used to provide analgesia with a narcotic infusion initially. After 24 hours, dilute bupivacaine (Marcaine) is added to the epidural mix and this infusion continues for several days after the patient leaves the ICU.

OPERATIVE TECHNIQUE

Irrespective of individual preferences about various technical components of the operation, an essential requirement for a successful technical operation is the provision of broad continuous exposure of the entire left posterolateral aspect of the aorta. Particularly in extensive type II aneurysms, maneuvers that tend to improve proximal exposure can compromise distal exposure and vice versa. The patient is positioned on the operating table in the right lateral decubitus position. The location and extent of the thoracic portion of the incision are dictated by the proximal extent of the aneurysm. The posterior portion of a standard posterolateral thoracotomy is only necessary for type I and II aneurysms.

We keep the thoracic portion of the incision low and have found that a fifth or sixth interspace incision with posterior division of the sixth and seventh ribs provides adequate exposure for the majority of even the more proximal aneurysms. The costal margin is divided at the level of the sixth interspace, and a self-retaining retractor system is essential to have continuous exposure of the entire operative field. An eighth interspace thoracoabdominal incision usually suffices for type IV aneurysms, and a double-lumen tube for deflation of the left lung is generally not necessary in these cases. The abdominal portion of the incision is transperitoneal as this allows for direct inspection and assessment of the visceral circulation at the conclusion of the operation.

The surgeon gains exposure of the left posterolateral aspect of the abdominal aorta by entering the plane posterior to the spleen, left kidney, and left colon with the electrocautery. All intra-abdominal contents are reflected to the patient's right side, and the left ureter is identified and protected under laparotomy pads. In addition to the retroperitoneal fatty and lymphatic tissues overlying the aorta, a large posterior branch of the left renal vein typically courses across the aorta and requires division. Located topographically close to this structure is the left renal artery, and a key point in the dissection is identifying the renal artery and dissecting it back to its aortic origin. This is a convenient starting point for division of the retroperitoneal tissues cephalad and caudad over the aorta inferiorly and division of the median arcuate ligament and diaphragmatic crura superiorly.

The incision in the diaphragm can be managed by one of several methods. There is little question that direct radial division of the diaphragm from underneath the costal margin to the aortic hiatus is the quickest and simplest and affords excellent exposure. However, such radial division of the diaphragm irrevocably paralyzes the left hemidiaphragm and contributes to postoperative respiratory compromise. Some surgeons prefer a circumferential division of the diaphragm through its muscular portion, leaving a few centimeters attached laterally to the chest wall.

Engle and colleagues[50] have emphasized the benefit of preservation of the phrenic innervation of the left hemidiaphragm by dividing only a portion of the diaphragm lateral to the phrenic nerve insertion, taking down the muscular fibers at aortic hiatus, but leaving the central portion intact. A large Penrose drain can thus be passed around the remaining diaphragm pedicle for retracting superiorly and inferiorly during different stages of the subsequent reconstruction. We apply this method of diaphragm preservation liberally, particularly in patients with evidence of preoperative pulmonary compromise.

After the left lung is deflated, the thoracic component of the dissection is usually straightforward. The mediastinal pleura over the aneurysm and proximal aorta are divided with electrocautery. For type I and II aneurysms, proximal

control of the aorta in the region of the left subclavian artery origin is necessary. Additional mobility of the vagus nerve can be obtained by dividing it distal to the origin of the left recurrent nerve, which is identified and preserved. If more proximal control is necessary, the ligamentum arteriosum is divided on the aorta. In this region, care is taken to keep dissection directly on the underside of the aortic arch to avoid injury to the left main pulmonary artery. In patients with degenerative aneurysm, dissection in this area is generally straightforward.

When chronic dissection is the pathologic feature, the prior inflammation from the dissecting process makes dissection more difficult. The aorta is surrounded with a vessel tape on either side of the left subclavian artery, depending on the proximal extent of the aneurysm. Sufficient normal aorta should be cleared with blunt dissection on the posterior aspect of the aorta to allow room for clamp placement and an accurate proximal aortic anastomosis. External control of the left subclavian artery is not necessary because intraluminal balloon control can be obtained if the cross-clamp needs to be placed proximal to the left subclavian artery.

The aortic prosthesis is next prepared by attaching a side-arm graft of 6 mm polytetrafluoroethylene (PTFE), which is our preferred technique for reconstruction of the left renal artery. As noted previously, a more proximal 10 mm side-arm graft is used as inflow for the in-line mesenteric shunt (see Fig. 92–4). For the aortic graft, we prefer a Dacron prosthesis, although in the circumstance of mycotic aneurysm, a PTFE aortic graft is used because of its decreased susceptibility to infection. At this point, the clamping sequence is begun in close cooperation with the anesthesiologist. The intent is to avoid abrupt, severe increases in afterload coincident with proximal thoracic aortic cross-clamping by the judicious use of pharmacologic afterload reduction in anticipation of cross-clamp placement. If atrial-femoral bypass is utilized, flow can gradually be increased in the pump circuit at this point to produce the desired afterload reduction, with the goal of keeping pressures equalized proximal to the aortic cross-clamp and equally in the distal aortic perfusion circuit, as monitored by a femoral arterial line. Abrupt and severe increases in afterload coincident with proximal aortic cross-clamping can cause undue left ventricular strain, myocardial ischemia, and abrupt increases in CSF pressure.

The aneurysm is opened initially in the abdomen, atherothrombotic debris is evacuated, and back-bleeding from the right iliac or distal aorta is controlled with a balloon catheter. When the entire descending thoracic aorta is resected, proximal intercostal vessel orifices between T4 and T8 are typically vigorously back-bleeding and these are rapidly oversewn. Intercostal vessels in the critical T9 to L1 aortic segment are evaluated for potential reimplantation into the main body of the graft. These vessels are balloon occluded to prevent both back-bleeding and the negative "sump" effect on net spinal cord perfusion that can result from these vessel orifices being exposed only to atmospheric pressure.[131]

For the proximal aortic anastomosis, we leave the posterior wall intact unless chronic dissection is present in the aortic wall. Some surgeons advocate routine complete transection of the aorta in proximal aneurysms to avoid the late complication of anastomotic esophageal erosion, but blunt finger dissection posteriorly on the aorta generally suffices to adequately separate the esophagus from the aortic suture line. Using the Creech technique with an intact posterior wall of the aorta is more expeditious and facilitates a secure proximal aortic anastomosis, which is then verified for hemostasis. A clamp is placed on the main aortic graft distal to the mesenteric shunt side-arm, flow is established in the shunt, and good perfusion to the mesentery is verified by checking for arterial back-bleeding from the other mesenteric vessel origin.

Reconstruction of intercostal vessels in the T9 to L1 segment is usually the next step in the operation. The most common technique utilized is an inclusion button anastomosis. Intercostal arteries in the region of a proximal or distal aortic anastomosis can be reconstructed by using a long beveled suture line. Alternate methods of intercostal artery reanastomosis include the attachment of other short side-arm grafts to the main aortic graft, or in certain cases in which the intercostal origins have been rotated superiorly and to the patient's left side, it may be feasible to simply anastomose Carrel's patches of aorta containing the intercostal vessels to the main aortic graft.

Depending on the topography of intercostal origins, it may be possible to defer intercostal artery reconstruction until after completion of the visceral artery anastomosis by then using partial occluding clamps on the main aortic graft. Because we have the protective effect of regional spinal cord hypothermia until all aspects of the reconstruction have been completed, there is no urgency to reestablish intercostal blood flow. The important intercostal arteries are those in the T9 to L1 segment. Therefore, it is common for the intercostal inclusion button to nearly overlap (on the opposite side of the aorta) the inclusion button for reconstruction of the visceral vessels. Because of their proximity, clamping the aortic graft distal to an intercostal inclusion button can interfere with reconstruction of the visceral vessels, obviating a sequential clamping technique.

Visceral and renal artery reconstruction is carried out next. Significant occlusive lesions of the right renal and superior mesenteric arteries should be treated with orificial endarterectomy. This method involves incising the diseased intima and media, entering the correct endarterectomy plane typically evidenced by the pink color of the inner aspect of the aortic adventitia, and completing a circumferential button around the vessel origin. Sufficient length of the superior mesenteric and celiac arteries should be dissected out to facilitate countertraction from the external side of the vessel, although this is not possible with the right renal artery. Should the calcified end of the obstructing lesion not break off easily, sharp division under direct vision is the preferred method.

The most common method of visceral-renal artery reconstruction, which has been applied in the overwhelming majority of our cases, is a single inclusion button to encompass the origins of the celiac, superior mesenteric, and right renal arteries (see Fig. 92–4). If the aneurysm is excessively large in the visceral aortic segment, wide separation of the visceral-renal ostia may necessitate multiple individual anastomoses. The aortic graft is placed under tension, and an elliptical side island is excised from the main aortic graft. Typically, this ellipse begins on the lateral aspect of

the graft and then spirals more posteriorly in the region of the right renal artery reconstruction.

By placing the graft on traction, the surgeon can usually perform the posterior aspect of this suture line using single bites of the suture passing through the aorta and the Dacron graft. Suture bites should be close to the visceral vessel origins to avoid leaving too much aneurysmal aortic wall. Since the posterior aspect of this suture line courses around the inferior border of the right renal artery, we exchange the 6 Fr. perfusion catheter for a 12 Fr. perfusion catheter to serve as a stent of sorts in the right renal artery origin. This catheter is gently agitated up and down as the suture line moves around the renal artery to ensure that the latter is not compromised by the suture bites as they pass outside of the aorta.

The topography and course of the right renal artery should be interrogated with this indwelling catheter because in circumstances where the right renal artery drapes over a large infrarenal component of the aneurysm, occlusion of the right renal artery is a definite technical complication of operation (Fig. 92–6). Just prior to completion of this suture line, back-bleeding and patency of the celiac, superior mesenteric, and right renal arteries are verified and the in-line mesenteric shunt is clamped and removed. A single flush of the proximal aortic cross-clamp is carried out to ensure that no clot or debris has collected in the graft. Reconstruction of the left renal artery is now accomplished, which we prefer to perform in nearly all cases with a separate side-arm graft of 6 mm of PTFE. This allows a direct deliberate anastomosis in end-to-end fashion as well as flexibility to deal with the spectrum of occlusive lesions and multiple renal arteries that may be encountered.

As noted in Figure 92–7, care must be taken to place this side-arm graft in an orientation where it will not kink when the left renal artery is returned to its anatomic position. Some surgeons prefer to use a single inclusion button to encompass both renal arteries along with the visceral vessels. In our experience, this includes too great an area of aneurysmal aorta unless the aneurysm is exceedingly small in the visceral aortic segment. The clamp is then moved again to a position inferior to the origin of the left renal artery graft, and the distal aortic anastomosis is carried out to complete the reconstruction. We make every effort to perform tube type reconstructions to the aortic bifurcation unless there is gross aneurysmal disease of the proximal common iliac arteries. Extending the reconstruction to separate iliac artery reconstructions or tunneling to an aortofemoral graft configuration is only performed when no other technical alternative exists.

After reestablishment of flow to the lower extremities and verification of adequate lower extremity perfusion by intraoperative pulse volume recordings. Doppler signals in the left renal, celiac, and superior mesenteric vessels are checked in addition to palpation of the superior mesenteric artery pulse in the root of the mesentery. Hemostasis is usually adequate, but infusions of platelets and fresh frozen plasma are typically increased at this point, when a final check for hemostasis is made. Careful inspection of the inferior aspect of the aneurysm sac in both the chest and abdomen is necessary to detect back-bleeding lumbar or intercostal arteries, which can be an important source of postoperative hemorrhage. The redundant aneurysm sac is

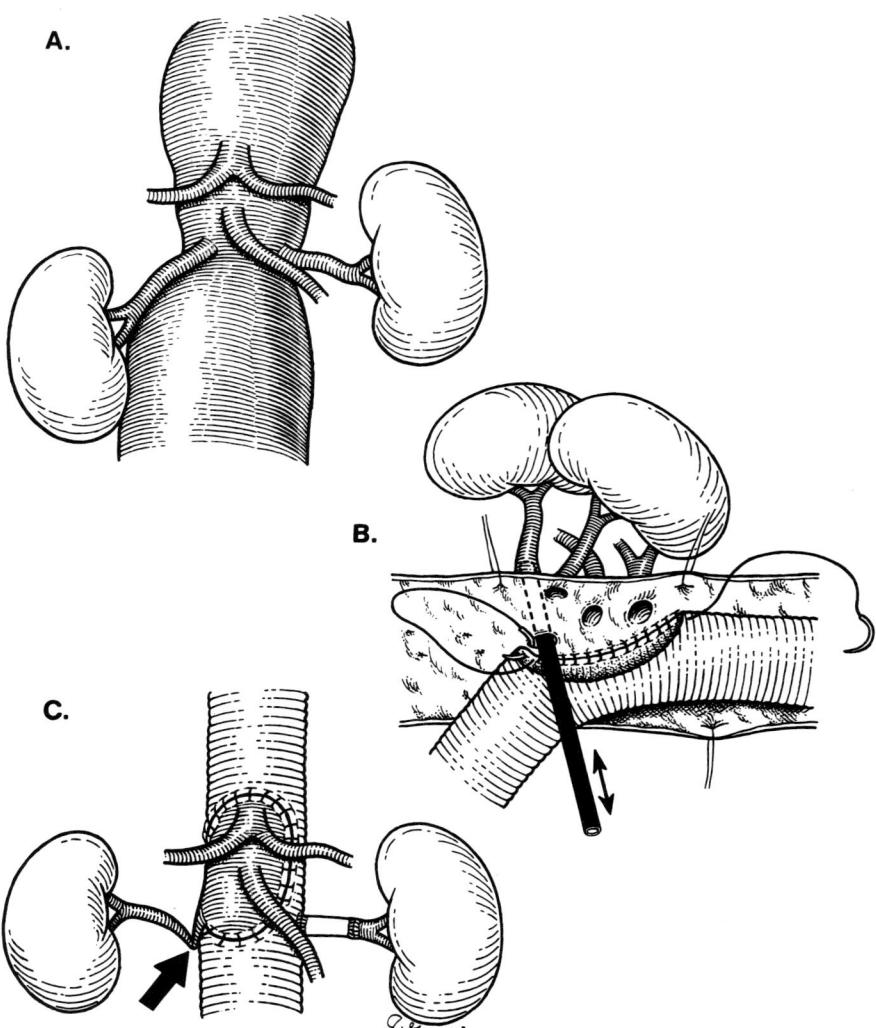

FIGURE 92–6. *A–C,* Pitfalls in renal artery reconstruction during thoracoabdominal aortic aneurysm repair. Commonly encountered anatomy with right renal artery draping over large infrarenal component of aneurysm *(A)* is depicted. During inclusion button reconstruction of visceral-renal vessel origins, a 12 French catheter is used to stent the right renal origin as the suture line courses around it. This catheter is agitated to ensure that the right renal artery origin is not compromised *(B).* As displayed in *C,* kinking and obstruction *(arrow)* of the proximal right renal artery can result from failure to appreciate the orientation of the renal artery to the inclusion button suture line.

then sutured securely over the aortic prosthesis in the abdomen and the chest. The left kidney is returned to its anatomic position to verify the orientation of the left renal artery reconstruction. Occasionally, in patients with modest-sized aneurysms, chronic dissections, or prior proximal thoracic aortic grafts, there is insufficient aneurysm wall to totally cover the proximal suture line and aortic graft.

In selected cases, we have used a PTFE patch to exclude the aortic prosthesis from the left lung. The perinephric fat as the left kidney is returned to its bed usually suffices to provide adequate coverage of the aortic graft in the region of the visceral aortic segment. Reapproximation of the diaphragmatic crura over the aortic prosthesis and the divided portion of the diaphragm is carried out with interrupted 2-0 silk sutures. A single chest tube is placed and a closed suction drain may be left in the retroperitoneum if hemostasis is not secure. Closure of extensive incisions typically takes nearly an hour, so that two teams are utilized. As displayed in Table 92–3, clamp times, blood turnover, and blood component replacement vary as a function of aneurysm extent, but overall operative time can be kept at 5 to 6 hours for most patients.

RESULTS OF SURGICAL TREATMENT

Spinal Cord Ischemic Complications

Spinal cord ischemic complications, manifest clinically as flaccid paraplegia or lesser degrees of lower extremity paraparesis, are the most feared and devastating nonfatal complication of TAA. A variety of surgical and adjunctive techniques notwithstanding, spinal cord ischemia remains an unsolved problem despite considerable improvements in the overall incidence of this complication. Efforts to minimize this complication have been the principal driving force in the application of the variety of general operative approaches discussed previously.

Svensson and associates,[122] in reviewing Crawford's experience with more than 1500 patients treated for TAA between 1960 and 1991, reported a 16% incidence of lower extremity neurologic deficits. Approximately half of these patients suffered total paraplegia without the prospect of any meaningful recovery. Patients treated for the most extensive type II TAAs sustained a 31% incidence of spinal cord ischemic complications. As indicated in Table 92–4,

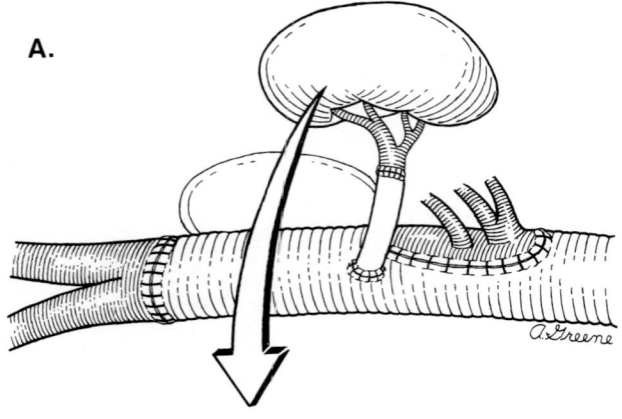

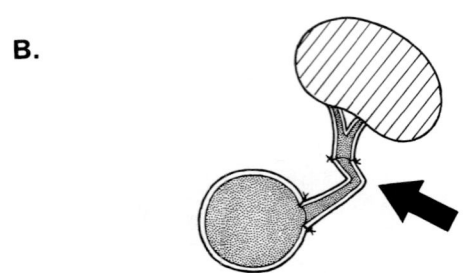

FIGURE 92–7. Side-arm graft reconstruction of left renal artery (A), is displayed. Care must be taken in the orientation of this graft because kinking and obstruction (arrow) can occur as the left kidney is returned to its bed (B), irrespective of the technique of left renal artery reconstruction.

thoracic region is provided by branches of the vertebral arteries, whereas the thoracolumbar cord is supplied by intercostal and lumbar arteries; the conus is supplied by the lateral sacral branches of the hypogastric vessels.

Two factors referable to human spinal cord circulation explain the nature of ischemic risk to the cord during TAA repair. The first factor concerns the vagaries of anatomy of the anterior spinal artery, which varies in caliber and continuity. If the anterior spinal artery were of adequate caliber and continuity in all individuals, there would be no risk of ischemic cord complications by clamping the descending thoracic aorta or sacrifice of intercostal vessels. However, angiographic studies have shown that the anterior spinal artery may be anatomically discontinuous and the typical pattern of the anterior spinal artery is that its caliber becomes extremely narrow cephalad to its anastomosis with the greater radicular artery. Svensson and coworkers[124, 126] attempted to overcome this caliber limitation of the anterior spinal artery by administering intrathecal papavarine, demonstrating benefit at least in experimental systems.

Second, the human spinal cord is irregularly supplied by radiculomedullary arteries. Although radicular arteries are contributed at each segmental level, only a few of these arteries actually go on to reach the cord components. The cervical thoracic territory is richly supplied with radiculomedullary arteries, but the middle thoracic segment has but one or two such arteries. Typically, however, the anterior spinal artery in the upper thoracic region continues to be well developed. The thoracolumbar region is at the most risk for ischemic injury, because this region is typically supplied by a single radiculomedullary artery, referred to as the artery of Adamkiewicz or the greater radicular artery. This artery enters the vertebral canal between the 9th to 12th thoracic vertebral segments in 75% to 80% of individuals, and angiographic studies have shown that one or more intercostal arteries can contribute to it.[110]

In addition to these variations in normal anatomy, patients with TAAs may have the added variable of mural thrombus, potentially obliterating many or all of the intercostal arteries. Such gradual obliteration of intercostal vessels in a chronic degenerative aneurysm serves to establish antecedent collateral circulation prior to surgical correction, and most authors agree that the risk of cord injury is considerably less when intercostal vessels in the critical T9 to L1 zone have been obliterated by mural thrombus.[104, 121, 123] Alternatively, in aneurysms in which chronic dissection is the etiologic mechanism, a typical pattern is that aneurysmal dilatation occurs in the outer wall of the false lumen,

contemporary results from centers of excellence show an approximate halving of the incidence of spinal cord ischemia detailed in Crawford's summary report.

A review of spinal cord circulation and its considerable variation is essential to understand the pathogenesis of spinal cord ischemia during TAA repair. The arterial circulation of the human spinal cord consists of its intrinsic blood supply composed of a single anterior spinal artery coursing along the central sulcus of the ventral aspect of the cord and ultimately supplying the bulk of the cord's substance via its penetrating arteries. Paired posterior spinal arteries supply the remainder of the posterior columns. This intrinsic circulation of the cord is in turn supplied by the more variable extrinsic "feeder" radiculomedullary arteries. The principal extrinsic blood supply in the cervical and upper

TABLE 92–3. INTRAOPERATIVE DATA FOR 160 THORACOABDOMINAL ANEURYSM OPERATIONS

VARIABLE (MEAN ± SD)	TYPES I AND II TAA (N = 75)	TYPES III AND IV TAA (N = 85)	p
Operative time (min)	323 ± 97	304 ± 109	.25
Visceral ischemic time* (min)	53 ± 16	41 ± 11	.001
Reperfusion of legs (min)	66 ± 24	74 ± 24	.03
Total blood transfusion† (cc)	3170 ± 1973	2496 ± 2376	.07
Fresh frozen plasma (units)	6 ± 4	4 ± 4	.01
Platelets (units)	10 ± 6	6 ± 6	.01

*Reperfusion of celiac, superior mesenteric, and right renal arteries.
†Sum of banked and autotransfused blood.
TAA = thoracoabdominal aneurysm; SD = standard deviation.

TABLE 92–4. OPERATIVE COMPLICATIONS IN MAJOR SERIES OF THORACOABDOMINAL AORTIC ANEURYSM REPAIR

REFERENCE	YEAR	STUDY INTERVAL	NO. OF PATIENTS	OPERATIVE TECHNIQUE	MORTALITY NO. (%)	PARAPLEGIA/ PARAPARESIS NO. (%)	RENAL FAILURE NO. (%)
Svensson et al[122]	1993	1960–91	1509	c/s (83%)‖	155 (10)	234 (16)	269 (18)
Coselli et al[31]	1999	1986–98	1220	c/s (72%)‖	89 (7.3)	56 (4.6)	133 (11)
Grabitz et al[66]	1996	1981–95	260	c/s	37 (14.2)	39 (15)	27 (10.4)‡
Acher et al[3]	1998	1984–96	217†	c/s	21 (9.7)	17 (7.8)	4 (3.8)‡
Safi et al[108]	1997	1991–96	343†	AFBP (67%)	43 (13)	33 (10)	99 (29)§
Hollier et al[72]	1992	1980–91	150	c/s	15 (10)	6 (4)	14 (9.3)
Cambria et al[13]*	1997	1986–97	210	c/s	17 (8)	15 (7.2)	22 (10.6)
Totals	—	—	3909	—	377 (9.8)	400 (10.8)	568 (14.7)

*Updated.
†Includes some descending thoracic aneurysm repairs (Acher[3] 19% and Safi[108] 15%).
‡Only those requiring dialysis.
§Stringent definition of "renal failure," i.e., 1 mg/dl ↑ in creatinine for 2 consecutive days.
‖Balance of procedures done with atriofemoral bypass.
AFBP = atriofemoral bypass for distal aortic perfusion; c/s = clamp and sew.

whereas a narrow compressed true lumen may give rise to multiple patent intercostal vessels (Fig. 92–8). Furthermore, obliteration of intercostal vessels in a chronic degenerative aneurysm is virtually never accompanied by spontaneous cord injury, whereas sudden obliteration of multiple intercostal vessels as might be seen in an acute aortic dissection can cause acute paraplegia. The variation in patency of intercostal arteries between degenerative and dissected aneurysms accounts for the higher risks of cord injury in patients treated with aneurysms in which dissection is the cause.

The pathogenesis of spinal cord injury after aortic replacement is likely multifactorial but ultimately results from the ischemic insult caused by temporary or permanent interruption of spinal cord blood supply. Debate continues regarding the relative importance of the initial ischemic insult versus reperfusion injury. The clinical observation of delayed deficits has led some authors to speculate that swelling in the rigid bony spinal canal, accompanied by relative increases in cerebrospinal fluid, is the pathogenesis of such delayed deficits.[107] Others have speculated that the initial ischemic insult in the operating room creates the milieu for programmed neuronal cell death as an inevitable consequence of the intraoperative ischemic insult.[101]

The author and others have noted the striking correlation between perioperative hypotension and delayed onset neurologic deficit, suggesting that the principal and collateral circulation to the cord may be in a delicate balance for some time after operation. Svensson and colleagues[121] reported that 10 of 31 neurologic deficits in a series of 98 prospectively studied patients occurred in delayed fashion and that such delayed deficits were correlated with postop-

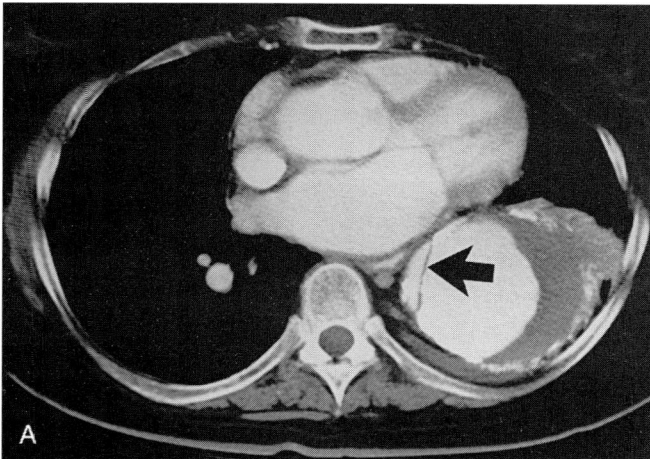
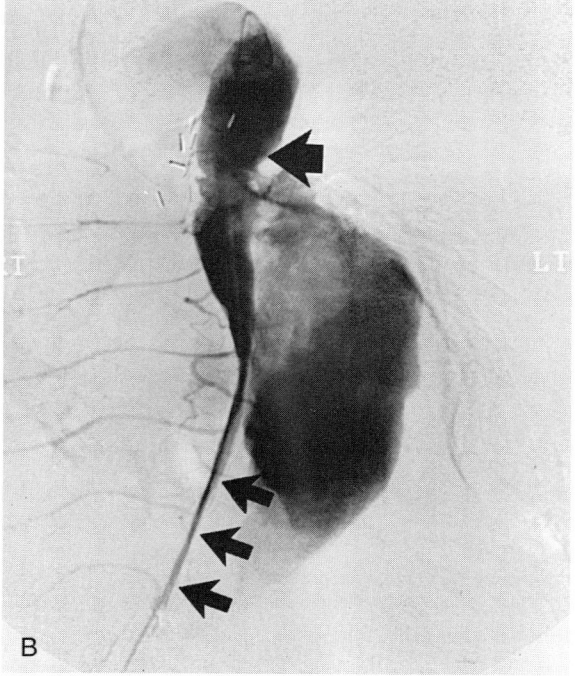

FIGURE 92–8. CT scan and arteriogram of type I thoracoabdominal aortic aneurysm of chronic dissection etiology treated 22 years after short proximal descending thoracic aortic graft performed in setting of acute distal aortic dissection. A, CT scan demonstrates "septum" (*arrow*) between the narrow compressed "true lumen" and the partly opacified aneurysmal false lumen. B, Corresponding arteriogram demonstrates region of prior distal anastomosis (*single arrow*) and multiple patent intercostal vessels arising from slit-like true lumen (*triple arrows*).

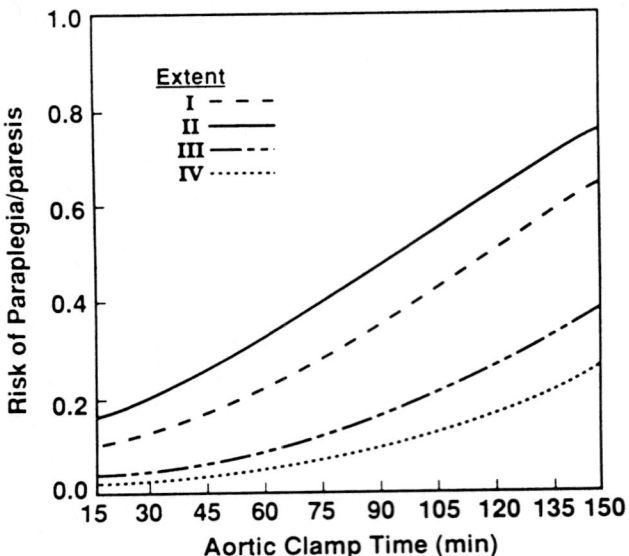

FIGURE 92–9. Risk of spinal cord ischemic complications as a function of thoracoabdominal aortic aneurysm extent and total aortic cross-clamp duration after multivariate analysis in more than 1500 patients. Risk is greatest for extent II aneurysms, but for each extent the overall risk increases substantially as clamp times exceed 45 minutes. (From Svensson LG, Crawford ES, Hess KR, et al: Experience with 1509 patients undergoing thoracoabdominal aortic operations. J Vasc Surg 17:357–370, 1993.)

erative hypotension. Careful attention to maintain adequate perfusion pressure in the days following TAA repair is important in limiting the occurrence of delayed spinal cord deficit, although other mechanisms such as thrombosis of reconstructed vessels and microembolization may contribute.

It is agreed that the clinical variables of aortic cross-clamp duration, TAA aneurysm extent, emergency operations, and operations in which dissection is the pathology increase the risks of spinal cord injury, although the latter has recently been disputed.[3, 13, 30, 105] Increasing age and diabetes have also been implicated as risk factors in development of paraplegia. Svensson and coworkers[122] demonstrated that for each extent of TAA, the risk of cord injury increased with increased duration of aortic cross-clamping (Fig. 92–9). Similarly, we reported that a visceral cross-clamp time longer than 60 minutes was significantly associated ($p = .02$) with ischemic cord injury.[17] Risk of cord injury clearly increases in treatment for the more extensive types I and II TAAs. Svensson and associates,[122] in reporting Crawford's summary experience with more than 1500 patients, noted a 24% incidence of cord injury in the treatment of types I and II TAAs as opposed to a 5.5% incidence for types III and IV TAAs. Griepp and colleagues[67] noted that cord injury increased dramatically when 10 or more pairs of intercostal arteries were sacrificed, which is when repair of the entire descending thoracic aorta was required.

The circumstances of the clinical presentation also greatly affect the risk of cord injury. In Crawford's experience, cord injury rates doubled for treatment of ruptured versus intact aneurysms.[122] In our patients, operation for acute presentation (half for frank rupture or dissection) was independently associated with postoperative lower extremity neurologic deficit (relative risk, 7.9; 95% confidence interval, 1.7

to 37.7; $p = .009$).[13] Acher and coworkers[1] incorporated these clinical variables into the formulation of a predictive model for neurologic deficit after TAA repair. These authors demonstrated excellent correlation ($r = .997$) between the predicted incidence of neurologic deficits from their model and that actually reported in 16 series published prior to 1993. Perhaps related to increased experience or the application of multiple adjuncts to prevent the complication of cord injury, contemporary series from centers of excellence typically report cord injury rates substantially less than that predicted from the Acher model (see Table 92–4).

A variety of clinical strategies and adjuncts have been applied in an effort to prevent ischemic spinal cord injury, and these have been extensively reviewed elsewhere.[16, 87] As displayed in Table 92–5, these methods can be divided into two general categories.

The first of these are surgical or adjunctive methods designed to preserve relative spinal cord perfusion pressure. Localization techniques (preoperative angiography and intraoperative evoked potential or polarographic measurements) act as guides for the surgeon to preserve or reconstruct critical intercostal arteries. Preoperative spinal arteriography can demonstrate the location and intercostal feeder vessels to the greater radicular artery in some 65% of patients with TAAs. However, except for predicting the risk of cord injury when the resection needs to encompass the critical aortic segment, the clinical benefit of preoperative spinal arteriography has been elusive.[78, 110, 132] The *hydrogen ion polarographic technique* described by Svensson and associates[125] has been elegantly documented with post-

TABLE 92–5. STRATEGIES TO PREVENT SPINAL CORD ISCHEMIA DURING THORACOABDOMINAL ANEURYSM REPAIR

Maintenance of Spinal Cord Blood Supply

Identification of critical segmental (intercostal) vessels
   Preoperative selective angiography
   Intraoperative hydrogen ion method
   Intraoperative evoked potential monitoring
Shunts and bypasses, distal aortic perfusion
   Passive internal (Gott) or external (axillofemoral) shunt
   Atriofemoral or femoral-femoral bypass (partial cardiopulmonary
    bypass)
   Complete cardiopulmonary bypass (with or without circulatory
    arrest/profound hypothermia)
Cerebrospinal fluid drainage
Intercostal or lumbar vessel reanastomosis
Intrathecal vasodilators

Neuroprotective Adjuncts

Hypothermia
   Systemic
    Passive (moderate)
    Active (moderate or profound, with cardiopulmonary bypass)
   Regional (moderate)
    Epidural or intrathecal infusion (closed or drained)
    Isolated aortic segment perfusion
Pharmacologic agents
   Neurotransmitter inhibition (naloxone)
   Nonspecific neuroprotective agents (steroids, barbiturate,
    magnesium)
   Calcium channel blockers
   Oxygen free radical scavengers
   Artificial oxygen delivery (Fluosol-DA)

operative angiographic studies and has significant research promise but has not been applied clinically in other centers.

Evoked potential monitoring evaluates the ability of the long tracks of the spinal cord to conduct an impulse during the cross-clamp period. Variations in the latency and amplitude of recorded potentials imply ischemia of the cord. The original technique used somatosensory evoked potentials, but this method has been plagued by lack of sensitivity and specificity, likely related to the fact that the peripheral nerve recording electrode is located distal to the cross-clamp.[42] Newer techniques for evoked potential monitoring, such as direct spinal cord stimulation with epidural electrodes and measurement of motor evoked potentials, have shown promise in both the correlation of cord deficits with intraoperative evoked potential monitoring and as a guide to the surgeon to apply intraoperative adjuncts when cord ischemia is detected with initial cross-clamping.[48, 66, 80, 86]

The rationale for CSF pressure monitoring and drainage relates to the concept of spinal cord perfusion pressure as the difference between distal arterial pressure below the clamp and CSF pressure.[9, 68, 91] Thoracic aortic clamping can result in an abrupt increase in intracerebral blood flow, which is likely the principal mechanism of the increase in CSF pressure that can accompany such clamping; however, the absolute degree of this rise is typically modest.[6, 124] Kazama and coworkers[77] found that CSF drainage favorably influenced spinal cord blood flow only when CSF pressure was experimentally elevated to four times the baseline values. Thus, the assumptions on which the theoretical benefit of CSF drainage are based may not be valid, and several studies have failed to demonstrate the benefit for CSF drainage.[39, 93] However, elevated CSF pressure has been correlated in particular with delayed onset neurologic deficit, and many authors continue to use CSF drainage either alone or more typically in combination with other strategies[2, 3, 105] because it is simple and safe and has shown promise in a variety of experimental studies.[10, 89] Furthermore, reversal of delayed deficits by CSF drainage has been reported.[71, 107]

In the category of maintaining spinal cord blood supply, intercostal artery reanastomosis is the most commonly applied surgical maneuver. Most authors contend that sacrifice of critical intercostal vessels and the inability to reperfuse these arteries in a timely fashion are important factors in the pathogenesis of ischemic cord injury. The author and others have demonstrated that sacrifice of intercostal arteries in the critical T9 to L1 zone correlates with postoperative cord injury.[13, 30, 104, 121] Reattachment of critical intercostal vessels can be technically impossible if excessive atheroma or acute dissection surrounds the intercostal artery origins.

Intraoperatively, the surgeon typically faces the management dilemma of expending aortic cross-clamp time to reattach intercostal vessels. Because the critical intercostal zone lies topographically close to the visceral aortic segment, it is generally not possible to separate reconstruction in the critical intercostal segment from the visceral aortic segment with a distal perfusion and sequential clamping technique. Some authors have suggested that expending aortic clamp time for intercostal vessel reanastomosis is a worthless maneuver and routinely oversew or occlude all intercostal vessels, often with the use of other adjuncts directed against spinal cord ischemia.[3, 67]

Where should efforts at intercostal artery reattachment be directed? Based on the previous discussion of the anatomy of the spinal cord circulation and on the angiographic evidence in humans indicating that the greater radicular artery originates between T8 and L1 in most patients, most agree that reattachment of intercostal arteries should be directed toward this region. Several investigative studies support the theory that freely back-bleeding intercostal arteries exposed only to atmosphere pressure can create a steal phenomenon and decrease spinal cord perfusion pressure.[44, 131] We rapidly oversew the typically vigorously back-bleeding intercostals in the T4 to T8 region. In addition, those intercostals selected for reconstruction in the T9 to T12 zone are balloon occluded until reconstructed.

Svensson and colleagues[121] and Safi and associates[104] have reported detailed studies of specific levels of intercostal artery management during operation. These reports and others have noted a significant increase in neurologic deficits when arteries in the T9 to T12 zone were sacrificed instead of being reconstructed or occluded by mural thrombus preoperatively.[17, 30] Intercostal artery reattachment, however, is a "blind" maneuver unless a reliable method of preoperative or intraoperative localization of critical vessels is applied.[116]

Perhaps the best documentation of the worth of intercostal artery reattachment was provided by Grabitz and coworkers[66] using direct spinal cord somatosensory evoked potential (SSEP) monitoring. These investigators reported increased neurologic deficits when rapid loss of spinal cord SSEPs was noted after aortic cross-clamping. Furthermore, neurologic outcome for each group of spinal cord SSEP responses was correlated with the ability to achieve rapid return of the evoked potentials with early intercostal vessel reimplantation. Jacobs and associates,[73] using motor evoked potentials to guide intercostal artery reconstruction or sacrifice, have demonstrated that this modality can provide rapid detection of intraoperative spinal cord ischemia and its reversal by either hemodynamic manipulations or intercostal artery reconstruction. However, restoration of intercostal perfusion may be inadequate as a stand-alone adjunct simply because it cannot be performed rapidly enough.

Neuroprotective adjuncts are intended to increase the tolerance of the spinal cord to ischemia during the cross-clamp interval. There are two general categories of such adjuncts, hypothermia and a variety of pharmacologic agents. The latter can be classified according to their intended mechanisms of actions:

1. Nonspecific neuroprotective agents, such as steroids, prostaglandins, magnesium, and barbiturates.[56, 57, 72, 81, 96, 118]
2. Excitatory neurotransmitter inhibitors, such as naloxone[2, 53, 55]; calcium channel blockers.[61]
3. Oxygen free radical scavengers, which act at different points on the cascade of reperfusion injury.[4, 6, 82]

Determining the benefit of any of these agents in the clinical setting is difficult because they are typically used in combination with other strategies. The preeminent clinical experience involving this general strategy has been reported by Acher and associates[3] applying endorphin receptor blockade with naloxone in combination with CSF drainage and a policy of routine intercostal artery ligation. These authors reported overall spinal cord ischemic injury rates of 3.5%, equivalent or superior to that achieved using other strategies.

The protective effect of hypothermia is presumed to be secondary to decreased tissue metabolism; however, the mechanism may be more complex, involving membrane stabilization and reduced release of excitatory neurotransmitters.[102] Hypothermic protection of the cord may ablate the typically seen hyperemic phase of cord reperfusion, possibly decreasing edema during the period after circulation is established to the cord.[5, 100] Oxygen requirements in central nervous symptom tissue are known to decrease 6% to 7% for each degree centigrade decrement in cord temperature.

Hypothermia for purposes of cord protection during TAA surgery can be either regional (i.e., confined to the spinal cord itself) or systemic. The techniques of applying hypothermic protection range from a modest degree of systemic hypothermia achieved passively by simply cooling the operating room and allowing evaporative and respiratory heat losses to profound hypothermia (15° to 18°C) achieved with complete cardiopulmonary bypass and temporary circulatory arrest. Lesser degrees of systemic hypothermia can be achieved actively by adding a heat exchanger to a partial cardiopulmonary bypass circuit. This provides for active systemic hypothermia, the extent of which is limited by the potential for cardiac arrhythmia.[58, 112, 126]

Regional hypothermic methods have the distinct advantage of avoiding *systemic* hypothermia, a concept we believe is important to the overall operative management of patients with TAAs. Systemic hypothermia has been independently associated with the development of complications after elective abdominal aortic surgery.[11] Regional hypothermia can be administered indirectly through the doubly clamped thoracic aorta[23, 24, 54] or directly onto the spinal cord.[45, 129] Given our experience with the rate and volumes of cooled epidural perfusate necessary to achieve moderate levels of regional cord hypothermia, it is doubtful that effective cooling can be achieved indirectly through the intercostal arteries in the excluded aneurysm sac. Clinical application of regional hypothermic techniques was based on convincing experimental data wherein a 100% protective effect against cord injury was demonstrated.[5, 7, 94, 100, 109, 127, 128, 133]

Marsala and coworkers[84] demonstrated that a clinically applicable closed epidural infusion system that achieved moderate (26° to 28°C) levels of cord hypothermia could be 100% effective against spinal cord ischemia induced by double thoracic aortic clamping in a dog model. We adopted this strategy and have applied it in patients since 1993. The mechanics of this clinically applicable system (see Fig. 92–4) are straightforward, with an epidural catheter used for infusion of 4°C saline and a separate intrathecal catheter used to measure CSF temperature and pressure. It is necessary to maintain a continuous infusion to achieve moderate (~25°C) levels of cord hypothermia. The infusion must be initiated some 45 minutes before the anticipated application of the cross-clamp.

The principal technical limitation of the epidural infusion system is related to the fact that CSF pressures rise during the epidural infusion, averaging twice the baseline in our patients, which is a significant concern relative to spinal

cord perfusion. It therefore is necessary to maintain an arbitrary gradient of 30 to 40 mmHg between mean arterial pressure and mean CSF pressure by either decreasing the epidural infusion rate or increasing systemic arterial pressure. Neurologic outcome in our first 70 patients treated with this method was significantly improved when compared with institutional controls operated in the 3-year period prior to adoption of the epidural cooling technique. Neurologic deficits after elective resections of types I, II, and III TAAs have been reduced to the 3% range in elective operations with the adjunctive use of epidural cooling.[17]

Operative Mortality and Other Major Complications

As displayed in Table 92–4, operative mortality in large clinical series averages about 10%[3, 13, 31, 66, 72, 108, 122]; other reports detail considerably higher perioperative mortality.[33, 64] Not surprisingly, the circumstances of the clinical presentation are the dominant factor with respect to the preoperative variables associated with operative mortality. In our material, operations for ruptured TAA or urgent operations (versus elective operation) were highly predictive ($p <$ .001) of perioperative mortality. Similar data have been reported by others.[3, 30, 33] Some contemporary series have demonstrated an increased risk of operative mortality in elderly patients.[3, 30, 31, 122] Increasing numbers of co-morbid conditions can naturally be expected to increase overall operative risk.

Individual series variously demonstrate increased operative risks in patients with antecedent coronary artery disease, significant COPD, and in particular preoperative renal insufficiency.[3, 13, 31, 33, 64, 111, 122] Stated differently, the presence of significant dysfunction in these respective organ systems clearly increases the risks of organ-specific complications after operation and these, in turn, increase operative mortality. In fact, aside from the dominant influence of emergency operation and TAA rupture the major correlates of operative mortality are the major postoperative complications. Patients who sustain major neurologic deficits, postoperative renal failure, and cardiopulmonary complications have a significantly increased risk of operative mortality.[3, 13, 30, 31, 108, 122] In our experience, this risk was increased more than sixfold in patients with postoperative renal failure and increased by a factor of 16 in those with paraplegia,[13] findings similar to those of Svensson and colleagues.[122] These data emphasize the importance of minimizing such complications.

Perioperative Hemorrhage

Intraoperative bleeding complications can occur from technical mishaps or dilutional coagulopathy caused by excessive blood turnover and previously were an important source of early mortality.[14] Blood loss during repair of extensive aneurysms is significant because large type II aneurysms, for example, can contain up to several liters of blood in the aneurysm sac alone. In our own experience, approximately half the blood loss during TAA repair is returned to the patient by autotransfusion methods. Total blood transfusion for repair of the more extensive type I and II aneurysms averages more than 3 L. Not surprisingly this figure varies with the extent of aortic replacement (see Table 92–3).

Coselli and associates[30] documented that blood and plasma transfusions increased with the use of partial cardiopulmonary bypass. Anticipatory use of blood component replacement in the form of fresh frozen plasma (and especially platelet transfusions), once perfusion to the abdominal viscera and lower extremities has been restored, is an important component of avoiding coagulopathic bleeding in the operating room. With this policy, plus avoidance of systemic heparin and careful attention to hemostasis throughout the course of operation, significant coagulopathic bleeding in the operating room has been observed rarely in contemporary practice.

Considerable attention has been focused on hepatic and mesenteric ischemia as contributory or principally responsible for the development of intraoperative coagulopathic bleeding.[20–22] We and others have documented the significant depletion of coagulation factors that occur intraoperatively in the course of a supraceliac aortic clamp and the fact that these changes are quantitatively more severe than with an infrarenal aortic cross-clamp.[62] Although such coagulation factor depletion is clearly demonstrable with laboratory testing, the clinical complication of coagulopathic bleeding has been distinctly uncommon. Irrespective of whether the mechanism of coagulopathic bleeding is hepatic ischemia or bacterial translocation in ischemic gut, the available experimental data and clinical observations suggest that minimizing mesenteric ischemia is an important component of avoiding coagulopathic bleeding.[22] As displayed in Figure 92–4, we prefer to reestablish mesenteric perfusion early by means of an in-line mesenteric shunt placed immediately after completion of the proximal aortic anastomosis and have demonstrated that this technique can reduce the coagulation defect seen with supraceliac clamping.[18, 63]

Reexploration for bleeding complications had a major impact on overall operative mortality in Crawford's summary experience.[122] Reoperation for bleeding was required in 7% of Crawford's patients but is currently done in fewer than 3% of patients.[13, 30] Postoperative splenic bleeding and undetected back-bleeding from intercostal or lumbar arteries have been the principal sources of postoperative hemorrhage. A careful search of the entire aneurysm sac after all suture lines have been completed for back-bleeding lumbar and intercostal vessels, and an aggressive posture toward splenectomy for even apparently trivial splenic tears should prevent these complications.

Perioperative Respiratory Insufficiency

Despite the more evident focus on spinal cord ischemic complications and renal failure, respiratory failure is the single most common complication after TAA repair in most clinical series, affecting in 25% to 45% of patients.[13, 31, 72, 122] There may be confusion as to how this is defined, because the term "prolonged" ventilatory support (the most common complication) may be variably interpreted. A slow weaning from ventilatory support, often planned to proceed over several days, is appropriate management in certain patients after extensive TAA repair, particularly those with baseline pulmonary insufficiency. Despite varying definitions, postoperative respiratory insufficiency occurs commonly and the variables predictive of this complication include active cigarette smoking, baseline COPD (especially those with significant reductions in FEV_1), and cardiac, renal, or bleeding complications.[13, 92, 120]

In the circumstance of elective operation, it is vital for patients to discontinue tobacco use for a minimum of 1 month before surgery. Preoperative consultation with a pulmonologist for optimization of bronchodilator therapy is an important component in the management of patients with significant COPD. Preoperative steroid therapy with the intent of improving respiratory function is contraindicated, however, because we have observed that this maneuver precipitates aneurysm rupture. It is logical that paralysis of the left hemidiaphragm by its radial division to the aortic hiatus contributes significantly to postoperative respiratory failure. Accordingly, a diaphragm sparing operative technique should be routinely applied in contemporary practice.[50]

Perioperative Renal Insufficiency

Postoperative renal failure has traditionally been an important factor in the overall morbidity of extensive aortic surgery. The summary experience of Crawford reinforced this fact: Svensson reported that among more than 1500 patients undergoing TAA repair, significant postoperative renal failure occurred in 18% of patients, with dialysis being required in half of these. The risk of operative mortality increased fivefold in patients sustaining postoperative renal failure.[122] Our data are consistent with the significant impact of postoperative renal failure on operative mortality. Reviewing more than 180 TAA operations, we found that in the 8% of patients who sustained significant postoperative renal failure, the risk of mortality was increased almost 10 times (odds ratio, 9.2; 95% confidence interval, 2.6 to 33; $p < .005$).[76]

Various criteria have been used to define postoperative renal failure. We define it as both a doubling of the baseline serum creatinine level and an absolute postoperative creatinine level of more than 3 mg/dl, a definition applied in most major clinical series. The important etiologic factors in the development of postoperative renal failure include the duration of renal ischemia, baseline renal dysfunction, cholesterol embolization from surgical manipulation of the aneurysm in the region of the renal artery orifices, and failure of a renal artery reconstruction. Transient and modest decreases in overall excretory function are the inevitable consequence of some obligatory period of renal ischemia; in most patients, this is both nonoliguric and reverses rapidly with appropriate maintenance of intravascular volume.

Not surprisingly, the risk of significant renal dysfunction increases as a function of total aortic cross-clamp time. In addition, virtually all reports that examine this complication have indicated that the most powerful predictive variable for the development of postoperative renal failure is the presence of preoperative renal insufficiency. We found that an abnormal preoperative serum creatinine level and a prolonged aortic cross-clamp time both increased the risk of postoperative renal failure by a factor of 4, findings consistent with those reported by others.[3, 31, 106, 122]

The most important maneuver to minimize the risk of postoperative renal failure is, of course, minimizing renal ischemic time. Some authors prefer the use of *distal aortic perfusion* and a sequential clamping technique so that the renal arteries can be perfused during construction of the proximal aortic anastomosis. The addition of individual visceral-renal perfusion catheters from the atrial-femoral bypass circuit, at least in theory, can provide for continuous renal artery perfusion during all phases of the operation (see Fig. 92–5). However, the size of such catheters may not permit adequate perfusion pressure or flow to the renal vessels, and at least two reports of this method suggest an apparent paradoxical detrimental effect on overall renal function.[31, 106]

The other frequently applied intraoperative adjunct, and the one we prefer, is selective *hypothermic renal artery perfusion*, as detailed previously (see Fig. 92–4). Although such regional renal hypothermia is likely unnecessary in patients with normal renal function preoperatively and with renal ischemic times less than 1 hour, it can provide a margin of safety in circumstances of either technical difficulty or prolongation of renal ischemia. An additional intraoperative adjunct employed to minimize the risk of postoperative renal failure is an aggressive posture toward the treatment of renal artery occlusive disease.[31]

Management of perioperative renal failure is usually conservative if the patient remains nonoliguric. Patients taking diuretic medications preoperatively generally require these postoperatively, and renal-dose dopamine infusions can also help to maintain an appropriate diuresis. We prefer to avoid the use of hemodialysis therapy unless clear-cut indications for its use exist. Conventional hemodialysis is accompanied by a substantial risk of hemodynamic instability in the patient after TAA repair, and such hypotension has precipitated spinal cord ischemic events even weeks after surgery. The availability of continuous venovenous hemodialysis therapy has obviated this consideration somewhat and provides for a smoother hemodynamic course than conventional hemodialysis does. Nonetheless, the need for anticoagulation, the potential complications of vascular access devices, and the threat of hemodynamic instability make hemodialysis therapy undesirable unless it is absolutely necessary.

Late Survival

The most extensive review of late survival in patients after TAA repair was reported by Svensson and coworkers.[122] These investigators reported Kaplan-Meier survival projections in the range of 60% at 5 years after operation, figures almost identical with our results in 160 patients (Fig. 92–10). This survival curve is also identical to that from a population-based study of Mayo Clinic patients who underwent elective AAA repair.[13, 69] These data indicate that the substantial resource investment required to bring these patients through successful operation and recovery is an appropriate expenditure of such resources. Most operative survivors return to their preoperative independent living status.[64, 111] Rupture of another aneurysm has accounted for approximately 10% of late deaths.[111, 122] This fact indicates the desirability of ongoing aortic surveillance after successful operative treatment of TAA. Cardiac events are the most

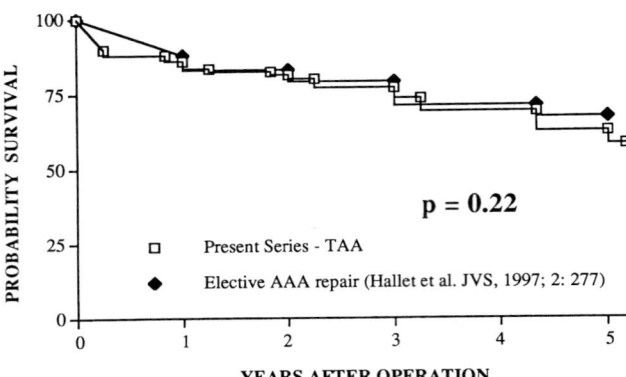

FIGURE 92–10. Probability of survival by the Kaplan-Meier method after resection of thoracoabdominal aortic aneurysm in the author's patients (□ = "present series"). Five years after operation, actuarial survival is 62% ± 6%. Also displayed are late survival data in a population-based series of patients after elective repair.[69] There is no difference (log-rank) in late survival between these two cohorts. (From Cambria R, Davison JK, Zannetti S, et al: Thoracoabdominal aneurysm repair: Perspectives over a decade with the clamp-and-sew technique. Ann Surg 226:294–305, 1997.)

common cause of late mortality.[111, 122] Similar to the negative effect on early postoperative survival, patients who sustained postoperative lower extremity neurologic deficits or who become dependent on dialysis have distinctly inferior late survival rates.[122]

SUMMARY

Considerable progress has been demonstrated in the overall results of surgical treatment for TAA. Given the unfavorable natural history data reviewed in this chapter, aggressive posture toward graft replacement is clearly justified when demonstrated surgical expertise is available. The multiplicity of surgical strategies and adjuncts applied in efforts to minimize the principal complications of operation indicates that the evolution of surgical sophistication is still incomplete. Similar to the evolution of surgical treatment for infrarenal AAA, an increase in the percentage of patients treated in elective circumstances will improve overall results in the future.

REFERENCES

1. Acher CW, Wynn MM, Hoch JR, et al: Combined use of cerebral spinal fluid drainage and naloxone reduces the risk of paraplegia in thoracoabdominal aneurysm repair. J Vasc Surg 19:236–248, 1994.
2. Acher CW, Wynn MM, Archibald J: Naloxone and spinal fluid drainage as adjuncts in the surgical treatment of thoracoabdominal and thoracic aneurysms. Surgery 108:755–762, 1990.
3. Acher CW, Wynn MM, Hoch JR, Kranner PW: Cardiac function is a risk factor for paralysis in thoracoabdominal aortic replacement. J Vasc Surg 27:821–830, 1998.
4. Agee JM, Flanagan T, Blackbourne LH, et al: Reducing postischemic paraplegia using conjugated superoxide dismutase. Ann Thorac Surg 51:911–914, 1991; discussion 914–915.
5. Allen BT, Davis C, Osborne D, Karl I: Spinal cord ischemia and reperfusion metabolism: The effect of hypothermia. J Vasc Surg 19:332–340, 1994.

6. Berendes J, Bredee J, Schipperheyn J, Mashhour Y: Mechanism of spinal cord injury after cross-clamping of the descending thoracic aorta. Circulation 66 (Suppl 1): 112–116, 1982.

7. Berguer R, Porto J, Fedoronko B, Dragovic L: Selective deep hypothermia of the spinal cord prevents paraplegia after aortic cross-clamping in the dog model. J Vasc Surg 15:62–72, 1992.

8. Bickerstaff LK, Pairolero PC, Hollier LH, et al: Thoracic aortic aneurysms: A population-based study. Surgery 92:1103–1108, 1982.

9. Blaisdell FW, Cooley DA: The mechanism of paraplegia after temporary aortic occlusion and its relationship to spinal fluid pressure. Surgery 57:351–355, 1962.

10. Bower TC, Murray MJ, Gloviczki P, et al: Effects of thoracic aortic occlusion and cerebrospinal fluid drainage on regional spinal cord blood flow in dogs: Correlation with neurologic outcome. J Vasc Surg 9:135–144, 1989.

11. Bush H, Hydo LJ, Fischer E, et al: Hypothermia during elective abdominal aortic aneurysm repair: The high risk of avoidable morbidity. J Vasc Surg 21:392–400, 1995.

12. Cambria RP, Brewster DC, Moncure AC, et al: Spontaneous aortic dissection in the presence of coexistent or previously repaired atherosclerotic aortic aneurysm. Ann Surg 208:619–624, 1988.

13. Cambria R, Davison JK, Zannetti S, et al: Thoracoabdominal aneurysm repair: Perspectives over a decade with the clamp-and-sew technique. Ann Surg 226:294–305, 1997.

14. Cambria R, Brewster D, Moncure A, et al: Recent experience with thoracoabdominal aneurysm repair. Arch Surg 124:620–624, 1989.

15. Cambria RA, Gloviczki P, Stanson A, et al: Outcome and expansion rate of 57 thoracoabdominal aortic aneurysms managed nonoperatively. Am J Surg 170:213–217, 1995.

16. Cambria RP, Giglia J: Prevention of spinal cord ischemic complications after thoracoabdominal aortic surgery. Eur J Vasc Endovasc Surg 15:96–109, 1998.

17. Cambria RP, Davison JK, Zannetti S, et al: Clinical experience with epidural cooling for spinal cord protection during thoracic and thoracoabdominal aneurysm repair. J Vasc Surg 25:234–243, 1997.

18. Cambria RP, Davison JK, Giglia JS, Gertler JP: Mesenteric shunting decreases visceral ischemic time during thoracoabdominal aneurysm repair. J Vasc Surg 27:745–749, 1998.

19. Cernaianu A, Olah A, Cilley JJ, et al: Effect of sodium nitroprusside on paraplegia during cross-clamping of the thoracic aorta. Ann Thorac Surg 56:1035–1038, 1993.

20. Cohen JR, Angus L, Asher A, et al: Disseminated intravascular coagulation as a result of supraceliac clamping: Implications for thoracoabdominal aneurysm repair. Ann Vasc Surg 1:552–557, 1987.

21. Cohen JR, Sardari F, Paul J, et al: Increased intestinal permeability: Implications for thoracoabdominal aneurysm repair. Ann Vasc Surg 6:433–437, 1991.

22. Cohen JR, Schroder W, Leal J, Wise L: Mesenteric shunting during thoracoabdominal aortic clamping to prevent disseminated intravascular coagulation in dogs. Ann Vasc Surg 2:261–267, 1988.

23. Coles J, Wilson G, Sima A, et al: Intraoperative management of thoracic aortic aneurysm: Experimental evaluation of perfusion cooling of the spinal cord. J Thorac Cardiovasc Surg 85:292–299, 1983.

24. Colon R, Frazier O, Cooley D, McAllister H: Hypothermic regional perfusion or protection of spinal cord during periods of ischemia. Ann Thorac Surg 43:639–643, 1987.

25. Comerota AJ, White JV: Reducing morbidity of thoracoabdominal aneurysm repair by preliminary axillofemoral bypass. Am J Surg 170:218–222, 1995.

26. Connolly J, Wakabayashi A, German J, et al: Clinical experience with pulsatile left heart bypass without anticoagulation for thoracic aneurysms. J Thorac Cardiovasc Surg 62:568–576, 1971.

27. Cooke J, Cambria RP: Simultaneous tracheobronchial and esophageal obstruction secondary to thoracoabdominal aneurysm. J Vasc Surg 18:90–94, 1993.

28. Coselli JS: Thoracoabdominal aortic aneurysms: Experience with 372 patients. J Card Surg 9:638–647, 1994.

29. Coselli JS, LeMaire SA, Buket S, Berzin E: Subsequent proximal aortic operations in 123 patients with previous infrarenal abdominal aortic aneurysm surgery. J Vasc Surg 22:59–67, 1995.

30. Coselli JS, LeMaire SA, Poli de Figueiredo L, Kirby RP: Paraplegia after thoracoabdominal aortic aneurysm repair: Is dissection a risk factor? Ann Thorac Surg 63:28–36, 1997.

31. Coselli JS, LeMaire SA, Miller CC III, et al: Mortality and paraplegia after thoracoabdominal aneurysm repair: A risk factor analysis. Ann Thorac Surg (in press).

32. Coselli JS, Poli de Figueiredo LF, LeMaire SA: Impact of previous thoracic aneurysm repair on thoracoabdominal aortic aneurysm management. Ann Thorac Surg 64:639–650, 1997.

33. Cox GS, O'Hara PJ, Hertzer N, et al: Thoracoabdominal aneurysm repair: A representative experience. J Vasc Surg 15:780–788, 1992.

34. Crawford ES: Thoracoabdominal and abdominal aortic aneurysm involving renal, superior mesenteric and celiac arteries. Ann Surg 179:763–772, 1974.

35. Crawford ES, Hess KR, Cohen JS, Safi HJ: Ruptured aneurysm of the descending thoracic and thoracoabdominal aorta. Ann Surg 213:417–426, 1991.

36. Crawford ES, DeNatale RW: Thoracoabdominal aortic aneurysm: Observations regarding the natural course of the disease. J Vasc Surg 3:578–582, 1986.

37. Crawford ES, Crawford JL, Safi H, et al: Thoracoabdominal aortic aneurysms: Preoperative and intraoperative factors determining immediate and long term results of operation in 605 patients. J Vasc Surg 3:389–404, 1986.

38. Crawford ES, Mizrahi EM, Hess KR, et al: The impact of distal perfusion and somatosensory evoked potential monitoring on prevention of paraplegia after aortic aneurysm operation. J Thorac Cardiovasc Surg 95:357–366, 1988.

39. Crawford ES, Svensson LG, Hess KR, et al: A prospective randomized study of cerebrospinal fluid drainage to prevent paraplegia after high risk surgery on the thoracoabdominal aorta. J Vasc Surg 13:36–46, 1991.

40. Crawford ES, Cohen ES: Aortic aneurysm: A multifocal disease. Arch Surg 117:1393–1400, 1982.

41. Cronenwett JL, Sargent SK, Wall MH, et al: Variables that affect the expansion rate and outcome of small abdominal aortic aneurysms. J Vasc Surg 11:260–269, 1990.

42. Cunningham JJ, Laschinger JC, Spencer FC: Monitoring of somatosensory evoked potentials during surgical procedures on the thoracoabdominal aorta: IV. Clinical observations and results. J Thorac Cardiovasc Surg 94:275–285, 1987.

43. Dake MD, Miller DC, Semba CP, et al: Transluminal placement of endovascular stent-grafts for the treatment of descending thoracic aortic aneurysms. N Engl J Med 331:1729–1734, 1994.

44. Dapunt O, Midulla PS, Sadeghi AM, et al: Pathogenesis of spinal cord injury during simulated aneurysm repair in a chronic animal model. Ann Thorac Surg 58:689–696, 1994.

45. Davison J, Cambria R, Vierra D, et al: Epidural cooling for regional spinal cord hypothermia during thoracoabdominal aneurysm repair. J Vasc Surg 20:304–310, 1994.

46. DeBakey ME, Creech O Jr, Morris CG: Aneurysms of the thoracoabdominal aorta involving the celiac, superior mesenteric, and renal arteries: Report of four cases treated by resection and homograft replacement. Ann Surg 44:549–573, 1956.

47. DeBakey ME, McCollum CH, Crawford ES, et al: Dissection and dissecting aneurysms of the aorta: Twenty-year follow-up of five hundred twenty-seven patients treated surgically. Surgery 92:1118–1134, 1982.

48. deHaan P, Kalkman CJ, De Mol BA, et al: Efficacy of transcranial motor-evoked myogenic potentials to detect spinal cord ischemia during operations for thoracoabdominal aneurysms. J Thorac Cardiovasc Surg 113:87–101, 1997.

49. Donahoo JS, Brawley RK, Gott VL: The heparin-coated vascular shunt for thoracic and great vessel procedures: A ten year experience. Ann Thorac Surg 23:507–513, 1977.

50. Engle J, Safi HJ, Miller CC III, et al: The impact of diaphragm management on prolonged ventilator support following thoracoabdominal aortic repair. J Vasc Surg 29:150–156, 1999.

51. Estes JE Jr: Abdominal aortic aneurysm: A study of one hundred and two cases. Circulation 2:258–264, 1950.

52. Etheredge SN, Yee J, Smith JV, et al: Successful resection of large aneurysm of the upper abdominal aorta and replacement with homograft. Surgery 38:1071–1081, 1955.

53. Faden A, Jacobs T, Smith M, Zivin J: Naloxone in experimental spinal cord ischemia: Dose-response studies. Eur J Pharmacol 103:115–120, 1984.

54. Fehrenbacher J, McCready R, Hormuth D, et al: One-stage segmental resection of extensive thoracoabdominal aneurysms with left-sided heart bypass. J Vasc Surg 18:366–371, 1993.

55. Follis F, Miller K, Scremin O, et al: NMDA receptor blockade and spinal cord ischemia due to aortic cross-clamping in the rat model. Can J Neurol Sci 21:227–232, 1994.

56. Fowl R, Patterson R, Gewirtz R, Anderson D: Protection against postischemic spinal cord injury using a new 21-aminosteroid. J Surg Res 48:597–600, 1990.

57. Francel P, Long B, Malik J, et al: Limiting ischemic spinal cord injury using a free radical scavenger 21-aminosteroid and/or cerebrospinal fluid drainage. J Neurosurg 79:742–751, 1993.

58. Frank S, Parker S, Rock P, et al: Moderate hypothermia, with partial bypass and segmental sequential repair for thoracoabdominal aortic aneurysm. J Vasc Surg 19:687–697, 1994.

59. Gadowski GR, Pilcher DB, Ricci MA: Abdominal aortic aneurysm expansion rate: Effects of size and beta-adrenergic blockade. J Vasc Surg 19:727–731, 1994.

60. Galla JD, Ergin MA, Lansman SL, et al: Identification of risk factors in patients undergoing thoracoabdominal aneurysm repair. J Card Surg 12:292–299, 1997.

61. Gelbfish J, Phillips T, Rose D, et al: Acute spinal cord ischemia: Prevention of paraplegia with verapamil. Circulation 74:15–10, 1986.

62. Gertler JP, Cambria RP, Laposata M, Abbott WM: Coagulation changes during thoracoabdominal aneurysm repair. J Vasc Surg 24:936–945, 1996.

63. Gertler JP, Cambria RP, Makary MA, et al: Correction of coagulation defect in thoracoabdominal aneurysm repair by mesenteric shunting. Surgery (in press).

64. Gilling-Smith GL, Worswick OL, Knight PF, et al: Surgical repair of thoracoabdominal aortic aneurysm: 10 years experience. Br J Surg 82:624–629, 1995.

65. Gloviczki P, Pairolero P, Welch T, et al: Multiple aortic aneurysms: The results of surgical management. J Vasc Surg 11:19–28, 1990.

66. Grabitz K, Sandmann W, Stuhmeirer K, et al: The risk of ischemic spinal cord injury in patients undergoing graft replacement for thoracoabdominal aortic aneurysms. J Vasc Surg 23:230–240, 1996.

67. Griepp RB, Ergen MA, Galla JD, et al: Looking for the artery of Adamkiewicz: A quest to minimize paraplegia after operations for aneurysm of the descending thoracic and thoracoabdominal aorta. J Thorac Cardiovasc Surg 112:1202–1215, 1996.

68. Grubbs PJ, Marini C, Toporoff B, et al: Somatosensory evoked potentials and spinal cord perfusion pressure are significant predictors of postoperative neurologic dysfunction. Surgery 104:216–223, 1988.

69. Hallett JW, Marshall DM, Petterson TM, et al: Graft-related complications after abdominal aortic aneurysm repair: Reassurance from a 36 year population-based experience. J Vasc Surg 25:277–286, 1997.

70. Heineman MK, Buehner B, Jurmann MJ, Borst HG: Use of "elephant trunk technique" in aortic surgery. Ann Thorac Surg 60:2–7, 1995.

71. Hill A, Kalman P, Johnston K, Vosu H: Reversal of delayed-onset paraplegia after thoracic aortic surgery with cerebrospinal fluid drainage. J Vasc Surg 20:315–317, 1994.

72. Hollier L, Money SR, Naslund TC, et al: Risk of spinal cord dysfunction in patients undergoing thoracoabdominal aortic replacement. Am J Surg 164:210–213, 1992.

73. Jacobs M, Meylaerts S, deHaan P, et al: Strategies to prevent neurologic deficit based on motor-evoked potentials in types I and II thoracoabdominal aortic aneurysm repair. J Vasc Surg 29:48–59, 1999.

74. Johansson G, Markstrom U, Swedenborg J: Ruptured thoracic aortic aneurysms: A study of incidence and mortality rates. J Vasc Surg 21:985–988, 1995.

75. Juvonen T, Ergin MA, Galla JD, et al: Prospective study of the natural history of thoracic aortic aneurysms. Ann Thorac Surg 63:1533–1545, 1997.

76. Kashyap VS, Cambria RP, Davison JK, L'Italien GJ: Renal failure after thoracoabdominal aortic surgery. J Vasc Surg 26:949–957, 1997.

77. Kazama S, Masaki Y, Maruyama S, Ishihara A: Effect of altering cerebrospinal fluid pressure on spinal cord blood flow. Ann Thorac Surg 58:112–115, 1994.

78. Kieffer E, Richard T, Chiras J, et al: Preoperative spinal cord arteriography in aneurysmal disease of the descending thoracic and thoracoabdominal aorta: Preliminary results in 45 patients. Ann Vasc Surg 3:34–46, 1989.

79. Kouchoukos N, Daily BB, Rokkas CK, et al: Hypothermic bypass and circulatory arrest for operations on the descending thoracic and thoracoabdominal aorta. Ann Thorac Surg 60:67–77, 1995.

80. Laschinger J, Owen J, Rosenbloom M, et al: Direct noninvasive monitoring of spinal cord motor function during thoracic aortic occlusion: Use of motor evoked potentials. J Vasc Surg 7:161–171, 1988.

81. Laschinger J, Cunningham JJ, Cooper MM, et al: Prevention of ischemic spinal cord injury following aortic cross-clamping: Use of corticosteroids. Ann Thorac Surg 38:500–507, 1984.

82. Lim K, Connolly M, Rose D, et al: Prevention of reperfusion injury of the ischemic spinal cord: Use of recombinant superoxide dismutase. Ann Thorac Surg 42:282–286, 1986.

83. Lobato AC, Puech-Leao P: Predictive factors for rupture of thoracoabdominal aortic aneurysm. J Vasc Surg 27:446–453, 1998.

84. Marsala M, Vanicky I, Galik J, et al: Panmyelic epidural cooling protects against ischemic spinal cord damage. J Surg Res 55:21–31, 1993.

85. Masuda Y, Takanashi K, Takasu J, et al: Expansion rate of thoracic aortic aneurysms and influencing factors. Chest 102:461–466, 1992.

86. Matsui Y, Goh K, Shiiya N, et al: Clinical application of evoked spinal cord potentials elicited by direct stimulation of the cord during temporary occlusion of the thoracic aorta. J Thorac Cardiovasc Surg 107:1519–1527, 1994.

87. Mauney M, Blackbourne L, Langenburg S, et al: Prevention of spinal cord injury after repair of the thoracic or thoracoabdominal aorta. Ann Thorac Surg 59:245–252, 1995.

88. Mauney M, Tribble C, Cope J, et al: Is clamp and sew still viable for thoracic aortic resection? Ann Surg 223:534–543, 1996.

89. McCullough J, Hollier L, Nugent M: Paraplegia after thoracic aortic occlusion: Influence of cerebrospinal fluid drainage. J Vasc Surg 7:153–160, 1988.

90. McNamara JJ, Pressler VM: Natural history of arteriosclerotic thoracic aortic aneurysms. Ann Thorac Surg 26:468–473, 1978.

91. Miyamoto K, Ueno A, Wada T, Kimoto S: A new and simple method of preventing spinal cord damage following temporary occlusion of the thoracic aorta by draining the cerebrospinal fluid. J Cardiovasc Surg 1:188–197, 1960.

92. Money SR, Rice K, Crockett D, et al: Risk of respiratory failure after repair of thoracoabdominal aortic aneurysms. Am J Surg 168:152–155, 1994.

93. Murray MJ, Bower TC, Oliver WCJ, et al: Effects of cerebrospinal fluid drainage in patients undergoing thoracic and thoracoabdominal aortic surgery. J Cardiothorac Vasc Anesth 7:266–272, 1993.

94. Naslund T, Hollier L, Money S, et al: Protecting the ischemic spinal cord during aortic clamping: The influence of anesthetics and hypothermia. Ann Surg 215:409–416, 1992.

95. Neya K, Omoto R, Kyo S: Outcome of Stanford type B acute aortic dissection. Circulation 86 (Suppl II): 1–7, 1992.

96. Nylander W, Plunkett RJ, Hammon JW Jr, et al: Thiopental modification of ischemic spinal cord injury in the dog. Ann Thorac Surg 33:64–68, 1982.

97. Panneton JM, Hollier LM: Basic data underlying clinical decision making: Non-dissecting thoracoabdominal aortic aneurysms: Part I. Ann Vasc Surg 9:503–514, 1995.

98. Perko MJ, Norgaard M, Herzog TM, et al: Unoperated aortic aneurysm: A survey of 170 patients. Ann Thorac Surg 59:1204–1209, 1995.

99. Rieumont MJ, Kaufman JA, Geller SC, et al: Evaluation of renal artery stenosis with dynamic gadolinium-enhanced magnetic resonance angiography. Am J Radiol 169:39–44, 1997.

100. Rokkas CK, Sundaresan S, Shuman TA, et al: Profound systemic hypothermia protects the spinal cord in a primate model of spinal cord ischemia. J Thorac Cardiovasc Surg 106:1024–1035, 1993.

101. Rokkas CK, Kouchoukos NT: Profound hypothermia for spinal cord protection in operations on the descending and thoracoabdominal aorta. Semin Thorac Cardiovasc Surg 10:57–60, 1998.

102. Rokkas CK, Cronin C, Nitta T, et al: Profound systemic hypothermia inhibits the release of neurotransmitter amino acids in spinal cord ischemia. J Thorac Cardiovasc Surg 110:27–35, 1995.

103. Safi HJ, Muller CC, Subramanian MH, et al: Thoracic and thoracoabdominal aortic aneurysm repair using cardiopulmonary bypass, profound hypothermia and circulatory arrest via left side of the chest incision. J Vasc Surg 28:591–598, 1998.

104. Safi HJ, Miller CC III, Carr C, et al: Importance of intercostal artery reattachment during thoracoabdominal aortic aneurysm repair. J Vasc Surg 27:58–68, 1998.

105. Safi HJ, Hess KR, Randel M, et al: Cerebrospinal fluid drainage and

distal aortic perfusion: Reducing neurologic complications in repair of thoracoabdominal aortic. aneurysms, type I and type II. J Vasc Surg 23:223–228, 1996.

106. Safi HJ, Harlin SA, Miller CC: Predictive factors for acute renal failure in thoracic and thoracoabdominal aortic aneurysm surgery. J Vasc Surg 24:338–345, 1996.

107. Safi HJ, Miller CC, Azizzadeh H, et al: Observations on delayed neurologic deficit after thoracoabdominal aneurysm repair. J Vasc Surg 26:616–622, 1997.

108. Safi HJ, Campbell MP, Miller CC, et al: Cerebral spinal fluid drainage and distal aortic perfusion decrease the incidence of neurological deficit: The results of 343 descending and thoracoabdominal aortic aneurysm repairs. Eur J Vasc Endovasc Surg 14:118–124, 1997.

109. Salzano R, Ellison LH, Altonji PF, et al: Regional deep hypothermia of the spinal cord protects against ischemic injury during thoracic aortic cross-clamping. Ann Thorac Surg 57:65–70, 1994.

110. Savader SJ, Williams GM, Trerotola SO, et al: Preoperative spinal artery localization and its relationship to postoperative neurologic complications. Radiology 189:165–171, 1993.

111. Schepens MA, Dekker E, Hamerlijnck RP, Vermeulen FE: Survival and aortic events after graft replacement for thoracoabdominal aortic aneurysm. Cardiovasc Surg 4:713–719, 1996.

112. Schepens MA, Defauw J, Hamerlijnck R, Vermeulen F: Use of left heart bypass in the surgical repair of thoracoabdominal aortic aneurysms. Ann Vasc Surg 9:327, 1995.

113. Schor JS, Yerlioghu ME, Galla JD, et al: Selective management of acute type B aortic dissection: Long-term follow-up. Ann Thorac Surg 61:1339–1341, 1996.

114. Schwartz LB, Belkin M, Donaldson M, et al: Improvements in results of repair of type IV thoracoabdominal aortic aneurysms. J Vasc Surg 24:74–81, 1996.

115. Shine T, Nugent M: Sodium nitroprusside decreases spinal cord perfusion pressure during descending thoracic aortic cross-clamping in the dog. J Cardiothorac Anesth 4:185–193, 1990.

116. Shiiya N, Yasuda K, Matsui Y, et al: Spinal cord protection during thoracoabdominal aortic aneurysm repair: Results of selective reconstruction of the critical segmental arteries guided by evoked spinal cord potential monitoring. J Vasc Surg 21:970–975, 1995.

117. Simpson JI, Eide T, Schiff G, et al: Isoflurane versus sodium nitroprusside for the control of proximal hypertension during thoracic aortic cross-clamping: Effects on spinal cord ischemia. J Cardiothorac Vasc Anesth 9:491–496, 1995.

118. Simpson JI, Eide T, Schiff G, et al: Intrathecal magnesium sulfate protects the spinal cord from ischemic injury during thoracic aortic cross-clamping. Anesthesiology 81:1493–1499, 1994.

119. Svensjö S, Bengtsson H, Bergqvist D: Thoracic and thoracoabdomi-nal aortic aneurysm and dissection: An investigation based on autopsy. Br J Surg 83:68–71, 1996.

120. Svensson LG, Hess KR, Coselli JS, et al: A prospective study of respiratory failure after high-risk surgery on the thoracoabdominal aorta. J Vasc Surg 14:271–282, 1991.

121. Svensson LG, Hess KR, Coselli JS, Safi HJ: Influence of segmental arteries, extent and atriofemoral bypass on postoperative paraplegia after thoracoabdominal aortic operations. J Vasc Surg 20:255–262, 1994.

122. Svensson LG, Crawford ES, Hess KR, et al: Experience with 1509 patients undergoing thoracoabdominal aortic operations. J Vasc Surg 17:357–370, 1993.

123. Svensson LG, Rickards E, Coull A, et al: Relationship of spinal cord blood flow to vascular anatomy during thoracic aortic cross-clamping and shunting. J Thorac Cardiovasc Surg 91:71–78, 1986.

124. Svensson LG, Grum DF, Bednarski M, et al: Appraisal of cerebrospinal fluid alterations during aortic surgery with intrathecal papaverine administration and cerebrospinal fluid drainage. J Vasc Surg 11:423–429, 1990.

125. Svensson LG, Patel V, Robinson MF, et al: Influence of preservation or perfusion of intraoperatively identified spinal cord blood supply on spinal motor evoked potentials and paraplegia after aortic surgery. J Vasc Surg 13:355–365, 1991.

126. Svensson LG, D'Agostino RS, et al: Reduction of neurologic injury after high-risk thoracoabdominal aortic surgery. Ann Thorac Surg 66:132–138, 1998.

127. Ueno T, Itoh T, Hirahara K, et al: Protection against spinal cord ischaemia: One-shot infusion of hypothermic solution. Cardiovasc Surg 2:374–378, 1994.

128. Ueno T, Furukawa K, Katayama Y, et al: Spinal cord protection: Development of a paraplegia-preventive solution. Ann Thorac Surg 58:116–120, 1994.

129. Vanicky I, Marsala M, Galik J, Marsala J: Epidural perfusion cooling protection against protracted spinal cord ischemia in rabbits. J Neurosurg 79:736–741, 1993.

130. von Oppell U, Dunne T, DeGroot K, Zilla P: Spinal cord protection in the absence of collateral circulation: Meta-analysis of mortality and paraplegia. J Card Surg 9:685–691, 1994.

131. Wadouh F, Arndt C, Oppermann E, et al: The mechanism of spinal cord injury after simple and double aortic cross-clamping. J Thorac Cardiovasc Surg 92:121–127, 1986.

132. Williams GM, Perler BA, Burdick JF, et al: Angiographic localization of spinal cord blood supply and its relationship to postoperative paraplegia. J Vasc Surg 13:23–35, 1991.

133. Wisselink W, Becker M, Nguyen J, et al: Protecting the ischemic spinal cord during aortic clamping: The influence of selective hypothermia and spinal cord perfusion pressure. J Vasc Surg 19:788–796, 1994.

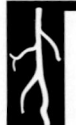

C H A P T E R   9 3

Dissection of the Descending Thoracic Aorta

Edouard Kieffer, M.D.

Aortic dissection is characterized by separation of the aortic wall layers by extraluminal blood that usually enters the aortic wall through an intimal tear.[1] Although it is recognized as one of the most common catastrophic events affecting the aorta, its true incidence is difficult to determine. It was found two to three times more frequently than rupture of abdominal aortic aneurysms in older reports.[2] Recent population-based reports, however, indicate that mortality from thoracic aortic dissection is now less than mortality from ruptured abdominal aortic aneurysms. Over the past 30 years in the United States, mortality from thoracic aortic dissection has steadily decreased, presumably due to better medical and surgical treatment. In 1990, the mortality rate per 100,000 was 1.5 in black men, 1.2 in white men, 0.8 in black women, and 0.5 in white women.[2a] Most series have reported that thoracic dissection is twofold to threefold more frequent in men than in women, although one population-based study from Sweden found that mortality from dissection had equivalent incidence in men and women.[2b] Although thoracic aortic dissection has been reported in patients as young as 13 years of age, it rarely occurs before age 50 years, after which time it increases dramatically in incidence.[1] It typically occurs 10 years earlier in men (median age, 69 years) than in women (median age, 76 years).[2b]

Most investigators had agreed for several decades that clinical presentation, prognosis, and therapeutic choices depend largely on the site and extent of aortic dissection.[3-18] Aortic dissection involves the proximal (ascending) aorta in roughly two thirds of patients, and in the other one third of patients, dissection is limited to the descending thoracic/thoracoabdominal aorta. A significant number of untreated patients who experience dissection of the descending thoracic aorta die within a year from aortic rupture or, more specifically, from branch vessel occlusion, although they have a distinctly better overall prognosis than patients with proximal aortic dissection.[1]

This chapter reviews the classification, anatomy, natural history, clinical presentation, and diagnosis as well as contemporary management and results of dissection of the descending thoracic aorta.

CLASSIFICATION

Acuity

Conventionally, aortic dissections are classified as acute if patients are seen within 14 days after the onset of symp-

toms, and as chronic if they are seen beyond 14 days.[9] The reason for this distinction is that the risk of life-threatening complications (especially rupture) is greatest in the first days following dissection.[19] De Bakey and colleagues[8] proposed an intermediate group of subacute dissection cases that are seen between 2 weeks and 2 months to take into account the persistence of extremely friable, inflammatory aortic tissues well beyond the first two weeks. However, most authors consider this distinction to be unnecessary.

Anatomy

Although classification systems based on the site of the aortic intimal tear have been described,[12, 20] most investigators have found that these have little clinical relevance and use one of two classification systems based on the extent of aortic dissection (Fig. 93–1).

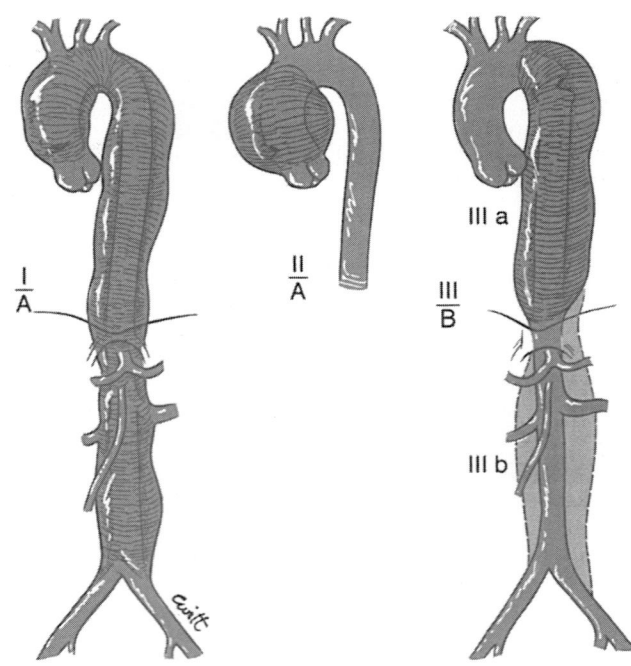

FIGURE 93–1. Anatomic classifications of aortic dissection. Shown are types I, II, and III as used in the DeBakey classification (see DeBakey ME, Henly WS, Cooley DA, et al: Surgical management of dissecting aneurysms of the aorta. J Thorac Cardiovasc Surg 19:130–149, 1965) and types A and B as used in the Stanford classification system. (From Daily PO, Trueblood HW, Stinson EB, et al: Management of acute aortic dissections. Ann Thorac Surg 10:237–247, 1970. Reprinted with permission from the Society of Thoracic Surgeons.)

TABLE 93–1. CLASSIFICATION SYSTEMS OF AORTIC DISSECTION

AUTHOR	YEAR	INSTITUTION	INVOLVEMENT OF ASCENDING AORTA Present	Absent
De Bakey et al[7]	1965	Baylor University	Types I and II	Type III
Applebaum et al[3]	1967	University of Alabama	Ascending	Descending
Daily et al[6]	1970	Stanford University	Type A	Type B
Slater and DeSanctis[22]	1976	Massachusetts General Hospital	Proximal	Distal
Meng et al[23]	1981	Rush Medical College	Anterior	Posterior

The best known and probably most widely used system is the one described by DeBakey and colleagues[7] in 1965, which distinguishes three types of aortic dissection:

- *Type I* dissection, involving the ascending aorta and a variable extent on the descending thoracic or thoracoabdominal aorta
- *Type II* dissection, limited to the ascending aorta
- *Type III* dissection, involving the descending thoracic aorta without (*type IIIa*) or with (*type IIIb*) extension to the abdominal aorta

Although not widely accepted, further subdivision by Reul and colleagues[21] of DeBakey type III dissection into four subgroups has the merit of emphasizing the possibility of retrograde dissection to the proximal aorta from an intimal tear in the descending thoracic aorta.

In 1970, Daily and colleagues[6] proposed a simpler classification of acute dissection known as the Stanford classification system, which differentiates type A dissection involving the ascending aorta and type B with no involvement of the ascending aorta. Type I and type II dissections of the DeBakey classification correspond to Stanford type A, whereas type III of the DeBakey classification corresponds to Stanford type B. Other classification systems based on the extent of aortic dissection[3, 22, 23] have been proposed using different terminology, but involvement of the ascending aorta remains the main criterion of classification (Table 93–1). Because they were established at a time when surgery for aortic dissection was limited to prosthetic replacement of limited portions of the ascending or descending thoracic aorta, these classification systems ignore the occasional "non-A non-B" dissection extending retrograde to involve or arising from the transverse aortic arch[24, 25] while sparing the ascending aorta.

This chapter uses the conventional DeBakey classification system. I shall not discuss the surgical management of dissection involving the aortic arch and dissecting aneurysms of the descending thoracic aorta developing late after surgery of the ascending aorta in patients with type I dissection.

ANATOMY OF LESIONS

Although dissection can result from an intramural hematoma with no connection to the aortic lumen,[26–31] most dissections have an entry site because of a localized intimal tear, and one or more reentry sites, allowing blood to circulate between the normal aortic lumen (true lumen) and the abnormal channel formed by the dissected zone (false lumen).[32] The inner lining of the aorta separating both lumina is referred to as the septum. The most common entry site in type III dissection is at the aortic isthmus. Location in the middle (Fig. 93–2) or lower part of the descending aorta is much less common, and location in the abdominal aorta is exceedingly rare.[33] Although it is usually transverse, the intimal tear can be round, straight, or curved. It does not generally involve the complete circumference of the aorta. At the level of the isthmus, it is usually limited to the upper aspect of the aorta, a few centimeters distal to the origin of the left subclavian artery.

Dissection can progress in retrograde fashion, antegrade fashion, or both. Progression usually takes place within seconds after the intimal tear, but delayed progression is possible, especially in patients with poorly controlled hy-

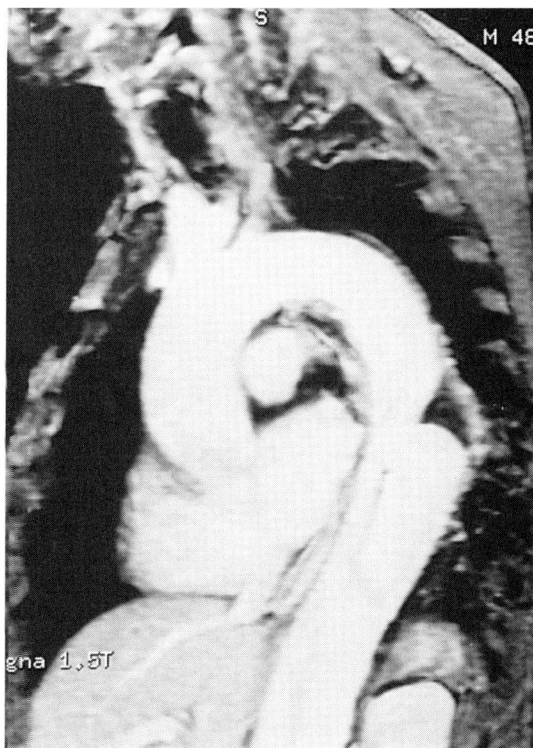

FIGURE 93–2. A magnetic resonance image demonstrating type III aortic dissection, with the entry site in the middle part of the descending thoracic aorta.

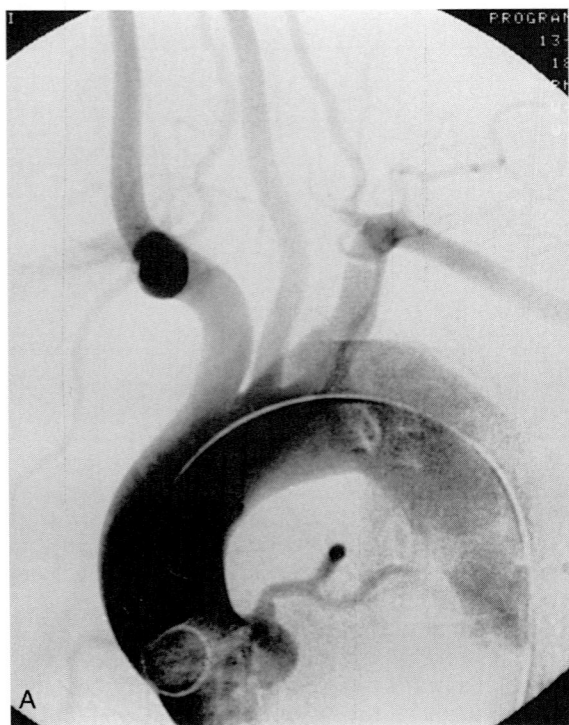
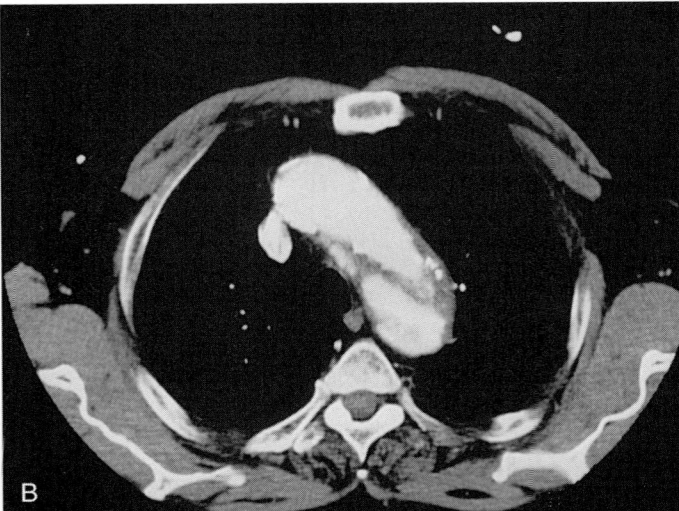

FIGURE 93–3. *A*, Aortography, *B*, computed tomography scanning demonstrating retrograde extension to the transverse aortic arch in a patient with type III aortic dissection.

pertension. Retrograde progression of type III aortic dissection is rarely more than a few centimeters, stopping at the origin of the left subclavian artery. However, retrograde extension involving the posterior aspect of the distal transverse aortic arch occurs in 10% to 15% of cases[5, 25] and poses a significant surgical challenge, especially since diagnosis using aortography (Fig. 93–3A), computed tomography (CT) scanning (Fig. 93–3B), or even transesophageal echocardiography (TEE) may be difficult.

Antegrade progression usually follows a spiral path involving between one half and two thirds of the left lateral aspect of the descending thoracic aorta. It is rarely limited to the upper part of the descending thoracic aorta. Dissection can stop at the diaphragm, where the aortic orifice has a stiff, fibrous consistency (type IIIa), but in most cases the whole abdominal aorta and even the iliac arteries are involved (type IIIb). Dissection may also stop immediately distal to the renal arteries in patients with preexisting degenerative infrarenal aortic aneurysms or previous aortic reconstruction.[34, 35] Dissection of the thoracoabdominal aorta usually involves the left posterolateral aspect of the aorta, with the visceral and right renal arteries branching from the true lumen and the left renal artery from the false lumen. Exit (reentry) sites may correspond to the ostia of disrupted collaterals (intercostal, lumbar, or visceral arteries) or occur at the distal end of dissection—that is, the aortic bifurcation, the iliac bifurcation, and even the femoral bifurcation. Flow rate in the false lumen is probably one of the main determining factors for rupture, ischemic complications, and thrombosis.

NATURAL HISTORY

The natural history of dissection of the ascending and descending aorta is different (Fig. 93–4). It is generally acknowledged that the risk of early death is much greater for type I and II than for type III dissections which tend to have a more chronic course.[3–18] In contrast to proximal aortic dissection, type III dissection is not associated with the major risks of intrapericardial rupture, acute aortic insufficiency, or occlusion of the coronary arteries. Although the dismal early and late evolution of types I and II aortic dissection have been underlined in most reports, knowledge about the natural history of type III dissection is still incomplete. Most data come from early clinical or autopsy studies,[14, 36–39] since observations made after current medical treatment can hardly be considered as indicative of the natural course of the disease.

As a rule, the potential complications of acute as well as chronic type III aortic dissection combine those of aneurysmal aortic disease with those of occlusive disease of the aortic branches.

Acute Dissection

The main risks of acute type III aortic dissection are rupture and ischemic complications. Both are usually lethal, accounting for mortality rates of up to 30% in the acute phase of dissection[14] unless successful emergency treatment is applied.

Rupture

Although the adventitia is the most resistant layer of the aorta, the incidence of rupture of the false lumen is high. Predisposing factors for rupture include poorly controlled hypertension, high flow rate within the false lumen, absence or small size of the reentry site(s), and increase in aortic diameter.

The usual configuration of the entry site and false lumen explains why most ruptures complicating acute type III

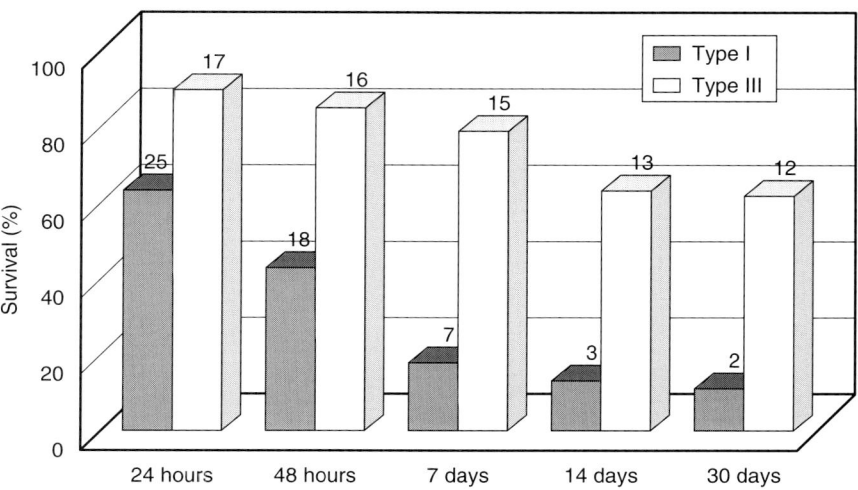

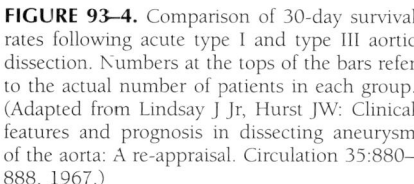

FIGURE 93–4. Comparison of 30-day survival rates following acute type I and type III aortic dissection. Numbers at the tops of the bars refer to the actual number of patients in each group. (Adapted from Lindsay J Jr, Hurst JW: Clinical features and prognosis in dissecting aneurysm of the aorta: A re-appraisal. Circulation 35:880–888, 1967.)

dissections occur in the left pleural cavity.[19, 32] Because of associated rupture of the pleura, massive hemothorax ensues, and death is usually prompt. This evolution is in distinct contrast to the more benign course of progressive and generally low-volume hemothorax due to transudation through the intact adventitia and pleura. Rupture can also occur into the mediastinum, the right pleural cavity, the retroperitoneal space, or the peritoneal cavity. A few cases have been reported involving rupture into the pericardial cavity, the esophagus, the tracheobronchial tree, and the lung.

Ischemic Complications

Ischemic complications are common in patients presenting with acute type III dissection involving the abdominal aorta (type IIIb).[5, 19, 40–42] In some cases, ischemic manifestations may be the main clinical and prognostic features (Fig. 93–5). Any branch of the descending thoracic and abdominal aorta as well as the aorta itself can be affected, and a variety of mechanisms can be involved.

Occurrence of high-grade stenosis or occlusion of the dissected aorta is rarely due to detachment of an intimal flap distal to an extensive intimal tear. If the tear is circumferential, intussusception of the intima can cause aortic obstruction.[43] In most cases, however, aortic obstruction is due to compression of the true lumen by the false lumen (Fig. 93–6)[44] and is usually located at the thoracoabdominal junction.[45] In such cases, an acute, coarctation-like process can lead to proximal hypertension, with an enhanced risk of rupture and distal ischemia affecting the spinal cord, kidneys, digestive tract, and lower extremities. Spontaneous resolution can occur if a reentry site of sufficient size develops and flow is reestablished to the abdoman and lower extremities. If this does not occur, therapeutic choices include surgical replacement of the descending thoracic aorta with reconstruction of the distal true lumen or creation of a reentry by fenestration of the septum separating the two lumina.

Although narrowing of the abdominal branches of the aorta and the iliofemoral arteries is often due to compression of the true lumen by the false lumen at the origin of the vessel, other mechanisms can be observed (Fig. 93–7).[5, 40, 46] Dissection can extend into the artery, resulting in a

reduction of the lumen. Dissection can disrupt the aortic intima at the origin of the artery and result in a waving intimal flap that blocks flow into the artery. Regardless of the mechanism, arterial stenosis can be complicated by extensive thrombosis, with further reduction in the patency of the lumen.

Occurrence of ischemia symptoms due to occlusion of the aortic branches depends on the degree of obstruction, the duration of ischemia, the availability of sufficient collateral circulation, and the susceptibility of the organ system

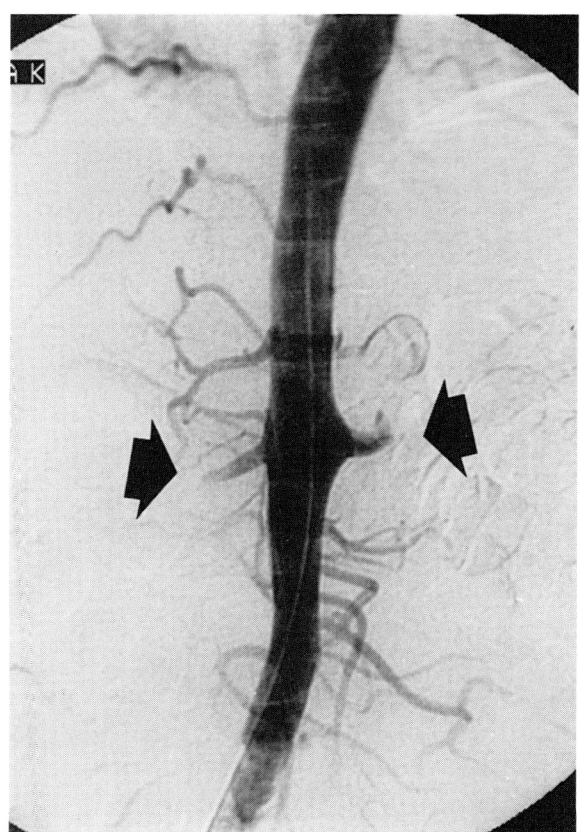

FIGURE 93–5. Aortogram showing bilateral renal artery occlusion (arrows) causing sudden anuria in a patient with a painless, acute type III aortic dissection.

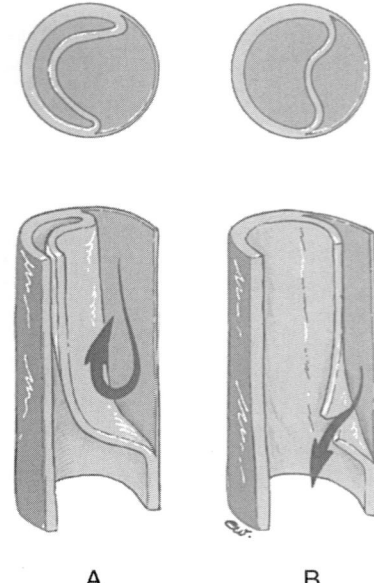

FIGURE 93–6. *A,* Aortic obstruction due to compression of the true lumen by the false lumen. *B,* Spontaneous resolution may occur if a reentry site of sufficient size develops, allowing reestablishment of flow to the abdomen and lower extremities.

or extremity to ischemia. This multifactorial etiology probably explains the discrepancy between the incidences of aortic branch lesions reported in autopsy and clinical studies.

In the autopsy series of Hirst and colleagues,[19] in which most patients died from rupture, aortic dissection involving

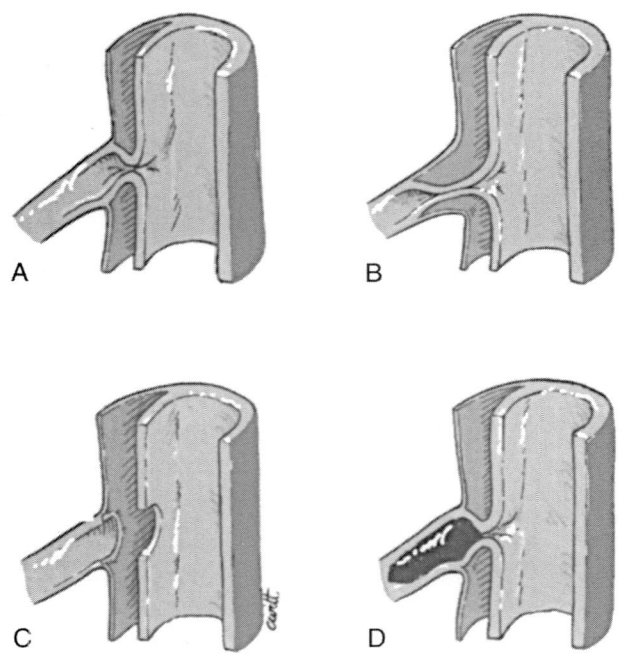

FIGURE 93–7. Occlusion of aortic branches may be due to compression of the true lumen by the false lumen at the origin of the artery *(A),* extension of dissection into the artery *(B),* disruption of the aortic intima at the origin of the artery *(C),* or extensive arterial thrombosis *(D).*

the abdominal aorta was associated with lesions of the visceral arteries in 27.7% of cases and with lesions involving the arteries supplying the lower extremities in 26.1% of cases. In the clinical series of Cambria and associates,[40] the corresponding incidences were only 8.7% and 11.7%, respectively. The increasing use of TEE may be an explanation for lower estimates in recent clinical reports since this diagnostic procedure does not examine the abdominal aorta and its branches.[47] Likewise, CT scanning and magnetic resonance imaging (MRI) are less sensitive for peripheral vascular lesions than is aortography.

Clinical symptoms depend on the affected organ. Spinal cord ischemia can lead to paraplegia, paraparesis, and partial neurologic deficits such as Brown-Séquard syndrome or isolated sphincter disturbances. These manifestations are uncommon but usually irreversible. Ischemia of the lower extremities is also uncommon. It is usually limited to a loss of one or both femoral pulses. Loss of pulse in the left upper extremity is also possible after retrograde extension of type III dissection or compression of the left subclavian artery by the aortic false lumen.[41] Ischemia involving the digestive tract may be associated with minor or no symptoms if only one of the main visceral arteries (celiac artery or superior mesenteric artery) is affected. However, since limited involvement is uncommon, intestinal infarction is a major life-threatening complication that may warrant exploratory laparotomy before or after replacement of the proximal aorta in suspicious cases.

Renal ischemia can also be asymptomatic if the arterial lesion is unilateral and function of the contralateral kidney is normal. Interpretation of hypertension or renal insufficiency in patients with acute dissection can be confounded by a number of factors, including the preexisting status of the kidneys and renal arteries and the renal effects of hypotensive drugs administered to prevent aortic rupture. Cardiopulmonary bypass used during reconstruction of the proximal aorta also may interfere with the visceral or renal circulation.

Chronic Dissection

Following initial medical management, most patients with acute type III aortic dissection survive long enough to reach the chronic phase of the disease. On the other hand, emergency surgical treatment of aortic dissection is usually palliative since complete removal of the dissected aorta is rarely possible. As a result, careful surveillance is necessary in all patients to avoid the risk of late aneurysm formation and aortic rupture.

Aneurysm Formation

Several cases of spontaneous cure of type III aortic dissection, documented by CT scanning, have been reported in the literature. However, these cases are rare and have always involved patients with complete thrombosis of the false lumen and moderate aortic dilatation. In nearly 85% of cases, the false lumen remains at least partially patent.[48] The risk of progressive dilatation of the false lumen leading to aneurysm formation has been estimated to be about 35%.[49]

Aneurysm formation is usually limited to either the upper part of the descending thoracic aorta opposite the entry site or the infrarenal abdominal aorta. The rate of expansion of dissecting thoracic aortic aneurysms has been studied only recently. Dapunt and associates[50] reported on 17 patients with chronic type III aortic dissection studied by serial CT scanning with 3-dimensional (3-D) reconstruction. The mean increase in diameter was 0.59 cm/year while the probably more relevant increase in volume was 94.1 ml/year. Evaluation of the risk of rupture and appropriate surgical indications will benefit from additional studies such as these in the future. In most cases, aneurysms involving the infrarenal abdominal aorta probably occur in patients with preexisting degenerative lesions of the media. Less often, aortic dilatation progresses to extensive thoracoabdominal aneurysm.

Aneurysm formation accounts for the risk of late rupture, which has been described as a major cause of late mortality following dissection of the descending thoracic aorta.[14, 19, 32, 36–38, 50] Complete thrombosis of the false lumen, once considered a favorable prognostic factor,[51, 52] does not protect against rupture since the diseased aorta may redissect or follow the same evolution as a degenerative aneurysm.[53, 54]

Ischemic Complications

When initial ischemia has been transient or partial because of adequate collateral circulation, aortic branches involved in acute dissection can remain patent beyond proximal occlusive lesions. This can lead to chronic ischemia, with intermittent claudication of the lower extremities, intestinal angina, renovascular hypertension, or ischemic renal insufficiency.[40–42] These ischemic complications are often, but not always, associated with aneurysm formation.

CLINICAL PRESENTATION AND DIAGNOSIS

Acute Dissection

In most patients with acute type III aortic dissection, onset of dissection is marked by a sudden, unexpected, intense, sometimes excruciating pain typically located in the interscapular area and rapidly migrating to the lower back, abdomen, or both.[22, 55] Pain may subside for a few hours or days, only to recur as a chronic, localized pain presumably due to distention of the false lumen, or as a more distal pain, caused by progression of the dissecting process.[1] Any unexplained chest pain, especially when associated with back or abdominal pain, in a middle-aged or elderly patient with a history of hypertension[55] should raise the suspicion of an aortic dissection in addition to other causes such as myocardial ischemia, expanding or ruptured aortic aneurysm, and penetrating atherosclerotic ulcer.[56–60] Painless dissection is unusual[61] except in patients undergoing corticosteroid therapy. It may be revealed by isolated, acute ischemia of the lower limb, kidney, intestine, or spinal cord, often resulting in diagnostic delay and sometimes inappropriate management until proper diagnosis is established. In rare patients, a delayed inflammatory syndrome with low-grade fever may be the only clinical manifestation of an acute aortic dissection.[62–64] Although it is inconstant and sometimes transitory, a pulse deficit in the lower limb, left upper extremity, or both may be helpful to increase the suspicion of a vascular problem.

Posteroanterior chest radiographs typically show enlargement of the aortic knob, sometimes with displacement of the calcified aortic intima inside the aortic shadow.[22, 55] Other suggestive findings include mediastinal widening, left pleural effusion, downward displacement of the left main bronchus, and deviation to the right of a nasogastric tube. A negative chest radiograph or equivocal findings, however, are seen in up to 20% of patients with acute type III dissection and should not rule out the diagnosis in the presence of other suggestive symptoms.[55, 65]

During the past decade, TEE has emerged as the most practical diagnostic modality in the emergency evaluation of patients with suspected aortic dissection.[52, 66–68] This safe, noninvasive technique is readily available in many centers. It has very good sensitivity and specificity when compared with aortography,[69] allowing rapid diagnosis of aortic dissection, including intramural hematoma without a detectable intimal tear,[70] and determination of whether or not the ascending aorta is involved. In some community hospitals, however, the only available option may be CT scanning, which is also acceptable as an emergency diagnostic procedure.[68] Although it has been used extensively in some centers,[69] MRI is not always available on an emergency basis and may not be desirable in unstable patients requiring close monitoring.[1, 68]

Any of these diagnostic modalities provides sufficient data to operate on a patient with impending rupture or acute expansion of the descending thoracic or thoracoabdominal aorta. However, most patients with acute type III aortic dissection will be stabilized initially with medical treatment. Whether or not ischemic symptoms occur in the first few days following admission, it has been the practice of my group and other groups[31] to perform aortography in most patients in order to evaluate visceral perfusion as well as possible retrograde extension to the transverse aortic arch. Aortography is also routinely performed in patients with indications for secondary aortic replacement or endovascular procedures. It should include the entire aorta and branches, and this usually calls for separate catheterization of both true and false lumina.[44, 71–75]

Chronic Dissection

Although large, expanding, chronic dissecting aneurysms may be responsible for chronic pain or compression of adjacent thoracic or abdominal structures, the chronic type III aortic dissection of many patients will remain clinically silent until rupture. Diagnosis is typically made during investigation of an abnormal chest radiograph or a pulsatile abdominal mass. Chronic ischemia due to branch involvement, as manifested by intermittent claudication, renovascular hypertension, renal insufficiency, or abdominal angina, is infrequent.

More often in recent years, aortic surveillance by CT scanning or MRI has demonstrated progressive, clinically silent enlargement of the false lumen and eventual aneurysm formation in patients treated medically in the acute phase of a type III aortic dissection, allowing consideration of elective surgery.

SURGICAL TECHNIQUES

A wide range of surgical techniques have been proposed for management of type III aortic dissection. Some are directed at the aortic lesion itself, some at the ischemic complications, and some at both lesions and complications. These methods can be used singly or in combination. In most cases, only palliative repair is possible due to the extent of dissection or the high risks of complete aortic replacement during the acute phase.

Graft Replacement

The optimal goals of aortic replacement, especially in patients with acute type III aortic dissection, are as follows:

1. Removing the most threatening area.
2. Closing the entry site of the dissection
3. Maintaining or reestablishing blood flow in the distal aorta and its branches.

The upper part of the descending thoracic aorta is the most frequently replaced segment in type III aortic dissection. In such limited operations, the risk of spinal cord ischemia is low, provided that blood supply to the distal aorta is satisfactorily maintained intraoperatively.[5, 76–78] In patients with an extensive aneurysm involving the lower part of the descending thoracic aorta, total replacement of the descending thoracic aorta may be necessary. Construction of the lower anastomosis near the diaphragm can require thoracoabdominal incision. Although rarely indicated in patients with acute aortic dissection, replacement of the entire thoracoabdominal aorta, using Crawford's inclusion graft technique,[79] is often indicated in patients with chronic dissection since these lesions usually lead to formation of Crawford type I and II thoracoabdominal aneurysms.

Limited aortic replacement may also be indicated for lesions of the infrarenal aorta (rupture, expansion, or aneurysm)[80] but also during fenestration to reestablish circulation to the branches of the aorta. In rare cases, replacement of the entire abdominal aorta is performed in combination with reimplantation of the visceral arteries directly or via an autogenous or prosthetic graft in order to treat visceral and/or renal ischemia.[81]

Replacement of the descending thoracic or thoracoabdominal aorta in patients with type III aortic dissection poses several technical problems. Preservation of the blood supply to the spinal cord and digestive tract is not a problem specific to management of aortic dissection. Extensive discussion of the indications and advantages of the various methods used for distal aortic perfusion is beyond the scope of this chapter. However, it should be emphasized that replacement of a dissected descending thoracic or thoracoabdominal aorta is a delicate procedure in which clamping time is unpredictable and often longer than in operations for degenerative aneurysms.

Svensson and associates[82] reported a high incidence (up to 24%) of spinal cord complications associated with simple aortic cross-clamping during thoracoabdominal aortic replacement for extensive dissecting aneurysm. The efficacy of distal aortic perfusion in protecting the spinal cord, kidneys, and digestive tract has been well documented.[77, 83] Distal perfusion also provides more effective decompression of the proximal aorta than pharmacologic manipulation during simple aortic cross-clamping. Decompression is important to avoid clamp injury, aortic rupture, or both during clamping.

The choice of distal aortic perfusion technique depends on personal preference. Excellent clinical results have been obtained using an in-line Gott shunt[78] or a left atriofemoral shunt with a centrifugal pump.[76, 83, 84] Despite the need for high-dose heparinization, the preference of my group is for partial cardiopulmonary bypass (femoral vein or pulmonary artery to femoral artery).[11, 12, 15, 17, 85] The main advantages of partial cardiopulmonary bypass[17] are:

1. Its ability to allow circulatory assistance before opening the chest and retrieval of blood in patients with intrapleural rupture.
2. Ensurance of maximal oxygenation by compensating for exclusion of the left lung.
3. Its easy convertibility to *total* cardiopulmonary bypass if necessary.

Regardless of the method of distal aortic perfusion used, there is a small but certain risk of intraoperative visceral and spinal cord ischemia due to selective perfusion of the false lumen in the absence of a reentry site beyond the distal aortic clamp. This risk must be borne in mind from the beginning of the operation so that an alternative arterial perfusion site can be chosen promptly if necessary. In some cases, perfusion of the distal aorta must be preceded by fenestration of the infrarenal aorta or, more conveniently, by graft replacement of the aortic bifurcation in combination with proximal fenestration. The left limb of the bifurcated graft can then be used for retrograde aortic perfusion.[86]

The poor quality of the aortic wall is a specific problem of surgical treatment of type III aortic dissection, in particular in patients presenting with acute dissection or dissection associated with preexisting conditions such as Marfan's syndrome. Aortoprosthetic anastomoses must be made after complete transection of the aorta[10, 87] in order to enable proper placement of sutures, including the aortic adventitia. Polytetrafluoroethylene (Teflon) pledgets are almost always used to reinforce the aortic edges and enable the anastomosis to withstand the shearing effect of each systolic thrust after clamp removal. Alternative suture reinforcement techniques recommended by other groups include application of glutaraldehyde[88] or fibrin glue on the transected edges of the aorta before suturing the graft, aortic banding with a (polyester) Dacron tube graft in the immediate vicinity of both anastomoses,[89] and adventitial inversion.[90]

Construction of the proximal anastomosis in a healthy zone is important to successful repair and nearly always feasible. If dissection extends beyond the limit of resection, which is usually the case distally, two anastomotic techniques can be used, depending on whether the dissection is acute or chronic (Fig. 93–8). In patients with acute dissection, dilatation of the aorta is moderate, and the two

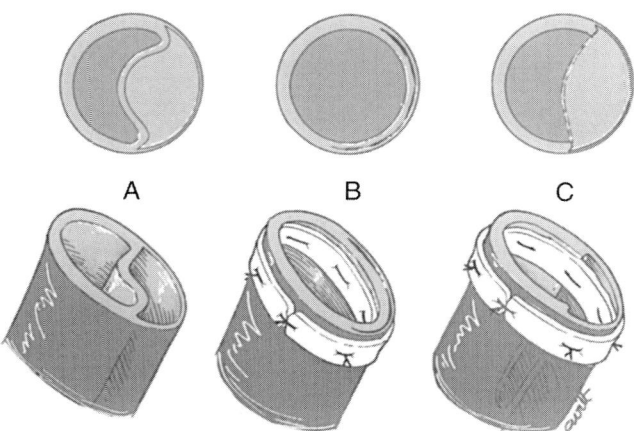

FIGURE 93–8. Graft anastomosis to the dissected distal aorta (A) may be performed using one of two techniques: Following reassembly of the two lumina, directing flow into the true lumen (B), or following fenestration of the septum immediately below the future anastomosis (C), directing flow into both lumina.

lumina can be reassembled, closing the false lumen and maintaining or reestablishing satisfactory flow through the true lumen. In patients with chronic dissection and a patent false lumen, the preferred technique consists of fenestration of the septum immediately below the future anastomosis, followed by graft anastomosis to the two lumina in order to insure that both remain patent. In this regard it should be understood that the false lumen often feeds one or more visceral or renal arteries, and diverting flow only into the true lumen would compromise supply to these arteries.

Another important precaution for successful outcome of surgical repair of aortic dissection is to avoid aortic injury during clamp placement. Although complete transection of the dissected aorta has been reported following clamp placement,[91] the most frequent clamp-induced aortic lesion is an intimal tear, which can have serious consequences. In patients with acute dissection, occurrence of an intimal tear distal to the distal anastomosis rules out any prospect of reassembly of the two lumina. As in surgical repair of dissection involving the ascending aorta, distal aortic clamping can be avoided easily by using the "open" anastomosis technique. This is done by temporarily discontinuing distal aortic perfusion after construction of the proximal anastomosis and dividing the distal aorta beyond the distal aortic clamp before constructing the distal anastomosis.

An intimal tear involving the aortic arch after clamp placement between the common carotid and left subclavian arteries also can lead to dire complications. Retrograde dissection is nearly always rapidly fatal (Fig. 93–9), [4, 15, 21, 78] unless deep hypothermia can be quickly instituted to achieve circulatory arrest and repair of the proximal aorta.[92, 93] At best, an intimal tear involving the aortic arch will lead only to formation of a juxta-anastomotic false aneurysm and require reoperation. The use of ringed prosthetic grafts has been fraught with technical difficulties and has not eliminated anastomotic problems.

With these clamp-related complications in mind, our group and others[94–97] have advocated performing surgical correction of type III aortic dissection under elective deep hypothermic circulatory arrest (Fig. 93–10). This technique

provides a blood-free operative field and allows precise aortic repair without clamping. Another important advantage of this technique is to allow better protection of the spinal cord during aortic clamping.[98] However, the etiology of spinal cord complications after surgery on the thoracoabdominal aorta is multifactorial, and deep hypothermia is not a panacea. Before undertaking surgery for chronic type III aortic dissection, we routinely perform selective preoperative arteriography of the intercostal and lumbar arteries to map spinal circulation so that we can preserve or reimplant critical arteries during surgery.[99]

Aortoplasty

In view of the high operative mortality associated with aortic replacement, various investigators have proposed more conservative aortic repairs. A variety of techniques have been described, but the common feature shared by all is suture of the intimal tear at the entry site. Reassembly of the two lumina is achieved in different ways.

Several years ago, Berger[100] revived the old transverse suture technique that had been used previously by several operators.[16, 77, 101–103] Tanabe and associates[104] proposed injection of Ivalon into the false lumen to induce thrombosis. More recently, Kawashima and colleagues[105] and Williams[106] described the so-called "tailored aortoplasty" technique designed to avoid graft replacement of the distal descending thoracic aorta and proximal abdominal aorta and thus minimize spinal cord complications associated with extensive aortic replacement. In 1989, Fabiani and associates[107] reported one case of "glue aortoplasty" in which early follow-up aortography was normal. Experience with these techniques is limited, and long-term results have not been clearly documented.

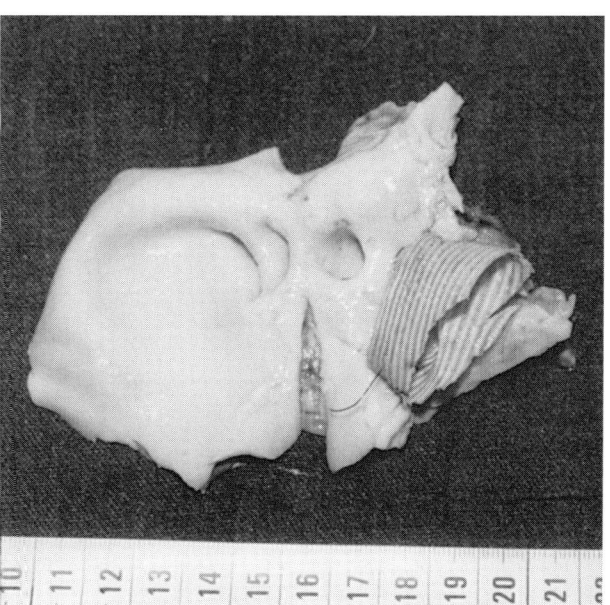

FIGURE 93–9. Clamp injury to the distal transverse aortic arch causing lethal intraoperative retrograde dissection and rupture of the proximal aorta.

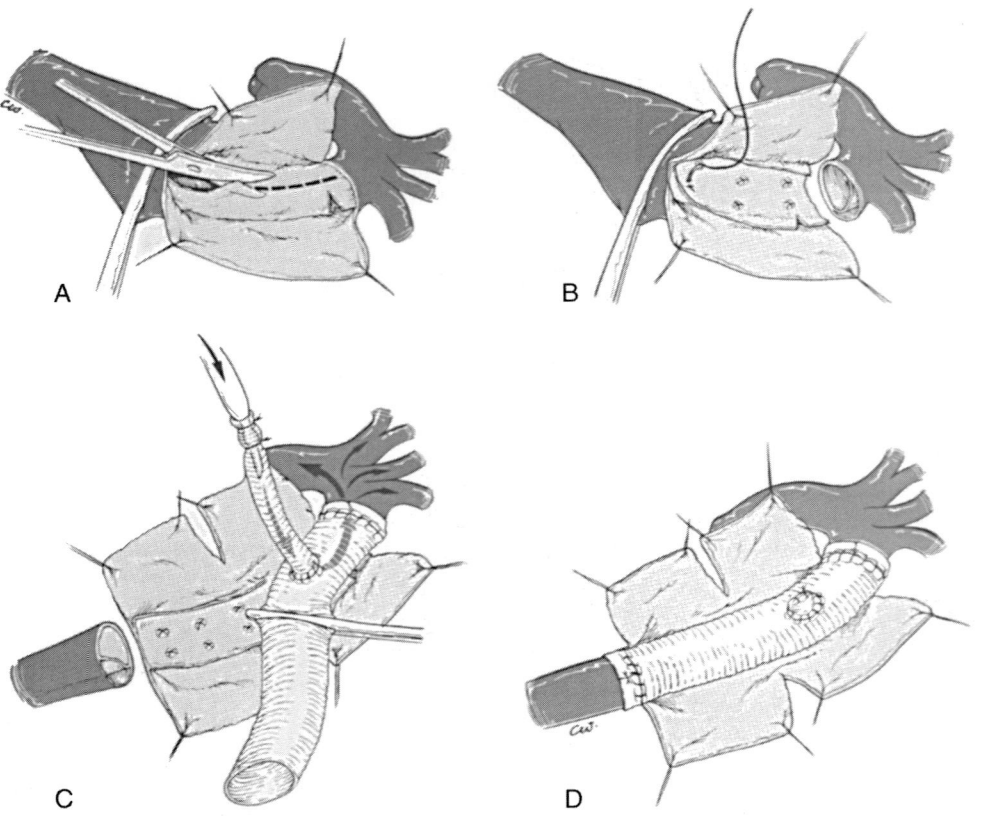

FIGURE 93–10. *A–D,* Graft replacement of the upper portion of the descending thoracic aorta under deep hypothermic circulatory arrest.

Thromboexclusion

Thromboexclusion, as described by Carpentier[108] in 1979, is based on a different principle from that of aortic replacement (Fig. 93–11). The first stage of the procedure consists of placing a prosthetic bypass graft between the ascending and abdominal aorta via median sternolaparotomy. The second stage consists of interrupting the aorta distal to the left subclavian artery. The true and false lumina are reassembled as a result of the reversed flow in the upper abdominal and descending thoracic aorta. The proximal part of the descending thoracic aorta, including the site of entry and the most proximal portion of the dissected aorta, are excluded by progressive thrombosis, theoretically with minimal risk for the blood supply to the spinal cord.

Although several investigators have used this new technique with reasonably good clinical results,[109–112] its apparent simplicity has been deceptive. The special metal clamp used by Carpentier and colleagues[109] to achieve aortic interruption is the source of several difficulties. The first is placement. Exposure of the aorta distal to the left subclavian artery is often difficult and entails a low but certain risk of injury to the proximal part of the false lumen.[110, 111] Another problem is clamp migration, which can lead to compression of the left subclavian artery[109] or pulmonary artery. Clamp-induced aortic lesions can lead to fatal complications owing to retrograde aortic dissection.[113]

To avoid these complications, some investigators have proposed using sutures[114] or staples[112] in association with Dacron or Teflon pledgets instead of the clamp. Moreover, all investigators agree that interruption should be carried out on a flaccid aorta, which can be obtained either by proximal clamping, administration of hypotensive drugs, or brief cardiac inflow occlusion by clamping of both venae cavae. Some investigators have also proposed interruption of the aorta between the left common carotid and subclavian arteries, but this raises the need either for bypass from the ascending aorta–abdominal aorta bypass to the

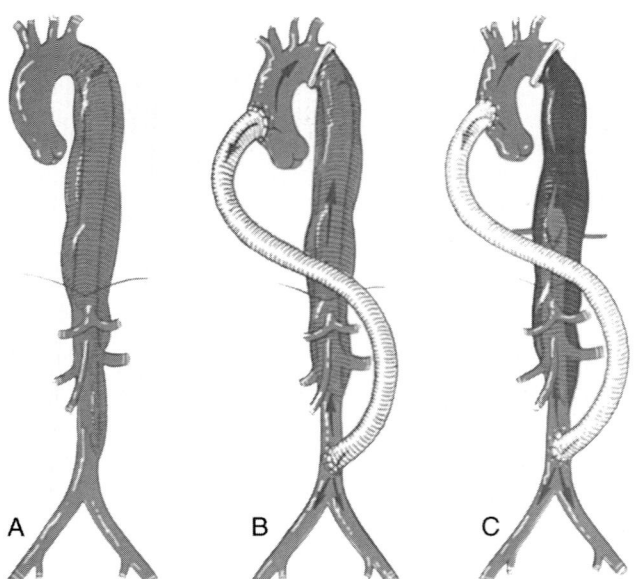

FIGURE 93–11. *A–C,* Thromboexclusion technique for type III aortic dissection.

subclavian artery[112] or for transposition of the subclavian artery into the common carotid artery.[114]

The main issues raised by the thromboexclusion technique involve its risk and efficacy. In comparison with aortic replacement, thromboexclusion reduces but does not rule out the risk of aortic rupture[80] or spinal cord complications.[110–112] Moreover, there are no large series with sufficient follow-up to document the long-term fate of the aortic lesions left in place. To avoid late aneurysmal formation involving the descending thoracic aorta, Robicsek[115] and our group[114] tried a variant technique, including complete interruption of the distal thoracic aorta either during the same procedure via the same anterior approach used for ascending aorta–abdominal aorta bypass or during a second procedure via left thoracotomy a few days later. However, we stopped using this technique several years ago since we found it as complicated and risky as aortic replacement.

"Elephant Trunk" Technique

The elephant trunk technique, as described by Borst and associates in 1983,[116] is widely used in the surgical management of extensive chronic thoracic aortic aneurysms, including type I aortic dissections,[31, 117, 118] because it has the distinct advantage of avoiding the potential technical difficulties and risks of the proximal anastomosis during second-stage graft replacement of the descending thoracic aorta. It has recently been proposed in the management of type III aortic dissection.[96, 119–122]

The technique is rather straightforward (Fig. 93–12). With use of a median sternotomy incision and deep hypothermic circulatory arrest, it is a relatively easy and quick matter to insert a prosthetic graft in the descending thoracic aorta and anchor it in a healthy portion of its proximal part. This can be accomplished using a longitudinal incision in the aortic arch[121] or, preferably, a transection of the aortic isthmus or distal transverse aortic arch.[96] The distal part of a 10- to 15-cm-long prosthetic graft is then inserted into the descending thoracic aorta. In most acute dissections, the true lumen is large enough to accommodate the graft and restore normal distal aortic flow, provided the septum is kept intact and the false lumen is not perfused by large distal reentry sites.

Anatomic conditions are quite different in chronic dissection.[121] The true lumen is usually compressed by the false lumen and rendered undistensible by chronic fibrosis. Moreover, flow in one or several distal aortic branches may originate from the false lumen, making resection of the septum necessary for perfusion of both lumina. Proximal anchoring to the aortic isthmus or transverse aortic arch is performed either from within the aorta[121] or, preferably, following complete aortic transection, which allows safe, full-thickness anastomosis.[96, 122] Provided that the graft is long enough to overpass the entry site of the dissection and complete thrombosis of the nonaneurysmal false lumen has occurred, one may be tempted to avoid distal anchoring of the graft. However, whenever the distal false lumen remains even partially patent, distal anchoring with or without extension of the graft should be performed either surgically, using a posterolateral thoracotomy incision, or by endovascular techniques, using stenting or stent-grafting. The latter technique can be used intraoperatively, from the aortic arch, or in a second-stage procedure from within the femoral artery.

Although the elephant trunk technique is not applicable to patients with aortic rupture, is not entirely protective against spinal cord complications,[121] and has little long-term follow-up, it certainly deserves further evaluation in the management of acute type III aortic dissection. However, we have found few indications for the elephant trunk technique in chronic type III aortic dissection. In this setting, resection of the septum allowing persistent flow in the false lumen renders a second-stage operation necessary in all cases, whereas a one-stage operation can be performed safely using a left thoracotomy incision and deep hypothermic circulatory arrest, even in patients with an intimal tear in the transverse aortic arch.[95] Only in the unusual patient with an indication for a concomitant cardiac procedure would we consider using this technique in chronic type III aortic dissection.

Fenestration

Although fenestration is now only rarely mentioned in discussions of surgical techniques, it was the first surgical technique proposed for treatment of acute aortic dissection[123] and the first to achieve long-term survival in a patient.[124] The principle of fenestration is simple. It consists of creating a large reentry from the false lumen into the true lumen. The dissected aorta is exposed, clamped, and opened. The septum is then resected with scissors up to the proximal clamp and the aortotomy is closed.

From analyses of the spontaneous course of aortic dissection, it was initially speculated that equilibrating flow in

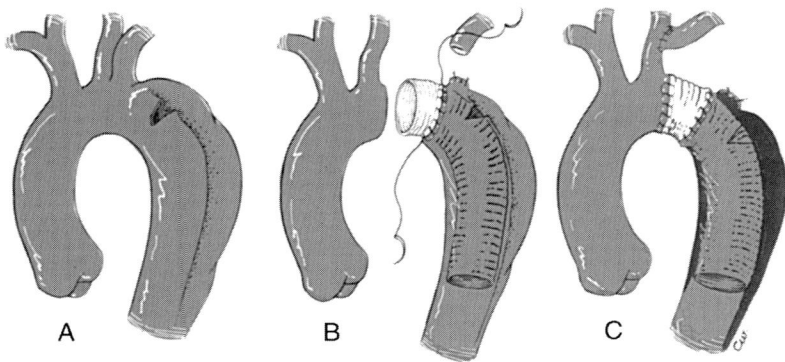

FIGURE 93–12. A–C, Elephant trunk technique for type III aortic dissection.

the two lumina would be a simple and effective means of avoiding aortic rupture. This hypothesis proved to be wrong, and we now know that the only way to prevent impending rupture is by aortic replacement. However, fenestration provides an effective means of treating the ischemic complications of aortic dissection by reestablishing flow to the collateral and terminal branches of the abdominal aorta (Fig. 93–13).[42, 45, 111, 125, 126] For this purpose, fenestration still has a place in the surgeon's arsenal of techniques for management of aortic dissection.

Elefteriades and colleagues[127] have described a simple technique for fenestration of the abdominal aorta. The infrarenal aorta is exposed by the retroperitoneal approach, clamped, and divided transversely in its midportion. The septum in the proximal segment is resected up to the proximal aortic clamp. The two lumina in the distal segment are reassembled, using a circular suture, and aortic continuity is reestablished by end-to-end anastomosis of the two aortic segments.

Like others,[5, 45, 128] my group prefers to perform fenestration via median laparotomy because this allows visual inspection of abdominal organs and bypass to any particular visceral or renal artery if the fenestration procedure fails to reestablish flow.[125] In this regard, it is important to emphasize that aortic fenestration cannot achieve effective revascularization in patients with extensive dissection, intimal flaps, or thrombosis of aortic branches.[5]

Additional problems associated with fenestration are that aorto-aortic anastomosis can be difficult, and leaving the infrarenal abdominal aorta unreplaced may lead to late aneurysm formation. For these reasons, our preference is to replace the infrarenal abdominal aorta.[80, 125] A tube graft is usually sufficient and has the advantage of facilitating anastomosis to the distal true lumen. However, use of a bifurcated graft with distal anastomoses to the iliac arteries or, more frequently, the femoral arteries may be indicated in patients presenting with distal thrombotic occlusion or preexisting atherosclerotic lesions as well as in cases in which reassembly of the two lumina in the distal aortic segment is either unfeasible or unreliable.

Some investigators have recommended clamping the supraceliac aorta to allow resection of the septum at the level of the visceral arteries.[5, 128–130] Our opinion is that this technique can be dangerous and is usually unnecessary, since resection of the infrarenal septum is nearly always sufficient to reestablish satisfactory retrograde flow in the aortic branches (Fig. 93–14).

Isolated Revascularization of Aortic Branches

In case of contraindications to or failure of fenestration, isolated revascularization of the branches of the aorta is an alternative. Since the donor artery ideally should be located proximal to dissection, some investigators have recommended long bypass either from the subclavian or axillary artery or from the ascending aorta. As a result, isolated revascularization of aortic branches may become a complicated technique, often with poor long-term patency rates. In most cases, the revascularization procedure can proceed from a nondissected iliac artery (crossover femorofemoral bypass, iliorenal bypass, or iliosuperior mesenteric bypass) or another visceral artery (renomesenteric or mesentericorenal bypass, left splenorenal or renosplenic anastomosis, or right hepatorenal or renohepatic bypass).[131] A prosthetic graft used for fenestration of the infrarenal abdominal aorta can serve as the origin of a bypass, especially if fenestration fails to achieve revascularization.[45, 125]

ENDOVASCULAR PROCEDURES

Like management of many types of vascular disease, treatment of aortic dissection has benefited from the introduction of endovascular techniques. Various endovascular procedures have been used for treatment of both the aortic lesions and ischemic complications. Two methods have been studied experimentally for endovascular treatment of aortic lesions: (1) stenting or stent-grafting,[132–138] and (2) placement of a balloon into the false lumen to close the entry site and promote thrombosis.[139]

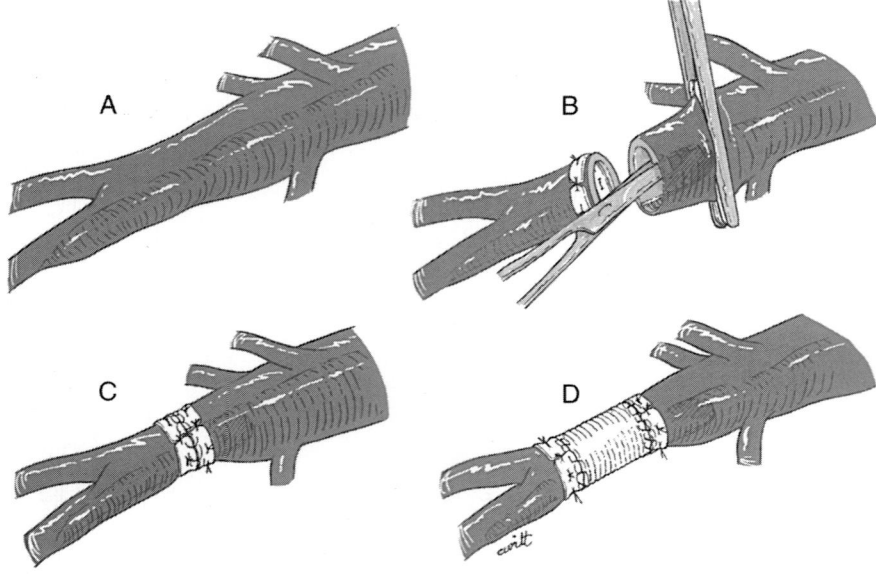

FIGURE 93–13. A–D, Surgical fenestration of infrarenal abdominal aorta for type III aortic dissection.

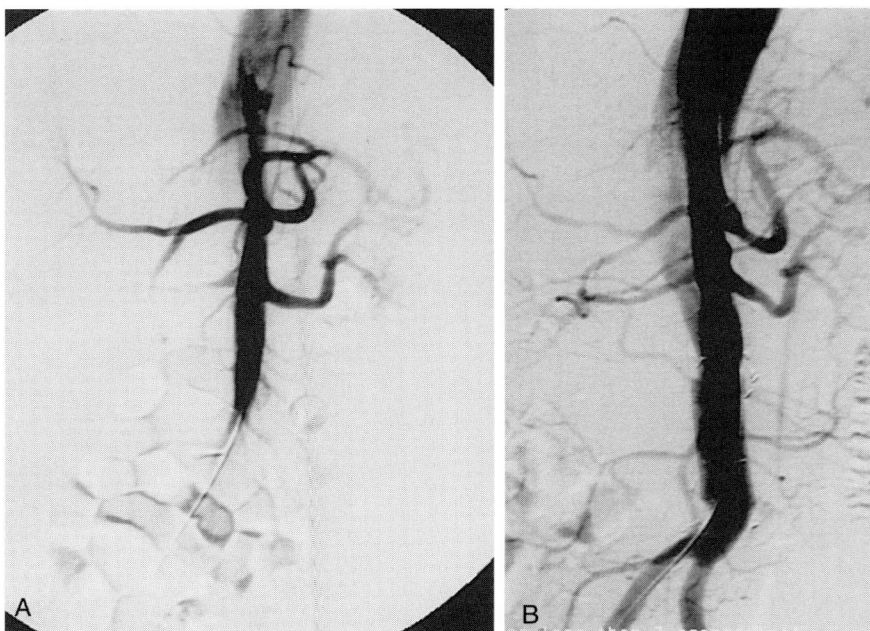

FIGURE 93–14. Preoperative (A) and postoperative (B) aortograms demonstrating revascularization of visceral branches following fenestration of the infrarenal abdominal aorta.

The clinical applicability of stent-grafting in the surgical management of dissection of the descending thoracic aorta is probably limited because of the usual mismatch between the limited elasticity of the dissection septum and the dimensions of the dilated false lumen,[75] especially in chronic dissection. Preliminary clinical experience with small numbers of patients has been reported from only two centers. Although analysis of their data concerning type III aortic dissection is somewhat confusing, the Stanford group[71, 140] has had at least one technical failure, followed by sudden death at 13 months. In the report by Inoue and associates[141] six patients had stent-grafting of type III aortic dissection, with three technical failures. Although technical improvements can be expected in the future, stent-grafting presently cannot be considered a standard option in the management of type III aortic dissection.

Endovascular techniques have been much more successful for treatment of the ischemic complications of aortic dissection. The Stanford group[44, 71, 72] has accumulated considerable experience with balloon fenestration (Fig. 93–15) and stenting of the thoracoabdominal aorta and its visceral branches. In their latest study,[71] they reported on 53 patients with 59 percutaneous procedures for the endovascular management of peripheral ischemic complications of aortic dissection. Technical complications (perinephric hematoma due to guidewire perforation of a distal renal branch, transient ischemic attack, and thrombosis of a stented renal artery) occurred in three patients, intestinal complications in four patients (including one death from peritonitis), and acute renal failure requiring hemodialysis in four patients (including three deaths from multiorgan failure). Overall 30-day mortality was 15% (eight patients). Delayed diagnosis probably accounted for persisting malfunction of the kidney, intestine, or both in several patients. In addition to the uncommonly high skills of the reporting radiology group, the main factors in achieving these excellent technical results were high-quality imaging facilities,

catheterization of both lumina, and intravascular manometry and ultrasonography.[47, 71–73] Careful preoperative evaluation is indeed necessary to identify the mechanism underlying ischemic complications and to choose the most suitable technique (i.e., fenestration of the dissection septum or aortic stenting if occlusion involves the aorta, and stenting of the branch if occlusion involves the branch itself).

INDICATIONS

Acute Dissection

Most agree that patients in whom type III acute aortic dissection is suspected or diagnosed should be given antihypertensive and negative inotropic treatment and kept under close clinical, hemodynamic, and radiologic surveillance in a surgical or cardiac intensive care unit, as originally described by Wheat and associates.[142] The main goal of initial assessment is to determine whether the ascending aorta is intact, since involvement of the ascending aorta would be an indication for immediate surgery. However, there is little agreement concerning the role of surgery in the management of acute type III aortic dissection.

Type of Approach

Three approaches have been proposed:

- Conservative treatment
- Routine elective surgery
- Intermediate approach

Conservative Approach

Most centers traditionally have adopted a conservative approach toward the management of acute type III aortic dissection, with surgery being performed only if there is

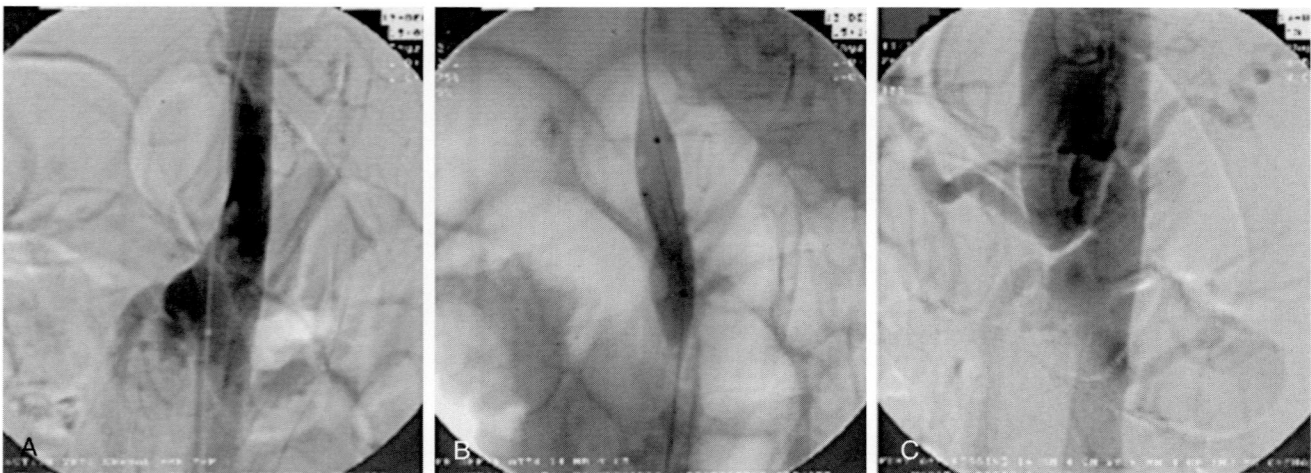

FIGURE 93–15. Aortograms demonstrating successful aortic balloon fenestration for intestinal ischemia owing to occlusion of aortic branches originating from the compressed true lumen.

demonstrable evidence of failure of medical therapy.[5, 11, 66, 77, 81, 102, 126, 127, 143–147] As summarized by Miller,[87, 148] this approach is based on three main assumptions:

1. Early death usually can be avoided by medical therapy.
2. Operative mortality is relatively high.
3. Long-term outcome is comparable after medical therapy and surgical treatment.

The main compulsory indications for surgery are rupture or expansion of the aorta; uncontrollable pain, hypertension, or both; successive chest radiographs showing progressive mediastinal enlargement, progressive hemothorax, or both; and occurrence of ischemic complications involving the digestive tract, kidneys, spinal cord, or lower extremities. With the conservative approach, most surgical procedures are performed under emergency conditions in unselected patients, and postoperative mortality rates above 50% are still reported.[11, 66, 103, 146] Limiting indications to surgery in such a selected group of poor-risk patients would also mean a higher incidence of rupture and reoperation in patients treated medically.

Routine Surgery

In contrast, the Stanford group[87, 148, 149] is recommending routine elective surgery in low-risk patients with type III acute aortic dissection. This rather aggressive attitude is based on reports showing a dramatic improvement in surgical results.[78, 82, 84, 145, 147, 155, 156] The main advantage of this approach is that procedures are performed under much more favorable conditions. The late prognosis in survivors is probably better, with fewer ruptures and reoperations.[148, 149] However, up to two thirds of patients with type III dissection are elderly and present cardiovascular, cerebrovascular, pulmonary, and renal problems.[18] Although these factors may not constitute absolute contraindications to surgery, they do worsen the postoperative prognosis (Fig. 93–16).[148, 150] Furthermore, this approach exposes some patients not at risk for aneurysm formation to unnecessary operative mortality and morbidity.

Intermediate Approach

The third approach, the one advocated by our group, is an intermediate approach between the conservative and surgical approach. It is intended to offer the best hope of

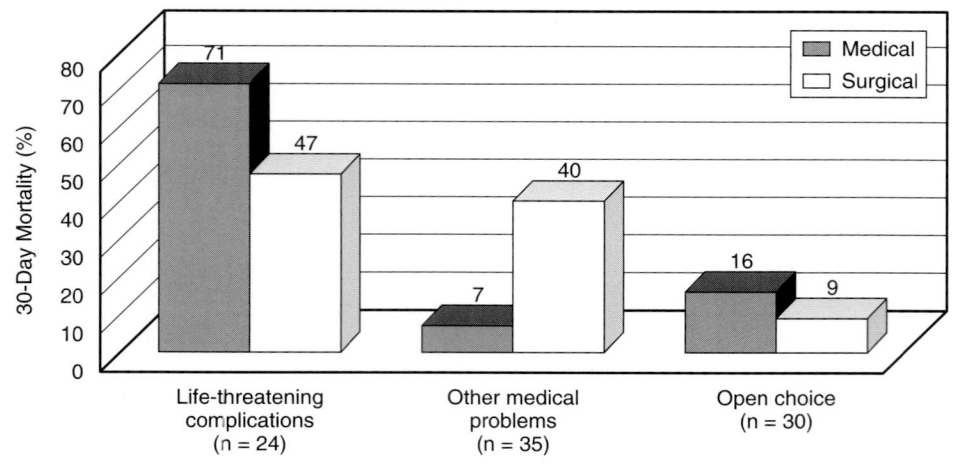

FIGURE 93–16. Comparison of 30-day mortality rates in three different groups of patients with acute type III aortic dissection who received either medical or surgical treatment. (Adapted from Miller DC: Acute dissection of the descending thoracic aorta. Chest Surg Clin North Am 2:347–378, 1992.)

avoiding uncontrollable late aortic complications while limiting the number of unnecessary early surgical procedures. This approach calls for an operation not only in patients presenting the previously mentioned compulsory indications but also in good-risk patients identified as being at risk for late rupture and aneurysm formation. Risk factors for rupture empirically accepted by most investigators include an aortic diameter greater than 5 cm, Marfan's disease or other connective tissue disorders, long-term corticosteroid therapy, and preexisting aortic abnormalities such as coarctation or pseudocoarctation of the aortic isthmus, aberrant subclavian artery, and dystrophic aneurysm.

Kato and colleagues[134] recently reported clinical data favoring indications for early surgery in selected low-risk patients with uncomplicated type III acute aortic dissection. With CT scans, they studied 41 patients with type III aortic dissection who had been successfully treated medically during the acute phase. Aortic enlargement was defined as:

- Maximum diameter of the dissected aorta 60 mm or more
- Rapid enlargement of the dissected aorta greater than 10 mm/year
- Rupture of the dissected aorta

Multivariate analysis identified two strongly significant predictors of late aortic enlargement: (1) a maximum aortic diameter of 40 mm or more during the acute phase and (2) a patent primary entry site in the thoracic aorta. No aortic enlargement was observed in the other patients. Provided the operative risk is low, these investigators advocate early surgery in this well-defined group of patients in order to avoid the added risks of rupture during medical therapy in the acute phase and a higher incidence of postoperative complications following surgery in the chronic phase.

Type of Procedure

Once the decision to operate has been made, the next question is what type of procedure should be used. The choice depends on the surgical indication. In patients presenting aortic complications (rupture, expansion, and aneurysm), direct exposure and aortic replacement are mandatory. The extent of emergency graft replacement should be as limited as possible. In most cases of acute type III aortic dissections, replacement can be limited to the upper part of the descending thoracic aorta or, more rarely, the infrarenal abdominal aorta.[80]

Management of ischemic complications is more controversial. Most cardiovascular surgeons recommend replacement of the proximal aorta as a reliable method of reestablishing flow to the branches of the aorta.[82, 149] With few exceptions, vascular surgeons have questioned the reliability of this technique[40] and argue that more conservative procedures, such as surgical fenestration of the abdominal aorta or current endovascular techniques, achieve the same results more economically. For patients undergoing elective surgical correction for uncomplicated acute aortic dissection, we feel that replacement of the proximal aorta, with removal of the site of entry and reassembly of the two lumina, using either a conventional left thoracotomy approach or the elephant trunk technique, is a more logical choice than thromboexclusion.

Whether or not surgery is performed during the acute phase of dissection, patients must be kept under strict, long-term surveillance. The first goal of therapy is control of hypertension, which is a statistically significant risk factor for aortic complications and late mortality.[8, 148] Even in normotensive patients, beta-blockers should be administered because of their demonstrated protective effect against aortic dilatation. The second goal of postoperative surveillance is to allow CT scan or MRI surveillance every 6 months. The relatively high incidence of late aneurysm formation justifies the inconvenience and cost involved in long-term surveillance.

Chronic Dissection

In some patients with chronic type III aortic dissection, chronic ischemic complications develop owing to stenosis or occlusion of the aorta and/or renal, visceral, or iliac arteries. When ischemic complications are not associated with aortic aneurysm, or in poor surgical candidates, conservative techniques such as surgical bypass grafting or endovascular procedures can be used.[5, 40, 42, 45, 71, 72, 126, 131] When dissection is associated with aortic aneurysm, aortic replacement is necessary and separate bypasses to the involved aortic branches can be performed from the aortic graft.

The surgical indications for chronic dissecting aneurysm are the same as those for degenerative aneurysm of the descending thoracic or thoracoabdominal aorta.[5, 8, 82, 149, 151] Surgery is indicated in patients with complicated or symptomatic aneurysm, patients with evidence of progression on successive CT scans, and asymptomatic good-risk patients with aneurysms larger than 5 cm in diameter.

In patients with asymptomatic aneurysms, careful workup is needed to evaluate the operative risk. In our group, this evaluation includes echocardiography, coronary arteriography, duplex ultrasonography of arteries to the brain, and respiratory function testing. Depending on the results of these investigations, it may be necessary to perform other interventional or surgical procedures first (myocardial revascularization, carotid endarterectomy, or, more rarely, cardiac valvular replacement) or otherwise prepare the patient for aortic surgery (respiratory physiotherapy). Another important feature of the preoperative evaluation is spinal cord arteriography. Visualization of the spinal cord blood supply significantly reduces the risk of postoperative spinal cord complications.[99, 152, 153] Conversely, failure to visualize the spinal cord blood supply may favor nonoperative management and close surveillance of a medium-sized aneurysm.

The extent of aortic replacement in patients with chronic type III dissecting aneurysm is variable. A cautious and often feasible approach consists of replacement of only the aneurysmal zone (generally all or part of the descending thoracic aorta) and careful postoperative surveillance of the remaining dissected but nonaneurysmal aorta. However, extensive replacement is unavoidable in patients with thoracoabdominal aneurysm. Extensive aortic replacement is associated with a higher risk of spinal cord complications, which must be weighed against the possibly fatal consequences of aneurysm rupture.

CURRENT RESULTS

Early Results

Acute Dissection

Table 93–2 summarizes 30-day results of surgical management of acute type III aortic dissection in 12 series reported from 1988 to 1998 in the English medical literature,[66, 78, 82, 84, 121, 126, 143, 146, 147, 154-156] to which we have added our own recent experience. Most patients in these series had graft replacement of the upper part of the descending thoracic aorta. Mortality rates ranged from 0%[147] to 69% (9/13).[146]

Interpretation of such conflicting data obviously should take into account important differences in referral patterns and indications for surgery from one institution to another. Schor and colleagues[147] acknowledged the fact that their outstanding surgical results (zero mortality) may well be explained by self-selection of the patients in a tertiary referral center. Although the same may apply to other studies reporting similarly good results,[78, 82, 84, 145, 154, 155] the fact remains that substantial improvement in mortality rates following surgery for acute type III aortic dissection has occurred since the mid-1980s, at least in selected patients operated upon in selected medical centers.

On the other hand, the poor results reported in other series are obviously related to operations being performed only in the most desperate situations. In the report by Neya and associates,[146] nine patients (69%) were operated on for aortic rupture and seven patients (50%) were in hemor-rhagic shock at the time of hospital admission. Adachi and associates[66] similarly reported a series of 39 patients in whom early surgery had been performed only for acute rupture. Of 10 patients operated under emergency conditions because of massive bleeding, six (60%) died intraoperatively or postoperatively. These series my reflect more closely the medical practice in the community setting.

In an attempt to compare medical and surgical therapy for uncomplicated type III aortic dissection, Glower and associates[150] reported the combined experience of Stanford and Duke Universities. Miller[87] subsequently reanalyzed their data concerning acute type III aortic dissection (see Fig. 93–16), clearly demonstrating the influence of surgical indications on postoperative results. Although mortality was high (47%) in patients operated on for life-threatening complications, it was still higher (71%) whenever those patients were treated medically. Patients without compelling indications for emergency surgery who had serious coexistent medical illnesses obviously did better following medical therapy. Finally, low-risk patients without compelling indications for emergency surgery or serious coexistent medical illnesses had low, equivalent mortality rates following either medical or surgical therapy (16% versus 9%).

It has also been reported by Fradet and associates[143] that mortality following early surgery for acute type III aortic dissection is much higher when surgery is performed because of the failure of medical therapy rather than as an initial therapy.

Ischemic complications involving the spinal cord, kidneys, digestive tract, or lower extremities have a significant influence on early mortality following graft replacement for

TABLE 93–2. CURRENT 30-DAY RESULTS OF SURGICAL MANAGEMENT OF ACUTE TYPE III AORTIC DISSECTION

AUTHOR	PERIOD	SURGICAL MANAGEMENT	NO. OF PATIENTS	DEATHS (%)	PARAPLEGIA/ PARAPARESIS (%)
Verdant et al[78]	1974–1994	Aortic replacement	52	12	0
Neya et al[146]	1979–1991	Aortic replacement	13	69	NA
Masuda et al[154]	1979–1989	Aortic replacement	27	19	NA
Fradet et al[143]	1980–1986	Aortic replacement			
		Initial	11	27	NA
		Secondary	6	83	NA
Grabitz et al[126]	1981–1995	Aortic replacement	7	43	14
		Fenestration	7	14	0
		Extra-anatomic bypass	11	0	0
Svensson et al[82]	1984–1989	Aortic replacement			
		Limited	17	6	NA
		Extensive	19	5	NA
Schor et al[147]	1985–1995	Initial aortic replacement	17	0	0
		Secondary operations*	12	0	0
Adachi et al[66]	1985–1989	Aortic replacement	10	60	NA
Coselli et al		Aortic replacement			
155	1987–1995	Limited	28	14	7
156	1986–1994	Extensive	16	6	13
Safi et al[84]	1991–1996	Aortic replacement	22	14	32
Palma et al[122]	1988–1995	Elephant trunk	70	20	3
Kieffer	1990–1998	Aortic replacement	27	11	0

*Includes three palliative procedures.
NA = not available.

TABLE 93–3. CURRENT 30-DAY RESULTS OF AORTIC REPLACEMENT FOR CHRONIC TYPE III DISSECTING AORTIC ANEURYSM OF THE DESCENDING THORACIC/THORACOABDOMINAL AORTA

AUTHOR	PERIOD	NO. OF PATIENTS	EXTENT OF REPLACEMENT	DEATHS (%)	PARAPLEGIA/ PARAPARESIS (%)
Verdant et al[78]	1974–1994	31	Thoracic	23	0
Kawashima et al[105]	1977–1991	13	Thoracic	31	0
		15	Thoracoabdominal*	20	0
Grabitz et al[126]	1981–1995	13	Thoracic	0	8
		24	Thoracoabdominal	29	21
Svensson et al[82]	1984–1989	96	Thoracic	4	NA
		100	Thoracoabdominal	5	NA
Coselli et al					
155	1987–1995	55	Thoracic	0	2
156	1986–1994	77	Thoracoabdominal	5	3
Kitamura et al[83]	1987–1993	15	Thoracic	9*	
		17	Thoracoabdominal		3*
Dudra et al[85]	1991–1994	10	Thoracoabdominal	10	50
Safi et al[84]	1991–1996	18	Thoracic	10*	
		74	Thoracoabdominal		0
Kieffer	1990–1998	37	Thoracic	5	5
		63	Thoracoabdominal	14	11

*Combined results.
NA = Not available.

acute type III aortic dissection. In the series of Fann and associates[41] operative mortality was 64% (7/11) in patients with vascular complications as opposed to 31% (9/29) in patients without vascular complications ($p < .002$). Mortality was 100% for patients with spinal cord ischemia, 67% for patients with renal ischemia, and 50% for patients with ischemia involving the lower extremities or compromised visceral perfusion. The fact that only renal ischemia showed independent predictive value for postoperative death at statistical analysis was probably due to the small number of patients.

The low rate of paraplegia/paraparesis in these series is probably explained by the usually limited extent of aortic replacement in the acute phase of dissection. In two series reporting results of extensive aortic replacement for acute type III aortic dissection, the rate of paraplegia or paraparesis was 29% (8/28).

Chronic Dissection

Table 93–3 summarizes late results of surgical management of chronic type III aortic dissection in eight series reported

from 1990 to 1998 in the English medical literature,[78, 82–85, 105, 126, 155, 156] to which we have added our own recent experience. Comparison with earlier series[6, 8, 15, 21] demonstrates substantial improvement in mortality and paraplegia/paraparesis rates. Refinements in operative indications, surgical techniques and perioperative care obviously have benefited those patients, the great majority of whom are operated on electively. Despite many efforts in different directions, elimination of spinal cord complications has not been achieved and remains an important goal for future research.

Late Results

Detailed analysis of late results following surgery for acute type III aortic dissection has been published by several groups.[8, 77, 82, 146, 147, 149] Actuarial 5-year survival rates (including perioperative mortality) are in the 50% to 70% range (Table 93–4). Late deaths following surgical management of type III aortic dissection may be caused by cardiovascular disease, aortic complications, or unrelated causes. In these patients, aneurysmal formation or redissection in

TABLE 93–4. LATE ACTUARIAL SURVIVAL RATES (INCLUDING PERIOPERATIVE MORTALITY) AFTER SURGICAL MANAGEMENT OF TYPE III AORTIC DISSECTION

AUTHOR	ACUTE VERSUS CHRONIC	NO. OF PATIENTS	SURVIVAL (%)					
			1 Yr	3 Yr	5 Yr	8 Yr	10 Yr	15 Yr
Jex et al[77]	Both	64	—	—	49	30	—	—
Svensson et al[82]	Both	232	81	71	—	—	—	—
Kitamura et al[83]	Both	65	—	—	70	—	70	—
Schor et al[147]	Acute	17	93	—	68	—	—	—
Fann et al[41]	Acute	46	56	—	48	—	29	11
	Chronic	34	78	—	59	—	45	27

untreated parts of the thoracic or abdominal aorta should be looked for by routine periodic surveillance of the entire aorta, using CT scanning, MRI, or aortography. Elective reoperation should be offered to most good-risk patients in order to avoid late aortic rupture and reduce late mortality rates.

In most patients, aortic dissection is nothing but an episode in the evolution of generalized aortic disease. Patients (and their physicians) should understand the lifelong nature of their disease in order to comply with the mandatory long-term aortic surveillance.

REFERENCES

1. Crawford ES: The diagnosis and management of aortic dissection. JAMA 264:2537–2541, 1990.
2. Sorenson HR, Olsen H: Ruptured and dissecting aneurysms of the aorta: Incidence and prospects of surgery. Acta Chir Scand 128:644–650, 1964.
2a. Gillum RF: Epidemiology of aortic aneurysms in the United States. J Clin Epidemiol 11:1289–1298, 1995.
2b. Svensjo S, Bengtsson H, Bergquist D: Thoracic and thoracoabdominal aortic aneurysm and dissection: An investigation based on autopsy. Br J Surg 83:68–71, 1996.
3. Applebaum A, Karp RB, Kirklin JW: Ascending vs descending aortic dissections. Am Surg 183:296–300, 1976.
4. Austen WG, DeSanctis RW: Surgical treatment of dissecting aneurysm of the thoracic aorta. N Engl J Med 272:1314–1318, 1965.
5. Borst HG, Heinemann MK, Stone CD: Surgical Treatment of Aortic Dissection. New York, Churchill Livingstone, 1996.
6. Daily PO, Trueblood HW, Stinson EB, et al: Management of acute aortic dissections. Ann Thorac Surg 10:237–247, 1970.
7. DeBakey ME, Henly WS, Cooley DA, et al: Surgical management of dissecting aneurysms of the aorta. J Thorac Cardiovasc Surg 19:130–149, 1965.
8. DeBakey ME, McCollum OH, Crawford ES, et al: Dissection and dissecting aneurysms of the aorta: Twenty-year follow-up of five hundred twenty-seven patients treated surgically. Surgery 92:1118–1134, 1982.
9. DeSanctis RW, Doroghazi RM, Austen WG, Buckley MJ: Aortic dissection. N Engl J Med 317:1060–1067, 1987.
10. Ergin MA, Galla JD, Lansman S, Griepp RB: Acute dissections of the aorta: Current surgical treatment. Surg Clin North Am 65:721–741, 1985.
11. Glower DD, Speier RH, White WD, et al: Management and long-term outcome of aortic dissection. Ann Surg 214:31–41, 1991.
12. Guilmet D, Bachet J, Goudot B, et al: Aortic dissection: Anatomic types and surgical approaches. J Cardiovasc Surg 34:23–32, 1993.
13. Kouchoukos NT, Dougenis D: Surgery of the thoracic aorta. N Engl J Med 26:1876–1888, 1997.
14. Lindsay J Jr, Hurst JW: Clinical features and prognosis in dissecting aneurysm of the aorta: A re-appraisal. Circulation 35:880–888, 1967.
15. Miller DC, Stinson EB, Oyer PE, et al: Operative treatment of aortic dissections: Experience with 125 patients over a sixteen-year period. J Thorac Cardiovasc Surg 78:365–382, 1979.
16. Parker FB Jr, Neville JF Jr, Hanson EL, et al: Management of acute aortic dissection. Ann Thorac Surg 19:436–442, 1975.
17. Pate JW, Richardson RL, Eastridge CE: Acute aortic dissections. Am Surg 42:395–404, 1976.
18. Williams GM: Aortic dissection: Clinical presentation, medical management, and indications for surgical intervention. In Perler BA, Becker GJ (eds): Vascular Intervention: A Clinical Approach. New York, Thieme, 1998, pp 377–385.
19. Hirst AE, Johns VJ, Kine SW: Dissecting aneurysm of the aorta: A review of 505 cases. Medicine 37:217–279, 1958.
20. Dubost C, Guilmet D, Soyer R: La Chirurgie des Anévrysmes de l'Aorte. Paris, Masson, 1970.
21. Reul GJ, Cooley DA, Hallman GL, et al: Dissecting aneurysm of the descending aorta: Improved surgical results in 91 patients. Arch Surg 110:632–640, 1975.

22. Slater EE, DeSanctis RW: The clinical recognition of dissecting aortic aneurysm. Am J Med 60:625–633, 1976.
23. Meng RL, Najafi H, Javid H, et al: Acute ascending aortic dissection: Surgical management. Circulation 64 (Suppl II):231, 1981.
24. Roberts CS, Roberts WC: Aortic dissection with the entrance tear in transverse aorta: Analysis of 12 autopsy patients. Ann Thorac Surg 50:762–766, 1990.
25. Von Segesser LK, Killer I, Ziswiler M, et al: Dissection of the descending thoracic aorta extending into the ascending aorta: A therapeutic challenge. J Thorac Cardiovasc Surg 108:755–761, 1994.
26. Harris KM, Braverman AC, Gutierrez FR, et al: Transesophageal echocardiographic and clinical features of aortic intramural hematoma. J Thorac Cardiovasc Surg 114:619–626, 1997.
27. Muluk SC, Kaufman JA, Torchiana DF, et al: Diagnosis and treatment of thoracic aortic intramural hematoma. J Vasc Surg 24:1022–1029, 1996.
28. Nienaber CA, von Kodolitsch Y, Petersen B, et al: Intramural hemorrhage of the thoracic aorta: Diagnostic and therapeutic implications. Circulation 92:1465–1472, 1995.
29. Robbins RC, McManus RP, Mitchell RS, et al: Management of patients with intramural hematoma of the thoracic aorta. Circulation 88 [part 2]:1–10, 1993.
30. Schappert T, Sadony V, Schoen F, et al: Diagnosis and therapeutic consequences of intramural aortic hematoma. J Card Surg 9:508–515, 1994.
31. Svensson LG, Crawford ES: Cardiovascular and Vascular Disease of the Aorta. Philadelphia, WB Saunders, 1997.
32. Roberts WC: Aortic dissection: Anatomy, consequences, and causes. Am Heart J 101:195–214, 1981.
33. Azodo MVU, Gutierrez OH, DeWeese JA: Abdominal aortic dissection with retrograde extension into the thoracic aorta. Cardiovasc Intervent Radiol 12:317–320, 1990.
34. Cambria RP, Brewster DC, Moncure AC, et al: Spontaneous aortic dissection in the presence of coexistent or previously repaired atherosclerotic aneurysm. Ann Surg 208:619–624, 1988.
35. Roberts CS, Roberts WC. Combined thoracic aortic dissection and abdominal aortic fusiform aneurysm. Ann Thorac Surg 52:537–540, 1991.
36. Bickerstaff LK, Pairolero PC, Hollier LH, et al: Thoracic aortic aneurysms: A population-based study. Surgery 92:1103–1108, 1982.
37. Crawford ES, DeNatale RW: Thoracoabdominal aortic aneurysm: Observations regarding the natural course of the disease. J Vasc Surg 3:578–582, 1986.
38. Pressler V, McNamara JS: Thoracic aortic aneurysm: Natural history and treatment. J Thorac Cardiovasc Surg 79:489–498, 1980.
39. Roberts CS, Roberts WC: Aortic dissection with the entrance tear in the descending thoracic aorta: Analysis of 40 necropsy patients. Ann Surg 213:356–368, 1991.
40. Cambria RP, Brewster DC, Gertler J, et al: Vascular complications associated with spontaneous aortic dissection. J Vasc Surg 7:199–209, 1988.
41. Fann JI, Sarris GE, Mitchell RS, et al: Treatment of patients with aortic dissection presenting with peripheral vascular complications. Ann Surg 212:705–713, 1990.
42. Okita Y, Takamoto S, Ando M, et al: Surgical strategies in managing organ malperfusion as a complication of aortic dissection. Eur J Cardiothorac Surg 9:242–247, 1995.
43. Heinemann MK, Buehner B, Schaefers HJ, et al: Malperfusion of the thoracoabdominal vasculature in aortic dissection. J Card Surg 9:748–755, 1994.
44. Slonim SM, Nyman UR, Semba CP, et al: True lumen obliteration in complicated aortic dissection: Endovascular treatment. Radiology 201:161–166, 1996.
45. Orend KH, Liewald F, Kirchdorfer B, Sunder-Plassmann L: Surgical management of descending aortic dissection. In Weimann S (ed): Thoracic and Thoracoabdominal Aortic Aneurysm. Bologna, Monduzzi, 1994, pp 103–108.
46. Walker PJ, Sarris GE, Miller DC: Peripheral vascular manifestations of acute aortic dissection. In Rutherford RB (ed): Vascular Surgery, 4th ed. Philadelphia, WB Saunders, 1995, pp 1087–1102.
47. Hughes JD, Bacha EA, Dodson TF, et al: Peripheral vascular complications of aortic dissection. Am J Surg 170:209–212, 1995.
48. Yamaguchi T, Naito H, Ohta M, et al: False lumens in type III aortic dissections: Progress CT study. Radiology 156:757–760, 1985.
49. Kato M, Bai H, Sato K, et al: Determining surgical indications for

acute type B dissection based on enlargement of aortic diameter during the chronic phase. Circulation 92 (Suppl II):107–112, 1995.
50. Dapunt OE, Galla JD, Sadeghi AM, et al: The natural history of thoracic aortic aneuryms. J Thorac Cardiovasc Surg 107:1323–1333, 1994.
51. Dinsmore RE, Willerson JT, Buckley MJ: Dissecting aneurysm of the aorta: Aortographic features affecting prognosis. Radiology 105:567–572, 1972.
52. Erbel R, Oelert H, Meyer J, et al: Effect of medical and surgical therapy on aortic dissection evaluated by transesophageal echocardiography: Implications for prognosis and therapy. Circulation 87:1604–1615, 1993.
53. Moriyama Y, Toyohira H, Koga M, et al: The management of patients with dissection of the descending thoracic aorta: A comparison between closing and nonclosing dissections. Jpn J Surg 27:910–914, 1997.
54. Sanderson CJ, Rich S, Beere PA, et al: Clotted false lumen: Reappraisal of indications for medical management of acute aortic dissection. Thorax 36:194–199, 1981.
55. Spittell PC, Spittell JA Jr, Joyce JW, et al: Clinical features and differential diagnosis of aortic dissection: Experience with 236 cases (1980 through 1990). Mayo Clin Proc 68:642–651, 1993.
56. Eagle KA, Quertermous T, Kritzer GA, et al: Spectrum of conditions initially suggesting acute aortic dissection but with negative aortograms. Am J Cardiol 57:322–326, 1986.
57. Braverman AC: Penetrating atherosclerotic ulcers of the aorta. Curr Opin Cardiol 9:591–597, 1994.
58. Coady MA, Rizzo JA, Hammond GL, et al: Penetrating ulcer of the thoracic aorta: What is it? How do we recognize it? How do we manage it? J Vasc Surg 27:1006–1016, 1998.
59. Movsowitz HD, Lampert C, Jacobs LE, Kotler MN: Penetrating atherosclerotic aortic ulcers. Am Heart J 128:1210–1217, 1994.
60. Stanson AW, Kasmer FJ, Hollier LH, et al: Penetrating atherosclerotic ulcers of the thoracic aorta: Natural history and clinicopathologic correlations. Ann Vasc Surg 1:15–23, 1986.
61. Cohen S, Littmann D: Painless dissecting aneurysm of the aorta. New Engl J Med 271:143–145, 1964.
62. Giladi M, Fines A, Averbuch M, et al: Aortic dissection manifested as fever of unknown origin. Cardiology 78:78–80, 1991.
63. Murray HW, Mann JJ, Genecin A, McKusick VA: Fever with dissecting aneurysm of the aorta. Am J Med 61:140–144, 1976.
64. Turner N, Fusey CD: Aortic dissection masquerading as systemic disease: The post-dissection syndrome. Q J Med 277:525–531, 1990.
65. Kaufman SL, White RI Jr: Aortic dissection with "normal" chest roentgenogram. Cardiovasc Intervent Radiol 3:103–106, 1980.
66. Adachi H, Kyo S, Takamoto S, et al: Early diagnosis and surgical intervention of acute aortic dissection by transesophageal color flow mapping. Circulation 82 (Suppl IV):19–23, 1990.
67. Ballal RS, Nanda NC, Gatewood R, et al: Usefulness of transesophageal echocardiography in assessment of aortic dissection. Circulation 84:1903–1914, 1991.
68. Cigarroa JE, Isselbacher EM, DeSanctis RW, Eagle KA: Diagnostic imaging in the evaluation of suspected aortic dissection. N Engl J Med 328:35–43, 1993.
69. Nienaber CA, von Kodolitsch Y, Nicolas V, et al: The diagnosis of thoracic aortic dissection by noninvasive imaging procedures. N Engl J Med 328:1–9, 1993.
70. O'Gara PT, DeSanctis RW: Acute aortic dissection and its variants: Toward a common diagnostic and therapeutic approach. Circulation 92:1376–1378, 1995.
71. Dake MD, Semba CP, Razavi MK, et al: Endovascular procedures for the treatment of aortic dissection: Techniques and results. J Cardiovasc Surg 39 (Suppl 1):45–52, 1998.
72. Slonim SM, Nyman U, Semba CP, et al: Aortic dissection: Percutaneous management of ischemic complications with endovascular stents and balloon fenestration. J Vasc Surg 23:214–253, 1996.
73. Williams DM, Lee DY, Hamilton BH, et al: The dissected aorta: Percutaneous treatment of ischemic complications. Principles and results. J Vasc Interv Radiol 8:605–625, 1997.
74. Williams DM, Lee DY, Hamilton BH, et al: The dissected aorta: Part III. Anatomy and radiologic diagnosis of branch-vessel compromise. Radiology 203:37–44, 1997.
75. Lee DY, Williams DM, Abrams GD: The dissected aorta. Part II: Differentiation of the true from the false lumen with intravascular US. Radiology 203:32–36, 1997.

76. Borst HG, Jurmann M, Bühner B, Laas J: Risk of replacement of descending aorta with a standardized left heart bypass technique. J Thorac Cardiovasc Surg 107:126–133, 1994.
77. Jex RK, Schaff HV, Piehler JM, et al: Early and late results following repair of dissections of the descending thoracic aorta. J Vasc Surg 3:226–237, 1986.
78. Verdant A, Cossette R, Pagé A, et al: Aneurysms of the descending thoracic aorta: Three hundred sixty-six consecutive cases resected without paraplegia. J Vasc Surg 21:385–391, 1995.
79. Crawford ES: Thoracoabdominal and abdominal aortic aneurysms involving renal, superior mesenteric, and celiac arteries. Ann Surg 179:763–772, 1974.
80. Hunter JA, Dye WS, Javid H, et al: Abdominal aortic resection in thoracic dissection. Arch Surg 111:1258–1262, 1976.
81. Kasprzak PM, Raithel D: Surgical concepts for treatment of aortic dissections type B. In Weimann S (ed): Thoracic and Thoracoabdominal Aortic Aneurysm. Bologna, Monduzzi, 1994, pp 95–102.
82. Svensson LG, Crawford ES, Hess KR, et al: Dissection of the aorta and dissecting aortic aneurysms: Improving early and long-term surgical results. Circulation 82 (Suppl IV):24–38, 1990.
83. Kitamura M, Hashimoto A, Tagusari O, et al: Operation for type B aortic dissection: Introduction of left heart bypass. Ann Thorac Surg 59:1200–1203, 1995.
84. Safi HJ, Miller CC III, Reardon MJ, et al: Operation of acute and chronic aortic dissection: Recent outcome with regard to neurologic deficit and early death. Ann Thorac Surg 66:402–411, 1998.
85. Dudra J, Shiiya N, Matsui Y, et al: Operative results of thoracoabdominal repair for chronic type B aortic dissection. J Cardiovasc Surg 38:147–151, 1997.
86. Coselli JS, Crawford ES: Femoral artery perfusion for cardiopulmonary bypass in patients with aortoiliac obstruction. Ann Thorac Surg 43:437–439, 1987.
87. Miller DC: Acute dissection of the descending thoracic aorta. Chest Surg Clin North Am 2:347–378, 1992.
88. Chen YF, Chou SH, Chiu CC, et al: Use of glutaraldehyde solution in the treatment of acute aortic dissections. Ann Thorac Surg 58:833–836, 1994.
89. Reul GJ Jr: New technique for surgical hemostasis of aorto-prosthetic anastomoses. Cardiovasc Dis Bull Texas Heart Inst 1:120–122, 1974.
90. Floten HS, Ravichandran PS, Furnary AP, et al: Adventitial inversion technique in repair of aortic dissection. Ann Thorac Surg 59:771–772, 1995.
91. Hume DM, Porter RR: Acute dissecting aortic aneurysms. Surgery 53:122–154, 1963.
92. Graham JM, Stinnett DM: Operative management of acute aortic arch dissection using profound hypothermia and circulatory arrest. Ann Thorac Surg 44:192–198, 1987.
93. Shiiya N, Yasuda K, Murashita T, et al: Simultaneous total aortic replacement without a sternotomy incision. Ann Thorac Surg 65:546–548, 1998.
94. Caramutti VM, Dantur JR, Favaloro MR, et al: Deep hypothermia and circulatory arrest as an elective technique in the treatment of type B dissecting aneuryms of the aorta. J Card Surg 4:206–215, 1989.
95. Kieffer E, Koskas F, Walden R, et al: Hypothermic circulatory arrest for thoracic aneurysmectomy through left-sided thoracotomy. J Vasc Surg 19:457–464, 1994.
96. Kieffer E: Chirurgie de l'aorte thoracique descendante. Encyclopédie Médico-Chirurgicale. Techniques Chirurgicales. 1997.
97. Tayama K, Akashi H, Fukunaga S, et al: Operation for type B aortic dissection using hypothermic selective cerebral perfusion. Ann Thorac Surg 63:535–537, 1997.
98. Kouchoukos NT, Daily BB, Rokkas CK, et al: Hypothermic bypass and circulatory arrest for operations on the descending thoracic and thoracoabdominal aorta. Ann Thorac Surg 60:67–77, 1995.
99. Kieffer E, Richard T, Chiras J, et al: Preoperative spinal cord arteriography in aneurysmal disease of the descending thoracic and thoracoabdominal aorta: Preliminary results in 45 patients. Ann Vasc Surg 3:34–46, 1989.
100. Berger RL: A simplified plastic repair for aortic dissection. Ann Thorac Surg 25:250–253, 1978.
101. Doroghazi RH, Slater EE, DeSanctis RM, et al: Long-term survival of patients with treated aortic dissections. J Am Coll Cardiol 3:1026–1034, 1984.
102. Ruberti U, Odero A, Arpesani A, et al: Acute aortic dissection: Personal experience. J Cardiovasc Surg 29:70–79, 1988.

103. Viljanen T, Luosto R, Jarvinen A, Sariola H: Surgical treatment of aortic dissection in 60 patients. Scand J Thorac Cardiovasc Surg 20:193–201, 1986.

104. Tanabe T, Hashimoto M, Sakai K, et al: Surgical treatment of aortic dissection: Application of Ivalon sponge to the dissected lumen. Ann Thorac Surg 41:169–175, 1986.

105. Kawashima Y, Shirakura R, Nakano S, et al: Long-term results of entry closure and aneurysmal wall plication with axillofemoral bypass: A new procedure for repair of DeBakey type III dissecting aneurysm. Surgery 113:59–64, 1993.

106. Williams GM: Treatment of chronic expanding dissecting aneurysms of the descending thoracic and upper abdominal aorta by extended aortotomy, removal of the dissected intima, and closure. J Vasc Surg 18:441–449, 1993.

107. Fabiani JN, Jebara VA, Carpentier A: Use of glue in treatment of type B aortic dissection (Letter). Lancet 2:1041, 1989.

108. Carpentier A: New approach to treatment of aortic dissections. Lancet 15:1291–1292, 1979.

109. Carpentier A, Deloche A, Fabiani JN et al: New surgical approach to aortic dissection: Flow reversal and thromboexclusion. J Thorac Cardiovasc Surg 81:659–668, 1981.

110. Carpentier A: Thromboexclusion: An alternative for type B dissection. Semin Thorac Cardiovasc Surg 3:242–244, 1991.

111. Elefteriades JA, Hartleroad J, Gusberg RJ, et al: Long-term experience with descending aortic dissection: The complication-specific approach. Ann Thorac Surg 53:11–21, 1992.

112. Odagiri S, Shimazu A, Shimokawaji M, et al: Use of a new stapling instrument for permanent occlusion of the aorta in the surgical procedure for thromboexclusion. Ann Thorac Surg 47:466–469, 1989.

113. Patra P, Petiot JM, Mainguene C, et al: Retrograde dissection of the aortic arch after exclusion-bypass of the descending thoracic aorta: A report of three cases. Ann Vasc Surg 3:341–344, 1989.

114. Kieffer E, Petitjean C, Richard T, et al; Exclusion-bypass for aneurysms of the descending thoracic and thoracoabdominal aorta. Ann Vasc Surg 1:182–195, 1986.

115. Robicsek F: "Very long" aortic grafts. Eur J Cardiothorac Surg 6:536–541, 1992.

116. Borst HG, Walterbusch G, Schaps D: Extensive aortic replacement using "elephant trunk" prosthesis. Thorac Cardiovasc Surg 31:37–40, 1983.

117. Crawford ES, Coselli JS, Svensson LG, et al: Diffuse aneurysmal disease (chronic aortic dissection, Marfan, and mega aorta syndromes) and multiple aneurysm: Treatment by subtotal and total aorta replacement emphasizing the elephant trunk operation. Ann Surg 211:521–537, 1990.

118. Heinemann MK, Buehner B, Jurmann MJ, Borst HG: Use of the "elephant trunk technique" in aortic surgery. Ann Thorac Surg 60:2–7, 1995.

119. Ando M, Takamoto S, Okita Y, et al: Elephant trunk procedure for surgical treatment of aortic dissection. Ann Thorac Surg 66:82–87, 1998.

120. Kato M, Ohnishi K, Kaneko M, et al: New graft-implanting method for thoracic aortic aneurysm or dissection with a stented graft. Circulation 94 (Suppl II):188–193, 1996.

121. Morota T, Ando M, Takamoto S, Okita Y: Modified "elephant trunk" procedure obliterating the false lumen in aortic dissection. J Cardiovasc Surg 38:487–488, 1997.

122. Palma JH, Almeida DR, Carvalho AC, et al: Surgical treatment of acute type B aortic dissection using an endoprosthesis (elephant trunk). Ann Thorac Surg 63:1081–1084, 1997.

123. Gurin D, Bulmer JW, Derby R: Dissecting aneurysm of the aorta: Diagnosis and operative relief of acute arterial obstruction due to this cause. NY State Med J 35:1200–1202, 1935.

124. DeBakey ME, Cooley DA, Creech O Jr: Surgical considerations of dissecting aneurysm of the aorta. Ann Surg 142:586–612, 1955.

125. Dinis da Gama A: The surgical management of aortic dissection: From uniformity to diversity, a continuous challenge. J Cardiovasc Surg 32:141–153, 1991.

126. Grabitz K, Sandmann W, Kniemeyer HW, Torsello G: Surgical management of complications in patients with acute and chronic dissection of the descending aorta. In Weimann S (ed): Thoracic and Thoracoabdominal Aortic Aneurysm. Bologna, Monduzzi, 1994, pp 227–234.

127. Elefteriades JA, Hammond GL, Gusberg RJ, et al: Fenestration revis-ited: A safe and effective procedure for descending aortic dissection. Arch Surg 125:786–790, 125.

128. Harms J, Hess U, Cavallaro A, et al: The abdominal aortic fenestration procedure in acute thoraco-abdominal aortic dissection with aortic branch artery ischemia. J Cardiovasc Surg 39:273–280, 1998.

129. Howell JF, Lemaire SA, Kirby RP: Thoracoabdominal fenestration for aortic dissection with ischemic colonic perforation. Ann Thorac Surg 64:242–244, 1997.

130. Webb TH, Williams GM: Abdominal aortic tailoring for renal, visceral, and lower extremity malperfusion resulting from acute aortic dissection. J Vasc Surg 26:474–480, 1997.

131. Andréassian B, Nussaume O, Kitzis M, et al: Dissection de l'aorte thoracique: Chirurgie "ad hoc" des branches de l'aorte et de l'aorte à distance de l'entrée. In Kieffer E (ed): Chirurgie de l'Aorte Thoracique Descendante et Thoraco-Abdominale. Paris, Expansion Scientifique, 1986, pp 252–264.

132. Boudghene F, Sapoval M, Bigot JM, Michel JB Endovascular graft placement in experimental dissection of the thoracic aorta. J Vasc Interv Radiol 6:501–507, 1995.

133. Charnsangavej C, Wallace S, Wright KC, et al: Endovascular stent for use in aortic dissection: An in vitro experiment. Radiology 157:323–325, 1985.

134. Kato N, Hirano T, Mizumoto T, et al: Experimental study for treatment of aortic dissection with expandable metallic stents. J Vasc Interv Radiol 5:417–423, 1994.

135. Marty-Ané C, Serres-Cousiné O, Laborde JC, et al: Use of endovascular stents for acute aortic dissection: An experimental study. Ann Vasc Surg 8:434–442, 1994.

136. Moon MR, Dake MD, Pelc LR, et al: Intravascular stenting of acute experimental type B dissection. J Surg Res 54:381–388, 1993.

137. Trent MS, Parsonnet V, Shoenfeld R, et al: A balloon-expandable intravascular stent for obliterating experimental aortic dissection. J Vasc Surg 11:707–717, 1990.

138. Yoshida H, Kakino T, Kajitani M, et al: Transcatheter placement of an intraluminal prosthesis for the thoracic aorta: A new approach to aortic dissection. ASAIO J 37:272–273, 1991.

139. Akaba N, Ujue U, Umezarva K, et al: Management of acute aortic dissection with a cylinder-type balloon to close the entry. J Vasc Surg 3:890–894, 1986.

140. Dake MD, Miller DC, Semba CP, et al: Transluminal placement of endovascular stent-grafts for the treatment of descending thoracic aortic aneurysms. N Engl J Med 331:1729–1734, 1994.

141. Inoue K, Iwase T, Sato M, et al: Clinical application of transluminal endovascular graft placement for aortic aneurysms. Ann Thorac Surg 63:522–528, 1997.

142. Wheat MW Jr, Palmer RF, Bartley TD, et al: Treatment of dissecting aneurysms of the aorta without surgery. J Thorac Cardiovasc Surg 50:364–371, 1965.

143. Fradet G, Jamieson WRE, Janusz MT, et al: Aortic dissection: A six-year experience with 117 patients. Am J Surg 155:697–700, 1988.

144. Genoni M, von Segesser LK, Carrel T, et al: Aorten-dissektionen typ B: Operations, technick und resultate. Helv Chir Acta 60:1151–1157, 1994.

145. Gysi J, Schaffner T, Mohacsi P, et al: Early and late outcome of operated and non-operated acute dissection of the descending aorta. Eur J Cardiothorac Surg 11:1163–1170, 1997.

146. Neya K, Omoto R, Kyo S, et al: Outcome of Stanford type B acute aortic dissection. Circulation 86 (Suppl I):1–7, 1992.

147. Schor JS, Yerlioglu ME, Galla JD, et al: Selective management of acute type B aortic dissection: Long-term follow-up. Ann Thorac Surg 61:1339–1341, 1996.

148. Miller DC. The continuing dilemma concerning medical versus surgical management of patients with acute type B dissections. Semin Thorac Cardiovasc Surg 5:33–46, 1993.

149. Fann JI, Smith JA, Miller DC, et al: Surgical management of aortic dissection during a 30-year period. Circulation 92 (Suppl II):113–121, 1995.

150. Glower DD, Fann JI, Speier RH, et al: Comparison of medical and surgical therapy for uncomplicated descending aortic dissection. Circulation 82 (Suppl IV):39–46, 1990.

151. Svensson LG, Crawford ES, Hess KR, et al: Experience with 1509 patients undergoing thoracoabdominal aortic operations. J Vasc Surg 17:357–370, 1993.

152. Heinemann MK, Brassel F, Herzog T, et al: The role of spinal angiography in operations on the thoracic aorta: Myth or reality? Ann Thorac Surg 65:346–351, 1998.

153. Williams GM, Perler BA, Burdick JF, et al: Angiographic localization of spinal cord blood supply and its relationship to postoperative paraplegia. J Vasc Surg 13:23–25, 1991.
154. Masuda Y, Yamada Z, Morooka N, et al: Prognosis of patients with medically treated aortic dissections. Circulation 84 (Suppl III):7–13, 1991.
155. Coselli JS, Plestis KA, La Francisca S, Cohen S: Results of contemporary surgical treatment of descending thoracic aortic aneurysms: Experience in 198 patients. Ann Vasc Surg 10:131–137, 1996.
156. Coselli JS: Thoracoabdominal aortic aneurysms: Experience with 372 patients. J Card Surg 9:638–647, 1994.

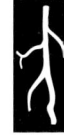

CHAPTER 94

Femoral and Popliteal Aneurysms

Linda M. Graham, M.D.

Femoral and popliteal artery aneurysms constitute the great majority of peripheral aneurysms. When first recognized centuries ago, these aneurysms were primarily mycotic, syphilitic, or traumatic in origin. Now most true aneurysms in these locations are of nonspecific etiology, reflecting their multifactorial pathogenesis (see Chapter 22). False aneurysms, which are actually encapsulated hematomas that communicate with the arterial lumen, are often associated with trauma (sometimes iatrogenic) or surgery and most frequently involve the femoral artery.

Femoral and popliteal aneurysms seem to be increasing in frequency. The incidence of all types of these aneurysms in hospitalized men is 7.39 per 100,000 population and in hospitalized women is 1.00 per 100,000 population.[19] An increase in nonspecific peripheral aneurysms seems to be coincident with the aging population, and these aneurysms are being recognized more frequently with the increased use of imaging modalities. In a series reported in 1972, the ratio of peripheral atherosclerotic aneurysms to abdominal aortic aneurysms (AAAs) identified in a single institution was 1:23.[15] In more recent series, the ratio of popliteal aneurysms to AAAs was 1:15 and 1:8.[25, 32] False aneurysms (pseudoaneurysms) are also occurring more frequently as bypass surgery and catheter-based diagnostic and therapeutic procedures become more common in the care of the patient with cardiovascular disease. In fact, this accounts for false aneurysms now being the most frequently recognized type of femoral artery aneurysm (see Chapters 48 and 97).

Femoral and popliteal artery aneurysms are important clinical entities because of their potential for limb-threatening complications. These aneurysms may be accompanied by symptoms of local pain owing to enlargement or pressure on the adjacent nerve, limb edema and venous distention due to compression of the adjacent vein, or lower extremity ischemia with intermittent claudication, rest pain, or gangrene secondary to complications of the aneurysm. As with all aneurysms, complications include rupture, thrombosis, embolization, and compression of adjacent structures, especially accompanying veins. The incidence of these complications, however, varies dramatically, depending on the site and etiology of the aneurysm. For example, nonspecific femoral artery aneurysms have a much more benign natural history than do popliteal artery aneurysms, which frequently develop limb-threatening complications.

The association of nonspecific femoral and popliteal artery aneurysms with AAAs is an important consideration. In a series of nearly 1500 patients, 3.1% of patients with aortoiliac aneurysms had peripheral aneurysms[15]; yet more than 70% of patients with peripheral aneurysms had concomitant AAAs, of which less than 50% were appreciated on physical examination.[15] Patients with a peripheral aneurysm must be evaluated for an AAA by an imaging modality.

Men are afflicted with nonspecific femoral and popliteal artery aneurysms far more frequently than women are; the male:female ratio is greater than 30:1.[12, 17] This predilection for men is markedly different from the usual incidence of aortic aneurysmal disease, in which the male:female patient ratio is approximately 5:1.[18]

The pathogenesis of nonspecific femoral and popliteal aneurysms is not clear. Factors believed to contribute to aneurysm formation include turbulent flow beyond a relative stenosis. At the groin, the inguinal ligament may form a constricting band, whereas at the popliteal level the tendinous hiatus of the adductor magnus or the arcuate popliteal ligament and the heads of the gastrocnemius muscle may compress the artery. Alterations in the arterial wall due to vibration and turbulence proximal to a major branching or due to stress and kinking during hip and knee flexion might contribute to aneurysm formation. None of these factors, however, explains the multiplicity of aneurysms in these patients or the male predilection for the disease. A genetic abnormality carried on the X chromosome could explain the distinct male predominance, and this is seen in the aneurysm-prone blotchy mouse in which an X chromosome mutation affects cross-linking of collagen and elastin.[8] However, there is no direct evidence of this in humans.

The multiplicity of peripheral aneurysms seems to reflect a systemic abnormality in the arterial wall. The presence of an inflammatory infiltrate has been documented in the wall of femoral and popliteal artery aneurysms,[16] just as in AAAs, but the role of the inflammatory cells in the pathogenesis of aneurysms remains speculative. In aortic aneurysm walls, the disrupted elastic lamellae, decreased elastin content, accelerated collagen turnover, and enhanced metalloproteinase production are accompanied by a relative decrease in the smooth muscle cell number and evidence of smooth muscle cell apoptosis.[35] Thus, because the cells that normally are capable of matrix synthesis are reduced, the capacity of the arterial wall to respond to the aneurysmal degenerative process may be limited.

False aneurysms result from loss of integrity of the arterial wall. Iatrogenic false aneurysms most commonly result from failed hemostasis at the site of arterial catheter insertion. Such pseudoaneurysms occur in 0.2% of diagnostic cardiac catheterizations and 0.6% of interventional catheterizations.[21] Larger catheters, longer procedures, the use of anticoagulation or thrombolytic therapy, and inability to maintain effective digital compression of the puncture site after removal of the catheter increase the incidence of these pseudoaneurysms. Anastomotic aneurysms result from a disrupted suture line between a graft and the host artery, and nearly 80% of all anastomotic aneurysms occur at the femoral artery. Approximately 3% of all femoral anastomoses, or 5.75% of femoral anastomoses after aortofemoral bypass, develop this complication, compared with 0.2% of aortic anastomoses.[31, 33] The incidence of anastomotic aneurysms is higher when prosthetic grafts are used: 5.5% of femoral anastomoses with polyester (Dacron) grafts compared with 0.9% with vein.[33] Anastomotic aneurysms are a late complication of bypass procedures; the mean interval from primary procedure to recognition is over 6 years.[14, 30]

Infected or mycotic aneurysms can follow any type of arterial trauma, including invasive diagnostic and therapeutic procedures, but they are often a complication of parenteral drug abuse. The femoral artery is now the most common site for a mycotic aneurysm, and central mycotic aneurysms have become rare.[2, 9] The importance of mycotic aneurysms is due to their propensity to rupture.

Regardless of the etiology, the principles for aneurysm treatment are the same. The life-threatening lesions should be addressed first, followed by the limb-threatening lesions. The surgical principles are also the same for aneurysms in any location. The aneurysm must be excluded from the circulation and arterial circulation restored. Unique characteristics and aspects of treatment of femoral and popliteal aneurysms are presented in the following sections.

FEMORAL ARTERY ANEURYSMS

The femoral artery is the most common site for a peripheral aneurysm. Femoral artery aneurysms are potentially limb-threatening lesions and may jeopardize the viability of the leg if thrombosis, embolization, or rupture occurs. The great majority of true aneurysms are of nonspecific etiology,

although rarely femoral aneurysms develop secondary to connective tissue disorders. False aneurysms include (1) anastomotic, (2) traumatic, (3) catheter-induced, and (4) infected lesions. As noted earlier, the femoral region is the most common site for anastomotic aneurysms, catheter-induced aneurysms, and mycotic aneurysms associated with trauma. Since the clinical manifestations and surgical repair of these lesions are presented in other chapters (see Chapters 48 and 97), the following review focuses on true femoral artery aneurysms of nonspecific etiology.

Common Femoral Artery Aneurysms

The frequency of femoral artery aneurysms in the general population is poorly defined, but they are closely associated with other nonspecific aneurysms, and their incidence can be defined on this basis. More than 3% of all patients with AAAs have femoral artery aneurysms.[15] In 100 patients with an atherosclerotic femoral artery aneurysm seen at a single institution, 85% of the patients also had an AAA, 72% had bilateral femoral artery aneurysms, 44% had popliteal artery aneurysms, and 6% had thoracic aortic aneurysms.[17]

Femoral aneurysms usually involve the common femoral artery, with the disease process including the femoral artery bifurcation in approximately half the cases. Femoral artery aneurysms may be classified as type I, those limited to the common femoral artery, or type II, those involving the orifice of the profunda femoris artery.[11] This classification provides a convenient reference system regarding vascular reconstructive procedures, since type II aneurysms usually require more complex reconstructions. Aneurysmal degeneration of the external iliac artery proximal to a femoral aneurysm is rare. Isolated profunda femoris artery aneurysms that begin distal to the artery's origin are unusual and constitute only 2% of all femoral artery aneurysms. Similarly, isolated superficial femoral artery aneurysms are rare, but aneurysmal degeneration of the entire artery may accompany common femoral and popliteal artery aneurysms.

Like all peripheral aneurysms, complications of femoral artery aneurysms can be limb-threatening, but this is unusual. The importance of femoral artery aneurysms lies in their frequent association with AAAs, which are potentially life-threatening, and with popliteal aneurysms, which are more frequently limb-threatening.

Clinical Manifestations

Patients with femoral artery aneurysms may be asymptomatic, with a pulsatile mass discovered on physical examination, or they may present with local pain, symptoms related to nerve or vein compression, or symptoms of lower extremity ischemia (Table 94–1). Although 40% of patients are asymptomatic at the time of diagnosis, most present with local symptoms or complaints of lower extremity ischemia.[17] Local pain or appreciation of a groin mass is the only symptom in nearly 20% of patients. Since femoral artery aneurysms tend to enlarge slowly, the local symptoms tend to be chronic and mild. Pressure on the femoral nerve may cause pain in the groin or anterior thigh. Neuropathic pain with distal radiation and paresis of distal muscle groups, although common in rapidly expanding false aneu-

TABLE 94-1. CLINICAL PRESENTATION OF FEMORAL ANEURYSMS

AUTHOR	PATIENTS	ANEURYSMS	MALE : FEMALE	BILATERAL (%)	AAA/PAA-ASSOCIATED (%/%)	ASYMPTOMATIC (%)	PRESENTING SYMPTOMS	COMPLICATIONS AT PRESENTATION
Pappas et al (1964)[24]*	89	115	86:3	36	28/38	—		Acute thrombosis/embolization, 13% Chronic thrombosis/embolization, 13% Rupture, 5%
Cutler and Darling (1973)[11]	45	63	40:5	47	51/27	29	Local, 29%	Acute thrombosis, 16% Chronic thrombosis, 16% Rupture, 14%
Adiseshiah and Bailey (1977)[1]	16	27	15:1	62	25/31	70		Embolization, 4% Thrombosis, 7% Rupture, 15%
Baird et al (1977)[+]	30	36	30:0	20	40/17	27	Local, 23% Ischemic, 50%	Acute thrombosis/embolization, 13% Rupture, 0%
Graham et al (1980)[17]	100	172	100:0	72	85/44	40	Local pain, 11% Mass, 16% Venous, 8% Ischemic, 42%	Embolization, 8% Acute thrombosis, 1% Chronic thrombosis, 1% Rupture, 2%
Sapienza et al (1996)[29]	22	31	21:1	41	50/—	64	Local, 5% Ischemic, 35%	

*Includes false aneurysms.
AAA = abdominal aortic aneurysm; FAA = femoral artery aneurysm; PAA = popliteal artery aneurysm.

rysms, is distinctly unusual in atherosclerotic femoral artery aneurysms. Compression of the femoral vein may produce lower extremity edema and changes suggestive of venous stasis, and this is present in nearly 10% of patients, being attributable to venous outflow obstruction by the femoral artery aneurysm in half the cases. Venous obstruction is rarely the only sign of a femoral aneurysm. Lower extremity ischemic symptoms of claudication, rest pain, or gangrene are present in more than 40% of patients and often lead to the diagnosis of femoral aortic aneurysm, but the symptoms usually are due to concomitant arterial occlusive disease rather than to the aneurysm itself.

Femoral artery aneurysms can be complicated by embolization, thrombosis, or rupture. The complication rate varies among reported series and tends to be higher in the series composed primarily of surgical patients. Peripheral embolization may be silent and detected only at angiography, or it may produce mild symptoms such as livedo reticularis or spotty discoloration on toes; it can result in severe peripheral gangrene and is one cause of "blue toe syndrome" when embolic material lodges in and occludes digital arteries. Embolization is reported in approximately 10% of extremities with a femoral aneurysm, but the femoral aneurysm is not necessarily the source of these emboli, since many patients have a concomitant popliteal aneurysm.[17]

Thrombosis of a femoral artery aneurysm usually produces severe, acute ischemia because flow through both the superficial femoral artery and the profunda femoris artery, with its potential collateral circulation, is disrupted. In larger clinical series, 1% to 16% of patients with atherosclerotic femoral artery aneurysms present with an acutely thrombosed aneurysm.[11, 17] Distinguishing between an acutely thrombosed aneurysm and a femoral artery embolus may be difficult, since both may present as an acutely ischemic leg with pulses absent below the femoral artery. The presence of a pulseless mass on physical examination may be appreciated, but ultrasonography demonstrating a thrombosed aneurysm may be necessary to establish the diagnosis.

In these same series, 1% to 16% of patients with femoral artery aneurysms have a chronically thrombosed lesion.[11, 17] Establishing the diagnosis of a chronically thrombosed aneurysm, as opposed to occlusive disease of the femoral artery, is also difficult. Again, the presence of a pulseless mass in the femoral region is suggestive, but use of imaging modalities is usually required to establish the diagnosis. Rupture of femoral artery aneurysms seems to be less common than embolization or thrombosis, and rates of 1% to 14% have been reported.[11, 17]

The typical patient with a femoral artery aneurysm is a man in his seventh decade of life; femoral artery aneurysms are distinctly unusual in women. These patients have many risk factors for atherosclerosis, with the majority being cigarette smokers, over one third having hypertension, and 14% having diabetes mellitus.[17] Associated cardiovascular disease is common. One third have clinical manifestations of coronary artery disease, and 7% have symptoms of cerebrovascular disease.

Diagnosis

The diagnosis of femoral artery aneurysm is usually made on routine physical examination or during evaluation for vascular disease when a pulsatile groin mass is discovered. The femoral artery is easily examined, so the diagnosis of a patent femoral artery aneurysm on physical examination is usually accurate in all but obese patients. The detection of a small aneurysm or a thrombosed femoral artery aneurysm, however, is difficult. Occasionally, the diagnosis is made by a roentgenogram of the region that shows the calcified rim of the aneurysm. Ultrasonography or duplex scanning is useful to establish the diagnosis and define the size of the aneurysm accurately. Furthermore, ultrasonography, computed tomography (CT), or magnetic resonance imaging (MRI) is essential to evaluate the infrarenal aorta and popliteal regions for the presence of associated aneurysmal disease. The accuracy of arteriography for the diagnosis of aneurysms is limited, because smooth intraluminal thrombus often fills much of the aneurysmal sac and the contrast material delineates only the residual lumen (Fig. 94–1). Arteriography, however, is essential to define the arterial anatomy to allow planning of indicated operative therapy.

Indications for Surgical Therapy

Operative treatment is indicated for all complicated or symptomatic aneurysms. Patients presenting with limb-threatening complications (embolization, thrombosis, or rupture) should undergo expeditious repair. Aneurysms that are enlarging or causing local symptoms (pain, venous

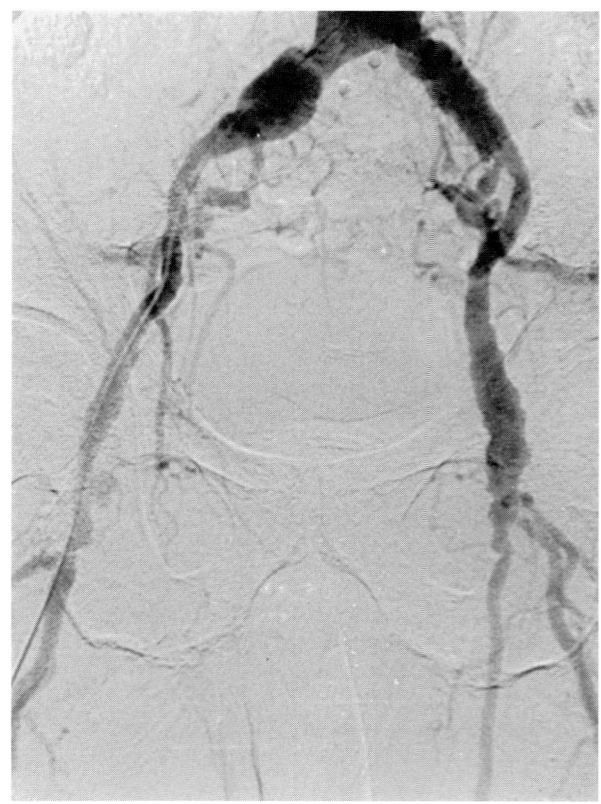

FIGURE 94–1. Arteriogram demonstrating bilateral femoral artery aneurysms. Although not apparent on the arteriogram the right femoral artery aneurysm is larger than the left one but has more luminal thrombus. Like many patients with femoral artery aneurysms, this patient has associated aortic and iliac aneurysms.

or neural compression) are best treated surgically. Although local symptoms are more frequently associated with larger lesions, and aneurysms with complications tend to be larger than those that are asymptomatic, there is no strong evidence that the incidence of limb-threatening complications increases with the aneurysm size. No specific aneurysm size has been identified at which the incidence of complications changes. This is a reflection of the propensity for femoral artery aneurysms to thrombose rather than rupture, and the risk of thrombosis is not directly related to the size of the aneurysm. The size at which surgical intervention is indicated in asymptomatic aneurysms has not been defined, but many surgeons suggest that a femoral artery aneurysm greater than 2.5 cm in diameter should also be repaired unless the patient is at high risk for operative intervention.

The indications for surgery in patients with asymptomatic lesions are best defined in the context of the natural history of femoral artery aneurysms; unfortunately, this is poorly defined because most publications focus on patients who presented for surgical repair. The number of series in which more than 10 aneurysms have been followed without surgery is severely limited. In one series, limb-threatening complications were documented in only 3% of 105 aneurysms observed for an average of 28 months.[17] In another series, no complications were encountered in 19 patients followed up for an average of 52 months.[1] These two series suggest that a small, asymptomatic femoral artery aneurysm does not pose the same threat to the limb as a popliteal artery aneurysm does. The development of complications in patients with asymptomatic aneurysms is sufficiently low to justify nonoperative management, particularly in the patient with multiple medical problems who would be at high risk for surgery and has a limited life expectancy.

If nonoperative management is selected, the size of the aneurysm should be documented by ultrasonography and follow-up evaluation should include repeated ultrasonography and careful examination for occult complications. Serial duplex scans to evaluate the extent of intraluminal thrombus are not of proven benefit but may be useful in predicting patients prone to developing complications. The presence of intraluminal thrombus is thought to be associated with the development of complications in popliteal artery aneurysms. Operative treatment should be undertaken without undue delay if the femoral aneurysm enlarges, produces symptoms, or is complicated by embolization, thrombosis, or rupture. The appropriate treatment of asymptomatic aneurysms is not clearly defined.

Operative Technique

Because patients often have multiple aneurysms, surgical intervention must be individualized based on symptoms, concomitant aneurysms, and the extent of the femoral aneurysm. If the patient presents with a symptomatic aneurysm, this lesion is addressed first. In patients with asymptomatic aortic, femoral, and popliteal lesions, a staged approach is used. The potentially life-threatening aortic lesion is usually treated first, followed by bypass grafting for limb-threatening popliteal lesions, and, finally, by femoral artery aneurysm repair as appropriate. When an aortofemoral bypass is necessary in a patient with aortoiliac and femoral aneurysms, the femoral anastomosis should not be sewn into a femoral aneurysm because of the high incidence of anastomotic aneurysm formation. The distal anastomosis is usually performed beyond the aneurysm or into an interposition graft that has replaced the femoral aneurysm.

The surgical treatment of an isolated femoral artery aneurysm is determined primarily by aneurysmal involvement of the superficial and deep femoral arteries. The surgeon usually approaches the femoral artery aneurysm through a vertical groin incision, although an unusually large or ruptured aneurysm can be approached more safely after controlling the external iliac artery through a retroperitoneal approach. After proximal and distal arterial flow is controlled, the aneurysmal sac is opened and the atheromatous debris is removed. Small aneurysms may be resected, but total excision of large aneurysms adherent to the adjacent vein and nerve is unnecessary and hazardous.

Type I aneurysms are replaced with an interposition graft of Dacron or expanded polytetrafluoroethylene (ePTFE) (usually 8 or 10 mm in diameter) anastomosed end-to-end to the distal external iliac or proximal common femoral artery above the aneurysm and to the distal common femoral artery above the femoral bifurcation (Fig. 94–2). Saphenous vein can be used as the graft if it is of adequate caliber, but it does not have any distinct advantage over prosthetic material in this location. The graft is usually sewn to the artery from within the aneurysmal cavity and the aneurysmal sac is closed over the graft.

Type II aneurysms with patent superficial and profunda femoris arteries are usually replaced with an interposition graft to the superficial femoral artery or the profunda femoris artery, with reimplantation of the other artery (Fig. 94–3). Alternatively, a prosthetic graft side limb can be used between the femoral interposition graft and the profunda femoris artery. Another option is "syndactylization," or suturing of the superficial and profunda femoris arteries together to form a common lumen. An interposition graft is then used to replace the aneurysm.

Treatment of a femoral aneurysm may be indicated because the femoral artery will be used as the origin of an infrainguinal graft to treat severe lower extremity occlusive disease or aneurysmal disease of the superficial femoral and popliteal arteries. In such cases, the femoral aneurysm should be addressed, even when it is a small, asymptomatic lesion. If the superficial femoral artery is chronically oc-

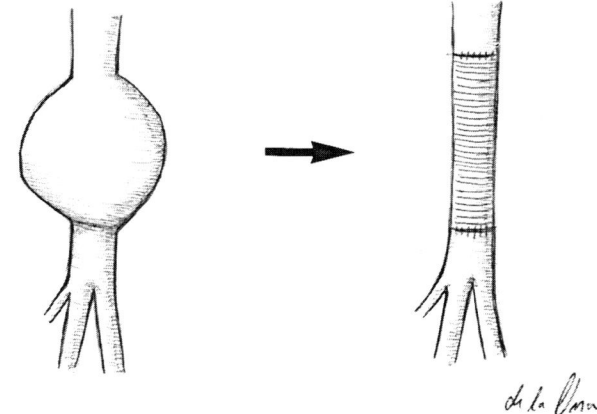

FIGURE 94–2. Diagram demonstrating options for operative repair of a type I femoral artery aneurysm that is confined to the common femoral artery.

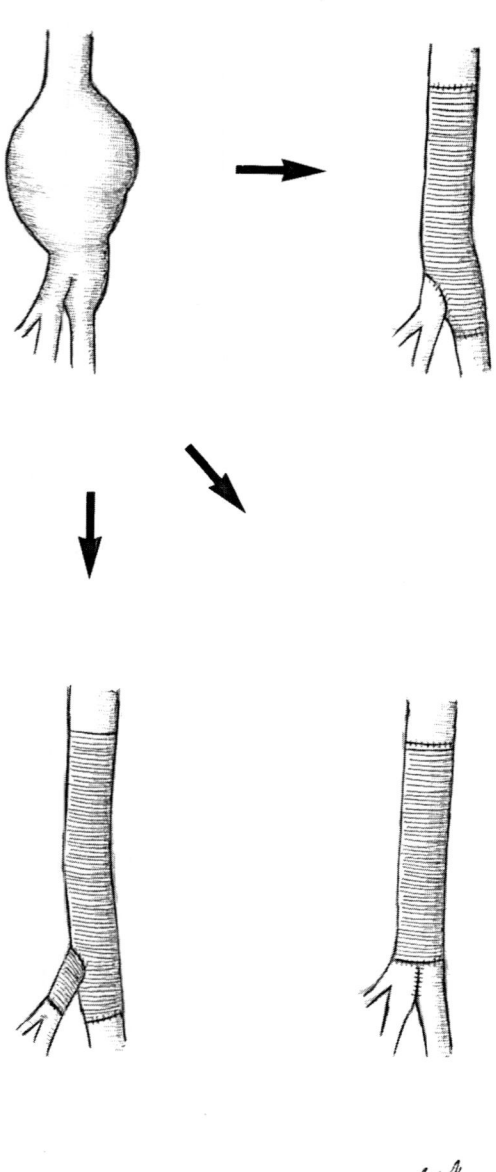

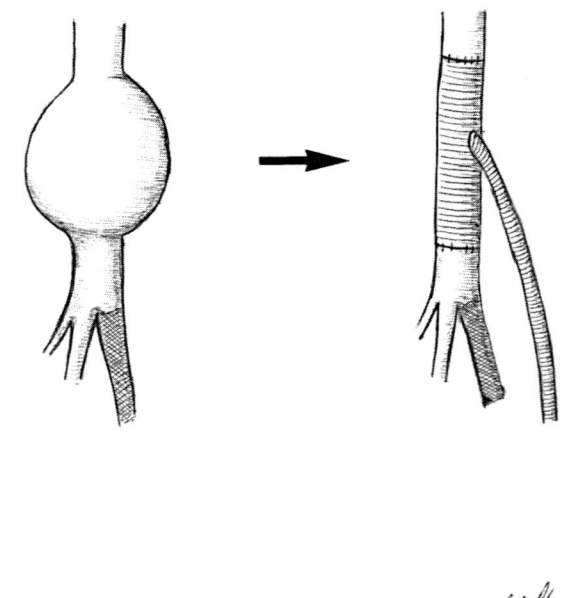

FIGURE 94–4. Diagram demonstrating repair of a femoral aneurysm followed by femoropopliteal bypass graft placement for treatment of occlusive disease.

mortality rate for repair of an isolated, uncomplicated femoral artery aneurysm approaches that of administering anesthesia to that patient. Mortality rates of up to 4%, however, reflect concomitant aortic reconstruction in many patients.[17] Long-term graft patency is excellent in asymptom-

FIGURE 94–3. Diagram demonstrating options for operative repair of a type II femoral artery aneurysm that involves the orifices of the superficial and profunda femoris arteries. Arterial continuity is restored with an interposition graft with reimplantation of the profunda femoris artery, a side limb to the profunda femoris artery, or syndactylization of the superficial and profunda femoris arteries.

cluded, a femoral interposition graft is placed, and a standard femoropopliteal or femorotibial bypass with saphenous vein is then performed, with an end-to-side proximal anastomosis to the interposition graft (Fig. 94–4). Patients with extensive aneurysmal degeneration of the superficial femoral and popliteal arteries, as well as the femoral artery, usually require a femoral interposition graft to the profunda femoris artery, with a saphenous vein bypass graft to the below-knee popliteal or tibial artery and ligation of the intervening aneurysmal segment (Fig. 94–5).

Results

Results of surgical therapy depend upon the concomitant vascular disease. In asymptomatic patients, the operative

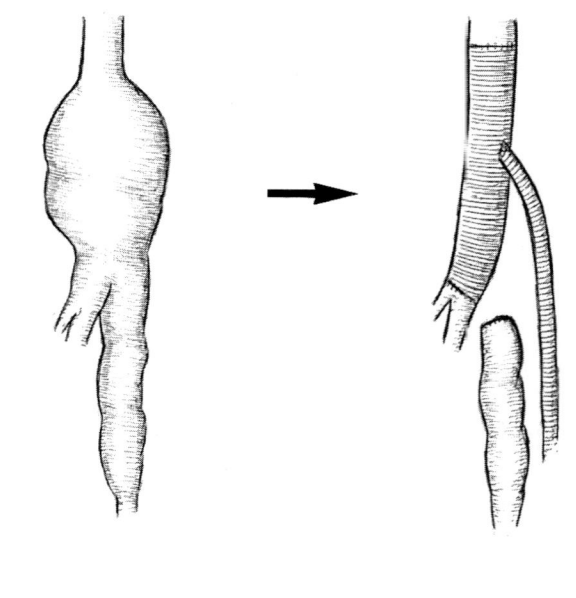

FIGURE 94–5. Diagram demonstrating repair of a femoral aneurysm followed by femoropopliteal bypass graft placement for treatment of diffuse aneurysmal degeneration of the superficial femoral and popliteal arteries.

atic patients. In those presenting with lower extremity ischemia, 68% achieve satisfactory long-term outcomes.[17]

Profunda Femoris Artery Aneurysms

Aneurysms of the profunda femoris artery are unusual, perhaps due to its protected location beneath the adductor magnus and its resistance to atherosclerotic degeneration. Most of these aneurysms are traumatic in origin, usually from penetrating, orthopedic, or iatrogenic trauma. Nonspecific aneurysms of the profunda femoris artery are rare (comprising only 2% of femoral artery aneurysms), and most are found in association with common femoral aneurysms, although isolated profunda femoris aneurysms are occasionally encountered.

The natural history of profunda femoris artery aneurysms is not known, since most reports consist of only one or two cases treated surgically. The lesions are rarely identified on routine physical examination because of their deep location; they are usually discovered as an incidental finding on an imaging study or after they become symptomatic because of a complication, such as rupture.

Rupture is a common presentation, affecting nearly one third of patients (six of 20 cases) in the sporadic case reports.[34, 39] This has led to the idea that these lesions are uniquely prone to rupture, but this is more likely a reflection of the difficulty in identifying asymptomatic lesions. Rapid enlargement producing local symptoms is also a common presentation (four of 20 cases), with thrombosis (one of 20 cases) and distal embolization (one of 20 cases) being less frequent. The remainder of reported cases (eight of 20 cases) are asymptomatic.[34] The incidence of thrombosis may be underestimated because of the lack of clinical consequences if the superficial femoral artery is patent.

Like common femoral aneurysms, multiple peripheral aneurysms and AAAs are often encountered in these patients. The diagnosis of a profunda femoris aneurysm is often made with ultrasound or CT scan; each of these modalities is also useful for identifying concomitant aneurysms. Arteriography is helpful in planning the surgical approach.

Treatment consists of aneurysm exclusion with restoration of blood flow. Replacement with an interposition graft, if possible, is the preferred method. If extensive aneurysmal degeneration of the profunda femoris artery precludes revascularization and the superficial femoral artery is disease-free, therapeutic options include ligation of the aneurysm proximally and distally, oversewing of branches and the profunda femoris from within the aneurysm, and angiographic obliteration. If the superficial femoral artery is not patent, a femoropopliteal or femorotibial bypass is undertaken in conjunction with profunda femoris ligation if collateral blood flow to the thigh is adequate.

Superficial Femoral Artery Aneurysms

Isolated aneurysms of the superficial femoral artery are rare. Most are traumatic or mycotic in origin. Nonspecific aneurysms of the superficial femoral artery are usually found in association with aneurysms in other locations, especially the popliteal artery, as diffuse aneurysmal degeneration of the entire superficial femoral artery, or in patients with arteriomegaly. Associated aneurysms are common, with at least 40% of patients having concomitant AAAs.[27] As with common femoral artery aneurysms, it is important to identify other potentially life-threatening or limb-threatening aneurysms in these patients.

A superficial femoral artery aneurysm usually presents as a pulsatile mass in the medial aspect of the thigh, which may be painful. Since the superficial femoral artery is relatively deep in the thigh, the aneurysm has usually attained significant size before it is recognized. Because of the difficulty in recognizing asymptomatic lesions, many superficial artery aneurysms are not found until a complication occurs. In their review of 17 superficial femoral artery aneurysms, Rigdon and Monajjem[27] report that 65% have complications at presentation: rupture in 35%, thrombosis in 18%, and distal emboli in 12%. Embolization and thrombosis seem to be less common than with popliteal aneurysms, making limb salvage possible in most cases.

The natural history of superficial femoral artery aneurysms is not clear because no large series have been reported, but surgical treatment is recommended for all symptomatic aneurysms. Asymptomatic aneurysms over 2.5 cm in diameter should also be treated surgically in all but the highest-risk patients. Superficial femoral artery aneurysms are often continuous with popliteal artery aneurysms and are repaired concomitantly with them. The usual approach is a bypass with saphenous vein, followed by proximal and distal ligation of the aneurysm. The limb salvage rate is 94%.[27]

POPLITEAL ARTERY ANEURYSMS

Popliteal artery aneurysms are important because of their propensity to develop limb-threatening complications. Most of these lesions are of nonspecific etiology. Anastomotic or traumatic aneurysms are unusual, and mycotic aneurysms are distinctly rare in current practice. Therefore, this discussion focuses on nonspecific popliteal aneurysms.

Popliteal artery aneurysms are the most commonly encountered nonspecific peripheral aneurysm, occurring slightly more frequently than femoral artery lesions. Compared with AAAs, however, they are relatively unusual. AAAs are diagnosed with 15 times the frequency of popliteal aneurysms.[32]

Multiple aneurysms are frequent in patients with popliteal aneurysms; Table 94–2 summarizes the larger series of popliteal aneurysms. Approximately 50% to 70% of patients have bilateral popliteal aneurysms, 40% to 50% have AAAs, and nearly 40% have femoral artery aneurysms.[3, 37, 38] Patients with bilateral popliteal aneurysms are particularly likely to have extrapopliteal aneurysms, and 70% of these patients have an AAA.[38] The importance of the associated aneurysms lies in the life-threatening nature of AAAs that may be missed on physical examination. The presence or absence of associated aneurysms must be documented by appropriate imaging studies, such as ultrasonography or CT, in every patient with a popliteal artery aneurysm. This allows potentially life-threatening AAAs and other limb-threatening lesions to be identified and managed appropriately.

TABLE 94–2. CLINICAL PRESENTATION OF POPLITEAL ANEURYSMS

AUTHOR	PATIENTS	ANEURYSMS	MALE : FEMALE	BILATERAL FAA (%)	AAA/FAA-ASSOCIATED (%/%)	ASYMPTOMATIC (%)	SYMPTOMS AT PRESENTATION	COMPLICATIONS AT PRESENTATION
Wychulis et al (1970)[39]	152	233	148:4	59	35/26	45	Local pain, 6% Venous symptoms, 18% Ischemic symptoms, 7% Tissue loss, 12%	Emboli, 10% Thrombosis, 28% Rupture, 2.5%
Bouhoutsos and Martin (1974)[6]	84	116	76:8	38	32/25		Venous symptoms, 6% Claudication, 73% Rest pain, 26% Gangrene, 6%	Emboli, 20% Thrombosis, 58% Rupture, 0%
Vermilion et al (1981)[37]	87	147	84:3	68	40/43	33	Local pain, 8% Venous symptoms, 7% Claudication, 45% Rest pain, 31% Gangrene, 6%	Emboli, 23% Thrombosis, 45% Rupture, 3%
Reilly et al (1983)[26]	159	244	149:10	53		46	Local symptoms, 5%	Emboli, 13% Acute thrombosis, 27% Chronic thrombosis, 9%
Anton et al (1986)[3]	110	160	108:2	45	32/12	48	Claudication, 41% Severe ischemia, 11%	Thromboemboli, 44% Rupture, 0.6%
Roggo et al (1993)[28]	167	252	159:8	51	38	25	Local symptoms, 4% Claudication, 30% Rest pain, 24% Gangrene, 17%	Emboli, 23% Thrombosis, 45% Rupture, 2%
Varga et al (1994)[36]	137	200	134:3	54	33/19	22	Local symptoms, 16% Claudication, 29% Severe ischemia, 28%	Atheroemboli, 6% Acute limb-threatening ischemia, 31%
Lowell et al (1994)[20]	106	161	103:3	53	51/27	58	Ischemic symptoms, 42%	Acute ischemia, 9%
Dawson et al (1997)[12] (review)	1673	2445	97:3	50	37	37	Local symptoms, 6.5% Ischemic symptoms, 55%	Rupture, 1.4%

AAA = abdominal aortic aneurysm; FAA = femoral artery aneurysm.

Popliteal aneurysms are confined to the popliteal artery in approximately 50% of cases; nearly 40% involve the origins of the anterior tibial artery and tibioperoneal trunk.[10] Approximately 10% of popliteal aneurysms are associated with aneurysmal degeneration of the superficial femoral artery.

Clinical Manifestations

The clinical manifestations of popliteal artery aneurysms span the spectrum from an asymptomatic pulsatile mass to severe lower extremity ischemia. Approximately 45% of patients are asymptomatic at the time of diagnosis (see Table 94–2).[3, 38] The majority of patients present with symptoms of limb ischemia, usually claudication, but severe ischemia with rest pain and gangrene may follow distal embolization or thrombosis. Local symptoms, including awareness of a popliteal mass, local pain, and leg swelling or phlebitis secondary to popliteal vein compression, account for the remainder of symptoms.

Popliteal artery aneurysms may be complicated by thrombosis, embolization, or rupture. Thrombosis is documented in approximately 40% of patients and embolization in 25%.[37] The incidence of embolization, however, varies with the care used in looking for the angiographic evidence. Thrombosis may result from multiple embolic events that occlude the tibial vessels, compromising outflow and precipitating thrombosis of the popliteal aneurysm. Severe ischemia usually results, but in some patients this process has proceeded slowly and allowed the development of collateral circulation so that extremity viability is not threatened when thrombosis occurs. Fewer than 5% of popliteal aneurysms present with rupture.[3, 37] Hemorrhage from rupture is usually confined to the popliteal space and does not preclude successful arterial reconstruction.

The typical patient with a popliteal aneurysm is a man in the seventh decade of life. The male:female ratio in patients with popliteal aneurysms is nearly 30:1, and as Reilly and colleagues[26] pointed out, the woman with a popliteal aneurysm is usually in her 80s, which is older than the typical patient with a popliteal aneurysm. Risk factors for atherosclerosis are common in these patients, 50% to 75% being smokers, 40% to 60% having hypertension, and approximately 15% having diabetes mellitus.[3, 20, 37, 38] As expected, there is a high incidence of other cardiovascular diseases in these patients. More than 40% have evidence of significant cardiac disease, and 10% have manifestations of cerebrovascular disease.[3]

Diagnosis

The diagnosis of a popliteal aneurysm is usually suspected on a careful physical examination. Palpation of the popliteal space with the knee slightly flexed identifies a prominent pulsatile mass in patients with patent aneurysms. Small aneurysms may not be palpable on physical examination. If thrombosis has occurred, the correct identity of a firm, nonpulsatile mass still may be suspected on physical examination, especially when a patent popliteal aneurysm is present in the contralateral leg. Roentgenograms of the knee may demonstrate calcium in the wall of the aneurysm, suggesting the diagnosis of popliteal artery aneurysm.

Once the diagnosis is suspected, it must be confirmed by ultrasonography, CT, or MRI. In addition to defining the true nature of a popliteal fossa mass and distinguishing it from other pathology such as a Baker's cyst, these modalities are useful in confirming the presence or absence of associated aneurysms, particularly AAAs. Angiography may be helpful in the diagnosis of aneurysms, but it may be misleading in the presence of intraluminal thrombus. Angiography, however, is essential prior to surgery to define the arterial anatomy, the extent of aneurysmal disease, and the patency of distal vasculature. This allows the appropriate operative procedure to be planned.

Indications for Surgical Treatment

Surgical treatment is indicated for all symptomatic or complicated aneurysms. Aneurysms that are enlarging or causing local symptoms (pain, venous or neural compression) should be treated without undue delay. Patients presenting with limb-threatening complications (embolization, thrombosis, or rupture) should undergo expeditious repair.

Controversy exists over the optimal management of the patient with an asymptomatic popliteal artery aneurysm. Ideally, recommendations for these patients should be based on the natural history of popliteal artery aneurysms, but this is not well defined. Most published series are composed primarily of aneurysms treated surgically. No large series is available to define complication rates or limb loss in the contemporary period with the availability of balloon catheter embolectomy and thrombolytic therapy. Dawson and colleagues,[12] however, reviewed 29 reports in the English medical literature published between 1980 and 1994, which included 1673 patients with 2445 popliteal aneurysms, and found that a mean of 35% of patients followed conservatively developed ischemic complications. This was associated with a mean amputation rate of 25% despite attempted repair when feasible.

The percentage of aneurysms that develops complications increases with time followed. Roggo and colleagues[28] reported that all patients with 45 aneurysms treated "conservatively" developed ischemic symptoms and required surgery at a mean of 4.2 years after diagnosis—half within the first 2 years. Because of the high incidence of complications, the inability to predict complications based on size of the aneurysm, the high amputation rate after the development of complications, and the lower graft patency rate after bypassing complicated aneurysms compared with asymptomatic lesions, most surgeons recommend operative treatment for asymptomatic popliteal aneurysms except in high-risk patients.

Some recommend conservative management of the asymptomatic aneurysm because of the limited life expectancy of patients with popliteal aneurysms.[7] In addition, they point to the high success rate of thrombolytic therapy combined with bypass surgery in patients who present with an acutely thrombosed popliteal aneurysm and limb-threatening ischemia. Vermilion and colleagues[37] found that patients with popliteal aneurysms had a 50% survival at 5.7 years compared with 14 years for an age-matched general population. Lowell and colleagues[20] found that the overall actuarial patient survival at 5 and 10 years was 67% and 38%, compared with approximately 77% and 55% in the normal matched population. The survival of patients with multiple aneurysms was particularly compromised, with a 10-year survival rate of only 16% compared with 66% for patients with a solitary aneurysm at the initial examination.[13]

Michaels and Galland[22] employed a *Markov decision tree* to model the problem and determine the criteria for a conservative approach. Their results suggested that elective operation produced better results than conservative management at 1 to 2 years after presentation. Thus, when life expectancy is severely compromised by another disease or operative risk is inordinately high, a conservative approach is warranted. Otherwise, elective treatment of asymptomatic aneurysms is appropriate until comparable outcomes from elective repair and emergency repair of symptomatic or complicated aneurysms are demonstrated.

Another approach to the management of patients with an asymptomatic popliteal aneurysm is to identify patients at high or low risk for the development of complications. A variety of factors have been suggested as risk factors for thrombosis, such as size greater than 2 cm, intraluminal thrombus, and poor runoff. Lowell and colleagues[20] found at least one of these three risk factors in 11 of 12 patients with popliteal aneurysms that became symptomatic during follow-up, compared with 9 of 24 aneurysms that remained asymptomatic, leading to their recommendation that aneurysms with any of these characteristics should be repaired electively if patients are expected to have a reasonable long-term survival. Ramesh and colleagues[25] found that size of the aneurysm, distortion within the aneurysm, or distortion of the popliteal artery above or below the aneurysm was associated with thrombosis, but that distortion was a more sensitive predictor of thrombosis than size alone (Fig. 94–6). Identification of aneurysms at high risk for thrombosis would be useful in selecting those patients who should undergo elective surgery, but these criteria have not been evaluated in a prospective manner.

Operative Technique

The treatment goals in patients with popliteal aneurysms are to (1) preserve life, (2) eliminate potential limb-threatening lesions, and (3) restore adequate blood flow to the limb. The operative approach must be individualized because these patients often have multiple aneurysms. In general, an aortic aneurysm is treated first, because it is a life-threatening lesion. Repair of the popliteal aneurysm follows. However, if a limb-threatening complication has occurred, the popliteal aneurysm may require expeditious treatment, with delay of the AAA repair.

One of the most important advances in the treatment of popliteal aneurysms is the use of thrombolytic therapy in the patient who presents with an acutely thrombosed aneurysm and thrombus extending into the runoff vessels. In this case, intra-arterial thrombolytic therapy should be directed at lysing thrombus in the distal runoff vessels to identify a suitable target for bypass surgery. This may be difficult because of the large amount of thrombus within the aneurysm, the potential for embolization, and the chronic nature of the distal atheroemboli precluding successful restoration of blood flow to the foot. Results with thrombolytic therapy followed by bypass of the aneurysm,

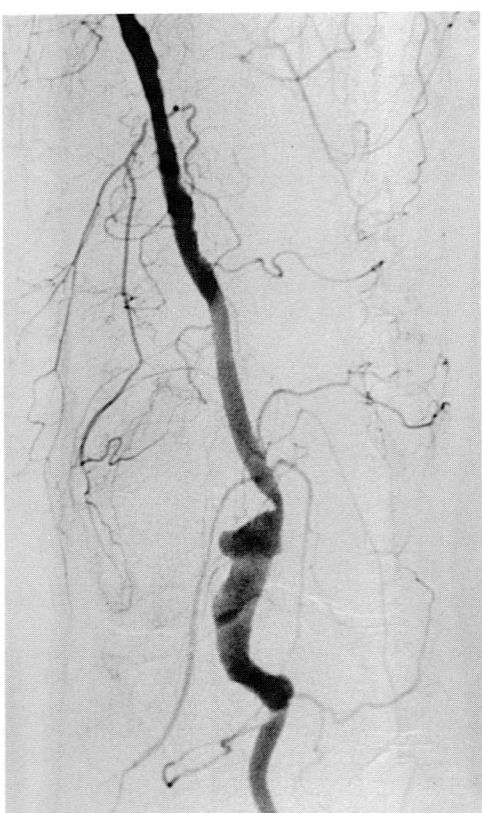

FIGURE 94–6. Arteriogram demonstrating a popliteal aneurysm with significant distortion of the artery. Distortion within, above, or below the aneurysm may be a more sensitive predictor of thrombosis than size alone.[25]

however, have been surprisingly good compared with an isolated operative approach.

Treatment of fusiform popliteal artery aneurysms is directed at eliminating an embolic source and bypassing the lesion. The medial operative approach is used most frequently (Fig. 94–7). The proximal popliteal artery is exposed through a medial incision in the distal thigh. The distal popliteal artery is approached through a medial leg incision that is parallel and just posterior to the tibia. Most aneurysms are left in situ to avoid injury to adjacent vein and nerve that may be firmly adherent. The surgeon bypasses the aneurysm using a segment of saphenous vein that is harvested and positioned along the course of the popliteal artery. The proximal anastomosis is to the common femoral or distal superficial femoral artery, depending on the extent of aneurysmal degeneration. The artery just proximal to the aneurysm is usually ligated to prevent late rupture, but some surgeons prefer to preserve potentially valuable collaterals if superior geniculate arteries are patent.

The distal anastomosis is performed end-to-end or end-to-side, with ligation of the popliteal artery proximal to the anastomosis to prevent embolization. The aneurysm usually thromboses proximally to the level of the geniculate arteries or proximal ligature. Late expansion and rupture of a bypassed and ligated popliteal aneurysm, even when ligated both proximally and distally, can occur secondary to continued perfusion of the aneurysm through patent genicu-

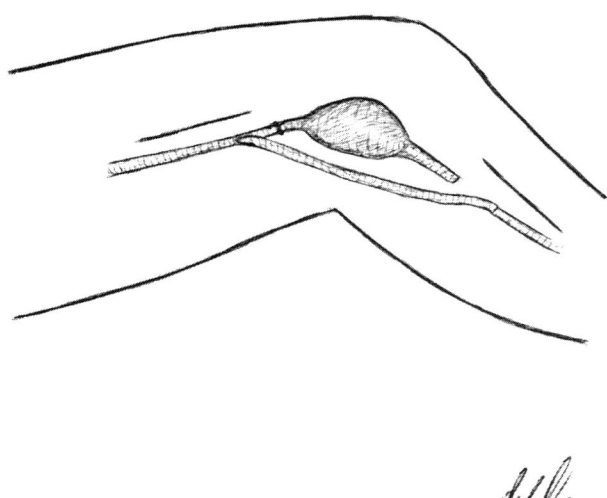

FIGURE 94–7. Diagram demonstrating the medial approach to a popliteal aneurysm. A bypass, usually with saphenous vein, is performed, followed by ligation of the popliteal artery immediately above and below the aneurysm.

lates. When the distal popliteal and proximal tibial arteries are occluded with emboli, balloon catheter embolectomy or infusion of thrombolytic therapy is a useful intraoperative adjuvant. Frequently, bypass grafts must be carried to the distal tibial vessels.

A posterior approach is sometimes preferred for large, saccular aneurysms causing local symptoms. The posterior approach has the disadvantage of requiring a separate incision for vein harvest unless the lesser saphenous vein is of adequate caliber. After proximal and distal control, the sac is opened, the thrombus evacuated and the redundant portion of the wall removed or an obliterative endoaneurysmorrhaphy is performed, avoiding trauma to the popliteal veins. A bypass graft is placed within the aneurysm sac.

Results

Results depend on the preoperative status of the popliteal aneurysm. Perioperative mortality is low: 1.5% in a report of the Joint Vascular Research Group from the United Kingdom,[36] but mortality is influenced by presentation. Reilly and colleagues[26] report operative mortality rates for asymptomatic and symptomatic aneurysms of 0% and 2.1%, respectively, presumably a reflection of emergency procedures required for acutely symptomatic lesions. Results are excellent in asymptomatic aneurysms with intact distal vasculature, with 5- and 10-year graft patency rates of greater than 80% and limb salvage of 93% to 98%[3, 28]; however, patients with thrombosed aneurysms or severely compromised outflow due to multiple embolic episodes have less optimal results. Graft patency rates at 5 and 10 years are 60% and 48%, respectively, and limb salvage rates are 60% and 80%.[3, 13, 28] Long-term patency of vein grafts is excellent and surpasses that of other graft materials, with 10-year patency rates of 94% and 27%, respectively.[3]

TIBIAL ARTERY ANEURYSMS

Aneurysms of the tibial arteries are distinctly uncommon, and references to these entities usually consist of case

reports. Tibial artery aneurysms are often pseudoaneurysms secondary to infection or trauma, either blunt or penetrating, and may result from balloon catheter injuries. Tibial artery aneurysms have also been reported as a result of polyarteritis nodosa, but most true tibial artery aneurysms are of nonspecific etiology.

These aneurysms may be asymptomatic and identified incidentally on an imaging study undertaken for another reason, or they may present as a calf mass, with leg ischemia, or with digital ischemia secondary to emboli from the aneurysm.[5, 23] The diagnosis is usually obvious on an arteriogram.

Therapeutic options depend upon the presentation and the anatomy. Small, asymptomatic lesions may be followed. Large or symptomatic aneurysms of a single tibial artery may be ligated or occluded angiographically if the remaining tibial arteries are normal. If concomitant aneurysmal or occlusive disease is present in the other tibial arteries, the aneurysms should be bypassed with saphenous vein and the aneurysm ligated or excised, depending on local symptoms.

REFERENCES

1. Adiseshiah M, Bailey DA: Aneurysms of the femoral artery. Br J Surg 64:174, 1977.
2. Anderson CB, Butcher HR Jr, Ballinger WF: Mycotic aneurysms. Arch Surg 109:712. 1974.
3. Anton GE, Hertzer NR, Beven EG, et al: Surgical management of popliteal aneurysms: Trends in presentation, treatment, and results from 1952 to 1984. J Vasc Surg 3:125, 1986.
4. Baird RJ, Gurry JF, Kellam J, et al: Arteriosclerotic femoral artery aneurysms. Can Med Assoc J 117:1306, 1977.
5. Borozan PG, Walker HSJ III, Peterson GJ: True tibial artery aneurysms: Case report and literature review. J Vasc Surg 10:457, 1989.
6. Bouhoutsos J, Martin P: Popliteal aneurysm: A review of 116 cases. Br J Surg 61:469, 1974.
7. Bowyer RC, Cawthorn SJ, Walker WJ, et al: Conservative management of asymptomatic popliteal aneurysm. Br J Surg 77:1132, 1990.
8. Brophy CM, Tilson JE, Braverman IM, et al: Age of onset, pattern of distribution, and histology of aneurysm development in a genetically predisposed mouse model. J Vasc Surg 8:45, 1988.
9. Brown SL, Busuttil RW, Baker JD, et al: Bacteriologic and surgical determinants of survival in patients with mycotic aneurysms. J Vasc Surg 1:541, 1984.
10. Buda JA, Weber CJ, McAllister FF, et al: The results of treatment of popliteal artery aneurysms: A follow-up study of 86 aneurysms. J Cardiovasc Surg 15:615, 1974.
11. Cutler BS, Darling RC: Surgical management of arteriosclerotic femoral aneurysms. Surgery 74:764, 1973.
12. Dawson I, Sie RB, Van Bockel JH: Atherosclerotic popliteal aneurysm. Br J Surg 84:293, 1997.
13. Dawson I, Van Bockel JH, Brand R, et al: Popliteal artery aneurysms: Long-term follow-up of aneurysmal disease and results of surgical treatment. J Vasc Surg 13:398, 1991.
14. Dennis JW, Littooy FN, Greisler HP, et al: Anastomotic pseudoaneurysms: A continuing late complication of vascular reconstructive procedures. Arch Surg 121:314, 1986.
15. Dent TL, Lindenauer SM, Ernst CB, et al: Multiple arteriosclerotic artery aneurysms. Arch Surg 105:338, 1972.
16. Faggioli GL, Gargiulo M, Bertoni F, et al: Parietal inflammatory infiltrate in peripheral aneurysms of atherosclerotic origin. J Cardiovasc Surg 33:331, 1992.
17. Graham LM, Zelenock GB, Whitehouse WM Jr, et al: Clinical significance of arteriosclerotic femoral artery aneurysms. Arch Surg 115:502, 1980.
18. Katz DJ, Stanley JC, Zelenock GB: Gender differences in abdominal aortic aneurysm prevalence, treatment, and outcome. J Vasc Surg 25:561, 1997.

19. Lawrence PF, Lorenzo-Rivero S, Lyon JL: The incidence of iliac, femoral, and popliteal artery aneurysms in hospitalized patients. J Vasc Surg 22:409, 1995.
20. Lowell RC, Gloviczki P, Hallett JW Jr, et al: Popliteal artery aneurysms: The risk of nonoperative management. Ann Vasc Surg 8:14, 1994.
21. Messina LM, Brothers TE, Wakefield TW, et al: Clinical characteristics and surgical management of vascular complications in patients undergoing cardiac catheterization: Interventional versus diagnostic procedures. J Vasc Surg 13:593, 1991.
22. Michaels JA, Galland RB: Management of asymptomatic popliteal aneurysms: The use of a Markov decision tree to determine the criteria for a conservative approach. Eur J Vasc Surg 7:136, 1993.
23. Monig SP, Walter M, Sorgatz S, et al: True infrapopliteal artery aneurysms: Report of two cases and literature review. J Vasc Surg 24:276, 1996.
24. Pappas G, Janes JM, Bernatz PE, et al: Femoral aneurysms. Review of surgical management. JAMA 190:97, 1964.
25. Ramesh S, Michaels JA, Galland RB: Popliteal aneurysm: Morphology and management. Br J Surg 80:1531, 1993.
26. Reilly MK, Abbott WM, Darling RC: Aggressive surgical management of popliteal artery aneurysms. Am J Surg 145:498, 1983.
27. Rigdon EE, Monajjem N: Aneurysms of the superficial femoral artery: A report of two cases and review of the literature. J Vasc Surg 16:790, 1992.
28. Roggo A, Brunner U, Ottinger LW, et al: The continuing challenge of aneurysms of the popliteal artery. Surg Gynecol Obstet 177:565, 1993.
29. Sapienza P, Mingoli A, Feldhaus RJ, et al: Femoral artery aneurysms: Long-term follow-up and results of surgical treatment. Cardiovasc Surg 4:181, 1996.
30. Seabrook GR, Schmitt DD, Bandyk DF, et al: Anastomotic femoral pseudoaneurysm: An investigation of occult infection as an etiologic factor. J Vasc Surg 11:629, 1990.
31. Szilagyi DE, Elliott JP Jr, Smith RF, et al: A thirty-year survey of the reconstructive surgical treatment of aortoiliac occlusive disease. J Vasc Surg 3:421, 1986.
32. Szilagyi DE, Schwartz RL, Reddy DJ: Popliteal arterial aneurysms. Their natural history and management. Arch Surg 116:723, 1981.
33. Szilagyi DE, Smith RF, Elliott JP, et al: Anastomotic aneurysms after vascular reconstruction: Problems of incidence, etiology, and treatment. Surgery 78:800, 1975.
34. Tait WF, Vohra RK, Carp HM, et al: True profunda femoris aneurysms: Are they more dangerous than other atherosclerotic aneurysms of the femoropopliteal segment? Ann Vasc Surg 5:92, 1991.
35. Thompson RW, Liao SX, Curci JA: Vascular smooth muscle cell apoptosis in abdominal aortic aneurysms. Coron Artery Dis 8:623, 1997.
36. Varga ZA, Locke-Edmunds JC, Baird RN, et al: A multicenter study of popliteal aneurysms. J Vasc Surg 20:171, 1994.
37. Vermilion BD, Kimmins SA, Pace WG, et al: A review of one hundred forty-seven popliteal aneurysms with long-term follow-up. Surgery 90:1009, 1981.
38. Whitehouse WM Jr, Wakefield TW, Graham LM, et al: Limb-threatening potential of arteriosclerotic popliteal artery aneurysms. Surgery 93:694, 1983.
39. Wychulis AR, Spittell JA, Wallace RB: Popliteal aneurysms. Surgery 68:942, 1970.

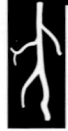

CHAPTER 9 5
Upper Extremity Aneurysms

G. Patrick Clagett, M.D.

Upper extremity aneurysms are relatively rare in comparison with other peripheral arterial aneurysms.[1] Their recognition and treatment are important, however, because these aneurysms can cause major disability, lead to limb and digit loss, and, in the case of proximal aneurysms of the subclavian artery, result in death from rupture and exsanguination. In addition to rupture, proximal aneurysms are complicated by thromboembolism with ischemic upper extremity signs and symptoms (including gangrene), neuromuscular and sensory dysfunction from brachial plexus compression, and central neurologic deficits due to retrograde thromboembolism in the vertebral and right carotid circulations. In contrast, more distally located upper extremity aneurysms are almost exclusively manifested by thromboembolic complications of the hand and digits.

Because of the relative rarity of upper extremity aneurysms, the natural history and the overall incidence of associated complications are unknown; however, in reviewing the reported cases in the literature, one is impressed by the serious morbidity encountered with the first manifestations of these aneurysms. Because of this, optimal surgical treatment should be carried out early, preferably before symptoms arise.

SUBCLAVIAN ARTERY ANEURYSMS

Subclavian artery aneurysms arise from degenerative disease, thoracic outlet obstruction, or trauma. Aneurysms involving the proximal and mid-subclavian artery are usually nonspecific, atherosclerosis-associated,[2, 9] or, less commonly, associated with syphilis,[3] cystic medial necrosis,[4] invasion of the wall by contiguous tuberculous lymphadenitis,[5] and idiopathic congenital causes.[6, 7] From 30% to 50% of patients with nonspecific, atherosclerosis-associated subclavian aneurysms have aortoiliac or other peripheral aneurysms.[8, 10] Therefore, patients presenting with subclavian aneurysms should be thoroughly evaluated for associated aneurysms. These aneurysms usually occur in patients over 60 years of age of either sex but appear to be more common in men. Aneurysms of the distal subclavian artery, frequently with extension into the first portion of the axillary artery, are appropriately considered aneurysms of the subclavian-axillary arteries and are most commonly associated with a thoracic outlet obstruction, cervical rib, and other bony abnormalities.[8]

Clinical Presentation

Presenting symptoms of subclavian aneurysms include (1) chest, neck, and shoulder pain from acute expansion or rupture; (2) upper extremity acute and chronic ischemic symptoms from thromboembolism; (3) upper extremity pain and neurologic dysfunction from brachial plexus compression; (4) hoarseness from compression of the right recurrent laryngeal nerve; (5) respiratory insufficiency from tracheal compression; (6) transient ischemic attacks and stroke from retrograde thromboembolism in the vertebral and right carotid circulations; and (7) hemoptysis from erosion into the apex of the lung. Patients without symptoms may note the presence of a supraclavicular pulsatile mass. Most frequently, asymptomatic pulsatile masses in this area represent tortuous common carotid and subclavian arteries. These can usually be distinguished from true aneurysms by duplex ultrasonography; however, on occasion arteriography is necessary (Fig. 95–1). In addition to a supraclavicular mass, physical signs may include (1) a supraclavicular bruit, (2) absent or diminished pulses in the upper extremity, (3) normal pulses with signs of microembolization (blue finger syndrome), (4) sensory and motor signs of brachial plexus compression, (5) vocal cord paralysis, and (6) Horner's syndrome due to compression

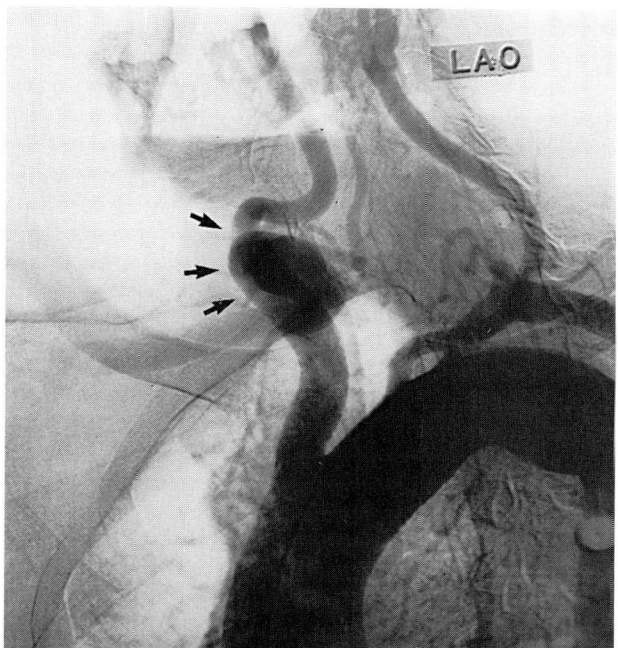

FIGURE 95–1. The confluence of elongated and tortuous innominate, subclavian, and common carotid arteries gives rise to a pulsatile mass in the right supraclavicular fossa and base of neck (*arrows*). This common condition is harmless but is frequently confused on physical examination with a subclavian or common carotid aneurysm. Ultrasonography can usually differentiate between these; however, arteriography is sometimes required. LAO = left anterior oblique view.

of the stellate ganglion and other contributions to the cervical sympathetic chain at the base of the neck.[11]

Plain films of the chest may reveal a superior mediastinal mass that can be confused with a neoplasm. Ultrasonography or CT establishes the diagnosis. Complete arch and upper extremity angiography is mandatory to delineate the extent of the aneurysm, to assess the sites of vascular occlusion in cases complicated by thromboembolism, and to note the competency of the contralateral vertebral circulation if the ipsilateral vertebral artery originates from an aneurysmal vessel. These points are crucial in planning appropriate surgical reconstruction.

Surgical Repair

The first attempted surgical correction of a proximal subclavian artery aneurysm was performed in 1818 by Valentine Mott of New York, who ligated the innominate artery.[3] The first successful treatment of a subclavian artery aneurysm was achieved in 1864 by Smyth of New Orleans, who ligated the right common carotid as well as the innominate artery.[3] Unfortunately, the aneurysm recurred and ruptured 10 years later. Halsted was the first to successfully combine ligation with resection of a subclavian artery aneurysm in 1892 at the Johns Hopkins Hospital.[12] In 1913, Matas reported 225 cases of treatment of aneurysms by endoaneurysmorrhaphy, and seven of these were subclavian aneurysms.[13]

Contemporary surgical repair of proximal and mid–subclavian artery aneurysms involves resection and reestablishment of arterial continuity with an end-to-end anastomosis (for very small aneurysms) or, more commonly, an interposition arterial prosthesis. Although proximal and distal ligation of subclavian aneurysms has occasionally been successful in the past, ligation without reconstruction should generally not be performed because ischemic symptoms develop in 25% of cases so treated.[8] For proximal right subclavian aneurysms, median sternotomy with extension into the supraclavicular fossa is usually necessary to gain adequate exposure for proximal control.[10] Resection of the clavicle also offers excellent exposure of the subclavian artery. In cases of proximal left subclavian aneurysms, a left thoracotomy may be necessary.

Extra-anatomic reconstruction combined with proximal and distal aneurysm ligation has also been described in unusual circumstances.[14] For aneurysms involving the mid–subclavian artery and the distal subclavian artery, a supraclavicular incision often gives adequate exposure and may be complemented by an infraclavicular incision for distal control. Division or resection of the mid-portion of the clavicle may be necessary to gain additional exposure,[9] and, if so, the clavicle may be reconstructed at the completion of the operation. If the aneurysm involves the origin of the vertebral artery, reconstruction by reimplantation or other means is appropriate, particularly if the contralateral vertebral artery is hypoplastic or diseased.

SUBCLAVIAN-AXILLARY ARTERY ANEURYSM: POST-STENOTIC DILATATION FROM THORACIC OUTLET COMPRESSION

Subclavian-axillary artery aneurysms are most frequently encountered in younger patients and appear to be more common in females. Although the first case of upper extremity ischemic complications associated with a cervical rib was reported by Hodgson in 1815, it is not clear that the presence of an underlying subclavian-axillary artery aneurysm was recognized.[15] Mayo, in 1813, described a subclavian aneurysm in association with thoracic outlet syndrome caused by exostosis of the first rib.[16] A cervical rib causing compression of the subclavian artery with resulting ischemia of the arm was reported in 1861 by Coote, who successfully performed the first decompressive operation by removing the cervical rib.[17]

In 1916, Halsted reported 27 cases of cervical rib in association with subclavian artery aneurysm and, based on experimental observation in dogs, hypothesized the rheologic mechanisms leading to post-stenotic dilatation and aneurysm formation.[18] The demonstration of thromboembolic complications emanating from cervical rib compression of the subclavian artery was made by Symonds in 1927, who reported two cases of contralateral hemiplegia from retrograde embolization in the carotid territory.[19] In 1934, Lewis and Pickering described the much more frequent occurrence of upper extremity thromboembolic complications.[20] The first case of arterial reconstruction for treatment of the thromboembolic complications from cervical rib was described by Schein and colleagues in 1956, who replaced the subclavian artery with a homograft.[21]

Aneurysms of the distal subclavian artery and proximal axillary artery are almost always associated with cervical ribs.[9, 22] Rarely, anomalous first ribs, nonunion of the clavicle, and other anatomic abnormalities of the thoracic outlet have been associated with subclavian-axillary aneurysms (see Chapter 70).[23–26] Although cervical ribs are estimated to occur in 0.6% of the population,[27] most are asymptomatic, and arterial lesions are uncommon. In reviewing 716 patients with cervical ribs, Halsted found 27 cases (3.8%) of associated subclavian aneurysms.[18] Six of these patients (0.8%) suffered from gangrene of the fingers. Because cervical ribs are bilateral in 50% to 80% of individuals with this anomaly,[27, 28] subclavian-axillary aneurysms in association with cervical ribs may also be bilateral[29]

Women may be more susceptible to arterial complications from cervical ribs (Fig. 95–2); in reviewing the literature, one is impressed with the female predominance among reported cases. This may be because cervical ribs are more common in women.[27] The right-sided predominance of arterial complications is also evident, perhaps because more frequent muscular activity with the dominant upper extremity leads to earlier and more pronounced changes in the artery on that side.

Cervical ribs may compress the subclavian artery at the point where the vessel crosses the first rib (Fig. 95–3). This is most often the case with complete cervical ribs that join the first rib lateral to the subclavian artery.[24] In this region, the anterior end of the rib may unite with the first rib by a fibrous band, a diarthrodial joint, or a synostosis.[24, 30] The resulting upward, medial, and anterior displacement of the subclavian artery against the tendinous portion of the scalenus anterior muscle causes trauma to the vessel by extrinsic compression and angulation. Post-stenotic dilatation leads to aneurysmal changes, which begin in the distal subclavian artery and extend into the proximal axillary artery. Intraluminal thrombus, engendered by aneurysm

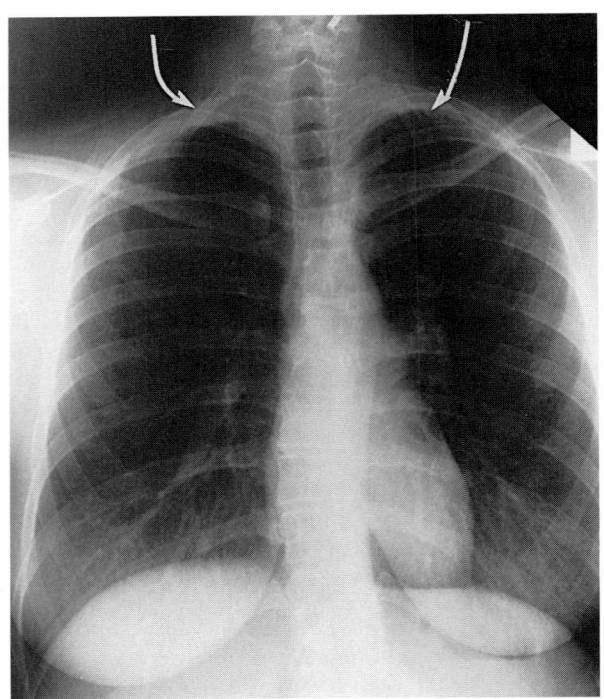

FIGURE 95–2. Bilateral, complete cervical ribs in a young female (*curved arrows*). Only the right cervical rib was associated with arterial dilatation and complications (complete thrombosis of the subclavian artery, as seen in the arteriogram of this patient shown in Figure 95–5).

formation and intimal damage, may become dislodged and embolize distally (Fig. 95–4). In some cases, the aneurysm may completely thrombose, and retrograde propagation may result in emboli in the vertebral circulation and, on the right side, in the common carotid artery (Fig. 95–5).[24, 31, 32] Central neurologic sequelae can result from vertebral or carotid artery involvement.

Patients with subclavian-axillary aneurysms associated with thoracic outlet syndrome may present with acute or chronic symptoms of upper extremity ischemia. On occasion, Raynaud's phenomenon may occur.[26] In some cases, neurologic symptoms typical of thoracic outlet obstruction predominate. On physical examination, a cervical rib may be palpated in the supraclavicular fossa along with the prominent subclavian artery pulsation that results from the anterior and upward displacement of this vessel. A loud, harsh subclavian bruit is usually present unless the artery is thrombosed, and a thrill is common. Patients with cervical ribs or other symptoms of thoracic outlet syndrome who present with any ischemic symptoms need expeditious and complete upper extremity angiography. The urgency of diagnosis is mandated by the imminent threat of limb or digit loss, a point emphasized by most authors.[26, 33–39]

Surgical treatment of subclavian-axillary aneurysms associated with thoracic outlet syndrome depends on the size of the aneurysm, the symptomatic status of the patient, and the presence and extent of thromboembolic complications.[28] In asymptomatic individuals who are found to have a cervical rib with a prominent supraclavicular pulse and bruit, arteriography is recommended to assess the degree of post-stenotic dilation of the subclavian artery (Fig. 95–6). Duplex ultrasonography may also allow partial visualization

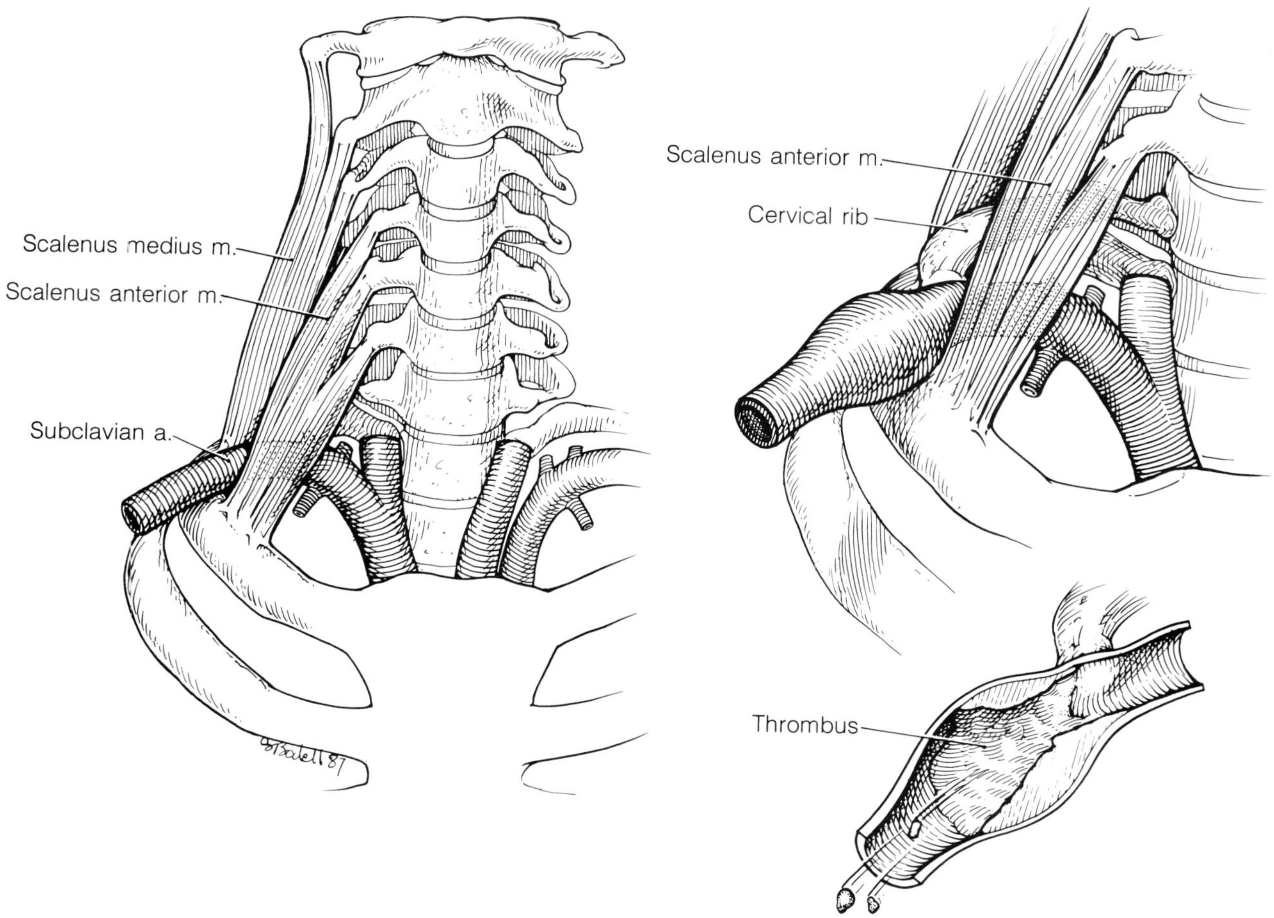

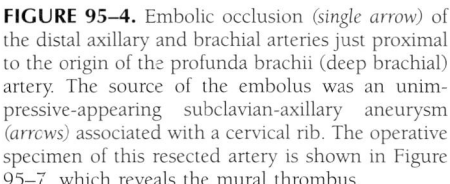

FIGURE 95–3. Pathologic anatomy of a cervical rib giving rise to subclavian-axillary aneurysm with mural thrombus and distal embolization.

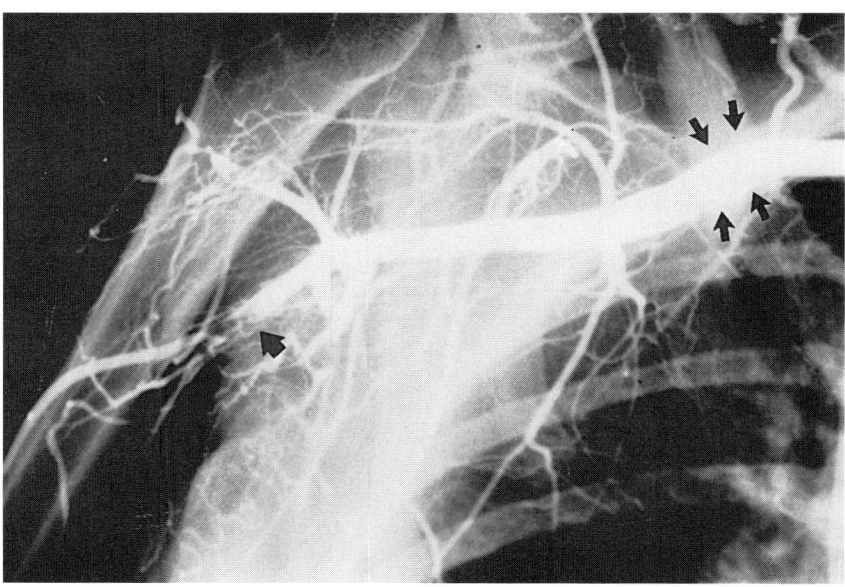

FIGURE 95–4. Embolic occlusion (*single arrow*) of the distal axillary and brachial arteries just proximal to the origin of the profunda brachii (deep brachial) artery. The source of the embolus was an unimpressive-appearing subclavian-axillary aneurysm (*arrows*) associated with a cervical rib. The operative specimen of this resected artery is shown in Figure 95–7, which reveals the mural thrombus.

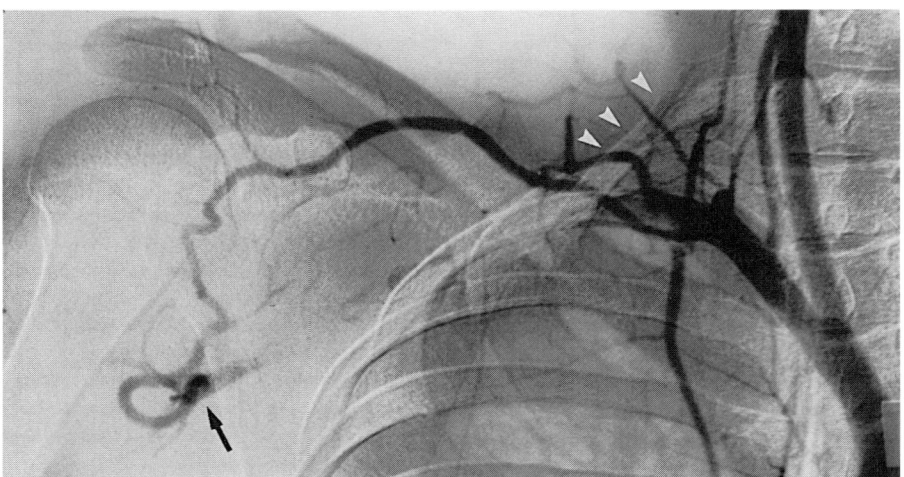

FIGURE 95–5. Arteriogram of the patient whose chest film is shown in Figure 95–2. There is complete occlusion of the subclavian artery with filling of the distal axillary artery (*arrow*) via the suprascapular branch of the subclavian artery to the circumflex scapular branch of the subscapular artery collateral pathway. The cervical rib is outlined by the *arrowheads*. Continued retrograde thrombosis of the subclavian artery would render the right vertebral and common carotid arteries susceptible to thromboembolism.

of this portion of the subclavian artery and has been used to document dilation.[40] If significant dilation is present and the patient has an acceptable surgical risk, thoracic outlet decompression with cervical rib removal is indicated. In the early stage, if only mild arterial dilation is present, relief of compression by removal of the rib may result in return to normal arterial caliber.[28] More often, an aneurysm is already present at initial evaluation, and arterial repair is also indicated (see later).

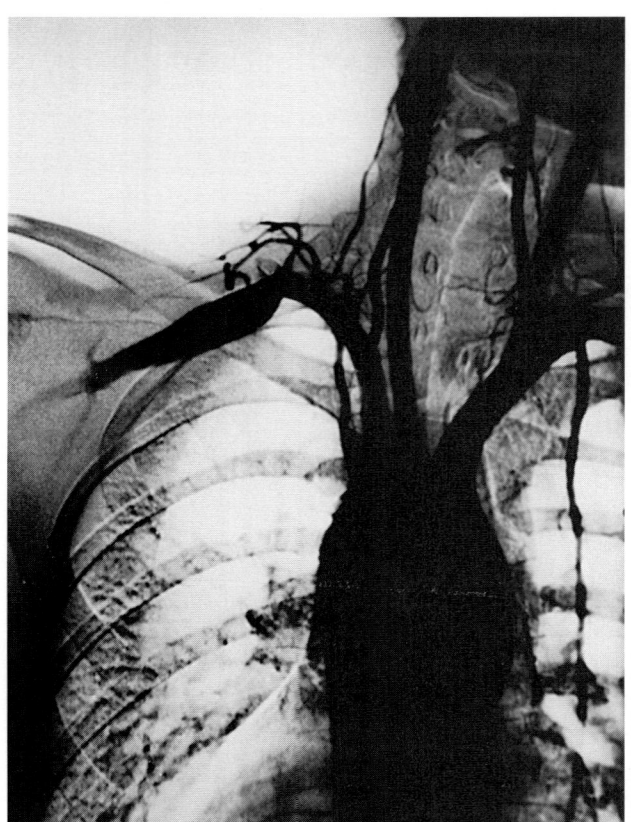

FIGURE 95–6. Large, asymptomatic subclavian-axillary aneurysm with a cervical rib in a young woman in whom a pulsatile right supraclavicular mass was found incidentally on physical examination. A harsh bruit and thrill were also present.

Although it is unknown how many patients in the asymptomatic stage will go on to develop complications if untreated, the natural history of the disorder appears to be progressive with the eventual development of thromboembolic complications. Because the first manifestations may be limb or digit threatening, an aggressive approach is warranted. In asymptomatic individuals with more extensive aneurysmal change (more than two times the normal artery diameter), repair of the subclavian aneurysm in addition to cervical rib removal should usually be performed. Scher and associates observed that these aneurysms frequently contain thrombus, even in asymptomatic patients, and it is unlikely that regression to normal size will occur because of irreversible wall changes.[22] Others have reported delayed embolic events occurring months to years after removal of a cervical rib without repair of the dilated subclavian artery.[26, 39] Operative inspection of the artery to assess its size accurately and, in selected cases, its luminal aspect to look for mural irregularity and thrombus may be useful to determine the need for repair.[36, 40] Evidence of thromboembolism mandates repair of the aneurysm.

In patients with thromboembolic complications associated with a cervical rib, the subclavian artery aneurysm should be repaired regardless of its size. The extent of intimal damage and thrombus in the aneurysm is frequently underestimated by angiography (see Fig. 95–4); invariably, mural thrombus is found in the aneurysm, usually along the inferior wall (Fig. 95–7). In rare cases, vascular reconstruction can be accomplished by proximal and distal mobilization of the ends of the artery and end-to-end anastomosis. Most cases, however, require a short interposition vein or prosthetic graft. In most cases, small subclavian aneurysms are resected and the graft interposed. Occasionally, large or very adherent aneurysms may be opened but left in place and treated with the graft inclusion technique. In view of the relatively young age of affected patients and the need for long-term graft function, a proximal saphenous vein of suitable size would be the optimal conduit for this reconstruction.[26] To best accomplish this, supraclavicular and infraclavicular incisions are used to mobilize the distal subclavian and proximal axillary arteries, respectively.[22] Resection of the clavicle is unnecessary. If present, the cervical rib is resected through the supraclavicular incision by standard techniques.[30]

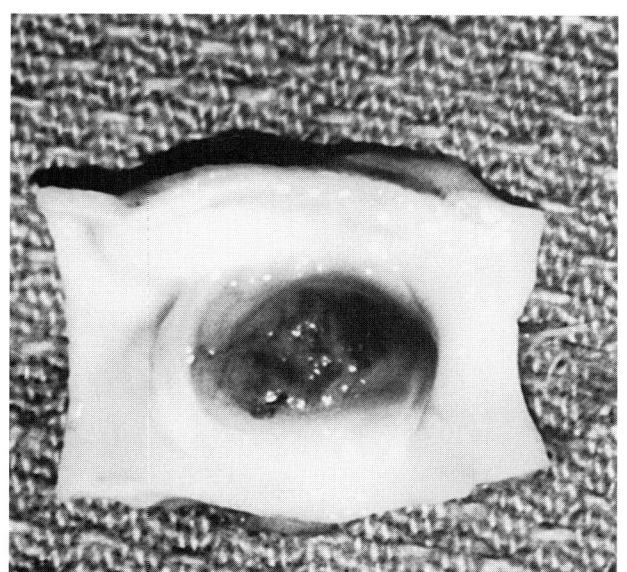

FIGURE 95–7. Mural thrombus within a minimally dilated segment of the subclavian artery distal to the cervical rib in a patient who presented with upper extremity rest pain and digital tip necrosis. The arteriogram of this patient is shown in Figure 95–4.

Key points in effectively relieving arterial compression include (1) complete resection of bony, cartilaginous, and fibrous parts of the anterior portion of the cervical rib where it attaches to or articulates with the first rib and (2) complete resection of the scalenus anterior muscle at the scalene tubercle on the first rib. Resection of most of the posterior portion of the cervical rib should also be performed so that it is free of the brachial plexus, which is usually draped over the rib. Surprisingly, most patients with arterial complications of cervical ribs do not have neurologic symptoms of the thoracic outlet syndrome, and complete resection of the cervical rib along with arterial reconstruction is all that is needed.[28] Although concomitant first rib resection has been advocated by some with either the transaxillary or the supraclavicular approach,[40, 41] this should rarely be necessary. Adequate decompression of the artery and the brachial plexus can almost always be accomplished by near-complete resection of the cervical rib and scalenus anterior muscle. In the less common cases where no cervical rib is present, however, first rib resection is advisable to adequately decompress the thoracic outlet.

Balloon catheter thromboembolectomy is necessary to restore patency to recently occluded distal arteries critical to limb viability. This may require separate exposure of the brachial and forearm arteries to effect complete thrombectomy. Unfortunately, many patients have suffered chronic repetitive embolic episodes, and the occluding thrombi may be partially organized and impossible to extract. In such cases, vein graft bypasses to arm and forearm arteries may be necessary to relieve critical ischemia and to promote healing of digital tip gangrene and ischemic ulcerations. Because of the inferior patency of prosthetic bypasses in this more distal region, vein grafts are required for optimal results.[26, 42] Adjunctive cervicodorsal sympathectomy has been advocated in the past, but most experts believe that this is unnecessary and that the emphasis should be placed

on adequate arterial reconstruction.[22, 26, 40] Sympathectomy might be considered for selected patients in whom vasospastic symptoms are prominent and complete restoration of pulsatile flow at the level of the hand is not possible.

ANEURYSM OF ABERRANT SUBCLAVIAN ARTERY: KOMMERELL'S DIVERTICULUM

Aneurysms of an aberrant subclavian artery are encountered most frequently in adults of either sex over age 50 years. An aberrant right subclavian artery arising from the proximal portion of the descending thoracic aorta is the most common congenital anomaly of the aortic arch.[43] Most patients with this anomaly are asymptomatic, and the aberrant subclavian artery is of no clinical consequence. Rarely, the vessel compresses the esophagus against the posterior trachea and gives rise to difficulty in swallowing, a condition termed *dysphagia lusoria*.[44] Even more rarely, degenerative aneurysmal change occurs in the anomalous vessel. This condition has been termed *Kommerell's diverticulum* after Kommerell, who in 1936 described a diverticulum of the aorta at the origin of the anomalous subclavian artery.[43] McCallen and Schaff first called attention to the clinical significance of aneurysmal change in an anomalous right subclavian artery in a report of 1956.[45] The largest experience to date with this condition was reported by Kieffer et al, who surgically treated 33 adult patients with aberrant subclavian arteries, 17 of whom had a Kommerell's diverticulum or aneurysmal change of the thoracic aorta at the origin of the aberrant subclavian artery.[46]

Patients with aneurysm of an aberrant right subclavian artery may present with dysphagia from esophageal compression, dyspnea and coughing from tracheal compression, chest pain from expansion or rupture, or symptoms of right upper extremity ischemia due to thromboembolism. Death from rupture has been reported and appears to be unrelated to the size of the aneurysm.[43] Many reported cases were in asymptomatic patients whose aneurysm was found on chest radiography and interpreted as a superior mediastinal mass. Chest CT can detect this condition noninvasively, but angiography is necessary to plan surgical treatment. Approximately one fifth of reported patients with this anomaly have an associated abdominal aortic aneurysm.[43]

Because of the propensity of these aneurysms to cause symptoms and because of the possibility of lethal rupture, resection of the aneurysmal artery with vascular reconstruction of the subclavian artery is recommended. This may be accomplished via a right or left posterolateral thoracotomy[43, 47, 48] or a median sternotomy.[46] The subclavian artery is reconstructed by an interposition arterial prosthesis anastomosed proximally to the ascending arch of the aorta. Alternatively, a left posterolateral thoracotomy for proximal resection of the aneurysm coupled with a right supraclavicular incision for reconstruction of the subclavian artery by end-to-side anastomosis to the right common carotid artery has been described.[49] A staged approach with right carotid–subclavian bypass or transposition (end-subclavian to side-carotid) preceding left thoracotomy and aneurysm resection with oversewing of the origin from the aortic arch is attractive because the risk of cerebral and right upper extremity embolization is minimized.[50]

Extra-anatomic reconstruction of the right subclavian artery has also been described.[51] Because it is necessary to resect the aneurysmal vessel near its origin from the aorta, the modified extrathoracic approach described for treatment of dysphagia lusoria would not be effective.[44]

AXILLARY ARTERY ANEURYSMS

Except for rare congenital causes,[6, 52] axillary aneurysms are caused by blunt or penetrating trauma (Fig. 95–8).[53] They occur typically in young males. Crutch-induced blunt trauma producing aneurysmal dilatation of the axillary artery occurs in older patients and was first described by Rob and Standeven[54] in 1956, with subsequent cases reported by Brooks and Fowler[55] and Abbott and Darling.[56] Pathologic examination of these aneurysms reveals markedly thickened walls and wrinkled, roughened intima. Instead of the typical intimal changes of atherosclerosis, severe fragmentation of medial elastic fibers and marked periadventitial fibrosis are present, suggesting chronic trauma.[56] Thrombus, usually loosely adherent to the damaged intima, may become dislodged by further trauma from crutches and is the source of acute, chronic, or repetitive emboli. In many cases, the aneurysm thromboses completely when symptoms begin. The most common presenting complaints relate to upper extremity ischemia, and these aneurysms should be suspected when a patient who has been using crutches for a prolonged period presents with an absent brachial pulse.[56]

False aneurysms of the axillary artery usually occur with penetrating trauma but may also occur with blunt trauma in the form of humeral fractures and anterior dislocation of the shoulder.[57–59] In the latter instance, the mechanism may be avulsion of the tethered thoracoacromial, subscapular, or circumflex humeral vessels at the time of dislocation. These aneurysms often present late as chronic false aneurysms because diagnosis is often delayed. This is especially true after blunt trauma, when lack of recognition is fostered by the difficulty of obtaining an adequate examination of the axillary artery because of the surrounding bone and muscles of the shoulder and the considerable pain and muscle spasm that prevent arm abduction to allow examination of the axilla.[57] Furthermore, because of the excellent collateral circulation in this area, distal perfusion may be adequate despite extensive axillary artery injury. These aneurysms can lead to serious and permanent neurologic disability, however, because of hemorrhage into the axillary sheath and compression of the brachial plexus.

Because of these possibilities, arteriography should be considered in all cases of significant penetrating trauma to the shoulder or arm, blunt trauma with abnormal pulse examination, and blunt trauma with normal pulse examination but brachial plexus palsy, since the likelihood of concomitant vascular injury is high in these cases. Duplex ultrasonography may also allow accurate diagnosis. Also, arteriography should be performed in patients with blunt trauma to the shoulder or axilla with a normal neurovascular examination initially but with signs of brachial plexus neuropathy on follow-up. The presence of an expanding chronic false aneurysm should be suspected in such cases.[57]

Surgical treatment of axillary artery aneurysms is straightforward and involves resection of the aneurysm and interposition of a vein graft. One must be careful to protect the brachial plexus and its major branches during dissection of the aneurysm. Prosthetic reconstruction of the axillary artery has been successful; however, because of the superior patency of vein grafts in upper extremity reconstructions,[42] these are preferred. On occasion, an adjacent segment of the axillary or brachial vein has been used to reconstruct the artery (Fig. 95–9). This vein is extremely thin walled, however, and may itself become aneurysmal with time (Figs. 95–10 and 95–11). For this reason, a segment of saphenous vein is the conduit of choice. Endovascular stent-grafts have also been successfully used to treat these aneurysms.[60]

ULNAR ARTERY ANEURYSM: THE HYPOTHENAR HAMMER SYNDROME

Ulnar artery aneurysms are most commonly seen in men younger than 50 years of age, but they can occur in older patients and in females. Although rare, ulnar artery aneurysms are one of the most common causes of ischemia

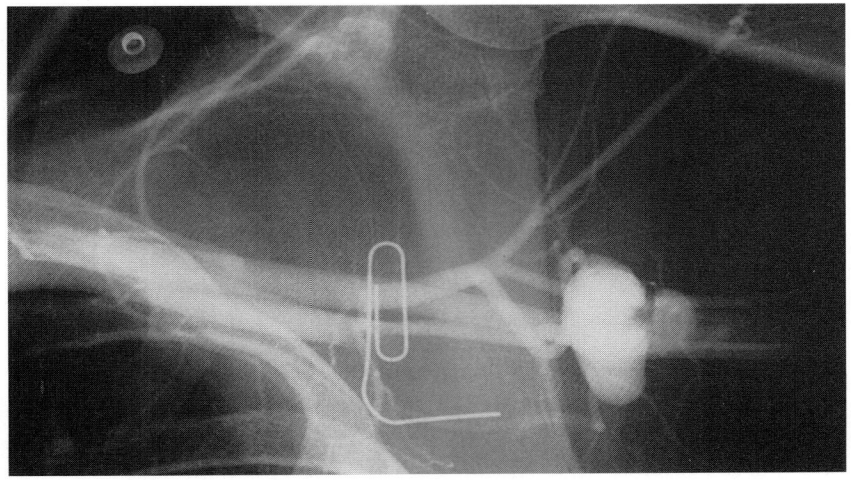

FIGURE 95–8. False aneurysm of the axillary artery as a result of a stab injury.

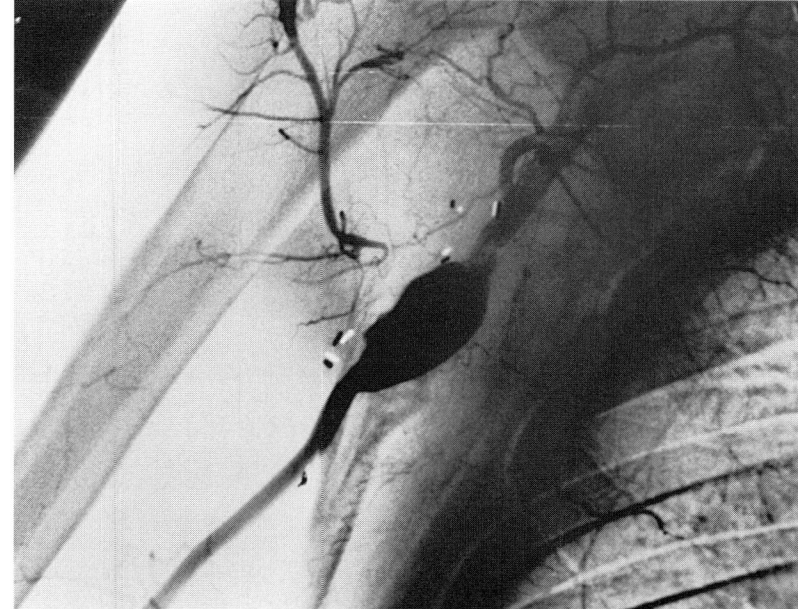

FIGURE 95–9. Aneurysmal dilatation of an interposition brachial vein graft used to reconstruct the axillary artery at the time of penetrating trauma 4 years previously.

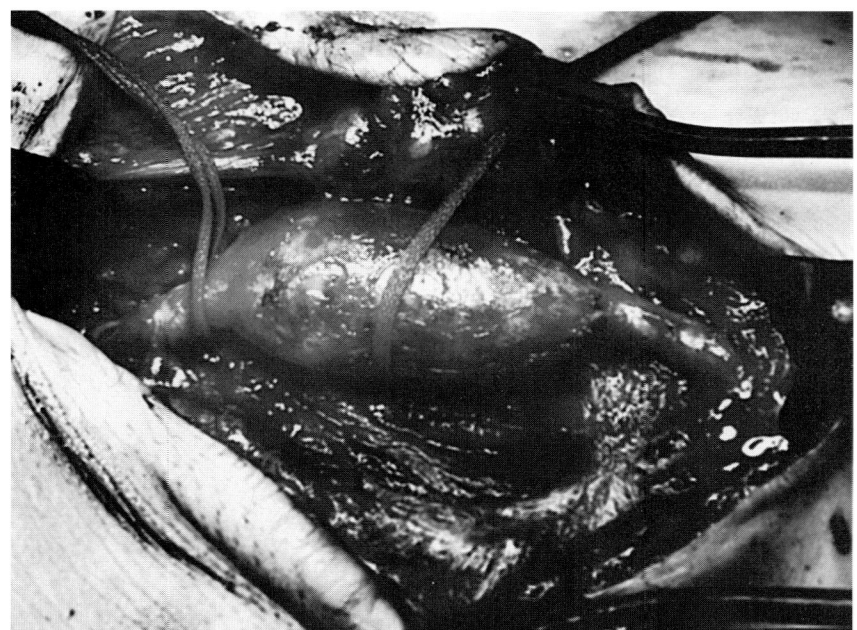

FIGURE 95–10. Operative dissection of the aneurysmal interposition brachial vein graft shown in Figure 95–9.

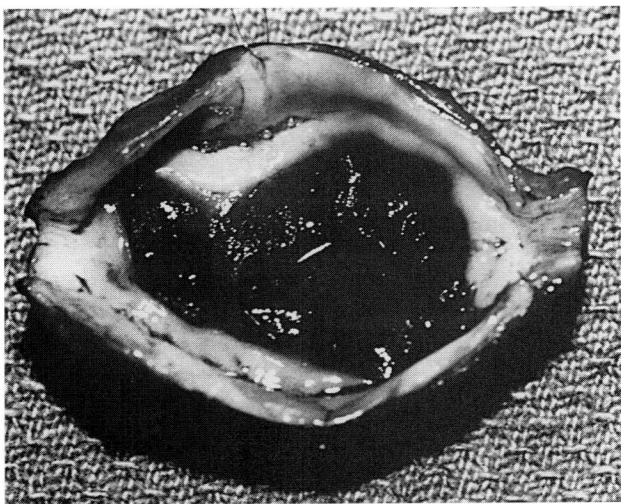

FIGURE 95–11. Mural thrombus lining the aneurysmal interposition brachial vein graft shown in Figures 95–9 and 95–10.

limited solely to the digits.[61, 62] It is important to recognize this disorder because ischemia arising from these aneurysms is frequently correctable and, if untreated, may lead to digital necrosis and severe disability. Diagnosis and treatment are all the more urgent when one considers that most individuals with the hypothenar hammer syndrome are middle-aged working men whose livelihood depends on using their dominant hand, which is invariably involved.

The first reported case occurred in a Roman coachman and was described by Guattani in 1772[63]; Middleton, in 1993, reported 16 cases,[64] Smith, in 1962, described 35 cases,[65] and Pineda and colleagues, in 1985, reviewed 53 cases.[66] All authors have identified trauma to the hand as

the cause of this disorder, and in 1970 Conn and associates coined the term "hypothenar hammer syndrome."[67]

The syndrome develops in people who use the palms of their hands for pushing, pounding, or twisting. The practice of repeatedly striking with the dominant hand is common in many industries. The hypothenar hammer syndrome has been most often described in mechanics, automobile repairmen, lathe operators, pipe fitters, tire braiders, carpenters, and machinists. The disorder has also been described in individuals with hobbies (sculpting) and athletic pursuits (volleyball, skiing, and karate) that involve repetitive trauma to the hand.[68–74]

The incidence is probably much higher than one would suspect from the number of patients reported in the literature (<150 cases). Little and Ferguson used noninvasive means to screen a population at risk.[75] Among 79 automobile repairmen who habitually used their hands as a hammer, 11 (14%) showed some evidence of digital ischemia and were deemed to have the hypothenar hammer syndrome. Duration of employment was positively correlated with the syndrome, and there was no evidence of the syndrome in workers who did not use their hands as hammers.[75] Many authors have stressed the importance of accuracy of diagnosis and its relationships to work activities because of insurance and workers' compensation considerations.[67, 75, 76]

The pathophysiology is based on the unique vascular anatomy of the hand (Fig. 95–12).[65] The ulnar artery and nerve enter the hand by traversing Guyon's canal, bounded medially (ulnarly) by the pisiform bone, dorsally by the transverse carpal ligament, and superficially by the volar carpal ligament. Within this tunnel, the artery and the nerve each bifurcates into deep and superficial branches. The deep branch of the artery along with the motor branch of the ulnar nerve penetrates the hypothenar muscle mass

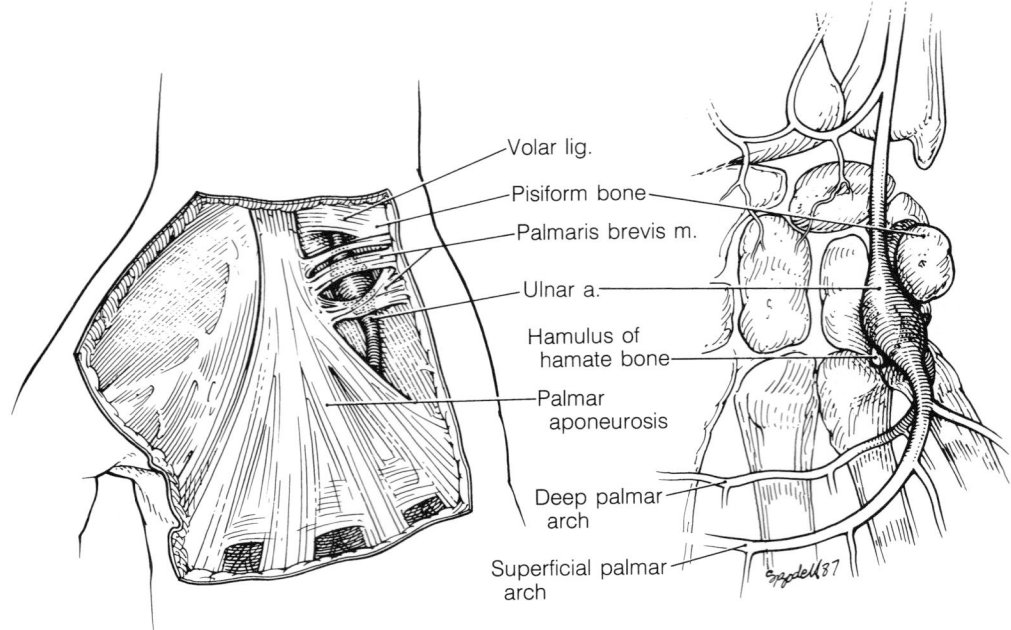

FIGURE 95–12. Pathologic anatomy of the hypothenar hammer syndrome. The distal ulnar artery is particularly vulnerable to external trauma in the 2-cm distance between its exit point from Guyon's canal (the roof of which is the volar carpal ligament) and the point where the artery dives under the tough palmar aponeurosis. In this short distance, the ulnar artery courses on top of the hook of the hamate bone and is covered incompletely by the thin palmaris brevis muscle and skin and subcutaneous tissue.

where the artery becomes the deep palmar arch. The superficial division of the ulnar artery remains superficial to the hypothenar musculature and penetrates the palmar aponeurosis to form the superficial palmar arch, the main blood supply to the fingers via the common palmar digital arteries. Over this short distance of approximately 2 cm between the distal margin of Guyon's canal and the palmar aponeurosis, the artery lies just anterior to the hook of the hamate bone and is covered only by the slight palmaris brevis muscle, overlying skin, and subcutaneous tissue.

With little protection above and the bony floor below, the artery is vulnerable to trauma. Fixation of the artery by the course of its deep branch allows little movement to escape blunt forces. In addition, the hook of the hamate may function as an anvil, accentuating the untoward results of repeated trauma. Similar vulnerable conditions exist for a short segment of the superficial branch of the radial artery at the base of the thenar eminence, a much less frequent site of vessel trauma.[65] In an extensive study of arterial patterns of the hand, Coleman and Anson found that in 78% of dissections, the superficial palmar arch was complete.[77] In approximately three fourths of these, the ulnar artery was the dominant component. In 22% of dissections, the arch was incomplete and there were diverse contributions to digital blood supply from the radial, ulnar, and, rarely, a persistent median artery. These anatomic variations are responsible for the diverse distribution of digital ischemic signs and symptoms in patients with the hypothenar hammer syndrome.

Trauma to the ulnar artery in this vulnerable area causes mural degeneration.[78] Damage to the intima alone results in thrombosis, whereas injury of the media leads to a true arterial aneurysm. Thrombosis of the ulnar artery or aneurysm is associated with downstream embolization. Pathologic studies of ulnar artery aneurysms have documented organizing thrombus adherent to the intimal surface and absence or severe fragmentation of the internal elastic lamina.[79] Fibrosis and focal intramural hemorrhage are also present, along with variable amounts of acute and chronic inflammation.[66] Although most authors have described true aneurysms with no loss in continuity of the arterial wall, some have reported false aneurysms of the ulnar artery, usually in association with penetrating trauma.[80–82]

Although the syndrome most often follows chronic, repetitive trauma, it may result from a single, acute episode.[66] The syndrome usually has a slow, insidious onset.[62] At the time of injury, many patients report episodes of severe lacerating pain over the hypothenar eminence. Typically, dull aching pain and tenderness are present over the hypothenar area after these episodes, and ischemic symptoms develop weeks or months later. A variety of ischemic signs and symptoms may be present and often include pain, cold sensation, paresthesias, cyanosis, and mottling of the digits. The fourth and fifth fingers are most frequently symptomatic, but any digit or any combination of digits may be involved with the exception of the thumb, which is invariably spared because of its radial blood supply. *Raynaud's phenomenon* may be the chief presenting symptom and is distinguished from "typical" Raynaud's phenomenon, in that it is unilateral, the thumb is not involved, and there is an absence of the classic triphasic color changes[66] because reactive hyperemia would not be expected to occur in the presence of fixed arterial obstruction.

On physical examination, in addition to the ischemic changes of the fingers, localized tenderness over the hypothenar eminence may be present with a pulsatile or nonpulsatile mass. A hypothenar callus may also be present. Atrophy and softening of the distal finger pads, ischemic fingertip ulcers, and subungual hemorrhages are sometimes evident. An abnormal Allen's test suggests occlusion or incomplete development of the superficial palmar arch or the distal ulnar artery and is present in the majority of patients with the hypothenar hammer syndrome.[66] Some patients may have an ulnar sensory deficit due to compression of the superficial ulnar sensory branch by the aneurysm.[83]

Noninvasive studies helpful in diagnosis include digital plethysmography, Doppler-derived digital pressures, and duplex ultrasonography. However, angiography is mandatory for patients thought to have this disorder, and the angiographic features are virtually pathognomonic (Fig. 95–13).[84–86] These include irregularity, aneurysmal change, or occlusion of the ulnar artery segment overlying the hook of the hamate bone with occasional extension of these changes into the superficial palmar arch, embolic occlusion of the proper digital arteries in the distribution of the ulnar artery, and normal proximal and contralateral arteries (Fig. 95–14). Magnification views and pharmacoangiography are

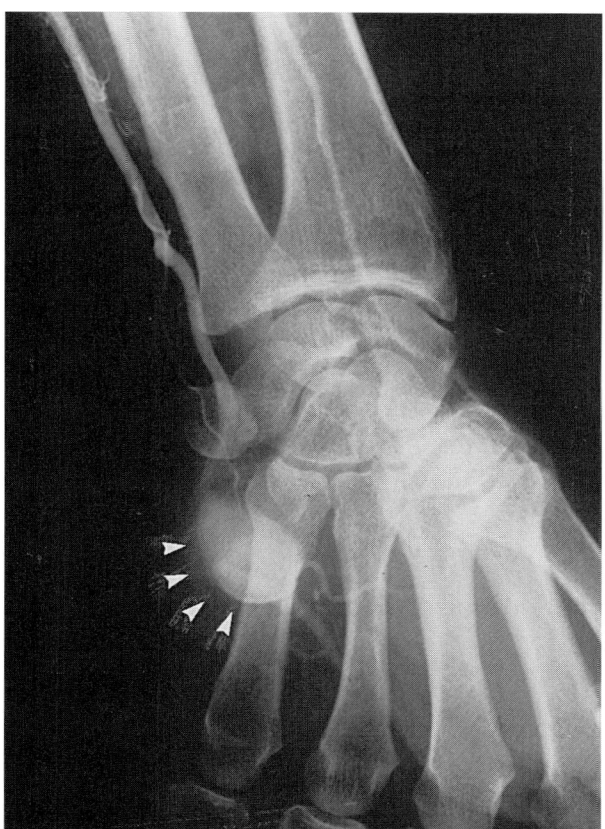

FIGURE 95–13. Large distal ulnar artery aneurysm *(arrowheads)* in a middle-aged man who frequently used his hand as a hammer in his work as an automobile repairman.

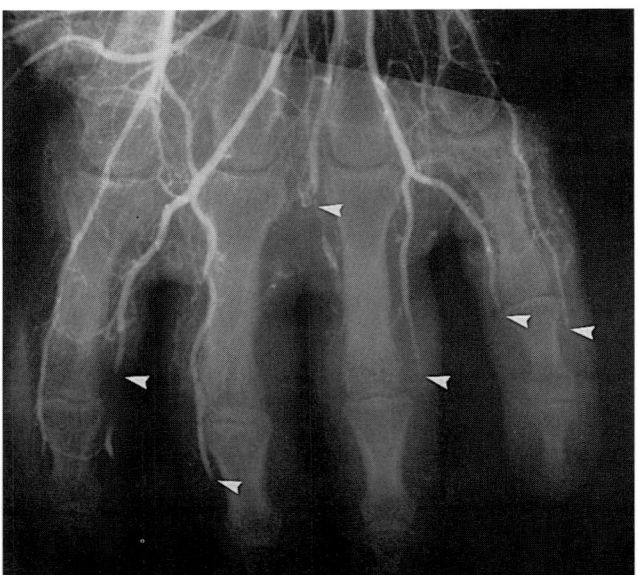

FIGURE 95–14. Delayed magnification views of the hand following papaverine injection, demonstrating multiple embolic occlusions (*arrowheads*) of the digital arteries in the patient whose initial arteriogram in Figure 95–15 showed only occlusion of the ulnar artery.

helpful in defining these features.[86] Frequently, distal ulnar artery occlusion is the only finding on initial arteriography (Fig. 95–15). Proximal angiography of the innominate, subclavian, and axillary arteries is important to rule out potential embolic sources.

Surgical therapy for the hypothenar hammer syndrome has included cervicodorsal sympathectomy, excision of the ulnar artery aneurysm with ligation of the ulnar artery, and aneurysmectomy with microsurgical reconstruction of the ulnar artery by reanastomosis or interposition vein graft (Fig. 95–16).[66] Although it is not clear which of these approaches is superior, most authors recommend microsurgical vascular reconstruction because it eliminates the thromboembolic source, removes the painful aneurysmal mass that may cause ulnar nerve compression, adds the vasodilatory benefits of a local periarterial sympathectomy, and improves digital perfusion.[61, 62, 78, 87–90] Resection of the aneurysm and placement of a vein interposition graft is the optimal treatment for either a patent ulnar aneurysm with clinical or radiographic evidence of distal embolization or a thrombosed ulnar aneurysm that has resulted in profound digital ischemia (Fig. 95–17).

Patients with minimal symptoms and no threat of digit loss after ulnar aneurysm thrombosis may not require revascularization.[50, 91, 92] Adjunctive preoperative thrombolytic therapy has been reported with excellent results (Fig. 95–18).[93, 94] The principal benefit of thrombolytic therapy is the restoration of patency to digital arteries, thus reducing adverse sequelae and improving distal runoff, theoretically enhancing patency of the reconstruction. When the ulnar artery and superficial palmar arch are chronically thrombosed and thrombolytic therapy is unsuccessful in restoring flow, medical therapy with calcium channel blockers may be helpful if vasospastic symptoms are prominent.[66] All patients with this disorder should be counseled to stop smoking and to avoid further hand trauma.

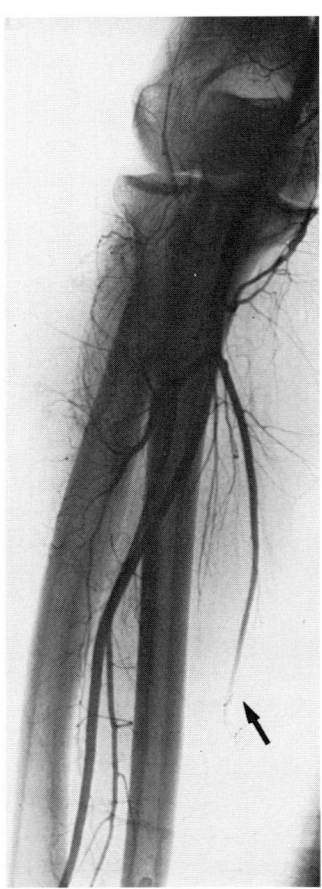

FIGURE 95–15. Initial arteriogram in a patient presenting with signs of small vessel embolism in the digits ("blue finger" syndrome). The arteriogram shows ulnar artery occlusion (*arrow*).

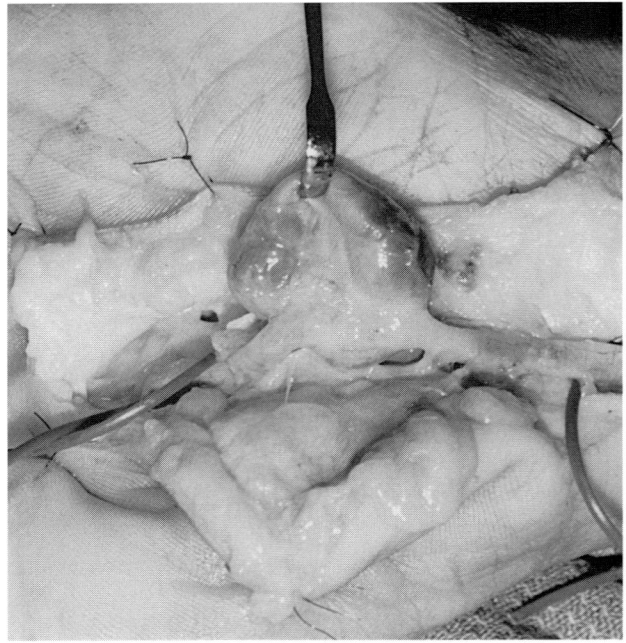

FIGURE 95–16. Operative exposure of an embolizing ulnar artery aneurysm in the right hand treated with resection and vein graft replacement.

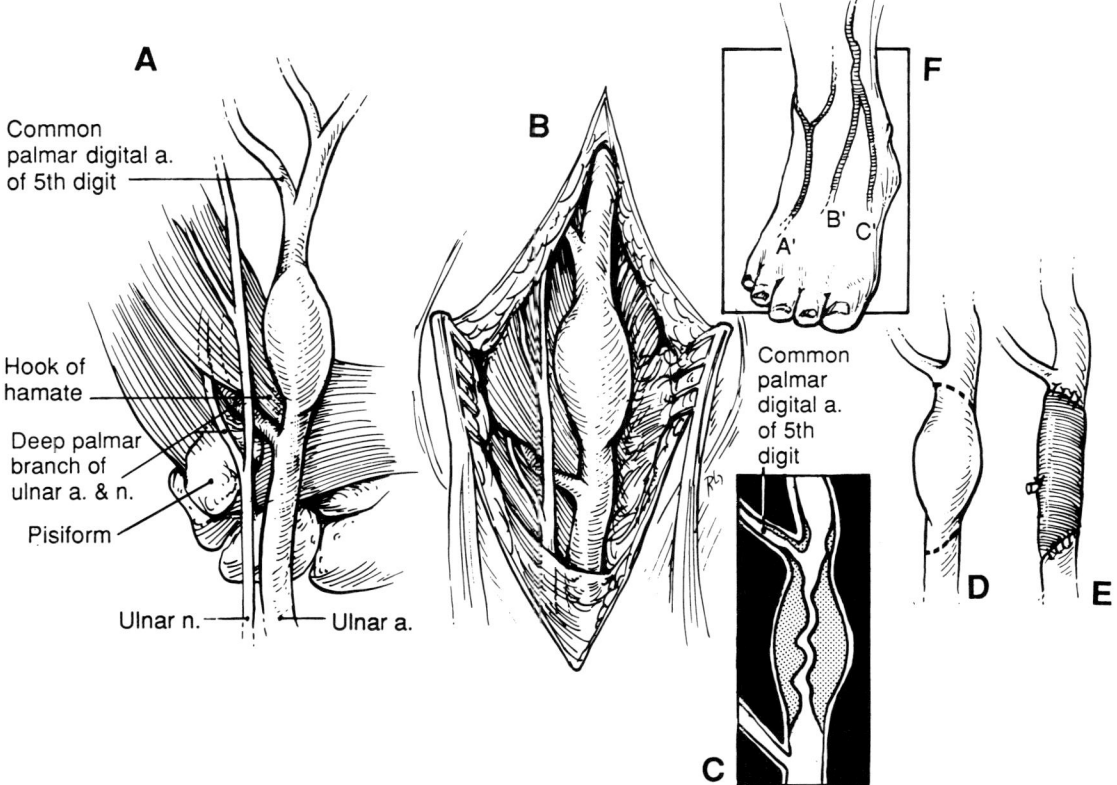

FIGURE 95–17. *A*, Detail of post-traumatic ulnar artery aneurysm, located distal to the pisiform bone at the wrist and distal to the deep palmar branch of the ulnar artery, but typically proximal to or just involving the common digital artery of the fifth digit. *B*, Operative exposure via longitudinal incision directly over the palpable ulnar artery pulse. *C*, Schematic of the arteriographic appearance of fusiform post-traumatic ulnar aneurysms. Frequently, the artery appears irregular or serpiginous, characteristically described as having a "corkscrew" appearance. *D*, Repair usually involves excision of the aneurysm, with interposition repair with reversed autogenous vein. *E* and *F*, Ideally, the dorsal foot vein provides the appropriate-sized match.

FIGURE 95–18. *A*, Urokinase was infused regionally for 24 hours in same patient whose initial arteriograms are shown in Figures 95–14 and 95–15. Near-complete lysis of thromboemboli restored patency to the distal ulnar artery, the superficial palmar arch, and some of the common digital arteries in addition to demonstrating the underlying ulnar artery aneurysm. *B*, A repeated arteriogram in the same patient after microvascular resection of the ulnar artery aneurysm and reconstruction with an interposition vein graft (*arrowheads*) harvested from the forearm. Complete circulation to the digits has been restored, and all digital arteries have been cleared of thrombus by the adjunctive preoperative use of regional urokinase infusion.

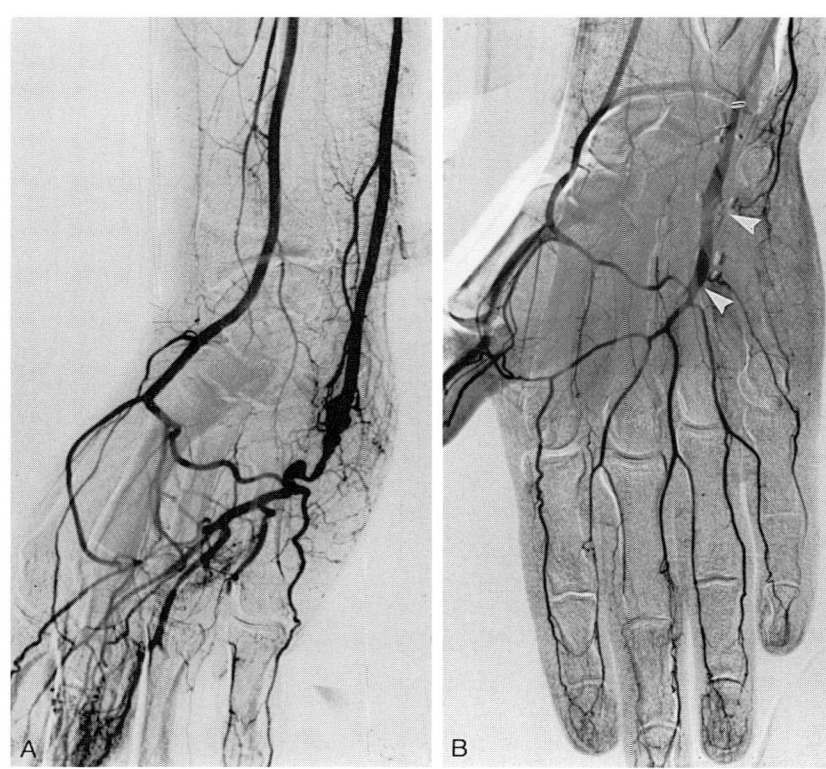

REFERENCES

1. Dent TL, Ernst CB: Multiple arteriosclerotic arterial aneurysms. Arch Surg 105:338, 1972.
2. Hobson RW II, Sarkaria J, O'Donnell JA, et al: Atherosclerotic aneurysms of the subclavian artery. Surgery 85:368, 1979.
3. Bjork VO: Aneurysm and occlusion of the right subclavian artery. Acta Chir Scand (Suppl)356:103, 1965.
4. Persaud V: Subclavian artery aneurysm and idiopathic cystic medionecrosis. Br Heart J 30:436, 1968.
5. Hara M, Bransford RM: Aneurysm of the subclavian artery associated with contiguous pulmonary tuberculosis. J Thorac Cardiovasc Surg 46:256, 1963.
6. Applebaum RE, Caniano DA, Sun C-C, et al: Synchronous left subclavian and axillary artery aneurysms associated with melorheostosis. Surgery 99:249, 1986.
7. Dobbins WO: Bilateral calcified subclavian arterial aneurysms in a young adult male. N Engl J Med 265:537, 1961.
8. Pairolero PC, Walls JT, Payne WS, et al: Subclavian-axillary artery aneurysms. Surgery 90:757, 1981.
9. Hobson RW II, Israel MR, Lynch TG: Axillosubclavian arterial aneurysms. In Bergan JJ, Yao JST (eds): Aneurysms: Diagnosis and Treatment. New York, Grune & Stratton, 1982, p 435.
10. McCollum CH, Da Gama AD, Noon GP, et al: Aneurysm of the subclavian artery. J Cardiovasc Surg 20:159, 1979.
11. Temple LJ: Aneurysm of the first part of the left subclavian artery: A review of the literature and a case history. J Thorac Surg 19:412, 1950.
12. Halsted WS: Ligation of the first portion of the left subclavian artery and excision of a subclavio-axillary aneurysm. Johns Hopkins Hosp Bull 24:93, 1892.
13. Muller GP: Subclavian aneurysm with report of a case. Ann Surg 101:568, 1935.
14. Elefteriades JA, Kay HA, Stansel HC Jr, et al: Extra-anatomical reconstruction for bilateral intrathoracic subclavian artery aneurysms. Ann Thorac Surg 35:188, 1983.
15. Hodgson J: Diseases of the Arteries and Veins. London, 1815, p 262.
16. Mayo H: Exostosis of the first rib with strong pulsations of the subclavian artery. Lond Med Phys J (NS) 11:40, 1831.
17. Coote H: Pressure on the axillary vessels and nerve by an exostosis from a cervical rib. Interference with the circulation of the arm. Removal of the rib in exostosis. Recovery. Med Times Gaz 2:108, 1861.
18. Halsted WS: An experimental study of circumscribed dilation of an artery immediately distal to a partially occluding band, and its bearing on the dilation of the subclavian artery observed in certain cases of cervical rib. J Exp Med 24:271, 1916.
19. Symonds CP: Two cases of thrombosis of subclavian artery, with contralateral hemiplegia of sudden onset, probably embolic. Brain 50:259, 1927.
20. Lewis T, Pickering GW: Observations upon maladies in which the blood supply to digits ceases intermittently or permanently, and upon bilateral gangrene of digits: Observations relevant to so-called "Raynaud's disease." Clin Sci 1:327, 1934.
21. Schein CJ, Haimovici H, Young H: Arterial thrombosis associated with cervical ribs: Surgical considerations. Surgery 40:428, 1956.
22. Scher LA, Veith FJ, Samson RH, et al: Vascular complications of thoracic outlet syndrome. J Vasc Surg 3:565, 1986.
23. Fidler MW, Helal B, Barwegen GMH, et al: Subclavian artery aneurysm due to costoclavicular compression. J Hand Surg 9B:282, 1984.
24. Matsumura JS, Yao JST: Thoracic outlet arterial compression: Clinical features and surgical management. Semin Vasc Surg 9:125, 1996.
25. Whelan TJ Jr: Management of vascular disease of the upper extremity. Surg Clin North Am 62:373, 1982.
26. Nehler MR, Taylor LM Jr, Moneta GL, et al: Upper extremity ischemia from subclavian artery aneurysm caused by bony abnormalities of the thoracic outlet. Arch Surg 132:527, 1997.
27. Adson AW: Cervical ribs: Symptoms, differential diagnosis and indications for section of the insertion of the scalenus anticus muscle. J Int Coll Surg 16:546, 1951.
28. Scher LA, Veith FJ, Haimovici H, et al: Staging of arterial complications of cervical rib: Guidelines for surgical management. Surgery 95:644, 1984.
29. Siu K, Ferguson I: Bilateral cervical rib and subclavian aneurysm. Aust NZ J Surg 42:245, 1973.
30. Schein CJ: A technic for cervical rib resection. Am J Surg 121:623, 1971.
31. Blank RH, Connar RG: Arterial complications associated with thoracic outlet compression syndrome. Ann Thorac Surg 17 315, 1974.
32. Fields WS, Lemak NA, Ben-Menachem Y: Thoracic outlet syndrome: Review and reference to stroke in a major league pitcher. Am J Roentgenol 146:809, 1986.
33. Banis JC, Rich N, Whelan TJ Jr: Ischemia of the upper extremity due to noncardiac emboli. Am J Surg 134:131, 1977.
34. Bertelsen S, Mathiesen RR, Ohlenschlaeger HH: Vascular complications of cervical rib. Scand J Thorac Cardiovasc Surg 2:133, 1968.
35. Dorazio RA, Ezzet F: Arterial complications of the thoracic outlet syndrome. Am J Surg 138:246, 1979.
36. Judy KL, Heymann RL: Vascular complications of thoracic outlet syndrome. Am J Surg 123:521, 1972.
37. Martin J, Gaspard DJ, Johnston PW, et al: Vascular manifestations of the thoracic outlet syndrome: A surgical urgency. Arch Surg 111:779, 1976.
38. Mathes SJ, Salam AA: Subclavian artery aneurysm: Sequela of thoracic outlet syndrome. Surgery 76:506, 1974.
39. Desai Y, Robbs JV: Arterial complications of the thoracic outlet syndrome. Eur J Vasc Endovasc Surg 10:362, 1995.
40. Kieffer E: Arterial complications of thoracic outlet syndrome. In Bergan JJ, Yao JST (eds): Evaluation and Treatment of Upper and Lower Extremity Circulatory Disorders. Orlando, Fla, Grune & Stratton, 1984, p 249.
41. Fantini GA: Reserving supraclavicular first rib resection for vascular complications of thoracic outlet syndrome. Am J Surg 172:200, 1996.
42. McCarthy WJ, Flinn WR, Yao JST, et al: Result of bypass grafting for upper limb ischemia. J Vasc Surg 3:741, 1986.
43. Austin EH, Wolfe WG: Aneurysm of aberrant subclavian artery with a review of the literature. J Vasc Surg 2:571, 1985
44. Valentine RJ, Carter DJ, Clagett GP: A modified extrathoracic approach to the treatment of dysphagia lusoria. J Vasc Surg 5:498, 1987.
45. McCallen AM, Schaff B: Aneurysm of an anomalous right subclavian artery. Radiology 66:561, 1956.
46. Kieffer E, Bahnini A, Koskas F: Aberrant subclavian artery: Surgical treatment in thirty-three adult patients. J Vasc Surg 19:100, 1994.
46. Campbell CF: Repair of an aneurysm of an aberrant retroesophageal right subclavian artery arising from Kommerel's diverticulum. J Thorac Cardiovasc Surg 62:330, 1971.
48. Hunter JA, Dye WS, Javid H, et al: Arteriosclerotic aneurysm of anomalous right subclavian artery. J Thorac Cardiovasc Surg 59:754, 1970.
49. Stoney WS, Alford WC Jr, Burrus GR, et al: Aberrant right subclavian artery aneurysm. Ann Thorac Surg 19:460, 1975.
50. Rothkopf DM, Bryan DJ, Cuadros CL, et al: Surgical management of ulnar artery aneurysms. J Hand Surg 15A:891, 1990.
51. Esquivel CO, Miller GE Jr: Aneurysm of anomalous right subclavian artery. Contemp Surg 24:81, 1984.
52. Perry SP, Massey CW: Bilateral aneurysms of the subclavian and axillary arteries. Radiology 61:53, 1953.
53. Ho PK, Weiland AJ, McClinton MA, et al: Aneurysms of the upper extremity. J Hand Surg 12A:39, 1978.
54. Rob CG, Standeven A: Closed traumatic lesions of the axillary and brachial arteries. Lancet 1:597, 1956.
55. Brooks A, Fowler B: Axillary artery thrombosis after prolonged use of crutches. J Bone Joint Surg 46-A:863, 1964.
56. Abbott WM, Darling RC: Axillary artery aneurysms secondary to crutch trauma. Am J Surg 125:515, 1973.
57. Gallen J, Wiss DA, Cantelmo N, et al: Traumatic pseudoaneurysm of the axillary artery: Report of three cases and literature review. J Trauma 24:350, 1984.
58. Majeed L: Pulsatile haemarthrosis of the shoulder joint associated with false aneurysm of the axillary artery as a late complication of anterior dislocation of the shoulder. Injury 16:565, 1985.
59. Stein E: Case report 374. Skeletal Radiol 15:391, 1986.
60. Sullivan TM, Bacharach JM, Perl J, et al: Endovascular management of unusual aneurysms of the axillary and subclavian arteries. J Endovasc Surg 3:389, 1996.
61. Silcott GR, Polich VL: Palmar arch arterial reconstruction for the salvage of ischemic fingers. Am J Surg 142:219, 1981.
62. Dalman RL: Upper extremity arterial bypass distal to the wrist. Ann Vasc Surg 11:550, 1997.
63. Guattani C: De externis aneurysmaibus, manu chirurgica methodice

perctrandis. Rome, 1771. [Translated by JE Erischsen.] London, London Sydenham Society, 1844, p 268.

64. Middleton DS: Occupational aneurysm of the palmar arteries. Br J Surg 21:215, 1933.

65. Smith JW: True aneurysms of traumatic origin in the palm. Am J Surg 104:7, 1962.

66. Pineda CJ, Weisman MH, Bookstein JJ, et al: Hypothenar hammer syndrome: Form of reversible Raynaud's phenomenon. Am J Med 79:561, 1985.

67. Conn J Jr, Bergan JJ, Bell JL: Hypothenar hammer syndrome: Posttraumatic digital ischemia. Surgery 68:1122, 1970.

68. Annetts DL, Graham AR: Traumatic aneurysm of the palmar arch Lemon squeezer's hand. Aust NZ J Surg 52:584, 1982.

69. Aulicino PL, Hutton PMJ, Du Puy TE: True palmar aneurysms: A case report and literature review. J Hand Surg 7:613, 1982.

70. Bayle E, Tran K, Benslamia H, et al: Ulnar artery aneurysm of the hand. Int Surg 68:215, 1983.

71. Foster DR, Cameron DC: Hypothenar hammer syndrome. Br J Radiol 54:995, 1981.

72. Gaylis H, Kushlick AR: The hypothenar hammer syndrome. S Afr Med J 50:125, 1976.

73. Ho PK, Dellon AL, Wilgis EFS: True aneurysms of the hand resulting from athletic injury. Report of two cases. Am J Sports Med 13:136, 1985.

74. Little JM, Grant AF: Hypothenar hammer syndrome. Med J Aust 1:49, 1972.

75. Little JM, Ferguson DA: The incidence of the hypothenar hammer syndrome. Arch Surg 105:684, 1972.

76. Ettien JT, Allen JT, Vargas C: Hypothenar hammer syndrome. South Med J 74:491, 1981.

77. Coleman SS, Anson BJ: Arterial patterns in the hand based upon a study of 650 specimens. Surg Gynecol Obstet 113:409, 1961.

78. Vayssairat M, Debure C, Cormier J-M, et al: Hypothenar hammer syndrome: Seventeen cases with long-term follow-up. J Vasc Surg 5:838, 1987.

79. Von Kuster L, Abt AB: Traumatic aneurysms of the ulnar artery. Arch Pathol Lab Med 104:75, 1980.

80. Green DP: True and false traumatic aneurysms in the hand. J Bone Joint Surg 55-A:120, 1973.

81. Sanchez A, Archer S, Levine NS, et al: Traumatic aneurysm of a common digital artery: A case report. J Hand Surg 7:619, 1982.

82. Walsh MJ, Conolly WB: False aneurysms due to trauma to the hand. Hand 14:177, 1982.

83. Kalisman M, Laborde K, Wolff TW: Ulnar nerve compression secondary to ulnar artery false aneurysm at the Guyon's canal. J Hand Surg 7:137, 1982.

84. Benedict KT, Chang W, McCready FJ: The hypothenar hammer syndrome. Radiology 111:57, 1974.

85. Dubois P, Stephen D: Angiographic findings in the hypothenar hammer syndrome. Aust Radiol 19:370, 1975.

86. Maiman MH, Bookstein JJ, Bernstein EF: Digital ischemia: Angiographic differentiation of embolism from primary arterial disease. Am J Roentgenol 137:1183, 1982.

87. Given KS, Puckett CL, Kleinert HE: Ulnar artery thrombosis. Plast Reconstr Surg 61:405, 1978.

88. Martin RD, Manktelow RT: Management of ulnar artery aneurysm in the hand: A case report. Can J Surg 25:97, 1982.

89. May JW Jr, Grossman JAI, Costas B: Cyanotic painful index and long fingers associated with an asymptomatic ulnar artery aneurysm: Case report. J Hand Surg 7:622, 1982.

90. Millender LH, Nalebuff EA, Kasdon E: Aneurysms and thromboses of the ulnar artery in the hand. Arch Surg 105:686, 1972.

91. Nehler MR, Dalman RL, Harris EJ, et al: Upper extremity arterial bypass distal to the wrist. J Vasc Surg 16:633, 1992.

92. Mehlhoff TL, Wood MB: Ulnar artery thrombosis and the role of interposition vein grafting: Patency with microsurgical technique. J Hand Surg 16A:274, 1991.

93. Lawhorne TW Jr, Sanders RA: Ulnar artery aneurysm complicated by distal embolization: Management with regional thrombolysis and resection. J Vasc Surg 3:663, 1986.

94. Kartchner MM, Wilcox WC: Thrombolysis of palmar and digital arterial thrombosis by intra-arterial thrombolysin. J Hand Surg 1:67, 1976.

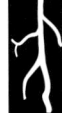

C H A P T E R   9 6
Splanchnic Artery Aneurysms

Gerald B. Zelenock, M.D., and
James C. Stanley, M.D.

Aneurysms of splanchnic arteries represent an uncommon but important vascular disease, since nearly 22% present as clinical emergencies, including 8.5% that result in death.[100] The pathogenesis and natural history of these aneurysms have been reassessed, and in most instances redefined, within the past three decades as advances in imaging technology and endovascular and laparoscopic treatments have begun to influence diagnostic and management strategies. There has been an increased recognition of splanchnic aneurysms because of the greater availability of advanced imaging capabilities such as high-resolution computed tomography (CT) scanning, magnetic resonance angiography (MRA), sophisticated ultrasound, and angiography. Furthermore, although surgery remains the mainstay

of therapy for many splanchnic aneurysms, certain smaller aneurysms, particularly those involving the second- and third-order branches of the main splanchnic arteries, are being treated with catheter-based obliteration.

Emergent endovascular control of bleeding accompanying aneurysm rupture has been advocated, and prophylactic treatment of incidentally discovered small aneurysms has become common,[88] particularly of those imbedded in pancreatic or hepatic parenchyma with their extensive collateral vascular beds. Although the long-term results of such therapies are lacking, their performance has been an important contributing factor to the increasing reports on this subject.

More than 3000 splanchnic artery aneurysms have been

documented in the literature. The increasing discovery of these lesions supports the contention that they are more common than previously claimed.[68] Distribution of aneurysms among splanchnic arteries has varied little from that noted in earlier reviews (Fig. 96–1).[21, 51, 52, 105] Vessels affected, in descending order of involvement, include the splenic (60%), hepatic (20%), superior mesenteric (5.5%), celiac (4%), gastric and gastroepiploic (4%), intestinal (jejunal, ileal, colic; 3%), pancreaticoduodenal and pancreatic (2%), gastroduodenal (1.5%), and inferior mesenteric arteries (rare). Anomalous arteries in the splanchnic circulation such as a common celiacomesenteric trunk or replaced hepatic artery may become aneurysmal but there does not appear to be a predilection for such to occur.[5, 93] Cumulative experience with some aneurysms is so meager that discussion of them is anecdotal. In other instances, evidence is sufficient to develop a rational basis for treatment.[17] Specific biologic differences between individual aneurysms make it imperative to comment on them separately rather than collectively.

SPLENIC ARTERY ANEURYSMS

The most common abdominal visceral vessel affected by aneurysmal disease is the splenic artery. Aneurysms of this vessel make up 60% of all splanchnic artery aneurysms. More than 1800 patients with splenic artery aneurysms have been described in previous publications, yet very few clinical series of more than 20 patients from a single institution exist in the English literature.[72, 103, 107] The incidence of these lesions remains ill defined,[56] ranging from 0.098% among nearly 195,000 necropsies[71] to 10.4% in a careful autopsy study of the splenic vessels in elderly patients.[9] Incidental demonstration of splenic aneurysms in 0.78% of nearly 3600 abdominal arteriographic studies at the authors' institution may be a relatively accurate approximation of the actual frequency of these lesions in the general population.[103] Macroaneurysms of the splenic artery usually are saccular. These lesions occur most often at bifurcations and are multiple in approximately 20% of patients.

In sharp contrast to aneurysms of the abdominal aorta and lower extremity arteries, splenic artery aneurysms exhibit an unusual sex predilection, with a female-to-male ratio of 4:1. The propensity for aneurysm development in the splenic artery rather than in other splanchnic arteries has been attributed to acquired derangements of the vessel wall, including elastic fiber fragmentation, loss of smooth muscle, and internal elastic lamina disruption. Three distinct phenomena may contribute to these changes.

The first contributing factor to splenic artery aneurysms is the presence of systemic arterial fibrodysplasia. The recognized disruption of arterial wall architecture by medial dysplastic processes[104] is a logical forerunner of aneurysms. In fact, patients with medial fibrodysplasia exhibit splenic artery aneurysms with a frequency six times greater than that seen in the normal population.[103]

The second contributing factor to the development of these splenic artery aneurysms is portal hypertension with splenomegaly.[10, 25, 66, 91, 103] Splenic artery aneurysms have been encountered in 10% to 30% of patients with portal hypertension and splenomegaly.[21, 83, 100] In these instances, aneurysms may have been sequelae of the apparent hyperkinetic process that causes increased splenic artery diameters in portal hypertension.[66, 74, 77] Whatever process underlies dilation of the artery, a similar process at vessel bifurcations would increase the likelihood of aneurysm formation. In this regard, aneurysm size in patients with portal hypertension has been directly correlated with splenic artery diameter.[83] These aneurysms are recognized often in patients who have undergone orthotopic liver transplantation.[3]

The third contributing factor relevant to the evolution of splenic artery aneurysms is the vascular effects of repeated pregnancy.[21, 103, 107] Forty percent of female patients de-

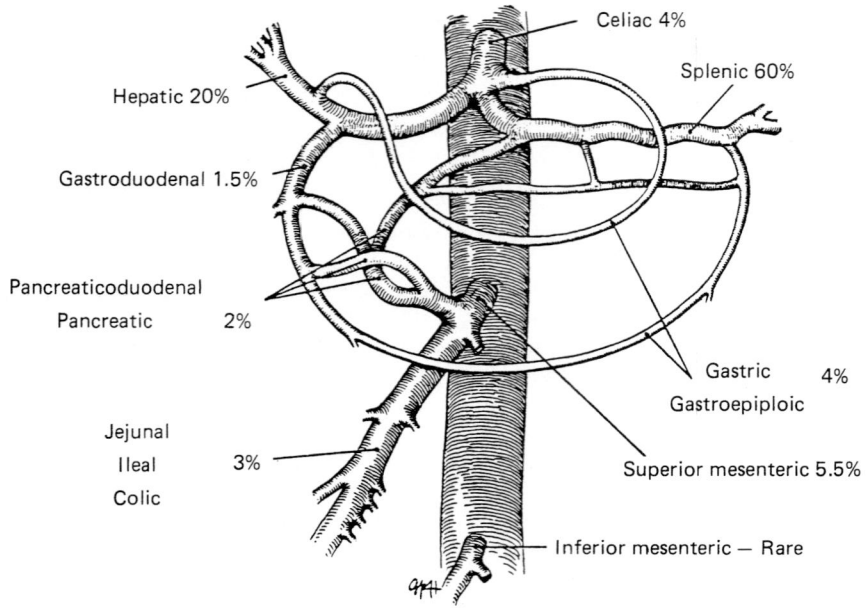

FIGURE 96–1. Relative incidence of aneurysms described in the literature affecting the visceral arteries of the splanchnic circulation.

scribed in a large series from our institution, with nc obvious cause of their aneurysms, had completed six or more pregnancies.[103] The importance of pregnancy in the genesis of these lesions receives further support from the fact that 45% of female patients with splenic artery aneurysms reported in the English-language literature from 1960 to 1970 in whom parity was stated were grand multiparous.[105] Gestational alterations in the vessel wall that are due to hormonal and local hemodynamic events may have a causal relation to medial defects and aneurysmal formation. Such effects may be similar to those underlying the vascular complications of pregnancy associated with Marfan's syndrome. The predilection for aneurysms to occur in the splenic artery instead of in other similar-sized muscular vessels may reflect increased splenic arteriovenous shunting during pregnancy with excessive blood flow, or it may represent preexisting structural abnormalities inherent to the splenic artery.

Certain splenic artery aneurysms appear to have evolved with arteriosclerotic weakening of the vessel wall.[79] However, frequent localization of calcific arteriosclerotic changes to aneurysms, without involvement of the adjacent artery (Fig. 96–2), supports the contention that arteriosclerosis often occurs as a secondary process rather than a primary etiologic event. Calcific arteriosclerotic changes in some but not all aneurysms where multiple lesions occur (Fig. 96–3) lend further credence to this hypothesis.

Inflammatory processes adjacent to the splenic artery, particularly chronic pancreatitis with associated pseudocysts, are also known to cause aneurysms. In fact, peripancreatic pseudoaneurysms occur in more than 10% of patients with chronic pancreatitis, and many of these involve the splenic artery.[46] Similarly, penetrating and blunt trauma may precipitate aneurysmal development. Infected (mycotic) lesions, often associated with subacute bacterial endocarditis in intravenous drug addicts, are being encoun-

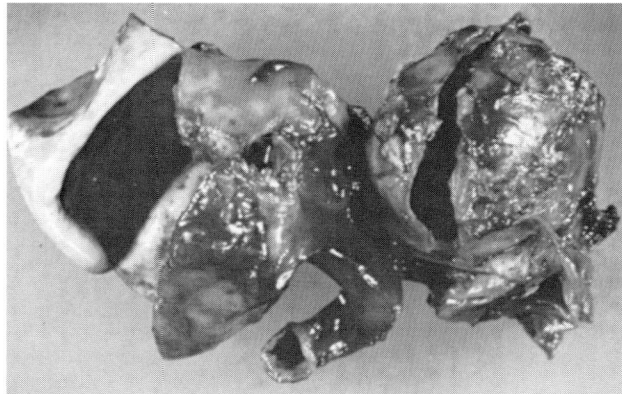

FIGURE 96–3. Splenic artery aneurysms. Multiple aneurysms involving a splenic artery with extensive arteriosclerosis and calcium deposition involving one aneurysm (left), immediately adjacent to a thin nonatherosclerotic aneurysm (right). Arteriosclerosis is considered a secondary event, not a primary factor in initiating splenic artery aneurysms.

tered more frequently in contemporary times. Microaneurysms of intrasplenic vessels are usually a manifestation of a connective tissue disease such as periarteritis nodosa and are of less surgical importance than macroaneurysms that are due to other causes.

The presence of a splenic artery aneurysm may be suspected with radiographic demonstration of curvilinear, signet ring–like calcifications in the left upper quadrant (Fig. 96–4). Such findings have been reported in as many as 70% of cases.[85] However, diagnoses of these aneurysms are most often the result of conventional arteriography, ultrasonography, computed tomography (CT), or magnetic resonance imaging (MRI)[53] in patients among whom there were no prior suspicions of the lesion's presence (Fig. 96–5).[94, 103]

Splenic artery aneurysms usually are asymptomatic, al-

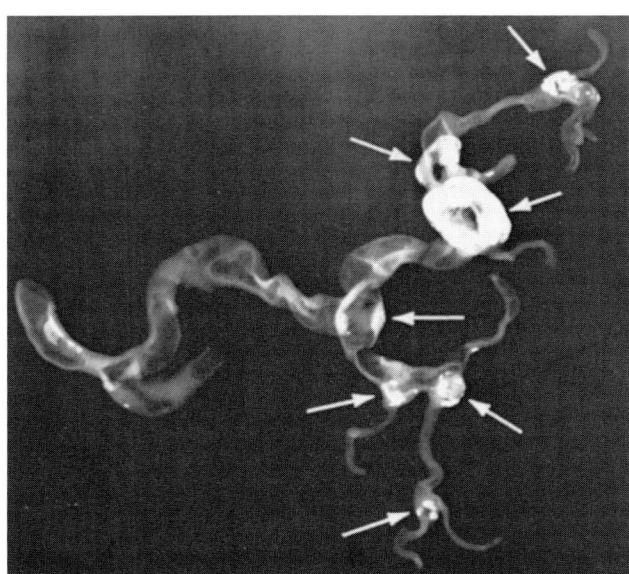

FIGURE 96–2. Splenic artery aneurysms (specimen roentgenogram). Marked calcific arteriosclerosis limited to splenic artery aneurysms occurring at vessel bifurcations (arrows). Intervening arterial segments are unaffected by advanced arteriosclerotic changes.

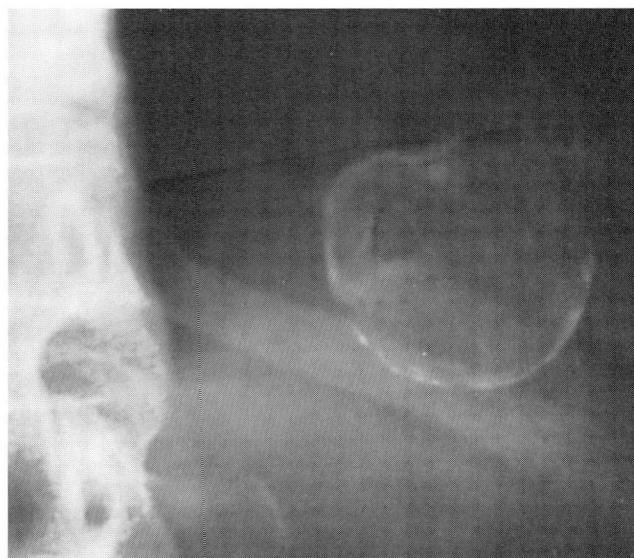

FIGURE 96–4. Splenic artery aneurysm. Curvilinear, signet ring–like calcifications in the left upper quadrant are characteristic of splenic artery aneurysms.

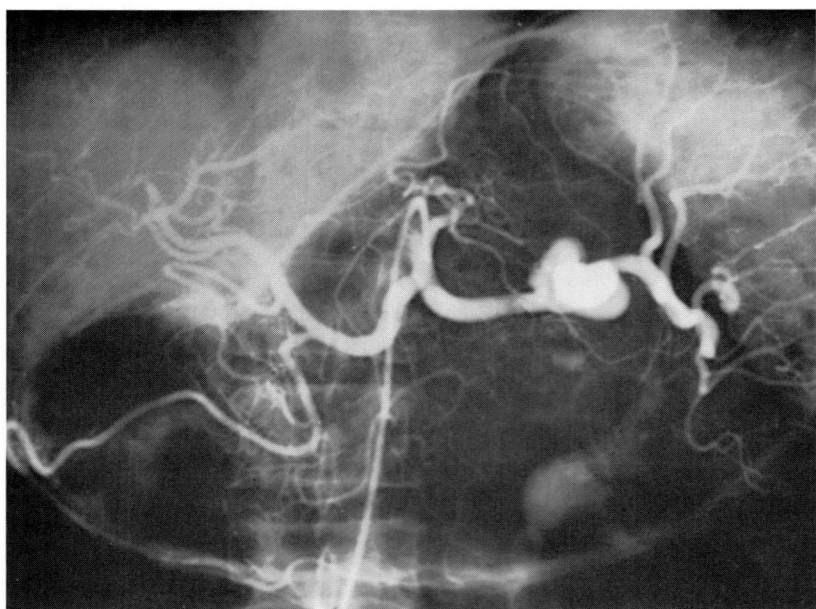

FIGURE 96–5. Splenic artery aneurysm. Arteriographic documentation of a pancreatitis-related aneurysm affecting the mid-splenic artery.

though 17% and 20%, respectively, of patients in two large series allegedly had symptoms referable to these lesions.[81, 85] Others have reported even higher incidences of symptomatic aneurysms. A common complaint among symptomatic patients is vague left upper quadrant or epigastric discomfort with occasional radiation to the left subscapular area. Acute expansion of splenic artery aneurysms intensifies these symptoms. Abdominal tenderness is an unlikely accompaniment of an intact aneurysm. A bruit ascribed to these lesions is more likely to arise from turbulent blood flow through the aorta and its branches than from splenic aneurysmal disease. Most splenic artery aneurysms are smaller than 2 cm in diameter. Accordingly, pulsatile abdominal masses associated with these lesions are palpated infrequently.

Aneurysmal rupture with intraperitoneal hemorrhage accounts for the most dramatic clinical presentation of a splenic artery aneurysm. In nonpregnant patients, rupture often presents as an acute intra-abdominal catastrophe with associated cardiovascular collapse. In most cases, bleeding initially occurs into the retrogastric area. Symptoms distant from the left upper quadrant and epigastrium may follow as blood escapes through the foramen of Winslow. Hemorrhage invariably proceeds to severe intraperitoneal bleeding as lesser sac containment is lost. Such a "double rupture phenomenon" occurs in nearly 25% of cases and often provides an opportunity for treatment before the onset of fatal hemorrhage. In pregnant patients, aneurysmal rupture often mimics common obstetric emergencies such as placental abruption, amniotic fluid embolization, or uterine rupture.[1, 7, 16, 60, 76]

Occasionally, intermittent gastrointestinal bleeding may reflect a communication between a splenic artery aneurysm and the intestinal tract or pancreatic ductal system.[112] These latter lesions usually are products of an inflammatory process, and the communication most often occurs directly, as with penetrating gastric ulcers. In cases associated with pancreatitis, bleeding may occur through the pancreatic ducts.[41] Splenic arteriovenous fistulae are an even more uncommon complication of aneurysmal rupture, but when they do occur they are often associated with secondary portal hypertension.[13]

Life-threatening rupture appears to affect fewer than 2% of bland splenic artery aneurysms.[103] Factors contributing to rupture of previously asymptomatic splenic artery aneurysms remain poorly defined. There is no basis for the contention that rupture is less likely to occur in patients with calcified aneurysms, in normotensive as opposed to hypertensive patients, or in patients older than 60 years of age. Aneurysms in patients who have received orthotopic liver transplants may be at greater risk of rupture than other bland aneurysms.[3, 12] The highest incidence of aneurysmal rupture occurs in young women during pregnancy. More than 95% of aneurysms discovered during pregnancy have ruptured.[1, 16, 60, 103] Despite this observation, it is logical to believe that many splenic artery aneurysms develop during pregnancy and that the majority of these do not rupture during the pregnancy.

Indications for surgical therapy of splenic aneurysms have become better defined in recent years.[6, 103, 107] Symptomatic aneurysms warrant early surgical therapy. Operative intervention appears to be justified for splenic artery aneurysms encountered in pregnant patients or in females of childbearing age who subsequently may conceive. Maternal mortality of aneurysmal rupture during pregnancy is approximately 70%, and fetal mortality exceeds 75%.[1, 7, 16, 76, 103] Survival of both mother and child following rupture of a splenic artery aneurysm, as of 1993, had been reported only 12 times.[1, 16, 58, 90] In nonpregnant patients, operative mortality following surgical treatment for aneurysmal rupture is less than 25%.[105]

Although rupture has been reported to occur in 3% to 9.6% of all patients with splenic artery aneurysms,[98, 103, 107] it is important to recall that disruption of bland lesions probably occurs in no more than 2% of cases. Thus, elective operation for bland splenic artery aneurysms is appropriate only when the predicted surgical mortality rate is no greater than 0.5%. This latter figure represents the product of the reported 2% incidence of rupture and the 25% mortality rate accompanying operative treatment of patients with ruptured aneurysms. In most instances, elective operation is recommended for good risk patients with splenic artery aneurysms greater than 2 cm in diameter. In certain patients in whom operative therapy entails a prohibitively high risk, transcatheter embolization of the aneurysm may be the preferred treatment.[64, 82] Several authors suggest that this may be the procedure of choice for splenic and indeed all splanchnic aneurysms. Temporizing enthusiasm for this approach is its 10% to 15% failure rate, the recognized complication of embolization, and continued enlargement of the aneurysm with potential for subsequent rupture.

Surgical techniques for treating splenic artery aneurysms have become standardized. Aneurysms of the proximal vessel may be treated by aneurysmectomy or simple ligation-exclusion without arterial reconstruction. In fact, restoration of splenic artery continuity when treating aneurysms of this vessel is rarely indicated. Proximal splenic artery aneurysms are easily exposed through the lesser sac after the gastrohepatic ligament has been incised. Entering and exiting vessels are ligated, and these lesions usually are excised if they are not embedded within pancreatic tissue. Certain mid-splenic artery aneurysms, especially those occurring as a result of pancreatic inflammatory disease, may not be removed so easily. Such false aneurysms, which often occur as a consequence of pancreatic pseudocyst erosion into the splenic artery, may be treated by arterial ligation from within the aneurysmal sac. Monofilament suture, such as polypropylene, is used to ligate vessels in this situation to lessen the risk of chronic infection that might occur in the presence of bacterial contamination of pseudocyst contents. Proximal splenic artery ligation or clamping, if easily accomplished, is recommended to lessen bleeding encountered upon opening the false aneurysm. Internal or external drainage of associated pseudocysts is often necessary following arterial ligation, and later extirpation of the diseased pancreas is frequently required. Distal pancreatectomy including the affected artery is preferred when treating inflammatory false aneurysms involving the distal body and tail regions of the pancreas.

In the past, surgical therapy of aneurysms within the hilus of the spleen usually has entailed a conventional splenectomy. Given the importance of splenic preservation in maintaining host resistance, simple suture obliteration, aneurysmorrhaphy, or excision of distal aneurysms may become favored over traditional splenectomy. Mortality following surgical therapy for pancreatitis-related bleeding arterial aneurysms, most commonly affecting the splenic artery, approaches 30%.[98] On the other hand, operative mortality following elective surgical treatment of bland noninflammatory splenic artery aneurysms, without concomitant vascular or gastrointestinal tract operations, has not been described among cases reported in the recent literature.[103, 105, 107] Laparoscopic ligation of these aneurysms is likely to lessen the expected morbidity accompanying conventional open procedures.[43] Endovascular occlusion of splenic artery aneurysms provides an alternative to operative intervention,[61] but splenic infarction and the inability

to ensure durable obliteration of the aneurysm mandate careful follow-up of patients treated in this fashion.

HEPATIC ARTERY ANEURYSMS

Aneurysmal disease of the hepatic artery accounts for 20% of aneurysms affecting splanchnic vessels.[59] Mycotic aneurysms, previously considered the most common type of hepatic artery aneurysm,[37] accounted for 16% of lesions described in the literature from 1960 to 1970.[105] At present, they represent only 10% of known hepatic artery aneurysms, occurring most often as a complication of illicit intravenous drug use. Atheromatous changes have been encountered in approximately 32% of hepatic artery aneurysms. In most instances, however, atherosclerosis is not considered an etiologic process but, rather, a secondary phenomenon.

Medial degeneration, including alterations similar to those encountered in many splenic artery aneurysms, has been documented in approximately 24% of these lesions. Medial defects appear to be acquired and are seemingly unrelated to congenital abnormalities. Specific events leading to the development of aneurysms in this latter setting are unknown. True aneurysms or pseudoaneurysms developing as a consequence of trauma represent an additional 22% of reported hepatic artery aneurysms, and the frequency of such lesions is increasing. Central hepatic rupture and deep parenchymal fractures subsequent to blunt abdominal injury or gunshot wounds are responsible for most traumatic aneurysms (Fig. 96–6). Polyarteritis nodosa, cystic medial necrosis, and other more unusual arteriopathies have been associated with a very small number of these aneurysms. A possible association between excessive oral amphetamine use and multiple visceral aneurysms has been reported. Both patients had hepatic and superior mesenteric artery aneurysms, and one also had a splenic artery aneurysm.[114] Last, periarterial inflammation, such as occurs with cholecystitis or pancreatitis, is a recognized but uncommon cause of hepatic artery aneurysms.

Hepatic artery aneurysms larger than 2 cm in diameter usually are saccular in character (Fig. 96–7). Smaller nontraumatic aneurysms tend to be fusiform. Of these lesions, 80% involve the extrahepatic vessels. Twenty per cent occur within the substance of the liver, with traumatic aneurysms dominating this latter group. A review of 163 aneurysms in which the specific site of the lesion could be ascertained revealed the following locations: common hepatic, 63%; right hepatic, 28%; left hepatic, 5%; and both right and left hepatic arteries, 4%.[105] Excluding multiple microaneurysms associated with inflammatory arteriopathies, such as polyarteritis nodosa,[80] most hepatic artery aneurysms are solitary.

Men with hepatic artery aneurysms outnumber women 2:1. Most of these lesions, excluding traumatic aneurysms, occur in patients who have entered their sixth decade of life. Most aneurysms remain asymptomatic. Among symptomatic patients with intact aneurysms, the most common complaint is right upper quadrant or epigastric pain. Discomfort, although frequently vague, usually is persistent and is often attributed to cholecystitis. In most instances, this pain is not related to meals. Expanding hepatic artery

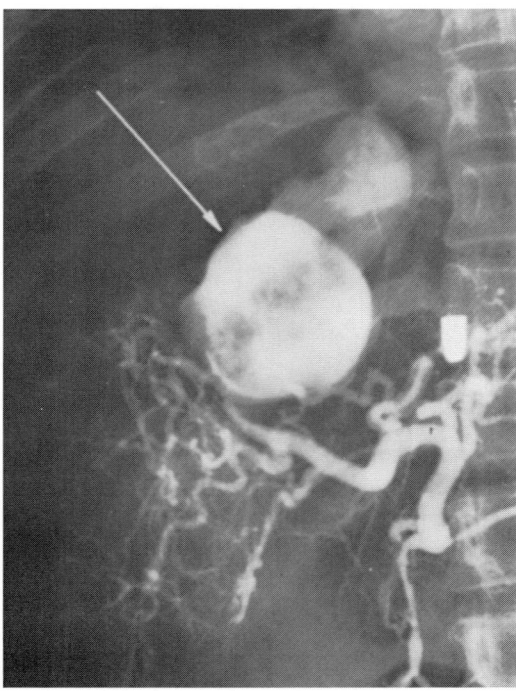

FIGURE 96–6. Traumatic hepatic artery aneurysm. Blunt abdominal injury and gunshot wounds cause most traumatic lesions. (From Whitehouse WM Jr, Graham LM, Stanley JC: Aneurysms of the celiac, hepatic, and splenic arteries. *In* Bergan JJ, Yao JST [eds]: Aneurysms, Diagnosis and Treatment. New York, Grune & Stratton, 1981, pp 405–415.)

aneurysms usually cause severe upper abdominal discomfort, often with radiation to the back, similar to that accompanying pancreatitis. Exceedingly large aneurysms may compress the biliary tree and result in clinical manifestations similar to other forms of extrinsic extrahepatic bile duct obstruction. Pulsatile masses and abdominal bruits are uncommon findings in the presence of intact aneurysms.

Rupture of hepatic artery aneurysms occurs into the hepatobiliary tract and the peritoneal cavity with equal

frequency. Rupture into bile ducts often is responsible for the characteristic findings of hematobilia.[24, 40, 49] In such a setting, patients may complain of intermittent abdominal pain similar to that of biliary colic. The majority exhibit massive gastrointestinal bleeding with periodic hematemesis.[85] More than half of these patients become jaundiced when blood clots obstruct their biliary ducts.

Most patients with hematobilia are febrile at some time during their illness. Symptoms of chronic anemia associated with insidious bleeding and melena are less common manifestations of aneurysmal communication with the biliary tree. Hematobilia occurs most often in the presence of traumatic intrahepatic pseudoaneurysms. Erosion of nontraumatic hepatic artery aneurysms into the stomach, duodenum, common bile duct, pancreatic duct, or portal vein is a recognized, but relatively rare, complication of these lesions. Intraperitoneal bleeding and exsanguinating hemorrhage, producing clinical signs of abdominal apoplexy, frequently accompany extrahepatic aneurysmal rupture.[85] In this regard, aneurysms associated with polyarteritis nodosa that rupture into the intraperitoneal cavity are most likely to arise from the hepatic artery.[73] Unfortunately, many patients destined to develop such catastrophes do not exhibit prior symptoms.

In the past, the diagnosis of hepatic artery aneurysms was made most often at autopsy or at times of surgical exploration for major complications of these lesions. Vascular calcifications in the upper abdomen and displacement of contiguous structures evident on barium studies or cholecystography may suggest the presence of these aneurysms. More recently, arteriographic studies in patients with unknown causes of gastrointestinal hemorrhage and in those with major abdominal trauma have led to an increased recognition of hepatic artery aneurysms. Ultrasonography and computed tomography may be valuable in screening patients for suspected hepatic artery aneurysms and in maintaining noninvasive follow-up.[2]

Excision or obliteration of all hepatic artery aneurysms appears justified unless unusual risks preclude operation. Although not every aneurysm eventually ruptures, rupture occurred in 44% of the lesions described in the literature

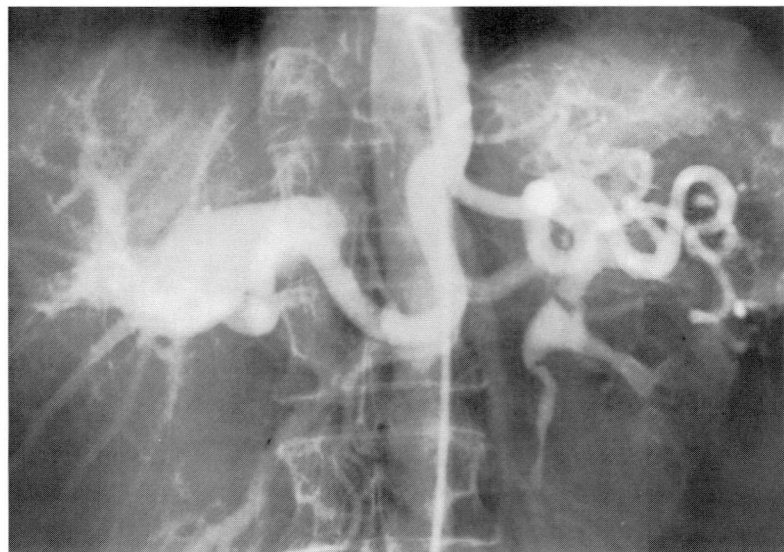

FIGURE 96–7. Hepatic artery aneurysms. Selective celiac arteriogram demonstrating a large saccular aneurysm at the bifurcation of the proper hepatic artery. Of all hepatic artery aneurysms, 80% are extrahepatic.

from 1960 to 1970.[105] In some isolated experiences, high incidences of rupture have been reported[89]; in general, however, the overall rupture rate is probably less than 20%. Mortality associated with rupture continues to be exceedingly high and certainly is not less than the 35% previously reported.[15] An aggressive approach to managing these aneurysms seems appropriate.

Preoperative arteriographic delineation of the foregut and midgut arterial circulation is essential in planning optimal surgical therapy of these aneurysms.[113] Common hepatic artery aneurysms may often be treated by aneurysmectomy or aneurysmal exclusion without arterial reconstruction. Extensive foregut collateral circulation to the liver through the gastroduodenal and right gastric arteries frequently provides adequate hepatic blood flow despite common hepatic artery interruption. However, if blood flow to the liver appears compromised following a 5-minute trial of intraoperative hepatic artery occlusion, then aneurysmorrhaphy or formal hepatic revascularization should be pursued. Similarly, coexisting liver parenchymal disease makes ligation of the proximal hepatic artery less advisable and arterial reconstruction much more preferable.

Restoration of normal hepatic blood flow is important in the management of aneurysms involving the proper hepatic artery and its extrahepatic branches. Aneurysms of the hepatic artery are usually approached through an extended right subcostal or a vertical midline incision. Intact common hepatic artery aneurysms are easily isolated. However, proximal proper hepatic artery aneurysms should be cautiously dissected, especially near the gastroduodenal artery and its pancreaticoduodenal artery branch, which often cross over the common bile duct inferiorly. Similarly, distal proper hepatic or hepatic artery branch aneurysms must be carefully dissected to avoid bile duct injuries. Expeditious vascular control of entering and exiting vessels from within an aneurysm may be safer than dissecting the adjacent arteries when treating large or inflammatory aneurysms.

A number of therapeutic alternatives exist in repairing aneurysmal hepatic arteries.[59] Aneurysmorrhaphy, with or without a vein patch closure, may be appropriate in managing select traumatic aneurysms. Fusiform and large saccular aneurysms that involve greater arterial circumferences are best treated by resection and arterial reconstruction. The use of an autogenous saphenous vein, despite occasional failures,[87] is preferred over synthetic prostheses in most circumstances. Anastomoses are best undertaken by spatulation of both the hepatic artery and vein graft to provide an ovoid anastomosis that will be less likely to become narrowed with healing. Interposition grafts within the hepatic arterial circulation are often possible, and when not, an aortohepatic bypass may be undertaken. An extended Kocher's maneuver with medial visceral rotation allows exposure of the vena cava and aorta. A vein graft from the anterolateral aspect of the infrarenal aorta may then be carried behind the duodenum to the porta hepatis. After the aneurysmectomy has been performed, the spatulated vein is anastomosed in an end-to-end fashion to either the common or proper hepatic artery.

Resection of liver parenchyma for intrahepatic aneurysms that are not amenable to reconstruction is occasionally necessary. Control of bleeding intrahepatic aneurysms by means of simple ligation of the proximal vessel, despite the possibility of subsequent liver necrosis, may be preferable to undertaking a major liver resection in a critically ill patient. Similarly, percutaneous transcatheter balloon embolization with occlusion of hepatic artery aneurysms in high-risk cases may be an acceptable alternative to operative therapy.[6, 31, 50, 78] This may be the preferred treatment for small intrahepatic pseudoaneurysms. Noteworthy is a reported 42% recanalization rate following hepatic artery embolocclusion, mandating careful follow-up. The potential for migration of embolic material with central lobular necrosis and abscess formation is also a recognized complication of transcatheter balloon embolization of these aneurysms.

SUPERIOR MESENTERIC ARTERY ANEURYSMS

The third most common splanchnic artery aneurysm, accounting for 5.5% of these lesions, involves the main trunk of the superior mesenteric artery. These lesions, affecting the proximal 5 cm of this vessel, are most often infectious in etiology.[26] Mycotic aneurysms account for more than half those lesions.[20, 105] In this regard, the superior mesenteric artery harbors more infectious aneurysms than any other muscular artery. Nonhemolytic *Streptococcus,* related to left-sided bacterial endocarditis, has been the organism reported most often in these lesions. A variety of other pathogens, especially staphylococcal organisms, have been described in aneurysms associated with noncardiac septicemia. Syphilitic aneurysms, frequently described in very early reports, have not been observed in contemporary times. Dissecting aneurysms associated with medial defects are rare[19] but affect this vessel more than any other splanchnic artery (Fig. 96–8).[38] Arteriosclerosis, most likely representing a secondary event, is evident in approximately 20% of reported superior mesenteric artery aneurysms. Trauma is a rare cause of these aneurysms.

Intermittent upper abdominal discomfort that progresses to persistent and severe epigastric pain often accompanies symptomatic mycotic superior mesenteric artery aneurysms. In certain cases, it may be difficult to distinguish symptomatology that is due to mesenteric ischemia from that due to aneurysmal expansion. It is noteworthy that a tender pulsatile abdominal mass that is not rigidly fixed has been discovered in nearly half of these patients.

Female patients were predominant in earlier series of superior mesenteric artery aneurysms. More recent experience has not confirmed such a sex predilection, and men and women are affected equally. Most studies reported mycotic aneurysms occur in patients under 50 years of age. Subacute bacterial endocarditis is usually present in these cases. Nonmycotic aneurysms of the superior mesenteric artery most often affect patients after the sixth decade of life. This older subgroup of patients often experiences prodromata of intestinal angina prior to aneurysm rupture.

Aneurysmal expansion with dissection, or propagation of intraluminal thrombus, beyond the vessel's inferior pancreaticoduodenal and middle colic branches, effectively isolates the superior mesenteric artery from the collaterals of the celiac and inferior mesenteric artery circulations. In

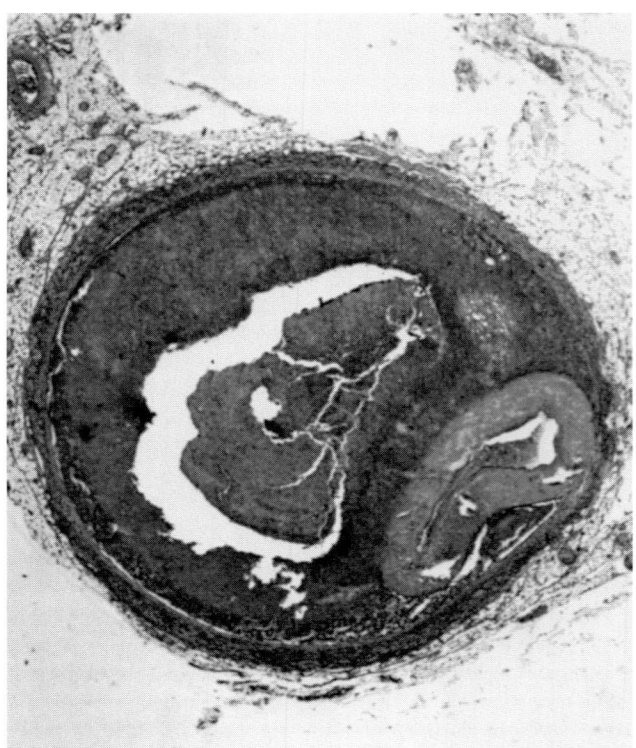

FIGURE 96–8. Superior mesenteric artery aneurysm. Microscopic cross section of a dissecting aneurysm affecting the proximal superior mesenteric artery. (H&E.)

such circumstances, any compromise of blood flow through the superior mesenteric artery may cause intestinal angina. Because of the critical location of most superior mesenteric artery aneurysms, the existence of asymptomatic lesions is not as common as with many other splanchnic aneurysms. Antemortem diagnosis of uncomplicated superior mesenteric artery aneurysms is uncommon. In fact, recognition of asymptomatic solitary dissecting superior mesenteric artery aneurysms has not been reported.[19] Radiographic evidence of calcified mycotic aneurysms and abdominal angiograms made during studies for unrelated disease have been responsible for the majority of antemortem diagnoses.

Surgical treatment of most superior mesenteric artery aneurysms appears justified in light of the seemingly common occurrence of rupture or arterial occlusion. Nearly a third of reported superior mesenteric artery aneurysms have been successfully treated by operation.[62] This includes fewer than 20 mycotic aneurysms of this vessel.[26] Operative exposure for more distal lesions may be obtained by a transmesenteric route, or for proximal lesions by a retroperitoneal approach after the lateral parietes are incised, allowing the colon, pancreas, and spleen to be reflected medially. Since the first successful surgical treatment of a superior mesenteric artery aneurysm was reported nearly five decades ago,[20, 54] the most common procedures attempted have been aneurysmorrhaphy and simple ligation, the latter having been undertaken in over a third of cases. Ligation of the vessels entering and exiting these aneurysms without arterial reconstruction has proved to be an acceptable, simple means of treatment.[30, 105] The existence of preformed collaterals involving the inferior pancreaticoduo-

denal and middle colic arteries allows this approach usually to be successful. Temporary occlusion of the superior mesenteric artery with intraoperative assessment of bowel viability offers a means of identifying cases in which mesenteric revascularization is necessary.

Superior mesenteric artery aneurysmectomy may prove hazardous because of the close proximity of neighboring structures such as the superior mesenteric vein and the pancreas. Endoaneurysmorrhaphy in selected patients with saccular aneurysms may be possible. Arterial reconstruction, with an interposition graft or aortomesenteric bypass after exclusion or excision of the aneurysm, has been rarely accomplished.[62, 111, 118] Use of synthetic prostheses, taking origin from the anterior aorta or intact proximal superior mesenteric artery and carried to the normal vessel beyond the aneurysm, is acceptable in the absence of a mycotic aneurysm or infarcted bowel. In the presence of infection, an autogenous saphenous vein is a more appropriate conduit for reconstruction. In such cases, long-term antibiotic therapy is also recommended. Contemporary surgical intervention for all types of superior mesenteric artery aneurysms carries a mortality of less than 15%. Transcatheter occlusion of saccular aneurysms with discrete necks arising from the side of the superior mesenteric artery may occasionally be justified.[6]

CELIAC ARTERY ANEURYSMS

Aneurysms of the celiac artery are unusual lesions that account for 4% of all splanchnic aneurysms. In 1985, only 108 celiac artery aneurysms had been described in the literature.[33] Arteriosclerosis and medial degeneration were the most common histologic changes observed in these aneurysms. The former, noted in 27% of patients, probably represents a secondary rather than a primary causative process. A preexisting paucity of elastic tissue and smooth muscle at major branchings appears to be a contributing factor in an additional 17% of patients in whom developmental aneurysms were suspected.

Traumatic aneurysms caused by penetrating injuries are uncommon. Post-stenotic dilatation occasionally progresses to frank aneurysmal change but is an uncommon cause of these lesions. Mycotic celiac artery aneurysms are very rare,[115] and in recent times syphilitic and tuberculous lesions have not been encountered. Associated aortic aneurysms were noted in 18% of patients with celiac artery aneurysms, and other splanchnic artery aneurysms affected 38% of these patients.[35]

Most celiac artery aneurysms are asymptomatic. Although males outnumber females among all reported cases, there has been no sex predilection in patients reported since the 1960s. The average age of patients reported prior to 1950 was 40 years, in contrast to an average age of 52 years reported since then.[35]

Abdominal discomfort localized to the epigastrium accompanies more than 60% of symptomatic celiac artery aneurysms. Intense discomfort, often with radiation to the back, as well as nausea and vomiting, has been attributed to aneurysmal expansion and may be confused with pancreatitis. Abdominal bruits are frequently heard in patients with celiac artery aneurysms. Nevertheless, such bruits are rarely directly due to the aneurysm. Celiac artery aneurysms are apparent as pulsatile abdominal masses in nearly 30% of cases.[35] Symptomatology suggestive of intestinal angina is a rare accompaniment of celiac artery aneurysms and, when present, is usually due to significant coexisting arteriosclerotic occlusive disease affecting the superior mesenteric and inferior mesenteric arteries.

The most serious clinical complication of celiac artery aneurysmal disease is rupture. Although nearly 80% of all previously reported lesions had ruptured, clinical experience in the past 25 years has documented the risk of rupture as 13%.[35] The contemporary incidence of rupture may be even lower. Aneurysmal disruption is most often associated with intraperitoneal hemorrhage, although communication with the gastrointestinal tract can occur.

Recognition of most celiac artery aneurysms encountered before 1950 occurred at the time of autopsy. Currently, unexpected discovery of aneurysms during angiography accounts for the diagnosis in nearly 65% of cases (Fig. 96–9).[35] Calcification of the aneurysm, which affects 20% of these lesions, and displacement of contiguous structures are occasional radiographic findings that suggest the diagnosis. Nearly 20% of celiac artery aneurysms recognized before death were encountered at the authors' institution.[39, 105] Ultrasonography and computed tomography (CT) may be of diagnostic use in assessing certain lesions[39, 44] and should be useful in longitudinal follow-up of nonoperative cases.

Surgical treatment of celiac artery aneurysms is warranted except when operative risks contraindicate an abdominal operation.[35] Successful operations in more than 90% of cases reported since the first successful surgical treatment 40 years ago support such a therapeutic approach.[96]

Most patients, especially those with small bland aneurysms, can be treated by the abdominal route alone. This approach is particularly applicable if there is a broad costal margin. In these instances, a transverse supraumbilical inci-

sion and subsequent medial visceral rotation of the left colon, spleen, and pancreas allow exposure of the aorta at the diaphragmatic hiatus. Transection of the crus and median arcuate ligament provides access to the origin of the celiac artery and adjacent aorta. Exposure of celiac artery aneurysms for symptomatic or large lesions is more difficult and may require a thoracoabdominal approach with the incision extending from the mid-axillary line on the left, usually in the seventh intercostal space, across the costal margin into the abdomen.

Aneurysmorrhaphy has been advocated in select cases. It is favored only for discrete saccular aneurysms in which the integrity of the remaining arterial wall appears normal. Aneurysmectomy with arterial reconstruction accounts for 50% of reported operations.[35] Aneurysmectomy and primary reanastomosis of the celiac artery trunk are sometimes possible but should be undertaken only in the presence of a relatively normal and lengthy proximal celiac artery. When reanastomosis is not feasible, an aortoceliac bypass with a synthetic prosthesis or autogenous vein graft should be performed, originating from the supraceliac aorta.

Celiac axis ligation with interruption of antegrade blood flow through the common hepatic, left gastric, and splenic vessels has been undertaken in 35% of reported operations.[35] Although celiac artery ligation rarely results in hepatic necrosis, it should be undertaken only when intraoperative findings suggest that liver blood flow will not be severely compromised.[33] Arterial ligation is not advised in patients with known liver disease. Mortality for operative treatment of patients with ruptured celiac artery aneurysms is 40% compared with only 5% for those with nonruptured celiac artery aneurysms.[35]

GASTRIC AND GASTROEPIPLOIC ARTERY ANEURYSMS

Aneurysms of gastric and gastroepiploic arteries account for approximately 4% of splanchnic aneurysms. These lesions

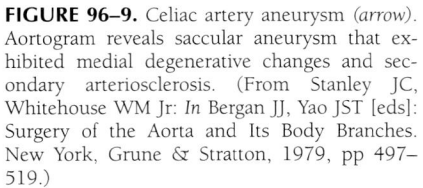

FIGURE 96–9. Celiac artery aneurysm *(arrow).* Aortogram reveals saccular aneurysm that exhibited medial degenerative changes and secondary arteriosclerosis. (From Stanley JC, Whitehouse WM Jr: *In* Bergan JJ, Yao JST [eds]: Surgery of the Aorta and Its Body Branches. New York, Grune & Stratton, 1979, pp 497–519.)

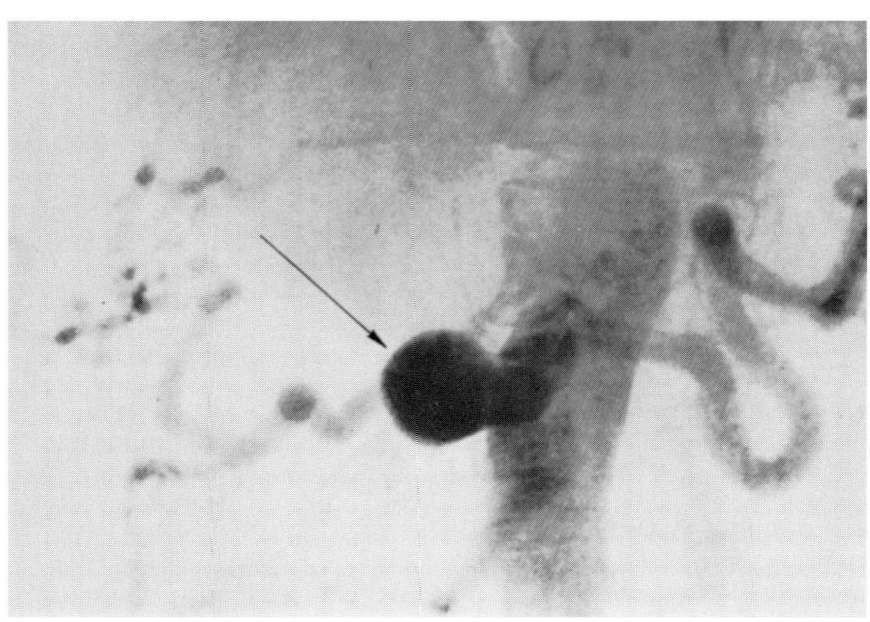

appear to be acquired, although their exact cause often remains undefined.[109] Histologic evidence of arteriosclerosis in many aneurysms led to an earlier belief that this was an important etiologic factor.[70] It is more likely that medial degeneration of undetermined origin or degeneration resulting from periarterial inflammation precedes most arteriosclerotic changes, which are considered a secondary event. Most clinically important aneurysms involving vessels to the stomach are solitary. Aneurysms of gastric arteries are nearly 10 times more common than those of gastroepiploic arteries. They are considered together because their natural history and management are similar.

Asymptomatic aneurysms of the gastric and gastroepiploic arteries have not been commonly reported. Most aneurysms described in the literature have presented as vascular emergencies, with rupture at the time of diagnosis occurring in more than 90% of cases. Nearly 70% were associated with serious gastrointestinal bleeding. A small number of patients describe antecedent dyspeptic epigastric discomfort, but the majority have no abdominal pain prior to aneurysmal rupture. Intestinal bleeding in these cases usually is manifest by acute massive hematemesis,[65] although a small number of patients experience chronic occult gastrointestinal bleeding. Rupture of gastric and gastroepiploic artery aneurysms causes life-threatening intraperitoneal bleeding in approximately 30% of cases.[48, 106] As is the case with intestinal bleeding, most patients are asymptomatic prior to the occurrence of acute intraperitoneal aneurysmal disruption. The majority of cases affect individuals in their sixth and seventh decades of life. Men outnumber women approximately 3:1.

Antemortem diagnosis of gastric and gastroepiploic artery aneurysms most often occurs during urgent operation for gastrointestinal or intraperitoneal bleeding. Intraoperative search for gastric and gastroepiploic aneurysms requires careful palpation and transillumination of the entire stomach. Arteriographic studies for unexplained gastrointestinal bleeding result in occasional preoperative recognition of these lesions (Fig. 96–10). Mucosal alterations associated with these aneurysms are often minimal, and endoscopic

recognition is difficult. Larger lesions may be mistaken for gastric ulcers or malignancies.

Treatment of gastric and gastroepiploic aneurysms is directed at controlling life-threatening hemorrhage. Approximately 70% of patients reported to have these lesions succumb following aneurysm rupture.[105] Early diagnosis and urgent operative intervention are necessary to improve survival. Ligation of aneurysmal vessels, with or without excision of the aneurysm, is appropriate treatment for extraintestinal lesions and for those aneurysms associated with inflammatory processes adjacent to the stomach. Intramural aneurysms and those associated with bleeding into the gastrointestinal tract should be excised with portions of the involved gastric tissue.

JEJUNAL, ILEAL, AND COLIC ARTERY ANEURYSMS

Small intramural and intramesenteric aneurysms of jejunal, ileal, and colic arteries are uncommon, accounting for only 3% of reported splanchnic aneurysms.[45, 63, 75, 86] Excluding aneurysms associated with connective tissue disorders, 90% of these intestinal branch aneurysms are solitary and range from a few millimeters to a centimeter in size. Occasionally, patients have two or three lesions, often in the same region of the intestinal circulation. The pathogenesis of these aneurysms is poorly understood. Most appear to be the result of congenital or acquired medial defects. Arteriosclerotic changes exist in approximately 20% of these lesions,[63] being most often a secondary process. Multiple lesions may represent late sequelae of an endarteritis associated with an immunologic injury or septic emboli from subacute bacterial endocarditis.[108] Necrotizing vasculitides, such as polyarteritis nodosa, are another recognized cause of multiple mesenteric branch microaneurysms.[92]

There does not appear to be any gender predilection in the development of mesenteric branch aneurysms. The peak age of involvement is during the seventh decade of life. Intact aneurysms are rarely symptomatic. Most aneurysms are recognized at operation for complications of rupture into the mesentery, intestinal lumen, or peritoneal cavity. Rupture of aneurysms affecting the jejunal arteries is relatively rare.[22] Abdominal pain associated with aneurysmal rupture, the presence of a tender mass, or the development of uncontained hemorrhage have been the initial manifestations of these lesions in 70% of reported cases.[62] Mortality following rupture approaches 20%.[105] Contemporary recognition of intestinal artery aneurysms is increasingly the result of more frequent abdominal arteriographic studies for nonvascular disease (Fig. 96–11),[42, 68] often during assessment of insidious gastrointestinal bleeding or massive rectal hemorrhage. Preoperative arteriographic localization of these small aneurysms is often essential for successful operative intervention.

Surgical therapy of mesenteric branch aneurysms necessitates arterial ligation, aneurysmectomy, and resection of the affected bowel if the intestinal blood supply is compromised. An intraoperative search should be undertaken for multiple aneurysms of the jejunal and ileal arteries. The risk of aneurysmal rupture remains undefined in the case

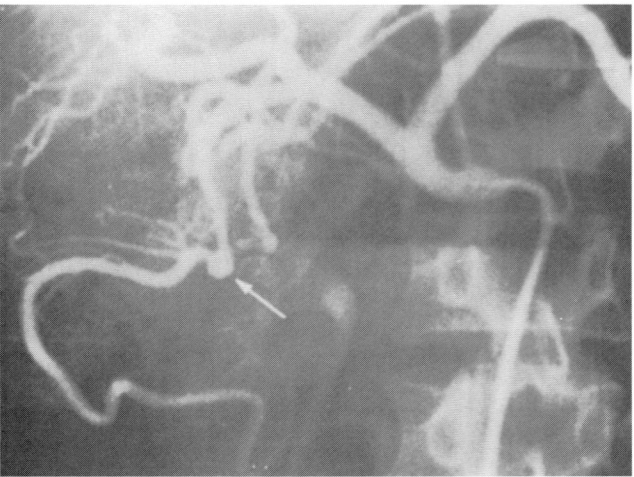

FIGURE 96–10. Gastroepiploic artery aneurysms. Selective celiac arteriogram. This saccular aneurysm (*arrow*) was responsible for massive gastrointestinal hemorrhage.

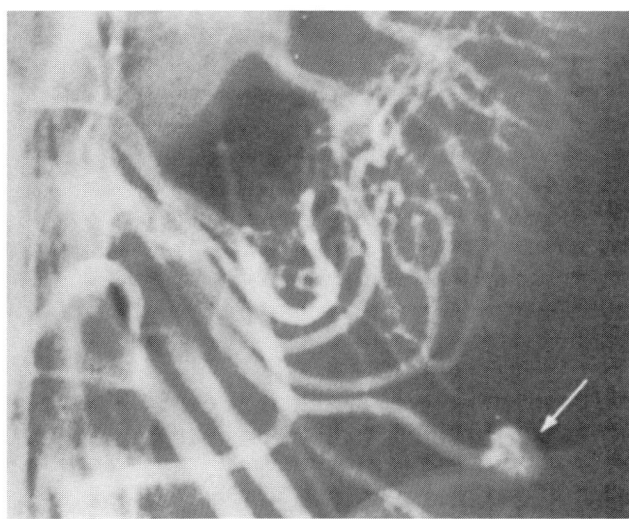

FIGURE 96–11. Ileal artery aneurysm. Mesenteric arteriogram documenting the presence of a saccular aneurysm (arrow) of a distal ileal artery.

of uncomplicated intestinal aneurysms. However, the seriousness of rupture and the limited risks of operative intervention support the contention that these lesions usually should be treated once their existence becomes known.

Aneurysms of the proximal inferior mesenteric artery or its branches are exceedingly rare (Fig. 96–12). As of 1985, only 13 of these lesions had been described in the literature.[34] Aneurysms of this vessel have diverse causes and varied clinical manifestations. Although their natural history remains poorly defined, operative intervention appears justified in most instances.

GASTRODUODENAL, PANCREATICODUODENAL, AND PANCREATIC ARTERY ANEURYSMS

Periduodenal and peripancreatic aneurysmal disease of the communicating vessels between the celiac and superior

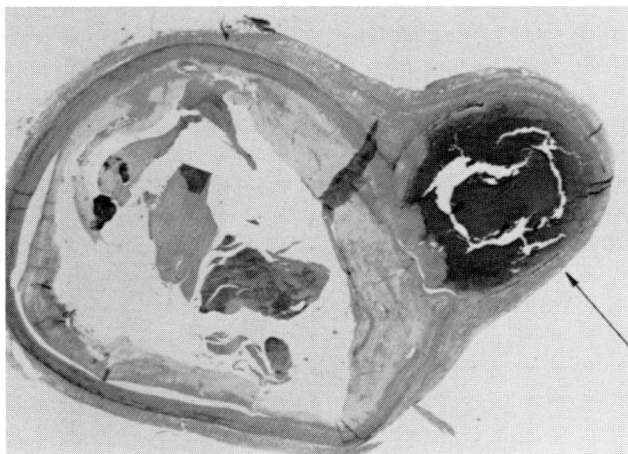

FIGURE 96–12. Inferior mesenteric artery aneurysm. Microscopic cross section of aorta and a thrombus containing aneurysm (arrow) of the inferior mesenteric artery trunk. (H&E.)

mesenteric artery circulations is uncommon.[18, 47] Gastroduodenal artery aneurysms account for 1.5% of all splanchnic artery aneurysms. These cases have all been reported since 1960.[95] Aneurysms of pancreaticoduodenal and pancreatic vessels account for an additional 2% of splanchnic artery aneurysms. Eighty-eight such aneurysms had been reported as of 1995, of which 53 presented with rupture carrying an attendant 49% mortality. The most common age of involvement is the sixth decade. Men are affected more often than women by nearly 4:1. This reflects the increased incidence of alcoholic pancreatitis in men and the fact that the majority of these lesions evolve as complications of acute or chronic pancreatitis.[23, 42, 102, 117]

Periarterial inflammation, actual vascular necrosis, and erosion by expanding pancreatic pseudocysts may produce both true and false aneurysms, the latter of which are by far the most common type.[28, 101] Pancreaticoduodenal artery pseudoaneurysms have been noted following liver transplantation.[119] Noninflammatory pancreaticoduodenal artery aneurysms appear to have no gender predilection.[36] Increased blood flow through these vessels, such as occurs with celiac artery or occlusion, may be an important etiologic factor.[32, 84] Arteriosclerosis used to be considered the most common cause of these aneurysms[105] but is now usually considered a secondary rather than a primary etiologic process.

Most patients with aneurysms involving the gastroduodenal, pancreaticoduodenal, or pancreatic arteries are symptomatic at the time of diagnosis. Epigastric pain, frequently with radiation to the back, is common. Silent inflammatory

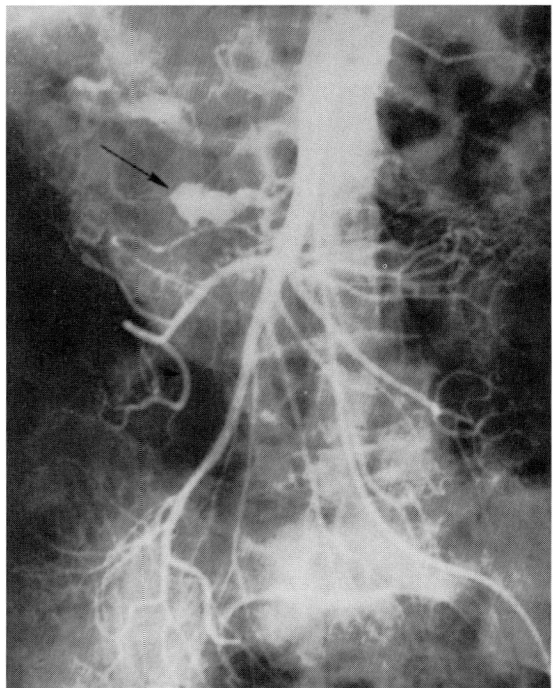

FIGURE 96–13. Inferior pancreaticoduodenal artery aneurysm. Aortogram demonstrating false aneurysm (arrow) that evolved as a complication of pancreatitis. (From Stanley JC, Frey CF, Miller TA, et al: Major arterial hemorrhage: A complication of pancreatic pseudocysts and chronic pancreatitis. Arch Surg 111:435, 1976. Copyright 1976, American Medical Association.)

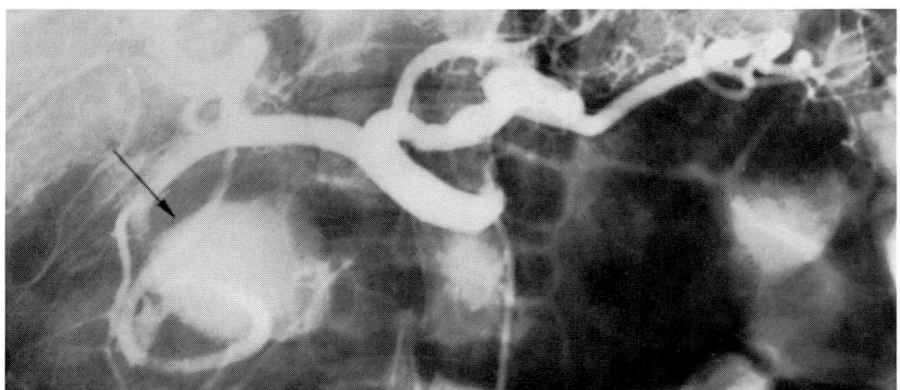

FIGURE 96–14. Gastroduodenal artery aneurysm *(arrow)*. Selective celiac arteriogram. (From Eckhauser FE, Stanley JC, Zelenock GB, et al: Gastroduodenal and pancreaticoduodenal artery aneurysms: A complication of pancreatitis causing spontaneous gastrointestinal hemorrhage. Surgery 88:335, 1980.)

aneurysms are very uncommon. In some cases, this discomfort is indistinguishable from that caused by underlying pancreatitis. This fact is particularly important because nearly 60% of all gastroduodenal artery aneurysms and 30% of all pancreaticoduodenal aneurysms are pancreatitis related.[23] Aneurysmal rupture is second only to abdominal pain as the most frequent manifestation of these lesions. Gastrointestinal hemorrhage affects nearly 75% of these inflammatory aneurysms. Bleeding in these circumstances occurs most often into the stomach or duodenum and less often into the biliary or pancreatic ductal system.[29, 101] An occasional patient becomes jaundiced,[8] but a direct association with aneurysmal disease and bilirubin elevations is not always easily documented. Rupture affects approximately 50% of noninflammatory aneurysms, occurring into the intestinal tract and peritoneal cavity with equal frequency.

Arteriographic studies are essential in evaluating patients suspected of symptomatic gastroduodenal, pancreaticoduodenal, or pancreatic arterial aneurysms, especially those associated with pancreatitis (Figs. 96–13 and 96–14).[11,]

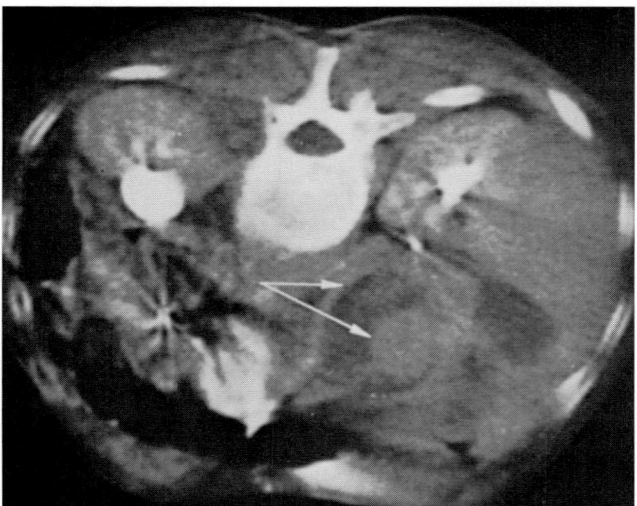

FIGURE 96–15. Gastroduodenal artery aneurysm. Computed axial tomography of a pancreatic pseudocyst *(short arrow)* containing an aneurysmal gastroduodenal artery *(long arrow)*. (From Eckhauser FE, Stanley JC, Zelenock GB, et al: Gastroduodenal and pancreaticoduodenal artery aneurysms: A complication of pancreatitis causing spontaneous gastrointestinal hemorrhage. Surgery 88:335, 1980.)

[23, 102] Endoscopic examinations, barium contrast studies, and ultrasonography may demonstrate coexisting gastroduodenal or pancreatic disease, but their usefulness in directly identifying these aneurysms is limited. CT has greater value as a means of evaluating these aneurysms (Fig. 96–15).[23]

Reported mortality following rupture of gastroduodenal artery aneurysms approaches 50%. Mortality is somewhat less for ruptured pancreaticoduodenal artery aneurysms and is approximately 20% for rupture of nonpancreatitis-related lesions.[36] Surgical intervention for aneurysms of the gastroduodenal or pancreaticoduodenal arteries is justified in all but the poorest risk patients.[23, 36, 101, 110]

In general, pancreaticoduodenal and pancreatic artery aneurysms are more difficult to manage operatively than gastroduodenal artery aneurysms.[23, 116] The multiple vessels that communicate with these smaller aneurysms and the difficulty of identifying them within the substance of the pancreas limit the efficacy of aneurysmal exclusion by simple ligature alone. Intraoperative arteriography may prove useful when lesions involve the proximal pancreas or other critical structures.[97] Suture ligature of entering and exiting vessels from within the aneurysmal sac rather than extra-aneurysmal dissection and arterial ligation is a more appropriate means of treating most gastroduodenal or pancreaticoduodenal artery aneurysms imbedded within the pancreas. When aneurysms involve pancreatic pseudocysts, some manner of cyst decompression should be undertaken. The choice between external or internal drainage is usually determined on the basis of intraoperative findings. Major resections of pancreatic tissue, including pancreaticoduodenectomy, may be necessary for adequate treatment of some patients exhibiting extensive aneurysmal involvement of the pancreatic arteries.[81]

Transcatheter embolization may be performed to ablate certain aneurysms.[64, 73] Rebleeding and rupture may complicate this type of therapy.[57] Although embolization may prove a reasonable alternative to operation in some critically ill patients, it is perhaps better to view that as a temporizing intervention before definitive surgical therapy is undertaken.

REFERENCES

1. Angelakis EJ, Bair WE, Barone JE, Lincer RM: Splenic artery aneurysm rupture during pregnancy. Obstet Gynecol Surv 48:145–148, 1993.
2. Athey PA, Sax SL, Lamki N, Cadavid G: Sonography in the diagnosis of hepatic artery aneurysms. Am J Roentgenol 147:725, 1986.

3. Ayalon A, Wiesner RH, Perkins JD, et al: Splenic artery aneurysms in liver transplant patients. Transplantation 45:386, 1988.
4. Babb RR: Aneurysm of the splenic artery. Arch Surg 111:924, 1976.
5. Bailey RW, Riles TS, Rosen RJ, Sullivan LP: Celiacomesenteric anomaly and aneurysm: Clinical and etiologic features. J Vasc Surg 14:229–234, 1991.
6. Baker JS, Tisnado J, Cho SR, Beachley MC: Splanchnic artery aneurysms and pseudoaneurysms: Transcatheter embolization. Radiology 163:135, 1987.
7. Barrett JM, Caldwell BH: Association of portal hypertension and ruptured splenic artery aneurysm in pregnancy. Obstet Gynecol 57:255, 1981.
8. Bassaly I, Schwartz IR, Pinchuck A, Lerner R: Aneurysm of the gastroduodenal artery presenting as common duct obstruction with jaundice. Am J Gastroenterol 59:435, 1973.
9. Bedford PD, Lodge B: Aneurysm of the splenic artery. Gut 1:321, 1960.
10. Boijsen E, Efsing HO: Aneurysm of the splenic artery. Acta Radiol [Diagn] (Stockh) 8:29, 1969.
11. Boijsen E, Gothlin J, Hallbook, T, Sandblom P: Preoperative angiographic diagnosis of bleeding aneurysms of abdominal visceral arteries. Radiology 93:781, 1969.
12. Bronsther O, Merhav H, Van Thiel D, Starzl TE: Splenic artery aneurysms occurring in liver transplant recipients. Transplantation 52:723, 1991.
13. Brothers TE, Stanley JC, Zelenock GB: Splenic arteriovenous fistula. Int Surg 80:189, 1995.
14. Buehler PK, Dailey TH, Lazarevic B: Spontaneous rupture of colic-artery aneurysms. Dis Colon Rectum 19:671, 1976.
15. Busuttil RW, Brin BJ: The diagnosis and management of visceral artery aneurysms. Surgery 88:619, 1980.
16. Caillouette JC, Merchant EB: Ruptured splenic artery aneurysm in pregnancy: Twelfth reported case with maternal and fetal survival. Am J Obstet Gynecol 168:1810, 1993.
17. Carr SC, Pearce WH, Vogelzang RL, et al: Current management of visceral artery aneurysms. Surgery 120:627–634, 1996.
18. Chiou AC, Josephs LG, Menzoian JO: Inferior pancreaticoduodenal artery aneurysms: Report of a case and review of the literature. J Vasc Surg 17:784, 1993.
19. Cormier F, Ferry J, Artru B, et al: Dissecting aneurysms of the main trunk of the superior mesenteric artery. J Vasc Surg 15:424, 1992.
20. DeBakey ME, Cooley DA: Successful resection of mycotic aneurysm of superior mesenteric artery: Case report and review of the literature. Am Surg 19:202, 1953.
21. Deterling RA: Aneurysm of the visceral arteries. J Cardiovasc Surg (Torino) 12:309, 1971.
22. Diettrich NA, Cacioppo JC, Ying DPW: Massive gastrointestinal hemorrhage caused by rupture of a jejunal branch artery aneurysm. J Vasc Surg 8:187, 1988.
23. Eckhauser FE, Stanley JC, Zelenock GB, et al: Gastroduodenal and pancreaticoduodenal artery aneurysms: A complication of pancreatitis causing spontaneous gastrointestinal hemorrhage. Surgery 88:335, 1980.
24. Erskine JM: Hepatic artery aneurysms. Vasc Surg 7:106, 1973.
25. Feist JH, Gajaraj A: Extra and intrasplenic artery aneurysms in portal hypertension. Radiology 125:331, 1977.
26. Friedman SG, Pogo GJ, Moccio CG: Mycotic aneurysm of the superior mesenteric artery. J Vasc Surg 6:87, 1987.
27. Fukunaga Y, Usui N, Hirohashi K, et al: Clinical courses and treatment of splenic artery aneurysms: Report of 3 cases and review of literature in Japan. Osaka City Med J 36:161, 1990.
28. Gadacz TR, Trunkey D, Kieffer RF: Visceral vessel erosion associated with pancreatitis: Case reports and a review of the literature. Arch Surg 113:1438, 1978.
29. Gangaher DM, Carveth SW, Reese HE, et al: True aneurysm of the pancreaticoduodenal artery: A case report and review of the literature. J Vasc Surg 2:741, 1985.
30. Geelkerken RH, van Bockel JH, de Roos WK, Hermans J: Surgical treatment of intestinal artery aneurysms. Eur J Vasc Surg 4:563, 1990.
31. Goldblatt M, Goldin AR, Shaff MI: Percutaneous embolization for the management of hepatic artery aneurysms. Gastroenterology 73:1142, 1977.
32. Gouny P, Fukui S, Aymard A, et al: Aneurysm of the gastroduodenal artery associated with stenosis of the superior mesenteric artery. Ann Vasc Surg 8:281, 1994.

33. Graham JM, McCollum CH, DeBakey ME: Aneurysms of the splanchnic arteries. Am J Surg 140:797, 1980.
34. Graham LM, Hay MR, Cho KJ, Stanley JC: Inferior mesenteric artery aneurysms. Surgery 97:158, 1985.
35. Graham LM, Stanley JC, Whitehouse WM Jr, et al: Celiac artery aneurysms: Historic (1745–1949) versus contemporary (1950–1984) differences in etiology and clinical importance. J Vasc Surg 5:757, 1985.
36. Granke K, Hollier LH, Bowen JC: Pancreaticoduodenal artery aneurysms: Changing patterns. South Med J 83:918, 1990.
37. Guida PM, Moore SW: Aneurysm of the hepatic artery: Report of five cases with a brief review of the previously reported cases. Surgery 60:299, 1966.
38. Guthrie W, Maclean H: Dissecting aneurysms of arteries other than the aorta. J Pathol 108:219, 1972.
39. Haimovici H, Sprayregen S, Eckstein P, Veith FJ: Celiac artery aneurysmectomy: Case report with review of the literature. Surgery 79:592, 1976.
40. Harlaftis NN, Akin JT: Hemobilia from ruptured hepatic artery aneurysm: Report of a case and review of the literature. Am J Surg 133:229, 1977.
41. Harper PC, Gamelli RL, Kaye MD: Recurrent hemorrhage into the pancreatic duct from a splenic artery aneurysm. Gastroenterology 87:417, 1984.
42. Harris RD, Anderson JE, Coel MN: Aneurysms of the small pancreatic arteries: A cause of upper abdominal pain and intestinal bleeding. Radiology 115:17, 1975.
43. Hashizume M, Ohta M, Ueno K, et al: Laparoscopic ligation of splenic artery aneurysm. Surgery 113:352, 1993.
44. Herzler GM, Silver TM, Graham LM, Stanley JC: Celiac artery aneurysm. J Clin Ultrasound 9:141, 1981.
45. Hoehn JG, Bartholomew LG, Osmundson PJ, Wallace RB: Aneurysms of the mesenteric artery. Am J Surg 115:832, 1968.
46. Hofer BO, Ryan JA Jr, Freeny PC: Surgical significance of vascular changes in chronic pancreatitis. Surg Gynecol Obstet 164:499, 1987.
47. Iyomasa S, Matsuzaki Y, Hiei K, et al: Pancreaticoduodenal artery aneurysm: A case report and review of the literature. J Vasc Surg 22:161, 1995.
48. Jacobs PPM, Croiset van Ughelen FAAM, Bruyninckx CMA, Hoefsloot F: Haemoperitoneum caused by a dissecting aneurysm of the gastroepiploic artery. Eur J Vasc Surg 8:236, 1994.
49. Jeans PL: Hepatic artery aneurysms and biliary surgery: Two cases and a literature review. Aust NZ J Surg 58:889, 1988.
50. Jonsson K, Bjernstad A, Eriksson B: Treatment of a hepatic artery aneurysm by coil occlusion of the hepatic artery. Am J Roentgenol 134:1245, 1980.
51. Jorgensen BA: Visceral artery aneurysms: A review. Dan Med Bull 32:237, 1985.
52. Kanazawa S, Inada H, Murakami T, et al: The diagnosis and management of splanchnic artery aneurysms: Report of 8 cases. J Cardiovasc Surg 38:479, 1997.
53. Keehan MF, Kistner RL, Banis J: Angiography as an aid in extranteric gastrointestinal bleeding due to visceral artery aneurysm. Ann Surg 187:357, 1978.
54. Kopatsis A, D'Anna JA, Sithian N, Sabido F: Superior mesenteric artery aneurysm: 45 years later. Am Surg 64:263, 1998.
55. Kraft RO, Fry WJ: Aneurysms of the celiac artery. Surg Gynecol Obstet 117:563, 1963.
56. Kreel L: The recognition and incidence of splenic artery aneurysms: A historical review. Australas Radiol 16:126, 1972.
57. Lina JR, Jaques P, Mandell V: Aneurysm rupture secondary to transcatheter embolization. Am J Roentgenol 132:553, 1979.
58. Lowry SM, O'Dea TP, Gallagher DI, Mozenter R: Splenic artery aneurysm rupture: The seventh instance of maternal and fetal survival. Obstet Gynecol 67:291, 1986.
59. Lumsden AB, Mattar SG, Allen RC, Bacha EA: Hepatic artery aneurysms: The management of 22 patients. J Surg Res 60:345–350, 1996.
60. MacFarlane JR, Thorbjarnason B: Rupture of splenic artery aneurysm during pregnancy. Am J Obstet Gynecol 95:1025, 1966.
61. McDermott VG, Shlansky-Goldberg R, Cope C: Endovascular management of splenic artery aneurysms and pseudoaneurysms. Cardiovasc Intervent Radiol 17:179, 1994.
62. McNamara MF, Bakshi KR: Mesenteric artery aneurysms. In Bergan JJ, Yao JST (eds): Aneurysms: Diagnosis and Treatment. New York, Grune & Stratton, 1981, pp 285–403.

63. McNamara MF, Griska LB: Superior mesenteric artery branch aneurysms. Surgery 88:625, 1980.
64. Mandel SR, Jaques PF, Mauro MA, Sanofsky S: Nonoperative management of peripancreatic arterial aneurysms: A 10-year experience. Ann Surg 205:126, 1987.
65. Mandelbaum I, Kaiser GD, Lemple RE: Gastric intramural aneurysm as a cause for massive gastrointestinal hemorrhage. Ann Surg 155:199, 1962.
66. Manenti F, Williams R: Injection studies of the splenic vasculature in portal hypertension. Gut 7:175, 1966.
67. Martin KW, Morian JP, Lee JKT, Scharp DW: Demonstration of a splenic artery pseudoaneurysm by MR imaging. J Comput Assist Tomogr 9:190, 1985.
68. Miani S, Arpesani A, Giorgetti PL, et al: Splanchnic artery aneurysms. J Cardiovasc Surg 34:221, 1993.
69. Michels NA: Collateral arterial pathways to the liver after ligation of the hepatic artery and removal of the celiac axis. Cancer 6:708, 1953.
70. Millard M: Fatal rupture of gastric aneurysm. Arch Pathol 59:363, 1955.
71. Moore SW, Guida PM, Schumacher HW: Splenic artery aneurysm. Bull Soc Int Chir 29:210, 1970.
72. Moore SW, Lewis RJ: Splenic artery aneurysm. Ann Surg 153:1033, 1961.
73. Naito A, Toyota N, Ito K: Embolization of a ruptured middle colic artery aneurysm. Cardiovasc Intervent Radiol 18:56, 1995.
74. Nishida O, Moriyasu F, Nakamura T, et al: Hemodynamics of splenic artery aneurysm. Gastroenterology 90:1042, 1986.
75. Nordenstoft EL, Larsen EA: Rupture of a jejunal intramural aneurysm causing massive intestinal bleeding. Acta Chir Scand 133:256, 1967.
76. O'Grady JP, Day EJ, Toole AL, Paust JC: Splenic artery aneurysm rupture in pregnancy: A review and case report. Obstet Gynecol 50:627, 1977.
77. Ohta M, Hashizume M, Ueno K, et al: Hemodynamic study of splenic artery aneurysm in portal hypertension. Hepatogastroenterology 41:181, 1994.
78. Okazaki M, Higashihara H, Ono H, et al: Percutaneous embolization of ruptured splanchnic artery pseudoaneurysms. Acta Radiol 32:349, 1991.
79. Owens JC, Coffey RJ: Aneurysm of the splenic artery including a report of six additional cases. Int Abstr Surg 97:313, 1953.
80. Parangi S, Oz MC, Blume RS, et al: Hepatobiliary complications of polyarteritis nodosa. Arch Surg 126:909, 1991.
81. Pitkaranta P, Haapiainen R, Kivisaari L, Schroder T: Diagnostic evaluation and aggressive surgical approach in bleeding pseudoaneurysms associated with pancreatic pseudocysts. Scand J Gastroenterol 26:58, 1991.
82. Probst P, Castaneda-Zuniga WR, Gomes AS, et al: Nonsurgical treatment of splenic-artery aneurysms. Radiology 128:619, 1978.
83. Puttini M, Aseni P, Brambilla G, Belli L: Splenic artery aneurysm in portal hypertension. J Cardiovasc Surg 23:490, 1982.
84. Quandalle P, Chambon JP, Marache P, et al: Pancreaticoduodenal artery aneurysms associated with celiac axis stenosis: Report of two cases and review of the literature. Ann Vasc Surg 4:540, 1990.
85. Reber PU, Baer HU, Patel AG, et al: Life-threatening upper gastrointestinal tract bleeding caused by ruptured extrahepatic pseudoaneurysm after pancreatoduodenectomy. Surgery 124:114, 1998.
86. Reuter SR, Fry WJ, Bookstein JJ: Mesenteric artery branch aneurysms. Arch Surg 97:497, 1968.
87. Rutten APM, Sikkenk PJH: Aneurysm of the hepatic artery: Reconstruction with saphenous vein graft. Br J Surg 58:262, 1971.
88. Salam TA, Lumsden AB, Martin LG, Smith RB III: Nonoperative management of visceral aneurysms and pseudoaneurysms. Am J Surg 164:215–219, 1992.
89. Salo JA, Aarnio PT, Jarvinen AA, Kivilaakso EO: Aneurysms of the hepatic arteries. Am Surg 55:705, 1989.
90. Salo JA, Salmenkivi K, Tenhunen A, Kivilaakso EO: Rupture of splanchnic artery aneurysms. World J Surg 10:123, 1986.
91. Scheinin TM, Vanttinen E: Aneurysms of the splenic artery in portal hypertension. Ann Clin Res 1:165, 1969.
92. Sellke FM, Williams GB, Donovan DL, Clarke RE: Management of intra-abdominal aneurysms associated with periarteritis nodosa. J Vasc Surg 4:294, 1986.
93. Settembrini PG, Jausseran J-M, Roveri S, et al: Aneurysms of anomalous splenomesenteric trunk: Clinical features and surgical management in two cases. J Vasc Surg 24:687, 1996.
94. Shanley CJ, Shah NL, Messina LM: Common splanchnic artery aneurysms: Splenic, hepatic and celiac. Ann Vasc Surg 10:315, 1996.
95. Shanley CJ, Shah NL, Messina LM: Uncommon splanchnic artery aneurysms: Pancreaticoduodenal, gastroduodenal, superior mesenteric, inferior mesenteric, and colic. Ann Vasc Surg 10:506, 1996.
96. Shumacker HB Jr, Siderys H: Excisional treatment of aneurysms of celiac artery. Ann Surg 148:885, 1958.
97. Spanos PK, Kloppedal EA, Murray CA: Aneurysms of the gastroduodenal and pancreaticoduodenal arteries. Am J Surg 127:345, 1974.
98. Spittell JA, Fairbairn JF, Kincaid CW, ReMine WH: Aneurysm of the splenic artery. JAMA 175:452, 1961.
99. Stabile BE, Wilson SE, Debas HT: Reduced mortality from bleeding pseudocysts and pseudoaneurysms caused by pancreatitis. Arch Surg 118:45, 1983.
100. Stanley JC: Abdominal visceral aneurysms. In Haimovici H (ed): Vascular Emergencies. New York, Appleton-Century-Crofts, 1981, pp 387–396.
101. Stanley JC, Eckhauser FE, Whitehouse WM Jr, Zelenock GB: Pancreatitis related splanchnic arterial microaneurysms and macroaneurysms. In Dent TL, Eckhauser FE, Vinik AI, Turcotte JG (eds): Pancreatic Disease. New York, Grune & Stratton, 1981, pp 325–341.
102. Stanley JC, Frey CF, Miller TA, et al: Major arterial hemorrhage: A complication of pancreatic pseudocysts and chronic pancreatitis. Arch Surg 111:435, 1976.
103. Stanley JC, Fry WJ: Pathogenesis and clinical significance of splenic artery aneurysms. Surgery 76:898, 1974.
104. Stanley JC, Gewertz BL, Bove EL, et al: Arterial fibrodysplasia: Histopathologic character and current etiologic concepts. Arch Surg 110:561, 1975.
105. Stanley JC, Thompson NW, Fry WJ: Splanchnic artery aneurysms. Arch Surg 101:689, 1970.
106. Thomford NR, Yurko JE, Smith EJ: Aneurysm of gastric arteries as a cause of intraperitoneal hemorrhage: Review of literature. Ann Surg 168:294, 1968.
107. Trastek VF, Pairolero PC, Joyce JW, et al: Splenic artery aneurysms. Surgery 91:694, 1982.
108. Trevisani MF, Ricci MA, Michaels RM, Meyer KK: Multiple mesenteric aneurysms complicating subacute bacterial endocarditis. Arch Surg 122:823, 1987.
109. Varekamp AP, Minder WH, VanNoort G, Wassenaar HA: Rupture of a submucosal gastric aneurysm, a rare cause of gastric hemorrhage. Neth J Surg 35:100, 1983.
110. Verta MJ Jr, Dean RH, Yao JST, et al: Pancreaticoduodenal artery aneurysms. Ann Surg 186:111, 1977.
111. Violago FC, Downs AR: Ruptured atherosclerotic aneurysm of the superior mesenteric artery with celiac axis occlusion. Ann Surg 174:207, 1971.
112. Wagner WH, Cossman DV, Treiman RL, et al: Hemosuccus pancreaticus from intraductal rupture of a primary splenic artery aneurysm. J Vasc Surg 19:158, 1994.
113. Weaver DH, Fleming RJ, Barnes WA: Aneurysm of the hepatic artery: The value of arteriography in surgical management. Surgery 64:891, 1968.
114. Welling TH, Williams DM, Stanley JC: Excessive oral amphetamine use as a possible cause of renal and splanchnic arterial aneurysms: A report of two cases. J Vasc Surg 28(4):727, 1998.
115. Werner K, Tarasoutchi F, Lunardi W, et al: Mycotic aneurysm of the celiac trunk and superior mesenteric artery in a case of infective endocarditis. J Cardiovasc Surg 32:380, 1991.
116. West JE, Bernhardt H, Bowers RF: Aneurysms of the pancreaticoduodenal artery. Am J Surg 115:835, 1968.
117. White AF, Baum S, Buranasiri S: Aneurysms secondary to pancreatitis. Am J Roentgenol 127:393, 1976.
118. Wright CB, Schoepfle J, Kurtock SB, et al: Gastrointestinal bleeding and mycotic superior mesenteric aneurysm. Surgery 92:40, 1982.
119. Zajko AB, Bron KM, Starzl TE, et al: Angiography of liver transplantation patients. Radiology 157:305, 1985.

C H A P T E R   9 7

Infected Aneurysms

Daniel J. Reddy, M.D., and
Calvin B. Ernst, M.D.

HISTORICAL BACKGROUND

Although aneurysmal disease was reported in Western literature in ancient times by Galen, 14 centuries passed until Ambroise Paré, writing in the mid-16th century, first noted the association between an aneurysm and infection. He described the fatal outcome and autopsy findings of a patient who suffered rupture of a syphilitic aneurysm of the descending thoracic aorta.[99]

During the 19th century, Rokitansky in Austria, Virkow and Koch in Germany, and Tufnell in Ireland predated Osler's landmark work with case reports associating endocarditis, septic emboli, arterial abscesses, and ruptured infected aneurysms of the superior mesenteric and popliteal arteries.[67, 117, 148, 151] Sir William Osler, in 1885, presented the first comprehensive discussion of an infected aneurysm, remarking on the "anatomical characters . . . , clinical features, and . . . etiological and pathological relations."[95] He used the term *mycotic aneurysm* to describe these infected aneurysms, which had developed as complications of bacterial endocarditis. Since there was no apparent association with fungal disease, Osler's choice of the term "mycotic" has been a source of discussion and confusion in the literature. Some have used this term when referring to an "infected" aneurysm regardless of pathogenesis.[3, 4, 9, 16, 20, 32, 45, 93, 101, 106, 146, 157, 159] Fungal infection is *not* implied when this designation is used. Strictly speaking, the term mycotic aneurysm should be used only to describe an infected aneurysm resulting from bacterial endocarditis complicated by septic arterial emboli or an infected aneurysm of the sinus of Valsalva resulting from contiguous spread from an infected aortic valve. Following Osler by 2 years, Eppinger provided evidence supporting the embolic etiology of a mycotic aneurysm when he documented identical strains of bacteria in both the peripheral embolus and the valvular vegetations of a patient with a mycotic aneurysm.[38]

At the beginning of the 20th century, Lewis and Schrager reviewed several cases of mycotic aneurysm occurring in young patients with endocarditis.[75] They commented on a case reported by Ruge involving a streptococcal coronary artery aneurysm in a 12-year-old boy with streptococcal osteomyelitis and hypothesized that not all infected aneurysms were "embolomycotic" in origin.

In 1923, Stengel and Wolferth described four patients and reviewed another 213 with a total of 382 bacterial aneurysms of intravascular origin.[140] Multiple aneurysms were found in 49 patients. Although aortic, mesenteric, and intracranial mycotic aneurysms predominated, virtually every other named vessel in the arterial tree was also involved. Of greater significance in the evolving understanding of the pathogenesis of infected aneurysms was the finding that in 30 patients (14%) there was no evidence of bacterial endocarditis, thereby demonstrating that infected aneurysms occur in connection with a variety of other septic conditions.

In 1937, Crane[27] presented the clinical course and autopsy findings of a 35-year-old man with a primary multilocular infected aortic arch aneurysm in association with a hypoplastic aorta and an infected superior mesenterial aneurysm. He postulated that in arteries predisposed by disease, blood-borne bacteria could settle and produce infected aneurysms. Six years later, this hypothesis—that bacteremia unassociated with endocarditis could cause an infected aneurysm—was confirmed by Revell.[115] Later authors reported that atherosclerotic vessels were susceptible to bacterial infection, particularly by various *Salmonella* species.[12, 20, 33, 52, 56, 96, 101, 112, 136, 145, 147, 164] Such arterial infections are considered to be examples of microbial arteritis starting in nonaneurysmal arteries and producing infected aneurysms after the vessel wall has been destroyed by infection.

The classification of infected aneurysm was further refined by the 1959 report of Sommerville and colleagues[135] of more than 20,000 Mayo Clinic autopsies as they related to atherosclerotic abdominal aortic aneurysms (AAAs). In all, 178 aneurysms (0.8%) were found. Of these, 172 were bland (97%) and six were infected (3%); four of the six infected aneurysms had ruptured. This report established the existence of a third type of arterial infection: one occurring in a preexisting atherosclerotic aneurysm. Bennett and Cherry in 1967,[11] Mundth in 1969,[91] and Jarrett in 1975[61] and their associates all reported series detailing the clinical course, bacteriology, treatment, and outcome for patients with this type of infected aneurysm. With the advent of antibiotic therapy, the overall incidence of arterial infection declined, paralleling the successful treatment of bacterial endocarditis.[147]

In more recent years, however, the incidence of arterial infections and infected aneurysms has increased in response to the increasing prevalence of immunosuppressed hosts,[52, 62, 71] invasive hemodynamic monitoring,[134] angiography,[7, 40] and drug addiction.[3, 64, 97, 105, 109] This change in pathogenesis has been noted by other authors, who emphasize that a fourth type of infected aneurysm has emerged as a significant clinical entity: namely, the *post-traumatic infected false aneurysm (pseudoaneurysm)*.[162] Although the greatest number of such infected aneurysms has been associated with intravenous or intra-arterial drug injections, the trend away from parenteral drug use in favor of smoking "crack" has

TABLE 97–1. CLINICAL CHARACTERISTICS OF INFECTED ANEURYSMS

	MYCOTIC ANEURYSM	MICROBIAL ARTERITIS	INFECTION OF EXISTING ANEURYSM	POST-TRAUMATIC INFECTED FALSE ANEURYSM
Etiology	Endocarditis	Bacteremia	Bacteremia	Narcotic addiction Trauma
Age	30–50 yr	>50 yr	>50 yr	<30 yr
Incidence	Rare	Common	Unusual	Very common
Location	Aorta Visceral Intracranial Peripheral	Atherosclerotic Aortoiliac Intimal defects	Infrarenal Aorta	Femoral Carotid
Bacteriology	Gram-positive cocci	*Salmonella* Others	*Staphylococcus* Others	*Staphylococcus aureus* Polymicrobial
Mortality	25%	75%	90%	5%

From Wilson SE, Van Wagenen P, Passaro E Jr: Arterial infection. Curr Probl Surg 15:5, 1978. Reproduced with permission of Year Book Medical Publishers, Inc.

resulted in a decline in incidence in recent years.[64] Owing to developing treatment modalities that employ catheter-based percutaneous approaches for a variety of occlusive or aneurysmal vascular lesions, iatrogenic infected false aneurysms seem to be increasing in frequency.[124]

CLASSIFICATION

On the basis of the foregoing historical review and the classifications suggested by others,[82, 162] this chapter considers four types of infected aneurysm:

- Mycotic aneurysms (i.e., from septic arterial emboli)
- Microbial arteritis with aneurysm
- Infected preexisting aneurysms
- Post-traumatic infected false aneurysms

Excluded are aneurysms resulting from contiguous infection, spontaneous aortoenteric fistulae, and infections of synthetic vascular prostheses (Table 97–1).

Mycotic Aneurysms

Incidence

Mycotic aneurysms develop when septic emboli of cardiac origin lodge in the lumen or the vasa vasorum of peripheral arteries. This can occur in both normal and abnormal arteries.

In the preantibiotic era, approximately 90% of all infected aneurysms were mycotic aneurysms.[75, 115, 140] They occurred in virtually every named artery intracranially, in the great vessels, the thoracoabdominal aorta, and the visceral, extremity, pulmonary, and coronary arteries. The century following Osler's initial description of this entity saw antibiotic therapy, the advancement of microbiologic techniques allowing identification and treatment of specific bacterial infections, and the development of open heart surgery to permit replacement of the infected cardiac valve. These advances have sharply lowered the incidence of

mycotic aneurysms occurring as embolic complications of infective endocarditis.[78]

In 1951, Cates and Christie reported the results of penicillin treatment of 442 patients with endocarditis[18]; 145 patients (35%) suffered a major arterial embolization, and 20 (4.5%) died after hemorrhage from a mycotic aneurysm, a marked improvement over previously quoted embolism rates of 80%.[95] In a comprehensive review of infected aneurysms, Brown and associates found that endocarditis was implicated in the pathogenesis of only 16% of all reported infected aneurysms and in only 10% of cases since 1965.[14]

The relationship between bacterial endocarditis and peripheral arterial embolization has been reported from the Henry Ford Hospital.[35, 36, 77, 133] Patient admissions for peripheral (extracranial) embolization during the period 1950 to 1964 were 23.1 per 100,000 and during the period 1960 to 1979 were 50.4 per 100,000. During this interval (1950 to 1979), 225 patients were admitted for 337 individual emboli.[78] In only two patients from this group did a mycotic aneurysm develop from these emboli,[35] and both patients were treated between 1957 and 1961, giving a hospital incidence of mycotic aneurysm of 1 per 35,000 during those 5 years. Since 1962, mycotic aneurysms occurring as an embolic complication of endocarditis have been encountered in only eight patients. Six of these eight aneurysms involved the intracranial arteries.[77]

From 1971 to 1983, Johansen and Devin reported that nine patients with infective endocarditis were treated for 14 episodes of mycotic embolization resulting in 17 individual emboli.[62] Six of these nine patients required cardiac valve replacement, but no mycotic aneurysm developed. From 1972 to 1984, 91 patients underwent cardiac valve replacement for endocarditis, and a mycotic cerebral aneurysm developed in five.[78] Other authors have noted this decreasing incidence of mycotic aneurysms, both in absolute terms and as a percentage of infected aneurysms.[3, 61, 75, 78, 135, 162]

Location

Even though mycotic aneurysms may occur in multiple sites in a given patient, certain anatomic locations predominate,[95] namely, the aorta and the intracranial, superior mesenteric, and femoral arteries (Table 97–2).[78, 140] The predilection of mycotic aneurysms for certain anatomic sites relates to their pathogenesis. In larger arteries, such as the aorta, infected emboli may lodge in the relatively large vasa vasorum, causing vessel wall ischemia and infection. As the media is destroyed by this process, an aneurysm forms. In smaller arteries, the infected macroscopic emboli may lodge in the vessel lumen or wall and may initiate a similar pathologic process. Sites predisposed to the formation of mycotic aneurysms are bifurcations, arteriovenous fistulae, and coarctations.[75, 113] Several reports of mycotic aneurysms occurring in the tibioperoneal trunk, the common hepatic artery, the ascending aorta, the carotid artery, and the cerebral artery represent the variety of arterial segments in which mycotic aneurysms are found.[1, 21, 31, 60, 129, 159]

Bacteriology

In 1923, Stengel and Wolferth reported that the predominant organisms were nonhemolytic streptococci, pneumococci, and staphylococci.[140] In 1986, Magilligan and Quinn reported that the dominant infecting organisms in patients with no history of drug abuse (n = 55) with native valve endocarditis were *Streptococcus viridans* (22%), *Staphylococcus aureus* (20%), *Streptococcus faecalis* (14%), and *Staphylococcus epidermidis* (11%). Exotic bacteria, such as *Eikenella corrodens* and *Propionibacterium acnes,* and the fungus *Aspergillus* were also noted. In narcotic addicts (n = 36), the infecting organisms were *S. aureus* (36%), *Pseudomonas* (16%), polymicrobial species (15%), *S. faecalis* (13%), and *S. viridans* (11%). Exotic organisms, such as *Micrococcus, Corynebacterium,* and *Candida albicans,* were also isolated.[78] The responsible organism in each of the six intracerebral mycotic aneurysms among these 91 patients was *S. faecalis* (3), *S. viridans* (1), *Pseudomonas* (1), and *C. albicans* (1).[78] In 1984, Brown and colleagues reported that *S. aureus* and various streptococcal species accounted for 38% of infected aneurysms of all types (Table 97–3).[14]

Microbial Arteritis with Aneurysm

Prevalence and Location

In the preantibiotic era, microbial arteritis with aneurysm occurred in approximately 14% of patients.[140] In modern times, owing to the decline in rheumatic fever and bacterial endocarditis, microbial arteritis with aneurysm is becoming more prevalent than mycotic aneurysm.[14] This increase is due to the aging of the population and the corresponding increase in atherosclerosis, an important factor predisposing arteries to infection.

The prevalence in adults of infected aneurysms produced by microbial arteritis is estimated to be 0.06% to 0.65%.[12, 112] Diseased intima, which, when normal, is highly resistant to infection, allows blood-borne bacteria to inoculate the arterial wall. Once infection is established, suppuration, localized perforation, and false aneurysm formation follow (Fig. 97–1). Supporting atherosclerosis as

TABLE 97–2. FREQUENCY DISTRIBUTION OF INFECTED ANEURYSMS

ARTERY	PREANTIBIOTIC ERA (1909–1943)			1968–1986	
Pulmonary	11	(3%)			
Coronary	8	(2%)			
Aorta	87	(25%)	Aorta	20	(12%)
Iliac	14	(4%)	Iliac	9	(5%)
Gluteal	2	(<1%)			
Upper extremity	35	(10%)	Upper extremity	12	(13%)
Subclavian (3)			Subclavian (3)		
Axillary (1)			Axillary (2)		
Brachial (8)			Brachial (3)		
Radial (1)			Radial (4)		
Ulnar (2)					
Lower extremity	40	(12%)	Lower extremity	69	(63%)
Femoral (10)			Femoral (69)		
Popliteal (2)					
Visceral	87	(25%)	Visceral	3	(2%)
Celiac (1)			Superior mesenteric (2)		
Hepatic (15)			Renal (1)		
Superior mesenteric (47)					
Splenic (18)					
Renal (5)					
Gastroepiploic (1)					
Extracranial cerebral vascular	3	(<1%)	Extracranial cerebral vascular	2	(1%)
Innominate (1)			Carotid (2)		
Carotid (1)					
Vertebral (1)					
Intracranial cerebral	50	(15%)	Intracranial cerebral	6	(4%)
Other	7	(2%)			
TOTAL	344	(100%)		121	(100%)

Data from Anderson CB, et al: Arch Surg 109:712, 1974[3]; Johnson JR, et al: Arch Surg 118:577, 1983[64]; Lewis D, Schrager J: JAMA 63:1808, 1909[75]; Mundth ED, et al: Am J Surg 117:460, 1969[91]; Reddy DJ, et al: J Vasc Surg 3:718, 1986[109]; and Stengel A, Wolferth CC: Arch Intern Med 31:527, 1923.[140]

TABLE 97–3. ORGANISMS CULTURED FROM INFECTED ANEURYSMS: COLLECTED SERIES FROM REVIEW OF ENGLISH LANGUAGE LITERATURE

ORGANISMS	PRIOR TO 1965	AFTER 1965	TOTAL
Salmonella species	14 (38%)	15 (10%)	29 (15%)
Staphylococcus aureus	7 (19%)	47 (30%)	54 (28%)
Streptococcus species	5 (14%)	15 (10%)	20 (10%)
Pseudomonas species	1	6	7
Staphylococcus epidermidis	1	5	6
Escherichia coli	—	4	4
Proteus species	2	1	3
Serratia species	—	3	3
Enterobacter species	—	3	3
Neisseria species	—	3	3
Clostridium species	—	2	2
Enterococcus group	—	2	2
Bacteroides species	—	2	2
Candida species	—	2	2
Klebsiella species	—	2	2
Bacteroides fragilis	—	1	1
Peptostreptococcus species	—	1	1
Corynebacterium species	—	1	1
Arizona hinshawii	—	1	1
Citrobacter freundii	—	1	1
Culture negative	7 (19%)	41 (25%)	48 (25%)
Total	37	158	195

From Brown SL, Busutill RW, Baker JD, et al: Bacteriologic and surgical determinants of survival in patients with mycotic aneurysms. J Vasc Surg 1:541, 1984.

the principal predisposing factor in the pathogenesis of microbial arteritis is the fact that the aorta, the most frequent site of atherosclerosis, is also the most frequent location of these lesions (by a 3:1 margin over peripheral sites).[11, 20, 91, 93, 106] In the authors' series, microbial arteritis accounted for 77% of infected aortoiliac aneurysms (Table 97–4).[112]

It has been thought that patients with the acquired immunodeficiency syndrome (AIDS) may be susceptible to infectious aortitis. These patients might thus represent a large cohort that will increase the incidence and alter the microbiology of this pathologic entity in the future.[33, 52]

Patients undergoing hemodialysis are thought to be particularly vulnerable to *Staphylococcus* bacteremia and resulting microbial arteritis.[127] Microbial arteritis of the subclavian artery after irradiation for breast cancer,[55] aortic infection after gastrointestinal endoscopy in an immunosuppressed patient, and appendicitis and lumbar osteomyelitis have been reported.[46, 120, 122]

Bacteriology

The predominant microorganisms associated with microbial arteritis leading to aneurysm are *Escherichia coli* and *Salmo-*

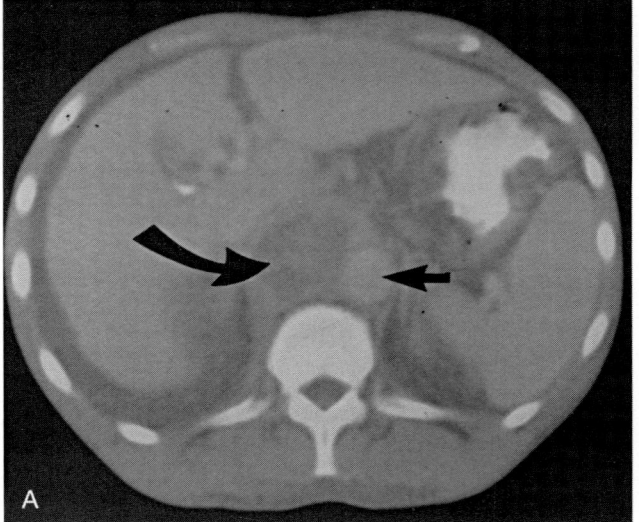
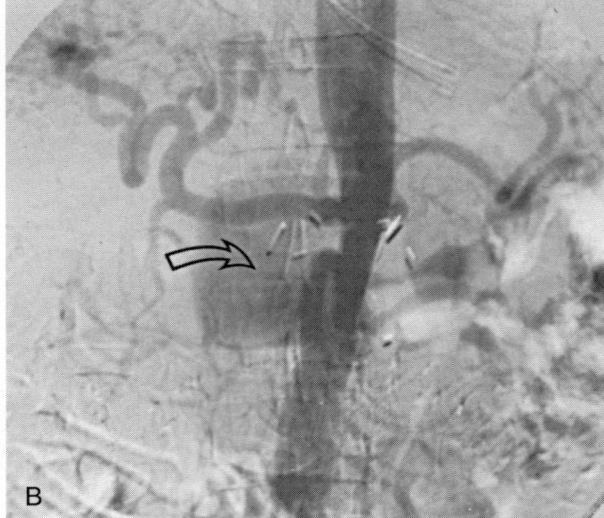

FIGURE 97–1. Diagnostic radiology studies of a patient with *Staphylococcus aureus* microbial aortitis with aneurysm. *A,* Contrast-enhanced computed tomogram demonstrates contained rupture of infected aneurysm *(curved arrow)* and the adjacent aorta *(straight arrow). B,* Digital subtraction aortogram demonstrates saccular eccentric infected aneurysm of the infrarenal aorta *(arrow).*

TABLE 97–4. ANATOMIC LOCATION AND TYPE OF INFECTED ANEURYSMS

| TYPE OF ANEURYSMS | NO. OF ANEURYSMS* | | | TOTAL NO. (%) OF ANEURYSMS |
	SRAA	IRAA	CIA	
Microbial arteritis	3	5	2	10 (77)
Mycotic aneurysm	0	0	1	1 (7.7)
Infection in preexisting aneurysms	0	1	0	1 (7.7)
Adjacent soft tissue infection	0	1	0	1 (7.7)
Total (%)	3 (23)	7 (54)	3 (23)	13 (100)

From Reddy DJ, Shepard AD, Evans JR, et al: Management of infected aortoiliac aneurysms. Arch Surg 126:873–879, 1991. Copyright 1991, American Medical Association.

*SRAA = suprarenal abdominal aorta; IRAA = infrarenal abdominal aorta; CIA = common iliac artery.

nella and *Staphylococcus* species.[162] *Bacteroides fragilis* aneurysms of the suprarenal aorta have also been reported, highlighting the necessity of culturing for anaerobes in these cases.[112, 141] The overall 25% culture-negative rate may indicate a deficiency in obtaining anaerobic cultures (see Table 97–3).

The importance of *Salmonella* species in microbial arteritis, particularly microbial aortitis, has been mentioned in many reports and confirmed in our own review at the Henry Ford Hospital.[112] The diseased aorta has a unique vulnerability to *Salmonella* (Fig. 97–2). The most virulent species are *S. choleraesuis* and *S. typhimurium*, which account for 62% of the reported cases of *Salmonella* arteritis.[162] Although *Salmonella* species are the predominant organisms reported worldwide,[19, 43, 79, 94] other organisms (e.g., *Listeria monocytogenes*,[47, 72] *Klebsiella pneumoniae*,[144] *Clostridium septicum*[88, 92, 123]) and fungal species (e.g., *Aspergillus niger*[132]) have also been reported.

Infected Preexisting Aneurysms

Prevalence and Location

The prevalence of infection in preexisting atherosclerotic aneurysms was estimated by Sommerville and associates to be 3.4%.[135] Bennett and Cherry[11] and Jarrett and coauthors[61] reported parallel findings, noting the relative rarity of this lesion as well as its propensity for rupture.

The related entity of aortic aneurysms colonized by bacteria has been identified in two nearly simultaneous reports by Ernst and colleagues[39] and Williams and Fisher.[160] Patients undergoing abdominal aortic aneurysmectomy were studied prospectively with operative bacterial cultures taken from the aneurysm wall and contents and from bowel bag fluid. Overall, 15% of cultures yielded positive results.[39] There was a higher prevalence of positive cultures among patients with ruptured aneurysms (38%) compared with those with asymptomatic (9%) and symptomatic (13%) aneurysms.[39] Even though the clinical significance of these findings is unknown, it appears that colonized aneurysms do not pose the same threat to patients as infected aneurysms. Steed and colleagues concluded that significant contamination of intraluminal thrombus in aneurysms is rare.[139] Others have confirmed this report and advise that routine culture of aneurysm contents or wall is not necessary when the clinical picture does not suggest aneurysm infection.[44]

The abdominal aorta is the predominant site reported for secondary infection of aneurysms. Lesions have been discovered in other locations, and in earlier times, bacterial overgrowth in luetic aneurysms of the thoracic aorta was encountered.[162]

Bacteriology

Some authors have noted that the index of suspicion for infected AAAs is generally low, and consequently these lesions may have been underreported.[160] The Jarrett study of infected preexisting AAAs documented a predominance

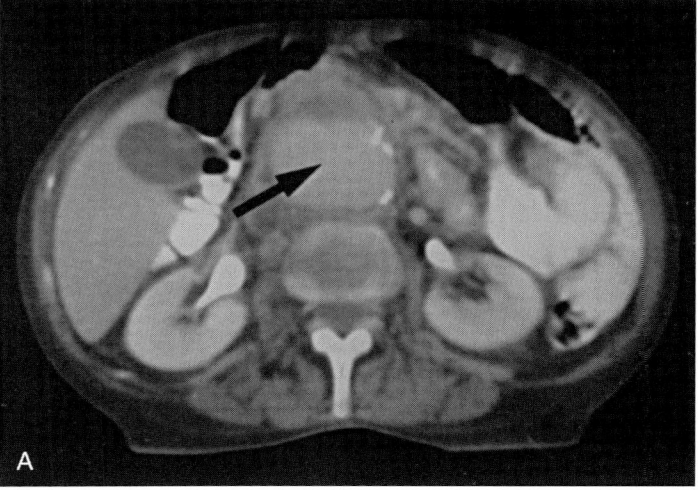
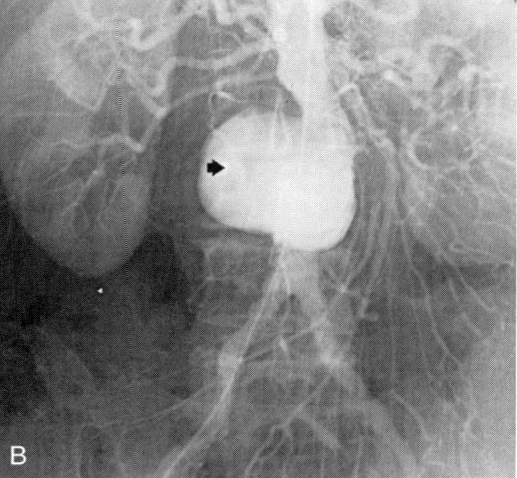

FIGURE 97–2. Diagnostic radiology studies of a patient with *Salmonella* infection of a preexisting small atherosclerotic aneurysm. *A,* Contrast-enhanced computed tomogram demonstrates saccular aneurysm with calcification (*arrow*). *B,* Transfemoral aortogram demonstrates saccular atherosclerotic infrarenal aneurysm (*arrow*).

TABLE 97–5. ETIOLOGY OF INFECTED ANEURYSMS: COLLECTED SERIES FROM A PUBLISHED REVIEW OF ENGLISH LITERATURE

ETIOLOGY	PRIOR TO 1965	AFTER 1965	TOTAL
Arterial trauma	4 (10%)	71 (51%)	75 (42%)
Endocarditis	15 (37%)	14 (10%)	29 (16%)
Local infection	3 (7%)	6 (4%)	9 (5%)
Bacteremia	—	9 (6%)	9 (5%)
Retroperitoneal abscess	2 (5%)	2 (1%)	4 (2%)
Gastrointestinal tract	1 (2%)	3 (2%)	4 (2%)
Oropharynx	—	3 (2%)	3 (2%)
Pneumonia	1 (2%)	—	1 (<1%)
Carcinoma	—	1 (1%)	1 (<1%)
Unknown	15 (36%)	30 (22%)	45 (25%)
TOTAL	41	139	180

From Brown SL, Busutill RW, Baker JD, et al: Bacteriologic and surgical determinants of survival in patients with mycotic aneurysms. J Vasc Surg 1:541, 1984.

of gram-positive organisms (59%) over gram-negative organisms (35%).[61] The most prevalent organism was *Staphylococcus* (41%). Though less common, gram-negative infections were more virulent than gram-positive infections from the standpoints of aneurysm rupture (84% versus 10%) and patient mortality (84% versus 50%).

In another study,[39] colonized aneurysms yielded 81% gram-positive and 19% gram-negative organisms. The most prevalent organism was *S. epidermidis*, accounting for 53% of positive cultures. Coliform sepsis in a preexisting AAA has been associated with an appendiceal abscess.[90]

As emerging technologies based on percutaneous or minimally invasive endovascular repairs gain popularity,[100] infection in a previously existing aneurysm and microbial arteritis may be associated with post-implantation infection, particularly when synthetic prostheses are employed. Unintentionally, grafts may be placed in a septic field that otherwise would have been subject to débridement in the course of a conventional open procedure.

Post-traumatic Infected False Aneurysms

Prevalence and Location

Post-traumatic infected false aneurysms have become the most prevalent type of infected aneurysm in recent decades (Table 97–5). The primary factor in this shifting emphasis in pathogenesis is drug addiction. In the 25 years following Huebl and Read's initial report of two infected femoral artery false aneurysms in narcotic addicts,[60] an additional 195 such cases have been reported.[3, 42, 45, 48, 60, 64, 97, 105, 109, 164]

The femoral artery, used by narcotic addicts for repeated groin injections, is the most common site in which these lesions occur (Fig. 97–3). Other locations, such as the external iliac and carotid arteries, have also been reported (Fig. 97–4).[64, 75, 87]

Another factor contributing to the increasing incidence of these lesions is the proliferation of various invasive testing and monitoring procedures. In susceptible individuals, percutaneous arterial puncture may result in an iatrogenic post-traumatic infected false aneurysm.[7, 134]

Malanoski and coworkers reported that 55 of 102 patients (54%) with blood cultures positive for *S. aureus* at

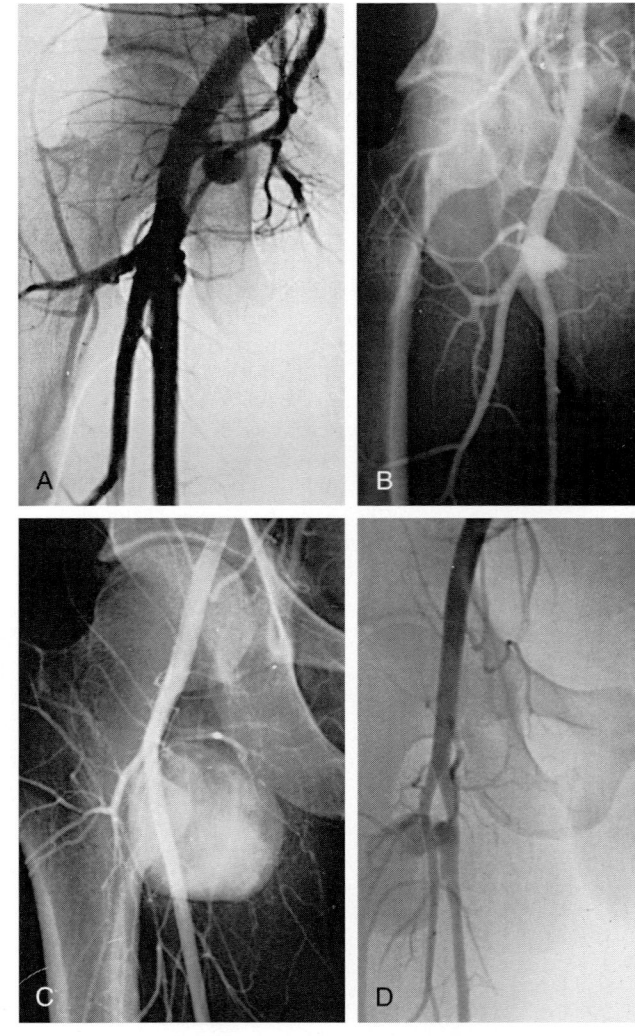

FIGURE 97–3. Arteriograms demonstrate the appearance of an infected femoral artery false aneurysm in each of four locations. *A,* Common femoral artery. *B,* Common femoral bifurcation. *C,* Deep femoral artery. *D,* Superficial femoral artery. (*A, B,* and *D,* From Reddy DJ, Smith RF, Elliott JP Jr, et al: Infected femoral artery false aneurysms in drug addicts: Evolution of selective vascular reconstruction. J Vasc Surg 3:718, 1986.)

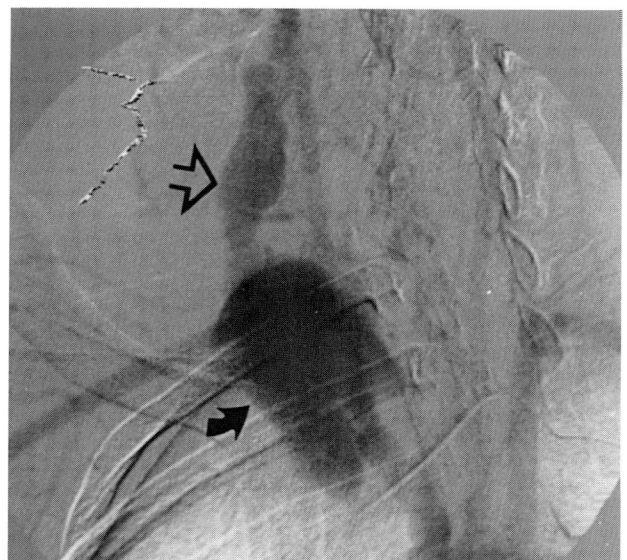

FIGURE 97-4. Digital subtraction angiogram of a patient with polymicrobial post-traumatic false aneurysm of the innominate artery caused by repeated cervical injections of narcotics *(closed arrow)*. There was an associated arteriovenous fistula to the internal jugular vein *(open arrow)* and a right recurrent laryngeal nerve paralysis.

the New England Deaconess Hospital over 2 years had bacteremia attributable to an intravascular catheter.[79] Five of these patients experienced the *Staphylococcus* sepsis after percutaneous transluminal coronary angioplasty (PTCA). Additionally, two of the five patients also manifested a post-traumatic infected false aneurysm of the accessed femoral artery.

Samore and colleagues, reporting on catheter-related bacteremia in 3473 PTCA patients from the Beth Israel Deaconess Medical Center, noted a low frequency (0.24%) of PTCA-related bacteremia. They reported significant morbidity, however, including post-traumatic infected false aneurysms of the punctured femoral artery.[124] Independent risk factors for development of septic complications of PTCA were noted as follows:

- Duration of the procedure
- Number of catheterizations at the same site
- Difficult vascular access
- Arterial sheath in place more than 1 day
- Congestive heart failure

Bacteriology

Since 1965, when the most prevalent form of infected aneurysm has been post-traumatic infected false aneurysm, the predominant infecting organism has been *S. aureus* (30%).[14, 50] In one report of infected femoral artery false aneurysms in drug addicts, 35 of 54 patients (65%) had pure cultures of *S. aureus* from the aneurysm. Seventeen of these 35 staphylococcal cultures (48%) were found to be methicillin resistant. An additional eight patients (33%) had mixed polymicrobial cultures, including *S. aureus, E. coli, S. faecalis, Pseudomonas aeruginosa,* and various *Enterobacter* organisms.[109] Johnson and coworkers, reporting on

drug-related infected false aneurysms in a variety of anatomic locations, isolated *S. aureus* from a high percentage of blood (71%) and wound (76%) cultures.[64]

CLINICAL PRESENTATION

The clinical presentation of infected aneurysms depends on the etiologic mechanism and the anatomic site involved. Clinical characteristics of various aneurysm types are summarized in Table 97-1.

Although infected aneurysms occur in all age groups, including neonates [29, 146] and children,[85] when there is no antecedent history of arterial injury, the typical patient is older with atherosclerosis.[10, 135] The principal signs and symptoms of an aneurysm and sepsis may be subtle (Table 97-6). Infection in an AAA may be difficult to detect. Patients with infected aortic aneurysms usually present with fever of unknown origin. Because of the insidious signs and symptoms of infected aneurysms, a high index of suspicion is needed in the following situations[16, 20, 61, 152]:

- A positive blood specimen
- Erosion of lumbar vertebrae
- Female sex
- Presence of uncalcified aneurysms
- First presentation of an aneurysm after bacterial sepsis

As many as 40% of infected AAAs may not be palpable and may go unrecognized until rupture.[91, 149, 163, 166] However, infected aneurysms of the femoral or carotid arteries or other superficial peripheral locations are readily appreciated, and up to 90% are palpable.[91] Infected femoral false aneurysms, for example, present with either a tender groin mass, indicating contained rupture; with some other manifestation of sepsis; or with bleeding in almost every patient.[97, 105, 109]

Fungal arterial infections are rare but characteristically occur in patients with chronic immune suppression[71] or diabetes mellitus[83] or after treatment for a disseminated fungal disease.[86] The clinical presentation of these rare infections may be limited to fever or malaise or may be more apparent, with gangrene in an extremity following distal embolization.

Even though infected aneurysms can occur in virtually

TABLE 97-6. INFECTED ANEURYSMS: CLINICAL PRESENTATION

CLINICAL MARKER	NO. (%) OF PATIENTS
Abdominal pain	12 (92)
Fever	10 (77)
Leukocytosis*	9 (69)
Positive blood cultures	9 (69)
Palpable abdominal mass	6 (46)
Rupture	4 (31)

From Reddy DJ, Shepard AD, Evans JR, et al: Management of infected aortoiliac aneurysms. Arch Surg 126:873–879, 1991. Copyright 1991, American Medical Association.
*Leukocyte count >10.0 × 10⁹/L.

any artery and may present with a variety of clinical signs and symptoms, they are similar in that they all eventually lead to sepsis or hemorrhage. Consequently, whenever the surgeon suspects this diagnosis, it must be assumed that the patient's life or limb is in jeopardy and confirmation of the diagnosis and urgent surgical therapy are required.

DIAGNOSIS

Laboratory Studies

In most patients, leukocytosis is a sensitive but nonspecific indicator of an infected aneurysm.[12, 61, 109, 112, 145] The sensitivity of this finding, however, may be limited by intercurrent antimicrobial therapy that has suppressed but not cured the infection.[86] A lack of specificity is also underscored by reports of sealed ruptures of bland, uninfected, atherosclerotic aneurysms that may simulate sepsis and exhibit leukocytosis.[142] Likewise, an elevated erythrocyte sedimentation rate (ESR) is often present but nonspecific. These limitations underscore the need for more specific and sensitive tests to confirm the presence of an infected aneurysm (see Table 97–6).

Positive blood specimens in a patient with an aneurysm are considered specific for an infected aneurysm until proven otherwise, although positive cultures lack sensitivity. Anderson and colleagues found positive cultures in only 50% of such patients.[3] It follows that negative blood cultures alone are not sufficiently sensitive to rule out the diagnosis of an infected aneurysm.

When the diagnosis of an infected aneurysm is first entertained during operation, samples of the aneurysm wall and contents should be obtained for culture with a search for aerobic and anaerobic bacteria and fungi. Additional information may be gained by Gram's stains. However, these studies should not be considered sufficient to ensure that the aneurysm is not infected because neither negative blood cultures nor intraoperative Gram's stains are sufficiently sensitive to exclude the diagnosis of infected aneurysm.[14] Moreover, aneurysm wall and contents culture results are not available during the operation and can be used only to direct postoperative antimicrobial therapy; even final culture results may be misleading in patients treated with antibiotics. Some authors have advocated wider use of aneurysm content and wall cultures in routine operations for aortic aneurysm.[39, 61] In our experience with infected aortoiliac aneurysms, 69% of patients had positive preoperative blood cultures and 92% had positive aneurysm wall cultures. Operative Gram's stains were positive in 50% of those with ruptured infected aneurysms but in only 11% of those with unruptured but infected aneurysms.[112]

Radiologic Studies

Aortic aneurysms associated with vertebral body erosion or those devoid of calcification should raise the suspicion of an infected aneurysm. Plain films are not sufficiently sensitive to confirm the diagnosis, and additional studies are needed. Of value are computed tomography (CT) and either conventional or digital subtraction angiography (DSA). Although ultrasonography of the abdominal aorta provides general information about aneurysm size and location, it is less reliable for detecting the presence or extent of arterial infection. Ultrasonography has proven utility in the diagnosis of femoral artery false aneurysm, but the ability of duplex scanning to detect infection is uncertain and the authors do not employ it for this purpose.[109]

In contrast, the utility of intravenous DSA in evaluating the femoral artery for infected aneurysm has been established.[131] DSA is particularly valuable for screening in drug addicts and for similar lesions in the great vessels and the arteries of both the upper and lower extremities. DSA is of comparable diagnostic accuracy and may be less expensive and more easily accomplished than cut-film arteriography.[131]

Arteriography, either digital subtraction or conventional, is indispensable in the evaluation of patients with a suspected infected aneurysm. The arteriographic criteria for infection in an aneurysm are (Figs. 97–1 to 97–5):

- Saccular aneurysm in an otherwise normal-appearing vessel
- Multilobulated aneurysm
- Eccentric aneurysm with a relatively narrow neck

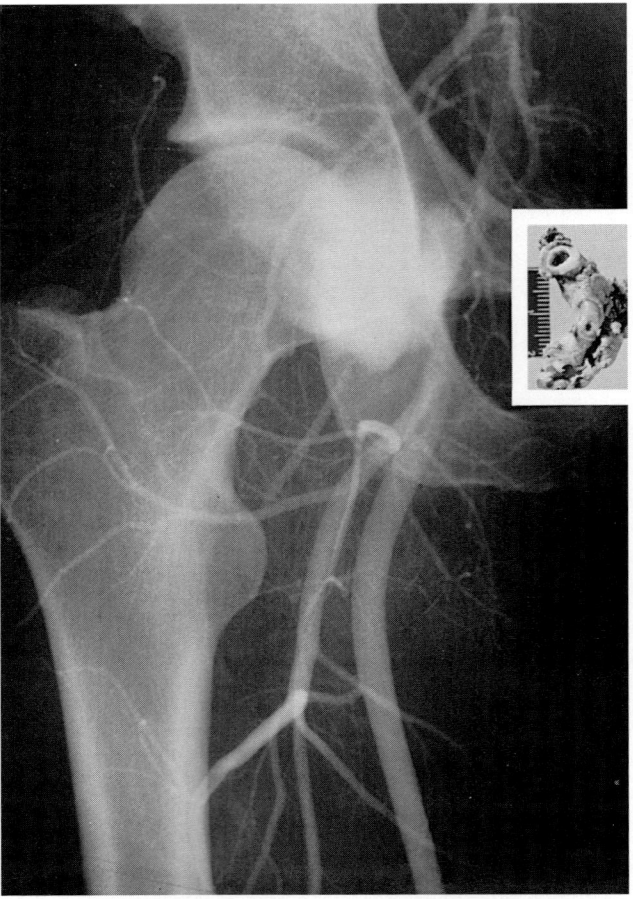

FIGURE 97–5. Femoral arteriogram of patient with a post-traumatic infected false aneurysm of the common femoral artery demonstrates a lobulated aneurysm. *Inset,* Resected femoral artery specimen showing the injured and infected artery.

However, an infected aneurysm may not exhibit any arteriographic characteristics indicative of infection.[157]

Contrast-enhanced CT is of value in determining etiology and assessing the presence or absence of aneurysm rupture (see Figs. 97–1 and 97–2) but often fails to give specific information about the presence or absence of infection.[49, 51, 73, 119] Case reports documenting the potential utility of CT performed early in the clinical course of infected aortic aneurysms suggest subtle diagnostic features and have also documented the rapidly deteriorating clinical course often experienced by such patients.[17, 51]

Magnetic resonance imaging (MRI) may prove helpful for screening certain anatomic sites or when radiography or contrast media are contraindicated. The use of MRI is being reported with increasing frequency.[89, 156]

Although some investigators have found indium 111–labeled white blood cell scanning useful in diagnosing prosthetic graft infection, this modality has not always been accurate in confirming the diagnosis of an infected aneurysm.[15, 22]

MANAGEMENT

Preoperative Care

When an infected aneurysm is suspected but efforts to identify the specific organisms are unsuccessful, broad-spectrum antibiotic therapy should be initiated. Chloramphenicol, ampicillin, a quinolone, or a third-generation cephalosporin should be included to combat *Salmonella* species. Drug therapy is begun before operation and continued postoperatively and, in certain circumstances, for life.[20, 28]

Treatment of narcotic addicts should include active and passive tetanus prophylaxis. Even though organism-specific antibiotic therapy is an essential element of successful surgical management of an infected aneurysm, patient survival depends on prompt diagnosis and operation.[61, 112] Ruptures of infected aneurysms have been reported in patients undergoing antibiotic therapy while awaiting operation or in those who have completed antibiotic therapy and are thought, erroneously, to have bland aneurysms, sterilized by antibiotics.[18, 25, 135] Undue delay in operative intervention must be avoided. Reported spontaneous cures of infected aneurysms are exceptions.[40] In cases of a ruptured or symptomatic aneurysm, operation should be undertaken urgently.

Operation

General Principles

Six general principles apply in the operative management of infected aneurysms:

1. Control of hemorrhage.
2. Confirmation of the diagnosis, including tissue smears for Gram stains and culture specimens for aerobic and anaerobic bacteria and fungi.
3. Operative control of sepsis, including aneurysm resection and ligation of healthy artery followed by wide débridement of all surrounding infected tissue with antibiotic irrigation and placement of drains when needed.
4. Thorough postoperative wound care, including frequent dressing changes and necessary débridement.
5. Continuation of antibiotics for a prolonged period after operation.
6. Arterial reconstruction of vital arteries through uninfected tissue planes with selected use of interposition grafting through the bed of the resected aneurysm and use of autologous tissue for reconstruction.

The first five principles are established, uncontroversial surgical tenets. Controversy exists, however, about the selection of patients for arterial reconstruction and the timing and methods of reconstruction, particularly when the infected aneurysm involves the aorta, the femoral artery, or the carotid artery.[4, 14, 20, 41, 42, 63, 64, 96, 97, 101, 109, 111, 145, 147]

Aorta

The classic approach to management of an infected aneurysm of the abdominal aorta is similar to the treatment of

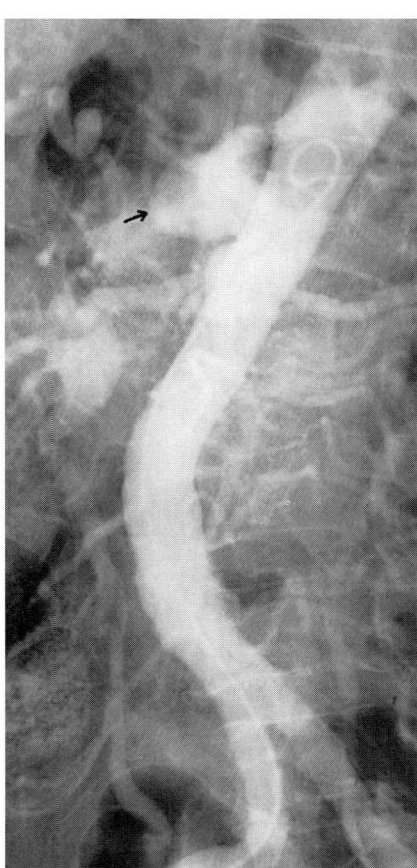

FIGURE 97–6. Aortogram of 72-year-old man with a methicillin-resistant *Staphylococcus aureus*–infected aneurysm of the periceliac aorta (*arrow*) caused by microbial arteritis. The presumed cause of the antecedent bacteremia was a mediastinal infection with the same organism following stenotomy for coronary artery bypass graft months earlier. Repair through the bed of the débrided aorta was required.

an infected aortic prosthesis. The entire aneurysm is resected, the infected tissues are thoroughly débrided, drainage is established, and arterial reconstruction is carried out through uninfected planes by an axillobifemoral bypass.[36, 41, 61, 145] This conservative approach avoids the risks associated with the placement of a graft in the infected retroperitoneum, reported to be associated with an overall 23% reoperation rate, which increases to 63% when the infecting organism is gram-negative.[41] Axillofemoral bypass, however, is a less durable reconstruction than successful interposition aortic grafting.[108, 112, 147] Moreover, some surgeons advocate "in situ" interposition aortic grafts after resection of an infected aortic aneurysm.[14, 20, 63, 96, 147]

The adjunctive use of antibiotic-releasing beads implanted in the perigraft tissue, omental coverage, and rifampin-bonded polyester (Dacron) grafts has been reported.[53, 101, 165] Others have speculated about the use of aortic homografts, but unfavorable previous experience with the late fate of homografts in noninfected sites argues against their use.[6, 143]

Experimental data in a canine model suggest that in situ arterial allografts are less vulnerable to infection than commonly available synthetic prostheses.[69] If this is true, this decreased infectibility may make arterial allografts an appropriate choice when circumstances require reestablishment of aortic continuity in a contaminated field. Eight recent clinical reports from Europe have detailed the use of cryopreserved arterial homografts for in situ replacement of infected aneurysms of various aortic segments.[2, 68, 70, 98, 103, 153–155] It appears that in situ repair through the bed of the resected aneurysm may be justified in favorable lesions with little or no gross sepsis, but it should be avoided when the retroperitoneum is grossly purulent.[104, 130] Even

complex reconstruction of the suprarenal aorta may be accomplished with extra-anatomic techniques.[80, 108]

Some reports have emphasized that recognition of organism virulence and the severity and extent of the aortic infection are more important than strict adherence to any single operative approach or method of arterial reconstruction.[23, 116, 137] Hence, proper patient selection and surgical judgment are among the prime determinants of management success. In infected aneurysms of the aortic arch, thoracic aorta, thoracoabdominal aorta, and suprarenal abdominal aorta, interposition grafting may be the only feasible approach (Fig. 97–6).[4, 20, 26, 58, 102]

Clagett and colleagues reported a prospective study suggesting the feasibility and durability of autogenous aortoiliac or aortofemoral vein grafts to treat prosthetic infections.[24] This method may have application in the treatment of infected aneurysms and awaits further clinical experience.

Femoral Artery

Management options in the treatment of infected femoral artery aneurysms are (1) arterial excision alone and (2) arterial excision followed by arterial reconstruction. The various operative techniques for arterial reconstruction are illustrated in Figure 97–7.

If the cause of the infected aneurysm is other than drug injection, obturator bypass or interposition grafting usually appears to be the preferred treatment.[57] Drug addicts are unsuitable candidates for arterial reconstruction with synthetic arterial prostheses because continued drug use carries a very high risk of graft infection (Table 97–7).[3, 97, 109] In this select group of patients, when reconstruction of the

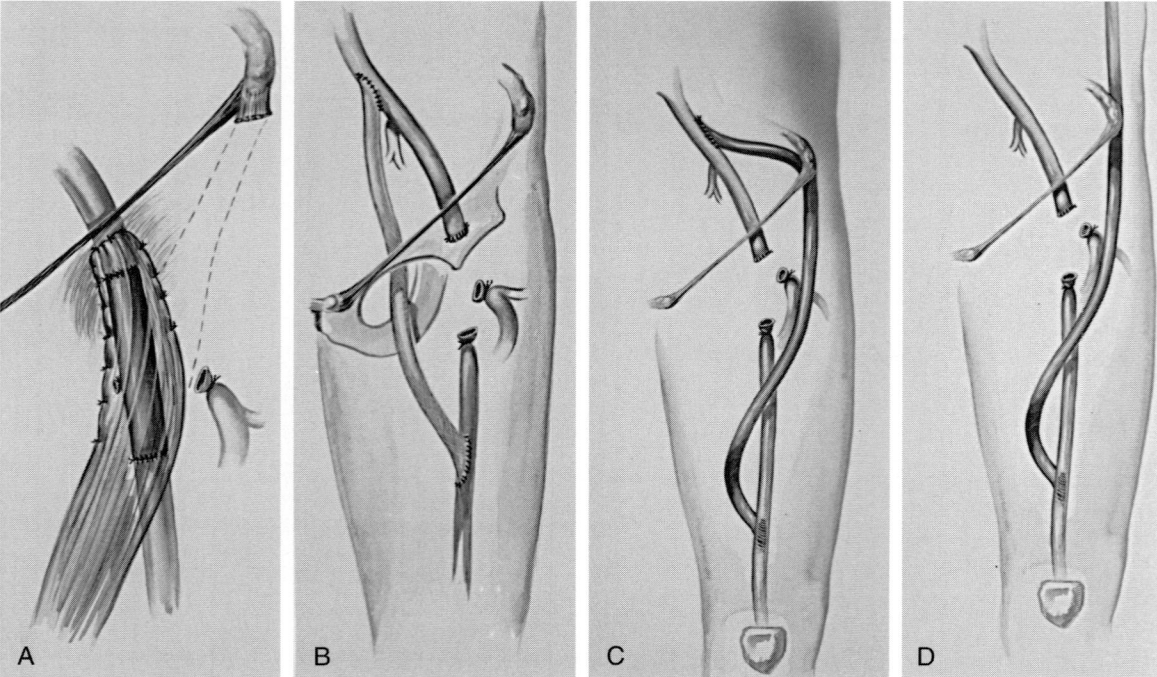

FIGURE 97–7. Methods of femoral artery reconstruction. A, Interposition vein autograft covered by rotated sartorius muscle. B, Obturator bypass. C, Lateral femoral bypass. D, Axillodistal femoral bypass. (A, B, and D, From Reddy DJ, Smith RF, Elliott JP Jr, et al: Infected femoral artery false aneurysms in drug addicts: Evolution of selective vascular reconstruction. J Vasc Surg 3:718, 1986.)

femoral artery is considered desirable, it is necessary to control groin sepsis and to use autogenous grafts. Surprisingly, greater saphenous vein from the mid-thigh usually is available even in patients with a long history of drug abuse (Fig. 97–8).[109]

Although selection criteria and methods of femoral arterial reconstruction in drug addicts are controversial, there is general agreement that most patients do not require reconstruction to avoid amputation.[42, 64, 97, 101, 109] Collateral circulation is usually sufficient to maintain limb viability even after the femoral artery bifurcation has been ligated (Fig. 97–9). In fact, amputation is almost never necessary when femoral artery ligation-excision is limited to a single femoral artery segment—the common, superficial, or deep femoral artery (see Table 97–7).

Patients at risk for amputation are those in whom the femoral artery bifurcation must be excised. Under these circumstances, autogenous vein interposition reconstruction may be considered when local wound conditions are favorable, although experience with this technique is limited.[109] When ligation of the femoral bifurcation is required but reconstruction is not feasible, we empirically instill a concentrated heparin-sodium solution antegrade into the ligated femoral artery in an effort to preserve all possible arterial collaterals. Unless there is a specific indication, however, anticoagulation therapy is not continued in the postoperative period.

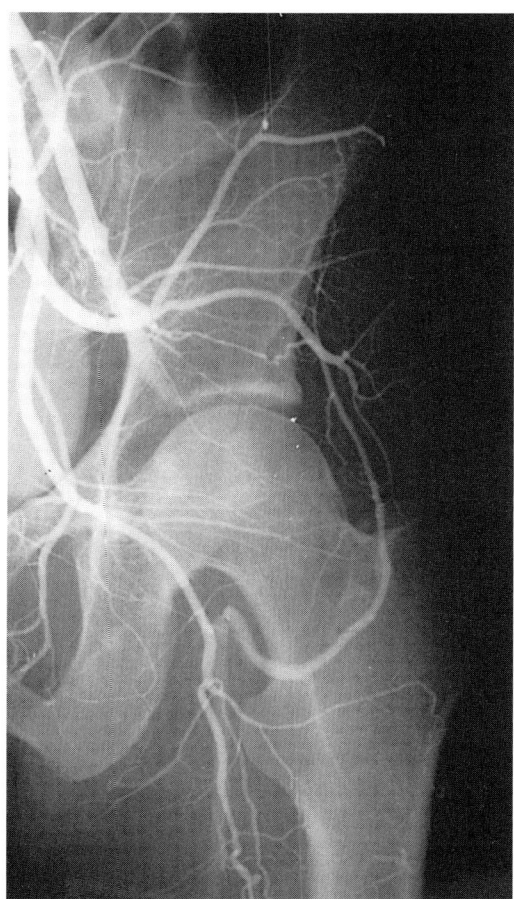

FIGURE 97–9. Arteriogram following ligation of femoral artery bifurcation demonstrates reconstitution of superficial femoral artery beyond the occlusion by numerous collaterals.

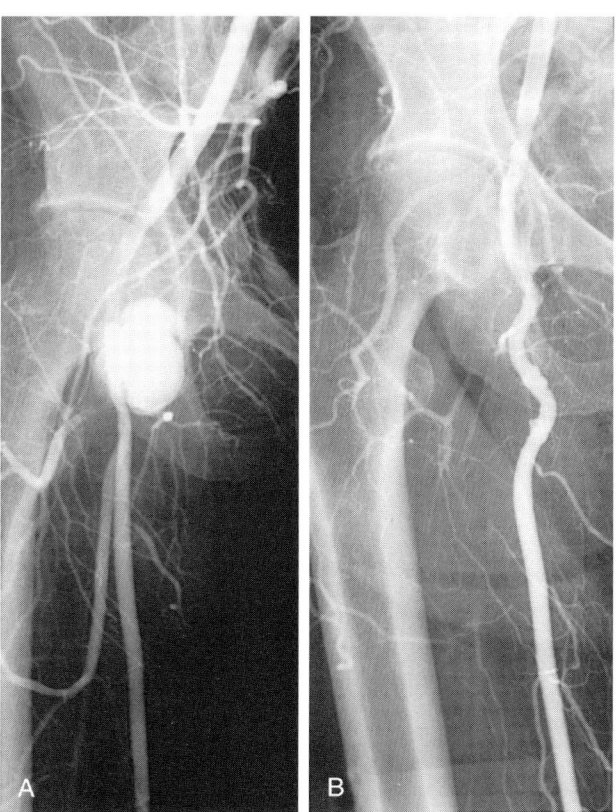

FIGURE 97–8. Angiographic sequence demonstrates preoperative appearance of infected false aneurysm of femoral bifurcation (A) and postoperative appearance of patent interposition vein graft after arterial reconstruction (B). (A and B, From Reddy DJ, Smith RF, Elliott JP Jr, et al: Infected femoral artery false aneurysms in drug addicts: Evolution of selective vascular reconstruction. J Vasc Surg 3:718, 1986.)

TABLE 97–7. TREATMENT METHOD AND RESULTS FOR INFECTED FEMORAL ARTERY FALSE ANEURYSMS RESULTING FROM DRUG ADDICTION

	NO.	VIABLE LIMB	GRAFT SEPSIS	AMPUTATION
Common femoral artery				
Ligation-excision	14	14	—	0
Deep femoral artery				
Ligation-excision	11	11	—	0
Superficial femoral artery				
Ligation-excision	4	4	—	0
Common femoral bifurcation				
Ligation-excision	21	14	—	7 (33%)
Reconstruction with autogenous vein	6	6	1	0
Reconstruction with synthetic prosthesis	3	3	3 (100%)	0
Reconstruction by primary anastomosis	1	1	0	0
TOTAL	60	53	4	7 (12%)

From Reddy DJ, Smith RF, Elliott JP Jr, et al: Infected femoral artery false aneurysms in drug addicts: Evolution of selective vascular reconstruction. J Vasc Surg 3:718, 1986.

The optimal management of these lesions is a matter of debate.[101, 105, 109–111] It is generally agreed that surgical therapy is required, and prolonged use of antibiotics is inappropriate.

Carotid Artery

Although ligation without arterial reconstruction is often safe in the treatment of infected aneurysms of the innominate, common carotid, or upper extremity vessels, there is a major risk of stroke or death after ligation of the cervical internal carotid artery. Although ligation-excision without reconstruction is controversial, many authors favor it, preferring to avoid the potential disastrous consequences of post-reconstruction graft sepsis and hemorrhage.[59, 74] Others favor primary reconstruction of the carotid artery with autogenous vein[87, 125] or progressive clamp occlusion of the internal carotid artery while observing the awake patient for clinical signs of cerebral ischemia.[5]

Data providing a rational basis for selection of patients for carotid artery ligation versus reconstruction have been reported by Ehrenfeld and colleagues.[34] They found carotid ligation to be safe if carotid stump pressure exceeded 70 mmHg systolic pressure. This was a selected group of patients who had received anticoagulation therapy and in whom systemic blood pressures had been maintained at defined levels, but this may not be a representative group. The rarity of these lesions highlights the need for individualized patient management.[66, 84, 159]

In the special circumstance of cerebral mycotic aneurysms, stereoscopic synthesized brain-surface imaging with magnetic resonance angiography (MRA) for anatomic localization has emerged as a useful modality.[31, 65]

Visceral Arteries

Although visceral arterial aneurysms are uncommon, a high percentage are infected.[138] Treatment must be individualized and directed by angiography. When feasible, aneurysm ligation-excision is desirable, but arterial reconstruction with saphenous autografts or other innovations may be required to preserve organ or bowel viability.[56, 150, 159]

Results

Successful surgical management of an infected aneurysm depends on the following factors:

- Type of aneurysm
- Location of the aneurysm
- The microorganism responsible
- Patient's general condition
- Patient's clinical presentation

In general, results following treatment of infected aneurysms have steadily improved because of prompt diagnosis, better surgical techniques, and modern antimicrobial therapy. In 1967, Bennett and Cherry reported that infected aneurysms of the abdominal aorta were invariably fatal.[11] Since then, rates of 74% survival among 96 cases have been reported in 26 series from 1978 to 1992, although management remains challenging.[4, 8, 12, 14, 16, 20, 30, 32, 33, 41, 52, 63, 81–83, 96, 101, 108, 112, 121, 126, 141, 147, 149, 161, 163] Although some

reports have tended to emphasize the improved outlook for patient survival, most authors believe that infectious aneurysms of all types, particularly those that do not respond to therapy, are underreported. To this end, Wilson and coworkers estimated, from a literature review, that mycotic aneurysms in treated patients had a mortality rate of 25%; microbial arteritis with aneurysm, 75%; infected preexisting aneurysms, 75%; and post-traumatic infected false aneurysms, 10% (see Table 97–1).[162]

Lower extremity amputation rates following treatment for infected femoral artery false aneurysms have ranged from 11% to 25%.[3, 42, 64, 97, 101, 109] The above-knee amputation rate following ligation-excision of the femoral artery bifurcation in drug addicts approximates 33%. When groin sepsis is not controlled, revascularization in an attempt to prevent amputation may pose an unnecessary and potentially lethal risk of graft sepsis and should be undertaken with caution. Amputation may be unavoidable among patients with infected femoral false aneurysms.

REFERENCES

1. Akers DL Jr, Fowl RJ, Kempczinski RF: Mycotic aneurysm of the tibioperoneal trunk: Case report and review of the literature. J Vasc Surg 16:71, 1992.
2. Alonso M, Caeiro S, Cachaldora J: Infected abdominal aortic aneurysm: In situ replacement with cryopreserved arterial homograft. J Cardiovasc Surg 38:371, 1997.
3. Anderson CB, Butcher HR Jr, Ballinger WF, et al: Mycotic aneurysms. Arch Surg 109:712, 1974.
4. Atnip RG: Mycotic aneurysms of the suprarenal abdominal aorta: Prolonged survival after in situ aortic and visceral reconstruction. J Vasc Surg 10:635, 1989.
5. Avellone JC, Ahmad MY: Cervical internal carotid aneurysm from syphilis: An alternative to resection. JAMA 241:238, 1979.
6. Bahnini A, Ruoyolo C, Koskas F, Kieffer E: In situ fresh allograft replacement of an infected aortic prosthetic graft: Eighteen months' follow-up. J Vasc Surg 14:98, 1991.
7. Baker WH, Moran JM, Dormer DB: Infected aortic aneurysm following arteriography. J Cardiovasc Surg 20:313, 1979.
8. Bardin JA, Collins GM, Devin JB, et al: Nonaneurysmal suppurative aortitis. Arch Surg 116:954, 1981.
9. Barker WF: Mycotic aneurysms. Ann Surg 139:84, 1954.
10. Bennett DE: Primary mycotic aneurysms of the aorta. Arch Surg 94:758, 1967.
11. Bennett DE, Cherry JK: Bacterial infection of aortic aneurysms: A clinicopathologic study. Am J Surg 113:321, 1967.
12. Bitseff EL, Edwards WA, Mulherin JL Jr, Kaiser AB: Infected abdominal aortic aneurysms. South Med J 80:309, 1987.
13. Blum L, Keefer E: Cryptogenic mycotic aneurysm. Ann Surg 155:398, 1962.
14. Brown SL, Busutill RW, Baker JD, et al: Bacteriologic and surgical determinants of survival in patients with mycotic aneurysms. J Vasc Surg 1:541, 1984.
15. Brunner MC, Mitchell RS, Baldwin JC, et al: Prosthetic graft infection: Limitations of indium white blood cell scanning. J Vasc Surg 3:42, 1986.
16. Byard RW, Leduc JR, Chambers J, Walley VM: The rapid evolution of a large mycotic aneurysm of the abdominal aorta. J Can Assoc Radiol 39:62, 1988.
17. Carreras M, Larena JA, Tabernero G, et al: Evolution of Salmonella aortitis towards the formation of abdominal aneurysm. Eur Radiol 1:54, 1997.
18. Cates JE, Christie RV: Subacute bacterial endocarditis. Q J Med 24:93, 1951.
19. Chan P, Tsai CW, Huang JJ, et al: Salmonellosis and mycotic aneurysm of the aorta: A report of 10 cases. J Infect 30:129, 1995.
20. Chan YF, Crawford ES, Coselli JS, et al: In situ prosthetic graft

replacement for mycotic aneurysms of the aorta. Ann Thorac Surg 47:193, 1989.

21. Chen YF, Lin PY, Yen HW, et al: Double mycotic aneurysm of the ascending aorta. Ann Thorac Surg 63; 529, 1997.

22. Chen P, Lamski, Raval B: Indium-111 leukocyte appearance of *Salmonella* mycotic aneurysm. Clin Nucl Med 19:646, 1994.

23. Chiba Y, Muraoka R, Ihaya A, et al: Surgical treatment of infected thoracic and abdominal aortic aneurysms. Cardiovasc Surg 4:476, 1996.

24. Clagett GP, Valentine RJ, Hagino RT: Autogenous aortoiliac/femoral reconstruction from superficial femoral-popliteal veins: Feasibility and durability. J Vasc Surg 25:255, 1997.

25. Cooke PA, Ehrenfeld WK: Successful management of mycotic aortic aneurysm: Report of a case. Surgery 75:132, 1974.

26. Cordero JA Jr, Darling RC 3rd, Chang BB, et al: In situ prosthetic graft replacement for mycotic thoracoabdominal aneurysms. Ann Surg 62:35, 1996.

27. Crane AR: Primary multilocular mycotic aneurysm of the aorta. Arch Pathol 24:634, 1937.

28. Crawford ES, Crawford JL (eds): Diseases of the Aorta Including an Atlas of Angiographic Pathology and Surgical Techniques. Baltimore, Williams & Wilkins, 1984.

29. Cribari C, Meadors FA, Crawford ES, et al: Thoracoabdominal aortic aneurysm associated with umbilical artery catheterization: Case report and review of the literature. J Vasc Surg 16:75, 1992.

30. Cull DL, Winter RP, Wheller JR, et al: Mycotic aneurysm of the suprarenal aorta. J Cardiovasc Surg 33:181, 1992.

31. D'Angelo V, Fiumara E, Gorgoglione L, et al: Surgical treatment of a cerebral mycotic aneurysm using the stereo-angiographic localizer. Surg Neurol 44:263, 1995.

32. Davies OG, Thorburn JD, Powell P: Cryptic mycotic abdominal aortic aneurysms. Am J Surg 136:96, 1978.

33. Dupont JR, Bonavita JA, DiGiovanni RJ, et al: Acquired immunodeficiency syndrome and mycotic abdominal aortic aneurysms: A new challenge? Report of a case. J Vasc Surg 10:254, 1989.

34. Ehrenfeld WR, Stoney RJ, Wylie EJ: Relation of carotid stump pressure to safety of carotid arterial ligation. Surgery 93:299, 1983.

35. Elliott JP, Hageman JH, Szilagyi DE, et al: Arterial embolization: Problems of source, multiplicity, recurrence, and delayed treatment. Surgery 88:833, 1980.

36. Elliott JP, Smith RF, Szilagyi DE: Aortoenteric and paraprosthetic-enteric fistulas. Arch Surg 114:1041, 1974.

37. Elliott JP, Smith RF: Peripheral embolization. *In* Magilligan DJ, Quinn EL (eds): Endocarditis: Medical and Surgical Management. New York, Marcel Dekker, 1986, p 164.

38. Eppinger H: Pathogenesis (histogenesis und aetiologie) der anerysmen eimschliesslich des aneurysma equi verminosum. Arch Klin Chir 35:404, 1887.

39. Ernst CB, Campbell C Jr, Daugherty ME, et al: Incidence and significance of intra-operative bacterial cultures during abdominal aortic aneurysmectomy. Ann Surg 185:626, 1977.

40. Eshaghy B, Scanlon RJ, Amirparviz F, et al: Mycotic aneurysm of brachial artery: A complication of retrograde catheterization. JAMA 228:1871, 1974.

41. Ewart JM, Burke ML, Bunt TJ: Spontaneous abdominal aortic infections: Essentials of diagnosis and management. Am Surg 49:37, 1983.

42. Feldman AJ, Berguer R: Management of an infected aneurysm of the groin secondary to drug abuse. Surg Gynecol Obstet 157:519, 1983.

43. Flamand F, Harris KA, DeRose G, et al: Arteritis due to *Salmonella* with aneurysm formation: Two cases. Can J Surg 35:248, 1992.

44. Fourneau I, Nevelsteen, Lacroix H, et al: Microbiological monitoring of aortic aneurysm sac contents during abdominal aneurysmectomy: Results in 176 patients and review of the literature. Acta Chir Belg 96:119, 1996.

45. Fromm SH, Lucas CE: Obturator bypass for mycotic aneurysm of the drug addict. Arch Surg 100:82, 1970.

46. Garb M: Appendicitis: An unusual cause of infected abdominal aortic aneurysm. Australas Radiol 38: 68, 1994.

47. Gauto AR, Cone LA, Woodard DR, et al: Arterial infections due to *Listeria monocytogenes*: Report of four cases and review of world literature. Clin Infect Dis 14:23, 1992.

48. Geelhoed GW, Joseph WL: Surgical sequelae of drug abuse. Surg Gynecol Obstet 139:749, 1974.

49. Gomes MN, Schellinger D, Hufnagel CA: Abdominal aortic aneurysms: Diagnostic review and new techniques. Ann Thorac Surg 27:479, 1979.

50. Gomes MN, Choyke PL, Wallace RB: Infected aortic aneurysms: A changing entity. Ann Surg 215:435, 1992.

51. Gomes MH, Choyke PL: Infected aortic aneurysms: CT diagnosis. J Cardiovasc Surg 33:684, 1992.

52. Gouny P, Valverde A, Vincent D: Human immunodeficiency virus and infected aneurysm of the abdominal aorta: Report of three cases. Ann Vasc Surg 6:239, 1992.

53. Gupta AK, Bandyk DF, Johnson BL: In situ repair of mycotic abdominal aortic aneurysms with rifampin-bonded gelatin impregnated Dacron grafts: A preliminary case report. J Vasc Surg 24:472, 1996.

54. Hankins JR, Yeager GH: Primary mycotic aneurysm. Surgery 40:747, 1956.

55. Har Shai Y, Schein M, Molek AD, et al: Ruptured mycotic aneurysm of the subclavian artery after irradiation: A case report. Eur J Surg 159:59, 1993.

56. Hashemi HA, Comerota AJ, Dempsey DT: Foregut revascularization via retrograde splenic artery perfusion after resection of a juxtaceliac mycotic aneurysm: Complicated by pancreatic infarction because of cholesterol emboli. J Vasc Surg 21:530, 1995.

57. Hegenscheid M, Alveizacos P, Hepp W: Autogene Rekonstruktion bei mykotischem inquinalem Aneurysma—Langzeitsergebnis. Vasa 23:159, 1994.

58. Hollier LH, Money SR, Creely B, et al: Direct repair of mycotic thoracoabdominal aneurysms. J Vasc Surg 18:477, 1993.

59. Howell HS, Barburao T, Graziano J: Mycotic cervical carotid aneurysm. Surgery 81:357, 1977.

60. Huebl HC, Read RC: Aneurysmal abscess. Minn Med 49:11, 1966.

61. Jarrett F, Darling RC, Mundth ED, et al: Experience with infected aneurysms of the abdominal aorta. Arch Surg 10:1281, 1975.

62. Johansen K, Devin J: Spontaneous healing of mycotic aortic aneurysm. J Cardiovasc Surg 21:625, 1980.

63. Johansen K, Devin J: Mycotic aortic aneurysms: A reappraisal. Arch Surg 118:583, 1983.

64. Johnson JR, Ledgerwood AM, Lucas CE: Mycotic aneurysm: New concepts in surgery. Arch Surg 118:577, 1983.

65. Kato Y, Yamaguchi S, Sano H, et al: Stereoscopic synthesized brain surface imaging with MR angiography for localization of a peripheral mycotic aneurysm: Case report. Minim Invasive Neurosurg 39:113, 1996.

66. Khalil I, Nawfal G: Mycotic aneurysms of the carotid artery: Ligation vs. reconstruction—case report and review of the literature. Eur J Vasc Surg 7:588, 1993.

67. Koch R: Ueber aneurysma der arteria mesenterica superior [About an aneurysm of the superior mesenteric artery]. *In* Erlangen JJ (ed): Inaug Dural-Abhandlung. Barfus'schen Universitaets-Buchdruckerei, 1851.

68. Koskas F, Plissonnier D, Bahnini A, et al: In situ arterial allografting graft infection: A 6-year experience. Cardiovasc Surg 4:495, 1996.

69. Koskas F, Goeau-Brissoniere O, Nicolas MH, et al: Arteries from human beings are less infectible by *Staphylococcus aureus* than polytetrafluoroethylene in an aortic dog model. J Vasc Surg 23:472, 1996.

70. Knosalla C, Weng Y, Yanakh AC, et al: Using aortic allograft material to treat mycotic aneurysms of the thoracic aorta. Ann Thorac Surg 61:1053, 1996.

71. Kyriakides GK, Simmons RL, Najarian JS: Mycotic aneurysms in transplant patients. Arch Surg 111:472, 1976.

72. Lamothe M, Simmons B, Gelfand M, et al: *Listeria monocytogenes* causing endovascular infection. South Med J 85:193, 1992.

73. Lee MH, Chan P, Chiou HJ, et al: Diagnostic imaging of *Salmonella*-related mycotic aneurysm of aorta by CT. Clin Imaging 20:26, 1996.

74. Ledgerwood AM, Lucas CE: Mycotic aneurysm of the carotid artery. Arch Surg 109:496, 1974.

75. Lewis D, Schrager J: Embolomycotic aneurysms. JAMA 63:1808, 1909.

76. Lou CY, Yang YJ: Surgical experience with *Salmonella*-infected aneurysms of the abdominal aorta. J Formos Med Assoc 96:346, 1997.

77. Magilligan DJ: Neurologic complications. *In* Magilligan DJ Jr, Quinn EL (eds): Endocarditis: Medical and Surgical Management. New York, Marcel Dekker, 1986, p 187.

78. Magilligan DJ, Quinn EL: Active infective endocarditis. *In* Magilligan DJ Jr, Quinn EL (eds): Endocarditis: Medical and Surgical Management. New York, Marcel Dekker, 1986, p 207.

79. Malanoski GJ, Samore MH, Pefanis A, et al: *Staphylococcus aureus* catheter-associated bacteremia: Minimal effective therapy and unusual infectious complications associated with arterial sheath catheters. Arch Intern Med 155:1161, 1995.

80. Marty Ane C, Alric P, Prudhoomme M, et al: Bilateral splenorenal bypass and axillofemoral graft for management of juxtarenal mycotic aneurysm. Cadiovasc Surg 4:331, 1996.

81. McIntyre KE, Malone JM, Richards E, et al: Mycotic aortic pseudoaneurysm with aortoenteric fistula caused by *Arizona hinshawii*. Surgery 91:173, 1982.

82. McNamara MF, Roberts AB, Bakshi KR: Gram-negative bacterial infection of aortic aneurysms. J Cardiovasc Surg 28:453, 1987.

83. Mendelowitz DS, Ramstedt R, Yao JST, et al: Abdominal aortic salmonellosis. Surgery 85:514, 1979.

84. Michielsen D, Van Hee R, Discart H: Mycotic aneurysm of the carotid artery: A case report and review of the literature. Acta Chir Belg 97:44, 1997.

85. Millar AJ, Gilbert RD, Brown RA, et al: Abdominal aortic aneurysms in children. J Pediatr Surg 31:1624, 1996.

86. Miller BM, Waterhouse G, Alford RH, et al: *Histoplasma* infection of abdominal aortic aneurysms. Ann Surg 197:57, 1983.

87. Monson RL, Alexander RH: Vein reconstruction of a mycotic internal carotid aneurysm. Ann Surg 191:47, 1980.

88. Montoya FJ, Weinstein-Moreno LF, Johnson CC: Mycotic thoracic aneurysm due to *Clostridium septicum* and occult adenocarcinoma of the cecum. Clin Infect Dis 24:785, 1997.

89. Moriarity JA, Edelman RR, Tumeh SS: CT and MRI mycotic aneurysms of the abdominal aorta. J Comput Assist Tomogr 16:941, 1992.

90. Mostovych M, Johnson L, Cambria RP: Aortic sepsis from an appendiceal abscess. Cardiovasc Surg 2:67, 1994.

91. Mundth ED, Darling RC, Alvarado RH, et al: Surgical management of mycotic aneurysms and the complications of infection in vascular reconstructive surgery. Am J Surg 117:460, 1969.

92. Murphy DP, Glazier DB, Krause TJ: Mycotic aneurysm of the thoracic aorta caused by *Clostridium septicum*. Ann Thorac Surg 62:1835, 1996.

93. Nabseth DC, Deterling RA: Surgical management of mycotic aneurysms. Surgery 50:347, 1961.

94. Oskoui R, Davis WA, Gomes MN: *Salmonella* aortitis: A report of a successfully treated case with a comprehensive review of the literature. Arch Intern Med 153:517, 1993.

95. Osler W: The Gulstonian lectures on malignant endocarditis. Br Med J 1:467, 1885.

96. Oz MC, Brener BJ, Buda JA, et al: A ten-year experience with bacterial aortitis. J Vasc Surg 10:439, 1989.

97. Padberg F, Hobson R II, Lee B, et al: Femoral pseudoaneurysm from drugs of abuse: Ligation or reconstruction? J Vasc Surg 15:642, 1992.

98. Pagano D, Guest P, Bonser RS: Homograft replacement of thoracoabdominal segment of the aorta for leaking mycotic aneurysm. Eur J Cardiothorac Surg 10:383, 1996.

99. Paré A: Of aneurismas. *In* The Apologie and Treatise Containing the Voyages Made into Divers Places with Many of His Writings upon Surgery. Birmingham, Ala, The Classics of Surgery Library, 1984.

100. Parodi JC: Endovascular repair of abdominal aortic aneurysms and other arterial lesions. J Vasc Surg 21:549, 1995.

101. Pasic M, Segesser L, Turina M: Implantation of antibiotic-releasing carriers and in situ reconstruction for treatment of mycotic aneurysm. Arch Surg 127:745, 1992.

102. Pasic M, Carrel T, Vogt M, et al: Treatment of mycotic aneurysms of the aorta and its branches: The location determines the operative technique. Eur J Vasc Surg 6:419, 1992.

103. Pasic M, Carrel T, von Segesser L, et al: In situ repair of mycotic aneurysm of the ascending aorta. J Thorac Cardiovasc Surg 105:321, 1993.

104. Pasic M, Carrel T, Tonz M, et al: Mycotic aneurysm of the abdominal aorta: Extra-anatomic versus in situ reconstruction. Cardiovasc Surg 1:48, 1993.

105. Patel KR, Semel L, Clauss RH: Routine revascularization with resection of infected femoral pseudoaneurysms from substance abuse. J Vasc Surg 8:321, 1988.

106. Patel S, Johnson KW: Classification and management of mycotic aneurysm. Surg Gynecol Obstet 144:691, 1977.

107. Perdue GD, Smith RB III: Surgical treatment of mycotic aneurysms. South Med J 60:848, 1967.

108. Reddy DJ, Lee RE, Oh HK: Suprarenal mycotic aortic aneurysm: Surgical management and follow-up. J Vasc Surg 3:917, 1986.

109. Reddy DJ, Smith RF, Elliott JP Jr, et al: Infected femoral artery false aneurysms in drug addicts: Evolution of selective vascular reconstruction. J Vasc Surg 3:718, 1986.

110. Reddy DJ: Treatment of drug-related infected false aneurysms of the femoral artery: Is routine revascularization justified? J Vasc Surg 8:344, 1988.

111. Reddy DJ: Letter to editor. J Vasc Surg 10:358, 1989.

112. Reddy DJ, Shepard AD, Evans JR, et al: Management of infected aortoiliac aneurysms. Arch Surg 126:873, 1991.

113. Reid MR: Studies on abnormal arteriovenous communications, acquired and congenital: I. Report of a series of cases. Arch Surg 10:601, 1925.

114. Reister WH, Serrano A: Infrarenal mycotic pseudoaneurysm. J Thorac Cardiovasc Surg 71:633, 1975.

115. Revell STR: Primary mycotic aneurysms. Ann Intern Med 22:431, 1943.

116. Robinson JA, Johansen K: Aortic sepsis: Is there a role for in situ graft reconstruction? J Vasc Surg 13:677, 1991.

117. Rokitansky CF: Handbuch der Pathologischen Anatomie, 2nd ed. Austria, 1844, p 55.

118. Rose HD, Stuart JL: Mycotic aneurysm of the thoracic aorta due to *Aspergillus fumigatus*. Chest 70:81, 1976.

119. Rozenblit A, Bennett J, Suggs W: Evolution of the infected abdominal aneurysm: CT observation of early aortitis. Abdom Imaging 21:512, 1996.

120. Rubery PT, Smith MD, Cammisa FP, et al: Mycotic aortic aneurysm in patients who have lumbar vertebral osteomyelitis: A report of two cases. J Bone Joint Surg Am 77:1729, 1995.

121. Rutherford EJ, Eakins JW, Maxwell JG, et al: Abdominal aortic aneurysm infected with *Campylobacter fetus* subspecies *fetus*. J Vasc Surg 10:193, 1989.

122. Sailors DM, Barone GW, Gagne PJ, et al: *Candida* arteritis: Are GI endoscopic procedures a source of vascular infections? Am Surg 62:472, 1996.

123. Sailors DM, Eidt JF, Gagne PJ, et al: Primary *Clostridium septicum* aortitis: A rare cause of necrotizing suprarenal aortic infection. A case report a review of the literature. J Vasc Surg 23:714, 1996.

124. Samore MH, Wessolossky MA, Lewis SM, et al: Frequency, risk factors, and outcome for bacteremia after percutaneous transluminal coronary angioplasty. Am J Cardiol 79:873, 1997.

125. Samson DS, Gewertz BL, Beyer CW Jr, et al: Saphenous vein interposition grafts in the microsurgical treatment of cerebral ischemia. Arch Surg 116:1578, 1981.

126. Scher A, Brener B, Goldendranz RJ, et al: Infected aneurysms of the abdominal aorta. Surgery 115:975, 1980.

127. Schrander-van de Meer AM, Guit GL, van Bockel JH: Mycotic aneurysm of the suprarenal abdominal aorta. Neth J Med 44:23, 1994.

128. Schumacker HB: Aneurysm development and degenerative changes in dilated artery proximal to arteriovenous fistula. Surg Gynecol Obstet 130:636, 1970.

129. Senocak F, Cekirge S, Senocak ME, et al: Hepatic artery aneurysm in a 10-year-old boy as a complication of infective endocarditis. J Pediatr Surg 31:1570, 1996.

130. Sessa C, Farah I, Voirin L, et al: Infected aneurysms of the infrarenal abdominal aorta: Diagnostic criteria and therapeutic strategy. Ann Vasc Surg 11:453, 1997.

131. Shetty PC, Krasicky GA, Sharma RP, et al: Mycotic aneurysms in intravenous drug abusers: The utility of intravenous digital subtraction angiography. Radiology 155:319, 1985.

132. Smith FC, Rees E, Elliott TS, et al: A hazard of immunosuppression: *Aspergillus niger* infection of abdominal aortic aneurysm. Eur J Vasc Surg 8:369, 1994.

133. Smith RF, Szilagyi DE, Colville JM: Surgical treatment of mycotic aneurysms. Arch Surg 85:663, 1967.

134. Soderstrom CA, Wasserman DJ, Ransom KJ, et al: Infected false femoral artery aneurysms secondary to monitoring catheters. J Cardiovasc Surg 24:63, 1983.

135. Sommerville RI, Allen EV, Edwards JE: Bland and infected arteriosclerotic abdominal aortic aneurysms: A clinicopathologic study. Medicine 38:207, 1959.

136. Sower ND, Whelan TJ: Suppurative arteritis due to *Salmonella*. Surgery 52:851, 1967.

137. Sriussadaporn S: Infected abdominal aortic aneurysms: Experience with 14 consecutive cases. Int Surg 81:395, 1996.

138. Stanley JC, Thompson NW, Fry WJ: Splanchnic artery aneurysms. Arch Surg 101:689, 1970.

139. Steed DL, Higgins RS, Pasculle A, et al: Culture of intraluminal thrombus during abdominal aortic aneurysm resection: Significant contamination is rare. Cardiovasc Surg 1:494, 1993.

140. Stengel A, Wolferth CC: Mycotic (bacterial) aneurysms of intravascular origin. Arch Intern Med 31:527, 1923.

141. Suddleson EA, Katz SG, Kohl RD: Mycotic suprarenal aortic aneurysm. Ann Vasc Surg 1:426, 1987.

142. Szilagyi DE, Elliott JP, Smith RF: Ruptured abdominal aneurysms simulating sepsis. Arch Surg 91:263, 1965.

143. Szilagyi DE, Rodriquez FT, Smith RF, Elliott JP: Late fate of arterial allografts: Observations 6 to 15 years after implantation. Arch Surg 101:721, 1970.

144. Tatebe S, Kanazawa H, Yamazaki Y, et al: Mycotic aneurysm of the internal iliac artery caused by *Klebsiella pneumoniae*. Vasa 25:184, 1996.

145. Taylor LM Jr, Deitz DM, McConnell DB, Porter JM: Treatment of infected abdominal aneurysms by extra-anatomic bypass, aneurysm excision, and drainage. Am J Surg 155:655, 1988.

146. Thompson TR, Tilleli J, Johnson DE, et al: Umbilical artery catheterization complicated by mycotic aortic aneurysm in neonates. Adv Pediatr 27:275, 1980.

147. Trairatvorakul P, Sriphojanart S, Sathapatayavongs B: Abdominal aortic aneurysms infected with *Salmonella*: Problems of treatment. J Vasc Surg 12:16, 1990.

148. Tufnell J: On the influence of vegetation of the valves of the heart in the production of secondary arterial disease. Dublin Q J Med 15:371, 1885.

149. Van Damme H, Belachew M, Damas P, et al: Mycotic aneurysm of the upper abdominal aorta ruptured into the stomach. Arch Surg 127:478, 1992.

150. Viglione G, Younes GA, Coste P, et al: Mycotic aneurysm of the celiac trunk: Radical resection and reconstruction without prosthetic material. J Cadiovasc Surg 34:73, 1993

151. Virkow R: Ueber die akute entzuendung der arterian. Virchows Arch Pathol 1:272, 1847.

152. Vogelzang RL, Sohaey R: Infected aortic aneurysms: CT appearance. J Comput Assist Tomogr 12:109, 1988.

153. Vogt PR, von Segesser LK, Goffin Y: Cryopreserved arterial homografts for in situ reconstruction of mycotic aneurysms and prosthetic graft infections. Eur J Cardiothorac Surg 9:502, 1995.

154. Vogt PR, von Segesser LK, Goffin Y: Eradication of aortic infections with the use of cryopreserved arterial homografts. Ann Thorac Surg 62:640, 1996.

155. von Segesser LK, Vogt P, Genoni M, et al: The infected aorta. J Card Surg 12:256, 1997.

156. Walsh DW, Ho VB, Haggerty MF: Mycotic aneurysm of the aorta: MRI and MRA features. J Magn Reson Imaging 7:312, 1997.

157. Weintraub RA, Abrams HL: Mycotic aneurysm. Am J Roentgenol 102:354, 1968.

158. Werner K, Tarasoutchi F, Lunardi W, et al: Mycotic aneurysm of the celiac trunk and superior mesenteric artery in a case of infective endocarditis. J Cardiovasc Surg 32:380, 1991.

159. Willemsen P, De Roover D, Kockx M, et al: Mycotic common carotid artery aneurysm in an immunosuppressed pediatric patient: Case report. J Vasc Surg 25:784, 1997.

160. Williams RD, Fisher FW: Aneurysm contents as a source of graft infection. Arch Surg 112:415, 1977.

161. Wilson SE, Gordon E, Van Wagenen PB: *Salmonella* arteritis. Arch Surg 113:1163, 1978.

162. Wilson SE, Van Wagenen P, Passaro E Jr: Arterial infection. Curr Probl Surg 15:5, 1978.

163. Yao JST, McCarthy WJ: Contained rupture of a thoracoabdominal aneurysm. Contemp Surg 33:47, 1988.

164. Yellin AE: Ruptured mycotic aneurysm. Arch Surg 112:981, 1977.

165. Yokoyama H, Maida K, Takahashi S, et al: Purulently infected abdominal aortic aneurysm: In situ reconstruction with transmesocolic omental transposition technique. Cardiovasc Surg 2:78, 1994.

166. Zak FG, Strauss L, Saphra I: Rupture of diseased large arteries in the course of enterobacterial (*Salmonella*) infection. N Engl J Med 258:824, 1958.

SECTION XIII

ARTERIOVENOUS COMMUNICATIONS AND CONGENITAL VASCULAR MALFORMATIONS

THOMAS S. RILES, M.D.

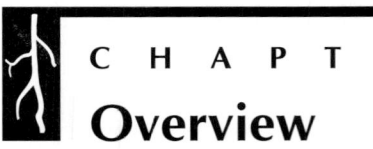

CHAPTER 98
Overview

Thomas S. Riles, M.D.

The management of abnormal arteriovenous communications is one of the greatest challenges to the clinician. Unlike atherosclerotic vascular occlusive or aneurysmal disease, which tends to occur in recognized anatomic patterns, producing well-defined clinical syndromes, the etiology, distribution, and presentation of arteriovenous communications are far more varied. Their relative infrequency accounts for the fact that few physicians have encountered a sufficient number of patients with these disorders to qualify as experts in their management. Relatively few basic experimental studies have addressed the problem of congenital malformations of the arterial and venous systems and their associated communications. A notable exception is the classic work of Woolard,[15] discussed in Chapter 103. The physiology of shunting has been studied in more detail, with laboratory animal models having been used as far back as Vignolo.[13]

Most of the information concerning human arteriovenous communications has come from two and a half centuries of observations by clinicians from all parts of the world who have carefully recorded the details of their patients' symptoms and physical findings. So many have shared in this heritage that it is possible to mention but a few of the more recognizable names: William Hunter,[4] Rudolf Virchow,[14] Sir William Osler,[9] Rudolph Matas,[7] and Mont Reid.[11, 12] For an excellent review and an account of the hundreds of contributors to this field, the reader is referred to the works of Emile Holman[3] and Ernardo Malan.[6]

The subject of arteriovenous communications includes a vast array of conditions, most of which are abnormal but some of which are essential to normal development. Some of these abnormalities are congenital anomalies, traumatic fistulae, erosions between an artery and a vein from infection or tumor, and even surgically created shunts. "Arteriovenous communication," a very general term, refers to any connection between the arterial and the venous systems other than the pulmonary and systemic capillary beds. Communications can be multiple or single. A wide range of physiologic responses may result, depending on the location of the communication, the amount of blood per unit of time that passes from the artery to the vein, and the duration of the communication.

A discussion of arteriovenous communications is often hampered by an inadequate vocabulary and an unsatisfactory classification of the many varied conditions that share this common description. Unfortunately, no single system of classification is suitable for all purposes. Many of the traditional systems, rich with descriptive terms and eponyms, have not been used in this section in order to avoid confusion with current terminology.

For the student and the diagnostician, a classification based on the etiology of the communication is quite helpful. Such a system is presented in Figure 98–1. Among the congenital lesions, those that are *single* communications are distinguished from those that have *multiple* channels. Multiple channels usually result from the persistence of communications that normally exist at the earliest stages of development of arteriovenous systems. Although not truly arteriovenous communications, venous anomalies (e.g., those found in the Klippel-Trenaunay syndrome) are often included in this category because of their appearance and etiologic similarities (see Chapter 103). Although single fistulae may result from early developmental abnormalities, they may also be normal fetal communications that have failed to close at birth (patent ductus and septal defects).

Acquired communications are almost always single. One of the first descriptions of an acquired fistula involved a patient whose lesion resulted from blood-letting, and medical procedures still account for the majority of traumatic fistulae. In addition to trauma, other etiologic factors such as infection, aneurysm (congenital and atherosclerotic), and neoplasm must be considered in any evaluation of acquired fistulae. Occasionally, spontaneous fistulae occur without an obvious underlying cause.

A special category of therapeutic arteriovenous fistulae has evolved with modern surgery; it includes (1) surgical fistulae for the correction of congenital defects of the heart and great vessels, (2) access procedures for dialysis and

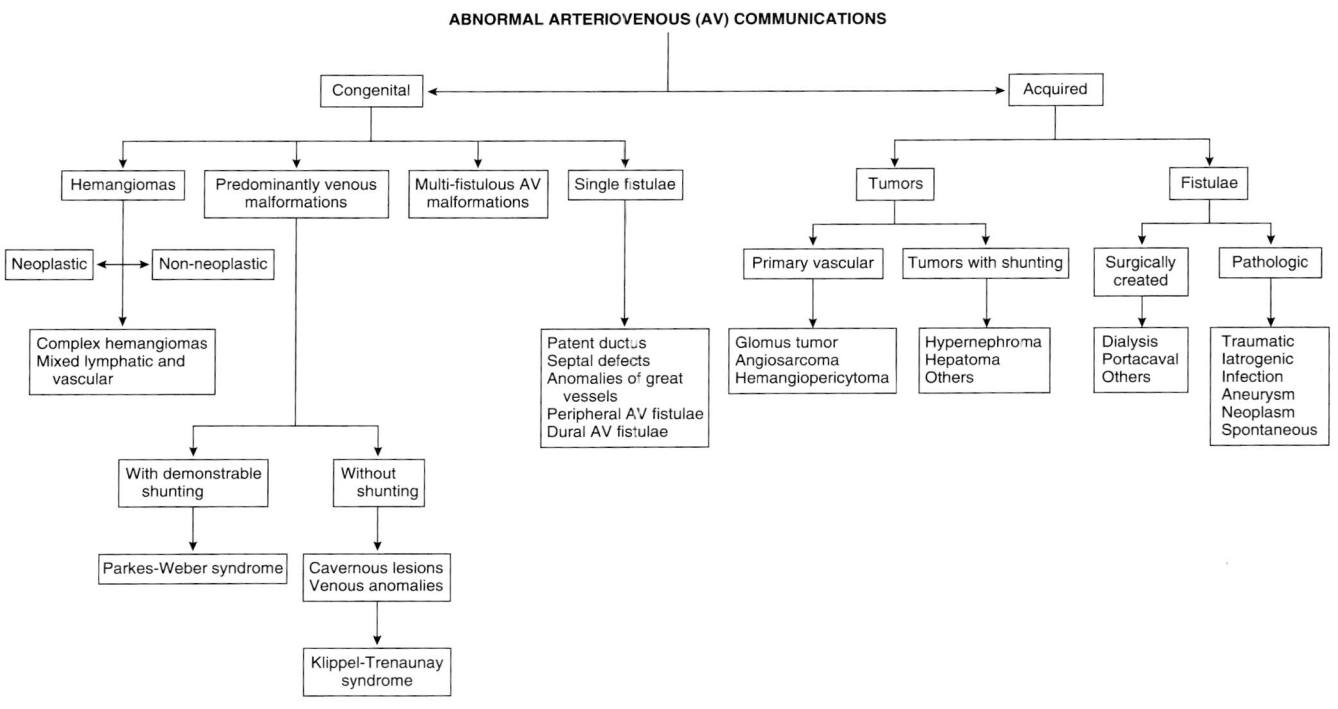

FIGURE 98–1. Classification of abnormal arteriovenous communications.

chemotherapy, and (3) fistulae created as an adjunct to other vascular operations, such as a femorotibial bypass or iliac vein thrombectomy (see Section XIV, Angioaccess).

The location, size, and physiologic effect of an abnormal arteriovenous communication are often more important than the etiology when a course of management is planned. For example, the treatment of a spontaneous carotid–cavernous sinus fistula may be similar to that of a traumatic fistula of the kidney. As an aid to the clinician who must manage these lesions, the chapters covering therapy have been organized into treatment-oriented groups. The arteriovenous fistulae are discussed in two chapters: one on the aorta and its major branches (see Chapter 101), the other on the smaller vessels, in which both surgical and radiologic techniques have a role (see Chapter 102). Congenital vascular malformations are described in Chapter 103.

A major advance since the late 1970s is the development of percutaneous occlusion of arteriovenous communications. With the emergence of interventional radiology, new skills and techniques have evolved. This development has produced a renewed interest in the entire field of arteriovenous communications. Malformations and fistulae previously considered untreatable have been skillfully managed by the use of embolic materials, balloons, glues, and other occlusive devices.[5] More recently, endovascular covered stents have been effective for treating arteriovenous fistulas.[10]

As experience grows, it is becoming clear that the best chance for cure of these complicated lesions is to coordinate the skills of many specialists from various disciplines. In one memorable case—high-output cardiac failure and bleeding from a pelvic arteriovenous malformation—success was achieved only with the sustained efforts of interventional radiologists, gynecologists, urologists, and vascular surgeons. Perhaps the greatest error in the han-

dling of complicated arteriovenous communications is unnecessary ligation of the major feeding vessels as the initial step. This seldom works and hampers further therapy. In some cases, ligated vessels have had to be reconstructed to allow embolization of the lesion. It is essential that radiologists and surgical specialists cooperate in order to avoid costly errors that may be disastrous for the patient or that would prevent successful therapy in the future.

Embolization followed by surgical resection sometimes produces excellent cosmetic results. Otolaryngologists and plastic surgeons have worked closely with interventional radiologists and vascular surgeons to plan therapy for head and neck lesions or extremity malformations with minimal risk. Brain malformations or fistulae previously considered inoperable can now be treated successfully with catheter embolization or balloon occlusion. Larger vessel fistulas have been treated with endovascular covered stents.[1, 2, 8, 10] Clearly, this is the dawn of a new era in the management of arteriovenous communications.

Chapters 99 to 103 explore the many facets of this interesting and challenging aspect of vascular disease. Few problems encountered by a vascular surgeon will be as complex with regard to anatomy, physiology, diagnosis, and therapy. The contributors to this fifth edition of *Vascular Surgery* have provided an excellent review of the basic physiology as well as a guide to the management of abnormal arteriovenous communications.

REFERENCES

1. Criado E, Marston WA, Ligush J, et al: Endovascular repair of peripheral aneurysms, pseudoaneurysms, and arteriovenous fistulas. Ann Vasc Surg 11:256–263, 1997.
2. Dorros G, Joseph G: Closure of a popliteal arteriovenous fistula

using an autologous vein-covered Palmaz stent. J Endovasc Surg 2:177–181, 1995.
3. Holman E: Arteriovenous Aneurysm: Abnormal Communications Between the Arterial and Venous Circulations. New York, Macmillan, 1937.
4. Hunter W: The history of an aneurysm of the aorta, with some remarks on aneurysms in general. Med Observ Inquiry 1:323, 1757.
5. Lasjaunias P, Berenstein A: Surgical Neuroangiography. Vol II. Heidelberg, Springer-Verlag, 1987.
6. Malan E: Vascular Malformations (Angiodysplasias). Milan, Italy, Carlo Erba Foundation, 1974.
7. Matas R: On the systemic or cardiovascular effects of arteriovenous fistulae. Trans South Surg Assoc 36:623, 1923.
8. Ohki T, Veith FJ, Marin ML, et al: Endovascular approaches for arterial trauma. Semin Vasc Surg 10:272–285, 1997.
9. Osler W: Care of arteriovenous aneurysm of the axillary artery and vein of 14 years' duration. Ann Surg 17:37, 1893.
10. Parodi JC: Endovascular repair of abdominal aortic aneurysms and other arterial lesions. J Vasc Surg 21:549–557, 1995.
11. Reid MR: Studies on abnormal arteriovenous communications, acquired and congenital: I. Report of a series of cases. Arch Surg 10:601, 1925.
12. Reid MR, McGuire J: Arteriovenous aneurysms. Ann Surg 108:643, 1938.
13. Vignolo O: Un contributo sperimentale all'anatomia e fisiopatologia dell'aneurisma arterio-venoso. Policlinico [Chir] 9:197, 1902.
14. Virchow R: Pathologis des Tumeurs. Paris, Germer-Balliere, 1876.
15. Woolard HH: The development of the principal arterial system in the forelimb of the pig. Cont Embriol Carnegie Inst 14:139, 1922.

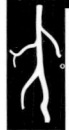

C H A P T E R   9 9

Hemodynamics and Pathophysiology of Arteriovenous Fistulae

David S. Sumner, M.D.

The "short circuit" between the high-pressure arterial system and the low-pressure venous system accounts for most of the symptoms and signs typical of an arteriovenous fistula. An electrical analogy is particularly apropos to the understanding of physiologic aberrations produced by arteriovenous fistulae. Let us suppose, for example, that a short circuit develops in the cord leading to a three-way floor lamp of a student intent on completing his or her evening studies (Fig. 99–1). Three problems may interfere with the completion of the work. First, the light may dim because the electrons have found a more direct route with less resistance back to the socket than that provided by the light bulb. Our enterprising student overcomes this difficulty by turning the switch to the high-intensity setting. However, just after the studies are again under way, all the lights go out. Too much current has burned out the fuse, which must be replaced. After the fuse has been replaced with one having a higher ampere rating, the student again begins work, only to be disturbed by the unmistakable odor of rubber burning. At last, the trouble is discovered: the local disruption of insulation, the overheated cord, and the threatened fire.

In a similar fashion, patients with arteriovenous fistulae may experience three problems that parallel those of the electrical circuit:

1. Ischemia may develop in portions of the limb distal to the fistula.
2. Even when peripheral vasodilatation is able to avert ischemia by compensating for the short circuit produced

by the fistula, the demands on the heart may be excessive, resulting in cardiac failure.

3. The blood vessels leading to and draining the fistula suffer degenerative changes.

Thus, the pathophysiologic changes associated with arteriovenous fistula may be considered under the following three headings: (1) *peripheral*, (2) *central*, and (3) *local* effects.

The magnitude and location of the leak determine the

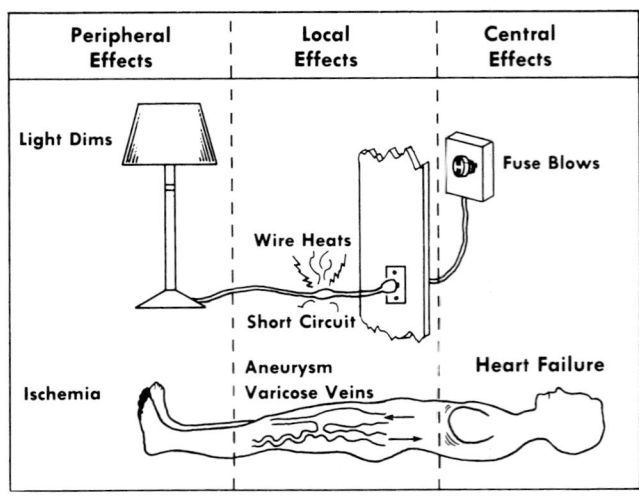

FIGURE 99–1. Like a short circuit in an electrical cord, arteriovenous fistulae produce peripheral, local, and central effects.

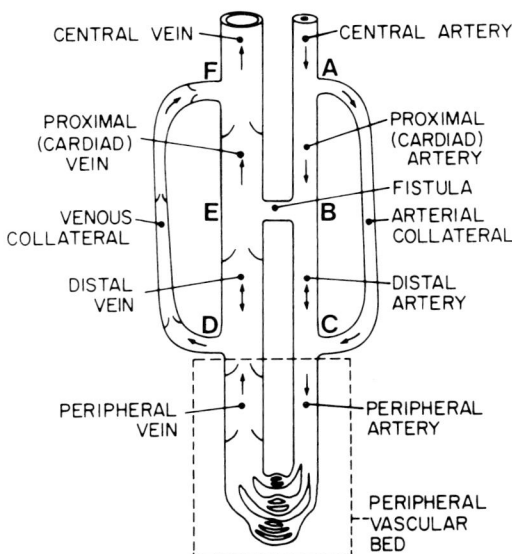

FIGURE 99–2. Diagram of a side-to-side arteriovenous fistula showing its relationship to collateral circulation and the peripheral vascular bed. (From Strandness DE Jr, Sumner DS: Arteriovenous fistulas. *In* Hemodynamics for Surgeons. New York, Grune & Stratton, 1975, pp 621–663.)

severity of the pathophysiologic changes. Whereas fistulae located centrally, near the heart, are more likely to produce cardiac failure, those located distally, in the extremities, are more likely to cause ischemia. Basically, the congenital and acquired forms of arteriovenous fistula are similar in principle from a hemodynamic point of view; however, the anatomy of the congenital fistula is far more complex. Instead of one major arteriovenous communication, there are usually many small, frequently innumerable, connections in parallel array. As a result, the central (cardiac) and the peripheral (ischemic) effects of congenital arteriovenous malformations are usually considerably less severe than those associated with acquired fistulae, and local effects (e.g., venous hypertension, secondary varicosities, and limb hypertrophy) predominate. This is apparent from detailed discussions in Chapter 103. Because of these facts, it is much simpler to use the acquired form as a prototype for illustrating the hemodynamic features of arteriovenous fistulae.

This chapter reviews the local, peripheral, and central effects of arteriovenous fistulae and explains how these effects dictate therapy and the design of fistulae for angioaccess. A brief discussion of naturally occurring arteriovenous communications is also included.

HEMODYNAMICS

Figure 99–2 illustrates the essential features of a typical side-to-side or **H**-type arteriovenous fistula. There is a *proximal* or *cardiad* artery and vein and a *distal* artery and vein. *Collateral arteries* connecting the proximal and distal arteries bypass the fistula. Similarly, *collateral venous channels* connect the distal vein with the proximal vein. A *peripheral vascular bed* that is supplied, at least in part, by the involved artery and drained by the involved vein lies

distal to the fistula. Completing the circuit are the heart and the vessels that feed and drain the fistula.

Resistance of the Fistula

All the effects of an arteriovenous fistula (local, peripheral, and central) are inversely related to its hemodynamic resistance. As in all blood conduits, the greater the diameter of the fistula and the shorter its length, the less its resistance becomes. Side-to-side arteriovenous fistulae, such as those constructed between the radial artery and the cephalic vein or those that occur when an aortic aneurysm ruptures into the vena cava, have virtually no length. Although Poiseuille's law (see Equation 7.13) suggests that a fistula with "zero" length should offer no resistance, some resistance is always present, owing to the inertial factors discussed in Chapter 7. Energy losses related to inertial factors, like those due to viscosity, are inversely proportional to the diameter of the opening. Consequently, small openings between contiguous arteries and veins may have a relatively high resistance despite their short length; however, beyond a certain critical diameter, the resistance becomes negligible in comparison with that of the other components of the fistulous circuit.

When the transverse diameter of an elliptically shaped fistula approaches that of the proximal artery, extension of the longitudinal diameter has little effect on blood flow through the parasitic circuit. Even though this may seem paradoxical in view of the lower resistance offered by the larger opening, the resistance of a fistula whose transverse diameter is near that of the proximal artery is so low that any further reduction in resistance will have essentially no effect on the total resistance of the entire circuit.[271]

On the other hand, the resistance of fistulous communications with a finite length—such as the **H** type, illustrated in Figure 99–2, or those constructed for hemodialysis with a graft interposed between the artery and vein—is affected by both length and diameter. Both length and diameter influence viscous and inertial energy losses, and geometric factors, such as the compliance and curvature of the graft and the configuration of the proximal and distal anastomoses, affect inertial losses. As a result, **H**-type fistulae always have a greater resistance than side-to-side fistulae of equal diameter.

In an **H**-type fistula, most of the pressure is lost between the donor artery and the arterial end of the graft and between the venous end of the graft and the recipient vein.[273] Fillinger and associates reported that 50% to 65% of the pressure drop occurred at the arterial end of nontapered loop grafts, 25% to 30% occurred at the venous end, and 11% to 18% occurred along the grafts themselves.[86] When grafts were tapered with the larger diameter at the arterial end and the smaller diameter at the venous end, pressure drops at the arterial anastomosis were minimized, whereas those at the venous anastomosis were increased.[87] Reversing the taper changed these relationships in the opposite direction. The direction of the taper had little effect on the pressure drop within the grafts. Thus, flow disturbances at the junctions exact a greater toll in terms of fluid energy than viscous effects do in the main body of the graft, where the decline in pressure is gradual (see Chapter 7).

Experimentally, flow increases through an **H**-type fistula until its diameter exceeds twice that of the proximal artery.[169] Beyond this point, further increases in diameter may or may not have a discernible effect.

The combined resistance of fistulae in parallel equals the reciprocal of the sum of the reciprocals of their individual resistances (see Equation 7.15). Therefore, the combined resistance must be less than the resistance of the fistula with the least resistance. Two parallel fistulae of equal size would have half the resistance of each fistula taken separately, but total blood flow through the two fistulae, although greatly increased, is seldom doubled.[167] Because of the increased flow, pressure at the proximal end of each fistula is reduced by opening the other; therefore, flow through each individual fistula is somewhat reduced. This explains why flow is more nearly doubled when the two fistulae are small than it is when they are large.

Local Effects

Blood Flow

Blood flow in the proximal artery is always increased (Fig. 99–3). The increase may be imperceptible when the fistula is small but is multiplied manyfold when the fistula is large.[169] Although the size of the fistula is the main determinant of the magnitude of proximal artery blood flow, other factors (e.g., the resistance of the venous outflow, the collateral arteries, and the peripheral vascular bed) also play a role.

Because the fistula markedly reduces the resistance "seen" by the proximal artery, diastolic flow is greatly increased. At times, diastolic flow may approach 80% to 90% of the maximal flow rate during systole.[140, 239] This flow pattern is distinctly different from that observed in normal peripheral arteries. Under resting conditions, flow in normal arteries falls toward zero during diastole and often reverses for a brief period (see Fig. 99–3). Thus, the fistula not only increases the flow rate in the proximal artery but may also reduce its pulsatility.

Blood flow in the proximal vein not only is greatly increased but also becomes more pulsatile, with peak flow

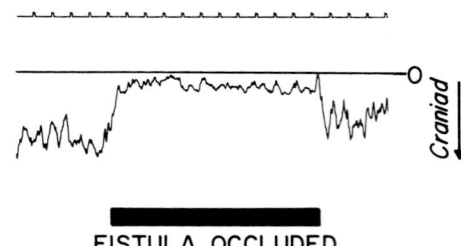

FISTULA OCCLUDED

FIGURE 99–4. Blood flow in the cephalic vein proximal to a side-to-side radial artery–cephalic vein fistula. Because the Doppler probe was pointed craniad, flow in the normal direction is indicated by a downward deflection of the tracing. Note the large volume and pulsatile nature of the flow while the fistula is open and the low-volume, nonpulsatile flow with the fistula occluded.

rates coinciding with arterial systole (Fig. 99–4). Because of the great compliance and low resistance of the proximal vein and its outflow channels, however, pulsations are rapidly damped out, usually within a few centimeters of the fistula. Pulsations are prominent only when the proximal vein is stenotic or occluded.

The direction of blood flow in the various components of the fistulous circuit is the key to understanding the essential hemodynamic features of this most interesting lesion (see Fig. 99–2). Flow in the proximal artery is always directed toward the fistula, and flow in the proximal vein is always directed centrally, toward the heart. Arterial collateral flow always travels peripherally, bypassing the fistula, and venous collateral flow always travels centrally, also bypassing the fistula. Blood in the distal artery and vein, however, may flow either toward or away from the fistula or may even be stagnant, depending on various anatomic and hemodynamic factors.

If the fistula is quite small, blood in the distal vein will continue to flow in the normal direction, past the fistula toward the heart (Fig. 99–5).[138, 239] This situation can occur only when the venous pressure at the nearest collateral junction exceeds that at the fistula site (see Fig. 99–2D and

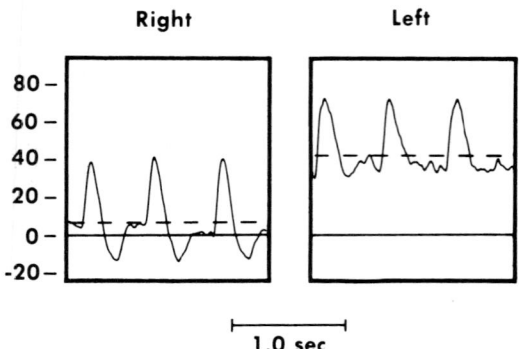

FIGURE 99–3. Blood flow in the common femoral arteries of a 25-year-old man with an acute traumatic fistula between the left superficial femoral artery and vein. Mean velocity is indicated by the *broken line*. Calculated flow in the left common femoral artery (diameter, 9.0 mm) was 1680 ml/min, whereas the flow in the right common femoral artery (same diameter) was only 217 ml/min. Contrast the reversal of flow during diastole on the right (normal) side with the high diastolic flow on the left (fistulous) side. The pulse pressure is reduced on the side of the fistula.

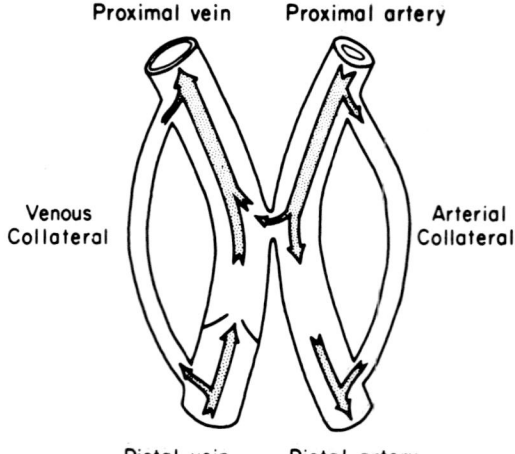

FIGURE 99–5. Flow patterns in a small arteriovenous fistula. The direction of flow is normal in all parts of the circuit. (From Sumner DS: Arteriovenous fistula. *In* Strandness DE Jr: Collateral Circulation in Clinical Surgery. Philadelphia, WB Saunders, 1969, pp 27–90.)

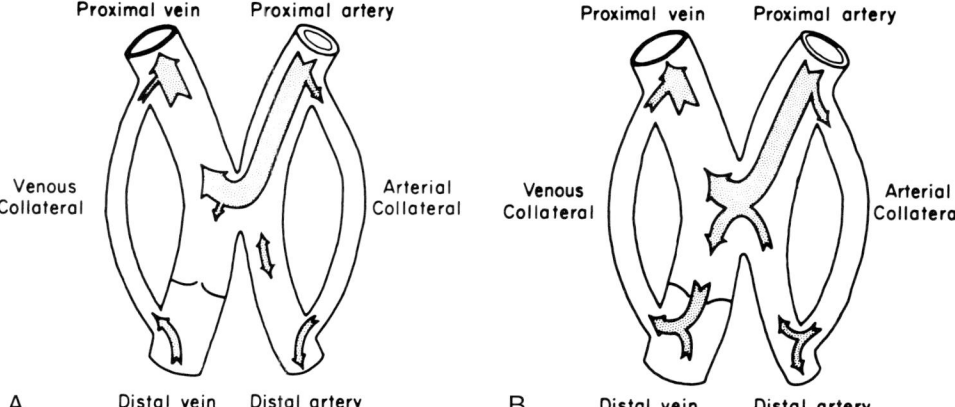

FIGURE 99–6. Flow patterns in large arteriovenous fistulae. *A*, Acute. *B*, Chronic. (*A* and *B*, From Sumner DS: Arteriovenous fistula. *In* Strandness DE Jr: Collateral Circulation in Clinical Surgery. Philadephia, WB Saunders, 1969, pp 27–90.)

E); if the fistula is large, the pressure in the vein at the site of the fistula (see Fig. 99–2*E*) will exceed that farther distally in the vein (see Fig. 99–2*D*). This situation favors retrograde flow in the distal vein.[271] Even in large acute fistulae, however, the presence of a single competent valve between the orifice of the fistula and the first venous collateral will prevent retrograde flow (Fig. 99–6*A*). Owing to increased pressure, the distal vein gradually becomes more distended so that the valves no longer coapt properly. Therefore, in large chronic fistulae, blood flows retrograde through incompetent valves down the distal vein until it is diverted into collateral venous channels (see Fig. 99–6*B*).[117, 147, 271] At some point, the excess pressure is completely dissipated and retrograde flow ceases (see peripheral vein, Fig. 99–2).

The direction and quantity of blood flow in the distal artery depend on the relative magnitude of the pressure at the arterial end of the fistula and that at the site of collateral inflow (Fig. 99–2*B* and *C*).[271, 274] As shown in Figure 99–7, the fistula circuit can be compared to a Wheatstone bridge. In this model, the distal artery corresponds to the cross-arm of the bridge. The ratio of the resistance of the proximal artery to that of the fistula determines the pressure in the artery at the level of the fistula. Similarly, the ratio of the resistance of the collateral arteries to that of the distal vascular bed determines the pressure in the peripheral portion of the distal artery at the site of collateral inflow.

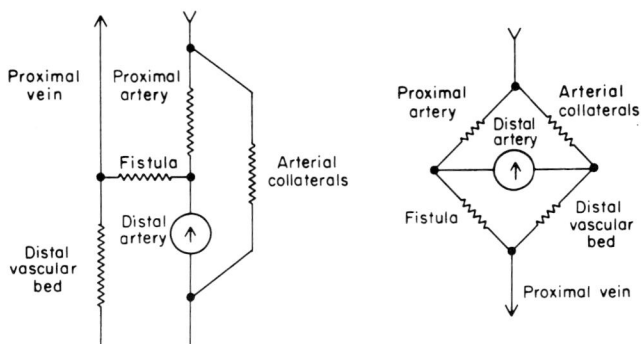

FIGURE 99–7. A Wheatstone bridge model of an arteriovenous fistula. The distal artery corresponds to the cross-arm of the bridge. (From Sumner DS: Arteriovenous fistula. *In* Strandness DE Jr: Collateral Circulation in Clinical Surgery. Philadelphia, WB Saunders, 1969, pp 27–90.)

There are three possibilities for flow in the distal artery:

1. Flow in the normal peripheral direction will occur when the ratio of the fistula resistance to the proximal artery resistance exceeds that of the distal vascular bed to the arterial collaterals. This is most likely to occur in a small, high-resistance fistula (see Figure 99–5), in which the arterial collaterals are not well developed and consequently have a high resistance.[117, 127, 138, 169, 179]

2. Flow in a retrograde direction will occur when the distal vascular bed resistance to the arterial collateral resistance ratio exceeds that of the fistula to the proximal artery. Typically, this occurs in large, chronic, low-resistance fistulae (see Fig. 99–6*B*) when the arterial collaterals are well developed.[6, 117, 127, 138, 165, 169, 179]

3. Stagnant flow exists only when the ratios are equal. This balance seldom occurs, but it can be seen in large acute fistulae before the collateral arteries are well developed. In this case, blood may flow in the normal peripheral direction during systole but reverse during diastole (see Fig. 99–6*A*).[239]

Retrograde flow in the distal artery can deprive the peripheral vascular bed of nutrition and also increase the burden on the heart.

Pressure Levels

Blood pressure in the proximal artery is usually well maintained. Both systolic and diastolic pressures may be somewhat depressed, however, in the presence of a large acute fistula, owing to the energy losses associated with increased blood flow through a normal-sized artery.[142, 168, 196] When the proximal artery becomes dilated, as in a chronic fistula, pressures may even exceed those in comparable normal arteries at the same anatomic level.[137, 142]

In contrast, blood pressure in the distal artery is always reduced (Fig. 99–8). At any given distance from the fistula, both the mean and the pulse pressures will be lower than in the proximal artery.[23, 169, 239] When the fistula is small, pressure will gradually decrease from the proximal artery, past the fistula opening, to the distal artery (Fig. 99–9*A*). If the fistula is large, a pressure "sink" will exist at its opening. Thus, pressures decrease from the proximal artery to the fistula but rise again from the fistula to the distal artery (see Fig. 99–9*B*).[138] This reversal of the pressure

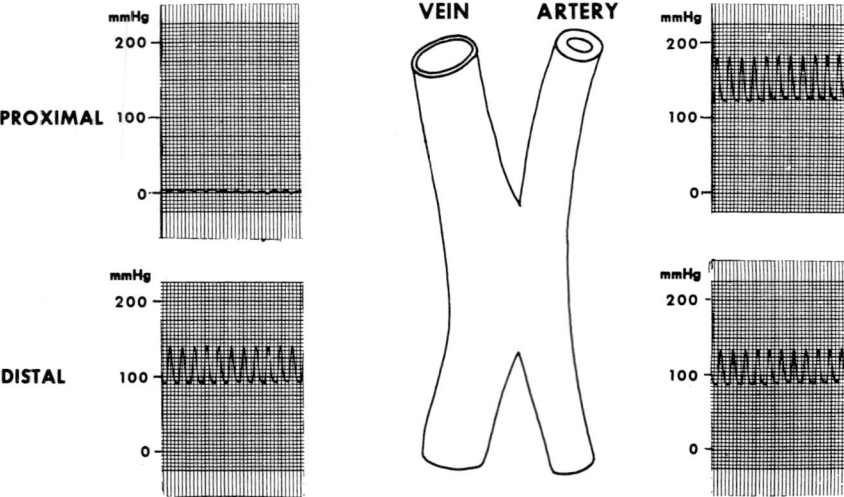

FIGURE 99–8. Blood pressures in the arteries and veins contributing to a large acute femoral arteriovenous fistula in a dog. Pressures were measured 1 cm away from the fistula. (From Sumner DS: Arteriovenous fistula. *In* Strandness DE Jr: Collateral Circulation in Clinical Surgery. Philadelphia, WB Saunders, 1969, pp 27–90.)

gradient in the distal artery occurs in conjunction with reversal of blood flow and depends on the resistance relationships discussed earlier. In chronic fistulae, as collateral arteries increase in size, pressure in the distal artery tends to rise.[127, 240] This has the dual effect of encouraging retrograde flow in the distal artery and of facilitating flow to the peripheral tissues.

Blood pressure in the proximal vein usually remains quite low despite the additional influx of blood from the fistula (compare Figs. 99–8 and 99–9). One centimeter proximal to the fistula, the mean pressure ranges between 0 and 15 mmHg, and the pulse pressure seldom exceeds 5 mmHg.[138, 168, 239, 240] The low outflow resistance of the proximal vein, together with the remarkable compliance of the venous wall, accounts for the ability of the proximal vein to accommodate the increased flow rate with little change in pressure. If the proximal vein is compressed or becomes obstructed, however, venous pressure will rise markedly, approaching that on the arterial side of the fistula.

The level of blood pressure in the distal vein depends on the size of the fistula and on the resistance offered to retrograde flow.[169] As mentioned previously, when the fistula is small, a normal pressure gradient will persist along the distal vein (see Fig. 99–9A); that is, there will be a slight but progressive fall in pressure from the periphery toward the fistula.[138, 239] When the fistula is large, venous pressure in the region of the fistula will be greatly increased (see Fig. 99–9B). This is especially true in acute fistulae when the venous valves are competent, prohibiting retrograde flow.[274] In such cases, the distal venous pressure may equal or even exceed that in the distal artery (see Fig. 99–8).[115, 116, 239, 288]

With the passage of time, resistance to retrograde flow diminishes as a result of the dilatation of the distal vein, the resulting incompetence of the venous valves, and the expansion of the venous collateral channels. Thus, blood pressure in distal venous segments tends to decrease as fistulae enter the chronic stage.[240]

Input Impedance

As one would predict, input impedance measured proximal to a large arteriovenous fistula is very low for the mean pressure-flow component (zero harmonic), reflecting the low outflow resistance.[245] The impedance curve remains flat across the spectrum of frequencies that correspond to

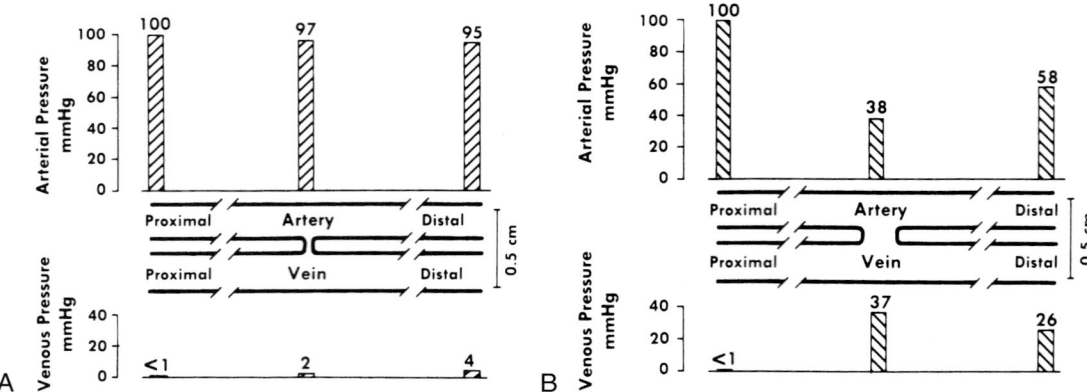

FIGURE 99–9. Theoretical blood pressures in the limbs of an arteriovenous fistula. The arterial diameter is 0.21 cm, and the venous diameter 0.24 cm. Proximal and distal pressures are measured 15 cm from the fistula. *A*, Small fistula, 0.02 cm in diameter. *B*, Large fistula, 0.20 cm in diameter. (*A* and *B*, Data from Strandness DE Jr, Sumner DS: Arteriovenous fistulas. *In* Hemodynamics for Surgeons. New York, Grune & Stratton, 1975, pp 621–663.)

higher harmonics, and the sine waves representing pressure and flow at each harmonic are roughly in phase. That pressure and flow are in phase is largely due to the absence of reflected waves from the low-resistance circuit. In contrast, the first harmonic of the input impedance in normal arteries is many orders of magnitude greater than that in arteries with distal arteriovenous fistulae, and phase angles for the higher harmonics are usually negative, indicating that the sine waves representing flow lead those representing pressure. Any impediment to the outflow of a fistula shifts the impedance curve toward that of normal arteries.

Turbulence

The bruit and thrill so characteristic of an arteriovenous fistula are the result of turbulent or disturbed flow patterns that cause vibrations in the walls of the associated blood vessels.[133, 170, 254] Several factors conspire to create these flow disturbances.

Increased velocity of blood flow elevates the tube Reynolds number (see Equation 7.11). Although the Reynolds number seldom reaches the critical value for turbulence in a smooth, straight pipe, it does reach that required for various geometric features to produce flow instability.[84, 87, 199] It is well known that bifurcations, bends, aneurysms, and sudden changes in the lumen of the blood vessel are responsible for flow disturbances.[8, 84, 199, 241, 262, 280] The circuit of an H-type fistula contains all these features. For example, the arterial flow stream either bifurcates at the entrance to the fistula—part flowing into the fistula and part into the distal artery—or, alternatively, is entirely diverted into the fistula, having been met head-on by a stream flowing proximally in the distal artery. The diameter of the lumen changes abruptly at the entrance to the fistula and again at its exit. This is particularly true if there is an intervening false aneurysm. As the flow stream emerges from the fistula, it may bifurcate into proximal and distal streams, swirl around in the distal vein, or join the proximally directed flow from the distal vein. Thus, there is little wonder that the flow pattern is markedly disturbed or that vibrations are set up in the walls of the contributing vascular channels.[86, 87]

Anatomic Changes

With the exception of early traumatic fistulae, aortocaval fistulae that develop as a result of aneurysmal rupture, residual fistulae associated with in situ bypass grafting, and those created for hemodialysis, most fistulae that come to the attention of the surgeon are of the chronic variety. Even fistulae created for hemodialysis are usually allowed to "mature" for some time before use. Because of the increased arterial and venous blood flow, morphologic changes typically occur in the contributing vessels of chronic fistulae.

In general, the size of the opening between artery and vein increases with time; few fistulae close spontaneously or become smaller.*

One of the most characteristic developments is the progressive elongation and distention of the proximal artery

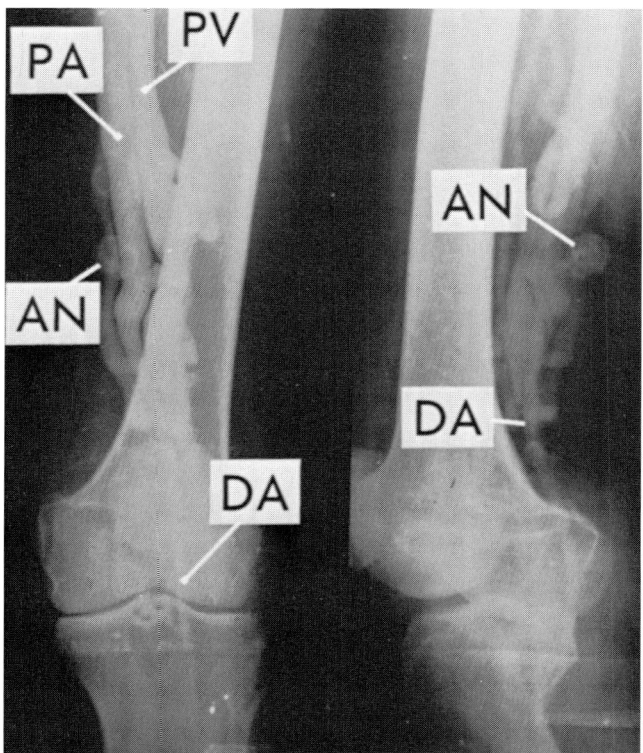

FIGURE 99–10. Chronic arteriovenous fistula of traumatic origin. It is interesting to compare the dilatation of the proximal artery (PA) and vein (PV) with the normal dimensions of the distal artery (DA). One might also note the increased density of contrast medium in the proximal vessels compared with the faint visualization of the distal artery. Calcium occurs in the wall of the aneurysm. AN = associated aneurysm.

(Fig. 99–10).[33, 99, 119, 133, 142, 143, 218, 240] Indeed, many of these arteries become very tortuous and aneurysmal.[133, 176, 217, 234, 251] Although the arterial wall may initially become somewhat thickened, it eventually undergoes degenerative changes, with atrophy of smooth muscle, decrease in the quantity of elastic tissue, and formation of atheromatous plaques.* These changes may be irreversible if the fistula is allowed to persist for more than 1 or 2 years.[100, 176, 234]

Hemodynamic factors probably account for the changes observed in the proximal artery. It appears that the increased velocity of blood is in some way responsible.[143, 175, 282] Investigators now believe that the arterial endothelium senses the increased hydrodynamic drag produced by the interaction of the bloodstream on the interior surface of the artery. This, in turn, induces a reorganization of the structural elements of the arterial wall in an effort to reduce the effect of the wall shear stress.[97, 159, 228] The resulting dilatation, which begins almost immediately,[180] is probably mediated through the release of endothelium-derived relaxing factor (nitric oxide).[152, 189, 190] Another less likely possibility is the effect of vibration on the arterial wall.[143, 208, 254] The fact that the enlargement is most marked in the immediate vicinity of the fistula lends credence to this idea.[143] Vibration plays a role in post-stenotic dilatation, an

---

*See references 125 and 127 for size that increases with time; see references 68, 130, 225, and 250 for fistulae that close or become smaller .

*See reference 255 for arterial wall that becomes thickened; see references 176, 217, 234, 251, and 263 for arterial wall that undergoes degenerative changes.

anatomic change not dissimilar to aneurysm formation in the proximal artery.[123, 224]

Elongation and tortuosity of the proximal artery are also related to similar hemodynamic factors. The force that tends to stretch the artery along its long axis is directly proportional to the longitudinal pressure gradient, which is a function of the velocity of blood flow.[139, 166]

Similar changes are observed in the proximal vein, which also becomes dilated and tortuous (compare Fig. 99–10).[99] Not only does the wall become irregularly thickened, owing to intimal proliferation and fibrosis, but also degenerative changes, such as atherosclerosis and aneurysms, may occur.* The internal elastic lamina tends to fragment and disappear. For these reasons, the term *arterialization,* often used to describe the changes in the venous wall, is inappropriate. Additional endothelial damage is produced in that portion of the vein wall immediately opposite the fistulous opening, presumably owing to the force of the jet of blood or to vibrations set up in the venous wall.[80, 254] Experiments with prosthetic graft fistulae in dogs suggest that thickening of the venous intima and media is correlated with turbulence at the distal anastomosis and kinetic energy transfer into the adjacent tissues.[86]

As mentioned earlier in the chapter, with the passage of time the distal vein dilates and elongates and its valves become incompetent. As the collateral veins develop, more and more of the fistula flow is carried distally by this vein, which suffers, albeit to a lesser degree, the same degenerative changes experienced by the proximal vein.[99, 117, 147]

The distal artery, in contrast to the proximal artery and the proximal and distal veins, tends to remain the same size, perhaps even shrinking a little (see Fig. 99–10).

About 60% of traumatic fistulae will have an associated false aneurysm.[74] Calcium deposits, commonly found in the walls of these structures, can be seen in Figure 99–10.[88] As shown in Figure 99–11, the aneurysm may be a part of the fistulous tract itself, or it may be an outgrowth of either artery, vein, or both.[74, 181]

Collateral Development

Arteriovenous fistulae constitute the most powerful known stimuli to collateral artery development.[122, 154, 217] The extent of the collateral bed far exceeds that associated with an atherosclerotic occlusion of a comparable artery.

What factors are responsible for the remarkable growth? Two major theories have been proposed:

1. Collateral development is a function of an increased velocity of blood flow.
2. There is an increased pressure differential across the collateral bed.†

The weight of the evidence appears to favor the first theory. For example, Holman[122] and Reid[217] observed that collateral artery development after ligation of the femoral artery in dogs was less extensive than it was when a large femoral arteriovenous fistula had been created, even though the reduction in pressure in the artery distal to the obstruc-

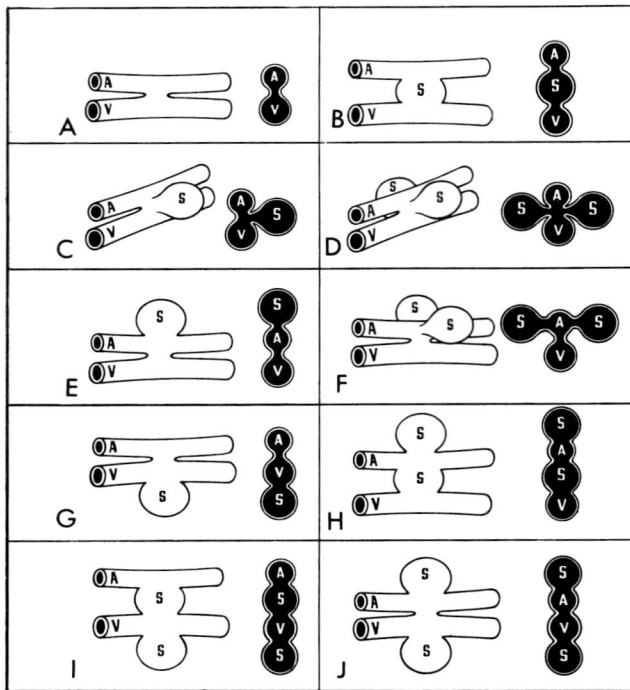

FIGURE 99–11. Relationship of aneurysmal sac to arteriovenous fistula. A, = artery; V = vein; S = aneurysmal sac. (From Elkin DC, Shumacker HB Jr: Arterial aneurysms and arteriovenous fistulas: General considerations. *In* Elkin DC, DeBakey ME: Surgery in World War II: Vascular Surgery. Washington, DC, Office of the Surgeon General, Department of the Army, 1955, pp 149–180.)

tion or fistula was the same. An obvious difference between the two circuits is that flow through the arterial collaterals bypassing an arteriovenous fistula usually exceeds that through the collaterals bypassing an occlusion. In the presence of a fistula, blood may flow retrograde in the distal artery toward the fistula; thus, the outflow resistance faced by the collateral channels is markedly reduced. In contrast, when the artery is obstructed, the collaterals empty into the relatively high resistance offered by the peripheral vascular bed. As a result, when there is reversed flow in the distal artery, collateral flow will always be higher in a limb containing a fistula than it will be in a limb with an arterial obstruction.

In a series of elegant experiments, Holman demonstrated clearly the importance of retrograde flow in the distal artery.[122] He found that collateral artery development was markedly reduced when the fistula was constructed at the end of the proximal artery or when the distal artery was ligated just beyond the fistula. These preparations permitted no retrograde flow. When the distal artery was ligated beyond a single branch, however, collateral development was extensive.

As mentioned earlier in this chapter, other investigators have shown convincingly that increased flow through a blood vessel stimulates the vessel to dilate, possibly as a result of increased shear stress on the endothelium (see Chapter 7).* Again, nitric oxide released from the endothelium has been implicated in this process.

---

*See references 88, 263, and 264 for proliferation and fibrosis; see references 209 and 265 for atherosclerosis and aneurysms.

†See references 69, 175, 228, and 283 for velocity of blood flow: see references 122, 125, and 154 for pressure differential.

---

*See references 69, 143, 175, and 283, stimulation of dilatation; see references 159 and 228, result of shear stress.

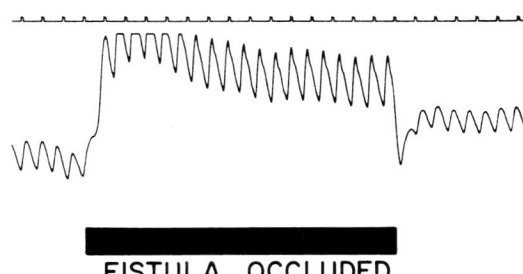

FIGURE 99–12. Plethysmographic pulses from the tip of the index finger in a patient with a side-to-side radial artery–cephalic vein fistula. Pulse volume and fingertip volume are markedly increased when the fistula is occluded. (From Strandness DE Jr, Sumner DS: Arteriovenous fistulas. *In* Hemodynamics for Surgeons. New York, Grune & Stratton, 1975, pp 621–663.)

Several investigators have observed that the growth of venous collaterals may even exceed that of arterial collaterals.[63, 64, 117] As with arterial collaterals, the mechanism of development is probably related to increased velocity of blood flow. Lengthening and tortuosity are more pronounced in venous collaterals than in arterial collaterals. The superficial veins resemble primary varicose veins. Indeed, the presence of unilateral varicose veins should alert the clinician to the possible presence of an arteriovenous fistula.

Venous collaterals are required in large acute fistulae to transport blood around the distal venous segment, the valves of which are closed to prevent retrograde flow. As the fistula ages and the valves in the distal vein become incompetent, additional venous collaterals are recruited to handle the retrograde flow. Maximal venous collateral development is observed when the proximal vein is occluded, forcing all the fistula flow to travel retrograde in the distal vein.

Peripheral Circulation

Arteriovenous fistulae always constitute a threat to the blood supply of the peripheral tissues. Weak peripheral pulses, pallor, cyanosis, and edema are frequently observed.[75, 133, 217] Plethysmographic pulses may be reduced in amplitude but usually retain a normal contour (Fig. 99–12).[31, 75, 272] Near the fistula, where arterial blood rapidly enters superficial and deep veins, the temperature of the skin, muscle, and bone is frequently elevated. Distal to the fistula, these tissues tend to be cooler than normal.[63, 64, 75, 110, 116, 141, 147, 160, 217] Oxygen tension within the peripheral muscles and bones may be decreased.[141] Likewise, the venous blood draining these tissues may show a decreased oxygen saturation and an increased concentration of lactic acid, implying marginal perfusion.[141, 182] Some patients describe pain and paresthesias of the digits distal to a fistula.[31, 71] Others may have painful ulcerations or gangrene of the fingers or toes.[44, 51, 71, 219] A few patients may complain of intermittent claudication when the fistula is located proximally in the limb.[217]

Blood Flow and Blood Pressure

When the fistula is small, blood flowing in the normal peripheral direction within the distal artery will be joined by blood from the collateral arteries to supply the peripheral arteries and their recipient tissues (see Figs. 99–2 and 99–5). Even when the fistula is large and flow in the distal artery is retrograde, at one of the distal collateral junctions, flow must again turn toward the periphery to supply the tissues of the vascular bed (see Figs. 99–2 and 99–6). In other words, at some point toward the periphery, arterial flow always regains its normal peripheral orientation.[138, 271] For example, in patients with large radial artery–cephalic vein fistulae, flow in the digital artery, which is beyond any major collateral input, is peripherally directed even though flow in the distal radial artery is reversed (Fig. 99–13). In such cases, the point of division between retrograde and antegrade flow is in the superficial palmar arch.

When the fistula is small and the collateral arteries are large, there may be little or no decrease in peripheral blood flow because arteriolar dilatation will be sufficient to compensate for the leak. When the fistula is large and the collaterals are poorly developed, arteriolar dilatation may not be adequate to maintain tissue nutrition. This is particularly likely to happen when there is a great deal of retrograde flow in the distal artery. In other cases, nutrition does not suffer but there is a relative reduction of blood flow in the distal portions of the involved extremity as compared with the uninvolved extremity.[31, 211, 227, 229, 271, 275, 290]

Although reduction in arteriolar resistance may permit blood flow to remain relatively normal, peripheral pressure is always more or less reduced because of the obligatory energy losses associated with the fistula.* Of the patients with side-to-side radial artery–cephalic vein fistulae whom the author studied, 88% had reduced digital artery pressures on the ipsilateral side. The average ratio of the pressure in the digital arteries to that in the brachial artery was 0.64 ± 0.24.[271, 275] As in the case of obstructive arterial disease, the drop in pressure is the most sensitive and reliable indicator of the hemodynamic severity of the lesion (see Chapters 7 and 10).[177]

Effect of Occluding the Fistula and Its Associated Vessels

Figure 99–14 illustrates the changes in finger blood pressure and blood flow produced by manual compression of

---

*See reference 229, blood flow normal; see references 177, 271, and 272, peripheral pressure reduced.

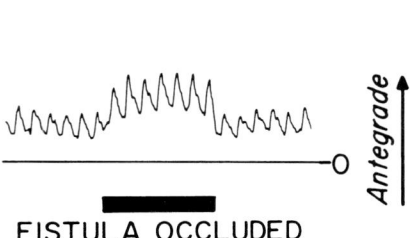

FIGURE 99–13. Blood flow in the digital artery of the middle finger in a patient with a radial artery–cephalic vein fistula on the same side. Blood flows in the normal distal direction even though flow in the distal radial artery is reversed. Temporary occlusion of the fistula increases the velocity of blood flow. The Doppler probe was pointed craniad. (From Strandness DE Jr, Sumner DS: Arteriovenous fistula. *In* Hemodynamics for Surgeons. New York, Grune & Stratton, 1975, pp 621–663.)

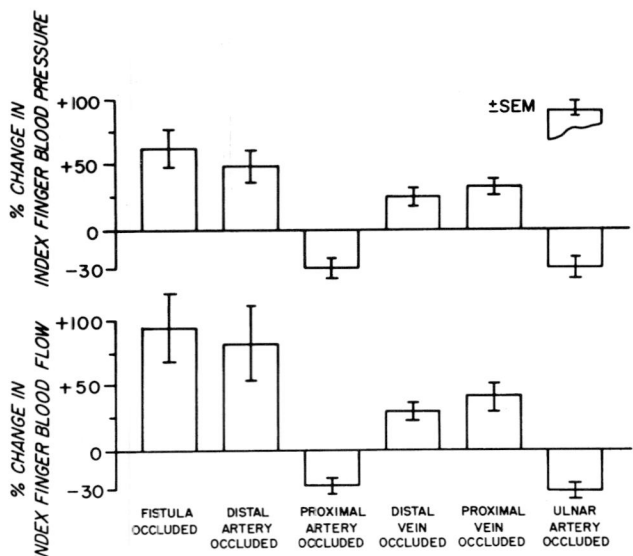

FIGURE 99–14. Effect of compressing various portions of the arteriovenous fistula circuit on peripheral blood flow and blood pressure. Values represent the average percentage change in index finger blood pressure and blood flow. (From Strandness DE Jr, Sumner DS: Arteriovenous fistulas. *In* Hemodynamics for Surgeons. New York, Grune & Stratton, 1975, pp 621–663.)

a radial artery–cephalic vein fistula and the contributing vessels.[271, 275]

Peripheral pressure and flow are decreased when the proximal radial artery is occluded. This occurs no matter what the size of the fistula is. When the fistula is small, proximal artery compression eliminates the antegrade flow in the distal radial artery but permits blood to flow retrograde in the distal radial artery toward the fistula; in other words, flow in the distal radial artery reverses. When the fistula is large, proximal artery compression serves to increase the retrograde flow in the distal radial artery. Thus, proximal artery compression increases the "steal" of blood from the collateral channels bypassing the fistula and further deprives the peripheral tissues of nutritive flow.

Compression of the major collateral channel, the ulnar artery, also results in a marked decrease in digital artery pressure and flow. Although this maneuver may cause flow in the distal radial artery to switch from retrograde to antegrade when the fistula is large or to increase the antegrade flow when the fistula is small, so much blood passes through the low-resistance fistula that peripheral perfusion is decreased. In fact, compression of the collateral arteries may produce a more severe deprivation of nutritive flow than does compression of the proximal artery.

Occlusion of any of the outflow channels of the fistula, such as the proximal or distal vein, increases the effective resistance of the fistula and increases the digital artery pressure and flow. However, a more striking increase in peripheral perfusion occurs when the radial artery distal to a large fistula is compressed. This eliminates retrograde flow through the distal artery, thereby permitting all the collateral flow to supply the distal tissues. If the fistula is small with antegrade flow in the distal artery, compression of the distal artery may decrease peripheral perfusion. The

extent of the decrease depends on the capacity of the collateral arteries.

Total occlusion of the fistula plus the proximal and distal arteries and veins may increase or decrease peripheral perfusion, depending on the size of the fistula and the functional capacity of the collateral vessels. If both the fistula and the collaterals are large, occlusion of the fistula and the four contributing vessels will increase the peripheral pressure and flow (see Fig. 99–14). If the fistula is small and the collaterals are poorly developed, this maneuver results in decreased peripheral perfusion.

How these responses apply to the design of arteriovenous fistulae for hemodialysis and to therapy for congenital and acquired fistulae is discussed later.

Systemic Effects

The introduction of an abnormal communication between the arterial and venous sides of the circulation produces a drop in *total peripheral resistance*. This is the essential pathophysiologic change responsible for all the systemic effects attributable to arteriovenous fistulae. In order to discuss these effects, some definitions are necessary.

Total peripheral resistance refers to the total resistance encountered by the left side of the heart. Its reciprocal equals the sum of the reciprocal of the *resistance of the fistula* plus the reciprocal of the *systemic resistance* offered by the peripheral vascular beds (see Equation 7.15).

Systemic blood flow is that part of the cardiac output that perfuses the peripheral tissues, and *fistula flow* is that part that passes exclusively through the parasitic circuit. Together, systemic blood flow and fistula flow equal the cardiac output.

If no circulatory adjustments were made, the reduction in total peripheral resistance accompanying an arteriovenous fistula would cause the arterial pressure to fall, the venous pressure to rise, and blood to be diverted from the peripheral tissues into the parasitic circuit. Arterial pressure could be maintained by increasing the systemic resistance, but this mechanism would further reduce flow to the peripheral tissues and would therefore be self-defeating. A more appropriate adjustment would be to augment the cardiac output by increasing heart rate and stroke volume. An increased cardiac output would maintain arterial pressure, reduce venous pressure, and supply enough blood to nourish the peripheral tissues. For stroke volume to increase, venous return must become more efficient, blood volume must increase, or both must occur.

All of these mechanisms are called into play in patients with arteriovenous fistulae. Thus, heart rate, stroke volume, cardiac output, and blood volume are usually increased. In large fistulae in which compensatory mechanisms are inadequate, arterial blood pressure and systemic blood flow may be reduced and systemic resistance, central venous pressure, and left and right atrial pressure may be elevated.

Arterial and Left Ventricular Pressure

When an acute arteriovenous fistula is suddenly opened, there is a precipitous drop in arterial pressure as a result of the marked decrease in peripheral resistance (Fig. 99–15).[119, 195, 288] As the cardiac output increases and systemic

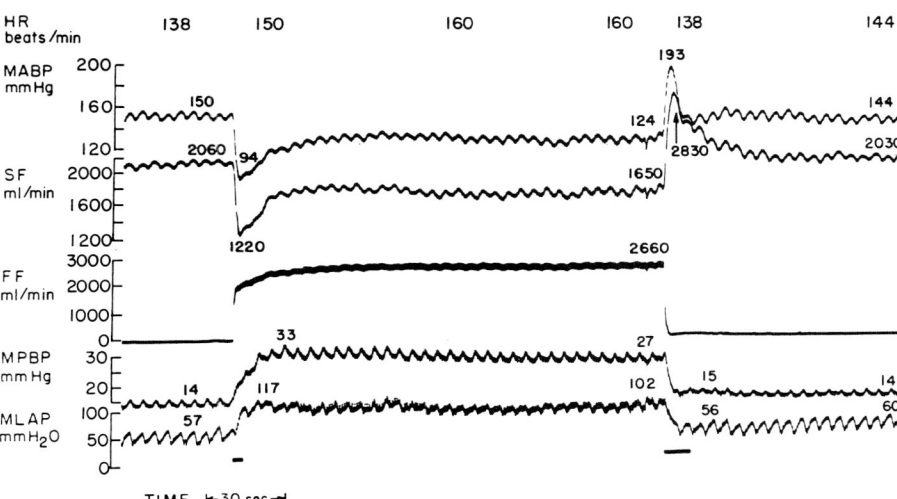

FIGURE 99–15. Effects of opening and closing a large acute arteriovenous fistula in an anesthetized dog. The fistula was opened at the *first bar* (base of graph) and closed at the second bar. HR = heart rate; MABP = mean systemic arterial blood pressure; SF = systemic (blood) flow; FF = fistula flow; MPBP = mean pulmonary arterial blood pressure; MLAP = mean left atrial blood pressure. (From Nakano J, DeSchryver C: Effects of arteriovenous fistula on systemic and pulmonary circulations. Am J Physiol 207:1319, 1964.)

resistance rises, the pressure rapidly returns toward baseline levels. Depending on the size of the fistula, however, the mean pressure often remains somewhat depressed.[195] In addition, the pulse pressure may increase because of a tendency for the diastolic pressure to be more depressed than the systolic, but this change is not consistently observed.* Closure of an acute fistula causes a sudden increase in arterial pressure to levels exceeding baseline values, as shown in Figure 99–15.[195] As the cardiac output and systemic resistance fall, the pressure rapidly returns to pre-fistula levels.[90, 195, 231, 288]

In most patients with chronic fistulae, the mean arterial pressure is maintained within normal limits but the diastolic pressure may be decreased, producing an increased pulse pressure (water-hammer pulse).[77, 174] The responses to compression or surgical closure of chronic fistulae are similar to those described for acute fistulae. Depending on the size of the fistula, there may be no perceptible rise in pressure, or there may be an immediate increase, particularly in the diastolic pressure.†

Left ventricular systolic and end-diastolic pressures drop on opening of an acute arteriovenous fistula, but the end-diastolic pressure rapidly returns to near pre-fistula levels.[195] Closure of the fistula causes a momentary increase in systolic and end-diastolic pressures before they return to control values. In the presence of large chronic fistulae, left ventricular end-diastolic pressure gradually rises and may reach remarkably high levels in patients in whom cardiac failure is severe enough to cause death.[233]

Venous Pressure

Because the central venous pressure rises only a few millimeters of water (a fraction of a millimeter of mercury) when an arteriovenous fistula is opened, this change cannot be detected unless careful serial measurements are made.[90, 103, 155, 195] Because the increased cardiac output serves to decompress the venous reservoir and because the compliant

nature of the venous circulation easily absorbs the increased venous volume, central venous pressures ordinarily remain within normal limits.[155, 169, 218, 288]

Atrial, Right Ventricular, and Pulmonary Arterial Pressure

Opening an arteriovenous fistula causes a rise in right and left atrial pressures and in mean pulmonary arterial pressure (see Fig. 99–15).[103, 129, 195, 196, 231] The absolute magnitudes of these increases are small and are related to the quantity of blood flowing through the fistula.

The resistance of the pulmonary vascular bed tends to drop, paralleling the increase in fistula flow.[195] This has the effect of maintaining the same pressure drop across the pulmonary circuit. When flow through the fistula becomes very large, however, a minimal level of pulmonary resistance is reached. Increasing the flow beyond this level causes a rise in the pressure gradient across the lung and an increase in mean pulmonary arterial pressure.[195]

Right ventricular systolic and end-diastolic pressures increase when an arteriovenous fistula is first opened, but the diastolic pressure rapidly returns to pre-fistula levels.[195] Closure of the fistula reverses this sequence.

Cardiac Output, Systemic Blood Flow, and Flow Through the Fistula

Cardiac output increases immediately after an acute arteriovenous fistula is opened, and peak flow is achieved within a few seconds. As a consequence of the rapid increase in fistula flow from zero to near maximal levels, there is an initial drop in blood flow through the systemic vascular beds, coinciding with the initial fall in mean arterial pressure. With the increase in cardiac output, systemic blood flow rises to stabilize at or somewhat below that existing before the introduction of the fistula into the circuit (see Fig. 99–15).[129, 195, 196]

Sudden closure of an acute arteriovenous fistula reverses the sequence. Fistula flow drops to zero, systemic blood flow is momentarily increased above pre-fistula levels, and cardiac output rapidly falls, as shown in Figure 99–15. The

---

*See reference 195 for diastolic pressure depressed more than systolic; see references 239 and 288 for change not consistent.

†See references 155 and 256 for no perceptible rise; see references 101, 118, 120, 121, 198, and 200 for immediate increase.

brief increase in systemic blood flow coincides with a temporary rise in systemic blood pressure and reflects the adjustment period during which excess cardiac output is forced to find egress through high-resistance peripheral vascular beds rather than through the low-resistance fistula.[90, 195]

When fistulae are small, the increase in cardiac output equals the blood flow through the fistula; consequently, there is no decrease in systemic blood flow. When fistulae are large and fistula flows exceed 27% to 40% of the control (pre-fistula) cardiac output, the increase in cardiac output may not equal the fistula flow.[90, 171] In such cases, blood is "stolen" from the peripheral vascular beds and systemic blood flow decreases. A fall in the mean arterial pressure may be prevented by compensatory peripheral vasoconstriction until fistula flows exceed 60% of the control cardiac output.[90, 195, 196, 288] Beyond this point, compensation is inadequate and systemic blood pressure falls. This situation develops clinically when an aortic aneurysm ruptures into the inferior vena cava, creating a massive arteriovenous fistula. Cardiac failure is rapid and death follows shortly unless the aneurysm is expeditiously removed and the fistula closed.[10, 12, 54, 58, 72, 226]

The percentage rise in systemic resistance always lags behind the percentage rise in fistula flow. Therefore, changes in systemic resistance can never fully compensate for the decrease in total peripheral resistance that follows the opening of an arteriovenous fistula. Were it not for the concomitant increase in cardiac output, blood pressure would fall to some extent in all cases.[196] Sympathoadrenal stimulation and increased levels of circulating catecholamines appear to be responsible for the increased systemic resistance.[195-197] As time passes and compensatory mechanisms are called into play, systemic resistance returns to normal levels.[129]

In most clinical cases, the increase in cardiac output is sufficient to prevent decreased blood flow to the systemic vascular beds. Depending on the size of the fistula, the cardiac output at rest may not be perceptibly elevated or it may be greatly increased.[14, 40, 79, 109, 155, 161, 194, 235, 242, 256, 261] Fistulae of moderate size do not appear to have an adverse effect on the increase in cardiac output induced by exercise.[66] Closure of a chronic arteriovenous fistula results in a decrease in cardiac output in 50% to 80% of patients.[155, 200, 256, 293]

Heart Rate and Stroke Volume

Cardiac output can be increased in two ways: (1) by an increase in heart rate and (2) by an increase in stroke volume. Both of these mechanisms are operational in the patient with an arteriovenous fistula, but an increase in stroke volume is the more significant of the two.[14, 82, 103, 195, 293]

Opening an acute arteriovenous fistula may produce a transient rise in pulse rate, but this response does not always occur. Closure of an acute fistula may cause the pulse rate to drop below control (pre-fistula) levels for a brief period before it returns to normal levels (see Fig. 99-15).[90, 103, 195, 196, 231, 288]

In patients with chronic arteriovenous fistulae, the heart rate is usually within normal limits. Slowing of the pulse rate with compression of the fistula or the proximal artery was reported first by Nicoladoni in 1875[183] and then by Branham in 1890.[22] In the majority of patients, the decrease is more than 4 beats/min, averaging 3 ± 4 beats/min.[155, 200] This response appears to follow the temporary rise in systemic arterial pressure and is abolished by large doses of atropine, which suggests that it is initiated by the baroreceptors in the carotid sinus and aortic arch and that it is mediated through the vagus nerve.[118, 119, 174, 200] A more recent study has shown that tachycardia induced by opening an arteriovenous fistula may occur despite a controlled arterial pressure and that changes in heart rate do not necessarily depend on arterial baroreceptor reflexes.[102] The receptors mediating the cardioacceleratory reflexes may be in the heart or lung, and the vagus nerves appear to constitute the afferent and efferent pathways. The Bezold-Jarisch reflex, which causes bradycardia by stimulation of baroreceptors in the left ventricle, may also play a role in producing Branham's sign.[295]

Although increasing the heart rate has little effect on cardiac output when venous return is normal, it does augment cardiac output in the presence of an arteriovenous fistula when venous return is elevated. This is especially true in the presence of increased catecholamine levels and heightened sympathetic activity, which accompany the opening of an arteriovenous fistula.[45]

Nevertheless, increased stroke volume alone accounts for 80% to 90% of the rise in cardiac output associated with an acute or chronic arteriovenous fistula.[103, 129, 195, 231] The elevated stroke volume has been attributed to the Frank-Starling mechanism, which is initiated by a slight rise in atrial pressure.[103] It may also reflect an increase in myocardial contractility that develops in response to increased sympathetic adrenergic outflow and elevated levels of circulating catecholamines.[195-197]

Normally, the subendocardium exhibits greater oxygen extraction, coronary blood flow, and oxygen consumption than the subepicardium. These differences are not observed in the presence of a moderate-volume arteriovenous fistula, suggesting a relative decrease in subendocardial oxygen demand in response to an increase in volume work, especially at the apex of the left ventricle.[27]

Heart Size

Cardiac enlargement is frequently seen in patients with chronic arteriovenous fistulae. This well-known association has been recognized for more than 75 years.[216, 217, 268] The increase in heart size ranges from a small percentage in patients with small fistulae to nearly 80% in those with large fistulae.[14]

A gradual enlargement of the heart begins immediately after the fistula is created and continues for several months.* When the fistula is large and uncompensated, the heart may initially decrease in size as a result of the displacement of blood into the capacious venous system.[120]

Closure of a chronic fistula may result in transient enlargement of the aorta and left ventricle together with a reduction in volume of the right atrium and pulmonary conus.[121] These effects are due to incomplete emptying of the left side of the heart and diminution of venous return to

---

*See references 174 and 218, begins immediately; see reference 148, continues for months.

the heart. Permanent correction of a chronic fistula causes the heart to decrease steadily in size, frequently returning to normal dimensions within a few weeks.[148, 253, 293]

The increase in cardiac size may represent either dilatation or hypertrophy. Volume overload, like that which accompanies an arteriovenous fistula, causes both of these effects.[19, 65] Experimental studies suggest that the hearts of adult dogs respond primarily by dilatation, whereas the hearts of growing puppies tend to hypertrophy.[120] In rats with chronic aortocaval fistulae, an increase in heart weight of 86% at 1 month has been shown to be due to hypertrophy of the individual myocytes rather than to hyperplasia.[178]

Blood Volume

Blood volume is often increased in the presence of a chronic arteriovenous fistula.[77, 121, 125, 161, 233, 242, 256, 292] In one series, the increase ranged from 200 ml/m² to more than 1000 ml/m² of body surface.[292]

The excess blood is accommodated in all parts of the expanded fistulous circuit, including proximal arteries and veins, cardiac chambers, central veins, and collateral vessels.[125, 256] It aids peripheral perfusion by permitting the cardiac output to rise sufficiently to accommodate both the fistula and the systemic circulation, thus avoiding a steal.[90, 103] Indeed, transfusion may be necessary to preserve life in the presence of a large arteriovenous fistula.[52] It appears that the major factor limiting cardiac output in the presence of an acute fistula is an insufficient blood volume and not an inadequate cardiac reserve.[90] The organism tends to correct this volume deficit as the fistula becomes chronic.

Expansion of plasma volume, which accounts for most of the increase in blood volume,[55] is largely a result of sodium-retaining and water-retaining mechanisms that are activated by the presence of a fistula.* This process appears to be triggered by a reduction in mean arterial pressure.[226] In response to the decreased perfusion pressure, renal blood flow and glomerular filtration rate decrease and reabsorption from the renal tubules increases. As a result, urine output falls, extracellular fluid accumulates, and blood volume expands.[129] In addition, decreased renal blood flow activates the renin-angiotensin-aldosterone system, which further increases renal sodium and fluid reabsorption.† Renal nerves evidently play an important role.[131] Once the proper volume elevation has been achieved, sodium and water excretion returns to normal.[56]

In experimental animals with large arteriovenous fistulae, right atrial pressure rises in response to the elevated blood volume. The increase in right atrial pressure is accompanied by a marked increase in the level of circulating atrial natriuretic peptide (ANP).[129, 220] This substance augments glomerular filtration rate, inhibits sodium reabsorption in the medullary collecting duct, and opposes the antinatriuretic activity of the renin-angiotensin-aldosterone system. Although it is attractive to postulate that ANP plays a role in achieving volume homeostasis in the presence of a chronic

arteriovenous fistula, studies have cast doubt on this mechanism.[220]

In chronic cases, occlusion of the fistula results in increased sodium excretion.[78, 131] In addition to retention of sodium, protein stores are mobilized, thus maintaining the oncotic pressure of the plasma.[243] Without this mechanism, the intravascular volume could not expand.

Cardiac Failure

Cardiac failure rapidly develops when there is a massive leak of blood from the arterial to the venous side of the circulation.[226, 261] This is particularly true with large aorta–inferior vena cava fistulae, which are highly lethal.[10, 12, 52, 54, 72, 226, 233] On the other hand, failure may never occur or may be delayed for many years if the fistula is small.[67, 93] In experimental animals, a direct relationship between increased cardiac output and the development of heart failure has been demonstrated.[52] In humans, the situation is more complex, depending not only on the size of the fistula and the cardiac output but also on the presence of preexisting coronary or myocardial disease.[94] Children, with their generally healthy hearts, are able to sustain the increased circulatory load for prolonged periods without lapsing into cardiac failure.[26]

The continued expansion of the entire fistulous circuit that occurs with the passage of time results in a gradual increase in cardiac output and the delayed appearance of cardiac failure in some patients who initially were able to tolerate the fistula without evident physiologic strain.[126] In patients with congenital fistulae, an elevated cardiac output is less likely and heart failure seldom develops.[15, 51, 161, 212, 278] Infants with massive congenital fistulae of the brain or liver are an exception to this rule. These large arteriovenous malformations may cause life-threatening cardiac failure, necessitating early operative intervention.[47, 98, 172, 291] Widely distributed arteriovenous malformations involving multiple organs are also known to cause greatly increased cardiac output and heart failure.[38] Treatment of these malformations is exceedingly difficult.

Edema formation in acute arteriovenous fistulae may be related to local elevation of venous pressure; however, when cardiac failure ensues, the full clinical picture of fluid retention appears, including peripheral edema, pulmonary edema, ascites, and weight gain.[5] Increased aldosterone secretion probably plays an important role at this stage.[56, 260, 286] Closure of chronic arteriovenous fistulae may result in massive diuresis.[143] Eiseman and Hughes reported that a patient lost 61 pounds (41.5% of his body weight) in the first 12 days after repair of an aorta–vena cava fistula.[72]

Effect of Fistula Location

Arteriovenous fistulae involving vessels close to the heart have a more profound systemic effect than do those located in the periphery.[120, 124, 126] This is quite simply explained on the basis of the comparative resistance of the parasitic circuits. When the fistula lies between major central vessels (e.g., the aorta and the inferior vena cava), the proximal arteries and veins have an extremely low resistance because of their wide diameter and short length; when the fistula involves vessels in an extremity, the resistance of the circuit

---

*See reference 77 for expansion of plasma volume; see reference 114 for mechanisms activated by fistula.

†See reference 281, triggered by pressure changes; see references 56, 129, 204, 220, and 286, mediated by renin-angiotensin-aldosterone system.

is much higher because of the smaller diameter of the vessels and the greater distance from the heart.[52, 75] Moreover, the diameter of the fistula itself can be much larger in central vessels than it can be in peripheral vessels, where its diameter is limited by the size of the involved artery and vein.

Fistulae of the pelvis and legs are said to exert a greater systemic effect than those of the head, neck, and arm.[253] This may be due to the hydrostatic effect of gravity, which tends to distend the involved vessels, thereby lowering their resistance.[91] However, there is no confirmatory evidence for this supposition.[171]

It is often stated that fistulae involving branches of the portal system have fewer systemic effects than would be expected from fistulae of similar size in other parts of the body. This may be related to the high outflow resistance offered by the hepatic sinusoids.[132, 192, 232, 269, 276] Nevertheless, some patients with fistulae between the superior mesenteric artery and vein do have significantly elevated cardiac outputs.[29, 257]

Outline of Systemic Effects

Opening an arteriovenous fistula produces an immediate reduction in total peripheral resistance. This causes the central arterial pressure to drop, the central venous pressure to rise, the systemic blood flow to decrease, and blood to be transferred from the arterial to the venous side of the circulation. A number of compensatory mechanisms are called into play to correct these physiologic aberrations.

The rise in central venous pressure distends the cardiac chambers, increasing the end-diastolic stretch of the myocardial fibers. The Frank-Starling mechanism, thus initiated, acts to increase stroke volume. Baroreceptor reflexes, responding to the fall in arterial pressure, cause the heart rate to rise, and myocardial contractility is strengthened through the effects of circulating catecholamines and sympathetic discharges on the cardiac muscle. Sympathoadrenal effects also stimulate systemic arteriolar constriction, which helps to maintain central arterial pressure but further decreases peripheral blood flow. Constriction of the central veins, however, facilitates venous return. Together these mechanisms cause the cardiac output and central aortic pressure to rise.

If compensation is adequate, as it usually is in most patients with good cardiac function, the cardiac output will increase sufficiently to permit central aortic pressure to approach normal pre-fistula values. Baroreceptor effects are thereby decreased, allowing the pulse rate to return to near-normal levels and the peripheral vascular constriction to be alleviated. Systemic blood flow returns to an adequate, although somewhat reduced, level. If, however, the fistula is massive or if the myocardium is damaged, compensation will be incomplete. Cardiac output, although increased, will not be sufficient to maintain peripheral blood flow in the face of the great leak between the two sides of the circulation. Cardiac failure ensues, and early death may result.

Activation of the renin-angiotensin-aldosterone system causes retention of sodium and water. Together with mobilization of protein stores, retention of sodium and water acts to increase the plasma volume. The resulting increase in blood volume allows the heart to enlarge and the remainder of the fistulous circuit to expand. This facilitates venous return, thereby improving the cardiac output. In the well-compensated system, systemic blood flow rises to pre-fistula levels and electrolyte metabolism returns to normal.

As time passes, the fistulous circuit often continues to expand as a result of the dilatation of the proximal arteries and veins as well as dilatation of the fistula itself. In addition, both arterial and venous collaterals may continue to develop. The end result is a further drop in total peripheral resistance and increased cardiac output. Sooner or later, depending on the presence or absence of coronary or myocardial disease, the cardiac reserve may be depleted and cardiac failure occurs.

A detailed study of aortocaval fistulae in rats by Huang and colleagues[129] provides an excellent summary of the acute and chronic systemic effects of large arteriovenous fistulae and confirms the mechanisms outlined previously.

HEMODYNAMIC CONSIDERATIONS IN TREATMENT

The indications for surgical therapy and the technical aspects of the various procedures are discussed in subsequent chapters. All modern operations are designed to eradicate the leak and, if possible, to restore the circulatory pattern to that which would normally exist in the absence of an arteriovenous fistula. Incomplete operations (i.e., those that merely decrease fistula flow) are avoided if at all possible.

Proximal Artery Ligation

Ligation of the artery leading to a fistula (the so-called Hunter operation) is a completely unsatisfactory and often dangerous procedure.[28] It has long been known that gangrene may result from this operation.[24]

Figure 99–16 shows the theoretical results of various operations in a model fistulous circuit in which the collateral artery resistance is no greater than that of the main arterial channel. In this illustration, proximal artery ligation would have little effect on the reduced peripheral blood flow and would further decrease peripheral blood pressure (see Fig. 99–16B). Although flow through the fistula would be reduced, it would still be appreciable. In many (perhaps most) cases, proximal arterial occlusion reduces both peripheral blood pressure and flow (see Fig. 99–14).

Thus, this operation not only decreases peripheral perfusion but also fails to eradicate flow through the fistula. When collateral channels are poorly developed, proximal arterial ligation can be expected to have devastating peripheral effects.[119] Because the fistula remains open, blood supplied by collateral arteries is further diverted into the distal artery, where it flows retrograde toward the fistula, thereby increasing the steal from the peripheral tissues.

It is probably safe to say that few surgeons today would knowingly treat an acquired arteriovenous fistula with proximal arterial ligation.[155] Unfortunately, physiologically similar procedures are sometimes performed inadvertently in the course of treating congenital arteriovenous fistulae. Most congenital fistulae are complex structures with many

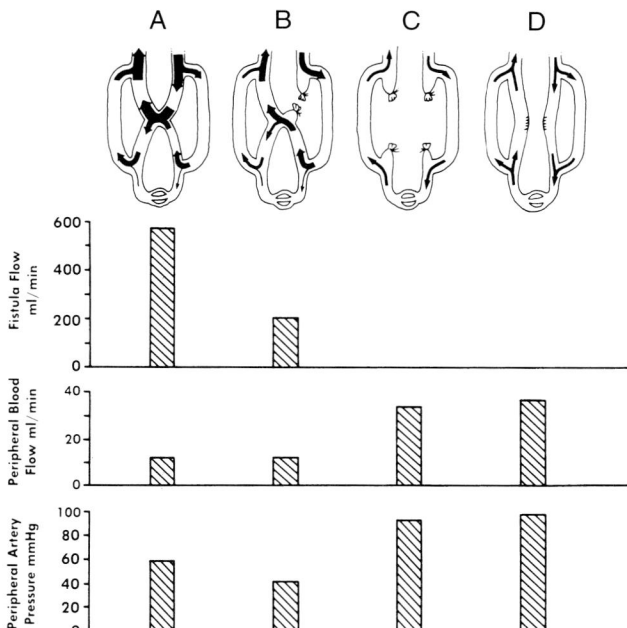

FIGURE 99–16. Effects of proximal artery ligation (B), quadruple ligation and excision (C), and total reconstructive surgery (D) on flow through the fistula, peripheral arterial pressure, and peripheral blood flow. A, Intact fistula. These theoretical results are based on a model with low-resistance arterial collaterals.

contributing arteries and veins and multiple arteriovenous communications, many of which are of microscopic size. Unless the fistula is very well localized, residual fistulae will be left behind after excisional therapy. With time, these residual fistulae and their communicating channels enlarge until the arteriovenous leak approaches that of the original lesion.[215]

When any of the major arteries feeding the fistula are also responsible for supplying tissues peripheral to the lesion, their ligation jeopardizes tissue nutrition in the same way that ligation of the proximal artery does in cases of acquired fistula. Not only do the terminal tissues have to depend on collateral blood flow; retrograde flow through residual fistulous communication creates a steal, thus further reducing peripheral flow. For these reasons, a conservative, nonoperative approach is advocated for most congenital arteriovenous fistulae unless they are well localized and readily accessible.[234, 278, 279]

When treatment is required because of skin ulceration, bleeding, excessive limb growth, or cardiac failure, embolic occlusion of the multiple arteriovenous communications in theory is appealing.[38, 158, 206] This procedure should obliterate the leak while preserving the major arteries, veins, and collateral channels on which the peripheral tissues depend for their nutrition.

Quadruple Ligation and Excision

The advantages of ligating all communicating vessels together with total excision of the arteriovenous fistula were first recognized by Bramann more than a century ago.[21] This operation remained the treatment most commonly employed before and even during World War II.[73]

Quadruple ligation is a physiologically sound procedure. By ligating the proximal artery and vein as well as the distal artery and vein and excising the fistula, the surgeon converts a complex hemodynamic circuit into one that is far more simple (see Fig. 99–16C). Because the distal artery and the fistula are eliminated, a steal can no longer occur. The afferent channels to the periphery consist of the collateral arteries, and the efferent channels are composed of the collateral veins. Thus, the success of quadruple ligation and excision depends on the resistance of the preexisting collateral vessels.

For optimal collateral development, it was formerly customary to delay operation for several months after injury.[73] A number of tests were devised to help the surgeon recognize adequate collateral flow. In the Moschcowitz hyperemia test, blood flow to the involved limb was obstructed by a pneumatic cuff for 5 minutes. After the fistula had been occluded by external pressure, the cuff was suddenly deflated. As blood returned to the limb, a visible flush began proximally and extended distally. If the flush reached the end of the limb within 2 minutes, the collateral circulation was assumed to be satisfactory.[249]

The presence of pulsations in the distal artery after the proximal artery has been occluded (the *Henle-Coenen phenomenon*) also confirms that the collateral circulation is adequate. Perhaps a better method for estimating the functional capacity of the collaterals is to note whether the distal portion of the limb retains its normal color and warmth after the involved vessels have been occluded for 20 minutes.[252] Other somewhat more objective tests that depend on measurement of pressure and flow have been devised (see Chapter 100).

Figure 99–16C illustrates an optimal response to quadruple ligation and excision. In this model, flow through the fistula is totally eliminated and peripheral artery pressure and flow return to nearly normal levels. A similar response to compression of radial artery-cephalic vein fistulae is shown in Figure 99–14. In both of these examples, the collateral artery resistance is quite low. In many clinical situations, however, collaterals are not as well developed and the results may not be as good. Although few patients treated in this way develop gangrene (none in Elkin's series), about 40% to 50% will have symptoms of arterial insufficiency, usually intermittent claudication.[13, 73, 88, 92, 96, 111, 130, 246] Clearly, the collateral arteries in these cases, although well developed, do not appear to be functionally superior to those that bypass chronic localized arterial obstructions in the lower limb.

Reconstructive Surgery

Although Matas had advocated total reconstruction of arteriovenous fistulae as early as 1922,[183] this approach was not widely adopted until after World War II. During this war, a few innovative surgeons clearly demonstrated the superiority of reconstructive surgery over quadruple ligation and excision, and by the time of the Korean conflict, reconstructive surgery became the rule.* These developments were made possible by the availability of antibiotics,

---

*See references 92 and 248 for demonstrated superiority; see references 146, 246, and 259 for having become the rule.

blood transfusions, improved vascular suture and instruments, autografts, and surgeons who were skilled in the disciplines required.

Obviously, successful elimination of the fistula and repair of the involved artery and vein return the circulation to normal (see Fig. 99–16D). Although some surgeons have adopted a cavalier approach to the vein, making no attempt at repair, more recent investigators have emphasized the importance of restoring venous continuity.[130, 222, 259] Ligation of the vein leads to varicose veins, chronic venous insufficiency, and sometimes gangrene.

Systemic Response

Elimination of the fistula, whether by reconstructive surgery or by quadruple ligation and excision, reverses the hemodynamic consequences of the leak from the arterial to the venous side of the circulation. Cardiac output falls to normal levels; blood pressure and pulse, if abnormal, return to pre-fistula values; and the heart, if enlarged, shrinks to normal size.[148, 194, 253, 256, 293] Blood volume decreases, and excess body fluid is eliminated.[72, 194, 256] In most cases, cardiac failure is rapidly cured.[94, 194, 261]

HEMODYNAMIC FACTORS IN THE DESIGN OF FISTULAE FOR VASCULAR ACCESS

The most important therapeutic application of arteriovenous fistulae is to provide a convenient access to the circulation in patients with chronic renal failure. Introduced in 1966 by Brescia and associates, this technique has rapidly supplanted the use of external shunts for long-term hemodialysis.[25] Chapter 104 discusses the technical aspects of these procedures.

Several constraints have been placed on the design of fistulae to be used for hemodialysis:

1. The fistula should transmit enough blood at sufficient pressure to permit a relatively high flow through the dialysis machine.
2. In order to avoid cardiac strain, fistula flow should not be excessively great.
3. Circulation to the tissues peripheral to the fistula should not be jeopardized.
4. Congestion of the peripheral venous bed should be avoided.
5. Percutaneous access to the fistula output should be easily accomplished.

Diameter of the Fistula

Based on theoretical considerations, there would be no advantage to making a side-to-side anastomosis between the artery and vein any larger than the diameter of the proximal artery. Provided the fistula diameter is 60% to 80% of the arterial diameter, its resistance is infinitesimally small in comparison with that of the artery.[271] Small fistulae, however, are difficult to construct, are prone to early occlusion as a result of fibrosis or thrombosis, and offer no

advantages over large fistulae. Therefore, for practical purposes, most radial artery–cephalic vein fistulae are constructed with an anastomotic length of 6 to 10 mm—several times the diameter of the proximal artery.[32, 34, 71, 282, 284]

When the fistula itself is relatively long, as in H-type arrangements constructed with prosthetic grafts or autogenous vein, the diameter of the fistula makes a difference.[165, 169] In order to minimize resistance, the fistula should be at least as large as the proximal artery and probably should have a diameter equal to that of the venous drainage. Aside from the question of flow, the graft must be large enough to avoid clotting and to facilitate percutaneous cannulation.

Common complications of polytetrafluoroethylene arteriovenous fistulae have been platelet deposition, intimal hyperplasia, and fibrosis in the runoff vein at the site of the anastomosis.[151] These complications occur with both end-to-end and end-to-side anastomoses.[86] Progressive stenosis causes rising pressure in the venous dialysis line and eventual failure of the fistula.[273] Although the cause of the fibrosis is unknown, it appears to be related to hemodynamic factors similar to those discussed earlier (see Anatomic Changes). Animal experiments have shown that venous hyperplasia is decreased when tapered grafts are used and the larger end is anastomosed to the vein.[87] This configuration appears to minimize turbulence and kinetic energy transfer to the perivascular tissues.

Advantages and Disadvantages of Various Types of Fistulae

Radial Artery–Cephalic Vein Fistulae

Radial artery–cephalic vein fistulae are well adapted to therapeutic use because they fulfill most of the requirements previously enumerated. Although these fistulae are capable of transmitting sufficient flow, they are situated far enough peripherally so that flow ordinarily is not excessive. Moreover, the ulnar artery provides an excellent collateral channel, fully capable of sustaining the circulation to the hand, thereby minimizing the risk of peripheral ischemia. Finally, the veins of the forearm are large, prominent, relatively straight, and easily punctured.

Several varieties of radial artery–cephalic vein anastomosis have been used (i.e., the classic side-to-side, the end of proximal artery–side of vein, the side of artery–end of proximal vein, and the end of proximal artery–end of vein). In addition, various H-type fistulae have been constructed. In these operations, autogenous vein or prosthetic grafts are used to link the artery with the vein.[2, 30, 41, 55, 71, 104, 156, 173, 185, 188, 284]

The hemodynamics described next are illustrated by theoretical values listed in Table 99–1. These results were obtained by analogy with electrical circuit theory. They are based on Kirchhoff's laws and published values of flow and pressure in the various components of the fistula circuit. (Results of a similar analysis by van Gemert and Bruyninckx were consistent with clinical experience.[287])

Because blood can enter the anastomosis from both the proximal and the distal radial arteries and exit through both the proximal and the distal cephalic veins, the side-to-side fistula transmits more blood than other fistulae of similar size.[31, 34, 134] The high flow rate keeps the anastomo-

TABLE 99–1. HEMODYNAMIC PROPERTIES OF VARIOUS RADIAL ARTERY–CEPHALIC VEIN FISTULAE (THEORETICAL VALUES BASED ON A STANDARD MODEL SYSTEM)

	FISTULA FLOW (ml/min)	PROXIMAL VEIN FLOW (ml/min)	ARTERIAL BLOOD PRESSURE IN HAND (mmHg)	VENOUS BLOOD PRESSURE IN HAND (mmHg)
No fistula	—	18	95	3
Side-to-side	571	434	58	26
End of proximal artery–side of vein (or distal artery ligated)	474	369	92	23
Side of artery–end of proximal vein (or distal vein ligated)	507	507	61	4
End-to-end proximal artery–proximal vein	435	435	91	6
Side-to-side (proximal vein occluded)	265	—	79	48
Side-to-side (proximal artery occluded)	194	152	41	9

From Strandness DE Jr, Summer DS: Arteriovenous fistulas. In Hemodynamics for Surgeons. New York, Grune & Stratton, 1975, pp 621–663.

sis open and facilitates hemodialysis. For these reasons, the side-to-side fistula is preferred by many surgeons.[32, 34, 41, 282] However, there are some problems associated with this arrangement.

Because the distal artery remains open, carrying blood in a retrograde fashion, the possibility of a steal exists.[23, 177] Indeed, the author's group found that the majority of such fistulae (88%) were associated with decreased digital artery pressures.[271] In one series, hand claudication occurred in 42% of the patients.[163] Fortunately, serious symptoms seldom develop unless there is concomitant obstructive disease of the digital arteries, the palmar arch, or the ulnar artery.[20, 31, 34, 41, 42, 71, 105, 188, 270, 284] Although ligation of the distal artery or construction of an end of artery-side of vein fistula eliminates the possibility of a steal, fistula flow is decreased somewhat.[20, 31, 271]

Another potential drawback of the side-to-side fistula is the relatively high pressure in the distal vein, as shown in Table 99–1. Although this is usually of little significance,[34] if the proximal vein becomes occluded, all the fistula flow will be diverted retrograde into the distal vein.[99] In such cases, the hand and fingers may become painful and swollen and may even develop ulcerations.[20, 62, 105, 191, 270] Moreover, blood flow in the distal vein, which seldom approaches that in the proximal vein, is rapidly dissipated into numerous venous collaterals. Thus, a vein capable of supplying enough blood for dialysis becomes difficult to find. When proximal vein thrombosis or narrowing occurs, the shunt must be reconstructed.[20, 62, 105] In rare instances in which the proximal vein remains patent, ligation of the distal vein has been curative.[62]

In an effort to avoid distal venous hypertension, many surgeons perform a side of artery-end of proximal vein anastomosis.[6, 37, 57, 62, 71, 104, 191, 207, 284] As indicated by the values in Table 99–1, this procedure has much to recommend it. Fistula flow is high, and distal venous pressure is low. Because all the fistula output is diverted through the proximal vein, more flow is available for hemodialysis. Although the potential for a peripheral arterial steal exists, it is no worse than that associated with side-to-side fistulae.[6]

End-to-end fistulae have many theoretical advantages. Fistula flow and proximal vein flow are very good, distal venous pressure is low, and peripheral perfusion is main-

tained at near-normal levels. Because of these features, there has been some support for end-to-end fistulae.[9, 42, 62, 104, 193] Unfortunately, they have a tendency to thrombose in the early postoperative period.[284]

H grafts and other makeshift shunts are usually employed only when a radial artery–cephalic vein fistula cannot be fashioned or has failed.[282] In practice, up to two thirds of all fistulae are of this variety.[205, 244] Most interposition grafts are constructed of polytetrafluoroethylene, have a straight or looped configuration, and connect the radial or brachial artery to the antecubital, cephalic, basilic, or axillary veins. The hemodynamics of these fistulae depend on the resistances of the fistula and the proximal and distal arterial and venous channels. In general, they fit one of the patterns already described.

Proximal Arteriovenous Fistulae

Because of their more proximal location, brachial fistulae have a higher blood flow than those toward the wrist.[5, 165] Although they function well, providing a good flow of blood through the fistula, they tend to shunt blood away from the peripheral tissues.[23, 32, 42, 271, 284] Patients with these fistulae may develop edema, skin ulcers, paresthesias, and pain.[105, 271, 284]

The major physiologic difference between the brachial artery and the radial artery locations is the quality of the collaterals that bypass the fistula. Although the brachial artery has several prominent collateral arteries, none compares with the ulnar artery. Therefore, in some cases the peripheral tissues must be supplied, at least in part, by blood flowing past the fistula into the distal artery, where it continues in a normal centrifugal direction toward the hand. The total quantity of blood reaching the hand depends on the magnitude of the leak through the fistula and the capacity of the collaterals.

Even when the collaterals are moderately well developed, there may be significant distal flow deprivation. In this event, flow in the distal brachial artery may be reversed so that only a small portion of the collateral flow is available to nourish the hand and distal forearm. Nevertheless, the development of peripheral ischemia—and its severity—is less closely related to the magnitude of reversed flow than it is to the extent of peripheral arterial occlusive disease.[165]

This is especially true in diabetic patients.[42] As time passes, the collateral arteries enlarge, the digital pressures tend to rise, and flow deprivation is usually alleviated.[23, 238]

When ischemic symptoms persist, reduction of fistula flow by plicating (or otherwise narrowing) the graft may be tried. Because the borderline between adequate reduction in flow and maintenance of graft patency is narrow, this approach often proves unsatisfactory. Monitoring digital pulses during the procedure has been advocated as a method of determining the point at which adequate reduction of the lumen has been achieved.[205, 223] When preservation of the hand requires fistula ligation, replacing the fistula with one using a branch of the axillary artery as the donor vessel has been advocated.[150] Because of the small size of the donor artery (3 mm in diameter), fistula flow is limited and a symptomatic steal no longer occurs.

Another method of alleviating ischemia associated with brachial fistulae is to ligate the artery distal to the fistula (thus eliminating reversed flow in the distal artery).[238] This must be accompanied by the insertion of a bypass graft from a normal segment of the artery proximal to the fistula into the artery distal to the site of the ligature, thereby creating an additional low-resistance collateral to supply the peripheral tissues.

Serious steal phenomena have also been reported with femoral arteriovenous fistulae using bovine grafts, but they seem to occur infrequently.[11, 81] Even though blood flow through these fistulae is high, the arterial collaterals in the femoral area are good and the input through the iliofemoral system is less limited than it is in the brachial area. Resting ankle pressure may be reduced, but the ankle pressure response to exercise does not seem to be affected.[11]

Systemic Effects

Flow through upper extremity arteriovenous fistulae used for hemodialysis varies widely, ranging from 100 to 3000 ml/min, with an average level of about 200 to 400 ml/min.[4, 6, 71, 155, 219] Values as high as 3600 ml/min have been reported in the absence of cardiac failure.[4, 284]

High-output cardiac failure, although rare, does occur with fistulae in the arm.[1, 4, 34, 76, 83, 94, 155, 186, 284] In these cases, fistula flows, measured intraoperatively, have ranged from 600 to 2900 ml/min. The decrease in cardiac output with fistula occlusion averages 2900 ml/min, although in one individual an 11 L/min decrease was reported.[4]

(Apparently, high-output congestive heart failure is much more common with lower extremity fistulae. According to one report, 59% of patients with femoral arteriovenous bovine shunts developed heart failure within the first year.[82] Presumably, this is due to the high rate of flow through these "proximal" fistulae.)

Most cases of cardiac failure occurring in patients on hemodialysis can be attributed to anemia, hypertension, and excessive sodium and water retention. Even in the absence of these complications, patients with coronary arterial insufficiency or myocardial disease may not be able to sustain the increased circulatory load imposed by the fistula.[4, 284] Cardiac failure in these patients tends to be resistant to medical therapy. Reduction in fistula flow by surgical revision of the fistula or by narrowing of the involved vessels is necessary to correct the cardiac failure. If it is no longer needed (e.g., after renal transplantation), the fistula can be eliminated. Results have usually been good with these procedures.[4, 73] There are, however, exceptions. In certain patients in whom left ventricular disease is primarily responsible for heart failure, occluding the fistula, which increases afterload, may have a detrimental effect on cardiac dynamics.[35, 285]

Several surgeons have reported success with banding procedures as a means of reducing fistula flow. In these operations, a 1-cm polytetrafluoroethylene (Teflon) band is placed around the proximal artery or vein (or the fistula, when a graft is used) and tightened gradually until the desired flow rate is achieved.[3, 83] It is mandatory that flow be monitored with an electromagnetic flowmeter as the band is tightened because little reduction in flow will be achieved until the vessel has been narrowed to about 50% of its original diameter, the "point of critical stenosis" (see Chapter 7). Beyond this point, flow drops off rapidly (see Fig. 7–9). Flow should be fixed between 400 and 700 ml/min in upper extremity fistulae and between 300 and 900 ml/min in lower extremity fistulae.* In practice, this is often difficult to accomplish.

THERAPEUTIC USES OF ARTERIOVENOUS FISTULAE

In addition to their widespread use for vascular access, arteriovenous fistulae have been employed to enhance limb growth, to ensure the patency of vascular anastomoses, and to revascularize ischemic extremities.

Enhancement of Limb Growth

The presence of a congenital arteriovenous fistula or a traumatic fistula in a limb before epiphyseal closure appears to stimulate bone growth.[128] This same phenomenon has been demonstrated experimentally in puppies with iliac arteriovenous fistulae.[149] Because of these observations, surgeons have constructed superficial femoral arteriovenous fistulae in children in an effort to increase the length of legs shortened as a result of poliomyelitis or congenital absence of a hip joint. In about 75% of these cases, there has been either no change or a relative increase in the length of the limb.[46, 113, 148] In rare instances, unfortunately, a serious complication, such as edema, venous distention, stasis ulceration, hemorrhage, endarteritis, cystic degeneration of the femoral vein, or cardiac enlargement, may develop.[26, 113]

It is difficult to explain why an acquired arteriovenous fistula should stimulate bone growth. Ingebrigtsen and colleagues noted that the oxygen tension was decreased in the tibial metaphysis of canine limbs with femoral arteriovenous fistulae.[141] Rogers and Aust found that blood flow in bones distal to arteriovenous fistulae was reduced.[229] Moreover, Henrie and associates were unable to demonstrate increased rates of healing of femoral or fibular fractures in animals with iliac arteriovenous fistulae.[110] These

*See reference 3 for upper extremity; see reference 83 for lower extremity.

observations are consistent with the dynamics of flow distal to acquired arteriovenous fistulae, as outlined previously. Ordinarily, flow in the peripheral tissues ranges from normal to severely reduced, and blood pressure is inevitably decreased.

Other investigators, however, have reported experimental data suggesting increased perfusion of bony tissues distal to an arteriovenous fistula. These findings include:

- Elevated temperature on the surface and within the intramedullary portion of the bone*
- Increased intramedullary pressure
- Hypervascularity of the intramedullary small vessels and capillaries

Apparently, vessels in the vicinity or within the bone contribute to the collateral pathways bypassing the fistula. Another explanation for increased bone growth involves the increased peripheral venous pressure that accompanies a proximally located fistula. Venous stasis has been shown to stimulate bone growth.[135]

The mechanism by which congenital fistulae accelerate bone growth is somewhat easier to comprehend. Typically, these lesions are diffuse, and the arteriovenous communications often involve bone. Increased blood flow through these communications sometimes stimulates bone growth as a result of the associated high oxygen tensions and elevated temperatures.

Use in Reconstructive Vascular Surgery

Among the frequently reported causes of early failure of vascular operations is sluggish blood flow. Placing an arteriovenous fistula distal to the reconstructed segment increases the rate of flow through the critical area, thereby decreasing the likelihood of thrombosis.

This method has been used successfully to maintain the patency of endarterectomies and bypass grafts in ischemic limbs with poor runoff.[16, 17, 136, 164] Initially, the use of an arteriovenous fistula for this purpose might seem counterproductive because all arteriovenous communications tend to "steal" blood from the periphery. Indeed, the creation of a fistula between a distal artery (e.g., the posterior tibial artery in the lower leg) and an adjacent vein would be quite detrimental to the blood supply to the foot in the presence of severe obstructive disease in the inflow arteries. Diversion of blood away from the posterior tibial artery would further reduce the already low pressure perfusing the distal vascular bed. However, when all proximal obstructions have been bypassed by a graft of sufficiently large caliber to carry the augmented blood flow without a significant pressure drop, the pressure in the posterior tibial artery at the site of the anastomosis will be increased.

Thus, patency of the graft is protected by the more rapidly flowing blood, and peripheral perfusion is improved by the increased pressure head. Placing the fistula at the site of the graft-artery anastomosis best fulfills the hemodynamic requirements outlined earlier.[53, 145] Although some surgeons have reported good clinical results when arteriovenous fistulae are constructed at some distance below the graft-artery anastomosis,[210, 221] there are theoretical arguments against this approach. If the intervening artery is widely patent, there is no problem; however, if this segment is or becomes stenotic, the increased blood flow supplying the fistula causes an additional drop in blood pressure and, consequently a reduction in the pressure head perfusing the distal tissues. In this situation, graft patency would be preserved and flow would be augmented in the intervening segment, but the tissues distal to the fistula would suffer.

Failure to ligate all of the tributaries of the saphenous vein during infrainguinal in situ bypass grafting often leads to the development of arteriovenous fistulae. A significant proportion of the blood entering the graft at its proximal end may be diverted into these fistulae. As long as the caliber of the vein is good, this rarely has an adverse effect on graft patency or function[36, 203]; however, when there is a stenosis in the graft above one or more large fistulae, the augmented blood flow may increase the pressure drop across the stenosis, which in turn may have a detrimental effect on peripheral perfusion.[202]

Arteriovenous fistulae have also been used to increase blood flow through reconstructed venous segments.[70, 115, 157, 214] That this surgical ploy improves long-term patency after femoral venous thrombectomy or venous bypass grafting is well accepted. To avoid peripheral venous hypertension, the surgeon must ensure that the fistula is not too large relative to the diameter of the reconstructed segment.[187] Venous hypertension would thwart the purpose of the reconstruction, which is to alleviate congestion in the peripheral veins by restoring venous outflow.

By constructing an arteriovenous fistula in the forearm, surgeons have been able to convert cephalic veins, which were previously too narrow and thin-walled to serve as satisfactory bypass grafts, into conduits of adequate thickness and diameter.[112] These "arterialized" veins are suitable for distal tibial and peroneal reconstruction in the absence of a suitable saphenous vein. This approach, however, is seldom used.

Revascularization of Ischemic Extremities

Surgeons have long entertained the hope that arterialization of the venous system might be used to improve the circulation to ischemic extremities.[236] Most of these attempts have met with only limited success.[267] In an early review of the literature, only three of 42 patients who received arteriovenous fistulae for the treatment of threatened or existing gangrene of the extremity experienced any prolonged benefits from the procedure.[108] Szilagyi and associates, in 1951, reported nine consecutive failures of femoral arteriovenous fistulae used for treating occlusive arterial disease.[277] Nevertheless, sporadic reports of good results continue to appear in the literature.[43, 89, 144] Sheil described the use of the saphenous vein, in situ, to transport blood retrograde from a proximal arterial anastomosis at the femoral level to the dorsum of the foot.[247] He believed that this procedure avoided amputation in three of six limbs with severe ischemia.

Several groups have reported favorable results in experimental preparations with a Y-type arteriovenous fistula.[39, 95, 153, 184, 230, 289] Basically, a Y-type fistula consists of an end

---

*See reference 160 for elevated temperature; see reference 266 for increased intramedullary pressure and vascularity.

of proximal artery–side of vein anastomosis with the distal artery tied off. In most of these studies, enhanced limb survival associated with the construction of an arteriovenous fistula has been the major criterion for improved circulation. However, the paper by Gerard and colleagues does provide objective documentation of improved nutrition of previously ischemic tissues.[95] These investigators showed that (1) the Y-type fistula increased intramuscular PO_2 in ischemic dog limbs from 5.3 mmHg to a nearly normal value of 45.5 mmHg, (2) the pH of the muscle surface increased from 7.06 to 7.40, (3) segmental blood pressures returned to normal, (4) toe pulse reappearance times decreased, and (5) toe plethysmograms approached normal volumes and configurations.

The following mechanisms have been postulated to explain the rationale for using this procedure:

1. Arteriovenous fistulae constitute a powerful stimulus for the development of collateral circulation.
2. Retrograde arterial flow in the distal venous limb may be able to nourish the peripheral tissues.

Based on current knowledge of the physiology of arteriovenous fistulae, it is difficult to understand how these changes would benefit the peripheral circulation. As Reid stated in 1925, "It would seem mere folly to expect any benefit from a fistula made between large vessels far removed from the part you are trying to help."[217] Although arteriovenous fistulae stimulate collateral development to a greater degree than simple occlusions do, the increased size of the collaterals is due to their role in supplying retrograde flow to the distal artery rather than antegrade flow to the peripheral tissues. Indeed, collateral development is markedly impaired when the artery is ligated just distal to the fistula, as it is in the Y-type anastomosis.[122] Therefore, there is little justification for believing that collaterals developed after such an anastomosis would significantly augment peripheral blood flow.[17] It is true that the Y-type fistula would have *fewer detrimental* effects than an H-type fistula because there would be no reversal of flow in the distal arterial limb and less steal from the peripheral tissues.

Although reversal of flow in the distal vein has been clearly demonstrated with Y- or H-type fistulae, it has never been shown that the blood flow in the capillary bed is reversed or even that this "arterialized" blood ever reaches the capillary bed. In fact, angiograms show that all of the blood containing enough contrast to be visible is transferred directly back to the heart by way of numerous venous collaterals. Some of the blood, however, might reach the venules and flow retrograde through the capillary bed and high-resistance terminal arterioles into the obstructed arteries of the ischemic extremity, which also would have a very high resistance. Once in these obstructed arteries, the blood would not flow retrograde into the major arteries but would have to be diverted back again to the venous system through terminal arterioles, capillaries, and venules.

Clearly, the only way in which such a system could work is for the reversed venous flow to find its way into the terminal arterioles through low-resistance peripheral arteriovenous shunts and then back through the capillaries proper into *another* nonarterialized vein.[144] Furthermore, most clinical and experimental observations have shown

that high distal venous pressure is actually detrimental to the peripheral circulation.[17, 20, 62, 105, 191, 270] It is well known, for example, that large residual subcutaneous fistulae associated with in situ bypass grafting may cause localized edema, inflammation, and possibly even skin necrosis. If, indeed, arterialization of the venous system does improve tissue nutrition, the mechanism remains obscure. For these reasons, a healthy skepticism toward the use of arteriovenous fistulae for revascularization of ischemic limbs seems justified.[294]

ARTERIOVENOUS ANASTOMOSES

The preceding portions of this chapter have covered *abnormal* communications between arteries and veins. There are, however, *normally* occurring connections between arteries and veins, called arteriovenous anastomoses. Arteriovenous anastomoses are situated proximal to the capillary bed, have no connections with the capillaries, and shunt blood away from the capillaries. Most are short, thick-walled structures, but some are long and tortuous. The arteriovenous glomus is a complex form, consisting of multiple channels composed of epithelioid cells surrounded by a connective tissue sheath.

All arteriovenous anastomoses are richly innervated by sympathetic nerve fibers. Because of their thick walls, it is unlikely that any exchange of nutrients or gases takes place between the anastomoses and the interstitial fluid. Unlike capillaries, which have a luminal diameter of about 7 μm and are composed of endothelial cells only, arteriovenous anastomoses commonly have an internal diameter of 20 to 40 μm (some exceed 100 μm) and have walls that are heavily invested with smooth muscle cells.

Arteriovenous anastomoses should be distinguished from *thoroughfare* or *preferential channels*, which have been described in some microvascular beds. Basically, these channels are enlarged capillaries that traverse a more direct route between arterioles and venules than true capillaries do. They have a few muscle fibers scattered in their walls, serve as the origin for most of the true capillaries, and probably function to regulate blood flow in the capillaries.

Although arteriovenous anastomoses have been found in most of the major vascular beds, those with diameters exceeding 20 μm are sparse or absent in the lung, liver, kidney, stomach, and intestine.[59] In muscles, they are confined to the intramuscular septa and tendons. They are most common in the nailbeds and occur frequently in the volar or plantar surfaces of the fingers, toes, hands, and feet; they are virtually absent in the skin of the calf or forearm. They are also found in the skin of the nose and ears. In the canine hindlimb, removal of the paw and skin virtually eliminates arteriovenous shunting.

Although one can estimate the volume of blood flowing through arteriovenous anastomoses by measuring the "nutrient" or capillary blood flow with xenon 133 or sodium radioiodide (iodine 131) and then subtracting this value from the total organ blood flow measured with a plethysmograph or an electromagnetic flowmeter, a more direct estimation can be obtained by using radionuclide-labeled microspheres (see Chapter 100). Intra-arterially injected microspheres with a diameter of about 20 to 30 μm will be trapped in the peripheral capillaries but will pass unimpeded through arteriovenous anastomoses to the lungs, where they will be filtered out. If the radioactivity of the injected microspheres is known and the radioactivity of the lungs is measured, it is a relatively simple matter to calculate the fraction of blood that is diverted through arteriovenous shunts. Under normal circumstances, only 1% to 5% of the total blood flow to the limb passes through these anastomoses.

Arteriovenous anastomoses are surgically important, in that they may exert a detrimental effect on cellular nutrition in ischemic tissues, may divert blood away from the capillaries in septic areas, may contribute to the formation of varicose veins, and may provide a rational explanation for the conflicting opinions regarding the efficacy of sympathectomy. Moreover, when one attempts to estimate the physiologic significance of congenital or acquired arteriovenous fistulae, it is necessary to distinguish normal arteriovenous shunting from pathologic shunting (see Chapter 100).

Physiology

Arteriovenous anastomoses dilate in response to warmth and constrict in response to cold. They seem to serve a thermoregulatory function. Whereas local application of heat to the peripheral tissues has little effect on the degree of shunting, central body heating increases the fraction of blood shunted through arteriovenous anastomoses from a few per cent to about 25% of the total blood flowing through the extremity.[296] Cooling, both central and peripheral, diminishes anastomotic flow almost to zero. It is postulated that the central nervous system senses the temperature of the arriving blood. When the temperature is elevated, sympathetic tone is relaxed and the arteriovenous anastomoses, which are innervated by sympathetic fibers, dilate. Because these structures are almost entirely confined to the skin and acral regions of the body, their dilatation acts to shunt blood from the deeper tissues into the superficial veins, where the excess heat can be radiated from the body. Closure of the anastomoses in response to cold conserves heat by reducing surface flow and by diverting blood into the deeper tissues.

Responses to various drugs indicate that the innervation of arteriovenous anastomoses is exclusively sympathetic and that the receptors are alpha-adrenergic. Administration of phenoxybenzamine and phentolamine, both alpha-receptor blockers, greatly increases shunting,[48, 61, 258] although propranolol, a beta-blocker, and isoproterenol, a beta-stimulator, have no effect.[61, 258] Papaverine dilates both capillaries and arteriovenous anastomoses, but adenosine triphosphate (ATP) increases only capillary flow and has no effect on shunt flow.[61] Anesthetic agents, both general and regional, augment arteriovenous shunting—an important consideration when one measures flow through arteriovenous fistulae in the anesthetized patient.

Short periods of ischemia (5 minutes) apparently have no effect on arteriovenous anastomoses.[48] Reactive hyperemia is therefore a manifestation of increased capillary blood flow. Long periods of ischemia (2 hours), likewise, have no immediate effect on arteriovenous anastomoses, but 24 hours later shunting is greatly increased.[162] Thus,

increased shunting is in part responsible for the delayed hyperemia that occurs when tourniquets are used to produce a bloodless field in certain operations.

Pathophysiology

Hypoxia greatly increases the flow of blood through arteriovenous anastomoses. Approximately one third of the blood flowing through an extremity may be shunted away from the capillary bed under the influence of hypoxia. Hypoventilation, which creates respiratory acidosis, hypercarbia, and mild hypoxia, has a similar effect. Both metabolic acidosis and pure hypercarbia increase flow through arteriovenous anastomoses, but the effect is less than that caused by hypoxia.[59]

Ischemic tissues are hypoxic, probably acidotic, and hypercarbic. Therefore, local ischemia, such as that occurring in conjunction with severe arterial disease, most likely increases arteriovenous shunting. This in turn would have a further detrimental effect on tissue nutrition because blood diverted away from the capillaries would serve no metabolic function. The observations of Delaney provide some support for this concept. In two of seven severely ischemic human limbs, he found that 13% and 25% of the total limb blood flow, respectively, was being shunted.[59]

The effect of sepsis on flow through arteriovenous anastomoses remains controversial. It is known that oxygen utilization within septic tissues is not increased despite an increase in blood flow. The difference between oxygen saturation of the arterial blood entering the affected region and that of the venous blood leaving the region is reduced. Using radionuclide-labeled microspheres, Cronenwett and Lindenauer demonstrated that 22% of the blood entering the septic hindlimbs of dogs was being shunted through arteriovenous anastomoses.[49] On the other hand, Archie observed little change in the shunt fraction in dogs with septic, or endotoxin-induced, shock, except in areas of local inflammation.[7]

For many years, it has been suspected that arteriovenous anastomoses play a role in the genesis of varicose veins. Blalock reported increased oxygen tension in varicose veins,[18] and Haimovici and associates demonstrated numerous arteriovenous maculae in the soles of the feet of patients with varicose veins.[107] Using the operating microscope, Schalin visualized direct connections between arteries with a diameter of 100 μm and varicosities.[210] That arterial flow signals can be detected with Doppler flowmetry along the course of varicose veins lends some support to these observations,[106] but the possibility that these signals may represent hyperemic flow in inflamed tissues has not been excluded.

Increased flow through arteriovenous anastomoses occurs in patients with hypertrophic pulmonary osteopathy and cirrhosis but not in patients with Paget's disease. In decompensated cirrhotic patients, precapillary arteriovenous shunting occurs in the lower extremities as demonstrated by radionuclide labeled microsphere studies, a reduction in the difference between femoral arterial and venous oxygen content, increase in femoral arterial blood flow, and a decrease in femoral and systemic vascular resistance.[85] An associated increase in vascular capacitance may diminish the effective blood volume, thus setting the stage for renal sodium retention by elevating plasma renin and aldosterone levels.

Sympathectomy

Because arteriovenous anastomoses are controlled by the sympathetic nervous system, it is not surprising to find that surgical sympathectomy increases the fraction of shunt flow to 20% to 30% of the total flow through the limb.[48, 50, 60] In ischemic canine hindlimbs, sympathectomy increases flow through arteriovenous anastomoses but has no effect on capillary perfusion, results in no increase in oxygen consumption, and causes no increase in tissue oxygen tension.[50, 213] All of the increased blood flow is confined to the skin and terminal regions of the extremities.[59, 60] There is no increase in blood flow through muscles, either at rest or during exercise.

Therefore, these results question the rationale for using sympathectomy in the treatment of peripheral arterial disease (see Chapter 7). Any apparent relief of claudication must not be a function of increased muscle blood flow. Likewise, there is little evidence that the increased peripheral blood flow has any effect on tissue nutrition because most of the increased flow is diverted through arteriovenous anastomoses, where it serves no nutritive purpose.

REFERENCES

1. Ahearn DJ, Maher JF: Heart failure as a complication of hemodialysis arteriovenous fistula. Ann Intern Med 77:201, 1972.
2. Alvarez JJP, Vargas-Rosendo R, Gutierrez-Bosque R, et al: A new type of subcutaneous arteriovenous fistula for chronic hemodialysis in children. Surgery 67:355, 1970.
3. Anderson CB, Groce MA: Banding of arteriovenous dialysis fistulas to correct high-output cardiac failure. Surgery 78:552, 1975.
4. Anderson CB, Codd JR, Graff RA, et al: Cardiac failure and upper extremity arteriovenous dialysis fistulas: Case reports and a review of the literature. Arch Intern Med 136:292, 1976.
5. Anderson CB, Etheredge EE, Harter HR, et al: Blood flow measurements in arteriovenous dialysis fistulas. Surgery 81:459, 1977.
6. Anderson CB, Etheredge EE, Harter HR, et al: Local blood flow characteristics of arteriovenous fistulas in the forearm for dialysis. Surg Gynecol Obstet 144:531, 1977.
7. Archie JP Jr: Anatomic arterial-venous shunting in endotoxic and septic shock in dogs. Ann Surg 186:171, 1977.
8. Attinger EO, Sugawara H, Navarro A, et al: Pulsatile flow patterns in distensible tubes. Circ Res 18:447, 1966.
9. Baker CRF Jr: Complications and management of methods of dialysis access for renal failure. Am Surg 42:859, 1976.
10. Baker WH, Sharzer LA, Ehrenhaft JL: Aortocaval fistula as a complication of abdominal aortic aneurysms. Surgery 72:933, 1972.
11. Baur GM, Porter JM, Fletcher WS: Human umbilical cord vein allograft arteriovenous fistula for chemotherapy access. Am J Surg 138:238, 1979.
12. Beall AC Jr, Cooley DA, Morris GC Jr, et al: Perforation of arteriosclerotic aneurysms into inferior vena cava. Arch Surg 86:809, 1963.
13. Bigger IA: Treatment of traumatic aneurysms and arteriovenous fistulas. Arch Surg 49:170, 1944.
14. Binak K, Regan TJ, Christensen RC, et al: Arteriovenous fistula: Hemodynamic effects of occlusion and exercise. Am Heart J 60:495, 1960.
15. Bjorkholm M, Aschberg S: Hemodynamic influence of multiple congenital arteriovenous fistulas. Acta Med Scand 200:333, 1976.
16. Blaisdell FW, Lim RC Jr, Hall AD: Reconstruction of small arteries with an arteriovenous fistula, an experimental study. Arch Surg 92:206, 1966.
17. Blaisdell FW, Lim RC Jr, Hall AD, et al: Revascularization of severely

18. Blalock A: Oxygen content of blood in patients with varicose veins. Arch Surg 19:898, 1929.
19. Blundell PE, Tobin JR Jr, Swan HJC: Effect of right ventricular hypertrophy on infundibular pressure gradients in dogs. Am J Physiol 209:513, 1965.
20. Blutt KMH, Friedman EA, Kountz SL: Angioaccess. Curr Probl Surg 13:1, 1976.
21. Bramann F: Arterio-venous aneurism. Arch Klin Chir 33:1, 1886.
22. Branham HH: Aneurismal varix of the femoral artery and vein following a gunshot wound. Int J Surg 3:250, 1890.
23. Brener BJ, Brief DK, Alpert J, et al: The effect of vascular access procedures on digital hemodynamics. In Diethrich EB (ed): Noninvasive Cardiovascular Diagnosis. Current Concepts. Baltimore, University Park Press, 1978, pp 189–203.
24. Breschet G: Mémorie sur les aneurysmes. Mem Acad R Med Paris 3:101, 1833.
25. Brescia MJ, Cimino JE, Appel K, et al: Chronic hemodialysis using venipuncture and surgically created arteriovenous fistula. N Engl J Med 275:1089, 1966.
26. Breslau RC: Complications of arteriovenous fistula induced for augmentation of limb growth. Surgery 63:1012, 1968.
27. Briden KL, Weiss HR: Effect of moderate arterio-venous shunt on regional extraction, blood flow, and oxygen consumption in the dog heart. Cardiovasc Res 15:206, 1981.
28. Brooks B: The treatment of traumatic arteriovenous fistula. South Med J 23:100, 1930.
29. Brunner JH, Stanley RJ: Superior mesenteric arteriovenous fistula. JAMA 223:316, 1973.
30. Buselmeier TJ, Rattazzi LC, Kjellstrand CM, et al: A modified arteriovenous fistula applicable where there is thrombosis of standard Brescia-Cimino fistula vasculature. Surgery 74:551, 1973.
31. Bussell JA, Abbott JA, Lim RC: A radial steal syndrome with arteriovenous fistula for hemodialysis. Ann Intern Med 75:387, 1971.
32. Byrne JP, Stevens LE, Weaver DH, et al: Advantages of surgical arteriovenous fistulas for hemodialysis. Arch Surg 102:359, 1971.
33. Callander CL: Study of arterio-venous fistulae with analysis of 447 cases. Ann Surg 71:428, 1920.
34. Cerilli J, Limbert JG: Technique and results of the construction of arteriovenous fistulas for hemodialysis. Surg Gynecol Obstet 137:922, 1973.
35. Cerra FB, Shapiro RI, Anthone S, et al: Clinically significant arteriovenous fistulas: Physiologic response to acute occlusion. Surg Forum 28:208, 1977.
36. Chang BB, Leopold PW, Kupinski AM, et al: In situ bypass hemodynamics: The effect of residual A-V fistulae. J Cardiovasc Surg 30:843, 1989.
37. Cheek RC, Messina JJ, Acchiardo SR, et al: Arteriovenous fistulas for hemodialysis: Experience with 100 cases. Am Surg 42:386, 1976.
38. Coel MN, Alksne JF: Embolization to diminish high output failure secondary to systemic angiomatosis (Ullman's syndrome). Vasc Surg 12:336, 1978.
39. Cohen SE, Matolo NM, Wolfman EF Jr: Arteriovenous fistula for revascularization of the ischemic extremity. Vasc Surg 10:238, 1976.
40. Cohen SM, Edholm OG, Howarth S, et al: Cardiac output and peripheral blood flow in arteriovenous aneurysms. Clin Sci 7:35, 1948.
41. Cohn HE, Solit RW: Arteriovenous fistulas for chronic hemodialysis. Surg Clin North Am 53:673, 1973.
42. Corry RJ, Patel NP, West JC: Surgical management of complications of vascular access for hemodialysis. Surg Gynecol Obstet 151:49, 1980.
43. Courbier R, Jausseran JM, Reggi M: Le shunt saphéno-fémoral dans les ischémies sévères des membres inférieurs. J Chir (Paris) 105:441, 1973.
44. Coursley G, Ivins JC, Barker NW: Congenital arteriovenous fistulas in the extremities: An analysis of 69 cases. Angiology 7:201, 1956.
45. Cowley AW Jr, Guyton AC: Heart rate as a determinant of cardiac output in dogs with arteriovenous fistula. Am J Cardiol 28:321, 1971.
46. Cranley JJ: Arteriovenous fistulas. In Vascular Surgery. Peripheral Arterial Diseases. Vol I. Hagerstown, Md, Harper and Row, 1972, pp 171–185.
47. Crocker DW, Cleland RS: Infantile hemangioendothelioma of the liver: Report of three cases. Pediatrics 19:596, 1957.

48. Cronenwett JL, Lindenauer SM: Direct measurement of arteriovenous anastomotic blood flow after lumbar sympathectomy. Surgery 82:82, 1977.
49. Cronenwett JL, Lindenauer SM: Direct measurement of arteriovenous anastomotic blood flow in septic canine hind limb. Surgery 85:275, 1979.
50. Cronenwett JL, Lindenauer SM: Hemodynamic effects of sympathectomy in ischemic canine hind limbs. Surgery 87:417, 1980.
51. Cross FS, Glover DM, Simeone FA, et al: Congenital arteriovenous aneurysms. Ann Surg 148:649, 1958.
52. Crowe CP, Schenk WG Jr: Massive experimental arteriovenous fistulas. J Trauma 3:13, 1963.
53. Dardik H, Berry SM, Dardik A, et al: Infrapopliteal prosthetic graft patency by use of the distal adjunctive arteriovenous fistula. J Vasc Surg 13:685, 1991.
54. Dardik H, Dardik I, Strom MG, et al: Intravenous rupture of arteriosclerotic aneurysms of the abdominal aorta. Surgery 80:647, 1976.
55. Dardik H, Ibrahim IM, Dardik I: Arteriovenous fistulas constructed with modified umbilical cord vein graft. Arch Surg 111:60, 1976.
56. Davis JO, Urquhart J, Higgins JT Jr, et al: Hypersecretion of aldosterone in dogs with a chronic aortic-caval fistula and high output heart failure. Circ Res 14:471, 1964.
57. Dawkins HG Jr, Vargish T, James PM Jr: Comparable hemodynamics of surgical arteriovenous fistulae in dogs. J Surg Res 18:169, 1975.
58. DeBakey ME, Cooley DA, Morris GC Jr, et al: Arteriovenous fistulae involving the abdominal aorta: Report of four cases with successful repair. Ann Surg 147:646, 1958.
59. Delaney JP: Control of arteriovenous anastomoses in the limb. In Rutherford RB (ed): Vascular Surgery. Philadelphia, WB Saunders, 1977, pp 785–791.
60. Delaney JP, Scarpino J: Limb arteriovenous shunting following sympathetic denervation. Surgery 73:202, 1973.
61. Delaney JP, Zanick DC, Scarpino JH: Control of arteriovenous shunting. Surg Forum 23:241, 1972.
62. Delpin EAS: Swelling of the hand after arteriovenous fistula for hemodialysis. Am J Surg 132:373, 1976.
63. Deterling RA Jr, Essex HE, Waugh JM: Arteriovenous fistula: Experimental study of influence of sympathetic nervous system on the development of collateral circulation. Surg Gynecol Obstet 84:629, 1947.
64. Deterling RA Jr, Essex HE, Waugh JM: Experimental studies of arteriovenous fistula with regard to the development of collateral circulation. Mayo Clin Proc 22:495, 1947.
65. Dodge HT, Kennedy JW, Petersen JL: Quantitative angiocardiographic methods in the evaluation of valvular heart disease. Prog Cardiovasc Dis 16:1, 1973.
66. Dongradi G, Rocha P, Baron B, et al: Hemodynamic effects of arteriovenous fistulae in chronic hemodialysis patients at rest and during exercise. Clin Nephrol 15:75, 1981.
67. Dorney ER: Peripheral A-V fistula of fifty-seven years' duration with refractory heart failure. Am Heart J 54:778, 1957.
68. Dry TJ, Horton BT: Traumatic arteriovenous fistula involving the right femoral artery and vein: Spontaneous closure. Arch Surg 33:248, 1936.
69. D'Silva J, Fouché RF: The effect of changes in flow on the caliber of the large arteries. J Physiol 150:23P, 1960.
70. Edwards WS: A-V fistula after venous reconstruction: A simplified method of producing and obliterating the shunt. Ann Surg 196:669, 1982.
71. Ehrenfeld WK, Grausz H, Wylie EJ: Subcutaneous arteriovenous fistulas for hemodialysis. Am J Surg 124:200, 1972.
72. Eiseman B, Hughes RH: Repair of an abdominal aortic vena caval fistula caused by rupture of an atherosclerotic aneurysm. Surgery 39:498, 1956.
73. Elkin DC: Operative treatment of aneurysm and arteriovenous fistula. South Med J 39:311, 1946.
74. Elkin DC, Shumacker HB Jr: Arterial aneurysms and arteriovenous fistulas: General considerations. In Elkin DC, DeBakey ME (eds): Surgery in World War II: Vascular Surgery. Washington, DC, Office of the Surgeon General, Department of the Army, 1955, pp 149–180.
75. Elkin DC, Warren JV: Arteriovenous fistulas: Their effect on the circulation. JAMA 134:1524, 1947.
76. Engelberts I, Tordoir JH, Boon ES, Schreij G: High-output cardiac failure due to excessive shunting in a hemodialysis access fistula: an easily overlooked diagnosis. Am J Nephrol 15:323, 1995.
77. Epstein FH, Ferguson TB: The effect of the formation of an arteriovenous fistula upon blood volume. J Clin Invest 34:434, 1955.
78. Epstein FH, Post RS, McDowell M: The effect of an arteriovenous fistula on renal hemodynamics and electrolyte excretion. J Clin Invest 32:233, 1953.
79. Epstein FH, Shadle OW, Ferguson TB, et al: Cardiac output and intracardiac pressures in patients with arteriovenous fistulas. J Clin Invest 32:543, 1953.
80. Fallon JT, Stehbens WE: Venous endothelium of experimental arteriovenous fistulas in rabbits. Circ Res 31:546, 1972.
81. Fee HJ Jr, Golding AL: Lower extremity ischemia after femoral arteriovenous bovine shunts. Ann Surg 183:42, 1976.
82. Fee HJ Jr, Levisman JA, Dickmeyer JP, et al: Hemodynamic consequences of femoral arteriovenous bovine shunts. Ann Surg 184:103, 1976.
83. Fee HJ, Levisman J, Doud RB, et al: High-output congestive failure from femoral arteriovenous shunts for vascular access. Ann Surg 183:321, 1976.
84. Ferguson GG, Roach MR: Flow conditions at bifurcations as determined in glass models with reference to the focal distribution of vascular lesions. In Bergel DH (ed): Cardiovascular Fluid Dynamics. Vol 2. London, Academic Press, 1972, pp 141–156.
85. Fernández-Rodriguez CM, Prieto J, Zozaya JM, et al: Arteriovenous shunting, hemodynamic changes, and renal sodium retention in liver cirrhosis. Gastroenterology 104:1139, 1993.
86. Fillinger MF, Kerns DB, Bruch D, et al: Does the end-to-end venous anastomosis offer a functional advantage over the end-to-side venous anastomosis in high-output arteriovenous grafts? J Vasc Surg 12:676, 1990.
87. Fillinger MF, Reinitz ER, Schwartz RA, et al: Graft geometry and venous intimal-medial hyperplasia in arteriovenous loop grafts. J Vasc Surg 11:556, 1990.
88. Foley PJ, Allen EV, Janes JM: Surgical treatment of acquired arteriovenous fistulas. Am J Surg 91:611, 1956.
89. Fontaine R, Kim M, Kieny R, et al: Resultats obtenus par 39 derivations artério-veineuses pour oblitérations artérielles périphériques. J Chir (Paris) 83:321, 1962.
90. Frank CW, Wang H, Lammerant J, et al: An experimental study of the immediate hemodynamic adjustments to acute arteriovenous fistulae of various sizes. J Clin Invest 34:772, 1955.
91. Freeman LW, Shumacker HB Jr, Finneran JC, et al: Studies with arteriovenous fistulas: II. Influence of posture upon volume flow. Surgery 31:180, 1952.
92. Freeman NE: Arterial repair in the treatment of aneurysms and arteriovenous fistulae: A report of eighteen successful restorations. Ann Surg 124:888, 1946.
93. Frishman W, Epstein AM, Kulick S, et al: Heart failure 63 years after traumatic arteriovenous fistula. Am J Cardiol 34:733, 1974.
94. George CRP, May J, Schieb M, et al: Heart failure due to an arteriovenous fistula for hemodialysis. Med J Aust 1:696, 1973.
95. Gerard DF, Gausewitz SM, Dilley RB, et al: Acute physiologic effects of arteriovenous anastomosis and fistula in revascularizing the ischemic canine hind limb. Surgery 89:485, 1981.
96. Gerbode F, Holman E, Dickenson EH, et al: Arteriovenous fistulas and arterial aneurysms: The repair of major arteries injured in warfare, and the treatment of an arterial aneurysm with a vein graft inlay. Surgery 32:259, 1952.
97. Girerd X, London G, Boutouyrie P, et al: Remodeling of the radial artery in response to a chronic increase in shear stress. Part 2. Hypertension 27:799, 1996.
98. Glass IH, Rowe RD, Duckworth JWA: Congenital arteriovenous fistula between the left internal mammary artery and the ductus venosus: Unusual cause of congestive heart failure in the new born infant. Pediatrics 26:604, 1960.
99. Göthlin J, Lindstedt E: Angiographic features of Cimino-Brescia fistulas. AJR 125:582, 1975.
100. Graham JM, McCollum CH, Crawford ES, et al: Extensive arterial aneurysm formation proximal to ligated arteriovenous fistula. Ann Surg 191:200, 1980.
101. Gunderman W: Cited in Allen EV, Barker NW, Hines EA Jr: Peripheral Vascular Diseases, 3rd ed. Philadelphia, WB Saunders, 1962, p 476.
102. Gupta PD, Singh M: Neural mechanism underlying tachycardia induced by nonhypotensive a-v shunt. Am J Physiol 236:H35, 1979.
103. Guyton AC, Sagawa K: Compensations of cardiac output and other

circulatory functions in areflex dogs with large A-V fistulas. Am J Physiol 200:1157, 1961.

104. Haimov M, Singer A, Schupak E: Access to blood vessels for hemodialysis: Experience with 87 patients on chronic hemodialysis. Surgery 69:834, 1971.

105. Haimov M, Baez A, Neff M, et al: Complications of arteriovenous fistulas for hemodialysis. Arch Surg 110:708, 1975.

106. Haimovici H: Arteriovenous shunting in varicose veins: Its diagnosis by Doppler ultrasound flow detector. J Vasc Surg 2:684, 1985.

107. Haimovici H, Steinman C, Caplan LH: Role of arteriovenous anastomoses in vascular disease of the lower extremity. Ann Surg 164:990, 1966.

108. Halstead AE, Vaugh RT: Arteriovenous anastomosis in the treatment of gangrene of the extremities. Surg Gynecol Obstet 14:1, 1912.

109. Harrison TR, Dock W, Holman E: Experimental studies in arteriovenous fistulae: Cardiac output. Heart 11:337, 1924.

110. Henrie JN, Johnson EW Jr, Wakim KG, et al: The influence of experimental arteriovenous fistula on the healing of fractures and on the blood flow distal to the fistula. Surg Gynecol Obstet 108:591, 1959.

111. Herringman EC, Rives JD, Davis HA: The repair of arteriovenous fistulas, evaluation of operative procedures, and analysis of fifty-three cases. JAMA 133:633, 1947.

112. Hertzer NR, Abud-Ortega AR: Cephalic vein arteriovenous fistula preceding lower-extremity arterial bypass. Vasc Diag Ther 2:57, 1981.

113. Hieronni T: Arteriovenous fistula for discrepancy in length of lower extremities. Acta Orthop Scand 31:25, 1961.

114. Hilton JG, Kanter DM, Hays DR, et al: The effect of acute arteriovenous fistula on renal functions. J Clin Invest 34:732, 1955.

115. Hobson RW II, Wright CB: Peripheral side-to-side arteriovenous fistula: Hemodialysis and application in venous reconstruction. Am J Surg 126:411, 1973.

116. Hobson RW II, Croom RD III, Swan KG: Hemodynamics of the distal arteriovenous fistula in venous reconstruction. J Surg Res 14:483, 1973.

117. Hol R, Ingebrigtsen R: Experimental arteriovenous fistulae. Acta Radiol 55:337, 1961.

118. Holman E: Arteriovenous aneurysm: Clinical evidence correlating size of fistula with changes in the heart and proximal vessels. Ann Surg 80:801, 1924.

119. Holman E: Arteriovenous Aneurysm: Abnormal Communications Between the Arterial and Venous Circulations. New York, Macmillan, 1937.

120. Holman E: The anatomic and physiologic effects of an arteriovenous fistula. Surgery 8:362, 1940.

121. Holman E: Roentgenologic kymographic studies of the heart in the presence of an arteriovenous fistula and their interpretation. Ann Surg 124:920, 1946.

122. Holman E: Problems in the dynamics of blood flow: I. Conditions controlling collateral circulation in the presence of an arteriovenous fistula, following the ligation of an artery. Surgery 26:880, 1949.

123. Holman E: New Concepts in Surgery of the Vascular System. Springfield, Ill, Charles C Thomas, 1955.

124. Holman E: Contributions to cardiovascular physiology gleaned from clinical and experimental observations of abnormal arteriovenous communications. J Cardiovasc Surg 3:48, 1962.

125. Holman E: The vicissitudes of an idea: The significance of total blood volume in the story of arteriovenous fistula. Rev Surg 20:153, 1963.

126. Holman E: Abnormal arteriovenous communications: Great variability of effects with particular reference to delayed development of cardiac failure. Circulation 32:1001, 1965.

127. Holman E, Taylor G: Problems in the dynamics of blood flow: II. Pressure relations at site of an arteriovenous fistula. Angiology 3:415, 1952.

128. Horton BT: Hemihypertrophy of extremities associated with congenital arteriovenous fistula. JAMA 98:373, 1932.

129. Huang M, Hester RL, Guyton AC: Hemodynamic changes in rats after opening an arteriovenous fistula. Am J Physiol 262:H846, 1992.

130. Hughes CW, Jahnke EJ Jr: The surgery of traumatic arteriovenous fistulas and aneurysms: A five-year follow-up study of 215 lesions. Ann Surg 148:790, 1958.

131. Humphreys MH, Al-Bander H, Eneas JF, et al: Factors determining electrolyte excretion and renin secretion after closure of an arteriovenous fistula in the dog. J Lab Clin Med 98:89, 1981.

132. Hunt TK, Leeds FH, Wanebo HJ, et al: Arteriovenous fistulas of major vessels in the abdomen. J Trauma 11:483, 1971.

133. Hunter W: Further observations upon a particular species of aneurysm. Med Observ Inquiry 2:390, 1764.

134. Hurwich BJ: Brachial arteriography of the surgically created radial arteriovenous fistula in patients undergoing chronic intermittent hemodialysis by venipuncture technique. AJR 104:394, 1968.

135. Hutchinson WJ, Bordeaux BD Jr: The influence of stasis on bone growth. Surg Gynecol Obstet 99:413, 1954.

136. Ibrahim IM, Sussman B, Dardik I, et al: Adjunctive arteriovenous fistula with tibial and peroneal reconstruction for limb salvage. Am J Surg 140:246, 1980.

137. Ingebrigtsen R, Husom O: Local blood pressure in congenital arteriovenous fistulae. Acta Med Scand 163:169, 1959.

138. Ingebrigtsen R, Wehn PS: Local blood pressure and direction of flow in experimental arteriovenous fistula. Acta Chir Scand 120:142, 1960.

139. Ingebrigtsen R, Fönstelien E, Solberg LA: Measurement of forces producing longitudinal stretching of the arterial wall, examined in the artery proximal to an arteriovenous fistula. Acta Chir Scand 136:569, 1970.

140. Ingebrigtsen R, Krog J, Leraand S: Velocity and flow of blood in the femoral artery proximal to an experimental arteriovenous fistula. Acta Chir Scand 124:45, 1962.

141. Ingebrigtsen R, Krog J, Leraand S: Circulation distal to experimental arterio-venous fistulas of the extremities: A polarographic study. Acta Chir Scand 125:308, 1963.

142. Ingebrigtsen R, Johansen K, Müller O, et al: Blood pressure of the proximal artery in experimental arterio-venous fistulas of long standing. Acta Chir Scand 253(Suppl):134, 1950.

143. Ingebrigtsen R, Lie M, Hol R, et al: Dilatation of the iliofemoral artery following the opening of an experimental arteriovenous fistula in the dog. Scand J Clin Lab Invest 31:255, 1973.

144. Inoue G, Tamura Y: The use of an afferent arteriovenous fistula in digit replantation surgery: A report of two cases. Br J Plast Surg 44:230, 1991.

145. Jacobs MJHM, Gregoric ID, Reul GJ: Prosthetic graft placement and creation of a distal arteriovenous fistula for secondary vascular reconstruction in patients with severe limb ischemia. J Vasc Surg 15:612, 1992.

146. Jahnke EJ Jr, Howard JM: Primary repair of major arterial injuries: A report of fifty-eight battle casualties. Arch Surg 66:646, 1953.

147. Jamison JP, Wallace WFM: The pattern of venous drainage of surgically created side-to-side arteriovenous fistulae in the human forearm. Clin Sci Mol Med 50:37, 1976.

148. Janes JM, Jennings WK Jr: Effect of induced arteriovenous fistula on leg length: 10-year observations. Mayo Clin Proc 36:1, 1961.

149. Janes JM, Musgrove JE: Effect of arteriovenous fistula on growth of bone: An experimental study. Surg Clin North Am 30:1191, 1950.

150. Jendrisak MD, Anderson CB: Vascular access in patients with arterial insufficiency: Construction of proximal bridge fistulae based on inflow from axillary branch arteries. Ann Surg 212:187, 1990.

151. Jenkins A McL, Buist TAS, Glover SD: Medium-term follow-up of forty autogenous vein and forty polytetrafluoroethylene (Gore-Tex) grafts for vascular access. Surgery 88:667, 1980.

152. Joannides R, Haefeli WE, Linder L, et al: Nitric oxide is responsible for flow-dependent dilatation of human peripheral conduit arteries in vivo. Circulation 91:1314, 1995.

153. Johansen K, Bernstein EF: Revascularization of the ischemic canine hind limb by arteriovenous reversal. Ann Surg 190:243, 1979.

154. John HT, Warren R: The stimulus to collateral circulation. Surgery 49:14, 1961.

155. Johnson G Jr, Blythe WB: Hemodynamic effects of arteriovenous shunts used for hemodialysis. Ann Surg 171:715, 1970.

156. Johnson JM, Kenoyer MR, Johnson KE, et al: The modified bovine heterograft in vascular access for chronic hemodialysis. Ann Surg 183:62, 1976.

157. Johnson V, Eiseman B: Evaluation of arteriovenous shunt to maintain patency of venous autograft. Am J Surg 118:915, 1969.

158. Joyce PF, Sundaram M, Riaz MA, et al: Embolization of extensive peripheral angiodysplasias. Arch Surg 115:665, 1980.

159. Kamiya A, Togawa T: Adaptive regulation of wall shear stress to flow change in the canine carotid artery. Am J Physiol 239:H14, 1980.

160. Kelly PJ, Janes JM, Peterson LFA: The effect of arteriovenous fistulae on the vascular pattern of the femora of immature dogs, a microangiographic study. J Bone Joint Surg 41:1101, 1959.

161. Kennedy JA, Burwell CS: Measurement of the circulation in a patient with multiple arteriovenous communications. Am Heart J 28:133, 1944.
162. Kennedy TJ, Miller SH, Nellis SH, et al: Effects of transient ischemia on nutrient and arteriovenous shunting in canine hind limbs. Ann Surg 193:255, 1981.
163. Kinnaert P, Struyven J, Mathieu J, et al: Intermittent claudication of the hand after creation of an arteriovenous fistula in the forearm. Am J Surg 139:838, 1980.
164. Kusaba A, Inokuchi K, Furuyama M, et al: A new revascularization procedure for extensive arterial occlusions of lower extremity: A-V shunt procedure. J Cardiovasc Surg 23:99, 1982.
165. Kwun KB, Schanzer H, Finkler N, et al: Hemodynamic evaluation of angioaccess procedures for hemodialysis. Vasc Surg 13:170, 1979.
166. Lamport H, Baez S: Physical properties of small arterial vessels. Physiol Rev 42(Suppl 5):328, 1962.
167. Lavigne JE, Kerr JC, Swan KG: Hemodynamic effects of multiple arteriovenous fistulae in the canine hind limb. J Surg Res 20:571, 1976.
168. Lavigne JE, Brown CS, Fewel J, et al: Hemodynamics within a canine femoral arteriovenous fistula. Surgery 77:439, 1975.
169. Lavigne JE, Mesinna LM, Golding MR, et al: Fistula size and hemodynamic events within and about canine femoral arteriovenous fistulas. J Thorac Cardiovasc Surg 74:551, 1977.
170. Lees RS, Dewey CF Jr: Phonoangiography: A new noninvasive method for studying arterial disease. Proc Natl Acad Sci U S A 67:935, 1970.
171. Leslie MB, Portin BA, Schenk WG: Cardiac output and posture studies in chronic experimental arteriovenous fistulas. Arch Surg 81:123, 1960.
172. Levine OR, Jameson AG, Nellkaus G, et al: Cardiac complications of cerebral arteriovenous fistula in infancy. Pediatrics 30:563, 1962.
173. Levowitz BS, Flores L, Dunn I, et al: Prosthetic arteriovenous fistula for vascular access in hemodialysis. Am J Surg 132:368, 1976.
174. Lewis T, Drury AN: Observations relating to arteriovenous aneurism. Heart 10:301, 1923.
175. Lie M, Sejersted OM, Kiil F: Local regulation of vascular cross-section during changes in femoral arterial blood flow in dogs. Circ Res 27:727, 1970.
176. Lindenauer SM, Thompson NW, Kraft RO, et al: Late complications of traumatic arteriovenous fistulas. Surg Gynecol Obstet 129:525, 1969.
177. Lindstedt E, Westling H: Effects of an antebrachial Cimino-Brescia arteriovenous fistula on the local circulation in the hand. Scand J Urol Nephrol 9:119, 1975.
178. Liu Z, Hilbelink DR, Crokett WB, Gerdes AM: Regional changes in hemodynamics and cardiac myocyte size in rats with aortocaval fistulas: 1. Developing and established hypertrophy. Circ Res 69:52, 1991.
179. Lough FC, Giordano JM, Hobson RW II: Regional hemodynamics of large and small femoral arteriovenous fistulas in dogs. Surgery 79:346, 1976.
180. Mahmutyazicioglu K, Kesenci M, Fitoz S, et al: Hemodynamic changes in the early phase of artificially created arteriovenous fistula: color Doppler ultrasonographic findings. J Ultrasound Med 16:813, 1997.
181. Makins GH: The Bradshaw lecture on gunshot injuries of the arteries. Lancet 2:1743, 1913.
182. Marinescu V, Pâusescu E, Fâgâãsanu D, et al: Metabolic factors in the cardiac insufficiency of arteriovenous fistula. Ann Surg 164:1027, 1966.
183. Matas R: Arteriovenous fistula of the femoral vessels (aneurysmal varix) on a level with the origin of the profunda. War injury of two years' duration: Dissection and mobilization of the femoral vessels with division and detachment of the anastomosis followed by separate lateral suture of the artery and vein, with perfect functional restoration of the circulation. Details of technic and commentaries. Surg Clin North Am 2:1165, 1922.
184. Matolo NM, Cohen SE, Wolfman EF Jr: Use of an arteriovenous fistula for treatment of the severely ischemic extremity: Experimental evaluation. Ann Surg 184:622, 1976.
185. May J, Tiller D, Johnson J, et al: Saphenous vein arteriovenous fistula in regular dialysis treatment. N Engl J Med 280:770, 1969.
186. McMillan R, Evans DB: Experience with three Brescia-Cimino shunts. Br Med J 3:781, 1968.
187. Menawat SS, Gloviczki P, Mozes G, et al: Effect of femoral arteriovenous fistula on lower extremity venous hemodynamics after femorocaval reconstruction. J Vasc Surg 24:793, 1996.
188. Merickel JH, Andersen RC, Knutson R, et al: Bovine carotid artery shunts in vascular access surgery: Complications in the chronic hemodialysis patient. Arch Surg 109:245, 1974.
189. Miller VM, Burnett JC Jr: Modulation of NO and endothelin by chronic increases in blood flow in canine femoral arteries. Am J Physiol 263: H108, 1992.
190. Miller VM, Vanhoutte PM: Enhanced release of endothelium-derived factor(s) by chronic increases in blood flow. Am J Physiol 255: H446, 1988.
191. Mindich B, Dunn I, Frumkin E, et al: Proximal venous thrombosis after side-to-side arteriovenous fistula. Arch Surg 108:227, 1974.
192. Mooney CS, Honaker AD, Griffen WO Jr: Influence of the liver on arteriovenous fistulas. Arch Surg 100:154, 1970.
193. Mozes M, Adar R, Eliahou HE, et al: Internal arteriovenous anastomoses for hemodialysis: Technical modifications and results of two years' experience. Vasc Surg 5:21, 1971.
194. Muenster JJ, Graettinger JS, Campbell JA: Correlation of clinical and hemodynamic findings in patients with systemic arteriovenous fistulas. Circulation 20:1079, 1959.
195. Nakano J: Effect of arteriovenous fistula on the cardiovascular dynamics. Jpn Heart J 12:392, 1971.
196. Nakano J, DeSchryver C: Effects of arteriovenous fistula on systemic and pulmonary circulations. Am J Physiol 207:1319, 1964.
197. Nakano J, Zekert H, Griege CW, et al: Effect of ventricular tachycardia and arteriovenous fistula on catecholamine blood level. Am J Physiol 200:413, 1961.
198. Nanu I, Alexandrescu-Dersca C, Lazeanu E: Les troubles cardiaques consécutifs. Aux anévrismes artério-veineux. Arch Mal Coeur 15:829, 1922.
199. Newman DL, Gosling RG, King DH, et al: Turbulence in bifurcation grafts. J Surg Res 13:63, 1972.
200. Nickerson JL, Elkin DC, Warren JV: The effect of temporary occlusion of arteriovenous fistulas on heart rate, stroke volume, and cardiac output. J Clin Invest 30:215, 1951.
201. Nicoladoni C: Phlebarteriectasie der rechten oberen Extremität. Arch Klin Chir 18:252, 1875.
202. Nielsen TG, Djurhuus C, Pedersen EM, et al: Arteriovenous fistulas aggravate the hemodynamic effect of vein bypass stenoses: An in vitro study. J Vasc Surg 24:1043, 1996.
203. Nielsen TG, Vogt K, Sillesen H, Schroeder TV: The haemodynamic effect of residual arteriovenous fistulae in in situ saphenous vein bypasses. J Vasc Invest 1:135, 1995.
204. Nishikimi T, Frohlich ED: Glomerular hemodynamics in aortocaval fistula rats: Role of renin-angiotensin system. Am J Physiol 264:R681, 1993.
205. Odland MD, Kelly PH, Ney AL, et al: Management of dialysis-associated steal syndrome complicating upper extremity arteriovenous fistulas: Use of intraoperative digital photoplethysmography. Surgery 110:664, 1991.
206. Olcott C, Newton TH, Stoney RJ, et al: Intra-arterial embolization in the management of arteriovenous malformations. Surgery 79:3, 1976.
207. Paruk S, Koenig M, Levitt S, et al: Arteriovenous fistulas for hemodialysis in 100 consecutive patients. Am J Surg 131:552, 1976.
208. Pasch TH, Bauer RD, Von der Emde J: Hemodynamic effects of an experimental chronic arteriovenous fistula. Res Exp Med 161:110, 1973.
209. Patel KR, Chan FA, Batista RJ, Clauss RH: True venous aneurysms and arterial "steal" secondary to arteriovenous fistulae dialysis. J Cardiovasc Surg 33:185, 1992.
210. Paty PSK, Shah DM, Saifi J, et al: Remote distal arteriovenous fistula to improve infrapopliteal bypass patency. J Vasc Surg 11:171, 1990.
211. Pauporte J, Lowenstein JM, Richards V, et al: Blood turnover rates distal to an arteriovenous fistula. Surgery 43:828, 1958.
212. Pemberton J de J, Saint JH: Congenital arteriovenous communications. Surg Gynecol Obstet 46:470, 1928.
213. Perry MO, Horton J: Muscle and subcutaneous oxygen tension: Measurements by mass spectrometry after sympathectomy. Arch Surg 113:176, 1978.
214. Rabinowitz R, Goldfarb D: Surgical treatment of axillosubclavian venous thrombosis: A case report. Surgery 70:703, 1971.
215. Ravitch MM, Gaertner RA: Congenital arteriovenous fistula in the

neck: 48-year follow-up of a patient operated upon by Dr. Halsted in 1911. Bull Johns Hopkins Hosp 107:31, 1960.

216. Reid MR: The effect of arteriovenous fistula upon the heart and blood-vessels: An experimental and clinical study. Bull Johns Hopkins Hosp 31:43, 1920.

217. Reid MR: Abnormal arteriovenous communications, acquired and congenital: III. The effects of abnormal arteriovenous communications on the heart, blood vessels, and other structures. Arch Surg 11:25, 1925.

218. Reid MR, McGuire J: Arteriovenous aneurysms. Ann Surg 108:643, 1938.

219. Reilly DT, Wood RFM, Bell PRF: Arteriovenous fistulas for dialysis: Blood flow, viscosity, and long-term patency. World J Surg 6:628, 1982.

220. Reiser IW, Chou S-Y, Porush JG: Failure of atrial natriuretic peptide to induce natriuresis in aortocaval fistula dogs. Kidney Int 42:867, 1992.

221. Ricco JB, Gauthier JB, Richer J-P, et al: Remote arteriovenous fistula with infrapopliteal polytetrafluoroethylene bypass for critical ischemia. Ann Vasc Surg 5:525, 1991.

222. Rich NM, Hughes CW, Baugh JH: Management of venous injuries. Ann Surg 171:724, 1970.

223. Rivers SP, Scher LA, Veith FJ: Correction of steal syndrome secondary to hemodialysis access fistulas: A simplified quantitative technique. Surgery 112:593, 1992.

224. Roach MR: An experimental study of the production and time course of post-stenotic dilatation in the femoral and carotid arteries of adult dogs. Circ Res 13:537, 1963.

225. Rob C, Eastcott HHG: Five unusual arteriovenous fistulae. Br J Surg 42:63, 1954.

226. Robertson MG: Spontaneous rupture of an abdominal aortic aneurysm into the inferior vena cava. Am J Med 42:1011, 1967.

227. Robertson RL, Dennis EW, Elkin DC: Collateral circulation in the presence of experimental arteriovenous fistula, determination by direct measurement of extremity blood flow. Surgery 27:1, 1950.

228. Rockard S, Ikeda K, Montes M: An analysis of mechanisms of post stenotic dilatation. Angiology 18:348, 1967.

229. Rogers W, Aust JB: The effect of arteriovenous fistula on tissue blood flow in the canine limb. Vasc Surg 8:238, 1974.

230. Root HD, Cruz AB Jr: Effects of an arteriovenous fistula on the devascularized limb. JAMA 191:645, 1965.

231. Rowe GG, Castillo CA, Afonso S, et al: The systemic and coronary hemodynamic effects of arteriovenous fistulas. Am Heart J 64:44, 1962.

232. Ryan KG, Lorber SH: Traumatic fistula between hepatic artery and portal vein. Report of a case. N Engl J Med 279:1215, 1968.

233. Sabiston DC Jr, Theilen EO, Gregg DE: Physiologic studies in experimental high output cardiac failure produced by aortic-caval fistula. Surg Forum 6:233, 1955.

234. Sako Y, Varco RL: Arteriovenous fistula: Results of management of congenital and acquired forms, blood flow measurements, and observations on proximal arterial degeneration. Surgery 67:40, 1970.

235. Samet P, Berstein WH, Jacobs W, et al: Indicator-dilution curves in systemic arteriovenous fistulas. Am J Cardiol 13:176, 1964.

236. San Martin y Satrustegui A: Anastomose arterioveineuse pour remedier à obliteration des artères des membres. Bull Med 16:451, 1902.

237. Schalin L: Arteriovenous communications in varicose veins localized by thermography and identified by operative microscopy. Acta Chir Scand 147:409, 1981.

238. Schanzer H, Schwartz M, Harrington E, Haimov M: Treatment of ischemia due to "steal" by arteriovenous fistula with distal artery ligation and revascularization. J Vasc Surg 7:770, 1988.

239. Schenk WG Jr, Bahn RA, Cordell AR, et al: The regional hemodynamics of experimental acute arteriovenous fistulas. Surg Gynecol Obstet 105:733, 1957.

240. Schenk WG Jr, Martin JW, Leslie MB, et al: The regional hemodynamics of chronic experimental arteriovenous fistulas. Surg Gynecol Obstet 110:44, 1960.

241. Scherer PW: Flow in axisymmetrical glass model aneurysms. J Biomech 6:695, 1973.

242. Schreiner GE, Freinkel N, Athens JW, et al: Cardiac output, central volume and dye injection curves in traumatic arteriovenous fistulas in man. Circulation 7:718, 1953.

243. Schreiner GE, Freinkel N, Athens JW, et al: Dynamics of T-1824 distribution in patients with traumatic arteriovenous fistulas. Circ Res 1:548, 1953.

244. Schuman ES, Gross GF, Hayes JF, et al: Long-term patency of polytetrafluoroethylene graft fistulas. Am J Surg 155:644, 1988.

245. Schwartz LB, Purut CM, O'Donohoe MK, et al: Quantitation of vascular outflow by measurement of impedance. J Vasc Surg 14:353, 1991.

246. Seeley SF, Hughes CW, Cook FN, et al: Traumatic arteriovenous fistulas and aneurysms in war wounded: A study of 101 cases. Am J Surg 83:471, 1952.

247. Sheil AGR: Treatment of critical ischemia of the lower limb by venous arterialization: An interim report. Br J Surg 64:197, 1977.

248. Shumacker HB Jr: The problem of maintaining the continuity of the artery in the surgery of aneurysms and arteriovenous fistulae: Notes on the development and clinical application of methods of arterial suture. Ann Surg 127:207, 1948.

249. Shumacker HB Jr: Test for and means of improving the collateral circulation in cases of aneurysm and arteriovenous fistula of the extremities. Angiology 5:167, 1954.

250. Shumacker HB Jr: Arterial aneurysms and arteriovenous fistulas: Spontaneous cures. In Elkin DC, DeBakey ME (eds): Surgery in World War II: Vascular Surgery. Washington, DC, Office of the Surgeon General, Department of the Army, 1955, pp 361–374.

251. Shumacker HB Jr: Aneurysm development and degenerative changes in dilated artery proximal to arteriovenous fistula. Surg Gynecol Obstet 130:636, 1970.

252. Shumacker HB Jr, Carter KL: Tests for collateral circulation in the extremities. Arch Surg 53:359, 1946.

253. Shumacker HB Jr, Stahl NMD: A study of the cardiac frontal area in patients with arteriovenous fistulas. Surgery 26:928, 1949.

254. Simkins TE, Stehbens WE: Vibrations recorded from the adventitial surface of experimental aneurysms and arteriovenous fistulas. Vasc Surg 8:153, 1974.

255. Solberg LA, Harkness RD, Ingebrigtsen R: Hypertrophy of the median coat of the artery in experimental arteriovenous fistula. Acta Chir Scand 136:575, 1970.

256. Solti F, Soltész L, Bodor E: Hemodynamic changes of systemic and limb circulation in extremital arteriovenous fistula. Angiologica 9:69, 1972.

257. Spellman MW, Mandal A, Freeman HP, et al: Successful repair of an arteriovenous fistula between the superior mesenteric vessels secondary to a gunshot wound. Ann Surg 165:458, 1967.

258. Spence RJ, Rhodes BA, Wagner HN Jr: Regulation of arteriovenous anastomotic and capillary blood flow in the dog leg. Am J Physiol 222:326, 1972.

259. Spencer FC, Grewe RV: Management of arterial injuries in battle casualties. Ann Surg 141:304, 1955.

260. Spielman WS, Davis JO, Gotshall RW: Hypersecretion of renin in dogs with a chronic aortic-caval fistula and high-output heart failure. Proc Soc Exp Biol Med 143:479, 1973.

261. Spurny OM, Pierce JA: Cardiac output in systemic arteriovenous fistulas complicated by heart failure. Am Heart J 61:21, 1961.

262. Stehbens WE: Turbulence of blood flow in the vascular system of man. In Copley AL, Stainsby G (eds): Flow Properties of Blood. London, Pergamon Press, 1960, pp 137–140.

263. Stehbens WE: Blood vessel changes in chronic experimental arteriovenous fistulas. Surg Gynecol Obstet 127:327, 1968.

264. Stehbens WE: The ultrastructure of the anastomosed vein of experimental arteriovenous fistulae in sheep. Am J Pathol 76:377, 1974.

265. Stehbens WE, Karmody AM: Venous atherosclerosis associated with arteriovenous fistulas for hemodialysis. Arch Surg 110:176, 1975.

266. Stein AH, Morgan HC, Porras R: The effect of an arteriovenous fistula on intramedullary bone pressure. Surg Gynecol Obstet 109:287, 1959.

267. Stetton D: The futility of arteriovenous anastomosis in the treatment of impending gangrene of the lower extremity. Surg Gynecol Obstet 20:381, 1915.

268. Stewart FT: Arteriovenous aneurysm treated by angiorrhaphy. Ann Surg 57:574, 1913.

269. Stone HH, Jordan WD, Acker JJ, et al: Portal arteriovenous fistulas: Review and case report. Am J Surg 109:191, 1965.

270. Storey BG, George CRP, Stewart JH, et al: Embolic and ischemic complications after anastomosis of radial artery to cephalic vein. Surgery 66:325, 1969.

271. Strandness DE Jr, Sumner DS: Arteriovenous fistulas. In Hemodynamics for Surgeons. New York, Grune & Stratton, 1975, pp 621–663.

272. Strandness DE Jr, Gibbons GE, Bell JW: Mercury strain gauge plethysmography: Evaluation of patients with acquired arteriovenous fistula. Arch Surg 85:215, 1962.
273. Sullivan KL, Besarab A, Dorrell S, Moritz MJ: The relationship between dialysis graft pressure and stenosis. Invest Radiol 27:352, 1992.
274. Sumner DS: Arteriovenous fistula. In Strandness DE Jr (ed): Collateral Circulation in Clinical Surgery. Philadelphia, WB Saunders, 1969, pp 27–90.
275. Sumner DS, Wilcox MW, Strandness DE Jr: Physiological studies of arteriovenous fistulas constructed for hemodialysis. Unpublished data.
276. Sumner RG, Kistler PC, Barry WF Jr, et al: Recognition and surgical repair of superior mesenteric arteriovenous fistula. Circulation 27:943, 1963.
277. Szilagyi DE, Jay GE, Munnel ED: Femoral arteriovenous anastomosis in the treatment of occlusive arterial disease. Arch Surg 63:435, 1951.
278. Szilagyi DE, Elliott JP, DeRusso FJ, et al: Peripheral congenital arteriovenous fistulas. Surgery 57:61, 1965.
279. Szilagyi DE, Smith RF, Elliott JP, et al: Congenital arteriovenous anomalies of the limbs. Arch Surg 111:423, 1976.
280. Szilagyi DE, Whitcomb JG, Schenker W, et al: The laws of fluid flow and arterial grafting. Surgery 47:55, 1960.
281. Taylor RR, Covell JW, Ross J Jr: Left ventricular function in experimental aorto-caval fistula with circulatory congestion and fluid retention. J Clin Invest 47:1333, 1968.
282. Tellis VA, Veith FJ, Soberman RJ, et al: Internal arteriovenous fistula for hemodialysis. Surg Gynecol Obstet 132:866, 1971.
283. Thoma R: Untersuchungen; auuber die Histogenese und Histomechanik des Gefassystems. Stuttgart, Enke, 1893.

284. Thompson BW, Barbour G, Bissett J: Internal arteriovenous fistula for hemodialysis. Am J Surg 124:785, 1972.
285. Timmis AD, McGonigle RJS, Weston MJ, et al: The influence of hemodialysis fistulas on circulating dynamics and left ventricular function. Int J Artif Organs 5:101, 1982.
286. Urquhart J, Davis JO, Higgins JT: Simulation of spontaneous secondary hyperaldosteronism by intravenous infusion of angiotensin II in dogs with an arteriovenous fistula. J Clin Invest 43:1355, 1964.
287. van Gemert MJC, Bruyninckx CMA: Simulated hemodynamic comparison of arteriovenous fistulas. J Vasc Surg 6:39, 1987.
288. Van Loo A, Heringman EC: Circulatory changes in the dog produced by acute arteriovenous fistula. Am J Physiol 158:103, 1949.
289. Vetto RM, Belzer FO: Use of an arterio-bone fistula in advanced ischemia. Surg Forum 16:131, 1965.
290. Wakim KG, Janes JM: Influence of arteriovenous fistula on the distal circulation in the involved extremity. Arch Phys Med 39:413, 1958.
291. Walker WJ, Mullins CE, Knovick GC: Cyanosis, cardiomegaly, and weak pulses: A manifestation of massive congenital systemic arteriovenous fistula. Circulation 24:777, 1964.
292. Warren JV, Elkins DC, Nickerson JL: The blood volume in patients with arteriovenous fistulas. J Clin Invest 30:220, 1951.
293. Warren JV, Nickerson JL, Elkins DC: The cardiac output in patients with arteriovenous fistulas. J Clin Invest 30:210, 1951.
294. Warren R: Can the venous system be made to act in situ for the arterial system? Arch Surg 112:1238, 1977.
295. Wattanasirichaigoon S, Pomposelli FB Jr: Branham's sign is an exaggerated Bezold-Jarisch reflex of arteriovenous fistula. J Vasc Surg 26:171, 1997.
296. Zanick DC, Delaney JP: Temperature influences on arteriovenous anastomoses. Proc Soc Exp Biol Med 144:616, 1973.

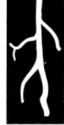

CHAPTER 100

Diagnostic Evaluation of Arteriovenous Fistulae

Robert B. Rutherford, M.D., and
David S. Sumner, M.D.

The clinical features that play a role in the diagnosis of acquired and congenital arteriovenous fistulae are discussed in Chapters 102 and 103 and are not described here. This chapter reviews a variety of methods that may assist the clinician in making the diagnosis, in evaluating the hemodynamic effects of the lesion, and in planning a therapeutic approach. Some have broad applications; others are useful only in certain settings.

PRESSURE MEASUREMENTS AND COMPRESSION TESTING

The mean arterial blood pressure distal to an arteriovenous fistula is always reduced to some degree (see Chapter 99*).

*The reader is also referred to various figures in Chapter 99.

This is the result of shunting of blood away from the peripheral vascular bed into the low-resistance pathway offered by the arteriovenous communication.[56] The reduction in pressure is particularly severe when the fistula is large and the arterial collaterals are small. Even when collaterals are well developed, reversal of flow in the distal artery further decreases peripheral arterial pressure because much of the collateral flow is diverted back into the fistulous circuit and never reaches the periphery (the basis for a distal steal); however, when the fistula is small and the collaterals are large, there may be little or no perceptible effect on the peripheral pressure. Thus, the magnitude of the pressure drop across a fistula can provide the surgeon with an objective assessment of its hemodynamic consequences (Fig. 100–1).[4, 11, 29, 47, 56, 57]

Although arterial pressures can be measured most accu-

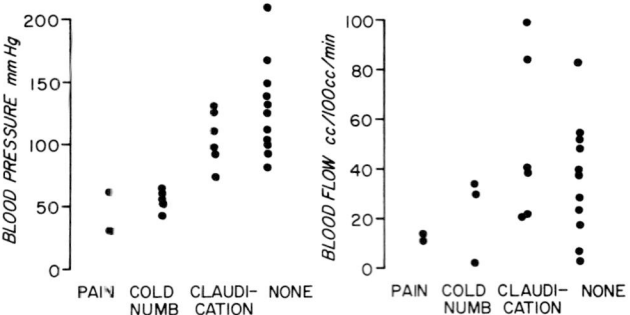

FIGURE 100–1. Relationship between symptoms and hemodynamic measurements in the index fingers of patients with side-to-side radial artery–cephalic vein fistulae. Blood pressure was measured at the proximal phalanx, and blood flow was measured in the distal phalanx. Note that pressure measurements correlate well with the patient's symptoms, whereas flow measurements do not.

rately with a transducer, this technique requires percutaneous puncture of the vessel, a rather sophisticated apparatus, and some technical skill. Noninvasive methods of measuring systolic blood pressure are usually sufficiently accurate and are painless, rapid, and much less cumbersome. A pneumatic cuff is placed around the part at the selected site and inflated above systolic pressure. As the cuff is deflated, the point at which blood flow returns distal to the cuff is noted on an aneroid or mercury manometer. Return of flow can be detected with a Doppler flowmeter, a mercury-in-Silastic (rubber silicone) strain-gauge, a photoplethysmograph, or a pulse volume recorder (see Chapter 10). In the upper extremity, pressure measurements can be made at the upper arm, forearm, wrist, or finger level; in the lower extremity, they can be made at the thigh, calf, ankle, foot, or toe.

Of course, low peripheral pressure does not necessarily imply the presence of an arteriovenous fistula because low pressures in limbs or digits are far more often due to obstructive arterial disease. If, however, compression of a pulsatile mass, the artery distal to a suspicious lesion, or a large proximal or distal vein causes the peripheral pressure to rise, the diagnosis of an arteriovenous fistula is established (see Chapter 99, Fig. 99–14). No other lesion of the arterial or venous tree behaves in this fashion. Compression of these vessels in aneurysmal disease, in obstructive arterial disease, or in venous disorders either causes no change in the pressure or, as is usually the case, causes it to *fall*.

On the other hand, a drop in peripheral blood pressure with compression of a suspected lesion does not rule out the possibility that it is a fistula. In most cases, it is impossible to exert pressure on a localized fistula without also narrowing the lumen of the associated artery. Therefore, when the peripheral tissues continue to depend on antegrade flow in the artery distal to the arteriovenous communication, compression of the fistula, because it interferes with this flow, causes peripheral blood pressure to drop (see Fig. 99–5). This is especially likely when the fistula is small or the collateral arteries are poor.

It must also be pointed out that a normal peripheral pressure does not rule out the presence of a congenital arteriovenous fistula. In fact, the *systolic* pressure may even be elevated in comparison with that of the opposite limb

at the same level.[48] This apparent paradox occurs when the pressure cuff has been placed over the site of the fistula or its afferent tributaries. Because the arteries supplying the fistula are dilated, and thus have reduced resistance to blood flow, the segmental pressure drop near the fistula is less than what would normally be expected at the same anatomic level. This same phenomenon has been noted in the proximal artery leading to an acquired fistula. In addition, the pressure may normally be elevated if it is measured *proximal* to the fistula and only *systolic* pressure is measured. Even though mean pressure is reduced in the arterial tree as one approaches an arteriovenous fistula, the pressure swings between systolic and diastolic (i.e., the pulse pressure) may be greater, so that systolic pressure may, in fact, be elevated proximal to a fistula.

By noting the effect on peripheral blood pressure produced by compression of the various vessels that make up the fistulous circuit, we can obtain a clear idea of their contribution to fistula flow.[11, 56] If compression of the distal or proximal veins produces little or no change in peripheral pressure, it is probable that only a small amount of the total fistula flow is exiting through that particular vein. If there is a distinct rise in pressure at the periphery, however, it is safe to assume that the vein constitutes an important outflow channel for the fistula. If compression of the distal artery causes a rise in peripheral pressure, it is likely that there is retrograde flow in this vessel. If compression causes a drop in peripheral pressure, the distal arterial flow is almost certainly antegrade.

Compression of the proximal artery always causes some decrease in peripheral pressure. When flow in the distal artery is derived entirely from the proximal artery, compression of proximal arterial flow causes a decrease in peripheral perfusion. Antegrade flow in the distal artery comes to a halt and may even be replaced by retrograde flow. When flow in the distal artery is already retrograde, compression of the proximal artery produces a relative increase in this retrograde flow, further aggravating the peripheral steal.

Compression of collateral arteries gives some idea of the extent to which they contribute to the nutrition of the peripheral tissues.[11, 56] Obviously, if blocking flow in these vessels causes a marked drop in peripheral pressure, it can be assumed that they play a vital role in supplying blood to the distal portions of the extremity.

One may also evaluate collateral arteries by noting the effect on peripheral pressure of compressing the fistula and the immediately associated vessels.[4, 11, 56, 57] If the pressure rises or does not change significantly with occlusion of the fistula and of the proximal and distal arteries and veins, the limb will certainly tolerate quadruple ligation and excision. If the peripheral pressure falls markedly, excisional surgery would be hazardous, and some sort of arterial reconstruction must be performed to ensure viability of the limb.

Pressure measurements are also useful in assessing the physiologic results of surgical therapy. Successful reconstruction should return peripheral pressures to normal levels.[29, 57] Pressures should improve (or at least not fall) after quadruple ligation and excision, provided that the collateral input is adequate. Finally, the efficacy of ligating individual component vessels of a surgically created arteriovenous fistula to decrease steal or restrict retrograde venous flow can be evaluated by pressure measurement. Testing this is extremely important when one is dealing with a symptomatic distal steal associated with an angioaccess arteriovenous fistula (see Chapter 104).

Invasive pressure measurements during surgery may be useful to determine the magnitude of the steal.[10] Swan-Ganz catheterization provides valuable hemodynamic data that not only facilitate the diagnosis of massive fistulae, such as those that develop between the aorta and the inferior vena cava or renal veins, but also aid in their perioperative management.[27, 34]

PLETHYSMOGRAPHY

Examination of plethysmographic pulse-volume tracings in the arms, legs, fingers, or toes may be helpful in making the diagnosis of arteriovenous fistula and in assessing its hemodynamic significance. Air-filled cuffs (e.g., the pulse volume recorder), photoplethysmographs, or mercury-in-Silastic strain-gauges (see Chapter 10) can be used.

Although the pulse contour may be normal (or nearly so) in a limb distal to an arteriovenous fistula, its volume is frequently reduced, particularly in the presence of a steal (Fig. 100–2).[4, 8, 11, 47, 56, 57] As with peripheral pressure measurements, the reduction in pulse volume depends on the size of the fistula and the adequacy of the collateral arteries. Successful reconstruction returns the pulse volume and contour to normal values.[8, 57] Although the volume of the pulse may increase after quadruple ligation and excision, the pulse usually has an "obstructive" contour.

When the pulse-sensing device is placed over the fistula or just proximal to it, the pulse volume may actually increase.[47, 48] This is commonly seen in limbs with congenital arteriovenous malformations, the increased pulsation being almost diagnostic (Fig. 100–3).

If compression of a lesion suspected of being an arteriovenous fistula—or of the distal artery or venous drainage—causes an immediate increase in pulse volume, the diagnosis of arteriovenous fistula is virtually confirmed (see Fig. 99–12). Although it is true that a similar reaction might be observed in other situations involving arterial steal (e.g., in the donor limb when a cross-pubic femoro-femoral graft is compressed), it does not occur with other spontaneous or traumatic lesions.

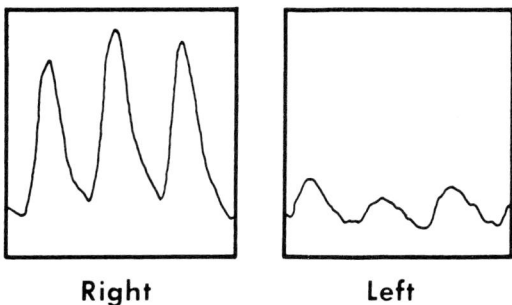

FIGURE 100–2. Plethysmographic pulses from the second toes of a patient with an acute fistula between the left superficial femoral artery and vein.

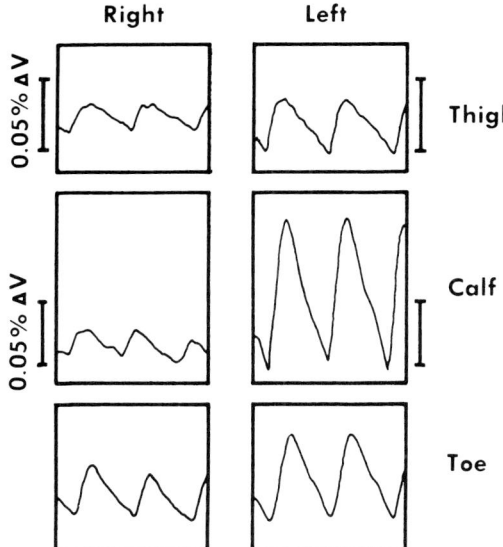

FIGURE 100–3. Plethysmographic pulses obtained with a mercury-in-Silastic strain-gauge at thigh, calf, and toe levels in a 4-year-old girl with a congenital arteriovenous fistula of the left pelvic region. The pulses measured: right thigh, 0.02% ΔV; left thigh, 0.04% ΔV; right calf, 0.03% ΔV; and left calf, 0.11% ΔV. Increased pulses on the left side suggest the presence of further arteriovenous malformations at multiple levels in the leg. ΔV = difference in velocity.

VOLUME FLOW MEASUREMENTS

It might seem that volume flow measurements would be a valuable component of the diagnostic assessment of arteriovenous fistulae; however, depending on the technique and the location of the fistula, they may be either difficult to perform or inaccurate and not reproducible.

Measurement of blood flow with venous occlusion plethysmography may be used to estimate the quantity of blood flowing through a limb that harbors an arteriovenous fistula.[24, 59] Unfortunately, the accuracy of this technique is compromised when the occluding cuff is proximal to the fistula because the venous pressure rises almost immediately to equal cuff pressure. This causes the limb volume to increase so rapidly that a good slope is difficult to obtain. Nevertheless, venous occlusion plethysmography can be used to measure flow distal to the fistula with a fair degree of accuracy.[4, 56] It has also been used to measure flow through wrist fistulae created for angioaccess, by comparing the difference between the flow determined by a volume plethysmograph encompassing the hand and forearm with similar measurements on the contralateral, normal side.[63]

With the use of the Doppler principle, volume measurements can be made in individual vessels, whereas venous occlusion plethysmography measures total flow to a limb segment. Doppler technique requires the measurement of mean velocity, the angle of the ultrasound beam, and the cross-sectional area. This technique of measuring flow can be done with a modern duplex scanner. Early attempts were confounded because they sought to measure flow in the fistula itself, where very turbulent flow and measuring the angle of insonation created difficulties. These drawbacks have been overcome by monitoring flow upstream over a major inflow artery in the affected and the contralateral unaffected limbs, the difference being equivalent to fistula flow

The absolute accuracy of this approach was once not very good, but the technique has been improved by better software and other modifications. Now cross-sectional area can be integrated using one mode and mean velocity integrated from all the velocity signals obtained by another, and these data can be analyzed by a computer using special software programs. A major stimulus has been its potential clinical application in evaluating the function of angioaccess arteriovenous fistulas and shunts.

Zeirler and coworkers tested the accuracy of duplex scanning in a canine model against timed blood collections over a large range of arterial flows and found an error of 13% ± 8%.[68] Willink and Evans tested a real-time duplex system for estimating flow in arteries by simultaneous processing of the audio Doppler velocity output and the video output of a lateral view of the artery, but they found that the need to tilt the transducer to get the correct angle of insonation for velocity information interfered with image measurements of arterial diameter. This and the low production rate of B-mode images and the limited computing power were the major limitations.[66] For that reason, most investigations now accept a single measurement of arterial diameter (for estimation of cross-sectional area) that is obtained before velocity information is collected at an appropriate angle of insonation. In the case of arteriovenous shunts created for angioaccess, the diameter of the graft is known, and this value can be used. Because the results of these flow measurements are often no more revealing than those obtained much more easily by means of pressure measurements (see Fig. 100–1), however, they tend to be applied more selectively, as in monitoring the flow of angioaccess fistulae and shunts (see later).

DOPPLER VELOCITY DETECTION

For many if not most clinical purposes, a *qualitative* estimate of flow velocity and pulse contour obtained with a directional Doppler velocity detector with analog tracings or "waveforms" provides sufficient information for clinical decision making. Finding a high-velocity flow pattern in an artery that leads to a suspicious lesion is good evidence that the lesion is an arteriovenous fistula (Fig. 100–4; compare Fig. 99–3).[4, 48, 54, 56] Increased venous velocity with damping of the respiratory variation in the draining vein provides confirmatory evidence. Although increased flow velocities are encountered when a part is inflamed, this problem is usually evident on clinical examination. Hyperdynamic flow associated with conditions such as beriberi and thyrotoxicosis is generalized and therefore should cause no confusion. Other causes of hyperemia isolated to an individual vessel or limb (e.g., exercise or reactive hyperemia following a period of ischemia) last only a few minutes. Externally applied heat, local infection (e.g., cellulitis or abscess), or sympathetic blockade can also increase flow.

The character of the audible flow signal is informative. Flow in an artery feeding an arteriovenous fistula is pulsatile but lacks the three sounds typical of the normal arterial

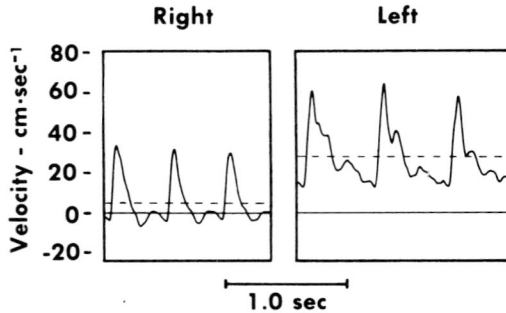

FIGURE 100–4. Blood flow in the common femoral arteries of a 4-year-old girl with a left iliofemoral arteriovenous fistula. The Doppler probe was held at a 45-degree angle to the underlying vessel. The right common femoral artery measured 0.45 cm in diameter, and the left one measured 0.55 cm (see Fig. 100–15). Mean flow velocity (*dashed line*) was 5 cm/sec on the right and 28 cm/sec on the left. Total flow was estimated to be 48 ml/min on the right and 397 ml/min on the left. Contrast the reversal of flow on the right during diastole with the high velocity of flow throughout diastole on the left.

signal (see Chapter 10). The first sound of a *normal* signal coincides with the rapid forward surge of blood during systole; the second reflects a period of reversed flow during early diastole; and the third represents a second diastolic forward-flow phase of much reduced volume. In the presence of an arteriovenous fistula, the proximal arterial signal is louder than normal, higher-pitched, and more continuous. These changes are due to an elevation of diastolic flow and to the absence of any reversed flow component (see Figs. 99–3 and 99–4).

The signal heard over veins draining a fistula is increased in volume and may be pulsatile if the probe is near the fistula (see Fig. 99–4).[4, 54, 56] These findings are often helpful in detecting and localizing arteriovenous fistulae in patients with unilateral varicose veins (Fig. 100–5).[58]

All of these audible Doppler signals have characteristic equivalents when seen on analog tracings obtained using a zero-crossing or some other frequency-to-voltage converter. This feature is not present on the simpler bedside Doppler units but is a standard feature of the Doppler instruments used in most vascular diagnostic laboratories. The characteristic arterial pattern (see Fig. 100–4) consists of an elimination of end-systolic reversal and a marked increase in diastolic velocity, which "elevates" the entire tracing above the zero-velocity baseline. The degree of elevation in end-diastolic velocity correlates directly with the flow increase caused by the arteriovenous fistula.[47, 48]

Using these characteristic arterial and venous flow signals as a guide, one can detect and localize congenital or traumatic arteriovenous communications that otherwise might escape detection.[9, 42, 58] Care must be taken to compare the signal from one limb with that from the other at the same anatomic site. Also, the physician must keep in mind that similar signals can be heard in hyperemic tissues. For example, pulsatile flow is often detected in inflamed skin, like that associated, for example, with bacterial infection, superficial thrombophlebitis, or lymphangitis.

The Doppler probe may also be used during operation to help locate the fistula (or fistulae) and to assess the "completeness" of the surgery.[8, 16, 29, 33, 39, 54] After a successful

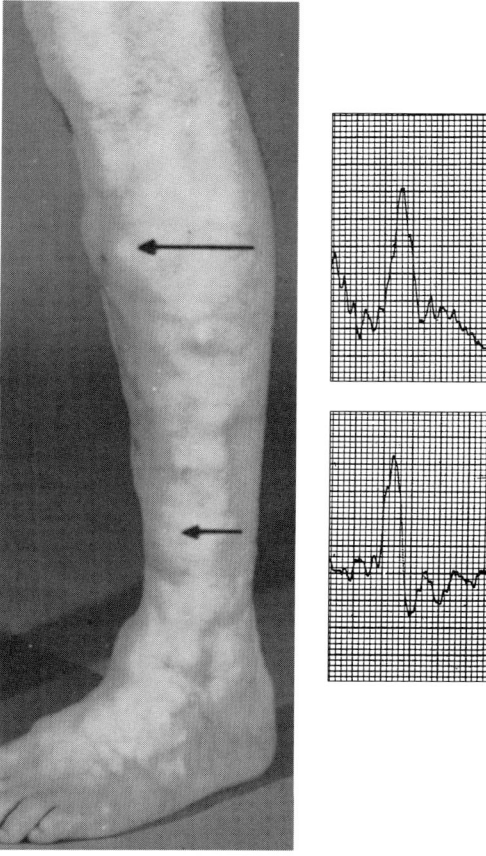

FIGURE 100–5. Tender unilateral varicose veins in a 33-year-old man who had sustained an injury to the lower part of the leg several years earlier. Pulsatile venous flow was heard over two subcutaneous venous "lakes" (*arrows*). Arteriovenous fistulae were found at these two sites. (From Strandness DE Jr, Schultz RD, Sumner DS, Rushmer RF: Ultrasonic flow detection: A useful technic in the evaluation of peripheral vascular disease. Am J Surg 113:311, 1967.)

operation, the arterial and venous flow signals should regain their normal character.

The direction of blood flow in the various arteries and veins that contribute to the fistulous circuit can be determined with a direction-sensing Doppler velocity detector.[4, 56] For example, reversed flow in the distal artery unequivocally establishes the diagnosis of a steal (Fig. 100–6). One can also estimate the contribution of the collateral

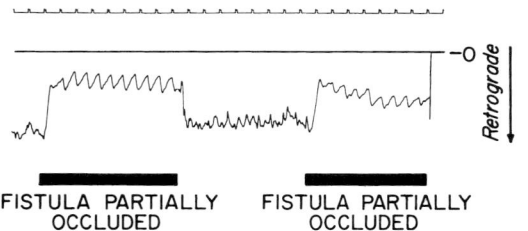

FIGURE 100–6. Velocity of blood flow in the radial artery distal to a side-to-side radial artery–cephalic vein fistula. Note that flow is reversed and the partial compression of the fistula decreases the volume of retrograde flow. The Doppler probe was pointed craniad. (From Strandness DE Jr, Sumner DS: Arteriovenous fistula. *In* Hemodynamics for Surgeons. New York, Grune & Stratton, 1975, pp 621–663.)

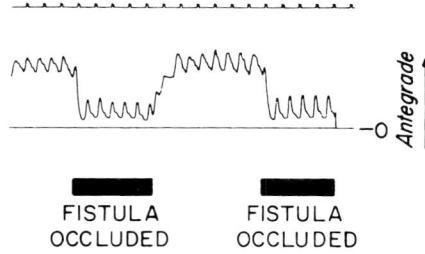

FIGURE 100–7. Velocity of blood flow in the ulnar artery of a patient with a side-to-side radial artery–cephalic vein fistula. Note the large volume of antegrade flow and the marked reduction in flow that occurs when the fistula is occluded. The excess flow was finding its way back through the fistula via the distal radial artery. The Doppler probe was pointed craniad. (From Strandness DE Jr, Sumner DS: Arteriovenous fistula. *In* Hemodynamics for Surgeons. New York, Grune & Stratton, 1975, pp 621–663.)

arteries to flow through the fistula by noting the decrease in flow through these arteries when the fistula is compressed (Fig. 100–7). The direction of blood flow and its course back to the heart can be mapped in the distal vein (Fig. 100–8). Examinations such as these may help to identify the cause of venous hypertension in the hand of the patient with a radial artery–cephalic vein fistula.

The Doppler signal in arteries far distal to an arteriovenous fistula may be reduced in volume if flow steal is significant.[4, 29, 54, 56] When the collateral arteries are good, compressing the fistula increases flow in these peripheral arteries (see Fig. 99–13). Examples of many of these applications are presented later.

DUPLEX SCANNING

The duplex scanner has simplified many of the Doppler methods described earlier. In turn, color coding of velocity signals has simplified the use of the duplex scanner and has provided color images that in themselves are diagnostic. Its application in obtaining volume flow measurements has already been described, as have the characteristic velocity changes detected by the Doppler probe. Duplex scanning simply allows the Doppler beam to be more precisely localized at a point in the vessel visualized on the B-mode image. In addition, the duplex scan obtains its signal by a range-gated pulsed Doppler probe focused on a small area

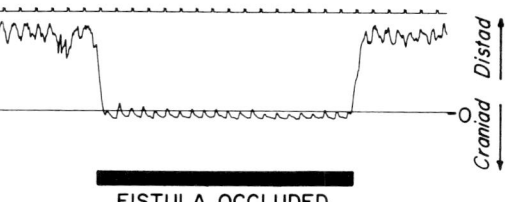

FIGURE 100–8. Blood flow in the cephalic vein distal to a side-to-side radial artery–cephalic vein fistula. Note the great volume of reversed, highly pulsatile flow when the fistula is open. When the fistula is compressed, flow decreases markedly and regains its normal cephalad orientation. The Doppler probe was pointed craniad. (From Strandness DE Jr, Sumner DS: Arteriovenous fistula. *In* Hemodynamics for Surgeons. New York, Grune & Stratton, 1975, pp 621–663.)

of insonation (rather than on the entire vessel when interrogated by a continuous wave instrument). Furthermore, the display on the duplex scan is adapted for spectral analysis rather than using simple analog velocity tracings. Nevertheless, the same basic information can be obtained using the same interpretive principles described for the Doppler velocity detector.

The images obtained with color duplex scanning afford an entirely new diagnostic dimension. Traumatic arteriovenous fistulae, particularly iatrogenic ones produced by percutaneous introduction of catheters via the femoral vessels, are readily seen as multicolored, orange to white "flashes" between the red artery and the blue vein. The nearby tissues transmitting the thrill appear to "light up" with each cardiac cycle because of a motion artefact. Congenital arteriovenous fistulae are more complex, but their high-flow patterns are readily recognized and the nature and extent of the more localized lesions can be well characterized. After this initial evaluation, duplex scanning can be used to follow up and evaluate the results of interventional therapy, whether embolization or surgical resection. Channels thrombosed by embolotherapy or sclerotherapy lose "color" (i.e., their velocity signal) and are not compressible when pressure is applied by the duplex scanner head. This approach is ideal for superficial, localized congenital vascular malformations, whereas magnetic resonance imaging (MRI) is better for follow-up of deeper, more extensive lesions.

TEMPERATURE MEASUREMENTS

Direct measurement of skin temperature with a thermistor or detection of "hot spots" with a thermograph may help to locate the site of arteriovenous fistulae (Table 100–1). Temperatures are usually elevated over the fistula and over the veins that drain it.[1, 20] Because retrograde flow in distal veins is common, the area of increased skin temperature may extend for a considerable distance down the limb, away from the fistula.[64] Similarly, temperatures are elevated proximal to the fistula as a result of the arterial blood that has been diverted into the proximal vein. In contrast, temperatures in the distal part of a limb containing a proximal arteriovenous fistula are often decreased,[18] especially when there is a significant flow steal.

Because of the diffuse nature of the temperature elevation, this technique cannot be relied on for precise localization of the fistula, and with advances in other noninvasive techniques, the use of thermography has greatly diminished.

VENOUS OXYGEN TENSION

The oxygen saturation of the venous blood draining a limb containing an arteriovenous fistula is always more or less elevated in comparison with that of the opposite, normal, limb.[1, 62] This finding may be very helpful in the diagnosis of congenital arteriovenous fistula, particularly for lesions that are difficult to localize and diagnose. Because the concentration of oxygen in the venous blood is directly related to the quantity of blood leaked from the arterial to the venous side of the circulation, this test aids in assessing the hemodynamic significance of the fistula; however, it is much less helpful in congenital vascular malformations, in which lesions are more diffuse and single sampling sites less representative. Furthermore, these lesions are usually associated with varicose veins, and the blood in even simple varicose veins is known to have higher oxygen saturation. Nevertheless, transcutaneous techniques (e.g., pulse oximetry) may restore the practical value of this approach in certain settings.

CARDIAC OUTPUT

Cardiac output can be measured by the direct oxygen–Fick method, indicator dilution methods, thermodilution, ballistocardiography, echocardiography, or another technique. Currently, echocardiography is the most popular noninvasive method. Using an ultrasound beam aimed at the aortic root from the suprasternal notch, cardiac output (minus coronary flow) can readily be monitored. Although many patients with arteriovenous fistulae have little or no perceptible increase in cardiac output, in others the cardiac output may be quite high. By noting how much cardiac output decreases with fistula compression, the clinician can estimate the quantity of blood flowing through the fistula.[3, 6, 25, 38, 45, 52, 61] In addition, we can assess the efficacy of surgical therapy by measuring the decrease in cardiac output.[14, 19, 36, 65]

From a diagnostic point of view, an exceptionally high cardiac output should alert the physician to the possibility of an arteriovenous fistula.[34] When indicator dilution methods are employed, early recirculation of dye in the systemic arterial tree and early appearance in right-sided heart samples are typical observations in the presence of arteriovenous fistulae.[50] Manual compression of the fistula corrects these abnormalities temporarily.

RADIONUCLIDE ASSESSMENT

Radionuclide-labeled microspheres can be used to detect and quantitate arteriovenous shunting. The rationale is simple. Microspheres too large to pass through capillaries are introduced into an artery; those passing through arteriovenous communications are trapped in the capillaries of

TABLE 100–1. TEMPERATURE MEASUREMENTS AT VARIOUS SITES ALONG THE LEGS

SITE	TEMPERATURE (°C)*	
	Right	Left
Thigh	31.6	32.4
Knee	31.1	35.8
Calf	30.6	33.0
Foot	31.0	31.9

*Room temperature was 26°C.

the lung, and the fraction of microspheres that reach the lung is determined. When the microspheres are thoroughly mixed with the arterial inflow, the fraction of the total quantity injected that reach the lung is proportional to the fraction of blood flow to the extremity that passes through the arteriovenous shunt. Although naturally occurring arteriovenous shunts are present in normal human extremities, less than 3.0% of the total blood flow (and usually much less) is diverted through these communications.[44] When the fraction of microspheres reaching the lung exceeds this value, abnormal shunting is present.

The method described by Rhodes and Rutherford and their colleagues is as follows: With the patient lying supine, the lungs are monitored by means of a gamma camera or a rectilinear scintillation scanner held in a fixed position over a limited pulmonary field.[44, 46, 47] The patient is instructed not to move during the period of study. The agent used consists of a suspension of 35-μm human albumin microspheres labeled with technetium 99m (similar to that commonly used in lung scintigraphy). To obtain a background counting rate for unbound technetium 99m, a sample of the suspending solution is initially injected through a cannula inserted into the major inflow artery of the extremity being studied. This is followed by one or more intra-arterial injections of the suspended microspheres, each of which has a volume of about 1.0 ml and radioactivity of 2 to 4 mCi.

After each injection, counting is continued for 3 to 5 minutes until a plateau is reached. Finally, a dose of microspheres is administered through a superficial vein in another extremity. Because 100% of the intravenously injected microspheres reach and are trapped by the lungs, the counts obtained after the venous injection represent the baseline situation of no shunting. To ensure similar counting efficiencies, the suspension injected into the vein has one fourth to one third of the activity of that injected into the artery, approximately 0.5 to 1.0 mCi. The relative radioactivity of the microsphere suspensions is measured by scintillation counting of the syringes before and after the microspheres have been administered. It is important that no microspheres be lost by extravasation.

The formula used to estimate the percentage of arteriovenous shunting is as follows:

$$\% \text{ shunt} = \frac{(Pa - Bg)}{(Pv - Pa)} \cdot \frac{(Iv_i - Iv_r)}{(Ia_i - Ia_r)}$$

where Bg is background pulmonary counts per unit of time, Pa is pulmonary counts per unit of time after the arterial injection, Pv is pulmonary counts per unit of time after the venous injection, Iv_i is counts per unit of time of the venous syringe before injection, Iv_r is residual counts per unit of time of the venous syringe after injection, Ia_i is counts per unit of time of the arterial syringe before injection, and Ia_r is residual counts per unit of time of the arterial syringe after injection.[44, 47]

For example, if the pulmonary radioactivity after the arterial injection (Pa − Bg) was half that measured after the venous injection (Pv − Pa) and the ratio of the activity of the venous injectate ($Iv_i - Iv_r$) to that of the arterial injectate ($Ia_i - Ia_r$) was one fourth, the estimated shunt volume would be 12.5% of the total flow to the extremity, or

$$(\tfrac{1}{2}) (\tfrac{1}{4}) (100) = 12.5\%$$

Although the study is minimally invasive, it is relatively simple to perform, causes little discomfort, and carries negligible risk. It can be undertaken as a separate procedure in conjunction with arteriography or during operation. When measurements are made during operation, it is necessary to obtain baseline estimations of arteriovenous shunting because anesthesia, general or regional, increases shunting through naturally occurring arteriovenous communications. Moreover, the percentage of blood shunted through such communications can reach 40% in the limbs of patients with sympathetic denervation, cirrhosis, or hypertrophic pulmonary osteopathy.[46] The examiner must be aware of these potential pitfalls and must make the proper allowances when interpreting test results.

Radionuclide-labeled microspheres are most useful for investigating suspected congenital arteriovenous fistulae.[46–48] As a diagnostic modality, the test can be performed before arteriography in patients with "hemangiomas," limb overgrowth, or atypical varicose veins as well as in those with obvious congenital vascular malformations in whom the presence and degree of arteriovenous shunting are in doubt. Arteriography occasionally fails to demonstrate the fistula or fistulae, either because they are too small or because the flow is too rapid. Early venous filling may be the only clue. In such cases, injection of microspheres in conjunction with arteriography can be used to establish the diagnosis. With diffuse or extensive congenital vascular malformations, it may be difficult to distinguish clinically between the so-called microfistulous lesions, in which the arteriovenous communications cannot be visualized angiographically, and the predominantly venous malformations. The labeled microsphere study solves this dilemma.

Because shunt flow can be quantified, the results have prognostic value.[46–48] The physician can estimate the hemodynamic significance of the lesion and the likelihood that it will cause heart failure, limb overgrowth, distal arterial insufficiency, ulceration, or skin changes. With this knowledge, the surgeon or interventional radiologist is better equipped to determine the need for intervention. By applying occlusive pneumatic tourniquets at different levels of the limb and repeating the microsphere injections, one can locate multiple fistulae and compare their hemodynamic significance. Arteriovenous fistulae that persist after excisional operations or embolotherapy may be detected and quantified by this approach. However, with MRI (discussed later) as available as it is today, this particular application has less unique value.

During operation, after all overt lesions have been excised, the injections can be repeated to determine whether residual communications have been overlooked. Follow-up studies may be used to evaluate the results of therapeutic procedures such as ablative surgery or embolotherapy. Finally, serial measurements indicate whether the fistula is following a stable or a progressive course and whether previously dormant arteriovenous communications have begun to open up or to grow.

COMPUTED TOMOGRAPHY AND MAGNETIC RESONANCE IMAGING

Angiographic studies tend to underestimate the full anatomic extent of vascular malformations. Computed tomography (CT) usually demonstrates the location and extent of the lesion and even the involvement of specific muscle groups and bone.[7, 43, 67] Deep intramuscular lesions have a mottled appearance, and with bolus administration of contrast medium, the enhancement depends on the rate of arteriovenous shunting in, and the degree of cellularity of, the lesion. Offsetting these desirable features are the need for contrast, the lack of an optimal protocol for administration, and the practical limitation of having to use multiple transverse images to reconstruct the anatomy of the lesion.

MRI possesses a number of distinct advantages over CT for evaluating congenital vascular malformations (CVMs). There is no need for contrast medium, the anatomic extent of the lesion is more clearly demonstrated, longitudinal as well as transverse sections may be obtained, and the flow patterns in the CVM can be characterized. As a result, MRI has become the *pivotal* diagnostic study of choice in the evaluation of most CVMs. MRI signal intensity depends on the proton density, magnetic relaxation time (T1 or T2), and the bulk proton flux (which reflects blood flow). If an image is obtained after the pulsed protons (in rapidly moving blood) have left the field, a (black) flow void on T2-weighted scans identifies high-flow vascular spaces and their feeding arteries and draining veins. In contrast, a predominantly venous malformation with its slow flow would appear white.

Another MRI technique, even-echo rephasing, identifies vessels where laminar flow is slow. Hemorrhage into soft tissues can be seen and roughly "aged." Cellularity can be appreciated because stromal tissues "relax" at different rates. Thus, cellularity produces a higher-intensity signal than blood-filled spaces.[35] Magnetic resonance angiography (MRA), which uses the time-of-flight principle, is being applied to the study of both acquired and congenital arteriovenous fistulae. It holds the promise of three-dimensional reconstruction. Clinical examples of the value of MRI in the setting of CVMs are illustrated in Figures 100–9 to 100–11.

Because of favorable experiences with MRI in evaluating patients with CVMs,[39] one of the authors (R.B.R.) now uses a combination of MRI and the noninvasive tests described earlier as the initial diagnostic approach in children with CVMs, avoiding angiography unless and until therapeutic intervention is indicated. An algorithm of this approach appears in Figure 100–12.

Finally, one can *selectively* combine the different studies described earlier in a logical manner to arrive at a definitive categorical diagnosis of CVM. This approach, shown algorithmically in Figure 100–13, allows CVMs to be separated into macrofistulous and microfistulous arteriovenous malformations, venous dysplasias, lymphatic abnormalities, and capillary-cavernous hemangiomas.

ANGIOGRAPHY

Since the advent of MRI, angiography is no longer necessary in the diagnosis of CVMs or even in managing most of the low-flow lesions. This is particularly important in children, who require general anesthesia for angiography. Fortunately, noninvasive tests allow parents to be given an accurate diagnosis and prognosis and at least guide initial therapy. Duplex scanning can identify most iatrogenic arteriovenous fistulae and serves as the instrument for compression therapy; however, angiography is necessary for most other acquired (e.g., traumatic) arteriovenous fistulae and with "intent to treat" CVMs, in which one may proceed with embolotherapy at the same time. These techniques are explained in Chapters 102 and 103.[12, 22, 53] Cineangiography or serial films (two or three per second) made with a rapid changer are necessary to visualize the fistula and to time the appearance of the radiopaque medium in the venous channels.[5]

CLINICAL APPLICATIONS

Acquired Arteriovenous Fistulae

The actual communication between artery and vein may be apparent in radiographs of acquired fistulae; otherwise, the site of the fistula is indicated by the point of initial venous opacification (Fig. 100–14). Not uncommonly, aneurysms are noted in the vicinity of the fistula (see Fig. 99–10). Flow in the proximal artery and proximal vein is usually quite rapid. When the fistula is large, flow in the distal artery is sluggish or entirely absent, and there may be retrograde opacification of the distal vein. As a rule, the proximal artery is dilated, sometimes to aneurysmal dimensions, and it may be tortuous if the fistula is of long standing. Similarly, the proximal vein is dilated, especially adjacent to the fistula. Valvular incompetence may be demonstrated for a variable distance when the distal vein is distended. If the fistula is small, opacification of the peripheral arteries may not be appreciably delayed and the appearance of dye in the communicating veins will be relatively slow.

Congenital Arteriovenous Fistulae

The radiographic appearance of congenital arteriovenous fistulae is much more complicated compared with acquired fistulae (Fig. 100–15).[37, 60] Indirect signs of an abnormal arteriovenous communication (i.e., increased flow in the afferent arteries, decreased flow in the peripheral arteries, and rapid venous filling) are nearly always present. The fistula or, more commonly, the multiple fistulae may not be visible, however, because they may be microscopic. In one large series, failure to visualize the arteriovenous fistulae themselves occurred in close to 30%.[60] Furthermore, the array of overlying arteries and veins adds to the complexity. Numerous arteries may feed and numerous veins may drain a single arteriovenous malformation. For this reason, selective angiography of the afferent artery, by reducing the number of opacified vessels, may be helpful in delineating the extent of the fistula.

Sometimes, localized dilated, contrast-filled spaces indicate the site of the fistula with some precision. On other occasions, small fistulae are revealed as faint, diffuse opacifications between major arterial and venous channels. Other clues include abnormal vessels arising from the parent artery, horizontal branches connecting parallel vessels, and venous retia.[37]

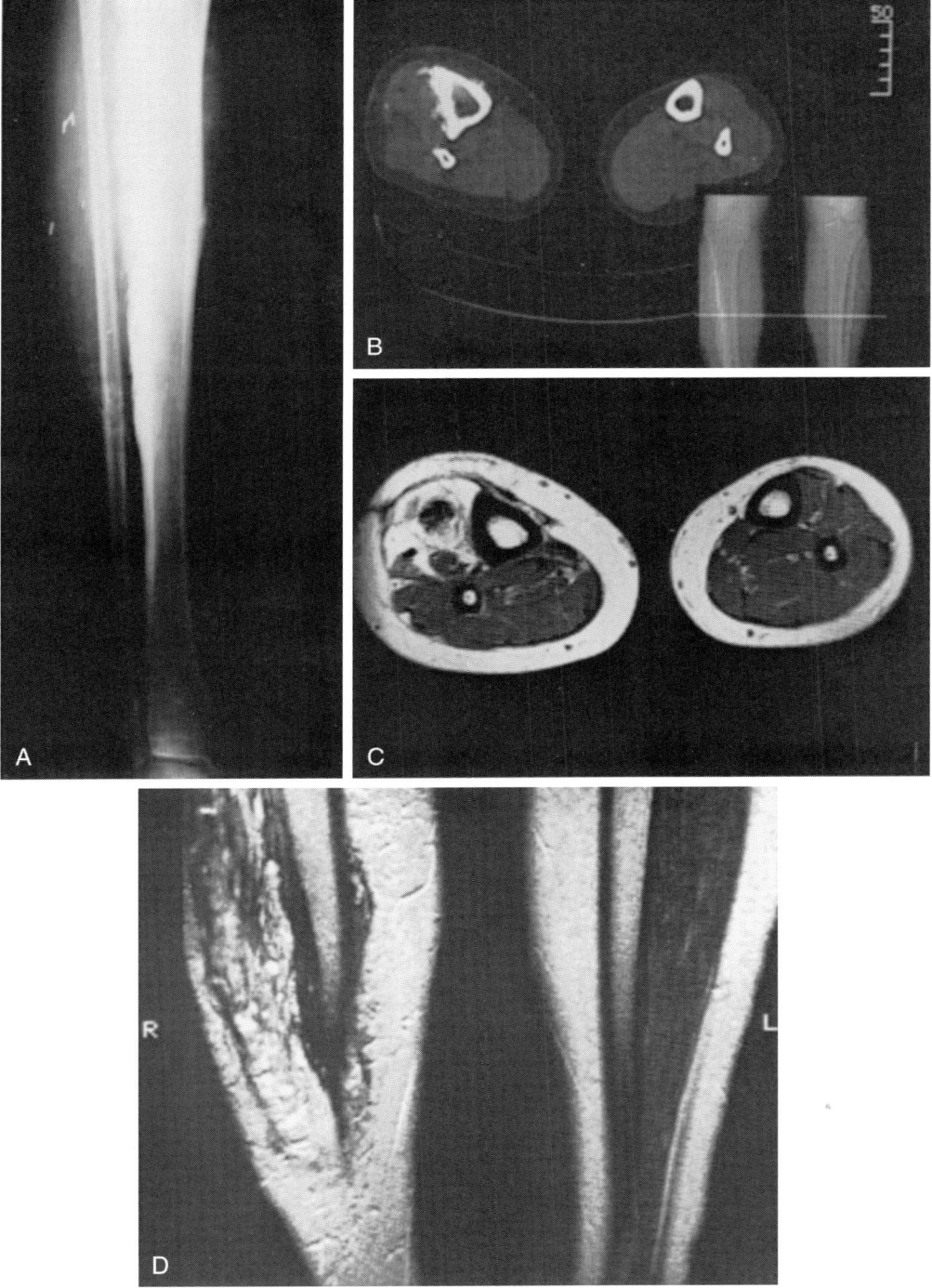

FIGURE 100–9. *A,* Radiograph of the lower leg of a 29-year-old woman with a right anterior tibial mass present since birth shows speckled calcifications, metal clips from multiple previous operations, and tibial cortical irregularities. An arteriogram (not shown) revealed "hypervascularity and one area of early venous filling." *B,* Computed tomographic scan also suggests bone involvement. *C,* Transverse magnetic resonance imaging (MRI) view shows lesion filling the anterior tibial compartment, but the margins of the tibia are clean. *D,* Longitudinal MRI view also demonstrates the lack of fast-flow voids. Total excision of the lesion was performed without difficulty or significant blood loss. Histologic study revealed a "highly cellular and fibrotic cavernous (venous) malformation." (*A–D,* From Pearce WH, Rutherford RB, Whitehill TA, Davis K: Nuclear magnetic resonance imaging: Its diagnostic value in patients with congenital vascular malformations of the limbs. J Vasc Surg 8:64, 1988.)

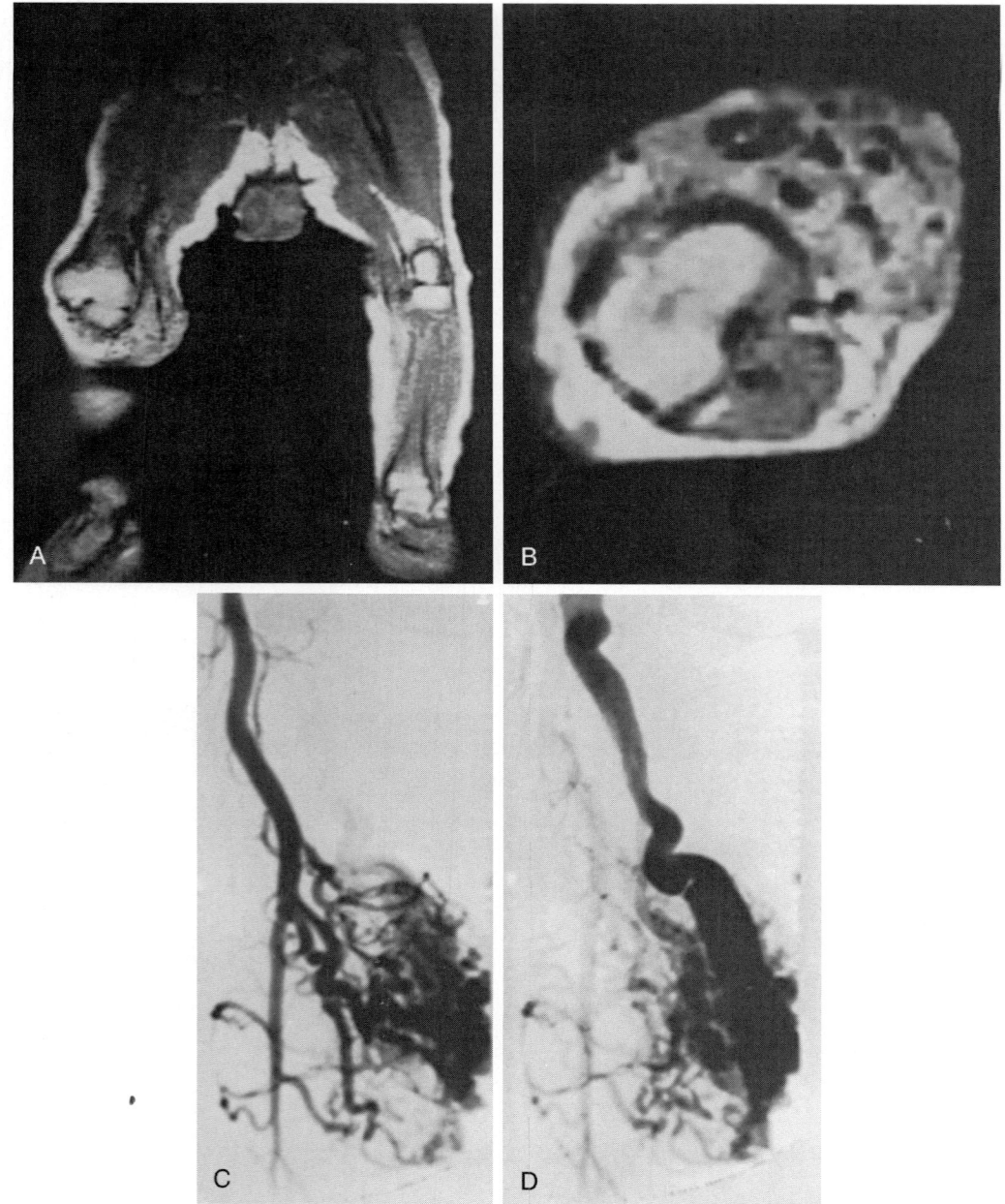

FIGURE 100–10. A 4-day-old infant presented with a medial lower thigh mass with palpable thrill. *A,* Longitudinal magnetic resonance imaging (MRI) view shows the mass with a large, high-flow draining vein. *B,* Transverse MRI view shows multiple fast-flow voids with involvement of muscle and bone. *C,* After several months, this arteriogram was obtained because of the onset of high-output heart failure. *D,* Later-phase view shows the same large draining vein seen on MRI. Therapeutic embolization was carried out, resulting in transient disseminated intravascular coagulation but with a diminution of the mass and control of heart failure. (*A–D,* From Pearce WH, Rutherford RB, Whitehill TA, Davis K: Nuclear magnetic resonance imaging: Its diagnostic value in patients with congenital vascular malformations of the limbs. J Vasc Surg 8:64, 1988.)

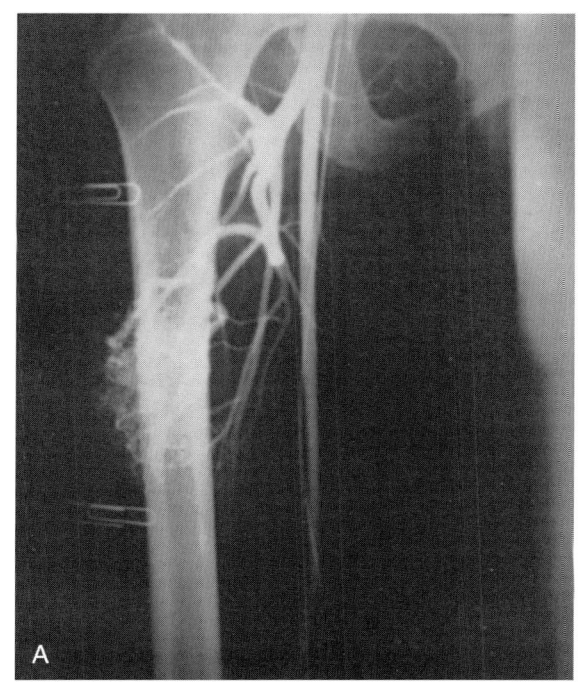

FIGURE 100–11. A 24-year-old man had been aware of a painless soft mass on his upper anterolateral thigh for many years. *A*, An arteriogram was obtained, which showed a localized arteriovenous malformation fed by the profunda femoris artery. The patient was referred for operation. *B*, Sagittal magnetic resonance imaging (MRI) view shows high-flow voids and large draining veins. *C*, Transverse MRI view shows not only the high-flow voids but also diffuse involvement of the anterior thigh muscles. Operation was withheld in this asymptomatic man because excision would have produced immediate neuromuscular disability. There was no distal steal or cardiac embarrassment.

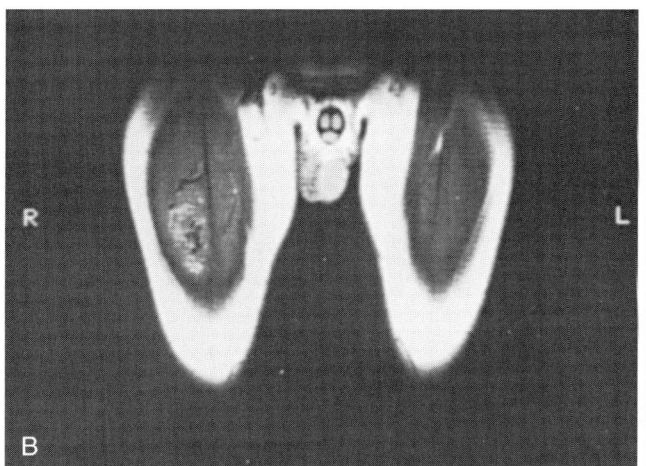

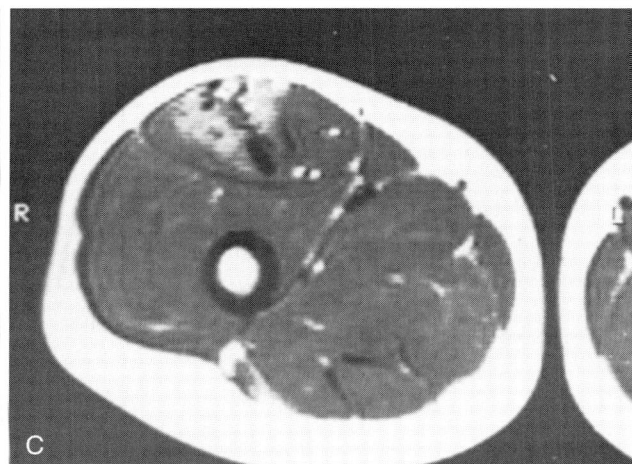

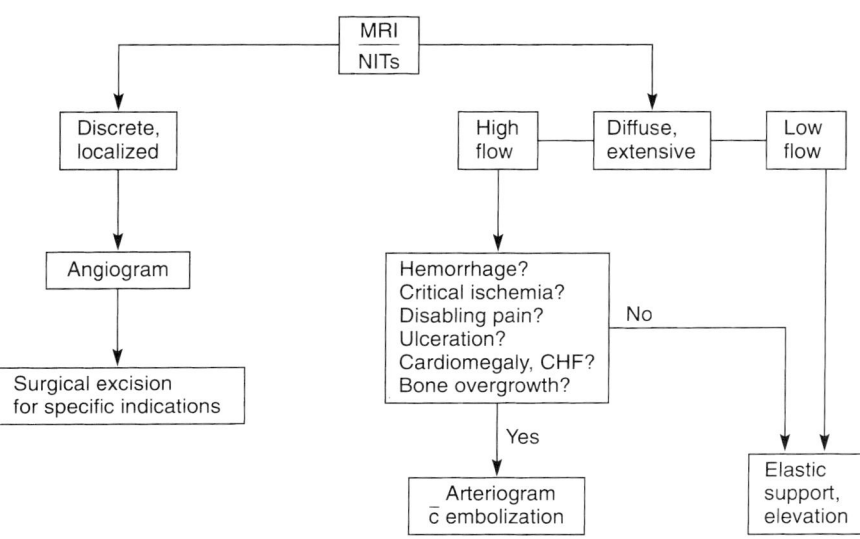

FIGURE 100–12. Algorithm showing how the use of noninvasive tests (NITs), including magnetic resonance imaging (MRI), can help guide the management of peripheral congenital vascular malformations. The treatment options and indications are oversimplified here (see Chapter 103). CHF = congestive heart failure.

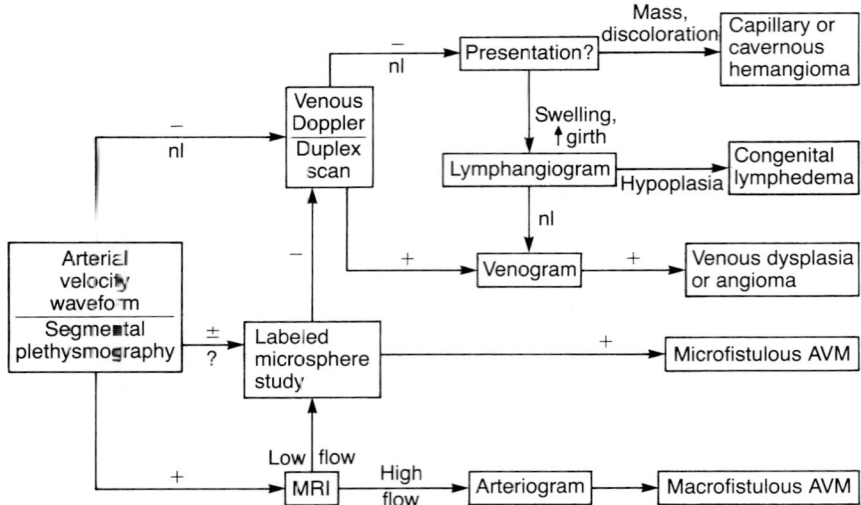

FIGURE 100–13. Algorithm of the diagnostic approach for categorizing peripheral congenital vascular malformations. In most cases, lymphoscintigraphy would be used before or instead of lymphangiography, and in each instance angiography would be withheld if there were no indications for therapeutic intervention, because it is not needed just to confirm the diagnosis. Magnetic resonance imaging (MRI) would be used in its place. AVM = arteriovenous malformation; nl = normal.

Because the radiopaque medium tends to seek out the fistulae that are most proximal and those that carry the greatest volume of flow, smaller and more distal communications may escape detection.[15] This is particularly unfortunate in cases of congenital arteriovenous malformations because multiple sites tend to be involved. MRI has overcome this problem.

Phlebography

Phlebography may be helpful in some cases of CVM.[60] Lindenauer found that deep veins in the popliteal and superficial femoral regions were absent in a number of limbs involved in the Klippel-Trenaunay syndrome (characterized by "hemangioma," varicose veins, and unilateral increase in leg size).[30] Typically, arteriographic findings are normal with this condition; no arteriovenous fistulae are evident.

Phlebography, as commonly used to identify deep venous thrombosis (DVT), often underestimates venous malformations because of grape-like clusters of venous "angiomas" that lie outside the mainstream of venous flow. Selective catheterization, direct percutaneous puncture, or passive filling under inflow occlusion (much like that used for Bier's block) may be necessary for proper visualization. Again, MRI is best for diagnosis; phlebography is needed only to guide therapy (e.g., sclerotherapy with absolute alcohol or sodium tetradecyl sulfate [Sotradecol]).

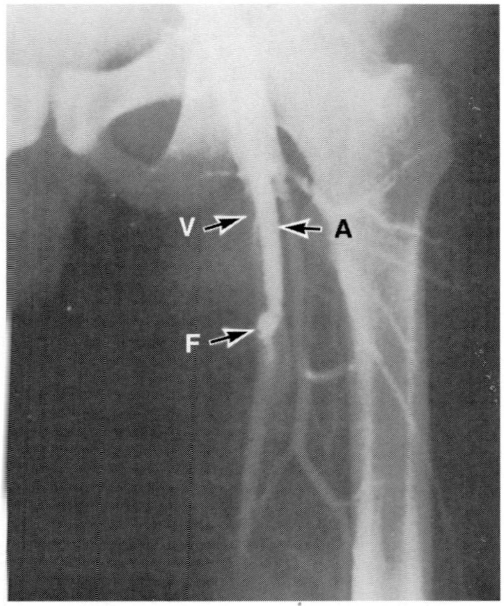

FIGURE 100–14. Acute traumatic arteriovenous fistula (F) between the left superficial femoral artery (A) and vein (V). Note the large, well-developed profunda femoris artery.

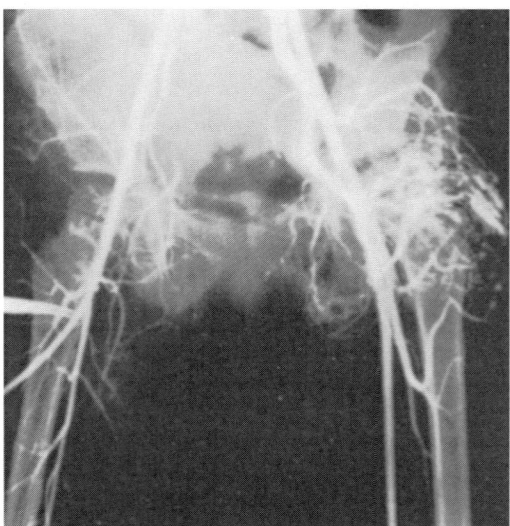

FIGURE 100–15. Arteriogram showing a large arteriovenous malformation in a 4-year-old girl. Branches of the hypogastric and profunda femoris arteries are involved. Note the pronounced enlargement of the hypogastric, external iliac, common femoral, and profunda femoris arteries.

ARTERIOVENOUS FISTULAE FOR HEMODIALYSIS: DIAGNOSTIC CONSIDERATIONS

Although the topic of arteriovenous fistulae for hemodialysis access is covered in detail in the next section of this book (see Chapter 104), most of the diagnostic studies are discussed in this chapter. To avoid repetition, the applications of the previously described studies in this particular setting are detailed here.

Preoperative Studies

For primary hemodialysis access procedures, or the initial procedure in a given limb, normal arteries and adequate veins may be assumed from palpation of bounding peripheral pulses and distention of adequate veins with tourniquet application. If this is not the case or if this is a reoperation, complicated by previous diagnostic or therapeutic procedures or evidence of preexisting vascular disease, the arterial tree may be better studied first noninvasively by segmental pressure measurements and plethysmography. This can be augmented by duplex scanning if results of the other studies are positive,[31, 47, 48, 51] and the adequacy of superficial veins can be determined primarily by duplex scanning.[28, 49] On the basis of these findings, and particularly in complicated cases or reoperations, arteriography and phlebography may still be required. Patients with long-standing azotemia and/or diabetes often have significant distal arterial occlusive disease, which may be occult. Patients with debilitating diseases require frequent hospital admissions, during which intravenous infusions may have produced obliterative phlebitis of the superficial arm veins. Those who previously underwent dialysis through proximal sites in the neck or groin may have occult thrombosis there, which may seriously complicate attempts to create an arteriovenous fistula distally in the same extremity.[41, 55] With this approach, Silva and coworkers[51] not only increased the proportion of patients in whom autogenous fistulas (rather than prosthetic bypasses) could be created but also improved primary patency rates for fistulae (83% versus 48%).

Postoperative Studies

Palpation of a prominent thrill over the outflow vein after creation of an arteriovenous fistula or a shunt may suffice, but Doppler investigation offers more objective evidence of adequate fistula flow in the perioperative period. Actual flow rates may be estimated as described earlier (see Volume Flow Measurements), and even though this has been shown to correlate with patency and function, it cannot be justified, on a cost-effectiveness basis, for routine serial study. Further improvements in software to provide reliable real-time flow rates as part of duplex surveillance might change this, but flow rates observed during dialysis are now the day-to-day index of function. Other late complications, usually producing persistent symptoms such as extremity pain or swelling, however, deserve investigation, and they are described and illustrated.

Late complications of radial artery–cephalic vein fistulae are relatively rare; however, some patients complain of ischemic symptoms in the hand or fingers, and others suffer from the effects of elevated peripheral venous pressure.[13, 17, 26] In addition, a few patients have markedly increased cardiac outputs, and in some of them cardiac failure may develop.

Pressure, flow, and plethysmographic measurements of the digital circulation often elucidate the cause of the patient's discomfort, ruling ischemia in or out (see Fig. 100–1). Selective compression of the vessels contributing to the fistulous circuit usually permits identification of the problem area: there may be reversed flow in the distal radial artery, retrograde flow in the distal cephalic vein, or an obstructed proximal cephalic vein (Fig. 99–14).[56] Directional Doppler ultrasound studies are valuable supplements to the foregoing information because they can be used to determine the direction of flow in the various vessels (see Figs. 99–4, 99–13, 100–6, 100–7, and 100–8). Findings derived from these studies often pinpoint the problem and enable the surgeon to correct it. Moreover, after surgical correction the benefits can also be assessed objectively.

When the problem is inadequate blood supply to the dialysis machine, noninvasive studies may be helpful. Obstruction of the proximal vein (perhaps related to repeated venipuncture or intimal hyperplasia) and excessive diversion of flow into the distal vein are easily recognized. If there is little or no reduction in digital blood pressure or if compression of the fistula produces no rise in pressure, it is likely that the problem is poor fistula flow. (On the other hand, when compression of the fistula causes the digital pressure to fall, the collateral arteries—usually the ulnar artery and its branches—are inadequate.) Stenoses of the fistula or afferent artery are among the causes of inadequate fistula flow. Sometimes the obstruction can be localized with the Doppler scanner or flowmeter.[5] Confirmation by arteriography may be necessary.[2, 21]

Cardiac output studies are useful in patients experiencing

TABLE 100–2. CASE 1: RADIAL STEAL: EFFECT OF LIGATING DISTAL RADIAL ARTERY ON BLOOD PRESSURE IN INDEX FINGER IPSILATERAL TO RADIAL ARTERY–CEPHALIC VEIN FISTULA

	BEFORE LIGATION OF DISTAL RADIAL ARTERY (mmHg)	AFTER LIGATION OF DISTAL RADIAL ARTERY (mmHg)
Brachial pressure	100	100
Index finger pressure		
Fistula open	32	80
Fistula occluded	68	92
Distal artery occluded	60	—
Ulnar artery occluded	0	0

TABLE 100–3. CASE 2: DISTAL VENOUS HYPERTENSION: EFFECT OF LIGATING DISTAL VEIN ON BLOOD PRESSURE IN INDEX FINGER IPSILATERAL TO RADIAL ARTERY–CEPHALIC VEIN FISTULA

	BEFORE LIGATION OF DISTAL VEIN (mmHg)	AFTER LIGATION OF DISTAL VEIN (mmHg)
Brachial pressure	156	160
Index finger pressure		
Fistula open	100	110
Fistula occluded	160	186
Distal artery occluded	140	178
Proximal vein occluded	110	140
Distal vein occluded	152	110

heart failure (see Cardiac Output, earlier), more often in those known to have cardiac disease and in association with larger-flow proximal shunts. The change in cardiac output with compression of the fistula also can be used to give an estimate of fistula flow.[3, 25] Such information is important to discovering the cause of cardiac failure in patients undergoing hemodialysis, since cardiac failure frequently results from causes other than high output (e.g., fluid overload). Again, the success or failure of any surgical procedure designed to correct the excess fistula flow can be assayed by cardiac output measurements in the postoperative period.[3]

Case Histories

The following cases are presented as examples of how the previously described studies give valuable information about patients with angioaccess fistulas who present with pain or discomfort in the hand of the involved extremity.

Case 1. A 29-year-old man with a side-to-side radial artery–cephalic vein fistula complained of pain in the thumb and index finger that was especially severe during dialysis. Although his brachial systolic pressure was 100 mmHg, his index finger pressure was only 32 mmHg (Table 100–2). When the fistula was compressed, the index finger pressure rose to 68 mmHg. Compression of the radial artery distal to the fistula caused the index finger pressure to rise to 60 mmHg. Directional Doppler studies revealed reversal of flow in the distal radial artery. Compression of the ulnar artery caused the index finger pressure to drop to zero. Doppler flow signals in the ulnar artery decreased markedly with compression of the fistula.

These data were interpreted as showing steal of blood from the finger by the fistula and retrograde flow through the distal radial artery. In addition, they indicated that the ulnar artery was the sole supplier of blood to the finger and that much of the ulnar flow was being siphoned off to feed the fistulous circuit. In light of this information, the distal radial artery was ligated. Postoperatively, the index finger pressure rose to 80 mmHg, even though the arm pressure remained at 100 mmHg. Although compression of the fistula continued to increase the pressure (to 92 mmHg), the percentage of change was reduced as compared with that obtained preoperatively, a finding that implied that the steal had been appreciably reduced (see Table 100–2). The patient's symptoms were distinctly improved: he no longer had pain while off dialysis, and pain during dialysis appeared only after about 5 hours.

Comment: Although this patient's symptoms were typical of radial steal, confirmation of the role of the distal radial artery by pressure measurement in the index finger and by Doppler flow studies helped to establish the diagnosis. Additionally, the low pressure in the index finger when the fistula was open provided objective proof that the fistula was severely restricting blood flow to the hand. The finding is important because most patients with chronic fistulas have some degree of distal steal. The efficacy of distal artery ligation was shown by the rise of the index finger pressure out of the ischemic range and by the fact that compression of the fistula had less effect on distal blood pressure.

Case 2. Three-and-a-half years after a side-to-side radial artery–cephalic vein fistula had been constructed in the left wrist of a 40-year-old man, he began to experience increasing swelling and pain in the hand. Index finger pressures were lower than the arm or wrist pressures, indicating a significant steal that could be corrected by manual compression of the fistula and partially corrected by compression of the distal radial artery (Table 100–3). The digital artery pressure, however, was well above the ischemic range. Although manual compression of the proximal vein had little effect on digital pressure, compression of the distended distal vein returned digital pressures to nearly normal levels (see Table 100–3). This fact implied that the *distal* vein was the major outflow tract of the fistula, which indeed was confirmed by directional Doppler studies.

The patient's symptoms were relieved by ligation of the distal vein followed by carpal tunnel release.[23, 32] Flow to the dialysis machine, obtained from cannulated proximal veins, was improved. Postoperatively, arterial blood pressure in the index finger was essentially unchanged, but manual compression of the proximal vein raised the pressure in the finger appreciably, indicating that this vein was now the major outflow tract of the fistula. Compression of distal veins no longer had an effect.

Comment: Measurements of digital pressure in this patient revealed that the cause of the patient's hand pain was not ischemia. They also demonstrated that the distal vein was carrying most of the venous outflow, which created painful venous hypertension in the hand and caused congestion in the carpal tunnel. Correction of these defects produced circulatory dynamics that were more favorable to dialysis and relieved the pain in the hand.

REFERENCES

1. Allen EV, Barker NW, Hines EA Jr: Arteriovenous fistulas. *In* Peripheral Vascular Diseases, 3rd ed. Philadelphia, WB Saunders, 1965, pp 475–494.
2. Anderson CB, Gilula LA, Harter HR, et al: Venous angiography and the surgical management of subcutaneous hemodialysis fistulas. Ann Surg 187:194, 1978.
3. Anderson CB, Codd JR, Graff RA, et al: Cardiac failure and upper extremity arteriovenous dialysis fistulas. Arch Intern Med 136:292, 1976.

4. Barnes RW: Noninvasive assessment of arteriovenous fistula. Angiology 29:691, 1978.
5. Bell D, Cockshott WP: Angiography of traumatic arteriovenous fistulae. Clin Radiol 16:241, 1965.
6. Bergrem H, Flatmark A, Simonsen S: Dialysis fistulas and cardiac failure. Acta Med Scand 204:191, 1978.
7. Bernardino ME, Jing BS, Thomas JL, et al: The extremity soft-tissue lesion: A comparative study of ultrasound, computed tomography, and xeroradiography. Radiology 189:53, 1981.
8. Bingham HG, Lichti E: Use of ultrasound transducer (Doppler) to localize peripheral arteriovenous fistulae. Plast Reconstr Surg 46:151, 1970.
9. Bingham HG, Lichti EL: The Doppler as an aid in predicting the behavior of congenital cutaneous hemangioma. Plast Reconstr Surg 47:580, 1971.
10. Boley SJ, Sammartano R, Brandt LJ, et al: Vascular ectasias of the colon. Surg Gynecol Obstet 149:353, 1979.
11. Brener BJ, Brief DK, Alpert J, et al: The effect of vascular access procedures on digital hemodynamics. In Diethrich EB (ed): Noninvasive Cardiovascular Diagnosis: Current Concepts. Baltimore, University Park Press, 1978, pp 189–203.
12. Bron KM: Femoral arteriography. In Abrams HL (ed): Angiography, 2nd ed. Vol II. Boston, Little, Brown, 1971, pp 1221–1249.
13. Bussell JA, Abbott JA, Lim RC: A radial steal syndrome with arteriovenous fistula for hemodialysis. Ann Intern Med 75:387, 1971.
14. Cantelmo NL, Alpert JS, Cutler BS, et al: Arteriovenous fistula masquerading as valvular heart disease. JAMA 245:1936, 1981.
15. Coleman CC: Diagnosis and treatment of congenital arteriovenous fistulas of the head and neck. Am J Surg 126:557, 1973.
16. Cooperman M, Martin EW Jr, Evans WE, et al: Use of Doppler ultrasound in intraoperative localization of intestinal arteriovenous malformation. Ann Surg 190:24, 1979.
17. Delpin EAS: Swelling of the hand after arteriovenous fistula for hemodialysis. Am J Surg 132:373, 1976.
18. Elkin DC, Warren JV: Arteriovenous fistulas: Their effect on the circulation. JAMA 134:1524, 1947.
19. Fee HJ, Levisman J, Doud RB, et al: High-output congestive failure from femoral arteriovenous shunts for vascular access. Ann Surg 183:321, 1976.
20. Galera GR, Martinez CA: Thermography in the management of carotid-cavernous fistulas. J Neurosurg 43:352, 1975.
21. Göthlin J, Lindstedt E: Angiographic features of Cimino-Brescia fistulas. Am J Roentgenol Radium Ther Nucl Med 125:582, 1975.
22. Hewitt RL, Smith AD, Drapanas T: Acute traumatic arteriovenous fistulas. J Trauma 13:901, 1973.
23. Holtmann B, Anderson CB: Carpal tunnel syndrome following vascular shunts for hemodialysis. Arch Surg 112:65, 1977.
24. Hurwich BJ: Plethysmographic forearm blood flow studies in maintenance patients with radial arteriovenous fistulae. Nephron 6:673, 1969.
25. Johnson G Jr, Blythe WB: Hemodynamic effects of arteriovenous shunts used for hemodialysis. Ann Surg 171:715, 1970.
26. Kinnaert P, Struyven J, Mathieu J, et al: Intermittent claudication of the hand after creation of an arteriovenous fistula in the forearm. Am J Surg 139:838, 1980.
27. Kwaan JHM, McCart PM, Jones SA, et al: Aortocaval fistula detection using a Swan-Ganz catheter. Surg Gynecol Obstet 144:919, 1977.
28. Leather RP, Kupinski AM: Preoperative evaluation of the saphenous vein as a suitable graft. Semin Vasc Surg 1:51, 1988.
29. Lichti EL, Erickson TG: Traumatic arteriovenous fistula: Clinical evaluation and intraoperative monitoring with the Doppler ultrasonic flowmeter. Am J Surg 127:333, 1974.
30. Lindenauer SM: The Klippel-Trenaunay syndrome: Varicosity, hypertrophy, and hemangioma with no arteriovenous fistula. Ann Surg 162:303, 1965.
31. Malorvh M: Noninvasive evaluation of vessels by duplex sonography prior to construction of arteriovenous fistulas for haemodialysis. Nephrol Dial Transplant 13:125, 1998.
32. Mancusi-Ungaro A, Corres JJ, DiSpaltro F: Median carpal tunnel syndrome following a vascular shunt procedure in the forearm. Plast Reconstr Surg 57:96, 1976.
33. Matjasko MJ, Williams JP, Fontanilla M: Intraoperative use of Doppler to detect successful obliteration of carotid-cavernous fistulas. J Neurosurg 43:634, 1975.
34. Merrill WH, Ernst C: Aorta-left renal vein fistula: Hemodynamic monitoring and timing of operation. Surgery 89:678, 1981.
35. Mills CM, Brant-Zawadzki M, Crooks LE: Nuclear magnetic resonance: Principles of blood flow imaging. AJR 142:165, 1984.
36. Muenster JJ, Graettinger JS, Campbell JA: Correlation of clinical and hemodynamic findings in patients with systemic arteriovenous fistulas. Circulation 20:1079, 1959.
37. Murphy TO, Margulis AR: Roentgenographic manifestations of congenital peripheral arteriovenous communications. Radiology 67:26, 1956.
38. Nickerson JL, Elkin DC, Warren JV: The effect of temporary occlusion of arteriovenous fistulas on heart rate, stroke volume, and cardiac output. J Clin Invest 30:215, 1951.
39. Pearce WH, Rutherford RB, Whitehill TA, Davis K: Nuclear magnetic resonance imaging: Its diagnostic value in patients with congenital vascular malformations of the limbs. J Vasc Surg 8:64, 1988.
40. Pinkerton JE Jr: Intraoperative Doppler localization of intestinal arteriovenous malformation. Surgery 85:472, 1979.
41. Piotrowski JJ, Rutherford RB: Proximal vein thrombosis secondary to hemodialysis catheterization complicated by arteriovenous fistula. J Vasc Surg 5:876, 1987.
42. Pisko-Dubienski ZA, Baird RJ, Bayliss CE, et al: Identification and successful treatment of congenital microfistulas with the aid of directional Doppler. Surgery 78:564, 1975.
43. Rauch RF, Silverman PM, Korobkin M, et al: Computed tomography of benign angiomatous lesions of the extremities. J Comput Assist Tomogr 8:1143, 1984.
44. Rhodes BA, Rutherford RB, Lopez-Majano V, et al: Arteriovenous shunt measurement in extremities. J Nucl Med 13:357, 1972.
45. Riley SM, Blackstone EH, Sterling WA, et al: Echocardiographic assessment of cardiac performance in patients with arteriovenous fistulas. Surg Gynecol Obstet 146:203, 1978.
46. Rutherford RB: Clinical applications of a method of quantitating arteriovenous shunting in extremities. In Rutherford RB (ed): Vascular Surgery. Philadelphia, WB Saunders, 1977, pp 781–783.
47. Rutherford RB: Noninvasive testing in the diagnosis and assessment of arteriovenous fistula. In Bernstein EF (ed): Noninvasive Diagnostic Techniques in Vascular Disease. St. Louis, CV Mosby, 1982, pp 430–442.
48. Rutherford RB, Fleming PW, McLeod FD: Vascular diagnostic methods for evaluating patients with arteriovenous fistulas. In Diethrich EB (ed): Noninvasive Cardiovascular Diagnosis: Current Concepts. Baltimore, University Park Press, 1978, pp 189–203.
49. Salles-Cunha SX, Andros G, Harris RW, et al: Preoperative noninvasive assessment of arm veins to be used as bypass grafts in the lower extremities. J Vasc Surg 3:813, 1986.
50. Samet P, Berstein WH, Jacobs W, et al: Indicator-dilution curves in systemic arteriovenous fistulas. Am J Cardiol 13:176, 1964.
51. Silva MB Jr, Hobson RW II, Pappas PJ, et al: A strategy for increasing use of autogenous hemodialysis access procedures: Impact of preoperative noninvasive evaluation. J Vasc Surg 27:302, 1998.
52. Solti F, Soltész L, Bodor E: Hemodynamic changes of systemic and limb circulation in extremity arteriovenous fistula. Angiologica 9:69, 1972.
53. Steinberg I, Tillotson PM, Halpern M: Roentgenography of systemic (congenital and traumatic) arteriovenous fistulas. AJR 89:343, 1963.
54. Stella A, Pedrini LD, Curti T: Use of ultrasound technique in diagnosis and therapy of congenital arteriovenous fistulas. Vasc Surg 15:77, 1981.
55. Stone WJ, Wall MN, Powers TA: Massive upper extremity edema with arteriovenous fistula for hemodialysis: A complication of previous pacemaker insertion. Nephron 31:184, 1982.
56. Strandness DE Jr, Sumner DS: Arteriovenous fistula. In Hemodynamics for Surgeons. New York, Grune & Stratton, 1975, pp 621–663.
57. Strandness DE Jr, Gibbons GE, Bell JW: Mercury strain gauge plethysmography: Evaluation of patients with acquired arteriovenous fistula. Arch Surg 85:215, 1962.
58. Strandness DE Jr, Schultz RD, Sumner DS, Rushmer RF: Ultrasonic flow detection: A useful technic in the evaluation of peripheral vascular disease. Am J Surg 113:311, 1967.
59. Sumner DS: Mercury strain-gauge plethysmography. In Bernstein EF (ed): Noninvasive Diagnostic Techniques in Vascular Disease. St. Louis, CV Mosby, 1982, pp 117–135.
60. Szilagyi DE, Smith RF, Elliott JP, et al: Congenital arteriovenous anomalies of the limbs. Arch Surg 111:423, 1976.

61. Timmis AD, McGonigle RJS, Weston MJ, et al: The influence of hemodialysis fistulas on circulatory dynamics and left ventricular function. Int J Artif Organs 5:101, 1982.

62. Veal JR, McCord WM: Congenital abnormal arteriovenous anastomoses of the extremities with special reference to diagnosis by arteriography and by the oxygen saturation test. Arch Surg 33:848, 1936.

63. Wallace WF, Jamison JP: Measurement by venous occlusion plethysmography of blood flow through surgically created arteriovenous fistulae in the human forearm. Clin Sci Mol Med 50:43, 1976.

64. Wallace WFM, Jamison JP: Effect of a surgically created side-to-side arteriovenous fistula on heat elimination from the human hand and forearm: Evidence for a critical role of venous resistance in determining fistular flow. Clin Sci Mol Med 55:349, 1978.

65. Warren JV, Nickerson JL, Elkins DC: The cardiac output in patients with arteriovenous fistulas. J Clin Invest 30:210, 1951.

66. Willink R, Evans DH: Volumetric blood flow measurement by simultaneous Doppler signal and B-mode processing: A feasibility study. Clin Phys Physiol Meas 11:1, 1990.

67. Wilson JS, Korobkin M, Genant HK, et al: Computed tomography of musculoskeletal disorders. Am J Roentgenol 131:55, 1978.

68. Zeirler BK, Kirkman TR, Kraiss LW, et al: Accuracy of duplex scanning for measurement of arterial flow. J Vasc Surg 16:520, 1992.

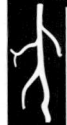

C H A P T E R   1 0 1

Arteriovenous Fistulae of the Aorta and Its Major Branches

William H. Baker, M.D., F.A.C.S., and
M. Ashraf Mansour, M.D., F.A.C.S.

The diagnosis and management of arteriovenous fistulae of the aorta and its major branches present an unparalleled challenge in patient care. Because of their central location, blood flow through these fistulae may be massive; the associated complications are usually dramatic, resulting in severe refractory congestive heart failure, massive venous hypertension, or extensive hemorrhage during an ill-fated surgical repair.

The average vascular surgeon does not have extensive experience with this disorder owing to its relative rarity. For this reason, it behooves the surgeon to become well acquainted with the problem in order to avoid complications and, therefore, to ensure optimal patient care.

ETIOLOGY

Arteriovenous fistulae of the aorta and its major branches may be *congenital* or *acquired*. The congenital types are briefly considered here; they are discussed more extensively in Chapter 103.

Any disease that spontaneously weakens the wall of the aorta or one of its major branches might logically lead to the formation of an arteriovenous fistula. Rare causes are erosion of false aneurysms secondary to sepsis and specific aortitis. There has been one report of a mesenchymal tumor between the aorta and inferior vena cava leading to an aorta–vena cava fistula, but arteriovenous fistulae secondary to tumors are most often reported with hypernephromas.[3, 6] Rupture of an atherosclerotic aneurysm is a relatively common cause of acquired fistulae.

Trauma is the major cause of arteriovenous fistulae. Low-velocity trauma from a knife or small-caliber missile, for example, leads to fistula formation, whereas higher-velocity wounds made by large-caliber missiles tend to disrupt the major vessels, leading to more immediate exsanguination.

The surgeon may unwittingly be another source of trauma. If, during lumbar disc operations, the rongeur penetrates the anterior longitudinal ligament, the immobile major vessels may be injured. The aorta and inferior vena cava are injured opposite the L4–L5 disc space, whereas the iliac vessels are injured opposite the L5–S1 space. Lumbar arteries and veins can be injured at any level. The popularity of microdiscectomy seems to have decreased the incidence of this complication.

Closure of the mesentery following gastrectomy and small bowel resections has damaged adjacent arteries and veins and has led to arterioportal venous fistulae. Mass ligations of major arteries and veins, such as the renal and splenic pedicle, have produced fistulae. Finally, needle biopsy of the kidney has led to renal arteriovenous fistulae.

DIAGNOSIS

The diagnosis of a major arteriovenous fistula is not usually difficult for the wary physician but may escape the casual examiner. The patient will often complain of a noise or a thrill over the fistula. There may be a pulsating mass caused by a false aneurysm. If there is a large flow of blood through the fistula, congestive heart failure may be evident. There may be symptoms related to the "stealing" of blood from a variety of end organs, producing renal ischemia and hypertension, visceral ischemia and abdominal angina, cerebrovascular insufficiency, and intermittent claudication.

The classic signs of increased pulse pressure, a bruit over the fistula, pulsating veins, venous hypertension and edema, and diminished distal pulses may or may not be present. In addition, renal function may be impaired, either because of reduced arterial flow through the kidney or because of venous hypertension leading to lower glomerular filtration rates. Hematuria, microscopic or gross, is a common finding with aorta to left renal vein fistulae.[12] However, hematuria is not commonly present with aortocaval fistulae unless venous engorgement of the bladder occurs.[4, 14]

Many of these arteriovenous fistulae have an associated false aneurysm or are secondary to aneurysm rupture. These aneurysms notoriously are partially filled with thrombus. The thrombus may partially, completely, or intermittently cover the fistula, and symptoms may be intermittently present or totally absent.[1] The surgeon may be unaware of this until the clot is removed in the operating room and the surgical field is flooded with venous blood.

The diagnosis can be made by noninvasive testing. With color flow duplex scanning, the presence and location of the fistula can be confirmed (Fig. 101–1). Doppler interrogation of the inferior vena cava shows the characteristic high-flow signals and turbulence typically associated with a fistula. Groin venous flow will be pulsatile.

The precise site of any arteriovenous fistula is best identified by arteriography, although both computed tomography (CT)[15] and ultrasonography[11] have been helpful in detecting this condition (Fig. 101–2). Frequent films must be taken because of the increased velocity of flow through the fistula.

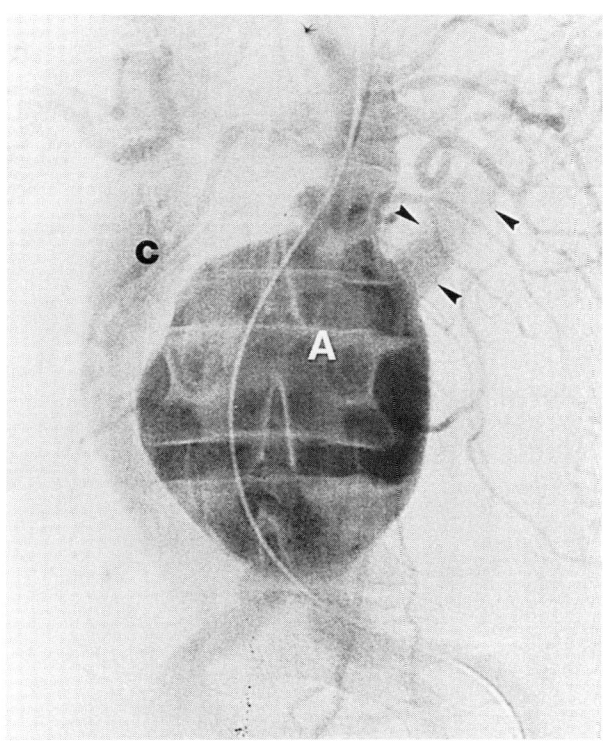

FIGURE 101–2. Angiogram showing a large abdominal aortic aneurysm (A) with early filling of the inferior vena cava (C) and the retroaortic left renal vein (*straight arrowheads*). (From Mansour MA, Russ PD, Subber SW, Pearce WH: Aorto–left renal vein fistula: Diagnosis by duplex sonography. AJR Am J Roentgenol 152:1107, 1989.)

In a patient who is bleeding actively from either trauma or ruptured aneurysm, there is not enough time to obtain arteriograms; thus the diagnosis must, of necessity, be made in the operating room. In elective cases, arteriography not only informs the surgeon of the exact arterial site (suprarenal or infrarenal aorta) but also yields information concerning venous drainage (left renal vein or inferior vena cava) (Fig. 101–3).

PRINCIPLES OF THERAPY

Preoperative recognition of an arteriovenous fistula of the aorta or its major branches is of paramount importance. It is an absolute necessity that the surgeon spend the extra time needed to examine the patient completely, with the following questions kept in mind: Is there a to-and-fro bruit over the aneurysm? Does the patient with penetrating abdominal trauma have distended leg veins? If the diagnosis is delayed until the patient is going into congestive heart failure from overtransfusion or until the thrill of the fistula is first felt through an inadequate or misplaced incision, the patient ultimately will suffer.

The fluid dynamics in patients with arteriovenous fistulae are reviewed in Chapter 99. Patients with acute fistulae may have associated blood loss and may be hypovolemic despite the presence of pulsating veins. Individuals with chronic fistulae are usually hypervolemic. In general, they do not need volume-for-volume blood replacement;

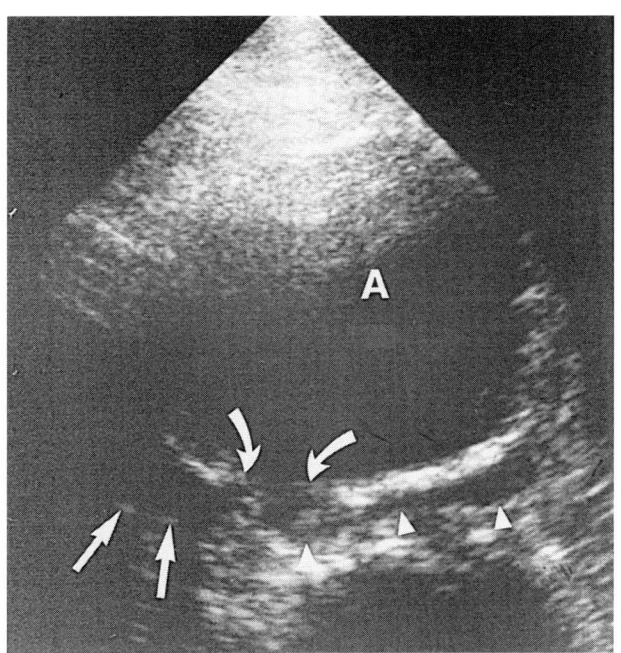

FIGURE 101–1. Duplex ultrasonography demonstrating an abdominal aortic aneurysm (A), with a fistulous communication in posterior wall (*curved arrows*) to a retroaortic left renal vein (*small arrowheads*), and a normal vena cava (*straight arrows*). (From Mansour MA, Russ PD, Subber SW, Pearce WH: Aorto–left renal vein fistula: Diagnosis by duplex sonography. AJR Am J Roentgenol 152:1107, 1989.)

thus, the surgeon should beware of overtransfusion if overloading would occur when the fistula is closed.

The central venous pressure is abnormally elevated in the patient with a central arteriovenous fistula, and this measurement cannot be used to guide fluid administration. A pulmonary artery (Swan-Ganz) catheter, however, facilitates fluid management and allows the surgical team to measure the pulmonary wedge pressure and cardiac output and, thereby, to assess the function of the left ventricle. The cardiac output may be elevated owing to the hyperdynamic circulation resulting from the fistula. The oxygen saturation of mixed venous blood is elevated secondary to direct infusion of arterial blood into the vena cava.[9]

Transesophageal echocardiography should also be helpful in assessment of cardiac performance. Although these principles are well known to the modern surgical team, when hypotension and hemorrhage occur during the hurried repair of these fistulae, fluid administration is both difficult and critical.

Whenever surgery is to be undertaken, enough blood must be available in case of hemorrhagic catastrophes. Acute fistulae are easily entered. Chronic fistulae have thinned, large arteries and bulging veins and are encased in a fibrotic or inflammatory mass. The dissection may be extremely difficult and bloody. *Autotransfusion* is an ideal way to replace large amounts of blood lost by hemorrhage in a clean surgical field and has been used successfully in patients with aorta–vena cava fistulae.[5] Total circulatory arrest has also been successfully used in patients with large central arteriovenous fistulae.[7]

The goals of surgical therapy for a major arteriovenous fistula are to close the fistula, thereby restoring normal hemodynamics, and to reestablish or maintain vascular continuity. There is little place in modern surgery for qua-

druple ligation of a major fistula involving the aorta or its major branches.

Before the patient is brought to the operating room, some care must be taken in planning the incision. It is always best to prepare an extensive area so that an adequate incision can be made to control major bleeding. For example, if the wound is at the base of the neck, the thorax is always prepared so that a thoracotomy or sternotomy can be performed for control of the major vessels as they come off the aortic arch. For treating high abdominal fistulae, the thorax is prepared so that the descending thoracic aorta can be controlled if major bleeding is encountered.

It is imperative that the surgeon obtain proximal and distal control of the artery involved. If arterial control is obtained at some distance from the fistula, the uncontrolled branches should then be individually isolated.

Occlusion of the aorta from the level of the aortic arch to the level of the renal arteries may cause significant hypertension. Elevated blood pressure can usually be tolerated by a young, vigorous heart, but the increased afterload may cause cardiac failure with diminished cardiac output and hypoperfusion. In this situation, the pressure and peripheral resistance should be pharmacologically controlled until the afterload caused by the occluding clamp is removed. At the time of clamp removal, the administration of antihypertensive drugs must be carefully stopped lest profound hypotension ensue.

Ideally, proximal and distal venous control should be obtained, but often this maneuver is most difficult to accomplish. The veins are distended from the increased pressure and the increased volume of blood. Blood under arterial pressure gushes forth from every small venous tributary that ordinarily retracts and bleeds but a few drops. If, indeed, venous control is obtained, it is facilitated by intermittent clamping of the proximal and distal artery. This maneuver diminishes the flow through the fistula, reduces the venous hypertension, and thereby makes dissection easier. Fogarty and Foley balloon catheters can be passed both proximally and distally in the vein as an alternative to digital occlusion until the fistulous communication is repaired.[4, 8]

When venous control is obtained, the surgeon must have careful communication with the anesthesiologists. Control of the inferior vena cava may seriously diminish the venous return to the heart, and this may cause dire cardiac effects in an already hypovolemic patient. In many cases, the patient can tolerate this hemodynamic insult for only a few seconds, and intermittent flow through the vena cava may be necessary to maintain acceptable hemodynamics.

More often, the vein is not encircled, but proximal and distal arterial control is obtained and the artery is opened. The fistula can be controlled by a finger or thumb placed over the communication. Compression with sponge sticks caudad and cephalad to the fistula will diminish blood flow through the vein (Fig. 101–4; see Fig. 101–2). This maneuver ordinarily takes but a few seconds and disturbs the patient's venous return only temporarily. If the surgeon is careful in sewing under his or her finger, blood loss can be kept at a minimum. Repair of the fistula should be performed from within the aneurysm sac. Polytetrafluoroethylene (Teflon) pledgets may be helpful; rarely, a synthetic patch of polyester (Dacron) or polytetrafluoroethylene

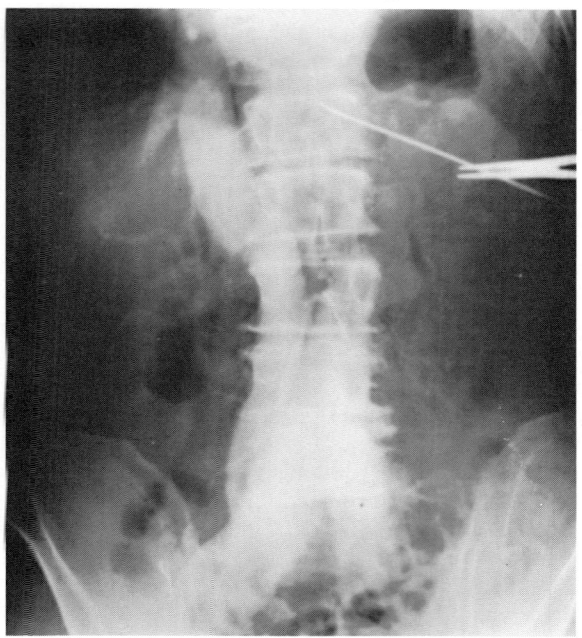

FIGURE 101–3. A translumbar aortogram reveals that this abdominal aortic aneurysm has eroded into the distal inferior vena cava. (From Baker WH, Sharzer LA, Ehrenhaft JL: Aortocaval fistula as a complication of abdominal aortic aneurysms. Surgery 72:933, 1972.)

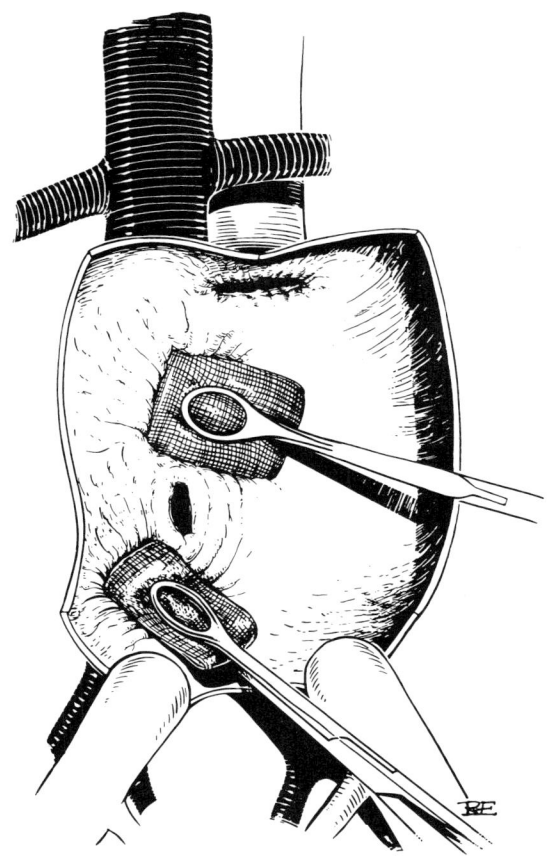

FIGURE 101–4. Sponge stick control of the inferior vena cava, as seen through the open aortic aneurysm. (From Baker WH, Sharzer LA, Ehrenhaft JL: Aortocaval fistula as a complication of abdominal aortic aneurysms. Surgery 72:933, 1972.)

(PTFE) is used to close a large defect and avoid narrowing of the vein.[4]

After the vein is repaired, the preferred method for restoring arterial continuity is with a graft. Ordinarily, a Dacron graft is used to bridge the deficit. If the surgical field is contaminated by concomitant injury to the adjacent viscera or by a wounding missile, however, the care becomes much more complicated. These patients should be managed in the same way as those with arterial infections. That is, the area of sepsis should be débrided, the artery should be closed proximally and distally, and arterial continuity should be restored extra-anatomically. After the abdomen is closed, a subcutaneous bypass can be performed in a clean surgical field to maintain viability of the extremities.

An alternative approach is to place a prosthetic graft into the potentially contaminated field. The operative area is completely débrided and irrigated with saline or antibiotic solution. After the prosthetic graft is sutured into place, it is isolated from the contaminated peritoneal cavity with an omental pedicle if necessary. Patients should be given massive doses of antibiotics, and they must be followed up continuously for many months to ensure that graft infection, false aneurysm formation, and exsanguination do not result.

Endovascular repair of arteriovenous fistulae and aneurysms is being performed successfully with stented grafts and endoluminal grafts (see Chapter 90) There have been isolated reports using these new devices.[18] Homografts and autogenous superficial femoral veins have been used in contaminated fields with reported success.

FISTULAE AT SPECIFIC SITES

Base of the Neck

It is rare to find an arteriovenous fistula that involves the thoracic aorta and superior vena cava or the great vessels as they come off the thoracic arch. Thoracic aortic aneurysms tend to dissect rather than form saccular aneurysms that erode into adjacent veins. Wounds of this area are usually explored immediately, before a fistula has had a chance to develop. Direct puncture of the carotid and vertebral arteries for arteriography is an uncommon cause of fistulae.

Subclavian artery and vein fistulae present with the symptoms that are discussed in Chapter 102 and with local symptoms of a palpable mass and thrill. They may be secondary to trauma (penetrating or blunt, causing fractures of the thoracic outlet) or congenital. Associated brachial plexus symptoms may be present, depending on the size of the aneurysm or the extent of the trauma.

A fistula between the carotid artery and the internal jugular vein may divert enough blood from the carotid system to create symptoms of cerebrovascular insufficiency. In addition, thrombus from the false aneurysm may embolize cephalad to the eye or brain. The patient usually complains of a mass in the neck, which represents the false aneurysm. In addition, a thrill or bruit is present over the fistula.

If the fistula is low in the base of the neck, the surgeon should plan to gain proximal control by thoracotomy or median sternotomy. The left common carotid artery and the innominate artery can be controlled through a full or limited median sternotomy (trapdoor incision), but the left subclavian artery is best controlled through a left anterior thoracotomy because of its posterior position on the arch. In most patients, the artery is opened, the fistula is closed from the arterial side, and the divided artery is repaired with an end-to-end anastomosis. If too much artery is resected to allow reanastomosis without undue tension, an interposition graft of vein or prosthetic material can be used with good results.

When the carotid circulation is interrupted during repair of a fistula involving the great vessels of the neck, an indwelling shunt may be used to ensure adequate cerebral circulation. The use of these shunts is a debatable topic. Ordinarily, at the base of the neck there is enough collateral circulation so that a shunt is unnecessary most, if not all, of the time.

There is little place for nonoperative therapy in the management of acquired arteriovenous fistulae at the base of the neck. Their natural history is that they will continue to grow, and the patient will experience either rupture of the false aneurysm or symptoms of cerebrovascular insufficiency. The risk of repair is related to cerebral complications and blood loss. Because these risks can be kept to a minimum, surgical repair is the treatment of choice.

Aorta and Vena Cava

Fistulae of the aorta and vena cava are most commonly due to rupture of aortic abdominal aneurysms (AAAs) of atherosclerotic origin. There have been more than 250 cases of aortocaval fistulae reported in the literature. The incidence is slightly higher in association with ruptured aortic aneurysms. In a series of six patients with aortocaval fistulae from the University of Iowa, classic symptoms (abdominal bruit, widened pulse pressure, venous hypertension, edema, arterial insufficiency, and congestive heart failure) were present in three, and a proper preoperative diagnosis was made in one.[1] Proximal and distal control of the aortic aneurysm was obtained in the usual manner. Venous control was not attempted, but the aneurysm was opened and the fistula controlled with compression, as mentioned earlier. The fistula was closed and the aneurysm replaced with a graft.

In a subsequent series from Boston of perhaps less urgent cases, 75% were correctly diagnosed preoperatively and the mortality rate was reduced from 50% to 10%.[2] A recent report from the Mayo Clinic identified 18 patients over a 27-year period (0.3% of all aortoiliac aneurysms performed in that institution). Although 94% of patients were symptomatic at presentation, only 17% had the classic triad of pain, pulsatile mass, and abdominal bruit.[4]

The surgeon should take special care to manipulate the aortic aneurysm as little as possible before closing the fistula. These aneurysms are notoriously filled with thrombus, and if this clot becomes dislodged, it will embolize through the fistula and return via the inferior vena cava to the right side of the heart and the pulmonary artery (Fig. 101–5) This complication can be avoided by careful surgical technique.

Traumatic fistulae between the aorta and the inferior vena cava are less common. Direct trauma usually causes massive blood loss, and most patients do not make it to the operating room.

The formation of arteriovenous fistulae between the aorta and the vena cava or the iliac vein after a total discectomy, fortunately, is uncommon. About 50% of these patients do not have extreme blood loss during the operation, although many have unexplained hypotension during the discectomy. However, the blood loss is into the retroperitoneum and may not be obvious to the operating surgeon posteriorly through the disc space. The treatment of these fistulae is surgical because they will continue to grow. They are located relatively caudad in the abdominal aorta, and thus exposure is usually not difficult. It is safer to close the fistula through the artery, because dissection at the confluence of the iliac veins and the inferior vena cava can be extremely hazardous in the presence of arterialized venous pressure. When covered stents and endoluminal grafts become more widely available, endovascular repair may very well be the preferred method of treatment. Because these devices are relatively new, no long-term results have yet been reported (see Chapter 90).

Aorta and Renal Vein

AAAs can rupture anteriorly into the left renal vein as it crosses in its normal position over the aorta, but they most

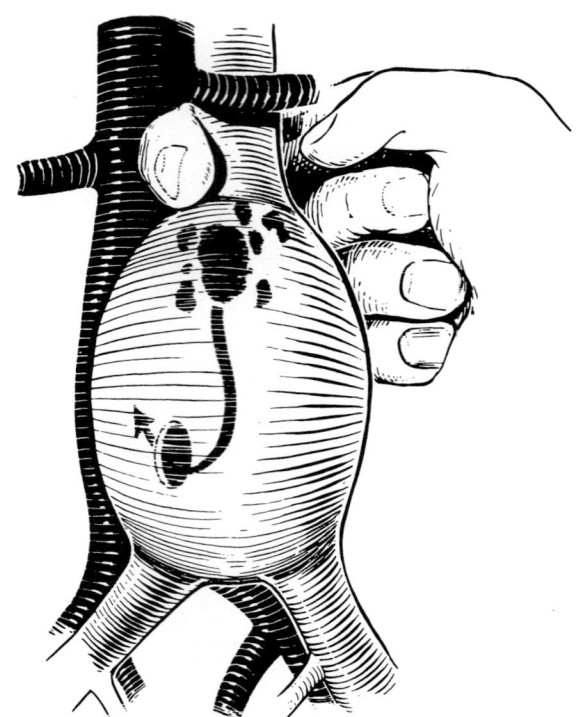

FIGURE 101–5. Dissection of the clot-containing aneurysm must be delicate lest the thrombus become dislodged, enter the inferior vena cava, and embolize to the pulmonary artery. (From Baker WH, Sharzer LA, Ehrenhaft JL: Aortocaval fistula as a complication of abdominal aortic aneurysms. Surgery 72:933, 1972.)

often rupture into a retroaortic left renal vein. There have been 20 reports of aorta to left renal vein fistula in the English literature; in all but one, the left renal vein was retroaortic.[9, 12, 17] AAAs should be treated as other aorta–inferior vena cava fistulae. The vein is closed from within the artery, and a graft is used to replace the AAA. Sacrifice of the vein is possible without sequelae if the adrenal or gonadal vein is left intact to provide collateral venous circulation.

Renal Artery and Vein

Renal arteriovenous fistulae are covered separately in Chapter 125. Suffice it to say that most are secondary to mass ligation of the renal hilum during nephrectomy.[13] Traumatic fistulae are caused by knife and missile wounds. The renal biopsy needle is a cause of intrarenal arteriovenous fistulization. Hypernephromas commonly grow caudad through the renal veins. Such a tumor has been reported to grow into the renal artery, producing a major arteriovenous fistula.[10] The indication for repair is usually the presence of a fistula. Rarely will a fistula be small and fail to enlarge. Hypertension, if present, is usually poorly controlled until the fistula is repaired or until the kidney is removed.

Portal Vein and Systemic Artery

Systemic artery–portal vein fistulae are extremely rare.[16] They may occur after surgical procedures, sepsis that erodes adjacent arteries and veins, rupture of aneurysms, and trauma. Splenic arteriovenous fistulae occur when splenic artery aneurysms rupture into the splenic vein. Congenital fistulae are reported to occur most commonly between the hepatic artery and the portal vein and are associated with hemangiomas and telangiectasia.

These fistulae characteristically do not cause symptoms of congestive heart failure, presumably because of the buffer of the hepatic venous circulation. Portal venous hypertension is produced, however, and esophageal, gastric, or small bowel varices may lead to gastrointestinal hemorrhage, ascites, or both.

The treatment of these fistulae depends on the vessels involved. Splenic fistulae may be excised by splenectomy. Peripheral mesenteric fistulae may be simply excised, but more centrally located fistulae should be excised, the arterial flow restored to maintain bowel viability, and the portal venous flow restored to correct the portal hypertension and to avoid venous infarction of the bowel. Peripheral hepatic aneurysms and fistulae may be treated by percutaneous embolization.

REFERENCES

1. Baker WH, Sharzer LA, Ehrenhaft JL: Aortocaval fistula as a complication of abdominal aortic aneurysms. Surgery 72:933, 1972.
2. Brewster DC, Cambria RP, Moncure AC, et al: Aortocaval and iliac arteriovenous fistulas: Recognition and treatment. J Vasc Surg 13:253, 1991.
3. Crawford ES, Turrell DJ, Alexander JK: Aorto-inferior vena caval fistula of neoplastic origin. Circulation 27:414, 1963.
4. Davis PM, Gloviczki P, Cherry KJ, et al: Aorto-caval and ilio-iliac arteriovenous fistulae: Rare and challenging problems. Am J Surg 176:115, 1998.
5. Doty DB, Wright CB, Lamberth WC, et al: Aortocaval fistula associated with aneurysm of the abdominal aorta: Current management using autotransfusion techniques. Surgery 84:250, 1978.
6. Gomes MMR, Bernatz PE: Arteriovenous fistulas: A review and ten-year experience. Mayo Clin Proc 45:81, 1970.
7. Griffin LH Jr, Fishback ME, Galloway RF, et al: Traumatic aortorenal vein fistula: Repair using total circulatory arrest. Surgery 81:480, 1977.
8. Ingoldby CJ, Case WG, Primrose JN: Aortocaval fistulas and the use of transvenous balloon tamponade. Ann R Coll Surg Engl 72:335, 1990.
9. Jabbour N, Radulescu OV, Flogiates T, Stahl W: Hemodynamics of an aorta–left renal vein fistula: A case report and a review of the literature. Crit Care Med 21:1092, 1993.
10. Jantet GH, Foot EC, Kenyon JR: Rupture of an intrarenal arteriovenous fistula secondary to carcinoma: A case report. Br J Surg 49:404, 1962.
11. Mansour MA, Russ PD, Subber SW, Pearce WH: Aorto–left renal vein fistula: Diagnosis by duplex sonography. AJR Am J Roentgenol 152:1107, 1989.
12. Mansour MA, Rutherford RB, Metcalf RK, Pearce WH: Spontaneous aorto–left renal vein fistula: The "abdominal pain, hematuria, silent left kidney" syndrome. Surgery 109:101, 1991.
13. Matos A, Moreira A, Mendonca M: Renal arteriovenous fistula after nephrectomy. Ann Vasc Surg 6:378, 1992.
14. Salo JA, Verkkala KA, Ala-Kulju KV, et al: Hematuria is an indication of rupture of an abdominal aortic aneurysm into the vena cava. J Vasc Surg 12:41, 1990.
15. Sheward SE, Spencer RR, Hinton RT, et al: Computed tomography of primary aortocaval fistula. Comput Med Imaging Graph 16:121, 1992.
16. Strodel WE, Eckhauser FE, Lemmer JH, et al: Presentation and perioperative management of arterioportal fistulas. Arch Surg 127:563, 1987.
17. Thompson RW, Yee LF, Natuzzi ES, Stoney RJ: Aorta-left renal vein fistula syndrome caused by rupture of a juxtarenal abdominal aortic aneurysm: Novel pathologic mechanism for a unique clinical entity. J Vasc Surg 18:310, 1993.
18. Zajko AB, Little AF, Steed DL, Curtiss EI: Endovascular stent-graft repair of common iliac artery to inferior vena cava fistula. J Vasc Interv Radiol 6:803, 1995.

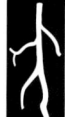

CHAPTER   1   0   2
Peripheral Arteriovenous Fistulae

Thomas S. Riles, M.D., Robert J. Rosen, M.D., and Glenn R. Jacobowitz, M.D.

PATHOGENESIS

The causes of an arteriovenous fistula, which is simply defined as an abnormal single communication between the arterial and venous systems, may be quite varied. Acquired fistulae most often result from trauma. Penetrating injuries from knives, bullets, needles, and catheters injure adjacent arteries and veins, opening communications between the two vascular systems. Blunt trauma that causes fracture or joint disarticulation may also lead to development of an arteriovenous fistula. Carotid-cavernous fistulae from facial trauma and hypogastric artery fistulae from pelvic injuries are examples. Arteriovenous fistulae may also result from neoplasm, infection, and atherosclerotic aneurysms, although they do so quite rarely.

Congenital arteriovenous fistulae are usually associated with malformations of the great vessels or result from failure of the fetal arteriovenous communications of the atrial septum and patent ductus arteriosus to close. Congenital fistulae may also occur in the peripheral circulation. First cousins of the multifistulous congenital arteriovenous

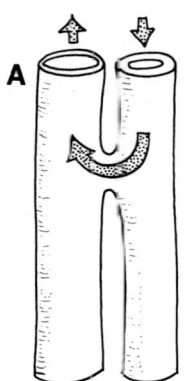
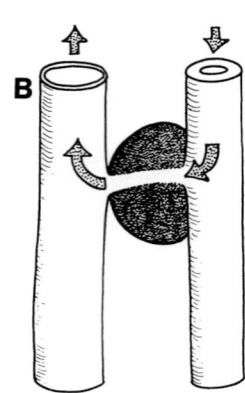

FIGURE 102–1. *A*, Arteriovenous fistula between two adjacent vessels. *B*, Arteriovenous fistula with an intervening false aneurysm.

malformations discussed in Chapter 103, congenital fistulae also result from failure of the embryonic vascular network to differentiate into separate arterial and venous systems with an intervening capillary network. Although congenital arteriovenous fistulae have long been noted to exist and occasionally have been observed on routine angiography, they are seldom of clinical significance. The diagnosis is usually made by exclusion of other, more common, causes. Arteriovenous fistulae for therapeutic purposes, such as dialysis, or for maintenance of arterial bypasses and venous repairs are discussed in Section XIV.

In some instances, the distance between the artery and the vein may be quite short, with the fistula consisting of no more than the walls of the adjacent vessels. In other cases, a fibrotic channel may separate the artery and the vein. False aneurysms are frequently found in association with fistulae, particularly with those that result from trauma (Fig. 102–1). Of the 195 patients with traumatic arteriovenous fistulae examined by Elkin and Shumacker, 60% had an associated false aneurysm.[12] Although most of the aneurysms were interposed between artery and vein, the remainder were at various locations separate from or on the venous side of the fistula (see Fig. 99–11).

PHYSIOLOGY AND CLINICAL MANIFESTATIONS

The physiology of arteriovenous fistulae is reviewed extensively in Chapter 99. In brief, a peripheral arteriovenous fistula may lead to local changes in the region of the abnormal communication, to central changes secondary to the stress on the entire cardiovascular system, or to both local and central changes. The extent of the clinical manifestations is related to the size of the fistula, its duration, and its precise location. For example, a small-caliber fistula of recent onset in an extremity may be appreciated only by an audible bruit or a palpable thrill. A chronic fistula in the same location may create venous hypertension and valvular incompetence. Fistulae of long standing are typically associated with dilatation and elongation of the feeding artery.[22] The venous system proximal to the fistula similarly dilates. Venous hypertension, incompetence, and hypertrophy commonly lead to distal swelling. A large fistula, acute or chronic, in the same area may result in

extensive shunting (steal) of peripheral blood flow, loss of pulse, and ischemia of the distal tissues.

In addition to the local changes, the heart and the remainder of the vascular system may be profoundly affected. The major determinant of the systemic response is the size of the shunt, which is measured in terms of the percentage of cardiac output that passes through the fistula. Other factors include the duration of the shunt and associated medical conditions, such as coronary artery disease, valvular incompetence, and myocardial dysfunction. Smaller shunts that have persisted longer may lead to ventricular dilatation, myocardial hypertrophy, and congestive heart failure. Massive shunts may quickly lead to hypotension, heart failure, and death.

DIAGNOSIS

Although many imaginative studies have been described for the diagnosis of arteriovenous fistulae, most fistulae are easily detected after a careful history taking and physical examination. An arteriovenous fistula should be considered with any penetrating injury in a trauma patient. A stethoscope placed over the site of injury may detect the continuous murmur characteristic of an arteriovenous fistula. If surgery is not immediately indicated for patients with deep wounds, arteriography may be indicated to rule out an arteriovenous fistula or another arterial lesion.

Patients who have a chronic arteriovenous fistula usually report a history of penetrating injury. The patient usually complains of a pulsatile mass, a buzzing sound, or a vibrating sensation. Swelling may also be present. It is rare that the diagnosis is not made before symptoms of ischemia and heart failure develop.

Examination reveals a site of recent injury or a scar from an old injury over the course of an artery. A to-and-fro ("machinery") murmur is usually best heard directly over the fistula and is often associated with a thrill. It is to be distinguished from the loud systolic and separate, faint diastolic murmurs of the false aneurysm and from the systolic murmur of arterial stenosis. The temperature of the skin overlying the arteriovenous fistula may be elevated, whereas distally, the skin temperature is often decreased. Veins, especially those peripheral to the fistula, are distended and at times tortuous and varicose. With long-standing fistula, chronic venous hypertension may cause dermatitis and ulceration similar to that seen in the post-phlebitic state. The tachycardia observed in some patients may decrease when the artery leading to the fistula or the fistula itself is occluded (Branham's sign).[6] Studies to document the increase in cardiac output and blood volume that accompanies some fistulae, although of physiologic interest, rarely aid the diagnosis or in treating these patients. The use of a Doppler probe and other noninvasive diagnostic methods is described in Chapter 100.

Angiography should be performed in most patients thought to have arteriovenous fistula to confirm the diagnosis and to localize the abnormal vascular communication. It may be difficult to demonstrate the actual site of communication because of the very high flow in and dilatation of the venous system. The diagnostic study should be as selective as possible. Rapid contrast injection and very rapid imaging are often essential for visualizing the communication. Even more difficult are chronic arteriovenous fistulae in patients who have undergone unsuccessful surgical or radiologic attempts at closure. After arterial ligation or embolization, complex patterns of collateral inflow obscure the view of the fistula. The use of balloon catheters to retard or arrest flow may greatly aid in localizing the lesion.[3] False aneurysms and secondary changes, such as dilatation and tortuosity of the feeding artery and reversal of venous flow distal to the fistula, may also be seen on angiography. Identification of these related changes may be important in planning therapy.

TREATMENT

Historical Perspective

The history of the treatment of arteriovenous fistulae is a fascinating tale of clinical frustration, scientific observation, and surgical ingenuity. Hunter's vivid description of an arteriovenous fistula, presented in 1762, was apparently the first to be recorded.[19] With the frequent use of bloodletting in the mid-1800s, surgeons had the opportunity to deal with numerous fistulae involving the brachial artery and vein. The debate over whether to do nothing, ligate the proximal and distal arteries, or use the "ancient method" of opening the sac and tying off the feeding vessels continued into the 1900s.[26]

In 1833, Breschet recognized that proximal artery ligation of an arteriovenous fistula was ill advised because the development of collateral circulation allowed the abnormal communication to persist (Fig. 102–2B).[7] Dupuytren, in 1854, continued to recommend proximal arterial ligation.[11] In 1843, Norris, while attempting proximal and distal arterial ligation, experienced many complications that, he reported, "Were such as would prevent my ever again having recourse to it" and recommended the "old operation of laying open the sac and securing the vessel above and below the wounded point."[26]

In 1897, Murphy closed a small hole in the vein of an arteriovenous fistula and then performed the first end-to-end anastomosis of the artery (Fig. 102–2C).[25] Despite this, Matas, in 1902, after extensive review of arteriovenous fistulae involving the subclavian vessels, concluded that "the old rule of non-intervention is still in order and should

be followed."[23] He added, however, that when the lesion is not tolerated well, it is justifiable to operate with a view to extirpating the lesion.

After 1902, when Carrel demonstrated the ability to create a vascular anastomosis, extirpation of the arteriovenous fistula with end-to-end anastomosis gradually became the treatment of choice for fistulas of short duration.[8] By 1922, Matas believed that "quadruple ligation with resection of both vessels has become an almost obsolete practice"[24] (Fig. 102–2D).

It is interesting that in a report by Elkin and Shumacker of 585 arteriovenous fistulae treated during World War II, 526 were treated by quadruple ligation and excision.[12] Despite this, extirpation of the lesion with maintenance or restoration of the continuity of the artery was considered to be the ideal treatment.[12, 14]

Foley and associates noted in 1956 that "postoperative arterial insufficiency" developed in 50% of all patients at the Mayo Clinic whose arterial continuity of the lower extremity was interrupted for treatment of arteriovenous communications.[13] As a result of this observation, Foley's group made a plea for early surgical treatment of traumatic arteriovenous fistulae and an attempt to reestablish arterial and venous continuity. This advice was echoed by Beall and associates in 1963.[2] Spencer and Grewe[32] and Hughes and Jahnke[18] urged simultaneous venous repair to prevent swelling of the distal extremity. Reports from Vietnam in 1966 and 1969 noted that arteriovenous fistulae were infrequently encountered when early repair of arterial injuries was the policy.[17, 31]

Thus, the repair of arteriovenous fistulae has evolved from simple arterial ligation through extirpation of the fistula to the currently recommended treatment of reconstructive surgery. Added to this now is the possibility of closure of fistulae with percutaneous catheters (Fig. 102–2I to K) and endoluminal stent grafts.[9, 30] With the techniques currently available, there should be few chronic traumatic arteriovenous fistulae in the practice of vascular surgery.

Current Therapy

Except in rare instances, the goal of treatment should be complete closure of an arteriovenous fistula, regardless of its cause. Proximal arterial ligation has repeatedly failed and should be avoided at all costs. In addition to the persistence of the fistula, the patient's condition usually deteriorates because of ischemia of the distal tissues. Percutaneous endovascular closure, which may be the procedure of choice, is virtually impossible after proximal arterial ligation has been performed.

After the location of the fistula is determined by angiography, a decision must be made as to how it might best be managed. Alternatives include various surgical options as well as a selection of catheter occlusion techniques that have been developed with the evolution of modern interventional radiology. In addition, recently developed endovascular covered stents (endografts) may prove to be valuable in treating arteriovenous fistulas. Endografts effectively exclude the arteriovenous connection when placed across the fistula tract from within the artery.[1, 9, 10, 16, 27, 28, 29] Early results show excellent patency, particularly in larger vessels such as the subclavian, iliac, and superficial femoral arter-

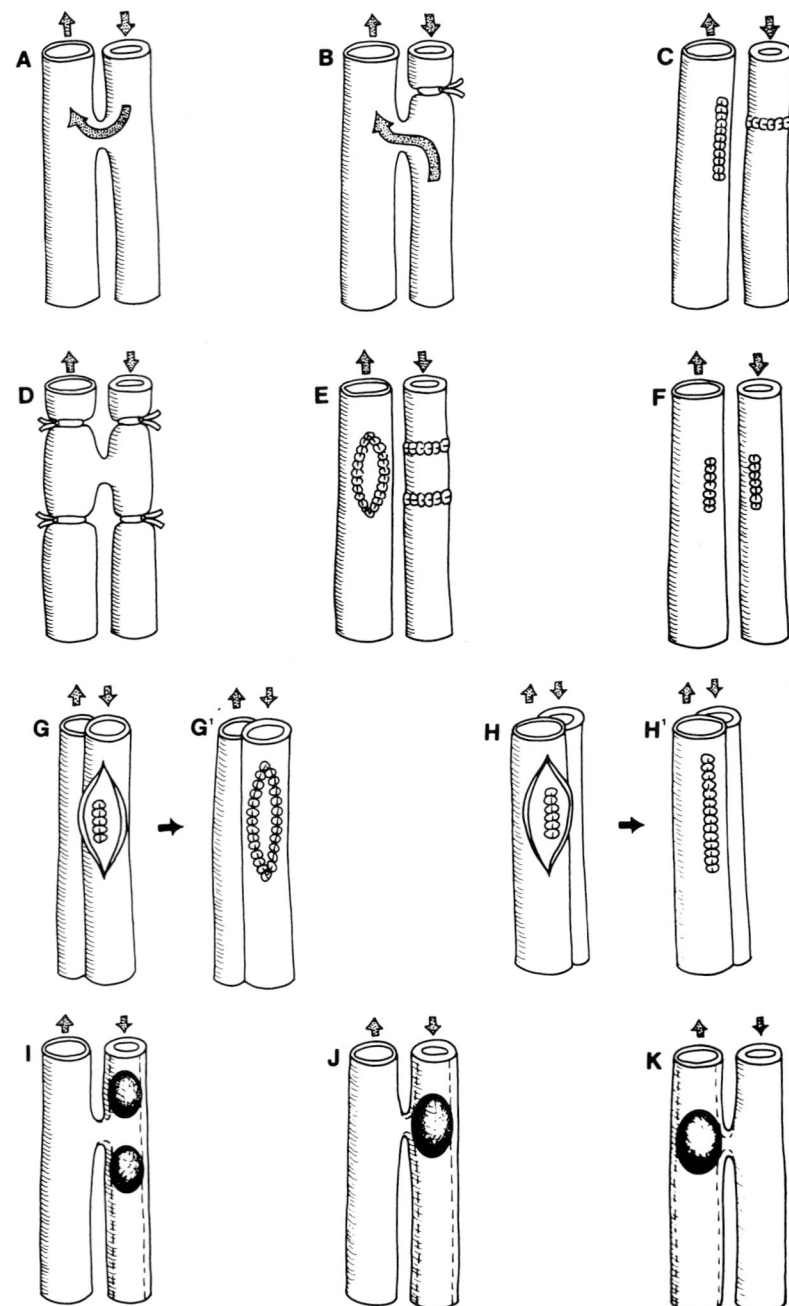

FIGURE 102–2. Methods of surgical and percutaneous treatment of arteriovenous fistulae. *A,* Arteriovenous fistula. *B,* Proximal ligation fails to control the fistula because of collateral circulation to the distal artery. *C,* Resection of the fistula with end-to-end reanastomosis of the artery and primary vessel closure. *D,* Quadruple ligation without reconstruction, which is reserved for small fistulae. *E,* Resection of the fistula with an interposition graft to reconstruct the artery and patch angioplasty repair of the vein. *F,* Simple division of the fistula and primary closure of the artery and the vein. *G,* Closure of the fistula through an arteriotomy, with patch closure of the arteriotomy, *G¹*. *H,* Closure of the fistula through a venotomy, with primary closure of the venotomy, *H¹*. *I* and *J,* Closure of the fistula by percutaneous placement of detachable balloons, which is an acceptable method for small fistulae with adequate collateral circulation around the site of communication. *K,* Closure of the fistula by percutaneous placement of a balloon on the venous side of the fistula.

ies.[27] The choice of technique is largely determined by the size, the accessibility, and the cause of the fistula. Other factors include the relative risks of the percutaneous and the surgical approaches. It is essential that the interventional radiologist and the surgeon together review the various possibilities and develop a unified plan with alternatives and contingencies. With very complex communications, both must be prepared for the unexpected.

As mentioned, most peripheral arteriovenous fistulae are the result of trauma.[15, 28] If a fistula arises from a branch artery or a nonessential one, simple obliteration of the fistula without concern for maintenance of arterial continuity may be the treatment of choice. The fistula may be obliterated by surgical ligation of the artery above and below the fistula. The addition of venous (quadruple) ligation is historically important but is seldom necessary as long as occlusion of the arterial component is properly performed. Failure to obliterate the artery exactly at the site of the fistula may lead to recurrence as collateral blood flow finds its way to the fistula. Exclusion of the arteriovenous connection by a covered endovascular stent separates the arterial and venous components of the fistula and restores normal hemodynamics. This particular method has been used effectively in the trauma setting.[16, 27]

The same result may be obtained by percutaneous placement of embolic materials or devices at the site of the fistula.[3–5, 30] Vessels amenable to this occlusion-obliteration technique include branches of the profunda femoris (deep femoral) or hypogastric artery; tibial or peroneal arteries; and subclavian, vertebral, and small branch arteries (Fig. 102–3). Rapid-polymerizing agents, such as the cyanoacrylate tissue adhesives, are most suitable for very small vessels. These agents polymerize in 1 to 2 seconds after contact with blood, hardening almost instantaneously to form an occlusive cast of the artery. Whether the fistula is closed by surgery or by a percutaneous technique, one must ensure that the remaining collateral circulation is sufficient to sustain the distal tissues.

When major vessels are involved, sacrificing the artery is not an option and direct surgical repair has most often been the treatment of choice. However, as endovascular techniques improve, endoluminal covered stents may become the preferred treatment. In addition to arteriography, preoperative measures include prophylactic administration of antibiotics. During surgery or endovascular stent placement, catheters for monitoring central venous pressure and blood replacement are placed. Preparation should be made for harvesting saphenous vein if vascular reconstruction is anticipated.

It is generally recommended that the surgical dissection begin with the artery proximal and distal to the fistula to allow for clamping if early bleeding is encountered. With chronic fistulae, it may be necessary to dissect the proximal and distal vein as well. With recent fistulae of small caliber, such as those caused by catheters and needles, this step may not be necessary. Heparin may be given if prolonged vascular occlusion is expected.

Once the vessels have been controlled and clamped, the repair may be as simple as separating the artery and vein and suture ligating the holes in the respective vessels. An alternative is to incise the artery opposite the fistula, repair the hole by suture ligation of the back wall of the artery, and then close the front wall by direct suture or patch angioplasty. Alternatively, the fistula may be approached through the vein. Care must be taken to avoid air emboli during these procedures.[20] More extensive injuries may require end-to-end reanastomosis of the artery, patching, or replacing segments of it or the vein, or both, with interposition grafts.

Saphenous vein is the preferred conduit for reconstruction. Completion angiography should be performed if any question remains about the integrity of the arterial repair. The authors generally recommend repair for all major veins the size of the popliteal vein or larger. Tibia-sized veins may simply be ligated. Venous repairs are associated with a high rate of thrombosis. Heparin or dextran therapy has

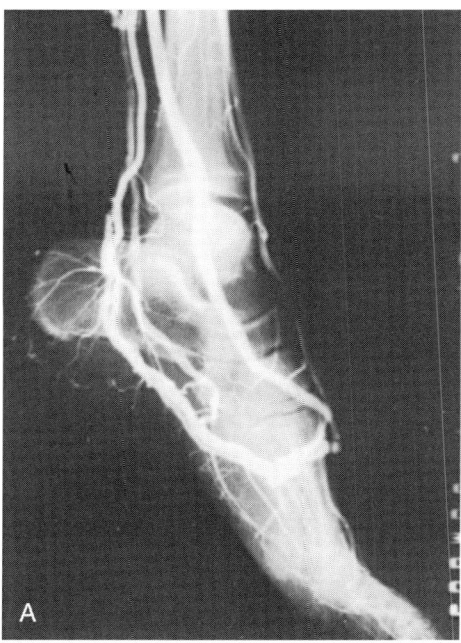
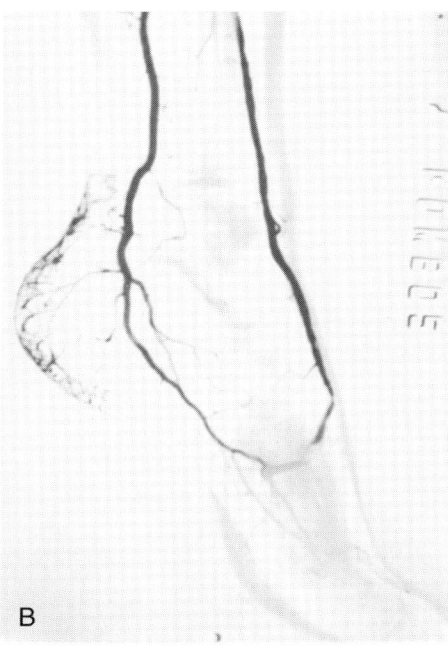

FIGURE 102–3. *A,* Arteriovenous fistula of the dorsalis pedis artery secondary to a surgically placed screw for fracture. *B,* Subtraction angiogram of the same patient after successful closure of the fistula with a liquid embolic agent placed by percutaneous catheter.

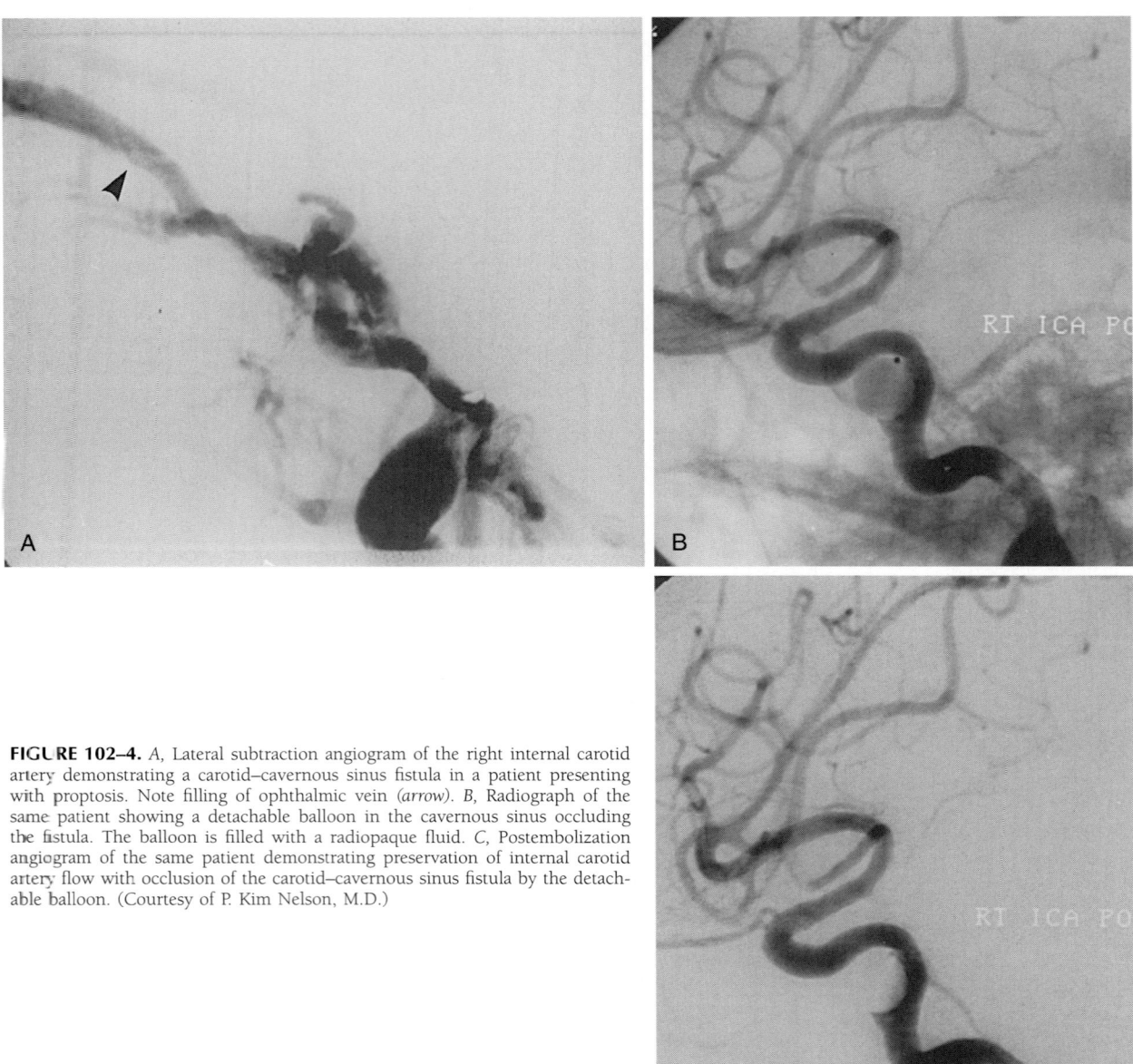

FIGURE 102–4. *A,* Lateral subtraction angiogram of the right internal carotid artery demonstrating a carotid–cavernous sinus fistula in a patient presenting with proptosis. Note filling of ophthalmic vein *(arrow).* *B,* Radiograph of the same patient showing a detachable balloon in the cavernous sinus occluding the fistula. The balloon is filled with a radiopaque fluid. *C,* Postembolization angiogram of the same patient demonstrating preservation of internal carotid artery flow with occlusion of the carotid–cavernous sinus fistula by the detachable balloon. (Courtesy of P. Kim Nelson, M.D.)

been recommended by some clinicians to try to minimize this problem. These issues are detailed in the section on venous surgery (see also Chapter 26).

Finally, some arteriovenous fistulae occur in vessels that are surgically inaccessible and too small to achieve reliable patency of a covered endovascular stent. An example is the carotid-cavernous fistula. In these cases, it is obviously preferable to maintain carotid artery continuity while closing the fistula. The technique that has evolved for managing this problem is percutaneous placement of balloons through the fistula and detaching them on the venous side of the communication (Fig. 102–4).[21, 23] This maneuver has provided excellent results, allowing preservation of the carotid artery while the fistula is being closed. The management of fistulae between large vessels (e.g., aortocaval fistula) is discussed in Chapter 101.

Acknowledgment: The authors acknowledge the earlier contributions to this text by Dr. George Johnson, Jr., particularly the historical section, which was borrowed almost verbatim from his writings in the third edition of *Vascular Surgery.*

REFERENCES

1. Allgayer B, Theiss W, Naundorf M: Percutaneous closure of an arteriovenous fistula with a Cragg endoluminal graft. AJR Am J Roentgenol 166:673, 1996.
2. Beall AC, Harrington DB, Crawford ES, et al: Surgical management of traumatic arteriovenous aneurysms. Am J Surg 106:610, 1963.
3. Berenstein A, Kricheff II: Balloon catheters for the investigation of carotid cavernous fistulas. Radiology 132:762, 1979.
4. Berenstein A, Scott J, Choi IS, Persky M: Percutaneous embolization of arteriovenous fistulas of the external carotid artery. AJNR 7:937, 1986.

5. Berenstein A, Kricheff II: Catheter and material selection for transarterial embolization. Technical considerations: II. Materials. Radiology 132(3):631, 1979.
6. Branham HH: Aneurysmal varix of the femoral artery and vein following a gunshot wound. Int J Surg 3:250, 1890.
7. Breschet G: Memoire sur les aneurysmes. Mem Acad R Med (Paris) 3:101, 1833.
8. Carrel A: La technique operatoire des anatomoses vasculaires et la transplantation des visceres. Lyon Med 98:859, 1902.
9. Criado E, Marston WA, Ligush J, et al: Endovascular repair of peripheral aneurysms, pseudoaneurysms, and arteriovenous fistulas. Ann Vasc Surg 11:256, 1997.
10. Dorros G, Joseph G: Closure of a popliteal arteriovenous fistula using an autologous vein–covered Palmaz stent. J Endovasc Surg 2:177, 1995.
11. Dupuytren G: False aneurysm of the brachial artery and varicose aneurysm. In Lesions of the Vascular System, Diseases of the Rectum, and Other Surgical Complaints, Part I, Section IV. London, Sydenham Society, 1854.
12. Elkin DC, Shumacker HB Jr: Arterial aneurysms and arteriovenous fistula. In Elkin DC, DeBakey ME (eds): Surgery in World War II: Vascular Surgery. Washington, DC, Office of the Surgeon General, Department of the Army, 1955.
13. Foley PJ, Allen EV, Janes JM: Surgical treatment of acquired arteriovenous fistulas. Am J Surg 91:611, 1956.
14. Freeman NE, Shumacker HB Jr: Arterial aneurysms and arteriovenous fistulas: Maintenance of arterial continuity. In Elkin DC, DeBakey ME (eds): Surgery in World War II: Vascular Surgery. Washington, DC, Office of the Surgeon General, Department of the Army, 1955.
15. Glaser RL, McKellar D, Sher KS: Arteriovenous fistulas after cardiac catheterization. Arch Surg 124:1313, 1989.
16. Gomez-Jorge J, Guerra J, Scagnelli T, et al: Endovascular management of a traumatic subclavian artery arteriovenous fistula. J Vasc Interv Radiol 7:599, 1996.
17. Heaton LD, Hughes CW, Rosegay H, et al: Military surgical practices of the United States Army in Viet Nam. Curr Probl Surg November 1966, p 1.
18. Hughes CW, Jahnke EJ Jr: Surgery of traumatic arteriovenous fistulas and aneurysms: A five-year follow-up study of 215 lesions. Ann Surg 148:790, 1958.
19. Hunter W: Further observations upon a particular species of aneurysm. Med Observ Inquiries 2:390, 1762.
20. Johnson G Jr, Dart CH, Peters RM, et al: The importance of venous circulation in arteriovenous fistula. Surg Gynecol Obstet 123:995, 1966.
21. Lasjaunias P, Berenstein A: Surgical Neuroangiography. Vol II. Heidelberg, Springer-Verlag, 1987, p 175.
22. Lindenauer SM, Thompson NW, Kraft RO, et al: Late complications of traumatic arteriovenous fistulas. Surg Gynecol Obstet 129:525, 1969.
23. Matas R: Traumatic arteriovenous aneurysms of the subclavian vessels, with an analytical study of fifteen reported cases, including one operated upon. JAMA 38:103, 1902.
24. Matas R: Arteriovenous fistula of the femoral vessels (aneurysmal varix) on a level with the origin of the profunda. (War injury of two years' duration. Dissection and mobilization of the femoral vessels with division and detachment of the anastomosis followed by separate lateral suture of the artery and vein, with perfect functional restoration of the circulation. Details of technic and commentaries.) Surg Clin North Am 2:1165, 1922.
25. Murphy JB: Resection of arteries and veins injured in continuity, end to end suture. Med Rec 1073, 1897.
26. Norris GW: Varicose aneurysm at the bend of the arm (ligature of the artery above and below the sac; secondary hemorrhages with a return of the aneurysmal thrill on the tenth day); care. Am J Med Sci 5:27, 1843.
27. Ohki T, Veith FJ, Marin ML, et al: Endovascular approaches for arterial trauma. Semin Vasc Surg 10(4):272–285, 1997.
28. Oweida SW, Roubin GS, Smith RB III, et al: Postcatheterization vascular complications associated with percutaneous transluminal coronary angioplasty. J Vasc Surg 12:310, 1990.
29. Parodi JC: Endovascular repair of abdominal aortic aneurysm and other arterial lesions. J Vasc Surg 21:549–557, 1995.
30. Peters FLM, Kromhout JG, Reekers JA, et al: Treatment of solitary arteriovenous fistulas. Surgery 109:220, 1991.
31. Rich NM, Baugh JH, Hughes CW: Popliteal artery injuries in Vietnam. Am J Surg 118:531, 1969.
32. Spencer FC, Grewe RB: Management of arterial injuries in battle casualties. Ann Surg 141:304, 1955.

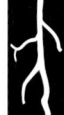

CHAPTER 103
Congenital Vascular Malformations

Robert J. Rosen, M.D., and Thomas S. Riles, M.D.

Although vascular malformations have been recognized as clinical entities for more than 100 years, they continue to be a source of confusion, in terms of diagnosis, classification, and treatment. It is impossible to precisely categorize every lesion encountered clinically, but "arteriovenous lesions" can be divided into four major types:

- Infantile hemangiomas, which are benign neoplasms
- Arteriovenous fistulas, which are usually acquired lesions and are discussed elsewhere in Section XIII
- True arteriovenous malformations (AVMs), which are congenital anomalies

- Predominantly venous lesions, including dysplasias and cavernous venous malformations

INFANTILE HEMANGIOMAS

General Considerations

Over the years, application of the term *hemangioma* to a wide variety of vascular lesions has caused considerable confusion in the literature regarding diagnosis and treatment.[1] It is now generally agreed that the term should be used to refer only to the benign vascular neoplasm usually encountered in infants and children, lesions that are present at birth in 30% of cases and otherwise appear in the first few months of life. Typically, these lesions exhibit a period of rapid growth in the first 6 months of life, demonstrating marked proliferation of endothelial cells on pathologic examination. The proliferative phase is generally followed by spontaneous, gradual involution beginning at about age 1 year and continuing to resolution by age 7 years in 95% of patients. The distinction between the pathologic appearance and the clinical behavior of this lesion and those of true congenital vascular malformations is emphasized in the classification of Mulliken and Glowacki (Table 103–1).[2]

Clinical Aspects

Hemangiomas can occur anywhere in the body. Most typically, they are red or reddish blue, flat or slightly raised skin lesions. They are generally isolated lesions but in 30% of cases are multiple. Most represent a purely cosmetic problem, but during the proliferative phase, endothelial proliferation is manifested clinically by rapid growth that can be not only disfiguring but also life-threatening in extreme cases owing to respiratory or gastrointestinal involvement. Extensive lesions, especially those in the liver, can be associated with high-output congestive heart failure.[3-7] These hepatic lesions carry significant risk of mortality, but when the infant is supported through the early stages, involution occurs, as in other hemangiomas.

Thrombocytopenia and consequent hemorrhagic complications have been associated with hemangiomas, a phenomenon called *Kasabach-Merritt syndrome*. It now appears that these findings are confined to a different pathologic entity with a more aggressive course, termed *kaposiform hemangioendothelioma*.[8, 9]

Treatment

The management of hemangiomas has long been a controversial subject.[10] While it is true that the majority of lesions

TABLE 103–1. DISTINGUISHING FEATURES OF HEMANGIOMAS AND ARTERIOVENOUS MALFORMATIONS

HEMANGIOMA	ARTERIOVENOUS MALFORMATION
Neoplasm	Congenital anomaly
30% present at birth; remainder present in first 3 months; proliferative phase: 1st year	90% present at birth, although many not manifested
Female: male ratio 5:1	Female: male ratio 1:1
Endothelial proliferation	No cellular proliferation
Growth in tissue culture	No growth in tissue culture
Cellular stroma	No mast cells
Increased mast cells	No spontaneous involution; growth with individual
Spontaneous involution in 95% by age 7 yr	Treatment sometimes required
No treatment required in most patients	

Data from Mulliken JB, Glowacki J: Hemangiomas and vascular malformations in infants and children: A classification based on endothelial characteristics. Plast Reconstr Surg 69:412, 1982.

involute spontaneously and require no specific treatment, in a certain number of patients either cosmetic or functional complications will develop. It is easy to counsel watchful waiting, but the psychosocial trauma of a large, visible hemangioma affects both parents and child. It has also been pointed out that "results considered cosmetically acceptable in 1955 are not necessarily acceptable [now]."[10]

It is generally agreed that the most common small superficial lesions should be managed conservatively, as they are likely to involute with minimal or no residua. It is also apparent that extremely large, disfiguring or life-threatening lesions require specific treatment.

Treatment options include systemic corticosteroids, pulsed dye laser, intralesional injection, interferon, embolization, and surgery. Before undertaking any of these approaches, a careful risk-benefit analysis is in order. Steroid therapy, while effective and usually well tolerated, may be associated with problems such as interference with growth and development, immune suppression, and behavioral changes. Interferon treatment has been reported to be associated with the development of spastic diplegia in some children.[11] Generally, laser treatment is effective only for superficial lesions, which also tend to show the most complete spontaneous involution.

Transcatheter embolization has a limited role, but it can be life-saving with extensive hepatic hemangiomatosis.[7] Death from this lesion is largely due to massive shunting, which results in high-output congestive failure. Particulate embolization has been used successfully to reduce the degree of shunting and allow the infant to survive until the lesion involutes.

Surgical management of hemangiomas is generally reserved for aggressive lesions that interfere with the respiratory tract or ocular structures, or those that tend to have a poor cosmetic outcome even after involution, such as those on the lips or nose and pedunculated or ulcerated lesions. Large superficial lesions are often associated with areas of epidermal atrophy and telangiectasia after involution; deeper lesions may leave behind abnormal excess skin or fibrofatty tissue. Both of these may require cosmetic surgery for an optimal result (Fig. 103–1A and B).

CONGENITAL VASCULAR MALFORMATIONS

General Considerations

AVMs are congenital anomalies that result from maldevelopment of arterial, capillary, venous, or lymphatic structures. These lesions are thought to be present at birth and are not neoplasms. Most occur sporadically in otherwise healthy individuals, although there are rare but well-known syndromes (among them, Rendu-Osler-Weber) that are clearly familial. New evidence also suggests that there may be a less well-defined genetic component to both hemangiomas and vascular malformations in certain families.[12]

The early work of Woollard on the embryology of the vascular system provides some insight into the developmental origin of these lesions (Fig. 103–2).[13] The embryonic vascular system initially consists of interlacing blood spaces in the primitive mesenchyme. Subsequent differenti-

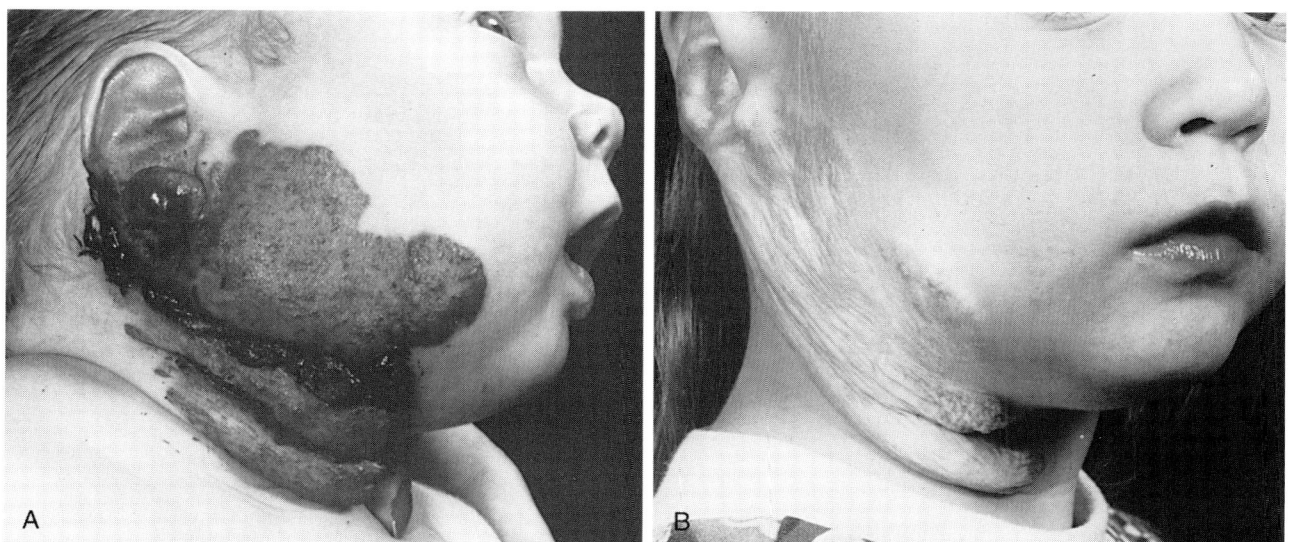

FIGURE 103–1. *A,* A 6-month-old infant demonstrating extensive hemangioma of face and neck during proliferative phase. *B,* Same child at age 5 years demonstrating involution of hemangioma but residual fibrofatty excess skin, which was treated surgically.

ation involves development of a primitive capillary network (*stage 1*), followed by a "retiform stage," when the primitive capillaries coalesce into large plexiform structures (*stage 2*). Through a process that is not totally understood, blood

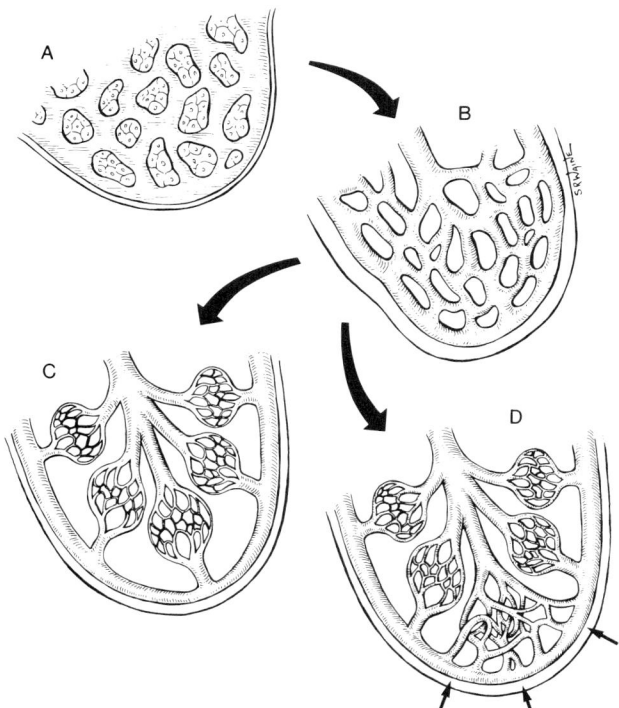

FIGURE 103–2. Stages of embryonic vascular development. *A,* Interlacing blood spaces in the primitive mesenchyme differentiate into a primitive capillary network (stage 1). *B,* Primitive capillaries coalesce into large plexiform structures (stage 2). *C,* Disappearance of primitive elements and the appearance of mature vascular stems and capillary beds (stage 3). *D,* Focal failure of the developmental sequence with the persistence of primitive vascular structures, resulting in an arteriovenous malformation (*small arrows*).

begins to flow through the retiform plexus from an "arterial" to a "venous" side. In the maturation phase (*stage 3*), the primitive elements are replaced by mature vascular stems, the remodeling apparently being influenced by blood flow. Congenital vascular malformations are presumed to represent focal persistence of primitive vascular elements. Depending on the stage at which this failure occurs, the abnormal communication may range from just above capillary level to large vessel (macrofistulous) communications.

Although AVMs generally occur as isolated anomalies in otherwise healthy persons, associated abnormalities in regional anatomic structures may occur. Some of these seem to be coexistent congenital anomalies, whereas others occur in response to abnormal local blood flow (e.g., overgrowth, undergrowth, focal gigantism) (Fig. 103–3). The observed association between AVMs and regional autonomic dysfunction (e.g., hyperhidrosis) and the common presence of café au lait spots also suggests connections between abnormal development of vascular and neural tissues. It has been suggested that some vascular malformations, particularly the venous and lymphatic types, may develop in response to acquired vascular obstructions occurring in utero.[14]

Vascular malformations differ from true hemangiomas in that they are not neoplasms. The work of Folkman[15] and of Mulliken and associates[2, 16] has shown that there is no endothelial proliferation and no cellular stroma in these lesions; nor do they show growth in tissue culture. These lesions do not exhibit the sequence of rapid proliferation followed by spontaneous involution that is characteristic of hemangiomas of infancy and childhood.

In general, congenital AVMs, like other congenital anomalies, remain incompletely understood in terms of pathogenesis. From a clinical standpoint, patients can be assured of the following:

1. These are malformations, not neoplasms.
2. They are usually isolated anomalies.

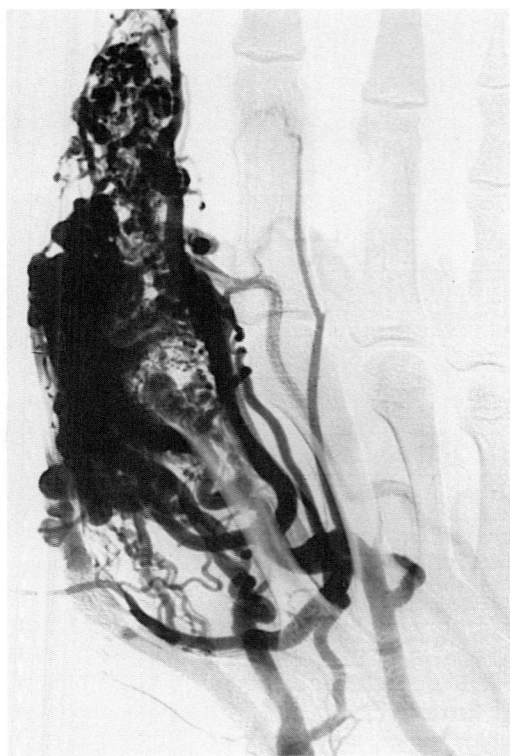

FIGURE 103–3. Angiogram of right hand demonstrating high-flow arteriovenous malformation causing hypertrophy of entire digit, including bones and soft tissues.

3. They are rarely genetically transmitted.

4. AVMs are often stable lesions that require no specific treatment.

Clinical Aspects

The clinical behavior of AVMs is quite variable. They can remain "dormant" for years, and many undoubtedly go undetected throughout life. There is no apparent sex predominance, as there is with infantile hemangiomas.[2] Gradual enlargement of the malformation occurs in proportion to the growth of the individual. Detection may result from the observation of a skin discoloration, palpation of a mass, or recognition of secondary effects of the lesion on adjacent normal structures, or the lesion may be discovered because of complications such as hemorrhage, ulceration, or regional ischemia of tissues. Some lesions become apparent after trauma or during periods of hormonal stimulation, such as in menarche and pregnancy. A history of trauma is sometimes elicited in patients with AVMs, but the relationship is unclear. In the majority of these cases, the lesion is actually a traumatic arteriovenous fistula or a preexisting congenital lesion discovered because of the trauma. It does appear that true congenital AVMs occasionally can be "activated" by trauma through creation of new arteriovenous communications or by disturbing a previously stable pattern of collateral circulation.[17] It should be emphasized that growth of lesions is due to enlargement of existing vascular channels and recruitment of collaterals rather than to any pathologically observable proliferation of cellular elements.[2]

Vascular malformations can occur anywhere in the body, although certain anatomic sites seem to be affected more often, such as the pelvis, the extremities, and the intracranial circulation. The vast majority of AVMs are isolated lesions, or at least are confined to one anatomic region. Multiple lesions may be encountered in some congenital syndromes, such as Rendu-Osler-Weber syndrome. Even extensive malformations may be clinically silent if they are located in deep structures and do not cause any functional impairment. These lesions seldom cause pain and rarely bleed spontaneously, although we have encountered patients who presented with hemoptysis, gastrointestinal bleeding, and hematuria.

Measured cardiac output may be increased in patients with arteriovenous malformations, but clinically significant cardiovascular effects are uncommon, in contrast with acquired arteriovenous fistulas. In our series of 215 patients with congenital AVMs, only three showed evidence of a clinically significant high-output state. The relative rarity of high-output failure is not fully understood, since the degree of angiographically observed shunting in some lesions is striking. Some authors have postulated that the multiple tortuous vessels that compose these lesions may allow peripheral resistance to be maintained, despite a large total cross-sectional area of arteriovenous communication.[18] Clinically significant high-output states associated with AVMs tend to occur in two settings: (1) lesions in infancy and (2) extremely large (usually pelvic) lesions in adults (Fig. 103–4A and B). A lesion that is relatively asymptomatic or even clinically silent may thus require treatment for its generalized cardiovascular effects.

AVMs in sites accessible to physical examination may or may not show associated pigment changes in the overlying skin. When a mass is palpable, it is usually firm, spongy, and not compressible, except for purely venous lesions. Prominent pulsations or a thrill are characteristic findings, and auscultation usually reveals a continuous or oscillating bruit. Enlarged draining veins are characteristic, and these veins may or may not be pulsatile.

Over time, the increased flow and pressure in the draining veins may result in varicosities that can be extremely troublesome. Superficial phlebitis, manifested by localized pain, tenderness, and inflammatory changes in the overlying skin, may complicate the situation; thrombosed veins may also be palpable. Ischemic ulcerations or areas of tissue breakdown with bleeding are sometimes seen in association with extremity lesions. This problem, which can be intractable, is due to both arterial ischemia (by a proximal steal through the AVM) and venous hypertension. The ulcerations and other skin changes associated with AVMs are strikingly similar to the chronic ulcers seen with long-standing venous disease of the legs. The pathophysiologic changes that develop in response to an abnormal arteriovenous communication were outlined in 1936 by Holman (Fig. 103–5).[19]

Extremity lesions presenting in childhood may be associated with overgrowth of bones and soft tissues that can be extreme and disfiguring. Leg length discrepancies may not be apparent until late in childhood, when limping or scoliosis is observed. Often, the limb is not only longer but larger overall; recording serial measurements may help to

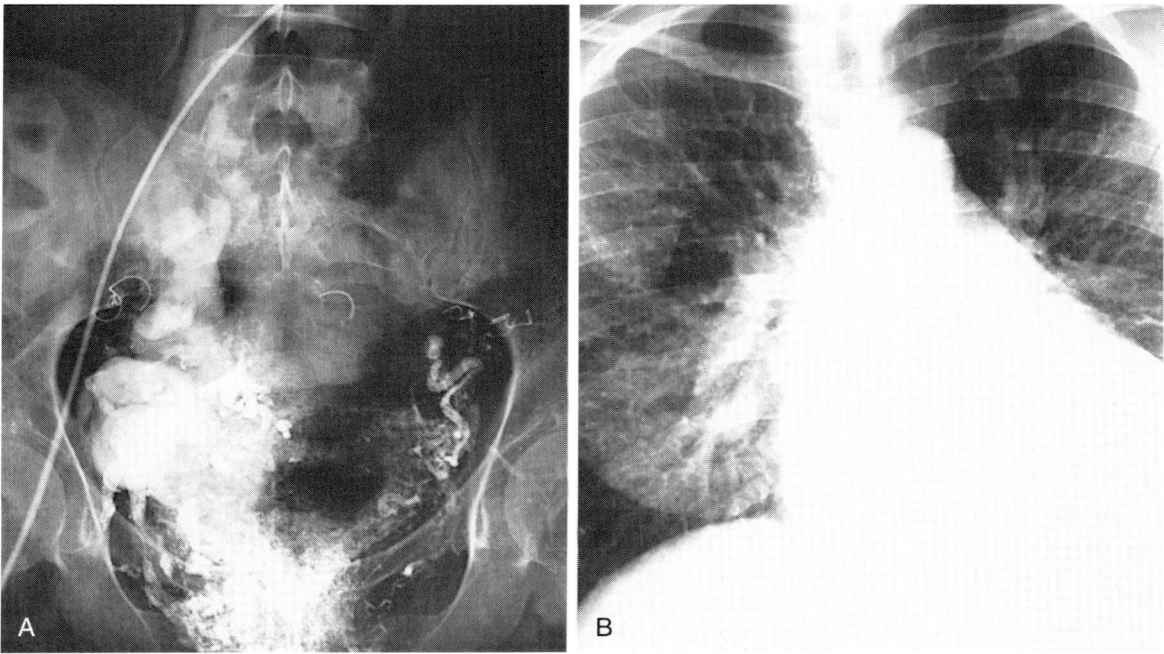

FIGURE 103–4. *A*, Extensive high-flow pelvic arteriovenous malformation in 28-year-old woman who had undergone previous surgical resection and embolization. Patient was also status post two pregnancies. *B*, A chest film of the same patient demonstrates high-output state. Patient ultimately succumbed to intractable congestive failure, an extremely rare event.

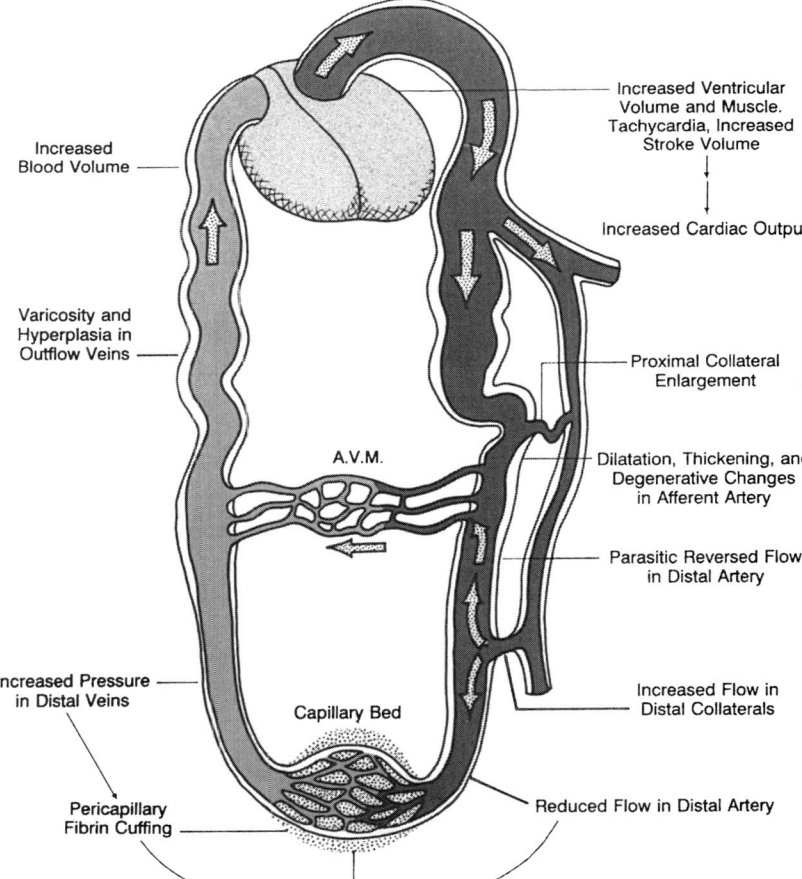

FIGURE 103–5. Pathophysiologic changes that occur in response to an abnormal arteriovenous communication, as first described by Holman in 1936. (From Young AE: Arteriovenous malformations. *In* Mulliken JB, Young AE [eds]: Vascular Birthmarks, Hemangiomas and Malformations. Philadelphia, WB Saunders, 1988, p 234.)

Increased Blood Volume

Varicosity and Hyperplasia in Outflow Veins

Increased Pressure in Distal Veins

Pericapillary Fibrin Cuffing

Capillary Bed

A.V.M.

Tissue Ischemia

Increased Ventricular Volume and Muscle. Tachycardia, Increased Stroke Volume

Increased Cardiac Output

Proximal Collateral Enlargement

Dilatation, Thickening, and Degenerative Changes in Afferent Artery

Parasitic Reversed Flow in Distal Artery

Increased Flow in Distal Collaterals

Reduced Flow in Distal Artery

determine the rate of growth and the need for intervention, whose timing may be critical.

The pelvis is one of the more common sites of vascular malformation. The lesions may be asymptomatic and be discovered incidentally, but they may also produce pelvic pain, pain referred to the leg, sexual dysfunction, pressure effects on pelvic organs, high-output failure, and occasionally hemorrhage. In female patients, these malformations tend to be complex, with multiple feeding arteries (Fig. 103–6). Although the primary supply is generally from one or both hypogastric arteries, additional supply is often noted from the inferior mesenteric artery, middle sacral artery, lumbar arteries, and common femoral and profunda femoral branches (Fig. 103–7). Because of their complex supply, these lesions are extremely difficult to eradicate completely, and recurrences are common. Patients must be aware of this, and symptoms must be severe enough to warrant initial intervention.

On occasion, the vascular malformation is confined to the uterus and presents as menorrhagia. These lesions can be cured by hysterectomy, but they have also been managed successfully with selective embolization, preserving fertility in women of childbearing age (Fig. 103–8).

In male patients we have encountered a distinctive pattern of pelvic vascular malformation characterized by supply from only one hypogastric artery and massively dilated

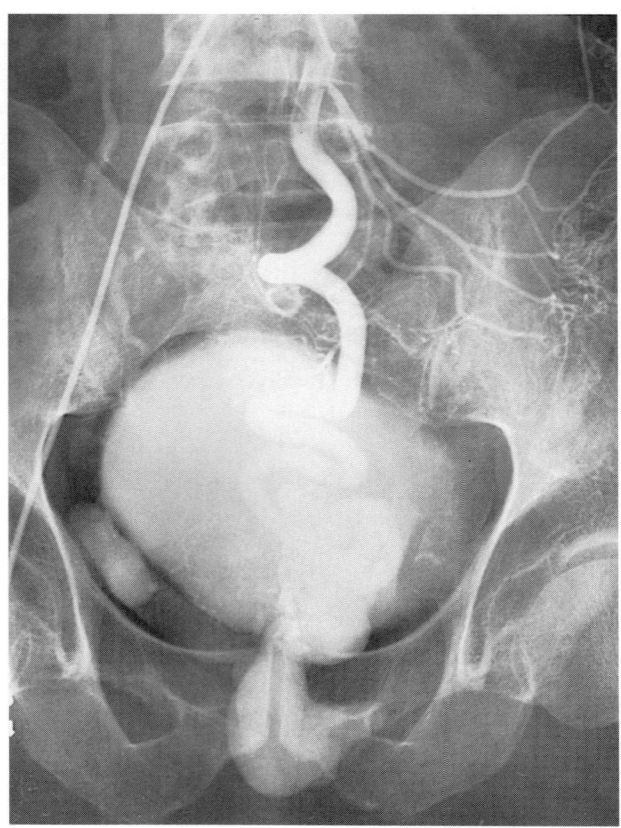

FIGURE 103–7. Selective inferior mesenteric arteriogram demonstrating marked hypertrophy of the branch that supplies part of a large pelvic arteriovenous malformation. The enlargement in caliber of the vessel, as well as its tortuosity, is a typical finding.

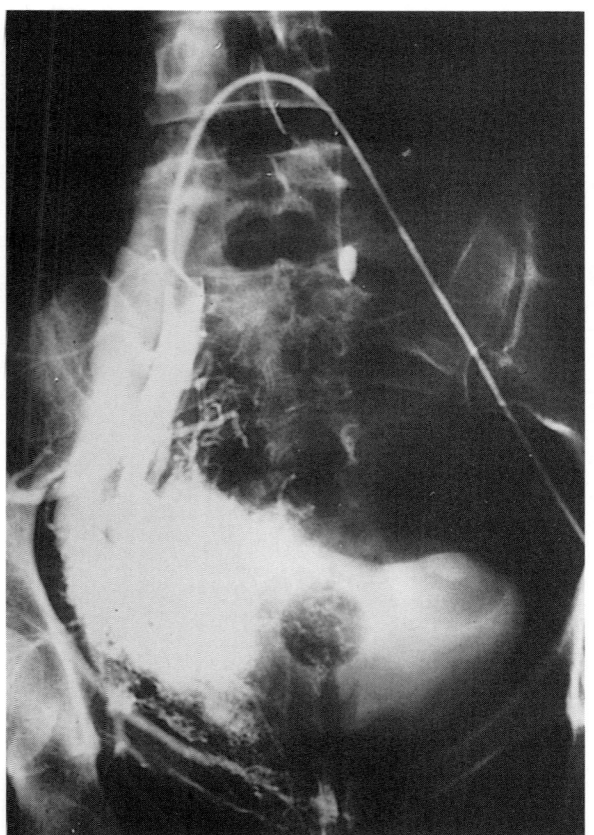

FIGURE 103–6. Selective right hypogastric arteriogram of 35-year-old woman with high-flow pelvic arteriovenous malformation (AVM). The lesion was also supplied by the opposite hypogastric artery and the inferior mesenteric artery. Pelvic AVMs in female patients are generally supplied by multiple trunks.

draining veins (Fig. 103–9). The venous component of the lesion is usually the cause of symptoms, which are related to pressure on surrounding structures. Presenting complaints have commonly included pelvic pain, lower gastrointestinal tract bleeding, and urinary outlet obstruction. These lesions tend to respond to embolization much more favorably, owing to their simpler blood supply.

A unique type of congenital vascular malformation is the *pulmonary AVM*, which consists of a fistula-like connection between a pulmonary artery branch and a pulmonary vein (Fig. 103–10A). Such lesions can be single or multiple and may be sporadic lesions or found in patients with Rendu-Osler-Weber syndrome, who generally have a strong family history. Unlike most vascular malformations, these represent right-to-left shunting and therefore pose specific, and sometimes life-threatening risks. The two major risks are (1) *paradoxical embolization,* which can result in stroke or brain abscess, and (2) *arterial desaturation.* The latter may be clinically manifested by decreased exercise tolerance and, in extreme cases, cyanosis. Even when the lesions are detected incidentally, as often they are, treatment is generally recommended to eliminate the risk of paradoxical embolization.

Isolated lesions can be treated by surgical resection of the involved lung segment or lobe. A less invasive approach is embolization to occlude the arteriovenous communication, which can generally be performed with minimal risk

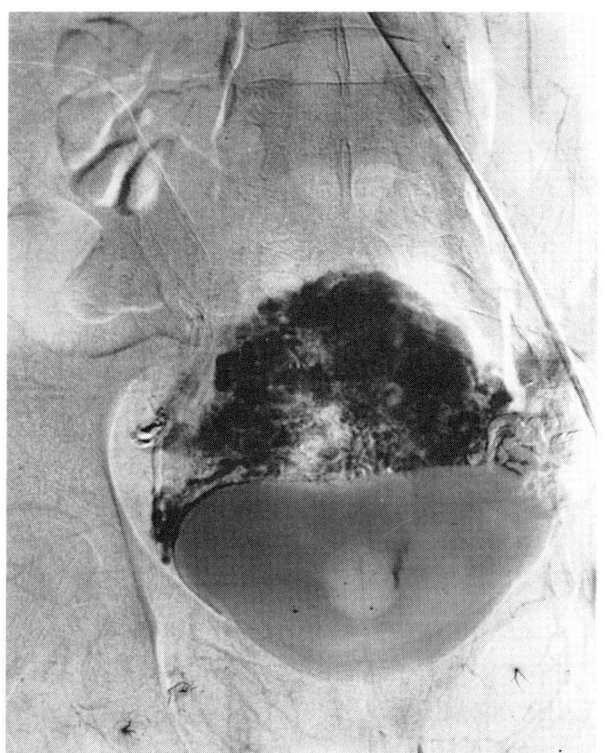

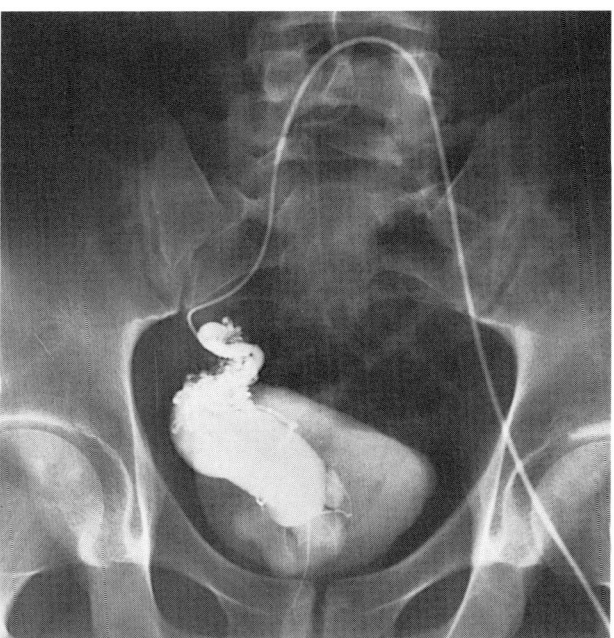

FIGURE 103–9. Selective right hypogastric arteriogram in 22-year-old man with typical "male pattern" arteriovenous malformation demonstrating supply entirely from one hypogastric artery with a dense arterial nidus draining into massively enlarged draining veins. These enlarged draining veins are generally the cause of presenting symptoms.

FIGURE 103–8. High-flow arteriovenous malformation confined to the body of the uterus. While curable with hysterectomy, many such lesions can be treated by embolization, thus preserving fertility.

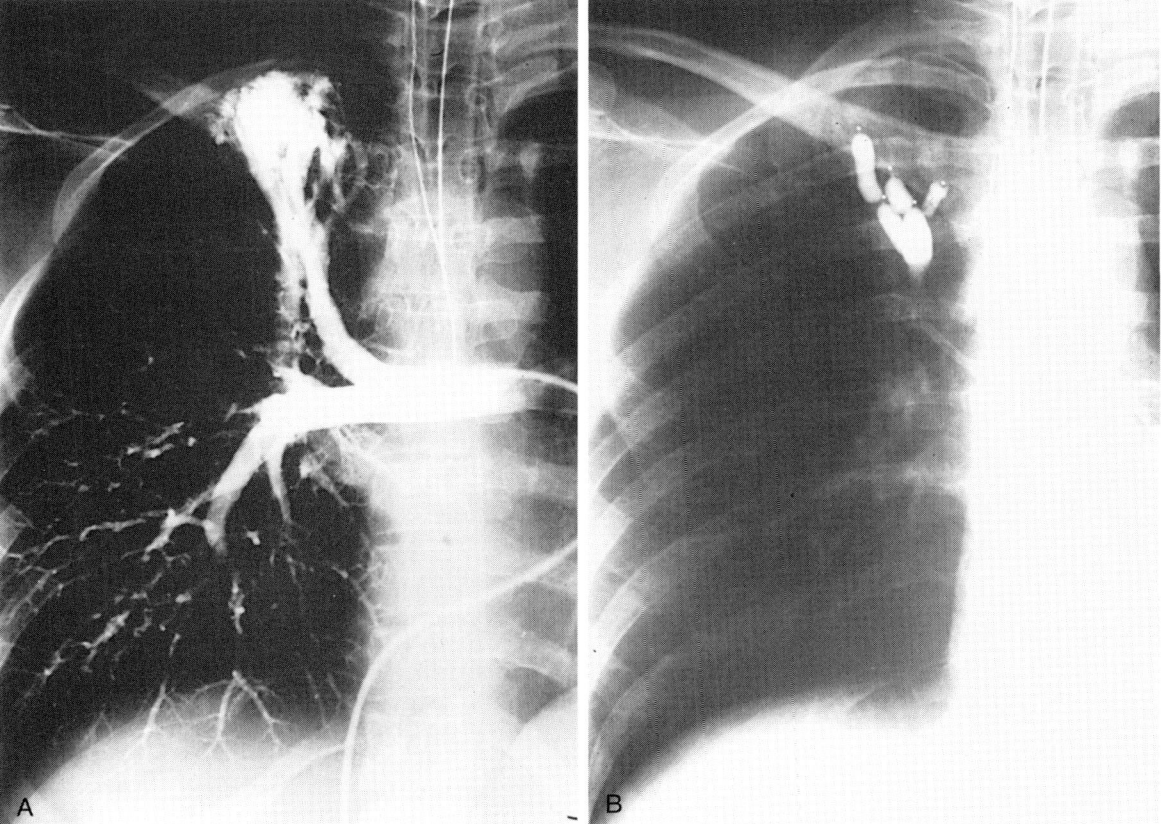

FIGURE 103–10. A, Right pulmonary arteriogram in patient with pulmonary arteriovenous malformation at right lung apex. This type of malformation presents the unique risk of paradoxical systemic embolization. B, Multiple detachable balloons were used to occlude the malformation completely.

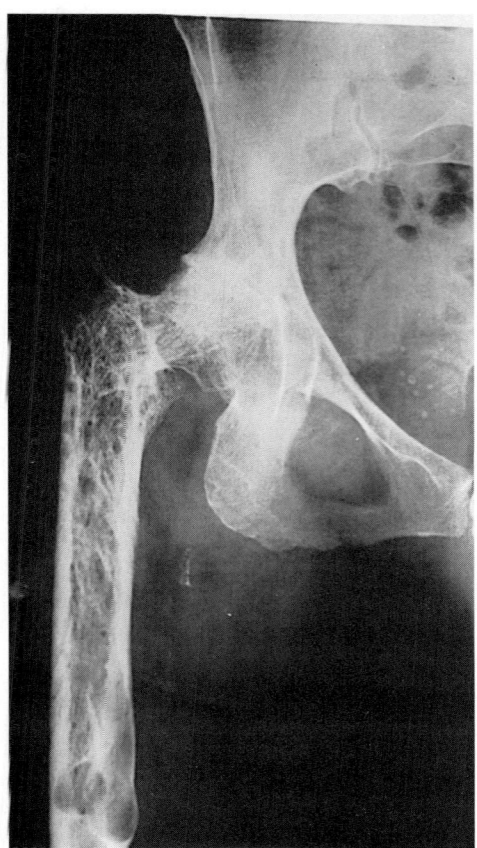

FIGURE 103–11. Plain film of 32-year-old woman with high-flow arteriovenous malformation of right thigh demonstrating unusual bone involvement. This patient had experienced two pathologic fractures.

using stainless steel coils or detachable balloons. The fairly simple fistulous architecture of these lesions, unlike that of most AVMs, allows them to be completely eradicated by selectively occluding the feeding pulmonary arterial branch (Fig. 103–10B).[20, 21]

Laboratory and Radiologic Findings

In patients with congenital AVMs, routine laboratory studies are usually unrevealing. Plain radiographs generally show no abnormality, but they may demonstrate bone and soft tissue hypertrophy, and limb length discrepancies when extremity lesions present in childhood. Regional bone demineralization or, more rarely, bone destruction may be seen in high-flow lesions in adults (Fig. 103–11). Phleboliths may be seen in lesions with a cavernous venous component (Fig. 103–12A and B). Color flow Doppler imaging has proved an extremely useful tool for evaluating vascular malformations. Flow patterns (arterial versus venous) are readily characterized and the extent of the lesion demonstrated. This noninvasive modality is particularly useful in the pediatric population and for follow-up after surgery or embolization.

Computed tomography (CT) and magnetic resonance imaging (MRI) are both extremely helpful in delineating the true extent of these lesions.[22–24] The lesion itself and the involvement of adjacent structures, including muscle and bone, are usually well demonstrated (Fig. 103–13). MRI also distinguishes between high-flow and low-flow components. Often, these studies show the lesion to be much more extensive than was expected on the basis of clinical, or even angiographic, findings. Magnetic resonance

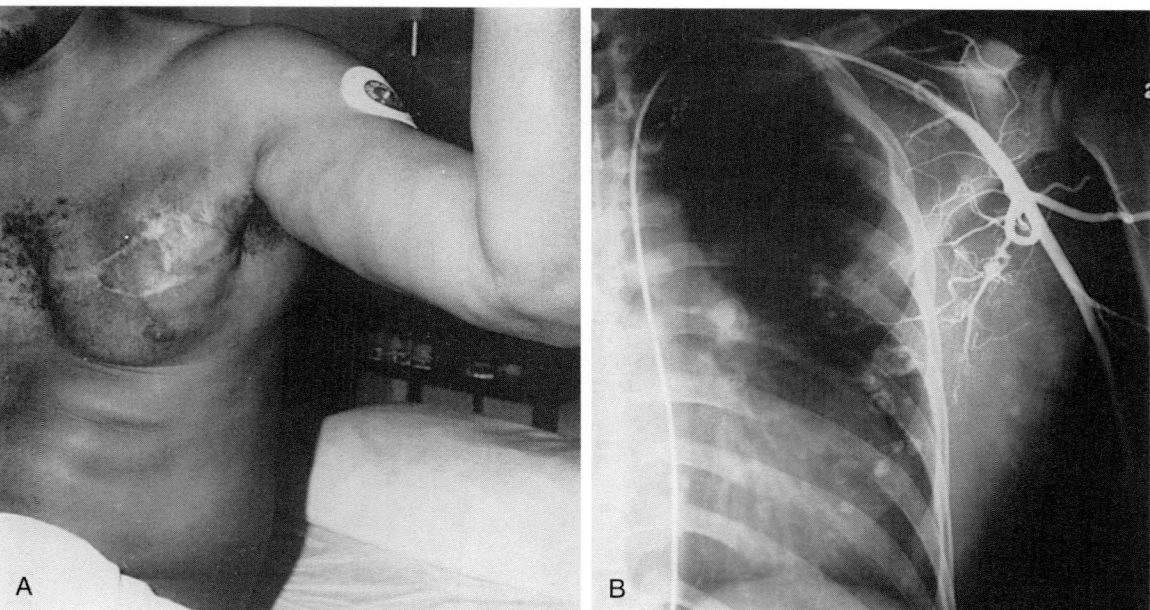

FIGURE 103–12. *A,* A 26-year-old man with extensive cavernous venous malformation of left chest wall who had undergone two previous attempts at resection. *B,* Arteriogram demonstrating no significant arterial supply and numerous phleboliths scattered in the soft tissues, typical of purely venous lesions.

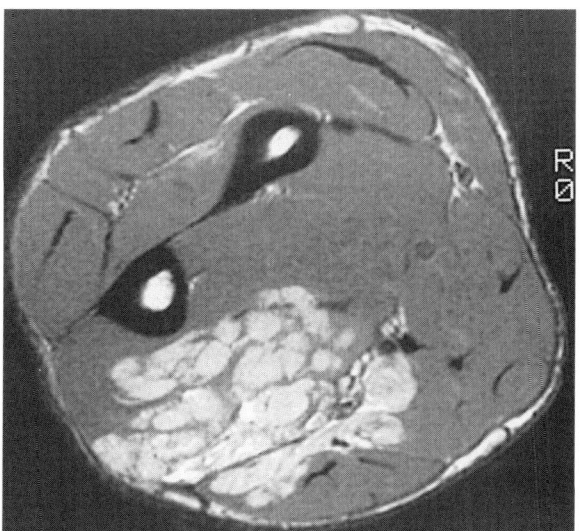

FIGURE 103–13. Cross-sectional magnetic resonance image of forearm arteriovenous malformation clearly demonstrating the lesion and its relation to surrounding soft tissue structures.

angiography (MRA), using intravenous gadolinium contrast agents and specific imaging sequences, is a major advance in imaging vascular malformations. With this noninvasive technique, accurate images of the involved vessels and their relations to surrounding structures can be routinely obtained (Fig. 103–14). We have now adopted MRA as the preferred imaging modality, both for the initial evaluation of vascular malformations and for follow-up studies.

Any lesion of significant size that is symptomatic enough to warrant therapeutic intervention should be evaluated by angiography. Angiography confirms the presence of a vascular lesion and generally distinguishes it from a vascular tumor. The study demonstrates the flow characteristics of the lesion and delineates feeding arteries and draining veins and their relationships to the normal circulation of the region. A characteristic finding is marked hypertrophy and tortuosity of the feeding arteries, which may enlarge to several times their normal diameter. The appearance of the nidus (center) of the lesion ranges from large, tortuous channels to innumerable small vessels appearing as an intense blush. In either case, arteriovenous shunting may be rapid and massive, with almost immediate opacification of the draining veins. Extensive collateral arteries are often demonstrated, particularly when the patient has been previously treated with surgical ligation or embolization (Fig. 103–15). While collateral vessels tend to have a characteristic "corkscrew" appearance and do not show shunting, it may be impossible to reliably distinguish between extensive collaterals and areas of vascular malformation.

Treatment

Congenital vascular malformations present an extremely difficult therapeutic challenge. Asymptomatic or mildly symptomatic lesions do not require treatment once the nature of the mass has been confirmed.

Absolute indications for treatment include hemorrhage, secondary ischemic complications, and congestive heart failure from arteriovenous shunting. Relative indications include pain, functional impairment, and cosmetic deformity, including limb asymmetry associated with extremity lesions. Hemorrhage is uncommon, but may occur when the lesion is in an area that is subject to trauma or when there is a potential communication between the lesion and a mucosal surface, such as the gastrointestinal tract or urinary bladder. Bleeding from a high-flow AVM may be

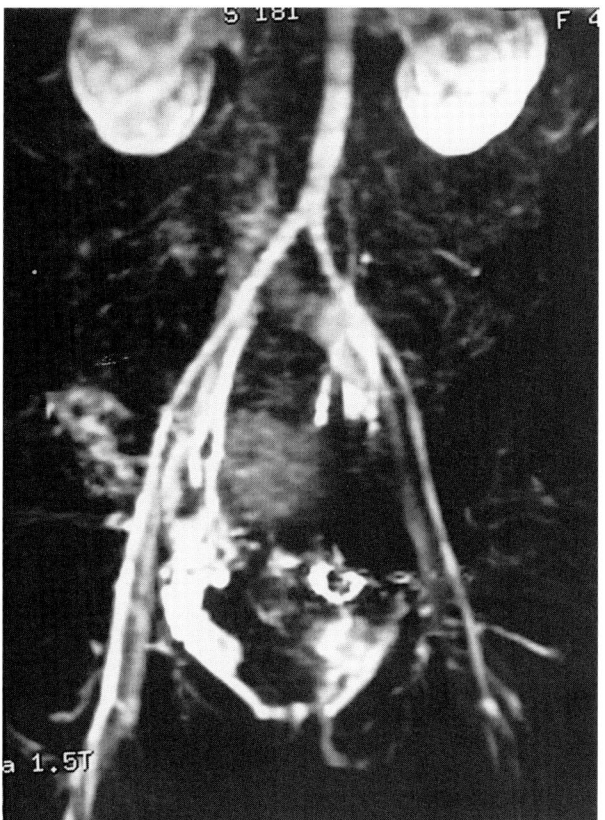

FIGURE 103–14. Magnetic resonance angiogram using gadolinium contrast demonstrates high-flow pelvic arteriovenous malformation (AVM) on right side supplied predominantly by right hypogastric artery. Magnetic resonance angiography is an excellent noninvasive technique for evaluating AVMs.

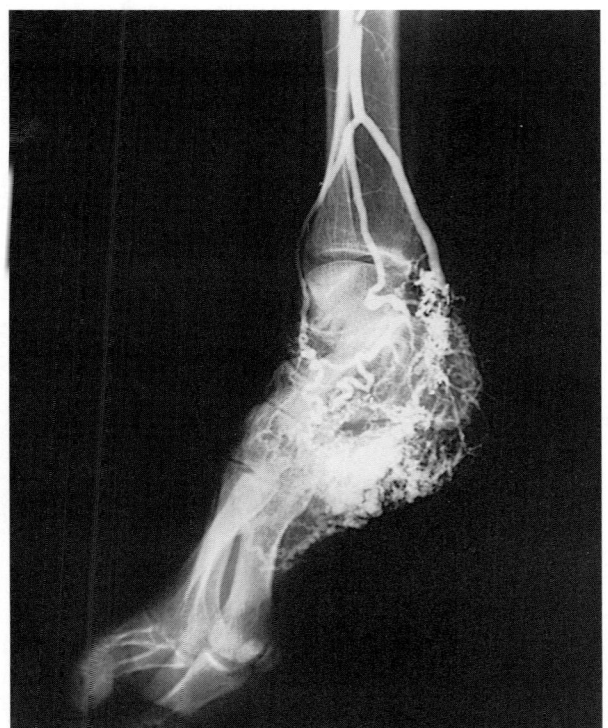

FIGURE 103–15. Right foot arteriogram in young woman who had undergone previous ligation of the posterior tibial artery to treat a high-flow arteriovenous malformation (AVM) involving the plantar aspect of the foot. Note recurrence of the AVM supplied by tortuous collaterals from peroneal and anterior tibial branches.

profuse and is notoriously difficult to control surgically. In this setting, emergency ligation of feeding vessels, or surgical packing when there is a closed space, may be effective, if only temporarily. Transcatheter embolization is a valuable approach in this setting, since control can often be obtained nonsurgically and there is less likelihood of making subsequent therapy more difficult, as can occur after proximal ligation.

Ischemic complications result from the "steal" of flow from normal structures and can be manifested by pain and ulceration in extremity lesions, and by neurologic symptoms when the lesion involves the central nervous system. These ischemic complications often improve significantly when the magnitude of arteriovenous shunting is reduced, even if the lesion cannot be eradicated completely (Fig. 103–16). It should be noted that pain and ulceration may also be related to chronic venous hypertension. In this situation, the usual measures used for chronic venous lesions (local wound care, elastic compression, elevation, removal of specific symptomatic veins) can be employed, in addition to efforts to treat the underlying problem.

If treatment is required, careful planning is mandatory. A team approach is often required that involves participation of appropriate specialists to achieve the optimal result. The patient must be made aware of the complex nature of the problem and the considerable uncertainties involved in treatment.

Patients with symptomatic lesions that are judged to be resectable by careful preoperative evaluation should proba-

bly undergo surgery, because complete removal provides the best chance for cure. This is most suitable for superficial lesions of the trunk, scalp, face, and extremities (Fig. 103–17). The goal of surgery should be complete resection of the lesion. Ligation of feeding arteries is only temporarily effective, and the rapid recruitment of collateral channels makes further treatment, especially embolization, difficult or impossible.

Surgical "skeletonization" of complex lesions has been performed in some cases. This treatment consist of meticulous dissection and ligation of all branches feeding the lesion; it often appears more feasible preoperatively than in the operating room. Moreover, even meticulous clipping or ligation of every regional branch generally has no lasting benefit, as collaterals from adjacent anatomic regions are rapidly recruited (Fig. 103–18A and B).

Resection of large lesions may be associated with significant blood loss. In anticipation of this possibility, provisions should be made to replace large volumes of blood. Intraoperative hypotension, autotransfusion, and proximal tourniquets have been successfully employed.[25, 25] Complete circulatory arrest or extracorporeal bypass has occasionally been necessary.[27] Preoperative embolization can facilitate surgical resection and reduce operative blood loss. In such cases, embolization should be performed as near to the time of surgery as is feasible to prevent recurrence or enlargement of collateral vessels.

Transcatheter embolization now plays a significant role in the treatment of many vascular malformations.[28–32] Advances in instrumentation and imaging over the past decade now routinely permit superselective catheterization to be performed with a high degree of control and safety. Numerous embolic materials have been employed, including foam pledgets, plastic particles, stainless steel and platinum coils, ethanol, sclerosing agents, and rapidly polymerizing adhesives. None of these agents is entirely satisfactory, but certain principles have been established to maximize results and minimize complications. Temporary occlusion materials such as reabsorbable foams and collagen preparations may be acceptable for preoperative devascularization but are unsuitable for long-term or definitive therapy, as recanalization and recurrence develop within weeks or months.

Macroscopic occlusion with devices such as coils and detachable balloons are equivalent to surgical ligation of arterial feeders and, in general, should not be used. Proximal occlusion, whether performed surgically or with embolization, may produce an impressive result initially, but nearly always recurrence should be anticipated. Recurrences after proximal ligation or embolization are extremely difficult to treat, owing to recruitment of multiple new blood vessels to the lesion. We have encountered patients whose mildly symptomatic lesions became severely symptomatic or even life-threatening because of hemorrhage or ischemia after proximal occlusion.

At least theoretically, deeply penetrating particulate or liquid embolic agents offer the possibility of eradicating the nidus of the lesion. These materials include plastic particles, ethanol and sclerosing agents, and liquid adhesives.[31] Polyvinyl alcohol foam particles are available in graded sizes from 50 to 1000 μm in diameter. They are injected in suspension and become lodged in the small vessels of the malformation. While a good initial angiographic result can

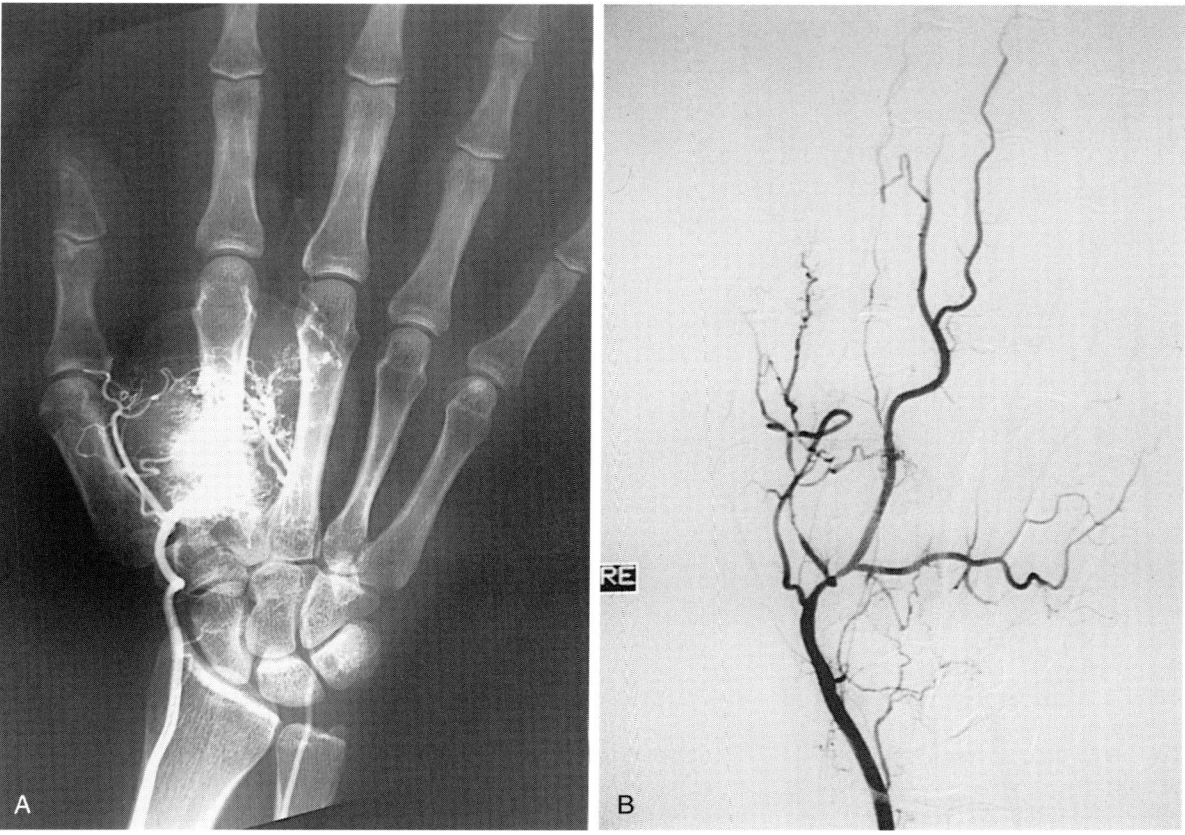

FIGURE 103–16. *A*, A 21-year-old man with high-flow arteriovenous malformation involving palmar aspect of hand causing primarily ischemic symptoms in the first and second digits secondary to proximal steal. *B*, A subsequent arteriogram following embolization of the lesion showing eradication of the nidus and improved distal flow.

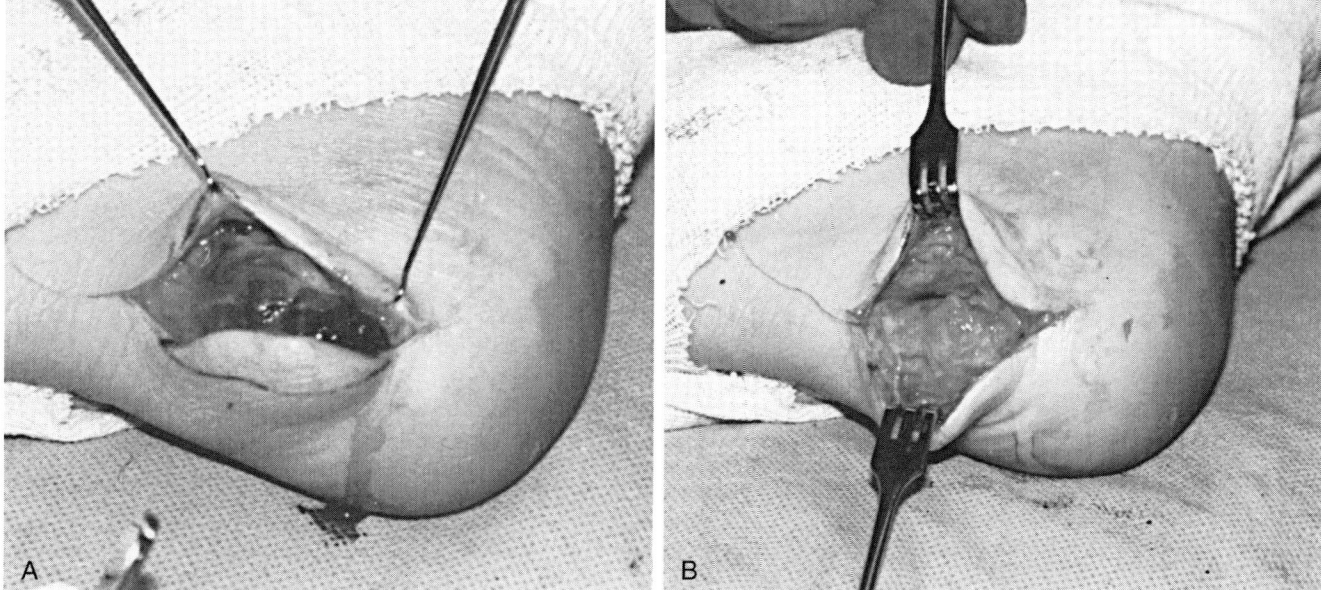

FIGURE 103–17. Rarely, arteriovenous malformations are localized enough to permit complete resection. This lesion on the heel of an 8-year-old boy was initially embolized and then resected en bloc. (Courtesy of Nolan Karp, M.D.)

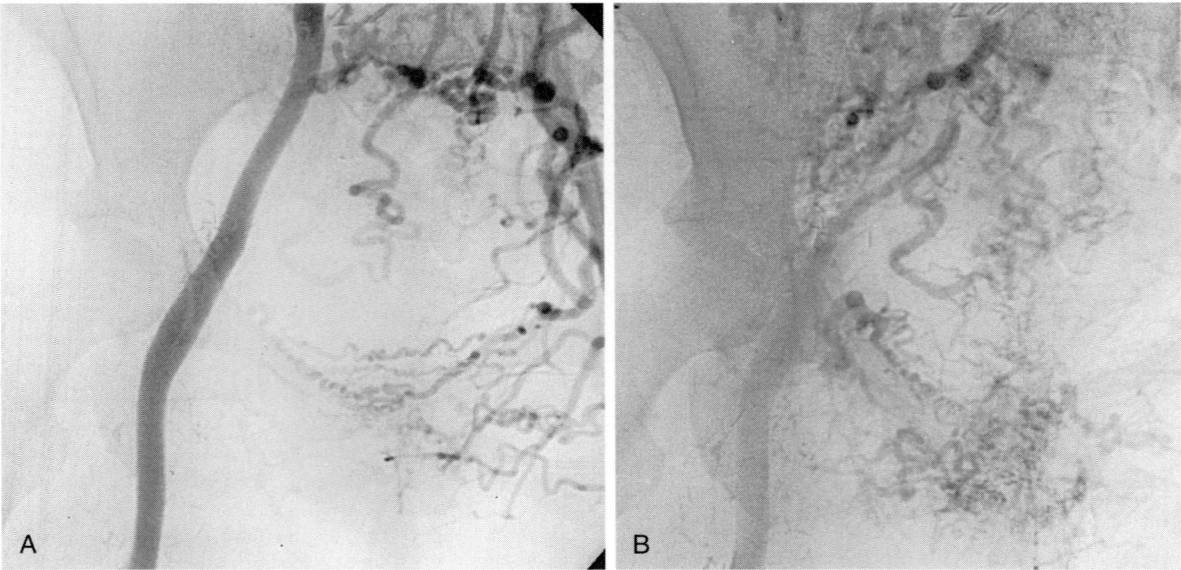

FIGURE 103–18. The patient is a young woman with a long history of extensive high-flow pelvic arteriovenous malformation who underwent surgical "skeletonization," including ligation of hypogastric artery, profunda femoris artery, and all femoral branches 1 year earlier. *A,* Early-phase arteriogram demonstrates complete skeletonization of the right iliac and common femoral segments with no filling of branches. *B,* Image taken a few seconds later demonstrates extensive collaterals resupplying the lesion. This type of recurrence is common.

be obtained, recanalization of vessels around the particles frequently results in early recurrence.

Some authors have advocated intra-arterial absolute ethanol as the agent of choice for treating high-flow AVMs.[33, 34] This agent is unquestionably effective in permanently occluding vessels but is very toxic to tissues and may produce complications such as nerve injury and necrosis of normal tissues.[35]

Rapidly polymerizing acrylic adhesives and other investigational agents have also been used in efforts to obliterate high-flow vascular malformations. Despite the technical complexity of delivering these agents superselectively, long-term results have been excellent.

Potential complications of any embolization procedure include tissue necrosis, inadvertent embolization of normal tissues, and passage of embolic materials through arteriovenous communications, resulting in pulmonary embolization. In our series of 215 patients with congenital vascular malformations outside the central nervous system who were treated by transcatheter embolization over an 18-year period, the overall incidence of complications was 6%. Three patients had major complications—temporary hemiparesis in two patients with thoracic lesions and intractable hematuria in a patient with an extensive pelvic malformation. In three patients, embolization of embolic materials to the lungs was documented radiographically. None of these patients demonstrated any clinical sequelae or changes in pulmonary function studies. No procedural deaths occurred in our series.

Because many therapeutic interventions produce an early response but are followed by recurrence, the efficacy of any given treatment must be judged by its long-term results. Of the 215 patients in our series, 25% are asymptomatic and have no radiographic evidence of residual or recurrent malformation at least 3 years after treatment. Thirty per cent are asymptomatic but show evidence of residual or recurrent malformation, clinically or on CT, MRI, or angiography. Another 21% are significantly improved but still symptomatic; 20% have had little or no change in symptoms, and 4% are more symptomatic or have different but more severe symptoms related to a complication of the procedure. Thus, it is apparent that although a significant number of patients (76% in our series) can be helped, these malformations remain extremely difficult to treat and only a minority can be eradicated completely.

Although it is impossible to compare results of different series directly when dealing with such a disparate group of patients, the results of embolization therapy compare favorably with those reported by Szilagyi and coworkers in 18 patients treated surgically, of whom 55% improved, 11% remained the same, and 33% were worse after treatment.[36] Obviously, treatment must be individualized, and in many cases a combination of embolization and subsequent surgery may provide the best long-term result.

VENOUS MALFORMATIONS

Clinical Aspects

Venous malformations are most often composed of large venous spaces under low pressure and have no clinical or angiographic evidence of significant arteriovenous shunting. They may occur anywhere in the body. When close to the skin surface, they have a distinct bluish color, and the overlying skin may be thinned, even to the extent that ulceration and spontaneous bleeding occur. Cavernous lesions can often be emptied by manual compression or elevation, showing slow refilling when pressure is released or the lesion is placed in a dependent position.

Venous lesions are often asymptomatic but may be disfiguring when large or in an exposed area (Fig. 103–19).

Pain may occur with venous distention or when the lesion is in a dependent position. Some venous lesions infiltrate an individual muscle or compartment, causing diffuse swelling and pain after exertion. Localized pain and tenderness can also result from focal areas of thrombosis in a lesion; findings are similar to those of superficial phlebitis on physical examination.

Klippel-Trenaunay syndrome, a specific complex of congenital abnormalities that affects one or more limbs, consists of extensive varicosities, venous anomalies and malformations, capillary malformations (port-wine stains), limb hypertrophy, and, in some cases, lymphatic abnormalities (Fig. 103–20).[14, 37, 38] While this is an uncommon syndrome, it is probably the one most frequently encountered in clinical practice. The cause of this syndrome remains obscure. Some authors postulate fetal venous obstruction; others invoke microscopic arteriovenous communications; and still others attribute the syndrome to mixed mesodermal and ectodermal dysplasia. Similar findings of unilateral varicosities, limb hypertrophy, and cutaneous pigmentation may be seen with AVMs. The distinction is based on angiographic absence of shunting.

Radiologic Findings

Plain films often demonstrate phleboliths (bead-like calcifications), which are pathognomonic for venous lesions. These lesions are often more extensive than they appear on clinical examination, having irregular extensions into deep tissues and infiltrating muscle planes. For this reason, evaluation of their true extent often requires CT or MRI.

Arteriography is generally unrevealing, demonstrating normal-caliber arteries and no significant shunting. If large boluses of contrast medium are injected, small "puddles" may be seen on late-phase films, which represent stasis

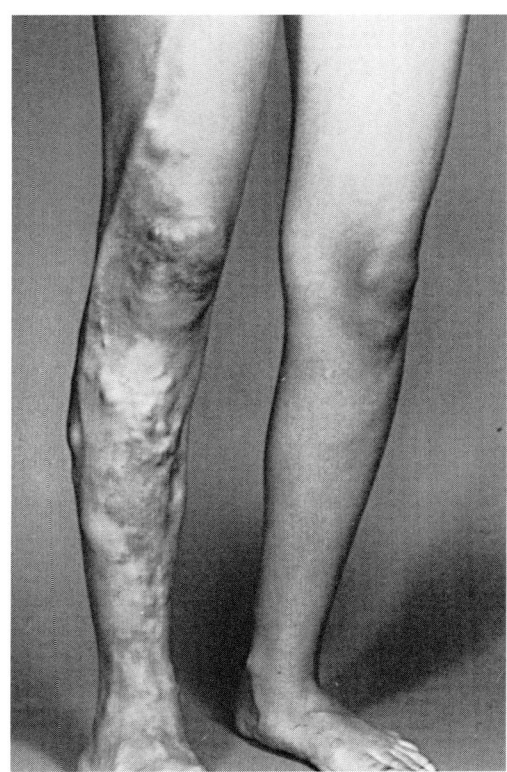

FIGURE 103–20. Typical Klippel-Trenaunay syndrome involving right lower extremity in a young woman. Findings include overgrowth of the extremity, a cutaneous birthmark, and extensive unilateral varicosities. Venography should be performed before any venous stripping in these patients.

in venous spaces. This contrast staining may persist for several minutes.

Venography may or may not demonstrate communication between the deep veins and a venous malformation. In Klippel-Trenaunay syndrome, venography typically demonstrates dysplastic veins, often including a persistent lateral embryonic avalvular vein (Fig. 103–21). Hypoplasia or aplasia of the deep venous system is often found in these patients, and it is a contraindication to removal of large superficial veins.

An effective method of studying cavernous venous malformations is direct puncture angiography (Fig. 103–22), which is performed by entering the lesion directly with a small-caliber, sheathed needle.[39] The needle is introduced through adjacent normal skin and enters the lesion subcutaneously to avoid bleeding. Slow contrast injection under fluoroscopic control demonstrates filling of irregular venous spaces and, in most cases, eventual opacification of draining veins. Because these lesions may be compartmentalized, more than one injection may be required to study the entire lesion. A small amount of a collagen suspension is injected through the sheath as it is withdrawn, to seal the tract and prevent bleeding.

Treatment

Localized symptomatic lesions may be treated by excision, although, as mentioned previously, they may be more ex-

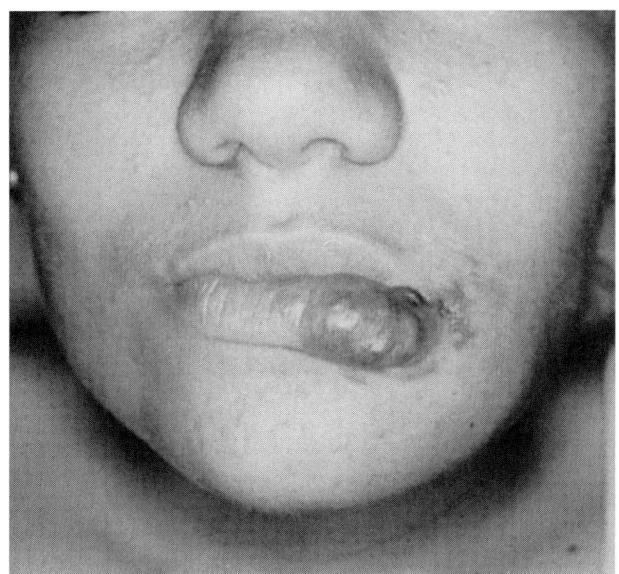

FIGURE 103–19. Typical cavernous venous malformation demonstrating soft tissue swelling and discoloration. When these lesions are compressed, they can be completely emptied and then show slow refilling. This type of lesion is best treated with direct puncture venography and embolization using ethanol.

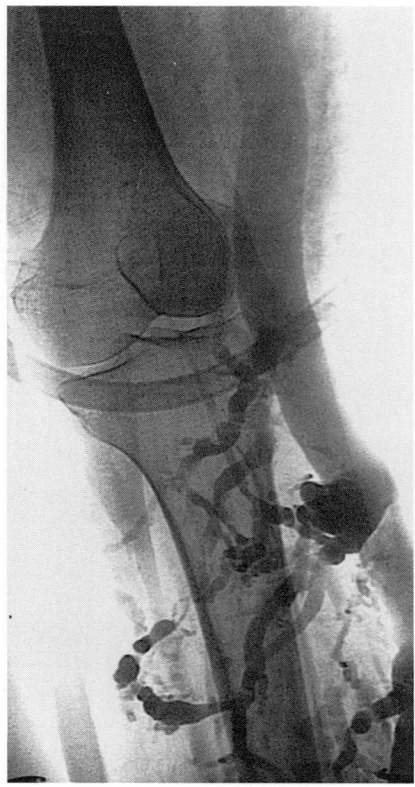

FIGURE 103–21. Venogram of leg vessels of a patient with Klippel-Trenaunay syndrome demonstrates anomalous venous development with large lateral embryonic vein, which is typical of this syndrome. Note the markedly hypoplastic deep system.

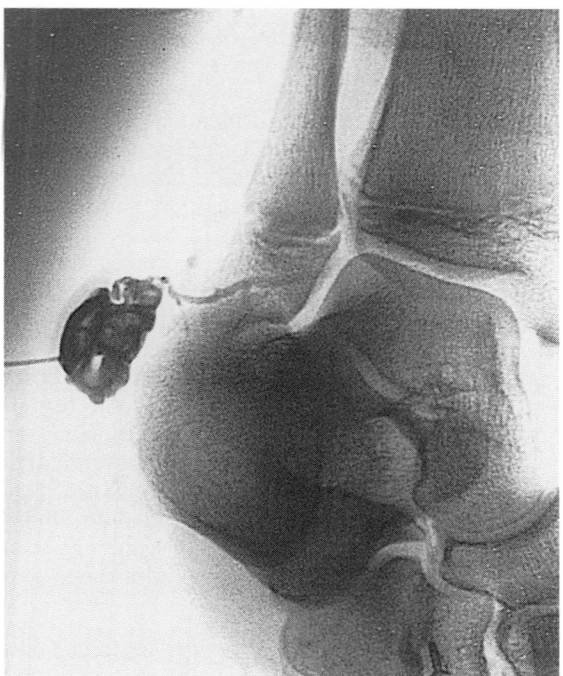

FIGURE 103–22. Direct puncture study of cavernous venous malformation of the heel. Note opacification of the draining vein from the superior aspect of the lesion once capacity is reached.

tensive than clinical signs suggest. Considerable cosmetic deformity may also result from the excision.

Embolization of arterial branches supplying the lesion has been attempted with disappointing results, as might be anticipated from the fact that the lesion does not contain significant arteriovenous communications. Direct puncture, as described above, followed by sclerosis with absolute ethanol, has been much more effective, resulting in marked shrinkage of the lesion in many cases.[40]

The treatment of Klippel-Trenaunay syndrome is controversial, but most authors advocate conservative management with support stockings, epiphysiodesis in the case of marked leg length discrepancy, and vein stripping only for specific veins that are causing discomfort.[38, 41] Before any vein-stripping procedure, contrast venography should be performed to evaluate the adequacy of the deep veins. Extensive venous stripping often markedly exacerbates symptoms.[38, 41] Servelle reported good clinical results after operations to repair sites of venous obstruction, which he postulated to be the primary cause of the entire syndrome.[14] The syndrome generally follows a benign but troublesome course in the majority of patients.

SUMMARY

Congenital vascular malformations include a wide range of lesions, most of which can be traced to a focal failure of embryonic vascular development. They must be distinguished from hemangiomas and acquired arteriovenous fistulae.

Hemangiomas are benign neoplasms of infancy. They characteristically have a proliferative phase followed by spontaneous involution during early childhood, so that specific treatment generally is not required. Acquired arteriovenous fistulae usually result from trauma and in most cases consist of simple shunts associated with high flow. They respond well to closure of the fistula, which is often necessary, owing to complications such as hemorrhage, high-output failure, or ischemia of regional tissues.

Congenital AVMs are complex lesions with multiple feeding arteries and draining veins. Clinically, they range from asymptomatic to life-threatening. Treatment is extremely difficult and is not indicated for asymptomatic lesions. Proximal ligation of feeding vessels, whether performed surgically or with embolization, has been shown to be ineffective, at best, and potentially deleterious. When treatment is indicated, it should be directed at eradicating the nidus of the lesion by surgical resection, transcatheter embolization, or a combination of the two.

Venous malformations are composed of large venous spaces with slow flow. The true anatomic extent is often greater than would be expected from clinical findings. Treatment options include surgical resection and, more recently, direct injection of sclerosing agents.

REFERENCES

1. Eichenfield LF: Evolving knowledge of hemangiomas and vascular malformations. Arch Dermatol 134:740–742, 1998.

2. Mulliken JB, Glowacki J: Hemangiomas and vascular malformations in infants and children: A classification based on endothelial characteristics. Plast Reconstr Surg 69:412, 1982.
3. Crocker DW, Cleland RS: Infantile hemangioendothelioma of the liver. Pediatrics 19:596, 1957.
4. Stanley P, Gates GF, Eto RS, et al: Hepatic cavernous hemangiomas and hemangioendotheliomas in infancy. Am J Roentgenol 129:317, 1977.
5. Jackson C, Greene H, O'Neill J, et al: Hepatic hemangioendothelioma: Angiographic appearances and apparent prednisone responsiveness. Am J Dis Child 131:74, 1977.
6. Rotan M, John M, Stowe S, et al: Radiation treatment of pediatric hepatic hemangiomatosis and coexisting cardiac failure. N Engl J Med 302:852, 1980.
7. Stanley P, Grinnell VS, Stanton RE, et al: Therapeutic embolization of infantile hepatic hemangioma with polyvinyl alcohol. Am J Roentgenol 141:1047, 1983.
8. Enjolras O, Wassef M, Mazoyer E, et al: Infants with Kasabach-Merritt syndrome do not have "true" hemangiomas. J Pediatr 130:631–640, 1997.
9. Sarkar M, Mulliken JB, Kozakewich HPW, et al: Thrombocytopenic coagulopathy (Kasabach-Merritt phenomenon) is associated with kaposiform hemangioendothelioma and not with common infantile hemangioma. Plast Reconstr Surg 100:1377–1381, 1997.
10. Frieden IJ (ed): Special symposium—management of hemangiomas. Pediatr Dermatol 14:57–83, 1997.
11. Barlow CF, Priebe CJ, Mulliken JB, et al: Spastic diplegia as a complication of interferon alfa-2a treatment of hemangiomas of infancy. J Pediatr 132:527–530, 1998.
12. Blei F, Walter J, Orlow S, et al: Familial segregation of hemangiomas and vascular malformations as an autosomal-dominant trait. Arch Dermatol 134:718–722, 1998.
13. Woollard HH: The development of the principal arterial stems in the forelimb of the pig. Contemp Embryol 14:139, 1922.
14. Servelle M: Klippel and Trenaunay's syndrome: 768 operated cases. Ann Surg 201:365, 1985.
15. Folkman J: Toward a new understanding of vascular proliferative disease in children. Pediatrics 74:850, 1984.
16. Mulliken JB, Zetter BR, Folkman J: In vitro characteristics of endothelium from hemangiomas and vascular malformations. Surgery 92:348, 1982.
17. Lawton RC, Tidrick RT, Brintnall ES: A clinico-pathological study of multiple congenital arteriovenous fistulae of the lower extremities. Angiology 8:161, 1957.
18. Szilagyi DE, Elliott JP, DeRusso FJ, et al: Peripheral congenital arteriovenous fistulas. Surgery 57:61, 1965.
19. Holman E: Abnormal Arteriovenous Communications, 2nd ed. Springfield, Ill, Charles C Thomas, 1968.
20. Lee DW, White RI, Egglin TK, et al: Embolotherapy of large pulmonary arteriovenous malformations: Long-term results. Ann Thorac Surg 64:930–939, 1997.
21. White RI, Pollak JS, Wirth JA: Pulmonary arteriovenous malformations: Diagnosis and transcatheter embolotherapy. J Vasc Intervent Radiol 7:787–804, 1996.
22. Cohen JM, Weinreb JC, Redman HC: Arteriovenous malformations of the extremities: MR imaging. Radiology 158:475, 1986.
23. Amparo EG, Higgins CB, Hricak H: Primary diagnosis of abdominal arteriovenous fistulae by MR imaging. J Comput Assist Tomogr 8:1140, 1984.
24. Rauch RF, Silverman PM, Korobkin M, et al: Computed tomography of benign angiomatous lesions of the extremities. J Comput Assist Tomogr 8:1143, 1984.
25. Trout HH, McAllister HA, Giordano JM, et al: Vascular malformations. Surgery 97:36, 1985.
26. Natali J, Jue-Denis P, Kieffer E, et al: Arteriovenous fistulae of the internal iliac vessels. J Cardiovasc Surg 25:165, 1984.
27. Polsen C, Anous M, Netscher D, et al: Hypothermia and cardiopulmonary bypass during resection of extensive arteriovenous malformation followed by microvascular reconstruction. Ann Plast Surg 34:642–649, 1995.
28. Kaufman SL, Kumar AAJ, Roland JA, et al: Transcatheter embolization in the management of congenital arteriovenous malformations. Radiology 137:21, 1980.
29. Palmaz JC, Newton TH, Reuter SR, et al: Particulate intraarterial embolization in pelvic arteriovenous malformations. Am J Roentgenol 137:117, 1981.
30. Gomes AS, Mali WP, Oppenheim WL: Embolization therapy in the management of congenital arteriovenous malformations. Radiology 144:41, 1982.
31. Berenstein A, Kricheff II: Catheter and material selection for transarterial embolization: II. Materials. Radiology 132:631, 1979.
32. Rosen RJ: Embolization in the treatment of arteriovenous malformations. In Goldberg HI, Higgins CB, Ring EJ (eds): Contemporary Imaging. San Francisco, University of California Press, 1985, p 153.
33. Yakes WF, Luethke JM, Merland JJ, et al: Ethanol embolization of arteriovenous fistulas: A primary model of therapy. J Vasc Interv Radiol 1:89, 1990.
34. Yakes WF, Rossi P, Odink H: How I do it: Arteriovenous malformation management. Cardiovasc Intervent Radiol 19:65–71, 1996.
35. Dickey KW, Pollak JS, Meier GH, et al: Management of large high-flow arteriovenous malformations of the shoulder and upper extremity with transcatheter embolotherapy. J Vasc Interv Radiol 6:765–773, 1995.
36. Szilagyi DE, Smith RF, Elliott JP, et al: Congenital arteriovenous anomalies of the limbs. Arch Surg 111:423, 1976.
37. Klippel M, Trenaunay P: Du naevus variqueux osteohypertrophique. Arch Gen Med (Paris) 3:611, 1900.
38. Jacob AG, Driscoll DJ, Shaughnessy WJ: Klippel-Trenaunay syndrome: Spectrum and management. Mayo Clin Proc 73:28–36, 1998.
39. Boxt LM, Levin DC, Fellows KE: Direct puncture angiography in congenital venous malformations. Am J Roentgenol 140:135, 1983.
40. Lasjaunias P, Berenstein A: Surgical Neuroangiography, Vol 2. Heidelberg, Springer-Verlag, 1987.
41. Lindenauer SM: Congenital arteriovenous fistula and the Klippel-Trenaunay syndrome. Ann Surg 174:248, 1971.

SECTION XIV

ANGIOACCESS

JULIE A. FREISCHLAG, M.D.

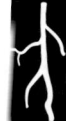

CHAPTER 1 0 4

Hemodialysis Access

Hugh A. Gelabert, M.D., and
Julie A. Freischlag, M.D.

Hemodialysis for chronic renal insufficiency has transformed American medicine. Patients who once were consigned to death from renal failure are now routinely maintained on hemodialysis with quite reasonable lives. The Medicare dialysis programs are unique in their availability. The number of patients on chronic hemodialysis is increasing dramatically. Currently, the population of dialysis patients has been increasing at a rate of 10% per year[2] and exceeds a total of 180,000 persons.[44] Dialysis access is now the most common vascular operation.[64] As a consequence, dialysis access surgery may account for as much as 40% to 50% of the practice of a busy general vascular surgeon.

The cornerstone of hemodialysis is the set of operations known collectively as *dialysis access surgery.* Included with these are hemodialysis catheter procedures, arteriovenous (AV) fistulae, and arteriovenous bridge grafts. The goal of dialysis access surgery is to provide the most durable access in a timely manner and to manage the complications of these fistulae and grafts with minimal disruption of the patient's dialysis routine.

HISTORICAL ELEMENTS

The first clinical report of hemodialysis is credited to Kolff.[33] Using hemodialysis, he managed a patient with acute renal failure in 1944. His patient died after 12 hemodialysis treatments; however, the dialysis was effective in controlling azotemia. Access for the dialysis was a significant problem, since it required surgically exposing and ligating the arteries and veins during each dialysis session. By the time the patient died, virtually all access sites had been exhausted. Vascular access remained the rate-limiting step in the clinical development of hemodialysis programs.

The Scribner shunt was developed in 1960.[57] It allowed a reliable means of dialyzing patients for prolonged periods of time. Patients could be dialyzed repeatedly without the necessity of a surgical cannulation of vessels. The shunts were designed to pass through the skin and thus could be placed at bedside. The original cannulas were made of polytetrafluoroethylene (Teflon) and rarely could be used for more than 3 months because of problems with infection and thrombosis.

In the same year, 1960, the first percutaneous dialysis catheter was developed by Shaldon and associates.[63] This cannula was also made of Teflon and was designed as a single-lumen percutaneous catheter. Typically, an arterial and a venous catheter were placed at the time of each dialysis session and removed once the session was completed. Refinements brought the use of softer materials and dual-lumen catheters. At present, the techniques of catheter-based dialysis are the mainstays of acute hemodialysis care.

The introduction of the Brescia-Cimino fistula in 1966 allowed long-term hemodialysis access, with a dramatic reduction in complications of thrombosis, infection, and bleeding.[14] The Brescia-Cimino fistula became the gold standard for hemodialysis access. Subsequent development of the "bridge" fistula, initially with saphenous vein and later with synthetic materials, further expanded the availability of hemodialysis to a larger population. The introduction of polytetrafluoroethylene (PTFE) for bridge fistulae in 1976 was another milestone in dialysis access surgery. Since its introduction, it has become the most popular graft for creation of bridge fistulae.

DIALYSIS ACCESS

Clinical Goals

The goal of hemodialysis access is to provide a reliable means of effective dialysis. This implies the ability to remove and return a sufficient volume of blood over a given period of time so as to allow efficient hemodialysis. The choice of methods used to achieve this goal forms the crux of clinical decision making in hemodialysis care. The principles of durability and availability often play against each other in choosing a method of establishing chronic hemodialysis. A more durable access site such as a proximal fistula may be deferred in favor of a more peripheral site (such as a radial artery fistula) in order to maximize available sites. The ultimate selection of methods frequently relies on a familiarity with both patient factors and available resources. It is imperative that vascular surgeons be well versed in the full range of dialysis access options.

Patient Assessment

The demographics of the dialysis patient are changing. The average age of dialysis patients is increasing as are the number and significance of co-morbid conditions,[7] which signifies that the surgical risk involved in managing hemodialysis access in these patients is increasing. The number of patients who die within the first year of initial hemodialysis has been recorded as between 17% and 35%.[66] For these reasons, assessing the patients and the timing of their dialysis are of greatest importance.

Patients requiring dialysis access may be stratified into three groups according to the urgency of their situation: (1) those in need of emergency dialysis (within hours); (2) those in need of prompt dialysis (within 48 hours); and (3) those whose dialysis need is anticipated within several months. The urgency of hemodialysis need generally determines what type of access should be provided. Those with immediate need for dialysis should have a percutaneous dialysis catheter placed. They may proceed directly to dialysis, and subsequent issues can be dealt with in a less urgent setting. Patients with less urgent dialysis needs usually may be assessed and scheduled for permanent access.

The decision regarding immediate need for dialysis is based on the presence of uremic symptoms, hyperkalemia, metabolic acidosis, or congestive failure from volume overload. The detection of fluid overload and uremia may be established by physical examination. The simple measurement of weight may detect significant fluid accumulation. Additional testing usually will include blood samples for the clinical laboratory (blood urea nitrogen, creatinine, potassium, bicarbonate), a chest radiograph, and an electrocardiogram.

Evaluation of the patient's general medical condition includes a careful review of cardiovascular factors, such as the presence of atherosclerotic risk factors like diabetes, hypertension, lipid abnormalities, coronary disease, and cigarette smoking. Recently, Barrett and colleagues reviewed the incidence of concomitant illness in their dialysis patients and noted that 36% were diabetic, 35% had some degree of heart failure, and 25.8% had subnormal serum albumin levels.[7] The impact of cigarette smoking on the success of dialysis access has been recognized as a significant factor in graft patency.[24]

Review of Access History

A review of prior access operations is essential since it will reveal potentially difficult problems that may be avoided. Such a review also helps direct the use of adjunctive testing modalities, such as venography or duplex ultrasonography, to establish patency of the vasculature. Of particular concern is the central venous system, since previous adjunctive use of percutaneous dialysis catheters frequently results in unrecognized central venous stenosis.

Examination

As in planning any operative procedure, attention must be given to examination of the patient. The examination addresses the presence of advanced renal failure and the possible need for emergency dialysis. Signs of volume overload, such as ankle and leg edema, jugular venous distention, rales, and orthopnea, are important and should be sought specifically. A search for signs of chronic peripheral vascular insufficiency, as well as evaluation of pulses and collateral circulatory pathways (e.g., Allen's test), is mandatory. The examination seeks specific evidence of venous collateralization or venous prominence in the area of the shoulders, as this may indicate the presence of an unknown subclavian vein stenosis or occlusion. Finally, it is important to review the scars from prior surgical procedures to confirm the nature of prior access operations. Frequently, patients may not have an exact understanding of prior surgery and in such instances the evaluation of surgical scars may provide valuable insight.

Preoperative Testing

The use of some form of preoperative testing to assess the patency of central venous structures is important in patients who have had repeated failures of dialysis access, or in those who have a history of multiple central venous catheterizations. The goal of these tests is to demonstrate an unobstructed venous system from the arms through the right atrium. The most common tests for this purpose include a duplex scan, a venogram, and a contrast-enhanced spiral computed tomography (CT) scan.[35] The widespread availability of the duplex scan has made it of considerable value in assessing the diameter and patency of peripheral venous sites and in detecting subclavian stenosis. Unfortunately, duplex scans cannot image vessels reliably inside the thoracic cage, and this limits their value to a degree. For this reason, contrast imaging, primarily venography, remains the definitive test.[19, 61]

Selection of Sites for Chronic Dialysis Access

The most common approach to chronic dialysis access is to choose the nondominant distal upper extremity as the first site for access. The hierarchy of choices is nondominant arm before dominant arm; forearm before upper arm; arms before legs. Thus the second-choice location is the nondominant upper arm, the third-choice location is the dominant forearm, and the fourth would be the dominant upper arm. The next sites are the lower extremities. Unfortunately, thigh AV grafts are attended by a slightly increased rate of sepsis.[9, 32, 49] Occasionally this sequence will be altered because of prior conditions, anatomic restrictions (e.g., very small vessels in the forearm or a prior subclavian vein thrombosis), or patient preferences.

Once the site of the chronic access has been chosen, consideration may be given to the site of an acute dialysis catheter, should one be required. Generally, it is placed in the side opposite the chronic access site. It is placed in a jugular vein rather than the subclavian vein because of concerns with causing either chronic subclavian vein stenosis or thrombosis and thus losing a potential later site for chronic dialysis.

Technical Requirements

The ideal dialysis access is easy to use, has good flow, is curable, and is dependable. From a technical perspective, this means that the catheter or fistula should be in a location that allows blood flows of at least 200 ml/min. The fistula should be easy to cannulate. If the grafts or the fistula veins are too deep to the skin, then they will not be useful. Deep veins may be transposed to a more superficial location. Deep grafts are best replaced with a new graft in a more superficial location. Although reliability of a graft or a catheter depends on some elements beyond the control of the surgeon (patient's coagulability, cardiac reserve, reaction to foreign bodies), other factors affecting reliability should be optimized (choosing optimal locations and vessels).

OPTIONS AND TERMINOLOGY

Acute Dialysis Access: Catheter access for urgent dialysis. The term implies that catheter devices are to be used for a relatively urgent, short period of time.

Chronic Dialysis Access: The term used to designate AV fistulas and AV grafts, used for long-term hemodialysis access. The name suggests that these devices are permanently implanted and are expected to be used as long as the patient requires dialysis.

Percutaneous Dialysis Catheter: One of the polyurethane or plastic catheters that may be placed at the bedside using a guide wire and dilator technique to permit catheter-based dialysis. In contrast to the permanently implanted catheters, these catheters do not have polyester (Dacron) cuffs. They are relatively stiff and are usually used for short periods of time (weeks to months). They may be either single-lumen catheters or, more commonly, double-lumen devices. Because of the relative rigidity of these devices, they are attended by problems of kinking and erosion, with perforation of central venous structures. They also expose the patients to a significant risk of catheter sepsis and venous thrombosis. Finally, because these catheters are firm, they may be more uncomfortable than the softer, cuffed catheters. Their principal advantage is that they may be placed at bedside with local anesthesia, thus allowing the establishment of emergency or urgent dialysis access in a matter of minutes.

Permanently Implanted Dialysis Catheter: These permanent or cuffed catheters are designed for long-term use. They are made of rubber-like silicone (Silastic) polymers that tend to be supple and accommodate readily to the patient's contour. Attached to the neck of the catheter is a Dacron cuff designed to allow fibroblast ingrowth. This ingrowth of fibroblasts leads to scar tissue, which both holds the catheter in place and forms an effective barrier against bacterial colonization along the catheter tract.

These catheters are usually placed in a patient in an operating room where sterile conditions prevail. However, they can be removed in an office setting with local anesthesia. The principal advantage of these catheters is their durability and comfort. The resistance to infection conferred by the Dacron cuff means that some catheters may last for periods of up to several years. These features make the cuffed catheters attractive adjuncts to the creation of new AV fistulae in patients who may have an urgent need for dialysis.

Arteriovenous Fistula: The union of a vein and artery in such a way as to allow blood to flow from the artery into the vein, returning blood to the central venous circulation. The most common location for fistulae is in the upper extremity, specifically the forearm. In this location, the most common fistula is one that joins the cephalic vein to the radial artery (Fig. 104–1). The principal attraction of the AV fistula is its durability and ability to resist infection. For these reasons, fistulae are considered the first choice for dialysis access. The main drawback of these fistulae is the need to allow 4 to 8 weeks for maturation before the fistula may be used. Additionally, not all patients have veins adequate to support the blood flow required for hemodialysis. In all, about 10% to 20% of AV fistulae will fail before the end of their first year. The long-term success rate for AV fistulae is considered quite good, with an anticipated average of 75% patency at 4 years.

Arteriovenous Bridge Fistula or Graft: Terms commonly used to denote a graft placed in a subcutaneous position, as a conduit or bridge between a donor artery and a recipient vein. They may be made of synthetic materials such as Dacron or PTFE, or they may be biologic grafts such as saphenous veins or bovine arteries.[6, 36, 42, 43, 54, 55, 68] These conduits may join virtually any two arteries and veins. Most commonly they are placed between the brachial artery and antecubital vein as a forearm graft, the brachial artery and the axillary vein as an upper arm graft, or the superficial femoral artery and the saphenous

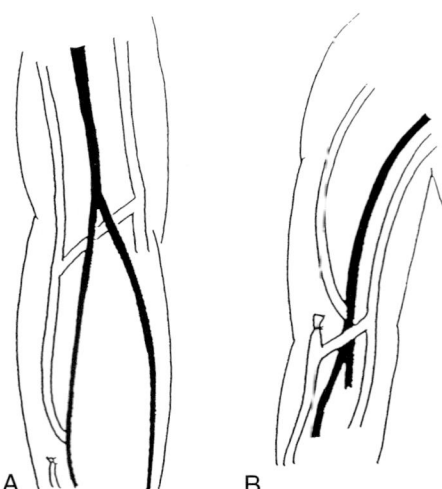

FIGURE 104–1. Common arteriovenous fistulae. *A,* Brescia-Cimino type of fistula between the radial artery and the cephalic vein, constructed at the wrist. *B,* Brachial artery to cephalic vein fistula constructed at the antecubital fossa.

vein as a thigh graft (Fig. 104–2). The principal benefit is that these grafts can usually be placed even in the absence of a large cephalic or basilic vein. They require only 10 to 14 days to mature before they can be used. However, grafts are more susceptible to thrombosis and infection than are fistulae and therefore are considered the second choice for hemodialysis. An average of 30% to 40% of AV grafts suffer a thrombotic event before the completion of the first year.

Anatomic Nomenclature

In naming AV fistulae, an anatomic nomenclature is most appropriate. This specifies the linked donor artery and the recipient vein. Although some AV fistulae are designated by the name of their originators (e.g., Brescia-Cimino fistulae), the anatomic nomenclature has the benefit of clearly designating the principal elements involved in the fistula and helps to reduce confusion as to the source and direction of blood flow.

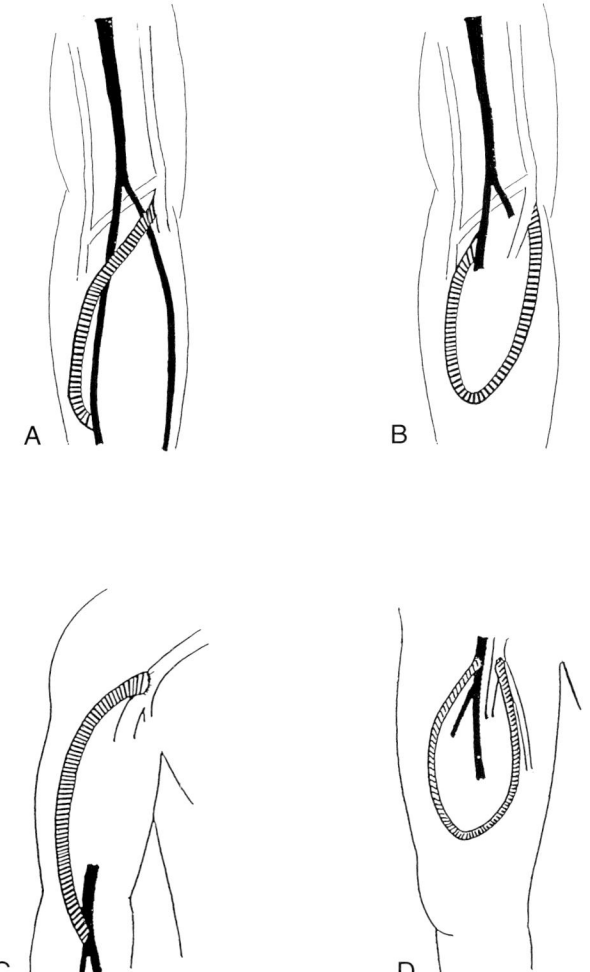

FIGURE 104–2. Common arteriovenous (AV) grafts. *A,* Straight forearm AV graft: radial artery to basilic vein (at the antecubital fossa). *B,* Forearm loop AV graft: brachial artery to basilic vein (at the antecubital fossa). *C,* Straight upper arm AV graft: brachial artery (above the antecubital fossa) to the axillary vein. *D,* Thigh loop AV graft: femoral artery to femoral vein.

Materials

Bridge fistulae may be constructed from a number of graft materials: autogenous conduits such as saphenous vein,[36, 41, 43] exogenous biologic conduits such as bovine graft[58] or preserved human saphenous vein,[55] and synthetic grafts made of Dacron or PTFE.[5, 18, 58] Unfortunately, the saphenous vein patency is less successful than anticipated. In clinical trials, the average patency was shown to be about 51% at 1 year. The use of cadaveric saphenous veins has been reported by Adar and colleagues.[1] Although the patency was reasonable (as high as 70% at 3 years), the grafts tended to develop aneurysms.[54] Similar results were obtained with vessel segments of bovine heterografts and human umbilical vein grafts denatured in dialdehyde, to be used as fistula conduits.[22, 31] Both Dacron and PTFE have been used for dialysis grafts. Although Dacron is widely used for arterial bypass, its use in dialysis access was accompanied by significant fibrous encapsulation of the graft, making it more difficult to puncture. Greater ease of puncture and handling ultimately favored PTFE.

Hemodynamics of Arteriovenous Fistulae

The size of artery and veins used in AV fistulae has a dramatic impact on the flow in the fistula. Blood flow in an AV fistula is minimal until the vein diameter exceeds that of the donor artery by 20%. If the vein diameter exceeds that of the artery by more than 75%, the fistula flow is restricted principally by the size of the feeding artery. In diameters of between 20% and 75%, the blood flow increases dramatically but remains primarily limited by the venous resistance.[28, 29, 62] Blood flow in a radial artery–based fistula commonly ranges between 150 and 400 ml/min. The larger brachial and femoral arteries may allow flows as high as 500 to 1500 ml/min.

Rittgers and colleagues reported a series of flow measurements using Doppler techniques. They noted that chronic fistulae based on the *radial* artery have an average blood flow of 650 ml/min.[59] Those based on the *distal* brachial artery have a blood flow approximating 900 ml/min, and those based on the *proximal* brachial artery have flows averaging 1100 ml/min. This in part explains the increased risk of steal syndrome associated with the more proximal AV fistulae.

The usual hemodynamic response to a large AV fistula is a decreasing total systemic peripheral resistance and an elevation of cardiac output. Elevated cardiac output is produced by an increase in both heart rate and stroke volume.[3] The occurrence of a reduction heart rate with occlusion and AV fistula is referred to as the Nicoladoni-Branham sign.[13, 51] The hemodynamic sequela of a large-volume AV fistula may be significant: Cardiac failure may develop in those with limited cardiac reserve, and extremity ischemia may develop in patients with clinical steal syndrome.

"Maturation" of an AV fistula refers to the progressive increase in the diameter of the vein, with attendant thickening of the vein wall (arterialization).[8] The process usually requires 4 to 8 weeks after the establishment of the fistula. It involves dilation of the runoff vein, thickening of its walls, and eventually enlargement of the afferent artery. Concomitant arterial changes consist primarily of dilation of the inflow artery up to the point of the fistula. Beyond the fistula, the artery will remain of normal caliber.

ACUTE HEMODIALYSIS ACCESS

Technique

Percutaneous catheter-based dialysis is accomplished with either rigid catheters or cuffed soft catheters. The rigid catheters have the advantage of being easier to place. They may be implanted at the bedside and used as soon as their location is confirmed. Their use may be limited by infection or thrombosis. The softer Silastic catheters are considered permanently implanted devices since they are constructed with a Dacron cuff that allows tissue healing to affix the catheter to the patient permanently. Technical details regarding the placement of these two types of catheters share similarities and have some significant differences.

Placing Percutaneous Catheters

Hemodialysis access in acute situations is accomplished most readily when catheter-based techniques are used. The elements of the technique involve use of a needle and syringe to identify the location of the central veins. Seldinger's technique then is used to cannulate the central veins with a guide wire. The guide wire is passed through the lumen of a large-bore needle into the central veins. This is followed by dilators to make a passage for the catheter. In the case of noncuffed catheters, these are then passed over the guide wire into position within the central venous circulation.

Although the technique is commonly used and well described, several precautions need mentioning. The technique of implantation must be sterile to avoid serious, potentially lethal infections. The patient must be positioned in a Trendelenburg position to reduce the risk of air embolization and distend the brachiocephalic veins. A common error is accidental puncture of an adjacent artery or the pleura. This may result in either a hematoma, hemothorax, or pneumothorax. For this reason, every patient should undergo chest radiography after a central catheter is placed.

Placing Cuffed Catheters

Cuffed catheters may be placed using a technique similar to that for noncuffed catheters. The principal difference is dictated by the catheter's supple nature, which requires the use of an introducer to allow passage of the catheter into the central venous system. Percutaneous catheters, being rigid, can pass over a guide wire. Cuffed catheters made of Silastic do not have sufficient axial strength to allow this technique and require the use of a rigid introducer that is later removed, leaving the catheter in place.

Alternatively, some surgeons prefer using a cutdown technique to gain access to the central venous system for cuffed catheters. In this case, a central vein or a major tributary (e.g., jugular or cephalic vein) is exposed and ligated distally. A venotomy allows the passage of the catheter directly into the vein. A concern with this technique is the loss of venous access sites, since each operation requires

ligation of a central venous site. To reduce this likelihood, an alternative technique uses purse-string sutures on the anterior vein wall to attain hemostasis and obviate the need to ligate the vessel. It should be noted that ligation of the jugular vein is attended with potential injury to the vagus nerve as well as the thoracic duct.

The use of intraoperative fluoroscopy is recommended because it facilitates the proper placement of the catheter. It is used to confirm the presence of the guide wire within the venous circulation. It is also used to observe the course of vein dilators and introducers as they are passed into the central veins. Finally, it is used to observe the passage of the catheters into the vena cava. If the catheter is misplaced initially, fluoroscopy will assist repositioning.

Surgeons performing these procedures should be familiar with the anatomic landmarks of the central venous circulation as well as the correct and incorrect trajectories of guide wires and catheters within these vessels. The passage of a guide wire into the pleural cavity may not result in a pneumothorax; however, the passage of a large introducer into the same space is of greater concern. Correct passage of a guide wire should lead the wire to enter the vena cava and the right atrium. Occasionally, the wire may pass through the atrium into the inferior vena cava. The transit through these areas confirms the intravenous placement of the guide wire.

Once the catheter has been placed, intraoperative transcatheter venography can further confirm the intravenous location of the catheter should any doubt remain. Injection of a few milliliters of contrast material under fluoroscopy serves this purpose. The same maneuver also serves to visualize the tip of the catheter if it is obscured by overlying bony structures.

At the conclusion of the procedure, an *upright* chest radiograph is obtained. This serves to document the absence of pneumothorax or hemothorax. It also confirms the location of the catheter tip. This is important since one of the most common causes for failure of the catheters to perform adequately is incorrect positioning of the catheter tip. Ideally, the tip of a catheter placed in the upper torso resides at the junction of the right atrium and superior vena cava.

The main complications of catheter access are hemothorax, pneumothorax, and infection. These are covered in a later chapter.

CHRONIC HEMODIALYSIS ACCESS

Technique

Arteriovenous Fistulae

The creation of an AV fistula obviously requires the presence of a good inflow artery as well as a satisfactory outflow vein. Preoperative evaluation includes palpation of pulses as well as Allen's test of palmar arch continuity. The brachial blood pressure is routinely measured in both arms. If the patient has weak brachial pulses, it may be instructive to compare upper extremity with lower extremity blood pressures to exclude the rare instance of bilateral subclavian stenosis.

Examination of the venous system includes observation

for obvious injuries or scars that may suggest loss of venous continuity. The presence of intravenous lines, hematomas, or prior phlebitis may limit an extremity's use. Conversely, if the veins in the chosen extremity have not been injured, then they should be protected until they may be used for construction of the dialysis access fistula. As soon as the decision to proceed with dialysis has been made, the patient is advised not to allow venipuncture or intravenous cannulation in the chosen limb. Instructions are given to nursing and clinical staff to the same effect by means of a prominent note in the patient's chart.

The operative procedure involves creation of an anastomosis between the chosen artery and vein. Generally, veins smaller than 3 mm will not be likely to succeed or mature to the point of allowing dialysis. Similarly, arteries smaller than 1.5 mm are less likely to succeed in providing sufficient flow for the fistula.

The anesthesia requirements for an AV fistula are fairly simple. The procedure may be performed comfortably under local anesthesia in the majority of patients. General anesthesia is required principally for those who have difficulty in cooperating with the procedure, or by preference of the patient or surgeon. The impact of anesthesia on the success of the fistula may be significant.[46] General anesthesia may depress cardiac output and reduce fistula flow. Brachial or supraclavicular regional anesthesia may increase arterial blood flow by allowing peripheral vasodilatation.

Following sterile preparation and draping, the limb is compressed with a tourniquet or blood pressure cuff to distend the superficial veins and allow marking of these for later identification. An incision is made in the distal forearm over the radial artery. Through this, the artery is mobilized and prepared for anastomosis. Through the same incision, the cephalic vein is identified and ligated just below the wrist. The vein is marked with a surgical scribe before division to prevent inadvertent twisting. It is then mobilized in the proximity of the artery and positioned to allow a tension-free anastomosis.

Four types of anastomosis have been employed in the radial-cephalic fistula: side-to-side, end of vein–to–side of artery, end-to-end, and end of artery–to–side of vein (Fig. 104–3). Of these, the side-to-side anastomosis is potentially complicated by venous hypertension of the hand. Although this is rarely a problem at the outset of the fistula, as the

fistula matures blood in the venous system may achieve sufficient pressure to defeat the venous valves that would protect the hand, and a painful, cyanotic, swollen hand may result. Correction requires ligation of the distal vein, stopping the transmission of elevated pressure into the hand. Failure to correct this will result in progressive edema and cyanosis, with ultimate infection and disuse atrophy.

The end of artery–to–side of vein anastomosis offers a reduced risk of the arterial steal phenomenon, but still it presents a risk of venous hypertension. It also has the disadvantage of a reduced fistula flow when compared with techniques in which the radial artery remains unobstructed and in continuity with the palmar arch. The end of artery–to–end of vein variation reduces the risk of venous hypertension of the hand but similarly has a lower fistula flow.

The end of vein–to–side of artery anastomosis is most commonly used. It has the advantage of avoiding venous hypertension of the hand, allowing for maximal fistula blood flow. The ulnar artery and distal radial artery contribute approximately 30% of the flow to the fistula by a retrograde route. This presents a significant increase in the fistula blood flow, at the same time that it exposes the fistula to the potential problem of the steal phenomenon. Such instances present with a range of symptoms from cool, pallid hand to paresthesia or paresis. Ligation of the distal radial artery corrects the steal phenomenon in most instances.

The anastomotic technique is similar to that employed in tibial artery bypass grafting. The anastomosis is constructed with a fine monofilament suture (6-0 or 7-0 polypropylene) in a continuous suture line. Prior to completion of the anastomosis, the vein and artery are gently probed with a small coronary dilator to ensure that the vein has not twisted and to overcome any spasm that may have occurred at the points of dissection and clamping.

On completion of the fistula and release of the clamps, there is an evident thrill in the fistula and beyond. Doppler examination reveals a continuous flow, with a pulsatile increase in flow in systole. Harsh pulsation to the Doppler interrogation and palpable pulsation in the fistula suggest distal obstruction. Should these be present, the fistula is examined with intravenous contrast and fluoroscopy or by gently passing a balloon catheter through the vein to seek an area of stenosis that could be corrected. Failure to

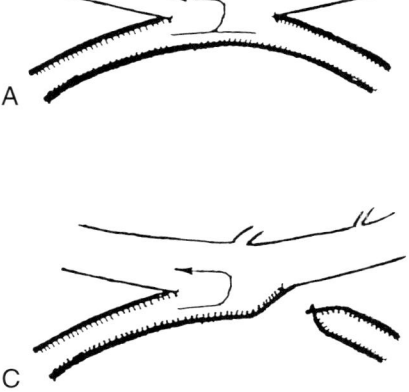

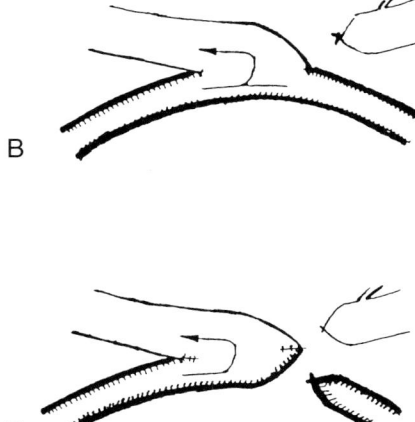

FIGURE 104–3. Variations of anastomosis for arteriovenous fistulae at the wrist. *A*, Side of artery to side of vein. *B*, End of vein to side of artery. *C*, End of artery to side of vein. *D*, End of artery to end of vein.

correct such a situation will almost certainly result in thrombosis of the fistula.

Postoperatively, patients are instructed about monitoring the thrill of the fistula and are warned about the potential problems of venous hypertension or steal phenomenon. Maturation of these fistulae requires a period of 6 to 8 weeks. During this time, the vein wall becomes arterialized and the fistula flow increases. Premature access of the fistula frequently results in hematoma and possibly thrombosis of the fistula. Patient exercise to overcome mild steal phenomena or to mature a fistula has been recommended widely by practitioners. Clinical trials have not indicated an improved result with this practice.[48]

Arteriovenous Grafts

The technique for creating a dialysis graft is similar to that used in arterial bypass with a prosthetic graft; there is a proximal anastomosis and a distal anastomosis, and the graft between these is tunneled in a precise manner. Exposure of the donor artery and target vein is carried out in a standard manner. First operations to place a new graft frequently can be accomplished with local anesthesia and intravenous sedation. Reoperation on thrombosed grafts may require a more durable anesthetic technique, such as regional block or general anesthesia—particularly if the surgical site is encased in dense scar tissue.

Once the vessels are exposed, a tunneling device is used to place a graft in the subcutaneous tissue just below the dermis. The vessels are controlled with occluding clamps, and anastomoses are constructed in an end-to-side manner to both artery and vein. When the anastomoses are completed, the clamps are removed and the fistula is allowed to flow. The graft should have a palpable thrill, and the Doppler examination should indicate a continuous flow through systole and diastole, with a pulsatile systolic increase of flow.

Postoperatively, the patient is advised that the arm will tend to swell and that arm elevation is the most effective method to reduce the edema and pain. Instruction is given regarding the possible development of a steal phenomenon or thrombosis of the fistula.

The ideal graft would be resistant to infection, would promote neoendothelialization, and would resist thrombosis. Unfortunately, none of the currently available prosthetic grafts fulfill these requirements. On occasion, autogenous tissue may be used for construction of a bridge graft. The requisite process of vein harvesting, however, is frequently a deterrent to the use of such conduits. Thus the use of a translocated saphenous vein for construction of a bridge fistula is most commonly practiced in areas of the world where the cost of prosthetic grafts make them prohibitive.

Of the synthetic grafts available for hemodialysis, PTFE has become the most common one. The reasons relate, in part, to convenience and ease of use. Patency, infection, and durability are not significantly different among the major prosthetic grafts. Other grafts that have been once popular are the bovine heterografts, umbilical vein grafts, and Dacron grafts.

The patency of AV fistulae and AV grafts remains disappointingly low. In a prospective study Hodges and colleagues noted the primary patency of fistulae at 1 year to be 43%.[29a] The 1-year primary patency for AV grafts was 41%. The 1-year secondary patency for these fistulae and grafts was 46% and 59%. The long-term patency of fistulae, however, is superior to that of AV grafts. These findings agree with a large number of retrospective studies. The failure rate of AV fistulae ranges from 30% to 50% in the first 3 months following construction.[38, 53, 69]

Complications

Thrombosis

Thrombosis remains the most common complication attending hemodialysis access surgery. The causes for graft thrombosis include stenosis-reducing graft flow, coagulation abnormalities, and cardiac insufficiency. The most common cause of graft thrombosis is venous outflow stenosis caused by neointimal hyperplasia. Almost 80% to 90% of graft thrombosis is due to stenosis at the venous anastomosis.

Intense efforts have been directed toward the early identification of these lesions in order to afford opportunity for elective repair before thrombosis occurs. Surveillance with duplex scanning,[38, 39] analysis of recirculation coefficient,[12, 34] and measurement of venous outflow pressures have resulted in modest improvements in patency. Prophylactic angioplasty of stenotic lesions has not resulted in a significant improvement in patency. The use of intravascular stents to maintain postangioplasty patency has had only modest success.[37]

Once graft thrombosis has occurred, removal of the thrombus and restoration of fistula flow may be achieved either by surgical thrombectomy or with endovascular techniques including thrombolysis. Reoperative surgery often involves revision of the venous anastomosis with patch angioplasty or segmental graft interposition.

Surgical exploration of a thrombosed AV graft requires exposure of the venous and arterial anastomosis. The venous anastomosis is opened with a longitudinal venotomy across the anastomosis, allowing direct visual inspection of the graft and vein. Attention is given to the presence of hyperplasia within the anastomotic region. Repair includes patch angioplasty to correct the anastomotic stenosis. A balloon catheter may be used to clear the graft of thrombus. The thrombus removed from the arterial anastomosis must be reviewed carefully. Typically, the portion of the thrombus that faces the arterial bloodstream will be compacted and firm. It forms a concave cap over the arterial anastomosis. It is inspected to ensure that the entire compacted cap of thrombus has been removed. Failure to remove this cap is frequently associated with early rethrombosis of the graft. If the entire cap of thrombus cannot be retrieved with a balloon catheter, the arterial anastomosis is opened and the thrombus removed under direct vision.

It is important to give systemic heparin to patients in the course of graft thrombectomy. The residual lining of thrombus along the graft walls after balloon thrombectomy is highly thrombogenic and may lead to repeated accumulation of clot within the graft. Flushing the graft with heparin and administering intravenous heparin reduce the risk of thrombosis.

Thrombosis of an AV fistula presents a different set of

considerations than thrombosis of a graft does. Fistula thrombosis most commonly is associated with one of three events:

- Development of a fistula aneurysm
- Development of a stenosis within the fistula
- Recent transplantation of a kidney into the patient

The extent of thrombosis of a fistula varies considerably. The thrombus may be a small obstruction at an area of stenosis, or it may propagate throughout the length of the fistula. Prompt thrombectomy and revision offer the best results. Delay that allows propagation of thrombus throughout the fistula may result in an unsalvageable situation.

If the thrombosis results from association with a fistula aneurysm, it is frequently necessary to open the aneurysm to remove the large thrombus that fills the vessel lumen. At the same time, the aneurysm should be repaired in a way to prevent future thrombosis. If fistula thrombosis is associated with renal transplantation, the principal question revolves around the function of the transplant. If further hemodialysis is required despite the transplant, the fistula should be repaired as soon as possible. If the thrombosis occurred in the absence of a mechanical lesion (such as stenosis or aneurysm), then consider some form of modulation of the patient's coagulation system to offset the procoagulative state associated with the recent transplant.

Endovascular techniques being used include thrombolytic therapy, mechanical clot disruption, percutaneous clot aspiration, angioplasty, and percutaneous thrombectomy. Although it is effective in dissolving clot, thrombolytic therapy has the disadvantage of being expensive. Additionally, by itself thrombolytic therapy does not address the mechanical reason leading to thrombosis: the anastomotic stenosis. Thus, angioplasty is frequently required as an adjunct to thrombolysis. The success rate for this approach is similar to that of surgical repair. The duration of patency is also similar, varying between 25% and 50% after 6 months.[11, 15, 23, 65] In comparison with surgical treatment, the incidence of complications as well as the cost of the thrombolysis favors surgery.[40, 65] In a recent prospective randomized study comparing surgery with thrombolysis, Marston and colleagues reported that surgical management resulted in significantly improved early graft function as well as longer primary patency.[40]

Other reasons for thrombosis of dialysis grafts are episodic hypotension and hypercoagulable states.[16, 21] Although unusual, these causes of graft thrombosis are notable in that they have no underlying mechanical lesion that would account for the thrombotic event. These conditions are most commonly detected when graft thrombosis is unaccompanied by a stenotic lesion. These situations are best managed by chronic anticoagulation therapy. The acute thrombotic event is managed either surgically or percutaneously with thrombolysis and angioplasty.

Venous Hypertension

Venous hypertension occurs when the venous outflow of the limb is impeded by stenosis or by increased arterial flow.[8] The result is painful swelling of the extremity. If untreated, necrosis, sepsis, and gangrene of the limb may ensue. The two most common settings leading to venous

hypertension are the presence of a side-to-side arteriovenous fistula, or subclavian vein stenosis. The venous hypertension from the side-to-side anastomotic technique is most commonly associated with a Brescia-Cimino fistula constructed in this manner. The problem develops gradually as the fistula matures. Back-pressure from the arterial outflow results in painful swelling and congestion of the hand. The problem is readily resolved by ligation of the distal aspect of the cephalic vein, thus eliminating the back-flow and pressure into the hand. It is an infrequent event now that most surgeons employ an end of vein–to–side of artery surgical technique.

Currently, the most common cause of venous hypertension presenting as a swollen, painful arm is a subclavian vein stenosis. This presentation frequently is of gradual onset, accompanied by engorgement of the superficial veins of the shoulder. It gradually becomes more dramatic as the graft or fistula matures and the flow in the vessel increases. Occasionally, the subclavian vein may be occluded prior to placement of the AV fistula. In such instances, the arm becomes acutely swollen immediately following establishment of the fistula.

Patients who have a subclavian vein stenosis are considered to be at great risk for progression of the stenosis to occlusion since increased flow in the subclavian vein is thought to accelerate the development of hyperplastic scar tissue, leading to progressive accentuation of the stenosis. These strictures usually arise as a consequence of subclavian venous cannulas placed earlier for acute hemodialysis. For this reason, subclavian vein cannulation should be assiduously avoided in favor of jugular cannulas.

When a patient presents with venous hypertension affecting the entire arm, the diagnosis is readily made by examination alone. Characteristic findings include edema extending from the upper arm down to the dorsum of the hand. The edema will improve only slightly with arm elevation. The presence of a palpable thrill indicates a functioning AV fistula. In advanced cases, the arm may be mottled or ulcerated. Venous collateralization can be noted in the distention of veins across the shoulder girdle. Occasionally, the edema may extend to the base of the neck.

The diagnosis is confirmed by ultrasonography, which demonstrates either a high-grade stenosis or occlusion of the subclavian vein, at or just proximal to the first rib. Venography may be preferred since it offers a more detailed view of the venous lesion and potentially offers the opportunity for thrombolysis, or angioplasty, or both.

Therapeutic interventions for a subclavian stenosis or occlusion are not necessary if the patient remains asymptomatic. These lesions often come to light after an AV graft has been placed and progressive arm edema develops. If unattended, this edema may become massive, leading to maceration and ulceration of the arm. If the AV graft can be moved to another limb, the simplest and most expeditious means of resolving the arm edema is ligation of the AV fistula. The arm edema will resolve promptly in virtually all cases. If the fistula must be preserved because of prior difficulty with access or because of other central venous occlusions, resolution of the arm edema will require reestablishing venous patency or continuity. To accomplish this, several approaches have been described. Percutaneous methods include balloon angioplasty and stenting.

Angioplasty offers an immediate means of reducing the arm swelling. If the angioplasty is successful in correcting the stenosis, there is a dramatic and prompt reduction in the arm edema. The durability of this improvement, however, may be limited because the lesions tend to recur as long as the fistula remains patent. Stenting does not appear to confer a significant improvement in patency either.[10, 56] Although repeated angioplasty and redilation of the stents are possible, the long-term prospect for venous patency is poor.[23]

The alternative course of treatment focuses on improved venous drainage. This may be obtained by surgically bypassing the venous lesion. The operations that may accomplish this include extending an interposition graft (usually ring-reenforced PTFE) from the subclavian or cephalic vein to the jugular vein. The PTFE bypass of the venous obstruction has the advantage of less dissection; however, the supraclavicular position of the graft is a concern from practical (graft compression) and cosmetic (visibility) perspective.

Another option is a jugular transposition or turndown operation in which the distal jugular vein is transected, mobilized, and anastomosed to the subclavian vein proximal to the stenosis. This venous transposition bypasses the obstructing venous lesion. Given the complexity of venous bypass procedures, most surgeons will choose to ligate the fistula and create a new fistula in the contralateral arm, thus reserving the venous bypass operation for patients whose particular situation demands preservation of the fistula in the hypertensive arm.[56] These operations are usually reserved for cases in which the contralateral arm has already been used for dialysis access.

Aneurysmal Degeneration

With repeated use, the walls of grafts and fistulae may become weakened and may lead to the formation of pseudoaneurysms. Aneurysms develop in about 5% to 8% of AV fistulae.[45] The aneurysms pose a problem in that they may be the source of embolization and thrombosis. They may also erode through the skin, causing infection or bleeding. Finally, the aneurysms may disfigure a patient's extremity, leading some inappropriately to avoid or delay the onset of hemodialysis.

The causes of aneurysmal degeneration lie in the materials used for the fistulae and the manner in which these are employed.[19, 22, 31, 52] Arterial and venous heterografts and allografts frequently develop aneurysms as the collagen matrix in the vessel wall degenerates. Prosthetic grafts and autogenous vein fistulae develop aneurysms primarily from suboptimal dialysis technique. The surgeon can delay or avoid aneurysmal degeneration by rotating the puncture sites, since repeated punctures at the same location weaken the vessel wall more rapidly. Periodic puncture, which occurs with rotating the puncture sites, is less destructive and allows longer use of the graft or fistula.[60]

Aneurysms that develop in AV fistulae may be repaired by either plication or resection with vein interposition. Plication alone frequently results in early recurrence of the aneurysm as the vein walls continue to weaken and dilate with time. Interposition of a small segment of vein is preferable, since the new vein segment will become arterialized and will be able to withstand repeated cannulation.

Repair of an aneurysmal graft is a more complicated procedure because the graft itself is frequently destroyed and needs replacement. Removing the old graft is rarely necessary and is not advisable, since the grafts tend to be densely adherent to the dermis. Removal frequently requires excision of the grafted surrounding tissues, resulting in a significant loss of blood and disfiguring scarring. In most instances, the new graft segment can be placed adjacent to the old graft and will function well.

Indications for repairing a fistula or replacing a graft include the presence of a "significant" aneurysm, tenderness of the aneurysm, thrombosis of the graft or fistula, the presence of a large thrombus within the aneurysm, and erosion of the aneurysm through the skin. What constitutes a significant aneurysm depends on several factors, such as the patient's general health and the patient's concern with the aneurysm. Generally, large aneurysms should be repaired *before* they become symptomatic.

Steal Phenomenon

Ischemia in the distal extremity after placement of a dialysis graft or fistula is called a vascular steal. Although some reduction in distal arterial pressures occurs in almost all high-flow shunts or fistulae, symptomatic steal occurs in less than 10% of patients with either AV grafts or fistulae.[26] Steal frequency appears to be associated with the inflow vessel, being more common with upper arm grafts than with more distal grafts; it is also seen more frequently with upper arm grafts than with fistulae.[20, 26] The manifestation of steal phenomena may be immediate or may require the maturation of the fistula. The symptoms vary from mild coolness and pallor of the hand to pain, neuropraxia, or ischemic gangrene. A well-described complication is the development of a Volkmann's ischemic contracture of the forearm following an upper extremity graft.

Factors that may predispose to the development of an ischemic syndrome include (1) diabetes, (2) arterial stenosis within the extremity, (3) grafts located in the proximal extremity, and (4) large-diameter grafts.[17, 20, 26, 30, 50] Noninvasive laboratory testing can identify patients at risk for development of a steal both preoperatively and intraoperatively. The use of digital plethysmography or digital pressures has been advocated by interested surgeons. Unfortunately, these techniques have not lent themselves to widespread use.

The development of ischemic symptoms following an AV graft or fistula is evaluated with digital pressures or plethysmography. If the symptoms are mild, the patient may be encouraged to tolerate coolness or pallor as long as no further ischemic signs appear. These symptoms usually resolve in 1 or 2 months. If the patient experiences pain or paresthesia, urgent revision of the fistula is required.

The four alternatives for resolution of the steal include:

1. Reducing the diameter of the arterial anastomosis.
2. Ligating the distal radial artery (only in the event of a Brescia-Cimino fistula).
3. Ligating the fistula entirely.
4. Ligating the distal artery and then bypassing the fistula.

Reducing the arterial anastomosis can be achieved by externally banding the fistula or replacing the anastomosis with a small-diameter (4-mm) PTFE graft segment. Alternatively, the fistula may be banded by wrapping it with a segment of small-diameter graft or suture plication of the vessel wall to reduce its size. An adequate revision usually results in immediate relief of symptoms and improvement of distal perfusion. This can be assessed by plethysmography, digital pressures, and physical examination. Unfortunately, reduction of the anastomotic area often results in thrombosis of the entire graft. The ligation and bypass technique has been described by Haimov as successful in reversing symptoms of steal in all 23 of his reported cases.[25] In essence, the artery is ligated just beyond the anastomosis to prevent steal from the distal artery. The surgeon then perfuses the distal hand by constructing a bypass from 5 cm above the fistula into the lower extremity.

In the event of ischemia associated with a Brescia-Cimino fistula, it has been observed that approximately 30% of the fistula's flow is derived via retrograde perfusion from the distal radial artery. Ligation of the artery distal to the anastomosis prevents the retrograde flow of blood out of the hand and usually corrects the steal phenomenon.

Congestive Heart Failure

Congestive heart failure associated with a hyperdynamic fistula is an unusual event. It has been estimated that fistula flow approximating 20% to 50% of total cardiac output may be required to produce this phenomenon.[3] Patients have been reported with cardiac outputs as high as 16 L/min.[4] The patient's underlying cardiac condition may be equally important in the development of congestive failure under these circumstances. Patients with limited cardiac reserve may be at greater risk. The finding of a decrease in heart rate with compression of the fistula (Branham's sign) has not been correlated with the development of congestive heart failure. Echocardiography has been successful in identifying patients who would not tolerate high-output AV fistulae.[67]

The development of congestive failure associated with a high-volume fistula may be readily corrected by reduction of its diameter. Use of an electromagnetic or ultrasonic flow probe allows quantification of the flow as the fistula or graft is constricted. Interposition of a small-diameter segment of graft has been advocated as a simple method of reducing flow in a hyperdynamic graft. In patients whose cardiac function remains marginal, peritoneal dialysis may offer a better alternative.

Infection

Infection is an uncommon problem with autogenous tissue fistulae, but it remains a particularly significant problem for AV grafts.[47] Given the frequent access with needles and the inherent vulnerability of prosthetic materials to infection, it is not an unexpected complication. Additionally, the effect of renal failure on the host immune system results in a relative weakening of host defenses.[41] The incidence of infection of AV bridge grafts is about 10% within the first year.[45] The most common infecting organism is *Staphylococcus aureus*.

Diagnosis of a graft infection may be made by seeing cellulitis around the graft. Erythema, edema, and tenderness are characteristic. Identification of a graft infection in the early postoperative period may be difficult because swelling, tenderness, and erythema frequently accompany the acute inflammatory process seen with implantation of an AV graft. In such instances, empirical treatment is frequently instituted. Resolution of the postoperative edema often coincides with decreasing pain and decreased erythema.

Cellulitis occurring in an established graft is considered a clear indication of a graft infection and merits aggressive intravenous antibiotic treatment. If the cellulitis does not resolve with antibiotic therapy, excision of the graft may be required. The incidence of infection of AV grafts is between 2.5% and 10%. Most episodes of cellulitis can be treated successfully with antibiotics so that removing a graft for infection remains an unusual event.

If a graft requires excision because of sepsis, it is important to recognize that any residual portion of the graft may become infected and give rise to further sepsis. This presents a problem in removing a graft from the arterial and venous anastomosis. The defect resulting from removal of the graft frequently requires repair of the vessel with a vein patch angioplasty. This is especially true for the arterial limb of the graft. The venous limb often may be ligated without adverse consequence. Failure to excise the entire graft has been noted to result in the development of an infected pseudoaneurysm at the site of the arterial anastomosis.

RECENT TRENDS

One recent trend in hemodialysis access centers on modification of the PTFE graft. Plasma coatings, carbon polymer coatings, endothelial seeded grafts, and changes in the graft venous anastomotic configuration have all been proposed and tested. None of these has resulted in a significant improvement. Similarly, recent applications of endovascular technologies to the issues of anastomotic stenosis and graft thrombosis have yet to yield a significantly improved outcome.

The most significant of recent advances is the increased use of autogenous fistulae. Upper extremity fistulae and vein translocation for fistula construction have been recently advocated. In 1998, Hakaim and colleagues reported significantly improved primary patency with upper arm fistulae (78%) when compared with Brescia-Cimino fistulae (33%) after 18 months.[27]

REFERENCES

1. Adar R, Siegal A, Bogodowisky H, et al: The use of arteriovenous autograft and allograft fistulas for chronic hemodialysis. Surg Gynecol Obstet 136:941–944, 1973.
2. Agodoa L, Eggers P: Renal replacement therapy in the United States: Data from the United States Renal Data System. Am J Kidney Dis 25:119–133, 1995.
3. Ahern D, Maher J: Heart failure as a complication of hemodialysis arteriovenous fistula. Ann Intern Med 77:201–204, 1972.

4. Anderson C, Codd J, Raff R, et al: Cardiac failure and upper extremity arteriovenous dialysis fistulas. Arch Intern Med 136:292–297, 1976.
5. Baker L, Johnson J, Goldfarb D: Expanded polytetrafluoroethylene (PTFE) subcutaneous arteriovenous conduit: An improved vascular access for chronic hemodialysis. Trans Am Soc Intern Organs 26:382–387, 1976.
6. Baraldi A, Manenti A, Di Felice A, et al: Absence of rejection in cryopreserved saphenous vein allografts for hemodialysis. ASAIO J 35:196–199, 1989.
7. Barret B, Parfrey P, Morgan J, et al: Prediction of early death in end-stage renal disease patients starting dialysis. Am J Kidney Dis 29:214–222, 1997.
8. Bennion R, Williams R: The radiocephalic fistula. Contempt Dial 3:12–16, 1982.
9. Bhandari S, Wilkinson A, Sellars L: Saphenous vein forearm grafts and Gortex thigh grafts as alternative forms of vascular access. Clin Nephrol 44:325–328, 1995.
10. Bhatla D, Money S, Ochsner J, et al: Comparison of surgical bypass and percutaneous balloon dilatation with primary stent placement in the treatment of central venous obstruction in the dialysis patient: One-year follow-up. Ann Vasc Surg 10:452–455, 1996.
11. Bitar G, Yang S, Badosa F: Balloon versus patch angioplasty as an adjuvant treatment to surgical thrombectomy of hemodialysis grafts. Am J Surg 174:140–142, 1997.
12. Bosc J, LeBlanc M, Garred L, et al: Direct determination of blood recirculation rate in hemodialysis by a conductivity method. ASAIO J 44:68–73, 1998.
13. Branham H: Aneurismal varis of the femoral artery and vein following a gunshot wound. Int J Surg 3:250, 1890.
14. Brescia M, Cimino J, Appel K, et al: Chronic hemodialysis using venipuncture and a surgically created arteriovenous fistula. N Engl J Med 275:1089–1092, 1966.
15. Brooks J, Sigley R, May KJ, et al: Transluminal angioplasty versus surgical repair for stenosis of hemodialysis grafts. Am J Surg 153:530–531, 1987.
16. Brunet P, Aillaud M, San Marco M, et al: Antiphospholipids in hemodialysis patients: Relationship between lupus anticoagulant and thrombosis. Kidney Int 48:794–800, 1995.
17. Bussell J, Abbott J, Lim R: A radial steal syndrome with arteriovenous fistula for hemodialysis. Ann Intern Med 75:387–394, 1971.
18. Butler H, Baker L, Johnson J: Vascular access for chronic hemodialysis: Polytetrafluoroethylene (PTFE) versus bovine heterograft. Am J Surg 134:791–793, 1977.
19. Criado E, Marston W, Ligush J, et al: Endovascular repair of peripheral aneurysms, pseudoaneurysms, and arteriovenous fistulas. Ann Vasc Surg 11:256–263, 1997.
20. Duncan H, Ferguson L, Faris I: Incidence of the radial steal syndrome in patients with Brescia fistula for hemodialysis: Its clinical significance. J Vasc Surg 4:144–147, 1986.
21. Fodinger M, Mannhalter C, Pabinger I, et al: Resistance to activated protein C (APC): Mutation at Arg506 of coagulation factor V and vascular access thrombosis in haemodialysis patients. Nephrol Dial Transplant 11:668–672, 1996.
22. Garvin P, Casteneda M, Codd J: Etiology and management of bovine graft aneurysms. Arch Surg 117:281–284, 1982.
23. Goodwin S, Arora L, Razavi M, et al: Dialysis access graft thrombolysis: Randomized study of pulse-spray versus continuous urokinase infusion. Cardiovasc Intervent Radiol 21:135–137, 1998.
24. Griffin P, Davies F, Salaman J, et al: Effects of smoking on long-term patency of artiovenous fistulas. Br Med J 286:685–686, 1983.
25. Haimov M: Vascular access for hemodialysis. Surg Gynecol Obstet 141:619–625, 1975.
26. Haimov M, Schanzer H, Skladani M: Pathogenesis and management of upper-extremity ischemia following angioaccess surgery. Blood Purif 14:350–354, 1996.
27. Hakaim A, Nalbandian M, Scott T: Superior maturation and patency of primary brachiocephalic and transposed basilic vein arteriovenous fistulae in patients with diabetes. J Vasc Surg 27:154–157, 1998.
28. Hobson R, Croom R, Swan K: Hemodynamics of the distal arteriovenous fistula in venous reconstruction. J Surg Res 14:483–489, 1973.
29. Hobson R, Wright C: Peripheral side to side arteriovenous fistula: Hemodynamics and application in venous reconstruction. Am J Surg 126:411–414, 1973.
29a. Hodges T, Fillinger M, Zwolak R, et al: Longitudinal comparison of dialysis access methods: Risk factors for failure. J Vasc Surg 26:1009–1019, 1997.
30. Johnson G, Blythe W: Hemodynamic effects of arteriovenous shunts used for hemodialysis. Ann Surg 171:715–721, 1970.
31. Karkow W, Cranley J, Cranley R, et al: Extended study of aneurysm formation in umbilical vein grafts. J Vasc Surg 4:486–492, 1986.
32. Khadra M, Dwyer A, Thompson J: Advantages of polytetrafluoroethylene arteriovenous loops in the thigh for hemodialysis access. Am J Surg 173:280–283, 1997.
33. Kolff W: The first clinical experience with the artificial kidney. Ann Intern Med 62:609–619, 1965.
34. Leblanc M, Fedak S, Mokris G, et al: Blood recirculation in temporary central catheters for acute hemodialysis. Clin Nephrol 45:315–319, 1996.
35. Lin Y, Wu M, Ng Y, et al: Spiral computed tomographic angiography—a new technique for evaluation of vascular access in hemodialysis patients. Am J Nephrol 18:117–122, 1998.
36. Lornoy W, Becans I, Gillardin J, et al: Autogenous saphenous vein AV fistula for hemodialysis: Eight years' experience with 30 patients. Proc Eur Dial Transplant Assoc 19:227–233, 1982.
37. Lumsden A, MacDonald M, Isiklar H, et al: Central venous stenosis in the hemodialysis patient: Incidence and efficacy of endovascular treatment. Cardiovas Surg 5:504–509, 1997.
38. Lumsden A, MacDonald M, Kikeri D, et al: Prophylactic balloon angioplasty fails to prolong the patency of expanded polytetrafluoroethylene arteriovenous grafts: Results of a prospective randomized study. J Vasc Surg 26:382–390, 1997.
39. Lumsden A, MacDonald M, Kikeri D, et al: Cost efficacy of duplex surveillance and prophylactic angioplasty of arteriovenous ePTFE grafts. Ann Vasc Surg 12:138–142, 1998.
40. Marston W, Criado E, Jaques P, et al: Prospective randomized comparison of surgical versus endovascular management of thrombosed dialysis access grafts. J Vasc Surg 26:373–380, 1997.
41. Martin R, Eknoyan G, Sacnz C, et al: Effects of renal failure on leukotaxis. J Med 10:267–278, 1979.
42. May J, Harris J, Fletcher J: Long-term results of saphenous vein graft arteriovenous fistulas. Am J Surg 140:387–390, 1980.
43. May J, Tiller D, Johnson J: Saphenous-vein arteriovenous fistula in regular dialysis treatment. N Engl J Med 280:770–773, 1969.
44. McCann R: Axillary grafts for difficult hemodialysis access: J Vasc Surg 24:457–461, 1996.
45. Mennes P, Gilula L, Anderson C, et al: Complications associated with arteriovenous fistulas in patients undergoing chronic hemodialysis. Arch Intern Med 138:1117–1121, 1978.
46. Monquet C, Bitker M, Bailliart O, et al: Anesthesia for creation of a forearm fistula in patients with endstage renal failure. Anesthesiology 70:909–914, 1989.
47. Montgomerie J, Kalmanson G, Guze L: Renal failure and infection. Medicine 47:1–32, 1963.
48. Rodriguez Moran M, Almazan Enriquez A, Ramos Boyero M, et al: Hand exercise effect in maturation and blood flow of dialysis arteriovenous fistulas ultrasound study. Angiology 35:641–644, 1984.
49. Morgan AP, Knight DC, Tilney NL, Lazarus JM: Femoral triangle sepsis in dialysis patients: Frequency, management, and outcome. Ann Surg 191: 460–464, 1980.
50. Morsy A, Kulbaski M, Chen C, et al: Incidence and characteristics of patients with hand ischemia after a hemodialysis access procedure. J Surg Res 74:8–10, 1988.
51. Nicoladoni C: Phlebarteriectasie der rechten oberen Extomotat. Arch Klein Chir 18:252–274, 1875.
52. Owens M, Shinaberger J, Wilson S, et al: Aneurysmal enlargement of e-PTFE fistulas. Dial Transplant 7:692–694, 1978.
53. Palder S, Kirkman R, Whittemore A, et al: Vascular access for hemodialysis. Ann Surg 202:235–239, 1985.
54. Piccone V, Lee H, Ramos S, et al: Preserved allografts of dilated saphenous vein for vascular access in hemodialysis: An initial experience. Ann Surg 182:727–732, 1975.
55. Piccone V, Sika J, Ahmed N, et al: Preserved saphenous vein allografts for vascular access. Surg Gynecol Obstet 147:385–390, 1978.
56. Puskas J, Gertler J: Internal jugular to axillary vein bypass for subclavian vein thrombosis in the setting of brachial arteriovenous fistula. J Vasc Surg 19:939–942, 1994.
57. Quinton W, Dillar D, Scribner B: Cannulation of blood vessels for prolonged hemodialysis. Trans Am Soc Artif Intern Organs 6:104–113, 1960.
58. Raju S: PTFE grafts for hemodialysis access: Techniques for insertion and management of complications. Ann Surg 206:666–673, 1987.

59. Rittgers S, Garcia-Valdez C, McCormick J, et al: Noninvasive blood flow measurement in expanded polytetrafluoroethylene graft for hemodialysis access. J Vasc Surg 3:635–642, 1986.
60. Rossi G, Munteau F, Padula G, et al: Non-anastomotic aneurysm formation in umbilical vein grafts. J Vasc Surg 4:486–492, 1986.
61. Rutherford R: The value of noninvasive testing before and after hemodialysis access in the prevention and management of complications. Semin Vasc Surg 10:157–161, 1997.
62. Schenk WJ, Bohn R, Stephens J: The regional hemodynamics of experimental acute arteriovenous fistulas. Surg Gynecol Obstet 105:733–735, 1957.
63. Shaldon S, Chiandussi L, Higgins B: Hemodialysis by percutaneous catheterization of the femoral artery and vein with regional heparinization. Lancet 2:857, 1961.
64. Stanley J, Barnes R, Ernst C, et al: Vascular Surgery in the United States: Workforce Issues. Report of the Society for Vascular Surgery and International Society for Cardiovascular Surgery, North American Chapter, Committee on Workforce Issues. J Vasc Surg 23:172–181, 1996.
65. Summers S, Drazan K, Gomes A, et al: Urokinase therapy for thrombosed hemodialysis access grafts. Surg Gynecol Obstet 176:534–538, 1993.
66. U.S. Renal Data System (USRDS): 1994 Annual Data Report. In The National Institutes of Health, National Institute of Diabetes and Digestive and Kidney Diseases, Bethesda Md, 1994.
67. von Bibra H, Castro L, Autenieth G, et al: The effects of arteriovenous shunts on cardiac function in renal dialysis patients: An echocardiographic evaluation. Clin Nephrol 9:205–209, 1978.
68. Wilson S, Hillman M, Owens M: Hemodynamic effects of bovine femorosaphenous fistula. Dial Transplant 6:84–89, 1977.
69. Winsett O, Wolma F: Complications of vascular access for hemodialysis. South Med J 78:513–517, 1985.

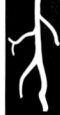

CHAPTER 1 0 5
Peritoneal Dialysis

Michael M. Farooq, M.D., and
Julie A. Freischlag, M.D.

An understanding of peritoneal dialysis principles and indications is often underemphasized among the armamentaria of vascular access surgeons. Patients with diminishing vascular access who might be alternatively supported by peritoneal dialysis are often overlooked. The informed surgeon can assist the nephrologist in determining the feasibility of peritoneal dialysis. This chapter presents the history, physiologic mechanisms, indications, and contraindications for peritoneal dialysis. Traditional catheter placement techniques are reviewed, and newer laparoscopic catheter placement strategies are described. The prompt identification and management of complications are emphasized.

HISTORY

The origins of peritoneal dialysis date back to 1923, when Ganter[1] first accomplished the modality in rabbits and guinea pigs that had undergone ureteral ligation. In this uremic model, peritoneal fluid exchanges lasting 2 to 4 hours were analyzed. He subsequently treated a patient with obstructive uropathy in a similar manner. In 1938, Rhoads[2] used intermittent peritoneal dialysis to treat two nephrotic patients with some success. Attention was directed toward the problem of maintenance peritoneal dialysis with the observation that dialysis would need to be performed frequently in a sterile setting. Other patient problems, including dietary restrictions and nutritional supplementation, were recognized as essential for patient survival.

In 1965, Weston and Roberts[3] reported the use of a catheter for acute peritoneal dialysis. Palmer and associates[4, 5] were the first to describe the concept of an indwelling peritoneal catheter, in 1964, and performed intermittent peritoneal dialysis for the first time. Unfortunately, the dialysis was inadequate because of this technique, and the procedure was complicated by peritonitis. In 1968, Tenckhoff and Schecter[6] devised a silicone catheter with two polyester (Dacron) cuffs for use in patients who would require long-term peritoneal dialysis. This catheter in a modified form is still the one most commonly used.[7–10] In 1976, Popovich and associates[12] first reported the use of a portable equilibrium method of peritoneal dialysis. Their technique has evolved to the present *continuous ambulatory peritoneal dialysis* (CAPD) regimen used by many patients today.[11–13]

According to the Report of the National Institutes of Health (NIH) National CAPD Registry, approximately 35,000 patients throughout the world are being treated with peritoneal dialysis.[14] Approximately 17% of the patients in the United States use peritoneal dialysis as opposed to hemodialysis. Physician bias attributable to a lack of familiarity with peritoneal dialysis is thought to explain this observation.

Benefits of peritoneal dialysis include[15]:

- Better hemodynamic stability
- More efficient maintenance of blood pressure
- Increased preservation of residual renal function
- Higher average hemoglobin levels
- Better lipoprotein profiles

Survival of patients treated with CAPD is similar to that of patients treated with hemodialysis, 3-year survival rates being 60%. Of the survivors, 60% continue to be maintained with peritoneal dialysis. CAPD has a higher relative risk for death only in older diabetic patients, probably related to peritonitis.[16] The cost of peritoneal dialysis is less than that of hemodialysis, and the procedure can be performed at home by most patients.[17]

PHYSIOLOGY

The peritoneum acts as a biologic membrane that is available for the exchange of solutes and fluid volume.[18–20] The capillary endothelium, endothelial basement membrane, interstitium, and mesothelium act as the surface membranes that permit this exchange. Smaller molecules, such as urea, equilibrate in 4 hours or less, whereas larger molecules take up to twice that long.[21] Protein losses occur with peritoneal dialysis at an average of 6 to 12 gm/day, depending on the size of the patient and the frequency of the exchanges.[22, 23] Amino acids are lost at a rate of 2.0 to 3.5 gm/day.[24–26] Serum levels of vitamins C, B_1, and B_6 and folic acid are decreased in patients being treated with peritoneal dialysis.[27, 28] Glucose absorption from the dialysate is substantial in these patients, approaching 100 to 200 gm/day; it can lead to obesity, impaired glucose tolerance, and hypertriglyceridemia if the patient's diet is not closely monitored.[29–32]

Glucose acts as an osmotic agent that facilitates the removal of fluid through the peritoneal cavity. The pH of the dialysate must be acidic to prevent caramelization of the glucose.[33] The low pH can cause pain as the solution is instilled into the peritoneal cavity. There is evidence that the low pH can inhibit the function of the peritoneal white blood cells and permit the development of bacterial peritonitis.[34]

Other substances have been utilized as osmotic agents in the dialysate fluid that may prove to be better than glucose. They include amino acids,[35, 36] glycerol,[37] xylitol,[38, 39] sorbitol,[40, 41] mannitol,[42] fructose,[43, 44] dextran,[45, 46] and other glucose polymers.[47] Amino acids may be as effective as glucose in their osmotic action and may provide better nutrition. Glycerol has a higher pH than glucose and delivers a lower caloric load to the patient; however, its osmotic action is not as good.

INDICATIONS

Short-Term Peritoneal Dialysis

Short-term peritoneal dialysis is an easy procedure to perform, especially in children.[48–51] Indications include[52–55]:

- Hyperkalemia
- Metabolic acidosis
- Electrolyte disorders
- Congestive heart failure due to fluid overload

Patients with a contraindication to heparinization, which is required for hemodialysis, are ideal candidates for short-term peritoneal dialysis, which does not require hepariniza-

tion. Also, patients with poor venous access can undergo short-term peritoneal dialysis. If the patient's cardiovascular status is borderline, peritoneal dialysis can be performed with fewer hemodynamic consequences than hemodialysis.[56]

Drug intoxication can also be treated with short-term peritoneal dialysis. Hemodialysis is typically utilized for drug intoxication; however, if it is unavailable or is contraindicated, peritoneal dialysis can be substituted.[57, 58] The pH of the peritoneal dialysate can be altered to enhance anion diffusion. Exogenous albumin can bind with the drug and prevent its absorption. Intraperitoneal administration of other agents can facilitate their absorption through the peritoneal cavity.[59–61]

Other indications for short-term peritoneal dialysis are profound hypothermia,[62–64] hypoglycemia from the long-term use of oral hypoglycemic agents, poisoning, congenital lactic acidosis,[65, 66] maple syrup urine disease, urea cycle defects, severe hyperuricemia associated with gouty nephropathy,[67–69] hepatic coma, and psoriasis.[70] Intraperitoneal deferoxamine has been used to chelate aluminum.[71, 72] Acute pancreatitis can be treated with short-term peritoneal dialysis,[73, 74] but results for this indication are not very encouraging, according to reviews of controlled clinical trials. The dialysate cannot reach the retroperitoneal area, where most of the damaging enzymes and debris from the necrotizing pancreas reside.

Long-Term Peritoneal Dialysis

Candidates for long-term peritoneal dialysis include patients with end-stage renal disease who can manage the catheter and exchanger themselves or with the aid of a motivated family member. Patients with diabetes or congestive heart failure can do well with peritoneal dialysis.[75–77] Those with a contraindication to heparinization (i.e., retinal or vitreous hemorrhages) can undergo dialysis with this modality. Children are ideal candidates for long-term peritoneal dialysis; those weighing less than 10 kg have very small arteries and veins, making creation of a hemodialysis fistula technically difficult.[78–81]

Timing Regimens

Intermittent peritoneal dialysis (IPD) can be used effectively in patients needing acute care but is not adequate for long-term use. Malnutrition, acidosis, anemia, and poor control of the patient's hydration are seen after the first year.[82, 83] IPD is usually offered to patients who have some residual renal function or who refuse other methods of peritoneal dialysis for whatever reason. IPD uses 2 to 3 L of dialysate with peritoneal cavity dwell times of 20 to 30 minutes between drainage of the peritoneal cavity. Ten-hour sessions every other night or three sessions per week are usually performed. IPD can be done manually or by means of an automated reverse-osmosis delivery system.

CAPD is a low-flow rate continuous dialysis technique that utilizes 2 L of dialysate with peritoneal cavity dwell times of 4 to 8 hours before drainage of the peritoneal cavity.[84–92] The cycle is continuous throughout all 24 hours of the day.

Continuous cycling peritoneal dialysis (CCPD) is similar to

CAPD, except that most of the cycles occur at night; there is only one diurnal cycle with a prolonged dwell time during the day using 1500 to 2000 ml of dialysate.[93, 94] Patients undergoing CCPD experience fewer peritoneal infections than patients undergoing CAPD because of fewer disconnections per day for exchanges.

Nocturnal peritoneal dialysis (NPD) is another method whereby the cycles occur primarily during the night, with 20- to 60-minute cycles occurring over 8 to 10 hours. High dialysate flows are required to maintain such exchange rates, and this type of peritoneal dialysis is best for patients who (1) have high peritoneal transfer rates or (2) cannot tolerate large peritoneal volumes because of pain or discomfort from the increased abdominal pressure.[95] Therefore, patients with abdominal leaks, hernias, bladder prolapse, low back pain, and restrictive lung disease may benefit from this form of peritoneal dialysis. Alternatively, clearances of urea and creatinine are lower with NPD, and the procedure is more expensive because of the need for higher flows from the exchanger.

Tidal peritoneal dialysis (TPD) is a fairly new experimental method that keeps the dialysate in contact with the peritoneal cavity at all times. A larger reservoir of fluid is kept in the peritoneal cavity and exchanges smaller volumes.[96–98] A special automated cycler is modified by volume rather than by time. No real benefit from this type of peritoneal dialysis has been shown.

No matter which form of peritoneal dialysis is chosen, its success is determined primarily by patient education and motivation. Training sessions are required prior to the institution of peritoneal dialysis at home. Between five and 15 sessions may be required to reduce the risks of contamination and other technical problems associated with the technique.[99] Patients undergoing peritoneal dialysis remain viable candidates for renal transplantation without increased risk of peritonitis or graft failure.[100]

CONTRAINDICATIONS

Major contraindications to peritoneal dialysis include:

- Recent abdominal surgery
- Inflammatory bowel disease
- Presence of a colostomy, ileostomy, or ileal conduit
- Extensive peritoneal fibrosis
- Immunosuppression

Patients with a significant neurologic deficit, psychosis, or poor intellect, and patients who are not motivated should not be considered for long-term peritoneal dialysis. Patients who are blind or who have crippling arthritis of the hands cannot be treated with long-term peritoneal dialysis unless a family member can help with the procedure.

Minor contraindications include severe chronic obstructive pulmonary disease, diverticulosis, polycystic kidney disease, hyperlipidemia, obesity, lumbar disc disease, and protein malnutrition. Patients who need short-term dialysis immediately after surgery may not be candidates for peritoneal dialysis owing to the presence of surgical wounds and drains. Previous abdominal surgery may lead to the formation of adhesions, which may prevent adequate dialysis. Diaphragmatic, abdominal, or inguinal hernias may become more symptomatic during peritoneal dialysis and therefore may need repair prior to institution of the treatment.[101–103] Severe gastroesophageal reflux may be exacerbated by peritoneal dialysis in some patients.

TYPES OF CATHETERS

Early Catheters

One of the first peritoneal dialysis catheters was made of latex rubber by Boen and colleagues[104] in 1961. Weston and Roberts[3] devised a nylon catheter for peritoneal dialysis in 1965. This short-term peritoneal dialysis catheter demonstrated outflow problems in 8% to 69% of patients in all series evaluated. Gutch[105, 106] first introduced silicone as the material of choice for use in peritoneal dialysis catheters because of its biocompatibility.

Tenckhoff Catheter

The most frequently used peritoneal access device is the Tenckhoff catheter.[6, 7] It is a soft, nonreactive polymeric silicone (Silastic) tube with multiple side holes along the distal peritoneal portion of the tube as well as a hole in the end of the catheter. Experiments have shown that the peritoneal cavity is more difficult to drain than to fill; therefore, during outflow, the majority of the dialysate returns via the side holes and not through the tip of the catheter. Catheters with a singular end hole have a higher incidence of outflow drainage malfunction.

The Tenckhoff catheter has two Dacron cuffs that help to fix it in place. The inner cuff prevents leakage around the catheter from the peritoneal cavity. Initially, the Dacron cuff initiates an inflammatory reaction, with formation of a fibrin clot. This is followed by infiltration of granulocytes and fibroblasts with giant cells. Simple squamous epithelium grows around the inner cuff over time to seal the peritoneal cavity. The outer cuff is placed in the subcutaneous space, where fibrous tissue ingrowth occurs, preventing bacterial contamination of the catheter. Stratified squamous epithelium grows around the skin exit site, helping to seal the catheter.[107] Single-cuff catheters are associated with a lower 1-year survival rate and a higher infection rate than double-cuff catheters.[108] Curled-tip catheters have no clear advantage over straight-tipped catheters.

Swan-Neck and Polytetrafluoroethylene Catheters

Newer types of catheters have been developed but do not appear to have particular advantage over the Tenckhoff catheter. Twardowski and coworkers[109, 110] have described a swan-neck catheter that is similar to the Tenckhoff catheter. The subcutaneous portion of the catheter is formed with a sharp arc, as in the neck of a swan. The subcutaneous tunnel is made at the same angle, with the catheter retaining its shape. It was thought that such a configuration might prevent tunnel infections; however, no such improvement has yet been documented.

A polytetrafluoroethylene catheter has also been developed, but it is associated with a higher number of tunnel infections than the Tenckhoff catheter.

Polyurethane Catheter

A polyurethane catheter (Corpak catheter, Thermedics) has an inner diameter 1.5 times that of the Tenckhoff catheter and demonstrates good tissue ingrowth.[111] Polyurethane catheters may possess more strength, remain patent longer, and resist infection better than polymeric silicone (Silastic) catheters. Silicone catheters become impregnated with a protein biofilm that inhibits bacterial destruction by white blood cells.[112] This phenomenon may lead to a higher catheter infection rate compared with polyurethane catheters.

Goldberg Catheter

The Goldberg catheter has a saline-filled balloon, which was devised to keep the catheter positioned within the lower abdomen.[113] It has shown no real advantage, however, in preventing catheter migration.

Silicone Disc Catheters

The Toronto Western Hospital has promoted the use of a catheter with two silicone discs perpendicular to the catheter tube that were devised to hold the catheter in place.[114] A 10% outflow failure rate due to obstruction from either bowel or omentum has been shown despite the presence of these silicone discs.

For a newer type of catheter, the *Lifecath*, an intraperitoneal silicone disc is placed just under the abdominal wall within the peritoneal cavity.[115] This catheter shows a 6% outflow failure rate owing to omental obstruction. The half-life of this catheter may be a bit longer than that of the Tenckhoff catheter because of reduced migration and infection; however, a higher leakage rate has been reported.[116]

CATHETER PLACEMENT

Percutaneous Technique

Short-term peritoneal dialysis catheters can be placed percutaneously, a method that is more efficient and less expensive. Most physicians choose to place the catheter at McBurney's point or its mirror image on the left. Preparation includes placement of a Foley catheter (if the patients still makes urine), administration of an enema, and the intravenous infusion of antistaphylococcal antibiotics. Xylocaine is infiltrated in the skin, and intravenous sedation can be used for patient comfort. A stylet or guide wire is then used to advance the catheter into the peritoneal cavity.[117]

Open Technique

Catheters for long-term peritoneal dialysis should be inserted in the operating room for maximum patient comfort and sterility. Local, regional, or general anesthesia should be utilized, depending on the patient. General anesthesia is preferred in children because relaxation of the abdominal musculature facilitates placement of the catheter. The preferred method is an open operative technique, which allows direct vision for positioning the catheter and viewing the contents of the peritoneal cavity. Preoperatively, the patient fasts from midnight the night before, and an enema is given. Systemic antibiotic prophylaxis with a cephalosporin or vancomycin is given for adequate antistaphylococcal coverage.

Many types of incisions have been used for insertion of peritoneal dialysis catheters, including the paramedian, the infraumbilical midline, and the transverse incision in either lower quadrant. The method preferred by the authors is a small longitudinal incision placed below the umbilicus, which allows excellent exposure. This incision is carried down through the anterior rectus fascia, and the muscle is split bluntly to expose the peritoneum. The peritoneum is grasped between clamps, lifted, and incised with a scalpel. Care must be taken if there are adhesions to the parietal peritoneum from previous procedures. Some surgeons recommend omentectomy to prevent later envelopment of the catheter by the omentum, which would lead to catheter occlusion. The authors do not routinely perform this procedure.

The catheter is introduced through the peritoneal opening and directed toward the pelvis, which is the most dependent area of the peritoneal cavity in both the upright and supine positions. A guide wire placed through the lumen of the catheter may help facilitate placement of the catheter. A nonabsorbable polypropylene suture is placed on the internal aspect of the anterior abdominal wall and tied loosely around the catheter to secure it in place in the pelvis. A pursestring suture is placed to secure the edges of the peritoneal opening to the first Dacron cuff; this ensures a watertight closure so that peritoneal dialysis can be started early in the postoperative period. The suture is reinforced with a second pursestring suture that incorporates the transversalis fascia around the cuff to further strengthen the seal.

The catheter exit site is chosen preoperatively and is positioned below the belt line for patient comfort. The catheter should be positioned through the rectus muscle to prevent migration. A small stab incision is made in the skin, and either a long clamp or a tunneling device is used to create a tunnel in the subcutaneous plane that is brought out medially through the midline incision.[118] The catheter is advanced through the tunnel and is positioned so that the second Dacron cuff lies at least 2 cm from the skin exit opening in the subcutaneous space. No suture is placed at the exit site, so as not to create an inflammatory reaction that might lead to infection. Irrigation of the catheter with heparinized saline documents patency of the catheter at the time of the operation, flushes out any debris or blood clots, and ensures that there is no leakage from around the first cuff. The instilled fluid should drain out of the abdominal cavity spontaneously with gravity.

The rectus fascia is closed with the use of interrupted 2-0 or 1-0 nonabsorbable sutures, and the skin is closed with 3-0 nylon sutures or skin staples. The catheter is connected to a bag of dialysate in the operating room, and peritoneal dialysis is begun with a small volume. The fluid should flow freely, and there should be no demonstrable leaks. A sterile gauze dressing is placed over the midline wound, and a clear, semipermeable dressing, such as Op-Site dressing, is placed over the catheter exit site.

If peritoneal dialysis does not need to be started immediately, daily flushes of the catheter should be performed in a sterile manner to maintain patency. If peritoneal dialysis needs to begin immediately, small volumes should be exchanged at frequent intervals with the patient in a supine and inactive position to prevent leakage from the wounds. The patient should not lift more than 30 pounds for 2 weeks after catheter placement so that proper healing can take place.

Laparoscopic Technique

Since its introduction by Ash and colleagues[119, 120] in 1981, the performance of laparoscopy (peritoneoscopy) to assist in peritoneal catheter placement has become more commonplace. Many surgeons have become familiar with the laparoscopic technique because of the rapid expansion of its use in general surgery.

The peritoneum is ideally exposed through an infraumbilical incision as described by Hasson. After inducing an adequate pneumoperitoneum with the patient under general anesthesia, the surgeon introduces a laparoscope through a blunt trocar secured in this location. In this manner, complications of visceral or vascular injury by an insufflation needle can be avoided.[121] This procedure permits documentation of appropriate peritoneal catheter placement with the use of the closed trocar technique through a lateral rectus insertion site. A second contralateral trocar can be placed under direct vision to permit entry of a grasper if catheter positioning is required.

The first cuff can be placed at the level of the peritoneum, and the remaining catheter is tunneled in the subcutaneous tissue lateral to the rectus muscle. After partial decompression of the pneumoperitoneum, saline is instilled into the peritoneum and allowed to egress spontaneously to confirm catheter patency. Even though the inner cuff is left unsutured with this technique, sequelae of leakage or migration have been infrequent, perhaps because of the small stab incision required with the laparoscopic technique. A reported lower incidence of wound infection is thought to be due to minimized tissue trauma at the catheter insertion site. However, repair of laparoscopic trocar site hernias is required on occasion.[122]

COMPLICATIONS

Catheter-Related Complications

Interestingly, there has been no change in the incidence of early and late complications following Tenckhoff catheter placement since 1977. During the first months after placement of a Tenckhoff catheter, the major complication is outflow failure, which in reported series occurs in 1% to 20% of cases.[123] Early catheter infections are rare.

During the first month, outflow failure can be caused by catheter malposition or side hole obstruction by omentum;

these events occur over days or weeks, respectively. A kink or clot is the usual cause of early inflow obstruction.

Inflow pain may indicate poor catheter position or sensitivity to the low pH of the dialysate. The addition of bicarbonate to the dialysate can relieve the discomfort in this instance. Persistence of pain despite this maneuver is suggestive of a mechanical problem. Usually, the catheter has become dislodged and shifted into a poor position, most commonly under the diaphragm. Using radiographic dye to delineate the catheter position can be helpful. In most cases, the catheter must be repositioned surgically. A laparoscopic approach can be used to effectively reposition the catheter or free obstructing omentum as needed, with reduced morbidity and discomfort.[121]

Outflow failure after 1 month is often due to a fibrin clot. The incidence ranges from 5% to 20%. If the catheter is obstructed, streptokinase or urokinase can be instilled into the catheter to dissolve the fibrin clot.[124, 125] If this maneuver is successful, heparin should be used in the dialysate for the next few days to ensure catheter patency.[126] Alternatively, laparoscopy can be helpful to document whether outflow failure is due to obstruction of the catheter side holes by bowel or omentum. Repositioning of the catheter under fluoroscopic guidance can be attempted but is not usually successful unless the catheter was recently placed.

Intraperitoneal bleeding can occur immediately following placement of the catheter. The most common sites are small visceral or abdominal wall vessels. If the hematocrit of the effluent is less than 2 ml/dl or if the red blood cell count is less than 60,000/cm³, the bleeding is insignificant and can be managed expectantly with good results. Heparin (1000 U/2 L dialysate) should be added while the effluent remains bloody to prevent clotting of the catheter.[127] If bleeding is noted more than 1 month after placement of the peritoneal dialysis catheter, one must suspect other causes. These include inflammation, perforated viscus, and immunoglobulin A (IgA) glomerulonephritis, which often occurs in association with upper respiratory tract infections. Bleeding may be seen in female patients secondary to endometriosis or at the time of a normal menstrual period.[128, 129] Diagnostic evaluation should be performed to determine the cause of late bleeding associated with peritoneal dialysis catheters.[130]

Leakage of dialysate from around the catheter exit site or from the midline wound can occur immediately after the operation.[131] Leakage may be manifested by edema in the abdominal wall, legs, or scrotum.[132] It usually occurs because the volume of dialysate is too large. Decreasing the amount of dialysate and increasing the number of exchanges allows the leak to seal without reoperation. Only if the inner Dacron cuff has been extruded from its original position does the pericatheter leak persist despite conservative management.

Pericatheter hernias may occur during the course of peritoneal dialysis.[133–135] They occur more frequently in older patients, multiparous women, and patients who experienced leakage from the abdominal wound in the immediate postoperative period. Most pericatheter hernias need to be surgically repaired. Other preexisting hernias may become enlarged during peritoneal dialysis because of the increased intra-abdominal pressure and volume[136]; they include (1) *inguinal* hernias (especially if there is a patent processus vaginalis), (2) *umbilical* hernias, and (3) *incisional* hernias. Acute hydrothorax on either side can occur early in the course of peritoneal dialysis if the pleuroperitoneal communication is still patent.[137, 138] In children, an asymptomatic Bochdalek or Morgagni hernia may be revealed after peritoneal dialysis has begun.

Visceral perforation may be seen early or late in the course of peritoneal dialysis.[139, 140] The catheter may have penetrated the hollow viscera, solid organs, pelvic wall, or retroperitoneal space.[141] Visceral perforation may be manifested by:

- Feculent effluent from the catheter
- Diarrhea after dialysate infusion
- High volumes of urine after dialysate infusion
- Bloody effluent from the catheter
- Retention of dialysate after infusion

Peritonitis due to enteric perforation can be confirmed by the predominance of polymicrobial flora on Gram's stain and culture of effluent. Visceral perforation is addressed surgically, followed by removal of the catheter to allow the peritonitis to clear.[142]

Local infectious complications of the catheter are common and lead to failure of 5% to 20% of catheters placed.[143] It is estimated that patients undergoing peritoneal dialysis experience one tunnel infection episode for every 16 patient-months of treatment.[144] Data collected from the NIH National Registry documented 4.6 episodes of infection per year per patient in 1978 and 1.7 episodes in 1982.[14] The 12-month period risk rate of infection in peritoneal dialysis patients is 65%.[145] The most common catheter infections are exit site infections, deep cuff infections, and unresolving peritonitis.[146, 147] Catheter tunnel infections may lead to peritonitis or may remain localized infections confined to the catheter.

An increased number of tunnel infections is associated with inadequate surgical technique, poor catheter maintenance, exit site skin irritation from tape and dressings, and undue tension placed on the catheter to cause protrusion of the outer Dacron cuff. If the exit site and the tract are erythematous but not purulent, the tunnel infection can be treated by means of local cleansing with hydrogen peroxide or povidone-iodine.[148, 149] Topical antibiotic ointment as well as systemic antibiotics can be administered. If there is frank purulence, catheter removal is indicated. Removal of the outer Dacron cuff to help eradicate the tunnel infection is rarely successful.[150–152] The use of Y-site catheter handling techniques to minimize contamination may decrease future infection rates.

Peritonitis

It is estimated that one third of hospitalizations of patients undergoing peritoneal dialysis are due to peritonitis.[133] Most patients stop using peritoneal dialysis because of frequent recurrent peritonitis, which occurs in 25% to 60% of cases.[153, 154] It is estimated that 15% of deaths of patients being treated with CAPD are due to peritonitis.[155] These infections are common because the catheter itself provides a direct route for contamination of the peritoneal cavity. The infused dialysate dilutes the concentrations of opsonins

(IgG and C3) and peritoneal macrophages, which are needed to fight intra-abdominal infection.[156] Phagocytic and bactericidal white blood cell activity is diminished by the hypertonicity and acidic nature of the dialysate.[157, 158] The fluid within the abdominal cavity impairs the ability of the omentum to localize infection.

Peritonitis is most commonly manifested by abdominal discomfort accompanied by the presence of a cloudy effluent.[159] The white blood cell count of the effluent increases to more than 100 white blood cells/cm³ with neutrophil predominance.[160, 161] Some patients experience nausea and vomiting (27%), rebound tenderness (40%), fever (27%), and peripheral leukocytosis (23%).[145, 162]

The pathogen often can be cultured from the catheter fluid; the result directs appropriate antibiotic therapy.[118] The pathogens most commonly responsible for catheter-related peritonitis are coagulase-negative *Staphylococcus* (55% to 80%) and *Staphylococcus aureus* (17% to 30%).[163, 164] Fungus can also cause peritonitis in patients undergoing peritoneal dialysis.[165–169] These contaminants originate from the patient's own skin flora, nasal flora, catheter exit site colonization, and, sometimes, transmural contamination from the bowel. As mentioned previously, a perforated viscus can cause signs and symptoms of peritonitis. Cultures of effluent obtained from patients with a perforated viscus reveal a polymicrobial flora with a predominance of enteric organisms rather than staphylococcal organisms.

Peritonitis that is due to one predominant organism and is not associated with a perforated viscus can be treated initially with antimicrobial therapy, which can be instilled through the peritoneal catheter itself.[170] Eradication of the organisms, as proven by culture and resolution of the patient's symptoms, should be apparent in 3 to 5 days. Organisms that produce slime, an amorphous glycocalyx that can adhere to plastic surfaces, may make eradication more difficult.[171] The slime protects the bacteria from opsonization, preventing white blood cells from engulfing them. Organisms that produce slime include coagulase-negative *Staphylococcus, S. aureus, Candida albicans,* and *Pseudomonas aeruginosa.*[172]

Most patients with peritonitis can be treated at home initially. Hospitalization is reserved for those with gram-negative infections, anaerobic infections, *Pseudomonas* infections, fungal infections, or symptoms of toxicity. Antimicrobial therapy should be selected to treat the offending organism cultured from the peritoneal cavity.[173] Initially, antibiotic coverage should be a cephalosporin plus an aminoglycoside, or vancomycin. If the peritonitis does not resolve, the catheter needs to be removed. Recurrent episodes of peritonitis suggest that the catheter itself may harbor the organisms causing the peritonitis.

A novel use of laparoscopy is for the diagnosis and treatment of catheter-related peritonitis.[174] Persistent toxicity despite adequate therapy and catheter removal can be evaluated with a laparoscopic examination. In the absence of visceral disease, the abdomen can be thoroughly irrigated and additional specimens for culture obtained. The insertion of multiple catheters has been performed at the same setting to permit more continuous peritoneal irrigation.

Dialysate Effects

Increased intra-abdominal pressure during peritoneal dialysis may induce delayed gastric emptying and may lead to gastroesophageal reflux.[175] Patients with impaired pulmonary function may find that the impairment worsens when the peritoneal cavity is filled with dialysate fluid.[176] Cardiac output and stroke volume in patients undergoing peritoneal dialysis are decreased owing to the reduced preload that results from compression of the inferior vena cava. This can critically alter the already tenuous hemodynamic stability of patients with significant congestive heart failure. Decreasing the volume of dialysate can help to lessen symptoms in these cases.

Metabolic complications can occur in patients receiving peritoneal dialysis. They include dehydration, which can be treated by decreasing the osmolarity of the dialysate, and overhydration, which can be treated by shortening the dwell time and raising the dialysate glucose concentration. Severe hyperglycemia and a hyperosmolar state can occur in diabetic patients.[30, 155] Protein malnutrition can occur owing to the daily obligatory losses of protein and amino acids through the dialysis process.[20, 22] Malnutrition can be treated with dietary supplements but peritoneal dialysis may have to be terminated if refractory.

The increased caloric load resulting from glucose absorption can result in obesity, uncontrolled hyperglycemia, or hypertriglyceridemia in some patients.[32] Changing to an osmotic agent other than glucose may help, but often, peritoneal dialysis must be stopped. Important vitamins that are depleted can be replenished through dietary supplements.[27, 28] Renal osteodystrophy, including osteitis fibrosis and osteomalacia, may be seen in patients undergoing peritoneal dialysis.[177, 178] Electrolyte alterations, such as hyponatremia, hypernatremia, hypokalemia, and hyperkalemia, can be avoided with appropriate changes in dialysate mixtures.[179]

The disequilibrium syndrome is incited by cerebral edema. It is characterized by headaches, nausea, vomiting, hypertension, seizures, and, rarely, coma.[180] This syndrome is thought to develop when a rapid osmotic gradient is created between the brain and the extracellular compartment as a result of the delayed removal of urea across the blood-brain barrier. Treatment of this syndrome is symptomatic; the syndrome can be avoided by decreasing the osmolality of the dialysate.

Peritoneal membrane dysfunction is characterized by increased peritoneal permeability, which results in rapid absorption of the dialysate. This alters the osmotic gradient needed for adequate dialysis. The transport of solutes remains the same, but transfer of water does not occur. This phenomenon may result from the use of acetate in the dialysate solutions.[181] Treatment consists of the use of shorter dwell times with higher flow rates and elimination of long diurnal dwell times.

Soon after the initiation of peritoneal dialysis, the peritoneum can become acutely thickened, leading to a loss of ultrafiltration capacity.[182] Silicone and aluminum inclusions have been found within the peritoneal membrane as well.[183] Peripheral eosinophilia may be seen in the first few days after catheter placement, and in some patients, eosinophilic peritonitis can ensue.[184–186] The pathophysiology of the eosinophilic peritonitis is unknown but has been linked to talc found in surgical gloves, air exposure alone, peritoneal administration of antibiotics, and perhaps, an allergic response to the silicone or aluminum polymers that are

deposited over time.[187, 188] No treatment is required for eosinophilic peritonitis.

Peritoneal sclerosis can lead to abandonment of peritoneal dialysis owing to the inability to achieve adequate dialysis.[189–194] A thickened peritoneal scar develops and envelops the intra-abdominal organs. The surface area available for dialysis is thus decreased.[195] The cause is unknown but may be related to repeated bouts of peritonitis, to hyperosmolar dialysate solutions, or to particulate matter or acetate in the dialysate.[196, 197] The process can be fatal if bowel obstruction or strangulation occurs. No treatment is known to aid in preventing or improving this complication.

SUMMARY

Vascular access surgeons should be familiar with peritoneal dialysis applications and consider them in concert with hemodialysis access strategies. Benefits of peritoneal dialysis include (1) increased hemodynamic stability, (2) better blood pressure control, (3) improved residual renal function, (4) higher average hemoglobin levels, and (5) reduced lipoprotein profiles. Patient satisfaction with peritoneal dialysis is due to increased independence, and this technique is preferentially used in children.

Laparoscopically assisted placement of a Tenckhoff catheter can reduce discomfort, catheter malpositioning, and wound complications. Complications such as obstruction, malposition, and peritonitis can be assessed and corrected with laparoscopic approaches as well. Although catheter tunnel infections and peritonitis are not uncommon, successful treatment strategies permit long-term peritoneal dialysis in many patients.

REFERENCES

1. Ganter G: Ueber die Beseitigung giftiger Stoffe aus dem Blute durch Dialyse. Munch Med Wochenschr 70-II:1478, 1923.
2. Rhoads JE: Peritoneal lavage in the treatment of renal insufficiency. Am J Med Sci 192:642, 1938.
3. Weston RE, Roberts M: Clinical use of stylet-catheter for peritoneal dialysis. Arch Intern Med 115:659, 1965.
4. Palmer RA, Quinton W, Gray JE: Prolonged peritoneal dialysis for chronic renal failure. Lancet 1:700, 1964.
5. Oreopoulos DG, Robson M, Faller B, et al: CAPD: A new era in the treatment of chronic renal failure. Clin Nephrol 11:125, 1979.
6. Tenckhoff H, Schecter H: A bacteriologically safe peritoneal access device. Trans Am Soc Artif Intern Organs 14:181, 1968.
7. Tenckhoff H, Shilipetar G, Boen ST: One year's experience with home peritoneal dialysis. Trans Am Soc Artif Intern Organs 11:11, 1965.
8. Striker GE, Tenckhoff H: A transcutaneous prosthesis for prolonged access to the peritoneal cavity. Surgery 69:70, 1971.
9. Tenckhoff H: Catheter implantation. Dial Transplant 1:18, 1972.
10. Bullmaster JR, Miller SF, Finley RK, et al: Surgical aspects of the Tenckhoff peritoneal dialysis catheter: A seven-year experience. Am J Surg 149:339, 1985.
11. Gutman RA: Automatic peritoneal dialysis for home use. Q J Med 47:261, 1978.
12. Popovich RP, Moncrief JW, Decherd JF, et al: The definition of a portable-wearable equilibrium peritoneal technique. Abstr Am Soc Artif Intern Organs 5:64, 1976.
13. Moncrief JW, Sorrels PAJ, Druger VG, et al: Development of training programs for continuous ambulatory peritoneal dialysis—Historical

review. *In* M Legrain (ed): Continuous Ambulatory Peritoneal Dialysis. Amsterdam, Excerpta Medica, 1980, pp 149–151.

14. Steinberg SM, Cutler SJ, Novak JW, et al: Report of the National CAPD Registry of the National Institutes of Health. Washington, DC, National Institutes of Health, 1986.

15. La Greca, G, Chiaramonte, S, Feriani, M, et al: Substitutive treatments in end-stage renal disease. Contrib Nephrol 109:45, 1994.

16. Nolph, KD: What's new in peritoneal dialysis—an overview. Kidney Int 42(Suppl 38):S148, 1992.

17. Roxe DM, del Greco F, Krumlovsky F, et al: A comparison of maintenance hemodialysis to maintenance peritoneal dialysis in the maintenance of end-stage renal disease. Trans Am Soc Artif Intern Organs 25:81, 1979.

18. Clark AJ: Absorption from the peritoneal cavity. J Pharmacol 16:415, 1921.

19. Putnam TJ: The living peritoneum as a dialyzing membrane. Am J Physiol 63:548, 1922.

20. Gjessing J: Absorption of amino acids and fat from the peritoneum. Opuscula Medica 13:251, 1968.

21. Nolph KD, Twardowski ZJ, Popovich RV, Rubin J: Equilibration of peritoneal dialysis solutions during long dwell exchanges. J Lab Clin Med 93:246, 1979.

22. Rubin J, Nolph KD, Arfania D, et al: Protein losses in continuous ambulatory peritoneal dialysis. Nephron 28:218, 1981.

23. Blumenkrantz MJ, Gahl GM, Kopple JD, et al: Protein losses during peritoneal dialysis. Kidney Int 19:593, 1981.

24. Dombros N, Oren A, Marliss EB, et al: Plasma amino acid profiles and amino acid losses in patients undergoing CAPD. Perit Dial Bull 2:27, 1982.

25. Giordano C, De Santo NG, Capodicasa G, et al: Amino acid losses during CAPD. Clin Nephrol 14:230, 1980.

26. Kopple JD, Blumenkrantz MJ, Jones MR, et al: Plasma amino acid levels and amino acid losses during continuous ambulatory peritoneal dialysis. Am J Clin Nutr 36:395, 1982.

27. Blumberg A, Hanck A, Sander G: Vitamin nutrition in patients on continuous ambulatory peritoneal dialysis. Clin Nephrol 20:244, 1983.

28. Henderson IS, Leung ACT, Shenkin A: Vitamin status in continuous ambulatory peritoneal dialysis. Perit Dial Bull 4:143, 1984.

29. Robson MD, Levi J, Rosenfeld JB: Hyperglycaemia and hyperosmolarity in peritoneal dialysis: Its prevention by the use of fructose. Proc Eur Dial Transplant Assoc 6:300, 1969.

30. Grodstein GP, Blumenkrantz MJ, Kopple JD, et al: Glucose absorption during continuous ambulatory peritoneal dialysis. Kidney Int 19:564, 1981.

31. Alvestrand A, Ahlberg M, Furst P, Bergstrom J: Clinical results of long-term treatment with a low protein diet and a new amino acid preparation in patients with chronic uremia. Clin Nephrol 19:67, 1982.

32. Shen FH, Sherrard DJ, Scollard D, et al: Thirst, relative hypernatremia, and excessive weight gain in maintenance peritoneal dialysis. Trans Am Soc Artif Intern Organs 24:142, 1978.

33. Nolph KD, Rubin J, Wiegman DL, et al: Peritoneal clearances with three types of commercially available peritoneal dialysis solutions: Effects of pH adjustment and intraperitoneal nitroprusside. Nephron 24:35, 1979.

34. Vas SI, Suwe A, Weatherhead J: Natural defense mechanisms of the peritoneum: The effect of peritoneal dialysis fluid on polymorphonuclear cells. *In* Atkins RC, Thomson NM, Farrell PC (eds): Peritoneal Dialysis. Edinburgh, Churchill Livingstone, 1981, pp 41–51.

35. Williams PF, Marliss E, Anderson GH, et al: Amino acid absorption following intraperitoneal administration in CAPD patients. Perit Dial Bull 2:124, 1982.

36. Gjessing J: Addition of amino acids to peritoneal dialysis fluid. Lancet 2:812, 1968.

37. Matthys E, Dolkart R, Lameire N: Extended use of glycerol-containing dialysate in diabetic CAPD patients. Perit Dial Bull 7:10, 1987.

38. Buoncristiani U, Carobi C, Cozzari M, et al: Xylitol as osmotic agent in CAPD: A reappraisal. Perit Dial Bull 7:S11, 1987.

39. Bazzato G, Coli U, Landini S, et al: Xylitol and low doses of insulin: New perspectives for diabetic uremic patients on CAPD. Perit Dial Bull 2:161, 1982.

40. Yutuc W, Ward G, Shilipetar G, Tenckhoff H: Substitution of sorbitol for dextrose in peritoneal irrigation fluid: A preliminary report. Trans Am Soc Artif Intern Organs 13:168, 1967.

41. Mailloux L, Allerhand J: Comparison of glucose and sorbitol peritoneal dialysis. Abstr Am Soc Nephrol p 52, 1970.

42. Olmstead WH: The metabolism of mannitol and sorbitol. Diabetes 2:132, 1953.

43. Raja RM, Kramer MS, Manchanda R, et al: Peritoneal dialysis with fructose dialysate. Ann Intern Med 79:511, 1973.

44. Robson M, Rosenfeld JB: Fructose for dialysis. Ann Intern Med 75:975, 1971.

45. Gjessing J: The use of dextran as a dialyzing fluid in peritoneal dialysis. Acta Med Scand 185:237, 1969.

46. Jirka J, Kotkova E: Peritoneal dialysis in iso-oncotic dextran solution in anesthetized dogs: Intraperitoneal fluid volume and protein concentration in the irrigation fluid. Proc Eur Dial Transplant Assoc 4:141, 1967.

47. Twardowski ZJ, Nolph KD, McGary TJ, Moore HL: Polyanions and glucose as osmotic agents in simulated peritoneal dialysis. Artif Organs 7:420, 1983.

48. Posen GA, Luiscello J: Continuous equilibration peritoneal dialysis in the treatment of acute renal failure. Perit Dial Bull 1:6, 1980.

49. Firmat J, Zucchini A: Peritoneal dialysis in acute renal failure. Contrib Nephrol 17:33, 1979.

50. Segar WE, Gibson RK, Rhamy R: Peritoneal dialysis in infants and small children. Pediatrics 27:603, 1961.

51. Chan JCM, Campbell RA: Peritoneal dialysis in children: A survey of its indications and applications. Clin Pediatr 12:131, 1973.

52. Raja RM, Krasnoff SO, Moros JG, et al: Repeated peritoneal dialysis in treatment of heart failure. JAMA 213:2268, 1970.

53. Shapira J, Lang R, Jutrin I, et al: Peritoneal dialysis in refractory congestive heart failure: Part I. Intermittent peritoneal dialysis. Perit Dial Bull 3:130, 1983.

54. Chopra MP, Gulati RB, Portal RW, Aber CP: Peritoneal dialysis for pulmonary edema after acute myocardial infarction. Br Med J 3:77, 1970.

55. Mailloux LU, Swartz CD, Onesti GO, et al: Peritoneal dialysis for refractory congestive heart failure. JAMA 199:873, 1967.

56. Rubin J, Ball R: Continuous ambulatory peritoneal dialysis as treatment of severe congestive heart failure in the face of chronic renal failure. Arch Intern Med 146:1533, 1986.

57. Winchester JF, Gelfand MC, Knepshield JH, Schreiner GE: Dialysis and hemoperfusion of poisons and drugs—Update. Trans Am Soc Artif Intern Organs 23:762, 1977.

58. Maher JF: Principles of dialysis and dialysis of drugs. Am J Med 62:475, 1977.

59. Di Paolo N, Capotondo L, De Mia M, et al: Phosphatidylcholine: Physiological modulator of peritoneal transport. Perit Dial Bull 7:S23, 1987.

60. Dombros N, Balaskas E, Savidis N, et al: Phosphatidylcholine increases ultrafiltration in CAPD patients. Perit Dial Bull 7:S24, 1987.

61. Miller FN, Wiegman DL, Joshua JG, et al: Effects of vasodilators and peritoneal dialysis solution on the microcirculation of the rat cecum. Proc Soc Exp Biol Med 161:605, 1979.

62. Reuler JB, Parker RA: Peritoneal dialysis in the management of hypothermia. JAMA 240:2289, 1978.

63. Zawada ET Jr: Treatment of profound hypothermia with peritoneal dialysis. Dial Transplant 9:255, 1980.

64. O'Connor J: The treatment of profound hypothermia with peritoneal dialysis. Perit Dial Bull 2:171, 1982.

65. Sheppard JM, Lawrence JR, Oon RCS, et al: Lactic acidosis: Recovery associated with the use of peritoneal dialysate. Aust N Z J Med 4:389, 1972.

66. Hayat JC: The treatment of lactic acidosis in the diabetic patient by peritoneal dialysis using sodium acetate: A report of two cases. Diabetologia 10:485, 1974.

67. Knochel JP, Mason AD: Effect of alkalinization on peritoneal diffusion of uric acid. Am J Physiol 210:1160, 1966.

68. Maher JF, Rath CE, Schreiner GE: Hyperuricemia complicating leukemia: Treatment with allopurinol and dialysis. Arch Intern Med 123:198, 1969.

69. Molitoris BA, Alfrey PS, Miller NL, et al: Efficacy of intramuscular and intraperitoneal deferoxamine for aluminum chelation. Kidney Int 31:986, 1987.

70. Twardowski ZJ, Nolph KD, Rubin J, Anderson PC: Peritoneal dialysis for psoriasis, an uncontrolled study. Ann Intern Med 88:349, 1978.

71. Sorkin MI, Nolph KD, Anderson HO, et al: Aluminum mass transfer during continuous ambulatory peritoneal dialysis. Perit Dial Bull 1:91, 1981.

72. Bertholf RL, Roman JM, Brown S, et al: Aluminum hydroxide induced osteomalacia, encephalopathy and hyperaluminemia in CAPD treatment with desferrioxamine. Perit Dial Bull 4:30, 1984.

73. Wall AJ: Peritoneal dialysis in the treatment of severe acute pancreatitis. Med J Aust 52:281, 1965.

74. Glenn LD, Nolph KD: Treatment of pancreatitis with peritoneal dialysis. Perit Dial Bull 2:63, 1982.

75. White N, Snowden SA, Parsons U, et al: The management of terminal renal failure in diabetic patients by regular dialysis therapy. Nephron 11:261, 1973.

76. Blumenkrantz MJ, Shapiro DJ, Mimura N, et al: Maintenance peritoneal dialysis as an alternative in the patient with diabetes mellitus and end-stage uremia. Kidney Int 6:S108, 1974.

77. Amair P, Khanna R, Leibel B, et al: Continuous ambulatory peritoneal dialysis in diabetics with end-stage renal disease. N Engl J Med 306:625, 1982.

78. Stefanidis C, Balfe JW, Arbus GS, et al: Renal transplantation in children treated with continuous ambulatory peritoneal dialysis. Perit Dial Bull 1:5, 1983.

79. Diaz-Buxo JA: CCPD is even better than CAPD. Kidney Int 28:S26, 1985.

80. Fine RN, Salusky IB: CAPD/CCPD in children: Four years' experience. Kidney Int 30:S7, 1986.

81. Leichter HE, Salusky IB, Fine RN: Renal transplantation in patients on CAPD and CCPD—special focus in pediatrics. Perspect Perit Dial 4:12, 1986.

82. Ahmad S, Gallagher N, Shen F: Intermittent peritoneal dialysis: Status reassessed. Trans Am Soc Artif Intern Organs 25:86, 1979.

83. Diaz-Buxo JA, Walker PJ, Chandler JT, et al: Experience with intermittent peritoneal dialysis and continuous cyclic peritoneal dialysis. Am J Kidney Dis 4:242, 1984.

84. Popovich RP, Moncrief JW, Nolph KD, et al: Continuous ambulatory peritoneal dialysis. Ann Intern Med 88:449, 1978.

85. Oreopoulos DG, Robson M, Izatt S, et al: A simple and safe technique for continuous ambulatory peritoneal dialysis. Trans Am Soc Artif Intern Organs 24:484, 1978.

86. Nolph KD, Sorkin M, Rubin J, et al: Continuous ambulatory peritoneal dialysis: Three-year experience at one center. Ann Intern Med 92:609, 1980.

87. Diaz-Buxo JA, Walker PJ, Farmer CD, et al: Continuous cyclic peritoneal dialysis—a preliminary report. Artif Organs 5:157, 1981.

88. Twardowski Z, Ksiazek A, Majdan M, et al: Kinetics of continuous ambulatory peritoneal dialysis (CAPD) with four exchanges per day. Clin Nephrol 15:119, 1981.

89. Oren A, Wu G, Anderson GH, et al: Effective use of amino acid dialysate over four weeks in CAPD patients. Perit Dial Bull 3:66, 1983.

90. Nolph KD, Ryan L, Moore H, et al: Factors affecting ultrafiltration in continuous ambulatory peritoneal dialysis: First report of an international cooperative study. Perit Dial Bull 4:14, 1984.

91. Nolph KD, Cutler SJ, Steinberg SM, Novak JW: Continuous ambulatory peritoneal dialysis in the United States: A three-year study. Kidney Int 28:198, 1985.

92. Nolph KD: Continuous ambulatory peritoneal dialysis (CAPD) 1987: A therapy in evolution. Contemp Dial Nephrol 8:26, 1987.

93. Diaz-Buxo JA, Farmer CD, Walker PJ, et al: Continuous cyclic peritoneal dialysis: A preliminary report. Artif Organs 5:157, 1981.

94. Diaz-Buxo JA, Farmer CD, Chandler JT, et al: Continuous cycling peritoneal dialysis (CCPD)—"wet" is better than "dry." Perit Dial Bull 7:S22, 1987.

95. Twardowski ZJ, Nolph KD, Khanna R, et al: Choice of peritoneal dialysis regimen based on peritoneal transfer rates. Perit Dial Bull 7:S79, 1987.

96. Frock J, Twardowski Z, Nolph K, et al: Tidal peritoneal dialysis. Kidney Int 31:250, 1987.

97. Twardowski ZJ, Nolph KD, Khanna R, et al: Eight hour tidal peritoneal dialysis matches 24-hour CAPD and surpasses 8 hour nightly intermittent peritoneal dialysis clearances. Perit Dial Bull 7:S79, 1987.

98. Twardowski ZJ, Prowant BF, Nolph KD, et al: High volume, low frequency continuous ambulatory peritoneal dialysis. Kidney Int 23:64, 1983.

99. Clayton S, Quinton C, Oreopoulos D: Training technique for continuous ambulatory peritoneal dialysis. Perit Dial Bull 1:S23, 1981.

100. Cardella CJ, Izatt SJ: What should one do with the peritoneal

101. Digenis GE, Khanna R, Mathews R, et al: Abdominal hernias in patients undergoing CAPD. Perit Dial Bull 2:115, 1982.

102. Rubin J, Raju S, Teal N, et al: Abdominal hernia in patients undergoing continuous ambulatory peritoneal dialysis. Arch Intern Med 142:1453, 1982.

103. Rocco MV, Stone WJ: Abdominal hernias in chronic peritoneal dialysis patients: A review. Perit Dial Bull 5:171, 1985.

104. Boen ST, Mulinari AS, Dillard DH, et al: Periodic peritoneal dialysis in the treatment of chronic uremia. Trans Am Soc Artif Intern Organs 8:256, 1962.

105. Gutch CF: Peritoneal dialysis. Trans Am Soc Artif Intern Organs 10:406, 1964.

106. Gutch CF, Stevens SC: Silastic catheter for peritoneal dialysis. Trans Am Soc Artif Intern Organs 12:106, 1966.

107. Diaz-Buxo JA, Chandler JT, Farmer CD, et al: Long-term observations of peritoneal clearances in patients undergoing peritoneal dialysis. ASAIO J 5:21, 1983.

108. Diaz-Buxo JA, Geissinger WT: Single cuff versus double cuff Tenckhoff catheter. Perit Dial Bull 4:S100, 1984.

109. Twardowski ZJ, Nolph KD, Khanna R, et al: The need for a "swan neck" permanently bent, arcuate peritoneal dialysis catheter. Perit Dial Bull 5:219, 1985.

110. Twardowski ZJ, Khanna R, Nolph KD, et al: Preliminary experience with the swan neck peritoneal dialysis catheters. Trans Am Soc Artif Intern Organs 32:64, 1986.

111. Oreopoulos DG, Zellerman G, Izatt S, Gotloib L: Catheters and connectors for chronic peritoneal dialysis: Present and future. In Atkins RC, Thomson NM, Farrel PC (eds): Peritoneal Dialysis. New York, Churchill Livingstone, 1981, pp 313–319.

112. Keane WF, Peterson PK: Host defense mechanisms of the peritoneal cavity and continuous ambulatory peritoneal dialysis. Perit Dial Bull 4:122, 1984.

113. Goldberg EM, Hill W: A new peritoneal access prosthesis. Proc Clin Dial Transplant Forum 3:122, 1973.

114. Khanna R, Izatt S, Burke D, et al: Experience with the Toronto Western Hospital permanent peritoneal catheter. Perit Dial Bull 4:95, 1984.

115. Thornhill JA, Dhein CR, Johnson H, Ash SR: Drainage characteristics of the column disc catheter: A new chronic peritoneal access catheter. Proc Clin Dial Transplant Forum 10:119, 1980.

116. Ash SR, Slingeneyer A, Schardin KE: Further clinical experience with the Lifecath peritoneal implant. Perspect Perit Dial 1:9, 1983.

117. Olcott C, Feldman CA, Coplon NS, et al: Continuous ambulatory peritoneal dialysis: Technique of catheter insertion and management of associated surgical complications. Am J Surg 146:98, 1983.

118. Oreopoulous DG, Baird-Helfrich G, Khanna R, et al: Peritoneal catheters and exit-site practices: Current recommendations. Perit Dial Bull 7:130, 1987.

119. Ash SR, Wolf GC, Bloch R: Placement of the Tenckhoff peritoneal dialysis catheter under peritoneoscopic visualization. Dial Transplant 10:383, 1981.

120. Ash SR, Handt AE, Bloch R: Peritoneoscopic placement of the Tenckhoff catheter: Further clinical experience. Perit Dial Bull 3:8, 1983.

121. Brownlee, J, Elkhairi, S: Laparoscopic-assisted placement of peritoneal dialysis catheter: A preliminary experience. Clin Nephrol 47(2):122, 1997.

122. Krug, F, Herold, A, Jochims, H, et al: Laparoscopic implantation of Oreopoulos-Zellermann catheters for peritoneal dialysis. Nephron 75:272, 1997.

123. Khanna R, Wu G, Vas S, Oreopoulos DG: Mortality and morbidity on continuous ambulatory peritoneal dialysis. ASAIO J 6:197, 1983.

124. Palacios M, Schley W, Dougherty J: Use of streptokinase to clear peritoneal catheters. Dial Transplant 11:172, 1982.

125. Wiegmann TB, Stuewe B, Duncan KA, et al: Effective use of streptokinase for peritoneal catheter failure. Am J Kidney Dis 6:119, 1985.

126. Thayssen P, Pindborg T: Peritoneal dialysis and heparin. Scand J Urol Nephrol 12:73, 1978.

127. Furman KL, Gomperts ED, Hockle J: Activity of intraperitoneal heparin during peritoneal dialysis. Clin Nephrol 9:15, 1978.

128. Blumenkrantz MJ, Gallagher N, Bashore RA, Tenckhoff H: Retrograde menstruation in women undergoing chronic peritoneal dialysis. Obstet Gynecol 57:667, 1981.

129. Coronel F, Marenjo P, Torrente J, Pratts D: The risk of retrograde menstruation in CAPD patients. Perit Dial Bull 4:190, 1984.

130. Twardowski ZJ, Tully RJ, Nichols WK, Sunderrajan S: Computerized tomography (CT) in the diagnosis of subcutaneous leak sites during continuous ambulatory peritoneal dialysis. Perit Dial Bull 4:163, 1984.

131. Nolph KD, Cutler SJ, Steinberg SM, et al: Factors associated with morbidity and mortality among patients on CAPD. Trans Am Soc Artif Intern Organs 33:57, 1987.

132. Orfei R, Seybold K, Blumberg A: Genital edema in patients undergoing continuous ambulatory peritoneal dialysis. Perit Dial Bull 4:251, 1984.

133. Chan MK, Baillod RA, Tanner A, et al: Abdominal hernias in patients receiving continuous ambulatory peritoneal dialysis. Br Med J 283:826, 1981.

134. Digenis GE, Khanna R, Oreopoulos DG: Abdominal hernias in patients undergoing continuous ambulatory peritoneal dialysis. Perit Dial Bull 2:115, 1982.

135. Jorkasky D, Goldfarb S: Abdominal wall hernia complicating chronic ambulatory peritoneal dialysis. Am J Nephrol 2:323, 1982.

136. Wetherington GM, Leapman SB, Robison RJ, Filo RS: Abdominal wall and inguinal hernias in continuous ambulatory peritoneal dialysis patients. Am J Surg 150:357, 1985.

137. Singh S, Vaidya P, Dale A, et al: Massive hydrothorax complicating continuous ambulatory peritoneal dialysis. Nephron 34:168, 1983.

138. Greberg N, Danielson BG, Benson L, et al: Right-sided hydrothorax complicating peritoneal dialysis. Nephron 34:130, 1983.

139. Watson LC, Thompson JC: Erosion of the colon by a long-dwelling peritoneal dialysis catheter. JAMA 243:2156, 1980.

140. Rubin J, Oreopoulos DG, Lio TT, et al: Management of peritonitis and bowel perforation during chronic peritoneal dialysis. Nephron 16:220, 1976.

141. Coward RA, Gokal R, Wise M, et al: Peritonitis associated with vaginal leakage of dialysis fluid in continuous ambulatory peritoneal dialysis. Br Med J 284:1529, 1982.

142. Vas SI: Indications for removal of the peritoneal catheter. Perit Dial Bull 1:149, 1981.

143. Steigbigel RT, Cross AS: Infections associated with hemodialysis and chronic peritoneal dialysis. In Remington JS, Swarts MN (eds): Current Clinical Topics in Infectious Diseases. New York, McGraw-Hill, 1987, pp 124–145.

144. Montgomerie JZ, Kalmanson GM, Guze LB: Renal failure and infection. Medicine 47:1, 1968.

145. Gokal R, Ramos JM, Francis DMA, et al: Peritonitis in continuous ambulatory peritoneal dialysis. Lancet 2:1388, 1982.

146. Prowant B, Nolph K, Ryan L, et al: Peritonitis in continuous ambulatory peritoneal dialysis: Analysis of an 8 year experience. Nephron 43:105, 1986.

147. Rubin J, Rogers WA, Taylor HM, et al: Peritonitis during continuous ambulatory peritoneal dialysis. Ann Intern Med 92:7, 1980.

148. Nichols WK, Nolph KD: A technique for managing exit site and cuff infection in Tenckhoff catheters. Perit Dial Bull Suppl 3:S4, 1983.

149. Andreoli SP, West KW, Grosfeld JL, Bengstein JM: A technique to eradicate tunnel infection without peritoneal dialysis catheter removal. Perit Dial Bull 4:156, 1984.

150. Poirier VL, Daly BDT, Dasse KA, et al: Elimination of tunnel infection. In Maher JF, Winchester JF (eds): Frontiers in Peritoneal Dialysis. New York, Field, Rich and Associates, 1986, pp 210–217.

151. Helfrich GB, Winchester JF: Shaving of external cuff of peritoneal catheter. Perit Dial Bull 2:183, 1982.

152. Piraino B, Bernardini J, Peitzman A, Sorkin M: Failure of peritoneal catheter cuff shaving to eradicate infection. Perit Dial Bull 7:179, 1987.

153. Wu G: A review of peritonitis episodes that caused interruption of continuous ambulatory peritoneal dialysis. Perit Dial Bull Suppl 3:S11, 1983.

154. Piraino B, Bernardini J, Sorkin M: The influence of peritoneal catheter exit-site infections on peritonitis, tunnel infections and catheter loss in patients on CAPD. Am J Kidney Dis 8:436, 1986.

155. Rottembourg J, Gahl GM, Poignet JL, et al: Severe abdominal complications in patients undergoing continuous ambulatory peritoneal dialysis. Proc Eur Dial Transplant Assoc 20:236, 1983.

156. Keane WF, Comty CM, Verbrugh HA, et al: Opsonic deficiency of peritoneal dialysis effluent in continuous ambulatory peritoneal dialysis. Kidney Int 25:539, 1984.

157. Verbrugh HA, Keane WF, Hoidal JR, et al: Peritoneal macrophage and opsonins: Antibacterial defense in patients on chronic peritoneal dialysis. J Infect Dis 147:1018, 1983.

158. Peresecenschi G, Blum M, Aviram A, Spirer ZH: Impaired neutrophil response to acute bacterial infection in dialyzed patients. Arch Intern Med 141:1301, 1982.

159. Prowant BF, Nolph KD: Clinical criteria for diagnosis of peritonitis. In Atkins RC, Thomson NM, Farrel PC (eds): Peritoneal Dialysis. Edinburgh, Churchill Livingstone, 1981, pp 257–263.

160. Males BM, Walshe JJ, Amsterdam D: Laboratory indices of clinical peritonitis, total leukocyte count, microscopy and microbiological culture of peritoneal dialysis effluent. J Clin Microbiol 25:2367, 1987.

161. Williams P, Pantalony D, Vas ST, et al: The value of dialysate cell count in the diagnosis of peritonitis in patients on continuous ambulatory peritoneal dialysis. Perit Dial Bull 1:59, 1981.

162. Keane WF, Everett ED, Fine RN, et al: CAPD related peritonitis management and antibiotic therapy recommendations. Perit Dial Bull 7:55, 1987.

163. Eisenberg ES, Ambalu M, Szylagi G, et al: Colonization of skin and development of peritonitis due to coagulase-negative staphylococci in patients undergoing peritoneal dialysis. J Infect Dis 156:478, 1987.

164. West TE, Walshe JJ, Krol CP, et al: Staphylococcal peritonitis in patients on continuous peritoneal dialysis. J Clin Microbiol 23:809, 1986.

165. Rault R: Candida peritonitis complicating peritoneal dialysis: A report of five cases and review of the literature. Am J Kidney Dis 2:544, 1983.

166. Johnson RJ, Ramsey PJ, Gallagher N, et al: Fungal peritonitis in patients on peritoneal dialysis: Incidence, clinical features and prognosis. Am J Nephrol 5:169, 1985.

167. Rubin J: Management of fungal peritonitis. Perspect Perit Dial 4:10, 1986.

168. Khanna R, McNeely DJ, Oreopoulos DG, et al: Treating fungal infections: Fungal peritonitis in CAPD. Br Med J 280:1147, 1980.

169. Kerr CM, Perfect JR, Craven PC, et al: Fungal peritonitis in patients on continuous ambulatory peritoneal dialysis. Ann Intern Med 99:334, 1983.

170. Digenis GE, Khanna R, Pierratos A, et al: Morbidity and mortality after treatment of peritonitis with prolonged exchanges and intraperitoneal antibiotics. Perit Dial Bull 2:45, 1982.

171. Reed WP, Light PD, Newman KA: Biofilm on Tenckhoff catheters: A possible source for peritonitis. In Proceedings of Third International Symposium on Peritoneal Dialysis, Washington, DC, June 1984, p 176.

172. Kilmos HJ, Anderson KEH: Peritonitis with Pseudomonas aeruginosa in hospitalized patients treated with peritoneal dialysis. Scand J Infect Dis 11:207, 1979.

173. Williams P, Khanna R, Vas SI, et al: The treatment of peritonitis in patients on CAPD: To lavage or not. Perit Dial Bull 1:12, 1980.

174. Chiu, CK, Karmakar, MG, Yang, HK, et al: Laparoscopic management of peritonitis in the setting of an infected Tenckhoff catheter: A case report and description of technique. J Am Coll Surg 183:640, 1996.

175. Brown-Cartwright D, Smith HJ, Feldman M: Delayed gastric emptying: A common problem in patients on continuous ambulatory peritoneal dialysis. Perit Dial Bull 7:S10, 1987.

176. Berlyne GM, Lee HA, Ralston AJ, Woodlock JA: Pulmonary complications of peritoneal dialysis. Lancet 2:75, 1966.

177. Buccianti G, Bianchi ML, Valenti G: Progress of renal osteodystrophy during continuous ambulatory peritoneal dialysis. Clin Nephrol 22:279, 1984.

178. Delmez JA, Fallon MD, Bergfeld MA, et al: Continuous ambulatory peritoneal dialysis and bone. Kidney Int 30:379, 1986.

179. Gault MH, Fergusson EL, Sidhu JS, Corbin RP: Fluid and electrolyte complications of peritoneal dialysis: Choice of dialysis solutions. Ann Intern Med 75:253, 1971.

180. Port F, Johnson WJ, Klass DW: Prevention of dialysis disequilibrium syndrome by use of high sodium concentration in the dialysate. Kidney Int 3:327, 1973.

181. Katirtzoglou A, Digenis GE, Kontensis P, et al: Is peritoneal ultrafiltration influenced by acetate of lactate buffers? In Maher JF, Winchester JF (eds): Frontiers in Peritoneal Dialysis. New York, Field, Rich and Associates, 1986, pp 270–273.

182. Faller B, Marichal JF: Loss of ultrafiltration in continuous ambulatory peritoneal dialysis: A role for acetate. Perit Dial Bull 4:10, 1984.

183. Taber T, Hageman T, York S, Miller R: Removal of aluminum with intraperitoneal deferoxamine. Perit Dial Bull 6:213, 1986.

184. Gokal R, Ramos JM, Ward MK, et al: Eosinophilic peritonitis in continuous ambulatory peritoneal dialysis. Clin Nephrol 15:328, 1981.

185. Nolph KD, Sorkin MI, Prowant BF, et al: Asymptomatic eosinophilic peritonitis in continuous ambulatory peritoneal dialysis. Dial Transplant 11:309, 1982.

186. Digenis GE, Khanna R, Pantalony D: Eosinophilia after implantation of the peritoneal catheter. Perit Dial Bull 2:98, 1982.

187. Daugirdas JT, Leehey DJ, Popli S, et al: Induction of peritoneal fluid eosinophilia by intraperitoneal air in patients on continuous ambulatory peritoneal dialysis. N Engl J Med 313:1481, 1985.

188. Daugirdas JT, Leehey DJ, Popli S, et al: Induction of peritoneal fluid eosinophilia and/or monocytosis by intraperitoneal air injection. Am J Nephrol 7:116, 1987.

189. Gandhi VC, Ing TS, Jablokow JT, et al: Thickened peritoneal membrane in maintenance peritoneal dialysis patients. Kidney Int 14:675, 1978.

190. Gandhi VC, Humayun HM, Ing TS, et al: Sclerotic thickening of the peritoneal membrane in maintenance peritoneal dialysis patients. Arch Intern Med 140:1201, 1980.

191. Slingeneyer A, Faller B, Beraud JT: Progressive sclerosing peritonitis: Late and severe complication of maintenance peritoneal dialysis. Trans Am Soc Artif Intern Organs 29:633, 1983.

192. Bradley JA, McWhinnie DL, Hamilton DNH, et al: Sclerosing obstructive peritonitis after continuous ambulatory peritoneal dialysis. Lancet 2:113, 1983.

193. Ing TS, Daugirdas JT, Gandhi VC: Peritoneal sclerosis in peritoneal dialysis patients. Am J Nephrol 4:173, 1984.

194. Novello AC, Port FK: Sclerosing encapsulating peritonitis. Int J Artif Organs 9:393, 1986.

195. Verger C, Brunschvicg O, Le Charpentier Y, et al: Structural and ultrastructural peritoneal membrane changes and permeability alterations during CAPD. Proc Eur Dial Transplant Assoc 18:199, 1981.

196. Nielsen LH, Nolph KD, Khanna R, Moore H: Sclerosing peritonitis on CAPD; The acetate-lactate controversy. Am J Nephrol 17:82A, 1984.

197. Junor BJR, Briggs JD, Forwell MA, et al: Sclerosing peritonitis: Role of chlorhexidine alcohol. Perit Dial Bull 5:101, 1985.

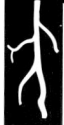

C H A P T E R 1 0 6
Long-Term Venous Access

Thomas M. Bergamini, M.D.,
Scott W. Taber, M.D.,
and John R. Hoch, M.D.

Advances in patient management and biotechnology, and the need for more cost-effective outpatient treatment, have greatly increased the use of long-term venous access. Current management often involves antibiotics for infection, total parenteral nutrition, hemodialysis, plasmapheresis, or chemotherapy. The administration of chemotherapeutic agents via catheter access through *peripheral veins* can be done only in the short term because the high-flow administration of hyperosmolar solutions causes arm pain, sclerosis of the peripheral veins, and extravasation of the infusate into the subcutaneous tissues. For long-term treatment, *central venous* access is necessary. The manufacturing of catheters that are compliant and infection-resistant and thrombosis-resistant, combined with advances in catheter and guide wire techniques for central venous access, has permitted safe and effective long-term use of venous access.

Central venous access is achieved using Seldinger's technique,[51] with peripheral insertion of a long central catheter, as originally described in 1929, or central insertion of a catheter into the internal jugular or subclavian vein, as described in the 1950s.[3, 36] Regardless of whether central venous access is gained through a peripheral or a central vein, the success of the chosen catheter device is determined by its ability to permit administration of medications and chemotherapeutic agents for the desired treatment period without complications. This chapter reviews the indications, types of catheters, insertion techniques, and complications associated with long-term venous access.

INDICATIONS AND PREOPERATIVE PATIENT EVALUATION

Central venous catheters were developed in the 1970s, principally for administration of total parenteral nutrition (TPN) and for recipients of bone marrow transplantation.[8, 29] Currently, long-term venous access is indicated for treatment of many diseases and conditions, such as infection, malignancy, renal failure, blood disorders, and malnutrition. Patients who need intravenous antibiotics for an infection are commonly managed with brief hospitalization, followed on an outpatient basis by continued administration of antibiotics, using long-term central venous access. For cancer patients long-term central venous access affords administration of chemotherapy and drugs to treat complications such as pain, nausea, vomiting, and dehydration. Patients with renal failure use central venous access for acute-phase hemodialysis while they await maturation of an arteriovenous fistula or placement of an arteriovenous shunt or for long-term dialysis while they undergo treatment for shunt thrombosis, infection, or other complications. Patients with an underlying blood disorder, such as sickle cell disease or hemophilia, often receive multiple transfusions or plasmapheresis through long-term central venous access routes. Malnourished patients with contraindications for enteral feeding receive long-term hypertonic parenteral nutrition via central venous access.[14, 15]

A thorough review of the patient's history, medications, laboratory test results, x-ray films, and a physical examination before insertion of the catheter minimize the risk of complications and maximize the success of catheter placement (Table 106–1). The successful insertion of a central venous catheter, without complications, depends on the venous anatomy at the site of cannulation. The body mass index of the patient, history of central venous cannulations, and number of attempts at catheter insertion are independent risk factors for perioperative complications.[41] Knowing the sites of earlier episodes of upper extremity deep venous thromboembolism, catheter insertions, anatomic anomalies, head and neck operations, or tumors or masses involving the mediastinum or upper extremity veins permits the clinician to select the "best site" for central venous access.

The risks associated with central venous catheter insertion are increased in patients with coagulopathy, thrombocytopenia, and leukopenia. Patients with coagulopathy secondary to warfarin or heparin should have the effects of those medications reversed, if possible, before the catheter is inserted to reduce the risk of bleeding. If coagulopathy cannot be reversed safely, the posterior approach to the internal jugular vein or the femoral vein, which permits direct pressure to be applied to the catheter insertion site or cutdown of the cephalic or external jugular vein, can minimize the risk of bleeding. Thrombocytopenia secondary to chemotherapy or bone marrow transplantation, for example, also increases the risk of bleeding. Patients with

TABLE 106–1. PATIENT EVALUATION FOR CENTRAL VENOUS ACCESS

History
- Chronic upper extremity deep venous thromboembolism
- Sites of prior catheter, pacemaker, or vascular access device placement
- Sites of current venous catheters
- Antecedent complications of venous access, such as arrhythmias, thrombosis, or infection
- Known bleeding or coagulation disorder

Examination
- Upper extremity swelling, infections, trauma, surgery, or venous thrombosis
- Anomalies of the chest wall or veins
- Tumors or masses of the upper mediastinum, pleural cavity, lung, or supraclavicular areas

Medications
- Antiplatelets (e.g., aspirin, ibuprofen)
- Anticoagulants (e.g., warfarin, subcutaneous or intravenous heparin)
- Chemotherapeutic agents

Laboratory or X-Ray Studies
- White blood cell count
- Platelet count
- Prothrombin time, partial thromboplastin time
- Chest radiograph

TABLE 106–2. LONG-TERM VENOUS ACCESS CATHETERS

CENTRAL CATHETER TYPE	SELECTION OF DEVICE: DETERMINANT FACTORS
Peripherally inserted	Inserted at bedside by skilled nurses Risks of central venous approach avoided Added risks of superficial phlebitis and mechanical failure
Centrally inserted External port	Single-, double-, or triple-lumen Patient compliance with flushing and local care Risk of infection and axillosubclavian thrombosis High-flow, large-diameter catheters for rapid transfusion, hemodialysis, plasmapheresis
Implantable port	More durable and cosmetically acceptable Less maintenance needed but special skill required to access Multiple skin punctures and added risk of fluid extravasation

platelet counts less than 50,000/mm³ should undergo platelet transfusion immediately before and during catheter placement.[61, 62] Neutropenia in cancer patients undergoing chemotherapy, for example, confers increased risk of fever and bacteremia,[1] but not of catheter-related infection.[58]

CATHETER DEVICES AND SELECTION

Advances in biotechnology led to the development of the silicone catheter, which is more flexible and remains patent longer than catheters made of polyethylene, polyvinyl chloride, and polyfluorotetraethylene (Teflon).[60] The Broviac and Hickman multilumen silicone catheters are centrally inserted external-port catheters that are radiopaque (Table 106–2). These catheters are placed with a polyester (Dacron) cuff in the subcutaneous tissue tunnel, the object being to decrease the risk of catheter infections that might result from bacterial migration along the catheter from the insertion point at the skin.

Dimethicone (Silastic) catheters with valves and implantable ports were developed later than external port catheters and required less frequent flushing and maintenance. Groshong's catheter, a centrally inserted catheter with a three-way valve, requires flushes only once weekly. Central venous catheters with implantable ports require flushing every 4 weeks when not used and are more cosmetically acceptable.[20, 39] The ports of these Silastic catheters are implanted in the subcutaneous tissue and are "accessed" by percutaneous placement of a Huber needle into the silicone septum of the port.[45] Further advances in catheter development have led to larger-diameter and higher-flow central venous catheters, which can be used for plasmapheresis and hemodialysis; examples are the port-A-Cath and Tesio catheters.

More recently, central venous catheters inserted through a peripheral vein have been the object of renewed attention.

The peripherally inserted central catheters avoid the risks attendant on central insertion, and skilled clinicians can insert them at patient's bedside. These catheters may be *less costly,* but they also have more complications with infection and phlebitis, since they exit around the elbow crease, making them susceptible to traumatic injury.[9, 40]

The choice of the appropriate catheter device for a particular clinical situation should be based on the function of long-term venous access, patient compliance, veins available for access, and the ability of the catheter to function for the duration of therapy. Patients who need long-term venous access for TPN, chemotherapy, or antibiotics can receive the requisite agents via centrally inserted external-port Silastic catheters, implantable port catheters, or peripherally inserted central catheters (see Table 106–2). External port catheters, inserted peripherally or centrally, require patients to flush the device frequently and to provide local care to the insertion sites at the skin. Patients who cannot comply with catheter maintenance may best be treated with implantable ports that require less maintenance.

Patients with active infections, trauma, or prior surgeries and those who are to receive radiation to the head and neck may suffer from conditions that prohibit central insertion of the venous catheter. If access to the subclavian or internal jugular veins is difficult because of anomalies, tumor, or a history of thrombophlebitis, peripherally inserted central catheters may be best. Patients who require therapy of longer duration may best be treated with implantable ports that are more durable and more cosmetically acceptable than external port catheters; however, the risk of fluid extravasation and multiple punctures of the skin, resulting in skin breakdown, must be considered when these implantable ports are used.[46] Patients who require hemodialysis or plasmapheresis should have high-flow, large-diameter catheters with external ports. Those who need intravenous fluids or blood samples drawn during the treatment with chemotherapeutic agents should have multiple-lumen catheters.

CATHETER INSERTION

Central venous access catheters can be placed percutaneously or by venous cutdown.[10, 26, 33, 42] Percutaneous insertion of central venous catheters by Seldinger's technique is less time-consuming and as safe as the open cutdown technique. The cutdown technique is preferred for patients whose body habitus or venous anatomy limits percutaneous access, for those whose percutaneous attempt at placement failed, and for those with coagulopathy or thrombocytopenia that increases their risk of bleeding. Placement of venous access catheters by the percutaneous or cutdown method can be performed with local anesthesia and conscious sedation or with general anesthesia. The choice of anesthetic is based on the risk posed to the patient and the difficulty of placing the central venous catheter. We prefer to place long-term venous access devices in the operating room under fluoroscopic guidance with local anesthesia and conscious sedation using the percutaneous technique.

The veins of choice for access into the superior vena cava system are the internal jugular, the external jugular, the cephalic, and the subclavian veins. These tributaries of the superior vena cava can be cannulated by percutaneous vein puncture or a cutdown technique, and, because they lie directly underneath the skin, analgesia can be provided by local/regional block and conscious sedation.

Several technical features of long-term subclavian catheter insertion need to be emphasized to ensure that venous access will last, that it is "user-friendly" for both the health care worker and the home caregiver, and that it is convenient and comfortable for the patient. The catheter exit site from the skin is located on the anterior chest wall, a flat and stable surface that supports the catheter hubs. In women, breast tissue should be avoided. The fibrous cuff is located proximally, approximately 2 cm from the exit site, to prevent it from eroding through the skin. What is the most effective length of the subcutaneous tunnel is controversial. Studies report that in adult patients the incidence of inadvertent catheter dislodgment is higher when the tunnel is shorter than 10 cm and the cuff is placed less than 2 cm from the exit site.[25] Wiener and coworkers[63] reported similar findings in a study of multilumen external catheters placed in children. The implantable port is positioned in a similar fashion, with a tunnel 10 cm long and the cuff at least 2 cm from the exit site. The port is carefully implanted into a subcutaneous pocket on the anterior chest wall, where it is more stable and accessible for use.

Proper placement of the catheter into the subclavian vein is important. The costoclavicular ligament (Halsted's) holds the first rib and the head of the clavicle in proximity and affords a narrow space through which the dilator and sheath can be passed. If obstructed they can be impossible to advance into the superior vena cava, or the catheter can become compressed and cause a partial obstruction or kink. Use of this site represents a potential for catheter obstruction. The entry point into the subclavian vein should be at a point farther distal than one for short-term venous access.[2] A site 2 cm proximal to the deltoid and pectoralis major muscle intersection and 2 to 4 cm inferior to the clavicle can allow more space between the clavicle and first rib.

The final step in catheter insertion is to position the catheter tip for long-term use as an infusion device and for collecting blood samples. The ideal position for the tip is a subject of controversy, but the literature suggests that early thrombosis is more likely when it is located at the bifurcation of the brachycephalic veins.

Stanislav and associates[53] reported a series of 113 patients who had long-term central venous catheters placed. In 31 patients, the tip of the catheter was placed in the right atrium under fluoroscopic guidance. There was no thrombosis and no instance of cardiac tamponade from catheter erosion. This patient series also illustrated the incidence of catheter thrombosis in relation to the location of the catheter tip in the superior vena cava. The incidence of thrombosis was greater when the catheter tip was located above the superior vena cava. No thrombosis was reported when the catheter tip was located in the lower superior vena cava or in the right atrium. In contrast, several case studies have reported catheter erosion and subsequent cardiac tamponade when the catheter tip was located in the right atrium.[11] We recommend that the catheter tip be located at the junction of the right atrium and the superior vena cava for long-term catheter placement.

ALTERNATIVE TECHNIQUES FOR CENTRAL VENOUS ACCESS

Because of the rapidly growing use of long-term venous access, it is not uncommon for patients to have had multiple catheters placed in the past and for the standard sites of catheter placement to have been already utilized and thrombosed. For this reason, techniques to provide alternative sites have been developed. Two alternative techniques for access into the superior vena cava are cannulation of the azygos vein and direct cannulation of the right atrium. These routes of central venous access require thoracotomy and general anesthesia.

The inferior vena cava, like the superior vena cava, has several tributaries that can be used to gain access into the central venous system. The greater saphenous, the femoral, and the inferior epigastric veins are tributaries of the inferior vena cava, located superficially and accessible by percutaneous venipuncture or open cutdown technique. Local or regional anesthesia, combined with conscious sedation, is adequate for placing central venous access through these tributaries. The inferior vena cava can be cannulated directly through the right gonadal vein or through the lumbar veins. These three techniques require general anesthesia, and, like the transthoracic approach, carry the risks associated with general anesthesia.

Techniques of percutaneous catheter placement into the inferior vena cava follow the same general principles as does percutaneous placement of a catheter into the superior vena cava. The preferred catheter exit site is on the anterior abdominal wall, a flat surface where the external hubs of the multilumen catheter or the well of the implantable port can be stabilized. Like the anterior chest, this site affords easier maintenance of the central venous access device for all involved. More important, the risk of bacterial contamination of the catheter is lower when the exit site is remote from the groin.[12, 18]

The ideal position of the catheter tip in the inferior vena cava has not been well elucidated. Fonkalsrud and coworkers[17] reported on a series of 151 catheters inserted in the inferior vena cava through the greater saphenous vein. The catheters remained in place for a combined total of 13,288 days, but they were later removed from 11 patients because of infection and from four because of subsequent occlusion of the inferior vena cava. We recommend that the catheter tip be free-standing in the inferior vena cava. The renal vein junction of the inferior vena cava and the side wall of the inferior vena cava are locations where the catheter tip can become obstructed, thus resulting in catheter failure. Fluoroscopic guidance for positioning the catheter tip helps to prevent catheter occlusion.

COMPLICATIONS

Complications associated with long-term access devices increase patient morbidity and significantly decrease cost-effectiveness and durability of the catheter. Complications that occur at the time of catheter insertion are secondary to inexperience, pneumothorax, cardiopulmonary complications, mechanical failure, thrombosis, or infection (Table 106–3).

Complication risk is also related to the experience of the clinician who is inserting the catheter. Bernard and Stahl[5] reported an 8.1% complication rate when catheters were inserted by clinicians who had performed fewer than 50 catheterizations; this compared with no complications among 90 venous access catheter insertions by physicians who had performed more than 50 catheterization procedures. Patients with thrombosis of the central veins as detected by duplex ultrasonography have a higher failure rate for catheter insertion.[22] Duplex scanning is very specific in identifying subclavian vein thrombosis and in determining successful central venous insertion.[22, 23, 37] Duplex scanning of the internal jugular and subclavian veins is recommended for patients with a history of central venous catheter insertion and a history of thromboembolism.

Pneumothorax follows insertion of the central venous catheter in 1% to 6% of cases.[5, 27, 28, 49, 52, 55, 56] Small apical pneumothoraces in asymptomatic patients can be followed with repeat radiographs or they can be "aspirated." Pneumothoraces that enlarge or cause symptoms should be treated with a chest tube. Hemothorax and hemomediastinum are unusual complications of percutaneous subclavian insertions (prevalence ≤ 3.8%). They are very important to recognize, however, and should alert the clinician to a potential life-threatening subclavian artery injury. Similarly, carotid or innominate artery injury can occur during the internal jugular approach with central venous access. When recognized immediately, most arterial sticks at the time of catheter insertion can be managed, with removal of the catheter and direct pressure.

Cardiopulmonary complications associated with catheter insertion include cardiac arrhythmias, cardiac puncture, and air embolism. Stuart and coworkers[54] reported atrial arrhythmias in 41% of patients and ventricular arrhythmias in 11% of patients during central venous access placement. The incidence of arrhythmias that require cardioversion, however, is less than 1%.[7] Life-threatening cardiac compli-

TABLE 106–3. COMPLICATIONS OF LONG-TERM VENOUS ACCESS

Catheter Insertion
  Hematoma, multiple skin punctures
  Catheter malposition
  Unsuccessful venous catheterization
  Pneumothorax, hemothorax, chylothorax, hemomediastinum
  Air embolism
  Arterial/venous injury
  Brachial plexus/phrenic nerve injury
  Cardiac arrhythmia, tamponade
Mechanical
  Catheter kinking, migration, breaking, embolism
  Catheter dislodgment, removal
  Catheter thrombosis
  Central venous thromboembolism
Infection
  Local catheter site infection
  Sepsis, bacteremia, fungemia
  Septic thrombophlebitis

cations from arrhythmias or cardiac puncture resulting in tamponade are extremely rare, but they must be immediately recognized and treated. Air embolism is also a potentially life-threatening, but extremely rare, complication at the time of catheter insertion. Air embolism more often occurs when long-term central venous catheters with external ports become dislodged or disconnected at the hub. Management of the patient with air embolism and respiratory failure includes reconnecting the catheter and placing the patient in the left lateral decubitus position with the head down for positive venous pressure.[59]

Mechanical complications such as kinking, migration, breaking, and embolization occur in only 1% to 2% of patients[7, 27, 49]; however, mechanical failure is the most common complication of peripherally inserted central venous catheters: incidence of catheter breakage 6% to 10%; of inadvertent catheter removal 6% to 17%.[6, 9, 38, 40] Catheter thrombosis is the most common mechanical complication associated with long-term venous access devices, occurring in as many as one third of patients with intraluminal or extraluminal thrombus or with deep venous thrombosis of the recipient vein.[7, 27, 49, 55, 56] Most catheter thromboses not related to central deep venous thrombosis (DVT) can be managed successfully with urokinase,[4, 21, 57] with thrombolysis of catheters in 32% of adults and in 76% of children. A bolus injection into the catheter of 5000 U of urokinase per ml of injectate should be given, followed for as long as 1 hour by attempts to withdraw blood from the catheter. A similar bolus of urokinase can be repeated after 1 hour for an additional hour. If after 2 hours thrombolysis still has not been achieved, continuous infusion of urokinase, 40,000 U/hr, over 6 hours can restore catheter patency. If the catheter is still thrombosed after 6 hours, the continuous infusion of urokinase can be extended to 12 hours. Haire and Lieberman[21] reported successful thrombolysis with continuous urokinase infusion in 19 catheters after bolus urokinase therapy had failed. Fifteen catheters were successfully treated with thrombolysis after 6 hours of urokinase, and two more were rendered patent after a total of 12 hours of continuous urokinase infusion.

Subclavian vein thrombosis secondary to central venous catheters is the most common cause of DVT of the upper extremities (currently "replacing" Paget-Schroetter axillosubclavian thrombosis).[31] Venographically proven upper extremity DVT has been reported to occur in as many as one third of patients with central venous catheters.[31, 35] Clinically symptomatic axillosubclavian vein thrombosis, however, occurs in 3% to 16% of patients with centrally inserted catheters and in 0.3% to 4% of patients with peripherally inserted central catheters.[6, 28, 32, 40, 56] Infection, malignancy, and long-term use of catheters are associated with increased risks of DVT. Patients with central venous thrombosis have a 12% risk of pulmonary embolism and a 19% risk of postphlebitic syndrome of the upper extremity characterized by chronic arm swelling and pain.[35] The diagnosis of upper extremity DVT can be made with duplex scanning in most cases.[16]

The optimal management of patients with catheter-related upper extremity deep vein thrombosis is not known, because no prospective comparison of treatment options has been performed. Treatment should be based on the severity of the patient's symptoms and the availability of alternative venous access sites. Patients with minimal symptoms and alternative venous access sites can be managed by simple catheter removal. The addition of heparin anticoagulation does not afford the patient any more protection against pulmonary embolism than does simple catheter removal.[13, 43]

Catheter removal and heparin anticoagulation are the initial treatment options for patients with catheter-related deep vein thrombosis who present with significant upper extremity symptoms of swelling and pain. The incidence of post-phlebitic syndrome is lower when patients are treated with heparin and warfarin, as compared with catheter removal alone (19% versus 50%).[31, 35] Because of the higher risk of hemorrhage with thrombolysis, compared with heparin, and the low incidence of upper extremity postphlebitic syndrome, thrombolysis is reserved for patients with catheter-related upper extremity deep vein thrombosis who have no alternatives for venous access.[13, 31, 35, 39]

The incidence of infection for long-term central venous catheters is as high as 30% to 40%. The most common cause of catheter-related infection is gram-positive bacteria, principally *Staphylococcus epidermidis* and *Staphylococcus aureus*. Catheter infections can be secondary to local site migration of skin pathogens or to bacteremia from a distant source of infection.[19, 48]

Local infections of the catheter where it exits the skin can be successfully treated with local care and systemic antibiotics in 70% to 80% of cases.[19, 47] Catheter-related infections that demonstrate no clinical improvement at the skin insertion site after 2 days are best treated with catheter removal. Infections of central venous catheters with implantable ports tend to be more resistant to antibiotic treatment, and in more than half of the patients the catheter and port must be removed.[24] Systemic bacterial or fungal infections secondary to long-term venous catheterization can in 70% of cases be treated successfully with intravenous antibiotics administered through the catheter.[19, 44] Catheter-related thrombus has been associated with the development of catheter infections. The combination of urokinase and antibiotics to treat catheter-related infections has improved outcome: more than 90% of catheter-related infections resolved.[34, 50] Recurrent catheter infection, however, remains a risk. It develops in as many as 40% of catheters treated with antibiotics alone and in 5% of catheters treated with thrombolytics and antibiotics.[34, 44]

Systemic sepsis secondary to catheter-related infection and central venous thrombosis can result in suppurative phlebitis. Unlike excision of peripheral veins, excision of central veins with suppurative thrombophlebitis is associated with significant morbidity. Treatment of suppurative thrombophlebitis with catheter removal, heparin, and systemic antibiotics can be successful in more than half of patients. Those who do not respond to this treatment can be treated with vena cava filter placement and central venous thrombectomy.[30] The use of thrombolytic therapy for the treatment of suppurative thrombophlebitis of the central veins has not been reported.

SUMMARY

Long-term venous access has improved the treatment of patients with a variety of diseases. A thorough knowledge of patient evaluation, catheter devices and selection, indications, standard and alternative catheter insertion techniques, and catheter management can minimize complications and maximize the effective use of long-term venous access devices for the duration of therapy.

REFERENCES

1. Alexander HR: Infectious complications associated with long-term venous access devices. In Alexander HR (ed): Vascular Access in the Cancer Patient. Philadelphia, JB Lippincott, 1994, p 113.
2. Alexander HR: Insertion techniques for long-term venous access catheters. In Alexander HR (ed): Vascular Access in the Cancer Patient. Philadelphia, JB Lippincott, 1994, p 39.
3. Aubania R: L'injection intraveincuse sous-claviculaire: Advantages et technique. Presse Med 60:1456, 1952.
4. Bagnall HA, Comperts E, Atkinson JB: Continuous infusion of low-dose urokinase in the treatment of central venous catheter thrombosis in infants and children. Pediatrics 83:963, 1989.
5. Bernard RW, Stahl WM: Subclavian vein catheters: A prospective study: I. Noninfectious complications. Ann Surg 173:184, 1971.
6. Bottino J, McCredie KB, Gorschel DHM, et al: Long-term intravenous therapy with peripherally inserted silicone elastomer central venous catheters in patients with malignant diseases. Cancer 43:1937, 1979.
7. Brothers JE, Von Moll LK, Niederhuber JE, et al: Experience with subcutaneous infusion ports in three hundred patients. Surg Gynecol Obstet 166:295, 1988.
8. Broviac JW, Cole JJ, Schribner BH: A silicone rubber atrial catheter for prolonged parenteral alimentation. Surg Gynecol Obstet 136:602, 1973.
9. Cardella JF, Cardella K, Bacci N, et al: Cumulative experience with 1,273 peripherally inserted central catheters at a single institution. J Vasc Intervent Radiol 7:5, 1996.
10. Cohen AM, Wood WC: Simplified technique for placement of long-term central venous silicone catheters. Surg Gynecol Obstet 154:721, 1982.
11. Collier PE, Goodman GB: Cardiac tamponade caused by central venous catheter perforation of the heart: A preventable complication. J Am Coll Surg 181:459, 1995.
12. Curtas S, Bonaventure M, Meguid MM: Cannulation of inferior vena cava for long-term central venous access. Surg Gynecol Obstet 168:120, 1989.
13. Donayre CE, White GH, Mahringer SM, et al: Pathogenesis determines late morbidity of axillosubclavian vein thrombosis. Am J Surg 152:179, 1986.
14. Dudrick JJ, Wilmore DW, Vars HM, et al: Long-term total parenteral nutrition with growth, development, and positive nitrogen balance. Surgery 64:134, 1968.
15. Dudrick SJ, Ruberg RL: Principles and practice of parenteral nutrition. Gastroenterology 61:901, 1971.
16. Falk RL, Smith DF: Thrombosis of upper extremity thoracic inlet veins: Diagnosis with duplex Doppler sonography. Am J Roentgenol 149:677, 1987.
17. Fonkalsrud EW, Ament ME, Berquist WE, et al: Occlusion of the vena cava in infants receiving central venous hyperalimentation. Surg Gynecol Obstet 154:189, 1982.
18. Fonkalsrud EW, Berquist WE, Burke M, et al: Long-term hyperalimentation in children through saphenous central venous catheterization. Am J Surg 143:209, 1982.
19. Groeger JS, Lucas AB, Thaler HT, et al: Infectious morbidity associated with long-term use of venous access devices in patients with cancer. Ann Intern Med 119:1168, 1993.
20. Gyves JW, Ensminger WD, Niederhuber JE, et al: A totally implanted injection port system for blood sampling and chemotherapy administration. JAMA 251:2538, 1984.
21. Haire WD, Lieberman RP: Thrombosed central venous catheters: Restoring function with 6-hour urokinase infusion after failure of bolus urokinase. JPEN J Parenter Enteral Nutr 16:129, 1992.
22. Haire WD, Lynch TM, Lieberman RP, et al: Duplex scans before subclavian vein catheterization predict unsuccessful catheter placement. Arch Surg 127:229, 1992.
23. Haire WD, Lynch TH, Lund GB, et al: Limitations of magnetic resonance imaging and ultrasound-directed (duplex) scanning in the diagnosis of subclavian vein thrombosis. J Vasc Surg 12:391, 1991.
24. Harvey WH, Pick TE, Reed K, et al: A prospective evaluation of the Port-a-cath implantable venous access system in chronically ill adults and children. Surg Gynecol Obstet 169:495, 1989.
25. Hayward SR, Ledgerwood AM, Lucas CE: The fate of 100 prolonged venous access devices. Am Surg 56:515, 1990.
26. Heimbach DM, Ivey TM: Technique for placement of a permanent home hyperalimentation catheter. Surg Gynecol Obstet 143:634, 1976.
27. Henriques H, Karmy-Jones R, Knoll SM, et al: Avoiding complications of long-term venous access. Am Surg 59:555, 1993.
28. Herbst CA: Indications, management, and complications of percutaneous subclavian catheters. Arch Surg 113:1421, 1978.
29. Hickman RO, Buckner CD, Clift RA, et al: A modified right atrial catheter for access to the venous system in marrow transplant recipients. Surg Gynecol Obstet 148:871, 1979.
30. Hoffman MJ, Greenfield LJ: Central venous septic thrombosis managed by superior vena cava Greenfield filter and venous thrombectomy: A case report. J Vasc Surg 4:606, 1986.
31. Horattas MC, Wright DJ, Fenton AH, et al: Changing concepts of deep venous thrombosis of the upper extremity: Report of a series and review of the literature. Surgery 104:561, 1988.
32. Hughes CJ, Rumsey-Stewart G, Storey DW: Percutaneous infraclavicular insertion of long-term central venous Hickman catheters. Aust N Z J Surg 59:889, 1989.
33. Jansen RFM, Wiggers T, van Geel BN, et al: Assessment of insertion techniques and complication rates of dual lumen central venous catheters in patients with hematological malignancies. World J Surg 14:101, 1990.
34. Jones GR, Konsler GK, Dunaway RP, et al: Prospective analysis of urokinase in the treatment of catheter sepsis in pediatric hematology-oncology patients. J Pediatr Surg 28:350, 1993.
35. Kerr TM, Lutter KS, Moeller DM, et al: Upper extremity venous thrombosis diagnosed by duplex scanning. Am J Surg 160:202, 1990.
36. Kerri-Szantu M: The subclavian vein, a constant and convenient intravenous injection site. Arch Surg 72:179, 1956.
37. Kraybill WG, Allen BT: Preoperative duplex venous imaging in the assessment of patients with venous access. J Surg Oncol 52:244, 1993.
38. Lam S, Scannell R, Roessler D, et al: Peripherally inserted central catheters in an acute-care hospital. Arch Intern Med 154:1833, 1994.
39. Lokich JJ, Bothe A, Benotti P, et al: Complications and management of implanted venous access catheters. J Clin Oncol 3:710, 1985.
40. Loughran SC, Borzatta M: Peripherally inserted central catheters: A report of 2,506 catheter days. JPEN J Parenter Enteral Nutr 19:133, 1995.
41. Mansfield PE, Hohn DC, Fornage BD, et al: Complications and failures of subclavian-vein catheterization. N Engl J Med 331:1735, 1994.
42. Mirro J Jr, Rao BN, Kumar M, et al: A comparison of placement techniques and complication of externalized catheters and implantable port use in children with cancer. J Pediatr Surg 25:120, 1990.
43. Monreal M, Raventos A, Lerma R, et al: Pulmonary embolism in patients with upper extremity DVT associated to venous central lines: A prospective study. Thromb Haemost 72:548, 1994.
44. Mukau L, Talamini MA, Sitzmann JV, et al: Long-term central venous access vs. other home therapies: Complications in patients with acquired immunodeficiency syndrome. JPEN J Parenter Enteral Nutr 16:455, 1992.
45. Niederhuber JE, Ensminger W, Gyves JW, et al: Totally implanted venous and arterial access system to replace external catheters in cancer treatment. Surgery 92:706, 1982.
46. Pomp A, Caldwell MD, Albina JE: Subcutaneous infusion ports for administration of parenteral nutrition at home. Surg Gynecol Obstet 169:329, 1989.
47. Press OW, Ramsey PG, Larson EG, et al: Hickman catheter infections in patients with malignancies. Medicine 63:189, 1984.
48. Raad II, Luna M, Khalil S-AM, et al: The relationship between the thrombotic and infectious complications of central venous catheters. JAMA 271:1014, 1994.
49. Sariego J, Bootorabi B, Matsumoto T, et al: Major long-term complications in 1,422 permanent venous access devices. Am J Surg 165:249, 1993.
50. Schuman ES, Winters V, Gross GF, et al: Management of Hickman catheter sepsis. Am J Surg 149:627, 1985.

51. Seldinger SI: Catheter replacement of the needle in percutaneous arteriography. Acta Radiol (Stockh) 39:368, 1953.
52. Sitzmann JV, Townsend TR, Siler MC, et al: Septic and technical complications of central venous catheterizations: A prospective study of 200 consecutive patients. Am Surg 202:766, 1995.
53. Stanislav GV, Fitzgibbons RJ Jr, Bailey RT Jr, et al: Reliability of implantable central venous access devices in patients with cancer. Arch Surg 122:1280, 1991.
54. Stuart RK, Shikora SA, Akerman P, et al: Incidence of arrhythmia with central venous catheter insertion and exchange. JPEN J Parenter Enteral Nutr 14:152, 1990.
55. Takasugi JK, O'Connell TX: Prevention of complications in permanent central venous catheters. Surg Gynecol Obstet 167:6, 1988.
56. Torramade JR, Cienfuegos JA, Hernandez J-L, et al: The complications of central venous access systems: A study of 218 patients. Eur J Surg 159:323, 1993.

57. Tschirhart JM, Rao MK: Mechanism and management of persistent withdrawal occlusion. Am Surg 54:326, 1988.
58. Viscoli C: Aspects of infections in children with cancer. Recent Results Cancer Res 108:71, 1988.
59. Waggoner SE: Case report: Venous air embolism through a Groshong catheter. Gynecol Oncol 48:394, 1993.
60. Welch GW, McKeel DW Jr, Silverstein P, et al: The role of catheter composition in the development of thrombophlebitis. Surg Gynecol Obstet 138:421, 1974.
61. Whitman ED: Complications associated with the use of central venous access devices. Curr Probl Surg 33:324, 1996.
62. Whitman ED, Ruppel LJ: Safe effective strategy to subclavian venous access in severely thrombocytopenic cancer patients (Abstract). Proc Am Soc Clin Oncol 1679, 1994.
63. Wiener ES, McGuire P, Stolar CJH, et al: The CCSG prospective study of venous access devices: An analysis of insertions and causes for removal. J Pediatr Surg 27:155, 1992.

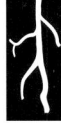

C H A P T E R   1 0 7

Iatrogenic Complications of Arterial and Venous Catheterizations

Robert A. Cambria, M.D., F.A.C.S., and
John W. Hallett, Jr., M.D., F.A.C.S.

Percutaneous catheterization of arteries and veins has become commonplace in the diagnosis and treatment of a variety of ailments. Peripheral arteriography was pioneered by dos Santos in 1929, who developed the translumbar needle cannulation of the abdominal aorta.[11] Although other investigators had inserted catheters into various arteries for the injection of contrast material, it was Seldinger in 1953 who described catheter exchange over a guide wire and who revolutionized percutaneous access to the intravascular space.[34] This technique has been adopted for nearly all procedures requiring cannulation of an artery or vein. Today, critically ill patients frequently require multiple catheters for fluid resuscitation, hemodynamic monitoring, parenteral nutrition, hemodialysis, chemotherapy, cardiac pacemakers, and intra-aortic balloon pumps.

With technologic advances in intravascular catheters and devices, an increasing number of coronary and peripheral angiograms as well as interventional procedures, such as thrombolytic therapy, angioplasty, and placement of intravascular devices, are being performed. The prevalence of iatrogenic vascular injuries is rising as well[3] and is directly related to the number and complexity of endovascular procedures performed.[29] Since the sheaths required for these interventions range from 7 to 12 French (diameter 2 to 4 mm), it is not be surprising that the number of iatrogenic complications of arterial and venous access has reached near-epidemic proportions. Each of these procedures, from the most simple placement of an intravenous catheter to the most complicated of endovascular prosthetic devices, can be associated with complications, some of which may threaten life or limb. This chapter provides an analysis of the incidence, presentation, and treatment of the most common iatrogenic complications of arterial and venous catheterization.

PREPROCEDURAL AND TECHNICAL CONSIDERATIONS

Careful consideration should be given before invasive monitoring catheters are employed. Although knowledge of central filling pressures provides a certain sense of security in the perioperative management of patients undergoing major surgery, the risks of such monitoring devices may outweigh their advantages. In a prospective randomized trial, routine placement of a pulmonary artery catheter did not reduce the morbidity or mortality associated with elective vascular surgery.[1] Although these catheters may be invaluable in certain circumstances, their routine application should be avoided. Similarly, the indications for any diagnostic or interventional procedure that involves cannulation of an artery or vein should be rigorously reviewed, and these procedures should not be recommended with complacency.

The first and most important step in the treatment of

iatrogenic complications of vascular access is an awareness of their possibility before the procedure, and dedication to their prevention. In patients with preexisting vascular disease, the pulse and the appearance of the extremity should be well documented before treatment proceeds. In patients without palpable pulses, Doppler-derived pressures in the distal extremity should be recorded. If there is a question of vascular injury after the procedure, evaluation of the extremity will be much easier if preprocedural data are available.

In all anatomic locations, strict adherence to anatomic landmarks and standard technique maximizes the chances for successful access and minimizes technical misadventure. In one study, for example, use of a rolled towel between the scapulae resulted in a higher likelihood of successful central venous catheter placement.[5] The use of adjunctive imaging for the choice of catheter insertion sites is frequently helpful. Fluorographic imaging of the femoral head assists in the placement of common femoral artery puncture, preventing inadvertent cannulation of the superficial femoral or profunda femoris arteries, which are more likely to result in the formation of a pseudoaneurysm or arteriovenous fistula.[22, 28] Similarly, the use of ultrasonographic imaging is frequently helpful for the placement of catheters in a variety of vascular structures[13] and avoids injury to adjacent structures.[37]

Removal of intravascular catheters should be performed as carefully as their insertion. Constant direct finger pressure should be applied for 20 to 30 minutes after removal of arterial catheters. Patients need to keep the involved area immobile for 6 to 8 hours to prevent late hemorrhage. New devices designed to prevent hemorrhage from the puncture site and to allow for early mobilization after arterial catheterizations are now available, but their efficacy is not certain.[14] Continued anticoagulation is associated with a higher risk of complications and should be used with caution. In most instances and for most indications, anticoagulation can be stopped temporarily immediately before and after removal of intravascular catheters without an undue risk of thrombosis.

COMPLICATIONS

Arterial Catheterizations

The incidence and type of complications that occur following arterial catheterization vary with anatomic location (Table 107–1). In this chapter, each specific anatomic location is addressed in turn, but first an overview of the various complications is provided.

In general, the most frequent complication of arterial

TABLE 107–1. COMPLICATION RATES FOR DIAGNOSTIC ANGIOGRAPHY FROM DIFFERENT ANATOMIC ACCESS SITES

Femoral access	1.7%
Translumbar access	2.9%
Axillary access	3.3%

From Hessel SJ, Adams DF, Abrams HL: Complications of angiography. Radiology 138: 273, 1981. Courtesy of the Radiological Society of North America.

cannulation is *bleeding*.[35] This may present as external hemorrhage, or with an expanding or occult hematoma formation. A special case of this type of injury is the pulsatile hematoma or *pseudoaneurysm* formation.

Thrombosis was once the most common complication following aortography,[24] but it is now less common than bleeding complications. This change has likely occurred because of the increased diameters of catheters utilized, more frequent use of anticoagulation, and increased recognition of arterial pathology at the insertion site at the time of angiography.

Dissection can occur as a result of the false passage of wires or catheters outside of the arterial lumen or from intimal disruption after balloon angioplasty. *Emboli* originating from intraluminal atherosclerotic debris, or thrombus adherent to the catheters themselves can be showered in the more distal arterial circulation, resulting in fixed occlusion of distal vessels. This complication, fortunately, is rare but can result in devastating and irreversible ischemia in the distal extremity or visceral circulation.

Finally, *arteriovenous fistulae* can result from simultaneous injury to the artery and vein, which heal in direct communication.

Injuries Following Catheterization of the Femoral Artery

The common femoral artery has become the access site of choice for nearly every intra-arterial procedure. This artery has several advantages over alternate sites, including:

- A large caliber, allowing for the passage of sizable catheters if necessary
- Its superficial location, allowing for ease of cannulation
- Its location over the femoral head, allowing for adequate compression after removal of the catheter

Despite these advantages, consideration should be given to alternate access sites if the femoral pulses are not palpable or if significant aortoiliac occlusive disease is suggested on preprocedural evaluation. When aortofemoral or femoropopliteal grafts are present, their puncture should be avoided whenever possible. If they must be punctured, prophylactic intravenous antibiotics (e.g., cefazolin 1 gm) should be given before the catheter is inserted.

Catheter complications can be minimized by use of correct anatomic landmarks to locate and cannulate the common femoral artery.[22, 28] The common femoral artery begins at the inguinal ligament, which spans a line between the anterior superior iliac spine and the pubic tubercle. The groin fat crease is inferior to the inguinal ligament and is sometimes mistaken for it. Puncture at the fat crease often results in puncture of the superficial femoral or deep femoral artery, both of which are more difficult to compress adequately after catheter removal.

Some angiographers use fluoroscopy to identify the head of the femur, which is generally deep to the common femoral artery. Despite the proper use of these landmarks, improper catheter angulation can place the puncture site above the inguinal ligament, in the external iliac artery, where compression after catheter removal can also be difficult. The importance of point compression with direct finger pressure cannot be overemphasized. Compression bandages, sandbags, and various hardware that attaches to the bed or patient to provide compression are not as effective as manual compression and should be used sparingly following hemostasis obtained by finger pressure.

Despite careful attention to technique and adequate compression after catheter removal, complications can occur. Of all arterial access sites, the femoral artery is associated with the fewest complications, and these complications are directly related to the complexity of the procedure performed.[29] Diagnostic angiography via the transfemoral route has been associated with a complication rate below 1% in many series,[28, 29] and this rate appears to have decreased since the 1970s. However, complication rates for interventional procedures have been reported to range from 3% to 18% because of the need for larger sheaths and use of anticoagulation.[6, 29]

As noted above, bleeding complications are the most common and can result in a number of groin complications. Any complaints of groin or lower extremity pain, coolness, or numbness must be immediately evaluated. Most frequently, the patient complains of pain at the catheterization site, and examination reveals a mass that may be stable, expanding, or pulsatile. A bruit may be audible in a minority of patients. Symptoms usually occur within 12 hours of the procedure, either immediately following catheter removal or as the patient resumes normal activity. An experienced health care provider should monitor the puncture site before the patient is discharged from the angiography suite or hospital.

Expanding hematomas or *ongoing uncontrolled hemorrhage* after catheter removal affects about 10% to 15% of patients with catheter injuries and may rapidly progress to shock. Fluid resuscitation with Ringer's lactate solution should be started while blood is typed and cross-matched. Anticoagulant therapy should be stopped and coagulation parameters corrected with protamine, vitamin K, or blood products as required. If the bleeding is originating from the groin puncture site, direct pressure for 20 to 30 minutes may suffice. If local compression fails after 30 to 40 minutes, operative exposure and closure are required (see later).

More commonly, a stable mass with or without a pulsatile component is present. Physical examination alone is unreliable to distinguish between hematoma and pseudoaneurysm. In a recent study, only one third of patients referred for evaluation were found to have a femoral pseudoaneurysm.[20] Therefore, in the absence of expansion or hemodynamic instability, evaluation of the mass and underlying femoral artery with color flow Doppler ultrasonography should be performed. This test is quite sensitive and specific for detection of flow outside of the arterial lumen and can thus identify pulsatile hematomas and pseudoaneurysms with a high degree of accuracy (Fig. 107–1).[26] In addition, compression of these pseudoaneurysms under ultrasound guidance is now recognized as an effective method of treatment.[15]

In 1991, ultrasound-guided compression of acute pseudoaneurysms following catheterization injuries was introduced by Fellmeth and colleagues,[12] and this technique has been well described. Several investigators have reported success rates ranging from 75% to more than 90%,[7, 15, 20, 33] with median time of compression required to thrombose aneurysms reported as 30 minutes when 10-minute com-

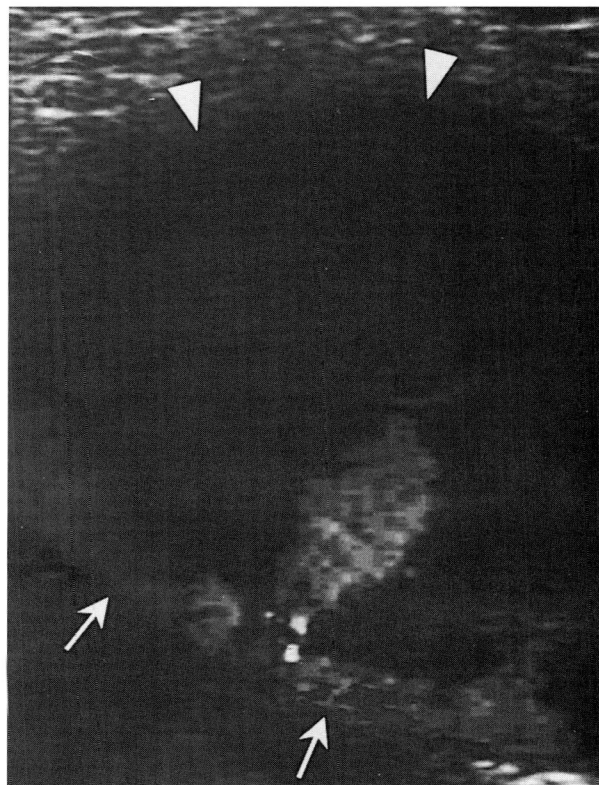

FIGURE 107–1. Duplex scan of a pseudoaneurysm after femoral artery catheterization. The wall of the pseudoaneurysm is clearly depicted (*arrowheads*), and the short neck with an area of high velocity flow can be seen arising from the femoral artery (*arrows*).

pression intervals are used. Intravenous sedation and analgesics may be necessary because of the proximity and potential involvement of the femoral nerve, causing this procedure to be relatively uncomfortable for some patients (Fig. 107–2).[16, 20]

After successful compression, bed rest overnight with a compression bandage is advisable. The area should be reevaluated before discharge and on late follow-up, since the aneurysm may recur in up to 10% of patients,[7, 15] and rupture of a recurrent aneurysm following successful compression therapy has been reported.[4] Aneurysms that do recur can usually be treated successfully with additional compression. Although individual studies have identified aneurysm age,[41] size,[10] anticoagulation,[15] and sheath size[17] as predictors for failure of compression therapy, none of these factors has been identified consistently to correlate with outcome. In a study from the Cleveland Clinic,[10] ultrasound-guided compression of femoral pseudoaneurysms was successful in 73% of patients despite continued anticoagulation therapy.

The natural history of iatrogenic femoral pseudoaneurysms is unknown, although rupture has been reported in 3% of one series.[20] Spontaneous thrombosis, however, is much more common. Of 147 patients, 86% who were observed with femoral pseudoaneurysms or arteriovenous fistulae experienced spontaneous resolution of these lesions within a mean of 23 days.[38] In a small series of 11 patients, 100% became thrombosed spontaneously, but an average

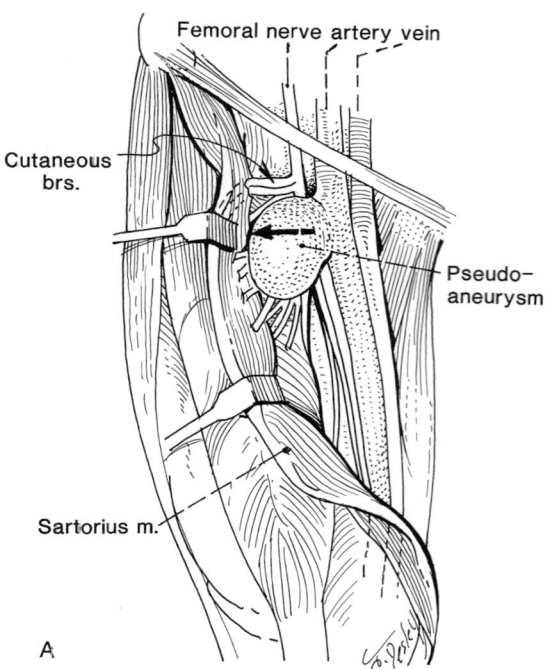

Femoral nerve artery vein

Cutaneous brs.

Pseudo-aneurysm

Sartorius m.

A

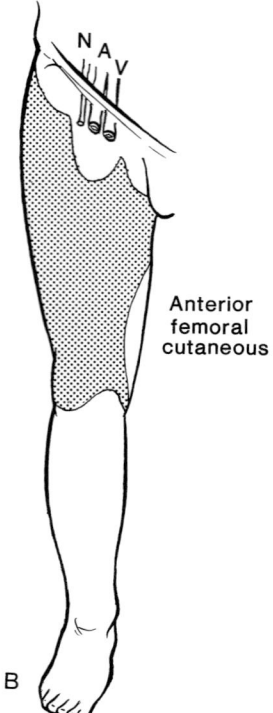

N A V

Anterior femoral cutaneous

B

FIGURE 107-2. Mechanism (A) and cutaneous distribution (B) of femoral cutaneous neuralgia syndrome after catheter-induced pseudoaneurysm. Compression, stretching, or suture entrapment may disturb cutaneous branches (brs.) of the femoral nerve. (A and B, From Hallett JW, Wolk SW, Cherry KJ, et al: The femoral neuralgia syndrome after arterial catheter trauma. J Vasc Surg 11:702, 1990.)

of 52 days was required for aneurysms with a tract smaller than 0.9 cm in length.[32] Therefore, indications for ultrasound-guided compression of these aneurysms remain to be defined, and some authors have often advocated initial observation.[18, 25]

Contraindications to ultrasound-guided compression include local infection, skin ischemia, and severe local pain, which exist in approximately 15% to 20% of patients. Although percutaneous installation of thrombin[27] or coils[30] to promote thrombosis of femoral pseudoaneurysms have been reported, the advantage of these procedures over direct surgical repair has not been documented.

The surgical approach to the femoral arteries for a pseudoaneurysm or for uncontrolled hemorrhage should be direct and gentle. A longitudinal groin incision over the femoral pulse is best. Instead of entering the hematoma, the surgeon should carry the dissection directly to the inguinal ligament, where the femoral artery or distal external iliac artery can be exposed and controlled. Further dissection should be minimized because hematoma may obscure the femoral nerve branches and the deep and superficial femoral arteries.

If *femoral artery thrombosis* has occurred or if arterial repair with a graft or patch angioplasty appears necessary (Fig. 107-3), a low dose of intravenous heparin (2000 to 3000 units) should be considered. After the femoral artery is clamped at the inguinal ligament, the hematoma can be incised and evacuated. The puncture site can be identified and controlled with finger pressure. Usually, a simple suture suffices. Large hematoma cavities should be drained with a closed suction catheter. Vigorous use of retractors and large closing sutures should be avoided because they can overstretch or entrap fibers of the femoral cutaneous nerve, resulting in a painful femoral neuralgia (Fig. 107-2).[16]

Occasionally, femoral catheterization can result in injury to the external or common iliac artery and may lead to *retroperitoneal hemorrhage*. Most patients with a large hematoma present with suprainguinal fullness and abdominal or back pain. Other presentations may include shock, a drop in hematocrit without apparent source of hemorrhage, or a

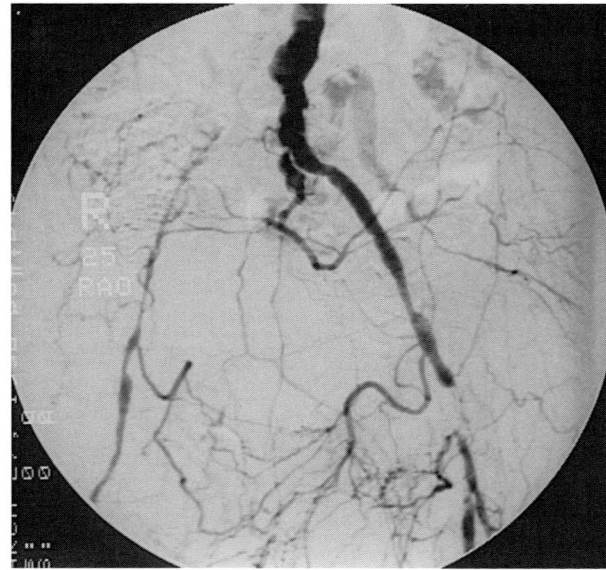

FIGURE 107-3. Aortogram from a patient who presented with numbness and tingling of his left lower extremity after cardiac catheterization via a left femoral puncture. Focal occlusion of the left common femoral artery, in addition to a chronic right iliac occlusion, is noted. At operation, both intraluminal and intraplaque thrombi were identified in the left common femoral artery. Patch angioplasty repair resulted in a marked improvement in perfusion and resolution of symptoms in the extremity.

femoral neuralgia and leg pain. Patients frequently hold their hip in flexion to reduce traction on the nerve roots. The incidence of this complication ranges from less than 1% of diagnostic angiographic procedures to as many as 3% of more complex endovascular interventions.[21] Computed tomography (CT) of the abdomen is accurate in the diagnosis of this problem. Most of the patients can be managed with observation and transfusion as needed; in one series of 45 such patients, only seven (16%) required operation because of hypotension unresponsive to resuscitation or because of a progressive decline in hematocrit over several days.[21]

As with pseudoaneurysms, *arteriovenous fistulae* are more likely to occur when arterial puncture has been placed below the femoral bifurcation (Fig. 107–4). Usually, a fistula is created between the superficial or deep femoral artery and its adjacent vein. These fistulas are usually asymptomatic and may be noted incidentally on angiography or duplex examination for other groin pathology. A palpable thrill or bruit may be present. Many of these fistulae close spontaneously, and others can be occluded with ultrasound-guided compression. For symptomatic or large chronic fistulae, endovascular exclusion or surgical repair is required.

Iatrogenic dissection can occur after catheterization of any artery, but it is most common in the iliac arteries owing to the high incidence of atherosclerotic occlusive disease and the tortuosity of these vessels. Paying careful attention to technique, advancing sheaths and catheters only over appropriate guide wires, and using test injections prior to power injection of contrast material help to minimize the occurrence of this complication. If dissection occurs, the operator should recognize and evaluate the extent of the injury immediately. Removal of malpositioned catheters and wires usually allows spontaneous resolution of the dissec-

tion; however, endoluminal stenting may be required to stabilize the injury. This type of injury, when recognized immediately, rarely warrants any measures other than endovascular management.

Embolic complications after catheterization of the femoral artery are rare, but as with most complications, they are more likely following endovascular intervention. The presence of mobile aortic plaque, identified by transesophageal sonography, may predict an increased risk of embolic complications. When possible, some authors have advocated altering the approach for vascular access based on the distribution of these plaques.[19] Because emboli tend to lodge in smaller vessels located more peripherally, ischemia resulting in tissue loss is not uncommon. Direct reconstruction of these vessels may not be possible, and therapeutic options may be limited to catheter-directed thrombolysis. In some cases of larger emboli, thromboembolectomy may be therapeutic.

Injuries Following Catheterization of Arteries in the Upper Extremity

If access from the femoral site is not available, the axillary or brachial arteries may be used for arterial access, depending on the region of interest and the complexity of the contemplated procedure. There are several disadvantages to accessing the arteries of the upper extremity however, and these procedures should be employed only by technicians with appropriate training and experience. Utilization of the upper extremity is less convenient for the patient; when the axillary artery is used for access, patients may experience a significant degree of discomfort. Access to the upper extremity arteries is more difficult because of the smaller size and greater mobility of these vessels; in addition, a cutdown may be required for access to the brachial artery.

The bleeding and thrombotic complications detailed for the femoral access site also occur in arteries of the upper extremity (axillary or brachial). However, thrombosis is relatively more common in these arteries because of their smaller size. Doppler ultrasound screening has demonstrated thrombosis in up to 17% of cannulated brachial arteries.[2] An extensive collateral network exists around both the shoulder and elbow, and thrombosis of the upper extremity arteries may be well tolerated and may even be asymptomatic initially. As these patients again begin to use the upper extremity, however, most experience claudication or hand coolness and discomfort with exercise, resulting in substantial disability. Therefore, if a pulse deficit or other ischemic symptoms suggest thrombosis after cannulation of an upper extremity artery, surgical exploration with thrombectomy and repair of the injured artery are recommended.[40]

Local thrombectomy and brachial artery repair can be easily performed with local anesthesia. In a consecutive series of 532 (1.5%) brachial artery repairs after 34,291 transbrachial cardiac catheterizations at the Cleveland Clinic, 97% of patients were discharged with a normal radial pulse.[23] Delay of operative repair for more than 1 day increased the risk of rethrombosis to 12%, in contrast to 2% in patients treated within 24 hours. Although some practitioners argue against repair of asymptomatic brachial

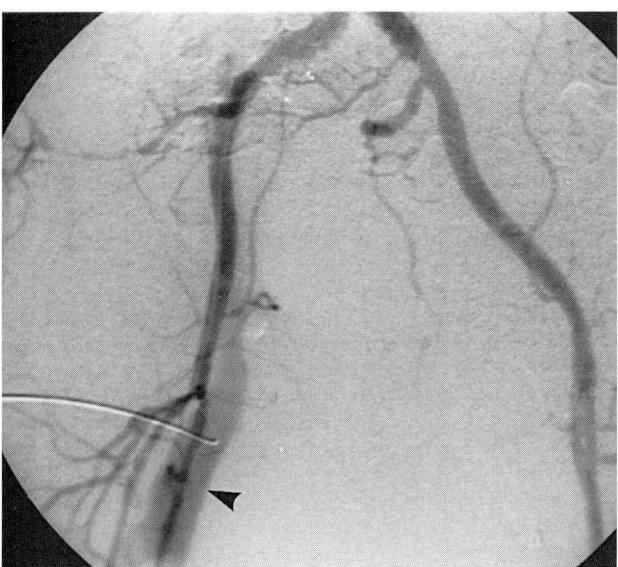

FIGURE 107–4. This angiogram obtained for left lower extremity ischemic symptoms demonstrated an arteriovenous fistula after a cardiac catheterization that had been performed several weeks earlier. A jet of contrast can be seen exiting the right superficial femoral artery and filling the right femoral vein (*arrowhead*). Suture repair of the artery and vein was performed without complication.

artery occlusions, this viewpoint is difficult to defend in light of the late limb disability and the ease of most brachial artery repairs.

Special attention must be paid to axillary puncture sites, where even small amounts of bleeding within the axillary sheath can lead to compression injury of the brachial plexus. After cannulation of the axillary artery, patients should be monitored closely for any neurologic symptoms in the upper extremity. Compression of the brachial plexus usually presents as paresthesias and numbness initially, followed by progression to hand weakness. Because only a small amount of blood can result in compression of the nerves, the access site itself may not be suggestive of bleeding, and other signs such as swelling and mass effect are frequently absent. If neurologic symptoms occur and do not resolve within a very short time, immediate operative exploration of the axillary sheath with release and drainage of the hematoma is mandatory. Chronic neurologic deficit is likely to result if these symptoms are not managed in a timely fashion.

Cannulation of the radial artery is frequently employed for continuous monitoring of systemic blood pressure in the intensive care unit. This procedure is very well tolerated and is rarely problematic. As with any invasive technique

however, complications can occur and should be kept in mind *before* the artery is cannulated. Assessment of collateral circulation to the hand with the Allen test should be routinely performed before placement of a radial artery catheter.

Venous Catheterizations

Cannulation of the central venous system via the internal jugular or subclavian veins remains the most common vascular access procedure. Because of the low pressure in the venous system, bleeding complications from the veins themselves are rare. Rather, complications of these procedures result from injury to adjacent structures. As with all of the procedures mentioned in this chapter, adherence to anatomic landmarks and proper technique can minimize, but can never completely prevent, the development of complications.

The large veins of the neck and upper thorax lie in close proximity to major arterial structures, and inadvertent puncture of the carotid, vertebral, thyrocervical, or subclavian arteries is not uncommon. Finger pressure for 15 to 20 minutes is usually sufficient to prevent continued bleeding, and complications requiring intervention are rare, oc-

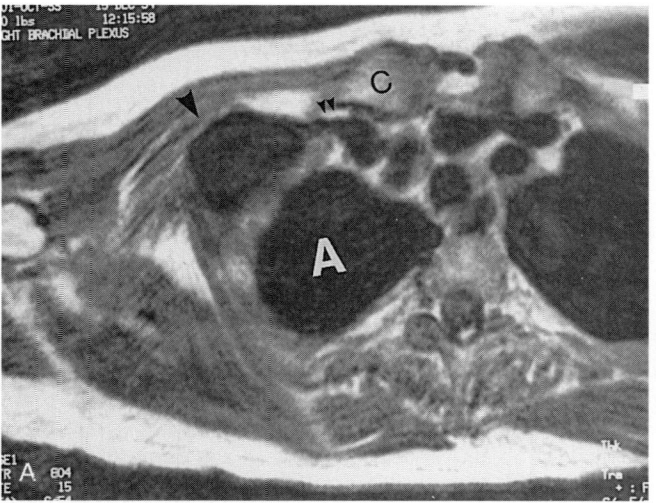
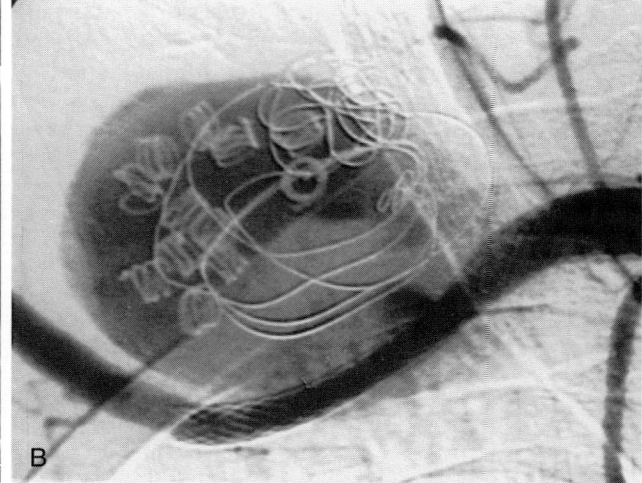
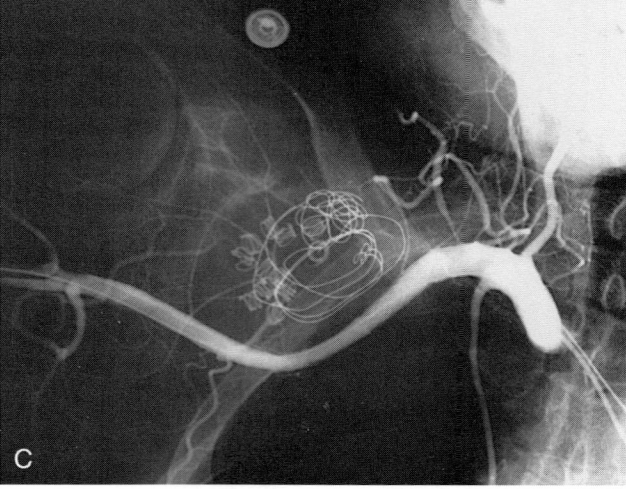

FIGURE 107–5. Pseudoaneurysm of the right subclavian artery following inadvertent puncture of this structure during placement of a temporary hemodialysis catheter. This patient presented with a pulsatile mass and brachial plexopathy several weeks following catheter placement. *A,* Axial magnetic resonance image demonstrating the pseudoaneurysm (*large arrowhead*) arising from the subclavian artery (*small double arrowheads*), beneath the head of the clavicle (C). The proximity of the lung apex (A) to the subclavian vessels can also be appreciated. *B,* Angiogram of the pseudoaneurysm. Attempts to thrombose the pseudoaneurysm via catheter directed delivery of wires and coils and placement of an intraluminal stent were unsuccessful. *C,* Delivery of a covered stent via brachial artery cutdown successfully excluded the aneurysm.

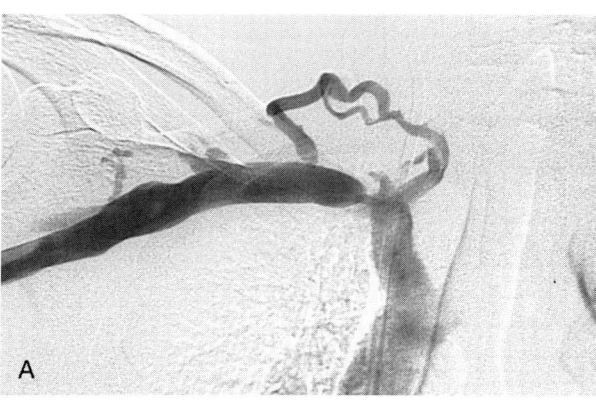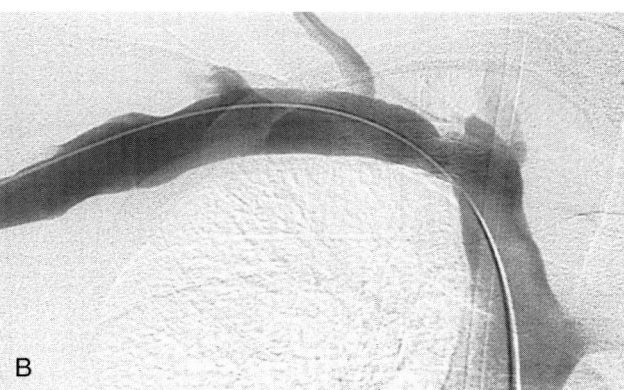

FIGURE 107–6. *A,* Stenotic right subclavian vein following multiple catheterizations for dialysis access. The patient presented with arm swelling and low flows on dialysis. *B,* Balloon angioplasty with stent placement resulted in resolution of arm swelling and salvaged the ipsilateral arteriovenous fistula for continued use in dialysis access.

curring with an incidence of less than 1%. For continued bleeding and pseudoaneurysm formation, however, repair is necessary (Fig. 107–5).[31] Neurologic complications caused by compression of the nearby brachial plexus may be the presenting symptom and are frequently associated with long-term morbidity.[36, 39] Surgical repair calls for considerable technical prowess; in areas where direct surgical exposure is difficult, endovascular repair with covered stents is likely to become the treatment of choice as these techniques and devices become more widely available.[8]

Injury to the visceral pleura may result in the development of a *pneumothorax.* Close examination of a chest radiograph following cannulation of the central veins should reveal a pneumothorax if it is present and should confirm the correct placement of the catheter. A small collection of air may be managed expectantly or treated with percutaneous aspiration. For larger collections, chest tube placement is required.

A *tension pneumothorax* may develop in a small percentage of patients, most frequently in those receiving positive pressure ventilation. A tension pneumothorax is heralded by rapid hemodynamic decompensation. Tube thoracostomy can be life-saving in this situation. Ongoing hemorrhage from the chest tube may indicate subclavian artery injury, which necessitates either direct or endovascular repair.

The most common complication of long-term central venous access is thrombosis of the subclavian vein. In one study, the majority of cancer patients with an indwelling catheter were found to have thrombus in the central veins, although only a small number of these patients were symptomatic.[9] Classically, these patients present with swelling of the upper extremity. This can be quite problematic in patients who continue to require access either for the chronic administration of pharmacologic agents or for hemodialysis. Subclavian vein thrombosis should initially be treated by removal of the offending line. If the subclavian veins are scarred by multiple previous catheters and the patient now has venous hypertension central to a hemoaccess fistula in the arm, balloon angioplasty with or without stenting of the subclavian vein may be attempted. With these techniques, the hemoaccess site can frequently be salvaged (Fig. 107–6).

Swan-Ganz catheters have become commonplace in the intensive care unit, and they are an integral component in the management of complex critically ill patients. These long intravascular catheters have some unique risks associated with their use, in addition to those of other central venous catheters. Ventricular arrhythmias, frequently noted during passage of the catheter through the chambers of the heart, may become symptomatic and require treatment. In some patients with irritable myocardium, arrhythmias persist until the catheter is removed.

The most life-threatening risk of the Swan-Ganz pulmonary artery catheter is perforation of the pulmonary artery with massive hemoptysis. Fortunately, this life-threatening catastrophe is very rare, occurring in about 1 in 1000 pulmonary artery catheter placements.[2] Whenever hemoptysis (>15 to 30 ml) occurs after pulmonary artery catheter insertion, a pulmonary artery perforation should be suspected. The diagnosis can be made by a "wedge angiogram" demonstrating contrast extravasation. A double-lumen endotracheal tube should be placed immediately to facilitate ventilation and prevent aspiration of the noninvolved lung. Emergency pneumonectomy or lobectomy may be life-saving.

REFERENCES

1. Bender JS, Smith-Meek MA, Jones CE: Routine pulmonary artery catheterization does not reduce morbidity and mortality of elective vascular surgery: Results of a prospective, randomized trial. Ann Surg 226:229, 1997.
2. Bergentz SE, Berquist D: Iatrogenic vascular injuries. Berlin, Springer-Verlag, 1989.
3. Bergqvist D, Helfer M, Jensen N, et al: Trends in civilian vascular trauma during 30 years: A Swedish perspective. Acta Chir Scand 153:417, 1987.
4. Birchall D, Fields JM, Chalmers N, et al: Case report: Delayed superficial femoral artery pseudoaneurysm rupture following successful compression therapy. Clin Radiol 52:629, 1997.
5. Boyd R, Saxe A, Phillips E: Effect of patient position upon success in placing central venous catheters. Am J Surg 172:380, 1996.
6. Cambria RA, Farooq MM, Freischlag JA, et al: Endovascular therapy of the iliac arteries: Routine application of endovascular stents does not improve clinical patency. Ann Vasc Surg (Submitted).
7. Cox GS, Young JR, Gray BR, et al: Ultrasound-guided compression repair of postcatheterization pseudoaneurysms: Results of treatment in one hundred cases. J Vasc Surg 19:683, 1994.
8. Criado E, Marston WA, Ligush J, et al: Endovascular repair of periph-

eral aneurysms, pseudoaneurysms, and arteriovenous fistulas. Ann Vasc Surg 11:256, 1997.

9. De Cicco M, Matovic M, Balestreri L, et al: Central venous thrombosis: An early and frequent complication in cancer patients bearing long-term Silastic catheter: A prospective study. Thromb Res 86:101, 1997.

10. Dean SM, Olin JW, Piedmonte M, et al: Ultrasound-guided compression closure of postcatheterization pseudoaneurysms during concurrent anticoagulation: A review of seventy-seven patients. J Vasc Surg 23:28, 1996.

11. dos Santos R, Lamas A, Pereira-Caldas J: Arteriografia da aorta e dos vasos abdominais. Med Contemp 47:93, 1929.

12. Fellmeth BD, Roberts AC, Bookstein JJ, et al: Postangiographic femoral artery injuries: Nonsurgical repair with US-guided compression. Radiology 178:671, 1991.

13. Gualtieri E, Deppe SA, Sipperly ME, et al: Subclavian venous catheterization: Greater success rate for less experienced operators using ultrasound guidance. Crit Care Med 23:692, 1995.

14. Gwechenberger M, Katzenschlager R, Heinz G, et al: Use of a collagen plug versus manual compression for sealing arterial puncture site after cardiac catheterization. Angiology 48:121, 1997.

15. Hajarizadeh H, LaRosa CR, Cardullo P, et al: Ultrasound-guided compression of iatrogenic femoral pseudoaneurysm failure, recurrence, and long-term results. J Vasc Surg 22:425, 1995.

16. Hallett JW, Wolk SW, Cherry KJ, et al: The femoral neuralgia syndrome after arterial catheter trauma. J Vasc Surg 11:702, 1990.

17. Hertz SM, Brener BJ: Ultrasound-guided pseudoaneurysm compression: Efficacy after coronary stenting and angioplasty. J Vasc Surg 26:913, 1997.

18. Johns JP, Pupa LE, Bailey SR: Spontaneous thrombosis of iatrogenic femoral artery pseudoaneurysms: Documentation with color Doppler and two-dimensional ultrasonography. J Vasc Surg 14:24, 1991.

19. Karalis DG, Quinn V, Victor MF, et al: Risk of catheter-related emboli in patients with atherosclerotic debris in the thoracic aorta. Am Heart J 131:1149, 1996.

20. Kazmers A, Meeker C, Nofz K, et al: Nonoperative therapy for postcatheterization femoral artery pseudoaneurysms. Am Surg 63:199, 1997.

21. Kent KC, Moscucci M, Mansour KA, et al: Retroperitoneal hematoma after cardiac catheterization: Prevalence, risk factors, and optimal management. J Vasc Surg 20:905, 1994.

22. Kim D, Orron DE, Skillman JJ, et al: Role of superficial femoral artery puncture in the development of pseudoaneurysm and arteriovenous fistula complicating percutaneous transfemoral cardiac catheterization. Cathet Cardiovasc Diagn 25:91, 1992.

23. Kline RM, Hertzer NR, Beven EG, et al: Surgical treatment of brachial artery injuries after cardiac catheterization. J Vasc Surg 12:20, 1990.

24. Kottke BA, Fairbairn JF, Davis GD: Complications of aortography. Circulation 30:843, 1964.

25. Kresowik TF, Khoury MD, Miller BV, et al: A prospective study of the incidence and natural history of femoral vascular complications after percutaneous transluminal coronary angioplasty. J Vasc Surg 13:328, 1991.

26. Lacy JH, Box JM, Connotes D, et al: Pseudoaneurysm: Diagnosis with color Doppler ultrasound. Cardiovasc Surg 31:727, 1990.

27. Liau CS, Ho FM, Chen MF, et al: Treatment of iatrogenic femoral artery pseudoaneurysm with percutaneous thrombin injection. J Vasc Surg 26:18, 1997.

28. Lilly MP, Reichman W, Sarazen AA, et al: Anatomic and clinical factors associated with complications of transfemoral arteriography. Ann Vasc Surg 4:264, 1990.

29. Messina LM, Brothers TE, Wakefield TW, et al: Clinical characteristics and surgical management of vascular complications in patients undergoing cardiac catheterization: Interventional versus diagnostic procedures. J Vasc Surg 13:593, 1991.

30. Pan M, Medina A, de Lezo JS, et al: Obliteration of femoral pseudoaneurysm complicating coronary intervention by direct puncture and permanent or removable coil insertion. Am J Cardiol 80:786, 1997.

31. Robinson JF, Robinson WA, Cohn A, et al: Perforation of the great vessels during central line placement. Arch Intern Med 155:1225, 1995.

32. Samuels D, Orron DE, Kessler A, et al: Femoral artery pseudoaneurysm: Doppler sonographic features predictive for spontaneous thrombosis. J Clin Ultrasound 25:497, 1997.

33. Schaub F, Theiss W, Busch R, et al: Management of 219 consecutive cases of postcatheterization pseudoaneurysm. J Am Coll Cardiol 30:670, 1997.

34. Seldinger S: Catheter replacement of the needle in percutaneous arteriography. Acta Radiol 39:368, 1953.

35. Skillman JJ, Kim D, Baim DS: Vascular complications of percutaneous femoral cardiac catheterization. Arch Surg 123:1207, 1988.

36. Sustic A, Stancic M, Eskinja N, et al: Iatrogenic pseudoaneurysm of the axillary artery: The role of color Doppler sonography. J Clin Ultrasound 24:323, 1996.

37. Teichgraber UK, Benter T, Gebel M, et al: A sonographically guided technique for central venous access. AJR Am J Roentgenol 169:731, 1997.

38. Toursarkissian B, Allen BT, Petrinec D, et al: Spontaneous closure of selected iatrogenic pseudoaneurysms and arteriovenous fistulae. J Vasc Surg 25:803, 1997.

39. Walden FM: Subclavian aneurysm causing brachial plexus injury after removal of a subclavian catheter. Br J Anesth 79:807, 1997.

40. Walton J, Greenhalgh RM: Brachial artery damage following cardiac catheterization: When to re-explore. Eur J Vasc Surg 4:219, 1990.

41. Weatherford DA, Taylor SM, Langan EM, et al: Ultrasound-guided compression for the treatment of iatrogenic femoral pseudoaneurysms. South Med J 90:223, 1997.

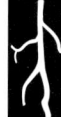

C H A P T E R   1 0 8

Diagnosis of Intestinal Ischemia

Gregory L. Moneta, M.D.

The clinical importance of vascular pain in the abdomen lies in the fact that it may be the precursor of fatal mesenteric vascular occlusion.
— *J. E. Dunphy*

There is surely no greater wisdom than well to time the beginning and onsets of things.
— *Bacon, Essay on "Delay"*

The quotations from Dunphy[1] and Bacon[2] summarize the two most important points in any discussion of intestinal ischemia. First, missed or delayed diagnosis of intestinal ischemia may result in fatal intestinal infarction. Second, even with improved understanding of the pathophysiology of intestinal ischemia and new diagnostic methods, intestinal arterial insufficiency remains primarily a clinical diagnosis that depends on proper performance and interpretation of the history and physical examination.

This section of *Vascular Surgery* focuses on gut ischemia. This chapter emphasizes the diagnosis of the surgically important causes of chronic, acute occlusive, and acute nonocclusive intestinal ischemia caused by arterial insufficiency. The diagnosis of intestinal ischemia caused by venous thrombosis and the treatment of intestinal ischemia are considered in other chapters in this section.

CHRONIC INTESTINAL ISCHEMIA

Differential Diagnosis

A number of conditions may produce chronic intestinal ischemia. These conditions, which may affect large or small arteries, are listed in Table 108–1.[3–19] The majority of cases of chronic intestinal ischemia, however, result from atherosclerotic occlusion or severe stenosis of the proximal (ostial) portion of the axial splanchnic arteries.

Failure to achieve normal postprandial hyperemic intestinal arterial flow is the basic pathophysiologic mechanism of chronic intestinal ischemia. Selected aspects of intestinal

anatomy and physiology are therefore relevant to the diagnosis of chronic intestinal ischemia.

Visceral Atherosclerosis and Collateral Circulation

Symptomatic intestinal ischemia is rare, but atherosclerotic stenosis or occlusion of the intestinal arteries is common. Six per cent to 10% of unselected autopsy specimens demonstrate 50% or greater stenosis of at least one of the three main intestinal arterial trunks.[20] The prevalence of atherosclerosis in visceral arteries increases with age and is higher in patients with other forms of symptomatic peripheral artery atherosclerosis. In one study, 27% of patients undergoing aortography before peripheral vascular surgery were found to have an asymptomatic stenosis of 50% or more of either the celiac artery or the superior mesenteric artery (SMA).[21] These observations illustrate the ability of the visceral arterial circulation to collateralize efficiently under most circumstances.

The importance of the intestinal collateral circulation has

TABLE 108–1. CONDITIONS ASSOCIATED WITH MESENTERIC ISCHEMIA

Visceral artery atherosclerosis	Systemic lupus erythematosus
Neurofibromatosis	
Visceral artery dissection	Polyarteritis nodosa
Fibromuscular hyperplasia	Cogan's syndrome
Buerger's disease	Coarctation repair
Radiation injury	Ergot poisoning
Rheumatoid arthritis	Cocaine abuse

been recognized for more than 100 years. In 1868, the autopsy of a 65-year-old woman revealed complete occlusion of the SMA and the celiac artery. The patient had died of causes unrelated to intestinal circulation. The bowel, which appeared normal, derived its arterial supply from a hypertrophied superior hemorrhoidal artery.[22]

A number of collateral pathways provide intestinal arterial supply when either the celiac artery or the SMA is significantly stenotic or is occluded.[23] When one of these arteries is narrowed and the other remains patent, the pancreaticoduodenal arteries are the most important collateral vessels. With stenosis or occlusion of the SMA, flow proceeds from the hepatic artery to the gastroduodenal artery and into the SMA distribution via the superior and inferior pancreaticoduodenal arteries. Narrowing of the celiac artery in the presence of a patent SMA leads to flow along the same pathway but in the opposite direction (Fig. 108–1).

If both the SMA and the celiac artery are severely diseased, the inferior mesenteric artery (IMA) serves as the source of collateral blood supply to the small intestine and the organs of the upper abdomen. Blood proceeds from the IMA through the arch of Riolan (basically an ascending branch of the left colic artery) to marginal anastomotic arteries and then to the middle colic and pancreaticoduodenal arteries to supply areas normally perfused via the celiac artery or the SMA (Fig. 108–2). The colon can be supplied by flow in the opposite direction when the IMA is occluded and the SMA remains patent. The internal iliac arteries may also serve as collateral sources of intestinal circulation through branches of the IMA contiguous with a patent IMA and marginal and pancreaticoduodenal arteries. When the

IMA is occluded, however, the principal source of collateral circulation to the left colon is the SMA rather than the internal iliac arteries.[24]

Undoubtedly, the ability of the visceral circulation to tolerate atherosclerotic occlusions and stenoses of its major arterial trunks reflects the slow progression of the atherosclerotic process, providing time for the gradual enlargement of collateral circulation pathways. For the rare patient with clinically evident intestinal ischemia, symptoms are not usually present until at least two of the three major splanchnic arteries are highly stenotic or are occluded.[25, 26] Symptoms of chronic intestinal ischemia occasionally result, however, from atherosclerotic occlusion of a single vessel, usually the SMA. This situation can occur in patients who have undergone previous abdominal surgery that has interrupted important collateral vessels. In contrast, isolated narrowing or occlusion of the celiac artery or the IMA is virtually always well tolerated.

Postprandial Intestinal Hyperemia

An appreciation of the dynamic metabolic requirements of the gut is important to an understanding of the pathophysiology of chronic intestinal ischemia. Intestinal arterial blood flow increases markedly after a meal.[27] Postprandial hyperemia varies in duration and magnitude, depending on the size and nutrient composition of the meal as well as on the species studied.[28, 29] Although small changes in intestinal blood flow may occur in anticipation of feeding, the presence of food in the stomach and intestine is required to achieve the greatest magnitude of increase in intestinal blood flow over baseline. Most of this hyperemic flow is

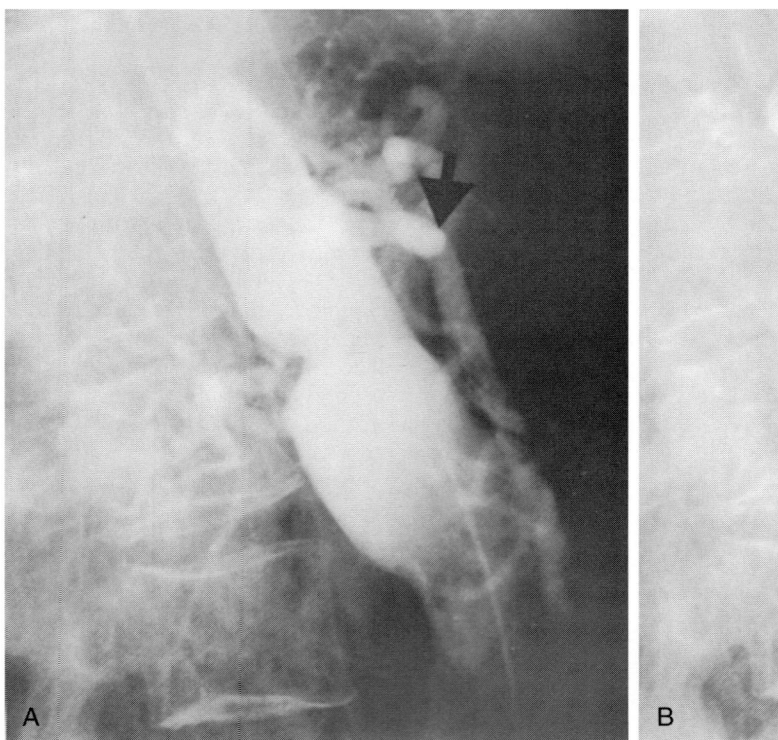
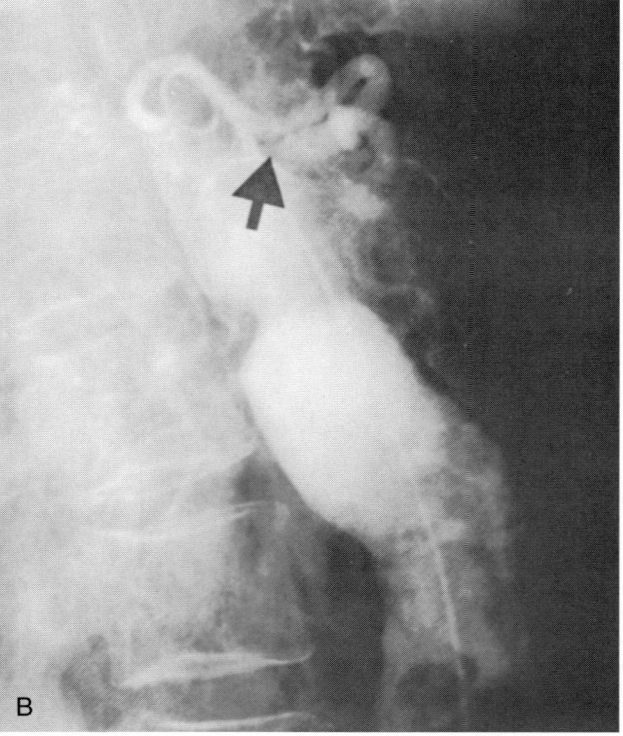

FIGURE 108–1. *A,* In this aortogram from a patient with a juxtarenal aortic aneurysm, the superior mesenteric artery *(arrow)* fills before the celiac artery, suggesting a high-grade celiac artery stenosis. *B,* In a later film from the same injection, the celiac artery lesion is well seen *(arrow)* and little contrast agent remains in the superior mesenteric artery, indicating celiac artery filling via superior mesenteric artery collaterals.

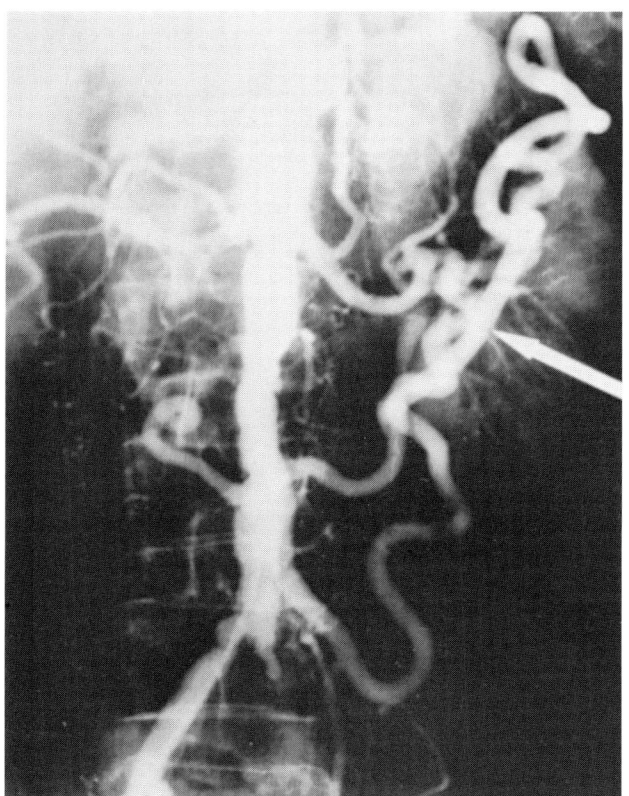

FIGURE 108–2. Angiogram from an asymptomatic patient with proximal occlusion of the celiac and superior mesenteric arteries. The arterial supply to the foregut and mid-gut is via a large collateral vessel of the inferior mesenteric artery, the arch of Riolan (arrow).

distributed to the small intestine and pancreas, with little or no increase in stomach or colonic arterial flow.[30] Total hepatic flow increases, but this change is secondary to an increase in portal venous flow. Hepatic artery flow does not change.[31, 32] In humans, intestinal hyperemia is maximal 30 to 90 minutes after food reaches the intestine. The duration of the hyperemic response is 4 to 6 hours.[29]

The mechanism of postprandial intestinal hyperemia is complex and incompletely understood. Humoral, metabolic, and, possibly, neural factors all appear to participate in its production.[33, 34] Gastrin, secretin, and especially cholecystokinin all clearly mediate postprandial intestinal hyperemia to some extent. Other intestinal hormones, such as neurotensin, glucagon, vasoactive intestinal peptide, substance P, and somatostatin, have also been observed to influence intestinal blood flow when given in pharmacologic doses.[33, 35, 36] Because the various gastrointestinal hormones probably act in a paracrine fashion, these substances may also be of physiologic importance, even though in experiments in animals, large peripheral doses are required to demonstrate an effect on intestinal arterial blood flow.

Duplex ultrasound scanning has provided a means of studying human visceral arterial blood flow regulation in vivo. Duplex scanning–derived SMA waveforms from a fasting subject are usually triphasic, reflecting high vascular resistance of the fasting intestinal circulation.[29, 35, 37, 38]

After feeding, the SMA waveform demonstrates a large increase in end-diastolic velocity, indicating a decrease in intestinal vascular resistance. Systolic velocities also increase significantly.[29, 35, 37] As in animal studies, the intestinal blood flow response depends on the composition of the test meal. Higher blood flow response is seen after a mixed-nutrient meal than after meals of pure protein, fat, or carbohydrate of equal caloric content, osmolality, and volume (Fig. 108–3).[29]

Fasting celiac artery velocity waveforms reflect the relatively low but constant vascular resistance of the splenic and hepatic arterial circulations. Celiac artery waveforms therefore demonstrate higher levels of diastolic flow than SMA waveforms.[39]

Mesenteric Ischemic Pain

Mesenteric ischemic pain represents an imbalance between oxygen supply and oxygen demand. The pain associated with eating in patients with chronic intestinal ischemia is analogous to that of angina pectoris. It is known that the active absorption of nutrients and the greater motor activity of the postprandial bowel require higher intestinal oxygen consumption.[40] The metabolic demands of nutrient absorption and intestinal motility in the setting of significant arterial obstruction may lead to the production of one or many anaerobic metabolic by-products, which may be the source of postprandial pain in patients with chronic intestinal ischemia.

An alternative hypothesis for the abdominal pain of chronic intestinal ischemia has been suggested. It is postulated that in the presence of SMA obstruction, increased blood flow in the distal small intestinal branches is achieved at the expense of flow to the stomach (gastric steal). Reduced gastric blood flow then results in higher gastric acid production, transient peptic ulceration, and abdominal pain.[41] Although the theory is supported by endoscopic observations of superficial gastric ulcerations in some patients with chronic intestinal ischemia, patients with chronic intestinal ischemia have usually been initially treated with histamine H_2-blocking agents or other antiulcer medications without symptom improvement. However, patients with chronic intestinal ischemia who undergo revascularization procedures show a significant increase in gastric mucosal pH compared with preoperative values.[42]

Although intestinal infarction is frequently marked by acidosis, leukocytosis, and hyperamylasemia, these findings are not markers of the reversible ischemic abdominal pain encountered in patients with chronic intestinal ischemia. Currently, abdominal pain in patients with acute or chronic intestinal ischemia without intestinal infarction has not been attributed to any specific metabolite. As a result, no serum or intraluminal marker is currently available to aid definitively in the diagnosis of intestinal ischemia.

Symptoms and Signs

The usual patient with chronic intestinal ischemia is a woman (female:male ratio of 3:1) between 40 and 70 years of age (mean age, 59) who has undergone an extensive evaluation for long-standing abdominal pain.[43] In one series, patients with chronic intestinal ischemia were symptomatic for an average of 18 months before diagnosis.[44]

The pain of chronic intestinal ischemia is mid-abdominal or epigastric and may be described as colicky or as a dull, deep, intense ache occasionally radiating to the back. It

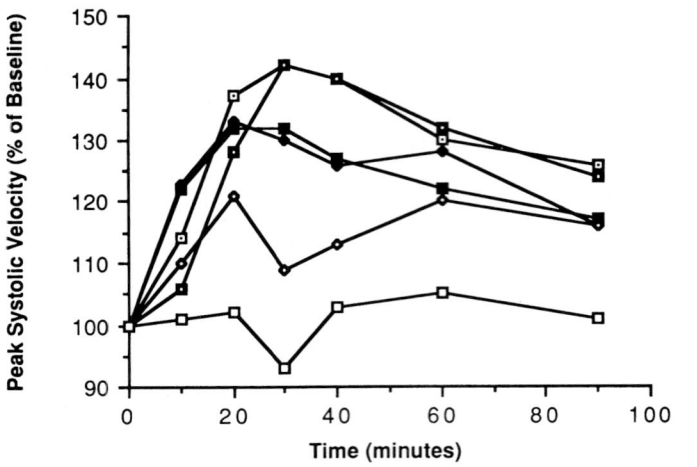

FIGURE 108–3. Increases in superior mesenteric artery duplex scanning–derived peak systolic velocities following equal-caloric test meals of varying compositions, with mannitol and water controls for osmolality and volume. (From Moneta GL, Taylor DC, Helton WS, et al: Duplex ultrasound measurement of postprandial intestinal blood flow: Effect of meal composition. Gastroenterology 95:1294, 1988.)

begins 15 to 30 minutes after eating, lasts 1 to 3 hours (often less), is not associated with signs of peritonitis, and usually varies in intensity with the size of the meal ingested.

Early in the course of chronic intestinal ischemia, patients may consume some meals without pain. Partially because of this feature, as well as the rarity of chronic intestinal ischemia, many physicians mistake the pain of chronic intestinal ischemia for that associated with abdominal malignancy. An ulcer diathesis or cholelithiasis may also be suspected. As the disease progresses, patients gradually come to associate eating with abdominal pain and begin to limit their meals. This fear of food and the resultant weight loss are invariably present in well-established cases of chronic intestinal ischemia. Weight loss is often so great that an advanced and incurable malignancy is diagnosed. Although frequently suspected, malabsorption is not a consistent feature of chronic intestinal ischemia; the weight loss in patients with chronic intestinal ischemia has been shown to result entirely from decreased nutritional intake.[45]

On occasion, severely symptomatic patients with chronic intestinal ischemia complain of constant mild, generalized abdominal discomfort not associated with eating that ultimately disappears with intestinal revascularization. Physical examination reveals no signs of peritonitis or intestinal infarction. Although the discomfort may represent critical resting ischemia or a preintestinal infarction state, this theory has not been proved.

Other than a history of recurring postprandial abdominal pain and weight loss, no symptoms or signs are reliably associated with chronic intestinal ischemia. Physical examination and history most often reveal atherosclerotic involvement of other organ systems, but occasional patients with chronic intestinal ischemia do not have widespread detectable atherosclerosis. Most patients with chronic intestinal ischemia have abdominal bruits, but this finding is so nonspecific that it is not useful. No pattern of bowel evacuation is constant. Diarrhea, constipation, and normal bowel habits have all been described in patients with well-documented chronic intestinal ischemia.

Diagnostic Tests

Diagnostic tests in patients with suspected chronic intestinal ischemia have included tests of intestinal absorptive and excretory function, arteriography, duplex scanning, and

magnetic resonance imaging (MRI) or angiography (MRA) to evaluate visceral artery stenosis noninvasively.

Tests of Intestinal Absorption and Excretion

Tests of intestinal function have not been found useful for diagnosing possible chronic intestinal ischemia. A number have been evaluated. The results are inconsistent and correlate so poorly with the presence of arterial lesions that these tests are not recommended in the evaluation of possible chronic intestinal ischemia.[46]

The most widely publicized test was the measurement of urinary D-xylose levels after oral administration of D-xylose. Urine is collected from the patient for 5 hours after an oral dose of 25 gm of D-xylose. Malabsorption is present if less than 5 gm of D-xylose can be recovered from the urine over 5 hours.[47] A modification of this test involved oral administration of 5 gm of D-xylose, with subsequent hourly determination of blood levels of D-xylose corrected for body surface area.[48] When results are positive, the D-xylose test indicates malabsorption but, unfortunately, not chronic intestinal ischemia.

Arteriography

Arteriography is the primary diagnostic procedure in patients with suspected chronic intestinal ischemia (Fig. 108–4). Lateral and anteroposterior views of the aorta are required to evaluate fully the severity of visceral stenosis and the extent of collateral vessel development. A transfemoral Seldinger technique suffices in most cases. Iliofemoral occlusive disease occasionally necessitates a transaxillary or translumbar approach. Contrast material, 60 to 100 ml, is required for appropriate lateral and anteroposterior views of the abdominal aorta. Because visceral arterial lesions are usually ostial, selective catheterization of the main intestinal arteries is neither necessary nor advisable. Most surgeons prefer full-sized cut films, but intra-arterial digital subtraction techniques are usually adequate for lateral views and require less contrast medium. Arteriography also demonstrates coexisting lesions of the aorta and of the renal and iliac arteries, knowledge of which aids in the planning of revascularization.

Some investigators believe that arteriographically demonstrated visceral artery collateral vessels indicate hemodynamic significance of visceral artery lesions.[49] The presence or absence of demonstrable collateral vessels is not useful, however in ascribing abdominal symptoms to mesenteric ischemia. Poor collateralization may indicate that the visceral artery lesion is either hemodynamically insignificant or poorly compensated. A technically inadequate arteriographic study secondary to poor timing of the contrast injection or injection at sites distal to collateral vessel origins may also explain poor angiographic demonstration of collateral vessels. Extensive collateralization found in association with visceral artery stenosis may reflect either an adequate collateral blood supply to the intestine or a vigorous but insufficient attempt at collateralization. Like peripheral and renal arteriography, visceral arteriography should be regarded as a means of demonstrating lesions that are compatible with arterial insufficiency, not as a means of ascribing symptoms to specific lesions (Fig. 108–5).

Duplex Scanning

Duplex ultrasonography has been advocated as a possible method of identifying high-grade visceral arterial lesions in

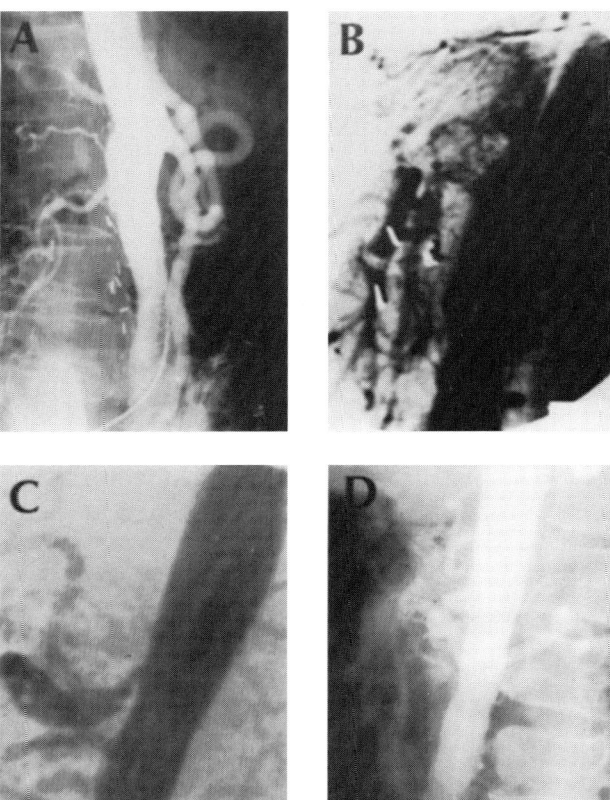

FIGURE 108–5. Lateral aortograms from four different patients demonstrating the often poor correlation between visceral artery stenoses and symptoms of chronic intestinal ischemia. A, Patient with normal celiac and superior mesenteric arteries despite symptoms of weight loss and postprandial abdominal pain. B and C, Despite celiac artery occlusion and superior mesenteric artery occlusion in B and superior mesenteric artery occlusion with high-grade celiac artery stenosis in C, both patients were asymptomatic. D, Patient with severe chronic mesenteric ischemia relieved by visceral artery bypass. (A–D, From Moneta GL: Diagnosis of chronic intestinal ischemia. Semin Vasc Surg 3:176, 1990.)

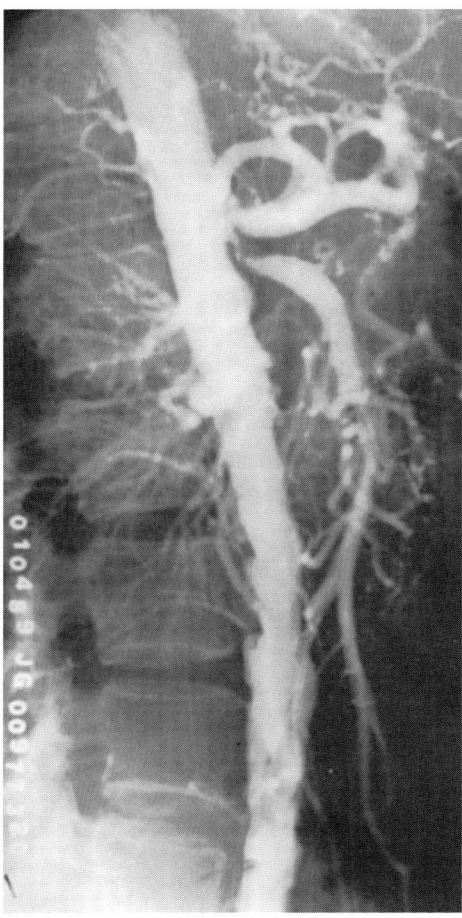

FIGURE 108–4. Lateral aortogram demonstrating high-grade stenoses of the celiac and superior mesenteric arteries. Symptoms of postprandial abdominal pain were relieved with splanchnic artery bypass. (From Moneta GL: Diagnosis of chronic intestinal ischemia. Semin Vasc Surg 3:176, 1990.)

patients thought to have chronic intestinal ischemia (Fig. 108–6).[50–52] Some investigators have speculated that the availability of a noninvasive method of screening patients for possible visceral artery stenosis would lead to earlier diagnosis of chronic intestinal ischemia in selected patients. Given the small numbers of patients with recognized chronic intestinal ischemia, the number of patients with chronic intestinal ischemia thus far studied with duplex scanning is small. Investigators have therefore focused on developing criteria for duplex scanning detection of high-grade celiac artery and SMA stenosis.

The first duplex scanning criteria for splanchnic artery stenosis were proposed in 1991.[52] Investigators at the Oregon Health Sciences University retrospectively reviewed 34 lateral aortograms and correlated them with splanchnic artery duplex scans. On the basis of these data, an SMA peak systolic velocity of greater than 275 cm/sec and a celiac artery peak systolic velocity of greater than 200 cm/sec appeared to be good predictors of 70% stenosis of the SMA and the celiac artery, respectively.

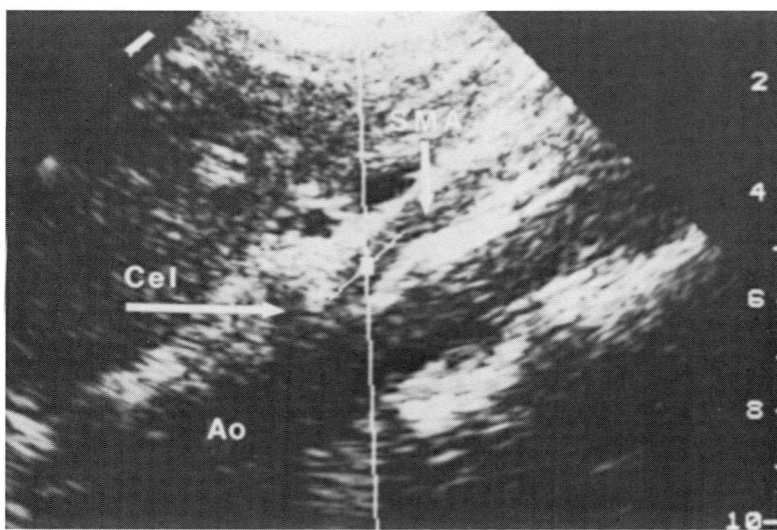

FIGURE 108–6. B-mode ultrasound image of the abdominal aorta (Ao). The celiac (Cel) and superior mesenteric (SMA) arteries are shown.

These retrospectively derived criteria were subsequently evaluated in a blinded, prospective study of 100 patients undergoing visceral artery duplex scanning and lateral aortography.[53] The results of this study showed that either a fasting SMA peak systolic velocity higher than 275 cm/sec or no flow signal predicted more than 70% angiographic stenosis with a sensitivity of 92%, a specificity of 96%, a positive predictive value of 80%, and a negative predictive value of 99%. For the ability of a fasting celiac artery peak systolic velocity of greater than 200 cm/sec to predict 70% angiographic stenosis in the celiac artery, the values were 87%, 80%, 63%, and 94%, respectively (Fig. 108–7).

Other investigators have proposed end-diastolic velocity criteria for detecting SMA stenosis. On the basis of retrospective data, it has been suggested that an SMA end-diastolic velocity higher than 45 cm/sec is predictive of 50% angiographic SMA stenosis.[54] A second study from the same institution confirmed the ability of an end-diastolic velocity higher than 45 cm/sec to identify a greater than 50% SMA stenosis.[55] Reversal of the normal flow direction in the hepatic and splenic arteries also appears to provide an important indirect clue to the presence of a high-grade stenosis or occlusion of the celiac axis.[56] It is also possible to examine the IMA with duplex scanning in more than 90% of patients with vascular disease.[57] To date, however, there are no large prospective studies assessing the accuracy of duplex scanning in detecting and quantifying IMA stenosis or occlusion.

Duplex scanning of the splanchnic arteries is technically demanding, with respiratory motion, depth of the vessels, and intra-abdominal gas all combining to make insonation of the visceral arteries difficult. Indeed, even with careful patient preparation (overnight fast, morning examinations, and pre-examination oral simethicone), the vessels cannot always be satisfactorily visualized. It is also critical to perform the examination with the Doppler angle as near as possible to 60 degrees. Doppler angles of more than 70 degrees result in falsely elevated peak systolic velocities and therefore contribute to false-positive results.[58]

As is true with arteriography, ascribing a patient's symptoms to visceral artery stenoses detected by duplex scanning is not advisable. Intestinal blood flow studies using indocyanine green have suggested that total intestinal blood flow does not increase following a test meal in patients with abdominal angina.[59] Because it is known that SMA peak systolic velocity and end-diastolic velocity normally increase after feeding (see Fig. 108–3),[29, 37] it has been suggested that preprandial versus postprandial SMA and celiac blood flow velocities determined by duplex scanning might aid in detecting splanchnic artery stenoses or confirming a diagnosis of chronic intestinal ischemia.[60] A prospective study of 25 control patients and 80 patients with vascular disease, including nine with 70% to 99% SMA stenosis concluded that SMA peak systolic velocities were higher and increased less postprandially in patients with greater than 70% to 99% SMA stenosis than in control patients and patients with vascular disease who had less than 70% SMA stenosis.

Failure of SMA peak systolic velocity to rise with feeding, however, did not substantially increase the ability of duplex scanning to detect high-grade SMA stenosis over that of fasting studies alone.[61] Failure of SMA blood flow to increase with feeding has also not been proven to be a confirmatory test for chronic intestinal ischemia. Certainly, there may be greater postprandial flow to the intestine via collateral vessels without significant increases in proximal SMA flow. Duplex scanning has detected increased postprandial flow within the hypertrophied IMA after a test meal in patients with both SMA and celiac artery occlusion.[62] Therefore, although visceral artery duplex scanning clearly can be used to demonstrate mesenteric postprandial blood flow changes, it currently cannot be used to distinguish physiologically appropriate from inadequate blood flow responses. No true "stress test" of the intestinal circulation with definite end-points currently exists.

MAGNETIC RESONANCE TECHNIQUES

Magnetic resonance techniques are now under evaluation as alternative methods for noninvasive evaluation of patients with possible chronic mesenteric ischemia. These techniques are not yet routinely used in clinical practice

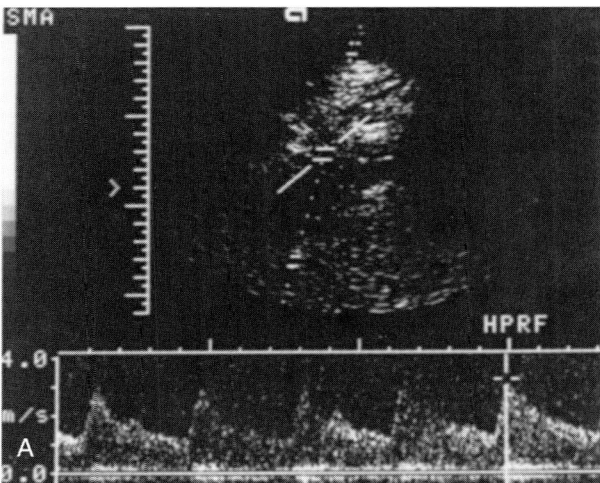

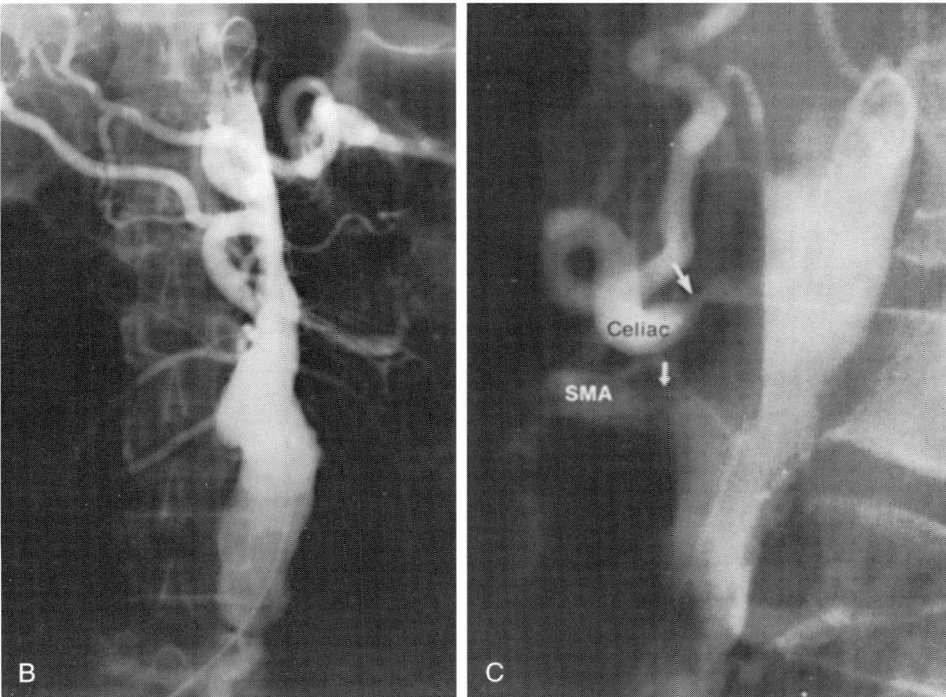

FIGURE 108–7. *A,* The Doppler sample volume is positioned in the proximal portion of the superior mesenteric artery (SMA) in this patient with persistent postprandial abdominal pain following repair of a thoracic aortic dissection. The greater than 300 cm/sec peak systolic velocity indicates a more than 70% diameter reducing superior mesenteric artery stenosis. *B* and *C,* Anteroposterior and lateral aortograms confirm the presence of splanchnic artery stenosis. Not demonstrated is the patient's 8-cm infrarenal aortic aneurysm. Postprandial abdominal pain was relieved by aneurysm repair coupled with superior mesenteric artery bypass.

but are theoretically attractive. Limitations of duplex scanning, such as operator dependence, bowel gas, and difficult body habitus, are largely circumvented with MR techniques. In addition to the generation of MR angiograms, MRI has been used to demonstrate postprandial retrograde flow in the SMA in a patient with symptoms of chronic mesenteric ischemia and an 80% SMA stenosis.[63]

Postprandial hyperemia in the superior mesenteric vein (SMV) has also been studied with phase contrast cine MRI. This technique combines flow-dependent phase contrast MRI with the ability to produce images throughout the cardiac cycle. In a study comparing asymptomatic volunteers and patients with symptoms of chronic mesenteric ischemia, postprandial augmentation of peak flow in the SMV was significantly less in the symptomatic patients.[64] Perhaps measurement of postprandial SMV blood flow will prove to be a useful discriminatory technique in assessing the adequacy of overall splanchnic arterial inflow.

CELIAC AXIS COMPRESSION SYNDROME

External compression of the celiac artery by the median arcuate ligament of the diaphragm has been reported to result in a variant of chronic intestinal ischemia.[65, 66] Diaphragmatic compression of the celiac axis is frequently reversible and varies with respiration. During inspiration, the aorta and the celiac axis move downward with the abdominal viscera, whereas in expiration, the vessels move upward to result in maximal external compression (Fig. 108–8). Reversible celiac axis compression can be demonstrated with both angiography and duplex scanning in many asymptomatic individuals.[67] Indeed, autopsy studies have indicated that the median arcuate ligament significantly compresses the celiac axis in up to one third of persons.[68] Patients described as having symptomatic celiac

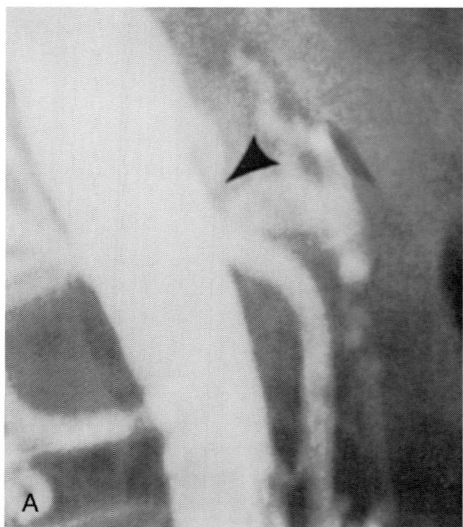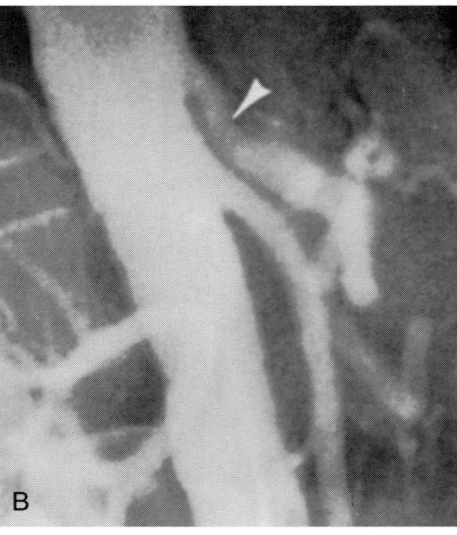

FIGURE 108–8. Lateral aortograms showing extrinsic compression of the celiac artery (*arrowhead*) in expiration (*A*) and compression relief with deep inspiration (*B*).

axis compression have manifested poorly defined symptoms and signs. These include cramping epigastric pain that changes with body position, nausea, vomiting, and diarrhea. Many patients treated surgically have had a known psychiatric disorder or a history of substance abuse or have undergone previous abdominal surgery. In only one third of patients was the abdominal pain clearly postprandial. Weight loss was often not present.[69]

Postprandial studies of the celiac artery using duplex scanning demonstrate little if any increase in celiac artery blood flow following a test meal.[29] This finding is inconsistent with the concept of isolated celiac artery occlusive disease or external compression of the celiac artery producing postprandial abdominal pain solely on the basis of impaired celiac artery blood flow. Some investigators have argued that angiographically demonstrated celiac artery compression is simply a marker of excessive celiac ganglion splanchnic nerve fiber entrapment. In this theory, pain relief with decompression of the celiac artery results not from improvement in postprandial flow but from destruction of the splanchnic nerves during the surgical exposure of the artery.[70]

Given the nonspecific nature of this syndrome and the inconsistent surgical results reported for celiac artery decompression, Reilly and colleagues evaluated the experience at the University of California, San Francisco.[71] They subsequently developed a group of positive and negative criteria believed to predict good relief of symptoms with celiac axis decompression:

- Female gender
- Postprandial pain
- Age 40 to 60 years
- Weight loss of more than 20 pounds
- Absence of a psychiatric or drug abuse history
- Arteriographic findings of celiac artery compression with post-stenotic dilatation or collateral flow

Symptomatic external compression of the visceral vessels is possible. A well-documented case reported by Lawson and Ochsner of concurrent celiac artery and SMA compression serves as an example.[72] It is obvious, however that isolated symptomatic celiac artery compression has an un-

certain pathophysiology. The diagnosis remains one of exclusion and should be made only with very careful deliberation. Only a single case, with unclear surgical benefit, has come to operation at the author's institution in the last 20 years. During the same period, more than 85 operations have been performed for symptomatic atherosclerotic occlusive disease of the celiac artery or the SMA.

OCCLUSIVE ACUTE INTESTINAL ISCHEMIA

Acute intestinal ischemia is defined as a sudden, symptomatic reduction in intestinal blood flow of sufficient magnitude to potentially result in intestinal infarction. In this part of the chapter, the term means abrupt occlusion of the proximal portion of a major splanchnic arterial trunk. The diagnosis of *nonocclusive* acute intestinal ischemia is discussed later in this chapter.

Acute intestinal ischemia is usually caused by embolism of organized thrombi to the SMA or from its thrombotic occlusion. Acute intestinal ischemia has, however, been reported to occur (1) from thrombotic emboli to the celiac trunk,[73] (2) from tumor emboli,[74] and (3) from iatrogenically induced cholesterol emboli. SMA thrombosis usually occurs as an end result of proximal SMA atherosclerotic stenosis and can be regarded as a complication of untreated chronic intestinal ischemia.

The mortality rate for occlusive acute intestinal ischemia exceeds 70% in most series.[75, 76] Occlusive acute intestinal ischemia secondary to SMA embolism has a more favorable prognosis than that resulting from SMA thrombosis. Survival following acute intestinal ischemia due to SMA thrombosis is, in fact, quite uncommon. The more favorable prognosis with embolism results from the fact that emboli characteristically lodge distally in the SMA (beyond the origin of the middle colic artery), thus allowing partial perfusion of the proximal intestine via middle colic and jejunal artery branches. Thrombotic occlusion of the SMA occurs proximal to the middle colic artery and therefore virtually totally interrupts mid-gut arterial perfusion in patients with poorly developed celiac artery or IMA collateral flow.

Clinical Presentation

Approximately two thirds of patients with acute intestinal ischemia are women. The median age is 70 years. Abdominal pain is present in all cases of acute intestinal ischemia. The nature, location, and duration of the pain vary. The usual presentation is sudden onset of steady abdominal pain referred to the anterior abdomen that is of sufficient severity that the patient usually seeks immediate medical attention. Presentation may be delayed for up to several days, however, and the pain may be felt most severely in the epigastrium or suprapubic areas. Interestingly, the duration of symptoms does not appear to correlate with the reversibility of intestinal injury.[75]

Physical examination usually reveals at least some degree of abdominal distention. Vomiting is present in more than half the patients, and diarrhea in about one third. The presence or absence of bowel sounds is not of any significant diagnostic value. Signs of peritoneal irritation are frequently striking by their absence; this is a well-known feature of acute intestinal ischemia, referred to as "pain out of proportion to physical findings." Occult gastric or rectal blood is found in 25% of patients.[75]

Laboratory Evaluation

Routine laboratory evaluation is not helpful. Most patients have a moderate to marked leukocytosis, but about 10% have a normal white blood cell count (<10,000/mm³). Serum amylase levels are mildly but not strikingly elevated in about 50% of patients.[75–77] Plain abdominal radiographs usually reveal only distended loops of bowel.

A number of serum markers have been evaluated as potentially useful diagnostic aids early in the course of acute intestinal ischemia. They include familiar seromuscular enzymes, such as lactic dehydrogenase, creatine phosphokinase, and alkaline phosphatase as well as hexosaminidase and serum phosphate.[78–82] Their low specificity and failure to identify acute intestinal ischemia before the development of intestinal infarction have limited their clinical utility. Because the intestinal mucosa is most sensitive to ischemia and the intestine can survive with ischemia-induced mucosal sloughing, enzymes such as diamine oxidase, which is present primarily in intestinal mucosa, have also been evaluated as suitable early serum markers in patients with acute intestinal ischemia.[83] Unfortunately, intestinal mucosal enzymes offer no advantage in detection over the seromuscular enzymes noted earlier. As with chronic intestinal ischemia, thus far no reliable serum marker for acute intestinal ischemia has been found.

Arteriography

The proper use of arteriography in the diagnosis of acute intestinal ischemia is controversial. Preoperative arteriography requires time and can result in unnecessary delay before laparotomy. Advocates suggest that liberal use of arteriography in patients with abdominal pain and possible acute intestinal ischemia may actually result in a more rapid diagnosis of acute intestinal ischemia by identifying

patients with acute abdominal pain who have visceral artery occlusions.[84] In addition, arteriography may help avoid operation in some patients without peritoneal signs, because intestinal ischemia resulting from nonocclusive causes (see later) and occasionally from both proximal and distal SMA embolism has been treated successfully with systemic anticoagulation or the selective infusion of vasodilating agents into the SMA.[85, 86] At the time of laparotomy, knowledge of the extent and distribution of atherosclerosis, emboli, or both, in the abdominal vasculature aids in the performance of optimal revascularization.

No randomized trial of patients with acute intestinal ischemia managed with and without preoperative arteriography exists, nor is one ever likely to be performed. The decision to employ arteriography in patients with possible acute intestinal ischemia before emergency laparotomy is best made on a case-by-case basis. Patients whose clinical history suggests embolic or thrombotic SMA occlusion rather than nonocclusive intestinal ischemia and who truly present acutely, so that there is a real possibility of saving threatened but not infarcted intestine, are probably best managed with prompt operation by a surgeon capable of rapidly correcting either embolic or thrombotic occlusion of the SMA. Patients who have a more delayed presentation or who are likely to have nonocclusive mesenteric ischemia (discussed later) should be considered for angiography before laparotomy. In such cases, the potential advantages of the added information provided by angiography probably outweigh the risk of further intestinal infarction resulting from the time required to perform angiography.

Ultrasonography

Duplex scanning is a theoretically attractive and more rapid alternative to angiography in patients with abdominal pain and possible acute intestinal ischemia. The technical limitations of duplex scanning imposed by abdominal distention and excessive intraluminal gas, however, make it less useful in patients with possible acute intestinal ischemia than in those examined for possible chronic intestinal ischemia.

NONOCCLUSIVE MESENTERIC ISCHEMIA

Acute intestinal ischemia may occur without actual occlusion of the mesenteric vessels, a condition termed "nonocclusive mesenteric ischemia." Infarction of the intestine in the absence of arterial or venous occlusion has been documented in the American medical literature since 1943.[87] The cause of this condition is severe and prolonged intestinal arterial spasm to the point that infarction occurs. Although a hypoperfusion state is present in most patients with nonocclusive mesenteric ischemia, some have nonocclusive mesenteric ischemia from visceral vasoconstriction alone, as is the case with cocaine or ergot intoxication.[14, 15]

The largest proportion of patients with nonocclusive mesenteric ischemia have severe cardiac failure.[88–90] The precise circumstances surrounding the cardiac decompensation are not as important as the associated hypoperfusion itself. Nonocclusive mesenteric ischemia is clearly associated with acute exacerbation of chronic congestive heart failure and acute congestive heart failure following myocardial infarction. Many cases have appeared in patients who have had cardiac surgery and whose postoperative course was marked by prolonged vasopressor dependency.[91-93] Nonocclusive mesenteric ischemia has also been reported as a complication of gastroenteritis, pneumonia, hemoconcentration, spinal shock, perforated appendicitis, and placenta previa.[89, 94, 95]

Many patients with nonocclusive mesenteric ischemia have received long-term treatment with digitalis preparations.[90] In animal experiments, baseline intestinal arterial resistance is not altered by digitalis; however, arterial resistance in animals treated with digitalis is higher in response to intestinal venous hypertension compared with that in controls not given digitalis.[96] Thus, a patient given digitalis with increases in portal pressure, such as occurs with worsening heart failure, may be more susceptible to nonocclusive mesenteric ischemia as a result of arterial mesenteric vasoconstriction. The availability and preferential use of medications other than digitalis for the treatment of congestive heart failure may in part explain the anecdotal impression of many clinicians that the incidence of nonocclusive mesenteric ischemia is decreasing.

No findings on physical examination or laboratory evaluation can confirm the diagnosis of nonocclusive mesenteric ischemia. With the exception of the presence of a preexisting shock state induced by severe cardiac or multisystem organ failure, the signs and symptoms of nonocclusive mesenteric ischemia are similar to those encountered in patients with the occlusive forms of acute mesenteric ischemia discussed previously. The diagnosis is often delayed because patients afflicted with this disease are generally severely ill, making history and physical examination more difficult. Nonocclusive mesenteric ischemia should therefore be considered in severely ill patients who demonstrate further deterioration accompanied by any new signs or symptoms referable to the abdomen.

Arteriography is required to confirm the diagnosis, which can be confirmed by the demonstration of patent mesenteric arterial trunks with tapering spastic narrowing of the visceral artery branches. Arteriography may also be used for therapy in many patients.[85] It should be liberally employed in seriously ill patients with a clinical picture suggestive of acute intestinal ischemia.

REFERENCES

1. Dunphy JE: Abdominal pain of vascular origin. Am J Med 192:109, 1936.
2. Cope Z: The Early Diagnosis of the Acute Abdomen, 14th ed. London, Oxford University Press, 1972.
3. Snyder MS, Mahoney EB, Rob CG: Symptomatic celiac artery stenosis due to constriction by the neurofibrous tissue of the celiac ganglion. Surgery 61:372, 1967.
4. Krupski WC, Effency DJ, Ehrenfeld WK: Spontaneous dissection of the superior mesenteric artery. J Vasc Surg 2:731, 1985.
5. Ripley HR, Levin SR: Abdominal angina associated with fibromuscular hyperplasia of the celiac and superior mesenteric arteries. Angiology 17:297, 1966.
6. Wylie EJ, Binkley FM, Palubinskas AJ: Extrarenal fibromuscular hyperplasia. Am J Surg 112:149, 1966.
7. Wolf EA, Sumner DS, Strandness DE Jr: Disease of the mesenteric circulation in patients with thromboangiitis obliterans. Vasc Surg 6:218, 1972.
8. Deucker H, Hison-Holmdahl K, Lunderquist A, et al: Mesenteric angiography in patients with radiation injury of the bowel after pelvis irradiation. AJR 114:476, 1972.
9. Williams LF Jr: Vascular insufficiency of the intestines. Gastroenterology 61:757, 1971.
10. McCauley RL, Johnston MR, Fauci AS: Surgical aspects of systemic necrotizing vasculitis. Surgery 97:104, 1985.
11. LaRaja RD: Cogan syndrome associated with mesenteric vascular insufficiency. Arch Surg 111:1028, 1976.
12. Sealy WC: Indications for surgical treatment of coarctation of the aorta. Surg Gynecol Obstet 97:301, 1953.
13. Mays ET, Sergeant CK: Postcoarctectomy syndrome. Arch Surg 91:58, 1965.
14. Green FL, Ariyan S, Stausel HC Jr: Mesenteric and peripheral vascular ischemia secondary to ergotism. Surgery 81:176, 1977.
15. Myers SI, Clagett GP, Valentine RJ, et al: Chronic intestinal ischemia caused by intravenous cocaine use: Report of two cases and review of the literature. J Vasc Surg 23:724, 1996.
16. Heresbach D, Pagenault M, Gueret P, et al: Leiden factor V mutation in four patients with small bowel infarctions. Gastroenterology 113:322, 1997.
17. Battarbee HD, Grisham MB, Johnson GG, et al: Superior mesenteric artery blood flow and indomethacin-induced intestinal injury and inflamation. Am J Physiol 271:G605, 1996.
18. Golino A, Crawford EM, Gathe JC, et al: Recurrent small bowel infarction associated with antithrombin deficiency. Am J Gastroenterol 92:323, 1997.
19. Hsiao C-H, Lee W-I, Chang S-L, et al: Angiocentric T-cell lymphoma of the intestine: A distinct etiology of ischemic bowel disease. Gastroenterology 110:985, 1996.
20. Croft RJ, Menon GP, Marston A: Does intestinal angina exist? A critical study of obstructed visceral arteries. Br J Surg 68:316, 1981.
21. Valentine RJ, Martin JD, Myers SI, et al: Asymptomatic celiac and superior mesenteric artery stenoses are more prevalent among patients with unsuspected renal artery stenoses. J Vasc Surg 14:195, 1991.
22. Chiene J: Complete obliteration of the celiac and mesenteric arteries. J Anat Physiol 3:65, 1869.
23. Olofsson PA, Connelly DP, Stoney RJ: Surgery of the celiac and mesenteric arteries. In Haimovici H (ed): Vascular Surgery: Principles and Techniques. Norwalk, Conn, Appleton Lange, 1989, p 750.
24. Iliopoulos JI, Pierce GE, Hermreck AS, et al: Hemodynamics of the inferior mesenteric arterial circulation. J Vasc Surg 11:120, 1990.
25. Mikkelsen WP, Berne CJ: Intestinal angina: Its surgical significance. Am J Surg 94:262, 1957.
26. Hansen HJB: Abdominal angina. Acta Chir Scand 142:319, 1976.
27. Fara JW: Postprandial mesenteric hyperemia. In Shephard AP, Granger DN (eds): Physiology of the Intestinal Circulation. New York, Raven Press, 1984, p 99.
28. Siregar H, Chou CC: Relative contribution of fat, protein, carbohydrate and ethanol to intestinal hyperemia. Am J Physiol 242:G27, 1982.
29. Moneta GL, Taylor DC, Helton WS, et al: Duplex ultrasound measurement of postprandial intestinal blood flow: Effect of meal composition. Gastroenterology 95:1294, 1988.
30. Bond JH, Prentiss RA, Levitt MD: The effects of feeding on blood flow to the stomach, small bowel, and colon of the conscious dog. J Lab Clin Med 93:594, 1979.
31. Dobson A, Barnes RJ, Comeline RS: Changes in the sources of hepatic portal blood flow with feeding in the sheep. Physiologist 24:15, 1981.
32. Gallavan RH, Chou CC, Kvietys PR, et al: Regional blood flow during digestion in the conscious dog. Am J Physiol 238:H220, 1980.
33. Chou CC, Mangino MJ, Sawmiller DR: Gastrointestinal hormones and intestinal blood flow. In Shephard AP, Granger DN (eds): Physiology of the Intestinal Circulation. New York, Raven Press, 1984, p 121.
34. Greenway CV: Neural control and autoregulatory escape. In Shephard AP, Granger DN (eds): Physiology of the Intestinal Circulation. New York, Raven Press, 1984, p 61.
35. Lilly MP, Harwood TRS, Flinn WR, et al: Duplex ultrasound measurement of changes in mesenteric flow velocity with pharmacologic and physiologic alteration of intestinal blood flow in man. J Vasc Surg 9:18, 1989.
36. Mulholland MW, Sarpa MS, Delvalle J, et al: Splanchnic and cerebral vasodilatory effects of calcitonin gene related peptide I in humans. Ann Surg 214:440, 1991.
37. Jager K, Bollinger A, Valli C, et al: Measurement of mesenteric blood flow by duplex scanning. J Vasc Surg 3:462, 1986.
38. Quamar MI, Read AE, Skidmore R, et al: Transcutaneous Doppler

ultrasound measurement of superior mesenteric artery blood flow in man. Gut 27:100, 1986.

39. Quamar MI, Read AE, Skidmore R, et al: Transcutaneous Doppler ultrasound measurement of coeliac axis blood flow in man. Br J Surg 72:391, 1985.

40. Chou CC: Relationship between intestinal blood flow and motility. Ann Rev Physiol 44:29, 1982.

41. Poole JW, Sammartano RJ, Boley SJ: Hemodynamic basis of pain of chronic mesenteric ischemia. Am J Surg 153:171, 1987.

42. Fiddian-Green RG, Stanley JC, Nostrant T, et al: Chronic gastric ischemia: A cause of abdominal pain or bleeding identified from the presence of gastric mucosal acidosis. J Cardiovasc Surg 30:852, 1989.

43. Olofsson PA, Connelly DP, Stoney RJ: Surgery of the celiac and mesenteric arteries. In Haimovici H (ed): Vascular Surgery: Principles and Techniques. Norwalk, Conn, Appleton Lange, 1989, p 750.

44. Schneider PA, Ehrenfeld WK, Cunningham CG, et al: Recurrent chronic visceral ischemia. J Vasc Surg (in press).

45. Marston A, Clarke JMF, Garcia J, et al: Intestinal function and intestinal blood supply. Gut 26:656, 1985.

46. Marston A: Chronic intestinal ischemia. In Vascular Disease of the Gastrointestinal Tract: Pathophysiology, Recognition and Management. Baltimore, Williams & Wilkins, 1986, p 116.

47. Farmer RG: Tests for intestinal absorption. In Brown CH (ed): Diagnostic Procedures in Gastroenterology. St. Louis, CV Mosby, 1967, p 143.

48. Haeney MR, Culank LS, Montgomery RD, et al: Evaluation of xylose absorption as measured in blood and urine: A one hour blood xylose screening test in malabsorption. Gastroenterology 75:393, 1978.

49. Pollak AA, Beckmann CF: Angiographic diagnosis of visceral vascular disease. In Persson AV, Skudder PA Jr (eds): Visceral Vascular Surgery. New York, Marcel Dekker, 1987, p 17.

50. Nicholls SC, Kohler TR, Martin RL, et al: Use of hemodynamic parameters in the diagnosis of mesenteric insufficiency. J Vasc Surg 3:507, 1986.

51. Taylor DC, Moneta GL: Duplex ultrasound scanning of the renal and mesenteric circulations. Semin Vasc Surg 1:23, 1988.

52. Moneta GL, Yeager RA, Dalman R, et al: Duplex ultrasound criteria for diagnosis of splanchnic artery stenosis or occlusion. J Vasc Surg 14:511, 1991.

53. Lee RW, Moneta GL, Yeager RA, et al: Mesenteric artery duplex scanning: A blinded, prospective study. J Vasc Surg 17:79, 1993.

54. Bowersox JC, Zwalak RM, Walsh DB, et al: Duplex ultrasonography in the diagnosis of celiac and mesenteric artery occlusive disease. J Vasc Surg 14:780, 1991.

55. Zwolak RM, Fillinger MF, Walsh DB, et al. Mesenteric and celiac duplex scanning: A validation study. J Vasc Surg 27:1078, 1998.

56. LaBombard FE, Musson A, Bowersox JC, et al: Hepatic artery duplex as an adjunct in the evaluation of chronic mesenteric ischemia. J Vasc Tech 16:7, 1992.

57. Denys AL, Lafortune M, Aubin B, et al: Doppler sonography of the inferior mesenteric artery: A preliminary study. J Ultrasound Med 14:435, 1995.

58. Rizzo RJ, Sandager G, Astleford P, et al: Mesenteric flow velocities as a function of angle of insonation. J Vasc Surg 11:688, 1990.

59. Hansen HJB, Engell HC, Ring-Larsen H: Splanchnic blood flow in patients with abdominal angina before and after arterial reconstruction: A proposal for a diagnostic test. Ann Surg 186:216, 1977.

60. Muller AF: Role of duplex Doppler ultrasound in the assessment of patients with postprandial abdominal pain. Gut 33:460, 1992.

61. Gentile AT, Moneta GL, Lee RW, et al: Usefulness of fasting and postprandial duplex ultrasound examinations for predicting high-grade superior mesenteric artery stenosis. Am J Surg 169:476, 1995.

62. Moneta GL, Cummings C, Castor J, et al: Duplex ultrasound demonstration of postprandial mesenteric hyperemia in splanchnic circulation collateral vessels. J Vasc Tech 15:37, 1991.

63. Li KCP, Whitney WS, McDonnell CH, et al: Chronic mesenteric ischemia: Evaluation with phase-contrast cine MR imaging. Radiology 190:175, 1994.

64. Burkart DJ, Johnson CD, Reading CC, et al: MR measurements of mesenteric venous flow: Prospective evaluation in healthy volunteers and patients with suspected chronic mesenteric ischemia. Radiology 194:801, 1995.

65. Curl JH, Thompson NW, Stanley JC: Medial arcuate ligament compression of the celiac and superior mesenteric arteries. Ann Surg 173:314, 1981.

66. Dunbar JD, Molnar W, Beman FF, et al: Compression of the celiac trunk and abdominal angina: Preliminary report of 15 cases. Am J Roentgenol 95:731, 1965.

67. Taylor DC, Moneta GL, Cramer MM, et al: Extrinsic compression of the celiac artery by the median arcuate ligament of the diaphragm: Diagnosis by duplex ultrasound. J Vasc Tech 11:236, 1987.

68. Linder HH, Kemprud E: A clinicoanatomical study of the arcuate ligament of the diaphragm. Arch Surg 103:600, 1971.

69. Taylor LM, Porter JM: Nonatherosclerotic diseases of the visceral vasculature. In Persson AV, Skudder PA Jr (eds): Visceral Vascular Surgery. New York, Marcel Dekker, 1987, p 101.

70. Carey JP, Stemmer EA, Connolly JE: Median arcuate ligament syndrome. Arch Surg 99:441, 1969.

71. Reilly LM, Ammar AD, Stoney RJ, et al: Late results following operative repair for celiac artery compression syndrome. J Vasc Surg 2:79, 1985.

72. Lawson JD, Ochsner JL: Median arcuate ligament syndrome with severe two-vessel involvement. Arch Surg 119:226, 1984.

73. Fratesi SJ, Barber GG: Celiac artery embolism: Case report. Can J Surg 24:512, 1981.

74. Low DE, Frenkel VJ, Manley PN, et al: Embolic mesenteric infarction: A unique initial manifestation of renal cell carcinoma. Surgery 106:925, 1989.

75. Ottinger LW: The surgical management of acute occlusion of the superior mesenteric artery. Ann Surg 188:72L, 1978.

76. Buchardt Hansen HJ, Oigaard A: Embolization to the superior mesenteric artery. Acta Chir Scand 142:451, 1976.

77. Wittenberg J, Athanasoulis CA, Shapiro JH: A radiological approach to the patient with acute, extensive bowel ischemia. Radiology 106:13, 1973.

78. Graeber GM, Cafferty PJ, Wolf RE: An analysis of creatinine phosphokinase in the mucosa and muscularis of the gastrointestinal tract. J Surg Res 37:376, 1984.

79. Graeber GM, Wolf RE, Harmon JW: Serum creatinine kinase and alkaline phosphatase in experimental small bowel infarction. J Surg Res 37:25, 1984.

80. Marks WH, Salvino C, Newell K, et al: Circulating concentrations of porcine ileal peptide but not hexosaminidase are elevated following one hour of mesenteric ischemia. J Surg Res 45:134, 1988.

81. Jamiesen WG, Lozon A, Durand D, et al: Changes in serum phosphate levels associated with intestinal infarction and necrosis. Surg Gynecol Obstet 140:19, 1975.

82. Leo PJ, Simonian HG: The role of serum phosphate level and acute ischemic bowel disease. Am J Emer Med 14:377, 1996.

83. Thompson JS, Bragg LE, West WW: Serum enzyme levels during intestinal ischemia. Ann Surg 211:369, 1990.

84. Boley SJ, Feinstein FR, Sammartano R, et al: New concepts in the management of emboli of the superior mesenteric artery. Surg Gynecol Obstet 153:561, 1981.

85. Boley SJ, Sprayregan S, Siegelman SS: Initial results from an aggressive roentgenological and surgical approach to acute mesenteric ischemia. Surgery 82:848, 1977.

86. Kaufman SL, Harrington DP, Siegelman SS: Superior mesenteric artery embolization: An angiographic emergency. Radiology 124:625, 1977.

87. Thorek M: Surgical Errors and Safeguards, 4th ed. Philadelphia, JB Lippincott, 1943, p 478.

88. Aldrete JS, Hansy SY, Laws HL, et al: Intestinal infarction complicating low cardiac output states. Surg Gynecol Obstet 144:371, 1977.

89. Williams LF, Anastasia LF, Hasiotis CA: Nonocclusive mesenteric infarction. Am J Surg 114:376, 1967.

90. Britt LG, Cheek RC: Nonocclusive mesenteric vascular disease: Clinical and experimental observations. Ann Surg 169:704, 1969.

91. Moneta GL, Misbach GA, Ivey TD: Hypoperfusion as a possible factor in the development of gastrointestinal complications after cardiac surgery. Am J Surg 149:648, 1985.

92. Rosemurgy AS, McAllister E, Karl RC: The acute surgical abdomen after cardiac surgery involving extracorporeal circulation. Ann Surg 207:323, 1988.

93. Allen KB, Salam AA, Lumsden AB: Acute mesenteric ischemia following cardiopulmonary bypass. J Vasc Surg 16:391, 1992.

94. Landreueau RJ, Fry WJ: The right colon as a target organ of nonocclusive mesenteric ischemia. Arch Surg 125:591, 1990.

95. Howard TJ, Plaskon LA, Wiebke EA, et al: Nonocclusive mesenteric ischemia remains a diagnostic dilemma. Am J Surg 171:405, 1996.

96. Kim EH, Gewertz BL: Chronic digitalis administration alters mesenteric vascular reactivity. J Vasc Surg 5:382, 1987.

CHAPTER 109

Treatment of Acute Intestinal Ischemia Caused by Arterial Occlusions

Lloyd M. Taylor, Jr., M.D., Gregory L. Moneta, M.D., and John M. Porter, M.D.

The clinical course of acute intestinal ischemia sufficiently severe to produce intestinal infarction is familiar to most surgeons. An elderly person complaining of severe abdominal pain is admitted to the hospital. Initially, there is a lack of accompanying physical findings, leading to an orderly diagnostic evaluation. Within a few hours, tachycardia, hypotension, acidosis, and marked abdominal tenderness occur, leading to emergency laparotomy. Extensive necrosis of the intestine is discovered. Despite treatment, the outcome is nearly always fatal. For the few patients who survive after extensive intestinal resection, a lifetime need for parenteral nutrition is nearly inescapable.

Although considerable advances have been made in the overall diagnosis and treatment of intestinal ischemia since the 1960s, as outlined in the other chapters of this section, the same cannot be said for the results of treatment of acute intestinal ischemia caused by arterial obstructions. Even the briefest literature review reveals prohibitive mortality rates, little changed from those of historical reports and averaging 75% to 80%, as shown in Table 109–1.[1-8] The reason for this grim prognosis is found in the time course of the clinical signs of the disease. The pain of intestinal ischemia is intially unaccompanied by physical signs, leading to an almost inevitable delay in diagnosis. By the time physical signs are prominent and the diagnosis of surgical abdominal disease becomes obvious, the pathology is typically so advanced that survival is doubtful. For the few patients fortunate enough to encounter an appropriately suspicious surgeon early, major abdominal arterial surgery in the emergency setting is required, often with the resection of various but significant lengths of bowel.

These considerations suggest that the mortality rate for patients with acute intestinal ischemia will probably always remain high. Nevertheless, there is potential for salvage with patients seen sufficiently early in the course of the disease and with those in whom the extent of the intestinal ischemia is limited. An approach to the management of such patients is the basis for this chapter. Systematic management of patients with acute intestinal ischemia caused by arterial obstructions requires the physician to confirm the diagnosis, to determine the cause and location of the arterial obstruction, and to perform appropriate treatment. The acute nature of the disease process means that for the majority of patients, each of these steps will be conducted during the course of an operation.

CONFIRMATION OF THE DIAGNOSIS OF ACUTE INTESTINAL ISCHEMIA

The diagnosis of intestinal ischemia is discussed in detail in Chapter 108. With regard to acute intestinal ischemia, the factor most essential to correct diagnosis is a *high index of suspicion* on the part of the examining physician. The foundation of this suspicion is recognition of the pattern of presentation of acute intestinal ischemia. The clinical presentations of acute intestinal ischemia caused by venous disease and that resulting from nonocclusive causes are discussed in Chapters 110 and 111. Acute intestinal ischemia caused by arterial obstructions most often results from thrombosis or embolism of the superior mesenteric artery, each of which is briefly described. In a few patients with chronic occlusion or stenosis of the superior mesenteric artery, acute intestinal ischemia may result from occlusion of collaterals.

Large Artery Thrombosis

An unknown number of patients with severe stenosis of the superior mesenteric artery develop thrombosis of this vessel, with resulting acute intestinal ischemia. Most of these patients are female, have evidence of symptomatic vascular disease at other sites, and have often had previous vascular surgery. About half have a history of chronic abdominal pain and weight loss suggestive of chronic visceral ischemia.[1-8] Acute severe abdominal pain out of proportion to physical findings in such a patient is strongly suggestive of acute intestinal ischemia.

TABLE 109–1. MORTALITY ASSOCIATED WITH TREATMENT OF ACUTE INTESTINAL ISCHEMIA FROM ARTERIAL OBSTRUCTIONS

STUDY	NO. OF PATIENTS	MORTALITY (%)
Ottinger and Austen, 1967[1]	51	43 (84)
Slater and Elliott, 1972[2]	4	4 (100)
Singh et al, 1975[3]	30	24 (81)
Smith and Patterson, 1976[4]	23	21 (91)
Kairaluoma et al, 1977[5]	44	31 (70)
Hertzer et al, 1978[6]	10	7 (70)
Sachs et al, 1982[7]	30	23 (77)
Levy et al, 1990[8]	45	20 (44)

Intestinal Artery Embolism

In the past, most arterial emboli were cardiac in origin. About 5% of cardiac emboli lodge within visceral vessels.[9] The likelihood of cardiac embolism to intestinal arteries should be considered when patients with known cardiac disease (e.g., atrial arrhythmias, cardiomyopathy, acute myocardial infarction, rheumatic valvular disease) experience the sudden onset of severe abdominal pain. The proportion of arterial emboli arising from the heart is decreasing in association with more widespread anticoagulant treatment of heart disease, especially atrial fibrillation, and the decrease in the prevalence of rheumatic heart disease. Proximal arterial sites have become an increasingly important source of emboli. Arterioarterial emboli can arise from ulcerated atherosclerotic plaques or from arterial aneurysms. A particularly important source of arterioarterial embolism has become diagnostic or interventional arteriographic catheter manipulation. Embolism occurs when atherothrombotic material is dislodged during manipulation of guide wires and catheters within the arterial lumen. Severe abdominal pain after cardiac catheterization or other diagnostic or interventional proximal aortic arteriographic procedures should lead to immediate suspicion of intestinal ischemia resulting from intestinal artery embolism.

The Decision to Perform Arteriography

Although the diagnosis of acute intestinal ischemia caused by arterial obstructions is facilitated by arteriography, the treatment of intestinal ischemia is a true surgical emergency, and performing visceral arteriography typically requires several hours—hours that may be crucial to successful treatment of a critically ill patient. The authors obtain arteriograms for patients thought to have intestinal ischemia based on the presence of *pain alone* in the typical clinical setting. In these patients, a diagnosis is necessary because pain alone is usually not an indication for surgery. For patients with typical pain and physical findings such as rebound tenderness or abdominal rigidity clearly indicating the need for operation, arteriography is contraindicated.

A typical arteriogram obtained from a patient with acute intestinal ischemia caused by superior mesenteric artery thrombosis is seen in Figure 109–1. Because the arteriosclerotic stenosis causing the thrombosis is almost always located at or near the origin of the artery, the entire superior mesenteric artery fails to visualize. An arteriogram from a patient with superior mesenteric artery embolism is seen in Figure 109–2. The vessel is occluded beyond the origin of several proximal branches, there is a sharp cutoff of a normal-appearing artery, and thrombus is visible at the site of the occlusion, all of which are angiographic signs of embolism.

INTERVENTIONAL ARTERIOGRAPHIC TREATMENT OF ACUTE INTESTINAL ISCHEMIA

Acute intestinal ischemia from arterial obstruction is usually caused by localized arterial thrombus occurring at the site

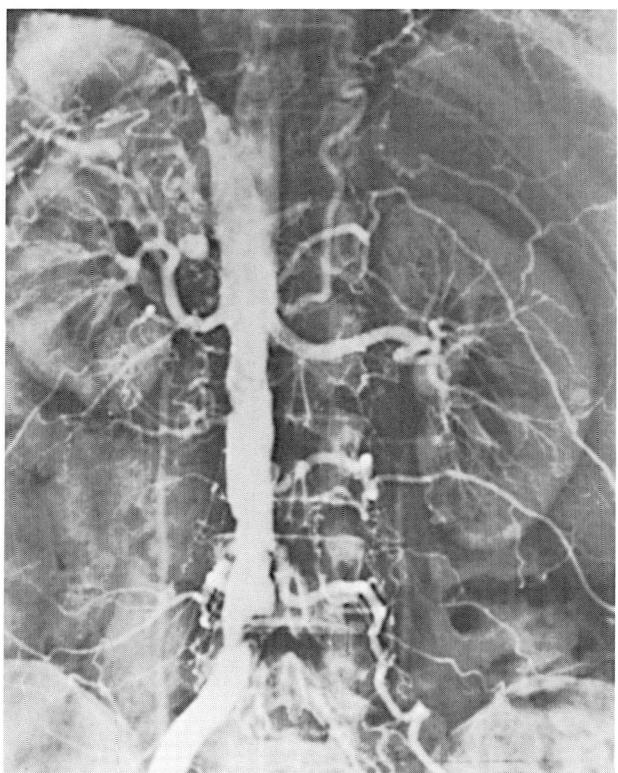

FIGURE 109–1. Aortogram from a patient with acute intestinal ischemia caused by superior mesenteric artery thrombosis. Note the complete absence of filling of any intestinal arteries as well as evidence of severe arterial disease in the aorta and the iliac arteries.

of atherosclerotic stenosis or by localized arterial embolism. It appears reasonable to consider the potential roles of thrombolytic treatment, balloon angioplasty, or both as definitive treatments. This may be especially true in patients undergoing arteriography in whom the arterial occlusion causing acute intestinal ischemia has just been visualized. The high mortality associated with conventional surgical

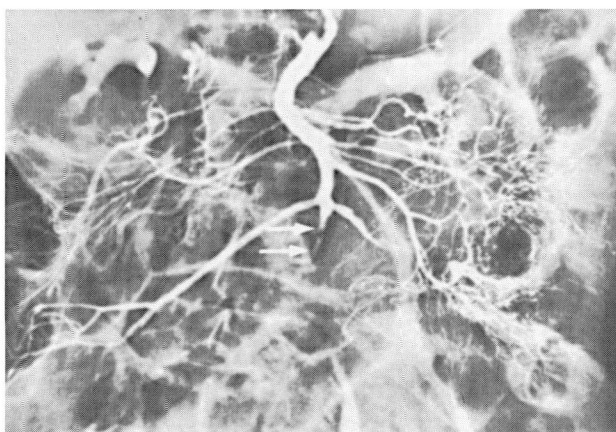

FIGURE 109–2. Selective arteriogram of the superior mesenteric artery in a patient with embolism. Note the patent proximal branches, the sharp cutoff at the site of the occlusion, and the visible thrombus (*arrows*) at the site of the occlusion.

treatment of acute intestinal ischemia indicates considerable room for improvement (see Table 109–1). It seems logical to consider correction of the underlying arterial obstruction by interventional means, with the need for acute surgery thereby reduced to resection of unsalvageable intestine.

Several reports of percutaneous interventional treatment of superior mesenteric artery obstruction causing acute intestinal ischemia have been published.[10–12] Although some cases have been successfully treated by percutaneous intervention alone, the extent and degree of intestinal ischemia cannot be predicted from physical examination or from any known laboratory or diagnostic test short of laparotomy. Although thrombolytic or catheter interventional therapy may restore arterial vascular supply to ischemic intestine, most patients with acute intestinal ischemia have at least some intestine that is frankly necrotic at the time of diagnosis. Most patients with acute intestinal ischemia caused by arterial obstructions still require laparotomy, even if arterial circulation has been successfully restored by interventional means.

Persistence of any symptoms of abdominal pain after revascularization is a clear indication for laparotomy and resection of residual ischemic bowel. Whether the approach of acute restoration of superior mesenteric artery patency by interventional means followed by bowel resection, if necessary, will result in lower morbidity or mortality than the standard surgical approach is not known. Nevertheless, the high mortality associated with the standard approach means that exploration of alternate therapies is reasonable.

OPERATIVE TREATMENT

Findings at Operation

At laparotomy, the etiology and appropriate treatment of intestinal ischemia are determined by the appearance of the intestines and the status of the circulation in the superior mesenteric artery. Acutely ischemic bowel that is not yet necrotic may be deceptively normal in appearance. The physical appearance of ischemic intestine includes loss of normal sheen, dull-gray discoloration (which may be especially difficult to detect if global), and lack of peristalsis. These subjective signs may be overlooked. Objective signs of intestinal ischemia include absence of palpable pulse in the proximal superior mesenteric artery (in the case of thrombosis) or in its more distal branches (in the case of embolism), lack of visible pulsations in mesenteric arcade vessels, and absence of pulsatile flow detected by Doppler examination of these vessels and of the intestine itself. Fluid is present within the abdomen in advanced cases, and it may be foul smelling even in the absence of intestinal perforation.

The distribution of the ischemic intestine provides important information about the cause of ischemia (Fig. 109–3).[13] In superior mesenteric artery thrombosis, the small intestine is usually ischemic throughout its length, with sparing of only the stomach, duodenum, and distal portion of the colon. In embolic occlusions of the superior mesenteric artery, the proximal jejunum frequently remains normal, reflecting the propensity of cardiac emboli to lodge beyond the first few branches of the superior mesenteric artery. Arterioarterial embolism may produce a patchy distribution of ischemia, with multiple areas of involvement and skipped sections of normal-appearing intestine.

The plan for operative treatment is based on these findings and is illustrated in Figures 109–4 through 109–6. Regardless of the etiology of ischemia, the goals of therapy are to ensure normal pulsatile flow to the superior mesenteric artery, restoration of adequate arterial inflow to ischemic but viable intestine, and resection of nonviable intestine. These steps in treatment are discussed next.

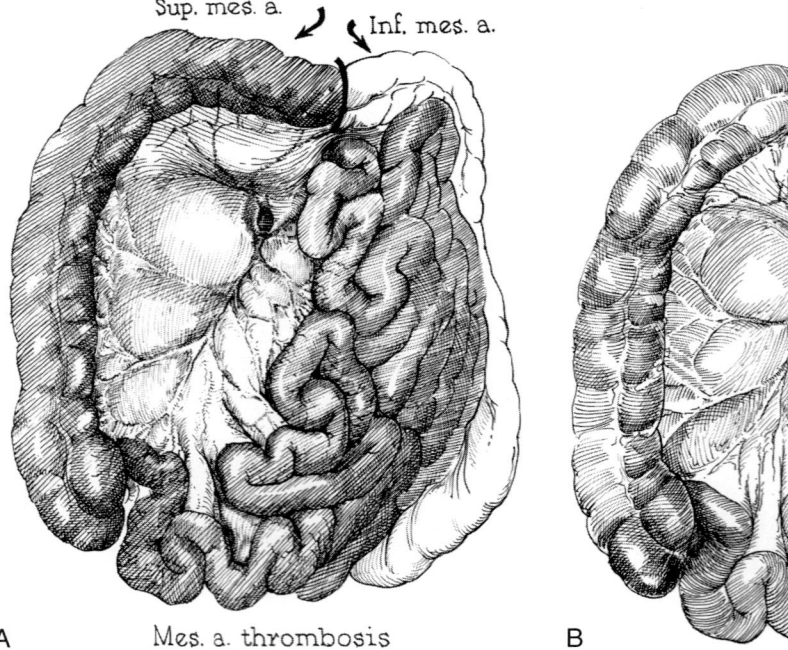
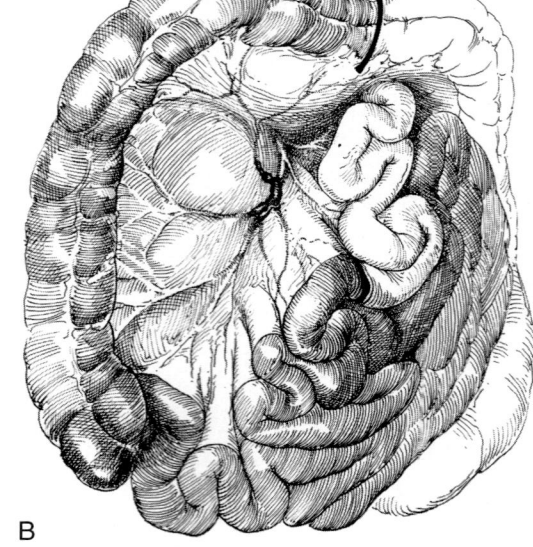

FIGURE 109–3. *A*, Distribution of intestinal ischemia with superior mesenteric artery thrombosis. The entire small bowel and the proximal colon are ischemic. *B*, Distribution of intestinal ischemia with superior mesenteric artery embolism. The proximal jejunum is spared. (From Bergan JJ: Recognition and treatment of intestinal ischemia. Surg Clin North Am 47:109, 1967.)

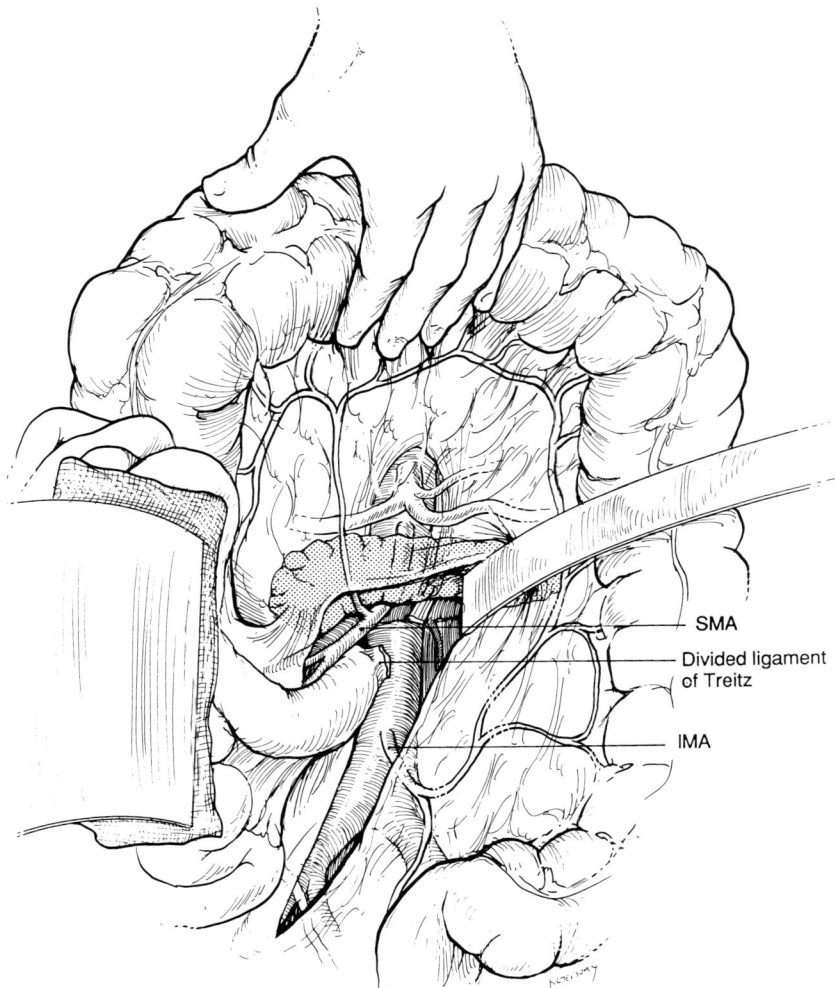

FIGURE 109–4. Exposure of infrarenal aorta, proximal right common iliac artery, and proximal superior mesenteric artery (SMA) achieved by intestinal retraction and division of posterior peritoneum, ligament of Treitz, and base of small bowel mesentery. IMA = inferior mesenteric artery. (From Kazmirs A: Operative management of acute mesenteric ischemia. Ann Vasc Surg 12:187–197, 1998.)

SMA
Divided ligament
of Treitz
IMA

Revascularization of the Acutely Ischemic Intestine

In patients with advanced intestinal ischemia, bowel necrosis may be widespread and obvious. The systemic effects of such a lesion are catastrophic and rapidly fatal. This means that most patients undergoing surgery for intestinal ischemia are in an earlier stage of the evolution of necrosis and that at least a portion of the bowel is of questionable viability. This has important implications for treatment. It is not possible to rapidly or accurately predict the potential for revascularization to restore viability to ischemia-appearing intestine. Thus, except in the most advanced cases, *revascularization should precede resection.* Restoration of pulsatile flow to the superior mesenteric artery may produce a remarkable change in the bowel that appeared hopelessly ischemic at first inspection. One of two techniques is used: mesenteric artery embolectomy or intestinal artery bypass. The choice of technique depends on the cause of the ischemia.

Superior Mesenteric Artery Embolectomy

For embolectomy, the superior mesenteric artery is exposed from within the abdomen, at the base of the junction of the small bowel and transverse colon mesenteries (see Fig. 109–

4). The authors prefer to open the artery with a longitudinal incision because its size in most patients prevents adequate visualization of the lumen through a transverse incision, although the latter approach is used by many surgeons for removal of emboli. Proximal embolectomy (see Fig. 109–5) is performed with a balloon catheter (size 3 or 4 French [Fr.]). Failure to establish copious pulsatile inflow from the aorta should lead to a diagnosis of mesenteric artery thrombosis and the performance of a bypass procedure.

Distal embolectomy of the superior mesenteric artery and its branches is difficult because of the size of the vessels, their fragility, and their multiplicity. The authors believe it is best performed with a size 2 Fr. balloon catheter, and the technique must be quite gentle in comparison to that used in the less fragile arteries of the extremities. Once all possible thrombus has been removed, the arteriotomy is closed primarily or with a patch of autogenous vein, if this is necessary to preserve the lumen after longitudinal arteriotomy. If adequate pulsatile inflow cannot be restored, the arteriotomy becomes the site of anastomosis for a bypass graft.

Superior Mesenteric Artery Bypass

For patients with mesenteric artery thrombosis seen early in whom the entire intestine appears salvageable by revas-

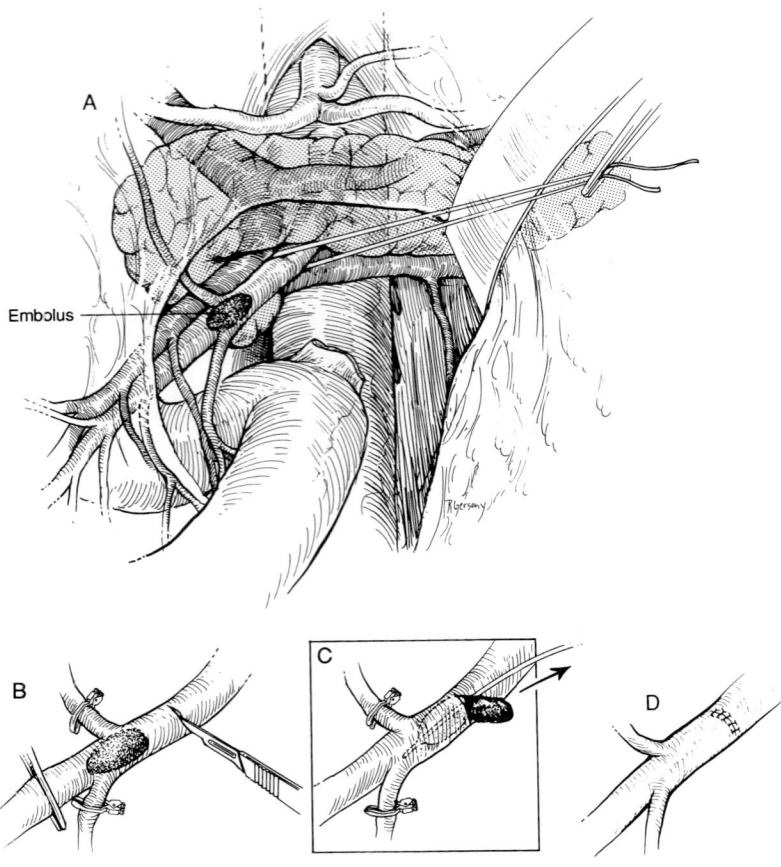

Embolus

FIGURE 109–5. *A*, Superior mesenteric artery embolectomy. Transverse *(B)* or longitudinal arteriotomy is followed by balloon catheter embolus extraction *(C)* and arteriotomy closure *(D)*. Primary closure suffices for a transverse arteriotomy, whereas a vein patch is usually required to close a longitudinal arteriotomy. (From Kazmers A: Operative management of acute mesenteric ischemia. Ann Vasc Surg 12:187–197, 1998.)

cularization, superior mesenteric artery bypass with a prosthetic graft is used to restore arterial flow (see Fig. 109–6A). In some patients, this degree of intestinal ischemia is accompanied by the presence of a foul odor within the abdomen in the absence of intestinal perforation or of obvious intestinal necrosis. This finding is not a contraindication to a prosthetic bypass.

In most patients with acute intestinal ischemia from mesenteric artery thrombosis, at least some of the intestine is obviously necrotic, requiring resection, and in some patients perforation has occurred. For these patients, the authors believe that prosthetic bypass is contraindicated. In this situation, a bypass to the superior mesenteric artery using the proximal greater saphenous vein in reversed fashion is used (see Fig. 109–6B). If the iliac artery and infrarenal aorta are too diseased to use for graft origin, the supraceliac aorta is a reasonable alternate.

For patients with arterioarterial embolism, the very small particle size of the embolic material means that a number of emboli lodge in peripheral arteries. Embolectomy is usually not possible, and bypass beyond the point of embolic obstruction is also not possible. For these patients, resection of nonviable intestine is the only practical operative therapy.

Determination of Intestinal Viability

Once revascularization is completed, the need for intestinal resection must be determined. In early cases, restoration of

pulsatile flow may be the only therapy necessary. In most, however, the bowel contains obviously necrotic areas, obviously viable areas, and areas of questionable viability. Multiple techniques have been proposed to aid in differentiating bowel that will remain viable and recover from bowel that will become frankly necrotic despite the restoration of flow. These techniques include clinical judgment based on inspection and palpation, Doppler ultrasound, intravenous fluorescein, infrared photoplethysmography, surface oximetry, and laser Doppler velocimetry.

Clinical inspection of viable intestine reveals visible pulsations in the mesenteric arcade vessels, bleeding from cut surfaces, a normal color, and peristaltic motions. None of these criteria is absolute, all are inherently subjective, and none is easily quantitated. Despite this, clinical inspection by experienced surgeons enables viable bowel to be distinguished from nonviable bowel in most cases. In the prospective study reported on by Bulkley and associates,[14] this method had a sensitivity of 82% and a specificity of 91%.

The use of a sterilized, continuous wave Doppler ultrasound flow detector (9 to 10 MHz) for determining intestinal viability was first reported in a canine model by Wright and Hobson.[15] With this method, pulsatile Doppler signals are sought on the intestinal surface. Segments with absent signals are deemed nonviable. Successful clinical use of this method has been reported in humans.[16, 17] This method has the distinct advantage of using instrumentation that is available sterile in most vascular surgery operating rooms.

With the fluorescein fluorescence method, 10 to 15 mg/kg

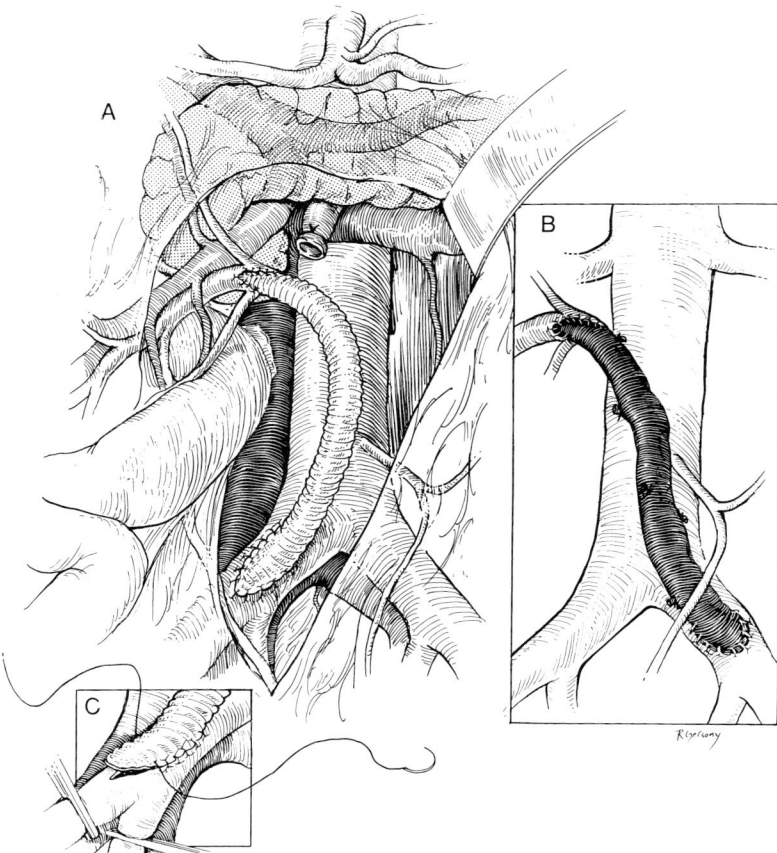

FIGURE 109–6. *A*, Iliac to superior mesenteric artery bypass using prosthetic for cases in which superior mesenteric artery thrombosis produces ischemic but salvageable bowel. *B*, Iliac to superior mesenteric artery bypass using saphenous vein for cases in which some segments of necrotic or perforated bowel must be resected. *C*, Detail of distal anastomosis. (From Kazmers A: Operative management of acute mesenteric ischemia. Ann Vasc Surg 12:187–197, 1998.)

of fluorescein is injected intravenously and the intestine is inspected using Wood's lamp. A complete absence of fluorescence is diagnostic of nonviability, whereas rapid, confluent, bright fluorescence is diagnostic of viability. There is a large area between these two extremes, however, and interpretation of the pattern and intensity of fluorescence is inherently subjective.

Carter and coworkers[18] described the use of a quantitative method of fluorescein testing using a perfusion fluorometer. In their experimental setting, the quantitative method had a sensitivity and specificity of 100% for detecting nonviable segments of intestine, compared with a sensitivity of 11% and a specificity of 100% for qualitative visual inspection. The requirement for special equipment and the possibility of serious allergic reactions resulting from the injection of this medication into patients who are already critically ill are significant drawbacks to the clinical use of this method.

Locke and colleagues[19] used surface oximetry and demonstrated in a canine model that abnormal PO_2 values from intestine with various degrees of ischemia were predictive of failure of anastomotic healing. The feasibility of this method for detecting nonviable segments of bowel using simpler equipment (the pulse oximeter) was demonstrated in dogs by Ferrara and associates[20] and by DeNobile and coworkers.[21]

Infrared photoplethysmography uses a small probe to detect changes in tissue blood volume resulting from changes in reflected infrared light. Sensitivity and specificity for this method comparable to those achieved with Doppler ultrasonography and with the fluorescein method were demonstrated by Pearce and colleagues.[22]

Yet another method with experimental success in detecting ischemic intestinal segments was demonstrated by Oohata and coworkers.[23] These authors used laser Doppler velocimetry of the surface of the intestine and showed excellent correlation with the results of hydrogen gas clearance testing in the same intestinal segments. The hydrogen gas method is extremely accurate in quantifying blood flow in the intestine but is not applicable in the clinical setting.

To date, only one study has evaluated various methods of determining intestinal viability in prospective, controlled fashion. Bulkley and associates[14] compared clinical judgment, Doppler ultrasound, and fluorescein injection in 78 intestinal segments of 28 consecutive patients with intestinal ischemia. The results of this study are shown in Table 109–2. Interestingly, standard clinical judgment proved to be very reliable, at least as reliable as the other two methods. Although these authors found perfect reliability for the fluorescein method, this has not been duplicated by other investigators.

Whitehill and colleagues[24] explained why the various techniques for determining bowel viability are less than perfect. These authors evaluated Doppler ultrasound, photoplethysmography, and fluorescein injection and discovered that each was capable of detecting intestinal blood

TABLE 109–2. DIAGNOSTIC ABILITY OF REPORTED TECHNIQUES FOR DETERMINING THE VIABILITY OF ACUTELY ISCHEMIC INTESTINE

TECHNIQUE	SENSITIVITY (%)	SPECIFICITY (%)	ACCURACY (%)
Clinical judgment	82	91	89
Fluorescein injection (qualitative)	100	100	100
Doppler ultrasound	63	88	84

Adapted from Bulkley GB, Zuidema GD, Hamilton SR, et al: Intraoperative determination of small intestinal viability following ischemic injury. Ann Surg 193:628, 1981.

flow at levels below the minimum required for viability. This means that each method has the potential for false-negative testing—the most dangerous incorrect result for patients.

Given the vagaries of these methods and the documented high reliability of clinical judgment, we rely on a combination of clinical judgment and Doppler ultrasound to determine intestinal viability. Our choice is based on the lack of documented superiority of any method and the ready availability of sterile Doppler probes in our operating room. In the decision as to which bowel to resect, the choices are clearly influenced by the length of the obviously viable segment remaining. If this segment is large and clearly adequate for life (>6 feet of small intestine), the resection of remaining bowel should be quite liberal, with removal of any questionably viable segments. If the length of obviously viable bowel is limited, however, the resection of questionably viable segments should be deferred to a "second-look" operation. Resection of multiple segments of necrotic bowel separated by skipped areas of normal viability is appropriate if the overall remaining bowel is limited, even if multiple anastomoses are required.

Our preference for treatment of the remaining bowel is to perform anastomoses to restore bowel continuity. Our reasoning is that segments of intestine used for stomas are rarely functional in an absorptive capacity, additional bowel is invariably lost during reanastomosis, and the stoma segment is more ischemic than adjacent bowel by virtue of detachment from the mesentery, compression by the body wall, and so on.

Second-Look Surgery

Because it is usually advisable to avoid resection of questionably viable bowel at the time of the initial operation, second-look operations are frequently performed after revascularization for acute intestinal ischemia. The decision to perform such surgery must be made at the time of the original operation, and the second procedure must be performed as planned *regardless of the condition of the patient*. The desperate condition of patients with severe acute intestinal ischemia may deceptively and dramatically improve after resection of the majority of ischemic bowel. Despite this, a small segment of remaining necrotic bowel will ultimately prove just as fatal as the original large segment if it is not detected and treated.

At the second-look operation, performed 18 to 36 hours after the first, any remaining nonviable bowel is resected,

the integrity of vascular repairs is ensured, and the anastomoses are checked. In some cases, especially when precarious anastomoses are made in revascularized intestine, we have used a "third-look" procedure, 4 to 6 days after the first procedure, in order to detect and treat any anastomotic leaks before the occurrence of peritonitis and sepsis.

PERIOPERATIVE CARE

Acute intestinal ischemia is a life-threatening condition that most frequently affects older patients with serious underlying medical conditions. The only hope for survival lies in the skilled performance of early treatment to revascularize ischemic intestine and to resect nonviable segments. Both the ischemic intestine and the surgical treatment required contribute to major hemodynamic instability and dysfunction of multiple organ systems. The most intensive care possible, including full hemodynamic monitoring, is required for maximal safety.

If patients recover from the acute illness and surgery, prolonged parenteral nutrition is an integral part of postoperative management. There is frequently severe ischemic damage to the remaining viable intestine, and motility and absorptive function may be compromised, requiring a prolonged recovery period that may extend for months. In our experience, most patients do not require lifelong parenteral nutrition if the remaining small bowel is at least a few feet in length and has been revascularized.

SUMMARY

We have emphasized that acute intestinal ischemia caused by arterial obstructions is associated with a very high patient mortality rate because severe symptoms occur only when disease is advanced and because the patient population affected is often elderly, with preexisting multisystem disease. Early diagnosis that is based on a high index of suspicion is the key to achieving survival in some patients seen early in the course of the disease. The differences between arterial thrombosis and arterial embolism are described, since each has a different treatment. The steps in therapy are detailed, with an emphasis on revascularization of intestine, resection of necrotic bowel, and second-look surgery to determine the viability of questionable segments. The importance of intensive perioperative care using hemodynamic monitoring and parenteral nutrition is also emphasized.

With the use of these principles, it should be possible to achieve survival in some patients with acute intestinal ischemia who are seen sufficiently early in the course of disease that some viable small bowel remains.

REFERENCES

1. Ottinger L, Austen WG: A study of 136 patients with mesenteric infarction. Surg Gynecol Obstet 124:1251, 1967.
2. Slater H, Elliott PW: Primary mesenteric infarction. Am J Surg 123:309, 1972.

3. Singh RP, Shah RC, Lee ST: Acute mesenteric vascular occlusion: A review of thirty-two patients. Surgery 78:613, 1975.
4. Smith JS Jr, Patterson LT: Acute mesenteric infarction. Am Surg 42:562, 1976.
5. Kairaluoma MI, Karkola P, Heikkinen E, et al: Mesenteric infarction. Am J Surg 133:188, 1977.
6. Hertzer NR, Beven EG, Humphries AW: Acute intestinal ischemia. Am Surg 44:744, 1978.
7. Sachs SM, Morton JH, Schwartz SI: Acute mesenteric ischemia. Surgery 92:646, 1982.
8. Levy PJ, Krausz MM, Manny J: Acute mesenteric ischemia: Improved results: A retrospective analysis of ninety-two patients. Surgery 107:372, 1990.
9. Elliott JP Jr, Hageman JH, Szilagyi E, et al: Arterial embolization: Problems of source, multiplicity, recurrence, and delayed treatment. Surgery 88:833, 1980.
10. Gallego AM, Ramirez P, Rodriguez JM, et al: Role of urokinase in the superior mesenteric artery embolism. Surgery 120:111, 1996.
11. Schoenbaum SW, Pena C, Koenigsberg P, Katzen BT: Superior mesenteric artery embolism: Treatment with intraarterial urokinase. J Vasc Interv Radiol 3:485, 1992.
12. McBride KD, Gaines PA: Thrombolysis of a partially occluding superior mesenteric artery thromboembolus by infusion of streptokinase. Cardiovasc Intervent Radiol 17:164, 1994.
13. Bergan JJ: Recognition and treatment of intestinal ischemia. Surg Clin North Am 47:109, 1967.
14. Bulkley GB, Zuidema GD, Hamilton SR, et al: Intraoperative determination of small intestinal viability following ischemic injury. Ann Surg 193:628, 1981.
15. Wright CB, Hobson RW: Prediction of intestinal viability using Doppler ultrasound technique. Am J Surg 129:642, 1975.
16. O'Donnell JA, Hobson RW: Operative confirmation of Doppler ultrasound evaluation of intestinal ischemia. Surgery 87:109, 1980.
17. Cooperman M, Paca WG, Martin EW, et al: Determination of viability of ischemic intestine by Doppler ultrasound. Surgery 83:705, 1978.
18. Carter MS, Fantini GA, Sammartano RJ, et al: Qualitative and quantitative fluorescein fluorescence in determining intestinal viability. Am J Surg 147:117, 1984.
19. Locke R, Hauser CJ, Shoemaker WC: The use of surface oximetry to assess bowel viability. Arch Surg 119:1252, 1984.
20. Ferrara J, Dyess D, Lasecki M, et al: Surface oximetry: A new method to evaluate intestinal perfusion. Am Surg 54:10, 1988.
21. DeNobile J, Guzzetta P, Patterson K: Pulse oximetry as a means of assessing bowel viability. J Surg Res 48:21, 1990.
22. Pearce WH, Jones DN, Warren GH, et al: The use of infrared photoplethysmography in identifying early intestinal ischemia. Arch Surg 122:108, 1987.
23. Oohata Y, Mibu R, Hotokezaka M, et al: Comparison of blood flow assessment between laser Doppler velocimetry and the hydrogen gas clearance method in ischemic intestine in dogs. Am J Surg 160:511, 1990.
24. Whitehill TA, Pearce WH, Rosales C, et al: Detection thresholds of nonocclusive intestinal hypoperfusion by Doppler ultrasound, photoplethysmography, and fluorescein. J Vasc Surg 8:28, 1988.

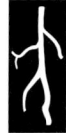

C H A P T E R   1 1 0
Nonocclusive Mesenteric Ischemia

Steven P. Rivers, M.D., and
Frank J. Veith, M.D.

Although embolic or thrombotic obstruction of the arterial or venous circulation is the usual source of acute mesenteric vascular insufficiency, intestinal ischemia also occurs in the absence of mechanical vascular obstruction. The most frequent clinical setting producing nonocclusive mesenteric ischemia is severe systemic illness with circulatory insufficiency and end-organ shock.[1, 2] In this setting, the cause of the ischemia that occurs has been demonstrated to be severe and prolonged visceral arterial vasospasm, frequently resulting in intestinal necrosis. Severe intestinal arterial vasospasm also occurs in response to drug intoxication, as with cocaine and ergot derivatives, and after repair of aortic coarctations. Each of these conditions is described in this chapter.

The true prevalence of nonocclusive mesenteric ischemia is unknown, because mesenteric ischemia without infarction undoubtedly occurs and resolves in some patients in whom the diagnosis is never confirmed. At the authors' institution, a policy of liberal use of angiography for all suspected cases of intestinal ischemia has produced a large number of arteriograms for review. On the basis of this experience, it is estimated that nonocclusive mesenteric ischemia may be responsible for up to 20% of all cases of splanchnic vascular insufficiency (Fig. 110–1). This incidence is lower than that previously reported by others,[3] when nonocclusive mesenteric ischemia was responsible for approximately 50% of mesenteric infarctions. In the authors' opinion, this declining incidence has resulted directly from improved treatment of critically ill patients in the intensive care setting. Specifically, the widespread use of invasive hemodynamic monitoring and a shift in emphasis from the use of peripheral vasoconstrictors to the use of peripheral vasodilatation for the treatment of refractory congestive heart failure and cardiogenic shock are probably

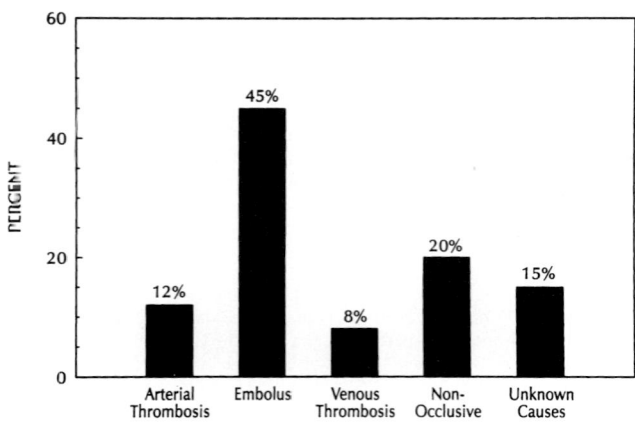

FIGURE 110–1. Etiology of mesenteric ischemia, 1980 to 1990. (From Rivers S: Acute nonocclusive mesenteric ischemia. Semin Vasc Surg 3:172, 1990.)

responsible for much of the decline in the prevalence of nonocclusive mesenteric ischemia.

PATHOPHYSIOLOGY

Mesenteric vasoconstriction occurs normally in response to both normovolemic and hypovolemic shock states and may persist for several hours after the reversal of all other manifestations of shock.[4] Intestinal mucosal permeability increases in direct proportion to the duration and severity of the vascular insult, although greater permeability is found with total occlusion than with a low but persistent flow of blood.[5] In the normal setting, the increasing local ischemia resulting from this vasoconstriction eventually leads to vasodilatation and restoration of adequate blood flow before the occurrence of necrosis. The specific reasons this sequence does not occur in some cases of shock have been difficult to ascertain.

Angiographically demonstrated hypoperfusion from vasospasm does not always result in mucosal damage and in fact correlates poorly with histologic evidence of ischemia in a dog model.[6] It has been suggested that autoregulatory vasodilatation, which usually results from local ischemia, requires a normal perfusion pressure,[7] a circumstance not usually present in the standard clinical setting for nonocclusive mesenteric ischemia. This may explain the failure of normal autoregulation to permit reperfusion before the occurrence of intestinal necrosis in the shock setting. In patients with cocaine or ergot poisoning, the mechanism of persistent vasospasm that is due to the persistence of extrinsic vasoconstrictor overriding local autoregulatory control seems clear. Whether the mechanism is centrally mediated decreased perfusion (as with shock), locally induced vasospasm (as with drug intoxication), or a combination of the two (as when shock is treated with vasoconstrictors), it is clear that vasoconstriction is the source of the ischemia sufficient to produce intestinal necrosis in patients with nonocclusive mesenteric ischemia.

Interestingly, the renin-angiotensin axis appears to be an important mediator of vasospasm in nonocclusive mesenteric ischemia. Experimentally, bilateral nephrectomy or

the administration of angiotensin-converting enzyme (ACE) inhibitors before the onset of shock will alleviate the ischemic response in the visceral circulation. Surprisingly, blockade of the alpha-adrenergic system before an episode of hypoperfusion does not seem to alter the incidence or severity of nonocclusive mesenteric ischemia.[8, 9]

The etiology of mesenteric ischemia may be multifactorial in some patients in whom no single lesion would be sufficient to cause symptoms. For example, in patients with intestinal distention, previously asymptomatic proximal mesenteric artery stenoses, or both, intestinal ischemia and necrosis may develop when a systemic low-flow state is superimposed.[10, 11]

PRESENTATION

Nonocclusive mesenteric ischemia appears in clinical settings in which severe, often multisystemic illnesses result in low-flow states and visceral vasoconstriction. Congestive heart failure, with or without other manifestations of cardiogenic shock, is by far the most frequent isolated etiology. Sepsis, dehydration, and renal or hepatic disease may occasionally be sufficiently severe to produce the necessary low-flow state and splanchnic vasospasm, but nonocclusive mesenteric ischemia is rarely seen in the absence of significant, clinically apparent cardiac dysfunction, vasoconstrictor drug administration (including self-administration), or both.

The signs and symptoms of nonocclusive mesenteric ischemia are similar to those of other forms of acute intestinal ischemia. Abdominal pain is the most common symptom, noted in at least 75% of patients. However, pain may be undetected or unreported in the critically ill patient. For this reason, a high index of suspicion is required for the diagnosis of nonocclusive mesenteric ischemia when isolated findings, such as abdominal distention, gastrointestinal bleeding, fever, or leukocytosis, occur in the appropriate clinical setting. Mild cases of nonocclusive mesenteric ischemia that are never clearly diagnosed probably occur frequently. These cases present as localized or intermittent abdominal pain secondary to fluctuating local perfusion, and they resolve spontaneously as the overall condition improves. The presentation of severe cases with impending or actual intestinal necrosis is indistinguishable from the presentations of the other types of acute mesenteric ischemia discussed in Chapters 109, 111, and 113.

Postcoarctectomy Syndrome

Nonocclusive mesenteric ischemia has been reported in as many as 4% of patients after repair of an aortic coarctation.[12] The syndrome is thought to be related to the paradoxical postoperative hypertension seen in many patients, with the sudden increase in pressure below the coarctation causing a necrotizing vasculitis of the mesenteric vessels.[13] Angiographic studies demonstrate mesenteric arterial spasm, which rapidly reverses in response to local intra-arterial papaverine infusion or treatment of hypertension with systemic vasodilating agents.[13] The problem occurs more frequently in the youngest patients and is one reason surgery is usually postponed whenever possible until the child reaches 3 to 5 years of age.[12, 14]

Drug-Induced Mesenteric Ischemia

Digoxin and vasopressor agents used to treat patients with multiorgan system failure have also been implicated in the development of nonocclusive mesenteric ischemia. In therapeutic doses, these medications do not usually cause significant intestinal ischemia. However, their vasoconstrictive effect on the splanchnic circulation undoubtedly contributes to the development of mesenteric ischemia in patients already suffering from a low-flow situation. The shift away from the use of these medications and the corresponding decrease in the incidence of nonocclusive mesenteric ischemia provide strong evidence of the contributory role of these medications.

Nonocclusive mesenteric ischemia from ergot poisoning or cocaine abuse may rarely develop in otherwise healthy patients,[15, 16] and in this setting abdominal pain and intestinal ischemia may be the presenting symptoms of these drug intoxications. The vasoactive properties of the various ergot alkaloids differ in intensity. Ergonovine has only a slight vasoconstrictive effect, dihydroergotamine has a much more active one, and ergotamine tartrate has the most severely vasoconstrictive effect.[17] The diagnosis of ergot-induced mesenteric ischemia is not difficult, because ergotism today is almost entirely the result of the medicinal use of ergot alkaloids for migraine headaches. Cocaine poisoning may be somewhat more difficult to establish if the history of ingestion is withheld.

Vasospasm Following Mesenteric Revascularization

A syndrome of diffuse vasospasm and persistent intestinal ischemia following antegrade revascularization for chronic mesenteric occlusive disease has been described.[18] The cause is unknown but has been postulated to occur as a consequence of reperfusion edema, myogenic responses to undampened antegrade pressure waves, or possible injury to the celiac neural plexus. Awareness of this potential complication has resulted in successful treatment by the methods discussed later.

DIAGNOSIS

Certain confirmation of the diagnosis of nonocclusive mesenteric ischemia would require actual observation of ischemic bowel in the absence of any organic vascular occlusion. In practice, the angiographic demonstration of intestinal arterial vasospasm in symptomatic patients at risk is acceptable for diagnosis. The radiologic signs of splanchnic arterial vasoconstriction include narrowed origins of major branches of the superior mesenteric artery; beading, tapering, or segmental narrowing of intestinal branches; spasm of intestinal arcades; and reduced or absent filling of intramural vessels.[19] The arteriographic findings are similar for any etiology of nonocclusive mesenteric ischemia; they are relatively specific only for the complication of mesenteric insufficiency.

In symptomatic patients at risk for nonocclusive mesenteric ischemia, plain abdominal radiographs are obtained first to rule out other causes of abdominal pain. Aortography and selective mesenteric arteriography may then be performed. On completion of the study, the catheter can be secured in place with the tip in the orifice of the superior mesenteric artery for subsequent papaverine infusion. This technique is useful even for patients requiring surgery for thrombotic or embolic occlusions because postoperative vasospasm may still occur.

A critical issue in patients with suspected intestinal ischemia and possible infarction is the requisite delay in operative intervention imposed by angiography. In the authors' opinion, the decision to perform arteriography or to proceed directly to surgery should be individualized. Patients with mild or intermittent abdominal pain thought to be ischemic in nature might not require angiography at all. Prompt correction of the low-flow state and bowel decompression may resolve the problem and eliminate the need for invasive studies. At the other end of the clinical spectrum, patients with peritoneal signs and a high probability of intestinal infarction can ill afford a significant delay in laparotomy. Even in the most well prepared centers, the transport of an intensive care unit patient with infusion pumps, monitors, and respirators and the need for selective and biplanar angiography are time-consuming and risk further intestinal necrosis or acidosis.

Nevertheless, arteriography is clearly a useful diagnostic tool and should be considered whenever feasible. Of the first 50 patients with suspected acute mesenteric ischemia examined angiographically at the authors' institution, the diagnosis was confirmed in 35 patients (70%), 15 of whom had nonocclusive mesenteric ischemia. Of the 15 patients with other causes of abdominal pain, arteriography facilitated the correct diagnosis in eight.[20] Furthermore, some patients with early signs of peritoneal irritation show improvement after the institution of intra-arterial papaverine therapy and are able to avoid laparotomy. Only patients with physical findings that mandate urgent exploration should forego this critical study. After thrombectomy, resection of gangrenous bowel, or both, adjunctive vasodilator therapy can be initiated intraoperatively or postoperatively.

Several interesting new diagnostic approaches developed to address the risks and limitations of angiography are currently being evaluated. These include duplex scanning,[21, 22] phosphorus magnetic resonance imaging,[23] radiolabeled leukocyte scintigraphy,[24] and intraperitoneal xenon injection.[25] Duplex scanning, in particular, has evolved into a valuable screening examination for patients with proximal large vessel stenoses or occlusions. However, the inability to assess the terminal mesenteric vasculature clearly limits the usefulness of this modality in vasospastic disease of the visceral circulation. Limitations of resolution have also limited the effectiveness of magnetic resonance angiography, although continuous improvements in imaging technique suggest a promising future alternative to conventional aortography.[26]

Although the more direct approach of diagnostic laparoscopy has also been proposed for patients for whom arteriography is unsuitable,[27] this modality detects only grossly ischemic bowel and has no therapeutic capability. Furthermore, the attendant increase in intraperitoneal pressure risks a further decrease in mesenteric blood flow.[28]

TREATMENT

In contrast to the reversal of intestinal ischemia caused by mesenteric arterial occlusions, the reversal of nonocclusive mesenteric ischemia essentially depends on nonoperative methods of increasing mesenteric blood flow. Measures such as pulmonary artery catheterization to optimize fluid therapy and improve cardiac output, the reduction or elimination of digitalis or vasopressor agents, and the management of cardiogenic shock with vasodilators have all contributed to both the prevention and the treatment of nonocclusive mesenteric ischemia. In particular, agents such as captopril are valuable because of the sensitivity of the mesenteric vasculature to the renin-angiotensin axis.

Treatment of the underlying disease process is also crucial for patients with a noncardiac source of nonocclusive mesenteric ischemia. Patients with post-coarctectomy syndrome should respond to prompt and adequate control of postoperative hypertension. Although the treatment of cocaine and ergot poisoning is not significantly different from that of the usual nonocclusive mesenteric ischemia in patients with multiorgan system failure, the response of patients with ergotism to vasodilators or sympatholytic drugs is noteworthy because experimental attempts to displace ergotamine from alpha-receptors have not been successful. In this setting, the adjunctive use of anticoagulants has been recommended.[17]

Direct superior mesenteric artery infusion of vasodilators has been recommended for the optimal management of nonocclusive mesenteric ischemia. Although the effective-

ness of this therapy has been difficult to confirm experimentally and clinically, papaverine is unequivocally able to reverse mesenteric artery vasoconstriction, even in low-flow states.[19] The relative contribution of intra-arterial infusion to ultimate patient outcome is hard to assess because treatment of the underlying shock state occurs simultaneously. The most impressive clinical data come from the observation of affected patients with severe abdominal pain and vasospasm whose symptoms and angiographic abnormalities resolve within hours of intra-arterial papaverine infusion (Fig. 110–2). Direct mesenteric drug administration should clearly be regarded as complementary to, rather than competitive with, systemic correction of hypoperfusion.

The authors' protocol for papaverine administration involves a constant infusion of 30 to 60 mg/hr directly into the superior mesenteric artery as soon as the diagnostic study is completed. The infusion is continued for at least 24 hours, after which arteriography is repeated. Obviously, patient physical findings are also closely monitored throughout the treatment period. Additional 24-hour treatment intervals are determined by the clinical and radiologic reassessment. However, most favorable responses occur within the first 24 hours. As an adjunct to laparotomy for mesenteric thrombosis or bowel resection, the infusion may be continued during and after surgery to maximize the perfusion of ischemic but viable segments of intestine. Although other medications such as nitroglycerine, tolazoline, and prostaglandin E_1 would logically be expected to produce similar results, most of the clinical experience has been obtained with papaverine.

A new approach to the treatment of intestinal ischemia uses intraluminal instillation of oxygenated perfluorocarbons.[29, 30] Although the concept is intriguing, its clinical application has not yet been established. Intravenous gluca-

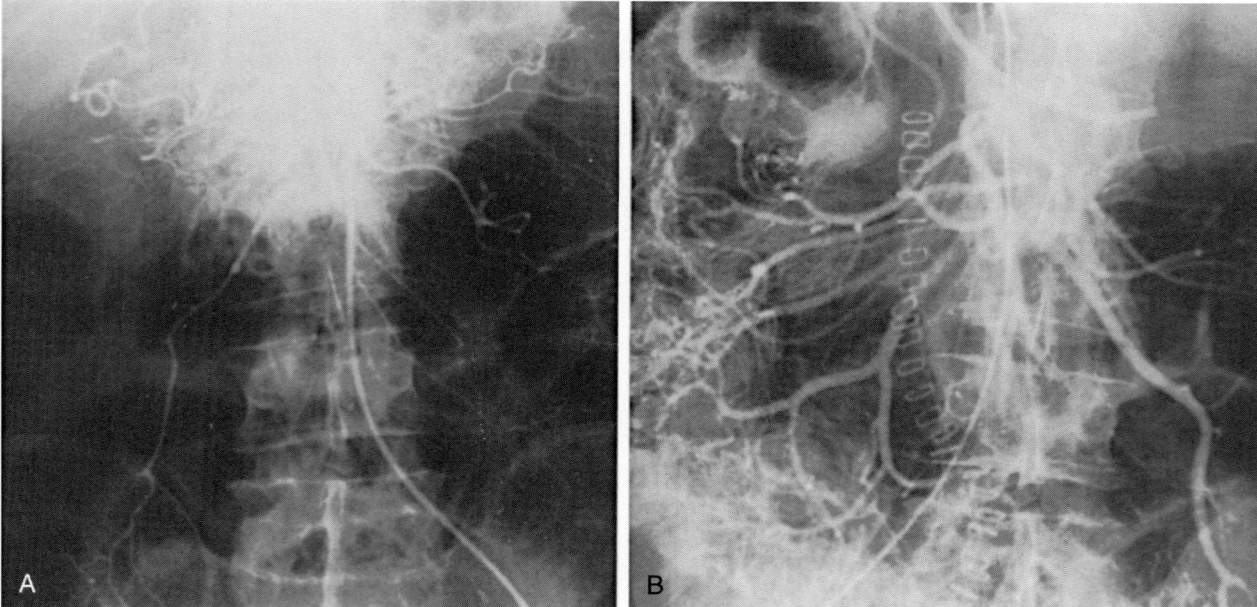

FIGURE 110–2. *A*, Nonocclusive mesenteric ischemia diagnosed arteriographically. There is diffuse spasm of the intestinal arcades with poor filling of intramural vessels. *B*, Relief of spasm and filling of distal vessels are observed after several hours of intra-arterial papaverine infusion. A laparotomy was performed for early peritoneal irritation, but no resection was required after the initiation of vasodilator therapy. (*A* and *B*, From Rivers S: Acute nonocclusive mesenteric ischemia. Semin Vasc Surg 3:172, 1990.)

gon administered during the early phase of reperfusion of ischemic intestinal segments has been shown experimentally to improve mucosal recovery, suggesting possible adjunctive use in the clinical setting.[31]

The role of surgical treatment in nonocclusive mesenteric ischemia is limited to the identification and resection of nonviable segments of bowel. Initial resection should be limited to clearly gangrenous segments because vasodilator therapy and treatment of the underlying disease may improve areas of uncertain viability.

The survival of patients with an established diagnosis of nonocclusive mesenteric ischemia has been reported to be as low as 0% to 29%, with or without papaverine infusion.[32–34] The results in the authors' institution have been somewhat better, probably because of an aggressive posture regarding early angiography of high-risk patients. The cause of death in most cases is irreversible shock or advanced intestinal necrosis at the time of diagnosis. The high mortality rate is a reflection of the seriousness of the underlying diseases and of the failure to recognize nonocclusive mesenteric ischemia in its earlier, treatable phase. Beneficial measures such as intra-arterial papaverine infusion directed toward specific end-organ damage remain entirely appropriate and are probably effective, despite the generally high mortality.

Acknowledgment: This chapter was supported in part by the Manning Foundation, the Anna S. Brown Trust, and the New York Institute for Vascular Studies.

REFERENCES

1. Wilson R, Qualheim RD: A form of acute hemorrhagic enterocolitis affecting chronically ill individuals: A description of twenty cases. Gastroenterology 27:431, 1954.
2. Ende N: Infarction of the bowel in cardiac failure. N Engl J Med 258:879, 1958.
3. Ottinger LW, Austen WG: A study of 136 patients with mesenteric infarction. Surg Gynecol Obstet 124:251, 1967.
4. Boley SJ, Regan JA, Tunick PA, et al: Persistent vasoconstriction: A major factor in nonocclusive intestinal ischemic injury. Curr Top Surg Res 3:435, 1971.
5. Parks DA, Grogaard B, Granger DN: Comparison of partial and complete arterial occlusion models for studying intestinal ischemia. Surgery 92:896, 1982.
6. Bookstein JJ, Goldberger L, Niwayama G, et al: Angiographic aspects of experimental nonocclusive intestinal ischemic injury. Am J Roentgenol 128:923, 1971.
7. Mellander S, Johansson B: Control of resistance, exchange, and capacitance functions in the peripheral circulation. Pharmacol Rev 20:117, 1968.
8. Bailey RW, Bulkley GB, Hamilton SR, et al: Protection of the small intestine from nonocclusive mesenteric ischemic injury due to cardiogenic shock. Am J Surg 153:108, 1987.
9. Bailey RW, Hamilton SR, Morris JB, et al: Pathogenesis of nonocclusive ischemic colitis. Am Surg 203:590, 1986.
10. Boley SJ, Agarwal GP, Warren AR, et al: Pathophysiologic effects of bowel distension on intestinal blood flow. Am J Surg 117:228, 1969.
11. Russ JE, Haid SP, Yao JST, et al: Surgical treatment of nonocclusive mesenteric infarction. Am J Surg 134:38, 1977.
12. Cheatham JE Jr, Williams GR, Thompson WM, et al: Coarctation: A review of 80 children and adolescents. Am J Surg 138:889, 1979.
13. Kawauchi M, Tada Y, Asano K, et al: Angiographic demonstration of mesenteric arterial changes in postcoartectomy syndrome. Surgery 98:602, 1985.
14. Behl PR, Sante P, Blesovsky A: Isolated coarctation of the aorta: Surgical treatment and late results: Eighteen years' experience. J Cardiovasc Surge (Torino) 29:509, 1988.
15. Greene FL, Ariyan S, Stansel HC Jr: Mesenteric and peripheral vascular ischemia secondary to ergotism. Surgery 81:176, 1977.
16. Nalbandian H, Sheth N, Dietrich R, et al: Intestinal ischemia caused by cocaine ingestion: Report of two cases. Surgery 97:374, 1985.
17. Merhoff GC, Porter JM: Ergot intoxication: Historical review and description of unusual clinical manifestations. Ann Surg 180:773, 1974.
18. Gewertz BL, Zarins CK: Postoperative vasospasm after antegrade mesenteric revascularization: A report of three cases. J Vasc Surg 14:382, 1991.
19. Siegelman SS, Sprayregan S, Boley SJ: Angiographic diagnosis of mesenteric arterial vasoconstriction. Diagn Radiol 112:533, 1974.
20. Boley SJ, Sprayregan S, Siegelman SS, et al: Initial results from an aggressive roentgenological and surgical approach to acute mesenteric ischemia. Surgery 82:848, 1977.
21. Jager K, Bollinger A, Valli C, et al: Measurement of mesenteric blood flow by duplex scanning. J Vasc Surg 3:462, 1986.
22. Lilly MP, Harward TRS, Flinn WR, et al: Duplex ultrasound measurement of changes in mesenteric flow velocity with pharmacologic and physiologic alteration of intestinal blood flow in man. J Vasc Surg 9:18, 1989.
23. Blum H, Barlow C, Chance B, et al: Acute intestinal ischemia studies by phosphorus nuclear magnetic resonance spectroscopy. Ann Surg 204:83, 1986.
24. Bardfeld PA, Boley SJ, Sammartano RJ, et al: Scintigraphic diagnosis of ischemic intestine with technetium 99m sulfur colloid labelled leukocytes. Radiology 124:439, 1977.
25. Gharagozloo F, Bulkley GB, Zuidema GD, et al: The use of intraperitoneal xenon for early diagnosis of acute mesenteric ischemia. Surgery 95:404, 1984.
26. Geelkerken RH, van Bockel JH: Mesenteric vascular disease: A review of diagnostic methods and therapies. Cardiovasc Surg 3:247, 1995.
27. Serreyn RF, Schoofs PR, Baetens PR, et al: Laparoscopic diagnosis of mesenteric venous thrombosis. Endoscopy 18:249, 1986.
28. Kleinhaus S, Sammartano RJ, Boley SJ: Variations in blood flow during laparoscopy. Physiologist 19:255, 1976.
29. Ricci JL, Sloviter HA, Ziegler MM: Intestinal ischemia: Reduction of mortality utilizing intraluminal perfluorochemical. Am J Surg 149:84, 1985.
30. Oldham KT, Guice KS, Gore D, et al: Treatment of intestinal ischemia with oxygenated intraluminal perfluorocarbons. Am J Surg 153:291, 1987.
31. Gangadharan SP, Wagner RJ, Cronenwett JL: Effect of intravenous glucagon on intestinal viability after segmental mesenteric ischemia. J Vasc Surg 21:900, 1995.
32. Sachs SM, Morton JH, Schwartz SI: Acute mesenteric ischemia. Surgery 92:646, 1982.
33. Hildebrand HD, Zierler RE: Mesenteric vascular disease. Am J Surg 139:188, 1980.
34. Bergan JJ, McCarthy WJ, Flinn WR, et al: Nontraumatic mesenteric vascular emergencies. J Vasc Surg 5:903, 1987.

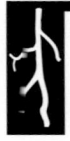

Intestinal Ischemia Caused by Venous Thrombosis

Andris Kazmers, M.D., M.S.P.H.

Splanchnic venous occlusions are a relatively infrequent, though important, cause of acute mesenteric ischemia (AMI).[1–17] Resection of infarcted intestine was the standard treatment for intestinal infarction from venous thrombosis even before 1935, when Warren and Eberhard reported a 34% mortality rate.[1] The availability of antibiotics and subsequent improvements in surgical care have not markedly improved mortality rates after intestinal resection for venous infarction.[16, 17] Anticoagulants, however, may reduce the frequency of recurrence and may have a beneficial effect on overall survival after mesenteric venous thrombosis.[2, 16, 17] Warren and Eberhard reported that only 5% of patients with intestinal ischemia from venous thrombosis left the hospital alive if they did not undergo surgery.[1] It is now understood that many cases of mesenteric venous thrombosis do not result in gut infarction and can be managed nonoperatively.[7, 8, 17]

EPIDEMIOLOGY

Warren and Eberhard reported that mesenteric venous thrombosis was present in 0.003% of the general hospital population and in 0.05% of autopsies.[1] More recently, splanchnic venous occlusions constituted 0.006% of hospital admissions and were present in fewer than 0.2% of autopsies.[12] As of 1984, only 372 patients with mesenteric venous thrombosis had been reported.[2] AMI is uncommon, and mesenteric venous thrombosis has been responsible for 5% to 15% of cases. One study reported that 0.38% of laparotomies performed for "acute abdomen" revealed mesenteric infarction, and only 17% of these cases were due to venous thrombosis.[14]

Older views of the natural history and incidence of mesenteric venous thrombosis were biased because most cases were detected at laparotomy or autopsy.[1, 8, 18, 19] Duplex ultrasonography, computed tomography (CT), and magnetic resonance imaging (MRI), and the aggressive use of diagnostic arteriography for evaluation of patients with possible AMI facilitate preoperative and antemortem diagnoses of mesenteric venous thrombosis.[20–59]

Acute intestinal ischemia from venous thrombosis occurs in either sex and at any age, although it is more common in those over 50 years old. The probability that a given patient with abdominal pain has mesenteric venous thrombosis is so low, however, that it is usually not considered in the differential diagnosis. A history of previous portomesenteric or lower extremity venous thrombosis in a patient who has unexplained abdominal pain, however, warrants inclusion of mesenteric venous thrombosis in the differential diagnosis.[4]

ETIOLOGY

Splanchnic venous occlusions have been categorized as *primary* or *secondary*. Primary occlusions have no known underlying cause, whereas secondary thromboses, which are more common, are associated with other disorders. Patients with secondary thromboses characteristically have conditions that act as variants of Virchow's triad.[60–98] These conditions may promote portal venous stasis (e.g., liver cirrhosis), splanchnic venous injury (e.g., after splenectomy), or hypercoagulability. Splanchnic venous thrombosis has been associated with protein C and protein S deficiencies, protein C resistance, antithrombin III deficiency, presence of anticardiolipin antibody, polycythemia vera, and certain malignancies. It is likely that a number of "primary" venous occlusions are due to yet undefined coagulation disturbances. When most clinical studies of splanchnic venous thrombosis were published, many of the underlying coagulation disturbances were unknown. More recent studies suggest that approximately half of patients with mesenteric venous thrombosis have underlying coagulation disorders.[4, 16, 17]

Secondary portomesenteric thrombosis may also be associated with intra-abdominal infection, particularly in children.[3] Thrombosis complicating infectious processes, such as appendicitis, may proceed to pyelophlebitis. In patients with malignancies, splanchnic venous thrombosis can result from venous invasion or external compression and hypercoagulability.

Those undergoing splenectomy are prone to portomesenteric venous thrombosis, which may be due to a combination of factors, including trauma to the splenic vein, stasis in the splenic vein stump, reduced portomesenteric venous flow, and perhaps thrombocytosis. When splenectomy is performed for hematologic disease, the underlying disorder may contribute to the thrombosis. Patients with myeloid metaplasia are particularly at risk for portomesenteric venous thrombosis after splenectomy. Portomesenteric venous thrombosis may complicate the course of patients with cirrhosis and portal hypertension. Splanchnic venous thromboses can occur spontaneously and have occurred after sclerotherapy for esophageal varices, selective transhepatic portal angiography, liver transplantation, and endovascular transvenous portosystemic shunt procedures.[73, 81, 82, 99]

CLINICAL PRESENTATION

The clinical presentation of mesenteric venous thrombosis may range from an asymptomatic state to a catastrophic acute illness. Prolonged abdominal discomfort is more common with visceral venous thrombosis than with the other disorders causing AMI. Symptoms tend to develop less rapidly than with acute arterial insufficiency of the intestines but may occasionally be as precipitous. Abdominal pain is typically generalized. Rebound tenderness is expected with transmural bowel injury.

Abdominal distention is commonly present and may be disproportionate to the expected degree of tympany on physical examination. This distention is due to bowel edema, sequestration of intraluminal and intraperitoneal fluid, and, in the case of intestinal infarction, blood. The presence of bloody peritoneal fluid has adverse prognostic significance.[9]

Occult gastrointestinal (GI) hemorrhage associated with mesenteric venous thrombosis is common, whereas upper GI bleeding from venous infarction that requires transfusion is less common.[100, 101] When significant GI bleeding occurs, it is likely to be due to variceal hemorrhage. In patients with preexisting hepatic cirrhosis, splanchnic venous thrombosis may be heralded by worsening ascites or variceal bleeding.

Recurrent thrombosis is not unusual, particularly in patients who have not received anticoagulation therapy.[2] A small percentage of patients may present with late intestinal stricture during prolonged follow-up in the absence of recurrent thrombosis.[102] Late hemorrhage may also rarely result from mesenteric varices that follow mesenteric venous thrombosis even in the absence of cirrhosis or portal venous occlusion.[100]

PATHOPHYSIOLOGY

Acute portomesenteric venous occlusions may increase portal venous pressure, which promotes the formation of varicies.[100, 101] Variceal hemorrhage may be the presenting sign of splanchnic venous thrombosis. Portal vein thrombosis is commonly associated with portal hypertension, varices, and splenomegaly, with or without hypersplenism. If the thrombotic process involves the portal vein, ascites may develop or worsen. Such portal vein occlusions may result in intestinal ischemia by obstruction of superior mesenteric venous outflow or by direct extension into the superior mesenteric vein (SMV). Isolated splenic vein thrombosis, usually associated with pancreatic disease, may result in upper GI bleeding from isolated gastric varices, a condition called *sinistral portal hypertension*.[76] When such venous thromboses are confined to the splenic vein, intestinal ischemia is not expected.

Thrombosis involving the SMV alone or the SMV and other associated portomesenteric venous thrombi may result in hemorrhagic gut infarction that is typically confined to the small intestine. Colon infarction has been reported but occurs much less commonly after venous thrombosis.[16, 17] The clinical manifestations relate to the extent, location, and rapidity of venous occlusion.[103] Though splanchnic venous thrombosis may present with worsening ascites, variceal hemorrhage, or intestinal ischemia, occlusion of the portal or superior mesenteric venous trunks can be asymptomatic. Isolated occlusions of the inferior mesenteric vein are usually asymptomatic.

Acute ligation of the inferior mesenteric vein is well tolerated.[104–108] Acute ligation of the portal vein or SMV is less well tolerated. It has been suggested, however, that portal vein ligation may be appropriate in managing irreparable portal vein injuries. Similarly, acute ligation of the SMV has been advocated for unstable patients with severe venous injuries. Not everyone, however, will tolerate such portal or SMV ligations. It is not currently possible to predict the consequences of ligation of these major splanchnic venous trunks in a given patient. Splanchnic venous reconstructions have been performed only rarely for venous hypertension in the SMV circulation.[109]

Advances in the understanding of portomesenteric venous thrombosis have resulted from the availability of CT, abdominal duplex ultrasound scanning, and MRI, which allow preoperative and antemortem diagnosis. Many cases of mesenteric venous thrombosis are detected incidentally by CT scanning before they become clinically evident. Autopsy series suggest that as many as 50% of patients who die with portomesenteric venous thrombosis do not develop bowel infarction.[110]

Extensive acute mesenteric venous obstruction results in massive intestinal fluid sequestration and hypovolemia with hemoconcentration.[111–118] Intestinal arteriolar vasoconstriction results from elevations of portal venous pressure. In addition, reduction of intestinal perfusion may follow in a fashion similar to that witnessed in phlegmasia cerulea dolens. In both situations, massive obstruction of venous outflow impairs arterial inflow. Hemorrhagic intestinal infarction may result.

Other adverse physiologic consequences follow intestinal ischemia. Ischemia impairs the ability of the GI tract to protect itself from its own luminal contents.[119–121] A loss of intestinal wall integrity results, which is associated with the release of vasoactive agents from intestinal cells as well as loss of boundary function for intestinal organisms that may be associated with the development of multiple organ failure.

The discussion of mesenteric venous thrombosis has thus far addressed the thrombotic process in the large visceral veins. A variant of splanchnic venous disease has recently been described, named *mesenteric inflammatory veno-occlusive disease* (MIVOD).[122–126] This disorder is more common in men and occurs in adults of all ages. Those with MIVOD present with unexplained acute intestinal ischemia. The patients do not have known connective tissue disorders or vasculitis, but MIVOD was reported to follow cytomegalovirus infection in one patient and was associated with the antiphospholipid syndrome in another. The diagnosis can be made with certainty only after careful histologic evaluation of resected intestine. There is no arterial involvement, and phlebitis or venulitis occurs transmurally in the gut wall. The inflammatory infiltrate may be lymphocytic, necrotizing, granulomatous, or mixed. There may be myointimal venous proliferation in a more chronic phase of inflammation that may coexist with acute inflammation.

The thrombotic component may overshadow the presence of the underlying phlebitis. It is therefore possible that this microscopic thrombotic process involving the small veins of the intestine has been overlooked in the past and is more common than appreciated. Imaging modalities useful for the diagnosis of mesenteric venous thrombosis would not be likely to facilitate the diagnosis of MIVOD. At present, the diagnosis can be made only after pathologic review of the infarcted intestine. After intestinal resection, patients with MIVOD have done well.

DIAGNOSIS

Laboratory tests or plain abdominal x-ray findings cannot identify intestinal ischemia caused by mesenteric venous thrombosis. Hemoconcentration and leukocytosis are expected, nonspecific findings. Elevations of serum phosphate or lactate levels may be found but are not diagnostic. Thumbprinting or gas in the portal venous system can be seen on abdominal roentgenographs. Barium contrast GI studies interfere with angiographic evaluation and should not be performed in the evaluation of patients who may have AMI.

When the differential diagnosis suggests that mesenteric venous thrombosis is likely, arteriography, CT with contrast enhancement, or abdominal duplex scanning may confirm the diagnosis. Duplex scanning is less sensitive than CT for detection of portomesenteric venous thrombosis, particularly for assessment of the superior mesenteric and splenic veins. Thrombus in the portal and hepatic veins may be difficult to distinguish from surrounding liver tissue by ultrasound examination. Inability to image the portal vein should raise the suspicion for portal venous thrombosis when failure of insonation is not due to overlying bowel gas or hepatic parenchymal abnormalities. Presence of worm-like vascular channels in the area of the portal vein suggests cavernomatous transformation from prior portal vein thrombosis.

Findings suggestive of splanchnic venous thrombosis include enlargement of the splanchnic vein, intravenous echogenic thrombus, abnormal or absent flow within the vein, and lack of compressibility or respiratory variation in vein size. Ultrasound studies cannot differentiate clot from tumor thrombus. The portal vein is less than 13 mm in diameter in normal adults, whereas the size of thrombosed portal veins ranges from 15 to 26 mm. Massive venous enlargement has been mistaken for pancreatic masses, including pancreatic pseudocyst.

The typical CT appearance of superior mesenteric venous thrombosis reveals enlargement of the thrombosed vein with a central area of low attenuation associated with clot within the lumen that is surrounded by well-defined, contrast-enhanced venous wall opacification. Such vein wall enhancement is not always present. In portomesenteric venous thrombosis, multivein occlusion is common.[103] The triad of hypodensity in the SMV, thickening of the small intestinal wall, and presence of peritoneal fluid found on CT scanning suggests that laparotomy should be performed because bowel infarction is likely.[9] The presence of peritoneal fluid indicates greater severity of intestinal ischemia from mesenteric venous occlusion and has prompted some to recommend laparotomy. The absence of peritoneal fluid has been a reassuring finding that would support a decision to treat a patient with mesenteric venous thrombosis nonoperatively.

Other important CT findings may include presence of gas in the intestinal wall, in the venous system, or in an extraluminal location. Pneumatosis intestinalis is more easily detected by CT than by plain film. Portal or mesenteric venous gas strongly suggests the presence of bowel infarction. MRI may also confirm the diagnosis of portomesenteric venous thrombosis. The role of MRI for establishing the diagnosis of intestinal ischemia from venous thrombosis is evolving. The addition of gadolinium as a contrast agent for more extensive evaluation of the visceral arterial and venous circulation appears promising.[99, 126]

Transhepatic portography may be used diagnostically. One complication associated with this technique, however, has been portal vein thrombosis. Transhepatic, transvenous selective clot lysis has been used to successfully manage portomesenteric venous thrombosis.[128] This approach, whether transhepatic or transjugular, may prove useful for selected patients.[128, 129]

Arterial portography was the preferred nonoperative method to confirm the diagnosis of portomesenteric venous thrombosis in the past. Visualization of the portomesenteric venous system requires prolonged infusion of contrast material into the celiac and superior mesenteric arteries followed by delayed filming. Such angiographic studies may reveal intraluminal thrombus or venous occlusion. Superior mesenteric arterial spasm, prolongation of the arterial angiographic phase, and other subtle findings result from superior mesenteric venous occlusion. Selective infusion of thrombolytic agents into the superior mesenteric artery has anecdotally been used to clear superior mesenteric venous thrombi.[130] The effectiveness of such an approach should be questioned because infusion of contrast into the superior mesenteric artery does not always result in visualization of the SMV. It is possible that lytic agents are not effective in such patients unless systemic lysis is achieved.

Abdominal duplex scanning is operator-dependent, may be unavailable at all hours or in all hospitals, and may be difficult to perform in those with acute intestinal ischemia from mesenteric venous thrombosis due to associated abdominal discomfort. Greater sensitivity for detection of splanchnic venous thrombosis, the ability to detect bowel wall thickening and other associated findings, and greater availability render CT superior to duplex ultrasonography and MRI for evaluation of patients with possible splanchnic venous thrombosis. In patients with mesenteric venous thrombosis, the CT scan will be abnormal. Angiography and CT can serve as complementary studies in difficult cases.

Abdominal paracentesis may provide *indirect* evidence (bloody ascites) and laparoscopy may provide *direct* evidence of intestinal ischemia from portomesenteric venous thrombosis (hemorrhagic infarction).[131, 132] In some cases, celiotomy is an appropriate and necessary diagnostic procedure. In venous gut infarction, the middle of the small intestine, which eludes colonoscopy and esophagogastro-duodenoscopy (EGD), is usually involved. Although EGD may not provide important diagnostic information in the absence of upper GI bleeding, it is reasonable to perform EGD in patients with portal or splenic vein thrombosis to assess the presence of gastroesophageal varices, particularly in patients who may be candidates for long-term anticoagulation therapy. EGD is indicated for evaluation of upper GI bleeding to determine whether the source is varices.

When the diagnosis of visceral infarction is made at laparotomy, systematic evaluation can help define the cause.[8] The intestine is discolored and edematous with portomesenteric venous thrombosis, and the mesentery may be thickened. Serosanguineous fluid is consistent with, but not specific for, venous infarction. Infarction from mesenteric venous thrombosis commonly involves the middle segment of the small intestine, and the colon is usually not affected. Duodenal involvement suggests that gut infarction is not venous in origin. If venous thrombi extrude when the mesentery is divided, especially in the absence of thrombus in the mesenteric arterioles, intestinal infarction from venous thrombosis is the most likely diagnosis.

MANAGEMENT

Patients with intestinal ischemia due to mesenteric venous thrombosis require vigorous resuscitation and broad-spectrum antibiotic coverage. The utility of mesenteric vasodilators is not established, although they have been used anecdotally. Anticoagulation is absolutely necessary to limit the thrombotic process and to reduce the likelihood of recurrence. If not begun preoperatively, anticoagulation should begin intraoperatively. Experimental studies have shown that either heparin or low-molecular-weight dextran can be used, but heparin is preferable.

Recurrent thrombosis can be expected in approximately one third of those with mesenteric venous thrombosis.[133, 134] Naitove and Weissman reported that no deaths occurred in patients with primary mesenteric venous thrombosis who received anticoagulants postoperatively, whereas 50% of those who did not receive postoperative anticoagulation died.[6] A review of mesenteric venous thrombosis reported that recurrence was significantly lower in the heparin-treated group than in untreated patients. Of those with recurrence, 22% treated with anticoagulants died, whereas 59% of those not treated with heparin died.[2]

Anticoagulation therapy should be continued indefinitely unless there is a contraindication or the factor responsible for the venous thrombosis has been corrected. If a bleeding complication results, it is difficult to justify continuation of anticoagulation even though the patients may be at greater risk for recurrent splanchnic venous thrombosis. The required duration of anticoagulation therapy is unknown. All patients with thrombosis of the portomesenteric venous circulation should undergo a complete evaluation of their coagulation system.

For patients with coagulation disorders, anticoagulation should be continued indefinitely. Only when such findings are normal can the patient be considered to have primary venous occlusion. Perhaps patients with primary mesen-

teric venous thrombosis should also receive anticoagulation indefinitely because they may harbor yet undefined coagulation disorders. Management plans for secondary splanchnic venous occlusion must consider the underlying disorder. For patients with splanchnic venous injury, the discontinuation of anticoagulation can be considered, particularly if varices develop during late follow-up. Anticoagulation in the presence of cirrhosis or gastrointestinal varices is problematic.

Lytic therapy with urokinase, streptokinase, or tissue plasminogen activator (t-PA) has been used in patients with mesenteric venous thrombosis.[135, 136] The risk of hemorrhage from fibrinolytic agents in someone with an acute abdominal process is considerable. Successful lysis of superior mesenteric venous thrombosis with recombinant tissue-type plasminogen activator (rt-PA) has been reported.[135] The presence of gastroesophageal varices was not a contraindication to lytic therapy. Interestingly, gastroesophageal varices have disappeared after clot lysis. It is not possible to compare the outcomes from thrombolytic therapy with the natural history of the disorder. Fibrinolytic agents have had increasing anecdotal clinical success in the splanchnic venous circulation. Problems with access to the splanchnic venous system have prompted a number of interesting approaches to infusion of lytic agents.[128–130]

At surgery, infarcted intestine should be resected with wide margins if possible. The thrombotic process may involve the mesentery of viable intestine adjacent to the infarcted intestine. Intestinal reanastomosis is permissible in stable patients when gut infarction is focal and confined to the small intestine if the remaining gut looks normal. Exteriorization of the intestine after resection is appropriate when conditions are not optimal for primary anastomosis.

If the initial infarction is extensive, limited resection of necrotic bowel should be done. Recurrent infarction from repeated venous thrombosis involves the area adjacent to the anastomosis in 60% of patients. Second-look procedures are not mandatory for patients who have segmental venous infarction that has been widely resected, who are stable, and who have received anticoagulation therapy with heparin. Intraoperative assessment of gut viability may be difficult, and the accuracy of Doppler and fluorescein techniques is not as great for intestinal ischemia from mesenteric venous thrombosis.[138, 139] These considerations should lead to the use of second-look procedures when the viability of unresected intestine is in question or when massive intestinal resection would otherwise be required.

Second-look operations might also be useful for the rare patient who undergoes portomesenteric venous thrombectomy. Anecdotal reports suggest that portomesenteric venous thrombectomy may be useful, particularly when it might prevent massive intestinal resection.[140–148] Removal of thrombus from the smaller veins is not likely, and continued patency of the main venous trunks after thrombectomy has not proved responsible for clinical improvement. Portomesenteric venous thrombectomy has been successful for reestablishing venous outflow to sustain liver transplants and for patients with acute intestinal ischemia from venous thrombosis. It is likely that venous thrombectomy has been underutilized in the management of patients with portomesenteric venous thromboses.

Surgeons may not be familiar with the operative ap-

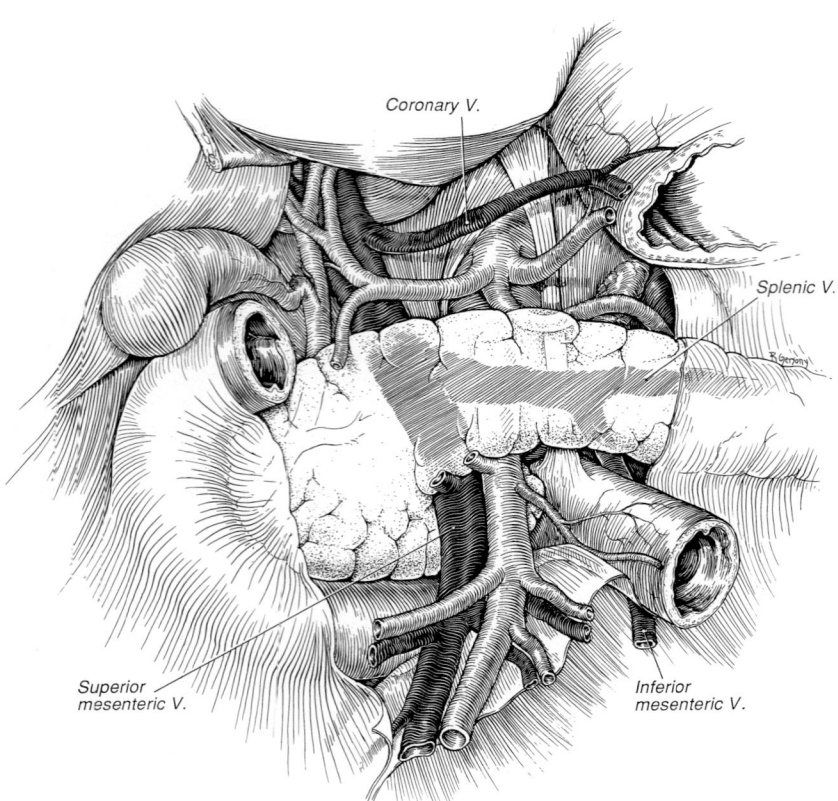

FIGURE 111–1. Regional anatomy of surgically accessible superior mesenteric vein.

proach to portomesenteric venous thrombectomy (Fig. 111–1). The approach to the SMV would be similar to that for superior mesenteric artery embolectomy.[149] The vein is to the right of the artery and is much more fragile. The surgeon obtains access to a segment of SMV by elevating the transverse mesocolon, displacing the small intestine to the right, and completely dividing the ligament of Treitz. This dissection proceeds onto the mesentery of the small intestine, past the superior mesenteric artery, and over the SMV.

Inahara isolated the SMV, performed linear venotomy, and removed the small clots from the peripheral veins by milking the bowel and mesentery (Fig. 111–2).[141] Both

linear and transverse venotomies in the SMV have been used. A Fogarty catheter can be used to retrieve more centrally located thrombus in the proximal superior mesenteric and portal veins (Fig. 111–3). The surgical approach used by Inahara is reasonable and comparable with that used by others.

SUMMARY

The improved ability to make the preoperative or antemortem diagnosis of portomesenteric venous thrombosis has

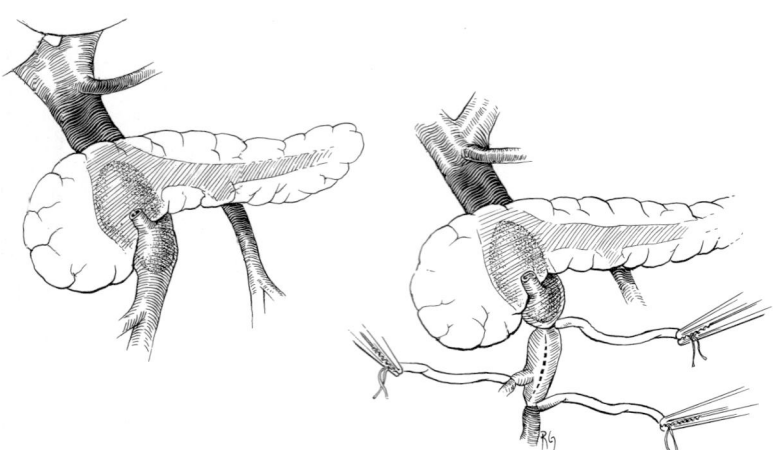

FIGURE 111–2. Infrapancreatic control of the superior mesenteric vein is achieved.

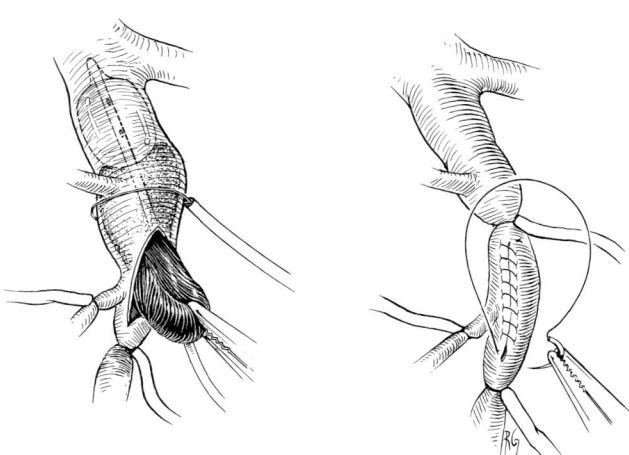

FIGURE 111–3. Venous thrombectomy is performed, and the venotomy is closed.

resulted in the realization that this disorder does not invariably proceed to intestinal infarction or death without operative intervention. Nonoperative management with anticoagulation is appropriate when intestinal ischemia from venous thrombosis has not progressed to transmural infarction. The continued absence of peritoneal fluid on CT scanning and the absence of peritoneal signs are favorable findings that allow continued nonoperative management in those with splanchnic venous thrombosis.

As an adjunct to surgical therapy, anticoagulation can reduce recurrent thrombosis and overall mortality rate for patients with intestinal infarction from venous thrombosis. Lytic therapy and thrombectomy have historically been less important in managing splanchnic venous thrombosis, but both techniques have been associated with anecdotal success. With the improved ability to diagnose and study intestinal ischemia from portomesenteric venous thrombosis, further improvements in the treatment of mesenteric venous thrombosis can be anticipated.

REFERENCES

1. Warren S, Eberhard TP: Mesenteric venous thrombosis. Surg Gynecol Obstet 61:102–121, 1935.
2. Abdu RA, Zakhour BJ, Dallis DJ: Mesenteric venous thrombosis 1911 to 1984. Surgery 101:383–388, 1987.
3. Grendell JH, Ockner RH: Mesenteric venous thrombosis. Gastroenterology 82:358–373, 1982.
4. Harward RS, Green D, Bergan JJ, et al: Mesenteric venous thrombosis. J Vasc Surg 9:328–333, 1989.
5. Mathews JE, White RR: Primary mesenteric venous occlusive disease. Am J Surg 122:579–583, 1971.
6. Naitove A, Weissman RE: Primary mesenteric venous thrombosis. Ann Surg 161:516–523, 1965.
7. Kispert JF, Kazmers A: Acute intestinal ischemia caused by mesenteric venous thrombosis. Semin Vasc Surg 3:157–171, 1990.
8. Kazmers A: Mesenteric venous occlusion. In Current Therapy in Vascular Surgery. Philadelphia, BC Decker, 1987, pp 230–323.
9. Clavien PA, Durig M, Harder F: Venous mesenteric infarction, a particular entity. Br J Surg 75:252–255, 1988.
10. Clavien PA, Muller C, Harder F: Treatment of mesenteric infarction. Br J Surg 74:500–503, 1987.
11. Montany PF, Finley RK: Mesenteric venous thrombosis. Am Surg 54:161–166, 1988.
12. Ottinger LW, Austen WG: A study of 136 patients with mesenteric infarction. Surg Gynecol Obstet 124:251–261, 1967.
13. Picardi E, Peoples JB: Mesenteric venous thrombosis: Ten year record review and evaluation of difficulties with the ICD coding system. S D J Med 44:33–37, 1991.
14. Rius X, Escalante JF, et al: Mesenteric infarction. World J Surg 3:489–496, 1979.
15. Umpleby HC: Thrombosis of the superior mesenteric vein. Br J Surg 74:694–696, 1987.
16. Rhee RY, Gloviczki P, Mendonca CT, et al: Mesenteric venous thrombosis: Still a lethal disease in the 1990s. J Vasc Surg 20(5):688–697, 1994.
17. Rhee RY, Gloviczki P: Mesenteric venous thrombosis. Surg Clin North Am 77(2):327–338, 1997.
18. Johnson CC, Baggenstoss AH: Mesenteric venous occlusion: Study of 99 cases of occlusion of veins. Mayo Clin Proc 24:628–636, 1949.
19. Donaldson JK, Stout BF: Mesenteric thrombosis: Arterial and venous types as separate clinical entities: A clinical and experimental study. Am J Surg 29:208–217, 1935.
20. Tomchik FS, Wittenberg J, Ottinger LW: The roentgenographic spectrum of bowel infarction. Radiology 96:249–260, 1970.
21. Clemett AR, Chung J: The radiologic diagnosis of spontaneous mesenteric venous thrombosis. Am J Gastroenterol 63:209–215, 1975.
22. Bolondi L, Mazziotti A, Arienti V, et al: Ultrasonographic study of portal venous system in portal hypertension and after portasystemic shunt operations. Surgery 95:261–269, 1984.
23. Miller VE, Berland LL: Pulsed Doppler duplex sonography and CT scan of portal venous thrombosis. Am J Roentgenol 145:73–76, 1985.
24. Friedenberg MJ, Polk HC, McAlister WH, et al: Superior mesenteric arteriography in experimental mesenteric venous thrombosis. Radiology 85:38–45, 1965.
25. Siegelman SS, Sprayregen S, Boley SJ: Angiographic diagnosis of mesenteric arterial vasoconstriction. Radiology 112:533–542, 1974.
26. Rosen A, Korobkin M, Silverman PM, et al: Mesenteric vein thrombosis: CT identification. Am J Roentgenol 143:83–86, 1984.
27. Clavien PA, Huber O, Mirescu D, Rohner A: Contrast enhanced CT scan as a diagnostic procedure in mesenteric ischaemia due to mesenteric venous thrombosis. Br J Surg 76:93–94, 1989.
28. Williams DM, Eckhauser FE, Aisen A, et al: Assessment of portosystemic shunt patency and function with magnetic resonance imaging. Surgery 102:602–607, 1987.
29. Johansen K, Paun M: Duplex ultrasonography of the portal vein. Surg Clin North Am 70:181–190, 1990.
30. Alpern MB, Glazer GM, Francis IR: Ischemic or infarcted bowel: CT findings. Radiology 166:149–152, 1988.
31. Federle MP, Chun G, Jeffrey RB, Rayor R: Computed tomographic findings in bowel infarction. Am J Roentgenol 142:91–95, 1984.
32. Harch JM, Radin RD, Yellin AE, Donovan AJ: Pylethrombosis: Serendipitous radiologic diagnosis. Arch Surg 122:1116–1119, 1987.
33. Kane RA, Katz SG: The spectrum of sonographic findings in portal hypertension: A subject review and new observations. Radiology 142:453–458, 1982.
34. Levy HM, Newhouse JH: MR imaging of portal vein thrombosis. Am J Roentgenol 151:283–286, 1988.
35. Martin K, Balfe DM, Lee JKT: Computed tomography of portal vein thrombosis: Unusual appearances and pitfalls in diagnosis. J Comput Assist Tomogr 13:811–816, 1989.
36. Mori H, Hayashi K, Uetani M, et al: High-attenuation recent thrombus of the portal vein: CT demonstration and clinical significance. Radiology 163:353–356, 1987.
37. Nordback I, Sisto T: Ultrasonography and computed tomography in the diagnosis of portomesenteric vein thrombosis. Int Surg 76:179–182, 1991.
38. Schwerk WB: Portal vein thrombosis: Real-time sonographic demonstration and follow-up. Gastrointest Radiol 11:312–318, 1986.
39. Tessler FN, Gehring BJ, Gomes AS, et al: Diagnosis of portal vein thrombosis: Value of color Doppler imaging. Am J Roentgenol 157:293–296, 1991.
40. Tey H, Sprayregen S, Ahmed A, Chan KF: Mesenteric vein thrombosis: Angiography in two cases. Am J Roentgenol 136:809–811, 1981.
41. Vogelzang RL, Gore RM, Anschuetz SL, Blei AT: Thrombosis of the splanchnic veins: CT diagnosis. Am J Roentgenol 150:93–96, 1988.
42. Vujic I, Rogers CI, LeVeen HH: Computed tomographic detection of portal vein thrombosis. Radiology 135:697–698, 1980.

43. Webb L, Berger LA, Sherlock S: Grey-scale ultrasonography of portal vein. Lancet 2:675–677, 1977.
44. Weinreb J, Kumari S, Phillips G, Pochaczevsky R: Portal vein measurements by real-time sonography. Am J Roentgenol 139:497–500, 1982.
45. Zerhouni EA, Barth KH, Siegelman SS: Demonstration of venous thrombosis by computed tomography. Am J Roentgenol 134:753–758, 1980.
46. Ivatury RR, Nallathambi M, Lankin DH, et al: Portal vein injuries: Noninvasive follow-up of venorraphy. Ann Surg 206:733–737, 1987.
47. Al Karawi MA, Quaiz M, Clark D, et al: Mesenteric vein thrombosis, non-invasive diagnosis and follow-up (US + MRI), and non-invasive therapy by streptokinase and anticoagulants. Hepatogastroenterology 37:507–509, 1990.
48. Subramanyam BR, Balthazar J, Lefleur RS, et al: Portal venous thrombosis: Correlative analysis of sonography, CT, and angiography. Am J Gastroenterol 79:773–776, 1984.
49. Verbanck JJ, Rutgeerts LJ, Haerens MH: Partial splenoportal and superior mesenteric venous thrombosis. Gastroenterology 86:949–954, 1984.
50. Matos C, Van-Gansbeke D, Zalcman M, et al: Mesenteric vein thrombosis: Early CT and US diagnosis and conservative management. Gastrointest Radiol 11:322–325, 1986.
51. Hricak H, Amparo E, Fisher MR, et al: Abdominal venous system: Assessment using MR. Radiology 156:415–422, 1985.
52. Haddad MC, Clark DC, Sharif HS, et al: MR, CT, and ultrasonography of splanchnic venous thrombosis. Gastrointest Radiol 17(1):34–40, 1992.
53. Farin P, Paajanen H, Miettinen P: Intraoperative US diagnosis of pylephlebitis (portal vein thrombosis) as a complication of appendicitis: A case report. Abdom Imaging 22(4):401–403, 1997.
54. Shirkhoda A, Konez O, Shetty AN, et al: Mesenteric circulation: Three-dimensional MR angiography with a gadolinium-enhanced multiecho gradient-echo technique. Radiology 202(1):257–261, 1997.
55. Ghisletta N, von Flue M, Eichlisberger E, et al: [Mesenteric venous thrombosis (MVT): A problem in diagnosis and management.] Swiss Surg 2(5):223–229, 1996.
56. Wiersema MJ, Chak A, Kopecky KK, Wiersema LM: Duplex Doppler endosonography in the diagnosis of splenic vein, portal vein, and portosystemic shunt thrombosis. Gastrointest Endosc 42(1):19–26, 1995.
57. Stringer MD, Heaton ND, Karani J, et al: Patterns of portal vein occlusion and their aetiological significance. Br J Surg 81(9):1328–1331, 1994.
58. Kim JY, Ha HK, Byun JY, et al: Intestinal infarction secondary to mesenteric venous thrombosis: CT-pathologic correlation. J Comput Assist Tomogr 17(3):382–385, 1993.
59. Rahmouni A, Mathieu D, Golli M, et al: Value of CT and sonography in the conservative management of acute splenoportal and superior mesenteric venous thrombosis. Gastrointest Radiol 17(2):135–140, 1992.
60. Broe RJ, Conley CL, Cameron JL: Thrombosis of the portal vein following splenectomy for myeloid metaplasia. Surg Gynecol Obstet 152:488–492, 1981.
61. Witte CL, Brewer ML, Witte MH, et al: Protean manifestations of pylethrombosis. Ann Surg 202:191–202, 1985.
62. Ashida H, Kotoura Y, Nishioka A, et al: Portal and mesenteric venous thrombosis as a complication of endoscopic sclerotherapy. Am J Gastroenterol 84:306–310, 1989.
63. Keith RG, Mustard RA, Saibil EA: Gastric variceal bleeding due to occlusion of splenic vein in pancreatic disease. Can J Surg 25:301–304, 1982.
64. Mergenthaler FW, Harris MN: Superior mesenteric vein thrombosis complicating pancreaticoduodenectomy: Successful treatment by thrombectomy. Ann Surg 167:106–111, 1986.
65. Belli L, Romani F, Sansalone CV, et al: Portal thrombosis in cirrhotics. Ann Surg 203:286–291, 1986.
66. Belli L, Romani F, Riolo F, et al: Thrombosis of portal vein in absence of hepatic disease. SG&O 169:46–49, 1989.
67. Bemelman WA, Butzelaar RMJM, Khargi K, Keeman JN: Mesenteric venous thrombosis caused by deficiency of physiologic anticoagulants: Report of a case. Neth J Surg 42-I:6–19, 1990.
68. Brown KM, Kaplan MM, Donowitz M: Extrahepatic portal venous thrombosis: Frequent recognition of associated diseases. J Clin Gastroenterol 7(2):153–159, 1985.
69. Cohen D, Johansen K, Cottingham K, et al: Trauma to major visceral veins: An underemphasized cause of accident mortality. J Trauma 20:928–932, 1980.
70. Cohen J, Edelman RR, Chopra S: Portal vein thrombosis: A review. Am J Med 92:173–182, 1992.
71. Collins GJ, Zuck TF, Zajtchuk R, Heymann RL: Hypercoagulability in mesenteric venous occlusion. Am J Surg 132:389–391, 1976.
72. Courcy PA, Brotman S, et al: Superior mesenteric artery and vein injuries from blunt abdominal trauma. J Trauma 24(9):843–845, 1984.
73. Deboever G, Elegeert I, Defloor E: Portal and mesenteric venous thrombosis after endoscopic injection sclerotherapy. Am J Gastroenterol 84:1336–1337, 1989.
74. De Clerck LS, Michielsen PP, Ramael MR, et al: Portal and pulmonary vessel thrombosis associated with systemic lupus erythematosus and anticardiolipin antibodies. J Rheumatol 18:1919–1921, 1991.
75. Engelhardt TC, Kerstein MD: Pregnancy and mesenteric venous thrombosis. South Med J 82:1441–1443, 1989.
76. Evans G, Yellin AE, Weaver FA, Stain SC: Sinistral (left-sided) portal hypertension. Am J Surg 56:758–763, 1990.
77. Hansen HJ, Christoffersen JK: Occlusive mesenteric infarction. Acta Chir Scand 472:103–108, 1976.
78. Hickman A, Wilson SK, et al: Portal and superior mesenteric venous thrombosis following splenectomy. J Tenn Med Assoc 84:329–330, 1991.
79. Ikeda N, Umetsu K, et al: Sudden unexpected death from a superior mesenteric venous thrombosis after a gastrectomy. Jpn J Legal Med 43:328–331, 1989.
80. Jaffe V, Lygidakis NJ, Blumgart LH: Acute portal vein thrombosis after right hepatic lobectomy: Successful treatment by thrombectomy. Br J Surg 69:211, 1982.
81. Korula J, Yellin A, Kanel GC, Nichols P: Portal vein thrombosis complicating endoscopic variceal sclerotherapy. Dig Dis Sci 36:1164–1167, 1991.
82. Leach SD, Meier GH, Gusberg RJ: Endoscopic sclerotherapy: A risk factor for splanchnic venous thrombosis. J Vasc Surg 10:9–13, 1989.
83. Mattox KL, Guinn GA: Mesenteric infarction. Am J Surg 126:332–335, 1973.
84. Britton BJ, Royle G: Mesenteric venous thrombosis: Br J Surg 69:118, 1982.
85. Olson JF, Steuber CP, Hawkins E, Mahoney DH: Functional deficiency of protein C associated with mesenteric venous thrombosis and splenic infarction. Am J Pediatr Hematol Oncol 13:168–171, 1991.
86. Orozco H, Guraieb E, et al: Deficiency of protein C in patients with portal vein thrombosis. Hepatology 8:1110–1111, 1988.
87. Berry FB, Bougas JA: Agnogenic venous mesenteric thrombosis. Ann Surg 132:450–474, 1950.
88. Tollefson D, Friedman KD: Protein C deficiency. Arch Surg 123:881–884, 1988.
89. Valla D, Casadevall N, et al: Etiology of portal vein thrombosis in adults. Gastroenterology 94:1063–1069, 1988.
90. Valla D, Denninger MH, et al: Portal vein thrombosis with ruptured oesophageal varices as presenting manifestation of hereditary protein C deficiency. Gut 29:856–859, 1988.
91. Webb L, Sherlock S: The aetiology, presentation and natural history of extra-hepatic portal venous obstruction. Q J Med 192:627–639, 1979.
92. Yates P, Cumber PM, Sanderson S, Harrison MS: Mesenteric venous thrombosis due to protein C deficiency. Clin Lab Haematol 13:137–139, 1991.
93. Maung R, Kelly JK, Schneider MP, et al: Mesenteric venous thrombosis due to antithrombin III deficiency. Arch Pathol Lab Med 112:37–39, 1988.
94. Green D, Ganger DR, Blei AT: Protein C deficiency in splanchnic venous thrombosis. Am J Med 82:1171–1174, 1987.
95. Broekmans AW, van Rooyen W, Westerveld BD, et al: Mesenteric vein thrombosis as presenting manifestation of hereditary protein S deficiency. Gastroenterology 92:240–242, 1987.
96. Sahdev P, Wolff M, Widmann WD: Mesenteric venous thrombosis associated with estrogen therapy for treatment of prostatic carcinoma. J Urol 134:563–564, 1985.
97. Heresbach D, Pagenault M, Gueret P, et al: Leiden factor V mutation in four patients with small bowel infarctions. Gastroenterology 113(1):322–325, 1997.

98. Ostermiller W Jr, Carter R: Mesenteric venous thrombosis secondary to polycythemia vera. Am Surg 35(6):40, 1969.

99. Stafford-Johnson DB, Hamilton BH, Dong Q, et al: Vascular complications of liver transplantation: Evaluation with gadolinium-enhanced MR angiography. Radiology 207(1):153–160, 1998.

100. Soper NJ, Rikkers LF, Miller FJ: Gastrointestinal hemorrhage associated with chronic mesenteric venous occlusion. Gastroenterology 88:1964–1967, 1985.

101. Miyaki CT, Park YS, Gopalswamy N: Upper gastrointestinal bleeding in acute mesenteric thrombosis. J Clin Gastroenterol 10(1):84–87, 1988.

102. Eugene C, Valla D, Wesenfelder L, et al: Small intestinal stricture complicating superior mesenteric vein thrombosis: A study of three cases. Gut 37:292–295, 1995.

103. Gertsch P, Matthews J, et al: Acute thrombosis of the splanchnic veins. Arch Surg 128(3):341–345, 1993.

104. Mattox KL: Abdominal venous injuries. Surgery 91:497–501, 1982.

105. Donahue TK, Strauch GO: Ligation as definitive management of injury to the superior mesenteric vein. J Trauma 28:541–543, 1988.

106. Patterson RB, Fowl RJ, et al: Letters to the editors. J Trauma 25:1684, 1988.

107. Sheldon GF, Lim RC, Yee ES, Petersen SR: Management of injuries to the porta hepatis. Ann Surg 202:539–545, 1985.

108. Sirinek KR, Levine BA: Traumatic injury to the proximal superior mesenteric vessels. Surgery 98:831–835, 1985.

109. Silvestri F, Dardik H, Vasquez R, et al: Mesoportal bypass: A unique operation for mesenteric hypertension. J Vasc Surg 22(6):764–768, 1995.

110. Laufman H, Scheinberg S: Arterial and venous mesenteric occlusion. Am J Surg 58:84–92, 1942.

111. Polk H: Experimental mesenteric venous occlusion. Ann Surg 163:432–444, 1966.

112. Turner MD, Neely WA, Barnett WO: The effects of temporary arterial, venous, and arteriovenous occlusion upon intestinal blood flow. Surg Gynecol Obstet 108:347–350, 1959.

113. Laufman H, Method H: Role of vascular spasm in recovery of strangulated intestine: Experimental study. Surg Gynecol Obstet 85:675–686, 1943.

114. Nelson LE, Kremen AJ: Experimental occlusion of the superior mesenteric vessels with special reference to the role of intravascular thrombosis and its prevention by heparin. Surgery 28:819–826, 1950.

115. Khanna SD: An experimental study of mesenteric occlusion. J Pathol Bacteriol 77:575–590, 1959.

116. Khodadadi J, Rozencwajg J, et al: Mesenteric vein thrombosis. Arch Surg 115:315–317, 1980.

117. Lepley D, Mani CJ, Ellison EH: Superior mesenteric venous occlusion: A study using low molecular weight dextran to prevent infarction. J Surg Res 2:403–406, 1962.

118. Granger DN, Richardson PDI, Kvietys PR, Mortillaro NA: Intestinal blood flow. Gastroenterology 78:837–863, 1980.

119. Montgomery A, Borgstrom A, Haglund U: Pancreatic proteases and intestinal mucosal injury after ischemia and reperfusion in the pig. Gastroenterology 102:216–222, 1992.

120. Kazmers A, Zwolak R, Appleman HD, et al: Pharmacologic interventions in acute mesenteric ischemia: Improved survival with intravenous glucagon, methylprednisolone, and prostacyclin. J Vasc Surg 1:472–481, 1984.

121. Zhi-Young S, Yuan-Lin D, Xiao-Hong W: Bacterial translocation and multiple system organ failure in bowel ischemia and reperfusion. J Trauma 32:148–153, 1992.

122. Corsi A, Ribaldi S, Coletti M, Bosman C: Intramural mesenteric venulitis: A new cause of intestinal ischaemia. Virchows Arch 427(1):65–69, 1995. .

123. Lie JT: Mesenteric inflammatory veno-occlusive disease (MIVOD): An emerging and unsuspected cause of digestive tract ischemia. Vasa 26:91–96, 1997.

124. Ailani RK, Simms R, Caracioni AA, West BC: Extensive mesenteric inflammatory veno-occlusive disease of unknown etiology after primary cytomegalovirus infection: First case. Am J Gastroenterol 92:1216–1218, 1997.

125. Flaherty MJ, Lie JT, Haggitt RC: Mesenteric inflammatory veno-occlusive disease. Am J Surg Pathol 18:779–784, 1994.

126. Gul A, Inanc M, Ocal L, et al: Primary antiphospholipid syndrome associated with mesenteric inflammatory veno-occlusive disease. Clin Rheumatol 15:207–210, 1996.

127. Shirkhoda A, Konez O, et al: Mesenteric circulation: Three-dimensional MR angiography with a gadolinium-enhanced multiecho gradient-echo technique. Radiology 202(1):257–261, 1997.

128. Bilbao JI, Rodriguez-Cabello J, Longo J, et al: Portal thrombosis: Percutaneous transhepatic treatment with urokinase—a case report. Gastrointest Radiol 14:326–328, 1989.

129. Rivitz SM, Geller SC, Hahn C, Waltman AC: Treatment of acute mesenteric venous thrombosis with transjugular intramesenteric urokinase infusion. J Vasc Intervent Radiol 6:219–223, 1995.

130. Poplausky MR, Kaufman JA, Geller SG, Waltman AC: Mesenteric venous thrombosis treated with urokinase via the superior mesenteric artery. Gastroenterology 110:1633–1635, 1996.

131. Serreyn RF, Schoofs PR, Baetens PR, et al: Laparoscopic diagnosis of mesenteric venous thrombosis. Endoscopy 18:249–250, 1986.

132. Jabbari M, Cherry R, Goresky CA: The endoscopic diagnosis of mesenteric venous thrombosis. Gastrointest Endosc 31:405–406, 1985.

133. Jona J, Cummins GM, Head HB, et al: Recurrent primary mesenteric venous thrombosis. JAMA 227:1033–1035, 1974.

134. Dada FB, Balan AD, Newark D: Recurrent primary mesenteric venous thrombosis. South Med J 80:1329–1330, 1987.

135. Robin P, Gruel Y, Lang M, et al: Complete thrombolysis of mesenteric vein occlusion with recombinant tissue-type plasminogen activator. Lancet 1(2):1391, 1988.

136. Picardi E, Rundell WK, Peoples JB: Effects of streptokinase on experimental mesenteric venous thrombosis in a feline model. Curr Surg Sept–Oct:378–380, 1989.

137. Levy PJ, Krausz MM, Manny J: The role of second-look procedure in improving survival time for patients with mesenteric venous thrombosis. Surg Gynecol Obstet 170:287–291, 1990.

138. Bulkley GB, Zuidema GD, Hamilton SR, et al: Intraoperative determination of small intestinal viability following ischemic injury: A prospective controlled trial of two adjuvant methods (Doppler and fluorescein) compared with standard clinical judgement. Ann Surg 193:628–637, 1981.

139. Cooperman M, Martin EW, Carey LC: Determination of intestinal viability by Doppler ultrasonography in venous infarction. Ann Surg 191:57–58, 1980.

140. Bergentz SE, Ericsson B, Hedner U, et al: Thrombosis in the superior mesenteric and portal veins: Report of a case treated with thrombectomy. Surgery 76:286–290, 1974.

141. Inahara T: Acute superior mesenteric venous thrombosis treatment by thrombectomy. Ann Surg 174:956–961, 1971.

142. Fontaine R, Pietri J, Masson JC, et al: 2 recent cases of intestino-mesenteric infarct of venous origin: The place of thrombectomy in the treatment. J Chir 97:145–148, 1969.

143. Ghaly M, Frawley JE: Superior mesenteric vein thrombosis. Aust N Z J Surg 56:277–279, 1986.

144. Harrison TA: Portal phlebothrombosis: The role of thrombectomy. Ann R Coll Surg Engl 60:320–323, 1978.

145. Langnas AN, Marujo WC, Stratta RJ, et al: A selective approach to preexisting portal vein thrombosis in patients undergoing liver transplantation. Am J Surg 163:132–136, 1992.

146. Shaked A, Busuttil RW: Liver transplantation in patients with portal vein thrombosis and central portacaval shunts. Ann Surg 214:696–702, 1991.

147. Neuhas P, Bechstein WO, Blumhardt G, Steffen R: Management of portal venous thrombosis in hepatic transplant recipients. Surg Gynecol Obstet 171:251–252, 1990.

148. Klempnauer J, Grothues F, Bektas H, Pichlmayr R: Results of portal thrombectomy and splanchnic thrombolysis for the surgical management of acute mesentericoportal thrombosis. Br J Surg 84(1):129–132, 1997.

149. Kazmers A: Operative management of acute mesenteric ischemia. Ann Vasc Surg 12:187–197, 1998.

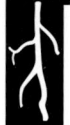

C H A P T E R 1 1 2
Treatment of Chronic Visceral Ischemia

Lloyd M. Taylor, Jr., M.D., Gregory L. Moneta, M.D.,
and John M. Porter, M.D.

Vascular surgeons become accustomed to diagnosing and treating disorders of the circulation caused by atherosclerosis, the most frequently encountered pathologic process in our aging population. This means that most atherosclerotic syndromes are encountered in large numbers, and individual surgeons quickly accumulate large personal case experiences. Similarly, the medical literature contains many articles describing the natural history and clinical outcome of patient series composed of hundreds or even thousands of individuals. Chronic intestinal ischemia, in contrast, is quite rare. All authorities agree that the clinical syndrome produced by inadequate blood supply to the intestines is encountered infrequently. Even major institutions with the accumulated experience of many thousands of arterial reconstructions rarely report an institutional experience exceeding 100 cases of chronic intestinal ischemia.[1-6] It is clear that few surgeons will accumulate sufficient case material to develop principles of treatment based on personal experience.

The available literature describing chronic intestinal ischemia includes no large-scale natural history studies and no randomized or controlled clinical trials. Published anecdotal clinical reports do not present consistent recommendations for operative treatment, and in many reports technical details of operative procedures are simply not described. Others describe technically demanding procedures requiring extensive dissections in areas not frequently approached by most vascular surgeons.[7, 8] For all these reasons, there is no consensus regarding the treatment of chronic visceral ischemia.

This chapter summarizes available information on chronic visceral ischemia. The topics addressed include the natural history, indications for treatment, and treatment options, among them nonoperative therapy, percutaneous interventional therapy, and surgical revascularization. The operations discussed are (1) arterial bypass, both antegrade and retrograde and using vein or prosthetic grafts, (2) visceral artery endarterectomy, and (3) visceral artery reimplantation. The recommendations for treatment in this chapter are based on the patient experience accumulated by the vascular surgery service at Oregon Health Sciences University. This service was founded by the senior author (J.M.P.) in 1971, allowing some conclusions to be drawn from the long-term follow-up of patients treated with standardized methods.

NATURAL HISTORY OF CHRONIC INTESTINAL ISCHEMIA

It is interesting that the existence of a clinical syndrome in which chronic episodic abdominal pain results from the obstruction of intestinal arteries was postulated before it was clinically recognized. Conner speculated in 1933 that some patients with fatal intestinal infarction might have suffered earlier from misdiagnosed abdominal pain.[9] This speculation was confirmed by the important study conducted by Dunphy.[10] He reviewed the case records of 12 patients who died of intestinal infarction at the Peter Bent Brigham Hospital and found that 7 (58%) had well-documented histories of "chronic recurrent abdominal pain preceding the fatal attack by weeks, months, or years."

After Dunphy's report, it was generally accepted that patients with "intestinal angina" existed and that, untreated, at least some of these patients progressed to fatal intestinal infarction.[11, 12] The possibility that surgical treatment might relieve the symptoms and prevent these deaths was proposed by Mikkelsen in 1957.[13] He described the typical orificial atherosclerotic lesions of the celiac and superior mesenteric artery that led to mesenteric thrombosis. Mikkelsen also noted that most frequently the distal arteries were spared in the atherosclerotic process and that this feature made surgical reconstruction before intestinal infarction feasible. In the next year, Shaw and Maynard performed the first reported arterial reconstructive surgery for the treatment of chronic intestinal ischemia.[14] Since then, many papers have documented successful surgical relief of the symptoms of chronic intestinal ischemia, including abdominal pain, food fear, and weight loss.[1-8]

Important questions about the natural history of chronic intestinal ischemia include the following:

1. How frequently do the typical arterial lesions occur?
2. How often are symptoms associated with the lesions?
3. How often do symptomatic or asymptomatic individuals with intestinal arterial obstructions develop intestinal infarction?

Although there is considerable information suggesting that atherosclerotic obstruction of the intestinal arteries is quite frequent, there is little information on the implications of these lesions in asymptomatic patients.

Significant atherosclerotic obstruction of the visceral arteries is present in 6% to 10% of unselected autopsy cases.[15] In the more selected population undergoing abdominal aortography, significant stenosis of the celiac artery, the superior mesenteric artery, or both is present in 14% to 24%.[16] An aortogram showing superior mesenteric artery occlusion in an asymptomatic patient is seen in Figure 112–1. Despite the frequency of visceral artery stenosis, symptomatic chronic intestinal ischemia is rare because of the excellent collateral circulatory network supplying the intestine. It is widely believed that intestinal collaterals are

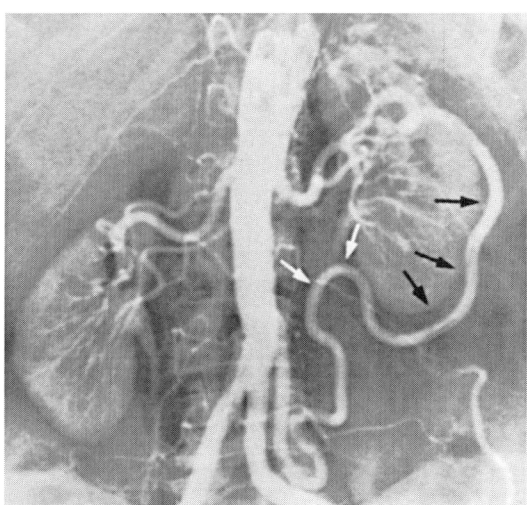

FIGURE 112–1. Aortogram of a patient with superior mesenteric and celiac artery occlusions. A meandering mesenteric artery collateral is prominent (*arrows*). The patient had no symptoms of intestinal ischemia. (From Taylor LM Jr, Porter JM: Treatment of chronic intestinal ischemia. Semin Vasc Surg 3:187, 1990.)

so extensive that at least two of the three intestinal vessels (the celiac, superior mesenteric, and inferior mesenteric arteries) must be stenotic or occluded for symptoms to occur.[13, 17] Although this aphorism serves to illustrate the principle, it is not true. Cases of bona fide symptomatic chronic intestinal ischemia to the point of infarction caused by single-vessel disease have occurred in our experience and in the reported experience of others.[18] Single-vessel obstructions producing symptoms are almost always limited to the superior mesenteric artery. Isolated occlusions of the celiac artery or the inferior mesenteric artery appear to be well tolerated.

A single study has addressed the issue of how many patients with asymptomatic intestinal arterial occlusions become symptomatic. Thomas and colleagues[19] looked at 980 consecutive aortograms performed from 1989–1995 and identified 60 (6%) with significant visceral arterial stenoses/occlusions. Fifteen patients had severe stenoses or occlusions of all three visceral vessels, and after a mean follow-up of 2.6 years, four of the 15 had symptomatic intestinal ischemia (one fatal intestinal infarction, three intestinal angina attacks). No patients with less than three vessels involved developed intestinal ischemia. If these findings are confirmed by other studies, they may provide strong rationale for recommending repair of asymptomatic occlusive disease involving all three intestinal arteries.

Some information suggests caution with regard to the prognosis for individuals with asymptomatic mesenteric arterial obstructions or patients who must undergo abdominal vascular surgery for other indications, such as aortoiliac or renal artery occlusive disease. Shaw and Maynard reported a patient in whom acute intestinal ischemia developed after aortic surgery for lower extremity ischemia.[14] Connolly and Stemmer later reported a series of patients who developed severe intestinal ischemia following aortic surgery.[20] Preoperatively, the patients had had no symptoms of intestinal ischemia. Connolly and Stemmer attributed this to a "steal" syndrome, although it appears more likely

that the ischemia resulted from the disruption of vital retroperitoneal collaterals coincident with the aortic surgery. These reports, however, clearly indicate that individuals with asymptomatic superior mesenteric artery obstruction are at risk for postoperative intestinal ischemia when they undergo aortic surgery.

The natural history of symptomatic chronic intestinal ischemia appears to be well documented. Patients suffer intermittent abdominal pain and progressive weight loss resulting from voluntary food avoidance. The usual outcome following what may be a prolonged period of symptoms, ranging from months to years, is death from inanition or from intestinal infarction. Presently, there are insufficient data from which to predict the anticipated duration of illness, the likelihood of remission, and the frequency of the development of infarction.

NONOPERATIVE TREATMENT OF CHRONIC INTESTINAL ISCHEMIA

Because the symptoms of chronic visceral ischemia occur with food ingestion, it is logical that cessation of oral intake will eliminate the pain. This is indeed the case, and most patients voluntarily or involuntarily limit food intake, which inevitably results in the profound weight loss characteristic of chronic intestinal ischemia. It is possible to offset this by the administration of parenteral nutrition and to achieve both reversal of weight loss and relief of symptoms. This treatment is impractical as a solution to chronic visceral ischemia but may be of value in preparation for more definitive treatment.

Patients with chronic visceral ischemia are inevitably severely malnourished as a result of simple starvation. The increased operative risk associated with malnutrition in elderly atherosclerotic patients is well documented.[21] It is not known whether this risk can be reduced by a period of preoperative nutritional supplementation.[22] It is our practice to treat patients who have chronic visceral ischemia with cessation of oral intake and total parenteral nutrition beginning prior to revascularization and continuing uninterrupted through the perioperative and postoperative course until oral intake adequate for nutrition can be resumed.

PERCUTANEOUS INTERVENTIONAL TREATMENT OF CHRONIC INTESTINAL ISCHEMIA

Surgical reconstruction of obstructed intestinal arteries usually requires a major operative procedure on an elderly patient, who usually has both multisystem disease and profound recent weight loss. Minimally invasive percutaneous treatment is obviously an attractive alternative. Balloon angioplasty of the superior mesenteric artery was first reported by Furrer and coworkers in 1980.[23] Since this initial report appeared, many others have described the technical feasibility and the anecdotal results of visceral angioplasty.[24–31]

As described by Mikkelsen,[13] a frequent feature of athero-sclerotic lesions producing intestinal artery obstruction is their location at the origin of the artery from the aorta. These "orificial" lesions are in fact composed mostly of aortic plaque, a portion of which extends into the visceral vessel. This location of plaque is the feature that makes visceral stenoses quite amenable to surgical repair but relatively unattractive for balloon angioplasty.[32]

For patients in whom balloon angioplasty has been successful, initial reports described frequent early recurrence of stenosis. Tegtmeyer and Selby summarized the results of several reported series.[33] Of the procedures described, follow-up information was available on 35 patients. These patients were selected for their suitability for angioplasty, which means that most patients with typical orificial lesions were not selected for treatment. For example, the series of Odurry and associates, the largest of those reviewed, included only 1 patient (of a total of 10) with an orificial lesion.[25] Angioplasty was initially successful, as judged by angiographic appearance and relief of symptoms in 28 patients (80%). The mean follow-up period was 28 months. During this interval, 8 patients (29% of those with successful procedures) required surgery or repeated dilatation for recurrence of symptoms. More importantly, 7 of the 18 patients with follow-up intervals of greater than 12 months experienced a recurrence (39%). Thus, the overall success rate of the procedure for patients with at least 12 months of follow-up was only 48% (61% of 80%). A more recent, larger series described by Allen and colleagues,[31] reported initial success in 18 of 19 (95%) patients, with recurrence in 3 (20%) after a mean follow-up of 28 months. Arteriograms of a patient with superior mesenteric artery stenosis before and after successful balloon angioplasty are shown in Figure 112–2. This patient experienced initial relief of symptoms associated with the angiographic improvement demonstrated in the figure. The symptoms and the stenosis recurred after 3 months, at which time the patient had successful surgical repair.

The use of expandable endovascular stents has been proposed to improve the results of dilatation of aortic orificial lesions involving the renal arteries. A preliminary trial has reported initial success in some patients.[34] A similar use of stents has also been proposed for intestinal arterial ostial stenoses. To date, the results of such procedures have not been reported.

The authors reserve balloon angioplasty and/or stenting for symptomatic visceral ischemia for lesions with a high likelihood of success. Examples include rare lesions such as those caused by fibromuscular disease[24] or isolated, short-segment atherosclerotic lesions beyond the first 1 to 2 cm of the superior mesenteric artery. Standard surgical reconstruction as described in the following section has sufficiently high success and low recurrence that it remains the procedure of choice for most patients with typical orificial lesions of the mesenteric arteries.

SURGICAL TREATMENT OF CHRONIC INTESTINAL ISCHEMIA

Indications for Surgery

In the majority of cases, patients with a diagnosis of chronic intestinal ischemia will have been subjected to extensive diagnostic evaluation before surgical referral. Occasionally, however, vascular surgeons encounter patients with abdominal pain in whom only angiography showing typical lesions has been performed. It is wise to remember that

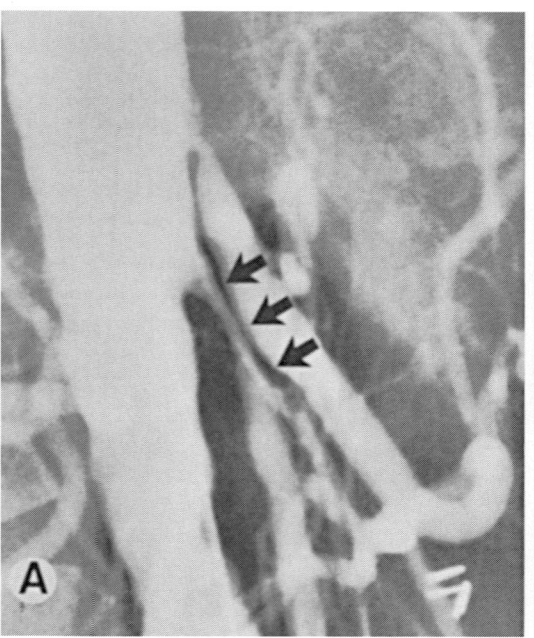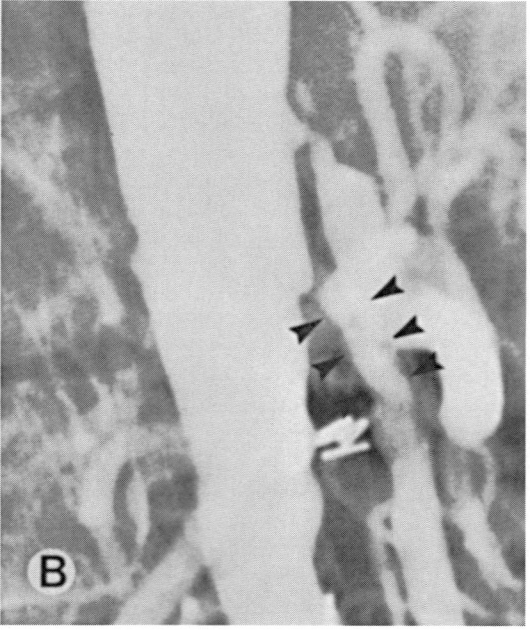

FIGURE 112–2. *A*, Lateral aortogram of a patient with intestinal ischemia and stenosis of the celiac and superior mesenteric arteries. Note that the superior mesenteric stenosis is distal to the aortic orifice (*arrows*). *B*, After balloon angioplasty, the lumen is considerably larger (*arrows*). The patient became asymptomatic for 3 months, when the symptoms and stenosis recurred. She was treated with bypass surgery. (From Taylor LM Jr, Porter JM: Treatment of chronic intestinal ischemia. Semin Vasc Surg 3:189, 1990.)

chronic visceral ischemia is rare, and other conditions producing abdominal pain and weight loss occur much more frequently, especially visceral malignancy. In view of this relationship, it seems prudent to perform at least a gastrointestinal examination with endoscopy or radiology and abdominal computed tomography (CT) before elective visceral revascularization.

At present, no information justifies visceral revascularization for asymptomatic lesions, with the important exception of patients with asymptomatic stenoses or occlusions of the superior mesenteric artery who must undergo other indicated aortic or renal artery operations. The occurrence of acute intestinal ischemia following such procedures is sufficiently well documented[14, 20] that we routinely perform superior mesenteric artery grafting at the time of the aortic surgery. Asymptomatic obstructions of the celiac artery do not require surgery.

Operative Techniques

A wide variety of operative techniques to revascularize obstructed superior mesenteric and celiac arteries have been reported, which serves as an ongoing source of confusion to surgeons with little experience in this field. Given the rarity of the clinical syndrome, a majority of surgeons are included in this category. Even a brief perusal of the literature yields techniques ranging from visceral artery reimplantation[35] to endarterectomy to bypass. Bypass grafting has been performed with vein or prosthetics, originating from almost any imaginable abdominal vessel.[1–8, 14, 36–48] A partial list of described techniques of visceral revascularization is given in Table 112–1. It is interesting that some authoritative reports on visceral revascularization have failed to describe operative technique beyond enumerating the visceral vessels revascularized, further compounding the difficulty of analyzing the suitability of different operations.[3, 42–48]

Although it is tempting to conclude that the lack of technical detail in many reports, combined with the wide variety of described procedures, means that operative technique is not critical, this is clearly not the case. Meticulous operative technique is the foundation of successful vascular surgery. Many of the operations described for visceral revascularization have been performed only in small numbers, and little long-term follow-up information is available. Three basic operations have been widely described for the treatment of visceral ischemia, and each of these is discussed. They include endarterectomy, vein bypass grafting, and prosthetic bypass grafting.

TABLE 112–1. TECHNIQUES OF INTESTINAL ARTERIAL REVASCULARIZATION

SMA or celiac reimplantation
Retrograde endarterectomy ("blind")
Direct vision endarterectomy
Transaortic endarterectomy
Antegrade infrarenal aorta–SMA vein graft
Retrograde infrarenal aorta–SMA or celiac artery vein graft or both
Retrograde infrarenal aorta–SMA or celiac artery prosthetic graft or both
Antegrade supraceliac aorta–SMA or celiac artery prosthetic graft or both

SMA = superior mesenteric artery.

Visceral Endarterectomy

As has been the history of most operations for atherosclerotic occlusive disease, the initial reports of surgery for visceral ischemia described the use of endarterectomy. Endarterectomy of the superior mesenteric artery can be accomplished in a blind retrograde fashion through a distal arteriotomy in the superior mesenteric artery,[14] although this approach is primarily of historical interest. A more reliable approach is surgery performed under direct vision with control of the suprarenal aorta and incision across the origin of the superior mesenteric artery.[44] A third technique of visceral endarterectomy, termed *transaortic endarterectomy*[7] by its developers at the University of California at San Francisco, involves a posterolateral approach to the aorta and a "trap-door" aortic incision, with subsequent visceral-origin endarterectomy through the opened aorta. This approach allows for simultaneous endarterectomy of the renal arteries and of the suprarenal aorta in selected patients.

Although significant numbers of patients have undergone visceral arterial endarterectomy, particularly transaortic endarterectomy, with excellent published results, most surgeons choose to use various forms of arterial bypass to treat chronic intestinal ischemia. There are multiple reasons for this decision. Surgical exposure of the proximal visceral vessels and the portion of the aorta from which they arise is infrequently performed by most surgeons and requires extensive dissection. The risks of suprarenal aortic clamping and direct operation on the origins of the visceral vessels include renal and lower extremity embolization, renal ischemia, and paraplegia, as well as a significantly increased risk of cardiac complications. Given the lack of familiarity with the required dissection on the part of most surgeons, as well as the significant inherent risks of the procedure, the choice of bypass by most surgeons is easily understood.

Infrarenal Aorta–Visceral Artery Vein Bypass

If not severely diseased, the infrarenal aorta may serve as the origin for visceral bypass grafts. If it is diseased, replacement with a prosthesis may be indicated, and this may obviously serve as a site for mesenteric graft origin. A technique shown as standard for these bypasses in many reference works consists of placement of a very short saphenous vein from the cephalad portion of the anterior wall of the infrarenal aorta to the superior mesenteric artery just below the inferior border of the pancreas.[49] Although this graft configuration is diagrammatically simple, there are several problems with it. When the patient is in the recumbent position, the proximal superior mesenteric artery is directly anterior to the aorta. The mass of the mesentery and the intestines normally rests on the retroperitoneum containing the aorta. Saphenous vein grafts from the infrarenal aorta to the superior mesenteric artery must be at right angles to both vessels if they are short. If the graft is lengthened, in an effort to avoid acute angulation, the origin must be more distal and the anastomoses remain acutely angulated. Thus, short grafts are particularly prone to kinking, and longer grafts do little to reduce this ten-

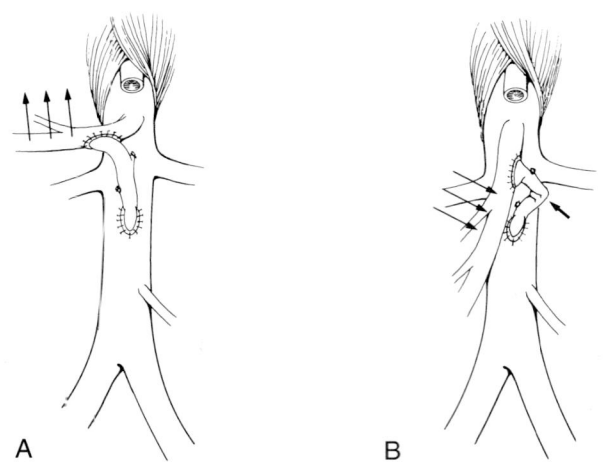

FIGURE 112–3. The potential for kinking that occurs with the use of short saphenous vein grafts from the infrarenal aorta to the superior mesenteric artery.

dency (Fig. 112–3). Besides being subject to kinking and compression, saphenous vein grafts of average size rarely carry more than 500 ml of blood per minute at physiologic pressures. Electromagnetic and noninvasive flow measurements indicate normal superior mesenteric artery flow in excess of 750 ml/min.[50]

Given these considerations, it is not surprising that several investigators have found saphenous vein grafts generally unsatisfactory for use as visceral bypass grafts.[2, 7, 51] We prefer prosthetic grafts, usually 6- to 7-mm double-velour

Dacron. An exception is made in cases in which perforation or necrosis of bowel has occurred, and intestinal resection is required. In these cases, surgical judgment suggests avoiding prosthetics. The saphenous vein grafts are placed, using the configuration described in the next section and illustrated in Figure 112–4.

Current Approach to Visceral Revascularization

The procedure chosen for visceral revascularization for individual patients is based on the extent and location of aortic disease and on the need for other vascular procedures, such as infrarenal aortic grafting. Our clear first choice for the origin of a visceral artery bypass graft is the infrarenal aorta. There are several reasons for this choice. The exposure is familiar. The risks associated with dissection and clamping are less than those with the suprarenal or supraceliac aorta, and the procedure can be readily combined with other intra-abdominal procedures.

Avoiding the problems of kinking associated with saphenous vein grafts requires careful attention to graft configuration. Our preference for the origin of the graft is from the junction of the aorta and the right common iliac artery. Crimped woven Dacron bifurcation grafts (12 × 7 mm) are used if both the superior mesenteric and the celiac arteries are to be revascularized. For superior mesenteric revascularization alone, a single limb is cut from a bifurcation graft in the manner described by Wylie and colleagues[52] to create a "flange" for sewing and to prevent constriction of the proximal anastomosis. The ligament of

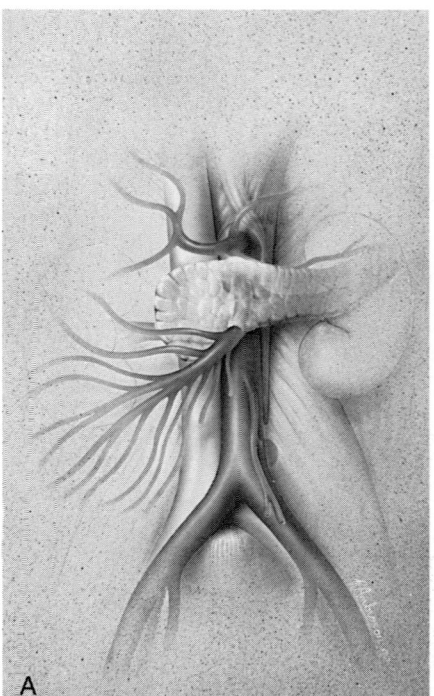
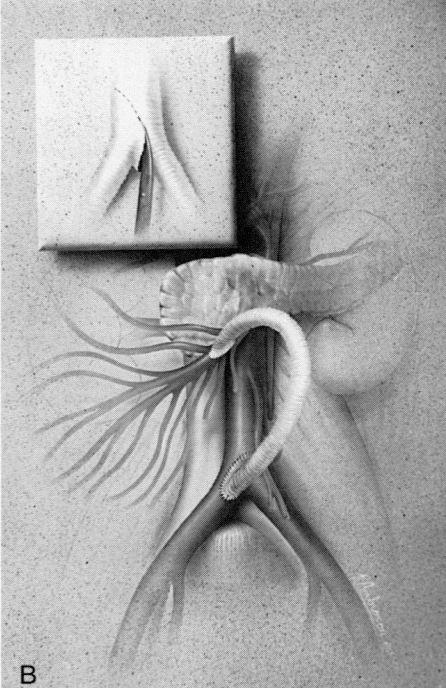
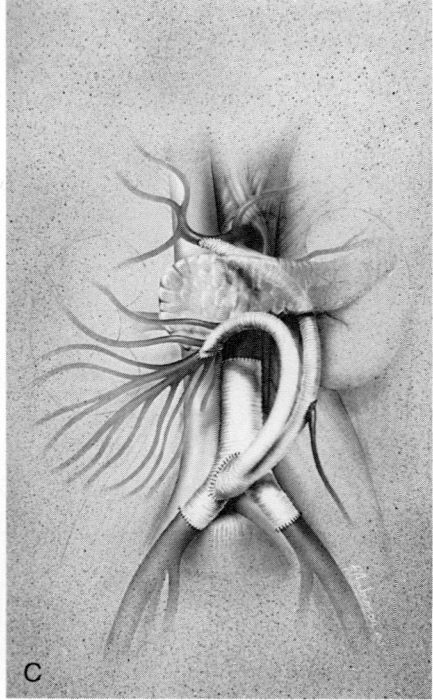

FIGURE 112–4. *A,* Exposure of the infrarenal aorta and the superior mesenteric and celiac arteries. *B,* Method of infrarenal aorta–superior mesenteric artery bypass. *Inset,* Method of forming the graft origin. *C,* Method of infrarenal aortic graft placement with bypass to the superior mesenteric and hepatic arteries. Note the reimplantation of the inferior mesenteric artery. (From Taylor LM Jr, Porter JM: Treatment of chronic intestinal ischemia. Semin Vasc Surg 3:193, 1990.)

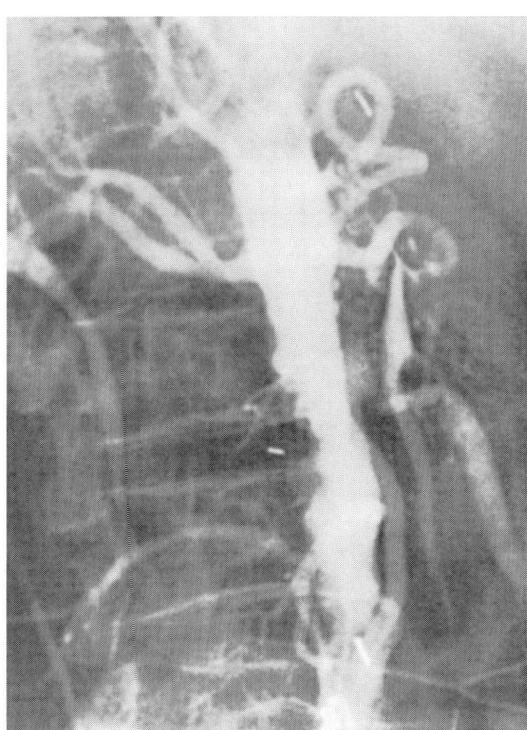

FIGURE 112–5. Severe disease of the infrarenal aorta in a patient with intestinal ischemia without symptoms of lower extremity ischemia. The supraceliac aorta was used for the visceral bypass origin. (From Taylor LM Jr, Porter JM: Treatment of chronic intestinal ischemia. Semin Vasc Surg 3:194, 1990.)

Treitz is dissected. The graft to the superior mesenteric artery is then passed, as illustrated in Figure 112–4: first cephalad, then turning anteriorly and inferiorly a full 180 degrees to terminate in an antegrade anastomosis to the anterior wall of the superior mesenteric artery just beyond the inferior border of the pancreas. Exclusion of the graft from the peritoneal cavity and contact with the intestine is performed by closing the posterior parietal peritoneum, the ligament of Treitz, and the mesenteric peritoneum. When a celiac artery limb is included, the course is retropancreatic, with anastomosis to the hepatic or (rarely) the splenic artery. Obviously, an infrarenal aortic graft serves equally well as the origin for this configuration.

Infrarenal aorta–visceral artery grafting serves the majority of patients requiring operation. Occasionally, patients have contraindications to the use of the infrarenal aorta. These include severe atherosclerotic disease of the infrarenal aorta for which concomitant aortic grafting is not indicated. An example is shown in Figure 112–5. Another relative contraindication to the use of the infrarenal aorta is previous surgery in this area, with resultant scarring and hazardous redissection. In these cases, bypass grafts from the supraceliac aorta to the visceral arteries are an excellent alternative.

Some surgeons have advocated the use of the supraceliac aortic graft origin as the procedure of choice for visceral artery bypass, based on a perception of improved results with this procedure.[5, 8] Such a conclusion is not justified by these reports. All based their conclusions of improved results on comparisons with historical control patients

treated by other methods. Obviously, much has changed over time, not just operative methods. In particular, the results of prosthetic supraceliac aorta–visceral artery bypass grafting have been compared with those achieved with vein grafts or with prosthetic grafts from the infrarenal aorta that had a disadvantageous graft configuration, which is hardly an appropriate comparison.

We reserve the use of the supraceliac graft origin for special indications because of the added potential risks associated with supraceliac surgery, which include proximal aortic clamping and possible renal, hepatic, and lower extremity embolization or prolonged ischemia. These are obviously relative risks. Visceral bypass grafts can be anastomosed to most supraceliac aortas with partial-occlusion clamping. Hepatic, intestinal, and renal ischemias are usually well tolerated, in part because well-formed collaterals already exist. To minimize the risks associated with supraceliac aortic surgery, the procedure should be reserved for patients in whom this arterial segment is *angiographically normal*. Severely diseased supraceliac aortas are not suitable for partial-occlusion clamping or for use as visceral artery bypass origins.[53] An example of such an aorta is seen in Figure 112–6.

Supraceliac aorta–visceral artery bypass is performed through a midline abdominal incision, with the use of a self-retaining retractor. The gastrohepatic ligament is incised; this is followed by incision of the diaphragmatic crus and exposure of the anterior surface of the aorta (Fig. 112–7). Woven Dacron bifurcation grafts or single limbs cut from a bifurcation graft are used (12 × 7 mm or 10 × 6 mm). After completion of the proximal anastomosis, celiac revascularization is accomplished by end-to-side anastomosis to the common hepatic artery. Grafts to the superior mesenteric artery are normally tunneled behind the pancreas and anastomosed to the anterior wall of the superior mesenteric artery in end-to-side fashion. In some

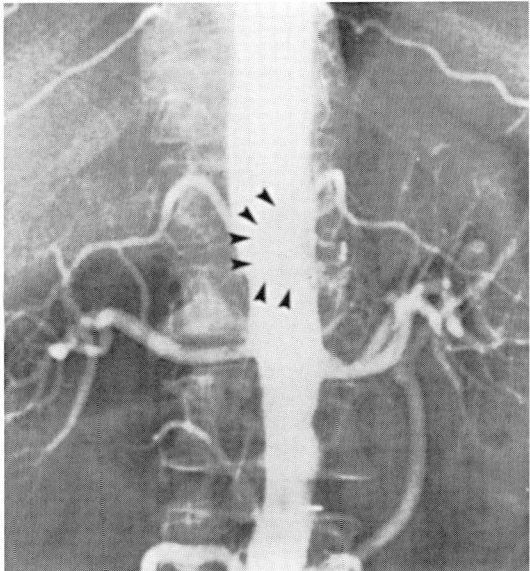

FIGURE 112–6. Extensive plaque (*arrows*) in the supraceliac aorta, making it unsuitable for safe clamping or for use as the origin of visceral bypass grafts. (From Taylor LM Jr, Porter JM: Treatment of chronic intestinal ischemia. Semin Vasc Surg 3:194, 1990.)

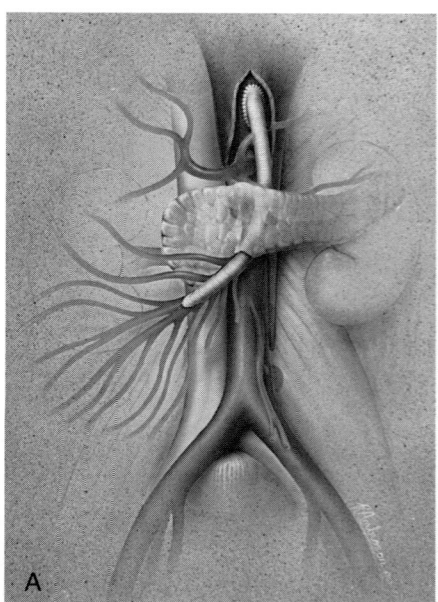
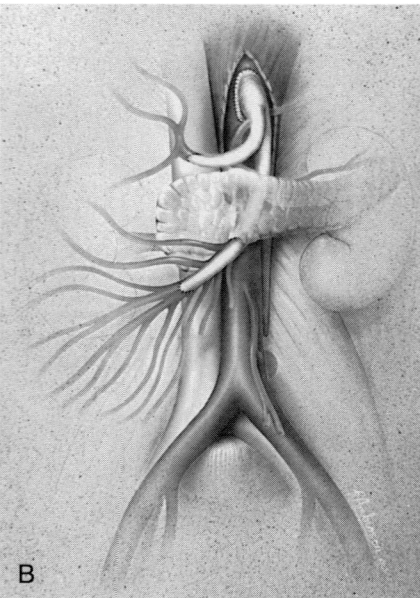

FIGURE 112–7. *A*, Supraceliac aorta–superior mesenteric artery bypass. The graft origin is best cut from a bifurcation graft, as illustrated in Figure 112–4*B*. *B*, Supraceliac aorta–superior mesenteric and hepatic bypass. (From Taylor LM Jr, Porter JM: Treatment of chronic intestinal ischemia. Semin Vasc Surg 3 195, 1990.)

patients, the retropancreatic space is narrow, and great care is necessary with the tunneling. Some surgeons advocate prepancreatic tunneling to avoid possible compression.[54]

Currently, the surgical literature favors revascularization of multiple visceral vessels over single-vessel repairs.[52, 55] There are no controlled or randomized studies to support this widely held opinion. Investigators advocating this position have invariably performed more multiple-vessel operations in their more recent experience, leaving comparison to historical controls as the basis for this recommendation. We believe that the critical vessel in chronic intestinal ischemia is the superior mesenteric artery, and adequate revascularization of this vessel will provide durable relief of symptoms in most patients. Published results from our institution and those of others are equivalent to recent reports achieved using multivessel repairs.[35, 56] At present,

we reserve multiple-vessel revascularization for patients in whom the superior mesenteric artery is diffusely diseased and there is a question about the durability of bypass to this vessel or for patients in whom previous surgery (especially gastrectomy or colectomy) has disrupted the normal collateral connections between the superior mesenteric and celiac beds.

Assurance of Technical Success

Electromagnetic flow measurement is helpful to ensure unobstructed intestinal revascularization. Flow below 400 ml/min in either celiac or superior mesenteric grafts is cause for concern. The majority of grafts have flow of between 500 and 800 ml/min. Occasional grafts have flow exceeding 1000 ml/min. It is important that flow measure-

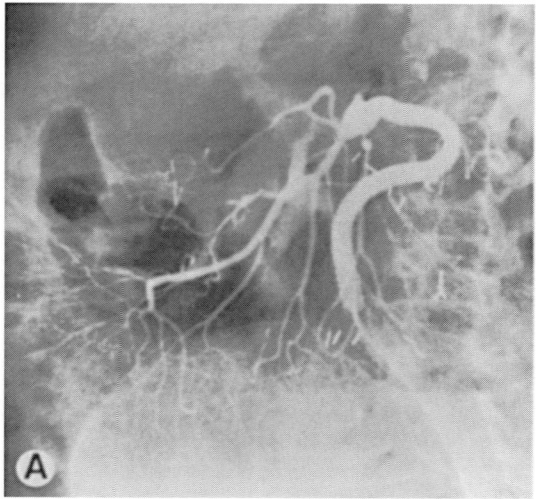
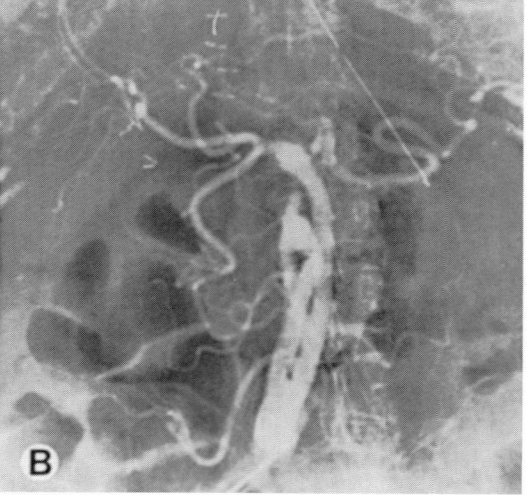

FIGURE 112–8. *A*, Selective postoperative arteriogram of an infrarenal aorta–superior mesenteric artery bypass. *B*, Postoperative arteriogram of an infrarenal aorta–superior mesenteric and hepatic bypass. (From Taylor LM Jr, Porter JM: Treatment of chronic intestinal ischemia. Semin Vasc Surg 3:196, 1990.)

TABLE 112–2. RESULTS OF REVASCULARIZATION FOR CHRONIC INTESTINAL ISCHEMIA

STUDY	NO. OF PATIENTS	OPERATIVE MORTALITY (%)	FEMALE (%)	FOLLOW-UP (YR)	LATE SUCCESS (%)
McAfee et al (1992)[53]	58	10	79	5*	90
Cunningham et al (1991)[57]	74	12	82	5*	85
Rheudasil et al (1988)[59]	41	5	51	3.5	84
Current series	84	11	67	11	95
Moawad et al (1997)[61]	24	4	76	2.4*	78
Johnston et al (1995)[60]	21	0	48	NA	86

*Life table follow-up.
NA = not available.

ments be performed after all packs and retractors have been removed and after the viscera have returned to their normal position of repose. This approach should minimize technical failures from graft kinking.

In contrast to the situation with most other vascular repairs, continuous postoperative monitoring of the patency of visceral revascularizations is impossible, and early postoperative duplex scanning is difficult or impossible. Because most patients with chronic visceral ischemia have symptoms only with eating, it is quite possible for postoperative occlusion of bypass grafts to go unrecognized. Because of the normal incisional pain, fluid shifts, leukocytosis, and temperature elevation characteristic of the postoperative state, diagnosis of acute graft occlusion is difficult or impossible in the early postoperative period. When symptoms do occur with resumption of oral intake, reoperation may be difficult because of postoperative inflammatory scarring. Because of this, we routinely obtain arteriograms 5 to 7 days postoperatively to confirm visceral revascularization patency. Examples of these arteriograms are seen in Figure 112–8. If graft occlusion is discovered, reoperation and restoration of patency are mandatory.

Postoperative Care

Patients with chronic visceral ischemia often have significant ischemic bowel injury, which requires time for recovery. In addition, the preoperative symptom of "food fear" is in part a learned behavior that does not resolve rapidly postoperatively. Prolonged periods of inability to achieve adequate oral nutrition are frequent following visceral revascularization. For this reason, total parenteral nutrition is continued postoperatively.

Some patients with severe preoperative ischemia develop a "revascularization syndrome" consisting of abdominal pain, tachycardia, leukocytosis, and intestinal edema. Gewertz and Zarins described postoperative abdominal pain caused by intestinal vasospasm after revascularization.[58] Any deviation from a totally normal postoperative course should suggest the need for arteriography, re-exploration, or both. Problems are usually readily corrected if discovered early. Delayed diagnosis of graft occlusion or intestinal necrosis is invariably fatal. Even in the face of a totally normal postoperative course, angiography before hospital discharge is mandatory in our opinion.

RESULTS OF REVASCULARIZATION FOR CHRONIC INTESTINAL ISCHEMIA

Table 112–2 lists the reported results of several large series of operations for the treatment of chronic intestinal ischemia. These results represent the outcome of revascularization with multiple operative methods, including bypass by antegrade and retrograde techniques and endarterectomy. The reported results are quite similar to those achieved by the vascular surgery service at Oregon Health Sciences University.

From 1972 to mid-1998, 84 patients with chronic visceral ischemia were operated on by the vascular surgery service at Oregon Health Sciences University. The mean age of the patients was 60 years (range, 13 to 87 years), and the majority were female (67%). It is interesting that no patients had diabetes. Most had had previous vascular surgery at some other site (63%). These details are given in Table 112–3.

Of the 84 patients, 21 (25%) had symptoms of acute visceral ischemia at the time of their operations, in addition to the clear history of chronic symptoms. Ten patients (12%) had no symptoms of visceral ischemia. Their superior mesenteric artery occlusions were repaired at the time of indicated aortic or renal artery surgery. Thirty operations (36%) included aortic grafting, renal artery grafting, or both.

All 84 patients had occlusion or severe stenosis of the superior mesenteric artery, emphasizing the central role of this vessel in chronic intestinal ischemia. Stenosis or occlusion of the celiac artery was present in 61 patients (71%), and stenosis or occlusion of the inferior mesenteric artery was present in 50 patients (60%). Only seven patients had occlusions of the superior mesenteric artery without stenosis or occlusion of at least one other vessel. These angiographic results are summarized in Table 112–4.

Patients were treated with arterial bypass grafting proce-

TABLE 112–3. CHRONIC INTESTINAL ISCHEMIA: PATIENT DATA

Number	84
Age	60 yr (mean); 13–87 yr (range)
Sex	67% female
Diabetes	0
Previous vascular surgery	64%

TABLE 112–4. CHRONIC INTESTINAL ISCHEMIA: ANGIOGRAPHIC FINDINGS

	%
SMA stenosis or occlusion	100
Celiac stenosis or occlusion	71
IMA stenosis or occlusion	60
Single-vessel stenosis or occlusion (all SMA)	8

SMA = superior mesenteric artery; IMA = inferior mesenteric artery.

dures, 56 (68%) of which were retrograde, from the infrarenal aorta, and 26 (31%) of which were antegrade, from the supraceliac aorta, or by trap-door transaortic endarterectomy (two procedures, 2%). Repair of the superior mesenteric artery was performed in all cases. The celiac artery was revascularized in 34 (40%), and the inferior mesenteric artery was revascularized in 11 (13%). Renal artery revascularization was performed simultaneously in six patients in this group. The operations performed are listed in Table 112–5.

Nine patients (11%) died postoperatively. All deaths occurred in patients with acute intestinal ischemia; four were from myocardial infarction, one was from extensive intestinal infarction, which in retrospect was irreversible, the others were from multiple organ system failure. There were no operative deaths in patients with chronic symptoms only and no operative deaths in patients without symptoms.

Postoperative complications included two hemorrhages requiring reoperation, one stroke, and four graft limb thromboses. All thromboses were asymptomatic, were discovered by routine postoperative arteriography, and were corrected by reoperation. There were no episodes of postoperative bowel necrosis.

The follow-up for these patients ranged from 6 months to 13 years (mean follow-up, 4.5 years). Late complications include one graft infection occurring 3 years postoperatively in a patient whose initial operation was complicated by gangrenous cholecystitis, the complications of which were fatal. There were three late graft occlusions, all occurring in retrograde grafts to the superior mesenteric artery, at intervals ranging from 1 to 11 years postoperatively.

SUMMARY

Chronic intestinal ischemia is a rare, symptomatic manifestation of atherosclerosis, and there are important gaps in

TABLE 112–5. CHRONIC INTESTINAL ISCHEMIA: OPERATIONS PERFORMED

OPERATION	NO. OF PATIENTS (%)
Retrograde bypass	56 (68)
Antegrade bypass	26 (31)
Trap-door endarterectomy	2 (2%)
SMA revascularization	84 (100)
Celiac artery revascularized	34 (40)
IMA revascularized	11 (13)
Simultaneous aortic graft, renal graft, or both	30 (36)

SMA = superior mesenteric artery; IMA = inferior mesenteric artery.

our knowledge of the natural history of this condition. When it does occur, the results given in Table 112–2 and those described from our service demonstrate that when it is properly diagnosed, chronic intestinal ischemia is amenable to surgical treatment by standard techniques, with predictably good immediate and long-term results. Although some unusual intestinal arterial lesions are amenable to treatment by balloon angioplasty, the anatomic nature of the most frequently encountered stenoses and occlusions means that for the foreseeable future, most patients will require surgery.

Our clear preference for surgical technique involves prosthetic bypass from the infrarenal aorta to the superior mesenteric artery, with antegrade bypass and multiple vessel revascularization reserved for special indications. We believe that aggressive postoperative care and angiographic confirmation of technical success are important for optimal results.

REFERENCES

1. Crawford ES, Morris GC Jr, Myhre HO, Roehm JOF Jr: Celiac axis, superior mesenteric artery, and inferior mesenteric artery occlusion: Surgical considerations. Surgery 82:856, 1977.
2. Zelenock GB, Graham LM, Whitehouse WM, et al: Splanchnic arteriosclerotic disease and intestinal angina. Arch Surg 115:497, 1980.
3. MacFarlane SD, Beebe HG: Progress in chronic mesenteric arterial ischemia. J Cardiovasc Surg 30:178, 1989.
4. Baur GM, Millay DJ, Taylor LM Jr, Porter JM: Treatment of chronic visceral ischemia. Am J Surg 148:138, 1984.
5. Rapp JH, Reilly LM, Qvarfordt PG, et al: Durability of endarterectomy and antegrade grafts in the treatment of chronic visceral ischemia. J Vasc Surg 3:799, 1986.
6. Hollier LH, Bernatz PE, Pairolero PC, et al: Surgical management of chronic intestinal ischemia: A reappraisal. Surgery 90:940, 1981.
7. Stoney RJ, Ehrenfeld WK, Wylie EJ: Revascularization methods in chronic visceral ischemia. Ann Surg 186:468, 1977.
8. Beebe HG, MacFarlane S, Raker EJ: Supraceliac aortomesenteric bypass for intestinal ischemia. J Vasc Surg 5:749, 1987.
9. Conner LA: A discussion of the role of arterial thrombosis in the visceral diseases of middle life, based upon analogies drawn from coronary thrombosis. Am J Med Sci 185:13, 1933.
10. Dunphy JE: Abdominal pain of vascular origin. Am J Med Sci 192:109, 1936.
11. Benjamin D: Mesenteric thrombosis. Am J Surg 76:338, 1948.
12. McClenahan JE, Fisher B: Mesenteric thrombosis. Surgery 23:778, 1948.
13. Mikkelsen WP: Intestinal angina: Its surgical significance. Am J Surg 94:262, 1957.
14. Shaw RS, Maynard EP III: Acute and chronic thrombosis of the mesenteric arteries associated with malabsorption: A report of two cases successfully treated by thromboendarterectomy. N Engl J Med 258:874, 1958.
15. Croft RJ, Menon GP, Marston A: Does intestinal angina exist? A critical study of obstructed visceral arteries. Br J Surg 68:316, 1981.
16. Moneta GL, Lee RW, Yeager RA, et al: Mesenteric duplex scanning: A blinded prospective study. J Vasc Surg 17:79, 1993.
17. Hansen HJB: Abdominal angina. Acta Chir Scand 142:319, 1976.
18. Bergan JJ, Yao JST: Chronic intestinal ischemia. In Rutherford RB (ed): Vascular Surgery, 3rd ed. Philadelphia, WB Saunders, 1989, pp 1097–1103.
19. Thomas JH, Blake K, Pierce GE, et al: The clinical course of asymptomatic mesenteric arterial stenosis. J Vasc Surg 27:840–844, 1998.
20. Connolly JE, Stemmer EA: Intestinal gangrene as the result of mesenteric arterial steal. Am J Surg 126:197, 1973.
21. Christou NV, Meakins JL: Neutrophil function in anergic surgical patients: Neutrophil adherence and chemotaxis. Ann Surg 190:557, 1979.
22. Fischer JE: Metabolism in surgical patients. In Sabiston DC Jr (ed):

Textbook of Surgery, 14th ed. Philadelphia, WB Saunders, 1991, pp 103–140.

23. Furrer J, Gruntzig A, Kugelmeier J, Goebel N: Treatment of abdominal angina with percutaneous dilation of an arteria mesenterica superior stenosis. Cardiovasc Intervent Radiol 3:43, 1980.

24. Golden DA, Ring EJ, McLean GK, Freiman DB: Percutaneous angioplasty in the treatment of abdominal angina. AJR Am J Roentgenol 139:247, 1982.

25. Odurny A, Sniderman KW, Colapinto RF: Intestinal angina: Percutaneous transluminal angioplasty of the celiac and superior mesenteric arteries. Radiology 167:59, 1988.

26. Birch SJ, Colapinto RF: Transluminal dilatation in the management of mesenteric angina: A report of two cases. J Can Assoc Radiol 33:46, 1982.

27. Roberts L, Wertman DA, Mills SR, et al: Transluminal angioplasty of the superior mesenteric artery: An alternative to surgical revascularization. AJR Am J Roentgenol 141:1039, 1983.

28. Wilms G, Baert AL: Transluminal angioplasty of superior mesenteric artery and celiac trunk. Ann Radiol 29:535, 1986.

29. Levy PJ, Haskell L, Gordon RL: Percutaneous transluminal angioplasty of splanchnic arteries: An alternative method to elective revascularization in chronic visceral ischaemia. Eur J Radiol 7:239, 1987.

30. McShane MD, Proctor A, Spencer P, et al: Mesenteric angioplasty for chronic intestinal ischaemia. Eur J Vasc Surg 6:333–336, 1992.

31. Allen RC, Martin GH, Rees CR, et al: Mesenteric angioplasty in the treatment of chronic intestinal ischemia. J Vasc Surg 24:415–423, 1996.

32. Cicuto KP, McLean GK, Oleaga JA, et al: Renal artery stenosis: Anatomic classification for percutaneous transluminal angioplasty. AJR Am J Roentgenol 137:599, 1981.

33. Tegtmeyer CJ, Selby JB: Balloon angioplasty of the visceral arteries (renal and mesenteric circulation): Indications, results, and complications. In Moore WS, Ahn SS (eds): Endovascular Surgery. Philadelphia, WB Saunders, 1989, pp 223–257.

34. Rees CR, Palmaz JC, Becker GJ, et al: Palmaz stent in atherosclerotic stenoses involving the ostia of the renal arteries: Preliminary report of a multicenter study. Radiology 181:507, 1991.

35. Gentile AT, Moneta GL, Taylor LM Jr, et al: Isolated bypass to the superior mesenteric artery for intestinal ischemia. Arch Surg 129:926–932, 1994.

36. Bergan JJ, Dean RH, Conn J Jr, Yao JST: Revascularization in treatment of mesenteric infarction. Ann Surg 182:430, 1975.

37. Nunn DB: Chronic intestinal angina: A report of two patients treated successfully by operation. Ann Surg 175:523, 1972.

38. Eidemiller LR, Nelson JC, Porter JM: Surgical treatment of chronic visceral ischemia. Am J Surg 138:264, 1979.

39. Jaxheimer EC, Jewell ER, Persson AV: Chronic intestinal ischemia. Surg Clin North Am 64:123, 1985.

40. Hollier LH: Revascularization of the visceral artery using the pantaloon vein graft. Surg Gynecol Obstet 155:415, 1982.

41. Daily PO, Fogarty TJ: Simplified revascularization of the celiac and superior mesenteric arteries. Am J Surg 131:762, 1976.

42. Rogers DM, Thompson JE, Garrett WV, et al: Mesenteric vascular problems. Ann Surg 195:554, 1982.

43. Rob C: Stenosis and thrombosis of the celiac and superior mesenteric arteries. Am J Surg 114:363, 1967.

44. Hansen HJB: Abdominal angina: Results of arterial reconstruction in 12 patients. Acta Chir Scand 142:319, 1976.

45. McCollum CH, Graham JM, DeBakey ME: Chronic mesenteric arterial insufficiency: Results of revascularization in 33 cases. South Med J 69:1266, 1976.

46. Reul GJ Jr, Wukasch DC, Sandiford FM, et al: Surgical treatment of abdominal angina: Review of 25 patients. Surgery 75:682, 1974.

47. Pokrovsky AV, Kasantchjan PO: Surgical treatment of chronic occlusive disease of the enteric branches of the abdominal aorta. Ann Surg 191:51, 1980.

48. Hollier LH, Bernatz PE, Pairolero PC, et al: Surgical management of chronic intestinal ischemia: A reappraisal. Surgery 90:940, 1981.

49. Stanton PE Jr, Hollier PA, Seidel TW, et al: Chronic intestinal ischemia: Diagnosis and therapy. J Vasc Surg 4:338, 1986.

50. Bergan JJ, Yao JST: Chronic intestinal ischemia. In Rutherford RB (ed): Vascular Surgery, 3rd ed. Philadelphia, WB Saunders, 1989, pp 1097–1103.

51. Moneta GL, Taylor DC, Helton WS, et al: Duplex ultrasound measurement of postprandial intestinal blood flow: Effect of meal composition. Gastroenterology 95:1294, 1988.

52. Wylie EJ, Stoney RJ, Ehrenfeld WK: Visceral atherosclerosis. In Manual of Vascular Surgery. New York, Springer-Verlag, 1980, p 211.

53. McAfee MK, Cherry KJ Jr, Naessens JM, et al: Influence of complete revascularization on chronic mesenteric ischemia. Am J Surg 164:220, 1992.

54. Taylor LM Jr, Porter JM: Supraceliac aortic bypass. In Bergan JJ, Yao JST (eds): Aortic Surgery. Orlando, Fla, Grune & Stratton, 1988, pp 195–210.

55. Cooley DA, Wukasch DC: Techniques in Vascular Surgery. Philadelphia, WB Saunders, 1979, p 120.

56. Kieny R, Batellier J, Kretz JG: Aortic reimplantation of the superior mesenteric artery for atherosclerotic lesions of the visceral arteries: Sixty cases. Ann Vasc Surg 4:122–125, 1990.

57. Cunningham CG, Reilly LM, Rapp JH, et al: Chronic visceral ischemia. Ann Surg 214:276, 1991.

58. Gewertz BL, Zarins CK: Postoperative vasospasm after antegrade mesenteric revascularization: A report of three cases. J Vasc Surg 14:382, 1991.

59. Rheudasil JM, Stewart MT, Schellack JV, et al: Surgical treatment of chronic mesenteric arterial insufficiency. J Vasc Surg 8:495, 1988.

60. Johnston KW, Lindsay TF, Walker PM, Kalman PG: Mesenteric arterial bypass grafts: early and late results and suggested surgical approach for chronic and acute mesenteric ischemia. Surgery 118:1–7, 1995.

61. Moawad J, McKinsey JF, Wyble CW, et al: Current results of surgical therapy for chronic mesenteric ischemia. Arch Surg 132:613–619, 1997.

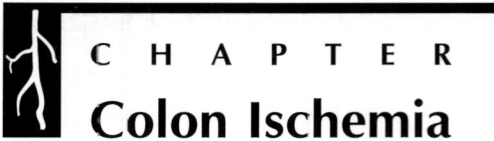

C H A P T E R   1 1 3

Colon Ischemia Following Aortic Reconstruction

Calvin B. Ernst, M.D.

Refinements in operative technique, improved preoperative and postoperative care, and sophisticated perioperative monitoring methods have contributed to a progressive reduction in mortality and morbidity for abdominal aortic reconstruction. This steady decline since the late 1950s to an operative death rate of about 4% for aortic aneurysmectomy has been gratifying.[13, 54, 55, 66] Achievement of better results and reduction of operative deaths and morbidity to the ideal minimum of zero depend not only on prevention but also on recognition and appropriate treatment of morbid and potentially lethal events after operation. Intestinal ischemia, particularly colonic, is such a complication. Identification of patients at risk should aid in its prevention. Furthermore, prediction may preclude its occurrence by identifying which patients require reconstruction of the inferior or the superior mesenteric artery during aortic reconstruction.

The overall mortality rate for colon ischemia approximates 5%, and it approaches 90% with transmural involvement.[5, 16, 28, 35, 42, 49, 51, 56, 64] Conservative estimates of the number of aortic reconstructions for aneurysmal disease performed in 1992 in the United States placed the number at 46,000. Added to this were about 31,000 aortic reconstructions for occlusive disease, for a total of 77,000 aortic reconstructive procedures performed annually.[18] If the accepted incidence of 2% for ischemic colitis developing after aortic reconstruction is assumed, with an attendant mortality rate of 50%, it is clear that colon ischemia contributes significantly to the total operative deaths from aortic reconstruction. Prevention of this complication should therefore improve results of aortic reconstruction and thereby help realize the ideal operative death rate of zero.

CLASSIFICATION AND INCIDENCE

Colon ischemia may follow abdominal aortic reconstruction for aneurysmal or occlusive disease.[6, 15, 23, 28, 37, 42, 56, 60, 67] Reports of clinically manifest cases after aneurysmectomy predominate. Almost all reports describe arterial ischemia. Venous ischemia is so rare after aortic reconstruction that for practical purposes it may be ignored.

Depending on the severity of ischemia and the thickness of bowel wall involved, three forms of ischemic colitis have been recognized: mucosal ischemia, which is transient and mild; mucosal and muscularis involvement, which may result in healing with fibrosis and stricture; and transmural ischemia, which results in gangrene and perforation (Table 113–1). More than 60% of reported cases describe transmural ischemia. The most commonly encountered type of intestinal ischemia after aortic reconstruction involves the sigmoid colon after aneurysmectomy with inferior mesenteric artery ligation.[3–6, 20, 23, 28, 35, 41, 42, 45, 46, 51, 56, 60]

The incidence of ischemic colitis after aortic reconstruction varies from 0.2% to 10%.[3–5, 16, 23, 27, 28, 37, 42, 46, 47, 51, 56, 60, 68, 69] Several authors have suggested that the actual incidence may be greater than the commonly accepted 2% because most reports in the literature are retrospective studies of clinically manifest cases. In such reports, ischemic colitis is three to four times as common after aneurysmectomy as it is after reconstruction for occlusive disease.[28]

In a prospective study of abdominal aortic reconstructive procedures for both aneurysmal and occlusive disease, the overall incidence of ischemic colitis, identified by routine postoperative colonoscopy, was 6%.[16] Ischemic changes were noted in 4.3% of patients who underwent reconstruction for occlusive disease and in 7.4% of those who underwent aneurysmectomy. When aneurysmectomy for ruptured aneurysm was included, the overall incidence of ischemic colitis approached 12%. Among patients studied after reconstruction for ruptured aneurysm, the incidence of ischemic colitis was 60%.[23] Other authors have confirmed a high incidence of ischemic colitis after aneurysm rupture.[1, 30, 67–69]

ANATOMY AND PATHOPHYSIOLOGY

The inferior mesenteric artery and its branches are connecting links between the superior mesenteric artery and hypogastric artery circulations. Among these three circuits, the inferior mesenteric artery provides the chief blood supply to the left colon. After arising at a 30-degree angle from the left anterolateral aspect of the aorta, the inferior mesenteric branches into the left colic artery, three to four sigmoid vessels, and the superior rectal artery. Inferior mesenteric branching occurs 3 to 4 cm from its aortic origin.

The marginal artery of Drummond, originally described by von Haller in 1786, is an important connecting link between the superior and inferior mesenteric arteries. At the splenic flexure, the left colic branch of the superior mesenteric artery and the left colic artery from the inferior mesenteric artery anastomose to provide marginal artery of Drummond continuity; this is *Griffiths' point*.[22] Griffiths noted a critical area in the region of the splenic flexure

TABLE 113–1. CLASSIFICATION AND CLINICAL COURSE

TYPE	PATHOLOGIC FINDINGS	CLINICAL FINDINGS	CLINICAL OUTCOME
I	Mucosal ischemia, submucosal edema or hemorrhage; mucosal slough ulceration may follow	Diarrhea with or without blood; presence or absence of fever; onset usually in 24–48 hr	Reversible; no sequelae; near-zero mortality
II	As above, with penetration of muscularis	Symptoms vary between type I and type II	Reversible; residual ischemic stricture possible
III	Transmural bowel involvement	Profound physiologic changes; sepsis, acidosis, cardiovascular collapse; may develop feculent peritonitis or late fecal fistula	Irreversible; mortality = 70 ± 10%

From Tollefson DFJ, Ernst CB: Colon ischemia following aortic reconstruction. Ann Vasc Surg 5:485–489, 1991. Reprinted by permission of Blackwell Scientific Publications, Inc.

where functional anastomoses may be marginal or lacking in 5% of individuals. In addition to noting the absence of the middle colic artery in 20% of individuals, he emphasized the importance of both the right colic branch from the superior mesenteric artery and the hypogastric arteries when ligating the inferior mesenteric artery in such patients.

The meandering mesenteric artery is a large, continuous communicating link between the left branch of the middle colic and the left colic arteries (Fig. 113–1). The meandering mesenteric artery has also been termed the central anastomotic artery of the colon, the marginal artery, the mesomesenteric artery, the middle-left colic collateral, the artery of Drummond, the arc of Riolan, and the arch of Treves. Such a profusion of names has caused confusion about colonic collateral circulation in general and the meandering mesenteric artery in particular. The preferred term for this vital collateral channel between the superior and inferior mesenteric arterial circuits is the *meandering mesenteric artery*.[40] This vessel is *potentially* present in about two thirds of normal individuals. It has been identified on routine preoperative aortography in 35% and 27% of patients with aortoiliac occlusive disease and aneurysmal disease, respectively.[16]

The hypogastric arteries through the middle and inferior rectal branches provide a communication between the systemic and visceral circulations to the left colon by way of the superior rectal branch of the inferior mesenteric artery.

The superior mesenteric artery provides blood to the small bowel and the right half of the colon. If the small bowel derives a significant amount of its blood supply from the inferior mesenteric by way of the meandering mesenteric artery because of occlusion or stenosis of the superior mesenteric artery, interruption of the meandering mesenteric artery during aortic reconstruction may eventuate in mid-gut gangrene.[4, 12, 21, 28, 50, 58]

Data suggest, however, that after acute occlusion of the inferior mesenteric artery, branches of the superior mesenteric artery provide the major collateral blood flow to the inferior mesenteric artery circulation and collateral contributions from the hypogastric arteries are insignificant.[61] However, hypogastric collateral blood flow cannot be completely ignored, particularly among patients with celiac and superior mesenteric artery stenoses in whom gut circulation depends on meandering mesenteric artery blood flow contributed by the hypogastric vessels.

Precise knowledge of anatomic pathways of collateral circulation to the bowel becomes important when the vascular surgeon undertakes aortic reconstruction. Preservation of as many collateral circuits and restoration of blood flow to as many vital arterial branches as possible are imperative to prevent ischemic colitis.

Development of colon ischemia after aortic reconstruction is multifactorial. Among the factors are (1) caliber of the vessel occluded, (2) duration and degree of ischemia, (3) rapidity of onset of the ischemic process, (4) adequacy and efficiency of collateral circulation, (5) state of the general circulation, (6) metabolic requirements of the affected bowel, (7) presence of bacteria within the bowel lumen, and (8) associated conditions, such as colonic distention.[7] Although ligation of the inferior mesenteric artery is the main factor in the development of ischemic colitis in most reports, other causes are also cited.

Identifiable predisposing factors include (1) improper ligation of the inferior mesenteric artery, (2) failure to restore inferior mesenteric or hypogastric artery blood flow,

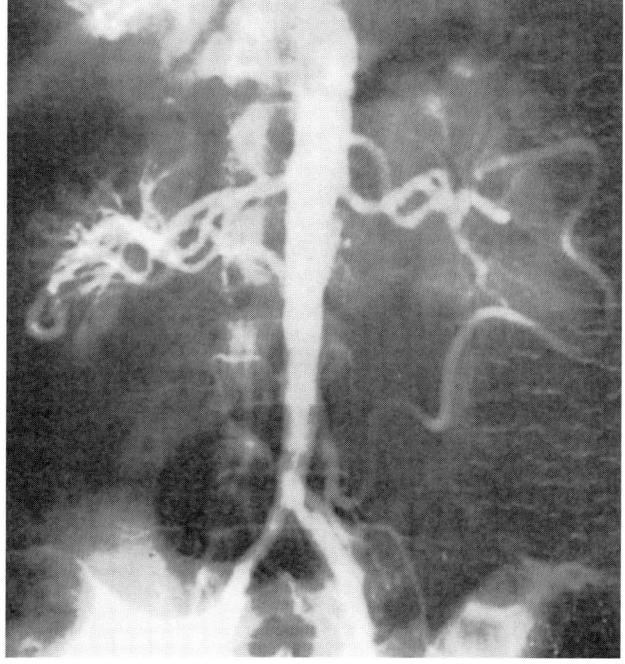

FIGURE 113–1. Aortographic documentation of a large meandering mesenteric artery.

(3) ruptured aneurysm with mesenteric compression by hematoma, (4) manipulative trauma to the colon by retractors, (5) persistent hypotension and hypoperfusion, (6) congenitally inadequate collateral communications between mesenteric circulations, and (7) damage of vital existing collateral vessels, such as the meandering mesenteric artery (Table 113–2).

Ischemia and reperfusion result in the release of toxic metabolites of molecular oxygen, superoxide, and hydroxyl free radicals.[59] Xanthine oxidase is a source of the superoxide radical. Superoxide species are very toxic to the intracellular matrix and cell membranes. Such ischemia-reperfusion injury may be responsible for a decline in sigmoid mucosal pH, as measured by operative tonometry, which appears to be most profound 4 to 6 hours after release of an aortic clamp.[70]

The abundance in intestinal mucosa of xanthine dehydrogenase, which is rapidly converted to xanthine oxidase during ischemia, provides a potential mechanism for free radical generation and subsequent cellular destruction with loss of integrity of the mucosal barrier. Loss of the mucosal barrier results in translocation of bacteria into the systemic circulation. The ensuing systemic sepsis and endotoxemia may exacerbate or eventuate in multiple organ system failure, the adult respiratory distress syndrome, hepatic failure, and renal failure. The precise clinical application of inhibitors of the conversion of xanthine dehydrogenase to xanthine oxidase (e.g., superoxide dismutase, catalase, allopurinol, soybean trypsin inhibitor, mannitol, and dimethyl sulfoxide) to prevent or treat colonic ischemia has not yet been delineated.

CLINICAL MANIFESTATIONS AND DIAGNOSIS

Awareness of the potential development of ischemic colitis after aortic reconstruction should alert the surgeon to early diagnosis. Knowledge of the predisposing factors cited earlier enhances this awareness. The reported overall 50% mortality rate from this complication suggests that delay in diagnosis may preclude effective therapy.[28] A high index of suspicion for patients at greatest risk for developing ischemic colitis is mandatory to reduce deaths and morbidity.

Depending on the degree of bowel ischemia, clinical manifestations vary from the subclinical form to bowel gangrene with perforation, peritonitis, and death (see Table 113–1). Undoubtedly, among many patients, minor degrees

TABLE 113–2. PREDISPOSING FACTORS FOR THE DEVELOPMENT OF ISCHEMIC COLITIS AFTER AORTIC RECONSTRUCTION

Improper IMA ligation
Loss of IMA-hypogastric blood flow
Ruptured aneurysm
Perioperative hypotension and hypoperfusion
Manipulative trauma
Inadequate collateral development and recruitment
IMA to SMA flow in the meandering mesenteric artery

IMA = inferior mesenteric artery; SMA = superior mesenteric artery.

of ischemia go unrecognized and the patients recover.[5, 16, 42, 46] Some minor and all major episodes of ischemia produce symptoms.

Clinical manifestations of colonic ischemia may be masked or complicated by the systemic responses and altered abdominal findings that normally follow major operations. The most common symptom is diarrhea, either brown liquid or bloody.[3, 5, 28, 31, 35, 46, 49, 51, 56, 67] Although its onset may occur as long as 14 days after operation, diarrhea usually begins within 24 to 48 hours of operation in 75% of patients. Bloody diarrhea has been reported to be more ominous than nonbloody diarrhea.[5] Some investigators, however, have noted no correlation between extent of ischemic injury, prognosis, and presence of bloody diarrhea.[42] Any diarrhea, bloody or not, should prompt immediate endoscopic evaluation.

Other symptoms include extraordinary postoperative pain, particularly in the left side of the abdomen. Progressive abdominal distention not relieved by intestinal decompression and accompanied by signs of peritoneal irritation points to bowel perforation. Signs and symptoms of sepsis, such as unexplained leukocytosis of 20,000 to 30,000 cells/mm³, severe or refractory acidosis, progressive oliguria, and elevated temperature, should cause the surgeon to consider colon ischemia. Unexplained metabolic acidosis, unusual requirements for crystalloid and colloid solutions, and development of hypotension in the absence of sepsis or hypovolemia are not specific for, but should suggest, bowel infarction. Severe thrombocytopenia (<90,000 platelets/mm³) has been suggested as a marker of bowel necrosis and should arouse suspicion of ischemic colitis in symptomatic patients.[31]

Biochemical markers such as serum phosphorus, urea, uric acid, lactic dehydrogenase, creatine phosphokinase, alkaline phosphatase, aspartate aminotransferase, alanine aminotransferase, hexosaminidase, and vasoactive intestinal polypeptide have not proved to be specific for documentation of ischemic colitis. Nevertheless, with normal liver and renal function, marked elevations in any of these markers should alert the clinician to possible colonic ischemia.

Endoscopy, employing the fiberoptic colonoscope, is the most reliable diagnostic modality available.[17, 23, 67, 68] Repeated studies over several days are required to document resolution or progression of the ischemic process. Passage of the colonoscope up to 40 cm is usually sufficient to detect ischemic colitis, with identification of ischemic lesions in up to 95% of patients.[68] Ischemia in other segments of the colon without left colon involvement is rare.[23, 68] If colonic ischemia is identified, colonoscopy must be terminated. Passage of the instrument beyond the involved bowel segment should be avoided lest perforation occur.

Flexible colonoscopy may be performed at the bedside and does not necessitate transport to a specialized area. Early changes include circumferential petechial hemorrhages and edema. The presence of pseudomembranes, erosions, and ulcers documents advanced stages of ischemia. A yellowish-green, necrotic, noncontractile surface defines gangrene.

Bedside laparoscopy has been anecdotally reported to be helpful in identifying small bowel infarction after aortic aneurysm repair.[71] The role of laparoscopy, however, is undefined when evaluating large bowel ischemia.

Barium contrast studies, although helpful in documenting late sequelae of ischemic colitis, are usually not required for diagnosis in the immediate postoperative period. Hazards of barium enema include those involved in moving a critically ill patient from the intensive care unit to the radiology suite and possible perforation with barium peritonitis.

Frequent reexamination of the abdomen; repeated colonoscopy; and monitoring of blood gases, urine output, fluid requirements, and vital signs are required when ischemic colitis has been identified. Progression of the ischemic process, documented by deteriorating clinical signs and worsening of symptoms, necessitates prompt operation. Increasing abdominal tenderness, fever, leukocytosis, and thrombocytopenia and worsening diarrhea that may progress from nonbloody to bloody indicate progression. Colonoscopy under these circumstances must be performed cautiously.

For progressive clinical deterioration associated with advancing colonic ischemia, such as described earlier, reoperation is necessary. For ischemia of the colon, all compromised bowel must be resected. Preoperative colonoscopy may be helpful to determine the extent of resection necessary. Primary anastomosis after bowel resection is contraindicated. Colostomy with Hartmann's pouch or distal mucous fistula construction is necessary. During bowel resection, isolation of the retroperitoneum and the recently placed aortic prosthesis is necessary to prevent graft contamination. The presence of rectal necrosis necessitates removal of the rectum and perineal drainage, but wide excision of the rectal segment as employed for treatment of rectal cancer is not necessary. Removal of the necrotic muscular and mucosal elements is all that is required to achieve pelvic débridement. Under these circumstances, every effort must be made to avoid exposing the aortic prosthesis. During reperitonealization of the pelvic floor, the area of the prosthesis must be isolated from the open perineum. An omental graft sutured into the pelvis may be required to achieve this objective.

Improvement, evidenced by subsidence of symptoms (e.g., lessening of diarrhea), stabilization of or improvement in laboratory parameters, and resolution of the ischemic process documented by repeated colonoscopy, permits nonoperative treatment. Under such circumstances, bowel rest must be maintained by nasogastric tube decompression. Broad-spectrum bacteriocidal antibiotics are administered intravenously.

Reversible lesions should improve within 7 to 10 days.[7, 17] Continued bleeding and diarrhea beyond 2 weeks strongly suggest walled-off colonic perforation requiring operation.

A minimally symptomatic or asymptomatic patient with a colonic stricture does not require operation. Such strictures usually occur 6 to 10 weeks after the acute process. Some of these may respond to dilatation, but many symptomatic strictures require bowel resection.

PREVENTION

Although both awareness that patients are at risk for developing ischemic colitis and early diagnosis allow effective therapy, prevention of this catastrophe is eminently more successful in minimizing mortality and morbidity than is therapy for clinically manifest disease. Prediction of the development of ischemic colitis may prevent this complication altogether by identifying patients who require reconstruction of the inferior mesenteric artery. Prediction, however, may prove challenging because of the many diverse predisposing factors (see Table 113–2). Thorough preoperative assessment, including aortography, and attention to operative technical details greatly assist in avoiding the development of ischemic bowel complications after aortic reconstruction.

Aortography

Preoperative aortography has proved useful in identifying patients at risk for developing ischemic bowel disorders.[2, 6, 8, 16, 17, 28, 48, 67] This is particularly true when the history and physical examination findings suggest intestinal angina. Under such circumstances, aortography is needed to document precarious visceral circulation dependent on the inferior mesenteric artery.[12, 21, 67]

Aortographic documentation of a meandering mesenteric artery signals concomitant superior or inferior mesenteric artery arteriosclerosis (see Fig. 113–1).[12, 16, 21] Inferior mesenteric artery opacification from the superior mesenteric by the meandering mesenteric artery is predictive of minimal risk of ischemic colitis developing after aortic reconstruction, provided that this important collateral vessel is preserved. Documentation of reversal of blood flow in the meandering mesenteric artery from the inferior to the superior mesenteric artery demands lateral filming after a second contrast medium injection to document occlusion or stenosis of the superior mesenteric artery. Under such conditions, prophylactic revascularization of the superior mesenteric artery or reconstruction of the inferior mesenteric artery during aortic reconstruction is required to prevent catastrophic small bowel ischemia.[12, 28, 67]

Arteriographic identification of the presence or absence of hypogastric artery patency is helpful in the planning of aortic reconstruction so that pelvic blood flow may be preserved or restored. When the inferior mesenteric artery is ligated, the hypogastric arteries assume an important role in collateral circulation to the rectum.

Operative Technical Details

Strict attention to operative technical details is probably more influential in avoiding the development of ischemic colitis than preoperative or postoperative factors are. Common to almost all instances of ischemic colitis after aneurysmectomy is ligation of the inferior mesenteric artery. Improper ligation interrupts communications between the ascending left colic artery and the descending sigmoid branches. To preserve these branches, the surgeon must dissect and ligate the inferior mesenteric artery at its origin: better yet, its orifice may be sutured closed from within the aneurysm after it has been opened.

Gentleness during dissection of the aorta minimizes dispersion of embolic debris and prevents "trash colon." Manipulative trauma from overly vigorous retraction or packing may occlude mesenteric collateral channels, particularly in the left colon mesentery and mesosigmoid. In managing a ruptured aneurysm with its associated mesocolic hematoma, avoidance of such manipulation or opening and evacuating the mesentery may prove critical in preserving tenuous collateral blood flow.

Operative or postoperative hypotension and hypoperfusion must be prevented by proper administration of blood and fluids. In critically ill patients, analysis of central venous pressure and pulmonary wedge pressure data is essential to balance fluid therapy properly. Colonic circulation that relies on collateral blood flow after ligation of the inferior mesenteric artery may be more susceptible to hypotension and hypoperfusion than if the artery were intact. Intact collateral circuits maintain inferior mesenteric artery blood pressure near preligation levels.[17] Using inferior mesenteric artery stump blood pressure measurements as an index of the adequacy of inferior mesenteric artery collateral blood flow, the author has found that 54% of patients had greater inferior mesenteric artery stump pressures recorded after aneurysmectomy. If postoperative hypotension occurs, however, collateral perfusion may be jeopardized, with the resultant development of ischemic colitis. Preservation of vital pelvic collateral circulation by the restoration of pulsatile flow to one or both hypogastric arteries is required to minimize the development of ischemic colitis or proctitis.[3, 17, 32, 36, 51, 52]

Adequate perfusion of at least one hypogastric artery may be accomplished in more than 90% of patients. If hypogastric blood flow cannot be restored without complex reconstructive techniques, inferior mesenteric stump pressure measurements may document that hypogastric reconstruction may not be required, as discussed later.

Clinical prediction of the viability of bowel, in particular the colon, is notoriously unreliable. Predictive criteria of viability based on color, arterial pulsations, and peristalsis

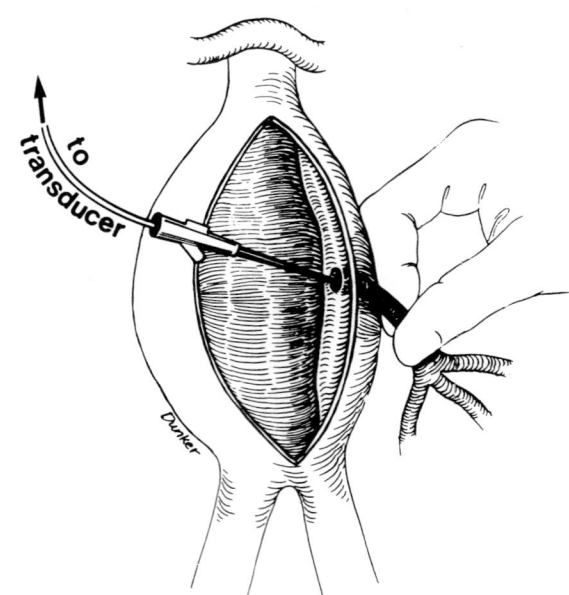

FIGURE 113–3. Inferior mesenteric artery (IMA) stump blood pressure measurement. The cannula is threaded into the IMA orifice through the opened aneurysm sac. The cannula is secured into the arterial lumen by compression of the IMA and adjacent mesentery between the thumb and forefinger. (From Ernst CB: Prevention of intestinal ischemia following abdominal aortic reconstruction. Surgery 93:102, 1983. Reprinted by permission.)

have proved unsatisfactory in distinguishing viable from nonviable bowel.[7, 10, 29, 38, 42, 46] Several techniques for predicting gut viability have been described, including radioisotope scanning, surface temperature determinations, electromyographic findings, and dye injection and detection techniques.[9, 10, 29, 38, 44, 53, 57] Such studies require specially designed equipment and may be time-consuming, cumbersome, and complex.

As they pertain to colonic viability, two techniques for determining when the inferior mesenteric artery may be safely ligated and when reconstruction is required have merit.[17, 25, 26] One technique employs Doppler ultrasonography to document arterial blood flow in the inferior mesenteric artery, in the large bowel mesentery, and on the serosal surface of the colon before and after occlusion of the artery (Fig. 113–2).[25, 26, 33] The other technique uses measurement of inferior mesenteric stump blood pressure (Fig. 113–3).[17]

Two other techniques, neither of which has undergone adequate clinical trials, have appeal.[19, 43, 70, 72] One employs indirect measurements of intramural pH by a silicone tonometer to measure P_{CO_2} changes in the lumen of the colon. Intramural pH measurements of less than 6.86 suggest colon ischemia.[19] That sigmoid tonometry may prove useful has been suggested by other investigators studying a limited number of patients. Sigmoid mucosal pH declines during aortic clamping, but in uncomplicated cases it returns to normal within 4 to 6 hours of aortic declamping.[70] Indirect intramural sigmoid pH monitoring has appeal because it may be applicable to both occlusive and aneurysmal diseases. More important, it may provide continuing postoperative monitoring of colon viability in the recovery room or intensive care unit.[72] The other technique employs a photoplethysmographic method based on a sterile pulse

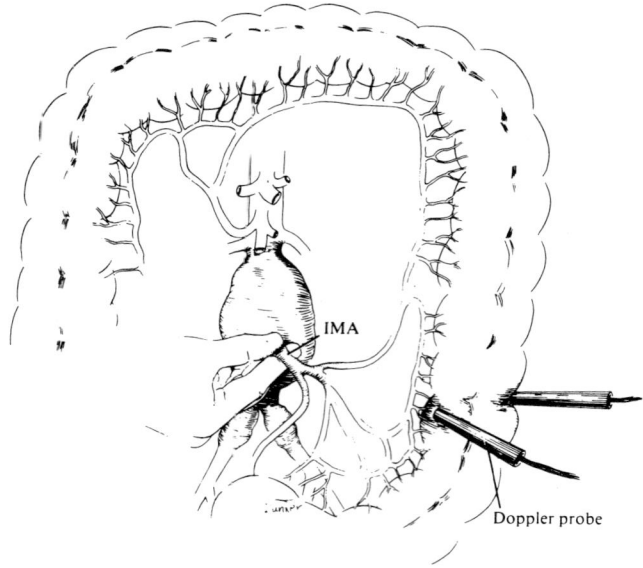

FIGURE 113–2. Application of a Doppler probe to the antimesenteric and mesenteric borders of the left colon during digital compression of the inferior mesenteric artery (IMA) documents the presence or absence of collateral blood flow. (From Bernhard VM, Towne JB: Complications in Vascular Surgery. New York, Grune & Stratton, 1980, p 398.)

oximeter probe to detect arterial pulsatility and transcolonic oxygen saturation. Unmeasurable transcolonic oxygen saturations and loss of pulsatility suggest colon ischemia.[43]

Hobson and colleagues, employing the Doppler technique, concluded that the presence of arterial flow sounds along the left colon confirmed adequacy of collateral flow, whereas the absence of Doppler sounds during inferior mesenteric artery occlusion suggested potential colon ischemia.[26] Whether reconstruction of the artery is necessary when Doppler signals are lost, however, cannot be determined from this study because control data were not presented. Furthermore, routine postoperative colonoscopy to detect colon ischemia was not employed. The Doppler technique may be used for both occlusive and aneurysmal disease.

Inferior mesenteric artery stump pressure measurements are obtained by cannulating the divided distal artery with an 18-gauge polytetrafluoroethylene (Teflon) catheter. Alternatively, and consistent with the author's preference, the catheter may be threaded into the arterial orifice from inside the open aneurysmal sac (see Fig. 113–3).[15] When mean stump blood pressures measure greater than 40 mmHg, the inferior mesenteric artery may be safely ligated, even when hypogastric pulsatile flow cannot be detected.[15, 17] Mean pressures of less than 40 mmHg forewarn of the possible development of ischemic colitis. It must be emphasized that reliance on stump pressure measurements assumes that systemic blood pressure and regional perfusion are maintained in the postoperative period at levels at least as high as when the operative measurements were determined. Impugning the usefulness of inferior mesenteric artery stump pressure measurements when postoperative bleeding and hypotension occur as a result of technical misadventures is not appropriate.[34] Even the best predictive test is not infallible under such circumstances.

Although intravenous fluorescein dye has been reported as helpful in assessing small bowel viability, there has been only limited application in evaluation of the sigmoid colon. In a study of 186 patients, the investigators concluded that among 15, use of intravenous fluorescein seemed valuable and they endorsed its selective use.[73]

Controlled data are still insufficient to endorse any of these techniques as foolproof predictors of the development of ischemic colitis or the need for inferior mesenteric artery reconstruction. Except for tonometric pH monitoring, all

techniques to predict colon ischemia have the shortcoming that they are single intraoperative measurements that may not reflect subsequent ischemic events. Table 113–3 summarizes methods of operative assessment of colon viability.

Routine, rather than *selective*, reconstruction of all patent inferior mesenteric arteries may be justified but only if the rate of complications after routine reconstruction is acceptably low. In a multicenter study, inferior mesenteric artery reconstruction was associated with an increased frequency of postoperative bleeding.[62] However, two reports in which 75 inferior mesenteric arteries were reconstructed provide support for routine reconstruction.[63, 65] Nevertheless, it could not be proved that routine inferior mesenteric artery reconstruction was superior to selective ligation, particularly when the safety of ligation was documented by objective evaluation of the adequacy of colonic collateral circulation with the use of the tests previously described.

INFERIOR MESENTERIC ARTERY RECONSTRUCTION

When to reconstruct the inferior mesenteric artery cannot be conclusively determined from reports in the literature. Some surgeons use objective data,[17, 26] whereas others rely on clinical intuitive methods.[3, 21, 24, 28, 39, 42] Nonetheless, the following techniques have proved effective (Figs. 113–4 and 113–5)[11, 14]:

- Reimplantation of the inferior mesenteric origin as a button from the aorta into the prosthesis (the Carrel patch technique)
- Anastomosis of a portion of the aneurysmal sac, including the orifice of the artery into the prosthesis (the inclusion technique, popularized by Crawford)

Alternative methods include (1) reimplantation of the inferior mesenteric artery without an aortic button and (2) interposition grafting of prosthetic material or autogenous tissue from the aortic graft to the artery.

SUMMARY

The prevention of ischemic colitis after aortic reconstruction is preferable to its successful management. Avoidance of this complication hinges on:

TABLE 113–3. OPERATIVE ASSESSMENT OF COLON VIABILITY

TEST	ADVANTAGES	DISADVANTAGES
Inspection	Easy	Inaccurate
Second look	Accurate	Second operation
Doppler ultrasound	Easy; inexpensive; 80% accurate	Limited bowel area sampled (2 cm²); one-time measurement during operation only
IMA stump pressure	Easy; inexpensive; highly accurate	One-time measurement during operation only; IMA must be cannulated
Colonic intramural pH	Able to monitor colonic blood flow operatively and postoperatively	Requires preoperative catheter placement in colon through rectum
Photoplethysmography with transcolonic oxygen saturation	Relatively easy; moderately accurate	Limited bowel area sampled; one-time measurement during operation only

From Tollefson DFJ, Ernst CB: Colon ischemia following aortic reconstruction. Ann Vasc Surg 5:485–489, 1991. Reprinted by permission of Blackwell Scientific Publications, Inc.
IMA = inferior mesenteric artery.

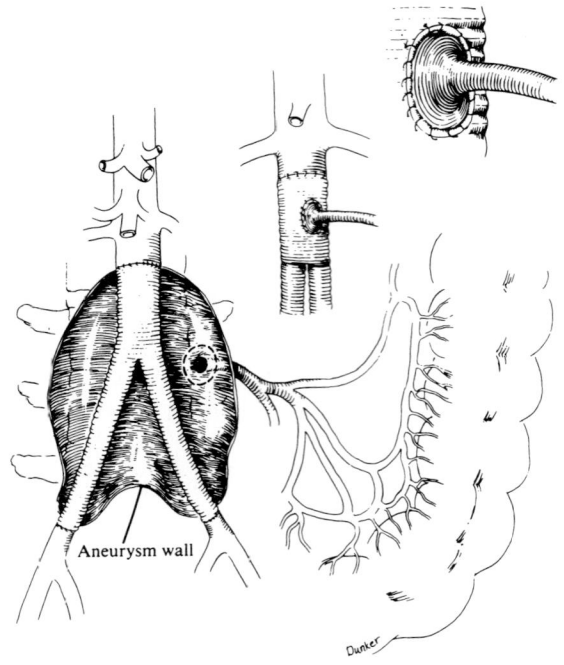

FIGURE 113–4. Carrel patch technique for reconstruction of the inferior mesenteric artery (IMA). Excision of a button of aneurysm wall surrounding the artery's orifice facilitates repair. (From Bernhard VM, Towne JB: Complications in Vascular Surgery. New York, Grune & Stratton, 1980, p 402.)

- Identification of the high-risk patient
- Precise, gentle, meticulous operative technique
- Knowledge of bowel blood supply
- Methods to prevent damage to the blood supply or to preserve it by inferior mesenteric artery reconstruction

Patients at greatest risk for development of ischemic colitis after aortic reconstruction include those with (1) ruptured aneurysms, (2) a patent inferior mesenteric artery,

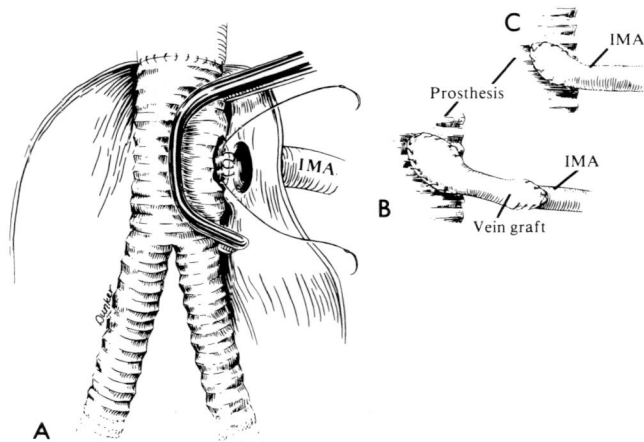

FIGURE 113–5. Reconstruction of the inferior mesenteric artery (IMA). *A*, Anastomosis of the rim of the aneurysmal sac, including the arterial orifice to the prosthesis (suture of hole-to-hole technique). *B*, Reconstruction with autogenous saphenous vein graft. *C*, Implantation of the large artery into the prosthesis. A button of prosthesis must be excised to ensure a patulous anastomosis.

TABLE 113–4. RISK PREDICTION FOR BOWEL ISCHEMIA AFTER AORTIC RECONSTRUCTION

Greatest risk
   Symptoms of visceral ischemia
   Aortic aneurysm (ruptured)
   Patent IMA
   No operative Doppler flow
   IMA stump pressure <40 mmHg
   Critical intramural pH decrease
   Loss of photoplethysmographic pulsatility and transcolonic oxygen
      saturation
   IMA to SMA flow in the meandering mesenteric artery

IMA = inferior mesenteric artery; SMA = superior mesenteric artery.

(3) post–aortic reconstruction mean inferior mesenteric stump pressures below 40 mmHg, (4) Doppler arterial flow signals that cease after division or occlusion of the inferior mesenteric artery, and (5) a damaged meandering mesenteric artery that has gone unrecognized (Table 113–4).

Diagnosis of ischemic colitis depends on early recognition of variable symptoms and on prompt fiberoptic colonoscopy. Aggressive management, at times employing colon resection, provides the only chance for successful outcome once the process has been established.

REFERENCES

1. Bandyk DF, Florence MG, Johansen KH: Colon ischemia accompanying ruptured abdominal aortic aneurysm. J Surg Res 30:297, 1981.
2. Baur GM, Porter JM, Eidemiller LR, et al: The role of arteriography in abdominal aortic aneurysm. Am J Surg 136:184, 1978.
3. Bernatz PE: Necrosis of the colon following resection for abdominal aortic aneurysms. Arch Surg 81:373, 1960.
4. Bernstein WC, Bernstein EF: Ischemic ulcerative colitis following inferior mesenteric arterial ligation. Dis Colon Rectum 6:54, 1963.
5. Bicks RO, Bale GF, Howard H, et al: Acute and delayed colon ischemia after aorta aneurysm surgery. Arch Intern Med 122:249, 1968.
6. Birnbaum W, Rudy L, Wylie EJ: Colonic and rectal ischemia following abdominal aneurysmectomy. Dis Colon Rectum 7:293, 1964.
7. Boley SJ, Brandt LJ, Veith FJ: Ischemic disorders of the intestines. Curr Probl Surg 15:1, 1978.
8. Brewster DC, Retana A, Waltman AC, et al: Angiography in the management of aneurysms of the abdominal aorta. N Engl J Med 292:822, 1975.
9. Bulkley GB, Zuidema GD, Hamilton SR, et al: Intraoperative determination of small intestinal viability following ischemic injury: A prospective, controlled trial of two adjuvant methods (Doppler and fluorescein) compared with standard clinical judgment. Ann Surg 193:628, 1981.
10. Bussemaker JB, Lindeman J: Comparison of methods to determine viability of small intestine. Ann Surg 176:97, 1972.
11. Carrel A: Technique and remote results of vascular anastomoses. Surg Gynecol Obstet 14:246, 1912.
12. Connolly JE, Kwaan JHM: Prophylactic revascularization of the gut. Ann Surg 190:514, 1979.
13. Crawford ES, Saleh SA, Babb JW III, et al: Infrarenal abdominal aortic aneurysm: Factors influencing survival after operation performed over a 25-year period. Ann Surg 193:699, 1981.
14. Crawford ES, Snyder DM, Cho GC, et al: Progress in treatment of thoracoabdominal and abdominal aortic aneurysms involving celiac, superior mesenteric, and renal arteries. Ann Surg 188:404, 1978.
15. Ernst CB: Prevention of intestinal ischemia following abdominal aortic reconstruction. Surgery 93:102, 1983.
16. Ernst CB, Hagihara PF, Daugherty ME, et al: Ischemic colitis incidence following abdominal aortic reconstruction: A prospective study. Surgery 80:417, 1976.
17. Ernst CB, Hagihara PF, Daugherty ME, Griffen WO Jr: Inferior mesen-

teric artery stump pressure: A reliable index for safe IMA ligation during abdominal aortic aneurysmectomy. Ann Surg 187:641, 1978.

18. Stanley JC, Barnes RW, Ernst CB, et al: Vascular surgery in the United States: Workforce issues. J Vasc Surg 23:172, 1996.
19. Fiddian-Green RG, Amelin PM, Herrimann JB, et al: Prediction of the development of sigmoid ischemia on the day of aortic operations. Arch Surg 121:654, 1986.
20. Gibson WE III, Pearce CW, Creech O Jr: Infarction of the left hemicolon due to primary vascular occlusion. Dis Colon Rectum 12:323, 1969.
21. Gonzalez LL, Jaffe MS: Mesenteric arterial insufficiency following abdominal aortic resection. Arch Surg 93:10, 1966.
22. Griffiths JD: Surgical anatomy of the blood supply of the distal colon. Ann R Coll Surg Engl 19:241, 1956.
23. Hagihara PF, Ernst CB, Griffen WO Jr: Incidence of ischemic colitis following abdominal aortic reconstruction. Surg Gynecol Obstet 149:571, 1979.
24. Hardy JD: Preservation of accessory arterial supply in abdominal aneurysm resection. Surg Gynecol Obstet 123:1317, 1966.
25. Hobson RW II, Wright CB, O'Donnell JA, et al: Determination of intestinal viability by Doppler ultrasound. Arch Surg 114:165, 1979.
26. Hobson RW II, Wright CB, Rich NM, et al: Assessment of colonic ischemia during aortic surgery by Doppler ultrasound. J Surg Res 20:231, 1976.
27. Javid H, Julian OC, Dye WS, et al: Complications of abdominal aortic grafts. Arch Surg 85:142, 1962.
28. Johnson WC, Nabseth DC: Visceral infarction following aortic surgery. Ann Surg 180:312, 1974.
29. Katz S, Wahab A, Murray W, et al: New parameters of viability in ischemic bowel disease. Am J Surg 127:136, 1974.
30. Kim MW, Hundahl SA, Dang CR, et al: Ischemic colitis after aortic aneurysmectomy. Am J Surg 141:392, 1983.
31. Lannerstad O, Bergentz SE, Bergqvist D, et al: Ischemic intestinal complications after aortic surgery. Acta Chir Scand 151:599, 1985.
32. Launer DP, Miscall BG, Beil AR Jr: Colorectal infarction following resection of abdominal aortic aneurysms. Dis Colon Rectum 21:613, 1978.
33. Lee BY, Trainor FS, Kavner D, et al: Intraoperative assessment of intestinal viability with Doppler ultrasound. Surg Gynecol Obstet 149:671, 1979.
34. Lie M, Normann E, Ovrum E: Necrosis of distal colon after abdominal aneurysmectomy despite high retrograde pressure in inferior mesenteric artery. Ann Chir Gynaecol 71:347, 1982.
35. McBurney RP, Howard H, Bicks RO, et al: Ischemia and gangrene of the colon following abdominal aortic resection. Am Surg 36:205, 1970.
36. McKain J, Shumacker HB Jr: Ischemia of the left colon associated with abdominal aortic aneurysms and their treatment. Arch Surg 76:355, 1958.
37. Miller RE, Knox WG: Colon ischemia following infrarenal aorta surgery: Report of four cases. Ann Surg 163:639, 1966.
38. Moosa AR, Skinner DB, Stark V, et al: Assessment of bowel viability using ^{99m}technetium-tagged albumin microspheres. J Surg Res 16:466, 1974.
39. Morris GC Jr: In discussion of Ernst CB, Hagihara PF, Daugherty ME, Griffen WO Jr: Inferior mesenteric artery stump pressure: A reliable index for safe IMA ligation during abdominal aortic aneurysmectomy. Ann Surg 187:641, 1978.
40. Moskowitz M, Zimmerman H, Felson B: The meandering mesenteric artery of the colon. Am J Roentgenol 92:1088, 1964.
41. Movius HJ II: Resection of abdominal arteriosclerotic aneurysm. Am J Surg 90:298, 1955.
42. Ottinger LW, Darling RC, Nathan MJ, Linton RR: Left colon ischemia complicating aortoiliac reconstruction. Arch Surg 105:841, 1972.
43. Ouriel K, Fiore WM, Geary JE: Detection of occult colonic ischemia during aortic procedures: Use of an intraoperative photoplethysmographic technique. J Vasc Surg 7:5, 1988.
44. Papachristou D, Fortner JG: Prediction of intestinal viability by intraarterial dye injection: A simple test. Am J Surg 132:572, 1976.
45. Papadopoulos CD, Mancini HW, Marino AWM Jr: Ischemic necrosis of the colon following aortic aneurysmectomy. J Cardiovasc Surg 15:494, 1974.
46. Perdue GD, Lowry K: Arterial insufficiency to the colon following

47. Rob C, Snyder M: Chronic intestinal ischemia: A complication of surgery of the abdominal aorta. Surgery 60:1141, 1966.
48. Robicsek F: In discussion of Ottinger LW, Darling RC, Nathan MJ, Linton RR: Left colon ischemia complicating aortoiliac reconstruction. Arch Surg 105:841, 1972.
49. Schroeder T, Christoffersen JK, Andersen J, et al: Ischemic colitis complicating reconstruction of the abdominal aorta. Surg Gynecol Obstet 160:299, 1985.
50. Shaw RS, Green TH: Massive mesenteric infarction following inferior mesenteric artery ligation in resection of the colon for carcinoma. N Engl J Med 248:890, 1953.
51. Smith RF, Szilagyi DE: Ischemia of the colon as a complication in the surgery of the abdominal aorta. Arch Surg 80:806, 1960.
52. Steward JA, Rankin FW: Blood supply of large intestine: Its surgical considerations. Arch Surg 26:843, 1933.
53. Stolar CJH, Randolph JG: Evaluation of ischemic bowel viability with a fluorescent technique. J Pediatr Surg 13:221, 1978.
54. Volpetti G, Barker CF, Berkowitz HD, et al: A twenty-two year review of elective resection of abdominal aortic aneurysms. Surg Gynecol Obstet 142:321, 1976.
55. Whittemore AD, Clowes AW, Hechtman HB, et al: Aortic aneurysm repair: Reduced operative mortality associated with maintenance of optimal cardiac performance. Ann Surg 192:414, 1980.
56. Young JR, Humphries AW, deWolfe VG, et al: Complications of aortic surgery. Part II: Intestinal ischemia. Arch Surg 86:65, 1963.
57. Zarins CK, Skinner DB, Rhodes HA, et al: Predictions of the viability of revascularized intestine with radioactive microspheres. Surg Gynecol Obstet 138:578, 1974.
58. Zimberg YH, Sullivan JM: Midgut gangrene after resection of an infrarenal aortic aneurysm. Am J Surg 107:785, 1964.
59. Bulkley GB: Pathophysiology of free-radical mediated reperfusion injury. J Vasc Surg 5:512, 1987.
60. Farkas JC, Calvo-Verjat N, Laurain C, et al: Acute colorectal ischemia after aortic surgery: Pathophysiology and prognostic criteria. Ann Vasc Surg 6:11, 1992.
61. Iliopoulos JI, Pierce GE, Hermreck AS: Hemodynamics of the inferior mesenteric arterial circulation. J Vasc Surg 11:120, 1990.
62. Johnson KW, Scobie TK: Multicenter prospective study of nonruptured abdominal aortic aneurysms: I. Population and operative management. J Vasc Surg 7:69, 1988.
63. Seeger JM, Coe DA, Kaelin LD, et al: Routine reimplantation of patent inferior mesenteric arteries limits colon infarction after aortic reconstruction. J Vasc Surg 15:635, 1992.
64. Tollefson DFJ, Ernst CB: Colon ischemia following aortic reconstruction. Ann Vasc Surg 5:485, 1991.
65. Zelenock GB, Strodel WE, Knoll JA, et al: A prospective study of clinically and endoscopically documented colonic ischemia in 100 patients undergoing aortic reconstructive surgery with aggressive colonic and direct pelvic revascularization, compared with historic controls. Surgery 106:771, 1989.
66. Ernst CB: Abdominal aortic aneurysm. N Engl J Med 328:1167, 1993.
67. Brewster DC, Franklin DP, Cambria RP, et al: Intestinal ischemia complicating abdominal aortic surgery. Surgery 109:447, 1991.
68. Bjorek M, Bergqvist D, Troeng T: Incidence and clinical presentation of bowel ischemia after aortoiliac surgery—2930 operations from a population-based registry in Sweden. Eur J Endovasc Surg 12:139, 1996.
69. Longo WE, Lee TC, Barnett, MG, et al: Ischemic colitis complicating abdominal aortic aneurysm surgery in the U.S. veteran. J Surg Res 60:351, 1996.
70. Kuttilak K, Perttila J, Vanttinen E, Niinikoski J: Tonometric assessment of sigmoid perfusion during aortobifemoral reconstruction for arteriosclerosis. Eur J Surg 160:491, 1994.
71. Iberti TJ, Salky BA, Onofrey D: Use of bedside laparoscopy to identify intestinal ischemia in postoperative cases of aortic reconstruction. Surgery 105:686, 1989.
72. Ernst CB: Discussion of Avino AJ, Oldenburg WA, Gloviczck P, et al: Inferior mesenteric venous sampling to detect colonic ischemia: A comparison with laser Doppler flowmetry and photoplethysmography. J Vasc Surg 22:271, 1995.
73. Bergman KT, Gloviczki P, Welch TJ, et al: The role of intravenous fluorescein in the detection of colon ischemia during aortic reconstruction. Ann Vasc Surg 6:74, 1992.

SECTION XVI

MANAGEMENT OF PORTAL HYPERTENSION

KAJ H. JOHANSEN, M.D., Ph.D.

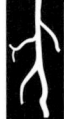

CHAPTER 114

Portal Hypertension: An Overview

Kaj H. Johansen, M.D., Ph.D.

Whether a consequence of alcoholic cirrhosis (most common in industrialized Western countries) or the result of any of a number of postviral, parasitic, or hepatotoxic conditions (common in developing countries), portal hypertension has medical and surgical implications of cost, morbidity, and frequently death. In this chapter, the epidemiology and natural history, pathologic anatomy and physiology, and clinical presentation of the various manifestations of this condition are discussed, and a diagnostic and therapeutic algorithm—to be applied as early as possible in the evaluation of such patients—is proposed. In Chapter 115, emergency management—how to resuscitate, stabilize, and diagnose patients with portal hypertension—is discussed. The appropriate role of endoscopic techniques for controlling both acute and chronic variceal hemorrhage is reviewed. Chapter 116 critically analyzes various nonoperative interventional techniques for management of the complications of portal hypertension. Finally, Chapter 117 discusses various operative techniques to treat bleeding esophageal varices, including the proper role of liver transplantation.

The fact that, depending on an individual patient's status, appropriate management may vary from pharmacologic to endoscopic to radiographic to operative means has resulted in a voluminous and sometimes contradictory literature. Interested readers are referred to several recent reviews of this topic for different perspectives and more detailed discussion.[1–3]

ANATOMY AND PATHOPHYSIOLOGY

Normally, the portal vein carries 75% of the total volume of hepatic blood flow, the remainder being provided by the hepatic artery. In a healthy adult, the portal vein conducts 1000 to 1500 ml of blood per minute from the splanchnic viscera to the hepatic sinusoids. Despite this high rate of flow and the density of the liver parenchyma, resistance to flow within the liver is normally very low, as manifested by a pressure differential between the portal vein and the suprahepatic vena cava (the portacaval pressure gradient) that rarely exceeds 5 to 7 mmHg. Under normal physiologic conditions, portal collateral flow is negligible.

Obstruction to portal venous flow before (presinusoidal, either extrahepatic or intrahepatic), within (perisinusoidal), or beyond (postsinusoidal) the liver, however, increases resistance to flow, portal venous pressure, and portal collateral flow. Portal hypertension is present when the corrected portal pressure (the portacaval pressure gradient) exceeds 15 mmHg or when absolute portal venous pressure exceeds 25 mmHg. Pressures as high as 50 mmHg may be recorded.

Collateral routes to decompress the hypertensive portal vein are numerous (Fig. 114–1). Many, such as those in the retroperitoneum and around the left renal vein, are clinically silent. Others are of clinical importance or interest, either as diagnostic markers for the underlying condition (dilated abdominal wall veins, resulting in a caput medusae) or as potential sites for major bleeding (esophagogastric, rectal, or stomal varices; portal hypertensive gastropathy).

In portal hypertension, portal venous flow falls precipitously as portal collateral flow increases. Depending on the nature and severity of the obstruction, portal venous flow may stagnate or even reverse; in other words, resistance to flow in the portal vein may exceed that in the portal collateral bed, in which case the portal vein reverses flow and becomes a venous outflow tract for the liver. As portal vein flow diminishes, compensatory increases in hepatic arterial flow occur. In fact, the capacity to increase hepatic arterial flow may be an independent determinant of hepatic survival when portal venous perfusion of the liver is lost,[4] for example when spontaneous reversal of flow occurs in the portal vein or after portal vein thrombosis or "total" portosystemic shunt.

The chronic liver dysfunction associated with most manifestations of portal hypertension must constantly be considered in the evaluation and management of persons with this condition. At one time or another, the majority of such patients display various disorders of hepatocellular malfunction—clotting abnormalities, extracellular fluid overload, jaundice, hepatic encephalopathy, hypoprothrom-

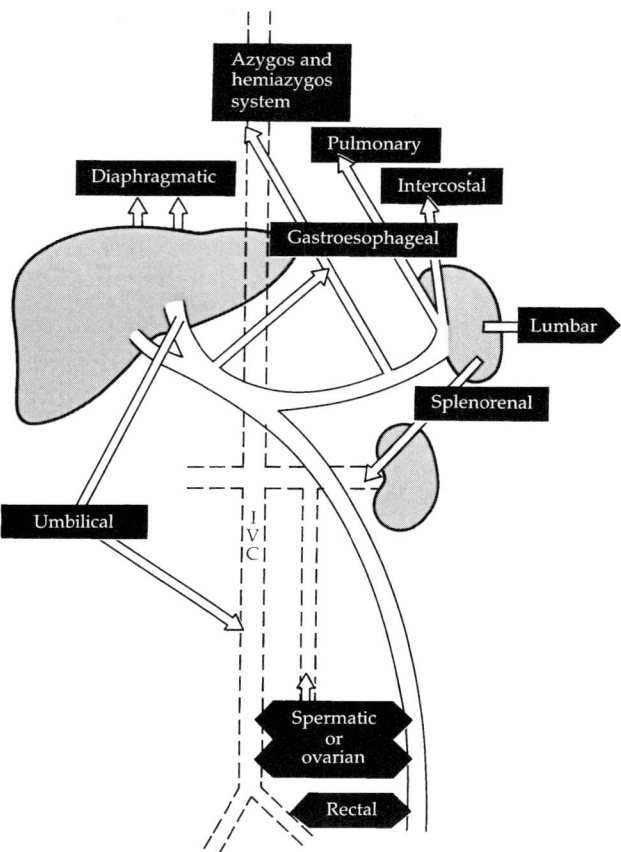

FIGURE 114–1. Multiple collateral pathways arise in response to the development of portal hypertension. Most important clinically, from the perspective of variceal hemorrhage, are pathways from the portal vein to the azygos or hemiazygos system via the gastroesophageal variceal plexus, and those communicating with hemorrhoidal tributaries of the hypogastric venous circuit. IVC = inferior vena cava. (From Sherlock S: The portal venous system and portal hypertension. *In* Diseases of the Liver and Biliary System, 8th ed. Oxford, Blackwell, 1989, p 166.)

binemia, malnutrition. The Child-Pugh classification (see later) is a clinical scoring system that takes into account many of these variables. Certain other implications of these patients' disease states must be confronted as well; for example, pancreatitis or acute alcohol withdrawal in patients with Laennec's cirrhosis, hepatitis virus seropositivity, a sharply increased risk of hepatoma in patients with postviral cirrhosis, and alcoholic or schistosomal cardiomyopathy.

Extrahepatic manifestations of severe liver dysfunction are manifold. The first clinical sign of portal hypertension is splenomegaly, and the hematologic manifestations of hypersplenism, especially thrombocytopenia and leukopenia, are commonplace. For reasons incompletely understood, advanced liver disease is associated with a hyperdynamic circulatory state, including elevated cardiac output and diminished peripheral resistance. The clinical picture may initially be mistaken for sepsis; but sepsis is characterized by high calculated pulmonary vascular resistance, whereas hepatic failure is accompanied by low resistance in both the systemic and the pulmonary circuits. In fact, the same opening of precapillary arteriovenous communi-

cations that leads to "spider" angiomas and palmar erythema in patients with advanced liver disease can be found in the pulmonary circulation; hypoxemia due to a physiologic shunt is frequently observed in cirrhotic subjects.

A poorly characterized but stereotypical neuropsychiatric disorder, hepatic or portal systemic encephalopathy, is frequently observed in those with far advanced cirrhosis. Both portosystemic shunting (spontaneous or secondary to a portal decompressive procedure) and hepatocellular dysfunction must be present for hepatic encephalopathy to be manifested. The underlying pathogenesis probably relates to excessive systemic levels of ammonia and other products of bacterial peptide metabolism in the gut.[5] That conclusion is derived in part from the observation that encephalopathy can be "improved" by oral antibiotics, colon resection or bypass, cathartics, liver transplantation, or portosystemic shunt occlusion.

Ascites, a common presentation in patients with portal hypertension, is found almost universally in those with decompensated or terminal liver failure.[6] The pathogenesis of ascites remains incompletely understood. It is known to be based primarily on the superimposition of a disordered Starling's equilibrium (increased hepatic sinusoidal hydrostatic pressure and reduced serum oncotic pressure resulting from hypoalbuminemia) on hepatic lymphatic obstruction, which produces excessive extracellular fluid. Hepatic lymph clearance, for which the threshold volume is 1000 mL/day, is overwhelmed, and excess fluid flows from the liver into the peritoneal cavity. Secondary hyperaldosteronism resulting from the diseased liver's inability to metabolize endogenous steroids further complicates normal removal of ascites. Other fluid and electrolyte disturbances in cirrhotic patients may include, besides extracellular volume overload and intravascular volume depletion, sodium excess and extreme total-body potassium deficit (with resulting metabolic alkalosis).

Renal dysfunction frequently accompanies decompensated liver failure.[7] The hepatorenal syndrome is characterized by oliguria and rising serum creatinine values in the absence of evidence for prerenal or renal parenchymal disease: hepatic dysfunction is advanced, and urine sodium levels are less than 10 mEq/L. Redistribution of regional blood flow in the kidneys, with extreme renal cortical vasoconstriction, has been documented: recent observations suggest that elevated serum endothelin levels may play a pathogenetic role.[8] The mortality rate of established hepatorenal failure exceeds 90%; the only predictably effective therapy is liver transplantation, which, when successful, can result in return of normal renal function.

EPIDEMIOLOGY, RISK FACTORS, AND NATURAL HISTORY

Although portal hypertension and its complications may arise from various disease states (Table 114–1), cirrhosis due to alcoholic liver disease predominates in Western and industrialized countries. In the United States, alcoholic liver disease accounts for about 90% of cases of portal hypertension. Worldwide, hepatic dysfunction leading to portal hypertension most commonly arises from an earlier

TABLE 114–1. CAUSES OF PORTAL HYPERTENSION

Presinusoidal

Extrahepatic
  Portal vein thrombosis
  Splenic vein occlusion
  Increased splenic blood flow (e.g., myelofibrosis)
Intrahepatic
  Schistosomiasis
  Congenital hepatic fibrosis
  Portal zone infiltrations (reticulosis, sarcoidosis)
  Primary portal hypertension (Indian childhood cirrhosis)

Sinusoidal

Cirrhosis
Sinusoidal occlusion (vitamin A toxicity, Gaucher's disease, myeloid
  metaplasia)
Alcoholic hepatitis

Postsinusoidal

Hepatic vein occlusion (vascular occlusion due to malignancy, Budd-
  Chiari syndrome)
Veno-occlusive disease
Alcoholic central hyaline necrosis

*Other Causes Not Defined by Presinusoidal, Intrasinusoidal, or
  Postsinusoidal Terminology*

Hematologic disorders (lymphoma, leukemia, myeloproliferative
  disorders)
Hemodynamic causes (increased splanchnic blood flow [e.g., splenic
  arteriovenous or hepatic arterioportal fistula])
Hepatic parenchymal abnormalities (partial nodular transformation,
  regenerative hyperplasia)
Idiopathic (portal phlebosclerosis, Banti's syndrome)

infection, either postnecrotic (hepatitis B virus) or secondary to schistosomal involvement of the liver. Other less common but clinically important causes of portal hypertension—congenital, toxic, inflammatory, and vascular—are enumerated in Table 114–1. Because of its predominance in Western and industrialized countries, cirrhosis arising from alcoholic liver disease will be the focus of much of the discussion here.

Conservative estimates suggest that 7.5% (World Health Organization criteria) to almost 20% (National Institute on Alcohol Abuse and Alcoholism criteria) of American adults manifest drinking behavior considered "at risk" for chronic alcoholism.[9] Accordingly, although only 10% of alcoholics develop hepatic cirrhosis, and of that group only 30% develop signs and symptoms of portal hypertension, alcoholic liver disease is clearly a major public health problem. It is little surprise that hepatic cirrhosis ranks 10th among all causes of death in the United States.[10] In some developing countries, variceal hemorrhage is one of the major nontraumatic causes of death in adults. Bleeding from varices is the leading cause of death from gastrointestinal hemorrhage worldwide and a major cause of disability and death between the ages of 35 and 59 years, when employment and child rearing are particularly important. The personal, public health, and societal costs of alcoholic liver disease are substantial.

The natural history of cirrhosis and portal hypertension relates primarily to the persistence and severity of the underlying hepatic dysfunction. For example, abstinence from alcohol frequently results in stabilization of the scarring-regenerating process that characterizes Laennec's cir-

rhosis. Bleeding from esophageal varices most often occurs in persons with cirrhosis who continue to consume alcohol, whereas it is unusual in those who have been abstinent from alcohol for more than 1 year. For patients with postnecrotic cirrhosis, the hepatic inflammation and fibrosis resulting from the underlying process may slow or halt; this phenomenon explains these patients' somewhat better long-term prognosis as compared with those with alcoholic cirrhosis. On the other hand, viral hepatitis may persist as a chronic relapsing infection, and affected patients also have a substantial risk of developing hepatocellular carcinoma.[11]

The outcome of untreated hepatic cirrhosis is poor. Classic studies demonstrate the natural history of the condition, since today medical or surgical intervention is the norm. The famous Boston Interhospital Liver Group studies demonstrated that cirrhotic patients who had ascites had only a 10% 1-year survival rate.[12] The development of jaundice was even more ominous, with a median survival time of 4 months. Before the liver transplantation era, Orloff demonstrated that patients who displayed the tetrad of jaundice, ascites, encephalopathy, and severe muscle wasting had a mortality rate approaching 100% at 1 year, notwithstanding optimal medical and surgical therapy.[13] In schistosomal disease of the liver, because hepatocellular function is relatively better preserved than in cirrhosis, the mortality rate is less. Nevertheless, the development of gastrointestinal hemorrhage is commonplace and frequently lethal.

The stereotypical nature of advanced liver disease makes possible semi-objective quantitation of hepatocellular dysfunction. The scoring systems of Child[14] and Pugh and colleagues[15] (Table 114–2), originally established to predict outcome after, respectively, emergency portacaval shunt and esophageal transection to treat bleeding esophageal varices, can also be used to classify such patients in numerous other therapeutic and prognostic settings. Child's system

TABLE 114–2. CHILD-PUGH CLASSIFICATIONS

CHILD CLASSIFICATION	Class		
	A	*B*	*C*
Bilirubin (mg/dl)	<2.0	2.0–3.0	>3.0
Albumin (mg/dl)	>3.5	3.0–3.5	<3.0
Ascites	None	Reversible	Refractory
Encephalopathy	None	Minimal	Spontaneous
Nutrition (muscle mass)	Normal	Fair	Poor

PUGH CLASSIFICATION	Points Scored for Increasing Abnormality		
	1	*2*	*3*
Encephalopathy (grade)	Normal	1 or 2	3 or 4
Albumin (mg/dl)	>3.5	2.8–3.5	<2.8
Bilirubin (mg/dl)	1.0–2.0	2.0–3.0	>3.0
Ascites	Absent	Slight	Significant
Prothrombin time (seconds prolonged)	1–4	4–6	>6
Grade A		5 or 6	
Grade B		7, 8, or 9	
Grade C		10–15	

From Child CG: Surgery and portal hypertension. *In* Dunphy JE (ed): The Liver and Portal Hypertension. Philadelphia, WB Saunders, 1964; and Pugh RNH, Murray-Lyon IM, Dawson JL, Williams R: Transection of the oesophagus for bleeding oesophageal varices. Br J Surg 60:646, 1973, by permission of Butterworth Heinemann, Ltd, Oxford, publisher.

includes assessment of ascites, encephalopathy, muscle wasting, and levels of serum albumin and bilirubin. Pugh's scale deletes nutritional status but considers, in addition, prothrombin time. A certain degree of controversy attends the use of these classifications[16]; nevertheless, they are simple, reproducible, and remain remarkably useful in predicting ultimate outcomes for cirrhotic patients.

Because the complications of portal hypertension—variceal hemorrhage, ascites, hypersplenism, and hepatic encephalopathy—always occur in the setting of advanced liver dysfunction (and, not infrequently, with major medical co-morbidities), hospitalization, and even intensive care unit admission, is usually required for these patients. The likelihood of various complications and of prolonged hospitalization is high as well. The mortality risk associated with hospitalization for a first episode of bleeding from esophageal varices approaches 50%.[17]

The optimal solution to the excessive mortality and other societal costs incurred by patients with cirrhosis and portal hypertension ultimately revolves around prevention. Unfortunately, alcoholism (and abuse of other substances) appears to be an unavoidable feature of the human condition; prohibition, taxation, education, and other attempts at mitigation have produced only minimal success. Alcohol treatment programs are notoriously unsuccessful; critical analysis suggests that their effect is brief, their costs substantial, and recidivism common. Other maneuvers, such as widespread hepatitis B vaccination, screening of community blood supplies, and more controversial measures such as needle-exchange programs for intravenous drug abusers, may have some prophylactic impact. Attempts to develop an anti-*Schistosoma* vaccine are ongoing.[18]

APPROACH TO THE PATIENT

A number of therapeutic options—pharmacologic, endoscopic, interventional radiologic, and operative—may be considered for patients who manifest the complications of portal hypertension. Which approach is pursued depends on the patient's clinical and physical status, on the underlying cause of the hepatic dysfunction being treated, and (to a degree) on the availability of various therapies. Whether such a patient is best managed in a major medical center or can be effectively cared for in the community setting is not clear. When a patient with bleeding esophageal varices or intractable ascites is being managed in a setting where all contemporary modes of therapy are available, optimal management can be determined by answering the following questions.

Is the Patient a Liver Transplantation Candidate?

As will be noted in Chapter 117, candidacy for liver transplantation generally implies end-stage liver disease in a patient younger than 60 years who manifests no other significant medical co-morbidity. Abstinence from alcohol for a minimum of 6 months should be documented. The portal vein should be patent, and scarring from right upper quadrant operations should be minimal or absent. Trans-plantation is much more difficult in patients with portal or diffuse splanchnic venous thrombosis as well as in those who have had right upper quadrant operations, especially portosystemic shunts.[19] A patient with variceal hemorrhage who is considered to be a transplant candidate should be managed medically (intravenous vasoconstrictor therapy, balloon tamponade, beta blockers), endoscopically (variceal sclerotherapy or banding), or by angiographic shunt. If operative portal decompression is required, it is best done as a splenorenal or mesocaval shunt, which avoids dissection and subsequent adhesions in the right upper quadrant and the hepatic hilum. Outcomes of liver transplantation are as good in patients with variceal hemorrhage as those of transplants for other reasons.[20]

Patients with cirrhosis and portal hypertension whose liver function is relatively preserved (Child-Pugh class A or B) should be considered for nontransplant therapies, as should those who are actively consuming alcohol, have advanced cardiopulmonary or other medical co-morbidity, are elderly, or are seropositive for hepatitis B. Most patients with variceal hemorrhage or other complications of portal hypertension fit into one of these categories.

Is the Patient Compliant and Responsible?

Some patients—for example, many of those who are actively drinking alcohol—are noncompliant. Their ability to be available for the long-term follow-up required by various palliative treatments for portal hypertension is limited. In such circumstances *definitive* therapy—operative shunt or liver transplantation—is preferable.

For some patients, substituting a definitive treatment for repeated palliative measures removes anxiety about future recurrent variceal hemorrhage. Still others who live at some distance from the medical center are placed at grave risk when drug or endoscopic therapy fails.[21] Conversely, compliant patients living near the medical center, especially those with nonalcoholic liver disease, may do well with *palliative* therapies such as chronic endoscopic variceal banding or sclerotherapy or beta-blocker administration.

Are There Anatomic, Physiologic, or Other Clinical Abnormalities That Might Affect Certain Therapies?

Operative or angiographic portacaval shunt is rarely possible in the presence of chronic portal vein thrombosis. Presence of a diminutive splenic vein or one anatomically distant from the renal vein is a contraindication to distal splenorenal shunt, as is the presence of significant ascites or hepatofugal portal vein flow. Significant preoperative encephalopathy often is worse after an otherwise successful portosystemic shunt (whether by operative or angiographic means). Endoscopic sclerotherapy is dangerous in the presence of significant esophageal ulceration secondary to earlier sclerotherapy. Beta-blocker administration to reduce portal hypertension pharmacologically may be relatively contraindicated in the presence of asthma or congestive heart failure. General anesthetics and operations are poorly tolerated by patients with decompensated cirrhosis.

SUMMARY

Portal hypertension, usually arising from some form of advanced chronic liver disease, is a complicated and lethal condition. In its most dramatic presentation, gastrointestinal hemorrhage, sometimes torrential, occurs against a backdrop of chronic hepatocellular dysfunction and, not infrequently, other medical co-morbidities. Related problems may include hypersplenism, ascites, and hepatic encephalopathy.

Therapy for the complications of portal hypertension depends on the nature and extent of the underlying liver disease and on other clinical factors such as the availability of various treatment modalities, patient compliance, and proximity to a major medical center. Subsequent chapters detail selection of the appropriate diagnostic and therapeutic approaches for patients with portal hypertension.

REFERENCES

1. D'Amico G, Pagliaro L, Bosch J: The treatment of portal hypertension: A meta-analytic review. Hepatology 22:332–354, 1995.
2. Bosch J: Portal hypertension. Baillieres Clin Gastroenterol 11:1–407, 1997.
3. Henderson JM, Barnes DS, Geisinger MA: Portal hypertension (Review). Curr Probl Surg 35:379–452, 1998.
4. Burchell AR, Moreno AH, Panke WF, Nealon TF: Hepatic artery flow improvement after portacaval shunt: A single hemodynamic clinical correlate. Ann Surg 192:9–18, 1976.
5. Jurgens P: New aspects on etiology, biochemistry, and therapy of portal systemic encephalopathy: A critical survey. Nutrition 13:560–570, 1997.
6. Gines P, Fernandez-Esparrach G, Arroyo V, Rodes J: Pathogenesis of ascites in cirrhosis (Review). Semin Liver Dis 17:175–189, 1997.
7. Epstein M: Hepatorenal syndrome: Emerging perspectives of pathophysiology and therapy (Review). J Am Soc Nephrol 4:1735–1753, 1994.
8. Soper CP, Latif AB, Bending MR: Amelioration of hepatorenal syndrome with selective endothelin-A antagonist (Letter). Lancet 347:1842–1843, 1996.
9. Fleming MF, Manwell LB, Barry KL, Johnson K: At-risk drinking in an HMO primary care sample: Prevalence and health policy implications. Am J Public Health 88:90–93, 1998.
10. Mortality patterns—preliminary data. MMWR Morb Mortal Wkly Rep 46:941–944, 1997.
11. Craig JR: Cirrhosis, hepatocellular carcinoma, and survival. Hepatology 26:798–799, 1997.
12. Garceau AJ and the Boston Interhospital Liver Group: The natural history of cirrhosis: I. Survival with esophageal varices. N Engl J Med 268:469–473, 1962.
13. Orloff MJ, Chandler JG, Charters AL, et al: Comparison of end-to-side and side-to-side portacaval shunt in dogs and humans with cirrhosis and portal hypertension. Am J Surg 128:195–201, 1974.
14. Child CG: Surgery and portal hypertension. In Dunphy JE (ed): The Liver and Portal Hypertension. Philadelphia, WB Saunders, 1964.
15. Pugh RNH, Murray-Lyon IM, Dawson JL, Williams R: Transection of the oesophagus for bleeding oesophageal varices. Br J Surg 60:646–649, 1973.
16. Conn HO: A peek at the Child-Turcotte classification. Hepatology 1:673–676, 1981.
17. Burroughs AK: The management of bleeding due to portal hypertension: Part 1. The management of acute bleeding episodes. Q J Med 67:447–458, 1988. Part 2. Prevention of variceal bleeding and prevention of the first bleeding episode in patients with portal hypertension. Q J Med 68:507–516, 1988.
18. Wynn TA: Development of an antipathology vaccine for schistosomiasis (Review). Ann N Y Acad Sci 797:191–195, 1996.
19. Aboujaoude M, Grant D, Ghent C, et al: Effect of portosystemic shunts on subsequent liver transplantation. Surg Gynecol Obstet 172:215–219, 1991.
20. Iwatsuki S, Starzl TE, Todo S, et al: Liver transplantation in the treatment of bleeding esophageal varices. Surgery 104:697–705, 1988.
21. Rikkers LF, Burnett DA, Valentine GD, et al: Shunt surgery versus endoscopic sclerotherapy for long-term treatment of variceal bleeding: Early results of a randomized trial. Ann Surg 206:261–271, 1987.

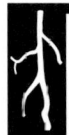

CHAPTER 115

Initial Management of Upper Gastrointestinal Hemorrhage in Patients with Portal Hypertension

Thomas O. G. Kovacs, M.D., and Dennis M. Jensen, M.D.

Severe upper gastrointestinal (GI) bleeding is a common and serious medical-surgical problem that, in most cases, requires the patient to be hospitalized for proper treatment. It has been estimated that more than 350,000 patients are admitted annually with acute upper GI bleeding in the United States.[1] It is a major cause of morbidity and mortal-ity, especially in elderly patients with serious underlying medical conditions. Mortality for patients with upper GI hemorrhage in the United States has remained at about 10% during the past 40 years, despite marked improvements in intensive care support, blood product replacement, endoscopy, and surgical techniques. These advances have been offset by the increasing proportion of these patients who are elderly or who have severe underlying medical illness.[1, 2]

Patients with underlying portal hypertension are just such a group. Variceal hemorrhage is the most lethal complication of portal hypertension, and bleeding from esophagogastric varices accounts for a third of all deaths of patients with cirrhosis and portal hypertension.[3] Between 40% and 70% of cirrhotic patients manifest esophageal varices during their lifetime, and 30% to 40% of them have hemorrhage. The risk of bleeding from esophagogastric varices is about 25% to 35%, regardless of the cause of cirrhosis, and most first bleeding episodes occur within the first year after diagnosis.[4] Depending on the clinical status of the patient, the risk of death with each episode of variceal hemorrhage is 30% to 50%.[5] For patients who survive the initial GI bleeding episode, the risk of recurrent hemorrhage is about 70%, and most recurrences occur within the next 6 months. Since hemorrhage associated with portal hypertension frequently recurs and frequently is fatal, prompt and effective management of variceal hemorrhage is essential.

DIAGNOSIS

Initial Approach to the Patient

The initial assessment of the patient with upper GI bleeding should include simultaneous evaluation of severity of the hemorrhage, resuscitation, a brief history and physical examination, and consideration of possible interventions. The main objective of the initial clinical assessment is to determine the patient's hemodynamic state. Rapid evaluation of the patient's circulatory status takes priority over all other measures, including those designed to locate the site of the bleeding. If the patient is not hypotensive, vital signs should be measured in both recumbent and upright positions. A brief account of presenting complaints, recent medications (including anticoagulants, nonsteroidal anti-inflammatory drugs [NSAIDs], and beta-blockers), and past history should be obtained. A brief physical examination should be done to evaluate the patient's mental status, skin, mucous membranes, neck veins, chest, and abdomen. Esophagogastric varices may be suggested by the finding of ascites or splenomegaly or other stigmata of chronic liver disease. In patients with marked abdominal pain or peritoneal signs, abdominal films should be ordered to exclude a perforated viscus. Blood should be sent for typing and cross-match for transfusion of red blood cells (RBC), fresh frozen plasma (FFP) and/or platelets, hemoglobin and hematocrit, prothrombin time, partial thromboplastin time, platelets, electrolytes, creatinine, blood urea nitrogen, and liver function tests. An electrocardiogram is indicated for patients with shock or chest pain or a history of cardiac disease and for elderly persons.

Patients with acute upper GI bleeding should be admitted to an intensive care unit, where the major cause of mortality—further bleeding—and underlying medical problems can best be managed.[6] It is essential that appropriate consultation be obtained soon after the patient presents. A gastroenterologist and a surgeon should be notified

of the patient's admission and should participate actively in management and therapeutic decisions. A consistent, planned approach to the diagnosis and treatment of upper GI bleeding, and close communication among consultants and the primary care physician, optimize patient management and improve outcomes.[1, 2]

Assessment of Severity of Upper Gastrointestinal Tract Bleeding

Assessment of the amount of blood loss includes review of the clinical presentation, the hemodynamic status, and the hemoglobin or hematocrit level. Upper GI bleeding may present with hematemesis, melena, or hematochezia. Occasionally, syncope or angina is the only symptom (i.e., without overt signs of GI blood loss). In general, hematemesis or hematochezia suggests serious upper GI bleeding.

The most accurate information on the severity of upper GI bleeding comes from assessment of the hemodynamic status. Blood pressure and heart rate reflect the amount of blood lost and the body's compensation for that loss. Orthostatic hypotension with a postural decrease of 10 mmHg in the systolic blood pressure or an increase in the pulse of 20 beats/minute indicates about 20% blood loss acutely. Shock is defined as a "supine" systolic blood pressure below 90 to 100 mmHg in a previously normotensive patient and suggests rapid loss of about 40% of blood volume. Some elderly or diabetic patients with poor vascular compensatory mechanisms may have orthostatic hypotension without volume loss, whereas some young patients may lose much blood without exhibiting orthostatic hypotension because of better cardiovascular compensation.

With acute hemorrhage both hemoglobin and hematocrit values may initially be falsely "normal." Since the acute hemorrhage results in loss of both plasma and RBCs, hemoglobin and hematocrit decrease only after extravascular fluid enters the circulation or fluid is given intravenously. Therefore, after acute upper GI hemorrhage, management decisions about blood transfusions are directed mainly by the physical examination findings and patient presentation, rather than initial hemoglobin or hematocrit values.

Resuscitation of the Patient

Resuscitation of the bleeding patient should start during the initial assessment. The critical elements include (1) correctly evaluating the amount of blood loss, (2) obtaining adequate intravenous (IV) access, and (3) aggressively administering fluids and blood products when necessary. IV access devices should include at least one 16-gauge catheter in patients with acute GI bleeding. If the patient is hypotensive, at least two 16-gauge or larger IV lines are recommended so that adequate volumes of fluid can be given quickly. For severe hypotension, central venous access for both fluid administration and monitoring purposes is recommended. Flow rates through catheters depend on their diameter and how short they are, not their location. Therefore, a 16-gauge peripheral IV line can administer more volume per unit of time than an 18-gauge central venous catheter does.

The initial aim of therapy is to restore blood volume through fluid replacement so that tissue perfusion and oxygen delivery are not further compromised. Improving perfusion pressure alone frequently restores oxygen delivery, despite the presence of anemia, since there is considerable reserve in the oxygen delivery system. Normal saline solution, administered rapidly and in appropriate volumes, usually corrects volume deficits associated with mild to moderate shock. An adequate volume of saline may be all that is necessary to avoid blood transfusion, even after loss of as much as 1 L of blood.

To hypotensive patients, normal saline should be given as rapidly as possible until systolic pressure is greater than 100 mmHg. If hypotension persists after 2 L of saline has been given, blood transfusions should be started. For these patients with severe upper GI bleeding, continuous blood pressure monitoring with an arterial line or frequent evaluation with an automated blood pressure cuff is recommended.

For patients with ongoing hematemesis or altered mental status, endotracheal intubation should be seriously considered to prevent aspiration and to prepare for emergency endoscopy. Aspiration is a critical cause of endoscopy-associated hypoxia and an important cause of bleeding-related morbidity and mortality. For example, in a nonrandomized study of patients with acute upper GI bleeding, respiratory complications were associated with 22% of bleeding episodes.[7] Some of the risk factors for respiratory complications were advanced liver disease, esophageal bleeding, and age older than 70 years. Mortality was much higher in patients who had respiratory complications (70%) than in those who did not (4%).

Blood Transfusion

The aim of blood product transfusions is to increase RBC mass, which improves tissue oxygenation, and to correct associated coagulopathy. The use of transfused blood products should be individualized. Rigid guidelines such as maintenance of the hematocrit at 30% at all times should be avoided, lest they encourage unnecessary use of blood products with their associated morbidity. In general, patients with underlying portal hypertension should be slightly undertransfused, to maintain a hematocrit value in "the low 30s," since overaggressive restoration of blood volume could enlarge the esophagogastric varices and precipitate more bleeding.

Patients with associated chronic liver disease may have coagulopathies (with prolonged prothrombin time or partial thromboplastin time) secondary to poor hepatic synthetic function as well as thrombocytopenia associated with hypersplenism. These hematologic problems should be corrected with FFP or platelet transfusion, as necessary. For patients whose prolonged prothrombin time or partial thromboplastin time is the result of anticoagulation with warfarin, for example, 2 to 4 units of FFP may be adequate. In contrast, cirrhotic patients with impaired hepatic synthesis of clotting factors may require several more units. A platelet count less than 50,000 to 60,000 or an abnormal bleeding time should be documented before platelets are transfused. Correction of associated coagulopathies may, on its own, reduce or stop portal hypertensive bleeding. These measures may have only minimal effect if there is ongoing concurrent disseminated intravascular coagulation.

Nasogastric Lavage

Gastric lavage is usually reserved for removing blood from the stomach in preparation for endoscopy. Although some endoscopists avoid routine nasogastric lavage, since it may delay endoscopy and create artifacts that are difficult to distinguish from vascular malformations or other lesions, selective gastric lavage still serves a useful function. It usually allows better visualization during upper endoscopy. It also provides a crude estimate of bleeding activity. In cirrhotic patients, removing the blood from the stomach may also reduce the risk of hepatic encephalopathy. Nasogastric lavage, however, has no therapeutic value in controlling hemorrhage, even when vasoconstricting agents are added to the gastric perfusate or instilled directly into the stomach.

If lavage is performed, a large oral gastric lavage tube (Ewald) should be used. Room-temperature tap water should be instilled, since it has been found to have no adverse effects and is cheaper than saline solution. Another technique for clearing stomach contents is giving an intravenous prokinetic agent, such as metoclopramide or erythromycin.

Endoscopy and Upper Gastrointestinal Tract Bleeding

After the patient has been stabilized, the next step is determining the specific diagnosis. Since as many as 50% of patients with underlying portal hypertension have a nonvariceal source of bleeding, diagnostic endoscopy should be performed to determine the specific cause of the GI hemorrhage. Upper GI endoscopy is the procedure of choice for cirrhotic patients with upper GI hemorrhage for several reasons[1, 2]:

1. Its diagnostic capability in determining the cause of bleeding, whether esophageal or gastric varices, portal hypertensive gastropathy, or another source, such as peptic ulcer disease or Mallory-Weiss tear.
2. Its prognostic capability, since it not only shows lesions that have bled actively by stigmata such as clot or "white nipple sign" but also identifies esophageal or gastric varices which are likely to bleed.
3. It affords endoscopic therapeutic intervention.

Barium studies should not be attempted in patients with GI bleeding for several reasons:

1. They interfere with other possible diagnostic and therapeutic modalities, such as endoscopy and angiography.
2. They lack sensitivity in identifying superficial mucosal bleeding sites.
3. They may fail to show the site of hemorrhage in patients with more than one potential bleeding lesion.

Endoscopy should be performed only after adequate resuscitation. In a patient with upper GI bleeding, emergency endoscopy requires a trained assistant, careful airway protection, and hemodynamic monitoring.

Contraindications to emergency endoscopy include GI tract perforation, severe hemodynamic instability, lack of expertise, an uncooperative patient, or lack of informed consent. Severe, irreversible coagulopathy is a relative contraindication. For upper GI bleeding, endoscopy is usually done within 12 hours after admission once hemodynamic stability is restored. Endoscopy is performed sooner for patients with chronic liver disease who continue to bleed despite appropriate resuscitative measures or rebleed while in the hospital.

Early endoscopy in cirrhotic patients with upper GI hemorrhage may show either variceal or nonvariceal sources of bleeding. Varices, collateral venous channels associated with portal hypertension, are most commonly seen in the distal esophagus and proximal stomach, but they may occur throughout the GI tract, including the small intestine, colon, and rectum, and at sites of earlier surgery (ectopic varices). Portal hypertensive mucosal changes may also be seen in the stomach (gastropathy), small intestine (enteropathy), or colon (colopathy).

Possible nonvariceal causes of upper GI bleeding in cirrhotic patients include peptic ulcer disease, stress-related mucosal disease, Mallory-Weiss tears, portal hypertensive gastropathy, upper GI tumor, and hemobilia.[8-10] In a recent UCLA Center for Ulcer Research and Education (CURE) prospective study evaluating the causes of severe upper GI hemorrhage in 103 patients with end-stage liver disease, 31% of the patients had nonvariceal causes (Table 115-1).[11]

The diagnosis of esophagogastric varices is best made by endoscopy. Several different grading systems have been suggested, but inter-observer agreement is usually limited to the presence of varices and their size (small, medium, large).[12] Endoscopic risk factors for bleeding esophageal varices include the size of the varices and endoscopic "red color" signs (cherry-red spots, red wale markings, hematocystic spots). Several studies have suggested a correlation between variceal size and the potential for bleeding. Large varices are more likely to bleed than small ones[13]; however, variceal size may change with blood volume. Changes to higher or lower grades, and even disappearance of varices after acute bleeding, have been described. Red color signs have also been used to predict bleeding in varices that have never bled. For example, a retrospective study showed that variceal bleeding occurred in about 60% of cirrhotic patients with red color signs, in contrast to 9% of those without red color signs.[4]

A prospective study has shown that large varices, red color signs, and the degree of hepatic disease are independent risk factors for variceal hemorrhage.[4] Although endoscopic classifications have been successful in identifying subgroups of cirrhotic patients at high risk for variceal hemorrhage, they do not identify the many patients who have variceal bleeding and are at the lower end of their risk classes.

THERAPY

The treatment of bleeding esophageal varices includes (1) initial management of the acute hemorrhage, (2) elective therapy to reduce the risk of recurrent bleeding, and (3) strategies to prevent the initial bleeding episode. The therapies may be endoscopic or non-endoscopic. This chapter focuses principally on endoscopic methods of treating bleeding esophagogastric varices.

Pharmacologic Therapy

Acute Management

Pharmacologic therapy is an important noninvasive treatment that can be administered before endoscopic therapy. The goal of any emergency drug therapy for acute variceal bleeding is to reduce portal pressure and thereby reduce bleeding from the esophageal and gastric varices.[14, 15] The initial enthusiasm for pharmacologic therapy with vasopressin was limited by its side effect profile. Newer agents, such as somatostatin, octreotide, and terlipressin, have been developed, and clinical trials have evaluated them. Vasopressin, somatostatin, octreotide, and terlipressin are all vasoconstrictors that decrease splanchnic arterial blood flow and subsequently reduce portal venous blood flow and pressure. Vasodilators act mainly by decreasing intrahepatic vascular resistance or by dilating the portal collateral circulation. Vasodilators may also produce reflex splanchnic vasoconstriction and decrease blood flow.

Vasopressin

Despite long-standing clinical use, vasopressin's role in the treatment of acute variceal bleeding is still controversial. Vasopressin is a synthetic peptide of nine amino acids that induces smooth muscle contraction and splanchnic vasoconstriction. It has a very short half-life (10 to 20 minutes) and must be given by continuous IV infusion. Randomized controlled trials have shown that vasopressin controlled acute variceal hemorrhage in about 50% of patients, as compared with 18% for placebo.[16-20] Rebleeding occurred in about 45%. Vasopressin treatment was not associated with a survival advantage, and it results in complications. It may cause systemic vasoconstriction producing bradycardia, hypertension, myocardial and peripheral ischemia, hyponatremia, and fluid retention.[14, 15]

To minimize side effects, selective vasopressin infusion into the superior mesenteric artery has been attempted. This technique showed bleeding control and side effects similar to those of peripheral administration.[20]

Vasopressin plus Nitroglycerin

Concomitant use of a vasodilator, such as nitroglycerin, reduces the vasoconstrictive complications of vasopressin.

TABLE 115–1. ENDOSCOPIC FINDINGS IN 103 CIRRHOTIC PATIENTS WITH SEVERE UPPER GASTROINTESTINAL HEMORRHAGE

FINDING	PATIENTS (NO.)
Esophageal varices	53
Gastric varices	18
Esophagitis	8
Mallory-Weiss tear	4
Gastroduodenal erosions	2
Gastric ulcer	7
Duodenal ulcer	5
Other lesions	6

Modified from Jensen DM, Kovacs TOG, Jutabha R, et al: Prospective study of the causes and outcomes of severe UGI hemorrhage in cirrhotics (Abstract). Gastrointest Endosc 49:AB167, 1997.

Three controlled trials showed that vasopressin plus nitroglycerin (by IV infusion or the sublingual route) decreased the systemic complications of vasopressin and increased control of acute bleeding.[21–23] This combination treatment is inconvenient, however, and in most centers has been supplanted by the use of octreotide.

Somatostatin and Octreotide

Somatostatin is a naturally occurring 14–amino acid peptide that has a very short half-life (2 to 3 minutes). Octreotide is a synthetic octopeptide analogue of somatostatin with a long half-life (up to 100 minutes). Octreotide can be administered as an IV bolus injection, IV infusion, or subcutaneous injection.[14, 15]

Randomized controlled trials have shown somatostatin to be equal to[24] or superior to control therapies for acute variceal hemorrhage, including vasopressin,[25] glypressin,[26] balloon tamponade,[27, 28] and sclerotherapy.[29–31] Meta-analysis did not show any survival advantage.[32] Somatostatin consistently had fewer side effects than vasopressin.[14, 15, 33]

Two reports showed that octreotide's efficacy was similar to that of vasopressin[34] or balloon tamponade[35] and that octreotide produced fewer side effects. For these reasons, octreotide has become the drug of choice for early prehospital and emergency management of variceal hemorrhage.[14, 15] In our own hospital, where we see many patients with end-stage liver disease, patients with upper GI hemorrhage are most often given an octreotide bolus (50 μg) and an octreotide infusion (50 μg/hour) during resuscitation and before emergency endoscopy.

Octreotide plus endoscopic therapy has also been evaluated for prevention of early rebleeding of esophageal varices. Three randomized controlled trials compared octreotide plus sclerotherapy to sclerotherapy alone. Two of them showed no benefit,[36, 37] whereas one reported significant reduction of variceal rebleeding with combination therapy.[38] In another trial, octreotide after endoscopic ligation reduced recurrent bleeding and the need for balloon tamponade when compared with ligation alone.[39]

Terlipressin

Terlipressin is a synthetic analogue of vasopressin that is converted to its active form by removing three glycine residues. This prolongs terlipressin's action to 3 to 4 hours, which allows bolus IV injection.[14, 15] In trials comparing terlipressin and vasopressin, the delayed release produced lower blood levels and, subsequently, diminished vasoconstriction and cardiotoxicity. Results to date suggest that terlipressin has fewer side effects than vasopressin and may be comparable to somatostatin and octreotide.[14, 15] Terlipressin is not yet available in the United States.

Miscellaneous Medications

Both metoclopramide and domperidone have been reported to reduce azygos blood flow and distal esophageal submucosal venous plexus blood flow. Small controlled studies suggest a role for metoclopramide in acute variceal hemorrhage.

Chronic Pharmacologic Management

Pharmacologic therapy has also been effective in preventing recurrent variceal bleeding. In comparison to placebo, nonselective beta-adrenergic blockers (propranolol, nadolol) significantly reduced rebleeding.[32, 40] This significant reduction in rebleeding risk was not, however, associated with significant mortality reduction.[32, 40] Despite the potential utility, many cirrhotic patients are unable to take beta-blockers owing to adverse side effects or relative contraindications.

Balloon Tamponade Tubes

Tamponade tubes aim to reduce esophagogastric blood flow by compressing esophageal or upper gastric varices with air-inflated balloons. Balloon tamponade can be used alone or in combination with other therapies. Several tubes are available. The Sengstaken-Blakemore (SB) tube has three lumina, one for aspirating gastric contents and one each for inflating the esophageal and gastric balloons. The Minnesota tube is a four-lumen tube similar to the SB but with an additional aspiration port above the esophageal balloon. Major complications occurred in 14% and lethal complications occurred in 3% of patients using tamponade tubes in 10 published series.[41]

Balloon tamponade can effectively control active bleeding. Alone, it controls variceal hemorrhage in 42% to 94% of patients; however, control is often only temporary, with rebleeding frequency and mortality both about 50%.[41] The high rebleeding rates imply that balloon tamponade should be used only as a temporary measure during resuscitation until more definitive maneuvers may be initiated. A comparison of two different tubes suggested that the SB tube was superior for esophageal varices and that the Linton tube was more effective for gastric varices.

A prospective randomized trial compared esophageal tamponade with the SB tube to esophageal sclerotherapy in the treatment of variceal hemorrhage. The SB tube was significantly less effective than sclerotherapy in producing definitive control of bleeding (52% versus 90%) and in reducing mortality (27% versus 10%).[42] In most centers, including ours, octreotide and emergency endoscopy with variceal hemostasis, either alone or in combination, have replaced balloon tamponade.

Endoscopic Hemostasis
Injection Sclerotherapy of Esophageal Varices

Variceal sclerotherapy was initially described in 1939, but it was not until 1973 that it became widely used for hemostasis of esophageal varices. Randomized controlled trials have shown that sclerotherapy is one of the most effective treatments for control of acute variceal hemorrhage and prevention of rebleeding. Injection sclerotherapy was superior to vasopressin and balloon tamponade, with initial success rates ranging from 60% to 90% (Tables 115–2 and 115–3).[32] In Burroughs' study of emergency sclerotherapy, 62% of patients were free of bleeding for 5 days after a single sclerotherapy session and 78% were without bleeding after two sessions.[43]

One report of patients with active variceal hemorrhage

TABLE 115-2. COMPARISON OF PHARMACOLOGIC HEMOSTASIS WITH SCLEROTHERAPY

STUDY	NO. OF PATIENTS	HEMOSTASIS OF VARICEAL BLEEDING (%)				
		Vasopressin	Somatostatin	Octreotide	Sclerotherapy	p Value
Westaby, 1989	64	65			88	<.05
Shields, 1992	80		97		98	N/S
Sung, 1993	100			84	90	N/S
Planas, 1994	70		80		83	N/S
Baxter, 1994	80		77		83	N/S
Jenkins, 1997	50			85	82	N/S

N/S = not significant.

showed that in comparison with sham treatment, sclerotherapy stopped active bleeding and decreased rebleeding, transfusion requirements, shunt surgery rate, and deaths.[44] Two other randomized studies using polidocanol injections failed to demonstrate a statistically significant advantage for acute sclerotherapy, either in controlling the initial variceal bleeding or in reducing mortality. In one of the reports, however, varices were not eliminated in seven of 41 patients.[45] For sclerotherapy to be effective in preventing early rebleeding, all the variceal columns must be obliterated with aggressive initial injections and follow-up treatment.

Other studies of acute bleeding comparing sclerotherapy to somatostatin[29, 30] or octreotide[31] found similar initial efficacy (see Table 115-2) but higher complication rates in endoscopically treated patients. Sclerotherapy complications include esophageal ulceration, stricture formation, bleeding, perforation, mediastinitis, pleural effusion, and bacteremia. Strictures, which may be associated with impaired esophageal motility, are usually managed by esophageal dilation. Complications occur in 10% to 30% of patients treated with sclerotherapy, esophageal ulcers and strictures being the most frequent ones.

Sclerotherapy has also been effective in preventing recurrent variceal hemorrhage.[46-53] Some randomized, controlled trials comparing sclerotherapy with medical control groups demonstrated that both rebleeding and mortality were decreased in sclerotherapy-treated patients. Other trials, however, reported that sclerotherapy reduced the rate of rebleeding from varices, transfusion requirements, and the need for shunt surgery without improving survival. Overall, results of these long-term trials suggest a lower recurrent bleeding rate with sclerotherapy and, possibly, prolonged survival.[32]

Sclerotherapy Versus Beta-Blockade

Several studies have compared sclerotherapy with propranolol for prevention of recurrent variceal bleeding.[55-60] For prevention of recurrent variceal hemorrhage, sclerotherapy

was superior in three trials,[55, 56, 60] similar in three,[54, 58, 59] and inferior to propranolol in one.[57] Sclerotherapy provided a survival advantage in only one study, although meta-analysis did not show a survival benefit for either treatment.[32]

Combination Sclerotherapy and Pharmacologic Therapy

The combination of sclerotherapy and nonselective beta-blockers theoretically would have the advantages of combining local variceal obliteration with agents that reduce portal pressure, thereby decreasing recurrent variceal hemorrhage. Several trials have compared sclerotherapy plus propranolol to sclerotherapy alone for preventing recurrent variceal hemorrhage. Four studies found similar efficacy,[61-64] and three showed combination therapy to be superior to sclerotherapy alone.[65-67] Neither treatment provided a survival advantage. Combination sclerotherapy has also been compared with propranolol alone. One trial did show a significant reduction in recurrent variceal hemorrhage associated with combination treatment.[64] Another randomized controlled trial found combination pharmacologic therapy with nadolol and isosorbide-5-mononitrate to be superior to sclerotherapy for preventing recurrent variceal bleeding.[68]

Sclerotherapy and Shunt Therapy

Sclerotherapy has been compared to shunt surgery in patients whose acute bleeding was controlled. A trial from Emory University compared distal splenorenal shunt to sclerotherapy and reported a significantly higher rate of rebleeding in the sclerotherapy group (53%) than in the surgical group (3%). Only 31% of sclerotherapy patients, however, were resistant to repeat sclerotherapy and required shunt surgery. Despite the greater frequency of rebleeding, significantly better 2-year survival was observed in the 31% of patients undergoing sclerotherapy and "res-

TABLE 115-3. COMPARISON OF BALLOON TAMPONADE WITH SCLEROTHERAPY

STUDY	NO. OF PATIENTS	HEMOSTASIS OF VARICEAL BLEEDING (%)		p Value
		Tamponade	Sclerotherapy	
Barsoum, 1982	100	42	74	<.05
Paquet, 1985	43	52	90	<.01
Moreto, 1988	43	45	83	<.05

cue" shunt than in the distal splenorenal shunt group (84% versus 59%).[69]

A randomized, comparative trial from Italy of sclerotherapy and distal splenorenal shunt in Child class A and B patients also showed significantly lower rates of rebleeding after surgical therapy than after sclerotherapy (14% versus 38%). Two-year survival rates were similar, but hepatic encephalopathy was significantly more frequent after shunting (24%) than after sclerotherapy (8%).[70]

The majority of the treatment failures and deaths in these studies occurred in Child class C patients. Cello and colleagues prospectively randomized Child class C patients with variceal hemorrhage who required at least 6 units of blood to treatment with acute-phase and long-term sclerotherapy or to urgent portacaval shunting (within 6 hours of enrollment).[71, 72] They observed that sclerotherapy treatment significantly reduced the initial hospital length of stay and the blood transfusion requirements.[71] Subsequently, however, rates of rebleeding, transfusion requirements, and rehospitalizations were significantly less in the shunted group.[72] Only 50% of the sclerotherapy group and 44% of the shunted group survived their initial hospitalization.[71] Over long-term follow-up neither treatment was found to afford any survival or economic advantage.[72]

In another high-risk group, the results of sclerotherapy were similar to those of esophageal staple transection in terms of permanent hemostasis and long-term survival.[43] Sclerotherapy caused fewer complications, a finding that led the authors to recommend it as the treatment of choice for patients at high risk.

These controlled trials suggest that sclerotherapy and shunt surgery are associated with similar survival rates. However, hepatic encephalopathy occurs less frequently, liver function is less compromised, and sclerotherapy is faster and easier to perform than shunt surgery. Therefore, it seems reasonable to treat patients with esophageal variceal hemorrhage first with sclerotherapy, and then to intervene with shunt surgery (or transjugular intrahepatic portosystemic shunt [TIPS]) if an aggressive sclerotherapy program fails.

Sclerotherapy Technique for Esophageal Varices

These studies also emphasize the importance of obliterating varices, since endoscopic therapy is effective in reducing rebleeding only when all varices are eradicated. The best method of achieving this is controversial, and some of the different outcomes of the controlled trials are clearly due to variability in techniques, sclerotherapy agents, treatment intervals, number of injections, use of tamponade or overtubes, and injection sites.

Sclerotherapy injections may be aimed directly into the varix (intravariceal) or into the submucosa adjacent to the varix (paravariceal). Intravariceal injections are thought to obliterate the lumen directly, paravariceal ones to induce inflammation that eventually produces a fibrotic covering over the varix. Intravariceal injections have been found to be significantly more effective than paravariceal injections in achieving primary hemostasis, in reducing the time to variceal obliteration, and in decreasing rebleeding. Varices were more likely to recur after the intravariceal technique, but mortality rates were similar. Except for a higher incidence of paravariceal injection–associated retrosternal pain, there was no difference in complications.

Although these results are impressive and confirm those of earlier studies, intravariceal injections may not always go where they are aimed. When a radiopaque dye was used as a marker, 44% of intended intravariceal injections were found to be paravariceal. In another study, one in five injections into a large varix and one in three into a small varix were paravariceal. Despite these limitations, it appears that intravariceal injections are preferable to paravariceal ones, especially for actively bleeding varices. The injections should be made in the distal 5 to 6 cm of the esophagus, where the majority of esophageal varices bleed.

When an actively bleeding varix is seen, injections are placed first about 1 cm distal to the site of active bleeding and then about 1 cm proximal (Table 115–4). The same varix is then injected 2 to 3 cm and about 5 cm proximal to the gastroesophageal junction (GEJ) (Fig. 115–1). Other varices are then injected in similar fashion, with the aim of injecting all those in the distal 5 cm of the esophagus during the initial treatment session in the hope of sclerosing and obliterating them. Gastric varices situated within a hiatal hernia are treated likewise and respond as esophageal varices do.

There is no major advantage to using a flexible sheath over the endoscope. Weekly injections are preferable to longer intervals. Animal studies have shown that 1.5% tetradecyl sulfate and 5% sodium morrhuate (both commercially available in the United States) are effective and less injurious than 95% ethanol. A combination of equal proportions of tetradecyl sulfate, ethanol, and normal saline solution (TES) has been shown to provide the best ratio of efficacy to safety in our animal studies. Polidocanol, which is used for paravariceal injections mainly in Europe, is not currently available in the United States.

The principal complications of sclerotherapy were recently reviewed. The most common ones are esophageal ulceration and stricture formation. Fortunately, perforation and mediastinitis are rare complications. Ulceration occurs in 20% to 75% of patients, depending on the type and volume of sclerosant, the site of delivery (intravariceal or paravariceal), and the proportion of Child class C patients in the study. Esophageal strictures develop in 5% to 10% of patients, usually as a late complication of multiple injection sessions, and usually they are amenable to esophageal dilation. Perforation occurs in 1% to 4% of patients. Diagnosis is often delayed from 2 to 14 days after injection and is more frequent in Child class C patients. Perforation caused by chemical necrosis of the esophageal wall represents a serious complication. Transient fever and chest pain may also occur in the absence of perforation.

Sclerotherapy-related bacteremia has been related to sclerotherapy injector needle length. Injector needles 6 to 8 mm long had a 39% incidence of bacteremia, as compared with 11% for 3- or 4-mm needles.

Our sclerotherapy techniques for esophageal and gastric varices are summarized in Table 115–4. To obliterate the varices, it is necessary to inject each variceal column in the distal 5 to 6 cm of the esophagus. In the past, we used a free-hand method for injecting the varix with a solution containing TES. This combination produced excellent hemostasis rates (75%) and few side effects (ulcer rate <10%)

TABLE 115–4. ENDOSCOPIC INJECTION SCLEROTHERAPY TECHNIQUE FOR BLEEDING ESOPHAGEAL AND GASTRIC VARICES

	ESOPHAGEAL VARICES	GASTRIC VARICES
Needle gauge	25	25
Needle length (mm)	5	5
Sclerosant		
Agent	TES	TEE
Injection dose (ml)	2	2–4
Maximum volume (ml)	<50*	<30†
Injection site		
Initial treatment	Bleeding focus	Bleeding focus
Concomitant treatment	Each esophageal varix at the GEJ, then 2.5 and 5 cm above the GEJ	Two adjacent gastric varices
Follow-up treatment	Residual esophageal varix in the distal 5 cm	Residual gastric varix at previous treatment site
Adjuvant therapy	PPI twice daily	PPI twice daily
Treatment intervals until obliteration	One week after initial treatment, then every 2–3 wk	One week after initial treatment, then every 2–3 wk

*Volume to inject all distal esophageal varices at the GEJ and 2.5 cm and 5 cm above the GEJ during first sclerotherapy session.
†Total volume to control the active bleeding of one gastric varix and to inject the two adjacent gastric varices.
TES = equal-volume mixture of 3% tetradecyl sulfate, 98% ethanol, 0.9 saline; TEE = mixture of 9.5 ml of TES and 0.5 ml of 1:1,000 epinephrine (final concentration 1% tetradecyl sulfate, 33% ethanol, 0.3 normal saline, and 1:20,000 epinephrine); GEJ = gastroesophageal junction; PPI = proton pump inhibitor (omeprazole, lansoprazole).

in a canine model, and these results were similar to those for cirrhotic humans with bleeding esophageal varices. We currently use a sclerosant solution of 3.4% ethanolamine and 33% ethyl alcohol (⅔ to ⅓), since tetradecyl sulfate is no longer commercially available in the United States. In the treatment of several hundred high-risk patients, these techniques produced 100% control of acute hemorrhage from bleeding esophageal varices and only a 7% stricture rate following emergency sclerotherapy.

Multiple studies have confirmed the efficacy and safety of sclerotherapy both for treating acute esophageal variceal hemorrhages and preventing rebleeding. Sclerotherapy is widely available, simple and quick to perform, inexpensive, and feasible for both emergency and elective therapy.[73, 74] It may be used in combination with other treatments. The potential complications are relatively mild, infrequent, and, when they occur, readily treatable.[73, 74]

Sclerotherapy of Gastric Varices

Achieving endoscopic hemostasis of bleeding gastric varices is a greater challenge than controlling bleeding from esoph-

ageal varices, since the source of bleeding may be more difficult to identify and hemorrhage is often torrential.[75] Gastric varices are found in 6% to 78% of patients with portal hypertension and are five times more common in patients with esophageal varices that have bled.[76] Gastric varices account for 20% to 30% of variceal bleeding in most large endoscopic series, including our own prospective studies.[76] They occur most often in the cardia or fundus but may involve any part of the stomach.[77, 78]

Kim and colleagues suggested that large size, presence of red spots, and poor hepatic functional reserve were predictors of gastric variceal hemorrhage.[79] Earlier reports of sclerotherapy for gastric varices documented either poor primary hemostasis or very high rebleeding rates (Table 115–5).[80–84] More recently, Chang and coworkers described 95% primary hemostasis and 3% rebleeding using a 50% glucose solution.[85] Our sclerotherapy technique for gastric varices is described in Table 115–4.

Endoscopic Variceal Ligation
General Results for Esophageal Varices

Endoscopic variceal ligation is the placement of rubber bands on varices with a special ligating device attached to the end of an endoscope. The technique, similar in principle to hemorrhoid banding, was developed by Steigmann as an endoscopic alternative to sclerotherapy. This method permits ligation of individual varices in the distal 5 cm of the esophagus. The banded varices thrombose and the bands fall off within 5 to 10 days and are passed spontaneously.

Although variceal ligation and sclerotherapy have been compared in several randomized controlled clinical trials, only a few of the studies specifically addressed control of acute variceal hemorrhage. In Steigmann's original controlled trial,[86] endoscopic ligation controlled active esophageal variceal bleeding in 86% of 13 patients, as compared with 77% of 14 patients treated with sclerotherapy. Subsequently, some studies found similar efficacy for ligation and sclerotherapy in acute variceal bleeding (range 89% to

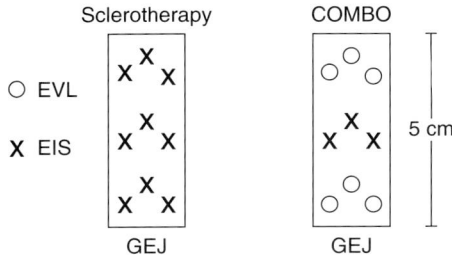

FIGURE 115–1. UCLA CURE Hemostasis Research Group technique of sclerotherapy (*left*) and combination therapy (*right*). After initial control of active bleeding is achieved with sclerotherapy, each esophageal varix is banded distally at the gastroesophageal junction and 5 cm proximally. Subsequently, sclerotherapy is done between the bands on each variceal column. EVL = endoscopic varix ligation; EIS = endoscopic injection sclerotherapy; GEJ = gastroesophageal junction.

TABLE 115–5. STUDIES OF SCLEROTHERAPY FOR ACUTE GASTRIC VARICEAL BLEEDING

	SARIN, 1988[80]	TRUDEAU, 1986[81]	BRETAGNE, 1986[82]	YASSIN, 1985[83]	GIMSON, 1991[84]
No. patients	8	9	10	35	41
Sclerosant	Alcohol	1.5% TDS	1.5% POLI	?	Ethanolamine
Hemostasis (%)	75	100	60	17	40
Rebleed (%)	25	89	50	87	68
Exsanguination (%)	25	55	32	23	24
Secondary gastric ulcer (%)	38	88	—	26	24

TDS = tetradecyl sulfate; POLI = polidocanol.

92%[87, 88]), whereas others reported 94% control of acute bleeding with sclerotherapy as compared with 80% with band ligation.[89] Complication rates were similar in one trial[87] but lower with ligation in four others.[86, 88–90]

In a randomized controlled trial comparing band ligation to sclerotherapy in cirrhotic patients with active variceal bleeding, sclerotherapy provided important benefits.[91] Rebleeding, TIPS, shunt surgery, and mortality rates were all lower in the sclerotherapy-treated group.[91] Treatment-related complications were similar in both groups.[91] These studies highlight the difficulty of performing band ligation for actively bleeding varices. The problems are that the endoscopic visualization is poor with the ligation device attached, suctioning of blood is inadequate because of partial blockage of the suction port with the ligation pull cord, and frequent flooding of the tip chamber with clots or blood renders banding of the bleeding point very difficult. Until the advent of the "multishot" band ligators, the technique of endoscopic banding was also relatively slow.

Several randomized controlled trials have compared variceal ligation with sclerotherapy for the prevention of recurrent variceal hemorrhage in patients without active bleeding.[86–90] A meta-analysis reported that band ligation reduced recurrent variceal bleeding, decreased deaths from bleeding, and diminished overall mortality when compared with sclerotherapy.[92] Some studies also reported that fewer variceal ligation sessions are necessary to obliterate varices, although treatment was skipped when ulcers or strictures were found after sclerotherapy. Ligation was reported to have a lower rate of serious complications than sclerotherapy. Since many of the comparative trials studied patients for less than 1 year, rebleeding following variceal ligation may be underestimated. Indeed, several authors have documented a higher esophageal variceal recurrence rate in patients who received band ligation than in those treated with sclerotherapy.[93] In a randomized controlled trial of cirrhotic patients without active variceal bleeding, sclerotherapy and band ligation provided similar benefits in terms of rebleeding, transfusion requirement, and survival.[94] Ligation required, on average, 3.3 sessions to obliterate the varices; sclerotherapy required 3.7 sessions.[94] Complications were arithmetically higher in the sclerotherapy-treated group.

Techniques of Rubber Band Ligation for Esophageal Varices

Initially, attempts are made to place a rubber band directly on the bleeding point to control hemorrhage. If control of active bleeding is not achieved by direct attack on the bleeding point, banding distal and adjacent to the bleeding point often results in control. Then, each variceal column is banded at the GEJ and again 4 to 5 cm above the GEJ.

Ligation is repeated weekly until the varices are obliterated or are too small to band. This usually requires three or four treatment sessions. Small varices often cannot be banded but enlarge with time and have the potential to bleed. This fact may account for the higher recurrence and bleeding rates reported for rubber band ligation in some long-term trials, as compared with endoscopic sclerotherapy or combination sclerotherapy and rubber band ligation.[93]

Techniques of Band Ligation for Gastric Varices

Band ligation has also been used to treat bleeding gastric varices.[94] Our approach includes first placing a band on the bleeding point of the gastric varix, followed by band placement 2 to 3 cm away on each side of the same varix. At least two bands are placed on each of two adjacent varices. Ligation is repeated weekly until the varices are obliterated.

Omeprazole, 20 mg twice daily, is also given to prevent ulceration. The authors have successfully treated actively bleeding gastric varices with this technique as well as those with platelet plugs or adherent clots. Some gastric varices are not amenable to this endoscopic band ligation as monotherapy, however, since they are too large and nodular or cannot be treated safely because they are in the gastric fundus. Significantly higher complication and rebleeding rates from banding of gastric varices (with active bleeding, platelet plug, or adherent clot), as compared with sclerotherapy, were reported in a randomized trial.[95] Therefore, we no longer use banding alone for gastric varices.

Recently, a modified gastric varix–ligating technique using a detachable loop device was described.[96] Although the preliminary results are encouraging, no comparative trials have been performed of this new technique for either esophageal or gastric varices.

Why Rubber Band Ligation Works

Whether in the esophagus or the stomach, rubber band ligation causes venous obstruction, mucosal inflammation, local necrosis, and scarring. The ulcers formed by ligating esophageal varices are smaller, shallower, and often less likely to bleed than those secondary to sclerotherapy. Possible complications of rubber band ligation include superficial ulceration of the esophagus, dysphagia, esophageal stricture, and sometimes transient chest pain secondary to esophageal spasm. Perforations associated with overtube use and single-shot band ligation have been reported. With large gastric varices, ulceration and fistulization into the varices have been reported.

In general, band ligation has been considered by some authors to be the endoscopic treatment of choice for esophageal variceal hemorrhage, based on lower rates of rebleeding, mortality, and complications, and the need for fewer treatment sessions. However, as with sclerotherapy, all esophageal varices must be treated before the risk of recurrent hemorrhage is reduced. Spurting varices, small varices, and varices in retroflexion are difficult to treat, and very large ones may not be amenable to banding.

Combination Sclerotherapy and Rubber Band Ligation

Sclerotherapy plus rubber band ligation for esophageal varices has been described and has potential advantages over either treatment alone, since it may accelerate variceal obliteration and limit complications (Table 115–6). Accelerating variceal obliteration would improve patient acceptance and reduce costs. Combination therapy has been provided during a single endoscopic session or sequentially, with one endoscopic technique done initially, followed by a different one later.

In a randomized trial in cirrhotic patients with documented esophageal variceal hemorrhage, 28 patients received sclerotherapy alone and 30 received combination therapy.[97] Combination treatment consisted of (1) initially controlling active bleeding with sclerotherapy, (2) band ligation on each esophageal varix distally at the gastroesophageal junction and 5 cm proximal, and (3) sclerotherapy applied between the bands on each variceal column (see Fig. 115–1). Combination therapy required significantly fewer sessions than sclerotherapy (median, three versus five) to obliterate esophageal varices. Furthermore, combination treatment required significantly smaller mean sclerosant volumes than sclerotherapy alone (10 ml versus 28 ml) for the first session. Complication rates were higher with sclerotherapy than with combination therapy (43% versus 20%). Similar rates of rebleeding, transfusion requirements, hospital stay, and survival were reported for both groups. Thus, in this trial combination therapy accel-

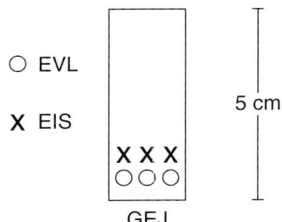

Esophageal varices

FIGURE 115–2. Combination therapy as described by Saeed and Laine. Bands are first placed distally on each variceal column at the level of the GEJ, and one injection is placed just above each band. EVL = endoscopic varix ligation; EIS = endoscopic injection sclerotherapy; GEJ = gastroesophageal junction.

erated esophageal variceal obliteration without increasing complications. Another report confirmed these results.[98]

However, two other randomized studies that compared combination sclerotherapy and band ligation to band ligation alone did not report any advantage for combination treatment in accelerating variceal obliteration or reducing rebleeding.[99, 100] The authors found that combined treatment prolonged therapy and produced more complications.[99, 100] The divergent results are probably related to different techniques of combination treatment or different comparison groups. The authors of each report described placing one band and one injection per variceal column during all sessions (Fig. 115–2). No attempt was made to place two bands on each column to block blood flow and then to inject between them.

ECONOMIC IMPACT OF VARICEAL HEMORRHAGE AND ENDOSCOPIC THERAPY

Since variceal hemorrhage is a common cause of upper GI bleeding and requires hospital admission (usually to an intensive care unit), multiple blood product transfusions, immediate and follow-up endoscopic therapy, and other possible interventions, management of these patients may consume substantial health care resources. The estimated direct and indirect medical costs of care for esophageal

TABLE 115–6. RANDOMIZED TRIALS OF COMBINATION THERAPY VERSUS MONOTHERAPY FOR ESOPHAGEAL VARICES

INVESTIGATOR	TREATMENTS	NO. OF PATIENTS	REBLEEDING RATE (%)	SESSIONS TO OBLITERATE	COMPLICATIONS (%)	DEATHS (%)
Jensen, 1996[97]	EVL + EIS	24	7 (29)	2*	6 (25)	7 (29)
	EIS	24	8 (33)	4	5 (21)	7 (29)
Koutsomanis, 1992[98]	EVL + EIS	9	N/R	1.2	0	0
	EIS	7	N/R	4.4	0	0
Laine, 1996[99]	EVL + EIS	21	6 (29)	4.9 + 0.6*	6 (29)	3 (14)
	EVL	20	6 (30)	2.7 + 0.4	2 (10)	3 (15)
Saeed, 1997[100]	EVL + EIS	22	8 (36)	4.1 + 0.6	23* (65) ulcer 7 (30) dysphagia	8 (36)
	EVL	25	6 (25)	3.3 + 0.4	5 (20) ulcer 0 (0) dysphagia	4 (16)

*$p \leq .05$.
EVL = endoscopic variceal ligation; EIS = endoscopic injection sclerotherapy; N/R = Not reported; however, authors stated that there were no significant differences in rebleeding between the two groups.

variceal hemorrhage are staggering. In 1985, direct costs of medical care for esophageal varices were estimated to be $78.2 million, including hospital charges, physicians' fees, and outpatient care. During that time, the diagnosis of esophageal variceal hemorrhage accounted for about 62,000 total hospital days in the United States and was the most expensive of all digestive diseases in terms of average daily cost of hospitalization ($1091 per day).[101] The indirect costs of esophageal varices were estimated to be $47.5 million.

From our group, Gralnek and coworkers reported the results of a cost analysis for acute hospital care of 39 patients with active esophagogastric varix bleeding in a randomized trial of emergency endoscopic sclerotherapy versus band ligation.[102] The mean total postrandomization direct costs were higher with band ligation ($13,390) than with sclerotherapy ($11,520). These higher costs were associated with longer stays in the intensive care unit, higher rates of transfusion, TIPS, variceal rebleeding, and complications.[102]

A similar cost analysis was reported for patients treated with either sclerotherapy or band ligation for prevention of recurrent variceal hemorrhage. We showed that mean total postrandomization direct costs were similar for the two groups: sclerotherapy $14,479 and band ligation $10,585.[103] Sclerotherapy-related stricture formation and the subsequent need for esophageal dilation contributed to the higher costs associated with sclerotherapy.[103] These studies suggest that sclerotherapy may be the better choice of endoscopic treatment for actively bleeding esophageal varices, whereas rubber band ligation is the better choice for nonbleeding varices.

ENDOSCOPIC POLYMER (GLUE) INJECTION

Endoscopic polymer injection has been used successfully to control bleeding esophageal, gastric, and duodenal varices.[104] Cyanoacrylate, which is not available in the United States, solidifies almost instantaneously on contact with proteinaceous or aqueous media. Anecdotal reports suggest that intravariceal injection of cyanoacrylate produces variceal hemostasis by mechanical plugging of the bleeding site. Both control of active bleeding and prevention of rebleeding from esophageal and gastric varices have been described.[105]

TREATMENTS FOR FAILURES OF THERAPY

Although both endoscopic and pharmacologic therapy decrease the rates of recurrent variceal hemorrhage, 30% to 40% of patients still have clinically significant rebleeding.[106] Other procedures available to these patients include angiographically (TIPS) or surgically created shunts and liver transplantation.[106] These interventions are discussed elsewhere.

SUMMARY

Improvements in pharmacologic and endoscopic therapy have greatly benefited patients with portal hypertension and upper GI hemorrhage. Beta-adrenergic blockers are effective in preventing recurrent variceal bleeding. The advent of endoscopic band ligation has provided another valuable therapeutic option. Sclerotherapy remains an important treatment alternative, especially in the setting of active bleeding and in cases of small varices that cannot be adequately treated with band ligation. Long-term prevention of variceal hemorrhage is possible only if obliteration is sustained. Regular endoscopic surveillance and retreatment are critical, since varices may recur regardless of which endoscopic method is used.

REFERENCES

1. Kovacs TOG, Jensen DM: Endoscopic control of gastroduodenal hemorrhage. Annu Rev Med 38:267–277, 1987.
2. Kovacs TOG, Jensen DM: Therapeutic endoscopy in upper gastrointestinal bleeding. In Taylor MB, Gollan JL, Steer ML, Wolfe MM (eds): Gastrointestinal Emergencies, 2nd ed. Baltimore, Williams & Wilkins, 1997, pp 181–198.
3. Garceau AJ, Chalmers TC, Boston Inter-Hospital Liver Group: The natural history of cirrhosis: I. Survival with esophageal varices. N Engl J Med 268:469–473, 1963.
4. The North Italian Endoscopic Club for the Study and Treatment of Esophageal Varices: Prediction of the first variceal hemorrhage in patients with cirrhosis of the liver and esophageal varices. A prospective multicenter study. N Engl J Med 319:983–989, 1988.
5. Graham D, Smith JL: The course of patients after variceal hemorrhage. Gastroenterology 80:800–809, 1981.
6. Lee H, Hawker FH, Selby W, et al: Intensive care treatment of patients with bleeding esophageal varices: Results, predictors of mortality, and predictors of the adult respiratory distress syndrome. Crit Care Med 20:1555–1563, 1992.
7. Liebler JM, Benner K, Putnam T, et al: Respiratory complications in critically ill medical patients with acute upper gastrointestinal bleeding. Crit Care Med 19:1152–1157, 1991.
8. Sutton R: Upper gastrointestinal bleeding in patients with esophageal varices: What is the most common source? Am J Med 83:273–275, 1987.
9. Tabibian N, Graham DY: Source of upper gastrointestinal bleeding in patients with esophageal varices seen at endoscopy. J Clin Gastroenterol 9:279–282, 1987.
10. Buset M, Des Marez B, Baise M, et al: Bleeding esophagogastric varices: An endoscopic study. Am J Gastroenterol 82:241–244, 1987.
11. Jensen DM, Kovacs TOG, Jutabha R, et al: Prospective study of the causes and outcomes of severe UGI hemorrhage in cirrhotics (Abstract). Gastrointest Endosc 49:AB167, 1999.
12. Cales P, Zabotto B, Meskens C, et al: Gastroesophageal endoscopic features in cirrhosis: Observer variability, interassociations, and relationships to hepatic dysfunction. Gastroenterology 98:156–162, 1990.
13. Lebrec D, DeFleury P, Rueff B, et al: Portal hypertension, size of esophageal varices, and risk of gastrointestinal bleeding in alcoholic cirrhosis. Gastroenterology 79:1139–1144, 1980.
14. Chan LY, Sung JJY: Review article: The role of pharmaco-therapy for acute variceal hemorrhage in the era of endoscopic hemostasis. Aliment Pharmacol Ther 11:45–50, 1997.
15. Bosch J: Medical treatment of portal hypertension. Digestion 59:547–555, 1998.
16. Conn HO, Ramsby GR, Starer EM, et al: Intra-arterial vasopressin in the treatment of upper gastrointestinal hemorrhage: A prospective controlled trial. Gastroenterology 68:211–221, 1975.
17. Mallory A, Schaeffer JU, Cohen JR, et al: Selective intra-arterial vasopressin infusion for upper gastrointestinal tract hemorrhage: A controlled trial. Arch Surg 115:30–32, 1980.

18. Fogel MR, Knauer CM, Andres LL, et al: Continuous intravenous vasopressin in active upper gastrointestinal bleeding: A placebo-controlled trial. Ann Intern Med 96:565–569, 1982.
19. Merigan TP, Plotkin GR, Davidson CS: Effect of intravenously administered posterior pituitary extract on hemorrhage from bleeding esophageal varices. N Engl J Med 266:134–135, 1962.
20. Chojkier M. Groszmann RJ, Atterburg CE, et al: A controlled comparison of continuous intra-arterial and intravenous infusions of vasopressin in hemorrhage from esophageal varices. Gastroenterology 77:540–546, 1979.
21. Gimson AE, Westaby D, Hegarty J, et al: A randomized trial of vasopressin and vasopressin plus nitroglycerin in the control of acute variceal hemorrhage. Hepatology 6:410–413, 1986.
22. Tsai YT, Lay CS, Lai KH, et al: Controlled trial of vasopressin plus nitroglycerin versus vasopressin alone in the treatment of bleeding esophageal varices. Hepatology 6:406–409, 1986.
23. Bosch J, Groszmann RJ, Garcia-Pagan JC, et al: Association of trans-dermal nitroglycerin to vasopressin infusion in the treatment of variceal hemorrhage: A placebo-controlled trial. Hepatology 10:962–968, 1989.
24. Kravetz D, Bosch J, Teres J, et al: Comparison of intravenous somato-statin and vasopressin infusions in treatment of acute variceal hemor-rhage. Hepatology 4:442–446, 1984.
25. Jenkins SA, Baxter JN, Corbett W, et al: A prospective randomized controlled clinical trial comparing somatostatin and vasopressin in controlling acute variceal hemorrhage. Br Med J 290:275–278, 1985.
26. Walker S, Kreichgauer HP, Bode JC: Terlipressin versus somatostatin in bleeding esophageal varices: A controlled, double blind study. Hepatology 15:1023–1030, 1992.
27. Jaramillo JL, de la Mata M, Mino G, et al: Somatostatin versus Sengstaken balloon tamponade for primary hemostasis of bleeding esophageal varices: A randomized pilot study. J Hepatol 12:100–105, 1991.
28. Avgerinos A, Klonis C, Rekoumis G, et al: A prospective randomized trial comparing somatostatin, balloon tamponade and the combination of both methods in the management of acute variceal hemor-rhage. J Hepatol 13:78–83, 1991.
29. Planas R, Quer JC, Boix J, et al: A prospective randomized trial comparing somatostatin and sclerotherapy in the treatment of acute variceal bleeding. Hepatology 20:370–375, 1994.
30. Shields R, Jenkins SA, Baxter JN, et al: A prospective randomized controlled trial comparing the efficacy of somatostatin with injection sclerotherapy in the control of bleeding esophageal varices. J Hepatol 15:128–137, 1992.
31. Sung JJY, Chung SCS, Lai CW, et al: Octreotide infusion or emer-gency sclerotherapy for variceal hemorrhage. Lancet 342:637–641, 1993.
32. D'Amico G, Pagliaro L, Bosch J: The treatment of portal hyperten-sion: A meta-analytic review. Hepatology 22:332–354, 1995.
33. Tarnasky PR, Kovacs TOG, Leung F, et al: Octreotide decreases gastric mucosal blood flow: A controlled assessment by endoscopic reflectance spectrophotometry. Gastrointest Endosc 40:56–61, 1994.
34. Hwang SJ, Lin HC, Chang CF, et al: A randomized controlled trial comparing octreotide and vasopressin in the control of acute esophageal variceal bleeding. J Hepatol 16:320–325, 1992.
35. McKee R: A study of octreotide in esophageal varices. Digestion 45:60–65, 1990.
36. Primignani M, Andreoni B, Carpinelli L, et al: Sclerotherapy plus octreotide versus sclerotherapy alone in the prevention of early rebleeding from esophageal varices: A randomized double-blind placebo-controlled multicenter trial. Hepatology 21:1322–1327, 1995.
37. Jenkins SA, Shields R, Davies M, et al: A multicenter randomized trial comparing octreotide and injection sclerotherapy in the man-agement and outcome of acute variceal hemorrhage. Gut 41:526–533, 1997.
38. Besson I, Ingrand P, Person B, et al: Sclerotherapy with or without octreotide for acute variceal bleeding. N Engl J Med 333:555–560, 1995.
39. Sung JJY, Chung SC, Yung MY: Prospective randomized study of effects of octreotide on rebleeding from esophageal varices after endoscopic ligation. Lancet 346:1666–1669, 1995.
40. Bernard B, Lebrec D, Mathurin P, et al: Beta-adrenergic antagonists in the prevention of gastrointestinal rebleeding in patients with cirrhosis: A meta-analysis. Hepatology 25:63–70, 1997.
41. Avgerinos A, Armonis A: Balloon tamponade technique and efficacy in variceal haemorrhage. Scand J Gastroenterol 207(Suppl):11–16, 1994.
42. Lo GH, Lai KH, Ng WW, et al: Injection sclerotherapy preceded by esophageal tamponade versus immediate sclerotherapy in arresting active variceal bleeding: A prospective randomized trial. Gastrointest Endosc 38:421–424, 1992.
43. Burroughs AK, Hamilton G, Phillips A, et al: A comparison of sclerotherapy with staple transection of the esophagus for emergency control of bleeding from esophageal varices. N Engl J Med 321:857–862, 1989.
44. Hartigan PM, Gebhard RL, Gregory PB, et al: Sclerotherapy for actively bleeding esophageal varices in male patients with cirrhosis. Gastrointest Endosc 46:1–7, 1997.
45. Terblanche J, Burroughs AK, Hobbs K: Controversies in the manage-ment of bleeding esophageal varices. N Engl J Med 320:1393–1398; 1469–1475, 1989.
46. Barsoum MS, Bolous FI, El-Rooby AA, et al: Tamponade and injec-tion sclerotherapy in the management of bleeding esophageal varices. Br J Surg 69:76–78, 1982.
47. Burroughs AK, McCormick PA, Siringo S, et al: Prospective random-ized trial of long term sclerotherapy for variceal rebleeding using the same protocol to treat rebleeding in all patients: Final report (Abstract). Hepatology 10:579, 1989.
48. The Copenhagen Esophageal Varices Sclerotherapy Project: Sclero-therapy after first variceal hemorrhage in cirrhosis: A randomized multicenter trial. N Engl J Med 311:1594–1600, 1984.
49. Gregory PB, The VA Cooperative Variceal Sclerotherapy Group, et al: Sclerotherapy for male alcoholics with cirrhosis who have bled from esophageal varices: Results of a randomized multicenter trial. Hepatology 20:618–625, 1994.
50. Korula J, Balart LA, Radvan G, et al: A prospective randomized controlled trial of chronic esophageal variceal sclerotherapy. Hepatol-ogy 5:584–589, 1985.
51. Soderlund C, Ihre T: Endoscopic sclerotherapy versus conservative management of bleeding esophageal varices: A 5 year prospective controlled trial of emergency and long term treatment. Acta Chir Scand 151:449–456, 1985.
52. Terblanche J, Bornman PC, Kahn D, et al: Failure of repeated injection sclerotherapy to improve long-term survival after esopha-geal variceal bleeding: A five year prospective controlled clinical trial. Lancet 2:1328–1332, 1983.
53. Westaby D, MacDougall BR, Williams R: Improved survival following injection sclerotherapy for esophageal varices: Final analysis of a controlled trial. Hepatology 5:827–830, 1985.
54. Rossi V, Cales P, Pascal B, et al: Prevention of recurrent variceal bleeding in alcoholic cirrhotic patients: Prospective controlled trial of propranolol and sclerotherapy. J Hepatol 12:283–289, 1991.
55. Dasarathy S, Divinedi M, Bharagava DK, et al: A prospective ran-domized trial comparing repeated endoscopic sclerotherapy and propranolol in decompensated (Child class B and C) cirrhosis pa-tients. Hepatology, 16:89–94, 1992.
56. Teres J, Bosch J, Bordas JM: Propranolol versus sclerotherapy in preventing variceal rebleeding: A randomized controlled trial. Gas-troenterology 105:1508–1514, 1993.
57. Dollet JM, Champigneulle B, Patgris A. et al: Sclérothérapie endo-scopique contre propranolol après hémorragie, par rupture de vari-ces oesophagiennes chez le cirrhotique: Resultats a 4 ans d'une étude randomisée. Gastroenterol Clin Biol 12:234–239, 1988.
58. Westaby D, Polson RJ, Gimson AES, et al: A controlled trial of oral propranolol compared with injection sclerotherapy for long term management of variceal bleeding. Hepatology 11:353–359, 1990.
59. Fleig WE, Stange EF, Hunecke R, et al: Prevention of recurrent bleeding in cirrhosis with recent variceal hemorrhage: Prospective randomized comparison of propranolol and sclerotherapy. Hepatol-ogy 7:355–361, 1987.
60. Alexandrino PT, Alves MM, Correia JP: Propranolol or endoscopic sclerotherapy in the prevention of recurrence of variceal bleeding: A prospective randomized controlled trial. J Hepatol 7:175–185, 1988.
61. Lundell L, Leth R, Lind T, et al: Evaluation of propranolol for prevention of recurrent bleeding from esophageal varices between sclerotherapy sessions. Acta Chir Scand 156:711–715, 1990.
62. Vicker C, Rhodes J, Chesner I, et al: Prevention of rebleeding from oesophageal varices: Two-year follow-up of a prospective controlled trial of propranolol in addition to sclerotherapy. J Hepatol 21:81–87, 1994.

63. Acharya KS, Dasarathy S, Saksena S, et al: A prospective randomized study to evaluate propranolol in patients undergoing long-term endoscopic sclerotherapy. J Hepatol 19:291–300, 1993.

64. O'Connor KW, Lehman G, Yune H, et al: Comparison of three nonsurgical treatments for bleeding esophageal varices. Gastroenterology 96:899–906, 1989.

65. Vinel JP, Lamouliate H, Cales P, et al: Propranolol reduces the rebleeding rate during endoscopic sclerotherapy before variceal obliteration. Gastroenterology 102:1760–1763, 1992.

66. Avgerinos A, Rekoumis G, Klonis C, et al: Propranolol in the prevention of recurrent upper gastrointestinal bleeding in patients with cirrhosis undergoing endoscopic sclerotherapy: A randomized controlled trial. J Hepatol 19:301–311, 1993.

67. Westaby D, Melia W, Hegarty J, et al: Use of propranolol to reduce the rebleeding rate during injection sclerotherapy prior to variceal obliteration. Hepatology 6:673–675, 1986.

68. Ink O, Martin T, Poynard T, et al: Does elective sclerotherapy improve the efficacy of longterm propranolol for prevention of recurrent bleeding in patients with severe cirrhosis? A prospective multicenter randomized trial. Hepatology 16:912–919, 1992.

69. Henderson JM, Kutner MH, Millileau W Jr, et al: Endoscopic variceal sclerosis compared with distal splenorenal shunt to prevent recurrent variceal bleeding in cirrhosis: A prospective randomized trial. Ann Intern Med 112:262–269, 1990.

70. Spina GP, Santambrogio R, Opocher E, et al: Distal splenorenal shunt versus endoscopic sclerotherapy in the prevention of variceal rebleeding: First stage of a randomized controlled trial. Ann Surg 211:178–186, 1990.

71. Cello JP, Grendell JH, Crass RA: Endoscopic sclerotherapy versus portacaval shunt in patients with severe cirrhosis and variceal hemorrhage. N Engl J Med 311:1589–1594, 1984.

72. Cello JP, Grendell JH, Crass RA, et al: Endoscopic sclerotherapy versus portacaval shunt in patients with severe cirrhosis and acute variceal hemorrhage: Long term follow-up. N Engl J Med 316:11–15, 1987.

73. Sauerbruch T, Schepke M: Sclerotherapy is out—nearly. Endoscopy 29:281–282, 1997.

74. Soehendra N, Binmoeller KF: Is sclerotherapy out? Endoscopy 29:283–284, 1997.

75. Sarin S: Long-term follow-up of gastric variceal sclerotherapy: An eleven year experience. Gastrointest Endosc 46:8–14, 1997.

76. Sarin SK: Prevalence, classification and natural history of gastric varices: A long term follow-up study in 568 portal hypertension patients. Hepatology 16:1343–1349, 1992.

77. Hosking SW, Johnson AG: Gastric varices: A proposed classification leading to management. Br J Surg 75:195–196, 1988.

78. Hashizume M, Kitano S, Yamaga H, et al: Endoscopic classification of gastric varices. Gastrointest Endosc 36:276–280, 1990.

79. Kim T, Shijo H, Kokawa H, et al: Risk factors for hemorrhage from gastric fundal varices. Hepatology 25:307–312, 1997.

80. Sarin SK, Sachdeu G, Nanda R, et al: Endoscopic sclerotherapy in the treatment of gastric varices. Br J Surg 75:747–750, 1988.

81. Trudeau W, Priniville T: Endoscopic injection sclerosis in bleeding gastric varices. Gastrointest Endosc 32:264–268, 1986.

82. Bretagne JF, Dudicourt JL, Moriscot D, et al: Is endoscopic variceal sclerotherapy effective for the treatment of gastric varices (Abstract)? Dig Dis Sci 31:5055, 1986.

83. Yassin MY, Eita MS, Hussein AMT: Endoscopic sclerotherapy for bleeding gastric varices (Abstract). Gut 26:A1105, 1985.

84. Gimson AES, Westaby D, Williams R: Endoscopic sclerotherapy in the management of gastric variceal hemorrhage. J Hepatol 13:274–278, 1991.

85. Chang KY, Wu CS, Chen PL: Prospective randomized trial of hypertonic glucose water and sodium tetradecyl sulfate for gastric variceal bleeding in patients with advanced liver cirrhosis. Endoscopy 28:481–486, 1996.

86. Stiegmann GV, Goff JS, Michaletz-Onody PA, et al: Endoscopic sclerotherapy as compared with endoscopic ligation for bleeding esophageal varices. N Engl J Med 326:1527–1532, 1992.

87. Gimson AES, Ramage JK, Panos MZ, et al: Randomized trial of variceal banding ligation versus injection sclerotherapy for bleeding esophageal varices. Lancet 342:391–394, 1993.

88. Laine L, El-Newihi HM, Migikovsky B, et al: Endoscopic ligation compared with sclerotherapy for the treatment of bleeding esophageal varices. Ann Intern Med 119:1–7, 1993.

89. Lo GH, Lai KH, Cheng JS, et al: A prospective randomized trial of sclerotherapy versus ligation in the management of bleeding esophageal varices. 22:466–471, 1995.

90. Hou MC, Liu HC, Kuo BIT, et al: Comparison of endoscopic variceal injection sclerotherapy and ligation for the treatment of esophageal variceal hemorrhage: A prospective randomized trial. Hepatology 21:1517–1522, 1995.

91. Jensen DM, Kovacs TOG, Randall GM, et al: Emergency sclerotherapy versus rubber band ligation for actively bleeding esophagogastric varices in a randomized, prospective study (Abstract). Gastrointest Endosc 40:77, 1994.

92. Laine L, Cook D: Endoscopic ligation compared with sclerotherapy for treatment of esophageal variceal bleeding: A meta-analysis. Ann Intern Med 123:280–287, 1995.

93. Baroncini D, Milandri G, Borioni D, et al: A prospective randomized trial of sclerotherapy versus ligation in the elective treatment of bleeding esophageal varices. Endoscopy 29:235–240, 1997.

94. Jensen DM, Kovacs TOG, Randall GM, et al: A randomized prospective study of emergency sclerotherapy versus banding for bleeding gastric varices: Initial results (Abstract). Am J Gastroenterology 88:150, 1993.

95. Jensen DM, Jutabha R, Kovacs TOG, et al: Endoscopic hemostasis of severe gastric varix hemorrhage in a randomized prospective blinded study of rubber band ligation versus sclerotherapy (Abstract). Gastrointest Endosc 41:365, 1995.

96. Sung JJY, Chung SCS: The use of a detachable mini-loop for the treatment of esophageal varices. Gastrointest Endosc 47:178–181, 1998.

97. Jensen DM, Kovacs TOG, Jutabha R: Final results of a randomized prospective trial of combination rubber band ligation and sclerotherapy versus sclerotherapy alone for hemostasis of bleeding esophageal varices (Abstract). Gastroenterology 110:A1222, 1996.

98. Koutsomanis D: Endoscopic variceal ligation combined with low-volume sclerotherapy (Abstract). Gastroenterology 102:A835, 1992.

99. Laine L, Stein C, Sharma V: Randomized comparison of ligation versus ligation plus sclerotherapy in patients with bleeding esophageal varices. Gastroenterology 110:529–533, 1996.

100. Saeed ZA, Stiegmann GV, Ramirez RC, et al: Endoscopic variceal ligation is superior to combined ligation and sclerotherapy: A multicenter prospective randomized trial. Hepatology 25:71–74, 1997.

101. Gralnek IM, Jensen DM: Cost assessment in the management of variceal bleeding. Clin Liver Dis 1:45–58, 1997.

102. Gralnek IM, Jensen DM, Jensen ME, et al: Direct costs of hospital care in patients with active esophagogastric variceal hemorrhage treated with emergency endoscopic sclerotherapy or rubber band ligation in a prospective randomized trial (Abstract). Gastroenterology 110:A1200, 1996.

103. Gralnek IM, Jensen DM, Jensen ME, et al: Assessment of direct costs of medical care in a prospective, randomized blinded study of banding versus sclerotherapy for preventing recurrent variceal hemorrhage for patients without active bleeding at endoscopy (Abstract). Gastrointest Endosc 43:A89, 1996.

104. Gotlib JP. Endoscopic obturation of esophageal and gastric varices with a cyanoacrylic tissue adhesive. Can J Gastroenterol 4:637–638, 1990.

105. Lux G, Retterspitz M, Stabenow-Lahbauer U, et al: Treatment of bleeding esophageal varices with cyanoacrylate and polidocanol, or polidocanol alone: Results of a prospective study of an unselected group of patients with cirrhosis of the liver. Endoscopy 29:241–246, 1997.

106. Grace ND: Diagnosis and treatment of gastrointestinal bleeding secondary to portal hypertension. Am J Gastroenterol 92:1081–1091, 1997.

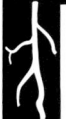

C H A P T E R   1 1 6

Percutaneous Interventions in Portal Hypertension

Robert K. Kerlan, Jr., M.D., and Jeanne M. LaBerge, M.D.

In 1974, Lunderquist and Vang[31] described a percutaneous transhepatic technique for placing catheters in the portal vein. With this method, the portal tributaries could be selectively catheterized and variceal hemorrhage treated by embolization of the bleeding varices (Fig. 116–1). Though this procedure was initially accepted with enthusiasm, it soon became apparent that rebleeding rates were unacceptably high, and transhepatic obliteration of varices has been abandoned as a primary therapeutic alternative. This work stimulated the development of other interventional radiologic procedures, however, that have become indispensable in the management of patients with complications related to portal hypertension. These procedures can be divided into two groups: (1) those performed to modify a surgically created shunt and (2) those used as primary treatment for portal hypertension.

PROCEDURES PERFORMED IN PATIENTS WITH SURGICAL SHUNTS

After portosystemic shunt surgery, it is usually not difficult to advance an angiographic catheter from the inferior vena cava across the shunt into the portal venous system to perform a variety of therapeutic interventions. In many cases, these procedures can be accomplished as outpatient procedures through a femoral venous puncture and with the use of local anesthesia. In some circumstances, however, a transjugular or transhepatic approach is required.

Embolization of Varices

Once a catheter has been manipulated through a shunt, it can be used to occlude flow in any residual varices. This technique is most commonly used in patients who have received small, partially decompressive shunts (Fig. 116–2). Surgeons who advocate the use of small-diameter shunts to reduce the incidence of post-shunt encephalopathy recommend routine postoperative catheterization and the use of transcatheter embolization if any residual varices are demonstrated.[8, 50] Occluding competing collateral veins after placement of a small-diameter shunt not only may reduce the risk of subsequent variceal hemorrhage and increase shunt flow but also may further elevate the residual mesenteric venous pressure. This increase in pressure could conceivably improve portal perfusion of the liver, further reducing the incidence of postoperative encephalopathy.

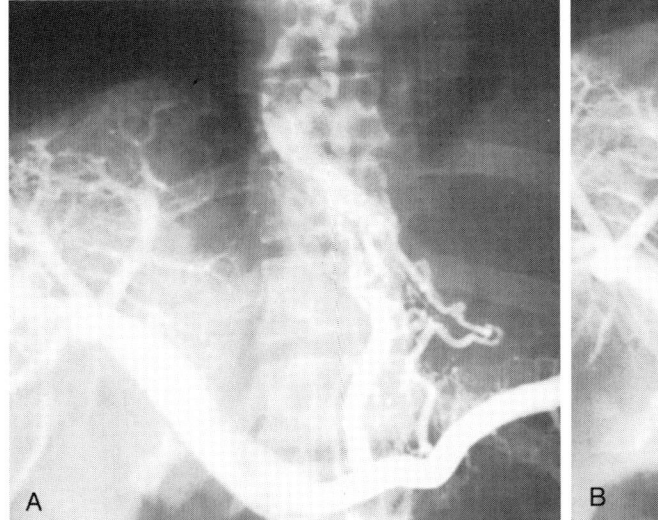 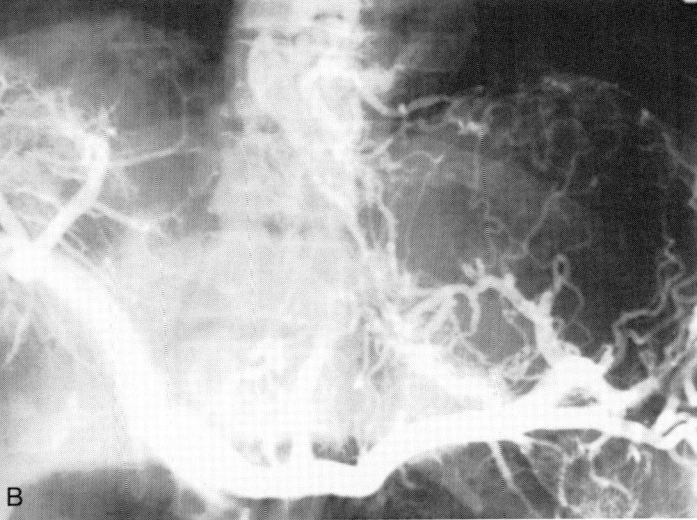

FIGURE 116–1. Recurrent variceal bleeding through collateral vessels following transhepatic embolization. *A,* A splenic venogram performed percutaneously via a transhepatic approach demonstrates two large veins supplying the esophageal varices. *B,* Both of the gastric veins supplying the varices were selectively catheterized and embolized. This resulted in immediate cessation of bleeding. However, 3 days later the bleeding recurred, and the portal vein was again catheterized. A second splenic venogram shows persistent occlusion of the gastric veins but filling of the esophageal varices through multiple short gastric collaterals.

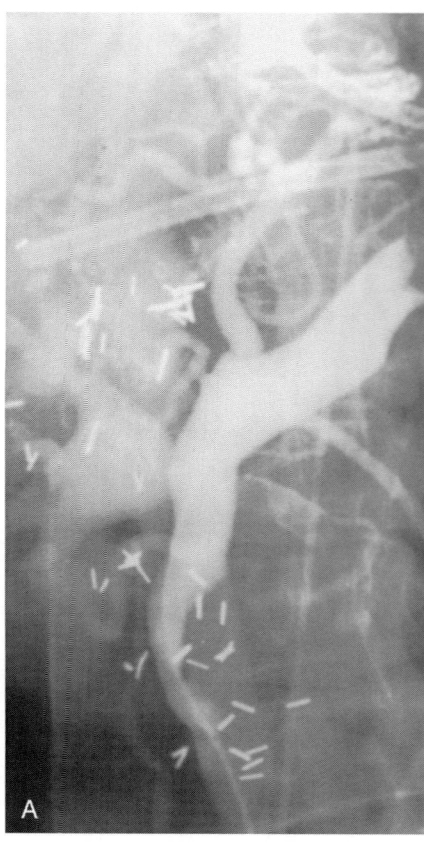 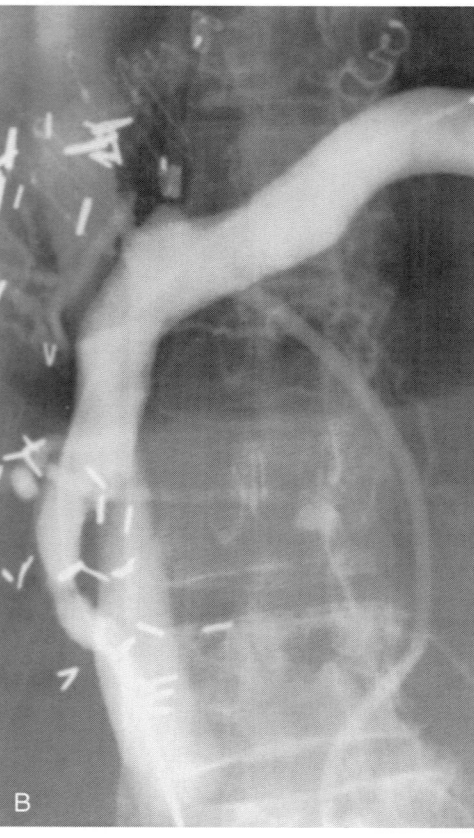

FIGURE 116–2. Trans-shunt catheterization and embolization for continued bleeding following a small-caliber mesocaval shunt. *A,* A catheter was advanced from the inferior vena cava through the shunt into the splenic vein. A splenic venogram demonstrates filling of the coronary vein. The mesocaval shunt is patent, but the channel is quite narrow. *B,* Following selective catheterization of the coronary vein and occlusion with ethanol and stainless steel coils, another splenic venogram was obtained. The varices no longer fill and there is improved flow through the shunt, as evidenced by the increased caval opacification.

Dilatation of Stenotic Shunts

Anastomotic stenoses are very uncommon following placement of large-diameter portosystemic shunts. With small-caliber shunts, however, particularly mesocaval shunts constructed with prosthetic grafts, a significant narrowing occasionally develops at one of the venous anastomoses. Several reports have described the use of balloon angioplasty to enlarge narrow shunt anastomoses; unfortunately, recurrent stenoses are common, and repeated dilatations are frequently necessary to maintain shunt patency.[9, 10, 58] The advent of expandable metallic stents will likely improve the durability of percutaneous dilatation.[58] However, sufficient literature documenting this improved durability is currently lacking.

Recanalization of Occluded Shunts

Percutaneous techniques can also be used to reopen occluded shunts. Unfortunately the success rate of recanalization is less because of the added difficulty one encounters in advancing a catheter through a shunt that is completely obstructed. Catheterization of occluded portocaval shunts is particularly difficult because there is nothing visible angiographically to identify the site of the anastomosis. Usually, however, catheters can be advanced through occluded mesocaval or splenorenal shunts. The success of shunt catheterization is much greater when the procedure is attempted soon after the occlusion and the clot is still soft enough to permit unencumbered passage of a guide wire.

Once a catheter has been advanced across an occluded shunt, patency can be reestablished in several ways. Cope[9] reported success with the use of urokinase to restore flow through occluded mesocaval shunts. To avoid the use of fibrinolytic drugs in a patient at risk for bleeding, balloon catheters can be used to fragment and dislodge the clot from the shunt. The clot either is pushed by the balloon into a portal vein branch or an outflow varix, such as the coronary vein, or is pulled into the inferior vena cava. The resulting pulmonary embolization is not without risk, but this approach has been used by us in several patients without any clinical manifestations of the emboli. None of the patients so treated experienced pulmonary complications or demonstrated any clinical evidence that pulmonary embolization had occurred.

As an alternative, a number of mechanical thrombectomy catheters have been developed to pulverize thrombus. These instruments include the Amplatz thrombectomy device (Microvena), the Possus Angiojet (Possus Medical), the Trerotola rotating basket, and a variety of suction catheters. Although currently no literature documents the effectiveness of these devices in the setting of an acutely occluded surgical portosystemic shunt, there are reports of successful applications in other clinical circumstances.[21, 62, 63]

Occlusion of Patent Shunts

Although the incidence of encephalopathy following conventional portacaval shunt surgery varies considerably in different series, it may be as high as 60%. In most cases, the symptoms are mild or episodic and are reasonably well controlled with medical therapy. Occasionally, however, the mental disturbance is so disabling that the patient is willing to forgo the shunt and risk further variceal bleeding. Stainless steel coils can be used to occlude flow through mesocaval shunts, successfully occluding the portosystemic communication.

PROCEDURES PERFORMED AS PRIMARY THERAPY FOR PORTAL HYPERTENSION

Improvements in catheter technology and imaging have allowed interventional radiologic procedures to emerge as primary therapeutic options for the treatment of selected patients with complications related to portal hypertension. These procedures are attractive because they usually do not require general anesthesia and do not alter the native portal venous anatomy. Leaving the portal venous anatomy intact has important ramifications if the patient is considered a potential candidate for orthotopic liver transplantation.

Transhepatic Embolization of Esophageal Varices

Although clearly not useful on a routine basis, transhepatic variceal embolization may still occasionally have a role in the management of specific clinical problems. Most often, it is used after distal splenorenal shunt to treat the late development of encephalopathy or recurrent variceal bleeding (Fig. 116–3). With this type of shunt, varices may recur when small or incompletely ligated gastric veins enlarge to become major collaterals between the high-pressure portal vein and the low-pressure splenic vein. These communications can be easily identified with transhepatic catheterization and portal venography, and selective catheterization with embolization can be used as an alternative to reoperation to occlude them. Embolization can be performed with stainless steel or platinum coils or with a liquid embolic agent, such as dehydrated alcohol or 2,3-isobutylcyanoacrylate.

Transjugular Intrahepatic Portosystemic Shunt

In 1969, Rosch and colleagues[45] reported a new method of decompressing the portal venous system through a percutaneously created shunt between the portal and hepatic veins. In a series of dog experiments, they showed the feasibility of passing a needle from the jugular vein into a hepatic vein and then advancing the needle through the liver parenchyma into a portal vein branch.

When balloon angioplasty catheters became available in the late 1970s, Burgener and Gutierrez[3] used them to establish intrahepatic shunts in dogs with portal hypertension. All of the initial shunts rapidly occluded, but when these researchers repeated the dilatations at weekly intervals (up to five times), some shunts remained patent for up to a year.

In 1983, Colapinto and associates[7] reported the first clinical use of the transjugular intrahepatic portosystemic shunt (TIPS). They kept a 9-mm balloon inflated across the parenchymal tract for 12 hours; with this method, they were able to lower portal pressure and control variceal bleeding in 15 patients. Unfortunately, the majority of their patients had rebleeding and died within a month, and only 2 patients survived for more than a year without experiencing rebleeding.

In 1985, Palmaz and colleagues[37] began investigating the use of expandable metallic stents for TIPS and found that in dogs with artificially created portal hypertension, shunts remained patent through 48 weeks when a stent was placed in the parenchymal tract. At necropsy, these investigators found a thin smooth layer of neo-intima covering the stents' luminal surface. In 1990, Richter and associates[42] used Palmaz stents to place TIPS in three patients with repeated failures to respond to endoscopic sclerotherapy; in a follow-up article, these investigators expanded the series to include nine patients.[43] In each case, rapid decompression of portal hypertension was achieved and bleeding was controlled. Subsequently, these results were reproduced at independent centers by other investigators,[44, 70] and interest in the procedure grew considerably.

Since these early reports, a number of technical refinements have been developed to facilitate the performance of the TIPS procedure. The flexible Wallstent emerged as a more suitable conduit to bridge the hepatic parenchymal tract.[27] Currently, the procedure is performed in most major medical centers, with a technical success rate of greater than 90% and a significant procedural complication rate of less than 10%.[27]

Technique

In the TIPS procedure, a stented channel is constructed within the liver to connect the portal and hepatic venous systems. This concept is illustrated in Figure 116–4 and explained in detail here.

Patient Preparation

Prior to a TIPS procedure, the patient is resuscitated or stabilized as much as possible with blood transfusions, intravenous vasopressin, and, if necessary, esophageal balloon tamponade. All patients undergo complete upper endoscopy prior to the procedure for confirmation of the diagnosis of variceal bleeding; duplex ultrasonography is performed to evaluate portal vein patency. Mesenteric angiography is performed only when ultrasound fails to demonstrate portal flow.

If significant coagulopathy is present, an attempt is made to correct it prior to the procedure. Although individual practices vary, platelets are given to patients with platelet counts less than 50,000/cc and fresh frozen plasma is given to patients with prothrombin times longer than 18 seconds or an International Normalized Ratio (INR) greater than 2.0.

Immediately prior to the procedure, a broad-spectrum antibiotic is administered, and intravenous sedation and analgesics are given as appropriate.

Shunt Creation

The right internal jugular vein is percutaneously punctured, and a 40-cm-long, 9 French (Fr.) angiographic sheath is advanced into the inferior vena cava. A curved angiographic catheter is manipulated under fluoroscopic guidance into a

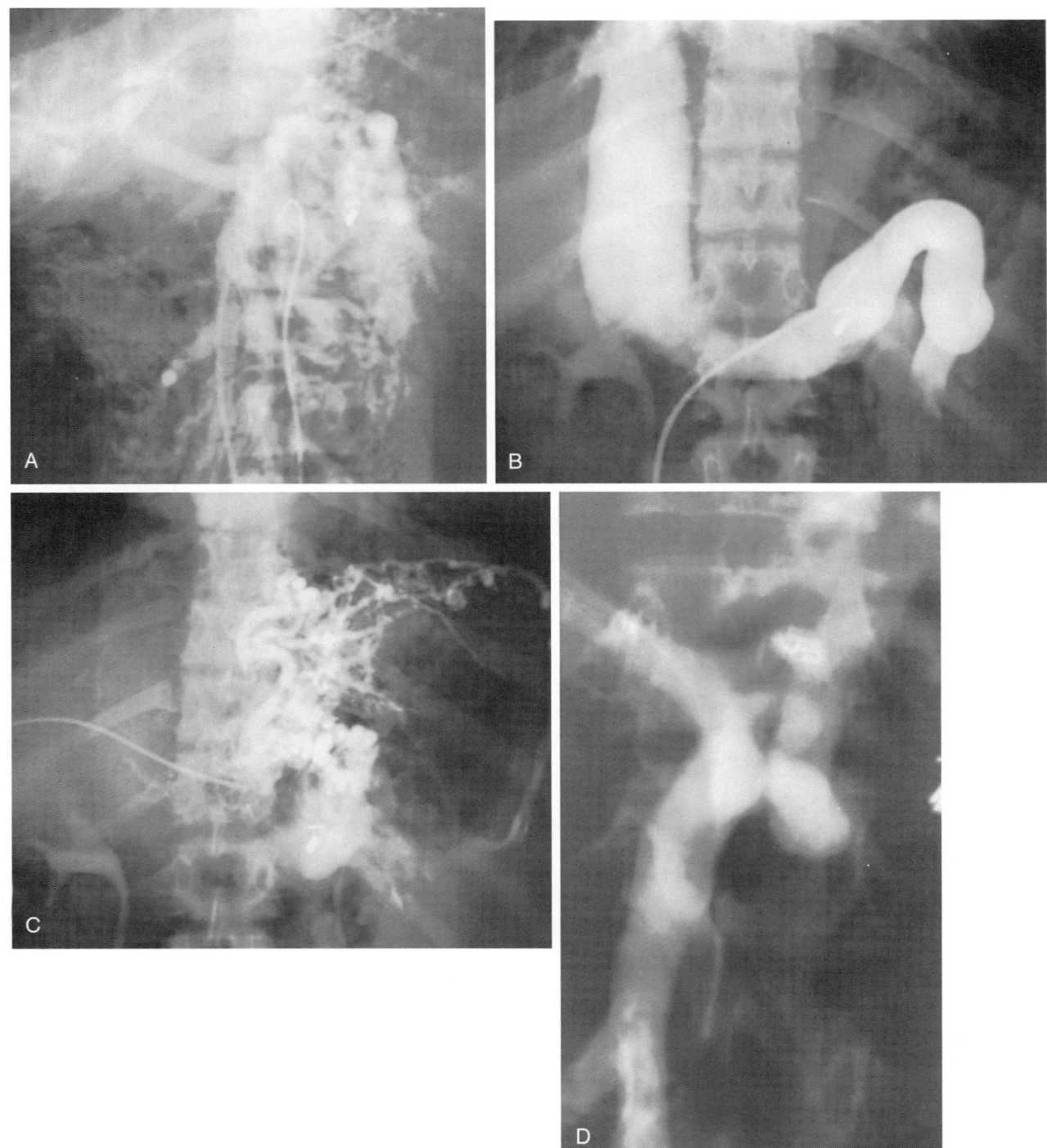

FIGURE 116–3. Recurrent variceal bleeding following distal splenorenal shunt surgery treated by transhepatic embolization of the portal collaterals. *A,* Several years after distal splenorenal shunt surgery, this patient presented with acute variceal hemorrhage. Arterial portography demonstrates large gastric varices filling from the portal vein. *B,* The shunt was catheterized through the renal vein, and a splenic venogram showed the shunt to be widely patent. *C,* The portal vein was entered transhepatically, and the coronary (left gastric) veins were selectively catheterized. Collaterals can be seen filling the renal vein. *D,* The collateral veins were occluded with the use of stainless steel coil emboli, and another portal venogram was obtained. It shows that all of the connections from the high-pressure portal side of the shunt have been occluded.

hepatic vein with a large enough diameter to form an adequate shunt. The right hepatic vein is generally preferred, but a TIPS can also be created from the middle or left hepatic vein.

In most patients, a digital subtraction wedged hepatic venogram is performed with carbon dioxide to delineate the position of the portal vein. This relatively simple and effective technique has replaced most other previously described methods for portal vein localization, including ultrasonographic guidance, percutaneous deposition of microcoils adjacent to the portal vein, hepatic arterial catheterization, and percutaneous transhepatic portal venous catheterization.

Once the appropriate hepatic vein has been catheterized, a transjugular needle is advanced through the sheath for transhepatic puncture of the portal vein. A number of needle systems have been designed for this purpose that vary in size, flexibility, and capability to be manipulated; they include Colapinto (Cook, Inc., Bloomington, Ind.), Rosch-Uchida (Cook), and Hawkins (Medi-tech, Boston Scientific, Watertown, Mass.).

The needle is rotated anteromedially and advanced caudally out of the right hepatic vein 4 to 5 cm into the liver parenchyma to the previously delineated position of the portal vein. A syringe is attached, and aspiration is performed as the needle is slowly withdrawn. When blood returns, contrast medium is injected to determine which vascular structure has been entered. When a portal vein branch is identified, a guide wire is passed through the needle and manipulated down the main portal vein into the splenic or superior mesenteric vein. The needle is removed, and a 5 Fr. catheter is advanced over the guide wire into the portal venous system.

Portal venography is performed to evaluate the anatomy and determine the direction of portal flow; an initial portal pressure is recorded. The 5 Fr. catheter is then exchanged for an 8-mm angioplasty balloon catheter, which is inflated in the tract between the hepatic and portal veins. The tract is then stented with a metallic endoprosthesis and expanded to 8 mm with the use of the angioplasty balloon. A second portal venogram is obtained, and the pressure is remeasured. If portal pressure remains elevated and there is continued rapid filling of varices, the stent is further distended to its maximum 10-mm diameter. The venogram and pressures are then obtained again. If varices are still filling briskly, they are selectively catheterized and embolized.

In about 10% of patients, a shunt 10-mm in diameter does not produce sufficient reduction in the portosystemic gradient to prevent recurrent bleeding (more than a 15 mmHg residual gradient). In these cases, the stent may be overdilated with a 12-mm balloon,[64] which often improves the gradient. If this maneuver fails to provide sufficient portal decompression, a second TIPS can be created from the middle or left hepatic vein to the left portal vein.

To avoid the problem of inadequate portal decompression with a single 10-mm stent, a larger-diameter stent (12 mm) can be placed initially and dilated only to the desired diameter. In the majority of patients, however, the 10-mm stent is adequate.

At the completion of the shunt, the jugular vein catheter is usually exchanged for a shorter 8.5 Fr. sheath through which fluid and blood can be administered when necessary.

Postprocedural Care

All patients are observed at least overnight in an intensive care unit. Serial hematocrit levels are obtained to identify residual bleeding or hemorrhage secondary to the procedure. In addition, liver function tests are performed to detect hepatic decompensation secondary to the shunt. Most patients are transferred to the ward on the following day.

Follow-up

Prior to a patient's discharge from the hospital, a baseline duplex ultrasonography examination is performed to evalu-

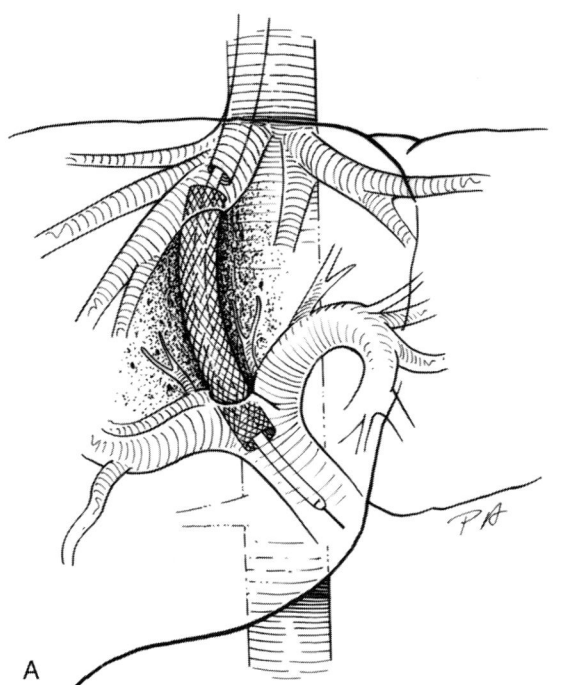
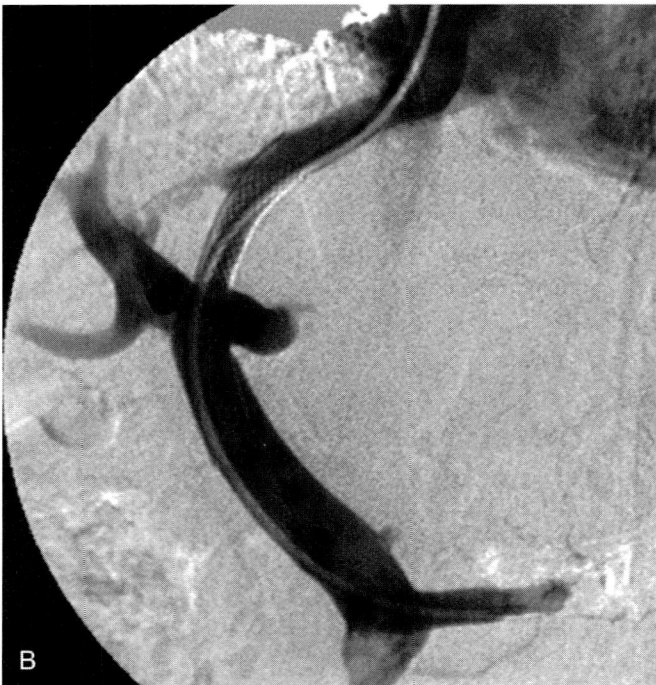

FIGURE 116–4. Transjugular intrahepatic portosystemic shunt (TIPS). *A,* This graphic illustration demonstrates the typical location of TIPS. A stented channel connects the right hepatic vein with the right portal vein. *B,* Completion portal venogram following TIPS implantation shows flow through the TIPS with persistent intrahepatic portal venous flow.

ate shunt flow. Duplex scanning is repeated at regular 3-month follow-up visits for the first year and at 6 month intervals thereafter.

Indications and Contraindications

Indications and contraindications for TIPS continue to be refined by the results of clinical trials. A summary of the indications and contraindications for this procedure in current practice is shown in Table 116–1.

Currently, the accepted indications for the procedure are acute variceal hemorrhage uncontrollable by sclerotherapy and recurrent variceal hemorrhage in patients who have undergone sclerotherapy.[54] Refractory ascites[36, 40, 56] and hepatic hydrothorax[14, 19, 61] also respond to TIPS in a substantial percentage of patients. The use of the procedure as the initial treatment for variceal hemorrhage or for the treatment of other disorders, including hepatorenal syndrome, hepatopulmonary syndrome, portal hypertensive gastropathy, and thrombocytopenia secondary to hypersplenism, remains investigational.

The TIPS procedure can be performed in almost any situation in which there is symptomatic portal hypertension requiring decompression. Polycystic liver disease appears to be the only absolute contraindication to attempting TIPS. However, patients with large, hypervascular neoplasms (such as hepatocellular carcinoma) that are interposed between the hepatic venous confluence and the portal vein are very poor candidates for the procedure. Patients who have tumors not in the projected path of the intrahepatic shunt may be considered candidates.

Anatomic problems making TIPS more difficult include right internal jugular vein occlusion (requiring a left internal jugular or external jugular approach) and biliary ductal dilatation. In addition, three other circumstances in which performance of TIPS can deserve special consideration:

- Portal vein occlusion
- Hepatic vein occlusion
- Portal hypertension in the pediatric patient

Portal Vein Occlusion

The TIPS procedure can be performed in patients with acute occlusion of the portal vein.[41] The thrombus can be easily crossed with a catheter and can be dislodged or macerated with thrombectomy devices. The success rate in patients with acute portal vein thrombosis appears to be nearly the same as that in patients without thrombus in the portal vein; it was reported to be 100% in a series of six patients.[41]

The creation of TIPS in patients with chronic portal vein occlusion is technically more challenging and often requires an adjunctive transhepatic approach to facilitate recanalization of the portal vein (Fig. 116–5). Because (1) the rate of the success of the procedure appears to be substantially lower in patients with chronic portal venous occlusion and (2) the risk of portal venous perforation is higher, conventional surgical portosystemic shunts may be more appropriate.

The presence of coexistent acute or chronic splenic or superior mesenteric vein thrombosis also diminishes the chance of a successful procedure. Although it is technically possible to manipulate catheters across these occlusions, the lack of inflow often leads to rapid reocclusion. In the patient with acute thrombosis, adjunctive treatment with urokinase might be considered, but the clinical success of this approach has yet to be established. As a general rule, anatomy that precludes any type of conventional surgical shunt also precludes the creation of a TIPS.

Budd-Chiari Syndrome

Although it is technically more difficult, TIPS can be established in patients with Budd-Chiari syndrome who have complete obliteration of the intraparenchymal hepatic veins.[38] In these cases, the shunt can be formed by connecting the right portal vein to a short stump of right hepatic vein near its junction with the inferior vena cava.

TIPS decompresses the portal venous system into the suprahepatic inferior vena cava. This may be clinically important in Budd-Chiari patients, whose enlarged caudate lobe may cause caval compression and elevated pressure in the inferior vena cava. The suprahepatic venous connection also may prove important in hypercoagulable patients with Budd-Chiari syndrome who have associated caval thrombosis; in these cases, TIPS can be used as an alternative to a mesoatrial shunt.

Portal Hypertension in the Pediatric Patient

TIPS creation in the pediatric patient has been reported in at least two series[16, 22] comprising a total of 21 patients. The

---

TABLE 116–1. INDICATIONS AND CONTRAINDICATIONS FOR TRANSJUGULAR INTRAHEPATIC PORTOSYSTEMIC SHUNT (TIPS)

Accepted Indications
Control of refractory acute variceal bleeding
Prevention of refractory recurrent variceal bleeding in patients with Child class B or C disease
Refractory hepatic hydrothorax

Promising but Unproven Indications
Refractory ascites
Hepatorenal syndrome
Budd-Chiari syndrome
Veno-occlusive disease

Unproven Indications
Prevention of refractory recurrent variceal bleeding in patients with Child class A disease
Initial therapy of acute variceal hemorrhage
Initial therapy to prevent recurrent variceal hemorrhage
Prevention of initial variceal hemorrhage
To reduce intraoperative morbidity during liver transplantation or other major surgery in patients with portal hypertension
Treatment of hepatopulmonary syndrome

Absolute Contraindications
Right-sided heart failure
Primary pulmonary hypertension
Polycystic liver disease
Severe hepatic failure
Cavernous obstruction of the portal vein

Relative Contraindications
Biliary obstruction
Active intrahepatic or systemic infection
Severe hepatic encephalopathy poorly controlled by medical therapy
Noncavernous obstruction of the portal vein

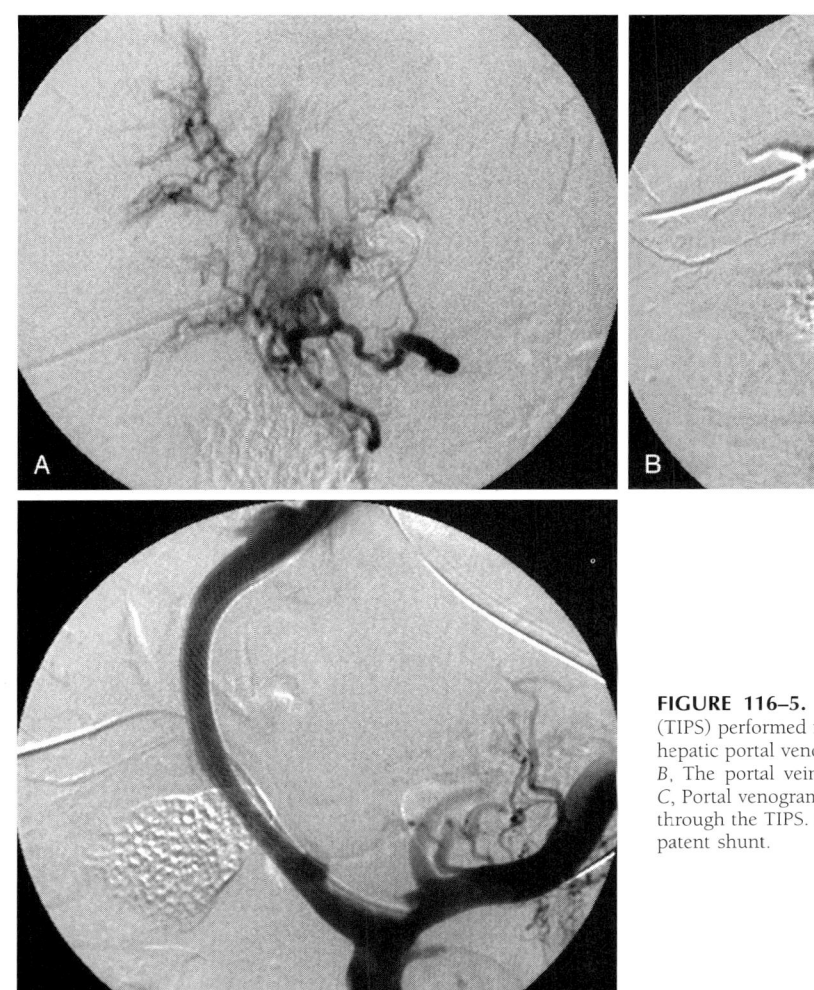

FIGURE 116–5. Transjugular intrahepatic portosystemic shunt (TIPS) performed in a patient with portal vein occlusion. *A*, Transhepatic portal venogram demonstrates occlusion of the portal vein. *B*, The portal vein was catheterized via a transhepatic approach. *C*, Portal venogram following completion of TIPS shows good flow through the TIPS. Follow-up venogram at 3 years showed a widely patent shunt.

youngest patient was 2 years and 5 months. Conventional instrumentation could be used in older children, but younger children required smaller shunts (6 mm in diameter) and catheters. All patients had successful control of acute variceal hemorrhage. As in adults is undergoing TIPS procedures, stunt stenosis and occlusion appear to be problematic, but the technique appears to be a useful bridge to transplantation. No follow-up data are currently available to give insight into problems created by growth in a child with a stent of fixed diameter and length.

Results

Management of Variceal Hemorrhage Not Controlled by Sclerotherapy

TIPS reduces the portosystemic gradient in the vast majority of patients, usually to a value less than 12 mmHg. More importantly, such a shunt controls acute bleeding refractory to endoscopic sclerotherapy in about 95% of cases. In fact, continued bleeding with a functioning TIPS should prompt a second endoscopy to look for another source of hemorrhage. As TIPS has generally been applied to sclerotherapy failures, prospective data comparing TIPS with endoscopic

therapy as primary therapy for variceal bleeding has been limited.

More data are available comparing TIPS with endoscopic therapy for prevention of recurrent bleeding following a variceal hemorrhage that either subsided spontaneously or was initially controlled by endoscopic methods. This so-called secondary prophylaxis has now been evaluated in nine randomized, controlled trials.[4, 5, 15, 23, 33, 39, 46, 49, 51] In some of the trials, TIPS was compared with endoscopic therapy plus beta-blocker administration.[15, 46, 51] One study compared TIPS with endoscopic banding,[39] and another compared TIPS with both sclerotherapy and banding.[46] The results of these studies have been remarkably consistent and can be summarized as follows:

1. TIPS reduces the incidence and magnitude of rebleeding as well as the number of hospital admissions for rebleeding.

2. Shunt insufficiency (stenosis, occlusion) and associated rebleeding are major problems with TIPS but are readily prevented if shunt surveillance is performed regularly.

3. A TIPS is associated with about a twofold higher incidence of hepatic encephalopathy, which is usually re-

versible with medical measures, compared with endoscopic therapy for bleeding varices.

4. TIPS procedures result in rates of survival similar to those for endoscopic therapy.

Not surprisingly, these results are consistent with previous data comparing surgical shunts and endoscopic sclerotherapy for the prevention of rebleeding. Meta-analyses of the outcomes of all randomized studies comparing surgical shunts with sclerotherapy have also shown that shunts are far more effective in controlling bleeding at the cost of a higher incidence of portosystemic encephalopathy and are no different from sclerotherapy in terms of survival outcome.[11, 59] The hope was that TIPS, with lower procedural morbidity and mortality compared with surgical shunts, would fare better against sclerotherapy in terms of survival benefit. Unfortunately, current data indicate that TIPS is no more effective than endoscopic therapy in prolonging life.

Refractory Ascites

Refractory ascites is defined as ascites that either fails to respond to maximal medical therapy or responds at the cost of debilitating complications. This disorder is associated with an extremely high mortality and often heralds the development of hepatorenal syndrome.[1] In patients who are appropriate candidates, liver transplantation is the optimal solution. Unfortunately, because resources for liver transplantation are limited, other therapeutic alternatives must often be used. These alternatives are:

* Repeated large-volume paracentesis
* Peritoneovenous (LeVeen or Denver) shunts
* TIPS

Paracentesis is usually the initial therapeutic alternative if the patient's symptoms can be controlled with procedures at acceptable intervals. Unfortunately, frequent taps may lead to protein depletion and intravascular hypovolemia. Therefore, alternative solutions are frequently sought.

Peritoneovenous shunting can lead to a dramatic short-term results, reducing the ascites while expanding intravascular volume and promoting diuresis.[66] The major disadvantages of this approach are a high frequency of shunt occlusion, coagulopathy, and infection.[66] Indeed, in many centers, these shortcomings have led to the abandonment of the technique.

Alternatively, the creation of a TIPS has been shown to be effective for the control of diuretic-refractory ascites in the majority of patients. Following TIPS, there are increases in urinary sodium excretion and, to a lesser extent, the glomerular filtration rate.[2, 67-69] Several uncontrolled studies of TIPS for refractory ascites have been reported. The rate of success (complete or partial resolution of ascites) ranges between 50% and 100%, with failures occurring primarily in patients with very severe liver disease or coexistent renal dysfunction. In a significant number of patients, the results have been dramatic, allowing complete withdrawal of diuretics.[34, 60]

The disadvantages of TIPS in the patient with intractable ascites include (1) the risk of encephalopathy and (2) accelerated hepatic failure.

The risk of encephalopathy may be reduced with the use of a smaller-diameter shunt. Because ascites is not immediately life-threatening, consideration should be given to placing an 8-mm stent to reduce the risk of encephalopathy.[55] Available data do not support the need to lower the portal pressure gradient below a certain "threshold" value (equivalent to the 12 mmHg threshold established for variceal bleeding) in order to acceptably improve refractory ascites in most patients.

The more important risk is the acceleration of hepatic failure. This ominous complication should not be confused with hepatic encephalopathy, which is treatable with medical measures and protein restriction or with interventional narrowing or occlusion of the TIPS. Hepatic failure is characterized by progressive and intractable jaundice, coagulopathy, and encephalopathy. This complication is most likely to occur in patients with advanced liver disease, manifested as a prolonged prothrombin time (>17.5 seconds) and hyperbilirubinemia prior to the procedure.[33, 47] Preexisting azotemia also appears to have an adverse effect on outcome.[33]

Hepatic hydrothorax is a complication of ascites in which the fluid tracks into the pleural space through defects in the diaphragm. If the condition fails to respond to diuretics, it can be very disabling and may require frequent thoracentesis. TIPS has been reported to be effective for this condition, which is now regarded as an accepted indication.[14, 19, 61]

On the basis of available data, TIPS appears to hold promise for the management of refractory ascites, but its place versus repeated paracentesis procedures and peritoneovenous shunting still needs to be established by randomized clinical trials.

Complications

The TIPS procedure is clearly versatile and can be performed safely in most clinical settings. Complications do occur, however. They can be divided into two groups: technical and functional.

The major technical complications of TIPS are:

* Bleeding
* Sepsis
* Contrast-induced renal failure

Bleeding can occur (1) into the gastrointestinal tract owing to hemobilia or (2) intraperitoneally because of puncture of the liver capsule or perforation of a mesenteric vein.[12, 13, 53] Though bleeding secondary to the procedure can be fatal, it is fortunately rare, occurring in less than 3% of patients.[27]

Fever is observed in 10% to 20% of patients following the procedure.[27] Bacterial contamination at the jugular vein entry site is most commonly considered the source. Routine prophylactic antibiotics to cover Staphylococcus should be used in most cases.

Renal failure attributable to contrast agent allergy is observed in 2% to 15% of patients. The amount of contrast agent should be limited in all patients. Carbon dioxide may be used as a contrast agent to minimize the dose of iodinated contrast agent in patients with preexisting renal insufficiency.

Other complications related to a TIPS procedure are cardiac dysrhythmias,[29] myocardial infarction, and stent dislodgment into the systemic circulation.[6, 48, 65]

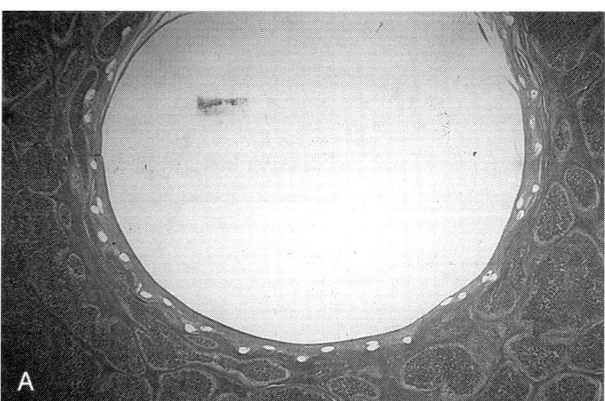
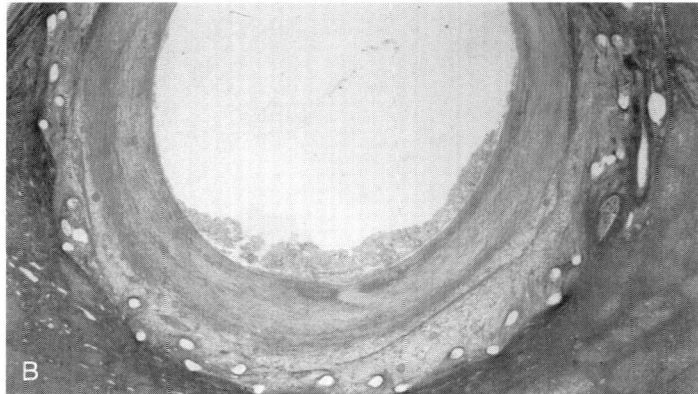

FIGURE 116–6. Histology of a transjugular intrahepatic portosystemic shunt (TIPS). *A*, Patent TIPS at 1 year. This patient received a transplant 1 year after TIPS. Histologic cross section of the shunt shows a widely patent shunt with a thin layer of neo-intima lining the metallic stent. The circular holes between the liver parenchyma and the neo-intima represent the spaces where the stent wires have been removed. *B*, Stenotic shunt at 6 months. This patient died of recurrent bleeding 6 months after TIPS. Note the exuberant neo-intima that has built up within the shunt channel, resulting in narrowing of the shunt lumen and hemodynamic compromise.

Functional complications of a TIPS procedure include

- Encephalopathy
- Shunt stenosis or occlusion

New or worsened encephalopathy is observed in about 25% of patients.[57] Elderly patients appear to be at more risk for TIPS-induced encephalopathy. Fortunately, the majority of such cases can be managed medically with protein restriction and lactulose therapy. In patients who experience disabling encephalopathy despite maximal medical therapy, expeditious liver transplantation is the optimal solution. Unfortunately, this solution is often impractical. As alternatives, the shunt can be occluded percutaneously[24] or shunt flow can be limited by a percutaneously placed "reducing" stent.[17, 20]

The most difficult problem with TIPS, however, is its lack of durability. All centers reporting experience with the procedure have indicated that significant stenosis and occlusions develop in at least a third of their patients within 1 year.[18, 28, 30] TIPS stenoses occur at points where the layer of neo-intima proliferates excessively (Fig. 116–6).[26] Stenoses occur either within the parenchymal segment of the shunt or in the hepatic vein cephalad to the stent (Fig. 116–7). Although these lesions are easily treated by balloon dilatation, there clearly is a need for ultrasonographic surveillance (performed initially at 3-month intervals) and repeated interventions to maintain patency.

It is likely that, as better technical methods such as covered stents are developed and the cause of neo-intimal stenosis is more clearly understood, this limitation of TIPS will be overcome. Early data from animal experiments and pilot clinical studies[35, 52] using these covered stents are encouraging, with a substantial decrease in restenosis. In a series reported by Saxon and colleagues,[52] six patients with recurrent TIPS stenosis underwent revision procedures for placement of a stent covered with polytetrafluoroethylene.

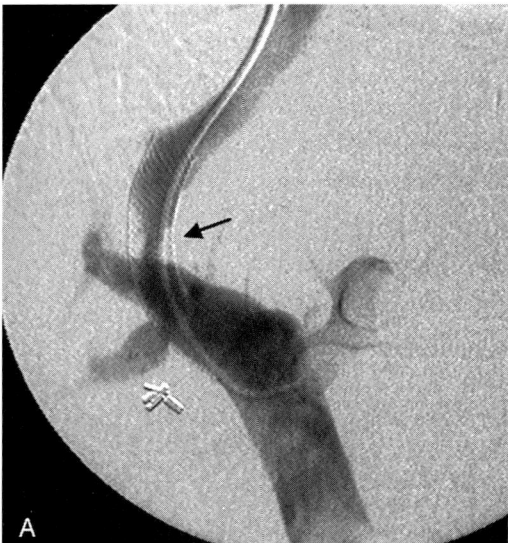
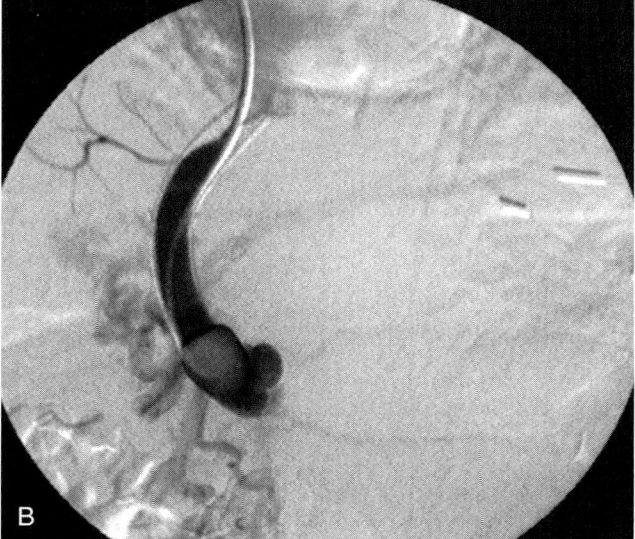

FIGURE 116–7. Transjugular intrahepatic portosystemic shunt (TIPS) stenosis may occur at the hepatic vein insertion site or within the shunt. *A*, Recurrent bleeding at 3 months is due to a intraparenchymal stenosis *(arrow)*. *B*, Recurrent bleeding at 8 months is due to a hepatic vein stenosis.

One patient died acutely of multiorgan failure, and one patient had stent occlusion at 1 month that was attributed to residual thrombus in a clotted portal vein. A single stenosis was encountered during follow-up of the four remaining patients, with a mean follow-up time of 315 days.

SUMMARY

Percutaneous procedures performed under fluoroscopic guidance have become an integral part of the management of patients with complications related to portal hypertension. In some situations, these procedures can be used to salvage a previously performed open surgical procedure.

In other circumstances, the open surgical procedure has been replaced by the percutaneous alternative. With the percutaneous method, the native anatomy can be preserved, thus simplifying subsequent orthotopic liver transplantation. Procedures such as TIPS, however, do carry some of the same risks, encountered with the analogous open surgical procedure, such as bleeding and encephalopathy, and cannot be looked upon as trivial undertakings. Moreover, durability of the TIPS procedure has been disappointing, and repeated interventions are often necessary to maintain patency. The clinical impact of the procedure will increase considerably if the problem of recurrent stenosis within the shunt or outflow vein can be solved.

REFERENCES

1. Arroyo V, Gines P, Gerbes AL, et al: Definition and diagnostic criteria of refractory ascites and hepatorenal syndrome in cirrhosis: International Ascites Club. Hepatology 23:164–176, 1996.
2. Azoulay D, Castaing D, Dennison A, et al: Transjugular intrahepatic portosystemic shunt worsens the hyperdynamic circulatory state of the cirrhotic patient: Preliminary report of a prospective study. Hepatology 19:129–132, 1994.
3. Burgener FA, Gutierrez OH: Nonsurgical production of intrahepatic portosystemic venous shunts in portal hypertension with the double lumen balloon catheter. Rofo Fortschr Gels Rontgenstr Neuen Bildgeb Verfahr 130:686, 1979.
4. Cabrera J, Maynar M, Granados R, et al: Transjugular intrahepatic portosystemic shunt versus sclerotherapy in the elective treatment of variceal hemorrhage. Gastroenterology 110:832–839, 1996.
5. Cello JP, Ring EJ, Olcott CW, et al: Endoscopic sclerotherapy compared with percutaneous transjugular intrahepatic portosystemic shunt after initial sclerotherapy in patients with acute variceal hemorrhage: A randomized, controlled trial. Ann Intern Med 126:858–865, 1997.
6. Cohen GS, Ball DS: Delayed Wallstent migration after a transjugular intrahepatic portosystemic shunt procedure: Relocation with a loop snare. J Vasc Interv Radiol 4:561–563, 1993.
7. Colapinto RF, Stronell RD, Gildiner M, et al: Formation of intrahepatic portosystemic shunts using a balloon dilatation catheter: Preliminary clinical experience. AJR 140:709, 1983.
8. Coldwell DM, Moore ADA, Ben-Menachem Y, Johansen KH: Bleeding gastroesophageal varices: Gastric vein embolization after partial portal decompression. Radiology 178:249, 1991.
9. Cope C: Balloon dilatation of closed mesocaval shunts. AJR 135:989, 1980.
10. Cope C: Dilation of mesocaval shunts. Ann Radiol 29:178, 1986.
11. D'Amico G, Pagliaro L, Bosch J: The treatment of portal hypertension: A meta-analytic review. Hepatology 22:332–354, 1995.
12. Davis AG, Haskal ZJ: Extrahepatic portal vein puncture and intraabdominal hemorrhage during transjugular intrahepatic portosystemic shunt creation. J Vasc Interv Radiol 7:863–866, 1996.
13. Freedman AM, Sanyal AJ, Tisnado J, et al: Complications of transjugular intrahepatic portosystemic shunt: A comprehensive review. RadioGraphics 13:1185–1210, 1993.
14. Gordon FD, Anastopoulos HT, Crenshaw W, et al: The successful treatment of symptomatic, refractory hepatic hydrothorax with transjugular intrahepatic portosystemic shunt. Hepatology 25:1366–1369, 1997.
15. Groupe d'Etude des Anastomoses Intra-Hépatiques: TIPS versus sclerotherapy and propranolol in the prevention of variceal rebleeding: Preliminary results of a multicenter randomized trial. Hepatology 22:297A, 1995.
16. Hackworth CA, Leef JA, Rosenblum JD, et al: Transjugular intrahepatic portosystemic shunt creation in children: Initial clinical experience. Radiology 206:109–114, 1998.
17. Haskal ZJ, Middlebrook MR: Creation of a stenotic stent to reduce flow through a transjugular intrahepatic portosystemic shunt. J Vasc Interv Radiol 5:827–830, 1994.
18. Haskal ZJ, Pentecost MJ, Soulen MC, et al: Transjugular intrahepatic portosystemic shunt stenosis and revision: Early and midterm results. AJR Am J Roentgenol 163:439–444, 1994.
19. Haskal ZJ, Zuckerman J: Resolution of hepatic hydrothorax after transjugular intrahepatic portosystentic shunt (TIPS) placement. Chest 106:1293–1295, 1994.
20. Hauenstein KH, Haag K, Ochs A, et al: The reducing stent: Treatment for transjugular intrahepatic portosystemic shunt induced refractory hepatic encephalopathy and liver failure. Radiology 194:175–179, 1995.
21. Henry M, Amor M, Henry I, Tricoche O, Allaoui M: The Hydrolyser thrombectomy catheter: A single-center experience. J Endovasc Surg 5:24–31, 1998.
22. Heyman MB, LaBerge JM, Somberg KA, et al: Transjugular intrahepatic portosystemic shunts (TIPS) in children. J Pediatr 131:914–919, 1997.
23. Jalan R, Forrest EH, Stanley AJ, et al: A randomized trial comparing transjugular intrahepatic portosystemic stent-shunt with variceal band ligation in the prevention of rebleeding from oesophageal varices. Hepatology 26:1115–1122, 1997.
24. Kerlan RK Jr, LaBerge JM, Baker EL, et al: Successful reversal of hepatic encephalopathy with intentional occlusion of transjugular intrahepatic portosystemic shunts. J Vasc Interv Radiol 6:917, 1995.
25. Kerlan RK Jr, LaBerge JM, Gordon RL, Ring EJ: TIPS: Current status. AJR Am J Roentgenol 164:1059, 1995.
26. LaBerge JM: Histology of transjugular intrahepatic portosystemic shunts. Semin Intervent Radiol 12:384–388, 1995.
27. LaBerge JM, Ring EJ, Gordon RL, et al: Creation of transjugular intrahepatic portosystemic shunts with the Wallstent endoprosthesis: Results in 100 patients. Radiology 187:413, 1993.
28. LaBerge JM, Somberg KA, Lake JR, et al: Two-year outcome following transjugular intrahepatic portosystemic shunt for variceal bleeding: Results in 90 patients. Gastroenterology 108:1143–1151, 1995.
29. Lee EN, Mankad S, Shaver J, et al: Transjugular intrahepatic portosystemic shunt (TIPS) complicated by complete heart block (Letter). Anaesth Intensive Care 25:312–313, 1997.
30. Lind CD, Malisch TW, Chong WK, et al: Incidence of shunt occlusion or stenosis following transjugular intrahepatic portosystemic shunt placement. Gastroenterology 106:1277–1283, 1994.
31. Lunderquist A, Vang J: Transhepatic catheterization and obliteration of the coronary vein in patients with portal hypertension and esophageal varices. N Engl J Med 291:646, 1974.
32. Merli M, Riggio O, Capocaccia L, et al: Transjugular intrahepatic portosystemic shunt (TIPS) vs endoscopic sclerotherapy in preventing variceal bleeding: Preliminary results of a controlled trial. Hepatology 20:107A, 1994.
33. Nazarian GK, Bjarnason H, Dietz CA, et al: Refractory ascites: Midterm results of treatment with a transjugular intrahepatic portosystemic shunt. Radiology 205:173–180, 1997.
34. Nazarian GK, Ferral H, Bjarnason H, et al: Effect of transjugular intrahepatic portosystemic shunt on quality of life. AJR Am J Roentgenol 167:963–969, 1996.
35. Nishimine K, Saxon R, Kichikawa K, et al: Improved TIPS patency using PTFE covered stent-grafts: Experimental results in swine. Radiology 196:341–347, 1995.
36. Ochs A, Rössle M, Haag K, et al: The transjugular intrahepatic portosystemic stent-shunt for refractory ascites. N Engl J Med 332:1192–1197, 1995.

37. Palmaz JC, Sibbitt RR, Reuter SR, et al: Expandable intrahepatic portacaval shunt stents: Early experience in the dog. Am J Roentgenol 145:821, 1985.
38. Peltzer MY, Ring EJ, LaBerge JM, et al: Treatment of Budd-Chiari by a transjugular intrahepatic portosystemic shunt. J Vasc Interv Radiol 4:263, 1993.
39. Pomier-Layrargues G, Dufresne MP, Bui B, et al: TIPS versus endoscopic variceal ligation in the prevention of variceal rebleeding in cirrhotic patients: A comparative randomized clinical trial (interim analysis). Hepatology 26:137A, 1997.
40. Quiroga J, Sangro B, Nunez M, et al: Transjugular intrahepatic portalsystemic shunt in the treatment for refractory ascites: Effect on clinical, renal, humoral, and hemodynamic parameters. Hepatology 21:986–994, 1995.
41. Radosevich PM, Ring EJ, LaBerge JM, et al: Transjugular intrahepatic portosystemic shunts in patients with portal vein occlusion. Radiology 186:523, 1993.
42. Richter GM, Noeldge G, Palmaz JC, Roessle M: The transjugular intrahepatic portosystemic stent-shunt (TIPSS): Result of a pilot study. Cardiovasc Intervent Radiol 13:200, 1990.
43. Richter GM, Noeldge G, Palmaz JC, et al: Transjugular intrahepatic portacaval stent shunt: Preliminary clinical results. Radiology 174:1027, 1990.
44. Ring EJ, Lake JR, Roberts JP, et al: Using percutaneous intrahepatic portosystemic shunts to control variceal bleeding prior to liver transplantation. Ann Intern Med 116:304, 1992.
45. Rosch J, Hanafee WN, Show H: Transjugular portal venography and radiologic portacaval shunt: An experimental study. Radiology 92:1112, 1969.
46. Rossle M, Deibert P, Haag K, et al: Randomised trial of transjugular-intrahepatic-portosystemic-shunt versus endoscopy plus propranolol for prevention of variceal rebleeding Lancet 349:1043–1049, 1997.
47. Rouillard SS, Bass NM, Roberts JP, et al: Severe hyperbilirubinemia after creation of transjugular intrahepatic portosystemic shunts: Natural history and predictors of outcome. Ann Intern Med 128:374–377, 1998.
48. Sanchez RB, Roberts AC, Valji K, et al: Wallstent misplaced during transjugular placement of an intrahepatic shunt: Retrieval with a loop snare. AJR Am J Roentgenol 159:129–130, 1992.
49. Sanyal AJ, Freedman AM, Luketic VA, et al: Transjugular intrahepatic portosystemic shunts compared with endoscopic sclerotherapy for the prevention of recurrent variceal hemorrhage: A randomized, controlled trial. Ann Intern Med 126:849–857, 1997.
50. Sarfeh IJ, Rypins EB, Fardi M, et al: Clinical implications of portal hemodynamics after small-diameter portacaval H graft. Surgery 96:223, 1984.
51. Sauer P, Thielmann L, Stremmel W, et al: Transjugular intrahepatic portosystemic stent shunt versus sclerotherapy plus propranolol for variceal bleeding. Gastroenterology 113:1623–1631, 1997.
52. Saxon RR, Timmermans HA, Uchida BT, et al: Stent-grafts for revision of TIPS stenoses and occlusions: A clinical pilot study. J Vasc Interv Radiol 8:539–544, 1997.
53. Semba CP, Saperstein L, Nyman U, Dake MD: Hepatic laceration from wedged venography performed before transjugular intrahepatic shunt placement. J Vasc Interv Radiol 7:143–146, 1996.
54. Shiffman ML, Jeffers L, Hoofnagle JH, Tralka TS: The role of transjugular intrahepatic portosystemic shunt for treatment of portal hypertension and its complications: A conference sponsored by the National Digestive Diseases Advisory Board. Hepatology 22:1591–1597, 1995.
55. Somberg KA: Transjugular intrahepatic portosystemic shunt for refractory ascites: Shunt diameter—optimizing risks and benefits. Hepatology 25:254–255, 1997.
56. Somberg KA, Lake JR, Tomlanovich SJ, et al: Transjugular intrahepatic portosystemic shunts for refractory ascites: Assessment of clinical and hormonal response and renal function. Hepatology 21:709–716, 1995.
57. Somberg KA, Riegler JL, Doherty M, et al: Hepatic encephalopathy following transjugular intrahepatic portosystemic shunts (TIPS): Incidence and risk factors. Hepatology 16:122A, 1992.
58. Soyer P, Levesque M, Zeitoun G: Treatment of mesocaval shunt stenosis with a metallic stent. AJR Am J Roentgenol 158:1251, 1992.
59. Spina GP, Henderson JM, Rikkers LF, et al: Distal spleno-renal shunt versus endoscopic sclerotherapy in the prevention of variceal rebleeding: A meta-analysis of 4 randomized clinical trials. J Hepatol 16:338–345, 1992.
60. Stanley AJ, Gilmour HM, Ghosh S, et al: Transjugular intrahepatic portosystemic shunt as a treatment for protein-losing enteropathy caused by portal hypertension. Gastroenterology 111:1679–1682, 1996.
61. Strauss RM, Martin LG, Kaufman SL, Boyer TD: Transjugular intrahepatic portal systemic shunt for the management of symptomatic cirrhotic hydrothorax. Am J Gastroenterol 89:1520–1522, 1994.
62. Trerotola SO, Vesely TM, Lund GB, et al: Treatment of thrombosed hemodialysis access grafts: Arrow-Trerotola percutaneous thrombolytic device versus pulse-spray thrombolysis: Arrow-Trerotola Percutaneous Thrombolytic Device Clinical Trial. Radiology 206:403–414, 1998.
63. Uflacker R: Mechanical thrombectomy in acute and subacute thrombosis with use of the Amplatz device: Arterial and venous applications. J Vasc Interv Radiol 8:923–932, 1997.
64. Valji K, Bookstein JJ, Roberts AC, et al: Overdilation of the Wallstent to optimize portal decompression during transjugular intrahepatic portosystemic shunt placement. Radiology 191:173–176, 1994.
65. Wilson MW, Gordon RL, LaBerge JM, et al: Liver transplantation complicated by malpositioned transjugular intrahepatic portosystemic shunts. J Vasc Interv Radiol 6:695–699, 1995.
66. Wong F, Blendis L: Peritoneovenous shunting in cirrhosis: Its role in the management of refractory ascites in the 1990s. Am J Gastroenterol 90:2086–2089, 1995.
67. Wong F, Blendis L: Transjugular intrahepatic portosystemic shunt for refractory ascites: Tipping the sodium balance. Hepatology 22:358–364, 1995.
68. Wong F, Blendis L: Transjugular intrahepatic portosystemic shunt: Is it the ultimate solution for refractory ascites? Hepatology 22:1613–1615, 1995.
69. Wong F, Sniderman K, Liu P, et al: Transjugular intrahepatic portosystemic stent shunt: Effects on hemodynamics and sodium homeostasis in cirrhosis and refractory ascites. Ann Intern Med 122:816–822, 1995.
70. Zemel G, Katzen BT, Becker GJ, et al: Percutaneous transjugular portosystemic shunt. JAMA 266:390, 1991.

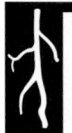

C H A P T E R   1 1 7

Operative Therapy for Portal Hypertension

Kaj H. Johansen, M.D., Ph.D., W. Scott Helton, M.D.,
and Layton F. Rikkers, M.D.

In a third or more of patients with hepatic cirrhosis, variceal hemorrhage results from underlying portal hypertension. Operative therapy for variceal bleeding is highly effective but is usually reserved for circumstances when all *nonoperative* therapies—risk factor modification, drugs, endoscopic treatment, angiographic intervention—either have failed or are contraindicated. The *other* major general indication for operative therapy—prophylactic intervention to forestall a catastrophic complication of a disease—has *not* been shown to be useful in the management of portal hypertension.

GENERAL PERIOPERATIVE CONSIDERATIONS

Patients with variceal hemorrhage are often both acutely and chronically ill and have multiple medical co-morbidities that complicate their hospital course and the conduct of operations. That stated, Child-Pugh class A and B patients whose variceal hemorrhaging has halted and who have been appropriately resuscitated constitute a majority of the cirrhotic "bleeders" seen in most clinical settings.

Because of its minimally invasive nature and excellent early success, angiographic shunt (transjugular intrahepatic portosystemic shunt [TIPS]) (see Chapter 116) has been utilized not only for poor-risk Child-Pugh class C patients awaiting liver transplantation, but increasingly also as "definitive" therapy for better-risk Child-Pugh class B and even A cirrhotic patients. Referrals for operative portal decompression have significantly declined. Yet TIPS's durability is demonstrably poor, with transhepatic stent channel primary patency and function rates only about 50% at 1 year.[1] Data from Helton's group demonstrate that TIPS results in markedly higher rates for 30-day mortality, repeat hospitalization, rebleeding episodes, and follow-up diagnostic studies than operative shunt in good-risk cirrhotic patients.[2] Clearly, it is premature to suggest that angiographic interventions have rendered operative portal decompression obsolete.

On the other hand, as noted in Chapter 114, anesthesia, major operation, significant blood loss, and diversion of hepatic portal blood flow are tolerated poorly by decompensated Child-Pugh class C cirrhotic patients. Therefore, when possible, patients with persistent jaundice, intractable ascites, spontaneous encephalopathy, and advanced muscle wasting should be managed by endoscopy, angiographic shunt, or, when appropriate, orthotopic liver transplantation. Not all such patients are terminally ill; temporary control of bleeding and vigorous nutritional and metabolic

resuscitation can frequently improve their Child-Pugh status and therefore their likelihood of surviving later definitive shunt therapy.[3] Similarly, documented abstinence from alcohol for 6 to 12 months in a previously refractory alcoholic patient with cirrhosis makes consideration of liver transplantation ethically reasonable.[4]

Another relative contraindication to operation is the presence of significant uncorrectable coagulopathy (e.g., a prothrombin time longer than 16 seconds, unresponsive to vitamin K). Such patients have excessive risks of intraoperative and postoperative hemorrhage, and operation should be withheld. Thrombocytopenia from hypersplenism is commonplace in patients with variceal hemorrhage, with platelet counts commonly in the region of 60,000/mm³; however, excessive bleeding is uncommon solely from platelet counts at these levels. Successful portosystemic shunting generally reverses hypersplenism and restores platelet counts to normal levels.[5]

Portal hypertension occurs in children usually because of extrahepatic portal vein thrombosis; hepatic function and coagulation status in this group are commonly normal, and bleeding can frequently be controlled with repeated endoscopic therapy. Pediatric patients with cirrhosis—for example, as a consequence of biliary atresia—are usually excellent candidates for liver transplantation. When interval portal decompression is required, a procedure that does not invade the right upper quadrant, such as a distal splenorenal shunt or a Clatworthy or prosthetic graft mesocaval shunt, should be considered.[6]

In the Budd-Chiari syndrome, congenital or thrombotic occlusion of the hepatic veins or the suprahepatic vena cava, or both, leads to acute hepatic congestion with severe right upper quadrant pain, massive ascites, and progressive hepatic dysfunction. It may occasionally be managed by interventional radiologic techniques, such as thrombolytic therapy or balloon dilatation (see Chapter 116). When such measures cannot be performed or are ineffective, operative therapy is warranted, since otherwise the condition is inevitably lethal. Bismuth and Sherlock have demonstrated that relatively early Budd-Chiari syndrome, without massive centrilobular necrosis or scarring noted on liver biopsy, can effectively be treated by portal decompression. In the presence of advanced hepatocellular destruction, optimal management is orthotopic liver transplantation.[7]

Angiography, including careful examination of the inferior vena cava, is crucial for patients with Budd-Chiari syndrome. If the inferior vena cava is patent, a side-to-side portacaval shunt (which converts the portal vein into an outflow tract for the congested liver) is curative.[7, 8] Others prefer a mesocaval shunt to avoid the subhepatic scarring that might complicate later liver transplantation.[9] In patients who have caval obstruction at or above the level of the liver, a portacaval shunt will not work; however, a mesoatrial shunt connecting the superior mesenteric vein to the right atrial appendage may satisfactorily decompress the portal system.[10] Patients in whom Budd-Chiari syndrome arises because of a hypercoagulable state may be at higher risk for treatment failure because of the greater risk of shunt or graft hepatic artery thrombosis.[11, 12]

Special concerns accompany the anesthetic management of patients with cirrhosis, especially those undergoing shunts or liver transplantation.[13, 14] Because generalized arteriovenous shunting seen in this condition may involve the pulmonary circulation, significant hypoxemia may be manifested.[15] Conduction anesthesia is imprudent in most patients because of the presence of coagulopathies and thrombocytopenia. Hepatocellular dysfunction slows clearance of anesthetic agents and sedatives ordinarily metabolized in the liver; cirrhosis is associated with upregulation of benzodiazepine receptors in the brain,[16] making such sedative agents relatively contraindicated. Fluid and electrolyte disorders—extracellular volume excess, respiratory alkalosis, total body potassium deficiency—can be anticipated. In actively bleeding patients, blood volume repletion results in many problems with volume shifts and dilutional coagulopathy. Endotracheal intubation of patients who have recently been bleeding is fraught with the risk of aspiration of gastric contents; this problem may be made more acute when ascites significantly raises intra-abdominal pressure.

Intraoperatively, intravenous vasopressin or octreotide may be administered, especially if the patient is bleeding; coronary vasoconstriction leading to myocardial ischemia (perhaps exacerbated by alcoholic cardiomyopathy) can result from administration of this agent. Concurrent administration of nitroglycerin may significantly reduce vasopressin's coronary vasoconstrictive side effects. Hypoalbuminemia and sodium excess in this group warrant consideration of volume repletion with a noncrystalloid extender such as plasma, albumin, or hetastarch.

EMERGENCY MANAGEMENT

Variceal hemorrhage can be torrential. Furthermore, a small percentage of patients may have early recurrence of bleeding or continued hemorrhage despite vasopressin administration and endoscopic variceal sclerotherapy or banding. As noted in Chapter 115, virtually all such early recurrent or persistent bleeding can be controlled with esophageal balloon tamponade. In fact, persistent bleeding in the face of these maneuvers should raise the possibility of a nonvariceal bleeding source—duodenal ulcer, esophageal ulceration secondary to sclerotherapy, or Mallory-Weiss tear. When bleeding is temporarily controlled by balloon tamponade, definitive management must be planned within the next 48 to 72 hours, by which time balloon tamponade must be discontinued.

In such a setting, angiographic shunt (TIPS) should be considered, if available; good short-term control of bleeding with this method has been demonstrated in about 90% of patients (see Chapter 116). TIPS is contraindicated in the hemodynamically unstable patient; Helton and colleagues demonstrated a 56% mortality, independent of Child classification, when TIPS was attempted in actively bleeding patients who had been inadequately resuscitated.[17]

Although general anesthesia and a major operation in a hypovolemic, malnourished, coagulopathic, chronically ill cirrhotic patient might seem to risk an overwhelmingly elevated morbidity and mortality, Orloff and Bell successfully performed emergency side-to-side portacaval shunts in more than 450 patients.[18] Although early mortality was 16% in patients undergoing emergency shunt, further variceal bleeding was eliminated and 5-year survival exceeded 70%. These remarkable results are ascribed to simplified diagnosis, operation within 8 hours, and aggressive lifelong follow-up; later demise correlated with return to alcohol consumption.[18]

If TIPS is unavailable and repeated endoscopic therapy is deemed imprudent (e.g., because of a recent course of variceal injections or banding), laparotomy and staple transection of the esophagus may be the optimal approach for emergency control of variceal bleeding.[19] Such a procedure is rapid, relatively straightforward, and effective (at least in the short term) and does not significantly interfere with consideration of a shunt or liver transplantation if the patient survives to be a candidate for either.

Thrombosis of the Portal Vein or Its Tributaries

Patients with variceal hemorrhage due to extrahepatic portal vein thrombosis generally cannot undergo TIPS. Liver transplantation, while possible,[20] is significantly more difficult. Portal decompression must be accomplished by splenorenal or mesocaval shunt. Because hepatic function in patients with portal vein thrombosis is frequently either normal or only minimally diminished, these subjects may have an excellent long-term prognosis.[21] Patients who suffer extrahepatic portal vein thrombosis and who have postnecrotic cirrhosis must be carefully screened for hepatocellular carcinoma by serum alpha-fetoprotein levels and hepatic imaging.[22]

Portal hypertension resulting from diffuse splanchnic venous thrombosis, commonly the result of a hematologic disorder,[23] may be difficult to treat. When the portal, splenic, and superior mesenteric veins are involved with diffuse thrombosis, the inferior mesenteric vein may sometimes be patent and can be anastomosed to the left renal vein, thereby effecting durable portosystemic decompression.[24] If this option is not available, devascularization by esophagogastrectomy[25] or a variant of the Sugiura procedure[26] may be the best option. In patients with cavernomatous transformation of the portal vein or diffuse mesenteric venous thrombosis, intra-abdominal variceal collaterals may be huge, but the temptation to anastomose one of these collaterals to the systemic venous circulation must be resisted; such "makeshift" shunts rarely remain patent.

The splenic vein may thrombose as a result of chronic pancreatic inflammation, usually secondary to alcoholic pancreatitis.[27] In such a setting, isolated "sinistral" or left upper quadrant venous hypertension may occur, manifested by massive splenomegaly, hypersplenism, and gastric varices. In such cases, splenectomy is curative. Polyvalent vaccine directed against encapsulated bacterial species

(Pneumococcus, Haemophilus influenzae, Neisseria meningitidis) must be administered to diminish the risk of postsplenectomy sepsis.

GENERAL OPERATIVE CONSIDERATIONS

Operations for managing the hemorrhagic complications of portal hypertension can be divided into two conceptual categories:

- Palliative procedures, which interrupt either the bleeding varices themselves or the venous channels leading to them.
- Definitive operations, which relieve the underlying portal hypertension either by a decompressive shunt or by liver transplantation.

Depending on the clinical circumstances, especially the urgency of treating variceal hemorrhage and the patient's clinical status, one or another of these treatment approaches may be warranted. Indeed, the patient's status may change significantly for better or worse, so that therapeutic options may develop or be eliminated by the passage of time and new clinical findings.

Devascularization Procedures

Direct operative attack on bleeding esophageal and gastric varices has been a well-established therapeutic concept for well over a century. Certain approaches, such as direct oversewing of variceal columns after thoracotomy and longitudinal esophagotomy,[28] are obsolete. Other devascularization procedures, usually variations of therapeutic themes combining splenectomy, gastroesophageal variceal plexus ligation, and occlusion of feeder channels such as the coronary, gastroepiploic, and short gastric veins, have been performed.[29, 30] While these procedures provide acceptable short-term protection against variceal rebleeding and may avoid the accelerated liver failure and encephalopathy resulting from portosystemic shunt procedures, intermediate and long-term follow-up show excessive rates of rebleeding. Accordingly, most of these procedures have fallen into disfavor.

An extremely aggressive devascularization procedure, including splenectomy, esophageal mucosal transection, and painstaking ligation of esophagogastric venous collaterals performed via staged thoracotomy and laparotomy, was originally promoted by Sugiura and Futagawa.[31] This procedure is relatively rarely performed outside Japan, although Orozco and colleagues[32] and Dagenais and Langer[33] have presented recent series with acceptable results. The relevance of this procedure to the management of alcoholic cirrhotic patients in Western cultures has been challenged.

The development of clinically usable surgical stapling devices led to the hope for simple, effective control of esophageal variceal hemorrhage by transection and reanastomosis of the terminal esophagus using the end-to-end anastomosis (EEA) stapling device.[34] Expectations that staple transection of the esophagus would prove to be a straightforward, rapid, and durable treatment for esopha-

geal variceal hemorrhage have not consistently been borne out by clinical experience[35]; however, as noted above, the approach may be an excellent "holding maneuver" while the patient is resuscitated to a state where more definitive therapy for variceal hemorrhage may be contemplated. In many major centers in Great Britain, staple transection of the esophagus is the initial operative approach for patients with variceal bleeding who are considered endoscopic therapy "failures."[19]

Portal Decompression

Because variceal hemorrhage results from underlying portal hypertension, reduction of portal pressure to normal physiologic levels invariably halts such bleeding. Bypassing splanchnic venous outflow obstruction by connecting the hypertensive portal system to the systemic venous circulation, either directly or by means of various autogenous or synthetic conduits, has proved a highly effective means of halting variceal hemorrhage.

Shunt operations appear to have been performed first in animals by Eck in 1885,[36] although the first substantive investigations of the metabolic effects of portosystemic shunts were performed in the 1890s in the laboratories of Pavlov,[37] also in imperial Russia. A resurgence of interest in portosystemic shunts paralleled the beginnings of arterial reconstructive surgery in the 1940s and 1950s,[38] and such procedures, usually end-to-side or side-to-side portacaval shunts, became commonplace therapy for variceal hemorrhage in the two decades after World War II.

Several complicating factors became evident. A characteristic neuropsychiatric disorder characterized by memory loss, altered levels of consciousness, behavioral changes, and (in its advanced stages) stupor, coma, and death, was noted to be a frequent and unpredictable result in patients who had undergone portosystemic shunt.[39] This syndrome, hepatic or portosystemic encephalopathy ("hepatic coma"), remains incompletely understood and has continued, in varying degrees, to complicate the subsequent course of all forms of portal decompression.

The nascent analytic tool of the prospective randomized clinical trial was used to investigate the effect on survival of portosystemic shunts both in variceal bleeders and in those whose varices had never bled. These studies showed that patients who survived a shunt operation rarely bled again. Those who had undergone a therapeutic shunt to treat previous variceal bleeding, however, were found to have, at best, only nonsignificant trends toward improved survival as compared with patients managed medically. Operated patients' sharply reduced risk of dying from bleeding was nearly equalized by a substantially increased likelihood of death from accelerated liver failure.[40-43] Patients who had undergone prophylactic shunting to prevent an initial episode of variceal bleeding were found to do worse than medically managed patients.[44] It is not surprising that a prophylactic operation would not help patients who had never bled, in view of the fact that only a third of cirrhotic patients with varices ever bleed from them.

More than a century ago, Pavlov's laboratory demonstrated that dogs subjected to portacaval shunting became listless and anorectic, suffered premature death, and at autopsy had hepatic atrophy.[37] Investigations in the 1950s and 1960s, summarized most elegantly by Starzl and colleagues,[45] suggested that an equivalent phenomenon in humans—accelerated hepatic atrophy and progressive loss of hepatocellular function—occurs because diversion of portal flow deprives the liver of a splanchnic venous factor (insulin seemed a likely candidate) necessary for normal hepatocellular function and regeneration. General acceptance of this "hepatotrophic theory,"[45] combined with the demonstration that portacaval shunts only minimally improved survival in prospective randomized trials, led to a significant decline in the performance of portacaval shunts and animated the basic and clinical investigations that led to the concept of the "selective" portosystemic shunt.

Drapanas and colleagues theorized that a conduit from a portal vein *tributary* (such as the superior mesenteric vein) to the systemic venous circulation might preserve prograde portal flow (and hepatic perfusion) while still effecting adequate portal decompression and protecting against further variceal hemorrhage. Development of the prosthetic interposition mesocaval shunt quickly followed.[46] Although mesocaval shunting continues to be performed, its long-term efficacy is questionable. Initially constructed using large-caliber polyester (Dacron) grafts, mesocaval shunts had an unacceptably high rate of thrombosis (about 10% per year),[47] undoubtedly because of slow flow through the highly thrombogenic synthetic conduit. Better results were reported in 1990 with a small-caliber expanded polytetrafluoroethylene (PTFE) interposition graft between the superior mesenteric vein and the infrarenal vena cava.[48] Interposition of autologous tissue (most commonly internal jugular vein) as a mesocaval graft probably has the best chance of long-term patency.[49] The underlying premise—that hepatic portal venous perfusion can be preserved by a mesocaval shunt—has *not* been borne out. Such patients have a risk of post-shunt complications equivalent to that of patients subjected to standard portacaval shunting.[47]

Decompressing the portal system while maintaining prograde portal flow seems a hemodynamic impossibility. A hypothesis of more enduring value has been that of the "selective" splanchnic-systemic shunt, most vigorously pursued in investigations of the distal splenorenal shunt by Warren and coworkers.[50–53] Warren based his concept on the premise that portal venous perfusion of the liver could be maintained only if pressure in the portal vein remained high enough to overcome the significant resistance to flow associated with the cirrhotic perisinusoidal block. On the other hand, if the gastrosplenic circulation, into which the gastroesophageal variceal plexus collateralizes via the short gastric veins, could be separated from the hypertensive portomesenteric venous system, the esophagogastric variceal plexus could be decompressed into the nearby left renal vein (or even the vena cava) without disturbing prograde portal venous flow to the liver. Thus, the concept of Warren's distal splenorenal shunt (Fig. 117–1) was developed. The operation consists of end-to-side anastomosis of the splenic vein to the left renal vein, combined with meticulous ligation of all collateral veins that connect, or might connect, the high-pressure portomesenteric and low-pressure gastrosplenic venous circuits.

Initial clinical trials of the distal splenorenal shunt appeared to bear out the theoretical rationale behind the procedure. Despite a number of relative or absolute contraindications (active variceal hemorrhage, ascites, Child-Pugh class C liver status, history of splenectomy, retrograde portal venous flow or portal vein thrombosis, unfavorable splenic or left renal venous anatomy), the procedure reliably protects against variceal rebleeding, and encephalopathy rates in most series are lower than those for standard portacaval shunts. Because the Warren shunt avoids the hepatic hilum, it is considered by many to be the optimal shunt for patients who may be liver transplantation candidates in the future. Distal splenorenal shunt became the portal decompressive approach of choice in many medical centers during the 1970s and 1980s.

Recent analyses, however, have clouded the validity of the selective shunt hypothesis. A gradual but predictable loss of selectivity of the distal splenorenal shunt,[54, 55] principally because of development of peripancreatic venous collaterals from the high-pressure portomesenteric circulation to the splenic vein, effectively converts the initially selective shunt to a total shunt.[33] Loss of prograde portal flow, or even portal vein thrombosis, can be demonstrated in as

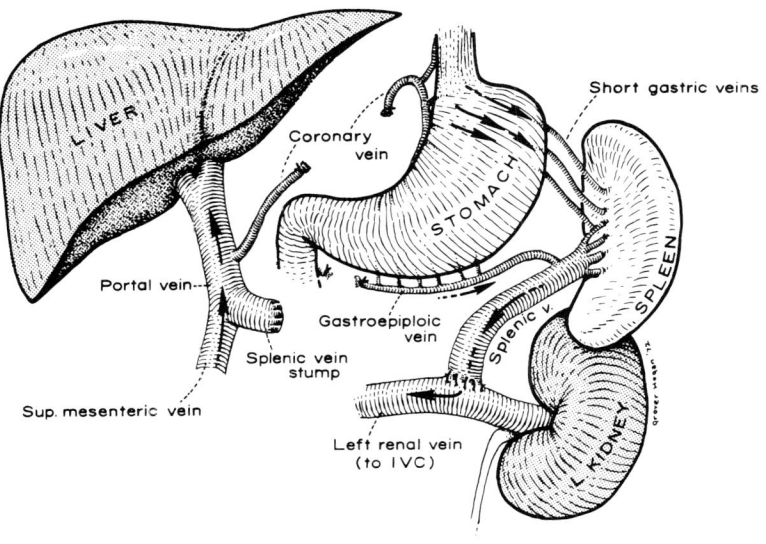

FIGURE 117–1. Conceptually, the distal splenorenal shunt of Warren and colleagues combines decompression of the esophagogastric variceal complex via the short gastric veins, the spleen, and the splenic vein into the left renal vein with maintenance of a high-pressure portomesenteric circulation. This latter state results from closure of the central end of the splenic vein as well as meticulous ligation of all potential right-to-left coronary and gastroepiploic venous collaterals. IVC = inferior vena cava.

many as 50% of distal splenorenal shunt patients at 1-year follow-up. For reasons that are unclear, this appears to be much more common in alcoholic cirrhotic patients than in those whose liver dysfunction is caused by other diseases.[56]

Warren and coworkers responded with a technical tactic—"splenopancreatic dissociation," complete dissection of the splenic vein out of its pancreatic bed—to obviate this inexorable collateralization.[53] Although clinical evidence supports the utility of this approach, splenopancreatic dissociation renders an already technically challenging operative procedure even more lengthy, tedious, and risky.

Long-term analyses of outcomes after distal splenorenal shunt with splenopancreatic dissociation show somewhat improved outcomes, but it has not been definitively demonstrated that this maneuver provides durable protection against loss of selectivity of the splenorenal shunt. Prospective randomized comparisons of selective and total shunts have not demonstrated a survival advantage for patients undergoing selective shunt.[57–59]

What may be the ultimate selective portal decompression technique is the coronary-caval shunt. This procedure re-routes the coronary vein flow into the infrahepatic vena cava, either by direct end-to-side anastomosis or by means of an interposed saphenous vein graft. Inokuchi and colleagues reported excellent results, with 2.2% operative mortality, 7.4% variceal rebleeding, and no new encephalopathy, in 146 patients followed for an average of 66 months.[60] The procedure is technically challenging and has rarely been performed outside Japan.

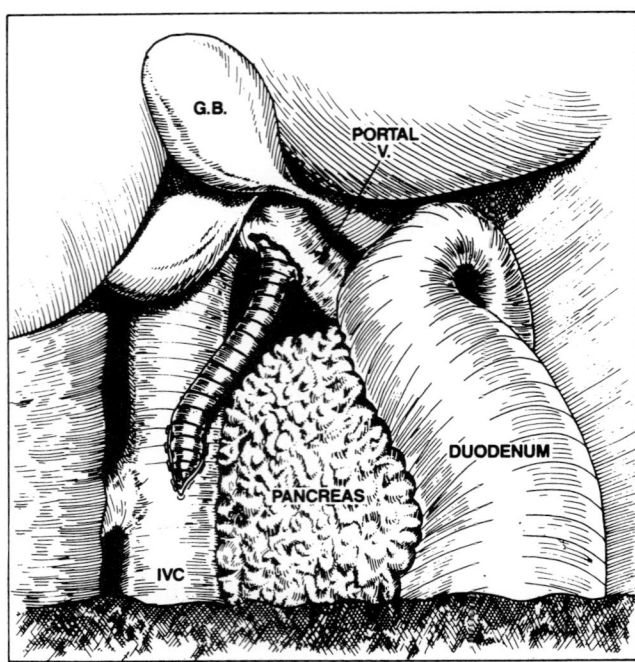

FIGURE 117–2. The portacaval H-graft shunt of Sarfeh and colleagues uses a 6-, 8-, or 10-mm externally reinforced polytetrafluoroethylene (PTFE) graft interposed between the inferior vena cava (left) and the portal vein (right). G.B. = gallbladder; IVC = inferior vena cava. (From Sarfeh IJ, Rypins EB, Mason GR: A systematic appraisal of portacaval H-graft diameters. Clinical and hemodynamic perspectives. Ann Surg 204:356, 1986.)

Partial Portal Decompression

Portal perfusion is lost after total shunt (end-to-side or side-to-side portacaval shunt, central splenorenal shunt, mesocaval shunt). Because resistance to flow is so much less through the shunt and into the systemic venous circulation than in the portal vein, hilar portal venous flow reverses and the vessel becomes a venous outflow tract toward the shunt. Hepatic perfusion is then provided entirely by the hepatic artery. In fact, it has been hypothesized that a patient's ability to tolerate a total portosystemic shunt is based on the capacity of the hepatic artery to enlarge in response to loss of hepatic portal perfusion.[61]

The possibility that prograde portal flow could be maintained by forming a smaller, higher-resistance portosystemic shunt was investigated initially by Marion[62] and by Bismuth and their respective colleagues.[63] In the 1980s, Sarfeh and colleagues introduced the concept of the small-caliber PTFE interposition portacaval graft (Fig. 117–2).[64] Although their study population was small and initial reports suggested a substantial risk of graft thrombosis, the procedure is technically straightforward and its protection against post-shunt encephalopathy seems satisfactory. Rypins and Sarfeh[65] and Collins and coworkers[66] ascribed this last favorable effect to preservation of hepatic portal perfusion, which they have demonstrated angiographically and by radionuclide techniques (although other studies of PTFE interposition portacaval grafts do not support this conclusion[67, 68]).

In 50 consecutive patients treated with direct side-to-side small-orifice portacaval shunt by Johansen, postoperative duplex ultrasonography[69] showed consistent loss of portal perfusion of the liver *despite* the relatively high resistance

of the shunt (10 mmHg portacaval pressure gradient).[70] However, an incidence of encephalopathy of only 6% in these patients suggested that the necessity of maintaining first-pass portal perfusion of the liver may not be relevant to the development of post-shunt encephalopathy. Studies in rats of end-to-side portacaval shunts suggest an inverse relation between splanchnic venous pressure and absorption of ammonia from the gut into the mesenteric circulation.[71] In a prospective comparison, patients treated with partial portal decompression had a late mortality risk of 13% and an encephalopathy rate of 8%, as compared with a late mortality risk of 39% ($p < .05$) and encephalopathy risk of 56% ($p < .0001$) in patients undergoing total shunt.[72] All patients in both groups had lost portal perfusion of the liver as demonstrated by postoperative duplex ultrasonography.

Whether partially decompressing portacaval shunts protect against encephalopathy and liver failure by preserving prograde portal flow[64–66] or by maintaining "physiologic" splanchnic venous pressures[67–73] remains unclear. The unacceptably high incidence of post-shunt complications with total portal decompression, and the ever-increasing technical complexity of the distal splenorenal shunt, have increased interest in the concept of partial portal decompression when an operative shunt is necessary.

OPERATIVE TECHNIQUES

Although this chapter is not intended to serve as a surgical atlas, certain elements of surgical technique for each of the commonly performed operations for complications of portal hypertension bear emphasis. More specific details on operative techniques may be found in several current surgical compendia.

Staple Transection of the Esophagus

EEA staple transection of the esophagus (Fig. 117–3) may provide effective short-term palliation for patients with persistent or recurrent esophageal variceal hemorrhage when definitive shunt surgery cannot or should not be attempted.[19]

Exploration is begun through an upper midline or left subcostal incision, and the proximal stomach and lower esophagus are mobilized. The stapler is inserted into the lower esophagus, in the open position through a high gastrotomy, a heavy suture around the outside of the distal esophagus is tied down snugly around the shaft of the stapler, and the device is closed. Firing the device then simultaneously divides and reanastomoses the distal esophagus, simultaneously dividing all variceal columns that traverse the lower esophagus.

Staple transection obviously does not treat gastric varices or portal hypertensive gastropathy; it may be rendered more difficult or impossible to perform if the esophagus is extensively edematous, inflamed, or scarred because of earlier endoscopic variceal therapy. Because the vagus nerves may unavoidably be divided during esophageal transection, pyloroplasty may be warranted to prevent postoperative gastric outlet obstruction.

Total Shunts

The goal of a total shunt is complete portal decompression. Theoretically, such shunts should be most likely to protect against further variceal rebleeding, and in general this expectation is borne out. Of more than 1700 portacaval shunts performed by Orloff, fewer than 10 (<0.1%) have been associated with proven variceal rebleeding (M. J. Orloff, personal communication). Shunt failure almost always results from an attempt to anastomose a partially or completely thrombosed portal vein to the vena cava rather than performing an alternative portal decompressive procedure.

Total shunts can conceptually be divided into the following categories:

- Portacaval shunts (end-to-side or side-to-side)
- Mesocaval shunts
- Proximal or central splenorenal shunts

Portacaval Shunts

The relative anatomic proximity of the portal vein and the inferior vena cava make creating a direct anastomosis between the two relatively straightforward, technically (Fig. 117–4). The patient should be placed in the left lateral decubitus position; many surgeons find "breaking" the patient with the kidney rest or a beanbag facilitates exposure to the intrahepatic vena cava and portal triad. An extended right Kocher's incision is made and carried laterally to the mid-axillary line. The general approach is from the lateral perspective (which enables portacaval shunting to be completed, even in the presence of adhesions from previous right upper quadrant operations). Extensive venous collaterals may be found in the subcutaneous tissue during the initial incision.

Abdominal exploration generally reveals ascites, substantial splenomegaly, fragile portosystemic venous collaterals in the retroperitoneum and at any sites of postoperative adhesions, and the cirrhotic liver in the right upper quadrant. The liver should be examined carefully for evidence of concurrent hepatocellular carcinoma (especially in patients with a history of hepatitis).

Attention is first turned to dissection of the inferior vena

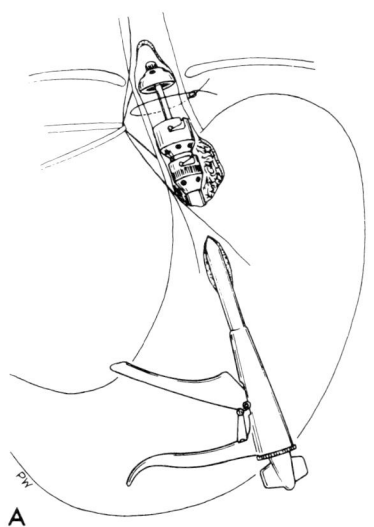
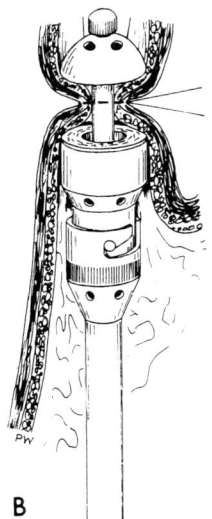
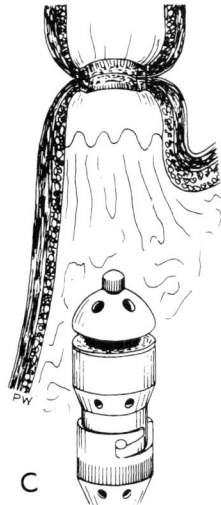

A   B   C

FIGURE 117–3. Esophageal transection using the end-to-end anastomosis (EEA) stapling device. *A,* Stapler introduced into the distal esophagus via a high gastrotomy. The distal esophagus is carefully dissected, and the vagus nerves are identified and preserved. *B,* A heavy monofilament suture is tied around the esophagus overlying the stapler's central rod in the "open" position. *C,* After firing, the stapler is removed, and the gastrotomy is closed in two layers. The area of esophageal transection and reanastomosis is carefully inspected, and the tissue "donut" from the stapler is checked for completeness.

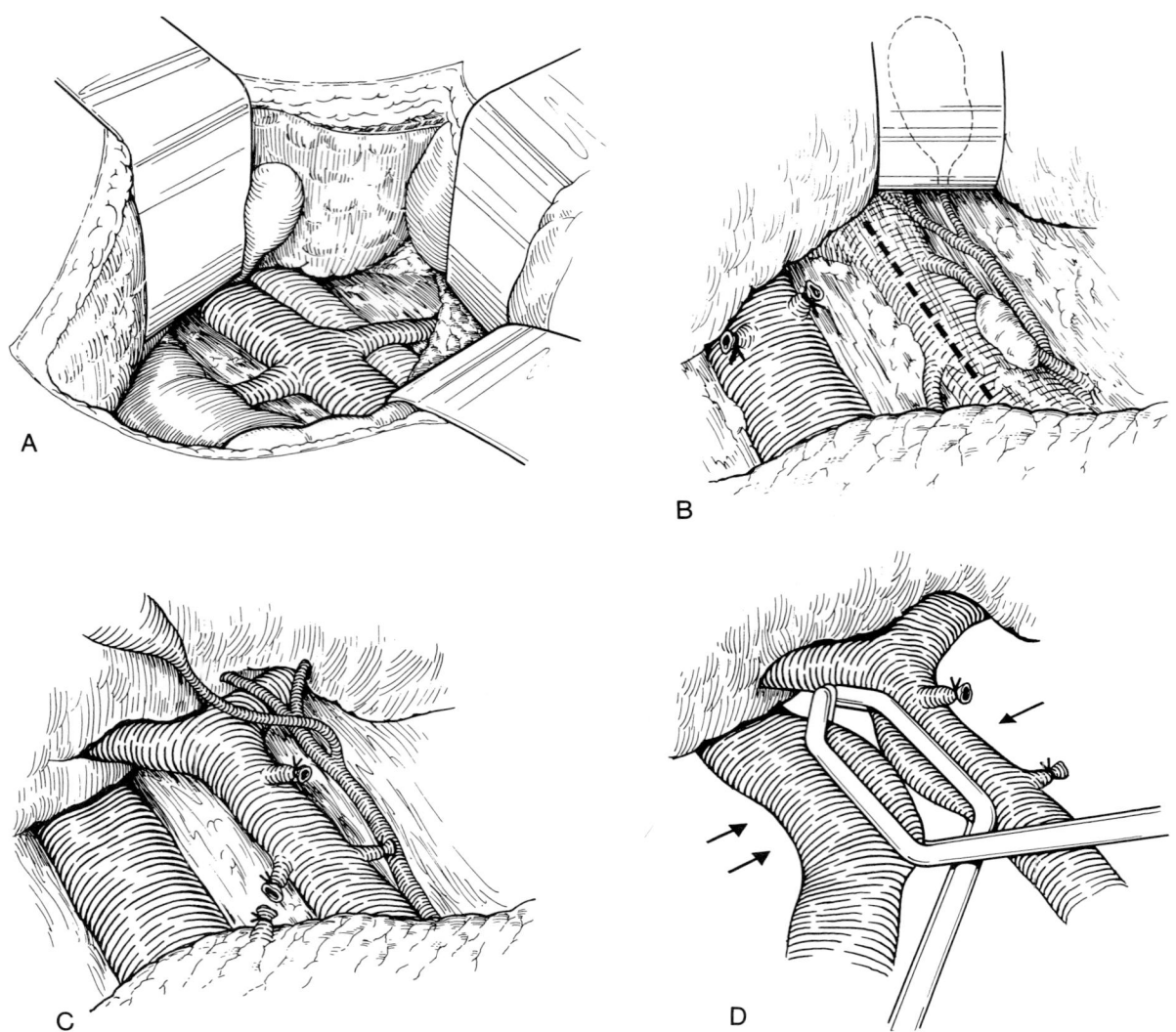

FIGURE 117–4. Portacaval shunt. *A,* An extensive Kocher maneuver is performed to expose the infrahepatic inferior vena cava caudally to a point just below the renal veins. *B,* Exposing the portal vein is best approached by incising the peritoneum over the lateral hepatoduodenal ligament *(hatched line);* alternatively, careful dissection of a prominent, anteriorly placed lymph node may expose the portal vein. *C,* Mobilization of the portal vein by careful ligature and division of one or more medially directed coronary veins (two are depicted here) and a constant, large posterolateral portal vein tributary from the head of the pancreas. *D,* Properly mobilized inferior vena cava and portal vein can be readily approximated for side-to-side anastomosis using apposing Satinsky clamps.

cava. After a generous Kocher maneuver, the vena cava is exposed in its entirety starting at its cephalad aspect where it is separated free from the caudate lobe of the liver (carefully dividing one to four caudate lobe veins) to a point just below the renal veins. No lumbar veins enter the vena cava cephalad to the renal veins; however, the right adrenal vein may be large, fragile, multiple, and located at any point from the retrohepatic inferior vena cava to the right renal vein. Careful and complete dissection of the inferior vena cava, including the central portions of the renal veins, is crucial because most of the mobilization that permits approximation of the inferior vena cava and the portal vein in the performance of a portacaval shunt is derived from careful caval dissection.

Attention then turns to exposure of the portal vein. The portal triad is palpated by passing a finger through the foramen of Winslow. Among other reasons, this maneuver ensures that there is no aberrant or replaced right hepatic artery in the lateral aspect of the structure (if it is present, it must be carefully preserved). Again, just as for the inferior vena cava, commencing the dissection cephalad near the hepatic hilum provides the best exposure to the portal vein. Incising the peritoneum overlying the portal vein, posterior and lateral to the common bile duct, usually exposes a substantial number of enlarged lymphatic channels and nodes. Removal of a characteristic large "sentinel" lymph node generally helps to expose the portal vein. This vessel is then carefully dissected from its bifurcation in the hepatic hilum caudad to a site where it disappears beneath the pancreas. *Extreme* caution must be exercised in dissecting medially beneath the common bile duct because one to four large, fragile, high-pressure coronary veins may

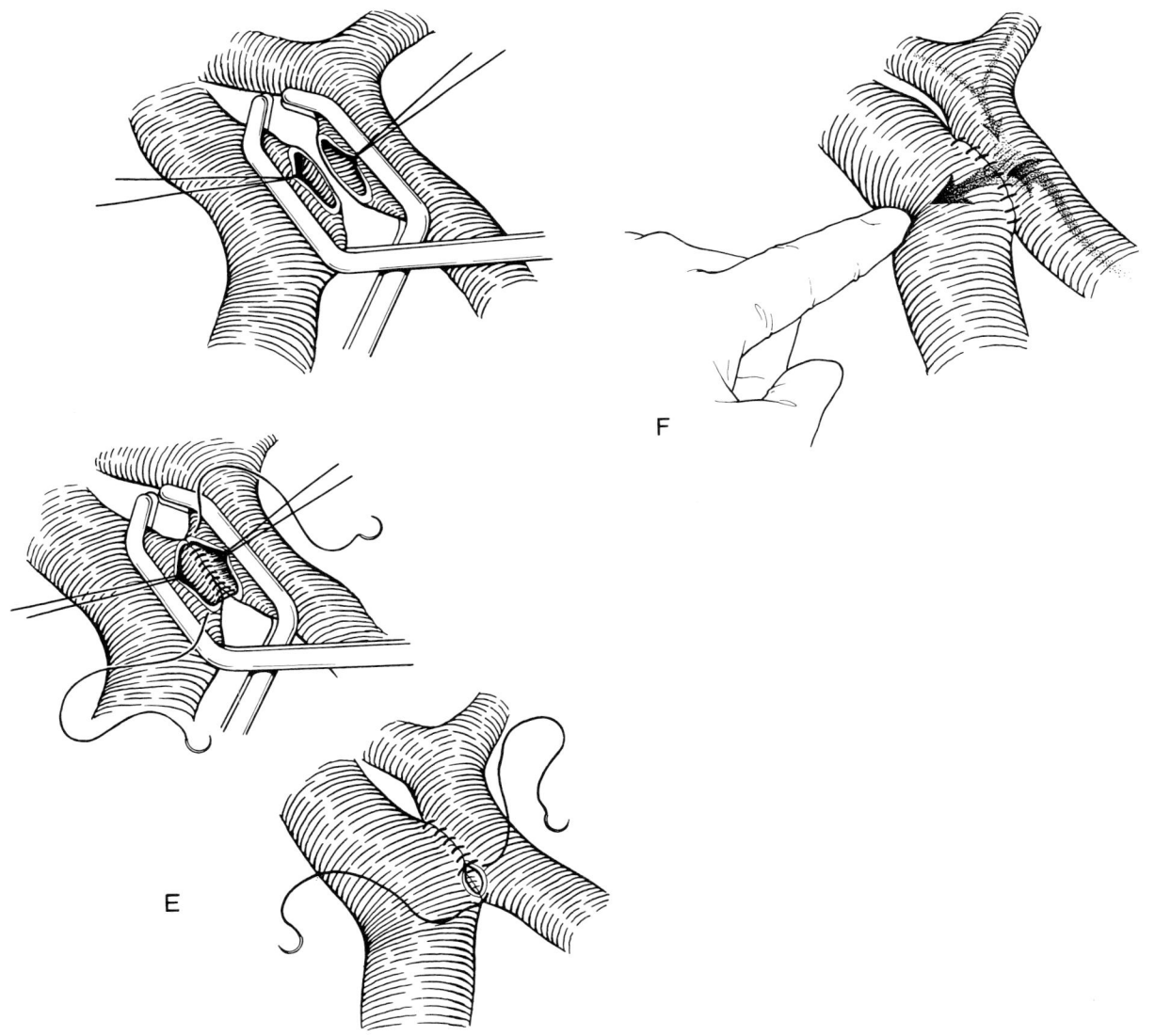

FIGURE 117–4. *Continued. E,* Completing the portacaval anastomosis. *Top,* A parallel cavotomy and portal venotomy are carried out, and stay sutures are placed as shown. *Middle,* After starting the anastomotic suture (a 4-0 or 5-0 monofilament stitch) at the top, the posterior walls are anastomosed from within using the first "arm" of the stitch. *Bottom,* The anterior closure is accomplished from the outside using the other arm of the stitch. *F,* Patency of the shunt can be assessed by palpation of the inferior vena cava wall opposite the shunt; a thrill is frequently noted. Pressures should be measured to ensure that portal decompression is adequate. (*A–F,* From Johansen K, Helton WS: The relief of portal hypertension. *In* Yao JST, Jamieson CW [Eds]: Rob and Smith's Operative Surgery, 5th ed. London, Chapman & Hall, 1994.)

reside there, and bleeding is extremely difficult to control if they are inadvertently avulsed.

End-to-side portacaval shunt is performed by dividing the portal vein as close to the hepatic hilum as possible, preferably even by dividing the right and left portal veins just cephalad to the portal vein bifurcation. This measure usually permits a relatively tension-free anastomosis to the side of the infrahepatic inferior vena cava. A Satinsky (or other partially occluding) vascular clamp is placed on the anteromedial surface of the vena cava. A linear cavotomy equivalent to the diameter of the portal vein is made, and the portacaval anastomosis is constructed between the end of the portal vein and the inferior vena cava using a 4-0 or 5-0 monofilament suture. Pressures should be measured in the portal vein and the inferior vena cava. If total

decompression is intended yet the portacaval pressure gradient (the difference between portal vein pressure and inferior vena cava pressure) exceeds 5 mmHg, the anastomosis should be dismantled and reconstructed.

Side-to-side portacaval shunting is thought by some surgeons to be technically more difficult than end-to-side shunting because increased tension between the two vessels to be anastomosed may result from the distance between them or by the intervening hypertrophic caudate lobe of the liver. In fact, it should rarely be a problem. *Complete* dissection of an adequate length of portal vein and inferior vena cava, and resection (if necessary) of a segment of caudate lobe (using the electrocautery or individual suture ligature of bleeding parenchymal vessels) should permit tension-free side-to-side portacaval anastomosis.

The shunt is constructed by clamping both vessels with Satinsky clamps, then making a longitudinal anteromedial cavotomy and a posterolateral portal venotomy, as close to the liver as possible. Each venotomy should be 2.5 to 3.0 cm long. The two venotomies are then anastomosed with fine monofilament vascular suture (4-0 or 5-0), "parachuting" down the posterior wall after placement of sutures.

On rare occasions, the gap between the portal vein and the inferior vena cava is too great to allow acceptable direct anastomosis. In this circumstance, interposition of a prosthetic vascular graft (see later) or, better, a segment of internal jugular vein or the left renal vein (divided over the aorta and anastomosed end-to-side to the portal vein) will suffice.

Mesocaval Shunt

Connecting the superior mesenteric vein and the inferior vena cava was initially thought to offer the possibility of variceal decompression while permitting continued portal perfusion of the liver.[46] This is now known not to be true; the mesocaval shunt is hemodynamically equivalent to a total portacaval shunt (Fig. 117–5). The mesocaval shunt has also been thought by some to be technically more straightforward than other portal decompressive procedures.

The operation is usually performed through a celiotomy incision. The inferior vena cava is generally exposed by leftward visceral rotation, including a Kocher maneuver. Alternatively, the inferior vena cava can be identified by dissecting dorsally through the root of the great mesentery, just to the right of the palpable aortic pulsation. The entire infrarenal inferior vena cava is dissected down to the iliac vein confluence, including ligature and division of several lumbar vein pairs (although the dissection need not be as extensive as that for portacaval anastomosis).

Attention is then turned to exposure of the superior

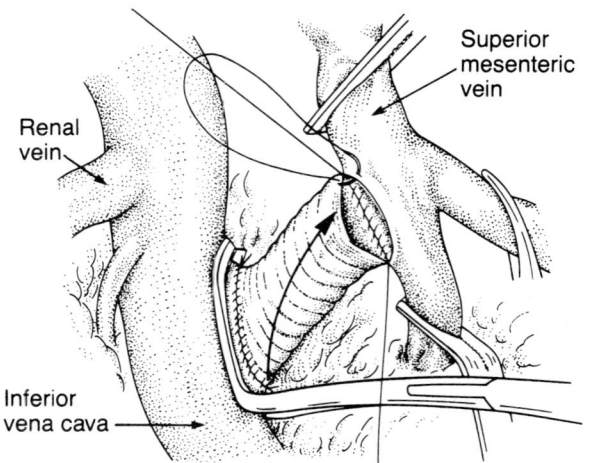

FIGURE 117–5. Mesocaval shunt. Anastomosis of a graft to the infrarenal inferior vena cava has been accomplished, and the anastomosis to the posterolateral superior mesenteric vein has been partially completed. Giving the prosthetic graft approximately a 30% clockwise twist (*solid arrow over graft*) accommodates the different vectors of the superior mesenteric vein and the inferior vena cava and eliminates any risk of kinking of the graft.

mesenteric vein. With the transverse colon retracted cephalad and the small intestine retracted to the right, a transverse incision is made at the base of the transverse mesocolon, near the ligament of Treitz. The peritoneum overlying the superior mesenteric vein is then incised longitudinally (best done with the electrocautery) for a distance of 5 cm, exposing the vein and several large branches. These tributaries may be ligated and divided to mobilize a 4- to 5-cm length of superior mesenteric vein.

An appropriate-sized graft—8- or 10-mm ringed PTFE or Dacron, or internal jugular vein—is then anastomosed end-to-side to an appropriate opening in the anteromedial surface of the inferior vena cava. The graft is then brought ventrally through the base of the mesentery, around the lower portion of the duodenum close to the superior mesenteric vein. The latter is clamped and rotated so that its right posterolateral aspect is anterior. A venotomy appropriate to the diameter of the graft is made, and the graft–superior mesenteric vein anastomosis is completed. When the clamps are removed, the graft should rest in a gentle curve below the duodenum.

Lower patency rates, and uncertainty about the proper graft material, make the indications for mesocaval shunt relatively limited. This procedure should be contemplated principally for patients with portal vein thrombosis or when the possibility of future liver transplantation favors avoidance of a right upper quadrant shunt. Relief of ascites and hypersplenism and acceleration of encephalopathy and liver decompensation are equivalent for mesocaval shunts and for other total portal decompressive procedures. The lower incidence of encephalopathy in some series probably relates to the higher likelihood of thrombosis of mesocaval shunts.

Central Splenorenal Shunt

Anastomosis of the splenic vein to the left renal vein decompresses the portal system, as in both central and distal splenorenal shunts (Fig. 117–6). Conceptually, however, the two procedures are substantially different. The central shunt is hemodynamically equivalent to a standard portacaval shunt and cannot preserve prograde portal flow.

The central splenorenal shunt is generally performed through a midline laparotomy or a transverse left upper quadrant incision. Splenectomy is performed, and the splenic vein is dissected centrally from its intimate attachment to the back of the pancreas. The left renal vein is exposed from beneath the pancreas and the transverse mesocolon. Gonadal or adrenal tributaries of the renal vein may be ligated and divided to free up this vessel. An end-to-side anastomosis of the splenic vein to the upper surface of the left renal vein is then accomplished, making sure that the splenic vein is not kinked at the lower border of the pancreas.

Like the mesocaval shunt, the central splenorenal shunt has the advantage of achieving effective portal decompression without involving the hilum of the liver. Early hopes to the contrary notwithstanding, this is a totally decompressing shunt that carries the same risks of encephalopathy and accelerated liver failure as any other total shunt. It is an excellent treatment for hypersplenism.

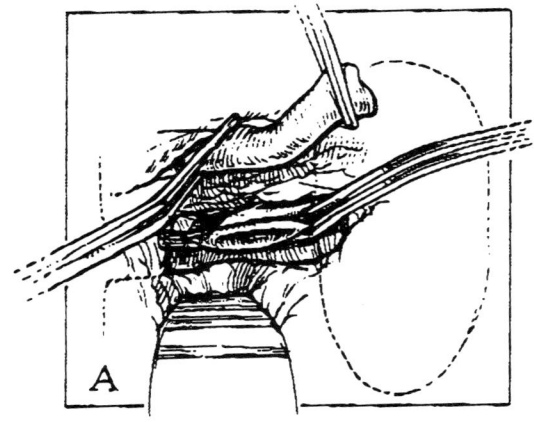

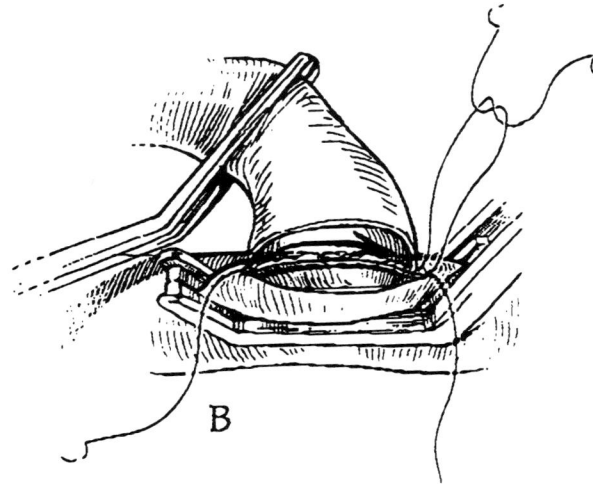

FIGURE 117–6. *A*, Proximal or central splenorenal shunt includes, after splenectomy, anastomosis of the mesenteric end of the splenic vein to the anterior-superior surface of the left renal vein. *B*, As for other portal decompressive shunts, suture of the posterior wall from within may facilitate anastomotic closure. (*A* and *B*, From Jones RS: Portal hypertension. *In* Jones RS [ed]: Atlas of Liver and Biliary Surgery. Chicago, Year Book Publishers, 1990, p 297. By permission of CV Mosby.)

Selective Shunt

Despite their excellent permanent protection against variceal rebleeding, totally decompressing shunts may result in accelerated liver failure and increased risk of portosystemic encephalopathy. Warren and colleagues designed the distal splenorenal shunt to provide isolated ("selective") decompression of the gastroesophageal variceal plexus while preserving portal perfusion of the liver.[50–53]

The distal splenorenal shunt (Fig. 117–7) is generally performed through an oblique left upper quadrant incision. It is composed of two parts: (1) anastomosis of the splenic end of the divided splenic vein to the left renal vein and (2) meticulous ligation and division of all potential venous collaterals between the portomesenteric and gastrosplenic venous beds.

The splenic vein is dissected away from the pancreas from above and behind (through the lesser sac) or from below the lower border of the pancreas. Initial reports

suggested dissection of just enough of the splenic vein to permit its anastomosis to the left renal vein. The subsequent finding that the low-pressure shunt attracts collaterals from the high-pressure portomesenteric circulation through the pancreatic "siphon" led to the concept of splenopancreatic dissociation—meticulous dissection, ligation, and division of all connections between the pancreas and the splenic vein throughout its entire length.[53] Extensive collateral ligation is performed by dividing the coronary vein (via a retrogastric approach), the gastroepiploic veins, the inferior mesenteric veins, and any other potential right-to-left collateral veins.

Distal splenorenal shunting cannot be performed in patients who have undergone splenectomy. It is also felt to be contraindicated in patients with ascites or with very poor hepatocellular function (Child class C), or when preoperative angiography demonstrates abnormalities of the splenic or left renal veins (unfavorable anatomic displacement, diminutive vessels, or areas of thrombosis). Because the procedure (especially with the addition of splenopancreatic dissociation) is a lengthy one, it is generally not indicated as an emergency decompressive operation.

Partial Portal Decompressive Shunts

Subtotal portal decompression has become an increasingly popular concept when operative shunting is required. In the approach utilizing direct side-to-side small-stoma portacaval anastomosis, complete vena cava and portal vein dissection and mobilization is accomplished, as described for a total shunt. Instead of a 2.5- to 3-cm anastomosis, however, a much smaller cavotomy and portal venotomy are created: 12- to 15-mm venotomies generally result in a portacaval pressure gradient of 7 to 12 mmHg.[72, 73] Collateral ligation is not considered important: persistently filling coronary veins can be readily embolized at postoperative trans-shunt angiography.[74]

In the interposition H-graft approach to partial portal decompression popularized by Sarfeh and colleagues,[64–65] initial operative exposure of the inferior vena cava and the portal vein is like that described earlier for total portacaval shunt. However, because the distance between the two vessels is bridged by an interposed synthetic graft, dissection of the two vessels need not be circumferential. Instead, it exposes only the anterior surface of the vena cava and the posterolateral surface of the portal vein. When side-biting clamps can be applied to both vessels, longitudinal venotomies are performed and a short, appropriately beveled 6-, 8-, or 10-mm segment of ringed PTFE is anastomosed end-to-side to both venotomies using fine (5-0 or 6-0) monofilament vascular suture (see Fig. 117–2). Sarfeh promotes the concept of assiduous collateral ligation to augment shunt flow and increase residual portal perfusion.

Liver Transplantation

Because it restores both portal pressure and hepatic functional reserve to normal, liver transplantation would appear to be the ideal therapy for variceal hemorrhage. In contrast to other operations described in this chapter that are directed specifically toward the treatment of portal hypertensive bleeding, transplantation is generally reserved for pa-

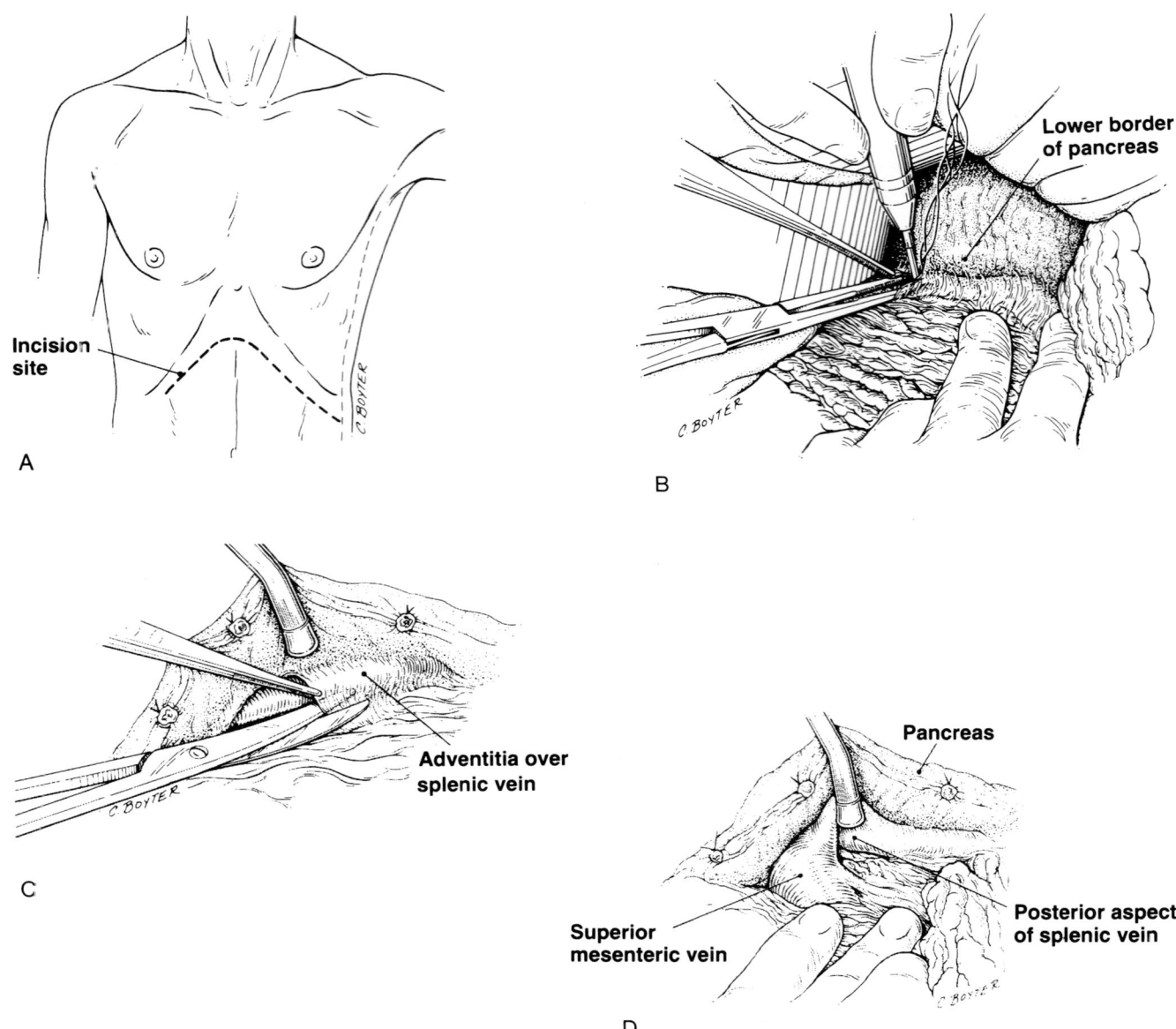

FIGURE 117–7. Steps in performing a distal splenorenal shunt. *A*, Exposure via a left subcostal incision, carried across the midline to the right side. *B*, Division of the gastrocolic omentum to expose the lower border of the pancreas. *C*, Exposure of the splenic vein caudal and dorsal to the lower border of the pancreas. *D*, Dissection of the splenic vein rightward to its junction with the superior mesenteric vein.

tients with end-stage liver disease, one symptom of which may be variceal hemorrhage. For example, although 28% of 652 adult patients who received liver transplants at one center between 1985 and 1992 had a history of variceal bleeding, only 34 (6%) had bled within a month of the transplant operation.[75] In the remaining transplant candidates, variceal bleeding had been successfully treated with either endoscopic sclerotherapy or portosystemic shunting, and the decision for transplantation had been forced by subsequent deterioration of hepatic function rather than by bleeding. During the same interval, 71 patients underwent shunt operations for treatment of variceal hemorrhage, either emergency or elective. Forty-four of these patients had been considered potential future liver transplant recipients, but to date only seven (16%) have required grafting because of the later onset of liver failure. Thus, in a referral

center for patients with chronic liver disease where sclerotherapy, TIPS, shunt surgery, and liver transplantation are all readily available, nontransplant operations are still performed more often than transplantation for definitive control of variceal hemorrhage.

Hepatic transplantation is rarely utilized as treatment for variceal bleeding per se. However, as noted in Chapter 114, the onset of variceal hemorrhage in a patient with chronic liver disease should always prompt the following questions:

- Is this patient a candidate for liver transplantation?
- If so, should the transplant be done in the near future or later in the course of the disease?
- What should be done to prevent recurrent bleeding until a transplant is indicated or a donor organ is available?

Most persons with variceal bleeding will never be transplant

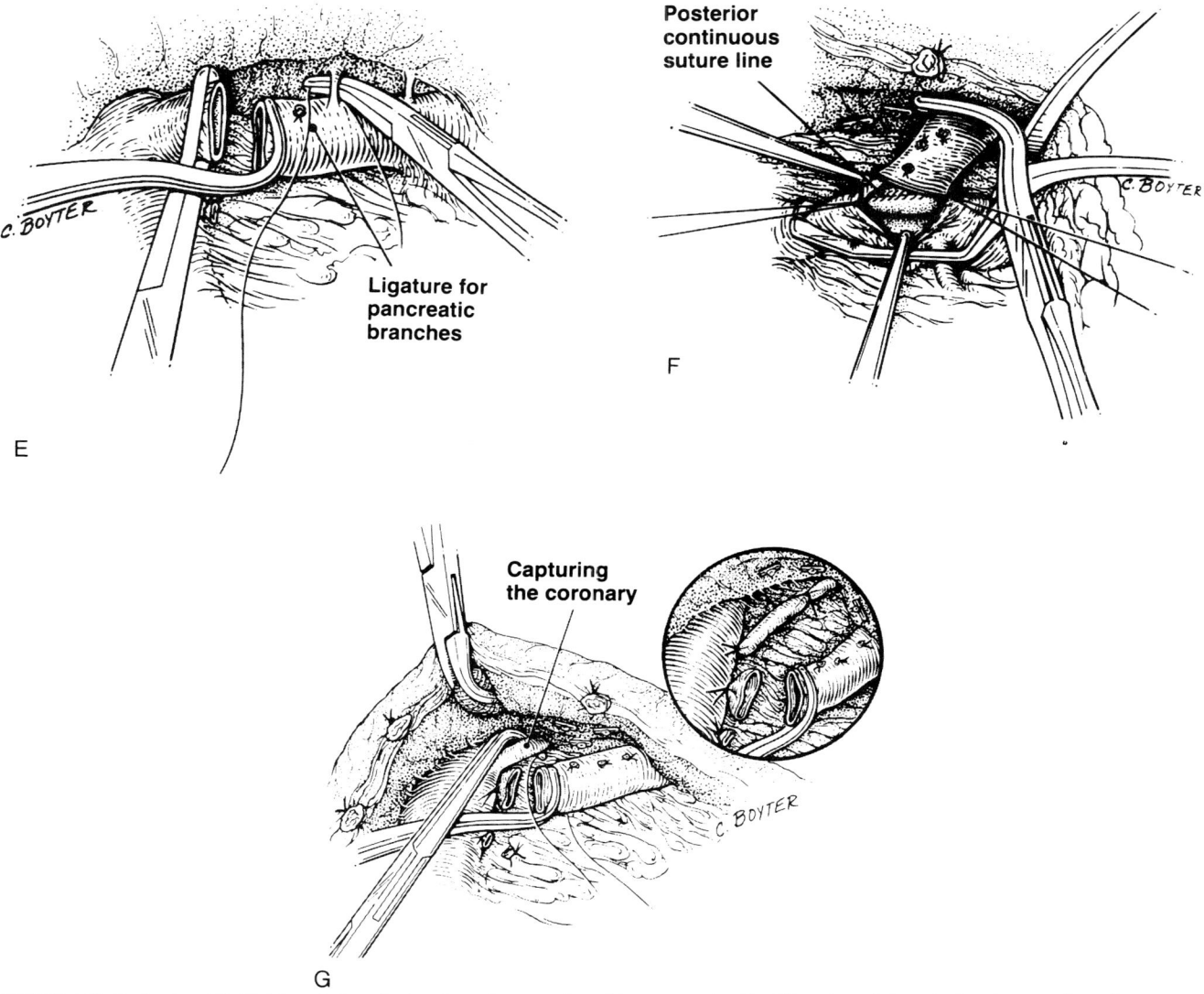

FIGURE 117–7. *Continued E,* Division of the splenic vein and oversewing of its mesenteric side. Dissection of the splenic vein away from the pancreas commences by painstaking ligation and division of multiple small, fragile pancreatic venous tributaries. *F,* After identification of the left renal vein, which lies behind and below, end-to-side anastomosis of the splenic and left renal veins is accomplished. The splenic vein may need to be shortened to avoid kinking of the shunt. *G,* Ligature of the coronary vein is a crucial component of the distal splenorenal shunt. It can be found exiting posteriorly from the hepatoduodenal ligament above the confluence of the splenic vein and the superior mesenteric vein. (*A–G,* from Warren WD, Millikan WJ: The distal splenorenal shunt. Contemp Surg 18:13, 1981.)

candidates. Even if they were, the limited donor organ supply would preclude transplantation for most of them. Persons with noncirrhotic portal hypertension (secondary to schistosomiasis, portal vein thrombosis, splanchnic arterioportal fistulae, or idiopathic portal hypertension) generally maintain their hepatic functional reserve indefinitely and have normal life spans when their bleeding can be successfully controlled by nontransplantation strategies.

In addition, a significant number of cirrhotic patients have one or more of the following contraindications to liver transplantation:

- Inoperability because of advanced dysfunction of another organ system (usually the pulmonary or cardiovascular system)
- Intractable medical noncompliance
- Acquired immunodeficiency syndrome
- Extrahepatic malignancy
- Active drug or alcohol abuse

Portal hypertensive bleeding can frequently be treated successfully in these patients by a single nontransplantation therapy or a sequence of treatments (e.g., chronic endoscopic therapy followed by TIPS or shunt when bleeding recurs).

The most controversial indication for liver transplantation is alcoholic cirrhosis, the leading cause of chronic liver disease and variceal bleeding in Western and industrialized countries. Several series have now demonstrated that short-term results of transplantation are at least as good in patients with alcoholic cirrhosis as in those with nonalcoholic liver disease. When alcoholic patients are carefully selected, based on either an interval of abstinence or an alcohol prognosis scale that takes into account numerous psychosocial factors, post-transplantation alcohol recidivism rates have been less than 20%.[76] Although the ethical issues surrounding expenditure of a limited resource on individuals with a self-induced disease continue to be debated,[4] a significant fraction of patients with alcoholic cirrhosis may be excellent candidates for hepatic transplantation.

Once candidacy for transplantation has been established for a variceal "bleeder," the timing of the operation must be determined. A key factor in this decision is the patient's hepatic functional reserve, which is most commonly assessed with the Child-Pugh classification (see Chapter 114). Patients who are Child-Pugh class C should undergo transplantation as soon as a donor organ can be located. Additionally, those with Child-Pugh class A or B disease whose symptoms adversely affect quality of life, such as extreme fatigue, encephalopathy, bone pain, or severe pruritus, should undergo transplantation rather than a palliative therapy directed only at preventing recurrent bleeding.

Most Child-Pugh class A patients should receive nontransplantation therapy for long-term control of portal hypertensive bleeding and should be seen at 6-month or 1-year intervals to assess the status of their liver disease. When it is apparent that the disease is progressive and is nearing end stage, they should be listed for transplantation. They should be treated with either chronic endoscopic therapy or a portosystemic shunt, depending on individual circumstances. Chronic endoscopic therapy is preferred for patients who have ready access to medical and surgical treatment so that recurrences of bleeding can be treated expeditiously. Patients who reside in a rural area, who bleed from gastric varices or lesions of portal hypertensive gastropathy, or who fail to respond to chronic endoscopic therapy are best treated with portal decompression.[77] Child-Pugh class B patients should be managed on a case-by-case basis after a comprehensive evaluation of their psychosocial situation, hepatic hemodynamics, and functional hepatic reserve to determine whether early or delayed transplantation is likely to produce the best overall results.

Owing to imprecisions inherent in the Child-Pugh classification,[78] quantitative tests of hepatic function (such as galactose elimination capacity and aminopyrine clearance) and estimation of hepatic mass by computed tomography have been used to determine the timing of hepatic transplantation in some center. The Emory group has proposed that variceal bleeders with a galactose elimination capacity less than 225 mg/min or liver volume less than 50% of the predicted value should undergo transplantation rather than shunting, because their hepatic reserve is insufficient to sustain life without transplantation.[79]

Patients with variceal hemorrhage who are early transplantation candidates can usually be treated successfully with one or more sessions of endoscopic variceal therapy (sclerosis or banding) until a donor liver becomes available. When bleeding persists or recurs repeatedly despite endoscopic therapy, portal decompression must be considered. The ideal procedure in this setting is TIPS because it does not require surgical intervention and does not usually interfere with later transplant operations. As noted previously, TIPS is less desirable for patients who are unlikely to require transplantation for several years because its durability is poor.[1,2] If expertise for TIPS is not available and urgent operation is required to prevent exsanguination, the operative procedure selected optimally should avoid the hepatic hilum so that future transplantation is not compromised.

That stated, most evidence indicates that a previous portosystemic shunt does not significantly compromise subsequent transplantation.[80,81] Post-transplantation survival rates are similar, regardless of history of portosystemic shunt; however, a previous shunt, especially when the portal vein is utilized, makes the transplantation more difficult and may increase the transfusion requirement.[81] Because they avoid the hepatic hilum, the distal splenorenal shunt and the interposition mesocaval shunts are probably the best alternative bridges to transplantation.

Contemporary results from major liver transplantation centers demonstrate operative mortality of 5% to 10%, 1- and 2-year survival rates exceeding 80%, and good to excellent quality of life in most graft recipients. Because chronic graft rejection cannot yet be predicted or prevented, liver transplant recipients may require another transplantation. Ongoing ethical debates about the suitability of liver transplantation for patients with alcoholic cirrhosis, as well as the procedure's extraordinary costs and the increasing deficit of donor organs, continue to limit transplantation for the great majority of patients with the complications of portal hypertension.

REFERENCES

1. Sanyal AJ, Freedman AM, Luketic VA, et al: The natural history of portal hypertension after transjugular intrahepatic portosystemic shunts. Gastroenterology 112:1040, 1997.
2. Helton WS, Maves R, Wicks K, Johansen K: Case control study comparing resource utilization after operative shunt or TIPS for variceal hemorrhage in Child A and B cirrhotics (Abstract). Gastroenterology 114:A1298, 1998.
3. Holman JM, Rikkers LF: Success of medical and surgical management of acute variceal hemorrhage. Am J Surg 140:816, 1980.
4. Moss AH, Siegler M: Should alcoholics compete equally for liver transplantation? JAMA 262:1295, 1991.
5. Soper NJ, Rikkers LF: Effect of operations for variceal hemorrhage on hypersplenism. Am J Surg 144:700, 1982.
6. Fonkalsrud EW: Surgical management of portal hypertension in childhood: Long-term results. Arch Surg 115:1042, 1980.
7. Bismuth H, Sherlock DJ: Portosystemic shunting versus liver transplantation for the Budd-Chiari syndrome. Ann Surg 214:581, 1991.
8. Orloff M, Gerard B: Long-term results of treatment of Budd-Chiari syndrome by side-to-side portacaval shunt. Surg Gynecol Obstet 168:33, 1989.
9. Hemming AW, Langer B, Greig P, et al: Treatment of Budd-Chiari syndrome with portosystemic shunt or liver transplantation. Am J Surg 171:176, 1996.
10. Tilamus HW: Budd-Chiari syndrome. Br J Surg 82:1023, 1995.
11. Halff G, Todo S, Tsakis A, et al: Liver transplantation for the Budd-Chiari syndrome. Ann Surg 211:43, 1990.
12. Campbell DA, Rolles K, Jamieson N, et al: Hepatic transplantation with perioperative and long-term anticoagulants as treatment for Budd-Chiari syndrome. Surg Gynecol Obstet 166:511, 1988.
13. Agarwal S: Anesthetic management during liver transplantation (Review). Transplant Proc 26:321, 1994.
14. Canton EG, Rettke SR, Plevak D, et al: Perioperative care of the liver transplant patient. Anesth Analg 28:120, 1994.
15. Yao EH, Kong MC, Hsue GL, et al: Pulmonary function changes in cirrhosis of the liver. Am J Gastroenterol 82:352, 1987.
16. Mullen KD, Martin JV, Mendelson WB, et al: Could an endogenous benzodiazepine ligand contribute to hepatic encephalopathy? Lancet 1:457, 1988.
17. Helton WS, Belshaw A, Althaus S, et al: Critical appraisal of the angiographic portacaval shunt (TIPS). Am J Surg 165:566, 1993.

18. Orloff MJ, Bell RH Jr: Long-term survival after emergency portacaval shunting for bleeding varices in patients with alcoholic cirrhosis. Am J Surg 151:176, 1986.

19. Burroughs AK, Hamilton G, Phillips A, et al: A comparison of sclerotherapy with staple transection of the esophagus for the emergency control of bleeding from esophageal varices. N Engl J Med 321:857, 1979.

20. Seu P, Shackleton CR, Shaked A, et al: Improved results of liver transplantation in patients with portal vein thrombosis. Arch Surg 131:840, 1996.

21. Webb LJ, Sherlock S: The etiology, presentation and natural history of extrahepatic portal venous obstruction. Q J Med 48:627, 1979.

22. Okuda K, Ohnishi K, Kimura K, et al: Incidence of portal vein thrombosis and liver cirrhosis: An angiographic study in 708 patients. Gastroenterology 89:279, 1985.

23. Schafer AL: The hypercoagulable state. Ann Intern Med 102;814, 1985.

24. Gorini P, Johansen K: Use of the inferior mesenteric vein for portal decompression. HPB Surg 10:365, 1998.

25. Orloff MJ, Orloff MS, Daily PO, Girard B: Long-term results of radical esophagogastrectomy for bleeding varices due to unshuntable extrahepatic portal hypertension. Am J Surg 167:96, 1994.

26. Caps MT, Helton WS, Johansen K: Left upper quadrant devascularization for "unshuntable" portal hypertension. Arch Surg 131:834, 1996.

27. Little AG, Moossa AR: Gastrointestinal hemorrhage from left-sided portal hypertension: An unappreciated complication of pancreatitis. Am J Surg 141:153, 1981.

28. Britton RC, Crile G: Late results of transesophageal suture of bleeding esophageal varices. Surg Gynecol Obstet 117:10, 1983.

29. Hassab MA: Gastroesophageal decongestion and splenectomy in the treatment of esophageal varices in bilharzial cirrhosis: Further studies with the report of 355 operations. Surgery 61:169, 1967.

30. Peters RM, Womack NA: Surgery of vascular distortions in cirrhosis of the liver. Ann Surg 154:432, 1961.

31. Sugiura M, Futagawa S: Results of 636 esophageal transections with paraesophagogastric devascularization in the treatment of esophageal varices. J Vasc Surg 1:254, 1984.

32. Orozco H, Takahashi T, Mercado MA, et al: The Sugiura procedure for patients with hemorrhagic portal hypertension secondary to extrahepatic portal vein thrombosis. Surg Gynecol Obstet 173:45–48, 1991.

33. Dagenais M, Langer B, Taylor B, Greig PD: Experience with radical esophagogastric devascularization procedures (Sugiura) for variceal bleeding outside Japan. World J Surg 18:222, 1994.

34. Wanamaker SR, Cooperman M, Carey L: Use of the EEA stapling instrument for control of bleeding esophageal varices. Surgery 94:620, 1983.

35. Durtschi M, Carrico CJ, Johansen KH: Esophageal transection fails to salvage high-risk patients with variceal bleeding. Am J Surg 150:18, 1985.

36. Eck NV: On the question of ligature of the portal vein. Voen Med J 130:1, 1877 annotated in Surg Gynecol Obstet 96:375, 1953.

37. Pavlov IP: On a modification of the Eck fistula between the portal vein and the inferior vena cava. Arch Sci Biol 2:580, 1893.

38. Whipple AO: The problem of portal hypertension in relation to the hepatosplenopathies. Ann Surg 122:499, 1945.

39. Sherlock S, Summerskill WHJ, White LP, et al: Portosystemic encephalopathy: Neurological complications of liver disease. Lancet 2:453, 1954.

40. Jackson FC, Perrin EB, Felix WR, et al: A clinical investigation of the portacaval shunt: V. Survival analysis of the therapeutic operation. Ann Surg 174:672, 1971.

41. Resnick RH, Iber FL, Ishihara AM, et al: A controlled study of the portacaval shunt. Gastroenterology 67:843, 1974.

42. Rueff B, Degos F, Degos JD, et al: A controlled study of therapeutic portacaval shunt in alcoholic cirrhosis. Lancet 1:655, 1976.

43. Reynolds TB, Donovan AJ, Mikkelson WP, et al: Results of a 12 year randomized trial of portacaval shunt in patients with alcoholic liver disease and bleeding varices. Gastroenterology 89:1005, 1981.

44. Conn HO, Lindemuth WW, May LJ, et al: Prophylactic portacaval anastomosis: A tale of two studies. Medicine 51:27, 1972.

45. Starzl TE, Porter KA, Francavilla JA: One Hundred Years of the Hepatotrophic Controversy: Hepatotrophic Factors. CIBA Symposium. Amsterdam, Elsevier Excerpta Medica, 1978.

46. Drapanas T, LoCicero J, Dowling JB: Hemodynamics of the interposition mesocaval shunt. Ann Surg 181:523, 1975.

47. Smith RB, Warren WD, Salam AA, et al: Dacron interposition shunts for portal hypertension: An analysis of morbidity correlates. Ann Surg 192:9, 1980.

48. Paquet K-J, Mercado MA, Gad HA: Surgical procedures for bleeding esophagogastric varices when sclerotherapy fails: A prospective study. Am J Surg 160:43, 1990.

49. Stipa S, Ziparo V, Anza M, et al: A randomized controlled trial of mesentericocaval shunt with autologous jugular vein. Surg Gynecol Obstet 153:353, 1981.

50. Warren WD, Zeppa R, Fomon JJ: Selective transsplenic decompression of gastroesophageal varices by distal splenorenal shunt. Arch Surg 168:437, 1967.

51. Warren WD: Control of variceal bleeding: Reassessment of rationale. Am J Surg 145:8, 1983.

52. Millikan WJ, Warren WD, Henderson JM, et al: The Emory prospective randomized trial: Selective vs. nonselective shunt to control variceal bleeding. Ten-year follow-up. Ann Surg 201:712, 1985.

53. Warren WD, Millikan WJ, Henderson JM, et al: Splenopancreatic disconnection: Improved selectivity of distal splenorenal shunt. Ann Surg 204:346, 1986.

54. Maillard GN, Flamant YM, Chandler JG: Selectivity of the distal splenorenal shunt. Surgery 86:663, 1979.

55. Belghiti J, Grenier P, Nouel O, et al: Long term loss of Warren's shunt selectivity: Angiographic demonstration. Arch Surg 116:1121, 1981.

56. Henderson JM, Millikan WJ Jr, Wright-Bacon L, et al: Hemodynamic differences between alcoholic and non-alcoholic cirrhotics following distal splenorenal shunt: Effect on survival? Ann Surg 201:346, 1983.

57. Harley HAJ, Morgan T, Redecker AG, et al: Results of a randomized trial of end-to-side portacaval shunt and distal splenorenal shunt in alcoholic liver disease and variceal bleeding. Gastroenterology 91:802, 1986.

58. Grace ND, Conn HO, Resnick RH, et al: Distal splenorenal vs. portal systemic shunts after hemorrhage from varices: A randomized controlled trial. Hepatology 8:1475, 1988.

59. Spina GP, Galeotti F, Opocher E, et al: Selective distal splenorenal shunt: Clinical results of a prospective controlled study. Am J Surg 155:564, 1988.

60. Inokuchi K, Beppu K, Koyanagi N, et al: Fifteen years experience with left gastric venous caval shunt for esophageal varices. World J Surg 8:716, 1984.

61. Burchell AR, Moreno AH, Panke WF, Nealon TF: Hepatic artery flow improvement after portacaval shunt: A single hemodynamic clinical correlate. Ann Surg 192:9, 1976.

62. Marion P, Balique JG, George M, et al: Anastomose portocave laterolaterale a debit minimum pour cirrhose haemorrhagique. Med Chir Dig 10:245, 1981.

63. Bismuth H, Franco D, Hepp J: Portal-systemic shunt in hepatic cirrhosis: Does the type of shunt decisively influence the clinical results? Ann Surg 179:209, 1974.

64. Sarfeh IJ, Rypins EB, Conroy RM, et al: Portacaval H-graft: Relationship of shunt diameter, portal flow patterns and encephalopathy. Ann Surg 197:422, 1988.

65. Rypins EB, Sarfeh IJ: Influence of portal hemodynamics on long-term survival of alcoholic patients after small diameter portocaval H-grafts. Am J Surg 155:152, 1988.

66. Collins JC, Ong MS, Rypins EB, Sarfeh IJ: Partial portacaval shunt for variceal hemorrhage: Longitudinal analysis of effectiveness. Arch Surg 133:590–592, 1998.

67. Rosemurgy AS, McAllister EW, Kearney RE: Prospective study of a prosthetic H-graft portacaval shunt. Am J Surg 161:159, 1991.

68. Zervos EE, Goode SE, Rosemurgy AS: Immediate and longterm portal hemodynamic consequences of small-diameter H-graft portacaval shunt. J Surg Res 74 71–75, 1998.

69. Helton WS, Montana M, Dwyer D, Johansen KH: Duplex sonography accurately assesses portacaval shunt patency. J Vasc Surg 8:657, 1988.

70. Johansen KH: Partial portal decompression for variceal hemorrhage. Am J Surg 157:479, 1989.

71. Johansen KH, Girod C, Lee SS, Lebrec D: Mesenteric venous stenosis reduces hyperammonemia in the portacaval-shunted rat. Eur Surg Res 22:170, 1990.

72. Johansen KH: Prospective comparison of partial versus total portal decompression for bleeding esophageal varices. Surg Gynecol Obstet 175:528, 1992.

73. Johansen K, Helton WS: Partial portal decompression for bleeding esophagogastric varices. Perspect Gen Laparos Surg 4:13–21, 1998.

74. Coldwell DM, Moore ADA, Ben-Menachem Y, Johansen KH: Bleeding gastroesophageal varices: Coronary vein embolization following partial portal decompression. Radiology 178:249–251, 1991.

75. Rikkers LF, Jin G, Langnas AN, Shaw BW Jr: Shunt surgery during the era of liver transplantation. Ann Surg 226:51, 1997.

76. Campbell DA Jr, Merion RM, McCurry KR, et al: The role of liver transplantation in the management of the patient with variceal hemorrhage. Probl Gen Surg 9:3, 1992.

77. Rikkers LF, Jin G, Burnett DA, et al: Shunt surgery versus endoscopic sclerotherapy for variceal hemorrhage: Late results of a randomized trial. Am J Surg 165:27, 1993.

78. Conn HO: A peek at the Child-Turcotte classification. Hepatology 1:673, 1981.

79. Millikan WJ, Henderson JM, Stewart MT, et al: Change in hepatic function, hemodynamics and morphology after liver transplant. Ann Surg 209:513, 1989.

80. Langnas AN, Marujo WC, Stratta RJ, et al: Influence of a prior portosystemic shunt on outcome after liver transplantation. Am J Gastroenterol 87:6, 1992.

81. Mazzaferro V, Todo S, Tzakis AG, et al: Liver transplantation in patients with previous portosystemic shunt. Am J Surg 160:111, 1990.

MANAGEMENT OF RENOVASCULAR DISORDERS

KIMBERLEY J. HANSEN, M.D.

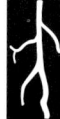

C H A P T E R   1 1 8

Renovascular Disease: An Overview

Kimberley J. Hansen, M.D.

HISTORICAL BACKGROUND

Renovascular Hypertension

Harry Goldblatt[1] defined a causal relationship between renovascular disease and hypertension through his innovative work published in 1934, but Richard Bright[2] of Guy's Hospital, London, first called attention to a potential association between hypertension and renal disease 100 years earlier. Bright observed that patients with "dropsy" and albuminuria during their lifetime had shrunken kidneys and an enlarged heart (cardiac hypertrophy) at autopsy. He suggested that the altered quality of the blood so affected the small circulation as to render greater action necessary to force the blood through the terminal divisions of the vascular system.

Although Bright failed to recognize the relationship between increased blood pressure and cardiac hypertrophy, his observations stimulated many theories. Among these theories was Traube's[3] speculation that the elevated blood pressure led to increased myocardial work and subsequent hypertrophy. Stimulated by Bright's observations and subsequent hypotheses, several investigators described experimental models intended to recreate the clinical lesions observed in the kidneys and heart. In 1879, Grawitz and Israel[4] produced acute occlusion of one renal artery and performed contralateral nephrectomy to decrease functioning renal mass. Although these investigators created what they thought to be cardiac hypertrophy in some animals, elevated blood pressures occurred in none.

Lewinski's findings[5] might well have predated Goldblatt's observations had his experiments included blood pressure measurements. In 1880, he reported that six of 25 dogs had cardiac hypertrophy after partial constriction of the renal arteries. In 1905, Katzenstein[6] created hypertension in dogs by producing partial occlusion of the renal arteries; complete occlusion after torsion of the renal pedicle did not, however, elevate blood pressures. Katzenstein demonstrated that the elevated pressures returned to normal when constricting rubber bands were removed, but he concluded, erroneously, that the blood pressure changes were not re-

lated to a chemically mediated mechanism. In 1898, Tigerstedt and Bergman[7] published the landmark description of a renal pressor substance in rabbits, a crude extract they called *renin*. Although their work was confirmed in 1911 by Senator,[8] these and other investigators did not consider renin to be central to the pathogenesis of hypertension.

In 1934, Goldblatt[1] demonstrated that constriction of the renal artery in dogs produced atrophy of the kidney and hypertension. A clinical pathologist, Goldblatt noticed that extensive vascular disease was often present at autopsy in patients with hypertension and was frequently severe in the renal arteries. In his own words, "Contrary, therefore, to what I had been taught, I began to suspect that the vascular disease comes first, and, when it involves the kidneys, the resultant impairment of the renal circulation probably, in some way, causes elevation of the blood pressure."[1] Goldblatt introduced a new era by demonstrating that renal artery stenosis could produce a form of hypertension that was correctable by nephrectomy.

Leadbetter and Burkland, in 1938, described the first successful treatment of this correctable form of hypertension.[9] They cured a 5-year-old child with severe hypertension by removing an ischemic ectopic kidney. The photomicrographs published from that renal artery specimen were the first documentation of a renovascular cause of hypertension. In subsequent years, numerous patients were treated by nephrectomy based on the findings of hypertension and a small kidney on intravenous pyelography.

Smith,[10] in 1956, reviewed 575 such cases and found that only 26% of patients were cured of hypertension by nephrectomy. This led him to suggest that nephrectomy should be limited to strictly urologic indications. Two years earlier, Freeman[11] reported aortic and bilateral renal artery thromboendarterectomies in a hypertensive patient, which resulted in resolution of the hypertension. This first cure of hypertension by renal revascularization, in combination with widespread use of aortography, was followed by enthusiastic reports of blood pressure benefits after renal revascularization.[12-15] Nevertheless, by 1960 it had become apparent that renal revascularization in hypertensive patients with renal artery stenosis was associated with benefi-

TABLE 118–1. PREVALENCE OF RENOVASCULAR HYPERTENSION IN 74 HYPERTENSIVE CHILDREN

	AGE 0–5 YEARS	AGE 6–10 YEARS	AGE 11–15 YEARS	AGE 16–20 YEARS
No. of children	9	9	29	27
Essential	2	5	24	21
Correctable	7 (78%)	4 (44%)	5 (17%)	6 (22%)

From Lawson JD, Boerth RF, Foster JH, et al: Diagnosis and management of renovascular hypertension in children. Arch Surg 112:1307, 1977. Copyright 1997, American Medical Association.

cial blood pressure response in fewer than half. These clinical results fostered general pessimism about the value of operative renal artery reconstruction for treatment of hypertension.

Contemporary operative management of renovascular hypertension began with the introduction of tests of split renal function by Howard and Conner[16] and by Stamey and associates.[17] As is described in Chapter 119, Page and Helmes[18] and others[19–21] identified the role of the renin-angiotensin system in blood pressure control, thus describing the pathophysiologic development of renovascular hypertension. After accurate assays for plasma renin activity became available, physicians could accurately predict which renal artery lesion was producing renovascular hypertension.

Renovascular Renal Insufficiency

Until the current era, the pathophysiology and management of renovascular disease focused solely on the associated hypertension; however, contemporary reports have emphasized the relationship between renovascular disease and renal insufficiency.[22–28]

The term *ischemic nephropathy* has been adopted to recognize this relationship. By definition, ischemic nephropathy is severe occlusive disease of the extraparenchymal renal artery in combination with excretory renal insufficiency. In 1962, Morris and associates reported on eight azotemic patients with global renal ischemia who exhibited improved blood pressure and renal function after renal revascularization.[29] Novick, Libertino, and Dean and their groups found similar beneficial functional responses when bilateral renal lesions were corrected in azotemic patients.[23, 25, 26] These early reports, and the ones that followed, suggested that ischemic nephropathy could mediate renal insufficiency that was rapidly progressive, contributing to end-stage renal disease. The diagnosis and management of renovascular disease contributing to renal insufficiency are discussed in Chapter 123.

PREVALENCE

Despite the proven benefit of renal artery repair in certain patients with hypertension or excretory renal insufficiency, the best method of screening for or treating renovascular disease remains uncertain. The low prevalence of renovascular hypertension and ischemic nephropathy in the general population, the expense of diagnostic and functional evaluations, the infrequent cure of hypertension, and the uncertain functional response after intervention are all perceived as reasons to avoid seeking and treating renovascular disease. In this overview, information on each of these issues is presented.

Renovascular disease is thought to account for approximately 3% of hypertension cases in the general population. Considering that 60 million persons in the United States demonstrate some degree of hypertension, the prevalence of renovascular hypertension is undoubtedly low in the general population. Since renovascular hypertension produces severe hypertension, its presence in the large number of patients with mild hypertension (diastolic blood pressure <105 mmHg) is probably negligible. In contrast, however, it is frequently the cause of hypertension in those persons who have severe systemic hypertension.

Severe hypertension, particularly at the two extremes of age, is most likely to be caused by renovascular disease. A review of 74 consecutive children evaluated for hypertension over a 5-year period showed that 78% of those younger than 5 years had a correctable renovascular condition (Table 118–1).[30] Interestingly, after childhood, the age group that is next most likely to have renovascular hypertension is elderly persons. In the 1996 academic year, the author's center screened 629 hypertensive individuals for renovascular disease (Table 118–2). Overall, 25% of subjects screened demonstrated significant renal artery disease; however, 52% of those older than 60 years whose diastolic pressure was greater than 110 mmHg had significant renal artery stenosis or occlusion. When serum creatinine was elevated in conjunction with these age and blood pressure findings, 71% of subjects demonstrated hemodynamically significant renovascular disease.

Among hypertensive patients with excretory renal insufficiency, the prevalence of renovascular disease (i.e., ischemic nephropathy) also varies. In a series of randomly selected patients 45 to 75 years of age with serum creatinine values greater than 2.0 mg/dL evaluated at the author's center, 14% were found to have unsuspected renovascular disease.[31] Moreover, among 90 consecutive patients older than 50 years with end-stage renal disease who presented for chronic renal replacement therapy, 22% demonstrated

TABLE 118–2. RENAL DUPLEX SONOGRAPHY FINDINGS IN 629 HYPERTENSIVE ADULTS

	RENOVASCULAR DISEASE PRESENT No. (%)	RENOVASCULAR DISEASE ABSENT No. (%)	TOTAL No. (%)
All patients	154 (24)	475 (76)	629 (100)
>60 yr and Diastolic BP ≥ 110 mmHg	98 (52)	91 (48)	189 (30)
Diastolic BP ≥ 110 mmHg and SCr ≥ 2.0 mg/dl	53 (71)	22 (29)	75 (12)

BP = blood pressure; SCr = serum creatinine value.

TABLE 118–3. PREVALENCE OF DIALYSIS-DEPENDENT ISCHEMIC NEPHROPATHY AMONG 45 PATIENTS WITH NEW END-STAGE RENAL DISEASE

	RENOVASCULAR DISEASE PRESENT	RENOVASCULAR DISEASE ABSENT
No. of patients (%)	10 (22%)	35 (78%)
Caucasians only	10 (40%)	15 (60%)
Type of disease		
Bilateral	5	
Unilateral	5	
Occlusion	4	
Mean age (years)*	69.4 ± 2.5	64.1 ± 1.5
Gender		
Male	5	15
Female	5	20
Ethnicity†		
African-American	0	20
Caucasian	10	15

Modified from Appel RG, Blyer AJ, Hansen KJ: Renovascular disease in older patients beginning renal replacement therapy. Kidney Int 48:171–176, 1995. Used with permission of Kidney International.

renal artery stenosis or occlusion.[32] Dialysis-dependent ischemic nephropathy demonstrated significant ethnic differences. Overall, 40% of white persons in the atherosclerotic age range who had end-stage renal failure had unsuspected renovascular disease, whereas 20% had global renal ischemia consistent with potentially reversible dialysis-dependent renal failure (Table 118–3).[32]

These data suggest that persons with hypertension or azotemia should not be regarded as a homogeneous group with respect to the prevalence of renovascular disease, renovascular hypertension, or ischemic nephropathy. Rather, the probability of finding clinically significant renal artery disease correlates with age, severity of hypertension, and the presence and severity of renal insufficiency. Consequently, the search for renovascular disease should be directed toward persons who are very young or in the atherosclerotic age range, and who have severe hypertension, especially when it is combined with excretory renal insufficiency. However, severity of hypertension refers to blood pressure *without medication* and is not related to the difficulty of medical control.

In attempts to discriminate between essential and renovascular hypertension, many reports have focused on the value of demographic factors and physical findings in guiding further diagnostic study. The Cooperative Study of Renovascular Hypertension remains the best study to date that compares the clinical characteristics of renovascular hypertension and of essential hypertension.[33] In that study, the prevalence of certain clinical characteristics in 339 patients with essential hypertension was compared with their prevalence in 175 patients with renovascular hypertension secondary to atherosclerotic lesions (91 patients) or fibromuscular dysplasia (84 patients). A summary of the significant differences identified in the Cooperative Study is presented in Table 118–4.[33] Several characteristics show statistically significant differences between the two varieties of hypertension; however, *none* has sufficient negative predictive value to exclude anyone from further investigation for renovascular disease.

Although the finding of an epigastric bruit in a young white woman with severe hypertension strongly suggests a renovascular cause for the elevated blood pressure, the absence of these clinical features does not rule out renovascular disease. Consequently, clinical criteria should not be used to eliminate patients from further diagnostic study.

The decision to search for renovascular disease should be based on the severity of the hypertension: mild hypertension has a minimal chance of being renovascular in origin, whereas, the more severe the hypertension is, the greater is the probability that it has a correctable renovascular cause. With this in mind, the author's center evaluates all persons with severe hypertension for renovascular disease, especially those at the extremes of age and especially when their hypertension is associated with excretory renal insufficiency.

EVALUATION AND DIAGNOSIS

The general evaluation of all hypertensive subjects should include a careful medical history, physical examination, serum electrolytes (including creatinine), and electrocardiography. Electrocardiography reveals the extent of secondary myocardial hypertrophy and associated ischemic heart disease. Serum electrolytes and serial serum potassium determinations can effectively exclude patients with primary aldosteronism if potassium levels are greater than 3.0 mEq/dl. Finally, estimation of renal function is mandatory for all patients. Primary renal parenchymal disease may mediate both renal dysfunction and hypertension. Conversely, hypertension from any cause may produce intrarenal arteriolar nephrosclerosis and mediate decreased excretory renal function.

A noninvasive screening test that accurately identifies renal artery disease in all individuals does not yet exist (a dilemma described more completely in Chapter 121).[34] Isotope-enhanced renography continues to be proposed as a valuable screening test, although the methods and the criteria for interpretation are continuously being modified in hope of improving its sensitivity and specificity.[35] Current isotope renography uses a variety of radiopharmaceuticals before and after exercise or converting enzyme inhibition (i.e., with captopril). As described in Chapter 119, only captopril renography has gained widespread use and acceptance as a screening tool for renovascular disease.

Currently available screening tests can be broadly characterized as *functional* (relying on some feature of the renin-angiotensin axis) or *anatomic* (providing a renal artery image or associated hemodynamic data). With the exception of captopril renography, studies that rely on the renin-angiotensin axis have been associated with unacceptable rates of false-negative results. Consequently, this author has emphasized direct screening methods.[36]

Of the direct screening methods currently in use (see Chapter 121), the author's center has chosen renal duplex sonography as the preliminary study of choice for both renovascular hypertension and ischemic nephropathy. Owing to continued improvements in software and probe design, duplex sonography has proven accurate for identifying hemodynamically significant renal artery occlusive disease. Moreover, it is ideally suited to the evaluation of anatomic renovascular disease in the contemporary patient

TABLE 118–4. CLINICAL CHARACTERISTICS OF ESSENTIAL HYPERTENSION AND RENOVASCULAR HYPERTENSION

| | ESSENTIAL HYPERTENSION (339 CASES) | | RENOVASCULAR HYPERTENSION | | | |
| | | | Arteriosclerotic (91 Cases) | | Fibromuscular (84 Cases) | |
	%	Years	%	Years	%	Years
History						
Average age		41		48		35
<20 yr	2		1		14	
Average duration		3.1		1.9		2.0
<1 yr	10		23		19	
>10 yr	23		12		10	
Average age at onset		35		46		33*
>50 yr	7		39		3*	
<20 yr	12		2		16*	
Sex (female)	40		34		81	
Race (black)	29		7		10	
Acceleration of hypertension	13		23		14	
Family History						
Hypertension	67		68*		41	
Stroke	37		44*		22	
Neither of foregoing	19		30*		46	
Symptoms						
Nocturia	38		55		35	
Weakness, fatigue	32		49		42*	
Angina						
Headache						
All of foregoing	0		14		10	
Previous vascular occlusive disease	10		20		6	
Physical Evaluation						
Body habitus						
Obese	38		17		11	
Thin	6		13*		30	
Fundi (grades 3 and 4)	12		26		10*	
Bruit						
Abdomen	6		38		55	
Flank	1		8		20	
Abdomen or flank	7		41		57	

From Simon N, Franklin SS, Bleifer KH, et al: Clinical characteristics of renovascular hypertension. JAMA 220:1209, 1972. Copyright 1972, American Medical Association.
*Differences are statistically significant at the 5% level, except where so designated.

populations.[37] When used as a screening study, preparation is minimal (an overnight fast) and there is no need to alter antihypertensive medications. The examination poses no risk to residual excretory renal function, and overall accuracy is not adversely affected by concomitant aortoiliac disease. These considerations are important since more than 70% of contemporary patients have at least mild renal insufficiency in combination with aortoiliac atherosclerosis.

During the past 10 years, the author's center has performed more than 8500 renal duplex studies to screen for renovascular disease in hypertensive subjects (age range 2 to 91 years). Overall, technically "satisfactory" studies (defined as complete main renal artery Doppler interrogation from aortic origin to renal hilum) were obtained for 92% of patients and for 96% of kidneys examined.[38] Although these success rates are not influenced by patient age, extent of disease, or renal insufficiency, these results require examination by a skilled sonographer.

The utility of renal duplex sonography is demonstrated by the results from our first prospective validity analysis in 74 consecutive patients who had 77 conventional cut-film angiograms to study 148 kidneys.[37] Renal duplex imaging correctly identified hemodynamically significant renal artery stenosis or occlusion in 41 of 44 patients with angiographically proven lesions and produced no false-positive findings. Among 122 kidneys with single renal arteries, renal duplex sonography provided 95% sensitivity, 98% specificity, 98% positive predictive value, 94% negative predictive value, and overall accuracy of 96%. These results were adversely affected among the 14 patients who had 20 kidneys with multiple renal arteries (Table 118–5).[37] Moreover, diastolic features of the renal artery spectral analysis correlated significantly and inversely with estimated glomerular filtration ($r = .30773$; $p = .009$); however, parameters from the Doppler spectral analysis did not correlate with hypertension or renal functional response in patients submitted to renovascular repair. The study provides accurate anatomic information, but Doppler parameters should not be used to predict response after renal artery intervention.

Judging from this experience, renal duplex sonography appears to be a valuable study for lesions of the main renal artery when the screened population demonstrates 20% to 40% prevalence of renovascular disease. A negative duplex

TABLE 118–5. RENAL DUPLEX SONOGRAPHY: COMPARATIVE ANALYSIS PARAMETER ESTIMATES AND THEIR 95% CONFIDENCE INTERVALS

GROUP	NO.	MEASURE	ESTIMATE	95% CI
All kidneys	142 (kidneys)	Sensitivity	0.88	(.84, .92)
		Specificity	0.99	(.97, 1.00)
		PPV	0.98†	(.96, .99)
		NPV	0.92‡	(.89, .95)
		Accuracy	0.91	(.87, .95)
Kidneys with single renal artery	122 (kidneys)	Sensitivity	0.93	(.90, .96)
		Specificity	0.98†	(.96, 1.00)
		PPV	0.98†	(.96, 1.00)
		NPV	0.94‡	(.91, .97)
	148 (kidneys)	Accuracy	0.91	(.87, .95)
Kidneys with multiple renal arteries	21 (arteries)	Sensitivity	0.67	(.53, .81)
		Specificity	1.00*	—
		PPV	1.00*†	—
		NPV	0.79‡	(.68, .90)
		Accuracy	0.86	(.76, .96)
All patients	74 (subjects)	Sensitivity	0.93	(.87, .99)
		Specificity	1.00*	—
		PPV	1.00*†	—
		NPV	0.91‡	(.84, .98)
		Accuracy	0.96	(.91, 1.00)

From Hansen KJ, Tribble RW, Reavis SW, et al: Renal duplex sonography: Evaluation of clinical utility. J Vasc Surg 12:227–236, 1990.
*Estimated standard error is zero, confidence level is inestimable.
†PPV = positive predictive value.
‡NPV = negative predictive value.
CI = confidence interval.

study effectively excludes ischemic nephropathy, since the primary consideration is global renal ischemia secondary to main renal artery disease. When duplex sonography is used to screen for renovascular hypertension, however, multiple or polar renal arteries and their associated disease are potential limitations. Despite enhanced recognition of multiple arteries provided by color flow Doppler scanning, only 40% of these accessory renal vessels are identified currently. Overall, 17% of patients treated for renovascular hypertension in the author's center have polar renal artery disease, and in 11% of patients polar disease is the sole cause of renovascular hypertension. This is important, particularly when children and young adults are considered. For these patients, the author's group proceeds with angiography when hypertension is severe or poorly controlled, despite negative duplex findings.

As a screening study for renovascular hypertension, angiography remains controversial (see Chapter 120). The author's group performs angiography as a screening study when renal duplex findings are technically incomplete or branch/polar renal artery disease is suspected in an individual with severe hypertension. Although intra-arterial digital subtraction angiography is used preferentially in many centers to evaluate the renal arteries, we have continued to rely on conventional cut-film angiography. In most instances, assessment of the renal vasculature and juxtarenal aorta requires multiple injections when intra-arterial digital subtraction angiography is used. By comparison, a single flush aortogram requires no more contrast material than do multiple intra-arterial digital subtraction studies. Moreover, conventional angiography provides information regarding cortical thickness and renal length and better images of the intrarenal arterial anatomy.

It is widely recognized that angiography can exacerbate renal failure in patients with severe renal insufficiency, especially those with diabetic nephropathy. Nevertheless, this risk appears justified in patients who have severe or accelerated hypertension and in those with positive renal duplex sonography results. In these circumstances, the benefit derived from the identification and correction of a functionally significant renovascular lesion outweighs the risks of conventional angiography. This clinical practice is supported by the fact that no patient at the author's center has been rendered permanently dialysis-dependent as a consequence of contrast-related renal failure.

When a unilateral renal artery lesion is confirmed by angiography, its functional significance should be defined. Both renal vein renin assays and split renal function studies have proven valuable in assessing the functional significance of renovascular disease. Neither has great value, however, when severe bilateral disease or disease in a solitary kidney is present. In these circumstances, the decision for intervention is based on the severity of the renal artery lesions, the severity of hypertension, and the degree of associated renal insufficiency.

Finally, split renal function studies are no longer performed (see earlier texts describing their use[39]). At present, renal vein renin assays (RVRAs) are most often used to establish the presumptive diagnosis of renovascular hypertension. Proper patient preparation and performance of RVRAs are critical to obtaining valid results (see Chapter 119).

MANAGEMENT OPTIONS

In recent years, what constitutes optimal management of renovascular disease contributing to hypertension or renal insufficiency has become increasingly controversial. In the absence of a prospective, randomized trial comparing treatment options, advocates of medical management, percutaneous transluminal renal angioplasty (PTRA), and operative intervention, respectively, cite clinical data selectively to support their particular views.

A majority of the medical community evaluate patients for renovascular hypertension only when medications are not tolerated or hypertension remains severe and poorly controlled. The study by Hunt and Strong[40] remains the most informative one available to assess the comparative value of medical therapy and operation. In this nonrandomized trial, the results of operative treatment in 100 patients were compared with the results of drug therapy in 114 similar patients. After 7 to 14 years of follow-up, 84% of the operated group were alive, as compared with 66% in the drug therapy group. Of the 84 patients alive in the operated group, 93% were cured or significantly improved in contrast to only 21% of those who were alive in the drug therapy group. As compared with surgical management, death during follow-up was twice as common in association with medical treatment; this fact resulted in differences that were statistically significant in patients with both atherosclerosis and fibromuscular dysplasia of the renal artery.

Additional prospective data on medical therapy for renovascular hypertension suggest that decreases in kidney size and renal function occur despite satisfactory blood pressure control. Dean and colleagues reported the results of serial renal function studies performed on 41 patients with renovascular hypertension (i. e., hypertension and positive functional studies) secondary to atherosclerotic renal artery disease who were randomly selected for nonoperative management (Table 118–6).[41] In 19 patients, serum creatinine levels increased between 25% and 120%. Glomerular filtration rates dropped 25% to 50% in 12 patients, and 14 others (37%) lost more than 10% of renal length. In four patients (12%), significant stenosis progressed to total occlusion. Overall, 17 patients (41%) experienced deterioration of renal function or a decrease in renal mass that led to operation, and one patient required removal of a "previously reconstructable" kidney. Of the 17 patients whose renal function deteriorated, 15 had had acceptable control of blood pressure during the period of nonoperative observation. This experience suggests that progressive decline of renal function in medically treated patients with atherosclerotic renovascular disease and renovascular hypertension occurs despite satisfactory blood pressure control.

TABLE 118–6. CHANGES IN EXCRETORY RENAL FUNCTION DURING MEDICAL MANAGEMENT OF RENOVASCULAR HYPERTENSION IN 41 PATIENTS

CHANGE	NO. AFFECTED (%)
Decreased by 25% to 49%	11 (37)
Decreased ≥ 50%	1 (3)
No change ± 24%	14 (47)
Improved ≥ 25%	4 (13)
Total	30 (100)

From Dean RH, Kieffer RW, Smith BM, et al: Renovascular hypertension: Anatomic and renal function changes during drug therapy. Arch Surg 166:1408, 1981. Copyright 1981, American Medical Association.

The detrimental changes associated with medical therapy alone, combined with the excellent contemporary results of operative management, argue for an aggressive surgical approach to renovascular disease that is causing hypertension or renal insufficiency.[42] The author's indications for interventional management include all cases of severe, refractory hypertension. This includes patients with complicating factors such as branch lesions and extrarenal atherosclerotic disease and those with associated cardiovascular disease that would improve with blood pressure reduction. Moreover, young patients whose hypertension is moderate, who have no associated end-organ disease, and who have easily correctable atherosclerotic or dysplastic main renal artery lesions are also candidates for operative intervention. The chance for cure of moderate hypertension is quite good in such patients, and it remains to be proved that medical blood pressure control is equivalent to cure of hypertension. In fact, it is plausible that reduction in perfusion pressure associated with the renovascular lesion during medical therapy may accelerate renal dysfunction by further reducing glomerular perfusion pressure.

Finally, no evidence exists to indicate that age, type of renovascular lesion (atherosclerotic or dysplastic), duration of hypertension, or bilateral lesions accurately estimates operative risk or of the likelihood of successful surgical management. Consequently, the presence or absence of these factors should not be determinants of operation.

Chapter 120 provides a comprehensive review of PTRA for renovascular disease. In this author's view, experience with liberal use of PTRA has helped to clarify its role as a therapeutic option for renovascular hypertension; however, the data argue for selective application. In this regard, PTRA of non-orificial atherosclerotic lesions and medial fibroplasia of the main renal artery yields results comparable to those of operative repair. In contrast, suboptimal lesions for PTRA include congenital lesions, fibrodysplastic lesions involving renal artery branches, and ostial atherosclerotic lesions. Treatment of these lesions with PTRA is associated with inferior results and increased risk of complications.

Endoluminal stenting of the renal artery as an adjunct to PTRA was first introduced in the United States in 1988 as part of a multicenter trial.[43] During the same period, the Palmaz stent and Wallstents were being used in Europe. Currently, no stent has been approved for renal use in this country; However, the most common indications appear to be (1) elastic recoil of the vessel immediately after angioplasty, (2) renal artery dissection after angioplasty, and (3) restenosis after angioplasty. With 263 patients entered, results from the multicenter trial demonstrated cure of or improvement hypertension in 61% of patients after 1 year. At follow-up earlier than 1 year, angiography demonstrated restenosis in 32.7% of patients. Given the poor results of PTRA alone for ostial atherosclerosis, primary placement of endoluminal stents has been recommended for these lesions.[44]

Table 118–7 summarizes single-center reports with renal function and angiographic follow-up after treatment of ostial atherosclerosis by PTRA in combination with endoluminal stents.[44–49] These studies differ in their criteria for ostial lesions, evaluation of the clinical response to intervention, and parameters for significant restenoses, but despite these

TABLE 118–7. PERCUTANEOUS TRANSLUMINAL RENAL ANGIOPLASTY WITH RENAL ARTERY STENT PLACEMENT FOR OSTIAL ATHEROSCLEROTIC RENAL ARTERY STENOSIS

INVESTIGATOR	PATIENTS WITH OSTIAL LESIONS (NO.)	PATIENTS WITH RENAL DYSFUNCTION (NO.)	FUNCTION RESPONSE (%)			HYPERTENSION RESPONSE (%)			RESTENOSIS (%)
			Improved	Unchanged	Worsened	Cured	Improved	Failed	
Rees CR (1991)[44]	28	14	36	36	29	11	54	36	39
Hennequin LM (1994)[45]	7	2	0	50	50	0	100	0	43
Raynaud AC (1994)[46]	4	3	0	33	67	0	50	50	33
MacLeod M (1995)[47]	22	13	15	85%		0	31	69	20
van de Ven PJG (1995)[48]	24	NR	33	58	8	0	73	27	13
Blum U (1997)[49]	68	20	0	100	0	16	62	22	17
Total	153	52	13	73	14	9	59	32	23

NR = not reported.

differences, the cumulative results provide the best available estimates of early hypertension response, change in renal function, and primary patency.

From these data, immediate technical success was observed in 99% of patients and beneficial blood pressure response (cure or improvement) was observed in 68%. However, only 13% of patients with renal insufficiency demonstrated improved excretory renal function, while renal function was worse in 14% of patients after intervention. During angiographic follow-up of 5.8 to 16.4 months, restenosis was observed in 13% to 39% of patients. Based on available data, PTRA with stenting of ostial atherosclerosis appears to yield blood pressure, renal function, and anatomic results that are inferior to those achieved with contemporary surgical approaches.[42] Moreover, no studies to date have examined long-term renal function after primary or secondary PTRA, with or without stents. For these reasons, the author believes that operation remains the initial treatment of choice for patients with ostial renal artery atherosclerosis, especially when hypertension is present in combination with renal insufficiency.

REFERENCES

1. Goldblatt H: Studies on experimental hypertension. J Exp Med 59:346, 1934.
2. Bright R: Cases and observations illustrative of renal disease accompanied with the secretion of albuminous urine. Guy's Hosp Rep 1:388, 1836.
3. Traube L: Über den Zusammenhang von Herz und nieren Krankheiten. In Gesammelte Beiträge zur Pathologie und Physiologie, vol 2, p 290. Berlin, A. Hirschwald, 1871.
4. Grawitz P, Israel O: Experimentelle Untersuchung über den Zusammenhang zwischen Nierenerkrankung und Herzhypertrophie. Arch Pathol Anat 77:315, 1879.
5. Lewinski L: Ueber den Zusammenhang zwischen Nierenschrumpfung und Herzhypertrophie. Z Klin Med 1:561, 1880.
6. Katzenstein M: Experimenteller Beitrag zur Erkenntnis der bei Nephritis auftretenden Hypertrophie des linken Herzens. Virchows Arch 182:327, 1905.
7. Tigerstedt R, Bergman PG: Niere und Kreislauf. Skand Arch Physiol 8:223, 1898.
8. Senator H: Ueber die Beziehungen des Nierenkreislaufs zum arteriellen Blutdruck und über die Ursachen der Herzhypertrophie bei Nierenkrankheiten. Z Klin Med 72:189, 1911.
9. Leadbetter WFG, Burkland CE: Hypertension in unilateral renal disease. J Urol 39:611, 1938.
10. Smith HW: Unilateral nephrectomy in hypertensive disease. J Urol 76:685, 1956.
11. Freeman N: Thromboendarterectomy for hypertension due to renal artery occlusion. JAMA 157:1077, 1954.
12. DeCamp PT, Birchall R: Recognition and treatment of renal arterial stenosis associated with hypertension. Surgery 43:134, 1958.
13. Morris GC Jr, Cooley DA, Crawford ES, et al: Renal revascularization for hypertension: Clinical and physiologic studies in 32 cases. Surgery 48:95, 1960.
14. Hurwitt ES, Seidenburg B, Hainovoco H, et al: Splenorenal arterial anastomosis. Circulation 14:537, 1956.
15. Luke JC, Levitan BA: Revascularization of the kidney in hypertension due to renal artery stenosis. Arch Surg 79:269, 1959.
16. Howard JE, Conner TB: Use of differential renal function studies in the diagnosis of renovascular hypertension. Am J Surg 107:58, 1964.
17. Stamey TA, Nudelman IJ, Good PH, et al: Functional characteristics of renovascular hypertension. Medicine (Baltimore) 40:347, 1961.
18. Page IH, Helmes OM: A crystalline pressor substance (angiotensin) resulting from the reaction between renin and renin activator. J Exp Med 71:29, 1940.
19. Bruan-Memendez E, Fasciolo JC, Lelois LF, et al: La substancia hypertensora de la sangre del rinon, isquemiado. Rev Soc Argent Biol 15:420, 1939.
20. Lentz KE, Skeggs LT Jr, Woods KR, et al: The amino acid composition of angiotensin II and its biochemical relationship to hypertension. Int J Exp Med 104:183, 1956.
21. Tobian L: Relationship of juxtaglomerular apparatus to renin and angiotensin. Circulation 25:189, 1962.
22. Bengtsson U, Bergentz S-E, Norback B: Surgical treatment of renal artery stenosis with impending uremia. Clin Nephrol 2:222, 1974.
23. Dean RH, Englund R, Dupont WD, et al: Retrieval of renal function by revascularization: Study of preoperative outcome predictors. Ann Surg 202:367, 1985.
24. Dean RH, Lawson JD, Hollifield JW, et al: Revascularization of the poorly functioning kidney. Surgery 85:44, 1979.
25. Libertino JA, Zinman L: Revascularization of the poorly functioning and nonfunctioning kidney. In Novick AC, Stratton RA (eds): Vascular Problems in Urologic Surgery. Philadelphia, WB Saunders, 1982, p 173.
26. Novick AC, Pohl MA, Schreiber M, et al: Revascularization for preservation of renal function in patients with atherosclerotic renovascular disease. J Urol 129:907, 1983.
27. Scoble JE, Maher ER, Hamilton G, Atherosclerotic renovascular disease causing renal impairment: A case for treatment. Clin Nephrol 31:119, 1989.
28. Zinman L, Libertino JA: Revascularization of the chronic totally occluded renal artery with restoration of renal function. J Urol 228:517, 1977.
29. Morris GC Jr, DeBakey ME, Cooley DA: Surgical treatment of renal failure of renovascular origin. JAMA 182:609, 1962.
30. Lawson JD, Boerth RF, Foster JH, et al: Diagnosis and management of renovascular hypertension in children. Arch Surg 112:1307, 1977.
31. O'Neal EA, Hansen KJ, Canzanello VJ, et al: Prevalence of ischemic nephropathy in patients with renal insufficiency. Am Surg 58:52, 1992.
32. Appel RG, Bleyer AJ, Reavis S, Hansen KJ: Renovascular disease in older patients beginning renal replacement therapy. Kidney Int 48:171, 1995.

33. Simon N, Franklin SS, Bleifer KH, et al: Clinical characteristics of renovascular hypertension. JAMA 220:1209, 1972.
34. Svetkey LP, Bollinger RR, Kozman PE, et al. Prospective analysis of strategies for diagnosing renovascular hypertension. Hypertension 14:242, 1989.
35. Nally JV Jr, Chen CC, Skakianakis G, et al: Diagnostic criteria of renovascular hypertension with captopril renography: A consensus statement. Am J Hypertens 4:749S, 1991.
36. Dean RH, Benjamin ME, Hansen KJ: Surgical management of renovascular hypertension. Curr Probl Surg 34:209, 1997.
37. Hansen KJ, Tribble RW, Reavis S, et al: Renal duplex sonography: Evaluation of clinical utility. J Vasc Surg 12:227, 1990.
38. Hansen KJ, Reavis SW, Dean RH: Duplex scanning in renovascular disease. Geriatr Nephrol Urol 6:89, 1996.
39. Dean RH, Rhamy RK: Split renal function studies in renovascular hypertension. In Stanley JC. Ernst CB, Fry WJ (eds): Renovascular Hypertension. Philadelphia, WB Saunders, 1984, p 135.
40. Hunt JC, Strong CG: Renovascular hypertension: Mechanism, natural history and treatment. Am J Cardiol 32:562, 1973.
41. Dean RH, Kieffer RW, Smith BM, et al: Renovascular hypertension: Anatomic and renal function changes during drug therapy. Arch Surg 166:1408, 1981.
42. Hansen KJ, Starr SM, Sands RE, et al: Contemporary surgical management of renovascular disease. J Vasc Surg 16:319, 1992.
43. Rees CR: Renovascular interventions. Twenty-first Annual Meeting Society of Cardiovascular and Interventional Radiology, Seattle, March 1996, p 311.
44. Rees CR, Palmaz JC, Beck GJ, et al: Palmaz stent in atherosclerotic stenoses involving the ostia of the renal arteries: Preliminary report of a multicenter study. Radiology 181:507, 1991.
45. Hennequin LM, Joffre FG, Rousseau HP, et al: Renal artery stent placement: Long-term results with the Wallstent endoprosthesis. Radiology 191:713, 1994.
46. Raynaud AC, Beyssen BM, Turmel-Rodrigues LE, et al: Renal, artery stent placement: Immediate and midterm technical and clinical results. J Vasc Interv Radiol 849, 1994.
47. MacLeod M, Taylor, AD, Baxter G, et al: Renal artery stenosis managed by Palmaz stent insertion: Technical and clinical outcome. J Hypertens 13:1791, 1995.
48. Van de Ven PJG, Beutler, JJ, Kaatee R, et al: Transluminal vascular stent for ostial atherosclerotic renal artery stenosis. Lancet 346:672, 1995.
49. Blum U, Krummer B, Flogel P, et al: Treatment of ostial renal-artery stenoses with vascular endoprostheses after unsuccessful balloon angioplasty. N Engl J Med 336:459, 1997.

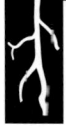

C H A P T E R   1 1 9

Pathophysiology, Functional Studies, and Medical Therapy of Renovascular Hypertension

Carlos M. Ferrario, M.D., and Pavel J. Levy, M.D

The role of the kidney in the pathogenesis of arterial hypertension remains a continual motif of medical research since Richard Bright first described in 1827 an association between heart size and the contracted kidney. One hundred years (1898) since Tigerstedt and Bergman observed that an aqueous extract from the rabbit kidney elevated the blood pressure of anesthetized animals the search for the mechanisms by which altered renal function affects blood pressure continues unabated. The pioneer studies initiated independently by Goldblatt and coworkers[46] and Page[80] strengthened the idea that a renal pressor system contributes to the pathogenesis of arterial hypertension, leading to some heroic approaches to the treatment of hypertension, including renal denervation, nephrectomy, and sympathectomy.[81, 82] Currently, Bianchi, from elegant studies in the Milan hypertensive rat, has provided the most cogent case for a primary contribution of the kidney in the pathogenesis of arterial hypertension.

Although this chapter focuses on the role of the kidney in the pathogenesis and medical management of renovascular hypertension (RVH), the lesson learned from the study of this problem undoubtedly continues to affect the analysis of the origin of essential hypertension. Strictly speaking,

the observation by Goldblatt and associates[46] that clamping of the canine renal artery caused a sustained elevation of blood pressure with a magnitude that correlated roughly with the degree of renal artery constriction was a turning point in the field of hypertension research. As a pathologist, Goldblatt duplicated in the living animal his precise observations of an association between enlarged left ventricles and narrowing of the renal arteries in autopsy materials. He deduced that chronic renal ischemia could stimulate the kidney to release a vasopressor material of the renin-like form described 36 years before by the Scandinavian investigators Tigerstedt and Bergman.

The Goldblatt studies made two major contributions to the field. First, the meticulously performed observations in the dog provided a reproducible model to study the mechanisms contributing to the pathogenesis of arterial hypertension. This included the analysis of the humoral factors that could be released by the kidney with a stenotic renal artery. Second, the work provided experimental evidence for the idea that essential hypertension may be produced by chronic renal ischemia, a possibility that science has still not been able to disprove.

Clinically, however, hypertension of renovascular origin

is a common cause of secondary hypertension. Although it may account for no more than 5% of all known causes of arterial hypertension,[54] the frequency of this entity in older people may be much greater than previously recognized. Atherosclerotic renal artery disease is becoming a frequently recognized ailment in subjects aged 65 years or older.[50] Epidemiologic studies suggest that atherosclerotic renal artery disease may be an important cause of end-stage renal disease (ESRD) in the elderly.[24, 72] An increased recognition of this problem may account for the perception that reports of the frequency of hypertension of renovascular origin vary from less than 1% in unselected populations to as many as 20% of patients referred to specialized centers.[54]

PATHOPHYSIOLOGY

Renovascular hypertension is an entity in which the blood pressure elevation is caused by hypoperfusion of the kidney with concomitant decreases in renal blood flow. Partial occlusion of the renal artery may affect a single kidney, but bilateral stenosis may also be found, particularly in subjects with atherosclerotic renal artery disease. In animals, silver clips or external constrictors can be applied to one or both renal artery to produce a chronic fall in intrarenal perfusion pressure. Another approach is to combine stenosis of the renal artery with removal of the opposite kidney. These various experimental conditions[40] have given rise to a nomenclature describing renal-induced forms of arterial hypertension (Table 119–1). Whereas these procedures are designed to elicit a drop in renal perfusion pressure, the mechanism by which blood pressure rises and hypertension is sustained in the various animal models may differ in its initiation, magnitude, and duration.

Because renal artery stenosis promotes growth of collateral vessels, the hypertension produced by clipping of one renal artery (*two-kidney, one-clip* renal hypertension) is often transient in nature. A more durable form of hypertension may be produced by clamping of both renal arteries (*two-kidney, two-clip* hypertension), the combination of clamping of one renal artery and removal of the contralateral kidney (*one-kidney, one-clip* hypertension), or the highly reproducible variation of a *two-step occlusion* of a renal artery described by Masaki and coauthors.[66] *Perinephritic hypertension*[80] is another experimental procedure in which renal ischemia results from the compression of the kidney by a cellophane or latex wrap.

The presence of a contralateral intact kidney has a significant effect on the mechanisms accounting for the evolution of experimental renal hypertension. In general, the mechanisms contributing to the initial rise in arterial pressure may be viewed in terms of the activation of volume and vasoconstrictor systems. The initial stimulus of renal hypoperfusion causes an activation of the renin-angiotensin system that translates to the release of renin with an attendant increase in the circulating levels of *angiotensin II (Ang II)*. Volume expansion due to Ang II–mediated sodium retention is partially counteracted by a natriuretic response from the intact kidney, which responds to the increase in blood pressure through the phenomenon of pressure natriuresis.[21, 48]

Thus, *two-kidney, one-clip* renal hypertension is considered a primary model for vasoconstriction hypertension, since the opposite kidney can effectively negate an important contribution from volume expansion. The removal of the contralateral kidney, however, eliminates the compensatory pressure-induced natriuresis; thus the *one-kidney, one-clip* model of hypertension is a prime example in which blood pressure rises by the combined effects of volume expansion and peripheral vasoconstriction.

The progression of hypertension over time reflects an overall adjustment of homeostatic mechanisms to the elevation of arterial pressure. The activation of neurogenic mechanisms by Ang II augments cardiac output but this effect is progressively replaced by a sustained increase in peripheral vascular resistance.[35] The cardiovascular system responds to the sustained increase in arterial pressure by adaptive structural changes of the heart and blood vessels. The restructuring of the cardiovascular system, in terms of left ventricular hypertrophy, vascular hypertrophy and vessel rarefaction, may become the predominant mechanism by which hypertension is sustained.[35] These mechanistic changes are mediated by the multiple actions of Ang II and the attendant activation of other vasopressor systems. These other systems include:

1. Activation of the sympathetic nervous system due to the stimulatory actions of Ang II on brain vasomotor centers, vascular noradrenergic nerve endings, and inhibition of baroreceptor reflexes.[37]

2. Increased secretion of vasopressin[59] and adrenal catecholamines.[83]

3. Alterations in anterior hypophysial hormones through activation of opioid-melanocorticoid hormones.[94]

4. Compensatory activation of prostanoid antihypertensive and hypertensive factors.[69, 78]

5. Vascular endothelial dysfunction primarily manifested by the reduction in the release of the endothelial derived relaxing factor, nitric oxide.[71]

It would be simplistic to think that the factors just enumerated provide an accurate description of the cohort of mechanisms activated by the onset of renal hypoperfusion. Two reviews are recommended for a thorough understanding of the mechanisms associated with the complex response of the cardiovascular system to the evolution of renal hypertension.[40, 49] The reader may also wish to peruse an ample and interesting literature describing the role of

TABLE 119–1. EXPERIMENTAL FORMS OF RENAL HYPERTENSION

TYPE	APPROACH
Two-kidney, one-clip renal hypertension	Clamping of one renal artery; opposite kidney untouched
One-kidney, one-clip hypertension	Partial occlusion of one renal artery; contralateral nephrectomy
Two-kidney, two-clip hypertension	Bilateral stenosis of the renal arteries
Perinephritic hypertension	Cellophane wrapping of one or both kidneys
Figure-of-8 hypertension	Silk wrapping of one or both kidneys
Aortic coarctation hypertension	Occlusion of aorta between ostium of renal arteries

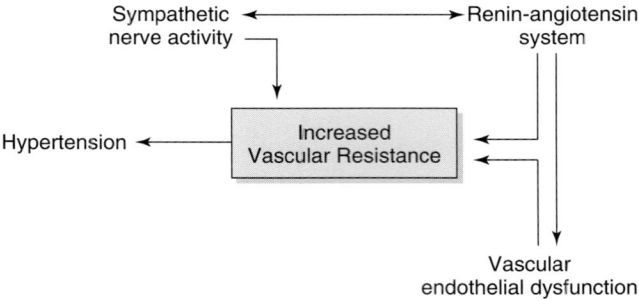

FIGURE 119–1. The increased vascular resistance in hypertension is a product of an unbalance between pressor and vasodepressor mechanisms. Vasoconstriction mediated by the dual actions of angiotensin II and norepinephrine is not appropriately buffered by the tonic vasodilator actions of endothelium-derived nitric oxide.

renal afferent nerves as a signal trigger for the activation of potent neurogenic mechanisms during the early stages of renal hypertension.[110] In the clinical context, however, the pathophysiology of renal hypertension may be summarized as illustrated in Figure 119–1.

Renal hypertension is characterized by a sustained elevation in peripheral vascular resistance that is mediated by activation of both the renin-angiotensin system and the sympathetic nervous system and their concomitant effects in causing vascular endothelial dysfunction. Although the contribution of increased secretion of renin and Ang II production is a sustaining trigger for the hemodynamic and hormonal response, the actions of Ang II on neurogenic mechanisms and the vascular endothelium may be of foremost importance in accounting for the persistence of the blood pressure elevation. A significant number of reports validates this interpretation.

Ablative procedures of vasomotor pathways in the brain effectively reversed the evolution of chronic experimental renal hypertension.[7, 36] Pharmacologic blockade of Ang II synthesis or action lowers blood pressure, restores endothelial dysfunction, and reverses hypertension-related structural changes in the heart and blood vessels. Thus, both the renin-angiotensin and sympathetic nervous system appear to act in concert to regulate the integrated hormonal response that operates to regulate sodium and potassium balance and arterial pressure simultaneously.

There is no denying that renal hypertension is caused by an increased activity of the renin-angiotensin system produced initially by hypersecretion of renin from the ischemic kidney. In the *two-kidney, one-clip* model, the increase in plasma Ang II may be sustained for the duration of the hypertension and may be associated with increased production of aldosterone. A decrease in intrarenal perfusion pressure beyond the obstruction is the stimulus for the increase in the renal release of renin. Sodium retention ensues as a result of the fall in renal blood flow and glomerular filtration rate (GFR) as well as the combined effect of the salt retaining actions of Ang II and aldosterone in renal tubular sodium transport.

The increase in production of circulating Ang II stimulates vasoconstriction through the mechanisms described. The phase of hypertension associated with a demonstrable increase in renin secretion or circulating Ang II may be quite variable because of ensuing activation of other factors.

Pressure natriuresis from the opposite kidney and partial restoration of intrarenal perfusion pressure through the growth of collateral capsular vessels are mechanisms that feed back to suppress renin hypersecretion.

As hypertension evolves into a chronic stage, vascular hypertrophy may become an essential mechanism for maintaining elevated blood pressure and peripheral vascular resistance. The effect of hypertension on the wall-to-lumen ratio of precapillary resistant vessels triggers a myogenic response that is evidenced by the combination of hypertrophy and hyperplasia of the vascular smooth muscle.[45, 85] The increase in bulk vascular smooth muscle augments vascular reactivity to pressor agents. There is also evidence that renin may be trapped in structural elements of the vascular wall.[93] Local production of tissue-borne Ang II may thus contribute to the remodeling of resistance vessels as angiotensinogen (Aogen) may be synthesized locally by vascular fibroblasts.[29]

Angiotensin-converting enzyme (ACE) exists in the plasma membrane of vascular endothelial and smooth muscle cells. Thus, the necessary components for the production of Ang II may be found in vascular and cardiac tissue. In the chronic phases of the hypertension process, hypersecretion of renin from the ischemic kidney may be supplanted by increased production of vascular Ang II as the mechanism that sustains the elevation in arterial pressure.

When abnormal renal renin secretion is demonstrable, the hypertension may be characterized as a curable form of renin-dependent RVH. Those forms of renovascular hypertension in which hypersecretion of renin from the hypoperfused kidney cannot be documented may be at a stage of hypertension in which vascular remodeling and tissue production of Ang II are the primary mechanisms maintaining the elevated blood pressure. Progression of RVH from a pure renal renin-dependent form to the peripheral vascular form of the disease is often a factor accounting for clinical errors of judgment in assessment of the prognosis of surgical intervention.

Experimentally, a positive response to the administration of ACE inhibitors in forms of renovascular hypertension coursing with normal levels of *plasma renin activity* (PRA) suggests activation of a tissue renin-angiotensin system. Clinically, however, a test of this form is not practical or even recommended because the drop in blood pressure produced by pharmacologic blockade of Ang II synthesis may further aggravate renal hypoperfusion, triggering an acute episode of renal failure.[5, 79]

RENIN-ANGIOTENSIN-ALDOSTERONE SYSTEM

The renin-angiotensin system is one of the mechanisms by which mammals regulate homeostasis. The active hormone products of the system act on the factors that regulate body fluid volumes, the electrolytic composition of the internal milieu, and tissue perfusion pressure. Physiologically, the renal renin-angiotensin system may function as a short-term regulator of arterial pressure and body fluid volumes.

Molecular biology has identified renin-angiotensin system genes in the cardiovascular and reproductive systems of mammals.[29] This tissue renin-angiotensin system may be primarily involved in the regulation of cell functions related to growth, neurotransmission, and cell-to-cell communication. The circulating renin-angiotensin system is an example of endocrine regulation, whereas the tissue renin-angiotensin system may manifest actions that conform closely to the action of paracrine, autocrine, and intracrine hormones.[43]

While there is no consensus as to the relative importance of the endocrine and paracrine functions of the circulating and tissue renin-angiotensin systems, emerging data favors an important participation of tissue-derived renin-angiotensin systems in cardiac and vascular pathology.[28, 43] This interpretation best suits accumulating evidence regarding the growth factor properties of Ang II.

Biochemistry

In parallel to other endocrine secretions, the production of the active hormones of the renin-angiotensin system requires sequential enzymatic cleavage of the bioactive peptide from a large molecular weight precursor polypeptide substrate. In recent years, the traditional concepts of the biochemical pathways characterizing the renin-angiotensin system have been revised as new biologically active peptides were characterized and alternate processing pathways were demonstrated. The current schematic outline of the biotransformation process of Aogen into the family of angiotensin peptides is illustrated in Figure 119–2. Each step in the processing of Aogen to the active forms of angiotensin peptides is described below.

Renin is an aspartyl protease which is stored and released by renal juxtaglomerular cells located in the afferent arterioles feeding the glomerulus. Changes in renal perfusion pressure stimulate the secretion of renin, whereas the contiguous region of the macula densa stimulates renin release by sensing changes in the tubular concentrations of Na$^+$ and possibly Cl$^-$.[1] Renin release may be also under the control of circulating Ang II and other cytocrines and transmitters.

Angiotensinogen is a large-molecular-weight polypeptide (α_2-globulin) produced primarily by the liver,[30] however, the messenger ribonucleic acid (mRNA) for Aogen has been

identified in fibroblasts, brown adipose fat, and glial cells. Tissue Aogen is thus a source for the local production of Ang II. Renin cleaves Ang I from Aogen. The second step in the process of biotransformation is the release of active angiotensin hormones from Ang I by specific carboxyl and endopeptidases. Ang II is cleaved from Ang I by a dipeptidyl-carboxypeptidase, known as ACE or *kininase II* (E.C. 3.4.15.1).[33] In humans, the somatic form of ACE contains two large homologous domains. Recent studies suggest that the C-domain of human somatic ACE is the catalytic site participating in the conversion of Ang I into Ang II and the degradation of bradykinin into inactive fragments.[14, 25]

Ang I is considered a circulating pro-hormone with no principal biologic activity. Conversion of Ang I into Ang II by ACE may occur in blood, but peptidase is found also in higher concentrations in the endothelium lining the vascular beds of the lung, kidney, visceral, and skeletal circulations and the choroid plexus. Inhibition of ACE increases the activity of renin in the plasma and concentrations of Ang I in blood. These changes are associated with a drop in plasma levels of Ang II and aldosterone.[53] Several investigators have noted, however, that plasma levels of Ang II may not remain consistently suppressed during chronic therapy with ACE inhibitors, even though blood pressure remains controlled.[15, 55] Dissociation between the therapeutic effects of these drugs and the level of plasma Ang II may indicate incomplete blockade or enhanced expression of the enzyme. Alternatively, the large increases in the circulating levels of Ang I may exceed the inhibitory capacity of the drugs in plasma or tissues.

In recent years, new studies suggest that production of Ang II may be explained by the processing of Ang I through alternate enzymatic pathways. Schiller and colleagues[90] first reported that Ang II could be produced from either the renin substrate tetradecapeptide or Ang I by an enzyme (*tonin*) initially purified from rat submandibular gland. Another enzyme (*chymase*), cloned from human heart, may form Ang II from Ang I.[100] Although the physiologic importance of these alternate Ang II–forming enzymes remains to be established, these proteases may limit the rate of Ang I accumulation in conditions of reduced availability or activity of ACE.

Also important are studies showing that Ang I is also

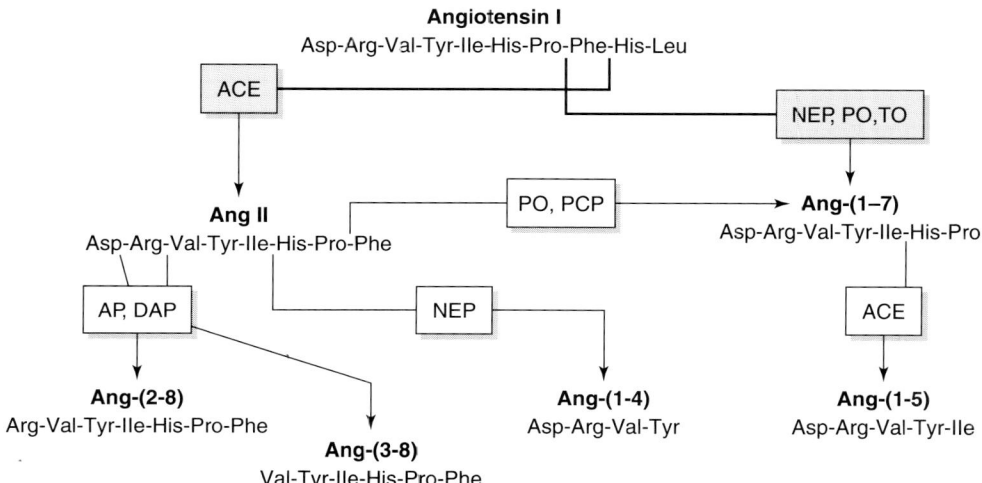

FIGURE 119–2. Biochemical pathways of angiotensin peptide formation and degradation.[104] ACE = angiotensin converting enzyme; NEP = neutral endopeptidase 24.11; PO = prolyl-endopeptidase 24.26; TO = thymet oligopeptidase (metalloendopeptidase 24.15); PCP = postproline carboxypeptidase; AP = aminopeptidase; DAP = diaminopeptidase.

Angiotensin I
Asp-Arg-Val-Tyr-Ile-His-Pro-Phe-His-Leu

ACE

NEP, PO, TO

Ang II
Asp-Arg-Val-Tyr-Ile-His-Pro-Phe

PO, PCP

Ang-(1–7)
Asp-Arg-Val-Tyr-Ile-His-Pro

AP, DAP

NEP

ACE

Ang-(2-8)
Arg-Val-Tyr-Ile-His-Pro-Phe

Ang-(1-4)
Asp-Arg-Val-Tyr

Ang-(1-5)
Asp-Arg-Val-Tyr-Ile

Ang-(3-8)
Val-Tyr-Ile-His-Pro-Phe

processed into novel biologically active forms of angiotensins by a family of endopeptidases. Traditionally, Ang II is known as the natural ligand for binding to angiotensin receptors. The recent discovery that an angiotensin fragment, the amino-terminal heptapeptide Ang-(1-7) ([des-Phe[8]]-Ang II), stimulates the release of vasopressin, acts as an excitatory neurotransmitter, and augments the synthesis and release of vasodilator prostaglandins demonstrated the existence of parallel enzymatic steps diverting peptide formation to selective biologically active peptides.[41] Furthermore, these findings reveal that the cellular actions of the renin-angiotensin system entail the interaction of specific molecular sequences of angiotensin peptides acting on specific types of membrane-bound angiotensin receptors.

Thus, post-transcriptional processing of Aogen is initiated by one or more of a group of *Aogen-processing enzymes*. This family of enzymes includes renin, other aspartyl proteases, and tonin. Additional Ang II–forming enzymes, such as chymotrypsin-like enzyme, kallikrein, and tissue plasminogen activator (t-PA), may be present in peripheral tissues. Since renin is cleaved from a precursor (*prorenin*), this enzymatic step precedes the initiation of the angiotensin system cascade. Prorenin is found both in the circulation and the adrenal gland and the ovary.[14] These findings have suggested that this protein may be a local reservoir of active renin. Recently, prorenin has been thought to have actions of its own as a local vasodilator hormone.[16]

Angiotensin I–processing enzymes comprise the next family of enzymes acting on Ang I to form Ang II and Ang-(1-7). Three endopeptidases have been identified to form Ang-(1-7) from Ang I[41]:

- Prolyl endopeptidase (E.C. 3.4.21.26)
- Neutral endopeptidase (NEP) 24.11 (E.C. 3.4.24.11)
- NEP 24.15 (E.C. 3.4.24.15)

Production of the vasodilator hormone Ang-(1-7) is augmented after inhibition of ACE.[109] These data illustrate a mechanism for diverting the metabolism of Ang I from ACE and the potential for Ang-(1-7) to participate in the vasodilator response elicited by ACE inhibitors.[52] Terminal steps in the biochemical map of the renin-angiotensin system entail the processing of Ang-(1-7) and Ang II into other smaller amino-terminal and carboxyl-terminal fragments. This function is accomplished in part by angiotensin *transformases* (*aminopeptidases*). Ang II may be converted to

Ang-(1-7) by prolyl endopeptidase and to Ang III ([des-Asp[1]]-Ang II) and Ang-(2-7) by aminopeptidases. Further hydrolysis of either Ang-(1-7) or Ang II by dipeptidyl aminopeptidases may produce Ang-(3-8) and Ang-(3-7). These smaller angiotensin fragments influence cyclic guanosine monophosphate (GMP) production and have psychoactive properties. New data, however, show that ACE is the primary route for the metabolism of circulating Ang-(1-7).[19]

Angiotensin peptides interact with receptors found in the plasma membrane of tissues. Two seven-transmembrane receptor proteins have been cloned.[106] The AT$_1$ receptor mediates the physiological actions of Ang II and may be involved in the proliferative actions of Ang II that account for the development of cellular hypertrophy and hyperplasia. The AT$_2$ receptor subtype participates in the regulation of cell differentiation and growth. Emerging data suggest that AT$_2$ receptors may be found in human renal vessels[47] and that they are reexpressed in the hypertrophied heart and in the neo-intima of injured vessels.[20, 60, 102] Additional information suggest that AT$_2$ receptors may negatively modulate the action of Ang II on AT$_1$ receptor subtypes.[20]

Mechanisms of Action of Angiotensin Peptides

Ang II is an ubiquitous hormone functioning to regulate blood pressure, volume, and growth. As a circulating hormone, Ang II has important effects as a vasoconstrictor and salt-retaining factor. Recently, the growth-promoting actions of Ang II have attracted great attention, since they may explain the role of the renin-angiotensin system in the development of cardiac and vascular remodeling (Fig. 119–3). The actions of Ang II at the AT$_1$ receptor initiate a cascade of cellular events that begin by activation of a G-protein/phospholipase second messenger system, causing the release of intracellular Ca^{2+} via the formation of inositol triphosphate and diacylglycerol.[4]

In contrast, Ang-(1-7) acts as a vasodilator, natriuretic, and antiproliferative agent, thus opposing the actions of Ang II.[41] Data derived from animal experiments and cells in culture suggest that Ang-(1-7) is a potent stimulus for the release of vasodilator prostaglandins and nitric oxide.[41] These effects explain the mechanisms by which Ang-(1-7) contributes to the antihypertensive action produced by ACE inhibitors and AT$_1$ receptor blockers. The receptor

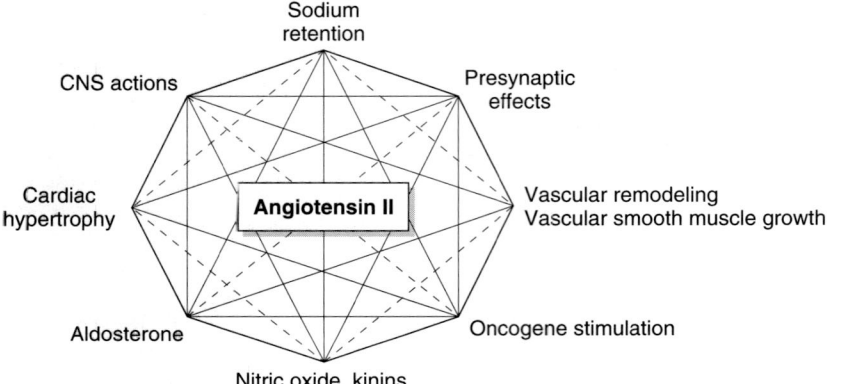

FIGURE 119–3. Mosaic of the multiple actions of angiotensin II in the pathogenesis of hypertension illustrates the effects of the hormone on the multiple systems that regulate arterial pressure.

TABLE 119–2. CLINICAL SYMPTOMS AND SIGNS SUGGESTIVE OF RENOVASCULAR HYPERTENSION

- Onset of hypertension before age of 20, or after age 55 years
- Loss of control of the blood pressure in patients with long standing hypertension
- Accelerated, or malignant hypertension in any age group
- Unexplained azotemia in elderly patients with diffuse atherosclerosis
- Acute renal failure following therapy with angiotensin-converting enzyme inhibitors
- Recurrent pulmonary edema in patients with poorly controlled hypertension
- Marked discrepancy in kidney size in adults, particularly with demonstration of atrophic kidney
- Hypokalemia in patients with severe hypertension not receiving diuretics, resulting from secondary hyperaldosteronism
- Presence of abdominal, epigastric, or flank bruit
- Grade III or IV hypertensive retinopathy

mediating the vasodepressor and antiproliferative actions of Ang-(1-7) has not yet been identified. Pharmacologic studies suggest that Ang-(1-7) binds to a novel receptor with pharmacologic characteristics distinct from either the AT_1 or AT_2 receptor subtype.[95]

DIAGNOSIS

Renovascular hypertension is among the leading causes of potentially curable elevated blood pressure; therefore, its timely diagnosis is crucial in the successful management and prevention of target organ damage. Over the past several decades, a wide range of noninvasive tests have been utilized in the diagnosis of RVH. Because their accuracy in identifying lesions that are amenable to surgical intervention remains questionable, only a few of these procedures are in wide use for the diagnosis of RVH.

Initial Steps

The initiation of a diagnostic evaluation typically follows recognition of clinical manifestations, which are suggestive of renovascular disease (Table 119–2). An active search for clinical and laboratory clues is a prerequisite to the initiation of problem-oriented diagnostic process aimed to exclude a renal origin of the hypertension. Noninvasive diagnostic tests include:

- Intravenous pyelography (IVP)
- Differential renal function studies
- Determination of renin activity
- Radionuclide renography

A complete description of renal duplex sonography appears in Chapter 116. With the introduction of ACE inhibitors (captopril, as a prototype), several stimulation tests have also been developed.

Functional Studies

Intravenous Pyelography

Rapid-sequence ("hypertensive") IVP together with nephrotomography was widely used in the 1960s and 1970s as a standard screening test for the diagnosis of renal artery stenosis (RAS). The following are diagnostic findings[86]:

1. A difference in kidney size greater than 1.5 cm.
2. More than a 1-minute delay in contrast medium appearance in the caliceal system during early sequence views.
3. Hyperconcentration of contrast material on delayed films (persistence nephrogram).

Among these, the last test (No. 3) was proposed as discriminative between RVH and essential hypertension.[6] In this study, however, patients with surgically proven *renal artery stenosis* showed an 11% false-positive and 17% false-negative rate of IVP. An especially low sensitivity was reported in patients with bilateral renal artery stenosis. In addition, the IVP was not reliable in predicting the blood pressure response to surgical revascularization. All of these factors contribute to the low utilization of this suboptimal screening test for RVH.[63] Yet IVP remains an important test in excluding other potential causes for renal dysfunction (i.e., obstructive uropathy and nephrolithiasis).

Differential Renal Function Studies

Split renal function tests were introduced to establish the existence of functional disparities in excretory capacity between the normal and stenosed kidneys. Renal artery stenosis is considered to be functionally significant if (1) urine flow is reduced by 40% to 60%, (2) urinary sodium concentration is decreased by 15%, or (3) the concentration of *non-reabsorbable* substances is increased by 50% to 100% on the stenotic kidney.[73]

Howard's test is based on experimental studies showing that a reduction in renal blood flow is associated with an increase in the fractional reabsorption of sodium and water in the affected kidney.[73] The *unabsorbable* concentration of substances rise in response to increased water and sodium reabsorption. Measurements of these variables in the clinical setting require catheterization of the ureters for the separate collections of urine.

The modification introduced by Stamey involves the concurrent determination of renal plasma flow by the intravenous infusion of both an osmotic diuretic and para-aminohippurate (PAH). Comparison of renal plasma flow values between the affected and unaffected kidneys provides additional information of the relative integrity in the function of the uninvolved kidney. The difficulties of performing these tests in the routine evaluation of hypertensive subjects have resulted in their rare inclusion for the diagnosis of RVH.

Renin Determinations

Plasma Renin Activity

A hallmark of RVH is unilateral hypersecretion of renin from the diseased kidney. Assessment of the degree of renal renin hypersecretion from measurements of renin activity in peripheral venous blood is of little value either as a screening or diagnostic test for RVH[17] because a large percentage of subjects may exhibit normal levels of PRA.[86] Furthermore, multiple factors may account for a detection of increased PRA levels; these include:

- Volume depletion
- Salt restriction
- Exercise
- Upright posture
- Therapy with antihypertensive agents, particularly vasodilators, ACE inhibitors, and diuretics

Accuracy of PRA determinations may be optimized if one indexes the variable to the amount of sodium excretion in urine.[11, 56] The accuracy of this procedure demands that strict pretest guidelines be followed. These guidelines include the use of antihypertensive medication, which should be withheld for up to 3 weeks. Almost 20% of patients with essential hypertension have increased PRA; false-positive and false-negative results may occur in 34% and 43%, respectively, in patients with confirmed RVH.[108] In the absence of antihypertensive medication, elevated PRA measured in the morning in the seated position and indexed against urinary sodium excretion was present in almost 75% of patients with RVH.[84] If patients are receiving an ACE inhibitor, low PRA levels may be considered to exclude RVH.

Stimulated Plasma Renin Activity

Among the attempts to improve the accuracy and predictive value of PRA, Muller and colleagues[74] introduced the provocative captopril test, which involves measurement of PRA 1 hour after administration of a standard dose of captopril. The blockade of ACE with subsequent decrease in Ang II production causes typically an increase in renin production in a negative feedback fashion. The following criteria for a captopril-induced renin response was proposed[89]:

1. Captopril stimulated PRA 12 mg/ml/hr.
2. An absolute increase in PRA amounting to 10 ng/ml/hr.
3. An increase above 150% in PRA or a 400% increase in PRA when baseline PRA is less than 3 ng/ml/hr.

Originally, the test was reported to have 100% sensitivity and specificity in untreated hypertensive patients with arteriographically documented renal artery stenosis.[74] A single-dose captopril test requires meticulous preparation that includes discontinuing antihypertensive medication for at least 2 weeks. Alternatively, patients may receive a beta-blocker, but they should avoid diuretics, ACE inhibitors, and nonsteroid anti-inflammatory drugs (NSAIDs) for at least 1 week. Also, patients should be taking a normal or high-sodium diet (a low-sodium intake may lead to false-positive results). A 24-hour urine collection is performed to measure sodium excretion. The reactive rise of PRA after captopril stimulation is expected to be higher in patients with RVH.

Since the introduction of this promising test, multiple prospective studies reported various test sensitivities and specificities, with sensitivity as low as 38%[87] to 40%[97] and a specificity of 58%.[31] It was demonstrated to be less reliable in subjects with underlying renal insufficiency and did not differentiate between unilateral versus bilateral renal artery stenosis.[74] Consequently, the usefulness of this test is limited.

Renal Vein Renin

A differential renal vein renin sampling is a relatively invasive procedure, introduced several decades ago to measure the ratio between ipsilateral and contralateral renal vein renin. Renal vein renin is elevated in the stenosed kidney, whereas it is suppressed in the contralateral normal one. A renal vein renin ratio greater that 1.5 (criterion for "lateralization" of renin secretion) is predictive of either cure or significant improvement following surgical revascularization.[65]

Marks and Maxwell,[65] in a large retrospective study, reported a 93% surgical success in subjects with unilateral renal artery stenosis and "lateralization" of renal vein renin. However, failure to demonstrate "lateralization" was not a predictive of failure, since 57% of such patients with hypertension and renal artery stenosis benefited from revascularization. Many other studies also demonstrated a high predictive value of renal vein renin lateralization and a high false-negative rate in case of nonlateralization.[92] This, in turn, constitutes a major limitation of the test.

The reasons for this discrepancy are unclear but may indicate technical error in placing the catheters in the renal vein or inadequate patient preparation. Several attempts were made to decrease the rate of false-negative results, such as administration of diuretics, sodium depletion, placing the patient in the upright position, or administering captopril. In a prospective study[89] the false-negative rate (35%) did not improve following pretreatment with captopril. Overall, demonstration of lateralization of renal vein renin in patients with unilateral renal artery stenosis has a high predictive value for beneficial results of renal revascularization.[86]

Captopril Test

Radionuclide Renography

The role of renal scintigraphy in the diagnosis of RVH is debatable. For many years, this method was widely used for the selection of candidates for renal arteriography. Radioisotopes used are ^{131}I-orthoiodohippuric acid (OIH) and ^{99m}Tc-diethylenetriamine pentaacetic acid (DTPA).

OIH serves as a marker for renal plasma flow, and DTPA is a marker for the GFR.[107] Recently, ^{99m}Tc-mercaptor acetyltriglycine (MAG_3) was introduced, and as OIH it is similarly excreted by kidney. The latter tracer provides images of comparable quality at lower radiation dose.

Radionuclide studies also provide a good estimate of kidney size. However, plain isotope renography was practically abandoned for the diagnosis of RVH because of the high incidence of false-negative results and the high frequency of abnormal results in patients with essential hypertension.[68] In addition, radionuclide renography has similar sensitivity and specificity to that for rapid-sequence IVP.[17]

Captopril Renography

The interest in radionuclide evaluation of RVH was rejuvenated with the introduction of ACE inhibitors and the development of a test procedure combining renal scintigraphy with the administration of captopril. The rationale for captopril stimulation is based on the fact that blockade of ACE decreases the vasoconstrictive effect of Ang II on the efferent arterioles. The decline in postglomerular resistance causes a decrease in GFR in the ischemic kidney, whereas GFR remains unchanged or even increases in the nonstenotic kidney.[75, 96] This differential lowering of GFR can be identified using the DTPA renogram. The diagnostic criteria for renal artery stenosis include[77]:

1. Prolonged uptake in the ischemic kidney (time to peak activity 11 minutes).
2. Delayed and decreased excretion (ratio of GFR between kidney 1.5).
3. Decreased size of kidney.

A radionuclide study should be performed in well-hydrated patients who have unlimited salt ingestion prior to the test. Typically, antihypertensive therapy should not be withheld (except for ACE inhibitors). After a baseline renogram is obtained, the patients receive a test dose of 25 to 50 mg of captopril orally, and a second renogram is performed 1 hour later.

Setaro and coauthors,[91] in a study of 90 patients, demonstrated a sensitivity of 91% and a specificity of 94% in the detection of renal artery stenosis greater than 50%. Several other studies reported similar results.[26, 64]

Results of captopril renography in patients with renal dysfunction are less impressive. In a large European trial, the positive predictive value of the test decreased from 88% to 57% when plasma creatinine was greater than 1.5 mg/dl.[76] Elliott and associates[31] reported a significantly higher accuracy of the captopril renogram compared with the captopril-stimulated PRA.

Currently, ACE inhibitor renography is widely used for screening of patients with suspected RVH. A normal captopril renogram makes the diagnosis of unilateral renal artery stenosis highly unlikely.[107] Erbsloh-Moller and colleagues[34] recommend captopril renogram with Hippuran and furosemide as an accurate modality to differentiate between ischemic nephropathy and intrinsic renal disease. Overall, a normal captopril renogram helps to exclude RVH with a reasonable degree of accuracy, whereas a positive finding suggests a high likelihood of RVH in subjects with preserved renal function. The accuracy of the ACE inhibitor renography is limited in subjects with excretory renal insufficiency.

MEDICAL THERAPY

Most patients with presumed RVH have a long-standing history of elevated blood pressure, which initially is typically diagnosed as essential hypertension and is treated accordingly. The availability of newer antihypertensive drugs (i.e., ACE inhibitors and specific angiotensin receptor antagonists) has contributed to the improved results of medical treatment of patients with RVH.

In general, when one is treating a hypertensive patient with severe renal artery stenosis, one would assume that the major dilemma in the management of such patient would be deciding whether to intervene or whether to continue with medical therapy. Until now, however, no large-scale prospective randomized trials have been available to verify the long-term benefits and risks of surgical intervention compared with medical therapy. Patients with severe atherosclerotic renal artery disease are typically elderly, have multiple medical and cardiovascular co-morbidities, and have specific problems related to the RVH (i.e.,

volume overload, progressive renal function impairment, or hypertensive cardiac dysfunction). Therefore, it is important to realize that in patients with renal artery stenosis, hypertension is not always caused by renovascular disease; as a result, not all patients with renal artery stenosis may benefit from renal revascularization. Consequently, several possible sequences of events should be considered:

1. True RVH may be caused solely by renal artery stenosis, or it may be associated with the presence of essential hypertension.
2. The hypertension may be of the essential type, but the renal arteries may be involved as an outcome of generalized vascular atherosclerosis.
3. Hypertensive glomerulosclerosis may be the major cause of the deterioration in renal function.

Thus, in many cases it may be difficult to differentiate which of these clinical categories is the primary cause of hypertension or renal insufficiency; assessment for the need of intervention when renal artery stenosis is discovered may be complex.

Main objectives of medical therapy are (1) to reduce blood pressure, (2) to control associated cardiovascular risk factors, and (3) to prevent target organ damage. Antihypertensive medications may control blood pressure in the majority of patients with RVH. Medical therapy should be closely monitored for blood pressure control, changes in the kidney size, anatomic progression of renal artery stenosis, development or worsening of renal dysfunction, and appearance of congestive heart failure.

Dustan's group[27] published the first large series of patients with RVH treated medically. Since then, a sizable number of similar nonrandomized studies were reported in the past three decades. Since the introduction of beta-blockers and ACE inhibitors, the results of pharmaceutical blood pressure control in RVH have improved dramatically, bringing the success rate from 40%[27] to between 80% and 90%.[18] In an early study, Dean and coauthors[23] evaluated 41 patients who had a presumed diagnosis of RVH initially treated medically, including 31 patients who had follow-up renal arteriograms. Blood pressure control was achieved in almost two thirds of those patients; renal artery occlusion developed in four patients (12%), and 17 patients (41%) underwent surgical revascularization after deterioration of renal function. Most of the studies unanimously reported high cardiovascular mortality in patients with atherosclerotic renal artery stenosis treated medically.

Recently, Webster's group,[103] from Scotland, reported results of the first prospective randomized trial that compared the effects of percutaneous renal artery angioplasty with medical therapy on blood pressure and renal function in 55 hypertensive patients with arteriographically severe (>50%) renal artery stenosis. During the short follow-up period, there was no significant difference between major cardiovascular events rate and renal function parameters. Only patients with bilateral renal artery stenosis who underwent angioplasty had a significant improvement in blood pressure control. No improvement in excretory renal function was observed.

PHARMACOLOGIC THERAPY

The mainstay of medical therapy in the patients with RVH involves primarily the use of pharmacologic agents that

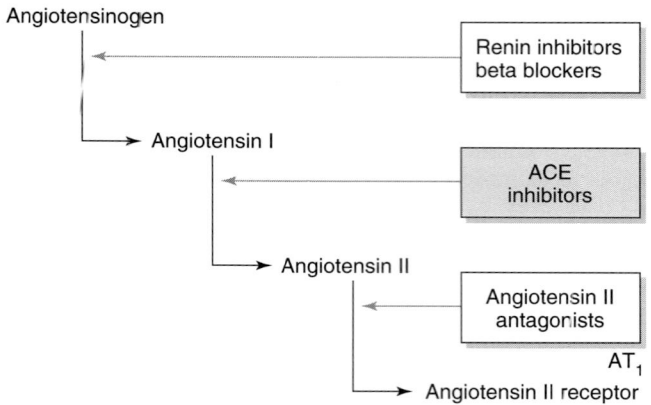

FIGURE 119–4. Principal site of action of antihypertensive agents with a mode of action affecting either the synthesis of angiotensin I and angiotensin II or the binding of the hormone to the AT_1 receptor. ACE = angiotensin-converting enzyme;

interfere with the components of the renin-angiotensin system. Figure 119–4 illustrates the effect of the antihypertensive activities of the three major groups of RVH. In addition to pharmacologic suppression of the renin-angiotensin system, volume control with the use of diuretics and salt restriction is important.[11, 57, 58]

Angiotensin-Converting Enzyme Inhibitors

The antihypertensive effects of ACE inhibitors are multifactorial and include the following mechanisms[2, 3, 3, 44, 88, 108]:

1. Inhibition of the conversion of Ang I to Ang II.
2. Inhibition of aldosterone secretion and induction of natriuresis.
3. Increased plasma concentration of vasodilator bradykinin.
4. Inhibition of local formation of Ang II in vascular tissue and myocardium.
5. Reduction of sympathetic reactivity.

ACE inhibitors were demonstrated to have a reno-protective effect resulting from an improved renal microcirculation.[51] The renal efferent arterioles are more sensitive to Ang II than the afferent and interlobular arterioles.[51] Thus, ACE inhibitors decrease efferent arteriolar resistance, which contributes to the lowering of glomerular capillary pressure. The protective effect of ACE inhibitors may also relate to blockade of the proliferative actions of Ang II on the renal mesangium and the arterial wall.[22] Although the short-term effect of ACE inhibition is related to the decrease in Ang II production, Ang II levels may remain above normal values during chronic therapy. The inability of chronic ACE therapy to suppress the production of Ang II may be the result of overflow from increased levels of Ang I or the activity of alternative pathways for the production of the peptide.[38] The renal-protective effects of ACE inhibition on renal function may also result from increases in the tissue activity of bradykinin and Ang-(1-7).[41]

ACE inhibitors (Table 119–3) differ in the chemical structure of their active moieties, in bioavailability, potency, plasma half-life, and the affinity to tissue-bound ACE.[53] Side effects include first-dose hypotension (especially in

the patients with high PRA), hyperkalemia (due to decrease in aldosterone levels), dry cough (attributed to increase in bradykinin effect), neutropenia, and angioedema.[9]

In patients with bilateral renal artery stenosis or in patients with unilateral renal artery stenosis limited to a solitary kidney, ACE inhibition may cause transient deterioration of renal function and acute renal failure, which typically resolve after discontinuation of the therapy. An increase in serum creatinine in these settings is due to decrease in the GFR following lowering of blood pressure and glomerular perfusion in the stenotic kidney.[88]

In an interesting study, van de Ven and coworkers summarized the results of the first prospective trial involving 108 hypertensive patients at risk for renovascular disease who received controlled exposure to ACE inhibition.[101] The authors correlated the follow-up serum creatinine and other renal function markers with renal arteriography findings. The increase in plasma creatinine correlated with the degree of renal artery stenosis ($r = .53$; $p < .001$). In this study, an increase greater than 25% in serum creatinine after ACE inhibition was 100% sensitive in detecting severe bilateral renal artery stenosis, but the specificity of the procedure was only 70%.

Angiotensin II Receptor Antagonists

The first peptide Ang II receptor blocker, saralasin, was abandoned from clinical use because of its agonist properties and poor bioavailability.[10] Recently, orally active selective Ang II receptor antagonists have been developed that are highly effective in binding to the AT_1 receptor.[98, 99] There are at least three advantages to the use of these substances:

1. Prolonged use of ACE inhibitors eventually leads to recovery of Ang II to above-normal levels.
2. ACE inhibitors interfere with the metabolism of other important vasoactive substances.[105]
3. Ang II receptor blockers do not interfere with ACE activity; therefore, their use is associated with no alterations in the endogenous function of bradykinin.

Ang II antagonists differ from other classes of antihypertensive agents in terms of being essentially devoid of side effects.[42] The smooth control of blood pressure achieved with this new class of agents is unrelated to the level of PRA. Ang II antagonists are contraindicated, however, in

TABLE 119–3. ANGIOTENSIN-CONVERTING ENZYME INHIBITORS AND ANGIOTENSIN II RECEPTOR BLOCKERS

CONVERTING ENZYME INHIBITORS		ANGIOTENSIN II ANTAGONISTS	
Drug	**Trade Name**	**Drug**	**Trade Name**
Captopril	Capoten	Losartan	Cozaar
Enalapril	Vasotec	Irbesartan	Avapro
Benazepril	Lotensin	Valsartan	Diovan
Fosinopril	Monopril	Candersartan	Atacan
Quinapril	Accupril	Eprosartan	
Ramipril	Altace	Telmisartan	
Lisinopril	Prinivil, Zestril	Tasosartan	
Trandolapril	Mavik		

patients with bilateral renal artery stenosis or with unilateral renal artery stenosis limited to a single kidney.

Beta-Blockers, Calcium-Channel Blockers, and Other Medications

The potential utilization of beta-blockade in the management of RVH is based on the suppression of renin release from the juxtaglomerular complex with subsequent decrease in conversion of Ang I to Ang II.[12] Beta-blockers have a greater antihypertensive effect in patients with high PRA than in those with low PRA.[13] Additional benefits of beta-blockade include:

1. Reduction of cardiac output and heart rate.
2. Decreased peripheral vascular resistance.
3. Blunted catecholamine response to stress.

Calcium antagonists are widely used in patients with RVH.[32, 62, 67, 70] Their effect is predominantly attributed to direct arteriolar vasodilation. The safety of these medications is also related to favorable effects on renal function. Particularly effective are dihydropyridine calcium-channel blockers.

From the practical standpoint, in patients with suspected RVH, initial medical therapy should include a combination of beta-blockers with ACE inhibitors, Ang II blockers, or calcium-channel antagonists. A combination of ACE and calcium channel inhibition is very potent. The use of diuretics should be reserved as a second tier of therapy.

REFERENCES

1. Abe K, Ito S: The kidney and hypertension. Hypertens Res 20:75–84, 1997.
2. Atlas SA, Rosendorf C: The renin-angiotensin system: From Tigerstedt to Goldblatt to ACE inhibition and beyond. Mt Sinai J Med 65:81–86, 1998.
3. Barbe F, Su JB, Guyene TT, et al: Bradykinin pathway is involved in acute hemodynamic effects of enalaprilat in dogs with heart failure. Am J Physiol 39:1985–1992, 1996.
4. Berk BC, Corson MA: Angiotensin II signal transduction in vascular smooth muscle: Role of tyrosine kinases. Circ Res 80:607–616, 1997.
5. Biollaz J, Brunner HR, Gavras I, et al: Antihypertensive therapy with MK 421: Angiotensin II–renin relationships to evaluate efficacy of converting enzyme blockade. J Cardiovasc Pharmacol 4:966–972, 1982.
6. Bookstein JJ, Abrams HL, Buenger RE, et al: Radiologic aspects or renovascular hypertension: 2. The role of urography in unilateral renovascular disease. JAMA 220:1225–1230, 1972.
7. Brody MJ, Fink GD, Buggy J, et al: The role of the anteroventral third ventricle (AV3V) region in experimental hypertension. Circ Res 43(Suppl I):I2–I13, 1978.
8. Brown NJ, Vaughan DE: Angiotensin-converting enzyme inhibitors. Circulation 97:1411–1420, 1998.
9. Brunner HR: ACE inhibitors in renal disease. Kidney Int 42:463–479, 1992.
10. Brunner HR, Gavras H, Laragh JH: Angiotensin-II blockade in man by Sar1-Ala8-angiotensin II for understanding and treatment of high blood-pressure. Lancet 10:1045–1048, 1973.
11. Brunner HR, Gavras H, Laragh JH, Keenan R: Hypertension in man: Exposure of the renin and sodium components using angiotensin II blockade. Circ Res XXXIV(Suppl I):I35–I46, 1974.
12. Brunner HR, Nussberger J, Waeber B: Angiotensin II blockade compared with other pharmacological methods of inhibiting the renin-angiotensin system. J Hypertens 11:S53–S58, 1993.
13. Buhler FR, Laragh JH, Baer L, et al: Propranolol inhibition of renin secretion. N Engl J Med 287:1209–1214, 1972.
14. Campbell DJ: Metabolism of prorenin, renin, angiotensinogen, and the angiotensins by tissues. In Robertson JIS, Nicholls MG (eds). The Renin-Angiotensin Sstem. London, Gower, 1993, pp 23.1–23.23.
15. Campbell DJ, Duncan AM, Kladis A, Harrap SB: Angiotensin peptides in spontaneously hypertensive and normotensive Donryu rats. Hypertension 25:928–934, 1995.
16. Campbell WG, Grahnem F, Catanzaro DF, et al: Plasma and renal prorenin/renin, renin mRNA, and blood pressure in Dahl salt-sensitive and salt-resistant rats. Hypertension 27:1121–1133, 1996.
17. Canzanello VJ, Textor SC: Noninvasive diagnosis of renovascular disease (Astract). Mayo Clin Proc 69:1172–1181, 1994.
18. Case DB, Atlas SA, Marion RM, et al: Long-term efficiency of captopril in renovascular and essential hypertension. Am J Cardiol 49:1440–1446, 1982.
19. Chappell MC, Pirro NT, Sykes A, Ferrario CM: Metabolism of angiotensin-(1–7) by angiotensin converting enzyme. Hypertension 31:362–367, 1998.
20. Chung O, Stoll M, Unger T: Physiologic and pharmacologic implications of AT1 versus AT2 receptors (Abstract). Blood Pressure 2:47–52, 1997.
21. Cowley AW, Jr, Roman RJ: The pressure-diuresis-natriuresis mechanism in normal and hypertensive states. In Zanchetti A, Tarazi RC (eds): Handbook of Hypertension. Vol 8. Pathophysiology of Hypertension—Regulatory Mechanisms. London, Elsevier, 1986, pp 295–314.
22. Daemen MJ, Lombardi DM, Boxman FT: Angiotensin II induces smooth muscle cell proliferation in the normal and injured rat arterial wall. Circ Res 68:450–456, 1991.
23. Dean RH, Kieffer RW, Smith BM, et al: Renovascular hypertension: Anatomic and renal function changes during drug therapy. Arch Surg 116:1408–1415, 1981.
24. Dean RH, Lawson JD, Hollifield JW, et al: Revascularization of the poorly functioning kidney. Surgery 85:44–52, 1979.
25. Deddish PA, Marcic B, Jackman HL, et al: N-domain specific substrate and C-domain inhibitors of angiotensin converting enzyme. Hypertension 31:912–917, 1998.
26. Dondi M: Captopril renal scintigraphy with 99mTc mercaptor acetyltriglycine (99mTc-MAG3) for detecting renal artery stenosis. Am J Hypertens 4:737S–740S, 1991.
27. Dustan HP, Page IH, Poutasse EF, et al: An evaluation of treatment of hypertension associated with occlusive renal arterial disease. Circulation 27:1018–1027, 1963.
28. Dzau VJ: Local expression and pathophysiological role of renin-angiotensin in the blood vessels and heart. Basic Res Cardiol 88:1–14, 1993.
29. Dzau VJ, Re R: Tissue angiotensin system in cardiovascular medicine. Circulation 89:493–498, 1994.
30. Eggena P, Barrett JD: Regulation and functional consequences of angiotensinogen gene expression. J Hypertens 10:1307–1311, 1992.
31. Elliott WJ, Martin WB, Murphy MB: Comparison of two noninvasive screening tests for renovascular hypertension. Arch Intern Med 153:755–764, 1993.
32. Epstein M: Calcium antagonists and the kidney: Implications for renal protection. Am J Hypertens 6:251S–259S, 1993.
33. Erdos EG: Angiotensin I converting enzyme. Circ Res 36:247–255, 1975.
34. Erbsloh-Moller B, Dumas A, Roth DR, et al: Furosemide 131I-hippuran renography after angiotensin-converting enzyme inhibition for the diagnosis of renovascular disease. Am J Med 90:23–29, 1991.
35. Ferrario CM: Contributions of cardiac output and peripheral resistance to experimental renal hypertension. Am J Physiol 226:711–717, 1974.
36. Ferrario CM: Central nervous system mechanisms of blood pressure control in normotensive and hypertensive states. Chest 83(Suppl):331–335, 1983.
37. Ferrario CM: Neurogenic actions of angiotensin II. Hypertension 5(Suppl V): V73–V79, 1983.
38. Ferrario CM: Biological roles of angiotensin-(1–7). Hypertens Res 15:61–66, 1992.
39. Ferrario CM, Blumle C, Nadzam GR, McCubbin JW: An externally adjustable renal artery clamp. J Appl Physiol 3:635–637, 1971.
40. Ferrario CM, Carretero OA: Hemodynamics of experimental renal hypertension. In DeJong W (ed): Handbook of Hypertension. Vol 4:

Experimental and Genetic Models of Hypertension. Amsterdam, Elsevier, 1984, pp 54–80.

41. Ferrario CM, Chappell MC, Tallant EA, et al: Counterregulatory actions of angiotensin-(1–7). Hypertension 30:535–541, 1997.
42. Ferrario CM, Flack JM: Pathologic consequences of increased angiotensin II activity. Cardiovasc Drugs Ther 10:511–518, 1996.
43. Ferrario CM, Moriguchi A, Brosnihan KB: Angiotensin mechanisms in hypertension. In Ganten, DeJong W (eds): Handbook of Hypertension. Amsterdam, Elsevier, 1998, pp 441–461.
44. Ferrario CM, Schiavone MT: The renin-angiotensin system: Importance in physiology and pathology. Cleve Clin J Med 56:439–446, 1989.
45. Folkow B: Physiological aspects of primary hypertension. Physiol Rev 62:347–504, 1982.
46. Goldblatt H, Lynch J, Hanzal RF, Summerville WW: Studies on experimental hypertension: I. The production of persistent elevation of systolic blood pressure by means of renal ischemia. J Exp Med 59:347–379, 1934.
47. Goldfarb DA, Diz DI, Tubbs RR, et al: Angiotensin II receptor subtypes in the human renal cortex and renal cell carcinoma. J Urol 151:208–213, 1994.
48. Guyton AC, Coleman TG, Cowrey AW, et al: A system analysis approach to understanding long-range arterial pressure control and hypertension. Circ Res 35:159–176, 1974.
49. Guyton AC, Coleman TG, Bower JD, Granger HJ: Circulatory control in hypertension. Circ Res XXVI and XXVII(Suppl II)]:II135–II147, 1970b.
50. Hansen KJ, Ditesheim JA, Metropol SH, et al: Management of renovascular hypertension in the elderly population. J Vasc Surg 10:266–273, 1989.
51. Inman SR, Stowe NT, Vidt DG: Role of the microcirculation in antihypertensive therapy. Cleve Clin J Med 61:356–361, 1994.
52. Iyer SN, Ferrario CM, Chappell MC: Angiotensin-(1–7) contributes to the antihypertensive effects of blockade of the renin-angiotensin system. Hypertension 31:356–361, 1998.
53. Johnston CI: Angiotensin-converting enzyme inhibitors. In Robertson JIS, Nicholls MG (eds): The Renin-Angiotensin System. London, Gower, 1993, pp 87.1–87.15.
54. Kaplan NM: Clinical Hypertension, 4th ed. Baltimore, Williams & Wilkins, 1986, pp 1–492.
55. Kohara K, Brosnihan KB, Ferrario CM: Angiotensin-(1–7) in the spontaneously hypertensive rat. Peptides 14:883–891, 1993.
56. Laragh JH: Curable renal hypertension—renin marker or cause? JAMA 218:733–734, 1971.
57. Laragh JH: Historical perspective on renin system blockade in the treatment of hypertension. Am J Hypertens 5:207S–208S, 1992.
58. Laragh JH, Baer L, Brunner HR, et al: Renin, angiotensin and aldosterone system in pathogenesis and management of hypertensive vascular disease. Am J Med 256:H1416–H1431, 1989.
59. Liard JF, Peters G: Role of the retention of water and sodium in two types of experimental renovascular hypertension in the rat. Pflugers Arch 344:93–108, 1973.
60. Liu Y-H, Yang X-P, Sharov VG, et al: Paracrine systems in the cardioprotective effect of angiotensin-converting enzyme inhibitors on myocardial ischemia/reperfusion injury in rats. Hypertension 27:7–13, 1996.
61. Lodwick D, Zagato L, Kaiser MA, et al: Genetic analysis of the S_A and Na^+/K^+-ATPase α_1 genes in the Milan hypertensive rat. J Hypertens 16:139–144, 1998.
62. Maher MJ, Dworkin LD: Calcium antagonists in the treatment of hypertension: Special clinical considerations. Curr Opin Nephrol Hypertens 5:437–441, 1996.
63. Mann SJ, Pickering TG: Detection of renovascular hypertension: State of the art: 1992. Ann Intern Med 117:845–853, 1992.
64. Mann SJ, Pickering TG, Sos TA, et al: Captopril renography in the diagnosis of renal artery stenosis: Accuracy and limitations. Am J Med 90:30–39, 1991.
65. Marks LS, Maxwell MH: Renal vein renin: Value and limitations in the prediction of operative results. Urol Clin North Am 2:311–325, 1975.
66. Masaki Z, Ferrario CM, Bumpus FM, et al: The course of arterial pressure and the effect of SAR2 Thr8-angiotensin II in a new model of two-kidney hypertension in conscious dogs. Clin Sci Mol Med 52:163–170, 1977.
67. Materson BJ, Reda DJ, Cushman WC, et al: Single-drug therapy for hypertension in men. N Engl J Med 328:914–921, 1993.
68. Maxwell MH, Lupu AN, Taplin GV: Radioisotope renogram in renal arterial hypertension. J Urol 100:376–383, 1968.
69. McGiff JC, Quilley CP: Thromboxane A_2 and prostaglandin mediators in hypertension. Clin Cardiol 12:IV-18–IV-22, 1989.
70. Mimran A, Ribstein J: Angiotensin-converting enzyme inhibitors versus calcium antagonists in the progression of renal diseases. Am J Hypertens 7:73S–81S, 1994.
71. Moncada S, Palmer RMJ, Higgs EA: Nitric oxide: Physiology, pathophysiology, and pharmacology. Pharmacol Rev 43:109–141, 1991.
72. Moore MA: End-stage kidney disease: A southern epidemic. South Med J 87:1013–1017, 1994.
73. Moser M, Goldman AG: Definitive diagnostic procedures. In Hypertensive Vascular Disease: Diagnosis and Treatment. Philadelphia, JB Lippincott, 1967, pp 56–67.
74. Muller FB, Sealey JE, Case DB, et al: The captopril test for identifying renovascular disease in hypertensive patients. Am J Med 80:633–644, 1986.
75. Nally JV: Renal physiology of renal artery stenosis. Am J Hypertens 4:669S–774S, 1991.
76. Nally JV: Provocative captopril testing in the diagnosis of renovascular hypertension (Abstract). Urol Clin North Am 21:227–234, 1994.
77. Nally JV, Chen C, Fine E, et al: Diagnostic criteria of renovascular hypertension with captopril renography—a consensus statement. Am J Hypertens 4:749S–752S, 1991.
78. Nasjletti A: The role of eicosanoids in angiotensin-dependent hypertension. Hypertension 31:194–200, 1997.
79. Olin JW, Vidt DG, Gifford RW Jr, Novick AC: Renovascular disease in the elderly: An analysis of 50 patients. J Am Coll Cardiol 5:1232–1238, 1985.
80. Page IH: A method for producing persistent hypertension by cellophane. Science 89:273–274, 1939.
81. Page IH, Heuer GJ: The effect of renal denervation on patients suffering from nephritis. J Clin Invest XIV:443–458, 1935.
82. Page IH, Heuer GJ: The effect of splanchnic nerves resection on patients suffering from hypertension. Am J Med Sci 193:820–842, 1937.
83. Page IH, Kaneko Y, McCubbin JW: Cardiovascular reactivity in acute and chronic renal hypertensive dogs. Circ Res 18:379–387, 1966.
84. Pickering TG, Sos TA, Vaughan ED, et al: Predictive value and changes of renin secretion in hypertensive patients with unilateral renovascular disease undergoing renal angioplasty. Am J Med 76:398–404, 1984.
85. Pipinos II, Nypaver TJ, Moshin SK, et al: Response to angiotensin inhibition in rats with sustained renovascular hypertension correlates with response to removing renal artery stenosis. J Vas Surg 28:167–177, 1998.
86. Pohl MA: Renal artery stenosis, renal vascular hypertension, and ischemic nephropathy. In Schrier RW, Gottoschalk CW (eds): Diseases of the Kidney, 6th ed. Boston, Little, Brown, 1997, pp 1367–423.
87. Postma CT, van der Steen PHM, Hoegnagels HL, et al: The captopril test in detection of renovascular disease in hypertensive patients. Arch Intern Med 150:625–628, 1990.
88. Rimmer JM, Gennari FJ: Atherosclerotic renovascular disease and progressive renal failure. Ann Intern Med 118:712–719, 1993.
89. Roubidoux MA, Dunnick NR, Cotman PE: Renal vein renins: Inability to predict response to revascularization in patients with hypertension. Radiology 178:819–822, 1991.
90. Schiller PW, Demassieux S, Boucher R: Substrate specificity of tonin from rat submaxillary gland. Circ Res 39 629–632, 1976.
91. Setaro JF, Saddler MC, Chen CC, et al: Simplified captopril renography in diagnosis and treatment of renal artery stenosis. Hypertension 18:289–298, 1991.
92. Smith MC, Dunn MJ: Renovascular and renal parenchymal hypertension. In Brenner BM, Rector FC Jr (eds): The Kidney, 3rd ed. Philadelphia, WB Saunders, 1986, p 1221.
93. Swales JD, Abramovici A, Beck F, et al: Arterial wall renin. J Hypertens 1:17–22, 1983.
94. Szilagyi JE, Chelly J, Doursout MF: Suppression of renin release by antagonism of endogenous opiates in the dog. Am J Physiol 250:R633–R637, 1986.
95. Tallant EA, Lu X, Weiss RB, et al: Bovine aortic endothelial cells contain an angiotensin-(1–7) receptor. Hypertension 29:388–392, 1997.
96. Textor SC, Tarazi RC, Novick AC, et al: Regulation of renal hemody-

namics and glomerular filtration in patients with renovascular hypertension during converting enzyme inhibition with captopril. Am J Med 76:29–37, 1984.

97. Thibonnier M, Sassano P, Joseph A, et al: Diagnostic value in a single dose of captopril in renin and aldosterone dependent surgically curable hypertension (Abstract). Cardiovasc Rev Rep 3:1659–1667, 1982.

98. Timmermans PBM, Duncia JV, Carini DJ, et al: Discovery of losartan, the first angiotensin II receptor antagonist. J Hum Hypertens 9:S3–S18, 1995.

99. Timmermans PB, Wong PC, Chiu AT, et al: Angiotensin II receptors and angiotensin II receptor antagonists. Pharmacol Rev 45:205–251, 1993.

100. Urata H, Kinoshita A, Misono KS, et al: Identification of a highly specific chymase as the major angiotensin II–forming enzyme in the human heart. J Biol Chem 265:22348–22357, 1990.

101. van de Ven PJG, Beutler JJ, Kaatee R, et al: Angiotensin converting enzyme inhibitor–induced renal dysfunction in atherosclerotic renovascular disease. Kidney Int 53:986–993, 1998.

102. Viswanathan M, Tsutsumi K, Correa FMA, Saavedra JM: Changes in expression of angiotensin receptor subtypes in the rat aorta during development. Biochem Biophys Res Commun 179:1361–1367, 1991.

103. Webster J, Marshall F, Abdalla M, et al: Randomized comparison of percutaneous angioplasty vs. continued medical therapy for hypertensive patients with atheromatous renal artery stenosis. J Hum Hypertens 12:329–334, 1998.

104. Welches WR, Brosnihan KB, Ferrario CM: A comparison of the properties, and enzymatic activity of three angiotensin processing enzymes: Angiotensin converting enzyme, prolyl endopeptidase and neutral endopeptidase 24.11. Life Sci 52:1461–1480, 1993.

105. Wexler RR, Carini DJ, Duncia JV, et al: Rationale for the chemical development of angiotensin II receptor antagonists. Am J Hypertens 5:209S–220S, 1992.

106. Wong PC, Hart SD, Chiu AT, et al: Pharmacology of DuP 532, a selective and noncompetitive AT, receptor antagonist. J Pharmacol Exp Ther 259:861–870, 1991.

107. Woolfson RG, Neild GH: Renal nuclear medicine: Can it survive the millennium? Nephrol Dial Transplant 13:12–14, 1998.

108. Working Group on Renovascular Hypertension: Detection, evaluation, and treatment of renovascular hypertension. Arch Intern Med 147:820–829, 1987.

109. Yamada K, Iyer SN, Chappell MC, et al: Converting enzyme determines the plasma clearance of angiotensin-(1–7). Hypertension (in press).

110. Zimmerman BG, Arendshortst WJ, Dibona GF, et al: Renal functional derangements in hypertension. Fed Proc 45:2661–2664, 1986.

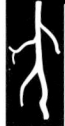

CHAPTER 1 2 0

Radiographic Evaluation and Treatment of Renovascular Disease

Suzanne M. Slonim, M.D., and Michael D. Dake, M.D.

Angiographic Evaluation

The recent technologic advances in diagnostic imaging have allowed the development of multiple noninvasive techniques for the evaluation of renal artery anatomy. These include ultrasonography with duplex scanning,[1-3] computed tomographic angiography (CTA),[4-7] and magnetic resonance angiography (MRA).[8-11] Several promising diagnostic tools also have emerged that may give important physiologic information about renal blood flow. These include captopril renal scintigraphy,[12, 13] renal artery blood flow quantitation with electron beam CT,[14] and magnetic resonance imaging (MRI).[15, 16]

Despite these advances, a definitive diagnosis of renal artery pathology continues to depend on visualization of renal artery anatomy with angiographic techniques. After a diagnosis of renal vascular disease is established, decisions regarding surgical or endovascular treatments are based in part on the arteriographic appearance of the lesion. Therefore, an understanding of angiographic techniques for evaluation of the renal arteries as well as the angiographic appearances of common renal arterial pathology are crucial.

ARTERIOGRAPHY

The "gold standard" of renal artery evaluation is arteriography. This can be performed with film-screen or digital subtraction techniques. In film-screen arteriography, multiple sequential x-ray images are recorded on 14 × 14 inch film during the intra-arterial injection of contrast material. The images are reviewed after the film is developed. During digital subtraction angiography (DSA), multiple sequential fluoroscopic images received by an image intensifier are electronically converted to digital form and stored. An image that contains no intravascular contrast material, the mask, is electronically subtracted from images containing contrast. In this manner, only the vessels filled with contrast material are visualized. The images are immediately displayed on a 1024 × 1024 matrix screen for review. Computer manipulation of the digital data allows modification of DSA images. Selected images can be stored on computer disk and printed on film for the patient record.

DSA is very sensitive to motion artifact because it involves the subtraction of one image from another. Any movement between images degrades image quality. Patient cooperation is necessary, and conscious sedation is often helpful. For patients with large amounts of bowel gas, the intravenous administration of glucagon (0.5 to 1.0 mg) before image acquisition also improves evaluation of the abdominal aorta and its branches by decreasing peristalsis. Small amounts of movement can usually be compensated for by computer manipulation of the images.

DSA has many advantages over film-screen arteriography. It has significantly higher contrast resolution, allowing the use of smaller volumes of contrast material. DSA provides significant cost savings related to reductions in film use, staffing needs, image acquisition time, and examination time.[17, 18] There was early interest in intravenous DSA (IV-DSA) to evaluate the renal arteries because of the lower cost and the potential to avoid an arterial puncture.[19-22] Inadequate examinations were fairly frequent, however, because of obscuration of the renal arteries by overlapping visceral vessels, movement of overlying bowel gas, and dilution resulting in inadequate opacification of the renal arteries. In a review of the IVDSA literature, the technique was found to produce a nondiagnostic study in approximately 7% of cases, with an average sensitivity of 87.6% and specificity of 89.5% compared with arteriography.[23] More recent studies have found IVDSA to be less accurate.[24-27] In addition, because patients thought to have renal vascular disease will likely require arteriography after IVDSA, the use of the technique has lost favor.[28-32]

Intra-arterial digital subtraction imaging, on the other hand, has proved very reliable. Specifically in the evaluation of the renal arteries, the reliability of intra-arterial DSA is considered equivalent to that of film-screen arteriography.[18, 28, 33-35] The three line pairs per millimeter spatial resolution of DSA is lower than the five line pairs per millimeter for the film-screen technique; however, digital technology is improving rapidly. The high contrast resolution, the convenience of immediate image availability and storage, the potential for manipulation of digital images after acquisition, and the cost savings all contribute to the probable replacement of film-screen arteriography with intra-arterial DSA.

During either film-screen arteriography or DSA, evaluation of the renal arteries usually begins with an aortic injection of contrast material. A 5 French (Fr.) multiple side-hole catheter is placed into the aorta through a femoral or brachial artery approach[36] with a modified Seldinger technique.[37] Contrast material is injected with an automatic power injector while sequential images are recorded. The rate and volume of contrast injection, as well as the rate of image acquisition, are determined for each patient based on flow seen during a manual injection of contrast material. In general, however, a contrast injection of between 15 and 20 ml per second for 2 seconds is usually adequate. Images usually are acquired at a rate of three per second for 3 to 5 seconds, followed by a rate of one to two images per second for the next 5 seconds. These images allow assessment of the arterial, the nephrographic, and occasionally the venous phases of flow.

For optimal visualization of the renal arteries, attention to several technical details is required. Multiple catheters have been designed to optimize opacification of the renal arteries during an injection into the aorta.[38, 39] The catheter should be positioned with the side holes at the level of the renal arteries, usually between the first and second lumbar vertebrae. Ideally, the catheter should be positioned low enough to avoid filling of the superior mesenteric artery and its branches, which may overlap the renal arteries and obscure them.[38]

The number of renal arteries is highly variable, with multiple arteries to a single kidney seen in 20% to 30% of patients.[40-42] The right renal artery usually arises cephalad to the left, and both the right and left renal arteries usually arise from the anterolateral surface of the aorta.[40, 43, 44] The proximal portions of the renal arteries, therefore, can be obscured by overlap with the contrast-filled aorta.

Because of the variability of the origins of the renal arteries in the sagital and coronal planes, many studies have attempted to establish the optimal rotational projection for acquiring images.[45-48] Most often, images are acquired in anteroposterior (AP) and shallow left anterior oblique (LAO) projections. Verschuyl and coworkers performed a detailed analysis of the angles at which the renal arteries originate from the aorta as seen on axial imaging with CT scans.[45] They found that a 15- to 20-degree LAO projection most frequently demonstrated the origins of the renal arteries without overlap of the contrast-filled aorta. The next most useful projections were the AP, followed by the 40-degree LAO view.[46] The maximum allowable projection error was 10 degrees before a significant length of vessel would be hidden. If a particular arteriographic view did not project the renal artery origin in profile, a subsequent projection change of at least 10 degrees was shown to be appropriate in most cases. If cross-sectional imaging is available for review before the arteriogram is performed, the exact projection that will best depict the renal arteries can be determined.

Aortography with optimized technique usually provides adequate evaluation of the main renal arteries and the segmental and subsegmental branches.[18, 30, 49, 50] In some cases, selective catheterization of the renal arteries[51] is necessary for visualization of the orifice and distal branches without overlap from the aorta or other vessels. Catheterization of the renal artery usually is performed with a preshaped Cobra- or Simmons-type catheter, with injection of 3 to 6 ml of contrast per second for 1 to 2 seconds. Selective renal arteriography allows limitation of the total volume of contrast material used for imaging in multiple obliquities.

CONTRAST MATERIAL

Except in the evaluation of a renal transplant donor, the indication for arteriographic evaluation of the renal arteries is usually suspicion of renal arterial vascular disease causing hypertension or renal functional impairment. Renal functional impairment associated with an elevated serum creatinine level is one of several clinical features in patients with a high likelihood of renal vascular disease.[52-54] Therefore, until there is a perfect alternative diagnostic tool, the need for renal arteriography in the setting of renal insufficiency is inevitable.

The intravascular administration of contrast material has been clearly established as a risk factor for the development of hospital-acquired renal insufficiency.[55, 56] The risk of acute contrast-induced nephrotoxicity ranges from 1% to 30%,[57–66] depending on the definition of nephrotoxicity and the risk level of the patients studied. Risk factors for the development of acute contrast-induced nephrotoxicity include dehydration,[67] renal insufficiency,[57, 61, 63, 65, 68] and diabetes mellitus.[59, 63, 65, 69] Diabetic patients with renal insufficiency have the highest risk and may occasionally require dialysis support.[70, 71] In patients who do not have risk factors, acute contrast-induced nephrotoxicity is usually transient.[58, 59, 65, 72–74] Additional risk factors include high volumes of contrast administration[69, 70, 75–77] and the use of high-osmolar contrast material in patients with renal insufficiency.[57, 78] Iodixanol, an isosmolar contrast agent available since the late 1990s, may provide the lowest renal risk,[79] but this remains to be proven.

Several measures to prevent acute contrast-induced nephrotoxicity have been tested, including infusion of mannitol, diuretics, calcium channel blockers, theophylline, and dopamine. No significant benefit of any of these agents over simple infusion of saline has yet been demonstrated.[80] Therefore, the risk of nephrotoxicity associated with arteriography can be minimized with adequate peri procedural hydration and use of limited volumes of low-osmolar contrast material.

For patients with significantly increased risk of contrast-induced nephrotoxicity, iodinated contrast material exposure can be drastically limited or entirely avoided when carbon dioxide gas is used as the contrast agent. Intravascular carbon dioxide was first used for diagnosis of pericardial effusion in the 1950s.[81] Extensive animal testing established its intravascular use to be safe, even with the administration of massive volumes.[82, 83] The gas passes rapidly through the capillary bed and is absorbed or passed through the venous system, back to the heart. It is eliminated through the lungs in a single pass.[84] Repeated carbon dioxide injections made at frequent intervals can produce a vapor lock phenomenon that rarely may cause transient ischemia.[84]

Resolution of intra-arterial carbon dioxide was inadequate for diagnostic imaging with film-screen techniques. Because DSA documents changes between the mask image and later images, however, it has much higher contrast resolution, allowing the use of carbon dioxide as a contrast agent.[85] Vessels filled with the gas stand out against the surrounding soft tissues, much like gas in the bowel is visible on an x-ray film of the abdomen. Imaging can be improved when the vessel of interest is positioned so that the buoyancy of carbon dioxide causes it to fill. For example, because the renal arteries generally arise from the lateral surface of the aorta, imaging of the left renal artery would be optimized by elevation of the patient's left side, allowing carbon dioxide to float into it. As in standard DSA imaging, it is essential to limit patient motion and peristalsis.

Advanced computer manipulation of the digital data, including electronic stacking of multiple images, allows enhancement of the diagnostic capabilities. Despite the lower resolution with carbon dioxide than with iodinated contrast, the use of optimized technique and computer manipulation of the data can produce diagnostic images of similar quality to those with iodinated contrast in more than 90% of cases.[86–93]

There is essentially no risk of nephrotoxicity resulting from intra-arterial carbon dioxide administration. Rigorous studies of the effects of direct carbon dioxide injection into the renal arteries of dogs demonstrated no significant effects on renal blood flow or function. There were no significant histologic changes except for the development of acute tubular necrosis in one dog in which a vapor lock phenomenon may have been created by the kidney being positioned vertically over the catheter during rapid, repeated injections.[94] There has not been a case reported in the literature of significant renal functional impairment in a patient who received only carbon dioxide as the contrast agent.[84–87, 90–92, 95–97] In many cases, sufficient diagnostic information can be attained solely with the use of carbon dioxide. If necessary, supplemental views with a limited volume of low-osmolar iodinated contrast material can be acquired after the optimal projection has been determined with carbon dioxide.[86, 89] In this manner, optimal high-quality images of the renal arteries can be obtained with as little as 2 to 10 ml of contrast material.

Another potential alternate contrast material is gadopentetate dimeglumine, which is the contrast agent routinely used during MRI. It has been used as a contrast agent for CT scan[98, 99] and angiography,[100, 101] including use to guide endovascular interventional procedures.[102] Gadopentetate dimeglumine does not pose a risk of nephrotoxicity[103–105]; however, it costs approximately four times more than low-osmolar iodinated contrast material. Given this fact and the availability of carbon dioxide arteriography, use of gadopentetate dimeglumine for arteriography is likely to be limited.

ADJUNCTIVE MEASURES

Arteriography provides the opportunity to use adjunctive measures to evaluate the renal arteries. Hemodynamic effects of a stenosis can be assessed with direct pressure measurements proximal and distal to the lesion.[106, 107] Intravascular ultrasonography can be used to help characterize renal artery pathology. The technique provides detailed structural information not shown by arteriography, including the morphology of a stenosis or the extent of a dissection flap.[108, 109] Newer techniques including direct intravascular determination of renal artery blood flow with a Doppler-tipped wire[110] and high-resolution MRI with an intravascular catheter receiver coil,[111] are being developed and may eventually become standard components in the arteriographic evaluation of renal vascular disease.

ARTERIOGRAPHIC FINDINGS

As mentioned earlier, the usual indication for arteriographic evaluation of the renal arteries is the search for renal artery stenosis. A culprit lesion is sought as a potential cause of renovascular hypertension or renal insufficiency (ischemic nephropathy).[112–114] Most renal artery stenoses are due to atherosclerosis or to fibromuscular dysplasia (FMD).[30, 115–120] It is well established that renal artery stenosis can occur in asymptomatic patients.[121–128]

Although many arteriographic signs, including asymmet-

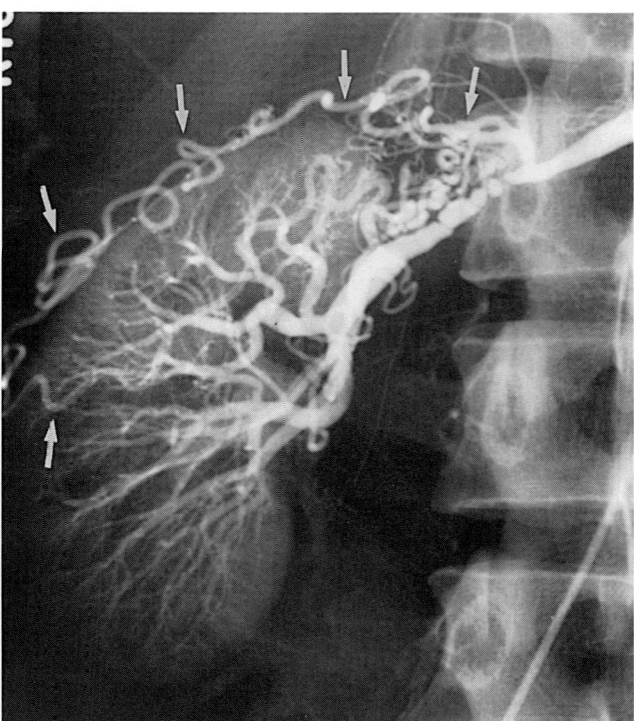

FIGURE 120–1. Arterial collaterals in renal artery stenosis. Selective right renal arteriogram demonstrates the classic "string of beads" appearance of fibromuscular dysplasia. Prominent filling of capsular collaterals (arrows) is seen.

ric kidney size,[115, 120, 123] unilaterally slowed blood flow,[129] severity of stenosis,[115, 116, 123, 129] presence of collaterals (Fig. 120–1),[115, 116, 129–133] and presence of post-stenotic dilatation (Fig. 120–2),[115, 116, 121, 123, 129] have been suggested as predictors of response to intervention, none has proved reliable. Consequently, the current definition of renovascular

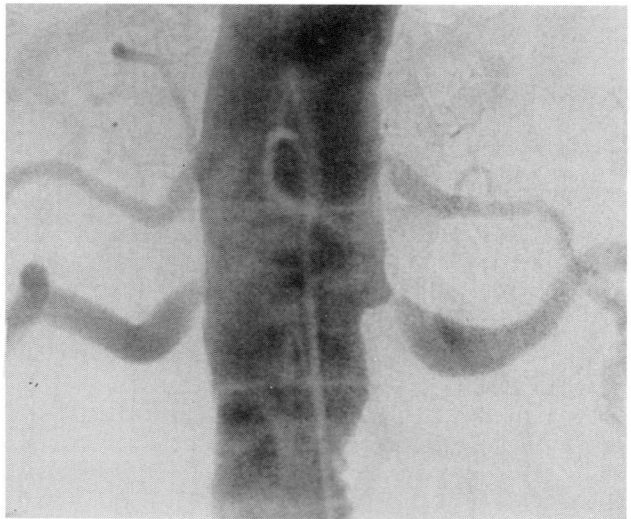

FIGURE 120–2. Post-stenotic dilatation. Subtracted image from an aortic injection demonstrates an atherosclerotic stenosis near the origin of the left renal artery. Post-stenotic dilatation increases the diameter of the vessel to nearly twice its expected size.

hypertension or ischemic nephropathy is the presence of renal vascular disease in a patient whose hypertension or renal insufficiency responds to surgical or endovascular treatment of the arterial lesion. Because atherosclerotic and fibromuscular lesions respond differently to intervention,[116, 134–139] arteriographic features of these entities as well as other less frequent causes of renal vascular disease are reviewed here.

ATHEROSCLEROSIS

Atherosclerosis is the most common cause of renal vascular disease, accounting for approximately two thirds of cases.[116, 120, 134, 140] Atherosclerotic renal artery stenosis is characterized by eccentric irregular narrowing at the ostium or in the proximal third of the vessel. While the distal main and branch arteries may occasionally be involved, the proximal segment is predominantly affected in approximately 80% of cases (see Fig. 120–2).[51, 116, 125, 141–143] Stenosis is unilateral in approximately 60% of cases,[116, 123, 141, 144] with similar distributions between right and left.[116]

A stenosis at the ostium can be related to atherosclerotic plaques in the aorta rather than in the renal artery,[145] significantly affecting results of endovascular intervention.[138, 145, 146] CT scanning has demonstrated that a stenosis within the first 10 mm of a renal artery originating from an atherosclerotic aorta on arteriography may actually be ostial.[147] Atherosclerotic renal artery stenosis is progressive in 30% to 70% of cases, leading to occlusion in approximately 15%.[119, 148–152]

FIBROMUSCULAR DYSPLASIA

FMD accounts for approximately one third of symptomatic renal vascular disease.[116, 120, 134, 140] Approximately three fourths of cases occur in women.[54, 117–120, 141, 153, 154] The process more frequently affects younger patients, between the second and fifth decades.[54, 117, 118, 141, 153, 154]. Renal artery involvement is often unilateral,[116, 123, 153, 154] usually affecting the right side[116, 141, 153, 154] and involving the middle and distal thirds of the vessel.[116, 117, 120, 141, 153] FMD progresses in 15 to 30% of cases.[119, 148, 149] This does not correlate, however, with worsened renal function or blood pressure control and rarely results in occlusion.[119]

Many classifications of the various types of FMD have been proposed based on the histology of the lesions.[141, 142, 155, 156] It is simplest to classify the disease by the region of the arterial wall predominantly involved. In this manner, lesions can be grouped into those that are (1) medial, (2) perimedial-adventitial, or (3) intimal.[142]

Medial fibroplasia is the most common type of FMD, accounting for 70% to 80% of cases.[30, 141, 142, 153] The arteriographic appearance is the characteristic "string of beads" (Fig. 120–3). This corrugated appearance is caused by luminal narrowings alternating with aneurysmal segments and is virtually pathognomonic.[141, 142] *Perimedial-adventitial* dysplasia accounts for approximately 15% of cases. The arteriographic appearance is of irregular, severe stenoses that may be beaded. The beads are not aneurysms,

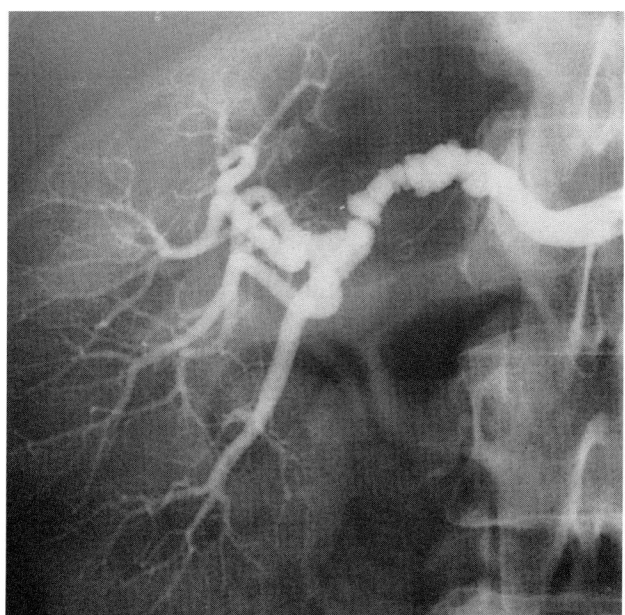

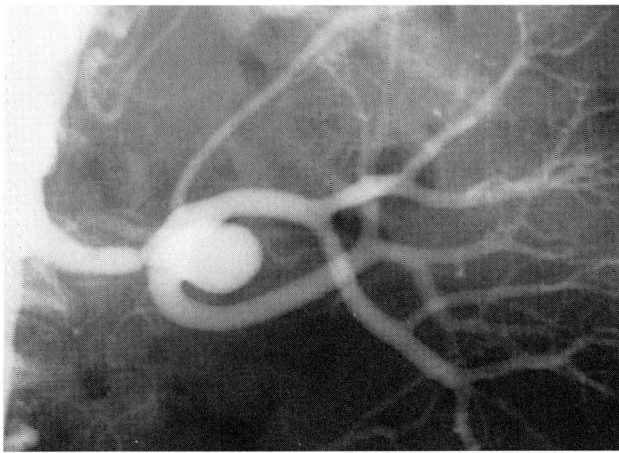

FIGURE 120–4. Renal artery aneurysm. Abdominal aortogram demonstrates a saccular aneurysm of the left renal artery. As in this case, renal artery aneurysms are commonly located at a branch point.

FIGURE 120–3. Medial fibroplasia form of fibromuscular dysplasia. Selective right renal arteriogram demonstrates the typical areas of luminal narrowing alternating with multiple dilated segments of greater diameter than the normal renal artery.

however, having a smaller diameter than the normal artery.[141, 142] *Intimal* fibroplasia accounts for approximately 5% of cases and appears arteriographically as a smooth concentric narrowing.[141, 142]

Less common arteriographic appearances of FMD include a web, a diaphragm-like stenosis, a dissection with luminal dilatation, a saccular aneurysm, a funnel-shaped tapering, and a short segmental narrowing that mimics an atherosclerotic lesion. Although arteriography is fairly accurate at distinguishing between FMD and atherosclerosis in the renal arteries, it is inaccurate at distinguishing between the individual types of FMD.[157]

OTHER RENAL ARTERIAL DISEASES

Many other causes of renal vascular hypertension or ischemic nephropathy have been reported, but they are rare.[30, 116] Renal artery aneurysms are seen in approximately 1% of patients undergoing renal arteriography (Fig. 120–4). They may be caused by atherosclerosis, FMD, arteritis, or trauma; or they may be congenital or mycotic. Atherosclerotic or congenital aneurysms are usually single and unilateral, while those associated with arteritis and FMD are usually multiple. They may involve the main renal artery or branch vessels and are often located near bifurcation points. Curvilinear calcifications may be seen in the wall. They may be saccular or fusiform and often demonstrate slow flow on arteriography. Renal artery aneurysms are usually asymptomatic, but may cause pain or hematuria. They are associated with hypertension in approximately 15% of cases, particularly when there is concurrent renal artery stenosis.[158–162]

Renal arteriovenous fistulae may be congenital or associ-

ated with renal biopsy, blunt trauma, carcinoma, rupture of an aneurysm into a vein, or FMD (Fig. 120–5). *Congenital* fistulae may present with hematuria and urinary obstruction related to clots. *Acquired* fistulae frequently present with hypertension, sometimes associated with signs of high-output cardiac failure. The hypertension is thought to be caused by segmental renal ischemia distal to the fistula.

Arteriographically, the classic finding is early opacification of the renal vein or inferior vena cava. The feeding artery or arteries and the draining renal vein may be dilated

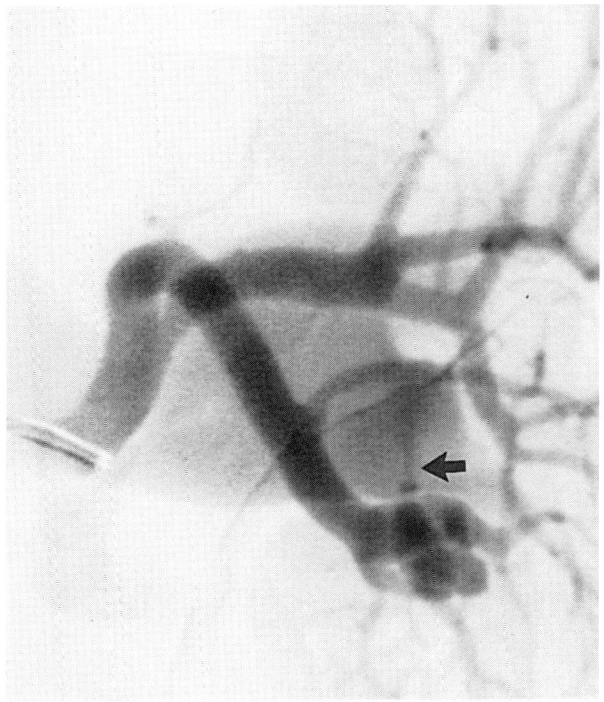

FIGURE 120–5. Renal arteriovenous fistula. Subtracted image from a selective left renal arteriogram demonstrates early filling of a markedly dilated left renal vein associated with a congenital arteriovenous malformation. A jet of contrast is seen filling the vein (*arrow*).

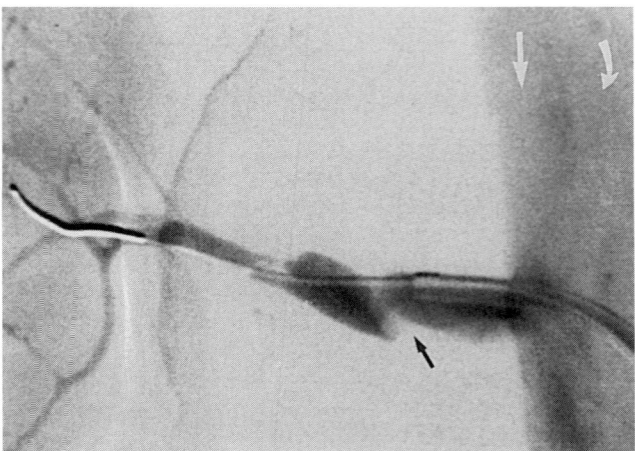

FIGURE 120–6. Renal artery involvement by an aortic dissection. Subtracted image from an arteriogram with the catheter at the orifice of the right renal artery demonstrates an irregular lumen with a prominent intimal flap (*black arrow*). Reflux of contrast into the aorta demonstrates differential opacification of the true (*straight arrow*) and false (*curved arrow*) lumens.

and tortuous. The site of arteriovenous communication can usually be delineated with selective arteriography.[163–166]

Dissection of the renal artery is usually associated with aortic dissection (Fig. 120–6). Isolated renal artery dissection is rare and may be seen in FMD, in blunt trauma (Fig. 120–7), in renal artery catheterization, or with physical exertion. Patients usually present with pain and hypertension. At arteriography an intimal flap, a narrowed true lumen, and a dilated irregular false lumen are usually seen. Branch vessels may be occluded by the dissection flap or by emboli from the flap, with resultant areas of hypoperfused renal parenchyma.[167–170]

Symptomatic renal vascular disease may be associated with several other rare processes, including Takayasu's arteritis,[171, 172] neurofibromatosis,[173, 174] thrombosis or embolic

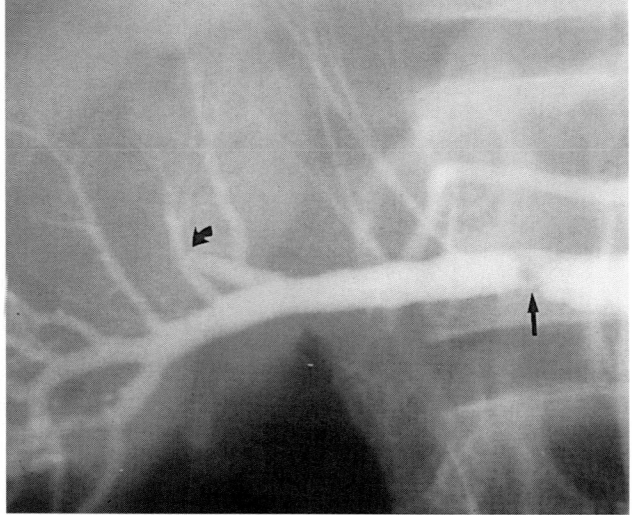

FIGURE 120–7. Renal artery dissection related to blunt trauma. Abdominal aortogram demonstrates an intimal flap within the proximal right renal artery (*straight arrow*). There is abrupt termination of an upper pole branch (*curved arrow*), likely due to an embolus from the intimal flap.

occlusion,[175–177] post-transplant stenosis,[34, 178, 179] post-renal bypass graft stenosis,[180] aortic coarctation,[174, 181, 182] post irradiation,[183] polyarteritis nodosa,[184, 185] necrotizing angiitis,[186] and congenital bands.[187]

SUMMARY

The diagnosis of renal arterial disease and decisions concerning surgical or endovascular management depend on arteriographic visualization of renal artery anatomy. Advances in arteriographic technique, including continued refinements in DSA, the correlation with cross-sectional imaging for appropriate angulation, the development of less nephrotoxic contrast agents, and the use of adjunctive intra-arterial techniques, allow optimal evaluation of the renal arteries.

Endovascular Treatment of Renovascular Diseases

No completely reliable test has yet been developed to determine in which patients the presence of a renal artery stenosis is responsible for hypertension or renal insufficiency.[188–190] Consequently, the only certain means to define the relationship of renovascular disease to hypertension or renal insufficiency is to observe benefit after successful intervention. Although an argument may be made for medical management of hypertension in patients with renal artery stenosis, this approach does not improve excretory renal insufficiency (i.e., ischemic nephropathy).[191]

Surgical treatment of renal artery stenosis has high technical and clinical success rates, usually with a low mortality rate and good long-term patency.[192–194] Endovascular techniques to treat renal artery stenosis and other renal artery pathology have the potential benefits of avoidance of general anesthesia, lower morbidity and mortality rates, shorter recovery time, shorter hospital stay, and lower cost. The rapid advancements in endovascular techniques have included the development and ongoing refinement of endovascular methods of treating renal artery stenosis and other renal artery pathology.

TECHNIQUES

Patient Management

Patient preparation for endovascular treatment of renal artery stenosis is similar to preparation for diagnostic arteriography. The patient should not eat solid foods after midnight the night before, although the intake of clear liquids may help prevent dehydration. Intravenous fluids are administered starting the evening before the procedure, with care taken to avoid fluid overload in patients with impaired cardiac function. In diabetic patients, insulin should be withheld the morning of the procedure, with the institution of sliding scale control of blood glucose after the procedure.

A unique feature of patient preparation for renal artery intervention is the cessation of antihypertensive medication. Because the intervention may cause a precipitous drop in blood pressure, patients should not take their routine medications the morning of the procedure. If necessary, hypertension can be controlled before and during the procedure with short-acting agents. In addition, many clinicians institute daily doses of aspirin or dipyridamole or both, usually starting the day before the procedure.

After renal artery intervention, the blood pressure must be closely monitored in the postprocedure period. The maximal decrease in blood pressure is usually seen in the first 48 hours after the procedure.[195, 196] Various pharmaceutical regimens to prevent thrombosis or restenosis are used after renal artery intervention.[197–203] Most frequently, aspirin is continued for 3 to 6 months, although some clinicians prescribe another antiplatelet agent, such as dipyridamole or ticlopidine. Anticoagulation with warfarin or low-molecular-weight heparin is also sometimes used for varying durations. The prescribed medications are similar to those used after coronary artery intervention, although there are few data regarding their effectiveness in the renal arteries.[204–206]

Angioplasty

Advancements in catheter and guide wire technology in the 1990s have allowed the development of techniques for renal artery access and intervention that are more stable and less traumatic to the vessel. Smaller-caliber catheters with high torque control and preshaped curves specific for renal artery anatomy have been developed. Several varieties of guide wires, including wires with hydrophilic coating, tapered wires with durometric transitions to provide support in the aorta yet an atraumatic tip, and wires with high torque control are available. There has been significant development in angioplasty balloon catheter design since the first renal interventions were performed. Today's angioplasty balloons have a low profile before inflation, track easily over a guide wire, allow high pressure inflation, and deflate to less traumatic shapes. Guiding catheters with pre-formed shapes specific for renal artery catheterization allow coaxial balloon dilatation as well as safe stent delivery to the renal arteries in the event of a flow-limiting dissection.

Percutaneous transluminal renal angioplasty (PTRA) usually can be performed from a femoral artery approach. If the renal artery is steeply down sloping, the brachial or axillary approach may facilitate catheterization. A cobra or sidewinder catheter is positioned at the renal artery origin, and a renal arteriogram may be performed. A bolus of heparin is given, after which a guide wire is gently manipulated past the stenosis. The catheter is advanced over the wire past the stenosis. A pressure gradient between the post-stenotic renal artery and the aorta can be measured. Some clinicians give intra-arterial antispasmodic medication at this point. The more frequently used agents include verapamil or nitroglycerin. Another common practice is to give an oral dose of verapamil or nifedipine before the procedure in order to minimize spasm in the renal artery.

The angioplasty balloon catheter is advanced to a position bridging the stenosis and is inflated. The interventionist chooses the balloon diameter by measuring the size of an adjacent segment of normal renal artery. The stenosis should optimally be dilated slightly larger than the normal vessel. This can be accomplished by not correcting for the approximately 10% to 15% magnification factor when the normal renal artery is measured. During inflation of the balloon, the patient may experience moderate pain, which should resolve when the balloon is deflated. Persistent pain may be an indication of dissection, occlusion, or rupture of the artery and requires additional diagnostic measures. Arteriography and pressure measurements are performed after the angioplasty.

Stent Placement

Significant advances in stent technology include the development of stents that are more easily visible with fluoroscopy and more suitably sized to the renal arteries. The ideal features of a renal artery stent include ease of visibility, low profile, ease of deployment, predictability of expansion, and negligible shortening. The ability for precise deployment is particularly important in the renal arteries, where the stenosis often involves the origin of the vessel from the aorta, and results depend on full coverage of the lesion.[202, 205–207]

Stent placement in the renal arteries was first used as a means to salvage technically unsuccessful angioplasty results or to treat restenosis after angioplasty.[208–210] A stent can be used to resist elastic recoil of the stenosis or to tack up a dissection flap (Fig. 120–8). Early success with stents has led to studies of their primary use in the treatment of lesions for which PTRA has been less effective.[199, 211] The Palmaz stent (Johnson & Johnson, Warren, N.J.) is most frequently used.[201–203, 205, 208, 211–217] Use of the Wallstent (Schneider, Minneapolis, Minn.)[206, 207, 209, 218] and Strecker stent (Boston Scientific, Watertown, Mass.)[210] has also been reported.

The technique for stent placement is similar to that for PTRA. From a femoral or axillary approach, the renal artery stenosis is gently crossed with a guide wire and catheter. For severe stenoses, predilatation with a balloon catheter is performed to allow room for passage of the stent.

For deployment of a Palmaz stent, the stent is crimped onto a balloon catheter and passed coaxially to the tip of a guide catheter. The guide catheter and stent are advanced over the guide wire across the stenosis.

The guide catheter is then retracted, uncovering the stent so that it bridges the stenosis. Optimal positioning of the stent is facilitated with multiple small injections of contrast material through the guide. Appropriate angulation of the fluoroscopy tube to see the renal artery origin in profile is crucial.[219, 220] For an ostial stenosis, the stent is deployed flush with the aortic wall in order to resist the recoil of the longitudinal aortic plaques surrounding the origin of the vessel.[221] Most authors prefer slight protrusion of the stent into the aortic lumen rather than allowing the ostial lesion to be unsupported.[201–203, 205–208, 211, 216] The stent is deployed when the balloon catheter on which it is mounted is inflated. A completion arteriogram and pressure measurements are performed at the conclusion of the procedure.

For the deployment of a Wallstent, the delivery catheter is positioned so that the stent is centered on the renal artery stenosis. As the outer membrane of the delivery catheter is withdrawn, the stent is released. Longitudinal shortening of this device, as it is deployed, makes positioning of the proximal end somewhat unpredictable. After deployment of the Wallstent, balloon dilatation of the device may be necessary for complete expansion, which may

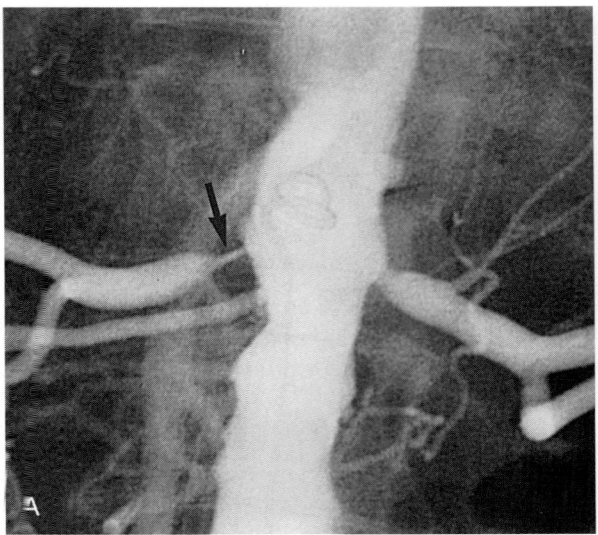
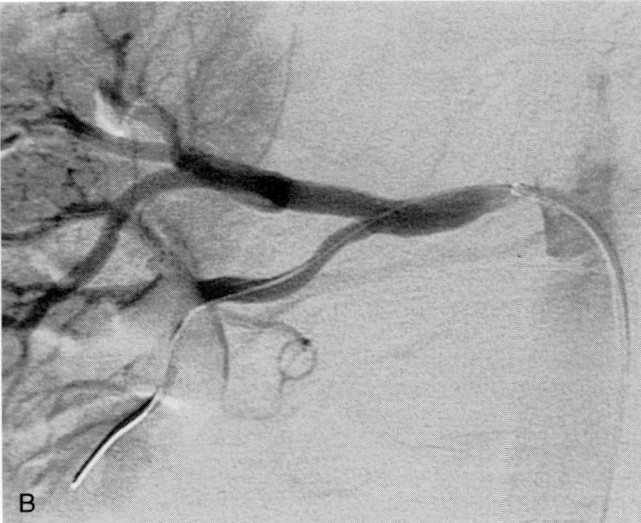
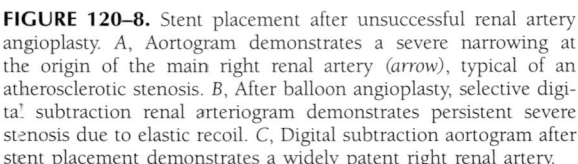

FIGURE 120–8. Stent placement after unsuccessful renal artery angioplasty. *A*, Aortogram demonstrates a severe narrowing at the origin of the main right renal artery *(arrow)*, typical of an atherosclerotic stenosis. *B*, After balloon angioplasty, selective digital subtraction renal arteriogram demonstrates persistent severe stenosis due to elastic recoil. *C*, Digital subtraction aortogram after stent placement demonstrates a widely patent right renal artery.

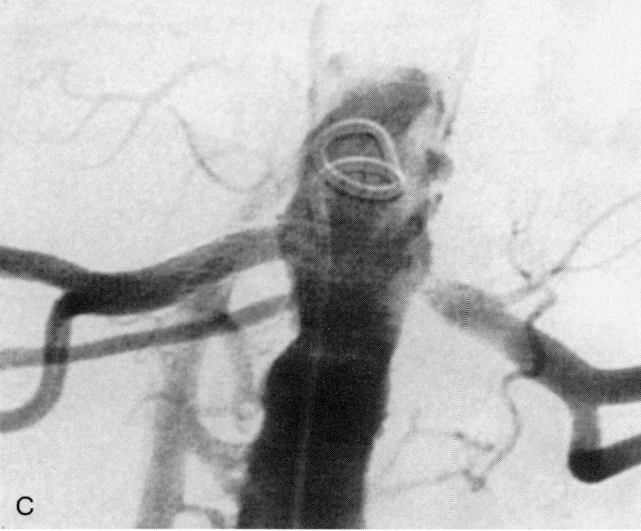

cause further shortening. Delayed shortening of the device has also been reported.[207, 209] A newly available version of the Wallstent is reconstrainable after partial deployment, allowing more precise adjustments of final stent position. This feature may add to its popularity for use in the renal arteries.

The Strecker stent has not been used in the United States; however, one report describes shortcomings that may limit its effectiveness, including difficulty with precise deployment and lack of sufficient radial strength to resist elastic recoil.[210]

Other Techniques

Anecdotal information on several other endovascular techniques used to treat renal arterial disease has been reported. Atherectomy has been performed to treat calcified[201] or eccentric stenoses.[222, 223] For hypertension caused by a renal arterial lesion that is not amenable to other endovascular treatments, selective infarction of the ischemic portion of the kidney may provide an alternative to nephrectomy. This can be accomplished by embolization of the blood supply

to the ischemic segments with particles or a chemical sclerosant.[224–230]

Endovascular occlusion of the renal artery with a detachable balloon has been reported to treat malignant hypertension.[231] Spontaneous renal artery dissection may be treated with stent placement.[207, 232] This technique has been used in a patient with a traumatic focal renal artery dissection as well.[233] Thrombosis of a renal artery aneurysm may be induced by coil embolization of the aneurysm.[234] Alternatively, the use of an endovascular stent graft to treat a renal artery aneurysm has been reported.[235]

Finally, thermal laser-assisted angioplasty of the renal artery has been reported as a treatment for renovascular hypertension.[236] It is evident that as new endovascular techniques become available, they will likely be applied to renal artery disease.

OUTCOMES

Various end-points can be used to evaluate outcomes of endovascular treatments for renovascular disease. These include immediate technical results, long-term patency, and clinical results. The outcomes depend in part on the cause of the stenosis, the clinical problem that is being treated, and the definition of success. Standards of reporting for renal artery interventions have not yet been established. Consequently, it can be difficult to make comparisons between studies. A review of published series, however, allows a general evaluation of the effectiveness of PTRA and stent placement for the treatment of renovascular disease.

Technical Results

Percutaneous Transluminal Renal Angioplasty

Technical success during PTRA has been variously defined as substantial relief of stenosis; less than 30%, 50%, 60%, or 70% residual stenosis; less than 20 mmHg residual gradient; or less than 10% residual gradient. With technologic advances and experience, technical success rates have improved.[237] Most technical failures are due to elastic recoil or flow-limiting dissections at the angioplasty site. Occasionally, a technical failure may be due to inability to pass a guide wire through a severe stenosis or occlusion.

Technical results of PTRA in patients with atherosclerotic disease are shown in Table 120–1.[188, 195, 200, 212, 242–244, 247, 248, 267, 280–282, 299–303] Table 120–1 includes studies that specify technical results in patients with atherosclerotic stenosis. Only studies published since 1988 and in which PTRA was performed in at least 20 patients are included. Table 120–2[195, 200, 226, 242, 244, 247, 290, 303] contains a similar summary of technical results of PTRA in patients with FMD. Thorough reviews of technical results of PTRA from earlier studies have been previously published.[238, 239]

The lower technical success rate of 77.4% in atherosclerotic disease compared with 91.8% in FMD is related to the greater severity of stenosis, the more frequent development of elastic recoil and the more frequent location at the ostium in atherosclerotic disease[240–242] The relatively low technical success rate in the study of Martin and coworkers[243] can be explained by the fact that 81% of the lesions were ostial. Although high technical success rates have been reported for ostial lesions,[244] the aortic plaques responsible for the stenosis generally respond worse to PTRA than does plaque truly within the renal artery.[221, 240, 245–247] In the study of Eldrup-Jorgensen and colleagues,[248] the authors believe that the relatively low technical success rate they had is related to their use of a retrospective blinded quantitative analysis of PTRA results rather than "qualitative and optimistic" assessments typically used in other published series. Early technical limitations, including the inability to dilate stenoses in small branch vessels[242, 249] or at bifurcation points, can be overcome with use of newer low-profile balloon catheters, balloons mounted on a wire instead of on a catheter, and a "kissing balloon" technique at branch points.[226, 250, 251]

In general, stenoses caused by FMD of the medial fibroplasia type and nonostial atherosclerotic lesions respond best to PTRA. Atherosclerotic occlusion, atherosclerotic ostial stenosis, and FMD types other than medial fibroplasia[226, 252, 253] have a lower technical success rate. Because most cases of technically unsuccessful PTRA can be salvaged by the placement of an endovascular stent, angio-

plasty should not be withheld for lesions with a less favorable morphology.

Stent Placement

Very high immediate technical success rates have been achieved for placement of stents in the renal arteries. Table 120–3[201–203, 205–218] summarizes the results of primary and secondary stent placement procedures for series in which at least 10 stents were placed. The data include all indications for renal artery intervention; however, the vast majority were placed for atherosclerotic disease. A secondary stent placement is defined as one after unsuccessful PTRA. The definitions of unsuccessful PTRA include 20%, 30%, 60%, or 75% residual stenosis; residual gradient of 5, 10, or 20 mmHg; dissection; acute occlusion; or delayed restenosis. The indication for primary stent placement was treatment of an ostial atherosclerotic stenosis in the series in which the indication was specified.[211, 214]

Long-Term Patency

Long-term patency of the renal artery after technically successful PTRA or stent placement is difficult to establish from available data. Although duplex ultrasonographic evaluation of the kidney and renal artery,[201–203, 254–256] spiral CTA,[257–260] and MRA[261–263] can suggest flow-limiting lesions, a precise assessment of restenosis depends on angiographic evaluation (Fig. 120–9). Routine arteriography is a rather invasive test to undergo if there is no clinical problem. Consequently, many published series include imaging follow-up only in patients with recurrent hypertension or worsening renal function. This practice may produce a bias toward a higher restenosis rate. Some published series, however, include routine imaging follow-up. Table 120–4[200, 226, 244, 249, 255, 268, 280, 281, 283, 301, 302] contains data on restenosis and secondary patency rates in PTRA, while Table 120–5[201–203, 205–211, 213–215, 217, 218, 304] contains similar information for stent placement procedures. The tables include studies in which at least 10 procedures were performed, with angiographic follow-up in at least 50% of the patients with a minimum or mean follow-up period of 6 months. Most studies define restenosis as greater than 50% reduction in luminal diameter, although a few use 30% or 60%. The 16.9% restenosis rate for PTRA, among a patient group including 20% with FMD, is similar to the 17.7% restenosis rate for renal artery stents applied for both ostial and nonostial atherosclerosis. These data demonstrate that although stent placement in the renal artery produces a higher immediate technical success rate, it has little effect on the rate of early restenosis.

Several factors influence restenosis after PTRA. Particularly during stent placement, technical aspects of the procedure play an important role. Incomplete coverage of the lesion by the stent is often considered to be the most important predictor of restenosis.[205, 208, 218] If this situation is recognized, a second stent can be easily placed to cover the lesion. Delayed shortening of a Wallstent leading to uncovering of a lesion and restenosis has been reported.[209] Incomplete dilatation of the artery and a smaller artery diameter also predispose to restenosis. In this regard, residual stenosis greater than 15% after stent placement,[208] stent

TABLE 120–1. TECHNICAL RESULTS OF PERCUTANEOUS TRANSLUMINAL RENAL ANGIOPLASTY FOR ATHEROSCLEROTIC STENOSIS

NO.	REF.	AUTHOR	YEAR	NO.		INDICATION		LESION TYPE		TECHNICAL SUCCESS		
				Patients	Arteries	HTN	RI	Ostial	Nonostial	Patients	(%)	Ostial (%)/Nonostial (%)
1	299	McDonald et al	1988	11	11	11	9	1	10	9	(81.8)	
2	267	Hayes et al	1988	55	55	49	42	41	14	38	(69.1)	27 (65.9)/11 (78.6)
3	300	Beebe et al	1988	38	49			43	6	22	(57.9)	
4	247	Klinge et al	1989	134		134				104	(77.6)	
5	282	Canzanello et al	1989	100	125	100	66	50	75	73	(73.0)	31* (62.0)/54 (72.0)
6	301	Julien et al	1989	66	70	66	16			60	(90.9)	
7	242	Baert et al	1990	165	207	165		37	170	172*	(83.1)	4† (28.6)/103† (94.5)
8	188	Postma et al	1991	22	23	22				22	(100.0)	
9	243	Martin et al	1992	110	160	110		129	31	39	(35.5)	
10	280	Weibull et al	1993	29	29	29		29		24	(82.8)	
11	302	Tykarski et al	1993	26	43	30	17			35*	(81.4)	
12	244	Losinno et al	1994	153		153	59	77	76‡	146	(95.4)	70 (90.9)/76 (100.0)
13	212	Pattynama et al	1994	40	58	35	40			51*	(87.9)	
14	303	Rodriguez-Perez et al	1994	37	50	37		24	13‡	29	(78.4)	
15	195	Bonelli et al	1995	190	242	190		53	189	155	(81.6)	
16	200	Jensen et al	1995	107	147	107		18	129	121*	(82.3)	13 (72.2)/108 (83.7)
17	248	Eldrup-Jorgensen et al	1995	52	60	52	42	14	31	18	(34.6)	4* (28.6)/13 (41.9)
18	281	Plouin et al	1998	23	23	23				23	(100.0)	
	TOTAL			1358	1352	1313	291	516	744	1141	(77.4)	149 (58.0) 365 (78.5)

*Number of arteries.
†Ostial and nonostial technical success rates tabulated only in 123 patients with unilateral stenosis (14 ostial and 109 nonostial).
‡Number of patients.
§Distribution of ostial versus nonostial lesions excludes five lesions through which the wire could not be passed, four arteries for which the arteriogram was lost, and six arteries with "indeterminate" lesions.
HTN = hypertension; RI = renal insufficiency.

TABLE 120–2. TECHNICAL RESULTS OF PERCUTANEOUS TRANSLUMINAL RENAL ANGIOPLASTY FOR STENOSIS DUE TO FIBROMUSCULAR DYSPLASIA

NO.	REF.	AUTHOR	YEAR	NO. Patients	NO. Arteries	INDICATION HTN	INDICATION RI	TECHNICAL SUCCESS Patients	TECHNICAL SUCCESS (%)
1	247	Klinge et al	1989	52		52		47	(90.4)
2	242	Baert et al	1990	22	28	22		24*	(85.7)
3	290	Tegtmeyer et al	1991	66	85	66	14	66	(100.0)
4	244	Losinno et al	1994	42		42	1	40	(95.2)
5	303	Rodriguez-Perez et al	1994	27	31	27		25	(92.6)
6	226	Cluzel et al	1994	20	35	20	1	17	(85.0)
7	195	Bonelli et al	1995	105	140	105		93	(88.6)
8	200	Jensen et al	1995	30	33	30		32*	(97.0)
		TOTAL		364	352	364	16	344	91.8

*Number of arteries.
HTN = hypertension; RI = renal insufficiency.

diameter less than 6 mm,[265] a smaller minimum luminal diameter immediately after stent placement,[214] and mild (< 60%) stenosis on duplex ultrasonographic examination the day after PTRA[255] have been found to increase the likelihood of restenosis in a statistically significant manner. Several authors have noted the importance of optimizing the luminal diameter after renal artery stent placement because deposition of a thin layer of tissue over the stent is inevitable and contributes to a reduction in the lumen diameter initially gained by stent deployment.[201, 203, 206, 208, 214] Finally, the specific stent used may be important. For example, a higher restenosis rate is attributed to the articulated Palmaz-Schatz stent than to the nonarticulated Palmaz stent.[208]

There is consensus that ostial lesions carry a worse patency prognosis after PTRA than non-ostial stenoses do.[221, 266, 267] Indeed, ostial or branch location was found to be a statistically significant predictor of restenosis after PTRA in a study of 92 hypertensive patients.[268] Ostial location, however, was found not to be a statistically significant predictor of restenosis after PTRA in a study of 50 hypertensive patients, 25 of whom had renal insufficiency.[255] A lack of a significant relationship between location of stenosis and restenosis rate has been found after stent placement.[206] The absence of adequate anatomic follow-up in many studies contributes to the lack of sufficient data concerning the true rate of restenosis in ostial lesions.

Many clinical features have been studied for potential association with restenosis after PTRA. Here, too, data are incomplete and conflicting. Age has a demonstrated significant association with restenosis after PTRA,[268] but not with restenosis after stent placement.[206] Widespread atherosclerotic disease increases the likelihood of restenosis after PTRA,[208, 269] statistically significantly so in patients with severe aortic atherosclerotic disease.[268] The presence of atherosclerotic risk factors does not appear to significantly affect restenosis rate after stent placement.[206] Stents placed in patients who have had restenosis after a previous angioplasty have a higher restenosis rate.[208, 270] Other factors that have shown no apparent association with restenosis include gender,[206, 213, 268] renal function,[206, 255] atherosclerotic versus FMD etiology,[255, 268] prolonged anticoagulation,[205, 206] smoking history,[268] serum cholesterol level,[268] and grade or length of stenosis.[268] Interestingly, improvement in luminal diameter on the follow-up angiogram compared with the

initial post-procedure arteriogram has been seen after PTRA for both FMD[226, 253] and atherosclerotic stenosis.[271]

Restenoses after PTRA[243] and after stent placement can be successfully treated with repeated PTRA.[201, 206, 208, 209, 211, 215] Treatment of restenosis within or at the margin of a stent by placement of an additional stent has also been reported in six patients.[202] With repeated intervention, very good secondary patency rates can be achieved. With life-table analysis, secondary patency rates of 94% at 12 months for PTRA,[253] 92% at 24 months for stent placement,[201] 92% at 60 months for stent placement,[202] and more than 80% at 10 years for PTRA[244] have been reported. These long-term secondary patency rates compare favorably with long-term surgical primary patency rates. In addition, there is still the potential to perform surgery if PTRA is unsuccessful,[272] although it may be more challenging.[273–275]

Clinical Results of Renal Artery Intervention

The clinical results of renal artery intervention are best evaluated separately for patients with atherosclerotic disease and FMD. Of patients with hypertension and renal artery stenosis, the older patients in the atherosclerotic group are more likely to have a component of essential hypertension than the younger patients with FMD. Although atherosclerotic disease is increasingly recognized as a cause of renal insufficiency,[276] FMD involvement of the renal arteries rarely induces a rise in serum creatinine level.[277] Consequently, these groups are considered separately.

Although reporting practices for blood pressure response after intervention are not standardized, most published studies use a variation of the criteria for cured or improved blood pressure defined by the Cooperative Study of Renovascular Hypertension.[278] The Cooperative Study defined *cure* as an average diastolic blood pressure of 90 mmHg or less, with at least 10 mmHg decrease from the preintervention level. Blood pressure *improvement* was defined as an average diastolic blood pressure of 90 to 110 mmHg, with a 15% or greater decrease from the preintervention level. Although the Cooperative Study definition does not consider antihypertensive medication, most current studies that report blood pressure response after renal artery interventions specify that all antihypertensive medications must have been discontinued in order for a patient to be classi-

TABLE 120–3. TECHNICAL RESULTS OF RENAL ARTERY STENT PLACEMENT

NO.	REF.	AUTHOR	YEAR	PATIENTS	NO. OF STENTED ARTERIES		STENT TYPE	INDICATION		ETIOLOGY			TECHNICAL SUCCESS	
					Primary	Secondary		HTN	RI	ASD	FMD	Other	Patients	%
1	208	Rees et al	1991	28		28	P, PS	28	14	28			27	96.4
2	209	Wilms et al	1991	11		12	WS	10	1	10		1	11	100.0
3	210	Kuhn et al	1991	10	2	12	Strk	9	10	6		4	8	80.0
4	218	Joffre et al	1992	16		16	WS	11	6	11	2	3	16	100.0
5	206	Hennequin et al	1994	21		25	WS	25	6	15	3	3	21	100.0
6	207	Raynaud et al	1994	18		18	WS	18	4	15		3	18	100.0
7	212	Pattynama et al	1994	40	3	10	P	35	40	40			13*	100.0
8	215	MacLeod et al	1995	29		32	P	16	17	28	1		29	100.0
9	211	van de Ven et al	1995	24	14	14	P	24	24	24			24	100.0
10	201	Henry et al	1996	59		64	P, PS	59	10	55	3	1	59	100.0
11	203	Rundback and Jacobs	1996	20		24	P	18	11	20			19	95.0
12	202	Blum et al	1997	68		74	P	68	20	68			68	100.0
13	216	Boisclair et al	1997	33		35	P	33	17	33			33	100.0
14	217	Harden et al	1997	32		32	P		32	32			32	100.0
15	205	Taylor et al	1997	29	1	31	P, PS	16	22	28	1		29	100.0
16	214	White et al	1997	100	107	26	P	100	44				99	99.0
17	213	Harjai et al	1997	66	78	10	P	66		65	1		66	100.0
TOTAL				604	205	463		536	278	478	11	15	572	98.3

*Number of arteries.

HTN = hypertension; RI = renal insufficiency; ASD = atherosclerotic disease; FMD = fibromuscular dysplasia; P = Palmaz; PS = Palmaz-Schatz; WS = Wallstent; Strk = Strecker.

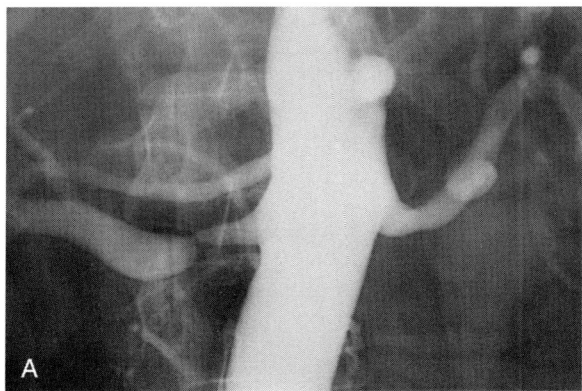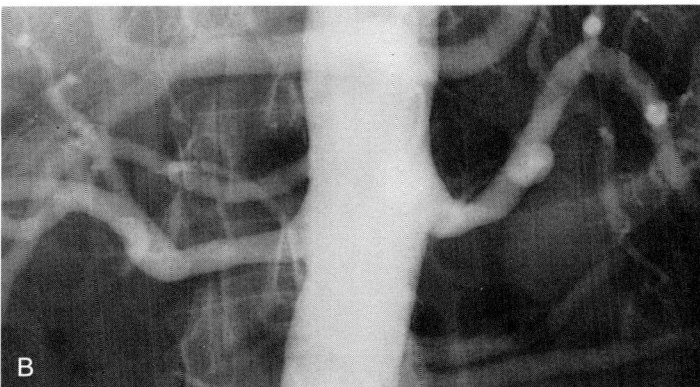

FIGURE 120–9. Long-term results of renal artery angioplasty. *A*, Aortogram demonstrates a severe atherosclerotic stenosis of the right renal artery with marked post-stenotic dilatation. *B*, Aortogram 1 year after balloon angioplasty demonstrates persistent absence of stenosis. There has been significant remodeling of the artery, with resolution of the post-stenotic dilatation.

fied as "cured." In addition, for most studies, the definition of "improvement" allows for a reduction in the number of antihypertensive medications. The category of those with blood pressure "benefit" includes all patients with cure or improvement. Clearly, there is room for many confounding variables, including changed doses and increased effectiveness of new classes of medications.

Renal function *response* after renal artery intervention has been variably defined as a 15% or 20% decrease in serum creatinine level or a 10% increase in creatinine clearance rate. Commonly, the category of those with renal function benefit includes all patients with improved or stabilized renal function.

Atherosclerotic Disease

The blood pressure responses in hypertensive patients with atherosclerotic renal artery stenosis who were treated with PTRA are shown in Table 120–6.[190, 195, 242–244, 247, 282, 301] The table includes series published since 1989 with at least 50 patients who had atherosclerotic stenosis.

Table 120–7[201–203, 205, 208, 211, 213, 215, 216, 304] shows similar information for patients who were treated with stent placement in the renal artery, including all series with a minimum of 20 patients with atherosclerotic stenosis. The benefit rate (i.e., cured and improved) of 68.4% for patients treated with PTRA is similar to the 65.6% benefit for patients treated with a stent. The lower cure rate for stent placement (8.2% versus 15.8%) is surprising given the similar restenosis and secondary patency rates. Among other explanations, the greater age (65.2 years versus 61.9 years) and the higher proportion of patients with renal impairment (42% versus 17%) in the group of patients treated with stents may partially account for this discrepancy.

In regard to the impact of ostial location of the stenosis on clinical outcome, Table 120–8[202, 203, 208, 211, 243, 280] shows the blood pressure responses in series of patients in whom at least 80% of the stenoses are ostial lesions. Although the large series of PTRA-treated patients of Martin and associates[243] has a somewhat lower benefit rate, overall blood pressure response in patients with ostial lesions is similar to that in patients for whom lesion location is not specified.

The renal function responses in patients with atherosclerotic stenosis who were treated with PTRA or stent placement in the renal artery are shown in Table 120–9.[201, 202, 205, 208, 211, 216, 243, 256, 280, 282, 302, 304] Series published since 1989 that define the number of atherosclerotic patients with renal insufficiency and that include follow-up in at least 10 patients are included. Approximately 33.6% of these patients have improved renal function. Cumulative anecdotal reports throughout the published series included 24 patients who were dependent on dialysis before intervention, 16 of whom were able to discontinue dialysis after intervention.[217, 248, 279]

Several series report the long-term clinical responses of patients with atherosclerotic renal artery stenosis treated with endovascular intervention. Only one prospective randomized trial, however, has compared endovascular with surgical treatment of renovascular disease.[280] This study did not represent the contemporary patient population because only nondiabetic, hypertensive patients younger than 70 years of age who had unilateral renal artery stenosis and a serum creatinine level of less than 300 mmol/L were included for randomization. Each of the surgical and endovascular groups included 29 patients. The study found a blood pressure benefit of 90% for PTRA versus 86% for surgery and a renal function benefit of 83% for PTRA versus 72% for surgery after 24 months of follow-up. The data are skewed, however, by the fact that four of five PTRA patient with an unsuccessful result underwent subsequent surgical treatment yet are included in the PTRA follow-up. The authors recommend PTRA as the first choice of therapy, with aggressive follow-up and reintervention, when necessary.

Another single prospective randomized trial has compared endovascular with medical treatment of renovascular hypertension.[281] This study includes hypertensive patients younger than 75 years of age with a creatinine clearance rate of at least 0.83 ml/sec who have unilateral renal artery stenosis. Patients with malignant hypertension or a history of stroke, pulmonary edema, or myocardial infarction in the previous 6 months were excluded. Antihypertensive medication regimens were standardized before the diagnostic arteriogram, at which point a patient entered the study. Diagnostic arteriogram and PTRA in 23 patients were compared with diagnostic arteriogram and medical manage-

Text continued on page 1631

TABLE 120-4. LONG-TERM PATENCY OF PERCUTANEOUS TRANSLUMINAL RENAL ANGIOPLASTY (PTRA) IN PATIENTS WITH ATHEROSCLEROTIC STENOSIS AND FIBROMUSCULAR DYSPLASIA (FMD)

NO.	REF.	AUTHOR	YEAR	NO. Patients	Procedures PTRA	Procedures Stent	LESION TYPE ASD	LESION TYPE FMD	INDICATION HTN	INDICATION RI	MEAN AGE (YR)	IMAGING ARTERIOGRAM	(%)	FOLLOW-UP MEAN (MO)	NO. OF RESTENOSIS PATIENTS	(%)	NO. OF SECONDARY PATENCIES	(%)
1	249	Kuhlmann et al	1985	60	60		35	25	60		48.0	33	(55.0)	6.8	12/33	(36.4)	26/33	(78.8)
2	283	Kremer Hovinga et al	1986	43	43		33	10	43	43	50.1	33	(76.7)	19	12/33	(36.4)	16/24	(66.7)
3	301	Julien et al	1989	66	70		66		66	16		49	(74.2)	6	5/49	(10.2)	45/49	(91.8)
4	268	Plouin et al	1993	92	92		59	33	92		51.7	92*	(100.0)	8.8	15/92	(16.3)		
5	280	Weibull et al	1993	29	29		29		29		60.0†	29	(100.0)	24	6/24	(25.0)	22/24	(91.7)
6	226	Cluzel et al	1994	20	35			20	20	1	30.5	16	(100.0)	6	3/30‡	(10.0)	29/30	(96.7)
7	244	Losinno et al	1994	195	246	1	153	42	195	60	56.0	145	(100.0)	6–102§	7/180‡	(3.9)		
8	200	Jensen et al	1995	137	180		107	30	137	22	58.0	144‡	(80.0)	12‖	34/144‡,¶	(23.6)		
9	255	Baumgartner et al	1997	50	63	8	37	13	50	25	60.0	29	(58.0)	11	16/59‡	(27.1)	60/63**	(95.2)
10	281	Plouin et al	1998	23	23	2	23		23		59.2	23#	(100.0)	6	3/23	(13.0)	22/23	(95.7)
	TOTAL			715	841	11	542	173	715	167	51.7	593		11.1	113/667	(16.9)	220/246	(89.4)

*Includes 21 intravenous digital subtraction angiograms (IVDSA).
†Median age.
‡Arteries.
§Range.
‖Minimum follow-up.
¶Includes technical failures.
**Secondary patency determined by duplex ultrasound.
#23 IVDSAs.
ASD = atherosclerotic disease; HTN = hypertension; RI = renal insufficiency.

TABLE 120–5. LONG-TERM PATENCY OF RENAL ARTERY STENTS IN PATIENTS WITH ATHEROSCLEROTIC STENOSIS AND FIBROMUSCULAR DYSPLASIA (FMD)

NO.	REF.	AUTHOR	YEAR	NO. OF Patients	NO. OF Stent	LESION TYPE ASD	LESION TYPE FMD	LESION TYPE Other	INDICATION HTN	INDICATION RI	MEAN AGE (YR)	IMAGING ARTERIOGRAM	(%)	FOLLOW-UP MEAN (MO)	NO. OF RESTENOSIS PATIENTS	(%)	SECONDARY PATENCY	(%)
1	210	Kuhn et al	1991	10	14	6		4	9	10	55	10	100.0	7.4	2/10	(20.0)	9/10	(90.0)
2	208	Rees et al	1991	28	28	28			28	14	66	18	64.3	7.5	7/18*	(38.9)	15/18	(83.3)
3	209	Wilms et al	1991	11	12	10		1	10	1	60.3	7	63.6	9	2/7	(28.6)	5/7	(71.4)
4	218	Joffre et al	1992	16	16	11		3	11	6		16	100	6	2/16	(12.5)	15/16	(93.8)
5	206	Hennequin et al	1994	21	25	15	2	3	25	6		20	95.2	29	4/20	(20.0)	19/20	(95.0)
6	207	Raynaud et al	1994	18	18	15	3	3	18	4	58	16†	88.9	11	2/16	(12.5)	15/16	(93.8)
7	304	Dorros et al	1995	76	92	76			76	48	67	45	59.2	7.1	14/56‡	(25.0)		
8	215	MacLeod et al	1995	29	32	28	1		16	17	63.6	24	82.8	7	4/24	(16.7)	23/24	(95.8)
9	211	van de Ven et al	1995	24	28	24			24	24	66	18	75.0	6	3/19	(15.8)	18/19	(94.7)
10	201	Henry et al	1996	59	64	55	3	1	59	10	65	51	91.5	6	5/54	(9.3)	54/54	(100.0)
11	203	Rundback and Jacobs	1996	20	24	20			18	11	70	12	60.0	6	3/16‡	(18.8)		
12	202	Blum et al	1997	68	74	68	0	0	68	20	60	48	70.6	12§	8/74||	(10.8)	72/74||	(97.3)
13	217	Harden et al	1997	32	32	32				32	67	24	75.0	6	3/24	(12.5)		
14	213	Harjai et al	1997	66	88	65	1		66		68	44	66.7	9.1	11/44	(25.0)		
15	205	Taylor et al	1997	29	32	28	1		16	22		25	86.2	6.7	4/25	(16.0)	24/25	(96.0)
16	214	White et al	1997	100	133				100	44	67	67	67.0	8.7	15/80‡	(18.8)		
		TOTAL		607	712	481	11	15	544	269	64.1	448	73.8	9.0	89/503	(17.7)	269/283	(95.1)

*Includes technical failures.
†Includes nine intravenous digital subtraction angiograms.
‡Arteries.
§Minimum follow-up period.
||Total restenosis and secondary patency rates determined by duplex ultrasonography.
ASD = atherosclerotic disease; HTN = hypertension; RI = renal insufficiency

TABLE 120–6. RESPONSE OF HYPERTENSION TO PERCUTANEOUS TRANSLUMINAL RENAL ANGIOPLASTY (PTRA) IN PATIENTS WITH ATHEROSCLEROTIC STENOSIS

			NO.		INDICATION		MEAN AGE (YR)	FOLLOW-UP MEAN (MO)	CLINICAL RESPONSE			
									HTN			
NO.	REF.	AUTHOR	YEAR	Patients	PTRA	HTN	RI			Cure	Benefit*	Cure (%)	Benefit* (%)
1	247	Klinge et al	1989	134	262†	134		63.7	0–60‡	13	103/115	11.3	89.6
2	282	Canzanello et al	1989	100	125	100	66	58.6	29	4	43/73	5.5	58.9
3	301	Julien et al	1989	66	70	66	16		7.5	5	42/53	9.4	79.2
4	242	Baert et al	1990	165	207	165			25.8§	71	109/141	50.4	77.3
5	243	Martin et al	1992	110	160	110		61.0	38	11	64/110	10.0	58.2
6	244	Losinno et al	1994	153	246‖	153	59	56.0	24–126‡	18	96/153	11.8	62.7
7	195	Bonelli et al	1995	190	242			63.8	33.3	16	133/190	8.4	70.0
8	200	Jensen et al	1995	107	147	107		62.5	12¶	11	47/74	14.9	63.5
9	248	Eldrup-Jorgensen et al	1995	52	60	52	42	68.0	28	3	20/52	5.8	38.5
		TOTAL		1077	1519	887	183	61.9	24.8	152	657/961	15.8	68.4

*Benefit includes patients who are cured and improved.
†Includes procedures in 79 patients with nonatherosclerotic stenoses.
‡Range.
§Follow-up period includes patients with nonatherosclerotic stenosis.
‖Includes one stent placement and procedures in 42 patients with nonatherosclerotic stenoses.
¶Minimum follow-up period.
HTN = hypertension; RI = renal insufficiency.

TABLE 120–7. RESPONSE OF HYPERTENSION TO STENT PLACEMENT IN PATIENTS WITH ATHEROSCLEROTIC STENOSIS

| | | | | NO. | | INDICATION | | MEAN AGE (YR) | FOLLOW-UP MEAN (MO) | CLINICAL RESPONSE | | | |
| | | | | | | | | | | HTN | | Cure (%) | Benefit* (%) |
NO.	REF.	AUTHOR	YEAR	Patients	Stent	HTN	RI			Cure	Benefit*		
1	208	Rees et al	1991	28	28	28	14	66.0	6.5	3	18/28	10.7	64.3
2	304	Dorros et al	1995	76	92	76	48	67.0	6	4	36/69	5.8	52.2
3	215	MacLeod et al	1995	29†	32	16	17	63.6	10.6		7/16		43.8
4	211	van de Ven et al	1995	24	28	24	24	66.0	9		16/22		72.7
5	201	Henry et al	1996	59‡	64	59	10	65.0	14	10	41/54	18.5	75.9
6	203	Rundback et al	1996	20	24	18	11	70.0	96		5/8		62.5
7	202	Blum et al	1997	68	74	68	20	60.0	27	11	53/68	16.2	77.9
8	216	Boisclair et al	1997	33	35	33	17	63.0	13.4	2	22/33	6.1	66.7
9	213	Harjai et al	1997	66†	88	66		68.0	18.6	1	42/64	1.6	65.6
10	205	Taylor et al	1997	29†	32	16	22	63.8	9.5		8/16		50.0
		TOTAL		432	497	404	183	65.2	21.1	31	248/378	8.2	65.6

*Benefit includes patients who are cured and improved.
†Includes one patient with nonatherosclerotic stenosis.
‡Includes four patients with nonatherosclerotic stenosis.
ASD = atherosclerotic disease; HTN = hypertension; RI = renal insufficiency.

TABLE 120-8. RESPONSE OF HYPERTENSION TO PERCUTANEOUS TRANSLUMINAL RENAL ANGIOPLASTY (PTRA) AND STENT PLACEMENT IN PATIENTS WITH OSTIAL ATHEROSCLEROTIC STENOSIS

NO.	REF.	AUTHOR	YEAR	Patients	PTRA	Stent	HTN	RI	OSTIAL	(%)	HTN Cure	HTN Benefit*	Cure (%)	Benefit* (%)
1	208	Rees et al	1991	28		28	28	14	28	(100)	3	18/28	10.7	64.3
2	243	Martin et al	1992	110	160		110		129	(81)	11	64/110	10.0	58.2
3	280	Weibull et al	1993	29	29		29		29	(100)	3	20/24	12.5	83.3
4	211	van de Ven et al	1995	24		28	24	24	28	(100)		16/22		72.7
5	203	Rundback and Jacobs	1996	20		24	18	11	22	(92)		5/8		62.5
6	202	Blum et al	1997	68		74	68	20	74	(100)	11	53/68	16.2	77.9
TOTAL				279	189	154	277	69	310	(90)	28	176/260	10.8	67.7

*Benefit includes patients who are cured and improved.
HTN = hypertension; RI = renal insufficiency.

TABLE 120–9. RENAL FUNCTION RESPONSE TO PERCUTANEOUS TRANSLUMINAL RENAL ANGIOPLASTY (PTRA) AND STENT PLACEMENT IN PATIENTS WITH ATHEROSCLEROTIC STENOSIS

NO.	REF.	AUTHOR	YEAR	NO. Patients	Procedures PTRA	Procedures Stent	INDICATION HTN	INDICATION RI	MEAN AGE (YR)	FOLLOW-UP MEAN (MO)	CLINICAL RESPONSE: RENAL INSUFFICIENCY Improved	Stable	Benefit*	(%)
1	282	Canzanello et al	1989	100	125		100	66	58.6	29	5		36/69	(52.2)
2	208	Rees et al	1991	28		28	28	14	66	6.5	5	5	10/14	(71.4)
3	243	Martin et al	1992	110	160		110		61	38	64		64/110	(58.2)
4	302	Tykarski et al	1993	26	43		30	17	58	10	11		11/16	(68.8)
5	280	Weibull et al	1993	29	29		29		60†	24	5	18	23/24	(95.8)
6	304	Dorros et al	1995	76		92	76	48	67	6	21	33	54/69	(78.3)
7	211	van de Ven et al	1995	24		28	24	24	66	9	8	14	22/22	(100.0)
8	201	Henry et al	1996	55		64	59	10	65	14	2		2/10	(20.0)
9	202	Blum et al	1997	68		74	68	20	60	27		20	20/20	(100.0)
10	216	Boisclair et al	1997	33		35	33	17	63	13.4	7	6	13/17	(76.5)
11	205	Taylor et al	1997	28		32	16	22	63.8	9.5	7	6	13/21	(61.9)
12	256	Tullis et al	1997	41	57	12	41	10	65	28	5	4	9/10	(90.0)
TOTAL				618	409	365	614	248	63.0	17.9	135	106	277/402	(68.9)

*Benefit includes patients who are improved and stabilized.
†Median age.
HTN = hypertension; RI = renal insufficiency.

TABLE 120–10. BLOOD PRESSURE RESPONSE TO PERCUTANEOUS TRANSLUMINAL RENAL ANGIOPLASTY (PTRA) IN PATIENTS WITH FIBROMUSCULAR DYSPLASIA (FMD)

NO.	REF.	AUTHOR	YEAR	NO. Patients	NO. PTRA	MEAN AGE (YR)	FOLLOW-UP MEAN (MO)	CLINICAL RESPONSE HTN Cure	CLINICAL RESPONSE HTN Benefit*	Cure (%)	Benefit* (%)
1	240	Sos et al	1983	31	31	30.9	16†	16	25/27	59.3	92.6
2	241	Tegtmeyer et al	1984	27	30	52.7†	23.7†	10	27/27	37.0	100.0
3	249	Kuhlmann et al	1985	25	25	37.6	21.6†	11	18/22	50.0	81.8
4	283	Kremer Hovinga et al	1986	10	10	47.0	0.5–48‡	7†	10/21	33.3	47.6
5	198	Greminger et al	1989	34	34	40.0	20.1	14	30/34	41.2	88.2
6	247	Klinge et al	1989	52	2628	33.8	0–60†,‡	18	44/47	38.3	93.6
7	242	Baert et al	1990	22	28	40.0	25.8†	18	18/19	94.7	94.7
8	290	Tegtmeyer et al	1991	66	85	45.0	39	26	65/66	39.4	98.5
9	226	Cluzel et al	1994	20	35	30.5	19	13	17/17	76.5	100.0
10	244	Losinno et al	1994	42	246‖	56.0	24–126†,‡	24	33/42	57.1	78.6
11	303	Rodriguez-Perez et al	1994	27	123¶	43.4	96	11	23/25	44.0	92.0
12	195	Bonelli et al	1995	105	140	50.5	42.7	23	66/105	21.9	62.9
13	200	Jensen et al	1995	30	33	43.0	12#	11	24/28	39.3	85.7
14	255	Baumgartner et al	1997	13	63**	49.0	13†	4	11/13	30.8	84.6
TOTAL				504	1145	42.8		206	411/493	41.8	83.4

*Benefit includes patients with cure or improved blood pressure.
†Includes atherosclerotic disease, FMD, and other.
‡Range.
§Includes procedures in 161 patients with stenosis not due to FMD.
‖Includes one stent placement procedure and procedures in 153 patients with atherosclerotic stenosis.
¶Includes procedures in 66 patients with stenosis not due to FMD.
#Minimum follow-up period.
**Includes eight stent placement procedures and procedures in 37 patients with atherosclerotic stenosis.
HTN = hypertension.

ment of hypertension in 26 patients. Although blood pressure did not differ in either treatment group, the study found that PTRA reduced the probability of requiring two or more medications for blood pressure control. However, the risk of complication was three times higher in the PTRA group (five hematomas and one dissection of a renal artery with segmental infarction) when compared with the medically treated group, who had two hematomas. The authors concluded that PTRA was a drug-sparing procedure that involved significant morbidity and that the benefit of PTRA for blood pressure management was overestimated.[281] They recommend weighing the risks and benefits of each case independently before renal artery intervention. Other authors have concluded that the predominant blood pressure benefit produced by PTRA is the ability to more easily control blood pressure with fewer medications.[195]

Several factors have been evaluated for an association with a beneficial response to endovascular intervention. Conflicting information has been published concerning the impact of technical results on clinical response. Sos and colleagues noted that *partial technical success*, defined as residual stenosis of 50% to 70% after PTRA, rarely improved blood pressure.[240] Other authors have reported the dependence of the clinical outcome on the anatomic result, both for PTRA[241] and stent placement.[208]

Contradictory data have been reported by Canzanello and coworkers, who found that blood pressure response was not significantly different between patients with less than 50% residual stenosis and those with 50% to 70% residual stenosis after PTRA.[282] Similarly, several other series found no relationship between technical and clinical success.[243, 247, 271] Adding to the confusion are the possibilities that there may be delayed blood pressure and renal function improvement,[244, 283, 284] restenosis may occur without the return of hypertension,[208, 249, 255, 266, 271] and there may be no blood pressure benefit despite a widely patent vessel.[201, 255]

The extent and location of atherosclerotic renovascular disease appear to affect the blood pressure benefit associated with PTRA. Superior blood pressure control has been reported with nonstial rather than ostial lesions[244, 247] as well as disease that is unilateral.[282, 283] In a study of 70 patients treated with PTRA,[285] dilatation of a unilateral stenosis demonstrated a significantly increased cure of hypertension than did angioplasty of bilateral stenosis. In patients with unilateral stenosis, the blood pressure benefit rate of 85.7% (18/21 patients) in patients with nonstial stenosis contrasted with a rate of 45.5% (5/11) in those with ostial stenosis—a significant difference.[282] Conversely, factors that have not demonstrated a significant association with blood pressure response include age,[195, 285] gender,[213, 236] duration of hypertension,[195] and renal function.[282, 285]

Factors associated with renal function response rates include patient age[203] and baseline renal function.[200, 203] As would be expected, one study found no renal function benefit after PTRA unless the patient had bilateral stenoses or a stenosis of a renal artery to a solitary kidney.[244]

Finally, the length of follow-up also affects interpretation of outcomes. In a study of 187 patients, 11.6% of the 80% with improved blood pressure at 6 months after PTRA experienced a recurrence of hypertension over the 8-year study period.[247] Although the patient numbers are small, blood pressure benefit rates of 80% have been reported for atherosclerotic renovascular disease at 5- and 10-year follow-ups after PTRA.[244, 247] Long-term blood pressure and renal function results are not yet available for patients treated with renal artery stents.

Fibromuscular Dysplasia

Blood pressure responses to renal artery intervention in patients with stenosis due to FMD are shown in Table 120–10.[195, 198, 200, 226, 240–242, 244, 247, 249, 255, 283, 290, 303] The table includes series with at least 10 patients with FMD. Clearly, this is the renal artery lesion and patient group for whom endovascular interventions perform best. The 83% benefit rate and the 42% cure rate make PTRA the treatment of choice for renovascular hypertension related to FMD of the medial fibroplasia type (Fig. 120–10). Beginning with early experience with PTRA, many studies have demonstrated better blood pressure outcomes for patients with FMD than with atherosclerotic renal artery stenosis.[240, 241, 249, 285, 287, 288] According to life-table analysis, the 5-year blood pressure

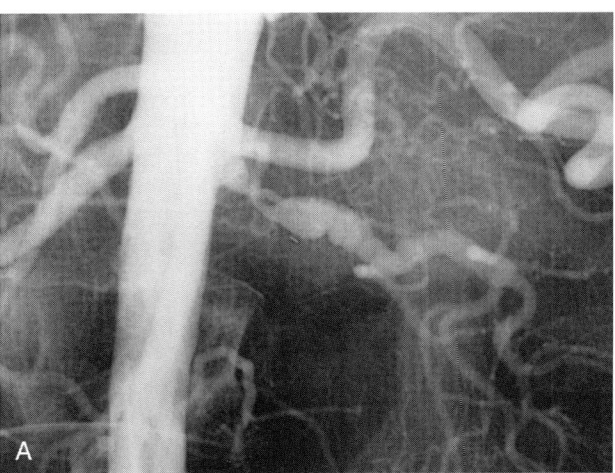
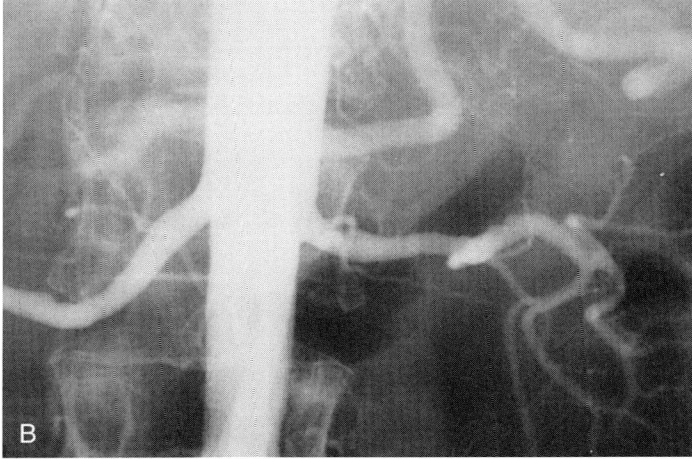

FIGURE 120–10. Response of fibromuscular disease to angioplasty. *A,* Aortogram demonstrates fibromuscular dysplasia of the left renal artery with a severe proximal stenosis. *B,* After angioplasty there is minimal residual irregularity of the renal artery, with resolution of the proximal stenosis.

benefit rate for renal artery stenosis due to FMD treated with PTRA has been reported to be 89%.[247] Because the response to PTRA is very good and because the arteries in these patients often show delayed remodeling with further improvement in residual stenoses,[226, 253] stents are usually reserved for patients in whom a flow-limiting dissection develops.

Data are very limited about the response of renal function to endovascular intervention in patients with FMD. In a series that included seven patients with FMD and renal insufficiency, improved renal function after PTRA was observed in only one patient.[289] In a larger series, 12 of the 14 patients with FMD and renal insufficiency had improved renal function after PTRA.[290] A significantly increased glomerular filtration rate was achieved in 89% of 30 patients treated with PTRA.[200] Additional data are needed before a conclusive statement regarding endovascular treatment for excretory renal insufficiency in patients with FMD can be made.

Complications

No discussion of procedural outcomes would be complete without mention of complications. Table 120–11[195, 199–203, 205, 206, 208–218, 226, 242–244, 247, 248, 255, 267, 268, 279–281, 290, 299–307] summarizes the complications that were reported in 44 series, including at least 10 patients published since 1988. The 17.2% complication rate is somewhat higher than the 9.3% complication rate found in a previous thorough analysis of patients treated with PTRA.[238] Part of this difference can be explained by the fact that the earlier analysis excluded renal failure. In addition, the inclusion of experience with stent placement likely increases the complication rate.[237, 291]

Complications have been tabulated according to those involving the renal artery or the puncture site, embolic phenomena, direct catheter-related complications, worsening renal function, and systemic complications. Although all are attributed to the renal artery intervention, many could easily be attributed instead to the diagnostic arteriography. Uncommon complications of renal artery intervention that have been reported but are not represented in Table 120–11 include renal arteriovenous fistula,[292, 293] flash pulmonary edema,[294] type B aortic dissection,[295] renal vein injury,[296] and stent infection.[297]

It is difficult to stratify the severity of complications because authors use widely varying definitions for minor or severe complications. For example, a renal artery dissection could be reported as a minor complication if it is not flow-limiting and if no further treatment is needed. A dissection that severely obstructs flow and requires surgical bypass or nephrectomy, however, clearly deserves classification as a severe complication. Mahler and associates recommended a classification system for reporting complications of PTRA, depending on the severity and the direct or indirect relationship to the PTRA procedure[298]; however, it has not been widely used. The rate of complications necessitating surgery, shown in Table 120–11, is slightly over 2% and includes puncture site complications and the 0.23% of complications requiring nephrectomy. The 1.27% 30-day mortality rate is similar to that found in other reviews of both PTRA and surgical reconstruction.[254, 274]

TABLE 120–11. COMPLICATIONS IN PATIENTS UNDERGOING PERCUTANEOUS TRANSLUMINAL RENAL ANGIOPLASTY (PTRA) OR RENAL ARTERY STENT PLACEMENT

COMPLICATION	NO.	%
Renal Artery Complications	**287**	**9.59**
Spasm	79	2.64
Dissection	73	2.44
Branch thrombosis/occlusion/perforation	31	1.04
Thrombosis/occlusion	29	0.97
Embolus	25	0.84
Segmental/complete infarction	23	0.77
Rupture	14	0.47
Pseudoaneurysm	9	0.30
Perirenal bleed	3	0.10
Stent thrombosis	1	0.03
Puncture Site Complications	**137**	**4.58**
Hematoma	81	2.71
Hematoma requiring transfusion	20	0.67
Hematoma requiring surgery	15	0.50
Pseudoaneurysm	15	0.50
Thrombosis	3	0.10
Infection	2	0.07
Brachial plexus injury	1	0.03
Embolic (Nonrenal) Complications	**28**	**0.94**
Distal embolization	21	0.70
Bowel infarction	3	0.10
Stroke*	4	0.13
Direct Catheter-Related Complication	**12**	**0.40**
Iliac/other dissection	10	0.33
Aortic dissection	1	0.03
Abdominal aortic aneurysm perforation	1	0.03
Renal Function Complication	**114**	**3.81**
Transient worsening of renal function	99	3.31
New dialysis requirement	15	0.50
Systemic	**39**	**1.30**
Myocardial infarction	9	0.30
Retroperitoneal bleed	8	0.27
Hypertensive crisis	5	0.17
Sepsis	5	0.17
Hemorrhage-related anemia	3	0.10
Pain	3	0.10
Transient ischemic attack	2	0.07
Vasovagal reaction	1	0.03
Pulmonary embolus	1	0.03
Pneumonia	1	0.03
Fever	1	0.03
Summary		
Patients reviewed	2993	
PTRA procedures	2872	
Stent procedures	792	
Patients with a complication	515	17.2
Complications requiring surgery†	63	2.10
Complications requiring nephrectomy	7	0.23
30-Day mortality rate‡	38	1.27

References: 8, 11–16, 18–31, 39, 55–57, 60, 61, 68, 80, 81, 92–95, 103, 112–120.
*One unrelated to catheter manipulation.
†Including nephrectomy and puncture site surgery.
‡Including mortality unrelated to renal artery intervention procedure.

SUMMARY

Endovascular treatments of renovascular disease have paralleled technical advancements in the field. PTRA has a moderate technical success rate, which can be raised to high immediate success if stent placement is used to salvage technical failures. For all lesions, the 6- to 12-month patency rates of PTRA and stents are similar, with a restenosis rate averaging 17% (3.9 to 36.4%). Restenosis is treatable with repeated PTRA, and secondary patency rates of above 90% have been reported for follow-up periods of 1 to 10 years.

Benefit in treatment of hypertension among patients with atherosclerotic disease can be achieved in approximately 65% of patients, with an approximately 10% cure rate. An improvement in renal function is observed in approximately one third of patients when all lesions are considered. Among patients with FMD of the medial fibroplasia type, PTRA achieves a remarkable 83% benefit rate and 42% cure rate.

Restoration of flow to an ischemic kidney provides the potential benefits of both lowering blood pressure and preventing progression of renal functional impairment. Endovascular treatment of renovascular disease produces acceptable results, with similar morbidity and mortality rates as surgical revascularization. In patients who often have several risk factors for surgery, PTRA and stent placement provide the options for a less invasive treatment.

REFERENCES

1. Helenon O, el Rody F, Correas JM, et al: Color Doppler US of renovascular disease in native kidneys. Radiographics 15(4):833–854, 1995; discussion, 854–865.
2. Miralles M, Cairols M, Cotillas J, et al: Value of Doppler parameters in the diagnosis of renal artery stenosis. J Vasc Surg 23(3):428–435, 1996.
3. Rene PC, Oliva VL, Bui BT, et al: Renal artery stenosis: Evaluation of Doppler US after inhibition of angiotensin-converting enzyme with captopril. Radiology 196(3):675–679, 1995.
4. Rubin GD, Dake MD, Napel S, et al: Spiral CT of renal artery stenosis: Comparison of three-dimensional rendering techniques. Radiology 190(1):181–189, 1994.
5. Beregi JP, Elkohen M, Deklunder G, et al: Helical CT angiography compared with arteriography in the detection of renal artery stenosis. AJR Am J Roentgenol 167(2):495–501, 1996.
6. Farres MT, Lammer J, Schima W, et al: Spiral computed tomographic angiography of the renal arteries: A prospective comparison with intravenous and intraarterial digital subtraction angiography. Cardiovasc Intervent Radiol 19(2):101–106, 1996.
7. Olbricht CJ, Paul K, Prokop M, et al: Minimally invasive diagnosis of renal artery stenosis by spiral computed tomography angiography. Kidney Int 48(4):1332–1337, 1995.
8. De Cobelli F, Mellone R, Salvioni M, et al: Renal artery stenosis: Value of screening with three-dimensional phase-contrast MR angiography with a phased-array multicoil. Radiology 201(3):697–703, 1996.
9. De Cobelli F, Vanzulli A, Sironi S, et al: Renal artery stenosis: Evaluation with breath-hold, three-dimensional, dynamic, gadolinium-enhanced versus three-dimensional, phase-contrast MR angiography. Radiology 205(3):689–695, 1997.
10. de Haan MW, Kouwenhoven M, Thelissen RP, et al: Renovascular disease in patients with hypertension: Detection with systolic and diastolic gating in three-dimensional, phase-contrast MR angiography. Radiology 198(2):449–456, 1996.
11. Prince MR, Schoenberg SO, Ward JS, et al: Hemodynamically significant atherosclerotic renal artery stenosis: MR angiographic features. Radiology 205(1):128–136, 1997.
12. Chen CC, Hoffer PB, Vahjen G, et al: Patients at high risk for renal artery stenosis: A simple method of renal scintigraphic analysis with Tc-99m DTPA and captopril. Radiology 176(2):365–370, 1990.
13. Schreij G, van Es PN, van Kroonenburgh MJ, et al: Baseline and postcaptopril renal blood flow measurements in hypertensives suspected of renal artery stenosis. J Nucl Med 37(10):1652–1655, 1996.
14. Lerman LO, Taler SJ, Textor SC, et al: Computed tomography-derived intrarenal blood flow in renovascular and essential hypertension. Kidney Int 49(3):846–854, 1996.
15. Schoenberg SO, Knopp MV, Bock M, et al: Renal artery stenosis: Grading of hemodynamic changes with cine phase-contrast MR blood flow measurements. Radiology 203(1):45–53, 1997.
16. Debatin JF, Ting RH, Wegmuller H, et al: Renal artery blood flow: Quantitation with phase-contrast MR imaging with and without breath holding. Radiology 190(2):371–378, 1994.
17. Norman D, Ulloa N, Brant-Zawadzki M, Gould RG: Intraarterial digital subtraction imaging cost considerations. Radiology 156(1):33–35, 1985.
18. Kaufman SL, Chang R, Kadir S, et al: Intraarterial digital subtraction angiography in diagnostic arteriography. Radiology 151(2):323–327, 1984.
19. Buonocore E, Meaney TF, Borkowski GP, et al: Digital subtraction angiography of the abdominal aorta and renal arteries: Comparison with conventional aortography. Radiology 139(2):281–286, 1986.
20. Smith CW, Winfield AC, Price RR, et al: Evaluation of digital venous angiography for the diagnosis of renovascular hypertension. Radiology 144(1):51–54, 1982.
21. Hillman BJ: Renovascular hypertension: Diagnosis of renal artery stenosis by digital video subtraction angiography. Urol Radiol 3(4):219–222, 1981.
22. Clark RA, Alexander ES: Digital subtraction angiography of the renal arteries: Prospective comparison with conventional arteriography. Invest Radiol 18(1):6–10, 1983.
23. Havey RJ, Krumlovsky F, delGreco F, Martin HG: Screening for renovascular hypertension: Is renal digital-subtraction angiography the preferred noninvasive test? JAMA 254(3):388–393, 1985.
24. Svetkey LP, Dunnick NR, Coffman TM, et al: Comparison of intravenous digital subtraction angiography and conventional arteriography in defining renal anatomy. Transplantation 45(1):56–58, 1988.
25. Wilms GE, Baert AL, Staessen JA, Amery AK: Renal artery stenosis: Evaluation with intravenous digital subtraction angiography. Radiology 160(3):713–715, 1986.
26. Shokeir AA, el-Diasty TA, Nabeeh A, et al: Digital subtraction angiography in potential live-kidney donors: A study of 1000 cases. Abdom Imaging 19(5):461–465, 1994.
27. Illescas FF, Braun SD, Cohan RH, et al: Fibromuscular dysplasia of renal arteries: Comparison of intravenous digital subtraction angiography with conventional angiography. Can Assoc Radiol J 39(3):167–171, 1988.
28. Hillman BJ: Imaging advances in the diagnosis of renovascular hypertension. AJR Am J Roentgenol 153(1):5–14, 1989.
29. Mann SJ, Pickering TG: Detection of renovascular hypertension: State of the art: 1992. Ann Intern Med 117(10):845–854, 1992.
30. Working Group on Renovascular Hypertension: Detection, evaluation, and treatment of renovascular hypertension: Final report. Arch Intern Med 147(5):820–829, 1987.
31. Derauf B, Goldberg ME: Angiographic assessment of potential renal transplant donors. Radiol Clin North Am 25(2):261–265, 1987.
32. Pickering TG: Diagnosis and evaluation of renovascular hypertension: Indications for therapy. Circulation 83(Suppl 2):I147–I154, 1991.
33. Kim D, Porter DH, Brown R, et al: Renal artery imaging: A prospective comparison of intra-arterial digital subtraction angiography with conventional angiography. Angiology 42(5):345–357, 1991.
34. Picus D, Neeley JP, McClennan BL, et al: Intraarterial digital subtraction angiography of renal transplants. AJR 145(1):93–96, 1985.
35. Petty W, Spigos DG, Abejo R, et al: Arterial digital angiography in the evaluation of potential renal donors. Invest Radiol 21(2):122–124, 1986.
36. Hawkins IF Jr: "Mini-catheter" technique for femoral run-off and abdominal arteriography. Am J Roentgenol Radium Ther Nucl Med 116(1):199–203, 1972.
37. Seldinger SI: Catheter replacement of the needle in percutaneous arteriography. Acta Radiol 39:368–376, 1953.
38. Ovitt TW, Amplatz K: Semiselective renal angiography. AJR 119:767–769, 1973.
39. Yedlicka JW Jr, Carlson JE, Hedlund LJ, et al: Nonselective and semiselective catheters for renal artery evaluation: Experimental study. J Vasc Interv Radiol 2(2):273–276, 1991.

40. Bauer FW, Robbins SL: A postmortem study comparing renal angiograms and renal artery casts in 58 patients. Arch Pathol 83(3):307–314, 1967.

41. Boijsen E: Angiographic studies of the anatomy of single and multiple renal arteries. Acta Radiol 183(Suppl):23–129, 1959.

42. Pick JW, Anson BJ: The renal vascular pedicle: An anatomical study of 430 body halves. J Urol 44:411–434, 1940.

43. Keen EN: Origin of renal arteries from the aorta. Acta Anat (Basel) 110(4):285–286, 1981.

44. Odman P, Ranniger K: The location of the renal arteries: An angiographic and postmortem study. Am J Roentgenol Radium Ther Nucl Med 104(2):283–286,

45. Verschuyl EJ, Kaatee R, Beek FJ, et al: Renal artery origins: Best angiographic projection angles. Radiology 205(1):115–120, 1997.

46. Verschuyl EJ, Kaatee R, Beek FJ, et al: Renal artery origins: Location and distribution in the transverse plane at CT. Radiology 203(1):71–75, 1997.

47. Gerlock AJ Jr, Goncharenko V, Sloan OM: Right posterior oblique: The projection of choice in aortography of hypertensive patients. Radiology 127(1):45–48, 1978.

48. Harrington DP, Levin DC, Garnic JD, et al: Compound angulation for the angiographic evaluation of renal artery stenosis. Radiology 146(3):829–831, 1983.

49. Caridi JG, Devane AM, Hawkins IF Jr, Newman R: Examination of renal donors as outpatients using intraarterial digital subtraction angiography and a pigtail catheter. AJR Am J Roentgenol 169(2):537–539, 1997.

50. Sherwood T, Ruutu M, Chisholm GD: Renal angiography problems in live kidney donors. Br J Radiol 51(602):99–105, 1978.

51. Meaney TF, Dustan HP: Selective renal arteriography in the diagnosis of renal hypertension. Circulation 28:1035–1041, 1963.

52. Horvath JS, Waugh RC, Tiller DJ, Duggin GG: The detection of renovascular hypertension: A study of 490 patients by renal angiography. Q J Med 51(202):139–146, 1982.

53. Scoble JE, Maher ER, Hamilton G, et al: Atherosclerotic renovascular disease causing renal impairment: A case for treatment. Clin Nephrol 31(3):119–122, 1989.

54. Simon N, Franklin SS, Bleifer KH, Maxwell MH: Clinical characteristics of renovascular hypertension. JAMA 220(9):1209–1218, 1972.

55. Hou SH, Bushinsky DA, Wish JB, et al: Hospital-acquired renal insufficiency: A prospective study. Am J Med 74(2):243–248, 1983.

56. Shusterman N, Strom BL, Murray TG, et al: Risk factors and outcome of hospital-acquired acute renal failure: Clinical epidemiologic study. Am J Med 83(1):65–71, 1987.

57. Rudnick MR, Goldfarb S, Wexler L, et al: Nephrotoxicity of ionic and nonionic contrast media in 1196 patients: A randomized trial. The Iohexol Cooperative Study. Kidney Int 47(1):254–261, 1995.

58. Schwab SJ, Hlatky MA, Pieper KS, et al: Contrast nephrotoxicity: A randomized controlled trial of a nonionic and an ionic radiographic contrast agent. N Engl J Med 320(3):149–153, 1989.

59. Barrett BJ, Parfrey PS, Vavasour HM, et al: Contrast nephropathy in patients with impaired renal function: High versus low osmolar media. Kidney Int 41(5):1274–1279, 1992.

60. Cramer BC, Parfrey PS, Hutchinson TA, et al: Renal function following infusion of radiologic contrast material: A prospective controlled study. Arch Intern Med 145(1):87–89, 1985.

61. D'Elia JA, Gleason RE, Alday M, et al: Nephrotoxicity from angiographic contrast material: A prospective study. Am J Med 72(5):719–725, 1982.

62. Davidson CJ, Hlatky M, Morris KG, et al: Cardiovascular and renal toxicity of a nonionic radiographic contrast agent after cardiac catheterization: A prospective trial. Ann Intern Med 110(2):119–124, 1989.

63. Lautin EM, Freeman NJ, Schoenfeld AH, et al: Radiocontrast-associated renal dysfunction: Incidence and risk factors. AJR Am J Roentgenol 157(1):49–58, 1991.

64. Moore RD, Steinberg EP, Powe NR, et al: Frequency and determinants of adverse reactions induced by high-osmolality contrast media. Radiology 170(3 Pt 1):727–732, 1989.

65. Moore RD, Steinberg EP, Powe NR, et al: Nephrotoxicity of high-osmolality versus low-osmolality contrast media: Randomized clinical trial. Radiology 182(3):649–655, 1992.

66. Rich MW, Crecelius CA: Incidence, risk factors, and clinical course of acute renal insufficiency after cardiac catheterization in patients 70 years of age or older: A prospective study. Arch Intern Med 150(6):1237–1242, 1990.

67. Eisenberg RL, Bank WO, Hedgock MW: Renal failure after major angiography can be avoided with hydration. AJR 136(5):859–861, 1981.

68. Berns AS: Nephrotoxicity of contrast media [clinical conference]. Kidney Int 36(4):730–740, 1989.

69. Taliercio CP, Vlietstra RE, Fisher LD, Burnett JC: Risks for renal dysfunction with cardiac angiography. Ann Intern Med 104(4):501–504, 1986.

70. Manske CL, Sprafka JM, Strony JT, Wang Y: Contrast nephropathy in azotemic diabetic patients undergoing coronary angiography. Am J Med 89(5):615–620, 1990.

71. Weinrauch LA, Healy RW, Leland OS Jr, et al: Coronary angiography and acute renal failure in diabetic azotemic nephropathy. Ann Intern Med 86(1):56–59, 1977.

72. Harris KG, Smith TP, Cragg AH, Lemke JH: Nephrotoxicity from contrast material in renal insufficiency: Ionic versus nonionic agents. Radiology 179(3):849–852, 1991.

73. Parfrey PS, Griffiths SM, Barrett BJ, et al: Contrast material-induced renal failure in patients with diabetes mellitus, renal insufficiency, or both: A prospective controlled study. N Engl J Med 320(3):143–149, 1989.

74. Taliercio CP, Vlietstra RE, Ilstrup DM, et al: A randomized comparison of the nephrotoxicity of iopamidol and diatrizoate in high risk patients undergoing cardiac angiography. J Am Coll Cardiol 17(2):384–390, 1991.

75. Cigarroa RG, Lange RA, Williams RH, Hillis LD: Dosing of contrast material to prevent contrast nephropathy in patients with renal disease. Am J Med 86(6 Pt 1):649–652, 1989.

76. Gomes AS, Baker JD, Martin-Paredero V, et al: Acute renal dysfunction after major arteriography. AJR 145(6):1249–1253, 1985.

77. Martin-Paredero V, Dixon SM, Baker JD, et al: Risk of renal failure after major angiography. Arch Surg 118(12):1417–1420, 1983.

78. Barrett BJ, Carlisle EJ: Meta-analysis of the relative nephrotoxicity of high- and low-osmolality iodinated contrast media. Radiology 188(1):171–178, 1993.

79. Jakobsen JA: Renal effects of iodixanol in healthy volunteers and patients with severe renal failure. Acta Radiol 36(Suppl 399):191–195, 1995.

80. Rudnick MR, Berns JS, Cohen RM, Goldfarb S: Nephrotoxic risks of renal angiography: Contrast media-associated nephrotoxicity and atheroembolism—a critical review. Am J Kidney Dis 24(4):713–727, 1994.

81. Paul RE, Durant TM, Oppenheimer MJ, Stauffer HM: Intravenous carbon dioxide for intracardiac gas contrast in the roentgen diagnosis of pericardial effusion and thickening. AJR 78:224–225, 1957.

82. Oppenheimer MJ, Durant DM, Stauffer H, et al: Cardiovascular-respiratory effects and associated changes in blood chemistry. Am J Physiol 186:325–334, 1956.

83. Moore RM, Braselton CW: Injections of air and carbon dioxide into a pulmonary vein. Ann Surg 112:212–218, 1940.

84. Hawkins IF Jr, Wilcox CS, Kerns SR, Sabatelli FW: CO_2 digital angiography: A safer contrast agent for renal vascular imaging? Am J Kidney Dis 24(4):685–694, 1994.

85. Hawkins IF: Carbon dioxide digital subtraction arteriography. AJR 139(1):19–24, 1982.

86. Seeger JM, Self S, Harward TR, et al: Carbon dioxide gas as an arterial contrast agent. Ann Surg 217(6):688–697, 1993; discussion, 697–698.

87. Harward TR, Smith S, Hawkins IF, Seeger JM: Follow-up evaluation after renal artery bypass surgery with use of carbon dioxide arteriography and color-flow duplex scanning. J Vasc Surg 18(1):23–30, 1993.

88. Schreier DZ, Weaver FA, Frankhouse J, et al: A prospective study of carbon dioxide-digital subtraction vs standard contrast arteriography in the evaluation of the renal arteries. Arch Surg 131(5):503–507, 1996; discussion, 507–508.

89. Kerns SR, Hawkins IF Jr: Carbon dioxide digital subtraction angiography: Expanding applications and technical evolution. AJR Am J Roentgenol 164(3):735–741, 1995.

90. Weaver FA, Pentecost MJ, Yellin AE, et al: Clinical applications of carbon dioxide/digital subtraction arteriography. J Vasc Surg 13(2):266–272, 1991; discussion, 272–273.

91. Hawkins IF, Caridi JG: Carbon dioxide (CO_2) digital subtraction angiography: 26-year experience at the University of Florida. Eur Radiol 8(3):391–402, 1998.

92. Miller FJ, Mineau DE, Koehler PR. et al: Clinical intra-arterial digital subtraction imaging: Use of small volumes of iodinated contrast material or carbon dioxide. Radiology 148(1):273–278, 1983.

93. Kriss VM, Cottrill CM, Gurley JC: Carbon dioxide (CO_2) angiography in children. Pediatr Radiol 27(10):807–810, 1997.

94. Hawkins IF Jr, Mladinich CR, Storm B, et al: Short-term effects of selective renal arterial carbon dioxide administration on the dog kidney. J Vasc Interv Radiol 5(1):149–154, 1994.

95. Sullivan KL, Bonn J, Shapiro MJ, Gardiner GA: Venography with carbon dioxide as a contrast agent. Cardiovasc Intervent Radiol 18(3):141–145, 1995.

96. Kuo PC, Petersen J, Semba C, et al: CO_2 angiography—a technique for vascular imaging in renal allograft dysfunction. Transplantation 61(4):652–654, 1996.

97. Frankhouse JH, Ryan MG, Papanicolaou G, et al: Carbon dioxide/digital subtraction arteriography-assisted transluminal angioplasty. Ann Vasc Surg 9(5):448–452, 1995.

98. Bloem JL, Wondergem J: Gd-DTPA as a contrast agent in CT. Radiology 171(2):578–579, 1989.

99. Quinn AD, O'Hare NJ, Wallis FJ, Wilson GF: Gd-DTPA: An alternative contrast medium for CT. J Comput Assist Tomogr 18(4):634–636, 1994.

100. Kinno Y, Odagiri K, Andoh K, et al: Gadopentetate dimeglumine as an alternative contrast material for use in angiography. AJR Am J Roentgenol 160(6):1293–1294, 1993.

101. Matchett WJ, McFarland DR, Russell DK, et al: Azotemia: Gadopentetate dimeglumine as contrast agent at digital subtraction angiography. Radiology 201(2):569–571, 1996.

102. Kaufman JA, Geller SC, Waltman AC: Renal insufficiency: Gadopentetate dimeglumine as a radiographic contrast agent during peripheral vascular interventional procedures. Radiology 198(2):579–581, 1996.

103. Prince MR, Arnoldus C, Frisoli JK: Nephrotoxicity of high-dose gadolinium compared with iodinated contrast. J Magn Reson Imaging 6(1):162–166, 1996.

104. Niendorf HP, Haustein J, Cornelius I, et al: Safety of gadolinium-DTPA: Extended clinical experience. Magn Reson Med 22(2):222–228, 1991; discussion, 229–232.

105. Haustein J, Niendorf HP, Krestin G, et al: Renal tolerance of gadolinium-DTPA/dimeglumine in patients with chronic renal failure. Invest Radiol 27(2):153–156, 1992.

106. Nahman NS Jr, Maniam P, Hernandez RA Jr, et al: Renal artery pressure gradients in patients with angiographic evidence of atherosclerotic renal artery stenosis. Am J Kidney Dis 24(4):695–699, 1994.

107. Carter SA, Ritchie GW: Measurement of renal artery pressures by catheterization in patients with and without renal artery stenosis. Circulation 33(3):443–449, 1966.

108. Sheikh KH, Davidson CJ, Newman GE, et al: Intravascular ultrasound assessment of the renal artery. Ann Intern Med 115(1):22–25, 1991.

109. Davidson CJ, Sheikh KH, Harrison JK, et al: Intravascular ultrasonography versus digital subtraction angiography: A human in vivo comparison of vessel size and morphology. J Am Coll Cardiol 16(3):633–636, 1990.

110. Savader SJ, Lund GB, Osterman FA Jr: Volumetric evaluation of blood flow in normal renal arteries with a Doppler flow wire: A feasibility study. J Vasc Interv Radiol 8(2):209–214, 1997.

111. Atalar E, Bottomley PA, Ocali O, et al: High resolution intravascular MRI and MRS by using a catheter receiver coil. Magn Reson Med 36(4):596–605, 1996.

112. Jacobson HR: Ischemic renal disease: An overlooked clinical entity? [clinical conference]. Kidney Int 34(5):729–743, 1988.

113. Hansen KJ: Prevalence of ischemic nephropathy in the atherosclerotic population. Am J Kidney Dis 24(4):615–621, 1994.

114. Dean RH, Tribble RW, Hansen KJ, et al: Evolution of renal insufficiency in ischemic nephropathy. Ann Surg 213(5):446–455, 1991; discussion, 455–456.

115. Andersson I, Bergentz SE, Ericsson BF, et al: Unilateral renal artery stenosis and hypertension. II. Angiographic findings correlated with blood pressure response after surgery. Acta Radiol [Diagn] (Stockh) 20(6):895–906, 1979.

116. Bookstein JJ, Abrams HL, Buenger RE, et al: Radiologic aspects of renovascular hypertension: 3. Appraisal of arteriography. JAMA 221(4):368–374, 1972.

117. Hunt JC, Sheps SG, Harrison EG Jr, et al: Renal and renovascular hypertension: A reasoned approach to diagnosis and management. Arch Intern Med 133(6):988–999, 1974.

118. Maxwell MH, Bleifer KH, Franklin SS, Varady PD: Cooperative study of renovascular hypertension: Demographic analysis of the study. JAMA 220(9):1195–1204, 1972.

119. Schreiber MJ, Pohl MA, Novick AC: The natural history of atherosclerotic and fibrous renal artery disease. Urol Clin North Am 11(3):383–392, 1984.

120. Sutton D: Arteriography and renal artery stenosis. Postgrad Med J 42(485):177–182, 1966.

121. Sutton D, Brunton FJ, Starer F: Renal artery stenosis. Clin Radiol 12:80–90, 1961.

122. Van Velzer DA, Burge CH, Morris GC: Arteriosclerotic narrowing of renal arteries associated with hypertension. AJR 86:807–818, 1961.

123. Eyler WR, Clark MD, Garman JE, et al: Angiography of the renal areas including a comparative study of renal arterial stenoses in patients with and without hypertension. Radiology 78:879–891, 1962.

124. Dustan HP, Humphries AW, DeWolfe VG, Page IH: Normal arterial pressure in patients with renal arterial stenosis. JAMA 187:1028–1029, 1964.

125. Holley KE, Hunt JC, Brown AL, et al: Renal artery stenosis: A clinical-pathologic study in normotensive and hypertensive patients. Am J Med 37:14–22, 1964.

126. Schwartz CJ, White TA: Stenosis of renal artery: An unselected necropsy study. Br Med J 2:1415–1421, 1964.

127. Choudhri AH, Cleland JG, Rowlands PC, et al: Unsuspected renal artery stenosis in peripheral vascular disease. BMJ 301(6762):1197–1198, 1990.

128. Valentine RJ, Clagett GP, Miller GL, et al: The coronary risk of unsuspected renal artery stenosis. J Vasc Surg 18(3):433–439, 1993; discussion, 439–440.

129. Bookstein JJ: Appraisal of arteriography in estimating the hemodynamic significance of renal artery stenoses. Invest Radiol 1(4):281–294, 1966.

130. Abrams HL, Cornell SH: Patterns of collateral flow in renal ischemia. Radiology 84(6):1001–1012, 1965.

131. Ernst CB, Bookstein JJ, Montie J, et al: Renal vein renin ratios and collateral vessels in renovascular hypertension. Arch Surg 104(4):496–502, 1972.

132. Brolin I: Renal artery changes in hypertension. Acta Radiol [Diagn] (Stockh) 6(5):401–423, 1967.

133. Paul RE, Ettinger A, et al: Angiographic visualization of renal collateral circulation as a means of detecting and delineating renal ischemia. Radiology 84:1013–1021, 1965.

134. Foster JH, Maxwell MH, Franklin SS, et al: Renovascular occlusive disease: Results of operative treatment. JAMA 231(10):1043–1048, 1975.

135. Bonelli FS, McKusick MA, Textor SC, et al: Renal artery angioplasty: Technical results and clinical outcome in 320 patients. Mayo Clin Proc 70(11):1041–1052, 1995.

136. Greminger P, Steiner A, Schneider E, et al: Cure and improvement of renovascular hypertension after percutaneous transluminal angioplasty of renal artery stenosis. Nephron 51(3):362–366, 1989.

137. Martin LG, Price RB, Casarella WJ, et al: Percutaneous angioplasty in clinical management of renovascular hypertension: Initial and long-term results. Radiology 155(3):629–633, 1985.

138. Sos TA, Pickering TG, Sniderman K, et al: Percutaneous transluminal renal angioplasty in renovascular hypertension due to atheroma or fibromuscular dysplasia. N Engl J Med 309(5):274–279, 1983.

139. Tegtmeyer CJ, Kellum CD, Ayers C: Percutaneous transluminal angioplasty of the renal artery: Results and long-term follow-up. Radiology 153(1):77–84, 1984.

140. National High Blood Pressure Education Program Working Group: 1995 update of the working group reports on chronic renal failure and renovascular hypertension. Arch Intern Med 156(17):1938–1947, 1996.

141. McCormack LJ, Poutasse EF, Meaney TF, et al: A pathologic-arteriographic correlation of renal arterial disease. Am Heart J 72(2):188–198, 1966.

142. Harrison EG, McCormack LJ: Pathologic classification of renal arterial disease in renovascular hypertension. Mayo Clin Proc 46:161–167, 1971.

143. McCormack LJ, Dustan HP, Meaney TF: Selected pathology of the renal artery. Semin Roentgenol 2:126–138, 1967.

144. Davis BA, Crook JE, Vestal RE, Oates JA: Prevalence of renovascular hypertension in patients with grade III or IV hypertensive retinopathy. N Engl J Med 301(23):1273–1276, 1979.

145. Cicuto KP, McLean GK, Oleaga JA, et al: Renal artery stenosis: Anatomic classification for percutaneous transluminal angioplasty. AJR 137(3):599–601, 1981.

146. Canzanello VJ, Millan VG, Spiegel JE, et al: Percutaneous transluminal renal angioplasty in management of atherosclerotic renovascular hypertension: Results in 100 patients. Hypertension 13(2):163–172, 1989.

147. Kaatee R, Beek FJ, Verschuyl EJ, et al: Atherosclerotic renal artery stenosis: Ostial or truncal? Radiology 199(3):637–640, 1996.

148. Wollenweber J, Sheps SG, Davis GD: Clinical course of atherosclerotic renovascular disease. Am J Cardiol 21(1):60–71, 1968.

149. Meaney TF, Dustan HP, McCormack LJ: Natural history of renal arterial disease. Radiology 91(5):881–887, 1968.

150. Dean RH, Kieffer RW, Smith BM, et al: Renovascular hypertension: Anatomic and renal function changes during drug therapy. Arch Surg 116(11):1408–1415, 1981.

151. Tollefson DF, Ernst CB: Natural history of atherosclerotic renal artery stenosis associated with aortic disease. J Vasc Surg 14(3):327–331, 1991.

152. Rimmer JM, Gennari FJ: Atherosclerotic renovascular disease and progressive renal failure. Ann Intern Med 118(9):712–719, 1993.

153. Kincaid OW, Davis GD, Hallermann FJ, Hunt JC: Fibromuscular dysplasia of the renal arteries: Arteriographic features, classification, and observations on natural history of the disease. Am J Roentgenol Radium Ther Nucl Med 104(2):271–282, 1968.

154. Foster JH, Dean RH, Pinkerton JA, Rhamy RK: Ten years experience with the surgical management of renovascular hypertension. Ann Surg 177(6):755–766, 1973.

155. Wylie EJ, Perloff D, Wellington JS: Fibromuscular hyperplasia of the renal arteries. Ann Surg 156:592, 1962.

156. Alimi Y, Mercier C, Pellissier JF, et al: Fibromuscular disease of the renal artery: A new histopathologic classification. Ann Vasc Surg 6(3):220–224, 1992.

157. Scott JA, Rabe FE, Becker GJ, et al: Angiographic assessment of renal artery pathology: How reliable? AJR 141(6):1299–1303, 1983.

158. Boijsen E, Kohler R: Renal artery aneurysms. Acta Radiol 1:1077–1090), 1963.

159. Bastounis E, Pikoulis E, Georgopoulos S, et al: Surgery for renal artery aneurysms: A combined series of two large centers. Eur Urol 33(1):22–27, 1998.

160. Cummings KB, Lecky JW, Kaufman JJ: Renal artery aneurysms and hypertension. J Urol 109(2):144–148, 1973.

161. Bulbul MA, Farrow GA: Renal artery aneurysms. Urology 40(2):124–126, 1992.

162. Tham G, Ekelund L, Herrlin K, et al: Renal artery aneurysms: Natural history and prognosis. Ann Surg 197(3):348–352, 1983.

163. Morin RP, Dunn EJ. Wright CB: Renal arteriovenous fistulas: A review of etiology, diagnosis, and management. Surgery 99(1):114–118, 1986.

164. Maldonado JE, Sheps SG, Bernatz PE, et al: Renal arteriovenous fistula: A reversible cause of hypertension and heart failure. Am J Med 37:499–513, 1964.

165. McAlhany JC Jr, Black HC Jr, Hanback LD Jr, Yarbrough DRD: Renal arteriovenous fistula as a cause of hypertension. Am J Surg 122(1):117–120, 1971.

166. Boijsen E, Kohler R: Renal arteriovenous fistula. Acta Radiol 57:433–445, 1962.

167. Rao CN, Blaivas JG: Primary renal artery dissecting aneurysm: A review. J Urol 118(5):716–719, 1977.

168. Gewertz BL, Stanley JC, Fry WJ: Renal artery dissections. Arch Surg 112(4):409–414, 1977.

169. Bakir AA, Patel SK, Schwartz MM, Lewis EJ: Isolated dissecting aneurysm of the renal artery. Am Heart J 96(1):92–96, 1978.

170. Alamir A, Middendorf DF, Baker P, et al: Renal artery dissection causing renal infarction in otherwise healthy men. Am J Kidney Dis 30(6):851–855, 1997.

171. Kerr GS, Hallahan CW, Giordano J, et al: Takayasu arteritis. Ann Intern Med 120(11):919–929, 1994.

172. Hall S, Barr W, Lie JT, et al: Takayasu arteritis: A study of 32 North American patients. Medicine (Baltimore) 64(2):89–99, 1985.

173. Itzchak Y, Katznelson D, Boichis H, et al: Angiographic features of arterial lesions in neurofibromatosis. Am J Roentgenol Radium Ther Nucl Med 122(3):643–647, 1974.

174. Stanley JC, Fry WJ: Pediatric renal artery occlusive disease and renovascular hypertension: Etiology, diagnosis, and operative treatment. Arch Surg 116(5):669–676, 1981.

175. Theiss M, Wirth MP, Dolken W, Frohmuller HG: Spontaneous thrombosis of the renal vessels: Rare entities to be considered in differential diagnosis of patients presenting with lumbar flank pain and hematuria. Urol Int 48(4):441–445, 1992.

176. Bouttier S, Valverde JP, Lacombe M, et al: Renal artery emboli: The role of surgical treatment. Ann Vasc Surg 2(2):161–168, 1988.

177. Gasparini M, Hofmann R, Stoller M: Renal artery embolism: Clinical features and therapeutic options. J Urol 147(3):567–572, 1992.

178. Jordan ML, Cook GT, Cardella CJ: Ten years of experience with vascular complications in renal transplantation. J Urol 128(4):689–692, 1982.

179. Lacombe M: Renal artery stenosis after renal transplantation. Ann Vasc Surg 2(2):155–160, 1988.

180. Ekelund L, Gerlock J Jr, Goncharenko V, Foster J: Angiographic findings following surgical treatment for renovascular hypertension. Radiology 126(2):345–349, 1978.

181. Cohen JR, Birnbaum E: Coarctation of the abdominal aorta. J Vasc Surg 8(2):160–164, 1988.

182. Vaccaro PS, Myers JC, Smead WL: Surgical correction of abdominal aortic coarctation and hypertension. J Vasc Surg 3(4):643–648, 1986.

183. Staab GE, Tegtmeyer CJ, Constable WC: Radiation-induced renovascular hypertension. Am J Roentgenol 126(3):634–637, 1976.

184. Bron KM, Strott CA, Shapiro AP: The diagnostic value of angiographic observations in polyarteritis nodosa. Arch Intern Med 116:450, 1965.

185. Fleming RJ, Stern LZ: Multiple intraparenchymal renal aneurysms in polyarteritis nodosa. Radiology 84:100, 1965.

186. Halpern M, Citron BP: Necrotizing angiitis associated with drug abuse. Am J Roentgenol Radium Ther Nucl Med 111(4):663–671, 1971.

187. Silver D, Clements JB: Renovascular hypertension from renal artery compression by congenital bands. Ann Surg 183(2):161–166, 1976.

188. Postma CT, van Oijen AH, Barentsz JO, et al: The value of tests predicting renovascular hypertension in patients with renal artery stenosis treated by angioplasty. Arch Intern Med 151(8):1531–1535, 1991.

189. Pickering TG: Diagnosis and evaluation of renovascular hypertension: Indications for therapy. Circulation 83(Suppl 2):I147–I154, 1991.

190. Mann SJ, Pickering TG: Detection of renovascular hypertension: State of the art: 1992. Ann Intern Med 117(10):845–853, 1992.

191. Rimmer JM, Gennari FJ: Atherosclerotic renovascular disease and progressive renal failure. Ann Intern Med 118(9):712–719, 1993.

192. Poulias GE, Skoutas B, Doundoulakis N, et al: Surgical treatment of renovascular hypertension and respective late results: A twenty years experience. J Cardiovasc Surg (Torino) 32(1):69–75, 1991.

193. McNeil JW, String ST, Pfeiffer RB Jr: Concomitant renal endarterectomy and aortic reconstruction. J Vasc Surg 20(3):331–336, 1994.

194. Cambria RP, Brewster DC, L'Italien GJ, et al: The durability of different reconstructive techniques for atherosclerotic renal artery disease. J Vasc Surg 20(1):76–85, 1994.

195. Bonelli FS, McKusick MA, Textor SC, et al: Renal artery angioplasty: Technical results and clinical outcome in 320 patients. Mayo Clin Proc 70(11):1041–1052, 1995.

196. Morganti A, Quorso P, Ferraris P, et al: Time-course of the changes in blood pressure and in plasma renin activity during the first week after dilation of renal artery stenosis. J Hypertens Suppl 7(6):S186–S187, 1989.

197. Tegtmeyer CJ, Sos TA: Techniques of renal angioplasty. Radiology 161(3):577–586, 1986.

198. Greminger P, Steiner A, Schneider E, et al: Cure and improvement of renovascular hypertension after percutaneous transluminal angioplasty of renal artery stenosis. Nephron. 51(3):362–366, 1989.

199. Dorros G, Prince C, Mathiak L: Stenting of a renal artery stenosis achieves better relief of the obstructive lesion than balloon angioplasty. Cathet Cardiovasc Diagn 29(3):191–198, 1993.

200. Jensen G, Zachrisson BF, Delin K, et al: Treatment of renovascular hypertension: One year results of renal angioplasty. Kidney Int 48(6):1936–1945, 1995.

201. Henry M, Amor M, Henry I, et al: Stent placement in the renal artery: Three-year experience with the Palmaz stent. J Vasc Intervent Radiol 7(3):343–350, 1996.

202. Blum U, Krumme B, Flugel P, et al: Treatment of ostial renal-artery stenoses with vascular endoprostheses after unsuccessful balloon angioplasty. N Engl J Med 336(7):459–465, 1997.

203. Rundback JH, Jacobs JM: Percutaneous renal artery stent placement for hypertension and azotemia: Pilot study. Am J Kidney Dis 28(2):214–219, 1996.

204. Becker GJ, Katzen BT, Dake MD: Noncoronary angioplasty. Radiology 170(3 Pt 2):921–940, 1989.

205. Taylor A, Sheppard D, Macleod MJ, et al: Renal artery stent placement in renal artery stenosis: Technical and early clinical results. Clin Radiol 52(6):451–457, 1997.

206. Hennequin LM, Joffre FG, Rousseau HP, et al: Renal artery stent placement: Long-term results with the Wallstent endoprosthesis. Radiology 191(3):713–719, 1994.

207. Raynaud AC, Beyssen BM, Turmel-Rodrigues LE, et al: Renal artery stent placement: Immediate and midterm technical and clinical results. J Vasc Interv Radiol 5(6):849–858, 1994.

208. Rees CR, Palmaz JC, Becker GJ, et al: Palmaz stent in atherosclerotic stenoses involving the ostia of the renal arteries: Preliminary report of a multicenter study. Radiology 181(2):507–514, 1991.

209. Wilms GE, Peene PT, Baert AL, et al: Renal artery stent placement with use of the Wallstent endoprosthesis. Radiology 179(2):457–462, 1991.

210. Kuhn FP, Kutkuhn B, Torsello G, Modder U: Renal artery stenosis: Preliminary results of treatment with the Strecker stent. Radiology 180(2):367–372, 1991.

211. van de Ven PJ, Beutler JJ, Kaatee R, et al: Transluminal vascular stent for ostial atherosclerotic renal artery stenosis. Lancet 346(8976):672–674, 1995.

212. Pattynama PM, Becker GJ, Brown J, et al: Percutaneous angioplasty for atherosclerotic renal artery disease: Effect on renal function in azotemic patients. Cardiovasc Intervent Radiol 17(3):143–146, 1994.

213. Harjai K, Khosla S, Shaw D, et al: Effect of gender on outcomes following renal artery stent placement for renovascular hypertension. Cathet Cardiovasc Diagn 42(4):381–386, 1997.

214. White CJ, Ramee SR, Collins TJ, et al: Renal artery stent placement: Utility in lesions difficult to treat with balloon angioplasty. J Am Coll Cardiol 30(6):1445–1450, 1997.

215. MacLeod M, Taylor AD, Baxter G, et al: Renal artery stenosis managed by Palmaz stent insertion: Technical and clinical outcome. J Hypertens 13(12 Pt 2):1791–1795, 1995.

216. Boisclair C, Therasse E, Oliva VL, et al: Treatment of renal angioplasty failure by percutaneous renal artery stenting with Palmaz stents: Midterm technical and clinical results. AJR Am J Roentgenol 168(1):245–251, 1997.

217. Harden PN, MacLeod MJ, Rodger RS, et al: Effect of renal-artery stenting on progression of renovascular renal failure. Lancet 349(9059):1133–1136, 1997.

218. Joffre F, Rousseau H, Bernadet P, et al: Midterm results of renal artery stenting. Cardiovasc Intervent Radiol 15(5):313–318, 1992.

219. Verschuyl EJ, Kaatee R, Beek FJ, et al: Renal artery origins: Best angiographic projection angles. Radiology 205(1):115–120, 1997.

220. Verschuyl EJ, Kaatee R, Beek FJ, et al: Renal artery origins: Location and distribution in the transverse plane at CT. Radiology 203(1):71–75, 1997.

221. Cicuto KP, McLean GK, Oleaga JA, et al: Renal artery stenosis: Anatomic classification for percutaneous transluminal angioplasty. AJR 137(3):599–601, 1981.

222. Dake MD, Oesterle SN, Robertson GC, et al: Percutaneous directional atherectomy for treatment of renal artery stenosis. Radiology 181(Suppl):295, 1991.

223. Kushner FG, Helm MJ: Successful directional atherectomy of eccentric renal artery stenosis using the Simpson directional coronary atherocath as a primary therapy. Cathet Cardiovasc Diagn 29(2):128–130, 1993.

224. Dal Canton A, Iaccarino V, Russo D, et al: Scleroembolization for treatment of hypertension caused by intrarenal arterial fibrodysplasia. Clin Nephrol 21(2):138–139, 1984.

225. Bachman DM, Casarella WJ, Spiegel R, Bregman D: Selective renal artery embolization: Treatment of acute renovascular hypertension. JAMA 238(14):1534–1535, 1977.

226. Cluzel P, Raynaud A, Beyssen B, et al: Stenoses of renal branch arteries in fibromuscular dysplasia: Results of percutaneous transluminal angioplasty. Radiology 193(1):227–232, 1994.

227. Teigen CL, Mitchell SE, Venbrux AC, et al: Segmental renal artery embolization for treatment of pediatric renovascular hypertension. J Vasc Intervent Radiol 3(1):111–117, 1992.

228. Ishijima H, Ishizaka H, Sakurai M, et al: Partial renal embolization for pediatric renovascular hypertension secondary to fibromuscular dysplasia. Cardiovasc Intervent Radiol 20(5):383–386, 1997.

229. Golwyn DH Jr, Routh WD, Chen MY, et al: Percutaneous transcatheter renal ablation with absolute ethanol for uncontrolled hypertension or nephrotic syndrome: Results in 11 patients with end-stage renal disease. J Vasc Intervent Radiol 8(4):527–533, 1997.

230. Reuter SR, Pomeroy PR, Chuang VP, Cho KJ: Embolic control of hypertension caused by segmental renal artery stenosis. Am J Roentgenol 127(3):389–392, 1976.

231. Grinnell VS, Hieshima GB, Mehringer CM, et al: Therapeutic renal artery occlusion with a detachable balloon. J Urol 126(2):233–237, 1981.

232. Mali WP, Geyskes GG, Thalman R: Dissecting renal artery aneurysm: Treatment with an endovascular stent. AJR Am J Roentgenol 153(3):623–624, 1989.

233. Whigham CJ Jr, Bodenhamer JR, Miller JK: Use of the Palmaz stent in primary treatment of renal artery intimal injury secondary to blunt trauma. J Vasc Interv Radiol 6(2):175–178, 1995.

234. Routh WD, Keller FS, Gross GM: Transcatheter thrombosis of a leaking saccular aneurysm of the main renal artery with preservation of renal blood flow. AJR Am J Roentgenol 154(5):1097–1099, 1990.

235. Bui BT, Oliva VL, Leclerc G, et al: Renal artery aneurysm: Treatment with percutaneous placement of a stent-graft. Radiology 195(1):181–182, 1995.

236. Tani M, Mizuno K, Midorikawa H, et al: Thermal laser-assisted angioplasty of renal artery stenosis for renovascular hypertension. Cardiovasc Intervent Radiol 16(1):52–54, 1993.

237. Martin LG, Casarella WJ, Alspaugh JP, Chuang VP: Renal artery angioplasty: Increased technical success and decreased complications in the second 100 patients. Radiology 159(3):631–634, 1986.

238. Martin LG, Rees CR, O'Bryant T: Percutaneous angioplasty of the renal arteries. In Strandness DE, van Breda A (eds): Vascular Diseases. Surgical and Interventional Therapy. Vol 2. New York, Churchill Livingstone, 1994, pp 721–741.

239. Tegtmeyer CJ, Matsumoto AH, Johnson AM: Renal angioplasty. In Baum S, Pentecost MJ (eds): Abram's Angiography. Vol 3. Boston, Little, Brown, 1997, pp 294–325.

240. Sos TA, Pickering TG, Sniderman K, et al: Percutaneous transluminal renal angioplasty in renovascular hypertension due to atheroma or fibromuscular dysplasia. N Engl J Med 309(5):274–279, 1983.

241. Tegtmeyer CJ, Kellum CD, Ayers C: Percutaneous transluminal angioplasty of the renal artery: Results and long-term follow-up. Radiology 153(1):77–84, 1984.

242. Baert AL, Wilms G, Amery A, et al: Percutaneous transluminal renal angioplasty: Initial results and long-term follow-up in 202 patients. Cardiovasc Intervent Radiol 13(1):22–28, 1990.

243. Martin LG, Cork RD, Kaufman SL: Long-term results of angioplasty in 110 patients with renal artery stenosis. J Vasc Intervent Radiol 3(4):619–626, 1992.

244. Losinno F, Zuccala A, Busato F, Zucchelli P: Renal artery angioplasty for renovascular hypertension and preservation of renal function: Long-term angiographic and clinical follow-up. AJR Am J Roentgenol 162(4):853–857, 1994.

245. Martin LG, Price RB, Casarella WJ, et al: Percutaneous angioplasty in clinical management of renovascular hypertension: Initial and long-term results. Radiology 155(3):629–633, 1985.

246. Miller GA, Ford KK, Braun SD, et al: Percutaneous transluminal angioplasty vs. surgery for renovascular hypertension. AJR 144(3):447–450,1985.

247. Klinge J, Mali WP, Puijlaert CB, et al: Percutaneous transluminal renal angioplasty: Initial and long-term results. Radiology 171(2):501–506, 1989.

248. Eldrup-Jorgensen J, Harvey HR, Sampson LN, et al: Should percutaneous transluminal renal artery angioplasty be applied to ostial renal artery atherosclerosis? J Vasc Surg 21(6):909–914, 1995.

249. Kuhlmann U, Greminger P, Gruntzig A, et al: Long-term experience in percutaneous transluminal dilatation of renal artery stenosis. Am J Med 79(6):692–698, 1985.

250. Chavan A, Galanski M, Jandeleit K, et al: The kissing balloons technique: Simultaneous dilatation of stenoses of branch arteries at the bifurcation of the renal artery. Acta Radiol 1993;34(5):486–488, 1993.

251. Baker KS, Sawyer RW, Tisnado J, Cho SR: Percutaneous transluminal angioplasty of the renal arteries: Double-catheter technique. Radiology 159(2):554–555, 1986.

252. Archibald GR, Beckmann CF, Libertino JA: Focal renal artery stenosis caused by fibromuscular dysplasia: Treatment by percutaneous transluminal angioplasty. AJR Am J Roentgenol 151(3):593–596, 1988.

253. Srur MF, Sos TA, Saddekni S, et al: Intimal fibromuscular dysplasia and Takayasu arteritis: Delayed response to percutaneous transluminal renal angioplasty. Radiology 157(3):657–660, 1985.

254. Hudspeth DA, Hansen KJ, Reavis SW, et al: Renal duplex sonography after treatment of renovascular disease. J Vasc Surg 18(3):381–388, 1993.

255. Baumgartner I, Triller J, Mahler F: Patency of percutaneous transluminal renal angioplasty: A prospective sonographic study. Kidney Int 51(3):798–803, 1997.

256. Tullis MJ, Zierler RE, Glickerman DJ, et al: Results of percutaneous transluminal angioplasty for atherosclerotic renal artery stenosis: A follow-up study with duplex ultrasonography. J Vasc Surg 25(1):46–54, 1997.

257. Rubin GD, Dake MD, Napel S, et al: Spiral CT of renal artery stenosis: Comparison of three-dimensional rendering techniques. Radiology 190(1):181–189, 1994.

258. Beregi JP, Elkohen M, Deklunder G, et al: Helical CT angiography compared with arteriography in the detection of renal artery stenosis. AJR Am J Roentgenol 167(2):495–501, 1996.

259. Farres MT, Lammer J, Schima W, et al: Spiral computed tomographic angiography of the renal arteries: A prospective comparison with intravenous and intraarterial digital subtraction angiography. Cardiovasc Intervent Radiol 19(2):101–106, 1996.

260. Olbricht CJ, Paul K, Prokop M, et al: Minimally invasive diagnosis of renal artery stenosis by spiral computed tomography angiography. Kidney Int 48(4):1332–1337, 1995.

261. De Cobelli F, Mellone R, Salvioni M, et al: Renal artery stenosis: Value of screening with three-dimensional phase-contrast MR angiography with a phased-array multicoil. Radiology 201(3):697–703, 1996.

262. De Cobelli F, Vanzulli A, Sironi S, et al: Renal artery stenosis: Evaluation with breath-hold, three-dimensional, dynamic, gadolinium-enhanced versus three-dimensional, phase-contrast MR angiography. Radiology 205(3):689–695, 1997.

263. de Haan MW, Kouwenhoven M, Thelissen RP, et al: Renovascular disease in patients with hypertension: Detection with systolic and diastolic gating in three-dimensional, phase-contrast MR angiography. Radiology 198(2):449–456, 1996.

264. Prince MR, Schoenberg SO, Ward JS, et al: Hemodynamically significant atherosclerotic renal artery stenosis: MR angiographic features. Radiology 205(1):128–136, 1997.

265. Rees CR, Niblett R, Snead D, and Multicenter Investigators: United States multicenter study of Palmaz-Schatz stents in the renal arteries. Cardiovasc Intervent Radiol 17(Suppl 2):S71, 1994.

266. Schwarten DE: Percutaneous transluminal angioplasty of the renal arteries: Intravenous digital subtraction angiography for follow-up. Radiology 150(2):369–373, 1984.

267. Hayes JM, Risius B, Novick AC, et al: Experience with percutaneous transluminal angioplasty for renal artery stenosis at the Cleveland Clinic. J Urol 139(3):488–492, 1988.

268. Plouin PF, Darne B, Chatellier G, et al: Restenosis after a first percutaneous transluminal renal angioplasty. Hypertension 21(1):89–96, 1993.

269. Flechner S, Novick AC, Vidt D, et al: The use of percutaneous transluminal angioplasty for renal artery stenosis in patients with generalized atherosclerosis. J Urol 127(6):1072–1075, 1982.

270. Ellis SG, Savage M, Fischman D, et al: Restenosis after placement of Palmaz-Schatz stents in native coronary arteries: Initial results of a multicenter experience. Circulation 86(6):1836–1844, 1992.

271. Wilms GE, Baert AL, Amery AK, et al: Short-term morphologic results of percutaneous transluminal renal angioplasty as determined with angiography. Radiology 170(3 Pt 2):1019–1021, 1989.

272. Martinez AG, Novick AC, Hayes JM: Surgical treatment of renal artery stenosis after failed percutaneous transluminal angioplasty. J Urol 144(5):1094–1096, 1990.

273. McCann RL, Bollinger RR, Newman GE: Surgical renal artery reconstruction after percutaneous transluminal angioplasty. J Vasc Surg 8(4):389–394, 1988.

274. Dean RH, Callis JT, Smith BM, Meacham PW: Failed percutaneous transluminal renal angioplasty: Experience with lesions requiring operative intervention. J Vasc Surg 6(3):301–307, 1987.

275. Guzzetta PC, Potter BM Kapur S, et al: Reconstruction of the renal artery after unsuccessful percutaneous transluminal angioplasty in children. Am J Surg 145(5):647–651, 1983.

276. Hansen KJ: Prevalence of ischemic nephropathy in the atherosclerotic population. Am J Kidney Dis 24(4):615–621, 1994.

277. Schreiber MJ, Pohl MA, Novick AC: The natural history of atherosclerotic and fibrous renal disease. Urol Clin North Am 11(3):383–392, 1984.

278. Maxwell MH, Bleifer KH, Franklin SS, Varady PD: Cooperative Study of Renovascular Hypertension: Demographic analysis of the study. JAMA 220(9):1195–1204, 1972.

279. Pattison JM, Reidy JF, Rafferty MJ, et al: Percutaneous transluminal renal angioplasty in patients with renal failure. Q J Med 85(307–308):883–888, 1992.

280. Weibull H, Bergqvist D, Bergentz SE, et al: Percutaneous transluminal renal angioplasty versus surgical reconstruction of atherosclerotic renal artery stenosis: A prospective randomized study. J Vasc Surg 18(5):841–850, 1993.

281. Plouin PF, Chatellier G, Darne B, Raynaud A: Blood pressure outcome of angioplasty in atherosclerotic renal artery stenosis: A randomized trial. Essai Multicentrique Medicaments vs Angioplastie (EMMA) Study Group. Hypertension 31(3):823–829, 1998.

282. Canzanello VJ, Millan VG, Spiegel JE, et al: Percutaneous transluminal renal angioplasty in management of atherosclerotic renovascular hypertension: Results in 100 patients. Hypertension 13(2):163–172, 1989.

283. Kremer Hovinga TK, de Jong PE, de Zeeuw D, et al: Restenosis prevalence and long-term effects on renal function after percutaneous transluminal renal angioplasty. Nephron 44(Suppl 1):64–67, 1986.

284. Tegtmeyer CJ, Teates CD, Crigler N, et al: Percutaneous transluminal angioplasty in patients with renal artery stenosis: Follow-up studies. Radiology 140(2):323–330, 1981.

285. Geyskes GG, Puylaert CB, Oei HY, Mees EJ: Follow up study of 70 patients with renal artery stenosis treated by percutaneous transluminal dilatation. Br Med J (Clin Res Ed) 287(6388):333–336, 1983.

286. Canzanello VJ, Textor SC: Noninvasive diagnosis of renovascular disease. Mayo Clin Proc 69(12):1172–1181, 1994.

287. Grim CE, Luft FC, Yune HY, et al: Percutaneous transluminal dilatation in the treatment of renal vascular hypertension. Ann Intern Med 95(4):439–442, 1981.

288. Mahler F, Probst P, Haertel M, et al: Lasting improvement of renovascular hypertension by transluminal dilatation of atherosclerotic and nonatherosclerotic renal artery stenoses: A follow-up study. Circulation 65(3):611–617, 1982.

289. Bell GM, Reid J, Buist TA: Percutaneous transluminal angioplasty improves blood pressure and renal function in renovascular hypertension. Q J Med 63(241):393–403, 1987.

290. Tegtmeyer CJ, Selby JB, Hartwell GD, et al: Results and complications of angioplasty in fibromuscular disease. Circulation 83(Suppl 2): I155–I161, 1991.

291. Beek FJ, Kaatee R, Beutler JJ, et al: Complications during renal artery stent placement for atherosclerotic ostial stenosis. Cardiovasc Intervent Radiol 20(3):184–190, 1997.

292. Oleaga JA, Grossman RA, McLean GK, et al: Arteriovenous fistula of a segmental renal artery branch as a complication of percutaneous angioplasty. AJR 136(5):988–989, 1981.

293. Mills SR, Wertman DE Jr, Grossman SH: Renal cortical arteriovenous fistula complicating percutaneous renal angioplasty. AJR 137(6):1251–1253, 1981.

294. Harker CP, Steed M, Althaus SJ, Coldwell D: Flash pulmonary edema: An acute and unusual complication of renal angioplasty. J Vasc Interv Radiol 6(1):130–132, 1995.

295. Gendler R, Mitty HA: Case report: Evolution of a type B aortic dissection following renal artery angioplasty. Mt Sinai J Med 60(4):330–332, 1993.

296. Sharma S, Arya S, Mehta SN, et al: Renal vein injury during percutaneous transluminal renal angioplasty in nonspecific aortoarteritis. Cardiovasc Intervent Radiol 16(2):114–116, 1993.

297. Gordon GI, Vogelzang RL, Curry RH, et al: Endovascular infection after renal artery stent placement. J Vasc Interv Radiol 7(5):669–672, 1996.

298. Mahler F, Triller J, Weidmann P, Nachbur B: Complications in percu-

taneous transluminal dilatation of renal arteries. Nephron 44(Suppl 1):60–63, 1986.

299. McDonald DN, Smith DC, Maloney MD: Percutaneous transluminal renal angioplasty in the patient with a solitary functioning kidney. AJR Am J Roentgenol 151(5):1041–1043, 1988.

300. Beebe HG, Chesebro K, Merchant F, Bush W: Results of renal artery balloon angioplasty limit its indications. J Vasc Surg 8(3):300–306, 1988.

301. Julien J, Jeunemaitre X, Raynaud A, et al: Influence of age on the outcome of percutaneous angioplasty in atheromatous renovascular disease. J Hypertens Suppl 7(6):S188–S189, 1989.

302. Tykarski A, Edwards R, Dominiczak AF, Reid JL: Percutaneous transluminal renal angioplasty in the management of hypertension and renal failure in patients with renal artery stenosis. J Hum Hypertens 7(5):491–496, 1993.

303. Rodriguez-Perez JC, Plaza C, Reyes R, et al: Treatment of renovascular hypertension with percutaneous transluminal angioplasty: Experience in Spain. J Vasc Interv Radiol 5(1):101–109, 1994.

304. Dorros G, Jaff M, Jain A, et al: Follow-up of primary Palmaz-Schatz stent placement for atherosclerotic renal artery stenosis. Am J Cardiol 75(15):1051–1055, 1995.

305. Nahman NS Jr, Maniam P, Hernandez RA Jr, et al: Renal artery pressure gradients in patients with angiographic evidence of atherosclerotic renal artery stenosis. Am J Kidney Dis 24(4):695–699, 1994.

306. Weibull H, Bergqvist D, Jendteg S, et al: Clinical outcome and health care costs in renal revascularization—percutaneous transluminal renal angioplasty versus reconstructive surgery. Br J Surg 78(5):620–624, 1991.

307. Kim PK, Spriggs DW, Rutecki GW, et al: Transluminal angioplasty in patients with bilateral renal artery stenosis or renal artery stenosis in a solitary functioning kidney. AJR Am J Roentgenol 153(6):1305–1308, 1989.

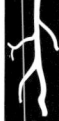

CHAPTER 1 2 1
Renal Artery Imaging: Alternatives to Angiography

Michael J. Bloch, M.D., and K. Craig Kent, M.D.

Renal artery disease is the most common cause of secondary hypertension; its prevalence in patients with hypertension is estimated to range from 1% to 5%.[1–5] In most cases, atherosclerosis or fibromuscular dysplasia is the cause. Effort has increasingly focused on the diagnosis and treatment of renovascular disease, since the resultant hypertension is potentially curable and subsequent reductions in morbidity and mortality would be substantial.

Owing to the advent of powerful new antihypertensive agents and the aging of the United States' population, patients with atherosclerotic *renal artery stenosis* (RAS) often present later in the course of their disease and with more advanced renal dysfunction. This trend has increased the incidence of ischemic nephropathy associated with RAS. It is estimated from angiographic studies that ischemic nephropathy may be a contributing factor in 10% to 20% of cases referred for dialysis or renal transplantation.[6–9]

Thus, it has become critically important to identify accurate methods for diagnosis of RAS. Although contrast angiography remains the "gold standard," because of its invasiveness and attendant risks it is not an appropriate screening test for all patients thought to have renovascular hypertension or ischemic nephropathy. As a consequence, many noninvasive modalities have been developed that can be used to evaluate this disease process. The noninvasive tests can be divided into those that rely on an evaluation of the *physiologic* sequelae of renal vascular disease (e.g., captopril test, captopril scintigraphy, renal vein renin values) and those that directly *image* the renal artery (duplex ultrasonography [DU], magnetic resonance angiography [MRA], and sequential helical computed tomography [spiral CT]).

Noninvasive studies that depend upon the *physiologic* evaluation of RAS are discussed in Chapter 119. Briefly, the accuracy of all such studies is impaired in the presence of significant renal insufficiency. Moreover, none of the studies has been shown to be predictive of improvement in renal function after intervention in azotemic patients.

In this chapter, current knowledge of available noninvasive *imaging* modalities for RAS is discussed. When one reviews the available data on noninvasive imaging tests, two themes become apparent. First, the accuracy and utility of noninvasive tests can vary significantly from one institution to another. Attaining acceptable accuracy with any of the noninvasive imaging modalities requires substantial institutional interest and dedication. Second, no noninvasive screening or imaging modality is acceptable for *all* patients. Instead, an individualized approach is necessary that relies largely on the clinician's index of suspicion for renovascular disease, the potential cause of the renal artery lesion, and the patient's anatomy and renal function.

CONVENTIONAL ANGIOGRAPHY: THE GOLD STANDARD?

As discussed in Chapter 120, conventional and digital subtraction arteriography have long been considered the gold standards for diagnosis and preoperative evaluation of renal artery disease.[10, 11] Properly, performed conventional angiography provides excellent resolution of the renal arteries and is highly predictive of the degree of stenosis that will be found at surgery.[12] It also allows for simultaneous measurement of a pressure gradient across the stenosis, additional information that is useful in determining the hemodynamic consequences of a renal artery lesion. Conventional angiography is invasive, however, and carries significant risk of morbidity, and even death.

The risks of aortography and selective renal arteriography can be substantial and may include complications related to the arterial puncture (e.g., hematoma, pseudoaneurysm), contrast-induced nephropathy, and cholesterol embolization. These risks increase in association with advanced atherosclerosis, severe hypertension, or renal insufficiency,[13] which frequently coexist in patients suspected to have atherosclerotic renal artery disease. The prevalence of these complications in this specific patient group is not well understood, since large published studies of conventional angiography generally include only "uncomplicated patients" who have renovascular hypertension and normal renal function. Furthermore, the complications of angiography are often insidious and difficult to assess accurately, especially retrospectively. Among 2374 patients who underwent contrast angiography as part of the Cooperative Study of Renovascular Hypertension,[14] a fatality rate of 0.11%, a nonfatal major complication rate of 1.2%, and a minor complications rate of 2.7% were observed. The authors of this study relied on self-reporting by radiologists at a number of different centers. Moreover, the subjects were principally patients who had normal renal function.

The incidence of contrast-induced nephropathy varies significantly and has been reported to range from zero to 7% with the largest studies reporting an average incidence of 3%.[15] The incidence increases substantially in patients with diabetes and renal insufficiency. Fortunately, contrast-induced renal dysfunction is usually reversible with conservative therapy.

Atheroembolism is an increasingly recognized complication of renal arteriography. It tends to be underdiagnosed, since it is an insidious disorder that is difficult to identify with certainty without performing a biopsy.[16] Only the most fulminant cases are recognized clinically. Although clinical studies have generally reported a low incidence, autopsy studies found evidence of atheroemboli in 25% to 30% of patients who died within 6 months after cardiac catheterization or aortography.[17] Patients with widespread atherosclerotic disease and preexisting renal insufficiency—precisely the population at risk for ischemic nephropathy—are those who are most susceptible to atheroembolism.

Although conventional angiography can detect the anatomic presence of a renal artery lesion, it does not provided data on its physiologic or hemodynamic significance. Thus, angiography cannot accurately differentiate between an incidental renal artery lesion and one that is producing potentially reversible renovascular hypertension or ischemic nephropathy. Also, since conventional angiography gives only a two-dimensional image and does not allow imaging of the renal artery in multiple planes, it can be difficult to determine the precise degree of stenosis, information that

is essential for making inferences about the hemodynamic significance of a renal artery lesion. Even when multiple views are obtained, it can be difficult to accurately identify the origin of a tortuous renal artery that arises from a severely diseased aorta.

Despite these limitations, if the index of suspicion for RAS is high and the patient has reasonably acceptable renal function, it may be appropriate in certain circumstances to proceed directly to conventional angiography without performing a noninvasive study.

NONINVASIVE RENAL ARTERY IMAGING

An ideal noninvasive imaging study would serve as both an accurate screening tool for RAS and a means for delineating renal anatomy before arterial reconstruction. Other attributes of the ideal imaging technique are minimal expense, great accuracy, good reproducibility, and a low rate of complications.

Over the past 10 years, a number of less invasive renal artery imaging strategies have been evaluated. Each has its advantages and disadvantages, but overall these studies are safer than conventional angiography. As opposed to the traditional screening tests that rely on physiologic criteria (i.e., captopril test, radionuclide renography, renal vein renin values), noninvasive imaging studies require no preprocedural adjustments in a patient's medication or diet. Also, their accuracy is not diminished by renal insufficiency. Noninvasive imaging techniques also can supply detailed anatomic information that might potentially obviate the need for preoperative angiography.

Unfortunately, in all investigations of noninvasive imaging modalities to date, contrast angiography has been used as the standard of comparison. Because of the previously mentioned limitations of conventional angiography, there is no true standard. Those who have worked extensively with noninvasive imaging modalities realize that, under some circumstances (particularly because of the three-dimensional capabilities of many of these techniques), these studies may be more revealing and accurate than contrast angiography. Of course, the ultimate test of any imaging technique designed to screen for RAS is its capability of identifying who will respond clinically to renal artery revascularization.

Multiple issues are encountered when one attempts to obtain a consensus on the diagnostic accuracy and utility of the various noninvasive methods of renal artery imaging. For each modality, investigators have employed a variety of approaches and techniques. Compounding this problem is the fact that the parameters of reporting often vary from one institution to another. For example, in many studies the threshold for determining significant RAS is 50%. Most clinicians, however, reserve intervention for renal artery lesions that are more than 70% stenotic.

Finally, patients entered into these studies are almost exclusively those who have been referred for angiography because of the results of other noninvasive tests. This very "selected" population tends to have a high prevalence of renal artery disease. It is therefore difficult to extrapolate from the results of these studies to a patient cohort that is being screened, since disease is much less prevalent in the latter group.

Duplex Ultrasonography

DU is the most investigated method of noninvasive imaging of the renal arteries. It combines direct visualization of the arteries through B-mode imaging with Doppler ultrasound measurement of the velocity of blood flow, affording both anatomic evaluation and hemodynamic assessment.[18] DU also allows for simultaneous measurement of kidney size, additional information that can be used to help determine the functional significance of a renal artery lesion.

Technical Considerations

Because of the depth of the renal arteries and their location in the retroperitoneum, B-mode imaging cannot be used to assess the luminal anatomy directly along the entire length of the renal artery and its branches. Instead, it is used to locate the main renal artery and to detect sites of turbulent flow. After the renal artery is identified, Doppler measurements can be sequentially sampled at regular intervals along the length of the main renal artery and in the kidney itself. These measurements are processed into spectral velocity waveforms using fast Fourier transform analysis (Fig. 121–1). Significant stenosis is indicated by an increase in velocity, which reflects acceleration of the blood as it crosses the area of stenosis. Alternatively, with indirect techniques proximal stenosis can be inferred from an abnormal Doppler waveform in the more distal segmental arteries of the kidney.

The main renal artery should be examined with the patient fasting to avoid interference from overlying bowel gas. A low-frequency transducer (in the range of 2 to 3.5 Hz) should be used and Doppler-shifted signals obtained at less than a 60-degree angle to the artery. It is essential to survey the entire renal artery, including the proximal, middle, and distal portions. If the artery is not examined carefully throughout its length, significant stenoses, especially those that are the consequence of fibromuscular disease (which can be focal and/or distal), may be missed. The examination can be performed without discontinuing antihypertensive medications and is appropriate even for patients who have advanced renal insufficiency.

A number of parameters have been reported for the identification of a hemodynamically significant main RAS.[19-23] The most widely accepted criteria are (1) a ratio of the peak systolic velocity in the renal artery to the peak systolic velocity in the adjacent aorta greater than 3.5:1 and (2) a peak systolic velocity in the renal artery greater than 180 cm/sec in association with post-stenotic turbulence. In numerous studies, these criteria have correlated with "angiographic stenosis" greater than 60%. The diagnosis of occlusion is made by absence of a flow signal in the renal artery. One of the disadvantages of DU is that criteria have yet to be developed that can more precisely measure stenoses that are in the 60% to 99% range.

Direct Examination

Direct interrogation of the renal arteries is a labor-intensive and time-consuming undertaking that requires a dedicated and experienced technologist and a cooperative patient. In centers where this test has been developed and studied

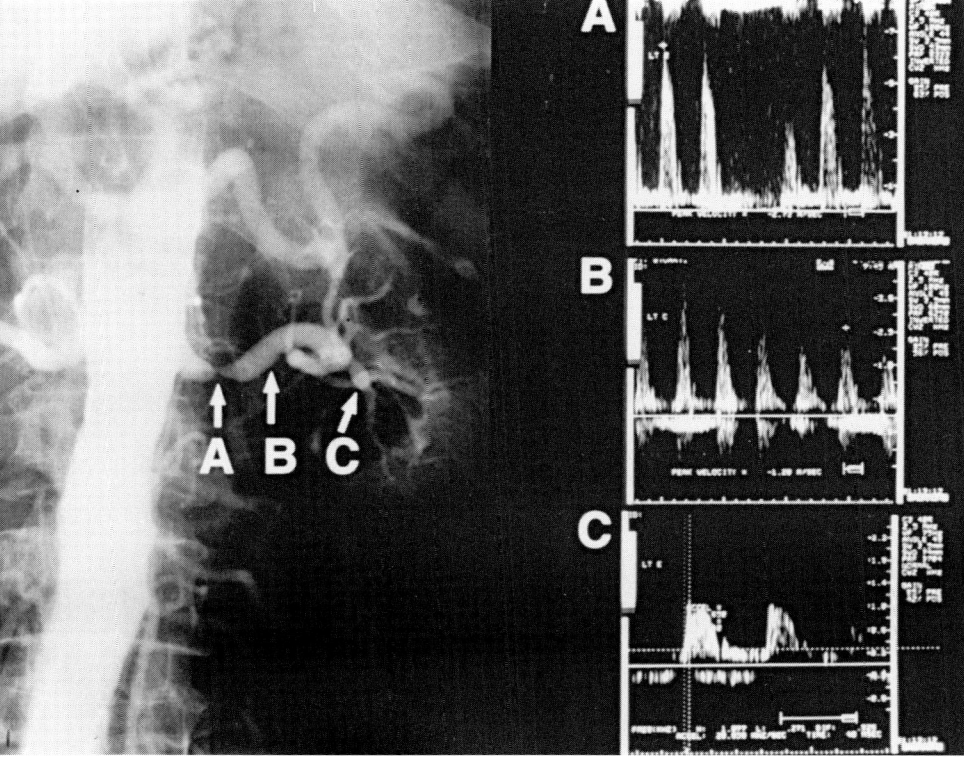

FIGURE 121–1. Duplex ultrasound spectral analysis and corresponding angiogram for patient with unilateral renal artery stenosis. Arrows A, B, and C indicate the approximate sites along the renal artery where the Doppler measurements were obtained.

extensively, excellent results have been obtained. In one of the earliest large studies, Hansen and coworkers[24] evaluated 74 consecutive patients with both DU and conventional angiography. DU predicted the presence of a main RAS more extensive than 60% with sensitivity of 93% and specificity of 98% when only kidneys with single renal arteries were evaluated. When patients with multiple renal arteries were also considered, the sensitivity decreased to 88%, although the specificity remained high (99%). Other centers have also reported sensitivities that range from 84% to 98% and specificities of 90% to 98% for the detection of angiographically significant main RAS.[25–29] The exact site of the renal artery lesion can be accurately ascertained in as many as 80% to 95% of patients.[27]

Many other investigators have been unable to duplicate these good results. Sensitivities as low as zero and rates of inadequate examinations as high as 40% have been reported.[30–33] There are a number of limitations to DU that may account for variations in accuracy. Frequently encountered technical difficulties include inability to identify the main renal artery owing to overlying fat or bowel gas, difficulty interrogating the entire length of the renal artery, and inability to hold the transducer at the optimal angle. Furthermore, traditional DU techniques do not allow accurate identification of accessory renal arteries, which may be present in as many as 20% of kidneys. This information may be clinically important, since stenosis of an accessory renal artery is a not infrequently a cause of reversible renovascular hypertension.

Indirect Examination

A number of attempts have been made to overcome these limitations. The most studied of these is a method of indirect Doppler evaluation of the distal renal arterial tree. Through a flank approach, segmental waveforms are obtained at the hilum and the upper, middle, and lower poles of the kidney. The presence of a more proximal high-grade renal artery lesion is inferred when a *tardus* or *parvus* waveform is observed in the distal vessels (Fig. 121–2). The hemodynamic significance of these lesions is determined by evaluating the acceleration time (normal value <0.07

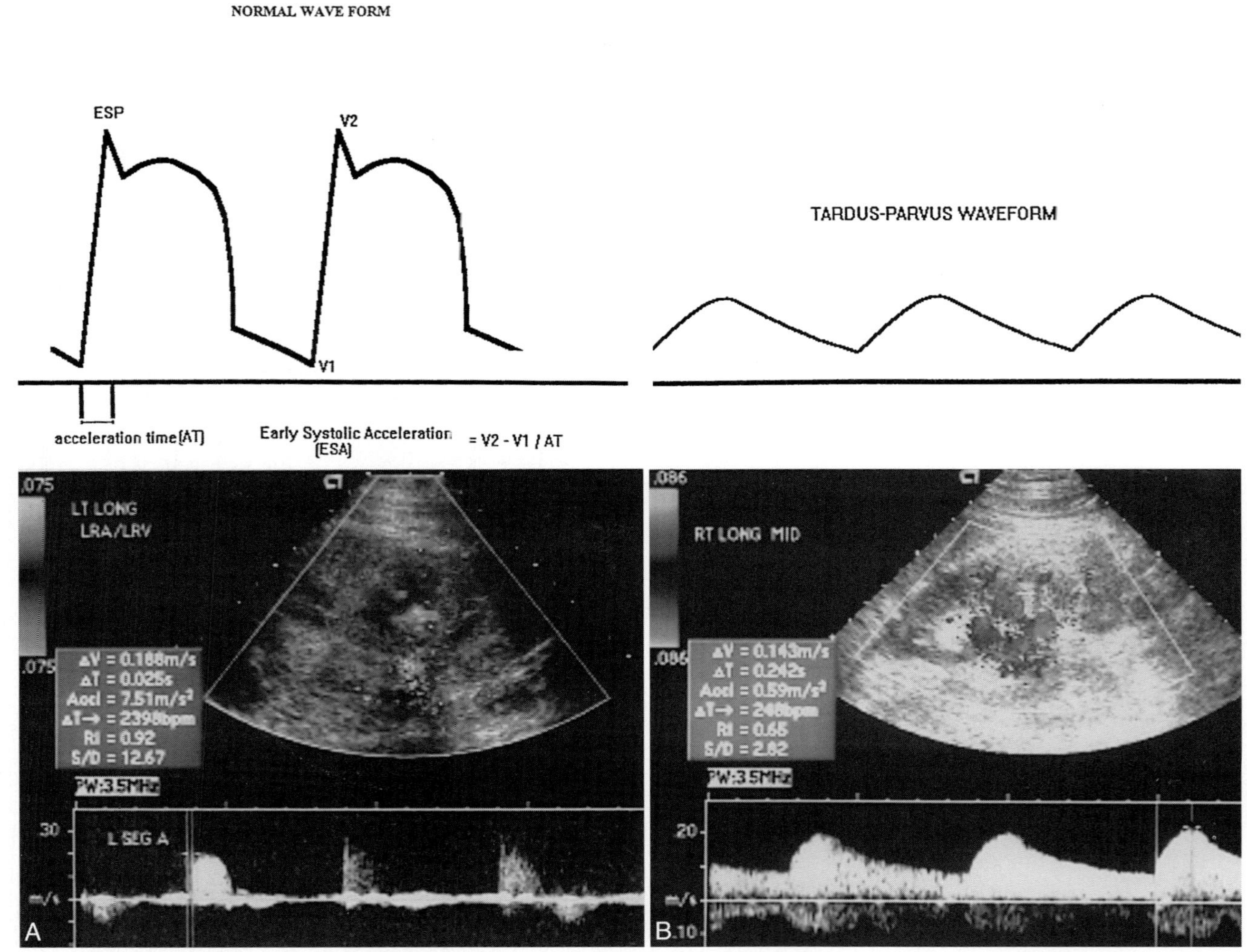

NORMAL WAVE FORM

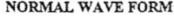

acceleration time [AT]   Early Systolic Acceleration = V2 - V1 / AT
[ESA]

TARDUS-PARVUS WAVEFORM

FIGURE 121–2. Waveforms obtained from indirect duplex ultrasound analysis of the distal renal arterial tree. *A,* Graphic representation of a normal waveform. *B,* Graphic representation of an abnormal waveform that would indicate the presence of significant renal artery stenosis. *C,* Waveform represents a normal study; the acceleration time (AT) was calculated to be 0.0025 sec (normal $<$ 0.07 sec), and the acceleration index (AI) was 7.51 m/sec² (normal $>$ 3.0 m/sec²). *D,* Waveform represents a highly abnormal study suggestive of renal artery stenosis with an AT of 0.242 sec, and AI 2.46 m/sec².

second), acceleration index (normal value >3.0 m/sec^2), and by waveform pattern recognition. A number of published series have shown this technique to have excellent accuracy in predicting angiographically significant RAS.[34–37]

In other studies using indirect Doppler techniques, a measurement called the *resistive index* (RI) has been used as a criterion for RAS (normal RI $<$ 0.70). This value, which estimates the state of renal arterial resistance, is defined as follows:

$$RI = \frac{\text{peak systolic shift} - \text{minimum diastolic shift}}{\text{peak systolic shift}}$$

Unfortunately, this measurement suffers from decreased specificity, since it can also be elevated in the presence of medical renal disease, decreased cardiac output, or perinephric or subcapsular fluid collections.

These indirect techniques have a number of potential advantages over direct interrogation of the renal artery. Segmental waveform analysis is much less time-consuming, and the results may be less dependent on operator experience than those derived from direct renal artery interrogation. Because the examination is performed from a lateral approach, adequate data can be obtained even in obese patients and those who have excessive bowel gas. Furthermore, accessory renal artery disease can be manifested by a damped waveform isolated to a kidney pole.[38]

Disadvantages of the indirect technique include the inability to distinguish a severe stenosis from an obstruction and the lack of information regarding the exact location of a stenotic lesion. Moreover, the systolic features of renal artery spectral analysis are affected by increased renovascular resistance (see Fig. 121–1). Increased resistance may change distal renal artery acceleration time or acceleration index in 40% of hemodynamically significant stenoses associated with renal insufficiency.[19, 24] In preliminary studies, some investigators have shown that the sensitivity of this technique can be enhanced by using an ultrasound contrast agent or by administration of captopril before the study.[39–41]

Many centers, including our own, have begun to routinely perform both direct examination of the renal arteries and indirect segmental waveform analysis.

Emerging Strategies

Other strategies have been employed to improve the accuracy of main renal artery interrogation. In a few preliminary studies, the use of intravenous contrast agents been found to significantly enhance the diagnostic accuracy of DU imaging. In a recent report,[42] one such agent was found to increase sensitivity for detecting RAS by 20% over that of non–contrast-enhanced studies. Other investigators have used color flow or power Doppler to facilitate the examination.[30, 43] Like contrast-enhanced ultrasound, these techniques may decrease examination time and increase accuracy by allowing (1) easier identification of the main renal artery and (2) detection of a larger percentage of accessory renal arteries. Although these strategies may prove to be powerful adjuncts in the evaluation of RAS by DU, larger and more thorough studies must be conducted to demonstrate their role definitively.

Other Clinical Applications

In addition to being a screening tool, DU has proved useful for a number of other clinical applications. Because it is noninvasive and can assess kidney size as well as the degree of stenosis, DU has become the procedure of choice for following patients with documented renal artery disease who are being treated medically.[44, 45] DU can also be used to monitor long-term patency after surgical reconstruction of the renal arteries. Studies have confirmed that a normal postoperative duplex scan is highly predictive of a patent bypass graft.[46, 47] Because of their size and position adjacent to the abdominal aorta, aortorenal grafts are often easier to assess than native renal arteries. Hepatorenal, splenorenal, and iliorenal bypasses are more difficult to study, but even these can often be successfully scanned by a skilled technician.

DU has also been used intraoperatively to detect and allow correction of technical problems that occasionally complicate renal artery bypass or endarterectomy.[43, 48] The superficial location of the transplanted kidney also makes this study well-suited for investigating suspected transplant RAS.[49–51] Finally, DU has been used to evaluate the results and long-term patency after percutaneous renal angioplasty and/or stenting.[52, 53]

One drawback of DU is that it does not provide the necessary anatomic information that would allow surgical intervention without first obtaining a contrast angiogram. However, DU is accurate in detecting celiac artery stenoses,[54] and this information may be useful in patients with severely diseased aortas when hepatorenal or splenorenal bypass is being considered.

In conclusion, renal artery DU is an excellent screening test for hemodynamically significant RAS in centers where the appropriate technical expertise is available. Of the various alternatives for noninvasive imaging, DU is clearly the least expensive. Adding indirect techniques and using contrast agents may further increase its accuracy and reproducibility, which would make it a more widely acceptable study for RAS screening.

Magnetic Resonance Angiography

MRA has also been extensively evaluated as a method for noninvasively evaluating RAS. MRA technology allows the demonstration of vascular anatomy and can generate an image that is similar in appearance to that obtained by conventional angiography (Fig. 121–3); Unlike conventional angiography, however, MRA does not require arterial puncture or any nephrotoxic agent. In contrast to the traditional physiologic studies for RAS, there is no need to discontinue antihypertensive medications which interfere with the renin-angiotensin system, and the accuracy of MRA does not diminish because of renal dysfunction. The similarity of the images generated by MRA and conventional angiograms increases the comfort level of clinicians, because the renal artery of interest can be visualized. However, there are significant differences between MRA and contrast angiography images and the interpretation of renal MRA requires specific expertise and experience.

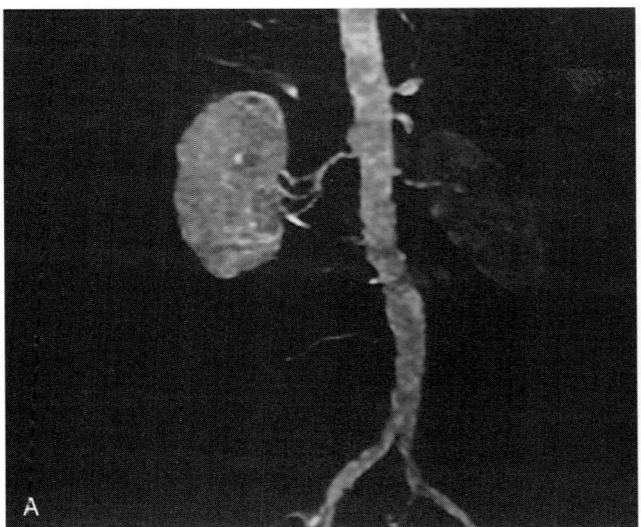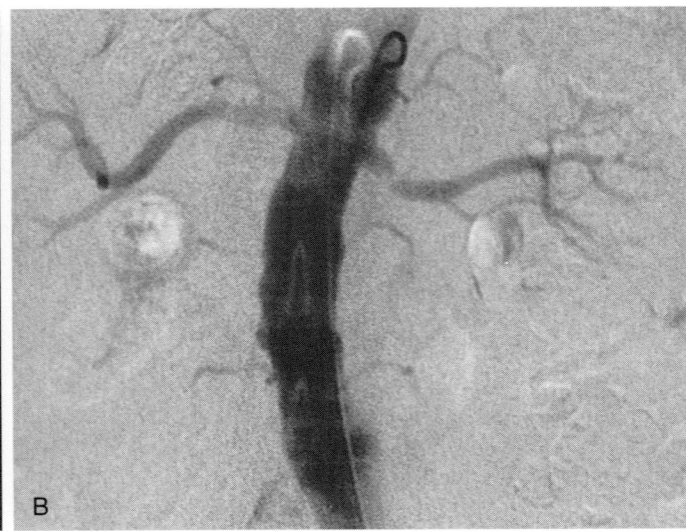

FIGURE 121–3. *A*, Three-dimensional gadolinium-enhanced magnetic resonance angiogram demonstrating severe left renal artery stenosis. *B*, The corresponding conventional contrast angiogram from the same patient.

Technical Considerations

The physics of MRA is complex, and a complete description of the technique is beyond the scope of this discussion. Yet, the clinician should have a basic understanding of the fundamental principles that underlie MRA in order to recognize its advantages and limitations. Any of a number of different MRA techniques can be used to image renal arteries.[55, 56] In early studies, two imaging techniques were employed: *time of flight* (TOF) and *phase contrast* (PC). With both, protons in tissue and blood are charged when the body is exposed to a magnetic field. The protons then emit a signal that is registered as a visual image.

TOF imaging relies on flow-related enhancement to image the renal arteries. With multiple magnetic pulses delivered at short intervals, stationary protons are "saturated" so that they no longer yield signal, whereas moving protons yield maximal signal. PC imaging relies on the differences in phase shift between moving and stationary protons.

Most recently, enthusiasm has increased for a third technique known as *three-dimensional gadolinium-enhanced MRA.* This technique attempts to overcome a number of the shortcomings of TOF and phase contrast MRA, including (1) saturation effects that can make vessels with relatively slow flow appear stenotic; (2) turbulence-induced signal loss, which results in overestimation of stenoses; and (3) long imaging times. Rather than image individual protons in flowing blood, this method allows direct visualization of the contrast agent filling the lumen much like conventional angiography. When this technique was initially developed, long acquisition times (~2 to 3 minutes) were necessary; however, distal and accessory arteries could not be accurately assessed owing to respiration artifact. More recently, rapid bolus injections used with suspended respiration have produced slightly poorer resolution but less pronounced respiratory artifact.

Data from MRA is compiled initially as multiple, thin, contiguous cross-sectional slices. The slices are then converted into a three-dimensional data set, which can be used to create projections in any orientation that look like conventional angiograms. The most commonly used reconstruction technique is called a *maximal intensity projection* (MIP).[57] Its great attribute is that it enhances the distinction between the blood vessel and background tissue.

Unlike conventional angiography, MRA allows data to be projected in multiple planes (axial, coronal, sagittal, oblique). This flexibility is particularly useful for investigating the renal ostium and tortuous renal arteries. To accurately assess the degree of stenosis it is necessary to examine the artery in multiple planes. It is also prudent to review the nonreformatted axial images, since the reformatting process, although it produces visually satisfying images, can often lead to overestimation or underestimation of the degree of stenosis.

Clinical Experience

Data from trials that compare MRA and conventional angiography are promising. Using a TOF protocol, Kent and coworkers[58] were able to predict the presence of stenoses greater than 50% with sensitivity of 100% and specificity of 94%. Moreover, MRA accurately classified lesions as mild, moderate, severe, or occluded in 91% of cases. Using a phase contrast technique, Gedroyc and coworkers[59] were able to predict angiographically significant renal artery disease with sensitivity of 84% and specificity of 91%. In several studies, TOF and phase contrast techniques have produced similar results with sensitivities ranging from 91% to 100% and specificities of 89% to 96%.[60–67]

Using a breath-holding, three-dimensional gadolinium-enhanced method, DeCobelli and coworkers[68] achieved 100% sensitivity and 97% specificity for RAS greater than 50%. Using these same techniques, they were also able to correctly identify significantly more accessory renal arteries than could be found using a phase contrast technique. A number of other investigators have also reported that three-dimensional gadolinium-enhanced MRA has high sensitivity and specificity and identifies accessory renal arteries better than other MRA techniques.[69–74]

Current Applications

Because of the high degree of accuracy associated with MRA and its ability to image arterial anatomy, in certain cases surgeons may proceed directly to operation for RAS without preoperative conventional contrast angiography.[75] As the accuracy of MRA improves, it may become increasingly unnecessary to subject patients to the risks of preoperative conventional angiography.

MRA has also been evaluated for detection of RAS in transplants, although not as thoroughly as has DU. Although accuracy has been satisfactory when MRA is used for this purpose, false-positive findings are not infrequent.[76–78]

Another potential advantage of MRA is its ability to obtain functional as well as anatomic data.[79] Several investigators have been able to accurately estimate split renal function with clearance of gadolinium contrast agents using a method similar to conventional radionuclide renography.[80–82] Others have used gated magnetic resonance techniques to accurately assess renal blood flow in patients with renal artery disease.[83, 84] It is also possible to obtain the rates of tissue diffusion and perfusion, both measures that may help to delineate the physiologic significance of RAS.[85]

Although the popularity of MRA for noninvasive imaging is increasing, it has a number of limitations. False-positive scans are not uncommon (Fig. 121–4). Also, MRA (especially using TOF or phase contrast imaging) has a general tendency to overestimate the degree of stenosis. Adequate standardized guidelines for determining the degree of stenosis have yet to be formulated.

Breath-holding, three-dimensional gadolinium-enhanced MRA is now the MRA technique most often used for imaging the renal vasculature. Although it appears to afford superior resolution of accessory and branch renal arteries, few patients with fibromuscular or other distal renal artery lesions have been studied. Thus, MRA is not the screening test of choice for patients who may harbor such lesions. Three-dimensional gadolinium-enhanced MRA also requires patients to hold their breath for a short time, which may be difficult for those with significant cardiac or pulmonary disease. Scanning times can be long, and patients must lie flat throughout the study, which may disqualify those with severe heart failure. Some patients are unable to tolerate the study because of claustrophobia. Regardless of the imaging technique, MRA is contraindicated in patients with pacemakers, cerebral aneurysm clips, or intraocular metal devices. Neighboring surgical clip artifact can produce signal voids and false-positive studies.

Finally, although it is not always evident when reviewing published reports, considerable expertise is required to obtain high quality images and proper interpretation.[11]

The most striking aspect of MRA, as used to detect proximal renovascular disease, is its extremely low false-negative rate, which makes it an excellent screening tool for suspected ischemic nephropathy secondary to atherosclerotic disease of the main renal artery. Because of this high negative predictive value, a clinician can be confident that with a normal MRA study, functionally significant renal artery disease is exceedingly unlikely. Because of its current tendency to overestimate the degree of stenosis, MRA is less accurate than conventional contrast angiography; however, MRA technology is continually evolving, and the images will certainly continue to improve.

Helical (Spiral) Computed Tomography

Helical CT has emerged as a promising technique for identifying RAS. Spiral CT employs a rotating gantry, which

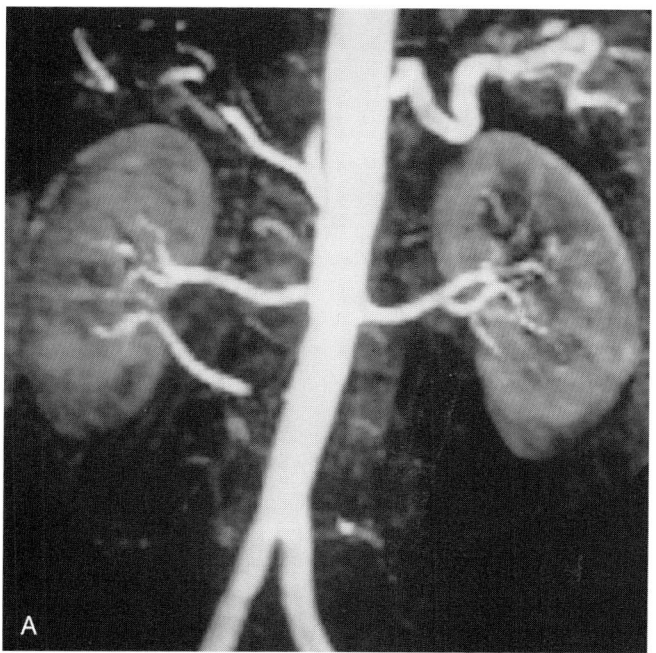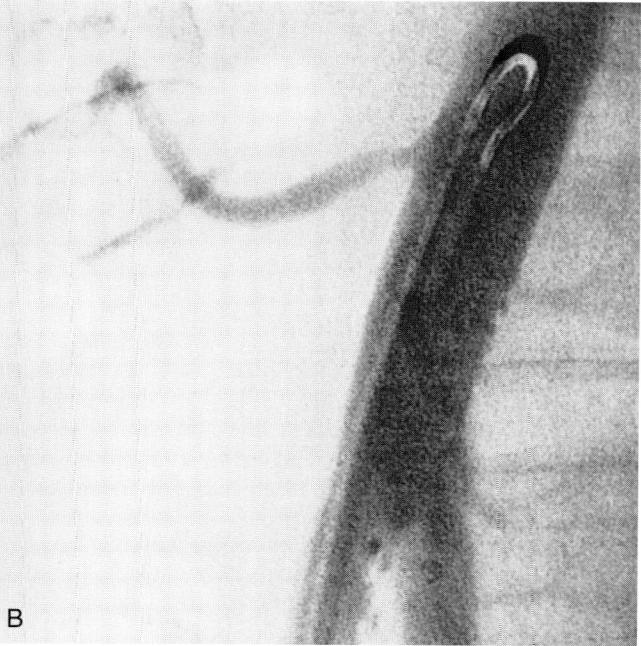

FIGURE 121–4. *A,* Three-dimensional gadolinium-enhanced magnetic resonance angiogram demonstrates severe ostial accessory renal artery stenosis. *B,* The conventional contrast angiogram of the same accessory renal artery reveals only a mild lesion. Pull-back pressures revealed no gradient across the ostium of this artery.

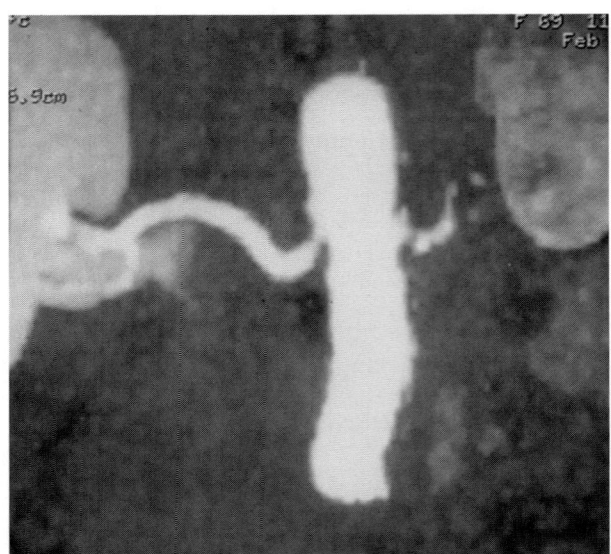

FIGURE 121–5. Helical computed tomogram postprocessed using the maximum intensity projection format reveals significant bilateral renal artery stenosis.

allows a large number of images to be acquired over a relatively brief time. For arterial imaging, intravenous iodinated contrast medium is injected through a peripheral vein. After appropriate delay to allow passage of contrast into the renal arterial circulation, a series of thin cuts are taken throughout the aorta at the level of the renal arteries. Rapid acquisition of data afforded by spiral CT allows multiple images to be made precisely at the moment when contrast medium passes through the renal arteries.

A number of technical variables must be optimized if the renal arteries are to be adequately imaged by spiral CT.[86] Several of these parameters (collimation, table speed, pitch) determine the intervals at which cuts are acquired. These variables are adjusted so that sections are taken at 2- to 3-mm intervals,[87] which afford spiral CT resolution of approximately 0.5 mm, whereas that for MRA is as poor as 1 to 1.5 mm.

It is also necessary to adjust the rate of injection and the interval between peripheral injection and renal artery imaging. Optimizing both of these timing variables allows maximal enhancement of the renal arteries by contrast medium. If the contrast bolus arrived in the renal arteries too early, the volume of contrast would be inadequate for complete visualization of the renal vessels. If the bolus arrived after imaging had begun, contrast returning from the renal vein could obscure the renal artery. The importance of precise timing of the interval has led many investigators to administer a test bolus using 15 to 20 ml of contrast medium. Interval imaging over 30 seconds then allows the physician to estimate when contrast enhancement of the renal vessels is maximal.

Breath-holding longer than 20 seconds is required during image acquisition. It is essential that patients remain immobile for these studies, since motion artifact reduces the quality of the images. The entire study takes only 20 to 30 minutes.

After the raw images are acquired, postprocessing is the next step. Initially, the spiral data are interpolated into axial sections, then reconstructed images are rendered. This time-consuming process takes 30 to 90 minutes of an experienced radiologist's or technician's time. Although many reconstruction techniques exist, those currently available on most commercial CT systems are MIP and surface-shaded display (SSD). Images provided by these two techniques differ much, as does the information they contain.[88]

MIP is a method wherein the raw data is reconstructed using the maximum-intensity signal along each ray through the data set (Fig. 121–5). MIP enhances visual distinction between the blood vessel and background tissue. The images are two-dimensional, however, and depth relationships are not apparent, nor are overlapping vessels clearly delineated. The lack of three-dimensional information inherent in a single MIP is minimized by displaying multiple MIP images. SSD has the advantage of three-dimensional representation of anatomic relationship (Fig. 121–6). Depending on the chosen threshold, however, SSD can exaggerate stenoses, and surrounding structures can produce artifacts that obscure arterial anatomy. Generally, MIP is the more accurate of the two techniques, although SSD is the more visually "pleasing."

When one is determining renal artery anatomy and degree of stenosis, images from all available modalities should be reviewed. In addition to the MIP and SSD reconstructions, much information can be obtained by examining the original axial data or by using multiplanar reformats. Such a complete analysis allows repeated confirmation of the degree of stenosis, which in turn improves diagnostic accuracy.

Regardless of which technique is used, the major hindrance of helical CT is arterial calcification. In MIP-formatted images, calcium obscures the vessel lumen. Atherosclerotic disease can be inferred by the presence of calcium, but the degree of stenosis cannot be gauged accurately. In SSD-formatted images, it is impossible to differentiate calcium from contrast medium. Thus, calcified atheromata blend with intraluminal contrast medium and create the image of a widely patent vessel. A number of calcium suppression techniques have been studied, but their utility remains to be confirmed.

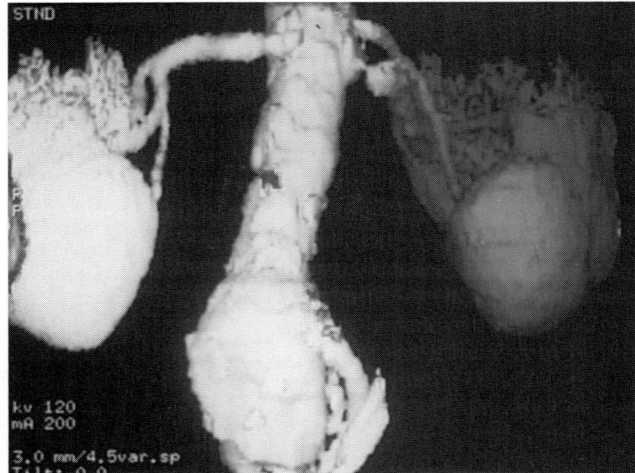

FIGURE 121–6. Helical computed tomogram postprocessed using surface-shaded display format reveals severe left renal artery stenosis, mild right renal artery stenosis, and an infrarenal abdominal aortic aneurysm.

Although helical CT has been less widely studied than MRA or DU, a number of centers with experience in helical CT have produced favorable results.[89–93] Olbricht and co-workers[94] prospectively compared helical CT and conventional angiography in 62 consecutive patients suspected to have renal artery disease. As compared to conventional angiography, helical CT detected stenoses greater than 50% with sensitivity of 98% and specificity of 94%. Helical CT underestimated the degree of stenosis in one artery and overestimated the degree of stenosis in six. In 50 patients with suspected renovascular disease, Beregi and coworkers[95] found helical CT to have sensitivity of 100% and specificity of 98% for main renal artery lesions more extensive than 50%. The two false-positive results in this study both were related to imaging of the right main renal artery adjacent to the vena cava. When accessory renal arteries were included, the sensitivity rate fell to 88%.

In addition to its great accuracy, other advantages of helical CT include the ability to determine renal size and, potentially, kidney perfusion.[96] It also affords simultaneous evaluation for aortic aneurysms and adrenal gland anatomy in patients suspected to have secondary hypertension.[97–99] Moreover, unlike MRA, helical CT can be used to assess the patency of renal arteries that have been treated with intravascular stents.

The principal drawback of spiral CT for imaging renal arteries is the necessity for iodinated contrast medium. For most studies, 120 to 150 ml of contrast agent is required. This is a quantity significantly greater than that required for digital subtraction angiography (15 to 20 ml if selective renal images need not be obtained). For this reason, helical CT may not be appropriate for the increasing number of patients with renal insufficiency who undergo screening for renal artery disease.

Like DU and MRA, helical CT does not produce satisfactory images of accessory renal arteries.[99] Although these arteries can often be identified, the extent of disease in them is difficult to assess owing to poor resolution. Since branch renal arteries tend to lie in a single plane, they, too, are often inadequately imaged by helical CT. Even given these limitations, CT may be more accurate than MRA for detecting lesions related to fibromuscular disease.

Other drawbacks of spiral CT include long postprocessing times, inability to image patients who weigh more than 125 kg, and a general tendency to produce false-positive results. False-positive images can result from incomplete opacification of the renal artery secondary to poor timing of a contrast bolus, overlying calcification, or artifact from adjacent tissue. Despite these limitations, for patients with relatively normal renal function and in centers with appropriate experience and expertise, spiral CT offers accurate, less invasive assessment of renal artery anatomy.

SUMMARY: SUGGESTED PARADIGM FOR DIAGNOSIS OF SUSPECTED RENAL ARTERY DISEASE

Renal artery disease is a complex disorder that can have a number of causes and different clinical presentations. Thus, a rigid diagnostic approach to suspected RAS is neither possible nor advisable. Instead, it is more prudent to adopt a flexible strategy that is based on each patient's clinical presentation and on "local expertise" with the various diagnostic modalities. Following are general recommendations for a diagnostic approach to patients thought to have RAS.

When there is strong clinical suspicion of renovascular hypertension and fibromuscular disease is the presumed cause, it may be appropriate to proceed directly to contrast angiography because of the relatively high incidence of distal and accessory renal artery lesions. No noninvasive imaging study currently available provides the necessary precision in detecting these lesions. In patients with suspected uncomplicated atherosclerotic renovascular hypertension who have normal renal function and who can tolerate temporary withdrawal of certain antihypertensive medications, a traditional functional or physiologic diagnostic test (e.g., radionuclide renography, renal vein renins) may be the most appropriate initial study.

The number of patients thought to have RAS who have impaired renal function or who cannot discontinue hypertensive medications is increasing. These patients are not optimal candidates for physiologic tests, and, for them, noninvasive renal artery imaging is advisable. Which noninvasive modality should be used is largely a matter of local expertise. If there is a vascular lab with a dedicated technician who has documented proficiency with renal artery DU, that would be the diagnostic modality of choice. Alternatively, if there is a radiologist with experience in three-dimensional gadolinium-enhanced MRA, MRA may be more appropriate. Experience with spiral CT is less extensive than with the other two modalities, but further development of this technique will make it a viable approach in selected patients with normal renal function. Although technologic advances will continue to improve the accuracy of noninvasive imaging for suspected RAS, sound clinical judgment is still paramount to the diagnosis and evaluation of this complicated disorder.

REFERENCES

1. Pickering TG: Diagnosis and evaluation of renovascular hypertension: Indications for therapy. Circulation 83(Suppl I):I-147–154, 1991.
2. Mann SJ, Pickering TG: Detection of renovascular hypertension: State of the art 1992. Ann Intern Med 117(10):845–853, 1992.
3. Lewin A, Blaufox MD, Castle H, et al: Apparent prevalence of curable hypertension in the hypertension detection and follow-up program. Arch Intern Med 145:451–455, 1985.
4. Berglund G, Andersson O, Wilhelmsen L: Prevalence of primary and secondary hypertension in a random population sample. Br Med J 2:554–556, 1976.
5. Bech K, Hilden T: The frequency of secondary hypertension. Acta Med Scand 195:65–79, 1975.
6. Greco BA, Breyer JA: Atherosclerotic ischemic renal disease. Am J Kidney Dis 29(2):167–187, 1997.
7. Scoble JE, Maher ER, Hamilton G: Atherosclerotic renovascular disease causing renal impairment—a case for treatment. Clin Nephrol 31:119–120, 1989.
8. Kahn IH, Catto GRD, Edward N: Influence of coexisting disease on survival on renal-replacement therapy. Lancet 341:415–418, 1993.
9. Mailloux LU, Napolitano B, Bellucci AG: Renal vascular disease causing end-stage renal disease, incidence, clinical correlates, and outcomes: A 20-year clinical experience. Am J Kidney Dis 24:622–629, 1994.
10. Hillman BJ, Oviatt TW, Capp MP, et al: Renal digital subtraction angiography: 100 cases. Radiology 145:643–646, 1982.

11. NHLBI workshop on renovascular disease: Summary report and recommendations. Hypertension 7:452–458, 1984.
12. King BF Jr: Diagnostic imaging evaluation of renovascular hypertension. Abdom Imaging 20:395–405, 1995.
13. Wilcox CS: Ischemic Nephropathy: Noninvasive testing. Semin Nephrol 16(1):43–52, 1996.
14. Reiss MD, Bookstein JJ, Bleifer KH: Radiologic aspects of renovascular hypertension: Part 4, Arteriographic complications. JAMA 221(4):374–378, 1972.
15. Rudnick MR, Berns JS, Cohen RM, Goldfarb S: Nephrotoxic risks of renal angiography: Contrast media–associated nephrotoxicity and atheroembolism—a critical review. Am J Kidney Dis 24(4):713–727, 1994.
16. Thadhani RI, Carnargo CA, Xavier RJ, et al: Atheroembolic renal failure after invasive procedures: Natural history based on 52 histologically proven cases. Medicine 74(6):350–358, 1995.
17. Ramirez G, O'Neill WM, Lambert R, Bloomer HA: Cholesterol embolization: A complication of angiography. Arch Intern Med 138:1430–32, 1978.
18. Burns PN: The physical principles of Doppler and spectral analysis. J Clin Ultrasound 15:567–590, 1987.
19. Clin JW: Role of duplex ultrasonography in screening for significant renal artery disease. Urol Clin North Am 21(2):215–226, 1994.
20. Schwerk WB, Restrepo IK, Stellwaag M, et al: Renal artery stenosis: Grading with image-directed Doppler US evaluation of renal resistive index. Radiology 190:785–790, 1994.
21. Potsma CT, van Aalen J, De Boo T, et al: Doppler ultrasound scanning in the detection of renal artery stenosis in hypertensive patients. Br J Radiol 65:857–860, 1992.
22. Bardilli M, Jensen G, Volkmann R, Aurell M: Non-invasive ultrasound assessment of renal artery stenosis by means of the Gosling pulsatility index. J Hypertens 10:985–999, 1992.
23. Kohler TR, Zierler RE, Martin RL, et al: Noninvasive diagnosis of renal artery stenosis by ultrasonic duplex scanning. J Vasc Surg 4:450–456, 1988.
24. Hansen KJ, Tribble RW, Reavis SW, et al: Renal duplex sonography: Evaluation of clinical utility. J Vasc Surg 12(3):227–236, 1990.
25. Olin JW, Piedmonte MA, Young JR, et al: The utility of duplex ultrasound scanning of the renal arteries for diagnosing significant renal artery stenosis. Ann Intern Med 122:833–838, 1995.
26. Taylor DC, Kettler MD, Moneta GL, et al: Duplex ultrasound scanning in the diagnosis of renal artery stenosis: A prospective evaluation. J Vasc Surg 7(2):363–369, 1988.
27. Hoffmann U, Edwards JM, Carter S, et al: Role of duplex scanning for the detection of atherosclerotic renal artery disease. Kidney Int 39:1232–1239, 1991.
28. Simoni C, Balestra G, Bandini A, Rusticali F: [Doppler ultrasound in the diagnosis of renal artery stenosis in hypertensive patients: A prospective study]. G Ital Cardiol 21(3):249–255, 1991.
29. Handa N, Fukunaga R, Etani H, et al: Efficacy of echo-Doppler examination for the evaluation of renovascular disease. Ultrasound Med Biol 14:1–5, 1988.
30. Desberg, AL, Paushter DM, Lammert GK, et al: Renal artery stenosis: Evaluation with color Doppler flow imaging. Radiology 177:749–753, 1990.
31. Lewis BD, James EM: Current applications of duplex and color Doppler ultrasound imaging: Abdomen. Mayo Clin Proc 643:1158–1169, 1984.
32. Robertson R, Murphy A, Dubbins PA: Renal artery stenosis: The use of duplex ultrasound as a screening technique. Br J Radiol 61:196–201, 1988.
33. Mollo M, Pelet V, Mouawad J, et al: Evaluation of colour duplex ultrasound scanning in diagnosis of renal artery stenosis, compared to angiography: A prospective study on 53 patients. Eur J Vasc Endovasc Surg 14(4)305–309, 1997.
34. Platt JF: Doppler ultrasound of the kidney. Semin Ultrasound CT MRI 18(1):22–32, 1997.
35. Stavros AT, Parker SH, Yakes WF, et al: Segmental stenosis of the renal artery: Pattern recognition of tardus and parvus abnormalities with duplex sonography. Genitourin Radiol 184:487–92, 1992.
36. Nazzal MMS, Hoballah JJ, Miller EV, et al: Renal hilar Doppler analysis is of value in the management of patients with renovascular disease. Am J Surg 174:164–168, 1997.
37. Halpern EJ, Needleman L, Nack TL, East SA: Renal artery stenosis: Should we study the main renal artery or segmental vessels? Radiology 195(3):799–804, 1995.
38. Hall NJ, Thorpe RJ, MacKechnie SG: Stenosis of the accessory renal artery: Doppler ultrasound findings. Australas Radiol 39(1):73–77, 1995.
39. Oliva VL, Soulez G, Lesage D, et al: Detection of renal artery stenosis with Doppler sonography after administration of captopril: Value of early systolic rise. AJR Am J Roentgenol 171(1):169–175, 1998.
40. Rene PC, Oliva VL, Bui BT, et al: Renal artery stenosis: Evaluation of Doppler US after inhibition of angiotensin-converting enzyme with captopril. Radiology 196(3):675–679, 1995.
41. Missouris CG, Allen CM, Balen FG, et al: Noninvasive screening for renal artery stenosis with ultrasound contrast enhancement. J Hypertens 14(4):519–524, 1996.
42. Melany ML, Grant EG, Duerinckx AJ, et al: Ability of phase shift US contrast agent to improve imaging of the main renal arteries. Radiology 205:147–152, 1997.
43. Dougherty MJ, Hallett JW, Naessens JM, et al: Optimizing technical success of renal revascularization: The impact of intraoperative color-flow duplex ultrasonography. J Vasc Surg 17(5):849–857, 1993.
44. Strandness DE: Natural history of renal artery stenosis. Am J Kidney Dis 24(4):630–635, 1994.
45. Guzman RP, Zierler RE, Isaacson JA, et al: Renal atrophy and arterial stenosis. Hypertension 23(3):346–350, 1994.
46. Taylor DC, Moneta GL, Strandness DE: Follow-up of renal artery stenosis by duplex ultrasound. J Vasc Surg 9(3):410–415, 1989.
47. Eidt JF, Fry RE, Clagett GP, et al: Postoperative follow-up of renal artery reconstruction with duplex ultrasound. J Vasc Surg 8(6):667–673, 1988.
48. Lantz EJ, Charboneau JW, Hallett JW, et al: Intraoperative color Doppler sonography during renal artery revascularization. AJR Am J Roentgenol 162(4):847–852, 1994.
49. Duda SH, Erley CM, Wakat JP, et al: Posttransplant renal artery stenosis—outpatient intrarterial DSA versus color aided duplex Doppler sonography. Eur J Radiol 16(2):95–101, 1993.
50. Sagalowsky A, McQuitty DM: The assessment and management of renal vascular hypertension after kidney transplantation. Semin Urol 12(3):211–223, 1994.
51. Snider JF, Hunter DW, Moradian GP, et al: Transplant renal artery stenosis: Evaluation with duplex sonography. Radiology 172:1027–1030, 1989.
52. Blum U, Drumme B, Flugel P, et al: Treatment of ostial renal artery stenosis with vascular endoprotheses after unsuccessful balloon angioplasty. N Engl J Med 336:459–465, 1997.
53. Guzman RP, Zierler RE, Isaacson JA, et al: Renal atrophy and arterial stenosis: A prospective study with duplex ultrasound. Hypertension 23(3):346–350, 1994.
54. Harward TRS, Smith S, Seeger JM: Detection of celiac axis and superior mesenteric artery occlusive disease with use of abdominal duplex scanning. J Vasc Surg 17:738–745, 1993.
55. Gedroyc WM: Magnetic resonance angiography of renal arteries. Urol Clin North Am 21(2):201–214, 1994.
56. Grist TM: Magnetic resonance angiography of renal artery stenosis. Am J Kidney Dis 24(4):700–712, 1994.
57. Borrello JA: Renal MR angiography. Genitourin Imaging 5(1):83–93, 1997.
58. Kent KC, Edelman RR, Kim D, et al: Magnetic resonance imaging: A reliable test for the evaluation of proximal atherosclerotic renal artery stenosis. J Vasc Surg 13(2):311–317, 1991.
59. Gedroyc WMW, Neerhut P, Negus R, et al: Magnetic resonance angiography of renal artery stenosis. Clin Radiol 50:436–439, 1995.
60. Fellner C, Strotzer M, Geissler A, et al: Renal arteries: Evaluation with optimized 2d and 3d Time of Flight MR angiography. Radiology 196:681–687, 1995.
61. De Cobelli F, Mellone R, Salvioni M, et al: Renal artery stenosis: Value of screening with three, dimensional phase contrast MR angiography with a phased array multicoil. Radiology 201:697–703, 1996.
62. Kim D, Edelman RR, Kent KC, et al: Abdominal aorta and renal artery stenosis: Evaluation with MR angiography. Radiology 174:727–731, 1990.
63. Postma CT, Joosten FB, Rosenbusch G, Thien T: Magnetic resonance angiography has a high reliability in the detection of renal artery stenosis. Am J Hypertens 10(9):957–963, 1997.
64. Laissy JP, Benyounes M, Limot O, et al: Screening of renal artery stenosis: Assessment with magnetic resonance angiography at 1.0 T. Magn Reson Imaging 14(9):1033–1041, 1996.
65. Silverman JM, Friedman ML, Van Allan RJ: Detection of main renal

artery stenosis using phase-contrast cine MR angiography. AJR Am J Roentgenol 166(5):1131–1137, 1996.

66. Hertz SM, Holland GA, Baum RA, et al: Evaluation of renal stenosis by magnetic resonance angiography. Am J Surg 168:140–143, 1994.

67. Smith HJ, Bakke SJ: Mr angiography of in situ and transplanted renal arteries: Early experience using a three-dimensional time of flight technique Acta Radiol 34:150–155, 1993.

68. DeCobelli F, Vanzuli A, Sironi S, et al: Renal artery stenosis: Evaluation with breath-hold, three-dimensional, dynamic, gadolinium-enhanced versus three-dimensional, phase-contrast MR angiography. Radiology 205:689–695, 1997.

69. Leung DA, Hany TF, Debatin JF: Three dimensional contrast enhanced magnetic resonance angiography of the abdominal arterial system. Cardiovasc Interv Radiol 21:1–10, 1998.

70. Prince MR, Narasimhan DL, Stanley JC, et al: Breath hold gadolinium enhanced MR angiography of the abdominal aorta and its branches. Radiology 197:785–792, 1995.

71. Steffens JC, Link J, Grassner J, et al: Contrast enhanced centered breath hold MR angiography of the renal arteries and the abdominal aorta. J Magn Reson Imaging 7:617–622, 1997.

72. Hany TF, Debatin JF, Leung DA, Pfammatter T: Evaluation of the aortoiliac and renal arteries: Comparison of breath-hold contrast-enhanced three-dimensional MR angiography with conventional catheter angiography. Radiology 204:357–362, 1997.

73. Rieumont MJ, Kaufman JA, Geller SC, et al: Evaluation of renal artery stenosis with dynamic gadolinium enhanced MR angiography. AJR Am J Roentgenol 169:39–44, 1997.

74. Holland GA, Dougherty L, Carpenter JP, et al: Breath hold ultrafast three dimensional gadolinium enhanced MR angiography of the aorta and the renal and other visceral abdominal arteries. Am J Roentgenol 166(4):971–981, 1996.

75. Prince MR: A Gadolinium enhanced MR aortography. Radiology 191:155–164, 1994.

76. Gedroyc WM, Negus R, Al-Kutoubi A, et al: Magnetic resonance angiography of renal transplants. Lancet 339:789–791, 1992.

77. Johnson DB, Lerner CA, Prince MR, et al: Gadolinium enhanced magnetic resonance angiography of renal transplants. Magn Reson Imaging 15(1):13–20, 1997.

78. Loubeyre P, Cahen R, Grozel F, et al: Transplant renal artery stenosis: Evaluation of diagnosis with magnetic resonance angiography compared with color duplex sonography and arteriography. Transplantation 62(4):446–450, 1996.

79. Bennett HF, Li D: MR imaging of renal function. MRI Clin North Am 5(1):107–126, 1997.

80. Taylor J, Summers PE, Keevil SF, et al: Magnetic resonance renography: Optimisation of pulse sequence parameters and Gd-DPTA dose, comparison with radionuclide renography. Magn Reson Imaging 15(6):637–649, 1997.

81. Grenier N, Trillaud H, Combe C, et al: Diagnosis of renovascular hypertension: Feasibility of captopril-sensitized dynamic MR imaging and comparison with captopril scintigraphy. AJR Am J Roentgenol 16(4):835–843, 1996.

82. Ros PR, Gauger J, Stoupis C, et al: Diagnosis of renal artery stenosis: Feasibility of combining MR angiography, MR renography, and gadopentetate based measurements of glomerular filtration rate. AJR Am J Roentgenol 165(6):1447–1451, 1995.

83. Cortsen M, Peterson LJ, Stahlberg F, et al: MR velocity mapping measurement of renal artery blood flow in patients with impaired kidney function. Acta Radiol 37(1):79–84, 1996.

84. Lundin B, Cooper TG, Meyer RA, Potchen J: Measurement of total and unilateral renal blood flow by oblique angle velocity encoded 2D–cine magnetic resonance angiography. Magn Reson Imaging 11:51–59, 1993.

85. Powers TA, Lorenz CH, Holburn GE, Price RK: Renal artery stenosis: In vivo perfusion MR imaging. Radiology 178:543–548, 1991.

86. Rubin GD: Spiral (helical) CT of the renal vasculature. Semin Ultrasound CT MR 17(4):374–397, 1996.

87. Brink JA, Lim JT, Wang G, et al: Technical optimization of spiral CT for depiction of renal artery stenosis: In vitro analysis. Radiology 194(1):157–163, 1995.

88. Rubin GD, Dake MD, Napel S, et al: Spiral CT of renal artery stenosis: Comparison of three-dimensional rendering techniques. Radiology 190(1):181–189, 1994.

89. Rubin GD, Dake MD, Napel SA, et al: Three dimensional spiral CT angiography of the abdomen: Initial clinical experience. Radiology 186:147–152, 1993.

90. Galanski M, Prokop M, Schaefer C, et al: Renal artery stenosis: Spiral CT angiography. Radiology 189:185–192, 1993.

91. Kaatee R, Beek FJ, de Lange EE, et al: Renal artery stenosis: Detection and quantification with spiral CT angiography versus optimized digital subtraction angiography. Radiology 205(1):121–127, 1997.

92. Farres MT, Lammer J, Schima W, et al: Spiral computed tomographic angiography of the renal arteries: A prospective comparison with intravenous and intraarterial digital subtraction angiography. Cardiovasc Interv Radiol 19(2):101–106, 1996.

93. Cikrit DF, Harris VJ, Hemmer CG, et al: Comparison of spiral CT scan and arteriography for evaluation of renal and visceral arteries. Ann Vasc Surg 10(2):109–116, 1996.

94. Olbricht CJ, Prokop M, Chavan A, et al: Minimally invasive diagnosis of renal artery stenosis by spiral computed tomography angiography. Kidney Int 48(4):1332–1337, 1995.

95. Beregi JP, Elkohen M, Deklunder G, et al: Helical CT angiography compared with arteriography in the detection of renal artery stenosis. AJR Am J Roentgenol 167(2):495–501, 1996.

96. Lerman LO, Taler SJ, Textor SC, et al: Computed tomography derived intrarenal blood flow in renovascular and essential hypertension. Kidney Int 49(3):846–854, 1996.

97. Gomes MN, Davros WJ, Zeman RK: Preoperative assessment of abdominal aortic aneurysm: The value of helical and three-dimensional computed tomography. J Vasc Surg 20(3):367–375, 1994.

98. Todd GJ, Nowygrod R, Benvenisty A, et al: The accuracy of CT scanning in the diagnosis of abdominal and thoracoabdominal aortic aneurysms. J Vasc Surg 13(2):302–310, 1991.

99. Elkohen M, Beregi JP, Deklunder G, et al: A prospective study of helical computed tomography angiography versus angiography for the detection of renal artery stenosis in hypertensive patients. J Hypertens 14(4):525–528, 1996.

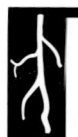

C H A P T E R   1 2 2

Renal Artery Fibrodysplasia and Renovascular Hypertension

Louis M. Messina, M.D., and James C. Stanley, M.D.

Arterial fibrodysplasia encompasses a heterogeneous group of arterial dysplastic lesions of unknown etiology that affect segments of small and medium muscular arteries.[70, 85] Fibrodysplastic lesions have been described in virtually every artery. The dysplastic process usually results in a stenosis, but it may cause aneurysm formation. The most commonly affected vessel is the renal artery, first reported by McCormick and colleagues, who used the term *fibromuscular dysplasia* in 1958 to describe renal artery stenoses in three patients with hypertension.[57] The renal artery stenosis affecting the first patient cured of renovascular hypertension, reported by Leadbetter and Burkland in 1938,[49a] was, in retrospect, fibromuscular dysplasia.

Occlusive renal artery lesions are the most common cause of surgically correctable hypertension. Although the precise incidence of renovascular hypertension has not been defined, its clinical importance has been clearly established. Fibrodysplastic renal artery stenoses, which affect up to 0.5% of the general population, are second only to atherosclerotic stenoses as the most frequent cause of renovascular hypertension. This overview of renal artery fibrodysplasia describes its pathology, clinical manifestations, indications for therapeutic intervention, drug therapy, percutaneous transluminal angioplasty, and the role of surgical therapy for lesions causing renovascular hypertension.

PATHOLOGY

Arterial dysplasia is categorized according to the principal layer of arterial wall involvement, and in these groupings it correlates with angiographic findings[30] and progression of renovascular disease. The four most commonly encountered dysplastic lesions of the renal arteries are (1) *intimal fibroplasia*, (2) *medial hyperplasia*, (3) *medial fibroplasia*, and (4) *perimedial dysplasia*.[36, 82] The first two represent distinctly different pathologic processes, whereas the latter two may be a continuum of the same disease. *Developmental stenoses* represent a fifth distinct and unusual form of renal artery dysplasia.[84]

Intimal Fibroplasia

Intimal fibroplasia accounts for 5% of all fibrodysplastic renal artery lesions. It affects children and young adults of both sexes equally. Intimal fibroplasia occurs morphologically as long, irregular tubular stenoses of the main renal artery in younger patients and as smooth focal stenoses in older patients.[83] Progression of intimal fibroplasia in most patients occurs more slowly than that of medial fibroplasia.

Medial Hyperplasia

Medial hyperplasia is found in fewer than 1% of fibrodysplastic renal artery lesions. It is angiographically similar to intimal hyperplasia, and is seen most often in women aged 30 to 50 years. Medial hyperplasia usually occurs as an isolated lesion in the mid-portion of the main renal artery. One study utilized the presence or absence of smooth muscle hyperplasia to classify fibrodysplastic lesions.[2] The presence of smooth muscle hyperplasia is associated with a shorter duration of hypertension, fewer aneurysms, and less extension of disease into branch vessels, as well as a better response to surgical intervention. This suggests that hyperplastic lesions may be precursors of advanced and more widespread fibrodysplastic lesions instead of representing a distinct pathologic process.

Medial Fibroplasia

Medial fibroplasia comprises approximately 85% of all dysplastic renal artery lesions and presents most commonly in white women in the third or fourth decades of life. It occurs most frequently in the renal arteries. Medial fibroplasia is bilateral in 55% of the patients; when it is unilateral, it affects the right side in 80% of cases.[83] Lesions usually affect the distal main renal artery, with extension into branch vessels in approximately 25% of cases.

The angiographic appearance of medial fibroplasia is the classic "string of beads." Aneurysms larger than the adjacent artery wall, alternating with luminal web-like projections, are responsible for this presentation. A pathologic study of isolated renal artery aneurysms demonstrated that most have evidence of fibrodysplastic disease, usually unaccompanied by a clinical presentation of renovascular hypertension.[37] Progression of medial fibroplasia appears to be less frequent than that of perimedial dysplasia.[30]

Perimedial Dysplasia

Perimedial dysplasia is characterized by accumulation of elastic tissue at the media-adventitia junction and is seen in 10% of arterial dysplastic lesions. Perimedial dysplasia is seen in younger women whose angiograms reveal either focal stenoses or multiple stenoses of the main renal artery, without the intervening aneurysmal dilations seen typically in medial fibroplasia. Perimedial dysplasia is usually associated with marked stenoses severe enough to cause renovascular hypertension.[30]

ETIOLOGY

Although the origin of arterial fibrodysplasia remains unclear, three factors appear to play important etiologic roles: (1) hormonal influences, (2) arterial wall ischemia, and (3) mechanical stresses.[83] The increased incidence of arterial dysplasia in women during their reproductive years contrasts with the protective effects of estrogen in human atherosclerosis. Similarly, the antiproliferative effect of estrogen on vascular smooth muscle at both the cellular[42] and arterial levels[101] is also contrary to the predilection for arterial dysplasia in women. Oral contraceptives and pregnancies are not significant risk factors for arterial fibrodysplasia,[83] although multiparity has been associated with other degenerative vascular lesions, such as splenic artery aneurysms.

Vessel wall ischemia may contribute to the development of arterial dysplasia.[70] Vasa vasorum of muscular arteries originate from branch points of the parent artery and supply oxygen and nutrients to the arterial wall. The most commonly affected vessels—the renal, internal carotid, and external iliac arteries—all have long segments that are free of branches and thus with few vasa vasorum. Arterial dysplasia may develop as a result of ischemia of the artery wall secondary to injury to the sparse vasa vasorum of these vessels. Animal studies demonstrate that occlusion of the vasa vasorum induces formation of dysplastic lesions.[74] The media-adventitia junction, where nutrient flow from vasa vasorum is most critical, is also the site of lesions of perimedial dysplasia and peripheral medial fibroplasia.

The unique stresses to which certain long muscular arteries (e.g., internal carotid artery, renal arteries) are subject suggests that mechanical forces may also play a role in development of arterial dysplasia. Repeated stretching of vessels may trigger a fibroproliferative response. This hypothesis is supported by the finding of predominantly right-sided lesions in unilateral fibromuscular disease. The right renal artery is longer than the left and may be subject to greater axial stretch, particularly because the right kidney is known to be subjected to ptosis more than the left, and ptosis in general is more common in women than men.

CLINICAL MANIFESTATIONS AND INDICATION FOR TREATMENT

The prevalence of renovascular hypertension in the population with elevated blood pressure is low, (~2% to 5%. Hypertension caused by arterial fibrodysplasia is even less common.[50] The first decision in a reasonable management algorithm depends on the ability to recognize clinical clues of renovascular hypertension secondary to fibrodysplasia (Fig. 122–1).[23] Hypertension in pediatric patients that is unaccompanied by obvious renal disease and the sudden onset of diastolic hypertension greater than 115 mmHg in women younger than 45 years of age are two dominant clinical features of renovascular hypertension. Elevated

blood pressure in this group of patients tends to be refractory to simple medical management. Furthermore, if arteries to both kidneys or if one artery to a solitary kidney is affected, impaired renal function may result from the use of angiotensin-converting enzyme (ACE) inhibitors. Renovascular hypertension secondary to arterial fibrodysplasia is rare in African Americans.[45]

Other clinical findings may be more common for patients with renovascular hypertension than for those with essential hypertension; unfortunately, they are not pathognomonic of this disease.[72] For instance, younger children and infants with renovascular hypertension frequently exhibit failure to thrive, whereas hyperkinesis, seizure disorders, cephalalgia, and easy fatigability often affect older children and adolescents.[103] Adults with renovascular hypertension secondary to fibrodysplasia often present with lethargy. Abdominal bruit and hypertensive retinal arteriolar changes may be common findings for patients with renal artery fibrodysplasia, but they are not specific enough to distinguish these patients from those with essential hypertension.

Certain characteristics of children with renal fibrodysplasia are noteworthy. In an earlier report reflecting the experience at the University of Michigan, renal arterial fibrodysplasia causing renovascular hypertension in children revealed atypical medial-perimedial dysplasia, often with secondary intimal fibroplasia, in 88% of the renal artery stenoses encountered.[87] The classic string-of-beads appearance of medial fibrodysplasia that occurs in adults was not observed in any child in that series. In a more recent series, 33 boys and 24 girls whose mean age was 9.5 and 12 years, respectively, presented with an average duration of hypertension of 14.2 months. The mean preoperative blood pressures were 181/117 mmHg without medication and 158/104 mmHg with drug therapy.[91]

In contrast, adults treated for renal artery fibrodysplasia at the same institution included 133 women and 11 men, with mean ages of 39.1 and 30.5 years, respectively.[87] The average duration of hypertension in this adult group was 42.5 months. Blood pressures without therapy averaged 206/122 mmHg, falling to 184/111 mmHg with drug treatment. More recent reports of adult patients undergoing treatment for renal fibrodysplasia show a distinct change in the presentation and outcome.[3, 66] Adult patients are now significantly older, experience a longer duration of hypertension, more frequently demonstrate extra renal atherosclerosis, and have branch vessel renal arterial fibrodysplasia. These changes in the presentation of the patient population has greatly influenced on treatment patterns and their outcome.

INDICATIONS FOR TREATMENT OF RENAL FIBRODYSPLASIA

Indications for treatment of renal fibrodysplasia depend largely on age at presentation. Because the incidence of essential hypertension is negligible in infants and children, most instances of hypertension in this patient population represent a renovascular etiology.[91] The presence of modest or severe blood pressure elevations in a pediatric patient is sufficient justification to undertake detailed diagnostic

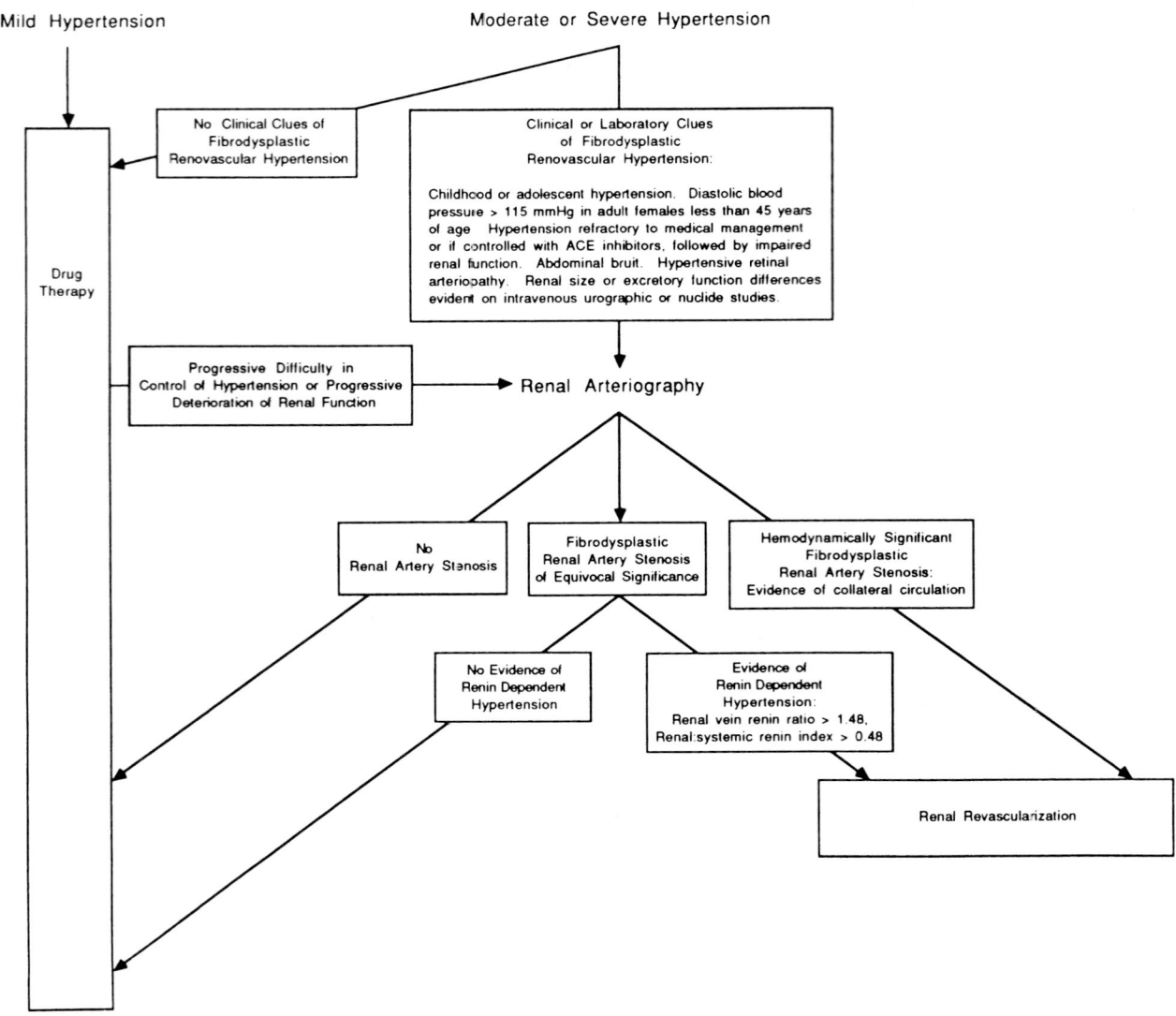

FIGURE 122–1. Management algorithm for fibrodysplastic renovascular hypertension.

studies in search of a correctable cause of hypertension. One exception is the occasional child who has evidence of significant underlying renal parenchymal disease. In pediatric patients, catheter angiography is the most important diagnostic study when renovascular hypertension is suspected.

Specific indications for intervention in adults include:

• Presence of moderate to severe hypertension
• A hemodynamically significant renal artery stenosis
• Evidence of its functional importance

The dramatic improvement of drug therapy for hypertension over the last two decades has increased the threshold for intervention for renovascular hypertension, most likely accounting for the observed increase in average age at presentation and duration of hypertension in these patients. However, this improvement often makes determination of the functional significance of renal fibrodysplasia more challenging because these older patients have a higher frequency of essential hypertension.[3] Nonetheless, clinical

clues provide the most cost effective manner in which to identify patients for screening for renovascular hypertension (see Fig. 122–1). The most commonly employed screening studies are renal duplex ultrasonography, magnetic resonance angiography (MRA), and radionuclide scans. Once a patient has been identified on the basis of clinical clues or the use of screening studies, catheter-angiography is the most useful test in assessing the hemodynamic and functional significance of renal artery dysplastic occlusive disease.[79–81]

A number of angiographic features can be used to determine the hemodynamic significance of dysplastic renal artery stenosis. Demonstration of collateral vessels as a manifestation of a significant stenosis has been important in this regard.[25] Development of collateral vessels circumventing a renal artery stenosis usually occurs when the pressure gradient across the stenosis approaches 10 mmHg. This same gradient is generally accepted to be associated with an increased release of renin from the juxtaglomerular apparatus of the kidney. In this way, demonstration of the nonparenchymal renal artery branches functioning as collateral vessels by pharmacoangiographic techniques with the use of epinephrine and acetylcholine has been useful in establishing the significance of many equivocal renal artery stenoses.[9] Intravenous digital subtraction angiography (IV DSA) has not been helpful in the evaluation of renal artery fibrodysplasia because of its inadequacy in demonstrating anything other than the most obvious main renal artery lesions.

Renin assays have also been important in determining functional significance of equivocal renal artery stenoses (see Fig. 122–1). Renin assays are most useful for patients who have medically controlled hypertension and in older patients with arterial fibrodysplasia and diffuse extrarenal atherosclerosis.[3] For young patients with poorly controlled hypertension or threatened ischemic nephropathy, such as those with arterial fibrodysplasia affecting a solitary kidney or those with severe bilateral stenoses, the diagnosis may also be made by renin profiling with the *renal systemic renin index* (RSRI).

The *renal vein renin ratio* (RVRR), which compares renin activity in the venous effluent from the ischemic and contralateral kidneys, has not been a highly predictive test, largely because of the frequent occurrence of bilateral disease, in which case the RVRR may revert toward 1.0.[25] Although the RRVRs are considered abnormal when they exceed 1.48, lower ratios occur in approximately 15% to 20% of patients eventually found to have a renovascular cause of their hypertension.[79, 83]

An alternative calculation of each kidney's renin secretory activity can be expressed as the RSRI.[51, 83] One can calculate this index by subtracting the systemic renin activity from renal vein renin activity and dividing the remainder by the systemic renin activity:

$$\frac{\text{renal vein renin} - \text{systemic renin}}{\text{systemic renin}}$$

Renin hypersecretion is defined as an RSRI above 0.48. *Suppression of renin secretion* by a kidney is defined as an RSRI below 0.24, usually approaching 0.0. This method of evaluating each kidney's renin secretory activity indexed to the systemic renin concentration provides a more accurate identification of patients likely to be improved or cured after operation.[79, 80] Absolute and relative renin activities do not appear to vary between pediatric or adult populations with renal arterial fibrodysplasia.[79, 95] ACE inhibitors have been used to enhance the sensitivity of these calculations in documenting the existence of renovascular hypertension.[62, 99]

Drug Therapy

As described in Chapter 119, improved antihypertensive drug therapy has had an important impact on the management of hypertension for patients with renovascular hypertension secondary to renal artery fibrodysplasia.[102, 105] Current principles underlying drug therapy for renovascular hypertension are based on the now well-known pathophysiology of hypertension secondary to a functionally significant renal artery stenosis. Renin-angiotensin–mediated vasoconstriction is the primary mechanism of hypertension in patients with unilateral renal artery stenosis and a normal contralateral kidney. Under these circumstances, the sodium retention and hypervolemia that results from the direct effect of angiotensin II, as well as angiotensin II–induced aldosterone secretion, is compensated by a natriuresis by the normal contralateral kidney. In the setting of bilateral renal artery stenoses—and thus an impaired capacity for natriuresis—renin-angiotensin-aldosterone–mediated sodium retention and hypervolemia are the dominant pathophysiologic mechanisms of hypertension. Similarly, sodium retention and hypervolemia is an important mechanism of hypertension in the presence of a unilateral stenosis and either contralateral parenchymal disease or renal absence as a result of agenesis or previous nephrectomy.

Hypertension in most patients with renal artery fibrodysplasia can be controlled with the appropriate pharmacologic intervention. Several issues may influence the long-term therapeutic effectiveness of drug therapy for hypertension:

1. Drug side effects.
2. Patient compliance.
3. Whether blood pressure control is achieved at the expense of diminished renal function, occurring as a direct affect of the drug or as unrecognized insidious progression of renal artery occlusive disease.

In this regard, ischemic nephropathy was not observed in earlier studies of young patients with renal artery fibrodysplasia. However, ischemic nephropathy has been reported in some recent studies of both surgical and angioplasty outcomes.[3, 68]

In patients with documented renovascular hypertension, a beta-blocking agent is often the first drug given. Inhibition in renin secretion by beta-blocking agents is the principal means of blood reduction in these patients.[11] Propranolol and atenolol are the drugs used most frequently, although many others, including metoprolol, nadolol, timolol, and pindolol, are also available. In instances of refractory hypertension, often as the result of bilateral renal artery stenoses, the addition of a diuretic agent may be used to compensate for the hypervolemic state that exists in these patients. A thiazide is usually used in this circumstance. In the subgroup of patients with impaired renal function, a loop diuretic, such as furosemide, maybe necessary to achieve an effective diuresis.

ACE inhibitors have become highly effective agents in the management of hypertension in general, and renovascular hypertension in particular.[1, 13, 28, 38] Captopril and enalapril are among the most commonly used ACE inhibitors. These agents may be supplemented by both beta-blockers and diuretics in instances of refractory hypertension. Calcium-channel blockers have been used to supplement ACE inhibitors in the management of renovascular hypertension. Finally, in the most cases of severe hypertension, vasodilators such as minoxidil are utilized.

It is recognized that when ACE inhibitors are used to treat renovascular hypertension, renal function may become impaired.[15] This occurs most often in patients with bilateral renal artery stenosis as well as in patients with a stenosis affecting a solitary kidney.[39] In these circumstances, a severe reduction in the glomerular filtration rate occurs, since the primary effect of the ACE inhibitors in the kidney is to mediate efferent arteriolar vasodilation, thereby reducing the effective driving pressure across the glomerulus.

Percutaneous Transluminal Renal Angioplasty

Although the first successful percutaneous transluminal angioplasty (PTA) reported by Gruntzig and colleagues[34] involved the dilation of an atherosclerotic renal artery stenosis, this technique was soon recognized to be effective in the treatment of fibrodysplastic lesion.[4, 32, 33, 55, 71, 97] For a variety of reasons, percutaneous transluminal renal angioplasty (PTRA) has become the dominant mode of treatment of renal arterial dysplasia at most institutions.

PTRA is performed after aortography and selective renal arteriographic studies have defined the severity and extent of renal artery stenosis. The renal artery itself is usually entered by means of a shepherd crook or a sidewinder catheter. This catheter is then exchanged over a guide wire for a balloon catheter of the appropriate size made of polyvinyl chloride or polyethylene. A balloon is positioned within the dysplastic lesions and inflated two to three times for brief periods to pressures ranging from 4 to 8 atmospheres (atm). Completion angiography is then undertaken. Angioplasty is deemed technically successful when preexisting pressure gradients across the stenosis are abolished and anatomic documentation of an adequate dilation is apparent.[73, 98]

The mechanism by which balloon angioplasty increases the diameter of fibrodysplastic arteries is similar to that used during dilation of atherosclerotic arteries. As the balloon is inflated, the artery wall is stretched, separating the intima from underlying structures, splitting the media, and stretching the adventitia beyond its elastic recoil. The dilated artery gradually undergoes a fibroproliferative reparative process, and a neointima is formed.

Approximately 85% of adult patients with renal artery fibrodysplasia and renovascular hypertension benefit from transluminal renal angioplasty (Table 122–1); however, the effectiveness and complication rates for this procedure vary widely. This may in part reflect differences in age and the type of renal artery fibrodysplasia that is being treated. For instance, PTRA is less effective for patients with intimal fibroplasia or perimedial dysplasia and for developmental lesions. The best results with transluminal renal angioplasty are obtained in adult patients who have unilateral medial fibroplasia.

The results of transluminal renal angioplasty for renal artery fibrodysplasia in pediatric patients are less salutary.[90] Most studies show that attempts to dilate proximal ostial lesions, especially those associated with neurofibromatosis or aortic anomalies, are likely to be unsuccessful.[48, 59, 60] In one series involving children, 60% of unsuccessful angioplasties resulted in nephrectomy.[103] However, more recent reports show a higher rate of short-term and long-term success.[12]

An overall complication rate after renal angioplasty, as reflected in review of 624 procedures, averaged 11%, ranging from 2.5% to 38.5%.[6, 54] In contrast to atherosclerosis, mortality after PTRA of renal arterial dysplasia is extremely rare.[8] However, certain complications are more common, in particular arterial dissection and perforation. Transluminal renal angioplasty is contraindicated in patients who have renal artery stenosis associated with macroaneurysms, extensive branch vessel disease, or complex dissections. In these latter circumstances, the frequency of angioplasty-related complications is high. Recent trends in outcome after PTRA parallel those after surgical management.[8, 3] Failures correlate with longer durations of hypertension and older age of patients at the time of presentation for treatment.

Surgical Therapy
Operative Technique

Adequate exposure is critical to the performance of successful arterial reconstructive surgery for the renal artery fibrodysplasia. Either a supraumbilical transverse or midline incision can be used.

TABLE 122–1. RESULTS OF PERCUTANEOUS TRANSLUMINAL ANGIOPLASTY FOR RENOVASCULAR HYPERTENSION DUE TO FIBRODYSPLASIA IN ADULTS

MEDICAL CENTER	NO. OF PATIENTS	POST-ANGIOPLASTY STATUS (%)*			LENGTH OF FOLLOW-UP (MONTHS)
		Cure	Improvement	Failure	
Mayo Clinic (1980–1993)[8]	105	22	41	37	43
University Hospital, Zurich (1978–1985)[52]	28	50	39	11	15
Hospital Nuestra Senora del Pino, Las Palmas, Canary Islands, Spain (1982–1990)[68]	27	43	48	10	60
Indiana University (1980–1985)[56]	26	58	35	8	60
Broussais Hospital, Paris (1984–1991)[16]	20	68	16	15	19
University of Florida, Gainesville (1986–1992)[17]	23	52	22	26	6
University Hospital, Uppsala, Sweden (1980–1985)[35]	18	33	22	44	36

*Criteria for blood pressure response are defined in cited publications. Data are expressed to nearest 1%.

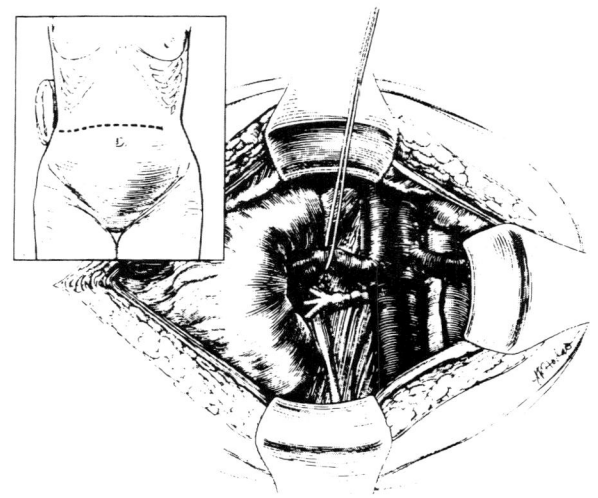

FIGURE 122–2. Operative approach through a transverse supraumbilical abdominal incision, with an extraperitoneal dissection and reflection of the colon and foregut structures providing exposure of the renal and great vessels.

The transverse incision extends from opposite the midclavicular line to the midaxillary line on the side of renal artery reconstruction. An advantage of a transverse abdominal incision is that the handling of instruments is perpendicular to the longitudinal access of the body.

Midline incisions extend from the xiphoid process to the pubic symphysis. After the peritoneal cavity has been entered and its contents explored, the intestines are displaced to the opposite side of the abdomen. In children and infants, proper exposure is more easily obtained if the intestines are eviscerated.

During *right-sided* reconstructions, the surgeon exposes the renal artery and vein as well as the inferior vena cava and aorta by incising the lateral attachments of the colon from the hepatic flexure to the cecum and by reflecting the right colon, duodenum, and pancreas medially in an extended Kocher-like maneuver. This measure provides excellent exposure of the mid-abdominal aorta, vena cava, and distal renal artery and vein (Fig. 122–2). Dissection of the renal artery should begin in its mid-portion just lateral to the vena cava, usually requiring retraction of the renal vein superiorly. The vein should be dissected carefully from surrounding tissues, and small venous branches, such as those to the adrenal gland, should be ligated and transected. If the more distal renal artery is dissected first, troublesome injury to small arterial and venous branches is more likely to occur. When one is treating developmental right-sided ostial lesions, the vena cava may be retracted laterally and the proximal renal artery exposed near its origin.

For *left-sided* reconstructions, the surgeon exposes the renal vessels using a retroperitoneal dissection similar to that performed on the right with reflection of the viscera, including the left colon, medially. Such a retroperitoneal approach offers better visualization of the middle and distal renal vessels than does an anterior exposure through the mesocolon at the root of the mesentery. Exposure of the left renal artery usually requires mobilization of the renal

vein with ligation and transection of the gonadal branch inferiorly and adrenal venous branches superiorly.

The infrarenal aorta is dissected circumferentially for approximately 5 cm, just below the origin of the renal arteries. A large-diameter aorta can be occluded partially, although in most instances total aortic occlusion is required. Systemic anticoagulation is accomplished by intravenous (IV) administration of heparin, 150 units/kg, prior to clamping the aorta. A linear aortotomy is created, with a length approximately two to three times the graft diameter. Whenever possible, the saphenous vein is harvested so that a branch is included at its caudal end. This branch is incised so that its orifice is connected to the lumen of the main trunk. A generous anastomotic circumference is created by this branch patch maneuver, which allows for a more perpendicular origin of the vein graft from the aorta (Fig. 122–3). To perform the vein graft-to-aorta anastomosis, the surgeon uses a 4-0 or 5-0 polypropylene suture. In certain patients, other sites of origin for renal grafts are preferable, with hepatic, splenic, and common iliac arteries being the most frequent non-aortic vessels from which grafts may originate.[14]

The graft is then positioned for the renal anastomosis. The most direct route for *right-sided* aortorenal grafts is in a retrocaval position originating from a lateral aortotomy. However, some grafts may be less likely to kink when taken from an anterolateral aortotomy and carried in front of the inferior vena cava and then posterior to the renal vessels. The choice of antecaval or retrocaval graft positioning must be individualized. Grafts to the *left kidney* are usually positioned beneath the left renal vein. The aortic clamp should be left in place during completion of the renal anastomosis. To remove it and to place an occluding device on a vein graft itself might injure the conduit.

Next, the renal anastomosis is performed. The proximal renal artery is clamped, transected, and ligated. Before antegrade renal artery blood flow is interrupted, a sustained diuresis should be established, usually by IV administration of 12.5 gm of mannitol. Preformed collateral vessels in these patients usually provide adequate blood flow to maintain kidney viability during renal artery occlusion. Microvascular clamps, developing tensions ranging from 30 to 70 gm, are favored over conventional vascular clamps or elastic slings for occluding distal renal vessels. They have less potential to cause vessel injury and, because of their very small size, do not obscure the operative field.

A graft-to-renal artery anastomosis, performed in an end-to-end fashion, is preferred to an end-to-side anastomosis. This is facilitated by spatulation of the graft posteriorly and the renal artery anteriorly (see Fig. 122–3). This allows visualization of the artery's interior, such that inclusion of intima with each stitch is easily accomplished. In adults, the surgeon completes the anastomosis using a continuous suture of 6-0 polypropylene. In pediatric patients, three or four sutures are interrupted to provide for anastomotic growth. If the vessels are smaller that 2 mm in diameter, the anastomosis is best completed with individual interrupted sutures about the entire circumference. Spatulated anastomoses are ovoid and with healing are less likely to develop strictures (Fig. 122–4).

After the aortic and renal anastomoses are completed, the vascular clamps are removed, antegrade renal blood

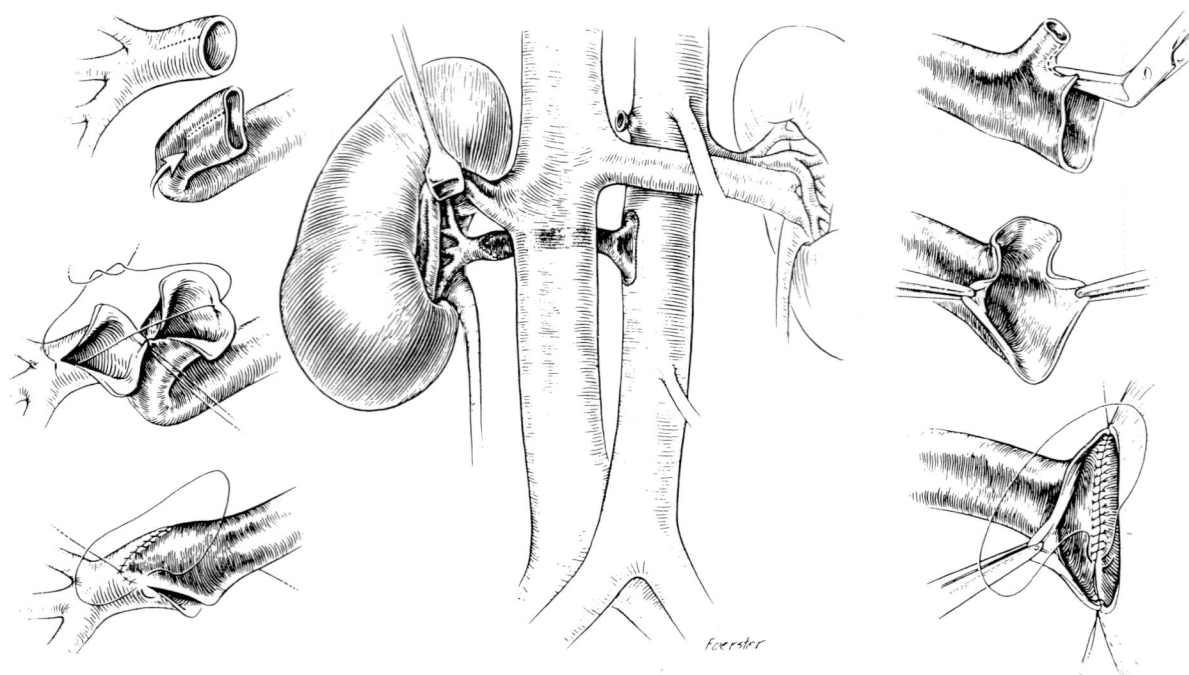

Foerster

FIGURE 122–3. Technique of end-to-end graft-renal artery anastomosis following spatulation of the artery anteriorly and the graft posteriorly, and end-to-side graft-aorta anastomosis following creation of a common orifice between a branch and the central lumen of the saphenous vein.

flow is reestablished, and the heparin effect is reversed with slow IV administration of 1.2 mg of protamine sulfate for each 100 units of heparin given previously. Assessment of the reconstruction is undertaken with duplex scanning or by evaluation of flow with a directional Doppler device. Although intraoperative arteriography is seldom necessary, all patients should undergo postoperative arteriography before discharge to establish the adequacy of the recon-

structive procedure and to provide a baseline for continued graft follow-up.

In the treatment of fibrodysplastic renovascular disease, autologous vein grafts are usually preferred for reconstructions in adults,[79] and autologous hypogastric artery grafts are favored when for bypass procedures in children (Fig. 122–5).[75, 92] The hypogastric artery may also be used in adult reconstructions.[44, 47] Vein grafts are procured carefully,

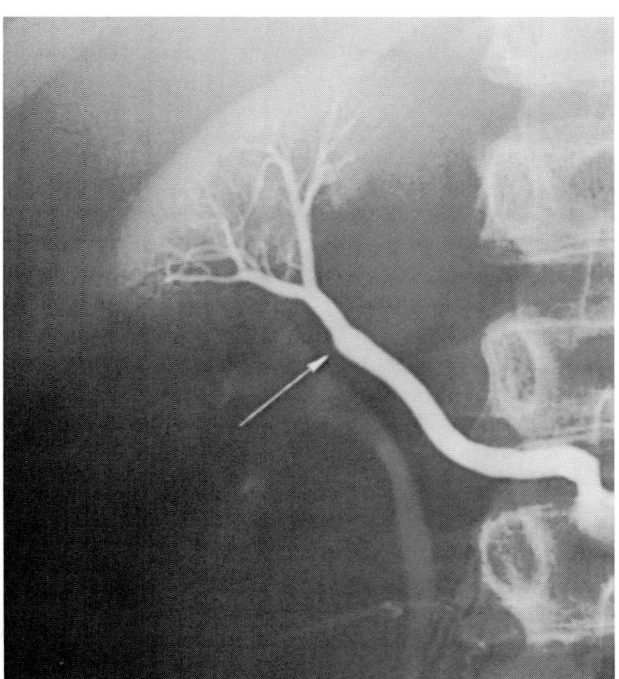

FIGURE 122–4. Autogenous saphenous vein aortcrenal bypass to a segmental artery. Note the ovoid appearance of the renal anastomosis (*arrow*). (From Fry WJ, Ernst CB, Stanley JC, Brink BE: Renovascular hypertension in the pediatric patient. Arch Surg 107:692–698, 1973. Copyright 1973, American Medical Association.)

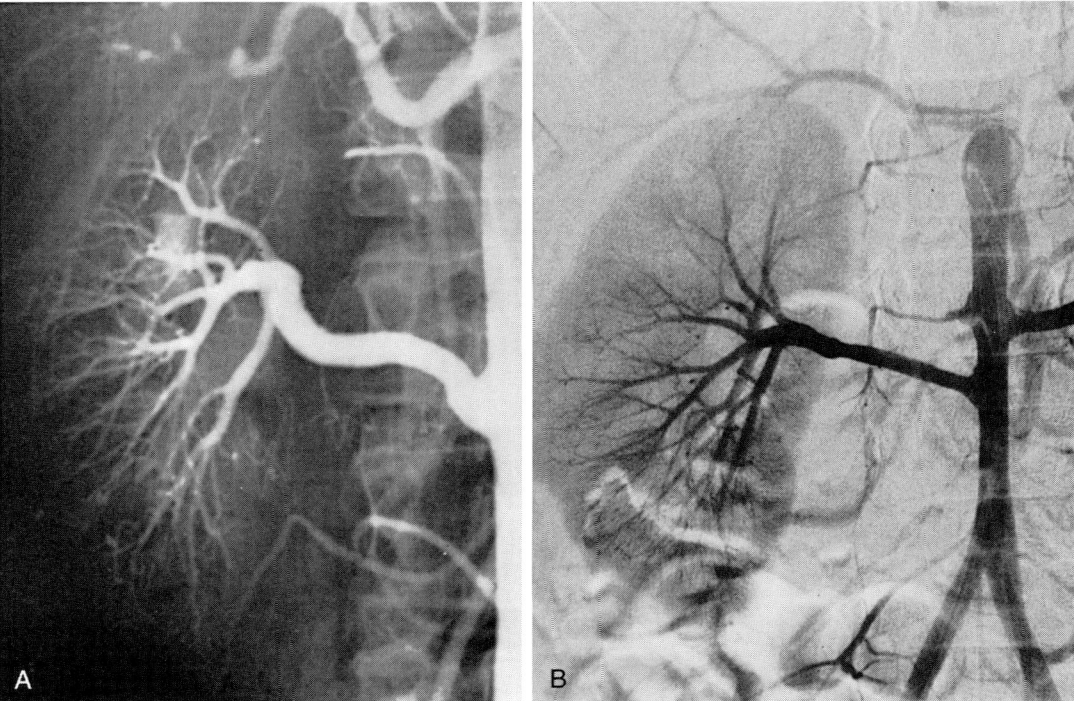

FIGURE 122–5. *A,* Autogenous saphenous vein aortorenal graft. *B,* Autogenous iliac artery aortorenal graft. (*A,* From Stanley JC, Graham LM: Renovascular hypertension. *In* Miller DC, Roon AJ [eds]: Diagnosis and Management of Peripheral Vascular Disease. Menlo Park, Calif., Addison-Wesley, 1981, pp 321–353. *B,* From Stanley JC, Zelenock GB, Messina LM, et al: Pediatric renovascular hypotension: A thirty-year experience of operative treatment. J Vasc Surg 21:212, 1995.)

handled gently, and irrigated cautiously with heparinized blood prior to implantation. Procurement of the hypogastric artery for use as an interposition graft proceeds in a similar manner, with the surgeon taking care not to cause excessive vessel wall trauma. Synthetic grafts of fabricated polyester (Dacron) or expanded polytetrafluoroethylene (PTFE) may also be used for main renal artery reconstructive procedures,[34, 37] but these conduits are less compliant and are technically more difficult to use when revascularizations involve small dysplastic segmental vessels.

Arterial dilation, alone or in conjunction with a bypass procedure, is sometimes used for treatment of intraparenchymal intimal and medial fibrodysplastic stenoses. After the renal artery is exposed in a manner similar to that noted previously, the patient receives systematic anticoagulation therapy, and rigid cylindrical-tipped dilators are advanced through a transverse arteriotomy in the main renal artery. Dilators are thoroughly lubricated with heparinized blood or a silicone solution to lessen intimal drag. The stenotic area is progressively dilated in increments of 0.5 mm by careful passage of increasingly larger dilators. Dilators 1.0 mm larger than the diameter of the normal proximal artery should not be used because they may disrupt the vessel wall. The role of operative dilation of fibrodysplastic renal artery stenoses using standard axial balloon catheters remains uncertain.

An increasing proportion of patients undergoing surgical management of renal artery fibrodysplasia display complex renal artery branch vessel disease.[63, 3] The method of repair depends upon whether the disease extends beyond the primary renal artery bifurcation. In situ repair can be ac-

complished for virtually all lesions that do not extend beyond the primary bifurcation into second or third order branches. Ex vivo repair is often used for more extensive patterns of complex disease.[2, 94, 100]

For the more proximal segmental disease pattern, three alternative methods of repair can be applied. The first calls for separate implantations of the renal arteries into a single conduit. This is usually accomplished with a proximal end-to-side anastomosis and a distal end-to-end anastomosis to an autograft. If a non-reversed branching segment of saphenous vein in which the valves have been cut or a hypogastric artery with its branches is used as the bypass conduit, separate graft-to-renal artery anastomoses may be undertaken in an end-to-end manner.

In the second method, an in situ anastomosis of the involved renal arteries is performed in a side-to-side manner so as to form a common orifice. The autograft is then anastomosed to the single channel created by this arterial union (Fig. 122–6).

The third method involves implantation of an affected artery, beyond its diseased segment, into an adjacent normal artery in an end-to-side manner. Such an anastomosis usually involves second-order branches of the renal artery (Fig. 122–7), but implantation may be undertaken into the main renal artery if the anastomosis can be fashioned without tension.

Ex vivo repairs require mobilization of the entire kidney, including the accompanying vasculature and ureter to the pelvis. The renal artery and vein are controlled with vascular clamps and transected, allowing the kidney to be placed on the abdominal wall. A tourniquet around the intact

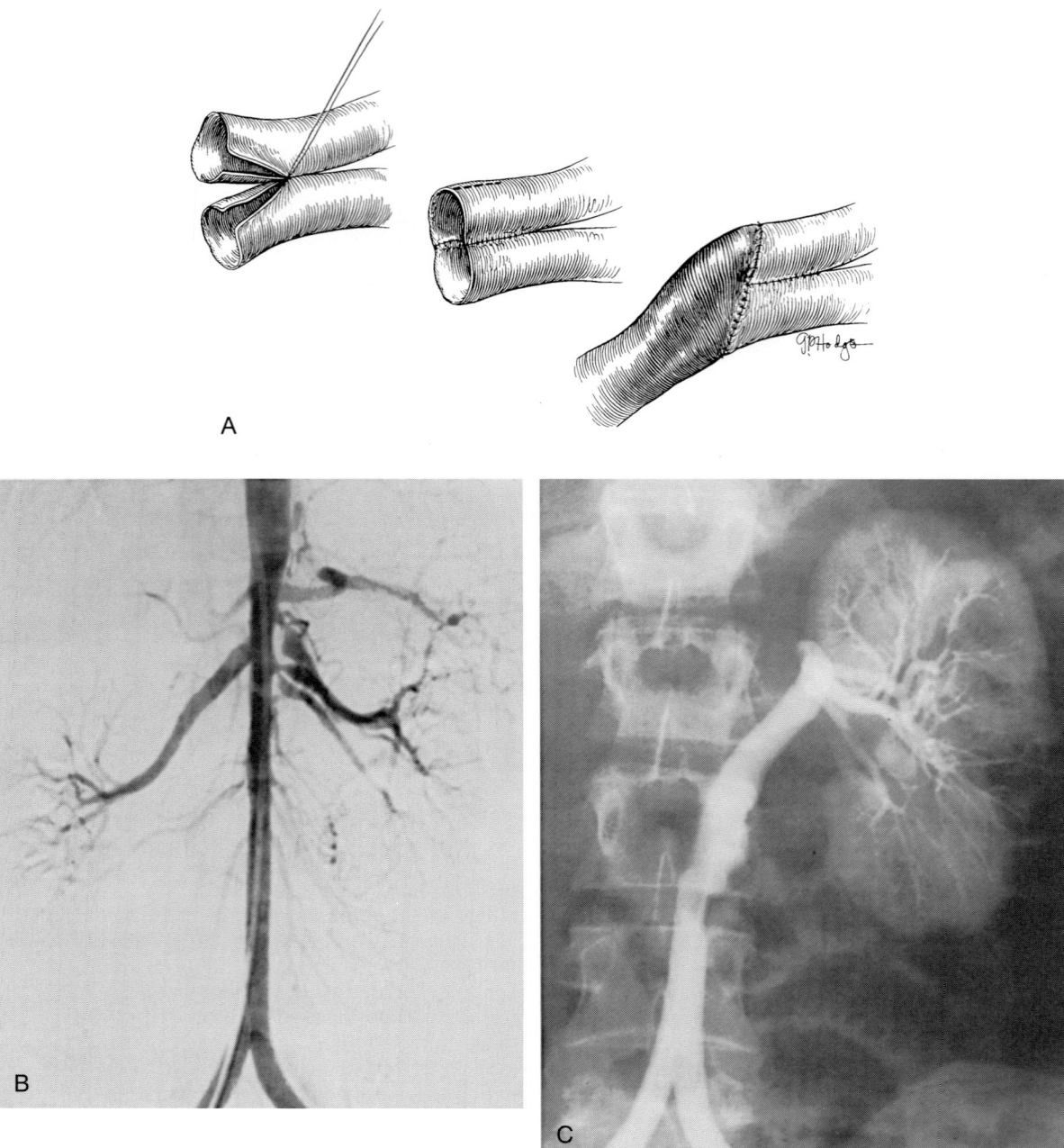

FIGURE 122–6. *A,* Revascularization of multiple renal arteries with side-to-side anastomoses of affected vessels followed by the anastomosis of a vein graft to their common orifice. *B* and *C,* Preoperative and postoperative arteriograms of this type of repair, with three vessels joined together before being anastomosed to a vein graft. (*A,* From Ernst BC, Fry WJ, Stanley JC: Surgical treatment of renovascular hypertension: Revascularization with autogenous vein. *In* Stanley JC, Ernst CB, Fry WJ [eds]: Renovascular Hypertension. Philadelphia, WB Saunders, 1984, p 284. *B* and *C,* From Stanley JC, Fry WJ: Pediatric renal artery occlusive disease and renovascular hypertension. Etiology, diagnosis and operative treatment. Arch Surg 116:669–676, 1981. Copyright 1981, American Medical Association.)

ureter prevents collateral blood flow to the kidney. Ringer's lactate solution at 4°C is used to flush the kidney until the venous effluent has cleared. The kidney is connected to the perfusion manifold of the dissecting platform, which has been placed on the lower abdominal wall (Fig. 122–8).[63] Hypothermic profusion is begun, monitored by a perfusionist, and the kidney surface is cooled to 8° to 12°C.

Meticulous dissection of the renal artery is undertaken to the distal level of visible and palpable disease. After the

renal artery branches are mobilized, an iliac artery arterial autograft is excised and flushed with Ringer's lactate solution. Sequential branch anastomoses are performed end-to-end with fine interrupted sutures (Fig. 122–9).[63] For vessels smaller than 2 mm in diameter, anastomoses are performed over a metal dilator to prevent an anastomotic narrowing. After the perfusion cannulas are disconnected, the reconstructed kidney is repositioned in the retroperitoneum. The proximal aortic anastomosis is performed in an end-to-

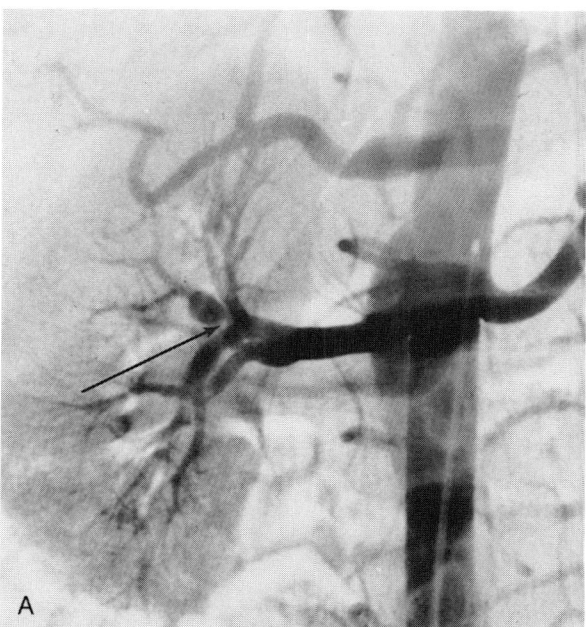
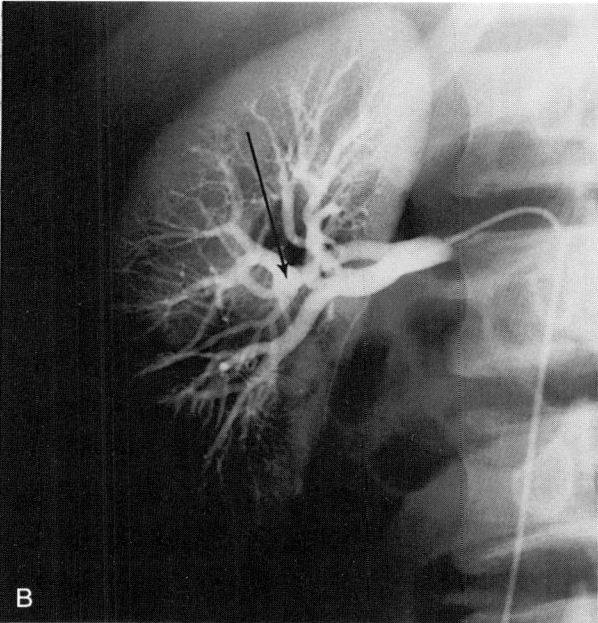

FIGURE 122–7. Reimplantation of segmental renal artery, beyond its stenosis, into the adjacent segmental renal artery. *A,* Preoperative arteriogram documenting stenosis and poststenotic dilation *(arrow). B,* Postoperative arteriogram demonstrates widely patent anastomosis *(arrow). (A* and *B,* from Stanley JC, Zelenock GB, Messina LM, et al: Pediatric renovascular hypertension: A thirty-year experience of operative treatment. J Vasc Surg 21:212, 1995.)

side manner, and the renal vein is reanastomosed to the transected proximal renal vein on the left or to a new site on the lateral vena cava on the right. The venous clamps, followed by the arterial clamps, are removed and the ureteral tourniquet released around the kidney can be reperfused.

Current indications for in situ versus ex vivo repair have become better defined. In general, in situ repair is appropriate when a patient has two kidneys requiring primary operation limited to the first renal bifurcation. Ex vivo repair with hypothermic perfusion has the advantage of uncompromised exposure beyond the limits of complex branch disease and should be applied for the following:

• Reoperation for failed prior renal arterial repairs
• Multiple branch artery lesions in a solitary kidney

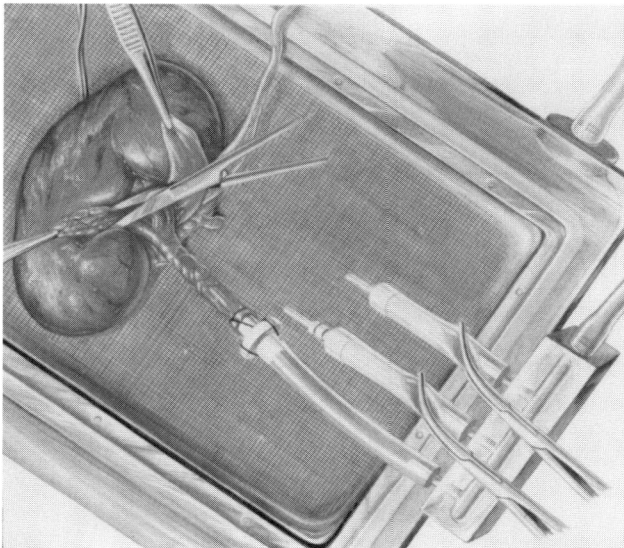

FIGURE 122–8. Illustration of dissection or renal hilus ex vivo. Kidney is perfused through one cannula on perfusion manifold of dissection platform. (From Murray SP, Kent C, Salvatierra O, et al: Complex branch renovascular disease: Management options and late results. J Vasc Surg 20:338, 1984.)

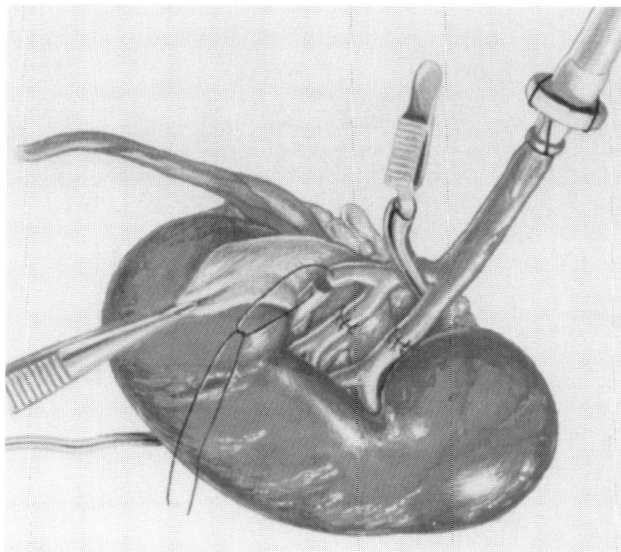

FIGURE 122–9. Ex vivo multi-branched arterial autograft repair. Two of three branch anastomoses are completed, and the lower one is being sutured. (From Murray SP, Kent C, Salvatierra O, et al: Complex branch renovascular disease: Management options and late results. J Vasc Surg 20:338, 1984.)

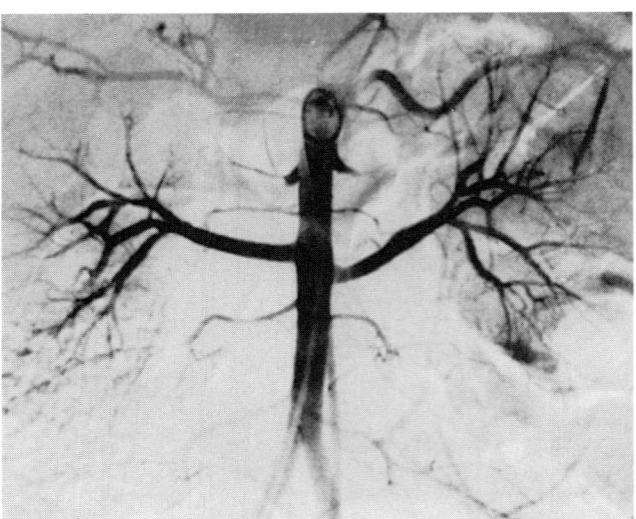

FIGURE 122–10. Reimplantation of main renal arteries beyond orificial stenosis into the aorta. (From Stanley JC, Zelenock GB, Messina LM, et al: Pediatric renovascular hypertension: A thirty-year experience of operative treatment. J Vasc Surg 21:212, 1995.)

- Extension of branch vessel disease into the renal hilus
- Certain branch artery stenoses in a children
- Traumatic injuries involving the renal hilus
- Stenoses involving multiple renal arteries

In these circumstances, the inserted branched arterial autograft allows the restoration of nearly normal renal artery anatomy. A durable repair, essential for the younger patients

affected by this pattern of disease who anticipate a normal life span after renal revascularization, is achieved.

Alternative means of revascularization may be appropriate in select circumstances. In the case of left-sided lesions in adults, an in situ splenorenal bypass offers an alternative to aortorenal bypass.[46, 61] However, before undertaking the latter, one must document that the proximal celiac artery is not involved with an occlusive lesion that might perpetuate the hypertensive state following such a bypass. Splenorenal bypasses for treatment of pediatric renovascular stenoses should be avoided. Results from this approach in these younger patients have been very poor.[65] This low success rate may reflect the small splenic artery caliber in children, but it is more likely due to proximal celiac artery stenoses.[84]

Treatment of pediatric orificial renal artery stenoses deserve comment, in that aortic reimplantation of the vessel beyond its disease has become favored over bypass procedures.[91] The vessel is transected beyond the stenotic segment and spatulated anteriorly and posteriorly so as to provide a generous patch for implantation (Fig. 122–10). For arteries 2 to 3 mm in diameter, the anastomosis should be performed with multiple interrupted sutures. The kidney may be mobilized medially during these reconstruction to reduce any potential tension on the reimplanted renal artery.

Operative treatment of fibrodysplastic renovascular hypertension associated with aortic hypoplasia or coarctation is often complex (Fig. 122–11). Thoracoabdominal bypasses and local aortoplasties are the most common aortic operations, with concomitant renal artery construction performed in a standard manner.[31, 35] The reported operative

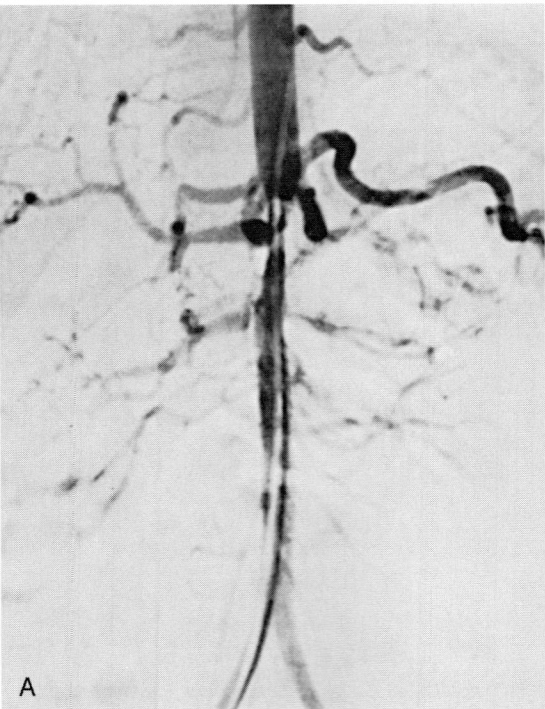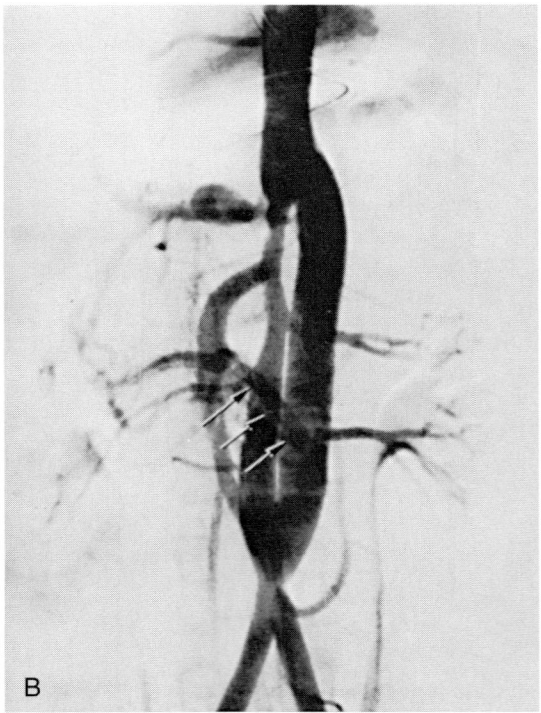

FIGURE 122–11. Complex renal reconstructive procedure for suprarenal aortic coarctation and stenosis (*arrow*) of the right superior renal artery (A) by thoracoabdominal bypass and saphenous vein bypass to the obstructed renal artery (B). (A and B, From Graham LM, Zelenock GB, Erlandson EE, et al: Abdominal aortic coarctation and segmental hypoplasia. Surgery 86:519, 1979.)

mortality rate for these extensive operations approaches 8%, but nearly 90% of the survivors benefit from such interventions.[31, 58]

Complications

The critical consequences of graft stenosis or occlusion, including loss of the kidney, attest to the importance of a properly planned and executed initial renal reconstructive procedure.[26, 31] Reoperations for complications of renal artery reconstructive surgery undertaken in pediatric and adult renal artery fibrodysplasia entail secondary nephrectomy rates up to 60% and 39%, respectively.[88]

The incidence of early postoperative aortorenal vein graft thrombosis is 2% to 7%.[3] Early postoperative thrombosis after arterial autografts appears to be less frequent.[53, 63, 93] Postoperative graft thrombosis occurs more frequently in small-diameter arteries and branch vessel reconstructions. Many experienced surgeons emphasize the importance of intraoperative duplex ultrasound assessment to determine the technical adequacy of the renal revascularization and early correction of significant defects at the time of primary procedure.[3]

Arteriography is essential to assess the status of small branch vessel reconstructions and equivocal reconstructions. When clinical circumstances suggest early postoperative graft occlusion, such as episodic hypertension, arteriography is the diagnostic study of choice. Radionuclide studies are of limited use in detecting postoperative graft occlusions, in that many kidneys have extensive preexisting collateral circulation that provides for relatively normal renal function and perfusion patterns despite acutely occluded grafts.

Late anastomotic stenoses have become less common with improved vascular surgical techniques. In particular, the creation of generous ovoid graft-to-renal artery anastomoses has reduced the frequency of this complication. Nevertheless late graft stenoses may be a consequence of intimal hyperplasia, clamp injury, and overzealous advancement of large dilators through stenoses or "sounding of segmental vessels." Overall, late vein graft stenoses can be encountered in up to 8% of aortorenal vein grafts.[24, 21] Late stenoses of aortorenal arterial autografts are rare.[43, 63, 93]

Late vein graft dilation, documented in 20% to 44% of aortorenal saphenous vein grafts, usually appears as a nonprogressive, uniform increase in vein graft diameter.[22, 77] Marked aneurysmal changes affect approximately 2% of aortorenal grafts in adults[77] and 20% of vein grafts placed in pediatric patients (Fig. 122–12).[81] Other investigators have reported a lower incidence of this complication.[22] The predisposition toward dilation of vein grafts in children may reflect anatomic variations in the number and distribution of the vasa vasorum in their veins. The veins in children may be particularly susceptible to ischemic injury during transplantation. Expansion and aneurysmal dilation have also occurred with renovascular reconstructions using autogenous arterial grafts, but the frequency of this complication is much lower than that affecting veins.[22, 93] Luminal thrombus formation and distal embolization of microthrombi can occur in aneurysmal veins and are the reason some advocate replacement or plication of dilated vein grafts.[86]

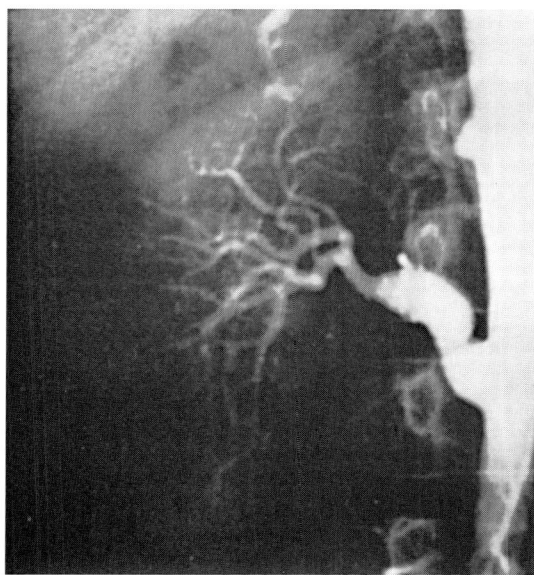

FIGURE 122–12. Aneurysmal dilatation of an autogenous saphenous vein aortorenal graft. This complication is most likely to affect pediatric patients. (From Stanley JC, Ernst CB, Fry WJ: Fate of 100 aortorenal vein grafts: Characteristics of late graft expansion, aneurysmal dilatation, and stenosis. Surgery 74:931, 1973.)

Outcome of Surgical Therapy

Beneficial outcomes after operative intervention for renovascular hypertension are directly proportional to the accurate identification of appropriate surgical candidates and performance of an appropriate reconstructive procedure. The Cooperative Study of Renovascular Hypertension was undertaken nearly three decades ago in an attempt to define the optimal diagnostic and therapeutic management of renal artery occlusive disease. The less than optimal results from the Study probably reflect errors in patient selection and early technical failures.[27, 29] The Study's overall results from 577 surgical procedures undertaken in 520 patients with all forms of renovascular hypertension included 51%, cure; 15%, improvement; and 34%, failure. As surgical techniques and new methods in patient selection evolved, overall results improved.[78] Patients with renal artery fibrodysplasia were more likely to respond favorably after operative intervention than those with atherosclerotic disease.

The results of surgical treatment of renal artery fibrodysplasia document excellent outcomes for control of arterial hypertension. During the 1980s and 1990s, between 90% and 95% of properly selected patients either are cured of or have gained more control of their renovascular hypertension (Tables 122–2 and 122–3). These results relate to the evolution of better reconstructive techniques, as evidenced by the reduction of primary nephrectomy rates.[80, 15] In addition, operative mortality rates approach 0% in most series of surgical treatment of renal arterial fibrodysplasia. Thus, the mortality rate of 3.4%, as noted for the surgical treatment of renal fibrodysplasia in the Cooperative Study, would be unacceptable in contemporary practice.

Finally, although renal failure secondary to renal artery fibrodysplasia is much less common than that seen secondary to atherosclerotic disease, long-term follow-up shows excellent preservation of renal function.[3, 20, 104]

TABLE 122–2. RESULTS OF SURGICAL THERAPY FOR RENOVASCULAR HYPERTENSION DUE TO FIBRODYSPLASIA IN ADULTS

MEDICAL CENTER	NO. OF PATIENTS	POSTOPERATIVE STATUS (%)*			OPERATIVE MORTALITY RATE (%)
		Cure	Improvement	Failure	
University of Michigan (1964–1980)[87]	114	55	39	6	0
Baylor College of Medicine (1959–1979)[46]	113	43	24	33	0†
Cleveland Clinic (1975–1984)[64]	104	63	30	7	0
University of California, San Francisco (1964–1980)[88]	77	66	32	1	0
University of Essen (1971–1979)[39]	75	63	24	13	0
Mayo Clinic (1965–1968)[37]	63	66	24	10	NA
Vanderbilt University (1977–1982)[19]	56	77	19	1	0
University of Leiden (1962–1982)[96]	53	53	34	11	1.9
Columbia University (1962–1976)[10]	42	76	14	10	NA
Wake Forest Medical Center, Winston-Salem, NC (1987–1994)[3]	40	33	57	10	0
University of Lund, Sweden (1971–1977)[7]	40	66	24	10	0

*Criteria for blood pressure response are defined in cited publications.
†No deaths in 100 isolated renal reconstructions; data on 13 patients with associated arteriosclerosis unavailable.
NA = Not available.

A distinct change in the clinical profile, clinical evaluation, and operative management of patients with renal arterial fibrodysplasia has been documented in many centers.[3, 63, 66] Patients presenting for treatment are significantly older, have had a longer duration of hypertension, and a have a higher prevalence of extrarenal atherosclerosis. Most significantly, a higher frequency of branch vessel involvement requiring complex repairs is found consistently. At the University of California, San Francisco, patients presenting with a complex branch vessel pattern secondary to arterial fibrodysplasia had solitary kidneys in 18% of cases; 9% required concomitant aortic replacement, and 10% represented failed previous operations. Thus, although the overall beneficial response rate remains similar to that in

earlier reports, the cure rate is generally lower, reflecting the changes in the overall clinical profile of the patient.

Outcome after management of complex branch renal artery disease deserves special comment. At the University of California, San Francisco, a recent report describing the outcome of 68 consecutive patients with complex branch vessel disease was notable for a renal salvage of 98.8%.[96, 97] No operative deaths occurred. Renal function and control of blood pressure was assessed at a mean follow-up of 7.5 years. Of the 68 patients, 46% underwent follow-up angiography at a mean of 52 months after operation. No evidence of late graft failure was documented. Hypertension was cured or improved in 51 of the 53 patients (96%) with a proven patent reconstruction. Renal function was

TABLE 122–3. RESULTS OF SURGICAL TREATMENT OF RENOVASCULAR HYPERTENSION DUE TO FIBRODYSPLASIA IN CHILDREN

MEDICAL CENTER	NO. OF PATIENTS	NO. OF PRIMARY PROCEDURES		NO. OF SECONDARY PROCEDURES	POSTOPERATIVE STATUS (%)*			OPERATIVE MORTALITY RATE (%)
		Arterial Reconstruction	Nephrectomy		Cure	Improvement	Failure	
University of Michigan (1963–1993)[78]†	57	50	7	14	79	19	2.0	0
Cleveland Clinic (1955–1977)[6,62]	27	22	11	5	59	18.5	18.5	4
University of California, Los Angeles[85] (1967–1977)	26	19		7	84.5	7.5	4	4
Vanderbilt University[47]‡ (1962–1977)	21	15	8	4	68	24	8	0
University of California, San Francisco[55] (1960–1974)	14	10	4	2	86	7	0	7

*Criteria for blood pressure response are defined in cited publications. Data are expressed to nearest 0.5%.
†Results include data from six patients treated at University of Texas Southwestern Medical Center at Dallas.
‡Results include data from four patients with parenchymal disease treated by nephrectomy. A more recent, but less detailed review includes 28 patients with cure, improvement, and failure rates of 72%, 21%, and 7%, respectively.[11]

improved in four patients with ex vivo repairs, unchanged in 59 patients, and worse in only three patients, all of whom had undergone in situ repair.

REFERENCES

1. Aldigier J. Plouin PF, Guyene TT, et al: Comparison of the hormonal and renal effects of captopril in severe essential and renovascular hypertension. Am J Cardiol 49:1447, 1982.
2. Alimi Y, Mercier C, Pellissier JF, et al: Fibromuscular disease of the renal artery: A new histopathologic classification. Ann Vasc Surg 6:220, 1992.
3. Anderson CA, Hansen JK, Benjamin ME, et al: Renal artery fibromuscular dysplasia: Results of current surgical therapy. J Vasc Surg 22:207, 1995.
4. Baumgartner I, Triller J, Mahler F: Patency of percutaneous transluminal renal angioplasty: A prospective sonographic study. Kidney Int 51:798, 1997.
5. Belzer FO, Raczkowski A: Ex vivo renal artery reconstruction with autotransplantation. Surgery 92:642, 1982.
6. Benjamin SP, Dustan HP, Gifford RW Jr, et al: Stenosing renal artery disease in children: Clinicopathologic correlation in 20 surgically treated cases. Cleve Clin Q 43:197, 1976.
7. Bergentz SE, Ericsson BF, Husberg B: Technique and complications in the surgical treatment of renovascular hypertension. Acta Chir Scand 145:143, 1979.
8. Bonelli FS, McKusick MA, Textor SC, et al: Renal artery angioplasty: Technical results and clinical outcome in 320 patients. Mayo Clin Proc 70:1041, 1995.
9. Bookstein JJ, Walter JF, Stanley JC, et al: Pharmacoangiographic manipulation of renal collateral blood flow. Circulation 54:328, 1976.
10. Buda JA, Baer L, Parra-Carrillo J, et al: Predictability of surgical response in renovascular hypertension. Arch Surg 111:1243, 1976.
11. Buhler FR, Laragh JH, Baer L, et al: Propranolol inhibition of renin secretion. N Engl J Med 287:1209, 1972.
12. Casalini E, Sfondrini M, Fossali E: Two-year clinical follow-up of children and adolescents after percutaneous transluminal angioplasty for renovascular hypertension. Invest Radiol 30:1, 1995.
13. Case DB, Atlas SA, Marion RM, et al: Long-term efficacy of captopril in renovascular and essential hypertension. Am J Cardiol 49:1440, 1982.
14. Chibaro EA, Libertino JA, Novick AC: Use of the hepatic circulation for renal revascularization. Ann Surg 199:406, 1984.
15. Chrysant SG, Dunn M, Marples M, et al: Severe reversible azotemia from captopril therapy: Report of three cases and review of the literature. Arch Intern Med 143:347,1983.
16. Cluzel P, Raynaud A, Beyssen B, et al: Stenoses of renal branch arteries in fibromuscular dysplasia: Results of percutaneous transluminal angioplasty. Radiology 193:227, 1994.
17. Davidson R, Barri Y, Wilcox CS: Predictors of cure of hypertension in fibromuscular renovascular disease. Am J Kidney Dis 28:334, 1996.
18. Dean RH: Renovascular hypertension during childhood. In Dean RH, O'Neil JA Jr (eds): Vascular Disorders of Childhood. Philadelphia, Lea & Febiger, 1983, pp 77–96.
19. Dean RH: Renovascular hypertension. Curr Probl Surg 22:1–67, 1985.
20. Dean RH, Englund R, Dupont WD, et al: Retrieval of renal function by revascularization: Study of preoperative outcome predictors. Ann Surg 202:367, 1985.
21. Dean RH, Krueger TC, Whiteneck JM, et al: Operative management of renovascular hypertension: Results after a follow-up of fifteen to twenty-three years. J Vasc Surg 1:234, 1984.
22. Dean RH, Wilson JP, Burko H, et al: Saphenous vein aortorenal bypass grafts: Serial arteriographic study. Ann Surg 130:469, 1974.
23. Detection, evaluation and treatment of renovascular hypertension: Final report. Working group on renovascular hypertension. Arch Intern Med 147:820, 1987.
24. Ekelund J, Gerlock J Jr, Goncharenko V, et al: Angiographic findings following surgical treatment for renovascular hypertension. Radiology 126:345, 1978.
25. Ernst CB, Bookstein JJ, Montie J, et al: Renal vein renin ratios and collateral vessels in renovascular hypertension. Arch Surg 104:496, 1972.
26. Foster JH, Dean RH, Pinkerton JA, et al: Ten years' experience with surgical management of renovascular hypertension. Ann Surg 177:755, 1973.
27. Foster JH, Maxwell SS, Bleifer KH, et al: Renovascular occlusive disease: Results of operative treatment. JAMA 231:1043, 1975.
28. Franklin SS, Smith RD: A comparison of enalapril plus hydrochlorothiazide with standard triple therapy in renovascular hypertension. Nephron 44(Suppl 1):73, 1986.
29. Franklin SS, Young JD Jr, Maxwell MH, et al: Operative morbidity and mortality in renovascular disease. JAMA 231:1148, 1975.
30. Goncharenko V, Gerlock AJ, Shaff MI, et al: Progression of renal artery fibromuscular dysplasia in 42 patients as seen on angiography. Radiology 139:45, 1981.
31. Graham LM, Zelenock GB, Erlandson EE, et al: Abdominal aortic coarctation and segmental hypoplasia. Surgery 86:519, 1979.
32. Grim CE, Luft FC, Yune HY, et al: Percutaneous transluminal dilatation in the treatment of renal vascular hypertension. Ann Intern Med 95:439, 1981.
33. Grim CE, Yune HY, Donahue JP, et al: Unilateral renal vascular hypertension: Surgery vs. dilation. Vasa 11:367, 1982.
34. Gruntzig A, Vetter W, Meier B, et al: Treatment of renovascular hypertension with percutaneous transluminal dilatation of a renal artery stenosis. Lancet 1:801, 1978.
35. Hagg A, Aberg H, Eriksson I, et al: Fibromuscular dysplasia of the renal artery-management and outcome. Acta Chir Scand 153:15, 1987.
36. Harrison EG, McCormack LJ: Pathologic classification of renal artery disease in renovascular hypertension. Mayo Clin Proc 46:161, 1971.
37. Henriksson C, Bjorkerud S, Nilson AE, Pettersson S: Natural history of renal artery aneurysm elucidated by repeated angiography and pathoanatomical studies. Eur Urol 11:244, 1985.
38. Hodsman GP, Brown JJ, Cummings AMM, et al: Enalapril in treatment of hypertension with renal artery stenosis: Changes in blood pressure, renin, angiotensin I and II, renal function, and body composition. Am J Med 77:52, 1984.
39. Hricik DE, Browning PK, Kopelman R, et al: Captopril-induced renal insufficiency in patients with bilateral renal-artery stenosis or renal-artery stenosis in a solitary kidney. N Engl J Med 308:373, 1983.
40. Hunt JC, Strong CG: Renovascular hypertension: Mechanisms, natural history and treatment. Am J Cardiol 32:562, 1973.
41. Jakubowski HD, Eigler FW, Montag H: Results of surgery in fibrodysplastic renal artery stenosis. World J Surg 5:859, 1981.
42. Karas RH, Caur W, Tassi L, Mendelsohn ME: Inhibition of vascular smooth muscle cell growth by estrogen. Circulation 88:I-325, 1993.
43. Kaufman JJ: Renovascular hypertension: The UCLA experience. J Urol 112:139, 1979.
44. Kaufmann JJ: Long-term results of aortorenal Dacron grafts in the treatment of renal artery stenosis. J Urol 111:298, 1974.
45. Keith TA III: Renovascular hypertension in black patients. Hypertension 4:438, 1982.
46. Khauli RB, Novick AC, Ziegelbaum M: Splenorenal bypass in the treatment of renal artery stenosis: Experience with sixty-nine cases. J Vasc Surg 2:547, 1985.
47. Lagneau P, Michel JB, Charrat JM: Use of polytetrafluoroethylene grafts for renal bypass. J Vasc Surg 5:738, 1987.
48. Lawrie GM, Morris GC Jr, Soussou ID, et al: Late results of reconstructive surgery for renovascular disease. Ann Surg 191:528, 1980.
49. Lawson JD, Boerth R, Foster JH, et al: Diagnosis and management of renovascular hypertension in children. Arch Surg 122:1307, 1977.
49a. Leadbetter WFG, Burkland CE: Hypertension in unilateral renal disease. J Urol 39:611, 1938.
50. Lewin A, Blaufox MD, Castle H, et al: Apparent prevalence of curable hypertension in the Hypertension Detection and Follow-up Program. Arch Intern Med 145:424, 1985.
51. Luscher TF, Greminger P, Kuhlmann TJ, et al: Renal venous renin determinations in renovascular hypertension: Diagnostic and prognostic value in unilateral renal artery stenosis treated by surgery or percutaneous transluminal angioplasty. Nephron 44(Suppl 1):17, 1986.
52. Luscher TF, Keller HM, Imhof HG, et al: Fibromuscular hyperplasia: Extension of the disease and therapeutic outcome. Results of the University Hospital Zurich Cooperative Study on Fibromuscular Hyperplasia. Nephron 44(Suppl 1):109, 1986.

53. Lye CR, String ST, Wylie EJ, et al: Aortorenal arterial auto-grafts: Late observations. Arch Surg 110:1321, 1975.

54. Mahler F, Triller J, Weidmarim P, et al: Complications in percutaneous transluminal dilation of renal arteries. Nephron 44(Suppl 1):60, 1986.

55. Martin EC, Diamond NG, Casarella WJ: Percutaneous transluminal angioplasty in non-atherosclerotic disease. Radiology 135:27, 1980.

56. Martin LG, Price RB, Casarella WJ, et al: Percutaneous angioplasty in clinical management of renovascular hypertension: Initial and long-term results. Radiology 155:629, 1985.

57. McCormick LJ, Hazard JB, Poutasse EF: Obstructive lesions of the renal artery associated with remediable hypertension. Am J Pathol 34:582,1958.

58. Messina LM, Reilly LM, Goldstone J, et al: Middle aortic syndrome: Effectiveness and durability of complex revascularization techniques. Ann Surg 204:331, 1986.

59. Millan VG, McCauley J, Kopelman RI, et al: Percutaneous transluminal renal angioplasty in nonatherosclerotic renovascular hypertension: Long-term results. Hypertension 7:668, 1985.

60. Miller GA, Ford KK, Braum SD, et al: Percutaneous transluminal angioplasty vs. surgery for renovascular hypertension. Am J Roentgenol 144:447, 1985.

61. Moncure AC, Brewster DC, Darling RC, et al: Use of the splenic and hepatic arteries for renal revascularization. J Vasc Surg 3:196, 1986.

62. Muller FB, Sealey JE, Case DB, et al: The captopril test for identifying disease in hypertensive patients. Am J Med 80:633, 1986.

63. Murray SP, Kent CK, Salvatierra O, et al: Complex branch renovascular disease: Management options and late results. J Vasc Surg 20:338, 1994.

64. Novick AC, Steward BH, Straffon RA, et al: Autogenous arterial grafts in the treatment of renal artery stenosis. J Urol 118:919, 1977.

65. Novick AC, Straffon RA, Steward BH, et al: Surgical treatment of renovascular hypertension in the pediatric patient. J Urol 119:794, 1978.

66. Novick AC, Ziegelbaum M, Vidt DG, et al: Trends in surgical revascularization for renal artery disease: Ten years' experience. JAMA 257:498, 1987.

67. Palubinskis AJ, Ripley HR: Fibromuscular hyperplasia in extra renal arteries. Radiology 82:451, 1964.

68. Rodriguez-Perez JC, Plaza C, Reyes R, et al: Treatment of renovascular hypertension with percutaneous transluminal angioplasty: Experience in Spain. J Vasc Interv Radiol 5:101, 1994.

69. Saffitz JE, Totty WG, McClennan BL, et al: Percutaneous transluminal angioplasty: Radiological-pathological correlation. Radiology 141:651, 1981.

70. Sarkar R, Messina LM: Renovascular disease: Pathology of renal artery occlusive Disease. In Ernst CB, Stanley JC (eds): Current Therapy of Vascular Surgery, 3rd ed. St. Louis, CV Mosby, 1985, pp 764–774.

71. Schwarten DE, Yune HY, Klatte EC, et al: Clinical experience with percutaneous transluminal angioplasty (PTA) of stenotic renal arteries. Radiology 135:601, 1980.

72. Simon N, Franklin SS, Bleifer KH, et al: Clinical characteristics of renovascular hypertension. JAMA 220:1209, 1972.

73. Sos TA, Saddekini S, Pickering TG, et al: Technical aspects of percutaneous transluminal angioplasty in renovascular disease. Nephron 44(Suppl 1):45, 1986.

74. Sottiurai V, Fry WJ, Stanley JC. Ultrastructural characteristic of experimental arterial medial fibroplasia induced by vasa vasorum occlusion. J Surg Res 24:169, 1978.

75. Stanley JC: Renal vascular disease and renovascular hypertension in children. Urol Clin 11:451, 1984.

76. Stanley JC: Surgery of failed percutaneous transluminal renal artery angioplasty. In Bergan JJ, Yao JST (eds): Reoperative Arterial Surgery. Orlando, Fla, Grune & Stratton, 1986, pp 441–454.

77. Stanley JC, Ernst CB, Fry WJ: Fate of 100 aortorenal vein grafts: Characteristics of late graft expansion, aneurysmal dilation, and stenosis. Surgery 74:931, 1973.

78. Stanley JC, Ernst CB, Fry WJ: Surgical treatment of renovascular hypertension: Results in Specific Patient Subgroups. In Stanley JC, Ernst CB, Fry WJ (eds): Renovascular Hypertension. Philadelphia, WB Saunders, 1984, pp 363–371.

79. Stanley JC, Fry WJ: Renovascular hypertension secondary to arterial fibrodysplasia in adults: Criteria for operation and results of surgical therapy. Arch Surg 110:922, 1975.

80. Stanley JC, Fry WJ: Surgical treatment of renovascular hypertension. Arch Surg 112:1291, 1977.

81. Stanley JC, Fry WJ: Pediatric renal artery occlusive disease and renovascular hypertension: Etiology, diagnosis and operative treatment. Arch Surg 116:669, 1981.

82. Stanley JC, Gewertz BL, Bove EL, et al: Arterial fibrodysplasia: Histopathologic character and current etiologic concepts. Arch Surg 110:561, 1975.

83. Stanley JC, Gewertz BL, Fry WJ: Renal systemic renin indices and renal vein renin ratios as prognostic indicators in remedial renovascular hypertension. J Surg Res 20:149, 1976.

84. Stanley JC, Graham LM, Whitehouse WM Jr, et al: Developmental occlusive disease of the abdominal aorta, splanchnic and renal arteries. Am J Surg 142:190, 1981.

85. Stanley JC, Wakefield TW: See Chapter 23, Arterial Fibrodysplasia, in Vol. 1 of this text.

86. Stanley JC, Whitehouse WM Jr, Graham LM: Complications of renal revascularization. In Bernhard VM, Towne JB (eds): Complications in Vascular Surgery. New York, Grune & Stratton, 1980, pp 189–218.

87. Stanley JC, Whitehouse WM Jr, Graham LM, et al: Operative therapy of renovascular hypertension. Br J Surg 69(Suppl):S63, 1982.

88. Stanley JC, Whitehouse WM Jr, Zelenock GB, et al: Re-operation for complications of renal artery reconstructive surgery undertaken for treatment of renovascular hypertension. J Vasc Surg 2:133, 1985.

89. Stanley P, Gyepes MT, Olson DL, et al: Renovascular hypertension in children and adolescents. Radiology 129:123, 1978.

90. Stanley P, Hieshima G, Mehringer M: Percutaneous transluminal angioplasty for pediatric renovascular hypertension. Radiology 153:101, 1984.

91. Stanley JC, Zelenock GB, Messina LM, et al: Pediatric renovascular hypertension: A thirty-year experience of operative treatment. J Vasc Surg 21:212, 1995.

92. Stoney RJ, Cooke PA, String ST: Surgical treatment of renovascular hypertension in children. J Pediatr Surg 10:631, 1975.

93. Stoney RJ, DeLuccia N, Ehrenfeld WK, et al: Aortorenal arterial autografts: Long-term assessment. Arch Surg 116:1416, 1981.

94. Stoney RJ, Silane M, Salvatierra O: Ex vivo renal artery reconstruction. Arch Surg 113:1272, 1978.

95. Stringer DA, deBruyn R, Dillion MJ, et al: Comparison of aortography, renal vein renin sampling, radionuclide scans, ultrasound and the IVU in the investigation of childhood renovascular hypertension. Br J Radiol 57:111,1984.

96. Surur MF, Sos Ta, Saddekni S, et al: Intimal fibromuscular dysplasia and Takayasu arteritis: Delayed response to percutaneous transluminal angioplasty. Radiology 157:657, 1985.

97. Tegtmeyer CJ, Elson J, Glass TA, et al: Percutaneous transluminal angioplasty: The treatment of choice for renovascular hypertension due to fibromuscular dysplasia. Radiology 143:631, 1982.

98. Tegtmeyer CJ, Sos TA: Techniques of renal angioplasty. Radiology 161:577, 1986.

99. Thibonnier M, Joseph A, Sassano P, et al: Improved diagnosis of unilateral renal artery lesions after captopril administration. JAMA 251:56, 1984.

100. vanBockel JH, van Schilfgaarde R, Felthuis W, et al: Long-term results of in situ and extracorporeal surgery for renovascular hypertension caused by fibrodysplasia. J Vasc Surg 6:355, 1987.

101. Vargas R, Wroblewska B, Rego A, et al: Oestradiol inhibits smooth muscle cell proliferation of pig coronary artery. Br J Pharm 09:612, 1993.

102. Vidt DG: Advances in the medical management of renovascular hypertension. Urol Clin 11:417, 1984.

103. Watson AR, Balfe JW, Hardy BE: Renovascular hypertension in childhood: A changing perspective in management. J Pediatr 106:366, 1985.

104. Whitehouse WM Jr, Kazmers A, Zelenock GB, et al: Chronic total renal artery occlusion: Effects of treatment on secondary hypertension and renal function. Surgery 89:753, 1981.

105. Zweifler AJ, Julius S: Medical treatment of renovascular hypertension. In Stanley JC, Ernst CB, Fry WJ (eds): Renovascular Hypertension. Philadelphia, WB Saunders, 1980, pp 231–245.

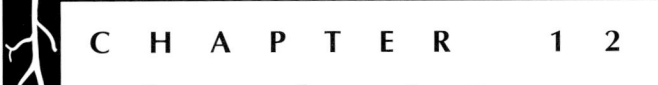

CHAPTER 123

Atherosclerotic Renovascular Disease: Evaluation and Management of Ischemic Nephropathy

Kimberley J. Hansen, M.D., and Richard H. Dean, M.D.

During the past two decades, the introduction of new antihypertensive agents and percutaneous transluminal renal angioplasty (PTRA) has changed many attitudes regarding the role of surgical intervention for atherosclerotic renovascular disease.[1-3] New treatment alternatives, combined with the increasingly older patient population seeking treatment for renovascular disease, have led many physicians to limit surgical intervention to patients (1) with severe hypertension despite maximal medical therapy, (2) with anatomic failures or disease patterns not amenable to balloon angioplasty, or (3) with renovascular disease complicated by renal excretory insufficiency.[4]

As a consequence of these changing attitudes and treatment strategies, the demography of the contemporary patient population has also changed.[5, 6] Current patient populations are characterized by diffuse extrarenal atherosclerosis complicated by site-specific, end-organ damage and renal insufficiency. Consequently, the current strategy and contemporary results of surgical management differ significantly from those described in earlier reported series.[1, 7-9] In addition to the traditional concerns about renovascular hypertension, these observations emphasize the relationship between renovascular occlusive disease and excretory renal dysfunction. This relationship, described by the term *ischemic nephropathy*, defines the presence of anatomically severe occlusive disease of the extraparenchymal renal artery in a patient with excretory renal insufficiency.

Three patient groups can be considered for reconstruction of atherosclerotic renovascular disease to improve renal function. The first group is represented by normal global renal function in a patient found to have a nonfunctioning kidney during evaluation for renovascular hypertension. Renal artery occlusion frequently characterizes this group. In this instance, overall renal function is maintained by the contralateral normal kidney, and the clinical question is whether to perform a nephrectomy or renal artery repair.

The second group consists of patients with azotemic ischemic nephropathy. In a patient in this group, the decision for renal artery intervention must balance the possibility of retrieving clinically significant excretory function with the risk of worsening residual function as well as the higher risk of operative morbidity and mortality.

Patients in the third group, with dialysis-dependent ischemic nephropathy, have end-stage, end-organ dysfunction. Despite general pessimism regarding recovery of renal function in this setting, patients who are dialysis-dependent enjoy the greatest potential benefit from successful renal artery intervention.

RENAL ARTERY OCCLUSION WITHOUT AZOTEMIA

The Patient with Hypertension

Hypertension in the patient with renal artery occlusion can be treated equally well by revascularization or nephrectomy. The most desirable management, however, would achieve benefits in both blood pressure and renal function. When the potential for improved renal function exists, the price of nephrectomy with the loss of functioning renal mass may be greater than the benefit despite a favorable blood pressure response. The practical value of this premise is demonstrated by progression of mild contralateral renal artery lesions to hemodynamically severe lesions in 35% of patients within 5 years of unilateral operative repair.[10] When such patients are treated with nephrectomy for renal artery occlusion and their contralateral renal disease progresses, global renal function is threatened and operative intervention must then be performed in azotemic patients who are at risk for dialysis-dependent renal failure. Moreover, the atherosclerotic renal artery disease in the remaining kidney may not develop in a manner that is clinically recognized, or it may occur at a site that is not amenable to surgical correction. Conversely, an overly aggressive approach to repair of renal artery occlusion sometimes leads to revascularization of a kidney in which no beneficial function or blood pressure response can be achieved. In this instance, primary nephrectomy would be simpler and safer than revascularization and would result in the control of hypertension.

Given these considerations, the authors have limited nephrectomy to patients with renal artery occlusion in whom the kidney contributing to severe hypertension has an unreconstructible renal artery and demonstrates negligible renal function. The value of this management philosophy is confirmed by the results obtained in 95 consecutive patients (52 women, 43 men; mean age, 63 years) treated for 100 atherosclerotic renal artery occlusions.[11] Cut-film angiography demonstrated distal renal artery reconstitution in 69% of kidneys and a nephrogram in 62%. Neither distal renal artery reconstitution nor nephrogram was demonstrated in 25% of kidneys. Overall, 75 renal artery occlu-

1665

TABLE 123–1. COMPARISON OF OPERATIVE RESULTS FOR PATIENT GROUPS TREATED FOR RENAL ARTERY OCCLUSION (RA-OCC) AND RENAL ARTERY STENOSIS (RAS)

	RA-OCC	RAS	*p* VALUE
No. of patients	95	302	
Perioperative mortality (%)	5.3	4.0	.59
Hypertension response (%)			.52
Cured	11	13	
Improved	80	74	
No change	9	13	
Renal function response (%)*			.20
Improved	49	41	
No change/worsened	51	59	

From Oskin TC, Hansen KJ, Dietch JS, et al: Chronic renal artery occlusion: Nephrectomy versus revascularization. J Vasc Surg 29:140–149, 1999.
*Preoperative serum creatinine ≥1.3 mg/dl.

sions were treated with direct aortorenal reconstruction, and 25 nephrectomies were performed.

After surgical renal artery repair, mortality rates were similar for renal artery revascularization and nephrectomy (2.8% and 12%, respectively; p = .11) and the total mortality rate (5.3%) did not differ from that in 302 patients treated during the same period for atherosclerotic renal artery stenosis (4.0%; p = .59; Table 123–1).[11] Hypertension among the 90 survivors of renal artery occlusion surgery was considered cured in 11% and improved in 80%; in 9% of patients, surgery failed to improve blood pressure. Importantly, beneficial blood pressure responses were equivalent after revascularization and nephrectomy (92% and 87%, respectively). However, significant improvement in estimated glomerular filtration rate (GFR) was observed only (1) after revascularization (p < .01) and (2) after nephrectomy if contralateral revascularization was included (p = .02). Not surprisingly, a significant increase in estimated GFR was not observed when nephrectomy alone was performed. Most important, improved excretory renal function had a significant and independent association with improved postoperative survival after operation (Fig. 123–1).

Absence of preoperative nephrogram or distal renal ar-

tery reconstitution did not preclude revascularization in half of these kidneys. In fact, eight of 21 patients (38%) with neither preoperative nephrogram nor distal renal artery reconstitution underwent operative reconstruction, and 75% showed beneficial blood pressure response and improved renal function. Preoperative kidney length was less in the nephrectomy patients (7.3 ± 1.4 cm) compared with the patients revascularized (8.2 ± 1.5 cm), but length alone did not preclude revascularization. Nine of 16 kidneys shorter than 7 cm were revascularized, with beneficial blood pressure response in all and improved renal function in 44%.

Because the lower limits of renal function retrieval are not well defined for renal artery occlusion, but progression of contralateral renal artery disease is common, these data suggest that nephrectomy should be limited to a subgroup of patients with severe hypertension in whom the kidney responsible for hypertension has a nonreconstructible vessel and negligible excretory renal function. This conservative use of nephrectomy is supported by the equivalent blood pressure response and improved renal function response observed after renal artery revascularization. Moreover, improved renal function after operation confers a survival advantage. In the patient in whom significant renal function exists in the occluded kidney, the price of nephrectomy with loss of functioning renal mass is greater than the benefit. Exception to this premise occurs only when hypertension is uncontrolled by maximal drug therapy and results in overt end-organ damage. In children, limited use of nephrectomy is of even greater importance because 50% of such patients demonstrate significant contralateral renal artery disease over time.[12]

Thus, the authors proceed with renal artery revascularization in the patient with renal artery occlusion and renovascular hypertension without azotemia whenever the distal vessel is identified and appears normal on angiography. If the vessel is not visualized by angiography, the distal vessel is explored prior to nephrectomy. When a normal distal vessel is demonstrated, renal revascularization is performed. With this practice, 40% of such patients undergo repair rather than nephrectomy. Conversely, if the distal renal artery and segmental branches demonstrate atherosclerosis

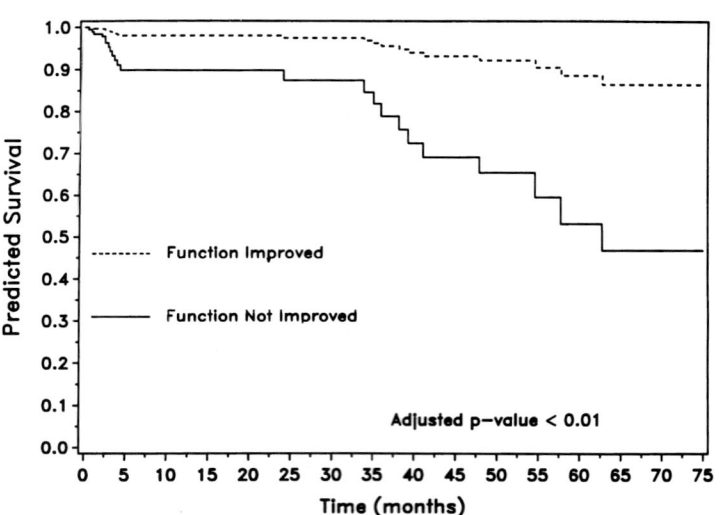

FIGURE 123–1. Predicted survival among patients with renal artery occlusion who had either improved or unimproved renal function after revascularization. (From Oskin TC, Hansen KJ, Deitch JS, et al: Chronic renal artery occlusion: Nephrectomy versus revascularization. J Vasc Surg 29:1409, 1999.)

during exploration, these findings correlate with intrarenal nephrosclerosis and poor hypertension response. In this instance, a primary nephrectomy is performed when renal function has been proven negligible by preoperative isotope renography.

The Patient Without Hypertension

This aggressive approach toward renal revascularization does not extend to prophylactic repair of renal artery disease in the normotensive patient. In this setting, the term *prophylactic repair* indicates that renal revascularization is performed prior to the appearance of any clinical sequelae related to the lesion. By definition, therefore, the patient considered for prophylactic renal artery repair has neither hypertension nor reduced excretory renal function. Correction of an atherosclerotic renal artery lesion in such patients is performed on the assumption that (1) a significant percentage of these asymptomatic patients would survive long enough for the renal lesion to cause hypertension or renal dysfunction and (2) preemptive correction is necessary to prevent an untreatable adverse event. On the basis of available data, the authors do not perform prophylactic renal artery repair as an isolated procedure or in combination with planned aortic repair.

Data from three series regarding the anatomic progression of atherosclerotic renovascular disease causing hypertension are summarized in Table 123–2.[13–15] Ipsilateral progression of renovascular atherosclerosis occurred in 44% of patients with renovascular hypertension, and 12% progressed to have total occlusion during medical management. Among these patients, however, only one (3%) lost a previously reconstructible renal artery.[15] In the absence of hypertension, one must assume that the renal artery lesion first progresses anatomically to become functionally significant (i.e, to produce hypertension). On the basis of preceding data, progression of a "silent" renal artery lesion to produce renovascular hypertension could be expected in approximately 44% of normotensive patients. If one also assumes that the subsequent development of renovascular hypertension is managed medically, the next consideration is the frequency of decline in renal function.

Among 30 patients with renovascular hypertension randomly assigned to receive medical management, significant loss of renal function, reflected by at least 25% decrease in

TABLE 123–2. ANGIOGRAPHIC PROGRESSION OF RENAL ARTERY ATHEROSCLEROSIS

| MEAN FOLLOW-UP (MO) | NO. | IPSILATERAL LESIONS | | CONTRALATERAL LESIONS |
		Exhibiting Progression	Progressing to Occlusion	Exhibiting Progression
29–35*	85	44%	16%	—
28†	35	—	12%	17%

*Data from Wollenweber J, Sheps SG, Davis GD: Clinical course of atherosclerotic renovascular disease. Am J Cardiol 21:60–71, 1968; and Schreiber MJ, Phol MA, Novick AC: The natural history of atherosclerotic fibrous renal artery disease. Urol Clin North Am 11:383–392, 1984.
†Data from Dean RH, Kieffer RW, Smith BM, et al: Renovascular hypertension: Anatomic and renal function changes during drug therapy. Arch Surg 166:1408–1415, 1981.

TABLE 123–3. COMPARISON OF RISK WITH ESTIMATED BENEFIT FOR PROPHYLACTIC RENAL REVASCULARIZATION IN 100 NORMOTENSIVE PATIENTS

BENEFIT OR RISK	NO. OF PATIENTS
Benefit	
Progression to renovascular hypertension (RVH) (44/100 or 44%)	44
Patients with RVH who lose renal function (16/44 or 36%)	16
Renal function restored by later operation (11/16 or 67%)	11
Renal function not restored by later operation (5/16 or 33%)	5
Unique benefit	5
Risk (Combined Aortorenal Reconstruction)	
Operative mortality (5.5%)	5
Early technical failure (0.5%)	1
Late failure of revascularization (4.0%)	4
Adverse outcome	10

GFR, occurred in 40% of patients during a 15- to 24-month follow-up period.[15] Medical management was considered to have failed in these patients, who then underwent operative renal artery repair. However, 13% of those patients who underwent operation continued to exhibit progressive deterioration in renal function. Therefore, in only 36% of patients with renovascular hypertension randomly assigned to receive medical management could an earlier operation have prevented loss of renal function. Moreover, one must consider how many of these patients with decline in kidney function during medical management could experience restoration of function with a subsequent operation. In this regard, Novick and colleagues[16] have reported that in 67% of properly selected patients, renal function is restored by renovascular repair.

The importance of these issues relative to the potential benefit of prophylactic renal revascularization can be demonstrated by considering 100 hypothetical patients without hypertension in whom a unsuspected renal artery lesions are demonstrated prior to aortic repair (Table 123–3). If the renal artery lesion are not repaired prophylactically, approximately 44 patients experience anatomic progression of disease and subsequently renovascular hypertension. Sixteen (36%) of the 44 patients experience a preventable reduction in renal function during follow-up. However, delayed operation restores function in 11 (67%) of the 16 patients. In theory, therefore, only 5 of the hypothetical 100 patients receive unique benefit from prophylactic intervention.

This unique benefit should be considered in terms of the associated morbidity and mortality of renal artery repair. In the authors' center, the operative mortality associated with the surgical treatment of isolated renal artery disease alone is approximately 1%; however, combined aortorenal reconstruction is associated with a 5% to 6% perioperative mortality.[1, 17] If direct aortorenal methods of reconstruction are employed in conjunction with intraoperative completion duplex ultrasonography, the early technical failure rate is 0.5% and late failures of reconstruction can be expected in 3% to 4% of renal artery repairs.[1] Therefore, adverse results could be expected in 10 of the 100 hypothetical patients after combined aortorenal repair.

Theoretically, then, prophylactic renal artery repair could provide unique benefit in only 5 patients but has the potential to produce an adverse outcome in up to 10 patients. On the basis of available data, the authors find no justification for prophylactic renal artery surgery either as an independent procedure or as a procedure performed in combination with aortic repair.

AZOTEMIC ISCHEMIC NEPHROPATHY

The azotemic patient with renovascular occlusive disease more clearly resembles the atherosclerotic patient with end-organ damage than does the patient with normal renal function. Retrieval of function has immediate practical significance in the azotemic patient; however, the hazard of aggravating renal failure to a dialysis-dependent level with ineffective intervention has limited enthusiasm for surgical treatment of such patients.

In 1962, Morris and associates[18] reported on eight azotemic patients with global renal ischemia who experienced improvements in blood pressure and renal function after renal revascularization. Novick and colleagues[16] found a similar beneficial renal function response when bilateral renal lesions were corrected in azotemic patients. Nevertheless, data regarding the prevalence, clinical presentation, and natural history of azotemic ischemic nephropathy are lacking or incomplete. Circumstantial evidence suggests that it may be a more common cause of renal insufficiency in the atherosclerotic age group (i.e., $\geq$ 50 years of age) than was previously recognized. In a 1992 study of randomly selected azotemic patients with serum creatinine levels 2 mg/dl or higher, 15% had unsuspected renovascular disease.[19] In comparison with patients without renal artery disease, patients who had azotemic ischemic nephropathy were significantly older and had greater prevalence of extrarenal atherosclerosis. Each of these clinical characteristics is compatible with the demographic features of patients with proven ischemic nephropathy.[20] In the authors' experience, patients treated for ischemic nephropathy are often elderly and demonstrate at least moderate hypertension, and only 14% have diabetes mellitus.[21] These data indicate that renovascular disease may be either the primary cause or an important secondary accelerant of renal insufficiency in more patients than is commonly recognized.[22]

The changes in renal function associated with azotemic ischemic nephropathy are demonstrated by a retrospective review of data collected from 58 consecutive patients with ischemic nephropathy who underwent operative renal artery repair.[20] The rate of decline in renal function during the period before and after intervention and the immediate effect of surgery on excretory function were examined. Patients with at least three sequential measurements for calculations of estimated GFR changes during the 6 months before operation (n = 32) were used to describe the preoperative rate of decline in estimated GFR, and postoperative rate of decline was determined in the operative survivors. Comparative analyses were performed for unilat-

TABLE 123–4. ESTIMATED GLOMERULAR FILTRATION RATE (GFR) RESPONSE VERSUS SITE OF OPERATION FOR AZOTEMIC ISCHEMIC NEPHROPATHY IN 53 PATIENTS

OPERATION	NO. OF PATIENTS	ESTIMATED GFR (ml/min/m³)		
		Preoperative	Postoperative	*p* Value†
Unilateral	12	25.94 ± 11.86	29.14 ± 14.34	.1633
Bilateral	41	21.38 ± 8.89	33.77 ± 18.39	.0001

From Dean RH, Tribble RW, Hansen KJ, et al: Evolution of renal insufficiency in ischemic nephropathy. Ann Surg 213:446, 1991.
*Values are mean ± S.D.
†The *p* values are for the paired *t* test.

eral versus bilateral lesions and patients classified as having improvement in estimated GFR versus those classified as having no improvement after operation.

Patient age ranged from 52 to 79 years (mean, 69 years). On the basis of serum creatinine values, preoperative estimated GFR averaged 23.9 ml/min/m². Comparison of the immediate preoperative estimated GFR with the immediate postoperative estimated GFR for the entire group demonstrated significant increase in response to operation (23.9 versus 32.7 ml/min/m²; p = .001). The immediate postoperative change in estimated GFR according to the site of disease and operation is summarized in Table 123–4.[20] For this analysis, lesions of (and procedures to) solitary kidneys and procedures consisting of unilateral revascularization with contralateral nephrectomy were considered along with bilateral repairs. As noted in Table 123–4, when the groups were considered according to the site of operation, the

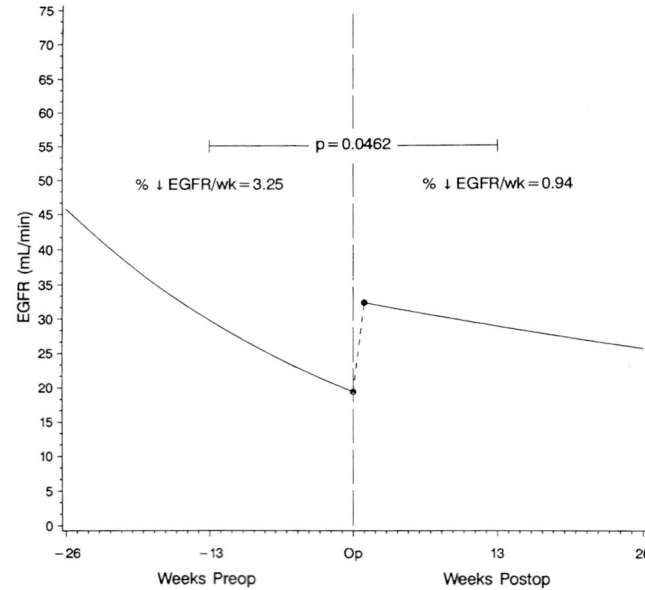

FIGURE 123–2. Per cent decrease in estimated glomerular filtration rate (EGFR) per week for the entire group of patients with azotemic ischemic nephropathy during the 6 months before (n = 5) and after (n = 32) renal artery repair. The immediate effect of operation on EGFR is also depicted. The *p* values for differences are determined with the use of the *t* test for unpaired data. Note the improvement in the slope of decline in EGFR after operation. (From Dean RH, Tribble RW, Hansen KJ, et al: Evolution of renal insufficiency in ischemic nephropathy. Ann Surg 213:446, 1991.)

bilateral repair group experienced a significant improvement in estimated GFR after operation (21.4 versus 33.8 ml/min/m²; p = .0001). Although four patients (33%) in the unilateral repair group had an improvement in estimated GFR (a 20% or greater increase) after operation, no statistically significant benefit was seen when all patients with unilateral disease were collectively examined (25.9 ml/min/m² preoperative versus 29.1 ml/min/m² postoperative.

Figure 123–2 demonstrates the preoperative and postoperative rates of change and immediate improvement in estimated GFR for the entire group. In all patients, a greater than 3.2% per week decrease in estimated GFR was observed, which differed significantly from the 0.9% per week decline after operation. However, this decrease in the rate of decline was observed *only* in patients who had immediate improvement in excretory renal function after operation (Figs. 123–2 and 123–3). Furthermore, immediate improvement was observed only in patients with rapid decline in estimated GFR in the 6 months preceding operative repair (see Fig. 123–3). Patients with slow preoperative decline in estimated GFR had no immediate improvement in renal function and had no change in the rate of decline in estimated GFR after intervention (Fig. 123–4). Unfortunately, the variance in individual slopes of change in estimated GFR prevents the determination of a critical rate of decline that would predict retrieval of renal function with operation; however, rapidly deteriorating renal function in a hypertensive patient should alert the physician to the possibility of ischemic nephropathy and supports the likelihood of renal function benefit after operation if ischemic nephropathy has been identified.

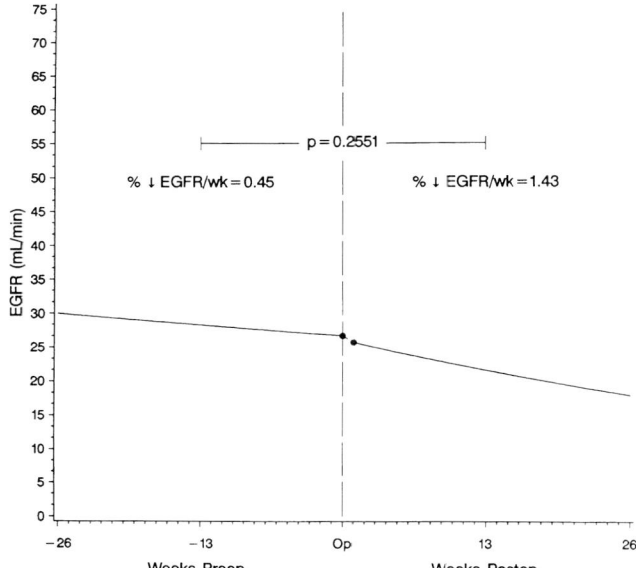

FIGURE 123–4. Per cent decline in estimated glomerular filtration rate (EGFR) per week during the 6 months before (n = 18) and after (n = 8) operation in the group of patients with azotemic ischemic nephropathy who had no significant immediate benefit in EGFR after renal artery repair. The p values for differences are determined using the t test for unpaired data. Note the absence of improvement in the rate of deterioration of EGFR after operation in this group. (From Dean RH, Tribble RW, Hansen KJ, et al: Evolution of renal insufficiency in ischemic nephropathy. Ann Surg 213:446, 1991.)

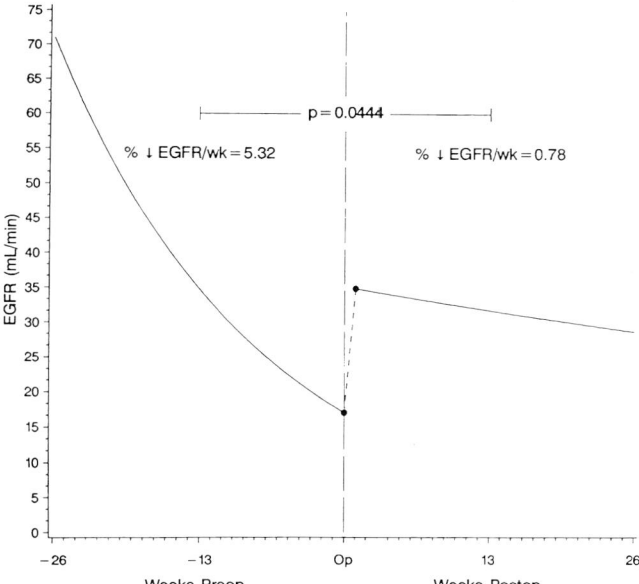

FIGURE 123–3. Per cent decline in estimated glomerular filtration rate (EGFR) per week during the 6 months before (n = 23) and after (n = 25) operation in the group of patients with azotemic nephropathy who had at least a 20% improvement in EGFR following renal artery repair. The immediate effect of operation on EGFR in this group is also depicted. The p values for differences are determined using the t test for unpaired data. Note the improvement in the slope of decline in EGFR after operation in this group. (From Dean RH, Tribble RW, Hansen KJ, et al: Evolution of renal insufficiency in ischemic nephropathy. Ann Surg 213:446, 1991.)

Among this patient group, renal artery repair had a beneficial effect on both immediate estimated GFR and the rate of decline in estimated GFR when data were analyzed collectively. When data were analyzed with respect to the individual subgroups, however, beneficial effect of operation on the rate of deterioration of estimated GFR was seen only in patients who experienced an immediate improvement in estimated GFR after operation. This observation may have important clinical significance because the detrimental effect of renovascular occlusive disease may arise from either of two causes: (1) the lesion may limit glomerular perfusion to a degree that it affects excretory function and (2) it may be the source of atheroembolism that destroys functioning renal parenchyma.

These data suggest that correction of renal artery atherosclerosis that is causing reversible ischemia will provide both an immediate improvement in estimated GFR and the slow postoperative rate of decline. Conversely, in patients in whom the lesion was not producing significant reversible ischemia, as evidenced by the absence of improvement in estimated GFR immediately after operation, no improvement in the rate of decline in estimated GFR was realized after operation. Moreover, these data suggest that it is false to classify patients with no immediate improvement in estimated GFR as having their renal function "preserved" by renal artery intervention. Patients without immediate increase in estimated GFR after operation continue to demonstrate decline in renal function unchanged after intervention.

This experience emphasizes the rapid decline in renal function among patients with proven ischemic nephropathy and demonstrates the benefit of operation on both estimated GFR and its rate of deterioration in azotemic patients. Although the biases inherent in this retrospective analysis limit the power of these observations, the rate of deterioration in estimated GFR was rapid and entirely consistent with early progression to end-stage renal disease (ESRD) and dialysis dependence for these patients.

DIALYSIS-DEPENDENT ISCHEMIC NEPHROPATHY

ESRD requiring long-term renal replacement therapy is the final clinical expression of ischemic nephropathy. In this instance, identification of dialysis-dependent ischemic nephropathy is a clinical imperative because both quality and quantity of life are adversely affected. Nevertheless, dialysis-dependent ischemic nephropathy is uncommonly discovered, and the associated renovascular disease less commonly corrected.[22-25] In part, this situation reflects the general pessimism regarding retrieval of excretory renal function and the risk associated with operative intervention in patients dependent on dialysis.

Despite the infrequent discovery of dialysis-dependent ischemic nephropathy, circumstantial evidence suggests that it is a more common cause of end-stage renal failure than previously recognized. In a 1986 survey, 73% of patients with ESRD were in the atherosclerotic age group.[26] In a report by Mailloux and coworkers,[27] ischemic nephropathy causing dialysis dependence increased from 6.7% for the period between 1978 and 1981 to 16.5% for the period between 1982 and 1985.[27] The median age of onset of ESRD for this latter group[82-85] was the highest among all groups.

These data are supported by a prospective study from the authors' center. During a 7-month period, all patients 50 years of age and older presenting for long-term renal replacement therapy were screened for occlusive renovascular disease by renal duplex ultrasonography. Of 90 consecutive patients, 53 agreed to undergo the study; among these patients, 45 studies were technically adequate to delineate the presence or absence of renovascular disease.[28] Nonparticipants were significantly older than participants (70.3 ± 1.7 years versus 65.0 ± 1.1 years, respectively; $p = .007$), but otherwise, the two groups demonstrated no significant differences in race, gender, or clinical diagnosis. A total of 103 kidneys were studied, and renal duplex scanning was complete in 92%.

Overall, significant renal artery disease was noted in 15 of 92 kidneys (16%), including four renal artery occlusions. Ten of 45 patients (22%) demonstrated renal artery stenosis or occlusion, including bilateral disease in 5 patients. When demographic characteristics were compared in participants with and without renal artery disease, age and race differed significantly. Older patients of white race presenting for long-term renal replacement therapy were significantly more likely to have renovascular disease. Among white participants, 40% demonstrated hemodynamically significant renal artery stenosis or occlusion, which involved both kidneys in 20%. Moreover, participants with renovascular disease had higher prevalences of tobacco abuse ($p = .04$)

and extrarenal atherosclerosis ($p = .005$) than those without renovascular disease. The results of this prospective study indicate that renovascular disease may exist in a significant minority of older patients beginning long-term renal replacement therapy. Advanced age, white race, tobacco abuse, and extrarenal atherosclerosis characterized the patients with dialysis-dependent ischemic nephropathy.[28]

The significance of these findings is demonstrated by both recovery of renal function and improved patient survival after operative renal artery repair. From January 1987 through June 1997, 37 of 534 patients treated at the authors' center were considered permanently dialysis-dependent if not improved by operation. Analysis of the rate of change in EGFR before and after operation and information about the impact of function retrieval are available for the first 20 consecutive patients.[23] This group of 20 patients (6 women, 14 men; mean age, 66 years) had been dialysis-dependent for 1 to 9 weeks (mean, 3.4 weeks) prior to operation. Each patient had severe hypertension and evidence of diffuse extrarenal atherosclerosis. Direct aortorenal reconstruction was performed in each patient without perioperative or in-hospital mortality. Sixteen of 20 patients (80%) were initially removed from hemodialysis. For these 16 patients, postoperative estimated GFR ranged from 9.0 to 56.1 ml/min/m^2 (mean, 32.4 ml/min/m^2). Two of the 16 patients resumed hemodialysis 4 and 6 months after surgery. Removal from dialysis was more likely after bilateral or complete renal artery repair (15 of 16 patients) than after unilateral repair (1 of 4 patients; $p = .01$). Permanent removal from dialysis was associated with a rapid preoperative rate of decline in EGFR (mean slope log$_e$ estimated GFR, -0.1393 ± 0.0340 off dialysis; -0.0188 ± 0.0464 on dialysis; $p = .04$). Immediate increase in estimated GFR after operation was inversely correlated with the severity of intrarenal atherosclerosis (rank correlation, -0.57; 95% confidence interval [CI] [-0.83, -0.10]). Death during follow-up was associated with dialysis dependence; two deaths occurred among 14 patients removed from dialysis, whereas 5 of 6 dialysis-dependent patients died ($p < .01$). The product-limit estimates for follow-up survival as a function of dialysis status are illustrated in Figure 123–5.

Applying the premise that significant renal artery disease is prevalent in the atherosclerotic age group and may cause excretory renal insufficiency that can progress to ESRD and dialysis dependence, the authors currently screen for ischemic nephropathy in all hypertensive patients older than 50 years who present with newly recognized renal insufficiency.[1, 21, 24, 25] As previously described, the preferred screening method is renal duplex ultrasonography.[21, 29] The authors' prospective experience with the use of this procedure as a screening technique was previously reported.[29] In this review, the authors found renal duplex ultrasonography to have an overall accuracy of 96% for establishing the presence or absence of main renal artery stenosis or occlusion.

Because the term *ischemic nephropathy* implies the presence of global renal ischemia, the authors believe that renal duplex ultrasonography, when performed by an experienced sonographer, is sufficient to guide further management of the patient with renal insufficiency. Through pre-

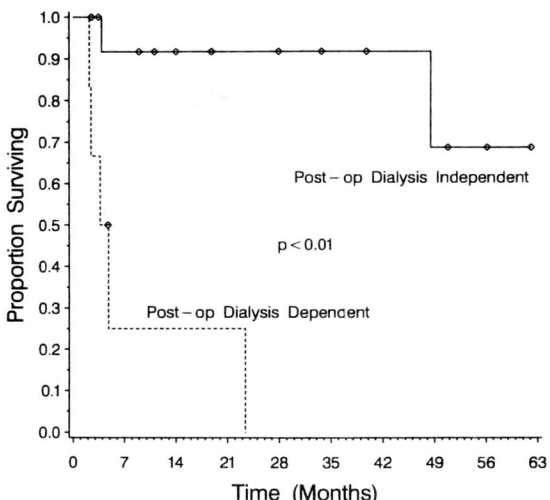

FIGURE 123–5. Product-limit estimate of patient survival according to dialysis status after operation for dialysis dependent ischemic nephropathy (n = 20). (From Hansen KJ, Thomason RB, Craven TE, et al: Surgical management of dialysis-dependent ischemic nephropathy. J Vasc Surg 21:197, 1995.)

liminary screening with renal duplex ultrasonography, the authors limit the use of conventional angiography in patients with renal insufficiency to those with either positive findings on renal duplex ultrasonography or severe, poorly controlled hypertension.

Unfortunately, once azotemic or dialysis-dependent ischemic nephropathy is identified, most issues regarding anticipated retrieval of renal function in a particular patient remain poorly defined.[20, 1, 30, 31] The authors observed that both the site of disease and operation and the rate of decline in preoperative EGFR differed between patients with improved renal function and those with unimproved renal function after operation. Although intrarenal atherosclerosis was inversely correlated with change in EGFR, this feature did not differ significantly between patients who still underwent and those who were free of dialysis after operation. In particular, the role of repair of unilateral renal artery stenosis in patients with renal insufficiency of any degree is uncertain. Even greater uncertainty surrounds the role of renal artery repair in the normotensive patient with renal insufficiency. In this instance, the issue is whether renovascular disease sufficient to cause renal failure can exist without raising the blood pressure.

This clinical scenario has the greatest practical importance for the patient who is normotensive as a consequence of antihypertensive agents. In the setting of renal artery disease, the contribution of potent diuretics and angiotensin-converting enzyme (ACE) inhibitors to renal dysfunction is widely recognized (see Chapter 119). Otherwise, in the complete absence of hypertension, the physiologic importance of renal artery disease as a cause of renal insufficiency must remain suspect.[25]

Finally, Zinman and Libertino[32] reported preoperative renal biopsy as a useful predictor of renal function retrieval in their series of patients, but the authors have not found the technique worthwhile. Having identified hyalinized glomeruli in open biopsy specimens of selected sections of kidneys with adequate renal function and in kidneys with

marked improvement in excretory function after operation, the authors abandoned renal biopsy because it was misleading and potentially hazardous.

CONTEMPORARY RESULTS OF OPERATIVE INTERVENTION

To examine the changes that have occurred in both the patient population presenting for operative management and the results of operation over the past three decades, the authors reviewed their recent (contemporary) operative experience. During one 10-year period (January 1987 through December 1997), more than 500 patients have undergone operative renal artery repair for renovascular hypertension, ischemic nephropathy, and renal artery aneurysms. The first 200 consecutive patients, treated from January 1987 through June 1991, included 43 patients with nonatherosclerotic renovascular disease ranging in age from 5 to 66 years (mean age, 38 ± 17 years), who demonstrated (1) fibromuscular dysplasia (FMD) (39 patients; 34 with medial fibroplasia, four with intimal fibroplasia, one with perimedial dysplasia); (2) renal artery dissection (three patients: two with traumatic dissection, one with spontaneous dissection); and (3) transplant renal artery stenosis (one patient).

The remaining 157 patients with atherosclerotic renovascular disease consisted of 80 men and 77 women ranging in age from 37 to 80 years (mean age, 62 ± 9 years). Ninety (57%) of these patients were older than 60 years, and 29 patients were in the eighth decade of life. Hypertension was present in 156 patients with atherosclerosis; blood pressure ranged from 178/90 to 300/178 mmHg (mean, 212/114 mmHg). Time since recognition of hypertension ranged from 1 to 30 years (mean duration, 15 ± 7 years), and drug regimens used to control hypertension before surgery employed an average of 2.8 agents. Overall, 62% of patients had been hypertensive for more than 5 years, and 59% of patients required three or more antihypertensive medications.

In addition to hypertension, 149 patients (95%) with atherosclerotic renovascular disease demonstrated one or more risk factors for atherosclerosis, including cigarette use (128 patients), hyperlipidemia (35 patients), and diabetes mellitus (26 patients). Evidence of at least one of the following manifestations of organ-specific atherosclerotic damage was present in 147 patients (94%) with atherosclerotic renovascular disease: cardiac disease (75%), cerebrovascular disease (33%), and renal disease (60%). Only eight patients were completely free of all organ-specific damage.

Defined as a serum creatinine level of 1.3 mg/dl or higher after the removal of high-dose diuretics and ACE inhibitors, renal insufficiency was present in 117 patients (75%) with atherosclerotic renal artery lesions.[1] Seventy patients (45%) were considered to have severe renal insufficiency (serum creatinine ≥ 2.0 mg/dl), and 23 patients had extreme renal insufficiency (serum creatinine ≥ 3.0 mg/dl), including 11 patients who were dependent on dialysis.

After operation, five patients with atherosclerotic renovascular disease died within 30 days of surgery, producing an overall operative mortality rate of 2.5% (0% for nonath-

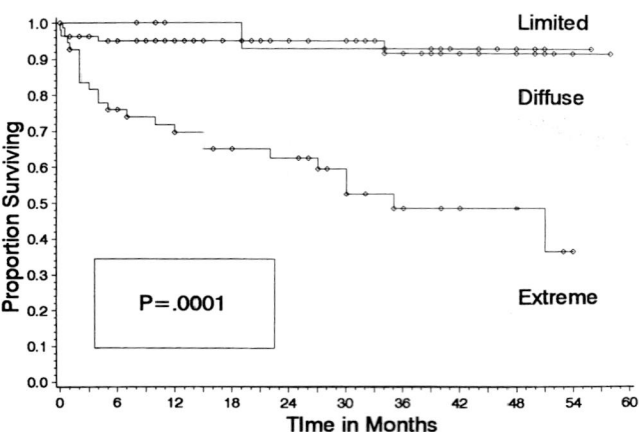

FIGURE 123–6. Kaplan-Meier life-table analysis showing estimated postoperative survival for patients with atherosclerotic renovascular disease according to whether they had limited, diffuse, or extreme atherosclerotic disease (n = 157). (From Hansen KJ, Starr SM, Sands RE, et al: Contemporary surgical management of renovascular disease. J Vasc Surg 16:319, 1992.)

erosclerotic renovascular disease and 3.1% for atherosclerotic renovascular disease).[1] Operative deaths occurred in association with diffuse disease (two patients) and extreme disease (three patients) requiring either intermediate repairs (three patients) or complex repairs (two patients). There were no operative deaths among patients with nonatherosclerotic renal artery disease, atherosclerotic patients with limited disease, or patients who had simple operative procedures. Two ex vivo reconstructions and two renal artery bypass grafts (1.4%) underwent thrombosis within 30 days of operation; in each case, the kidney could not be salvaged at reoperation, and a nephrectomy was required.

During mean follow-up of 24 months, there were 26 deaths among the 195 operative survivors observed for up to 58 months after operation.[1] All deaths occurred in patients with atherosclerotic renovascular disease (17.1%), and cardiovascular causes accounted for 92% of the deaths during follow-up. The likelihood of death during follow-up was significantly influenced by the extent of preoperative atherosclerosis and the presence of preoperative renal insufficiency (Fig. 123–6). Twenty-three of 26 deaths (88%) occurred in patients demonstrating extreme disease before surgery ($p = .0001$). Preoperative renal insufficiency demonstrated a significant and independent association with follow-up death ($p = .012$). Twenty-two of 26 deaths occurred in patients with serum creatinine of 2.0 mg/dl or greater (mean serum creatinine, 4.0 mg/dl). Preoperative evidence of left ventricular hypertrophy (11 patients) and congestive heart failure (eight patients) tended to be associated with deaths during follow-up; however these tendencies did not reach significance as determined by multivariate analysis in this group of 157 patients.

In addition to these preoperative parameters, postoperative renal function response and progression to dependence on dialysis demonstrated a significant association with death during follow-up. Of the 22 patients with renal insufficiency who died during follow-up, renal function was not improved in 20 patients (in 13 patients, no change; in 7 patients, worsened; $p = .0035$). Furthermore, 11 of

20 patients with unchanged or worsened EGFR progressed to eventual dialysis dependence before death ($p = .0001$). For all 534 patients treated from January 1987 through June 1997, multivariate analysis demonstrated that preoperative renal insufficiency ($p = .0001$), clinical congestive heart failure ($p = .0002$) diabetes mellitus ($p = .0001$), and unimproved renal function response after operation ($p = .001$) had significant and independent associations with eventual progression to dialysis dependence and postoperative death.[33]

On the basis of criteria encompassing blood pressure measurement and need for medication at least 8 weeks after surgery, hypertension among the 195 survivors of surgery was considered cured in 41 patients (21%), improved in 137 (70%), and unchanged in 17 (9%) (Table 123–5).[1] Overall, 91% of patients demonstrated a beneficial blood pressure response. Among the 43 patients with nonatherosclerotic renovascular disease, hypertension was considered cured in 43%, improved in 49%, and unchanged in 8%. In the 152 patients with atherosclerosis who survived operation, hypertension was considered cured in 15%, improved in 75%, and unchanged in 10%. Of the patients in whom renal vein renin assays were performed, 98% of patients with lateralizing renin activity had a beneficial blood pressure response, whereas 87% of patients treated empirically showed improvement. In this latter group, 10 of 24 patients demonstrated severe bilateral renovascular disease. Equivalent blood pressure benefit was observed irrespective of patient age, duration of hypertension, complexity of repair, and extent of associated atherosclerotic disease.

Table 123–6 summarizes the differences between contemporary patient demographics, surgical management, and response to operation and a previously reported experience.[1, 9] Clearly, the current patient population includes individuals who presented for treatment with more advanced disease. Specifically, patients in the current group with nonatherosclerotic lesions presented with hypertension almost 7 years longer in duration, and the subgroup with atherosclerotic disease had had hypertension for almost 10 years longer. Likewise, the current group presented at an older age for treatment than the patients in the previous experience. The much higher incidence of renal insufficiency (65% [contemporary] versus 8% [previous]) and the lower cure rates in both the atherosclerotic and

TABLE 123–5. BLOOD PRESSURE RESPONSE TO OPERATION FOR RENOVASCULAR DISEASE (RVD) IN 195 PATIENTS

RESPONSE	ALL PATIENTS (n = 195)		NONATHERO-SCLEROTIC RVD PATIENTS (n = 43)		ATHERO-SCLEROTIC RVD PATIENTS (n = 152)	
	No.	%	No.	%	No.	%
Cured	41	21	19	44	22	15
Improved	137	70	21	49	116	76
Failed	17	9	3	7	14	9
Total	195		43		152	

From Hansen KJ, Starr SM, Sands RE, et al: Contemporary surgical management of renovascular disease. J Vasc Surg 16:39, 1992.

TABLE 123–6. TREATMENT OF RENOVASCULAR DISEASE (RVD): EARLIER SURGICAL EXPERIENCE AND CONTEMPORARY EXPERIENCE

	1961–1972*	1987–1991†
No. of patients	122	200
Mean age (yr)		
Nonatherosclerotic RVD	33	38
Atherosclerotic RVD	50	62
Duration of hypertension (yr)		
Nonatherosclerotic RVD	4.6	11.2
Atherosclerotic RVD	5.1	15.0
Renal artery disease (%)		
Nonatherosclerotic RVD	35	21
Atherosclerotic RVD	65	79
Renal artery repair (%)		
Unilateral	80	60
Bilateral	20	40
Combined‡	13	32
Renal insufficiency (%)		
Not dependent on dialysis	8	65
Dependent on dialysis	0	6
Graft failure (%)	16	3
Hypertension response (%)		
Nonatherosclerotic RVD		
Cured	72§	43
Improved	24§	49
Atherosclerotic RVD		
Cured	53§	15
Improved	36§	75

Data from Foster JH, Dean RH, Pinkerston JA, et al: Ten years experience with the surgical management of renovascular hypertension. Ann Surg 177:755–766, 1973.
†Data from Hansen KJ, Starr SM, Sands RE, et al: Contemporary surgical management of renovascular disease. J Vasc Surg 16:319–331, 1992.
‡Combined aortic repair for occlusive or aneurysmal disease.
§Hypertension response, excluding technical failures.

nonatherosclerotic disease groups are probably influenced by this longer duration of drug therapy prior to intervention.

CONSEQUENCE OF FAILED RENAL ARTERY REPAIR

In the absence of a well-controlled, prospective, randomized trial comparing treatment modalities, advocates of medical management, percutaneous balloon angioplasty, and surgical reconstruction typically cite selected clinical results to support their respective views. Moreover, reports that examine failure of interventional management by either balloon angioplasty or operative repair emphasize the techniques required to reestablish renal artery patency and the immediate blood pressure response to secondary treatment.[34-37] For both angioplasty and operative repair, data regarding renal function response and event-free survival after remedial management of failed renal artery intervention are rarely presented and remain incomplete.

The consequences of failed renal artery repair in the 534 consecutive patients treated at the authors' center from

January 1987 to July 1997 provide additional information. Among the primary procedures, 80 were performed for congenital lesions or FMD and 454 were performed for atherosclerotic renovascular disease. Unilateral procedures were performed in 269 patients and bilateral procedures in 265, providing a total of 720 renal artery reconstructions during this period (Table 123–7).[33] During mean follow-up of 27 months, failure of renal artery repair was identified in 20 patients with either recurrent hypertension (12 patients) or recurrent hypertension with worsening excretory renal function (8 patients).[33]

This group of 20 patients with failed renal artery repair consisted of 9 women and 11 men ranging in age from 12 to 77 years (mean, 54 years) who were treated for either FMD (6 patients), atherosclerosis (13 patients), or coarctation of the abdominal aorta.[33] Prior to primary renovascular reconstruction, each patient had hypertension (mean blood pressure, 198/111 mmHg; mean number of medications, 3) and their preoperative serum creatinine levels ranged from 0.7 to 3.3 mg/dl (mean, 1.6 mg/dl). Renal dysfunction, diagnosed from serum creatinine value higher than 1.8 mg/dl after removal of high-dose diuretics and ACE inhibitors, was considered present in 7 patients, including one patient who was dialysis-dependent. Failed percutaneous balloon angioplasty preceded primary operative intervention in four patients (one with FMD; three with atherosclerosis). Twenty-two of 24 patients with failed primary reconstructions underwent secondary operative intervention. Four patients had bilateral procedures (including repair to a solitary kidney), 15 patients had unilateral procedures, and one patient declined reoperation. Secondary operative interventions consisted of five renal artery bypasses, five patch angioplasties, two hepatorenal bypasses, and 10 nephrectomies for unreconstructible disease.

Secondary management was influenced by the type of primary repair, the presence of postoperative stenosis or thrombosis, and whether clinical failure occurred early or late after primary operation.[33] All three early failures required nephrectomy. Of the remaining 21 repairs that failed between 2 and 36 months, nine failures were associated with thrombosis and 12 were secondary to stenosis. Thrombosis was significantly more common in the first postoperative year than recurrent stenosis (89% versus 33%, respectively; $p = .050$). Thrombosis developed in two ex vivo reconstructions 2 and 4 months after surgery. Each failure

TABLE 123–7. SUMMARY OF OPERATIVE MANAGEMENT OF RENOVASCULAR DISEASE FROM JANUARY 1987 THROUGH JUNE 1997 IN 534 PATIENTS

Total renal reconstructions			720
Aortorenal Bypass		445	
Vein	288		
Polytetrafluoroethylene (PTFE)	127		
Polyester (Dacron)	19		
Hypogastric artery	11		
Ex vivo	33		
Reimplantation		52	
Thromboendarterectomy		223	
Total nephrectomies			57
Total kidneys operated			777

From Hansen KJ, Deitch JA, Oskin TC, et al: Renal artery repair: Consequence of operative failures. Ann Surg 227:678–690, 1998.

led to renal infarction and recurrent hypertension requiring nephrectomy. Two ex vivo reconstructions failed after recurrent branch stenosis or degenerative change in a patch angioplasty (Fig. 123–7A and B). Each was treated with "redo" ex vivo repair and patch angioplasty (Fig. 123–7C). In the remaining seven primary repairs (six renal artery bypasses, one thromboendarterectomy) thrombosis developed 4 to 30 months after repair (mean, 9.8 months). Among the seven patients with repair failures, five nephrectomies were performed to control hypertension. In each case, the kidney was shown by isotope renography to be providing less than 5% renal function. Two repairs in one patient that had undergone thrombosis were revised with thrombectomy and patch angioplasty. This patient had been removed from dialysis after the primary operation and was returned to dialysis after the bilateral repair failure.

Blood pressure responses after primary and secondary operative interventions were equivalent. Among the 20 patients, had beneficial blood pressure response, and the repair in 1 patient (6%) was classified as *failed*. Beneficial blood pressure response (i.e., hypertension cured or improved) demonstrated no association with type of renovascular disease; however, three of six patients treated for FMD were cured, compared with none of 12 with atherosclerosis ($p = .031$). Secondary blood pressure response was equivalent for patients receiving nephrectomy and secondary renal artery reconstruction.

In contrast to blood pressure response, renal function responses after primary and secondary repair differed significantly. Renal function response after primary repair in 10 (59%) patients was *improved*; one patient was removed from dialysis dependence, status of five (29%) patients was *unchanged*, and renal function in two (12%) patients was classified as *worsened*. Eventual renal function response in all 20 patients after secondary operative intervention was classified as *improved* in 2 (10%) patients, *unchanged* in 10 (50%) patients, and *worse* in 8 (40%) patients, including 7 patients who were dialysis-dependent ($p = .015$). In the subgroup of patients with atherosclerotic renovascular disease, renal function one patient was *improved*, five were

unchanged, and seven were eventually dialysis-dependent. Eventual renal function response was not associated with the extent of primary renal artery disease or repair, presence of thrombosis or stenosis, or performance of secondary renal artery repair or nephrectomy. Eventual renal function response demonstrated a significant association, however, with the presence of preoperative ischemic nephropathy ($p = .039$) and bilateral failure of primary repair ($p = .007$).

Tables 123–8 and 123–9[33] compare the demographic features and results of surgical treatment for these 20 patients with those of 514 patients undergoing only primary renal artery reconstruction during the same period. There were no differences in gender, age distribution, or prevalence of end-organ disease between the two groups. Severity of hypertension, prevalence of preoperative renal insufficiency, and prevalence of diabetes mellitus were similar. However, patients requiring secondary intervention differed in the type of primary renovascular disease and the requirement for branch ex vivo repair (see Table 123–8). Fibromuscular dysplasia ($p = .020$) requiring ex vivo branch repair ($p = .001$) was significantly more common among patients with failed renovascular repairs. After primary renal artery repair, blood pressure and renal function responses were equivalent in the two groups (see Table 123–9).

Following secondary operation as well, blood pressure responses were equivalent, although eventual renal function responses differed significantly (see Table 123–9). Patients requiring secondary intervention had a significantly greater risk of worsened renal function (40% for secondary intervention versus 13% for primary intervention; $p = .015$), including eventual dialysis dependence (35% versus 4%, respectively; $p < .001$) In Figure 123–8, the product-limit estimates for dialysis-free survival for patients requiring secondary intervention (*solid line*) are compared with patients having only primary renovascular repair (*broken line*). Patients requiring secondary intervention demonstrated a significant and independent higher risk of eventual dialysis dependence (relative risk [RR]: 12.6; CI: 4.5, 34.9; $p = \leq$

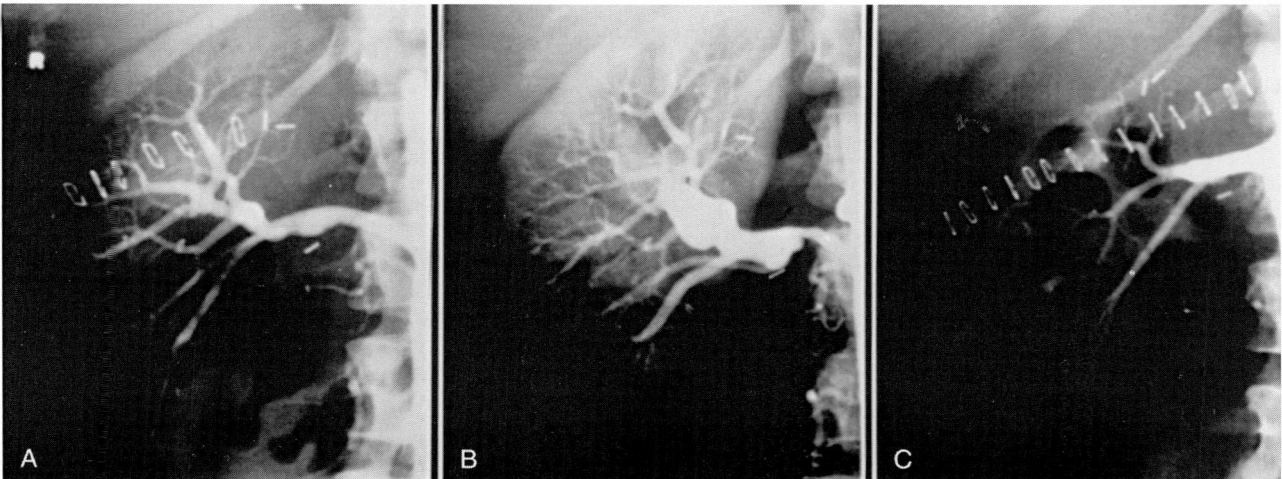

FIGURE 123–7. *A*, Angiogram 1 week after ex vivo renal artery branch repair with saphenous vein patch angioplasty. *B*, Angiographic appearance 28 months after primary renal artery repair and recurrent hypertension. *C*, Angiogram after "redo" ex vivo renal artery reconstruction. (From Hansen KJ, Deitch JS, Oskin TC, et al: Renal artery repair: Consequences of operative failures. Ann Surg 227:678, 1998.)

TABLE 123-8. COMPARATIVE ANALYSIS OF PATIENTS WITH AND WITHOUT NEED FOR SECONDARY OPERATIVE INTERVENTION FOR RENOVASCULAR DISEASE

	PRIMARY INTERVENTION ONLY	SECONDARY INTERVENTION	p VALUE
Sex			
Male	237/514 (46%)	11/20 (45%)	.434
Female	277/514 (54%)	9/20 (55%)	
Age—year (± S.D.)			
Mean	59.6 (±15.0)	54.2 (±15.9)	.114
Range	5–86	12–77	
Renal artery disease type			
Non-ASO	73/514 (14%)	7/20 (35%)	.020
ASO	441/514 (86%)	13/20 (65%)	
Mean BP (± S.D.)	196 (±36)/105 (±22)	197 (±30)/111 (±16)	.873*
Duration of HTN—months (± S.D.)	122 (±116)	106 (±97)	.569
Primary intervention			
Combined aortic repair	177/514 (34%)	6/20 (30%)	.682
Bilateral RA repair	254/514 (49%)	9/20 (45%)	.698
Number of kidneys			
Ex vivo	29/696 (4%)	6/24 (25%)	<.001
Bypass	427/696 (61%)	19/24 (79%)	.176
Thromboendarterectomy	218/696 (31%)	4/24 (17%)	.275
Reimplantation	51/696 (7%)	1/24 (4%)	.999
Azotemia (SCr > 1.8 mg/dl)	206/503 (41%)	7/20 (35%)	.595
Diabetes mellitus	67/514 (13%)	1/20 (5%)	.494
Congestive heart failure	89/514 (17%)	2/20 (10%)	.551

From Hansen KJ, Deitch JA, Oskin TC, et al: Renal artery repair: Consequence of operative failures. Ann Surg 227:678–690, 1998.
*p value for systolic pressure only.
ASO = atherosclerosis; HTN = hypertension; RA = renal artery; SCr = serum creatinine; S.D. = standard deviation; BP = blood pressure.

.001) and shortened dialysis-free survival (RR: 2.4; CI: 1.1, 5.4; p = .035).

The authors' methods for evaluation and treatment of renovascular disease are described earlier. However, this experience with failed renal artery repairs reinforces the following two important issues:

1. The irretrievable loss of excretory renal function observed after failed renal artery repair supports the view that renal revascularization should be performed for clear clinical indications but not as a "prophylactic" procedure in the absence of either hypertension or renal insufficiency.[1, 17]

2. The direct aortorenal reconstructions utilized in these patients are durable. The short length and high blood flow characterizing aortorenal repair favor prolonged patency. Consequently, most failures of repair reflect errors in surgical technique or judgment.

The role of percutaneous balloon angioplasty after failed renovascular repair is uncertain. In this series, balloon angioplasty was utilized in seven of 20 patients prior to either primary (four patients; six arteries) or secondary (three patients; five arteries) operative intervention. As a primary procedure for atherosclerotic lesions, balloon an-

TABLE 123-9. COMPARISON OF EVENTUAL RESULTS OF REOPERATION FOR FAILED RENAL ARTERY REPAIR (n = 20) WITH RESULTS FROM PRIMARY INTERVENTION ONLY (n = 514)

	PRIMARY INTERVENTION ONLY	SECONDARY INTERVENTION		p VALUE
		Initial	Eventual	
Perioperative mortality (%)	3.6	0	0	.999
Hypertension response (%)				
Cured	19	24	15	.808
Improved	71	70	80	
No Change	10	6	5	
Renal function response (%)				
Improved	34	59	10	.003
No Change	53	29	50	
Worsened	13	12	40	
Eventual dialysis dependence	4	0	35	<.001

From Hansen KJ, Deitch JA, Oskin TC, et al: Renal artery repair: Consequence of operative failures. Ann Surg 227:678–690, 1998.

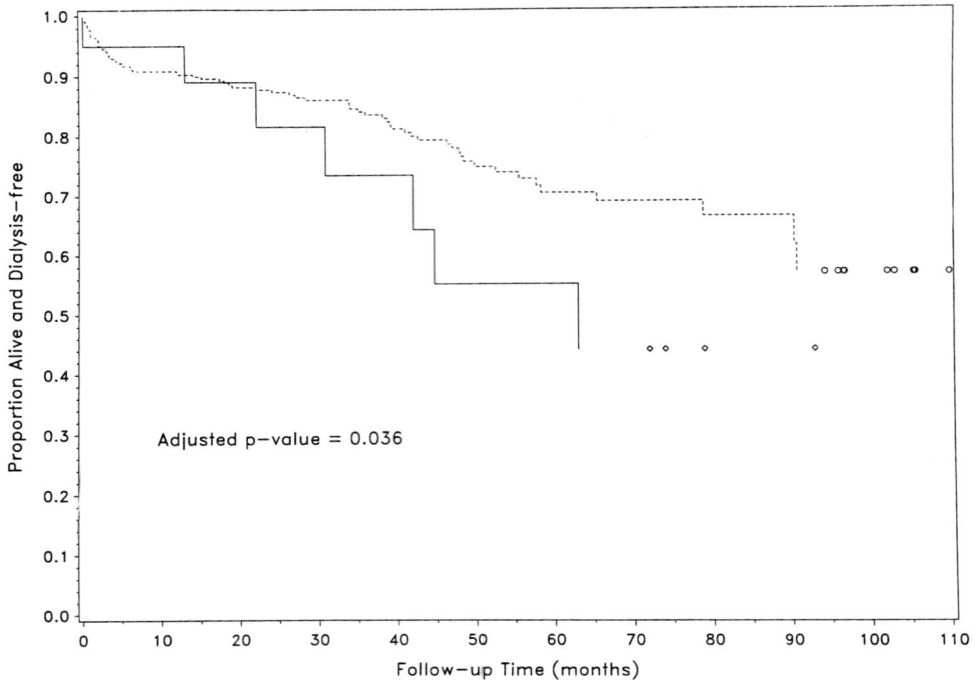

FIGURE 123–8. Product-limit estimates of dialysis-free survival for 20 patients requiring secondary renal artery operation (*solid line*) and 514 patients having primary renal artery repair only (*broken line*) with adjusted *p* value. Operative failure was associated with a significant and independent decrease in dialysis-free survival. (From Hansen KJ, Deitch JS, Oskin TC. et al: Renal artery repair: Consequences of operative failures. Ann Surg 227:678, 1998.)

gioplasty is frequently associated with focal plaque dissection and disruption of the intima and media. As a consequence of the resulting periarterial fibrosis, subsequent operative procedures often resemble secondary procedures after failed operative repair.[38] In the case of failed operative repair, the technical challenges posed by secondary operative intervention may make percutaneous treatment appealing.[39–41] In this group, balloon dilatation was applied to five renal arteries after stenosis of a primary operative repair due to a sclerotic venous valve (1), focal subendothelial fibrous proliferation (2), or recurrent disease at a site of endarterectomy (3). In each case, percutaneous angioplasty was considered immediately successful but failed 1 to 8 months later. Given the paucity of data regarding balloon angioplasty after failed operative repair, secondary operative intervention should be considered the preferred, albeit challenging, method of remedial management.

EFFECT OF BLOOD PRESSURE AND RENAL FUNCTION RESPONSE ON EVENT-FREE SURVIVAL

The rationale for treatment of renovascular disease is to improve event-free survival. For the authors' contemporary group of 534 patients reviewed previously, beneficial hypertension response has not improved the estimated survival.[33] This result contrasts sharply with the outcome of 71 patients who underwent operative management of renovascu-

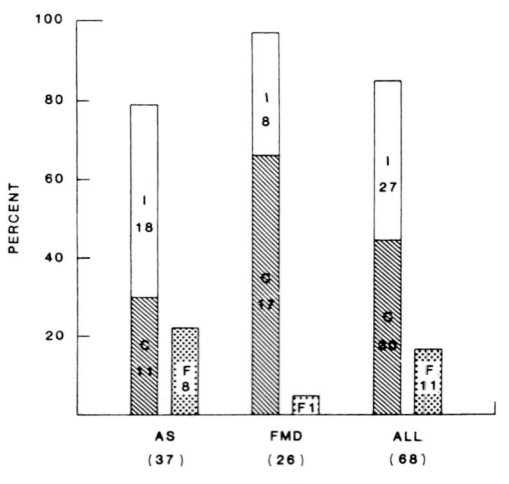

FIGURE 123–9. Bar graphs comparing initial benefit with late blood pressure response in the respective types of lesions. FMD = fibromuscular dysplasia. (From Dean RH, Krueger TC, Whiteneck JM, et al: Operative management of renovascular hypertension. J Vasc Surg 1:234, 1984.)

lar hypertension 15 to 23 years previously.[42] Complete follow-up was available in 66 of the 68 patients in this earlier group who survived operation. Comparison of the initial blood pressure response to operation (1 to 6 months postoperatively) with the blood pressure status at the time of death or the date of the study (up to 23 years later) showed that the effect of operative treatment was maintained over long-term follow-up (Fig. 123–9). In patients who required a second renovascular operation for recurrent hypertension during follow-up, the majority of the operations were performed for the management of contralateral renal artery lesions that had progressed to functional significance. For this latter group of patients, beneficial blood pressure response was associated with better estimated survival than failure of response. Although the subgroup of patients with response failures was small, it demonstrated a higher rate of death during follow-up (Fig. 123–10). This finding suggests that inadequate management of renovascular hypertension leaves the patient at higher risk of cardiovascular death over the long term.

There are several potential explantations for the failure of the authors' contemporary patient group to demonstrate a similar improvement in estimated survival after beneficial blood pressure response. First, the average follow-up for the contemporary group of 534 patients is much shorter (mean, 3 years, versus 17 years for the earlier group). During the period of follow-up, not a single death has been observed among the 80 patients with nonatherosclerotic renovascular disease. Second, the contemporary group was significantly older at the time of initial intervention (mean age, 68 years, versus 50 years for the earlier group) with significantly more extrarenal atherosclerotic disease (95%, versus 40% for the earlier group). Finally, and perhaps most important, 71% of the contemporary patients demonstrated at least mild excretory renal insufficiency and 41% had severe azotemia (i.e., serum creatinine >2.0 mg/dl).

In contrast to blood pressure response, renal function

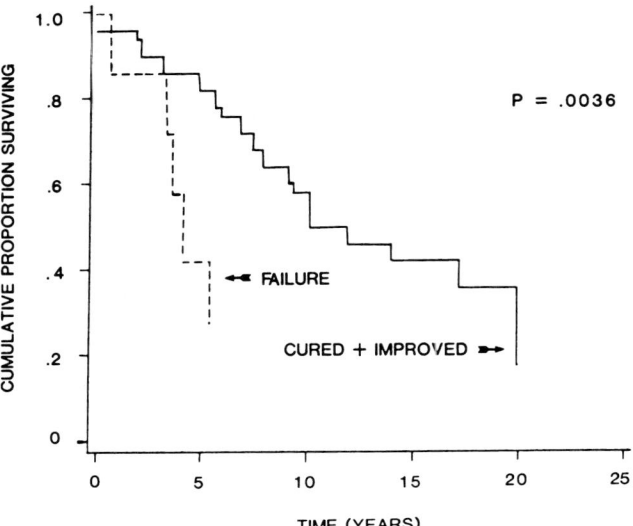

FIGURE 123–10. Kaplan-Meier life-table analysis showing estimated survival according to response to operation in 37 patients with arteriosclerosis. Deaths are from cardiovascular causes. (From Dean RH, Krueger TC, Whiteneck JM, et al: Operative management of renovascular hypertension. J Vasc Surg 1:234, 1984.)

response among contemporary patients demonstrated a significant and independent association with survival during follow-up.[33] Global renal disease treated with complete renal artery repair after rapid decline in excretory renal function is associated with the best opportunity for recovery of renal function.[1, 20, 23, 43] In addition, patients with improved renal function have demonstrated a significant decrease in the rate of decline in estimated GFR after renal artery repair.[20, 23] In the case of primary renal artery repair, only patients with ischemic nephropathy whose renal function is unimproved or worsened after repair remain at risk for dialysis dependence.[1, 33] The clinical significance of these observations is expressed in both the quality and quantity of the patient's life after intervention. Becoming dialysis-dependent after surgery exerts profound effect on a patient's vigor and independence and contributes significantly to a higher risk for death during follow-up.[1, 23, 27] In the contemporary patient population, the single strongest risk factor for death during follow-up has been progression to dialysis-dependent renal failure.

OPERATIVE STRATEGY

As discussed earlier, the authors do not recommend prophylactic renal revascularization; however, empiric renal artery repair is appropriate under selected circumstances. The term *empiric repair* implies that hypertension, renal dysfunction, or both are present, although a causal relationship between the renal artery lesion and these clinical sequelae has not been established. The specific circumstances in which empiric renal artery repair may be performed are summarized in the following discussion.

Repair of unilateral renal artery disease may be appropriate as an independent or combined procedure in the presence of negative functional studies when (1) hypertension remains severe and uncontrollable with maximal drug therapy, (2) the patient is relatively young and without significant surgical risk factors, and (3) the probability of technical success is greater than 95%. In these circumstances, correction of a renal artery lesion may be justified in order to eliminate all possible causes of hypertension before assigning a patient as having an increased risk for adverse cardiovascular events. However, because the probability of blood pressure benefit is low in such a patient, the morbidity of the procedure must also be predictably low. Although the authors have undertaken unilateral renal artery repair in patients with renal insufficiency who have not had positive functional test results, such procedures have been performed as a part of a clinical research study on ischemic nephropathy. The authors do not recommend this procedure as a clinically proven therapeutic intervention. Although the authors commonly correct bilateral renal artery disease without prior functional assessment in patients with severe hypertension, renal insufficiency, or both, the authors do not proceed with empiric renal artery repair as an independent procedure in patients with mild hypertension but without renal insufficiency.

The incidental finding of renal artery disease during angiographic evaluation of either occlusive or aneurysmal aortic disease frequently produces a therapeutic dilemma.

Although concern about leaving uncorrected anatomic disease in juxtaposition with an aortic reconstruction has led to a liberal approach to simultaneous renal reconstruction in many centers, the application of a selective approach to such combined procedures is more appropriate. As discussed earlier, the authors consider hypertension a prerequisite for renal artery repair. If the patient is normotensive, operation should be limited to the aortic procedure. If unilateral renal artery stenosis is found in a hypertensive patient, then simultaneous aortic and renal repair should be performed when the stenosis is found to have functional significance as demonstrated by positive renal vein renin assays. When hypertension is either severe or poorly controlled, renal revascularization may be undertaken without functional assessment even though the blood pressure benefit is less predictable.

When a patient has bilateral renal artery stenoses and hypertension, the decision to combine renal artery repair with correction of the aortic disease is based on the severity of both the hypertension and the renovascular lesions. When the two renal artery lesions consist of severe disease on one side and only mild or moderate disease on the other side, the patient is treated as having only a unilateral lesion. If both lesions are only moderately severe (stenosis reducing the diameter by 60% to 80%), renal revascularization is undertaken only if the hypertension is severe. If both renal artery lesions are severe (>80% stenosis) and the patient has drug-dependent hypertension, bilateral simultaneous renal revascularization is performed. In this instance, hypertension secondary to severe bilateral renal artery stenosis is particularly severe and difficult to control. Furthermore, at least mild renal insufficiency is often present.

Because azotemia usually parallels the severity of hypertension, a patient who presents with severe azotemia but only mild hypertension usually has renal parenchymal disease. Characteristically, renovascular hypertension associated with severe azotemia or dialysis dependence is associated with total renal artery occlusions or with very severe bilateral stenoses. When considering combined repair of incidentally identified bilateral renal artery disease with correction of aortic disease, one should evaluate the patient's clinical status with respect to this characteristic presentation. In such situations, combined renal artery repair at the time of aortic surgery is indicated to improve excretory renal function, with beneficial blood pressure response a secondary goal. Such indications appear justified in light of the observed increase in estimated survival associated with improved renal function despite the greater morbidity and mortality of a combined aortorenal procedure.

With application of this approach, the authors' operative mortality rate for "combined aortorenal procedures" compares well with that of other contemporary experiences (Table 123–10).[44–53] Review of the authors' operative mortality rates and clinical characteristics in this contemporary experience with "combined," "renal alone," and "aortic alone" surgical groups suggests that operative risk is affected by the patient's stage of atherosclerosis and the complexity of the procedure. The prevalence of end-organ damage, such as azotemia and heart disease, and the frequency of extrarenal atherosclerosis was greater in the "combined" and "renal alone" groups than in the "aortic alone" group.[17]

Although the operative mortality rate of the "combined" group was higher (5.3%) than that of the "renal alone" group (1.7%), the difference is not statistically significant; in contrast, it was statistically higher than the "aortic alone" operative death rate (0.7%). These two observations suggest that stage of disease and magnitude of operation both may affect operative risk, providing further support for empiric, but not prophylactic, renovascular repair.

SPECIAL ISSUES

Renovascular Disease in the Elderly Patient

Adults in the fifth decade of life with severe hypertension of recent onset are frequently considered representative of the population with renovascular hypertension. In contrast, many reported experiences have confirmed that hypertension of renal origin is most commonly caused by renovascular occlusive disease at the extremes of age.[54–56] However, the value of diagnostic evaluation and intervention for atherosclerotic renovascular disease in a patient beyond the seventh decade of life is debated. Some investigators suggest that renal artery disease in the elderly patient represents only one component of a widespread atherosclerotic process associated with advanced and irreversible renal and nonrenal atherosclerotic damage, which decreases the opportunity for improvement in blood pressure and increases the risks of surgical intervention.[54]

This pessimistic argument is amplified when one considers that contemporary patients in the seventh and eighth decades of life are characterized by hypertension of long duration, overt extrarenal atherosclerosis, and renal insufficiency.[57, 58] Consequently, elderly patients with hypertension are often systematically excluded from diagnostic evaluation and surgical management of significant renovascular disease.[54] When one considers that the population with atherosclerosis evaluated for renal artery disease is an increasingly older group, evaluation of the results of operation in elderly patients has importance.[8]

At the authors' center, 230 patients 60 years of age and older underwent operative renal artery repair from January 1987 through June 1995.[43] The group consisted of 117 men and 113 women in their seventh (153 patients), eighth (70 patients) or ninth (7 patients) decade of life (range, 60 to 86 years; mean age, 68 years). Significant hypertension was present in all patients, and blood pressure ranged from 280/190 mmHg to 178/90 mmHg (mean, 202/102 mmHg). Fifty patients had a normal serum creatinine (<1.2 mg/dl). Seventy-six patients had mild renal insufficiency as indicated by serum creatinine level (1.3–1.9 mg/dl) and 104 patients had severe insufficiency (>2.0 mg/dl), including 23 patients who were dialysis-dependent for 10 to 31 days prior to operation.

All patients underwent direct aortorenal reconstruction.[43] Simultaneous aortic reconstruction was required in 95 patients. All hemodynamically significant disease was corrected surgically. Among 366 kidneys operated, only six nephrectomies were performed. Thirteen patients died in the hospital or within 30 days of surgery, providing a perioperative mortality of 6%. Ten deaths occurred after complex vascular procedures combined with aortic recon-

TABLE 123–10. COMPARISON OF MAJOR SERIES OF COMBINED AORTORENAL RECONSTRUCTION

STUDY				PATIENTS		TYPE OF RENAL REPAIR (%)		HYPERTENSION RESPONSE* (%)	PERIOPERATIVE MORTALITY (%)
Author	Chapter Reference No.	City	Year	Mean Age (yr)	No.	Unilateral	Bilateral		
Perry	44	New York	1984	—	60	—	—	50	5
Sterpetti	45	Omaha	1986	61.8	39	64	36	65.6	10
Tarazi	46	Cleveland	1987	63	89	63	37	57.5	10
O'Mara	47	Jackson	1988	67	32	0	100	90	3
Atnip	48	Hershey	1990	66	27	79	21	64	10.3
Allen	49	St. Louis	1993	66.3	102	83	17	86	5
McNeil	50	Mobile	1994	64	101	64	36	74	1
Huber	51	Gainesville	1995	—	56	—	—	—	8.9
Brothers	52	Charleston	1995	63	70	59	41	—	16
Cambria	53	Boston	1995	67.5	100	81.5	18.5	68	6.5
Benjamin	17	Winston-Salem	1996	62.5	133	47	53	63	5.3

*Represents the total patients whose hypertension was *cured* and/or *improved*.

struction. No preoperative or operative parameters demonstrated a significant association with operative mortality. Significant perioperative (30-day) morbidity that extended hospitalization occurred in 61 patients (27%). During a mean follow-up of 29 months, 28 deaths occurred, 25 of which were from a presumed cardiovascular cause. Multivariate analysis demonstrated that a preoperative history of congestive heart failure and preoperative renal insufficiency were significant and independent predictors of death during follow-up among these elderly patients. Moreover, survival rate was significantly greater for patients with improved renal function after operation than in those with unimproved renal function ($p = .001$).

Blood pressure measurements and antihypertensive medication requirements at a point at least 8 weeks after operation were used for analysis of the hypertension response to operation. After a mean follow-up of 29 months (6 to 102 months), hypertension in 20 patients (9%) was classified as cured and in 167 patients (77%) as improved, for an overall beneficial blood pressure response rate of 86% among the 217 patients surviving surgery. Equivalent blood pressure benefit was realized for patients irrespective of age, duration of hypertension, or presence of severe renal or extrarenal organ-specific atherosclerotic damage. Among operative survivors in whom the serum creatinine level was higher than 1.3 mg/dl before operation, renal function was improved in 43%, including 18 of 23 patients removed from dialysis; renal function in 42% showed no change and in 15% was worsened. Advanced excretory renal insufficiency did not reduce the opportunity for favorable renal function response after operation. After the analysis was controlled for the level of preoperative EGFR, patients undergoing bilateral or global renal artery repair demonstrated a significant increase in EGFR compared with those undergoing unilateral repair. Overall, 47% of patients undergoing bilateral repair had at least a 20% increase in estimated GFR compared with 36% of patients undergoing unilateral repair.

Many of the controversies surrounding decisions for evaluation and surgical management of atherosclerotic renovascular disease causing hypertension and renal insufficiency are illustrated by this group of elderly patients and the results of the authors' management. As shown by this experience, elderly patients often have hypertension of long

duration and extensive extrarenal atherosclerosis. These features have been reported by others to diminish beneficial blood pressure response to renal revascularization.[54, 57] Similarly, nonrenal organ-specific atherosclerotic damage as a result of diffuse atherosclerosis has been recognized to significantly increase the risk of cardiovascular morbidity and mortality associated with surgery. In addition, renovascular hypertension associated with diffuse vascular disease, as seen in the authors' group of elderly patients, has been associated with decreased long-term survival in patients who have undergone surgery and in those who have not.[42, 59, 60]

As a result of these reports indicating smaller chance for cure of hypertension, higher risk for operative morbidity and mortality, and shorter long-term survival regardless of surgical intervention, many investigators have advised a conservative diagnostic and nonsurgical approach in patients with hypertension beyond the fifth or sixth decade of life.[8, 54, 57] Conversely, the authors evaluate every patient with severe hypertension regardless of chronologic age or associated atherosclerosis if the patient would otherwise be considered a candidate for correction of renal artery disease if a significant renal artery lesion were defined. Preoperative evaluation is designed to identify those parameters that contribute independently to increased postoperative mortality.

Renovascular Disease in the Diabetic Patient

Despite the recognized contribution of elevated blood pressure to cardiovascular morbidity and mortality, the value of surgical correction of atherosclerotic renovascular disease in the diabetic patient is uncertain. On the basis of a decreased rate of beneficial blood pressure response in diabetic patients, early reports cited diabetes mellitus as a relative contraindication to operative renal artery repair.[54, 61] Moreover, the results of surgical intervention to retrieve excretory renal function in the diabetic patient with renal insufficiency are often unpredictable because the relative contributions of ischemic nephropathy and renal parenchymal disease (e.g., diabetic nephropathy) are poorly defined.[25, 62]

Given the uncertainties regarding surgical intervention in this setting, the authors' operative experience with management of atherosclerotic renal artery disease in 54 consecutive diabetic adults is reviewed.[63] This patient group comprised 37 women and 17 men ranging in age from 52 to 78 years (mean, 64 ± 6.0 years). Each patient was hypertensive (mean blood pressure, 213 ± 29/103 ± 21 mmHg; mean number of medications, 3) and each was diabetic. Sixteen patients required insulin and 38 patients had required oral agents for control of hyperglycemia for 3 to 24 years (mean duration, 12.6 years); 11 patients had been diabetic for longer than 10 years. No patient had been found to have with diabetes mellitus prior to the fourth decade of life. Renal dysfunction, evidenced by a serum creatinine 1.8 mg/dl after removal of ACE inhibitors and high-dose diuretics, was present in 45 patients (82%; mean, 2.4 mg/dl; 3 patients dialysis-dependent).

On the basis of preoperative urinalysis from morning specimens, the presence of preoperative proteinuria was determined. Persistent proteinuria was present in 36 patients (67%). Thirteen patients had trace to 30 mg/dl protein levels, whereas 23 patients had levels higher than 100 mg/dl. Seven patients had persistent proteinuria exceeding 300 mg/dl and in each case demonstrated nephrosis-range proteinuria from a 24-hour urine collection.

Among the 50 patients who survived operation, 36 patients (72%) demonstrated a beneficial blood pressure response and in 14 patients (28%), blood pressure was considered unimproved.[63] Blood pressure response demonstrated no significant association with patient age, duration of hypertension or diabetes, or requirement for insulin. In the 42 operative survivors with preoperative serum creatinine values exceeding 1.8 mg/dl, renal function response was improved in 17 patients (40%), including three removed from dialysis; 18 patients (43%) showed *no change*; and renal function in seven patients (17%) was *worsened*. The increase in postoperative estimated GFR for patients considered to have improved renal function was significantly greater than that for patients whose renal function was considered unchanged or worsened ($p = \le .01$). In individual patients, however, a change in estimated GFR demonstrated no significant relationship to the site of disease or the extent of operation. Similarly, neither the presence or severity of preoperative proteinuria nor the angiographically determined grade of nephrosclerosis was significantly associated with change in estimated GFR after operation.

The product-limit estimates for this group of patients demonstrated that preoperative estimated GFR was significantly and inversely associated with time to dialysis or death during follow-up ($p = .03$).[63] Although hypertension response did not demonstrate a significant association with dialysis dependence or death during follow-up, renal function response to operation was important. Diabetic patients who demonstrated improved renal function after operation had a significantly lower risk of death or dialysis dependence than patients whose renal function was unchanged or worsened ($p = .01$). Diabetic patients demonstrated an operative mortality more than double (7.4%) that of 291 hypertensive nondiabetic patients (3.1%) who underwent renal artery repair during the same period; however, this difference did not reach statistical significance. No significant difference was observed in the rate of improved renal function response between the two groups (40% [diabetic]

versus 51% [nondiabetic]; $p = .21$), however, significantly fewer diabetic patients demonstrated a beneficial blood pressure response after renal artery repair than nondiabetic patients (72% versus 89% cured or improved, respectively; $p = \le 0.01$).

This experience suggests that the majority of selected diabetic patients demonstrate beneficial blood pressure response after operation, but significantly fewer diabetic patients are cured or improved compared with nondiabetic patients. Overall, renal function response was not statistically different for diabetic patients, but renal function response in diabetic patients was unpredictable. Contrary to findings for nondiabetic patients, neither the site of disease or operation nor the grade of nephrosclerosis was associated with renal function response in diabetic patients. In addition, the presence and level of preoperative proteinuria failed to demonstrate an association with excretory function either before or after renal revascularization.

Renovascular Disease in African Americans

Hypertension in African Americans differs in a quantitative sense from that observed in white patients. Hypertension in black patients occurs with greater frequency and severity and at a younger age.[64] In addition, elevated blood pressure at any level is associated with greater cardiovascular morbidity and renal disease in black patients.[65] Many putative mechanisms have been suggested to account for this aggressive form of hypertension, implying that hypertension in African Americans is intrinsically different from that in white patients.[66] Although these mechanisms remain speculative, it has generally been accepted that correctable renovascular disease and renovascular hypertension occur infrequently.[67–69] Moreover, the increased end-organ damage at any level of hypertension along with the perceived low prevalence of renovascular hypertension have limited enthusiasm for the investigation and treatment of renovascular disease in African Americans.

In a comparison of 28 African Americans with 370 white patients operated for atherosclerotic renovascular disease at the authors' center, no significant difference was observed in severity or duration of hypertension between the two groups.[70] Overall, black patients had a greater prevalence of clinically detectable cardiovascular disease and demonstrated a significantly higher rate of left ventricular hypertrophy than white patients ($p = .02$). Clinical congestive heart failure and significant aortoiliac occlusive disease were more common in African Americans but the rates did not differ significantly from those in white patients ($p = .09$). More extensive renovascular disease was noted among African Americans; bilateral disease was present in 68% of black patients compared with 54% of white patients ($p = .16$). Moreover, African Americans tended have more severe excretory renal dysfunction (mean serum creatinine 2.5 mg/dl for blacks versus 2.1 mg/dl for whites; $p = .25$). Fifty-seven per cent of African Americans, versus 40% of white patients, were determined to have severe renal dysfunction.

Despite the tendency for higher prevalence of cardiovascular disease, greater extent of renal disease, and more severe renal dysfunction in black patients, the beneficial blood pressure responses to operation were similar for

African Americans and white patients (70% versus 89%, respectively, benefited).[70] Although the proportion of patients with improved renal function after surgery did not differ significantly (59% [black] versus 42% [white] improved), African Americans demonstrated a significantly greater decline in serum creatinine level than white patients (0.74 mg/dl versus 0.14 mg/dl decrease, respectively; $p <$ .05). Unlike the white patients, equivalent and significant improvement was observed in African Americans regardless of the site of disease or extent of operation.

Compared with essential hypertension in white patients, hypertension in African Americans is approximately 40% more prevalent, tends to occur at an earlier age, is usually more severe within any age range, and is associated with a greater frequency of pressure-related end-organ damage.[64] For any given elevation in blood pressure, African Americans demonstrate a higher rate of death secondary to hypertensive heart disease, stroke, and renal disease.[65, 71] Considered in context of the genetic, physiologic, and socioeconomic explanations offered for these ethnic differences, hypertension and its associated morbidity are often regarded as inevitable in black patients.[72] For many investigators, this discouraging view also applies to renovascular hypertension.[73] Data derived from 7200 African American adults referred to a tertiary care hypertension clinic demonstrated that renovascular hypertension was present in only 0.2%.[68] A low prevalence of renovascular hypertension among hypertensive black patients was also suggested by the Cooperative Study of Renovascular Hypertension.[74] Although African Americans constituted 30% of the study sample, only 8% of the patients with renal artery stenosis were black. Foster and colleagues[69] described a lower prevalence of renal artery stenosis in black women than in white women; moreover, they found no case of advanced renovascular disease in black men, compared with a 30% prevalence in white men. Given the apparent rarity of renovascular disease and renovascular hypertension black patients, these investigators suggested that hypertensive African Americans should not be subjected to extensive investigation for renal artery disease.

In contrast, the authors believe that the presence of atherosclerotic renovascular disease is not determined by ethnicity. Preliminary results from an ongoing population-based study at the authors' center suggest that black and white patients demonstrate equivalent prevalences of hemodynamically significant renovascular disease (unpublished data). Renal artery disease may occur with equal frequency, but renovascular hypertension does not contribute equally to hypertension in black and white patients. In this regard, the authors reviewed the results from renal duplex ultrasonography studies obtained to screen for renovascular disease among 629 consecutive subjects, consisiting of 127 black patients (20%) and 502 white patients (80%). Twelve percent of black subjects and 28% of white subjects demonstrated renovascular disease according to the duplex ultrasonography criteria ($p <$ .001).[29] This highly significant difference between black and white patients should be considered in the context of the selection criteria for study. The primary clinical criterion prompting renal duplex ultrasonography for the entire group was severe or poorly controlled hypertension. Because severe essential hypertension occurs more commonly in African Americans than in white

patients, proportionately fewer black patients would be expected to demonstrate renovascular disease when screened according to these selection criteria.

On the basis of these findings, the authors believe that clinicians should search for a renovascular cause of severe hypertension without regard to race. Proportionately fewer black patients will demonstrate renovascular hypertension, but the beneficial effects of operative renovascular repair in black patients are demonstrated by the authors' operative experience. Especially gratifying is the observed improvement in excretory renal function in the black cohort. Both unilateral and bilateral renal reconstructions were associated with significantly improved renal function in black patients, which in turn was significantly greater than the improvement observed among white patients.

REFERENCES

1. Hansen KJ, Starr SM, Sands RE, et al: Contemporary surgical management of renovascular disease. J Vasc Surg 16:319, 1992.
2. Maxwell MH, Waks AU: Renovascular hypertension: Current approaches to management. Pract Cardiol 13:128, 1987.
3. Cumberland DC: Percutaneous transluminal angioplasty: A review. Clin Radiol 34:25, 1983.
4. Vaughan ED, Case DB, Pickering TG, et al: Indication for intervention in patients with renovascular hypertension. Am J Kidney Dis 5:A136, 1985.
5. Libertino JA, Flam TA, Zinman LN, et al: Changing concepts in surgical management of renovascular hypertension. Arch Intern Med 148:357, 1988.
6. Novick AC, Ziegelbaum M, Vidt DG, et al: Trends in surgical revascularization for renal artery disease. JAMA 257:498, 1987.
7. Stanley JC, Fry WJ: Surgical treatment of renovascular hypertension. Arch Surg 112:1291, 1977.
8. Hansen KJ, Ditesheim JA, Metropol SH, et al: Management of renovascular hypertension in the elderly population. J Vasc Surg 10:266, 1989.
9. Foster JH, Dean RH, Pinkerston JA, et al: Ten years experience with the surgical management of renovascular hypertension. Ann Surg 177:755, 1973.
10. Dean RH, Wilson JP, Burko H, Foster JH: Saphenous vein aortorenal bypass grafts: Serial arteriographic study. Ann Surg 180:469, 1974.
11. Oskin TC, Hansen KJ, Deitch JS, et al: Chronic renal artery occlusion: Nephrectomy versus revascularization. J Vasc Surg 29:140, 1999.
12. Lawson JD, Boerth RF, Foster JH, et al: Diagnosis and management of renovascular hypertension in children. Arch Surg 112:1307, 1977.
13. Wollenweber J, Sheps SG, Davis GD: Clinical course of atherosclerotic renovascular disease. Am J Cardiol 21:60, 1968.
14. Schreiber M, Phol MA, Novick AC: The natural history of atherosclerotic fibrous renal artery disease. Urol Clin North Am 11:383, 1984.
15. Dean RH, Kieffer RW, Smith BM, et al: Renovascular hypertension: Anatomic and renal function changes during drug therapy. Arch Surg 166:1408, 1981.
16. Novick AC, Pohl MA, Schreiber M, et al: Revascularization for preservation of renal function in patients with atherosclerotic renovascular disease. J Urol 129:907, 1983.
17. Benjamin ME, Hansen KJ, Craven TE, et al: Combined aortic and renal artery surgery: A contemporary experience. Ann Surg 233:555, 1996.
18. Morris GC Jr, DeBakey ME, Cooley DA: Surgical treatment of renal failure of renovascular origin. JAMA 182:609, 1962.
19. O'Neal EA, Hansen KJ, Conzarillo VJ, et al: Prevalence of ischemic nephropathy in patients with renal insufficiency. Am Surg 58:52, 1992.
20. Dean RH, Tribble RW, Hansen KJ, et al: Evolution of renal insufficiency in ischemic nephropathy. Ann Surg 213:446, 1991.
21. Hansen KJ, Reavis SW, Dean RH: Duplex scanning in renovascular disease. Geriatr Nephrol Urol 6:89, 1996.
22. Hansen KJ, Dean RH: Ischemic nephropathy: Clinical curiosity or

neglected imperative? *In* Ferrario CM (ed): Council for High Blood Pressure Newsletter. Vol 2, American Heart Association, 1993, p 7.

23. Hansen KJ, Thomason RB, Craven TE, et al: Surgical management of dialysis-dependent ischemic nephropathy. J Vasc Surg 21:197, 1995.

24. Jacobson HR: Ischemic renal disease: An overlooked clinical entity? Kidney Int 34:729, 1988.

25. Rimmer JM, Gennari FJ: Atherosclerotic renovascular disease and progressive renal failure. Ann Intern Med 118:712, 1993.

26. North Carolina Kidney Council: Annual Report. Raleigh, 1986.

27. Mailloux LU, Bellucci AG, Mossey RT, et al: Predictors of survival in patients undergoing dialysis. Am J Med 84:855, 1988.

28. Appel RG, Bleyer AJ, Reavis S, Hansen KJ: Renovascular disease in older patients beginning renal replacement therapy. Kidney Int 48:171, 1995.

29. Hansen KJ, Tribble RW, Reavis SW, et al: Renal duplex sonography: Evaluation of clinical utility. J Vasc Surg 12:227, 1990.

30. Dean RH, Lawson JD, Hollifield JW, et al: Revascularization of the poorly functioning kidney. Surgery 85:44, 1979.

31. Towne JB, Bernhard VM: Revascularization of the ischemic kidney. Arch Surg 113:216, 1978.

32. Zinman L, Libertino JA: Revascularization of the chronic totally occluded renal artery with restoration of renal function. J Urol 228:517, 1977.

33. Hansen KJ, Deitch JA, Oskin TC: Renal artery repair: Consequence of operative failures. Ann Surg 227:678, 1998.

34. Stanley JC, Whitehouse WM, Zelenock GB, et al: Reoperation for complications of renal artery reconstructive surgery undertaken for treatment of renovascular hypertension. J Vasc Surg 2:133, 1985.

35. Novick AC: Secondary renal vascular reconstruction for arterial disease in the native and transplant kidney. Urol Clin North Am 21:255, 1994.

36. Fowl RJ, Hollier LH, Bernatz PE, et al: Repeat revascularization versus nephrectomy in the treatment of recurrent renovascular hypertension. Surg Gynecol Obstet 162:37, 1986.

37. Erzuck E, Novick AC, Vidt DG, Cunnington R: Secondary renal revascularization for recurrent renal artery stenosis. Cleve Clin J Med 56:427, 1989.

38. Dean RH, Callis JT, Smith BM, Meacham PW: Failed percutaneous transluminal renal angioplasty: Experience with lesions requiring operative intervention. J Vasc Surg 6:301, 1987.

39. Libertino JA, Beckmann CF: Surgery and percutaneous angioplasty in the management of renovascular hypertension. Urol Clin North Am 21:235, 1994.

40. Novick AC: Percutaneous transluminal angioplasty and surgery of the renal artery. Eur J Vasc Surg 8:1, 1994.

41. Erdoes LS, Berman SS, Hunter GC, Mills JL: Comparative analysis of percutaneous transluminal angioplasty and operation for renal revascularization. Am J Kidney Dis 27:496, 1996.

42. Dean RH, Krueger TC, Whiteneck JM, et al: Operative management of renovascular hypertension: Results after 15–23 years follow-up. J Vasc Surg 1:234, 1984.

43. Hansen KJ, Benjamin ME, Appel RG, et al: Renovascular hypertension in the elderly: Results of surgical management. Geriatr Nephrol Urol 6:3, 1996.

44. Perry MO, Silane MF: Management of renovascular problems during aortic operations. Arch Surg 119:681, 1984.

45. Sterpetti AV, Schultz RD, Feldhaus RJ, et al: Aortic and renal atherosclerotic disease. Surg Gynecol Obstet 163:54, 1986.

46. Tarazi RY, Hertzer NR, Beven EG, et al: Simultaneous aortic reconstruction and renal revascularization: Risk factors and late results in eighty-nine patients. J Vasc Surg 5:707, 1987.

47. O'Mara CS, Maples MD, Kilgore TL, et al: Simultaneous aortic reconstruction and bilateral renal revascularization. J Vasc Surg 8:357, 1988.

48. Atnip RG, Neumyer MM, Healy DA, et al: Combined aortic and visceral arterial reconstruction: Risks and result. J Vasc Surg 12:705, 1990.

49. Allen BT, Rubin GG, Anderson CB, et al: Simultaneous surgical management of aortic and renovascular disease. Am J Surg 166:726, 1993.

50. McNeil JW, String ST, Pfeiffer RB: Concomitant renal endarterectomy and aortic reconstruction. J Vasc Surg 20:331, 1994.

51. Huber TS, Harward TRS, Flynn TC, et al: Operative mortality rates after elective infrarenal aortic reconstruction. J Vasc Surg 22:287, 1995.

52. Brothers TE, Elliott BM, Robison JG, et al: Stratification of mortality risk for renal artery surgery. Am Surg 61:45, 1995.

53. Cambria RP, Brewster DC, Italien GL, et al: Simultaneous aortic and renal artery reconstruction: Evolution of an 18 year experience. J Vasc Surg 21:916, 1995.

54. Shapiro AP, Perez-Stable E, Scheib ET, et al: Renal artery stenosis and hypertension: Observations on the current status of therapy from a study of 115 patients. Am J Med 47:175, 1969.

55. Foster JH, Maxwell MH, Franklin SS, et al: Renovascular occlusive disease. JAMA 231:1043, 1975.

56. Hunt JC, Strong CG: Renovascular hypertension: Mechanism, natural history and treatment. Am J Cardiol 32:562, 1973.

57. Ernst CB, Stanley JC, Marshall FF, Fry WJ: Renal revascularization for atherosclerotic renovascular hypertension: Prognostic implications for focal renal artery vs. overt generalized arteriosclerosis. Surgery 73:859, 1973.

58. Lawrie GM, Morris GC, Sousson ID, et al: Late results of reconstructive surgery for renovascular disease. Ann Surg 191:528, 1980.

59. van Bockel JH, van Schifgaarde MD, Felthuis W, et al: Surgical treatment of renovascular hypertension caused by arteriosclerosis: II. Influence of preoperative risk factors and postoperative blood pressure response on late patient survival. Surgery 4:468, 1987.

60. Delin K, Aurell M, Granerus G, et al: Surgical treatment of renovascular hypertension in the elderly patient. Acta Med Scand 211:169, 1982.

61. Shapiro AP, Perez-Stable E, Moutsos SE: Coexistence of renal arterial hypertension and diabetes mellitus. JAMA 192:813, 1965.

62. Connolly JO, Higgins RM, Walters HL, et al: Presentation, clinical features and outcome in different patterns of atherosclerotic renovascular disease. Q J Med 87:413, 1994.

63. Hansen KJ, Andrew HL, Benjamin ME, et al: Is renal revascularization in diabetic patients worthwhile? J Vasc Surg 24:383, 1996.

64. Calhoun DA, Oparil S: Racial differences in the pathogenesis of hypertension. Am J Med Sci 310(Suppl 1):S86, 1995.

65. Flack JM, Neaton, JD, Daniels, B, Esunge P: Ethnicity and renal Disease: Lessons from the multiple risk factor intervention trial and the treatment of mild hypertension study. Am J Kidney Dis 21:31, 1993.

66. Jamerson KA: Prevalence of complications and response to different treatments of hypertension in African Americans and white Americans in the US. Clin Exp Hypertens 15:979, 1993.

67. Albers FJ: Clinical characteristics of atherosclerotic renovascular disease. Am J Kidney Dis 24:636, 1994.

68. Working Group on Renovascular Hypertension: Detection, evaluation, and treatment of renovascular hypertension. Arch Intern Med 147:820, 1987.

69. Foster JH, Oates JA, Rhamy RK, et al: Detection and treatment of patients with renovascular hypertension. Surgery 60:240, 1966.

70. Deitch JS, Hansen KJ, Craven TE, et al: Renal artery repair in African-Americans. J Vasc Surg 26:465, 1997.

71. Levy SB, Talner LB, Coel MN, et al: Renal vasculature in essential hypertension: Racial differences. Ann Intern Med 88:12, 1978.

72. Rostand SG: Hypertension and renal disease in blacks: Role of genetic and/or environmental factors? Adv Nephrol 21:99, 1992.

73. Keith TA: Renovascular hypertension in black patients. Hypertension 4:438, 1982.

74. Simon N, Franklin SS, Bleifer KH, et al: Clinical characteristics of renovascular hypertension. JAMA 220:1209, 1972.

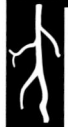

C H A P T E R 1 2 4

Techniques of Operative Management

Kimberley J. Hansen, M.D., Marshall E. Benjamin, M.D., and
Richard H. Dean, M.D.

A variety of operative techniques have been used to correct renal artery disease. From a practical standpoint, three basic operations have been most frequently utilized:

- Aortorenal bypass
- Renal artery thromboendarterectomy
- Renal artery reimplantation

Although each method may have its proponents, no single approach provides optimal repair for all types of renal disease. Aortorenal bypass using saphenous vein is probably the most versatile technique; however, thromboendarterectomy is especially useful for orificial atherosclerosis involving multiple renal arteries. Occasionally, the renal artery is sufficiently redundant to allow reimplantation, probably the simplest technique and one particularly appropriate to renal artery disease in children.

PREOPERATIVE PREPARATION

Antihypertensive medications are reduced during the preoperative period to the minimum necessary for blood pressure control. Frequently, patients who usually need large doses of multiple medications for hypertension management have significantly reduced requirements while hospitalized and placed at bed rest. If continued therapy is required, vasodilators (e.g., nifedipine) and selective beta-adrenergic blocking agents (i.e., atenolol, metoprolol) are useful. Adverse effects on hemodynamics are few when these agents are combined with general anesthesia. If an adult's diastolic blood pressure exceeds 120 mmHg, it is essential that the operative treatment be postponed until the pressure is brought under control. In this instance, the combination of intravenous sodium nitroprusside and esmolol is administered in an intensive care setting with continuous intra-arterial blood pressure monitoring. Similarly, in the patient with significant heart disease, pulmonary artery wedge pressure, cardiac index, and oxygen delivery are monitored to maintain optimal cardiac performance before and after operation.

Certain measures are used in almost all renal artery operations. Mannitol is administered intravenously in 12.5-gm doses early in the operation. Repeated doses are administered before and after periods of renal ischemia, up to a total dose of 1 gm/kg of patient body weight. Just prior to renal artery cross-clamping, 100 units of heparin per kilogram body weight are given intravenously, and systemic anticoagulation is verified with activated clotting time. Un-

less required for hemostasis, protamine is not routinely administered for reversal of heparin at the completion of the operation.

MOBILIZATION AND DISSECTION

A midline xiphoid-to-pubis abdominal incision is made for operative repair of atherosclerotic renal artery disease. The last 1 or 2 cm of the proximal end of the incision are made coursing to one side of the xiphoid to obtain full exposure of the upper abdominal aorta and renal branches. Some type of fixed mechanical retraction is also advantageous, particularly when combined aortorenal procedures are required. Otherwise, extended flank and subcostal incisions are reserved for unilateral fibrodysplastic lesions or splanchnorenal bypass.

When the supraceliac aorta is selected as an inflow source for unilateral aortorenal bypass, an extended flank incision is useful. With the ipsilateral flank elevated, the incision extends from the opposite semilunar line into the flank, bisecting the abdominal wall between the costal margin and iliac crest. A left or right visceral mobilization allows access to the renal vasculature and the aortic crus. If necessary, the crus can be divided and an extrapleural dissection of the descending thoracic aorta can provide access to the T9–T10 thoracic aorta for proximal control and anastomosis.[1, 2]

When the midline xiphoid-to-pubis incision is used, the posterior peritoneum overlying the aorta is incised longitudinally, and the duodenum is mobilized at the ligament of Treitz (Fig. 124–1). During this maneuver, it is important to identify visceral collaterals that course at this level. Finally, the duodenum is reflected to the patient's right to expose the left renal artery. By extending the posterior peritoneal incision to the left along the inferior border of the pancreas, the surgeon can enter an avascular plane posterior to the pancreas (see Fig. 124–1) to expose the entire left renal hilum. This exposure is of special significance when there are distal renal artery lesions to be managed (Fig. 124–2A). The left renal artery lies posterior to the left renal vein. In some cases, the vein can be retracted cephalad to expose the artery; in other cases, caudal retraction of the vein provides better access.

Usually, the gonadal and adrenal veins, which enter the left renal vein, must be ligated and divided to facilitate exposure of the distal artery. Frequently, a lumbar vein enters the posterior wall of the left renal vein, and it can

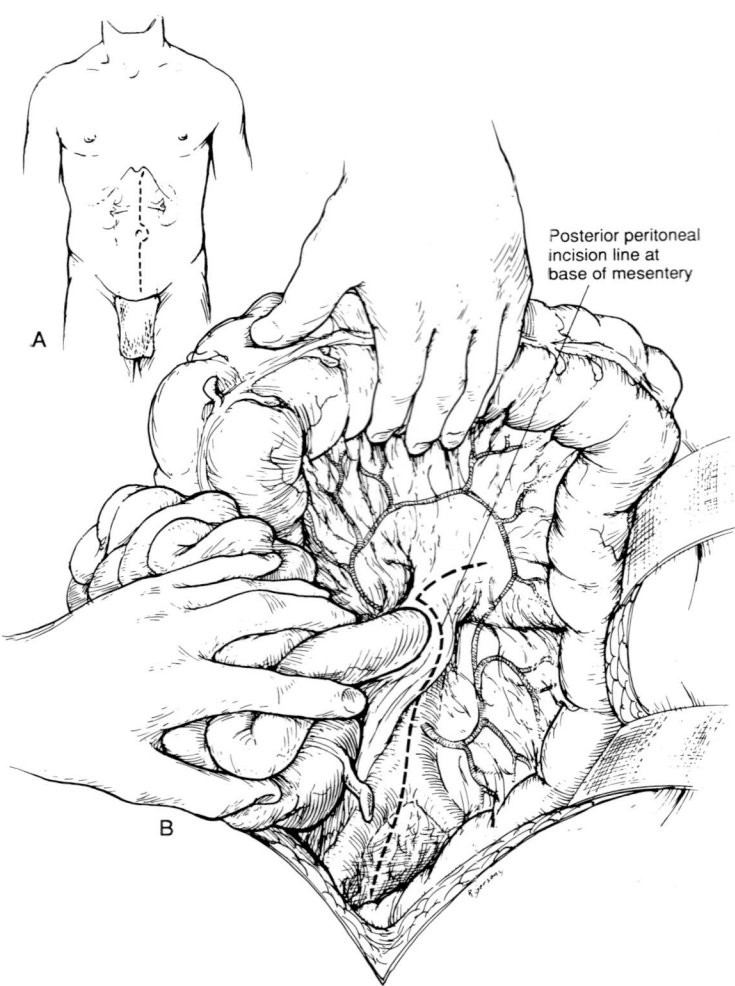

FIGURE 124-1. *A* and *B,* Exposure of the aorta and left renal hilum through the base of the mesentery. Extension of the posterior peritoneal incision to the left, along the inferior border of the pancreas, provides entry to an avascular plane behind the pancreas. This allows excellent exposure of the entire left renal hilum as well as the proximal right renal artery. (From Benjamin ME, Dean RH: Techniques in renal artery reconstruction: Part I. Ann Vasc Surg 10(3):306–314, 1996.)

be injured easily unless special care is taken (Fig. 124–2B). The surgeon can expose the proximal portion of the right renal artery through the base of the mesentery by ligating two or more pairs of lumbar veins and retracting the left renal vein cephalad and the vena cava to the patient's right (Fig. 124–2C). The distal portion of the right renal artery is best exposed, however, by medial mobilization of the duodenum and right colon; the right renal vein is mobilized and usually retracted cephalad in order to expose the artery.

Exposure of the distal right renal artery is achieved by colonic and duodenal mobilization. First, the hepatic flexure is mobilized at the peritoneal reflection (Fig. 124–3). With the right colon retracted medially and inferiorly, a Kocher maneuver mobilizes the duodenum and pancreatic head to expose the inferior vena cava and right renal vein (Fig. 124–4). Typically, the right renal artery is located just inferior to the accompanying vein, which can be retracted superiorly to provide the best exposure. Although accessory vessels may arise from the aorta or iliac vessels at any level, all arterial branches coursing anterior to the vena cava should be considered accessory right renal branches and should be carefully preserved (Fig. 124–5).

When bilateral renal artery lesions are to be corrected and when correction of a right renal artery lesion or bilateral lesions is combined with aortic reconstruction, these exposure techniques can be modified. The surgeon can extend the aortic exposure by mobilizing the base of the small bowel mesentery exposure to allow complete evisceration of the entire small bowel, right colon, and transverse colon. For this extended exposure, the posterior peritoneal incision begins with division of the ligament of Treitz and proceeds along the base of the mesentery to the cecum and then along the lateral gutter to the foramen of Winslow (Fig. 124–6A). The inferior border of the pancreas is fully mobilized to allow entry to a retropancreatic plane, thereby exposing the aorta to a point above the superior mesenteric artery. Through this modified exposure, simultaneous bilateral renal endarterectomies, aortorenal grafting, or renal artery attachment to the aortic graft can be performed with complete visualization of the entire area.

Another useful technique for suprarenal aortic exposure is partially dividing both diaphragmatic crura as they pass behind the renal arteries to their paravertebral attachments. Through this partial division of the crura, the aorta above the superior mesenteric artery is easily visualized and can be mobilized for suprarenal cross-clamping (Fig. 124–6B).

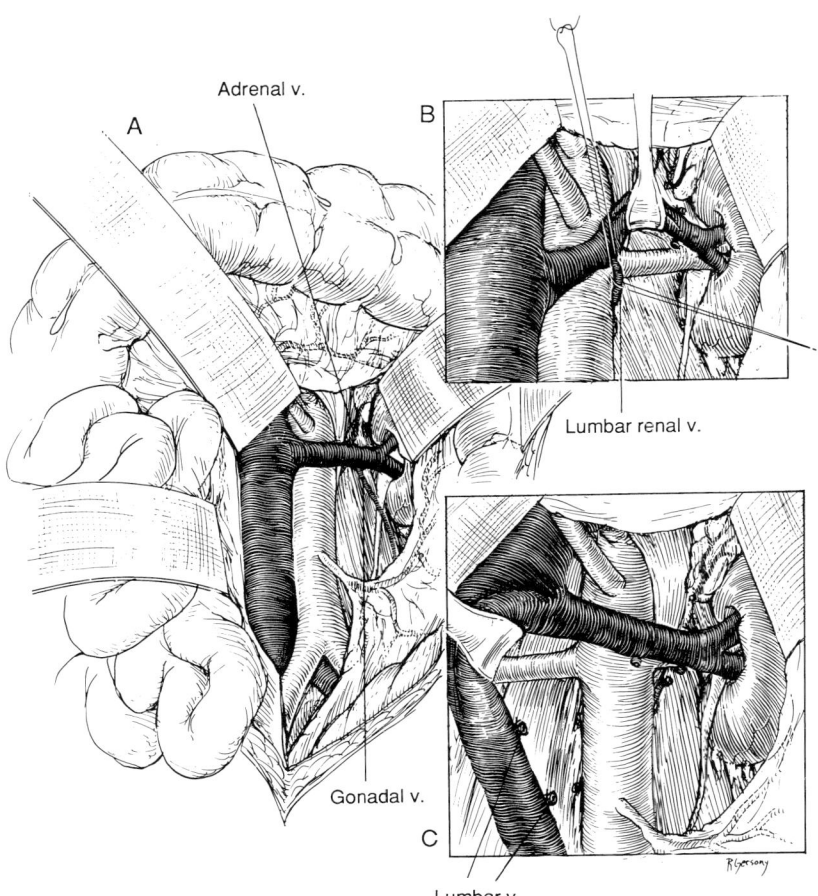

Adrenal v.

A

B

Lumbar renal v.

Gonadal v.

C

Lumbar v.

FIGURE 124–2. *A,* Exposure of the proximal right renal artery through the base of the mesentery. *B,* Mobilization of the left renal vein by ligation and division of the adrenal, gonadal, and lumbar-renal veins allows exposure of the entire left renal artery to the hilum. *C,* Two pairs of lumbar vessels have been ligated and divided to allow retraction of the vena cava to the right, revealing adequate exposure of the proximal renal artery disease. (From Benjamin ME, Dean RH: Techniques in renal artery reconstruction: Part I. Ann Vasc Surg 10(3):306–314, 1996.)

FIGURE 124–3. Exposure of the distal right renal artery begins with mobilization of the ascending colon. (From Benjamin ME, Dean RH: Techniques in renal artery reconstruction: Part I. Ann Vasc Surg 10(3):306–314, 1996.)

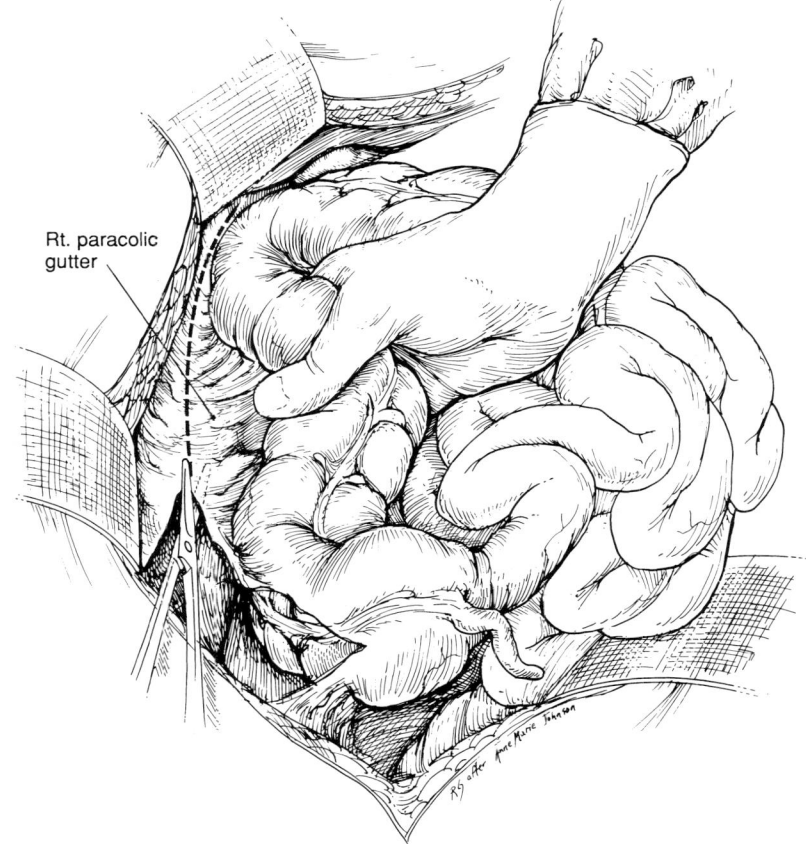

Rt. paracolic gutter

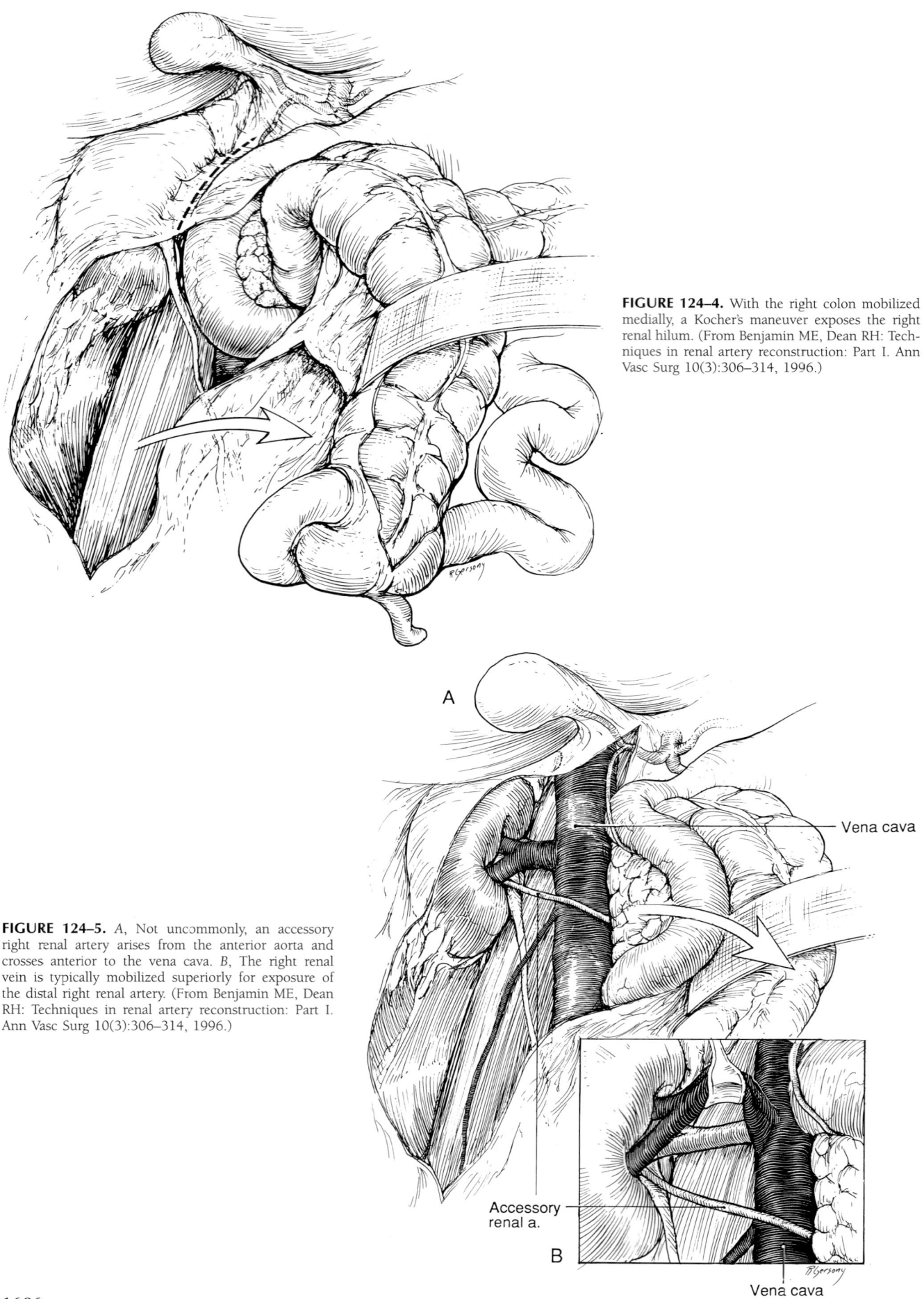

FIGURE 124–4. With the right colon mobilized medially, a Kocher's maneuver exposes the right renal hilum. (From Benjamin ME, Dean RH: Techniques in renal artery reconstruction: Part I. Ann Vasc Surg 10(3):306–314, 1996.)

FIGURE 124–5. *A*, Not uncommonly, an accessory right renal artery arises from the anterior aorta and crosses anterior to the vena cava. *B*, The right renal vein is typically mobilized superiorly for exposure of the distal right renal artery. (From Benjamin ME, Dean RH: Techniques in renal artery reconstruction: Part I. Ann Vasc Surg 10(3):306–314, 1996.)

Vena cava

Accessory renal a.

Vena cava

A

B

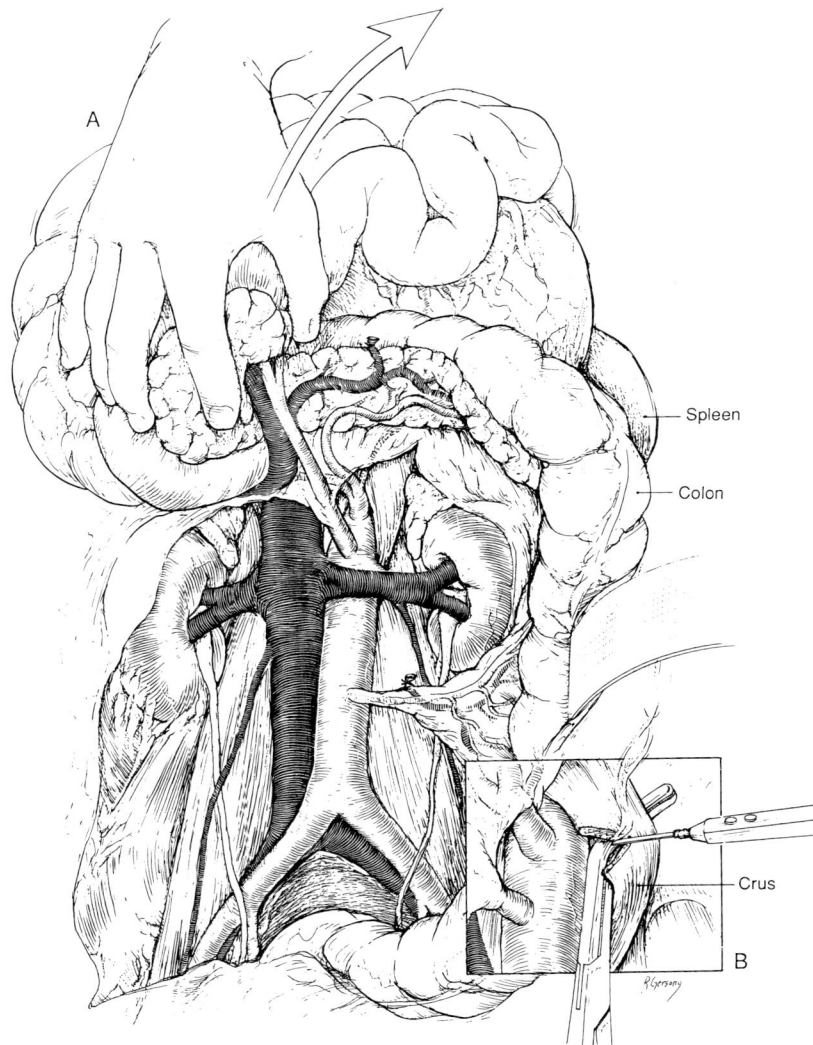

FIGURE 124–6. *A*, For bilateral renal artery reconstruction combined with aortic repair, extended exposure can be obtained with mobilization of the cecum and ascending colon. The entire small bowel and right colon are then mobilized to the right upper quadrant and placed onto the chest wall. *B*, Division of the diaphragmatic crura exposes the origin of the mesenteric vessels. (From Benjamin ME, Dean RH: Techniques in renal artery reconstruction: Part I Ann Vasc Surg 10(3):306–314, 1996.)

AORTORENAL BYPASS

Three types of materials are available for aortorenal bypass:

- Autologous saphenous vein
- Autologous hypogastric artery
- Synthetic prosthesis

The decision as to which graft should be used depends on a number of factors. In most instances, the authors use the saphenous vein preferentially. If the vein is small (<4 mm in diameter) or sclerotic, the hypogastric artery or a synthetic prosthesis may be preferable. A 6-mm, thin-walled polytetrafluoroethylene (PTFE) graft is quite satisfactory when the distal renal artery is of large caliber (≥4 mm). Hypogastric artery autograft is used for aortorenal bypass in children when reimplantation is not possible.[3, 4]

When an end-to-side renal artery bypass is performed, the anastomosis between the renal artery and the graft is performed first (Fig. 124–7A). Polymeric silicone (Silastic) vessel loops can be used to occlude the renal artery distally. This method of vessel occlusion has special application to renal reconstruction. In contrast to vascular clamps, these slings are essentially atraumatic to the delicate renal artery and avoid the presence of clamps in the operative field. Furthermore, when tension is applied to the slings, they lift the vessel out of the retroperitoneal soft tissue for better visualization. In creating the anastomosis, the surgeon should ensure that the length of the arteriotomy is at least three times the diameter of the smaller conduit to guard against late suture line stenosis (Fig. 124–7B). A 6-0 or 7-0 monofilament polypropylene continuous suture is employed with loop magnification.

After the renal artery anastomosis is completed, the occluding clamps and slings are removed from the artery, and a small bulldog clamp is placed across the vein graft adjacent to the anastomosis. The surgeon then performs the aortic anastomosis (Fig. 124–7C), removing an ellipse of the anterolateral aortic wall. If the graft is too long, kinking of the vein and subsequent thrombosis may result; the aortic anastomosis should be taken down and revised after appropriate orientation of the graft.

Sometimes, an end-to-end anastomosis between the graft and the renal artery provides a better reconstruction (Fig.

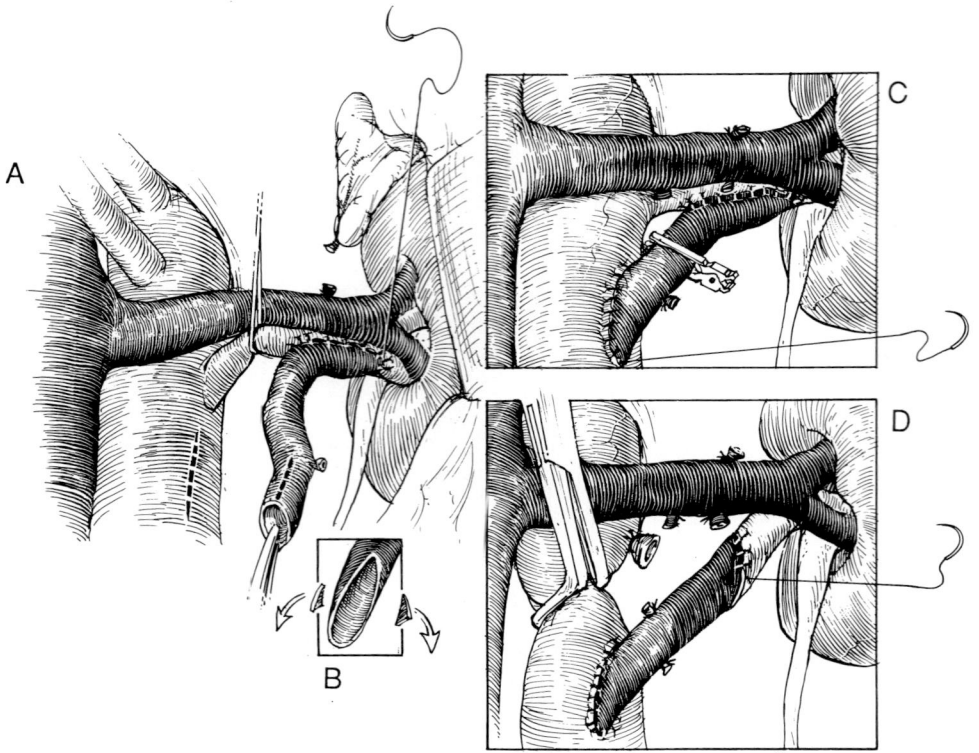

FIGURE 124–7. Technique for end-to-side (*A* to *C*) and end-to-end (*D*) aortorenal bypass grafting. The length of arteriotomy is at least three times the diameter of the artery to prevent recurrent anastomotic stenosis. For the anastomosis, 6-0 or 7-0 monofilament polypropylene sutures are placed in continuous fashion under loupe magnification. If the apex sutures are placed too deeply or with excess advancement, stenosis can be created, posing a risk of late graft thrombosis. (From Benjamin ME, Dean RH: Techniques in renal artery reconstruction: Part I. Ann Vasc Surg 10(3):306–314, 1996.)

124–7D). The authors routinely employ end-to-end renal artery anastomosis when combining aortic replacement with renal revascularization. In combined reconstructions, the proximal anastomosis is performed first and the distal renal anastomosis is performed second to limit renal ischemia. Regardless of the type of distal anastomosis, the proximal aortorenal anastomosis is best performed after excision of an ellipse of aortic wall. This is especially important when the aorta is relatively inflexible owing to atherosclerotic involvement.

THROMBOENDARTERECTOMY

In some cases of bilateral atherosclerotic involvement of the renal artery origins, simultaneous bilateral endarterectomy may be the most suitable procedure. Endarterectomy may be either transrenal or transaortic.

In *transrenal* endarterectomy, the aortotomy is made transversely and is carried across the aorta and into the renal artery to a point beyond the visible atheromatous disease (Fig. 124–8). With this method, the distal endarterectomy can be assessed and tacked down with mattress sutures under direct vision if necessary. After the endarterectomy is completed, the arteriotomy is closed. In most patients, this closure is performed with a prosthetic patch to ensure that the proximal renal artery is widely patent.

The *transaortic* endarterectomy technique is increasingly used. It is particularly applicable in patients with multiple renal arteries that demonstrate orificial disease. In this instance, all visible and palpable renal artery atheromas should end within 1 cm of their aortic origin. Transaortic

endarterectomy is performed through a longitudinal aortotomy with sleeve endarterectomy of the aorta and eversion endarterectomy of the renal arteries (Fig. 124–9). When combined aortic replacement is planned, the transaortic endarterectomy is performed through the transected aorta. With the transaortic technique, it is important to mobilize the renal arteries extensively to enable eversion of the vessel into the aorta. This eversion allows the distal end-point to be completed under direct vision. When the aortic atheroma is divided flush with the adventitia, tacking sutures are not required.

Like thromboendarterectomy at all sites, the procedure is contraindicated in renal artery disease by the presence of (1) preaneurysmal degeneration of the aorta and (2) transmural calcification. The latter condition is subtle and can be missed unless careful attention is given to gentle palpation of the aorta. Aortic atheroma complicated by transmural calcification feels like fine-grade sandpaper. Endarterectomy performed in this setting is characterized by numerous sites of punctate bleeding after blood flow is restored.

RENAL ARTERY REIMPLANTATION

After the renal artery has been dissected from the surrounding retroperitoneal tissue, the vessel may be somewhat redundant. When the renal artery stenosis is orificial and there is sufficient vessel length, the artery can be transected and reimplanted into the aorta at a slightly lower level. The renal artery must be spatulated, and a portion of the aortic wall removed, as in renal artery bypass (Fig.

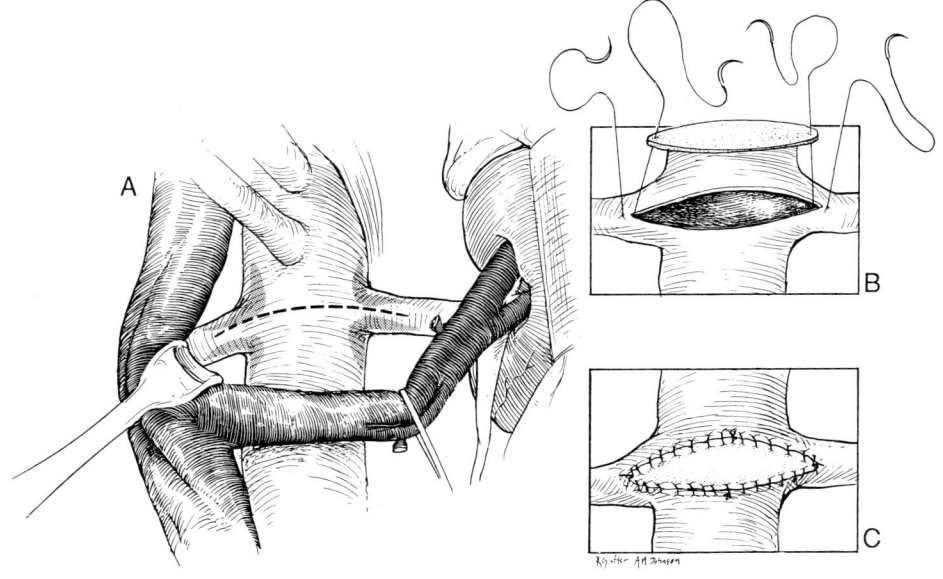

FIGURE 124–8. *A*, Exposure of the juxtarenal aorta and renal arteries in preparation for transrenal endarterectomy. *B*, Transverse aortotomy is used in some instances; the surgeon must be certain to carry the incision out onto the renal artery to a point beyond the stenosis. *C*, Following completion of the endarterectomy, the arteriotomy is usually closed with a polyester (Dacron) patch angioplasty to ensure that the newly repaired renal artery is left widely patent. (From Benjamin ME, Dean RH: Techniques in renal artery reconstruction: Part I. Ann Vasc Surg 10(3):306–314, 1996.)

124–10). This technique has particular application to children with orificial lesions in whom the need for graft material is avoided; however, it is suitable for selected atherosclerotic lesions as well.[5]

SPLANCHNORENAL BYPASS

Splanchnorenal bypass and other indirect revascularization procedures have received greater use as alternative methods for renal revascularization.[6] The authors do not believe that these procedures are as durable as direct aortorenal reconstructions, but they are useful in a highly selected subgroup of high-risk patients.[7]

Hepatorenal Bypass

A right subcostal incision is used to perform hepatorenal bypass.[6] The lesser omentum is incised to expose the hepatic artery both proximal and distal to the gastroduodenal artery (Fig. 124–11). Next, the descending duodenum is mobilized by a Kocher maneuver, the inferior vena cava is identified, the right renal vein is identified, and the right renal artery is encircled either immediately cephalad or caudad to the renal vein.

A greater saphenous vein graft is usually used to construct the bypass. The hepatic artery anastomosis of the vein graft can be placed at the site of the amputated stump of the gastroduodenal artery. This vessel may serve, however, as an important collateral for intestinal perfusion.

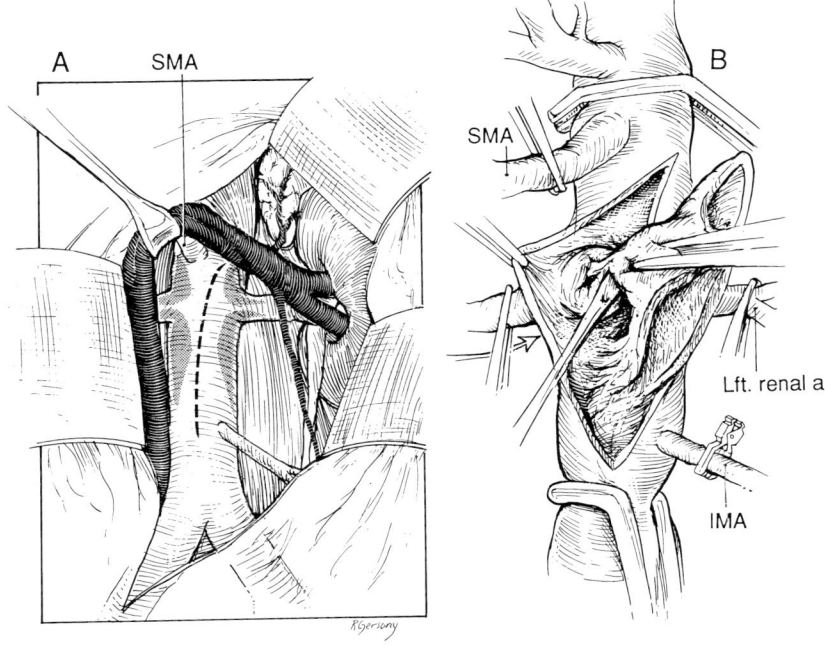

FIGURE 124–9. Exposure for a longitudinal transaortic endarterectomy is through the standard transperitoneal approach. The duodenum is mobilized from the aorta laterally in standard fashion or, for more complete exposure, the ascending colon and small bowel are mobilized. *A*, Dotted line shows the location of the aortotomy. SMA = superior mesenteric artery. *B*, The plaque is transected proximally and distally, and with eversion of the renal arteries, the atherosclerotic plaque is removed from each renal ostium. The aortotomy is typically closed with a running 4-0 or 5-0 polypropylene suture. IMA = inferior mesenteric artery. (From Benjamin ME, Dean RH: Techniques in renal artery reconstruction: Part I. Ann Vasc Surg 10(3):306–314, 1996.)

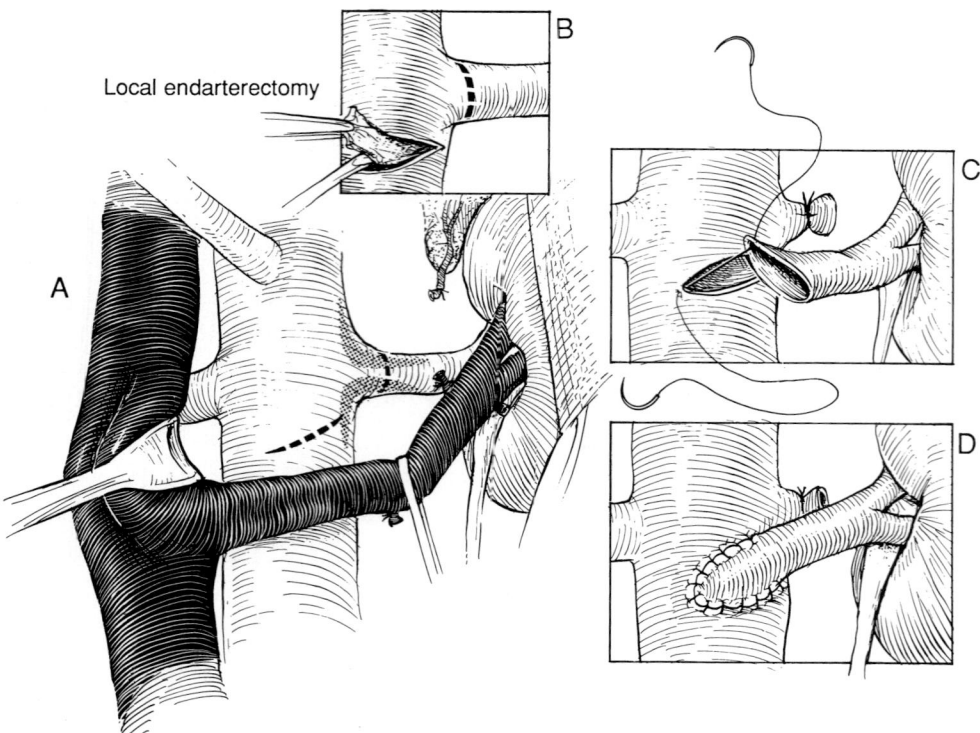

Local endarterectomy

FIGURE 124–10. *A*, When the renal artery is redundant and the disease orificial, the vessel usually can be reimplanted at a lower level. Local endarterectomy (*B*) allows for placement of the monofilament suture in the aortic wall (*C*). *D*, The native renal artery is then ligated, proximally spatulated, and reimplanted. (From Benjamin ME, Dean RH: Techniques in renal artery reconstruction: Part II. Ann Vasc Surg 10(4):409–414, 1996.)

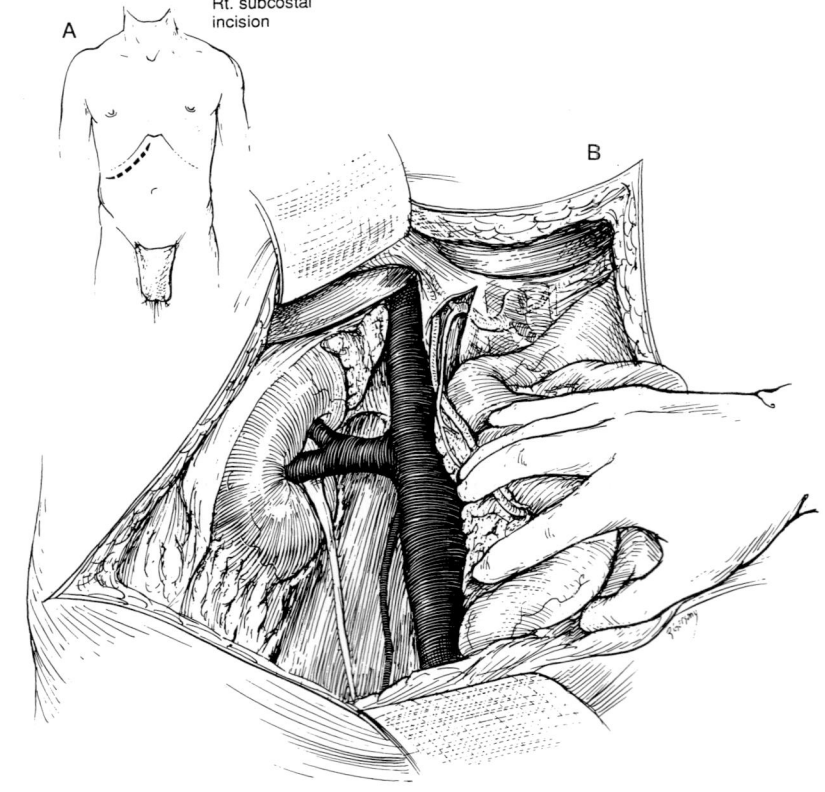

Rt. subcostal incision

FIGURE 124–11. In preparation for extra-anatomic reconstruction of the right renal artery, the common hepatic artery and proximal gastroduodenal artery are exposed in the hepatoduodenal ligament. Exposure (*B*) would typically be through a right subcostal skin incision (*A*). (From Benjamin ME, Dean RH: Techniques in renal artery reconstruction: Part II. Ann Vasc Surg 10(4):409–414, May 1996.)

Therefore, the proximal anastomosis is usually made to the common hepatic artery. After completion of this anastomosis, the renal artery is transected and brought anterior to the vena cava for end-to-end anastomosis to the graft (Fig. 124–12).

Splenorenal Bypass

Splenorenal bypass can be performed through a midline or a left subcostal incision.[6, 7] The posterior pancreas is mobilized by cephalad reflection of the inferior border. A retropancreatic plane is developed, and the splenic artery is mobilized from the left gastroepiploic artery to the level of its branches. The left renal artery is exposed cephalad to the left renal vein after division of the adrenal vein. After the splenic artery has been mobilized, it is divided distally, spatulated, and anastomosed end-to-end to the transacted renal artery (Fig. 124–13).

EX VIVO RECONSTRUCTION

In part, operative strategy for renal artery repair is determined by the exposure required and the anticipated period of renal ischemia. When reconstruction can be accomplished with less than 40 minutes of ischemia, an in situ repair is undertaken without special measures for renal preservation. When longer periods of ischemia are anticipated, one of two techniques for hypothermic preservation of the kidney is considered.[8]

• Renal mobilization without renal vein transection
• Ex vivo repair and anatomic replacement in the renal fossa

Ex vivo management is necessary when extensive expo-

sure is required for extended periods. Such a requirement exists in the following circumstances:

• Fibromuscular dysplasia and aneurysms or stenoses involving renal artery branches
• Fibromuscular dysplasia and renal artery dissection with branch occlusion
• Congenital arteriovenous fistulae of renal artery branches requiring partial resection
• Failure of a prior reconstruction to the distal renal artery

Several methods of ex vivo hypothermic perfusion and reconstruction are available. A midline xiphoid-to-pubic incision is used for most renovascular procedures and is preferred when autotransplantation of the reconstructed kidney or combined aortic reconstructions are to be performed. When isolated branch renal repair is planned, an extended flank incision is made parallel to the lower rib margin and carried to the posterior axillary line, as described earlier. This latter method is the authors' preferred approach for ex vivo reconstructions. The ureter is always partially mobilized, but left intact, and an elastic sling is placed around the ureter to prevent perfusion from ureteric collaterals and subsequent renal rewarming.

Gerota's fascia is opened with a cruciate incision, the kidney is mobilized, and the renal vessels are divided (Fig. 124–14). The kidney is placed on the abdominal wall and perfused with a chilled renal preservation solution. Continuous perfusion during the period of total renal ischemia is possible with perfusion pump systems and may be superior for prolonged renal preservation.[9] However, simple intermittent flushing with a chilled preservation solution provides equal protection during the shorter periods (2 to 3 hours) required for ex vivo dissection and branch renal artery reconstructions. For this technique, the authors refrigerate the preservative overnight, add components (Table 124–1) immediately before use to make up a liter of solu-

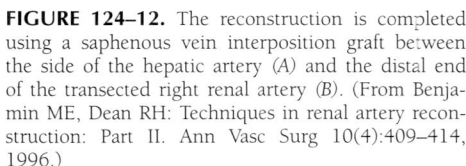
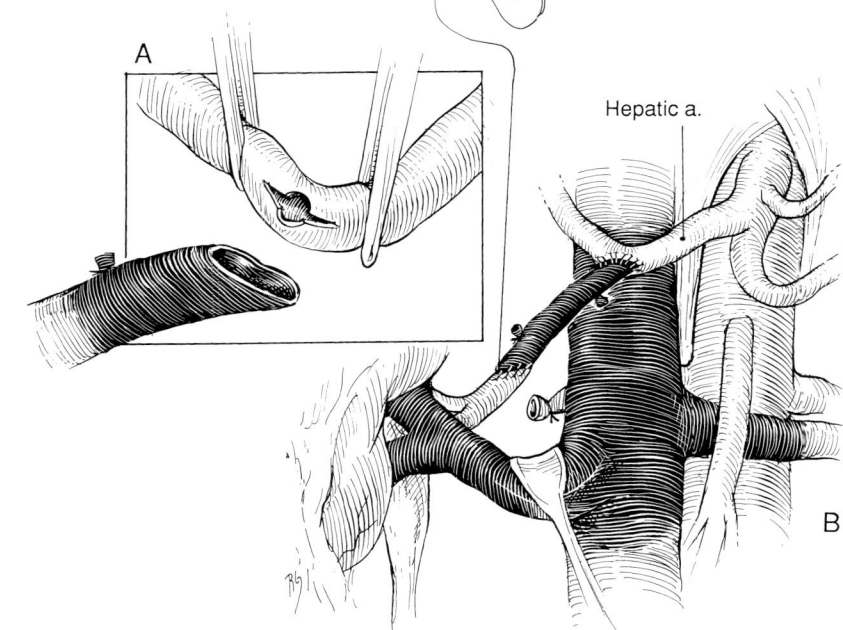

FIGURE 124–12. The reconstruction is completed using a saphenous vein interposition graft between the side of the hepatic artery (A) and the distal end of the transected right renal artery (B). (From Benjamin ME, Dean RH: Techniques in renal artery reconstruction: Part II. Ann Vasc Surg 10(4):409–414, 1996.)

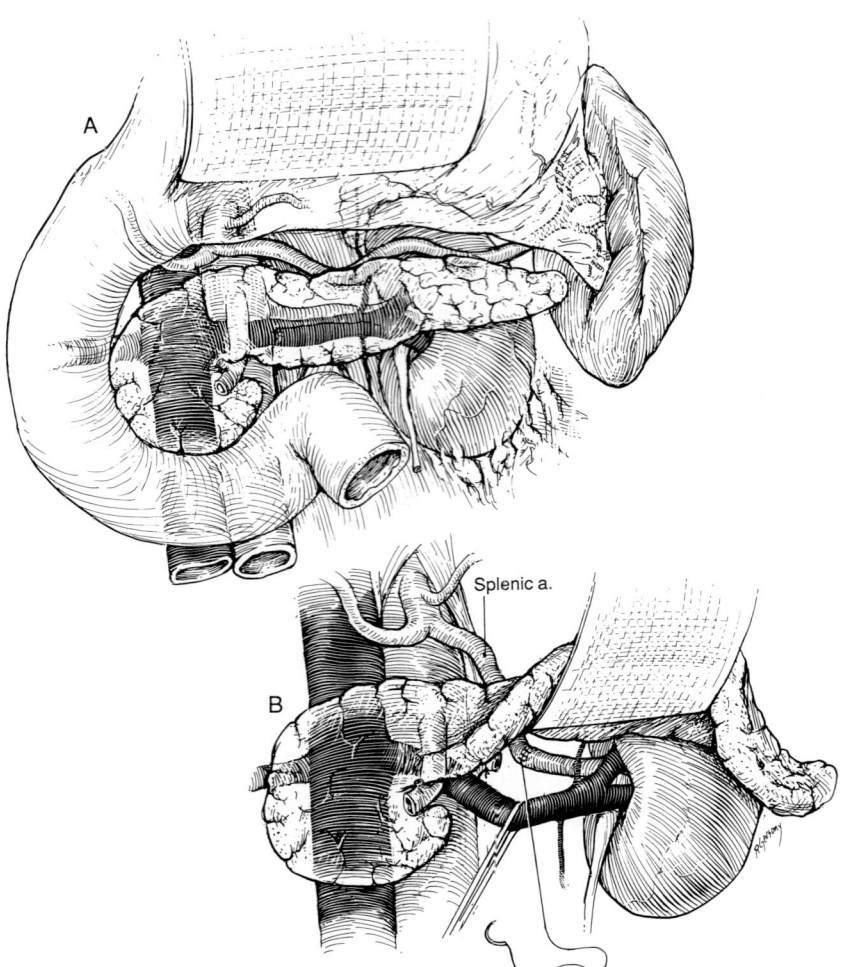

FIGURE 124–13. *A,* Exposure of the left renal hilum in preparation for splenorenal bypass. *B,* The pancreas has been mobilized along its inferior margin and retracted superiorly. The transected splenic artery is anastomosed end-to-end to the transected left renal artery. A splenectomy is not routinely performed. (From Benjamin ME, Dean RH: Techniques in renal artery reconstruction: Part II. Ann Vasc Surg 10(4): 409–414, May 1996.)

tion, and hang the chilled (5° to 10°C) solution at a height of at least 2 meters. From 300 to 500 ml of solution is flushed through the kidney immediately after its removal from the renal fossa, with flushing continued until the venous effluent is clear. As each anastomosis is completed, the kidney is perfused with an additional 150 to 200 ml of solution. In addition to maintaining satisfactory hypothermia, periodic perfusion demonstrates suture line leaks that can then be repaired prior to reimplantation.

As a supplement to perfusion, surface hypothermia is used during ex vivo renal artery reconstruction. Liter bot-

tles of normal saline solution are placed in ice slush overnight. When the kidney is elevated it is placed in a watertight plastic bag. Laparotomy pads are placed over the kidney, which is then kept cool and moist with a constant drip of the chilled saline solution. With this technique, renal core temperatures are maintained at 10°C or less throughout the period of reconstruction

Autotransplantation to the iliac fossa is unnecessary for most ex vivo reconstructions, even though it is an accepted method after ex vivo reconstruction. This technique was adopted from the renal transplant surgeon. Reduction in

TABLE 124–1. SOLUTION FOR COLD PERFUSION PRESERVATION OF THE KIDNEY

COMPOSITION (gm/L)		IONIC CONCENTRATION (mEq/L)		ADDITIVES AT TIME OF USE TO 930 ml OF SOLUTION
Component	Amount	Electrolyte	Concentration	
K_2HPO_4	7.4	Potassium	115	50% dextrose, 70 ml heparin sodium, 2000 units
KH_2PO_4	2.04	Sodium	10	
KCl	1.12	Phosphate (HPO_4^-)	85	
$NaHCO_3$	0.84	Phosphate ($H_2PO_4^-$)	15	
		Chlorideate	15	
		Bicarbonate	10	

*Electrolyte solution for kidney preservation supplied by Travenol Labs, Inc., Deerfield, Ill.

the magnitude of the operative exposure, manual palpation of the transplanted kidney, and ease of removal when treatment of rejection fails are all practical reasons for placing the transplanted kidney into the recipient's iliac fossa. However, none of these advantages apply to the patient requiring autogenous ex vivo reconstruction. In this latter patient group, the most important factors are those that improve the long-term patency after renal artery repair.

Because many ex vivo procedures are performed in relatively young patients, the durability of the operation must be measured in terms of decades. For this reason, attachment of the kidney to the iliac arterial system within or below sites that are susceptible to subsequent atherosclerotic occlusive disease subjects the repaired vessels to atherosclerotic disease that may threaten their long-term patency. Moreover, subsequent management of peripheral vascular disease may be complicated by the presence of the autotransplanted kidney. Finally, if the kidney is replaced in the renal fossa and the renal artery graft is properly attached to the aorta at a proximal infrarenal site, the result should mimic that of the standard aortorenal bypass and thus should carry a high probability of technical success and long-term durability.

INTRAOPERATIVE ASSESSMENT

Provided that the best method of reconstruction is chosen for renal artery repair, the short course and high blood flow rates characteristic of renal reconstructions favor their patency. Consequently, flawless technical repair plays a dominant role in determining postoperative success.[10–12] The negative impact of technical errors that go unrecog-

nized at operation is implied by the fact that the authors have observed no late thromboses of renovascular reconstructions that were free of disease after 1 year.[13]

Intraoperative assessment of most arterial reconstructions has been made with intraoperative angiography.[14, 15] This method has serious limitations, however, when applied to upper aortic and branch aortic reconstruction. At these locations, intraoperative angiography calls for additional suprarenal or supraceliac aortic occlusion. The study obtained provides static images in the absence of pulsatile blood flow and allows anatomic evaluation in only one projection.[16, 17] In addition, arteriolar vasospasm in response to cross-clamp ischemia and contrast injection may falsely suggest distal vascular occlusion. Finally, coexisting renal insufficiency is present in 75% of contemporary patients with atherosclerotic renovascular disease, increasing the risk of postoperative contrast nephropathy.

Intraoperative Duplex Sonography

These risks and the inherent limitations of completion angiography are not associated with intraoperative duplex sonography.[18] Because the ultrasound probe can be placed immediately adjacent to the vascular repair, high carrying frequencies may be used, which provide excellent B-scan detail sensitive to anatomic defects smaller than 1 mm. Once imaged, defects can be viewed in a multitude of projections during conditions of uninterrupted, pulsatile blood flow. Intimal flaps not apparent during static conditions are easily imaged with this technique, which avoids the adverse effects of additional renal ischemia required in angiography. In addition to excellent anatomic detail, important hemodynamic information is obtained from the

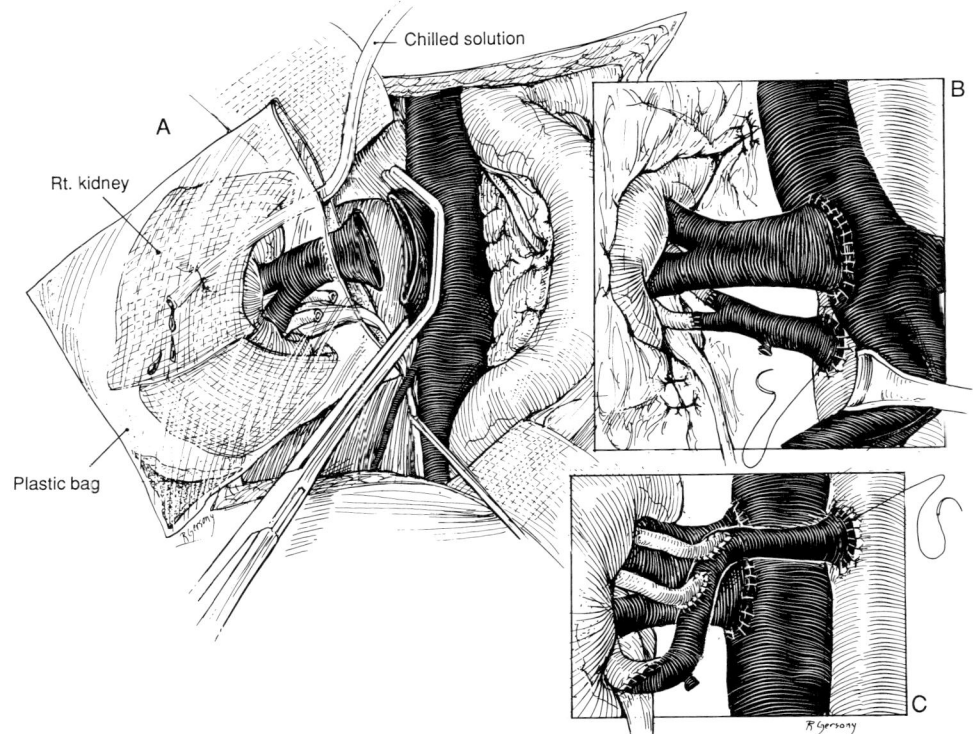

FIGURE 124–14. *A,* An ellipse of the vena cava containing the renal vein origin is excised by placement of a large partially occluding clamp. After ex vivo branch repair, the renal vein can then be reattached without risk of anastomotic stricture. *B,* The kidney is repositioned in its native bed after ex vivo repair. Gerota's fascia is reattached to provide stability to the replaced kidney. Arterial reconstruction can be accomplished via end-to-end anastomoses (as in *B*) or occasionally with a combination of end-to-end and end-to-side anastomoses (*C*). (From Benjamin ME, Dean RH: Techniques in renal artery reconstruction: Part II. Ann Vasc Surg 10(4):409–414, 1996.)

spectral analysis of the Doppler-shifted signal proximal and distal to the imaged defect.[18] Freedom from static projections, the absence of potentially nephrotoxic contrast material or additional ischemia, and the hemodynamic data provided by Doppler spectral analysis make duplex sonography a very useful intraoperative method for assessment of both renovascular and mesenteric repairs.

In order for these advantages of intraoperative duplex sonography to be realized, close cooperation between the vascular surgeon and the vascular technologist is required for accurate intraoperative assessment. Although the surgeon is responsible for manipulating the probe head to acquire optimal B-scan images of the vascular repair at likely sites of technical error, proper power and time gain adjustments are best made by an experienced vascular technologist. Close cooperation is also required to obtain complete pulsed Doppler sampling associated with abnormalities on B-scan. While the surgeon images areas of interest at an optimal insonating angle, the technologist sets the Doppler sample depth and volume and estimates blood flow velocities from the Doppler spectrum analyzer.

Finally, the participation of the vascular technologist during intraoperative assessment enhances his or her ability to obtain satisfactory surveillance duplex sonography studies during follow-up. In the authors' experience, intraoperative duplex sonography assessment and the routine participation of a vascular technologist has yielded a scan time of 5 to 10 minutes and a 98% study completion rate.[18, 19]

Technique

Currently, the authors use a 10/5.0 MHz compact linear array probe with Doppler color flow imaging designed specifically for intraoperative assessment. The probe is placed within a sterile sheath that has a latex tip containing sterile gel. After the operative field is flooded with warm saline, B-scan images are first obtained in longitudinal projection. Care is taken to image the entire upper abdominal aorta and renal artery origins along the full length of the repair. All defects seen in longitudinal projection are imaged in transverse projection to confirm their anatomic presence and to estimate associated luminal narrowing. Doppler samples are then obtained just proximal and distal to imaged lesions in longitudinal projection to determine their potential contribution to flow disturbance. The authors' criteria for major B-scan defects associated with a greater than 60% reduction in diameter by stenosis or occlusion have been validated in a canine model of graded renal artery stenosis (Table 124–2).[18] These criteria have also proved valid in a retrospective study in which preoperative radiographic studies were compared with intraoperative duplex sonography prior to surgical repair.[19]

Clinical Experience

In the first validity analysis of intraoperative duplex sonography, the authors used the technique to assess 57 renovascular reconstructions in 35 patients who underwent unilateral (13 patients) or bilateral (22 patients) repair.[18] Direct aortorenal methods of reconstruction included renal artery bypass (RAB) in 29 patients (20 saphenous vein, five PTFE, four Dacron [polyester]), reimplantation in 7 repairs,

TABLE 124–2. INTRAOPERATIVE DOPPLER VELOCITY CRITERIA FOR RENAL ARTERY REPAIR

B-SCAN DEFECT	DOPPLER CRITERIA
Minor	
<60% diameter-reducing stenosis	PSV from entire artery < 2.0 m/sec
Major	
≥60% diameter-reducing stenosis	Focal PSV ≥ 2.0 m/sec and distal turbulent waveform
Occlusion	No Doppler-shifted signal from renal artery B-scan image
Inadequate study	Failure to obtain Doppler samples from entire arterial repair

From Hansen KJ, O'Neill EA, Reavis SW, et al: Intraoperative duplex sonography during renal artery reconstruction. J Vasc Surg 14:364, 1991.
PSV = peak systolic velocity.

transrenal thromboendarterectomy (TEA) with PTFE patch angioplasty in 13 repairs, and transaortic TEA in 8 repairs. Branch renal artery repair was performed in six patients (five in vivo, one ex vivo), and combined aortic replacement in 14 patients.

Average time for intraoperative duplex sonography was 4.5 minutes, and the studies provided complete B-scan and Doppler information in 56 of 57 repairs (98%).[18] Results of duplex sonography were considered normal in 44 repairs (77%), but B-scan defects were found in 13 (23%). Six of these B-scan defects (11%) had Doppler spectra with focal increases in peak systolic velocity of 2.0 meters/second (m/sec) or more with post-stenotic turbulence. These defects were defined as "major," and each underwent immediate operative revision (Fig. 124–15). In each case, a significant defect was discovered during revision and was corrected. Seven B-scan defects without Doppler spectral abnormality were defined as minor and were not repaired.

At a mean follow-up of 12.4 months, the status of 55 renal artery reconstructions in 34 patients was determined by either surface renal duplex sonography or renal angiography. Forty-two of 43 renal artery repairs with normal intraoperative duplex sonography findings and six of six repairs with minor B-scan defects were found to be patent and free of critical stenosis. Of the six revisions prompted by abnormal B-scan and Doppler criteria for a major defect, four were patent without stenosis, stenosis had recurred in one, and one had become occluded. In the revision procedures for the restenosis and occlusion, duplex sonography was not repeated.

Intraoperative duplex sonography in this experience was 86% sensitive and 100% specific for technical defects associated with postoperative stenosis and occlusion of direct aortorenal repairs. These anatomic results were supported by the clinical response to operation. Eighty-six per cent of hypertensive patients demonstrated a favorable blood pressure response, whereas 63% of patients with renal insufficiency demonstrated improved renal function after surgery.

Since this initial evaluation, the authors have studied an additional 249 renal artery repairs with anatomic follow-up evaluation.[19] Complete B-scan and Doppler information was obtained in 241 of 249 renal artery repairs. Intraoperative assessment was normal in 157, and 84 (35%) repairs

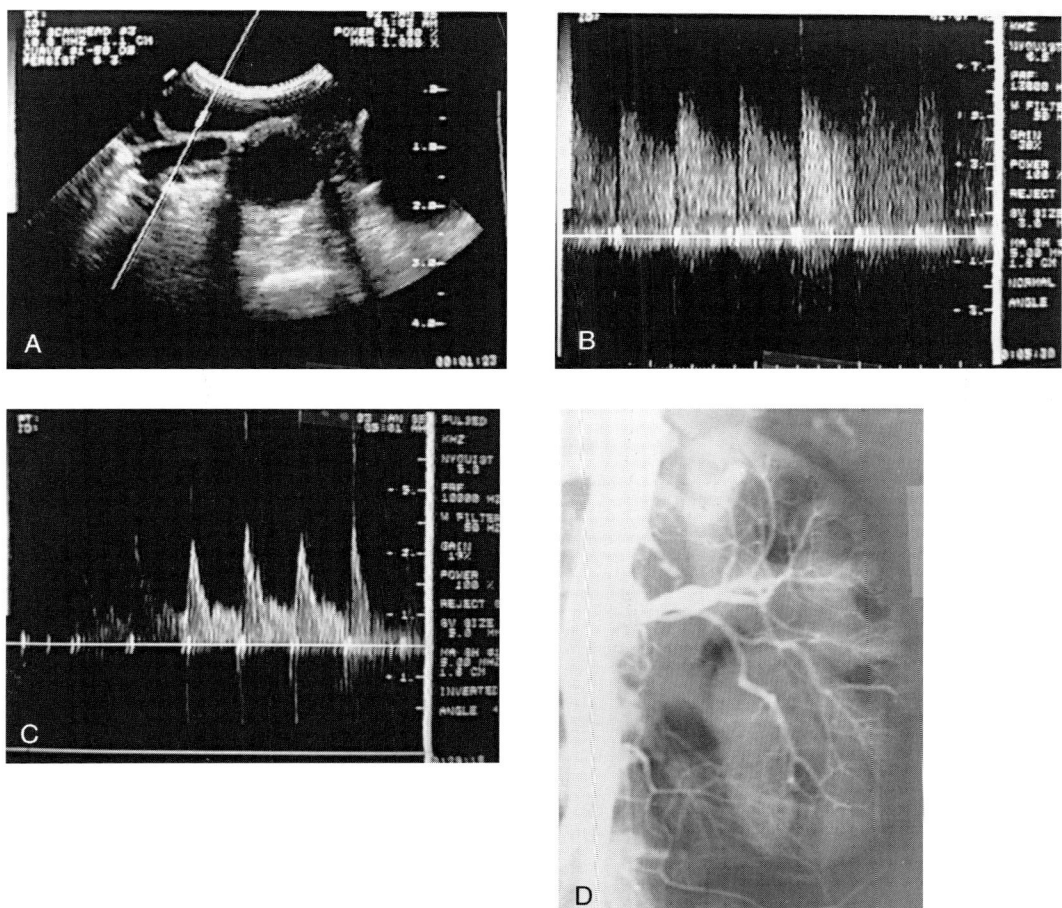

FIGURE 124–15. *A*, Sagittal image of a major B-scan defect (*heavy arrow*). *B*, The intimal flap at the proximal anastomosis demonstrated a focal increase in renal artery peak systolic velocity (3.1 m/sec). *C*, After revision, RA-PSV was decreased (1.1 m/sec). *D*, Follow-up angiogram demonstrated a widely patent anastomosis. This patient was cured of hypertension. (From Hansen KJ, O'Neil EA, Reavis SW, et al: Intraoperative duplex sonography during renal artery reconstruction. J Vasc Surg 14:364, 1991.)

demonstrated one or more B-scan defects. Of the defects, 25 (10%) had focal increases in peak systolic velocity of greater than 2.0 m/sec with turbulent distal waveform, and were defined as major. Each major B-scan defect prompted immediate operative revision, and in each case, a significant defect was discovered. B-scan defects defined as minor were not repaired. At 12-month follow-up, renal artery patency (free of critical stenosis) was demonstrated in 97% of normal studies, 100% of minor B-scan defects, and 88% of revised major B-scan defects, providing an overall patency rate of 97%. Of the five failures with normal B-scan studies, three failures occurred after ex vivo branch renal artery repair.

Special Considerations

Designation of B-scan defects according to Doppler peak systolic velocity criteria provides accurate information to guide decisions regarding intraoperative revision. Special circumstances deserve comment, however. Unlike surface duplex sonography, in which the Doppler sample volume is large relative to the renal artery diameter, a small Doppler sample volume can be accurately positioned within mid-center stream flow. Despite a small, centered Doppler sam-

ple, renal artery repairs demonstrate at least moderate spectral broadening, which gives the audible signal an oscillating characteristic. These findings seem inherent to normal renal artery reconstructions and they are not associated with anatomic defects.

An infrequent intraoperative study demonstrates peak systolic velocities that exceed criteria for critical stenosis when no anatomic defect exists. In these cases, the peak systolic velocities are elevated uniformly throughout the repair, with no focal velocity change and no distal turbulent waveform. This scenario is most commonly encountered after renal artery reconstruction for nonatherosclerotic renovascular disease. Moreover, renovascular repair to a solitary kidney frequently demonstrates increased velocities throughout.

Finally, an increase in peak systolic velocity is observed in transition from the main renal artery to the segmental renal vessels after branch renal artery repair but no distal turbulent waveform is observed. Given these velocity changes and the observed postoperative failures of ex vivo repairs despite normal intraoperative duplex sonography, the authors still rely on postoperative angiographic assessment of ex vivo branch renal artery reconstruction to define technical success.

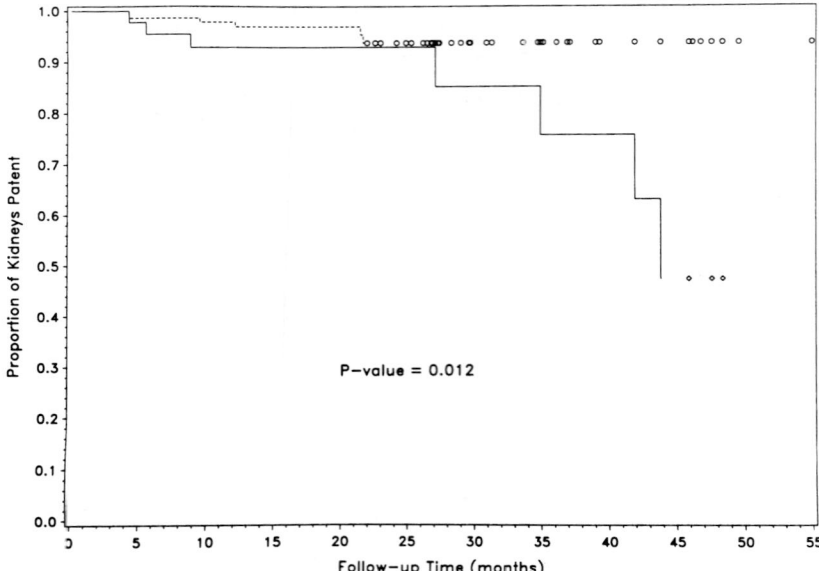

FIGURE 124–16. Comparison of product-limit estimates of patency of direct aortorenal repair (*broken line*) compared with development of significant disease in unrepaired native renal arteries (*solid line*). (From Hansen KJ, Deitch JS, Oskin TC, et al: Renal artery repair: Consequence of operative failures. Ann Surg 227:678, 1998.)

In addition to these systolic spectral abnormalities, changes may be observed in the diastolic features of the Doppler spectra in the absence of technical error. Abnormal diastolic spectra may be observed after revascularization for chronic renal ischemia. Reflecting increased vascular resistance in response to reperfusion, these spectra demonstrate abbreviated systolic flow, short systolic acceleration times, and virtually no diastolic flow. This picture can mimic distal embolic catastrophe; however, it can be distinguished from embolization by spectral changes observed after intra-arterial administration of a vasodilator. Given intra-arterially at the site of repair, 60 mg of papaverine relieves this reactive vasospasm. In this instance, the Doppler spectral signature characteristic for the renal artery usually appears within 5 minutes.

B-scan abnormalities observed in conjunction with renal endarterectomy deserve comment. Infrequently, an irregular B-scan abnormality evolves during performance of a completion scan. This B-scan finding may be associated with either increased or decreased (blunted) peak velocities but reflects formation of intra-arterial thrombus. Unlike acute venous thrombus, which is usually echolucent, the acute arterial event is characterized by irregular echogenic material. Regardless of the associated velocity estimates, the endarterectomy site is reopened and revised immediately. Also, a B-scan defect classified as minor according to velocity criteria may be surgically revised because of its location and appearance. A mobile flap greater than 2 mm in length at the distal end-point of an endarterectomy site is usually revised on the basis of its mere presence and potential for dissection or thrombosis.

ANATOMIC RESULT OF OPERATIVE MANAGEMENT

The cumulative operative experience from the authors' center is summarized in Chapter 123, Table 123–7.[20] During a 10.5-year period, the authors performed 720 renovascular reconstructions and 57 primary nephrectomies in 534 patients, applying the management philosophy and operative techniques described. Postoperative stenosis or thrombosis occurred in 3.3% of renal artery repairs, resulting in recurrent hypertension and declining renal function in 3.7% of patients during a mean follow-up of 36 months. However, because complete anatomic failure of repair (i.e., thrombosis) may result in blood pressure benefit equivalent to that of nephrectomy, anatomic failure is potentially more common than the rate of recurrent hypertension or reoperation.[18]

To examine the rate of anatomic failure, the authors reviewed the results of 227 postoperative duplex sonography studies in 128 consecutive patients.[20] During a 22-month mean follow-up period, six of 177 operative renal artery repairs (3.4%) became stenotic, whereas hemodynamically significant disease developed in 7 of 59 contralateral, unoperated arteries (11.9%). Overall, the incidence of stenosis during follow-up was significantly greater for unoperated renal arteries than for operative repairs (Fig. 124–16; $p = .020$). Compared with other reports describing failure of renovascular repair,[11, 21, 22] these results support the techniques of operative management described.

REFERENCES

1. Fry RE, Fry WJ: Suprailiac aortorenal bypass with saphenous vein for renovascular hypertrophy. Surg Gynecol Obstet 168:181–182, 1989.
2. Novick AL: Use of the thoracic aorta for renal arterial reconstruction. J Vasc Surg 19:605–609, 1994.
3. Dean RH, Benjamin ME, Hansen KJ: Surgical management of renovascular hypertension. Curr Probl Surg 34:209–316, 1997.
4. Stoney RJ, Olofsson PA: Aortorenal arterial autografts: The last two decades. Ann Vasc Surg 2:169–173, 1988.
5. Fry WJ, Ernst CB, Stanley JC, et al: Renovascular hypertension in the pediatric patient. Arch Surg 107:692–698, 1973.
6. Moncure AC, Brewster DC, Darling RC, et al: Use of the splenic and hepatic arteries for renal revascularization. J Vasc Surg 3:196–203, 1986.
7. Fergany A, Kolettis P, Novick AL: The contemporary role of extra-

anatomic surgical renal revascularization in patients with atherosclerotic renal artery disease. J Urol 153:1798–1802, 1995.

8. Dean RH, Meacham PW, Weaver FA: Ex vivo renal artery reconstructions: Indications and techniques. J Vasc Surg 49:546–552, 1986.

9. Salvatierra O Jr, Olcott C IV, Stoney RJ: Ex vivo renal artery reconstruction using perfusion preservation. J Urol 119:16–19, 1978.

10. Dean RH, Wilson JP, Burko H, et al: Saphenous vein aortorenal bypass grafts: Serial angiographic study. Ann Surg 180:469–478, 1974.

11. Stanley JC, Ernest CB, Fry WJ: Fate of 100 aortorenal vein grafts: Characteristics of late graft expansion, aneurysmal dilatation, and stenosis. Surgery 74:931–944, 1973.

12. Dean RH: Complications of renal revascularization. In Bernhard VM, Towne JB (eds): Complications in Vascular Surgery, 2nd ed. Orlando, Fla, Grune & Stratton, 1985, pp 229–246.

13. Dean RH, Krueger TC, Whiteneck JM, et al: Operative management of renovascular hypertension. J Vasc Surg 1:234–242, 1984.

14. Plecha FR, Pories WJ: Intraoperative angiography in the immediate assessment of arterial reconstruction. Arch Surg 105:902–907, 1972.

15. Courbier R, Jausseran JM, Reggi M: Detection complications of direct arterial surgery. Arch Surg 112:1115–1118, 1977.

16. Okuhn SP, Reilly LM, Bennett JR, et al: Intraoperative assessment of renal and visceral artery reconstruction: The role of duplex scanning and spectral analysis. J Vasc Surg 5:137–147, 1987.

17. Goldstone J: Intraoperative assessment of renal and visceral arterial reconstruction using Doppler and duplex imaging. In Ernst CB, Stanley JC (eds): Current Therapy In Vascular Surgery, 2nd ed. Philadelphia, BC Decker, 1991, p 872–875.

18. Hansen KJ, O'Neil EA, Reavis SW, et al: Intraoperative duplex sonography during renal artery reconstruction. J Vasc Surg 14:364–374, 1991.

19. Hansen KJ, Reavis SW, Dean RH: Duplex scanning in renovascular disease. Geriatr Nephrol Urol 6:89–97, 1996.

20. Hansen KJ, Deitch JA, Oskin TC: Renal artery repair: Consequence of operative failures. Ann Surg 227:678–690, 1998.

21. Stanley JC, Whitehouse WM, Zelenock GB, et al: Reoperation for complications of renal artery reconstructive surgery undertaken for treatment of renovascular hypertension. J Vasc Surg 2:133–144, 1985.

22. Svetkey LP, Kadir S, Dunnick NR, et al: Similar prevalence of renovascular hypertension in selected blacks and whites. Hypertension 17:678–683, 1991.

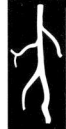

C H A P T E R   1 2 5

Renal Artery Aneurysms and Arteriovenous Fistulae

Keith D. Calligaro, M.D., and
Matthew J. Dougherty, M.D.

Although renal artery aneurysms and renal arteriovenous fistulae (AVFs) are rare, they are encountered frequently enough that vascular surgeons need to be well acquainted with the natural history, diagnosis, and management of these lesions. Aneurysms and AVFs are discussed separately because they rarely occur concomitantly and their clinical course and treatment differ.

RENAL ARTERY ANEURYSMS

Even in referral centers, very few vascular surgeons have extensive experience with the clinical management of renal artery aneurysms.[50, 77] Autopsy studies have revealed an incidence of renal artery aneurysms of 0.01% to 0.09%, which is probably an underestimation because these lesions may be small, intrarenal, or not specifically sought.[8, 50] In two studies, renal artery aneurysms were documented in 0.73% (7/965) to 0.97% (83/8525) of arteriograms.[18, 84] Conversely, these two reports may overestimate the prevalence of these lesions. If renal artery aneurysms were present in almost 1% of patients undergoing abdominal aortography, vascular surgeons would be expected to have a far greater experience diagnosing and treating these lesions

than has been reported to date. At Pennsylvania Hospital in Philadelphia, we have documented renal artery aneurysms in only 0.1% (1/845) of consecutive abdominal aortograms performed at our hospital (excluding patients referred with angiograms). Renal artery aneurysms are bilateral in about 10% of cases.[50, 84] If fibrodysplastic cases are omitted, there is an equal incidence in males and females.[11, 50, 77]

Because of the lack of controlled data, controversy persists regarding the indications for repair of asymptomatic renal artery aneurysms. The optimal method of repair is also controversial. Types of renal artery aneurysms, their clinical manifestations, indications for repair, and techniques of both traditional surgical and newer endovascular interventions are reviewed.

Types of Renal Artery Aneurysms

Types of renal artery aneurysms include (1) true (saccular and fusiform), (2) false, (3) dissecting, and (4) intrarenal.

True Aneurysms

More than 90% of true renal artery aneurysms are extraparenchymal.[20, 46, 77, 78] The peak incidence occurs in patients between the ages of 40 and 60 years. Stanley and colleagues have suggested that true aneurysms are probably due to either atherosclerosis or a congenital defect.[77, 78] Although arteriosclerotic changes have been identified in most aneurysms in patients with multiple lesions, this is not a uniform finding, suggesting that arteriosclerosis may not be the most important factor in the genesis of renal artery aneurysms. These aneurysms are more likely due to a congenital medial degenerative process with weakness of the elastic lamina.[11, 78] Lesions typically occur at the primary or secondary renal artery bifurcations and are rarely confined only to the main trunk of the renal artery. As discussed later, this finding makes surgical repair challenging.

Approximately 75% of true renal artery aneurysms are saccular. This type of renal artery aneurysm is usually less than 5 cm in diameter,[63] although some have been reported as large as 9 cm.[5, 17, 46] Saccular aneurysms occur almost invariably at the main renal artery bifurcation.[11] Fusiform aneurysms are usually associated with atherosclerosis or are a result of a post-stenotic dilatation distal to a hemodynamically significant renal artery stenosis, the latter occurring due to atherosclerosis or fibromuscular disease.[11, 20, 64, 65] Fusiform aneurysms are generally less than 2 cm in diameter and usually affect the main renal artery trunk.[20]

Arterial fibrodysplasia is often a direct contributor to the development of aneurysm.[77, 78] This disease is typically associated with multiple stenoses and post-stenotic dilatation of the distal two thirds of the renal artery. Renal artery aneurysms in association with fibromuscular dysplasia are generally only a few millimeters in diameter. The typical angiographic appearance of a renal artery involved with fibromuscular disease is a "string of beads." Larger aneurysms can also occur, however, and in one study renal artery macroaneurysms were found in 9.2% of adults with fibromuscular dysplasia.[78]

A very rare cause of renal artery aneurysms is Ehlers-Danlos syndrome. This disorder is associated with extreme arterial fragility and spontaneous rupture.[51]

False Aneurysms

False aneurysms of the renal artery arise from blunt or penetrating trauma and occasionally from iatrogenic causes. They represent contained ruptures of the renal artery, with only inflammatory and fibrous tissue encasing the leak.

Dissections

Spontaneous dissections confined to the renal artery that do not arise from the adjacent aorta are very rare; however, primary dissections causing pseudoaneurysms affect the renal arteries more than any other peripheral artery.[22, 25, 36, 49, 64, 77] Poutasse[64] and Stanley and coworkers[78] reported that 14 of 57 cases of renal artery aneurysms were due to spontaneous dissections. An intimal defect of the renal artery due to atherosclerosis is probably the underlying cause of spontaneous renal artery dissections causing aneurysms, along with dysplastic renovascular disease and trauma.[20] The incidence of dissection in patients with fibrodysplastic renal arteries ranges from 0.5% to 9.0%.[22, 77] Dissection often extends into the branches of the renal

artery and may pose particularly challenging reconstruction problems.

Traumatic renal artery dissections can occur secondary to blunt abdominal trauma or catheter-induced injury. Blunt trauma accounts for the higher prevalence of dissection in men and is more likely to result in right-sided injuries, possibly because of ptosis-related physical stresses affecting the renal pedicle.[77] Blunt trauma can cause renal artery dissections by either severe stretching of the artery with fracture of the intima or compression of the artery against the vertebra. Renal artery dissection caused by guide wires or catheters can occur but is rare, being observed in only four of 2200 selective renal artery arteriograms.[22]

Intrarenal Aneurysms

Fewer than 10% of renal artery aneurysms are intraparenchymal.[46, 78] Intrarenal aneurysms are usually multiple and may be congenital, associated with collagen vascular disease, or post-traumatic. They may be associated with AVFs, possibly as a result of spontaneous closure of a fistula. Intrarenal aneurysms can occur with polyarteritis nodosa and are usually in the renal cortex.[28, 75]

Clinical Manifestations

The vast majority of renal artery aneurysms are asymptomatic and found on imaging studies such as arteriography, ultrasonography, and computed tomography (CT) performed to investigate other intra-abdominal pathology.[17, 29, 77] Magnetic resonance angiography (MRA) can also delineate renal artery aneurysms.[82] Clinical manifestations of renal artery aneurysms include rupture, hypertension, pain, and hematuria. In one series, only 11 of 32 (34%) patients who underwent surgery for renal artery aneurysms presented with symptoms.[17]

Rupture

The most dreaded complication of renal artery aneurysm is rupture. Patients with this complication present with manifestations similar to other intra-abdominal arterial ruptures, including syncope, abdominal or flank pain, abdominal distention, and possibly a pulsatile mass. Occasionally, an intact renal artery aneurysm presents with abdominal or flank pain, discomfort, or fullness, symptoms that are presumed to reflect acute aneurysmal expansion.

Hypertension

Renal artery aneurysms may be associated with severe hypertension. Macroaneurysms were found in 2.5% of arteriograms performed for evaluation of hypertension.[78] Renal artery aneurysms may cause renovascular hypertension by distal embolization with segmental hypoperfusion and renin-mediated vasoconstriction and fluid retention. Compression of an adjacent renal artery branch or luminal stenosis due to extensive thrombus may also lead to renin-mediated hypertension. Frequently there is a significant renal artery stenosis causing a post-stenotic fusiform aneurysm, and the renal artery stenosis is responsible for the hypertension. Saccular and intrarenal aneurysms are much less likely to be associated with hypertension.

Dissection

Patients with renal artery aneurysms caused by dissection may present with severe flank pain, hematuria, or acute hypertension, although most dissections are asymptomatic. An intravenous pyelogram may reveal nonfunction or diminished function of the involved kidney but is rarely the first test ordered unless urolithiasis is considered likely to be causing the symptoms. Contrast or MRA is essential to detect dissection.

Hematuria

Intrarenal aneurysms may rupture into calyces.[8] In addition to pain, microscopic or gross hematuria may occur.

Collecting System Obstruction

Renal artery aneurysms rarely cause obstruction of the collecting system. Although main renal artery aneurysms may be large, they are usually not near enough to the caliceal system to cause obstruction. Intrarenal aneurysms tend to be too small to cause significant collecting duct obstruction. However, a 9-cm renal artery aneurysm has been documented to cause hydronephrosis.[5]

Indications for Intervention

Indications to repair a renal artery aneurysm are related to (1) the risk of rupture, (2) hypertension, (3) acute dissection, and (4) other clinical symptoms.

Rupture

Rupture of a renal artery aneurysm is an indication for emergency intervention, as with virtually any arterial aneurysm. Probably fewer than 3% of renal artery aneurysms rupture.[77, 78] This complication is associated with a mortality rate of approximately 10% in males and nonpregnant females.[24, 31, 77, 78] In a hemodynamically stable patient, an emergent CT scan may reveal the pathology and allow the surgeon to further plan the operative repair. However, if a hypotensive elderly patient presents to the emergency department with abdominal pain and a tender, distended abdomen and does not respond to fluid resuscitation, emergency exploration for a presumptive diagnosis of a ruptured abdominal aortic aneurysm may be indicated. In the case of a hypotensive patient with a known renal artery aneurysm and abdominal pain and distention who does not respond to fluid resuscitation, emergency surgery is also required.

Prevention of rupture is the most common indication for intervention of an asymptomatic renal artery aneurysm. Traditionally, repair of renal artery aneurysms has been recommended for aneurysms greater than 2.0 cm in diameter.[20, 65] The likelihood of rupture of a renal artery aneurysm is controversial as the natural history has yet to be delineated. Most reports are retrospective reviews of incidentally discovered intact renal artery aneurysms in autopsy series or collections of ruptured aneurysms without full details concerning their size and presence or the absence of calcification. Many authorities believe that there are no good data to support the belief that the larger the renal artery aneurysm, the more likely it is to rupture.[20, 50, 60, 77, 78] Harrow and Sloane reported one of the highest rates of rupture of renal artery aneurysms, noting 14 ruptures in 100 cases.[27] In another series of 126 renal artery aneurysms, 6 ruptured.[48]

Most other series of asymptomatic renal artery aneurysms in men and nonpregnant women report a much lower incidence of rupture. Only one of 62 patients with aneurysms less than or equal to 4.0 cm in diameter ruptured after follow-ups from 1 to 17 years.[31] None of 19 small aneurysms in another series ruptured.[24] A group of 21 patients were observed for an average of about 3 years without rupture.[29] In another report, of 18 patients with renal artery aneurysms less than 2.6 cm who were followed up for 1 to 16 years, none ruptured.[50]

There were no ruptures in a series of 32 patients (who eventually underwent surgery) of renal artery aneurysms, which ranged from 0.7 to 9.0 cm.[17] Of 83 renal artery aneurysms found on arteriography from a series in Sweden, 69 were followed up without surgery, and none ruptured or became symptomatic after a mean of 4.3 years of follow-up.[34] In a pooled analysis, there were no ruptures in more than 200 renal artery aneurysms observed for up to 17 years.[11] One must keep in mind that there was obvious selection bias in following up many of these aneurysms (i.e., small size and not recommending surgery) and that many of the larger aneurysms were operated on.

Besides aneurysm size, other factors may play a role in the consideration of elective surgery for asymptomatic renal artery aneurysms. Calcification of the aneurysm has been thought to protect from rupture. Poutasse suggested that a heavily calcified renal artery aneurysm may be less likely to rupture than a noncalcified or minimally calcified one.[65] In a review of cases through 1959, 14 of 100 noncalcified aneurysms ruptured.[27] In a more recent series, 15 of 18 ruptured renal artery aneurysms were noncalcified.[30] In a series of 62 solitary aneurysms less than 4.0 cm in diameter, however, one third were not calcified, and only one aneurysm in the entire series ruptured between 1 and 17 years of follow-up.[31] Because of these conflicting data, some authorities believe that presence or absence of calcification is not relevant to predict risk of rupture.[77]

Most authorities agree, however, that pregnancy is associated with a significant increased risk of rupture of a renal artery aneurysm.[12, 17, 77, 78] Pregnancy may increase the risk of rupture because of the hyperdynamic state with increased blood volume and cardiac output, hormonal influences on the aneurysm, and increased intra-abdominal pressure due to the gravid uterus.[50, 78] Cohen and Shamash reported 18 cases of rupture during pregnancy.[12] In a different series of 18 patients having surgery for renal artery aneurysms, the only two ruptures were in females at childbirth.[50] Both of these aneurysms measured only 1.0 cm in diameter.[50]

In a review of 43 ruptured renal artery aneurysms, 35 (81%) occurred in women.[30] Twenty-one of the 35 women in this series were younger than 40 years of age, and 18 were pregnant. Of the 18 aneurysms of known size, three ruptured when they were smaller than 2.0 cm.[30]

Of note, rupture of renal artery aneurysms in pregnancy has been associated with a maternal mortality rate of 55% and a fetal death rate of 85%.[12, 77] Risk of renal artery rupture is small, however, even in pregnant women. In a series of 19,600 autopsies of pregnant women, no ruptured renal artery aneurysms were found.[48] This report did not indicate the number of unruptured renal artery aneurysms in this population, however, so the risk of rupture remains uncertain. We agree with others that there are enough data to support an aggressive surgical approach for pregnant women with renal artery aneurysms of any size.

Essentially all false renal artery aneurysms of recent onset should be repaired because of the high likelihood of rupture.[20] In the rare instance when a chronic contained rupture of a small false aneurysm is found months or years later, however, and the pseudoaneurysm has thrombosed, careful follow-up is probably all that is warranted.

Renal artery aneurysms associated with fibrodysplastic disease may be associated with a higher risk of rupture because of the thin-walled nature of these aneurysms, although firm data supporting this concern are lacking.[20] Certainly, renal artery aneurysms in men or women beyond childbearing age that are less than 2.0 in diameter due to fibrodysplastic disease should be studied closely.[20]

Our recommendation concerning elective repair of asymptomatic renal artery aneurysms in men and women beyond childbearing age is based on the data just presented and on the well-documented history of other abdominal arterial aneurysms. General guidelines for repair of asymptomatic abdominal aneurysms include (1) infrarenal aortic aneurysms greater than 5.0 cm in diameter, (2) common iliac aneurysms greater than 3.0 cm, and (3) splenic artery aneurysms greater than 3.0 cm.[79] On the other hand, surgery is recommended for visceral artery aneurysms of any size.[79] Although various hemodynamic factors may play a role in other intra-abdominal aneurysms, and despite the relative paucity of data suggesting a high risk of rupture for renal artery aneurysms, it seems prudent to recommend repair of renal artery aneurysms greater than 3.0 cm in diameter in good-risk patients when there is reasonable certainty that nephrectomy will not be required.[46, 60] This suggested guideline remains controversial, as others have taken a more conservative approach, reserving repair for aneurysms larger than 4.0 cm.[89] As previously mentioned, any renal artery aneurysm in a women of childbearing age should be repaired.

Hypertension

Although the prevalence of hypertension in patients with renal artery aneurysms is approximately 80% in several series, there is no conclusive evidence that the aneurysms themselves are the direct cause of hypertension unless there is an associated stenosis or compression of an adjacent artery.[17, 50, 78] In a series of 39 patients with renal artery aneurysms, 33 had diastolic hypertension, but only nine (23%) proved to have a renovascular origin.[50] The indication for surgical intervention for renovascular hypertension due to renal artery stenosis secondary to atherosclerosis is failure of medical management, namely diastolic blood

pressure greater than 90 to 100 mmHg despite three antihypertensive medications. The same criteria for surgical intervention for renovascular hypertension secondary to atherosclerosis described in Chapter 123 should probably be applied when renal artery aneurysm is present. The stenotic artery along with the aneurysm must be repaired. The diagnosis of renovascular hypertension is discussed in another chapter. Our current evaluation of these patients rarely includes measurement of renal vein renin studies but instead primarily relies on the clinical picture, exclusion of other causes of secondary hypertension, documentation of significant renal artery stenoses, and the use of captropril renal scans.[87]

Dissection

Emergent intervention is required for dissections that cause renal artery aneurysms and threaten the viability of the kidney. Nephrectomies are frequently required in these cases, however, because of the extensive damage to the renal branch vessels and the limited time available to salvage a previously healthy kidney that will not tolerate prolonged periods of ischemia. If hypertension is the only manifestation of a chronic dissection, and the hypertension is well controlled by blood pressure medications, or if the patient is asymptomatic and a renal artery dissection if found incidentally (without an associated aneurysm), surgery is probably not justified.[77]

Other Clinical Manifestations

If a patient with an intact renal artery aneurysm, as documented by CT or magnetic resonance imaging (MRI), is symptomatic as manifested by abdominal or flank pain or fullness, then repair is indicated regardless of the previously mentioned criteria. Symptoms may be a harbinger of impending rupture, but even if not, medical treatment will not relieve these symptoms. Embolization to the renal parenchyma may also account for these symptoms.[46]

Treatment

Ruptured Renal Artery Aneurysm

If emergent surgery is required for a ruptured renal artery aneurysm, a midline approach and supraceliac aortic control are generally required. A sizable juxtarenal hematoma does not allow safe aortic exposure and clamping immediately above the renal arteries. If proximal control of the renal artery itself can be obtained, the supraceliac clamp can then be removed. If the bleeding is quickly controlled and the patient is clearly hemodynamically stable, and if the proximal and distal renal arteries lend themselves to a relatively quick and straightforward bypass, consideration can be given to salvaging the kidney.

In most cases, however, nephrectomy is required because of the instability of the patient, the prolonged ischemia of the kidney augmented by severe hypotension, and the technical and time-consuming nature of surgical repair with a bypass.[64, 77, 78, 91] If the aneurysm extends into the renal parenchyma or if a "bench" repair of the kidney is required, the patient is generally best treated by nephrectomy as long as the contralateral kidney is known to be intact with normal function. Of note, a stable patient with a ruptured true or false renal artery aneurysm may potentially be treated with newer endovascular techniques. Routh and associates reported thrombosis of a leaking saccular aneurysm using Gianturco coils, thrombin, and bucrylate.[70]

Elective Repair of Renal Artery Aneurysm

Even in the elective situation, repair of a renal artery aneurysm is usually more challenging than revascularization for a renal artery stenosis. Most renal artery aneurysms extend past the bifurcation of the main renal arteries and frequently extend into the renal parenchyma. An associated renal artery stenosis must be repaired in conjunction with the aneurysm. For in situ repairs of a renal artery aneurysm, exposure of the left kidney can be obtained through a retroperitoneal approach with a transverse left supraumbilical incision. The right kidney can be exposed through a transperitoneal approach with a Kocher maneuver to reflect the right colon and duodenum medially or occasionally with a subcostal incision.

Several methods have been used to repair renal artery aneurysms. The most straightforward technique for saccular aneurysms involves *aneurysmorrhaphy* with primary repair or patching. In three combined series of patients undergoing surgical repair for renal artery aneurysms, about one third (6/18, 3/10, 6/23) of renal artery aneurysms were able to be repaired in this manner.[17, 45, 50] If this technique is not possible, we and others prefer autologous tissue bypasses such as saphenous vein if the graft can be anastomosed to the distal part of the main trunk of the renal artery or to the most proximal branches.[17, 20]

Another method of in situ repair includes use of bifurcated internal iliac artery autograft.[56] The proximal anastomosis of the graft is usually the infrarenal aorta. Useful alternatives include a splenorenal bypass for a left-sided renal artery aneurysm and hepatorenal bypass for a right-sided aneurysm.

If multiple branch vessels are involved, and especially if the cause of the renal artery aneurysm is dissection resulting in a friable vessel, extracorporeal or "bench" surgery may be required.[6, 16] Ex vivo surgery requires nephrectomy, followed by hypothermic perfusion of the kidney with a heparinized renal preservation solution. The kidney can then be autotransplanted to its original bed, as Dean and associates prefer,[15] or the iliac fossa. Perfusion is carried out through the main renal artery to preserve the kidney while selected branches are individually repaired and other branches perfused. This technique is recommended when renal ischemia is projected to exceed 45 minutes or when exposure of small renal branches is required.

For renal autotransplantation into the iliac fossa, a flank incision with a retroperitoneal approach is used for exposure of the kidney, ureter, and iliac artery. Gonadal and adrenal veins are divided to obtain an adequate length of renal vein. If the reconstruction can be safely performed by placing the kidney on the anterior abdominal wall, the ureter does not need to be divided. The procedure is occasionally best performed at a separate table, however, after dividing the ureter and removing the kidney from the operative field. Ex vivo repair is also discussed in Chapter 124.

The kidney may be perfused with a heparinized crystalloid solution, such as Collins solution or lactated Ringer's solution with 1000 units of heparin/L with 12.5 gm of mannitol, while the kidney is wrapped with gauze and placed in a chilled solution at 4°C.[6, 20, 42] The use of continuous pulsatile perfusion is controversial.[6]

The most common arterial reconstruction is an end-to-side anastomosis of a small renal artery branch to the main renal artery or a side-to-side anastomosis of two small renal arteries to create a common inflow channel with a single lumen of larger diameter, which can then be anastomosed to the renal artery or vein. Because the small branches of the main renal artery are often involved with the aneurysm, an autologous graft is preferred to reconstruct these lesions. The internal iliac artery is an excellent choice in these reconstructions because of its multiple small side branches.[56, 60] The saphenous vein, however, also functions well. The renal artery and vein are then anastomosed end-to-side to the external iliac vessels or to the renal vein and aorta in the kidney's original bed.[6, 20] The clamps are removed from the venous anastomosis first. A ureteroneocystostomy is constructed if the ureter was divided after the vessels were anastomosed.

When performed for proper indications by well-trained surgeons, repair of renal artery aneurysms should be associated with low morbidity and mortality.[42, 46, 74, 77] In a series of 12 patients operated on for renal artery aneurysms, there was no mortality and only one patient required reoperation for a ureteral stenosis.[74] Ex vivo repairs have also been shown to be safe and effective by Dean[6] and others.[15] Murray and coworkers reported a series of 11 patients with renal artery aneurysms successfully treated using ex vivo repair.[56] Another series of eight aneurysms were all successfully repaired with the ex vivo technique without deaths or complications.[86] In a review of ex vivo repairs, postoperative mortality rates ranged from 0% to 9.6%.[76] Bifurcated internal iliac artery autograft was highly successful in a series of 11 patients, most with fibrodysplastic aneurysms, treated by in situ or bench repair.[56] In a series of 35 repairs of renal artery aneurysms treated by in situ repair, ex vivo repair, or nephrectomy, there was no mortality and only one postoperative graft occlusion.[17]

An exciting new approach to treat renal artery aneurysms includes use of endovascular techniques.[7, 60, 38, 83] One aneurysm was treated with transcatheter emobilization with detachable platinum coils, which occluded the aneurysm but maintained renal flow.[83] Another patient in whom a renal artery aneurysm occurred after percutaneous renal biopsy was successfully treated by embolization.[59] One patient with fibrodysplastic disease and a 1.5-cm saccular aneurysm was treated by percutaneous placement of a polytetrafluoroethylene (PTFE) stent-graft that remained patent at 1-year follow-up with normalization of blood pressure.[7]

In one of the largest series of endovascular repairs that has been reported, Klein and coworkers treated 12 renal artery aneurysms using endovascular selective embolization with nondetachable microcoils or Guglielmo's detachable coils.[38] Eight aneurysms were located in the bifurcation of the main renal artery, two were in the main renal artery, and two were intrarenal. All 12 aneurysms were successfully occluded with only two minor complications. The authors concluded that endovascular treatment of renal artery aneurysms with microcoils is as safe as but less invasive than surgical treatment.[38] It remains to be seen whether partial occlusion of renal artery aneurysms will prevent enlargement and later rupture, although early data are encouraging.

Fibromuscular Dysplasia

Post-stenotic dilatations resulting from fibromuscular disease can be treated by balloon angioplasty of the stenotic lesions, although in these cases the primary indication for treatment is the stenotic lesions. When the lesions extend into the branches of the main renal artery, surgery can yield excellent results. Dean and coworkers reported 24 patients with fibromuscular disease, many of whom had branch aneurysms, all but 1 of whom did well.[15]

Intrarenal Aneurysms

Intrarenal aneurysms represent particularly challenging lesions. Frequently a partial nephrectomy is required.[41] Intrarenal aneurysms in association with polyarteritis nodosa have also been successfully treated with renal artery embolization with preservation of the kidney.[71]

RENAL ARTERIOVENOUS MALFORMATIONS AND FISTULAE

Arteriovenous malformations (AVMs) and AVFs are uncommon lesions that can be associated with hematuria, hypertension and renal dysfunction, high-output congestive heart failure, and even rupture. More than 200 cases have been reported since the first description in 1928.[55] Fistulae may be congenital or acquired. Multiple diagnostic modalities are now available, although conventional selective arteriography remains the standard. Many asymptomatic lesions do not require treatment. Symptomatic lesions have previously been treated surgically, but endovascular treatment now supplants surgery in most cases.

Etiology

Congenital Arteriovenous Malformations

True congenital AVMs of the kidney are quite rare, with an incidence of only 0.04%.[10] In a large series, only one congenital AVM was noted in 30,000 autopsies.[14] These lesions represent approximately one fourth of all renal AVFs.[37, 47] The right kidney is more frequently involved than the left, and, although multiple lesions may occur, a single focus is more common.[19] The angiographic appearance of lesions is similar to AVMs elsewhere, with large coils of dilated vessels. Though Piquet and colleagues describe a single artery feeding all but advanced cases,[62] others describe multiple connections of arterial branches and venous tributaries.[55]

An early "blush" is noted and correlates with the degree of arteriovenous shunting, which is variable. These lesions have been described as "cirsoid," or varix-like, and are

generally focal and located in the renal medulla. AVMs are not neoplastic, but enlargement presumably can occur based on vessel dilatation and hypertrophy associated with high flow volume from arteriovenous shunting. Symptomatic AVMs have been reported in pregnancy,[23, 55] and it is thought that the hyperdynamic state of the gravida leads to increased AVM flow and symptoms.

Histologically, involved vessels have irregular fibrosis or intimal hyperplasia as well as medial hypertrophy. Focal intraparenchymal hemorrhage may be noted in the lamina propria beneath the transitional epithelium of the collecting system.[19]

Acquired Arteriovenous Fistula—Spontaneous

Acquired AVFs may occur spontaneously. Spontaneous AVFs have been documented in association with fibromuscular dysplasia[54] and are thought to develop when a dysplastic or aneurysmal renal artery erodes into a neighboring vein.[33] This may also occur with renal malignancy, and indeed significant arteriovenous shunting is a hallmark of renal cell carcinoma.[90] With arteriography, it can be difficult to differentiate a renal malignancy from a congenital or acquired AVF, although CT and MRI generally reveal a mass distinct from renal parenchyma in malignancy. As with AVMs, symptoms depend on the degree of shunting.

Acquired Arteriovenous Fistula—Traumatic

Traumatic AVFs are the most common lesions, accounting for more than 70% of all renal AVFs.[55] These lesions may occur after nephrectomy related to erosion of the arterial stump into the vein with mass ligature,[14, 68, 80] after renal artery angioplasty,[57] after blunt[88] or penetrating[68] trauma, nephrostomy,[32] and, most commonly, after percutaneous renal biopsy. With routine use of needle biopsy for the diagnosis of rejection in renal allografts, the incidence of acquired AVF has grown. Although only 1% to 2% of patients who undergo needle biopsy develop an symptomatic AVF,[43, 85] the true incidence of AVF is 15% to 18% when arteriography is routinely used.[52, 66]

Ozbek and colleagues[58] found AVFs in 8 of 64 patients (12.5%) monitored by color duplex ultrasonography, whereas only 5.0% developed AVFs in the study of Rollino and associates.[69] In the prospective study of Merkus and colleagues, who used routine color duplex surveillance, 10% of patients undergoing biopsy developed AVFs.[52] In their series, the development of AVFs correlated with bleeding dysfunction (elevated bleeding time or diminished platelet count), supporting the idea that inadequate intraparenchymal hemostasis leads to the development of a channel between artery and vein that subsequently enlarges. Others have reported fewer fistulae and bleeding complications with automated small-gauge needles rather than the standard 14-gauge core biopsy technique.[39, 67]

Clinical Presentation

The majority of both congenital and acquired AVFs do not produce clinical symptoms, and increasingly lesions are noted incidentally in studies done for other reasons. The most common symptom of congenital AVM is hematuria, occurring in 72% of cases.[14] Hematuria occurs when subepithelial varices erode transitional epithelium into the collecting system. Dramatic presentation with massive hematuria can occur,[9, 23] although minor or microscopic hematuria is more common.

Hypertension occurs in congenital AVM and is the primary abnormality in most acquired AVFs described as symptomatic. The hypertension is renin-mediated, based on diminished glomerular filtration pressure distal to the fistula because of arterial "steal."[32, 47, 73] Renal dysfunction is not usually noted except in transplant patients, where diminished parenchymal flow in the solitary kidney is not masked by a functional contralateral kidney.[26]

Some patients have been discovered to have AVF when undergoing radiographic evaluation for vague abdominal or flank symptoms. Although AVFs are generally painless, intermittent perilumbar discomfort has been reported in some patients.[80, 90] This discomfort has generally been associated with hematuria and may represent renal colic.

Dyspnea and other symptoms of congestive heart failure may be the primary complaint of some patients, more commonly with acquired lesions, and only those lesions with a large communication between artery and vein. This "high-output" type of heart failure is manifest by tachycardia, left ventricular hypertrophy and cardiomegaly, and a palpable thrill in the flank. A continuous abdominal bruit is a hallmark of acquired AVF and is frequently noted with congenital AVM as well.

Retroperitoneal or intra-abdominal hemorrhage occurs rarely with AVM and AVF.[4, 9] Patients present with severe abdominal and flank pain and shock, a clinical picture indistinguishable from rupture abdominal aortic aneurysm.

Diagnosis

Excretory urography has been performed in many patients presenting with hematuria or flank pain. A filling defect may be noted in the kidney, and dilated vessels can compress the collecting system, although these findings are not specific. Although helpful to exclude more common causes of hematuria such as nephrolithiasis, intravenous pyelography is of limited use in the diagnosis of AVF.

CT can usually define AVFs and AVMs within the kidney, but it is not always possible to differentiate these lesions from other hypervascular abnormalities such as renal cell carcinoma. Similarly, radionuclide imaging can demonstrate early augmented perfusion, but differentiation from malignancy is not possible.[93] Although newer tomography reconstruction techniques such as "CT angiography" are promising,[61] experience remains limited.

Color duplex imaging is of growing importance in the diagnosis of AVM and AVF. Because it is inexpensive and noninvasive, it is the ideal study for screening purposes. Color duplex imaging has been used liberally to assess for AVF after percutaneous renal biopsy.[21, 52, 58] Marked turbulence is noted on color examination, and Doppler spectral analysis reveals elevation of peak systolic flow velocity (PSV) and a larger increase in end-diastolic flow velocity (EDV) compared with the normal renal artery, with a resultant low "resistive index"[21, 58]:

$$\frac{PSV - EDV}{PSV}$$

Arteriography has been and remains the definitive diagnos-

tic modality for renal AVMs and AVFs. Rapid opacification of the inferior vena cava is noted. Depending on the size of the fistula, the nephrogram may be diminished distal to the AVF. With congenital AVM, multiple segmental and interlobar arteries communicate with varix-like veins, whereas a single arterial communication is generally present with acquired AVF.[14] Although a relatively expensive and invasive diagnostic study, unlike other modalities, arteriography alone offers the opportunity for definitive therapy.

Treatment: Medical, Surgical, and Endovascular

The majority of both congenital and acquired AVFs do not cause symptoms and do not require treatment. Patients may become symptomatic even many years after the occurrence or diagnosis of AVF and should be closely observed for the development of hypertension, hematuria, or high-output cardiac failure.

Most AVFs occurring after percutaneous renal biopsy close spontaneously.[3, 32, 52, 53, 58] This is particularly true of AVFs discovered early after biopsy by color duplex ultrasonography. Periodic duplex surveillance, along with clinical follow-up for the development of hypertension or renal insufficiency, is indicated. If a postbiopsy AVF persists at 1 year, it is unlikely to close spontaneously,[43] although intervention should still be reserved for the development of symptoms.[26, 52]

Although hypertension related to AVF may be readily controlled with angiotensin-converting enzyme (ACE) inhibitors,[54] as with renal artery stenosis, the long-term effect on renal function is not known. In most published reports, patients with hypertension have undergone surgical or endovascular therapy; thus, the natural history of medically treated patients with hypertension secondary to AVF remains undefined.

For patients with an symptomatic AVF, surgery had been the standard treatment for many years and may still be the best option for certain AVFs.[40, 81] Except for very peripheral lesions, a transperitoneal approach is preferred to establish proximal arterial and venous control at the renal pedicle. Owing to the frequent presence of thin-walled, dilated veins and channels, surgery can be challenging. Ligation of the feeding vessel or vessels alone is often not possible, and frequently partial or total nephrectomy is required. The resultant loss of functional renal mass, as well as the morbidity of the operation itself, make endovascular treatment a more attractive approach.

There are now more than two decades of experience with percutaneous arterial embolization therapy for congenital and acquired AVFs. Because renal arteries are "end-arteries," they are especially amenable to therapeutic occlusion. In earlier reports, autologous clot was used as the embolic material, but recanalization and recurrence of AVF are possible, and thrombus has been supplanted by other materials, including gelatins, glues, alcohols, silicon, steel and platinum coils, and detachable balloons.[3, 4, 31, 37, 92] The development of coaxial catheter systems has allowed for highly selective embolization, which can preserve renal function. Loss of functional renal parenchyma has been reported to be between 0% and 30% with modern techniques.

In general, smaller AVFs are treated with glues or macro-

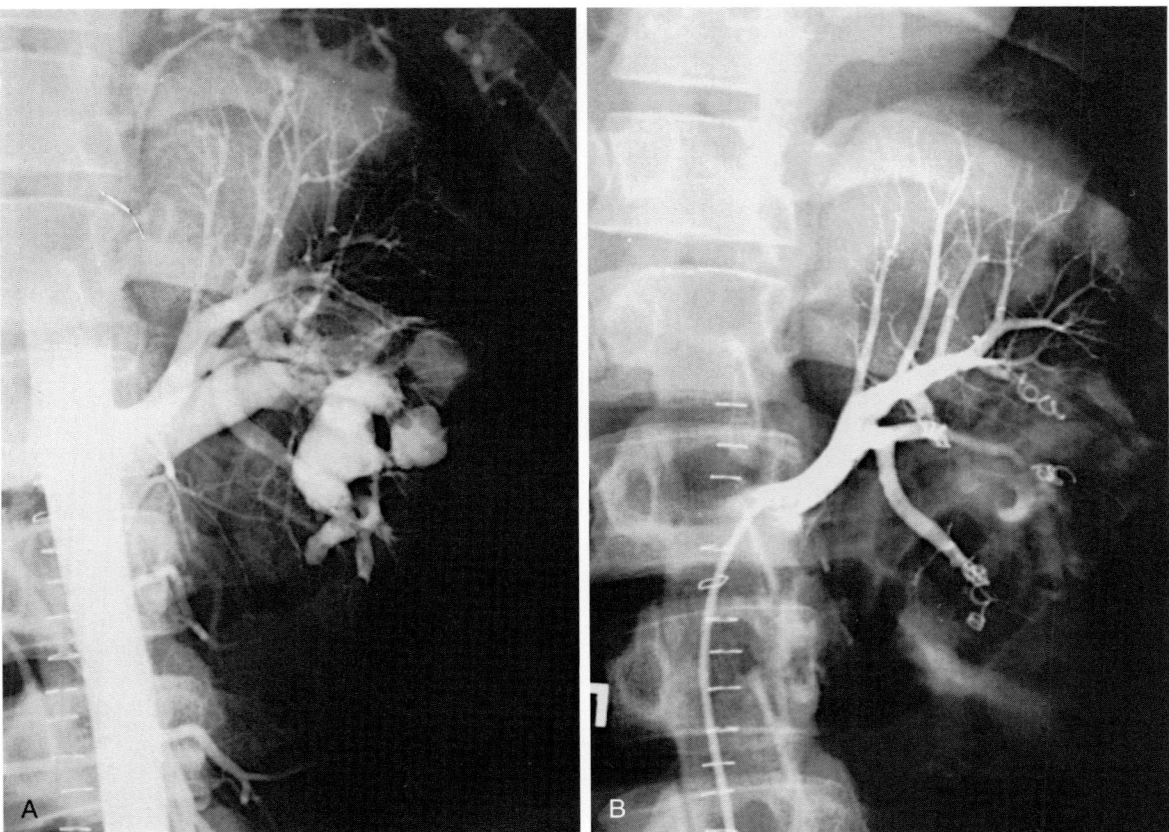

FIGURE 125–1. *A,* Arteriogram showing post-traumatic arteriovenous fistula. This patient suffered a stab wound to the flank and presented with hematuria. *B,* After Gianturco coil embolization of multiple arterial branches, venous communication is no longer present. Hematuria resolved, and the patient recovered uneventfully.

particles, while coils and balloons have been used for larger vessel fistulae (Fig. 125–1).[72] There is a trend away from the use of gelatinous sponge (Gelfoam) and glues in favor of microcoils even for smaller lesions because of a perception that the microcoils cause less indiscriminate embolization and less loss of functional renal parenchyma.[3, 4, 31]

Very large AVFs may present a technical challenge for treatment due to the risk of central embolization, and some authors recommend surgery in this setting.[40, 81] Others have reported success in this setting using the Amplatz "spider" device (Cook Inc., Bloomington, Ind.) to provide a scaffolding that can then engage other embolic materials.[37, 68] As very large arteriovenous communications tend to be at the renal pedicle rather than intraparenchymal, surgical treatment is feasible and probably preferable for good-risk patients.

Complications of embolization are unusual but not insignificant. In addition to arterial access site morbidity and contrast toxicity, pulmonary or peripheral arterial embolization can occur. This is usually related to improper selection and delivery of embolic materials. Large AVFs require large agents such as coils or detachable balloons, but even these can embolize centrally. Gelfoam, alcohol, and various glues may be more appropriate for very small communications, but delivery is less precise and more renal parenchymal infarction seems to occur with these material.[32] It is common for patients to have fever, leukocytosis, and even hypertension after embolization, which is transient and

presumed to be secondary to renal infarction.[66] Embolization itself was reported to cause massive collecting system hemorrhage in one case, but this was successfully managed with further embolization.[35] With modern techniques, success is achieved with endovascular treatment in more than 80% of patients[32] and clearly is the treatment of choice for symptomatic congenital or acquired AVF.

SUMMARY

Congenital renal AVMs and acquired AVFs are uncommon and often asymptomatic. When symptoms of hematuria, hypertension, renal dysfunction, high-output congestive heart failure, or rupture occur, treatment is mandated. Endovascular embolization is the treatment of choice, with surgical ligation or nephrectomy indicated only when embolization is unsafe or unsuccessful.

REFERENCES

1. Alcazar R, de la Torre M, Peces R: Symptomatic intrarenal arteriovenous fistula detected 25 years after percutaneous renal biopsy: Case report. Nephrol Dial Transplant 11:1346–1348, 1996.
2. Armstrong A, Birch B, Jenkins J: Renal arteriovenous fistula following blunt trauma: Case report. Br J Urol 73:321–322, 1994.
3. Beaujeux R, Boudjema K, Ellero B, et al: Endovascular treatment of

renal allograft postbiopsy arteriovenous fistula with platinum micro-coils. Transplantation 57(2):311–314, 1994.

4. Beaujeux R, Saussine C, Al-Fakir A, et al: Superselective endovascular treatment of renal vascular lesions. J Urol 153:14–17, 1995.

5. Bernhardt J, Zwicker C, Hering M, et al: A major renal artery aneurysm as the cause of a hydronephrosis with renovascular hypertension. Urol Int 57:237, 1996.

6. Brayman KL, Gincherman Y, Levy MM, et al: Ex vivo reconstruction of the renal artery for aneurysm and other abnormalities of renal vascular anatomy. In Calligaro KD, Dougherty MJ, Dean RH (eds): Modern Management of Renovascular Hypertension and Renal Salvage. Baltimore, Williams & Wilkins, 1996, p 269.

7. Bui BT, Oliva VL, Leclerc G, et al: Renal artery aneurysm: Treatment with percutaneous placement of a stent-graft. Radiology 195:181, 1995.

8. Charron J, Belanger R, Vauclair R, et al: Renal artery aneurysm: Polyaneurysmal lesion of kidney. Urology 5:1, 1975.

9. Chivate J, Blewitt R: Congenital renal arteriovenous fistula: Case report. Br J Urol 71:358–359, 1993.

10. Cho KJ, Stanley JC: Non-neoplastic congenital and acquired renal arteriovenous malformations and fistulas. Radiology 129:333–343, 1978.

11. Cinat M, Yoon P, Wilson SE: Management of renal artery aneurysms. Semin Vasc Surg 9:236, 1996.

12. Cohen JR, Shamash FS: Ruptured renal artery aneurysms during pregnancy. J Vasc Surg 6:51, 1987.

13. Coppes M, Anderson R, Mueller D, et al: Arteriovenous fistula: A complication following renal biopsy of suspected bilateral Wilms' tumor. Med Pediatr Oncol 28:455–461, 1997.

14. Crotty K, Orihuela E, Warren M: Recent advances in the diagnosis and treatment of renal arteriovenous malformations and fistulas. J Urol 150:1355–1359, 1993.

15. Dean RH, Meacham PW, Weaver FA: Ex vivo renal artery reconstructions: Indications and techniques. J Vasc Surg 4:546, 1986.

16. Dubernard JM, Martin X, Gelet A, et al: Aneurysms of the renal artery: Surgical management with special reference to extracorporeal surgery and autotransplantation. Eur Urol 11:26, 1985.

17. Dzsinich C, Gloviczki P, McKusick MA, et al: Fibromuscular dysplasia and surgical management of renal artery aneurysm. Cardiovasc Surg 1:243, 1993.

18. Erdsman G: Angionephrography and suprarenal angiography. Acta Radiol 155(Suppl):104, 1957.

19. Fogazzi G, Moriggi M, Fontanella U: Spontaneous renal arteriovenous fistula as a cause of haematuria. Nephrol Dial Transplant 12:350–356, 1997.

20. Fry WF: Renal artery aneurysm. In Ernst CB, Stanley JC (eds): Current Therapy in Vascular Surgery. Philadelphia, BC Decker, 1987, p 363.

21. Gainza F, Minguela I, Lopez-Vidaur I, et al: Evaluation of complications due to percutaneous renal biopsy in allografts and native kidneys with color-coded Doppler sonography. Clin Nephrol 43(5):303–308, 1995.

22. Gewertz BL, Stanley JC, Fry WJ: Renal artery dissections. Arch Surg 112:409, 1977.

23. Gopalakrishnan G, Al-Awadi K, Bhatia V, Mahmoud A: Renal arteriovenous malformation presenting as haematuria in pregnancy: Case report. Br J Urol 75:110–111, 1995.

24. Hageman JH, Smith RF, Szilagyi DD, et al: Aneurysms of the renal artery: Problems of prognosis and surgical management. Surgery 84:563, 1978.

25. Hare WSC, Kincaid-Smith P: Dissecting aneurysms of the renal artery. Radiology 97:255, 1970.

26. Harrison K, Nghiem H, Coldwell D, Davis C: Renal dysfunction due to an arteriovenous fistula in a transplant recipient. J Am Soc Nephrol 5(6):1300–1306, 1994.

27. Harrow BR, Sloane JA: Aneurysm of renal artery: Report of five cases. J Urol 81:35, 1959.

28. Hekali P, Kivisaara L, Standerskjold-Nordenstam CG, et al: Renal complications of polyarteritis nodosa: CT findings. J Comput Assist Tomogr 9:333, 1985.

29. Henriksson C, Bjorkerud S, Nilson AE, et al: Natural history of real artery aneurysm elucidated by repeated angiography and pathoanatomic studies. Eur Urol 11:244, 1985.

30. Hidai H, Kinoshita Y, Murayama T, et al: Rupture of renal artery aneurysm. Eur Urol 11:249, 1985.

31. Hubert JP Jr, Pairolero PC, Kazmier FJ: Solitary renal artery aneurysms. Surgery 88:557, 1980.

32. Huppert P, Duda S, Erley C, et al: Embolization of renal vascular lesions: Clinical experience with microsoils and tracker catheters. Cardiovasc Intervent Radiol 16:361–367, 1993.

33. Imray TJ, Cohen AJ, Hahn L: Renal arteriovenous fistula associated with fibromuscular dysplasia. Urology 23:378–381, 1989.

34. Kajbafzadeh A, Broumand B: Arteriovenous fistula following nephrectomy: Case report. Eur Urol 31:112–114, 1997.

35. Kamai T, Saito K, Hirokawa M, et al: A case of gross hematuria arising during embolization for renal arteriovenous malformation. Urol Int 58:55–57, 1997.

36. Kaufman JJ, Coulson WF, Lecky JW, et al: Primary dissecting aneurysms of renal artery: Report of a case causing reversible renal hypertension. Ann Surg 177:259, 1973.

37. Kearse W Jr, Joseph A, Sabanegh E Jr: Transcatheter embolization of large idiopathic renal arteriovenous fistula: Case report. J Urol 151:967–969, 1994.

38. Klein GE, Szolar DH, Breinl E, et al: Endovascular treatment of renal artery aneurysm with conventional non-detachable microcoils and Guglielmi detachable coils. Br J Urol 79:852, 1997.

39. Kolb L, Velosa J, Bergstralh E, Offord K: Percutaneous renal allograft biopsy: A comparison of two needle types and analysis of risk factors. Transplantation 57(12):1742–1746, 1994.

40. Kumar U, German K, Blackford H, Dux A: Per-operative use of a balloon-occluding arterial catheter in renal arteriovenous malformation. Br J Urol 77:312–313, 1996.

41. Kyle VN: Renal artery aneurysms. Can Med Assoc J 98:815, 1968.

42. Lacombe M: Ex situ repair of complex renal artery lesions. Cardiovasc Surg 2:767, 1994.

43. Lawen JD, van Buren CT, Lewis RM, Kahan BD: Arteriovenous fistulas after renal allograft biopsy: A serious complication in patients beyond one year. Clin Transplant 4:357–369, 1990.

44. Lee W, Lee E: Arteriovenous fistula and renal artery stenosis in a transplant kidney: Letter to editor. Nephron 69:190–192, 1995.

45. Leong K, Boey M, Feng P: Renal arteriovenous fistula following kidney biopsy in systemic lupus erythematosus. Singapore Med J 34:327–328, 1993.

46. Lumsden AB, Salam TA, Walton KG: Renal artery aneurysm: A report of 28 cases. Cardiovasc Surg 4:185, 1996.

47. McAlhany JC Jr, Black HC Jr, Hanback LD Jr, Yarbrough DR 3rd: Renal arteriovenous fistula as a cause of hypertension. Am J Surg 122:117–120, 1971.

48. McCarron JP Jr, Marshall VF, Whitsell JC II: Indications for surgery on renal artery aneurysms. J Urol 114:177, 1975.

49. McCormack LJ, Poutasse EF, Meaney TF, et al: A pathologic arteriographic correlation of real arterial disease. Am Heart J 72:188, 1966.

50. Martin RS III, Meacham PW, Ditesheim JA, et al: Renal artery aneurysm: Selective treatment for hypertension and prevention of rupture. J Vasc Surg 9:26, 1989.

51. Mattar SG, Kumar AG, Lumsden AB: Vascular complications in Ehlers-Danlos syndrome. Am Surg 60:827, 1994.

52. Merkus J, Zeebregts C, Hoitsma A, et al: High incidence of arteriovenous fistula after biopsy of kidney allografts. Br J Surg 80(3):310–312, 1993.

53. Messing E, Kessler R, Kavaney PB: Renal arteriovenous fistulas. Urology 8:101–103, 1976.

54. Morimoto A, Nakatani A, Matsui K, et al: A unique case of renovascular hypertension caused by combined renal artery disease: Case report. Hypertens Res 18(3):255–257, 1995.

55. Motta J, Breslin D, Vogel F, et al: Congenital renal arteriovenous malformation in pregnancy presenting with hypertension: Case report. Urology 44(6):911–914, 1994.

56. Murray SP, Kent C, Salvatierra O, et al: Complex branch renovascular disease: Management options and late results. J Vasc Surg 20:338, 1994.

57. Oleaga JA, Grossman RA, McLean GK, et al: Arteriovenous fistula of a segmental renal artery branch as a complication of percutaneous angioplasty. AJR 136:988–989, 1981.

58. Ozbek S, Memis A, Killi R, et al: Image-directed and color Doppler ultrasonography in the diagnosis of postbiopsy arteriovenous fistulas of native kidneys. J Clin Ultrasound 23(4):239–242, 1995.

59. Pall AA, Reid AW, Allsion MEM: Renal artery aneurysm six years after percutaneous renal biopsy: Successful treatment by embolization. Nephrol Dial Transplant 7:883, 1992.

60. Panayiotopoulos YP, Assadourian R, Taylor PR: Aneurysms of the visceral and renal arteries. Ann R Coll Surg Engl 78:412, 1996.

61. Peces R, Gorostidi M, Garcia-Gala J, et al: Giant saccular aneurysm of the renal artery presenting as malignant hypertension. J Hum Hypertens 5:455–466, 1991.

62. Piquet P, Trairier P, Garibotti F, et al: Aneurysmes des arteres renales et fistules arterioveineuses renales. In Kieffer E (ed): Chirurgie des Arteres Renales. Paris, AERCV, 1993, pp 237–250.

63. Pliskin MJ, Dresner ML, Hassell LH, et al: A giant renal artery aneurysm diagnosed post partum. J Urol 144:1459, 1990.

64. Poutasse EF: Renal artery aneurysms: Their natural history and surgery. J Urol 95:297, 1966.

65. Poutasse EF: Renal artery aneurysms. J Urol 43:113, 1975.

66. Reilly K, Shapiro M, Haskal Z: Angiographic embolization of a penetrating traumatic renal arteriovenous fistula. J Trauma 41(4):763–765, 1996.

67. Riehl J, Maigatter S, Kierdorf H, et al: Percutaneous renal biopsy: Comparison of manual and automated puncture techniques with native and transplant kidneys. Nephrol Dial Transplant 9:1568–1574, 1994.

68. Robinson D, Teitelbaum G, Pentecost M, et al: Transcatheter embolization of an aortocaval fistula caused by residual renal artery stump from previous nephrectomy: A case report. J Vasc Surg 17(4):794–797, 1993.

69. Rollino C, Garofalo G, Roccatello D, et al: Colour-coded Doppler sonography in monitoring native kidney biopsies. Nephrol Dial Transplant 9:1260–1263, 1994.

70. Routh WD, Keller FS, Gross GM: Transcatheter thrombosis of a leaking saccular aneurysm of the main renal artery with preservation of renal blood flow. AJR 154:1097, 1990.

71. Sachs D, Langevitz P, Moraq B, et al: Polyarteritis nodosa and familial Mediterranean fever. Br J Rheumatol 26:139, 1987.

72. Saliou C, Raynaud A, Blanc F, et al: Idiopathic renal arteriovenous fistula: Treatment with embolization. Ann Vasc Surg 12(1):75–77, 1998.

73. Schmid T, Sandbichler P, Ausserwinkler M, et al: Vascular lesions after percutaneous biopsies of renal allografts. Transplant Int 2:56–58, 1989.

74. Seki T, Koyanagi T, Togashi M, et al: Experience with revascularizing renal artery aneurysms: Is it feasible, safe and worth attempting? J Urol 158:357, 1997.

75. Sellar RJ, Mackay IG, Buist TA: The incidence of microaneurysms in polyarteritis nodosa. Cardiovasc Intervent Radiol 9:123, 1986.

76. Sicard GA, Reilly JM, Picus DD, et al: Alternatives in renal revascularization. Curr Probl Surg 32:569, 1995.

77. Stanley JC: Natural history of renal artery stenosis and aneurysms. In Calligaro KD, Dougherty MJ, Dean RH (eds): Modern Management of Renovascular Hypertension and Renal Salvage. Baltimore, Williams & Wilkins, 1996, p 15.

78. Stanley JC, Rhodes EL, Gewertz BL, et al: Renal artery aneurysms: Significance of macroaneurysms exclusive of dissections and fibrodysplastic mural dilations. Arch Surg 110:1327, 1975.

79. Stanley JC, Zelenock GB: Splanchnic artery aneurysms. In Rutherford RB (ed): Vascular Surgery, 4th ed. Philadelphia, WB Saunders, 1995, p 1124.

80. Steffens J, et al: Selective transcatheter embolization of a pediatric postnephrectomy arteriovenous fistula: Case report. Urol Int 53:99–101, 1994.

81. Takatera H, Nakamura M, Nakano E, et al: Renal arteriovenous fistula associated with a huge renal vain dilatation. J Urol 137:722, 1987.

82. Takebayashi S, Ohno T, Tanaka K, et al: MR angiography of renal vascular malformations. J Comp Assist Tomogr 18:596, 1994.

83. Tateno T, Kubota Y, Sasagawa I, et al: Successful embolization of a renal artery aneurysm with preservation of renal blood flow. Int Urol Nephrol 28:283, 1996.

84. Tham G, Ekelund L, Herrlin K, et al: Renal artery aneurysms: Natural history and prognosis. Ann Surg 197:348, 1983.

85. Thistlethwaite JR Jr, Woodle ES, Mayes JT, et al: Aggressive needle biopsy protocol prevents loss of renal allografts to undetected rejection during early post-transplant dysfunction. Transplant Proc 21:1890–1892, 1989.

86. Toshino A, Oka A, Kitajima K, et al: Ex vivo surgery for renal artery aneurysms. Int J Urol 3:421, 1996.

87. Turpin S, Lambert R, Querin S, et al: Radionuclide captopril renography in postpartum renal artery aneurysms. J Nucl Med 37:1368, 1996.

88. van der Zee J, van den Hoek J, Weerts J: Traumatic renal arteriovenous fistula in a 3-year-old girl, successfully treated by percutaneous transluminal embolization. J Pediatr Surg 30(10):1513–1514, 1995.

89. Van Way CW III: Renal artery aneurysms and arteriovenous fistulae. In Rutherford RB (ed): Vascular Surgery, 4th ed. Philadelphia, WB Saunders, 1995, p 1438.

90. Vasavada S, Manion S, Flanigan RC, et al: Renal arteriovenous malformations masquerading as renal cell carcinoma. Urology 46(5):716–721, 1995.

91. Vaughan TJ, Barry WF, Jeffords DL, et al: Renal artery aneurysms and hypertension. Radiology 99:287, 1971.

92. Wikholm G, Svendsen P, Herlitz H, et al: Superselective transarterial embolization of renal arteriovenous malformations of cryptogenic origin. Scand J Urol Nephrol 28:29–33, 1994.

93. Yeo E, Low J: Intrarenal arteriovenous fistula simulating a hypervascular renal tumor on radionuclide renal imaging. Clin Nucl Med 20(6):549–564, 1995.

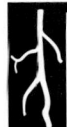

C H A P T E R 1 2 6
Acute Occlusive Events Involving the Renal Vessels

Navyash Gupta, M.D., and
Bruce L. Gewertz, M.D., F.A.C.S.

Acute events involving the renal vessels include renal artery trauma, renal artery occlusion from embolic events or thrombosis, renal artery dissections, and renal vein thrombosis. The clinical management of these entities is discussed less frequently than that of chronic renovascular disease and renovascular hypertension, yet proper decision making can lead to substantial differences in outcomes.

The diverse mechanisms involved in each presentation further complicate the clinical situation. For example, penetrating trauma of the renal vessels usually requires emergent operative repair to prevent life-threatening hemorrhage, whereas blunt injury to the renal artery from an impact or acceleration/deceleration phenomenon necessitates a more precise diagnostic approach directed toward salvage of renal function.

RENAL ARTERY EMBOLISM

Embolic occlusion of the renal artery is a relatively rare occurrence. Traube described a case of embolic renal artery occlusion in 1856,[1] but this entity gained notice in the modern era only in 1940 when Hoxie and Coggin reported 205 cases of renal infarction found at autopsy.[2] This study involved a total of 14,411 autopsies, yielding an incidence of 1.5% of renal infarction from either embolic or thrombotic events.

The majority of renal artery emboli originate from the left side of the heart in association with atrial fibrillation, mitral valvular disease, and acute myocardial infarction. Suprarenal aneurysms and ulcerative atherosclerotic plaques ("shaggy aorta") can also embolize to the renal arteries. Although embolization of aneurysmal contents can occur spontaneously, atheroemboli more frequently result from manipulation of angiographic catheters within the aorta. In these circumstances, the ischemic insult is intensified by the distal impaction of microscopic debris and the adverse effects of nephrotoxic contrast. As many as 30% of renal artery emboli of cardiac origin are bilateral. Simultaneous emboli to other visceral, extremity, and brachiocephalic vessels are also common. In instances of atheroembolization, bilateral embolization is even more common (>75%).

The classic clinical presentation of renal artery embolism may not be manifest until renal ischemia progresses to infarction.[3] Symptoms include flank, back, or abdominal pain, new-onset hypertension, hematuria, and nausea and vomiting. A low-grade fever may also be present. For the experienced clinician, the most compelling initial evidence for renal artery embolus is the association of these common symptoms with arrhythmia. Laboratory findings include leukocytosis and elevated lactate dehydrogenase levels. Urinalysis usually reveals erythrocytes, leukocytes, and proteinuria. The fact that these nonspecific symptoms are rarely ascribed to renal pathology accounts for the delays in diagnosis and overall low rate of renal salvage.

Intravenous pyelography may reveal absent or poor function, depending on the degree of renal artery obstruction (Fig. 126–1). Renal nuclear medicine studies also may demonstrate impaired renal perfusion. Unfortunately, both of these studies are not definitive and provide no anatomic information. Because any delay in diagnosis adversely affects renal salvage, renal arteriography is the better diagnostic test, yielding the most specific information. In particular, the degree of atherosclerotic disease and the pattern of collateral blood flow to the distal renal artery can help differentiate between renal artery embolus and thrombosis. In medical centers with superior diagnostic capabilities, urgent duplex ultrasonography before arteriography can be useful as a screening study.[4]

The decision regarding intervention depends on the du-

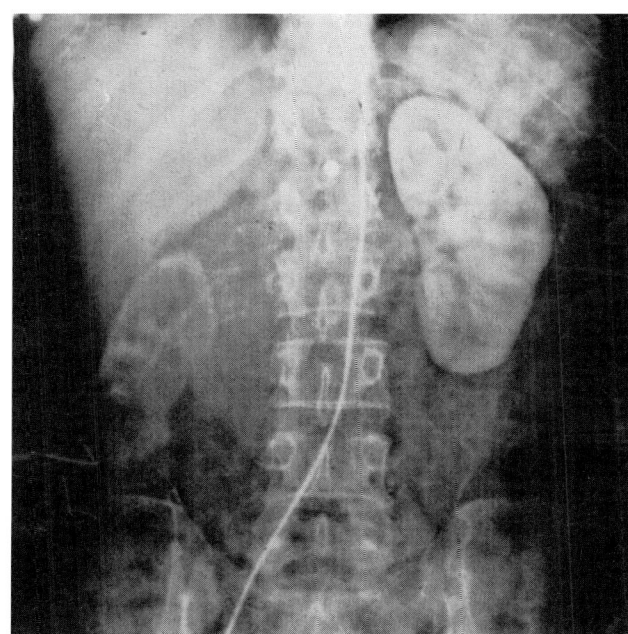

FIGURE 126–1. Nephrogram phase of arterial injection in a patient with embolus to right renal artery. Note delayed and incomplete nephrogram of involved right kidney.

ration and severity of renal ischemia, the site of the embolus, the status of the contralateral kidney, and underlying cardiopulmonary risk factors. In the past, renal salvage was thought unlikely in patients presenting with symptoms of prolonged duration (>12 hours) with no evidence of ipsilateral renal perfusion. In particular, patients with distal branch emboli or severe cardiopulmonary risk factors were rarely considered operative candidates; anticoagulation alone was recommended. More recently, the evolution of thrombolytic therapy and improvements in operative and perioperative management have allowed a much more aggressive approach to these patients.[5] In a recent report by Salam and colleagues, seven of 10 patients presenting with acute embolic or thrombotic occlusions were successfully treated by thrombolytics.[6] It is noteworthy that four of these patients presented with acute renal failure.

It is now accepted that most patients with early presentations of embolic occlusion should be considered for revascularization by operative embolectomy or catheter-directed thrombolytic therapy. Surgical intervention is preferable in good-risk patients with partial renal artery occlusion, bilateral renal artery emboli, or an embolus to a solitary kidney. Operative mortality is significantly reduced by preoperative correction of metabolic derangements and fluid resuscitation.

Exposure of the left kidney can be gained via a retroperitoneal approach through a transverse left supraumbilical incision. With some effort even the right renal artery can be exposed through this route, although most surgeons prefer a midline transperitoneal approach with an extended Kocher maneuver.[7] The renal vein is gently retracted and the renal artery dissected free. A transverse aortotomy is performed at the level of the renal artery, and an embolectomy catheter is passed distally and the thromboembolic debris cleared. The aortotomy can usually be closed primarily. If atherosclerotic disease of the renal artery is encountered, the aortotomy can be extended across the renal ostium, the endarterectomy is performed, and the arteriotomy is closed with a patch.

Complete extraction of embolic material can be difficult to assess in the operating room. Although arteriography can be performed, the nephrotoxicity of contrast and other technical difficulties in adequately visualizing the in situ kidney make this approach less attractive. Intraoperative duplex ultrasonography avoids these potential complications and has been utilized with some success. Diuretics, mannitol, and renal dose dopamine are all advisable after revascularization.[8] Finally, because the renal parenchyma can swell considerably after revascularization, partial renal decapsulation may be considered in extreme cases.[9] The precise indications for this adjunctive procedure are not clearly defined.

Thrombolytic therapy offers the advantage of avoiding operative stress in an acutely ill patient and may be preferable for a patient with distal branch emboli.[5] The disadvantages include the significant hemorrhagic complications associated with thrombolytic therapy regardless of the agent used or route of administration. This is a particular concern for patients with renal infarction or simultaneous cerebral emboli. Fibrinolytic agents are less likely to be effective when occlusions are due to mature organized thrombus, embolized valvular vegetations, and atheromatous debris.

Thus, renal infarction has often occurred by the time the diagnosis of renal artery embolus is made. Irrespective of treatment instituted at this late stage, parenchymal salvage rates are low. This is especially true in patients with complete embolic obstruction of a main renal artery. Although Lacombe in 1977 reported a salvage rate of 68% in patients with renal artery embolism treated surgically,[10] in a more recent report Ouriel and associates reported that they were unable to salvage any of 13 kidneys with emboli occluding the main renal artery.[11]

RENAL ARTERY DISSECTIONS EXCLUSIVE OF TRAUMA

Renal artery dissections can be broadly categorized into *primary* and *secondary* lesions. Primary dissections are associated with underlying renal artery disease, such as fibromuscular dysplasia (FMD) or atherosclerosis. Secondary dissections result from either blunt trauma or interventional procedures, such as selective renal artery catheterization and percutaneous renal artery angioplasty.

Renal artery dissections are often clinically silent, yet they can result in a broad spectrum of outcomes, including renal infarction and the acute onset of severe hypertension. The clinical course is largely dictated by the degree of renal artery obstruction and by the presence or absence of preformed arterial collateral vessels. Treatment is appropriately individualized based on the severity of symptoms and the anatomic nature of the lesion.

It is thought that renal arteries are the most common site of primary dissections involving peripheral vessels.[12] Nonetheless, spontaneous dissection of the renal artery is rare and usually occurs in the setting of FMD, advanced

atherosclerosis, or other arteritides (Fig. 126–2).[13] The demographics of the patient population suffering dissections parallels that of the underlying diseases; that is, young women with a dysplastic lesion and older individuals with generalized atherosclerosis. Because most spontaneous dissections are clinically silent, the precise incidence of complications relating to these lesions is difficult to assess. Symptomatic dissections typically present with upper abdominal or flank pain (92%), hematuria (33%), and onset of severe hypertension (100%).[14]

The hypertension produced by spontaneous dissection of the renal artery is difficult to control and usually requires multidrug therapy. Although there are isolated reports of spontaneous reversion to normal blood pressure, this phenomenon is far less common in localized dissections than in instances of aortic dissection extending into or excluding the renal arteries.[15] Histopathologic examination suggests, in fact, that, unlike typical aortic dissections, spontaneous renal artery dissection channels often do not communicate with the vessel lumen but rather represent intramural hematoma formation along a deeper medial plane.[16] Hence, true "reentry" is less likely. In contrast, post-traumatic dissections in previously normal vessels usually begin with an intimal tear and extend along subintimal or superficial medial planes.

Although isotope renography may be helpful in determining the presence of renal ischemia, this information does not aide in planning operative repair and may not define those patients with dissections who are most amenable to treatment (i.e., patent but stenosed renal arteries with adequate antegrade renal perfusion). Duplex ultraso-

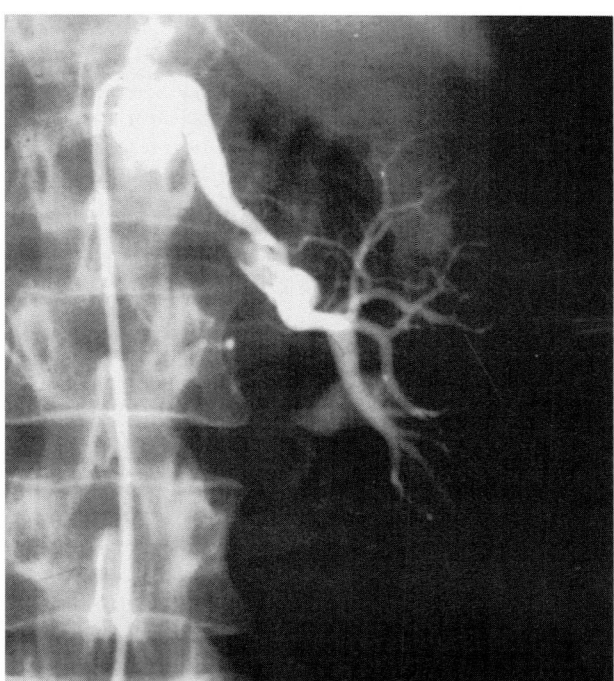

FIGURE 126–2. Spontaneous dissection in left renal artery in a patient with acute onset of severe hypertension. Such highly stenotic dissections require operative treatment. (From Gewertz BL, Stanley JC, Fry WJ: Renal artery dissections. Arch Surg 112:409–414, 1977. Copyright 1977, American Medical Association.)

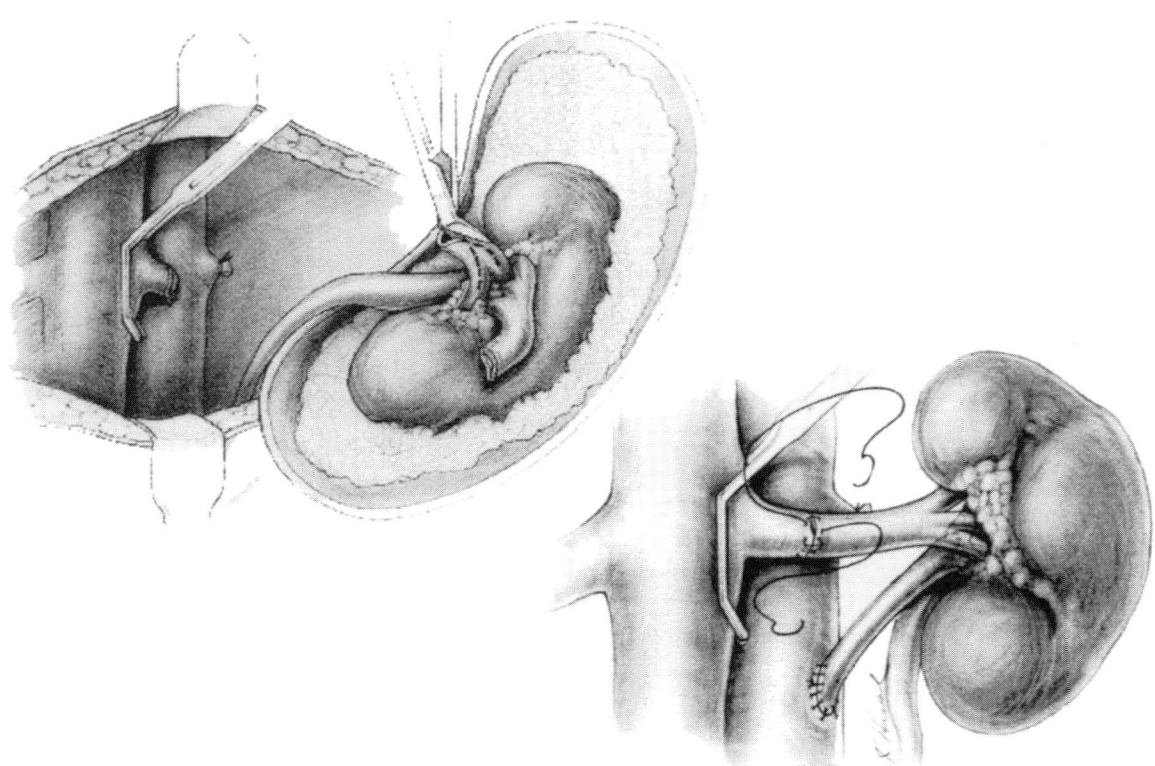

FIGURE 126–3. Technique for ex vivo repair of distal left renal artery dissection. The kidney is flushed with renal preservation solution and placed on ice during repair to minimize ischemic injury. Bypass with autologous vein or artery is completed *(lower right)*, and vein is reanatomosed.

nography can identify abnormalities of the renal arteries, but this technique is unlikely to reliably distinguish between intrinsic disease and dissection. Hence, selective renal arteriography remains the diagnostic test of choice and should be used in every case to define the nature and extent of the lesion and the suitability for repair.

Limited dissections without significant main renal artery stenoses and hypertension are best treated expectantly. For symptomatic patients with severe hypertension, however, most experienced surgeons advocate renal artery revascularization unless irreversible renal ischemia has occurred or if reconstruction cannot be performed because of extension of the dissection into renal artery parenchymal branches. Although partial or total nephrectomy usually results in resolution of the hypertension, the high incidences of bilateral renal artery dissection (>20%) as well as bilateral and related occlusive FMD (>50%) argue strongly for maximal renal salvage attempts.

Operative repair is challenging and invariably requires control of at least the primary branches of the renal artery regardless of the apparent limits of the dissection. When the dissection does not extend past the first branch point, in situ repair is almost always technically feasible. In contrast, repair of dissections extending into the secondary branches is best performed with ex vivo techniques (Fig. 126–3). In a series of patients with extensive dissections reported by Reilly and associates, temporary preservation with reimplantation was utilized successfully in six of seven reconstructions.[17] Intraoperative duplex ultrasonography is

most useful to assess the technical success of the repair in the small hilar branches.

Before the widespread application of percutaneous interventional procedures, the incidence of secondary (iatrogenic) dissections was very low. In 1976, Gewertz and associates from the University of Michigan documented only four instances among a total of 11,000 abdominal arteriograms, including more than 2000 selective renal catheterizations.[16] With more aggressive and successful transluminal treatments of diseased renal arteries, the frequency of secondary dissection has predictably increased, although the precise incidence is not known.[18] Virtually all balloon dilations create a controlled dissection when the plaque or dysplastic lesion is fractured; hence, the practical definition of a postangiographic dissection hinges on whether the vessel is occluded or significantly narrowed after the procedure. Using this criteria, authors of collected series estimate an incidence of approximately 4% of main and branch renal artery dissections, with less then half of these requiring surgery.[19–22]

In current practice, many limited dissections of the main renal artery are effectively managed with immediate stent placement and, in the absence of sequelae, may not even be recorded as a complication. In instances of extensive dissection with main renal artery or major branch occlusion, urgent operation is appropriate. Results are far less attractive than those seen with elective renal revascularizations but probably compare reasonably well with those associated with the operative treatment of spontaneous dissections. That said, highly experienced renovascular surgeons have noted the unique challenges of operating on dissected renal arteries, including the dense periarterial inflammatory response that greatly complicates distal repairs even with the ex vivo technique.[23]

ACUTE RENAL VEIN THROMBOSIS

Renal vein thrombosis is an unusual clinical entity that infrequently requires operative intervention and usually responds well to anticoagulation. Renal vein thrombosis is seen in two discrete patient populations: (1) adults with nephrotic syndrome and (2) neonates with severe dehydration.[24 25] It is noteworthy that the morbidity associated with renal vein thrombosis is primarily related to the underlying condition producing the coagulopathic state.

The nephrotic syndrome results in loss of low-molecular-weight proteins in the urine, decreased antithrombin III levels, and thrombocytosis, all of which contribute to a hypercoagulable state.[26] A contracted intravascular volume and hemoconcentration also lead to renal vein stasis. Other conditions occasionally associated with renal vein thrombosis in adults include pregnancy, use of oral contraceptives, neoplasms (especially renal cell carcinoma), sickle cell anemia, and trauma.

Adults with acute renal vein thrombosis present with acute onset of flank pain, hematuria, proteinuria, and decreased renal function. Very rarely, venous congestion of the kidney can cause hemorrhagic infarction and rupture. In these unusual cases, severe retroperitoneal hemorrhage may require urgent nephrectomy.

Neonatal renal vein thrombosis occurs in infants who are severely dehydrated secondary to diarrhea or vomiting or who are in septic states.[27] Infants of diabetic mothers may be predisposed to this disorder due to hyperglycemia and solute diuresis.[28] Children present with sudden onset of abdominal distention, flank mass, hematuria, and proteinuria. In advanced cases of bilateral renal vein thrombosis, infants can suffer progressive renal insufficiency.

Diagnosis can be established by duplex ultrasonography, which demonstrates renal enlargement with distortion of the parenchymal pattern, renal vein dilatation, and thrombus within the renal vein. Computed tomography (CT) may also be helpful in establishing the diagnosis, although it requires the administration of potentially nephrotoxic contrast agents. Magnetic resonance imaging avoids contrast administration and may prove in the future to be the test of choice, especially for adults.[29]

Treatment in both the adult and pediatric populations is primarily supportive and directed toward treatment of underlying metabolic abnormalities and correction of any potentially reversible hypercoagulable state. Hydration and immediate heparin anticoagulation followed by warfarin anticoagulation for 6 months is standard. A longer period of anticoagulation is indicated for patients with nephrotic syndrome. More recently, thrombolytic therapy has been used via either renal venous or arterial infusion. This approach is most attractive for patients with bilateral renal vein thrombosis or venous thrombosis of a solitary kidney. Operative thrombectomy of renal vein thrombosis is limited

to patients with rapidly declining renal function when thrombolytic therapy is contraindicated or unsuccessful.

Both the underlying hypercoagulable state and the presence of thrombus along the vena cava substantially increase the likelihood of pulmonary embolus in these patients. If pulmonary emboli are documented, strong consideration should be given to placement of a suprarenal filter in addition to anticoagulation. Although this has the theoretical disadvantage of predisposing to vena caval thrombosis, the incidence of this complication appears to be quite low.

RENAL ARTERY TRAUMA

Renal artery trauma is unusual. Penetrating abdominal or lower thoracic injuries result in renal pedicle laceration in fewer than 7% of cases, while it is estimated that blunt abdominal trauma leads to disruption, dissection, or occlusion of the renal artery in fewer than 4% of seriously injured patients.[30] Although management strategies for these two types of injuries are somewhat different, results from all treatments are not particularly good.

The mechanisms of renal artery injury with penetrating trauma are unambiguous. Nonetheless, for such gunshot and stab wounds, management is still complicated by the likelihood that the renal parenchyma and other vital structures are injured simultaneously. In contrast, diagnosis and management of blunt trauma reflect the two distinct patterns of injury.[31] In *direct injuries* from contact sports or motor vehicle accidents, anterior blows to the mid-abdomen compress the right renal artery as it crosses the vertebral column (Fig. 126–4). In *indirect injuries*, acceleration/deceleration forces accompanying high-speed collisions stretch both renal pedicles and can disrupt the vessels or

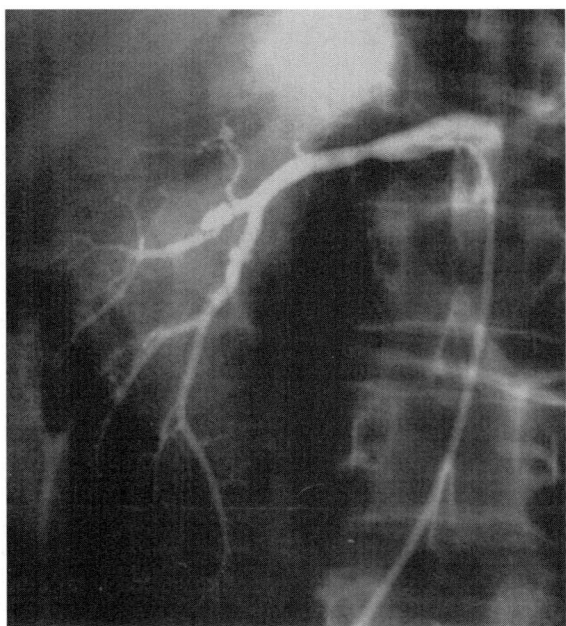

FIGURE 126–4. Right renal artery injury after blunt trauma demonstrates dissection of both main renal artery and both primary branches. (From Gewertz BL, Stanley JC, Fry WJ: Renal artery dissections. Arch Surg 112:409–414, 1977. Copyright 1977, American Medical Association.)

rupture the intima, the least elastic portion of vessel. Intimal tears can lead to acute renal artery thrombosis or a more stable, yet obstructive dissection.[16]

As a result of these divergent mechanisms of injury, the diagnosis and treatment of penetrating trauma and blunt trauma differ substantially. Patients with hypotension or exsanguinating hemorrhage from penetrating truncal injury require immediate operative exploration. In such situations, control of hepatic, splenic, and major vascular injury is mandatory. Surgical decision making relative to the kidneys is enhanced if the patient is stable enough to undergo a "single-shot" intravenous pyelogram in the operating room before any hematoma in the retroperitoneum is opened. Although such studies may not necessarily differentiate a renal parenchymal laceration from a pedicle injury, the presence of a functional contralateral kidney can be confirmed.

If nonrenal injuries are controlled and the patient's condition is stable, vascular repair of an injured renal pedicle can be considered. Most commonly, this will require an aortorenal bypass to the débrided distal renal artery. Unfortunately, circumstances usually do not allow for such repairs; renal artery lacerations or transections are rarely the only serious injury, and most of the time the patient's overall condition mandates the most rapid resolution for the problem, which is nephrectomy.

The diagnosis of renal artery injury after blunt trauma is based on the routine inclusion of thoracic and abdominal vascular imaging in the initial assessment of any patient suffering a high-speed accident. A history of such an injury is a more compelling indication for such an evaluation than any specific sign or symptom. In fact, up to 25% of patients with renal pedicle injuries have no urinary findings to support the observation that the presence of hematuria or flank pain reflects associated renal contusions, not the status of the renal vessels.[32] In the past, aggressive utilization of arteriography was the only reliable method of screening for such injuries.[33, 34] More recently, CT with helical scanning techniques have supplanted arteriography in many large medical centers.[35, 36]

Successful emergency reconstruction of renal artery injuries in the setting of blunt trauma is rare. Stables and associates reported that only two of 26 renal artery injuries could be successfully reconstructed.[37] Clark and colleagues reported only a 17% restoration of function in 12 kidneys revascularized after injury.[31] In truth, this dismal outlook more likely reflects the common association of other life-threatening injuries, especially of the aortic isthmus, spleen, and liver, that detract from the attention given renal artery injuries.

ACUTE RENAL ARTERY THROMBOSIS

Acute thrombosis of the renal artery occurs most commonly in patients with advanced atherosclerotic disease of the aorta and its branches. This event may be clinically silent if adequate collateral circulation to the distal renal artery from ureteral, lumbar, adrenal, or capsular vessels already exists.[38] In patients with only one functional kidney or poor renal reserve, however, renal artery thrombosis may present with both severe hypertension and the acute onset of oliguric renal failure.[39] Renal artery thrombosis may also complicate percutaneous transluminal renal angioplasty, which is being used more commonly to treat atherosclerotic renal artery stenosis.[23, 40] Patients at highest risk for periprocedural thrombosis are those with significant abdominal aortic atherosclerosis and associated ostial renal artery stenosis (Fig. 126–5).[41]

Both renal ultrasonography and angiography can aid in establishing the diagnosis. If adequate collateral arterial supply is present, arteriography may reveal retrograde filling of the distal renal arterial tree. This finding in combination with documentation of renal perfusion by isotope renography are excellent prognostic signs even if excretory function is markedly reduced.[41] Most important, unlike the treatment of renal artery embolism, correction of renal artery thrombosis superimposed on a preexistent severe occlusive lesion rarely mandates an urgent operative approach. Any metabolic derangements should be corrected, and the appropriate evaluation of cardiac and other risk factors should be carried out. Although patients may require dialysis during this period, it has been the experience at many medical centers that this does not preclude considerable recovery of renal function after revascularization, even if the procedure is delayed by weeks.[42, 43]

Surgical revascularization options include aortorenal bypass with saphenous vein or synthetic grafts.[44–46] For patients with severe atherosclerosis of the abdominal aorta, extra-anatomic bypasses, including hepatorenal bypass, splenorenal bypass, and ileorenal bypass, may be preferable. Revascularization can yield dramatic results with almost immediate recovery of renal function in a majority of appropriately selected patients.[42] It is also possible that fibrinolysis with angioplasty and stent placement may have

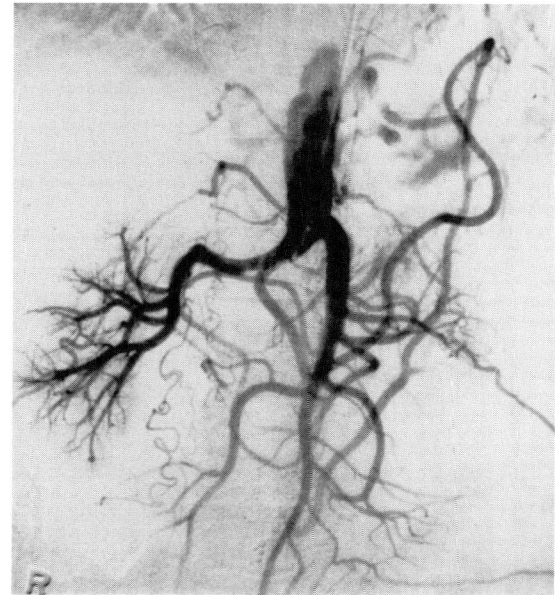

FIGURE 126–5. Patient with thrombotic occlusion of severely diseased aorta with proximal propagation of clot to left renal artery. Severe hypertension was a more prominent presenting symptom than lower limb ischemia, which was mitigated by collateral vessels to common femoral arteries.

a role in treatment of these patients.[47] To date, the reports of such treatments are anecdotal, and long-term patency and risks are unknown.

Acknowledgment: We gratefully acknowledge the assistance of Karen Hynes in the preparation of the manuscript.

REFERENCES

1. Traube L: Uber den Zusammenhang von Herz und Nieren Krakheiten. *In* Gesammelte Beitrage zur Pathologie und Physiologie. Berlin, A Hirschwald, 1856, p 77.
2. Hoxie HJ, Coggin CB: Renal infarction: Statistical study of two hundred and five cases and detailed report of an unusual case. Arch Intern Med 65:587, 1940.
3. Nicholas GG, De Muth WE Jr: Treatment of renal artery embolism. Arch Surg 119:278–281, 1984.
4. Platt JF: Duplex Doppler evaluation of acute renal obstruction. Semin Ultrasound CT MR 18:147–153, 1997.
5. Fischer CP, Konnak JW, Cho KJ, et al: Renal artery embolism: Therapy with intra-arterial streptokinase infusion. J Urol 125:402–405, 1981.
6. Salam TA, Lumdsen AB, Martin LG: Local infusion of fibrinolytic agents for acute renal artery thromboembolism: Report of ten cases. Ann Vasc Surg 7(1):21–26, 1993.
7. Shah DM, Darling RC 3rd, Chang BB, et al: Access to the right renal artery from the left retroperitoneal approach. Cardiovasc Surg 4:763–765, 1996.
8. Schwartz LB. BL Gewertz: The renal response to low dose dopamine: A review. J Surg Res 54:574–588, 1988.
9. Stone HH, Fulenwider JT: Renal decapsulation in the prevention of post-ischemic oliguria. Ann Surg 186:343–355, 1977.
10. Lacombe M: Surgical versus medical treatment of renal artery embolism. J Cardiovasc Surg 18:281–290, 1977.
11. Ouriel K, Andrus CH, Ricotta JJ, et al: Acute renal artery occlusion: When is revascularization justified? J Vasc Surg 5:348–355, 1987.
12. Foord AG, Lewis RD: Primary dissecting aneurysms of the peripheral and pulmonary arteries: Dissecting hemorrhage of the media. Arch Pathol 68:553–577, 1956.
13. Englund GW: Primary dissecting aneurysm of the renal artery: Report of a case and review of the literature. Am J Clin Pathol 45:472–479, 1966.
14. Smith BM, Holcomb GW, Richie RE, et al: Renal artery dissection. Ann Surg 200:134–146, 1984.
15. Park JH, Chung W, Cho YK, et al: Percutaneous fenestration of aortic dissection: Salvage of an ischemic solitary left kidney. Cardiovasc Intervent Radiol 20(2):146–148, 1997.
16. Gewertz BL, Stanley JC, Fry WJ: Renal artery dissections. Arch Surg 112:402–414, 1977.
17. Reilly LM, Cunningham CG, Maggisano R, et al: The role of arterial reconstruction in spontaneous renal artery dissection. J Vasc Surg 14:468–479, 1991.
18. Anwar YA. Sullivan ED, Chen HH, et al: Abrupt, severe hypertension associated with dissection of a renal artery during selective catheterization. J Hum Hypertens 11:533–536, 1997.
19. Martinez AG, Novick AC, Hayes JM: Surgical treatment of renal artery stenosis after failed percutaneous transluminal angioplasty. J Urol 144:1094–1096, 1990.
20. Tegtmeyer CJ, Selby JB, Hartwell GD, et al: Results and complications of angioplasty in fibromuscular disease. Circulation 83(Suppl 1):I155–I161, 1991.
21. Rees CR, Palmaz JC, Becker GJ, et al: Palmaz stent in the atherosclerotic stenoses involving the ostia of the renal arteries: Preliminary report of a multicenter study. Radiology 181:507–514, 1991.
22. Martin LG, Casarella WJ, Alspaugh JP, et al: Renal artery angioplasty: Increased technical success and decreased complications in the second 100 patients. Radiology 159:631–634, 1986.
23. Dean RH, Callis JT, Smith BM, et al: Failed percutaneous transluminal renal angioplasty: Experience with lesions requiring operative intervention. J Vasc Surg 6:301–307, 1987.
24. Baum NH, Moriel E, Carlton CE Jr: Renal vein thrombosis. J Urol 119:443–448, 1978.
25. Arneil GC, MacDonald AM, Murphy AV, et al: Renal venous thrombosis. Clin Nephrol 1:199–231, 1973.
26. Brumfitt W, O'Brien W: Renal vein thrombosis with nephrotic syndrome and renal failure. BMJ 2:751, 1956.
27. Jones JE, Reed JF: Renal vein thrombosis and thrombocytopenia in a newborn infant. J Pediatr 67:681, 1965.
28. Avery ME, Oppenheimer EH, Gordon HH: Renal vein thrombosis in newborn infants of diabetic mothers. N Engl J Med 256:1134, 1957.
29. Deitrich RB, Kangarloo H: Kidneys in infants and children: Evaluation with MR. Radiology 159:215–221, 1986.
30. Brown MF, Graham JM, Mattox KL, et al: Renovascular trauma. Am J Surg 140:802–805, 1980.
31. Clark DE, Georgitis JW, Ray FS: Renal arterial injuries caused by blunt trauma. Surgery 90:87–96, 1981.
32. Grablowsky OM, Weichert RF 3rd, Goff JB, et al: Renal artery thrombosis following blunt trauma: Report of four cases. Surgery 67:895–900, 1970.
33. Itzchak Y, Adar R, Moses M, et al: Occlusion of the renal and visceral arteries following blunt abdominal trauma: Angiographic observations. Cardiovasc Surg 15:383–388, 1973.
34. Marks LS, Brosman SA, Lindstrom RR, et al: Arteriography in penetrating renal trauma. Urology 3:18–22, 1974.
35. Nunez D Jr, Becerra JL, Fuentes D, et al: Traumatic occlusion of the renal artery: Helical CT diagnosis. AJR Am J Roentgenol 167(3):777–780, 1996.
36. Fang YC, Tiu CM, Chou YH, et al: A case of renal artery thrombosis caused by blunt trauma: Computed tomographic and Doppler ultrasonic findings. J Formos Med Assoc 92(4):356–358, 1993.
37. Stables DP, Fouche RF, de Villiers van Niekerk JP, et al: Traumatic renal artery occlusion: 21 cases. J Urol 115:229–233, 1976.
38. Abrams HL, Cornell SH: Patterns of collateral flow in renal ischemia. Radiology 84:1010–1012, 1965.
39. Hall SK: Acute renal vascular occlusion: An uncommon mimic. J Emerg Med 11(60):691–700, 1993.
40. Komeyama T: Successful fibrinolytic therapy using tissue plasminogen activator in acute renal failure due to thrombosis of bilateral renal arteries. Urol Int 51:177–180, 1993.
41. Gilbert LA, Katz N, Mandal AK, et al: Acute proximal occlusion of a nonaneurysmal abdominal aorta and renal arteries detected by renal imaging. Clin Nucl Med 22:231–234, 1997.
42. Dean RH, Tribble RW, Hansen KJ, et al: Evolution of renal insufficiency in ischemic nephropathy. Ann Surg 213:446–455, 1991.
43. Higgins EM, Goldsmith DJ, Charlesworth D, et al: Elective rather than emergency intervention for acute renal artery occlusion with anuria. Nephron 68:265–267, 1994.
44. Dean RH: Surgery for renovascular hypertension. *In* Bergen JJ, Yao JST (eds): Operative Techniques in Vascular Surgery. New York, Grune & Stratton, 1980, pp 81–87.
45. Chaikof EL: Revascularization of the occluded renal artery. Semin Vasc Surg 9:218–220, 1996.
46. Fujitani RM, Murray SP: Surgical methods for renal revascularization. Semin Vasc Surg 9:198–217, 1996.
47. Ellis D, Kaye RD, Bontempo FA: Aortic and renal artery thrombosis in a neonate: Recovery with thrombolytic therapy. Pediatr Nephrol 11:641–644, 1997.

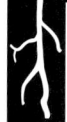

C H A P T E R   1 2 7

Fundamental Considerations in Cerebrovascular Disease

Wesley S. Moore, M.D.

Stroke is the third leading cause of death in the United States each year. It is the second leading cause of cardiovascular death and the most common cause of death as a result of neurologic disorders. The incidence of new stroke is approximately 160 per 100,000 population per year.[59, 63] In addition to death, the disability following cerebral infarction must be considered from the standpoint of the crippling effect on the patient as well as the socioeconomic burden on the patient, his or her family, and society. Reviews of the financial impact of stroke for calendar year 1999 were estimated to be $45.3 billion of direct and indirect cost.[2, 93a]

The earliest report linking stroke with extracranial vascular disease is credited to Gowers, who in 1875 described a patient with right hemiplegia and blindness in the left eye.[37] He attributed this syndrome to an occlusion of the left carotid artery in the neck. Several similar reports soon followed.[9, 12, 41] In 1914, Hunt emphasized that extracranial carotid artery occlusive disease was a possible cause of stroke.[54] He noted that the cervical portions of the carotid arteries were not examined routinely post mortem and urged that thorough examination of this portion of the circulatory system be carried out during autopsy. Furthermore, he believed that transient cerebral ischemia was tantamount to intermittent claudication of the brain and represented a prodrome to a major stroke.

In spite of these early reports, work in this field remained relatively dormant until Moniz and coworkers reported in 1937 that arteriography could be used to diagnose carotid artery occlusion.[76] Johnson and Walker reviewed 101 cases of carotid occlusion diagnosed by arteriography and advocated either carotid arterectomy or cervical ganglionectomy to relieve cerebral vasospasm, which they believed to be a major cause of subsequent disability following the initial stroke.[56] Strully and his associates are credited with the first attempt at endarterectomy of a totally occluded carotid artery; however, this was unsuccessful.[93]

The first report of a successful surgical procedure on the extracranial carotid artery appeared in 1954: Eastcott and colleagues described their experience with a patient who had episodes of transient hemispheric cerebral ischemic attacks.[22] She was found to have an atherosclerotic lesion at the carotid bifurcation that was treated with a resection and primary anastomosis. A later publication by DeBakey[16] and one of Carrea and coworkers[10] cite operative procedures reportedly performed at earlier dates, but the report of Eastcott and colleagues must be credited as the most influential in bringing the possibility of carotid artery repair to medical attention. Vascular surgery had progressed to a point at which surgical repair of this lesion was rapidly accepted, and subsequently carotid endarterectomy has become one of the most common and successful operations performed on the vascular system.

The surgical approach to cerebrovascular disease is predicated on the relief of symptoms of cerebral dysfunction and the prevention of cerebral infarction or stroke by excision of a critical lesion in the extracranial carotid artery. There was a major international debate concerning the efficacy of carotid endarterectomy in stroke prevention when one considers the combination of perioperative risk and late results. It has been shown that an aggressive surgical approach to cerebrovascular disease can be justified only when the operation can be performed with sufficiently low rates of morbidity and mortality for the longevity and quality of survival of patients with cerebrovascular atherosclerosis to be materially altered, when compared with the results of medical management alone.[26, 48, 80, 81, 94]

EPIDEMIOLOGY AND NATURAL HISTORY OF CEREBROVASCULAR DISEASE

Knowledge of the incidence and natural history of hemispheric transient ischemic attacks (TIAs) and strokes in a given population is of paramount importance, not only in understanding the magnitude of the problem but also in designing a program of diagnosis, treatment, and prevention. The magnitude of the problem will dictate its investigative priority, and knowledge of the natural history is fundamental in evaluating and comparing the impact of various therapeutic interventions.

The objective of all therapeutic intervention is to prevent cerebral infarction. Episodes of transient cerebral ischemia usually are considered benign events, but they are harbingers of subsequent stroke, neurologic disability, or death.

Cerebral Infarction

There is considerable variability concerning the incidence of stroke, depending on the year of reporting, geographic location, and racial and gender mix of patients. For example, there has been a steady decline in mortality from cerebrovascular disease in the United States dating back to 1915.[104] This decline in mortality may or may not translate into a true decline in stroke incidence. The reason for the decline in stroke mortality is difficult to ascertain. It may be something as simple as a more accurate diagnosis of stroke on a death certificate, or it may represent a true change in the incidence of the disease. Finally, various interventions, ranging from control of hypertension to the use of aspirin and other antiplatelet drugs to carotid endarterectomy, must be interpreted accordingly.

There have been several population studies designed to look at stroke incidence. The Rochester, Minnesota, population study (from 1955 to 1969) emphasized the influence of advancing age on the progressive incidence of cerebral infarction.[68] The age group of 55 to 64 years had a cerebral infarction rate of 276.8 per 100,000 population per year; the age group of 65 to 74 years had an incidence of 632 per 100,000 population per year; and the over-75 age group had a stroke rate of 1786.4 per 100,000 population per year. Analysis of the cerebral infarction rate divided by sex distribution indicated that in men the rate was approximately 1.5 times as great as that in women of the same age. Six months following survival from cerebral infarction, only 29% of the patients in the Rochester study had normal cerebral function; 71% continued to have manifestations of neurologic dysfunction. In the latter group, 4% required total nursing care, 18% were disabled but capable of contributing to self-care, and 10% were aphasic. Of those patients who suffered a fatal stroke, 38% died of the initial stroke, 10% died of a subsequent stroke, and 18% died from complications of coronary artery disease. The chance of a recurrent stroke within 1 year of the initial stroke was 10%, and the chance of a recurrent stroke within 5 years of the initial attack was 20%.

Wolfe and colleagues, in 1989, reported data from the Framingham study.[105] They reviewed the experience from three successive decades beginning in 1953. They noted a decline of *stroke fatality* in both men and women. However, the 10-year prevalence rate of stroke actually rose, and the *incidence* of stroke rose in men from 5.7% to 7.6% to 7.9% without any apparent change in women. The investigators suggested that the case fatality rates may result from changes in diagnostic criteria, a lessening in stroke severity, or improved care of stroke patients. Nonetheless, they clearly show that there was not a declining incidence.[105]

Wallace studied the natural history of stroke in 188

patients in the city of Goulburn, Australia.[100] The overall incidence of stroke for all ages was 330 per 100,000 population per year. During a 24-month interval, they accumulated 158 cases of stroke, of which 101 were presumed to be due to cerebral infarction. The mortality rate of the first attack was 37%, and the recurrence rate among survivors was 35%. The mortality rate with the first recurrence was 35%, but the mortality rate for subsequent recurrences in survivors of a first recurrence was 65%.

Baker and his colleagues reported a series of 430 hospitalized patients who survived their initial cerebral infarction.[4] The mortality rate from the initial stroke was not described. However, the overall mortality rate for the 430 survivors during the interval of study was 40%. On a life table, the mortality rate was 10% per year of patients at risk. The cumulative 5-year mortality rate was 50%. Twenty-three per cent of subsequent deaths were due to recurrent cerebral infarction. Of the 430 survivors of the initial stroke, 26% developed a subsequent recurrent cerebral infarction, and 20% experienced new TIAs. Because some patients have both TIA and stroke, a combined 38% were reported to develop a new neurologic event: stroke, transient cerebral ischemia, or both. Of the 113 patients who developed a new cerebral infarction, 62% died.

Sacco and coworkers, reviewing the stroke data from the Framingham, Massachusetts, population, noted an alarmingly high incidence of recurrent cerebral infarction in the same anatomic region.[89] Among 394 patients surviving an initial stroke, 84 second and 27 third strokes were reported. The cumulative 5-year recurrent stroke rate in the male population was 42%. Thus, the recurrent stroke rate, following an initial stroke, is approximately 9% per year.

These data indicate that cerebral infarction produces significant morbidity and mortality in the United States. Of particular interest is the remarkably high rate of recurrence of cerebral infarction in patients following their first stroke, if no intervention has taken place. Most of the recurrences appear to occur within the first year of the initial event. Not only is the rate of recurrence with progressive neurologic deterioration high, but also the death rate with subsequent infarction is considerable.

Transient Ischemic Attacks

In order to discuss the incidence and significance of TIAs, one must define the type and anatomic distribution of the event. Those reports that combine focal neurologic events with those of global symptoms such as dizziness and vertigo cloud the issue and lead to erroneous conclusions because the natural history and prognosis of the two types of attacks are quite different. Most investigators agree that TIAs producing focal neurologic deficits have a greater risk for subsequent cerebral infarction.[34] For purposes of this discussion, therefore, TIAs are considered those that produce transient focal neurologic deficit, in either the anterior or the posterior circulation.

Because many patients with attacks of transient ischemia never reach a hospital, studies of hospital populations are not an accurate reflection of the disease. Studies that review the overall incidence in *specific communities* give a far better view of the incidence and natural history of the event. There have been several such population studies, and these are cited in the text and among the references.[67] One of the most important studies has been carried out using Rochester, Minnesota, as a population base and reported by members of the staff of the Mayo Clinic. Their reports evaluated two time intervals: 1945 to 1954 and 1955 to 1969.[68, 102] In the Rochester, Minnesota, population, the incidence of TIAs amounted to 31 patients per 100,000 population per year for all ages, with a rapidly rising incidence associated with advancing age. The incidence of new attacks in the 65- to 74-year-old age group was 200 patients per 100,000 population per year. As in the instance of cerebral infarction, there was also a higher incidence of TIAs in men than in women of the same age group at a ratio of 1.3:1 Table 127–1 compares the average annual incidence of first TIA per 100,000 population in three population studies: Rochester, Minnesota; Framingham, Massachusetts; and Lehigh Valley, Pennsylvania.

Reviewing the natural history of patients with TIA reveals somewhat conflicting data. This is due, primarily, to the lack of definition of the underlying lesion present in the patient population manifesting transient cerebral ischemia. For example, if one population has a large preponderance of patients with high-grade stenoses, composed of soft plaque with ulceration, there is likely to be a much higher subsequent stroke rate than there would be if the population consisted of a large number of patients with low-grade to medium stenoses. Nonetheless, considerable information is to be gained by looking at some of the general population studies with regard to TIA outcome. In the Rochester, Minnesota study, the probability of surviving free of stroke 5 years after the onset of TIA was only 64%. Conversely, the incidence of stroke was 36% during follow-up. Fifty-one per cent of the strokes occurred within the first year after the onset of TIAs (Fig. 127–1). In the stroke population, the authors noted that, in addition to advancing age, the three major predisposing factors for cerebral infarction were transient ischemia, hypertension, and cardiac disease.

In an excellent review of the available literature, Wiebers and Whisnant noted that of the available studies, the reported annual stroke incidence in patients with TIA ranged from 5.3% to 8.6% per year for the first 5 years. They concluded that the average annual stroke rate among TIA patients was 7% per year for the first 5 years or that approximately one third of patients with TIA will suffer a stroke within 5 years of onset.[103]

The definition of transient ischemic attack as opposed to stroke is quite arbitrary. If the neurologic deficit lasts less than 24 hours, it is defined as a TIA. If it lasts more than 24 hours it is presumably a stroke. New data suggest that a large proportion of TIAs are actually small strokes. Toole,

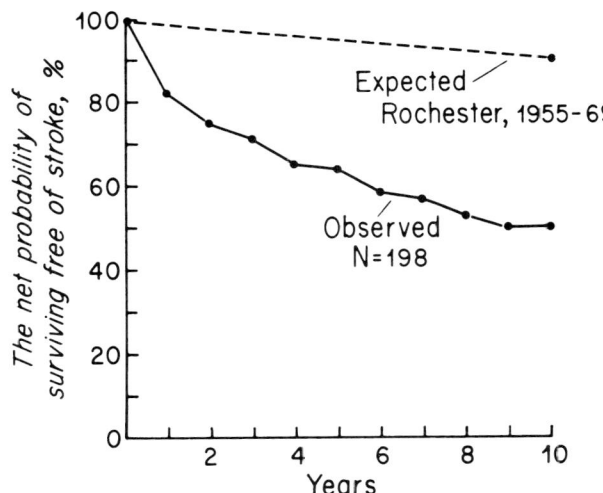

FIGURE 127–1. Conditional probability of surviving free of stroke after first transient ischemic attack (TIA), if the patients survive. Expected survivorship is for a population of the given age and sex and is based on the stroke incidence rates of the Rochester, Minnesota, study for 1955 through 1969. (From Whisnant JP, Matsumoto N, Elveback LR: Transient cerebral ischemic attacks in a community: Rochester, Minnesota, 1955 through 1969. Mayo Clin Proc 48:194, 1973.)

in his Willis lecture, reminded us that TIA patients suffer a large number of cerebral infarctions that go unrecognized from a clinical perspective. These lesions can now be identified by better brain-imaging techniques.[98] Further evidence suggesting that a TIA is actually a small stroke is provided by the observations of Grigg and colleagues, who correlated cerebral infarction and atrophy as a function of TIAs and per cent stenosis.[38] In patients who presented with transient episodes of monocular blindness, the incidence of cerebral infarction, as documented by CT scanning, rose from 2% in patients with mild stenoses to 58% in patients with high-grade, so-called asymptomatic stenoses. In addition, the incidence of cerebral atrophy showed a parallel increase.[38] With these observations, the benignity of transient cerebral ischemia is called into question. Thus, the need to identify so-called asymptomatic lesions and treat them before TIAs (probably small strokes) occur becomes more important.

Asymptomatic Lesions of the Carotid Artery

Asymptomatic, potentially critical lesions of the carotid bifurcation can be divided into two categories: preocclusive

TABLE 127–1. AVERAGE ANNUAL INCIDENCE OF NEW TRANSIENT ISCHEMIC ATTACKS IN A PREVIOUSLY ASYMPTOMATIC POPULATION*

AGE (YR)	ROCHESTER		FRAMINGHAM		LEHIGH VALLEY	
	Male	Female	Male	Female	Male	Female
45–54	21	12	56	15	85	48
55–64	96	50	114	49		
65–74	263	192	184	142	244	151

*Expressed in number/100,000 population.

stenoses resulting in hemodynamic compromise; and large, grossly irregular or ulcerative lesions, independent of hemodynamic compromise but with the potential of releasing emboli into the cerebral circulation. In the past few years, the natural history of these lesions has been better defined as a result of several retrospective studies as well as new prospective studies.

The asymptomatic carotid stenosis was the original asymptomatic lesion to be identified as a potential cause of stroke. Stenotic lesions now can be readily identified in screening programs that utilize noninvasive testing. The natural history of these lesions, however, remains variable and controversial. Three prospective randomized trials were initiated to determine the efficacy (or lack thereof) of carotid endarterectomy in patients with asymptomatic, hemodynamically significant carotid stenosis.

The European study (Casanova) reported no benefit of carotid endarterectomy when compared with medical management alone.[107] Unfortunately, the study was hampered by serious methodologic flaws in that a large number of patients in the control group were removed and operated on but were counted as medically managed in an intent-to-treat design. Furthermore, the reasons that the patients were removed from the control group, including TIAs, were not considered treatment failures.[107]

The Veterans Administration reported that the combined incidence of ipsilateral neurologic events (TIA plus stroke) was 8% in the surgery group in contrast to 20.6% in the medical group ($p < .001$). Unfortunately, the study was not designed to look for differences in stroke alone.[48]

The Asymptomatic Carotid Atherosclerosis Study (ACAS) is the largest of the trials on asymptomatic carotid stenosis. The trial is now complete and has provided definitive evidence to support the benefit of carotid endarterectomy versus medical management alone in patients with carotid stenosis that equals or exceeds 60% diameter reduction by angiography. In 1994, the Data Safety and Monitoring Committee called a halt to the study far earlier than anticipated and informed the investigators and the public that an end-point had been reached in favor of carotid endarterectomy. With a mean follow-up of 2.7 years (4657 patient-years of observation), the 5-year risk for ipsilateral stroke, any perioperative stroke, and death was 5.1% for the surgical patients and 11% for patients treated medically alone. This represents an absolute risk reduction of 5.9% and a relative risk reduction of 53% in favor of carotid endarterectomy.[94] The benefit of carotid endarterectomy compared with medical management alone was made possible by a low operative morbidity and mortality. Of patients actually undergoing carotid endarterectomy, the combined neurologic morbidity and mortality was 1.52%. Thus, careful selection of surgeons and institutions that participated in the study and that could perform this operation safely contributed in large part to the outcome favoring operation.[80]

Perhaps one of the most important arguments in favor of prophylactic repair of asymptomatic lesions is based on a review of various populations of stroke patients. Careful histories from patients who have suffered a stroke reveal that only 30% to 50% of patients had antecedent TIAs. That means that up to one half of patients who developed

stroke proceeded from an asymptomatic lesion one day to a stroke the next.

The early leaders in the aggressive surgical approach to the asymptomatic stenoses are Thompson and colleagues, who in 1978 described their experience with 138 patients who presented with asymptomatic bruits and who were followed without operation.[95–97] They noted that 37 of these patients developed TIAs and required endarterectomy. Another 24 patients, or 17% presented with stroke without antecedent TIA. From these data, the investigators argue that the imminence of stroke is significant in the asymptomatic patient, and they recommended prophylactic operation when an appropriate lesion is identified.[95–97] The weakness of this argument lies in the fact that the data do not have angiographic substantiation of the nature of the lesion that was present in the patients that were being followed, nor were noninvasive observations made to determine whether a hemodynamically significant stenosis was present. Perhaps a more impressive series was reported by Kartchner and McRae in 1977, in which they followed 147 patients who had oculoplethysmographic and phonoangiographic evidence of carotid stenosis.[60] Without carotid operation, 17 of these 147 patients, or approximately 12%, suffered an acute stroke.

Two fairly new prospective studies have been reported. Roederer and colleagues studied 167 asymptomatic patients with cervical bruit using duplex scanning.[85] They noted that progression of a lesion to compromise the lumen by 80% or more carried a 35% risk of stroke, TIA, or occlusion within 6 months and a 46% event rate at 12 months. Further, they noted that 89% of all events were preceded by a disease progression to greater than 80% stenosis. This probably represents an underestimate of risk in view of the fact that 96 of the 167 patients underwent carotid endarterectomy during the study interval.

The second important natural history study was carried out by Chambers and Norris.[11] These investigators have followed the natural history of 500 patients with asymptomatic carotid bruits in whom the carotid arteries were characterized by Doppler scanning. The patients were restudied every 6 months. In patients identified as having carotid stenoses in excess of 75%, the neurologic event rate was 18% per year and the completed stroke rate was 5% per year. The completed stroke rate without antecedent TIA was 3% per year.

The arguments against an aggressive approach to asymptomatic carotid stenosis are best exemplified in a report by Humphries and colleagues from the Cleveland Clinic.[53] They followed 168 patients with 182 carotid stenoses for an average of 32 months and noted that 26 patients developed TIAs and underwent surgical correction, whereas only four patients developed a stroke before operative intervention could be considered. This report suggested that asymptomatic stenosis is a relatively benign lesion and that an imminent stroke will usually be heralded by an antecedent TIA. It is of interest that Dr. Humphries' colleagues at the Cleveland Clinic, in spite of this report, continue to advocate prophylactic operation on the asymptomatic stenosis.

In addition to the asymptomatic stenosis, the asymptomatic ulceration in the absence of major concomitant stenosis has been identified as a lesion of potential stroke risk. The author's group has carried out a retrospective review of nonstenotic ulcerative lesions that were identified at the time of angiography as being performed for contralateral symptomatic lesions.[77] Because it had been this group's practice not to operate on the asymptomatic ulcer, we had the opportunity to examine the natural history of 67 patients with ulcerative lesions in 72 carotid arteries. The ulcer size was semiquantitatively described as small (group A), medium (group B), or large (group C). In the initial series, 40 lesions were classified as group A and 32 lesions were combined group B and group C. The follow-up of these patients was expressed in the life table format in which the event of stroke was looked at as a function of duration of follow-up. The author's follow-up extended for approximately 7 years. In this group, only one patient in the small ulcer series (group A) went on to have a stroke. There were, however, 10 strokes in the group with larger ulceration, and this produced a stroke rate that averaged 12.5% per year of follow-up.

The report was challenged by a retrospective review carried out by Kroener and colleagues, who confirmed the benign prognosis of small ulcers in group A but could not find a significant stroke risk in group B ulcers.[62] It is of interest that their series excluded patients with the large ulcers, group C, since it had been their practice to operate routinely on those with a very large carotid ulceration. More recently, the author's group reviewed yet another series and included data from their original report. This yielded 153 asymptomatic, nonstenotic ulcerative lesions of the carotid bifurcation in 141 patients. During the course of the study, with follow-up extending up to 10 years, 3% of patients in group A, 21% of patients in group B, and 19% of patients in group C had hemispheric strokes without antecedent transient ischemia on the side appropriate to the lesion. The interval stroke rates were 4.5% per year for group B and 7.5% per year for group C.[20] Because the interval stroke rate among patients with asymptomatic ulcers was comparable with the stroke rate among patients with TIA, the author and his associates have made the recommendation that prophylactic operation be carried out in patients who are good surgical candidates when they have an identifiable group B or C ulceration.

With the publication of the results of the ACAS study, the controversy concerning management of patients with asymptomatic high-grade carotid stenoses has been resolved. Provided that a surgeon can offer a patient a carotid endarterectomy with a stroke morbidity and mortality of less than 1.5%, those patients will clearly fare better than if they were treated with medical management alone. However, not every critic of asymptomatic carotid stenosis intervention has been satisfied. Currently, there is yet another prospective randomized trial in progress in Europe. This will be a large multicenter trial. The design of this trial has been published, but results are not yet available.[43]

PATHOLOGY

The primary pathologic entity responsible for disease in the extracranial cerebrovascular system is *atherosclerosis*, which accounts for approximately 90% of lesions in the extracranial system seen in the Western world. The remaining 10% include such entities as fibromuscular dysplasia, arterial kinking as a result of elongation, extrinsic compression, traumatic occlusion, intimal dissection, the inflammatory angiopathies, and migraine. Radiation-induced arteriosclerotic change of the extracranial carotid artery has become a recognized entity. Other rare entities, usually involving intracranial vessels, include fibrinoid necrosis, amyloidosis, polyarteritis, allergic angiitis, Wegener's granulomatosis, granulomatous angiitis, giant cell arteritis, amphetamine-associated arteritis, infectious arteritis, and moyamoya disease.[28] Embolization of cardiac origin is a major entity, but for purposes of this presentation it will not be considered a primary manifestation of arterial disease of the extracranial system.

Atherosclerosis

The atherosclerotic plaque consists of nodular deposition of fat, primarily cholesterol, in the arterial intima. An associated inflammatory response results in fibroblastic proliferation (Fig. 127–2). In addition, calcium salts may be precipitated in the primary fatty plaque, producing various degrees of calcification of the lesion. The lesion may enlarge as a result of progression of the atheromatous process, or it may be altered by a sudden intraplaque hemorrhage causing precipitous enlargement and possibly occlusion. With either slow or rapid enlargement, there may be a rupture of the intimal lining, with discharge of degenerative atheromatous debris into the lumen of the vessel. Following such an atheromatous discharge, an open cavity remains within the central portion of the lesion. This cavity, or so-called ulcer, can be the nidus for platelet aggregation or thrombus formation or the outlet for further degenerative plaque egress (Fig. 127–3). If the aggregates within the ulcer are only loosely attached, they can be swept into the arterial bloodstream as secondary arterial emboli.

Atheromatous lesions characteristically occur at branches or arterial bifurcations. The common sites include (1) the points of takeoff for the branches of the aortic arch; (2) the origins of the vertebral artery from the subclavian artery; (3) the bifurcation of the common carotid artery and, particularly, the carotid bulb; (4) the carotid siphon; and (5) the origins of the anterior and middle cerebral arteries. The course of the basilar artery may also be studded with atheromatous beads, often corresponding to the origins of major branches, including the posterior cerebral arteries. All these locations are of clinical importance, but the relative frequency of involvement of each potential site influences the frequency of occurrence of various clinical manifestations. The predilection of the carotid bifurcation for atheromatous plaquing has been extensively studied and appears to be related to arterial geometry, velocity profile, and wall shear stress.[106] The relative distribution has been studied both by angiography and at the time of autopsy (Figs. 127–4 to 127–6).

Without question, the most common location of significant lesions is the carotid bifurcation. The ratio of extracranial to intracranial lesions is in excess of 2:1. Blaisdell and associates, in a review of aortocranial angiograms of 300

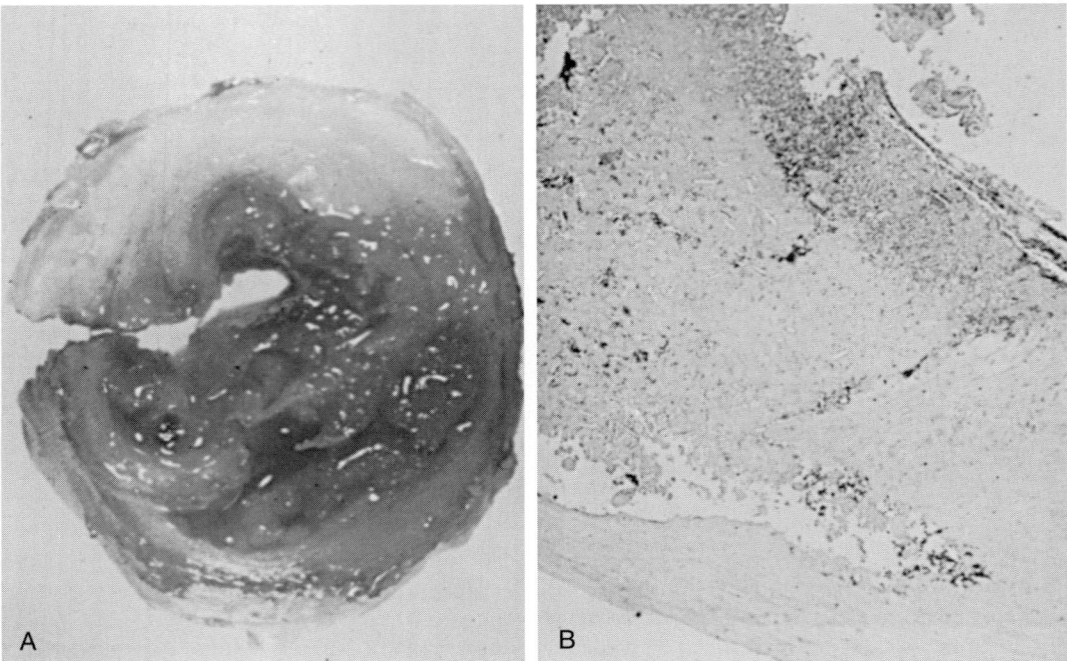

FIGURE 127–2. *A*, Cross section through a proliferative arteriosclerotic plaque taken at the bifurcation of the common carotid artery. Note the tiny lumen that remains. The material is glistening and consists primarily of cholesterol and necrotic atheromatous debris. *B*, Microscopic section at 10 × magnification. The atheromatous portion of the diseased intima is at the upper part of the photograph. The small spaces or clefts distributed throughout the intimal lesion represent cholesterol crystals.

patients, noted that 33% of lesions seen on angiography were distributed intracranially or in locations that were inaccessible to direct surgical repair.[7] The remaining 67% were extracranial, with 38% of all lesions located at the carotid bifurcation, 20% at vertebral origins, and 9% at the origin of the branches of the aortic arch. Hass and coworkers, reviewing the arteriograms of 4748 patients followed in the joint study of extracranial arterial occlusive disease, reported a similar distribution.[46]

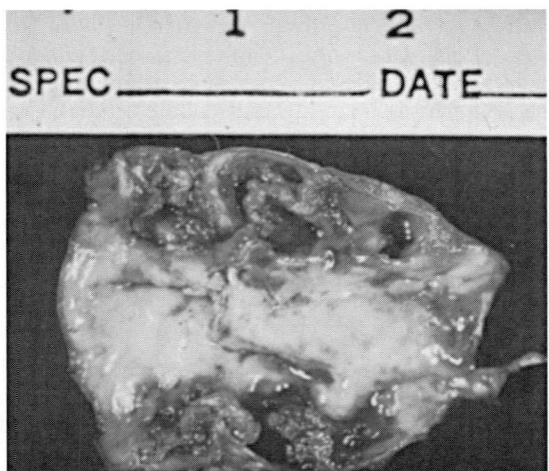

FIGURE 127–3. Atherosclerotic plaque removed from a carotid bifurcation and opened longitudinally to demonstrate the cavities, or ulcers, produced by evacuation of atheromatous debris. These ulcers continue to harbor degenerative atheromatous debris, platelet aggregate material, and thrombus.

Arterial Elongation, Tortuosity, and Kinking

Sixteen per cent to 21% of the carotid arteriograms of adults demonstrate some degree of elongation of the internal carotid artery in its cervical portion. The extent can vary from a mild tortuosity to as much as a 360-degree coil (Fig. 127–7). On occasion, excessive redundancy of the vessel produces kinking with apparent compromise of blood flow[84] (Fig. 127–8). These changes are attributed to either congenital or acquired factors. The carotid artery is formed from the third aortic arch and the dorsal aorta. During embryonic development, the carotid normally is redundant or kinked. As the heart descends into the thorax, the carotid artery is stretched and the redundancy is eliminated. Some redundancy may remain until further growth takes place, as evidenced by a redundancy rate as high as 43% seen in arteriograms of infants.[60, 101] The acquired form of carotid redundancy is attributed to a manifestation of atherosclerosis that produces lengthening of the affected vessels leading to redundancy and, ultimately, to anatomic kinking. Carotid tortuosity and kinkings are discussed in detail in Chapter 135.

Fibromuscular Dysplasia

The pathology of this entity is discussed in detail in Chapter 133.

Extrinsic Compression

Extrinsic compression of the cervical arteries carrying blood to the brain is seen most often in the vertebral arteries as

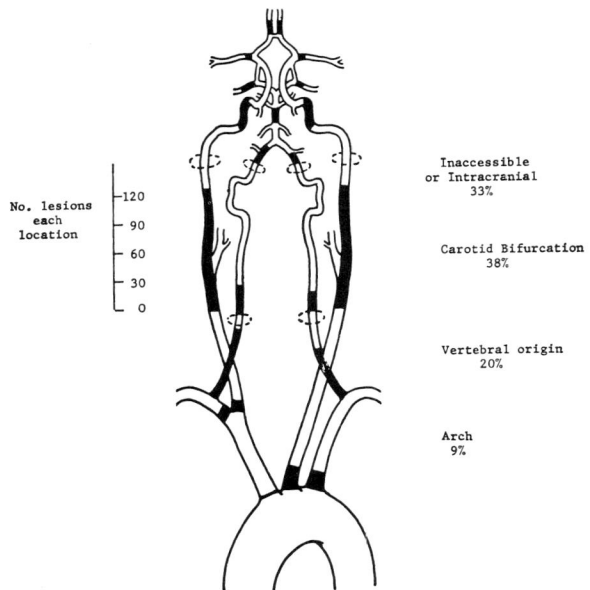

FIGURE 127–4. Location and incidence of significant atherosclerotic lesions. The length of the dark area at each location (measured against the scale at left) corresponds to the number of lesions detected by arteriography in this series. (Reprinted by permission of the Western Journal of Medicine: Blaisdell FW, Hall AD, Thomas AN, Ross SJ: Cerebrovascular occlusive disease: Experience with panarteriography in 300 consecutive cases. Calif Med 103:321, 1965.)

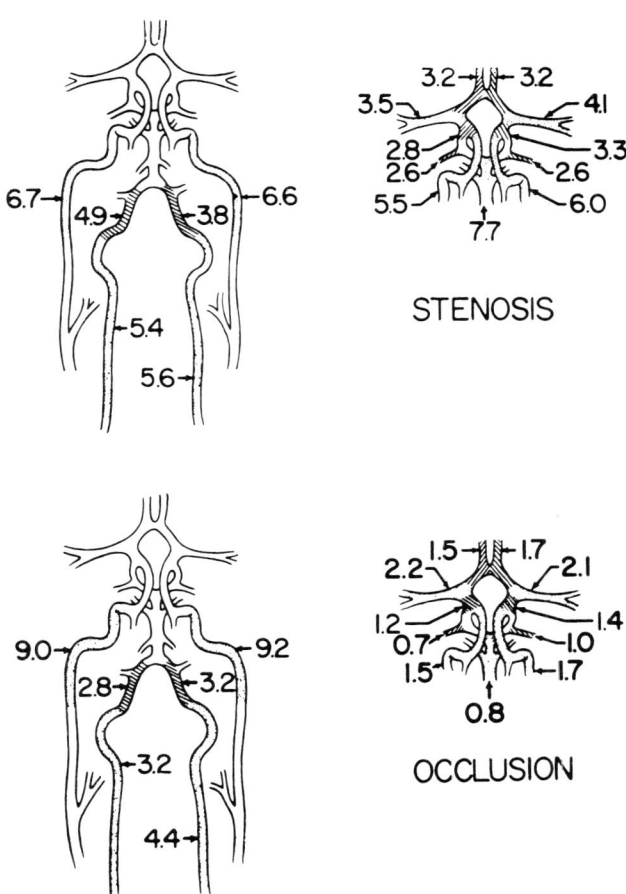

FIGURE 127–6. Frequency distribution of surgically inaccessible lesions. (From Hass WK, Fields WS, North RR, et al: Joint study of extracranial arterial occlusion: II. Arteriography, techniques, sites, and complications. JAMA 203:961. Copyright 1968, American Medical Association.)

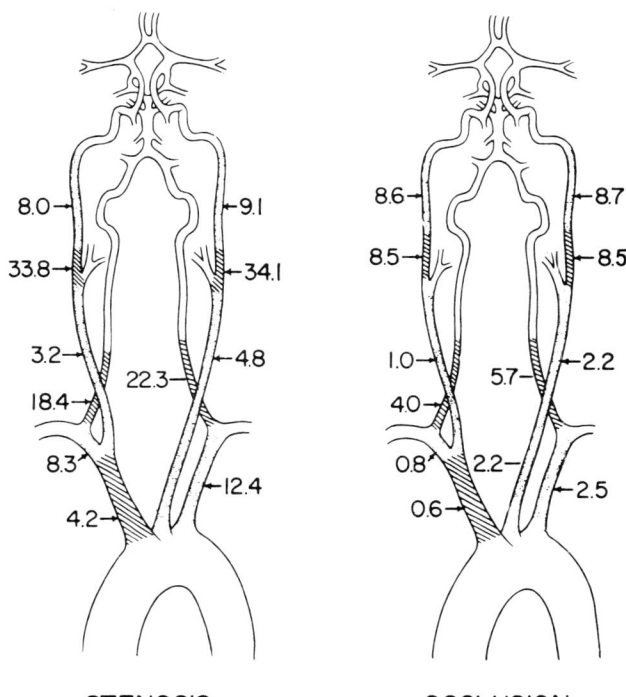

FIGURE 127–5. Frequency distribution of arterial lesions at surgically accessible sites (4748 patients). (From Hass WK, Fields WS, North RR, et al: Joint study of extracranial arterial occlusion: II. Arteriography, techniques, sites, and complications. JAMA 203:961–968. Copyright 1968, American Medical Association.)

they course through the bony vertebral canal. Hyperostoses, or bone spurs, related to the cervical transverse processes can impinge on the vertebral artery and result in compression.[3, 5, 45, 92]

Another source of external compression can be caused by neoplasms within the neck. Tumors can surround the carotid artery and invade its wall.

Radiation-Induced Carotid Stenosis

It has been long recognized experimentally that external radiation can produce an arterial injury.[66] With the increasing use of cervical radiation to treat neoplasia, we are now beginning to see patients with radiation-induced atherosclerotic change producing symptomatic carotid artery disease.[25, 70]

Postoperative Restenosis of the Carotid Artery

The pathology of this lesion is discussed in detail in Chapter 136.

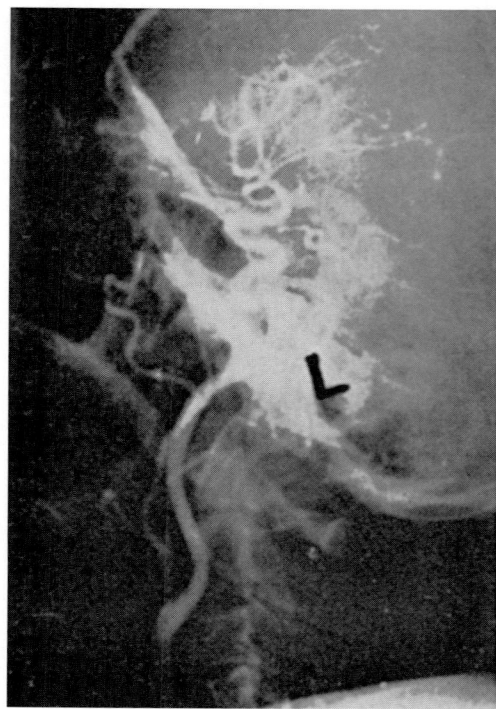
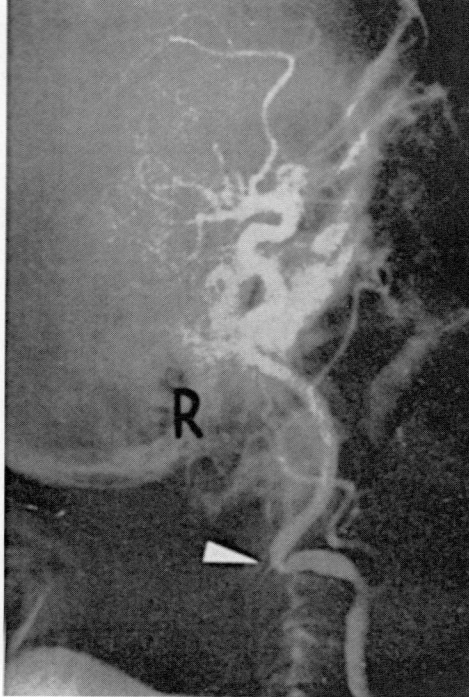

FIGURE 127–7. Carotid arteriograms showing bilateral coiling of circular configuration at level of base of skull (*arrow* shows 360-degree coil). No aneurysmal dilatation is present in the proximal segment of arteries. (From Weibel J, Fields WS: Tortuosity, coiling, and kinking of the internal carotid artery: I. Etiology and radiographic anatomy. Neurology 15:7, 1965.)

FIGURE 127–8. Carotid arteriograms demonstrating mild post-stenotic aneurysmal dilatation and kinking of the right internal carotid artery (*arrowheads*). The left internal carotid artery has S-shaped tortuosity. (From Weibel J, Fields WS: Tortuosity, coiling, and kinking of the internal carotid artery: I. Etiology and radiographic anatomy. Neurology 15:7, 1965.)

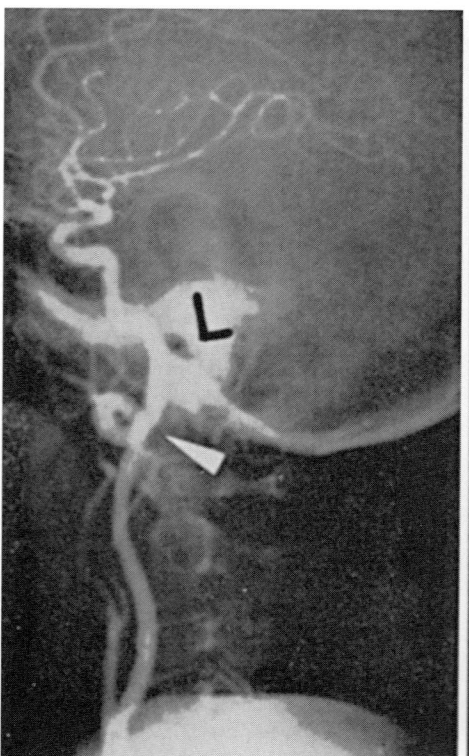
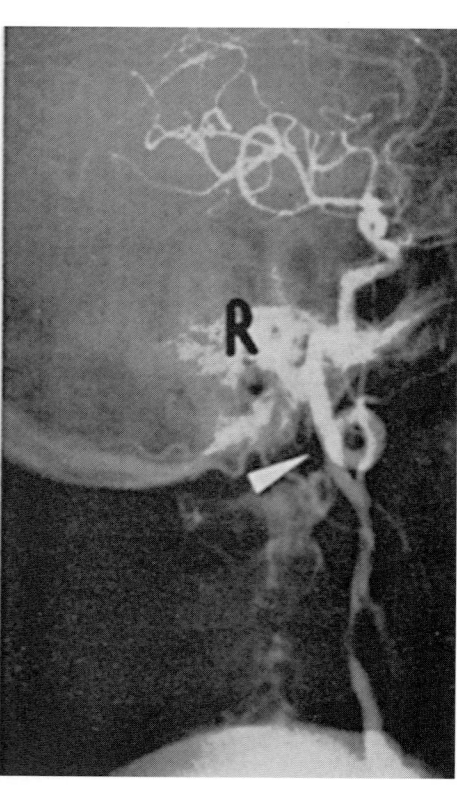

Traumatic Occlusion and Spontaneous Intimal Dissection

Blunt craniocervical trauma, as a result of either a direct blow or the indirect effect of sudden head and neck extension, has been reported to produce occlusion of the internal carotid artery.[32, 33, 52, 91] Angiographic and autopsy studies suggest that the most likely mechanism for this phenomenon is a tear of the intima followed by an acute intimal dissection, resulting in an occlusion of the lumen with secondary thrombosis. Spontaneous intimal dissection in the absence of trauma can also occur (Fig. 127–9).

Inflammatory Arteriopathies

Inflammatory conditions are rare, but they should be kept in mind during the evaluation of patients with cerebrovascular symptoms. Takayasu's disease is an inflammatory arteriopathy that involves the major trunks of the aortic arch. This is most frequently seen in women and occurs with greatest frequency in Asia and the Middle East. It has also been reported with some frequency in Latin America. It is less common in North America and Europe. The lesion produces occlusion of major branches of the aortic arch with the concomitant physical findings and varying symptomatic manifestations.[57] One dramatic finding on examination is often the total absence of extremity pulses; hence, the common synonym for this condition is "pulseless disease." The central nervous system may also be involved in the systemic collagen vascular diseases, which include periarteritis nodosa, lupus erythematosus, and temporal arteritis. Chapter 135 further discusses carotid arteriopathies.

Migraine

The vasospasm associated with migraine prodrome can cause transient neurologic dysfunction. The visual symptoms associated with the prodrome, the so-called scintillating scotoma, on occasion can be mistaken or misinterpreted as amaurosis fugax. There are also documented cases of permanent neurologic damage resulting from the prolonged phase of cerebral vasospastic prodrome.

PATHOGENETIC MECHANISMS OF CEREBRAL DYSFUNCTION

In addition to a knowledge of the various pathologic lesions that can affect the extracranial system, an understanding of the mechanism by which a lesion produces symptoms, either transient or permanent, is of particular importance when planning a diagnostic evaluation and selecting appropriate therapy.

Lateralizing Transient Ischemic Attacks

Several theories have been proposed to explain ischemic events that are transient in nature. These have included

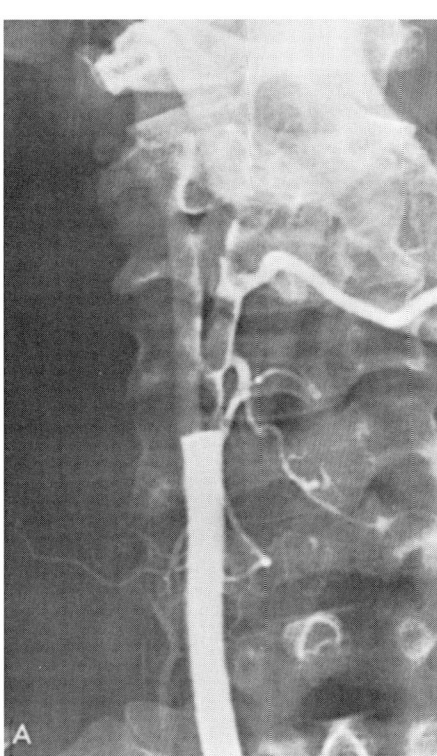
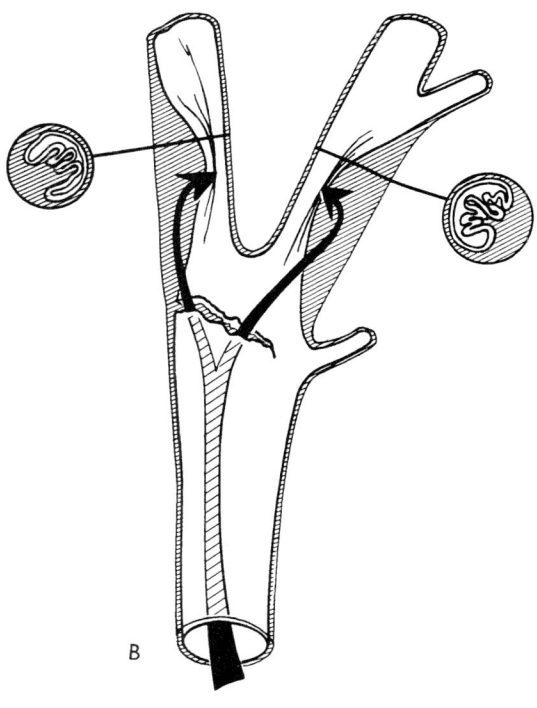

FIGURE 127–9. A, Right carotid arteriogram of a 32-year-old man who experienced a sudden episode of left hemiparesis. Carotid arteriography demonstrates a sharp cutoff contrast at the carotid bifurcation with faint visualization of the internal and external carotid arteries beyond. Subsequent exploration of this region revealed a spontaneous transverse intimal tear with subintimal dissection of blood and distal occlusion. B, Artist's concept of an intimal tear with subintimal dissection of blood and occlusion of the lumen. The insets of the internal and external carotid arteries in cross section graphically demonstrate luminal compromise by subintimal dissection.

cerebral angiospasm, mechanical reduction of cerebral blood flow secondary to a critical arterial lesion, cerebral emboli originating from arteriosclerotic plaques, cervical arterial kinking or compression, polycythemia, anemia, and the transient shunting of blood away from the brain such as is seen in the subclavian steal syndrome.[19, 72, 74] The theory of cerebral vasospasm was held to be an important mechanism in the not-too-distant past. Therapy that was advocated to treat symptoms that were due to cerebral vasospasm included carotid arterectomy or cervical sympathetic ganglionectomy.[56]

Eastcott and colleagues spoke out against the vasospastic theory, stating that it would be difficult to conceive of spasm involving just those few vessels that were required to produce repetitive ischemic attacks, while the remaining cerebral vessels were left unaffected.[22] Rothenberg and Corday[86] produced experimental evidence against the angiospasm theory, and Millikan[74] pointed out that such potent vasodilators as 5% carbon dioxide mixed with 95% oxygen and cervical sympathectomy were not effective in preventing or treating attacks of transient cerebral ischemia. Two theories emerged as the primary explanation for transient ischemic events: the arterial stenotic theory (mechanical flow reduction) and the cerebral embolic theory.

During the early experience with carotid artery disease, most surgeons accepted the concept that arterial stenosis, producing reduced cerebral blood flow, represented the mechanism for transient cerebral ischemia.[64] For example, Crawford and coworkers stated that the criterion for carotid endarterectomy should be the presence of a pressure gradient across a stenosis involving the internal carotid artery.[15] These workers measured the carotid artery pressure during operation; if a gradient was present across a stenotic lesion, an endarterectomy was performed. If no gradient could be documented, the artery was not opened, since it was assumed that the patient's symptoms might be due to something other than a lesion in the carotid artery. On the basis of this experience, the investigators stated that at least a 50% stenosis, as measured in one projection of an arteriogram, was necessary to justify operation on the carotid artery. In their opinion, a gradient indicated not only decreased flow in that artery but also a decrease in total cerebral blood flow.

This concept was affirmed by other investigators.[17, 18, 49] Haller and Turrell stated that cerebral ischemia as a result of carotid artery disease was purely the result of mechanical flow obstruction and that surgical treatment should be directed at relief of this obstruction.[42] They concluded that lesions that failed to produce a pressure gradient did not constitute a significant threat to the patient. The mechanical concept of transient cerebral ischemia is appealing, particularly when surgeons are used to treating stenotic or obstructive arteries in other locations. The concept of transient ischemia has been likened to intermittent claudication of the brain. However, with the advent of techniques for the measurement of cerebral blood flow, it has been determined that the cerebral perfusion rate is relatively constant due to autoregulation. For this reason, it is difficult to understand how a constant stenosis could produce intermittent reduction in blood flow. In an attempt to explain this inconsistency, several investigators suggested that TIAs may result from intermittent episodes of systemic hypotension or de-

creased cardiac output in patients with stenosed or occluded cerebral arteries.[14, 19, 55]

In spite of the wide acceptance of the hemodynamic theory, there appeared increasing evidence to dispute it. In 1963, Adams and associates studied cerebral blood flow in patients with carotid and vertebral artery stenoses.[1] They found that cerebral blood flow, prior to carotid artery surgery, was normal and that endarterectomy did not produce any change or increase in hemispheric cerebral blood flow. Brice and colleagues measured carotid artery blood flow at the time of ligation for intracranial aneurysm and found that blood flow was not reduced until a stenosis of 84% to 93% was produced.[8] In view of these observations, those who advocate operating on an artery that is only 50% stenotic would have to offer some justification other than the improvement of blood flow. Furthermore, the intermittent nature of ischemic attacks is difficult to reconcile with the presence of a constant stenosis, since there is no significant variation in the demand for cerebral blood flow.

Some workers state that transient reduction in blood pressure or cardiac output associated with a stenosis may cause neurologic symptoms. Kendall and Marshall studied 37 patients who had frequent TIAs.[61] They were unable to reproduce these symptoms with deliberately induced systemic hypotension. Similar experience was reported by others.[22, 27] Russell and Cranstone noted that ophthalmic pressures did not diminish in patients with associated ischemic attacks and carotid artery stenosis.[87] When total occlusion of the internal carotid artery occurred, the ophthalmic artery pressure fell transiently but then rapidly returned to normal levels as collateral circulation became effective. Several workers have noted that TIAs disappear at the time of carotid occlusion.[21, 88] It is unlikely that transient cerebral ischemia results from mechanical reduction of blood flow through a stenosed artery when the symptoms can be relieved by total occlusion of the same vessel. A similar phenomenon has been observed by surgeons who noted that occlusion of the common carotid artery under local anesthesia at the time of carotid endarterectomy is usually well tolerated.

Several investigators have stated that hemispheric TIAs can best be explained as a manifestation of cerebral embolization.[40, 41, 51, 74] Atheromatous plaques in the extracranial arteries can be a source of either atheromatous or platelet emboli. The fact that atheromatous plaques can be a source of emboli was first reported by Panum in 1862.[82] Flory reported a series of autopsies in which emboli from atheroma were detected in kidneys, spleen, and thyroid.[31] The presence of emboli, confirmed microscopically, produced areas of infarction in the affected organs. Although Chiari, in 1905, suggested that carotid artery lesions could produce cerebral emboli, this was not documented conclusively until 1947.[12, 73] Handler, studying embolization of atheromatous material in a series of autopsy cases, noted that there was a frequent occurrence of encephalomalacia in patients who demonstrated atheroma embolism to other parts of the body.[44] Prior support for the embolic cause of transient cerebral ischemia came from the reports of Millikan and associates in 1955[75] and Fisher in 1958,[29] who noted that TIAs could be virtually eliminated if the patients were placed on anticoagulant therapy. In examining the ocular fundus of patients with carotid artery stenosis, Fisher described a "boxcar" effect in the retinal arteries.[30] He did not arrive at a definite explanation for this phenomenon but suggested that it might represent embolic material in the retinal arteries and that transient cerebral ischemia might be due to the same type of embolism. Hollenhorst described a series of patients with "bright plaques" in the retinal vessels and suggested that these were cholesterol crystals from eroded atheromatous plaques.[50] Russell observed two patients presenting with transient monocular blindness and concluded that this phenomenon was due to retinal emboli composed of friable thrombus.[88] He stated that if this observation were correct, thrombotic microemboli carried to the brain might be responsible for the TIAs often associated with carotid artery disease.

McBrien and coworkers performed a histologic examination of retinal vessels of a patient who had been having transient monocular blindness.[69] These workers noted that the material within the vessels was indeed microembolic and consisted of platelets, a few leukocytes, and a small quantity of lipid material. Julian and associates reported a series of patients in whom ulceration was seen in carotid plaques at the time of operation.[58] They postulated that thrombotic material within the ulcer might embolize and cause episodes of transient cerebral ischemia. Ehrenfeld and colleagues reported a series of patients with carotid stenosis and intermittent monocular blindness.[23] They found that the ocular phenomenon as well as the cerebral ischemic attacks stopped following carotid endarterectomy.

Additional evidence for the embolic theory of transient cerebral ischemia comes from the fact that ischemic attacks stop abruptly when carotid stenosis progresses to occlusion, provided the patient does not go on to have a major stroke. The cessation of TIAs presumably occurs because the route for embolic material to the brain has been obstructed, not because of the establishment of collateral circulation.[21, 87] The relationship between transient cerebral ischemia and emboli has been difficult to prove on the basis of operative results, because the criterion for operation dictates that a hemodynamically significant carotid stenosis be present before an operation is performed.

After reviewing the overwhelming evidence in favor of the embolic theory, our group realized that the presence of a hemodynamically significant stenosis is probably not necessary for the release of embolic material. Rather, the nature of the plaque itself would be the important factor. Atherosclerotic plaques whose consistency leads to degeneration with atheromatous fragmentation or whose surface characteristics are irregular or ulcerated, thus forming a suitable nidus for platelet aggregation, are the necessary requirements for emboli. Our group began to operate on patients with so-called nonstenotic ulcerative lesions who were experiencing hemispheric TIAs. In two subsequent publications, we described prompt relief without recurrence of transient ischemic phenomena following removal of the low-profile or nonstenotic ulcerative lesion.[78, 79] These reports represented the first surgical series in which the lesions removed did not have associated stenosis or compromise in blood flow and in which, therefore, the relief of symptoms could be construed to be due not to the augmentation of blood flow but rather to the removal of the ulcerated plaque as a source of cerebral emboli.

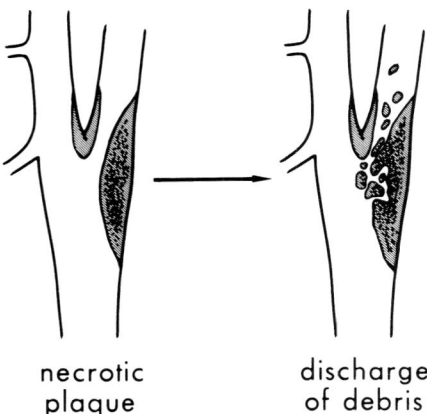

FIGURE 127–10. Graphic representation of the process by which a bulky atheromatous lesion undergoes central degeneration with subsequent discharge of atheromatous debris into the arterial lumen and embolization to the brain.

From this discussion, it seems evident that the primary mechanism responsible for episodes of transient monocular or hemispheric symptoms associated with atherosclerotic lesions is cerebral emboli originating from the plaque surface. These emboli may consist of atheromatous debris, platelet aggregates, or thrombus. Embolization may occur either at the time an atheromatous plaque ruptures into the luminal surface and dislodges atheromatous contents into the bloodstream, or from secondary platelet or thrombus aggregation within the irregularity or ulceration on the surface of the plaque (Figs. 127–10 to 127–16).

One question often posed by those who doubt the embolic theory is: "If these episodes are embolic, why is the same pattern of neurologic dysfunction frequently reproduced in a carbon-copy fashion? Shouldn't the recipient site be random if the cause is really embolization?" The answer to this question is related to the fluid mechanics associated with laminar blood flow. If the source of emboli from an ulcerated atheromatous plaque is located at one point on the arterial wall circumference, embolic discharge into the bloodstream will inevitably be carried to the same terminal branch because of the characteristics of laminar blood flow. This phenomenon was nicely demonstrated by Millikan.[74] During experiments on cerebral embolization, he introduced tiny metal beads through a needle placed in the internal carotid artery in monkeys. This method of introduction is analogous to a point source of atheromatous embolization. Autopsy studies of these experimental animals demonstrated that the metallic embolic beads would inevitably stack up, one behind the other, in the same cortical branch (Fig. 127–17).

Lateralizing Ischemic Attacks with Concomitant Internal Carotid Occlusion

Although the majority of territorial TIAs are probably caused by emboli of arterial origin that pass through a patent internal carotid artery, we do see patients who experience these symptoms in the presence of a known and totally occluded internal carotid artery. Two possible explanations for these phenomena exist: emboli may come from collateral sources; or marginally perfused brain tissue, distal

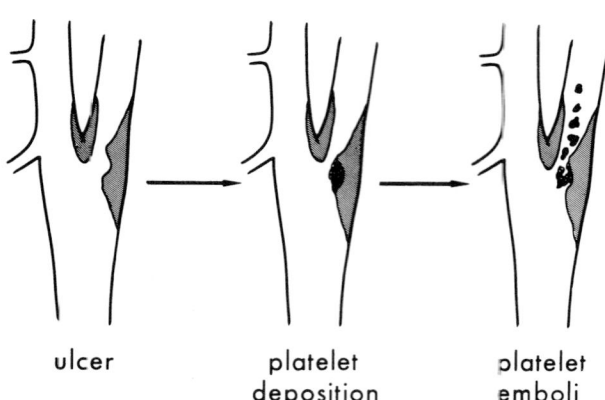

ulcer   platelet   platelet
               deposition   emboli

FIGURE 127–11. An irregular or ulcerated surface on an arterial sclerotic plaque can provide a nidus for deposition of platelet aggregate material. These platelet aggregates can be dislodged into the arterial lumen and can embolize to the intracranial circulation.

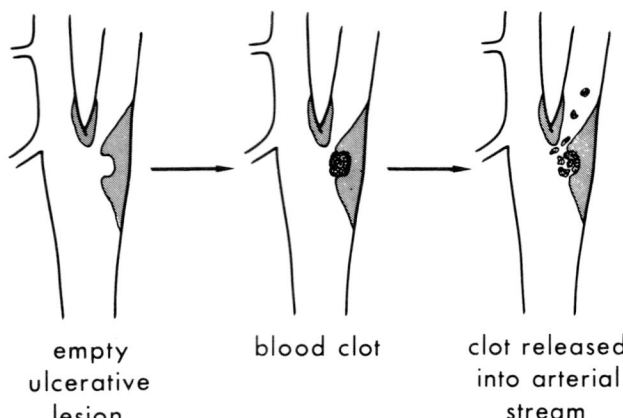

empty   blood clot   clot released
ulcerative   into arterial
lesion   stream

FIGURE 127–12. An empty ulcerative lesion can also be filled with mature thrombus material. The thrombus can be dislodged by the arterial stream or by manipulation, thus releasing clot into the arterial lumen with subsequent cerebral embolization.

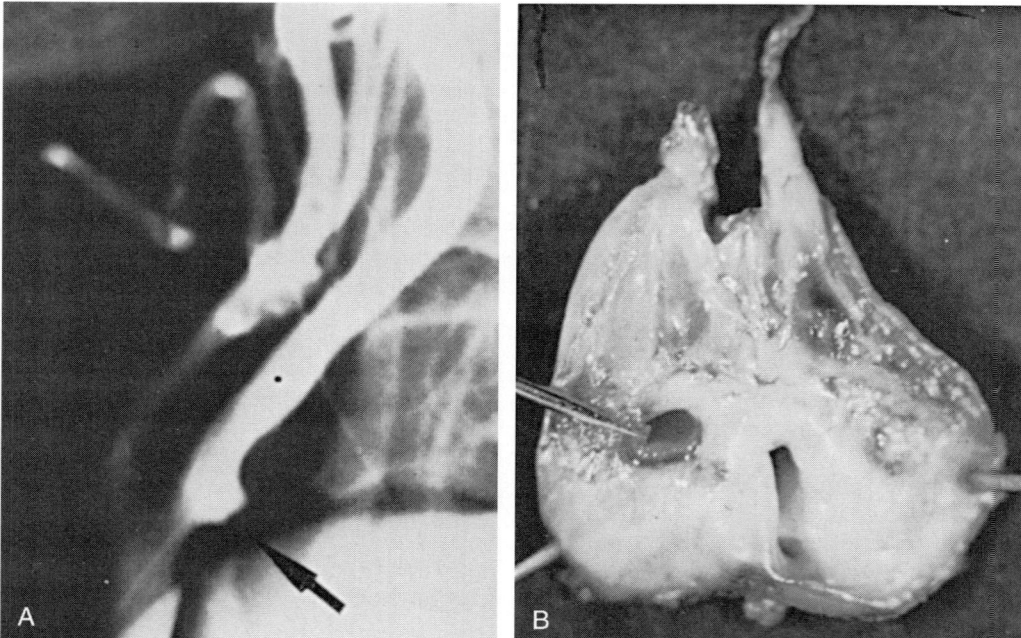

FIGURE 127–13. *A,* Left carotid arteriogram in a patient who was experiencing episodes of left hemispheric transient cerebral ischemia. The *arrow* points to a posterior outpouching of the internal carotid artery just beyond the bifurcation. This finding was interpreted as being an ulcerative atherosclerotic lesion. *B,* Atherosclerotic plaque that corresponds to the angiographically demonstrated lesion. It was removed from the carotid bifurcation, and the pointer indicates the ulcerative lesion containing remnants of mature thrombus.

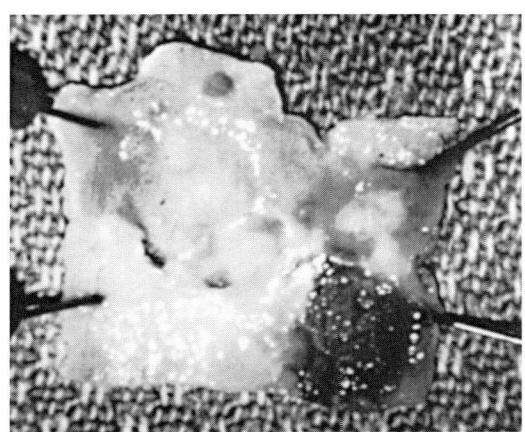

FIGURE 127–14. Example of an atherosclerotic plaque removed from the carotid bifurcation and opened out for visualization of the luminal surface. In the lower right-hand corner, a mature thrombus is loosely adherent to a very superficial ulceration.

to the internal carotid artery occlusion, may temporarily fall below the minimal threshold of perfusion to maintain function. The external carotid artery is a well-recognized source of collateral blood flow and a recently recognized source of emboli. Ulcerated plaques at the carotid bifurcation can release emboli into the external carotid artery, where they pass retrograde via collateral communications to the ophthalmic artery and subsequently to the carotid siphon and into branches of the middle cerebral artery.[13, 47] Barnett and colleagues have identified the "stump" of the occluded internal carotid artery as a source of emboli to the external carotid artery.[6] This stump serves as a functional ulcer feeding emboli to a major collateral branch.

Emboli can also reach the hemisphere ipsilateral to an internal carotid artery occlusion from the opposite carotid artery or from the vertebral-basilar system.

Finally, marginally perfused brain, distal to an internal carotid artery occlusion, will be more susceptible to temporary alterations in systemic blood pressure. In this instance, the cerebral vasculature is maximally vasodilated and therefore does not have the capacity to autoregulate in response to a drop in blood pressure. There will be a direct and linear relationship between blood pressure and perfusion.

Nonlateralizing Transient Ischemic Attacks

Nonlateralizing ischemic attacks, such as dizziness, vertigo, ataxia, or syncope, may represent symptoms that are associated with brain stem or posterior circulation dysfunction. Because these attacks are often precipitated by postural changes, the mechanism is presumed to be flow-related rather than a consequence of emboli. To make this connection between symptoms and lesions, it is necessary to have either occlusive lesions of several extracranial vessels involving both anterior and posterior circulation or a critical lesion in the vertebral-basilar distribution with an effective anatomic disconnection between anterior and posterior blood flow.

One variant of posterior circulation ischemia occurs with the subclavian steal syndrome. The anatomic lesion and the collateral circulatory response to arm ischemia have been described previously. It is easy to associate brain stem ischemic symptoms that occur with arm exercise in the presence of an ipsilateral subclavian artery occlusion; blood is diverted away from the vertebral-basilar system as a result of retrograde flow down the ipsilateral vertebral artery. This diversion occurs because the vertebral artery now functions as a collateral channel for the exercising upper extremity. For this to occur, however, the principal or dominant vertebral artery must be on the side of the subclavian stenosis or occlusion. If the dominant vertebral artery is on the opposite side and a smaller vertebral artery is on the side of subclavian occlusion, it is not physiologically possible for a small artery to steal a sufficient quantity

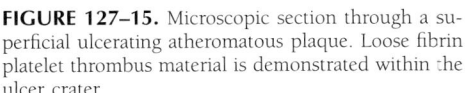

FIGURE 127–15. Microscopic section through a superficial ulcerating atheromatous plaque. Loose fibrin platelet thrombus material is demonstrated within the ulcer crater.

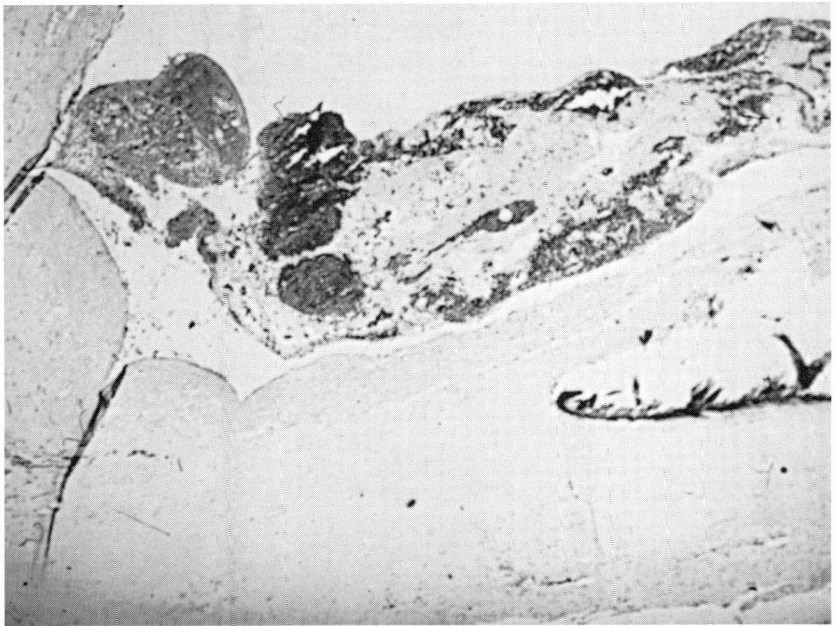

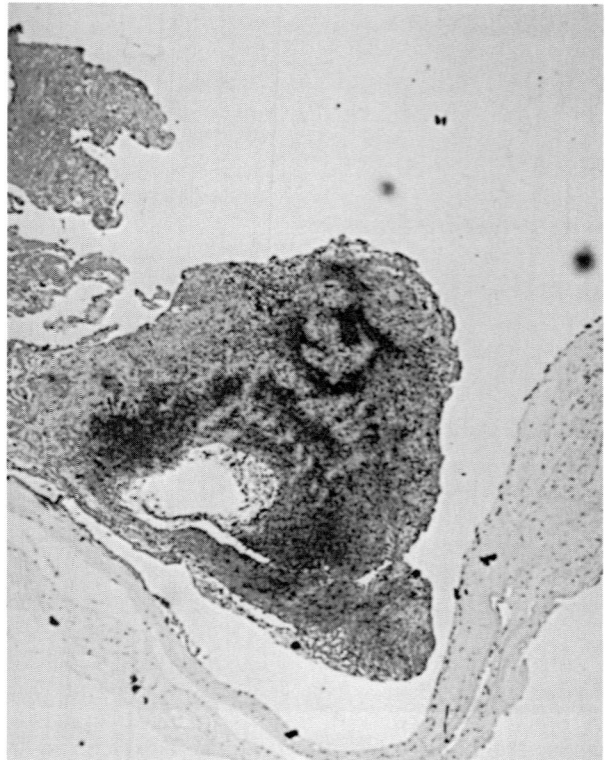

FIGURE 127–16. Microscopic section taken through a deeper ulcerating lesion of an atheromatous plaque removed from the carotid bifurcation. An organizing thrombus, only loosely attached, is seen partially filling the ulcer crater.

of blood from the posterior circulation because the opposite or dominant vertebral artery can more than make up the difference. Similarly, if the dominant vertebral artery is on the side of a total subclavian artery occlusion and the opposite vertebral artery is either small or absent, it is possible to have these symptoms in the absence of arm

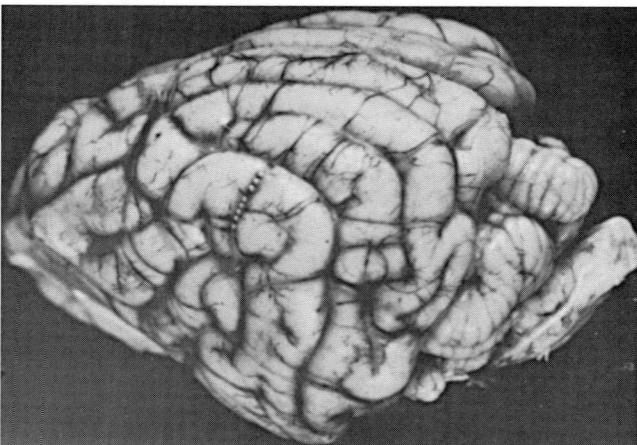

FIGURE 127–17. Brain of monkey removed following experimental embolization with ball bearings. The ball bearings were introduced from a point source in the carotid artery. Note that all the ball bearings lodged in a single cortical branch. (Courtesy of Clark Millikan, M.D., Department of Neurology, Mayo Clinic, Rochester, Minn.)

exercise because, in this instance, the subclavian artery stenosis or occlusion becomes a de facto vertebral artery stenosis or occlusion and compromises blood flow through this dominant vessel to the brain stem.[24, 71]

It is probable that emboli may occur in association with atherosclerotic plaques in the vertebral-basilar system, but the exact nature of the clinical consequences of such an event is not clear at present.

Completed Stroke

The completed stroke represents an area of brain infarction. Cerebral infarction can result from embolic occlusion of a critical vessel, thrombosis of an end-vessel, or an acute deprivation of blood flow as a result of proximal arterial occlusion with inadequate collateral contribution through the circle of Willis.[83]

The mechanism of embolic occlusion of a distal cerebral vessel is essentially the same as that of a hemispheric TIA. Why one embolic event results in transient symptoms on one occasion and produces an area of cerebral infarction at a later time is the subject of considerable speculation. Presumably, the variables that operate during any one embolic event must include the size of the embolus, the nature of the embolic material, and the final location of the embolic fragment. A large embolus clearly presents a major threat of infarction, since the likelihood of subsequent fragmentation or rapid clot lysis is reduced. Similarly, if the embolic material is composed of platelet aggregates or thrombus, the chances of fragmentation or lysis with prompt restoration of blood flow are good, whereas if the embolus is composed of an atheromatous fragment, the chances of permanent end-vessel occlusion and subsequent infarction are increased significantly. Finally, if the embolus lodges in a critical location such as the internal capsule, the time during which the ischemic changes are reversible is likely to be shorter and the neurologic dysfunction that occurs with such a critical embolization is likely to be more prominent.

Evidence using computed tomography (CT) scanning and magnetic resonance imaging (MRI) also indicates that what is clinically a transient ischemic event is actually cerebral infarction in a small focal zone that is compensated for function by adjacent tissue.

It is likely that intracerebral thrombosis is caused by one of two mechanisms. The first is related to intracranial atheromatosis, with branch vessel occlusion occurring in association with a critical stenotic lesion. The second mechanism results from propagation of thrombus from the internal carotid artery distal to the proximal atheromatous stenosis.

The top of the column of thrombus in the internal carotid artery can literally spill into the middle cerebral artery and cause occlusion and cerebral infarction. This mechanism has not been recognized uniformly, but it can be deduced from the sequence of events that takes place with carotid thrombosis.

An atheromatous lesion located at the origin of the internal carotid artery will slowly and progressively cause a reduction of blood flow as the lesion produces a further compromise of cross-sectional luminal area. Ultimately, the lesion approaches a critical compromise, following which

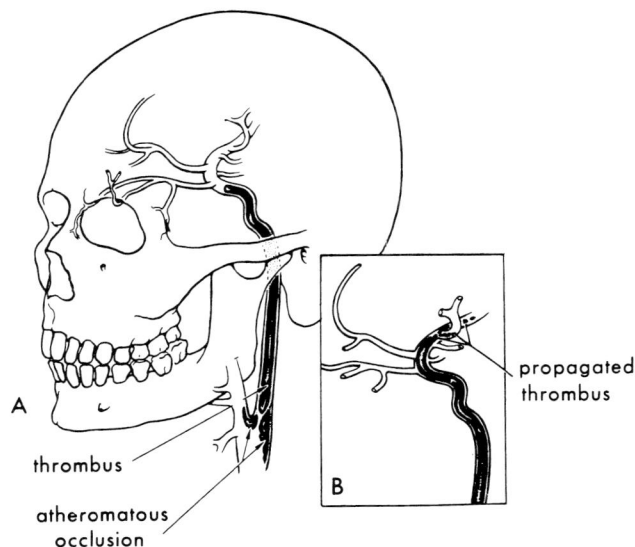

FIGURE 127–18. *A*, Artist's concept of the events following carotid occlusion. The thrombus within the internal carotid artery ascends to the first branch of that artery, the ophthalmic artery. At this point, the thrombus stops and the remaining portion of the intracranial circulation is not compromised. *B*, An alternative sequence of events in which the thrombus does not stop at the ophthalmic artery but progresses up to the terminal branches of the internal carotid artery, so that thrombus material spills over and propagates into the middle cerebral artery, producing cerebral infarction.

the flow is so reduced that thrombosis will occur. When this happens, there may be no sequelae, or the patient may suffer a cerebral infarction with major neurologic deficit.

Because flow is reduced just prior to occlusion, it is unreasonable to assume that the tiny flow through the vessel before occlusion is really that important and that the absence of this tiny flow will make the difference between live functioning brain and cerebral infarction. In some patients, when thrombosis occurs, the column of clot probably progresses up to the first major branch, such as the ophthalmic artery, and stops. In this instance, the clinical consequence of stroke is unlikely, and this sequence represents the events that occur in patients who later are found to have an asymptomatic carotid occlusion. In other patients, the clot may not stop at the siphon branches but may progress through the siphon to the takeoff of the

middle cerebral artery. If some of this clot "spills over" or is carried by collateral blood flow, thrombotic occlusion of a major intracranial artery will occur and cerebral infarction will be the consequence, resulting in a major stroke (Fig. 127–18). This phenomenon has been demonstrated at autopsy in patients who died shortly after a critical event. If the patient lives for a considerable time after the initial stroke, the propagated thrombus will usually undergo lysis back to the branches of the siphon and no clue will remain at subsequent autopsy to demonstrate the actual events that occurred.

On occasion, a modest atheromatous lesion of the internal carotid artery may undergo sudden intraplaque hemorrhage. This will produce an acute occlusion (Fig. 127–19). This precipitate event will cause an acute change in circulatory dynamics. Occlusion of this type will produce acute ischemia, and probably infarction, in the distribution of that artery. Likewise, thrombosis and propagation, as described earlier, may also take place with the same consequences.

Stroke-in-Evolution

The stroke-in-evolution, in contrast to a simple acute stroke, is one in which the resultant neurologic deficit progressively worsens by a series of discrete exacerbations occurring over a period of hours or days. The exact mechanism for this type of progression is unknown. Several hypotheses can be speculated on to explain this pattern. One might be a series of infarct-producing emboli from a bulky, friable, carotid bifurcation lesion. These emboli, occurring serially, would result in a series of events that produce a progressively worsening neurologic deficit.[35, 36] Another explanation might be a series of thromboemboli coming off the top of a thrombotic column in an occluded internal carotid artery. A third possibility might involve the dynamics of the infarct zone, such as secondary thrombosis or occlusion of a neighboring vessel in the brain substance as the result of edema, or expansion of the original infarct zone as a consequence of central hemorrhage, although this last mechanism is probably unlikely.

Deterioration of Intellectual Function

The relationship between intellectual dysfunction with cerebrovascular disease is a hotly debated issue among

FIGURE 127–19. *A*, Artist's concept of spontaneous hemorrhage within an atherosclerotic plaque resulting in sudden acute occlusion of the internal carotid artery. *B*, A similar phenomenon can occur within the depths of an atheromatous ulcer, producing acute cessation of blood flow.

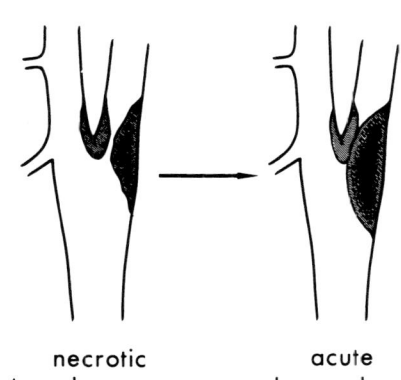

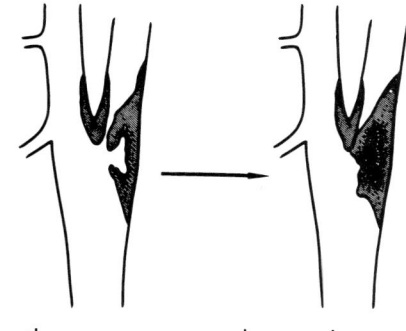

neurologists. Many believe that dementia is not a manifestation of vascular disease, but others do not share this concept. The subjective responses of patients following carotid thromboendarterectomy are interesting. Patients often will report an improvement in intellectual function following successful operation, which may be manifested as improved ability to carry out mathematical operations, improved reading comprehension, better conversational ability, and so forth. The patients' observations usually are shared by their friends or relatives.[99]

If we accept the notion that intellectual abilities are a function of cerebral performance, and that reduced blood flow, either from proximal arterial occlusive disease or from distal embolization, can impair cerebral function, it is reasonable to assume that multiple thromboembolic events in the areas of the brain, silent with regard to motor and sensory functions but important to intellectual function, may be affected adversely by decreased arterial perfusion. Areas that may be so affected include the frontal lobes. If the embolic or ischemic events persist, intellectual deterioration may result in time. The author's group has followed several such patients who, when arteriograms were finally performed, demonstrated loss of multiple branches in the distribution of the anterior cerebral artery. Our group has also had experience with patients who were somnolent when first examined, being aroused with great difficulty, and in whom there were multiple extracranial stenoses or occlusions. Repair or bypass of these lesions resulted in a prompt return to a normal level of consciousness and a resumption of previous intellectual function.

In evaluating the status of patients after cerebrovascular operations, the surgeon must be careful to avoid taking credit for seeming intellectual improvement as a result of the effect of operation. The patient who is told that a major occlusive lesion was removed from a critical artery going to his or her brain may, following operation, exhibit a brightness and jubilation because he or she believes that the brain is now going to work better. Improved intracranial function may be a sham effect of operation, but correction of multiple cerebral occlusive lesions with intellectual improvement is an undeniable observation.

REFERENCES

1. Adams JE, Smith MC, Wylie EJ: Cerebral blood flow and hemodynamics in extracranial vascular disease: Effect of endarterectomy. Surgery 53:449, 1963.
2. American Heart Association: 1999 Economic Cost of Cardiovascular Diseases.
3. Bakay L, Leslie EV: Surgical treatment of vertebral artery insufficiency caused by cervical spondylosis. J Neurosurg 23:596, 1965.
4. Baker RN, Schwartz WS, Ramseyer JC: Prognosis among survivors of ischemic stroke. Neurology (Minneap) 18:933, 1968.
5. Balla JI, Langford KH: Vertebral artery compression in cervical spondylosis. Med J Aust 1:284, 1967.
6. Barnett HJM, Peerless SJ, Kaufmann JCE: "Stump" on internal carotid artery—a source for further cerebral embolic ischemia. Stroke 9:448, 1978.
7. Blaisdell FW, Hall AD, Thomas AN, et al: Cerebrovascular occlusive disease: Experience with panarteriography in 300 consecutive cases. Calif Med 103:321, 1965.
8. Brice JG, Dowsett DJ, Lowe RD: Hemodynamic effects of carotid artery stenosis. Br Med J 3:1363, 1964.
9. Cadwalader WB: Unilateral optic atrophy and contralateral hemiplegia consequent on occlusion of the cerebral vessels. JAMA 59:2248, 1912.
10. Carrea R, Molins M, Murphy G: Surgical treatment of spontaneous thrombosis of the internal carotid artery in the neck. Carotid-carotid anastomosis: Report of a case. Acta Neurol Lat Am 1:71, 1955.
11. Chambers BR, Norris JW: Outcome in patients with asymptomatic neck bruits. N Engl J Med 315:860, 1986.
12. Chiari H: Ueber das Verhalten des Teilungswinkels der Carotid communis bei der Endarteriitis chronica deformans. Verh Dtsch Ges Pathol 9:326, 1905.
13. Connolly JE, Stemmer EA: Endarterectomy of the external carotid artery. Arch Surg 106:799, 1973.
14. Corday E, Rothenberg S, Weiner SM: Cerebral vascular insufficiency: An explanation of the transient stroke. Arch Intern Med 98:683, 1956.
15. Crawford ES, DeBakey ME, Blaisdell FW, et al: Hemodynamic alterations in patients with cerebral arterial insufficiency before and after operation. Surgery 48:76, 1960.
16. DeBakey ME: Successful carotid endarterectomy for cerebrovascular insufficiency: Nineteen-year follow-up. JAMA 233:1083, 1975.
17. DeBakey ME, Crawford ES, Fields WS: Surgical treatment of patients with cerebral arterial insufficiency associated with extracranial arterial occlusive lesions. Neurology (Minneap) 11:145, 1961.
18. DeBakey ME, Crawford ES, Cooley DA, et al: Cerebral arterial insufficiency: One- to 11-year results following arterial reconstructive operation. Ann Surg 161:921, 1965.
19. Denny-Brown D: Recurrent cerebrovascular episodes. Arch Neurol 2:194, 1960.
20. Dixon S, Pais SO, Raviola C, et al: Natural history of nonstenotic asymptomatic ulcerative lesions of the carotid artery: A further analysis. Arch Surg 117:1493, 1982.
21. Drake WE Jr, Drake MAL: Clinical and angiographic correlates of cerebrovascular insufficiency. Am J Med 45:253, 1968.
22. Eastcott HHG, Pickering GW, Robb CG: Reconstruction of internal carotid artery in a patient with intermittent attacks of hemiplegia. Lancet 2:994, 1954.
23. Ehrenfeld WK, Hoyt WF, Wylie EJ: Embolization and transient blindness from carotid atheroma. Surgical considerations. Arch Surg 93:787, 1966.
24. Eklof B, Schwartz SI: Effects of subclavian steal and compromised cephalic blood flow on cerebral circulation. Surgery 68:431, 1969.
25. Elerding SC, Fernandez RN, Grotta JC, et al: Carotid artery disease following external cervical irradiation. Ann Surg 194:609, 1981.
26. European Carotid Surgery Trialists' Collaborative Group: MRC European Carotid Surgery Trial: Interim results for symptomatic patients with severe (70–99%) or with mild (0–29%) carotid stenosis. Lancet 337:1235, 1991.
27. Fazekas JF, Alman RW: The role of hypotension in transitory focal cerebral ischemia. Am J Med Sci 248:567, 1964.
28. Feigin I, Budzilovich GN: The general pathology of cerebrovascular disease. In Vinken PJ, Bruyn GW (eds): Handbook of Clinical Neurology. Part I. Amsterdam, North-Holland Publishing Co, 1972.
29. Fisher CM: The use of anticoagulants in cerebral thrombosis. Neurology 8:311, 1958.
30. Fisher CM: Observations of the fundus oculi in transient monocular blindness. Neurology (Minneap) 9:333, 1959.
31. Flory CM: Arterial occlusions produced by emboli from eroded aortic atheromatous plaques. Am J Pathol 21:549, 1945.
32. Garg AG, Gordon DS, Taylor AR, et al: Internal carotid artery thrombosis secondary to closed craniocervical trauma. Br J Surg 55:4, 1968.
33. Gee W, Kaupp HA, McDonald KM, et al: Spontaneous dissection of internal carotid arteries. Arch Surg 115:944, 1980.
34. Goldner JC, Whisnant JP, Taylor WF: Long-term prognosis of transient cerebral ischemic attacks. Stroke 2:160, 1971.
35. Goldstone J, Moore WS: Emergency carotid artery surgery in neurologically unstable patients. Arch Surg 111:1284, 1976.
36. Goldstone J, Moore WS: A new look at emergency carotid artery operations for the treatment of cerebrovascular insufficiency. Stroke 9:599, 1978.
37. Gowers WR: On a case of simultaneous embolism of central retinal and middle cerebral arteries. Lancet 2:794, 1875.
38. Grigg MJ, Papadakas K, Nicolaides AM, et al: The significance of cerebral infarction and atrophy in patients with amaurosis fugax and

transient ischemic attacks in relation to internal carotid artery stenosis: A preliminary report. J Vasc Surg 7:215, 1988.

39. Grunnet ML: Cerebrovascular disease: Diabetes and cerebral atherosclerosis. Neurology (Minneap) 13:486, 1963.

40. Gunning AJ, Pickering GW, Robb-Smith AHT, et al: Mural thrombosis of the internal carotid artery and subsequent embolism. Q J Med 33:155, 1964.

41. Guthrie LG, Mayou S: Right hemiplegia and atrophy of left optic nerve. Proc R Soc Med 1:180, 1908.

42. Haller JA Jr, Turrell R: Studies on effectiveness of endarterectomy in treatment of carotid insufficiency. Arch Surg 85:637, 1962.

43. Halliday AM, Thomas D, Mansfield A: The Asymptomatic Carotid Surgery Trial (ACST): Rationale and design. Eur J Vasc Surg 8:703, 1994.

44. Handler FP: Clinical and pathological significance of atheromatous embolization, with emphasis on an etiology of renal hypertension. Am J Med 20:366, 1956.

45. Hardin CA, Williamson WP, Steegmann AT: Vertebral artery insufficiency produced by cervical osteoarthritic spurs. Neurology (Minneap) 10:855, 1960.

46. Hass WK, Fields WS, North RR, et al: Joint study of extracranial arterial occlusion: II. Arteriography, techniques, sites, and complications. JAMA 203:961, 1968.

47. Hertzer NR: External carotid endarterectomy. Surg Gynecol Obstet 153:186, 1981.

48. Hobson RW II, Weiss DG, Fields WS, et al: Efficacy of carotid endarterectomy for asymptomatic carotid stenosis, for The Veterans Affairs Asymptomatic Cooperative Study Group. N Engl J Med 328:221, 1993.

49. Hohf RP: The clinical evaluation and surgery of internal carotid insufficiency. Surg Clin North Am 47:1:71, 1967.

50. Hollenhorst RW: Significance of bright plaques in the retinal arteries. JAMA 178:23, 1961.

51. Hollenhorst RW: Vascular status of patients who have cholesterol emboli in the retina. Am J Ophthalmol 61:1159, 1966.

52. Houck WS, Jackson JR, Odom DL, et al: Occlusion of the internal carotid artery in the neck secondary to closed trauma to the head and neck: A report of two cases. Ann Surg 159:219, 1964.

53. Humphries AW, Young JR, Santilli PM, et al: Unoperated, asymptomatic significant internal carotid artery stenosis. Surgery 80:695, 1976.

54. Hunt JR: The role of the carotid arteries in the causation of vascular lesions of the brain, with remarks on certain special features of the symptomatology. Am J Med Sci 147:704, 1914.

55. Hutchinson EC, Yates PO: Caroticovertebral stenosis. Lancet 1:2, 1957.

56. Johnson HC, Walker AE: The angiographic diagnosis of spontaneous thrombosis of internal and common carotid arteries. J Neurosurg 8:631, 1951.

57. Judge RD, Currier RD, Gracie WA, et al: Takayasu's arteritis and the aortic arch syndrome. Am J Med 32:379, 1962.

58. Julian OC, Dye WS, Javid H, et al: Ulcerative lesions of the carotid artery bifurcation. Arch Surg 86:803, 1963.

59. Kannel WB: Epidemiology of cerebrovascular disease: An epidemiologic study of cerebrovascular disease. In American Neurological Association and American Heart Association: Cerebral Vascular Diseases. New York, Grune & Stratton, 1966, pp 53–66.

60. Kartchner MM, McRae LP: Noninvasive evaluation and management of the "asymptomatic" carotid bruit. Surgery 82:840, 1977.

61. Kendall RE, Marshall J: Role of hypertension in the genesis of transient focal cerebral ischemic attacks. Br Med J 2:344, 1963.

62. Kroener JM, Dorn PL, Shoor PM, et al: Prognosis of asymptomatic ulcerating carotid lesions. Arch Surg 115:1387, 1980.

63. Kuller LH, Cook LP, Friedman GD: Survey of stroke epidemiology studies. Stroke 3:579, 1972.

64. Landolt AM, Millikan CH: Pathogenesis of cerebral infarction secondary to mechanical carotid artery occlusion. Stroke 1:52, 1970.

65. LeNet M: Le cout des malaides cardio-vasculaires. Coeur et Santé 33(Suppl), Edition Medicale (Commission Paritaire No. 55920), Paris, 1982.

66. Lindsay S, Entenman C, Ellis EE, Geraci CL: Aortic arteriosclerosis in the dog after localized aortic irradiation with electrons. J Circ Res 10:61, 1962.

67. Marshall J: The natural history of transient cerebrovascular ischemic attacks. Q J Med 131:309, 1964.

68. Matsumoto N, Whisnant JP, Kurland LT, et al: Natural history of stroke in Rochester, Minnesota, 1955 through 1969: An extension of a previous study, 1945 through 1954. Stroke 4:20, 1973.

69. McBrien DJ, Bradley RD, Ashton N: The nature of retinal emboli in stenosis of the internal carotid artery. Lancet 1:697, 1963.

70. McCready RA, Hyde GL, Bivins BA, et al: Radiation-induced arterial injuries. Surgery 93:306, 1983.

71. McLaughlin JS, Linberg E, Attar A, et al: Cerebral vascular insufficiency: Syndromes of reversed blood flow in vessels supplying the brain. Am Surg 33:317, 1967.

72. Meyer JS: Occlusive cerebrovascular disease: Pathogenesis and treatment. Am J Med 30:577, 1961.

73. Meyer WW: Cholesterinkrystallembolie kleiner Organarterien und ihre Folgen. Virchows Arch Pathol Anat 314:616, 1947.

74. Millikan CH: The pathogenesis of transient focal cerebral ischemia. Circulation 32:438, 1965.

75. Millikan CH, Siekert RG, Shick RM: Studies in cerebrovascular disease: V. The use of anticoagulant drugs in the treatment of intermittent insufficiency of the internal carotid arterial system. Proc Staff Meeting Mayo Clin 30:578, 1955.

76. Moniz E, Lima A, deLacerda R: Hemiplegies par thrombose de la carotide interne. Presse Med 45:977, 1937.

77. Moore WS, Boren C, Malone JM, et al: Natural history of nonstenotic asymptomatic ulcerative lesions of the carotid artery. Arch Surg 113:1352, 1978.

78. Moore WS, Hall AD: Ulcerated atheroma of the carotid artery: A cause of transient cerebral ischemia. Am J Surg 116:237, 1968.

79. Moore WS, Hall AD: Importance of emboli from carotid bifurcation in pathogenesis of cerebral ischemic attacks. Arch Surg 101:708, 1970.

80. Moore WS, Young B, Baker WH, et al: Surgical results: A justification of the surgeon selection process from the ACAS trial. J Vasc Surg 23:323, 1996.

81. North American Symptomatic Carotid Endarterectomy Trial Collaborators: Beneficial effect of carotid endarterectomy in symptomatic patients with high-grade carotid stenosis. N Engl J Med 325:445, 1991.

82. Panum PL: Experimentelle Beitrage zur Lehre von der Embolie. Virchows Arch (Pathol Anat) 25:308, 1862.

83. Paulson OB: Cerebral apoplexy (stroke) pathogenesis, pathophysiology, and therapy as illustrated by regional blood flow measurements in the brain. Stroke 2:327, 1971.

84. Quattlebaum JK Jr, Wade JS, Whiddon CM: Stroke associated with elongation and kinking of the carotid artery: Long-term follow-up. Ann Surg 177:572, 1973.

85. Roederer GO, Langlois YE, Jager KA, et al: The natural history of carotid arterial disease in asymptomatic patients with cervical bruits. Stroke 15:605, 1984.

86. Rothenberg SF, Corday E: Etiology of the transient cerebral stroke. JAMA 164:2005, 1957.

87. Russell RW, Cranstone WI: Ophthalmodynamometry in carotid artery disease. J Neurol Neurosurg Psychiatry 24:281, 1961.

88. Russell RWR: Observations on the retinal blood-vessels in monocular blindness. Lancet 2:1422, 1961.

89. Sacco RL, Wolf PA, Kannel WB, et al: Survival and recurrence following stroke in the Framingham study. Stroke 13:290, 1982.

90. Sarkari NBS, Holmes JM, Bickerstaff ER: Neurological manifestations associated with internal carotid loops and kinks in children. J Neurol Neurosurg Psychiatry 33:194, 1970.

91. Schneider RC, Lemmen LJ: Traumatic internal carotid artery thrombosis secondary to nonpenetrating injuries to the neck: A problem in the differential diagnosis of craniocerebral trauma. J Neurosurg 9:495, 1952.

92. Sheehan S, Bauer RB, Meyer JS: Vertebral artery compression in cervical spondylosis. Arteriographic demonstration during life of vertebral artery insufficiency due to rotation and extension of the neck. Neurology (Minneap) 10:968, 1960.

93. Strully KJ, Hurwitt ES, Blankenberg HW: Thromboendarterectomy for thrombosis of the carotid artery in the neck. J Neurosurg 10:474, 1953.

93a. Taylor TN, Davis PH, Torner JC, et al: Lifetime cost of stroke in the United States. Stroke 27:1459, 1996.

94. The Executive Committee for the Asymptomatic Carotid Atherosclerosis (ACAS) Study: Endarterectomy for asymptomatic carotid artery stenosis. JAMA 273:1421, 1995.

95. Thompson JE, Austin DJ, Patman RD: Carotid endarterectomy for cerebrovascular insufficiency: Long-term results in 592 patients followed up to thirteen years. Ann Surg 172:663, 1970.

96. Thompson JE, Patman RD: Endarterectomy for asymptomatic carotid bruits. Surg Digest 7:9, 1972.
97. Thompson JE, Patman RD, Talkington CM: Asymptomatic carotid bruit. Ann Surg 188:308, 1978.
98. Toole JF: The Willis Lecture: Transient ischemic attacks, scientific method, and new realities. Stroke 22:99–104, 1991.
99. Vitale JH, Pulcs SM, Okada A, et al: Relationships of psychological dimensions to impairment in a population with cerebrovascular insufficiency. J Nerv Ment Dis 158:456, 1974.
100. Wallace DC: A study of the natural history of cerebral vascular disease. Med J Aust 1:90, 1967.
101. Weibel J, Fields WS: Tortuosity, coiling, and kinking of the internal carotid artery. I. Etiology and radiographic anatomy. Neurology (Minneap) 15:7, 1965.
102. Whisnant JP, Fitzgibbons JP, Kurland LT, et al: Natural history of stroke in Rochester, Minnesota, 1945 through 1954. Stroke 2:11, 1971.
103. Wiebers DO, Whisnant JP: In Warlow C, Morris PJ (eds): Transient Ischemic Attacks. New York, Marcel Dekker, 1982, p 8.
104. Wolfe PA, Kannel WB, McGee DL: Epidemiology of strokes in North America. Stroke 1:19, 1986.
105. Wolfe PA, O'Neal A, D'Agostino RV, et al: Declining mortality, not declining incidence of stroke: The Framingham Study. Stroke 20:29, 1989.
106. Zarins CK, Giddens DP, Bharadvaj BK, et al: Carotid bifurcation atherosclerosis: Quantitative correlation of plaque localization with flow velocity profiles and wall shear stress. J Circ Res 53:502, 1983.
107. The Casanova Study Group: Carotid surgery vs. medical therapy in asymptomatic carotid stenosis. Stroke 22:1229, 1991.

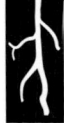

C H A P T E R   1 2 8

Diagnosis, Evaluation, and Medical Management of Patients with Ischemic Cerebrovascular Disease

Richard L. Hughes, M.D., C. Alan Anderson, M.D., and Gene Y. Sung, M.D.

Stroke is the third leading cause of death in the United States. Each year, approximately 500,000 Americans have strokes. Nearly 150,000 of these patients will die, and many of the survivors will have permanent cognitive, motor, and sensory impairments.[4] There are approximately 4 million stroke survivors living today; stroke is the leading cause of serious long-term disability in the nation. The estimated total financial cost of stroke in 1997 was $40 billion. This figure includes the direct cost of medical care in hospitals and nursing homes and the indirect cost of lost productivity resulting from stroke mortality and morbidity. The treatment of strokes has changed dramatically with the introduction of thrombolytic therapy. Early and aggressive diagnosis and treatment of cerebrovascular disease and stroke can reduce morbidity, mortality and the likelihood of recurrence.

NOMENCLATURE

The nomenclature for cerebrovascular disease is confusing and contains many archaic and imprecise terms, perhaps because of the evolution of knowledge about cerebrovascular disease and the use of different terms for various conditions by clinicians, radiologists, and pathologists. *Stroke* is a general term that refers to any vascular injury to the brain. *Ischemic stroke* (often shortened to "stroke") is an ischemic injury to the brain that causes a persistent clinical neurologic deficit at 24 hours. Even mild residual deficits are classified as strokes. The severity of the neurologic deficit is not the determinant for the diagnosis of stroke, only that the deficit is present at 24 hours.

Transient ischemic attacks (TIAs) are ischemic neurologic deficits that have *completely* resolved at 24 hours, regardless of their severity or relative duration (seconds or hours). Short TIAs that resolve within minutes usually do not cause permanent damage to the central nervous system (CNS), but a longer TIA that lasts for hours can be associated with cell death. Some patients who do not have a neurologic deficit on physical examination do have evidence of permanent ischemic brain injury as assessed by neuroimaging studies.

In the past, a variety of other terms were used to describe the clinical course of brain ischemia including *reversible ischemic neurologic deficit* (RIND). RIND describes a neurologic deficit that lasts beyond 24 hours but resolves in a way similar to that of a TIA. Like longer TIAs, RINDs invariably produce actual cell death. For this reason, the term has fallen into disfavor. In addition, patients may have strokes that steadily worsen over a period of hours. Because reembolization would typically produce stepwise deterioration and cerebral edema would not be expected for several days, this worsening is assumed to be from progressing thrombosis in the occluded artery in or around the affected brain. Such strokes are deemed "strokes in evolution" or "progressing strokes." Because appropriate therapy may include anticoagulation or thrombolysis, these terms still have clinical relevance.

Hemorrhages in the CNS are classified according to the anatomic areas in which the hemorrhage occurs. Thus, an *epidural* hemorrhage occurs between the skull and the dura; a *subdural* hemorrhage occurs between the dura and the thin arachnoid layer. *Intraparenchymal* hemorrhages include hematomas (formed blood clots that dissect into the brain) and hemorrhagic transformation of ischemic stroke (localized or multifocal regions of hemorrhage in an ischemic area.)

EPIDEMIOLOGY

There has been a decrease in the frequency of ischemic stroke in the past three decades, with a dramatic improvement in stroke survival.[9] This change has been attributed to better recognition and treatment of hypertension and improved management of complications in patients who suffer strokes. For reasons that remain unclear, stroke incidence and mortality have reached a plateau in the past decade.

Ischemic strokes occur more commonly in patients with coexistent medical conditions.[34, 68, 85] Atherosclerotic risk factors for ischemic stroke are essentially the same as those for coronary artery disease and peripheral vascular disease. Some, however, carry greater risk for stroke (Table 128–1).

Stroke incidence increases with age; 72% of ischemic strokes occur in individuals over age 65 years. Presumably, as the population ages, there will be a continued increase in the number of patients with ischemic strokes over the next 20 to 30 years.

The incidence of stroke averages about 100/100,000, varying from 10/100,000 in those younger than age 45 years to 100/100,000 for people aged 55 to 65 years. Those older than 75 years have an incidence of over 1000/100,000. Those over 65 years old have a 5% prevalence of stroke.

There are racial differences in the incidence, severity, mechanism and outcome from stroke. Extracranial large vessel (carotid bifurcation plaque or stenosis) disease is more common in whites. Asians have an increased rate of intracranial atherosclerotic cerebrovascular disease.[33, 76] African American men and women in the United States have a twofold to threefold increased incidence of ischemic stroke, with a stroke mortality more than twice that of whites.[4]

In addition, there are regional differences in the incidence of ischemic stroke. Because of increased stroke frequency and mortality, the southeast United States has been labeled the "stroke belt."[17, 33, 43, 51, 63] Residents in that region experience a stroke mortality rate that is 1.7 times the rate in other regions.[63] International differences have also been noted. Residents of Siberia, Russia, and Finland have had a threefold higher incidence of ischemic stroke compared with a similar population in Italy.[71] Possible reasons for the increased stroke incidence include ethnic, racial, and genetic differences as well as variable access to health care.

CLINICAL EVALUATION

Whereas ischemic stroke is a common cause of an acute focal neurologic deficit, a variety of non-stroke causes must be excluded.[52] The medical history, assessment of risk factors, a detailed review of symptom onset, the pattern of progression, associated signs and symptoms, laboratory studies, and neuroimaging all contribute to establishing the diagnosis of ischemic stroke. Many medical and neurologic conditions can mimic ischemic stroke (Table 128–2). Neuroimaging cannot differentiate many of these diagnoses from ischemic stroke.

When assessing a patient with stroke, one must answer two major questions:

- Where is the probable location of the lesion?
- What is the most likely mechanism?

The evaluation and management of the patient are guided by the initial determination of the anatomy and pathophysiology. All patients should have a thorough history, general physical examination, and neurologic examination. In the setting of acute stroke, time is critical. Decisions about thrombolytic therapy and other interventions must be made quickly, often with a limited amount of information.

Key questions in the history of the present illness include the following:

- When did the symptoms begin?
- What was the patient doing when the symptoms began?
- Was there progression of symptoms over time?
- Did the patient experience headache, seizures, vomiting, or a change in level of consciousness?
- Was there recent trauma?

Important questions in the medical history include the following:

- What are the patient's present and past illnesses and operations?
- Does the patient have any risk factors for stroke?
- What medications is the patient taking?
- Does the patient have any medication allergies?
- Is there any illicit drug use?

TABLE 128–1. RELATIVE RISK FOR ISCHEMIC STROKE

Age:
    100/100,000 overall
    10/100,000 ≤ 45 yr
    1000/100,000 ≥ 75 yr
Hypertension, 6×
Previous stroke or transient ischemic attack, 5×
Asymptomatic carotid bruit, 3×
Diabetes, 3×
Smoking, 2×
Rheumatic atrial fibrillation, 17×
Atrial fibrillation, 6×
Obesity, 1.5×
Elevated cholesterol and triglyceride levels, 2×
Elevated homocysteine, 2×

6. Gait (if possible)
7. Deep tendon reflexes and the plantar response

TABLE 128–2. DIFFERENTIAL DIAGNOSIS OF ACUTE ISCHEMIC STROKE

Seizure or Todd's paralysis	Hypertensive encephalopathy
Demyelinating disease	Complicated migraine
Toxic or metabolic disorders	Trauma
Meningoencephalitis	Peripheral nerve disease
Brain abscess	Transient global amnesia
Subdural or epidural hematoma	Multiple sclerosis
Systemic infections	Psychiatric illness

LOCALIZATION

The patient's symptoms and the findings on the neurologic examination determine the possible locations in the brain that have been affected by the stroke. Whereas there can be considerable variation among patients, common patterns of brain injury from ischemic stroke emerge. Rather than try to localize each individual abnormality, it is better to think in terms of pattern of injury and to match the constellation of findings in each patient.[15]

COMMON STROKE PATTERNS

Most major strokes present in reproducible constellations that follow either "large vessel" or "small vessel" patterns. Specific localization based on the occlusion and infarction of the territory of one of the large vessels of the cerebral hemisphere or brain stem include the (1) middle cerebral artery (MCA), (2) anterior cerebral artery (ACA), (3) posterior cerebral artery (PCA), (4) basilar artery, (5) vertebral arteries, and (6) branches to the cerebellum.[75] Similarly, the small penetrating vessels that coarse deep into the cortex, basal nuclei, white matter, brain stem, or feed the optic nerve and eye, result in typical patterns of deficit. These patterns can be useful historically and on examination to confirm TIA and stroke.

Middle Cerebral Artery

Of the large vessel patterns, the MCA is most often affected. With proximal MCA lesions and poor collateral support, the entire MCA can be lost with devastating consequences. In the dominant hemisphere, this would cause a contralateral hemiplegia, global aphasia, contralateral hemianopsia, and lateral eye deviation (toward the dominant hemisphere). Strokes of this size that do not show some early spontaneous recovery can lead to fatal brain herniation over the next few days.

Because the MCA tends to split into two main branches, a superior and inferior branch, slightly smaller emboli may progress past the proximal MCA and may lodge in those individual vessels. Infarctions in these MCA branch territories are common.

A stroke in the *superior* MCA branch causes a modest to severe weakness in the face and arm, and a Broca's (or nonfluent) aphasia. *Broca's aphasia* is characterized by good, but not perfect, comprehension and great difficulty with speech output. Patients transiently can be mute, then begin to speak in a slow, stuttering manner.

A stroke in the *inferior* branch of the MCA often causes transient or no motor weakness, mild visual field changes, but a dramatic Wernicke's (or fluent) aphasia. *Wernicke's aphasia* is characterized by very poor comprehension and nonsensical speech containing made up words, misused words, and unintelligible phrases. A contralateral hemi-

PHYSICAL EXAMINATION

Essential components of the general physical examination of the stroke patient are (1) the *vital signs* (temperature, pulse, respirations, and blood pressure), (2) the *heart examination* (with attention to rate, rhythm, heart sounds, and murmurs), and (3) the *vascular examination*. The carotid arteries, subclavian arteries, and orbits should be auscultated for bruits. The patient should be examined for signs of trauma or infection.

The neurologic examination is to be guided by the information in the history. For example, if the patient has problems with speech or language, a more detailed examination for dysarthria and aphasia must be performed. If there are complaints of numbness, additional time should be spent on a detailed examination of sensation. In general, the following parts of the neurologic examination should be evaluated in stroke patients.

1. Mental status
   a. Level of alertness
   b. Content
      (1) Test patient's ability to name objects, repeat spoken language, and read and write (aphasia, alexia, and agraphia)
      (2) Have patient copy a figure or draw a clock (visuospatial function)
      (3) Test patient's ability to remember three words and three objects in the room (verbal and visual memory)
2. Cranial nerves
   a. Visual fields (II) and pupils (II and III)
   b. Extraocular movements (III, IV, VI)
   c. Facial sensation (V) and strength (VII)
   d. Hearing (VIII)
   e. Ability to swallow a small amount of water and eat a cracker (IX and X)
   f. Shrugging of shoulders (XI) and protruding the tongue (XII)
3. Motor
   a. Muscle strength
   b. Muscle bulk
   c. Muscle tone
   d. Fine movements
4. Sensation
   a. Light touch, including double simultaneous stimulation
   b. Pin or temperature (nociception)
   c. Vibration or position sense (proprioception)
5. Coordination testing

anopsia, partial or complete, may be present with larger superior or inferior branch infarctions.

If the stroke extends into the *dominant parietal lobe*, the patient may also have *Gerstmann's syndrome*. This syndrome causes an inability to calculate, right/left disorientation, an inability to write (agraphia), and an inability to identify one's own fingers (*finger agnosia*).

The *nondominant* MCA similarly can be completely destroyed by a proximal MCA infarction with contralateral hemiplegia, contralateral hemianopsia, and eye deviation, but the patient would retain normal language without normal prosody. *Prosody* is the ability to express emotion by intonation in one's language. The patient with a large right hemisphere infarction often communicates in a monotone or "deadpan" manner. The larger nondominant infarctions show signs of neglect or inattentiveness. Some patients lie quietly with their eyes closed, despite being fully alert.

Specific infarction of the superior branch of the nondominant MCA causes contralateral weakness in the face and arm, with relative sparing of the leg. The ability to express emotions verbally by intonations (prosody) can be affected, causing patients to speak in a monotone. These patients are sometimes thought to be depressed when they actually are experiencing a symptom of stroke. Infarction of the *nondominant* MCA inferior branch produces difficulty in recognizing speech intonations (prosody recognition), double simultaneous sensory perception, and inattentiveness. Just as in the dominant hemisphere, the larger branch infarctions may have a contralateral hemianopsia, partial or complete. If the nondominant parietal lobe is included in the stroke, the inattentiveness and neglect are more obvious.

Anterior Cerebral Artery

Infarction of the ACA is much less common and typically results in weakness of the leg, with relative or complete sparing of the face and arm. These infarctions are relatively well tolerated unless bilateral infarction of ACA causes neurologic devastation from behavioral and cognitive impairment. Bilateral ACA infarction can produce a disinhibited state, not unlike head trauma, and can be severe enough to cause abulia or akinetic mutism. Such patients ignore their environment and resist interaction with others.

One of the small branches from the anterior cerebral artery, Heubner's artery, supplies the anterior limb and genu of the internal capsule and part of caudate nucleus.[75] Although typically well collateralized, infarctions in this area cause hemiparesis (from the internal capsule) or bradykinesia (from the caudate).

Posterior Cerebral Artery

Infarction in the PCA typically results in a contralateral homonymous hemianopsia that is congruous, which means that the visual field loss is similar in each eye when each eye is tested individually. Some stroke patients manage to spare the area of the visual cortex that is used for central vision, and thus they can retain more functional vision ("macular sparing") despite the loss of half the visual field. Because the PCA often supplies the cerebral peduncle of the midbrain, a hemiparesis can be included in PCA in-

farction. This obviously makes it difficult to distinguish PCA from MCA infarction. Visual field loss in the MCA territory tends to be less congruous and it is associated with other MCA signs. With better collateral circulation, smaller PCA infarctions can result in a partial homonymous hemianopsia and can cause bizarre disruptions in visual perception.

When both PCAs are involved, there is either a complete loss of vision ("cortical blindness") or a loss of functional vision when only the visual association areas are affected. Damage to the visual association areas with some retained visual perception can result in a number of strange syndromes, including Balint's syndrome and Anton's syndrome. *Balint's syndrome* causes optic ataxia and optic apraxia such that preserved areas of visual field cannot be used in a functional manner. Affected patients are unable to volitionally move their eyes to look at something and have difficulty in eye/hand coordination tasks. In *Anton's syndrome*, patients believe they are not blind; in reality, however, they have absolutely no functional vision.

Basilar Artery

The basilar artery runs with the pons, and when occluded can be rapidly fatal. With lesser degrees of pontine ischemia, alertness is preserved but essentially all other functions are lost, resulting in a "locked in" state. These patients can communicate only by blinking their eyes (a midbrain function). If the infarction is largely restricted to one of the cerebellar arteries that branch from the basilar, ipsilateral cranial nerve findings (e.g., facial weakness, numbness) are often combined with contralateral motor and sensory findings in the arm and leg. These "crossed" syndromes are the hallmarks of the brain stem localization.

The level of the infarction can be determined by the level of the ipsilateral cranial nerve functions. For example, midbrain infarctions affect the cranial nerve III or the red nucleus (tremor), and pontine infarctions affect cranial nerves V, VI, and VII. Since the pons is the center for lateral eye movements, pontine infarctions produce nystagmus (usually worse as one looks toward the side of infarction) or a lateral gaze palsy.

Vertebral Arteries

The vertebral arteries course to the base of the pons to create the basilar artery. Typically, the posterior inferior cerebellar arteries originate from the distal vertebral artery. Occlusion of either of these arteries results in the lateral medullary syndrome (*Wallenberg syndrome*). Patients usually present with an unusual pattern of nociception loss (pain and temperature) that affects the ipsilateral face and the contralateral body. In addition, a *Horner's syndrome* and limb ataxia often are found ipsilateral to the infarction. Generalized brain stem syndromes, including nystagmus, vertigo, nausea, vomiting, and dysphasia, are often present.

Small Vessel Infarction

Last, many patients have manifestations of ischemia from occlusion of the smaller vessels that penetrate the substance of the brain, brain stem, optic nerve, or eye. Although many syndromes have been described, the most typical presentations are focal loss of one neurologic system that affects the entire side of the body. For example, an isolated small infarction in the corticospinal tracts may create a pure motor hemiparesis (or hemiplegia) in the contralateral body. Occasionally, there is a mixture of both hemiparesis and ataxia (so-called ataxia hemiparesis). Often, the symptoms are fairly similar between face, arm, and leg, helping to distinguish small vessel infarctions from the MCA infarctions that relatively spare leg function. Similarly, patients with a thalamic infarction have an isolated dense sensory loss contralateral to the infarction.

Other Vessels

Although not technically part of the brain, the optic nerve and retina are common sites of ischemia. Patients typically present with a dense monocular loss of vision (amaurosis fugax). This is described as either a black shade or, sometimes, as a white or smoky shade. A variety of patterns can be present, including hemifield monocular vision loss in the inferior or superior field.

The mechanism of stroke in small vessel syndromes remains controversial. General thickening of the vessels from hypertension or age causes lipohyalinosis and subsequent ischemia. Platelet fibrin emboli and vasospasm[12] are also well-established mechanisms of ischemia, especially in the optic nerve and retina.

MECHANISMS OF ISCHEMIC STROKE

Once the diagnosis of ischemic stroke is made, it is necessary to determine the mechanism of the ischemic event. If the mechanism is known, appropriate intervention to prevent worsening or recurrent stroke is likely to be successful. Initial examination of the patient usually can determine whether the stroke follows a large vessel or small vessel pattern. *Large vessel ischemia* causes deficits in *multiple* systems. For example, a patient with a large vessel ischemic stroke has a hemiparesis, a hemisensory loss, and a homonymous hemianopsia contralateral to the ischemic side of the brain. A typical *small vessel stroke* produces an *isolated* motor (or isolated sensory) deficit on one side of the patient's body without affecting other neurologic systems. The distinction between large vessel and small vessel stroke determines immediate care for the patient and directs a focused evaluation during the patient's hospital stay.

Emboli

Large vessel strokes are generally caused by emboli[25, 55] from the heart, aorta, or carotid artery. A variety of cardiac conditions are associated with embolic stroke (Table 128–3). Occasionally, a patient may have a paradoxical embolus that originates from a thrombus in the venous system and passes through a patent foramen ovale or other intracardiac defect.[2, 36, 42]

Focal thrombotic occlusion of an intracranial artery is an unusual cause of stroke but can occur in the very elderly; it also is more common in Asian Americans and African

TABLE 128–3. HEART DISEASE ASSOCIATED WITH STROKE

Atrial fibrillation	Prosthetic heart valves
Rheumatic valvular disease	Endocarditis
Patent foramen ovale	Akinetic ventricular wall
Atrial septal aneurysm	segments
Atrial appendage thrombi	Cardiomyopathy
Mitral valve prolapse	Cardiac tumors (myxoma,
Left ventricular aneurysm	fibroelastoma)

Americans.[76] Small vessel infarctions typically are caused by occlusion of the small penetrating vessels which course from large arteries deep into the brain. These occlusions produce "lacunar" infarctions and contribute to the process of multi-infarct dementia in the older population.

Hypoperfusion

Hypoperfusion is a rare mechanism of stroke that can occur with or without stenotic or diseased arteries. Profound systemic hypotension, inadequate perfusion during cardiac arrest or cardiopulmonary bypass can cause a multifocal ischemic injury in the end-arterial zones or arterial border zones. Older people have a reduced ability to compensate for hypoperfusion, which places them at greater risk.

Injury

Primary injury to the arteries from trauma, radiation, or fibromuscular dysplasia may result in stenosis or occlusion of the carotid or vertebral arteries and cause ischemia. A history of trauma or radiation (to the area of the neck or head) suggests this diagnosis. In contrast, it is not unusual for patients to have little more than unexplained hypertension as a clue to fibromuscular dysplasia (because of coexistent renal artery involvement). Arterial dissection is associated with trauma, but may occur spontaneously from fibromuscular dysplasia, or collagen disorders.

Hypercoagulable States

Hypercoagulable states increase the risk of both thrombotic and embolic events. Homocysteinuria,[83] the antiphospholipid antibody syndrome,[53] protein C and S deficiency, and activated protein C resistance from the Leiden factor V genetic mutation, are examples. Many patients with malignancies have coagulation disturbances. Hemoglobinopathies, elevated fibrinogen, thrombocytosis, and polycythemia increase the viscosity of blood, hence increasing the risk of thrombosis.

Amyloid Angiopathy

Amyloid angiopathy is a poorly understood disorder of the small vessels in the central nervous system. It is distinct and unrelated to systemic amyloidosis, although amyloid protein is found in both disorders. Typically occurring in the elderly and rarely in younger patients, this disorder causes a slowly progressive dementia of probable vascular etiology and is characterized by episodes of cerebral hemorrhage in a lobar or cortical pattern. These hemorrhages are remarkably well tolerated. Often, the diagnosis is made by CT scan in the outpatient setting many days after the hemorrhage. Unfortunately, no specific treatment is available for amyloid angiopathy except control of hypertension (to reduce the risk of hemorrhage) and antiplatelet agents (to reduce the risk of ischemic injury). The characteristic presentation of these lesions usually makes neurosurgical biopsy unnecessary.

The "Four Vs"

Several other unusual mechanisms may need to be evaluated in the occasional patient, including the four "Vs":
• Vasculitis
• Vasculopathy
• Vasospasm
• Venous infarction

Vasculitis

Vasculitis of the central nervous system can occur either as a primary event without systemic involvement or in association with a systemic vasculitis. In either case, the diagnosis of vasculitis can be challenging to confirm and difficult to exclude. Patients typically have multiple events that can come and go or fluctuate, and they have evidence of infarction on neuroimaging studies (especially magnetic resonance imaging [MRI]). With rare exception, cerebrospinal fluid (CSF) findings are abnormal, demonstrating white blood cells and increased protein. Angiography is helpful to confirm vasculitis, but if only the very small vessels are affected, the larger vessels that are visualized by cerebral angiography may appear normal.

Although blood tests to establish an inflammatory condition can be useful to confirm or refute the presence of a systemic vasculitis that affects the CNS, an *isolated* CNS vasculitis will by definition have normal blood test. For this reason, the evaluation of the CSF is necessary when vasculitis is a possible etiology. A variety of bacterial, viral, and parasitic infections can cause an infectious arteritis that may be difficult to differentiate from noninfectious inflammatory conditions.

Temporal arteritis, a "giant cell arteritis," produces inflammation and, eventually, occlusion of small to medium arteries. Typical symptoms include headache, scalp tenderness, and jaw claudication. The sedimentation rate is typically, but not always, elevated. Ischemia to the retina, optic nerve, or brain can be prevented by appropriate treatment with steroids.

Vasculopathy

A variety of conditions, often referred to as "vasculitis" in the past, are actually noninflammatory abnormalities of the vessels and better classified as a vasculopathy. Most notable is fibromuscular dysplasia, but other entities such as radiation vasculopathy, Fabry's disease, familial recurrent arterial dissections, and malignant atrophic papulosis (Dego's disease)[23, 24, 62] are best classified together. The underlying pathophysiology and potential risk for stroke vary, and the best treatment is often unclear. However, definitive establishment of these diagnoses avoids the tendency to overtreat patients with potentially dangerous interventions (immunosuppression, anticoagulation).

Vasospasm

Although occurring mostly after subarachnoid hemorrhages, arterial vasospasm is a potential etiologic mechanism for ischemic stroke in a number of settings. Recently, patients with transient monocular visual loss were found to fail antithrombotic therapy but respond dramatically to calcium reentry blockers.[12] This observation has fueled the hypothesis that some small vessel infarctions, perhaps related to hypertension, may be mediated by vasospasm.

Unfortunately, there is no specific diagnostic test that will unequivocally establish vasospasm, and the only available confirmatory evidence is a beneficial response to an appropriate antivasospastic agent.

Venous Infarction

Venous infarctions typically cause hemorrhagic stroke in a brain distribution that is unusual for large vessel or embolic infarction. Often there is an infectious or hematologic predisposition for venous occlusion. Typically, venous infarction occurs post partum or it can complicate head trauma or CNS infection. Venous infarction is often readily apparent on neuroimaging studies (once the infarction is visualized) because of the tendency for venous infarctions to extend across more than one arterial territory.

Unfortunately, because most neuroimaging results are normal on the first day after stroke, the diagnosis of venous infarction is often delayed for several days. Venous infarctions tend to have more associated edema, more hemorrhagic changes, and more seizures than arterial infarctions. Although in the past angiography was necessary to confirm the diagnosis, both computed tomography (CT) and MRI scanning can noninvasively confirm most venous infarctions.

HEMORRHAGE

Cerebral hemorrhages also present with sudden onset of neurologic deficits but typically have associated headache, nausea, vomiting, and a depressed level of consciousness. The onset of subarachnoid hemorrhage is cataclysmic and typically described as a "light switch" or "firecracker" in the head, which creates a severe headache. Sudden death occurs in about one third of patients with subarachnoid hemorrhages. Intraparenchymal hematomas begin with a mild neurologic deficit and progress within a few minutes to include headache, nausea, and decreased level of consciousness. The patient's family often describes hemiparesis that steadily progresses to hemiplegia and a level of consciousness that quickly deteriorates to coma.

Given the wide range of medical conditions associated with stroke, some patients require additional tests, particularly patients with few risk factors for atherosclerosis, patients with known concomitant illness, and patients with atypical stroke symptoms (Table 128–4). Initial screening may include an echocardiogram to diagnose high-

TABLE 128–4. ADDITIONAL LABORATORY TESTS FOR SELECTED STROKE PATIENTS

Lipis tests	Rheumatologic tests
Diabetes tests	Hypercoagulability tests
Lumbar puncture	Blood cultures
Toxicology screening	Viral serology
Cardiac enzymes	Pregnancy tests
Erythrocyte sedimentation rate	Syphilis serology

risk cardiac structural (see Table 128–3) abnormalities, and carotid and vertebral ultrasound to exclude arterial stenosis or occlusion.

IMAGING

All patients with significant neurologic symptoms and signs require CT or MRI to determine whether the stroke is hemorrhagic or ischemic and to exclude other intracranial processes that can mimic stroke. In most centers, CT is the study of choice because of its availability and speed.[84] Compared with MRI, CT is better tolerated by critically ill patients because of shorter scan times and ease of monitoring patients in the scanner. CT is very good for imaging hemorrhage and can show most intracranial masses of consequence. In many instances, ischemic changes are not seen on the CT for 24 hours. Subtle changes including loss of gray-white differentiation, sulcal effacement, and hypodensity from edema may be seen within a few hours of symptom onset, especially with newer CT scanners.[67, 81]

Most patients may require additional imaging studies as part of their evaluation. Doppler duplex ultrasonography of the cervical and intracranial vessels, contrast angiography, echocardiography, and radionucleotide perfusion studies provide valuable information about the anatomy and mechanism of stroke but are not always available in the emergency setting. Diffusion and perfusion-weighted MRI studies, MR angiography, CT angiography, and bedside transcranial Doppler examination have potential for use in the acute setting, but their roles in the clinical management of stroke remain to be determined.

Although very useful for the study of the pathophysiology of stroke, cerebral blood flow (CBF) determination has not made its way into routine clinical use.[84] Available modalities to measure CBF include positron emission tomography (PET), xenon-CT, single photon emission computed tomography (SPECT), and magnetic resonance (MR) techniques. Each method has strengths and weaknesses. For example, PET scanning generates the highest level of technical information, but it is very expensive, available only at a few locations across North America, and cannot be performed quickly enough to direct acute therapy except in the exceptional case.[8] Xenon-CT generates CBF maps in a very short time, providing information for acute treatments, even within the first few hours after stroke.[31, 46] Now that a true resuscitative therapy is available, interest in xenon-CT is increasing.

SPECT generates a qualitative, not a quantitative blood flow map, which readily demonstrates areas of ischemia, but cannot differentiate ischemia from frank infarction.[40]

Magnetic resonance diffusion and perfusion images can determine very detailed and clear anatomy of infarction and may be able to differentiate reversible ischemia from infarction by diffusion-perfusion mismatch.[74, 78] This information is realistically available toward the very end of resuscitation windows and may be useful to identify "late" resuscitation cases beyond the usual "three hour window."

PREVENTION OF STROKE

The long-term prevention of stroke involves the treatment of the mechanism of the ischemia and any vascular risk factors. Prophylaxis for cerebrovascular events can be divided into three categories:

- Primary prevention
- Acute (temporary) prophylaxis
- Secondary prevention

Primary Prevention

Primary prevention is not performed often because physicians and patients wait until an ischemic event occurs somewhere in the body before considering intervention. Data from the Physicians Health Study[70] indicate that the widespread indiscriminate use of aspirin is perhaps not ideal, but the use of primary antiplatelet treatment has become popular in higher-risk subgroups. Most physicians try to customize an approach for the individual patient.

Recognition of the profound efficacy of warfarin to prevent complications of atrial fibrillation[72, 73] has fueled enthusiasm for other primary prevention strategies. With better understanding of emerging biochemical markers of atherosclerosis, such as homocysteine,[83] widespread prevention strategies may become available similar to those used in the treatment of hypercholesterolemia.[34, 65]

Acute Prophylaxis

Acute prophylaxis after stroke or TIA remains controversial. Available data are incomplete and do not reflect current use, case selection, agent choice, timing, or dosing. For example, results from recent trials indicate that aspirin has a very small effect and that heparin is ineffective in preventing strokes in patients who present with strokes or TIAs.[21, 47] Unfortunately, in these studies heparin was not restricted to patients with embolic strokes and was administered subcutaneously, perhaps in inadequate doses. In this setting, several smaller trials with better case selection indicate some advantage for acute administration of heparin to prevent stroke, deep venous thrombosis, pulmonary embolism, and death with only a slight increase in hemorrhagic transformation of the stroke.[19, 20, 66, 80] Heparin may even be safe when hemorrhagic changes are present.[61]

The theoretically safer low-molecular-weight heparins behave similarly to conventional heparin, at least for stroke prophylaxis.[54] By using heparin selectively in cases with higher stroke recurrence risks, avoiding excessive dosing, and by excluding or delaying anticoagulation in those patients at the highest risk for hemorrhage, the physician can consider acute anticoagulation a reasonable option for preventing recurrence.

Secondary Prophylaxis

Long-term medical therapies for prevention of atherosclerotic strokes include aspirin, ticlopidine, clopidogrel, and warfarin (Table 128–5). Aspirin has been demonstrated to reduce the risk of stroke and other vascular events by about 25% at 5 years.[5] Most studies have demonstrated that lower doses of aspirin are as effective as 1300 mg/day.[27, 79]

Ticlopidine is an antiplatelet agent that is more effective than aspirin (10% fewer ischemic end-points, including myocardial infarction, peripheral vascular disease, or other vascular deaths),[39] but its cost and toxicity (1% neutropenia, diarrhea) limit its utility. Clopidogrel, a thienopyridine like ticlopidine, has been shown to provide benefit in prevention of strokes, myocardial infarctions, and peripheral vascular disease.[14] This agent became available in 1998 and has no more toxicity than aspirin. Like ticlopidine, it has a modest advantage, about 10%, over aspirin.

Anticoagulation has been demonstrated repeatedly to reduce the risk of embolization from cardiac or other sources. This risk, however, must be weighed against the risk of hemorrhage (which can be fatal). Chronic warfarin clearly is efficacious for the patient with prosthetic heart valves,[77] and atrial fibrillation associated with mitral valve disease. Patients with ischemic and episodic atrial fibrillation also benefit from chronic warfarin.[60, 72, 73] Isolated atrial fibrillation (atrial fibrillation in the absence of other diseases) probably is not an indication for warfarin unless the patient is 65 years old or has early atherosclerosis.[48, 60] Warfarin should also be considered for short-term treatment in patients who have an embolus of unknown or unclear origin. Such short-term therapy theoretically is useful because the risk of recurrence of embolization is highest in the first few months after the initial embolic event. Therefore, administration of warfarin over 3 to 6 months may reduce this risk during the most dangerous time period, and thereafter it may be discontinued in favor of aspirin, ticlopidine, or clopidogrel to avoid the long-term complications of anticoagulation.

Recently, a sustained-release version of dipyridamole has been tested in Europe with promising results (ESPS-2).[26, 29] The addition of dipyridamole to aspirin was twice as effective as aspirin alone. Unfortunately, the reliability of the data has come under question because one center was discovered to have "fabricated" patients.[28a] Although these data were not used in the final analysis, serious questions remain about the validity of the trial. Additional criticisms include the small dose of aspirin used (25 mg twice daily) and the possibility that there is a specific aspirin-dipyridamole dose ratio that is needed to gain additive or synergistic effects. Since all prior antiplatelet treatment studies involving aspirin and an aspirin-dipyridamole combination indicate that there was absolutely no effect of dipyridamole when added to aspirin,[5] there is no satisfactory explanation for the positive results of ESPS-2.[28] Nonetheless, because of the safety of dipyridamole, the FDA may approve a combination dipyridamole and aspirin tablet sometime in 1999.

The optimal antiplatelet agent has become controversial.[7, 38, 49] The first demonstration of aspirin efficacy (at 1300 mg/day) generated a "standard" that is still adhered today.[14] Multiple studies have demonstrated the efficacy of lower doses of aspirin but without sufficient power to prove convincingly equivalent efficacy.[27, 79] As a result, there are proponents for higher doses of aspirin and for lower doses of aspirin based on interpretation of the same data. With the demonstration of about a 10% benefit to thienopyridine (ticlopidine and clopidogrel) over aspirin, the debate has shifted to low cost (aspirin) versus slightly better efficacy at substantially higher cost (thienopyridine). A resolution is not in sight at this time. Any of the choices, from low-dose aspirin to a thienopyridine, represent a substantial improvement over placebo, and the relative differences between agents is modest at best.

The most common paradigm for therapy includes the use of a 325-mg enteric coated aspirin as the basic standard

TABLE 128–5. ANTITHROMBOTIC AGENTS FOR STROKE PREVENTION

AGENT	DOSE	EFFICACY	ADVERSE EFFECTS	COMMENT
Aspirin	30–1350 mg	25%–30%	Gastric; allergic	Aspirin, in a 325 mg enteric coated tablet, is general standard for patients with average atherosclerotic risks; very low or very high dosing may have advantages for the occasional patient
Ticlopidine	250 mg bid	27%–32%	Neutropenia (1%); diarrhea	About 10% more effective than aspirin, ticlopine is a reasonable alternative, best tested in stroke; used with aspirin to maintain cardiac stent patency
Clopidogrel	75 mg	27%–32%	Diarrhea	A thienopyridine like ticlopidine but without the 1% risk of neutropenia; tested in patients with stroke, myocardial infarction, and peripheral vascular disease
Warfarin	To INR goal	70% in atrial fibrillation	Hemorrhage	For patients at highest risk of central nervous system embolization from either cardiac or arterial structural abnormalities, and/or due to hypercoagulable states

INR = International Normalized Ratio.

for most patients. Patients who are intolerant are allowed to take lower doses of aspirin or are switched to a thieno-pyridine. Patients who are considered to be at higher overall vascular risk because of sensitivity to aspirin, severe carotid stenosis, and failure of aspirin efficacy can be switched to a high dose of aspirin (1300 mg) or a thienopyridine. Provided that this does not preclude appropriate patients from treatment with warfarin[73] or carotid endarterectomy,[22, 30, 44, 57, 58] benefit-risk estimations of this type are the only satisfactory solution until definitive data are available.

Newer concepts of antiplatelet agent use include resurgence in research on combining antiplatelet agents. Recently, cardiac stent patency was enhanced by combining ticlopidine and aspirin.[35] This, along with ESPS-2 data on the use of dipyridamole with low dose aspirin, has resurrected interest in combination therapy.[28] If these or other approaches can be reproduced by others, it is likely that combination therapy will gain acceptance.

The optimal degree of anticoagulation induced by warfarin therapy always has been controversial. Greater anticoagulation (International Normalized Ratio [INR] of 3 to 4) is most effective, but more dangerous.[77] Such levels are appropriate for patients who are at very high risk for stroke. Examples include patients with congenital heart disease, severe mitral valve disease, and symptomatic antiphospholipid antibody syndrome. Less intense anticoagulation with warfarin (INR of 2 to 3) is appropriate for most stroke patients. This includes patients with atrial fibrillation (complicated by congestive heart failure, hypertension, or previous embolization) and patients with recent large vessel occlusion. Patients who have less risk may do as well with antiplatelet agents or a low dose of warfarin (INR 1.7 to 2.0). Unfortunately, it is not efficacy that usually determines the dose of warfarin but, rather, the risk of life-threatening intracranial or systemic hemorrhage that increases with INR.[72] For patients aged 75 years or older, the risks of warfarin escalate. In this situation, a lower than ideal intensity of warfarin is usually the best compromise. Further, patients who are older or fragile are often managed with lower INRs because intracranial hemorrhages are unusual when INRs are below 2.5.

The use of more sophisticated cardiac imaging has indicated that a variety of subgroups of stroke patients may benefit from warfarin treatment. Echocardiographic observations that suggest high risk of recurrent stroke include the appearance of spontaneous atrial contrast, "strands"[64] and redundant or large mitral valve prolapse. Additional studies should clarify the risk of these markers within the next few years.

CAROTID ENDARTERECTOMY

In the United States, the number of carotid endarterectomies peaked in the early 1980s at more than 100,000 procedures per year. In the middle 1980s, controversy concerning the appropriateness of the procedure, especially in the asymptomatic patient, resulted in fewer procedures (83,000 in 1986). After the publication of prospective randomized trials[30, 58] carotid endarterectomy became less controversial and more popular (150,000 in 1998). The following general principles help dictate who is an appropriate candidate:

1. After a successful endarterectomy, the risk of stroke in that vascular distribution is reduced for many years.

2. The risks of undergoing carotid endarterectomy increase as the severity of disease increases; that is, the patients likely to benefit the most from a carotid endarterectomy also have the highest risk in undergoing the operation.

3. The angiographic and surgical morbidity and mortality vary greatly between individual patients, institutions, and surgeons. This obviously makes comparison of different studies extremely difficult.

With the publication of the North American Symptomatic Carotid Endarterectomy (NASCET)[58] trial and the Asymptomatic Carotid Atherosclerosis Study (ACAS) trial,[30] there is finally reasonable data to select candidates for carotid endarterectomy. These trials used a precise method to measure stenosis (Fig. 128–1).

First, the symptomatic patient with carotid artery stenosis of 70% or greater benefits greatly by endarterectomy in the hands of an experienced surgeon. Because the benefit of endarterectomy (in addition to medical therapy) is statistically significant after a few months, older patients, if robust, are reasonable candidates for the procedure. Benefit of endarterectomy in symptomatic patients was confirmed by trials in Europe and by the Veterans Affairs Department.[57]

The 30% to 69% carotid artery stenosis group in NASCET has been completed with nearly 3000 patients. Preliminary presentations support a modest benefit (~30%) for surgery in the 50% to 69% group but no

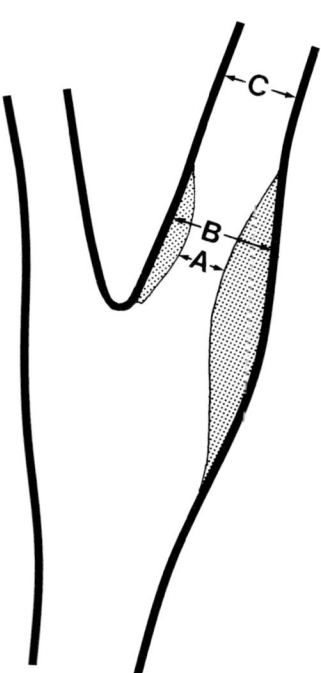

FIGURE 128–1. The method to measure stenosis that was used in the clinical trials demonstrating efficacy uses the narrowest part of the lumen (A) and the internal carotid size distal to the bifurcation and the atherosclerotic lesion (C). Using a theoretical bulb measurement (B) will overestimate the stenosis and prevent the use of North American Asymptomatic Carotid Endarterectomy Trial (NASCET) and Asymptomatic Carotid Atherosclerosis Study (ACAS) data for patient categorization.

benefit for patients with less than 50% stenosis. The choice for surgery must be individualized, especially in the lower stenosis categories.

The asymptomatic patient with stenosis of 60% or greater also benefits from surgery, but the details of case selection are less clear.[22, 44] The relatively healthy ACAS patients decreased their stroke risk by 55% over a 5-year period with endarterectomy by a qualified surgeon.[30] The overall risk of large stroke, with or without surgery, is not great, making the option to use medical therapy alone reasonable, if somewhat less effective. The 60% to 80% group fared the same as the 80% to 99% group, so that increasing stenosis was not a factor as it was in the NASCET trial. The VA Trial of carotid endarterectomy in patients with asymptomatic carotid artery stenosis demonstrated a significant reduction in TIAs, but not strokes, largely because of insufficient stroke end points in the study.[41] For patients who are fragile, elderly, and in poor health, the choice for medical therapy is certainly the best. For younger, healthier, and robust patients, endarterectomy is a reasonable option that should be offered and discussed.[48]

Since strokes from carotid artery disease are usually due to embolization, the use of angioplasty has been restricted because of the risks of iatrogenic embolization.[11] Carotid artery stenting may be a better solution than angioplasty if morbidity and mortality rates remain reasonable. Clinical trials to compare stenting to conventional surgery are being organized. Data may be available within the next several years to help guide the use of this technique in the prevention of stroke.

MANAGEMENT OF ACUTE ISCHEMIC STROKE

From the moment the stroke patient arrives in the emergency department, it is important to monitor the vital signs and sequentially examine the patient. Patients may rapidly deteriorate, and medical complications may develop.[1, 69] The airway should be assessed and protected from aspiration. The need for supplemental oxygen is guided by pulse oximetry. Some patients will require endotracheal intubation. Myocardial infarction, arrhythmias, congestive heart failure, and hypovolemia all cause global hypoperfusion with worsening of the ischemic injury and should be identified and promptly treated.

Thrombolysis

Recombinant tissue plasminogen activator (rt-PA) was approved for use in acute ischemic stroke in 1996. Approval of rt-PA therapy in acute stroke was based in large part on the results from the National Institute of Neurological Disorders and Stroke (NINDS) rt-PA Study Group.[59] The group evaluated the outcome in patients with acute ischemic stroke treated with intravenous rt-PA given within 3 hours from the onset of symptoms. These two double-blind studies included a total of 624 patients who were randomized to treatment with placebo or rt-PA, 0.9 mg/kg with 10% of the dose given as a bolus and the remainder infused over 1 hour. The number of patients recovering to

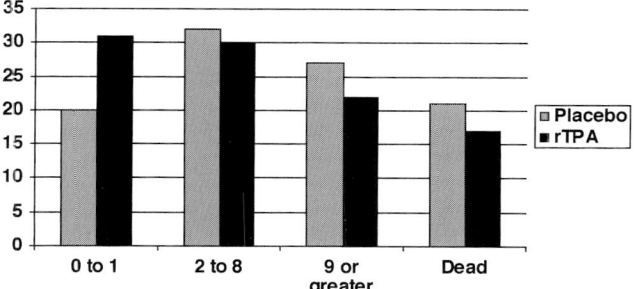

FIGURE 128–2. Outcome percentages at 3 months using the National Institutes of Health (NIH) Stroke Scale. Treatment with intravenous tissue plasminogen activator (t-PA) increases the number of patients with a NIH Stroke Scale (NIHSS) of 0 or 1, which is normal or essentially normal. Patients with a moderate deficit at their eventual outcome (NIHSS of 2 to 8) are relatively unchanged. Despite the chance of worsening the deficit with hemorrhage, the number of patients who end up with severe deficits (NIHSS 9 or above) or die is less.

"normal" increased from 20% to 36% (Fig. 128–2). With a global test statistic combining all of the outcome measures, the odds ratio for a favorable outcome with rt-PA was 1.7 ($p = .008$). There was no difference with respect to the patients' age, race, sex, location of the stroke, or stroke mechanism in terms of benefit from the drug. There was no significant difference between the rt-PA and placebo groups in mortality, with rt-PA patients faring slightly better. This was true despite a significantly higher incidence of symptomatic hemorrhage during the first 24 hours after treatment in the rt-PA group.

On the basis of these results, intravenous rt-PA is recommended if it can be given within 3 hours of onset of acute ischemic stroke.[59, 69] If the patient awakens from sleep with a deficit, the last time he or she was known to be well is used to calculate the time of the onset of stroke.

The diagnosis must be established by a physician with experience in diagnosis of acute stroke. Further, a physician with expertise in CT must review the study prior to administration of drug (Fig. 128–3). The use of rt-PA requires careful patient selection with specific exclusion criteria (Table 128–6). Studies with another thrombolytic agent, streptokinase, did not demonstrate benefit. A lower dose of streptokinase may eventually be shown to be worthwhile, but until that dose is demonstrated to be safe, intravenous streptokinase is contraindicated.

Data from the Colorado Acute Stroke Network (CASN) has shown that the use of rt-PA in a combination of rural, community, and urban hospitals produces benefits (and risks) similar to those in the NINDS study.[45]

A potential alternative to intravenous rt-PA in some patients may be the administration of thrombolytic agents via an angiographic catheter. This permits demonstration of the thrombus and the vascular anatomy, followed by delivery of the thrombolytic agent directly to the site of occlusion.[50] The total amount of lytic drug used is typically much less, about 30%, of the intravenous dose. Some interventional radiologists have added mechanical disruption of the thrombus using the catheter to rt-PA infusion. A better understanding of proper patient selection, contraindications, and the benefit of catheter-based thrombolytic ther-

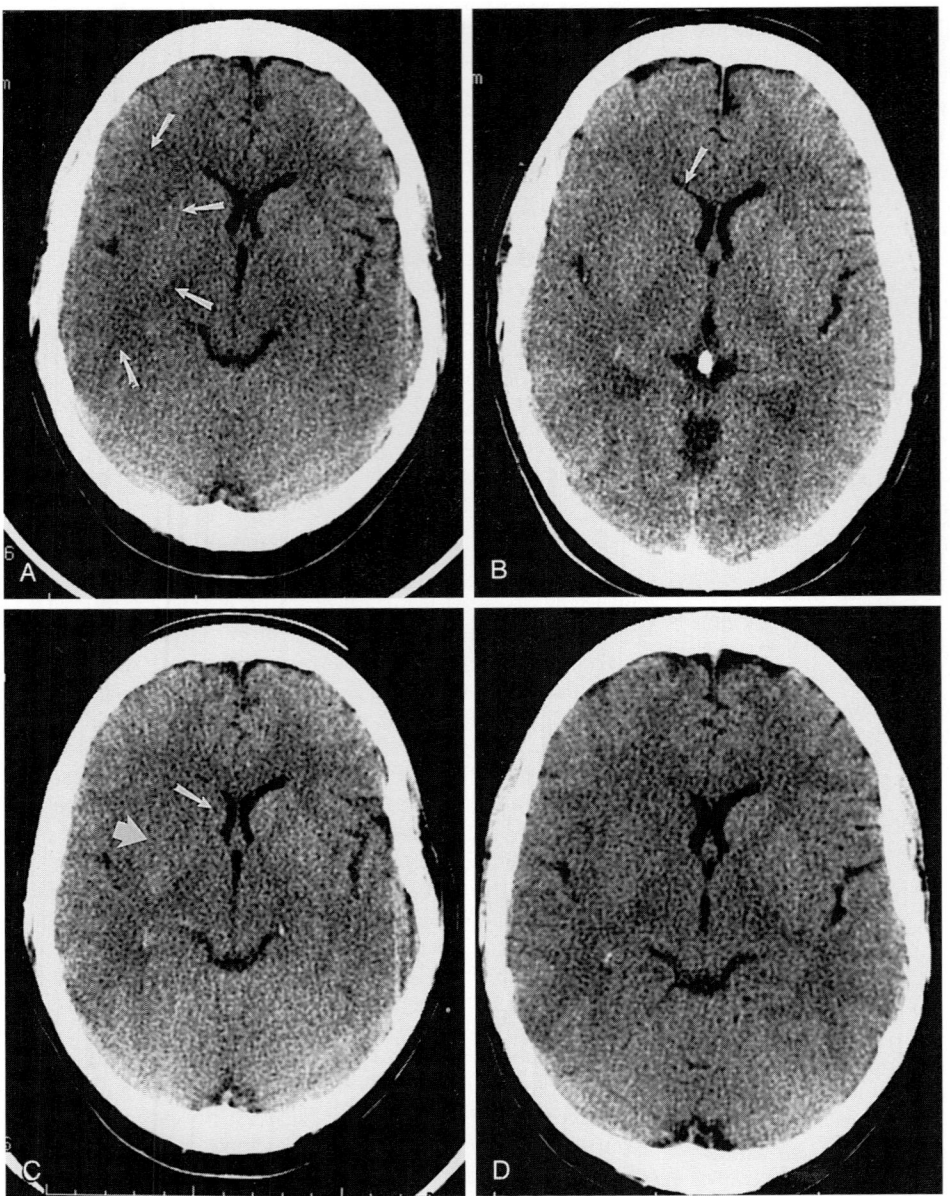

FIGURE 128–3. CT changes in acute ischemic stroke. The use of high-resolution CT scanning has become an effective means to help corroborate the relative age of an infarct and to help the appropriate selection of patients for thrombolysis. These four scans shown demonstrate the early CT changes and the evolution of changes in a stroke. Patients with symptomatic bleeding into the area of the stroke after thrombolytic agents typically have abnormal CT scans at the onset and very large deficits (NIHSS of 22 or greater). Although treatment of patients with very large strokes is clearly riskier, patients with thrombolytic treatment fare better than those without treatment. *A*, At 2½ hours from the onset of a stroke, there is loss of the cortical ribbon in the right cortex (*arrows*). *B*, At 8 hours, compression of the right lateral ventricle is obvious (*arrow*) in addition to the previous changes. This is due to diffuse swelling in the hemisphere. *C*, By 12 hours, the swelling has increased and the caudate nucleus (*arrow*) is now clearly infarcted as is part of the putamen and globus pallidus (*thick arrow*). *D*, By 30 hours after the stroke, continued swelling and loss of the cortical structures are obvious. The overall decrease in density of the right hemisphere is more apparent here than on earlier scans.

apy relative to intravenous thrombolytic therapy awaits the results of additional trials, but clearly this technique can recanalize occluded vessels and produce dramatic improvement in selected patients.[25] Generally, patients who meet intravenous rt-PA inclusion criteria but who have relative or absolute medical exclusions are the best candidates for catheter-based thrombolysis (Table 128–7).

Blood Pressure Management in Ischemic Stroke

A transient elevation in blood pressure (BP) occurs in most patients with ischemic stroke. Usually lasting several days, this hypertension spontaneously returns to normal in most patients. Whereas clinical trials have consistently demonstrated the benefit of long-term BP reduction in reducing the risk of stroke, there does not appear to be a similar benefit to reducing BP in the acute setting. In fact, even minor BP reductions in the first few hours after stroke can be harmful.[1, 10, 69]

An algorithm for emergency antihypertensive therapy for acute stroke follows[10]:

1. If diastolic BP is above 140 mmHg on two readings 5 minutes apart, start infusion of sodium nitroprusside (0.5 to 10 mg/kg/min).

2. If systolic BP is above 230 mmHg or diastolic BP is 121 to 140 mmHg on two readings 20 minutes apart, give 20 mg labetalol IV over 1 to 2 minutes. The labetalol dose may be repeated or doubled every 10 to 20 minutes until BP is reduced or until a cumulative dose of 300 mg has been administered via this minibolus technique. After the initial dosing schedule, labetalol doses may be administered every 6 to 8 hours as needed. Labetalol should be avoided for patients with asthma, cardiac failure, or severe cardiac conduction abnormalities.

TABLE 128–6. SOME EXCLUSION CRITERIA FOR INTRAVENOUS RECOMBINANT TISSUE PLASMINOGEN ACTIVATOR (rt-PA) THERAPY IN STROKE

- Onset more than 3 hours prior to therapy
- Rapidly improving deficit
- Isolated, mild neurologic deficits
- Possible hemorrhage revealed on CT scan
- Early changes of major infarction evident on CT scan
- Stroke in the previous 3 months
- Head trauma in the previous 3 months
- Major surgery within past 14 days
- Recent myocardial infarction
- Gastrointestinal or urinary tract bleeding within the prior 21 days

- Seizure at the onset of stroke
- Prior intracranial hemorrhage
- Use of oral anticoagulants
- INR greater than 1.7
- Use of heparin within last 48 hr and prolonged PTT
- Blood glucose <50 mg/dl or >400 mg/dl
- Platelet count <100,000/ml
- Sustained systolic blood pressure >185 mmHg
- Sustained diastolic blood pressure >110 mmHg

CT = computed tomography; INR = International Normalized Ratio; PTT = partial thromboplastin time.

3. If systolic BP is 180 to 230 mmHg or diastolic BP is 105 to 120 mmHg, emergency therapy should be deferred in the absence of documented intracerebral hemorrhage or left ventricular failure. If elevation persists with two readings 60 minutes apart, administer oral labetalol (200 to 300 mg) two to three times daily as needed. Satisfactory alternative treatments to labetalol are oral nifedipine (10 mg) every 6 hours or captopril (6.25 to 25 mg) every 8 hours. If oral monotherapy is unsuccessful or if medications cannot be given orally, give labetalol IV as outlined earlier.

4. For acute stroke patients with systolic BP below 180 mmHg or diastolic BP below 105 mmHg, antihypertensive therapy is not usually indicated. Patients requiring heparin acutely should receive anticoagulation therapy after BP has been cautiously lowered to an acceptable range. A target BP range of 150/85 to 150/95 mmHg for patients without previous hypertension or 160/90 to 170/100 mmHg in patients with a history of hypertension is recommended. Because the benefits of heparin are modest even when indicated, rapid lowering of BP cannot be justified.

Experimental Therapies for Acute Stroke

After an initial ischemic event, a surviving section of brain exists for a time, called the "ischemic penumbra." During

TABLE 128–7. CRITERIA FOR CATHETER-BASED THROMBOLYSIS

1. Identify candidates for IV thrombolytic therapy.
   a. Treat stroke within 3 hours from onset
   b. IV rt-PA (NINDS) inclusions/exclusions
   c. Treat immediately
2. Next, if the patient is not a candidate, consider IA thrombolysis for:
   a. IV rt-PA inclusions, with exclusions
   b. Can achieve lysis by hour 6, or stop
   c. Unclear onset with normal CT findings (presumed 0–3)
   d. Very large (NIHSS > 22) strokes
   e. Presumed basilar occlusion

IV = intravenous; IA = intra-arterial; rt-PA = recombinant tissue plasminogen activator; CT = computed tomography; NINDS = National Institute of Neurological Disorders and Stroke; NIHSS = National Institutes of Health Stroke Study.

this time and after reperfusion, a variety of metabolic processes inhibit recovery and exacerbate injury to the ischemic brain. The best-defined metabolic process is *excitotoxicity*, which is caused by excitatory neurotransmitters (e.g., glutamate), which are persistently elevated in progressive infarction.[18] Other parts of the ischemic cascade, including intracellular calcium elevation, membrane disintegration, free radical formation, nitric oxide inhibition, and leukocyte migration, have been identified and have been the subject of clinical trials to minimize ischemic injury after stroke.[32] Unfortunately, none of these agents has been beneficial (Table 128–8). The reasons for failure include drugs that are too toxic in the human to reproduce benefits seen in animal models, the lack of clinical trials sufficiently large and sophisticated to observe subtle improvements, and the need to utilize some agents in an unreasonable time frame (some within 30 minutes). Interest has now turned toward using some of these agents in combination with thrombolytics to show that subtle benefits can be enhanced in the setting of thrombolysis-induced reperfusion.

Hypothermia

Recent evidence that head injury patients may benefit from induced hypothermia[56] and the observation that hyperthermia is a predictor of poor outcome in ischemic stroke[6] have led to renewed interest in hypothermia as a potential treatment for stroke. This has been established in animal models of stroke.[13, 82] Although methods to rapidly cool patients who are sedated, paralyzed, and ventilated are feasible, the use of hypothermia in the awake and alert stroke victim remains problematic.[86]

Hemodilution

Although commonly used in the setting of post-subarachnoid hemorrhage vasospasm, hypertensive hypervolemic hemodilution has been tested in patients with general ischemic strokes without benefit.[2, 37] In these trials, a subgroup of patients seem to improve, but the tendency of hypervolemic hemodilution to exacerbate cerebral edema negated this benefit. More sophisticated cerebral blood flow testing to determine the viability of tissue may eventually define a role for hypertensive hypervolemic hemodilution.

Complications

Stroke patients are at risk for several complications. Many are preventable, and if they occur, they must be recognized and treated. Serial examination, monitoring vital signs, and close attention to fluid and electrolyte balance are important general principles. Stroke patients often are immobile and at risk for deep venous thrombosis and pulmonary embolism. Subcutaneous heparin or pneumatic compression stockings should be used. Early mobilization, variable pressure mattresses, and frequent turning and repositioning are effective prevention for decubitus ulcers.

Brain edema in ischemic stroke is predominantly cytotoxic. The typical scenario is the onset of drowsiness, changes in respiratory patterns, and worsening deficits 24 to 96 hours after an acute ischemic event. Therapy for increased intracranial pressure in the stroke patient in-

TABLE 128–8. RESUSCITATION AGENTS FOR STROKE PATIENTS

AGENT	TYPE	STATUS	COMMENT
IV rt-PA	Thrombolytic	FDA-approved	The only approved agent for ischemic stroke
IA lysis	Thrombolysis; mechanical disruption	Available in many centers	Not approved, but an alternative to IV rt-PA
Pro-Urokinase	Thrombolytic	In trial	Investigational drug
Ancrod	Fibrinogen depleater	In trial	Investigational drug
Clomethazole	GABA antagonist	In trial	Investigational drug
Magnesium	NMDA antagonist	In trial	Given IV
Lubeluzole	Nitric oxide	Abandoned	Investigational drug
Eliprodil	Glutamate antagonist	Abandoned in stroke	Investigational drug
Nalmefene	Opiate antagonist	Abandoned in stroke	Investigational drug
Naloxone	Opiate antagonist	Available	No benefit in earlier trials
Nimodipine	Ca²⁺ reentry blocker	FDA-approved for SAH vasospasm	No benefit in stroke trials
Citicoline	Membrane stabilizer	Abandoned in stroke	Investigational drug
Glycine	Glutamate	In trial	Investigational drug
Antagonists	Antagonists		
Tirilazad	Membrane stabilizer	Abandoned in stroke	Investigational drug
Various agents	NMDA antagonists	Abandoned in stroke	Selfotel, aptiganel, dextrophan
Volume expander	Hypervolemic hemodilution	Available, not approved	Dextran, albumin, others; benefits still theoretical, not demonstrated
Emlibmomab	Leukocyte inhibitor	Abandoned in stroke	Investigational drug
HU23F2G	Leukocyte inhibitor	In trial	Investigational drug
Hypothermia	Hypothermia	In trial	

IV rt-PA = intravenous recombinant tissue plasminogen activator; IA = Intra-arterial; NMDA = N-methyl-D-aspartate; FDA = Food and Drug Administration; GABA = gamma aminobutyric acid; SAH = subarachnoid hemorrhage.

cludes elevating the head of the bed to 30 degrees, limiting fluid intake, intravenous mannitol or furosemide, and intubation with mechanical hyperventilation. Neurosurgical consultation is suggested. Steroids are not effective in this setting.

Up to 15% to 20% of stroke patients experience seizure. Most of the early seizures are of partial onset with secondary generalization and occur in the first 24 hours after the ischemic event. Seventy-five per cent of patients with seizures after stroke have them in the first year. Most seizures that occur following a stroke are easily controlled by a single anticonvulsant medication. There is no evidence to support the routine use of prophylactic anticonvulsants in acute stroke.

All stroke patients should be considered at risk for aspiration. The risk is greater with large strokes, brain stem strokes, and a depressed level of consciousness. Many stroke victims have mild or transient aspirations in the first few hours or days. Patients should not be given food, liquids, or medications by mouth until their ability to swallow has been assessed. For some patients, a bedside evaluation and a glass of water with crackers is sufficient; others may require formal evaluation, including videofluoroscopic barium swallow. Some patients require nutritional support via nasogastric tubes until they have recovered their ability to protect the airway. Patients at long-term risk for aspiration benefit from percutaneous gastrostomy.

REFERENCES

1. Adams H, Brott T, Crowell R, et al: Guidelines for the management of patients with acute ischemic stroke: A statement for healthcare professionals from a special writing group of the Stroke Council. Stroke 25:1901–1903, 1994.
2. Aichner FT, Fazekas F, Brainin M, et al: Hypervolemic hemodilution in acute ischemic stroke: The Multicenter Austrian Hemodilution Stroke Trial (MAHST). Stroke 29:743–749, 1998.
3. Albers GW, Comess KA, DeRook FA, et al: Transesophageal echocardiographic findings in stroke subtypes. Stroke 25:23–28, 1994.
4. American Heart Association: Heart and Stroke Statistical Update. Dallas, Texas, 1997.
5. Antiplatelet Trialists Collaboration: Collaborative overview of randomized trials of antiplatelet therapy: I. Prevention of death, myocardial infarction, and stroke by prolonged antiplatelet therapy in various categories of patients. BMJ 308:87–106, 1994.
6. Albrecht RF II, Wass TC, Lanier WL: Occurrence of potentially detrimental temperature alterations in hospitalized patients at risk for brain injury. Mayo Clin Proc 73:629–635, 1998.
7. Barnett HJM, Kaste M, Meldrum H, et al: Aspirin dose in stroke prevention: Beautiful hypotheses slain by ugly facts. Stroke 27:588–592, 1996.
8. Baron JC: Positron emission tomography studies in ischemic stroke. In Barnett HJM (ed): Stroke: Pathophysiology, Diagnosis, and Management, 2nd ed., New York, Churchill Livingstone, 1992.
9. Broderick J, Phillips S, Whisnant J, et al: Incidence rates of stroke in the eighties: The end of decline in stroke? Stroke 20:577–582, 1989.
10. Brott T, Reed AL: Intensive care for acute stroke in the community hospital setting. Stroke 20:694–697, 1989.
11. Brown MM: Balloon angioplasty for extracranial carotid disease. In Whittemore AD (ed): Advances in Vascular Surgery. Vol 4. St. Louis, Mosby–Year Book, 1996, pp 53–69.

12. Burger SK, Saul RF, Selhorst JB, et al: Transient monocular blindness caused by vasospasm. N Engl J Med 325:870–873, 1991.

13. Busto R, Dietrich ED, Globus MY-T, et al: Small differences in intraischemic brain temperature critically determine the extent of ischemic neuronal injury. J Cereb Blood Flow Metabol 7:729–738, 1987.

14. Canadian Cooperative Study Group: A randomized trial of aspirin and sulfinpyrazone in the threatened stroke. N Engl J Med 299:53–59, 1978.

15. Caplan LR: Diagnosis and treatment of ischemic stroke. JAMA 266:2413–2418, 1991.

16. CAPRIE Steering Committee: A randomised, blinded, trial of clopidogrel versus aspirin in patients at risk of ischaemic events (CAPRIE). Lancet 348:1329–1339, 1996.

17. Casper ML: The shifting stroke belt: Changes in the geographic pattern of stroke mortality in the United States, 1962 to 1988. Stroke 26:755–760, 1995.

18. Castillo J, Davalos A, Noya M: Progression of ischaemic stroke and excitotoxic amino acids. Lancet 349:79–83, 1997.

19. Cerebral Embolism Study Group: Immediate anticoagulation of embolic stroke: Brain hemorrhage and management options. Stroke 15:779–789, 1984.

20. Chamorro A, Vila N, Saiz A, et al: Early anticoagulation after large cerebral embolic infarction: A safety study. Neurology 45:861–865, 1995.

21. Chen ZM: CAST: Randomized placebo-controlled trial of early aspirin use in 20,000 patients with ischemic stroke. Lancet 349:1641–1649, 1997.

22. Cohen SN: Carotid endarterectomy for asymptomatic disease. J Stroke Cerebrovascular Disease 6:180–184, 1997.

23. Dastur DK, Singhal BS, Shroff HJ, et al: CNS involvement in malignant atrophic papulosis (Kohlmeier-Degos): Vasculopathy and coagulopathy. J Neurol Neurosurg Psychiatry 44:156–160, 1981.

24. Degos R, Delort J, Tricot R: Dermatite papulosquameuse atrophiante. Bull Soc Franc Dermatol Syph 49:148–150, 1942.

25. Del Zoppo GJ, Higashida RT, Furlan AJ, et al: PROACT: A phase II randomized trial of recombinant pro-urokinase by direct arterial delivery in acute middle cerebral artery stroke. Stroke 29:4–11, 1998.

26. Diener H, Cunha L, Forbes C, et al: European Stroke Prevention Study 2: Dipyridamole and acetylsalicylic acid in the secondary prevention of stroke. J Neurosci 143:1–13, 1996.

27. The Dutch TIA Trial Study Group: A comparison of two doses of aspirin (30 mg vs. 283 mg a day) in patients after a transient ischemic attack or minor ischemic stroke. N Engl J Med 325:1261–1266, 1991.

28. Dyken ML, Barnett HJM, Easton JD, et al: Low-dose aspirin and stroke: 'It ain't necessarily so.' Stroke 23:1395–1399, 1992.

28a. Enserink M: Fraud and ethics charges hit stroke drug trial. Science 274:2004, 1996.

29. ESPS Group: European Stroke Prevention Study. Stroke 21:1122–1130, 1990.

30. Executive Committee for the Asymptomatic Carotid Atherosclerosis Study: Endarterectomy for asymptomatic carotid stenosis. JAMA 273:1421–1428, 1995.

31. Firlik AD, Rubin G, Yonas H, et al: Relation between cerebral blood flow and neurologic deficit resolution in acute ischemic stroke. Neurology 51:177–182, 1998.

32. Fisher M, Bogousslavsky J: Further evolution toward effective therapy for acute ischemic stroke. JAMA 279:1298–1303, 1998.

33. Gaines K: Regional and ethnic differences in stroke in the southeastern United States population (Review). Ethn Dis 7:150–164, 1997.

34. Gould AL, Rossouw JE, Santanello NC, et al: Cholesterol reduction yields clinical benefit: Impact of statin trials. Circulation 97:946–952, 1998.

35. Hall P, Nakamura S, Maiello L, et al: A randomized comparison of combined ticlopidine and aspirin therapy versus aspirin therapy alone after successful intravascular ultrasound-guided stent implantation. Circulation 93:215–222, 1996.

36. Hanna JP, Sun JP, Furlan AJ, et al: Patent foramen ovale and brain infarct: Echocardiographic predictors, recurrence, and prevention. Stroke 25:782–786, 1994.

37. Hypervolemic hemodilution treatment of acute stroke: Results of a randomized multicenter trial using pentastarch. Stroke 20:1286–1287, 1989.

38. Hart RG, Harrison M JG: Aspirin wars: The optimal dose of aspirin to prevent stroke. Stroke 27:585–587, 1996.

39. Hass WK, Easton JD, Adams HD, et al: A randomized trial comparing ticlopidine hydrochloride with aspirin for the prevention of stroke in high-risk patients. N Engl J Med 321:501–507, 1989.

40. Hayman AL, Taber KH, Jhingran SG, et al: Cerebral infarction: Diagnosis and assessment of prognosis by using ^{123}IMP-SPECT and CT. AJNR Am J Nueroradiol 10:557–562, 1989.

41. Hobson RW II, Weiss DG, Fields WF, et al; for the Veterans Affairs Cooperative Study Group: Efficacy of carotid endarterectomy for asymptomatic carotid stenosis. N Engl J Med 328:221–227, 1993.

42. Homma S, Tullio MDR, Sacco RL, et al: Surgical closure of patent foramen ovale in cryptogenic stroke patients. Am Heart Assoc 28:2376–2381, 1997.

43. Howard G: Is the stroke belt disappearing? An analysis of racial, temporal, and age effects. Stroke 26:1153–1158, 1995.

44. Hughes RL: Carotid endarterectomy for the asymptomatic patient. J La State Med Soc 148:474–478, 1996.

45. Hughes RL, Smith D, Smith R, et al: Creation of a regional organization to support stroke resuscitation: The Colorado Acute Stroke Network (CASN) (Abstract). Stroke Cerebrovasc Dis 6:471, 1997.

46. Hughes RL, Yonas H, Gur D, et al: Cerebral blood flow determination within the first 8 hours of cerebral infarction using stable xenon-enhanced computed tomography. Stroke 20:754–760, 1989.

47. International Stroke Trial Collaborative Group: The International Stroke Trial (IST): A randomized trial of aspirin, subcutaneous heparin, both, or neither among 19,435 patients with acute ischemic stroke. Lancet 349:1569–1581, 1997.

48. Kopecky SL, Gersh BJ, McGoon MD, et al: The natural history of lone atrial fibrillation: A population-based study over 3 decades. N Engl J Med 317:669–674, 1987.

49. Krupski WC, Weiss DG, Rapp JH, et al: Adverse effects of aspirin in the treatment of asymptomatic carotid artery stenosis. J Vasc Surg 16:558–600, 1992.

50. Kumpe DA, Hughes RL: Thrombolytic therapy for acute stroke. In Whittemore AD (ed): Advances in Vascular Surgery, Vol 4. St. Louis, Mosby–Year Book, 1996, pp 71–96.

51. Lanska DJ, Kuller LH: The geography of stroke mortality in the United States and the concept of a stroke belt (Editorial). Stroke 26:1145–1149, 1995.

52. Libman R: Conditions that mimic stroke in the emergency department. Arch Neurol 52:1119–1122, 1995.

53. Lockshin MD: Antiphospholipid antibody: Babies, blood clots, biology. JAMA 277:1549–1551, 1997.

54. Low molecular weight heparinoid, ORG 10172 (danaparoid), and outcome after acute ischemic stroke: A randomized controlled trial. JAMA 279:1265–1272, 1998.

55. Luigi B, Luigi MF, Stefano B, et al: Early collateral blood supply and late parenchymal brain damage in patients with middle cerebral artery occlusion. Stroke 20:735–740, 1989.

56. Marion DW, Penrod LE, Kelsey SF, et al: Treatment of traumatic brain injury with moderate hypothermia. N Engl J Med 336:540–546, 1997.

57. Mayberg MR, Winn HR: Endarterectomy for asymptomatic carotid stenosis: Resolving the controversy. JAMA 73:1459–1461, 1995.

58. North American Symptomatic Carotid Endarterectomy Trial (NASCET) Collaborators: Beneficial effect of carotid endarterectomy in symptomatic patients with high-grade carotid stenosis. N Engl J Med 325:445–453, 1991.

59. The National Institute of Neurological Diseases and Stroke rt-PA Stroke Study Group: Tissue plasminogen activator for acute ischemic stroke. N Engl J Med 333:1581–1587, 1995.

60. The SPAF III Writing Committee for the Stroke Prevention in Atrial Fibrillation III Study: Patients with nonvalvular atrial fibrillation at low risk of stroke during treatment with aspirin. JAMA 279:1273–1277, 1998.

61. Pessin MS, Estol CJ, Lafranchise F, et al: Safety of anticoagulation after hemorrhagic infarction. Neurology 43:1298–1303, 1993.

62. Petit WA Jr, Soso MJ, Higman H, et al: Degos disease: Neurologic complications and cerebral angiography. Neurology 32:1305–1309, 1982.

63. Pickle LW, Mungiole M, Gillum RF, et al: Geographic variation in stroke mortality in blacks and whites in the United States (Review). Stroke 28:1639–1647, 1997.

64. Roberts KJ, Omarali I, Di Tullio MR, et al: Valvular strands and cerebral ischemia: Effect of demographics and strand characteristics. Stroke 28:2185–2188, 1997.

65. Sacks FM, Pfeffer MA, Moye LA, et al: Effect of provastatin on coronary events after myocardial infarction in patients with average cholesterol levels. N Engl J Med 335:1001–1009, 1996.

66. Sandercrock PAG, Van Den Belt AGM, Lindley RI, et al: Anti-thrombotic therapy in acute ischemic stroke: An overview of the completed randomized trials. J Neurol Neurosurg Psychiatry 56:17–25, 1993.
67. Schriger DL, Kalafut M, Starkman S, et al: Cranial computed tomography interpretation in acute stroke: Physician accuracy in determining eligibility for thrombolytic therapy. JAMA 279:1293–1297, 1998.
68. Simons Leon A, McCallum J, Friedlander Y, et al: Risk factors for ischemic stroke: Dubbo study of the elderly. Stroke 29:1341–1346, 1998.
69. Special Writing Group of the Stroke Council, American Heart Association: Guidelines for thrombolytic therapy for acute stroke: A supplement to the guidelines for the management of patients with acute ischemic stroke. Circulation 94:1167–1174, 1996.
70. Steering Committee of the Physicians' Health Study Research Group: Final report on the aspirin component of the ongoing Physicians' Health Study. N Engl J Med 321:129–135, 1989.
71. Stegmayr B: Stroke incidence and mortality correlated to stroke risk factors in the WHO MONICA Project: An ecological study of 18 populations. Stroke 28:1367–1374, 1997.
72. Stroke Prevention in Atrial Fibrillation Investigators: Bleeding during antithrombotic therapy in patients with atrial fibrillation: Stroke Prevention in Atrial Fibrillation Study. Arch Intern Med 156:409–416, 1996.
73. Stroke Prevention in Atrial Fibrillation Study. Stroke prevention in atrial fibrillation. Circulation 84:527–539, 1991.
74. Takano K, Carano RAD, Tatlisumak T, et al: Efficacy of intra-arterial and intravenous pro-urokinase in an embolic stroke model evaluated by diffusion-perfusion MRI. Neurology 50:870–875, 1998.
75. Tatu L, Moulin T, Bogousslavsky J, et al: Arterial territories of the human brain: Cerebral hemispheres. Neurology 50:1699–1708, 1998.
76. Taveras JM: Multiple progressive intracranial arterial occlusion: A syndrome of children and young adults. Am J Roentgenol 106:235, 1969.
77. Tiede DJ, Nishimura RA, Gastineau DA, et al: Modern management of prosthetic valve anticoagulation. Mayo Clin Proc 73:665–680, 1998.
78. Tong DC, Yenari MA, Albers GW, et al: Correlation of perfusion and diffusion weighted MRI with NIH SS score in acute ischemic stroke. Neurology 50:864–870, 1998.
79. UK-TIA Study Group. The United Kingdom Ischemic Attack (UK-TIA) aspirin trial: Final results. J Neurol Neurosurg Psychiatry 54:1044–1054, 1991.
80. Van Den Berg E, Lohmann N, Friedburg, et al: Report of general temporary anticoagulation in the treatment of cerebral and retinal ischemia. Vasa 26:222–227, 1997.
81. Von Kummer R, Allen KL, Holle R, et al: Acute stroke: Usefulness of early CT findings before thrombolytic therapy. Radiology 205:327–333, 1997.
82. Wass CT, Lanier WL, Hofer RE, et al: Temperature changes of > or = 1°C alter functional neurologic outcome and histopathology in a canine model of complete cerebral ischemia. Anesthesiology 83:325–335, 1995.
83. Welch GN, Loscalzo J: Homocysteine and atherothrombosis. N Engl J Med 338:1042–1050, 1998.
84. Welch KMA, Levine SR, Ewing JR: Viewing stroke pathophysiology: An analysis of contemporary methods. Stroke 17:1071–1077, 1986.
85. Wolf PA, Agostino RB, Belanger AJ, et al: Probability of stroke: A risk profile from the Framingham Study. Stroke 22:312–318, 1991.
86. Zweifler RM: Mild induced hypothermia following ischemic stroke via surface cooling and intravenous meperidine. J Stroke Cerebrovasc Dis 6:460, 1997.

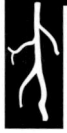

CHAPTER 1 2 9

Anatomy and Angiographic Diagnosis of Extracranial and Intracranial Vascular Disease

Larry-Stuart Deutsch, M.D., C.M., F.R.C.P. (C)

ARTERIAL ANATOMY: EXTRACRANIAL AND INTRACRANIAL VASCULAR SYSTEM

Aortic Arch and Its Branches

The surgical approach to the treatment of cerebrovascular disease requires an understanding of the vascular anatomy that begins with the aortic arch and ends with the principal intracranial arteries. The normal aortic arch curves smoothly upward into the superior mediastinum, running from right to left and anterior to posterior, with its apex at approximately the mid-manubrium. It passes to the left of the trachea, arching over the pulmonary artery bifurcation and the left mainstem bronchus, descending to the left of

the esophagus. The ligamentum arteriosum, the fibrous remnant of the fetal ductus arteriosus. tethers the concave undersurface of the aortic arch to the proximal left main pulmonary artery, attaching at a point usually just distal to the left subclavian artery.

In approximately 95% of all individuals, the aortic arch gives rise to three major branches: the right brachiocephalic trunk (formerly designated the innominate artery), the left common carotid artery, and the left subclavian artery (Fig. 129–1). One of the most common variants is a common ostial origin of the brachiocephalic and left common carotid arteries, which occurs in approximately 10% of individuals and has been termed a "bovine trunk" because of its occurrence in that animal. However, a true trunk of more than a few millimeters in length that then divides into the right brachiocephalic and left common carotid arteries is

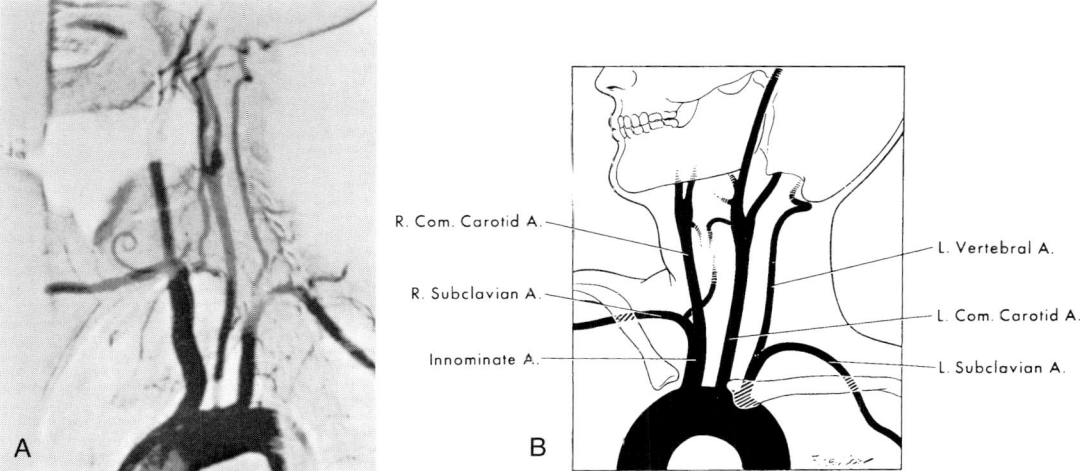

FIGURE 129–1. *A,* An arch aortogram demonstrating the three primary branches of the aortic arch: the innominate artery, the left common carotid artery, and the left subclavian artery. *B,* Artist's concept of an arch aortogram illustrating the three primary branches of the aortic arch and their pertinent anatomic relationships.

relatively rare. Origination of the left vertebral artery directly from the aorta proximal to the left subclavian artery is another common anatomic variant, occurring in approximately 5% of individuals (Fig. 129–2).

True anomalies of the aortic arch are actually rare, present in less than 2% of adults. Anomalies, such as double aortic arch; interrupted arch; right-sided arch, especially the mirror image branching form; and cervical arch, are often associated with complex congenital heart disease. Symptoms caused by pressure on the trachea or esophagus often require surgical correction in neonates or children. Because routine surgical correction of such anomalies is

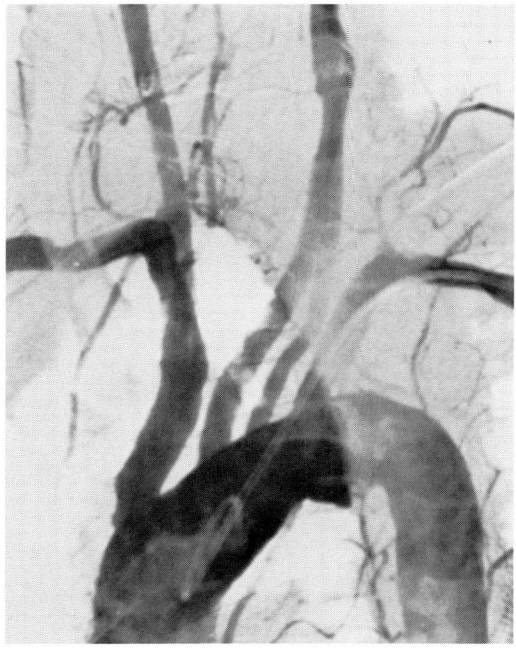

FIGURE 129–2. Arch aortogram obtained using an arterial catheter inserted via the left subclavian artery. Visualization of the primary branches of the aortic arch demonstrates that the left vertebral artery originates from the arch between the left common carotid and the left subclavian arteries.

relatively recent, few of these patients have reached adulthood, when they would be subject to the most common cerebrovascular disease, atherosclerosis. Indeed, even when these patients eventually do develop clinically significant cerebrovascular atherosclerosis, it is most likely to be simple carotid bifurcation disease requiring a standard surgical thromboendarterectomy, although the angiographic evaluation may be challenging.

The most common aortic arch anomaly compatible with long-term survival is the aberrant right subclavian artery that originates from the proximal descending thoracic aorta and passes posterior to the esophagus (Fig. 129–3). Unless this anomaly causes dysphagia in the neonatal period, it may escape detection until the patient is examined angiographically later in life. A diverticulum often accompanies the origin of an aberrant right subclavian artery, called Kommerelli's diverticulum; it can become aneurysmal, with rupture or compressive symptoms. Simple right aortic arches with normal branching, uncomplicated right arches with mirror image branching, and mirror image arches associated with thoracic situs inversus are sufficiently uncommon that many surgeons and angiographers will never actually encounter a case even in a busy clinical practice.

Right Brachiocephalic Trunk (Innominate Artery)

The right brachiocephalic trunk (innominate artery) is the first major branch of the thoracic aorta and the largest of its branches. It originates in the superior mediastinum posterior to the mid-point of the sternal manubrium and passes superiorly and posteriorly for a distance of 4 to 6 cm, then bifurcates into the right common carotid and right subclavian arteries in the root of the neck posterior to the right sternoclavicular joint. Whereas the proximal segments of the other major branches of the aortic arch are usually relatively straight, the right brachiocephalic trunk and the proximal segments of the right common carotid and subclavian arteries are often rather tortuous in elderly patients. Such tortuosity, especially when it involves the

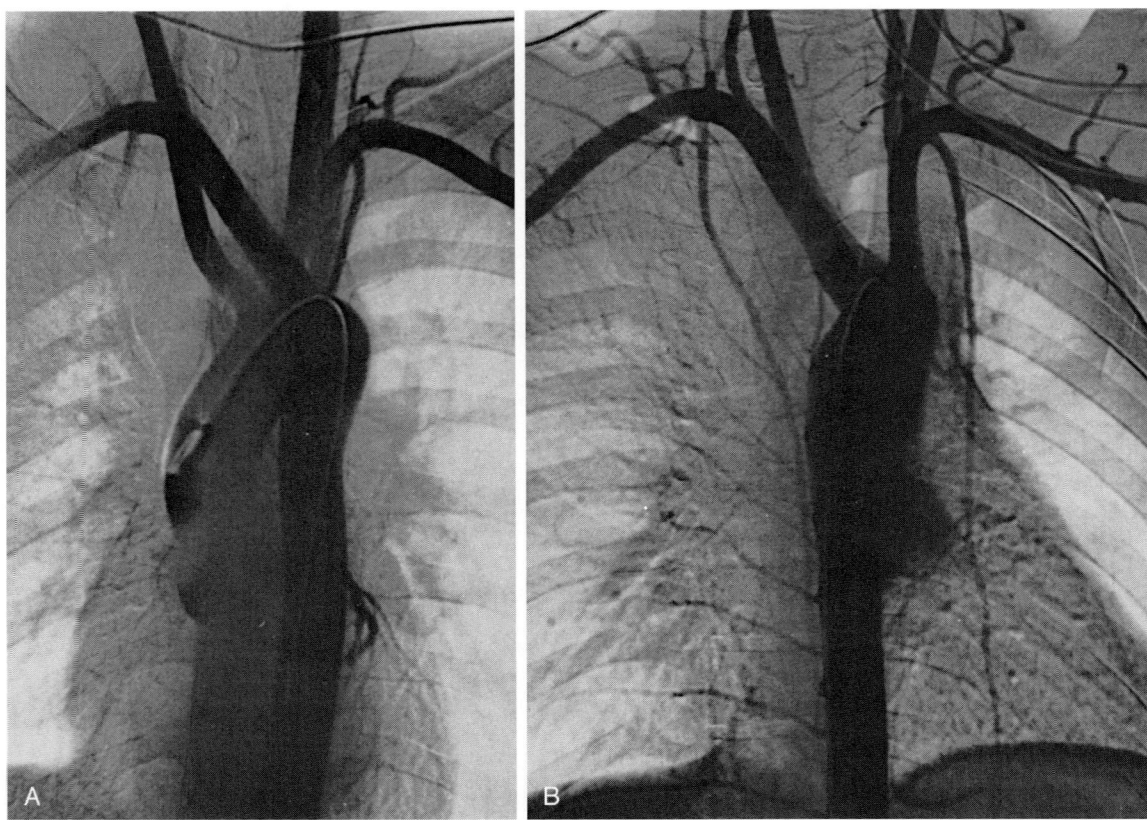

FIGURE 129–3. *A* and *B,* An arch aortogram demonstrating the first branch of the aortic arch to be an isolated right common carotid artery. An aberrant right subclavian artery originates just distal to the left subclavian artery and courses posterior to all of the other major branches of the aortic arch.

right subclavian artery at the base of the neck, often can mimic aneurysmal dilatation on physical examination and angiography.

Subclavian Arteries

The right subclavian artery originates from the right brachiocephalic trunk and arches laterally and posteriorly, passing behind the anterior scalene muscle. The left subclavian artery originates directly from the aorta and is usually its third branch. It ascends vertically within the mediastinum, then arches laterally in the root of the neck, also to pass behind the anterior scalene muscle. Both subclavian arteries pass immediately above the dome of the pleura. The principal branches of the subclavian arteries arise from the segment proximal to the medial border of the anterior scalen muscle and consist of the vertebral, internal mammary, thyrocervical, and costocervical arteries (Fig. 129–4).

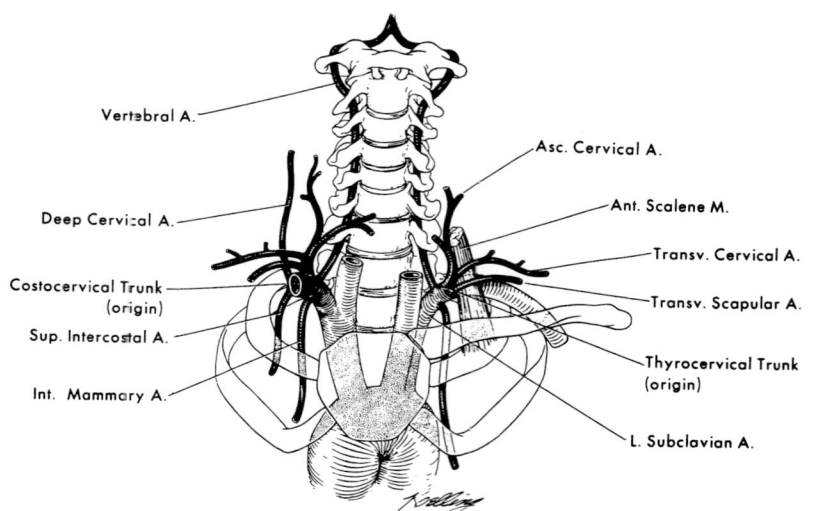

Vertebral A.

Deep Cervical A.

Costocervical Trunk (origin)

Sup. Intercostal A.

Int. Mammary A.

Asc. Cervical A.

Ant. Scalene M.

Transv. Cervical A.

Transv. Scapular A.

Thyrocervical Trunk (origin)

L. Subclavian A.

FIGURE 129–4. Artist's concept of the relationships of the subclavian arteries and their primary branches.

The vertebral and internal mammary arteries have a very constant relationship, originating directly opposite each other, with the vertebral artery arising from the cephalad aspect and the internal mammary artery arising from the anteroinferior aspect. The subclavian arteries then exit from the neck by passing over the superior surface of the first rib posterior to the clavicle, in close relationship to the lower portion of the brachial plexus. After they pass the lateral aspect of the first rib, these vessels are designated the axillary arteries. Although the vertebral artery is the primary subclavian branch that contributes to the cerebral circulation, the other branches may become important sources of collateral supply in the setting of vertebral artery stenoses.

Common Carotid Arteries

The right common carotid artery originates from the right brachiocephalic trunk in the base of the neck, whereas the left common carotid artery originates directly from the aortic arch in the mediastinum. However, the anatomy of the cervical segments is virtually identical on both sides (Fig. 129–5). The common carotid arteries ascend in the neck, running anterior to the transverse processes of the cervical vertebrae and separated from them by the anterior scalene, longus coli, and capitis muscles and by the sympathetic trunks. The common carotid artery usually bifurcates into the external and the internal carotid arteries near the superior horn of the thyroid cartilage (at approximately vertebrae C2–C3), although there is considerable variation in the level of this bifurcation. The carotid arteries bifurcate at the same level in only 28% of cases; in 50%, the left bifurcation is higher than the right one, whereas the reverse is present in the remaining 22%. Throughout their cervical course, the common and internal carotid arteries are en-

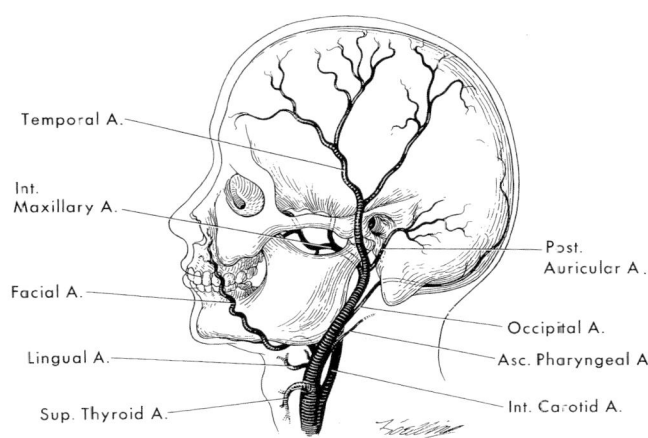

FIGURE 129–6. Artist's concept of the distribution of the external carotid artery with its major branches visualized.

closed in a fibrous sheath—deemed the carotid sheath, which also encompasses the internal jugular vein and the vagus nerve.

External Carotid Arteries

The external carotid artery is usually smaller than the internal carotid artery and originates anterior and medial to it, passing laterally to ascend just posterior to the ramus and neck of the mandible and superficial to the styloid process. It supplies the face, scalp, oronasopharynx, skull, and meninges through four major branch vessel groups: (1) anterior branches (superior thyroid, lingual, facial, transverse facial, (2) posterior branches (occipital and auricular), (3) ascending branches (ascending pharyngeal), and (4) terminal branches (superficial temporal, internal maxillary) (Fig. 129–6). These vessels are of significance to the cerebral circulation in the setting of carotid or vertebral artery occlusive disease, where they can become important sources of collateral blood supply.

One of the most common collateral routes involves distal anastomoses between the pterygopalatine branches of the internal maxillary artery and the ethmoidal branches of the ophthalmic artery system (Fig. 129–7). Other important collateral pathways include anastomoses between orbitonasal branches of the facial artery and orbital branches of the ophthalmic artery, anastomoses between anterior branches of the superficial temporal artery and ethmoidal branches of the ophthalmic artery, and anastomoses between ascending pharyngeal branches of the external carotid artery and muscular branches of the vertebral artery.

Internal Carotid Arteries

The internal carotid artery is divided into five major segments: carotid bulb, cervical, petrous, cavernous, and cerebral (Fig. 129–8). The *carotid bulb*, literally a focal bulbous dilation, is located at the origin of the internal carotid artery. It is a relatively constant feature, although its shape and size vary considerably among individuals. The *cervical* segment has no significant branches and ascends in the neck immediately anterior to the transverse processes of

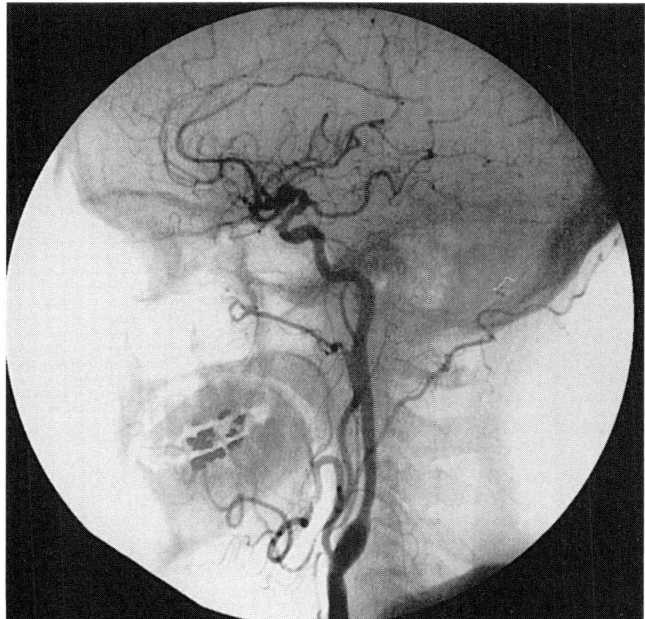

FIGURE 129–5. A selective injection of the left common carotid artery outlines the common carotid artery as it bifurcates into the internal and external carotid arteries within the mid-cervical region.

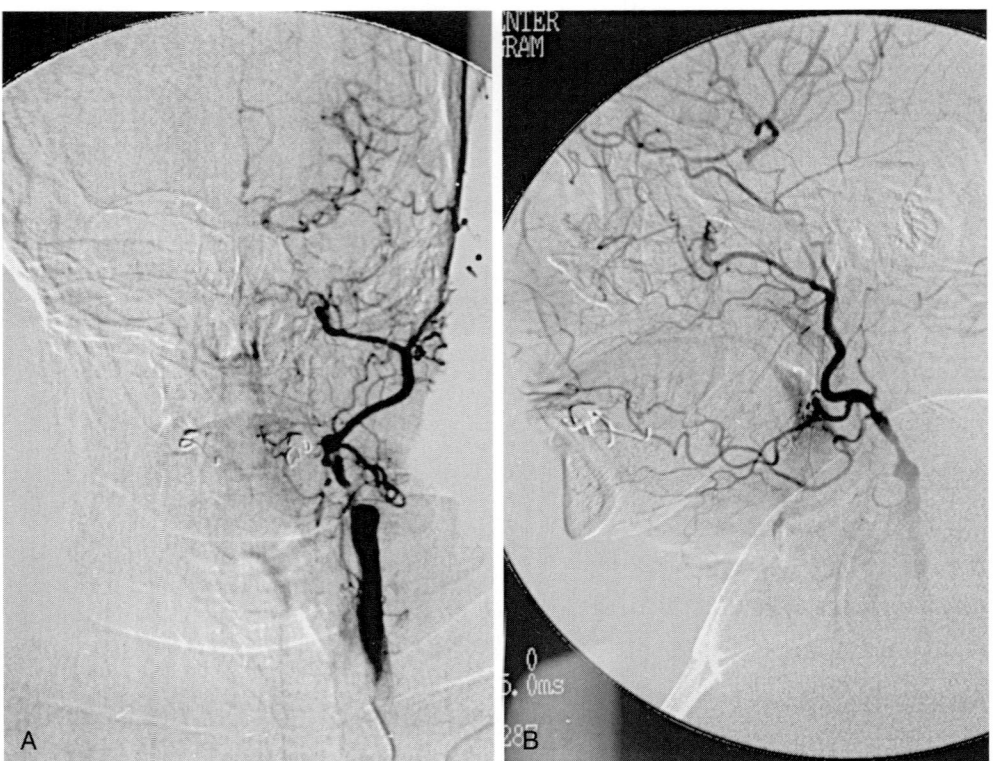

Figure 129–7. Anteroposterior AP (A) and lateral B) views of an angiogram showing occlusion of the left internal carotid artery at its origin, with filling of the intracranial carotid system via collateral vessels providing retrograde flow in the ophthalmic artery.

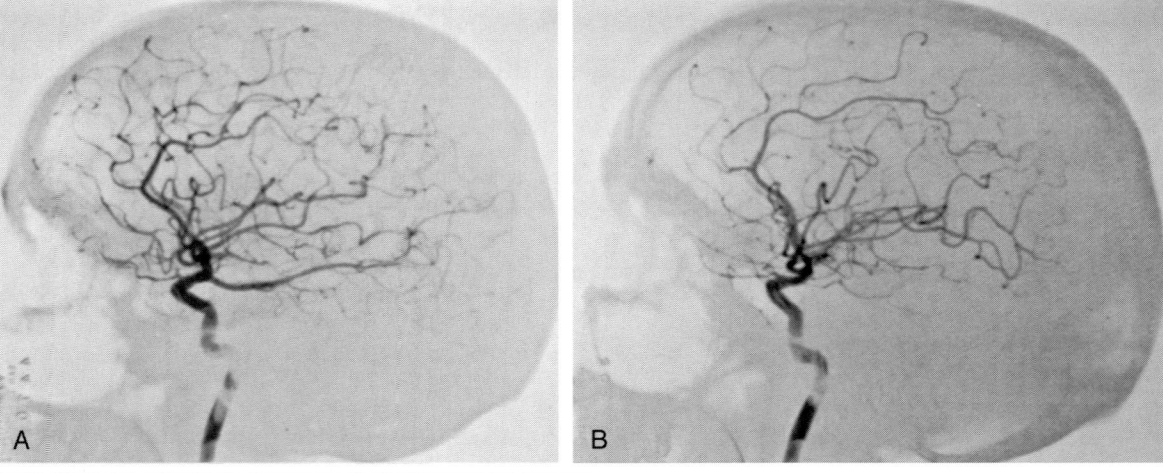

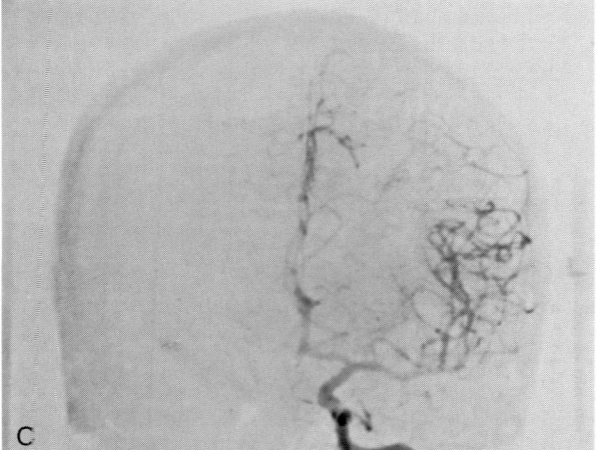

FIGURE 129–8. A, Left carotid arteriogram, shown in a lateral projection, demonstrating one variation, which is the primary takeoff of the posterior cerebral artery from the internal carotid artery. B, Right carotid arteriogram presented in a lateral projection and showing the terminal distribution into the anterior and middle cerebral branches. C, Anteroposterior projection of a left carotid arteriogram demonstrating filling of the anterior cerebral artery (ACA) in the midline and the branches of the middle cerebral artery (MCA) in the lateral or parietal region.

the cervical vertebrae and their associated muscles. The internal carotid artery then enters the skull via the carotid canal, traversing the *petrous* portion of the temporal bone in a slightly medial direction and separated from the middle ear structures by only a thin layer of bone. The petrous segment also has no major branches, although there are minor branches that anastomose with small pterygopalatine branches of the internal maxillary artery that can become sources of collateral supply in the setting of occlusive disease.

The *cavernous* segment of the internal carotid artery is called the carotid siphon because of its gentle, S-shaped configuration as it passes through the cavernous sinus along the sella turcica toward the anterior clinoid process. Along its course through the cavernous sinus it often indents the wall of the sphenoid sinus, sometimes separated from the sinus cavity by only dura and sinus mucosa. Although this segment has several minor branches, the ophthalmic artery is the cavernous segment branch of primary clinical significance since it can become an important collateral route to the intracranial circulation in the setting of extracranial occlusive disease of the internal carotid artery, and because hemodynamic or embolic phenomena can produce amaurosis fugax. Thus, the ophthalmic artery is the first branch of the internal carotid artery of major clinical importance.

The *cerebral* segment of the internal carotid artery is relatively short. After traversing the dura mater medial to the anterior clinoid process, it passes superolaterally to divide into the anterior and middle cerebral arteries.

Vertebral Arteries

The vertebral artery is the first branch of the subclavian artery. It takes a relatively straight course, entering the transverse foramen of C6 and passing cranially through the transverse foramina of C6–C1. Because the transverse foramen of the atlas is lateral to that of the axis, it passes laterally between the axis and the atlas. It then runs posteromedially along the arch of the atlas lateral to the atlanto-occipital joint. After passing the atlas, it turns sharply cephalad to enter the cranium via the foramen magnum. Within the skull, the paired vertebral arteries pass medially along the inferior surface of the brain stem to unite into a single midline vessel, the basilar artery (Fig. 129–9).

Although the carotid arteries are of similar size bilaterally, considerable asymmetry is frequent in the vertebral system, even including absence of one of the vertebral arteries. The left vertebral artery is dominant in approximately 50% of individuals, whereas the right one is dominant in 25%, and they are of roughly equal caliber in the remaining 25%. These variations are of little or no clinical significance except in cases of subclavian artery disease proximal to the vertebral origin. A moderate degree of tortuosity and smooth variation in caliber of the intracranial vertebral arteries is common even in young individuals and is also of no clinical significance.

The cervical portion of the vertebral arteries supplies multiple small segmental branches to the spinal cord, cervical vertebrae, and adjacent muscles. The anastomotic connections between these small vertebral artery branches and the occipital and ascending pharyngeal branches of the external carotid artery system form potential collateral

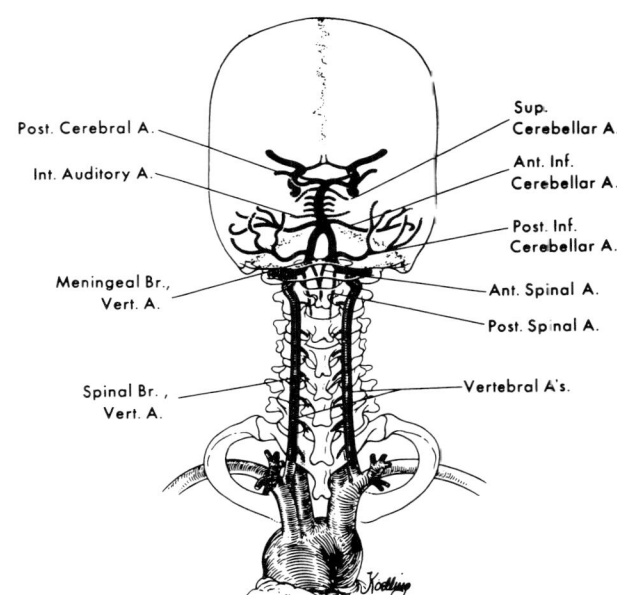

FIGURE 129–9. Artist's concept of the relationship of the vertebral arteries as they enter the root of the neck and ascend within the vertebral canal en route to joining at the brain stem to form the basilar artery. The significant cervical and cranial branches are labeled.

routes in the event of development of vertebral or carotid occlusive disease (Figs. 129–10, 129–11).

The intracranial portion of the vertebral artery gives rise to the anterior and posterior spinal arteries, the penetrating medullary arteries, and the complex posterior inferior cerebellar artery, which supplies the inferior surface of the cerebellum.

Basilar Artery

The basilar artery is a relatively short mid-line vessel formed by the union of the vertebral arteries along the inferior surface of the pons. It runs along the pons, dividing into the left and right posterior cerebral arteries. In its short course, it gives rise to several important paired sets of arteries, including the anterior inferior cerebellar arteries, the internal auditory arteries, multiple small pontine arteries, and the superior cerebellar arteries (Fig. 129–12). These branch vessels are important sources of blood supply to the brain and play important roles in the plethora of symptoms associated with vertebrobasilar insufficiency.

Middle Cerebral Artery

The middle cerebral artery (MCA) (Fig. 129–13) is generally larger in caliber than the anterior cerebral artery (ACA), and its initial segment forms a relatively straighter pathway from the internal carotid artery than the corresponding segment of the ACA. For this reason, most of the emboli originating in, or traversing, the carotid system lodge in branches of this vessel. The initial (M1) segment of the MCA is straight and runs laterally along the inferior surface of the anterior perforated substance of the brain toward the sylvian fissure, which separates the temporal lobe from the frontoparietal lobes. Numerous short, straight, vertical

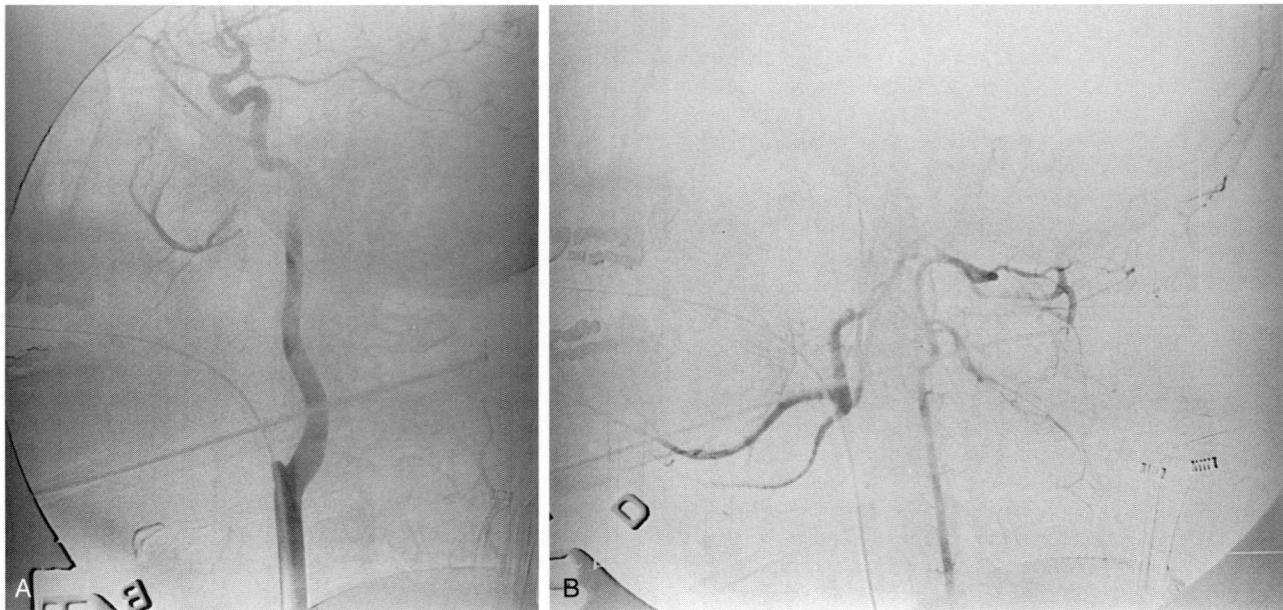

FIGURE 129–10. *A*, Carotid angiogram showing occlusion of the external carotid artery at its origin, with collateral flow to the internal maxillary artery system via orbital collaterals (not shown). *B*, Vertebral angiogram showing collateral flow to the external carotid artery system via anastomoses between deep muscular branches of the vertebral artery and the ascending pharyngeal artery and similar branches communicating with the occipital artery.

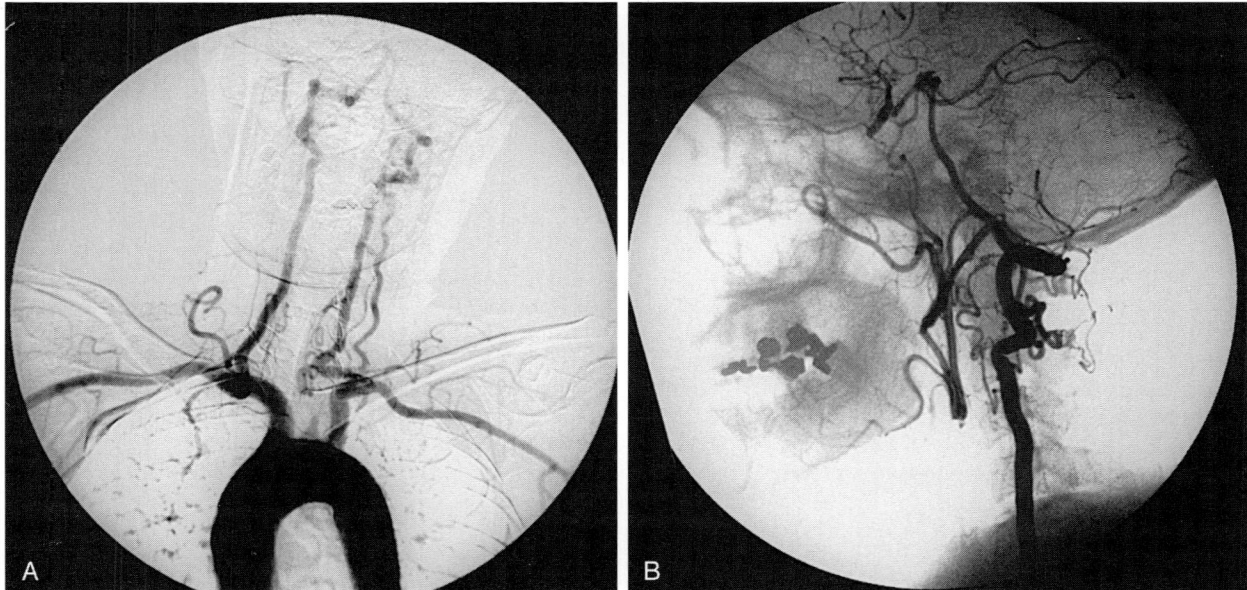

FIGURE 129–11. *A*, Thoracic aortogram showing total occlusion of both the right and left common carotid arteries. *B*, Selective injection of the right vertebral artery shows extensive collateral supply to the right external carotid artery via cervical branches of the vertebral artery. These vessels are normally so small that they are not routinely visualized on angiography. The large size of the vessels indicates that the occlusion is chronic, as it takes weeks to months for such small vessels to dilate to their present size. The intracranial portions of the right internal carotid artery fill via the posterior communicating artery, a key part of the circle of Willis. Although not documented by selective angiography, the collateral supply pattern is similar on the patient's left side.

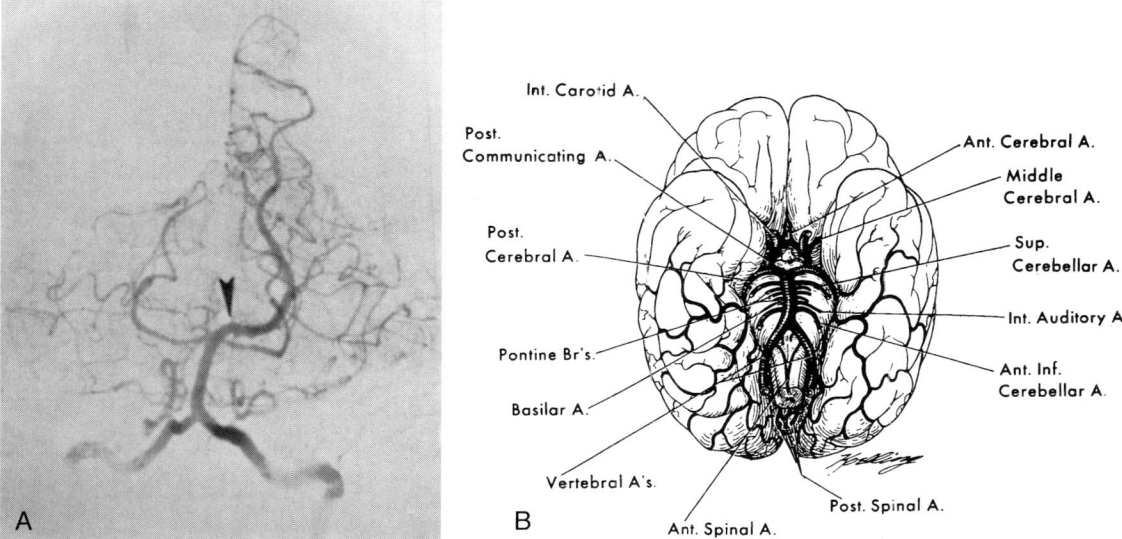

FIGURE 129–12. *A,* Vertebral-basilar arteriogram demonstrating the confluence of both vertebral arteries as they form the basilar artery running along the brain stem. Note that on the left side the basilar artery terminates in the posterior cerebral artery, but on the right side the terminal branch is the right superior cerebellar artery. This occurred because the right posterior cerebral artery originated from the carotid artery in this patient. *B,* Artist's concept of the relationship of the vertebral-basilar system to the brain stem. All the major branches of the terminal vertebral arteries and the extent of the basilar arteries are named.

lenticulostriate arteries arise from this segment to supply the basal ganglia and adjacent structures. The MCA branches in the sylvian fissure; its branches bend upward to run over the surface of the insula, then turn inferiorly again to emerge onto the cortical surfaces of the temporal and frontoparietal lobes. This pathway forms a characteristic, upwardly convex "genu," or knee-like curvature.

Although there is considerable variation in the course of the MCA branches as they emerge from the sylvian fissure, they form three general groups: (1) the anterior temporal artery; (2) the anterior group, including the orbitofrontal and operculofrontal arteries; and (3) the posterior group, including the posteroparietal, angular, and posterior temporal arteries. Although extracranial-intracranial (EC-IC) bypass procedures have fallen out of favor because of the unfavorable report of the EC/IC Bypass Study group in 1985 (see Chapter 135), these MCA branches do provide a fortuitously convenient bypass pathway because of their accessibility on the surface of the brain and the close proximity of the overlying superficial temporal artery branches of the external carotid system.

Anterior Cerebral Artery

The ACA begins at the bifurcation of the internal carotid artery (Fig. 129–14). Its initial segment is the short, straight (A1) segment that runs anteromedially just above the optic chiasm. Several medial lenticulostriate arteries originate from this segment. The A1 segment communicates with its

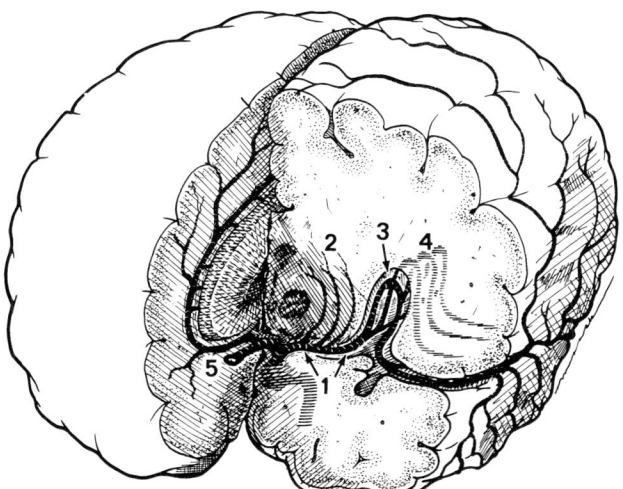

FIGURE 129–13. Artist's concept showing the relationship of the MCA to adjacent structures (the sylvian fissure has been exaggerated to emphasize that the MCA loops over the insula). 1, M1 (horizontal) segment. The "genu" is the upward curve of the MCA branches into the sylvian fissure. 2, Lateral lenticulostriate arteries. 3, Sylvian fissure. 4, MCA branches within the depths of the sylvian fissure. 5, ACA. (From Osborn AG: Introduction to Cerebral Angiography. Hagerstown, Md, Harper & Row, 1980.)

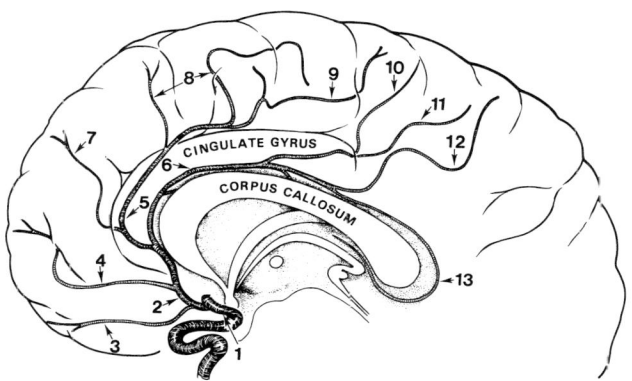

FIGURE 129–14. Artist's concept showing the relationship of the ACA to adjacent structures. 1, A1 (horizontal) segment. 2, ACA in front of lamina terminalis. 3, Orbitofrontal artery. 4, Frontopolar artery. 5, Callosomarginal artery. 6, Pericallosal artery. (From Osborn AG: Introduction to Cerebral Angiography. Hagerstown, Md, Harper & Row, 1980.)

opposite counterpart across the interhemispheric fissure via the short but important anterior communicating artery, the anterior component of the circle of Willis. A reciprocal size relationship between the A1 segment and the anterior communicating artery is common; a relatively hypoplastic A1 segment is usually accompanied by a large-caliber anterior communicating artery. In such cases, both ACAs are preferentially dependent on a single internal carotid system and thus are especially sensitive to flow disturbances and other abnormalities in the corresponding carotid artery.

Beyond the origin of the anterior communicating artery, the ACA turns abruptly upward to pass around the genu of the corpus callosum. As it passes the genu, it gives rise to the pericallosal artery, which runs posteriorly along the superior surface of the corpus callosum, and the callosomarginal artery, which runs along the cingulate sulcus roughly parallel to the pericallosal artery. The branches of these vessels supply the inner aspects of the frontal and parietal cortex in the interhemispheric fissure and end by passing over the superior margins of the interhemispheric fissure to supply a small band of cortical tissue along the anterior two thirds of the frontal and parietal lobes. Although the ACA and its branches are of considerable functional significance, they are largely inaccessible to the vascular surgeon because of their location deep within the interhemispheric fissure.

Circle of Willis

The circle of Willis is a unique vascular ring that encircles the diencephalon, including the sella turcica and pituitary. The A1 segments of the ACAs and the anterior communicating artery form the anterior portion of the ring and connect the internal carotid systems with each other. The short posterior communicating arteries originate from the internal carotid arteries at or near the bifurcation into anterior and middle cerebral arteries. The posterior communicating arteries run posteriorly to connect with the corresponding proximal segments of the posterior cerebral arteries (PCAs), thus connecting the internal carotid system, which is the anterior circulation, with the vertebral-basilar system, which is the posterior circulation (Fig. 129–15).

The circle of Willis, as described, effectively forms an arterial manifold that balances the inflow coming from the internal carotid and vertebral arteries with the outflow to the anterior, middle, and posterior cerebral arteries (see Fig. 129–11). However, only 20% of individuals actually have the "textbook" symmetric circle of Willis; hypoplasia of one or more components occurs in most individuals. Hypoplasia, or absence of one or both posterior communicating arteries, occurs in approximately 25% to 30% of cases, thus effectively isolating the anterior and posterior circulations. Anomalies of the anterior communicating artery, including hypoplasia, absence, or duplication, occur in approximately 10% of individuals. Hypoplasia of the A1 segments occurs in approximately 25% of cases, making both ACA systems preferentially dependent on a single internal carotid artery. Hypoplasia of the initial (P1) segment of the PCA, with primary or sole flow to the PCA via an enlarged posterior communicating artery from the internal carotid artery, occurs in approximately 15% to 20% of cases and is termed a fetal origin. Persistence of additional fetal communications between the carotid and the verte-

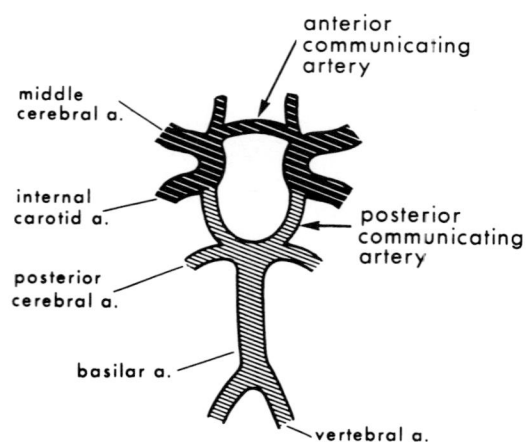

FIGURE 129–15. The classic intact circle of Willis forms a distribution manifold balancing the anterior (*dark shading*) inflow with the posterior (*light shading*) inflow; however, many variations occur, and the circle is often incomplete.

bral-basilar systems, including the trigeminal, otic, hypoglossal, and proatlantal intersegmental arteries, also occurs but is relatively rare.

The frequency of variations in the textbook arrangement of the circle of Willis often explains seemingly paradoxical ischemic or embolic neurovascular abnormalities. Such variations are also of considerable practical clinical significance because they imply that existence of the textbook collateral routes cannot be simply assumed before surgical interventions such as carotid endarterectomy are undertaken. Unless routine shunting is employed, adequate collateral supply must therefore be proved by preoperative angiography or intraoperative hemodynamic or electroencephalographic (EEG) monitoring or both. Even in the case of endovascular therapy, e.g., carotid artery angioplasty and stenting, with its very short inflation times and correspondingly short ischemic periods, knowledge of the collateral supply is essential for assessing procedural risk.

ANGIOGRAPHIC DIAGNOSIS AND TREATMENT

Noninvasive Alternatives to Cerebral Angiography

The surgical aphorism, "There is no such thing as a *little* operation," applies equally well to angiography and, indeed, to all invasive radiologic procedures. Although remarkably free of serious complications, angiography is not a simple laboratory test nor is it an inexpensive screening examination. Accordingly, the angiographer should function as a consultant specialist able to evaluate the indications and contraindications of the proposed procedure with regard to the patient's overall medical history and physical status, as well as the specific details of the present illness and the proposed treatment. Furthermore, the angiographer should also be able to provide guidance in the selection of appropriate noninvasive imaging prior to, or instead of, angiography.

Angiographic procedures, like surgical operations,

should also be tailored to the needs of the individual patient. Thus, optimal patient care involves a consultative relationship between the angiographer and the referring physician; angiography should not be "ordered" like a routine laboratory test. Furthermore, if the proposed therapy is surgical in nature, a surgeon should be involved in the patient's care prior to angiography. Conversely, basic risk/benefit analysis also suggests that there are few indications for angiography when surgical therapy is not contemplated.

The approach to investigation and management of intracranial vascular lesions has changed significantly over the past decade, largely as a result of dramatic advances in imaging technology. High-resolution x-ray computed tomography (CT) and magnetic resonance imaging (MRI) have virtually replaced angiography as primary diagnostic modalities. Nuclear medicine brain scanning for the investigation of mass lesions has been all but eliminated, whereas the radioisotope cerebral perfusion study has become an essential tool in the determination of brain death (Fig. 129–16, 129–17). Positron emission tomography (PET) scanning, with its ability to image and quantify regional metabolic function, now offers even greater insights, although at present the high cost and limited availability relegate PET scanning to a research tool.

Similarly, the approach to the investigation and management of extracranial cerebrovascular disease has also changed considerably. Noninvasive duplex Doppler screening evaluations of the cervical carotid circulation can now be performed effectively and inexpensively using a combination of high-resolution gray scale ultrasound imaging, to delineate anatomic detail, and color-coded pulsed Doppler ultrasound scanning, to determine the hemodynamic sig-

nificance of lesions identified by anatomic imaging (Fig. 129–18). Power Doppler imaging, a relative newcomer to the noninvasive imaging arsenal, creates a two-dimensional color-coded flow map by using the integrated power of the Doppler spectrum, rather than mean Doppler frequency, and is thus inherently more sensitive to low-flow states. This makes it a very useful adjunct to the conventional duplex Doppler examination in differentiating nearly occlusive stenoses from total occlusions, one of the more challenging and clinically significant tasks in noninvasive carotid imaging. (See Chapter 130 for more details on the use of ultrasound techniques in the evaluation of cerebrovascular disease.)

Although supraorbital and transcranial Doppler ultrasound examinations provide information about the state of the intracranial portions of the carotid circulation, the circle of Willis, and some of the common collateral circulation pathways not evaluated by duplex Doppler scanning, these examinations have a far steeper learning curve than does duplex Doppler ultrasound and they are far more operator-dependent. Accordingly, whereas they are indeed used to advantage in some noninvasive vascular laboratories, they are not routinely available in most centers. Similarly, oculoplethysmography, once a common examination, has been largely replaced by duplex Doppler scanning.

MRI is yet another noninvasive imaging technique that shows promise for use in evaluating the cerebrovascular circulation because of its inherent sensitivity to blood flow. By varying pulse sequences and signal sampling methods, images can be created that exploit various aspects of the differences between the physical properties of blood, especially flowing blood, and adjacent tissues.

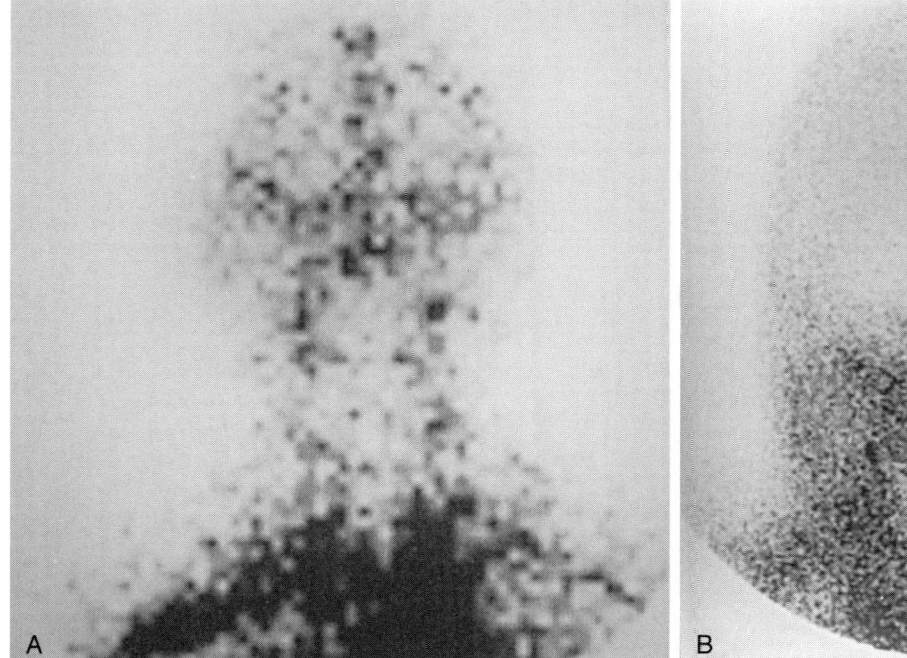
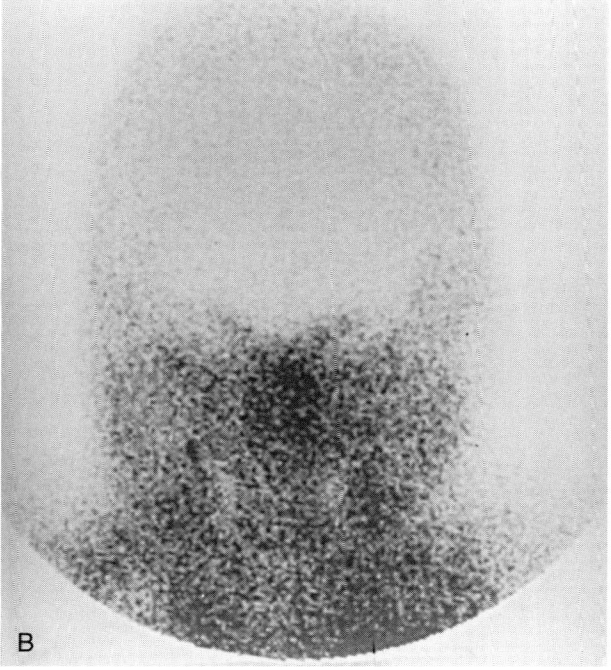

FIGURE 129–16. A, Normal isotope brain flow study showing filling of the internal carotid, anterior cerebral, and middle cerebral arteries. The relative paucity of flow to the facial regions is simply a reflection of preferential flow to the intracranial circulation. B, Abnormal isotope brain flow study with no detectable flow in the area of the anterior or middle cerebral arteries, indicating ischemic brain death, associated with severe cerebral edema. Increased isotope activity in the facial regions represents increased flow in the external carotid artery branches, which fill preferentially because there is no longer any significant flow to the intracranial vessels. (Courtesy of Felix Wang, M.D., Nuclear Medicine Section, University of California, Irvine Medical Center, Orange, Calif.)

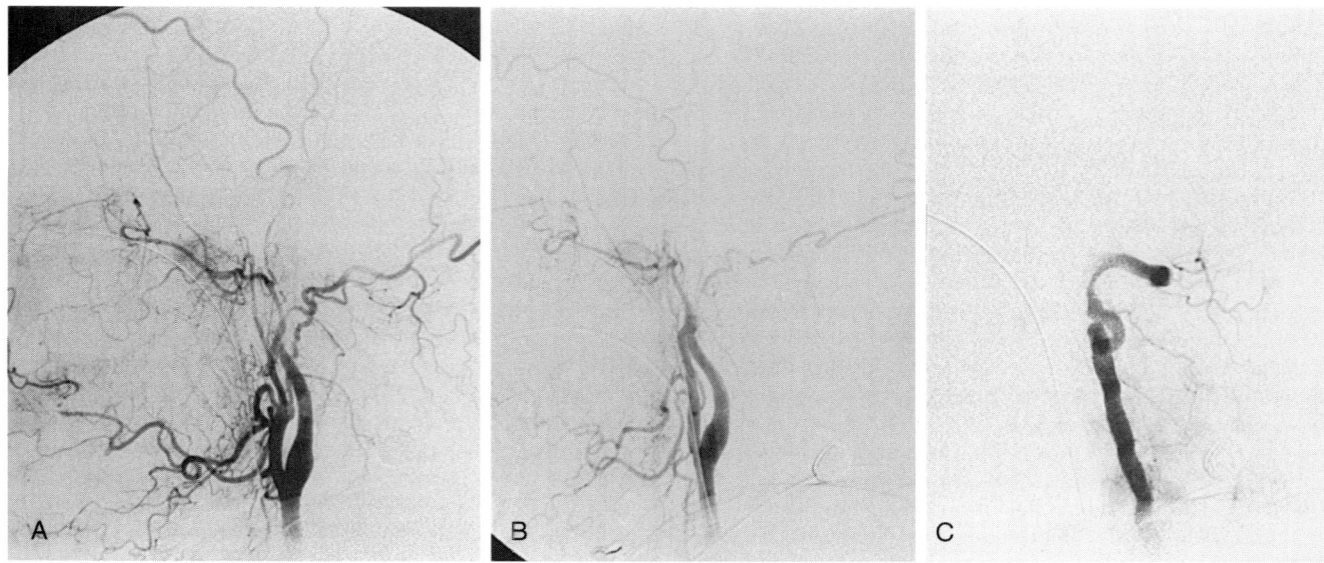

FIGURE 129–17. Angiograms of a 30-year-old female patient with intracranial hemorrhage that was thought to be due to a ruptured aneurysm or AVM. The patient was on a respirator and being maintained in barbiturate coma to minimize brain injury, which masked the occurrence of brain death. The angiogram shows no intracranial blood flow via (*A*) right internal carotid artery, (*B*) left internal carotid artery, or (*C*) left vertebral artery. (Courtesy of David D. Kidney, M.D., Vascular and Interventional Radiology Section, University of California, Irvine Medical Center, Orange, Calif.)

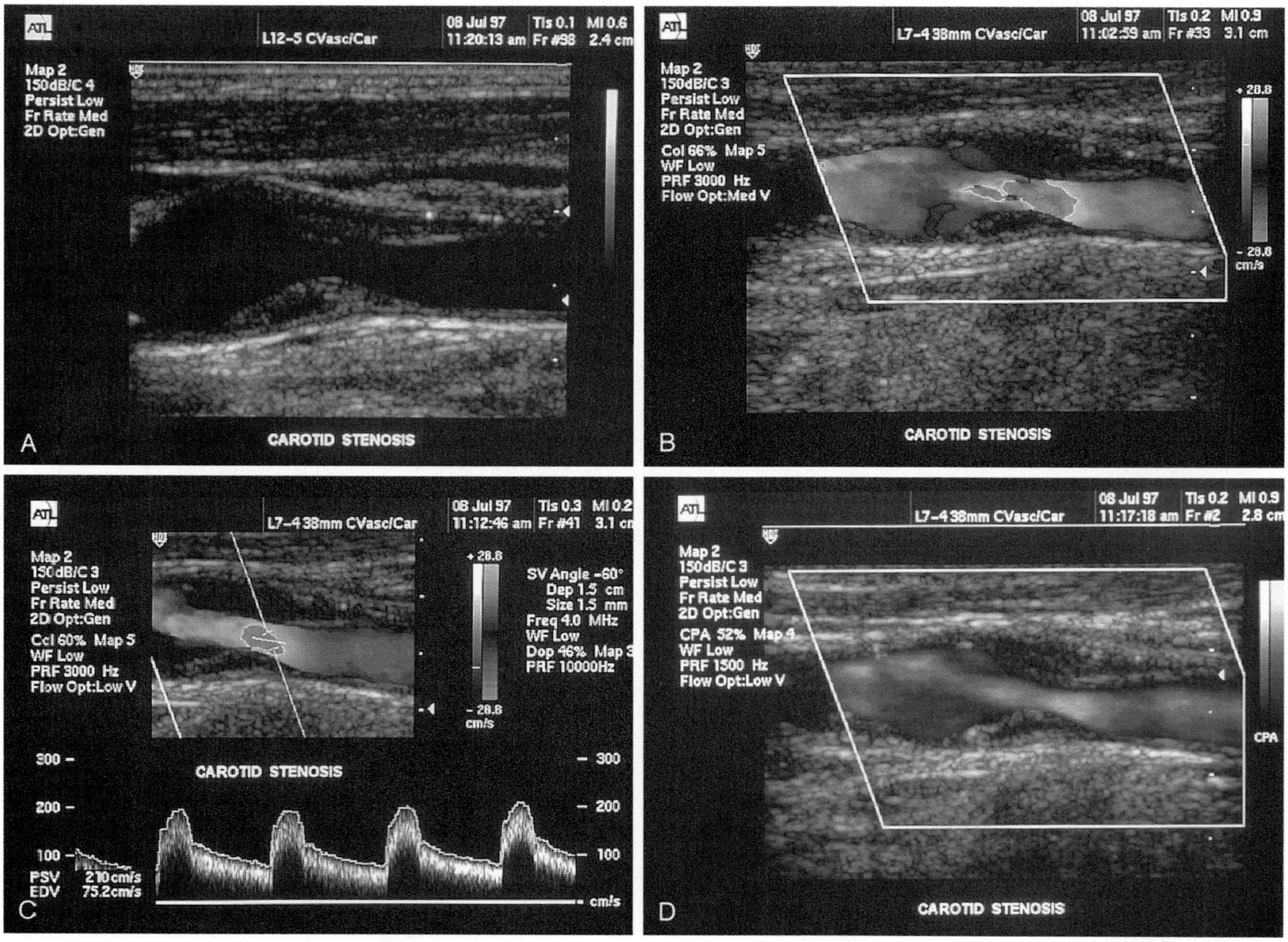

FIGURE 129–18. Ultrasound examination of the carotid artery. *A*, Gray scale view of stenosis. *B*, Color flow Doppler image of the same stenosis. *C*, Doppler flow velocity measurements used to grade the approximate severity of the stenosis. *D*, Power Doppler image of the same stenosis. See Color Plate for *B–D*. (Courtesy of ATL—Advanced Technology Laboratories, Bothell, Wash.)

Although most magnetic resonance angiography (MRA) techniques rely on the inherent differences between the physical properties of blood, especially flowing blood, and adjacent tissues, some methods also employ the use of intravenously injected contrast agents, exploiting differences in magnetic properties rather than x-ray absorption properties, as in the case of conventional angiographic contrast agents. Mathematically "stacking" multiple closely spaced cross-sectional "slice" images of a body region permits two- and three-dimensional depiction of vessels that can then be displayed in many different formats, some of which closely resemble conventional contrast angiograms (Fig. 129–19). However, it is important to remember that the physical basis of MRA is very different from that of conventional contrast angiography.

Factors affecting MRA image quality include flow direction, velocity, vessel size, turbulence (chaotic flow), vortices (localized areas of direction reversal), boundary layer flow separation, pulsatility, elasticity, capacitance, and peripheral impedance. Vessel tortuosity, as well as the intravascular disturbances of flow encountered in the region of a lesion such as a carotid bifurcation stenosis, includes complex and unpredictable combinations of most of these flow phenomena, leading to imaging artifacts that can be difficult to evaluate. Accordingly, although MRA is rapidly becoming a very sophisticated technique capable of impressive image quality, its utility as a screening technique remains to be determined. Nevertheless, one need only look at the incredible progress in MRI technology achieved since the crude images of orange slices and cadaver mice abdomens shown so proudly by MRI researchers in the early 1980s to appreciate the potential of this technology in the area of vascular imaging.

CT in the form of CT angiography (CTA) also can be applied to the task of noninvasive extracranial cerebrovascular examination (Fig. 129–20). Like MRA, it also employs the mathematical manipulation of multiple, closely spaced, cross-sectional "slice" images to reconstruct two-dimensional and three-dimensional depictions of vessels. Unlike many MRA techniques, most of which do not involve the administration of intravenous contrast media, CTA techniques do require the use of iodinated contrast agents of the same sort as those used for conventional angiography.

As the physics of CT imaging is essentially the same as that employed in conventional angiography (i.e., transmission x-ray absorption), the interpretation of CTA images and the understanding of artefacts is generally more straightforward than the interpretation of MRA images. However, although the artefacts due to the physics of CTA imaging are less troublesome than those of MRA, still significant artefacts can be introduced by the computational process used to assemble the displays.

Although there are definite differences in the applicability, sensitivity, specificity, spatial resolution, and ability to provide physiologic information, the ultimate choice of which noninvasive modality (ultrasound, MRA, or CTA) to employ is determined by technical factors, economics, and availability. Ultrasound currently has taken a commanding lead as a first-line noninvasive screening and evaluation modality, simply because of its relatively low cost and widespread availability.

Indications and Contraindications for Cerebral Angiography

The choice of whether to rely on noninvasive testing or angiography in the investigation and management of pa-

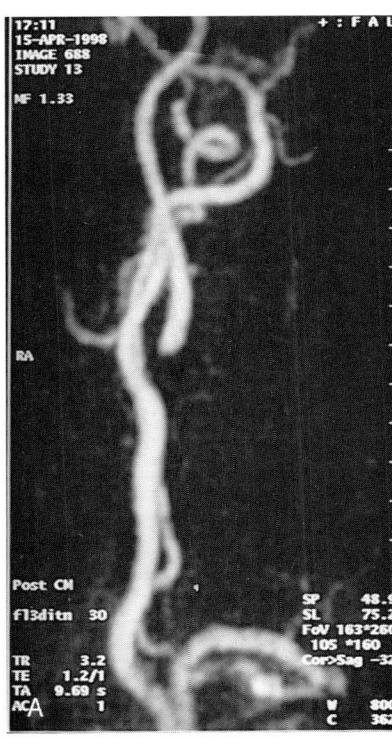
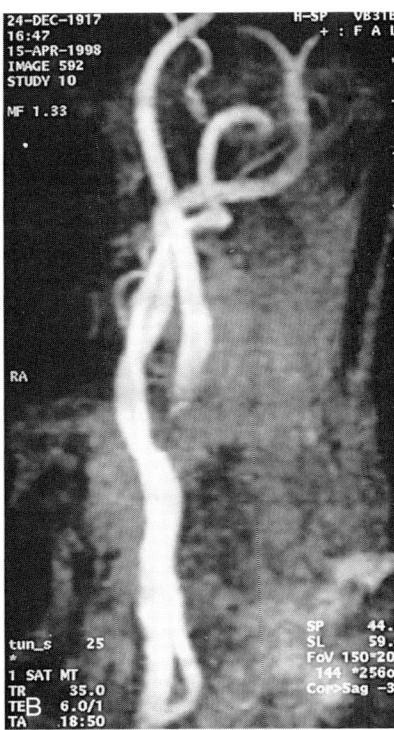

FIGURE 129–19. Magnetic resonance imaging (MRI) images of a near-occlusive internal carotid artery stenosis. *A* was acquired in 18 minutes using conventional time-of-flight technique (3D-TOF). *B* was acquired in 10 seconds using the newly developed first-pass gadolinium intravenous contrast-enhanced pass technique. Surgery was performed without further diagnostic imaging. (Courtesy of William G. Bradley, M.D., Long Beach Memorial Magnetic Resonance Imaging Center, Long Beach, Calif.)

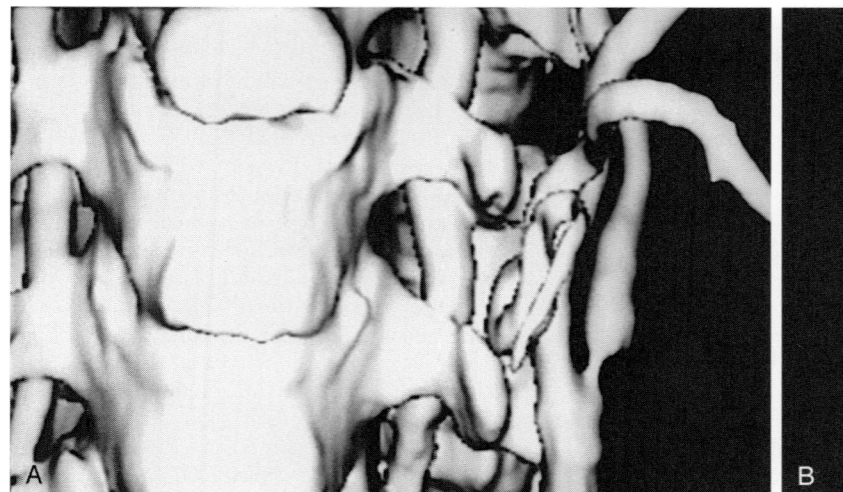
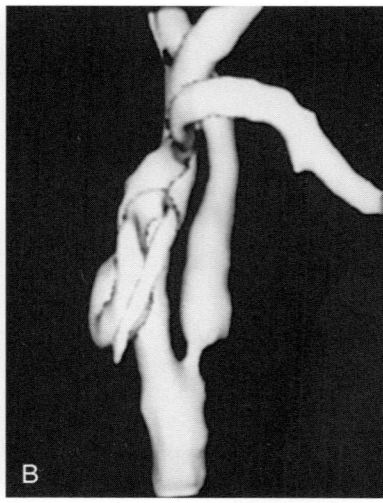

FIGURE 129-20. Three-dimensional images of a CT angiographic (CTA) study showing high-grade proximal left internal carotid artery stenosis with *A*, surrounding structures and with *B*, those structures removed by computer processing. (Courtesy of GE Medical Systems, Milwaukee, Wisconsin.)

tients with cerebrovascular lesions depends largely on the question of lesion type, location, and symptoms, together with local resources and expertise.

The incidence of asymptomatic nonvascular lesions of the intracranial central nervous system (e.g., tumors) is sufficiently low that routine noninvasive screening is rarely warranted. However, with the exception of systemic conditions known to be associated with intracranial vascular lesions such as the Osler-Weber-Rendu syndrome and carotid artery fibromuscular dysplasia, the true incidence of asymptomatic intracranial vascular lesions (e.g., arteriovenous malformations [AVMs] and aneurysms) is not well known. Generally, however, such patients do not come to medical attention until they have become symptomatic, often in a catastrophic manner associated with intracranial hemorrhage. In such patients, CT or MRI scanning is often useful as a guide to planning angiographic investigation, but prompt angiography is the definitive procedure for establishing the diagnosis and planning therapy.

In any event, noninvasive (CT and MRI) delineation and characterization of symptomatic intracranial mass lesions is generally so reliable that angiography is used primarily as a tool in planning or administering therapy rather than as a purely diagnostic tool. In the case of surgically treatable, intracranial lesions, mapping of the associated vascular supply and drainage can be vital to a successful outcome. Occasionally, transcatheter embolization of feeding vessels is a useful adjunct to surgery. For intracranial lesions not amenable to surgical treatment, angiographic embolization or regional infusion of chemotherapeutic agents may provide effective treatment for a number of benign and malignant lesions. Indeed, with recent advances in the microcatheter technologies, the endovascular approach to the treatment of AVMs and aneurysms is rapidly becoming the method of choice rather than surgical clipping or resection.

The ideal strategy to use in determining the relative roles of noninvasive testing and angiography when dealing with extracranial cerebrovascular disease is still controversial, although much of the intellectual dust has begun to settle. Angiographic *screening* of asymptomatic individuals even in specific high-risk groups is now unjustifiable, because the low cost, accuracy, and widespread availability of ultrasound examination make this noninvasive modality the logical choice for the initial imaging evaluation of asymptomatic patients. Unlike intracranial vascular lesions, asymptomatic extracranial lesions, specifically hemodynamically significant carotid stenoses, occur with sufficient frequency that selective noninvasive screening is reasonable in specific at-risk patient populations. Ultrasound techniques permit relatively inexpensive screening of asymptomatic patients in groups identified to be at risk for developing cerebrovascular symptoms by several prospective randomized studies.

The appropriate imaging evaluation for symptomatic patients, however, remains controversial. Many surgeons still lack confidence in the reliability of noninvasive testing, insisting on the "gold standard" of angiography before subjecting the patient to the risks of operative intervention. In contrast, many angiographers and surgeons feel that the risks of angiography, while admittedly low, do not justify adding the risks of preoperative angiography to those of the operative intervention when noninvasive imaging is able to provide an unequivocal diagnosis. When the noninvasive examination is either negative or equivocal in the face of appropriate symptoms and a high clinical index of suspicion, proceeding to contrast angiography is, at least for the present, the standard of care.

When a noninvasive modality is being chosen, selecting ultrasound, MRI, or CTA is a more complex issue and is largely a compromise between efficacy, cost, availability, and local expertise. Although ultrasound technology continues to progress, especially in the areas of automated error and artefact correction, as well as three-dimensional imaging, ultrasound is simply a more mature modality that MRA or CTA in which significant advances in quality and accuracy are likely in the near future.

The Basic Examination Plan

From the standpoint of the vascular surgeon, most angiography of the cerebrovascular system is performed for the evaluation of atheromatous (atherosclerotic) occlusive disease of the carotid system in the region of the carotid bifurcation because this is the most common location of this very common disease. Nevertheless, a complete examination must allow for the possibility that the disease process may not be confined to that region and that it may not even be atherosclerotic in nature.

Multi-view imaging and examination of the inflow and outflow are the basic principles in the angiographic evaluation of any vascular system. Therefore, a complete examination of the cerebrovascular system ideally should include delineation of the aortic arch origins of the great vessels and their major branches, the cervical and intracranial segments of the carotid and vertebral arteries, and the major intracranial branches of these vessels. This can be accomplished by first obtaining a nonselective arch aortogram to demonstrate the aortic arch origins of the great vessels and their major branches.

Omission of the preliminary nonselective aortic arch angiogram is unwise when investigating patients for occlusive vascular disease, even when selective angiography of the carotid arteries is planned. Ostial disease of the principal aortic arch branch vessels is sufficiently common that failure to detect such lesions prior to selective catheterization needlessly exposes patients to the risks of embolization associated with markedly irregular atheromatous plaques or cerebral ischemia associated with traversing high-grade stenoses (Fig. 129–21).

Failure to detect significant atherosclerotic lesions at the aortic origin of the great vessels, whether they be hemodynamically significant stenoses or sources of emboli, also exposes patients to the risk of undergoing operative procedures that may not fully address the cause of their problems. In addition, the aortogram serves as a road map for use in selective catheterization of the right and left common carotid arteries, which should then be examined at least to the level of the intracranial carotid bifurcation. Whether selective vertebral artery angiography or more detailed views of the intracranial circulation are also obtained depends on the specifics of the clinical situation.

Several variations of the basic examination have gained wide acceptance. High-quality, nonselective, biplanar oblique arch aortograms showing the cerebrovascular system from the level of the aortic arch to the level of the proximal major intracranial branches are often sufficient to evaluate the extracranial occlusive disease of the cerebrovascular system. Such examinations are usually adequate for the evaluation of atherosclerotic occlusive disease, because significant atherosclerotic disease distal to the carotid siphon is relatively uncommon, although disease at that level is not uncommon. Obviously, both carotid bifurcations must be well demonstrated; otherwise, the examination should be supplemented by selective angiography of one or both carotid arteries. Disease of the vertebral-basilar system may also require supplemental selective angiography with views designed to show the vertebral-basilar junction. Because the basilar artery is formed by the union of

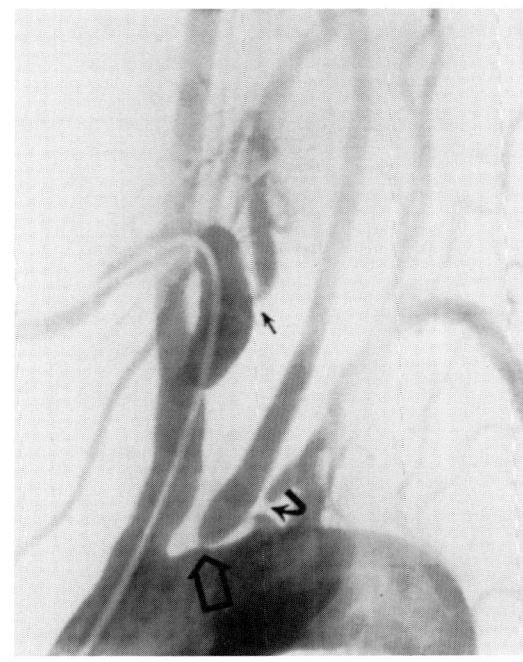

FIGURE 129–21. Arch aortogram (subtraction film). The right vertebral artery (straight arrow) and left common carotid artery (open arrow) are both stenotic. The left vertebral artery (curved arrow) arises from the aorta and is also stenotic. A decreased pulse in the left carotid artery was not recognized prior to this examination.

the right and left vertebral arteries, it is rarely necessary to perform selective angiography of both vertebral arteries.

Reporting Conventions

The criteria for reporting percentage stenosis is simple throughout the cerebral vascular system (i.e., comparison of residual lumen diameter with adjacent normal vessel diameter), except in the internal carotid artery where the variable configuration of the carotid bulb has been approached in a number of ways, not all of which make hemodynamic sense. The North American Symptomatic Carotid Endarterectomy Trial (NASCET) and the Asymptomatic Carotid Artery Study (ACAS) both confirmed the effectiveness of carotid endarterectomy for preventing stroke in patients who have significant carotid stenosis. These studies addressed both the clinical approach to treating occlusive carotid disease and methods of measuring stenoses. Specifically, both studies adopted the convention of reporting percentage stenoses by dividing the minimal diameter of the stenoses by the diameter of the normal carotid segment distal to the stenosis ($\times$ 100).

Before that strict definition was adopted, most radiologists reported percentage stenosis by comparing the stenosis to the *expected* maximal diameter of the carotid bulb—obviously an imagined estimate (truly a "guesstimate"). The NASCET/ACAS convention has been uniformly adopted in North America and, while not yet standard in Europe and elsewhere, it is certainly becoming common practice. The method makes physiologic sense, and it is based on precise measurements, not estimates.

RADIOGRAPHIC EQUIPMENT AND IMAGING TECHNIQUES

Specific Considerations for Cerebrovascular Angiography

High-resolution image-intensified video fluoroscopic units equipped with high-output x-ray generators and rapid-sequence imaging capabilities have become standard equipment in most angiographic laboratories, enabling angiographers to routinely visualize and manipulate small-caliber catheters with ease. However, simultaneous biplane angiographic imaging capability, while desirable because of the reduction in contrast dosage and procedure time achieved by simultaneous multiview imaging, is relatively uncommon even in larger institutions simply because of its expense and complexity. In fact, the decline in diagnostic neuroangiographic procedures occasioned by the advent of high-resolution CT and MRI often results in replacement of older biplane units by newer single-plane units because of significant cost differences and the lack of importance of simultaneous biplane angiography in other areas of the body.

One of the most significant technical advances in cerebrovascular angiography has been widespread deployment of modern digital imaging equipment since the early 1990s, including both digital angiography (DA) and digital subtraction angiography (DSA) capabilities. High-resolution digitized images are obtained directly from the fluoroscopic image intensifier; these images can then be manipulated by computer to enhance image contrast or subtract background detail from contrast-filled vessels. Both DA and DSA images are composed of a fixed number of pixels (picture elements), creating an important tradeoff between field of view and resolution. Because resolution is at least partially dependent on the pixel density per unit area, it can be improved by using the magnification modes of the image intensifier at the expense of reducing the field of view to a specific region of interest. In that manner, a given number of pixels span a smaller anatomic region, thus showing the region in greater detail.

Both DA and DSA images are available on the computer console immediately after contrast injection, unlike conventional photographic x-ray films, which require chemical processing; thus, DA and DSA techniques are much more convenient to use than conventional film technique and allow an examination to progress considerably faster.

DA images, unlike those of DSA, are basically conventional fluoroscopic images recorded digitally for storage and enhancement (Fig. 129–22). DSA, in contrast, is an image subtraction process conceptually similar to conventional film subtraction, which makes the appearance of an image dependent on the accuracy of the subtraction process, as well as the lack of motion between the initial noncontrast "mask" image and subsequent images. These are assumed to be identical except for the presence of intravascular contrast media. In the ideal situation, all structures not containing contrast agents are eliminated from the image after film or DSA subtraction processing, leaving an image composed solely of contrast-filled vessels.

In the case of film subtraction, the mask is actually a photographic reversal of an angiographic film taken prior

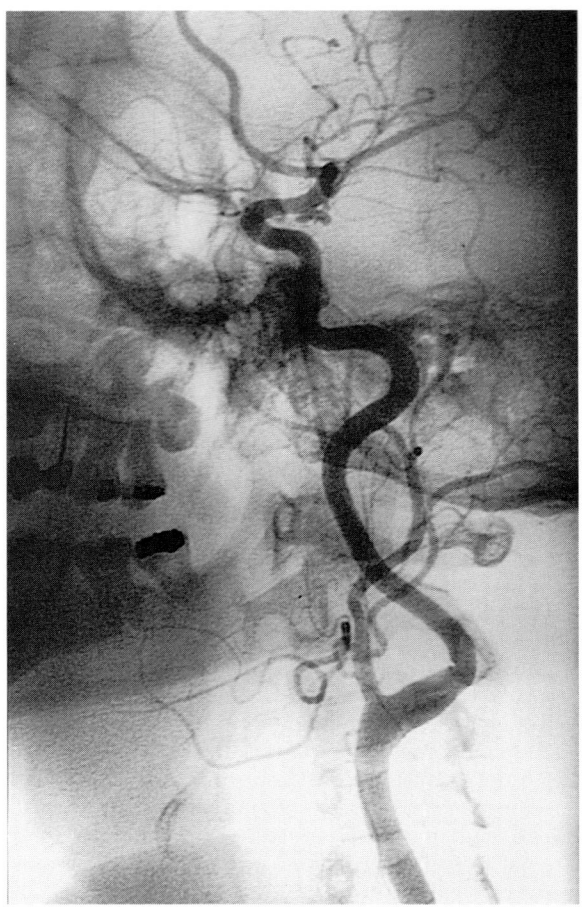

FIGURE 129–22. Digital angiography (DA) of the carotid artery. Because this is a nonsubtracted image, it is relatively immune to the sort of motion artefacts that can severely degrade a digital subtraction angiography (DSA) image. However, because it is also a digital image, the DA image can be manipulated to enhance various details using the viewing station computer system, just like a DSA image. (Courtesy of Julius Grollman, M.D., Little Company of Mary Hospital, Torrance, Calif.)

to the injection of contrast media, made by copying that film onto a special film that accurately renders the various shades of an image in the mathematically opposite shades of the gray scale. When the mask film is superimposed on a film containing contrast medium, the images cancel except for the contrast-filled vessels. In the case of DSA, the mask is simply a precontrast digital image, and subtraction is just a point-by-point mathematical process.

In practice, however, whether one uses film or digital subtraction techniques, slight differences between the precontrast mask and the contrast-filled images, caused primarily by motion, make the subtraction less than perfect, leaving faint residual images of bone and soft tissue. Although the presence of these faint images associated with imperfections in the subtraction process might at first seem undesirable, the residual background images are actually quite useful in providing a visual frame of reference for what would otherwise be a difficult-to-evaluate "disembodied" image of a vessel—allowing, for example, estimation of the location of the carotid bifurcation with respect to the cervical vertebrae or angle of the mandible. For that reason, most modern DSA systems now include the capability to subtract a variable percentage of the original image pixel values, thus leaving residual landmark images of whatever intensity the examiner desires (Fig. 129–23).

Because the basic assumption inherent in both DSA and film image subtraction is the absence of any change in the image other than the appearance of radiographic contrast material within the vascular system, these techniques require a considerable degree of patient cooperation. Motion such as simple head and neck movement, swallowing, or breathing creates artefacts in the subtraction process. Simple translational movement artefacts can be eliminated by shifting the precontrast and postcontrast injection images relative to each other to compensate for such movements. Artefacts that are due to complex motion, such as swallowing or breathing, are nonuniform across the image field of view and cannot be totally eliminated by simple image shifting. When such artefacts overlie an area of interest, they can cause significant diagnostic uncertainty. Although satisfactory results often can be obtained even in the presence of motion artefacts by simple correlation of the information obtained from different images in a sequence as well as images obtained in different views, this is not always possible, especially in patients unable to cooperate.

DSA provides far better contrast resolution than either DA or standard photographic x-ray film technique. Visualization of vessels is possible with much less contrast material (or much more dilute material) than that required by film technique, which was the basis for early efforts at intravenous DSA. Injection of contrast material through a small right atrial catheter, introduced via a percutaneous antecubital venipuncture, held out the promise of rapid,

low-cost, low-risk outpatient angiographic carotid artery screening. However, problems with motion artefacts are much more frequent with venous injection than with arterial injection because there is a much longer period between the onset of the subjective sensations resulting from the injection and filling of the vessels of interest than there is with arterial injection. Dispersal and dilution of the contrast bolus in patients with low cardiac output also tended to degrade image quality. For these reasons, the percentage of diagnostic quality studies proved to be disappointing, and the technique has been virtually abandoned. In addition, the advent of small-caliber (4 and 5 Fr.), high-flow arterial catheters has substantially reduced arterial puncture site complications; outpatient arterial angiography now carries little more risk than venous angiography.

Although intravenous DSA imaging of the cerebrovascular system has justifiably fallen out of favor in most applications, it does have utility in those rare circumstances that involve combined upper and lower extremity peripheral vascular disease of such severity that direct arterial access is impractical. IV DSA studies may well be prudent in this very small cohort of patients; however, direct translumbar aortic puncture with the patient in the prone position, a technique once popular for lower extremity angiography and now largely of historical interest, can still be used to gain direct arterial access for both selective and nonselective angiography of the head and neck vessels.

The choice between conventional photographic x-ray film and DSA or DA techniques involves theoretical as well as practical considerations. DSA provides contrast resolution far superior to that of standard photographic x-ray

FIGURE 129–23. *A* and *B*, Digital subtraction angiography (DSA) showing an ulcerated plaque that narrows the proximal internal carotid artery. Owing to the lack of motion artefact, background subtraction is virtually complete. Although this shows the lesion to advantage, it also makes orientation difficult. Reducing the degree of background subtraction in the same DSA image produces an image that contains useful background landmarks.

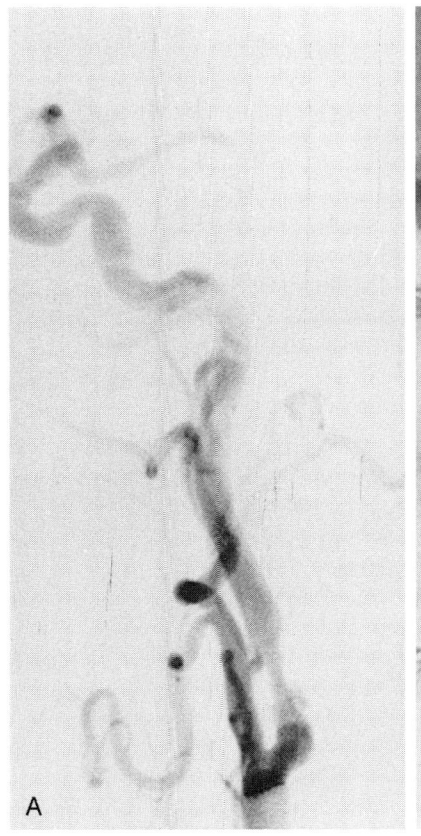
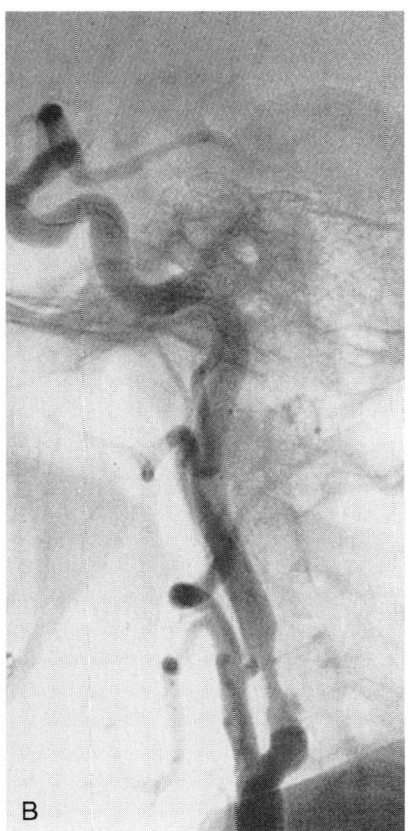

film, whereas film is capable of considerably better spatial resolution than either DA or DSA. In contrast, DA and DSA are far more efficient and convenient than film. In the early days of digital angiographic imaging, this was an important tradeoff. When very fine detail and the detection of nonocclusive disease, such as ulceration or fibromuscular dysplasia, was the principal concern, angiographers often opted for conventional film techniques in preference to digital imaging. However, the advent of high-resolution digital imaging systems and the use of supplemental high-magnification views when appropriate have made it practical to achieve spatial resolution with digital techniques that provide diagnostic accuracy equivalent to conventional film techniques. Indeed, it is the equivalence of diagnostic accuracy that has driven the shift toward digital imaging.

Although a comparison of these techniques based solely on the physics of imaging still shows that film provides better spatial resolution, the nature of the images, is such that the ability to detect disease is not significantly different when using either of these techniques. Now that the equivalence has been established with regard to spatial resolution, the differences in contrast resolution weigh even more in favor of digital imaging techniques. Perhaps the best example of this advantage is the classic problem of differentiating a total occlusion from a near-total occlusion in which distal flow cannot be shown with certainty on a conventional film angiogram but can be detected on a DSA study, owing to the superior contrast resolution of the DSA technique.

Technical Aspects of Cerebrovascular Angiography

Prior to the advent of selective catheterization via peripheral vascular access routes, direct puncture carotid angiography was routinely employed. The technique is simple, quick, and relatively safe, although, by definition, it limits the scope of examination, making assessment of the proximal vessel segment virtually impossible. Direct cannulation is accomplished by puncturing the common carotid artery low in the neck, using a thin-walled cannula equipped with a hollow stylet. Single-wall or double-wall (puncture and pull-back) techniques are acceptable. Once the vessel has been successfully punctured, as shown by brisk blood flow through the cannula, the cannula is advanced a short distance into the vessel over a soft-tipped guide wire. Between injections, the cannula is plugged with a blunt-tipped obturator to prevent thrombus formation in the cannula; frequent flushing and meticulous injection techniques are also essential. Numerous needle, cannula, and sheath combinations have been designed for this purpose, and most work well.

The development of small-caliber, high-torque catheters that can be introduced via remote access sites (e.g., femoral, axillary, or brachial arteries) and easily manipulated into the cerebral vessels has completely eliminated the use of direct puncture carotid angiography, as it allows the entire cerebrovascular system to be studied with a single puncture. In addition, usually less patient anxiety is associated with distal puncture than with the direct technique. A detailed discussion of the techniques and materials used for cerebrovascular angiography is beyond the scope of this text; however, just as there are strong personal preferences regarding surgical instruments among surgeons, catheter choice is often a matter of both technical and personal preference among radiologists. The development of small-caliber (4 and 5 Fr.), high-flow, high-torque preshaped catheters available in a wide range of curve shapes and sizes has virtually eliminated the use of "homemade" heat-shaped polyethylene catheters once popular among neuroradiologists.

Although the variety of catheter shapes is too numerous to discuss in detail, there are two basic classes of catheter shape: advancement and withdrawal (Fig. 129–24). Advancement catheters are designed to be advanced into the vessel of choice by a combination of torque and guide wire manipulations. Withdrawal catheters, typified by the shepherd's crook–shaped Simmons' sidewinder catheter, are used by advancing beyond the vessel ostium and withdrawing in order to engage the tip in the vessel ostium (Fig. 129–25). Thus, withdrawal catheters are advanced out of a vessel and withdrawn into it. The withdrawal catheters are particularly useful when the angulation of the proximal segment of the branch vessel makes direct advancement difficult. Although they are easy to use, withdrawal catheters have the disadvantage of requiring a re-forming maneuver to regain their special shape after being introduced into the vessel over a guide wire in a relatively straight configuration (Fig. 129–26). The choice of catheter shape depends largely on the anatomy and tortuosity of the vessels to be traversed (Fig. 129–27).

For reasons of convenience and safety, most angiographers prefer the percutaneous femoral artery approach popularized by Dr. Sven Seldinger. However, when that approach proves to be impractical because of severe ileofemoral vascular disease, cerebral angiography can be carried out successfully via percutaneous axillary (Fig. 129–28), brachial, or even translumbar catheterization. Withdrawal catheters are generally used as part of the transaxillary approach, and the right axillary artery is generally

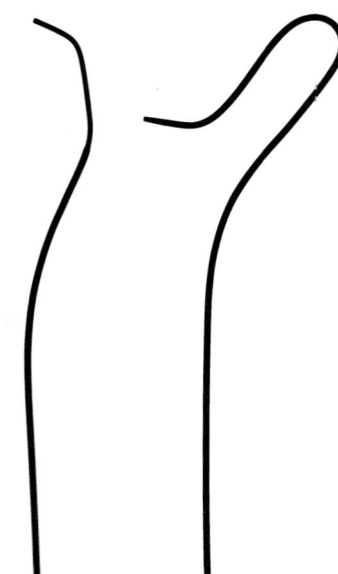

FIGURE 129–24. *Left,* Headhunter catheter—an advancement catheter. *Right,* Simmons' sidewinder catheter—a withdrawal catheter.

FIGURE 129–25. *A*, Headhunter catheter advanced into the left common carotid artery. *B*, Simmons' sidewinder catheter withdrawn into the left common carotid artery. Note that the angulation of this vessel would have made advancement catheterization with the headhunter catheter difficult.

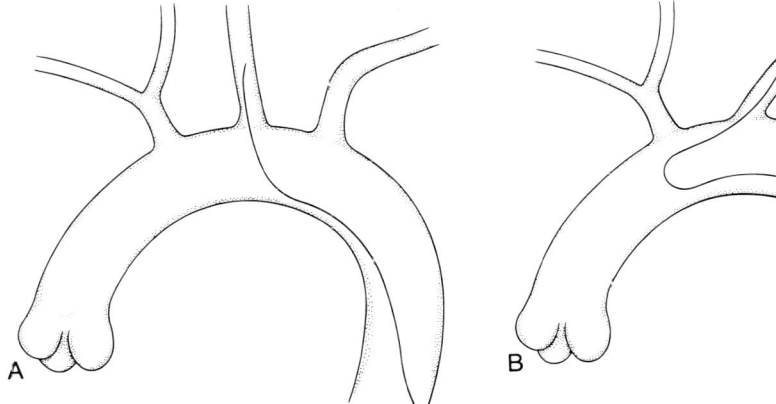

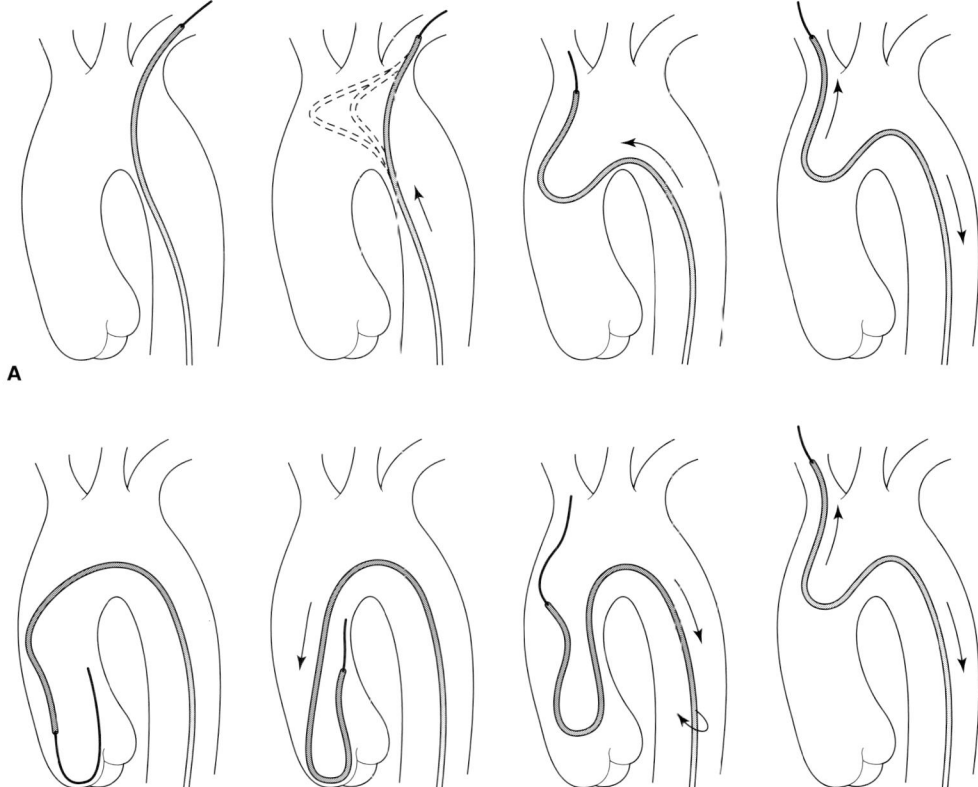

FIGURE 129–26. *A*, Simmons' sidewinder catheter re-formed, with the left subclavian artery used as a pivot point. *B*, Catheter re-formed using a guide wire looped on the aortic valve to redirect the catheter tip. This maneuver should be done rapidly to avoid prolapsing across the valve into the left ventricle. If prolapse occurs, the catheter is simply withdrawn and the maneuver repeated. Re-forming the catheter can also be done using the contralateral common iliac artery, the renal artery, or the superior mesenteric artery, although such maneuvers are somewhat more difficult than those shown.

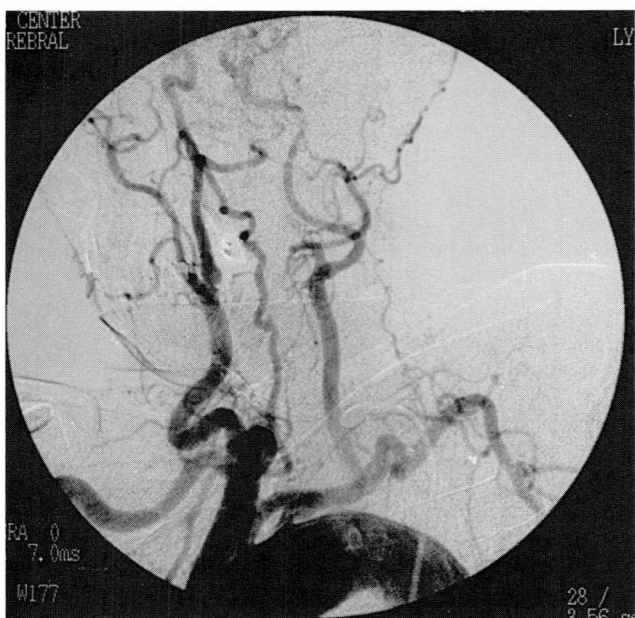

FIGURE 129–27. Marked tortuosity in this elderly patient makes selective catheterization of the internal carotid and vertebral arteries extremely difficult, requiring the use of a Simmons' sidewinder III catheter to negotiate the reverse curves encountered en route to the vessels. (Simmons' catheters are designated as I to III depending on the length of the reverse direction segment, with III being the longest.)

chosen because it greatly simplifies selective catheterization of the right common carotid artery.

Numerous acceptable radiographic contrast agents are available for use in cerebrovascular angiography. These agents fall into three broad categories:

- Ionic
- Low osmolarity (low dissociation)
- Non-ionic

In general, the negative chronotropic and inotropic cardiac effects, as well as the neurotoxicity, nephrotoxicity, allergic potential, and subjective discomfort associated with ionic agents, are greater than those associated with the low-osmolarity and non-ionic agents. Many angiographers continue to use ionic agents except in patients considered to be at increased risk for adverse events due to advanced age or a prior history of allergic reaction to contrast, or significant cardiac or renal disease due simply to the dramatic cost differences in these agents, but market forces have begun to drive down the cost of the non-ionic and low-osmolarity agents resulting in a shift toward use of these agents. It must be noted, however, that although these newer agents are safer than conventional ionic agents, they are not completely free of risk for the same types of adverse events.

COMPLICATIONS OF CEREBROVASCULAR ANGIOGRAPHY

Most complications are associated with the puncture site or the administration of radiographic contrast material and have already been discussed elsewhere in this text. Furthermore, most of the access site complications (e.g., hematoma as a result of ineffective postwithdrawal hemostasis or delayed puncture site bleeding and occlusion as a result of excessive postwithdrawal pressure on the vessel) can be avoided by careful technique and a refusal to delegate this important phase of the procedure to an assistant or a mechanical compression device.

Fortunately, neurologic complications are relatively uncommon during cerebral angiography. The incidence of major complications (e.g., death, stroke, access site problems requiring surgical intervention) has been quoted as being approximately 0.16% in one large study. Transient neurologic deficits (transient ischemic attacks, TIAs) were reported to occur with a frequency of approximately 0.9% in another study. It should be noted, however, that the angiography-related stroke rate in the multicenter, prospec-

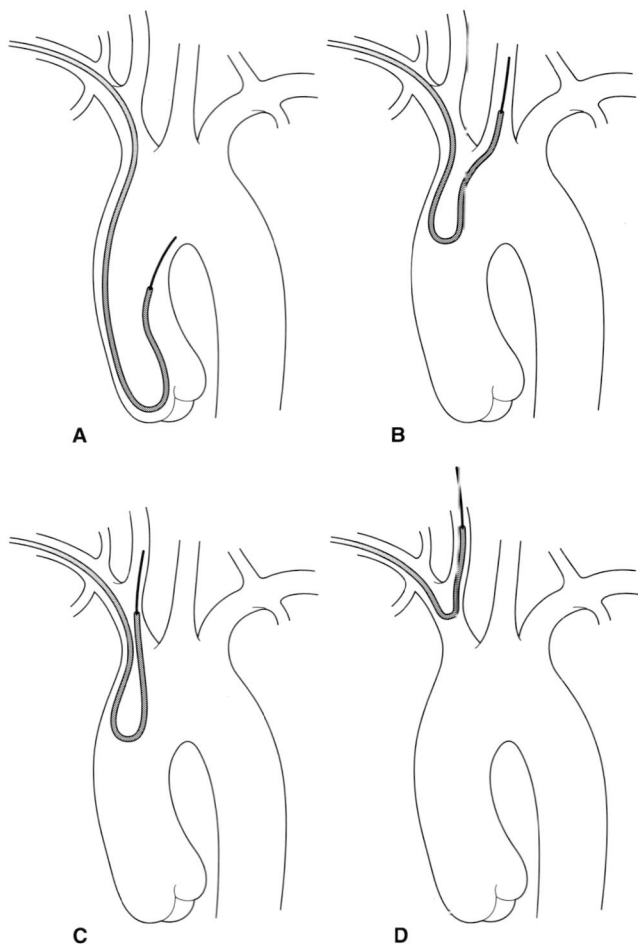

FIGURE 129–28. Selective catheterization of the cerebral vessels can be accomplished from the right brachial approach using a withdrawal type of catheter (Simmons' sidewinder II or III). *A,* The catheter is re-formed as usual, via the aortic valve (see also Fig. 129–22*B–D*). *B–D,* The catheter can then be directed toward any of the cerebral vessels by a combination of catheter and guide wire manipulations. Selective catheterization of the vertebral arteries is more difficult than catheterization of the carotids, especially on the left side. When selective catheterization of a vertebral artery cannot be accomplished, injection of radiographic contrast in the adjacent subclavian artery using an occlusive pressure cuff on the ipsilateral arm will usually yield a diagnostic quality angiogram.

tive and randomized ACAS study was 1.2%. Although some angiographers employ routine anticoagulation during cerebral angiography, no studies have shown a definite beneficial effect in reducing neurologic complications. Unlike the case in coronary angiography, anticoagulation is not routinely employed during diagnostic cerebral angiography. However, as is often the case for surgical procedures, there is a direct correlation between the duration of the procedure and the incidence of complications. This fact is of special relevance to academic institutions in which the educational requirements of the housestaff and the safety of the patient must be carefully balanced. The occurrence of a neurologic complication, even if relatively transient, generally should halt the angiographic study, at least until a complete neurologic assessment is performed and consultation with the referring physician obtained to determine whether the clinical situation justifies the risk of continuing the procedure.

Although there are varying opinions regarding the level of sedation desirable in noncerebral angiography, there is a general consensus that major sedation for most cerebrovascular angiographic procedures should be avoided so as not to mask neurologic complications.

GOAL-DIRECTED ANGIOGRAPHIC PROCEDURES

The precise design of an angiographic study must balance the information needs of the referring physician with the risks and benefits to the patient. Thus, the following discussion is divided into five major subgroups of patients:

- Asymptomatic
- Symptomatic
- Injured
- Stroke-in-evolution
- Postoperative

The Asymptomatic Patient

Asymptomatic patients are considered for cerebrovascular evaluation because they are at high risk for neurologic events. As previously discussed, angiography is rarely indicated as a first-line investigation in asymptomatic individuals. When noninvasive assessment yields equivocal results, simple nonselective multiview aortic arch angiography using either DSA, DA, or conventional x-ray film technique is generally adequate to determine the accuracy of the noninvasive findings. However, selective angiography may be required when the regional vascular anatomy cannot be adequately depicted because of overlapping vessel images and there is no contraindication to selective angiography, such as a high-grade ostial stenosis or a markedly irregular ostial plaque. Of course, performing angiography presupposes that the patient is a good surgical candidate.

The Symptomatic Patient

As indicated previously, many surgeons feel angiography is unnecessary in symptomatic patients with unequivocal duplex Doppler findings. Once it has been determined that angiography is indicated, however, comprehensive angiography is generally desirable; angiography limited solely to the suspect vessel is inadequate owing to the propensity for vascular occlusive disease of various etiologies (atherosclerosis, fibromuscular dysplasia, and arteritis) to occur at multiple sites. The general plan of examination is similar to that used in the asymptomatic patient; however, additional views of clinically suspect areas may be required to complete the examination, especially in the detection of nonocclusive ulcerative disease that might serve as a site of thrombus formation (Fig. 129–29). In symptomatic patients, absence of occlusive or ulcerative disease at the carotid bifurcation also necessitates a detailed examination of the aortic arch vessels and the intracranial vessels, particularly the region of the carotid siphon. Failure to find demonstrable anatomic disease then mandates a search for other sources of emboli and hemodynamic insufficiency, with particular attention to heart disease and arrhythmias.

The finding of a seemingly occluded carotid or vertebral artery, especially on nonselective arch angiography, is a special case. Because there is a major difference in the approach to a total occlusion and to a near-total occlusion, definitive resolution of the issue is essential. In such cases, selective injection of the vessel in question should be performed with imaging that provides both early and late views of the area in order to differentiate total occlusion from near-total occlusion with very slow faint antegrade filling of the distal vessel segment (Fig. 129–30) or retrograde collateral filling (Fig. 129–31).

Although image subtraction techniques applied to nonselective arch aortograms may be useful in evaluation of collateral filling patterns and the detection of low-volume filling distal to a near-total obstruction, they can also introduce motion artefacts that are difficult to evaluate. Selective injection presents a maximal opacification dose of undiluted contrast material to the suspect area, whereas nonselective arch angiography, of necessity, involves significant dilution of the contrast bolus (see Fig. 129–29). Once a near-total occlusion has been confirmed, prompt anticoagulation generally should be instituted because there is a definite, although poorly quantified, risk of occlusion of such lesions after angiography.

Patients who have recently had a completed stroke thought to be a consequence of atherosclerotic carotid disease constitute a special case of the symptomatic patient. Determining whether angiography is appropriate and when it should be performed depends on the determination of whether surgery would be of benefit in prevention of additional cerebral vascular events in that vascular territory. Basically, the decision involves assessment of the extent of the infarct in relation to the residual at-risk vascular territory. In the presence of a significant residual at-risk vascular territory, noninvasive assessment is the first logical step, with angiography reserved for situations in which the noninvasive testing fails to yield an unequivocal result.

The presence of a recent cerebral infarct implies a defect in the blood-brain barrier; thus, on principle, direct injection of a neurotoxic agent such as radiographic contrast material probably should be avoided unless benefit significantly outweighs the risk (although the actual magnitude of the risk in such circumstances has never been well

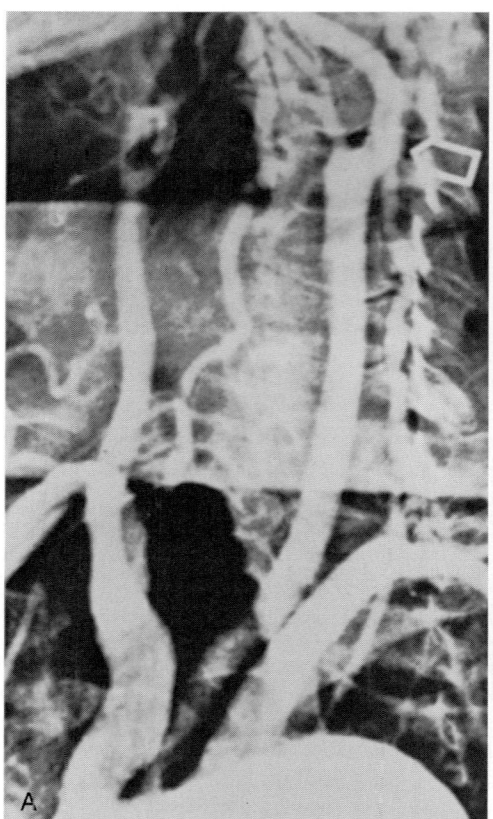

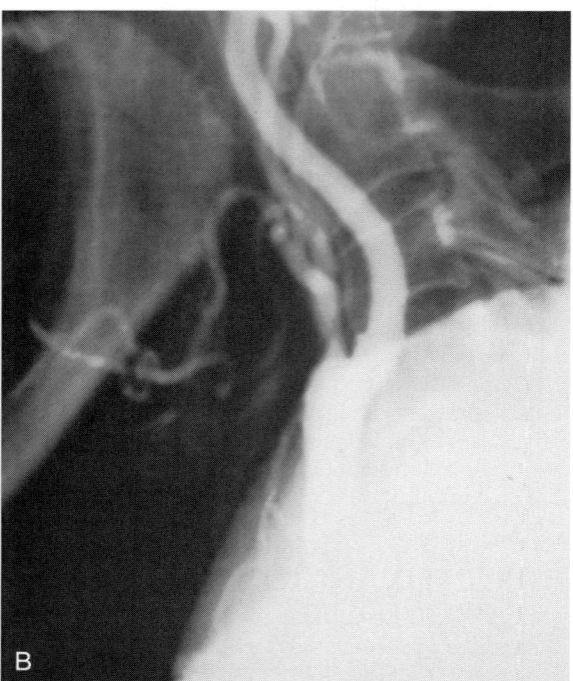

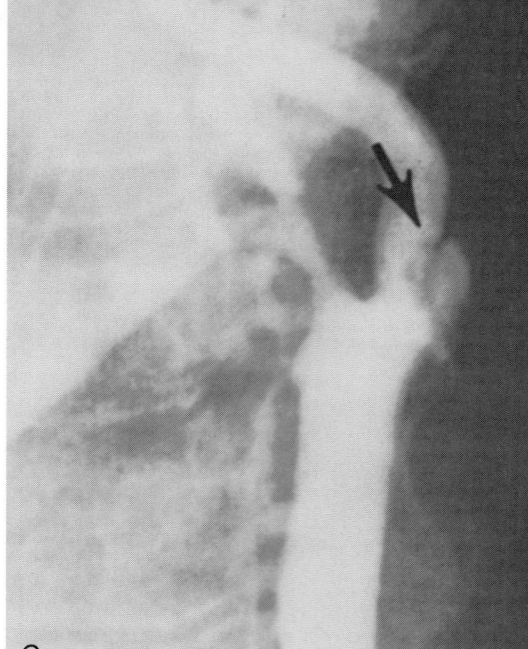

FIGURE 129–29. Ulcerated atheroma, left internal carotid. *A*, Arch aortogram. The diseased vessel is hidden by the superimposed left vertebral artery (*arrow*). *B*, Left carotid arteriogram, lateral view. The internal carotid is only slightly irregular. *C*, Left carotid arteriogram, frontal view. A large ulcer (*arrow*) is present.

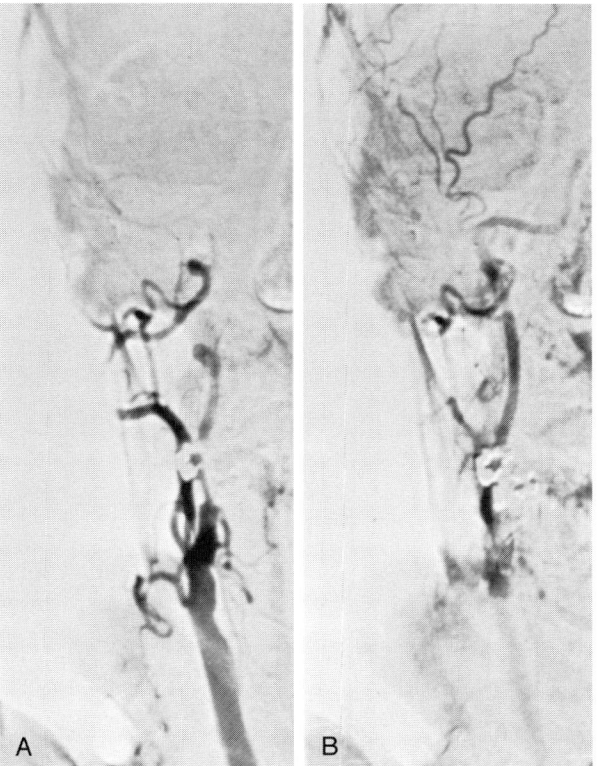

FIGURE 129–30. *A*, Early film from a right common carotid artery injection showing primarily the external carotid artery system. The proximal internal carotid artery and its high-grade ostial stenosis are actually visualized but difficult to detect (vertebral artery partly opacified by reflux flow from the common carotid to the right subclavian). *B*, Late film of the same angiogram clearly showing internal carotid artery and near-occlusive proximal stenosis.

established). Indeed, there are few definitive data as to when angiography can be safely performed in the post-stroke patient. The persistence of parenchymal CT contrast enhancement, which implies a defect in the blood-brain barrier, can last for as long as 6 weeks. Therefore, although the decision is based on anecdotal experience, a delay of about 6 weeks probably constitutes an appropriate waiting period, particularly in patients with substantial neurologic deficits.

The Injured Patient

Angiographic examination of the injured patient involving trauma to the extracranial or intracranial cerebral circulation, or both, constitutes an important exception to the rule of completeness because there is usually a premium on expeditious diagnosis and treatment. Even the so-called stable patient rapidly can become unstable. Because single-system injury is uncommon, the angiographer must participate in the radiologic and nonradiologic evaluation of the patient as a member of a team able to coordinate and prioritize various investigations and treatments. The need for angiographic evaluation depends on patient condition and the location and type of injury as well as the management approach of the trauma surgeons caring for the patient (Fig. 129–32). Angiography of superficial facial injur-

ies is not usually required, since physical examination is generally very accurate and surgical exploration is straightforward. Deep, penetrating facial injuries, in contrast, may well require angiography for both diagnosis and treatment involving transcatheter embolization because such injuries can involve relatively inaccessible structures.

Most surgeons agree as to the need for angiographic evaluation of neck injuries to zone I (angle of jaw—base of skull) and zone III (cricoid—clavicle) since these areas present significant problems in surgical exposure. The need for angiographic evaluation of injuries to zone II (cricoid—angle of jaw) is far more controversial, since this is an area relatively amenable to prompt surgical exploration. Despite the controversy, some of which is economic in nature, angiography of zone II injuries still seems like a worthwhile step in the stable patient because it can easily diagnose unsuspected vascular injuries or eliminate unnecessary explorations. Once the role of angiography in the overall management of the patient has been determined, a study plan for the areas subjected to trauma should be formulated on the basis of the anatomy and mode of injury.

The most common cerebrovascular injuries of interest to the vascular surgeon that require emergency angiographic evaluation are the penetrating injuries of the neck. Although stab wounds may at first seem relatively limited in scope, it is important to remember that a small entry wound can easily hide more extensive underlying trauma. For that reason, angiographic evaluation of a stab wound should involve at least selective angiography of the cervical segments of the ipsilateral carotid or vertebral arteries, or both. If an injury is detected, views of the intracranial circulation, including the contralateral supply, generally should be obtained to evaluate collateral flow pathways. Knowledge of the collateral flow becomes especially important when the injury occurs in a region where surgical access is difficult, such as the zone III area just below the base of the skull, in which case ligation of an injured vessel may be preferable to repair if the collateral flow patterns permit sacrificing the vessel in question (Fig. 129–33).

The trajectory of a bullet within tissue, especially in a complex area like the neck, is virtually impossible to reconstruct. Furthermore, the extent of both direct and shock wave injury is also difficult to determine simply by physical examination. If the path of injury is clearly confined to one side, ipsilateral selective angiography of the cervical segments of the carotid or vertebral arteries is usually sufficient; however, if there is any doubt as to whether the bullet crossed the mid-line, bilateral angiography should be performed. As in the case of stab wound injuries, the detection of a cervical segment injury strongly suggests the need for delineation of the intracranial circulation and potential collateral pathways.

The absence of an angiographically detectable abnormality or the presence of a minor irregularity such as localized bulging or indistinctness, which might be overlooked on routine diagnostic angiography, should be considered highly suspect in the traumatized patient, especially for high-velocity wounds, and the suspect area should be carefully evaluated with additional views as needed. This is especially true if there are clinical, physical, or radiographic findings suggesting significant trauma, such as hypotension or a soft tissue swelling indicating the presence of a hema-

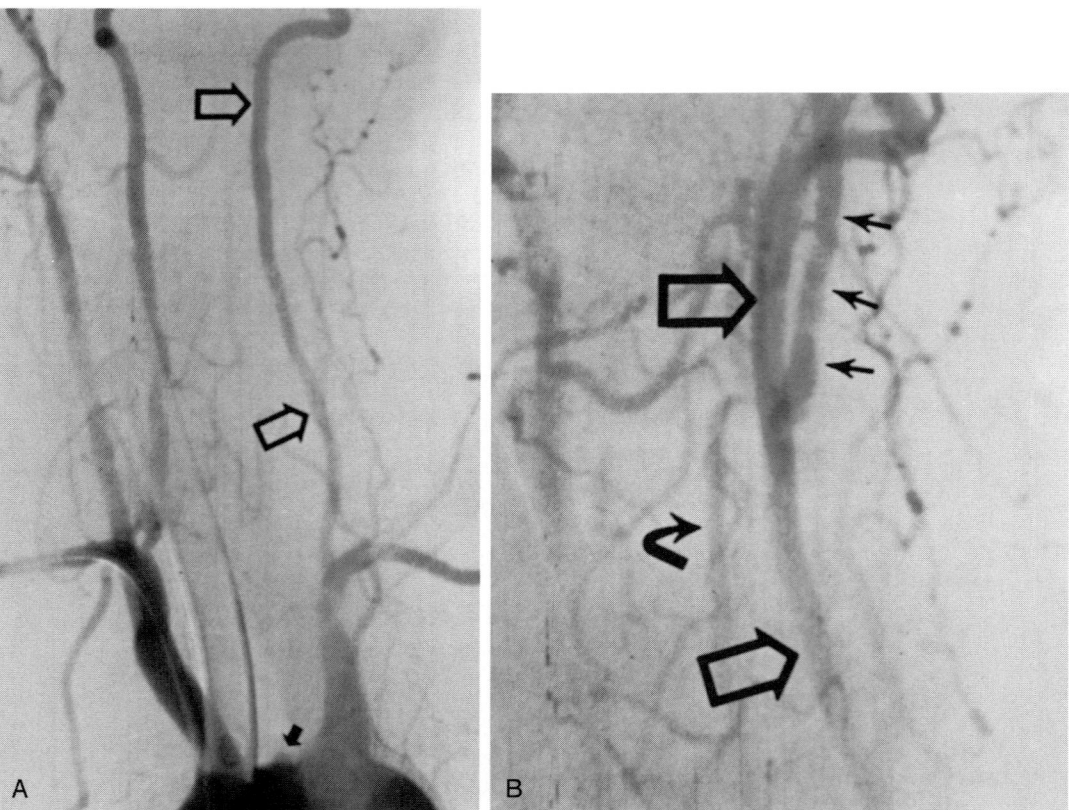

FIGURE 129–31. Occluded left common carotid artery with patent internal and external carotid branches. *A,* Arch aortogram, early film. The left common carotid is occluded *(solid arrow).* The left vertebral artery is outlined by *open arrows. B,* Arch aortogram, delayed film (close-up view). The vertebral artery is again outlined by *open arrows.* The internal carotid *(straight arrows)* is filled via the external carotid. The chief collateral pathway is the superior thyroid artery *(curved arrow).*

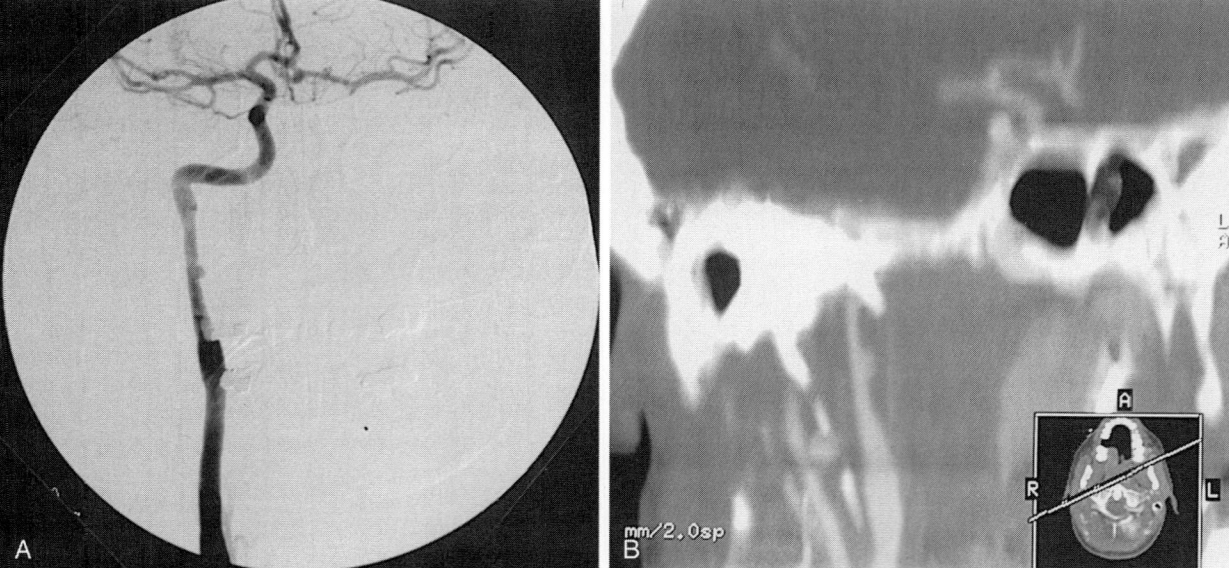

FIGURE 129–32. *A,* Angiogram of the right internal carotid artery, showing a dissection resulting from motor vehicle trauma. In view of the fact that the contralateral internal carotid artery sustained a total occlusion during the accident as well as the relatively inaccessible location of the lesion, which extended to the skull base behind the mandible, both operative and endovascular intervention were considered high-risk options. *B,* For that reason, the patient was anticoagulated and followed with serial computed tomographic angiography examinations.

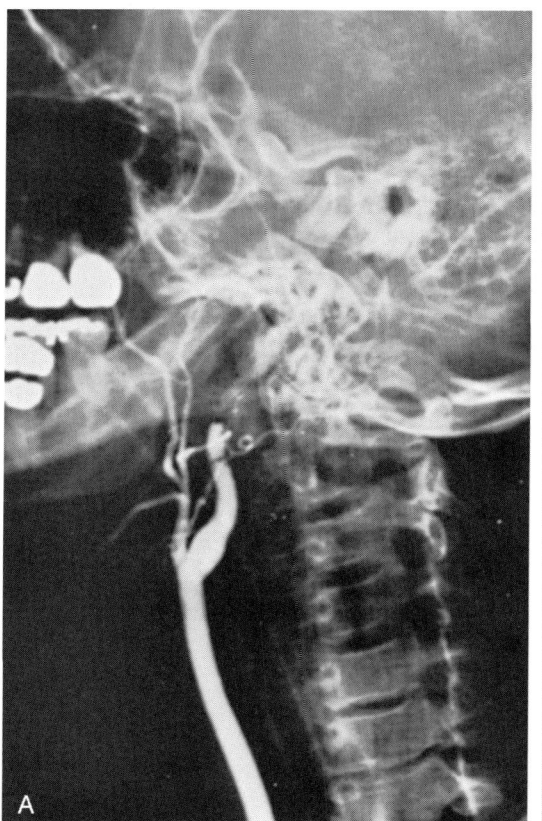

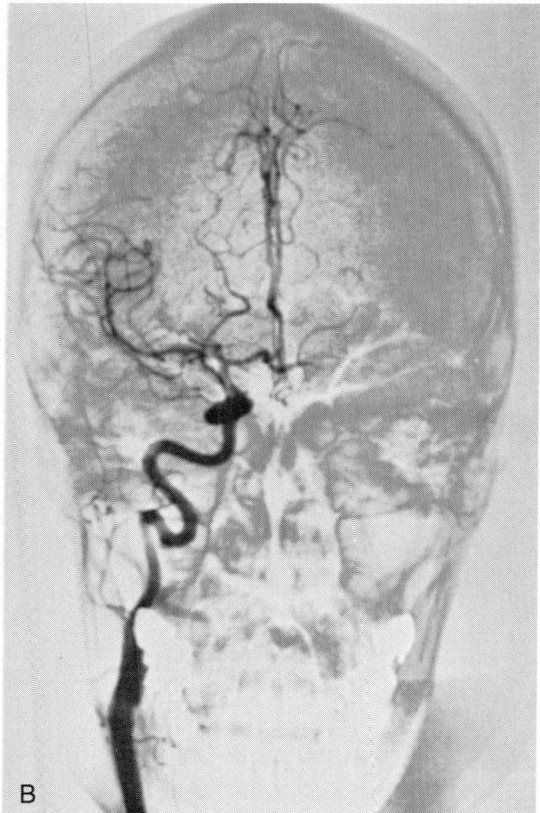

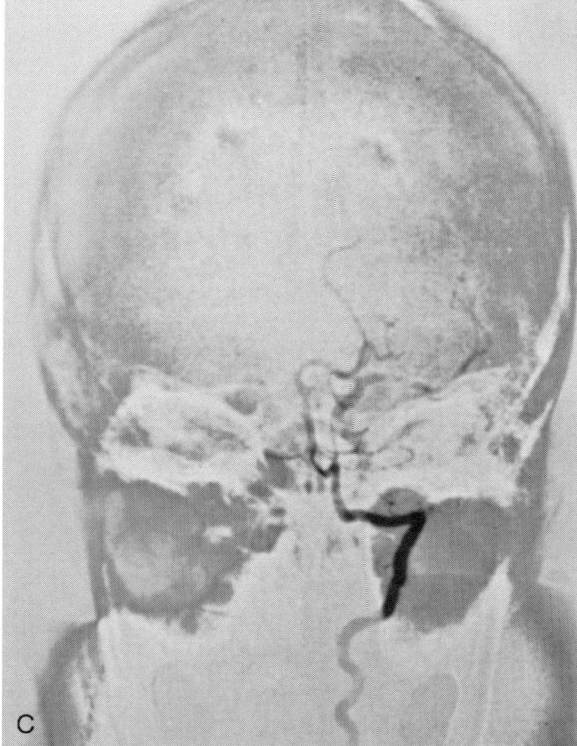

FIGURE 129–33. *A,* Selective left common carotid angiogram of a young woman stabbed in the neck just below the base of the skull during a violent rape assault. The left common carotid artery is totally occluded, but there is no evidence of extravasation. *B,* Selective right common carotid angiogram showing flow to right MCA as well as both right and left ACAs. The flow "pseudo-occlusion" of the left MCA is caused by inflow of unopacified blood to the left MCA arising from the posterior circulation. *C,* Selective left vertebral injection showing normal posterior circulation as well as supply to the left MCA. Demonstration of adequate flow from the contralateral and posterior circulations allowed safe ligation of the left internal carotid artery just below the base of the skull rather than a difficult reconstruction. (Examination of the vessel at surgery showed it to be occluded by thrombus, presumably as the result of an intimal disruption associated with violent neck motion and trauma to the vessel at the atlanto-occipital joint; no penetrating injury was found.)

toma (Fig. 129–34). Such findings should raise the examiner's "index of suspicion" as they may be the only evidence of a major vascular injury temporarily hidden by the tamponade of a precarious clot.

However, additional views and selective catheterization obviously should be undertaken with considerable care, as these maneuvers may well pinpoint the injury, revealing its true significance by initiating bleeding at the injury site and suddenly destabilizing the situation (Fig. 129–35). Urgent surgical intervention is required in such situations; however, simple local compression may be insufficient to stop bleeding long enough to transport the patient to the

operating room. Temporary hemostasis can often be obtained very quickly by catheterizing the injured vessel with either an angioplasty or soft occlusion balloon placed across the injury site and inflated to a low pressure sufficient to provide both proximal and distal vascular control. If ligation rather than primary repair is contemplated, the same effect can also be achieved in the angiography suite by placing either coil or detachable balloon occlusive devices proximal and distal to the injury site.

Zone I injuries add a special consideration to planning the angiographic evaluation, since these injuries may actually involve intrathoracic structures such as the arch origins

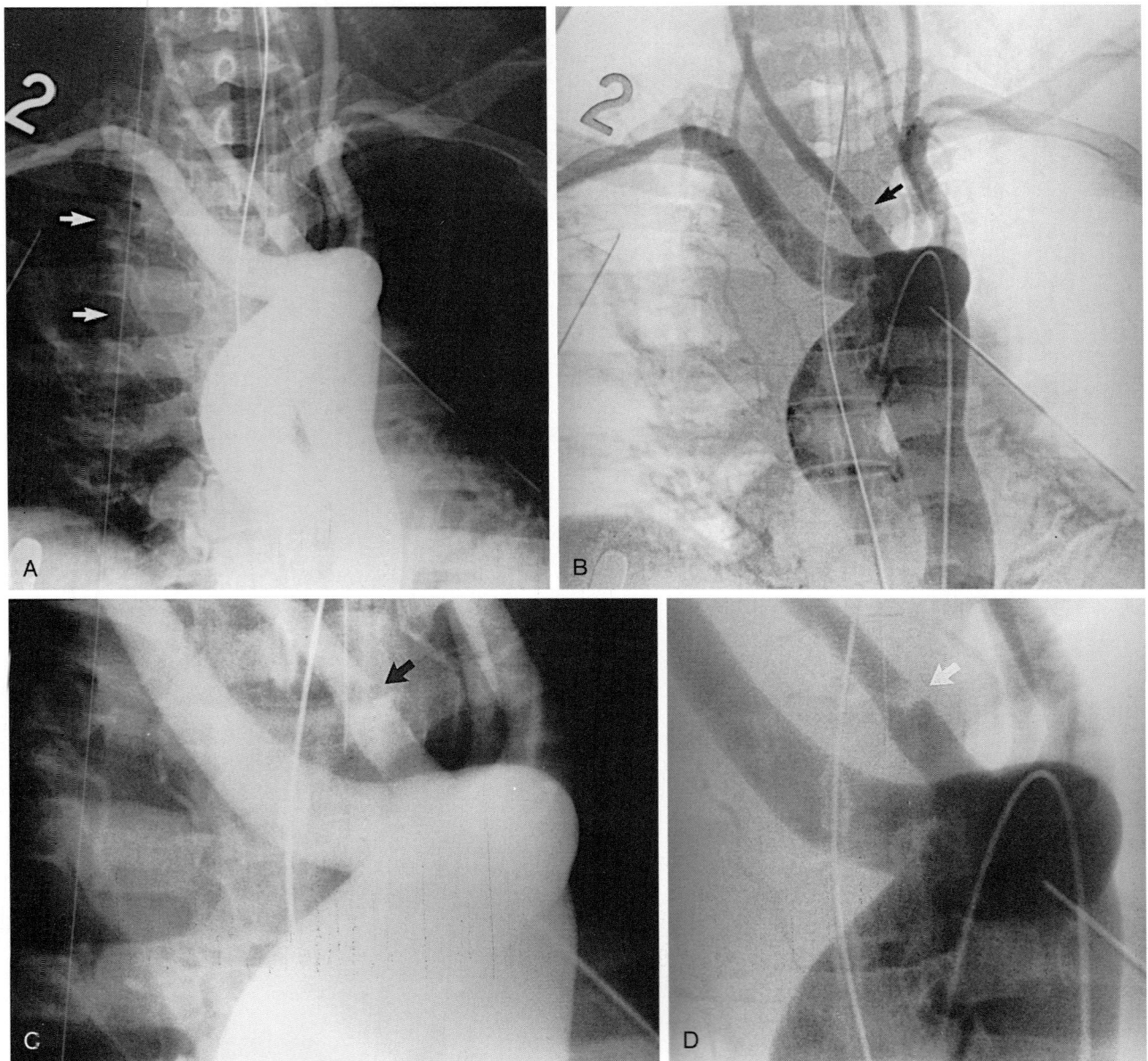

FIGURE 129–34. *A,* Nonselective aortic arch angiogram in patient with a gunshot wound, which was initially interpreted as showing no definite evidence of a major vascular injury despite the presence of a large right superior mediastinal soft tissue density indicating the presence of a large hematoma (*arrows*). (*Note:* The aberrant right subclavian artery is a normal anatomic variant.) *B,* Film subtraction of the same angiogram revealing partial transection of the right common carotid artery (*arrow*). Although, in retrospect, this lesion may indeed have been seen on the unsubtracted angiogram, the allowance made for radiographic shadows of underlying bony structures effectively desensitized the examiner, precluding detection of this very significant injury. *C,* Unsubtracted magnification view of the same area makes the injury (*arrow*) far more obvious, as does magnification film subtraction (*D*).

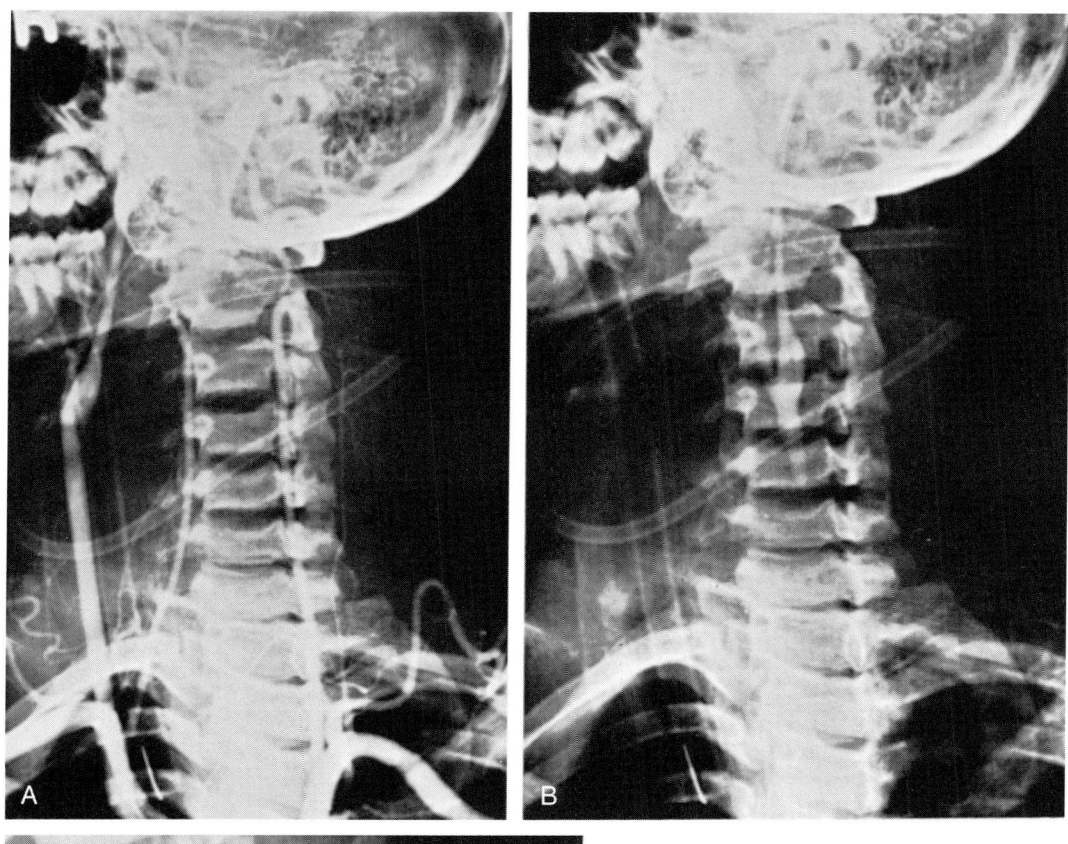

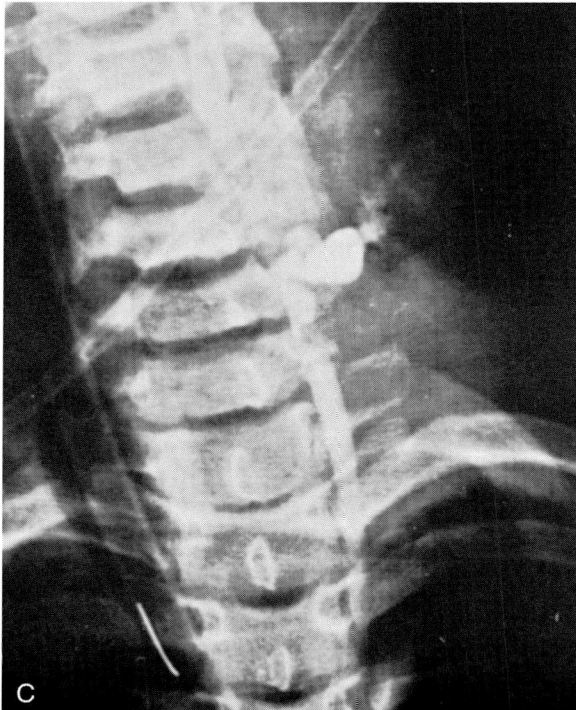

FIGURE 129–35. *A,* Arch aortogram showing apparent absence of the left common carotid artery. *B,* Late film from arch aortogram showing retrograde collateral filling of the left common carotid artery. *C,* Selective left common carotid angiogram demonstrating precise location of injury (stab wound) and unequivocal extravasation.

of the great vessels. Thus, a thoracic aortogram prior to selective catheterization should be obtained in low zone I injuries. Likewise, a thoracic aortogram prior to selective angiography is advisable in the elderly patient, in whom unsuspected atherosclerotic occlusive disease may make selective catheterization a greater risk.

Direct blunt trauma to the neck and acceleration-deceleration injuries such as those sustained in motor vehicle or pedestrian-vehicle accidents present a difficult clinical problem. If there are obvious physical signs of significant injury or neurologic signs that cannot be explained on the basis of head injury, angiography is usually indicated in the acute setting. Similarly, should the patient experience a delayed neurologic event that might be referable to traumatic vascular injury, prompt angiographic evaluation is also indicated.

In the case of intracranial vascular trauma, CT scanning is usually the primary evaluation modality, followed by angiography if the CT scan suggests that a salvageable situation still exists. Diagnosis and treatment of such injuries are usually the province of the neurosurgeon rather than the vascular surgeon and, as such, are beyond the scope of this discussion.

The Patient with Stroke-in-Evolution

The crescendo TIA syndrome, in which ischemic neurologic events occur with ominously increasing frequency although they completely resolve in the intervals between TIAs, should be considered an urgent presentation of the symptomatic patient. Stroke-in-evolution is another dangerous entity, consisting of an ongoing neurologic symptoms event that does not completely disappear but may wax and wane. Whereas many investigators have attempted to place arbitrary time limits on the strict definition of stroke-in-evolution, the distinction between it and crescendo TIAs is far from clear. Attempting to make that distinction may be counterproductive because waiting to determine whether the event will resolve also may forfeit the opportunity to provide timely therapy.

Treatment, and hence the angiographic approach to the stroke-in-evolution, is changing. Over the past several years, a new concept of the pathophysiology of ischemic stroke has gained acceptance, in which irreversible neurologic damage does not occur as an all-or-none phenomenon. In some instances, prompt restoration of flow can restore brain viability and neurologic function. Whether this represents the presence of an ischemic penumbra surrounding a smaller but irrevocably infarcted core of tissue, as opposed to a potentially viable but "stunned" volume of neurons, is unclear, but it may be that both of these mechanisms occur. In fact, while still unproved, it seems likely that progression from a stunned but completely viable state to the infarcted core with viable penumbra is the basic mode of evolution for all strokes. Indeed, an understanding of the factors affecting the time course would help explain the variation in the clinical course of individual patients. In any event, stroke-in-evolution seems to be analogous to a myocardial infarction (MI) in which a period of ischemic viability exists between the inciting event and irreversible infarction, during which restoration

of flow will restore function and either prevent or minimize the extent of myocardial damage.

The emergency treatment of stroke-in-evolution is a logical outgrowth of advances in the treatment of acute MI and peripheral vascular disease. Progress in the understanding of the pathophysiology of MI since 1980 has led to the establishment of regionalized acute care cardiac centers organized around the concept of providing rapid and effective treatment. Acute cardiac care at the dawn of a new millennium, based upon the concept of salvageable myocardium, represents a dramatic shift from the passive rest, recovery, and rehabilitation approach to MI of the 1970s that was predicated on the paradigm of irreversible damage. This strategy is now being applied to patients with acute strokes. We know that "time is myocardium"; we need to recognize that "time is brain." "Brain attacks" should engender similar connotation to "heart attacks." Prompt restoration of cerebral perfusion is critical to outcome; thus, every aspect of the treatment plan must be directed toward preserving neurons and restoring blood flow as rapidly as possible.

The one practical difference that exists between MI and cerebral infarction is the occurrence of both hemorrhagic and ischemic infarcts in the brain. Obviously, thrombolytic therapy must be avoided in the setting of hemorrhage, but this diagnosis can be made easily using CT scanning, because hemorrhage, unlike bland cerebral infarction, is detectable as soon as it occurs. Since ischemic infarction accounts for approximately 75% of all strokes, reperfusion induced by thrombolysis is widely applicable.

Although there are few data defining the so-called "window of opportunity" (i.e., the interval between onset of symptoms and irreversible damage), most authorities think that perfusion must be restored within 4 to 6 hours in order to provide maximal benefit. Indeed, although the interval of irreversible cerebral ischemia is still undetermined, there is evidence from both animal and human experiments that delayed thrombolysis is ineffective and also extends infarction due to hemorrhage.

Can intravenous thrombolysis produce results comparable to catheter-directed intra-arterial thrombolytic techniques (a question similar to the controversy encountered in the cardiac care arena)? Logistics and economics dictate that emergency treatment of stroke by simple IV infusion is more economical and available than are the specialized personnel and equipment needed to provide subselective cerebral angiography and catheter-directed thrombolysis. Prospective cost-effectiveness analyses will be required to answer this question.

Strategy for Thrombolytic Therapy

From a purely technical standpoint, subselective catheter-directed thrombolysis appears to be more effective than intravenous thrombolysis. Unlike endovascular occlusion of intracranial AVMs and aneurysms for which considerable experience and a knowledge of functional neuroanatomy (including the innumerable potential routes of collateral circulation) is required, restoring cerebral perfusion is far easier.

Preservation of normal neurons is another area of active research. Because it is not yet possible to differentiate ischemic from hemorrhagic infarcts before hospitalization, administration of IV thrombolytic agents is unsafe. Experiments in cardiac reperfusion models have shown that reperfusing myocardium with blood can produce cell damage that limits therapeutic benefit in proportion to the duration of the ischemia. Whether a conceptually similar neuroplegia is possible is another topic of active research.

The work done in catheter-directed thrombolysis explains why emergency surgery has had such disappointing results in the care of patients with the stroke-in-evolution syndrome. Until the advent of catheter-directed thrombolytic treatment for stroke-in-evolution, there had been little reason to perform cerebral angiography in the case of ischemic stroke. (Obviously, if one is dealing with stroke due to subarachnoid or certain specific types of intracerebral hemorrhage, there is a premium on obtaining prompt angiographic diagnosis in order to detect intracranial aneurysms or AVMs amenable to endovascular or surgical therapy.) As angiographic experience has grown in this area, it is clear that most ischemic infarcts are due to thrombi or emboli lodged in branches of the middle cerebral artery or, less commonly, the anterior cerebral artery, not thrombotic occlusion at the site of atheromatous carotid disease.

The Postoperative Patient

Routine intraoperative "completion angiography" following carotid endarterectomy has become very common, although there is still some controversy as to its indication. Irregularities of the endarterectomy margins and intimal fractures ("clamp defects") are common and are of little clinical significance. Furthermore, such irregularities are likely to disappear when the vessel heals. However, the presence of an unsuspected and potentially occlusive intimal flap or an endarterectomy that fails to traverse the area of stenosis fully is of considerable significance and therefore best detected when correction involves simply reopening an already exposed vessel and repairing the defect. Although completion angiography has become commonplace, some surgeons have chosen to employ routine angioscopic evaluation or intraoperative duplex ultrasonography, since these techniques may be even more sensitive than conventional angiography in the detection of correctable technical problems.

The occurrence of an acute neurologic event in the immediate postoperative period is best treated by prompt reexploration when it occurs in the same vascular territory rather than accepting the delays inherent in obtaining angiography even in the most efficient centers. If reexploration fails to reveal a correctable surgical problem, however, intraoperative angiography is essential. Once the immediate postoperative period has passed, the occurrence or recurrence of symptoms in a patient who has recently undergone carotid endarterectomy mandates angiographic evaluation of both the operative site and the downstream vascular territory subject to embolization from that area. If the surgery is not recent (>6 months ago), evaluation should be as thorough as in the case of a patient who has not yet had surgery, because of the possible development of new lesions or the exacerbation of previously mild lesions.

ENDOVASCULAR PROCEDURES

Until fairly recently, angiography was primarily a diagnostic modality in the management of cerebrovascular disease despite rapid advances in interventional radiology elsewhere in the body. However, interventional neuroradiologic techniques, notably intracranial embolization, have gained general acceptance owing to their high degree of success, as well as to the corresponding limitations of conventional surgical therapy in such cases. Indeed, endovascular treatment is now widely accepted as the appropriate first-line management for intracranial aneurysms and AVMs. Similarly, catheter-directed thrombolysis also may become important in the management of acute stroke. In contrast, the excellent results and low morbidity of extracranial cerebrovascular surgery, specifically carotid endarterectomy, at first would seem to make endovascular therapies nothing more than valuable adjunctive techniques, with specific but limited application. However, it is obvious that percutaneous carotid angioplasty and stenting are currently very controversial topics.

From a strictly technical point of view, percutaneous internal carotid angioplasty with stent implantation is a remarkably simple procedure. Indeed, it is far less technically demanding than either peripheral, visceral, or coronary angioplasty and can be accomplished with remarkable speed. The problem is that there has been a dramatic and rather uncontrolled surge in enthusiasm for this procedure. Numerous 1- and 2-day courses have been given as how-to sessions, with many of the proponents presenting their material in a "don't try this at home" manner that actually encourages exactly that sort of approach.

Unfortunately, much of the debate has broken down along specialty turf lines. Vascular surgeons, who generally stand ready to be convinced by real evidence, remain skeptical in view of the already well-documented favorable outcomes for conventional carotid endarterectomy. Interventional radiologists, usually strong proponents of endovascular alternatives to conventional open surgery, have also tended to remain skeptical, seeing carotid angioplasty as a technique with benefits in limited applications, such as recurrent stenosis following carotid endarterectomy, stenosis due to radiation-induced fibrosis, fibromuscular dysplasia (Fig. 129–36), carotid disease in the setting of a hostile surgical field associated with major prior head and neck surgery, and unusually high carotid bifurcations. The fact that carotid endarterectomy can be accomplished with either general anesthesia or local anesthesia and mild conscious sedation also means that almost no patients are too ill to undergo this procedure and reinforces the attitude of both the surgeons and the radiologists.

Interventional cardiologists, in contrast, have been the major proponents in this area, often to the dismay of their surgical and radiologic colleagues. Of particular concern to their colleagues is the fact that many patients are routed toward angioplasty and stenting simply as a result of referral patterns that do not include either surgeons or radiologists in the evaluation or management decisions.

Leaving the thorny, albeit very significant, turf issues aside, carotid angioplasty is certainly a technique that merits substantive critical evaluation (Fig. 129–37). In its pres-

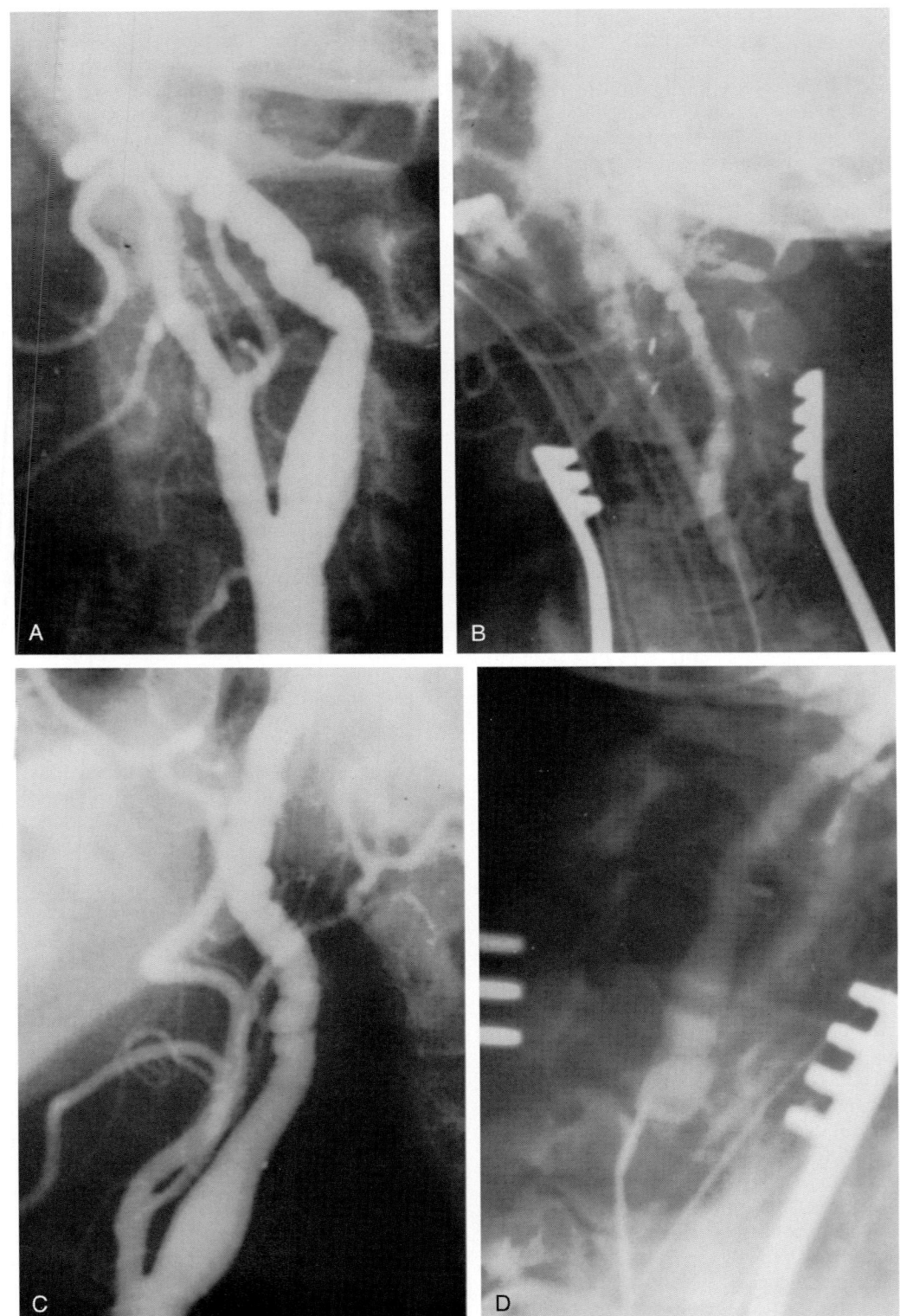

FIGURE 129–36. *A,* Preoperative left common carotid angiogram showing multiple diaphragm-like stenoses of fibromuscular dysplasia. *B,* Intraoperative completion angiogram following two attempts at dilatation using rigid DeBakey dilators, documenting the presence of residual stenoses and irregularities. *C,* Preoperative right common carotid angiogram documenting similar lesions. *D,* Intraoperative completion angiogram following dilatation using transluminal balloon angioplasty catheter, showing no significant residual stenoses.

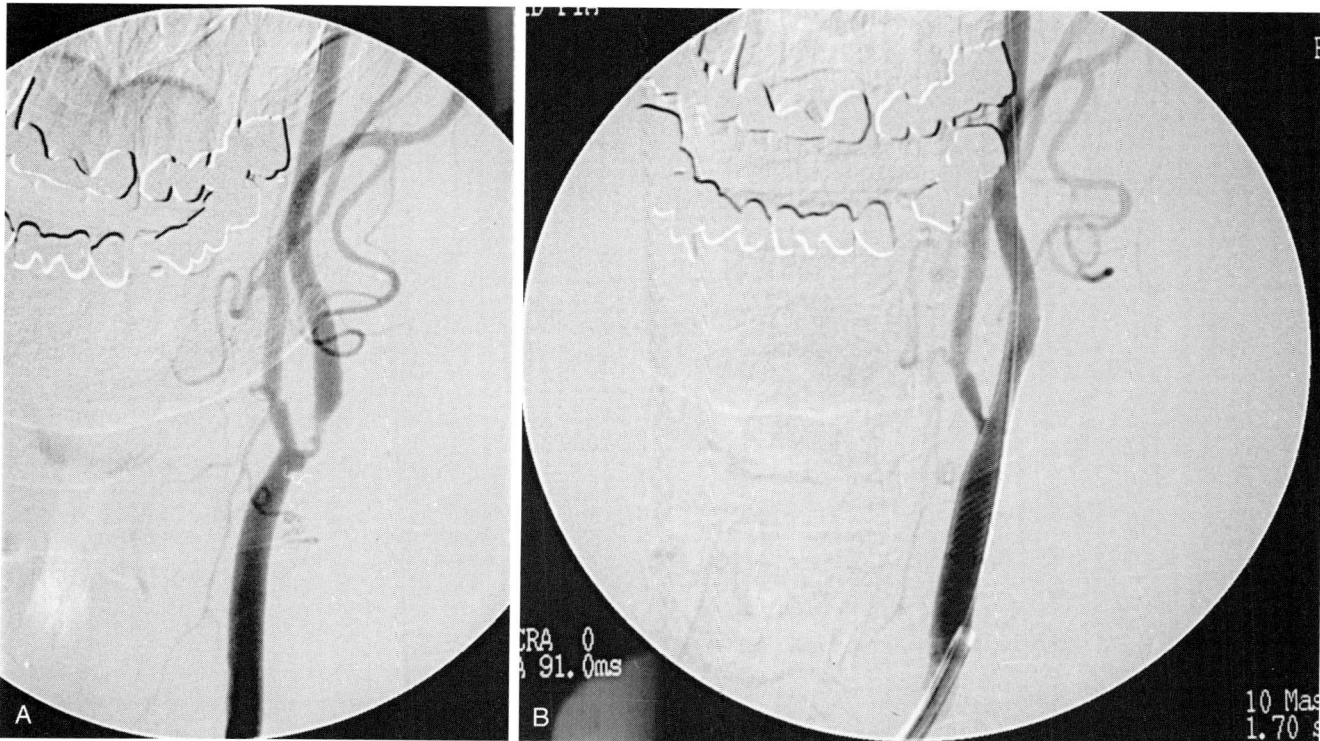

FIGURE 129–37. *A,* Left carotid angiogram showing high-grade stenosis in the proximal internal carotid artery, which recurred after two prior carotid endarterectomies. *B,* Angiogram following balloon catheter angioplasty and deployment of a self-expanding stent (Wallstent—Schneider USA, Minneapolis, Minn.)

ent iteration, it seems unlikely to be a technique that can compete solely on its technical merits. In addition, cost comparisons often fail to show significant differences, although such comparisons are difficult and subject to artificial manipulation. Reports from very capable individuals indicate complication rates (significant neurologic deficits and death) ranging from 5% to 7%, in contrast to surgical carotid endarterectomy in which complications of 1% to 2% are the norm. Furthermore, long-term follow-up data are just starting to become available, so that the durability of an initially favorable result is still unknown. Also, numerous technical improvements are being made in the procedure, making evaluation of older data of limited utility in evaluating current techniques. To that end, a number of prospective randomized trials are being undertaken in an effort to put the technique on a solid intellectual footing so that the real merits vis-à-vis conventional surgery can be determined scientifically. One can only speculate as to how this issue will be resolved and whether carotid angioplasty and stenting will merit a brief historical footnote or its own chapter in the next edition of this textbook.

SELECTED READINGS

1. Ahuja A, Blatt GL, Guterman LR, Hopkins LN: Angioplasty for symptomatic radiation-induced extracranial carotid artery stenosis: Case report. Neurosurgery 36(2):399–403, 1995.
2. Appleyard RF, Cohn LH: Myocardial stunning and reperfusion injury in cardiac surgery. J Card Surg 8(2 Suppl):316–324, 1993.
3. Arlart I, Bongartz GM: Magnetic Resonance Angiography. Darmstadt, Springer Verlag, 1996.
4. Babatasi G, Massetti M, Theron J, Khayat A: Asymptomatic carotid stenosis in patients undergoing major cardiac surgery: Can percutaneous carotid angioplasty be an alternative? Eur J Cardiothorac Surg 11(3):547–553, 1997.
5. Balousek PA, Knowles HJ, Higashida RT, del Zoppo GJ: New interventions in cerebrovascular disease: The role of thrombolytic therapy and balloon angioplasty. Opin Cardiol 11(5):550–557, 1996.
6. Baum S (ed), Abrams HL: Abrams Angiography: Vascular and Interventional Radiology. Philadelphia, Lippincott-Raven, 1996.
7. Ben-Menachem Y: Angiography in Trauma: A Work Atlas. Philadelphia, WB Saunders, 1981.
8. Bergeon P, Rudondy P, Benichou H, et al: Transluminal angioplasty for recurrent stenosis after carotid endarterectomy: Prognostic factors and indications. Int Angiol 12(3):256–259, 1993.
9. Bettmann MA, Katzen BT, Whisnant J, et al: Carotid stenting and angioplasty: A statement for healthcare professionals from the Councils on Cardiovascular Radiology, Stroke, Cardio-Thoracic and Vascular Surgery, Epidemiology, and Prevention, and Clinical Cardiology, American Heart Association. Stroke 29(1):336–338, 1998.
10. Buckberg GD: Update on current techniques of myocardial protection. Ann Thorac Surg 60(3):805–814, 1995.
11. Busch E, Kruger K, Allegrini PR, et al: Reperfusion after thrombolytic therapy of embolic stroke in the rat: Magnetic resonance and biochemical imaging. J Cereb Blood Flow Metab 18(4):407–418, 1998.
12. Chaturvedi S, Policherla PN, Femino L: Cerebral angiography practices at US teaching hospitals: Implications for carotid endarterectomy. Stroke 28(10):1895–1897, 1997.
13. Comerota AJ, Eze AR: Intraoperative high-dose regional urokinase infusion for cerebrovascular occlusion after carotid endarterectomy. J Vasc Surg 24(6):1008–1016, 1996.
14. del Zoppo GJ: Thrombolysis in acute stroke. Neurologia 10(Suppl) 2:37–47, 1995.
15. del Zoppo GJ, Higashida RT, Furlan AJ, et al: PROACT: A phase II randomized trial of recombinant pro-urokinase by direct arterial delivery in acute middle cerebral artery stroke. PROACT Investigators. Prolyse in Acute Cerebral Thromboembolism. Stroke 29(1):4–11, 1998.
16. Derdeyn CP, Powers WJ, Moran CJ, et al: Role of Doppler ultrasound

in screening for carotid atherosclerotic disease. Radiology 197(3):635–643, 1995.

17. Ferguson RD, Ferguson JG: Carotid angioplasty: In search of a worthy alternative to endarterectomy. Arch Neurol 53(7):696–698, 1996.

18. Gagne PJ, Matchett J, MacFarland D, et al: Can the NASCET technique for measuring carotid stenosis be reliably applied outside the trial? J Vasc Surg 24(3):449–455, 1996.

19. Gasecki AP, Ferguson GG, Eliasziw M, et al: Early endarterectomy for severe carotid artery stenosis after a nondisabling stroke: Results from the North American Symptomatic Carotid Endarterectomy Trial. J Vasc Surg 20(2):288–295, 1994.

20. Golledge J, Wright R, Pugh N, Lane IF: Colour-coded duplex assessment alone before carotid endarterectomy. Br J Surg 83(9):1234–1237, 1996.

21. Hacke W, Kaste M, Fieschi C, et al: Intravenous thrombolysis with recombinant tissue plasminogen activator for acute hemispheric stroke The European Cooperative Acute Stroke Study. JAMA; 274(13):1017–1025, 1995.

22. Higashida RT, Tsai FY, Halbach VV, et al: Interventional neurovascular techniques in the treatment of stroke: State-of-the-art therapy. Intern Med 237(1):105–115, 1995.

23. Jordan WD Jr, Roye GD, Fisher WS 3rd, et al: A cost comparison of balloon angioplasty and stenting versus endarterectomy for the treatment of carotid artery stenosis. J Vasc Surg 27(1):16–22, 1998.

24. Jordan WD Jr, Schroeder PT, Fisher WS, McDowell HA: A comparison of angioplasty with stenting versus endarterectomy for the treatment of carotid artery stenosis. Ann Vasc Surg 11(1):2–8, 1997.

25. Kachel R: Results of balloon angioplasty in the carotid arteries. J Endovasc Surg 3(1):22–30, 1996.

26. Kadir S: Diagnostic Angiography. Philadelphia, WB Saunders, 1986.

27. Kent KC, Kuntz KM, Patel MR, et al: Perioperative imaging strategies for carotid endarterectomy: An analysis of morbidity and cost-effectiveness in symptomatic patients. JAMA 274(11):888–893, 1995.

28. Landis DM, Tarr RW, Selman WR: Thrombolysis for acute ischemic stroke. Neurosurg Clin North Am 8(2):219–226, 1997.

29. Lanzer P, Rösch J: Vascular Diagnostics. Darmstadt, Springer-Verlag, 1994.

30. Lee TT, Solomon NA, Heidenreich PA, et al: Cost-effectiveness of screening for carotid stenosis in asymptomatic persons. Ann Intern Med 126(5):337–346, 1997.

31. Link J, Brossmann J, Grabener M, et al: Spiral CT angiography and selective digital subtraction angiography of internal carotid artery stenosis. AJNR Am J Neuroradiol 17(1):89–94, 1996.

32. Link J, Brossmann J, Penselin V, et al: Common carotid artery bifurcation: Preliminary results of CT angiography and color-coded duplex sonography compared with digital subtraction angiography. Am J Roentgenol 168(2):361–365, 1997.

33. Mani RL, Eisenberg RL, McDonald EJ, et al: Complications of catheter cerebral angiography: Analysis of 5000 procedures: I. Criteria and incidence. AJR 131:861, 1978.

34. Marek J, Mills JL, Harvich J, et al: Utility of routine carotid duplex screening in patients who have claudication. Vasc Surg 24(4):572–577, 1996.

35. Mathur A, Dorros G, Iyer SS, et al: Palmaz stent compression in patients following carotid artery stenting. Cathet Cardiovasc Diagn 41(2):137–140, 1997.

36. McMinn RMH, Hutchings RT, Logan BM: Color Atlas of Head and Neck Anatomy. St. Louis, Mosby–Year Book, Medical, 1994.

37. Mori E, Tabuchi M, Yoshida T, Yamadori A: Intracarotid urokinase with thromboembolic occlusion of the middle cerebral artery. Stroke 19(7):802–812, 1988.

38. Muller M, Bartylla K, Rolshausen A, et al: Influence of the angiographic internal carotid artery stenosis assessment method on indicating carotid surgery. Vasa 27(1):24–28, 1998.

39. Murphy KJ, Rubin JM: Power Doppler: It's a good thing. Semin Ultrasound CT MR 18(1):13–21, 1997.

40. Osborn AG: Diagnostic Neuroradiology. St. Louis, Mosby-Year Book, 1994.

41. Padayachee TS, Cox TC, Modaresi KB, et al: The measurement of internal carotid artery stenosis: Comparison of duplex with digital subtraction angiography. Eur J Vasc Endovasc Surg 13(2):180–185, 1997.

42. Paddock-Eliasziw LM, Eliasziw M, Barr HW, Barnett HJ: Long-term prognosis and the effect of carotid endarterectomy in patients with recurrent ipsilateral ischemic events. North American Symptomatic Carotid Endarterectomy Trial Group. Neurology 47(5):1158–1162, 1996.

43. Romanes GJ (ed): Cunningham's Manual of Practical Anatomy; Head, Neck, and Brain. London, Oxford University Press, 1986.

44. Roubin GS, Yadav S, Iyer SS, Vitek J: Carotid stent-supported angioplasty: A neurovascular intervention to prevent stroke. Am J Cardiol 78(3A):8–12, 1996.

45. Sivaguru A, Venables GS, Beard JD, Gaines PA: European carotid angioplasty trial. J Endovasc Surg 3(1):16–20, 1996.

46. Skolnick AA: Rapid clot-dissolving drugs promising for stroke. JAMA 269(2):195–198, 1993.

47. Smith DC, Smith LL, Hasso AN: Fibromuscular dysplasia of the internal carotid artery treated by operative transluminal balloon angioplasty. Radiology 155:645, 1985.

48. Stark DD, Bradley WG (eds): Magnetic Resonance Imaging. St. Louis, Mosby–Year Book, Medical, 1992.

49. Steinke W, Ries S, Artemis N, et al: Power Doppler imaging of carotid artery stenosis: Comparison with color Doppler flow imaging and angiography. Stroke 28(10):1981–1987, 1997.

50. Streifler JY, Eliasziw M, Fox AJ, et al: Angiographic detection of carotid plaque ulceration: Comparison with surgical observations in a multicenter study. North American Symptomatic Carotid Endarterectomy Trial. Stroke 25(6):1130–1132, 1994.

51. Theron JG, Payelle GG, Coskun O, et al: Carotid artery stenosis: Treatment with protected balloon angioplasty and stent placement. Radiology 201(3):627–636, 1996.

52. Vale FL, Fisher WS 3rd, Jordan WD Jr, et al: Carotid endarterectomy performed after progressive carotid stenosis following angioplasty and stent placement: Case report. J Neurosurg 87(6):940–943, 1997.

53. Vanninen RL, Manninen HI, Partanen PK, et al: How should we estimate carotid stenosis using magnetic resonance angiography? Neuroradiology 38(4):299–305, 1996.

54. Yin D, Carpenter JP: Cost-effectiveness of screening for asymptomatic carotid stenosis. J Vasc Surg 27(2):245–255, 1998.

55. Executive Committee for the Asymptomatic Carotid Atherosclerosis Study: Endarterectomy for asymptomatic carotid artery stenosis. JAMA 273(18):1421–1428, 1995.

56. The EC/IC Bypass Study Group: Failure of extracranial-intracranial arterial bypass to reduce the risk of ischemic stroke. N Engl J Med 313:1191, 1985.

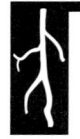

C H A P T E R   1 3 0

The Role of Noninvasive Studies in the Diagnosis and Management of Cerebrovascular Disease

Michael A. Ricci, M.D., and Steven J. Knight, R.V.T.

The benefits of carotid endarterectomy reported in randomized trials[30, 31, 58, 82] have brought to the forefront the need for accurate, safe diagnosis of carotid bifurcation disease.[40, 77] Concepts once thought to be unassailable, such as pre-endarterectomy contrast angiography, are now being challenged.[77] A multitude of diagnostic tests, combinations of tests, and diagnostic algorithms may leave the student of vascular diseases bewildered and frustrated.

HISTORY OF NONINVASIVE TESTING

Perhaps the best way to understand the current controversies is to understand how the field of noninvasive evaluation of cerebrovascular disease has developed. The interested reader is referred to a fascinating and complete history of the development of ultrasound technologies for cerebrovascular diagnosis provided by Strandness.[74]

The clinical use of ultrasound for vascular diagnosis began in the mid-1960s, when a continuous wave Doppler device was developed at the University of Washington and subsequently marketed as the "Dopotone."[74] The device had a single transducer connected to a speaker to produce an audible output of the detected frequency shift. The device could detect the presence or absence of blood flow, and, with some experience, the user could subjectively estimate the quality of the signal as normal or abnormal. However, (1) the listener could not be sure of which vessel was examined (because any vessel within the path of the ultrasound wave could be detected), (2) an objective analog display was lacking, and (3) direction of flow could not be determined.

The third of these shortcomings was solved by McLeod and colleagues at the University of Washington when changes in the direction of flow were recognized as positive and negative Doppler frequency shifts that were separated electronically.[74] The inability to detect flow direction is almost inconceivable 25 years later, but the use of this "pulsed Doppler" technique allowed the study of complex flow patterns, such as that seen at the carotid bulb, that ultimately had clinical diagnostic implications. Yet the early Doppler devices still lacked the ability to determine definitively which vessel was being examined and to produce an archivable analog recording.

Early clinical use of the *Doppler flowmeter* was introduced

by Brockenbrough in 1969.[14] Through a sequence of maneuvers, the periorbital Doppler examination evaluated the direction of flow in branches of the ophthalmic artery and collateral vessels to predict internal carotid artery (ICA) stenosis. Despite modifications,[11] this simple, inexpensive test did not prove reliable enough for all users and, when used today, is only an adjunct to other investigations. The fundamental principle is sound, however, and in fact forms the basis of today's transcranial Doppler (TCD) examinations.

Practical clinical applications of ultrasound technology required two additional innovations to gain widespread acceptance. The first was a successful means to convert Doppler frequency shifts to an analog form (fast-Fourier transformation [FFT] spectral analysis), and the second was accurate imaging of the vascular system with B-mode or gray scale ultrasound, forming the basis of the modern *duplex scanner*. Many technical electronic modifications followed that improved the image, Doppler ultrasound quality, and reproducibility of testing while clinicians defined diagnostic criteria and expanded indications for its use.[74]

The next significant advance, however, did not occur until the late 1970s, when color flow imaging was developed. Interestingly, the addition of color by itself does not improve the criteria for diagnosis but aids in defining complex flow patterns. Tortuous vessels, flow disturbances, and even "routine" examinations are facilitated by real-time color flow patterns within the vessel under investigation. The current iteration of the duplex scanner is the result of three decades of technical innovations and clinical experience that followed each innovation. Future enhancements may include power Doppler imaging[70] or extended field-of-view technology,[84] although the accuracy and utility of these technologies need to be validated.

Not all noninvasive cerebrovascular techniques have utilized ultrasound, however. Concurrent with introduction of the Doppler flowmeter, Kartchner and McRae reported that *carotid phonoangiography* could accurately evaluate the degree of ICA stenosis when a carotid bruit was present.[43] This technology employed a special microphone placed over the vessel and an oscilloscope recording of the bruit. A bruit extending throughout systole was determined to represent an ICA stenosis greater than 40% with 87% accuracy.[43] Despite initial enthusiasm, this technique was applicable only to a small percentage of patients and proved to be inaccurate for screening or diagnosis of carotid artery stenoses.

Ocular pneumoplethysmography (OPG) is another noninvasive test developed in the 1970s to diagnose indirectly
carotid artery stenosis. Two different OPG methods have
been developed.[38, 44] Kartchner and associates developed
the OPG-Kartchner method to quantitate the arrival of the
pulse wave in the eye.[44] A unilateral carotid stenosis would
produce a delay in the arrival of the pulse wave. With
fluid-filled eye cups held in place with 40 to 50 mmHg
suction and photodetectors on each earlobe, a delay in the
arrival of one pulse wave compared with that arriving in
the contralateral eye indicated an ipsilateral stenosis of
70%. Delay of pulse waves in both eyes compared with the
earlobes indicated bilateral stenosis. Although initial studies
were promising, the OPG-Kartchner was largely abandoned
because of inaccuracies inherent in most indirect tests.[44]

The second method of ocular pneumoplethysmography,
OPG-Gee, was developed contemporaneously with OPG-
Kartchner but utilized an entirely different methodology[38];
the ophthalmic artery pressure was measured directly by
applying sustained pressure to fluid-filled eye cups. The
OPG-Gee test result is abnormal if (1) there is a difference
in ophthalmic artery pressure of 5 mmHg or more between
the eyes; (2) the pressure difference is between 1 and 4
mmHg and the ratio of the ophthalmic artery pressure to
the brachial pressure is less than 0.66; or (3) the pressures
in each eye are equal and the ratio is less than 0.6. This
indirect evaluation also produced excellent initial results[7, 37]
and is still used for screening or for monitoring during
carotid surgery. Although OPG-Gee also suffers from the
inadequacies of indirect testing, it is still used as a research
tool for screening populations for carotid stenosis.

A minimally invasive angiographic technique also deserves mention in this section: intravenous digital subtraction angiography (IV DSA). Although this test may still be
performed in some hospitals, initial interest waned because
of large contrast loads and unsatisfactory images in most
patients.[21, 26] Because IV DSA avoided an arterial puncture,
outpatient examinations, lower costs, and decreased risk of
arterial complications were thought to be advantages. More
recent techniques of intra-arterial digital subtraction angiography have eliminated some of those potential advantages
with clearly superior images, and the reliability and low
cost of duplex scanning has supplanted the need for IV
DSA.

DUPLEX SCANNING

Equipment

The modern duplex scanner includes gray scale image
production, velocity spectral analysis, and color flow imaging and plays a pivotal role in cerebrovascular diagnosis.
As a bare minimum, an ultrasound system consists of a
computer processor to manage the huge volume of information and calculations generated by scanning, a color
monitor, and ultrasound transducers of different frequencies. Although most ultrasound systems automatically pre-
set the system settings to optimize performance based on
the selected transducer and the test to be performed, adjustments may be made to the *pulse repetition frequency*

(PRF), gain, and power, depending on circumstances. The
transducer's transmitting frequency may vary from 2.5 to
12 MHz, with the lower frequencies allowing greater tissue
penetration. For cerebrovascular examinations, usually a
5.0- or 7.5-MHz frequency is used.

Strandness[75] has listed the essential system elements for
cerebrovascular duplex scanning:

1. Good high-resolution image.
2. A small Doppler sample volume (~3 mm³ at an
operating range of 25 mm to allow sampling in four sites
across the vessel).
3. Real-time spectral analysis that allows a display from
−3 to +7 kHz.
4. Hard copy output for image and spectral analysis.
5. Automatic display of the angle of incidence of the
Doppler ultrasound beam.
6. Conversion of frequency to angle-adjusted velocity.

Technique

A thorough understanding of the carotid artery anatomy as
well as Doppler physics, hemodynamics (see Chapter 7),
and physiology (see Chapter 10) is necessary. Patients
should be positioned supine with their heads turned away
from the side being examined and with the examiner at the
head. Each step in the examination sequence should be
carried out in exactly the same way each time to ensure
that no step is overlooked. The examination should include
both longitudinal and transverse views throughout. Scanning with the 5.0- or 7.5-MHz transducer should begin
low in the neck with the common carotid artery (CCA)
and proceed distally to the carotid bulb, external carotid
artery (ECA), and ICA. After examination of the carotid
system, the transducer is positioned posteriorly to assess
the vertebral artery. The examination is then repeated on
the opposite side. At each level, the color flow pattern, the
gray scale image, and spectral analysis are assessed.

The color flow pattern accelerates the examination by
rapidly identifying "suspicious" areas. The presence of a
"jet," a focal color change indicating very high velocities,
can locate an area of stenosis to be interrogated with
Doppler spectral analysis. A color change indicating reversed flow at the end of systole is normal in the CCA,
ECA, and ICA bulb, but more pronounced color changes
may indicate turbulence in the region of a stenosis. Sometimes turbulence created by a stenosis may produce a "color
bruit" as tissue adjacent to the artery reverberates and
creates pixels of color (indicating movement) outside of the
vessel. In the vertebral system, reversal of flow may indicate
a pathologic obstruction of the subclavian artery. Simultaneously, the location of plaque should be noted, but estimates of the degree of stenosis based on the gray scale
image alone should be avoided.

Usually, the CCA is reasonably free of disease, but sometimes significant plaque may be identified. It is also important to identify the distal extent of the plaque in the
ICA, particularly if carotid endarterectomy (CEA) is to be
performed without angiography, to ensure that the lesion
is completely surgically accessible.

Ulcerations may sometimes be more easily seen with gray scale imaging, without color.[59] The ability to see ulcerations, however, is variable; many authors have found that duplex scanning is unreliable, with overall detection rates in the 50% to 60% range compared with the rate for surgical specimens.[20, 64] Color flow scanning has not improved the ability to visualize ulcerations.[72] Comerota and colleagues have suggested that ulcerations may be more reliably detected when the degree of stenosis is less than 50%.[20] Absence of ulceration on duplex scans does not mean that an ulcer does not exist because this is not a reliable method of detection (neither, as it turns out, is arteriography, which is equally poor in detecting ulceration).[27, 29] Additionally, the plaque characteristics (hard, calcific plaque; soft, hemorrhagic plaque; or heterogeneous plaque, which has elements of both) should be noted, although the significance of these findings remains undetermined. Calcific plaque may prevent the transmission of ultrasound waves, creating shadowing artifacts. Some authorities have suggested that plaque hemorrhage (producing "soft" plaque) places the patient at increased risk for stroke,[42] but whether the character of the plaque can predict the risk of stroke remains unproved.

Although each of the aforementioned details is important during the cerebrovascular duplex examination, the most important factor in diagnosis of carotid stenosis is the spectral analysis. The B-mode or color image serves to direct the placement of the Doppler beam for sampling. Multiple samples from the midstream of the vessel being interrogated are routinely obtained. The angle of incidence of the ultrasound beam should be 60 degrees or less. (Subsequent scans should be done at the same angle.) Spectral analysis should be obtained low in the CCA and in its middle and distal portions, in the ECA, through the carotid bulb, and throughout the ICA.

Specific parameters to be recorded include peak systolic velocity (PSV), end-diastolic velocity (EDV), the ratio of the PSV in the ICA and CCA (PSV ICA/CCA ratio), and the ratio of the EDV in the ICA and CCA (EDV ICA/CCA ratio). Obviously, any areas suggestive of stenosis on the basis of the color pattern should be thoroughly investigated. The spectral profile in the CCA typically demonstrates a mix of the low-resistance pattern seen in the ICA (flow during diastole) and the high-resistance pattern (no flow during diastole) of the ECA (Fig. 130–1). A high-resistance profile in the CCA may be the first clue to an ICA occlusion.

As previously noted, a brief flow reversal in the carotid bulb is a normal finding. In addition, there is normally a narrow spectra of velocities in undiseased vessels, known as a "spectral window" (Fig. 130–1). Stenosis within the bulb and ICA produces turbulence that diminishes or obliterates the window with "spectral broadening," one of the earlier signs of stenosis. Spectral broadening can also be artificially generated if the sample volume is too large or the sample is too close to the vessel wall (as opposed to mid-stream sample) or in tortuous vessels. In addition, if the gain is too high, the spectral window will be obliterated with artificially elevated velocities. The gain should be set so that there is a minimal but discernible amount of background noise.

Diagnostic Criteria

Various criteria have been developed for the duplex diagnosis of carotid artery disease, but the two most commonly used are those of Strandness[75] and Zwiebel[88, 89] (Table 130–1). Strandness has reported a sensitivity of 99% and a specificity of of 84%[75]; others have reported 96% accuracy with the same criteria to detect stenosis greater than 50% and 97% accuracy in the detection of occlusion.[10] Criteria for identifying normal and abnormal vertebral arteries have also been determined and are listed in Table 130–2.[12] It is important, however, that these criteria be validated in the vascular laboratory in which they are used.[4, 34, 57] Whether the same ultrasound system is used in different laboratories[4] or the same personnel use different systems,[34] it is clear that variations occur even when the same patients are scanned.[34]

One special situation exists that requires modification of the standard criteria: When a severe stenosis or complete ipsilateral occlusion is present, diagnostic criteria in the contralateral vessel must be altered. In this situation, flow through the contralateral carotid system may be increased to compensate for the obstruction.[36, 73] Spadone and colleagues first pointed out that the PSV and EDV were increased in the ICA contralateral to severe stenosis or occlusion.[73] The effect was most prominent in the 50% to 79% category. Subsequently, Fujitani and coworkers modified the standard Strandness criteria (Table 130–3) after reviewing the duplex scans of 154 patients who had angiographic evidence of unilateral ICA occlusion.[36] The modified criteria were 97.5% accurate in detecting 80% to 99% stenosis and 96.9% accurate in detecting 50% to 79% stenosis contralateral to ICA occlusion (Table 130–4).

Slightly different criteria were developed by AbuRahma and coworkers,[3] who evaluated the criteria of Strandness[75] and Fujitani and coworkers[36] and two modifications based on velocity or ICA/CCA ratios. They identified 356 arteries with more than 50% stenosis by duplex scanning. Angiography revealed stenoses of at least 50% in 247 arteries: 97 had 80% to 99% stenosis, and 39 had complete occlusion. They found that the Strandness criteria[75] were less reliable in the presence of contralateral severe stenosis or occlusion. (see Table 130–4). Their results were comparable with the criteria of Fujitani and coworkers,[36] but PSV ICA/CCA ratios were unreliable (see Table 130–4). For 50% to 79% stenoses, the criteria of Fujitani and coworkers[36] and the new criteria of AbuRhama and coworkers[3] were comparable with 97% accuracy and high sensitivity, specificity, and predictive values (see Table 130–3). For 80% to 99% stenoses, both sets of criteria were good, with a slight edge in accuracy with the criteria of AbuRahma and coworkers[3]: 96% versus 94%. It should be emphasized that AbuRahma and coworkers[3] included both hemodynamically significant stenoses and occlusions in contrast to Fujitani and coworkers,[36] who included only occlusions. The former approach may actually have greater clinical applicability. Adoption of the criteria of AbuRahma and coworkers[3] or Fujitani and coworkers[36] is recommended, but individual laboratories should correlate their results with angiography, as emphasized above.

Another special situation that has prompted modifications of the diagnostic criteria is the desire to correlate

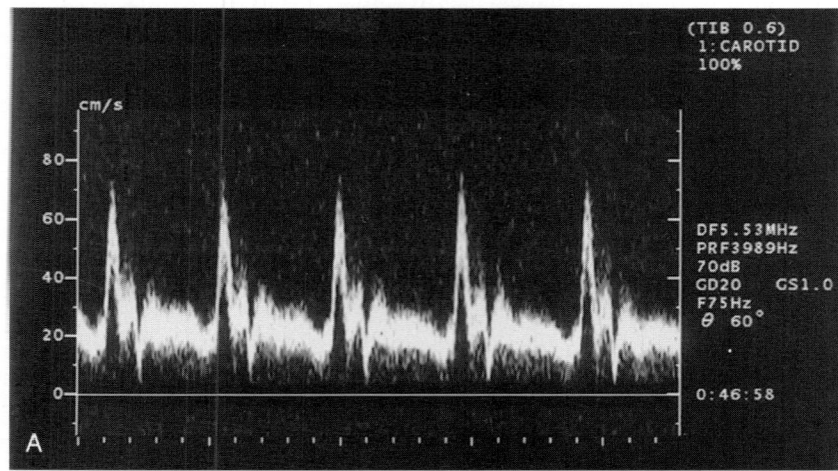

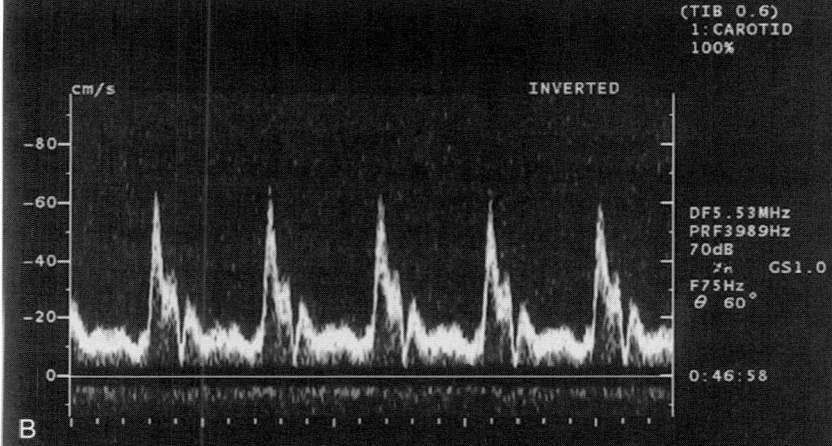

FIGURE 130–1. Normal fast-Fourier transformation spectral analysis patterns in the (A) common carotid artery (CCA), (B) external carotid artery (ECA), and (C) internal carotid artery (ICA). The ECA demonstrates minimal flow during diastole, indicating a high-resistance peripheral vascular bed, and a prominent dichrotic notch. The ICA supplies the low-resistance bed in the brain and demonstrates flow throughout diastole. The CCA demonstrates a mix of the patterns from the ICA and ECA. Note the absence of signals below the peak velocities recorded in the ICA, an area known as the "spectral window."

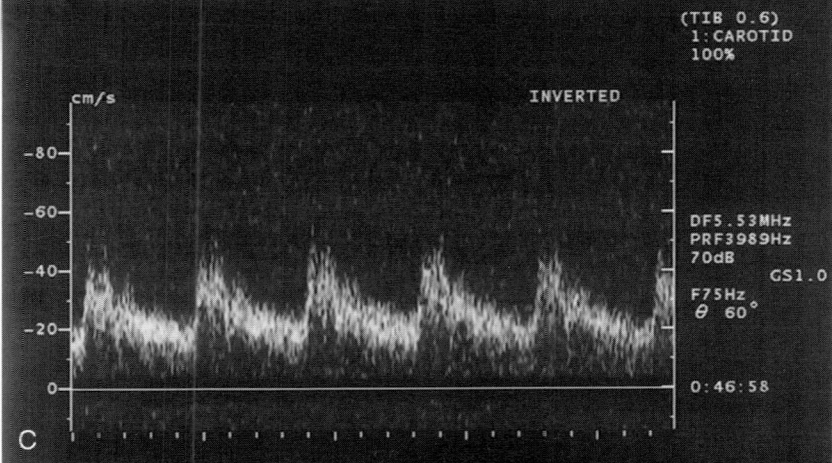

TABLE 130–1. CRITERIA FOR DUPLEX SCANNING DIAGNOSIS OF INTERNAL CAROTID ARTERY STENOSIS

STRANDNESS CRITERIA[75]		ZWIEBEL CRITERIA[89]	
Stenosis	Characteristics	Stenosis	Characteristics
Normal	PSV < 125 cm/sec No SB Flow reversal in bulb	0%	PSV < 110 cm/sec EDV < 40 cm/sec PSV ICA/CCA ratio < 1.8 EDV ICA/CCA < 2.4 SB < 30 cm/sec
1%–15%	PSV < 125 cm/sec No or minimal SB Flow reversal in bulb absent	1%–39%	PSV < 110 cm/sec EDV < 40 cm/sec PSV ICA/CCA ratio < 1.8 EDV ICA/CCA < 2.4 SB < 40 cm/sec
16%–49%	PSV > 125 cm/sec Marked SB	40%–59%	PSV < 130 cm/sec EDV < 40 cm/sec PSV ICA/CCA ratio < 1.8 EDV ICA/CCA < 2.4 SB < 40 cm/sec
50%–79%	PSV > 125 cm/sec EDV < 140 cm/sec	60%–79%	PSV > 130 cm/sec EDV > 40 cm/sec PSV ICA/CCA ratio > 1.8 EDV ICA/CCA > 2.4 SB > 40 cm/sec
80%–99%	PSV > 125 cm/sec EDV > 140 cm/sec	80%–99%	PSV > 250 cm/sec EDV > 100 cm/sec PSV ICA/CCA Ratio > 3.7 EDV ICA/CCA > 5.5 SB > 80 cm/sec
Occlusion	No flow	Occlusion	No flow

Data from Strandness DE Jr: Duplex Scanning in Vascular Disorders, 2nd ed. New York, Raven Press, 1993, pp 113–158; and Zweibel WJ (ed): Introduction to Vascular Ultrasonography, 3rd ed. Philadelphia, WB Saunders, 1992, pp 123–132.
SB = spectral broadening; PSV = peak systolic velocity; EDV = end-diastolic velocity; ICA = internal carotid artery; CCA = common carotid artery.

duplex scanning with clinical trials.[63] After large-scale clinical trials of CEA showed the benefit of the procedure in both symptomatic patients with greater than 70% ICA stenosis[30, 58] and asymptomatic patients with greater than 60% stenosis,[31] several groups have tried to corroborate duplex findings with these results.[33, 41, 53, 54, 57] An important point that should first be emphasized is that the North American Symptomatic Carotid Endarterectomy Trial (NASCET)[58] and European Carotid Surgery Trial (ECST),[30] which concluded that CEA was effective for symptomatic patients with ICA stenoses greater than or equal to 70%,

TABLE 130–2. CRITERIA FOR DUPLEX SCANNING DIAGNOSIS OF VERTEBRAL ARTERY STENOSIS

HEMODYNAMIC ASSESSMENT	DOPPLER SIGNAL QUALITY	SYSTOLIC VELOCITY (cm/sec)
Strong	Good	>40
Normal	Good	20–40
Moderately damped	Fair, systolic damping	12–20
Severely damped	Poor, nearly absent	<12
Occlusion	Absent	0
Subclavian steal	Fair to good, blood pressure cuff on ipsilateral arm reverses flow	Reversed

From Bendick PJ, Jackson VP: Evaluation of vertebral arteries with duplex ultrasonography. J Vasc Surg 3:523, 1986.

used different measurements of angiographic stenosis (Fig. 130–2). The Asymptomatic Carotid Atherosclerosis Study (ACAS) trial[31] of CEA in asymptomatic patients used the same measurement technique as NASCET did.

To reconcile these differences between angiographic measurements and duplex criteria, Moneta and coworkers reviewed 184 patent ICAs that had undergone duplex scanning within 1 week of angiography, with the degree of stenosis measured by the NASCET method.[53] The maximum accuracy (88%) to determine 70% to 99% ICA stenosis was PSV of at least 325 cm/sec or ICA/CCA ratio of at least 4.0. Of these, they recommended the ICA/CCA ratio of at least 4.0 as the best predictor of 70% to 99% angiographic stenosis because of the greater sensitivity (91% versus 83%). Faught and associates utilized a PSV of at least 130 cm/sec and an EDV of at least 100 cm/sec and found 95% accuracy with these criteria in a retrospective review of 770 carotid studies.[33] They validated these criteria in a prospective study as well.[41] Neale and coworkers used another set of criteria (PSV ≥270 cm/sec and EDV ≥110 cm/sec) and reported an accuracy of 93% and a sensitivity of 96%.[57] Because all of these authors have described excellent results, individual vascular laboratories must select and internally validate criteria.

To determine criteria that might best predict ICA stenoses of at least 60%, Moneta and coworkers evaluated 352 carotid bifurcations and found that a PSV of at least 260 cm/sec and an EDV of at least 70 cm/sec, together, were the best predictors because of the highest overall accuracy (90%), sensitivity (84%), and specificity (94%)[54] However,

TABLE 130–3. CRITERIA FOR DUPLEX SCANNING DIAGNOSIS OF INTERNAL CAROTID ARTERY STENOSIS WITH CONTRALATERAL SEVERE STENOSIS OR OCCLUSION

	CRITERIA			
	Strandness[75]	Fujitani et al[36]	AbuRahma et al[3]	Carotid Ratios[3]
Normal	PSV < 125 cm/sec No SB Flow reversal in bulb	PSV < 125 cm/sec No SB	PSV < 125 cm/sec No SB	PSV < 125 cm/sec No SB
1%–15%	PSV < 125 cm/sec No or minimal SB Flow reversal in bulb absent	PSV < 125 cm/sec Minimal SB	PSV < 125 cm/sec Minimal SB	ICA/CCA PSV Ratio < 1.5
16%–49%	PSV > 125 cm/sec Marked SB	PSV > 125 cm/sec EDV < 155 cm/sec Minimal SB	PSV < 140 cm/sec EDV < 140 cm/sec	ICA/CCA PSV Ratio < 1.5
50%–79%	PSV > 125 cm/sec EDV < 140 cm/sec	PSV > 140 cm/sec EDV < 155 cm/sec Marked SB	PSV ≥ 140 cm/sec EDV < 140 cm/sec	ICA/CCA PSV Ratio ≥ 1.5 EDV < 100 cm/sec
80%–99%	PSV > 125 cm/sec EDV > 140 cm/sec	PSV > 140 cm/sec EDV > 155 cm/sec Marked SB	PSV > 140 cm/sec EDV > 140 cm/sec	ICA/CCA PSV Ratio ≥ 1.8 EDV > 100 cm/sec
Occlusion	No flow	No flow	No flow	No flow

Modified from Ricci MA: The changing role of duplex scan in the management of carotid bifurcation disease and endarterectomy. Semin Vasc Surg 11:3, 1998.
SB = spectral broadening; PSV = peak systolic velocity; EDV = end-diastolic velocity; ICA = internal carotid artery; CCA = common carotid artery.

TABLE 130–4. ACCURACY OF MODIFIED DUPLEX SCANNING DIAGNOSTIC CRITERIA WITH CONTRALATERAL SEVERE STENOSIS OR OCCLUSION

REFERENCE	CRITERIA	ACCURACY (%)	SENSITIVITY (%)	SPECIFICITY (%)	PPV (%)	NPV (%)
50%–79% Stenosis						
36	Fujitani: PSV > 140 cm/sec, EDV < 155 cm/sec	71	84	70	28	97
3	Fujitani: PSV > 140 cm/sec, EDV < 155 cm/sec	97	99	98	98	95
3	Strandness: PSV > 125 cm/sec, EDV < 140 cm/sec	83	100	56	78	100
3	AbuRahma: PSV ≥ 140 cm/sec, EDV < 140 cm/sec	97	97	98	99	95
3	Ratios: ICA/CCA ≥ 1.5, EDV < 100 cm/sec	76	96	44	73	86
80%–99% Stenosis						
36	Fujitani: PSV > 140 cm/sec, EDV > 155 cm/sec	96	91	97	89	98
3	Fujitani: PSV > 140 cm/sec, EDV > 155 cm/sec	94	96	92	92	96
3	Strandness: PSV > 125 cm/sec, EDV > 140 cm/sec	76	100	53	68	100
3	AbuRahma: PSV > 140 cm/sec, EDV > 140 cm/sec	96	100	92	92	100
3	Ratios: ICA/CCA ≥ 1.8, EDV > 100 cm/sec	71	96	47	64	92
All > 50% Stenosis						
36	Fujitani	74	97	57	62	96
3	Fujitani	92	88	100	100	83
3	Strandness	74	100	33	71	100
3	AbuRahma	97	96	100	100	94
3	Ratios	77	100	40	73	100

Modified from Ricci MA: The changing role of duplex scan in the management of carotid bifurcation disease and endarterectomy. Semin Vasc Surg 11:3, 1998.
PSV = peak systolic velocity; EDV = end-diastolic velocity; ICA = internal carotid artery; CCA = common carotid artery.

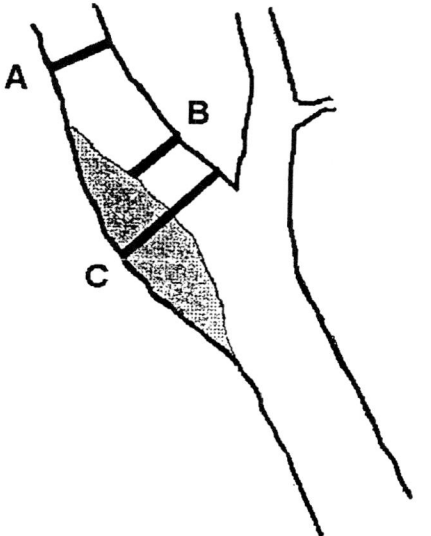

FIGURE 130–2. Degrees of carotid artery stenosis as measured in the North American Symptomatic Carotid Endarterectomy Trial (NASCET)[58] and European Carotid Surgery Trial (ECST).[30] The NASCET measured the residual lumen (B) and the normal distal internal carotid artery beyond the bulb (A). The ECST measured the residual lumen (B) compared with the estimated diameter of the carotid bulb (C). The same stenosis measured by the NASCET method would produce a more severe stenosis than the ECST method. (From Ricci MA: The changing role of duplex scan in the management of carotid bifurcation disease and endarterectomy. Semin Vasc Surg 11:3, 1998.)

if they turned the question around and first asked which criteria would produce a positive predictive value of 95%, a different result was found. In that case, a PSV of at least 290 cm/sec and an EDV of at least 80 cm/sec produced a positive predictive value of 95%, but with lower sensitivity (78%). To date, these are the best published results of modified criteria to predict greater than 60% stenosis.

Indications for Cerebrovascular Duplex Scanning

Generally accepted indications for cerebrovascular duplex examinations include:

1. Cervical bruit in asymptomatic patients.[76]
2. Amaurosis fugax.[76]
3. Focal transient ischemic attacks.[76]
4. Stroke in a potential candidate for CEA.[76]
5. Follow-up of known stenoses (>20%) in asymptomatic patients.[75, 76]
6. Follow-up after CEA.[19, 52, 66, 75, 76]
7. Intraoperative assessment of CEA.[8, 9, 45]
8. CEA without arteriography.[47, 55, 75]
9. Drop attacks (rare indications).[76]

Several of these indications merit further discussion. Strandness has recommended follow-up of stenoses that are asymptomatic (or lesions contralateral to an operated side).[75] For patients who have less than 50% stenosis, a follow-up duplex scan at yearly intervals is adequate. For those with moderate stenosis of 50% to 79%, a surveillance scan every 6 months is appropriate, although progression to more than 80% stenosis may prompt consideration for CEA.[69, 75]

Historically, vascular surgeons have observed their patients after CEA with regular duplex scans; however, extended follow-up examinations may not be necessary or cost-effective. Restenosis after CEA is uncommon, occurring in 10% or less of all cases.[19, 52, 66] Coe and colleagues found that only 15% of 88 CEAs had a restenosis of more than 50%, with symptoms in two patients.[19] Only 7.9% of 449 patients experienced severe restenosis in the study by Ricotta and coworkers, and 1.1% had symptoms.[66] Mackey and colleagues reviewed 1053 postoperative duplex scans of 348 carotid arteries in 258 patients with an average follow-up of 52.6 ± 2.3 months.[52] Only 56 arteries (16.1%) developed a restenosis greater than 50%. Of these, 46.4% occurred within 3 years of surgery, with 41% developing more than 5 years postoperatively. These authors recommended a single postoperative study at 6 to 12 months after surgery,[52] whereas Ricotta and associates suggested a single study at 1 to 2 months postoperatively.[66] Strandness has also recommended a single postoperative study at 3 months.[75] Thus, routine postoperative surveillance at 3- to 6-month intervals no longer seems warranted in the absence of a specific indication, such as contralateral stenosis.

Intraoperative assessment of the results of CEA may also reduce the likelihood of restenosis.[8, 9, 45] Surgeons performing such examinations should have the requisite skills with ultrasonography to perform and interpret the intraoperative examination. Bandyk and associates found that 68 of 250 CEAs had abnormal completion duplex findings.[9] The restenosis rate at 1 year in the group with duplex abnormalities was 21% compared with only 9% in those who had a normal duplex scan after CEA. Bandyk's group suggested that restenosis after CEA may actually be *residual* stenosis.[9]

Baker and coworkers had similar results: 17% of patients with abnormal completion duplex scans who had no corrective action taken developed restenoses (>75%) compared with 4.3% in those who had normal post-CEA duplex scans (p < .001).[8] These studies seem to indicate that uncorrected intraoperative duplex abnormalities after completion of CEA may cause restenosis.

The importance of intraoperative completion duplex scanning is demonstrated by the clinical outcomes reported by Kinney and colleagues.[45] These authors prospectively studied 461 CEAs and correlated the results of intraoperative assessment by ultrasonography, arteriography, or clinical inspection with stroke as an end-point. The CEA site was assessed by duplex scan alone in 142 cases, by duplex scan and arteriography in 268 cases, and by clinical inspection alone in 51 cases. Based on these intraoperative assessments, 5.6% of CEAs were revised. Perioperative morbidity was similar in cases with normal, mildly abnormal, or no duplex scans: six (1.3%) strokes, 12 (2.6%) transient neurologic deficits, and six deaths. The postoperative development of greater than 50% ICA stenosis or occlusion was increased (p < .007) in patients with residual duplex abnormalities or when no duplex was performed. For those patients with late restenosis or occlusion, the risk of stroke was increased (3/35) compared with patients without restenosis (3/426; p = .00016). Additionally, when a normal intraoperative duplex examination was obtained, patients had a significantly lower rate of *late* ipsilateral stroke compared with the other patients ($p = .04$). Thus, intraoperative duplex scanning may detect abnormalities that may lead to restenosis as well as stroke after CEA.

The performance of CEA without angiography has enhanced the importance of duplex scanning. As the reliability and reproducibility of duplex scanning increased, it became apparent that the duplex scan could provide all the information the surgeon needed to plan the operation, without the risks of arteriography, particularly stroke (see Chapter 129). Ricotta and associates reported that arteriography in patients with hemispheric symptoms did not add to the management of two thirds of their patients.[65] In a retrospective review, Dawson and coworkers found in 83 patients that the clinical presentation and duplex findings were adequate for patient management in 87%.[23] In the remaining 13%, arteriography was required for those who had (1) technically inadequate duplex scans, (2) an atypical disease pattern, or (3) an ICA stenosis of less than 50%. A subsequent prospective study by this group revealed that arteriography affected clinical management in only one of 94 cases (1%).[24]

Moore and coworkers also prospectively evaluated 85 patients with duplex scans and arteriograms.[55] Duplex scans correctly characterized 159 of 170 carotid arteries (93.5%); hemodynamically significant stenosis was determined correctly by duplex scans in 100%. These authors then performed 32 CEAs in 29 patients without angiography, confirming the duplex scan–predicted lesion in every case. There were no perioperative strokes. Kuntz and coworkers demonstrated a lower 5-year risk of stroke with duplex scanning as the sole preoperative test compared with angiography (6.35% versus 7.12%).[47]

The major issues that must be confronted when CEA is considered without preoperative arteriography are[75]:

1. Is the accuracy of carotid duplex scanning comparable with that of arteriography?
2. Can the risks and costs of arteriography safely be eliminated?

Surgeons planning CEA without arteriography should be well versed in the interpretation and pitfalls of carotid duplex scanning. It is our policy at the University of Vermont that the surgeon be present during the scan or review videotapes personally. Only vascular laboratories that have excellent, systematic quality assurance programs and proven track records should use duplex scanning as the sole preoperative test before CEA.[40]

If arteriography, which carries a 1% to 6% risk of stroke, is eliminated, the overall risk of treatment of carotid stenosis will be reduced. The possibility of a proximal source for emboli, however, must occasionally be considered, and the aortic arch or CCA in the chest cannot be accurately assessed by duplex scanning. In addition, duplex scans cannot detect carotid siphon stenosis, intracranial aneurysms, or a brain tumor that could be a source of hemispheric symptoms. Fortunately, carotid siphon disease is an unlikely source of symptoms, and a stenosis there does not have a significant impact on the clinical decision to perform CEA.[57, 68, 75] Likewise, intracranial aneurysms can be seen in 1% to 2% of patients undergoing arteriography,[50] but most of these aneurysms are small and are unlikely to be affected by CEA.[50, 60] Finally, advanced cerebral imaging

techniques make the concern about occult brain tumors less relevant.[55]

CEA without arteriography can be safely performed if the following criteria are met[24, 77]:

1. Vascular laboratory duplex accuracy is known (ongoing quality assurance).
2. The duplex scan is technically adequate.
3. Vascular anomalies, such as kinks or loops, are not present.
4. The CCA is free of significant disease.
5. The distal ICA is free of significant disease (i.e., disease is localized to the carotid bifurcation).

Potential pitfalls include patients with recurrent stenosis, nonhemispheric symptoms, or ICA stenosis less than 50%.[23, 24]

An emerging indication for carotid duplex scanning is diagnosis of and screening for blunt and penetrating wounds to the carotid artery.[22, 35] Carotid duplex examination after trauma can be difficult, however, because of edema, hematoma, uncooperative patients, and the bustling activity around a patient with multiple injuries. Only experienced examiners and interpreters should attempt this examination. Davis and coworkers, after experience with a small group of patients, suggested that duplex scanning should be the primary screening modality for suspected carotid injury and dissection.[22]

In a prospective evaluation, Fry and colleagues studied carotid duplex scanning after blunt and penetrating cervical trauma.[35] Fifteen patients had a duplex scan followed by arteriography. Of these, 11 patients had a region of interest in zone II and four had a region of interest in zone III. Duplex scans correctly identified both the single injury demonstrated by arteriography and the remaining 14 normal studies. Fry and colleagues then performed duplex scans for the next 85 patients, and arteriography was performed only when the duplex scan was abnormal. In this group, 62 patients had potential injuries in zone II and the remainder in zone III. Seven arterial injuries identified by duplex scan were confirmed by arteriography. The remaining 76 patients with normal duplex scans had no sequelae for up to 3 weeks after discharge. Savings of $1252 per case accrued when carotid duplex scanning was used instead of arteriography. The potential utility of duplex scanning in this clinical situation is comparable with the benefits reported when duplex scanning is used in the management of atherosclerotic carotid artery disease.

TRANSCRANIAL DOPPLER EXAMINATION

Transcranial Doppler (TCD) ultrasonography employs pulsed wave Doppler imaging ($\sim$2 to 3 MHz) to insonate a finite segment of the arteries of the intracranial circulation.[1] A region of the temporal bone is thin enough in most subjects[39] to allow adequate signal transmission. This transtemporal window allows the sonographer to measure flow in the middle cerebral artery (MCA), anterior cerebral artery (ACA), posterior cerebral artery (PCA), and the anterior and posterior communicating arteries (AcomA,

PComA) (Table 130–5). The sonographer can assess the vertebrobasilar circulation by insonating through the foramen magnum (suboccipital or transforaminal window). The carotid siphon and the ophthalmic artery (OA) are evaluated via the orbit bilaterally (transorbital window). The adept sonographer can sample the ACA via the contralateral transorbital window. The distal extracranial ICA is studied at the level of the jaw (submandibular). In the past, sonographers relied on manual dexterity and keen hearing alone to blindly study cranial arterial segments. With color duplex imaging, however, vascular anatomy is readily apparent, which reduces the time required to perform an examination and increases the diagnostic accuracy.

A Doppler angle of zero degrees is assumed for both blind (static) and color TCD. Most vessels insonated lie in an orientation within 15 degrees of the Doppler beam axis. This introduces a velocity estimation error of less than 10%. Even with an estimated error of 30 degrees off axis, the error is only 1% per 1 degree.[39] With the transtemporal window, only the PComA is oriented at an untenable angle for reasonable flow estimation. Flow velocity information in this segment is sought to determine its role as a collateral pathway, so the most useful data are direction of flow and existence of bruits rather than absolute velocity.[1]

Blind/Static Transcranial Doppler Technique

The fundamental steps in the TCD examination include location of the window, identification of the vessel, insonation in small increments, and documentation of spectral parameters. A good acoustic window is requisite to a successful examination. The best transtemporal window is usually found just above the zygomatic arch and adjacent to the ear. Correct vessel identification is essential. Four key elements are considered in the identification of a vessel: (1) depth, (2) flow direction, (3) spectral waveform profile, and (4) spatial position (traceability of the vessel throughout its length).

The most practical starting point of the study is identification of the MCA. It should be audible at a 45-mm depth with antegrade flow. Its spectral profile should be similar to that of the ICA. By moving the Doppler sample gate (sample volume) deeper in 2- to 5-mm increments, and with minute angulations of the transducer, the operator should be able to trace the path of the vessel from the distal trifurcation proximally to its origin at the bifurcation of the ICA. Once the sample gate encompasses part of the ACA, that flow information is superimposed onto the MCA spectrum. When the ACA flows in its usual retrograde course (away from the transducer), the spectral profile appears on the opposite side of the spectral trace baseline and in register with the cardiac cycle of the MCA. The profile may be slightly different. By demonstrating this "butterfly" pattern, the operator is assured that the sample gate has located the bifurcation of the ICA. The ACA can then be traced distally as far as possible. ACA mean flow velocities are usually less than those found in the MCA but greater than those in the PCA. If the signal is lost for whatever reason, the exercise may need to be repeated to rediscover the ACA confidently.

To insonate the supraclinoid portion of the ICA, the operator continues to increase the depth of the sample gate beyond the bifurcation. To insonate the PCA, the transducer is angled posteriorly and the sample gate positioned 60 to 70 mm in depth. The first (P1) segment of the PCA typically flows antegrade, whereas the second (P2) segment should flow away from the transducer. This technique is repeated on the contralateral side.

Vertebrobasilar values are obtained most easily when the patient lies on one side or sits with the head tipped down toward the chest. This acts to "open" the window. With sufficient gel the transducer is placed just below the inion and aimed at the nasion. The transducer is slowly slid to one side with the gate depth at approximately 60 to 70 mm. When a signal is found and optimized with minute adjustments, the contralateral vertebral artery is found in the reverse manner. Increasing gate depth incrementally allows the sonographer to follow a vertebral artery to its confluence and continue along the basilar artery. Ordinarily, the vertebral and basilar arteries flow away from the transducer. The basilar artery is usually found between 80 and 100 mm in depth. The degree of head tilt may need to be altered to optimize this window. This window can be insonated, with experience, on a patient in the supine position.

The carotid siphon and ophthalmic artery are investigated via the transorbital window. The patient is instructed to keep eyes closed with contact lenses removed. Power output level on the TCD equipment is reduced to 10%. Gel again is applied to the transducer, and, with a gate depth of 45 to 55 mm, the transducer is lightly applied to the eyelid and directed rostrad but slightly lateral to the

TABLE 130–5. NORMAL VELOCITY, DEPTH, AND DIRECTION OF TRANSCRANIAL DOPPLER–MEASURED BLOOD FLOW

WINDOW	ARTERY	MEAN VELOCITY (cm/sec)	DEPTH (mm)	FLOW DIRECTION
Transtemporal	MCA	62 ± 12	40–50	Toward
	ACA	50 ± 12	65–75	Away
	PCA	42 ± 10	60–70	P1 toward, P2 away
Transorbital	Terminal ICA	39 ± 9	55–65	Toward
	ICA siphon	42 ± 11	60–80	Bidirectional
	Ophthalmic	21 ± 5	46–55	Toward
Transforaminal	Vertebral	36 ± 10	60–70	Away
	Basilar	39 ± 10	80–100	Away
Submandibular	Extracranial ICA	Variable	50	Away

MCA = middle cerebral artery; ACA = anterior cerebral artery; PCA = posterior cerebral artery; ICA = internal carotid artery.

midline. The signal, once optimized, is traceable to greater depth until the bidirectional flow pattern of the carotid siphon is found. This is usually at a depth of 60 to 80 mm.

Color Transcranial Doppler Technique

The windows and angles of insonnation are the same as with the blind technique. The difference lies in optimizing the color Doppler sensitivity and display to suit the circumstances. Even when the quality of color Doppler data is only marginal, when this modality is used in conjunction with depth and flow direction, an otherwise indeterminate test may be salvaged to render usable information. Documentation of flow parameters such as direction, mean velocity, pulsatility index, PSV, EDV, and the presence of a bruit is essential. With modern-day TCD devices this is often accomplished with digital technology in conjunction with an electronically archivable summary report or video printout.

Pitfalls and Limitations

Ultrasound examinations through the skull are difficult to perform not only because of the mismatched impedance of sound transmission between bone and soft tissue but also because of the refraction of sound waves by the bone structure of the skull.[86] A knowledge of relevant anatomy and pathophysiology is essential. Misidentification of vessels is reduced when color Doppler imaging is available. Branch arteries, variable anatomy, and anomalous vessels are better visualized. With blind TCD, collateral channels or vasospasm may be mistaken for stenosis; if a vessel is displaced by a mass, it may not be located or it may be thought to be a different vessel altogether, with misleading flow characteristics. A poor acoustic window can make any examination daunting or impossible. Surprisingly, too good a window (such as after a craniotomy) can also handicap the study by the confusing addition of otherwise "silent" small vessels.

TCD typically uses fairly large sample volumes (≥ 7.5 mm^3) in order to improve the signal to noise ratio.[1] Large sample volumes (sample gate size) give rise to spectral broadening of the displayed waveform and are less specific for an individual vessel if another vessel is in close proximity to be detected simultaneously. Any flow detected in the gate will be displayed. If a neighboring vessel is stenotic, spastic, or tortuous, elevated velocities or bruits may be attributed to the wrong vessel. Color Doppler imaging may not help this. Unknown Doppler angles in blind TCD studies may result in velocity data that are inaccurate.

Interpretation Criteria

The "normal" mean velocity and its range are unique to individual laboratory due to patient demographics, interoperator and intraoperator variabilities, and differences with equipment. Although each vascular laboratory must validate its own normal velocity data, there are some general guidelines (see Table 130–5).

The detection of a focal elevation in velocity, limited to one to two sample depths with a drop in velocity distally or evidence of turbulence, is more likely to be caused by

stenosis than by vasospasm or collateral flow recruitment. Age,[6, 83] hyperventilation,[46] and blood pressure may affect velocity.

Collateralization through the circle of Willis is also common through the extracranial circulation to the basal vessels via retrograde flow within the periorbital vessels and the ophthalmic artery. Reversal of flow in a segment of the circle of Willis implies an obstruction of hemodynamic significance. Even the basilar artery can act as a collateral pathway to the arm via the vertebral artery in the case of subclavian steal. The recruitment of collateral pathways can be documented by reversal of flow of the insonated vessels and disruption of flow during strategic compression maneuvers of the extracranial supply vessels.[2]

Indications

The American Academy of Neurology has recommended use of TCD for the following clinical situations[15]:

1. Detection of severe stenosis (>65%) in the major basal intracranial arteries.
2. Assessment of the patterns and extent of collateral circulation in patients with known regions of severe stenosis or occlusion.
3. Evaluation and follow-up of patients with cerebral vasoconstriction of any cause (especially after subarachnoid hemorrhage).
4. Detection of arteriovenous malformations and study of their supply arteries and flow patterns.
5. Assessment of patients with suspected brain death.

Clinically, TCD is indicated when a patient complains of syncopal or vertebrobasilar symptoms or when a bruit is heard by the patient, especially when duplex Doppler examination does not suggest panhypoperfusion. Patients who have experienced transient ischemic attacks with no other source of emboli may also benefit from TCD. TCD can be used to monitor vasospasm after subarachnoid hemorrhage or closed head injury or serve as an indirect measure of intracranial pressure. TCD has also been utilized to evaluate the patency of cerebral shunts in patients with hydrocephalus.[17]

COMPUTED TOMOGRAPHY ANGIOGRAPHY

Spiral or helical computed tomography (CT) allows the acquisition of images from a large volume of tissue in a short time period as the system continuously moves the patient while rotating the x-ray tube within the gantry. This technique produces better vascular images than with conventional CT because the speed of data acquisition permits scanning to be completed when higher levels of circulating contrast material are present. Postprocessing of images with volume-rendering methods and three-dimensional (3-D) reconstructions allows image generation unavailable with conventional techniques.[56] CT angiography (CTA) has been applied as a minimally invasive method of diagnosis for cerebrovascular disease.

Technique and Results

Multiple variations of the technique, timing of image acquisition, contrast volume, and other factors have been published.[18, 25, 48, 71] In brief, the patient is supine while 2- to 3-mm section images are obtained from C2 to C6 with continuous data acquisition. Patients are asked to breathe quietly and avoid swallowing. Often a set of images without contrast is obtained first. A volume of contrast material (75 to 120 ml) is injected intravenously with a 20- to 25-second scan delay (or a delay determined by computer-assisted techniques) after contrast is administered. Axial images and 3-D reconstructions are produced on the CT workstation after the examination has been completed. Reconstructions are typically done with a maximum image projection (MIP) technique after bony structures are deleted.

Although the fast scanning technique minimizes motion artefacts, calcifications can produce imaging artefacts, particularly when MIP reconstruction is attempted. These artefacts may be incorrectly identified as stenoses. In addition, interpretation may be complicated by the numerous vascular structures in this region. Other factors that may produce suboptimal images are poor timing and inadequate volume of contrast.[18]

CTA has been favorably compared with contrast arteriography. Dillon and coworkers characterized the degree of stenosis as mild, moderate, severe, or occluded and found that there was agreement in 41 of 50 carotid arteries studied (82%).[25] Leclerc and coworkers, using six categories (normal, <30%, 30% to 70%, >70%, near occlusion, and occlusion), found agreement with contrast arteriography in 95%.[48] These authors also thought that MIP reconstructions, when technically possible, offered a more reliable estimate of stenosis. Unfortunately, 10 of the 40 arteries they evaluated could not be reconstructed because of calcifications.

Simeone and colleagues compared 80 arteries imaged with CTA to intra-arterial digital subtraction angiography (DSA).[71] When classified as normal, 1% to 29%, 30% to 69%, 70% to 99%, or occlusion, accuracy was 96% with 88% sensitivity and 100% specificity. Ulcerations are not shown well with CTA.[18] CTA has also been suggested as a reliable means of evaluating the vertebral arteries[32] or aortic arch,[62] although there are fewer data reported for these regions. Use of CTA for cerebrovascular diagnosis has diminished, in part, because of concern over the administration of contrast but also because it has been supplanted by magnetic resonance angiography (MRA).

MAGNETIC RESONANCE ANGIOGRAPHY

MRA has been developed as another noninvasive method to evaluate the cerebrovasculature. This technique does not require the use of contrast material, a major advantage over CTA and conventional angiography. MRA uses pulses of radiofrequency energy to excite protons of primarily hydrogen (water molecules) within a magnetic field. The characteristic spin produces a radiofrequency echo of the original signal. Tissue produces a signal, whereas air and bone do not. Many protocols can generate images of blood flow or flow velocity. The common clinical protocols utilize MIP technology to reconstruct images of vessels and frequently are combined with imaging studies of the brain. Though there are few contraindications to MRA, patients with implanted metallic or electronic devices, such as pacemakers, and those who are severely claustrophobic cannot undergo magnetic resonance imaging (MRI) or MRA.

Technique and Results

The usual clinical MRA technique is the time-of-flight (TOF) technique, which relies on "flow-related enhancement."[5] Stationary tissue becomes saturated with the radiofrequency pulses, while blood moving through the field of interest provides unsaturated echoes that produce a strong signal from the vessel. Through different methods, the signal in the vessel can be maximized.

Both two-dimensional (2-D) and 3-D techniques are utilized to acquire data. The 2-D technique acquires data with sequential thin transverse slices, whereas the 3-D TOF technique acquires data in any plane. The 2-D method allows blood to flow quickly through the scanning slice; thus, blood will not become saturated with radiofrequency signal as with a 3-D method that obtains images in a sagittal plane. The 2-D TOF method produces better visualization of slowly moving blood, which may be useful in attempting to distinguish between a tight stenosis and occlusion. On the other hand, the 3-D method can image vessels in any direction, is less susceptible to turbulence-generated artefacts, can image plaque, and has better image resolution.[5] The 3-D TOF method may also allow the injection of gadolinium, which may enhance areas of slow flow.

During the "first pass" of an injection of gadolinium (a non–contrast-enhancing agent), rapid acquisition of data with 3-D TOF techniques gives greater spatial resolution and reduces artefacts from low flow, radiofrequency saturation, and areas of turbulence.[13] This compound is primarily in the extracellular space but is not strictly intravascular, so that the timing of the initial bolus is critical to avoid more widespread distribution and venous overlay, obscuring the diagnosis.

Studies with MRA had good results when this technique was used to evaluate the carotid artery.[5, 85] MRA has the advantage of demonstrating the intracerebral vessels, if the clinician feels that is important information before CEA. Wesbey and coworkers found that MRA results agreed with contrast arteriography results in 86% of 36 ICAs and with surgical findings in 39 of 40 cases.[85] The tendency for MRA to overestimate the degree of stenosis is a well-recognized pitfall; a precise estimate of stenosis is difficult to obtain with MRA.[49, 79] MRA does not accurately reveal ulcerations. MRA has been reported to be a sensitive technique to determine the need for surgery. MRA may be utilized to evaluate the aortic arch,[16] carotid dissections,[78] or post-endarterectomy carotid arteries.[79] Individual institutions must correlate their MRA results with conventional angiography results, particularly because there are such variations in MRA techniques.

COMPARISONS BETWEEN IMAGING MODALITIES

It seems unlikely that any of these noninvasive tests will replace conventional contrast or DSA entirely, but several strategies have been recommended to limit use of arteriography and avoid its attendant expense and risk.[5, 47–49, 55, 75, 85, 87] Whereas contrast and DSA techniques are considered the "gold standard" for the diagnosis of cerebrovascular disease, arteriography may underestimate the degree of stenosis[61] and fail to detect ulceration.[27, 29] In addition, there are both interobserver and intraobserver variabilities in determination of the degree of stenosis.[87] For instance, an arteriogram reported as 78% stenosis when read by one radiologist could be read as a 71% to 85% stenosis by another based on the interobserver variability noted by Young and coworkers.[87] A duplex scan interpreted as 80% to 99% stenosis might be correlated as correct if one radiologist reads the arteriogram and incorrect if another reads it. Moreover, if the original 78% reading is correct, is that really *clinically* significantly different from a 80%–99% stenosis by duplex scan?

No studies have compared arteriography with all three noninvasive modalities (duplex scanning, CTA, and MRA). A unique attempt to compare arteriography, duplex scanning, and MRA with surgical specimen study was carried out by Pan and coworkers.[61] These authors studied 31 CEA specimens that were removed en bloc at the time of surgery with contrast DSA, 3-D MRA, and color-flow duplex imaging. They utilized the ECST method (see Fig. 130–2) to estimate stenosis because the distal ICA diameter could not be determined in the specimens. The gold standard for comparison was the surgical specimen itself, with the diameters determined by high-resolution MRI. Data were then analyzed by placing in vivo measurements from each modality and the specimen measurement in the following categories: 1% to 39%, 40% to 59%, 60% to 79%, 80% to 99%, and occluded.

The 31 measurements from the ex vivo specimens were found to be 40% to 59% in 2 specimens, 60% to 79% in 6, and 80% to 99% in the remaining 23. A diagnostic match was found in 76% of MRAs, 75% of duplex scans, and only 57% of arteriograms. MRA was more likely to overestimate stenosis (17%) than duplex (14%) or arteriography (6%). On the other hand, arteriography was most likely to *underestimate* the degree of stenosis (37% versus 11% for duplex and 7% for MRA). Of the 23 specimens with 80% to 99% stenosis, MRA was accurate in 95%, duplex in 90%, and arteriography in 52%. Overall, the correlation of the ex vivo measurement with the in vivo modalities was better for duplex ultrasound ($r = .80$) and MRA ($r = .76$) than for arteriography ($r = .56$). This study adds significant data to the growing body of evidence that confirms the reliability of duplex scanning and MRA to determine critical stenosis and the pitfalls in relying on arteriography as the gold standard. The risks, benefits, and disadvantages of each modality are outlined earlier in the text and in Table 130–6.

CLINICAL RECOMMENDATIONS

On the basis of the NASCET[58] experience with duplex ultrasonography, it has been suggested that contrast arteriography must be performed before CEA. Besides the significant methodologic problems with the use of duplex ultrasonography in that trial, the earlier discussion points out many of the problems and pitfalls with arteriography.

TABLE 130–6. COMPARISON OF ARTERIOGRAPHY, DUPLEX SCANNING, COMPUTED TOMOGRAPHY ANGIOGRAPHY (CTA), AND MAGNETIC RESONANCE ANGIOGRAPHY (MRA)

	CONTRAST ARTERIOGRAPHY*	DUPLEX SCAN	CTA	MRA
Stroke risk	1%–6%	0%	0%	0%
Other risks	Contrast-induced renal dysfunction, iatrogenic arterial injury, puncture site bleeding	No known biologic risks for diagnostic ultrasonography	Contrast-induced renal dysfunction	No known biologic risks for diagnostic radiofrequency
Contraindications	Renal dysfunction	None	Renal dysfunction	Claustrophobia, electronic or metal implants
Equipment cost	Very high	$60,000–$150,000	Very high	Very high
Test cost	High	Low	Moderate	Moderate
Sources of technical failure	Inability to do selective catheterization	Heavy calcifications	Heavy calcifications, wrong timing for contrast injection	Slow flow or areas of flow separation
Plaque characterization	No	Yes	No	Yes
Overall accuracy	Considered "gold standard," may underestimate disease, misses ulcerations	High, misses ulcerations	Moderately high, calcifications can obscure diagnosis, misses ulcerations	Overestimates disease, reliability of less than 50% stenosis has been questioned, misses ulcerations

*Including intra-arterial digital subtraction angiography.

It must be recognized that there is presently no clinical test that can give an absolute value for the degree of stenosis in every carotid artery. The mere fact that large, randomized clinical trials,[30, 31, 58, 82] measuring the degree of stenosis in different ways, all found a clinical benefit to CEA suggests that there is a range of stenoses at which point patients benefit from CEA. The surgeon's clinical judgment and familiarity with the accuracy and pitfalls of diagnostic modalities are the most important factors in determining the appropriateness of CEA. Although arteriography will continue to play a role in cerebrovascular diagnosis, it seems that currently the most appropriate role for that test should be resolution of conflicting noninvasive tests or confirmation of other diagnoses.

Combination of duplex scanning and MRA has been recommended at several medical centers.[49, 51, 81] With this strategy, the tendency of MRA to overestimate the degree of stenosis should be balanced by the ultrasound findings. This combination of tests has been reported to be accurate in selection of patients for surgery. Although this approach is more expensive than duplex scanning alone, the combination of duplex scanning and MRA remains less expensive than arteriography.[80, 81] As previously emphasized, rigorous quality assurance is essential for both studies.

Yet Erdoes and coworkers have suggested that MRA is rarely, if ever, indicated.[28] In their study of 103 patients who had duplex scanning and MRA, the MRA results did not alter the management of any patient, although some patients did need angiography. Many reports confirm that duplex scanning as the sole diagnostic test is safe and cost-effective.[24, 28, 77] As noted earlier, the accuracy of the laboratory must be known, the individual scan should be technically adequate, the CCA should be free of disease, and the ICA should be free of significant anomalies and free of disease in its distal portion. If these conditions are met, CEA can be carried out without the risk of arteriography or the expense of other invasive or noninvasive tests.

REFERENCES

1. Aaslid R: The Doppler principle applied to measurement of blood flow velocity in cerebral arteries. In Aaslid R (ed): Transcranial Doppler Sonography. New York, Springer-Verlag, 1986, pp 22–38.
2. Aaslid R, Markwalder MD, Nornes H: Noninvasive transcranial Doppler ultrasound recording of flow velocity in basal cerebral arteries. J Neurosurg 57:769, 1982.
3. AbuRahma AF, Richmond BK, Robinson PA, et al: Effect of contralateral severe stenosis or carotid occlusion on duplex criteria of ipsilateral stenoses: Comparative study of various duplex parameters. J Vasc Surg 22:751, 1995.
4. Alexandrov AV, Vital D, Brodie DS, et al: Grading carotid stenosis with ultrasound: An interlaboratory comparison. Stroke 28:1208, 1997.
5. Anderson CM, Haacke EM: Approaches to diagnostic magnetic resonance imaging. Semin Ultrasound CT MR 13:246, 1992.
6. Arnolds BJ, von Reutern GM: Transcranial Doppler sonography: Examination technique and normal reference values. Ultrasound Med Biol 16:115, 1986.
7. Baker JD, Barker WF, Machleder HI: Evaluation of extracranial cerebrovascular disease with ocular pneumoplethysmography. Am J Surg 136:206, 1978.
8. Baker WH, Koustas G, Burke K, et al: Intraoperative duplex scanning and late carotid artery stenosis. J Vasc Surg 19:829, 1994.
9. Bandyk DF, Kaebnick HW, Adams MB, Towne JB: Turbulence occurring after carotid bifurcation endarterectomy: A harbinger of residual and recurrent stenosis. J Vasc Surg 7:261, 1988.
10. Bandyk DF, Levine AW, Pohl L, Towne JB: Classification of carotid bifurcation disease using quantitative Doppler spectrum analysis. Arch Surg 120:306, 1985.
11. Barnes RW, Russell HE, Bone GE, Slaymaker EE: Doppler cerebrovascular examination: Improved results with refinements in technique. Stroke 8:468, 1974.
12. Bendick PJ, Jackson VP: Evaluation of vertebral arteries with duplex sonography. J Vasc Surg 3:523, 1986.
13. Bongartz GM, Boos M, Winter K, et al: Clinical utility of contrast-enhanced MR angiography. Eur Radiol 7:S178, 1997.
14. Brockenbrough EC: Screening for the prevention of stroke: Use of Doppler flowmeter. Brochure by Alaska/Washington Regional Medical Program, 1969.
15. Caplan L, Van den Noort S, Dyck P, et al: Transcranial Doppler: Report of the Therapeutics and Technology Assessment Subcommittee, American Academy of Neurology, Minneapolis, Minn, 1989.
16. Carpenter JP, Holland GA, Golden MA, et al: Magnetic resonance angiography of the aortic arch. J Vasc Surg 25:145, 1997.
17. Case T, Wald S, Ricci M, Pilcher D: Pediatric transcranial Doppler for surveillance of ventriculoperitoneal shunt malfunction (Abstract). J Vasc Tech 19:207, 1995.
18. Castillo M, Wilson JD: CT angiography of the common carotid artery bifurcation: Comparison between two techniques and conventional angiography. Neuroradiology 36:602, 1994.
19. Coe DA, Towne JB, Seabrook GR, et al: Duplex morphologic features of the reconstructed carotid artery: Changes occurring more than five years after endarterectomy. J Vasc Surg 25:850, 1997.
20. Comerota AJ, Katz ML, White JV, Grosh JD: The preoperative diagnosis of the ulcerated carotid atheroma. J Vasc Surg 11:505, 1990.
21. Crocker EF Jr, Tutton RH, Bowen JC: The role of intravenous digital subtraction angiography in the evaluation of extracranial carotid artery disease: Can the decision for carotid artery surgery be made solely on the basis of its findings? J Vasc Surg 4:157, 1986.
22. Davis JW, Holbrook TL, Hoyt DB, et al: Blunt carotid artery dissection: Incidence, associated injuries, screening, and treatment. J Trauma 30:1514, 1990.
23. Dawson DL, Zierler RE, Kohler TR: Role of arteriography in the preoperative evaluation of carotid artery disease. Am J Surg 161:619, 1991.
24. Dawson DL, Zierler RE, Strandness DE Jr, et al: The role of duplex scanning before carotid endarterectomy: A prospective study. J Vasc Surg 18:673, 1993.
25. Dillon EH, van Leeuwen MS, Fernandez MA, et al: CT angiography: Application to the evaluation of carotid artery stenosis. Radiology 189:211, 1993.
26. Earnest F IV, Houser OW, Forbes GS, et al: The accuracy and limitations of intravenous digital subtraction angiography in the evaluation of atherosclerotic cerebrovascular disease: Angiographic and surgical correction. Mayo Clin Proc 58:735, 1983.
27. Eikelboom BC, Riles TR, Mintzer R, et al: Inaccuracy of angiography in the diagnosis of carotid ulceration. Stroke 14:882, 1983.
28. Erdoes LS, Marek JM, Mills JL, et al: The relative contributions of carotid duplex scanning, magnetic resonance angiography, and cerebral angiography to clinical decision making: A prospective study in patients with carotid occlusive disease. J Vasc Surg 23:950, 1996.
29. Estol C, Claassen D, Hirsch W, et al: Correlative angiographic and pathologic findings in the diagnosis of ulcerated plaques in the carotid artery. Arch Neurol 48:692, 1991.
30. European Carotid Surgery Trialists' Collaborative Group: MRC European Surgery Trial: Interim results for symptomatic patients with severe (70–99%) carotid stenosis. Lancet 337:1235, 1991.
31. Executive Committee for the Asymptomatic Carotid Atherosclerosis Study: Endarterectomy for asymptomatic carotid artery stenosis. JAMA 273:1421, 1995.
32. Farrés MT, Grabenwöger F, Magometschnig H, et al: Spiral CT angiography: Study of stenoses and calcification at the origin of the vertebral artery. Neuroradiology 38:738, 1996.
33. Faught WE, Mattos MA, van Bemmelen PS, et al: Color-flow duplex scanning of carotid arteries: New velocity criteria based on receiver operator characteristics analysis for threshold stenoses used in the symptomatic and asymptomatic carotid trials. J Vasc Surg 19:818–828, 1994.
34. Fillinger MF, Baker RJ, Zwolak RM, et al: Carotid duplex criteria for a 60% or greater angiographic stenosis: Variation according to equipment. J Vasc Surg 24:856, 1996.

35. Fry WR, Dort JA, Smith RS, et al: Duplex scanning replaces arteriography and operative exploration in the diagnosis of potential cervical vascular injury. Am J Surg 168:693, 1994.

36. Fujitani RM, Mills JL, Wang LM, Taylor SM: The effect of unilateral internal carotid arterial occlusion upon contralateral duplex study: Criteria for accurate interpretation. J Vasc Surg 16:459, 1992.

37. Gee W, Oller DW, Amundsen DG, Goodreau JJ: The asymptomatic carotid bruit and the ocular pneumoplethysmography. Arch Surg 112:1381, 1977.

38. Gee W, Smith CA, Hinsen LE, Wylie EJ: Ocular plethysmography in carotid artery disease. Med Instrum 8:244, 1974.

39. Grolimund P: Transmission of ultrasound through the temporal bone. In Aaslid R (ed): Transcranial Doppler Sonography. New York, Springer-Verlag, 1986, pp 10–21.

40. Hachinski V: The issue is standards, not techniques. Arch Neurol 52:834, 1995.

41. Hood DB, Mattos MA, Mansour A, et al: Prospective evaluation of new duplex criteria to identify 70% internal carotid artery stenosis. J Vasc Surg 23:254–262, 1996.

42. Imparato AM, Riles TS, Mintzer R, Baumann FG: The importance of hemorrhage in the relationship between gross morphologic characteristics and cerebral symptoms in 376 carotid artery plaques. Ann Surg 197:195, 1983.

43. Kartchner MM, McRae LP: Auscultation for carotid bruits in cerebrovascular insufficiency. JAMA 210:494, 1969.

44. Kartchner MM, McRae LP, Morrison FD: Noninvasive detection and evaluation of carotid occlusive disease. Arch Surg 106:528, 1973.

45. Kinney EV, Seabrook GR, Kinney LY, et al: The importance of intraoperative detection of residual flow abnormalities after carotid artery endarterectomy. J Vasc Surg 17:912, 1993.

46. Kirkham FJ, Padayachee TS, Parsons S, et al: Transcranial measurement of blood velocities in the basal cerebral arteries using pulsed Doppler ultrasound: Velocity as an index of flow. Ultrasound Med Biol 12:15, 1986.

47. Kuntz KM, Skillman JJ, Whittemore AD, Kent KC: Carotid endarterectomy in asymptomatic patients—Is contrast angiography necessary? A morbidity analysis. J Vasc Surg 22:706, 1995.

48. Leclerc X, Godefroy O, Pruvo JP, Leys D: Computed tomographic angiography for the evaluation of carotid artery stenosis. Stroke 26:1577, 1995.

49. Lee KS: What workup should be required for a patient who has one TIA and demonstrates 80% carotid stenosis? J Neurosurg Anesthesiol 8:305, 1996.

50. Lord RSA: Relevance of siphon stenosis and intracranial aneurysm to results of carotid endarterectomy. In Ernst CB, Stanley JC (eds): Current Therapy in Vascular Surgery, 2nd ed. Philadelphia, BC Decker, 1991, pp 94–101.

51. Lustgarten JH, Soloman RA, Quest DO, et al: Carotid endarterectomy after noninvasive evaluation by duplex ultrasonography and magnetic resonance angiography. Neurosurgery 34:612, 1994.

52. Mackey WC, Belkin M, Sindhi R, et al: Routine postendarterectomy duplex surveillance: Does it prevent late stroke? J Vasc Surg 16:34, 1992.

53. Moneta GL, Edwards JM, Chitwood RW, et al: Correlation of North American Symptomatic Carotid Endarterectomy Trial (NASCET) angiographic definition of 70% to 99% internal carotid artery stenosis with duplex scanning. J Vasc Surg 17:152–159, 1993.

54. Moneta GL, Edwards JM, Papanicolaou G, et al: Screening for asymptomatic internal carotid artery stenosis: Duplex criteria for discriminating 60% to 99% stenosis. J Vasc Surg 21:989–994, 1995.

55. Moore WS, Ziomek S, Quinones-Baldrich WJ, et al: Can clinical evaluation and noninvasive testing substitute for arteriography in the evaluation of carotid artery disease? Ann Surg 208:91, 1988.

56. Napel S, Marks MP, Rubin GD, et al: CT angiography with spiral CT and maximum image projection. Radiology 185:607, 1992.

57. Neale ML, Chambers JL, Kelly AT, et al: Reappraisal of duplex criteria to assess significant carotid stenosis with special reference to reports from the North American Symptomatic Carotid Endarterectomy Trial and the European Carotid Surgery Trial. J Vasc Surg 20:642, 1994.

58. North American Symptomatic Carotid Endarterectomy Trial Collaborators: Beneficial effect of carotid endarterectomy in symptomatic patients with high-grade carotid stenosis. N Engl J Med 325:445, 1991.

59. O'Donnell TF Jr, Erodes L, Mackey WC, et al: Correlation of B-mode ultrasound imaging and arteriography with pathologic findings at carotid endarterectomy. Arch Surg 120:443, 1985.

60. Orecchia PM, Clagette GP, Youkey JR, et al: Management of patients with symptomatic extracranial carotid artery disease and incidental intracranial berry aneurysm. J Vasc Surg 2:158, 1985.

61. Pan XM, Saloner D, Reilly LM, et al: Assessment of carotid artery stenosis by ultrasonography, conventional angiography, and magnetic resonance angiography: Correlation with ex vivo measurement of plaque. J Vasc Surg 21:82, 1995.

62. Park JH, Chung JW, Lee KW, et al: CT angiography of Takayasu arteritis: Comparison with conventional angiography. J Vasc Interv Radiol 8:393, 1997.

63. Ricci MA: The changing role of duplex scan in the management of carotid bifurcation disease and endarterectomy. Semin Vasc Surg 11:3, 1998.

64. Ricotta JJ, Bryan FA, Bond MG, et al: Multicenter validation study of real-time (B-mode) ultrasound, arteriography, and pathological examination. J Vasc Surg 6:512, 1987.

65. Ricotta JJ, Holen J, Schenk E, et al: Is routine arteriography necessary prior to carotid endarterectomy? J Vasc Surg 1:96, 1984.

66. Ricotta JJ, O'Brien MS, DeWeese JA: Natural history of recurrent and residual stenosis after carotid endarterectomy: Implications for postoperative surveillance and surgical management. Surgery 112:656, 1992.

67. Roederer GO, Langois YE, Chan ATW, et al: Ultrasonic duplex scanning of the extracranial carotid arteries: Improved accuracy using new features from the common carotid artery. J Cardiovasc Ultrasonogr 1:373, 1982.

68. Roederer GO, Langlois YE, Chan AR, et al: Is siphon disease important in predicting outcome of carotid endarterectomy? Arch Surg 118:1177, 1983.

69. Roederer GO, Langlois YE, Lusiani L, et al: Natural history of carotid artery disease on the side contralateral to endarterectomy. J Vasc Surg 1:62, 1984.

70. Rubin J, Bude RO, Carson PL, et al: Power Doppler: A potentially useful alternative to mean frequency-based color Doppler ultrasound. Radiology 190:853, 1994.

71. Simeone A, Carriero A, Armillotta M, et al: Spiral CT angiography in the study of the carotid stenoses. J Neuroradiol 24:18, 1997.

72. Sitzer M, Müller W, Rademacher J, et al: Color-flow Doppler-assisted duplex imaging fails to detect ulceration in high-grade internal carotid artery stenosis. J Vasc Surg 23:461, 1996.

73. Spadone DP, Barkmeier LD, Hodgson KJ, et al: Contralateral internal carotid artery stenosis or occlusion: Pitfall of correct ipsilateral classification: A study performed with color-flow imaging. J Vasc Surg 11:42, 1990.

74. Strandness DE Jr: Historical aspects. In Strandness DE Jr (ed): Duplex Scanning in Vascular Disorders, 2nd ed. New York, Raven Press, 1993, pp 1–26.

75. Strandness DE Jr: Extracranial arterial disease. In Strandness DE Jr (ed): Duplex Scanning in Vascular Disorders, 2nd ed. New York, Raven Press, 1993, pp 113–158.

76. Strandness DE Jr: Indications for and frequency of noninvasive testing. Semin Vasc Surg 7:245, 1994.

77. Strandness DE Jr: Angiography before carotid endarterectomy—no. Arch Neurol 52:832, 1995.

78. Stringaris K, Liberopoulos K, Giaka E, et al: Three-dimensional time-of-flight MR angiography and MR imaging versus conventional angiography in carotid artery dissections. Int Angiol 15:20, 1996.

79. Stuckey SL, Gilford EJ, Smith PJ, Kean M: Magnetic resonance angiography findings in the early post-carotid endarterectomy period. Aust Radiol 39:350, 1995.

80. Turnipseed WD, Kennell TW, Turski PA, et al: Magnetic resonance angiography and duplex imaging: Noninvasive tests for selecting symptomatic carotid endarterectomy. Surgery 114:643, 1993.

81. Turnipseed WD, Kennell TW, Turski PA, et al: Combined use of duplex imaging and magnetic resonance angiography for evaluation of patients with symptomatic ipsilateral high-grade stenosis. J Vasc Surg 17:832, 1993.

82. Veterans Administration Cooperative Study: Role of carotid endarterectomy in asymptomatic carotid stenosis. Stroke 17:534, 1986.

83. Vriens EM, Kraaier V, Musbach M, et al: Transcranial pulsed Doppler measurements of blood velocity in the middle cerebral artery: Reference values at rest and during hyperventilation in healthy volunteers in relation to age and sex. Ultrasound Med Biol 15:1, 1989.

84. Weng L, Tirumalai AP, Lowery CM, et al: US extended-field-of-view imaging technology. Radiology 203:877, 1997.

85. Wesbey GE, Bergan JJ, Moreland SI, et al: Cerebrovascular magnetic resonance angiography: A critical verification. J Vasc Surg 16:619, 1992.
86. White DN, Curry GR, Stevenson RJ: The acoustic characteristics of the skull. Ultrasound Med Biol 4:225, 1978.
87. Young GR, Humphrey PRD, Shaw MDM, et al: Comparison of magnetic resonance angiography, duplex ultrasound, and digital subtrac-

tion angiography in assessment of extracranial carotid artery stenosis. J Neurol Neurosurg Psychiatry 57:1466, 1994.
88. Zwiebel WJ: Spectrum analysis in carotid sonography. Ultrasound Med Biol 13:625, 1987.
89. Zwiebel WJ: Doppler evaluation of carotid stenosis. In Zwiebel WJ (ed): Introduction to Vascular Ultrasonography, 3rd ed. Philadelphia, WB Saunders, 1992, pp 123–132.

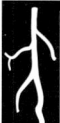

C H A P T E R   1 3 1

Indications, Surgical Technique, and Results for Repair of Extracranial Occlusive Lesions

Wesley S. Moore, M.D., William Quiñones-Baldrich, M.D., and William C. Krupski, M.D.

Prevention of stroke is the primary objective of surgery for extracranial lesions involving the cerebrovascular system. Carotid artery operations are warranted when surgery improves the natural history of the disease and provides a safe and more effective alternative to medical management.

Although the symptomatic manifestations of cerebrovascular lesions can be frightening and certainly annoying, opinions differ as to whether transient ischemic attacks (TIAs) produce irreversible brain injury. Thus, prevention or relief of TIAs is viewed as an important secondary objective.

Selecting patients for operation requires the identification of specific patient subsets who are at high risk for stroke.

INDICATIONS FOR OPERATIVE REPAIR

Indications for operation can be derived from three sources: (1) retrospective reviews, (2) prospective randomized trials, and (3) position/consensus statements.

Indications Based on Retrospective Reviews

Reports that document the natural history of disease, usually subdivided by symptomatic status, are compared with reports concerning immediate and long-term results of operation. If operative results, including 30-day morbidity/mortality and long-term reduction of amaurosis fugax, TIAs, and strokes, are less with operation than with medical treatment, then operation can be justified. The following is an analysis of operative indications by symptomatic status.

Transient Ischemic Attacks

When associated with an appropriate lesion, hemispheric or monocular TIAs have been the most readily accepted indications for carotid endarterectomy.

Most of the early natural history studies were performed without characterization of the underlying arterial lesion. Nevertheless, it is safe to say that the stroke risk in the untreated patient with TIAs is at least 10% within the first year of symptom onset and continues at the rate of about 6% per year, declining after 3 years.[75, 181] In contrast, the stroke risk in the hemisphere ipsilateral to carotid endarterectomy (CEA) in the same patient group falls to less than 1% per year.[13, 38, 54, 83, 85, 103, 162, 176] Provided that carotid endarterectomy by an individual surgeon can be performed with a low stroke morbidity and mortality, TIAs are a compelling indication for operation.

Stroke with Recovery

Because many patients who suffer strokes are only mildly disabled and often enjoy complete or nearly complete recovery, such patients require careful evaluation to discover a lesion that places them at risk for recurrent stroke. The natural history of this group of patients with respect to the annual recurrent stroke rate is approximately 9% per year.[5, 53, 146, 151] The risk for recurrent stroke does not decrease after 3 years as occurs in patients with a TIA. Antiplatelet drugs are relatively ineffective in reducing this recurrence rate.[86] In contrast, carotid endarterectomy has successfully lowered the recurrent stroke rate to under 2% per year.[106, 112, 165]

Patients who recover after completed strokes require careful assessment to determine the presence of a continuing unstable causative lesion. For example, a patient who has recovered from a left hemisphere stroke and is found to have a significant stenosis of the left internal carotid artery is at high risk for subsequent left hemispheric stroke. In contrast, if the same patient has total occlusion of that artery, carotid endarterectomy is no longer feasible.

Review of operative outcomes in patients operated on after strokes reveals that the operative morbidity and mortality rates will be higher in this group of patients; therefore, they require special management (see Operative Technique).

Whether a patient who has made an *incomplete* recovery from a prior stroke is a candidate for carotid endarterectomy requires considerable experience and prudent judgment. In general, the patient who has been devastated by a stroke is not a candidate for carotid endarterectomy. Conversely, the patient who has had a mild stroke with complete or nearly complete recovery is an excellent candidate. The decision for operation for the in-between categories depends on a variety of factors, including how much neurologic function the patient has left to lose, his or her general functional status, the presence of medical comorbidities, and the patient's life expectancy.

Stroke-in-Evolution

The patient with stroke-in-evolution represents the highest risk for either medical or surgical management. Appropriately timed and appropriately performed carotid endarterectomy in such patients who are carefully selected dramatically improves the natural history of this disorder. In contrast, the risk of mortality and the risk of major stroke are predictably high. Operation on these patients should be performed only by those teams that have had considerable experience in managing this category of patient and can accept the added risk in order to achieve an important benefit.[69, 115]

Global Ischemia

Patients who present with symptoms of global cerebral ischemia most often have these symptoms on the basis of decreased cardiac output secondary to arrhythmia or myocardial ischemia. Often the surgical dictum, "The dizzy surgeon operates on the dizzy patient for carotid disease," applies. However, a few patients who have *multiple* lesions involving the extracranial arteries manifest global ischemia and do benefit from correction of one or more of these lesions.[92]

Subclavian Steal Syndrome

Although many patients demonstrate an anatomic subclavian steal syndrome by angiography (i.e., reversed flow through the ipsilateral vertebral artery), only a few have symptoms produced by extremity exercise on the side of the subclavian artery stenosis or occlusion. Those patients who fall into the latter category or those who have a dominant vertebral artery on the side of the proximal subclavian lesion may be candidates for subclavian artery revascularization.[8]

Progressive Intellectual Dysfunction

Progressive intellectual dysfunction represents an extremely controversial indication for carotid endarterectomy. Nonetheless, many anecdotal cases document improved intellectual function after carotid endarterectomy. Decreased intellectual function can occur because of flow or as a summating effect of multiple emboli to centers of the brain responsible for cognitive abilities, independent of motor or sensory findings. In properly selected patients, intervention by carotid endarterectomy *may* improve intellectual function or prevent its further deterioration.

Asymptomatic Carotid Stenosis

Asymptomatic carotid stenosis is one of the most common indications for carotid endarterectomy. It is also the most controversial. Recently, several publications have provided surgeons with considerable natural history data that were previously unavailable. It is now safe to state that the risk of stroke in patients with a carotid artery stenosis in excess of 75% is about 3% to 5% per year of follow-up. Most of these strokes occur without warning symptoms.[29, 114] Many authorities have recommended that patients with carotid stenoses in excess of 75%, who are otherwise in satisfactory medical condition and have a reasonable life expectancy, undergo prophylactic carotid endarterectomy, if the operation can be performed safely in the hands of the individual surgeon.[82, 118] Operative morbidity and mortality rate for this indication should be less than 3%.

The average late stroke rate in the distribution of the operated artery is 0.3% per year.[168] In a 10-year experience at the University of California at Los Angeles (UCLA), there were no late strokes in the distribution of the operated artery, with a mean follow-up of 54 months.[62]

Asymptomatic Ulceration

Patients who are discovered by angiography to have ulcerative lesions of the carotid artery have an increased risk of subsequent stroke when treated expectantly.[121] This risk rises progressively as the size and complexity of the ulceration increases.

Retrospective natural history studies have divided ulcers into three categories: A, B, and C.[121] Quantitation of A, B, and C ulcers is performed by examining an unmagnified lateral projection of a carotid arteriogram.[42] If the product of the length and depth of the ulcer is obtained, an A ulcer is one that is 10 mm^2 or less; a B ulcer varies from 10 to 40 mm^2; and a C ulcer exceeds 40 mm^2 or is cavernous or compound.

Retrospective natural history studies suggest that the stroke rate in patients with asymptomatic A ulcers is insignificant. Of note, the stroke rate in patients with asymptomatic C ulcers exceeds 7.5% per year.[42] According to these retrospective data, patients with a C ulcer on arteriogram, who are acceptable surgical risks, warrant consideration for prophylactic CEA. The decision whether to operate on the patient with a B ulcer depends on the experience of the operating team and the individual conviction of the importance of this lesion. There is no place for surgery for patients with the asymptomatic A ulcer. These recommendations are somewhat controversial because the key studies originated from UCLA and have not been corroborated at other centers.

Prospective Randomized Trials
Symptomatic Patients

Three prospective randomized trials have provided definitive data concerning indications for carotid endarterectomy in symptomatic patients.[55, 109, 135] Patients with *hemispheric* or *monocular* TIAs or prior mild stroke with a 70% or greater stenosis have clear indications for carotid endarterectomy. Patients with *crescendo* TIAs in the presence of a 50% or greater stenosis benefit from operation. Symptomatic patients with stenoses of fewer than 30% showed no benefit from operation in one study.[55] Symptomatic patients with stenoses ranging from 30% to 69% are still being evaluated in two randomized trials.[55, 135] Preliminary results from the North American Symptomatic Carotid Endarterectomy Trial (NASCET) for symptomatic patients with 50% to 69% carotid stenoses were reported at the 1998 meeting of the American Heart Association (see Results).

Three prospective randomized trials in asymptomatic patients with carotid stenoses have been completed. The CASANOVA Study Group concluded that no benefit was to be derived from carotid endarterectomy in the asymptomatic patient.[28] High-risk patients were excluded, and 118 of 206 patients (57%) randomized to medicine were systematically withdrawn as they became "high-risk" and were treated surgically. In an intent-to-treat analysis, however, they were counted as if they were treated medically. Therefore, no conclusions can be drawn from this study.

The Veterans Affairs Cooperative Study has reported definitive results.[89] Carotid endarterectomy plus aspirin was more effective than aspirin alone in reducing the combined incidence of TIAs and stroke in patients with asymptomatic stenosis of 50% or more, which was the study's hypothesis. The number of patients randomized (n = 444) was insufficient to make a definitive statement about stroke prevention alone, although the trend was clearly in favor of operation.

Results of the Asymptomatic Carotid Atherosclerosis Study (ACAS) were published in 1995.[3] Acquisition of patients began in November 1987 and ended in December 1992, with randomization of 1622 men and women with asymptomatic carotid stenoses of between 60% and 99%. According to Kaplan-Meier projections at 5 years, the risk of ipsilateral stroke for the medical group was 11% and 5.1% for the surgical group. This represents a relative risk reduction of 53% and an absolute risk reduction of about 1% per year.

Consensus Statements Affecting Indications

Several organizations have published position papers or consensus statements based on the collective opinion of recognized experts. These include an ad hoc committee report from the Joint Council of the two national vascular societies[124] and the Rand Corporation.[107] Most recently, the American Heart Association convened a consensus conference, and its report has been published.[119a] Table 131–1 summarizes the current indications for carotid endarterectomy and compares the recommendations from retrospective reviews, the Rand panel, the Joint Council position statement, and the prospective randomized trials.[119]

CONTRAINDICATIONS TO OPERATIVE REPAIR

An aggressive surgical approach is contraindicated if the general condition of the patient includes a serious illness that will materially shorten the normal life expectancy. In addition to this general reservation, some patients have specific neurologic complications that prohibit operation or make its postponement advisable. These include the patient

TABLE 131–1. CURRENT INDICATIONS FOR CAROTID ENDARTERECTOMY

PATIENTS	SOURCE OF RECOMMENDATION			
	Retrospective Data Analysis	Rand Panel	Joint Council*	Randomized Trials
Symptomatic				
Single focal TIA (>70% stenosis)	Yes	Yes	Yes	Yes
Multiple focal TIAs with				
>70% stenosis	Yes	Yes	Yes	Yes
>50% stenosis with ulceration	Yes	Yes	Yes	NA
50% to 69% stenosis†	Yes	Yes	Yes	NA
30% to 49% stenosis†	Yes	Yes	Yes	NA
<30% stenosis with or without ulcer†	Yes	Yes	Yes	No
Previous stroke (mild), ipsilateral				
>70% stenosis	Yes	Yes	Yes	Yes
>50% with large ulcer	Yes	Yes	Yes	NA
30% to 69% with and without ulcer	Yes	Yes	Yes	NA
Evolving stroke				
>70% stenosis	Yes	Yes	Yes	NA
Global symptoms				
>70% carotid stenosis with uncorrectable vertebrobasilar disease	Yes	Yes	Yes	NA
Asymptomatic				
>70% stenosis with contralateral occlusion or high-grade stenosis	Yes	Yes	Yes	NA
>70% unilateral stenosis	Yes	No	Yes	NA
Large ulcer with >50% stenosis	Yes	No	NA	NA

Reprinted by permission of the Western Journal of Medicine, from Moore WS: Carotid endarterectomy for prevention of stroke. 1993, July, 159:37–43.
*Joint Council of the Society for Vascular Surgery and the International Society for Cardiovascular Surgery (North American Chapter).
†Patients receiving aspirin therapy.
NA = not available; TIA = transient ischemic attack.

who presents acutely with a major stroke and has not yet begun to recover. Another is one who has had a major stroke in the past and is so devastated by neurologic dysfunction or altered level of consciousness that operation is inadvisable.

During early experience with carotid surgery, emergency operation for acute stroke was relatively common.[145] However, emergency thromboendarterectomy in an acutely occluded carotid artery frequently resulted in conversion of an ischemic cerebral infarction to a hemorrhagic cerebral infarction, resulting in death. These findings were particularly dramatized in the first randomized cooperative study involving operation for carotid artery disease.[17] In addition, premature endarterectomy in a diseased but open internal carotid artery, prior to neurologic recovery, often resulted in an exacerbation of the neurologic deficit because of an increase in localized cerebral edema and its attendant adverse consequences. After recent major neurologic injury, it is better to wait for the patient to reach a plateau of recovery before proceeding with elective carotid endarterectomy.

OPERATIVE TECHNIQUE

Surgery of the Carotid Bifurcation

Anesthesia and Positioning of the Patient

Operations on the carotid bifurcation were originally, and often still are, performed using local or cervical block anesthesia. Local anesthesia has the advantage of allowing the surgeon to evaluate the patient's cerebral tolerance to trial carotid clamping. When the carotid clamp is temporarily applied, the patient is asked to speak and move the extremities of the appropriate side as evidence of adequate collateral cerebral circulation to support brain function during the time required to remove the lesion. For this reason, a number of surgeons continue to advocate local anesthesia as the anesthetic technique of choice.

The disadvantages of local anesthesia primarily relate to patient anxiety. If the patient becomes restless or agitated, this will also disturb the surgical team. Finally, when a difficult lesion is encountered, extended operating time may exceed the forbearance of the average patient under local anesthesia.

General anesthesia has three major advantages.

1. The anesthesiologist has better control of the patient's airway and ventilatory mechanics.

2. Halogenated anesthetic agents can increase cerebral blood flow and, at the same time, decrease cerebral metabolic demand.[31] This combined effect may increase tolerance to temporary carotid artery clamping.

3. The sleeping, anesthetized patient can undergo comfortably whichever exacting procedure is required without disturbing the operating field and the surgical team.

Positioning the patient is an important aspect of preparing for a carotid endarterectomy. The patient is placed supine on the operating table with the neck slightly hyperextended. This may be accomplished by placing a folded sheet under the shoulders. Excessive hypertension actually

makes exposure more difficult by tightening the sternocleidomastoid muscle and by restricting the mobility of the common carotid artery and carotid bifurcation. Once the head is extended, it is then gently turned to the side opposite that of operation.

Many patients in the age group appropriate for carotid artery disease may have a significant degree of cervical arthritis. Care must be taken to avoid neck injury with rotation. If the patient's blood pressure is stable, flexing the operating table and introducing a 10-degree reverse Trendelenburg inclination brings the patient's neck into best perspective, reducing venous pressure and minimizing incisional bleeding (Fig. 131–1).

Two incisions have been employed for exposure of the carotid bifurcation. The first is a vertical incision parallel to the anterior border of the sternocleidomastoid muscle, along a line connecting the sternoclavicular junction with the mastoid process. The surgeon decides its exact length and placement along this imaginary line by noting the position of the carotid bifurcation and the extent of the lesion on the lateral projection of the carotid arteriogram (Fig. 131–2). This determination is also made solely by the use of carotid duplex ultrasound scans. The incision is deepened through the platysmal layer to gain access to the investing fascia in the interval between the sternocleido-

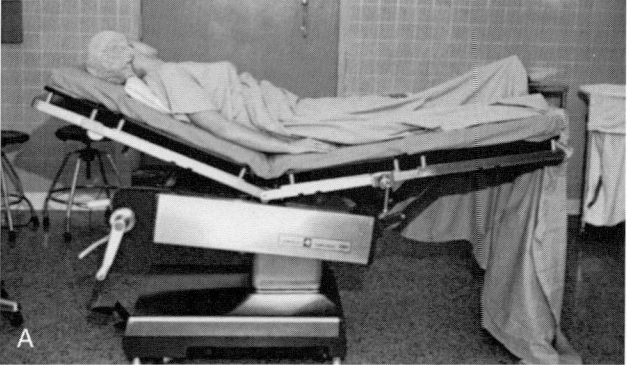
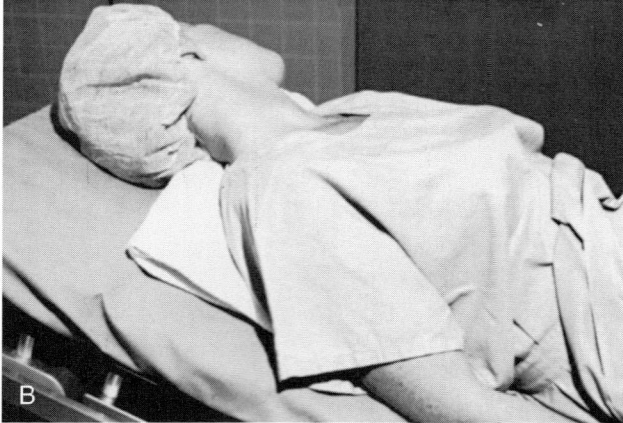

FIGURE 131–1. *A,* The optimal operating table adjustment for carotid bifurcation endarterectomy. The table is flexed approximately 20 degrees in the reverse Trendelenburg position in order to bring the patient into a semirecumbent position. *B,* The neck is mildly hyperextended by introducing a folded sheet under the patient's shoulders. Finally, the patient's head is turned to the side opposite the operation. The neck on the side of operation is now exposed to best surgical advantage.

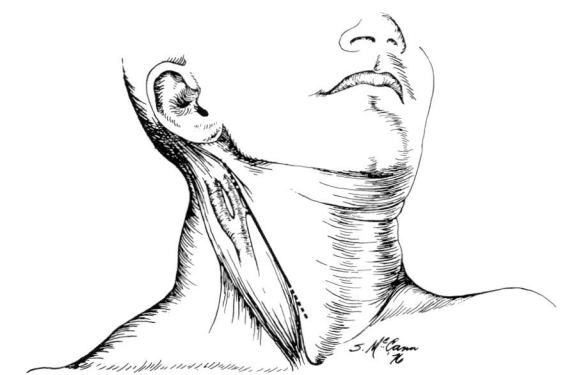

FIGURE 131–2. Placement of a vertical incision along the anterior border of the sternocleidomastoid muscle in relationship to the underlying carotid artery bifurcation.

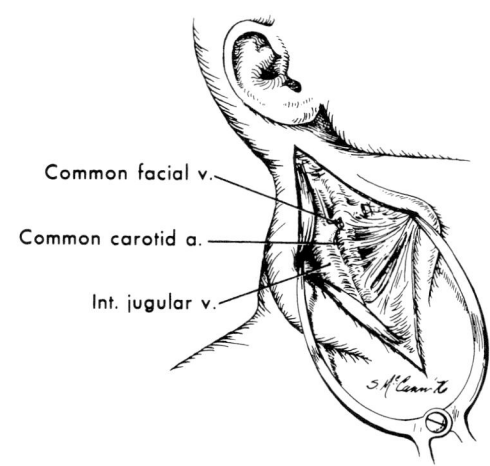

FIGURE 131–4. The relationship of the internal jugular vein and common carotid artery within the carotid sheath. The major tributary to the internal jugular vein at this level is the common facial vein. Division of the common facial vein consistently gives access to the carotid bifurcation.

mastoid muscle and the trachea. The authors prefer this incision because it parallels the carotid artery. If the surgeon needs to gain additional exposure of the proximal or distal part of the vessel, extension of the incision is simple and easy.

The second incision employed for exposure of the carotid bifurcation is oblique and is placed in one of the skin creases over the side of the neck (Fig. 131–3). It is deepened through the platysma, and the subplatysmal space between the sternocleidomastoid muscle and the trachea is mobilized. The advantage of this incision is that it may produce a more cosmetically acceptable scar than that resulting from the vertical incision. The disadvantages are that (1) it is necessary to raise skin flaps and (2) it is more difficult to gain additional proximal or distal arterial exposure because the direction of the incision is oblique to the direction of the artery.

After exposure, the investing fascia is incised along the anterior border of the sternocleidomastoid muscle, and the muscle is then mobilized to expose the underlying carotid sheath (Fig. 131–4). The carotid sheath is incised low on the neck, and the dissection is directed along the medial aspect of the internal jugular vein. The vein is retracted laterally to expose the common carotid artery (Fig. 131–5).

The vagus nerve is usually the most posterior occupant of the carotid sheath, but occasionally it may spiral to take an anterior position at the point where the sheath is opened. This anomaly should be anticipated, and the surgeon should take care to avoid injuring the nerve when the sheath is initially incised.

The medial aspect of the jugular vein is exposed until the common facial vein is seen coursing obliquely across the common carotid artery and draining into the jugular vein. The common facial vein is a constant landmark for the carotid bifurcation and represents the venous analogue of the external carotid artery. The vein is mobilized, suture-ligated, and divided (Fig. 131–6). When the vein is divided, the carotid artery can be appropriately visualized. The common carotid artery is mobilized circumferentially and encircled with polymeric silicone (Silastic) tape. The periarterial dissection continues superiorly to expose the ca-

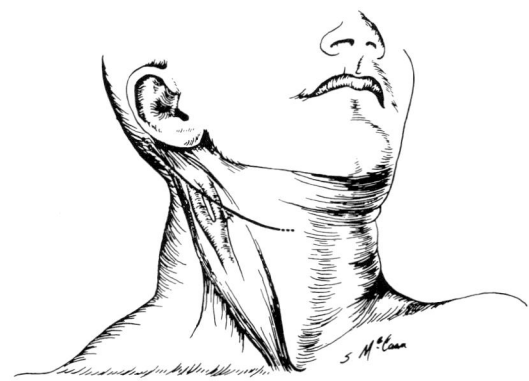

FIGURE 131–3. The alternative incision placed obliquely in a skin crease over the carotid bifurcation. The dissection is carried down through the platysma, and subplatysmal flaps are developed in the superior and inferior aspects of the incision to convert the exposure of the carotid bifurcation to a vertical approach.

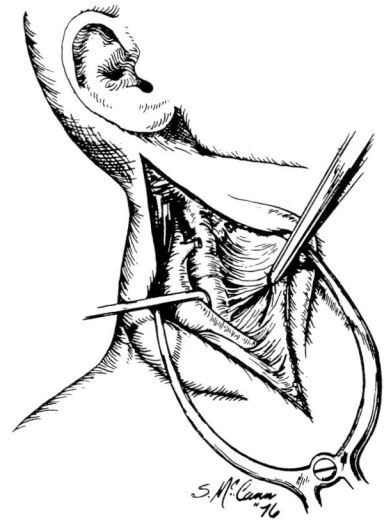

FIGURE 131–5. Following mobilization of its anteromedial aspect, the internal jugular vein is retracted laterally, giving clear exposure to the underlying common carotid artery.

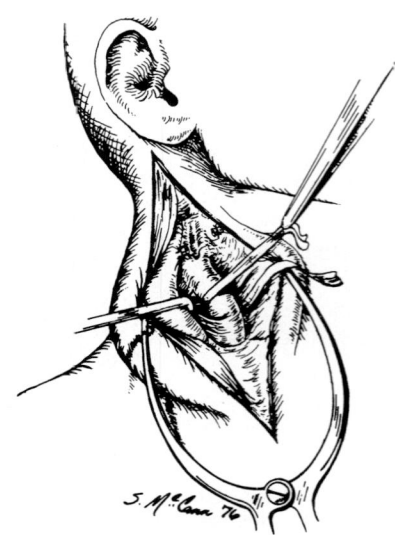

FIGURE 131–6. The mobilized common carotid artery with the surrounding umbilical tape. The dissection toward the internal and external carotid arteries has begun.

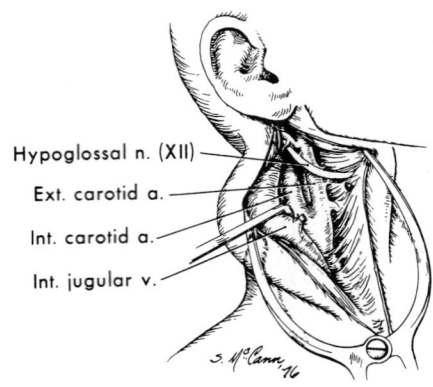

FIGURE 131–8. The relationship of the twelfth cranial nerve to the upper extent of the dissection of the carotid bifurcation.

rotid bifurcation. As soon as the bifurcation is identified, if a sinus bradycardia occurs, 1 to 2 ml of 1% lidocaine may be injected into the tissues between the external and the internal carotid arteries to block the nerves to the carotid sinus. Some surgeons routinely anesthetize the carotid sinus to prevent this phenomenon.

Particular care must be taken during this part of the dissection to avoid undue manipulation or palpation of the carotid bifurcation and bulb of the internal carotid artery. Because this is the location of the atheromatous lesion and because the lesion may be quite friable or contain thrombotic or atheromatous debris, manipulation may cause dislodgment with subsequent cerebral embolization and stroke. Some surgeons have described this requirement for gentleness as "dissecting the patient away from the carotid, not vice versa."

The internal carotid artery is mobilized to a point well above the palpable atheromatous lesion, where it is unques-

tionably soft and not diseased (Fig. 131–7). The same is done for the external carotid artery, with care taken not to injure the superior thyroid branch. In patients with a high carotid bifurcation or a lesion that goes relatively far up the internal carotid artery, the surgeon obtains additional exposure by carefully dividing the tissues in the crotch formed by the internal and the external carotid arteries. This maneuver should be performed between clamps because, on occasion, the ascending pharyngeal artery can be located in this position. The tissues in this crotch often act as a suspensory ligament of the carotid bifurcation and, once divided, allow the bifurcation to drop down, making further mobilization of the internal carotid artery possible.

The 12th cranial nerve should always be identified when the internal carotid artery is mobilized. It passes obliquely through the upper portion of the field, just superior to the bulb of the carotid artery, on its way to innervate the tongue (Fig. 131–8). Injury to this nerve causes a lateral deviation of the tongue toward the side of operation when the patient attempts to extrude the tongue. This also produces difficulty with initiation of swallowing. Should additional exposure of the internal carotid artery be necessary, mobilization and division of the posterior belly of the digastric muscle may be required (Fig. 131–9).

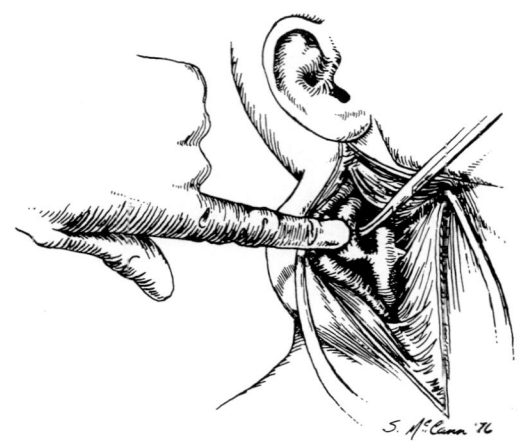

FIGURE 131–7. The internal carotid artery is mobilized well above the diseased intima. This fact is confirmed by careful palpation of the relatively normal internal carotid artery against the surface of the right-angle clamp.

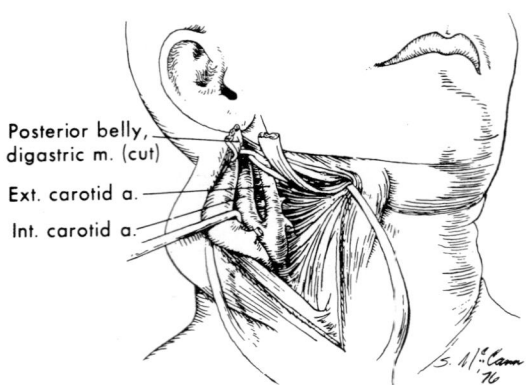

FIGURE 131–9. When the carotid bifurcation is high or when the lesion extends for an unusual distance up the internal carotid artery, additional distal exposure of the internal carotid artery can be obtained by division of the posterior belly of the digastric muscle.

Determination of Cerebral Tolerance to Carotid Cross-Clamping

Once the carotid bifurcation is exposed but before endarterectomy can be started, a decision must be made regarding the method of maintaining cerebral flow during carotid occlusion. The time-honored technique for determining the safety of temporary carotid clamping is trial occlusion with local anesthesia. The common, external, and internal carotid arteries are occluded for 3 minutes. During this time, the patient is asked to talk and move the arm and leg on the side affected by the carotid lesion. If there is no evidence of weakness or disturbance of consciousness, the intracranial circulation is judged to be adequate and operation can proceed without additional circulatory support. Adequate cerebral collateral circulation is found in approximately 85% to 90% of patients tested. In the 10% to 15% in whom circulation is inadequate, an internal shunt must be employed.

Local anesthesia and trial occlusion constitute a very satisfactory technique. If the surgeon prefers general anesthesia, an alternative method for determining the safety of temporary carotid occlusion must be employed. Many surgeons who use general anesthesia prefer to insert an internal shunt routinely. This does not identify selectively the individual patient who requires such circulatory support, but it has the advantage of "playing it safe" by providing additional flow to all patients.[169] The disadvantage is that the presence of an internal shunt makes the performance of endarterectomy somewhat more cumbersome. It also compromises precise visualization of the distal endpoint and introduces the potential complications inherent in the use of the shunt.

These complications include scuffing or disruption of the distal intima during shunt insertion and the possible introduction of air or thrombotic emboli through the shunt when flow is reconstituted (Fig. 131–10). In a personal series (W.S.M), surgical patients without a shunt had a postoperative neurologic complication rate of 1.5%, whereas those with a shunt had a neurologic complication rate of 5%. Because of such experiences, we prefer to reserve the use of an internal shunt for those selected few patients with inadequate collateral circulation when it is clearly indicated and justified. We prefer not to expose the remaining majority of patients to the small but finite increased risk of shunt use when there is no need to provide the additional cerebral blood flow.

The next question is how to identify inadequate collateral blood flow in patients undergoing general anesthesia. Several methods have been attempted, such as the measurement of ipsilateral jugular venous oxygen tension.[104] The hypothesis on which this test is based states that patients with adequate collateral blood flow would have a higher oxygen tension in the venous blood draining from that segment than those patients with inadequate blood flow. This test proved to be inexact because, owing to the anatomy of the venous-sinus system, the venous drainage from the brain is a mixture of blood from both hemispheres.[98]

Another suggested method is electroencephalographic monitoring during operation. Initial experience with this technique was disappointing, owing to the effect of general anesthesia on electroencephalographic tracing.[72] More re-

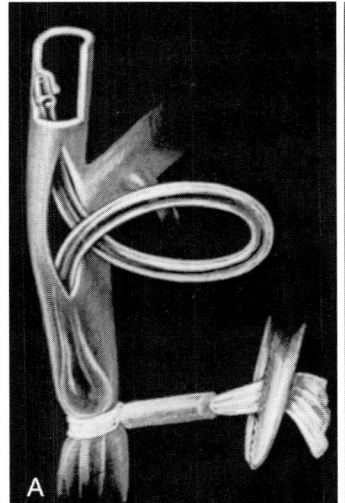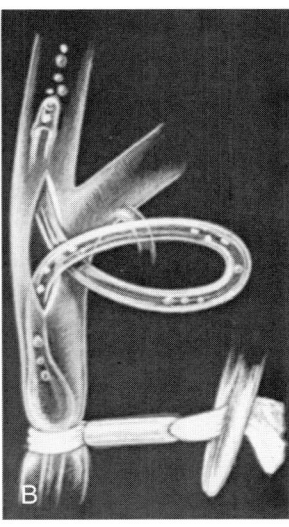

FIGURE 131–10. Two potential complications of internal shunt insertion. A, If the tip of the shunt is not carefully placed in the internal carotid artery, it is possible to scuff or elevate a flap of distal intima. B, Unless care is taken to evacuate air from the shunt or from the blind portion of the common carotid artery, it is possible to introduce air bubbles as cerebral emboli. Also, scuffing of an atherosclerotic plaque by the proximal portion of the shunt may scoop up atheromatous debris, which may also embolize to the distal cerebral circulation.

cently, however, the technique was reintroduced and has now become a standard method by which adequacy of cerebral blood flow is monitored.[4, 176] This test is somewhat cumbersome because of the instrumentation involved and the expertise needed to interpret the electroencephalographic tracing. Nonetheless, several centers use it with enthusiasm and with excellent results.

Many surgeons have noted that patients who tolerate carotid cross-clamping also have excellent back-bleeding from the internal carotid artery through the arteriotomy when the clamps are released. Some investigators have used this observation to determine the adequacy of collateral blood flow and shunt requirement. This method can work in the hands of the experienced surgeon who has developed the ability to judge back-flow; however, it is a qualitative rather than a quantitative observation, and as such cannot be taught.

Recognizing the validity of the observation of back-flow, in 1966 the author (W.S.M.) and his colleagues set about to develop a method of quantitation. The results of this clinical research have led to the introduction of the *internal carotid artery back-pressure determination* as a means of estimating collateral cerebral blood flow. These investigators reasoned that a relationship existed between the intracranial collateral blood flow and perfusion pressure. Measurement of the back-pressure down the proximally clamped internal carotid artery is an indirect measurement of the perfusion pressure that is present on the ipsilateral side of the circle of Willis (Fig. 131–11). Our group initially validated the technique by measuring back-pressure in a series of 36 patients undergoing 48 carotid thromboendarterectomies under local anesthesia. The patients' conscious response to trial occlusion was correlated with the measured value of internal carotid artery back-pressure. Of the 48 carotid arteries tested, 43 had back-pressures that ranged from 25

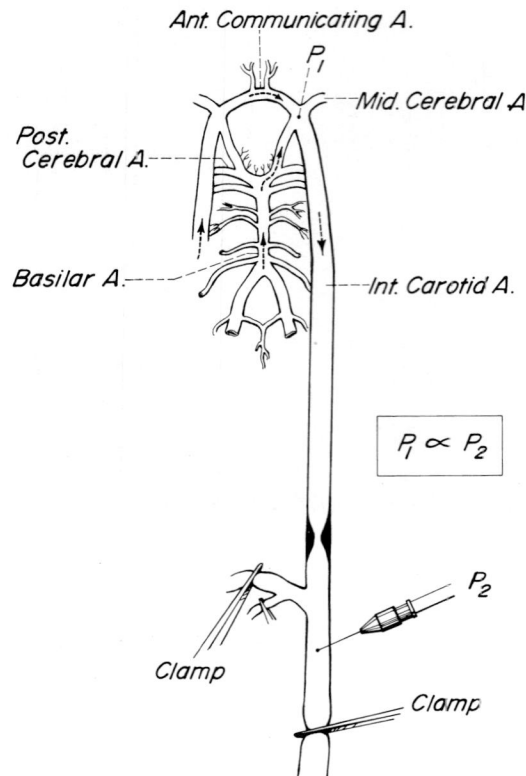

FIGURE 131–11. Pathways of collateral circulation about the circle of Willis. Perfusion pressure at the middle cerebral artery (P_1). Internal carotid back pressure as measured at the bifurcation (P_2). Being a closed, unbranched fluid system, P_2 is proportional to P_1. (From Moore WS, Hall AD: Carotid artery back pressure. Arch Surg 99:702, 1969. Copyright 1969, American Medical Association.)

to 88 mmHg. In each instance, the patient maintained full motor and intellectual function. Three patients were intolerant of trial occlusion, and their internal carotid artery back-pressure ranged from 12 to 24 mmHg. These observations led the investigators to conclude that 25 mmHg under ambient conditions of P_{CO_2} and the patient's normal blood pressure was the minimal safe level. All patients with back-pressures below 25 mmHg required an internal shunt, and the carotid arteries of those with pressures above 25 mmHg could be occluded temporarily without additional cerebral circulatory support.[122]

Other investigators reported similar results using carotid artery back-pressure of 40 mmHg.[50, 78] The validity of carotid back-pressure measurements to determine the need for temporary shunt placement in patients under general anesthesia has been confirmed, but one group of patients constitute an exception to the back-pressure criteria—those who have had a previous cerebral infarction. Patients who have suffered a previous stroke often experience a temporary exacerbation of neurologic deficit when a shunt is not used, because patients with a previous cerebral infarction have a surrounding zone of relative ischemia that is being perfused through collateral channels, the "ischemic penumbra." These collateral channels have a variably higher resistance to flow; therefore, this group of patients has a greater perfusion pressure requirement to maintain flow to the ischemic penumbra than those with normal circulatory patterns.[125]

In patients with a previous cerebral infarction, in the

authors' opinion, shunts should be used routinely regardless of the measured back-pressure. The temporary shunt is indicated for all patients with a prior history of cerebral infarction as well as for those with a back-pressure of less than 25 mmHg. Patients undergoing operations for TIAs or asymptomatic carotid stenosis in whom the back-pressure is greater than 25 to 40 mmHg do not require a shunt. Using these criteria, the author's group (W.S.M) then carried out a series of 172 carotid endarterectomies in 153 patients with a 0.6% overall neurologic morbidity rate that included postoperative TIAs as well as infarction. In 74% of cases, the operation was performed without an internal shunt, whereas 26% required internal shunt support.[93]

The technique for measuring internal carotid back-pressure is quite simple and has been validated by others.[78, 91] After the carotid bifurcation is mobilized, 5000 to 10,000 units of heparin is administered intravenously. A 22-gauge needle is bent at a 45-degree angle and is connected via rigid pressure tubing to a pressure transducer. The bent portion of the needle is then inserted into the common carotid artery so that it rests in a position that is axial to the artery and does not impinge on the posterior wall. Systemic arterial pressure is measured and compared with radial artery pressure. The common carotid artery, proximal to the needle, is then clamped.

A second clamp is placed on the external carotid artery. This leaves the needle in continuity with a static column of blood that is open to the internal carotid artery. Even though the needle is placed proximal to the carotid stenosis, pressure equalizes on both sides of the carotid stenosis because there is no blood flow. The residual pressure or internal carotid artery back-pressure is then recorded (Fig. 131–12).

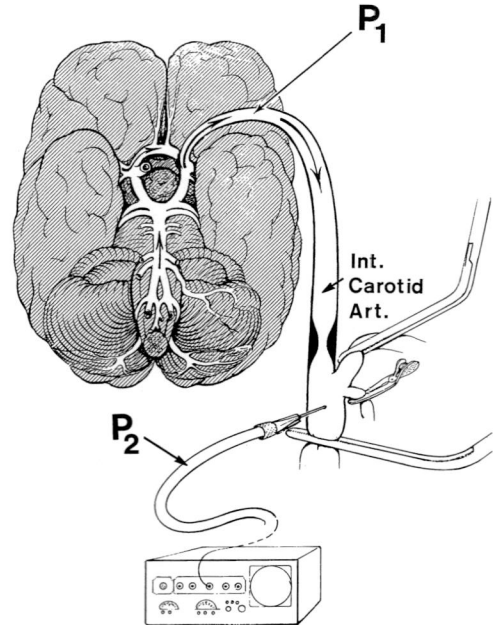

FIGURE 131–12. Relationship of middle cerebral to internal carotid perfusion pressure is represented. With common and external carotid arteries clamped, back pressure distal to the internal carotid artery is in direct continuity with the middle cerebral artery. Therefore, P_2 is essentially equal to P_1. (From Moore WS, Yee JM, Hall AD: Collateral cerebral blood pressure: An index of tolerance to temporary carotid occlusion. Arch Surg 106:520, 1973. Copyright 1973, American Medical Association.)

In an effort to reduce further the need for internal shunt, investigation was conducted into possible methods of increasing cerebral blood flow during carotid surgery. The methods attempted include inducing arterial hypertension and manipulating arterial P_{CO_2}.[51, 97, 180] Increasing arterial blood pressure by use of vasopressor drugs increases perfusion pressure in collateral channels and, presumably, increases collateral blood flow. There is, however, a price to be paid for this benefit in the form of increasing afterload on the myocardium. Because most of these patients have associated coronary artery disease, the net result may be increased myocardial damage. It is preferable to use an internal shunt in a few more patients rather than risk increasing the incidence of myocardial infarction.

Increasing P_{CO_2} (hypercapnia) effectively induces cerebral vasodilatation.[90, 140] For this reason, many surgeons employ hypercapnia in order to increase cerebral blood flow during carotid occlusion. However, there is evidence to suggest that the cerebral vasculature in areas of decreased cerebral perfusion is already maximally dilated. Hypercapnia not only fails to increase cerebral blood flow where it is needed but also, by producing cerebral vasodilatation in the opposite hemisphere, causes a redistribution of blood flow with a reduced collateral contribution from the normally perfused hemisphere. Therefore, some investigators have suggested that the reverse approach be employed (i.e., a reduction of P_{CO_2}, or hypocapnia), in order to cause cerebral vasoconstriction on the normally perfused side so that collateral redistribution will be from the normal to the ischemic side. The experimental data in the literature are contradictory, and the information is inadequate upon which to base a conclusion about the relative merits of hypocapnia versus hypercapnia. Because the back-pressure data originally were obtained using normocapnia, we prefer to continue using normocapnia to avoid confusing the interpretation of back-pressure values.

Internal Shunt Placement

A shunt is a valuable surgical adjunct that, properly used, can reduce the incidence of neurologic complications in those patients who depend on continued flow through the carotid artery that is undergoing repair. An improperly placed shunt, however, can be the source of several complications that may lead to permanent neurologic damage. Once it has been decided to use an internal shunt, the operating surgeon should take a few minutes to describe the technique to the team and make certain that the proper shunt and appropriate instruments are immediately available in order to minimize ischemia time between carotid clamping and shunt placement.

The *Javid shunt* is popular because of the appropriate diameter, length, and smooth finish of the ends to be inserted into the artery (Fig. 131–13). A modified Rumel tourniquet may be used to anchor the shunt, by drawing an umbilical tape encircling the common and internal carotid arteries through a short segment of rubber tubing, and "snugging down" on the rubber tube clamp in order to draw the umbilical sling firmly around the internal shunt within the artery (Fig. 131–14). Alternatively, specially fashioned Javid shunt clamps are available.

A longitudinal arteriotomy is begun on the posterior lateral part of the common carotid artery, well proximal to

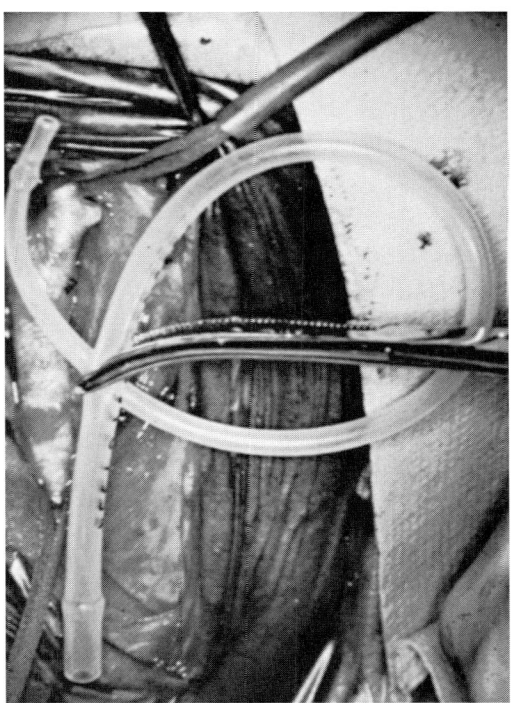

FIGURE 131–13. A Javid shunt prior to placement. The author's group prefers this type of inlying shunt because its size is appropriate to provide maximal flow, and the proximal and distal diameter expansions reduce the possibility of inadvertent displacement while the shunt is functioning.

the lesion. The arteriotomy is extended through the lesion, into the carotid bulb, and beyond into the internal carotid artery as far as necessary to clear the obvious diseased intima. The distal end of the shunt is placed in the internal carotid artery, which is then allowed to back-bleed and fill the shunt with blood. The proximal part of the shunt is passed into the common carotid artery. This passage is

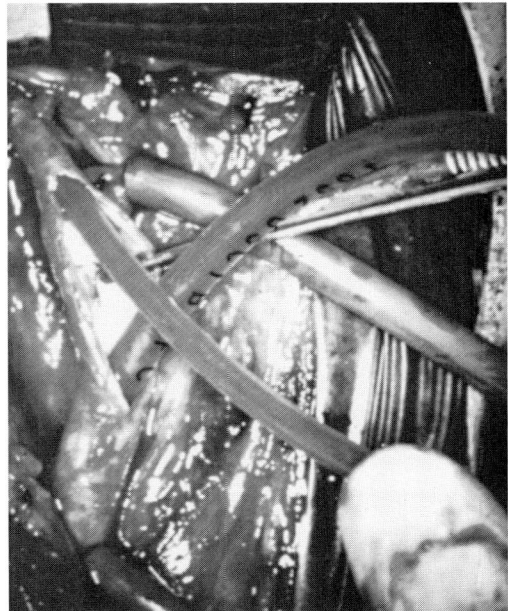

FIGURE 131–14. A functioning shunt in place. The shunt is held in position by a proximal and distal sling tourniquet.

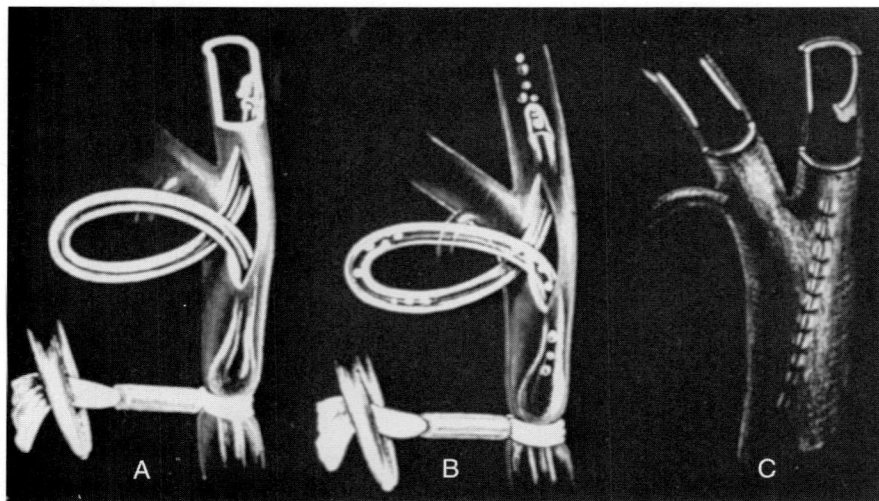

FIGURE 131–15. The three potential complications of an internal shunt. *A,* Scuffing of the distal intima. *B,* Embolization of air or atherothrombotic debris. *C,* Poor visualization of the distal end-point so that an intimal flap is left, producing the risk of subsequent thromboembolic complications.

made with the shunt actively back-bleeding in order to dissipate any air from the common carotid segment. Several insertions and withdrawals of the shunt may be required to flush all the air out of the blind segment.

The shunt is then clamped, the tourniquet about the shunt within the common carotid artery is tightened, and the clamp on the common carotid artery is released. At this point, the clamp on the shunt tubing is slowly opened and the translucent tubing is carefully observed for air bubbles and atheromatous debris. If no bubbles or debris is seen, the shunt is fully opened and the operation can proceed. The complications of an internal shunt include scuffing of the distal arterial intima, embolization of atheromatous debris or air, and poor distal end-point management (Fig. 131–15).

Scuffing of the intima can be minimized by using the polyethylene shunt tubing with a smooth, rounded tip specifically manufactured for this purpose. Atheroma embolization can be avoided by making an arteriotomy large enough to prevent scooping up of atheromatous debris at the time the proximal portion of the shunt is inserted into the common carotid artery. Air emboli can be prevented by careful evacuation of the air at the time of shunt insertion. Problems with distal end-point management can be reduced by opening the internal carotid artery as far as necessary to ensure direct visualization of a smooth end-point (Fig. 131–16).

In another technique of shunting, the distal end of the shunt is placed in the external rather than the internal carotid artery.[105] This method augments, to a variable degree, cerebral collateral blood flow through the external carotid artery–ophthalmic artery–internal carotid artery route, which has the advantage of keeping the shunt out of the internal carotid artery and reducing the problems with distal end-point management (Fig. 131–17).

Bifurcation Endarterectomy

One of the most critical details of endarterectomy is the selection of an appropriate endarterectomy plane. The optimal plane of dissection lies between the diseased intima and the circular fibers of the arterial media (Fig. 131–18).

A carotid endarterectomy performed in this plane allows for a smooth, distal tapering of end-point. It is easy to get into the plane between the arterial media and the adventitia. Although this is an easily dissectible plane, obtaining a smooth tapering end-point is more difficult because of the increased thickness of the relatively normal intima and media at the termination point of dissection in the internal carotid artery. Because of this thickness, there is often a shelf or a step-up in the internal carotid artery, which may require the use of sutures to tack down the end-point. The authors believe that it is disadvantageous to use tacking sutures and prefer to achieve a smooth, tapered end-point that occurs naturally within a proper dissection plane.

Once the proper plane is established in the common carotid artery, dissection is continued with a dissector circumferentially about the artery. The circumferential dissection is completed with a right-angle clamp, making it

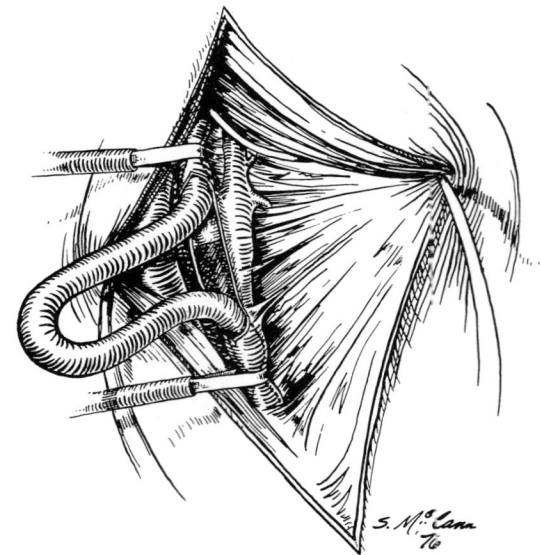

FIGURE 131–16. Appearance of the carotid bifurcation with the shunt in place following bifurcation endarterectomy. The distal portion of the arteriotomy extends far enough up the internal carotid artery to permit direct visualization of the distal end-point.

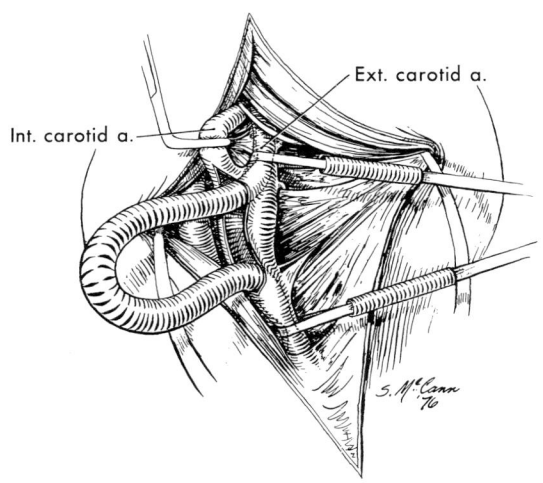

FIGURE 131–17. Technique of placing the distal end of the shunt in the external carotid artery to provide free access to the internal carotid artery. This is an alternative way to minimize problems with end-point management.

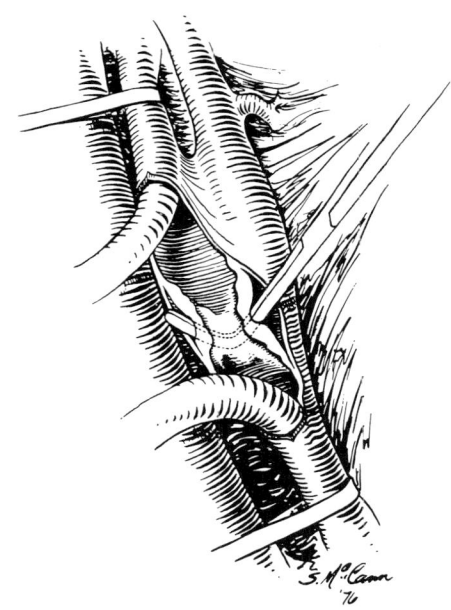

FIGURE 131–19. Technique of completing circumferential mobilization of the atheromatous lesion by utilizing the closed jaws of a right-angle clamp.

possible to identify the same dissection plane on the opposite side of the artery (Fig. 131–19). The atheromatous lesion is then sharply divided at its most proximal limit in the common carotid artery. The circumferential dissection is then carried to the external carotid artery, where a core of diseased intima is carefully developed by eversion of the artery and then gently removed.

The final and most important part of the dissection can now proceed up the internal carotid artery. Care is taken to advance equal distances circumferentially up the internal carotid artery. The specimen suddenly becomes free at a point where the intima becomes relatively normal, leaving a smooth, tapering end-point. The intimectomized surface of the carotid bifurcation is then generously irrigated with

heparinized saline solution, and any loose bits of debris or tiny strips of media are carefully removed. The proximal and distal end-points in the internal and external carotid arteries are irrigated under direct vision to make certain that there are no floating intimal flaps. A free edge of intima that floats is gently picked at with the tip of a fine clamp.

This part of the operation must not be hurried. If the patient has adequate collateral circulation, increased clamp time is not a problem. If collateral circulation is inadequate, a shunt should have been employed so that the operation can be done in a careful, unhurried fashion.

Once the endarterectomy is complete, the next step is closure. If a shunt has not been employed, a careful primary closure can be performed with 6–0 polypropylene suture. Tiny, closely placed, continuous stitches restore the normal contour of the artery without narrowing. If the arteriotomy was carried high up on a small or attenuated internal carotid artery, closure with a patch of vein or prosthetic material is desirable. Reports concerning recurrent carotid stenosis suggest that the use of a patch in patients with small arteries, particularly women, can minimize both early and late recurrence of stenosis.[81]

If an internal shunt has been employed, the closure is somewhat encumbered and the technique must be modified. A suture line is begun at the distal portion of the arteriotomy on the internal carotid artery and carried down to the common carotid artery. A second suture is then started proximally and is continued as far as the emergence of the plastic shunt will permit. The loop of the internal shunt then emerges between the two sutures (Fig. 131–20). The shunt is then removed, each vessel is carefully flushed, and a partially occluding pediatric vascular clamp is applied to approximate the remaining open portion of the arteriotomy. Flow is restored initially to the external carotid artery to flush any possible residual air or debris into that vessel. Flow is then restored to the internal carotid artery,

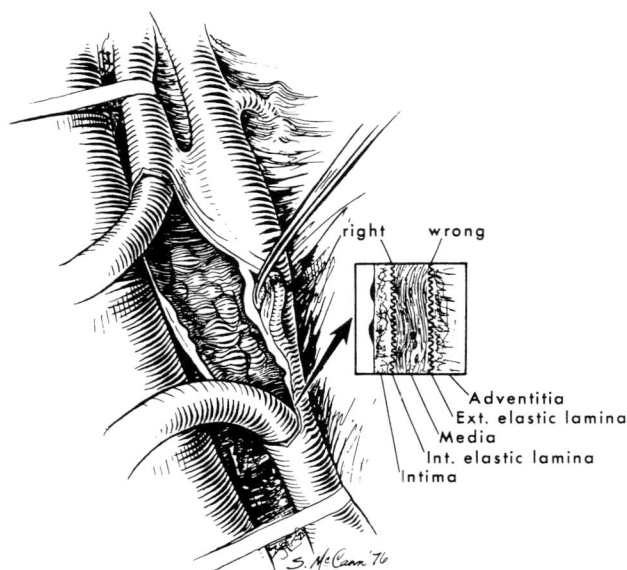

right   wrong

Adventitia
Ext. elastic lamina
Media
Int. elastic lamina
Intima

FIGURE 131–18. The proper endarterectomy dissection plane. The optimal plane lies between the diseased intima and the media at the level of the internal elastic lamina.

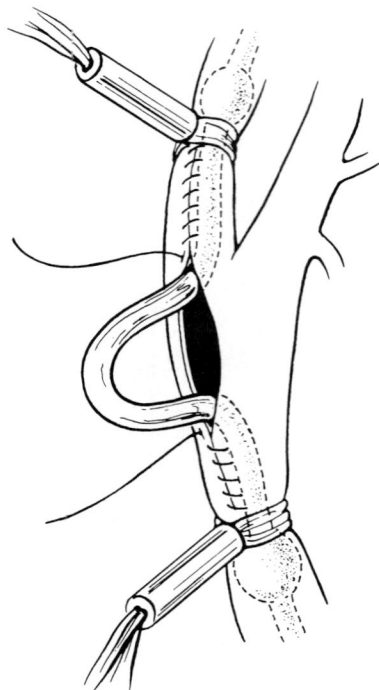

FIGURE 131–20. Partial closure of the arteriotomy with a suture beginning at each end. The arteriotomy is closed as far as the emergence of the internal shunt will permit.

and the surgeon makes a final closure of the arteriotomy by approximating the tissue held in place with the pediatric vascular clamp (Fig. 131–21).

Endarterectomy of an external carotid artery stenosis, in the presence of a totally occluded internal carotid artery, can be performed in the same manner as a carotid bifurcation endarterectomy.[32] In this instance, the arteriotomy ex-

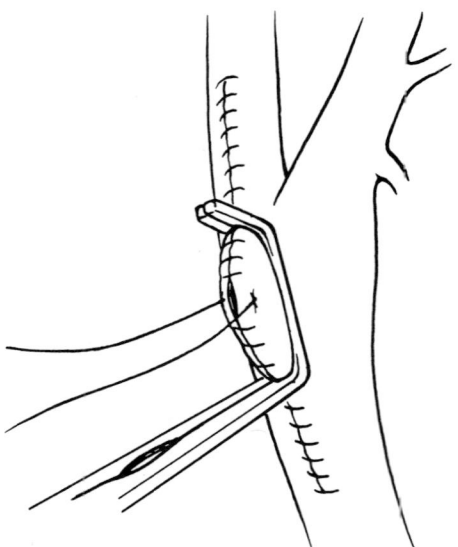

FIGURE 131–21. Application of a partially occluding pediatric vascular clamp permits restoration of blood flow to the internal and external carotid arteries while the final portion of the arteriotomy closure is completed after removal of the internal shunt.

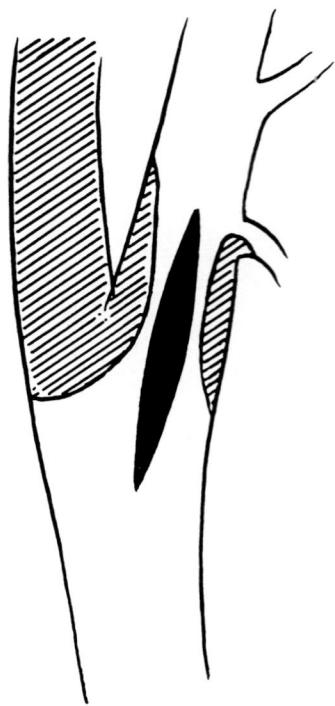

FIGURE 131–22. An endarterectomy of the external carotid artery can be carried out through an arteriotomy. It begins on the common carotid artery and extends through the stenotic lesion in the external carotid artery. Because the internal carotid artery is totally occluded, the lesion in this vessel can be ignored.

tends from the common carotid artery onto the external carotid artery (Fig. 131–22). It may be more convenient to detach the occluded internal carotid artery, in which case the arteriotomy passes through the opening left by this detachment. This has the advantage of eliminating the stump of the internal carotid artery at the time of arteriotomy closure.

Several techniques are available for the correction of coiling, kinking, or tortuosity of the internal carotid artery (see Chapter 135).[132] These include (1) resection of a segment of the internal carotid artery, (2) reimplantation of the internal carotid artery in a more proximal location, and (3) resection of a segment of the common carotid artery (Fig. 131–23). If an arteriosclerotic lesion is present in the carotid bifurcation, a thromboendarterectomy must be performed in combination with one of the shortening procedures.

Verification of the Technical Result

The surgeon who performs carotid endarterectomy has one chance to get it right. Thus, it is helpful to have some objective means of verifying the technical result. The most direct method is a *completion angiogram*. Other techniques include visualization with intraoperative *B-mode ultrasonography* and *waveform analysis* with continuous Doppler ultrasound.

The technique of operative completion angiography is both simple and effective. A 20-gauge needle is bent at a 45-degree angle so as to allow the needle to be placed into the artery and for it to lie axial to the direction of the

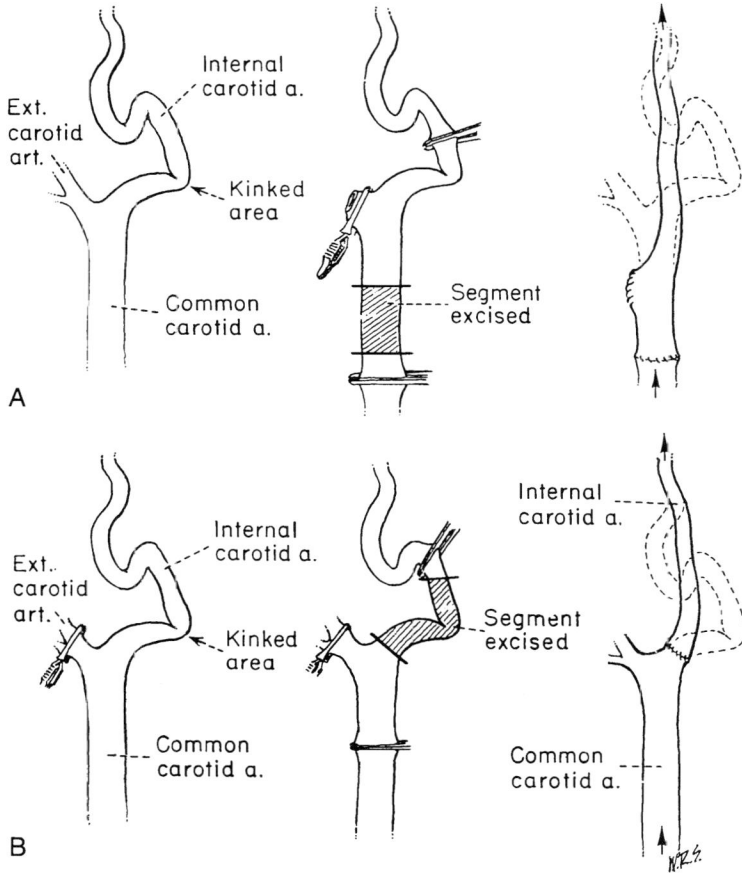

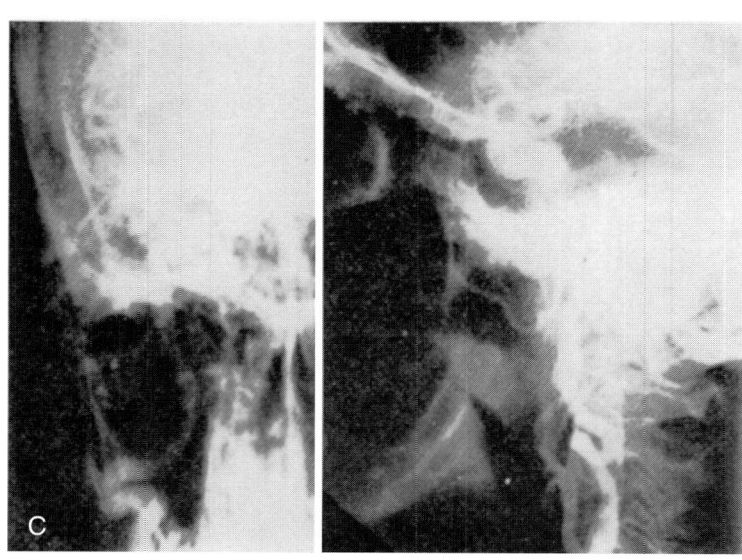

FIGURE 131–23. *A,* Indirect relief of a kinked internal carotid artery by resection of a portion of the common carotid artery. *B,* Direct relief of a kinked internal carotid artery by resection and end-to-end anastomosis. *C,* Markedly redundant and kinked left internal carotid artery in a 55-year-old man with intermittent attacks of right hemiparesis. (From Najafi H, Javid H, Dye WS, et al: Kinked internal carotid artery: Clinical evaluation and surgical correction. Arch Surg 89:134, 1964. Copyright 1964, American Medical Association.)

artery and minimize the risk of a subintimal injection. A 10-ml syringe is filled with angiographic contrast material and is connected to the needle with flexible tubing. A film is placed beneath the patient's head and neck, either in a sterile cassette holder or slid into the film slot of the operating table. A portable x-ray machine can be used, and the 10 ml of full-strength contrast material is rapidly injected at the time the film is exposed. This yields an excellent quality of image of the carotid bifurcation and the cervical carotid artery. The anatomic result of operation can thus be verified.

Any defect or intimal flap in the internal carotid artery can be corrected before a thromboembolic complication occurs. If an unsatisfactory end-point of the external carotid artery appears, it should be corrected as well. If the angiographic appearance is satisfactory, the heparin can be reversed with protamine prior to closure, although some surgeons do not reverse heparin with protamine because of potential adverse reactions to this drug.

Surgery of the Vertebral Artery

The clinical manifestations, indications, technique, and results of surgical repair of the vertebral artery are detailed in Chapter 132. For the sake of continuity, a brief discourse concerning the reconstruction of orificial lesions of the vertebral artery is presented here.

Most lesions involving the vertebral artery are atheromatous plaques of the subclavian artery that encroach on the lumen of the vertebral artery origin. This area is best exposed through a supraclavicular incision centered over the clavicular head of the sternocleidomastoid muscle. The incision is deepened through the platysmal layer, and the clavicular head of the sternocleidomastoid muscle is divided. The scalene fat pad is dissected along its inferior margin and retracted superiorly, together with the omohyoid muscle. The anterior scalene muscle is identified, and the phrenic nerve lies obliquely along this muscle. The phrenic nerve is mobilized, and the anterior scalene muscle is divided.

The subclavian artery is now identified. The vessel is

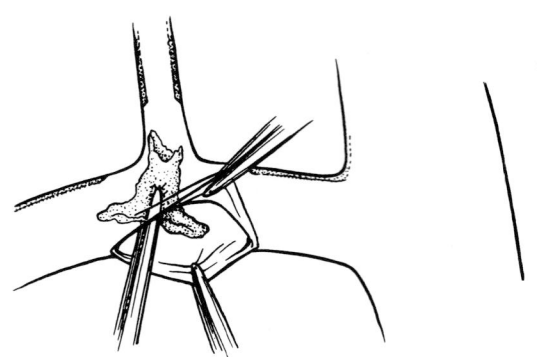

FIGURE 131-25. Separation of the atheromatous core from the distal intima within the vertebral artery and its dislocation into the subclavian artery as it is removed.

mobilized circumferentially, and an umbilical sling is applied. Mobilization of the subclavian artery continues proximally. At a point where the subclavian artery arches toward the mediastinum, the vertebral artery can be identified on the superior portion of the subclavian artery and the internal mammary artery identified on the inferior margin, opposite the takeoff of the vertebral artery. The vertebral artery branch can be mobilized carefully, and the proximal subclavian artery is dissected as far proximal as possible.

The atherosclerotic plaque, encroaching on the vertebral artery orifice, can be handled in one of two ways. If the plaque primarily involves the orifice and does not extend into the artery itself, a most satisfactory technique is a trans-subclavian artery endarterectomy. The subclavian artery is clamped proximally and distally, and a longitudinal incision is made along its anterior-inferior aspect approximately 3 mm from the vertebral artery. A thromboendarterectomy plane is established in the subclavian artery, and a circular intimal button is developed around the vertebral artery orifice (Fig. 131–24). The atheromatous lesion is then carefully cored out to achieve a clean distal end-point (Fig. 131–25). The area is flushed with saline solution, the artery is back-bled, and closure of the subclavian arteriotomy is accomplished with a simple running suture of 6–0 polypropylene (Fig. 131–26). After a completion angiogram, the wound is closed in layers.

If the lesion extends up the vertebral artery for a short distance or if it was not possible to achieve a clean end-

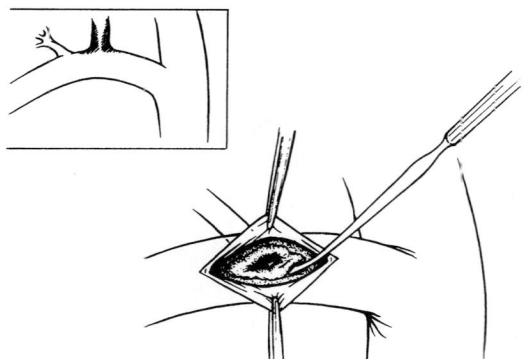

FIGURE 131–24. The trans-subclavian approach to vertebral artery endarterectomy. The inset demonstrates the vertebral artery stenosis in profile, emphasizing that the origin of the lesion is within the subclavian artery. A longitudinal arteriotomy is made on the posteroinferior aspect of the subclavian artery opposite the vertebral artery orifice. An endarterectomy is started at the base of the vertebral artery plaque within the subclavian artery.

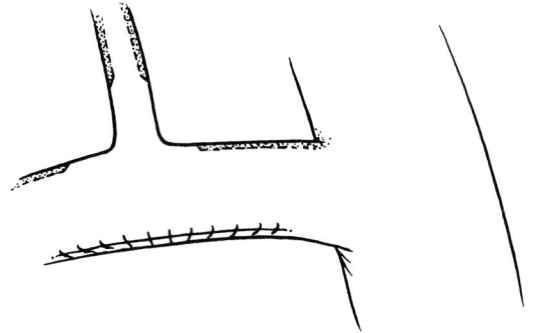

FIGURE 131–26. The final appearance following trans-subclavian endarterectomy, leaving a widely patent vertebral artery and showing the closure of the subclavian arteriotomy.

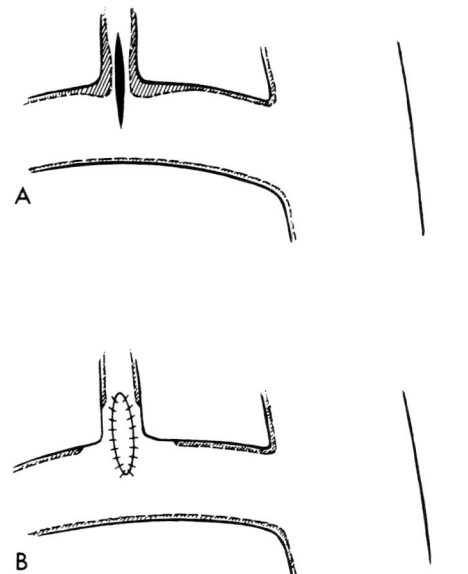

FIGURE 131–27. *A,* Technique of direct vertebral artery thromboendarterectomy through a vertical arteriotomy incision. *B,* Following endarterectomy, the arteriotomy in the vertebral artery is closed with a vein patch.

point with trans-subclavian endarterectomy, a direct vertebral thromboendarterectomy can be accomplished through a vertical arteriotomy extending from the subclavian artery through the vertebral artery orifice and up to a point distal to the atheromatous lesion. After the endarterectomy, the arteriotomy should be closed with vein patch angioplasty (Fig. 131–27).

Surgery of Occlusive Lesions of the Aortic Arch

Occlusive lesions at the level of the aortic arch account for fewer than 10% of operations on the extracranial vascular tree. Early in the experience with cerebrovascular surgery, these lesions were repaired by a transthoracic or transmediastinal approach.[33, 36, 50] These approaches utilized either endarterectomy of the affected vessel or bypass graft. These operations were occasionally associated with significant morbidity and mortality rates. Less direct techniques have been described that enabled the surgeon to revascularize a branch of the aortic arch without entering either the thorax or the mediastinum to expose its proximal extent.[123]

Stenoses or Occlusion of the Subclavian Artery

Lesions of the subclavian artery can be repaired in one of four ways:

1. Bypass graft from the ipsilateral common carotid artery to the subclavian artery distal to the site of an occlusive lesion.

2. Transposition of the subclavian artery to the side of the common carotid artery (the most preferable method).

3. Subcutaneous bypass graft extending from the opposite, unaffected axillary artery to the axillary artery distal to the subclavian lesion.[14, 34, 130]

4. Mediastinal approach to the subclavian artery, with

repair by either thromboendarterectomy or bypass graft from the ascending aorta to a point distal to the obstructing lesion.

Carotid-Subclavian Bypass

The carotid-subclavian bypass is best performed through a supraclavicular approach to the subclavian artery. Once the subclavian artery is mobilized, the common carotid artery is easily exposed through the same incision. The sternocleidomastoid muscle is mobilized along its posterior extent in order to visualize the carotid sheath, which is opened, and the common carotid artery is mobilized for a short distance. An 8-mm polyester (Dacron) graft or a 6-mm polytetrafluoroethylene (PTFE) graft can be used for bypass. The patient receives systemic anticoagulation with 5000 units of heparin. The back-pressure from the proximally clamped common carotid artery is measured. If the collateral back-pressure or residual pressure is greater than 25 mmHg, a second distal clamp is applied to the common carotid artery. A longitudinal incision is made and an anastomosis is constructed between the end of the graft and the side of the common carotid artery.

After appropriate flushing of the graft, a clamp is placed on the proximal portion of the graft and carotid artery blood flow is restored. The distal graft is then brought to the side of the subclavian artery at a convenient location, and an end-to-side anastomosis is constructed in a similar manner (Fig. 131–28). The wound is closed in layers, and the operation is complete. If carotid back-pressure is less than 25 mmHg, a carotid shunt can be used and subsequently withdrawn through the graft on completion of the anastomosis.

Subclavian Artery Transposition

Subclavian artery transposition has three advantages. It is an autogenous reconstruction, has only one anastomosis, and carries the best long-term patency. The common carotid and subclavian arteries are exposed and mobilized as described previously. The subclavian artery must be mobilized well proximal to the vertebral and internal mammary arteries, which are both carefully preserved. The subclavian artery is then divided proximally, and the proximal stump is oversewn. The distal end, proximal to the vertebral artery, is then sutured end-to-side to the common carotid artery.

Axillary-Axillary Bypass

The axillary-axillary bypass is an alternative procedure to the carotid-subclavian bypass. Both axillary arteries are exposed through infraclavicular incisions. The wound is deepened through the fascia. The sternal and clavicular portions of the pectoralis major muscle are split to expose the insertion of the pectoralis minor muscle. This muscle may be divided to provide additional access to the axillary artery (Fig. 131–29).

Thromboendarterectomy or Bypass Graft

A bypass graft is sutured end-to-side to the donor axillary artery, brought subcutaneously across the sternum, and

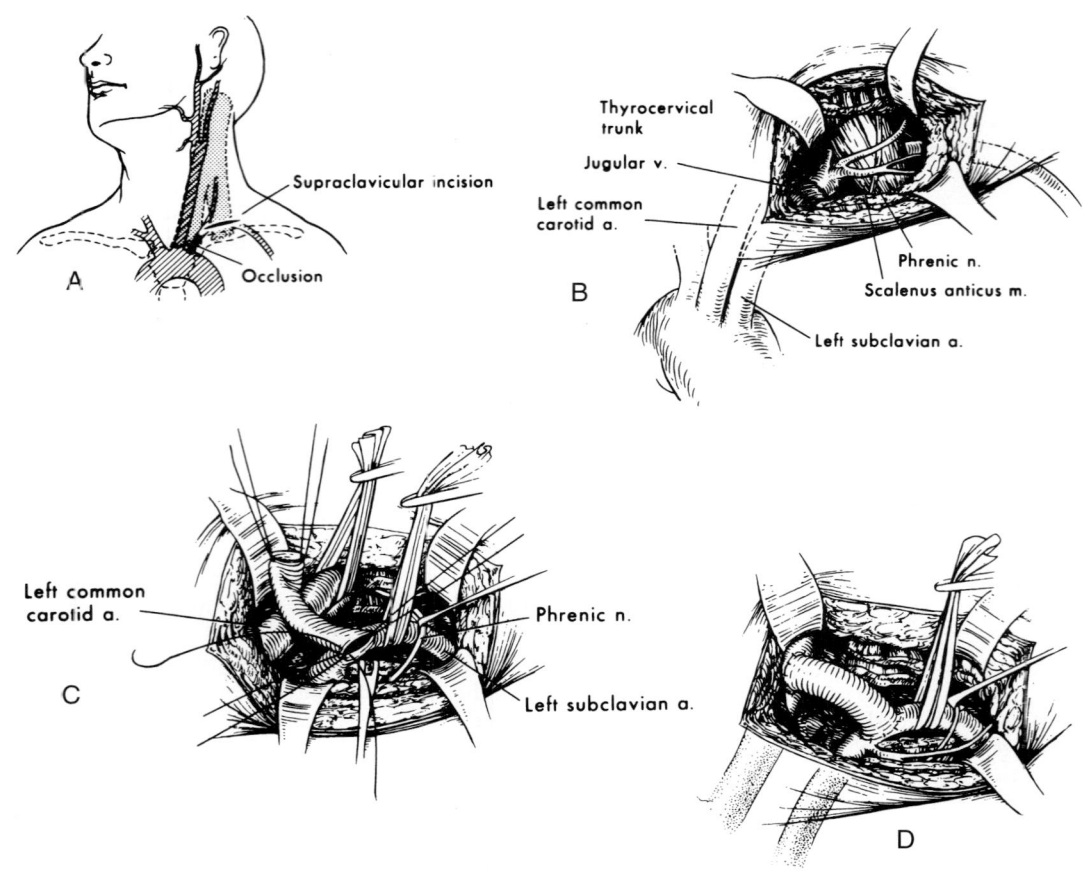

FIGURE 131–28. *A,* Placement of the supraclavicular incision. It is centered over the clavicular head of the sternocleidomastoid muscle. *B,* After division of the clavicular head of the sternocleidomastoid muscle, the relationships of the phrenic nerve, scalenus anticus, and subclavian artery are demonstrated. *C,* After mobilization of the carotid and subclavian arteries, preparation is made for a graft connection. *D,* Completion of the subclavian-carotid artery bypass is demonstrated and points out the close proximity of the two arteries and the short length of graft that is required. (From Moore WS, Malone JM, Goldstone J: Extrathoracic repair of branch occlusions of the aortic arch. Am J Surg 132:249, 1976.)

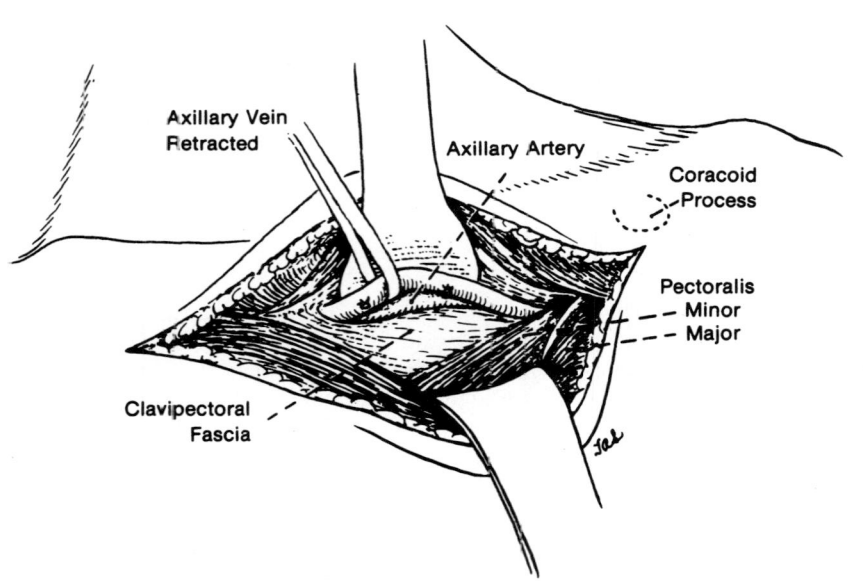

FIGURE 131–29. Surgical exposure of the axillary artery. (From Mozersky DJ, Sumner DS, Barnes RW, Strandness DE: Subclavian revascularization by means of a subcutaneous axillary-axillary graft. Arch Surg 106:20, 1973. Copyright 1973, American Medical Association.)

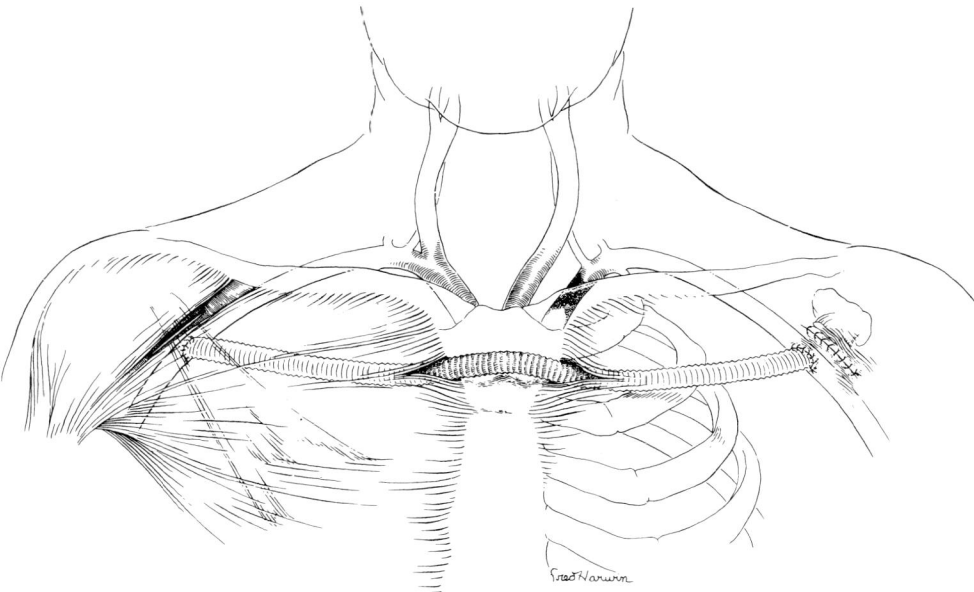

FIGURE 131–30. Diagrammatic representation of placement of the axillary-axillary graft. (From Snider RL, Porter JM, Eidemiller LR: Axillary-axillary artery bypass for the correction of subclavian artery occlusive disease. Ann Surg 180: 888, 1974.)

anastomosed end-to-side to the recipient axillary artery (Fig. 131–30). The advantage of this technique over subclavian-carotid bypass is that temporary interruption of common carotid artery blood flow is avoided; however, two incisions are needed, it utilizes a longer graft, and it is somewhat less cosmetically acceptable because the graft passes subcutaneously over the sternum.

Common Carotid Artery Occlusive Lesions

The primary cause of an occlusion of the common carotid artery is an atheromatous plaque involving its bifurcation with retrograde thrombosis. The thrombus extends down to the innominate artery bifurcation on the right side, or to the level of the aortic arch on the left side. Some common carotid artery occlusions are due to lesions that begin at the level of the aortic arch and produce an antegrade thrombosis. Finally, a few occlusions of the common carotid artery are due to lesions in its mid-portion, with both antegrade and retrograde propagation (Fig. 131–31).

Occlusions produced by retrograde thrombosis can be treated by late retrograde thrombectomy in combination with bifurcation endarterectomy.[120] Occlusions produced by more proximal lesions can be bypassed with a subclavian-to-carotid bypass or a carotid-to-carotid bypass. The authors approach these lesions by initially exposing the carotid bifurcation in the usual manner. A bulky atheromatous plaque at the carotid bifurcation will confirm the mechanism of carotid artery occlusion to be retrograde clot propagation. The internal carotid artery may be kept open by flow between the internal and the external carotid arteries.

If the internal carotid artery is occluded, one can depend on the external carotid artery to be patent beyond the superior thyroid branch. An arteriotomy should be made on the common carotid artery, proximal to the atheromatous lesion. By carefully opening the vessel, one can identify a plane that exists between the organized thrombus and the

intact intima of the common carotid artery. The organized thrombotic cord can be mobilized circumferentially and then divided at a convenient portion within the arteriotomy. A smooth loop endarterectomy stripper can be used to develop the plane between thrombus and intima in a retrograde fashion. Usually, several gentle passes frees the thrombus down to the level of the aortic arch or innominate bifurcation and will allow the thrombotic cord to be pushed out of the arteriotomy by pulsatile blood flow. A clamp is then applied to the common carotid artery, once inflow is established. A standard bifurcation endarterectomy is then performed.

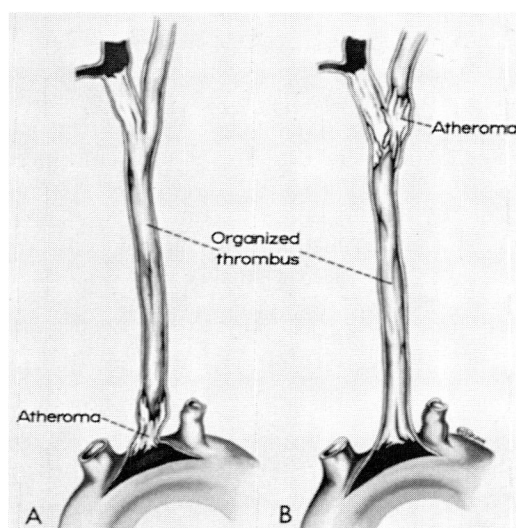

FIGURE 131–31. Occlusion of the common carotid artery can be produced by an atheromatous lesion at the origin of the common carotid artery (A), with antegrade thrombosis to involve the carotid bifurcation, or, more commonly, by an atheromatous lesion at the common carotid bifurcation (B) with retrograde thrombosis down to the level of the aortic arch.

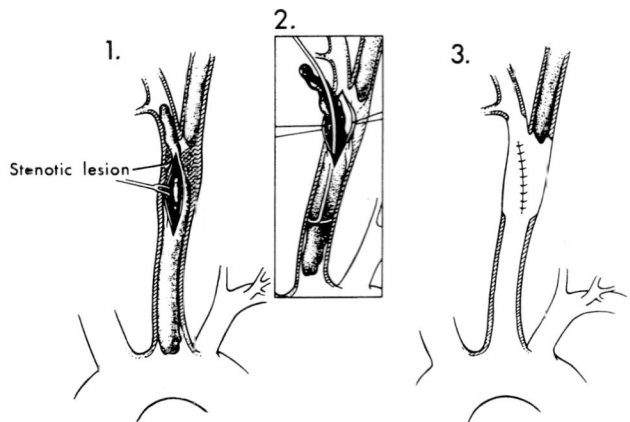

FIGURE 131–32. *Step 1,* An arteriotomy is made in the common carotid artery to begin separating the organized thrombus from the arterial wall. *Step 2,* A flexible wire loop stripper is passed over the organized thrombus in order to free its entire length. *Step 3,* After removal of the occlusive arteriosclerotic plaque at the carotid bifurcation, the outflow of the external carotid artery is restored and the arteriotomy is closed. (From Moore WS, Malone JM, Goldstone MD: Extrathoracic repair of branch occlusions of the aortic arch. Am J Surg 132:249, 1976.)

If the internal carotid artery is occluded, it should be removed in order to avoid a blind stump that may serve as a source of further emboli. The arteriotomy is closed, and flow is restored to the external carotid artery (Fig. 131–32).

If the lesion that produced common carotid artery occlusion is located at a more proximal location or if the thrombotic cord cannot be removed by retrograde thrombectomy, a subclavian-carotid bypass can be performed in a manner identical to that described for a carotid-subclavian bypass. If a lesion is also present in the ipsilateral subclavian artery, a bypass graft in the opposite common carotid artery can be used for inflow.

Occlusive Lesions of the Innominate Artery

Lesions of the innominate artery are best treated directly through a median sternotomy. This can be achieved with either an open endarterectomy or a bypass graft from the ascending aorta to the innominate artery bifurcation.[35]

If the patient's general condition is so poor as to prohibit a median sternotomy, occlusive lesions of the innominate artery can be treated by a carotid-carotid bypass (Fig. 131–33). Alternative methods include left subclavian–to–right carotid bypass, subclavian-subclavian bypass, or axillary-axillary arterial bypass.

Occlusive Lesions of All Three Arch Vessels

It is rare for a patient to present with occlusive lesions involving all three major arch trunks. When this occurs, the patient is at high risk for major complications associated either with the natural history of the disease or with revascularization. The temptation to carry out a total revascularization at one operative procedure should be avoided. In these patients, autoregulatory control of the cerebral circulation has been lost. A total revascularization places the patient at high risk for intracerebral hemorrhage as a result of hyperperfusion syndrome.

In general, it is much better to stage the reconstruction of patients with this complex series of lesions, using either a direct or an extrathoracic approach. A direct approach would consist of an aortic-innominate bypass or innominate endarterectomy. This then establishes reperfusion of the right carotid and right subclavian systems. Subsequent revascularization if required, can be achieved by various combinations of extrathoracic repair, such as carotid-carotid bypass or by axillary-axillary bypass in combination with subclavian-carotid bypass.

If the patient is not a suitable candidate for a mediastinal approach, revascularization can be carried out by means of a femoral-axillary bypass if there is an intact aortofemoral system.[120, 160] A subcutaneous bypass from the femoral artery to the right axillary artery will establish blood flow to the right vertebral and right carotid arteries through retrograde perfusion. If necessary, a subsequent right carotid–to–left carotid artery bypass can be added to complete the extrathoracic revascularization of the arch vessels (Fig. 131–34).

RESULTS

Medical Management

The principles of medical management of cerebrovascular disease are discussed in Chapter 128. Several important points, however, are emphasized here.

Anticoagulation

In patients with atrial fibrillation, anticoagulation has been of benefit in preventing strokes and other thromboembolic events. Five randomized clinical trials have been published documenting this effect.[73] Patients with atrial fibrillation randomized to placebo had an average ischemic stroke rate of 5% per year. In contrast, warfarin anticoagulation reduced the risk of thromboembolism substantially. Such results have revived interest in anticoagulation for the prevention of stroke in patients with extracranial cerebrovascular disease.

Initial clinical studies of oral anticoagulation for preven-

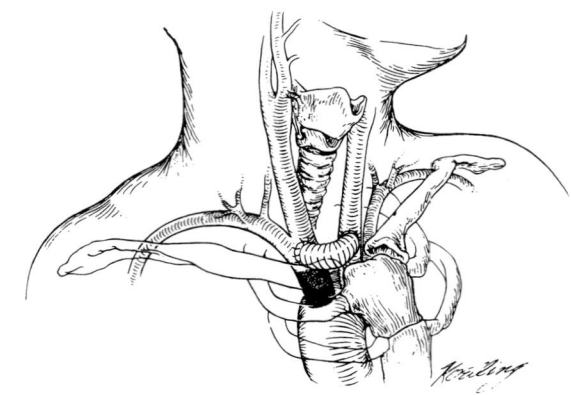

FIGURE 131–33. Bypass graft from the left carotid to the right carotid artery as a means of bypassing an innominate artery occlusion. (From Moore WS, Malone JM, Goldstone J: Extrathoracic repair of branch occlusions of the aortic arch. Am J Surg 132:249, 1976.)

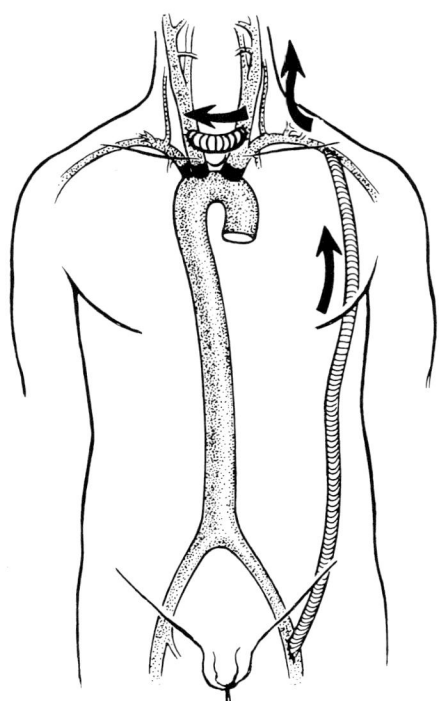

FIGURE 131–34. Artist's concept of subcutaneous bypass grafts from the right femoral to the right axillary arteries in combination with a graft from the right carotid to left carotid arteries. (From Moore WS, Malone JM, Goldstone J: Extrathoracic repair of branch occlusions of the aortic arch. Am J Surg 132:249, 1976.)

tion of anterior circulation strokes carried out in the 1970s showed little benefit. Whisnant and colleagues from the Mayo Clinic performed a retrospective study in 1973 that showed a reduction in strokes in patients treated with oral anticoagulation.[181] The risk of stroke within 5 years in control patients was approximately 40% and was reduced to 20% after anticoagulation. However, the stroke rate in treated patients is still higher than rates reported from both retrospective and prospective series of surgically treated patients.

Conflicting reports have come from Sweden regarding the efficacy of anticoagulation in cerebrovascular disease. Link and associates reported an increased incidence of stroke when anticoagulation therapy was discontinued in patients who presented with carotid territory TIAs; these results prompted a recommendation for long-term treatment with warfarin.[100] In contrast, Torrent and Anderson found more deaths in stroke patients treated with anticoagulants because of serious bleeding complications related to length of treatment, hypertension, and inadequate patient compliance.[174]

Five small prospective randomized trials compared anticoagulation (approximate International Normalized Ratio [INR], 1.7 to 4.0) to antiplatelet agents in patients with TIAs and minor strokes.[6, 25, 64, 138, 142] However, these trials were small, with poorly defined entry and outcome criteria and short follow-up. In part because of the low occurrence rate of strokes, none of these studies showed a clear reduction in the incidence of strokes by anticoagulation, and aggregate results remain inconclusive. Moreover, in two of

these studies,[6, 142] mortality was higher in the anticoagulated group of patients owing to bleeding complications. At present, chronic oral anticoagulation agents should not be the initial treatment for patients with carotid territory cerebrovascular disease.

Antiplatelet Treatment

At least 10 randomized trials have compared aspirin with placebo for prevention of stroke in patients with TIAs and minor and major strokes[1, 20, 26, 60, 61, 150, 159, 163, 178] (Table 131–2). The first of these studies was published in 1977 by Fields and colleagues.[60] This American trial randomized patients with cerebrovascular symptoms to 650 mg of aspirin twice daily versus placebo. Half the patients had operable carotid artery stenoses. After 6 months of follow-up, there was a statistically significant benefit for aspirin treatment when the end-points of death, cerebral or retinal infarction, and TIAs were combined. There was no significant difference in any single end-point, however. A second part of this trial involved aspirin treatment versus placebo in patients who eventually underwent endarterectomy.[61] With these same end-points, there was no significant benefit of aspirin treatment at 24-month follow-up. When non–stroke-related deaths were eliminated, aspirin was beneficial.

The Canadian Cooperative Study of aspirin versus placebo for patients with symptomatic extracranial cerebrovascular disease is perhaps the most widely quoted of the antiplatelet trials in which 585 patients were randomized.[26] About 65% had ischemic events in carotid artery territories, 25% had vertebral-basilar insufficiency, and 10% had both. After 12 to 57 months of follow-up, aspirin reduced the risk of continuing TIAs, stroke, or death by 19%, whereas sulfinpyrazone had no significant benefit. When male patients were analyzed separately, the risk reduction was even higher. In women, there was no significant reduction in stroke or death rates in any of the four treatment regimens.

In 1983, the French AICLA trial was published.[20] Six hundred four patients were randomized to aspirin (990 mg/day), placebo, or aspirin (990 mg/day) plus dipyridamole (225 mg/day). Most of these patients had completed minor strokes, and patients with severe carotid stenoses and women younger than 50 years of age were excluded from the study. End-points were fatal and nonfatal strokes. Both aspirin and aspirin-dipyridamole produced reduction in end-points compared with placebo by about 60% at 3-year follow-up (10.5% versus 18%). Although this trial shows a general benefit of antiplatelet treatment for cerebrovascular disease, its exclusion criteria calls into question its applicability to patients with significant carotid stenoses.

Also in 1983, the Danish Cooperative Study of aspirin in the prevention of stroke in patients with TIAs appeared.[159] Two-hundred-three patients with TIAs were treated with aspirin (n = 101) or placebo (n = 102). After an average follow-up of 25 months, there was no statistically significant difference between groups with respect to the primary end-points of stroke or death (aspirin, 20.8%; placebo, 16.7%). There was a trend toward fewer myocardial infarctions in the aspirin group, but statistical significance was not achieved because of the relatively small sample size.[46]

TABLE 131–2. RANDOMIZED, PROSPECTIVE TRIALS OF ANTIPLATELET AGENTS IN TREATMENT
OF CEREBROVASCULAR DISEASE

TRIAL	YEAR	ENTRY CRITERIA	END POINT (24 MO)	GROUPS	NO. OF PATIENTS	OUTCOME
Canadian Study[26]	1978	TIA	Stroke or death	Sulfinpyrazone, 200 mg qid	115	23%
						p = placebo
				ASA, 325 mg qid	98	15%
						p = .005
				Both	102	8%
						p = ASA alone
				Placebo	91	19%
Fields et al[60]	1976	TIA	Stroke or death	ASA, 650 mg bid	88	19%
				Placebo	90	27%
						p = .18
AICLA (French)*[20]	1983	TIA, stroke	Stroke	ASA, 330 mg tid	198	7%
						p = .05
				ASA (330 mg) + DP (75 mg) tid	202	8%
						p = ASA alone
				Placebo	204	13%
American-Canadian Study[1]	1985	TIA	Stroke or death	ASA, 325 mg qid	442	8.2%
				ASA (325 mg) + DP (75 mg) qid	448	8.6%
						p = n.s.

*Men only.

TIA = transient ischemic attack; DP = dipyridamole; ASA = aspirin; AICLA = Accidents, Ischemiques, Cerebraux Lies a l'Atherosclerose; n.s. = nonsignificant.

The American-Canadian Cooperative Study is one of the largest to examine aspirin treatment of symptomatic cerebrovascular disease.[1] Eight hundred ninety patients were randomized to aspirin (1300 mg/day) alone or aspirin (1300 mg/day) plus dipyridamole (300 mg/day). After 1 to 5 years of follow-up, end-points (stroke, retinal infarction, or death) were nearly identical in the two groups, leading investigators to conclude that the addition of dipyridamole to aspirin was of no supplemental benefit. The cumulative risk of stroke in both groups was about 20% at 4 years, averaging 5% per year.

In 1987, the Swedish Cooperative Study of high-dose aspirin after minor stroke was published.[163] Five hundred five patients were randomized to aspirin (1500 mg/day) or placebo within 3 weeks of stroke. After an average follow-up of 2 years, there was no difference in stroke recurrence rate or death between groups. Moreover, the risk of TIA or myocardial infarction was not reduced in the aspirin group.

Sze and colleagues reported a meta-analysis of these trials shortly after they had all appeared. These investigators concluded that aspirin produced a nonsignificant reduction in stroke rate of 15% compared with placebo.[164] When aspirin was combined with sulfinpyrazone or dipyridamole, a 39% reduction of stroke was observed, but there was a 250% increase in peptic ulcer or gastrointestinal hemorrhage. Men enjoyed a "trend" in stroke reduction with aspirin treatment, regardless of regimen, but a measurable decrease in the incidence of stroke by aspirin treatment alone or in combination could not be established.

Another meta-analysis examined additional studies of aspirin for treatment of patients with peripheral vascular disease, some of which used stroke as an end-point; this report was not limited to review of cerebrovascular trials. This publication reported an overall reduction in nonfatal strokes of 22% and a 25% reduction in the combined end-points of nonfatal stroke, myocardial infarctions, or vascular death.[2] Examination of individual series, however, shows several inconsistencies, which may in part be explained by methodologic differences and insufficient sample sizes producing Type II statistical errors. There appears to be a sex difference in responsiveness to aspirin, with men experiencing more therapeutic benefit than women.[26, 60, 61] This difference may also be artefactual due to the small number of women entered into the trials and their inherent lower event rates. More recent studies have shown equal therapeutic benefits in men and women.[155]

There is ongoing controversy regarding the optimal dose of aspirin for treatment of cerebrovascular disease. As indicated earlier, the large clinical trials all used relatively high doses of aspirin. However, we have shown that high doses of aspirin produce high complication rates (chiefly gastrointestinal bleeding and other gastrotoxicity), and patients assigned to high doses of aspirin have low compliance.[95] Aspirin also probably increases the risk of intracerebral hemorrhage.[111] Variability in the pharmacologic response to aspirin contributes to the debate regarding appropriate dosage. For example, as little as 20 mg of aspirin in some individuals completely acetylates platelet cyclooxygenase and ablates platelet aggregation,[179] whereas even 1300 mg in other individuals may not achieve this effect.[79] The factors inciting platelet aggregation may determine the efficacy of low-dose aspirin.[173] Moreover, in vitro measurement of platelet aggregation in patients taking aspirin may not correlate with prevention of in vivo cerebrovascular events.[79]

Several trials have examined lower doses of aspirin in patients with peripheral vascular and cerebrovascular disease. The Dutch TIA trial randomized 3131 patients with TIA or minor stroke to 283 mg or 30 mg of aspirin daily.[45] Using end-points of vascular death, stroke, or myocardial infarction, there was no difference between the two groups (15.2% in the 283-mg group versus 14.7% in the 30-mg group). Predictably, the incidence of major bleeding complications was low in both groups (3.2% and 2.6%, respectively).

The *Swedish Aspirin Low-Dose Trial* (SALT) showed a significant beneficial effect of a daily aspirin dose of 75 mg/day compared with placebo.[152] This dose of aspirin reduced the risk of vascular death, stroke, or myocardial infarction by 17% versus placebo. The incidence of significant hemorrhagic complications was low in the aspirin group (3%) but significantly higher than the placebo group (1.3%). Although low-dose aspirin is much safer than high-dose aspirin, bleeding complications are not eliminated.

The *United Kingdom-Transient Ischemic Attack* (UK-TIA) study compared medium-dose aspirin (300 mg/day) to high-dose aspirin (1200 mg/day).[178] The two doses were equally effective for prevention of strokes. High-dose aspirin was associated with a 5% risk of major bleeding complications, compared with 3% for the low-dose aspirin. Most American physicians seem to favor medium-dose aspirin (325 mg/day) for secondary stroke prevention, whereas Canadians endorse high-dose (>1000 mg/day) and Europeans advocate low-dose aspirin (30 to 75 mg/day).

Ticlopidine hydrochloride is a potent antiplatelet agent that does not inhibit the thromboxane A_2 pathway for platelet aggregation like aspirin does, nor does it affect prostacyclin production by vascular endothelium. Instead, it inhibits the adenosine diphosphate (ADP) pathway in platelet aggregation and adhesion.[113] It has no analgesic characteristics.[157] Maximal antiplatelet effect occurs after 5 days of treatment, and normal platelet activity returns 4 to 8 days after discontinuation.[101] Serious side effects are associated with administration of ticlopidine, including a 2.4% incidence of neutropenia, a 20% incidence of diarrhea, and a 10% incidence of rash.[66, 76]

Most cases of ticlopidine-induced neutropenia occur during the first 3 months of therapy; after the first 3 months of treatment, the incidences of mild and moderate neutropenia are no different for ticlopidine, aspirin, and placebo. It is impossible to predict which patients will develop neutropenia, so white blood cell differential counts must be performed every 2 weeks beginning from the second week to the end of the third month of therapy.[157] In contrast to ticlopidine, clopidogrel, which has an identical mechanism of action, does not produce neutropenia.[27]

Three large clinical trials have evaluated ticlopidine and clopidogrel for secondary prevention of stroke and vascular events (Table 131–3).[27, 66, 75] In the *Ticlopidine Aspirin Stroke Study* (TASS), 3069 patients with TIAs or minor strokes were randomized to ticlopidine or aspirin.[75] After an average follow-up of 3 years, 13% of patients taking aspirin (1300 mg/day) had strokes versus 10% of patients taking ticlopidine (500 mg/day). This results in a relative risk reduction of 21%, but the absolute reduction in risk of stroke is only 1% per year with ticlopidine therapy compared with aspirin therapy.[148] These data are confounded by including "aspirin failures" (i.e, patients whose initial qualifying event occurred while they were taking aspirin) in the ticlopidine group, thus potentially biasing the study against aspirin. In addition, a significantly elevated level of cholesterol was noted in patients taking ticlopidine.

In the *Canadian-American Ticlopidine Study* (CATS), patients with minor thromboembolic strokes were randomized to 250 mg of ticlopidine twice a day (n = 525) or placebo (n = 528) and followed for an average of 2 years.[66] Ticlopidine produced a relative risk of reduction for recurrent stroke of 30%; strokes occurred at a rate of 15.3% per year in the placebo group versus 10.8% per year in the ticlopidine group. The drug was equally effective in men and women. Severe neutropenia occurred in 4 patients taking ticlopidine (0.8%) and one patient taking placebo (0.2%).

Results of a randomized, blinded trial of *Clopidogrel* (75 mg once daily) *versus Aspirin* (325 mg once daily) in *Patients at Risk for Ischemic Events* (CAPRIE) were published in 1996.[27] This extremely large multicenter trial enrolled 19,185 patients with more than 6300 in clinical subgroups of those with atherosclerotic vascular disease manifested as either recent ischemic stroke, recent myocardial infarction, or symptomatic peripheral arterial disease. Patients were studied 1 to 3 years, with a mean follow-up of 1.9 years. In the entire group, ischemic stroke, myocardial infarction, or vascular death occurred in 939 patients taking clopidogrel (17,636 patient-years) and in 1021 patients taking aspirin (17,519 patient-years), for a relative risk reduction of 8.7% (p = .04).

In the subgroup of patients who were enrolled because they had suffered strokes, 6054 were assigned to aspirin treatment, and 5979 were assigned to clopidogrel. There were 315 versus 338 fatal and nonfatal recurrent strokes in

TABLE 131–3. RANDOMIZED, PROSPECTIVE TRIALS OF THIENOPYRIDINE DERIVATIVES IN THE TREATMENT OF CEREBROVASCULAR ISCHEMIC EVENTS

TRIAL	ENTRY CRITERIA	END-POINT (24 mo)	GROUPS	NO. OF PATIENTS	OUTCOME
Canadian-American Ticlopidine Study (CATS)[66]	Stroke	Stroke, MI, death	ASA (325 mg) + DP (75 mg) qid	448	8.6% p = n.s.
			Ticlopidine, 250 mg bid	525	18%
			Placebo	528	25% p = .006
TASS[75]	TIA, stroke	Stroke or death	Ticlopidine, 250 mg bid	1515	10%
			ASA, 650 mg bid	1519	12% p = .048
Clopidogrel versus Aspirin for the Prevention of Ischemic Events (CAPRIE)[27]	Stroke, MI, PVD	Stroke, MI Amputation Death	Clopidogrel, 75 mg qd	17636	10.6%
			ASA, 325 mg qd	17519	11.2% p = .043

DP = dipyridamole; ASA = aspirin; TIA = transient ischemic attack; MI = myocardial infarction; PVD = peripheral vascular disease; n.s. = nonsignificant.

the clopidogrel (n = 6054) versus aspirin (n = 5979) groups, respectively, for a relative risk reduction of 7.3% ($p = .26$). It is important to note that although the adverse side effects or rash or diarrhea were slightly more common in the clopidogrel group, gastrointestinal symptoms and bleeding and abnormal liver function studies occurred more commonly in patients taking aspirin. Moreover, there was no difference in major bleeding, intracranial hemorrhage, or neutropenia between the treatment groups. Thus, it appears that clopidogrel is at least as safe as medium-dose aspirin and is safer than ticlopidine, but the indications for preferential use of clopidogrel instead of aspirin are unclear at present—at least for patients with symptomatic cerebrovascular disease.

A combination of low-dose aspirin and ticlopidine has been reported in a small study.[177] Patients with symptomatic cerebrovascular disease were randomized to combination therapy (aspirin 81 mg/day plus ticlopidine 100 mg/day), medium-dose aspirin 300 mg/day), or placebo. Platelet aggregation by ADP, arachidonate, and platelet-activating factor (PAF) was markedly inhibited by combination therapy, and in vivo platelet activation was decreased, as evidenced by lowered plasma concentrations of beta-thromboglobulin and platelet factor IV (released by aggregating platelets). Bleeding time was significantly increased by combination therapy compared with the other groups. However, such profound platelet inhibition potentially could result in an increase in the risk of hemorrhagic complications.[37] The author (W.C.K.) has had anecdotal experience operating on patients who were taking both aspirin and ticlopidine preoperatively, and operative blood loss seemed substantially greater than in patients taking only aspirin or ticlopidine alone.

Surgical Management

Nonrandomized Studies of Carotid Endarterectomy

Symptomatic and Asymptomatic Carotid Artery Stenosis

Hertzer has nicely summarized the multitude of reports from individual and cooperative studies of carotid endarterectomy for various indications in Chapter 136. Tables 136-1, 136-3, 136-5, and 136-6 relate the operative morbidity and mortality described in these reports. It is readily apparent that results vary, but such nonrandomized studies provided important data to develop the hypothesis that underlies the prospective randomized trials of carotid endarterectomy for both symptomatic and asymptomatic carotid artery stenosis—namely, that this procedure is a safe and effective treatment for these disorders.

Analysis of the outcomes of carotid endarterectomy, as performed in nonrandomized studies, is crucial for the determination of the appropriateness of operation in any given institution or by any given surgeon. The importance of low perioperative morbidity and mortality for carotid endarterectomy cannot be overemphasized. For example, using retrospective chart reviews, Easton and Sherman reported surgical morbidity and mortality of 21% in community hospitals in Springfield, Illinois.[47] This unacceptably high rate is often quoted by opponents of surgical interven-

tion. Indeed, when 1 of every 5 patients undergoing carotid endarterectomy has an adverse outcome, the operation cannot be recommended. In contrast, operative morbidity and mortality rates as low as 0.1% have been reported (see Tables 136-3 and 136-5). Such differences in adverse outcomes underscore the importance of internal review to establish local morbidity and mortality rates. An updated review of the Springfield, Illinois, experience with carotid endarterectomy in 1983 revealed a reduction in stroke and death rate to 5%.[117]

Late follow-up provided by nonrandomized reports has confirmed that carotid endarterectomy is a durable procedure. One of the leaders in cerebrovascular surgery, Dr. J. E. Thompson, and colleagues, reviewed their own results of carotid endarterectomies in 592 patients followed for up to 13 years.[170] Operative mortality for the last 476 consecutive operations was 1.47%, and stroke rate was 2.7%. Overall, late mortality was 30%; half of deaths were due to cardiac disease, and only 3.9% occurred from stroke. Of those patients who had a preoperative stroke as an indication for carotid endarterectomy, 88.9% were normal or improved at follow-up. Of those patients who had TIAs preoperatively, 81% had no further attacks and only 7 patients (3.3%) eventually experienced permanent deficits. Two of these 7 patients suffered strokes on the side contralateral to the carotid endarterectomy.

In a later report, Thompson and colleagues described long-term results in 132 patients undergoing 167 carotid endarterectomies for asymptomatic carotid stenoses.[172] There were no perioperative deaths, and permanent neurologic deficits occurred in only two patients (1.2%). At a mean follow-up of 55 months, 90.9% of the patients remained asymptomatic. Six patients (4.5%) had TIAs—five from the unoperated side. Strokes occurred in 4.6%. Although not truly a "control" group (because many patients were denied surgery because of prohibitive operative risk and other factors), 1328 contemporaneous patients had asymptomatic stenoses and did not undergo carotid endarterectomy. Only 55.8% remained asymptomatic; 26.8% had TIAs; and 17.4% suffered strokes.

A Belgian series from 1980 reported late outcomes in 141 patients followed for up to 16 years after carotid endarterectomy.[154] Forty-three patients operated on for asymptomatic carotid stenoses were followed for an average of 5.4 years; there were no deaths and 1 stroke referable to the contralateral carotid artery. Twenty-five patients presented with symptomatic stenoses and contralateral carotid occlusions; in mean follow-up of 7.3 years, only two patients had strokes (8%). Of 70 symptomatic patients without contralateral occlusions, only 6 had strokes, for an overall rate of 8.6%. A similar stroke rate of less than 2% per year was reported by Field in a series of 400 endarterectomies.[58]

Riles and associates compared 146 patients who underwent unilateral carotid endarterectomy (with nonstenotic contralateral carotid arteries) with 86 patients who underwent bilateral carotid endarterectomy.[144] Both groups were followed for a mean of 4.3 years. No significant differences existed between groups with respect to age, gender, neurologic status, or associated illnesses, and all patients were treated with aspirin postoperatively. Seventeen new strokes occurred in the first group, of which only six involved the hemisphere ipsilateral to the carotid endarterectomy. In the second group, there were four new strokes. The cumulative stroke rates at 5 years by life-table analysis were 17.6% and 5.6%, respectively ($p < .05$).

Hertzer and Arison reported the Cleveland Clinic experience with 329 patients followed a minimum of 10 years after carotid endarterectomy.[80] In 126 patients who underwent carotid endarterectomy for asymptomatic stenoses, the incidence of stroke in the ipsilateral cerebral hemisphere was 9%, less than 1% per year. Two hundred three patients operated on for symptomatic carotid artery stenoses had a late ipsilateral stroke incidence of 6%. The overall ipsilateral stroke risk was 10% at 10 years. Late strokes were most common among hypertensive patients (31%), patients whose indication for carotid endarterectomy was stroke (31%), and patients with uncorrected contralateral stenosis (42%). Patients with uncorrected contralateral stenosis had a contralateral late stroke incidence of 36%, compared with 8% in patients who underwent elective staged bilateral carotid endarterectomies.

The Cleveland Clinic group also provided useful retrospective data regarding the late risk of stroke with respect to degree of stenosis.[82, 83] Two hundred eleven patients presented with symptomatic carotid artery stenosis; 126 were treated nonoperatively, and 85 underwent carotid endarterectomy. In patients with greater than 70% carotid artery stenosis treated medically, the stroke rate was 31% at 5 years, compared with 7% in similar patients treated surgically.[83] Surgically treated patients with 50% stenosis also enjoyed improved outcomes compared with medically treated patients (5-year stroke rate of 3% versus 28%, respectively). Of 290 asymptomatic patients, 195 were treated expectantly and 95 underwent carotid endarterectomy.[82] Five-year stroke incidence was 15% in the expectant group and 14% in the surgical group. However, patients with greater than 70% stenosis had a 24% to 33% 5-year stroke risk with nonoperative treatment versus 7% to 12% for those having prophylactic endarterectomies. Although neither of these studies was prospective or randomized, the results are consistent with findings from cooperative trials inspired by such descriptive data.

Completed Strokes

The natural history of patients with completed stroke and good neurologic recovery justifies therapeutic carotid endarterectomy, with most reports citing an annual risk of recurrent stroke between 6% and 12%. Carotid endarterectomy is beneficial in these patients. Rubin and colleagues reported no ipsilateral strokes in 95 patients studied from 6 to 72 months after surgery for completed strokes.[149] Operative morbidity and mortality was 2.7%; annual cumulative stroke risk was thus 0.64%. Not all reports have corroborated such favorable results, however. For example, Bardin and coworkers reported a cumulative stroke rate of 20% at 5 years in 127 patients who underwent carotid endarterectomy for minor strokes.[7] Perioperative morbidity and mortality was 7%. Almost one third of patients died or suffered a stroke as a result of or in spite of carotid endarterectomy.

The indication and timing of carotid endarterectomy for acute stroke remain controversial. Bruetman and colleagues[24a] first described disastrous results after carotid end-

arterectomy for acute stroke, describing autopsy findings of intracerebral hemorrhage with blood in the subarachnoid space and ventricles. Wylie and coworkers corroborated these adverse outcomes in an independent study 1 year later.[188] They reported nine patients operated on for acute stroke; catastrophic hemorrhages occurred in five of these patients (56%), three of whom had attempted revascularization after complete carotid artery occlusions.

In 1969, Rob described a 29% perioperative mortality rate following revascularization after carotid occlusions; only 21% of operated patients were benefited by surgery.[145] The mortality rate of operation during the acute phase of cerebral infarction was 42% in the Joint Study for Extracranial Arterial Disease, the first prospective multicenter study of carotid endarterectomy.[12, 17] Other investigators have noted similar findings.[68, 171] Of note, many of the reported unfavorable results occurred in patients who presented with profound neurologic deficits and diminished consciousness, and many operations of acutely occluded arteries were performed in patients with neurologic deficits who had diminished consciousness. In addition, many operations for acutely occluded arteries were performed after a prolonged interval. Nevertheless, dismal consequences after carotid endarterectomy for acute strokes led most authorities to recommend delaying operative intervention for at least 30 days or more.[59, 68, 137, 147]

The reasons for "conversion of a white to red infarction" (i.e., hemorrhage occurring in a bland thrombotic cerebral infarction) are multifactorial. Probably the most important principle is restoration of normotensive blood flow to vessels that have lost the ability to autoregulate.[159] This vasomotor paralysis with maximal vasodilatation regardless of perfusion pressures extends to vessels supplying peri-infarct tissue in the "ischemic penumbra."[70, 99] When the ability for blood vessels to autoregulate is lost, blood flow becomes passively dependent on blood pressure.[126] The combination of hypertension, which often accompanies acute stroke, and loss of autoregulation produces elevated perfusion pressures that are capable of precipitating small vessel disruption and hemorrhage both within and adjacent to the area of infarction. Several experimental animal studies support this hypothesis.[74, 116]

Currently, neither computed tomography (CT) nor magnetic resonance imaging (MRI) reliably distinguishes areas of reversible ischemia (penumbra) and irreversible brain cell death (infarction). Wing and associates reported that CT brain scan indicates loss of integrity of the blood-brain barrier, suggesting that the reperfusion produced by carotid endarterectomy may be associated with increased risk of hemorrhage transformation.[186] When the CT brain scans in patients did not show enhancement after strokes, Ricotta and colleagues found that only one (6%) of 17 patients deteriorated neurologically after carotid endarterectomy, whereas 15 of 17 (88%) improved.[143] In contrast, when the CT scan remained enhancing, only five (50%) patients improved, whereas four (40%) deteriorated. Similar findings were reported by the Cleveland Clinic group.[102]

Postponing operation until CT scans "normalize" has disadvantages, however. Dosick and colleagues found that waiting 4 to 6 weeks for observation after acute stroke resulted in a 21% incidence of recurrent stroke.[44] Based on these findings, these investigators proceeded directly to surgery (within 2 weeks of onset) in patients with acute strokes who had no bleeding, as shown on CT scans. This strategy resulted in no perioperative morbidity and mortality in 110 patients. Whitney and associates reported similar results in 28 patients who presented with small, fixed neurologic deficits undergoing endarterectomy an average of 11 days from onset of symptoms.[183] Only one postoperative death and no new neurologic deficits occurred in this small group of patients. Other studies have confirmed the relative safety of early endarterectomy after small, fixed deficits, but the ideal algorithm remains unsettled because reported series are small and nonrandomized.[124, 182]

Stroke-in-Evolution

Stroke-in-evolution is a variety of acute stroke in which the initial deficit is followed by varying degrees of resolution and deterioration. An Ad Hoc Committee to the Joint Council of the North American Chapter of the International Society for Cardiovascular Surgery defined this entity as a variation of acute stroke in which neurologic changes begin with "one level of deficit and in a progressive or stuttering fashion the deficit worsens."[124] After excluding intracranial hemorrhage by CT scans, heparin anticoagulation should be initiated, but despite medical management, the prognosis is poor.

Improved results have been reported in patients presenting with stroke-in-evolution treated surgically.[69, 115] Mentzer and associates reported 17 patients with stroke-in-evolution who underwent emergency carotid endarterectomy.[115] Seventy per cent had complete recovery, 24% remained unchanged, and none were worse after carotid endarterectomy.[115] One patient died, for an overall mortality rate of 6%. This compared favorably with a parallel group of 20 patients with stroke-in-evolution treated medically. Mortality in the medical group was 15% with 55% of the remaining patients having permanent moderate-to-severe neurologic deficits. In a review of the literature, 55% of patients having emergency carotid endarterectomy for stroke-in-evolution showed improvement, 25% showed no change, and 10% were worse after surgery.[124] Average mortality was about 10%.

Patients presenting with stroke-in-evolution should undergo emergency CT scans to exclude intracranial bleeding. After a high-risk carotid lesion has been identified in a patient with stroke-in-evolution or crescendo TIAs, well-performed carotid endarterectomy carries the best prognosis for neurologic recovery. However, the patient and the family must understand that the procedure has the highest mortality and morbidity for all carotid endarterectomy indications, and some patients' neurologic conditions will worsen in the perioperative period.

External Carotid Artery Revascularization

Surgical revascularization of the external carotid artery (ECA) is indicated in rare patients. The importance of the ECA as a major collateral pathway to the cerebral circulation has been well demonstrated, particularly in the presence of an ipsilateral internal carotid artery occlusion.[153, 190] Neurologic symptoms may arise owing to a stenosis at the origin of the ECA either from emboli or hemodynamic compromise. Emboli may also originate from the cul-de-sac created by an occluded internal stump.

The Cleveland Clinic group reported 42 ECA endarterectomies in 37 patients.[136] Temporary shunting and patch angioplasty were utilized in two thirds of the cases. Thirty procedures were primary ECA reconstructions (limited operations) and 12 were reoperations or were combined with subclavian or intracranial bypass (extended operations). There were significant differences in outcomes between these two groups. Four patients (33%) in the extended operations group suffered perioperative ipsilateral hemispheric strokes, versus none in the limited operations group. Three late strokes, one ipsilateral and two contralateral at 1, 16, and 33 months, respectively, occurred after ECA reconstruction. Five additional patients required further therapy (anticoagulation, reoperation, or bypass) for recurrent symptoms. Appropriately, the authors urged caution and careful patient selection for ECA revascularization.

Halstuk and colleagues analyzed the outcomes of 36 patients undergoing ECA revascularization, noting a 13.8% stroke rate and a 2.7% mortality rate.[71] In addition, 14.2% of patients suffered a late stroke on follow-up. The combination of bilateral carotid occlusion and preoperative fixed neurologic deficit was found to predict the highest perioperative morbidity (37%). In a literature review in this paper, the authors described perioperative neurologic morbidity of 14.3% in 126 reported patients.

In another literature review, Gertler and Cambria found 23 series reporting cases in which ECA reconstruction was undertaken.[67] Two hundred eighteen ECA revascularizations were performed in the 23 series. Of the patients, 83% enjoyed resolution of symptoms, with another 7% showing improvement. Perioperative mortality was 3%, with a 5% perioperative neurologic morbidity. Increased perioperative adverse outcomes were associated with a severely diseased contralateral carotid artery and in symptomatic patients with internal carotid artery occlusion. The best results were obtained when surgery was performed to relieve specific hemispheric or retinal symptoms, as opposed to nonspecific neurologic complaints or previous stroke. Vertebral artery occlusive disease did not affect outcome.

ECA reconstruction should be reserved for symptomatic patients with significant orificial ECA stenoses whose intracerebral circulation can be demonstrated by ipsilateral injection of contrast on arteriogram, thus providing a potential conduit for emboli or suitable anatomy for cerebral hemodynamic compromise. The presence of a fixed neurologic deficit, bilateral internal carotid artery occlusion, or severe intracranial arterial disease increases the morbidity of ECA revascularization, and medical therapy may be warranted in these cases.

RANDOMIZED STUDIES OF CAROTID ENDARTERECTOMY

Symptomatic Carotid Artery Stenosis

The first prospective randomized multicenter study of surgical versus medical treatment for extracranial carotid occlusive disease began in 1959.[12] The Joint Study of Extracranial Arterial Occlusion randomized 1225 patients, with 621 having carotid endarterectomy and 604 treated with "best medical therapy" (not necessarily including antiplatelet agents). In many but not all instances, best medical therapy included anticoagulation. The groups were well matched with respect to symptoms, demographics, associated diseases, and angiographic patterns of disease, but mortality rates, according to the patient's clinical presentation and the angiographic pattern of disease, revealed significant differences.

At 43 months of follow-up, the survival rate was above 80% in the surgical group, but only 50% in the medical group for patients who had unilateral carotid artery stenosis and no other surgically accessible lesion. In 316 patients who had hemispheric TIAs without residual deficit as an indication for entrance into the study (including patients with unilateral stenosis, bilateral stenosis, and unilateral stenosis with contralateral occlusion), the incidence of subsequent TIAs or strokes was lower in the surgical group. Moreover, most adverse neurologic events occurred in the ipsilateral hemisphere in medical patients and the contralateral hemisphere in surgical patients. These differences were all statistically significant. By today's standards, the perioperative neurologic morbidity and mortality were strikingly high at 8%. Nevertheless, this randomized study confirmed the beneficial effects of carotid endarterectomy described in nonrandomized series. The popularity of carotid endarterectomy rose so much that the number of these procedures performed in non-Veterans Hospitals increased from 15,000 in 1971 to 107,000 in 1985.[141]

Despite the overwhelming preponderance of evidence, mostly from nonrandomized studies as described earlier, that carotid endarterectomy is safe and effective therapy for symptomatic carotid artery stenosis, reports such as the one by Easton and Sherman[47] from Springfield, Illinois, and the failure of extracranial to intracranial bypasses to improve outcomes in symptomatic patients with complete carotid occlusions[48] led to an abundance of negative publicity concerning carotid endarterectomy in the late 1980s. In addition to alarm over high complication rates in community hospitals and suspected lack of efficacy, there was concern over indications for surgery and marked regional variations in the number of carotid endarterectomies performed.[21] Numerous editorials appeared appealing for more restrained treatment of carotid artery stenosis and for development of randomized clinical trials to resolve the question.[11, 30]

Three clinical trials of carotid endarterectomy in symptomatic patients have now been partially or fully completed; results were published in 1991.[55, 109, 135] These investigations are (1) The North American Symptomatic Carotid Endarterectomy Trial (NASCET), (2) The European Carotid Surgery Trial (ECST), and (3) The Department of Veterans Affairs Symptomatic Trial (VAST). The trial design and methods differed among studies. One of the shortcomings of all three trials is that they used nonstandardized ultrasound examinations and relied primarily on arteriographic findings to determine patient eligibility and degree of stenosis. In addition, the two largest studies used different methods of determining eligibility and measuring degree of carotid stenosis by arteriogram (see Chapter 128, Fig. 128–1). The formula for calculating per cent stenosis is

$$(1 - S/D) \times 100$$

where S is the diameter of the stenosis at the narrowest part of the artery and D is the diameter of the "normal artery."

In NASCET and VAST, the distal internal carotid artery just beyond the stenosis was used as the "denominator (D)" (i.e., the normal-sized artery) for determination of per cent stenosis; in ECST, determination of per cent stenosis was based on estimation of the diameter of the normal carotid bulb as the "denominator (D)." Thus, a lesion that NASCET measured as 70% was about 85% in ECST. A 50% stenosis in NASCET was 70% to 75% in ECST.

North American Symptomatic Carotid Endarterectomy Trial

NASCET was conducted at 50 clinical centers throughout the United States and Canada, stratifying patients into 30% to 69% carotid stenosis and 70% to 99% stenosis.[135] The surgical results of the vascular surgeons or neurosurgeons in NASCET were reviewed by the Surgical Committee before each center was certified as acceptable, and morbidity and mortality rates had to be 5% or less. Patients were eligible for randomization who had TIAs or minor strokes within 3 months of entry into the study. Aspirin (1300 mg/day or less if poorly tolerated) was the primary medical therapy, along with control of hypertension, hyperlipidemia, and diabetes. Aspirin was also given to surgical patients; the details of operative intervention were not standardized.

Follow-up protocol was rigorous. In addition to determinations by surgeons in the immediate postoperative period and at 30 days, an independent neurologic evaluation was performed by participating neurologists at 30 days, every 3 months for the first year, and every 4 months in ensuing years. Duplex ultrasonography was performed 1 month postoperatively and after neurologic symptoms. Repeat arteriograms were obtained if clinically indicated.

In the 70% to 99% carotid stenosis subset, between January, 1988, and February, 1991, 659 patients were randomized: 328 in the surgical group and 331 in the medical group. Table 131–4 describes the baseline characteristics of the two groups. In February, 1991, after only 18 months of mean follow-up, The Data and Safety Monitoring Board

TABLE 131–4. BASELINE CHARACTERISTICS OF THE NASCET STUDY

	MEDICAL (n = 331)	SURGICAL (n = 328)
Median age (years)	66	65
Sex		
Male	69%	68%
Female	31%	32%
Race		
White	89%	93%
Black	4%	2%
Other	7%	5%
Antithrombotic medications	85%	85%
TIA at entry	69%	67%
Stroke at entry	31%	33%
Ipsilateral stenosis		
70%–79%	43%	40%
80%–89%	33%	38%
90%–99%	24%	22%
Contralateral 70%–99% stenosis	9%	8%

NASCET = North American Symptomatic Carotid Endarterectomy Trial; TIA = transient ischemic attack.

TABLE 131–5. FIRST ADVERSE EVENTS FOR THE PATIENTS IN THE TWO ARMS OF THE NASCET STUDY AT TWO YEARS OF FOLLOW-UP

EVENT	Events (Event Rate, %)[a]		Absolute Difference (% ± SE)	Relative Risk Reduction
	Medical Patients (n = 331)	Surgical Patients (n = 328)		
Any ipsilateral stroke	61 (26)	26 (9)	17 ± 3.5[b]	65%
Any stroke	64 (27.6)	34 (12.6)	15 ± 3.8[b]	54%
Any stroke or death	73 (32.3)	41 (15.8)	16.5 ± 4.2[b]	51%
Major or fatal ipsilateral stroke	29 (13.1)	8 (2.5)	10.6 ± 2.6[b]	81%
Any major or fatal stroke	29 (13.1)	10 (3.7)	9.4 ± 2.7[b]	72%
Any major stroke or death	38 (18.1)	19 (8.0)	10.1 ± 3.5[c]	56%

[a]Event rates were determined by Kaplan-Meier estimates for survival. "Death" refers to mortality from all causes. All events from the time of randomization to the first 30 days in the surgical group and 32 days in the medical group are included, along with subsequent events defining treatment failure.
[b]$p < .001$ for the comparison of the treatment groups.
[c]$p < .01$ for the comparison of the treatment groups.
NASCET = North American Symptomatic Carotid Endarterectomy Trial.

prematurely stopped the enrollment of patients with 70% to 99% stenoses by invoking the predetermined stopping rule and the National Institutes of Health issued a Clinical Alert informing physicians of the results. Patients in the medical arm of this subset of the study were advised to undergo carotid endarterectomy. Altogether, these were highly unusual measures that emphasized the importance of findings.

Table 131–5 summarizes the results for patients in both NASCET groups.[135] The total adverse event rate for surgical patients was 5.8% during the first 30 days, compared with 3.3% in medically treated patients. The 30-day major stroke and death event rates were 2.1% and 0.9% in the surgical and medical groups, respectively. The cumulative risk of an ipsilateral stroke was 9% for surgically treated patients and 26% in those randomized to medical therapy, which represented an absolute risk reduction of 17% and a relative risk reduction of 65% ($p < .001$). The number of patients-needed-to-treat to prevent stroke in 2 years is 6. The risk of a major or fatal ipsilateral stroke in the surgical group was 2.5% versus 13.1% in the medical group, representing a relative risk reduction of 81% ($p < .001$). For patients who did not die or have a major stroke within 30 days of randomization, the 2-year stroke risk was 1.6% versus 12.2% in surgically versus medically treated patients, respectively.

The degree of stenosis correlated profoundly with the risk of stroke in NASCET. In a subset analysis, Morgenstern and colleagues showed progressively increasing surgical benefit in the eighth, ninth, and tenth deciles.[127] The results of this analysis are portrayed in Figure 131–35. Symptomatic patients with 90% to 94% stenoses have the greatest medical risk and the most surgical benefit. Less difference between medical and surgical treatment (only 4.4% at 1 year in those with a "string sign") is seen in patients with near-occlusion, presumably because excellent collateral development was relatively protective, and the conduit for large emboli is substantially narrowed (Fig. 131–36).

NASCET continued to randomize symptomatic patients with less than 70% carotid stenosis until December, 1996. All patients were then followed for 1 additional year. The results of this phase of the trial have been presented at the annual meeting of the American Heart Association, but publication of the manuscript is in press. In brief, there was

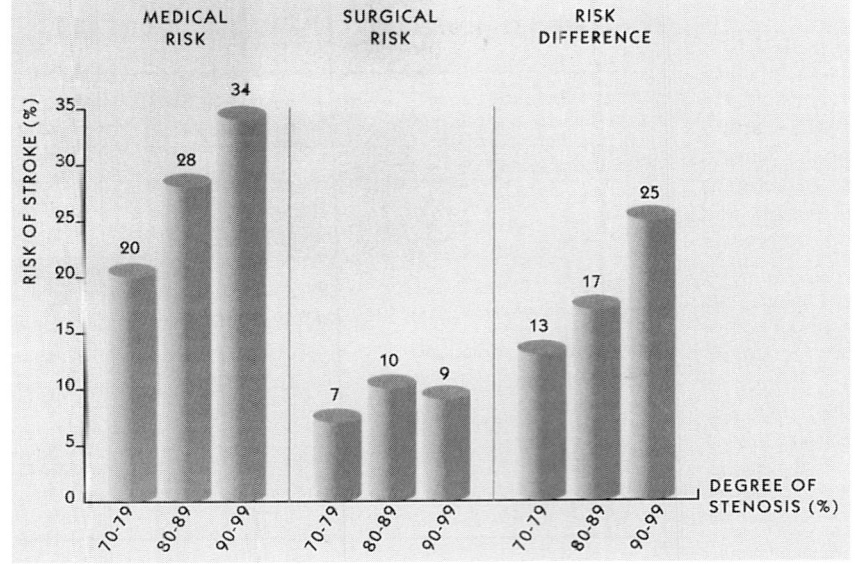

FIGURE 131–35. Estimates of risk of stroke at 2 years by degree of stenosis by deciles, as determined by Kaplan-Meier statistics from the North American Symptomatic Carotid Endarterectomy Trial (NASCET). The risk of stroke is similar for all deciles of stenosis in surgically treated patients; in contrast, the risk of stroke increases with deciles in medically treated patients. (From Barnett HJM, Meldrum HE, Elaiasziw M: Lessons from the symptomatic trials for the management of asymptomatic disease. In Caplan LR, Shifrin EG, Nicolaides AN, Moore WAS (eds): Cerebrovascular Ischaemia Investigation and Management. London, Med-Orion Publishing Company, 1996, p 385.)

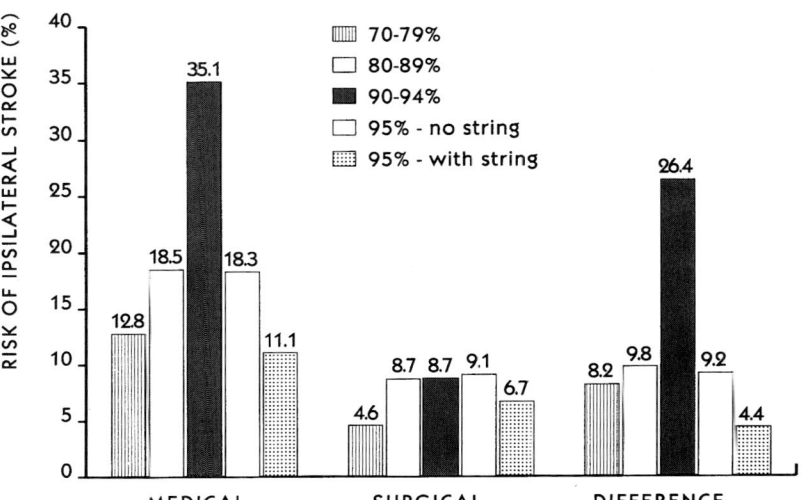

FIGURE 131–36. Estimates of ipsilateral stroke at 1 year by degree of stenosis according to Kaplan-Meier statistical analysis of NASCET data. 95% = near-occlusion. (From Morgenstern LB, Fox AJ, Sharpe BL, et al: The risks and benefits of carotid endarterectomy in patients with near-occlusion of the carotid artery. Neurology 48:911, 1997.)

definite but moderate benefit for carotid endarterectomy in symptomatic patients in this subset.[9] Although carotid endarterectomy was not associated with a reduction in major or fatal stroke, there was a statistically significant 39% relative risk reduction for any stroke in surgically treated patients with 50% to 69% carotid stenoses. The number-needed-to-treat to prevent 1 stroke in 5 years was 15 patients. There appeared to be no significant benefit of carotid endarterectomy in those with less than 50% stenoses. With respect to long-term survival, there was no significant benefit in (1) women or (2) those who presented with retinal symptoms compared with those with hemispheric events. There was little benefit in patients who were enrolled for hemispheric TIAs versus those with completed minor strokes.

Once again, it is important to emphasize that the NASCET results were not based on duplex ultrasound findings. NASCET's ultrasound/arteriography findings were subject to an error of approximately 15%.[52] In contrast to the Asymptomatic Carotid Atherosclerosis Study (ACAS, see later), the arteriographic complications in NASCET were low, occurring in only 0.6% of 2885 conventional cerebral angiograms.

European Carotid Surgery Trial

Over a 10-year period, a total of 2518 patients with carotid territory nonincapacitating strokes, TIAs, or retinal infarctions were randomized to either medical or surgical treatment with an average follow-up of nearly 3 years. The study was conducted in 80 medical centers in 14 countries. In contrast to NASCET, medical treatment was not specified but rather left to the discretion of the treating physician. In addition, in NASCET the qualifying event had to occur within 120 days of randomization, in comparison with a 6-month interval in ECST. Another major difference between ECST and NASCET is that ECST allowed participating centers to enter only the patients for whose treatment they had uncertainty, thus calling into question the true "randomized" status of ECST. A ratio of 1:2 of patients randomized into the medical:surgical arms also emphasizes the problematic design of ECST.

Finally, the arteriographic measurement differences between ECST and NASCET have been discussed. This difference "diluted" the ECST results so that about 350 patients who would be classified as having less than 70% stenosis by NASCET criteria were included in the "severe" ECST group.

Seven hundred seventy-eight patients with 70% to 99% carotid stenosis were randomized to carotid endarterectomy versus medical treatment in ECST.[55] There was a disappointing 30-day perioperative morbidity and mortality rate for surgical intervention of 7.5%, but despite this high rate of adverse outcomes, the results favored carotid endarterectomy for the severe stenosis subgroup. After 3 years of follow-up, the risk of an ipsilateral stroke was an additional 2.8% in the carotid endarterectomy group versus 16.8% in the medical group, for a sixfold risk reduction ($p < .0001$). The risk of death, ipsilateral stroke, or any other stroke was 12.3% in surgical patients compared with 21.9% of patients in the medical group ($p < .01$) at 3 years. Among those with severe stenosis, only 3.7% of surgical patients had disabling strokes, compared with an incidence of 8.4% in the medical arm. A total 3-year risk of any disabling or fatal stroke was 6% versus 11% in the surgical and medical groups, respectively.

Patients in the mild carotid stenosis category (0% to 29%) had a very small 3-year risk of ipsilateral stroke, so that the surgical risks were not outweighed by its benefits.[55] Thus, randomization in this group was stopped in 1991. More than 2000 patients with 30% to 69% carotid stenosis were enrolled in ECST. In a preliminary report of the results in this group, there was no significant benefit from endarterectomy, according to the measurement method used in this trial.[56] The perioperative complication rate was 7.6%. Again, it must be emphasized that a substantial number of patients in this subgroup would have had less than 50% stenoses by NASCET criteria.

Veterans Affairs Symptomatic Trial

The Department of Veterans Affairs randomized multicenter trial of carotid endarterectomy for patients with symptomatic carotid stenosis was terminated in 1991 after publication of the other trials described earlier.[109] Only 189 patients were randomized in 16 university-affiliated Veterans Affairs Medical Centers. In contrast to the other trial, TIAs were included as end-points in this trial. After a mean follow-up of 11.9 months, the risk of a neurologic event for patients in the surgical group was 7.7% compared with 19.4% in the medical group ($p = .011$).

Thus, all three randomized trials of symptomatic patients with high-grade stenoses showed significant benefit for carotid endarterectomy compared with nonsurgical treatment.

Asymptomatic Carotid Artery Stenosis

Through population-based studies, it has been well established that an asymptomatic carotid bruit is associated with a low risk of stroke.[84, 187] Norris and colleagues reported bruits in stenoses of only 20%; when the degree of stenosis was less than 50%, the annual percentage rate of stroke was only 1.3%. In contrast, when carotid stenosis was greater than 75%, the annual stroke rate was 3.3%; moreover, the combined TIA, stroke, cardiac, and vascular death event rate was 25.3% in this group. Based on such findings, investigators focused on functional stenosis, using noninvasive screening tests such as ocular pneumoplethysmography and duplex scanning.[16, 65]

Despite excellent results from nonrandomized series of carotid endarterectomy in asymptomatic patients, as discussed previously, even greater disagreement existed regarding carotid endarterectomy for asymptomatic stenoses than for symptomatic disease. This controversy gave rise to four randomized clinical trials, discussed next, on the efficacy of carotid endarterectomy in patients with asymptomatic carotid stenosis.[28, 56, 89, 110]

Carotid Surgery versus Medical Therapy in Asymptomatic Carotid Stenosis Trial

The first published results of a randomized controlled trial of carotid endarterectomy for asymptomatic carotid stenosis are those of the Carotid Surgery Versus Medical Therapy in Asymptomatic Carotid Stenosis (CASANOVA) Study Group.[28] This multicenter trial compared surgical and medical treatment in 410 patients with asymptomatic carotid stenosis ranging from 50% to 90%. Arteriography was performed in all patients. Two hundred six patients underwent carotid endarterectomy and received aspirin postoperatively; 204 patients received aspirin therapy alone. All patients also received 75 mg of dipyridamole three times daily. Patients in the medical group who had bilateral carotid stenoses of 90% or more were immediately referred for carotid endarterectomy, thus negating the influence of surgical management in patients most likely to experience neurologic events. In addition, carotid endarterectomy was performed in the medical group when the stenosis progressed to 90%, if bilateral internal carotid artery stenosis greater than 50% developed, or if the patient had TIAs in the brain supplied by the randomized internal carotid artery.

Minimum follow-up was 3 years. A total of 334 carotid endarterectomies were performed, including 118 in the medically treated patients who were analyzed by "intent to treat" in the medical group. Twenty per cent of patients randomized to the medical group underwent carotid endarterectomy immediately (30 patients as part of the protocol for bilateral lesions and 10 in violation of the protocol). An additional 20% of patients in the medical group underwent endarterectomy performed by protocol in follow-up. The authors concluded that there was no benefit of the procedure in patients with asymptomatic stenoses, but the many methodologic errors in this study invalidate the findings—as admitted by the authors in their response[39] to a critical editorial.[156] In the final analysis, the best thing about the CASANOVA Study is its catchy title.

Mayo Clinic Asymptomatic Carotid Endarterectomy Trial

In 1992, results of an attempted randomized trial of carotid endarterectomy for asymptomatic carotid stenoses at the Mayo Clinic were published.[110] Only 71 patients were randomized to carotid endarterectomy versus medical treatment during a 30-month period. Too few neurologic events occurred in this small group of patients to permit analysis of efficacy of these treatments. In addition, the trial was terminated because significantly more adverse cardiac events occurred in the surgical group. These cardiac events may have been related to absence of aspirin therapy in the patients undergoing carotid endarterectomy.

The Veterans Affairs Asymptomatic Trial

In 1986, the Department of Veterans Affairs launched the Cooperative Study on Asymptomatic Carotid Stenosis (Clinical Studies Program No. 167) to determine the role of carotid endarterectomy in the treatment of asymptomatic carotid stenosis.[89] The trial was conducted in 11 university-affiliated Veterans Affairs Medical Centers. End-points were TIAs, transient monocular blindness, and stroke. A total of 444 men (mean age, 64.5 years) with asymptomatic internal carotid stenoses of 50% or more (lumen diameter reduction on arteriogram as calculated by NASCET criteria) were randomized to optimal medical care, including aspirin plus carotid endarterectomy (n = 211, surgical group) or optimal medical care alone (n = 233, medical group). All patients initially received aspirin at a dose of 1300 mg/day, but this dose was lowered for many patients who were intolerant of aspirin.[87, 96] Patients were followed by a neurologist and a vascular surgeon for a mean follow-up of 47.9 months.

The 30-day operative mortality for the surgical group was 1.9% (4 of 211 patients). Three deaths occurred from MI, and one resulted from MI followed by stroke. The incidence of nonfatal perioperative stroke was 2.4% (five of 211 patients). Three nonfatal strokes occurred after arteriography (3 of 714, 0.4%). When all complications of arteriography were assigned to the surgical group, the permanent stroke and death rate within 30 days of randomization was 4.7% for patients randomized to carotid endarterectomy. In comparison, in the medical group, 1 patient committed suicide (0.4%) and 2 patients had neurologic events (one stroke, one TIA; 0.9%).

The combined incidence of ipsilateral neurologic events was 8% in the surgical group and 20.6% in the medical group ($p < .001$, Fig. 131–37). The incidence of ipsilateral stroke alone was 4.7% in the surgical group and 9.4% in the medical group ($p = .056$). While this 2:1 "trend" in stroke reduction by carotid endarterectomy in asymptomatic patients is interesting, the results of the study were unconvincing to many clinicians.[10] Nevertheless, the Veterans Affairs trial was the first to demonstrate a reduction in neurologic events in patients undergoing prophylactic carotid endarterectomy for significant asymptomatic carotid artery stenosis.

Asymptomatic Carotid Atherosclerosis Study

The Asymptomatic Carotid Atherosclerosis Study (ACAS) is the largest published randomized trial of carotid endarterectomy versus medical treatment for asymptomatic carotid stenosis.[56] This NIH-sponsored study is similar in design to the Veterans Affairs cooperative study. Arteriography was not absolutely mandated in ACAS if the participating institutions' noninvasive determination of degree of carotid stenosis had been validated. A 60% luminal reduction was considered significant in ACAS. The advantages of ACAS are inclusion of both men and women and enrollment of a large sample. Acquisition of patients began in November 1987, and was completed in December 1992. A total of 1662 men and women were randomized, nearly four times the sample size of the Veterans Affairs study. In the middle of the study, the ACAS trialists changed their statistical analysis to observe stroke alone rather than the combined end-points of stroke plus TIAs.

The results of ACAS were reported on September 28, 1994. The 30-day perioperative stroke and mortality rate was 2.3%. Of note, the risk of stroke from arteriography alone was a surprisingly high 1.2%. When data were extrapolated to 5 years using Kaplan-Meier projections, the primary outcome of ipsilateral stroke was 5.1% for the surgical group and 11% for the medical group, representing a relative risk reduction of 53% ($p = .006$). The absolute risk reduction was only about 1% per year; this was a much less dramatic reduction than that demonstrated in the symptomatic trials.

PERCUTANEOUS CAROTID ARTERY TRANSLUMINAL ANGIOPLASTY

There has been great controversy over the role of percutaneous transluminal angioplasty (PTA) for carotid artery stenoses in recent years. Initial interest in this procedure addressed PTA for fibromuscular dysplasia of the carotid artery.[77] In 1981, Mathias reported the first PTA for atherosclerotic carotid disease in Germany.[108] Numerous individual case reports and small series soon appeared in the world literature, but many contained a mixture of causes (e.g., Takayasu's disease, recurrent stenoses, radiation-induced stenoses, fibromuscular dysplasia, dissections), and angioplasties of vessels other than the internal carotid artery (e.g., common carotid, brachiocephalic, intracranial arteries, and so on).[19, 23, 63, 128, 175, 185] For example, in 1993 Motarjeme and Gordon described 131 angioplasties of the supra-aortic vessels, including 66 PTAs of the subclavian arteries.[129] In this series, PTA was performed on only 7 internal carotid arteries, each of which was afflicted with fibromuscular dysplasia. Likewise, Bergeron and colleagues reported 47 PTAs of the supra-aortic arteries, including 24 of the internal carotid arteries (ICAs).[15] The etiology of carotid disease in this series was fibromuscular dysplasia in one patient, atherosclerosis in eight, and post-CEA restenoses in 15. PTA with primary stenting was performed in most of the atherosclerotic lesions.

At least nine series have reported substantial numbers of patients undergoing ICA angioplasties (mostly with stenting) for atherosclerotic disease since 1994.[22, 41, 49, 85, 94, 131, 166, 184, 189] The results in these reports are summarized in Table 131–6. Analysis of the data is difficult for many

FIGURE 131–37. Event-free rates for ipsilateral stroke and transient ischemic attach (TIA) or amaurosis fugax in the Veterans Affairs Cooperative Study (Clinical Studies Program No. 167) by Kaplan-Meier analysis. The numbers of patients (N) remaining event-free and in the study at the beginning of each 12-month period are provided beneath the graph. Treatment group comparisons by the log-rank test showed significant differences in favor of the surgical group ($p<.001$). (From Hobson RW, Weiss DG, Fields WAS, et al: Efficacy of carotid endarterectomy for asymptomatic carotid stenosis. N Engl J Med 3288:221, 1993.)

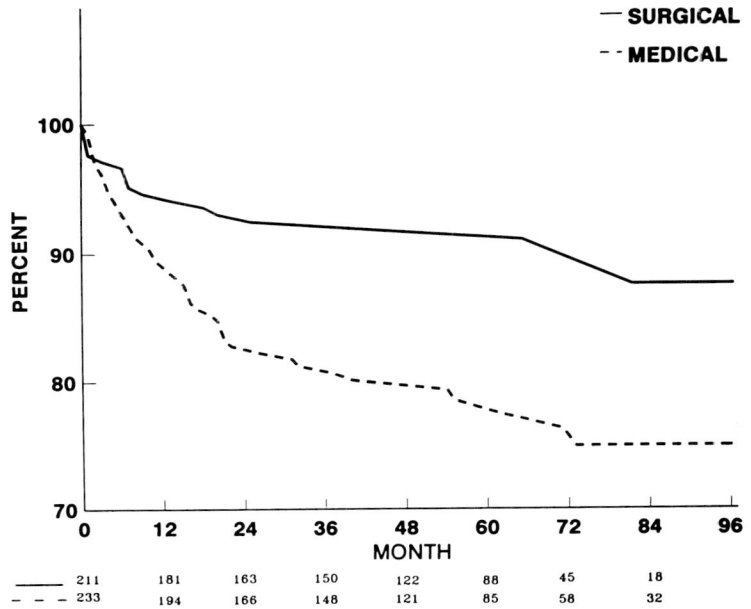

TABLE 131–6. SHORT-TERM RESULTS OF PUBLISHED SERIES OF CAROTID PERCUTANEOUS TRANSLUMINAL ANGIOPLASTY (PTA)

AUTHOR	YEAR	CAROTID PTA	TIA	STROKE	DEATH	% MORBIDITY AND MORTALITY
Munari et al[131]	1992	44	1	4	0	9.1
Brown[22]	1994	18	2	1	1	11.1
Higashida et al[85]	1994	42	5	1	0	2.4
Theron[166]	1996	174	0	7	1	4.6
Eckert et al[49]	1996	54	8	3	0	5.6
Diethrich et al[41]	1996	83	5	6	2	9.6
Wholey[184]	1996	61	2	3	0	4.9
Kachel[94]	1996	65	1	1	0	1.6
Yadav et al[189]	1997	126	0	9	1	7.9
TOTAL		667	24	35	5	6.0

reasons. As noted earlier, the patients described generally represent only a portion of the total number of PTAs reported for various indications and in various arteries. Many of the series are reported in foreign and obscure journals. In some series, the majority of patients had symptomatic stenoses, whereas in others many patients were asymptomatic. Several investigators failed to report interventional indications completely.[166, 184] Failure to maneuver a catheter across a carotid stenosis ranged from 7%[49] to 25%,[22] and such failures were not taken into account in calculating the complication rate; in other words, only successful PTAs were considered. Technique was not standardized; in most but not all cases, stents of different manufacturers were employed.

Exclusion criteria were variable; some investigators eliminated patients with calcific or ulcerated plaques.[41, 49, 94] Patient demographics varied widely: in some reports, patients were candidates for either PTA or conventional carotid endarterectomy,[41, 49] and in others they were considered prohibitive operative risks and offered PTA for compassionate use.[22, 85] Central neurologic complications were poorly described in most papers. Finally, none of the series reported long-term clinical follow-up, so the efficacy of PTA with or without stenting for the prevention of strokes is unknown.

Residual or recurrent stenoses are a problem in patients with carotid stenosis treated by PTA. In one series of 61 carotid PTAs in 58 symptomatic patients, for example, there were 5 residual stenoses of between 50% and 70%.[49] If persistent stenosis is considered a complication, the combined morbidity and mortality in this report increases from 5.6% to 20%. If the 7 catheterization failures are included, the adverse outcome rate is even higher! High restenosis rates have been reported by others.

Touho reported a 38% restenosis rate in 13 angioplasties with systematic angiographic follow-up.[175] Munari and colleagues reported a 16% restenosis at 1 year in 44 carotid angioplasties.[131] Theron described 18 restenoses in 119 cases (15%) before the routine use of stents and four in 93 cases after the use of Strecker stents.[166] In addition to restenosis, others have reported stent thrombosis.

In 1996, Diethrich and associates from the Arizona Heart Institute reported 83 carotid bifurcation PTAs with primary Palmaz stenting for atherosclerotic lesions in a series of 117 carotid angioplasties in 110 patients.[41] In a mean follow-up of only 7 months, there were seven strokes (6.4%), five TIAs (4.5%), and two deaths (1.8%), for a cumulative neurologic morbidity and death rate of 13% in the entire series. Three stents thrombosed asymptomatically in follow-up, two in the first month and one after 2 months. These events were not included in the reported complication rates.

The optimal method for prevention of cerebral embolization during carotid PTA is unsettled. Theron and associates recommend cerebral protection by placing a coaxial catheter with an inflated balloon in the distal carotid artery,[167] but this technique has been criticized as cumbersome and complex.[22, 131] Kachel[94] and Touho[175] used inflation of a balloon in the proximal common carotid artery to provide cerebral protection. Higashida and coworkers perfused the distal ICA with the patient's blood through the angioplasty catheter while the dilatation balloon was inflated.[85] Routine primary carotid stenting has been proposed as a means of protection against cerebral emboli.[15, 41, 166, 184, 189] The design of multicenter randomized trials of carotid PTA mandates primary stenting.

Only preliminary results are available for multicenter trials of percutaneous carotid artery angioplasty. The Carotid and Vertebral Artery Transluminal Angioplasty Study (CAVATAS) commenced in Great Britain in 1992.[95] There are two arms of this study: patients eligible for carotid endarterectomy are randomized to angioplasty versus surgery; patients considered a prohibitive risk for carotid endarterectomy are randomized to angioplasty versus medical treatment. Although results of this trial have not been published, criticism has already appeared in the literature.[24, 134]

The North American Cerebral Percutaneous Transluminal Angioplasty Register (NACPTAR) prospectively analyzed the results of carotid PTA in patients with contraindications to carotid endarterectomy. Two abstracts describing preliminary results in this study have been published. The first appeared in 1993.[57] There were two lethal strokes, eight nonlethal strokes, and four TIAs in 113 angioplasties in 113 patients for a combined morbidity and mortality rate of 9.8%. The second abstract appeared in 1995.[129] In the first month after PTA, the mortality rate was 3%, and the stroke rate was 6%, in 165 carotid PTAs.

Currently, three large multicenter randomized studies comparing carotid endarterectomy with carotid PTA are either underway or in the planning stage: one European study (Carotid Artery Stenting versus Carotid Endarterectomy Trial, CASCET) and two North American studies (Carotid Artery Stenting versus Endarterectomy Trial, CASET, and Carotid Revascularization Endarterectomy versus Stent Trial, CREST).[88, 161]

SUMMARY

Based on published data, carotid endarterectomy remains the treatment of choice for carotid artery stenosis in appropriate patients with atherosclerotic lesions. The low morbidity and mortality rates described in both nonrandomized and randomized series for both symptomatic and asymptomatic patients must be equaled in studies of PTA, and this is certainly not the case at present.[43] Data on PTA are insufficient to make knowledgeable recommendations about this experimental procedure. In the authors' opinion, it is unlikely—considering the low perioperative event rates for carotid endarterectomy—that enough patients can be enrolled in randomized controlled trials to prove equivalence of PTA to carotid endarterectomy for treatment of carotid stenosis.

REFERENCES

1. American-Canadian Cooperative Study Group: Persantine aspirin trial in cerebral ischemia: Part II: Endpoint results. Stroke 16:406, 1985.
2. Antiplatelet Trialists' Collaboration: Secondary prevention of vascular disease by prolonged antiplatelet treatment. Br Med J 296:320, 1988.
3. Asymptomatic Carotid Artery Stenosis Group: Study design for randomized prospective trial of carotid endarterectomy for asymptomatic atherosclerosis. Stroke 20:844, 1989.
4. Baker JD, Gluecklich B, Watson CW, et al: An evaluation of electroencephalographic monitoring for carotid artery study. Surgery 78:787, 1975.
5. Baker RN, Schwart WS, Ramseyer JC: Prognosis among survivors of ischemic stroke. Neurology 18:933, 1968.
6. Baker RN, Schwartz WS, Rose AS: Transient ischemic strokes: A report of a study of anticoagulant therapy. Neurology 16:841, 1964.
7. Bardin JA, Bernstein EF, Humber BB, et al: Is carotid endarterectomy beneficial in the prevention of recurrent stroke? Arch Surg 117:1401, 1982.
8. Barner HB, Rittenhouse EA, Willman VL: Carotid-subclavian bypass for "subclavian steal syndrome." J Thorac Cardiovasc Surg 55:773, 1968.
9. Barnett HJM: An update on NASCET and ECST. In Branchereau A, Jacobs M (eds): New Trends and Developments in Carotid Artery Disease. Armonk, NY, Futura Publishing Company, 1998, p 107.
10. Barnett HJM, Haines SJ: Carotid endarterectomy for asymptomatic carotid stenosis. N Engl J Med 328:276, 1993.
11. Barnett HJM, Plum F, Walton JN: Carotid endarterectomy: An expression of concern. Stroke 15:941, 1984.
12. Bauer RG, Meyer JS, Fields WAS, et al: Joint study of extracranial arterial occlusion: III. Progress report of controlled study of long-term survival in patients with and without operation. JAMA 208:509, 1969.
13. Bernstein EF, Humber PB, Collins GM, et al: Life expectancy and late stroke following carotid endarterectomy. Ann Surg 198:80, 1983.
14. Bergan JJ, Dean RH, Yao JS: Use of the axillary artery in complex cerebral revascularization. Surgery 77:338, 1975.
15. Bergeron P, Chambran P, Bianca S, et al: Traitement endovasculaire des arteres a destinée cerebrale: Echecs et limites. J Mal Vasc 21(Suppl):123, 1996.
16. Blackshear WM Jr, Phillips DJ, Thiele BL, et al: Detection of carotid occlusive disease by ultrasonic imaging and pulsed Doppler spectral analysis. Surgery 86:698, 1979.
17. Blaisdell FW, Clauss RH, Galbraith JG, et al: Joint study of extracranial artery occlusion: IV. A review of surgical considerations. JAMA 209:1889, 1969.
18. Blaisdell FW, Lim RJ Jr, Hall AD: Technical result of carotid endarterectomy: Arteriographic assessment. Am J Surg 114:239, 1967.
19. Bockenheimer SA, Mathias K: Percutaneous transluminal angioplasty in arteriosclerotic internal carotid artery stenosis. Am J Neuroradiol 4:791, 1983.
20. Bousser MG, Eschwege E, Haguenau M, et al: "AICLA" controlled trial of aspirin and dipyridamole in the secondary prevention of atherosclerothrombotic cerebral ischemia. Stroke 14:5, 1983.
21. Brooke R, Park E, Chassin M, et al: Carotid endarterectomy for elderly patients: Predicting complications. Ann Intern Med 113:747, 1990.
22. Brown MM: Angioplastie des arteres carotides et verterbrales: Des etudes randomisees sont encoare necessaires. Sang Thrombose Vaisseaux 6:227, 1994.
23. Brown MM, Butler P, Gibbs J, et al: Feasibility of percutaneous transluminal angioplasty for carotid artery stenosis. J Neurol Neurosurg Psychiatry 53:238, 1990.
24. Brown MM, Venables G, Clifton A, et al: Carotid endarterectomy vs carotid angioplasty. Lancet 349:880, 1997.
24a. Bruetman ME, Fields WS, Crawford ES, et al: Cerebral hemorrhage in carotid artery surgery. Arch Neurol 9:458, 1963.
25. Buren A, Ygge J: Treatment program and comparison between anticoagulants and platelet aggregation inhibitors after transient ischemic attack. Stroke 12:578, 1981.
26. Canadian Cooperative Study Group: A randomized trial of aspirin and sulfinpyrazone in threatened stroke. N Engl J Med 299:53, 1978.
27. CAPRIE Steering Committee: A randomized, blinded trial of Clopidogrel versus Aspirin in Patients at Risk of Ischaemic Events (CAPRIE). Lancet 348:1329, 1996.
28. The CASANOVA Study Group: Carotid surgery versus medical therapy for asymptomatic carotid stenosis. Stroke 22:1229, 1991.
29. Chambers BR, Norris JW: Outcome in patients with asymptomatic neck bruits. N Engl J Med 315:860, 1986.
30. Chambers BR, Norris JW: The case against surgery for asymptomatic carotid stenosis. Stroke 15:964, 1984.
31. Christensen MS, Hoedi-Rasmussen K, Lassen NA: Cerebral vasodilatation by halothane anesthesia in man and its potentiation by hypotension and hypercapnia. Br J Anaesth 39:927, 1967.
32. Connolly JE, Stemmer EA: Endarterectomy of the external carotid artery: Its importance in the surgical management of extracranial cerebrovascular occlusive disease. Surgery 106:799, 1973.
33. Crawford ES, DeBakey ME, Morris GC Jr, et al: Surgical treatment of occlusion of the innominate, common carotid, and subclavian arteries: A 10-year experience. Surgery 65:17, 1969.
34. Dardik H, Dardik I: Axillo-axillary bypass with cephalic vein for correction of subclavian steal syndrome. Surgery 76:143, 1974.
35. Davis JB, Grove WJ, Julian OC: Thrombotic occlusion of the branches of the aortic arch—Martorell's syndrome: Report of a case treated surgically. Ann Surg 144:124, 1956.
36. DeBakey ME, Crawford ES, Cooley DA, et al: Surgical considerations of occlusive disease of the innominate, carotid, subclavian, and vertebral arteries. Ann Surg 149:690, 1959.
37. DeCaterina R, Sicari R, Bernini W, et al: Benefit/risk profile of combined antiplatelet therapy with ticlopidine and aspirin. Thromb Haemost 65:504, 1991.
38. DeWeese JA, Rob CG, Satran R, et al: Results of carotid endarterectomy for transient ischemic attacks five years later. Ann Surg 178:258, 1973.
39. Diener HC: Response to Letter to the Editor. Stroke 23:918, 1992.
40. Diethrich EB, Garrett HE, Ameriso J, et al: Occlusive disease of the common carotid and subclavian arteries treated by carotid-subclavian bypass. Analysis of 125 cases. Am J Surg 113:800, 1967.
41. Diethrich EB, Ndiaye M, Reid DB: Stenting in the carotid artery: Initial experience in 110 patients. J Endovasc Surg 3:42, 1996.
42. Dixon S, Pais SO, Raviola C, et al: Natural history of nonstenotic asymptomatic ulcerative lesions of the carotid artery. Arch Surg 117:1493, 1982.

43. Dorros G: Carotid arterial obliterative disease: Should endovascular revascularization (stent supported angioplasty) today supplant carotid endarterectomy? J Intervent Cardiol 9:257, 1996.
44. Dosick SM, Whalen RC, Gale SS, Brown OW: Carotid endarterectomy in the stroke patient: Computerized axial tomography to determine timing. J Vasc Surg 2:214, 1985.
45. The Dutch TIA Study Group: A comparison of two doses of aspirin (30 mg vs 283 mg a day) in patients after a transient ischemic attack or minor ischemic stroke. N Engl J Med 325:1261, 1991.
46. Dyken ML: Transient ischemic attacks and aspirin, stroke, and death: Negative studies and type II error (Editorial). Stroke 14:2, 1983.
47. Easton JD, Sherman DG: Stroke and mortality rate in carotid endarterectomy: 228 consecutive operations. Stroke 8:565, 1977.
48. EC/IC Bypass Study Group: Failure of extracranial-intracranial arterial bypass to reduce the risk of ischemic stroke: Results of an international randomized trial. N Engl J Med 313:1191, 1985.
49. Eckert B, Zanella FE, Thie A, et al: Angioplasty of the internal carotid artery: Results, complications, and follow-up in 61 cases. Cerebrovasc Dis 6:97, 1996.
50. Ehrenfeld WK, Chapman ED, Wylie EJ: Management of occlusive lesions of the branches of the aortic arch. Am J Surg 118:236, 1969.
51. Ehrenfeld WK, Hamilton FN, Larson CP Jr, et al: Effect of CO_2 and systemic hypertension on downstream cerebral arterial pressure during carotid endarterectomy. Surgery 67:87, 1970.
52. Eliasziw M, Rankin RN, Fox AJ, et al: Accuracy and prognostic consequences of ultrasonography in identifying severe carotid artery stenosis. Stroke 26:1745, 1995.
53. Enger E, Boyesen S: Long-term anticoagulant therapy in patients with cerebral infarction: A controlled clinical study. Acta Med Scand 178(Suppl 438): 1, 1965.
54. Eriksson SE, Link H, Alm A, et al: Results from eighty-eight consecutive prophylactic carotid endarterectomies in cerebral infarction and transitory ischemic attacks. Acta Neurol Scand 63:209, 1981.
55. European Carotid Surgery Trialists' Collaborative Group: Medical Research Council European Carotid Surgery Trial: Interim results for symptomatic patients with severe (70–99%) or with mild (0–29%) carotid stenosis. Lancet 337:1235, 1991.
56. The Executive Committee for the Asymptomatic Carotid Atherosclerosis Study: Endarterectomy for asymptomatic carotid artery stenosis. JAMA 273:1421, 1995.
57. Ferguson R, Ferguson J, Schwarten D, et al: Immediate angiographic results and in-hospital central nervous system complications of cerebral percutaneous transluminal angioplasty (Abstract). Circulation 88 (Suppl I):393, 1993.
58. Field PL: Effective stroke prevention with carotid endarterectomy: A series of 400 cases with two-year follow-up. International Vascular Symposium Program and Abstracts. New York, Macmillan, 1981, p 528.
59. Fields WAS: Selection of stroke patients for arterial reconstructive surgery. Am J Surg 125:527, 1973.
60. Fields WAS, Lemak N, Frankowski RF, Hardy RJ: Controlled trial of aspirin in cerebral ischemia. Stroke 8:301, 1977.
61. Fields WAS, Lemak N, Frankowski RF, Hardy RJ: Controlled trial of aspirin in cerebral ischemia; Part II. Surgical results. Stroke 9:309, 1978.
62. Freischlag JA, Hanna D, Moore WS: Improved prognosis for asymptomatic carotid stenosis with prophylactic carotid endarterectomy. Stroke 23:479, 1992.
63. Freitag J, Koch RD, Wagemann W: Percutaneous transluminal angioplasty of the carotid artery stenoses. Neuroradiology 28:126, 1986.
64. Garde A, Samuelsson K, Fahlgran H, et al: Treatment after transient ischemic attacks: A comparison between anticoagulant drug and inhibition of platelet aggregation. Stroke 14:677, 1983.
65. Gee W, Mehigan JT, Wylie EJ: Measurement of collateral cerebral hemispheric blood pressure by ocular pneumoplethysmography. Am J Surg 130:121, 1975.
66. Gent M, Blakeley JA, Easton JC, and CATS Group: The Canadian-American Ticlopidine Study (CATS) in thromboembolic stroke. Lancet 1:1215, 1989.
67. Gertler JP, Cambria RP: The role of external carotid endarterectomy in the treatment of ipsilateral internal carotid occlusion: Collective review. J Vasc Surg 6:158, 1987.
68. Giordano JM, Trout HM III, Kozloff L, DePalma RG: Timing of carotid endarterectomy after stroke. J Vasc Surg 2:350, 1985.
69. Goldstone J, Moore WS: Emergency carotid artery surgery in neurologically unstable patients. Arch Surg 111:1284, 1976.
70. Hachinski V, Norris JW: The reversibility of cerebral ischemia. In Hachinski V, Norris JW: The Acute Stroke. Philadelphia, FA Davis, 1985, p 41.
71. Halstuk KS, Baker WH, Littooy FN: External carotid endarterectomy. J Vasc Surg 1:398, 1984.
72. Harris EJ, Brown WH, Pavy RN, et al: Continuous electroencephalographic monitoring during carotid artery endarterectomy. Surgery 62:441, 1967.
73. Hart RG: Cardiogenic embolism to the brain. Lancet 339:589, 1992.
74. Harvey J, Rasmussen T: Occlusion of the middle cerebral artery. Arch Neurol Psychiatry 66:20, 1951.
75. Hass WK, Easton JD, Adams HP Jr, et al: Ticlopidine Aspirin Stroke Study Group: A randomized trial comparing ticlopidine hydrochloride with aspirin for the prevention of stroke in high-risk patients. N Engl J Med 321:501, 1989.
76. Hass WK, Jonas S: Caution: Falling rock zone: An analysis of the medical and surgical management of threatened stroke. Proc Inst Med Chicago 33:80, 1980.
77. Hasso AN, Bird CR, Zinke DE, Thompson J: Fibromuscular dysplasia of the internal carotid artery: Percutaneous transluminal angioplasty. Am J Neuroradiol 2:175, 1981.
78. Hays RJ, Levinson SA, Wylie EJ: Intraoperative measurement of carotid back pressure as a guide to operative management for carotid endarterectomy. Surgery 72:953, 1972.
79. Helgason CM, Tortorice KL, Winkler SR, et al: Aspirin response and failure in cerebral infarction. Stroke 24:345, 1993.
80. Hertzer NR, Arison R: Cumulative stroke and survival ten years after carotid endarterectomy. J Vasc Surg 2:661, 1985.
81. Hertzer NR, Beven EG, O'Hara PJ, et al: A prospective study of vein patch angioplasty during carotid endarterectomy. Ann Surg 206:628, 1987.
82. Hertzer NR, Flanagan RA Jr, O'Hara PJ, et al: Surgical versus nonoperative treatment of asymptomatic carotid stenosis. Ann Surg 204:163, 1986.
83. Hertzer NR, Flanagan RA Jr, O'Hara PJ, et al: Surgical versus nonoperative treatment of symptomatic carotid stenosis. Ann Surg 204:154, 1986.
84. Heyman W, Wilkinson WE, Heyden S, et al: Risk of stroke in asymptomatic persons with cervical arterial bruits: A population study in Evans County, Georgia. N Engl J Med 302:838, 1980.
85. Higashida RT, Tsai FY, Halbach V, et al: Transluminal angioplasty, thrombolysis, and stenting for extracranial and intracranial cerebral vascular disease. J Intervent Cardiol 9:245, 1996.
86. High-dose acetylsalicylic acid after cerebral infarction: A Swedish Cooperative Study. Stroke 18:325, 1987.
87. Hobson RW, Krupski WC, Weiss DG, et al: Influence of aspirin in the management of asymptomatic carotid artery stenosis. J Vasc Surg 17:257, 1993.
88. Hobson RW II, Brott T, Ferguson R, et al: Regarding "Statement regarding carotid angioplasty and stenting." J Vasc Surg 25:1117, 1997.
89. Hobson RW II, Weiss DG, Fields WS, et al: Efficacy of carotid endarterectomy for asymptomatic carotid stenosis. N Engl J Med 328:221, 1993.
90. Homi J, Humphries AW, Young JR, et al: Hypercarbic anesthesia in cerebrovascular surgery. Surgery 59:57, 1966.
91. Hughes RK, Bustos M, Byrne JP Jr: Internal carotid artery pressures: A guide for use of shunt during carotid repair. Arch Surg 109:494, 1974.
92. Humphries AW, Young JR, Beven EG, et al: Relief of vertebrobasilar symptoms by carotid endarterectomy. Surgery 57:48, 1965.
93. Hunter GC, Sieffert G, Malone JM, et al: The accuracy of carotid back pressure as an index for shunt requirement: A reappraisal. Stroke 13:319, 1982.
94. Kachel R: Results of balloon angioplasty in the carotid arteries. J Endovasc Surg 3:22, 1996.
95. Kinoshita A, Itoh M, Takemoro O: Percutaneous transluminal angioplasty of internal carotid artery: A preliminary report of seesaw balloon technique. Neurol Res 15:356, 1993.
96. Krupski WC, Weiss DG, Rapp JH, et al: Adverse effects of aspirin in the treatment of asymptomatic carotid artery stenosis. J Vasc Surg 16:588, 1992.

97. Larson CP: Anesthesia and control of the cerebral circulation. *In* Wylie EJ, Ehrenfeld WK (eds): Extracranial Occlusive Cerebrovascular Disease. Philadelphia, WB Saunders, 1970.

98. Larson CP, Ehrenfeld WK, Wade JG, et al: Jugular venous oxygen saturation as an index of adequacy of cerebral oxygenation. Surgery 62:31, 1967.

99. Lassen WA: The luxury-perfusion syndrome and its possible relation to acute metabolic acidosis localized within the brain. Lancet 2:1113, 1996.

100. Link H, Lebram G, Johannson I, Radberg C: Prognosis in patients with infarction and TIA in carotid territory during and after anticoagulant therapy. Stroke 10:529, 1979.

101. Lips JPM, Sixma JJ, Schiphorst ME: The effect of ticlopidine administration to humans on binding of adenosine diphosphate to blood platelets. Thromb Res 17:19, 1980.

102. Little JR, Moufarrij NA, Furlan AJ: Early carotid endarterectomy after cerebral infarction. Neurosurgery 24:334, 1989.

103. Lord RSA: Later survival after carotid endarterectomy for transient ischemic attacks. J Vasc Surg 1:512, 1984.

104. Lyons C, Clark LC Jr, McDowell H, et al: Cerebral venous oxygen content during carotid thrombointimectomy. Ann Surg 106:561, 1964.

105. Machleder HI, Barker WF: External carotid artery shunting during carotid endarterectomy. Arch Surg 108:785, 1974.

106. Makhoul RG, Moore WS, Colburn MD, et al: Benefit of carotid endarterectomy following prior stroke. J Vasc Surg 18:666, 1993.

107. Matchar DB, Goldstein LB, McCory DC, et al: Carotid Endarterectomy: A Literature Review and Ratings of Appropriateness and Necessity. Santa Monica, Calif, Rand Corporation, 1992.

108. Mathias K: Perkutane transluminale katheterbehandlung supra-aortaler Arterionobstruktionen. Angio 3:47, 1981.

109. Mayberg MR, Wilson SE, Yatsu F, et al, for the Veterans Affairs Cooperative Studies Program 309 Trialist Group: Carotid endarterectomy and prevention of cerebral ischemia in symptomatic carotid stenosis. JAMA 266:3289, 1991.

110. The Mayo Asymptomatic Carotid Endarterectomy Study Group: Results of a randomized controlled trial of carotid endarterectomy for asymptomatic carotid stenosis. Mayo Clin Proc 67:513, 1992.

111. Mayo NE, Levy R, Goldberg MS: Aspirin and hemorrhagic stroke. Stroke 212:1213, 1991.

112. McCullough JL, Mentzer RM, Harman PK, et al: Carotid endarterectomy after a completed stroke: Reduction in long neurologic deterioration. J Vasc Surg 2:7, 1985.

113. McTavish D, Faulds D, Goa K: Ticlopidine A: An updated review of its pharmacology and therapeutic use in platelet-dependent disorders. Drugs 40:238, 1990.

114. Meissner I, Wiebers DO, Whisnant JP, et al: The natural history of asymptomatic carotid artery occlusive lesions. JAMA 258:2704, 1987.

115. Mentzer RN, Finkelmeir BA, Crosby LK, Wellons MA Jr: Emergency carotid endarterectomy for fluctuating neurologic deficits. Surgery 89:60, 1981.

116. Meyer JS: Importance of ischemic damage to small vessels in experimental cerebral infarcts. J Neuropathol Exp Neurol 17:571, 1958.

117. Modi JR, Finch WT, Sumner DS: Update of carotid endarterectomy in two community hospitals: Springfield revisited. Stroke 14:128, 1983.

118. Moneta GL, Taylor DC, Nicholls SC, et al: Operative versus nonoperative management of asymptomatic high-grade internal carotid artery stenosis: Improved results with endarterectomy. Stroke 18:1005, 1987.

119. Moore WS: Carotid endarterectomy for prevention of stroke. West J Med 159:37, 1993.

119a. Moore WS, Barnett MJ, Beebe HE, et al: Guidelines for carotid endarterectomy: A multidisciplinary consensus statement from the Ad Hoc Committee, American Heart Association. Stroke 26:188–201, 1995.

120. Moore WS, Blaisdell FW, Hall AD: Retrograde thrombectomy for chronic occlusion of the common carotid artery. Arch Surg 95:664, 1967.

121. Moore WS, Boren C, Malone JM, et al: Natural history of nonstenotic asymptomatic ulcerative lesions of the carotid artery. Arch Surg 113:1352, 1978.

122. Moore WS, Hall AD: Carotid artery back pressure. Arch Surg 99:702, 1969.

123. Moore WS, Malone JM, Goldstone J: Extrathoracic repair of branch occlusions of the aortic arch. Am J Surg 132:249, 1976.

124. Moore WS, Mohr JP, Najafi H, et al: Carotid endarterectomy: Practice guidelines. J Vasc Surg 15:469, 1992.

125. Moore WS, Yee JM, Hall AD: Collateral cerebral blood pressure: An index of tolerance to temporary carotid occlusion. Arch Surg 106:520, 1973.

126. Morasch MD, Baker WH: How soon can carotid endarterectomy be safely performed following an ischemic stroke? *In* Calligaro KD (ed): Management of Extracranial Cerebrovascular Disease. Philadelphia, Lipincott-Raven, 1997, p 73.

127. Morgenstern LB, Fox LJ, Sharpe BL, et al: The risks and benefits of carotid endarterectomy in patients with near occlusion of the carotid artery. Neurology 48:911, 1997.

128. Motarjeme A: Percutaneous transluminal angioplasty of the brachiocephalic, carotid, and vertebral arteries. J Intervent Cardiol 9:257, 1996.

129. Motarjeme A, Gordon GI: Percutaneous transluminal angioplasty of the brachiocephalic vessels: Guidelines for therapy. Int Angiol 12:260, 1995.

130. Mozersky DJ, Barnes RW, Sumner DS, et al: The hemodynamics of the axillary-axillary bypass. Surg Gynecol Obstet 135:925, 1972.

131. Munari LM, Belloni G, Perreti A, et al: Carotid percutaneous angioplasty. Neurol Res 14:(2 Suppl):156, 1992.

132. Najafi H, Javid H, Dye WS, et al: Kinked internal carotid artery: Clinical evaluation and surgical correction. Arch Surg 89:134, 1964.

133. The NACPTAR investigators: Update on the immediate angiographic results and in-hospital central nervous system complications of cerebral percutaneous transluminal angioplasty (Abstract). Circulation 92(Suppl I):I-383, 1995.

134. Naylor AR, London NJ, Bell PR: Carotid endarterectomy vs carotid angioplasty. Lancet 349:203, 1997.

135. North American Symptomatic Carotid Endarterectomy Trial Collaborators: Beneficial effect of carotid endarterectomy in symptomatic patients with high-grade carotid stenosis. N Engl J Med 325:445, 1991.

136. O'Hara PJ, Hertzer NR, Beven EG: External carotid revascularization: Review of a 10-year experience. J Vasc Surg 2:709, 1985.

137. Ojemman RG, Crowell RM, Robertson GH, Fisher CM: Surgical treatment of extracranial carotid disease. Clin Neurosurg 22:214, 1975.

138. Olsson JE, Brechter C, Backolund H, et al: Anticoagulant vs. antiplatelet therapy as prophylactic against cerebral infarction in transient ischemic attacks. Stroke 11:4, 1980.

139. Piotowski JJ, Bernhard VM, Rubin JR, et al: Timing of carotid endarterectomy after acute stroke. J Vasc Surg 11:45, 1990.

140. Pistolese GR, Citone G, Faraglia V: Effects of hypercapnia on cerebral blood flow during the clamping of the carotid arteries in surgical management of cerebrovascular insufficiency. Neurology (Minneap) 21:95, 1971.

141. Pokras JR, Dyken ML: Dramatic changes in the performance of endarterectomy for diseases of the extracranial arteries of the head. Stroke 10:1289, 1988.

142. Report of the Veterans Administration Cooperative Study of Arteriosclerosis: An evaluation of anticoagulant therapy in the treatment of cerebrovascular disease. Neurology 11:132, 1961.

143. Ricotta JJ, Ouriel K, Green RM, DeWeese JA: Use of computerized cerebral tomography in the selection of patients for elective and urgent carotid endarterectomy. Ann Surg 202:783, 1985.

144. Riles TS, Imparato AM, Mintzer R, Baumann FS: Comparison of results of bilateral and unilateral carotid endarterectomy five years after surgery. Surgery 91:258, 1982.

145. Rob CG: Operation for acute completed stroke due to thrombosis of the internal carotid artery. Surgery 65:862, 1969.

146. Robinson RW, Demirel M, LeBeau RJ: Natural history of cerebral thrombosis: Nine- to nineteen-year follow-up. J Chronic Dis 21:221, 1968.

147. Rosenthal D, Borrero E, Clark MD, et al: Carotid endarterectomy after reversible ischemic neurologic deficit or stroke: Is it of value? J Vasc Surg 8:527, 1988.

148. Rothrock JF, Hart RG: Ticlopidine use and threatened stroke: A clinical perspective. West J Med 160:43, 1994.

149. Rubin JR, Goldstone J, McIntyre KE, et al: The value of carotid endarterectomy in reducing the morbidity and mortality of recurrent stroke. J Vasc Surg 4:443, 1986.

150. Ruether R, Dorndorf W: Aspirin in patients with cerebral ischemia and normal angiograms or nonsurgical lesions: The results of a double-blind trial. In Breddin K, Dorndorf W, Lowe D, et al (eds): Acetylsalicylic Acid in Cerebral Ischemia and Coronary Heart Disease. Stuttgart, Schattauer, 1978, pp 97.

151. Sacco RL, Wolf PA, Kannel WB, et al: Survival and recurrence following stroke; The Framingham Study. Stroke 13:290, 1982.

152. The SALT Collaborative: Swedish aspirin low-dose trial (SALT) of 75 mg aspirin as secondary prophylaxis after cerebrovascular ischemic events. Lancet 338:1345, 1991.

153. Schuler JJ, Flanigan B, DeBord JR, et al: The treatment of cerebral ischemia by external carotid artery revascularization. Arch Surg 118:567, 1983.

154. Sergeant PT, Derom F, Berzsenyi G, et al: Carotid endarterectomy for cerebrovascular insufficiency: Long-term follow-up of 141 patients followed up to 16 years. Acta Chir Belg 79:309, 1980.

155. Silvenius J, Laakso M, Pentilla IM, et al: The European Stroke Prevention Study: Results according to sex. Neurology 41:1189, 1991.

156. Solis MM, Ranval TJ, Barone GW, et al: The CASANOVA Study: Immediate surgery versus delayed surgery for moderate carotid stenosis (Letter)? Stroke 23:917, 1992.

157. Solomon DH, Hart RG: Antithrombotic therapies to prevent stroke. In Zierler RE (ed): Surgical management of cerebrovascular disease. New York, McGraw-Hill, 1995, p 237.

158. Solomon RA, Loftus CM, Quest DO, Correll JW: Incidence and etiology of intracerebral hemorrhage following carotid endarterectomy. J Vasc Surg 64:29, 1986.

159. Sorenson PA, Pedersen H, Marquardsen J, et al: Acetylsalicylic acid in the prevention of stroke in patients with reversible cerebral ischemia attacks: A Danish cooperative study. Stroke 14:15, 1983.

160. Sproul G: Femoral-axillary bypass for cerebrovascular insufficiency. Arch Surg 103:746, 1971.

161. Stanley JC, Abbott WM, Towne JB, et al: Statement regarding carotid angioplasty and stenting. J Vasc Surg 24:900, 1996.

162. Stewart G, Ross-Russell RW, Browse NL: The long-term results of carotid endarterectomy for transient ischemic attacks. J Vasc Surg 4:600, 1986.

163. Swedish Cooperative Study: High-dose acetylsalicylic acid after cerebral infarction. Stroke 18:325, 1987.

164. Sze PC, Reitman D, Pincus MM, et al: Antiplatelet agents in the secondary prevention of stroke: Meta-analysis of the randomized control trials. Stroke 19:436, 1988.

165. Takolander RJ, Bergentz SE, Ericsson BF: Carotid artery surgery in patients with minor stroke. Br J Surg 70:13, 1982.

166. Theron J: Angioplastie carotidienne protegee et stents carotidiens. J Mal Vasc 21(Suppl A):113, 1996.

167. Theron J, Courtheoux P, Alachkar F, et al: New triple coaxial catheter system for carotid angioplasty with cerebral protection. Am J Neuroradiol 11:869, 1990.

168. Thompson JE: Carotid endarterectomy for asymptomatic carotid stenosis: An update. J Vasc Surg 13:669, 1991.

169. Thompson JE: Cerebral protection during carotid endarterectomy. JAMA 202:1046, 1967.

170. Thompson JE, Austen DJ, Patman RD: Carotid endarterectomy for cerebrovascular insufficiency: Long-term results in 592 patients followed up to 13 years. Ann Surg 172:663, 1970.

171. Thompson JE, Austen DJ, Patman RD: Endarterectomy of the totally occluded carotid artery for stroke. Arch Surg 95:791, 1967.

172. Thompson JE, Patman RD, Talkington CM: Asymptomatic carotid bruit: Long-term outcome of patients having endarterectomy compared with unoperated controls. Ann Surg 188:308, 1978.

173. Tohgi H, Konno S, Tamura K, et al: Effects of low-to-high doses of aspirin on platelet aggregatability and metabolites of thromboxane A_2 and prostacyclin. Stroke 23:1400, 1992.

174. Torrent A, Anderson B: The outcome of patients with transient ischemic attacks and stroke treated with anticoagulation. Acta Med Scand 208;359, 1980.

175. Touho H: Percutaneous transluminal angioplasty in the treatment of the anterior cerebral circulation and hemodynamic evaluation. J Neurosurg 82:953, 1995.

176. Trojaborg W, Boysen G: Relation between EEG, regional cerebral blood flow and internal carotid artery pressure during carotid endarterectomy. Electroencephalogr Clin Neurophysiol 34:61, 1973.

177. Uchiyama S, Sone R, Nagayama T, et al: Combination therapy with low-dose aspirin and ticlopidine in cerebral ischemia. Stroke 20:1643, 1989.

178. UK-TIA Study Group: United Kingdom transient ischaemic attack (UK-TIA) aspirin trial: Final results. J Neurol Neurosurg Psychiatry 54:1044, 1991.

179. Van Gijn J: Aspirin: Dose and indications in modern stroke. Neurol Clin 10:193, 1992.

180. Waltz AG: Effect of blood pressure on blood flow in ischemic and in nonischemic cerebral cortex. Neurology (Minneap) 18:613, 1968.

181. Whisnant JP, Matsumoto M, Elveback LR: The effect of anticoagulant therapy on the prognosis of patients with transient cerebral ischemic attacks in a community; Rochester, Minnesota, 1965–1969. Mayo Clin Proc 48:844, 1973.

182. Whitemore AD, Ruby ST, Couch MP, Mannick JA: Early carotid endarterectomy in patients with small, fixed neurologic deficits. J Vasc Surg 1:795, 1984.

183. Whitney DG, Kahn EM, Estes JW, Jones CE: Carotid artery surgery without a temporary indwelling shunt: 1917 consecutive procedures. Arch Surg 115:1393, 1980.

184. Wholey MH, Eles G, Jarmolowski CR, et al: Percutaneous transluminal angioplasty and stents in the treatment of extracranial circulation. J Interven Cardiol 9:225, 1996.

185. Wiggli U, Gratzl O: Transluminal angioplasty of stenotic carotid arteries: Case reports and protocol. Am J Neuroradiol 4:793, 1983.

186. Wing SD, Norman D, Pollock JA, Newton TH: Contrast enhancement of cerebral infarcts in computed tomography. Radiology 121:89, 1979.

187. Wolf PA, Kannel WB, Sorlie P, McNamara P: Asymptomatic carotid bruit and the risk of stroke. JAMA 245:1442, 1981.

188. Wylie EJ, Hein MF, Adams JE: Intracranial hemorrhage following surgical revascularization for treatment of acute stroke. J Neurosurg 21:212, 1964.

189. Yadav JS, Roubin GS, Iyer S, et al: Elective stenting of the extracranial carotid arteries. Circulation 95:376, 1997.

190. Zarins CK, DelBaccaro EJ, Johns L, et al: Increased cerebral blood flow after external carotid artery revascularization. Surgery 89:730, 1981.

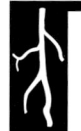

C H A P T E R   1 3 2

Vertebrobasilar Ischemia: Indications, Techniques, and Results of Surgical Repair

Ramon Berguer, M.D., Ph.D.

INDICATIONS

Direct surgery on the vertebral artery (VA) to correct stenosis or occlusion may be indicated for two types of patients: (1) those with vertebrobasilar ischemia (VBI), to increase blood flow to the basilar territory or to prevent further embolization and (2) those with extensive severe and symptomatic extracranial disease, to increase total brain blood flow.

VBI may be due to *microembolization* from the heart or, more frequently, from the arteries leading to the basilar artery (innominate, proximal subclavian, and vertebral arteries). These patients may present with transient ischemic attacks (TIAs) or infarctions in the territory supplied by the basilar artery. The importance of the *embolic* mechanism as a cause of vertebrobasilar symptoms has only recently been emphasized.[1, 2] This new information is derived from autopsy studies, from magnetic resonance imaging (MRI), which can identify small infarcts in the brain stem and cerebellum (previously not visualized by computed tomography [CT] scanning), and from selective arteriograms showing the embolic source in the subclavian or vertebral arteries. Patients with embolic VBI develop multiple infarcts in the brain stem, cerebellum, and, occasionally, posterior cerebral artery territory and have a high incidence of stroke. About 30% of patients with symptoms of VBI have microembolization as the cause.[1]

The *hemodynamic* mechanism of VBI is better recognized and more frequent than the embolic type. Patients with VBI present with TIAs in the territory of the basilar artery because of the lack of appropriate inflow from the VA and inadequate compensation from the carotid territory. Hemodynamic VBI, manifested as TIAs, is usually caused by stenosis or occlusion of the VA. Although the majority of these lesions are atherosclerotic plaques, the VA may also be compressed extrinsically by osteophytes adjacent to the VA canal. For patients with hemodynamic VBI, it is essential to rule out systemic causes of VBI before advising arteriography.

In the later years of life, VA stenosis is a frequent arteriographic finding, and dizziness is also a common symptom. The presence of both in a patient cannot be assumed to be a cause-and-effect relationship. Common systemic causes of VBI are orthostatic hypotension, poorly regulated antihypertensive therapy, arrhythmias, heart failure, malfunction of pacemakers, and anemia.

The evaluation of patients with VBI should include a number of specific steps. The precise circumstances associated with development of symptoms should be ascertained. Symptoms often appear on standing in older individuals with poor sympathetic control of their venous tone, which causes excessive pooling of blood in the veins of the leg. This is particularly common in patients with diabetes who have diminished sympathetic reflexes. We use an arbitrary 20-mmHg systolic pressure drop on rapid standing as the criterion for a diagnosis of orthostatic hypotension causing hypoperfusion of the vertebral arteries. The pressure drop in these cases triggers the symptoms of VBI.

Patients may relate symptoms to turning or extending their heads. Symptoms may appear only when turning the head to one side. Frequently, the mechanism here is extrinsic compression of the VA, usually the dominant or the only one, by arthritic bone spurs.[3] To differentiate this mechanism from VBI secondary to otologic labyrinthine disorders that may appear with head or body rotation, the patient should attempt to reproduce the symptoms by turning the head *slowly* and then repeating the maneuver, but this time briskly, as when shaking the head from side to side. In labyrinthine disease, the sudden inertial changes caused by the latter maneuver result in immediate symptoms and nystagmus. Conversely, in extrinsic VA compression, a short delay occurs before the patient fears for his or her balance.

Demonstration of extrinsic compression of the VA, usually by osteophytes, requires an arteriogram. This is performed either with the patient sitting up, by means of bilateral brachial injections, or with the patient supine in Trendelenburg's position with the head against a block if the femoral route is used. In these positions, intended to exert axial compression of the cervical vertebrae, the angiographer should request the specific rotation or extension of the head that provokes the symptoms. When the patient is rendered symptomatic, the arteriographic injection demonstrates the extrinsic compression. The reason for these positional requirements is that the weight of the head acting on the cervical spine changes its curvature and decreases the distance between C1 and C7. This longitudinal compression of the spine often enhances the extrinsic compression effects caused by osteophytic spurs.[4]

A CT scan is mandatory to rule out a brain tumor and to assess the integrity of the brain. Unsuspected hemispheric infarction may be found, but brain stem infarctions are often missed because they tend to be smaller in size and the resolution of the CT scan in this area is poor. For patients who are candidates for vertebral arterial reconstruction, MRI brain scans should routinely be performed to ascertain whether infarctions have taken place in the vertebrobasilar territory. Excessive use of antihypertensive medications can also cause hemodynamic VBI by decreasing the perfusion pressure and inducing severe orthostatic hypotension.

An ambulatory 24-hour electrocardiogram (ECG) (Holter monitor) is obtained in all patients evaluated for hemodynamic VBI. Sometimes patients with VBI secondary to arrhythmias recognize the association of palpitations with the appearance of VBI symptoms, the latter being secondary to decreased cardiac output resulting from the arrhythmia.

Physical examination can alert the physician to the possibility of a subclavian steal in patients with brachial pressure differences greater than 25 mmHg or with diminished or absent pulses in one arm. The diagnosis of reversal of VA flow can be made accurately by noninvasive indirect methods[5] and demonstrated directly by duplex imaging.

Any systemic mechanism that decreases the mean pressure of the basilar artery may be responsible for the syndrome of VBI. Affected individuals may or may not have concomitant VA stenosis or occlusion. For some patients, the cause of the drop in mean arterial pressure can be corrected by readjustment of their antihypertensive medication, by administration of antiarrhythmic drugs, or by insertion of a cardiac pacemaker. In patients with orthostatic hypotension, the problem may not respond to medical treatment and only the reconstruction of a diseased or occluded VA will render the patient asymptomatic in the face of persistent oscillations of blood pressure secondary to poor sympathetic venous tone. Rheologic factors, such as increased viscosity (polycythemia) and decreased oxygen-carrying capacity (anemia), may exacerbate or cause VBI in patients with severe VA occlusive disease.

The second major indication for VA reconstruction pertains to patients who have extensive extracranial disease with one or both internal carotid arteries occluded and who have global manifestations of cerebrovascular ischemia. In these patients the carotid arteries may be occluded or involved with severe siphon stenosis, making a direct revascularization via the internal carotid arteries impossible, and reconstruction of the VA may offer the best option for reestablishment of adequate cerebral blood flow. In patients with global ischemia, the VAs are important pathways for cerebral perfusion and they may be critically stenosed; if they are occluded, they can be revascularized at the skull base. In this latter group, demonstration of satisfactory posterior communicating arteries increases the likelihood of success.

In VA reconstructions done for hemodynamic symptoms, the minimal anatomic requirement to justify a VA reconstruction is bilateral stenosis of more than 60% diameter if both VAs are patent or a greater than 60% diameter stenosis in the dominant VA. It is assumed that a hypoplastic VA ending in a posteroinferior cerebellar artery is equivalent to an occluded VA. In addition, a normal VA is sufficient to perfuse adequately the basilar artery, regardless of a stenosis in the contralateral VA. In patients with embolic lesions in one vertebral (or subclavian) artery, the potential source of the embolus needs to be eliminated regardless of the status of the contralateral VA.

In our series of VA reconstructions, 96% of patients presented with neurologic symptoms (TIA or stroke) and 4% were asymptomatic. The neurologic symptoms were referable to the hemispheres in 4%, to the vertebrobasilar system in 60%, and were considered global in 30%.

ARTERIOGRAPHIC EVALUATION

The arteriographic investigation of VA pathology necessitates systematic positions and projections to evaluate the vertebrobasilar system from its origin to the top of the basilar artery. The VA is divided into four segments, each with specific radiologic and pathologic features (Fig. 132–1).

Arteriographic evaluation begins with an arch view, which will determine the presence or absence of VAs on each side; it will show whether one VA is dominant (generally the left) and whether one of the VAs has an abnormal origin. The most common anomalous origin is the left VA, originating from the arch (6%). A much rarer variant is the right VA arising from the innominate or right common carotid artery (Fig. 132–2); this is present in patients with a retroesophageal right subclavian artery. Arch views must be obtained in at least two projections: right and left posterior obliques. Usually these two views display well the *first segment* (V1) of the VA, from its origin to the transverse process of C6. Occasionally additional oblique views may be required (see below).

The most common atherosclerotic lesion of the VA is stenosis of its origin. This lesion may be missed in standard arch views because of superimposition of the subclavian

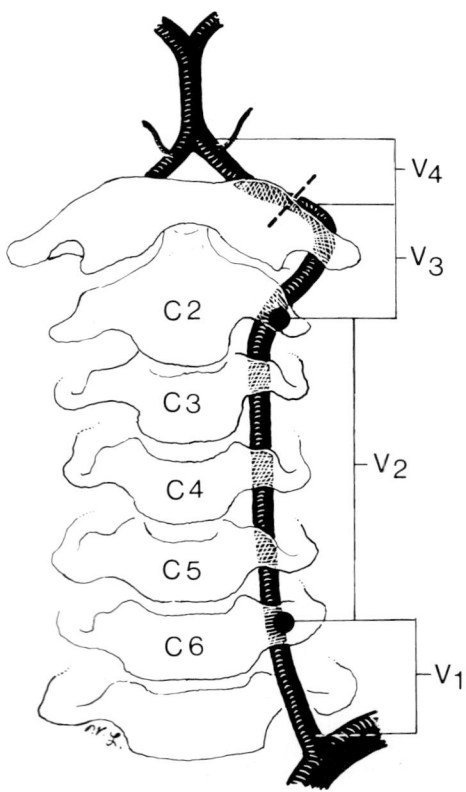

FIGURE 132–1. The four segments of the vertebral artery (VA). (From Berguer R: Surgical management of the vertebral artery. *In* Moore WS [ed]: Surgery for Cerebrovascular Disease. Reproduced by permission of Churchill Livingstone, Inc, New York, 1986.)

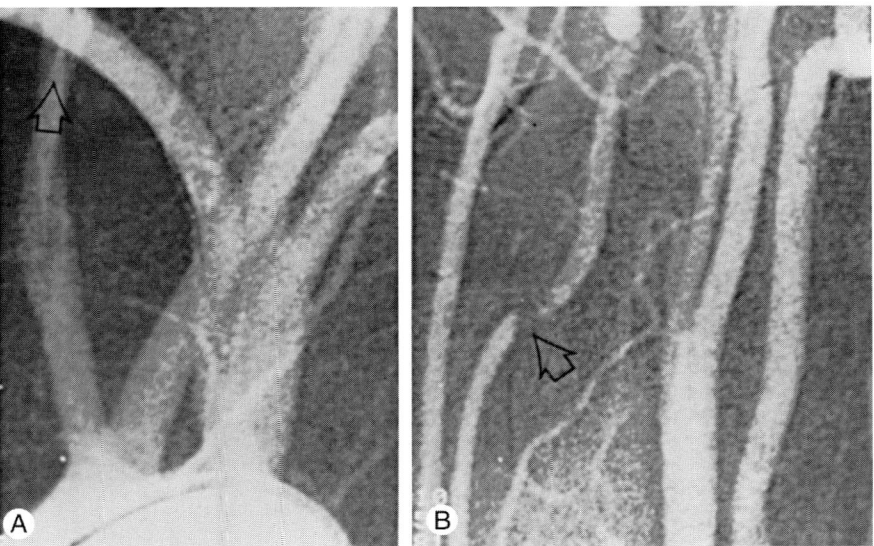

FIGURE 132–2. Arch injection in a 33-year-old woman with vertebrobasilar ischemia. *A,* The right vertebral artery (VA) and the right external carotid artery arise from a long common right carotid trunk (*arrow*). The right internal carotid artery is congenitally absent. The right subclavian arises as the last branch of the aorta. *B,* The right VA, which has an anomalous origin, enters the spine at a high level (C4) and is severely compressed (*arrow*) at this level on head rotation.

artery over the first segment of the VA. Additional oblique projections may be needed to "throw off" the subclavian artery in order to obtain a clear view of the origin of the VA (Fig. 132–3). The presence of a post-stenotic dilatation in the first centimeter of the VA suggests that there may be a significant stenosis at its origin that cannot be seen because of an overlying subclavian artery. Redundancy and kinks are common, but only very severe kinks associated with post-stenotic dilatations produce hemodynamic symptoms.

Visualization of the *second segment* (V2) of the VA. from C6 to the top of the transverse process of C2, can usually be accomplished in the oblique arch views in conjunction with selective subclavian injections. The point of entry of the artery in the spine is determined, and an abnormally low entry at the level of C7 instead of C6 should be noted.

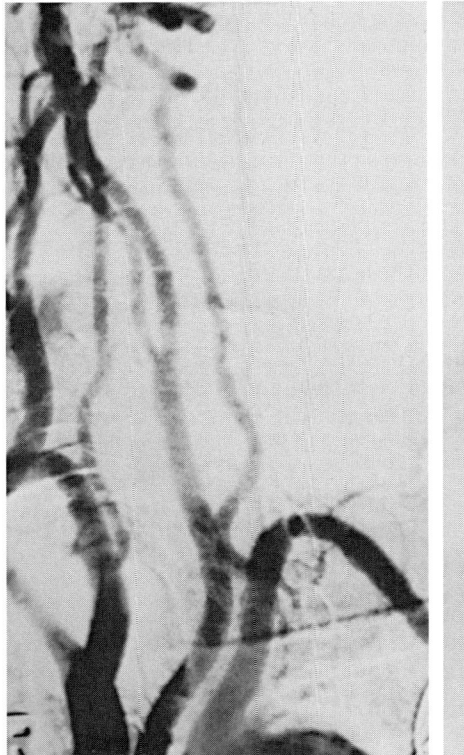
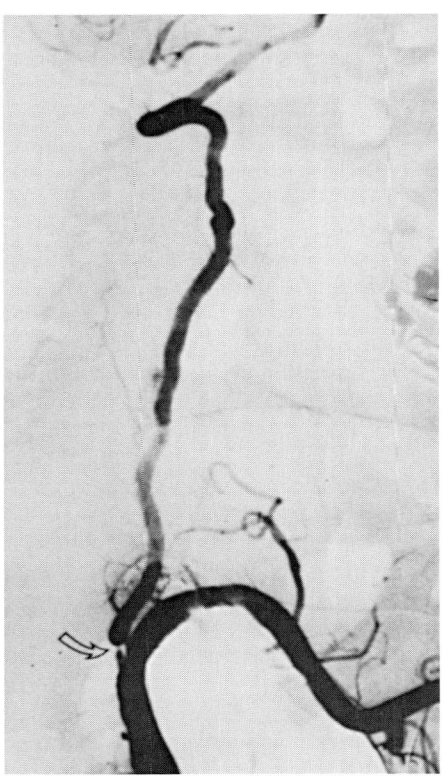

FIGURE 132–3. A severe stenosis (*arrow*) of a dominant left vertebral artery (VA) seen only after additional oblique rotation of the patient (*right*). (From Berguer R: Role of vertebral artery surgery after carotid endarterectomy. *In* Bergan JJ, Yao JST [eds]: Reoperative Arterial Surgery. Orlando, Fla, Grune & Stratton, 1986, pp 555–564.)

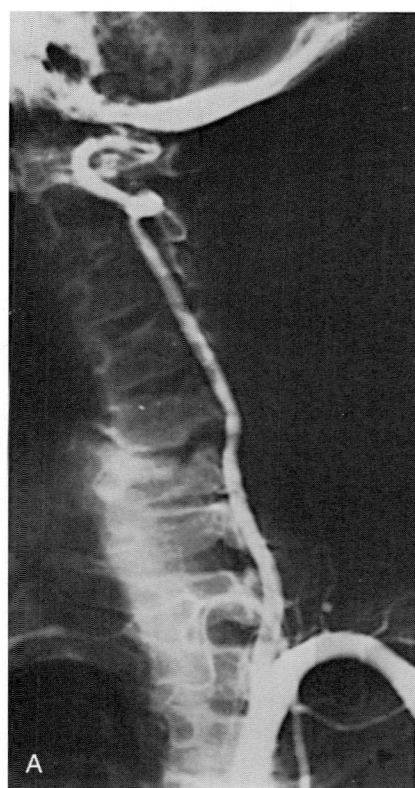
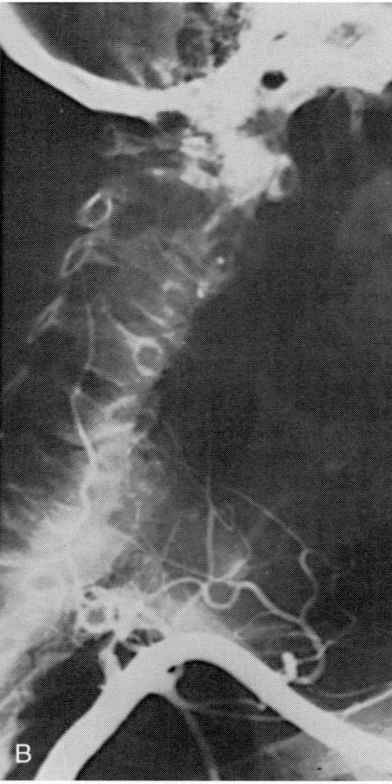

FIGURE 132–4. A patient with a single vertebral artery (VA) showing minimal extrinsic compression (A) when the neck is rotated to the right and occlusion (B) when the neck is rotated to the left. (From Berguer R: Surgical management of the vertebral artery. *In* Moore WS [ed]: Surgery for Cerebrovascular Disease. Reproduced by permission of Churchill Livingstone, Inc, New York, 1986.)

This finding is associated with a short V1 segment of the VA, which suggests inadequate length will be available to allow its transposition to the common carotid artery. The level of entry into the spine is best determined in unsubtracted views. Extrinsic compression by musculotendinous structures is common in a VA with an abnormally high level of entry into the spine, usually C4 or C5 (see Fig. 132–2). This is due to the sharp angulation resulting from the abnormal level of entry.

The most common pathology of the V2 segment is extrinsic compression of the VA by osteophytes.[3] In patients with symptoms prompted by neck rotation, the V2 segment must be evaluated with arteriograms taken with the neck in right and left rotation. The VA may be perfectly normal in one projection and be occluded in the other by extrinsic compression (Fig. 132–4). The compression perpetrator may be bone (an osteophyte) or tendon (longus colli). The V2 and V3 segments are frequent sites for traumatic or spontaneous arteriovenous fistulae because of the fixation of the adventitia of the VA to the periosteum of the vertebral foramina and the close proximity of the artery to its surrounding venous plexus. The VA may tear completely or incompletely (dissection) as a consequence of stretch injury after brisk rotation or hyperextension of the neck.

The *third segment* of the VA (V3) extends from the top of the transverse process of C2 to the atlanto-occipital membrane. After crossing this membrane, the artery enters the foramen magnum at the base of the skull and becomes intradural. The first two cervical vertebrae are the most mobile of the spine. About 50% of the neck rotation occurs between C1 and C2. The VA is redundant at this level to allow for the arc of displacement of the transverse process of the atlas (about 80 degrees) to which the VA is attached. The most common problems at this level are arterial dissection, arteriovenous fistulae, and arteriovenous aneurysms. Dissection may be associated with fibromuscular dysplasia or occur after trauma such as sudden rotation or extension in acceleration/deceleration trauma (Fig. 132–5). A dissection may produce stenosis, thrombosis, or aneurysmal dilatation. Arteriovenous fistula or arteriovenous aneurysm results from rupture of the wall of the VA into its surrounding venous plexus. In long-standing fistulae the pulsatile mass formed by the fistula and its dilated venous channels is called an *arteriovenous aneurysm.*

An anatomic finding crucial for surgical strategy is that when the VA is occluded proximally it usually reconstitutes at the V3 segment via collateral blood vessels linking the occipital artery with the VA at this level (Fig. 132–6). Because of this collateral network, the distal (V3 + V4) vertebral and basilar arteries usually remain patent despite a proximal VA occlusion.

The *fourth segment* (V4) is infrequently affected by atherosclerosis. Finally, the basilar artery (Fig. 132–7) should be clearly seen in lateral or oblique projection. Subtracted views are needed to eliminate the temporal bone density in the lateral projection. In the Towne anteroposterior view, routinely used in neuroradiology, the basilar artery is foreshortened and therefore the resolution is poor. Advanced atherosclerotic disease of the basilar artery contraindicates reconstruction of VA lesions.

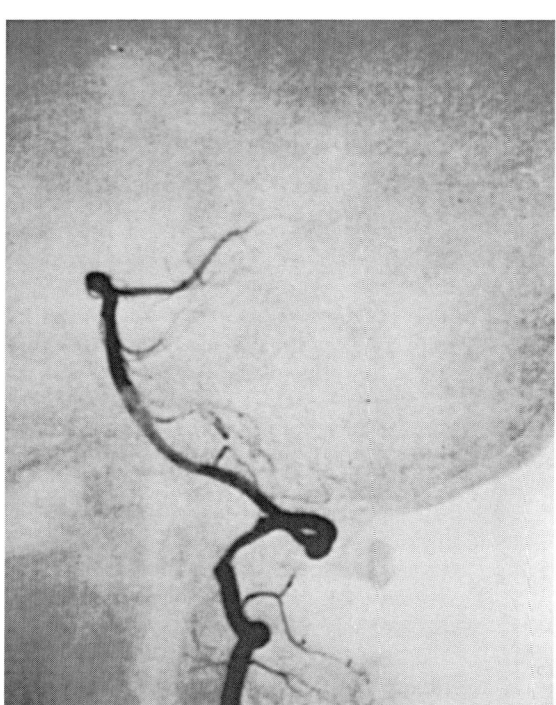

FIGURE 132-5. Intramural dissection of the vertebral artery at the V3 segment in a 40-year-old woman with Klippel-Feil syndrome and subluxation of the atlantoaxial joint.

SURGICAL TECHNIQUES

With rare exceptions, most reconstructions of the VA are performed to relieve either an orificial stenosis (V1 segment) or stenosis, dissection or occlusion of its intraspinal component (V2 and V3 segments).[6]

Although in the 1970s Berguer and colleagues advocated the correction of proximal VA disease by subclavian-vertebral bypass,[7, 8] they currently seldom use this technique, reserving it for uncommon anatomic circumstances such as (1) contralateral carotid occlusion that increases the risk of clamping the only carotid supply during VA-carotid transposition; (2) a short V1 segment; or (3) VA entrance into the foramen transversarium of C7. As previously noted, the latter anatomic variant provides inadequate length to transpose the VA to the common carotid artery. For disease involving the origin of the VA, we routinely perform a transposition of this vessel into the common carotid artery, which is a better and more durable operation than subclavian-VA bypass. The common carotid artery is more accessible than the subclavian artery, and this procedure needs only one anastomosis without a vein graft.

For disease involving any level at or above the transverse process of C6, we routinely carry the reconstruction to the C2 to C1 level (V3 segment). This is usually accomplished by a common carotid to distal VA bypass,[9–12] although other techniques (see later) may be required in specific circumstances. Bypasses above the level of C1 (suboccipital) are technically demanding and have been required in only 4% of cases of distal VA reconstruction. There is no reason to approach the VA for reconstruction in its V2 portion, where the exposure is poorer than that obtained in the V3

segment. In addition, reconstruction of the VA above the level of C2 bypasses most potential areas of extrinsic compression by osteophytes.

Transposition of the Vertebral Artery into the Common Carotid Artery

If the VA operation is performed as an isolated procedure, the incision is supraclavicular approaching the VA between the heads of the sternocleidomastoid muscle (Fig. 132–8). The omohyoid muscle is divided. The jugular vein and vagus nerve are retracted laterally, and the carotid sheath is entered. The carotid artery should be exposed proximally as far as possible; this is facilitated if the surgeon temporarily stands at the head of the patient and looks down into the mediastinum.

After the carotid artery is mobilized, the sympathetic chain is identified running behind and parallel to it. The thoracic duct is divided between ligatures, which avoids any transfixion sutures that may result in lymph leaks. The proximal end of the thoracic duct is doubly ligated. Accessory lymph ducts should be identified, ligated, and divided. The entire dissection is confined medial to the prescalene fat pad that covers the scalenus anticus muscle and phrenic nerve. These latter structures are left unexposed lateral to the field, thus avoiding potential phrenic

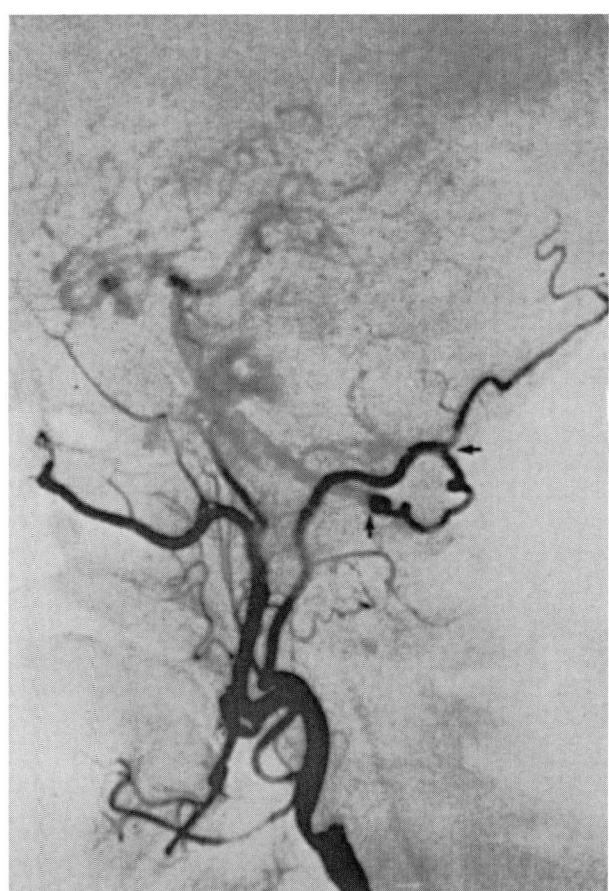

FIGURE 132-6. The distal vertebral and basilar artery being fed by an occipital collateral in a patient with proximal vertebral artery occlusion.

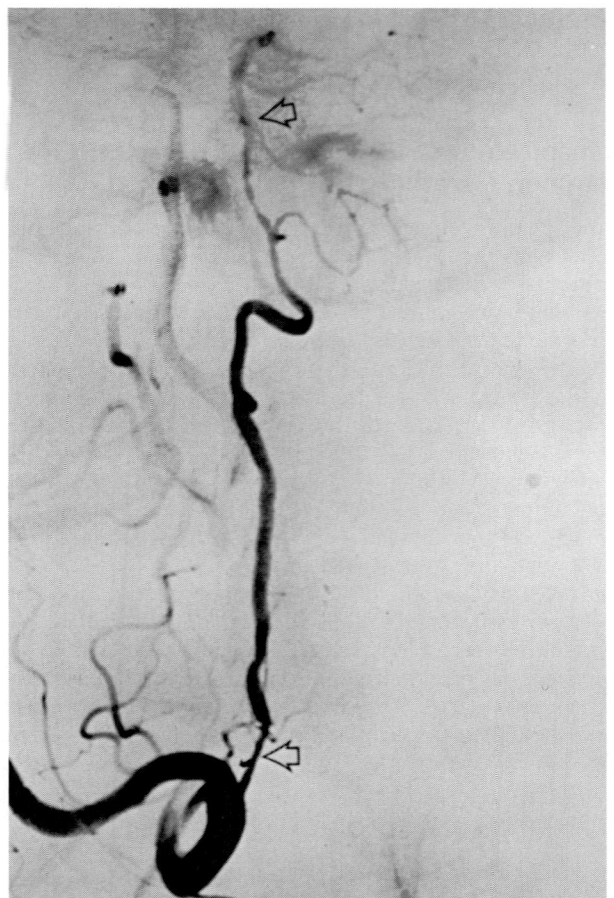

FIGURE 132–7. Arteriogram showing atheromatous disease of the V1 and V4 segments (*arrows*) of the vertebral artery and of the basilar artery.

nerve injury. The inferior thyroid artery runs transversely across the field, and it is ligated and divided.

The vertebral vein is next identified emerging from the angle formed by the longus colli and scalenus anticus and overlying the VA and, at the bottom of the field, the subclavian artery. Unlike its sister artery, the vertebral vein has branches. It is ligated in continuity and divided. Below the vertebral vein lies the VA. It is important to identify and avoid injury to the entire sympathetic chain. The VA is dissected superiorly to the tendon of the longus colli and interiorly to its origin in the subclavian artery. To preserve the sympathetic trunks and the stellate or intermediate ganglia resting on the artery, it may be necessary to isolate and loop the VA above and below these structures. The VA is freed from the sympathetic trunk resting on its anterior surface without damaging the trunk or the interganglionic connections.

Once the artery is fully exposed, an appropriate site for reimplantation in the common carotid artery is selected. The patient is given systemic heparin. The distal portion of the V1 segment of the VA is clamped below the edge of the longus colli with a microclip placed vertically to indicate the orientation of the artery and to avoid axial twisting during its transposition. The proximal VA, immediately above the stenosis at its origin, is occluded with a hemoclip, transected directly above it, and the stump is oversewn by

a transfixing polypropylene suture. The artery is then pulled from under the overlying sympathetic trunk and brought to the common carotid artery. The free end of the VA is spatulated for anastomosis.

The carotid artery is then cross-clamped. An elliptical defect of approximately 5 × 7 mm is created in the posterolateral wall of the common carotid artery with an aortic punch. The anastomosis is performed in open fashion with continuous 6-0 or 7-0 polypropylene suture, avoiding any tension on the VA, which tears easily. Before completion of the anastomosis, the suture slack is tightened appropriately with a nerve hook, standard flushing maneuvers are performed, and the suture is tied with reestablishment of flow.

When a simultaneous carotid endarterectomy is planned (Fig. 132–9), the VA is approached through the standard carotid incision extended inferiorly to the head of the clavicle. With this approach, the sternocleidomastoid muscle is lateral and the field is a bit narrower than when the VA is approached between the heads of the sternocleidomastoid. The remaining steps of the operation are as described previously.

Distal Vertebral Artery Reconstruction

Reconstruction of the distal VA is generally done at the C1 to C2 level. Rarely the reconstruction is done at the C0 to C1 level with a posterior neck approach. Various techniques can be applied to revascularize the VA in its V3 segment between the transverse processes of C1 and C2, but the approach to the VA at this level is the same for all procedures.[11–13]

The incision is anterior to the sternocleidomastoid muscle, the same as in a carotid operation, and is carried superiorly to immediately below the earlobe (Fig. 132–10). The dissection proceeds between the jugular vein and the anterior edge of the sternocleidomastoid, exposing the spinal accessory nerve. The nerve is followed distally as it joins the jugular vein and crosses in front of the transverse process of C1, which can be easily felt by the operator's finger. This necessitates freeing and retracting the digastric muscle upward or resecting it.

The next step involves the identification of the levator scapula muscle by removal of the fibrofatty tissue overlying it. With the anterior edge of the levator scapula identified, the surgeon searches for the anterior ramus of C2. With the ramus as a guide, a right-angle clamp is slid over the ramus, elevating the levator scapula muscle, which is transected (Fig. 132–11). The proximal stump of the levator is excised up to its insertion on the C1 transverse process. The C2 ramus divides into three branches after crossing the VA. The artery runs below, in contact with the nerve and perpendicular to it. The surgeon cuts the ramus (Fig. 132–12) before its branching; underneath it, the VA can be identified.

The dissection of the artery at this level is best accomplished with loupe magnification, advisable for all vertebral artery reconstruction. The artery is freed from the surrounding veins with extreme care because hemorrhage is difficult to control at this level. Before encircling the artery with polymeric silicone (Silastic) vessel loops, one must ensure that the occipital collateral artery does not join the

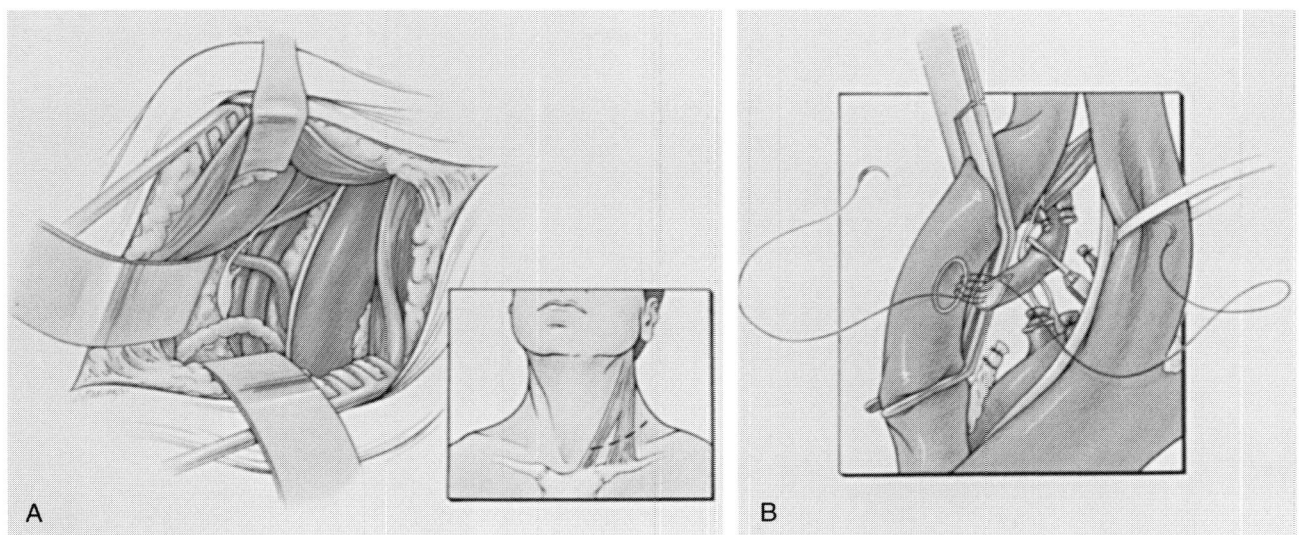

FIGURE 132–8. *A*, Access to the proximal vertebral artery (VA) between the sternocleidomastoid muscle bellies. *B*, Transposition of the proximal VA to the posterior wall of the common carotid artery. (*A* and *B*, from Berguer R, Kieffer E: Surgery of the Arteries to the Head. New York, Springer-Verlag, 1992.)

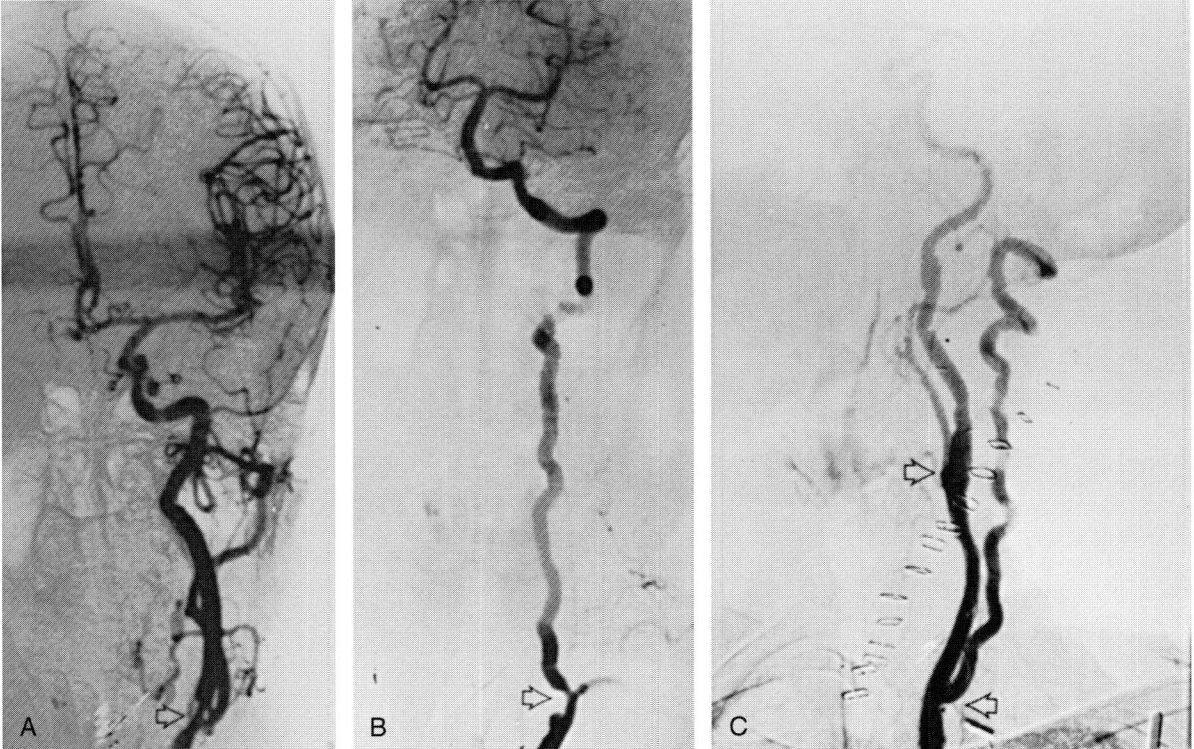

FIGURE 132–9. *A* and *B*, Arteriogram in a patient with left hemispheric transient symptoms showing carotid and vertebral (dominant) arterial stenoses (*arrows*). *C*, Arteriogram obtained 2 days after left carotid endarterectomy and transposition of the left vertebral artery into the left common carotid artery (*arrows*).

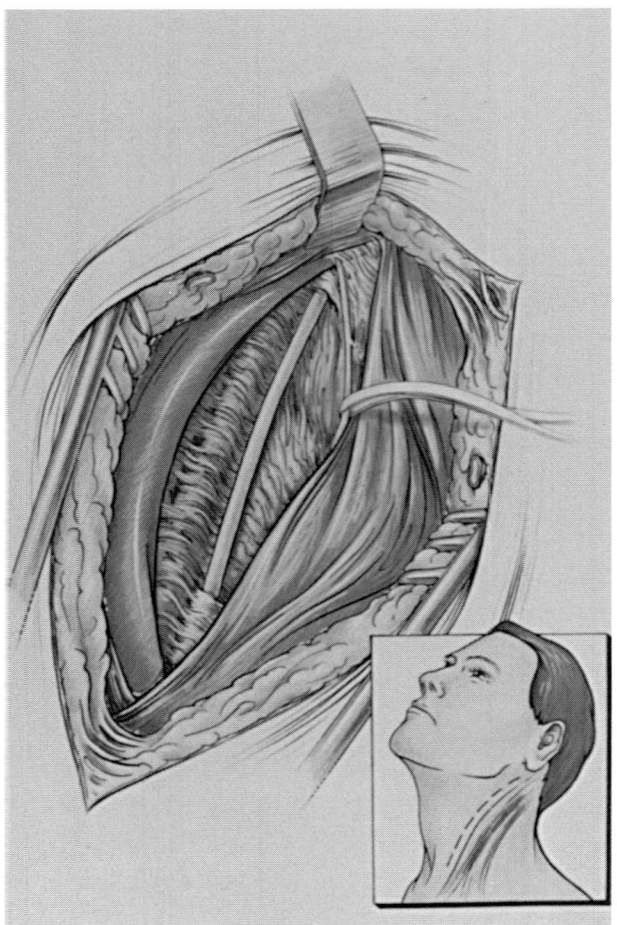

FIGURE 132–10. Retrojugular approach and isolation of the spinal accessory nerve. (From Berguer R, Kieffer E: Surgery of the Arteries to the Head. New York, Springer-Verlag, 1992.)

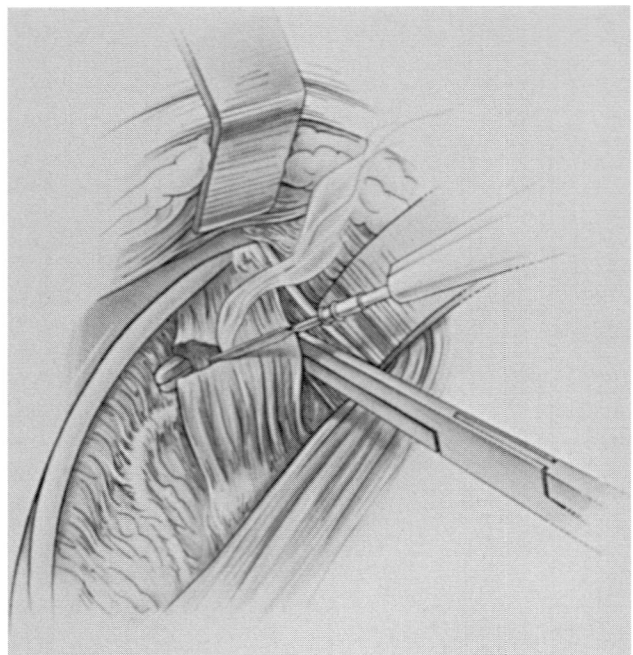

FIGURE 132–11. Dividing the levator scapula over the C2 ramus. The vagus, internal jugular vein, and internal carotid artery are anterior to the muscle. (From Berguer R, Kieffer E: Surgery of the Arteries to the Head. New York, Springer-Verlag, 1992.)

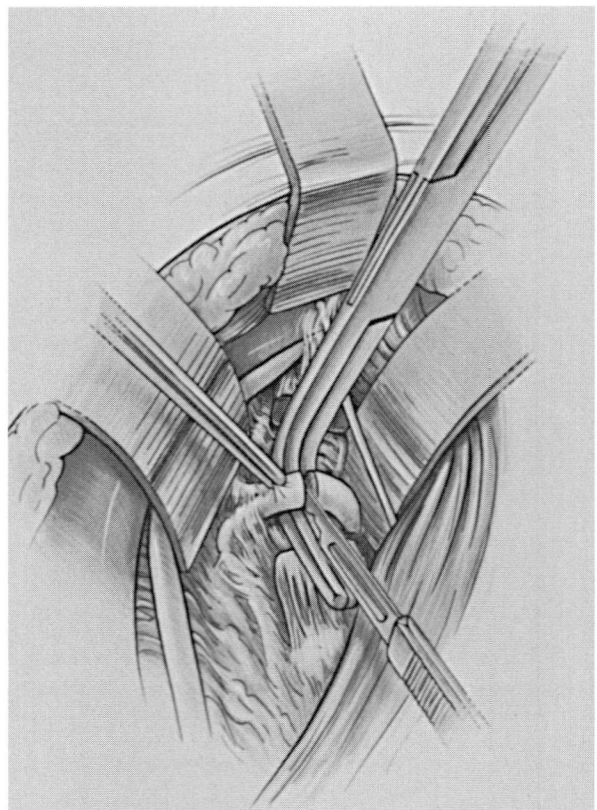

FIGURE 132–12. Dividing the anterior ramus of C2 to expose the underlying vertebral artery running perpendicular to the former. (From Berguer R, Kieffer E: Surgery of the Arteries to the Head. New York, Springer-Verlag, 1992.)

posterior aspect of the VA at the location at which the surgeon is dissecting to avoid tearing this important collateral vessel (Fig. 132–13). Once the VA is encircled, the distal common carotid artery is dissected and prepared to receive a saphenous vein graft. There is no need to dissect the carotid bifurcation. The location selected for the proximal anastomosis of the saphenous vein graft on the common carotid artery should not be too close to the bifurcation because cross-clamping at this level may fracture underlying atheroma.

A saphenous vein graft of appropriate length is obtained and prepared. A valveless segment facilitates back-bleeding of the VA after completion of the distal anastomosis. The patient is given intravenous heparin. The VA is elevated and occluded with a small J-clamp that will isolate this segment for an end-to-side anastomosis. The VA is opened longitudinally with a coronary knife for a length adequate to accommodate the spatulated end of the vein graft. The end-to-side anastomosis is done with continuous 7-0 polypropylene. The distal anastomosis is assessed for back-flow, and, if satisfactory, a Heifitz's clip is placed in the vein graft proximal to the anastomosis, resuming flow through the VA.

The proximal end of the graft is passed beneath the

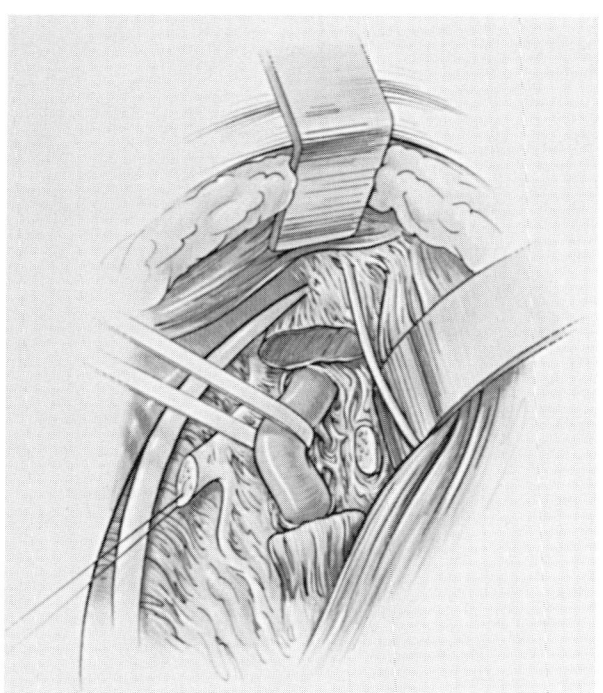

FIGURE 132–13. After the vertebral venous plexus is dissected away, the vertebral artery is slung with a polymeric silicone (Silastic) loop for clamping and anastomosis. (From Berguer R, Kieffer E: Surgery of the Arteries to the Head. New York, Springer-Verlag, 1992.)

jugular vein and in proximity to the side of the common carotid artery. The common carotid artery is then cross-clamped, an elliptical arteriotomy is made in its posterior wall with an aortic punch, and the proximal vein graft is anastomosed end-to-side to the common carotid artery with continuous 6-0 polypropylene (Fig. 132–14). Before the anastomosis is completed, standard flushing maneuvers are performed, the suture is tied, and flow is reestablished. Next, the proximal VA is occluded with a clip immediately below the anastomosis so as to avoid competitive flow and the potential for recurrent emboli.

Variations on Technique

The distal VA may also be revascularized via the external carotid artery (ECA) either directly by means of a transposition of the ECA to the distal VA or by anastomosis of the proximal end of a graft to the ECA. The transposition of the ECA to the distal VA (Figs. 132–15 and 132–16) requires a carotid bifurcation free of disease and a long ECA trunk. ECAs that divide early often are too small to match the caliber of the VA. If the trunk of the ECA is of adequate size and length to reach the VA, the ECA is skeletonized by dividing all its branches. The ECA is then rotated over the internal carotid artery and beneath the jugular vein to construct an end-to-side anastomosis to the distal VA at the C1 to C2 level. After completion of this anastomosis, the proximal VA, immediately below the anastomosis, is permanently occluded with a clip.

A patient may have a segment of saphenous vein that is of appropriate diameter but of insufficient length to bridge the distance between the common carotid artery and the distal VA. In this case, the proximal ECA can be used as

the inflow source for the vein graft. This technique is particularly useful when the contralateral internal carotid artery is occluded and avoidance of clamping the common carotid supplying the only patent internal carotid artery is desirable. If a vein bypass graft is used between the ECA and the distal VA, it should be placed with the proper amount of tension and assessed with the neck rotated back to the neutral position to avoid kinking.

In patients under 35 years of age without atherosclerosis, the cause of VA occlusion is usually trauma (subluxation, injury), fibromuscular dysplasia, or deliberate ligation (during a Blalock-Taussig procedure) (Fig. 132–17). These patients usually have patent internal carotid arteries, and collaterals to the distal VA develop via an enlarged ECA branch (occipital). These collaterals may nevertheless be too small to provide adequate flow into the basilar system. Under these circumstances, if the occipital artery is sufficiently enlarged, it can be directly anastomosed to the distal VA (Fig. 132–18). This strategy should also be considered in patients who do not have a satisfactory saphenous vein. If the patient is at risk for atherosclerosis, however, one should ensure that the origin of the ECA is not stenotic.

Another method of revascularization of the distal VA is the transposition of this vessel into the distal cervical internal carotid artery below the transverse process of C1 (Fig. 132–19). This technique is particularly applicable for patients with inadequate saphenous veins or in whom the ECA cannot be used because of unsuitable anatomy or disease in the carotid bifurcation. This is a straightforward end-to-side anastomosis between the distal VA and the

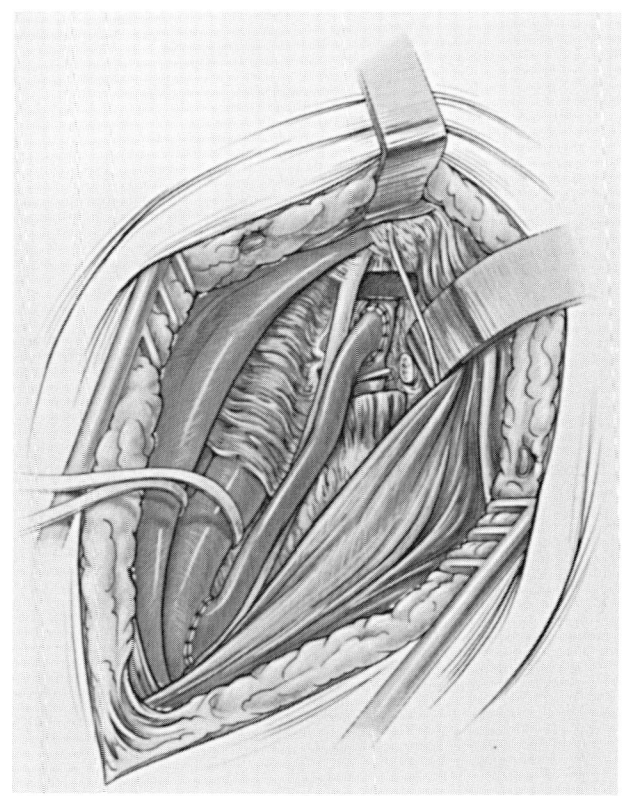

FIGURE 132–14. A completed common carotid artery to distal vertebral artery bypass using saphenous vein. (From Berguer R, Kieffer E: Surgery of the Arteries to the Head. New York, Springer-Verlag, 1992.)

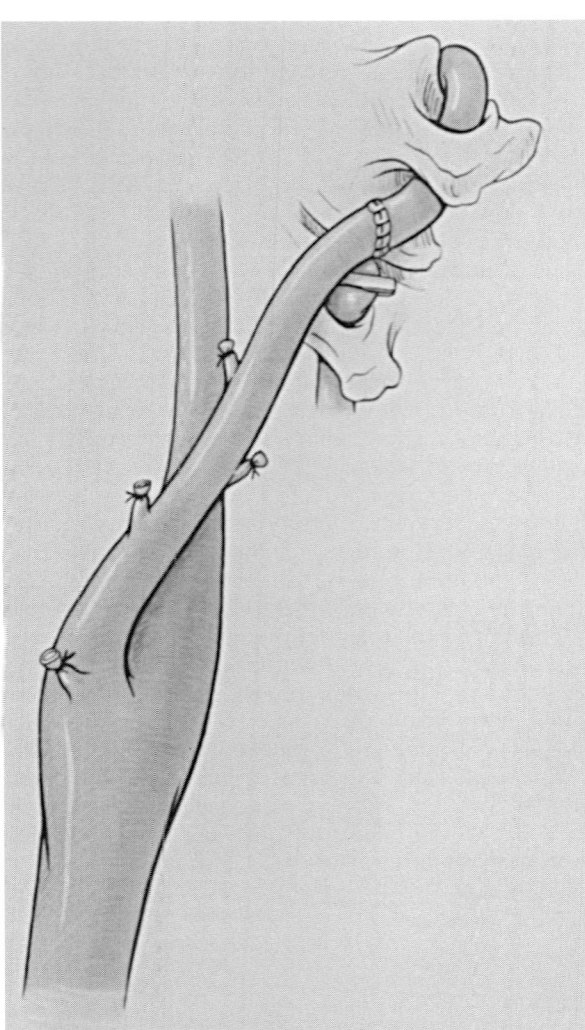

FIGURE 132–15. Transposition of external carotid artery to distal vertebral artery. (From Berguer R, Kieffer E: Surgery of the Arteries to the Head. New York, Springer-Verlag, 1992.)

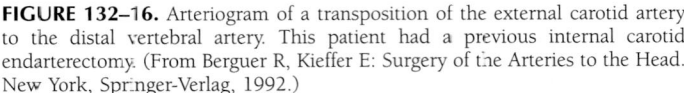
FIGURE 132–16. Arteriogram of a transposition of the external carotid artery to the distal vertebral artery. This patient had a previous internal carotid endarterectomy. (From Berguer R, Kieffer E: Surgery of the Arteries to the Head. New York, Springer-Verlag, 1992.)

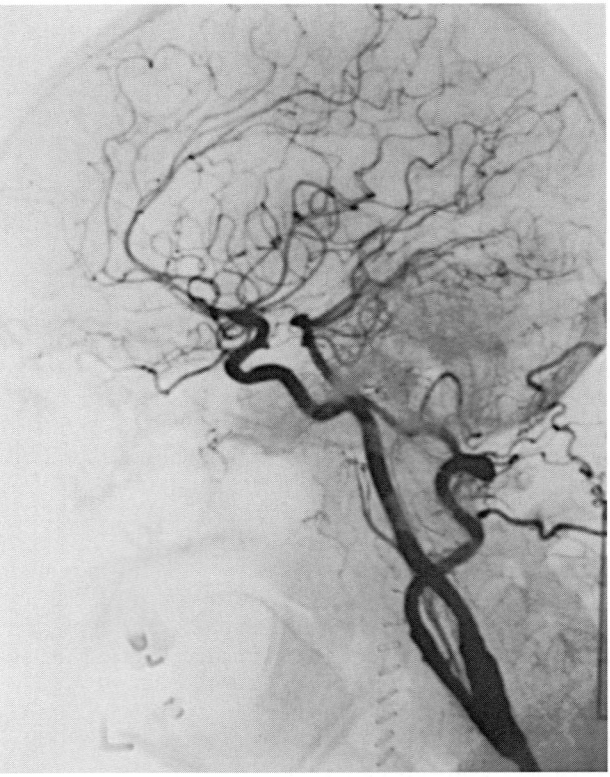

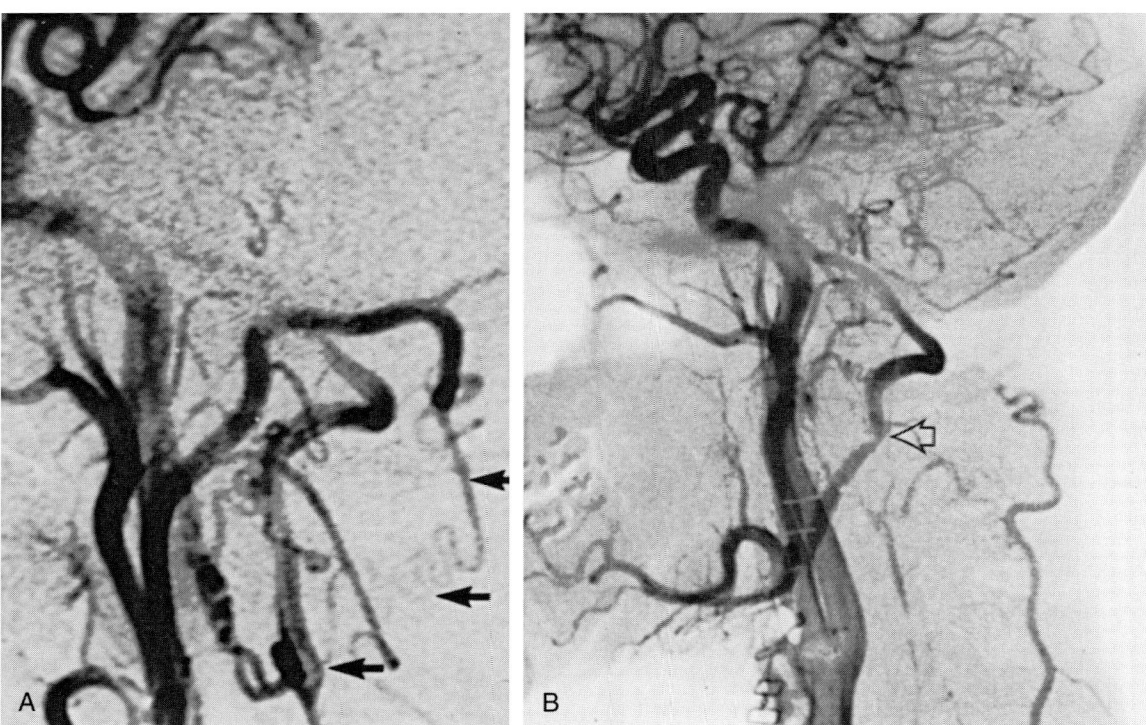

FIGURE 132–17. *A*, Occlusion of the proximal vertebral artery (bilaterally) in a young patient with congenital heart disease who underwent bilateral Blalock-Taussig procedures with ligation of both proximal VAs. *B*, Postoperative arteriogram showing an occipital to distal vertebral artery anastomosis.

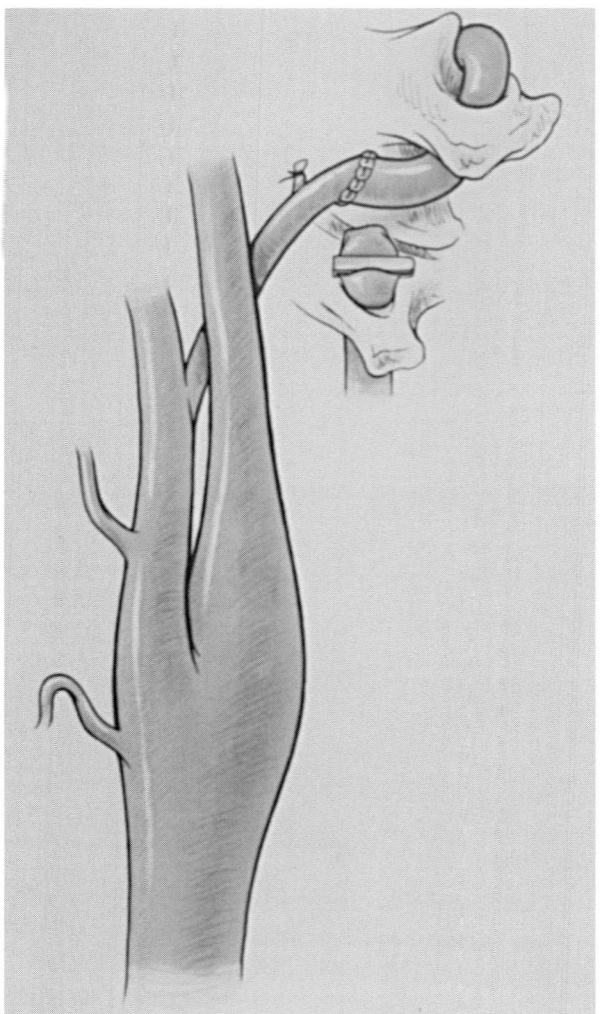

FIGURE 132–18. Transposition of the occipital artery to the distal vertebral artery. (From Berguer R, Kieffer E: Surgery of the Arteries to the Head. New York, Springer-Verlag, 1992.)

distal cervical internal carotid artery. This procedure, however, is contraindicated in patients with contralateral internal carotid artery occlusion in whom the risk of cerebral ischemia during the anastomosis would be prohibitive.

A small group of patients have disease up to the level of C1 and require revascularization in the last segment of extracranial VA.[14] To accomplish this, the VA must be exposed in its pars atlantica, where the artery runs parallel to the lamina of the atlas before entering the foramen magnum.

The approach to the suboccipital segment of the distal VA is posterior. The patient lies prone in the "park-bench" position. The incision is racket-shaped with a horizontal segment below the occipital bone from the midline laterally to the level of the sternocleidomastoid. There the incision becomes oblique and follows the posterior belly of the sternocleidomastoid muscle. The superficial nucchal muscle layer (splenius capitis and semispinalis) is transected (Fig. 132–20). The accessory spinal nerve is isolated laterally below the sternocleidomastoid muscle. The transverse process of C1 is located by palpation. The short posterior muscles between the atlas and occipital bone (obliquus

capitis and rectus capitis posterior major) are divided (Fig. 132–21). The artery can now be seen enveloped by a dense venous plexus (Fig. 132–22) from which it is extricated by bipolar coagulation and microligature of these veins. The artery can be exposed from its emergence at the top of C1 to the dura mater (Fig. 132–23). Through the same posterior approach, the internal carotid artery can be isolated posterior and medial to the sternocleidomastoid after mobilization and retraction of the hypoglossal and vagus nerves that, at this level, cover its posterior wall. The distal anastomosis of the vein graft to the VA is performed first. The vein is allowed to distend over the lamina of the atlas and into its site of anastomosis at the posterior wall of the internal carotid artery (Figs. 132–24 and 132–25).

RESULTS

The author's group's experience with reconstruction of the VA comprises 369 reconstructions, of which 252 were proximal and 117 were distal operations. Forty-eight VA reconstructions were performed in combination with a carotid operation.

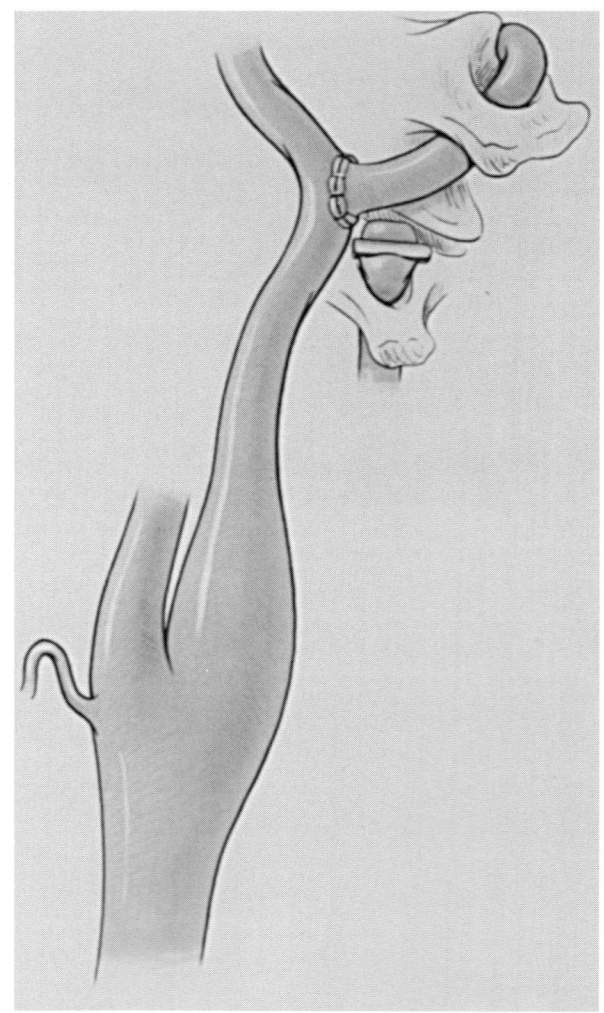

FIGURE 132–19. Transposition of the distal vertebral artery to the cervical internal carotid artery. (From Berguer R, Kieffer E: Surgery of the Arteries to the Head. New York, Springer-Verlag, 1992.)

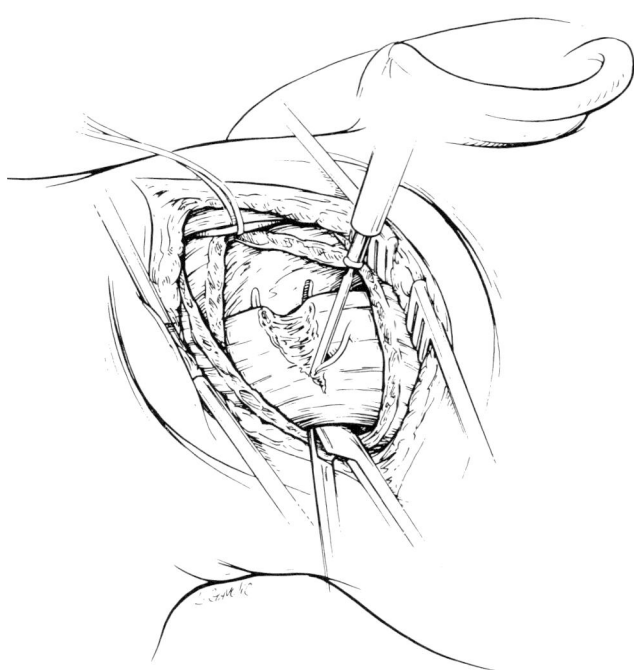

FIGURE 132–20. Posterior approach to the suboccipital segment of the distal vertebral artery: division of the splenius capitis and semispinalis.

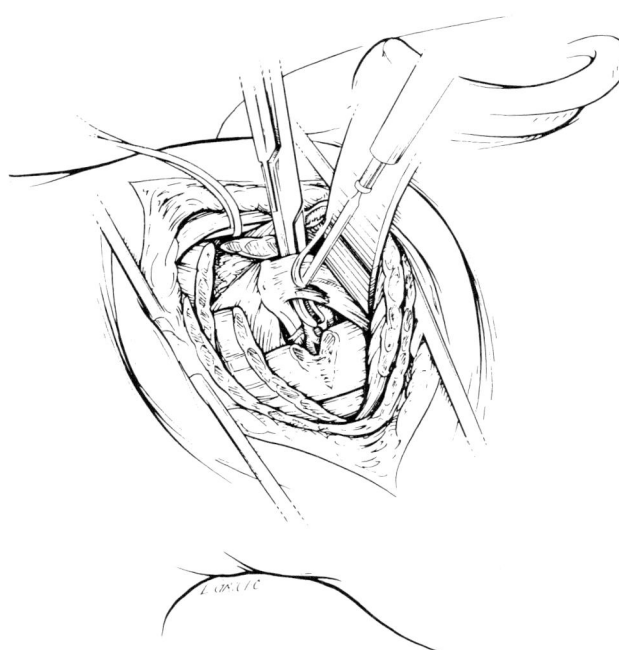

FIGURE 132–21. Posterior approach to the suboccipital vertebral artery: division of the obliquus and rectus capitis.

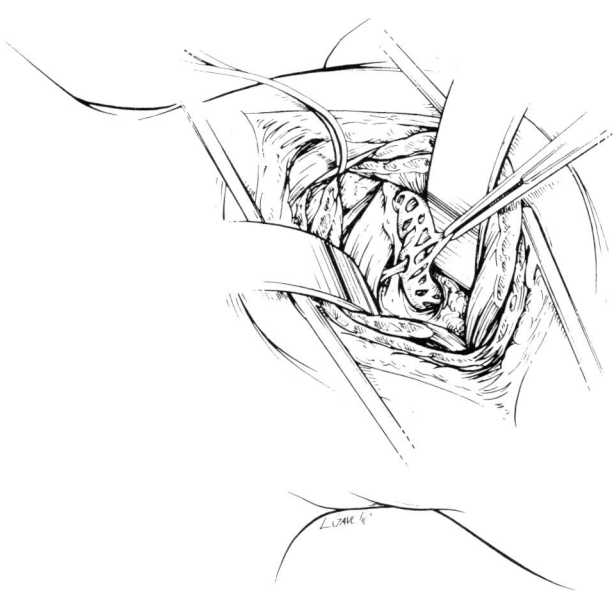

FIGURE 132–22. The pars atlantica of the distal vertebral artery exposed and surrounded by a dense venous plexus.

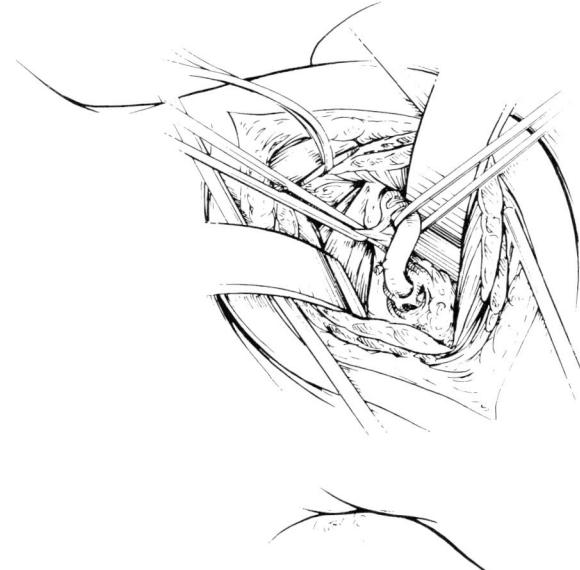

FIGURE 132–23. Exposure of the pars atlantica of the vertebral artery from its exit from the transverse foramen of C1 to its entrance in the dura mater.

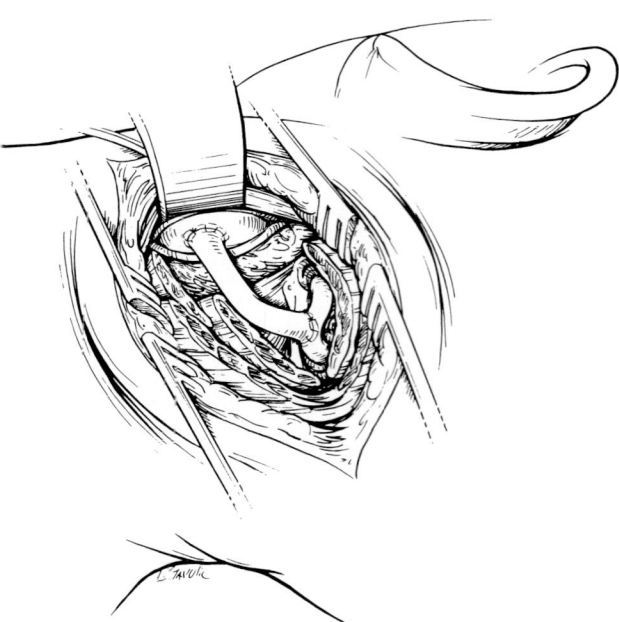

FIGURE 132–24. A distal cervical internal carotid to suboccipital vertebral bypass.

Proximal Vertebral Artery Reconstruction

Among patients undergoing proximal operations, there were no deaths or stroke in those who had only a vertebral reconstruction. When the proximal VA reconstruction was combined with a carotid operation, the observed stroke and death rates increased to 6%.

There were four instances of immediate postoperative thrombosis (1.5%). Three of the four patients had vein grafts interposed between the VA and the common carotid due to a short V1 segment. The grafts kinked and thrombosed. With better attention to avoidance of injury to the sympathetic chain, the incidence of Horner's syndrome has decreased to 10% in the last 90 patients.

Lymphocele was also a common complication early in our experience. By avoiding transfixion sutures and securely ligating the thoracic duct and any accessory ducts this complication practically has been eliminated. There was one postoperative hemorrhage necessitating reoperation in a patient in whom the origin of the VA was occluded with a hemoclip that became dislodged. A 5-0 transfixion ligature has been used routinely since then.

The cumulative patency rate of proximal VA reconstruction at 10 years was 92%.

Distal Vertebral Artery Reconstruction

Operations on the distal VA carry higher stroke and death rates than operations on the proximal VA (Table 132–1). Among 117 distal operations, there were seven strokes, five of which resulted in deaths: Three patients had brain stem strokes and deaths related to the procedure. Two died of a large hemispheric infarction.

Routine intraoperative postreconstruction arteriography was not used for the first part of our series. In the first 53 distal reconstructions done before January 1991, there were 3 stroke/deaths (4.5%) and an 11% rate of immediate

TABLE 132–1. RATES OF STROKE AND DEATH FOR ALL VERTEBRAL ARTERY RECONSTRUCTIONS BEFORE/SINCE JANUARY 1991

| | Before 1/91 (N:215) | | Since 1/91 (N:154) | |
	No.	%	No.	%
Stroke	9	4.1	3	1.9
Death	7	3.2	1	0.6
Death/stroke	11	5.1	3	1.9

postoperative thrombosis. After the introduction of routine intraoperative arteriography in 1991, we have performed an additional 64 distal vertebral reconstructions and, in this group, there was only one stroke/death (1.9%) and a 2% rate of immediate postoperative thrombosis. Although the improved results partly reflect a learning curve, they are primarily the consequence of correction of technical flaws that are identified by arteriography during the operation.

The cumulative patency rates for distal vertebral reconstruction at 5 years was 80%. Similar to patients undergoing standard carotid endarterectomies, 70% of the patients undergoing distal VA reconstruction are dead at 5-year follow-up, mostly from cardiac disease. Freedom from stroke among survivors at 5 years is 97%. In this group, symptoms were cured in 71% of patients and improved in 16% of patients.

It is appropriate to consider our experience in two periods. Before 1991, we were having problems linked to a learning curve for new procedures and unfamiliar territory. Our indications also changed during this time. In 1991, we started using routine intraoperative arteriography and we had the continuous availability of a dedicated vascular anesthesia team and of magnetic resonance technology. Our

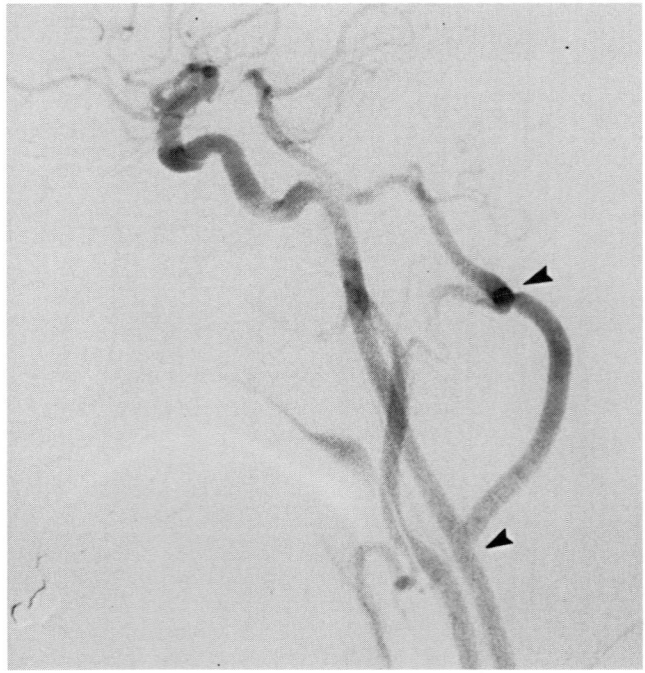

FIGURE 132–25. Bypass from mid-cervical internal carotid artery to suboccipital vertebral artery.

protocols and indications have not changed since then. The data corresponding to patients operated since 1991 reflect the immediate risk and outcomes of vertebral artery reconstruction today.

Table 132–1 shows the difference in the rates of strokes and deaths for this period. The period since January 1991 reflects the management risk and outcomes of VA reconstruction today.

SUMMARY

Vertebral artery reconstruction can be accomplished with minimal morbidity in its proximal segment and with a combined stroke/death rate of less than 2%. This operation achieved excellent protection from stroke in the posterior brain.

REFERENCES

1. Caplan LR, Tettenborn B: Embolism in the posterior circulation. In Berguer R, Caplan LR (eds): Vertebrobasilar Arterial Disease. St. Louis, Quality Medical Publishing, 1992, pp 52–65.
2. Pessin MS: Posterior cerebral artery disease and occipital ischemia. In Berguer R, Caplan LR (eds): Vertebrobasilar Arterial Disease. St. Louis, Quality Medical Publishing, 1992, pp 66–75.
3. Bauer RB: Mechanical compression of the vertebral arteries. In Berguer R, Bauer RB (eds): Vertebrobasilar Arterial Occlusive Disease: Medical and Surgical Management. New York, Raven Press, 1984, pp 45–71.
4. Ruotolo C, Hazan H, Rancurel G, Kieffer E: Dynamic arteriography. In Berguer R, Caplan LR (eds): Vertebrobasilar Arterial Disease. St. Louis, Quality Medical Publishers, 1992, pp 116–123.
5. Berguer R, Higgins RF, Nelson R: Noninvasive diagnosis of reversal of vertebral artery flow. N Engl J Med 302:1349, 1980.
6. Berguer R, Kieffer E: Surgery of the Arteries to the Head. New York, Springer-Verlag, 1992.
7. Berguer R, Andaya LV, Bauer RB: Vertebral artery bypass. Arch Surg 111:976, 1976.
8. Berguer R, Bauer RB: Vertebral artery reconstruction: A successful technique in selected patients. Ann Surg 193:441, 1981.
9. Edwards WH, Mulherin JL Jr: The surgical approach to significant stenosis of vertebral and subclavian arteries. Surgery 87:20, 1980.
10. Malone JM, Moore WS, Hamilton R, et al: Combined carotid-vertebral vascular disease. Arch Surg 115:783, 1980.
11. Roon AJ, Ehrenfeld WK, Cooke PB, et al: Vertebral artery reconstruction. Am J Surg 138:29, 1979.
12. Berguer R: Distal vertebral artery bypass: Technique, the occipital connection and potential uses. J Vasc Surg 2:621, 1985.
13. Kieffer E, Rancurel G, Richart T: Reconstruction of the distal cervical vertebral artery. In Berguer R, Bauer RB (eds): Vertebrobasilar Arterial Occlusive Disease: Medical and Surgical Management. New York, Raven Press, 1984, pp 265–289.
14. Berguer R: Revascularization of the vertebral arteries. In Nyhus L, Baker RJ, Fischer JE (eds): Mastery of Surgery. Boston, Little, Brown, 1997, p 1937.
15. Berguer R, Morasch M, Kline RA: A review of 100 consecutive reconstructions of the distal vertebral artery for embolic and hemodynamic disease. J Vasc Surg 27:852–859, 1998.

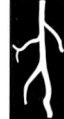

C H A P T E R   1 3 3
Extracranial Fibromuscular Arterial Dysplasia

Peter A. Schneider, M.D., and Robert B. Rutherford, M.D.

Fibromuscular dysplasia (FMD) is a nonatheromatous degenerative process of unknown etiology that involves long, unbranched segments of medium-sized arteries, such as the renal artery, the internal carotid artery, the external iliac artery, and the splenic and hepatic arteries (in order of frequency).[1, 2] Although this disease has been described in Chapter 23, certain aspects pertinent to its involvement of the extracranial cerebral arteries are summarized here.

FMD is found in 0.25% to 0.68% of consecutive cerebral arteriograms.[3, 4] In a series of 2000 carotid operations, it was the offending pathologic feature in 3.4% of cases.[5] Among the four distinct types, the internal carotid artery (like the renal) is involved predominantly with medial fibroplasia, which results in an arteriographic appearance resembling a "string of beads" (Fig. 133–1) and constitutes 80% to 95% of the lesions.[3, 5, 6, 7] In one large series,[3] this type was seen in 89%, with a fusiform narrowing in 7%

and an eccentric septum-like lesion in 4%. Except for the latter lesion, involvement tends to be more distal than that in arteriosclerosis, in the middle and upper thirds of the internal carotid artery. The artery is often elongated, tortuous, and occasionally kinked. Carotid FMD is bilateral in 39% to 86% of reported cases.[1, 3, 8, 9] Women predominate in most series and constitute 60% to 90% of patients.[1, 5, 8–13]

CLINICAL PRESENTATION

Extracranial cerebral artery FMD may present as either an incidental finding without symptoms or as the cause of neurologic events. Symptomatic presentations in large, contemporary series of treated patients demonstrate the capac-

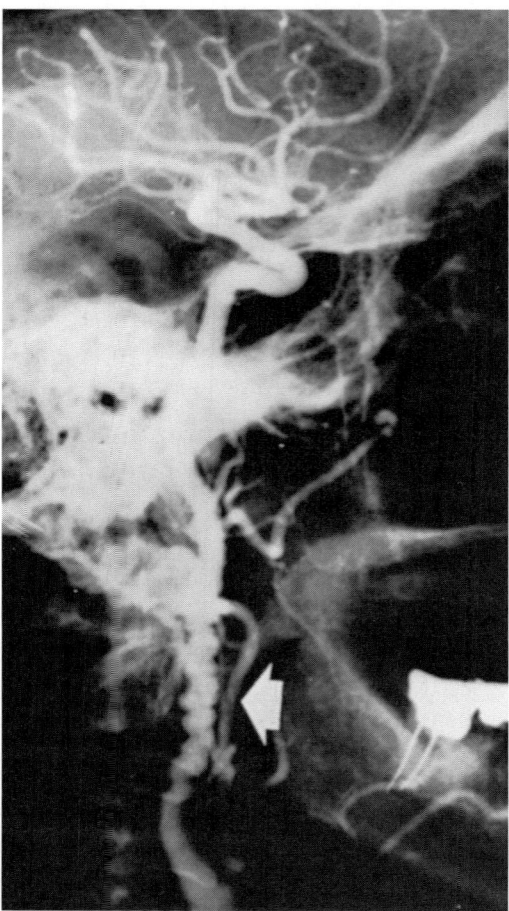

FIGURE 133–1. Carotid arteriogram demonstrating the classic appearance of fibromuscular dysplasia *(arrow)* in the usual location opposite the C1-C3 vertebral bodies and intervening discs. Note low bifurcation and long internal carotid artery.

ity of FMD to cause transient ischemic attack (TIA), stroke, and disability (Table 133–1). Stroke was the initial finding in 12% to 27% of patients, hemispheric TIA occurred in 31% to 42%, and amaurosis fugax was present in 22% to 28%.[5, 13, 14] Other series were similar with respect to presenting symptoms.[10, 15, 16] In an experience at the University of California, San Francisco, 9% of patients were left with a significant, permanent neurologic deficit.[1]

NATURAL HISTORY

Many series have documented the potential for carotid FMD to present with symptoms, but the natural history of asymptomatic lesions is not clear. In one series of 79 patients, most of whom were found to have carotid FMD incidentally on cerebral angiogram (0.6% of the total), only three patients (4%) *subsequently* suffered a cerebral ischemic event during an average follow-up of 5 years.[11] When small groups of asymptomatic patients were studied prospectively, fewer than 10% of patients went on to experience new neurologic symptoms.[2, 8, 11] Nevertheless, two series have shown that about a third of these lesions demonstrate significant angiographic progression with time.[2, 10] None of

these studies has followed a significant number of *high-grade* asymptomatic stenoses, in which the risk of stroke would be expected to be higher.

Most reported cases of symptomatic carotid FMD have been treated with dilatation of the corresponding artery. There is no study in which a large number of patients with carotid FMD who presented with focal cerebral ischemic events were observed expectantly. In one series, 13 patients who presented with either TIA (10 patients) or stroke (three patients) did not undergo surgical correction of carotid FMD but instead were observed. Only one patient remained symptomatic.[17]

Some investigators have suggested that symptomatic lesions should not be considered for operation until their natural history is better understood.[17, 18] This advice is not useful, since there is no way to define the natural history of these *rare* lesions. A multicenter study, in which patients are prospectively randomized to treatment, would be an acceptable approach; however, it is unlikely that this effort could gain funding or could gather sufficient data to allow meaningful conclusions. At present, we are left with a rare cause of focal cerebral ischemic events caused by extracranial carotid stenosis, which can be repaired with a fairly simple operation.

ASSOCIATED LESIONS

Concurrently presenting lesions that frequently complicate the management of carotid FMD, include (1) atherosclerotic occlusive disease at the carotid bifurcation, (2) extracranial carotid artery aneurysms, (3) carotid artery dissection, (4) vertebral artery FMD, (5) intracranial aneurysms, and (6) renal artery FMD.

Atherosclerotic Occlusive Disease

Ipsilateral atheromatous carotid bifurcation disease is present in as many as 20% of individuals.[5, 19] Although it may not always be possible to attribute symptoms to one lesion or the other, when atherosclerotic and fibromuscular dysplastic lesions present together in the same symptomatic artery, they are usually treated simultaneously. In a series

TABLE 133–1. PRESENTING SYMPTOMS IN PATIENTS WITH EXTRACRANIAL FIBROMUSCULAR ARTERIAL DYSPLASIA

	SCHNEIDER et al* (n = 115)	CHICHE et al† (n = 70)	MOREAU et al‡ (n = 58)
Hemispheric TIA (%)	42	36	31
Hemispheric stroke (%)	23	27	12
Amaurosis fugax (%)	22	NA	28
Vertebrobasilar TIA or stroke (%)	NA	45	22

*Data from Schneider PA, et al: *In* Veith FJ, et al (eds): Vascular Surgery: Principles and Practice. New York, McGraw-Hill, 1994, pp 711–717.
†Data from Chiche L, et al: Ann Vasc Surg 11:496–504, 1997.
‡Data from Moreau P, et al: J Cardiovasc Surg 34:465–472, 1993.
NA = not available.

of 72 operations for extracranial FMD, carotid endarterectomy was performed as part of a combined procedure in 14 patients (19%).[5]

Extracranial Carotid Artery Aneurysms

Extracranial carotid artery aneurysms are uncommon, and those associated with FMD are rare. Among 130 extracranial carotid aneurysms in one literature review, 2.3% were associated with FMD.[20] In a single institution series of 15 carotid aneurysms, one third were thought to be caused by FMD, and most were successfully managed with resection and replacement grafting.[21] In a case report from the Mayo Clinic, the arterial pathology in two such cases was medial fibrodyplasia.

Carotid Artery Dissection

FMD may play a role in the development of spontaneous dissection of the carotid artery. This often catastrophic event is responsible for 4% of strokes and is associated with fibrodysplasia in at least 15% of cases.[23, 24] FMD is often suggested among the potential etiologic mechanisms of spontaneous carotid dissection.[6, 25–27] However, reports of spontaneous dissection occurring subsequent to the identification of asymptomatic carotid FMD are not available. The structural abnormality of the arterial wall in FMD and its association with spontaneous dissection suggest that dilatation of the artery may pose an increased risk of perioperative dissection. Nevertheless, dissection is a rare complication of dilatation.[1, 5, 13, 28]

Vertebral Artery Disease

Vertebral artery FMD is identified in 7% to 38% of those with carotid lesions and occasionally presents as an isolated finding.[5, 10, 13] Vertebral artery disease is usually located at the level of the C2 vertebral body and does not extend intracranially.[7] Fortunately, it is rarely responsible for symptoms and does not usually complicate the management of the internal carotid lesion. One series reported 32 patients with vertebrobasilar TIA and stroke due to vertebral artery FMD.[13] Among 12 vertebral artery reconstructions performed, half were for isolated vertebral FMD and half were performed at the time of rigid dilatation of a carotid lesion. The most frequently employed operative approach was a vein bypass to the distal vertebral artery.

Intracranial Aneurysms

Intracranial aneurysms, another expression of the dysplastic process, are found in at least 10% and as many as 51% of patients with internal carotid FMD (~20% on average).[8, 10] Not only do these pose an independent threat of rupture and subarachnoid hemorrhage, but their natural history has the potential to be worsened by relieving a proximal stenosis. In one series, intracranial aneurysms and extracranial FMD each caused half the symptoms and in another, half the strokes were due to aneurysm rupture.[8, 17] In most studies, however, they produced one quarter to one third of the rate of neurologic symptoms caused by the cervical carotid lesion.[2]

Intracranial aneurysms should be treated on their own individual merits (e.g., size, presenting symptoms. coexistence of hypertension), just as the cervical fibrodysplastic lesions should, with primary attention directed toward the most threatening lesion. The presence of a small, asymptomatic intracranial aneurysm should not dissuade the vascular surgeon from operating on a threatening cervical lesion.

Renal Artery Disease

Renal artery FMD coexists in 8% to 40% of patients with carotid FMD.[2, 5, 14] It presents an additional threat in patients with intracranial aneurysms. Because renal artery FMD generally responds well to percutaneous balloon angioplasty, the possibility of coexistent renal artery involvement should be considered prior to the treatment of carotid stenosis (see Chapter 122).

DIAGNOSTIC EVALUATION

There is no highly accurate but noninvasive method of detecting extracranial arterial FMD. At present, most asymptomatic patients with a carotid bruit and those with hemispheric or nonfocal neurologic symptoms undergo carotid duplex scanning. Duplex may reveal velocity elevation resulting from FMD, but the lesion may be missed because it is located more distally than the usual atherosclerotic plaque.[7]

Catheter-based contrast arteriography remains the best way to evaluate FMD of the extracranial cerebral arteries. Many cases of carotid FMD are discovered during arteriography.[7, 29] When carotid FMD is identified, intracranial vascular anatomy should be evaluated arteriographically to check for the presence of intracranial aneurysms. Magnetic resonance angiography (MRA) has not been particularly useful in the diagnostic evaluation of FMD, but it may be beneficial for follow-up of known FMD.[29] Patients with symptomatic carotid FMD should undergo computed tomography (CT) or magnetic resonance imaging (MRI) of the brain and complete cerebral angiography.

TREATMENT

Controversies frequently arise in the management of carotid FMD and must be considered during the treatment planning stage. For example, it is not always possible to determine which of two concurrently presenting lesions is symptomatic. Occasionally, these lesions should be treated simultaneously, as in the case of carotid FMD with significant bifurcation atherosclerosis. The presence of an intracranial aneurysm may alter the treatment sequence or the surgical approach. PTA has been very successful for the treatment of renal artery FMD, but its early results and durability are not known for carotid FMD. Nevertheless, some patients may be better served with a percutaneous approach.

Indications for Intervention

On the basis of the relative safety and effectiveness of surgical intervention (see later), operative management is appropriate for lesions causing focal ischemic events (hemispheric or ocular) or episodes of cerebral hypoperfusion. The lesion that presents with a focal cerebral ischemic event has declared itself and remains a significant threat. Hypoperfusion is rare but can occur in the setting of critical bilateral carotid FMD or even unilateral disease when there is a significant defect in the circle of Willis.

Arterial Repair: Rationale and Results

The three main methods of mechanical intervention advocated for the treatment of carotid FMD include:

- Open, graduated, rigid dilatation
- Open transluminal balloon dilatation with outflow control
- PTA

The usual fibrodysplastic lesion encountered in the internal carotid artery responds to dilatation. Over the past three decades, this has been performed with relative success and safety by means of rigid dilators of progressively enlarging sizes passed antegrade into the internal carotid artery with outflow control.[1, 5, 12-16] This approach permits gentle disruption of the obstructive webs while allowing associated debris to be flushed out of the artery.

The results of three large, contemporary series of surgically managed patients are presented in Tables 133-2 and 133-3. These reports consist primarily of patients undergoing rigid carotid dilatation but also include some instances of carotid replacement and vertebral revascularization.[5, 13, 14] The risk of perioperative stroke for surgical treatment in these series ranged from 1.4% to 2.6%. TIA occurred in 1.4% to 7.7%, and perforation occurred twice in 318 operations (0.6%).[5, 14] Cranial nerve injuries, most of which were transient, resulted from extensive distal operative exposure of the internal carotid artery and were reported to occur in 5.1% to 16.7% of cases.[5, 13]

Excellent long-term follow-up data are available (see Table 133-3). Late stroke developed in 1.2% to 3.8% of patients, and nearly all late deaths (up to 22 years) were due to non-neurologic causes. In one series,[13] 94% of patients underwent duplex scanning (mean follow-up, 7 years). The actuarial rates of primary patency, survival, and

TABLE 133-2. RESULTS OF SURGICAL TREATMENT OF EXTRACRANIAL FIBROMUSCULAR ARTERIAL DYSPLASIA

	SCHNEIDER et al* (n = 115)	CHICHE et al† (n = 70)	MOREAU et al‡ (n = 58)
Operations	168	78	72
Operative stroke (%)	1.7	2.6	1.4
Operative TIA (%)	6.0	7.7	1.4
Operative death (%)	0	1.3	0

*Data from Schneider PA, et al: *In* Veith FJ, et al (eds): Vascular Surgery: Principles and Practice. New York, McGraw-Hill, 1994, pp 711–717.
†Data from Chiche L, et al: Ann Vasc Surg 11:496–504, 1997.
‡Data from Moreau P, et al: J Cardiovasc Surg 34:465–472, 1993.

TABLE 133-3. LATE FOLLOW-UP AFTER SURGICAL TREATMENT OF EXTRACRANIAL FIBROMUSCULAR ARTERIAL DYSPLASIA

	SCHNEIDER et al* (n = 115)	CHICHE et al† (n = 70)	MOREAU et al‡ (n = 58)
Follow-up (mean yrs.)	1–17	7 (1–15)	13 (6–22)
Recurrent stenosis (%)	2.3	0	0
Late occlusion (%)	0.6	0	2.8
Late stroke (%)	1.2	2.9	3.8
Death (other causes) (%)	NA	8.6	13.2

*Data from Schneider PA, et al: *In* Veith FJ, et al (eds): Vascular Surgery: Principles and Practice. New York, McGraw-Hill, 1994, pp 711–717.
†Data from Chiche L, et al: Ann Vasc Surg 11:496–504, 1997.
‡Data from Moreau P, et al: J Cardiovasc Surg 34:465–472, 1993.
NA = not available.

stroke-free survival were 94%, 96% and 94%, respectively, at 5 years and 94%, 82%, and 88%, respectively, at 10 years. When follow-up angiography is obtained, it usually demonstrates a normal-sized lumen (Fig. 133–2).

When the length of the diseased internal carotid artery extends too distally to be dissected out and ensure adequate control of manual dilatation, some authors have advised balloon angioplasty combined with open, outflow control.[30-33] The benefit of this approach is the opportunity for a controlled dilatation while maintaining the ability to back-bleed the artery and avoid embolization of debris from the dilated lesion. Among a small number of patients from different reports, it appears that early results with this approach may be comparable to those of rigid dilatation.

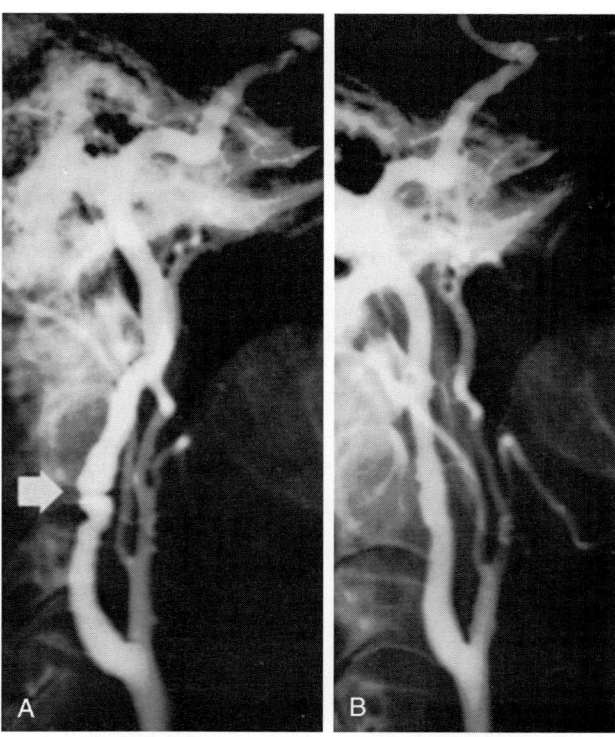

FIGURE 133–2. *A*, Preoperative right carotid arteriogram showing a localized zone of fibromuscular dysplasia characterized by an intraluminal diaphragm *(arrow)*. *B*, Postoperative right carotid arteriogram following graduated intraluminal dilatation. The carotid lumen is now widely patent.

Some authors have advocated PTA as the new treatment of choice for carotid FMD.[34, 35] The rationale for this approach is based upon the success of PTA in the treatment of renal artery FMD. Balloon angioplasty has fewer complications than open surgery of the renal artery and provides reasonable long-term results. However, it is not clear whether this approach can be readily applied to carotid FMD for the following reasons:

1. Carotid lesions for which intervention is justified will have already presented with embolic cerebral ischemic events, placing the patient at higher risk for this complication, whereas most renal lesions result in symptoms by renal hypoperfusion with secondary hypertension.

2. Embolism, which occurs in up to 10% of PTA procedures, may be of little clinical consequence after lower extremity angioplasty and tolerable, in view of the advantages of percutaneous treatment over a major abdominal operation for renal lesions, but it can be disastrous if it has occurred in the carotid artery distribution.

3. Surgical dilatation of the carotid lesion is a simple, safe operation in a generally younger population with fewer co-morbid conditions; it is considerably safer than carotid endarterectomy if proper technique is used.

Unfortunately, it is not possible to develop a balanced approach to treatment that includes this alternative therapy, since few data are available regarding perioperative complications or longer-term follow-up. Between 1981 and 1998, at least 20 patients were reported in the literature as having undergone balloon angioplasty for carotid FMD, usually as part of larger series of angioplasty patients.[28, 35–38] In one case report,[28] post-angioplasty carotid dissection resulted in a stroke; in other reports, however, no specific mention was made of periprocedural complications. No follow-up is available beyond the perioperative period.

SURGICAL TECHNIQUE

Exposure is similar to that for carotid endarterectomy except that *higher* internal carotid artery exposure is usually required to ensure that safe dilatation is carried out under direct vision. The posterior belly of the digastric muscle may be divided, but subluxation of the mandible is rarely required. The normal arterial segment above the highest point of involvement is apparent by inspection, and the internal carotid artery is encircled at this point.

The surgeon should take care not to manipulate the intervening segment of the internal carotid artery as it is gently exposed throughout its length. Stump pressures or electroencephalographic (EEG) monitoring is *not* ordinarily needed for this brief procedure but may be indicated if a more extensive procedure is planned (e.g., bifurcation endarterectomy, correction of redundancy, or interposition grafting). Except in such unusual circumstances, a shunt is unnecessary.

The authors prefer to give 75 to 100 U/kg of heparin prior to interrupting flow. A single 500-ml unit of dextran 40, at 25 ml/hr, beginning at the time of operation and continued during the immediate postoperative period may help prevent early deposition of thrombotic material on the inner surfaces of the arteriotomy and the fractured septa. The common carotid artery is cross-clamped. Traction on a polymeric silicone (Silastic) "sling" placed around the internal carotid artery just above the bifurcation is performed to straighten the artery. A short arteriotomy is made in the internal carotid artery at the base of the bulb. Graduated metal dilators are then gently passed up the straightened internal carotid artery, beginning with a 1.5-mm diameter probe and progressing up to a 3.5-mm, or, occasionally, a 4.0-mm diameter probe (Fig. 133–3). There is usually a series of "giving" sensations felt as each septal stenosis is gently fractured for the first time, but this is not felt thereafter.

The procedure is terminated after the segment has been seen to be gently stretched to full diameter throughout its course. It is important not to exceed this gentle stretching and, therefore, not to proceed beyond a 4-mm diameter. Back-bleeding following passage of the dilators prevents embolism, and the short arteriotomy is rapidly closed with a simple running suture of 6–0 polypropylene. Careful interrogation of the entire segment with a Doppler probe or duplex scanner after restoration of flow ensures patency without turbulence or residual defect.

The upper limits of the disease must be fully exposed. If not, as in lesions that extend into the upper third of the internal carotid artery, transluminal balloon dilatation is performed under fluoroscopic guidance.

When there is significant associated bifurcation atherosclerosis, a concomitant endarterectomy may be performed. In this case, the initial arteriotomy is *longitudinal.* If severe elongation and kinking are present, such that the kinking cannot be ruled out as a cause of hypoperfusion episodes (particularly position-related syncope), an oblique arteriotomy, initially placed anteriorly at the base of the carotid bulb at the bifurcation, can be extended circumferentially after the dilatation procedure; it is then carried longitudinally down the common carotid artery, allowing the internal carotid to be translocated downward until it is straightened and anastomosed at this lower position.

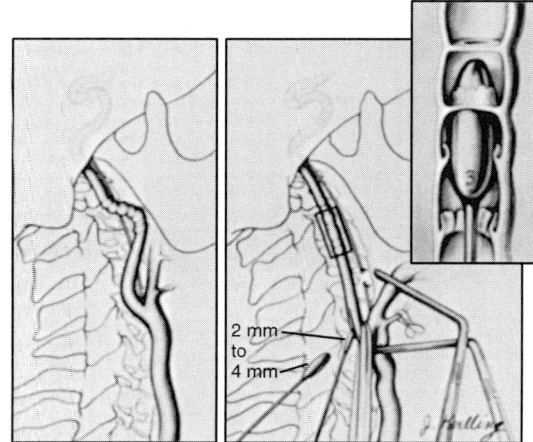

FIGURE 133–3. Drawing representing the main features of the operative technique. Straightening of the carotid artery from the preoperative state shown on the left and gentle graduated dilatation from 2 to 4 mm. *Inset,* The mechanism of rupture of the stenotic membranes. (From Effeney D, Ehrenfeld WK, Stoney RJ, Wylie EJ: Fibromuscular dysplasia of the internal carotid artery. World J Surg 3:179, 1979.)

SUMMARY

More than half the patients present with cerebral ischemic events. Fewer than half of these patients will have suffered infarcts, and only half of the latter will be left with significant neurologic deficits (i.e., ~10% of the total). The natural history of incidentally identified lesions is more benign, with one third showing angiographic progression but less than one tenth ultimately producing cerebral ischemic symptoms.

Surgical dilatation of carotid FMD is safe and effective, and any surgeon who obtains excellent results with carotid endarterectomy can expect even better results with this procedure. It is appropriate to operate on lesions producing focal hemispheric or ocular ischemic events or on critical stenoses that cause hypoperfusion symptoms. An aggressive posture with asymptomatic lesions, however, can be justified only for unusually threatening combinations of lesions (e.g., operating on one of two severe bilateral stenoses). Associated intracranial aneurysms should be managed according to their own merits and should not be allowed to compromise valid indications for operation on the cervical lesion. Balloon angioplasty carries a small but definite risk of thromboembolic events, and there are insufficient data to justify its routine use.

It is possible to develop a logical, selective management approach based on much that is known and to apply it to individual patients based on *their* clinical findings, operative risk, and longevity outlook.

REFERENCES

1. Effeney DJ: Surgery for fibromuscular dysplasia of the carotid artery: Indications, technique, and results. In Moore WS (ed): Surgery for Cerebrovascular Disease. New York, Churchill Livingstone, 1987, pp 525–533.
2. Stanley JC, Wakefield TW: Arterial fibrodysplasia. In Rutherford RB (ed): Vascular Surgery, 3rd ed. Philadelphia, WB Saunders, 1990, pp 245–265.
3. Osborn AG, Anderson RE: Angiographic spectrum of cervical and intracranial fibromuscular dysplasia. Stroke 8:617. 1977.
4. Houser OW, Baker HL: Fibrovascular dysplasia and other uncommon diseases of the cervical carotid artery: Angiographic aspects. Am J Roentgenol 104:201, 1968.
5. Moreau P, Albat B, Thevenet A: Fibromuscular dysplasia of the internal carotid artery: Long-term results. J Cardiovasc Surg 34:465–472, 1993.
6. Fisicaro M, Tonizzo M, Mucelli RP, et al: Fibromuscular dysplasia: A case report of multivessel vascular involvement. Int Angiol 13:347–350, 1994.
7. Furie DM, Tien RD: Fibromuscular dysplasia of arteries of the head and neck: Imaging findings. AJR Am J Roentgenol 162:1205–1209, 1994.
8. Mettinger KL, Ericson K: Fibromuscular dysplasia and the brain: I. Observations on angiographic, clinical and genetic characteristics. Stroke 13:46, 1982.
9. Schievink WI, Bjornsson J: Fibromuscular dysplasia of the internal carotid artery: A clinicopathological study. Clin Neuropathol 15:2–6, 1996.
10. So EL, Toole JF, Dalal P, et al: Cephalic fibromuscular dysplasia in 32 patients: Clinical findings and radiologic features. Arch Neurol 38:619, 1981.
11. Corrin LS, Sandok BA, Houser OW: Cerebral ischemic events in patients with carotid artery fibromuscular dysplasia. Arch Neurol 38:616, 1981.
12. Morris GC Jr, Lechter A, DeBakey ME: Surgical treatment of fibromuscular disease of the carotid arteries. Arch Surg 96:636, 1968.
13. Chiche L, Bahnini A, Koskas F, et al: Occlusive fibromuscular disease of the arteries supplying the brain: Results of surgical treatment. Ann Vasc Surg 11:496–504, 1997.
14. Schneider PA, Cunningham CG, Ehrenfeld WK, et al: Fibromuscular dysplasia of the carotid artery. In Veith FJ, Hobson RW, Williams RA, Wilson SE (eds): Vascular Surgery: Principles and Practice. New York, McGraw-Hill, 1994, pp 711–717.
15. Starr DS, Lawrie GM, Morris GC: Fibromuscular disease of carotid arteries: Long-term results of graduated internal dilatation. Stroke 12:196, 1981.
16. Collins GJ, Rich NM, Clagett GP, et al: Fibromuscular dysplasia of the internal carotid arteries: Clinical experience and follow-up. Ann Surg 194:89, 1981.
17. Stewart MT, Moritz MW, Smith RB, et al: The natural history of carotid fibromuscular dysplasia. J Vasc Surg 3:305, 1986.
18. Patman RD, Thompson JE, Talkington CM, et al: Natural history of fibromuscular dysplasia of the carotid artery. Stroke 2:135, 1980.
19. Effeney DJ, Ehrenfeld WK: Extracranial fibromuscular disease. In Rutherford RB (ed): Vascular Surgery, 3rd ed. Philadelphia, WB Saunders, 1990, pp 1412–1417.
20. Miyauchi M, Shionoya S: Aneurysm of the extracranial internal carotid artery caused by fibromuscular dysplasia. Eur J Vasc Surg 5:587–591, 1991.
21. Coffin O, Maiza D, Galateau-Salle F, et al: Results of surgical management of internal carotid artery aneurysm by the cervical approach. Ann Vasc Surg 11:482–490, 1997.
22. Rhee RY, Gloviczki P, Cherry KJ, et al: Two unusual variants of internal carotid artery aneurysms due to fibromuscular dysplasia. Ann Vasc Surg 10:481–485,1996.
23. Hart RG, Easton JD: Dissections of cervical and cerebral arteries. Neurol Clin 1:155, 1983.
24. Luscher TF, Lie JT, Stanson AW, et al: Arterial fibromuscular dysplasia. Mayo Clin Proc 62:931–952, 1987.
25. DeOcampo J, Brillman J, Levy DI: Stenting: A new approach to carotid dissection. J Neuroimag 7:187–190, 1997.
26. Manninen HU, Koivisto T, Saari T, et al: Dissecting aneurysms of all four cervicocranial arteries in fibromuscular dysplasia: Treatment with self-expanding endovascular stents, coil embolization and surgical ligation. AJNR Am J Neuroradiol 18:1216–1220, 1997.
27. Klufas RA, Hsu L, Barnes PD, et al: Dissection of the carotid and vertebral arteries: Imaging with MR angiography. AJR Am J Roentgenol 164:673–677, 1995.
28. Jooma R, Bradshaw JR, Griffith HB: Intimal dissection following percutaneous transluminal carotid angioplasty for fibromuscular hyperplasia. Neuroradiology 27:181–182, 1985.
29. Russo CP, Smoker WRK: Nonatheromatous carotid artery disease. Neuroimaging Clin North Am 6:811–830, 1996.
30. Smith LL, Smith DC, Killeen JD, et al: Operative balloon angioplasty in the treatment of internal carotid artery fibromuscular dysplasia. J Vasc Surg 6:482–487, 1987.
31. de Smul G, Bostoen H: Operative balloon dilatation of fibromuscular dysplasia of the internal carotid artery: Two case reports. Acta Chir Belg 95:139–141, 1995.
32. Ballard JL, Guinn JE, Killeen D, et al: Open operative balloon angioplasty of the internal carotid artery: A technique in evolution. Ann Vasc Surg 9:390–393, 1995.
33. Lord RSA, Graham AR, Benn IV: Radiologic control of operative carotid dilation: Aneurysm formation following balloon dilation. Cardiovasc Surg 27:158–161, 1986.
34. Brown MM: Balloon angioplasty for cerebrovascular disease. Neurol Res 14:159–163, 1992.
35. Motarjeme A: Percutaneous transluminal angioplasty of the supra-aortic vessels. J Endovasc Surg 3:171–181, 1996.
36. Hasso AN, Bird CR, Zinke DE, et al: Fibromuscular dysplasia of the internal carotid artery: Percutaneous transluminal angioplasty. Am J Neuroradiol 2:175–180, 1981.
37. Tsai FY, Matovich V, Hiesheima G, et al: Percutaneous transluminal angioplasty of the carotid artery. Am J Neuroradiol 7:349–358, 1986.
38. Theron JG, Payelle GG, Coskun O, et al: Carotid artery stenosis: Treatment with protected balloon angioplasty and stent placement. Radiology 201:627–636, 1996.

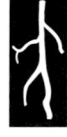

C H A P T E R   1 3 4

Aneurysms of the Extracranial Carotid Artery

Jerry Goldstone, M.D.

Occlusive and ulcerated atherosclerotic lesions of the cervical carotid arteries are extremely common. Aneurysms of these vessels are rare, particularly in comparison with the frequency of aneurysms involving the *intracranial* carotid arteries and their branches and the frequency of aneurysms that occur throughout the rest of the arterial system. From 1927 to 1947, only five cases of carotid aneurysm were encountered at the Hospital of the University of Pennsylvania, and Reid noted only 12 cases in a 30-year survey at the Johns Hopkins Hospital through 1922.[33, 53] The largest reported series from a single institution, that of McCollum and associates at Baylor University, consisted of only 37 aneurysms treated over a 21-year period during which approximately 8500 operations for arterial aneurysms of all types were performed in the same institution.[39] Similarly, only six extracranial carotid aneurysms were repaired by Painter and associates at the Cleveland Clinic over a 7-year interval during which more than 1500 patients were treated for carotid occlusive disease.[48]

Overall, about 2600 aneurysms of all types of the extracranial carotid arteries have been reported. Because of the rarity of these aneurysms, it is impossible to define their true incidence or to determine whether their frequency is increasing; however, with the widespread use of angiography and duplex ultrasound and other imaging modalities, they clearly are being recognized more often than before. This is borne out by two reports from the Mayo Clinic. The first included six carotid aneurysms identified between 1936 and 1963.[52] The second included 25 aneurysms treated from 1950 to 1990.[6] Although rare, extracranial carotid aneurysms should be considered in the differential diagnosis of a mass in the neck or posterior pharynx. Aneurysms of the intracranial carotid arteries are much more common but are the concern of neurosurgeons.

LOCATION

The common carotid artery, particularly at its bifurcation, is the most frequently reported site of true aneurysm formation in the extracranial carotid system; the internal carotid artery is the next most common; and the external carotid the least common (Figs. 134–1 to 134–9).[1, 20, 54, 56, 57] Location varies with etiology, and the relative proportion of the various causes of these aneurysms is changing. For example, atherosclerotic aneurysms usually occur at or near the carotid bifurcation, whereas those caused by blunt trauma usually involve the high cervical portion of the internal carotid artery.

ETIOLOGY

There are many causes of extracranial carotid aneurysms, and the relative frequency of each has changed over the years. Syphilis, tuberculosis, and other local infections were the most common causes 50 years ago, but they are rare today. Instead, dissection, atherosclerosis, trauma, and previous carotid surgery are the cause of most extracranial carotid aneurysms in current practice.

Atherosclerosis

Atherosclerosis has been attributed to be now the most frequently reported pathologic process associated with extracranial carotid artery aneurysms, occurring in up to 70% of the aneurysms in more recently published series.[13, 17, 19, 43, 48, 67, 70] These are *true aneurysms*. The histologic features are typically atherosclerotic (often termed "degenerative"), with disruption of the internal elastic lamina and thinning of the media. Grossly, these aneurysms tend to be fusiform rather than saccular and are most commonly located at the bifurcation of the common carotid artery or the proximal internal carotid artery, where occlusive atherosclerotic plaques are very common.

Aneurysms that do not involve the carotid bifurcation are frequently *saccular*. The majority of affected patients have severe arterial hypertension. Most bilateral, nontraumatic, extracranial carotid aneurysms are this type.

Trauma

Another major and increasingly frequent cause of carotid aneurysms is trauma,[15, 34, 59] both penetrating and blunt. The resulting transmural carotid disruption leads to the formation of *false aneurysm* ("pseudoaneurysm").

Penetrating Trauma

Penetrating wounds involving the carotid arteries can lead to two important sequelae: (1) arteriovenous fistula (aneurysm) and (2) false aneurysm. Arteriovenous fistula was more common[20] than false aneurysm in reports from World War II, although earlier reports indicated a higher incidence of false aneurysm, probably because the causative injuries

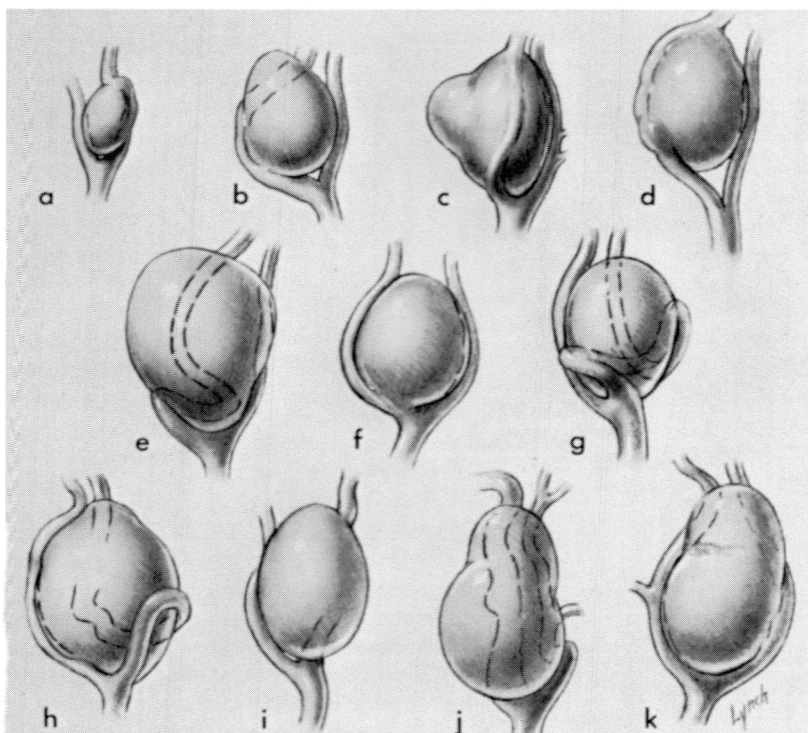

FIGURE 134–1. Artist's depiction of aneurysms of the extracranial internal carotid artery, showing variations in size and configuration. (From Alexander E Jr, Wigser SM, Davis CH: Bilateral extracranial aneurysms of the internal carotid artery. J Neurosurg 25:437, 1966.)

were produced by low-velocity, low-energy–releasing missiles or by penetrating hand-driven weapons.[68] The decreased number of such cases reported since the mid-1930s may be due to the high initial mortality rate associated

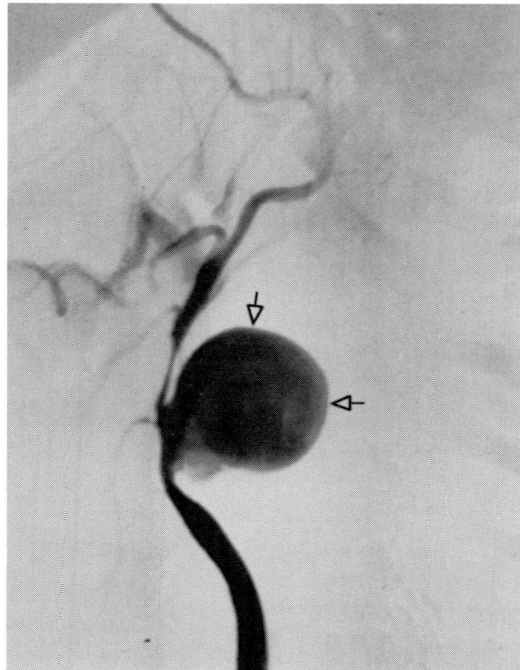

FIGURE 134–2. Left carotid arteriogram showing a 3.5 by 4.0 cm aneurysm arising from left carotid artery adjacent to common carotid bifurcation. The left internal carotid is occluded. (From Margolis MT, Stein RL, Newton TH: Extracranial aneurysms of the internal carotid artery. Neuroradiology 4:78, 1972.)

with neck wounds produced by modern high-velocity weapons when they involve the region of the internal carotid artery. Such injuries to an area so closely related anatomically to the base of the skull are often lethal. In the Vietnam conflict, nearly all of the patients who survived to be treated for carotid injuries were wounded by relatively low-velocity fragments from land mines, rockets, mortars, or grenades.

Direct carotid puncture for arteriography also can result in the formation of a false carotid aneurysm, but this technique is rarely used now for cerebral angiography. However, accidental puncture of the common carotid artery is a well-described complication of percutaneous cannulation of the internal jugular vein, and subsequent pseudoaneurysms have been reported.

Nonpenetrating Trauma

Blunt or nonpenetrating trauma, although more often the cause of thrombosis of the injured vessel, can be associated with the development of false aneurysms. Blunt injury of the carotid artery produces a spectrum of abnormalities, including spasm, intimal and medial tears, and partial or complete severance of the vessel.[66] Carotid false aneurysms are formed by the same sequence of events as false aneurysms elsewhere. Disruption of the continuity of the arterial wall is required to produce any false aneurysm. This results in formation of a periarterial hematoma that is contained by fascial planes. The center of the hematoma becomes a cavity composed of blood and laminated thrombus communicating with the arterial lumen. A fibrotic reaction is initiated in the surrounding tissues that assists in containing the aneurysm.

Hyperextension and rotation of the neck can cause

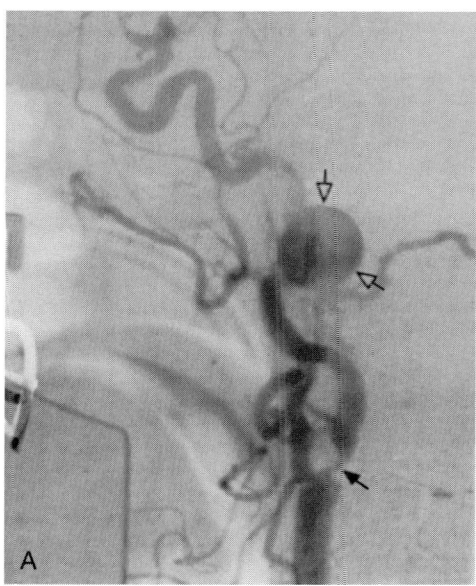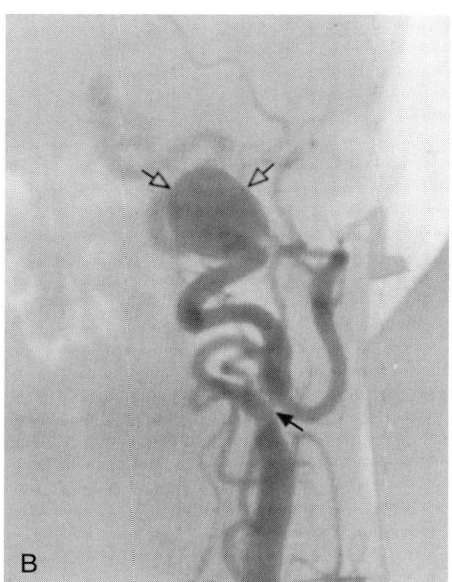

FIGURE 134–3. Left common carotid arteriogram showing a 1.8 by 2.0 cm aneurysm of the left internal carotid extending up to the base of the skull, associated with stenosis of the origin of the internal artery (closed arrows). A, Lateral projection. B, Anteroposterior projection. (From Margolis MT, Stein RL, Newton TH: Extracranial aneurysms of the internal carotid artery. Neuroradiology 4:78, 1972.)

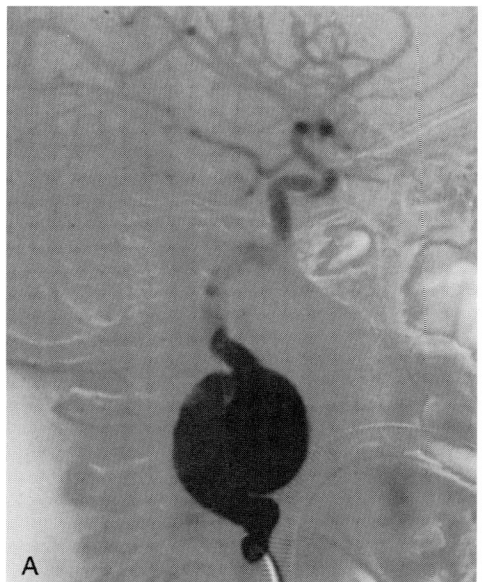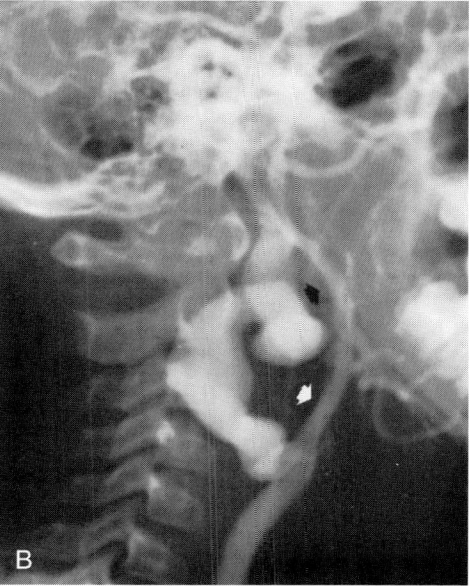

FIGURE 134–4. Right internal carotid arteriogram demonstrating fusiform aneurysm and looping of the proximal right internal carotid artery. (From Margolis MT, Stein RL, Newton TH: Extracranial aneurysms of the internal carotid artery. Neuroradiology 4:78, 1972.)

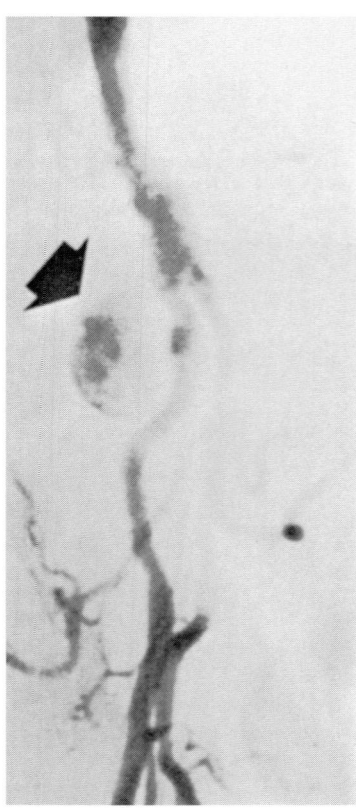

FIGURE 134–5. Left carotid arteriogram showing false aneurysm adjacent to carotid endarterectomy site (arrow). (From Ehrenfeld WK, Hays RJ: False aneurysm after carotid endarterectomy. Arch Surg 104:288, 1972. Copyright 1972, American Medical Association.)

stretching and compression of the distal extracranial internal carotid artery on the transverse process of the second and third cervical vertebrae, producing disruption of the wall and subsequent aneurysm formation, or intimal fracture and dissection or thrombosis.[54, 66] Similarly, the extreme displacement of the tissues of the neck that can occur during motor vehicle accidents and other trauma may stretch or disrupt the artery at its points of fixation to bone at the base of the skull.

The styloid process has been implicated in the pathophysiology of these blunt carotid injuries because it rotates with the skull on the dens, whereas the artery moves with the cervical spine.[61, 69] In addition, when mandibular fracture is associated with blunt cervical trauma, bone fragments may penetrate the arterial wall, with subsequent development of one or more false aneurysms. Most of these blunt injuries are located high in the neck near the base of the skull, making them difficult to approach surgically, in contrast to carotid aneurysms that are due to penetrating trauma, which most often involve the common carotid artery.

Dissection

Dissection of the extracranial internal carotid artery can occur after penetrating or blunt injury to the neck, inadvertent intraoperative trauma, percutaneous or catheter angi-

ography, and chiropractic manipulation or spontaneously without obvious cause (see Chapter 135).[4, 18, 22, 23, 27, 40, 42, 47, 69] Nearly 20% of patients with dissecting aneurysms of the carotid artery have fibromuscular dysplasia of the involved or contralateral carotid vessel, and in nearly 10% of patients they are bilateral. Many of the trauma-related dissections are associated with motor vehicle accidents.

Typical angiographic findings of dissection include a tapered narrowing in the mid or upper cervical internal carotid artery ("string sign") as well as a localized saccular aneurysm or cylindrical dilatation in the dissected segment. Very focal lesions and total occlusions can also occur. The vertebral artery can also be affected by dissection. These dissecting aneurysms develop as a result of a break in the intima followed by hemorrhage into the media, which enlarges the vessel wall and reduces the caliber of the true lumen. If the hemorrhage dissects into the plane between the media and the adventitia, an aneurysm forms. About 30% of carotid dissections are associated with aneurysm formation. These lesions are often associated with hemicrania and Horner's syndrome in addition to transient or fixed neurologic deficits.

Surgery

False aneurysms can also occur after carotid bifurcation endarterectomy for cerebrovascular insufficiency.[8, 13, 28, 45, 52] About 50% of the reported cases have occurred after endarterectomy in which a synthetic patch was used. Most often, these pseudoaneurysms have been attributed to the presence of infection or suture failure. However, pseudoaneurysms can also occur when a vein patch is used and after endarterectomy with primary closure. Although the incidence of false aneurysm is low, significant morbidity is associated with these pseudoaneurysms. Surgical trauma to the carotid artery during tonsillectomy or drainage of a

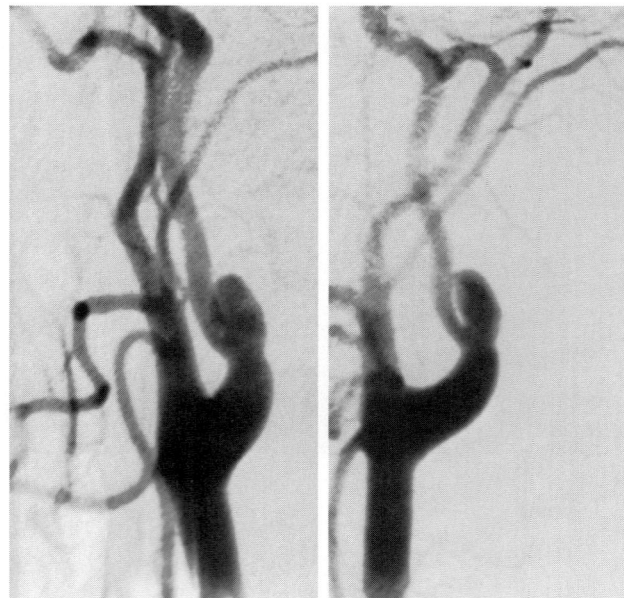

FIGURE 134–6. Left carotid arteriogram showing dissecting aneurysm of proximal internal carotid artery caused by arteriographic catheter injury.

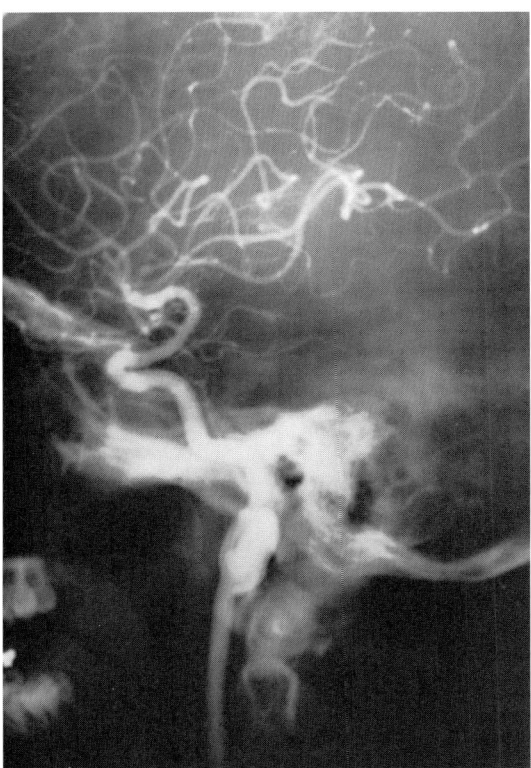

FIGURE 134–7. Left carotid arteriogram (lateral view) showing traumatic internal carotid pseudoaneurysm involving typical location in distal internal carotid artery.

peritonsillar abscess can also lead to pseudoaneurysm formation.

Infection

Prior to the development of antibiotics, most extracranial carotid aneurysms were caused by infection resulting from either syphilis or contiguous pharyngeal or cervical infection.[33, 60, 68] In fact, in their 1949 review, Kirby and associates stated that "at least 90% of all aneurysms of the common carotid artery are due to syphilis."[33] The near disappearance of syphilitic arteritis accounts for the rarity of syphilitic aneurysms today, but infectious or *mycotic* aneurysms caused by other organisms still occur.

In the 19th century, during streptococcal epidemics children were frequently seen with profuse oropharyngeal bleeding from infective aneurysms of the internal carotid artery. Cervical carotid aneurysms may protrude through the relatively thin pharyngeal constrictor muscles into the posterolateral pharyngeal wall, where they can rupture or where the true nature of these mycotic aneurysms may not be recognized until an unsuspecting physician drains a "peritonsillar abscess," only to be met with a gush of blood. *Staphylococcus aureus* has been the most frequent organism responsible for mycotic carotid aneurysms in recent years, but *Escherichia coli, Klebsiella, Corynebacterium* species, *Proteus mirabilis,* and *Yersinia enterocolitica* have also been reported. *Salmonella* species, which are a frequent pathogen in other arterial mycotic aneurysms, are less common in this location.[12, 21, 25, 31, 55]

The presence of a pulsatile neck mass associated with fever and pain should strongly suggest the diagnosis of a mycotic carotid artery aneurysm. Sources of infection include septicemia with involvement of the vasa vasorum, septic emboli within the lumen, and direct extension of infection from contiguous sites. This is obviously not a common problem today, although heroin addicts are especially susceptible to these nonsyphilitic, infectious aneurysms.[36, 39, 53]

Miscellaneous Causes

Other well-documented but even less common causes of carotid aneurysm include cystic medial necrosis, Marfan's syndrome, idiopathic medial arteriopathy, and fibromuscular dysplasia.[5, 35, 41, 55, 64, 65] Several carotid aneurysms have been thought to be congenital because of their occurrence early in life, bilaterality, their saccular shape, the presence of a defect in the media of the vessel similar to the "berry" type of intracranial aneurysm, and the absence of pathologic or clinical features characteristic of other entities.[26, 44] Thus, carotid aneurysm should be in the differential diagnosis of a painless neck mass in a young adult.[37]

NATURAL HISTORY

The natural history of extracranial carotid aneurysms is uncertain because these lesions are very rare and because no single institution has had a large clinical experience

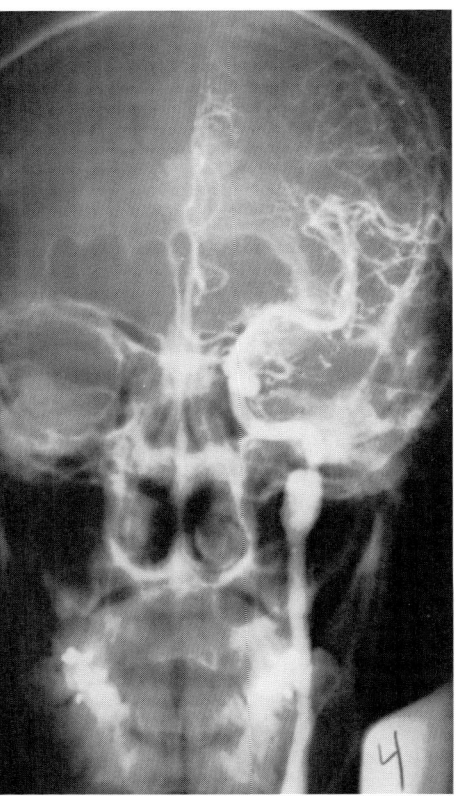

FIGURE 134–8. Left carotid arteriogram (anteroposterior view) of same patient as in Figure 134–7.

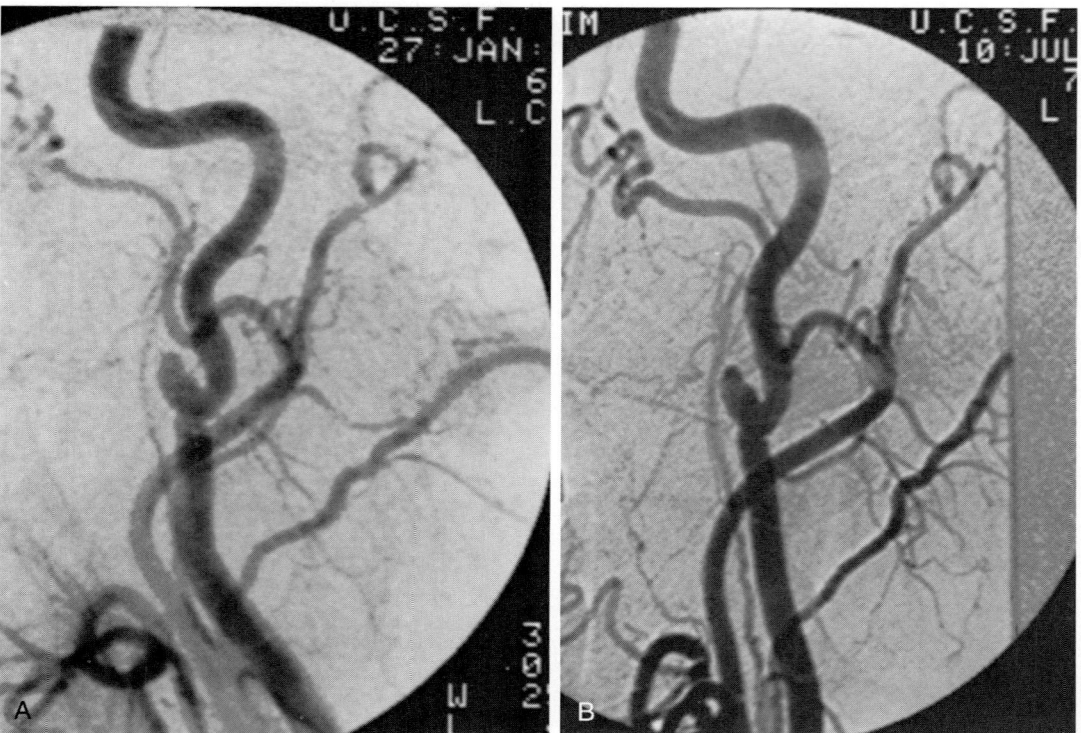

FIGURE 134–9. *A*, Left carotid arteriogram showing traumatic pseudoaneurysm of distal internal carotid artery. *B*, Left carotid arteriogram of same patient, 6 months later, showing no change in size of aneurysm.

with them. Thus, only estimates of natural history can be made, based on multiple case reports, small series, and collected reviews. Unfortunately, most of these include aneurysms of all types, and results have not always been correlated with specific causes; as a result, information regarding specific etiologic mechanisms is even more fragmentary. Furthermore, because these reports describe only aneurysms requiring medical attention, it is impossible to determine the number that were never detected. Although routine autopsy studies suggest the incidence is low, the available information suggests that the natural history of these lesions is generally unfavorable.

Winslow's 1926 report revealed a 71% mortality rate from rupture, thrombosis, or embolism in 35 untreated patients, compared with a 30% mortality rate in those patients who underwent proximal carotid ligation, the only surgical treatment available at that time.[68] More contemporary reviews have substantiated this poor prognosis of untreated patients[32, 55, 59] and have emphasized the high incidence of neurologic symptoms. For example, Zwolak and coworkers reported a stroke rate of 50% for atherosclerotic aneurysms followed up without surgery.[70] Aneurysm rupture is rare.

An especially high incidence of complications and death with mycotic and postsurgical pseudoaneurysms is documented in several reviews and case reports.[21, 25, 31, 37, 55] Conversely, some small, high cervical traumatic aneurysms remain stable or even become smaller when observed for long periods (see Fig. 134–9). Therapy must therefore be individualized, with the major objective being prevention of severe neurologic complications in atherosclerotic aneu-

rysms and hemorrhage and thrombosis from mycotic aneurysms.[46]

CLINICAL FEATURES

Pulsatile Mass

The symptoms of extracranial carotid aneurysms vary according to their location, size, and etiology. Small internal carotid aneurysms may be asymptomatic, but most cervical carotid aneurysms (30%) are identified by the finding of a pulsating mass in the neck just below the angle of the mandible. Systolic bruits are present in many of these patients, especially the elderly, but there is often no evidence of other atherosclerotic lesions. These aneurysms may be painful, tender, or asymptomatic. They are occasionally recognized as a pulsating tumor of the tonsillar fossa or pharynx, with little or no manifestation of their presence externally in the neck.

The classic paper by Shipley's group[60] emphasized that aneurysms of the internal carotid present inwardly into the throat, whereas those of the common carotid present outwardly in the neck. The absence of cervical swelling in the former is attributed to the dense, deep cervical fascia and muscles attached to the styloid process anteriorly and the cervical vertebrae posteriorly that crowd the gradually dilating aneurysm inward toward the tonsillar fossa, where the thin superior pharyngeal constrictor muscle and mucous membrane offer only minimal resistance to inward protrusion. The level at which the common carotid bifurcates also influences the point of appearance, for with a low bifurcation even an internal carotid aneurysm is likely to be visible and palpable externally in the neck.

Because aneurysms that arise at or proximal to the carotid bifurcation are readily palpable, they usually pose no diagnostic difficulty; however, those arising from the internal carotid near the base of the skull can and do cause diagnostic problems. A chronic unilateral swelling of the posterior pharynx should raise the level of suspicion, especially when other physical signs are lacking, bizarre, or atypical. Otolaryngologists often are the first to see these lesions. A high index of suspicion usually leads to computed tomography (CT), magnetic resonance imaging (MRI), or angiography, which are nearly always diagnostic when an aneurysm is present.

Most patients with extracranial carotid aneurysms are symptomatic. Although larger lesions tend to produce the most severe symptoms, even small carotid aneurysms can be symptomatic.

Pain

Overall, pain probably is the most common local symptom.[32] It was prominent in 40% of patients in a reported series from the Mayo Clinic.[6] Some patients have aching in the neck, retro-orbital pressure, or throbbing headaches. Glossopharyngeal compression can account for auricular pain, and radiation into the occipital area also occurs. Dissection can cause acute, severe cervical, retro-orbital or hemicranial pain.[59]

Dysphagia

The mass of an aneurysm can cause compression of adjacent structures. Dysphagia secondary to the bulk of the lesion or to compression of the nerve supply to the pharynx is a frequent symptom.

Cranial Nerve Compression

Aneurysms arising near the carotid canal may compress other nerves and produce severe recurrent facial pain, fifth and sixth cranial nerve palsies, deafness, and occasionally a Horner syndrome. Vagal compression may cause hoarseness. Oculosympathetic paresis and intermittent facial pain (Raeder's paratrigeminal syndrome) in some cases have been caused by a carotid aneurysm at the base of the skull.[34]

Central Nervous System Dysfunction

Reports indicate that central neurologic deficits are the most common symptoms produced by carotid aneurysms.[54] This reflects the high percentage of atherosclerotic aneurysms in several series.[6, 14, 50, 51] These lesions tend to produce either transient ischemic attacks or strokes occurring in more than 40% of patients. Transient neurologic deficits occur about twice as often as completed strokes.[43, 67, 70] Most neurologic events are due to embolization of thrombotic material emanating from the aneurysmal wall, but some are caused by diminished flow when a large aneurysm compresses the internal carotid artery when the head is turned to certain positions. Occasionally, concomitant carotid bifurcation occlusive disease accounts for neurologic events.

Hemorrhage

Hemorrhage is now a rare manifestation of carotid aneurysm. In earlier reports, many of these aneurysms were first noticed because of hemorrhage from the pharynx, ear, or nose. Bleeding of this type is usually from an internal carotid artery aneurysm or from infected false aneurysms after carotid endarterectomy. If rupture occurs into the oropharynx, the bleeding can be massive and can lead to suffocation and death. Most fatalities have usually been preceded by repeated episodes of hemorrhage that were improperly recognized or treated. Mycotic aneurysms are especially susceptible to rupture and bleeding.[46]

DIFFERENTIAL DIAGNOSIS

The most frequently encountered lesion that must be distinguished from an extracranial carotid aneurysm is a kinked or coiled carotid artery (see Chapter 135).[33, 49] This usually involves the common carotid artery, producing a pulsatile mass at the base of the neck, typically on the right side, in obese, hypertensive, older women. This lesion has been referred to by Bergan and Hoehn as "evanescent cervical pseudoaneurysm."[3] It is much more common than bona fide aneurysms in this location, from which it can be readily distinguished by the characteristic location and by the nature of the pulsation, which is parallel to the long axis of the vessel, in contrast to the pulsation of an aneurysm, which typically is expansile at right angles to the axis of the parent vessel. Soft tissue radiographs of the neck may reveal linear calcification in an atherosclerotic aneurysm, but not in a tortuous artery. Duplex ultrasonography readily defines the lesion.

Redundant length also causes sigmoid curves, loops, and coils of the internal carotid artery higher in the neck. These usually are discovered by angiography because their high cervical location renders them nonpalpable.

A prominent carotid bifurcation in a patient with a thin neck can also be mistaken for a carotid aneurysm, as are carotid body tumors, enlarged lymph nodes, branchial cleft cysts, and cystic hygromas. Careful physical examination should identify these entities correctly, but more objective modalities are useful in confirming the diagnosis.

Ultrasonography (B-mode with or without Doppler spectral analysis) should establish the correct diagnosis of those aneurysms low enough in the neck to be evaluated with this technique. Extracranial carotid aneurysms can also be demonstrated by CT.[17] The CT anatomy of the neck, nasopharynx, and parapharyngeal spaces is well known, and carotid aneurysms deforming these areas should be clearly differentiated from other mass lesions, particularly if bolus contrast injection and dynamic scanning are employed. MRI is equally effective and may be the method of choice when dissection is the suspected cause, owing to its unique ability to identify old blood in the dissection plane. Recently, ultra-fast (spiral) CT scans have also been shown to be very accurate for diagnosis of dissection.

Even if the diagnosis of extracranial carotid aneurysm is made by one of the imaging techniques described, angiography is necessary to obtain the detailed vascular anatomy necessary for the planning of surgical treatment; angiography should also be performed in virtually all patients in whom an aneurysm is suspected and cannot be excluded by other diagnostic methods.[38] Magnetic resonance angiography (MRA) can also provide definitive diagnostic information. Early experience with spiral CT with three-dimensional image reconstruction (CT angiography) has been favorable for other types of carotid lesions and may prove useful for aneurysms as well (see Chapters 14 and 15). As they do with aneurysms in other locations, conventional angiograms (including digital subtraction angiography) may underestimate the size of carotid aneurysms as a result of the presence of mural thrombus. High-quality, detailed views of both carotid arteries and both vertebral arteries as well as the intracranial vessels are essential for adequate angiographic evaluation.

TREATMENT

The treatment of extracranial carotid aneurysms has evolved with the specialty of vascular surgery. The choice of treatment depends on the size, location, and etiologic mechanism of the lesion in question, and it must be individualized. As noted previously, some small, traumatic, distal internal carotid aneurysms may remain stable or may even shrink when observed for a long period, whereas mycotic aneurysms are associated with a much poorer prognosis.[9]

For most patients, the primary objective of treatment is the prevention of permanent neurologic deficits that arise from atheroembolism or thromboembolism. This can best be accomplished by resection of the aneurysm and restoration of arterial continuity. Unfortunately, these goals are not always possible.

Ligation

In 1552, Ambroise Paré published the first account of operative ligation of the common carotid artery to control massive hemorrhage from a laceration of the artery. His patient had aphasia and a contralateral monoplegia. In 1805, Astley Cooper performed the first common carotid ligation for an aneurysm of the artery. Hemiplegia developed on the eighth postoperative day, and the patient died 13 days later. Cooper later accomplished the first successful treatment of a cervical carotid aneurysm by proximal ligation, and this, coupled occasionally with distal ligation and extirpation, remained the procedure of choice until Matas developed the technique of *endoaneurysmorrhaphy.*

In 1926, Winslow was able to report that the death rate from cervical carotid aneurysms had decreased from 71% with conservative therapy to 30% following ligation, and in 1951 ligation was still recommended as the treatment of choice despite the unpredictability of the outcome.[68] Modifications, such as the use of partially constricting bands rather than complete occlusion, were used by some surgeons to lessen the danger of cerebral ischemia. Kirby

and coworkers pointed out the dangers of such procedures, and made an unsuccessful attempt to resect a syphilitic carotid aneurysm in 1949.[33]

The subsequent development of reconstructive vascular techniques has eliminated ligation as a procedure of choice. Ligation now should be limited to aneurysms of the internal carotid artery that extend distally to the base of the skull so that distal control of the vessel cannot be obtained, making resection with arterial reconstruction impossible. Even then, however, successful reconstructions can be accomplished using special maneuvers to increase exposure, such as drilling away portions of the petrous and mastoid bones. Ligation of the vessel also may be necessary in emergency situations when rupture has occurred, especially if infection is the cause.

Ligation results in thrombosis from the level of the interruption up to the origin of the first major intracranial collateral artery, usually the ophthalmic artery, thereby obliterating the aneurysm. When this method is used, however, neurologic deficits occur in 30% to 60% of the patients, and half of such patients die.[7, 33] This may be the result of acute cerebrovascular insufficiency due to inadequate collateral circulation. Gradual carotid occlusion with devices such as the Selverstone clamp has not eliminated this problem.

In an effort to avoid this complication, numerous techniques have been developed for preoperative determination of the adequacy of cerebral collateral circulation. The *carotid compression tests* (Matas' test, and the like) have all proved unreliable, as has the observation of intracerebral cross-filling seen on angiography or by transcranial Doppler examination. Intraoperative measurement of the back-pressure in the temporarily occluded internal carotid artery has been shown by Moore and associates and by others to be an excellent predictor of tolerance of temporary carotid occlusion in patients with occlusive disease, and it can be applied similarly to patients with aneurysms. The oculopneumoplethysmograph (OPG-Gee), when used with carotid compression, also can be used to determine the internal carotid back-pressure and can provide this information preoperatively.[24] These instruments are no longer available in most medical centers. Alternatively, carotid artery back-pressure can be measured at the time of angiography by means of a catheter with an inflatable balloon proximal to a measuring port. Both methods correlate closely with carotid back-pressure measured intraoperatively. A carotid back-pressure in excess of 60 to 70 mmHg suggests the presence of sufficient collateral cerebral perfusion to enable a patient to withstand carotid ligation without development of an ischemic neurologic deficit.

Careful analysis of the results of carotid ligation reveals a substantial number of patients who experience hemiplegia hours to days after the procedure. Because this sequela most probably represents propagation of thrombus into the branches of the internal carotid artery rather than acute cerebrovascular insufficiency, heparin anticoagulation should be maintained for 7 to 10 days when carotid ligation is performed. When carotid ligation is required but collateral cerebral perfusion is inadequate, an extracranial-to-intracranial arterial bypass procedure should be considered. The superficial temporal-middle cerebral bypass was the most commonly performed procedure of this type, but concerns about the volume of flow through the superficial temporal artery has led to the use of saphenous vein grafts as the preferred method of minimizing the risk of irreversible cerebral ischemia.

Wrapping

External wrapping of the aneurysm, suggested by Thompson and Austin more than 40 years ago, is an alternative to ligation when resection is not feasible.[63] These authors used fascia lata, but prosthetic materials seem equally well suited. Wrapping may control the expansion of the aneurysm and may limit the risk of rupture, but it is not reliable for reducing the more significant risks of embolism or thrombosis. This method is not appropriate except in the most unusual circumstances. Of note, it was usually unsuccessful for treatment of abdominal aortic aneurysms.

Endoaneurysmorrhaphy

Originally described by Matas, endoaneurysmorrhaphy has largely been replaced by more modern reconstructive vascular techniques, but it still is useful for some fusiform aneurysms that are unresectable because they extend to the base of the skull. This technique can be performed over an internal shunt wedged into the carotid foramen to control back-bleeding. Some saccular aneurysms may also be treatable by localized arterial repair, and several mycotic aneurysms have been treated by a modification of this technique employing débridement of the arterial wall and autogenous patch angioplasty.[25, 31, 55]

Resection

Resection of the aneurysm with restoration of flow is the preferred method of treatment.[11, 44, 56, 59] It is indicated for accessible lesions of the common carotid and proximal third of the internal carotid artery. More distal lesions usually present difficulties in gaining distal control, and other methods often must be employed. A small saccular aneurysm with a narrow neck can be managed by aneurysmectomy and primary closure or patch angioplasty as previously described. Fusiform lesions and saccular lesions with large necks are not as suitable for this type of local repair. They should be resected, and arterial continuity reestablished.

The first report of resection of a carotid aneurysm with primary anastomosis was that of Shea and associates in 1955,[59a] although the first successful procedure of this type was performed by Dimtza in 1952.[16, 58] Beall and associates performed the first prosthetic graft replacement for this lesion in 1959.[2] In subsequent years, there have been numerous reports of successful carotid aneurysm resection with reestablishment of arterial continuity, and this should be the objective of all such procedures. Redundancy of the carotid vessels allows resection and primary anastomosis to be performed in more than 50% of cases, especially when the aneurysm is small.

Anastomosis of the proximal external carotid artery to the more distal internal carotid artery has been successfully used to bridge an internal carotid defect resulting from aneurysm excision. A spatulated anastomosis using inter-rupted suture technique diminishes the likelihood of anastomotic narrowing. When inadequate length of vessels precludes primary anastomosis, interposition grafts must be used. Prosthetic and autogenous (artery or vein) grafts have been used with equally good results, although an autogenous conduit is preferable whenever infection is a possibility.

Large aneurysms and aneurysms involving the most distal internal carotid artery are especially challenging technically. Exposure of the upper end of the internal carotid may be enhanced by several maneuvers, including:

1. Division of the sternocleidomastoid muscle from its mastoid attachment and elevation or resection of the parotid gland.
2. Division of the digastric muscle.
3. Removal of the styloid process and its attached muscles.
4. Use of intraluminal balloons (usually as an intraluminal shunt) to control distal internal carotid back-bleeding.

Subluxation of the mandible by any of several techniques can increase the width of exposure of the distal field at the base of the skull by approximately 1 cm.[10, 11, 14, 51, 59] Nearly equal advantage can be gained by using a nasotracheal rather than an endotracheal tube for administration of general anesthesia.

Complete excision of large lesions risks injury to cranial nerves, including the facial, vagus, spinal accessory, hypoglossal, and glossopharyngeal nerves. Profound disturbances in swallowing can occur as a result of injury to pharyngeal muscular branches arising from the vagus, superior laryngeal, and glossopharyngeal nerves. Although these are usually temporary deficits, they can be severely disturbing to affected patients and the cause of considerable postoperative morbidity. To minimize these problems, the surgeon must use extreme care when dissecting these structures, and a bipolar cautery should be employed for hemostasis. The surgeon should also pay attention to gentle handling of the aneurysm itself in order to prevent dislodgment and downstream embolization of mural thrombus.

Methods of cerebral protection during the period of carotid occlusion required for repair of carotid aneurysms are the same as those used during bifurcation endarterectomy for occlusive disease. Some surgeons employ electroencephalographic monitoring or cerebral blood flow measurements.[43, 59, 62] Others selectively use an internal shunt based on back-pressure criteria. Routine shunting is advocated by many surgeons because of the longer time required for this type of carotid reconstruction compared with that required for endarterectomy. The shunt may also be helpful by serving as a stent during construction of the anastomoses. Hypothermia, induced hypertension, and hypercapnia or hypocapnia are unnecessary and confusing adjuncts.

With modern vascular surgical techniques, correction of most extracranial carotid aneurysms should be possible with a high rate of success and an acceptable rate of neurologic complications. Results vary with the type, size, and location of the aneurysm. In general, surgical therapy is associated with a mortality rate of about 2%, although mortality rates as high as 40% have been reported for carotid ligation for infected post-endarterectomy false aneurysms. The central neurologic morbidity rate ranges from

6% to 20%; it is highest in atherosclerotic cases, and this rate is obviously higher than that with the treatment of occlusive carotid bifurcation atherosclerosis. Cranial nerve defects occur in about 20% of patients. Fortunately, most of these defects are transient.

Endovascular Therapy

The application of endovascular techniques to the management of cerebrovascular lesions is increasing rapidly. Higashida and colleagues have definitively treated several high-cervical true and false aneurysms with intravascular detachable silicone balloons and platinum coils inserted via a transfemoral route.[29, 30] This has resulted in obliteration of the aneurysm and preservation of cervical carotid patency and flow. In several other patients with acute pseudoaneurysms that were due to trauma or tumor erosion, these investigators obliterated the aneurysm by trapping it between two balloons; one was placed in the cavernous carotid artery below the ophthalmic artery but beyond the inferolateral and meningohypophyseal trunk, and a second one was placed just proximal to the aneurysm. As with surgical ligation, test occlusion to document tolerance to permanent carotid occlusion is obviously mandatory prior to this method of treatment.

Although neurologic complications have followed this form of therapy, the long-term results have been encouraging. This procedure should be considered in the treatment of carefully selected patients with difficult and dangerous aneurysms, especially those at the skull base. Despite the advances in skull base surgery, the associated morbidity may be substantial with some of the special techniques required to gain adequate exposure at that location. Endovascular treatment avoids such problems by reaching the lesion entirely through an intraluminal route.[27, 39] Endoluminal stents and stented grafts have also been used to treat these lesions, especially dissections. Stents can be placed across the neck of an aneurysm to promote aneurysm thrombosis while maintaining vessel patency. If thrombosis does not occur, thrombogenic coils can be placed into the aneurysm through the interstices of the stent.

REFERENCES

1. Agrifoglio M, Rona P, Spirito R, et al: External carotid artery aneurysms. J Cardiovasc Surg 30:942, 1989.
2. Beall AC, Crawford ES, Cooley DA, et al: Extracranial aneurysms of the carotid artery: Report of seven cases. Postgrad Med 32:93, 1962.
3. Bergan JJ, Hoehn JG: Evanescent cervical pseudoaneurysms. Ann Surg 162:213, 1965.
4. Biller J, Hingtgen WL, Adams HP Jr, et al: Cervicocephalic arterial dissections: A ten-year experience. Arch Neurol 43:1234, 1986.
5. Bour P, Taghavi I, Bracard S, et al: Aneurysms of the extracranial internal carotid artery due to fibromuscular dysplasia: Results of surgical management. Ann Vasc Surg 6:205, 1992.
6. Bower TC, Pairolero PC, Hallett JW Jr, et al: Brachiocephalic aneurysm: The case for early recognition and repair. Ann Vasc Surg 5:125, 1991.
7. Brackett CE Jr: The complications of carotid artery ligation in the neck. J Neurosurg 10:91, 1953.
8. Buscaglia LC, Moore WS, Hall AD: False aneurysm after carotid endarterectomy. JAMA 209:1529, 1969.
9. Busuttil RW, Davidson RK, Foley KT, et al: Selective management of extracranial carotid artery aneurysms. Am J Surg 140:35, 1980.
10. Carrel T, Bauer E, von Segesser L, et al: Surgical management of extracranial carotid-artery aneurysms: Analysis of 6 cases. Cerebrovasc Dis 1:49, 1991.
11. Coffin O, Maiza D, Galateau-Salle F, et al: Results of surgical management of internal carotid artery aneurysms by the cervical approach. Ann Vasc Surg 11:482, 1997.
12. Dawson KJ, Stansby G, Novell JR, Hamilton G: Mycotic aneurysm of the cervical carotid artery due to Salmonella enteritidis. Eur J Vasc Surg 6:327, 1992.
13. Dehn TCB, Taylor GW: Extracranial carotid artery aneurysms. Ann R Coll Surg Engl 66:247, 1984.
14. de Jong KP, Zondervan PE, van Urk H: Extracranial carotid artery aneurysms. Eur J Vasc Surg 3:557, 1989.
15. Deysine M, Adiga R, Wilder JR: Traumatic false aneurysm of the cervical internal carotid artery. Surgery 66:1004, 1969.
16. Dimtza A: Aneurysms of the carotid arteries: Report of two cases. Angiology 7:218, 1956.
17. Duvall ER, Gupta KL, Vitek JJ, et al: CT demonstration of extracranial carotid artery aneurysms. J Comput Assist Tomogr 10:404, 1986.
18. Ehrenfeld WK, Wylie EJ: Spontaneous dissection of the internal carotid artery. Arch Surg 111:1294, 1976.
19. Ekestrom S, Bergdahl L, Huttunen H: Extracranial carotid and vertebral artery aneurysms. Scand J Thorac Cardiovasc Surg 17:135, 1983.
20. Faggioli GL, Freyrie A, Stella A, et al: Extracranial internal carotid artery aneurysms: Results of a surgical series with long-term follow-up. J Vasc Surg 23:587, 1996.
21. Ferguson LJ, Fell G, Buxton B, Royle JP: Mycotic cervical carotid aneurysm. Br J Surg 71:245, 1984.
22. Fisher CM, Ojemann RG, Roberson GH: Spontaneous dissection of cervicocerebral arteries. J Can Sci Neurol 5:9, 1978.
23. Friedman WA, Day AK, Guisling RG, et al: Cervical carotid dissecting aneurysms. Neurosurgery 7:207, 1980.
24. Gee W, Mehigan JT, Wylie EJ: Measurement of collateral cerebral hemispheric blood pressure by ocular pneumoplethysmography. Am J Surg 130: 121, 1975.
25. Grossi RJ, Onofrey D, Tvetenstrand C, Blumenthal J: Mycotic carotid aneurysm. J Vasc Surg 6:81, 1987.
26. Hammon JW Jr, Silver D, Young WF Jr: Congenital aneurysm of the extracranial carotid arteries. Ann Surg 176:777, 1972.
27. Hacein-Bey L, Connolly ES Jr, Duong H: Treatment of inoperable carotid aneurysms with endovascular occlusion after extracranial-intracranial bypass surgery. Neurosurgery 41:1225, 1997.
28. Hejhal L, Hejhal J, Firt P, et al: Aneurysms following endarterectomy associated with patch graft angioplasty. J Cardiovasc Surg 15:620, 1974.
29. Higashida RT, Hieshima GB, Halbach VV, et al: Cervical carotid artery aneurysms and pseudoaneurysms. Acta Radiol 369:591, 1986.
30. Higashida RT, Hieshima GB, Halbach VV, et al: Intravascular detachable balloon embolization of intracranial aneurysms. Acta Radiol 369:594, 1986.
31. Jebara VA, Acar C, Dervanian P, et al: Mycotic aneurysms of the carotid arteries: Case report and review of the literature. J Vasc Surg 14:215, 1991.
32. Kaupp HA, Haid SP, Gurayj MN, et al: Aneurysms of the extracranial carotid artery. Surgery 72:946, 1972.
33. Kirby CK, Johnson J, Donald JG: Aneurysm of the common carotid artery. Ann Surg 130:913, 1949.
34. Klein GE, Szolar DH, Raith J: Posttraumatic extracranial aneurysm of the internal carotid artery: Combined endovascular treatment with coils and stents. Am J Neuroradiol 18:1261, 1997.
35. Latter DA, Ricci MA, Forbes RDC, Graham AM: Internal carotid artery aneurysm and Marfan's syndrome. Can J Surg 32:463, 1989.
36. Ledgerwood AM, Luca CE: Mycotic aneurysm of the carotid artery. Arch Surg 109:496, 1974.
37. Lueg EA, Awerbuck D, Forte V: Ligation of the common carotid artery for the management of a mycotic pseudoaneurysm of an extracranial carotid artery: A case report and review of the literature. Int J Pediatr Otorhinolaryngol 33:67, 1995.
38. Margolis MT, Stein RL, Newton TH: Extracranial aneurysms of the internal carotid artery. Neuroradiology 4:78, 1972.
39. McCollum CH, Wheeler WG, Noon GP, et al: Aneurysms of the extracranial carotid artery: Twenty-one years' experience. Am J Surg 137:196, 1979.
40. McNeill DH Jr, Driesbach J, Marsden RJ: Spontaneous dissection of the internal carotid artery: Its conservative management with heparin sodium. Arch Neurol 37:54, 1980.

41. Miyauchi M, Shionoya S: Aneurysm of the extracranial internal carotid artery caused by fibromuscular dysplasia. Eur J Vasc Surg 5:587, 1991.

42. Mokri B, Sundt TM Jr, Houser OW: Spontaneous internal carotid dissection, hemicrania, and Horner's syndrome. Arch Neurol 36:677, 1979.

43. Mokri B, Piepgras DG, Sundt TM, et al: Extracranial internal carotid artery aneurysms. Mayo Clin Proc 57:310, 1982.

44. Moreau P, Albat B, Thevent, A: Surgical treatment of extracranial internal carotid aneurysm. Ann Vasc Surg 8:409, 1994.

45. Motte S, Wautrecht JC, Bellens B, et al: Infected false aneurysm following carotid endarterectomy with vein patch angioplasty. J Cardiovasc Surg 28:734, 1987.

46. Nicholson ML, Horrocks M: Leaking carotid artery aneurysm. Eur J Vasc Surg 2:197, 1988.

47. O'Connell BK, Towfighi J, Brennan RW, et al: Dissecting aneurysms of head and neck. Neurology 35:993, 1985.

48. Painter TA, Hertzer NR, Beven EG, et al: Extracranial carotid aneurysms: Report of six cases and review of the literature. J Vasc Surg 2:312, 1985.

49. Perdue GD, Barreca JP, Smith RB III, et al: The significance of elongation and angulation of the carotid artery: A negative view. Surgery 77:45, 1975.

50. Petrovic P, Avramov S, Pfau J, et al: Surgical management of extracranial carotid artery aneurysms. Ann Vasc Surg 5:506, 1991.

51. Pratschke E, Schafer K, Reimer J, et al: Extracranial aneurysms of the carotid artery. Thorac Cardiovasc Surg 28:354, 1980.

52. Raptis S, Baker SR: Infected false aneurysms of the carotid arteries after carotid endarterectomy. Eur J Vasc Endovasc Surg 11:148, 1996.

53. Reid MR: Aneurysms in the Johns Hopkins Hospital. Arch Surg 12:1, 1926.

54. Rhodes EL, Stanley JC, Hoffman GL, et al: Aneurysms of extracranial carotid arteries. Arch Surg 111:339, 1976.

55. Rice HE, Arabi S, Kremer R, Needle D, Johansen K: Ruptured *Salmonella* mycotic aneurysm of the extracranial carotid artery. Ann Vasc Surg 11:416, 1997.

56. Rosset E, Roche PH, Magnan PE, Branchereau A: Surgical management of extracranial internal carotid aneurysms. Cardiovasc Surg 2:567, 1994.

57. Schechter DC: Cervical carotid aneurysms: I. N Y State J Med 79:892, 1979.

58. Schechter DC: Cervical carotid aneurysms: II. N Y State J Med 79:1042, 1979.

59. Schievink W, Piepgras D, McCaffrey TV, Mokri B: Surgical treatment of extracranial internal carotid artery dissecting aneurysms. Neurosurgery 35:809, 1994.

59a. Shea PC, Glass LG, Reid WA, et al: Anastomosis of common and internal carotid arteries following excision of mycotic aneurysm. Surgery 37:829, 1955.

60. Shipley AM, Winslow N, Walker WW: Aneurysm in the cervical portion of the internal carotid artery: An analytical study of the cases recorded in the literature between August 1, 1925, and July 31, 1936. Report of two new cases. Ann Surg 105:673, 1937.

61. Stonebridge PA, Clason AE, Jenkins AM: Traumatic aneurysm of the extracranial internal carotid artery due to hyperextension of the neck. Eur J Vasc Surg 4:423, 1990.

62. Sundt TM Jr, Pearson BW, Piepgras DG, et al: Surgical management of aneurysms of the distal extracranial internal carotid artery. J Neurosurg 64:169, 1986.

63. Thompson JE, Austin DJ: Surgical management of cervical carotid aneurysms. Arch Surg 74:80, 1957.

64. Un-Sup K, Friedman EW, Werther LJ, et al: Carotid artery aneurysm associated with nonbacterial suppurative arteritis. Arch Surg 106:865, 1973.

65. Webb JC, Barker WF: Aneurysms of the extracranial internal carotid artery. Arch Surg 99:501, 1969.

66. Welling RE, Kakkasseril JS, Peschiera J: Pseudoaneurysm of the cervical internal carotid artery secondary to blunt trauma. J Trauma 25:1108, 1985.

67. Welling RE, Taha A, Goel T, et al: Extracranial carotid artery aneurysms. Surgery 93:319, 1983.

68. Winslow N: Extracranial aneurysm of the internal carotid artery. Arch Surg 13:689, 1926.

69. Zelenock GB, Kazmers A, Whitehouse WM, et al: Extracranial internal carotid artery dissections. Arch Surg 117:425, 1982.

70. Zwolak RM, Whitehouse WM, Knake JE, et al: Atherosclerotic extracranial carotid artery aneurysms. J Vasc Surg 1:415, 1984.

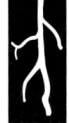

C H A P T E R   1 3 5

Uncommon Disorders Affecting the Carotid Arteries

Thomas A. Whitehill, M.D., and
William C. Krupski, M.D.

Never bet against atherosclerosis.

Edwin J. (Jack) Wylie

One of my (W.C.K.) beloved former mentors, Dr. Jack Wylie, was fond of using this aphorism. Indeed, atherosclerotic occlusive disease is the most common abnormality of the extracranial cerebrovasculature, but there are many other processes with which the surgeon dealing with cerebrovascular disorders must be familiar. Because these conditions are rare, large studies are unavailable and their management must be based on the experience of several select authorities and anecdotal reports. Several relatively uncommon extracranial disorders, including vertebrobasilar insufficiency, extracranial aneurysms, and extracranial fibromuscular disease, have been discussed in earlier chapters. This chapter discusses the clinical presentation and management of carotid artery coils and kinks, carotid body tumors, carotid sinus syndrome, carotid artery dissection, radiation-induced carotid arteritis and stenosis, adjacent malignancy and infection, vasculitis (including Takayasu's arteritis and temporal arteritis), and moyamoya disease. In addition, the current status of extracranial-intracranial bypass is briefly summarized.

CAROTID ARTERY KINKS AND COILS

Anatomists first described elongated and distorted carotid arteries in autopsy specimens in the mid-1700s.[201] In 1898, Kelly reported finding large, pulsating vessels in the pharynx in the proximity of tortuous internal carotid arteries.[110] In the early 1900s, there were numerous reports describing fatal hemorrhage after injury to tortuous carotid arteries during tonsillectomy or adenoidectomy.[39, 59, 102, 213] Riser and colleagues in France first described cerebrovascular symptoms related to redundant kinked carotid arteries in 1951.[191] These investigators described a patient with an elongated carotid artery that was straightened by affixing the artery to the sheath of the sternocleidomastoid muscle. Subsequently, the patient remained asymptomatic.

In 1956, Hsu and Kistin reported the first direct surgical repair of a kinked carotid artery.[97] In 1959, Quattlebaum and associates described 3 patients who presented with hemiplegia and kinked carotid arteries.[184] The patients were treated by resection and reanastomosis of the common carotid artery, with relief of symptoms.

There is no universal agreement regarding the potential for alleviation of cerebrovascular symptoms by surgical repair of tortuous kinked and coiled carotid arteries. Numerous angiographic and autopsy studies have shown that carotid redundancy is not uncommon and that most individuals with this anatomic variant remain asymptomatic.[92] Although most carotid kinks and coils are incidental findings with no clinical significance, there does appear to be a subset of patients whose anatomy produces cerebrovascular symptoms as a direct consequence of carotid angulation.

Pathophysiology

Kinks and coils of the internal carotid artery may be developmental or acquired. In both types, the carotid artery is excessively long in fixed space, resulting in redundancy and tortuosity of the vessel. The redundancy may occur in coronal, transverse, or sagittal planes. Usually the internal carotid artery is affected, but occasionally kinks and coils are seen in the common carotid artery as well. The internal carotid artery usually assumes an S shape, but single and even double complete loops have been described. When the elongation becomes acutely angulated, a carotid kink may be present; kinks are usually associated with atherosclerotic plaque or arterial stenoses (Fig. 135–1).

The congenital coils seen in children may result from faulty descent of the heart and great vessels within the mediastinum during embryologic development. The carotid artery is formed by the third aortic arch and the dorsal aorta. During embryologic development, there is a prominent bend at the junction of these vessels. The carotid artery is quite tortuous. As the heart descends into the thorax, these vessels straighten, but kinking can occur if the straightening process is incomplete. Alternatively, tortuosity may result from relative overgrowth of the lengthening process of the carotid as the cervical skeletal elongates. Normally, one process keeps pace with the other, establishing the correct length of the carotid artery. A greater frequency of bilateral carotid coiling in children (~50%) than in adults supports this hypothesis.

Carotid coils in adults occur more frequently in elderly people in whom atherosclerosis is also frequently present.

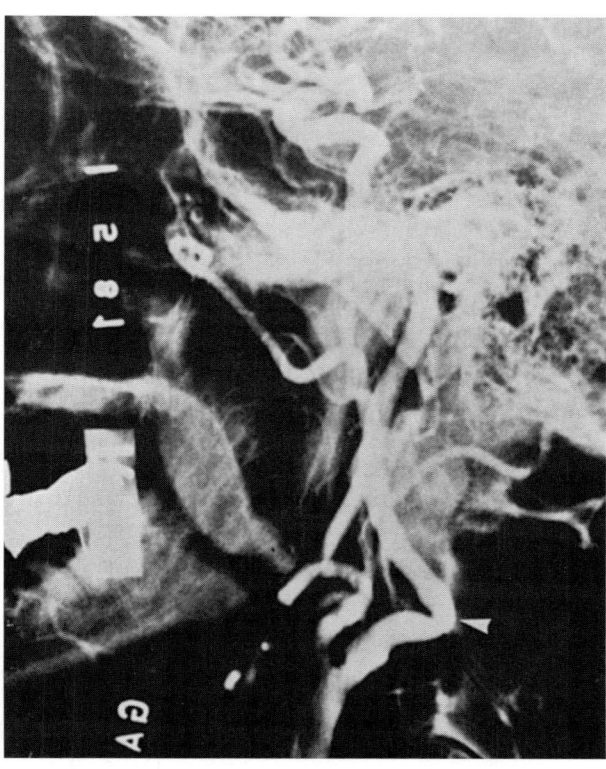

FIGURE 135–1. Lateral carotid arteriogram demonstrating a tight kink of the internal carotid artery (*arrowhead*). The external carotid artery is also elongated and tortuous.

Coiling may be acquired from excessive elongation of the artery with age, and the elongated artery may have thinning of the media and fragmentation of elastic lamina. Often, one carotid artery is more prominently coiled than the other; bilaterality occurs in only 25% of adults. A kink in the carotid artery may be a consequence of degeneration of the arterial wall, loss of elasticity, or hypertension-induced elongation due to increased intraluminal pressure. Support for this hypothesis is provided by the occurrence of kinks in older individuals who frequently have hypertension as well as atherosclerotic disease. In most instances, athero-sclerotic plaques are present proximal to internal carotid kinks, which can fix the vessel and promote tortuosity. Alternatively, fascial bands can tether the artery. These bands, which represent remnants of the embryonic aortic arch, cross the internal carotid artery at or above the bifurcation and become fibrotic with increasing age. As the involved carotid arteries elongate with age, they become fixed between two points by the arch and these external bands. Thus, a kink usually occurs in the internal carotid artery 2 to 3 cm beyond the bifurcation.

Vannix and associates have reported that carotid kinks are four times more common in women than in men.[234] This increased predominance in women may explain the greater frequency with which older hypertensive women, in contrast to men, are thought to have carotid aneurysms when they actually have tortuous carotid or subclavian vessels. Bergan and Hoen have described this physical finding as the "evanescent cervical pseudoaneurysm."[15]

Incidence

The true incidence of kinks and coils of the carotid artery is unknown because most patients with this anatomy remain asymptomatic. In a review of anatomic studies in patients who died of other causes, Cairney described a 30% preva-lence.[26] Most recent reports are based on arteriographic studies in elderly individuals with cerebrovascular symp-toms. One of the largest angiographic series was reported by Weibel and Fields from the Methodist Hospital in Hous-ton, Texas.[241] In 2453 carotid angiograms performed in 1438 patients, tortuosity of the carotid artery was observed in 489 (35%), coiling in 88 (6%), and kinking in 65 (5%). Among 76 patients with coiled carotid arteries, 40 (53%) had bilateral involvement, and 15 (28%) of 53 patients with kinked carotid arteries had bilateral disease.

In another large review, Metz and coworkers analyzed 1000 consecutive carotid arteriograms.[152] These investiga-tors defined a kink as angulation between two vessel seg-ments of 90 degrees or less, or formation of a complete loop. Kinked carotid arteries were found in patients of every decade examined (the first through the eighth), but most cases occurred between ages 41 and 70 years. In all, 161 patients (16%) had some degree of kinking. Sixty patients (6%) had severe kinking (angle less than 30 de-grees); of these, 14 (23%) had cerebrovascular symptoms (stroke, n = 8; single transient ischemic attack [TIA], n = 2; recurrent TIA, n = 4).

In a series of 308 patients who had undergone carotid artery operations, Najafi and associates reported a 5% inci-dence of carotid artery kinking.[168] Vannix and associates reported 15 cases of post-endarterectomy kinking in 312 carotid reconstructions, resulting in an incidence of

4.8%.[234] Busuttil and colleagues described kinks in 10 of 670 carotid operations (1.4%) in a 13-year period.[23] Ca-rotid kinks can occur after operations for carotid atheroscle-rosis.

Clinical Presentation

In children, carotid coils have rarely been associated with neurologic symptoms; but in adults, kinks are much more commonly responsible for neurologic manifestations in adult patients with elongated carotid arteries.[199] Because cerebrovascular flow is not compromised by carotid loops or coils, the finding is often of no clinical significance in adults. However, kinks in the carotid artery are more likely to produce luminal narrowing and flow abnormalities. In addition to hemodynamic abnormalities, carotid artery kinking may produce turbulent blood flow and subsequent intimal ulceration and embolization. Symptoms, therefore, are usually similar to those caused by atherosclerotic dis-ease of the carotid bifurcation, and patients may present with strokes, hemispheric TIAs, or amaurosis fugax. Verte-bral artery kinking may present with vertebrobasilar insuf-ficiency, and symptoms include ataxia, diplopia, bilateral paresthesias, vertigo, dysarthria, or drop attacks.

A peculiar feature of symptoms caused by carotid artery kinks is an association with head turning. Quattlebaum and associates have described occurrence of symptoms as patients turn their heads sideways.[185] Ipsilateral rotation produces greatest flow reduction, but even contralateral and neck flexion/extension may exaggerate the kink and reduce blood flow.[220] In some patients, head rotation pro-duces total occlusion of an otherwise patent, but redun-dant, carotid artery. Thus, when focal neurologic deficits of vertebral basilar insufficiency can be reproduced by head motion, the clinician should suspect a carotid kink.

Diagnosis

Carotid kinks and coils cannot be reliably diagnosed by physical examination, although occasionally a prominent pulsation suggestive of a carotid aneurysm may be palpated in the neck. The mass is due to the tissue volume occupied by the carotid kink or coil; it is accentuated by head rotation if the kink involves the internal carotid artery (ICA). Occasionally, the kink can be palpated intraorally in a tonsillar fossa.[201] A bruit may be present but may appear when the patient's head is turned to the side in the presence of a carotid kink.

Noninvasive studies historically have been used to iden-tify patients who might have carotid kinks that are hemody-namically significant. These include oculoplethysmography, technetium-pertechnetate brain scans, and electroencepha-lography.[91, 92, 131, 199, 220, 229] Although such positional testing might be helpful in identifying hemodynamically significant kinking, the incidence of false-positive studies has not been established; thus, all these tests must be corroborated by angiography.

The definitive diagnosis of carotid kinks and coils re-quires four-vessel cerebral arteriography. Multiple views are necessary, with patients in neutral, flexion, extension, and rotation positions. It is most important that the arteriogram be performed with the head in a position thought to pro-duce neurologic symptoms.

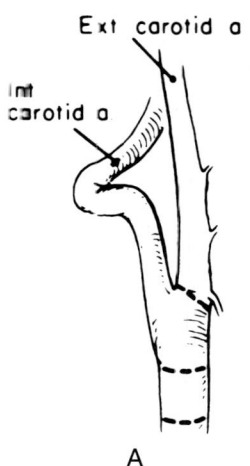
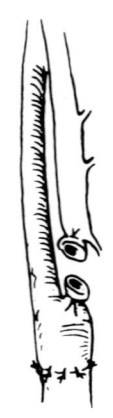

Ext carotid a

Int carotid a

A

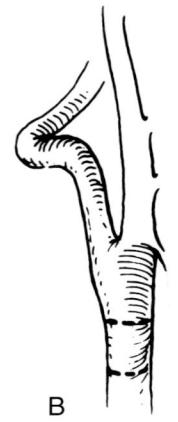
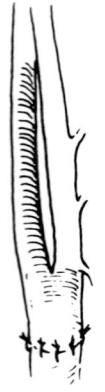

B

FIGURE 135–2. *A,* Resection of the common carotid artery with external carotid artery (ECA) ligation and division to remove a kink from the internal carotid artery. *B,* If the ECA is also redundant, as shown in Figure 135–1, it may not require ligation as part of this maneuver.

Treatment

Because the natural history of carotid kinks and coils is uncertain and because of the relatively small number of patients identified with symptomatic disease, most authorities recommend nonoperative management in asymptomatic patients. When symptoms are corroborated by arteriographic findings in symptomatic patients, hemodynamic alterations may be implicated, and surgical correction is indicated.[45, 180]

Although it has been described in the past, simple surgical tethering of the elongated redundant and tortuous kinked or coiled carotid artery (arteriopexy) is inadequate treatment because it does not correct the redundancy. There are several surgical options for the correction of the internal carotid kink: (1) a long patch angioplasty, (2) internal carotid resection and reanastomosis, (3) internal carotid resection and saphenous vein interposition, (4) internal carotid reimplantation into the side of the common carotid artery, and (5) resection and reanastomosis of a portion of the common carotid.[37, 67, 214, 220, 234] Although some investigators recommend ligation and division of the external carotid artery when performing common carotid resection, Poindexter and colleagues have advocated preservation of this potential collateral vessel[180] (Fig. 135–2).

A more anatomic procedure than common carotid resection involves resection of the kinked portion of the ICA and reanastomosis with or without patch angioplasty. The disadvantage of this technique is the use of the smaller ICA, a difficulty that is occasionally posed when the kink is close to the base of the skull (Fig. 135–3). Alternatively, the ICA may be detached from its bifurcation and reanastomosed more proximally to the common carotid artery (Fig. 135–4). During the operation, the patient's head should be turned to be sure that the new location will not produce a new kink.

Although there are no large individual series, the collective results of operations for carotid kinks in patients with symptomatic disease have been good. Approximately 80% of patients have been rendered asymptomatic, with an approximate 5% perioperative stroke and mortality rate.[91, 185, 220, 234] Patients operated on for lateralizing symptoms have better outcomes than patients operated on for global ischemic symptoms.

CAROTID BODY TUMORS

The controversy regarding the biologic behavior and surgical management of carotid body tumors is reflected in the voluminous literature on the subject. In 1743, Von Haller first described the carotid body.[238] Reigner first attempted resection of a carotid body tumor in 1880, but the patient did not survive.[188] Maydl was the first to remove a carotid body tumor successfully, in 1886, but the patient became aphasic and hemiplegic.[146] In 1903, Scudder performed the first successful removal of a carotid body tumor in the United States, with preservation of the carotid artery and avoidance of significant nerve injury.[206] As of this writing, more than 900 cases have been reported in the literature.[16, 42, 44, 62, 69, 98, 123, 149, 150, 189, 196, 244]

Physiology

The carotid body is a chemoreceptor located in the bifurcation of the common carotid artery, in the adventitia of its posterior medial surface. It is attached by a thin strand of adventitia known as Meyer's ligament, which also carries its blood supply that arises from the external carotid artery in most cases. The carotid body is derived from both

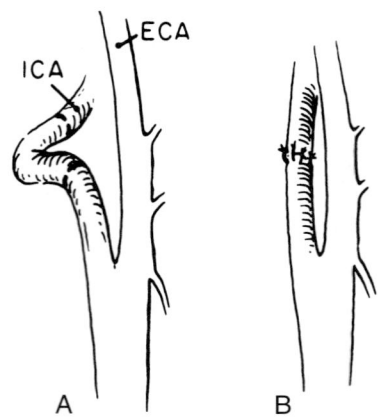

ECA

ICA

A

B

FIGURE 135–3. *A,* Segmental resection of a length of the internal carotid artery. *B,* Reanastomosis of the internal carotid artery using meticulous interrupted suture technique.

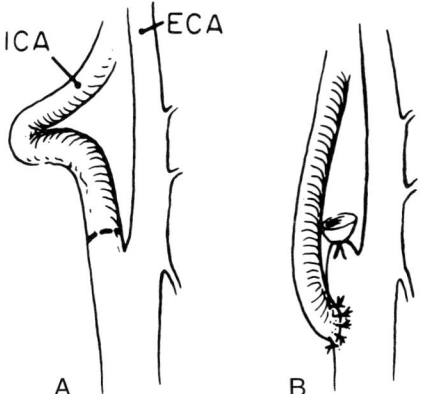

FIGURE 135–4. *A*, Transection of the kinked internal carotid artery (ICA) at its origin with the ECA. *B*, Reimplantation onto the more proximal common carotid artery.

mesodermal elements of the third branchial arch and neural elements originating from the neural crest ectoderm.[183] These neural crest cells further differentiate into forerunners of paraganglionic cells. Because cells in the neural crest migrate in close association with autonomic ganglion cells, neoplasms have been called "paragangliomas." Mulligan introduced the term "chemodectoma" from the Greek words *chemia* (infusion), *dechesthai* (to receive), and *oma* (tumor).[166] The terms paraganglioma and chemodectoma are often used interchangeably.

Histologically, cervical chemodectomas resemble the normal architecture of the carotid body. The tumors are highly vascular, and between the many capillaries are clusters of cells called *Zellballen* (cell balls) (Fig. 135–5). One is a "sustentacular" or supporting cell. The other is the epithelioid, or chief, cell, which has finely granular eosinophilic cytoplasm. Cytochemical techniques have demonstrated epinephrine, norepinephrine, and serotonin in these cells.[79] Although there are reports of functioning tumors producing hypertension in the carotid and jugular bodies[64, 133] this is clearly unusual. In contradistinction, retroperitoneal chemodectomas often secrete catecholamines, and more than 60% of patients with such tumors present with a *pressor-amine syndrome*.[27] In the absence of hypertension, screening studies for catecholamine metabolites in patients with cervical chemodectoma appear unwarranted.

Paragangliomas are classified as *chromaffin* and *non-chromaffin*. Chromaffin-positive cells possess the ability to produce catecholamines. Initially, carotid body tumors were thought to be non-chromaffin paragangliomas, but recent studies have demonstrated some chromaffin-positive secretory granules, suggesting that the carotid body is capable of secreting catecholamines.[183] At most, 5% of carotid body tumors are endocrinologically active.[41, 73, 130]

It has been suggested that carotid body tumors may be a part of the neurocristopathies that occur in various combinations, such as *multiple endocrine neoplasia* (MEN), types I and II. Secondary tumors are common in patients with carotid body tumors, including pheochromocytomas.

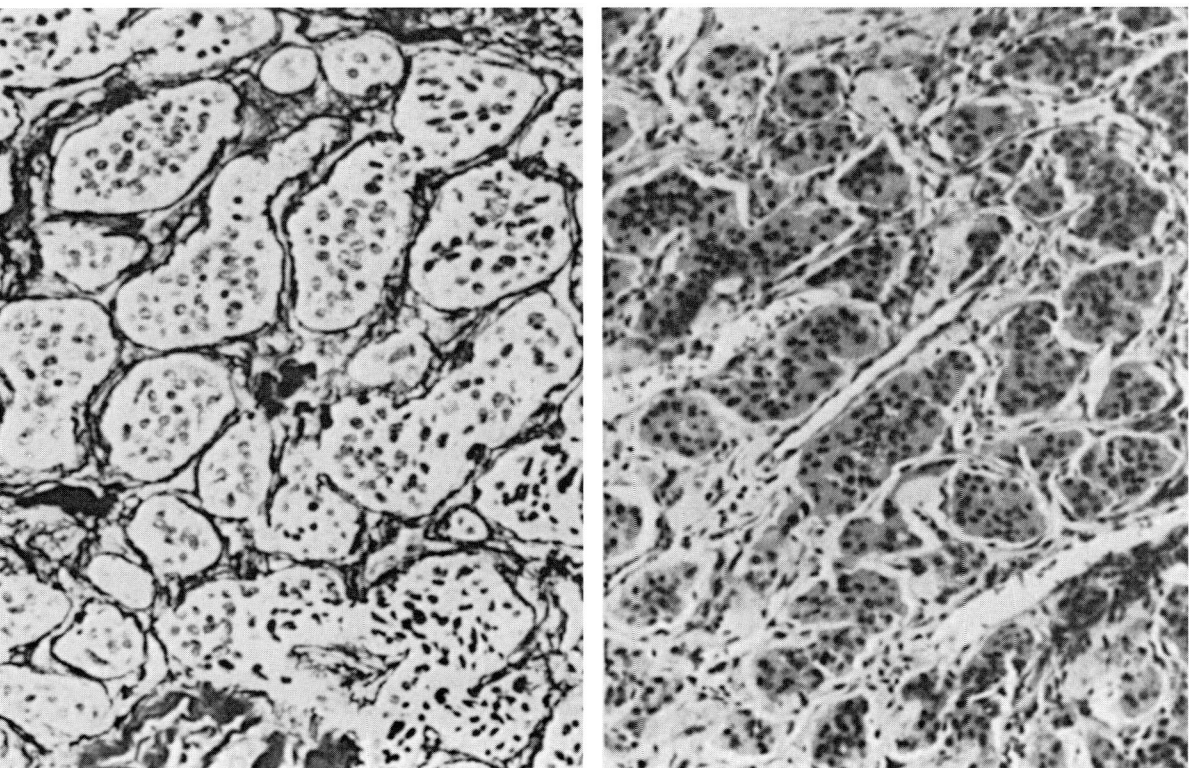

FIGURE 135–5. Cross-sectional photomicrographs of a carotid body tumor. *Left,* Reticulin stain accentuates the characteristic Zellballen (cell nests). Clusters of darkly stained red blood cells mark numerous small blood vessels. *Right,* On hematoxylin/eosin staining, the cell nests are shown to be separated by fibrous septa containing numerous small vascular spaces. The tumor cells have moderately abundant, finely granular eosinophilic cytoplasm, indistinct cell borders, and round-to-oval nuclei. (× 125.) (From Krupski WC, Effeney DJ, Ehrenfeld WK, Stoney RJ: Cervical chemodectoma: Technical considerations and management options. Am J Surg 144:218, 1982. With permission from Excerpta Medica Inc.)

MEN I and II involve tissues, such as the medulla of the thyroid, that are also derived from the neural crest.[19] The carotid body has extremely high blood flow and oxygen consumption, averaging approximately 0.2 L/gm/minute, which is more than is required by the thyroid, brain, and heart.[153]

The carotid body is responsive primarily to hypoxia and, to a lesser degree, to hypercapnia and acidosis. In addition, the incidence in carotid body tumors is increased in individuals living at high altitudes and in patients subjected to chronic hypoxia.[34, 197] Stimulation of the carotid body produces an increase in respiratory rate, tidal volume, heart rate, blood pressure together with vasoconstriction, and production of circulating catecholamines.[62] The afferent input to the carotid body is via the glossopharyngeal nerve to the reticular formation of the medulla.[30]

Pathology

The normal carotid body measures approximately 5 × 3 × 2 mm, approximately the size of a grain of wheat.[28, 153] Its only known pathology is neoplasia, which is the most common of the non-chromaffin paragangliomas. Paragangliomas are located at the base of the skull, in the nasopharynx, and throughout the body cavities. They are known as glomus jugulare, glomus intravagale, glomus aorticum, glomus ciliare, and Zuckerkandl bodies. They also are found in various locations in the retroperitoneum (Fig. 135–6). Synonyms for carotid body tumor include chemodectoma, endothelioma, glomus caroticum, perithelioma,

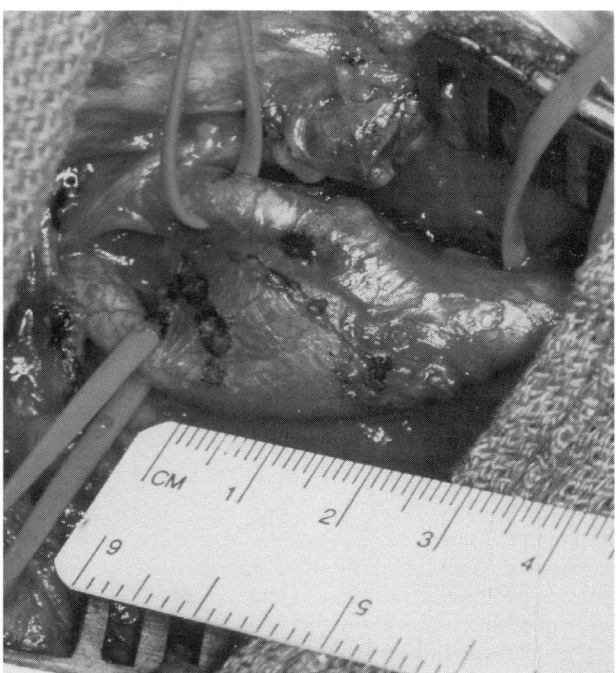

FIGURE 135–7. Operative photograph taken during resection of a small carotid body tumor. Vessel loops encircle the common (right), external (left upper), and internal (left lower) carotid arteries. (See Color Plate.)

chromaffinoma, and non-chromaffin paraganglioma. "Carotid body tumor" is the preferred term in current usage, however.

Macroscopically, carotid body tumors are well circumscribed, rubbery in consistency, and reddish brown in color. Their microscopic appearance has been described earlier. Despite the well-circumscribed nature of carotid body tumors, there is no true capsule.[105, 183] As the tumor grows, the carotid bifurcation is progressively distorted, and the internal and external carotid arteries are "splayed" (Fig. 135–7).

The renowned Mayo Clinic surgeon Shamblin and colleagues described three anatomic groups of carotid body tumors.[207]

Group I consists of relatively small tumors, which are minimally attached to the carotid vessels; surgical excision is not difficult.
Group II tumors are larger, with moderate attachments. These tumors can be resected, but many patients require a temporary intraluminal carotid shunt.
Group III tumors are very large neoplasms that encase the carotid arteries and often require arterial resection and grafting.

Biologic Behavior

Carotid body tumors may be sporadic or familial. In the more common *sporadic* form, there is a 5% incidence of bilateral carotid body tumors.[105, 150, 207] In the *familial* form of carotid body tumors, transmission is by an autosomal dominant pattern.[82] In the familial form, there is a 32% incidence of bilateral tumors.[82, 86] Screening of family mem-

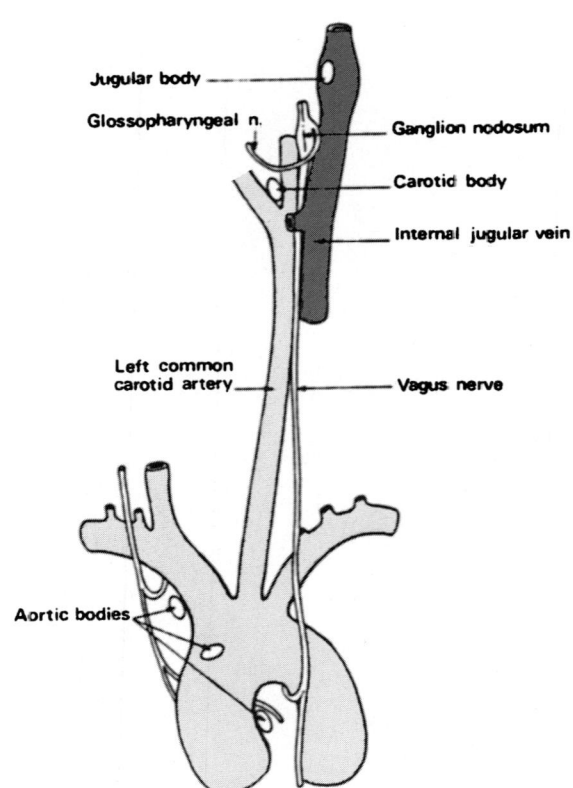

FIGURE 135–6. Anatomic location of chemoreceptive tissues. (From Krupski WC, Effeney DJ, Ehrenfeld WK, Stoney RJ: Cervical chemodectoma: Technical considerations and management options. Am J Surg 144:217, 1982. With permission from Excerpta Medica Inc.)

bers is strongly recommended in these cases, since the ease of resection is based on size of the tumor.

There has been considerable controversy over the malignant potential of carotid body tumors. The reported rates of malignancy range from 2% to 50% in the medical literature.[31, 69, 130, 186, 207, 218] Malignant potential cannot be predicted by nuclear pleomorphism or mitotic activity. Dissemination can become apparent many years after the initial diagnosis.[79, 207, 218] Because the malignant potential of carotid body tumors cannot be predicted by histologic markers, this determination can be made only by the presence of lymph nodes or distant metastases. Metastatic spread generally occurs in regional lymph nodes. Metastases have also been described to the kidney, thyroid, pancreas, cerebellum, lungs, bone, brachial plexus, abdomen, and breast.[56, 186, 193, 244] Metastases should not be confused with multicentricity of paragangliomas at other sites in the body.[47] Most authorities estimate that the metastatic rate of carotid body tumors is approximately 5%.[98, 130, 193, 207]

Most carotid body tumors grow slowly and exhibit benign characteristics. Many patients may survive for long periods without surgical treatment, but these tumors can cause significant disability and death, even without malignancy. Death due to asphyxia and intracranial extension of carotid body tumors has been described.[44, 142, 163] Martin and colleagues noted a death rate of about 8% in untreated patients.[142] Some authors have reported palliation using radiation therapy alone, but most agree that this is not acceptable primary treatment.[130, 142, 149, 207] Complications from radiation therapy include osteonecrosis of the mandible, carotid radiation arteritis, and laryngeal injury. Even after prolonged disease-free intervals, local recurrence following surgical resection has also been described.[142, 218] Predictors of future biologic behavior are the severity of symptoms and the size of the carotid body tumors at the time of diagnosis.[123]

Incidence

Because of the rarity of carotid body tumors, their incidence is difficult to determine. Hallett and associates reported one of the largest experiences in 1988, in which 153 cervical paragangliomas were treated over a 50-year period from 1935 to 1985 at the Mayo Clinic.[86] This experience far surpassed the experience at most busy centers, but accounted for only at most three to four patients with this disorder per year. There are conflicting reports with respect to gender prevalence; some citations show a male predominance whereas others note a 3:1 female predominance.[86] In familial carotid body tumors, there appears to be an equal distribution between men and women, thus supporting an autosomal mode of genetic transmission. Although cases have been reported in patients ranging in age from the second to the eighth decade, most tumors become apparent in the fifth decade of life.

Clinical Presentation

Most commonly, patients present with a painless swelling in the neck, located at the angle of the mandible. The mass has often been present for several years, and patients may first become aware of it because their shirt collars become

tight. Other nonspecific symptoms may include neck or ear pain, local tenderness, hoarseness, dysphasia, or tinnitus. Typically, many years may elapse between initial recognition of the mass and surgical treatment.[123, 207] Although cranial nerve dysfunction in unoperated carotid body tumors is unusual, symptoms from vagal, hypoglossal, and cervical sympathetic nerve impingement have been described.[42, 178] Patients rarely have lateralizing central neurologic symptoms or signs, although they may describe dizziness.[16] Because approximately 5% of tumors may have neurosecretory activity, some patients describe symptoms of dizziness, flushing, palpitations, tachycardia, arrhythmias, headache, diaphoresis, and photophobia. Neuroendocrine activity obviously has anesthetic implications.[250]

The most notable finding on physical examination is a neck mass located below the angle of the mandible, which is laterally mobile but vertically fixed because of its attachment to the carotid bifurcation. The mass is often pulsatile due to its close relationship to the carotid artery. A bruit may be audible due to impingement of the artery, but this is a nonspecific finding as atherosclerosis is frequently present in this location as well. Rarely, patients demonstrate neurologic abnormalities caused by vagal or hypoglossal nerve involvement; even more unusual is the patient who presents with Horner's syndrome. The mass is usually nontender, rubbery in consistency, firm in texture, and noncompressible. Because of the 5% incidence of bilaterality even in nonfamilial tumors, the opposite side of the neck should be carefully palpated as well; this is especially important when familial tumors are suspected.[86]

Diagnosis

Although history and physical findings are helpful, the diagnosis of carotid body tumor is included in the differential diagnosis of numerous other causes of neck masses, including lymphomas, metastatic tumors, carotid artery aneurysms, thyroid lesions, submandibular salivary gland tumors, and branchial cleft cysts. The vascularity of carotid body tumors is important in several ways. First, percutaneous needle aspiration or incisional biopsy is strongly contraindicated, as these procedures may result in massive hemorrhage, pseudoaneurysm formation, and carotid thrombosis.[178, 218] Duplex scanning with color flow imaging usually documents the highly vascularized mass in the area of the carotid bifurcation.[80, 221, 249] Characteristically, tumors separate the internal and external carotid arteries, widening the bifurcation (Fig. 135–8). The vascularity of carotid body tumors is readily shown by color flow imaging, which differentiates them from the relatively nonvascular masses listed earlier. In addition, duplex scanning can provide information on the tumor dimensions and demonstrate any coexistent carotid occlusive disease.

The carotid body normally obtains its blood supply from the external carotid artery, but as the tumor grows, contributions from the ICA, vertebral artery, and thyrocervical trunk can develop.[31, 251] Because patients may demonstrate such unusual blood supply, thereby complicating exposure and hemostasis, angiography remains the gold standard for the diagnosis of carotid body tumors. Bilateral angiography is important for the evaluation of concurrent atherosclerosis, collateral flow, and identification of multicentric disease.

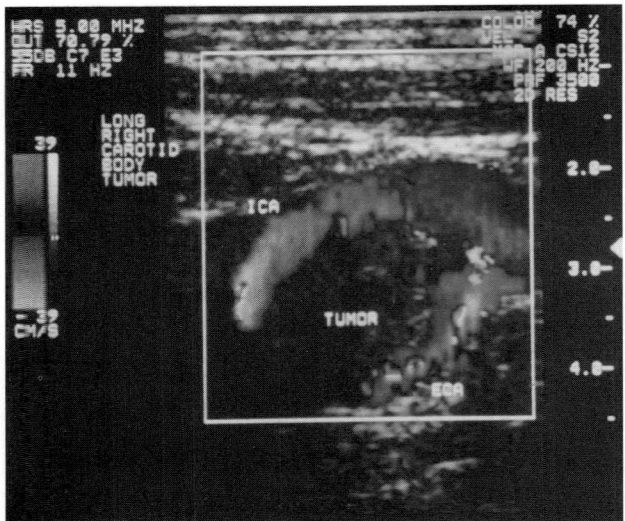

FIGURE 135–8. Characteristic duplex color flow image of a carotid body tumor. The internal and external carotid branches are splayed by the tumor mass. The tumor may exhibit a very active mixed-signal pattern representing the extensive vascularity of the tumor. (See Color Plate.)

Both computed tomography (CT) scans and magnetic resonance imaging (MRI) scans have been useful in evaluating cervical masses. Although differentiation between aneurysm and neoplasm may be difficult, dynamic or rapid sequencing CT improves this differentiation.[210] MRI may be superior to CT scanning for demonstrating the relationship of the carotid body tumors to adjacent structures.[177, 237] MRI can readily differentiate carotid body tumors from other soft tissue lesions at the base of the skull because of the highly vascular nature of these lesions. Both CT and MRI scans can demonstrate the size and extent of the tumor and help plan proper surgical exposure.

Treatment

Because of the 5% or greater incidence of metastases and the unrelenting growth of unresected tumors (which tends to encase the adjacent neurovascular structures, making delayed surgery more hazardous), the mainstay of treatment for carotid body tumors is complete surgical excision. Early removal of small, asymptomatic tumors decreases the incidence of cranial nerve and carotid artery injuries. Unfortunately, most carotid body tumors, when discovered, are in Shamblin's group II and III at the time of clinical presentation.[123] As indicated previously, radiation therapy for carotid body tumors has been largely unsatisfactory, except for local control of residual or recurrent disease.[204, 233] Radiotherapy prior to surgery makes operative treatment more difficult. Chemotherapy has no role.

The role of preoperative embolization of highly vascular carotid body tumors is controversial. Preoperative embolization has been reported by some to decrease vascularity and improve the safety of surgical excision, with lower operative blood loss and decreased technical difficulties.[127, 192, 215] However, percutaneous embolization may produce thrombosis of the ICA or cerebral embolization.[179]

Surgical Technique

As indicated, arteriography is essential for diagnosis and to provide information about carotid artery anatomy and the vascular supply of the carotid body tumor (Fig. 135–9). Cranial nerve function should be evaluated carefully prior to operation. Despite increased improvements in technique, the incidence of postoperative nerve damage has not been substantially reduced. Catecholamine screening should be reserved for those few individuals who present with a history suggesting endocrine activity and for those with bilateral tumors, even without clinical evidence of neurosecretory activity.

The anatomic and technical details of operations for carotid body tumors are similar to those for carotid endarterectomy. Because blood loss can be substantial, an autotransfusion device should be available, reducing the requirements for bank blood. Extremely large tumors extending toward the base of the skull may require subluxation of the temporal mandibular joint to facilitate distal carotid artery exposure. A suitable saphenous vein should be available, if a graft is required, since complicated arterial reconstruction is required in up to 25% of cases. Carotid shunts also should be available if clamping of the ICA is necessary because of low carotid back-pressure, intraopera-

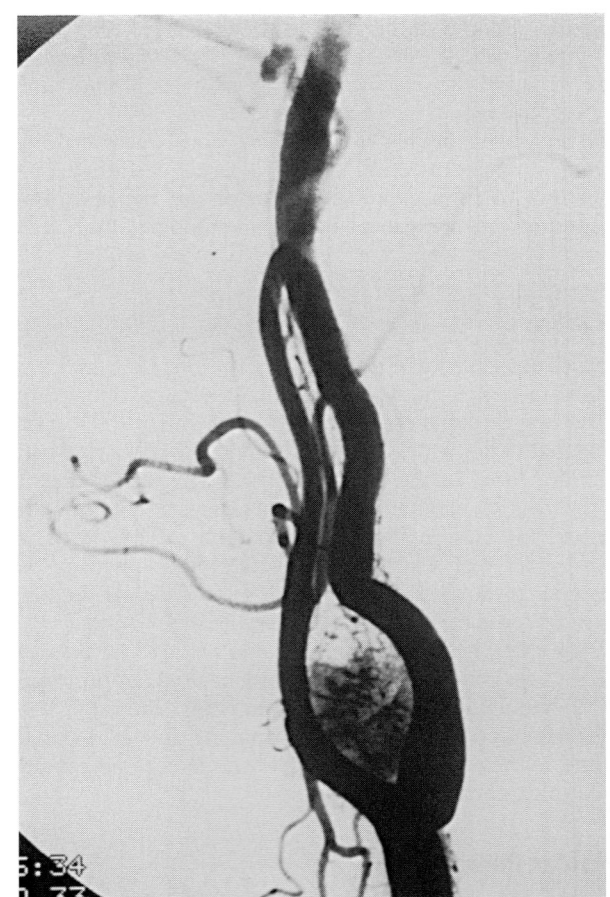

FIGURE 135–9. Selective carotid arteriogram demonstrating the classic characteristics of a carotid body tumor. The bifurcation is widened by the tumor; note the contrast density of the "tumor blush" that portrays the highly vascular nature of these tumors.

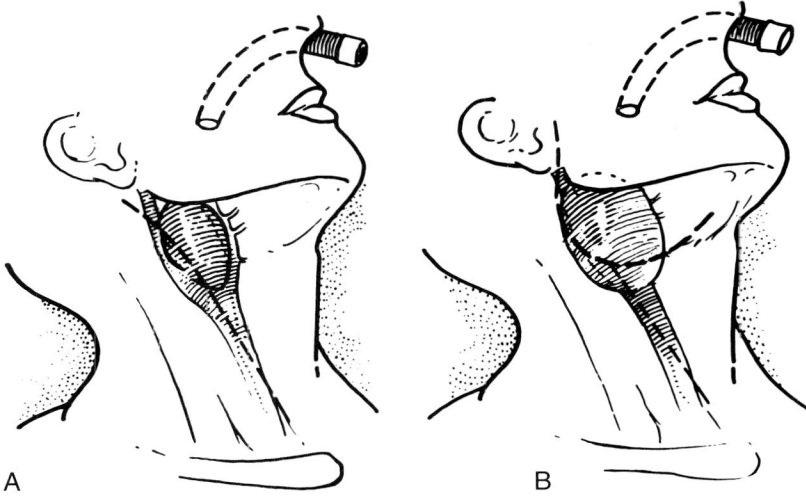

FIGURE 135–10. Operative incisions appropriate for carotid body tumor resection. The nasotracheal tube allows for greater distraction of the mandible, if required. *A*, Incision for small tumor (Shamblin I). *B*, Incision for medium and large tumors (Shamblin II and Shamblin III). (From Hallett JW: Carotid body tumor resection. *In* Bergan JJ, Yao JST [eds]: Techniques in Arterial Surgery. Philadelphia, WB Saunders, 1990, p 214.)

tive electroencephalographic (EEG) changes, or other indications of inadequate cerebral perfusion. Avoidance of cranial nerve injury may be achieved by meticulous dissection around the tumor and by the use of bipolar electrocautery to minimize conductive heat injury to adjacent nerves.

General endotracheal anesthesia is preferable. Nasotracheal intubation may be required if temporal mandibular subluxation is anticipated. Patient positioning is identical to that for carotid endarterectomy. A longitudinal incision along the anterior border of the sternocleidomastoid muscle curving behind the ear usually gives adequate exposure. However, large tumors are more easily excised with a modified T neck incision (Fig. 135–10). An alternative incision in front of the ear, with parotid gland mobilization and facial nerve preservation, can facilitate distal ICA exposure. The first tenet of vascular surgery, which is to obtain distal and proximal arterial control, should be followed. However, control of the external carotid artery may be especially difficult because it gives rise to the blood supply of the tumor.

Occasionally, with very large tumors, the distal ICA cannot be exposed and arterial reconstruction is impossible. In this case, sacrifice of the ICA may be required. However, ligation of the internal common carotid artery results in a postligation and stroke incidence ranging from 23% to 50% and a mortality rate of from 14% to 64%.[143, 164] When carotid ligation is anticipated preoperatively, the oculopneumoplethysmograph (OPG) may be useful in evaluating the cerebral collateral circulation and the patient's ability to tolerate carotid artery occlusion.[70]

After proximal and distal arterial control has been obtained, the tumor should be mobilized circumferentially to assess the extent of disease. The hypoglossal and vagus nerves must be identified and protected during this maneuver. Resection should not be carried out within the media of the vessels. This can lead to a weakened wall, predisposing the patient to intraoperative hemorrhage or postoperative carotid blowout. Instead, the plane of dissection should be periadventitial, in a so-called "white line" described by Gordon-Taylor.[75] Unfortunately, this white line is often difficult to find, particularly because carotid body tumors

do not have a true capsule and do not shave off the arterial wall easily.

The tumor should be removed beginning at the inferior extent and continuing cephalad. Two particular areas of difficulty are the carotid bifurcation and the posterior surface, which often encompasses the superior laryngeal nerve. Tumors may extend quite high. The posterior belly of the digastric muscle should then be divided, preferably at its insertion into the mastoid groove. The digastric muscle should also be divided to improve exposure and resection of the stylomandibular ligament when access to the most distal ICA is required.

If the proper plane between the tumor and the carotid artery cannot be developed because of transmural tumor invasion of the arterial wall, carotid resection may be required. When this occurs, a segment of greater saphenous vein harvested from the thigh can be used as an interposition graft. In some cases, earlier ligation and division of the external carotid artery may reduce blood flow and facilitate further resection of the tumor[123] (Fig. 135–11). The clamped external carotid artery can be used as a "handle" to assist in mobilization of the tumor. Reconstruction of the external carotid artery following tumor removal is not necessary, and the external carotid stump may be oversewn.

The liberal use of arteriography and modern surgical techniques have reduced the risk of postoperative stroke in carotid body tumor resection from approximately 30% to less than 5%. However, the incidence of cranial nerve injury remains strikingly high, ranging from 20% to 40%.[86, 123, 178] Because of the high incidence of cranial nerve injury, some have questioned the appropriateness of surgical treatment, because most of these tumors are small and slow growing. However, because the morbidity of surgical removal is lowest when the tumors are small, generally they should be removed soon after diagnosis to minimize the risk of postoperative nerve dysfunction (Fig. 135–12).

Most patients do well after curative resection of carotid body tumors. Survival of patients after tumor resection is equivalent to that of sex- and age-matched controls. Metastatic disease develops in fewer than 2% of patients, and only 6% of patients experience recurrence after complete

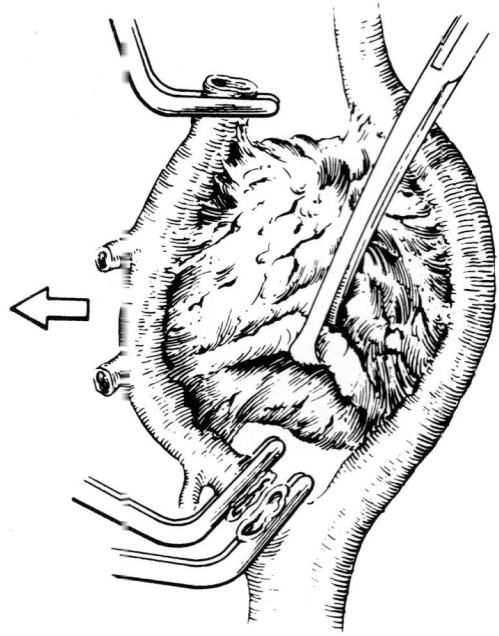

FIGURE 135–11. Ligation and division of the external carotid artery facilitates control of the carotid body tumor blood supply and aids in mobilizing large tumors. The vessel is removed with the tumor. (From Krupski WC, Effeney DJ, Ehrenfeld WK, Stoney RJ: Cervical chemodectoma: Technical considerations and management options. Am J Surg 144:219, 1982. With permission from Excerpta Medica, Inc.)

resection.[164] Periodic clinical observation is indicated in patients with carotid body tumors to detect multicentric or recurrent disease. Those with interposition grafts should undergo duplex scanning periodically to identify graft stenoses. Finally, examination of the patient's relatives is advisable in cases of suspected familial carotid body tumors.

CAROTID SINUS SYNDROME

The carotid sinus is located at the distal end of the common carotid artery as it branches into the internal and external carotid arteries. It is a localized area of dilatation where the tunica media is thinner and the adventitia thicker than elsewhere in the arterial wall. The *carotid sinus* must be differentiated from the *carotid bulb*. The carotid bulb is a fusiform enlargement of the first portion of the ICA, immediately adjacent to the bifurcation of the common carotid artery (Fig. 135–13). The carotid sinus is a collection of sensory nerve endings, with an unusual amount of elastic tissue where smooth muscle cells are scarce. The carotid sinus is baroreceptor tissue; when stimulated by increased intraluminal pressure, it produces reflex bradycardia and decreased blood pressure. The nerve of Hering arises from the glossopharyngeal nerve and has been designated "the carotid sinus nerve." It supplies the carotid sinus and the carotid body; it synapses with the cardioinhibitory and vasomotor centers in the medulla through efferent fibers that are carried in the vagus nerve. (Some anatomists have labeled this the nerve of de Castro.) The nerve of Hering may descend either on the surface of the ICA or between the internal and external carotid artery branches.

The *carotid sinus syndrome* (CSS) consists of syncope caused by carotid sinus hypersensitivity. Patients experience the sudden onset of bradycardia and hypotension. Although the syndrome has been attributed to a hypersensitive carotid sinus, the true pathophysiology is unknown. CSS occurs in elderly patients, most commonly men; it is associated with atherosclerosis, diabetes, hypertension, and coronary artery disease.[202, 243] The existence of this syndrome has been questioned, because denervation of one or both carotid sinuses does not produce prolonged and permanently increased blood pressure in patients who have undergone carotid endarterectomy. Thus, CSS must be differentiated from far more common causes of syncope in the elderly—arrhythmias, vertebrobasilar insufficiency, hypoglycemia, orthostatic hypotension, vasovagal attacks, aortic stenosis, and, probably most commonly, overmedication with antihypertensives. It has been estimated that fewer than 1% of elderly patients with syncope have CSS.[108]

A unique finding in patients with CSS is that direct carotid sinus massage or pressure at the carotid artery reproduces symptoms that may be related to both *heart rate–independent* factors and *heart rate–dependent* factors.[78] It is interesting that right-sided hypersensitivity is more frequent than left-sided hypersensitivity. One third of patients describe a prodrome before syncope, and one third have retrograde amnesia. In approximately half of patients, syncope may be precipitated by head movement.[113] Many patients are taking antihypertensive agents and other medications that block compensatory heart rate. If possible, discontinuation of these medications may be efficacious. Carotid body denervation has been suggested in the past for patients with CSS.[3, 35] Currently, carotid body denervation is not recommended because patients have better results when cardiac pacemakers are implanted.[21]

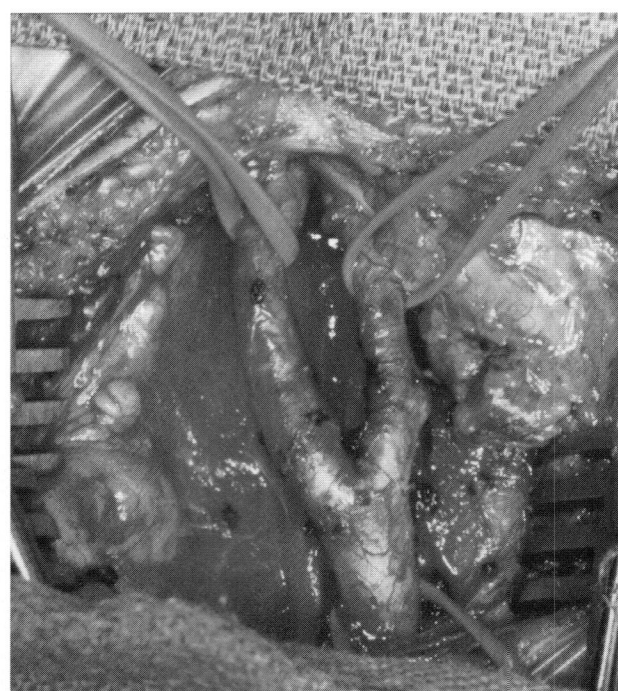

FIGURE 135–12. Postoperative photograph taken after resection of the carotid body tumor shown in Figure 135–7. The adventitia of the carotid arteries is intact; the external carotid artery is preserved. (See Color Plate.)

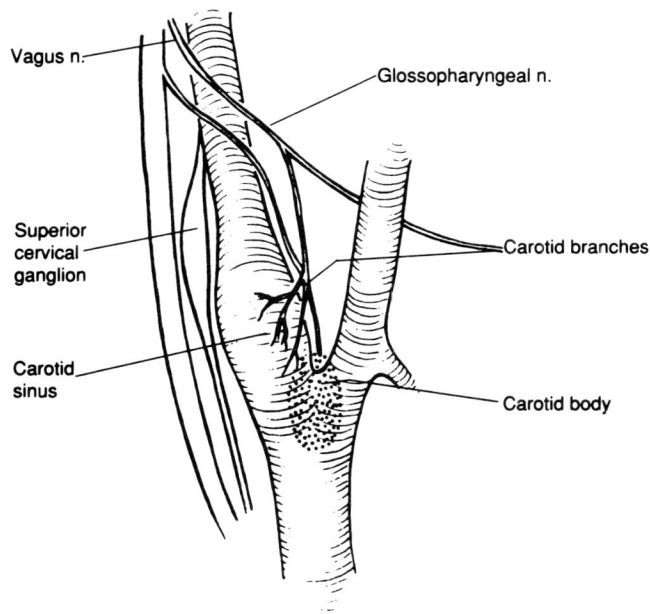

FIGURE 135–13. Diagram of the carotid sinus and the carotid body. The nerve of Hering is shown as it courses to the glossopharyngeal nerve. (From Hollinshead WH: Anatomy for surgeons. *In* The Head and Neck. Vol 1. New York, Hoeber and Harper, 1958.)

Of historical interest is a report by Nakayama that bilateral carotid body excision controlled carbon dioxide retention in patients with asthma.[169] Nakayama reported success in 65% of a staggering 3914 patients who underwent the procedure. Because chemoreceptive tissue exists throughout the body, however, partial excision would be expected to be of little benefit. Follow-up studies demonstrated deleterious effects of this procedure; it has subsequently been abandoned.[248]

CAROTID ARTERY DISSECTION

Arterial dissection consists of intimal disruption, with extravasation of blood into layers of the arterial wall pro-

ducing luminal stenosis, occlusion, or aneurysm formation (Fig. 135–14).[155] Carotid artery dissections are of two types: (1) "spontaneous" dissection, which occurs presumably without cause, and "all others," which include dissections for which a precipitating cause can be identified. However, distinction between these types is imprecise. Unquestionably, dissection of the cervical segment of the carotid artery may occur as a result of penetrating or blunt trauma. In fact, the first case of extracranial dissection of the ICA was described (more than a century ago) in a patient who sustained a blunt, nonpenetrating trauma.[235] Seventy years elapsed before the next case was reported.[27] Subsequently, many cases of both traumatic and spontaneous dissection of the carotid artery have been reported.[4, 12, 52, 60, 68, 76, 89, 94, 106, 137, 154, 156, 158, 175, 222, 230, 242, 253, 254]

In addition to blunt trauma associated with automobile accidents, other mechanisms have produced ICA dissections, including fist fights, boxing, falls, direct neck trauma, accidental hanging, diagnostic carotid compression, and chiropractic manipulative therapy.[157] Hyperextension and rotation of the neck may produce intimal tears by stretching the ICA against the transverse processes of the second and third cervical vertebrae (Fig. 135–15).[253]

Spontaneous carotid dissections were first described by Jentzer in 1954.[106] Five year later, Anderson and Schechter described a second case of spontaneous carotid dissection.[5] Since that time, almost 300 cases have been reported, but the true incidence is difficult to determine because the diagnosis is easily missed in patients who have minimal or no symptoms.[77] In an early series of carotid dissections reported by Ehrenfeld and Wylie, the term "spontaneous dissection" was popularized because a history of recent past cervical trauma or unusual head position or movement preceding the onset of symptoms was not described for any of their group of 19 patients.[52] Despite that publication, controversy continues as to whether or not carotid dissection truly occurs in a spontaneous fashion. In some cases, the role of trivial trauma cannot be entirely excluded. For example, carotid dissection has been described after "bottoms-up" drinking; whiplash injuries; head turning while leading a parade; diving into water; childbirth; paroxysms of coughing, retching, or vomiting; and "head banging" during punk rock dancing.[60, 89, 103, 230, 242]

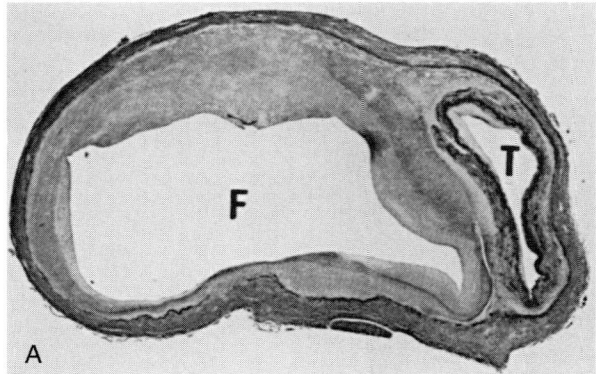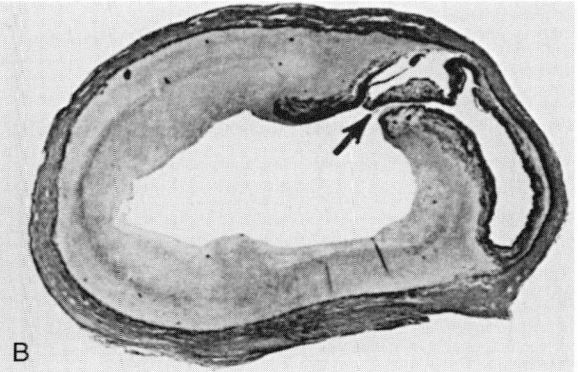

FIGURE 135–14. *A,* Cross section through an aneurysmal segment of a dissected extracranial internal carotid artery. Note the true lumen (*T*) with its surrounding intact internal elastic lamina. The false lumen (*F*) is formed within the media. The external elastic lamina and adventitia surround both lumina. Numerous blood vessel elements are present in the outer vessel wall. *B,* An adjacent cross section reveals the actual intimal tear (*arrow*) and an entry/reentry point of communication between the true and false lumina. (From Mokri M: Dissections of cervical and cephalic arteries. *In* Meyer FB [ed]: Sundt's Occlusive Cerebrovascular Disease. Philadelphia, WB Saunders, 1994, p 45.)

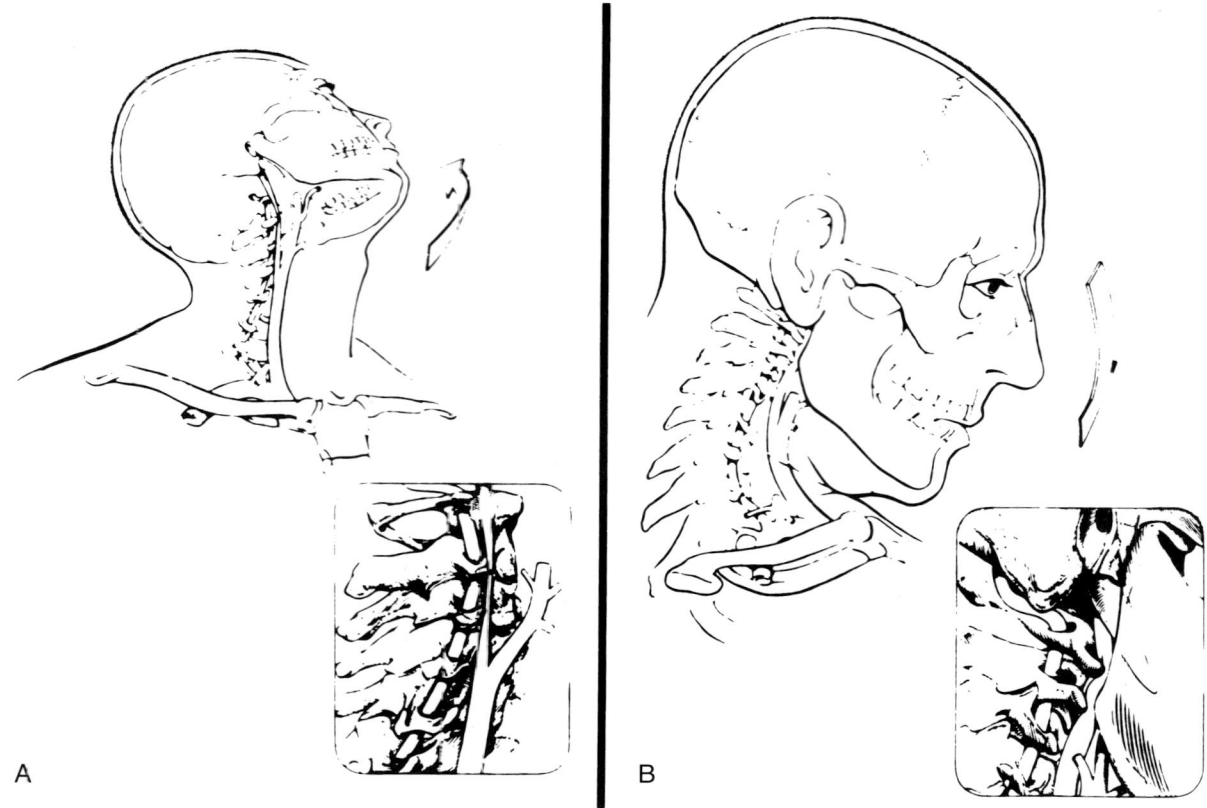

A

B

FIGURE 135–15. A, Hyperextension and rotation of the head subject the opposite carotid artery to stretching and compression injury (1) by the lateral mass of the first cervical vertebra (C-1) or the transverse processes of C-2 and C-3 (B), (2) by direct compression between the angle of the mandible and the transverse processes of C-2 and C-3 through extreme flexion of the head on the neck, or (3) by fracture or posterior dislocation of the mandible. (From Mokri M: Dissections of cervical and cephalic arteries. *In* Meyer FB [ed]: Sundt's Occlusive Cerebrovascular Disease. Philadelphia, WB Saunders, 1994, p 59.)

The misleading term *dissecting aneurysm* has often been applied to any arterial dissection with or without aneurysmal dilatation. In fact, aneurysmal dilatation in initial stages rarely is present. As the intramural hematoma dissects the vessel wall and expands toward the adventitia, aneurysmal dilatation can occur as a late complication.

Pathology

As the hematoma dissects into the vessel wall, it creates a false lumen within the media. Dissections may be in close proximity to the arterial lumen (*subintimal dissections*) or to the adventitia (*subadventitial dissections*). Occasionally, rupture occurs back into the arterial lumen, creating a "double lumen" or a "reentry phenomenon." The false lumen may compress and narrow the true lumen or may expand toward the adventitia, causing aneurysmal dilatation.[137]

In general, the pathogenesis of spontaneous dissection of the ICA artery is unclear in most patients. Atherosclerotic changes in the vessels of patients suffering this disorder are unusual. However, carotid artery dissections have been noted and are associated with Marfan's syndrome and fibromuscular dysplasia of the ICA.[4, 10, 156, 190, 252] The usual location of the intimal tear, the starting point of the dissection, is within 2 to 4 cm of the bifurcation. Thus, it arises

in the carotid bulb. In general, the dissection stops at the entrance of the carotid into the carotid canal, but exceptions do exist. Limited dissections into the cavernous and petrous portions of the ICA have been described.

In spontaneous dissection, histologic abnormalities of the artery are difficult to detect unless arterial resection is required because of extensive arterial pathology, such as in fibromuscular dysplasia (FMD) or Marfan's syndrome. As is usually encountered in dissections, direct communication between the hematoma and arterial lumen cannot be demonstrated. Subtle luminal irregularities remote from the site of dissection have been noted.[94] The significance of these irregularities is unclear, and they may represent an early form of FMD. This was substantiated when Wirth and coworkers described such irregularities, which ultimately proved to be a type of FMD.[247]

Epidemiology

The true incidence of carotid dissection is unknown. Internal carotid dissection occurs in all age groups, but it is more common in young adults. The mean patient age ranges from 41 to 51 years but tends to be lower in those sustaining known traumatic dissections.[18, 89] Hypertension is present in about 40% of patients, in contrast to the lower incidence (14% to 20%) found in the general population in age- and sex-matched controls.

Dissections are often multiple and involve both cervical and visceral arteries in some patients.[154] There is an increased incidence of intracranial aneurysms in patients with carotid artery dissections.[203] In addition, familial intracranial aneurysm and carotid artery dissections have been reported, suggesting the occurrence of a primary arteriopathy in some of these patients.[158] Preference for one gender or side has not been clearly demonstrated.[7, 151]

Clinical Presentation

Carotid artery dissections often produce multiple symptoms. This multiplicity of presentations makes the diagnosis difficult, and the disorder can easily be missed in trauma patients who present with an altered level of consciousness. The principal manifestation in patients with spontaneous carotid dissection is pain, which usually occurs as unilateral headache, particularly in the anterior aspect of the head or in the orbital and periorbital regions. Headaches may also be diffuse or bilateral; they are usually described as steady and nonthrobbing, with fluctuations in intensity. Neck pain occurs much less frequently than does headache. When it does occur, it is often associated with headache and is usually unilateral in the anterolateral aspect of the neck. Patients rarely report scalp tenderness ipsilateral to the headache.

There is discrepancy in the literature with respect to the frequency of central neurologic symptoms associated with carotid dissection. TIAs, stroke, or both have been reported in one third to three quarters of patients with this disorder.[18, 68, 89, 157] The most common combination of symptoms associated with spontaneous carotid dissection is unilateral headache followed by delayed cerebral ischemic symptoms.[162] Mechanisms for hemispheric neurologic deficits include emboli due to platelet aggregates and thrombus formation at sites of intimal damage. Flow reduction from luminal stenosis has also been postulated as a potential mechanism for neurologic symptoms. Subarachnoid hemorrhage can also occur in patients who suffer intracranial carotid artery dissection.[63]

The third most common clinical presentation in patients with spontaneous carotid dissection is *oculosympathetic paresis*, which may occur minutes to days after the onset of headaches. The oculosympathetic paresis of dissection of the ICA consists of incomplete Horner's syndrome, so that facial sweating is unaffected. The cause of this presentation is presumed to be involvement of the sympathetic fibers that accompany the ICA, with sparing of the external carotid plexus that produces facial sweating.

Palsies of other lower cranial nerves have also been described, with dysgeusia (involvement of the chorda tympani branch of cranial nerve VII), slurred speech (involvement of cranial nerve XII), and dysphagia (involvement of cranial nerves IX and X).[129, 154] The precise mechanism of lower cranial nerve palsies is unknown. Proposed mechanisms include direct compression of the lower cranial nerves below the jugular foramen by the dissected artery. Alternatively, an anomalous artery that originates from the petrous or extrapetrous ICA in the neck may be compromised, thus affecting the vascular supply to the nearby cranial nerves. A third proposed mechanism is compromise of an anomalous ascending pharyngeal artery, which arises from the cervical ICA that supplies the lower cranial nerves. Cranial nerve XII is most commonly involved.[159]

Headache, focal cerebral ischemic symptoms, oculosympathetic paresis, and peripheral nerve symptoms may occur in various combinations in patients with dissections of the ICA. Two more distinct syndromes are (1) unilateral headache associated with ipsilateral oculosympathetic paresis, and (2) unilateral headache accompanying delayed focal cerebral ischemic events. Involvement of lower cranial nerves is much less common.

Diagnosis

As with atherosclerotic carotid artery stenosis, evaluation of carotid dissections should begin with a carotid duplex scan. Although ICA dissections usually occur distal to the carotid bifurcation at about the second cervical (C2) vertebral level (beyond the range of carotid ultrasonography), the Doppler signal of the proximal ICA or of the common carotid artery is usually abnormal and suggestive of distal stenosis or occlusion.[12, 254] Because the patients are usually young, they do not often have significant coexistent atherosclerosis. Occasionally, the image demonstrates the intimal flap.

Recently, MRI has played an increasing role in the diagnosis of ICA and vertebral artery dissections. Diagnosis of arterial dissection is made when both the arterial lumen and the intramural hematoma are shown. The lumen appears as a dark, circular area resulting from flow void, which is usually smaller than the normal ICA caliber. The intramural hematoma appears hyperintense and bright in both T1 and T2 weighted images, surrounding the area of flow void as a bright crescent.[195, 205] Advances in magnetic resonance angiography (MRA) also have added to the diagnostic capabilities of MRI. MRI, in combination with MRA, eventually may be the modality of choice for most cases of carotid and vertebral artery dissections.

Despite advances in these newer modalities, angiography remains the "gold standard" for the diagnosis of carotid artery dissection. Arteriography demonstrates the origin of the dissection, the extent of dissection, the presence of distal embolization, and collateral blood flow. The arteriographic appearances of carotid dissections vary, depending on severity and extent. Typical features include luminal stenosis, decreased flow in the ICA and middle cerebral artery, tapered occlusion, distal branch occlusions, abrupt reconstitution of the lumen, intimal flaps, and aneurysm of the extracranial arterial segment.

Luminal stenosis is the most common angiographic finding. It is usually elongated, tapered, and irregular and usually extends to the base of the skull and the carotid canal. The length of dissection is usually 2 to 4 cm, localized to the level of the first and second cervical vertebral bodies.[162] Reconstitution of the lumen is also fairly common. This usually occurs at the entrance of the ICA into the carotid canal (Fig. 135–16). The elongated, tapered narrowing has been described as a "string sign" by Ojemann and colleagues.[175]

Aneurysms occur in about one third of ICAs involved by dissection. They are usually located in the upper cervical and subcranial regions[161] (Fig. 135–17). Emboli occluding

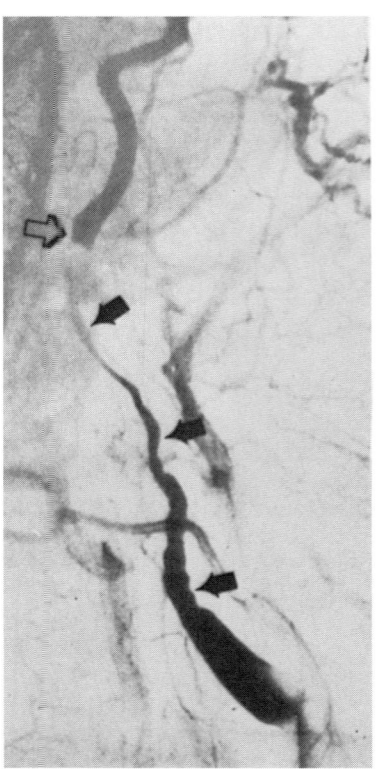

FIGURE 135–16. Dissection of the cervical segment of the internal carotid artery. Note the elongated, narrowed, and tapered luminal stenosis (*solid arrows*), a finding frequently seen in association with extracranial dissections. Another common feature of this entity, fairly abrupt reconstitution of the carotid lumen at the base of the skull (*open arrow*), is also shown. (From Mokri M: Dissections of cervical and cephalic arteries. *In* Meyer FB [ed]: Sundt's Occlusive Cerebrovascular Disease. Philadelphia, WB Saunders, p 51, 1994.)

distal cervical branches occur in about 10% of patients; in about 25% of cases, dissections of the ICAs are bilateral.

Natural History

Most patients who present with carotid dissection do well. Seventy-eight per cent to 92% of patients recover when they either had mild symptoms or were asymptomatic.[89, 151, 157] Those who present with fixed neurologic deficits do less well, with a 40% rate of return of good function.[18] Traumatic dissections are more likely to result in fixed neurologic deficits than are spontaneous dissections.

In contrast to neurologic signs, oculosympathetic paresis resolves less frequently. It persists in two thirds of patients as a result of permanent damage to the sympathetic fibers in the internal carotid plexus. Clinical Horner's syndrome, however, is usually quite mild and does not create significant functional or esthetic problems. Headaches resolve in 95% of patients, three quarters of whom recover within 3 months. Residual dissection with aneurysm formation may produce persistent headache. Angiographically, stenoses of the ICA either completely resolve or significantly improve in approximately 85% of patients; complete resolution occurs in more than half of patients, and significant improvement occurs in 30%.[94, 160] Although recanalization of a completely occluded vessel can occur, this is uncommon.

Aneurysms resolve or diminish in size in two thirds of involved vessels, and these aneurysms rarely rupture. Recurrence of dissection in the same vessel is extremely rare.

In summary, spontaneous dissection of the ICA is associated with a good prognosis. Complete or excellent clinical recovery occurs in 85% of patients, and stenotic lesions improve or completely resolve in 85% of vessels. Most aneurysms resulting from dissection resolve angiographically or diminish in size.

Treatment

Because carotid dissection is uncommon and there are no controlled studies regarding treatment, the proper therapy for extracranial dissection of the ICA has not been firmly established. Although Ehrenfeld and Wylie originally recommended operative treatment, they also recognized the unfavorable outcomes associated with surgical intervention in many cases.[52] In many instances, surgical revascularization was limited by technical difficulties involved in obtaining distal control. This discouraging early surgical experience, in conjunction with the remarkably favorable results of nonoperative therapy, has led most authorities to recommend anticoagulation as standard management. Surgical intervention is performed only when medical therapy fails and when the lesion is surgically accessible.[18] Surgical intervention may include thrombectomy, progressive intraluminal dilatation, endarterectomy, intimectomy, or graft interposition.

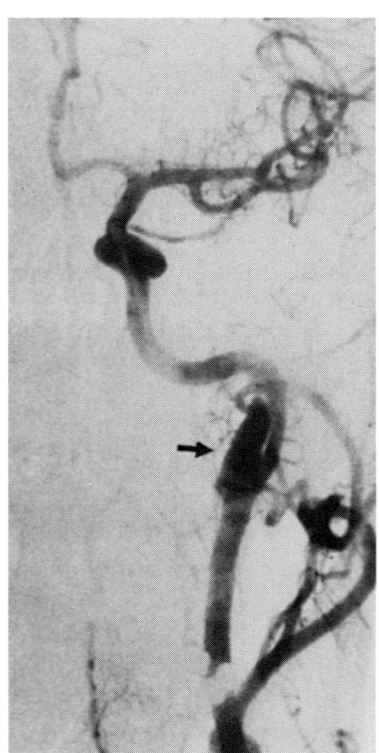

FIGURE 135–17. Finger-like aneurysm formation along a point of dissection of the cervical segment of the internal carotid artery (*arrow*) lying parallel to the course of the vessel. (From Mokri M: Dissections of cervical and cephalic arteries. *In* Meyer FB [ed]: Sundt's Occlusive Cerebrovascular Disease. Philadelphia, WB Saunders, 1994, p 51.)

Carotid ligation has also been suggested for patients with recurrent embolization, with or without concomitant extracranial-intracranial (EC-IC) bypass, depending on carotid back-pressure and collateral circulatory status. Carotid stump pressure at or above 70 mmHg is thought to be satisfactory to permit safe carotid ligation.[52] Most authorities recommend anticoagulation with heparin and then warfarin (Coumadin) for a period of 3 to 4 months, followed by antiplatelet treatment for a similar length of time.[89, 162]

Treatment of patients with traumatic carotid dissections is even less unequivocally established. Presentation and angiographic findings are similar to those of patients with spontaneous dissections of the ICA, with the exception that fixed neurologic symptoms are more common. This is thought to be due to an increased incidence of distal embolization. If there is apparent potential for thromboembolism in patients with traumatic ICA dissections, anticoagulation should be strongly considered. However, this may not be advisable because of hemorrhagic risk owing to concomitant traumatic injuries.

Most patients who survive the initial episode do well. Traumatic dissections result in aneurysms or chronic luminal irregularities more frequently than do spontaneous dissections.[154] Fewer patients with traumatic dissections are asymptomatic at follow-up compared with the spontaneous group. Although both traumatic and spontaneous dissections of the carotid arteries have a good prognosis, the outcome is less favorable in the traumatic group. Nevertheless, initial anticoagulation therapy followed by repeat angiography within a few months appears to be the most reasonable strategy for these patients.

VASCULITIS

Cerebral vasculitis—or arteritis—includes a spectrum of disorders, including lymphoid granuloma, collagen diseases, giant cell arteritis (temporal arteritis), Takayasu's disease, and Behçet's disease.[55, 95, 226, 239] Arteritis is an inflammatory process resulting in necrosis of the structural elements of the vessel wall. Obliteration of the lumen produces ischemia of dependent tissues as the terminal event. The course of vasculitis is usually quite variable, with unusual and varied clinical presentations. Vasculitis may affect blood vessels of any type, location, or size. The nomenclature and classification of vasculitis in the literature are quite confusing. Moreover, there is no definitive laboratory test or pathognomonic or clinical sign for most of these syndromes. The diagnosis depends on a combination of clinical, radiologic, laboratory, and histologic information.

Cerebrovascular arteritis is generally classified as *primary* or *secondary*. Primary vasculitis manifests only as vascular disease; secondary vasculitis complicates an underlying systemic primary illness.[118] Theories abound regarding the etiology of arteritis. Most authorities implicate humoral and cellular autoimmune mechanisms.[200] Circulating antibody complexes invade arterial walls, with triggering of the complement cascade. Polymorphonuclear leukocytes become activated and infiltrate the vessel wall, engulfing the immune complexes and producing damaging enzymes. Several primary types of vasculitis are characterized by granulomas; this finding weakens the immune complex model but does not exclude it, and it increases the likelihood of a cellular-mediated or combined mechanism.

Cerebral vasculitis can portray almost all central nervous signs and symptoms; the clinical presentation depends on whether the arteritis is primary or secondary. Women patients outnumber men by 2:1, and half of the patients are under 50 years of age. Focal neurologic deficits, including transient ischemic attacks and strokes, often result from focal cerebral vasculitis. Cranial nerve palsies, especially when multiple, simulate vertebrobasilar insufficiency, producing diplopia, visual changes, dysphagia, tinnitus, vertigo, syncope, and headache. Diagnosis is further confused by the frequent angiographic appearance of luminal "beading" suggestive of FMD or arterial dissections.[128] Because angiography has a resolution of only 100 to 200 mm or μm, vasculitis cannot reliably be excluded on the basis of a negative arteriogram.[111]

Treatment of arteritis usually requires steroids and anti-inflammatory drugs. However, because vasculitis is uncommon, nomenclature is unstandardized, diagnosis is empirical, and no control series exists regarding optimal treatment.

Giant Cell Arteritis

Giant cell arteritis is a generalized vasculitis that usually affects medium and large arteries in elderly patients, more commonly in women than men. Because granulomas typify the histology of this disorder, it has also been known as *granulomatous arteritis*. In addition, because it has been described in patients with rheumatoid arthritis, it has been called *polymyalgia rheumatica*. Classically, giant cell arteritis presents as temporal arteritis with headache, scalp tenderness, jaw claudication, and visual disturbances. Polymyalgia rheumatica, a systemic variety of giant cell arteritis, has been identified with increasing frequency due to a higher incidence of suspicion.

The lesions of giant cell arteritis occur in medium- to large-caliber arteries throughout the body. Most often, the aortic arch and the extracranial carotid arteries are involved. The inflammatory process consists of invasion of lymphocytes and plasma cells, with edema and fragmentation of the internal elastic lamina and deposition of multinucleated foreign body giant cells appearing late in the course of the disease. Gradually, the media is entirely replaced by connective tissue. The most prominent findings of giant cell arteritis are disruption of the elastic lamina and media, with foreign body reaction leading to granulomatous degeneration. Lesions are typically short and segmental, with normal artery between lesions. Biopsy confirms the diagnosis but is not always accurate because of inadequate sample size.[13]

Giant cell arteritis, temporal arteritis, and Takayasu's arteritis are all characterized by necrotizing changes within the vessel wall, with giant cell granuloma formation. In addition, mild fever, malaise, weight loss, and an elevated erythrocyte sedimentation rate (ESR) accompany these disorders. Approximately 25% to 50% of patients have fever and weight loss.[28] The demography of these disorders is quite different, however. *Temporal arteritis* affects the elderly and responds promptly to early treatment. *Takayasu's arteritis* occurs in young individuals (mostly women), but has a much poorer prognosis. Giant cell or granulomatous arteritis is confined primarily to the central nervous system. It occurs in all ages in both sexes, and the prognosis is poor. Temporal arteritis is usually classified as a form of giant cell arteritis, illustrating the confusing nomenclature.

Giant cell arteritis appears almost exclusively in whites.[14] Nordborg and Bengtsson reported the average incidence in Sweden of giant cell arteritis to be 6.7 per 100,000 inhabitants.[172] In individuals 50 years of age or older, the yearly incidence rose to 18.3 per 100,000 inhabitants, with 25 cases per 100,000 inhabitants in women and 9.4 per 100,000 in men.

Similar statistics were reported by investigators at the Mayo Clinic. In Olmstead County, Minnesota, giant cell arteritis occurred in 17 per 100,000 individuals over 50 years of age.[139] Women were three times more likely to have giant cell arteritis than men. In both the Swedish and American studies, the incidence of giant cell arteritis in women appears to be increasing, whereas in men the rate is stable or decreasing.

Clinical Presentation

Typically, giant cell arteritis (which most commonly presents as temporal arteritis) produces a flu-like syndrome, with low-grade fever, lassitude, and headache. After the initial event, patients often complain of jaw claudication, diffuse joint aches, and tender temporal arteries. In 20% to 60% of patients, amaurosis fugax, scintillating scotomata, diplopia, or permanent visual loss occurs in the second or third month. Laboratory findings are nonspecific. They may include an elevated ESR, mild thrombocytosis, leukocytosis, normocytic anemia, and elevations of prothrombin time, alkaline phosphotase, and transaminases. Patients with active disease may occasionally have a normal ESR. ESR elevation may be unmasked once anti-inflammatory drugs are discontinued.[107]

Temporal arteritis usually involves the branches of the external carotid artery, including the facial, occipital, internal maxillary, and especially the superficial temporal arteries. In addition, the posterior ciliary and ophthalmic arteries are frequently affected. Arteritis in the superficial temporal artery is probably responsible for the typical headache and ocular symptoms. Headache is a characteristic feature of those patients with temporal arteritis with external carotid artery involvement.

In the polymyalgia rheumatic variety, pain occurs in the muscles of the shoulder girdle in about 60% of patients.[28] When the superficial temporal artery or other external carotid branches are involved, the vessel is usually extremely tender to palpation, with spontaneous pain made worse by palpation. The vessel is often cord-like and difficult to compress, with reduced or absent pulsations. Often the overlying skin is swollen, erythematous, and warm. Pain may not be limited to the temporal area but may be facial, occipital, or diffuse. Duplex ultrasonography may be useful to localize a portion of the superficial temporal artery for biopsy, which is the preferred method for diagnosis.

Characteristically, the involved segment has abnormal flow velocities. Mumenthaler, however, reported a 62% incidence of sudden and complete visual loss.[167] The mechanism of blindness involves loss of blood supply to the optic nerve because of occlusion of branches of the ophthalmic artery, usually the posterior ciliary arteries. It is not uncommon for the clinical course to progress to blindness in less than 24 hours, and recovery of vision almost never occurs even after institution of steroids and anti-inflammatory agents.[76] Persistent blindness is likely due to the inability to stop progressive thrombosis of the involved artery. On funduscopic examination, the retina appears pale, with decreased flow in the retinal vessels, diminished vessel size, and papilledema.

The temporal artery biopsy should include a 4- to 7-cm-long specimen, particularly when the artery is grossly normal because of intermittent distribution of lesions. Some authorities have recommended contralateral biopsy when the first biopsy is negative and the clinical suspicion is high.[57, 85] Hall and Hunder reported a 14% incidence of positive contralateral biopsies.[85] In contrast, Klein and colleagues reported a series of 60 patients who underwent bilateral biopsies with only 3 cases of unilateral involvement.[120]

As indicated previously, angiography may miss lesions. When present, characteristic findings include tapered narrowings with post-stenotic dilatation, vessel occlusion, and collateral vessel formation. Despite localization to the head, many arteries throughout the body are often involved. The aorta is involved in one half of affected patients, and the carotid and vertebral arteries also show typical changes.[246] The coronary and visceral arteries are affected less commonly. Thoracic aortic dissection and aneurysm formation have also been reported.[107, 219]

Treatment

Because of the potential for rapid onset of permanent visual loss, temporal arteritis is considered to be a medical emergency. Steroids should be started immediately, followed by temporal artery biopsy. Positive biopsy results are not changed by 2 to 3 days of steroid treatment.[53, 57, 107] However, Allison and Gallagher reported that the positive biopsy rate fell from 60% to less than 10% after 1 week of steroid therapy.[2]

Arterial reconstruction is rarely necessary for patients with giant cell arteritis. Surgical indications may include aneurysm formation, aortic valvular incompetence, aortic dissection, or persistent ischemia after adequate medical therapy. Elective procedures ideally should be delayed until the disease becomes quiescent, because graft occlusion is common when operation is performed during the active phase of arteritis.[107]

The prognosis for patients with giant cell arteritis is good when they are treated expeditiously. The disease is generally self-limited and does not adversely influence life expectancy. Andersson and associates reported a survival rate similar to that of the general population in a series of 90 patients with giant cell arteritis followed for 9 to 16 years.[6]

Takayasu's Arteritis

A case of Takayasu's arteritis may have first been recognized as early as 1761, when Margagni reported the autopsy findings in a 40-year-old woman with absent radial pulses, a thickened proximal aorta, lower thoracic aortic stenoses, cardiac hypertrophy, and pulmonary edema.[46] In 1908, Takayasu, a Japanese ophthalmologist, described a young Japanese woman who presented with progressive visual loss, vertigo, syncope, conjunctival injection, retinal arteriovenous anastomoses, and alopecia.[226] A colleague of Takayasu, Onishi, noted that the retinal changes were associated with absent pulses in the upper extremities, and Takayasu's disease became known as "pulseless disease."[117] Currently, a preferred term is *obliterative brachiocephalic arteritis*, because involvement of the aortic arch and vessels is a prominent feature.

Although it was initially thought that there was a prediction for this condition in Asians, it is now clear that Takayasu's arteritis occurs in all races and age groups, but it is more common in women in the second and third decade of life.[72] It may occur as late as the fourth decade, however. In a 13-year population study at the Mayo Clinic of individuals of Olmstead County, Minnesota, three cases of Takayasu's disease were noted for an incidence of 2.6 per million per year.[83]

Takayasu's arteritis exclusively involves the aortic arch and great vessels. Cerebral ischemia, however, is generally considered to be the most life-threatening complication of this disorder.[101] Lupi-Herrera and colleagues and Ueno and colleagues have described four distinct classifications of Takayasu's disease[138, 232] (Fig. 135–18).

Type I is Takayasu's original description involving the aortic arch and great vessels; roughly 20% to 40% of patients have this distribution of disease, which results in signs and symptoms of cerebrovascular insufficiency, including visual abnormalities.

Another 20% to 40% of patients with Takayasu's disease have a middle aortic syndrome *(type II)* in which the distal thoracic and visceral abdominal aorta is affected; these patients present with mesenteric ischemia and symptoms of postprandial pain, fear of food, weight loss, and renal artery stenosis or occlusion (Fig. 135–19).

The majority of patients, 50% to 65%, have *type III*,

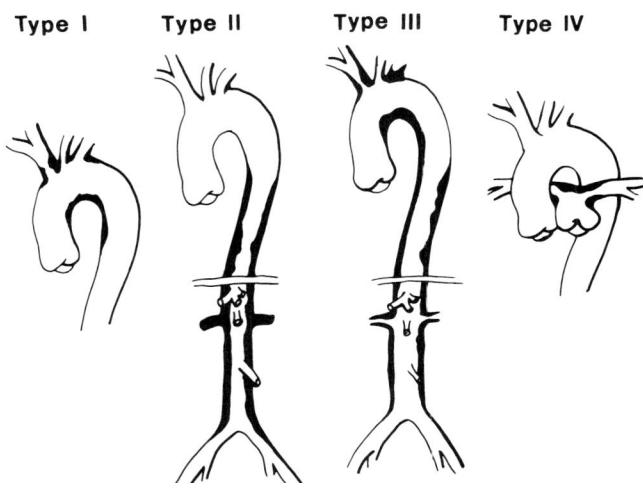

FIGURE 135–18. Classification system used to categorize the four types of arterial involvement in Takayasu's arteritis as determined by arteriography. (From Cottrell ED, Smith LL: Management of uncommon lesions affecting the extracranial vessels.

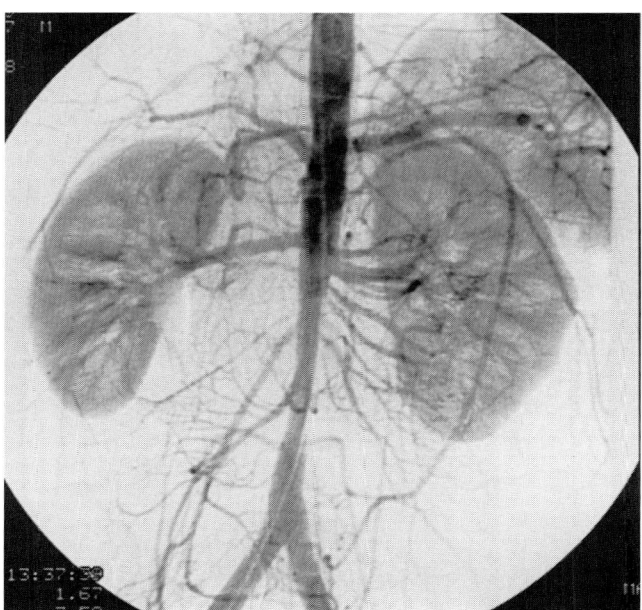

FIGURE 135–19. Abdominal aortogram demonstrating pathologic aortic anatomy as seen in a patient with Type III Takayasu's arteritis. Note the narrowed infrarenal aortic segment and the prominent meandering mesenteric artery (superior mesenteric artery to inferior mesenteric artery collateral). The patient had diminished femoral artery pulses and depressed bilateral lower extremity segmental limb pressures.

which involves both the aortic arch and the abdominal aorta. These patients may present with both cerebrovascular and lower extremity symptoms.

Only 10% of patients have *type IV* Takayasu's disease in which the pulmonary arteries are involved.

Pathophysiology

Patients with Takayasu's arteritis typically present with three distinct clinical phases. The *first phase* is characterized by prodromal symptoms that are primarily constitutional: malaise, anorexia, fatigue, weight loss, anemia, myalgias, fevers, and night sweats. Because of these vague symptoms, it was long thought that a causal relationship existed between Takayasu's arteritis and tuberculosis and other indolent chronic infections. This was particularly true in Third World countries, such as China, where large numbers of patients with this disorder were referred from rural areas with lower living standards, where infections were especially common.

The *second phase* revolves around inflammation of blood vessels, in which discomfort in the region of the involved arteries is described by patients. In the *third*, or "burned out" *phase*, patients present with symptoms of ischemia caused by arterial stenosis, embolization, or occlusion.

Pathologic changes of Takayasu's arteritis include inflammation of all three layers of the arterial wall (intima, media, and adventitia) (Fig. 135–20). In the inflammatory stage of the disease, macrophages and giant cells are abundant, and acute lesions show edema of the wall and lymphocytic infiltration. The elastic lamina becomes fragmented. However, despite the large number of giant cells, caseation and cavitation are absent. Patchy involvement of the vessel, with frequent "skip" areas, is characteristic, and

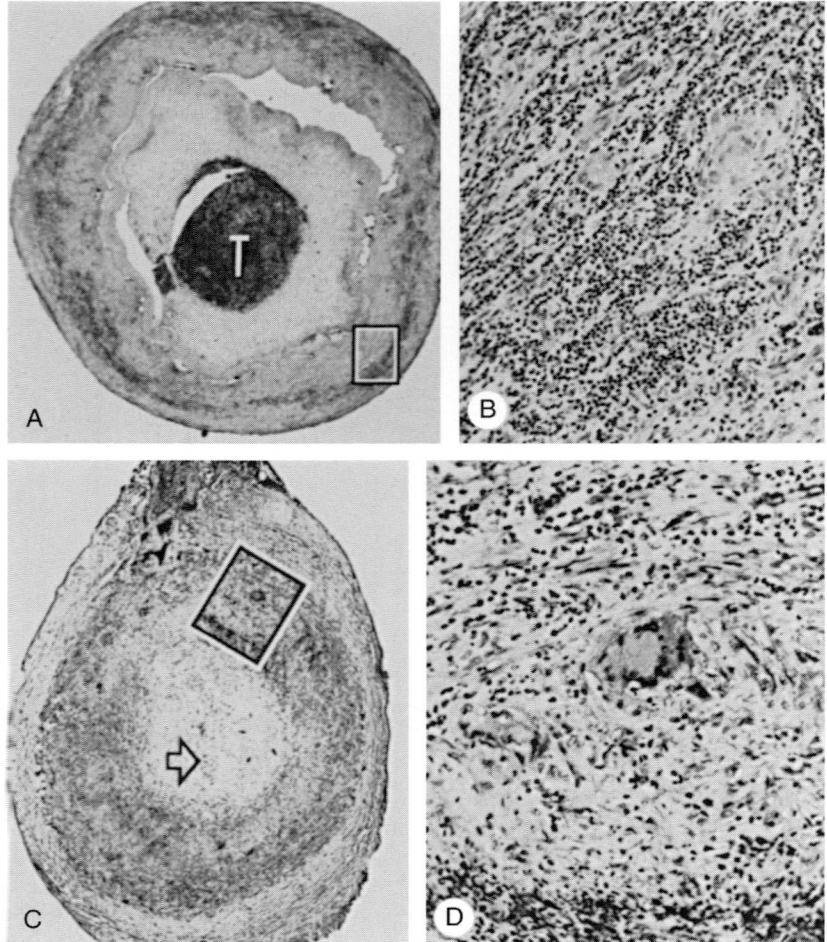

FIGURE 135–20. Photomicrographs of Takayasu's arteritis of the carotid artery (*A* and *B*) and temporal arteritis (*C* and *D*). (*A*, × 16; *B*, × 160; *C*, × 40; *D*, × 160.) Both are granulomatous giant cell arteritides, as shown in *B* (boxed area of *A*) and in *D* (boxed area of *C*) at higher magnifications. Thrombosis (T) and occlusive proliferation (*arrow*) are common complications. (H & E.) (From Lie JT: Pathology of occlusive disease of the extracranial arteries. *In* Meyer FB [ed]: Sundt's Occlusive Cerebrovascular Disease. Philadelphia, WB Saunders, 1994, p 39.)

diseased segments show varying amounts of intimal thickening and narrowing. In the latter stages of disease, fibrous scarring of the media and adventitia occurs along the length of the vessel in conjunction with degeneration of the media and deposition of ground substance in the intima.[46, 194, 236] Eventually, thrombosis occurs, occasionally followed by recanalization. Deterioration of the arterial wall with aneurysm formation also may develop.

Clinical Presentation

As would be expected from the distribution of lesions and phases of the clinical course, the clinical presentation of patients with Takayasu's disease can vary. Signs and symptoms of ischemia may occur early in the course or may not appear until many years after onset of systemic inflammatory symptoms. The patient's symptoms are completely dependent upon location of the lesions in Takayasu's arteritis. Aortic involvement may result in renovascular hypertension, mesenteric ischemia, and lower extremity insufficiency. Aortic arch and brachiocephalic involvement produces TIAs, visual impairment, stroke, and effort fatigue of the upper extremities. In the Mayo Clinic series of 32 patients with Takayasu's disease, 14 (45%) presented with symptoms of upper extremity vascular insufficiency, and 30 (94%) had multiple bruits.[83] Visual symptoms, including

amaurosis fugax, diplopia, and blurred vision, have been described in about one third of patients.[84] In patients with pulmonary involvement, pulmonary hypertension, dyspnea on exertion, and pleuritic chest pain may develop. Ascending aortic involvement may also produce aortic valvular insufficiency owing to aneurysm formation.

The diagnosis of Takayasu's disease relies upon a careful clinical evaluation and a high index of suspicion. The ESR is usually elevated in the inflammatory phase of the disease, but it may be normal in the burned out phase or when patients are treated with anti-inflammatory agents and steroids. Angiography is essential to document the extent of the disease and to confirm the diagnosis. Typically, angiograms show stenosis or occlusion of the proximal extracranial cerebral arteries in the vicinity of the aorta (Fig. 135–21). In a series of 244 angiograms reviewed by Liu, 85% of lesions were purely stenotic, 2% were aneurysmal, and the rest were a combination of both.[134]

Serial angiography may be necessary to determine the progress and extent of disease. Ultrasonography may also be used in the detection and follow-up of carotid lesions in patients with Takayasu's arteritis.[20, 22, 140] The so-called "macaroni sign" is characteristic of Takayasu's disease. This is described as diffuse, circumferential vessel thickening in the common carotid artery, which decreases as the disease becomes quiescent.[140]

Ishikawa has reviewed the clinical course of 96 Japanese patients with Takayasu's arteritis.[99] Diagnostic criteria included one *obligatory* criterion (age of 40 years or younger at diagnosis or at onset of characteristic signs and symptoms of 1 month's duration); two *major* criteria (left and right subclavian artery lesions); and nine *minor* criteria (elevated ESR, common carotid tenderness, hypertension, aortic regurgitation, and lesions of the pulmonary artery, left mid-common carotid artery, distal brachiocephalic trunk, descending thoracic aorta, and abdominal aorta). In 60 of 64 patients with active disease, these criteria were fulfilled. In 21 of the 32 patients with inactive disease they were not, producing an overall sensitivity of 84%. In addition to the obligatory criteria, the presence of two major criteria, or one major plus two or more minor criteria, or four or more minor criteria suggested the high possibility of Takayasu's disease.

Natural History

The course of Takayasu's arteritis is totally unpredictable. In his reviews of this disorder, Ishikawa noted that prognosis of Takayasu's arteritis was dependent on the presence of complications and the severity of disease.[99, 100] Patients with hypertension, retinopathy, aortic valvular insufficiency, and aneurysm formation, in conjunction with a progressive clinical course, had a 6-year survival rate of only 55%. Conversely, patients without these complications and with stable disease had a 6-year survival rate of 98%. In the Mayo Clinic study, Hall and colleagues reported a 5-year survival rate of 94%.[83] Death was most commonly due to congestive heart failure, stroke, myocardial infarction, or renal failure.

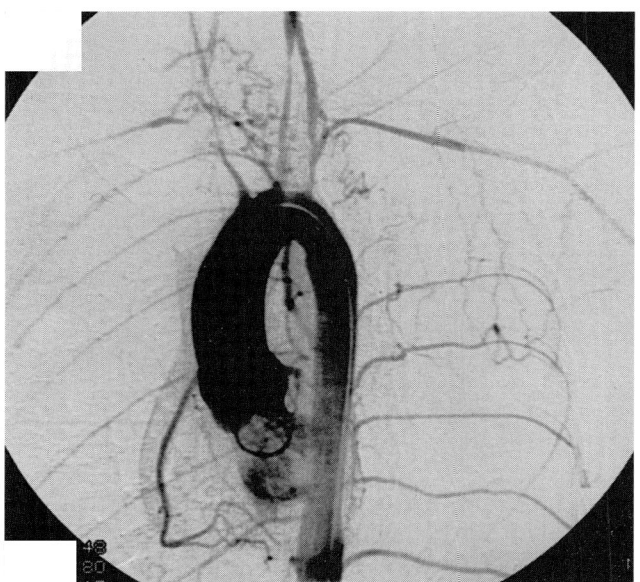

FIGURE 135–21. Arch aortogram from a young woman with Takayasu's arteritis. This demonstrates a critical uniform narrowing of the innominate artery, leading to a complete occlusion at its bifurcation. There is a tight stenosis of the left common carotid artery at its mid-portion; the left subclavian orifice is nearly occluded.

Treatment

Takayasu's arteritis is probably best managed by intensive treatment with steroids and anti-inflammatory agents, which should be given at a high initial dosage and then, depending on response, gradually tapered to a maintenance dose. Most patients can discontinue steroid therapy eventually, but others may require maintenance steroids for 5 years or more. In patients without any response to clinical steroids after 3 months, cyclophosphamide therapy should be added.[209]

Long-term anticoagulation therapy has also been recommended, but results are inconclusive and for the most part disappointing. In the Mayo Clinic series, 29 patients with active Takayasu's disease were treated with oral prednisone.[83] Substantial reduction in systemic inflammatory symptoms occurred in all patients within days to weeks. Eight of 16 patients with absent pulses had return of pulses, and 13 patients were able to discontinue steroids after duration of therapy of only 22 months. Not all studies have reported such dramatic improvement and regression of the lesion, as shown by angiography, by treatment with corticosteroids.[209, 212, 240]

Up to one third of patients with chronic advanced Takayasu's arteritis require surgery for palliation or prevention of ischemic complications. However, the role of surgical intervention is controversial, and multiple questions exist regarding timing, efficacy, and durability. Whenever possible, operative intervention should be delayed until the active phase of the disease has passed.[72, 83] Ideally, patients should not be taking corticosteroids or cyclophosphamide, but often discontinuation of these agents is impossible.

Transmural disease involves all layers of the vessel wall. Endarterectomy or patch angioplasty is not recommended. Instead, interposition grafting should be performed when necessary. Suture lines should not be placed in diseased segments in order to avoid false aneurysms and stenoses.[115, 181]

Giordano and coworkers reported excellent results in selected patients.[72] In 21 vascular surgery operations performed on 10 patients with Takayasu's arteritis, there were no deaths. Seven of these procedures were for cerebral revascularization; during an average follow-up of 5 years, no strokes occurred.

Multiple operations are often required in these patients.[209] All patients require close postoperative surveillance because of the frequent development of anastomotic stenoses, which can occur as early as 1 or 2 years after the initial operation.

Radiation-Induced Carotid Arteritis and Stenosis

In 1899, Gassman reported vascular endothelial edema and perforation with subsequent luminal narrowing after radiotherapy.[66] Cade described rupture of irradiated arteries in 1940.[25] Radiation-induced atherosclerosis in large blood vessels was reported by Thomas and Forbus in 1959.[228] In the mid-1970s, numerous reports associated cerebral ischemic cerebrovascular disease and cervical irradiation.[40, 132, 211] These reports highlighted the general absence of significant atherosclerotic risk factors in patients who developed carotid atherosclerosis after cervical irradiation. In addition, patients tended to be younger and had an unusual distribution of occlusive disease in that arterial lesions were limited to the field of radiation.

When irradiated, small vessels develop plaque-like thickening of the intima owing to the collection of fluid, with foam cells and hyaline material between the endothelium and the internal elastic membrane.[208] These plaques narrow the lumen and decrease perfusion to local tissue. Fonkalsrud and colleagues have divided changes that occur in irradiated arteries into *acute* and *chronic* phases, based on experiments in dogs.[61] After a 10-day total dose of 4000 cGy of radiation, endothelial injury was demonstrated within 48 hours. Changes included nuclear disruption, deposition of fibrin, and cell sloughing. The media was minimally affected, and the adventitia showed only mild fibrosis and hemorrhage. After 2 to 3 weeks, endothelium regenerated, whereas the media and adventitia demonstrated marked necrosis and hemorrhage. After 4 months, the endothelial surface became thickened and irregular, the media and adventitia continued to fibrose, and the regeneration of endothelium in conjunction with the fibrosis of the media-adventitia narrowed the lumen.

These pathologic changes predisposed vessels to thrombosis and lipid accumulation. This intimal cell injury model was similar to other studies involving direct endothelial injury to produce experimental atherosclerosis. A high-cholesterol diet administered after radiation therapy accelerates atheromatous changes in animal models.[74, 147] Later, pathologic changes to the media and adventitia are responsible for the total vessel involvement, which may be secondary to injury to the vasa vasorum. The common carotid artery has a predilection for radiation-induced changes, particularly in patients with hypercholesteremia.[135] Irradiation-induced occlusive vascular disease takes three patterns.[24] The first pattern consists of intimal damage producing mural thrombosis occurring within the first 5 years after irradiation. The second pattern occurs at about 10 years and consists of fibrotic occlusion. Twenty years after irradiation, periarterial fibrosis and accelerated atherosclerosis occur.

Although clinically and angiographically these lesions are indistinguishable from those of atherosclerosis, there are certain characteristic features of radiation-induced disease. Often, the narrowing is diffuse rather than focal, as is seen in standard atherosclerosis.[144] Symptoms often develop at an earlier age in patients with radiation-induced disease than with non–radiation-induced atherosclerosis, and patients are less likely to have associated coronary or other vascular disease, since irradiation injuries are localized to the irradiated areas.[17, 24, 54, 135]

Despite all this extensive investigation, it is still unclear whether radiation induces atherosclerosis or accelerates its formation in susceptible individuals. All studies using duplex scans of carotid arteries in patients who have received cervical radiation have shown significant progression of disease compared with controls.[58, 165] One MRI study has corroborated these findings.[36]

Clinical Presentation

McCready and associates described 20 patients with radiation-induced arterial injuries.[147] Two patterns of the disease were described: (1) luminal occlusion and (2) arterial disruption. Atypical stenoses or occlusions occurred in 6 patients from 7 to 24 years after radiation. Three of these patients presented with symptoms of cerebrovascular disease after neck irradiation, and 3 patients had iliofemoral disease with severe lower extremity ischemia after pelvic radiation. Carotid disruptions occurred in seven patients. All had undergone resection of the primary tumor and radical neck dissection 3 to 8 weeks following 5000 to 6500 cGy of cervical radiation. Infection was present in the vicinity of the carotid arteries in all patients, manifested by disrupted skin flaps or oral cutaneous fistulae. Arterial rupture occurred from 14 days to 16 weeks after the initial operation. A similar experience was reported by Marcial-Rojas and Castro, who described 6 patients with carotid artery rupture following treatment for head and neck carcinomas.[141] Necrosis of skin flaps in association with salivary fistulae preceded arterial ruptures.

Treatment

Several questions must be answered before surgical intervention for radiation-induced carotid artery occlusive disease is undertaken:

1. What is the estimated life expectancy with respect to the underlying malignancy?
2. Will an incision through irradiated skin heal primarily without added risk of infection?
3. To what extent are the carotid artery and neighboring nerves entrapped in postirradiation scar tissue?
4. Has the artery adjacent to the irradiated tumor been affected by radiation arteritis or accelerated atherosclerosis?[29]

If the probability of death from the malignancy outweighs the risk of a vascular event, surgical revascularization should be reconsidered. Because irradiated skin heals poorly, use of myocutaneous flaps for coverage is often warranted. Radiation may produce progressive small vessel and connective tissue changes in the epidermis that result in atrophy. The epidermis loses hair follicles, sebaceous glands, and sweat glands, and normal tissues are gradually replaced with dense fibrous tissue. Radiation dermatitis and hyperkeratosis may occur. The net result is thin, poorly nourished skin that heals unpredictably.

The transmural radiation damage to vessels obliterates the normal cleavage plane in the vessel wall, rendering endarterectomy very difficult.[17, 135] Thus, most authorities recommend bypass grafting of diseased segments. Reversed saphenous vein interposition grafts may be used, although extra-anatomic grafts or bypass grafts originating from the ascending aorta are required to avoid diseased segments. Autogenous tissue is preferable to prosthetic graft to avoid infection, but kinking of vein grafts in the neck may be a problem. After vascular repair, it is mandatory to have good tissue coverage, which may require rotational or advancement myocutaneous flaps.

In patients who present very late after irradiation, accelerated atherosclerosis may produce symptoms. These patients generally can undergo routine endarterectomy, but the surgeon must proceed with care through irradiated tissues.

Atkinson and coworkers concluded that carotid endarterectomy after cervical irradiation was technically more demanding, but feasible, and produced good long-term results.[8] They reported nine carotid endarterectomies, with an average follow-up of 49 months. One patient who underwent primary closure of the arteriotomy experienced TIAs postoperatively; two patients suffered transient cranial nerve palsies. The authors stated that the arterial dissection was more difficult because of periarterial fibrosis and that the endarterectomy was complicated by strong adherence of the plaque to the vessel wall. They also noted that after removal of the lesion, the arterial wall was attenuated more than usual, and segmental resection and reconstruction were required.[9] It is advisable to close the arteriotomy using a patch to help prevent future stenoses of the irradiated vessel.[96]

Predictably, patients who sustained carotid artery rupture after irradiation have a poor prognosis. In series reported by McCready and colleagues, ligation of the vessel resulted in stroke or death in five of nine patients.[148] Two of nine patients in the McCready study and two of six patients who suffered carotid rupture reported by Marcial-Rojas and Castro[141] presented with a sentinel bleed followed by exsanguinating hemorrhage. When a sentinel bleeding episode occurs, the authors recommend prompt surgical exploration and carotid ligation if no neurologic deficits are produced by carotid cross-clamping. Otherwise, extracranial-infracranial bypass with autogenous graft is recommended, with the subclavian artery used as the inflow source.

ADJACENT MALIGNANCY AND INFECTION

Patients with malignant tumors of the head and neck may present with primary or metastatic involvement of structures adjacent to the carotid artery. Fortunately, actual invasion of the carotid artery occurs in only 5% of these patients.[112] Because it provides only a two-dimensional view of the arterial lumen, arteriography cannot determine whether or not a malignancy has invaded the carotid artery. When the contrast column is narrowed, external compression, rather than invasion, may be present, whereas normal appearance can mislead the surgeon to think that there is no vessel wall involvement. When invasion is suspected, however, particularly with large, symptomatic tumors, angiography provides important anatomic information regarding coexistent carotid artery disease, collateral blood flow, and relevant anatomy. In addition, a stump pressure can be measured by inserting a balloon catheter in the proximal ICA.[176] CT scans show the proximity of lesions to the carotid artery but cannot identify invasion. MRI is promising and may best visualize tissue planes and give anatomic data in multiple projections.

Conley first reported resection of the carotid artery involved with tumor.[38] In 1981, Olcott and colleagues described six patients who presented with tumor invasion of the carotid artery.[176] The authors excised the carotid artery with the tumor and used saphenous vein interposition grafts for reconstructions. There were no operative deaths and no neurologic deficits in the immediate postoperative period, although hemiparesis developed in 1 patient on the fourth postoperative day and eventually cleared. Subsequent arteriography showed a patent graft with no obvious source of embolus in this patient.

In 1988, Biller and associates reported 26 patients who underwent carotid resection and graft replacement for recurrent cancer of the head and neck.[17] Seven per cent of patients who received grafts suffered postoperative neurologic events; the postoperative mortality rate was 15%. The authors stated that as of 1986, only 60 cases of carotid artery resection and graft placement had been reported in the English literature.

In 1989, McCready reported 16 patients with advanced cervical carcinomas, 3 of whom were treated with simple ligation of the carotid; each suffered postoperative TIAs that resolved.[148] Thirteen patients were treated with resection of the involved carotid and saphenous vein interposition grafting. There were two postoperative strokes and one postoperative death in the series. Preoperative cerebral angiography and a Javid shunt were used in all patients to determine collateral flow, and all arteries were closed with myocutaneous flaps using the greater pectoral muscle.[148]

Often carotid involvement can be assessed only at the time of operation. Occasionally, even when a carotid artery is not actually invaded, the dissection of tumor strips the vessel and weakens it beyond repair. In these cases as well as in those of carotid invasion, a saphenous vein interposition graft is advisable. Occasionally, reconstruction is impossible, and ligation is necessary. Measurement of the carotid back-pressure at operation can assist in determining tolerance of carotid interruption. Ehrenfeld and associates have shown that a back-pressure of 50 mmHg indicates acceptable collateral flow, but 70 mmHg is safer.[51] Patients with carotid back-pressure of less than this have significant neurologic morbidity. Many of the patients who sustain strokes after carotid ligation experience delayed neurologic symptoms.[51, 164] These delayed strokes are probably thromboembolic due to propagation of thrombus into the middle cerebral artery. Thus, when possible, after ligation of the ICA, the patient should receive anticoagulation therapy for at least 7 to 10 days. In contrast to the low stroke rate for atherosclerotic disease, after arterial reconstruction these patients have stroke rates ranging from 7% to 20%.[8, 38, 136, 176]

Infection of the carotid artery following head and neck surgery or after endarterectomy is a rare but potentially life-threatening problem. Hematogenous dissemination can also be a source for carotid artery infection.[116] Forty patients with carotid artery rupture sustained permanent neurologic damage, and 30% died despite rapid and prompt treatment.[87] Carotid artery blowouts occur in 3% of patients after operation for head and neck cancer.[114] Wound infection, salivary leaks, skin flap necrosis, and radiation are contributing factors to this postoperative problem. Again, a sentinel bleed is often present prior to massive sanguination.

Patients who present with carotid artery infection require rapid surgical intervention. Wound and blood cultures with directed antibiotic selection are advisable, but definitive operative intervention should not be postponed pending these results. If time permits, angiography is useful to identify relevant anatomy and document collateral circulation. Likewise, carotid back-pressure can be measured in preparation for possible carotid ligation. Reconstruction should employ autogenous tissue, thus avoiding proximity of interposition grafts within the area of infection. Wide débridement of infected tissue and flap coverage are also important.

MOYAMOYA DISEASE

Moyamoya disease is a rare cerebrovascular disorder in which there is progressive stenosis in the arteries of the circle of Willis. Initially, the disease involves the intracranial vessels of both cerebral hemispheres and then may progress to involve one or both of the middle cerebral and posterior cerebral arteries. As the disease progresses, an abnormal capillary network develops at the base of the brain. These vascular changes may result in ischemic strokes in children and cerebral hemorrhages in adults.

Moyamoya disease was first described by Takeuchi and Shimizu in 1957 as "bilateral hypogenesis of the internal carotid arteries."[227] In 1968, Kudo introduced this disorder in the English literature as "spontaneous occlusion of the circle of Willis, a disease apparently confined to the Japanese."[124] In that same year, Nishimoto and Takeuchi described 96 cases that occurred in Japanese individuals.[171] Suzuki and Takaku first coined the term "moyamoya disease" in 1969, employing the Japanese word *moyamoya* to describe the typical "puff of smoke" appearance of the abnormal capillary network at the base of the skull.[225]

The cause is unknown. There is no evidence that the disorder is inflammatory or autoimmune, but an episode of infection (often upper respiratory) is frequently antecedent. The disease does not affect large vessels and has no relationship to extracranial cervical arteries. The disease slowly and progressively occludes the major trunks of the intracerebral arteries, beginning at the carotid artery in the cavernous sinus. The formation of abnormally small moyamoya vessels distal to the carotid narrowings is now considered to be a secondary process that attempts to develop collateral circulation.[124, 231] At autopsy, characteristic findings include intimal thickening and medial thinning of affected intracranial arteries without inflammatory infiltrates.[87] There have been reports of familial cases and a higher incidence in individuals with Down's syndrome.[65, 119]

Because moyamoya disease does not affect large vessels and is unrelated to the extracranial cervical arteries, it is not amenable to treatment by the vascular surgeon. It is of interest, nevertheless, because it is occasionally visualized on angiograms brought to the attention of the vascular surgeon because it produces symptoms similar to those of extracranial carotid disease, and because of its unusual name.

Clinical Presentation

Moyamoya disease has a biphasic distribution of age of onset, affecting individuals in the first and fourth decades of life. In 1979, according to national statistics in Japan, 518 cases were registered; the overall female:male ratio was about 1:5.[170] The clinical presentations between juvenile and adult types are distinctly different. In the juvenile type, children usually present with ischemic events, such as repetitive TIAs or a completed stroke.

Typically, cerebral ischemia is induced by crying, coughing, or straining. Seizures are also common, oc-

curring in about 14% of affected individuals. In adults with moyamoya disease, hemorrhage from the fragile abnormal vessels is the most prominent clinical feature. In 70% to 80% of patients, bleeding occurs in the ventricles, thalamus, and basal ganglia. Hemorrhage may be either subarachnoid or intracerebral.

Adults have a slightly worse prognosis than children do. Nishimoto reported 39 deaths (7.5%) in the 518 patients previously cited.[170] Adults had a mortality rate of 10%; children, 4.3%. Intracranial bleeding was the cause of death in 56% of children and 63% of adults. Few have examined the natural history of patients who present with TIAs because most of these patients go on to treatment. In 1985, Kurokaw and colleagues observed 47 patients who presented with TIAs; in most, TIAs disappeared, but one half to two thirds of the patients showed deterioration in cognitive function over 5 to 10 years.[125] There is also an increased incidence of intracranial aneurysms in patients with moyamoya disease. The aneurysms are characteristically in the posterior circulation.[126]

Diagnosis

Imaging

CT and MRI may reveal multiple dilated abnormal vessels in the basal ganglia or thalamus, occlusion or narrowing of the major arteries of the circle of Willis, ischemic infarction (predominantly in the watershed of the brain parenchyma), or intra-cerebral hemorrhages.[32] Cerebral blood flow studies have also been described for diagnosis of this disorder. Ogawa and colleagues reported that the distribution of cerebral blood flow was greater to the occipital regions, whereas normally blood flow is predominantly to the frontal lobes.[173] In addition, the response to hypotension/hypocapnia, which requires vasodilatation, is severely impaired in contrast to a relatively preserved response to hypertension and hypercapnia.[174]

Stages

Arteriography is the standard for diagnosis of moyamoya disease (Fig. 135–22). Suzuki and Takaku have described six distinct stages.[225]

In *stage I*, stenosis of the carotid artery is present at its suprasellar portion, usually occurring bilaterally.

In *stage II*, the carotid artery is narrow, and moyamoya vessels begin to develop at the base of the brain.

In *stage III*, these abnormal moyamoya vessels become more prominent as major arteries in the anterior circulation become severely stenotic or occluded; at this stage, the diagnosis is usually confirmed.

In *stage IV*, the moyamoya vessels extend to all components of the circle of Willis, including the posterior cerebral arteries.

In *stage V*, the moyamoya vessels begin to diminish.

By *stage VI*, they disappear completely. In stage VI, the cerebral hemisphere receives blood through abnormal extracranial-intercranial anastomoses.

These changes are almost always bilateral, and if angiographic abnormalities are unilateral, the case is considered questionable.

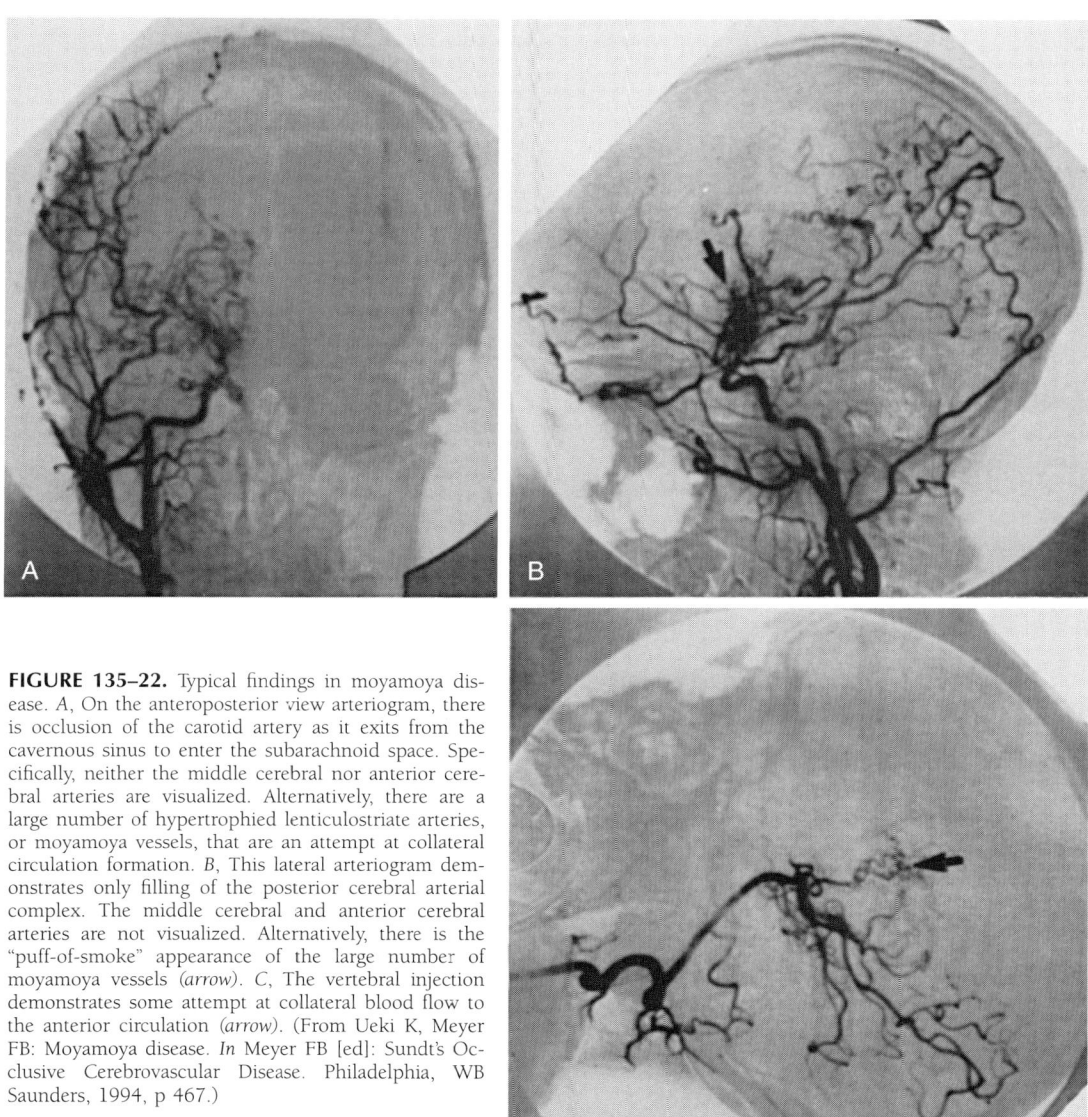

FIGURE 135–22. Typical findings in moyamoya disease. *A,* On the anteroposterior view arteriogram, there is occlusion of the carotid artery as it exits from the cavernous sinus to enter the subarachnoid space. Specifically, neither the middle cerebral nor anterior cerebral arteries are visualized. Alternatively, there are a large number of hypertrophied lenticulostriate arteries, or moyamoya vessels, that are an attempt at collateral circulation formation. *B,* This lateral arteriogram demonstrates only filling of the posterior cerebral arterial complex. The middle cerebral and anterior cerebral arteries are not visualized. Alternatively, there is the "puff-of-smoke" appearance of the large number of moyamoya vessels *(arrow)*. *C,* The vertebral injection demonstrates some attempt at collateral blood flow to the anterior circulation *(arrow)*. (From Ueki K, Meyer FB: Moyamoya disease. *In* Meyer FB [ed]: Sundt's Occlusive Cerebrovascular Disease. Philadelphia, WB Saunders, 1994, p 467.)

This "puff of smoke" angiographic pattern is mimicked in other conditions, including generalized atherosclerosis, radiation arteritis, trauma, sickle cell anemia, and even tuberculous meningitis.[88] In 1975, Debrun described moyamoya disease as the end-stage of a number of conditions that may result in this nonspecific angiographic pattern rather than representing a discrete clinical entity.[43]

Treatment

In 1983, Suzuki and Kodoma proposed perivascular sympathectomy and superior cervical ganglionectomy to produce both intracranial and extracranial vasodilation for treatment of moyamoya disease.[224] Currently, most surgeons use some sort of intracranial procedure to treat this rare disease. The most popular is *superficial temporal artery–to–middle cerebral artery* (STA-MCA) anastomosis, which was proposed by Krayenbuhl for treatment of moyamoya dis-

ease in 1975.[122] Additional procedures include *encephalomyosynangiosis* and *encephaloduroarteriosynangiosis*.

Encephalomyosynangiosis, proposed by Matsushima and coworkers in 1981, consists of suturing a patent superficial temporal artery along the longitudinal dural defect to approximate the artery to the brain surface.[145] Encephalomyosynangiosis, utilized by Karasawa in 1977, consists of suturing the temporalis muscle to surgical dural defects, approximating the muscles to the surface of the brain.[109] Most of the procedures are indirect anastomotic operations, the goal of which is developing neovascularization from the extracranial arterial and soft tissue systems to the ischemic brain. Reportedly, the operations are easier and safer to perform than STA-MCA bypass, especially in small children.

In general, results of operation in children are better than in adults because the primary purpose of these revascularization techniques is to prevent brain ischemia. When applied to the adult or hemorrhagic type of moyamoya disease, they are less likely to reduce the risk of bleeding despite the expectation of retarding development of abnormal moyamoya vessels.

EXTRACRANIAL-INTRACRANIAL BYPASS

Because the international multicenter randomized study of extracranial-intracranial (EC-IC) bypass failed to show improved outcome in the surgical group, this operation has largely fallen into disfavor.[50] Thus, this procedure is summarized only briefly in this chapter.

Microvascular anastomosis was first successfully performed in experimental models in the 1960s.[43, 104] The first EC-IC bypass was by Donaghy and Yasargil in 1967 when they performed an STA-MCA anastomosis.[48] In 1978, Samson and Boone introduced use of the occipital or middle meningeal artery when the superficial temporal artery is inadequate.[198] In 1987, Hopkins and colleagues developed bypass procedures for posterior circulation revascularization.[93] Spetzler and associates first used a saphenous vein graft from the external carotid artery, subclavian artery, or proximal superficial temporal artery to provide a high-flow conduit.[217]

EC-IC bypass was originally designed to treat patients with ICA occlusion or intracranial occlusive lesions, such as siphon stenosis or middle cerebral artery occlusion. These lesions are not amenable to standard extracranial carotid procedures.[223] Several nonrandomized studies suggested long-term resolution of ischemic symptoms after EC-IC bypass.[33, 90]

The EC-IC Bypass Study

Despite the apparent success of numerous uncontrolled and nonrandomized studies supporting the use of EC-IC bypass for cerebrovascular disease, the definitive study awaited funding by the National Institutes of Health, the results of which were initiated in 1977 and published in 1985.[50] This international, multicenter, randomized prospective study included patients who had one or more TIAs or minor completed strokes in the carotid distribution within 3 months of entering the study.

One of the following ipsilateral lesions was present: (1) occlusion of the ICA; (2) stenosis of the ICA at or above the C2 vertebral body; or (3) stenosis or occlusion of the middle cerebral artery. All patients received 325 mg of aspirin four times per day and were randomized to best medical care (aspirin plus risk factor control) or to the same regimen with the addition of EC-IC bypass. Mean follow-up was 55.8 months, and end-points included fatal or non-fatal stroke. Secondary analysis involved ipsilateral stroke, death from any cause, and functional status. A total of 1377 patients were randomized, 714 to best medical care and 663 to surgery.

Postoperative mortality was only 0.6%, and major stroke morbidity was 2.5%. The angiographically confirmed bypass patency rate was 96%. In the 5-year follow-up, perioperative nonfatal and fatal strokes occurred slightly more frequently and earlier in patients who had surgery compared with the best medical care group. Subset analysis did not identify a specific group that was preferentially benefited by EC-IC bypass, including those with bilateral carotid occlusion and middle cerebral artery occlusion. In fact, the group of patients with severe middle cerebral artery stenosis had a significantly worse outcome when treated operatively than those treated medically, suggesting that the bypass actually caused the strokes by precipitating proximal middle cerebral artery occlusion.

Unfortunately, the EC-IC bypass study was riddled with methodologic flaws.[11, 216] Two features of the study conspired to weaken its validity. First, there was a strikingly low stroke rate of the medically treated patients, suggesting that lower stroke risk patients were selected for randomization and inclusion. Second, and perhaps more important, a substantial number of patients had EC-IC bypasses at the participating medical centers without being offered randomization. Thus, it would appear that only relatively stable, low-risk patients were entered into the trial, whereas patients who might have benefited most from operative treatment were excluded, presumably because surgeons felt that they were at "excessive risk." Although these criticisms have been addressed by participants of the EC-IC bypass study, the conclusions of the study will forever be questioned by some. Nevertheless, after this international trial was published, there was a marked reduction in the number of EC-IC bypasses performed. For example, in one center in which 70 such cases were performed annually, only four have been performed annually in recent years.[217]

It is noteworthy that several important clinical categories of cerebrovascular disease were not included in the EC-IC bypass cohort. These included patients with ischemic ocular syndromes, moyamoya disease, vertebrobasilar insufficiency, and chronic low-perfusion syndromes.[109, 216] In addition, some authorities consider patients as candidates for this operation (1) who have persistent or progressive cerebrovascular symptoms despite maximal medical therapy and who have demonstrated cerebral hemodynamic insufficiency, and also (2) those with therapeutic carotid occlusion who failed temporary balloon test occlusion. Findings of those patients with "hemodynamic insufficiency" may be accomplished using a number of special studies, including xenon-computed tomography, transcranial Doppler, single photon emission tomography (SPECT), and positron emission tomography (PET).[49, 71, 81, 182, 245] Use of various vasodilator stimulants (CO_2, acetazolamide) has also been suggested to select patients for this procedure.[49, 121, 245] The technique of EC-IC bypass is beyond the scope of this chapter. Interested readers are referred to numerous treatises on this topic.

REFERENCES

1. Albert G, cited by Staats EF, Brown RL, Smith RR: Carotid body tumors, benign and malignant. Laryngoscope 76:907, 1966.
2. Allison MC, Gallagher PJ: Temporal artery biopsy and corticosteroid treatment. Ann Rheum Dis 43:416, 1984.
3. Almquist A, Gornick C, Benson DW Jr, et al: Carotid sinus hypersensitivity: Evaluation of the vasodepressor component. Circulation 71:927, 1985.

4. Anderson CA, Collins JG Jr, Rich HM, et al: Spontaneous dissection of the internal carotid artery associated with fibromuscular dysplasia. Am Surg 46:263, 1980.

5. Anderson RM, Schecter MM: A case of spontaneous dissecting aneurysm of the internal carotid artery. J Neurol Neurosurg Psychiaty 22:195, 1959.

6. Andersson R, Malmvall E, Bengtsson BA: Long-term survival in giant cell arteritis, including temporal arteritis and polymyalgia rheumatica: A follow-up study of 90 patients treated with corticosteroids. Acta Med Scand 220:361, 1986.

7. Anson J, Crowell RM: Cervicocranial arterial dissection. Neurosurgery 29:89, 1991.

8. Atkinson DP, Jacobs LA, Weaver AW: Elective carotid resection for squamous cell carcinomas of the head and neck. Am J Surg 148:483, 1984.

9. Atkinson JL, Sundt TM Jr, Dale AJ, et al: Radiation associated atheromatous disease of the cervical carotid artery: Report of 7 cases and review of the literature. Neurosurgery 24:171, 1989.

10. Austin MG, Schaefer RF: Marfan's syndrome with unusual blood vessel manifestations: Primary media necrosis dissection of right innominate, right carotid, and left carotid arteries. Arch Pathol 64:205, 1957.

11. Awad IA, Spetzler RF: Extracranial-intracranial arterial bypass surgery: A critical analysis in light of the International Cooperative Study. Neurosurgery 19:655, 1986.

12. Bashour TT, Crew JP, Dean M, et al: Ultrasonic imaging of common carotid artery dissection. J Clin Ultrasound 13:210, 1985.

13. Bengtsson BA: Incidence of giant cell arteritis. Acta Med Scand 658 (Suppl):15, 1987.

14. Bengtsson BA, Andersson R: Giant cell and Takayasu's arteritis. Curr Opin Rheumatol 3:15, 1991.

15. Bergan JJ, Hoen JG: Evanescent cervical pseudoaneurysm. Ann Surg 162:213, 1965.

16. Bergdahl L: Carotid body tumours. Scand J Thorac Cardiovasc Surg 12:275, 1978.

17. Biller HF, Urken M, Klawson W, Haimov M, et al: Carotid artery resection and bypass for neck carcinoma. Laryngoscope 98:181, 1988.

18. Bogousslavsky J, Despland PA, Regli F: Spontaneous carotid dissection with acute stroke. Arch Neurol 44:137, 1987.

19. Bolande RP: The neurocristopathies: A unifying concept of disease arising in the neural crest development. Hum Pathol 5:409, 1976.

20. Bond JR, Charboneau JW, Stanson AW: Takayasu's arteritis: Carotid duplex and sonographic appearance, including color Doppler imaging. J Ultrasound Med 9:625, 1990.

21. Brignole M, Menozzi C, Lolli G, et al: Long-term outcome of paced and non-paced patients with severe carotid sinus syndrome. Am J Cardiol 69:1039, 1992.

22. Buckley A, Southwood T, Culham G, et al: The role of ultrasound in the evaluation of Takayasu's arteritis. J Rheumatol 18:1073, 1991.

23. Busuttil RW, Memsic L, Thomas DS: Coiling and kinking of the carotid artery. In Rutherford RB (ed): Vascular Surgery, 4th ed. Philadelphia, WB Saunders, 1995, p 1588.

24. Butler MS, Lane RHS, Webster JHH: Irradiation injury to large arteries. Br J Surg 67:341, 1980.

25. Cade S: Malignant Disease and Its Treatment by Radium. Baltimore, Williams & Wilkins, 1940, p 161.

26. Cairney J: Tortuosity of the cervical segment of the internal carotid artery. J Anat 59:87, 1924.

27. Cairns H: Vascular aspects of head injuries. Lisboa Med 19:375, 1942.

28. Callow AD (ed): Surgery of the Carotid and Vertebral Arteries. Baltimore, Williams & Wilkins, 1996, p 152.

29. Callow AD (ed): Surgery of the Carotid and Vertebral Arteries. Baltimore, Williams & Wilkins, 1996, p 136.

30. Carpenter MB: Human Neuroanatomy, 7th ed. Baltimore, Williams & Wilkins, 1976, p 345.

31. Chambers RG, Mahoney WD: Carotid body tumors. Am J Surg 116:554, 1968.

32. Chang KH, Yi JG, Han MH, et al: MR imaging finding of moyamoya disease. J Korean Med Sci 5:85, 1990.

33. Chater N, Popp J: Microsurgical vascular bypass for occlusive cerebrovascular disease: Review of 100 cases. Surg Neurol 6:114, 1976.

34. Chedid A, Jao W: Hereditary tumors of the carotid bodies and chronic obstructive pulmonary disease. Cancer 33:1635, 1974.

35. Cheng LH, Norris CW: Surgical management of the carotid sinus syndrome. Arch Otolaryngol 97:395, 1973.

36. Chung TS, Yousem DM, Lexa FJ, Markiewicz DA: MRI of carotid angiopathy after therapeutic radiation. J Comput Assist Tomogr 18:533, 1994.

37. Collins PS, Orecchia P, Gomez E: A technique for correction of carotid kinks and coils following endarterectomy. Ann Vasc Surg 5:116, 1991.

38. Conley JJ: Free autogenous vein graft to the internal and common carotid arteries in the treatment of tumors of the neck. Ann Surg 137:205, 1953.

39. Connolly JH: Large pulsating vessels in the right portion of the posterior pharyngeal wall partially concealed behind the right tonsil in a boy aged five. Proc R Soc Med (Laryngol Sect) 7:25, 1913.

40. Conomy JP, Kellermeyer RW: Delayed cerebrovascular consequences of therapeutic radiation: A clinicopathologic study of a stroke associated with radiation-related carotid arteriopathy. Cancer 36:1702, 1975.

41. Crowell WT, Grizzle WE, Siegel AL: Functional carotid paragangliomas: Biomedical, ultrastructural, and histochemical correlation with clinical symptoms. Arch Pathol Lab Med 106:599, 1982.

42. Davidge-Pitts KJ, Pantanowitz D: Carotid body tumors. Surg Annu 16:203, 1984.

43. Debrun GT, Sauvegrain J, Goutieres F: Moyamoya, a nonspecific radiologic syndrome. Neuroradiology 8:241, 1975.

44. Dent TL, Thompson NW, Fry J: Carotid body tumors. Surgery 80:365, 1976.

45. Desai B, Toole JF: Kinks, coils, and carotids: A review. Stroke 6:649, 1975.

46. Di Giacomo V: A case of Takayasu's disease occurred over 200 years ago. Angiology 35:750, 1984.

47. Dockerty MB, Love JG, Patton MM: Non-chromaffin paraganglioma of the middle ear: Report of a case in which the clinical aspects were those of a brain tumor. Proc Staff Meet Mayo Clin 26:25, 1961.

48. Donaghy RMP, Yasargil MG: Microvascular Surgery. St. Louis, CV Mosby, 1967.

49. Durham SR, Smith HA, Rutigliano MJ, Yonas H: Assessment of cerebral vasoreactivity and stroke risk using Xe CT acetazolamide challenge. Stroke 22:138, 1991.

50. The EC-IC Bypass Study Group: Failure of extracranial-intracranial arterial bypass to reduce the risk of ischemia stroke: Results of an international randomized trial. N Engl J Med 313:1191, 1985.

51. Ehrenfeld WR, Stoney RJ, Wylie EJ: Relation of carotid stump pressure to safety of carotid arterial ligation. Surgery 93:299, 1983.

52. Ehrenfeld WR, Wylie EJ: Spontaneous dissection of the internal carotid artery. Arch Surg 111:1294, 1976.

53. Ehsan M, Lange RK, Waxman J: Overdiagnosis of temporal arteritis. South Med J 74:1198, 1981.

54. Elerding SC, Fernandez RN, Gotta JC, et al: Carotid artery disease following cervical irradiation. Ann Surg 194:609, 1981.

55. Faer MJ, Mead JH, Lynch RD: Cerebral granulomatous angiitis. Case report and literature review. AJR Am J Roentgenol 129:463, 1977.

56. Fanning JP, Woods FM, Christian HJ: Metastatic carotid body tumor: Report of a case with review of the literature. JAMA 185:49, 1963.

57. Fauchald P, Rygvold O, Oystese B: Temporal arteritis and polymyalgia rheumatica: Clinical and biopsy findings. Ann Intern Med 77:845, 1972.

58. Feehs RS, McGuirt WF, Bond MG, et al: Irradiation; A significant risk factor for carotid atherosclerosis. Arch Otolaryngol Head Neck Surg 117:1135, 1991.

59. Fisher AGT: Sigmoid tortuosity of the internal carotid artery and its relation to tonsil and pharynx. Lancet 2:128, 1915.

60. Fisher CM, Ojemann RG, Roberson GH: Spontaneous dissection of cervicocerebral arteries. Can J Neurol Sci 5:9, 1978.

61. Fonkalsrud EW, Sanchez M, Zerubavel R, et al: Serial changes in arterial structure following radiation therapy. Surg Gynecol Obstet 145:389, 1977.

62. Frey CF, Karoll RP: Management of chemodectomas. Am J Surg 111:536, 1966.

63. Friedman AH, Drake CG: Subarachnoid hemorrhage from intracranial dissecting aneurysm. J Neurosurg 60:325, 1984.

64. Fries JC, Chamberlin JA: Extra-adrenal pheochromocytoma: Literature review and report of a cervical pheochromocytoma. Surgery 63:268, 1968.

65. Fukushima Y, Kondo Y, Kuroki Y, et al: Are Down syndrome patients predisposed to moyamoya disease? Eur J Pediatr 144:516, 1986.

66. Gassman A: Zur Histologie der Röntgenulcera. Fortschr Geb Roentgenstr 2:199, 1899.

67. Gates JD, Murphy MP, Lipson WE: Autogenous patching of a kinked internal carotid artery. Surgery 123:483, 1998.

68. Gauthier G, Rohr J, Wildi E, Megret M: Spontaneous dissecting aneurysm of the internal carotid artery: General review of 205 published cases with ten personal cases. Schweiz Arch Neurol Psychiatr 136:53, 1985.

69. Gaylis H, Mieny CJ: The incidence of malignancy in carotid body tumours. Br J Surg 64:885, 1977.

70. Gee W, Mehigan JT, Wylie EJ: Measurement of collateral cerebral hemispheric blood pressure by ocular pneumoplethysmography. Am J Surg 130:121, 1975.

71. Gibbs JM, Leeders KL, Wiser RJS, Jones T: Evaluation of cerebral perfusion in patients with carotid artery occlusion. Lancet 2:310, 1984.

72. Giordano JM, Leavitt RY, Hoffman G, Fauci AS: Experience with surgical treatment of Takayasu's disease. Surgery 109:252, 1991.

73. Glenner GG, Crout JR, Roberts WC: A functional carotid body-like tumor secreting levarterenol. Arch Pathol 73:66, 1962.

74. Gold H: Production of atherosclerosis in the rat: Effect of x-ray and a high-fat diet. Arch Pathol 71:268, 1961.

75. Gordon-Taylor G: On carotid body tumours. Br J Surg 28:163, 1940.

76. Graham E, Holland A, Avery A, Russell RWR: Prognosis in giant cell arteritis. Br Med J 282:269, 1981.

77. Graham JM, Miller T, Stinnett DM: Spontaneous dissection of the common carotid artery: Case report and review of the literature. J Vasc Surg 7:811, 1988.

78. Griebenow R, Kramer L, Steffen HM, et al: Quantification of the heart rate–dependent vasopressor component in carotid sinus syndrome. Klin Wochenschr 67:1132, 1989.

79. Grimley PM, Glenner GG: Histology and ultra-structure of carotid body paragangliomas: Comparison with a normal gland. Cancer 20:473, 1967.

80. Gritzmann N, Herold C, Haller J, et al: Duplex sonography for tumors of the carotid body. Cardiovasc Intervent Radiol 10:280, 1987.

81. Grubb RL Jr, Ratcheson RA, Raichle MD, et al: Regional cerebral blood flow and oxygen utilization in superficial temporal middle cerebral artery anastomosis patients. J Neurosurg 50:733, 1979.

82. Grufferman S, Gillman AB, Pasternak LR, et al: Familial carotid body tumors: Case report and epidemiologic review. Cancer 46:2116, 1980.

83. Hall S, Barr W, Lie JT, et al: Takayasu's arteritis: A study of 32 North American patients. Medicine 64:89, 1985.

84. Hall S, Buchbinder R: Takayasu's arteritis. Rheum Dis Clin North Am 16:411, 1990.

85. Hall S, Hunder GG: Is temporal artery biopsy prudent? Mayo Clin Proc 59:793, 1984.

86. Hallett JW Jr, Nora JD, Hollier LH, et al: Trends in neurovascular complications of surgical management for carotid body and cervical paragangliomas: A 50-year experience with 153 tumors. J Vasc Surg 7:284, 1988.

87. Hanakita J, Kondo A, Ishikawa J, et al: An autopsy case of "Moyamoya" disease. No Shinkei Geka 10:531, 1982.

88. Hardy RC, Williams RG: Moyamoya disease and cerebral hemorrhage. Surg Neurol 21:507, 1984.

89. Hart RG, Easton JD: Dissections of the cervical and cerebral arteries. Neurol Clin 1:155, 1983.

90. Heilbrun MP, Reichman OH, Anderson RE, Roberts DW: Regional cerebral blood flow studies following middle cerebral artery anastomosis. J Neurosurg 43:706, 1975.

91. Henly WW, Cooley DA, Gordon WB, et al: Tortuosity of the internal carotid artery: Report of seven cases treated surgically. Postgrad Med 31:133, 1962.

92. Herrschaft P, Duus P, Glenn F, et al: Preoperative and postoperative cerebral flow in patients with carotid artery stenoses. In Lanfitt TW, McHenry LCM Jr, Reivich M (eds): Cerebral Circulation and Metabolism. New York, Springer-Verlag, 1975, p 275.

93. Hopkins L, Martin N, Hadley M, et al: Vertebrobasilar insufficiency: 2. Microsurgical treatment of intracranial vertebrobasilar disease. J Neurosurg 66:662, 1987.

94. Houser OW, Mokri B, Sundt TM Jr, et al: Spontaneous cervical cephalic arterial dissection and its residuum: Angiographic spectrum. Am J Neuroradiol 5:27, 1984.

95. Hunder GG: Giant cell (temporal) arteritis. Rheum Dis Clin North Am 16:399, 1990.

96. Hurley JJ, Nordestgaard AG, Woods JJ: Carotid endarterectomy with vein patch angioplasty for radiation-induced symptomatic atherosclerosis. J Vasc Surg 14:419, 1991.

97. Hsu I, Kistin AD: Buckling of the great vessels. Arch Intern Med 98:712, 1956.

98. Irons GB, Weiland LH, Brown WL: Paragangliomas of the neck: Clinical and pathological analysis of 116 cases. Surg Clin North Am 57:575, 1977.

99. Ishikawa K: Diagnostic approach and proposed criteria for the clinical diagnosis of Takayasu's arteriopathy. J Am Coll Cardiol 12:964, 1986.

100. Ishikawa K: Natural history and classification of occlusive thromboaortopathy (Takayasu's disease). Circulation 57:27, 1978.

101. Ishikawa K: Survival and morbidity after diagnosis of occlusive thromboarthropathy (Takayasu's disease). Am J Cardiol 47:1026, 1981.

102. Jackson JL: Tortuosity of the internal carotid artery in its relation to tonsillectomy. Can Med Assoc J 29:475, 1933.

103. Jackson MA, Hughes RC, Ward SP, McInnes EG: "Headbanging" and carotid dissection. Br Med J 287:1262, 1983.

104. Jacobson JH II, Suarez E: Microsurgery in anastomosis of small vessels. Surg Forum 11:243, 1960.

105. Javid H, Chawla SK, Dye WS, et al: Carotid body tumors: Resection or reflection. Arch Surg 111:344, 1976.

106. Jentzer A: Dissecting aneurysm of the left internal carotid artery. Angiology 5:232, 1954.

107. Joyce JW: Giant cell arteritis. In Ernst CB, Stanley JC (eds): Current Therapy in Vascular Surgery, 2nd ed. Philadelphia, BC Decker, 1991, p 173.

108. Kapoor WN, Karpf M, Wieand S: A prospective evaluation and follow-up of patients with syncope. N Engl J Med 309:197, 1983.

109. Karasawa J, Kikuchi H, Furuse S, et al: A surgical treatment of "moyamoya" disease, "encephalo-myo synangiosis." Neurol Med Chir 17:29, 1977.

110. Kelly AB: Large pulsating vessels in the pharynx. Glasgow Med J 49:28, 1898.

111. Kendall B: Vasculitis in the central nervous system: Contribution of angiography. Eur Neurol 23:472, 1984.

112. Kennedy JT, Krause CJ, Loevy S: The importance of tumor attachment to the carotid artery. Arch Otolaryngol 103:70, 1977.

113. Kenny RA, Traynor G: Carotid sinus syndrome—clinical characteristic in elderly patients. Age Ageing 20:449, 1991.

114. Ketcham AS, Hoyle RC: Spontaneous carotid artery hemorrhage after head and neck surgery. Am J Surg 110:649, 1965.

115. Kieffer E, Bahnini A: Aortic lesions in Takayasu's disease. In Bergan JJ, Yao JST (eds): Aortic Surgery. Philadelphia, WB Saunders, 1989, p 111.

116. Killeen JD, Smith LL: Management of contiguous malignancy, radiation damage, and infection involving the carotid artery. Semin Vasc Surg 4:123, 1991.

117. Kimoto S: The history and present status of aortic surgery in Japan, particularly for aortitis syndrome. J Cardiovasc Surg 20:107, 1979.

118. Kissel JT: Neurologic manifestations of vasculitis. Neurol Clin 7:655, 1989.

119. Kitahara T, Ariga N, Yamaura A, et al: Familial occurrence of moyamoya disease: Report of three Japanese families. J Neurol Neurosurg Psychiatry 42:208, 1979.

120. Klein RG, Campbell RJ, Hunder GG, Carney JA: Skip lesions in temporal arteritis. Mayo Clinic Proc 51:504, 1976.

121. Kleiser B, Widder B: Course of carotid occlusions with impaired cerebrovascular reactivity. Stroke 23:171, 1992.

122. Krayenbuhl HA: The moyamoya syndrome and the neurosurgeon. Surg Neurol 4:353, 1975.

123. Krupski WC, Effeney DJ, Ehrenfeld WK, Stoney RJ: Cervical chemodectoma: Technical considerations and management options. Am J Surg 144:215, 1982.

124. Kudo T: Spontaneous occlusion of the circle of Willis: A disease apparently confined to Japanese. Neurology 18:485, 1968.

125. Kurokawa T, Tomita S, Ueda K, et al: Prognosis of occlusive disease of the circle of Willis (moyamoya disease) in children. Pediatr Neurol 1:274, 1985.

126. Kwak R, Ito S, Yamamoto N, et al: Significance of intracranial

aneurysms associated with moyamoya disease (Part I). Neurol Med Chir (Tokyo) 24:97, 1984.

127. Lamuraglia GM, Fabian RL, Brewster DC, et al: The current surgical management of carotid body paragangliomas. J Vasc Surg 15:1038, 1992.

128. Launes J, Ivanainen M, Erkininjuntti T, et al: Isolated angiitis of the central nervous system. Acta Neurol Scand 74:108, 1986.

129. Lee NS, Jones HR Jr: Extracranial cerebrovascular disease. Cardiol Clin 9:523, 1991.

130. Lees CD, Levine HL, Beven EG, Tucker HM: Tumors of the carotid body: Experience with 41 operative cases. Am J Surg 142:362, 1981.

131. Leipzig TJ, Dohrmann GJ: The tortuous or kinked carotid artery: Pathogenesis and clinical considerations. Surg Neurol 25:478, 1986.

132. Levinson SA, Close MB, Ehrenfeld WK, Stoney RJ: Carotid artery occlusive disease following external cervical irradiation. Arch Surg 107:395, 1973.

133. Levit SA, Sheps SG, Espinosa RE, et al: Catecholamine-secreting paraganglioma of glomus-jugular region resembling pheochromocytoma. N Engl J Med 281:805, 1969.

134. Liu YQ: Radiology of aortoarteritis. Radiol Clin North Am 23:671, 1985.

135. Lofftus CM, Biller J, Hart MN, et al: Management of radiation-induced accelerated carotid atherosclerosis. Arch Neurol 44:711, 1987.

136. Lore JM, Boulos EJ: Resection and reconstruction of the carotid artery in metastatic squamous cell carcinoma. Am J Surg 142:437, 1981.

137. Luken MG III, Ascherl GF Jr, Correll JW, et al: Spontaneous dissecting aneurysms of the extracranial internal carotid artery. Clin Neurosurg 26:353, 1979.

138. Lupi-Herrera E, Sanchez GT, Horwitz S, et al: Pulmonary artery involvement in Takayasu's arteritis. Chest 63:69, 1975.

139. Machado EB, Michet CJ, Ballard DJ, et al: Trends and incidents and clinical presentation of temporal arteritis in Olmstead County, Minnesota, 1950–1985. Arthritis Rheum 31:745, 1988.

140. Maed H, Handa N, Matsumoto M, et al: Carotid lesions detected by B-mode ultrasonography in Takayasu's arteritis: "Macaroni sign" as an indicator of the disease. Ultrasound Med Biol 17:695, 1991.

141. Marcial-Rojas RA, Castro JR: Irradiation injury to elastic arteries in the course of treatment for neoplastic disease. Ann Otol 71:945, 1962.

142. Martin CE, Rosenfeld L, McSwain B: Carotid body tumors: A 16-year follow-up of seven malignant cases. South Med J 66:1236, 1973.

143. Martinez SA, Oller DW, Gee W, et al: Elective carotid artery resection. Arch Otolaryngol 101:744, 1975.

144. Mathes SJ, Alexander J: Radiation injury. Surg Oncol Clin North Am 5:809, 1996.

145. Matsushima Y, Fukai N, Tanaka K, et al: A new surgical treatment of moyamoya disease in children: A preliminary report. Surg Neurol 15:313, 1981.

146. Maydl: Cited by Byrne JJ: Carotid body and allied tumors. Am J Surg 95:371, 1958.

147. McCready RA, Hyde GL, Bivens BA, et al: Radiation-induced arterial injuries. Surgery 93:306, 1982.

148. McCready RA, Miller KS, Hamaker RC, et al: What is the role of carotid arterial resection in the management of advanced cervical cancer? J Vasc Surg 10:274, 1989.

149. McGuirt WF, Harker LA: Carotid body tumors. Arch Otolaryngol 101:58, 1975.

150. McIlrath DC, Remine WH: Carotid body tumors. Surg Clin North Am 43:1135, 1963.

151. Meissner I, Mokri B: Vascular diseases of the cervical carotid artery. Cardiovasc Clin 22:161, 1992.

152. Metz H, Murray-Leslie RM, Bannister RG, et al: Kinking of the internal carotid artery in relation to cerebrovascular disease. Lancet 1:424, 1961.

153. Meyer FB, Sundt TM Jr, Pearson BW: Carotid body tumors: A subject review and suggested surgical approach. J Neurosurg 64:377, 1986.

154. Mokri B: Traumatic and spontaneous extracranial internal carotid artery dissections. J Neurol 237:356, 1990.

155. Mokri B: Dissection of cervical and cephalic arteries. In Meyer FB (ed): Sundt's Occlusive Cerebrovascular Disease. Philadelphia, WB Saunders, 1994, p 46.

156. Mokri B, Okazaki H: Cystic medial necrosis and internal carotid

157. Mokri B, Piepgras DG, Houser OW: Traumatic dissections of the extracranial internal carotid artery. J Neurosurg 68:189, 1988.

158. Mokri B, Piepgras DG, Wiebers DO: Familial occurrence of spontaneous dissection of the internal carotid artery. Stroke 18:246, 1987.

159. Mokri B, Schievink WI, Olsen KD, Piepgras DG: Spontaneous dissection of the cervical internal carotid artery: Presentation with lower cranial nerve palsies. Arch Otolaryngol Head Neck Surg 118:431, 1992.

160. Mokri B, Houser OW, Sundt TM Jr, et al: Spontaneous dissection of the internal carotid arteries: Clinical presentation and angiographic features (Abstract). Ann Neurol 12:84, 1982.

161. Mokri B, Sundt TM Jr, Houser OW, et al: Spontaneous internal carotid dissection, hemicrania, and Horner's syndrome. Arch Neurol 36:677, 1979.

162. Mokri B, Sundt TM, Houser OW, et al: Spontaneous dissection of the cervical internal carotid artery. Ann Neurol 19:126, 1986.

163. Monro RS: Natural history of carotid body tumors and their diagnosis and treatment. Br J Surg 37:445, 1950.

164. Moore OS, Karlan M, Sigler L: Factors influencing the safety of carotid ligation. Am J Surg 118:666, 1969.

165. Moritz MW, Higgins RF, Jacobs JR: Duplex imaging and incidence of carotid radiation injury after high-dose radiotherapy for tumors of the head and neck. Arch Surg 125:1181, 1990.

166. Mulligan RM: Syllabus of Human Neoplasms. Philadelphia, Lea & Febiger 1950, p 98.

167. Mumenthaler M: Cranial arteritis. In Vinken PJ, Bruyn GD, Klawans HL, Toole JF (eds): Handbook of Clinical Neurology. Vol 5. Vascular Diseases, Part III. New York, Elsevier Science Publishers, 1986, p 341.

168. Najafi H, Javid H, Dye WS: Kinked internal carotid artery. Arch Surg 89:135, 1964.

169. Nakayama K: Surgical removal of the carotid body for bronchial asthma. Dis Chest 40:595, 1961.

170. Nishimoto A: Moyamoya disease. Neurol Med Chir (Tokyo) 19:221, 1979.

171. Nishimoto A, Takeuchi S: Abnormal cerebrovascular network related to the internal carotid arteries. J Neurosurg 29:255, 1968.

172. Nordborg E, Bengtsson BA: Epidemiology of biopsy-proven giant cell arteritis (GCA). J Intern Med 227:233, 1990.

173. Ogawa A, Nakamura N, Yoshimoto T, et al: Cerebral blood flow in moyamoya disease: Part I. Correlation with age and regional distribution. Acta Neurochir (Wien) 105:30, 1990.

174. Ogawa A, Nakamura N, Yoshimoto T, et al: Cerebral blood flow in moyamoya disease: Part II: Autoregulation and CO_2 response. Acta Neurochir (Wien) 105:107, 1990.

175. Ojemann RG, Fisher CM, Rich JC: Spontaneous dissecting aneurysm of the internal carotid artery. Stroke 3:434, 1972.

176. Olcott CN, Fee WE, Enzmann DR, et al: Planned approach to management of malignant invasion of the carotid artery. Am J Surg 142:123, 1981.

177. Olsen WL, Dillon WP, Kelly WM, et al: MR imaging of paragangliomas. Am J Roentgenol 148:201, 1987.

178. Padberg FT Jr, Cady B, Persson AV: Carotid body tumor: the Lahey Clinic experience. Am J Surg 145:526, 1983.

179. Pandya SK, Nagpal RD, Desai AP, Purohit AT: Death following external carotid arterial embolization for a functioning glomus jugular chemodectoma. J Neurosurg 48:1030, 1978.

180. Poindexter JM Jr, Patel KR, Clauss RH: Management of kinked extracranial cerebral arteries. J Vasc Surg 6:127, 1987.

181. Pokrovsky AV, Sultanaliev TA, Spiridonov AA: Surgical treatment of vasorenal hypertension in non-specific aorto-arteritis (Takayasu's disease). J Cardiovasc Surg 24:111, 1983.

182. Powers WJ, Tempel L, Grubb RL Jr: Influence of cerebral hemodynamics on stroke risk: One-year follow-up of 30 medically treated patients. Ann Neurol 25:325, 1989.

183. Pryse-Davies J, Dawson IMP, Westbury G: Some morphological histochemical and chemical observations on chemodectomas and the normal carotid body, including a study of the chromaffin reaction and possible ganglion cell elements. Cancer 17:185, 1964.

184. Quattlebaum JK Jr, Upson ET, Neville RL: Stroke associated with elongation and kinking of the internal carotid artery. Ann Surg 150:824, 1959.

185 Quattlebaum JK Jr, Wade JS, Whiddon CM: Stroke associated with elongation and kinking of the carotid artery: Long-term follow-up. Ann Surg 177:572, 1973.

186 Rangwala F, Sylvia LC, Becker SM: Soft tissue metastases of a chemodectoma: A case report and review of the literature. Cancer 42:2865, 1978.

187. Razack MS, Sako K: Carotid artery hemorrhage of ligation in head and neck cancer. J Surg Oncol 19:189, 1982.

188. Reigner: Cited by Lahey FH, Warren KW: A long-term appraisal of carotid tumors with remarks on their removal. Surg Gynecol Obstet 92:481, 1951.

189. Ridge BA, Brewster DC, Darling RC, et al: Familial carotid body tumors: Incidence and implications. Ann Vasc Surg 7:190, 1993.

190. Ringel SP, Harrison SH, Norenberg MD, et al: Fibromuscular dysplasia: Multiple "spontaneous" dissecting aneurysms of the major cervical arteries. Ann Neurol 1:301, 1977.

191. Riser MM, Gelraud J, Ducoudray J, et al: Dolicho-carotide interne avec syndrome vertigineux. Rev Neurol (Paris) 85:145, 1951.

192. Robison JG, Shagets FW, Beckett WC Jr, et al: A multidisciplinary approach to reducing morbidity and operative blood loss during resection of carotid body tumor. Surg Gynecol Obstet 168:166, 1989.

193. Romanski R: Chemodectoma (non-chromaffinic paraganglioma) of the carotid body with distant metastases with illustrative case. Am Pathol 30:1, 1954.

194. Rose G, Sinclair-Smith CC: Takayasu's arteritis: A study of 16 autopsy cases. Arch Pathol Lab Med 104:231, 1980.

195. Rothrock JF, Lim V, Press G, et al: Serial magnetic resonance and carotid duplex examinations in the management of carotid dissection. Neurology 39:686, 1989.

196. Rush BF: Familial bilateral carotid body tumors. Ann Surg 147:633, 1963.

197. Saldana MJ, Salem LE, Travezan R: High altitude hypoxia and chemodectomas. Hum Pathol 4:251, 1973.

198. Samson DS, Boone S: Extracranial-intracranial (EC/IC) arterial bypass: Past performance and current concepts. Neurosurgery 3:79, 1978.

199. Sarkari NBS, Holmes JM, Bickerstaff ER: Neurological manifestation associated with internal carotid loops and kinks in children. J Neurol Neurosurg Psychiaty 33:194, 1970.

200. Savage CO, Ng YC: The etiology and pathogenesis of major systemic vasculitides. Postgrad Med J 62:627, 1986.

201. Schechter DC: Dolichocarotid syndrome: Cerebral ischemia related to cervical carotid artery redundancy with kinking: I and II. Stat Med 79:1391, 1979.

202. Schellack J, Fulenwider JT, Olson RA, et al: The carotid sinus syndrome: A frequently overlooked cause of syncope in the elderly. J Vasc Surg 4:376, 1986.

203. Schevink WI, Mokri B, Piepgras DG: Angiographic frequency of saccular intracranial aneurysms in patients with spontaneous cervical artery dissection. J Neurosurg 76:62, 1992.

204. Schild SE, Foote RL, Buskirk S, et al: Results of radiotherapy for chemodectomas. Mayo Clin Proc 67:537, 1992.

205. Schwaighofer BW, Kline MV, Lynden PD, et al: MR imaging of vertebrobasilar vascular disease. J Comput Assist Tomogr 14:895, 1990.

206. Scudder CL: Tumor of the intercarotid body. A report of one case, together with all cases in literature. Am J Med Sci 126:1384, 1903.

207. Shamblin WR, ReMine WH, Sheps SG, et al: Carotid body tumor (chemodectoma): Clinicopathologic analysis of ninety cases. Am J Surg 122:732, 1971.

208. Shehan JF: Foam cell plaques in the interna elastica of irradiated small arteries. Arch Pathol 37:297, 1944.

209. Shelhamer JH, Volkman DJ, Parrillo JE, et al: Takayasu's arteritis and its therapy. Ann Intern Med 103:121, 1985.

210. Shugar MA, Mafee MF: Diagnosis of carotid body tumors by dynamic computerized tomography. Head Neck Surg 4:518, 1982.

211. Silverberg JD, Brit RH, Goffinet DR: Radiation-induced carotid artery disease. Cancer 41:130, 1978.

212. Sise MJ, Connihan CM, Shackford SR: The clinical spectrum of Takayasu's arteritis. Surgery 104:905, 1988.

213. Skillern PG: Anomalous internal carotid artery and its clinical significance in operations of the tonsils. JAMA 60:172, 1913.

214. Smith BM, Starnes VA, Maggart MA: Operative management of the kinked carotid artery. Surg Gynecol Obstet 162:70, 1986.

215. Smith RF, Shetty PC, Reddy DJ: Surgical treatment of carotid paragangliomas presenting unusual technical difficulties: The value of preoperative embolization. J Vasc Surg 7:631, 1988.

216. Spetzler R, Hadley M: Extracranial-intracranial bypass grafting: An update. In Wilkins R, Rengachary S (eds): Neurosurgery, Update II: Vascular, Spinal, Pediatric and Functional Neurosurgery. New York, McGraw-Hill, 1991, p 197.

217. Spetzler RF, Selman WR, Roski RA, et al: Cerebral revascularization during barbiturate coma in primates and humans. Surg Neurol 17:111, 1982.

218. Staats EF, Brown RL, Smith RR: Carotid body tumors, benign and malignant. Laryngoscope 76:907, 1966.

219. Stanson AW, Klein RG, Hunder GG: Extracranial angiographic findings in giant cell (temporal) arteritis. AJR Am J Roentgenol 127:957, 1976.

220. Stanton PE Jr, McClusky DA Jr, Lamis PA: Hemodynamic assessment and surgical correction of kinking of the internal carotid artery. Surgery 84:793, 1978.

221. Steinke W, Hennerici M, Aulich A: Doppler color flow imaging of carotid body tumors. Stroke 20:1574, 1989.

222. Stringer WL, Kelly DL Jr: Traumatic dissection of extracranial internal carotid artery. Neurosurgery 6:123, 1980.

223. Sundt TM, Whistman JP, Piepgras DG, et al: Techniques, results, complications, and follow-up in superficial temporal artery to middle cerebral artery bypass pedicles. In Meyer FB (ed): Sundt's Occlusive Cerebrovascular Disease, 2nd ed. Philadelphia, WB Saunders, 1994, p 436.

224. Suzuki J, Kodoma H: Moyamoya disease—a review. Stroke 14:104, 1983.

225. Suzuki J, Takaku A: Cerebrovascular "Moyamoya" disease: Disease showing abnormal net-like vessels in the base of brain. Arch Neurol 20:288, 1969.

226. Takayasu M: A case with peculiar changes of the central retinal vessels. Acta Soc Ophthalmol Japan 12:554, 1908.

227. Takeuchi K, Shimizu K: Hypoplasia of the bilateral internal carotid arteries. Brain Nerve (Tokyo) 9:37, 1957.

228. Thomas E, Forbus WB: Irradiation injury to the aorta and the lung. Arch Pathol 67:256, 1959.

229. Trackler RT, Mikulicich AG: Diminished cerebral perfusion resulting from kinking of the internal carotid artery. J Nucl Med 15:634, 1974.

230. Trosch RM, Hasbani M, Brass LM: "Bottoms-up" dissection (Letter). N Engl J Med 320:1564, 1989.

231. Ueki K, Meyer FB: Moyamoya disease. In Meyer FB (ed): Sundt's Occlusive Cerebrovascular Disease, 2nd ed. Philadelphia, WB Saunders, 1994, p 466.

232. Ueno A, Awane Y, Wakabayashi A, et al: Successfully operated obliterative brachiocephalic arteritis (Takayasu's) associated with elongated coarctation. Jpn Heart J 93:94, 1977.

233. Valdagni R, Amichetti M: Radiation therapy of carotid body tumors. Am J Clin Oncol 13:45, 1990.

234. Vannix RS, Joergenson FJ, Carter R: Kinking of the internal carotid artery: Clinical significance and surgical management. Am J Surg 134:82, 1977.

235. Verneuil M: Contusions multiples délire violate, hémiplégia àdroite, signes de compression cérébrale. Bull Acad Natl Med (Paris) 1:46, 1872.

236. Vinijchaikul K: Primary arteritis of the aorta and its main branches (Takayasu's arteriopathy): A clinicopathologic autopsy study of 8 cases. Am J Med 43:15, 1967.

237. Vogl T, Brunning R, Schedel H, et al: Paragangliomas of the jugular bulb and carotid body: MR imaging with short sequences and Gd-DTPA enhancement. AJR Am J Roentgenol 153:583, 1989.

238. Von Haller: Cited by Gratiot JH: Carotid tumors: A collective review. Abstr Surg VII:117, 1943.

239. Waddington MM, Ring BA: Syndromes of occlusions of middle cerebral artery branches: Angiographic and clinical correlation. Brain 91:685, 1968.

240. Weaver FA, Yellin AE, Campen DH: Surgical procedures in the management of Takayasu's arteritis. J Vasc Surg 12:429, 1990.

241. Weibel J, Fields WS: Tortuosity, coiling, and kinking of the internal carotid artery: Relationship of morphological variation to cerebrovascular insufficiency. Neurology 15:462, 1965.

242. Weibers DO, Mokri B: Internal carotid artery dissection after childbirth. Stroke 16: 956, 1988.

243. Weidemann G, Grotz J, Bewermeyer H, et al: High resolution real-time ultrasound of the carotid bifurcation in patients with hyperactive carotid sinus syndrome. J Neurol 232:318, 1985.
244. Westbrook KC, Guillamondequi OM, Medellin H, et al: Chemodectomas of the neck. Selective management. Am J Surg 124:760, 1972.
245. Widder B: The Doppler CO_2 test to exclude patients not in need of extracranial-intracranial bypass surgery. J Neurol Neurosurg Psychiatry 28:449, 1965.
246. Wilkinson IMS, Russell RWR: Arteries of the head and neck in giant cell arteritis: A pathological study to show the pattern of arterial involvement. Arch Neurol 27:378, 1972.
247. Wirth FP, Miller WA, Russell AP: Atypical fibromuscular hyperplasia: Report of two cases. J Neurosurg 54:685, 1981.
248. Wood JB, Frankland AW, Eastcott HHG: Bilateral removal of carotid bodies for asthma. Thorax 20:570, 1965.
249. Worsey MJ, Laborde AL, Bower T, et al: A evaluation of color duplex scanning in the primary diagnosis and management of carotid body tumors. Ann Vasc Surg 6:90, 1992.
250. Wright DJ, Pandya A, Noel F: Anesthesia for carotid body tumour resection. Anaesthesia 34:806, 1979.
251. Yaghami I, Shariat S, Shamloo M: Carotid body tumors. Radiology 97:559, 1970.
252. Youl BD, Coutlellier A, Dubois B, et al: Three cases of spontaneous extracranial vertebral artery dissection. Stroke 21:618, 1990.
253. Zelenock GB, Kazmers A, Whitehouse WM Jr, et al: Extracranial internal carotid artery dissections: Noniatrogenic traumatic lesions. Arch Surg 117:425, 1982.
254. Zirkel PK, Wheeler JR, Gregory RT, et al: Carotid involvement in aortic dissection diagnosed by duplex scanning. J Vasc Surg 1:700, 1984.

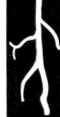

CHAPTER 136

Postoperative Management and Complications Following Carotid Endarterectomy

Norman R. Hertzer, M.D.

According to data from the National Center for Health Statistics, carotid endarterectomy has been the most common operation performed in the field of vascular surgery in the United States for nearly the past two decades.[80] The annual number of these procedures peaked at 107,000 in 1985, declined to 70,000 in 1989 during a period of uncertainty regarding their efficacy, then increased to 91,000 in 1992 after disclosures from the North American Symptomatic Carotid Endarterectomy Trial (NASCET),[132] the European Carotid Surgery Trial (ECST),[69] and the Veterans Administration (VA) trial on symptomatic carotid stenosis[127] reconfirmed the benefit of surgical treatment for severe (70% to 99%) carotid stenosis associated with previous transient ischemic attacks (TIAs) or prior strokes with good functional recovery. Now that the VA trial on asymptomatic stenosis[102] and the Asymptomatic Carotid Atherosclerosis Study (ACAS)[71] have strongly suggested that carotid endarterectomy also provides a reduction in relative stroke risk in patients found to have severe, asymptomatic carotid stenosis, the number of carotid operations can be expected to escalate even more dramatically in the future.

The results of these five influential trials are summarized in Table 136–1 and have become widely accepted as guidelines for the selection of surgical candidates. A number of reports have demonstrated, however, that the appropriateness of carotid endarterectomy can be determined only in the context of its early complications.[35, 36, 122, 192, 202] For example, whereas the superiority of surgical treatment was

sufficiently robust to compensate for a perioperative stroke and mortality rate of nearly 8% in the ECST, a risk of this magnitude would not justify intervention for asymptomatic carotid stenosis. The point is clear: There is no higher priority in vascular surgery than the safety of carotid endarterectomy.

POSTOPERATIVE MANAGEMENT

Although the elements of appropriate care may differ from one center to the next, the following approach has proved to be satisfactory at the Cleveland Clinic. Patients remain for 6 to 8 hours in the post-anesthesia care unit (recovery room), where wound bleeding or hematoma formation, hypoxia, labile blood pressure, and abrupt neurologic deterioration may be recognized more promptly than might be the case on a conventional hospital ward. Serious complications so rarely occur after this period that overnight admission to an intensive care unit represents an unnecessary expense in nearly 90% of patients.[8, 15, 101, 120, 156]

Hemoglobin, hematocrit, and serum electrolytes also are measured because many patients who undergo carotid endarterectomy are aged or need maintenance antihypertensive medication and may experience either hemodilution or hypokalemia during administration of intravenous fluids. Coronary artery disease (CAD) is prevalent among patients with carotid atherosclerosis, and a routine electrocardio-

TABLE 136–1. RESULTS OF MAJOR PROSPECTIVE RANDOMIZED TRIALS*

	NASCET[132]		ECST[69]		VETERANS AFFAIRS SYMPTOMATIC[127]		VETERANS AFFAIRS ASYMPTOMATIC[102]		ACAS[71]	
	Surg	Med	Surg	Med	Surg	Med	Surg	Med	Surg	Med
Severity of stenosis	70% to 99%		70% to 99%		70% to 99%		50% to 99%		60% to 99%	
Angiographic reference	Cervical ICA		Carotid bulb		Cervical ICA		Cervical ICA		Cervical ICA	
Surveillance										
Maximum	30 mo		10 yr		31 mo		7 yr		6 yr	
Mean	18 mo		3 yr		12 mo		4 yr		2.7 yr	
Patients	328	331	455	323	63	66	211	233	825	834
Hospital mortality	0.5%	—	1%	—	0	—	2%	—	0.1%	—
Stroke rates										
30-day	5%	3%	7%	NA	2%	NA	2%	0.5%	2%	0.5%
Late ipsilateral	7%	24%	12%	22%	8%	26%	5%	9%	5%	11%
	($p < .001$)		($p < .0001$)		($p = .01$)		($p = .06$)		($p = .004$)	

*End-points include stroke and crescendo transient ischemic attacks.
NASCET = North American Symptomatic Carotid Endarterectomy Trial; ECST = European Carotid Surgery Trial; ACAS = Asymptomatic Carotid Atherosclerosis Study; ICA = internal carotid artery; Surg = surgical treatment; Med = medical treatment; NA = data not available.
Source: Data from N Engl J Med 325:445, 1991[132]; Lancet 337:1235, 1991[69]; JAMA 266:3289, 1991[127]; N Engl J Med 328:221, 1993[102]; and JAMA 273:1421, 1995.[71]

gram is performed to exclude obvious myocardial ischemia. Patients who are recognized to have coronary involvement receive either sublingual or cutaneous nitroglycerin compounds until oral medication is resumed. Transient premature ventricular contractions are not uncommon and usually respond to potassium supplementation or the parenteral infusion of lidocaine hydrochloride.

An adequate neurologic examination is necessary to evaluate extremity strength, fine hand movements, articulate speech, visual acuity, and mentation. Provided that the external carotid artery was not occluded during bifurcation endarterectomy, the presence of a normal superficial temporal pulse indicates patency of the common carotid artery but does not reflect the status of the internal carotid artery. The neurologic evaluation is repeated frequently during the initial postoperative period by the nursing staff, and any new deficit is reported immediately to the responsible surgeon. Transient hypertension or hypotension is not unusual after carotid endarterectomy, and because extreme fluctuations in systemic blood pressure may provoke either cerebral hemorrhage or carotid thrombosis, a percutaneous radial or brachial artery catheter is used for continuous monitoring until all parameters have been stable for several hours.

Nothing is given by mouth until the patient leaves the recovery room because sudden neurologic deterioration or wound bleeding occasionally requires an urgent reoperation. A brief course of prophylactic antibiotics ordinarily is administered on the day of the operation but probably is superfluous unless prosthetic material was employed during the original procedure or an early reoperation is required. In an attempt to prevent platelet aggregation that may cause either internal carotid thrombosis or cerebral embolization, however, aspirin is given by rectal suppository in the recovery unit and is continued orally in a dosage of 5 grains twice daily for at least the first postoperative month. Edwards and colleagues[62] found that the preoperative use of antiplatelet agents reduced the incidence of post-endarterectomy internal carotid occlusion from 3.1%

to only 0.3%. An earlier study by French and Rewcastle[77] suggested that endothelial regeneration at the site of carotid endarterectomy is reasonably complete within an interval of 4 to 6 weeks.

If all parameters are satisfactory after 6 to 8 hours of observation, the patient is transferred to a regular nursing unit, where full activity is encouraged during only 1 or 2 days of hospital convalescence. An outpatient examination is performed approximately a month after suture removal for assessment of the neurologic results, the presence and quality of cervical pulses and residual bruits, and wound healing. Unless the patient is to undergo additional cardiovascular or other surgical procedures in the interim, an annual evaluation is scheduled. The Cleveland Clinic includes in postoperative management annual duplex scanning for at least 3 years to detect asymptomatic progression of other extracranial lesions or recurrent stenosis on the operated side. Finally, and perhaps most important, the patient is instructed to report any unexpected neurologic symptoms as soon as they occur.

COMPLICATIONS

Wound Complications
Cervical Hematoma

Although (1) carotid reconstruction ordinarily is performed with the use of full heparin anticoagulation and (2) many, if not most, surgical candidates have received preoperative antiplatelet therapy, the incidence of postoperative wound bleeding is surprisingly low. Reoperations for hemostasis following carotid endarterectomy were required in only 0.7% of a personal experience with 1022 patients reported by Thompson[190] and in 1.5% of a 3-year series of 917 operations at the Cleveland Clinic.[94] Sodium heparin may be predictably reversed with protamine sulfate at the conclusion of the original procedure, but because sodium warfarin (Coumadin) derivatives initiate a sustained elevation of the prothrombin time, formal oral anticoagulation should be corrected preoperatively with vitamin K and. if necessary, with fresh frozen plasma. The use of aspirin, dipyridamole, and related compounds is so ubiquitous among cerebrovascular patients that these agents probably are responsible for most troublesome blood losses. Capillary bleeding caused by these agents rarely may require platelet transfusions, but patience and conventional measures usually are sufficient because the standard approach to the carotid bifurcation through an incision parallel to the anterior border of the sternocleidomastoid muscle is relatively avascular.

A retrospective review of 697 carotid endarterectomies conducted by Treiman and associates[195] indicated that wound hematomas may occur less frequently when systemic heparin therapy is reversed with protamine sulfate at the conclusion of the operation (1.8%) than when it is not (6.5%). Some other reports have suggested, however, that the administration of protamine might be associated with a modest risk for carotid thrombosis and related stroke. In a retrospective review of 348 consecutive operations, Mauney and colleagues[126] encountered this particular complication in five (2.6%) of 193 patients receiving protamine, compared with none of the 155 patients in whom heparin corticoagulation was left unreversed ($p < .045$).

Fearn and associates[72] have reported a prospective randomized trial in which two (6.5%) of the 31 patients receiving protamine sustained carotid thrombosis and related strokes, and two (6.1%) of another 33 patients not receiving protamine experienced cervical hematomas. On the basis of their experience with another small series of 42 patients, Coyne and associates[45] have recommended that protamine be used only in the presence of troublesome bleeding or a documented elevation in the activated clotting time. With none of these data conclusive, however, this controversy remains unresolved.

It is axiomatic that the best method for obtaining hemostasis after an operation is to maintain it throughout the preliminary dissection. Nevertheless, postoperative bleeding from the edges of the incision sometimes occurs and may be controlled by light compression or the addition of a few superficial sutures incorporating the skin and the underlying platysma. Cervical hematomas often are discovered after Valsalva's maneuvers at the time the endotracheal tube is removed, a feature implicating transient arterial hypertension and venous distention as contributing factors. For this reason, suture ligatures are preferable to simple ligation for control of the facial vein and branches of the external carotid artery that may be divided to permit mobilization of the hypoglossal nerve. If an autogenous vein patch is applied to the arteriotomy, its branches should be transfixed with sutures or incorporated into the anastomosis. Low-molecular-weight dextran is administered to selected patients at the Cleveland Clinic in order to prevent immediate platelet aggregation when a subadventitial endarterectomy plane is entered during the removal of a deeply ulcerated plaque, but this precaution seems to cause no more bleeding than antiplatelet therapy alone.

A pliable vacuum drain customarily is employed at the Cleveland Clinic to detect continued bleeding during the first postoperative hours and to prevent the accumulation of a hematoma large enough to produce deviation of the trachea and airway obstruction. Even if ventilation is not impaired, however, a large cervical hematoma is undesirable because it may compress the internal carotid artery and adjacent cranial nerves, establish a potential nidus for infection, and foster a draining wound that is both uncomfortable and cosmetically unsatisfactory. Therefore, a postoperative cervical hematoma should be corrected by an elective reoperation on the same day as the original procedure. The incision should be completely opened to allow evacuation of the hematoma and to obtain adequate hemostasis. The wound should be thoroughly irrigated prior to primary closure, and a brief course of intravenous antibiotics also seems to be appropriate if wound exploration has been necessary for any reason.

Infection and False Aneurysm

Postoperative cervical infections almost never occur because the neck represents a clean surgical field with abundant circulation, and only anecdotal reports of carotid artery false aneurysms have been described.[150] Thompson[190] had encountered a single wound infection (0.09%) prior to 1979, and each of the seven false aneurysms (0.6%) in his series involved a prosthetic patch applied with silk suture several years earlier. Although polyester (Dacron) patch angioplasty has been employed during carotid endarterectomy without mycotic complications on countless occasions, any infection in the presence of prosthetic material can have disastrous consequences. The use of autogenous tissue has theoretical advantages in this respect, and if the local arterial supply is sufficient to heal a harvesting incision, a patch of saphenous vein may instead be removed from the thigh or, at least in men, from the lower leg with preservation of the proximal vein for subsequent coronary or lower extremity revascularization. Spontaneous rupture of an ankle vein patch is not impossible even in the absence of infection, but this unpredictable catastrophe appears to be limited to less than 1% of patients.[94, 135]

Infected false aneurysms occurred after only 4 (0.15%) of 2651 carotid reconstructions at the Cleveland Clinic from 1977 through 1984.[88] Because of suppuration and degeneration of the arterial wall, multiple ligation of the common carotid artery, the internal carotid artery, and the external carotid artery was the only alternative in one patient, who subsequently experienced TIAs in the ipsilateral cerebral hemisphere before these events were controlled with oral anticoagulation. The remaining three patients underwent vein patch angioplasty of their false aneurysms in conjunction with systemic antibiotic therapy. In each case, a recurrent false aneurysm developed that required carotid ligation, but none of the patients sustained a postoperative stroke. During the same study period, a chronic infection in a Dacron patch angioplasty performed at another center was treated successfully with resection of the carotid bifurcation and an interposition vein graft to the distal cervical segment of the internal carotid artery. These limited examples suggest that infected false aneurysms usually require multiple ligation unless it is feasible to excise the septic arterial wall and replace it with an uncontaminated autogenous graft.

Hypertension and Hypotension

Postoperative hypertension and hypotension may be caused by alterations in intravascular volume, peripheral vasoconstriction, or cardiac dysfunction following any major operation. They appear to be especially common, however, after carotid endarterectomy, and this observation has generated considerable interest in the possible contribution of the carotid sinus mechanism because of its perceived importance in blood pressure regulation and its proximity to the carotid bifurcation.

As illustrated in Figure 136–1, specialized neurons located in the adventitia of the carotid bulb monitor systemic blood pressure and respond to sustained elevations by initiating a reflex arc to the upper brain stem that is mediated by the sinus nerve of Hering, a branch of the glossopharyngeal nerve.[87, 88] Compensatory bradycardia and a reduction in blood pressure normally occur under these circumstances, but there is evidence that interruption of this negative-feedback system by injury to the sinus nerve during carotid endarterectomy may actually encourage a hypertensive response by simulating a hypotensive episode, particularly after bilateral carotid reconstruction has been performed.[28, 31, 174] Conversely, Angell-James and Lumley[9] also have postulated that the excision of a calcified, nondistensible atheroma may instead cause reflex hypotension in some patients by restoring compliance to the bifurcation and reactivating a dormant baroreceptor mechanism.

It is important to recognize the theoretical role of the sinus nerve in the etiology of abrupt changes in blood pressure, because unanticipated bradycardia and hypotension during surgical exposure of the carotid bifurcation often may be corrected by infiltration of the sinus with local anesthetic.[9, 31, 67] Nevertheless, Wade and colleagues[199] discovered that baroreceptor function may disappear entirely with advancing age, and Towne and Bernhard[194] were unable to demonstrate that either preservation or transection of the sinus nerve had any real influence on postoperative blood pressure in the clinical setting.

Because a consistent causal relationship between sinus nerve activity and perioperative blood pressure has not been established, other factors also deserve consideration. Davies and Cronin[53] found no correlation between preoperative and postoperative blood pressure, but both Bove and coworkers[28] and Towne and Bernhard[194] calculated that hypertensive patients had a statistically significant risk for severe postoperative hypertension, especially if preoperative medical control was inadequate. Moreover, Ranson and associates[148] concluded that an unsuspected deficit in intravascular volume was the critical feature of postoperative hypotension and that reflex bradycardia was a predictable complication only in the presence of hypovolemia.

Tarlov and colleagues[186] later restated this principle and reduced the incidence of postoperative hypotension from 54% to 18% in their patients by using colloid infusions to maintain adequate central venous pressures. Elegant studies by other investigators have suggested that postoperative hypertension may be related to the systemic release of either renin, vasopressin, or norepinephrine from obscure intracranial sources that remain poorly understood.[4, 119, 179]

Irrespective of their etiology, extreme fluctuations in postoperative blood pressure have been associated with an increase in surgical strokes and mortality.[28, 128, 148, 158, 160, 174, 194] Bove and coworkers[28] encountered postoperative hypertension in 19% and hypotension in 28% of 100 consecutive patients and found neurologic deficits in 9% of these two subsets, in comparison with none of the patients who remained normotensive. Similarly, Towne and Bernhard[194] reported operative strokes in 10% of their patients who experienced postoperative hypertension, compared with 3% of those who did not.

There are conflicting data concerning whether patients who require bilateral carotid reconstruction have a specific risk for hypertensive neurologic complications after the second operation if it is performed too soon after the first. In a small series of 56 patients described by Schroeder and associates,[176] hypertension occurred in 48% when the procedures were performed less than 3 weeks apart and in only 8% when the interval was longer. There was no conclusive correlation, however, between hypertension and neurologic deficits even though the stroke rate was 20% after the contralateral operations in this study.

Another investigation by Satiani and coworkers[173] suggested that the staging interval had no influence on the complication rate in patients with bilateral carotid disease. Darling and colleagues[51] encountered no perioperative strokes in a large series of 164 patients who underwent bilateral carotid procedures under regional anesthesia with

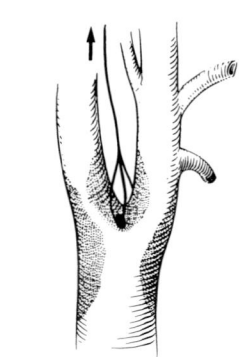

A. PREOPERATIVE

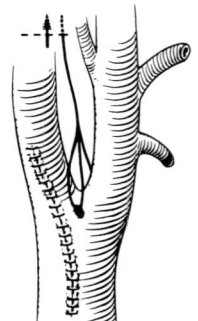

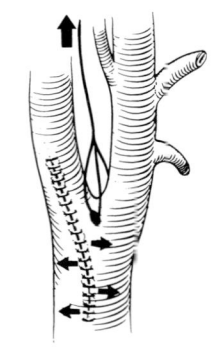

B. POSTOPERATIVE HYPERTENSION   C. POSTOPERATIVE HYPOTENSION

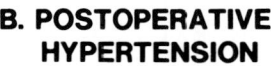

FIGURE 136–1. A–C, Schematic representation of the possible influence of the carotid sinus mechanism on blood pressure fluctuations at the time of bifurcation endarterectomy. (From Hertzer NR: Nonstroke complications of carotid endarterectomy. In Bernhard VM, Towne J [eds]: Complications in Vascular Surgery, 2nd ed. Orlando, Fla, Grune & Stratton, 1985.)

a staging interval of only 2 days, but the advantages of this approach are not entirely clear.[89]

Management

In light of this accumulated experience, either hypertension or hypotension should be prevented, when possible, and treated judiciously when it does occur. Chronic hypertension must be under medical control even if the operation is postponed in order to obtain it.[140] By the same token, perioperative rehydration with parenteral fluids may be necessary for aged patients receiving maintenance diuretic management. Although any precise definition of *hypertension* or *hypotension* is arbitrary, blood pressure generally should be supported at preoperative levels following carotid endarterectomy. At present, pharmacologic treatment is initiated at the Cleveland Clinic if the postoperative systolic blood pressure exceeds 180 mmHg or falls below 100 mmHg in patients who previously were normotensive. However, precipitous manipulation of the blood pressure may itself be associated with a potential risk for either myocardial infarction or stroke.[158, 174]

Sodium nitroprusside is an effective peripheral vasodilator that provides responsive control of hypertension when titrated with a mechanical infusion pump in a dosage of 50 mg in 250 to 500 ml of 5% dextrose in water (D_5W). Postoperative hypotension occurring in conjunction with bradycardia may resolve once the heart rate has been stimulated with a single intravenous bolus of 0.5 to 1.0 mg of atropine sulfate. Hypovolemia should be corrected before the use of vasoconstrictor agents if additional treatment is necessary, but provided that such traditional parameters as urine volume and central venous pressure are satisfactory, low blood pressure may be reversed by the continuous infusion of dopamine hydrochloride in a dosage of 200 to 400 mg in 250 ml of D_5W. In conjunction with their hypothesis that postoperative hypertension may be associated with the intracranial production of norepinephrine, Ahn and coworkers[4] also collected anecdotal evidence that it might be prevented by the administration of sympatholytic agents (e.g., clonidine).

Postoperative blood pressure complications nearly always are transient, and in most patients who experience them, immediate pharmacologic intervention may be withdrawn within a matter of hours. The critical aspect of both hypertension and hypotension is their recognition and management before other related complications occur.

Cranial Nerve Dysfunction

Although the stroke rate and operative mortality associated with carotid endarterectomy have been thoroughly documented for many years, the incidence of iatrogenic injury to cranial nerves near the bifurcation has received relatively little attention. Case reports and retrospective clinical investigations have suggested that symptomatic cranial nerve dysfunction is uncommon and involves the hypoglossal nerve in 5% to 8% of patients and all other cranial nerves in less than 2%.[16, 113, 123, 148] Nevertheless, other reports have demonstrated that the diagnosis of cranial nerve injury is more likely to be established by prospective studies, especially when they are performed in conjunction with objective postoperative testing. In a review of carotid reconstruction at three university, VA, and community hospitals, Krupski and colleagues[114] described at least transient injuries to the vagus or recurrent laryngeal nerves in 8% of patients, the hypoglossal nerve in 4%, and the marginal mandibular branch of the facial nerve in 2%. Evans and associates[70] and Liapis and coworkers[118] encountered early postoperative dysfunction of the vagus or recurrent laryngeal nerve in 15% of their patients and the hypoglossal nerve in 6%, but they also found that as many as 35% of patients had integrated motor deficits that could be detected by speech pathologists. Functional impairment was almost always temporary, however, and only a few of these patients still had persistent deficits as soon as 6 weeks later. Other researchers have made the same observation.[2, 48, 172, 175]

Direct otolaryngologic examinations were conducted after 450 consecutive carotid procedures at the Cleveland Clinic (Table 136–2).[88, 96] Sixty (13%) of these patients had a total of 72 cranial nerve injuries, corresponding to the vagus or recurrent laryngeal nerve in approximately 7%, the hypoglossal nerve in 6%, and the marginal mandibular

TABLE 136–2. CRANIAL NERVE DYSFUNCTION AFTER CAROTID ENDARTERECTOMY*

POSTOPERATIVE DYSFUNCTION	CRANIAL NERVES							
	Recurrent Laryngeal		Hypoglossal		Marginal Mandibular		Superior Laryngeal	
	No.	%	No.	%	No.	%	No.	%
Early incidence								
Symptomatic	21	4.7	16	3 6	8	1.8	3	0.7
Asymptomatic	9	2.0	10	2 2	0	—	5	1.1
Total	30	6.7	26	5 8	8	1.8	8	1.8
Late results								
Follow-up examinations	24	80	20	77	7	88	4	50
Complete recovery	20	83	17	85	6	86	2	50
Mean interval (mo)	3		2		3		2	
Incomplete	4	17	3	15	2	14	2	50
Maximal interval (mo)	14		12		9		2	

*Early incidence and late results of cranial nerve dysfunction following 450 carotid endarterectomies at the Cleveland Clinic. See Hertzer NR, 1985[88] and 1980.[96]

and the superior laryngeal nerves each in 2%. Perhaps the most important feature of this study is the fact that 24 (33%) of these injuries were asymptomatic and would not have been obvious without formal evaluation. Because simultaneous dysfunction of both recurrent laryngeal and hypoglossal nerves can have disastrous consequences, the tongue should be entirely normal and the integrity of the larynx should be established by direct inspection during the staging interval between operations in patients who require bilateral carotid endarterectomy. If either the tongue or the vocal cord is impaired, the contralateral procedure should be postponed until cranial nerve dysfunction has resolved unless there are compelling reasons to do otherwise.

As indicated in Table 136–2, 55 (76%) of the 72 iatrogenic injuries in this series were reassessed with additional examinations. Complete functional recovery occurred in most patients within 3 months after their operations, a finding that suggests that blunt trauma probably is responsible for the majority of cranial nerve complications. Temporary dysfunction may be unavoidable in some patients who have anomalous nerves or in whom exposure of the internal carotid artery near the base of the skull is required, but every surgeon who performs carotid endarterectomy

should be familiar with the normal anatomy of cranial nerves (Fig. 136–2).

Vagus Nerve

The vagus nerve usually pursues a course posterior or slightly lateral to the common carotid and internal carotid arteries, but it occasionally must be reflected from an anomalous anterior position in order to expose the carotid bifurcation. The recurrent laryngeal nerve customarily takes its origin from the vagus nerve within the mediastinum and loops around the subclavian artery on the right side and the aortic arch on the left before entering the tracheoesophageal groove posterior to the thyroid gland; however, it may rarely rise from the vagus nerve near the carotid bifurcation and cross behind the common carotid artery to enter the larynx. It is conceivable that the blades of self-retaining retractors that are placed too deeply in the wound may engage the recurrent laryngeal nerve where it is concealed by strap muscles behind the trachea, but because recurrent laryngeal dysfunction is the only clinical manifestation of unilateral vagal injury, it is probable that most vocal cord complications instead are caused by direct trauma to the vagus nerve itself. Whether the vagus nerve is stretched

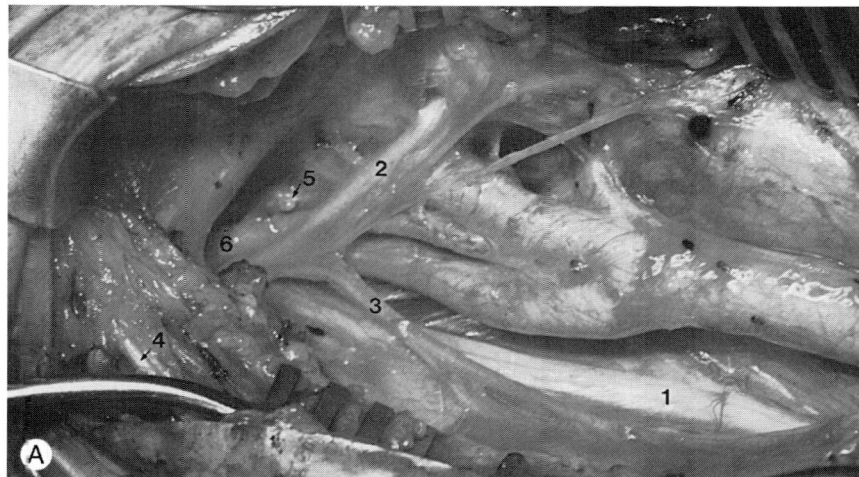

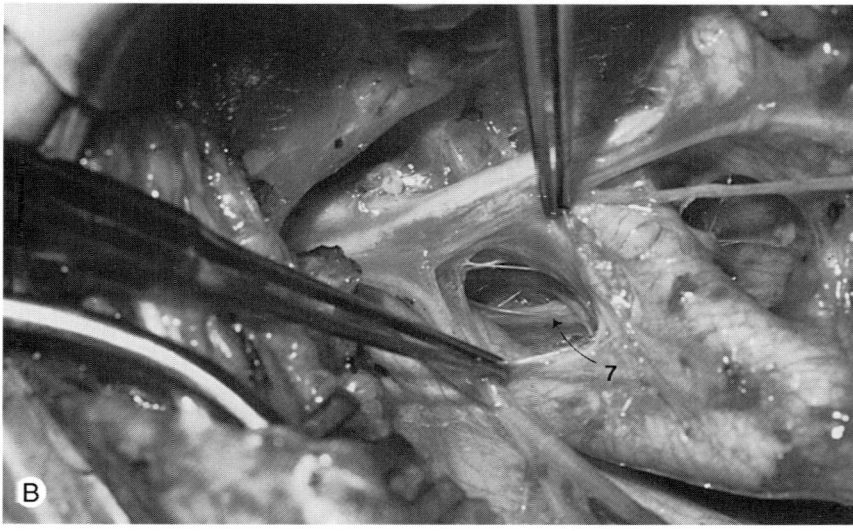

FIGURE 136–2. Surgical exposure of the carotid bifurcation. *A*, The vagus (1) and hypoglossal (2) nerves, the ansa hypoglossi (3), and the greater auricular nerve (4). The sternocleidomastoid artery and vein(s) have been divided, but the hypoglossal nerve (5) remains tethered by the ansa and the occipital artery (6). *B*, The superior laryngeal nerve (7).

within the carotid sheath or injured by forceps, electrocautery, or the application of arterial clamps, paralysis of the ipsilateral vocal cord in the paramedian position results in hoarseness and the loss of an effective cough mechanism.

Although these symptoms customarily resolve within several weeks, polytetrafluoroethylene (Teflon) may be injected into the cord to return it to the midline if the symptoms persist beyond 6 to 12 months. AbuRahma and Lim[2] have emphasized the importance of early injection or even cricopharyngeal myotomy in occasional patients who aspirate food or fluids because of their vagal injuries.

Hypoglossal Nerve

The hypoglossal nerve descends into the neck in a relatively constant position medial to the internal carotid artery and jugular vein before crossing anterior to the external carotid artery to enter the base of the tongue. Except in patients who have especially low carotid bifurcations, the hypoglossal nerve is a surgical landmark that may interfere with adequate exposure of the internal carotid artery because the nerve is tethered in place by the ansa hypoglossi, by the small artery and vein to the sternocleidomastoid muscle, and often by the occipital artery as well as the posterior belly of the digastric muscle. Any or all of these structures may be divided in order to elevate the hypoglossal nerve from the internal carotid artery, since the nerve is more likely to be injured by excessive retraction than by appropriate steps to mobilize it.[103, 190] Trauma to the hypoglossal nerve causes deviation of the tongue to the ipsilateral side, inarticulate speech, and clumsy mastication.

Superior Laryngeal Nerve

The superior laryngeal nerve arises from the vagus nerve near the jugular foramen and passes diagonally behind the internal and external carotid arteries before supplying sensation to the mucosa of the larynx as well as innervation to the cricothyroid muscle and the inferior pharyngeal constrictor muscle. Either the motor or the sensory branch of this nerve may be lacerated during dissection near the superior thyroid artery, and because the main trunk of the nerve is hidden by the carotid sinus, it may also be injured by the vascular clamp applied to the internal carotid artery. Voice fatigue and the loss of high-pitch phonation are the principal manifestations of superior laryngeal nerve trauma, but the impairment is relatively minor in patients who are neither vocalists nor public speakers.

Marginal Mandibular Nerve

The marginal mandibular branch of the facial nerve emerges from the anterior border of the parotid gland and extends across the masseter muscle and the ramus of the mandible before entering the perioral muscles in the lower lip. Although it lies between the platysma and the deep cervical fascia and is not visible within the surgical field, the nerve is drawn downward by rotation of the head to the opposite side. Unless the incision has been extended on a line posterior to the tragus, the nerve may be injured by retraction used to facilitate the exposure of a high carotid bifurcation. This example of blunt trauma imposes little functional disability and almost always is transient, but the inexperienced observer may sometimes misinterpret the resultant drooping at the corner of the mouth as representing an atypical stroke.

Glossopharyngeal Nerve

Motor filaments of the glossopharyngeal nerve cross the distal cervical segment of the internal carotid artery to innervate the middle pharyngeal constrictor muscle and the tensor muscle of the soft palate. Although glossopharyngeal nerve trauma is unlikely unless the internal carotid lesion is exceedingly high, its symptoms are among the most serious of all cranial nerve deficits. Solid food becomes difficult to swallow because of paralysis of the middle pharyngeal constrictor muscle. Oral fluids are tolerated even more poorly owing to nasopharyngeal reflux, and because simultaneous vagal dysfunction is not uncommon, they may be aspirated into the airway as a result of ipsilateral vocal cord palsy. Under these circumstances, intravenous hyperalimentation or enteric tube feeding may be required for at least a short period.

Because both the pharynx and the palate receive multiple motor fibers from the injured nerve as well as from the opposite nerve, nutritional support usually may be discontinued after 2 to 3 weeks with the anticipation that complete functional recovery will occur within the following month. Nevertheless, preservation of the glossopharyngeal nerve may well be one of the most important features of mandibular subluxation and detachment of the styloid process to enhance exposure of the internal carotid artery near the base of the skull.[123, 130]

Other Cervical Nerves

Tucker and associates[196] encountered four injuries to the spinal accessory nerve in a series of 850 carotid endarterectomies (0.5%), but they were able to collect only three other examples of this complication during their review of the previous literature. Horner's syndrome may occur if the superior cervical sympathetic chain is transected during mobilization of the internal carotid artery above the level of the digastric muscle, but this injury is also so rare as to be anecdotal.[198] However, virtually every patient who has an incision parallel to the anterior margin of the sternocleidomastoid muscle experiences temporary sensory loss caused by injury to cutaneous nerves entering the neck and lower mandible. The greater auricular nerve emerges from behind the superior border of the sternocleidomastoid to supply the skin of the scalp and the external ear. Blunt trauma from retractor blades at the upper extent of a standard incision may result in painful paresthesias in the distribution of this nerve that are particularly troublesome.

Operative Stroke

Carotid endarterectomy must be associated with a low incidence of iatrogenic stroke if it is to be considered a reasonable alternative to nonoperative management of cerebrovascular disease. Remarkable improvements have been made in this respect since the Joint Study of Extracranial Arterial Occlusion reported, for operations performed prior to 1969, an overall early mortality of 8% and determined that fatal complications occurred in 42% of patients who had sustained completed strokes within the 2 weeks preceding surgery.[21, 73] By the late 1980s, the combined morbidity and mortality for carotid reconstruction was well below 5% at most centers with a large experience in the procedure, largely because of refinements in patient selection and surgical technique.[87]

In recognition of this progress, a subcommittee of the American Heart Association stated in 1989 that the 30-day mortality rate for all carotid endarterectomies should not exceed 2% and established acceptable risks for perioperative stroke according to discrete surgical indications (asymptomatic stenosis, less than 3%; previous TIA, less than 5%; prior ischemic infarction, less than 7%; recurrent carotid stenosis, less than 10%).[22] Even before higher standards were established in the 1990s by the randomized trials (see Table 136–1), poor results in some geographic areas provoked speculation concerning the safety of the operation throughout the United States.[29, 60, 202] However unjustified, such criticism cannot be easily dismissed until the success of carotid reconstruction has been documented at every hospital in which it is performed.

Incidence

Table 136–3 contains a summary of early results for carotid endarterectomy in 15 large or academic series reported since 1984. Most of these series include a representative distribution of symptomatic and asymptomatic patients, but two of the studies were limited to patients in whom either nonspecific or cortical TIA was the indication for operation.[159, 180] Approximately 60% of the patients included in the most recent reports summarized in Table 136–3 had asymptomatic carotid stenosis,[50, 97] a feature that probably reflects contemporary trends at most centers in response to the ACAS disclosures.[71] Patient selection clearly influences the combined stroke and mortality rate (CSM) of carotid endarterectomy. For the past several years at the Cleveland Clinic, for instance, this overall rate has been 1.5% for patients with asymptomatic stenosis, 2.7% for those with previous TIAs, and 3.8% for those with prior strokes.[97] In a collective review of 25 series reported between 1980 and 1996, Rothwell and associates[166] calculated an aggregate CSM of 3.4% for asymptomatic patients and 5.2% for symptomatic patients.

Although regional anesthesia permits continuous assessment of the neurologic status and has been associated with excellent outcome at several centers, general inhalation anesthesia is more widely used because it reduces the cerebral oxygen requirement and provides complete control of ventilation as well as a comfortable setting for both the patient and the surgical team. Every conceivable approach has been employed to determine the indications for carotid artery shunting, including test clamping, measurement of internal carotid artery back-pressure, and operative electroencephalography (EEG) or cortical blood flow studies. None of these methods has an absolute correlation with stroke risk, however, and Thompson[190] long maintained that routine shunting was the safest and most expeditious alternative. In spite of a number of differences in intraoperative management, results from the 15 nonrandomized series summarized in Table 136–3 are reasonably similar and suggest that an overall stroke and mortality rate of 4% or less represents the contemporary standard of excellence with respect to early outcome of carotid endarterectomy.

TABLE 136–3. REPRESENTATIVE RESULTS OF CAROTID ENDARTERECTOMY REPORTED IN LARGE OR ACADEMIC SERIES SINCE 1984

| SERIES | YEAR | NO. | ANESTHESIA AND CEREBRAL MONITORING | CAROTID SHUNT | NEUROLOGIC COMPLICATIONS | | | |
					TIA (%)	Stroke (%)	Total (%)	Mortality (%)
Baker et al[18]	1984	940	General, back-pressure	None	2.2	2.4	4.7	0.6
Cleveland Vascular Registry[91]	1984	2646	Mixed	NA	NA	2.5	NA	1.2
Ouriel et al[138]	1984	402	General, EEG (35%)	17%	3.2	3.2	6.5	NA
Sachs et al[169]	1984	557	General	All	2.2	2.3	4.5	0.7
Green et al[84]	1985	562	General, EEG	18%	NA	2.7	NA	NA
Fode et al[76]	1986	2535	Mixed	NA	NA	4.2	NA	1.8
Sundt et al[184]	1986	1935	General, EEG	42%	1.8	1.8	3.6	1.3
Toronto Cerebrovascular Study Group[193]	1986	358	Mixed	NA	5.0	4.5	9.5	1.4
Cleveland Clinic[94]	1987	917	General	All	0.8	1.9	2.7	0.5
Cleveland Vascular Registry[167]	1988	8535	Mixed	NA	NA	2.1	NA	1.6
Edwards et al[61]	1989	3028	General	97%	1.3	1.0	2.3	1.5
Goldstein et al[80]	1994	1160	Mixed	NA	NA	4.3	NA	1.4
Riles et al[157]	1994	3062	Regional or local (89%)	19%	NA	2.1	NA	NA
Darling et al[50]	1996	802	Regional (83%)	5%	1.5	1.4	2.9	1.2
Cleveland Clinic[97]	1997	1924	General	All	NA	1.8	NA	0.5

EEG = operative electroencephalography; NA = data not available; TIA = transient ischemic attack.

TABLE 136–4. SPECIFIC CONSIDERATIONS CONCERNING THE INCIDENCE OF PERMANENT STROKE AFTER CAROTID ENDARTERECTOMY

	COMPOSITE RESULTS OF REPRESENTATIVE SERIES		
SPECIFIC CONSIDERATIONS	Data Available (No.)	Permanent Operative Strokes No.	%
Total	14,606	323	2.2
Surgical indications			
Asymptomatic carotid stenosis	1784	29	1.6
Previous neurologic symptoms	7712	194	2.5
Transient ischemia	3288	58	1.8
Prior strokes	933	36	3.9
Contralateral carotid status			
Patent	2276	26	1.1
Occluded	313	19	6.1
Anesthetic management			
General	7494	163	2.2
Local or regional	447	6	1.3
Cerebral protection			
Shunt	1973	37	1.9
No shunt	4479	80	1.8

From Hertzer NR: Early complications of carotid endarterectomy. *In* Moore WS (ed): Cerebrovascular Disease. New York, Churchill Livingstone, 1987.

In another large collected series of 22 publications from 1977 through 1984, sufficient data were available to make a number of comparisons regarding the influence of surgical indications, contralateral carotid disease, choice of anesthesia, and shunt protection on stroke risk (Table 136–4).[87] Permanent iatrogenic strokes occurred in 1.6% of patients with asymptomatic carotid stenosis, compared with 2.5% of those who had previous neurologic symptoms, and they were twice as common in patients having a history of prior strokes (3.9%) as in patients whose preoperative symptoms had been limited to TIAs (1.8%). Of 2589 patients for whom the angiographic status of the contralateral carotid system was designated, operative strokes occurred in 6.1%

of those with recognized contralateral internal carotid occlusion, in comparison with 1.1% of all others. Permanent deficits occurred in conjunction with general anesthesia in 2.2%, with local or regional anesthesia in 1.3%, and with shunting or nonshunting in 1.9% or 1.8%, respectively.

These figures cannot be interpreted to imply that shunts are unnecessary, because selective shunting was used for patients who had specific indications for cerebral protection throughout most of the reference studies. In a series of 940 operations performed without shunts, Baker and associates[18] found that the stroke rate was significantly higher among patients who had low back-pressure as well as contralateral carotid occlusion (11%) than in those having only one (2.8%) or neither (0.9%) of these risk factors. Greene and coworkers[84] described ischemic EEG changes after carotid clamping in 37% of patients who had contralateral internal carotid occlusion or a history of previous stroke, and Graham and associates[83] reported that an abnormal operative EEG was as much as 20 times more common in such patients than in all others.

Sundt and coworkers[184] followed an elegant protocol for intraoperative assessment with both EEG and cerebral blood flow measurements, and they still concluded that shunting was warranted in 42% of their patients. Alimi and colleagues[5] employed shunts in 32% of the 74 patients in their study group yet still discovered new silent infarcts on routine postoperative brain scans in five of the 50 patients who had received shunts. Interestingly, four of these five new strokes involved the contralateral cerebral hemisphere. The perpetual controversy concerning shunts probably will not be resolved in the foreseeable future, but it appears to be related to *when* (rather than *whether*) they should be used.

Community Hospital Results

Most operations in the United States are performed at community hospitals; Table 136–5 contains a summary of results for carotid reconstruction since 1984 in this generally unreported sector. Although the safety of carotid endarterectomy in several of these series was comparable with

TABLE 136–5. RESULTS OF CAROTID ENDARTERECTOMY REPORTED FROM COMMUNITY HOSPITALS SINCE 1984

SERIES	YEAR	NO.	ANESTHESIA AND CEREBRAL MONITORING	CAROTID SHUNT	NEUROLOGIC COMPLICATIONS			
					TIA (%)	Stroke (%)	Total (%)	Mortality (%)
Brott and Thalinger[29]	1984	431	Mixed	NA	4.8	7.9	12.7	2.8
Moore et al[129]	1984	510	General, back-pressure or EEG (33%)	75%	2.0	5.3	7.3	1.6
Slavish et al[178]	1984	743	General	All	3.5	1.8	5.3	2.7
Krupski et al[114]	1985	100	General, back-pressure	54%	1.0	3.0	4.0	NA
Cafferata and Gainey[30]	1986	390	Mixed	74%	NA	8.5	NA	3.1
Kempczinski et al[110]	1986	750	Mixed	34%	NA	NA	5.1	2.3
Kirshner et al[111]	1989	4035	Mixed	25%	2.3	4.3	6.7	1.4
Gibbs and Guzzetta[79]	1989	566	General	10%	1.6	1.6	3.2	0.5
Mattos et al[125]	1995	2243	NA	NA	NA	5.3	NA	1.6
Lawhorne et al[115]	1997	500	General	All	1.8	0.2	2.0	1.0

EEG = operative electroencephalography; NA = data not available; TIA = transient ischemic attack.

that at referral centers, Easton and Sherman[60] in Springfield, Illinois, and Brott and Thalinger[29] in Cincinnati earlier had reported excessive complication rates from pooled community data that galvanized opposition to surgical treatment at the time of their publication. Each of these two studies included a substantial number of patients with preoperative strokes as the indication for operation, and the data for both were collected retrospectively from many surgeons with undesignated training and limited personal experience in extracranial reconstruction.

Taylor and Porter[187] subsequently reviewed the surgical literature and found that the perioperative stroke rate was twice as high among patients with a history of previous strokes who were reported in community surveys rather than in large individual series. All of these data suggest that, at least in some areas, patients having acute or profound neurologic deficits still are being selected for immediate surgical treatment. Although Piotrowski and associates[146] have suggested that an arbitrary delay of 6 weeks or longer is not always necessary before carotid endarterectomy may be performed safely after a completed stroke, they strongly emphasized that patients must attain a stable neurologic plateau before earlier intervention can be seriously considered.

Additional data from the same two hospitals participating in one of these investigations now are available and indicate that unsatisfactory results may be improved provided that they are discovered in the first place. While studying a related issue, Moore and associates[129] incidentally reported on the 510 consecutive carotid procedures that followed the 228 operations described by Easton and Sherman in 1977. Prior stroke declined as an indication for carotid endarterectomy from 43% in the earlier series to 19% thereafter, and there also were impressive reductions in the operative stroke rate (from 14% to 5.3%) and mortality (from 6.6% to 1.6%).

Mattos and associates[125] subsequently updated the Springfield experience still further with their review of 2243 operations performed from 1976 through 1993. They found significant differences in perioperative stroke rates between surgeons who performed more than and fewer than 12 carotid procedures annually (4.1% versus 7.2%, respectively; $p = .009$), and between surgeons who had and had not acquired additional training in vascular surgery (2.7% versus 6.8%, respectively; $p = .0014$). Previous data from northeastern Ohio also suggested that surgeons who are trained in arterial reconstruction and maintain an active interest in their field can perform carotid endarterectomy with exemplary success.[91, 167] Other community series have failed to demonstrate that specialty training influences the neurologic outcome, usually because their results were either universally good or consistently poor among all participating surgeons.[30, 110, 114, 178] In any event, the information from southern Illinois is important because it illustrates so clearly that the recognition of unfavorable trends is essential to their correction.

Population Survey Results

Table 136–6 contains data from several statewide or Medicare population surveys in which sufficient information has been documented regarding the annual volume of carotid operations for either hospitals or surgeons that a few cautious conclusions appear to be justified. First, depending on the case mix of symptomatic and asymptomatic patients, which is unstated in nearly all of the surveys, the safety of carotid endarterectomy seems to be improving in comparison with its general level of risk in the 1970s and early 1980s. The report of Perler and coworkers[144] concerning the results in Maryland within the past decade is an encouraging example in this respect. Individually and collectively, however, these surveys substantiate an inverse relationship between caseload and complication rates that is especially evident between hospitals and surgeons having the most experience and those having the least.

Finally, although the number of hospitals at which exceedingly few carotid operations are performed may be declining, it must be noted that in the Connecticut database (1985 through 1991), 79% of the participating surgeons in that state had performed fewer than six carotid procedures per year, and 43% of the surgeons annually averaged only one carotid operation or less.

Management

Postoperative neurologic deficits may be caused by atheromatous embolization during the surgical exposure, by clamp ischemia, by delayed platelet emboli or thrombosis, and, rarely by cerebral hemorrhage occurring a few days after the procedure. Thus, the patient who experiences an ischemic event following carotid endarterectomy may have sustained one of the following:

1. An embolic TIA that will resolve without treatment.
2. An embolic stroke for which reoperation is contraindicated.
3. A stroke-in-evolution caused by thrombosis at the endarterectomy site, which may improve dramatically if prompt thrombectomy of the internal carotid artery is performed.

The cause of neurologic complications is not always immediately obvious, but the patency of the carotid bifurcation should be documented with urgent noninvasive testing, objective imaging, or cervical exploration whenever such complications occur.

A number of reports indicate that (1) preoperative cerebral infarction is more common than would be suspected on clinical grounds, (2) infarcts discovered on computed tomography (CT) scans often are associated with ulcerated lesions of the carotid bifurcation, and (3) atheromatous ulcers, in turn, carry a higher risk for postoperative stroke than nonulcerated lesions.[23, 82, 92, 207] Intraoperative neurologic deficits are recognized only after recovery from general anesthesia. Jernigan and coworkers[106] and Rosenthal and colleagues,[165] employing regional anesthesia, found that most of these events appeared to be embolic because they occurred in alert patients either during carotid manipulation or at the time flow was restored after an uneventful period of clamp occlusion. The severity of the postoperative symptoms and the circumstances encountered during the original operation inevitably influence the decision whether a patient who awakens with a neurologic deficit after general anesthesia should undergo immediate reoperation, carotid angiography, or close observation alone. For example,

TABLE 136–6. RESULTS OF CAROTID ENDARTERECTOMY IN POPULATION SURVEYS

SERIES	YEAR	POPULATION	ANNUAL VOLUME	NO.	STROKE (%)	MORTALITY (%)	STROKE OR MORTALITY (%)
Hospitals							
Fisher et al[74]	1986	New England Medicare	>40	457	NA	1.1	2.0
			21–40	561	NA	2.7	4.6
			6–20	913	NA	3.0	4.7
			≤5	158	NA	3.2	5.7
			Total	2089	NA	2.5	4.2
Perler et al[144]	1998	Maryland statewide	≥50	5615	1.8	0.8	NA
			11–49	4089	1.3	1.1	NA
			≤10	214	6.1	1.9	NA
			Total	9918	1.7	0.9	NA
Cebul et al[34]	1998	Ohio Medicare	>62	339	NA	NA	2.4
			≤62	339	NA	NA	7.1
			Total	678	2.9	1.8	4.7
Surgeons							
Richardson and Main[155]	1989	Kentucky Medicare	>12	504	2.3	NA	NA
			3–12	152	7.2	NA	NA
			<3	82	6.1	NA	NA
			Total	738	3.7	3.1	5.7
Edwards et al[64]	1991	Tennessee statewide	≥50	772	2.1	1.2	NA
			13–49	3876	3.7	1.7	NA
			≤12	5067	4.0	2.6	NA
			Total	9715	3.7	2.1	NA
Ruby et al[168]	1996	Connecticut statewide	>10	NA	NA	NA	4.3
			6–10	NA	NA	NA	4.8
			2–5	NA	NA	NA	6.2
			≤1	NA	NA	NA	10
			Total	3997	NA	NA	4.9

NA = data not available.

surgical exploration may be completely appropriate in the presence of a dense postoperative hemiparesis when there is a predictable risk of technical complications after a tedious reconstruction. Conversely, nonoperative assessment of the internal carotid artery may be the most that is necessary for a patient who is found to have a mild early deficit following routine endarterectomy for symptomatic, grossly ulcerated carotid disease.

According to experience at a number of centers, however, the majority of perioperative neurologic complications actually occur after a lucent interval during which functional recovery is satisfactory.[139, 193] Because it is difficult to attribute such delayed events to surgical manipulation or clamping, other contributing factors must also be considered. Carotid thrombosis and cerebral hemorrhage are the most serious of these, and at least in some cases, they may be anticipated in time to avoid irreversible consequences.

Carotid Thrombosis

In a comprehensive review of 3062 consecutive procedures at their center, Riles and associates[157] found that symptomatic carotid thrombosis occurred in only 0.8% of patients but caused 40% of the 66 strokes in their series. Otherwise, the incidence of postoperative internal carotid thrombosis has been reported to range from 2% to 18% in scattered prospective studies employing hemodynamic testing or objective imaging.[6, 93, 136] Although occlusion rates after endar-

terectomy almost certainly differ from one hospital and even one surgeon to the next, several reports have recommended the use of selective or routine operative angiography in an attempt to eliminate technical complications.[26, 44, 130] Alternatively, others have found that Doppler ultrasonography is a convenient method for intraoperative assessment that detects residual internal carotid lesions in 4% to 8% of patients.[19, 59, 75, 177] Using this approach, Zierler and colleagues[205] discovered fresh thrombus or iatrogenic defects actually requiring correction during 5% of their operations.

At the Cleveland Clinic, to discourage platelet aggregation, aspirin therapy (5 grains twice daily) is administered empirically on the preoperative evening and for at least the first month after carotid reconstruction. In addition, an infusion of low-molecular-weight dextran (35 to 50 ml per hour) is begun prior to closure of the arteriotomy and is continued until the following day in selected patients who have atheromatous ulceration extending into a deep endarterectomy plane. Both of these precautions are based on the principle that inhibition of platelets must precede their "first pass" across the endarterectomy surface to be effective.[87] In a total of 366 patients, Edwards and associates[62] calculated that this type of antiplatelet therapy was associated with significant improvement in the incidence of perioperative stroke and carotid thrombosis compared with incidence in a nonrandomized control group.

Because relatively few examples of early carotid thrombo-

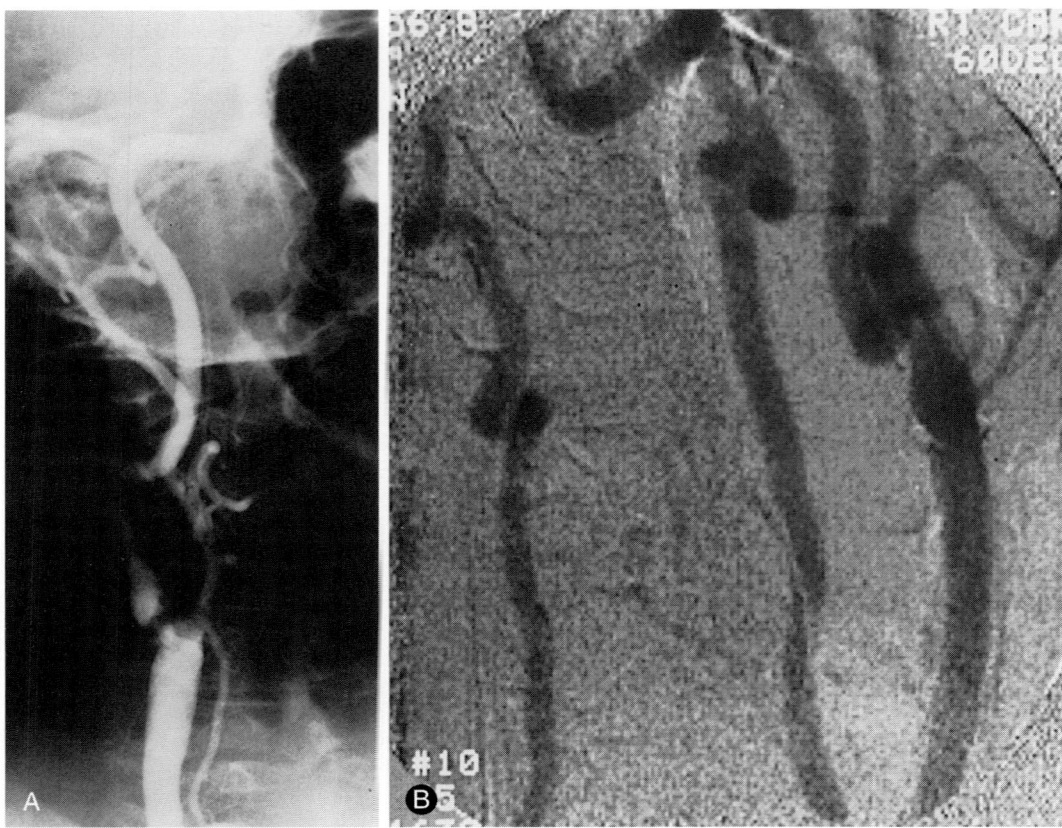

FIGURE 136–3. Preoperative (A) and postoperative (B) angiograms demonstrating an early occlusion of the right carotid system following proximal endarterectomy of a kinked internal carotid artery. An acute neurologic deficit improved after urgent thrombectomy, kink resection, and vein patch angioplasty. (From Painter TA, Hertzer NR, O'Hara PJ, et al: Symptomatic internal carotid thrombosis after carotid endarterectomy. J Vasc Surg 5:445, 1987.)

sis have been reported from any single center it is difficult to determine even from collected data whether patients in whom delayed postoperative deficits develop should undergo either preliminary investigation of internal carotid patency (Fig. 136–3) or immediate surgical exploration. Rosenthal and associates[165] and Perdue[145] have estimated that reoperations are indicated in only 20% of patients who sustain cerebral ischemia related to carotid endarterectomy. Also, there is no convincing evidence that the hour or so that is necessary to perform intravenous or conventional angiography in an adequate hospital setting influences the eventual outcome in patients who do have carotid thrombosis. Nevertheless, it is reasonable to return patients in whom this correctable complication is suspected directly to the operating room, and any decision *not* to perform a reoperation in the presence of a delayed neurologic event should be supported by some objective confirmation that the internal carotid artery has remained patent.

The surgical management of postendarterectomy thrombosis is illustrated in Figure 136–4.[141] Retrograde internal carotid artery bleeding may be restored by removal of platelet thrombus from the bifurcation, but if a balloon embolectomy catheter is used to retrieve propagated clot, it should be introduced cautiously in order not to cause a cavernous sinus fistula.[65, 108] After a shunt has been inserted to reestablish cerebral blood flow, the distal intima may be secured with tacking sutures prior to closure of the arteriotomy with a patch of saphenous vein.

Eleven (0.4%) of the 2651 patients who underwent carotid endarterectomy at the Cleveland Clinic from 1977 to 1984 required early reoperations because of symptomatic thrombosis of the internal carotid artery. Table 136–7 presents the results of urgent surgical treatment in these 11 patients as well as in 30 others already described in the literature.[141] All reoperations were performed within 4 hours after perioperative deficits were discovered, and the interval between the original procedure and the onset of symptoms was available for 36 of the 41 patients. Because only four patients recovered from their initial anesthesia with discrete deficits, some period of normal neurologic function was witnessed after endarterectomy in the remaining 32 (88%). Substantial improvement occurred in 61% of the composite series after thrombectomy, approximately half of whom had complete recovery, whereas neurologic function was unchanged in another 22%. The overall mortality rate was 17%, but a limited delay in intervention did not appear to compromise the outcome.

Peer and associates[142] subsequently reported on 21 patients who underwent reoperations for symptomatic postendarterectomy thrombosis, the majority performed within an hour of the onset of the neurologic deficits. Eleven (52%) of these patients improved, eight (38%) were unchanged, and two (10%) died. AbuRhama and colleagues[3] obtained similar results in 12 patients. This accumulated experience suggests that decisive surgical management is the preferred approach to postendarterectomy thrombosis

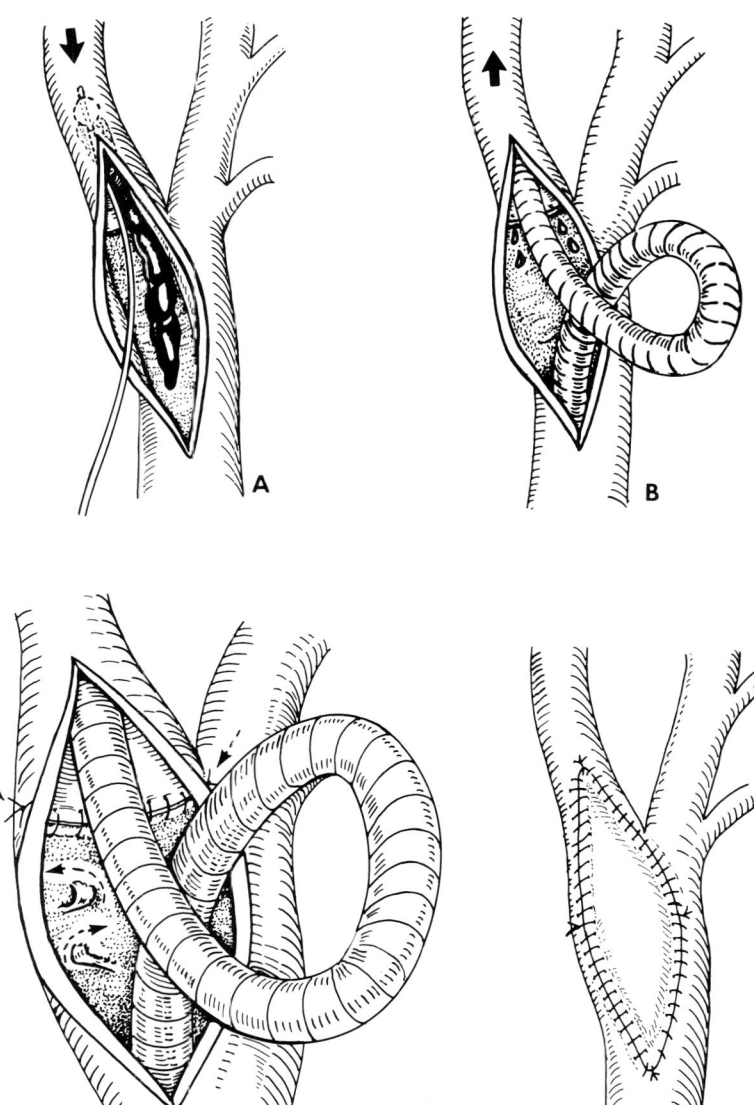

FIGURE 136–4. Technical features of urgent carotid reoperations. *A,* Careful thrombectomy. *B,* Immediate shunting. *C,* Removal of loose debris and suture fixation of the distal intima. *D,* Vein patch angioplasty. (From Painter TA, Hertzer NR, O'Hara PJ, et al: Symptomatic internal carotid thrombosis after carotid endarterectomy. J Vasc Surg 5:445, 1987.)

TABLE 136–7. URGENT THROMBECTOMY IN THE MANAGEMENT OF SYMPTOMATIC INTERNAL CAROTID OCCLUSION AFTER CAROTID ENDARTERECTOMY

| | | POSTOCCLUSION NEUROLOGIC DEFICIT | | | | | |
| | | Improved | | Unchanged | | Mortality | |
ELIGIBLE PATIENTS	NO.	No.	%	No.	%	No.	%
Collected series	41	25	61	9	22	7	17
Documented surgical delay							
<2 hr after symptoms	22	14	63	5	23	3	14
2–4 hr after symptoms	7	5	72	1	14	1	14

From Painter TA, Hertzer NR, O'Hara PJ, et al: Symptomatic internal carotid thrombosis after carotid endarterectomy. J Vasc Surg 5:445, 1987.

and is not associated with a higher mortality rate than might be anticipated with expectant care alone.

According to some preliminary reports, transcranial Doppler ultrasonography (TCD) may provide a means to recognize the accumulation of platelet debris or mural thrombus at the endarterectomy site in time to prevent its progression to either internal carotid artery occlusion or an embolic stroke. TCD has been shown to be a sensitive indicator of cerebral microembolization during surgical manipulation of the carotid artery, the sheer volume of emboli occasionally being associated with deterioration either in the intraoperative EEG waveform or in postoperative cognitive function.[78, 105] On the basis of their earlier work with TCD, Lennard and associates[78, 117] performed continuous monitoring for 6 hours after carotid endarterectomy in a prospective series of 100 patients. One or more asymptomatic emboli were detected in 48 of these patients, most of which occurred within the first 2 hours after operation and were presumed to represent platelet aggregates. Five patients had sustained periods of embolization, defined as a threshold of 25 particles detected during 10 minutes of observation, and received intravenous dextran 40 therapy (20 to 40 ml/hour) with prompt reduction of embolic activity. None of the 100 patients in this series had neurologic complications. This careful study demonstrates an interesting application of TCD technology. Perhaps just as importantly, it suggests that the use of low-molecular-weight dextran probably should be an empiric consideration in more patients than currently is the case at most centers, even if continuous TCD monitoring is not available.

In a related report, Barr and colleagues[20] have described selective catheterization of the middle cerebral artery with infusion thrombolysis of an intraoperative embolism. This approach requires the immediate availability of a skilled neuroradiology team, but it could have a specific role for the patient who continues to have a neurologic deficit following surgical thrombectomy of the internal carotid artery (see Fig. 136–4).

Cerebral Hemorrhage

Cerebral hemorrhage is the most lethal neurologic complication that can occur after any type of extracranial reconstruction. This rare, irreversible catastrophe usually occurs several days postoperatively, and because little can then be done to improve its prognosis, selected patients warrant close surveillance and even prophylactic treatment because of their risk of having a fragile intracranial capillary bed.

Caplan and associates[33] implicated hypertension as the principal etiologic feature of hemorrhagic infarction, but others have described additional contributing factors, such as the correction of severe internal carotid stenosis at the time of the original procedure, diffuse cerebrovascular disease with contralateral carotid occlusion, and the administration of anticoagulants.[85, 147] Excruciating unilateral headache may be a harbinger of both focal seizure activity and cerebral hemorrhage in patients who required carotid endarterectomy for high-grade lesions associated with previous strokes.[151, 185, 201, 204]

All of these observations suggest that cerebral edema, and ultimately hemorrhage, may be caused by regional hyperperfusion of a recipient capillary network accustomed to a state of relatively low blood flow. It is difficult to draw absolute conclusions concerning such an unusual syndrome, but patients who exhibit any evidence of cerebral edema clearly should be kept under close observation and probably should receive empirical management in an attempt to prevent subsequent motor seizures or intracranial bleeding. Bed rest, fluid restriction, and maintenance of the blood pressure at a level slightly lower than normal are appropriate precautions, and either formal anticoagulation or antiplatelet therapy seems to be contraindicated. The morbidity of cerebral edema, like that of swelling in a limb after extremity revascularization, undoubtedly declines as the integrity of the capillary bed is restored.[87]

Carotid Patch Angioplasty

Throughout their extensive experience, Imparato and colleagues[104] and Sundt and associates[183] encouraged the use of patch angioplasty to complement carotid endarterectomy. Stewart and coworkers[181] have since found that patch closure was associated with better early patency than primary arterial repair after intimal resection in animal models, and patching has virtually eliminated operative strokes and thrombosis in several other clinical reports.[1, 10, 56, 57, 109]

The merit of patch angioplasty was reconfirmed in a series of 801 consecutive patients who underwent 917 primary carotid endarterectomies at the Cleveland Clinic.[94] Conventional arteriotomy closure was performed during 483 operations in this 3-year study, whereas a patch of saphenous vein (usually harvested from the lower leg) was employed in 434. Otherwise, preoperative risk factors, surgical management, and antiplatelet therapy were equivalent in the patch and nonpatch groups, and the immediate technical result was documented by intravenous digital

TABLE 136–8. COMPLICATIONS RELATED TO VEIN PATCH ANGIOPLASTY DURING CAROTID ENDARTERECTOMY*

| | SURGICAL COHORTS | | | | | |
| RELATED COMPLICATIONS | Routine Closure | | Patch Angioplasty | | Total | |
	No.	%	No.	%	No.	%
Perioperative Period						
Total procedures	483	100	434	100	917	100
Neurologic events	19	3.9	8	1.8	27	2.9
Transient deficits	3	0.6	4	0.9	7	0.8
Completed strokes	15	3.1	3	0.7	18	2.0
Hemorrhagic infarcts	15	3.1	3	0.7	18	2.0
Carotid thrombosis	15	3.1	2	0.5	17	1.9
Symptomatic	9	1.9	0	—	—	1.0
Asymptomatic	6	1.2	2	0.5	8	0.9
Miscellaneous						
Cervical hematoma	7	1.4	7	1.6	14	1.5
Patch disruption	—	—	3	0.7	—	—
Late Interval (Mean, 21 mo)						
Reoperations for recurrent stenosis	7	1.4	3	0.7	10	1.1
Objective imaging	146	31	186	43	332	36
Documented internal carotid defects	21	14	9	4.8	30	9.0
<70% diameter	11	7.5	5	2.7	16	4.8
≥70% diameter	8	5.5	2	1.1	10	3.0
Occlusion	2	1.4	2	1.1	4	1.2

From Hertzer NR, Beven EG, O'Hara PJ, Krewjewski LP: A prospective study of vein patch angioplasty during carotid endarterectomy: Three-year results for 801 patients and 917 operations. Ann Surg 206:628, 1987.

*Perioperative and late results of a prospective study of vein patch angioplasty during carotid endarterectomy at the Cleveland Clinic.

subtraction angiography in a total of 715 patients (89%). As presented in Table 136–8, ischemic strokes or internal carotid thrombosis each occurred in approximately 2% of the entire series. Nevertheless, both the stroke rate (0.7% versus 3.1%; p = .0084, Fisher exact test) and the incidence of postoperative thrombosis (0.5% versus 3.1%; p = .0027) were significantly lower in the patched cohort. This favorable experience with vein patches has extended throughout the 1990s at the Cleveland Clinic, a study period in which vein patching was associated with an overall perioperative stroke rate of only 1.3% in 1437 operations (0.8% in 857 patients with asymptomatic carotid stenosis).[97] These results were statistically superior (p = .015) to the stroke risk (3.3%) for another 387 procedures employing either synthetic patching or primary arteriotomy closure.

Although it conserves the greater saphenous system for future coronary bypass or extremity revascularization, a distal vein patch may occasionally lack the tensile strength of a segment excised from the groin (Fig. 136–5). Urgent replacement was necessary for three (0.6%) of the initial 434 vein patches at the Cleveland Clinic (see Table 134–8), and a total of eight central patch ruptures (0.5%) have occurred in the overall series of 1691 patients who received vein patch angioplasty during carotid endarterectomy at this center from 1983 to 1990.[135] All of these complications occurred within 5 days of the primary procedure (including 4 during the first 24 hours) and involved ankle vein segments, a feature that also has been noted by other investigators.[27, 107, 159, 203] Archie and Green[13] subsequently confirmed in vitro that the hoop strength of small veins is substantially less than that of large veins, irrespective of the level at which they are harvested, and that the experimental bursting pressure for vein patches of similar size appears to be less in women than in men. These composite data strongly suggest that, at least in women, autogenous carotid patches should be constructed with the use of the greater saphenous vein in the upper thigh in order to avoid the low but serious risk of early postoperative rupture. With the use of this approach, no patch ruptures have occurred at the Cleveland Clinic since 1988.

Recurrent Carotid Stenosis

Although its true incidence and clinical implications still are controversial, recurrent stenosis can occur at any interval following carotid endarterectomy (Fig. 136–6). Early complications (intimal flaps or perioperative occlusions) may eventually be misinterpreted as representing recurrent disease unless immediate surgical results are assessed with objective testing, but most recurrent lesions undoubtedly are caused by either of two etiologic factors:

- Myointimal hyperplasia, a collagenous proliferation of the medial layer of the arterial wall that appears to be more prevalent in women and usually is discovered within the first 3 postoperative years
- Secondary atherosclerosis, occurring later in the follow-up period and more closely associated with smoking and hyperlipidemia[39, 42, 52, 55, 99, 133, 149, 152, 182]

As indicated in Figure 136–7, the essential features of recurrent stenosis in a series of 65 late carotid reoperations at the Cleveland Clinic[52] were consistent with those originally described by Stoney and String[182] several years earlier. Hyperplastic recurrences generally were asymptomatic and were suspected on the basis of routine noninvasive studies, whereas atherosclerotic lesions commonly were demonstrated by angiography after the onset of neurologic events.

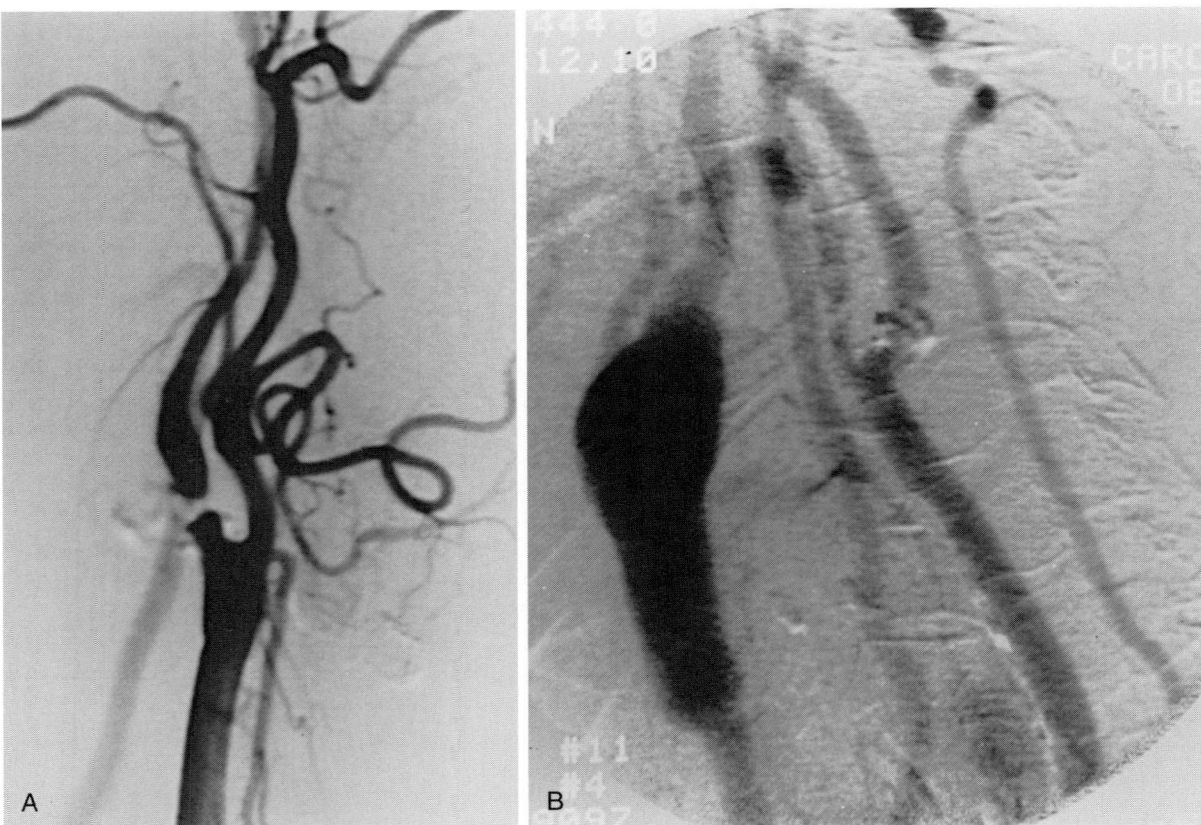

FIGURE 136–5. Preoperative *(A)* and postoperative *(E)* angiograms in a patient who sustained an acute false aneurysm 1 week after carotid endarterectomy and patch angioplasty using a segment cf saphenous vein harvested from the ankle. The patch appears dilated on the postoperative study and ruptured centrally the next day.

The mean recurrence interval for myointimal hyperplasia in this series was 21 months, compared with 57 months for atherosclerosis (*p* = .0007).

Because of the uncertain natural history of asymptomatic carotid stenosis, the possibility of recurrence has been cited as a relative contraindication to its surgical treatment.[40, 206] As a practical matter, however, the data necessary to establish this conclusion are highly contradictory (Table 136–9). The crude incidence of serious recurrent disease has been estimated to be only 1% to 4% among large, retrospective series in which follow-up angiography traditionally was restricted to patients who were found to have new neurologic symptoms or cervical bruits. Since the introduction of noninvasive cerebrovascular testing, a number of reports have suggested that recurrent lesions instead occur in as many as 9% to 15% of operated arteries and that the merit of carotid endarterectomy should be reconsidered on this basis. It should be noted from the information provided in Table 136–9, however, that all reoperation rates were less than 4%, irrespective of whether objective studies were employed, and that the vast majority of patients with evidence of recurrent stenosis on noninvasive examinations have remained asymptomatic. The unexpected results of objective tests clearly cannot be disregarded, but Healy and Zierler and colleagues[86, 206] have described regression of early recurrent lesions in about one third of the patients in whom they occur, an observation implying that at least some of the changes detected by Doppler ultrasonography may represent a normal sequence of arterial remodeling that simply was never documented before scanning was available.

Therefore, it seems likely that the actual incidence of recurrent stenosis probably strikes a balance between the figures generated from large series with incomplete follow-up and figures provided by prospective noninvasive testing without angiographic confirmation. Moreover, several considerations may influence the perceived recurrence rate even within a single study. As an example, late clinical information was obtained during a mean postoperative interval of 22 months for a total of 232 patients who underwent carotid endarterectomy (270 arteries) at the Cleveland Clinic in 1980 to 1981, and a subset of this group (113 patients, 129 arteries) subsequently was reassessed by intravenous digital angiography.[37] Five-year survival and the incidence of stroke, reoperation, and recurrence of at least 30% stenosis were calculated using both crude and cumulative methods. There were few late strokes as calculated by either approach, but the recurrence rate could arbitrarily be expressed throughout a wide range of 3% (reoperations in the entire series) to 34% (measurable defects on objective imaging). There were no strokes related to any of the recognized recurrences even though remedial procedures were performed only for lesions associated with severe (70% to 99%) stenosis.

In the final analysis, the clinical significance of mild to moderate recurrent stenosis identified by noninvasive test-

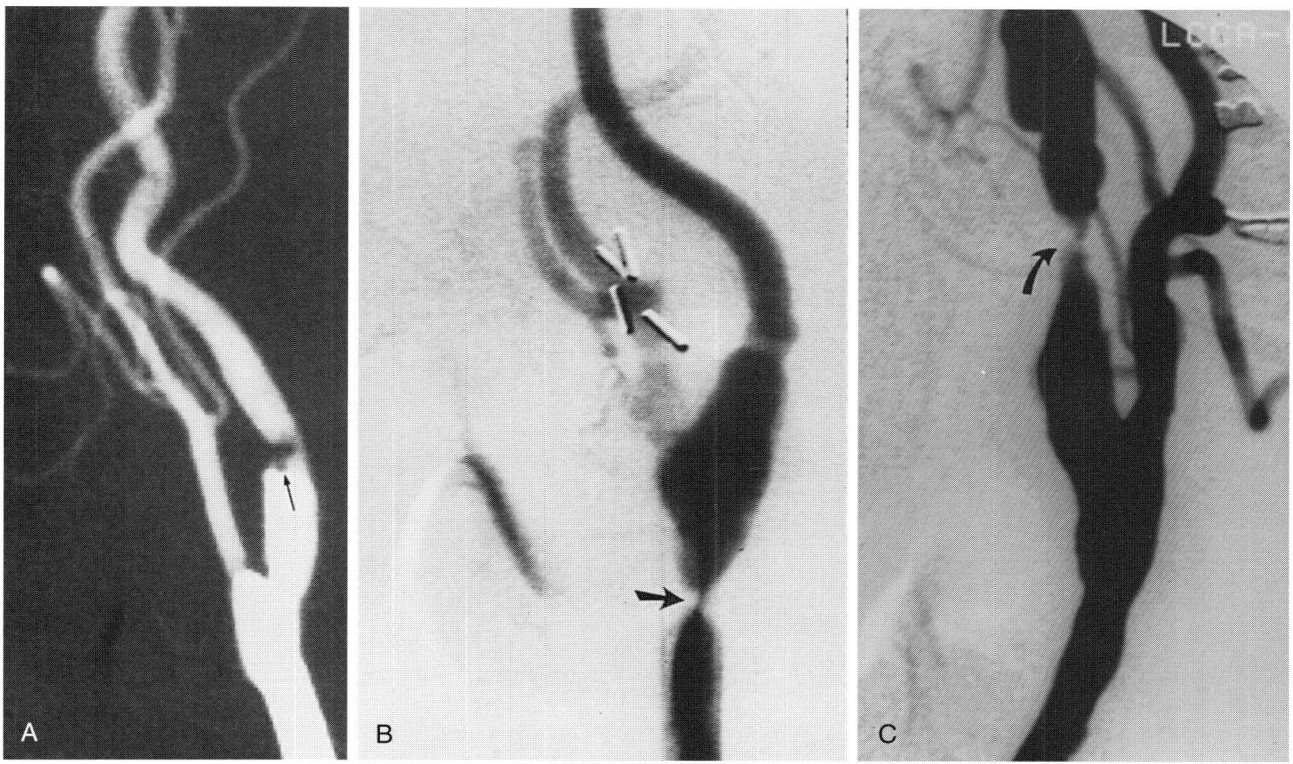

FIGURE 136–6. Similar angiographic features of different sources of recurrent carotid stenosis. *A,* An intimal flap *(arrow)* 1 month after the original endarterectomy. *B,* Hyperplastic lesion *(arrow)* discovered at 8 months. *C,* New atherosclerosis *(arrow)* in the 8th postoperative year.

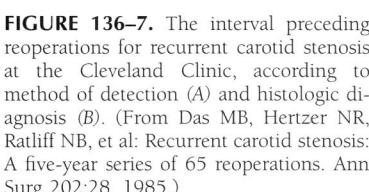

FIGURE 136–7. The interval preceding reoperations for recurrent carotid stenosis at the Cleveland Clinic, according to method of detection *(A)* and histologic diagnosis *(B)*. (From Das MB, Hertzer NR, Ratliff NB, et al: Recurrent carotid stenosis: A five-year series of 65 reoperations. Ann Surg 202:28, 1985.)

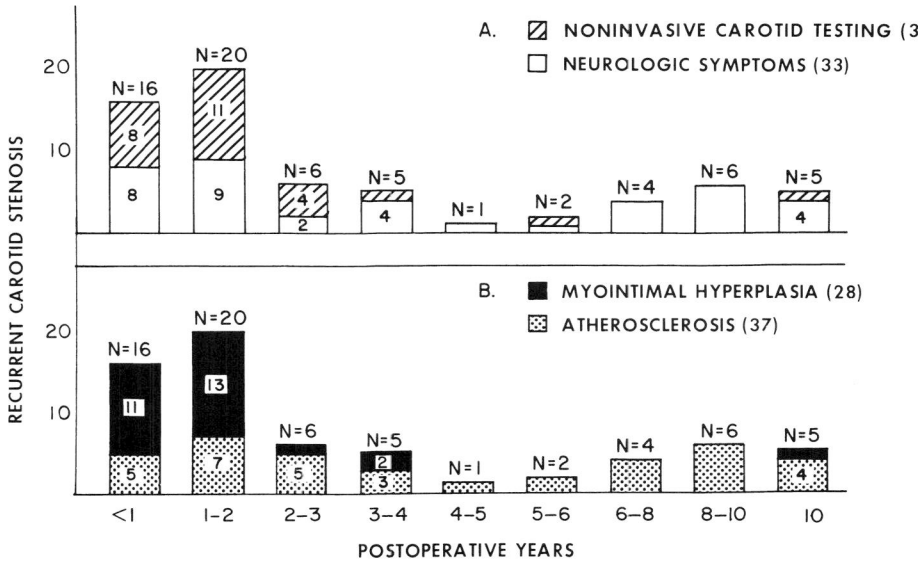

TABLE 136–9. RECURRENT CAROTID STENOSIS*

SERIES	YEAR	ORIGINAL OPERATIONS	MAXIMUM FOLLOW-UP (yr)	RECURRENT CAROTID STENOSIS		
				Incidence (%)	Asymptomatic (%)	Reoperation (%)
Clinical Assessment						
Stoney and String[182]	1976	1654	13	1.5	0.1	1.5
Cossman et al[42]	1978	361	2	3.6	—	3.6
Cleveland Clinic[52, 99]	1979, 1985	1250	13	1.2	0.2	1.2
Piepgras et al[145]	1986	1992	12	1.7	NA	1.7
Noninvasive Testing						
Kremen et al[112]	1979	173	12	9.8	8.1	2.3
Turnipseed et al[197]	1980	80	3	8.8	8.8	NA
Cantelmo et al[32]	1981	199	8	12.1	7.5	2.0
Zierler et al[206]	1982	89	4	14.6	5.6	NA
Baker et al[17]	1983	133	4	9.7	8.3	2.6
Colgan et al[40]	1984	80	4	12.5	11.2	NA
Thomas et al[189]	1984	257	5	14.8	13.2	2.3
O'Donnell et al[133]	1985	276	15	12.3	9.8	1.4
Healy et al[86]	1989	301	7	19.3	15.6	1.3
Mattos et al[124]	1993	409	14	10.8	8.1	1.7
Golledge et al[81]	1997	305	8	11.8	10.5	NA

*Representative data concerning recurrent carotid stenosis detected by clinical assessment or prospective objective testing.
NA = data not available.

ing currently is unknown. After finding that recurrent stenosis did not substantially influence the incidence of new neurologic symptoms in their experience, several reliable investigators have questioned the merit of long-term postoperative surveillance using duplex scanning.[41, 81, 86, 124] This is an important issue that is especially relevant in an era of cost containment in health care. Nevertheless, whereas both Bicotta and associates[153, 154] and O'Donnell and colleagues[134, 200] first proposed nonoperative management for recurrent carotid stenosis, they eventually found it necessary to expand their indications for reoperation when their own follow-up data indicated that these lesions were associated with higher risks for unheralded stroke or internal carotid occlusion than had been anticipated during shorter periods of observation.

Management

Unless there are compelling reasons otherwise, the management of recurrent stenosis probably should be determined by the same judicious principles that are applicable to primary carotid disease. Hyperplastic stenosis tends to be asymptomatic, possibly because its smooth, firm surface discourages cerebral embolization.[133] Accordingly, early recurrences of intermediate severity should be treated with empirical antiplatelet therapy while their progress is monitored with serial objective studies. Although some investigators might disagree, elective reoperation seems to be appropriate if high-grade stenosis occurs, especially if the contralateral internal carotid artery is occluded. Because late atherosclerotic lesions often are symptomatic by the time they are discovered, a conventional approach to their diagnosis and surgical correction appears to be completely justified. Although the risk for at least temporary cranial nerve dysfunction is slightly higher (~10%) following carotid reoperations, the incidence of major neurologic complications is 4% or less at centers with large experience.[52, 97, 145]

From a technical standpoint, reoperations are performed with the use of a vertical incision parallel to the anterior border of the sternocleidomastoid muscle, and sharp dissection is maintained within the plane of avascular scar tissue that leads directly to the bifurcation. The proximal common carotid may be isolated easily once the old arteriotomy has been identified as a landmark, but care must be taken not to injure the vagus nerve in this area. The surgeon usually begins dissection of the internal carotid artery along its lateral aspect in order to reflect the hypoglossal nerve medially. Tethering structures (the sternocleidomastoid artery and vein, digastric muscle, and occipital artery) may be divided to facilitate access to the distal artery. Patch angioplasty should always be performed in conjunction with reoperations, and if formal endarterectomy of hyperplastic stenosis proves to be difficult, the application of a vein patch alone may be the best option. Interposition grafts are rarely necessary, but they represent yet another alternative, especially in the setting of multiple recurrences.[163] Because of the extended period of clamp ischemia during most reoperations, temporary shunting warrants serious consideration.

Carotid Patch Angioplasty

Further recurrent stenosis very rarely occurs following reoperations performed with patch angioplasty, an observation that indirectly supports the opinion, long expressed by Sundt and colleagues[145, 183] and Imparato and associates,[104] that primary patching should routinely be performed in order to prevent this complication. Furthermore, other investigators have encountered no serious recurrences with the use of either venous or autogenous patches in small series of patients studied with objective imaging during a maximal follow-up interval of approximately 3 years.[10, 56, 109]

As indicated in Table 136–8, recurrent lesions (≥ 30% diameter) have been discovered on intravenous angiography or duplex scanning in only 4.8% of patients receiving vein patch angioplasty at the Cleveland Clinic, compared with 14% of those who underwent standard arteriotomy closure (p = .0137). Cumulative data for all 332 arteries evaluated with objective imaging in this investigation are illustrated in Figure 136–8.[94] Actuarial 3-year recurrence rates were 9% and 31% (p = .0066) for the patch and nonpatch groups, respectively, and this distinction (3.7% versus 39%, respectively) was especially significant (p = .0019) for patients in whom the original surgical indication was asymptomatic carotid stenosis.[49, 116] Although few reoperations have been necessary in either cohort, these results suggest that patching may enhance the long-term outcome of carotid endarterectomy.

Several prospective studies employing duplex scanning also have implied that recurrent carotid stenosis is approximately twice as common in women as in men, and both Eikelboom and colleagues[66] and Ten Holter and associates[188] have recommended the use of vein patch angioplasty as a means to reduce the incidence of this complication in patients of either sex (Table 136–10). There currently is no consensus concerning the perceived benefit of patch

angioplasty, however, because other published reports have failed to confirm that patching is associated with a reduction in the risks for either early postoperative thrombosis or late recurrent stenosis.[38, 47, 126] Clagett and associates,[38] conducting a prospectively randomized investigation, concluded that recurrent disease during a 4-year follow-up period actually was more common (13%) after the use of patches than following primary closure (1.7%). Nevertheless, it should be noted that just one woman was included in this series of 136 patients, and the randomization process was initiated only after the intraoperative exclusion of 30 patients who required "obligatory" vein patching because of the small size of their internal carotid arteries or subadventitial penetration of their atherosclerotic plaques. Rosenthal and colleagues[164] calculated no significant differences in the 5-year cumulative incidence of severe restenosis among patients who received vein patch angioplasty, synthetic patches, or primary closure (3.5%, 10% to 14%, or 9.6%, respectively), but vein patching was associated with the same low recurrence rate in this study that previously had encouraged others to advocate its routine use. Counsell and associates[43] performed a meta-analysis of six small prospective trials comparing patch angioplasty with primary arteriotomy repair, and concluded that patch angioplasty appears to be associated with significant reductions in the incidence of recurrent carotid stenosis, perioperative stroke or internal carotid thrombosis, and late stroke; nevertheless, they cautioned that a large definitive trial would be necessary to resolve this lingering controversy.

Both Archie[11] and Lord and associates[121] have noted that an element of dilatation predictably occurs in saphenous vein patches. Because this feature could eventually foster the accumulation of laminated thrombus within the carotid bifurcation, the surgeon must anticipate this occurrence by tailoring the width of the patch to no more than 5 mm at the time it is applied. On balance, although some of the data concerning carotid patching are contradictory, this method seems to deserve wider consideration than it traditionally has been accorded.

Cardiac Mortality

Largely because of a concomitant reduction in the incidence of profound perioperative stroke, the early mortality of carotid reconstruction has steadily declined since 1969, when Bauer and colleagues[21] reported an operative risk of 8.4% for the Joint Study of Extracranial Arterial Occlusion. The results summarized in Table 136–3 indicate that fatal complications at present should occur in less than 2% of patients; unless the stroke rate is high, most of these postoperative deaths are caused by incidental CAD. Riles and coworkers[158] found in the 1970s that 5% of all patients in whom CAD was suspected sustained perioperative myocardial infarctions despite the use of local or regional anesthesia, and other investigators historically have shown that surgical mortality may be correlated with predictable cardiac risk factors.[54, 68] In a series of 1546 carotid operations in 1238 patients, Ennix and associates[68] reported that the early mortality rate was 1.5% for patients who had no indications of ischemic heart disease, 3% for those with angina pectoris who also received simultaneous myocardial

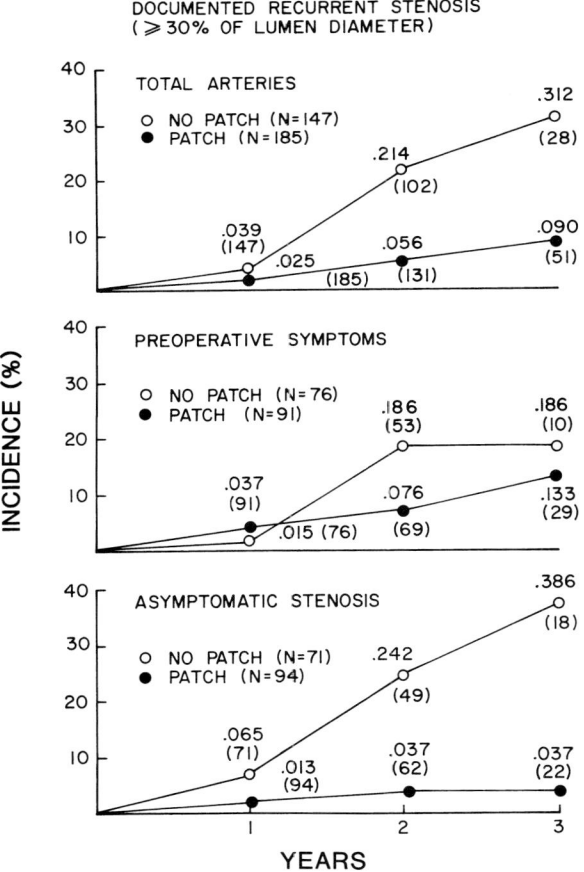

FIGURE 136–8. Cumulative incidence of recurrent carotid defects (30% diameter) documented by noninvasive imaging in a prospective study of vein patch angioplasty at the Cleveland Clinic. *A*, All arteries eligible for objective assessment. *B*, Original operations for symptomatic disease. *C*, Original operations for asymptomatic stenosis. (From Hertzer NR, Beven EG, O'Hara PJ, Krajewski LP: A prospective study of vein patch angioplasty during carotid endarterectomy: Three-year results for 801 patients and 917 operations. Ann Surg 206:628, 1987.)

TABLE 136–10. RECURRENT STENOSIS: SELECTED COMPARISONS*

SERIES	YEAR	LENGTH OF FOLLOW-UP	DATA ANALYSIS	MEN		WOMEN		TOTAL	
				No.	Recurrent Stenosis	No.	Recurrent Stenosis	No.	Recurrent Stenosis
Nonrandomized									
Thomas et al[189]	1984	20 mo (mean)	Crude	161	14 (9%)	96	24 (25%)	257	38 (15%)
Ouriel and Green[137]	1987	17 mo (mean)	Crude	61	5 (8%)	41	12 (29%)	102	17 (17%)
Sanders et al[170]	1987	24 mo	Crude	72	3 (4%)	27	4 (15%)	99	7 (7%)
Bernstein et al[25]	1990	42 mo (mean)	Crude	311	25 (8%)	173	24 (14%)	484	49 (10%)
Atnip et al[14]	1990	35 mo (mean)	Crude	128	10 (8%)	56	1 (2%)	184	11 (6%)
TOTAL				733	57 (8%)	393	65 (17%)	1126	122 (11%)
Randomized									
Eikelboom et al[66]	1988	12 mo; primary closure Patch angioplasty	Crude	37 43	4 (11%) 2 (5%)	11 14	6 (55%) 0	48 57	15 (31%) 2 (4%)
Ten Holter et al[188]	1990	36 mo; primary closure Patch angioplasty	Cumulative	124 118	17% 8%	45 47	27% 7%	169 165	NA NA

*Representative data concerning the incidence of recurrent stenosis following carotid endarterectomy.
NA = data not available.

revascularization, and a surprising 18% for those with angina pectoris who underwent carotid endarterectomy alone.

Although operative mortality may be limited by conservative patient selection and appropriate anesthetic precautions, neither of these measures appears to influence the impact of associated CAD on the long-term survival of patients with cerebrovascular disease. Fatal neurologic events are uncommon irrespective of whether medical or surgical treatment is advised, and several clinical studies have demonstrated that cardiac disease is the leading cause of late death after carotid reconstruction, especially in patients with completed strokes.[24, 58, 191] Most patients who require carotid endarterectomy eventually die because of myocardial infarctions, and the overall 5-year postoperative

survival rate has remained constant at approximately 70% for nearly two decades.[54, 90]

Crawford and colleagues[46] first demonstrated that the risk of peripheral vascular and other major procedures performed after previous coronary bypass was no higher than would be expected in patients who had no evidence of CAD. The mortality rate of subsequent operations was only 1.1% in this retrospective series of 358 patients, and less than 5% experienced fatal myocardial infarctions within the next 5 years. Figure 136–9 illustrates similar data for a total of 329 patients during a minimal follow-up period of 10 years after successful carotid endarterectomy at the Cleveland Clinic.[90] Ten-year survival (55%) in patients who incidentally underwent coronary bypass was equivalent to survival (48%) for patients who had no pre-

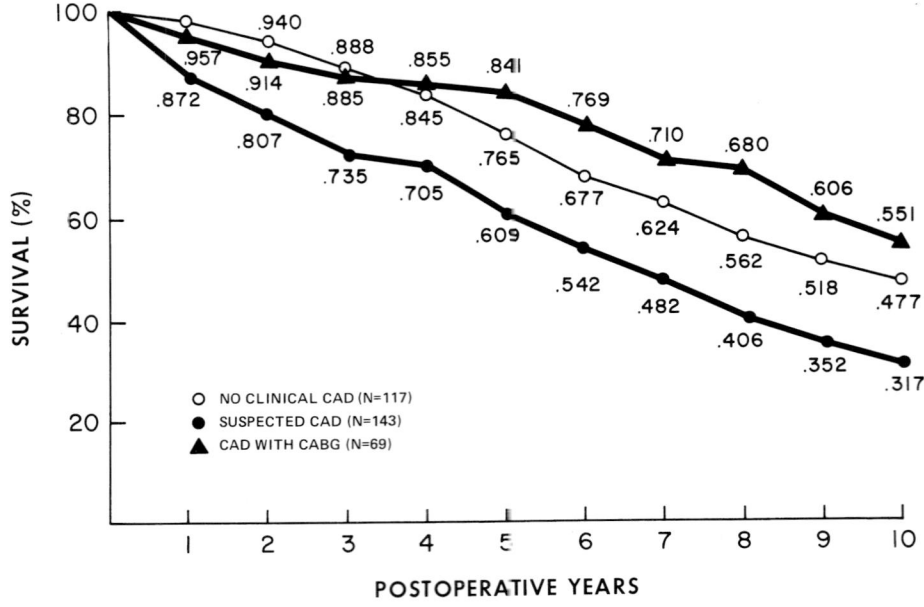

FIGURE 136–9. Cumulative 10-year survival after carotid endarterectomy at the Cleveland Clinic (1969–1973), according to conventional indications for associated coronary artery disease (CAD) and incidental coronary artery bypass grafting (CABG). (From Hertzer NR, Arison R: Cumulative stroke and survival ten years after carotid endarterectomy. J Vasc Surg 2:661, 1985.)

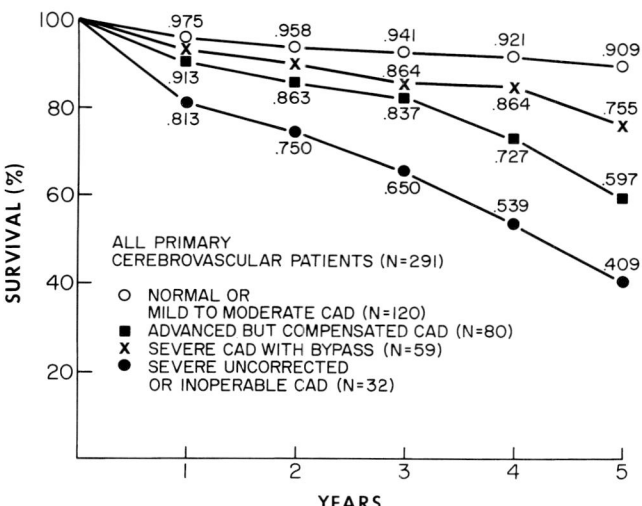

FIGURE 136–10. Cumulative 5-year survival in a prospective series of patients who presented to the Cleveland Clinic with primary extracranial lesions but also underwent survey coronary angiography and selective myocardial revascularization. CAD-coronary artery disease. (Data from Hertzer NR et al: Ann Surg 199:223, 1984; and Hertzer NR et al: Arch Intern Med 145:849, 1979. Copyright 1985, American Medical Association.)

operative indications of CAD and was superior to survival (32%) among patients in whom CAD was suspected on clinical grounds (p = .0001). The 5-year cumulative cardiac mortality in these three subsets was 7%, 8%, and 20% (p = .009), respectively. Furthermore, the 5-year survival rate (84%) for the 69 patients making up the coronary bypass subset in this study was virtually identical to that (83%) for 331 others who received combined carotid and coronary operations at this center during the following 8 years.[98]

Management

Obviously, the recognition of serious coronary disease is a prerequisite to its treatment. In 1984, Rokey and associates[161] reported nonspecific evidence of associated CAD in 29 (58%) of 50 patients with prior TIAs or strokes who underwent thallium myocardial imaging and exercise angiocardiography. That same year, the results of coronary angiography in a series of 1000 candidates for elective vascular

reconstruction were reported from the Cleveland Clinic.[95] The angiographic findings for 295 patients who were investigated primarily because of extracranial disease are presented in Table 136–11. According to a classification defined in earlier reports, 26% of those under consideration for carotid endarterectomy also were found to warrant myocardial revascularization.[95, 100] Severe, correctable CAD was identified in 33% of patients who had clinical indications of coronary involvement, but it also was present in 17% of those who did not. Of the 77 patients with CAD of this severity, 62 actually underwent coronary bypass surgery. Three (4.8%) had fatal complications after staged vascular procedures; actuarial survival (including the risk of coronary bypass itself) for the remaining 59 is illustrated in Figure 136–10. The 5-year survival rate in the bypass subset (75%) was surpassed only by that in patients having normal coronary arteries or mild to moderate CAD (91%) and was superior to the cumulative calculation for 32 others (41%) who had severe, uncorrected or inoperable coronary lesions (p = .0015).

Several technologic advances have influenced the investigation and treatment of incidental CAD in patients presenting with peripheral vascular disease since the Cleveland Clinic study was published in 1984. Coronary angiography largely has been supplanted as a primary diagnostic approach by pharmacologic stress testing and noninvasive myocardial imaging. The indications for coronary bypass surgery have been refined and, in many patients, replaced by modern medical management or catheter-based coronary intervention.

Finally, contemporary cost constraints discourage the use of cardiac screening studies in other than specific, high-risk patient populations. For all of these reasons, a joint task force of the American College of Cardiology and the American Heart Association has attempted to develop practical guidelines for the perioperative cardiovascular evaluation in candidates for noncardiac surgery.[6] An algorithm describing patients under consideration for elective vascular surgery is illustrated in Figure 136–11.

In summary, patients with surgical carotid lesions and no clinical predictors of cardiac risk can proceed directly to carotid endarterectomy without further investigation, whereas those who have unstable coronary syndromes should receive the same consideration for coronary angiography as any other patient with unstable heart disease.

TABLE 136–11. RESULTS OF CORONARY ANGIOGRAPHY*

| ANGIOGRAPHIC CLASSIFICATION | CLINICAL INDICATIONS OF CAD | | | | | |
| | None | | Suspected | | Total | |
	No.	%	No.	%	No.	%
Normal coronary arteries	19	15	8	5	27	9
Mild to moderate CAD	63	50	31	18	94	32
Advanced but compensated CAD	21	17	59	35	80	27
Severe, correctable CAD	22	17	55	33	77	26
Severe, inoperable CAD	1	1	16	9	17	6

From Hertzer NR, Beven EG, Young JR, et al: Coronary artery disease in peripheral vascular patients: A classification of 1000 coronary angiograms and results of surgical management. Ann Surg 199:223, 1984.

*Results of coronary angiography in a prospective series of 295 patients presenting with extracranial cerebrovascular disease at the Cleveland Clinic.

CAD = coronary artery disease.

Elective Vascular Patient

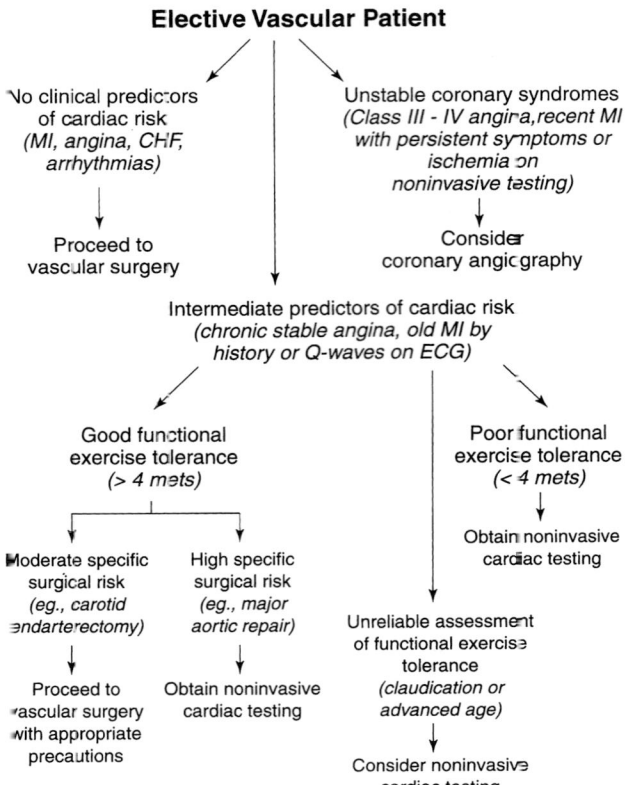

FIGURE 136–11. Algorithm describing the diagnostic approach to associated coronary artery disease (CAD) that has been suggested by a task force representing the American College of Cardiology and the American Heart Association for patients who required elective vascular surgery. MI = myocardial infarction; CHF = congestive heart failure; ECG = electrocardiogram. (Modified from American College of Cardiology/American Heart Association Task Force: Guidelines for perioperative cardiovascular evaluation for noncardiac surgery. J Am Coll Cardiol 27:910, 1996.)

Candidates for carotid surgery who have chronic stable angina or a remote history of myocardial infarction are selected for additional cardiac testing on the basis of their functional exercise tolerance; patients whose activities are unrestricted may safely undergo their carotid operations, whereas those who are seriously limited by other factors (including claudication) that could mask the true severity of their underlying CAD probably should undergo noninvasive cardiac screening preoperatively. These precautions generally are consistent with the thoughtful recommendations made by Nicolaides and associates[131] and are based on the accepted principle that stroke-free *survival* is the measure by which the benefit of carotid endarterectomy is determined.

REFERENCES

1. AbuRahma AF, Khan JH, Robinson PA, et al: Prospective randomized trial of carotid endarterectomy with primary closure and patch angioplasty with saphenous vein, jugular vein, and polytetrafluoroethylene: Perioperative (30-day) results. J Vasc Surg 24:998, 1996.
2. AbuRahma AF, Lim RY: Management of vagus nerve injury after carotid endarterectomy. Surgery 119:245, 1996.
3. AbuRahma AF, Robinson PA, Short YS: Management options for post carotid endarterectomy stroke. J Cardiovasc Surg 37:331, 1996.
4. Ahn SS, Marcus DR, Moore WS: Postcarotid endarterectomy hypertension: Association with elevated cranial norepinephrine. J Vasc Surg 9:351, 1989.
5. Alimi Y, Kallee K, Poncet M, et al: Silent brain infarct after carotid artery surgery: Incidence and prevention. Ann Vasc Surg 9:S76, 1995.
6. van Alphen HAM, Polman CH: Carotid endarterectomy: How does it work? A clinical and angiographic evaluation. Stroke 17:1251, 1986.
7. American College of Cardiology/American Heart Association Task Force: Guidelines for perioperative cardiovascular evaluation for noncardiac surgery. J Am Coll Cardiol 27:910, 1996.
8. Ammar AD: Cost-efficient carotid surgery: A comprehensive evaluation. J Vasc Surg 24:1050, 1996.
9. Angell-James JE, Lumley JSP: The effects of carotid endarterectomy on the mechanical properties of the carotid sinus and carotid sinus nerve activity in atherosclerotic patients. Br J Surg 61:805, 1974.
10. Archie JP Jr: Prevention of early restenosis and thrombosis-occlusion after carotid endarterectomy by saphenous vein patch angioplasty. Stroke 17:901, 1986.
11. Archie JP Jr: Early and late geometric changes after carotid endarterectomy patch reconstruction. J Vasc Surg 14:258, 1991.
12. Archie JP: Carotid endarterectomy saphenous vein patch rupture revisited: Selective use on the basis of vein diameter. J Vasc Surg 24:346, 1996.
13. Archie JP Jr, Green JJ Jr: Saphenous vein rupture pressure, rupture stress, and carotid endarterectomy vein patch reconstruction. Surgery 107:389, 1990.
14. Atnip RG, Wengrovitz M, Gifford RM, et al: A rational approach to recurrent carotid stenosis. J Vasc Surg 11:511, 1990.
15. Back MR, Harward TRS, Huber TS, et al: Improving the cost-effectiveness of carotid endarterectomy. J Vasc Surg 26:456, 1997.
16. Bageant TE, Tondini D, Lysons D: Bilateral hypoglossal-nerve palsy following a second carotid endarterectomy. Anesthesiology 43:595, 1975.
17. Baker WH, Hayes AC, Mahler D, et al: Durability of carotid endarterectomy. Surgery 94:112, 1983.
18. Baker WH, Littooy FN, Hayes AC, et al: Carotid endarterectomy without a shunt: The control series. J Vasc Surg 1:50, 1984.
19. Barnes RW, Nix ML, Nichols BT, et al: Recurrent versus residual carotid stenosis: Incidence detected by Doppler ultrasound. Ann Surg 203:652, 1986.
20. Barr JD, Horowitz MB, Mathis JM, et al: Intraoperative urokinase infusion for embolic stroke during carotid endarterectomy. Neurosurgery 36:611, 1995.
21. Bauer RB, Meyer JS, Fields WS, et al: Joint Study of Extracranial Arterial Occlusion: III. Progress report of controlled study of long-term survival in patients with and without operation. JAMA 208:509, 1969.
22. Beebe HG, Clagett GP, DeWeese JA, et al: Assessing risk associated with carotid endarterectomy. Circulation 79:472, 1989.
23. Berguer R, Sieggreen MY, Lazo A, et al: The silent brain infarct in carotid surgery. J Vasc Surg 3:442, 1986.
24. Bernstein EF, Humber RP, Collins GM, et al: Life expectancy and late stroke following carotid endarterectomy. Ann Surg 198:80, 1983.
25. Bernstein EF, Torem S, Dilley RB: Does carotid restenosis predict an increased risk of late symptoms, stroke, or death? Ann Surg 212:629, 1990.
26. Blaisdell FW, Lim R Jr, Hall AD: Technical result of carotid endarterectomy: Arteriographic assessment. Am J Surg 114:239, 1967.
27. Blok JG, Ultee JM, Voorwinde A, et al: Vein patch rupture: Early complication of carotid endarterectomy. Eur J Surg 161:519, 1995.
28. Bove EL, Fry WJ, Gross WS, et al: Hypotension and hypertension as consequences of baroreceptor dysfunction following carotid endarterectomy. Surgery 85:633, 1979.
29. Brott T, Thalinger K: The practice of carotid endarterectomy in a large metropolitan area. Stroke 15:950, 1984.
30. Cafferata HT, Gainey MD: Carotid endarterectomy in the community hospital: A continuing controversy. J Cardiovasc Surg 27:557, 1986.
31. Cafferata HT, Merchant RF, DePalma RG: Avoidance of postcarotid endarterectomy hypertension. Ann Surg 196:465, 1982.
32. Cantelmo NL, Cutler BS, Wheeler HB, et al: Noninvasive detection of carotid stenosis following endarterectomy. Arch Surg 116:1005, 1981.
33. Caplan LR, Skillman J, Ojemann R, et al: Intracerebral hemorrhage following carotid endarterectomy: A hypertensive complication? Stroke 9:457, 1978.

34. Cebul RD, Snow RJ, Pine R, et al: Indications, outcomes and provider volumes for carotid endarterectomy. JAMA 279:1282, 1998.
35. Chambers BR, Norris JW: The case against surgery for asymptomatic carotid stenosis. Stroke 15:964, 1984.
36. Chambers BR, Norris JW: Outcome in patients with asymptomatic neck bruits. N Engl J Med 315:860, 1986.
37. Civil ID, O'Hara PJ, Hertzer NR, et al: Late patency of the carotid artery after endarterectomy: Problems of definition, follow-up methodology and data analysis. J Vasc Surg 8:79, 1988.
38. Clagett GP, Patterson CB, Fisher DF Jr, et al: Vein patch versus primary closure for carotid endarterectomy: A randomized prospective study in a selected group of patients. J Vasc Surg 9:213, 1989.
39. Clagett GP, Rich NM, McDonald PT, et al: Etiologic factors for recurrent carotid artery stenosis. Surgery 93:313, 1982.
40. Colgan MP, Kingston V, Shanik G: Stenosis following carotid endarterectomy. Arch Surg 119:1033, 1984.
41. Cook JM, Thompson BW, Barnes RW: Is routine duplex examination after carotid endarterectomy justified? J Vasc Surg 12:334, 1990.
42. Cossman D, Callow AD, Stein A, et al: Early restenosis after carotid endarterectomy. Arch Surg 113:275, 1978.
43. Counsell CE, Salinas R, Naylor R, et al: A systematic review of the randomised trials of carotid patch angioplasty in carotid endarterectomy. Eur J Vasc Endovasc Surg 13:345, 1997.
44. Courbier MD, Jausseran JM, Reggi M, et al: Routine intraoperative carotid angiography: Its impact on operative morbidity and carotid restenosis. J Vasc Surg 3:343, 1986.
45. Coyne TJ, Wallace C, Benedict C: Peri-operative anticoagulant effects of heparinization for carotid endarterectomy. Aust N Z J Surg 64:679, 1994.
46. Crawford ES, Morris GC Jr, Howell JF, et al: Operative risk in patients with previous coronary artery bypass. Ann Thorac Surg 26:215, 1978.
47. Curley S, Edwards WS, Jacob TP: Recurrent carotid stenosis after autologous tissue patching. J Vasc Surg 6:350, 1987.
48. Curan AJ, Smyth D, Sheehan SJ, et al: Recurrent laryngeal nerve dysfunction following carotid endarterectomy. J R Coll Surg Edinb 42:168, 1997.
49. Cutler SJ, Ederer F: Maximum utilization of the life table method in analyzing survival. J Chronic Dis 8:699, 1958.
50. Darling RC III, Paty PSK, Shah DJM, et al: Eversion endarterectomy of the internal carotid artery: Technique and results in 449 procedures. Surgery 120:635, 1996.
51. Darling RC III, Kubaska S, Shah DM, et al: Bilateral carotid endarterectomy during the same hospital admission. Cardiovasc Surg 4:759, 1996.
52. Das MB, Hertzer NR, Ratliff NB, et al: Recurrent carotid stenosis: A five-year series of 65 reoperations. Ann Surg 202:28, 1985.
53. Davies MJ, Cronin KD: Post-carotid endarterectomy hypertension. Anaesth Intensive Care 8:190, 1980.
54. DeBakey ME, Crawford ES, Cooley DA, et al: Cerebral arterial insufficiency: One- to 11-year results following arterial reconstructive operation. Ann Surg 161:921, 1965.
55. DePalma RG, Chidi CC, Sternfeld WC, et al: Pathogenesis and prevention of trauma-provoked atheromas. Surgery 82:429, 1977.
56. Deriu GP, Ballotta E, Bonavina L, et al: The rationale for patch-graft angioplasty after carotid endarterectomy: Early and long-term follow-up. Stroke 15:972, 1984.
57. Désiron Q, Detry O, Van Damme H, et al: Comparison of results of carotid artery surgery after either direct closure or use of a vein patch. Cardiovasc Surg 5:295, 1997.
58. DeWeese JA, Rob CG, Satran R, et al: Results of carotid endarterectomies for transient ischemic attacks—five years later. Ann Surg 178:258, 1973.
59. Dilley RB, Bernstein EF: A comparison of B-mode real-time imaging and arteriography in the intraoperative assessment of carotid endarterectomy. J Vasc Surg 4:457, 1986.
60. Easton JD, Sherman DG: Stroke and mortality rate in carotid endarterectomy: 228 consecutive operations. Stroke 8:565, 1977.
61. Edwards WH, Edwards WH Jr, Jenkins JM, et al: Analysis of a decade of carotid reconstructive operations. J Cardiovasc Surg 30:424, 1989.
62. Edwards WH, Edwards WH Jr, Mulherin JL Jr, et al: The role of antiplatelet drugs in carotid reconstructive surgery. Ann Surg 201:765, 1984.
63. Edwards WH Jr, Edwards WH St, Mulherin JL Jr, et al: Recurrent

64. carotid artery stenosis: Resection with autogenous vein replacement. Ann Surg 209:662, 1989.
64. Edwards WH, Morris JA Jr, Jenkins JM, et al: Evaluating quality, cost-effective health care. Ann Surg 213:433, 1991.
65. Eggers F, Lukin R, Chambers AA, et al: Iatrogenic carotid cavernous fistula following Fogarty catheter thromboendarterectomy. J Neurosurg 51:543, 1979.
66. Eikelboom BC, Ackerstaff RGA, Hoeneveld H, et al: Benefits of carotid patching: A randomized study. J Vasc Surg 7:240, 1988.
67. Englund R, Dean RH: Blood pressure aberrations associated with carotid endarterectomy. Ann Vasc Surg 1:304, 1986.
68. Ennix CL Jr, Lawrie GM, Morris GC Jr, et al: Improved results of carotid endarterectomy in patients with symptomatic coronary disease: An analysis of 1,546 consecutive carotid operations. Stroke 10:122, 1979.
69. European Carotid Surgery Trialists' Collaborative Group: MRC European Carotid Surgery Trial: Interim results for symptomatic patients with severe (70–99%) or with mild (0–29%) carotid stenosis. Lancet 337:1235, 1991.
70. Evans WE, Mendelowitz DS, Liapis CW, et al: Motor speech deficit following carotid endarterectomy. Ann Surg 196:461, 1982.
71. Executive Committee for the Asymptomatic Carotid Atherosclerosis Study: Endarterectomy for asymptomatic carotid artery stenosis. JAMA 273:1421, 1995.
72. Fearn SJ, Parry AD, Picton AJ, et al: Should heparin be reversed after carotid endarterectomy? A randomised prospective trial. Eur J Vasc Endovasc Surg 13:394, 1997.
73. Fields WS, Maslenikov V, Meyer JS, et al: Joint Study of Extracranial Arterial Occlusion: V. Progress report of prognosis following surgery or nonsurgical treatment of transient cerebral ischemic attacks and cervical carotid artery lesions. JAMA 211:1993, 1970.
74. Fisher ES, Malenka DJ, Solomon NA, et al: Risk of carotid endarterectomy in the elderly. Am J Public Health 79:1617, 1989.
75. Flanigan DP, Douglas DJ, Machi J, et al: Intraoperative ultrasonic imaging of the carotid artery during carotid endarterectomy. Surgery 100:893, 1986.
76. Fode NC, Sundt TM Jr, Robertson JT, et al: Multicenter retrospective review of results and complications of carotid endarterectomy in 1981. Stroke 17:370, 1986.
77. French BN, Rewcastle NB: Sequential morphological changes at the site of carotid endarterectomy. J Neurosurg 41:745, 1974.
78. Gaunt ME, Martin PJ, Smith JL, et al: Clinical relevance of intraoperative embolization detected by transcranial Doppler ultrasonography during carotid endarterectomy: A prospective study of 100 patients. Br J Surg 81:1435, 1994.
79. Gibbs BF, Guzzetta VJ: Carotid endarterectomy in community practice: Surgeon-specific versus institutional results. Ann Vasc Surg 3:307, 1989.
80. Goldstein LB, McCrory DC, Landsman PB, et al: Multicenter review of preoperative risk factors for carotid endarterectomy in patients with ipsilateral symptoms. Stroke 25:1116, 1994.
81. Golledge J, Cuming R, Ellis M, et al: Clinical follow-up rather than duplex surveillance after carotid endarterectomy. J Vasc Surg 25:55, 1997.
82. Graber JN, Vollman RW, Johnson WC, et al: Stroke after carotid endarterectomy: Risk as predicted by preoperative computerized tomography. Am J Surg 147:492, 1984.
83. Graham AM, Gewertz BL, Zarins CK: Predicting cerebral ischemia during carotid endarterectomy. Arch Surg 121:595, 1986.
84. Green RM, Messick WJ, Ricotta JJ, et al: Benefits, shortcomings, and costs of EEG monitoring. Ann Surg 201:785, 1985.
85. Hafner DH, Smith RB, King OW, et al: Massive intracerebral hemorrhage following carotid endarterectomy. Arch Surg 122:305, 1987.
86. Healy DA, Zierler RD, Nicholls SC, et al: Long-term follow-up and clinical outcome of carotid restenosis. J Vasc Surg 10:662, 1989.
87. Hertzer NR: Early complications of carotid endarterectomy. In Moore WS (ed): Cerebrovascular Disease. New York, Churchill Livingstone, 1987.
88. Hertzer NR: Non-stroke complications of carotid endarterectomy. In Bernhard VM, Towne J (eds): Complications in Vascular Surgery, 2nd ed. Orlando, Fla, Grune & Stratton, 1985.
89. Hertzer NR: The staging interval for bilateral carotid endarterectomies. Cardiovasc Surg 4:687, 1996.
90. Hertzer NR, Arison R: Cumulative stroke and survival ten years after carotid endarterectomy. J Vasc Surg 2:661, 1985.

91. Hertzer NR, Avellone JC, Farrell CJ, et al: The risk of vascular surgery in a metropolitan community. J Vasc Surg 1:13, 1984.

92. Hertzer NR, Beven EG, Greenstreet RL, Humphries AW: Internal carotid back pressure, intraoperative shunting, ulcerated atheromata, and the incidence of stroke during carotid endarterectomy. Surgery 83:306, 1978.

93. Hertzer NR, Beven EG, Modic MT, et al: Early patency of the carotid artery after endarterectomy: Digital subtraction angiography after two hundred sixty-two operations. Surgery 92:1049, 1982.

94. Hertzer NR, Beven EG, O'Hara PJ, Krajewski LP: A prospective study of vein patch angioplasty during carotid endarterectomy: Three-year results for 801 patients and 917 operations. Ann Surg 206:628, 1987.

95. Hertzer NR, Beven EG, Young JR, et al: Coronary artery disease in peripheral vascular patients: A classification of 1000 coronary angiograms and results of surgical management. Ann Surg 199:223, 1984.

96. Hertzer NR, Feldman BJ, Beven EG, et al: A prospective study of the incidence of injury to the cranial nerves during carotid endarterectomy. Surg Gynecol Obstet 151:781, 1980.

97. Hertzer NR, O'Hara PJ, Mascha EJ, et al: Early outcome assessment for 2228 consecutive carotid endarterectomy procedures: The Cleveland Clinic experience from 1989 to 1995. J Vasc Surg 26:1, 1997.

98. Hertzer NR, Loop FD, Taylor PC, et al: Combined myocardial revascularization and carotid endarterectomy: Operative and late results in 331 patients. J Thorac Cardiovasc Surg 85:577, 1983.

99. Hertzer NR, Martinez BD, Benjamin SP, et al: Recurrent stenosis after carotid endarterectomy. Surg Gynecol Obstet 149:360, 1979.

100. Hertzer NR, Young JR, Beven EG, et al: Coronary angiography in 506 patients with extracranial cerebrovascular disease. Arch Intern Med 145:849, 1985.

101. Hirko MK, Mkorasch MD, Burke K, et al: The changing face of carotid endarterectomy. J Vasc Surg 23:622, 1996.

102. Hobson RW II, Weiss DG, Fields WS, et al: Efficacy of carotid endarterectomy for asymptomatic carotid stenosis. N Engl J Med 328:221, 1993.

103. Imparato AM, Bracco A, Kim GE, et al: The hypoglossal nerve in carotid arterial reconstructions. Stroke 3:576, 1972.

104. Imparato AM, Ramirez A, Riles T, et al: Cerebral protection in carotid surgery. Arch Surg 117:1073, 1982.

105. Jansen C, Moll FL, Vermeulen FEE, et al: Continuous transcranial Doppler ultrasonography and electroencephalography during carotid endarterectomy: A multimodal monitoring system to detect intraoperative ischemia. Ann Vasc Surg 7:95, 1993.

106. Jernigan WR, Fulton RL, Hamman JL, et al: The efficacy of routine completion operative angiography in reducing the incidence of perioperative stroke associated with carotid endarterectomy. Surgery 96:831, 1984.

107. John TG, Bradbury W, Ruckley CV: Vein-patch rupture after carotid endarterectomy: An avoidable catastrophe. Br J Surg 80:852, 1993.

108. Kakkasseril JS, Tomsick TA, Arbaugh JA, et al: Carotid cavernous fistula following Fogarty catheter thrombectomy. Arch Surg 119:1095, 1984.

109. Katz MM, Jones GT, Degenhardt J, et al: The use of patch angioplasty to alter the incidence of carotid restenosis following thromboendarterectomy. J Cardiovasc Surg 28:2, 1987.

110. Kempczinski RF, Brott TG, Labutta RJ: The influence of surgical specialty and caseload on the results of carotid endarterectomy. J Vasc Surg 3:911, 1986.

111. Kirshner DL, O'Brien MS, Ricotta JJ: Risk factors in a community experience with carotid endarterectomy. J Vasc Surg 10:178, 1989.

112. Kremen JR, Gee W, Kaupp HA, et al: Restenosis or occlusion after carotid endarterectomy: A survey with ocular pneumoplethysmography. Arch Surg 114:608, 1979.

113. Krennmair G, Moser G, Pachinger O, et al: Periphere Hirnnervenlähmungen als folge von operationen an der a. carotis. Wien Klin Wochenschr 10:309, 1995.

114. Krupski WC, Effeney DJ, Goldstone J, et al: Carotid endarterectomy in a metropolitan community: Comparison of results from three institutions. Surgery 98:492, 1985.

115. Lawhorne TW Jr, Brooks HB, Cunningham JM: Five hundred consecutive carotid endarterectomies: Emphasis on vein patch closure. Cardiovasc Surg 5:141, 1997.

116. Lee ET, Desu MM: A computer program for comparing K samples with right-censored data. Comput Programs Biomed 2:315, 1972.

117. Lennard N, Smith J, Dumville J, et al: Prevention of postoperative thrombotic stroke after carotid endarterectomy: The role of transcranial Doppler ultrasound. J Vasc Surg 26:579, 1997.

118. Liapis CD, Satiani B, Florance CL, et al: Motor speech malfunction following carotid endarterectomy. Surgery 89:56, 1981.

119. Lilly MP, Brunner MJ, Wehberg KE: Jugular venous vasopressin increases during carotid endarterectomy after cerebral reperfusion. J Vasc Surg 16:1, 1992.

120. Lipsett PA, Tierney S, Gordon TA, et al: Carotid endarterectomy: Is intensive care unit care necessary? J Vasc Surg 20:403, 1994.

121. Lord RSA, Raj B, Stary DL, et al: Comparison of saphenous vein patch, polytetrafluoroethylene patch, and direct arteriotomy closure after carotid endarterectomy: I. Perioperative results. J Vasc Surg 9:521, 1989.

122. Matchar DB, Oddone EZ, McCrory DC, et al: Influence of projected complication rates on estimated appropriate use rates for carotid endarterectomy. Health Serv Res 32:3, 1997.

123. Matsumoto GH, Cossman D, Callow AD: Hazards and safeguards during carotid endarterectomy: Technical considerations. Am J Surg 133:458, 1977.

124. Mattos MA, van Bemmelen PS, Barkmeier LD, et al: Routine surveillance after carotid endarterectomy: Does it affect clinical management? J Vasc Surg 17:819, 1993.

125. Mattos MA, Modi JR, Mansour A, et al: Evolution of carotid endarterectomy in two community hospitals: Springfield revisited—seventeen years and 2243 operations later. J Vasc Surg 21:719, 1995.

126. Mauney MC, Buchanan SA, Lawrence A, et al: Stroke rate is markedly reduced after carotid endarterectomy by avoidance of protamine. J Vasc Surg 22:264, 1995.

127. Mayberg MR, Wilson SE, Yatsu F, et al: Carotid endarterectomy and prevention of cerebral ischemia in symptomatic carotid stenosis. JAMA 266:3289, 1991.

128. McCrory DC, Goldstein LB, Samsa GP, et al: Predicting complications of carotid endarterectomy. Stroke 24:1285, 1993.

129. Moore DJ, Modi JR, Finch WT, et al: Influence of the contralateral carotid artery on neurologic complications following carotid endarterectomy. J Vasc Surg 1:409, 1984.

130. Moore WS, Martello JY, Quinones-Baldrich WJ, et al: Etiologic importance of the intimal flap of the external carotid artery in the development of postcarotid endarterectomy stroke. Stroke 21:1497, 1990.

131. Nicolaides AN, Salmasi AM, Sonecha TN: How should we investigate the arteriopath for coexisting lesions? J Cardiovasc Surg 27:515, 1986.

132. North American Symptomatic Carotid Endarterectomy Trial (NASCET) Collaborators: Beneficial effect of carotid endarterectomy in symptomatic patients with high-grade carotid stenosis. N Engl J Med 325:445, 1991.

133. O'Donnell TF Jr, Callow AD, Scott G, et al: Ultrasound characteristics of recurrent carotid disease: Hypothesis explaining the low incidence of symptomatic recurrence. J Vasc Surg 2:26, 1985.

134. O'Donnell TF, Rodriguez AA, Fortunato JE, et al: Management of recurrent carotid stenosis: Should asymptomatic lesions be treated surgically? J Vasc Surg 24:207, 1996.

135. O'Hara PJ, Hertzer NR, Krajewski LP, et al: Saphenous vein patch rupture after carotid endarterectomy. J Vasc Surg 15:504, 1992.

136. Ortega G, Gee W, Kaupp HA, et al: Postendarterectomy carotid occlusion. Surgery 90:1093, 1981.

137. Ouriel K, Green RM: Clinical and technical factors influencing recurrent carotid stenosis and occlusion after endarterectomy. J Vasc Surg 5:702, 1987.

138. Ouriel K, May AG, Ricotta JJ, et al: Carotid endarterectomy for nonhemispheric symptoms: Predictors of success. J Vasc Surg 1:339, 1984.

139. Owens ML, Atkinson JB, Wilson SE: Recurrent transient ischemic attacks after carotid endarterectomy. Arch Surg 115:482, 1980.

140. Owens ML, Wilson SE: Prevention of neurologic complications of carotid endarterectomy. Arch Surg 117:551, 1982.

141. Painter TA, Hertzer NR, O'Hara PJ, et al: Symptomatic internal carotid thrombosis after carotid endarterectomy. J Vasc Surg 5:445, 1987.

142. Peer RM, Shah RM, Upson JF, et al: Carotid exploration for acute postoperative thrombosis. Am J Surg 168:168, 1994.

143. Perdue GD: Management of postendarterectomy neurologic deficits. Arch Surg 117:1079, 1982.

144. Perler BA, Dardik A, Burleyson GP, et al: Influence of age and hospital volume on the results of carotid endarterectomy: A statewide analysis of 9918 cases. J Vasc Surg 27:25, 1998.

145. Piepgras DG, Sundt TM Jr, Marsh WR, et al: Recurrent carotid stenosis: Results and complications of 57 operations. Ann Surg 203:205, 1986.

146. Piotrowski JJ, Bernhard VM, Rubin JR, et al: Timing of carotid endarterectomy after acute stroke. J Vasc Surg 11:45, 1990.

147. Pomposelli FB, Lamparello PJ, Riles TS, et al: Intracranial hemorrhage after carotid endarterectomy. J Vasc Surg 7:8, 1988.

148. Ranson JHC, Imparato AM, Clauss RH, et al: Factors in the mortality and morbidity associated with surgical treatment of cerebrovascular insufficiency. Circulation 39(Suppl 1):I269, 1969.

149. Rapp JH, Zvarfordt P, Krupski WC, et al: Hypercholesterolemia and early restenosis after carotid endarterectomy. Surgery 101:277, 1987.

150. Raptis S, Baker SR: Infected false aneurysms of the carotid arteries after carotid endarterectomy. Eur J Vasc Endovasc Surg 11:148, 1996.

151. Reigel MM, Hollier LH, Sundt TM Jr, et al: Cerebral hyperperfusion syndrome: A cause of neurologic dysfunction after carotid endarterectomy. J Vasc Surg 5:628, 1987.

152. Reilly LM, Okuhn SP, Rapp JH, et al: Recurrent carotid stenosis: A consequence of local or systemic factors? The influence of unrepaired technical defects. J Vasc Surg 11:448, 1990.

153. Ricotta JJ, O'Brien-Irr MS: Conservative management of residual and recurrent lesions after carotid endarterectomy: Long-term results. J Vasc Surg 26:963, 1997.

154. Ricotta JJ, O'Brien MS, DeWeese JA: Natural history of recurrent and residual stenosis after carotid endarterectomy: Implications for postoperative surveillance and surgical management. Surgery 112:656, 1992.

155. Richardson JD, Main KA: Carotid endarterectomy in the elderly population: A statewide experience. J Vasc Surg 9:65, 1989.

156. Rigdon EE, Monajjem N, Rhodes RS: Criteria for selective utilization of the intensive care unit following carotid endarterectomy. Ann Vasc Surg 11:20, 1997.

157. Riles TS, Imparato AM, Jacobowitz GR, et al: The cause of perioperative stroke after carotid endarterectomy. J Vasc Surg 19:206, 1994.

158. Riles TS, Kopelman I, Imparato AM: Myocardial infarction following carotid endarterectomy: A review of 683 operations. Surgery 85:249, 1979.

159. Riles TS, Lamparello PJ, Giangola G, et al: Rupture of the vein patch: A rare complication of carotid endarterectomy. Surgery 107:10, 1990.

160. Rockman CB, Cappadona C, Riles TS, et al: Causes of the increased stroke rate after carotid endarterectomy in patients with previous strokes. Ann Vasc Surg 11:28, 1997.

161. Rokey R, Rolak LA, Harati H, et al: Coronary artery disease in patients with cerebrovascular disease: A prospective study. Ann Neurol 16:50, 1984.

162. Rosenbloom M, Friedman SG, Lamparello PJ, et al: Glossopharyngeal nerve injury complicating carotid endarterectomy. J Vasc Surg 5:468, 1987.

163. Rosenthal D, Archie JP, Avila MH, et al: Secondary recurrent carotid stenosis. J Vasc Surg 24:424, 1996.

164. Rosenthal D, Archie JP Jr, Garcia-Rinaldi R, et al: Carotid patch angioplasty: Immediate and long-term results. J Vasc Surg 12:326, 1990.

165. Rosenthal D, Zeichner WD, Lamis PA, et al: Neurologic deficit after carotid endarterectomy: Pathogenesis and management. Surgery 94:776, 1983.

166. Rothwell PM, Slattery J, Warlow CP: A systematic comparison of the risks of stroke and death due to endarterectomy for symptomatic and asymptomatic stenosis. Stroke 27:266, 1996.

167. Rubin JR Jr, Pitluk HC, King TA, et al: Carotid endarterectomy in a metropolitan community: The early results after 8635 operations. J Vasc Surg 7:256, 1988.

168. Ruby ST, Robinson D, Lynch JT, et al: Outcome analysis of carotid endarterectomy in Connecticut: The impact of volume and specialty. Ann Vasc Surg 10:22, 1996.

169. Sachs SM, Fulenwider JT, Smith RB, et al: Does contralateral carotid occlusion influence neurologic fate of carotid endarterectomy? Surgery 96:839, 1984.

170. Sanders EACM, Hoeneveld H, Eikelboom BC, et al: Residual lesions and early recurrent stenosis after carotid endarterectomy. J Vasc Surg 5:731, 1987.

171. Sandmann W, Hennerici M, Aulich A, et al: Progress in carotid artery surgery at the base of the skull. J Vasc Surg 1:734, 1984.

172. Sanella NA, Tober RL, Cipro RP, et al: Vocal cord paralysis following carotid endarterectomy: The paradox of return of function. Ann Vasc Surg 4:42, 1990.

173. Satiani B, Liapis C, Pflug B, et al: Role of staging in bilateral carotid endarterectomy. Surgery 84:784, 1978.

174. Satiani B, Vasko JS, Evans WE: Hypertension following carotid endarterectomy. Surg Neurol 11:357, 1979.

175. Schauber MD, Fontenelle LJ, Solomon JW, et al: Cranial/cervical nerve dysfunction after carotid endarterectomy. J Vasc Surg 25:481, 1997.

176. Schroeder T, Sillesen H, Engell HC: Staged bilateral carotid endarterectomy. J Vasc Surg 3:355, 1986.

177. Seifert KB, Blackshear WM Jr: Continuous-wave Doppler in the intraoperative assessment of carotid endarterectomy. J Vasc Surg 2:817, 1985.

178. Slavish LG, Nicholas GG, Gee W: Review of a community hospital experience with carotid endarterectomy. Stroke 15:956, 1984.

179. Smith BL: Hypertension following carotid endarterectomy: The role of cerebral renin production. J Vasc Surg 1:623, 1984.

180. Stanley JC, Barnes RW, Ernst CB, et al: Vascular surgery in the United States: Workforce issues. J Vasc Surg 23:172, 1996.

181. Stewart GW, Bandyk DF, Kaebnick HW, et al: Influence of vein-patch angioplasty on carotid endarterectomy healing. Arch Surg 122:364, 1987.

182. Stoney RJ, String SJ: Recurrent carotid stenosis. Surgery 80:705, 1976.

183. Sundt TM, Houser OW, Whisnant JP, et al: Correlation of postoperative and two-year follow-up angiography with neurologic function in 99 carotid endarterectomies in 86 consecutive patients. Ann Surg 203:90, 1986.

184. Sundt TM Jr, Sharbrough FW, Marsh WR, et al: The risk-benefit ratio of intraoperative shunting during carotid endarterectomy: Relevancy to operative and postoperative results and complications. Ann Surg 203:196, 1986.

185. Sundt TM Jr, Sharbrough FW, Piepgras DG, et al: Correlation of cerebral blood flow and electroencephalographic changes during carotid endarterectomy with results of surgery and hemodynamics of cerebral ischemia. Mayo Clin Proc 56:533, 1981.

186. Tarlov E, Schmidek H, Scott RM, et al: Reflex hypotension following carotid endarterectomy: Mechanism and management. J Neurosurg 39:323, 1973.

187. Taylor LM, Porter JM: Basic data related to carotid endarterectomy. Ann Vasc Surg 1:262, 1986.

188. Ten Holter JBM, Ackerstaff RGA, Schwartzenberg GWST, et al: The impact of vein patch angioplasty on long-term surgical outcome after carotid endarterectomy. J Cardiovasc Surg 31:58, 1990.

189. Thomas M, Otis SM, Rush M, et al: Recurrent carotid artery stenosis following endarterectomy. Ann Surg 200:74, 1984.

190. Thompson JE: Complications of carotid endarterectomy and their prevention. World J Surg 3:155, 1979.

191. Thompson JE, Austin DJ, Patman RD: Carotid endarterectomy for cerebrovascular insufficiency: Long-term results in 592 patients followed up to thirteen years. Ann Surg 172:663, 1970.

192. Toole JF, Yuson CP, Janeway R, et al: Transient ischemic attacks: A prospective study of 225 patients. Neurology 28:746, 1978.

193. Toronto Cerebrovascular Study Group: Risks of carotid endarterectomy. Stroke 17:848, 1986.

194. Towne JB, Bernhard VM: The relationship of postoperative hypertension to complications following carotid endarterectomy. Surgery 88:575, 1980.

195. Treiman RL, Cossman DV, Foran RF, et al: The influence of neutralizing heparin after carotid endarterectomy on postoperative stroke and wound hematoma. J Vasc Surg 12:440, 1990.

196. Tucker JA, Gee W, Nicholas GG, et al: Accessory nerve injury during carotid endarterectomy. J Vasc Surg 5:440, 1987.

197. Turnipseed WD, Berkoff HA, Crummy A: Postoperative occlusion after carotid endarterectomy. Arch Surg 115:573, 1980.

198. Verta MJ Jr, Applebaum EL, McClusky DA, et al: Cranial nerve injury during carotid endarterectomy. Ann Surg 185:192, 1977.

199. Wade JG, Larson CP Jr, Hickey RF, et al: Effect of carotid endarterectomy on carotid chemoreceptor and baroreceptor function in man. Ann Surg 185:192, 1977.

200. Washburn WK, Mackey WC, Belkin M, et al: Late stroke after

carotid endarterectomy: The role of recurrent stenosis. J Vasc Surg 15:1032, 1992.

201. Wilkinson JT, Adams HP Jr, Wright CB: Convulsions after carotid endarterectomy. JAMA 244:1827, 1980.

202. Winslow CM, Solomon DH, Chassin MR, et al: The appropriateness of carotid endarterectomy. N Engl J Med 318:721, 1988.

203. Yamamoto Y, Piepgras DG, Marsh WR, et al: Complications resulting from saphenous vein patch graft after carotid endarterectomy. Neurosurgery 39:670, 1996.

204. Youkey JR, Clagett GP, Jaffin JH, et al: Focal motor seizures complicating carotid endarterectomy. Arch Surg 119:1080, 1984.

205. Zierler RE, Bandyk DF, Thiele BL: Intraoperative assessment of carotid endarterectomy. J Vasc Surg 1:73, 1984.

206. Zierler RE, Bandyk DF, Thiele BL, et al: Carotid artery stenosis following endarterectomy. Arch Surg 117:1408, 1982.

207. Zukowski AJ, Nicolaides AN, Lewis RT, et al: The correlation between carotid plaque ulceration and cerebral infarction seen on CT scan. J Vasc Surg 1:782, 1984.

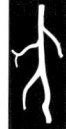

C H A P T E R   1 3 7

Venous Disease: An Overview

Peter Gloviczki, M.D.

Chronic ulceration of the lower extremity following deep venous thrombosis is a condition that undoubtedly has plagued the human race since man assumed the erect position.

Robert R. Linton, 1953

Acute and chronic venous diseases are among the most prevalent medical conditions worldwide. Acute venous thromboembolism is a serious and frequently lethal disease, whereas chronic venous insufficiency can be the source of considerable discomfort, disability, and loss of working days. Venous diseases of the lower limbs, as noted by Linton in 1953,[1] are greatly influenced by the erect position of the human race, and impairment of return of venous blood to the heart against gravity contributes to the development of both acute venous thrombosis and chronic venous insufficiency. Manifestations of venous disease, including varicosity, pain, swelling, skin changes, and leg ulcers, have long been known to humankind, and attempts to treat them date back thousands of years.

HISTORICAL BACKGROUND

1550 BC to 200 AD: Venous Discoveries

The fascinating history of venous surgery has been the subject of many reviews and monographs.[2–9] The first written record of varicose veins and suggestions on treatment were found in the Ebers papyrus around 1550 BC.[4] The first illustration of a varicose vein, discovered in Athens at the foot of the Acropolis, dates back to the 4th century BC. It is a commonly reproduced votive tablet that shows a large leg with a serpentine varicose vein on its medial aspect (Fig. 137–1). Extensive description of venous ulceration was found in the work of Hippocrates, entitled *De ulceribus*, in which he stated that "in the case of an ulcer, it is not expedient to stand, more especially if the ulcer is

situated in the leg."[10] Hippocrates recognized that incisions around large ulcers do not heal well, and he suggested puncturing the ulcer to stimulate healing. According to Browse and colleagues,[6] Hippocrates made the first reference to compressive dressing when he instructed, "if necessary, cut out the ulcer and then compress it to squeeze out the blood and humours."

The first ligation of blood vessels was described by members of the Alexandrian School of Medicine in Egypt around 270 BC.[3] Celsus,[11] a Roman physician in the 1st century, treated varicose veins by excision and cauterization and described ligation of bleeding veins and division of veins between ligatures. Galen, in the 2nd century, used silk ligature to tie off blood vessels and suggested that varicose veins should be treated by incision and avulsion with the use of hooks.[12] It was not until several centuries after Galen that major new discoveries in medicine were documented.

14th to 20th Century: Progress in Anatomy and Physiology

In the 14th century, Maitre Henri de Mondeville followed the advice of Hippocrates and successfully used bandages on limbs with ulcerations to "drive back the evil humours."[13] The 15th century brought new interest in venous anatomy, as illustrated in Leonardo da Vinci's drawings of the human body (Fig. 137–2), and in the 16th century the anatomy of the venous system was presented in great details in the works of Andreas Vesalius (Fig. 137–3). The presence of venous valves was probably first mentioned by J. B. Canano, who described the valvular fold in the azygos

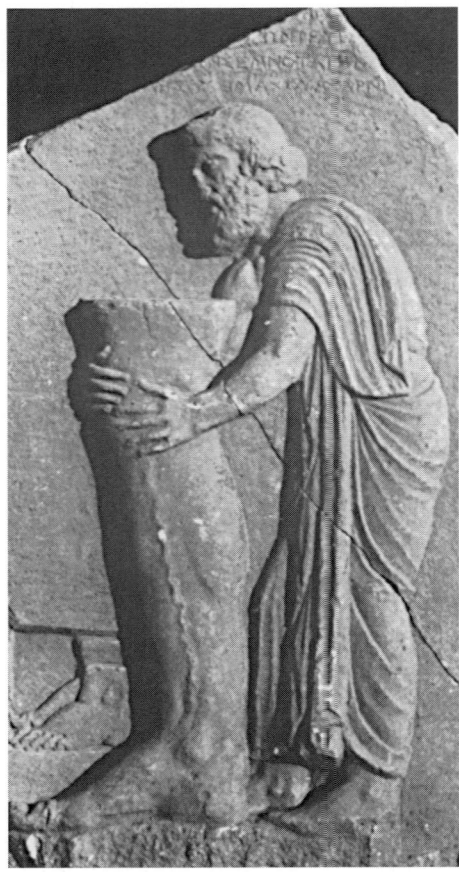

FIGURE 137–1. Votive tablet found at the base of the Acropolis in Athens, Greece, dating back to the 4th century. It was dedicated to Dr. Amynos by his patient, Lysimachidis of Acharnes. This is the earliest known illustration of a varicose vein.

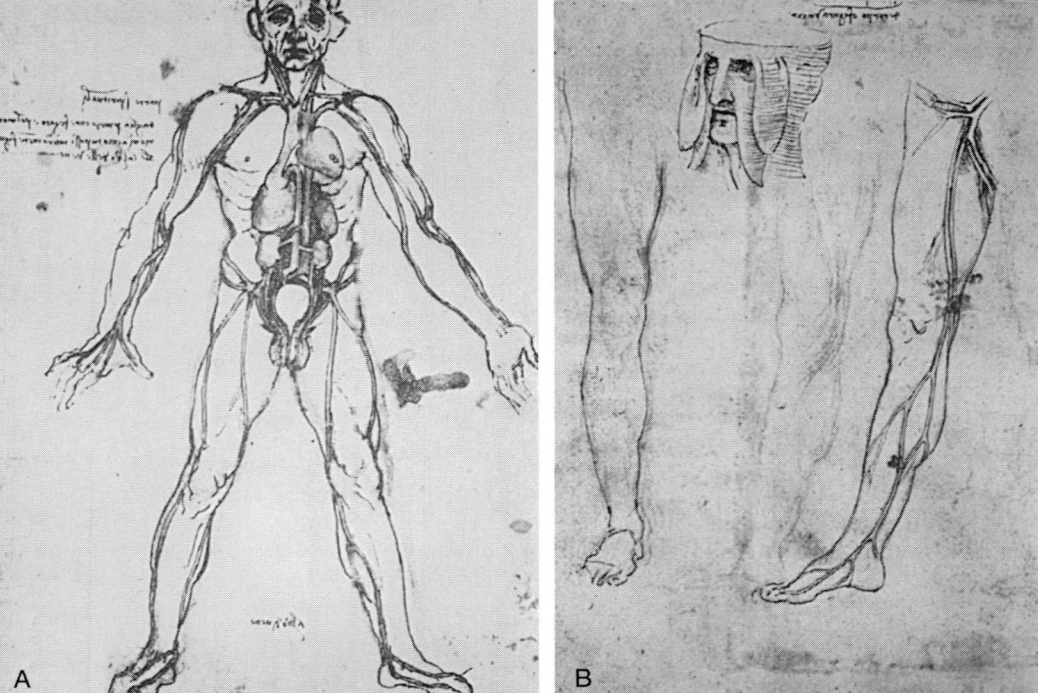

FIGURE 137–2. The anatomy of veins depicted by Leonardo da Vinci in the 15th century. *A*, The "tree of vessels." *B*, Superficial veins of the lower limb.

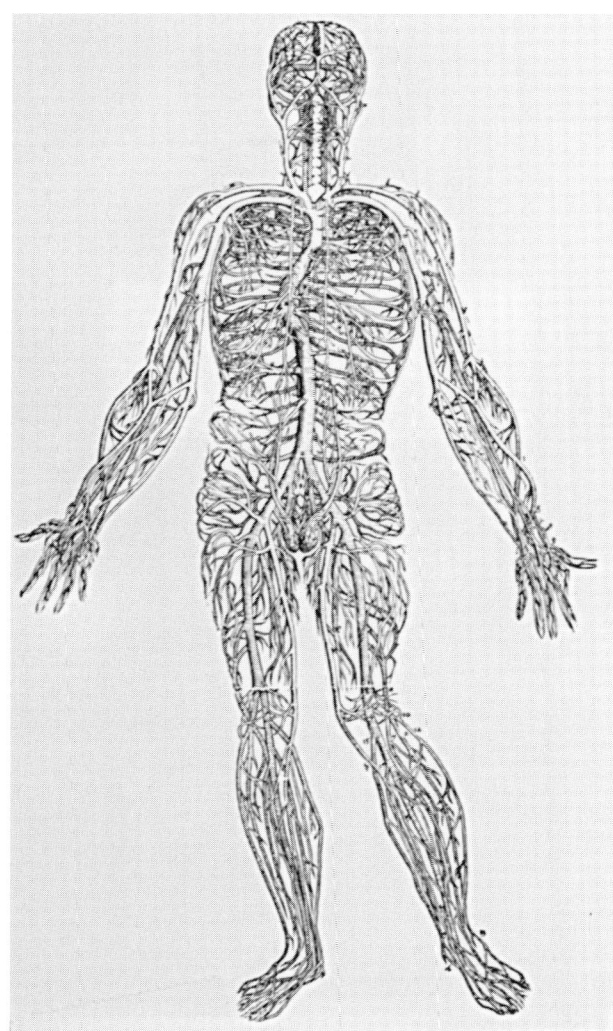

FIGURE 137–3. The venous system, as depicted by Andreas Vesalius in 1543. (From works of Andreas Vesalius of Brussels, World Publishing Co, Cleveland and New York, 1950.)

phlegmasia alba dolens, but he still presumed that the condition was caused by lymphatic obstruction. The relationship between phlegmasia alba dolens and acute *deep venous thrombosis* (DVT) was established by Davis[18] in 1822; he also recognized the relationship between venous thrombosis and childbirth. Anatomic studies on the venous system in the 1800s were definitive in most aspects (Figs. 137–7 through 137–9), and information on management of venous disease has also rapidly accumulated. Brodie,[19] in 1846, described his test of venous valvular incompetence and used compression bandages to treat venous ulcers. Unna's description of an elastic plaster dressing with a glycerine-gelatin mixture known as the Unna boot, in 1854 gave further impetus to nonoperative management.[20]

Virchow[21] described his revolutionary discovery of the three main causes of DVT—changes in the venous wall, stasis of venous blood, and changes in the blood coagulation—in his book *Die Cellular Pathologie*. His depiction of propagation of thrombus in the deep veins and pulmonary emboli changed our understanding of DVT (Fig. 137–10). In 1864, the French physician Pravaz initiated sclerotherapy and injected perchloride of iron to sclerose varicose veins using hypodermic needles, as described previously by Francis Rynd.[6] John Gay's Lettsomian lectures, published in 1868, are most important because they contain accurate descriptions of perforating veins in patients with varicosity and ulcerations and emphasize that treatment of varicose veins results in healing of ulcers (Fig. 137–11).[22] Gay clearly understood that permanent changes occur in the deep veins as a result of venous thrombosis.

20th Century Landmarks

Surgical treatment of DVT at the end of the 19th century included proximal ligation of the greater saphenous vein, as described by Trendelenburg[23] in 1891. In the early 20th century, stripping of the saphenous veins was added to proximal ligation. Keller[24] described an internal stripper in 1905, and Charles H. Mayo[25] used an external ringed

vein in 1547.[14] Browse and colleagues[6] give credit to Saloman Alberti in 1585 for the first drawing of a valve in a vein (Fig. 137–4), but the first full description of the valves was given by Hieronymus Fabricius de Aquapendente,[15] professor of anatomy of the renowned medical school of Padua, in 1603 (Fig. 137–5). Browse and colleagues[6] suggest, however, that Fabricius, a teacher of William Harvey, demonstrated the valves in public dissections as early as 1579. Fabricius also wrote on the surgical treatment of varicose veins in his book *Opera chirurgica*, published in 1593.

Stimulated by the work of Fabricius and by his own observations on the venous circulation of the arm (Fig. 137–6), William Harvey[16] published his monumental discovery of the circulation in 1628. He wrote that his demonstration "clearly established that the blood moves in the veins from parts below to those above and to the heart, and not in the opposite way."

Accurate reports on acute venous thrombosis were published much later than descriptions of varicosities. It was not until 1810 that Ferriar[17] described a patient with

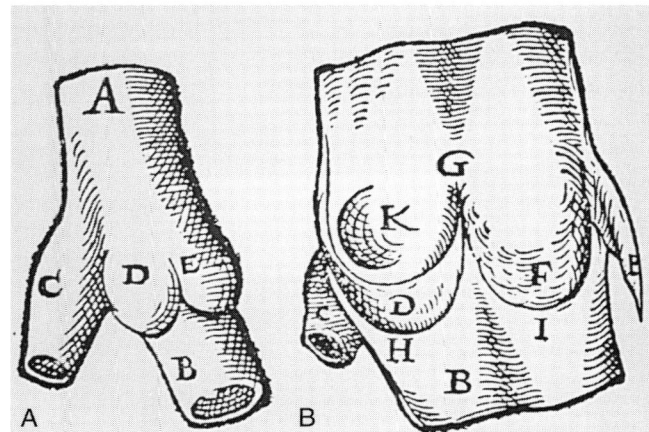

FIGURE 137–4. The first known depiction of venous valves. *A*, Outside depiction of a valve stationed just distal to the origin of a venous tributary. *B*, Inside drawing of a pair of valve leaflets. (From Alberti S: De valvulis membraneis quorundam vasorum: Tres orations. Norimb, 1585. Reprinted in Browse NL, Burnand KG, Thomas ML: Diseases of the Veins: Pathology, Diagnosis, and Treatment. London, Edward Arnold, 1988, p 5.)

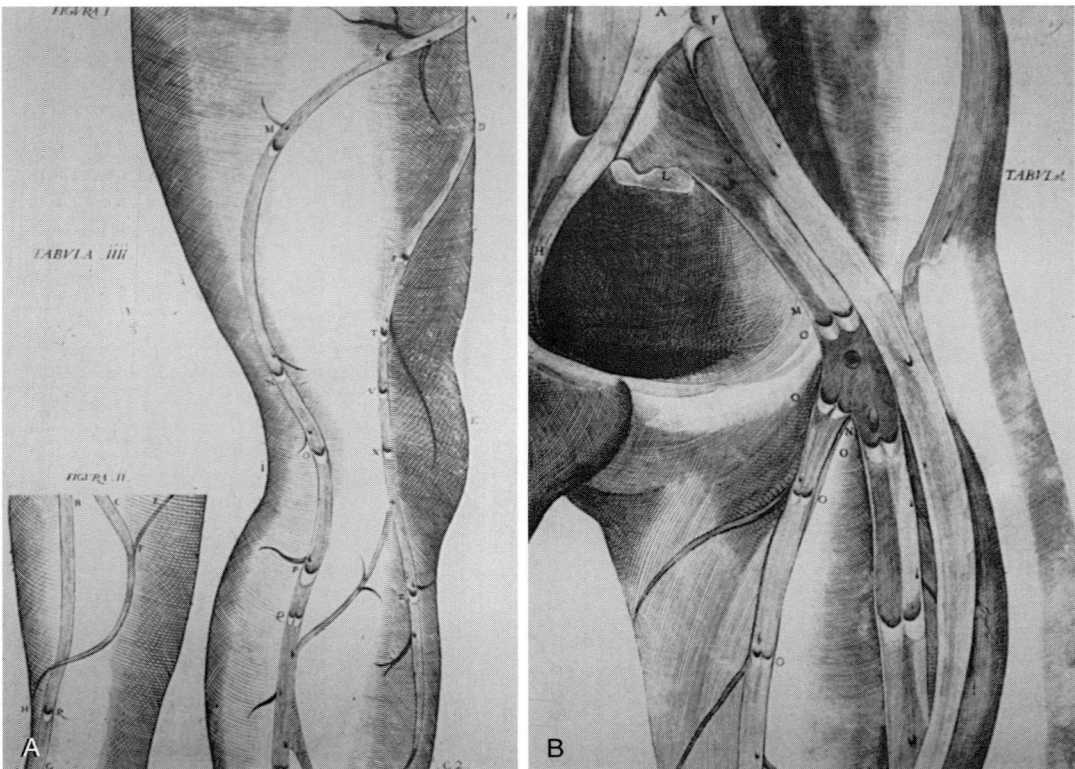

FIGURE 137–5. The first full description of venous valves by Hieronymus Fabricius de Aquapendente. *A*, Venous valves in the superficial veins of the lower limb. *B*, Venous valves in the superficial and deep veins of the lower limbs and pelvis. (From Fabricius Hieronymus de Aquapendente: Anatomici Patavini de Venarum Ostiolis [Valves of veins]. *In* Laufman H [ed]: The Veins. Austin, Tex, Silvergirl, Inc, 1986, pp 14–24.)

vein stripper in 1906. Babcock's[26] contribution was the development of a flexible internal saphenous stripper soon thereafter. Reconstructive venous surgery dates back to 1877, when Eck first performed anastomoses between the portal vein and the inferior vena cava; in 1906, Carrel and Guthrie[27] described their first attempts at venous anastomoses. John Homans[28] in 1917 introduced the terms *venous stasis* and *post-thrombotic syndrome* and classified varicose veins as primary and post-thrombotic.[28, 29]

The first attempts at phlebography by injection of strontium bromide were made by Berberich and Hirsch[30] in 1923, although it was not until 1938 that Dos Santos[31] in Lisbon described a usable technique of contrast phlebography in humans. Bauer[32–34] performed phlebographies regularly in patients to study DVT. The fibrinolytic effect of *Streptococcus* was first described in 1933 by Tillett and Garner,[35] and heparin was first used successfully in humans first by Crafoord[36, 37] in 1937. Bauer[33] also showed the beneficial effect of heparin on deep venous thrombosis already in 1941. Details of a coagulation cascade were first reported by MacFarlane and Biggs[38] in 1946, and the Hungarian-born Geza De Takats, practicing in Chicago, was the first to use low-dose heparin for the prevention of DVT.[39] Research by Tillet and colleagues[40] published in 1955, on the beneficial effect of streptokinase in venous thrombosis started the era of thrombolysis in the management of acute venous thromboembolism.

The first attempts at venous thrombectomy date back to 1926, when Basy[41] performed thrombectomy in a patient with axillary vein thrombosis. The technique of surgical

thrombectomy was described by Leriche[42] in 1939; in the same year, Oschner and DeBakey[43] suggested the terms *phlebothrombosis* and *thrombophlebitis* in a major review of the topic.

Prominent figures in perforating vein surgery included Robert R. Linton,[44] who described subfascial ligation of incompetent communicating veins in 1938 (Fig. 137–12), and Frank Cockett,[45] who suggested the term "ankle blowout syndrome" for varicose ulcers and described, with Jones, his technique of extrafascial ligation of incompetent perforators. Cockett's book, cowritten with Dodd, was the first standard textbook of the treatment of venous disease.[46] The work of the Austrian Robert May and colleagues[47] on perforating veins, along with May's description of the *iliac vein compression syndrome*, also has to be mentioned here.

Venous reconstructive surgery developed as a result of extensive experimental work in the middle of the 20th century. To improve patency of grafts placed in the venous system, Jean Kunlin and associates,[49] in France, suggested the use of a distal arteriovenous fistula (Fig. 137–13A) and ring suspension of venous anastomoses (Figure 137–13B).[48, 49] Deep venous reconstruction was first performed successfully in a patient with superficial femoral vein occlusion in 1954 by Warren and Thayer.[50] In 1958, Palma and colleagues[51] described an operation of a femorofemoral bypass using the greater saphenous vein to relieve an iliac vein obstruction. The pioneer work by Dale and coworkers[52] accelerated prosthetic replacement of large veins.

Kistner's[53] important contribution in 1968 began the era of venous valve reconstructions to treat deep venous

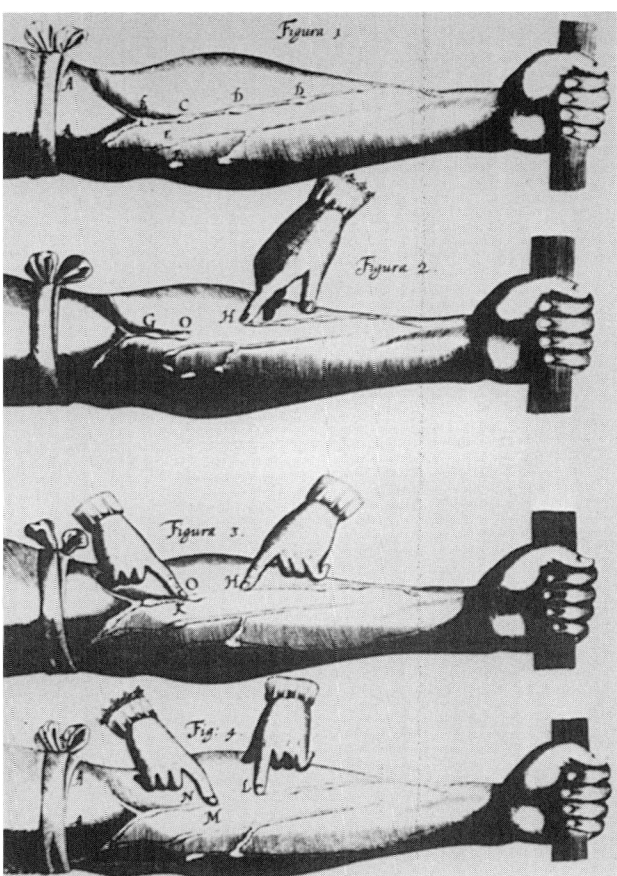

FIGURE 137–6. Illustrations from "De Motu Cordis" of William Harvey, published in 1628. The observations depicted in the drawings persuaded Harvey of unidirectional blood flow in the veins toward the heart. They are also the first known illustrations of the strip test to confirm valvular competence.

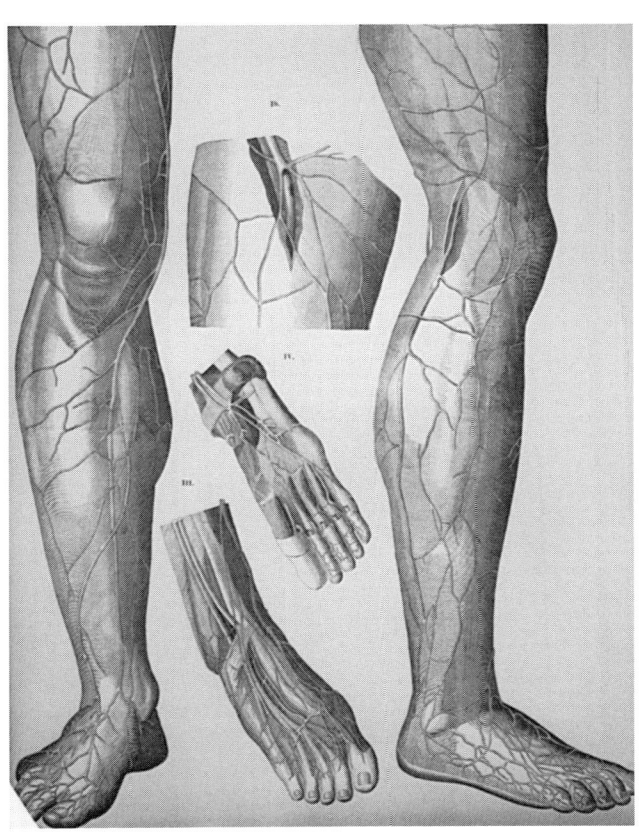

FIGURE 137–7. Illustrations of superficial veins of the legs from the 19th century. (From Oesterreicher JH: Atlas of Human Anatomy. Cincinnati, A. E. Wilde and Co, 1879.)

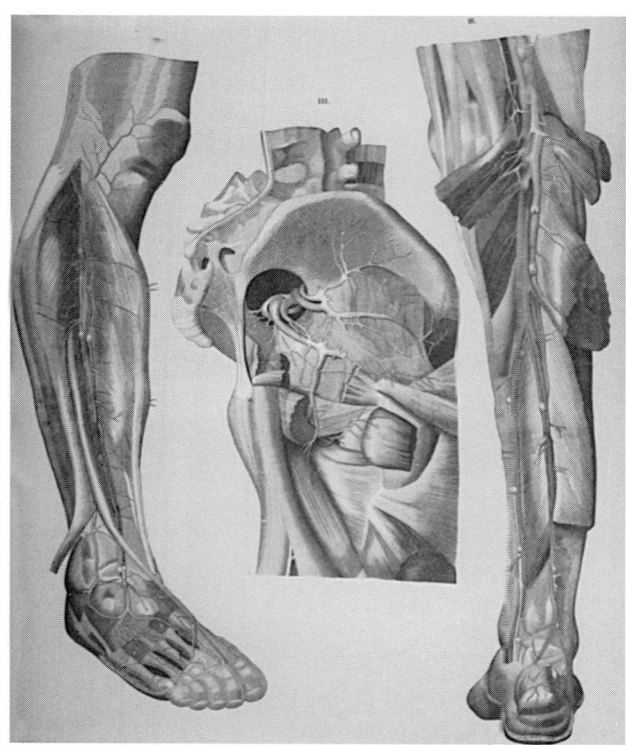

FIGURE 137–8. Illustration of the anatomy of deep veins of the hip, thigh, and leg. (From Oesterreicher JH: Atlas of Human Anatomy. Cincinnati, A. E. Wilde and Co, 1879.)

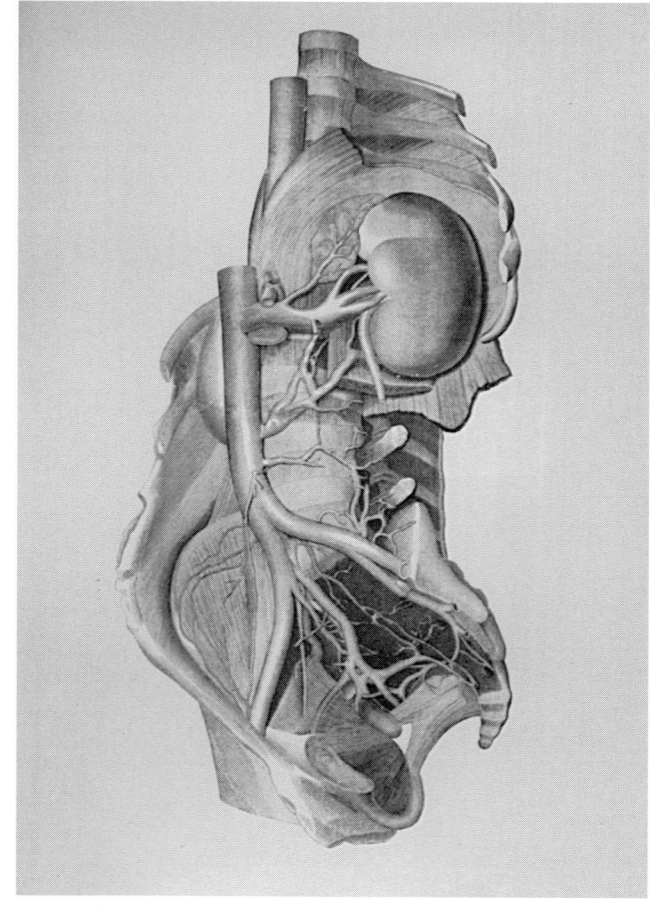

FIGURE 137–9. Anatomy of the common iliac vein and the vena cava. Note the "nutcracker" position of the left renal vein between the superior mesenteric artery and the aorta. (From Oesterreicher JH: Atlas of Human Anatomy. Cincinnati, A. E. Wilde and Co, 1879.)

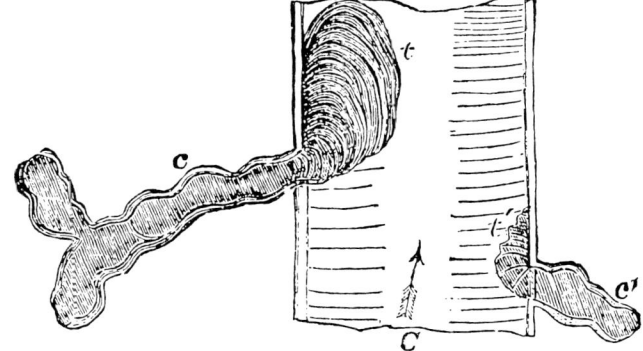

FIGURE 137–10. Venous thrombi protruding into a deep vein from side branches. (From Virchow's Die Cellular Pathologie, 1860.)

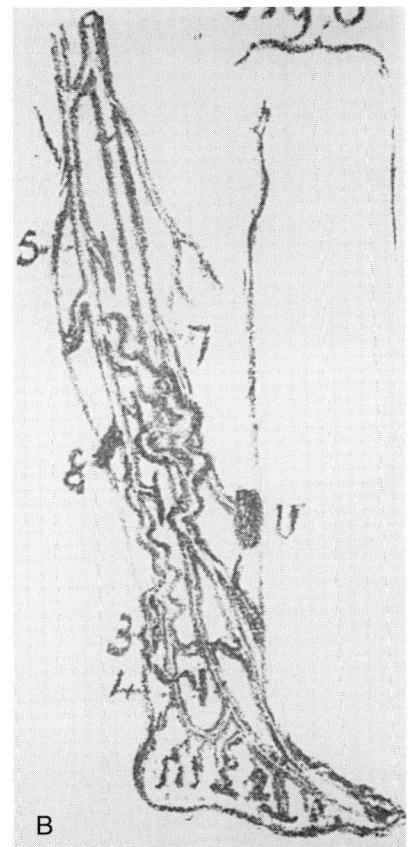

ON

VARICOSE DISEASE

OF THE

LOWER EXTREMITIES

AND ITS ALLIED DISORDERS :

SKIN DISCOLORATION,

INDURATION, AND ULCER:

BEING THE

LETTSOMIAN LECTURES...

DELIVERED BEFORE THE

MEDICAL SOCIETY OF LONDON

IN 1867, BY

JOHN GAY, F.R.C.S.,

SURGEON TO THE GREAT NORTHERN HOSPITAL, CONSULTING SURGEON TO THE
EARLSWOOD IDIOT ASYLUM, ETC., ETC.

" Disséquer en anatomie, faire des expériences en physiologie, suivre les
maladies, et ouvrir les cadavres en médicine, c'est la une triple voie hors
laquelle il ne peut y avoir d'anatomiste, de physiologiste, ni de médecin."
BRIQUET.

LONDON:
JOHN CHURCHILL AND SONS,
NEW BURLINGTON STREET.
1868.

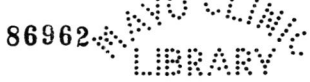

A

B

FIGURE 137–11. *A,* Front page of the Lettsomian Lectures of John Gay. *B,* Illustrations of the medial leg veins by John Gay. Note the posterior arch vein and three perforating veins (5, 8, and 4), which are clearly depicted. (From Gay J: On Varicose Disease of the Lower Extremities, Lettsomian Lecture, London, Churchill, 1868.)

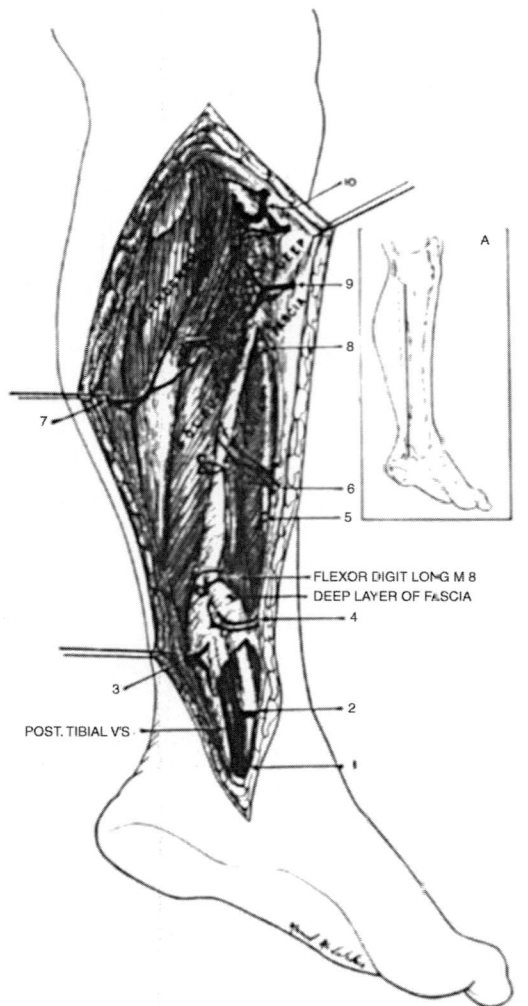

FIGURE 137–12. Linton's technique of ligation of the communicating veins. (From Linton RR: The communicating veins of the lower leg and the operative technic for their ligation. Ann Surg 107:582–593, 1938.)

incompetence (Fig. 137–14).[53] In the past three decades, the introductions of endovascular interventions, the use of thrombolysis, venous angioplasty, and stents have rapidly improved our ability to reconstruct the deep venous system.[54] Minimally invasive endoscopic surgical procedures (Fig. 137–15) have also been introduced and added to our armamentarium to treat patients with venous disease.[55]

STATE OF THE ART AT THE TURN OF THE 21ST CENTURY

In the United States each year, more than 250,000 people experience acute DVT and at least 50,000 suffer from pulmonary embolism.[56] High-probability lung scans document pulmonary emboli in 25% to 51% of the patients with DVT, even in the absence of respiratory symptoms.[57, 58]

Although new information on the pathophysiology of acute DVT has emerged, including venous thrombogenesis and the early course of the disease, the basic mechanism

of thrombosis, as described by Virchow[21] more than a century ago, has remained valid. In Chapter 138 of this book, Meissner and Strandness from the University of Washington, Seattle, summarize our current understanding of the pathophysiology of DVT, give an update on coagulation and fibrinolysis, and relay new data regarding the role of the venous endothelium. Our understanding of primary hypercoagulable states has advanced considerably in recent years with discovery of natural anticoagulants, including antithrombin III, protein C, protein S, and the tissue factor pathway inhibitors. Resistance to activated protein C has received increased attention recently. It is now recognized that factor V Leiden mutation is present in 94% of individuals with activated protein C resistance and that this mutation has an autosomal dominant mode of inheritance.[59] This is an important discovery, because approximately 25% of people with Leiden V mutation have venous thrombosis by age 50 years. In addition, the prevalence of activated protein C resistance in patients with DVT has varied from 10% to 65%.[59, 60]

Duplex scanning has extended our knowledge in many areas of venous disease, including the natural history of acute DVT. Multiple studies have confirmed that recanalization is early, with the greatest reduction in thrombus load occurring within 3 months and complete resolution in more than half of patients by 9 months. Recanalization of thrombus, however, can continue for months to years after the acute event.

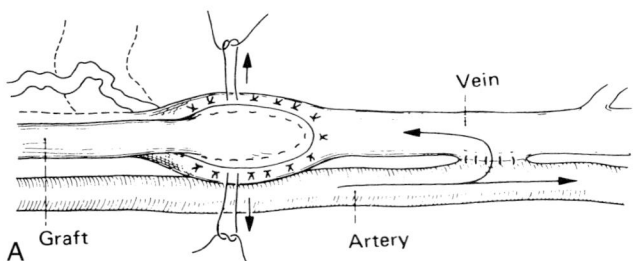

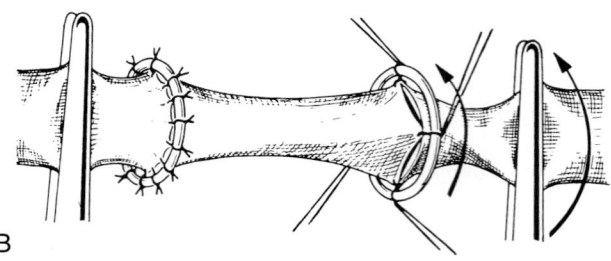

FIGURE 137–13. A, Kunlin's drawing on a distal arteriovenous fistula to improve blood flow in a graft placed in the venous system. (From Kunlin J: Les greffes veineuses. Lisbon, Congres Soc Internat de Chirurgie, September 1953.) B, External support of venous interposition graft by suspension of the anastomoses on rings, as suggested by Kunlin. (From Kunlin J, Kunlin A, Richard S, Tregouet T: Le remplacement et l'anastomose latero-laterale des veines par greffon avec sutures suspendue par des anneaux: Etude experimentale. J Chir (Paris) 85:305–337, 1953.)

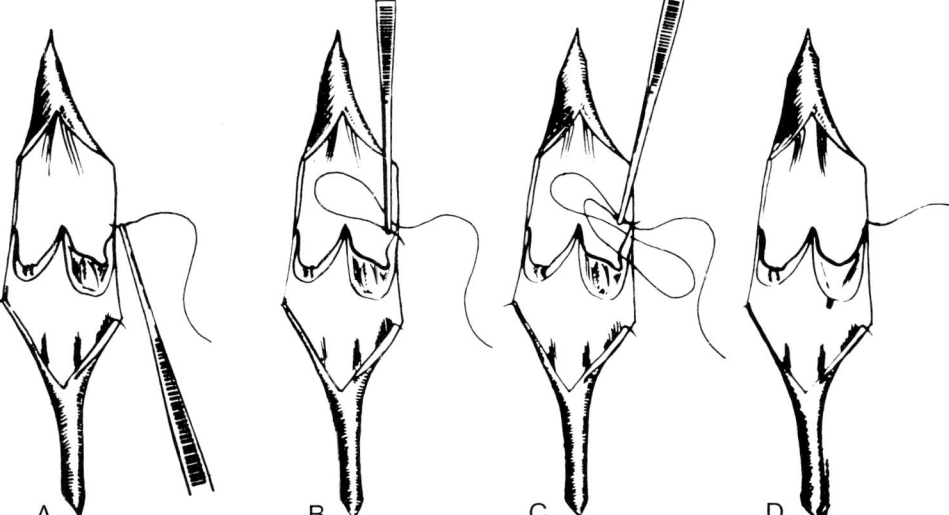

FIGURE 137–14. A–D, Illustrations of repair of incompetent femoral vein valves by Kistner.

Readers will benefit greatly from the expert overview by Comerota and colleagues,[62] from Temple University, who described the clinical presentation and risk factors of DVT and provide sound and practical guidelines for efficient and cost-effective diagnostic evaluation (Chapter 139). Advanced age, immobilization, history of venous thromboembolism, surgical treatment, and trauma have remained the most important risk factors for venous thrombosis. Comerota emphasizes the need for accurate and expeditious diagnosis so that immediate treatment can be initiated not only to provide relief of symptoms but also to decrease the two possible major complications of DVT, pulmonary embolism and post-thrombotic syndrome. Although history and physical examination complemented with hand-held Doppler examination are important to raise suspicion of DVT, venous duplex imaging is the current mainstay in the diagnosis of acute venous thrombosis, having excellent diagnostic accuracy.[61, 62] The role of contrast phlebography is limited, but magnetic resonance venography is emerging as a useful noninvasive diagnostic examination, with excellent sensitivity to diagnose proximal, pelvic, and vena caval thrombosis.[63] Still, availability, metallic implants, patient claustrophobia, and higher costs limit its application.

An important advance at the turn of the 21st century is that blood tests are now used with excellent results to exclude the diagnosis of acute venous thrombosis. In patients with acute DVT, elevated levels of D-dimer, a degradation product of fibrin, are measured in the blood. Although D-dimer levels are elevated in postoperative and acutely ill patients,[64] a negative test result has a high negative predictive value to exclude DVT.[65]

In the past two decades, evidence-based medicine has transformed clinical research and retrospective clinical reviews and nonrandomized trials have been replaced by large multicenter randomized studies to provide level I evidence of treatment efficacy. Such clinical trials are discussed by Pineo and Hull in Chapter 140, on the prevention and medical management of acute DVT. Credible evidence now supports the effectiveness of low-molecular-weight heparins in both the prevention and the treatment of DVT. Low-molecular-weight heparin given subcutaneously once or twice daily is as effective as or more effective than unfractionated heparin in preventing thrombosis[66–72] and superior in decreasing bleeding.[66, 67] The greater efficacy of outpatient treatment of acute DVT with low-molecular-weight heparin in comparison with conventional intravenous unfractionated heparin given in hospital also has been documented in several clinical studies.[73–75] There is every reason to believe that low-molecular-weight heparins will replace unfractionated heparin for both the prevention and treatment of acute DVT.

Progress in invasive management of acute DVT has also

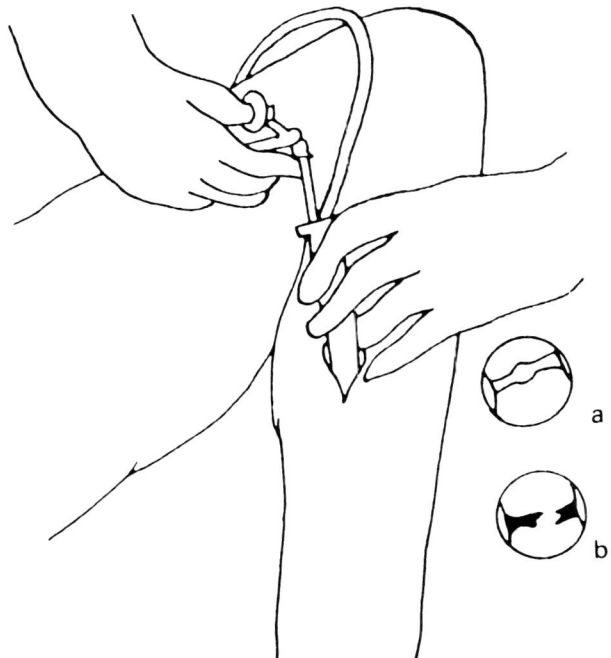

FIGURE 137–15. The first illustration of endoscopic subfascial perforator vein surgery by Hauer in 1985. (From Hauer G: The endoscopic subfascial division of the perforating veins—preliminary report [in German]. Vasa 14:59–61, 1985.)

been considerable. Additional evidence for both early and late efficacy of surgical thrombectomy has been collected, and in the last decade the popularity of minimally invasive endovascular techniques has rapidly transformed management algorithms of acute venous disease. In Chapter 141, a team of experts present the rationales for both surgical thrombectomy and catheter-directed thrombolysis, used with or without additional endovascular techniques, such as angioplasty and stents. In experience by Plate and colleagues with more than 200 operations, mortality was 1% and no fatal pulmonary embolism occurred. The long-term benefit of surgical treatment is supported by a prospective, randomized study from Sweden.[76, 77]

A multicenter venous registry for catheter-directed thrombolysis collected data on almost 500 patients.[78] Significant lysis with catheter-directed thrombolysis (>50%) was achieved in 80% of patients, and complete lysis in one third. Preliminary data indicate better results for (1) iliofemoral than for femoropopliteal thrombosis, (2) patients with acute (<10 days) presentation, and (3) patients with the first episode of DVT. Mortality (0.4%) and pulmonary embolism (1.2%) were rare. These data support the use of catheter-directed thrombolysis in carefully selected patients with iliofemoral DVT. In phlegmasia cerulea dolens, surgery is preferred, whereas in phlegmasia alba dolens, catheter-directed thrombolysis is attempted first, unless there are contraindications to fibrinolysis.

Prevention of pulmonary embolism by inferior vena caval filter placement (Chapter 142) remains an effective method in patients with DVT who cannot undergo anticoagulation or who had documented pulmonary embolism in spite of adequate anticoagulation. Indications for filter placement in trauma patients still are not fully defined, and level 1 evidence on routine filter placement is not available. The standard for comparison of all the devices remains the stainless steel Greenfield filter, which, in a study that observed nearly 500 patients over 12 years, had a 4% rate of recurrent embolism and a long-term filter patency rate of 98%.[79]

The management of superficial thrombophlebitis continues to be controversial, and most surgeons continue to be cautious and advocate high ligation in patients with proximal greater saphenous vein thrombophlebitis to prevent pulmonary embolism. Others, however, have collected valuable data to support full anticoagulation to prevent thrombus extension or development of new thrombi in the deep veins and avoid pulmonary embolism (Chapter 143). As emphasized by De Palma, recurrent thrombophlebitis clearly requires thorough investigation for an underlying thrombotic disorder, malignancy, or, in young smokers, Buerger's disease.

Post-thrombotic syndrome develops in 29% to 79% of patients after an acute episode of DVT.[80] Primary valvular incompetence and, less frequently, congenital venous anomalies are additional causes of chronic venous insufficiency. Recent epidemiologic studies are not available; in the United States, however, it is estimated that 25 million people have varicosities, 2 to 6 million have more advanced forms of chronic venous insufficiency (swelling, skin changes), and about 500,000 have venous ulcers.[81]

Current theories of the pathophysiology of chronic venous insufficiency are presented in Chapter 144 by the Oregon Group. Macrocirculatory and microcirculatory changes are described for the two main forms of chronic venous insufficiency, primary valvular incompetence and post-thrombotic syndrome. It has become evident in the past decade that a large percentage of patients with deep venous insufficiency do not have a known history of DVT. Arguments for and against the different theories, such as fibrin cuff, tissue hypoxia, local neural control, and white blood cell trapping, are presented.[82–85] The authors conclude that although venous hypertension is the main cause of chronic venous insufficiency, the complex relationships of cellular, microangiopathic, and functional abnormalities are not well-defined at present and remain a fertile area for further research.

In Chapter 145, Kistner and Masuda present a practical approach to definitive diagnosis of chronic venous disease using the updated CEAP (clinical, etiologic, anatomic, pathophysiologic) classification that has been accepted worldwide.[86, 87] Kistner and Masuda describe clinical presentations in each class and suggest different levels of diagnostic evaluation. As in the diagnosis of acute venous disease, duplex scanning has become important in diagnosis of chronic venous obstruction and in confirming the presence of superficial and deep venous valvular incompetence. It has also been used to localize perforating veins and confirm their incompetence. Ascending and descending venography is reserved now in chronic venous disease for patients who are candidates for endovascular or surgical intervention.[88]

Nonoperative management in patients who are compliant with therapy remains highly effective in controlling symptoms and promoting healing of venous ulcers.[89–91] Leg elevation, elastic and nonelastic bandages and stockings, paste gauze boots, and intermittent compression pumps are elements of compression therapy. Drug treatment in the United States awaits clinical trials; in Europe, the most frequently used drugs are fibrinolytic agents, flavonoids, pentoxifylline, and prostaglandin E_1. For topical ulcer treatment, a bioengineered product made from human foreskin has been reported to show effectiveness in inducing ulcer healing.[92] The authors of Chapter 146, Moneta and Porter from Oregon Health Sciences University, offer a critical analysis on nonoperative management, but admit that ulcer healing can be prolonged and in some cases painful and that recurrence of venous ulceration remains a significant problem.[93] Still, compression therapy continues to be the standard against which all other therapies for venous ulcer and chronic venous insufficiency should be compared.

Chapter 147, on the management of varicose veins, reflects the lifelong experience devoted to this subject by chapter author John Bergan, a noble scholar of venous surgery. Bergan guides us masterfully to find the appropriate balance between surgery and sclerotherapy, a technique that in the past decade has received increasing and well-deserved recognition. Greater saphenous reflux is best treated by inversion stripping of the segment that demonstrates reflux, usually from the groin to the knee. Care of axial veins (greater and lesser saphenous veins) that show reflux, varicosities above the knee, and large varicose clusters are best treated by removal. Other vessels, especially those with telangiectasia, may be subjected to sclerotherapy.

Chapter 148 discusses progress in perforating vein surgery with emphasis on a minimally invasive new technique, subfascial endoscopic perforator surgery (SEPS).[94, 95] The contributing role of perforating veins in the pathophysiology of venous ulcers remains a topic of debate.[96] Available studies documented that about two thirds of patients with chronic venous insufficiency have incompetent perforating veins, and about 70% of cases are of moderate to major hemodynamic significance.[97] Interruption of incompetent perforating veins in this group of patients contributes to improvement in ambulatory venous hypertension and calf muscle pump function. Two publications for the North American Registry confirmed safety of SEPS, but mid-term results also reflected increased ulcer recurrence in post-thrombotic patients.[98, 99] Level 1 evidence is still required not only to confirm the effectiveness of surgical treatment over medical management but also to ascertain the contributory role of perforators to the development of venous ulcers.

Current techniques and results of reconstruction of deep vein valves is presented in an expert review by Raju in Chapter 149. Patients with either post-thrombotic syndrome or primary valvular incompetence in whom venous ulcerations recurred in spite of nonoperative management or correction of superficial reflux are candidates for valve reconstruction. Currently used techniques include internal valvuloplasty, external and transcommissural valvuloplasty with or without angioscopic control, prosthetic sleeve in situ placed around the dilated valve station, and axillary vein transfer. The last remains the mainstay in patients with destroyed valves. The best results have been reported with internal valvuloplasty, which appeared to be durable with few recurrences 3 or 4 years after surgery.[100–103] Hemodynamic improvement using ambulatory venous pressure measurements and air plethysmography has also been documented following valve reconstructions.

Venous grafting for iliocaval occlusion has been performed with increasing frequency with the use of polytetrafluoroethylene grafts, frequently with an arteriovenous fistula (see Chapter 150).[104, 105] Still, the most popular venous reconstructive operation remains the Palma procedure.[106] The suprapubic saphenous femorofemoral bypass can be performed in patients with unilateral iliac vein occlusion. Clinical improvement following the Palma-Dale procedure has been observed in 75% to 86% of patients.[105–110] In one report on 50 consecutive cases, the cumulative 5-year patency rate was 75%.[108]

Advances made in the fields of thrombolysis, percutaneous transluminal angioplasty (PTA), and endoluminal stenting to recanalize chronic large vein occlusions is presented by the experienced Stanford group in Chapter 151. Lidell and Dake discuss advances made in radiologic imaging and catheter-based interventional procedures that now offer safe, less invasive, and effective treatment alternatives for patients with iliocaval or superior vena cava occlusion.[54] Advantages and disadvantages of the different stents, such as the Gianturco Z-stents, the Palmaz stent, and the Wallstent, used in large veins are discussed, and indications for each suggested. The role of transluminal angioplasty has changed; it is used now most frequently for predilatation before stenting.

With improvement of imaging techniques and the ability to detect abdominal, retroperitoneal, and pelvic tumors at an earlier stage,[109] vascular surgeons are faced more and more commonly with problems of primary and secondary tumors invading the inferior vena cava.[111–114] In Chapter 152, Bower and Stanson from the Mayo Clinic provide guidelines for diagnosis and management of primary venous leiomyosarcomas, renal cancers, and metastatic liver and adrenal tumors that invade the vena cava. Tumor resection can be combined with caval reconstruction, using polytetrafluoroethylene grafts with external ring support, with excellent early graft patency. Postoperative quality of life, even if survival in many patients is limited, can be improved by caval reconstruction.

The last chapter in this section discusses evaluation and surgical management of superior vena cava syndrome. It is appropriate to conclude with the treatment of this venous disease, because few areas of reconstructive venous surgery provide more satisfying experience than reconstruction of the superior vena cava or innominate veins, with the use of either autologous or prosthetic grafts. Relief from severe, frequently incapacitating symptoms of superior vena cava obstruction following surgery is instantaneous; the benefit, because of high flow and favorable conditions, is generally long-lasting.[115] Patients with nonmalignant disease have excellent long-term outcome; survival and graft patency in patients with malignant disease are determined by the nature of the underlying tumor.[116]

This entirely revised, new venous section of the 5th edition of *Vascular Surgery* brings the readers the very best that the 20th century can offer on management of acute and chronic venous diseases. An additional, noble goal of the authors has been to inspire investigators of the 21st century to intensify basic and clinical research in the evaluation and treatment of venous disease. Future editions of this volume will testify whether this mission has been accomplished.

REFERENCES

1. Linton RR: The post-thrombotic ulceration of the lower extremity: Its etiology and surgical treatment. Am J Surg 107:415–432, 1953.
2. Major RH: A History of Medicine. Vol 1. Oxford, Blackwell Scientific Publications, 1954.
3. Anning ST: Historical aspects. In Dodd H, Cockett FB (eds): The Pathophysiology and Surgery of Veins of the Lower Limb. Edinburgh, Livingstone, 1956.
4. Majno G: The Healing Hand. Cambridge, Mass, Harvard University Press, 1975.
5. Laufman H: The Veins. Austin, Tex, Silvergirl, Inc, 1986.
6. Browse NL, Burnand KG, Lea TM: Diseases of the Veins. London, EH Arnold, Publishers, 1988, pp 1–21.
7. Bergan JJ, Ballard JL: Historical perspectives. In Gloviczki P, Bergan JJ (eds): Atlas of Endoscopic Perforator Vein Surgery. London, Springer-Verlag, 1998, pp 5–13.
8. Bergan JJ, Cho JS, Weber J, Gloviczki P: Profiles. In Gloviczki P, Bergan JJ (eds): Atlas of Endoscopic Perforator Vein Surgery. London, Springer-Verlag, 1998.
9. Negus D: Leg Ulcers: A Practical Approach to Management. London, Butterworth-Heinemann, 1995, pp 3–10.
10. Hippocrates: The Genuine Works of Hippocrates. Adams EF, trans. Vol 2. New York, Wm Wood & Co, 1886, p 305.
11. Celsus AC: Of Medicine in Eight Books. Grieve J, trans. London, Wilson & Durham, 1756.

12. Walsh J: Galen's writings and influences inspiring them. Ann Med Hist Part I:14, 1934.

13. Mondeville H: de Chirurgie de Maitre Henri de Mondeville, Composé de 1306 à 1320. Nicalse A, trans. Paris, Alcan, 1893.

14. Friedenwald H. Amatus Lusitanus. Bull Inst Hist Med 5:644, 1937.

15. Hieronymus Fabricius de Aquapendente: Anatomici Patavini de Venarum Ostiolis [Valves of veins]. In Laufman H (ed): The Veins. Austin, Tex, Silvergirl, Inc, 1986, pp 14–24.

16. Harvey W: Exercitatio Anatomica de Motu Cordis et Sanguini in Animalibus. Frankfurt, W Fitzer, 1628.

17. Ferriar J: An affectation of the lymphatic vessels hitherto misunderstood. Medical Histories and Reflections 3:129, 1810

18. Davis DD: The proximate cause of phlegmasia dolens. Med Chir Trans 12:419, 1822.

19. Brodie BC: Lectures Illustrative of Various Subjects in Pathology and Surgery. London, Longman, Brown, Green & Longman, 1846.

20. Unna PG: Ueber Paraplaste eine neue Form Medikamentoser Pflaster. Wien Med Wochenschr 46:1854, 1896.

21. Virchow R: Die Cellular Pathologie. Berlin, Verlag von August Hirschwald, 1859.

22. Gay J: On Varicose Disease of the Lower Extremities. Lettsomian Lecture. London, Churchill, 1866.

23. Trendelenburg F: Uber die Unterbindung der Vena Saphena magna bie Unterschenkel Varicen. Beitr Z Clin Chir 7 195, 1891.

24. Keller WL: A new method of extirpating the internal saphenous and similar veins in varicose condition. N Y Med J 82:385, 1905.

25. Mayo CH: Treatment of varicose veins. Surg Gynecol Obstet 2:385, 1906.

26. Babcock WW: A new operation for extirpation of varicose veins of the leg. N Y Med J 86:153, 1907.

27. Carrel A, Guthrie CC: Uniterminal and biterminal venous transplantation. Surg Gynecol Obstet 2:266, 1906.

28. Homans J: The operative treatment of varicose veins and ulcers, based upon a classification of these lesions. Surg Gynecol Obstet 22:143, 1916.

29. Homans J: The aetiology and treatment of varicose ulcers of the leg. Surg Gynecol Obstet 24:300, 1917.

30. Berberich J, Hirsch S: Die roentgenographische Darstellung der Arterien und Venen am lebenden Menschen. Klin Wochenschr 2:2226, 1923.

31. Dos Santos JC: La phlébographie directe: Conception, technique, premier résultats. J Int Chir 3:625, 1938.

32. Bauer G: A venographic study of thromboembolic patients. Acta Chir Scand 84:Suppl 61, 1940.

33. Bauer G: Venous thrombosis: Early diagnosis with aid of phlebography and abortive treatment with heparin. Arch Surg 43:463, 1941.

34. Bauer G: A roentgenological and clinical study of the sequels of thrombosis. Acta Chir Scand 86:Suppl 74, 1942.

35. Tillett WS, Garner RL: The fibrinolytic activity of haemolytic streptococci. J Exp Med 58:485, 1933.

36. Crafoord C: Heparin and post-operative thrombosis. Acta Chir Scand 82:319, 1939.

37. Crafoord C, Jorpes E: Heparin as a prophylactic against thrombosis. JAMA 116:2831, 1941.

38. MacFarlane RG, Biggs R: Observations on fibrinolysis spontaneous activity associated with surgical operations and trauma. Lancet 2:862, 1946.

39. De Takats G: Anticoagulant therapy in surgery. JAMA 142:527, 1950.

40. Tillett WS, Johnson AJ, McCarty WR: The intravenous infusion of the streptococcal fibrinolytic principle (streptokinase) into patients. J Clin Invest 34:169, 1955.

41. Basy L: Thrombose de la veine axillaire droite (thrombo-phlébite par effort): Phlébotomie, ablation de caillots, suture de la veine. Mem Acad Chir 52:529, 1926.

42. Leriche R, Geisendorf W: Résultats d'une thrombectomie précoce avec résection veineuse dans une phlébite grave des deux membres inférieurs. Presse Med 47:1239, 1939.

43. Oschner A, DeBakey M: Therapy of phlebothrombosis and thrombophlebitis. South Surg 8:269, 1939.

44. Linton RR: The communicating veins of the lower leg and the operative technique for their ligation. Ann Surg 107:582, 1938.

45. Cockett FB, Jones DE: The ankle blow-out syndrome: A new approach of the varicose ulcer problem. Lancet 1:17, 1953.

46. Dodd H, Cockett FB (eds): The Pathophysiology and Surgery of Veins of the Lower Limb. Edinburgh, Livingstone, 1956.

47. May R, Partsch H, Staubesand J (eds): Perforating Veins. Munchen, Urban & Schwarzenberg, 1979.

48. Kunlin J: Les greffes veineuses. Lisbon, Congres Soc Internat de Chirurgie, September 1953.

49. Kunlin J, Kunlin A, Richard S, Tregouet T: Le remplacement et l'anastomose latéro-latérale des veines par greffon avec sutures suspendue par des anneaux: Etude expérimentale. J Chir (Paris) 85:305–337, 1953.

50. Warren R, Thayer T: Transplantation of the saphenous vein for postphlebitic stasis. Surgery 35:867, 1954.

51. Palma EC, Risi F, De Campo F: Tratamiento de los trastornos post-flebiticos mediante anastomosis venosa safeno-femoral contro-lateral. Bull Soc Surg Uruguay 29:135, 1958.

52. Dale WA, Harris J, Terry RB: Polytetrafluoroethylene reconstruction of the inferior vena cava. Surgery 95:625–630, 1984.

53. Kistner RL: Surgical repair of a venous valve. Straub Clin Proc 34:41–43, 1968.

54. Rosch J, Petersen BD, Lakin PC: Venous stents: Indications, techniques, results. In Perler BA, Becker GJ (eds): Vascular Intervention: A Clinical Approach. New York, Thieme, 1998, p 706.

55. Hauer G: The endoscopic subfascial division of the perforating veins—preliminary report (in German). Vasa 14:59–61, 1985.

56. Anderson FA Jr, Wheeler HB, Goldberg R, et al: A population-based perspective of the hospital incidence and case-fatality rates of deep vein thrombosis and pulmonary embolism: The Worcester Deep Venous Thrombosis Study. Arch Intern Med 151:933, 1991.

57. Jick H, Derby LE, Myers MW, et al: Risk of hospital admission for idiopathic venous thromboembolism among users of postmenopausal oestrogens. Lancet 348:981, 1996.

58. Nicolaides AN, Irving D: Clinical factors and the risk of deep venous thrombosis. In Nicolaides AN (ed): Thromboembolism: Aetiology, Advances in Prevention and Management. Lancaster, England, MTP Press, 1975.

59. Simioni P, Prandoni P, Lensing AW, et al: The risk of recurrent venous thromboembolism in patients with an Arg506→Gln mutation in the gene for factor V (factor V Leiden). N Engl J Med 336:399, 1997.

60. Ridker PM, Glynn RJ, Miletich JP, et al: Age-specific incidence rates of venous thromboembolism among heterozygous carriers of factor V Leiden mutation. Ann Intern Med 126:528, 1997.

61. Meissner MH, Manzo RA, Bergelin RO, et al: Deep venous insufficiency: The relationship between lysis and subsequent reflux. J Vasc Surg 18:596, 1993.

62. Comerota AJ, Katz ML, Greenwald LI, et al: Venous duplex imaging: Should it replace hemodynamic tests for deep venous thrombosis? J Vasc Surg 11:53, 1990.

63. Carpenter JP, Holland GA, Baum RA, Owen RS: Magnetic resonance venography for detection of deep venous thrombosis: Comparison with contrast venography and duplex Doppler ultrasonography. J Vasc Surg 18:734, 1993.

64. Rowbotham BJ, Carrol P, Whitaker AN, et al: Measurement of cross-linked fibrin derivatives: Use in the diagnosis of venous thrombosis. Thromb Haemost 57:59–61, 1987.

65. Ginsberg JS, Kearon C, Douketis J, et al: The use of D-dimer testing and impedance plethysmographic examination in patients with clinical indications of deep vein thrombosis. Arch Intern Med 157:1077, 1997.

66. Kakkar VV, Cohen AT, Edmonson RA, et al: Low molecular weight versus standard heparin for prevention of venous thromboembolism after major abdominal surgery. Lancet 341:259–265, 1993.

67. Kakkar VV, Boeckl O, Boneau B, et al: Efficacy and safety of a low molecular weight heparin and standard unfractionated heparin for prophylaxis of postoperative venous thromboembolism: European Multicenter Trial. World J Surg 21:2–9, 1997.

68. Bergqvist D, Matzsch T, Brumark U, et al: Low molecular weight heparin given the evening before surgery compared with conventional low dose heparin in prevention of thrombosis. Br J Surg 75:888–891, 1988.

69. Caen JP: A randomized double-blinded study between a low molecular weight heparin Kabi 2154 and standard heparin in the prevention of deep vein thrombosis in general surgery: A French Multicentre Trial. Thromb Haemost 59:216–220, 1988.

70. Bergqvist D, Burmark US, Flordal PA, et al: Low molecular weight heparin started before surgery as prophylaxis against deep vein thrombosis: 2500 versus 5000 XaI units in 2070 patients. Br J Surg 82:496–501, 1995.

71. Nurmohamed MT, Verhaeghe R, Haas S, et al: A comparative trial of a low molecular weight heparin (Enoxparin) versus standard heparin for the prophylaxis of postoperative deep vein thrombosis in general surgery. Am J Surg 169:567–571, 1995.

72. ENOXACAN Study Group: Efficacy and safety of enoxaparin versus unfractionated heparin for prevention of deep vein thrombosis in elective cancer surgery: A double-blind randomized multicentre trial with venographic assessment. Br J Surg 84:1099–1103, 1997.

73. Levine M, Gent M, Hirsh J, et al: A comparison of low molecular weight heparin administered primarily at home with unfractionated heparin administered in the hospital for proximal deep vein thrombosis. N Engl J Med 334:677–681, 1996.

74. Koopman MMW, Prandoni P, Piovella F, et al: Treatment of venous thrombosis with intravenous unfractionated heparin administered in the hospital as compared with subcutaneous low molecular weight heparin administered at home. N Engl J Med 334:682–687, 1996.

75. The Columbus Investigators: Low molecular weight heparin in the treatment of patients with venous thromboembolism. N Engl J Med 337:657–662, 1997.

76. Plate G, Einarsson E, Ohlin P, et al: Thrombectomy with temporary arteriovenous fistula: The treatment of choice in acute iliofemoral venous thrombosis. J Vasc Surg 1:867–876, 1984.

77. Plate G, Akesson H, Einarsson E, et al: Long-term results of venous thrombectomy combined with a temporary arteriovenous fistula. Eur J Vasc Surg 4:483–489, 1990.

78. Mewissen MW: Data presented at the Venous Registry Investigators Meeting, San Diego, September 1997.

79. Greenfield LJ, Michna BA: Twelve-year clinical experience with the Greenfield vena cava filter. Surgery 104:706, 1988.

80. Salzman EW, Hirsh J: The epidemiology, pathogenesis, and natural history of venous thrombosis. In Colman RW, Hirsh J, Mardr VJ, Salzman EW (eds): Hemostasis and Thrombosis: Basic Principles and Clinical Practice, 3rd ed. Philadelphia, JB Lippincott, 1994.

81. Coon WW, Willis PW, Keller JB: Venous thromboembolism and other venous disease in the Tecumseh Community Health Study. Circulation 48:839–846, 1973.

82. Burnand KG, Whimster I, Naidoo A, Browse NL: Pericapillary fibrin in the ulcer-bearing skin of the leg: The cause of lipodermatosclerosis and venous ulceration. Br Med J 285:1071, 1982.

83. Thomas PR, Nash GB, Dormandy JA: Increased white cell trapping in the dependent legs of patients with chronic venous insufficiency. J Mal Vasc 15:35, 1990.

84. Saharay M, Shields DA, Porter JB, et al: Leukocyte activity in the microcirculation of the leg in patients with chronic venous disease. J Vasc Surg 25:265, 1997.

85. Scott HJ, Coleridge Smith PD, Scurr JH: Histologic study of white blood cells and their association with lipodermatosclerosis and venous ulceration. Br J Surg 78:210, 1991.

86. Porter JM, Moneta GL, International Consensus Committee on Chronic Venous Disease: Reporting standards in venous disease: An update. J Vasc Surg 21:635–645, 1995.

87. The Consensus Group: Classification and grading of chronic venous disease in the lower limb: A consensus statement. Vasc Surg 30:5–11, 1996.

88. Kistner RL: Definitive diagnosis and definitive treatment in chronic venous disease: A concept whose time has come. J Vasc Surg 24:703–710, 1996.

89. Mayberry JC, Moneta GL, DeFrang RD, Porter JM: The influence of elastic compression stockings on deep venous hemodynamics. J Vasc Surg 13:91, 1991.

90. Mayberry JC, Moneta GL, Taylor LM, Porter JM: Fifteen-year results of ambulatory compression therapy for chronic venous ulcers. Surgery 109:575, 1991.

91. O'Donnell TF, Rosenthal DA, Callow AD, Ledig BL: The effect of elastic compression on venous hemodynamics in postphlebitic limbs. JAMA 242:2766, 1979.

92. Falanga V, Margolis D, Alvarez O, et al: Rapid healing of venous ulcers and lack of clinical rejection with an allogenic cultured human skin equivalent. Human Skin Equivalent Investigations Group. Arch Dermatol 134:293–300, 1998.

93. Erickson CA, Lanza DJ, Karp DL, et al: Healing of venous ulcers in an ambulatory care program: The roles of chronic venous insufficiency and patient compliance. J Vasc Surg 22:629–636, 1995.

94. Pierik EGJM, Wittens CHA, van Urk H: Subfascial endoscopic ligation in the treatment of incompetent perforating veins. Eur J Vasc Endovasc Surg 9:38–41, 1995.

95. Gloviczki P, Bergan JJ: Atlas of Endoscopic Perforator Vein Surgery. London, Springer-Verlag, 1998.

96. Burnand K, O'Donnell T, Lea MT, Browse NL: Relationship between post-phlebitic changes in deep veins and results of surgical treatment of venous ulcers. Lancet I:936–938, 1976.

97. Zukovsxky AJ, Nicolaides AN, Szendro G, et al: Haemodynamic significance of incompetent calf perforating vein. Br J Surg 78:625–629, 1991.

98. Gloviczki P, Bergan JJ, Menawat SS, et al: Safety, feasibility, and early efficacy of subfascial endoscopic perforator surgery (SEPS): A preliminary report from the North American Registry. J Vasc Surg 25:94–105, 1997.

99. Gloviczki P, Bergan JJ, Rhodes JM, et al: Mid-term results of endoscopic perforator vein interruption for chronic venous insufficiency: Lessons learned from the North American Subfascial Endoscopic Perforator Surgery (NASEPS) Registry. J Vasc Surg 1998. 29:489–499, 1999.

100. Masuda E, Kistner RL: Long-term results of venous valve reconstruction: A 14- to 21-year follow-up. J. Vasc Surg 19:391–403, 1994.

101. Raju S: New approaches to the diagnosis and treatment of venous obstruction. J Vasc Surg 4:42–54, 1986.

102. Raju S, Fredericks RK, Neglen PN, Bass JD: Durability of venous valve reconstruction techniques for "primary" and postthrombotic reflux. J Vasc Surg 23:357–367, 1996.

103. Sottiurai VS: Results of deep-vein reconstruction. Vasc Surg 31:276–278, 1997.

104. Gloviczki P, Pairolero PC, Toomey BJ, et al: Reconstruction of large veins for nonmalignant venous occlusive disease. J Vasc Surg 16:750, 1992.

105. Gruss JD: Venous bypass for chronic venous insufficiency. In Bergan JJ, Yao JT (eds): Venous Disorders. Philadelphia, WB Saunders, 1991, pp 316–330.

106. Palma EC, Esperon R: Vein transplants and grafts in the surgical treatment of the postphlebitic syndrome. J Cardiovasc Surg 1:94, 1960.

107. Dale WA, Harris J: Cross-over vein grafts for iliac and femoral venous occlusion. J Cardiovasc Surg 10:458, 1969.

108. Halliday P, Harris J, May J: Femoro-femoral crossover grafts (Palma operation): A long-term follow-up study. In Bergan JJ, Yao JST (ed): Surgery of the Veins. Orlando, Fla, Grune & Stratton, 1985, pp 241–254.

109. AbuRahma AF, Robinson PA, Boland JP: Clinical hemodynamic and anatomic predictors of long-term outcome of lower extremity veno-venous bypasses. J Vasc Surg 14:635, 1991.

110. Stanson AW, Breen JF: Computed tomography and magnetic resonance imaging. In Gloviczki P, Yao JST (eds): Handbook of Venous Disorders: Guidelines of the American Venous Forum. London, Chapman & Hall, 1996, pp 190–232.

111. Dzsinich C, Gloviczki P, van Heerden JA, et al: Primary venous leiomyosarcoma: A rare but lethal disease. J Vasc Surg 15:595–603, 1992.

112. Bower TC: Primary and secondary tumors of the inferior vena cava. In Gloviczki P, Yao JST (eds): Handbook of Venous Disorders: Guidelines of the American Venous Forum. pp 529–550.

113. Bower TC, Nagorney DM, Toomey BJ, et al: Vena cava replacement for malignant disease: Is there a role? Ann Surg 7:51–62, 1993.

114. Neves RJ, Zincke H: Surgical treatment of renal cancer with vena cava extension. Br J Urol 59:390–395, 1987.

115. Alimi YS, Gloviczki P, Vrtiska TJ, et al: Reconstruction of the superior vena cava: Benefits of postoperative surveillance and secondary endovascular interventions. J Vasc Surg 27:287–299, 1998.

116. Dartevelle PG, Chapelier AR, Pastorino U, et al: Long-term follow-up after prosthetic replacement of the superior vena cava combined with resection of mediastinal-pulmonary malignant tumors. J Thorac Cardiovasc Surg 102:259–265, 1991.

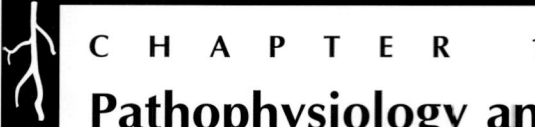

C H A P T E R   1 3 8

Pathophysiology and Natural History of Acute Deep Venous Thrombosis

Mark H. Meissner, M.D., and D. Eugene Strandness, Jr., M.D.

The complications of acute deep venous thrombosis (DVT), pulmonary embolism, and the post-thrombotic syndrome are important not only as the most common preventable cause of hospital death[89] but also as a source of substantial long-term morbidity.[11, 28, 197] An understanding of the underlying epidemiology, pathophysiology, and natural history of DVT is essential in guiding appropriate prophylaxis, diagnosis, and treatment. Recognition of the underlying risk factors and an appreciation of the multifactorial nature of DVT may facilitate the identification of situations likely to provoke thrombosis in high-risk individuals as well as the further evaluation of those with unexplained thromboembolism. An understanding of the natural history of DVT is similarly important in defining the relative risk and benefits of anticoagulation as well as the duration of treatment in individual patients.

Components of the pathophysiologic triad initially described by Rudolph Virchow remain applicable today. However, an improved understanding of the coagulation and fibrinolytic systems, as well as the role of the vascular endothelium in thrombosis and hemostasis, has led to the identification of new prethrombotic conditions and also a more thorough appreciation of previously recognized risk factors. Furthermore, accurate and repeatable noninvasive diagnostic methods, such as duplex ultrasonography, have allowed the pathophysiology to be related to the natural history of deep venous thrombosis. It now appears that many venous thrombi arise from the convergence of several risk factors against a background of imbalanced coagulation and fibrinolysis. Similar factors defining the balance between recanalization of the venous lumen and recurrent thrombotic events also may be important determinants of long-term outcome after an episode of acute DVT.

EPIDEMIOLOGY

Precise definition of the incidence of acute DVT is complicated by the clinically silent nature of most thromboses in hospitalized patients as well as the nonspecific signs and symptoms.[6, 31, 69, 94] The incidence depends on the population studied, the intensity of screening, and the accuracy of the diagnostic tests employed. Autopsy studies, which are biased by inclusion of the very sick and old, have reported the prevalence of DVT to be 35% to 52%.[61, 118] Most clinical trials and studies on the incidence of acute DVT have focused on specific inpatient groups such as postoperative patients. Although useful in defining risk

factors for acute DVT, such studies provide few data regarding the overall prevalence of acute DVT. Community-based studies may provide a better estimate of overall prevalence but frequently suffer from a lack of objective documentation of DVT. Extrapolating data from a longitudinal community-based study, Coon and associates calculated an incidence of 250,000 cases of acute DVT per year in the United States.[28] These results, however, were based largely on questionnaires and clinical findings suggestive of previous DVT. Community-based studies of venographically documented symptomatic DVT have reported a yearly incidence of 1.6 per 1000 residents.[153] Among men, the cumulative probability of suffering a thromboembolic event is estimated to be 10.7% by the age of 80 years.[72]

PATHOPHYSIOLOGY

Venous Thrombogenesis

As initially postulated by Virchow, three factors are of primary importance in the development of venous thrombosis: (1) abnormalities of blood flow, (2) abnormalities of blood, and (3) vascular injury. These tenets have subsequently been refined, and it currently appears that flow abnormalities determine the localization of venous thrombi, that abnormalities of blood may include aberrations of both the coagulation and fibrinolytic systems, and that biologic injury to the venous endothelium is potentially more important than gross trauma. It also clear, however, that the origin of DVT is frequently multifactorial, with components of Virchow's triad assuming variable importance in individual patients.

Mechanical venous injury clearly plays a role in thrombosis associated with direct venous trauma,[39, 207] hip arthroplasty,[193, 202] and central venous catheters.[235] Central venous cannulation is largely responsible for the increasing incidence of upper extremity thrombosis while similar venous injury is presumably responsible for the observation that 57% of thrombi following hip arthroplasty arise from the femoral vein rather than the usual site in the calf.[202] However, the importance of mechanical venous injury in other situations is questionable. Focal venous injury cannot account for the observations that thromboses in trauma patients are more commonly bilateral (77%) than unilateral (23%) and may be as frequent in an injured limb as in an uninjured limb.[192] Neither do mechanical crush injuries in animal models usually cause thrombosis, even when followed by stasis.[5, 212] Overt endothelial injury likely is neither necessary nor sufficient to cause thrombosis in the absence of other stimuli.[212, 231]

The potential role of biochemical injury to the venous endothelium has only recently become apparent.[125] The normal venous endothelium is antithrombotic, producing prostaglandin I_2 (PGI_2, prostacyclin), glycosaminoglycan cofactors of antithrombin, thrombomodulin, and tissue-type plasminogen activator (t-PA).[22] However, the endothelium may become prothrombotic under some conditions, producing tissue factor, von Willebrand factor, and fibronectin. It is conceivable that some thrombotic risk factors act through production of a procoagulant endothelium. Microscopic changes in the endothelial surface associated with increased endothelial permeability and leukocyte adhesion have been demonstrated in response to distant surgical injury.[204] Induction of procoagulant activity, suppression of anticoagulant mechanisms and exposure of neutrophil receptor ligands may accompany such endothelial perturbation.[147, 203]

Associated inflammatory cells may be capable of both initiating and amplifying thrombosis.[228] The importance of cytokine-mediated expression of tissue factor procoagulant activity under clinical conditions is unknown, but both interleukin-1 (IL-1) and tumor necrosis factor (TNF) may induce fibrin deposition through a combination of endothelial procoagulant expression and fibrinolytic depression.[138, 147, 210] TNF also may downregulate endothelial thrombomodulin expression, further converting the endothelium from an antithrombotic to a procoagulant state.[228] In such situations, Virchow's concept of venous injury may be more important at the molecular than the macroscopic level.

Regardless of etiology, most venous thrombi originate in areas of low blood flow, either in the soleal veins of the calf[61, 95, 150] or behind valve pockets.[191] Furthermore, many risk factors for acute DVT are associated with immobilization and slow venous flow, and several mechanisms have been advanced to explain the role of stasis in thrombogenesis. In comparison with pulsatile flow, static streamline flow is associated with profound hypoxia at the depths of the venous valve cusps and may induce endothelial injury.[70] The effects of hypoxia in cultured endothelial cells have been noted to include stimulation of cytokine production and leukocyte adhesion molecule expression,[194] perhaps accounting for the adhesion and migration of leukocytes observed in association with stasis.[211] Furthermore, stasis also allows the accumulation of activated coagulation factors and the consumption of inhibitors at sites prone to thrombosis. Stasis in the large veins may be particularly important, since the low surface-to-volume ratio may prevent interaction with endothelial inhibitory pathways, particularly the endothelium-bound thrombomodulin–protein C system.[210]

Despite these observations, there is little evidence that stasis can activate coagulation and in isolation appears to be an inadequate stimulus for thrombosis.[14, 211] Experimental ligation of the rabbit jugular vein for intervals of 10 to 60 minutes has consistently failed to cause thrombosis.[5, 211, 232] From a clinical perspective, activation of coagulation during hip arthroplasty is associated with manipulation of the femoral component rather than simply occlusion of the femoral vein.[193] Stasis should thus perhaps be viewed as a

permissive factor in venous thrombosis, localizing activated coagulation to thrombosis-prone sites.

Activation of coagulation appears to be of critical importance in the pathogenesis of DVT. The coagulation cascade functions through serial activation of zymogens in the intrinsic and tissue factor pathways, with the ultimate generation of thrombin by the prothrombinase complex. Antithrombin and the thrombomodulin–protein C systems are the primary inhibitors of coagulation, whereas the fibrinolytic system serves to further limit fibrin deposition. Although the hemostatic system is continuously active, thrombus formation is ordinarily confined to sites of local injury by a precise balance between activators and inhibitors of coagulation and fibrinolysis. A prethrombotic state may result either from imbalances in the regulatory and inhibitory systems or from activation exceeding antithrombotic capacity.[3]

Although measurement of zymogen levels and in vitro clotting assays has not proved fruitful in defining prethrombotic states, identification of activated coagulation has been facilitated by the development of sensitive assays for stable by-products of thrombin activation.[7] The most useful of these have included:

- Prothrombin fragment F1+2 generated by factor Xa in the cleavage of prothrombin to thrombin
- Fibrinopeptide A formed in the thrombin-mediated conversion of fibrinogen to fibrin
- Thrombin-antithrombin complex formed by the combination of thrombin with its primary inhibitor

Increased levels of these markers have been described in association with risk factors including surgery,[96, 103] oral contraceptives,[171, 226] and malignancy.[50]

Just as the combination of stasis and injury may be ineffective in causing thrombosis without low levels of activated coagulation factors,[5] activated coagulation alone may be insufficient to provoke thrombosis. Activated coagulation factors are ordinarily rapidly cleared from the circulation. When localized in regions of stasis, however, the coagulation cascade allows activated factors to rapidly amplify the thrombotic stimulus, leading to platelet aggregation and fibrin formation.[5, 210] DVT thus appears to be a multifactorial phenomenon, with convergence of several pathologic factors often required to produce a thrombotic event.[179]

Although infusion of activated coagulation factors alone may not cause thrombosis, infusion of TNF and antibody to protein C, combined with low flow and subtle catheter injury, consistently produces proximal venous thrombosis in a baboon model.[228] In a similar fashion, the thrombogenic potential of hip arthroplasty derives from the combination of injury to the femoral vein, venous occlusion, and measurable activation of coagulation during placement of the femoral component.[193] The existence of a prethrombotic state prior to the precipitation of overt thrombosis is also well recognized.[7, 159] Increased thrombin activity may precede the development of a positive leg scan in surgical patients by several days,[159] whereas thrombosis in patients with congenital thrombophilias is often precipitated by events such as injury, surgery, or pregnancy.[177]

Early Course

Against this pathophysiologic background, the factors contributing to clinically important thrombosis have been most thoroughly evaluated in the valve pockets of the lower extremity veins. In flow models, primary and secondary vortices are produced beyond the valve cusps, which tend to trap red cells in a low shear field near the apex of the cusp.[98] The early nidus for thrombus formation likely consists of red blood cell aggregates forming within these eddies; however, these aggregates are probably transient until stabilized by fibrin in the setting of locally activated coagulation. The further events in the evolution of these thrombi have been described by Sevitt in a series of detailed histologic studies.[190, 191]

Once formed in the valve pocket, early thrombi may become adherent to the endothelium near the apex of the valve cusp. These valve pocket thrombi appear to form on structurally normal endothelium and largely spare the valve cusp. Laminated appositional growth may then occur outward from the apex of the cusp, with propagation beyond the valve pocket likely depending on the relative balance between activated coagulation and thrombolysis. Once luminal flow is disturbed, prograde and retrograde propagation may occur.

Clinical symptoms, present in a minority of hospitalized patients, develop only when a sufficient fraction of the venous outflow is occluded. If present, such symptoms appear 24 to 36 hours after the first appearance of thrombus detectable by radioactive iodine (^{125}I)-fibrinogen scanning.[95] Conversely, early thrombi may fail to propagate, with evidence of aborted thrombi appearing as endothelialized fibrin fragments within the valve pockets.[190, 191] A significant number of these early thrombi spontaneously resolve after serial ^{125}I-fibrinogen scanning.[42, 94]

RISK FACTORS

DVT occurring in the setting of a recognized risk factor is often defined as *secondary*, whereas that occurring in the absence of risk factors is termed *primary* or *idiopathic*.[26] Recognized risk factors for DVT are listed in Table 138–1.

The high incidence of acute DVT in hospitalized patients, the availability of objective diagnostic tests, and the existence of clinical trials evaluating prophylactic measures have allowed identification of high-risk groups in this population. In contrast, the risk factors for acute DVT have been less well defined in population-based studies. Substantial differences, however, have been noted in the distribution of risk factors between inpatients and outpatients.[164] Malignancy, surgery, and trauma within the previous 3 months remain significant risk factors for outpatient thrombosis, whereas the frequency of surgery and malignancy are higher among inpatients with DVT.[26, 157] Approximately 47% of outpatients with a documented DVT have one or more recognized risk factors,[26] with the incidence of venous thromboembolism increasing with the number of risk factors.[4] Although some investigators[157] have found the risk of acute DVT to be significantly higher only for those with three or more risk factors, others[179] have reported the relative risk to increase progressively from 2.4 in those with

TABLE 138–1. RISK FACTORS FOR ACUTE DEEP VENOUS THROMBOSIS

RISK FACTOR	DEGREE OF SUPPORT*	REFERENCE
Advanced age	Epidemiologic	32, 78, 164
Immobilization	Epidemiologic	66, 208, 244
Previous venous thromboembolism	Epidemiologic	103, 164, 176, 211
Malignancy	Epidemiologic	150, 164, 176
Surgery	Epidemiologic	28
Trauma	Epidemiologic	63, 138, 205
Primary hypercoagulable states	Epidemiologic	132, 156, 198
Pregnancy	Epidemiologic	18, 32, 107, 131, 192, 230
Oral contraceptives and estrogen therapy	Epidemiologic	58, 74, 119, 174, 183, 194, 219, 237
Blood group	Epidemiologic	99, 155, 164
Geography and ethnicity	Circumstantial/ epidemiologic	27, 71, 226
Central venous catheters	Circumstantial	84, 89, 147
Inflammatory bowel disease	Circumstantial	97, 117
Systemic lupus erythematosus	Circumstantial	130, 241
Cardiac disease	Equivocal	120, 162, 212
Obesity	Equivocal	98, 160, 174

*Risk factors stratified based on consistent epidemiologic findings, a strong circumstantial association between the risk factor and venous thromboembolism, or equivocal results among epidemiologic studies.

1 risk factor to greater than 20 among subjects with three or more risk factors.

Age

Venous thromboembolism occurs in both the young and the elderly, although an increased incidence has consistently been associated with advanced age. Some investigators have identified precise cut-off points at which the risk of DVT is increased, whereas others have reported a progressive increase with advancing age. In a community-based study of phlebographically documented DVT, the yearly incidence of DVT was noted to increase progressively from almost 0 in childhood to 7.65 cases in men older than 80 years and 8.22 cases in women the same ages, per 1000.[153] The incidence of DVT increased 30-fold from age 30 years to 80 or more years. Rosendaal[179] similarly noted an incidence of 0.006 per 1000 children under age 14 years, increasing to 0.7 among adults 40 to 54 years of age, and Hansson and colleagues[72] found the prevalence of objectively documented thromboembolic events among men to increase from 0.5% at age 50 years to 3.8% at age 80 years.

The influence of age on the incidence of venous thromboembolism is likely multifactorial. The number of thrombotic risk factors increases with age, three or more risk factors being present in only 3% of hospitalized patients younger than age 40 years but in 30% of those aged 40 years and older.[4] Furthermore, it appears that the number of risk factors required to precipitate thrombosis decreases with age.[179] This may be related to an acquired prethrombotic state associated with aging, since increased levels of thrombin activation markers are found among older people.[209] Advanced age also has been associated with anatomic changes in the soleal veins and more pronounced stasis in the venous valve pockets.[61, 129]

Venous diseases, including venous thromboembolism, are usually regarded as rare in children younger than 10 years of age.[28] Population-based studies have suggested an incidence of 0.006 per 1000 children less than age 14 years,[179] whereas the incidence in hospitalized children under age 18 years has been estimated to be 0.05%.[178] Early mobilization and discharge may partially explain the lower incidence in children.[178] The diagnosis, however, is often not considered in pediatric patients, and few studies have systematically evaluated children for DVT.

Venous thromboembolism in children is almost always associated with recognized thrombotic risk factors,[17, 27, 179, 234] and multiple risk factors are often required to precipitate thrombosis.[179] Venous thrombosis is more common in some pediatric populations, such as children hospitalized in the intensive care unit, those with spinal cord injuries, and those with prolonged orthopedic immobilization, although the incidence is substantially less than in corresponding adult populations. DVT may occur in as many as 3.7% of pediatric patients immobilized in halo-femoral traction for preoperative treatment of scoliosis;[116] 4% of children hospitalized in the intensive care unit;[37] and 10% of children with spinal cord injuries.[128, 172] Symptomatic postoperative DVT is regarded as unusual in children, although there are few data from studies employing routine surveillance,[148] and autopsy-identified pulmonary embolism is approximately four times more frequent in postoperative patients than in the general pediatric medical population.[17] Other thrombotic risk factors in hospitalized children have been noted to include local infection and trauma, immobilization,[234] inherited hypercoagulable states,[179] oral contraceptive use,[9] lower limb paresis,[116] and the use of femoral venous catheters.[37]

Immobilization

Many of the clinical circumstances in which thromboembolism occurs support the role of immobilization as a risk factor. Stasis in the soleal veins and behind the valve cusps is exacerbated by advancing age and inactivity of the calf muscle pump,[129] both of which are associated with an increased risk of DVT. The prevalence of lower extremity DVT in autopsy studies also parallels the duration of bed rest, with an increase during the first 3 days of confinement rapidly rising to very high levels after 2 weeks. DVT was found in 15% of patients dying after 0 to 7 days of bed rest, in comparison with 79% to 94% of those dying after 2 to 12 weeks.[61] Preoperative immobilization is similarly associated with a twofold increased risk of postoperative DVT,[195] and DVT among stroke patients is significantly more common in paralyzed or paretic extremities (53% of limbs) than in nonparalyzed limbs (7%).[229]

Immobilization as a thrombotic risk factor has sometimes been extended to include prolonged travel, particularly the "economy class syndrome" arising after sitting in a cramped position during extended aircraft flights.[32] Several case series have reported the occurrence of pulmonary embolism in relation to extended travel,[32, 82, 115, 156, 182, 208] but none have rigorously examined the prevalence relative to that in the general population, and few have thoroughly reported the presence of coexisting risk factors. A high prevalence of preexisting venous disease and other thrombotic risk factors among this group has sometimes been noted.[208, 209] The questionable importance of prolonged travel is supported by observations that extreme degrees of venous stasis alone may fail to produce thrombosis[231] and that no consistent rheologic or prothrombotic changes have been demonstrated during prolonged travel.[113, 209] However, the observation that pulmonary embolism is the second leading cause of travel-related mortality, accounting for 18% of 61 deaths, suggests that such a relationship cannot be entirely excluded.[182]

History of Venous Thromboembolism

Approximately 23% to 26% of patients presenting with an acute DVT have a previous history of thrombosis,[153, 164] and histologic studies confirm that acute thrombi are often associated with fibrous remnants of previous thrombi in the same or nearby veins.[189] Depending on sex and age, population-based studies have demonstrated that recurrent thromboembolism occurs once in every 11 to 50 persons with a previous episode of thromboembolism.[28] The risk of recurrent thromboembolism is higher among patients with idiopathic DVT.[198] The relative importance of disordered venous hemodynamics, residual damage to the venous wall, and underlying abnormalities of the coagulation and fibrinolytic systems in recurrent thrombosis is unknown. However, primary hypercoagulability appears to have a significant role in many recurrences. The cumulative incidence of recurrent thrombosis among patients heterozygous for the factor V Leiden mutation is 40% at 8 years of follow-up, 2.4-fold higher than in those without the mutation.[198] Other investigators[38] estimated that 17% of recurrent thromboembolic events may be due to hyperhomocyst(e)inemia. A similar relationship between impaired fibrinolysis and recurrent DVT has been suggested by several investigators, although the methodologic validity of these findings has been questioned.[169]

Malignancy

A recognized malignancy is present in 19% to 30% of patients with DVT.[140, 153, 164] Approximately 15% of malignancies are complicated by venous thromboembolism, with a substantially higher prevalence in autopsy studies.[50] An association between mucin-secreting gastrointestinal tumors and thrombosis has long been recognized. However, carcinoma of the lung is more prevalent and is now the most common tumor associated with venous thromboembolism, accounting for one quarter of cases.[175] Although more than half the tumors underlying episodes of venous thromboembolism are located in the genitourinary and gastrointestinal systems,[153] thrombosis has been reported to accompany a wide variety of malignancies. The frequency of any individual malignancy likely depends on referral patterns, treatment, and intensity of screening.

DVT may also herald a previously undetected malignancy in 3% to 23% of patients with idiopathic thrombosis.[29, 140, 167] In another 5% to 11% of patients, malignancy appears within 1 to 2 years of presentation.[152, 153, 167] Although small studies have reported no difference between patients in whom diagnostic studies confirm or exclude thromboembolism,[29, 67] several other series have documented a significantly increased risk of malignancy in patients with idiopathic DVT. Among such patients, 7.6% have been noted to develop a malignancy during follow-up, with an odds ratio of 2:3 in comparison to those with secondary thrombosis.[167] The incidence of occult malignancy diagnosed within 6 to 12 months of an idiopathic DVT is 2.2 to 5.3 times higher than that expected from general population estimates.[152, 201] Recurrent idiopathic DVT is associated with a 9.8-fold increased risk in comparison to secondary thrombosis, a subsequent malignancy being identified in 17.1% of such patients.[167]

The thrombogenic mechanisms associated with cancer may be heterogeneous, but likely they involve release of substances that directly or indirectly activate coagulation. Tissue factor and cancer procoagulant, a cysteine protease activator of factor X, are the primary tumor cell procoagulants; associated macrophages may also produce procoagulants as well as inflammatory cytokines.[49, 176] As many as 90% of patients with cancer have abnormal coagulation results, including increased levels of coagulation factors, elevated fibrinogen or fibrin degradation products, and thrombocytosis.[48, 50, 176] Elevated fibrinogen levels and thrombocytosis are the most common abnormalities, perhaps reflecting an overcompensated form of intravascular coagulation.[45, 175] Levels of the coagulation inhibitors antithrombin, protein C, and protein S also may be reduced in malignancy.[176]

The clinical significance of these abnormalities is suggested by observations that markers of activated coagulation are elevated in the majority of patients with solid tumors and leukemia.[45, 50, 51, 176] Fibrinopeptide A levels reflect tumor activity, decreasing or increasing in response to treatment or progression of disease, suggesting that tumor growth and thrombin generation are intimately related.[45, 176] Furthermore, these levels may fail to normalize after administration of heparin to cancer patients with DVT, perhaps explaining why they may be refractory to anticoagulants.[175]

Venous thromboembolism is also associated with the treatment of some cancers. DVT complicates 29% of general surgical procedures for malignancy.[24] Preoperative activation of the coagulation system, as reflected by elevated thrombin-antithrombin complex levels, is associated with a 7.5-fold greater risk of postoperative DVT.[48, 51] Some chemotherapeutic regimens also predispose to DVT, and thrombotic complications may be as common as the more widely recognized infectious complications.[117] Venous thromboembolism has been reported in up to 6% of patients undergoing treatment for non-Hodgkin's lymphoma, 17.5% of those receiving therapy for breast cancer, and in patients being treated for germ cell tumors.[40] Among patients with stage II breast cancer, thrombosis was significantly more common among patients randomized to 36 weeks of chemotherapy (8.8%) than among those receiving only 12 weeks of treatment (4.9%).[117] Potential thrombogenic mechanisms associated with chemotherapy include

direct endothelial toxicity, induction of a hypercoagulable state, reduced fibrinolytic activity, tumor cell lysis, and use of central venous catheters.[25, 40] Some intravenous chemotherapeutic agents are associated with activation of coagulation and increased markers of thrombin generation, a response that is blocked by pretreatment with heparin.[44]

Surgery

The high incidence of postoperative DVT, as well as the availability of easily repeatable, noninvasive diagnostic tests such as ^{125}I-labeled fibrinogen scanning, have allowed a greater understanding of the risk factors associated with surgery than have most other conditions. Surgery constitutes a spectrum of risk that is influenced by patient age, coexistent thrombotic risk factors, type of procedure, extent of surgical trauma, length of procedure, and duration of postoperative immobilization.[23, 125] The type of surgical procedure is particularly important.[195] The overall incidence of DVT is approximately 19% in patients undergoing general surgical operations; 24% for elective neurosurgical procedures; and 48%, 51%, and 61% among those undergoing surgery for hip fracture, hip arthroplasty, and knee arthroplasty, respectively.[23] On the basis of these data, patients can be classified as being at low, moderate, or high risk for thromboembolic complications, as shown in Table 138–2.

Approximately half of postoperative lower extremity thrombi detected by ^{125}I-labeled fibrinogen scanning develop in the operating room, with the remainder occurring over the next 3 to 5 days.[95] However, the risk for development of DVT does not end uniformly at hospital discharge. Among gynecologic patients, 51% of thromboembolic events occurred after initial discharge.[122] Similarly, up to 25% of patients undergoing abdominal surgery have been noted to have DVT within 6 weeks of discharge.[187]

All components of Virchow's triad may be present in the surgical patient—perioperative immobilization, transient changes in coagulation and fibrinolysis, and the potential for gross venous injury, as exemplified by hip arthroplasty. Immobilization is associated with a reduction in venous outflow and capacitance during the early postoperative period.[218] Surgery is also accompanied by a transient, low-level hypercoagulable state, presumably mediated by the release of tissue factor, marked by a rise in thrombin

TABLE 138–2. RISK OF POSTOPERATIVE DEEP VENOUS THROMBOSIS

CATEGORY	CHARACTERISTICS
Low	Age < 40 years, no other risk factors, uncomplicated abdominal/thoracic surgery Age > 40 years, no other risk factors, minor elective abdominal/thoracic surgery < 30 min
Moderate	Age > 40 years, abdominal/thoracic surgery > 30 min
High	History of recent thromboembolism Abdominal or pelvic procedure for malignancy Major lower extremity orthopedic procedure

From Hull RD, Raskob GE, Hirsh J: Prophylaxis of venous thromboembolism. Chest 89(5) Suppl:374S–383S, 1986.

activation markers shortly after the procedure begins.[96] The thrombogenic potential of surgical procedures appears to differ, with greater rises in thrombin activation markers during hip arthroplasty than after laparotomy.[193] Increased plasminogen activator inhibitor (PAI)-1 levels are also associated with a decrease in fibrinolytic activity on the first postoperative day, the "postoperative fibrinolytic shutdown."[47, 103] The relationship between impaired fibrinolysis and postoperative DVT may be particularly important,[169] with elevated preoperative and early postoperative PAI-1 correlating with the development of thrombosis in orthopedic patients.[47]

Trauma

Despite improvements in trauma care and thromboembolism prophylaxis, DVT remains a significant source of morbidity and mortality in the injured patient. The prevalence of DVT among autopsied trauma casualties has been reported to be 62% to 65%,[71, 192] comparable to the 58% incidence among injured patients in modern venographic series.[58] Substantially lower DVT rates of 4% to 20%[19, 105, 106, 146, 183, 219] have been noted in series employing duplex ultrasonography, although many patients were receiving prophylaxis and the limitations of ultrasound in screening asymptomatic patients are well recognized.

Although the risk of DVT may be less than 20% in as few as 8% of injured patients,[58] certain subgroups are at particularly high risk. Age (odds ratio of 1.05 for each 1-year increment), blood transfusion (1.74), surgery (2.30), fracture of the femur or tibia (4.82), and spinal cord injury (8.59) have been significantly associated with the development of DVT in this population.[58] Other reported risk factors include a hospital stay of greater than 7 days,[146] increased Injury Severity Score (ISS),[76, 146] Trauma Injury Severity Score (TRISS) of 85 or less,[146] pelvic fractures,[106] major venous injury,[39, 207] femoral venous lines,[107] the duration of immobilization,[105, 106, 146] and prolongation of the partial thromboplastin time.[105]

As with postoperative DVT, several pathophysiologic elements may be responsible for the high incidence of DVT in trauma patients. Immobilization by skeletal fixation, paralysis, and critical illness are obviously associated with venous stasis, whereas mechanical injury is important following direct venous trauma and central venous cannulation. Less well appreciated may be the hypercoagulable state following depletion of coagulation inhibitors and components of the fibrinolytic system. Fibrinopeptide A levels increase following injury,[56] consistent with activation of coagulation, whereas fibrinolytic activity has been found to increase initially and then decrease.[57, 97]

Primary Hypercoagulable States

Primary hypercoagulable states represent discrete genetic mutations and include inherited deficiencies of the naturally occurring anticoagulants antithrombin (antithrombin III), protein C, and protein S; resistance to activated protein C (APC); hyperhomocyst(e)inemia; and several potential defects in fibrinolysis. Overall, 42% to 46% of patients with a lower extremity DVT can be characterized as thrombophilic on this basis, and a positive family history is

associated with a relative risk of 2.9 for venous thromboembolism.[15, 77] Most of the thrombotic events occurring in association with these disorders are venous in origin.[185] Although occasionally associated with thrombosis in unusual sites, hypercoagulable states appear to be less important as a risk factor for upper extremity thrombosis, with a prevalence (15%) similar to that in control populations.[78] Heterozygous protein C and protein S deficiency have also been associated with warfarin (Coumadin)-induced skin necrosis.[145]

The natural anticoagulation systems, including antithrombin, the protein C system, and tissue factor pathway inhibitor, are the primary inhibitors of thrombin generation and activity.[145] Antithrombin inhibits thrombin as well as factors Xa, IXa, XIa and XIIa, actions that are accelerated by heparin and heparin-like glycosaminoglycans on the endothelial surface. The protein C–protein S–thrombomodulin system is a negative feedback system initiated by the binding of thrombin to thrombomodulin at the endothelial surface, with subsequent activation of protein C and degradation of activated factors V and VIII. Factors Va and VIIIa function as critical cofactors for factors Xa and IXa, respectively, increasing their activity more than 1000-fold.[33] Protein S, approximately 60% of which is bound to C4b-binding protein, in its free form functions as a nonenzymatic cofactor of activated protein C. In addition to congenital deficiencies, acquired antithrombin, protein C, and protein S deficiencies may accompany liver disease, the nephrotic syndrome, disseminated intravascular coagulation (DIC), and chemotherapy with L-asparaginase.[145] Thrombotic tendencies caused by abnormal tissue factor pathway inhibitor have not yet been described.[185]

Primary deficiencies of the coagulation inhibitors antithrombin, protein C, and protein S are present in approximately 0.5% of healthy subjects.[233] Although these are generally regarded as autosomal dominant traits, the observation that some heterozygotes are minimally affected while homozygotes have severe thrombotic manifestations suggests a recessive component in some types of protein C deficiency.[33] In aggregate, these three deficiencies may be associated with 5% to 10% of thrombotic events.[33] Patients with heterozygous deficiency states often present with a first thrombotic event before age 40 years, approximately 50% of such events being related to predisposing situations such as surgery or trauma.[63] Associated thrombotic episodes are often recurrent and may occur at unusual sites, such as in the mesenteric and cerebral veins.[123]

However, the phenotypic expression of these deficiencies may vary both within and between families. A multitude of mutations in the genes coding for these proteins may lead to either quantitative (type I) or qualitative (type II) deficiencies.[1] A type III protein S deficiency is further characterized by low free-protein S levels with normal total antigen levels.[33] Although approximately 50% of individuals with these deficiencies may have a history of venous thrombosis,[63, 123] the frequency of thrombotic manifestations within different kindreds may range from 15% to 100% for antithrombin deficiency[185] and is less than 50% in some protein C–deficient families.[1, 185] It has been hypothesized that multigene interactions may be partially responsible for such phenotypic variability.[185] The factor V Leiden mutation may be particularly important in this regard, with a higher frequency of thrombotic manifestations among the 9.5% to 19% of protein C heterozygotes who also carry this mutation.[1, 123]

Resistance to activated protein C, characterized by the failure of exogenous activated protein C to prolong the activated partial thromboplastin time, was initially described in 1993. It is now recognized that a single point mutation in the factor V gene, resulting in replacement of arginine 506 with glutamine (factor V Leiden; FV:R506Q), is present in 94% of individuals with activated protein C resistance.[10, 33, 123] Factor Va is inactivated by protein C–mediated cleavage at the Arg 306 and Arg 506 sites; this mutation thus renders factor Va less sensitive to degradation by activated protein C. The factor V Leiden mutation has an autosomal dominant mode of inheritance and is at least ten times more common than other inheritable defects.[33, 109] The frequency of the mutation shows significant geographic variability, with 8.8% of Europeans being carriers.[174] Heterozygotes for the factor V Leiden mutation carry a fivefold to tenfold increased risk of thrombosis that is an additional ten times higher in homozygotes.[33, 123] Approximately 25% of individuals with the factor V Leiden mutation sustain a thrombosis by age 50 years, and the prevalence of activated protein C resistance among DVT patients has varied from 10% to 65%.[185]

Several other primary coagulation disorders may also be associated with heritable thrombophilia. A recently identified point mutation at position 20210 in the prothrombin gene (G to A) has been associated with increased prothrombin levels and a thrombotic tendency. This mutation, present in 7.1% of patients with confirmed DVT and 1.8% of controls, carries a fourfold increased risk of DVT.[77] Although less clearly established than for arterial disease, hyperhomocyst(e)inemia may be related to venous thromboembolism.[38, 52]

Finally, several disorders of plasmin generation, including dysplasminogenemia, hypoplasminogenemia, decreased synthesis or release of t-PA, and increased PAI-1 have been associated with recurrent familial thromboembolism.[145, 185] However, critical review of the literature has suggested that methodologic problems make this relationship inconclusive at present.[169]

Pregnancy

The frequency of venous thromboembolism in young women has been noted to be higher than that in men, with half of first episodes in women under age 40 years associated with pregnancy.[28] Although the absolute numbers may be small, thromboembolism during pregnancy and the puerperium is associated with higher rates of preterm delivery and perinatal mortality,[217] whereas pulmonary embolism is second only to abortion as a cause of maternal mortality.[99] Population-based studies, often relying on clinical diagnosis, have suggested that venous thromboembolism complicates 0.1% to 0.7% of pregnancies.[28, 122, 217] However, this incidence has been disputed, with studies employing objective documentation of clinically suspected thromboembolism suggesting a lower incidence of 0.013% to 0.029%.[15, 99] Recurrent thromboembolism may complicate 4% to 15% of subsequent pregnancies.[216]

Although the third trimester has often been associated with the greatest thrombotic risk,[216] some studies suggest that objectively documented thromboses are distributed among all three trimesters.[62] The risk of thrombosis appears to be two to three times greater during the puerperium, with a rate of 2.3 to 6.1 per 1000 deliveries.[179, 217]

The inherited thrombophilias constitute an additional risk for pregnancy-associated thromboembolism,[160, 179, 216, 222] complicating 4% of pregnancies in women with congenital anticoagulant deficiencies.[55] Anticoagulant factor deficiencies, lupus anticoagulant, or fibrinolytic deficiencies have been reported in 20% of patients with pregnancy-related thrombosis.[36] The factor V Leiden mutation may be particularly important in this regard, as resistance to activated protein C has been identified in up to 59% of patients with pregnancy-related thromboembolism.[74, 81] The risk of puerperal DVT also increases with maternal age, suppression of lactation, hypertension, and assisted delivery but not with the number of pregnancies.[122, 215, 217]

DVT in pregnancy has been attributed to an acquired prethrombotic state in combination with impaired venous outflow due to uterine compression; 81% to 97% of documented thromboses have been isolated to the left leg.[36, 62, 216] A variety of coagulation factors, including fibrinogen and factors II, VII, VIII, and X, are increased during pregnancy.[8] Perhaps more important, protein S levels are decreased by 50% to 60% early during pregnancy, with free protein S levels comparable to those in hereditary heterozygous protein S deficiency.[2, 124] Fibrinolytic activity has also been reported to decrease during pregnancy.[8]

Oral Contraceptives and Hormonal Therapy

As suggested by case reports in the early 1960s, case control and population-based studies have now established the use of oral contraceptives as an independent risk factor for the development of DVT. Most studies have reported odds ratios of 3.8 to 11.0 for idiopathic thrombosis,[170, 180, 181, 206] with an unweighted summary relative risk among 18 controlled studies of 2.9.[110] Approximately one quarter of idiopathic thromboembolic events among women of childbearing age have been attributed to oral contraceptives.[181] The risk of hospital admission for a thromboembolic event, including cerebral thrombosis, has been estimated to be 0.4 to 0.6 per 1000 for oral contraceptive users, in comparison to 0.05 to 0.06 for nonusers.[53, 170, 225] Early studies also suggested that thromboembolism is responsible for approximately 2% of deaths in young women, with contraceptive-associated mortality rates of 1.3 and 3.4 per 100,000 among women aged 20 to 34 and 35 to 44 years of age, respectively.[90] The increased risk of thromboembolism appears to diminish soon after oral contraceptives are discontinued and is independent of the duration of use.[66, 68, 158, 170, 181]

Risk is correspondingly increased when oral contraceptive use is combined with other factors, such as surgery[66] and inherited inhibitor deficiencies.[160] The factor V Leiden mutation may be particularly important in this regard; resistance to activated protein C has been reported in up to 30% of patients with contraceptive-associated thromboembolism.[74] The use of third-generation oral contraceptives may act synergistically with the factor V Leiden mutation, increasing thromboembolic risk 30- to 50-fold.[13, 75, 221]

Thromboembolic risk may be related both to the dose of estrogen and type of progestin in contraceptive preparations. Preparations containing less than 30 to 50 μg of estrogen are associated with less thrombotic risk; the relative risk of intermediate-dose (50 μg of estrogen) and high-dose (>50 μg of estrogen) contraceptives is 1.5 and 1.7 times that of low-dose preparations (<50 μg of estrogen).[59, 60] Although no clear dose-response relationship has been demonstrated for progestin potency and deep venous thrombosis, third-generation contraceptives containing the progestins desogestrel, norgestimate, or gestodene have been associated with a twofold higher risk of venous thromboembolism than have second-generation drugs.[75, 221] The risk of venous thromboembolism among users of third-generation oral contraceptives may be up to eight times that of young women who do not use oral contraceptives. However, the increased risk associated with third-generation progestins has been questioned based upon the possible confounding effects of age and other prescribing biases.[53]

Estrogenic compounds also increase the risk of venous thromboembolism when used for lactation suppression,[215] in treatment of carcinoma of the prostate, and as postmenopausal replacement therapy.[68] Although estrogen doses used for postmenopausal replacement therapy are approximately one sixth of those in oral contraceptives, recent data support an increased thromboembolic risk at these doses as well. Several studies have now reported a twofold to fourfold increased risk among women taking hormone replacement therapy.[35, 68, 92, 162, 223] This increased risk is greatest during the first year of treatment.[92, 162, 223] However, given the relative infrequency of thromboembolism, this risk represents only one to two additional cases of thromboembolism per year among 10,000 women of this age.

Estrogen in pharmacologic doses is associated with alterations in the coagulation system that may contribute to this thrombotic tendency. Such alterations may include decreases in PAI-1[184] and increases in blood viscosity, fibrinogen, plasma levels of factors VII and X, and platelet adhesion and aggregation.[170, 171, 226] An associated prethrombotic state is implied by increases in markers of activated coagulation occurring in conjunction with elevated levels of circulating factor VIIa[171] and decreases in antithrombin and protein S inhibitor activity.[124, 171, 226, 233] The degree to which antithrombin and protein S are depressed is significantly less with lower-estrogen preparations.[233]

Blood Group

There also appears to be a consistent relationship between thromboembolic risk and the ABO blood group, with a higher prevalence of blood group A and correspondingly lower prevalence of group O among patients with thromboembolism. In comparison to the types in blood donors, deficits of blood type O have been noted in both Belgian and Swedish patients with DVT.[153, 230] In reviewing the literature, Mourant and colleagues[144] similarly found the relative incidence of blood group A to be 1.41 times higher among patients with thromboembolism than among controls. The effect of blood group was greater in young women who were taking oral contraceptives or were pregnant—the relative incidence of blood group A among

thromboembolism patients was 3.12 and 1.85, respectively. Jick and colleagues[93] estimated the relative risk of thromboembolism among group A patients in comparison to group O to vary from 1.9 in medical patients to 3.2 in young women receiving oral contraceptives. A relationship between soluble endothelial cell markers and ABO blood group is known to exist, with significantly lower levels of von Willebrand's factor among those with type O blood.[12]

Geography and Ethnicity

Geographic differences in the frequency of venous thromboembolism do exist. The incidence of postoperative DVT in Europe has been noted to be approximately twice that in North America.[23, 24] Higher rates of thromboembolism have also been noted within the interior United States than on either coast.[104] Autopsy series suggest that while the prevalence of thromboembolism is identical among American black and white patients, it is significantly higher than in a matched Ugandan black population.[213] A similar autopsy series noted the prevalence of thromboembolism to be 40.6% in Boston compared with 13.9% in Kyushu, Japan.[65]

Unfortunately, regional variations in underlying medical and surgical conditions as well as in prophylactic measures and diagnostic methods may confound any apparent differences in the incidence of thromboembolism among different ethnic groups. However, it is certainly conceivable that true differences among ethnic groups might also arise from either genetic or environmental factors. Such differences seem likely based upon recognized geographic differences in the spectrum of mutations leading to congenital anticoagulant deficiencies.[1] Such theoretical concerns are also supported by geographic variability in the incidence of the factor V Leiden mutation. The factor V Leiden allele has a prevalence of 4.4% in Europeans, corresponding to a carrier rate of 8.8%, but the allele has not been identified in Southeast Asian or African populations.[174]

Central Venous Catheters

The use of central venous cannulation for hemodynamic monitoring, infusion catheters, and pacemakers has been associated with an increasing frequency of DVT. This is particularly true in the upper extremities, where as many as 65% of thrombi are related to central venous cannulation.[79] Although the incidence of symptomatic thrombosis may be low, studies employing objective surveillance have reported thrombosis to occur with a mean incidence of 28% following subclavian cannulation.[83] This risk also extends to femoral venous catheters, with ipsilateral thrombosis developing in 12% of patients undergoing placement of large-bore catheters for trauma resuscitation.[137]

Experimental studies in rats suggest that the catheter itself, associated vascular injury, and stasis contribute to the development of early perigraft thrombus in virtually all cases.[235] Catheter material appears to be an important determinant of thromboembolism;[131, 142] polytetrafluoroethylene (Teflon) and heparin-bonded catheters are associated with thrombosis in fewer than 10% of cases.[46] Other determinants of thrombosis have included catheter diameter, number of venipuncture attempts, duration of catheter placement, and composition of the infusate.[83]

Inflammatory Bowel Disease

Clinical series have reported venous thromboembolism to complicate inflammatory bowel disease in 1.2% to 7.1% of cases.[91, 108] Such thromboses frequently occur among young patients, are more common with active disease, and may include unusual sites such as the cerebral veins.[91, 108] Although there are anecdotal reports of cases occurring in patients with primary hypercoagulable states, most cases are not associated with inherited inhibitor deficiencies, antiphospholipid antibodies, or the factor V Leiden mutation. The significance of thrombocytosis and increased levels of factor V, VIII, and fibrinogen during active disease episodes is unclear, since all are acute-phase reactants.[108]

Other coagulation abnormalities, including depressed antithrombin levels, increased PAI-1 levels, and anticardiolipin antibodies, have been inconsistently reported.[224] However, increased fibrinopeptide A levels suggest that active inflammation is associated with activation of coagulation, possibly mediated by endotoxin-induced monocyte activation.[108, 224]

Systemic Lupus Erythematosus

The syndrome of arterial and venous thrombosis, recurrent abortion, thrombocytopenia, and neurologic disease may complicate systemic lupus erythematosus (SLE) when accompanied by antiphospholipid antibodies.[84] Lupus anticoagulant and anticardiolipin antibodies may be seen in association with SLE; other autoimmune disorders; nonautoimmune disorders, such as syphilis and acute infection; drugs, including chlorpromazine, procainamide, and hydralazine; and in elderly people.[121]

Lupus anticoagulant and anticardiolipin antibodies are present in 34% and 44% of patients with SLE in comparison with 2% and 0% to 7.5% of the general population.[121] Among patients with SLE, those with lupus anticoagulant are at a sixfold increased risk for venous thromboembolism, whereas those with anticardiolipin antibodies are at a twofold greater risk.[227] The incidence of arterial or venous thrombosis in these patients is 25% with lupus anticoagulant and 28% with anticardiolipin antibodies.[121] The relationship between antiphospholipid antibodies and thrombosis is much less clear in non-SLE disorders.

Other Risk Factors

Traditional risk factors for venous thromboembolism have included obesity, varicose veins, and cardiac disease; however, the evidence supporting these risk factors remains equivocal at present. Among postmenopausal women, a body mass index of greater than 25 to 30 kg/m^2 has been associated with a significantly increased risk,[92, 162] although, obesity has not proved uniformly to be an independent risk factor in high-risk situations. Some investigators have reported obesity to be associated with a twofold greater risk for postoperative DVT,[95] although multifactorial analysis by others has not shown obesity to constitute an independent

risk.[149] Obesity has not been proven to be a risk factor for the development of DVT after stroke.[229]

Varicose veins have also been included as a risk factor for acute DVT, presumably as a marker of either previous DVT or venous stasis.[149] Most studies evaluating thrombotic risk have been performed in inpatients with other major risk factors for DVT. Such studies have inconsistently supported varicose veins as a risk factor in postoperative DVT and following stroke or myocardial infarction.[127, 149, 180, 229] The importance of varicose veins in otherwise healthy outpatients is equally unclear and has been questioned.[20] The few studies evaluating outpatients have suggested that varicose veins are either not a risk factor for DVT[26] or are an independent risk factor only among women and those older than age 65 years.[157] Consistent with this observation, some studies of postmenopausal women have reported varicose veins or superficial thrombophlebitis to be associated with odds ratios of 3.6 to 6.9 for the development of thromboembolism.[162, 223] However, varicose veins have not been uniformly identified as an independent risk factor in studies of young women.[225] The importance of varicose veins in the general population is thus questionable, although their role in some higher-risk groups cannot be entirely excluded.

Systemic hypercoagulability, congestive heart failure, and enforced bed rest theoretically may predispose patients hospitalized with acute myocardial infarction to DVT. The incidence of DVT in this population has been reported to be 20% to 40%, with an overall average of 24%.[23, 111, 127] Some investigators have noted the incidence of DVT to be higher among patients in whom myocardial infarction was confirmed (34%) than in those in whom the diagnosis was excluded (7%). However, other workers[151] have found a high incidence of ^{125}I-fibrinogen–detected thrombosis both among patients with myocardial infarction (38%) and among those with other severe illnesses but without confirmed infarction (62%). The prevalence of pulmonary embolism among autopsied patients has also not differed substantially from that in other patients dying while hospitalized.[65, 213]

Although Kotilainen and colleagues[111] found the incidence of DVT to be similar among those in whom myocardial infarction was confirmed (21%) and excluded (25%), a substantially higher incidence was noted among those over 60 years of age with congestive heart failure (54%), a finding that has been confirmed by others.[199] However, the evidence supporting congestive heart failure as an independent risk factor for DVT is also conflicting. A variety of thromboembolic complications account for nearly half the deaths among patients not anticoagulated after hospitalization for congestive heart failure, but congestive heart failure has not been identified as an independent risk factor for postoperative DVT.[195] The balance of evidence suggests that severely ill medical patients are at significant risk for venous thromboembolism,[80] although it is difficult to define precisely the additional risk associated with cardiac disease in these patients.

NATURAL HISTORY

Histologic Evolution

Although once regarded as relatively static structures that changed little over time, it is now clear that venous thrombi undergo a dynamic evolution beginning soon after their formation. The venous lumen is most often reestablished after a thrombotic event, although the factors responsible for this and the nomenclature to be employed remain the subject of debate. Often referred to interchangeably as *recanalization* or *spontaneous lysis*, it is important to remember that this is a complex series of both cellular and humoral processes. Animal models afford an opportunity for serial evaluation of the histologic evolution of a thrombus, although artifacts introduced by a variety of injuries or generation in a static column of blood may limit correlation with that observed in humans.

Disappearance and early regeneration of the underlying endothelium has been reported in some experimental models,[154, 200] whereas other workers[186] have reported the endothelium to remain intact. In either case, this endothelium or neoendothelium appears to be fibrinolytically active, with clearing of the thrombus–vein wall interface within 4 days.[154] At this time, small, endothelium-lined clefts become visible between the thrombus and vein wall.[54, 186] As in the initial stages of thrombosis, white blood cells appear to be intimately involved in the process of recanalization.

An early neutrophil infiltrate is largely replaced by monocytes within 6 days of thrombosis.[43] This progressive monocyte infiltration is accompanied by early signs of organization at the vein wall interface as well as an increase in t-PA and urokinase-type plasminogen activator (u-PA) activity within the thrombus.[155] Although t-PA activity within distal vein walls also increases soon after thrombosis, the greatest t-PA activity is associated with the infiltrating monocytes rather than with the luminal endothelium.[155, 200] Thrombolysis is marked by a progressive thinning and loss of fibrin strands, with disappearance of red blood cells.[196] Complete resolution of experimental thrombi in the rat, leaving only an endothelialized subintimal streak, is observed within 21 days.[155] Rapid recanalization of experimental thrombi has been also observed in other animal models.[54, 186]

Although precise aging and serial histologic evaluation of human thrombi are difficult, they appear to follow a similar course. Thrombus organization begins in the attachment zone, with the infiltration of fibroblasts, monocytes, and capillary sprouts and the migration of surfacing cells over the thrombus.[30, 189, 190] These migrating endothelial cells have previously been regarded as important in recanalization, with endothelium-derived t-PA causing the activation of thrombus-bound plasminogen and contributing to peripheral fragmentation of the thrombus.[188] However, the animal models described earlier raise questions regarding the relative importance of monocytes and the endothelium as sources of plasminogen activator. Furthermore, the degree to which recanalization depends on cell-mediated local thrombolysis, versus systemic thrombolysis, has not been completely defined. Although changes in systemic t-PA levels have been observed to parallel the resolution of thrombus, increasing 1 to 2 weeks after presentation and returning to baseline within 24 to 36 weeks, these levels are not clearly related to the degree of thrombus resolution.[101]

Regardless of the mechanism, progressively enlarging pockets are formed between the thrombus and vein wall through a combination of fibrinolysis, thrombus retraction, and peripheral fragmentation.[189] These pockets are lined by flat cells, presumably derived from the endothelium, which invade the thrombus and may initiate organization and fragmentation in unattached zones.[188, 190] The primary factor limiting the extent of recanalization may be the extent of fibrous anchoring to the vein wall.[188] Although the most common outcome is a restored venous lumen with fibroelastic intimal thickening at the site of initial thrombus attachment, residual fibrous synechia may be present in 3% to 11% of specimens.[188]

Thrombus Evolution as Determined by Noninvasive Studies

Unlike animal models employing a transient stimulus to thrombosis, the relative balance between organization, thrombolysis, propagation, and rethrombosis determines outcome after human thrombosis. From a clinical perspective, the most important events following thrombosis are recanalization and recurrent thrombosis. However, the relative importance, frequency, and rate of these processes were not possible to define until the development of noninvasive technology, which permitted serial examination of patients.

Impedance plethysmography was the first widely available noninvasive test permitting serial evaluation of venous outflow obstruction due to an acute DVT. Although this test could not distinguish between recanalization and the development of collateral venous outflow, such studies were found to normalize in 67% of patients by 3 months and 92% of patients by 9 months.[85] Venous duplex ultrasonography, which permits individual venous segments to be observed over time, has further documented that recanalization does occur in most patients after an episode of acute DVT. Among 21 patients followed prospectively, recanalization was evident in 44% of patients at 7 days and in 100% of patients by 90 days after the acute event.[100] The percentage of initially involved segments that remained occluded decreased to a mean of 44% by 30 days and 14% by 90 days (Fig. 138–1).

Van Ramshorst and associates[220] similarly noted an exponential decrease in thrombus load over the first 6 months after femoropopliteal thrombosis. Most recanalization occurred within the first 6 weeks, with flow reestablished in 87% of 23 completely occluded segments during this interval. Killewich and colleagues[101] reported a linear decrease in thrombus load such that by 24 to 36 weeks, only 26% of the original thrombus remained. Using a somewhat different approach, measuring thrombus thickness when maximally compressed, Prandoni and colleagues[165] noted the most significant reduction in thrombus mass over the first 3 months after thrombosis—62% in the common femoral vein and 50% in the popliteal vein. In aggregate, these studies confirm the histologic findings that recanalization begins early after an episode of acute DVT, with the greatest reduction in thrombus load occurring within 3 months of the event. Complete thrombus resolution has been reported in 56% of patients followed up for 9 months.[101] However, recanalization may continue, albeit at a slower rate, for months to years after the acute event.[126, 165]

Recurrent thrombotic events appear to compete with recanalization early after an acute DVT. The importance of such events is well recognized clinically, although their frequency in patients studied prospectively has only recently been described. Most clinical studies have included

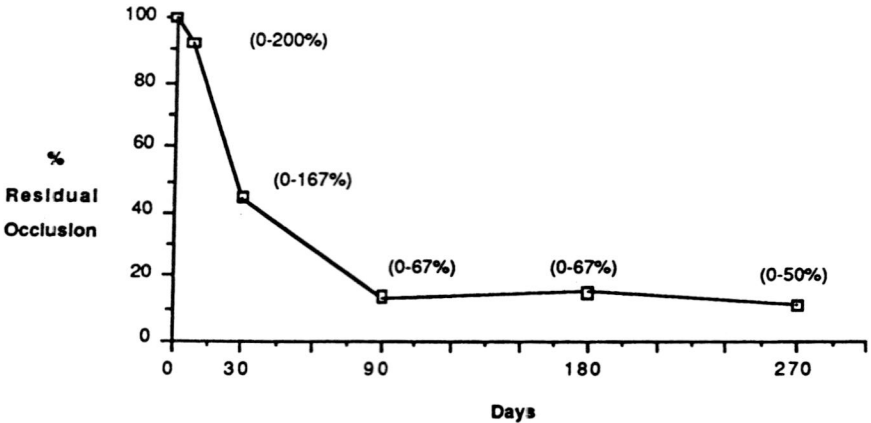

FIGURE 138–1. Mean percentage of initially occluded segments remaining occluded at follow-up among 21 patients with acute deep venous thrombosis (per cent residual occlusion = number of segments occluded at follow-up/number of segments occluded at presentation). Numbers in parentheses are the ranges for individual cases, with numbers greater than 100% indicating extension of the initial thrombus. (From Killewich LA, Bedford GR, Beach KW, et al: Spontaneous lysis of deep venous thrombi: Rate and outcome. J Vasc Surg 9:89, 1989.)

both recurrent DVT and pulmonary embolism, with rates depending on treatment, location of thrombus, and duration of follow-up. Among patients with proximal DVT, recurrent thromboembolic events have been reported in 5.2% of patients treated with standard anticoagulation measures for 3 months,[88] compared with 47% of patients inadequately treated with a 3-month course of low-dose subcutaneous heparin.[87] Proximal propagation may also complicate isolated calf vein thrombosis in up to 23% of untreated patients.[163]

Despite the significance of these observations, studies employing serial noninvasive follow-up examinations suggest that they may underestimate the incidence of new thrombotic events. In the acute setting, Krupski and colleagues[112] found ultrasound evidence of proximal propagation in 38% of 24 patients being treated with intravenous heparin. In a larger series of 177 patients, most of whom were treated with standard anticoagulation measures, recurrent thrombotic events were observed in 52% of patients.[133] New thrombi were observed in 6% of uninvolved contralateral extremities, while propagation to new segments occurred in 30% of involved limbs and rethrombosis of a partially occluded or recanalized segment in 31% of extremities. Propagation to new segments in the ipsilateral limb tended to occur as an early event at a median of less than 40 days after presentation, whereas rethrombosis and extension to the contralateral limb tended to occur sporadically as later events.

COMPLICATIONS

Pulmonary Embolism

Pulmonary embolism, with its attendant mortality, is the most devastating complication of acute DVT. Inadequate treatment of proximal lower extremity venous thrombosis is associated with a 20% to 50% risk of clinically significant recurrent thromboembolism,[173] with approximately 90% of thromboemboli arising from the lower extremity veins.[63, 89] Symptomatic pulmonary embolism may also complicate 7% to 17% of proximal upper extremity thrombi.[21, 41, 78, 79, 83] As for acute DVT, the majority of pulmonary emboli may be clinically silent. High-probability lung scans may occur in 25% to 51% of patients with documented DVT in

the absence of pulmonary symptoms,[86, 139] and some autopsy series have reported the combination of pulmonary embolism and DVT to be 1.8 times more common than proximal DVT alone.[118] The presence of symptomatic pulmonary embolism may depend not only on the amount of the pulmonary circulation occluded but also on the patients' underlying cardiopulmonary reserve.

Unfortunately, estimates of the prevalence of symptomatic pulmonary embolism are less reliable, since the diagnosis ante mortem is difficult to establish.[180] Studies of autopsied and hospitalized patients likely are overestimates and are significantly influenced by the detail of dissection, whereas community-based studies that exclude chronically and seriously ill individuals may be underestimates. Extrapolation from autopsy studies, to which pulmonary embolism causes or contributes approximately 15% of hospital deaths, suggests 150,000 to 200,000 deaths per year from pulmonary embolism in the United States.[27, 34] In contrast, community-based studies have suggested a lower prevalence of 64,000 cases per year in the United States.[28] Combining autopsy data and a number of observations concerning the natural history of pulmonary embolism, Dalen and Alpert[34] calculated an incidence of 630,000 episodes of symptomatic pulmonary embolism per year.

Among patients with symptomatic pulmonary embolism, death occurs within 1 hour of presentation in 11% and in 30% of those surviving 1 hour but in whom the diagnosis of pulmonary embolism is not made.[34] In contrast, the mortality among those with an appropriate diagnosis and treatment is only 8% to 9%. Among the survivors, early resolution of abnormal lung scans has been documented in several series employing routine follow-up studies.[86] Chronic cor pulmonale is rare after pulmonary embolism, generally occurring after repeated, often silent, emboli.[34]

The Post-thrombotic Syndrome

Although less dramatic than pulmonary embolism, development of the post-thrombotic syndrome is responsible for a greater degree of chronic socioeconomic morbidity. Data regarding the prevalence of the post-thrombotic syndrome may be more accurate than those for pulmonary embolism, which are largely derived from hospitalized patients.[27] As many as 29% to 79% of patients[119, 168, 205] may have long-term manifestations of pain, edema, hyperpigmentation, or ulceration after an episode of acute DVT. Coon and associates[28] have estimated that severe post-thrombotic changes are present in 5% of the United States population, corresponding to a prevalence of between 6 and 7 million individuals with stasis changes and 400,000 to 500,000 with leg ulcers.

Severe manifestations of the post-thrombotic syndrome are a consequence of ambulatory venous hypertension, which is determined by a number of factors, including valvular reflux, persistent venous obstruction, and the anatomic distribution of these abnormalities. The pathophysiology and natural history of chronic venous insufficiency are reviewed in Chapter 144. However, despite the importance of valvular reflux in post-thrombotic sequelae, valvular destruction does not appear to be universally associated with recanalization, and as many as one third of patients may remain free of chronic symptoms after an episode of acute DVT. Only 69% of involved extremities and 33% to 59% of initially thrombosed segments show evidence of reflux by duplex ultrasonography 1 year after the event.[126]

Such clinical observations are supported by histologic evidence that thrombus organization rarely involves the valve cusps. In most cases, the thrombus is separated from the valve cusp by a clear zone postulated to arise from the local fibrinolytic activity of the valvular endothelium.[64, 188, 190] This protective mechanism appears to fail in approximately 10% of cases in which thrombus adherence to the valve cusp is noted.[188, 190] Initial thrombus adherence presumably accounts for the histologic findings in established post-thrombotic syndrome; approximately 50% of popliteal valves in such extremities demonstrate thrombus formation on the valve leaflets, usually on the surface facing the valve sinus, with associated loss of the endothelium and basement membrane.[18]

Most investigators have not found a clear relationship between the extent of thrombus on initial presentation and ultimate clinical outcome.[16, 73, 134, 141, 166] However, several factors in the early natural history of a thrombotic event do appear to influence the ultimate development of valvular incompetence and eventual post-thrombotic manifestations.

Among these, the rate of recanalization and recurrent thrombotic events appear to be important determinants of valvular competence. Depending upon the segment involved, venous segments developing reflux have been noted to require 2.3 to 7.3 times longer for complete recanalization than segments in which valve function is preserved (Fig. 138–2).[135] Recurrent thrombotic events are also detrimental to valve competence. Reflux may develop in 36% to 73% of segments with rethrombosis, which is considerably higher than the rate in segments without rethrombosis (Fig. 138–3).[133] Consistent with these observations, Prandoni and associates[166] have noted a sixfold increased risk of the post-thrombotic syndrome among patients with recurrent thrombosis.

Mortality After Acute Deep Venous Thrombosis

DVT is associated with a high frequency of co-morbid medical conditions, and early mortality after a lower extremity thrombosis is substantial. Piccioli and coworkers[164] noted a 3-month mortality rate of 19%, with no deaths due to pulmonary embolism. Other workers[104] have confirmed similar mortality (21%) during the first year after an acute DVT but have noted that the survival curve after 1 year parallels that of an age-, sex-, and race-matched population. Higher short-term mortality rates have been noted in patients with upper extremity DVT, who tend to be more ill, with an increased prevalence of metastatic malignancy.[78, 214] Six-month mortality may be as high as 48% among those with upper extremity DVT, in comparison to 13% following a lower extremity thrombosis.[78]

CALF VEIN THROMBOSIS

Thrombosis isolated to the deep veins of the calf is often differentiated from that involving the proximal veins based upon perceived differences in the frequency of pulmonary

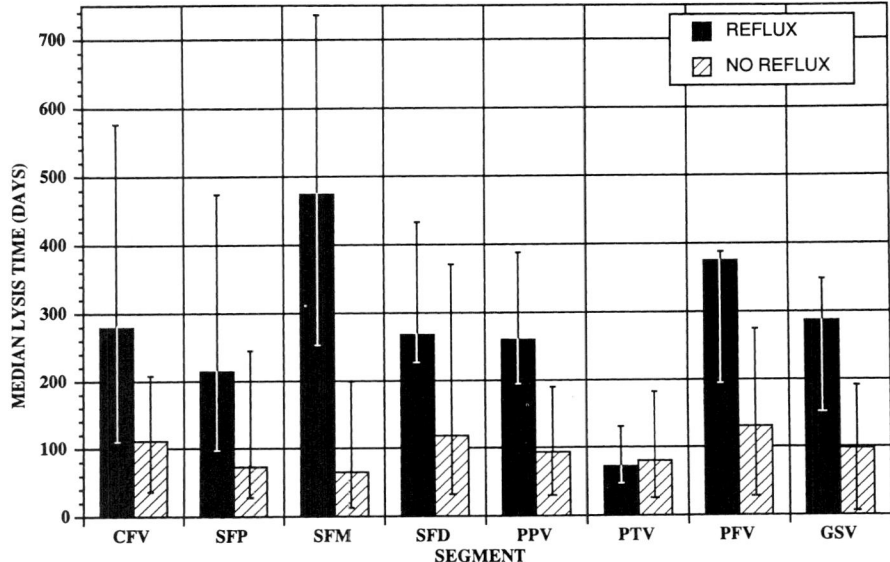

FIGURE 138–2. Median time (± interquartile range) from thrombosis to complete recanalization, stratified according to ultimate reflux status. Median times are 2.3 to 7.3 times longer among segments developing reflux in all but the posterior tibial veins. Segments: common femoral vein (CFV), proximal superficial femoral vein (SFP), mid-superficial femoral vein (SFM), distal superficial femoral vein (SFD), popliteal vein (PPV), posterior tibial vein (PTV), profunda femoris vein (PFV), and greater saphenous vein (GSV). (From Meissner MH, Manzo RA, Bergelin RO, et al: Deep venous insufficiency: The relationship between lysis and subsequent reflux. J Vasc Surg 18:596, 1993.)

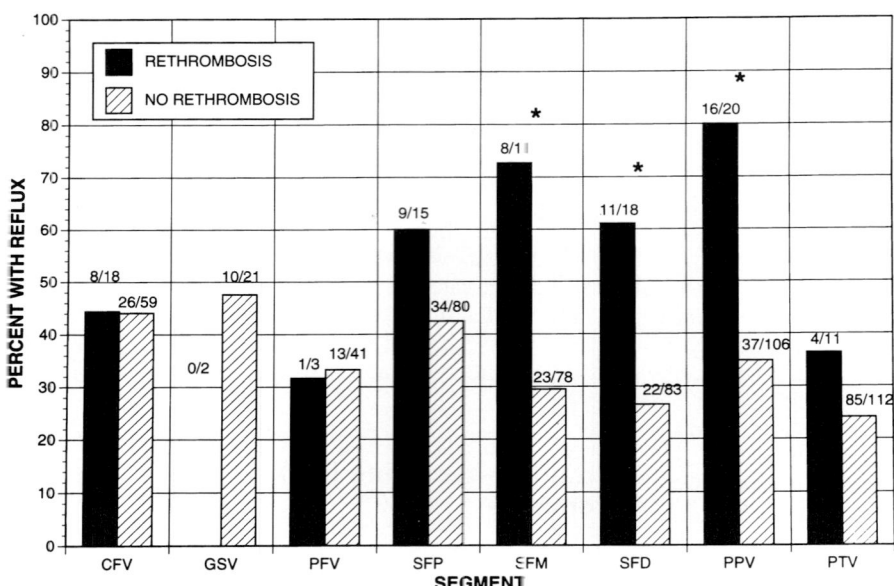

FIGURE 138–3. Reflux incidence in initially involved venous segments with and without subsequent rethrombosis. Numbers above bars indicate the number of segments in which reflux was observed over the number of segments in which reflux could be definitively assessed. Differences between segments with and without rethrombosis are statistically significant (*$p < .005$) for the SFM, SFD, and PPV segments. Segments: common femoral vein (CFV), greater saphenous vein (GSV), profunda femoris vein (PFV), proximal superficial femoral vein (SFP), mid-superficial femoral vein (SFM), distal superficial femoral vein (SFD), popliteal vein (PPV), and posterior tibial vein (PTV). (From Meissner MH, Caps MT, Bergelin RO, et al: Propagation, rethrombosis and new thrombus formation after acute deep venous thrombosis. J Vasc Surg 22:558, 1995.)

embolism and post-thrombotic complications. Noninvasive studies do suggest that such isolated thrombi recanalize more rapidly than proximal thrombi,[135] with a mean 50% reduction in thrombus load by 1 month and complete recanalization within 1 year.[132] The frequency of reflux in involved calf vein segments is also lower than in proximal venous segments.[135] However, propagation to more proximal segments also occurs in 15% to 23% of limbs with thrombosis confined to the calf veins.[94, 114, 120, 132]

Clinical data suggest that although the incidence of acute and long-term complications may be less than after proximal venous thrombosis, isolated calf vein thrombi are not entirely benign. Although prior embolization of more proximal thrombus cannot be excluded, concurrent pulmonary embolism has been noted in approximately 10% of patients with calf vein thrombosis when clinical suspicion is supplemented by objective tests[132, 136, 161] and in up to 33% of patients in series employing routine ventilation-perfusion lung scans.[102, 143] Even if clinically significant emboli are presumed to arise only from proximal thrombus extension, a 20% rate of proximal propagation in untreated calf vein thrombosis theoretically would be associated with a 2% risk of fatal pulmonary embolism and a 5% to 10% risk of symptomatic recurrent thromboembolism.[173]

Post-thrombotic symptoms, although perhaps less frequent than after proximal thrombosis, may also complicate isolated calf vein thrombosis. Persistent symptoms of pain and swelling at 1 year have been noted in 23% of extremities with calf vein thrombosis compared with 54% of those with proximal thrombosis and 9% of uninvolved limbs

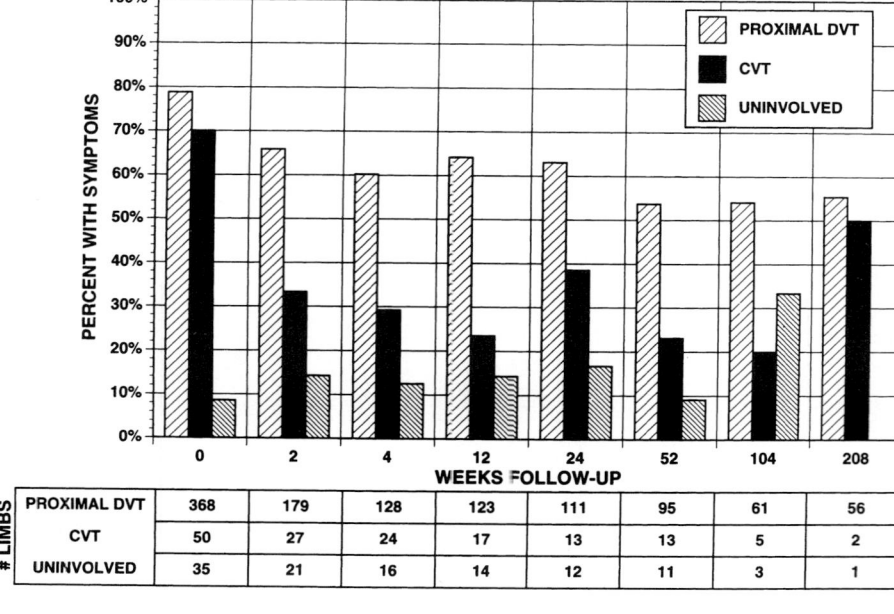

# LIMBS	0	2	4	12	24	52	104	208
PROXIMAL DVT	368	179	128	123	111	95	61	56
CVT	50	27	24	17	13	13	5	2
UNINVOLVED	35	21	16	14	12	11	3	1

FIGURE 138–4. Prevalence of symptoms (edema, pain, hyperpigmentation, or ulceration) during follow-up among extremities with proximal deep venous thrombosis, isolated calf vein thrombosis (CVT), and uninvolved limbs contralateral to a calf vein thrombosis. The prevalence of symptoms between the three groups is significantly different at 12 months ($p = .004$). The Table shows the total number of extremities within each group evaluated at each follow-up interval. (From Meissner MH, Caps MT, Bergelin RO, et al: Early outcome after isolated calf vein thrombosis. J Vasc Surg 26:749, 1997.)

(Fig. 138–4).[132] In contrast, Prandoni and colleagues[168] found the frequency of mild (21%) and severe (5%) post-thrombotic sequelae 45 months after the acute event to be similar among those with isolated calf and proximal venous thrombosis. Others have reported post-thrombotic symptoms in 38% of patients after a mean follow-up of 3.4 years[130] and 47% after 5 to 10 years.[119]

REFERENCES

1. Aiach M, Gandrille S, Emmerich J: A review of mutations causing deficiencies of antithrombin, protein C, and protein S. Thromb Haemost 74(1):81, 1995.
2. Alving BM, Comp PC: Recent advances in understanding clotting and evaluating patients with recurrent thrombosis. Am J Obstet Gynecol 167(4):1184, 1992.
3. Amiral J, Fareed J: Thromboembolic diseases: Biochemical mechanisms and new possibilities of biological diagnosis. Semin Thromb Hemost 22(Suppl 1):41, 1996.
4. Anderson FA, Wheeler HB, Goldberg RJ, et al: The prevalence of risk factors for venous thromboembolism among hospital patients. Arch Intern Med 152(8):1660, 1992.
5. Aronson DL, Thomas DP: Experimental studies on venous thrombosis: Effect of coagulants, procoagulants and vessel contusion. Thromb Haemost 54(4):866, 1985.
6. Barnes RW, Wu KK, Hoak JC: Fallability of the clinical diagnosis of venous thrombosis. JAMA 234(6):605, 1975.
7. Bauer KA, Rosenberg RD: The pathophysiology of the prethrombotic state in humans: Insights gained from studies using markers of hemostatic system activation. Blood 70(2):343, 1987.
8. Beller FK, Ebert C: The coagulation and fibrinolytic enzyme system in pregnancy and the puerperium. Eur J Obstet Gynecol Reprod Biol 13(3):177, 1982.
9. Bernstein D, Coupey S, Schonberg SK: Pulmonary embolism in adolescents. Am J Dis Child 140(7):667, 1986.
10. Bertina RM, Koeleman BPC, Koster T, et al: Mutation in blood coagulation factor V associated with resistance to activated protein C. Nature 369:64, 1994.
11. Biland L, Widmer LK: Varicose veins (VV) and chronic venous insufficiency (CVI). Medical and socioeconomic aspects, Basle study. Acta Chir Scand(Suppl) 544:9, 1988.
12. Blann AD, Daly RJ, Amiral J: The influence of age, gender, and ABO blood group on soluble endothelial cell markers and adhesion markers. Br J Haematol 92(2):498, 1996.
13. Bloemenkamp KWM, Rosendaal FR, Helmerhorst FM, et al: Enhancement by factor V Leiden mutation of risk of deep-vein thrombosis associated with oral contraceptives containing a third generation progestagen. Lancet 346(8990):1593, 1995.
14. Breddin HK: Thrombosis and Vichow's triad: What is established? Semin Thromb Hemost 15(3):237, 1989.
15. Brickner LA, Scannell KA, Ackerson L: Pregnancy-related thromboembolism (Letter). Ann Intern Med 127(2):164, 1997.
16. Browse NL, Clemenson G, Thomas ML: Is the postphlebitic leg always postphlebitic? Relation between phlebographic appearances of deep-vein thrombosis and late sequelae. Br Med J 281(6249):1167, 1980.
17. Buck JR, Connors RH, Coon WW, et al: Pulmonary embolism in children. J Pediatr Surg 16(3):385, 1981.
18. Budd TW, Meenaghan MA, Wirth J, et al: Histopathology of veins and venous valves of patients with venous insufficiency syndrome: Ultrastructure. J Med 21(3–4):181, 1990.
19. Burns GA, Cohn SM, Frumento RJ, et al: Prospective ultrasound evaluation of venous thrombosis in high-risk trauma patients. J Trauma 35(3):405, 1993.
20. Campbell B: Thrombosis, phlebitis, and varicose veins. Br Med J 312(7025):198, 1996.
21. Campbell CB, Chandler JG, Tegtmeyer CJ, et al: Axillary, subclavian, and brachiocephalic obstruction. Surgery 82(6):816, 1977.
22. Carter CJ, Anderson FA, Wheeler HB: Epidemiology and pathophysiology of venous thromboembolism. In Hull RD, Raskob GE, Pineo GF (eds): Venous Thromboembolism: An Evidence-based Atlas. Armonk, NY, Futura Publishing Company, 1996, p 3.
23. Clagett GP, Anderson FA, Heit J, et al: Prevention of venous thromboembolism. Chest 108(4 Suppl):312S, 1995.
24. Clagett GP, Reisch JS: Prevention of venous thromboembolism in general surgical patients: Results of meta-analysis. Ann Surg 208:(2)277, 1988.
25. Clarke CS, Otridge BW, Carney DN: Thromboembolism: A complication of weekly chemotherapy in the treatment of non-Hodgkin's lymphoma. Cancer 66(9):2027, 1990.
26. Cogo A, Bernardi E, Prandoni P, et al: Acquired risk factors for deep-vein thrombosis in symptomatic outpatients. Arch Intern Med 154(2):164, 1994.
27. Coon WW: Epidemiology of venous thromboembolism. Ann Surg 186(2):149, 1977.
28. Coon WW, Willis PW, Keller JB: Venous thromboembolism and other venous disease in the Tecumseh Community Health Study. Circulation 48(4):839, 1973.
29. Cornuz J, Pearson SD, Creager MA, et al: Importance of findings on the initial evaluation for cancer in patients with symptomatic idiopathic deep venous thrombosis. Ann Intern Med 125(10):785, 1996.
30. Cox JST: The maturation and canalization of thrombi. Surg Gynecol Obstet 116:593, 1963.
31. Cranley JJ, Canos AJ, Sull WJ: The diagnosis of deep venous thrombosis: Fallibility of clinical symptoms and signs. Arch Surg 111(1):34, 1976.
32. Cruickshank JM, Gorlin R, Jennett B: Air travel and thrombotic episodes: The economy class syndrome. Lancet 2(8609):497, 1988.
33. Dahlback B: Inherited thrombophilia: Resistance to activated protein C as a pathogenic factor of venous thromboembolism. Blood 85(3):607, 1995.
34. Dalen JE, Alpert JS: Natural history of pulmonary embolism. Prog Cardiovasc Dis 17(4):259, 1975.
35. Daly E, Vessey MP, Hawkins MM, et al: Risk of venous thromboembolism in users of hormone replacement therapy. Lancet 348(9033):977, 1996.
36. de Boer K, Buller HR, ten Cate JW, et al: Deep vein thrombosis in obstetric patients: Diagnosis and risk factors. Thromb Haemost 67(1):4, 1992.
37. DeAngelis GA, McIlhenny J, Willson DF, et al: Prevalence of deep venous thrombosis in the lower extremities of children in the intensive care unit. Pediatr Radiol 26(11):821, 1996.
38. den Heijer M, Blom HJ, Gerrits WB, et al: Is hyperhomocysteinaemia a risk factor for recurrent venous thrombosis? Lancet 345(8954):882, 1995.
39. Dennis JW, Menawat S, Von Thron J, et al: Efficacy of deep venous thrombosis prophylaxis in trauma patients and identification of high-risk groups. J Trauma 35(1):132, 1993.
40. Doll DC, Ringenberg QS, Yarbro JW: Vascular toxicity associated with antineoplastic agents. J Clin Oncol 4(9):1405, 1986.
41. Donayre CE, White GH, Mehringer SM, et al: Pathogenesis determines late morbidity of axillosubclavian vein thrombosis. Am J Surg 152(2):179, 1986.
42. Doouss TW: The clinical significance of venous thrombosis of the calf. Br J Surg 63(5):377, 1976.
43. Downing LJ, Streiter RM, Kadell AM, et al: Neutrophils are the initial cell type identified in deep venous thrombosis-induced vein wall inflammation. ASAIO J 42(5):M677, 1996.
44. Edwards RL, Klaus M, Matthews E, et al: Heparin abolishes the chemotherapy-induced increase in plasma fibrinopeptide A levels. Am J Med 89(1):25, 1990.
45. Edwards RL, Rickles FR, Moritz TE, et al: Abnormalities of blood coagulation tests in patients with cancer. Am J Clin Pathol 88(5):596, 1987.
46. Efsing HO, Lindblad B, Mark J, et al: Thromboembolic complications from central venous catheters: A comparison of three catheter materials. World J Surg 7(3):419, 1983.
47. Eriksson BI, Eriksson E, Risberg B: Impaired fibrinolysis and postoperative thromboembolism in orthopedic patients. Thromb Res 62(1/2):55, 1991.
48. Falanga A, Barbui T, Rickles FR, et al: Guidelines for clotting studies in cancer patients. For the Scientific and Standardization Committee of the Subcommittee on Haemostasis and Malignancy, International Society of Thrombosis and Haemostasis. Thromb Haemost 70(3):540, 1993.
49. Falanga A, Gordon SG: Isolation and characterization of cancer procoagulant: A cysteine proteinase from malignant tissue. Biochemistry 24(20):5558, 1985.

50. Falanga A, Ofosu FA, Oldani E, et al: The hypercoagulable state in cancer patients: Evidence for impaired thrombin inhibitions. Blood Coagul Fibrinolysis 5(Suppl 1):S19, 1994.

51. Falanga A, Ofosu FA, Cortelazzo S, et al: Preliminary study to identify cancer patients at high risk of venous thrombosis following major surgery. Br J Haematol 85(4):745, 1993.

52. Falcon CR, Cattaneo M, Panzeri D, et al: High prevalence of hyperhomocyst(e)inemia in patients with juvenile venous thrombosis. Arterioscler Thromb 14(7):1080, 1994.

53. Farmer RD, Lawrenson RA, Thompson CR, et al: Population-based study of risk of venous thromboembolism associated with various oral contraceptives. Lancet 349(9045):83, 1997.

54. Flanc C: An experimental study of the recanalization of arterial and venous thrombi. Br J Surg 55(7):519, 1968.

55. Friederich PW, Sanson B-J, Simioni P, et al: Frequency of pregnancy-related venous thromboembolism in anticoagulant factor–deficient women: Implications for prophylaxis. Ann Intern Med 125 (12):955, 1996.

56. Gando S, Tedo I, Kubota M: Posttrauma coagulation and fibrinolysis. Crit Care Med 20(5):594, 1992.

57. Garcia Frade LJ, Landin L, Avello AG, et al: Changes in fibrinolysis in the intensive care patient. Thromb Res 47(5):593, 1987.

58. Geerts WH, Code KI, Jay RM, et al: A prospective study of venous thromboembolism after major trauma. N Engl J Med 331 (24): 1601, 1994.

59. Gerstman BB, Piper JM, Freiman JP, et al: Oral contraceptive oestrogen and progestin potencies and the incidence of deep venous thromboembolism. Int J Epidemiol 19(4):931, 1990.

60. Gerstman BB, Piper JM, Tomita DK, et al: Oral contraceptive estrogen dose and the risk of deep venous thromboembolic disease. Am J Epidemiol 133(1):32, 1991.

61. Gibbs NM: Venous thrombosis of the lower limbs with particular reference to bed rest. Br J Surg 45(191):209, 1957.

62. Ginsberg JS, Brill-Edwards PB, Burrows RF, et al: Venous thrombosis during pregnancy: Leg and trimester of presentation. Thromb Haemost 67(5):519, 1992.

63. Girolami A, Prandoni P, Simioni P, et al: The pathogenesis of venous thromboembolism. Haematologica 80(2 Suppl):25, 1995.

64. Glas-Greenwalt P, Dalton BC, Astrup T: Localization of tissue plasminogen activator in relation to morphological changes in human saphenous veins used as coronary artery bypass autografts. Ann Surg 181(4):431, 1975.

65. Gore I, Hirst AE: Myocardial infarction and thromboembolism. Arch Intern Med 113:323, 1964.

66. Greene GR, Sartwell PE: Oral contraceptive use in patients with thromboembolism following surgery, trauma, or infection. Am J Public Health 62(5):680, 1972.

67. Griffin MR, Stanson AW, Brown ML, et al: Deep venous thrombosis and pulmonary embolism: Risk of subsequent malignant neoplasms. Arch Intern Med 147(11):1907, 1987.

68. Grodstein F, Stampfer MJ, Manson JE, et al: Prospective study of exogenous hormones and risk of pulmonary embolism in women. Lancet 348(9033):983, 1996.

69. Haeger K: Problems of acute deep venous thrombosis. Angiology 20(4):219, 1969.

70. Hamer JD, Malone PC, Silver IA: The PO2 in venous valve pockets: Its possible bearing on thrombogenesis. Br J Surg 68(3):166, 1981.

71. Hamilton T, Angevine D: Fatal pulmonary embolism in 100 battle casualties. Mil Surg 99:450, 1946.

72. Hansson PO, Welin L, Tibblin G, et al: Deep vein thrombosis and pulmonary embolism in the general population: 'The Study of Men Born in 1913.' Arch Intern Med 157(15):1665, 1997.

73. Heldal M, Seem E, Sandset PM, et al: Deep vein thrombosis: A 7-year follow-up study. J Intern Med 234(1):71, 1993.

74. Hellgren M, Svensson PJ, Dahlback B: Resistance to activated protein C as a basis for venous thromboembolism associated with pregnancy and oral contraceptives. Am J Obstet Gynecol 173(1):210, 1995.

75. Helmerhorst FM, Bloemkamp KWM, Rosendaal FR, et al: Oral contraceptives and thrombotic disease: Risk of venous thromboembolism. Thromb Haemost 78(1):327, 1997.

76. Hill SL, Berry RE, Ruiz AJ: Deep venous thrombosis in the trauma patient. Am Surg 60(6):405, 1994.

77. Hillarp A, Zoller B, Svensson PJ, et al: The 20210 A allele of the prothrombin gene is a common risk factor among Swedish outpatients with verified deep venous thrombosis. Thromb Haemost 78(3):990, 1997.

78. Hingorani A, Ascher E, Hanson J, et al: Upper extremity versus lower extremity deep venous thrombosis. Am J Surg 174(2):214, 1997.

79. Hingorani A, Ascher E, Lorenson E, et al: Upper extremity deep venous thrombosis and its impact on morbidity and mortality rates in a hospital-based population. J Vasc Surg 26(5):853, 1997.

80. Hirsch D, Ingenito E, Goldhaber S: Prevalence of deep venous thrombosis among patients in medical intensive care. JAMA 274(4):335, 1995.

81. Hirsch DR, Mikkola KM, Marks PW, et al: Pulmonary embolism and deep venous thrombosis during pregnancy or oral contraceptive use: Prevalence of factor V Leiden. Am Heart J 131(6):1145, 1996.

82. Homans J: Thrombosis of the deep leg veins due to prolonged sitting. N Engl J Med 250(4):148, 1954.

83. Horattas MC, Wright DJ, Fenton AH, et al: Changing concepts of deep venous thrombosis of the upper extremity: Report of a series and review of the literature. Surgery 104(3):561, 1988.

84. Hughes GR, Harris NN, Gharavi AE: The anticardiolipin syndrome. J Rheumatol 13(3):486, 1986.

85. Huisman MV, Buller HR, ten Cate JW: Utility of impedance plethysmography in the diagnosis of recurrent deep-vein thrombosis. Arch Intern Med 148(3):681, 1988.

86. Huisman MV, Buller HR, ten Cate JW, et al: Unexpected high prevalence of silent pulmonary embolism in patients with deep venous thrombosis. Chest 95(3):498, 1989.

87. Hull R, Delmore T, Genton E, et al: Warfarin sodium versus low-dose heparin in the treatment of venous thrombosis. N Engl J Med 301(16):855, 1979.

88. Hull RD, Raskob GE, Hirsch J, et al: Continuous intravenous heparin compared with intermittent subcutaneous heparin in the initial treatment of proximal-vein thrombosis. N Engl J Med 315(18): 1109, 1986.

89. Hull RD, Raskob GE, Hirsh J: Prophylaxis of venous thromboembolism: An overview. Chest 89(5 Suppl):374S, 1986.

90. Inman WHW, Vessey MP: Investigation of deaths from pulmonary, coronary, and cerebral thrombosis and embolism in women of child-bearing age. Br Med J 2(599):193, 1968.

91. Jackson LM, O'Gorman PJ, O'Connell J, et al: Thrombosis in inflammatory bowel disease: Clinical setting, procoagulant profile and factor V Leiden. Q J Med 90(3):183, 1997.

92. Jick H, Derby LE, Myers MW, et al: Risk of hospital admission for idiopathic venous thromboembolism among users of postmenopausal oestrogens. Lancet 348(9033):981, 1996.

93. Jick H, Westerholm B, Vessey MP, et al: Venous thromboembolic disease and ABO blood type. Lancet 1(7594):539, 1969.

94. Kakkar VV, Flanc C, Howe CT, et al: Natural history of postoperative deep-vein thrombosis. Lancet 2(7614):230, 1969.

95. Kakkar VV, Howe CT, Nicolaides AN, et al: Deep vein thrombosis of the leg: Is there a "high risk" group? Am J Surg 120(4):527, 1970.

96. Kambayashi J, Sakon M, Yokota M, et al: Activation of coagulation and fibrinolysis during surgery, analyzed by molecular markers. Thromb Res 60(2):157, 1990.

97. Kapsch DN, Metzler M, Harrington M, et al: Fibrinolytic response to trauma. Surgery 95(4):473, 1984.

98. Karino T, Motomiya M: Flow through a venous valve and its implications for thrombus formation. Thromb Res 36(3):245, 1984.

99. Kierkegaard A: Incidence and diagnosis of deep vein thrombosis associated with pregnancy. Acta Obstet Gynecol Scand 62(3):239, 1983.

100. Killewich LA, Bedford GR, Beach KW, et al: Spontaneous lysis of deep venous thrombi: Rate and outcome. J Vasc Surg 9(1)89, 1989.

101. Killewich LA, Macko RF, Cox K, et al: Regression of proximal deep venous thrombosis is associated with fibrinolytic enhancement. J Vasc Surg 26(5):861, 1997.

102. Kistner R, Ball J, Nordyke R, et al: Incidence of pulmonary embolism in the course of thrombophlebitis of the lower extremities. Am J Surg 124:169, 1972.

103. Kluft C, Verheijen JH, Jie AFH, et al: The post-operative fibrinolytic shutdown: A rapidly reverting acute phase pattern for the fast-acting inhibitor of tissue-type plasminogen activator after trauma. Scand J Clin Lab Invest 45(7):605, 1985.

104. Kniffen WD, Baron JA, Barrett J, et al: The epidemiology of diagnosed pulmonary embolism and deep venous thrombosis in the elderly. Arch Intern Med 154(8):861, 1994.

105. Knudson MM, Collins JA, Goodman SB, et al: Thromboembolism following multiple trauma. J Trauma 32(1):2, 1992.

106. Knudson MM, Lewis FR, Clinton A, et al: Prevention of venous thromboembolism in trauma patients. J Trauma 37(3):480, 1994.

107. Knudson MM, Morabito D, Paiement GD, et al: Use of low molecular weight heparin in preventing thromboembolism in trauma patients. J Trauma 41(3):446, 1996.

108. Koenigs KP, McPhedran P, Spiro HM: Thrombosis in inflammatory bowel disease. J Clin Gastroenterol 9(6):627, 1987.

109. Koster T, Rosendaal FR, Briet E, et al: Venous thrombosis due to poor anticoagulant response to activated protein C: Leiden thrombophilia study. Lancet 342:1503, 1993.

110. Koster T, Small R-A, Rosendaal FR, et al: Oral contraceptives and venous thromboembolism: A quantitative discussion of the uncertainties. J Intern Med 238(1):31, 1995.

111. Kotilainen M, Ristola P, Ikkala E, et al: Leg vein thrombosis diagnosed by ¹²⁵I-fibrinogen test after acute myocardial infarction. Ann Clin Res 5(6):365, 1973.

112. Krupski WC, Bass A, Dilley RB, et al: Propagation of deep venous thrombosis by duplex ultrasonography. J Vasc Surg 12(4):467, 1990.

113. Landgraf H, Vanselow B, Schulte-Huermann D, et al: Economy class syndrome: Rheology, fluid balance, and lower leg edema during a simulated 12-hour long distance flight. Aviat Space Environ Med 65(10,Part 1):930, 1994.

114. Lagerstedt CI, Olsson C, Fagher BO, et al: Need for long-term anticoagulant treatment in symptomatic calf vein thrombosis. Lancet 2(8454):515, 1985.

115. Lederman JA, Keshavarzian A: Acute pulmonary embolism following air travel. Postgrad Med J 59(688):104, 1983.

116. Leslie IJ, Dorgan JC, Bentley G, et al: A prospective study of deep vein thrombosis of the leg in children on halo-femoral traction. J Bone Joint Surg [Br] 63-B(2):168, 1981.

117. Levine MN, Gent M, Hirsh J, et al: The thrombogenic effect of anticancer drug therapy in women with stage II breast cancer. N Engl J Med 318(7):404, 1988.

118. Lindblad B, Sternby NH, Bergqvist D: Incidence of venous thromboembolism verified by necropsy over 30 years. Br Med J 302(6778):709, 1991.

119. Lindner D, Edwards J, Phinney E, et al: Long-term hemodynamic and clinical sequelae of lower extremity deep vein thrombosis. J Vasc Surg 4(5):436, 1986.

120. Lohr J, Kerr T, Lutter K, et al: Lower extremity calf thrombosis: To treat or not to treat? J Vasc Surg 14:618, 1991.

121. Love PE, Santoro SA: Antiphospholipid antibodies: Anticardiolipin and the lupus anticoagulant in systemic lupus erythematosus (SLE) and in non-SLE disorders. Ann Intern Med 112(9):682, 1990.

122. Macklon NS, Greer IA: Venous thromboembolic disease in obstetrics and gynaecology: The Scottish experience. Scot Med J 41(3):83, 1996.

123. Makris M, Rosendaal FR, Preston FE: Familial thrombophilia: Genetic risk factors and management. J Intern Med 242(Suppl 740):9, 1997.

124. Malm J, Laurell M, Dahlback B: Changes in plasma levels of vitamin K–dependent proteins C and S and of C4b-binding protein during pregnancy and oral contraception. Br J Haematol 68(4):437, 1988.

125. Mammen EF: Pathogenesis of venous thrombosis. Chest 102(6 Suppl):640S, 1992.

126. Markel A, Manzo RA, Bergelin RO, et al: Valvular reflux after deep vein thrombosis: Incidence and time of occurrence. J Vasc Surg 15(2):377, 1992.

127. Maurer BJ, Wray R, Shillingford JP: Frequency of venous thrombosis after myocardial infarction. Lancet 2(7739):1385, 1971.

128. McBride WJ, Gadowski GR, Keller MS, et al: Pulmonary embolism in pediatric trauma patients. J Trauma 37(6):913, 1994.

129. McLachlin AD, McLachlin JA, Jory TA, et al: Venous stasis in the lower extremities. Ann Surg 152(4):678, 1960.

130. McLafferty R, Moneta G, Passman M, et al: Late clinical and hemodynamic sequelae of isolated calf vein thrombosis. J Vasc Surg 27(1):50, 1998.

131. McLean Ross AH, Griffith CDM, Anderson JR, et al: Thromboembolic complications with silicone elastomer subclavian catheters. J Parenter Enteral Nutr 6(1):61, 1982.

132. Meissner MH, Caps MT, Bergelin RO, et al: Early outcome after isolated calf vein thrombosis. J Vasc Surg 26(5):749, 1997.

133. Meissner MH, Caps MT, Bergelin RO, et al: Propagation, rethrombosis, and new thrombus formation after acute deep venous thrombosis. J Vasc Surg 22(5):558, 1995.

134. Meissner MH, Caps MT, Zierler BK, et al: Determinants of chronic venous disease after acute deep venous thrombosis. J Vasc Surg 28(5):826, 1998.

135. Meissner MH, Manzo RA, Bergelin RO, et al: Deep venous insufficiency: The relationship between lysis and subsequent reflux. J Vasc Surg 18(4):596, 1993.

136. Menzoin JS, Sequeira J, Doyle J, et al: Therapeutic and clinical course of deep venous thrombosis. Am J Surg 146:581, 1983.

137. Meredith JW, Young JS, O'Neil EA, et al: Femoral catheters and deep venous thrombosis: A prospective evaluation with venous duplex sonography. J Trauma 35(2):187, 1993.

138. Merton RE, Hockley D, Gray EP, et al: The effect of interleukin 1 on venous endothelium—an ultrastructural study. Thromb Haemost 66(6):725, 1991.

139. Monreal M, Barroso R-J, Ruiz Manzano J, et al: Asymptomatic pulmonary embolism in patients with deep vein thrombosis: Is it useful to take a lung scan to rule out this condition? J Cardiovasc Surg 30(1):104, 1989.

140. Monreal M, Lafoz E, Casals A, et al: Occult cancer in patients with deep venous thrombosis: A systematic approach. Cancer 67(2):541, 1991.

141. Monreal M, Martorell A, Callejas J, et al: Venographic assessment of deep vein thrombosis and risk of developing post-thrombotic syndrome: A prospective trial. J Intern Med 233(3):233, 1993.

142. Monreal M, Raventos A, Lerma R, et al: Pulmonary embolism in patients with upper extremity DVT associated to venous central lines—a prospective study. Thromb Haemost 72(4):548, 1994.

143. Moreno-Cabral R, Kistner R, Nordyke R: Importance of calf vein thrombophlebitis. Surgery 80(6):735, 1976.

144. Mourant AE, Kopec AC, Domaniewska-Sobczak K: Blood groups and blood clotting. Lancet 1(7692):223, 1971.

145. Nachman RL, Silverstein R: Hypercoagulable states. Ann Intern Med 119(8):819, 1993.

146. Napolitano LM, Garlapati VS, Heard SO, et al: Asymptomatic deep venous thrombosis in the trauma patient: Is an aggressive screening protocol justified? J Trauma 39(4):651, 1995.

147. Nawroth PP, Handley DA, Esmon CT, et al: Interleukin 1 induces endothelial cell procoagulant while suppressing cell-surface anticoagulant activity. Proc Natl Acad Sci USA 83(10):3460, 1986.

148. Nguyen LT, Laberge JM, Guttman FMA: Spontaneous deep vein thrombosis in childhood and adolescence. J Pediatr Surg 21(7):640, 1986.

149. Nicolaides AN, Irving D: Clinical factors and the risk of deep venous thrombosis. In Nicolaides AN (ed): Thromboembolism: Aetiology, Advances in Prevention and Management. Lancaster, England, MTP Press, 1975.

150. Nicolaides AN, Kakkar VV, Field ES, et al: The origin of deep vein thrombosis: A venographic study. Br J Radiol 44(525):653, 1971.

151. Nicolaides AN, Kakkar VV, Renney JTG, et al: Myocardial infarction and deep venous thrombosis. Br Med J 1(746):432, 1971.

152. Nordstrom M, Lindblad B, Anderson H, et al: Deep venous thrombosis and occult malignancy: An epidemiological study. Br Med J 308(6933):891, 1994.

153. Nordstrom M, Lindblad B, Bergqvist D, et al: A prospective study of the incidence of deep-vein thrombosis within a defined urban population. J Intern Med 232(2):155, 1992.

154. Northeast AD, Burnand KG: The response of the vessel wall to thrombosis: The in vivo study of venous thrombolysis. Ann N Y Acad Sci 667:127, 1992.

155. Northeast AD, Soo KS, Bobrow LG, et al: The tissue plasminogen activator and urokinase response in vivo during natural resolution of venous thrombus. J Vasc Surg 22(5):573, 1995.

156. O'Donnell D: Thromboembolism and air travel (Letter). Lancet 797, 1988.

157. Oger E, Leroyer C, Le Moigne E, et al: The value of risk factor analysis in clinically suspected deep venous thrombosis. Respiration 64(5):326, 1997.

158. Olivieri O, Friso S, Manzato F, et al: Resistance to activated protein C, associated with oral contraceptive use: Effect of formulations, duration of assumption, and doses of oestro-progestins. Contraception 54(3):149, 1996.

159. Owen J, Kvam D, Nossel HL, et al: Thrombin and plasmin activity and platelet activation in the development of venous thrombosis. Blood 61(3):476, 1983.

160. Pabinger I, Schneider B, Inhibitors GS, Go N: Thrombotic risk of

women with hereditary antithrombin III-, protein C-, and protein S-deficiency taking oral contraceptive medication. Thromb Haemost 71(5):548, 1994.

161. Passman M, Moneta G, Taylor L, et al: Pulmonary embolism is associated with the combination of isolated calf vein thrombosis and respiratory symptoms. J Vasc Surg 25(1):39, 1997.

162. Perez Gutthann S, Garcia Rodriguez LA, Castellsague I, et al: Hormone replacement therapy and risk of venous thromboembolism: Population based case-control study. Br Med J 314(7083):796, 1997.

163. Philbrick JT, Becker DM: Calf deep venous thrombosis: A wolf in sheep's clothing? Arch Intern Med 148:(10):2131, 1983.

164. Piccioli A, Prandoni P, Goldhaber SZ: Epidemiologic characteristics, management, and outcome of deep venous thrombosis in a tertiary-care hospital: The Brigham and Women's Hospital DVT Registry. Am Heart J 132(5):1010, 1996.

165. Prandoni P, Cogo A, Bernardi E, et al: A simple ultrasound approach for detection of recurrent proximal vein thrombosis. Circulation 88 (Part 1):1730, 1993.

166. Prandoni P, Lensing A, Cogo A, et al: The long-term clinical course of acute deep venous thrombosis. Ann Intern Med 125(1):1, 1996.

167. Prandoni P, Lensing AW, Buller HR, et al: Deep-vein thrombosis and the incidence of subsequent symptomatic cancer. N Engl J Med 327(16):1128, 1992.

168. Prandoni P, Villalta S, Polistena P, et al: Symptomatic deep-vein thrombosis and the post-thrombotic syndrome. Haematologica 80(2 Suppl):42, 1995.

169. Prins MH, Hirsch J: A critical review of the evidence supporting a relationship between impaired fibrinolytic activity and venous thromboembolism. Arch Intern Med 151(9):1721, 1991.

170. Boston Collaborative Drug Surveillance Program: Oral contraceptive use and venous thromboembolic disease, surgically confirmed gallbladder disease, and breast tumors. Lancet 1(7817):1399, 1973.

171. Quehenberger P, Loner U, Kapiotis S, et al: Increased levels of activated factor VII and decreased plasma protein S activity and circulating thrombomodulin during use of oral contraceptives. Thromb Haemost 76(5):729, 1996.

172. Radecki RT, Gaebler-Spira D: Deep vein thrombosis in the disabled pediatric population. Arch Phys Med Rehabil 75(3):248, 1994.

173. Raskob G: Calf-vein thrombosis. In Hull RD, Raskob GE, Pineo GF (eds): Venous Thromboembolism: An Evidence-based Atlas. Armonk, NY, Futura Publishing Company, 1996, p 307.

174. Rees DC, Cox M, Clegg JB: World distribution of factor V Leiden. Lancet 346:1133, 1995.

175. Rickles FR, Edwards RL: Activation of blood coagulation in cancer: Trousseau's syndrome revisited. Blood 62(1):14, 1983.

176. Rickles FR, Levine M, Edwards RL: Hemostatic alterations in cancer patients. Cancer Metast Rev 11(3–4):237, 1992

177. Ridker PM, Glynn RJ, Miletich JP, et al: Age-specific incidence rates of venous thromboembolism among heterozygous carriers of factor V Leiden mutation. Ann Intern Med 126(7):528, 1997.

178. Rohrer MJ, Cutler BS, MacDougall E, et al: A prospective study of the incidence of deep venous thrombosis in hospitalized children. J Vasc Surg 24(1):46, 1996.

179. Rosendaal FR: Thrombosis in the young: Epidemiology and risk factors: A focus on venous thrombosis. Thromb Haemost 78(1):1, 1997.

180. Salzman EW, Hirsh J: The epidemiology, pathogenesis, and natural history of venous thrombosis. In Colman RW, Hirsh J, Marder VJ, Salzman EW (eds): Hemostasis and Thrombosis: Basic Principles and Clinical Practice, 3rd ed. Philadelphia, JB Lippincott, 1994, p 1275.

181. Sartwell PE, Masi AT, Arthes FG, et al: Thromboembolism and oral contraceptives: An epidemiologic case-control study. Am J Epidemiol 90(5):365, 1969.

182. Sarvesvaran R: Sudden natural deaths associated with commercial air travel. Med Sci Law 26(1):35, 1986.

183. Sattani B, Falcone R, Shook L, et al: Screening for major deep vein thrombosis in seriously injured patients: A prospective study. Ann Vasc Surg 11(6):626, 1997.

184. Scarabin P-Y, Plu-Bureau G, Zitoun D, et al: Changes in haemostatic variables induced by oral contraceptives containing 50 μg or 30 μg oestrogen: Absence of dose-dependent effect of PAI-1 activity. Thromb Haemost 74(3):928, 1995.

185. Schafer AI: Hypercoagulable states: Molecular genetics to clinical practice. Lancet 344(8939):1739, 1994.

186. Scott GBD: A quantitative study of the fate of occlusive red venous thrombi. Br J Exp Pathol 49(6):544, 1968.

187. Scurr JH: How long after surgery does the risk of thromboembolism persist? Acta Chir Scand (Suppl) 556:22, 1990.

188. Sevitt S: The mechanisms of canalisation in deep vein thrombosis. J Pathol 110(2):153, 1973.

189. Sevitt S: The vascularisation of deep-vein thrombi and their fibrous residue: A post-mortem angiographic study. J Pathol 111(1):1, 1973.

190. Sevitt S: Organization of valve pocket thrombi and the anomalies of double thrombi and valve cusp involvement. Br J Surg 61(8):641, 1974.

191. Sevitt S: The structure and growth of valve-pocket thrombi in femoral veins. J Clin Pathol 27(7):517, 1974.

192. Sevitt S, Gallagher N: Venous thrombosis and pulmonary embolism: A clinico-pathological study in injured and burned victims. Br J Surg 48:475, 1961.

193. Sharrock NE, Go G, Harpel PC, et al: The John Charnley Award: Thrombogenesis during total hip arthroplasty. Clin Orthop (319): 16, 1995.

194. Shreeniwas R, Koga S, Karakurum M, et al: Hypoxia-mediated induction of endothelial cell interleukin-1α: An autocrine mechanism promoting expression of leukocyte adhesion molecules on the vessel surface. J Clin Invest 90(6):2333, 1992.

195. Sigel B, Ipsen J, Felix WR: The epidemiology of lower extremity deep venous thrombosis in surgical patients. Ann Surg 179(3):278, 1974.

196. Sigel B, Swami V, Can A, et al: Intimal hyperplasia producing thrombus organization in an experimental venous thrombosis model. J Vasc Surg 19(2):350, 1994.

197. Silva MDC: Chronic venous insufficiency of the lower limbs and its socio-economic significance. Int Angiol 10(3):152, 1991.

198. Simioni P, Prandoni P, Lensing AW, et al: The risk of recurrent venous thromboembolism in patients with an Arg506→Gln mutation in the gene for factor V (factor V Leiden). N Engl J Med 336(6):399, 1997.

199. Simmons AV, Sheppard MA, Cox AF: Deep venous thrombosis after myocardial infarction: Predisposing factors. Br Heart J 35:623, 1973.

200. Soo KS, Northeast AD, Happerfield LC, et al: Tissue plasminogen activator production by monocytes in venous thrombolysis. J Pathol 178(2):190, 1996.

201. Sorensen HT, Mellemkjaer L, Steffensen FH, et al: The risk of a diagnosis of cancer after primary deep venous thrombosis or pulmonary embolism. N Engl J Med 338(17):1169, 1998.

202. Stamatakis JD, Kakkar VV, Sagar S, et al: Femoral vein thrombosis and total hip replacement. Br J Med 2(6081):223, 1977.

203. Stewart GJ: Neutrophils and deep venous thrombosis. Haemostasis 23(Suppl 1):127, 1993.

204. Stewart GJ, Stern HS, Lynch PR, et al: Responses of canine jugular veins and carotid arteries to hysterectomy: Increased permeability and leukocyte adhesions and invasion. Thromb Res 20(5–6):473, 1980.

205. Strandness DE, Langlois Y, Cramer M, et al: Long-term sequelae of acute venous thrombosis. JAMA 250(10):1289, 1983.

206. Strolley PD, Tonascia JA, Tockman MS, et al: Thrombosis with low-estrogen oral contraceptives. Am J Epidemiol 102(3):197, 1975.

207. Sue LP, Davis JW, Parks SN: Iliofemoral venous injuries: An indication for prophylactic caval filter placement. J Trauma 39(4):693, 1995.

208. Symington IS, Stack BHR: Pulmonary thromboembolism after travel. Br J Dis Chest 71(2):138, 1977.

209. Tardy B, Tardy-Poncet B, Bara L, et al: Effects of long travels in sitting position in elderly volunteers on biologic markers of coagulation activity and fibrinolysis. Thromb Res 83(2):153, 1996.

210. Thomas D: Venous thrombogenesis. Br Med Bull 50(4):803, 1994.

211. Thomas DP, Merton RE, Hockley DJ: The effect of stasis on the venous endothelium: An ultrastructural study. Br J Haematol 55(1):113, 1983.

212. Thomas DP, Merton RE, Wood RD, et al: The relationship between vessel wall injury and venous thrombosis: An experimental study. Br J Haematol 59(3):449, 1985.

213. Thomas WA, Davies JNP, O'Neal RM, et al: Incidence of myocardial infarction correlated with venous and pulmonary thrombosis and embolism. Am J Cardiol 5:41, 1960.

214. Tilney NL, Griffiths HJG, Edwards EA: Natural history of major venous thrombosis of the upper extremity. Arch Surg 101(6):792, 1970.

215. Tindall VR: Factors influencing puerperal thromboembolism. J Obstet Gynaecol Br Commonw 75(2):1324, 1968.
216. Toglia MR, Weg JG: Venous thromboembolism during pregnancy. N Engl J Med 335(2):108, 1996.
217. Treffers PE, Huidekoper BL, Weenink GH, et al: Epidemiological observations of thromboembolic disease during pregnancy and in the puerperium, in 56,022 women. Int J Gynaecol Obstet 21(4):327, 1983.
218. Tripolitis AJ, Bodily KC, Blackshear WM, et al: Venous capacitance and outflow in the post-operative patient. Ann Surg 190(5):634, 1979.
219. Upchurch GR Jr, Demling RH, Davies J, et al: Efficacy of subcutaneous heparin in prevention of venous thromboembolic events in trauma patients. Am Surg 61(9):749, 1995.
220. van Ramshorst B, van Bemmelen PS, Honeveld H, et al: Thrombus regression in deep venous thrombosis: Quantification of spontaneous thrombolysis with duplex scanning. Circulation 86(2):414, 1992.
221. Vandenbroucke JP, Helmerhorst FM, Bloemenkamp KW, et al: Third-generation oral contraceptive and deep venous thrombosis: From epidemiologic controversy to new insight in coagulation. Am J Obstet Gynecol 177(4):887, 1997.
222. Vandenbrouke JP, van der Meer FJM, Helmerhorst FM, et al: Factor V Leiden: Should we screen oral contraceptive users and pregnant women? BMJ 313(7065):1127, 1996.
223. Varas-Lorenzo C, Garcia-Rodriguez LA, Cattaruzzi C, et al: Hormone replacement therapy and the risk of hospitalization for venous thromboembolism: A population-based study in southern Europe. Am J Epidemiol 147(4):387, 1998.
224. Vecchi M, Cattaneo M, de Franchis R, et al: Risk of thromboembolic complications in patients with inflammatory bowel disease: Study of hemostasis measurements. Int J Clin Lab Res 21(2):165, 1991.
225. Vessey MP, Doll R: Investigation of relation between use of oral contraceptives and thromboembolic disease. Br Med J 2(599):199, 1968.
226. von Kaulla E, Droegemueller W, Aoki N, et al: Antithrombin III depression and thrombin generation acceleration in women taking oral contraceptives. Am J Obstet Gynecol 109(6):868, 1971.
227. Wahl DG, Guillemin F, de Maistre E, et al: Risk for venous thrombosis related to antiphospholipid antibodies in systemic lupus erythematosus—a meta-analysis. Lupus 6(5):467, 1997.
228. Wakefield TW, Greenfield LJ, Rolfe MW, et al: Inflammatory and procoagulant mediator interactions in an experimental baboon model of venous thrombosis. Thromb Haemost 69(2):164, 1993.
229. Warlow C, Ogston D, Douglas AS: Deep venous thrombosis of the legs after strokes: Part I—Incidence and predisposing factors. Br Med J 1(6019):1178, 1976.
230. Wautrecht JC, Galle C, Motte S, et al: The role of ABO blood groups in the incidence of deep vein thrombosis (Letter). Thromb Haemost 79(3):688, 1998.
231. Wessler S: Thrombosis in the presence of vascular stasis. Am J Med 33:648, 1962.
232. Wessler S, Reimer SM, Sheps MC: Biologic assay of a thrombosis-inducing activity in human serum. J Appl Physiol 14(6):943, 1959.
233. Winkler UH, Holscher T, Schulte H, et al: Ethinylestradiol 20 versus 30 μg combined with 150 μg desogestrel: A large comparative study of the effects of two low-dose oral contraceptives on the hemostatic system. Gynecol Endocrinol 10(4):265, 1996.
234. Wise RC: Spontaneous lower extremity venous thrombosis in children. Am J Dis Child 126(6):766, 1973.
235. Xiang DZ, Verbeken EK, Van Lommel ATL, et al: Composition and formation of the sleeve enveloping a central venous catheter. J Vasc Surg 28(2):260, 1998.

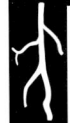

CHAPTER 1 3 9

Clinical and Diagnostic Evaluation of Deep Venous Thrombosis

Anthony J. Comerota, M.D., F.A.C.S.

BACKGROUND

Deep venous thrombosis (DVT) remains a common and serious medical condition, frequently complicating the postoperative recovery of surgical patients or manifesting de novo in patients with recognized (or unrecognized) risk factors. More than 1 million cases of DVT are diagnosed in the United States annually, resulting in approximately 50,000 to 200,000 deaths due to pulmonary emboli.[1, 17] The predilection for blood clots to form in the veins of the lower extremities has not been fully explained, although investigation of the pathophysiology of postoperative DVT has shed some light on this aspect.[12, 13, 31] A number of well-defined patient populations and high-risk factors have been identified.[21]

Pulmonary embolism remains the major early complica-

tion of DVT. The post-thrombotic syndrome is a costly and morbid long-term complication of DVT, resulting from venous valvular damage and persistent luminal obstruction.[24, 30] The risks for both pulmonary embolism and post-thrombotic syndrome escalate in patients with recurrent DVT. Recurrent DVT is more likely to occur in patients who are inadequately treated,[23] emphasizing the necessity of accurate diagnosis.

Arriving at an accurate evaluation of the patient at high risk for or suspected to have acute DVT can be challenging. Although some physicians rely on a single diagnostic test, others integrate imaging of the venous system with the known physiology of venous return and the pathophysiology that accompanies thrombotic obstruction of the venous system. Elements of the physiology of clot formation and lysis have been integrated into the diagnostic approach to these patients through the inclusion of markers of clot breakdown.[19, 29] Newer imaging techniques allow evaluation of the peripheral venous system, which was previously unavailable.[7]

This chapter focuses on the current approach to the diagnosis of DVT, which incorporates available diagnostic techniques to arrive at the most reliable evaluation of the patient. The available diagnostic techniques for DVT have been described in previous chapters. Certain elements of the various diagnostic methods are reviewed here to put the techniques in proper clinical perspective.

CLINICAL ASSESSMENT

It has been accepted that an objective diagnosis of DVT is mandatory because clinical evaluation is inaccurate.[15] Unfortunately, this observation has spawned the attitude that clinical assessment is never of any value in patients in whom DVT is suspected. The situation is unfortunate, since clinical features can be used to classify symptomatic patients with suspected DVT and to improve diagnostic strategies. Such patients are categorized as having either a high or low probability of DVT prior to diagnostic testing.

Studies have demonstrated that categorizing the patients' pretest probability of DVT into low, moderate, or high likelihood improves diagnostic precision.[32] Wells and associates[32] demonstrated that combining the use of a model of clinical probability of DVT with common femoral and popliteal vein compression ultrasound decreased the number of false-positive and false-negative diagnoses; they used ascending phlebography as the definitive diagnostic test. These investigators found that patients with a high clinical suspicion of DVT (Table 139–1) had an 85% chance of having phlebographically proven DVT. They suggested that patients with low pre-test probability and negative noninvasive test results do not require treatment or additional testing, and those with high pre-test probability and positive noninvasive test results should be treated. In patients with discordance between clinical assessment (pre-test probability) and diagnostic testing, additional evaluation is necessary. This approach parallels that used in the Prospective Investigation of Pulmonary Embolism Diagnosis (PIO-PED),[27] which demonstrated the value of the clinical assessment of a patient with suspected pulmonary embolism.

PHLEBOGRAPHY

Contrast ascending phlebography has been regarded as the diagnostic standard for lower extremity DVT. Its advantages and disadvantages are discussed in Chapter 17. Because of the numerous disadvantages of phlebography and the better results of venous duplex imaging, ascending phlebography is infrequently used today. Opinions expressing the value of phlebography are generally inflated and based on biased evaluation of selected patients. By that, I mean that phlebograms used for objective reports frequently are chosen after they are completed and the films judged to be of good quality rather than entering the diagnostic matrix at the "point of need." In my experience and that of others, phlebography could not be completed in more than 20%

TABLE 139–1. CLINICAL SIGNS, SYMPTOMS, AND RISK FACTORS OF DEEP VEIN THROMBOSIS (DVT)*

Major
  Acute cancer
  Paralysis/paresis
  Recent cast immobilization of lower extremities
  Bedridden × 3 days
  Major operation within 4 weeks
  Tenderness in distribution of the deep venous system
  Swelling of thigh or calf (>3 cm)
  Family history of DVT (≥first-degree relatives)

Minor
  History of recent trauma to symptomatic leg
  Unilateral pitting edema (symptomatic leg)
  Dilated (nonvaricose) superficial veins, symptomatic leg only
  Hospitalization within prior 6 months
  Erythema

Clinical probability
  High
    ≥3 major points and no alternative diagnosis
    ≥2 major points and >2 minor points and no alternative diagnosis
  Low
    1 major point and ≥2 minor points and an alternative diagnosis
    1 major point and ≥1 minor point and no alternative diagnosis
    0 major points and ≥3 minor points and an alternative diagnosis
    0 major points and ≥2 minor points and no alternative diagnosis
  Moderate
    All other combinations

*Used to develop clinical model for predicting pre-test probability of DVT.

of patients for whom it was requested.[4, 14] When venous access for contrast injection succeeds, good-quality biplanar visualization of the lower leg is frequently achieved; however, inadequate evaluation of the proximal venous system is common.[14]

INDIRECT PHYSIOLOGIC STUDIES

Physiologic studies have been used to evaluate the deep venous system as an indirect evaluation of DVT, with the assumption that reduction in maximal venous outflow (impedance plethysmography),[22, 33] phasic respiratory volume change, or abnormal augmentation maneuvers (phlebo-rheography)[8, 16] were the consequences of acute DVT. In patients with clinically suspected DVT, these tests proved reasonably reliable for detecting proximal DVT. The same physiologic studies were unreliable, however, in the screening of high-risk but asymptomatic patients.[11] Because many of the asymptomatic patients had nonocclusive thrombus, the physiologic parameters monitored were not sensitive enough to demonstrate abnormalities; therefore, unacceptably low sensitivities were observed.

VENOUS DUPLEX IMAGING

Venous duplex imaging is the current mainstay of the diagnosis of DVT. It has excellent diagnostic accuracy in patients with clinically suspected DVT.[9, 10] Some centers have reported very good results in high-risk asymptomatic patients,[10] but others have reported poor sensitivity in asymptomatic patients in surveillance programs.[18] Venous duplex imaging is more accurate than indirect physiologic tests for DVT[10, 20] and has essentially replaced them for the initial screening of patients and as the definitive diagnostic study.

MAGNETIC RESONANCE VENOGRAPHY

Magnetic resonance venography (MRV) has demonstrated excellent sensitivity for the diagnosis of proximal venous thrombosis in comparison with ascending phlebography.[7] Availability, cost, nonuse with metallic implants, and patient claustrophobia limit its application, however. The true value of MRV is likely to be in the patients with pelvic and vena caval thrombosis, for which traditional diagnostic studies are inadequate.

BLOOD TESTS

During the 1980s and 1990s, the use of blood tests has been investigated to assist with the diagnosis of acute DVT. Attempts were made to identify reliable markers that might indicate the presence of acute thrombus. Breakdown products of fibrinogen generated during thrombus formation and breakdown products of complexed fibrin generated during physiologic fibrinolysis have been studied.[2, 5] Prothrombin fragment and fibrinopeptides A and B are sensitive by-products of thrombus formation, but they have not been found to be clinically useful.

D-dimer, a degradation product resulting from fibrinolysis of complexed fibrin (fibrin acted upon by factor XIII), has proved to be useful in evaluating patients with suspected DVT. Although D-dimer levels are elevated in postoperative and acutely ill patients,[28] a negative D-dimer test result in patients with suspected DVT has demonstrated a high negative predictive value.[19] The conventional enzyme-linked immunosorbent assay (ELISA) determination is the best assay for D-dimer analysis; however it is time-consuming and is not practical for clinical use.[3, 6] A number of rapid assays have been found to yield results comparable to those of the ELISA determinations,[19, 20] indicating that the D-dimer blood test can be performed quickly and reliably enough to be used clinically. Although a D-dimer elevation cannot be used to make treatment decisions, a normal D-dimer value does reliably exclude DVT. Ginsberg and colleagues[19] showed that a normal D-dimer value had a negative predictive value of 97%; in the subgroup of patients in this study with a low pre-test likelihood of DVT, the negative predictive value of a normal D-dimer level was 99.4%.

SCINTIGRAPHIC TESTS

Radioisotopic tests have been used in selected patients with suspected DVT, and the radiolabeled fibrinogen uptake test (RFUT) has been the most popular.[25, 26] Unfortunately, because of concerns about transmission of blood-borne diseases from the pooled fibrinogen, RFUT is not available in the United States. As recombinant fibrinogen is developed, this test probably will be reintroduced and will be useful in selected patients.

Other isotopic techniques have used platelets, labeled with radioactive indium, and technetium Tc 99m labeled albumin and red blood cells. These tests have not been incorporated into clinical practice because of poor sensitivity and specificity.

DIAGNOSTIC STRATEGY

On the basis of the preceding information, a number of approaches can be applied to patients in whom DVT is suspected and that a single diagnostic test is not appropriate for all patients. With that assumption as background, venous duplex imaging has become the major tool for diagnosis. Therefore, in patients with the clinical suspicion of DVT, venous duplex imaging is the initial test (Fig. 139–1).

If the scan is positive, the patient is treated for DVT. If the scan is negative, the patient should be classified according to the level of clinical suspicion of DVT assigned prior to venous duplex imaging:

1. A low clinical suspicion of DVT accompanied by a negative duplex scan effectively excludes DVT, and no further evaluation is necessary.

2. For the patient with moderate clinical suspicion of DVT, a negative duplex scan should be followed by a second scan in 3 to 5 days or a D-dimer blood test. A negative D-dimer test result offers good assurance that the patient does not have DVT. A positive D-dimer test following a normal venous duplex scan requires further evaluation with MRV or ascending phlebography.

3. The patients with a high clinical suspicion of DVT despite a negative venous duplex scan should undergo additional investigation with MRV, ascending phlebography, or a second duplex scan.

Indeterminate venous duplex scans are infrequent but require additional evaluation:

1. In patients with a low clinical suspicion for DVT, a second duplex scan in 3 to 5 days is appropriate, assuming that the second scan has a better technical result.

2. For the patient with a moderate or high clinical suspicion of DVT, an indeterminate venous duplex scan should be followed by a D-dimer blood test or evaluation with MRV or ascending phlebography. If the D-dimer test result is negative, and if the patient's clinical status remains stable or improves, the patient can then be observed.

3. If clinical suspicion of DVT increases with time or if the D-dimer test is positive, MRV or ascending phlebography is indicated.

SUMMARY

The relatively straightforward approach to patients with suspected DVT presented here combines clinical acumen,

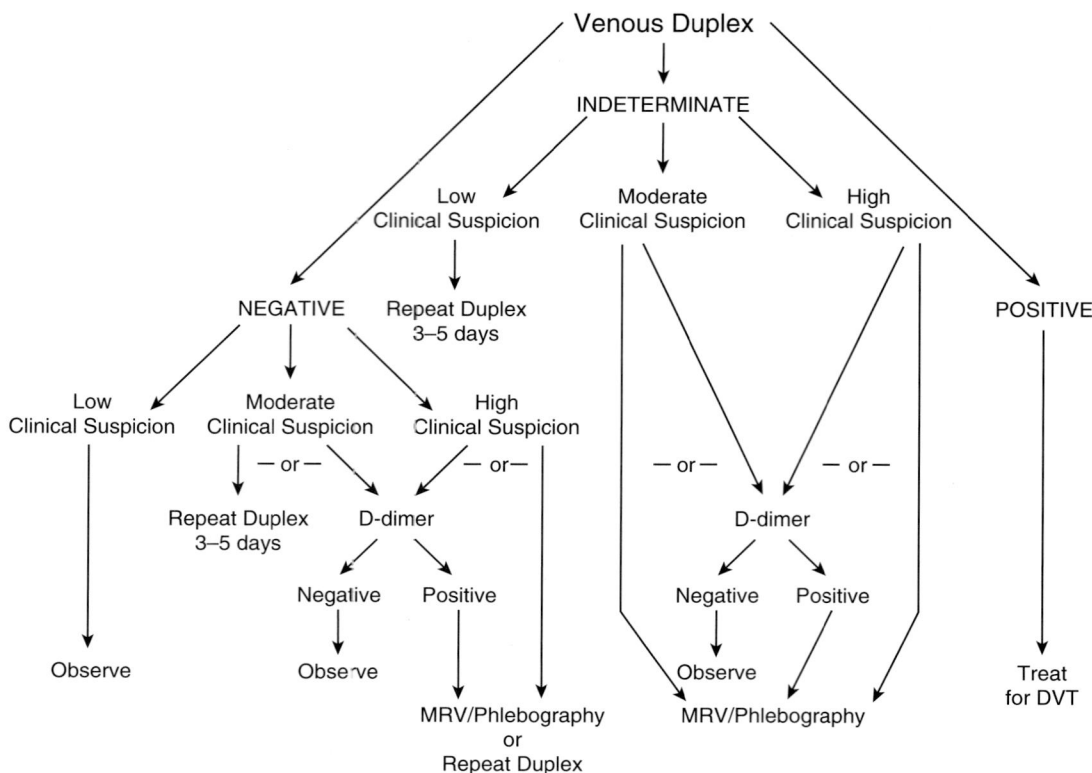

FIGURE 139–1. Algorithm for clinical suspicion of deep vein thrombosis (DVT). MRV = magnetic resonance venography.

the well-documented utility of modern ultrasound technology, the physiology of thrombus breakdown, and the new and traditional imaging modalities, MRV and ascending contrast phlebography, to achieve accurate assessment of patients with clinical suspicion of DVT.

REFERENCES

1. Anderson FA Jr, Wheeler HB, Goldberg R, et al: A population-based perspective of the hospital incidence and case-fatality rates of deep vein thrombosis and pulmonary embolism: The Worcester DVT Study. Arch Intern Med 151:933, 1991.
2. Bauer KA: Laboratory markers for coagulation activation. Arch Pathol Lab Med 177:71, 1993.
3. Becker DM, Philbrick JT, Bachhuber TL, Humphries JE: D-dimer testing and acute venous thromboembolism. Arch Intern Med 156:939, 1996.
4. Bergqvist D: Efficacy and safety of enoxaparin versus unfractionated heparin for prevention of deep vein thrombosis in elective cancer surgery: A double-blind randomized multicentre trial with venographic assessment. Br J Surg 84:1099, 1997.
5. Boneu B, Bes G, Pelzer H, et al: D-dimers, thrombin antithrombin III complexes and prothrombin fragments 1+2: Diagnostic value in clinically suspected deep vein thrombosis. Thromb Haemost 65:28, 1991.
6. Bounameaux H, De Moerloose P, Perrier A, Reber G: Plasma measurement of D-dimer as diagnostic aid in suspected venous thromboembolism: an overview. Thromb Haemost 71:1, 1994.
7. Carpenter JP, Holland GA, Baum RA, Owen RS: Magnetic resonance venography for detection of deep venous thrombosis: Comparison with contrast venography and duplex Doppler ultrasonography. J Vasc Surg 18:734, 1993.
8. Comerota AJ, Cranley JJ, Cook SE, et al: Phleborheography: Results of a ten-year experience. Surgery 91:573, 1982.
9. Comerota AJ, Katz ML: The diagnosis of acute deep venous thrombosis by duplex venous imaging. Semin Vasc Surg 1:32, 1988.
10. Comerota AJ, Katz ML, Greenwald LL, et al: Venous duplex imaging: Should it replace hemodynamic tests for deep venous thrombosis? J Vasc Surg 11:53, 1990.
11. Comerota AJ, Katz ML, Grossi RJ, et al: The comparative value of noninvasive testing for diagnosis and surveillance of deep venous thrombosis. J Vasc Surg 7:40, 1988.
12. Comerota AJ, Stewart GJ, Alburger PD, et al: Operative venodilation, a previously unsuspected factor in the cause of postoperative deep vein thrombosis. Surgery 106:301, 1989.
13. Comerota AJ, Stewart GJ, White JV: Combined dihydroergotamine and heparin prophylaxis of postoperative deep vein thrombosis: Proposed mechanism of action. Am J Surg 150:39, 1985.
14. Comerota AJ, White JV, Katz ML: Diagnostic methods for deep vein thrombosis: Venous Doppler examination, phleborheography, iodine-125 fibrinogen uptake and phlebography. Am J Surg 150:14, 1985.
15. Cranley JJ, Canos AJ, Sull WJ: The diagnosis of deep venous thrombosis: Fallibility of clinical symptoms and signs. Arch Surg 111:34, 1976.
16. Cranley JJ, Canos AJ, Sull WJ, Grass AM: Phleborheographic technique for diagnosis of deep vein thrombosis of the lower extremities. Surg Gynecol Obstet 141:331, 1975.
17. Dalen JE, Alpert JS: Natural history of pulmonary embolism. Progr Cardiovasc Dis 17:257, 1975.
18. Ginsberg JS, Caco CC, Brill-Edwards P, et al: Venous thrombosis in patients who have undergone major hip or knee surgery: Detection with compression US and impedance plethysmography. Radiology 181:651, 1991.
19. Ginsberg JS, Kearon C, Douketis J, et al: The use of D-dimer testing and impedance plethysmographic examination in patients with clinical indications of deep vein thrombosis. Arch Intern Med 157:1077, 1997.
20. Heijboer H, Buller HR, Lensing AWA, et al: A comparison of real-time compression ultrasonography with impedance plethysmography for the diagnosis of deep-vein thrombosis in symptomatic outpatients. N Engl J Med 329:1365, 1993.

21. Hirsh J, Hull RD: Pathogenesis of venous thromboembolism and clinical risk factors. *In* Hirsh H, Hull RD (eds): Venous Thromboembolism: Natural History, Diagnosis and Management. Boca Raton, Fla, CRC Press, 1987, p 5.

22. Hull RD, Hirsh J, Carter CJ, et al: Diagnostic efficacy of impedance plethysmography for clinically suspected deep-vein thrombosis: A randomized trial. Ann Intern Med 102:21, 1985.

23. Hull RD, Raskob GE, Hirsh J, et al: Continuous intravenous heparin compared with intermittent subcutaneous heparin in the initial treatment of proximal vein thrombosis. N Engl J Med 315:1109, 1986.

24. Johnson BF, Manzo RA, Bergelin RO, Strandness DE: Relationship between changes in the deep venous system and the development of the post thrombotic syndrome after an acute episode of lower limb deep vein thrombosis: A one-to-six year follow-up. J Vasc Surg 21:307, 1995.

25. Kakkar V: The diagnosis of deep vein thrombosis using the ^{125}I-fibrinogen test. Arch Surg 104:152, 1972.

26. Moser KM, Brach BB, Dolan GF: Clinically suspected deep venous thrombosis of the lower extremities: A comparison of venography, impedance plethysmography, and radiolabeled fibrinogen. JAMA 237:2195, 1977.

27. The PIOPED Investigators: Value of the ventilation/perfusion scan in acute pulmonary embolism: Results of the Prospective Investigation of Pulmonary Embolism Diagnosis (PIOPED). JAMA 268:2753, 1990.

28. Rowbotham BJ, Carrol P, Whitaker AN, et al: Measurement of cross-linked fibrin derivatives: Use in the diagnosis of venous thrombosis. Thromb Haemost 57:59, 1987.

29. Scarano L, Bernardi E, Prandoni P, et al: Accuracy of two newly described D-dimer tests in patients with suspected deep venous thrombosis. Thromb Res 86:93, 1997.

30. Shull KC, Nicolaides AN, Fernandez JF, et al: Significance of popliteal reflux in relation to ambulatory venous pressure and ulceration. Arch Surg 114:1304, 1979.

31. Stewart GJ, Alburger PD, Stone EA, Soszka TW: Total hip replacement induces injury to remote veins in a canine model. J Bone Joint Surg 65A:97, 1983.

32. Wells PS, Hirsh J, Anderson DR, et al: Accuracy of clinical assessment of deep vein thrombosis. Lancet 345:1326, 1995.

33. Wheeler HB, Anderson FA Jr, Cardullo PA, et al: Suspected deep vein thrombosis: Management by impedance plethysmography. Arch Surg 117 1206, 1982.

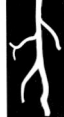

C H A P T E R   1 4 0

Prevention and Medical Treatment of Acute Deep Venous Thrombosis

Russell D. Hull, M.D., and Graham F. Pineo, M.D.

Unfractionated heparin is used widely for the prevention of venous thromboembolism in medical patients and in patients undergoing various surgical procedures. Furthermore, unfractionated heparin, given by a continuous intravenous infusion with laboratory monitoring using the activated partial thromboplastin time, and warfarin starting on day 1 or day 2 and continued for 3 months, has been the standard treatment of established venous thromboembolism. Heparin is used in a number of other clinical settings and constitutes one of the most frequently used agents in hospital medicine. Over the past 15 years, various low-molecular-weight heparins have been evaluated against a number of different controls, including unfractionated heparin for many of these clinical problems. In a number of countries, the low-molecular-weight heparins have replaced unfractionated heparin for both the prevention and treatment of venous thromboembolism. This chapter reviews the prevention and medical management of deep vein thrombosis with the agents that are currently available.

PATHOGENESIS OF VENOUS THROMBOEMBOLISM

Although the pathophysiology of acute deep venous thrombosis (DVT) is discussed in detail in Chapter 136, im-

portant aspects of pathogenesis should be reiterated here to understand the mode of action of different techniques and drugs used for prevention and treatment. In recent years, more information has become available on inherited and acquired defects predisposing to thrombosis, in particular, activated protein C resistance,[1–3] inherited or acquired defects of homocysteine metabolism,[4–6] and a new prothrombin mutant (2021A)[7] (Table 140–1).

Activated protein C resistance is commonly found in patients with idiopathic deep vein thrombosis or recurrent venous thromboembolism[8, 9] and in patients with venous thromboembolism complicating pregnancy or oral contraceptive therapy.[10] However, many patients with the heterozygous or homozygous form of activated protein C resistance have no problems with thrombosis, and many patients with activated protein C resistance who do have thrombosis have combined defects such as protein C deficiency or the antiphospholipid syndrome.[11, 12] Also, the incidence of activated protein C resistance and the prothrombin mutant varies widely in different ethnic groups.[13, 14] Many patients with familial thrombophilia have no detectable prothrombotic disorder, and further work is required before firm recommendations can be made regarding screening for these defects in patients in high-risk situations or the need for long-term anticoagulant therapy after a first episode of venous thromboembolism.

TABLE 140–1. CLINICAL RISK FACTORS PREDISPOSING TO THE DEVELOPMENT OF VENOUS THROMBOEMBOLISM

Surgical and nonsurgical trauma
Previous venous thromboembolism
Immobilization
Malignant disease
Congestive heart failure
Leg paralysis
Age (>40 yr)
Obesity
Estrogens and oral contraceptives
Inherited or acquired disorders
   Antithrombin III deficiency
   Protein C or S deficiency
   Activated protein C resistance
   Prothrombin mutant
   Homocysteinemia
   Heparin-induced thrombocytopenia
   Antiphospholipid syndrome

DVT most commonly arises in the deep veins of the calf muscles or, less commonly, in the proximal deep veins of the leg. DVT confined to the calf veins is associated with a low risk of clinically important pulmonary embolism.[15, 16] Without treatment, however, approximately 20% of calf vein thrombi extend into the proximal venous system, where they may pose a serious and potentially life-threatening disorder.[17–19] Untreated proximal venous thrombosis is associated with a 10% risk of fatal pulmonary embolism and at least a 50% risk of pulmonary embolism or recurrent venous thrombosis.[15–17] Furthermore, the post-phlebitic syndrome is associated with extensive proximal venous thrombosis and carries its own long-term morbidity.

It is now well established that clinically important pulmonary emboli arise from thrombi in the proximal deep veins of the legs.[17, 20–24] Other less common sources of pulmonary embolism include the deep pelvic veins, renal veins, inferior vena cava, right side of the heart, and, occasionally, axillary veins. The clinical significance of pulmonary embolism depends on the size of the embolus and the cardiorespiratory reserve of the patient.

Upper extremity DVT involving the subclavian, axillary, and brachial veins is seen more commonly in men than in women, and in many cases strenuous exercise is a triggering factor.[25, 26] Other risk factors include the use of central venous catheters and previous venous thrombosis, but limited studies have shown little relationship to the presence of hypercoagulable states. Unilateral swelling, distention of superficial veins, cyanosis, and a palpable cord in the axillary vein are common clinical manifestations. Diagnosis is best confirmed by compression ultrasonography and color flow Doppler imaging.

Superficial thrombophlebitis involves the superficial veins of the lower or sometimes upper extremity is commonly associated with the presence of varicose veins or pregnancy, and may be precipitated by trauma.[27, 28] Superficial thrombophlebitis is sometimes associated with DVT, especially when the more proximal superficial veins in the thigh are involved, and anticoagulant therapy is usually not necessary. However, if any doubt exists, objective tests for deep vein thrombosis should be carried out.

It is widely accepted that venous thromboembolism is a single disorder and, therefore, the treatment of venous thrombosis or pulmonary embolism is basically the same. The diagnostic approach may start with the legs or the lungs, beginning with the least invasive test and proceeding to the more invasive tests.

PREVENTION OF VENOUS THROMBOEMBOLISM

Without prophylaxis, the frequency of fatal pulmonary embolism ranges from 0.1% to 0.8% in patients undergoing elective general surgery,[29–31] 2% to 3% in patients undergoing elective hip replacement,[32] and 4% to 7% in patients undergoing surgery for a fractured hip.[33] The need for prophylaxis after elective hip replacement has been questioned because of the low incidence of fatal pulmonary embolism in patients participating in clinical trials.[34] However, review of data from the National Confidential Enquiry into Peri-operative Deaths (NCEPOD) indicates that pulmonary embolism continues to be the commonest cause of death following total hip replacement surgery; 35% of patients who died had pulmonary embolism confirmed at autopsy.[35] Factors increasing the risk of postoperative venous thrombosis include advanced age, malignancy, previous venous thromboembolism, obesity, heart failure, or paralysis.

There are two approaches to the prevention of fatal pulmonary embolism:

1. *Primary* prophylaxis is carried out using either drugs or physical methods that are effective for preventing DVT.

2. *Secondary* prevention involves the early detection and treatment of subclinical venous thrombosis by screening postoperative patients with objective tests that are sensitive for venous thrombosis.

Primary prophylaxis is preferred in most clinical circumstances. Furthermore, prevention of DVT and pulmonary embolism is more cost-effective than treatment of the complications when they occur.[36–40] Secondary prevention by case-finding studies should never replace primary prophylaxis. It should be reserved for patients in whom primary prophylaxis is either contraindicated or relatively ineffective.

The ideal prophylactic method is described in Table 140–2. Prophylactic measures most commonly used are low-dose or adjusted-dose unfractionated heparin, low-molecular-weight (LMW) heparin or heparinoid, oral anticoagulant (International Normalized Ratio, INR, 2.0 to 3.0), and intermittent pneumatic compression. Prevention of venous thrombosis following total hip replacement with the use

TABLE 140–2. FEATURES OF AN IDEAL PROPHYLACTIC METHOD FOR VENOUS THROMBOEMBOLISM

Effective compared with placebo or active approaches
Safe
Good compliance from patient, nurses, and physicians
Ease of administration
No need for laboratory monitoring
Cost-effective

of the specific antithrombin hirudin has been reported more recently.

The prevention of thrombosis can be directed toward three components of Virchow's triad: (1) blood flow, (2) factors within the blood itself, and (3) the vascular endothelium. Some methods act on all three components, resulting in a reduction of venous stasis, prevention of the hypercoagulable state induced by tissue trauma and other factors, and protection of the endothelium. Whichever method is used, prophylaxis probably should be initiated prior to induction of anesthesia, as it has been demonstrated that the thrombotic process commences intraoperatively.[41] Patterns of prophylaxis practice differ in Europe and North America. In Europe, prophylaxis prior to high-risk surgery is commenced preoperatively, whereas in North America, prophylaxis starts on the night of surgery.[42] These patterns of practice may account for the difference in the rates of postoperative venous thrombosis and bleeding in Europe and North America.

The duration of prophylaxis required after high-risk procedures such as total joint replacement is currently under study. Extended prophylaxis to days 28 to 35 has shown that the venographically proved venous thrombosis rates are lower with LMW heparin than with placebo.[43–45] Specific recommendations regarding the duration of prophylaxis are controversial because of outcome trials in 1996 and 1997.[46, 47]

There has been concern regarding the use of regional anesthesia in the form of intraspinal or epidural anesthesia or analgesia and the use of prophylactic anticoagulants. Spinal hematomas have been reported with the use of intravenous or subcutaneous heparin and warfarin treatment, but most of these complications occurred in patients with complex clinical problems.[48] With the advent of LMW heparin and the increased use of regional anesthesia, concern was raised regarding the potential risk of neuraxial damage because of bleeding when both procedures are used together. Surveys among anesthetists in Europe suggested that the likelihood of spinal hematoma in this setting was remote.[49, 50] However, recent experience in the United States with the use of neuraxial anesthesia and analgesia and the postoperative administration of LMW heparin has resulted in a number of case reports of spinal hematoma, many of which caused permanent neurologic damage.[51] Many of these occurred with continued epidural analgesia; many of the procedures were traumatic, and several patients were prescribed nonsteroidal anti-inflammatory drugs (NSAIDs).[51] Other risk factors appear to be age over 75 years and female gender. At this stage, the Food and Drug Administration (FDA) has recommended caution when neuraxial anesthesia is used in the presence of anticoagulant prophylaxis, and further recommendations will be forthcoming.

Patterns of clinical practice with respect to the prevention of venous thromboembolism and the appropriate use of anticoagulants for the treatment of thrombotic disease have been influenced very strongly by recent consensus conferences. Recommendations from the fourth American College of Chest Physicians Consensus Conference on Antithrombotic Therapy[52] (1995) and the International Consensus Statement on the Prevention of Venous Thromboembolism[53] (1997) have been published. Rules of evidence for assessing the literature were applied to all recommendations regarding prevention and treatment of venous thrombosis, thereby indicating which recommendations were based on rigorous randomized trials, which were based on extrapolation of evidence from related clinical disorders, and which were based only on nonrandomized clinical trials or case series.[54]

SPECIFIC PROPHYLACTIC MEASURES

Low-Dose Heparin

The effectiveness of low-dose unfractionated heparin for preventing DVT has been established by multiple randomized clinical trials. Low-dose subcutaneous heparin is usually given in a dose of 5000 U 2 hours preoperatively, and postoperatively every 8 or 12 hours. Most of the patients in these trials underwent abdominothoracic surgery, particularly for gastrointestinal disease, but patients having gynecologic and urologic surgery as well as mastectomies or vascular procedures, were also included. Pooled data from meta-analyses confirm that low-dose heparin significantly reduces the incidence of all DVT, proximal DVT, and all pulmonary emboli, including fatal pulmonary emboli.[54, 55] The International Multicentre Trial also established the effectiveness of low-dose heparin for preventing fatal pulmonary embolism, a clinically and significantly striking reduction from 0.7% to 0.1% ($p < .005$).[56]

The incidence of major bleeding complications is not increased by low-dose heparin, but there is an increase in minor wound hematomas. The platelet count should be monitored regularly in all patients on low-dose heparin to detect the rare but significant development of heparin-induced thrombocytopenia.

Adjusted-Dose Heparin

The use of adjusted-dose subcutaneous heparin has been effective for prophylaxis compared with low-dose heparin in patients undergoing total hip replacement.[57] Adjusted-dose heparin, however, has not become popular because of the time and expense required for laboratory monitoring.

Low-Molecular-Weight Heparin

A number of low-molecular-weight heparin fractions have been evaluated by randomized clinical trials in moderate-risk general surgical patients, including many who underwent cancer surgery.[58–64] In randomized clinical trials comparing LMW heparin with unfractionated heparin, the low-molecular-weight heparins given once or twice daily have been shown to be as effective as or more effective than unfractionated heparin in preventing thrombosis.[58–64] In most of the trials, similarly low frequencies of bleeding for low-molecular-weight heparin and low-dose unfractionated heparin were documented, although the incidence of bleeding was significantly lower in the LMW heparin group, as evidenced by a reduction in the incidence of wound hematoma and severe bleeding, and the number of patients requiring reoperation for bleeding.[58, 59]

A number of randomized control trials have been performed with low-molecular-weight heparin, comparing it with either placebo, intravenous dextran, unfractionated heparin, or warfarin for the prevention of venous thrombosis following total hip replacement (Table 140–3).[65–72] The drugs under investigation and their dosage schedules vary from one clinical trial to another, making comparisons across trials difficult. Furthermore, even within the same clinical trial there can be considerable intercenter variability.[70] Low-molecular-weight heparin is usually started the night before surgery in the European trials, in contrast to North American trials, in which it is started 12 to 24 hours postoperatively. Major bleeding rates and definitions of major bleeding vary across trials as well, making comparisons difficult.

Although the number of patients undergoing total knee replacement now equals those undergoing total hip replacement, there have been fewer trials in this patient population. Recent clinical trials comparing LMW heparin with either placebo or warfarin are shown in Table 140–4.[70, 71, 73–75] Although the rates of DVT with LMW heparin are significantly lower than those with warfarin, the rates continue to be high.

Multiple meta-analyses have shown that low-molecular-weight heparin and low-dose heparin are equally effective in preventing venous thrombosis in general surgery,[76–78] but LMW heparin is more effective in orthopedic surgery.[76–79] Bleeding rates were higher with low-dose heparin in patients undergoing general surgery.

Two recent decision analyses compared the cost-effectiveness of enoxaparin with warfarin in patients undergoing hip replacement.[80, 81] Although enoxaparin was more expensive than low-dose warfarin, its cost-effectiveness compared favorably with that of other medical interventions. A recent economic evaluation of LMW heparin versus warfarin prophylaxis after total hip or knee replacement identified that LMW heparin was cost-effective.[82]

Studies published in 1996 have shown that LMW heparin is superior to low-dose unfractionated heparin in patients suffering multiple trauma[83] and equally effective in medical patients.[84, 85]

The LMW heparinoid danaparoid (Organon) has been evaluated in patients undergoing surgery for cancer,[86] hip fractures,[87, 88] and total hip replacement.[89] The thrombosis rates were similar with danaparoid and unfractionated heparin in patients undergoing cancer surgery.[86] In patients undergoing surgery for hip fracture, the rates of DVT were significantly lower compared with intravenous dextran and with low-intensity warfarin.[87] More blood transfusions were required in the dextran group. Compared with placebo, the rates of DVT following total hip replacement were significantly lower.[89]

Oral Anticoagulants

For prophylaxis, oral anticoagulants (coumarin derivatives) can be commenced preoperatively, at the time of surgery, or in the early postoperative period. Oral anticoagulants begun at the time of surgery or in the early postoperative period may not prevent small venous thrombi from forming during or soon after surgery, because the antithrombotic effect is not achieved until the third or fourth postoperative day. However, oral anticoagulants are effective in inhibiting the extension of these thrombi, thereby preventing clinically important venous thromboembolism.

TABLE 140–3. RANDOMIZED TRIALS OF LOW-MOLECULAR-WEIGHT HEPARIN PROPHYLAXIS FOR DEEP VEIN THROMBOSIS FOLLOWING HIP REPLACEMENT SURGERY: TOTAL DEEP VEIN THROMBOSIS

STUDY	TREATMENT	NO. OF PATIENTS	TOTAL DEEP VEIN THROMBOSIS (%)	TOTAL BLEEDING (%)
Danish Enoxaparin Study Group[65] (1991)	Enoxaparin	108	6.5	13.9
	Dextran 70	111	21.6	23.4
Levine et al[66] (1991)	Enoxaparin	258	19.4	5.1
	Unfractionated heparin	263	23.2	9.3
Leyvraz et al[57] (1991)	Nadroparin	198	12.6	0.5
	Unfractionated heparin	199	16.0	1.5
Eriksson et al[67] (1991)	Dalteparin	67	30.2	1.5
	Unfractionated heparin	68	42.4	7.4
Planes et al[68] (1991)	Enoxaparin	120	12.5	2.4
	Heparin	108	25.0	1.8
Colwell et al[69] (1994)	Enoxaparin	136	21.0	10.0
	Enoxaparin	136	6.0	12.0
	Heparin	142	1.5	12.0
Hull et al[70] (1993)	Tinzaparin	332	21.0	4.1
	Warfarin	340	23.0	3.8
Hamulyak et al[71] (1995)	Nadroparin	195	13.8	2.4*
	Warfarin	196	13.8	5.2
Francis et al[72] (1997)	Dalteparin	192	15.0	2.0†
	Warfarin	190	26.0	1.0

*Clinically important, plus minor bleeding for combined hip and knee replacement patients.
†Major bleeding only.

TABLE 140–4. RANDOMIZED CONTROL TRIALS OF LOW-MOLECULAR-WEIGHT HEPARIN PROPHYLAXIS FOR DEEP VEIN THROMBOSIS FOLLOWING TOTAL KNEE REPLACEMENT: TOTAL DEEP VEIN THROMBOSIS AND MAJOR BLEEDING

STUDY	TREATMENT	NO. OF PATIENTS	TOTAL DEEP VEIN THROMBOSIS (%)	MAJOR BLEEDING (%)
Leclerc et al[73] (1992)	Enoxaparin	41	20.0	6.1*
	Placebo	54	65.0	6.2
Hull et al[70] (1993)	Tinzaparin	317	45.0	0.9
	Warfarin	324	54.0	2.0
Hamulyak et al[71] (1995)	Nadroparin	65	24.6	2.4†
	Warfarin	61	37.7	5.2
Leclerc et al[74] (1996)	Enoxaparin	206	37.0	2.1
	Warfarin	211	52.0	1.8
Heit et al‡[75] (1997)	Ardeparin	232	27.0	7.9§
	Warfarin	222	38.0	4.4

*Bleeding complications (major and minor).
†Overt bleeding—total.
‡Venogram on operated leg only.
§Clinically important and minor bleeding for combined hip and knee replacement patients.

The postoperative use of warfarin following total hip or total knee replacement surgery has been compared with LMW heparin[70, 72, 74, 75] or intermittent pneumatic compression,[90–92] with little or no difference in the incidence of postoperative venous thrombosis or bleeding.

When warfarin was initiated in small doses 7 to 10 days preoperatively to prolong prothrombin time 1.5 to 3.0 seconds and then less intense warfarin was started the night of surgery, the results were similar to those when warfarin was started the night before surgery.[92]

In patients with hip fractures, warfarin was more effective than either aspirin or placebo.[93] Compared with placebo, very low doses of oral anticoagulants (warfarin, 1 mg/day) decreased the postoperative thrombosis rate in patients undergoing gynecologic surgery[94] or major general surgery and decreased the thrombosis rate in indwelling central line catheters.[95] There was no increase in bleeding rates. Very-low-dose warfarin, however, did not provide protection against DVT following hip or knee replacement.[96]

Intermittent Leg Compression

The use of intermittent pneumatic leg compression prevents DVT by enhancing blood flow in the deep veins of the legs, thereby preventing venous stasis. It also increases blood fibrinolytic activity, which may contribute to its antithrombotic properties. Intermittent pneumatic leg compression is effective for preventing venous thrombosis in moderate-risk general surgical patients,[97] following cardiac surgery,[98] and in patients undergoing neurosurgery.[99–101] In patients undergoing hip surgery, intermittent pneumatic compression of the calf is effective for preventing calf vein thrombosis, but it is less effective against proximal vein thrombosis than is warfarin sodium.[52, 102] Intermittent pneumatic compression of the calf decreased venous thrombosis following knee replacement.[103, 104]

Intermittent pneumatic compression is virtually free of clinically important side effects and offers a valuable alternative for patients who have a high risk of bleeding. It may produce discomfort in an occasional patient, and it should not be used in patients with overt incidence of leg ischemia caused by peripheral vascular disease. A variety of well-accepted, comfortable, and effective intermittent pneumatic devices are available that may be applied preoperatively, at operation, or in the early postoperative period. These devices should be used for the entire period until the patient is fully ambulatory, with only temporary removal for nursing care or physiotherapy.

Graduated Compression Stockings

Graduated compression stockings are a simple, safe, and moderately effective form of thromboprophylaxis. It is by no means clear how graduated compression stockings achieve a thromboprophylactic effect. They increase the velocity of venous blood flow, and thus graduated compression stockings are recommended in low-risk patients and as an adjunct in those with medium and high risk.[53, 105, 106] The only major contraindication is peripheral vascular disease. The majority of studies in patients undergoing general abdominal and gynecologic procedures have shown a reduction in the incidence of DVT using these stockings. A comprehensive meta-analysis concluded that, in studies using sound methods, there was a highly significant risk reduction of 68% in patients at moderate risk of postoperative thromboembolism.[107] However, there is no conclusive evidence that graduated compression stockings are effective in reducing the incidence of fatal and nonfatal pulmonary embolism. It is not known whether wearing graduated compression stockings following discharge from hospital is efficacious.

Other Agents

Hirudin started preoperatively was superior to unfractionated heparin and LMW heparin in the prevention of venous thrombosis following total hip replacement.[108, 109]

Although meta-analyses indicate that aspirin decreases the frequency of venous thrombosis following general or orthopedic surgery, this reduction is significantly less than that obtained using other agents.[110] Aspirin, therefore, cannot be recommended for the prevention of venous thrombosis in high-risk patients. Also, although intravenous dextran has been shown to be effective in the prevention of venous thrombosis after major orthopedic surgery, it is cumbersome, expensive, and associated with significant side effects. It has, therefore, been replaced by other agents.

SPECIFIC RECOMMENDATIONS

The recommended primary prophylactic approach depends on the patient's risk category and the type of surgery. In the literature relating to the prevention of DVT, the rules of evidence, as defined by Cook and associates, have been used[54]:

Level I. Randomized trials with low false-positive (a) and low false-negative (b) errors.
Level II. Randomized trials with high false-positive (a) and high false-negative (b) errors.
Level III. Nonrandomized concurrent cohort studies.
Level IV. Nonrandomized historical cohort studies.
Level V. Case series.

Unless indicated, all recommendations in the following section are based on Level I evidence.[52, 53]

Low-Risk Patients

Apart from early ambulation, specific prophylaxis is usually not recommended.[51, 52] However, prophylaxis for low-risk patients is recommended in certain circumstances. It is the clinical custom in some countries to use graduated compression stockings, but this is not based on evidence from clinical trials.

Moderate-Risk Patients

General Abdominal, Thoracic, or Gynecologic Surgery

In moderate-risk patients, the use of subcutaneous low-dose unfractionated heparin (5000 units every 8 to 12 hours) or subcutaneous LMW heparin is recommended.[52, 53] Subcutaneous LMW heparin is as effective as subcutaneous heparin prophylaxis and has the advantage of a once-daily injection. An alternative recommendation is the use of intermittent pneumatic compression until the patient is ambulatory. This method is indicated in patients at high risk for bleeding. Pharmacologic methods may be combined with graduated compression stockings in selected patients.

Neurosurgery

Neurosurgical patients should receive intermittent pneumatic compression. This approach may be used in conjunction with graduated compression stockings. Low-dose heparin is an acceptable alternative.[52, 53]

High-Risk Patients

Elective Hip Replacement

Several approaches are effective. Subcutaneous LMW heparin given once or twice daily is effective and safe.[52, 53] Several such agents are approved for use in Europe and North America. At present in North America, these agents are approved for postoperative use only. Prophylaxis with oral anticoagulants adjusted to maintain an INR of 2.0 to 3.0 is effective and is associated with a low risk of bleeding.[52] Other effective approaches include adjusted-dose subcutaneous unfractionated heparin and intermittent pneumatic compression.[52] However, rates of proximal venous thrombosis are higher with intermittent pneumatic compression than with the other approaches.

Elective Knee Replacement

Although intermittent pneumatic compression was shown in earlier studies to be effective and to be a still useful alternative, the prophylaxis of choice today is LMW heparin given once or twice daily postoperatively.[52, 53] Oral anticoagulants are less effective than LMW heparin and cannot be recommended.

Hip Fractures

Two approaches to prophylaxis are available: (1) oral anticoagulation (INR, 2.0 to 3.0)[93] and (2) fixed-dose subcutaneous LMW heparin started preoperatively.[52, 53] The combined use of intermittent pneumatic compression with LMW heparin or warfarin may provide additional benefit in certain patients (not Level I).

Multiple Trauma

Multiple trauma represents a high risk for thrombosis. LMW heparin is the prophylaxis of choice.[83] Intermittent pneumatic compression has been recommended, when feasible, because it eliminates any risk for bleeding.[52] Other alternatives include low-dose unfractionated heparin or warfarin based on extrapolation from other high-risk situations, such as hip fracture and hip replacement surgery. Insertion of an inferior vena caval filter has been recommended for very-high-risk situations when anticoagulants may be contraindicated, but this recommendation is based on Level V data.

Acute Spinal Cord Injury Associated with Paralysis

LMW heparin is the most effective prophylaxis.[52] Adjusted-dose heparin has also been effective. Low-dose heparin and intermittent pneumatic compression are less effective. Combining intermittent pneumatic compression with LMW heparin or adjusted-dose heparin may provide additional benefit, but this is not supported by data.

Other Conditions

Medical Patients

These patients should be classified as at low, moderate, or high risk for venous thromboembolism, depending on their underlying medical condition and other co-morbid factors, such as immobility, previous DVT, cancer, and so on. Low-risk patients should be considered for graduated compression stockings. For patients having experienced myocardial infarction who have no other significant risk factors, anticoagulation with heparin or warfarin is recommended. In the presence of congestive heart failure, pulmonary infections, or both, either low-dose heparin or LMW heparin is recommended.[84, 85] For patients with ischemic strokes and lower limb paralysis, low-dose heparin or LMW heparin is recommended.[52] Intermittent pneumatic compression may be used for high-risk patients who are susceptible to bleeding, although this recommendation is not based on clinical trial data.[52]

Pregnancy

Subcutaneous low-dose heparin is the prophylaxis of choice for pregnant patients who are at high risk for DVT and pulmonary embolism, although data on efficacy from controlled trials are lacking.[111] For patients undergoing an emergency cesarean section, prophylaxis with low-dose unfractionated heparin or LMW heparin is recommended. LMW heparin has been studied in case series for the prevention of venous thrombosis in high-risk pregnancies, but there have been no prospective clinical trials to date. In most countries, LMW heparin has not been approved for use in pregnancy.

TREATMENT

The objectives of treatment in patients with venous thromboembolism are (1) to prevent death from pulmonary embolism, (2) to prevent recurrent venous thromboembolism, and (3) to prevent the postphlebitic syndrome. The anticoagulant drugs heparin, low-molecular-weight heparin, and warfarin constitute the mainstay of treatment of venous thrombosis. The use of graduated compression stockings for 24 months significantly decreases the incidence of the post-thrombotic syndrome.[112] Furthermore, the incidence of the post-thrombotic syndrome appears to have decreased in the 1990s, suggesting that the more efficient treatment of venous thromboembolism and the prevention of recurrent DVT are having a positive impact on this complication.[113]

Heparin Therapy

The anticoagulant activity of unfractionated heparin depends upon a unique pentasaccharide that binds to antithrombin III (AT III) and potentiates the inhibition of thrombin and activated factor X (Xa) by AT III.[114–116] About one third of all heparin molecules contain the unique pentasaccharide sequence, regardless of whether they are low- or high-molecular-weight fractions.[115–120] The pentasaccharide sequence confers the molecular high affinity for AT III.[115–120] In addition, heparin catalyzes the inactivation of thrombin by another plasma cofactor (cofactor II), which acts independently of AT III.[121]

Heparin has a number of other effects, such as (1)

release of tissue factor pathway inhibitor[122]; (2) binding to numerous plasma and platelet proteins, endothelial cells, and leukocytes[114, 119, 123]; (3) suppression of platelet function[120]; and (4) an increase in vascular permeability.[124] The anticoagulant response to a standard dose of heparin varies widely among patients. This makes it necessary to monitor the anticoagulant response of heparin, using either the activated partial thromboplastin time (aPTT) or heparin levels and to titrate the dose to the individual patient.

The accepted anticoagulant therapy for venous thromboembolism is a combination of continuous intravenous heparin and oral warfarin. The length of the initial intravenous heparin therapy has been reduced to 5 days, thus shortening the hospital stay and leading to significant cost savings.[125] The simultaneous use of initial heparin and warfarin has become clinical practice for all patients with venous thromboembolism who are medically stable.[125–127] Exceptions include patients who require immediate medical or surgical intervention, as in thrombolysis or insertion of a vena caval filter, or patients at very high risk of bleeding. Heparin is continued until the INR has been within the therapeutic range (2.0 to 3.0) for 2 consecutive days.[127]

It has been established from experimental studies and clinical trials that efficacy of heparin therapy depends on achieving a critical therapeutic level of heparin within the first 24 hours of treatment.[128–130] Data from three consecutive double-blind clinical trials indicate that failure to achieve the therapeutic aPTT threshold by 24 hours was associated with a 23.3% subsequent recurrent venous thromboembolism rate, compared with a rate of 4% to 6% for the patient group who achieved therapeutic levels at 24 hours.[129, 130] The recurrences occurred throughout the 3-month follow-up period and could not be attributed to inadequate oral anticoagulant therapy.[129] The critical therapeutic level of heparin, as measured by the aPTT, is 1.5 times the mean of the control value or the upper limit of the normal aPTT range.[128] This corresponds to a heparin blood level of 0.2 to 0.4 U/ml by the protamine sulfate titration assay, and 0.35 to 0.70 by the anti–factor Xa assay.

However, there is a wide variability in the aPTT and heparin blood levels with different reagents and even with different batches of the same reagent.[131] It is, therefore, vital for each laboratory to establish the minimal therapeutic level of heparin, as measured by the aPTT, that will provide a heparin blood level of at least 0.35 U/ml by the anti–factor Xa assay for each batch of thromboplastin reagent being used, particularly if the reagent is provided by a different manufacturer.[131]

Although there is a strong correlation between subtherapeutic aPTT values and recurrent thromboembolism, the relationship between supratherapeutic aPTT and bleeding (aPTT ratio of 2:5 or more) is less definite.[128] Indeed, bleeding during heparin therapy is more closely related to underlying clinical risk factors than to aPTT elevation above the therapeutic range.[128] Recent studies confirm that weight, gender, and age over 65 years are independent risk factors for bleeding during heparin therapy.[132–134]

Numerous audits of heparin therapy indicate that administration of intravenous heparin is fraught with difficulty and that the clinical practice of using an ad hoc approach to heparin dose titration frequently results in inadequate therapy.[135–137] For example, an audit of physician practices

TABLE 140–5. HEPARIN PROTOCOL

1. Administer initial intravenous heparin bolus: 5000 U
2. Administer continuous intravenous heparin infusion: commence at 42 ml/hr of 20,000 U (1680 U/hr) in 500 ml of two thirds dextrose and one third saline (a 24-hr heparin dose of 40,320 U), except in the following patients, in whom heparin infusion is commenced at a rate of 31 ml/hr (1240 U/hr, a 24-hr dose of 29,760 U):
   a. Patients who have undergone surgery within the previous 2 weeks
   b. Patients with a previous history of peptic ulcer disease or gastrointestinal or genitourinary bleeding
   c. Patients with recent stroke (i.e., thrombotic stroke within 2 weeks previously)
   d. Patients with a platelet count < 150* 10⁹/L
   e. Patients with miscellaneous reasons for a high risk of bleeding (e.g., hepatic failure, renal failure, or vitamin K deficiency)
3. Adjust heparin dose by use of the aPTT. The aPTT test is performed in all patients as follows:
   a. 4–6 hr after commencing heparin; the heparin dose is then adjusted
   b. 4–6 hr after the first dosage adjustment
   c. Then, as indicated by the nomogram, for the first 24 hr of therapy
   d. Thereafter, once daily, unless subtherapeutic,* in which case the aPTT test is repeated 4–6 hr after the heparin dose is increased

Adapted with permission from Hull RD, Raskob GE, Rosenbloom D, et al: Optimal therapeutic level of heparin therapy in patients with venous thrombosis. Arch Intern Med 152:1589–1595, 1992. Copyright 1992, American Medical Association.
*Subtherapeutic = aPTT < 1.5 times the mean normal control value for the thromboplastin reagent being used.
aPTT = activated partial thromboplastin time.

at three university-affiliated hospitals documented that 60% of patients failed to achieve an adequate aPTT response (ratio, 1:5) during the initial 24 hours of therapy and, further, that 30% to 40% of patients achieved only subtherapeutic levels over the next 3 to 4 days.[136]

Several practices were identified that led to inadequate therapy. The common theme that explains these practices is an exaggerated fear of bleeding complications on the part of clinicians.[136] Consequently, it has been common practice for many clinicians to start treatment with a low heparin dose and to increase this dose cautiously over several days to achieve the therapeutic range.

The use of a prescriptive approach or protocol for administering intravenous heparin therapy has been evaluated in two prospective studies in patients with venous thromboembolism.[128, 138]

In one clinical trial for the treatment of proximal venous thrombosis, patients were given either intravenous heparin alone followed by warfarin or intravenous heparin and simultaneous warfarin.[128] The heparin nomogram is summarized in Tables 140–5 and 140–6. Only 1% and 2% of the patients were undertreated for more than 24 hours in the heparin group and in the heparin and warfarin group, respectively. Recurrent venous thromboembolism (objectively documented) occurred infrequently in both groups (7%), a rate similar to those previously reported. These findings demonstrated that subtherapy was avoided in most patients and that the heparin protocol resulted in effective delivery of heparin therapy in both groups.

In the other clinical trial, a weight-based heparin-dosage nomogram was compared with a standard care nomogram (Table 140–7).[138] Patients on the weight-adjusted heparin nomogram received a starting dose of 80 U/kg as a bolus and 18 U/kg/hr as an infusion. The heparin dose was adjusted to maintain an aPTT of 1.5 to 2.3 times control. In the weight-adjusted group, 89% of patients achieved the therapeutic range within 24 hours, compared with 75% in the standard care group. The risk of recurrent thromboembolism was more frequent in the standard care group, supporting the previous observation that subtherapeutic heparin during the initial 24 hours is associated with a higher incidence of recurrences. This study included patients with unstable angina and arterial thromboembolism in addition to venous thromboembolism, which suggests that the principles applied to a heparin nomogram for the treatment of venous thromboembolism may be generalized to other clinical conditions. Continued use of the weight-based nomogram has also been effective.[139]

Complications of Heparin Therapy

The main adverse effects of heparin therapy include bleeding, thrombocytopenia, and osteoporosis. Patients at particular risk are those who have had recent surgery or trauma or who have other clinical factors that predispose to bleed-

TABLE 140–6. INTRAVENOUS HEPARIN DOSE TITRATION NOMOGRAM ACCORDING TO THE aPTT

aPTT (sec)	RATE CHANGE (ml/hr)	DOSE CHANGE (U/24 hr)*	ADDITIONAL ACTION
≤45	+6	+5760	Repeat aPTT† in 4–6 hr
46–54	+3	+2880	Repeat aPTT in 4–6 hr
55–85	0	0	None‡
86–110	−3	−2880	Stop heparin sodium treatment for 1 hr; repeat aPTT 4–6 hr after restarting heparin treatment
>110	−6	−5760	Stop heparin treatment for 1 hr; repeat aPTT 4–6 hr after restarting heparin treatment

Adapted with permission from Hull RD, Raskob GE, Rosenbloom D, et al: Optimal therapeutic level of heparin therapy in patients with venous thrombosis. Arch Intern Med 152:1589–1595, 1992. Copyright 1992, American Medical Association.
*Heparin sodium concentration, 20,000 IU in 500 ml = 40 IU/ml.
†With the use of Actin-FS thromboplastin reagent (Dade, Mississauga, Ontario, Canada).
‡During the first 24 hr, repeat aPTT in 4–6 hr. Thereafter, the aPTT will be determined once daily, unless subtherapeutic.
aPTT = activated partial thromboplastin time.

TABLE 140–7. WEIGHT-BASED NOMOGRAM FOR INITIAL INTRAVENOUS HEPARIN THERAPY: FIGURES IN PARENTHESES SHOW COMPARISON WITH CONTROL

	DOSE (U/kg)
Initial dose	80 U/kg bolus, then 18 U/kg/hr
aPTT <35 sec (<1.2 ×)	80 U/kg bolus, then 4 U/kg/hr
aPTT 35–45 sec (1.2–1.5 ×)	40 U/kg bolus, then 2 U/kg/hr
aPTT 46–70 sec (1.5–2.3 ×)	No change
aPTT 71–90 sec (2.3–3.0 ×)	Decrease infusion rate by 2/hr
aPTT > 90 sec (>3.0 ×)	Hold infusion 1 hr, then decrease infusion rate by 3 U/kg/hr

Adapted with permission from Raschke RA, Reilly BM, Guidry JR, et al: The weight-based heparin-dosing nomogram compared with a "standard-care" nomogram. Ann Intern Med 119:874–881, 1993.
aPTT = activated partial thromboplastin time.

ing on heparin dosage, such as peptic ulcer, occult malignancy, liver disease, hemostatic defects, weight, age over 65 years, and female gender.

The management of bleeding during heparin administration depends on the location and severity of bleeding, the risk of recurrent venous thromboembolism, and the aPTT. Heparin should be discontinued temporarily or permanently. Patients with recent venous thromboembolism may be candidates for insertion of an inferior vena caval filter. If urgent reversal of heparin effect is required, protamine sulfate can be administered.[140]

Heparin-induced thrombocytopenia is a well recognized complication of heparin therapy, usually occurring within 5 to 10 days after heparin treatment has started.[141–146] Approximately 1% to 2% of patients receiving unfractionated heparin experience a drop in platelet count to less than the normal range, or a 50% fall in the platelet count within the normal range. In most cases, this mild-to-moderate thrombocytopenia appears to be a direct effect of heparin on platelets and is of no consequence. However, approximately 0.1% to 0.2% of patients receiving heparin experience immune thrombocytopenia mediated by immunoglobulin G (IgG) antibody directed against a complex of platelet factor 4 (PF$_4$) and heparin.[144, 145]

The development of thrombocytopenia may be accompanied by arterial or venous thrombosis, which may lead to serious consequences such as death or limb amputation.[142] The diagnosis of heparin-induced thrombocytopenia, with or without thrombosis, must be made on clinical grounds, because the assays with the highest sensitivity and specificity are not readily available and have a slow turnaround time.

When the diagnosis of heparin-induced thrombocytopenia is made, heparin in all forms must be stopped immediately. In those patients requiring ongoing anticoagulation, several alternatives exist.[146] The agents most extensively used include the heparinoid danaproid,[147] hirudin,[148] and, most recently, the specific antithrombin argatroban.[149] Danaproid is available for limited use on compassionate grounds and are currently under review (1999) for approval by regulatory agencies. Hirudin has recently been approved by the Food and Drug Administration for this indication. Warfarin may be used but probably should not be started

until one of the aforementioned agents has been used for 3 to 4 days to suppress thrombin generation. The defibrinogenating snake venom ancrod (Arvin)[150] has been used extensively in the past but probably will be replaced by other agents, as will the use of plasmapheresis or intravenous gamma globulin infusion. Insertion of an inferior vena caval filter is often indicated.

Osteoporosis has been reported in patients receiving unfractionated heparin in dosages of 20,000 U/day (or more) for more than 6 months. Demineralization can progress to the fracture of vertebral bodies or long bones, and the defect may not be entirely reversible.[140]

Low-Molecular-Weight Heparin

Heparin currently in use clinically is polydispersed unmodified heparin, with a mean molecular weight ranging from 10 to 16 kD. In recent years, LMW derivatives of commercial heparin have been prepared that have a mean molecular weight of 4 to 5 kD.[151–159]

The LMW heparins commercially available are made by different processes (such as nitrous acid, alkaline, or enzymatic depolymerization), and they differ chemically and pharmacokinetically.[153–159] The clinical significance of these differences, however, is unclear, and very few studies have compared different LMW heparins with respect to clinical outcomes.[153] The doses of the different LMW heparins have been established empirically and are not necessarily interchangeable. Therefore, at this time the effectiveness and safety of each of the LMW heparins must be tested separately.[153]

The LMW heparins differ from unfractionated heparin in numerous ways. Of particular importance are increased bioavailability[156, 158] (>90% after subcutaneous injection), prolonged half-life[153, 158] and predictable clearance enabling once or twice daily injection, and predictable antithrombotic response based on body weight, permitting treatment without laboratory monitoring.[153] Other possible advantages are their ability to inactivate platelet-bound factor X$_a$,[153] resistance to inhibition by platelet factor IV,[120] and their decreased effect on platelet function[120] and vascular permeability[124] (possibly accounting for fewer hemorrhagic effects at comparable antithrombotic doses).[160–162]

There has been a hope that the LMW heparins will have fewer serious complications such as bleeding,[160–163] osteoporosis,[164–167] and heparin-induced thrombocytopenia,[168] when compared with unfractionated heparin. Evidence is accumulating that these complications are indeed less serious and less frequent with the use of LMW heparin. LMW heparin has not been approved for the prevention or treatment of venous thromboembolism in pregnancy. These drugs do not cross the placenta,[169–171] and small case series suggest they may be both effective and safe.[172–176] However, at this writing, the standard treatment for venous thromboembolism in pregnancy is adjusted-dose subcutaneous unfractionated heparin twice daily. The LMW heparins all cross-react with unfractionated heparin, and therefore they cannot be used as alternative therapy in patients in whom heparin-induced thrombocytopenia develops.[127] The heparinoid danaparoid possesses a 10% to 20% cross-reactivity with heparin, and it can be safely used in patients who have no cross-reactivity.

Several different LMW heparins and one heparinoid are available for the prevention and treatment of venous thromboembolism in various countries. Four LMW heparins are approved for clinical use in Canada and three LMW heparins and one heparinoid have been approved for use in the United States.

In a number of experimental[177, 178] and early clinical trials (some of which were dose finding), LMW heparin given by subcutaneous or intravenous injection was compared with continuous intravenous unfractionated heparin. In these clinical trials, the primary end-point was repeated venography at 7 to 10 days.[179-184] These studies demonstrated that LMW heparin was at least as effective as unfractionated heparin in preventing extension or increasing resolution of thrombi.

Subcutaneous unmonitored LMW heparin has been compared with continuous intravenous heparin in a number of clinical trials for the treatment of proximal venous thrombosis, using long-term follow-up as an outcome measure[185-190] (Table 140–8). These studies have shown that LMW heparin is at least as effective and safe as unfractionated heparin in the treatment of proximal venous thrombosis. Pooling of the most methodologically sound studies indicates a significant advantage for LMW heparin in the reduction of major bleeding and mortality. More recent studies have indicated that LMW used predominantly out of hospital was as effective and safe as intravenous unfractionated heparin given in hospital[191-193] (Table 140–9), and two clinical trials showed that LMW heparin was as effective as intravenous heparin in the treatment of patients presenting with pulmonary embolism.[193, 194] Economic analysis of treatment with LMW heparin versus intravenous heparin demonstrated that LMW heparin was cost-effective for treatment in hospital[195] as well as out of hospital.[195, 196] As these agents become more widely available for treatment, they will undoubtedly replace intravenous unfractionated heparin in the initial management of patients with venous thromboembolism.

Warfarin therapy is started on day 1 or 2, with the LMW heparin continuing for 4 to 5 days or until the INR is therapeutic for 2 consecutive days. Protamine sulfate reduces clinical bleeding if patients experience bleeding while receiving LMW heparins, presumably by neutralizing high molecular fractions of heparin that are thought to be most responsible for bleeding.

Oral Anticoagulant Therapy

There are two distinct chemical groups of oral anticoagulants: (1) the 4-hydroxy coumarin derivatives and (2) the indanedione derivatives (e.g., phenindione).[197] The coumarin derivatives are the oral anticoagulants of choice because they are associated with fewer nonhemorrhagic adverse effects than the indanedione derivatives.

The anticoagulant effect of warfarin is mediated by the inhibition of the vitamin K–dependent g-carboxylation of coagulation factors II, VII, IX, and X.[198, 199] This results in the synthesis of immunologically detectable but biologically inactive forms of these coagulation proteins. Warfarin also inhibits the vitamin K–dependent g-carboxylation of proteins C and S.[199] Protein C circulates as a proenzyme that is activated on endothelial cells by the thrombin/thrombomodulin complex to form activated protein C. Activated protein C in the presence of protein S inhibits activated factors VIII and V activity.[198] Therefore, vitamin K antagonists such as warfarin create a biochemical paradox by producing an anticoagulant effect owing to the inhibition of procoagulants (factors II, VII, IX, and X) and a potentially thrombogenic effect by impairing the synthesis of naturally occurring inhibitors of coagulation (proteins C and S).[199] Heparin and warfarin treatment should overlap by 4 to 5 days when warfarin treatment is initiated in patients with thrombotic disease.

The anticoagulant effect of warfarin is delayed until the normal clotting factors are cleared from the circulation, and the peak effect does not occur until 36 to 72 hours after

TABLE 140–8. RANDOMIZED TRIALS OF LOW-MOLECULAR-WEIGHT HEPARIN VERSUS UNFRACTIONATED HEPARIN FOR THE IN-HOSPITAL TREATMENT OF PROXIMAL DEEP VEIN THROMBOSIS OR ACUTE PULMONARY EMBOLISM: RESULTS OF LONG-TERM FOLLOW-UP

STUDY	TREATMENT	RECURRENT VENOUS THROMBOEMBOLISM No. (%)	MAJOR BLEEDING No. (%)	MORTALITY No. (%)
Hull et al[185] (1992)	Tinzaparin	6/213 (2.8)	1/213 (0.5)	10/213 (4.7)
	Heparin	15/219 (6.8)	11/219 (5.0)	21/219 (9.6)
Prandoni et al[186] (1992)	Nadroparin	6/85 (7.1)	1/85 (1.2)	6/85 (7.1)
	Heparin	12/85 (14.1)	3/85 (3.8)	12/85 (14.1)
Lopaciuk et al[187] (1992)	Nadroparin	0/74 (0)	0/74	0/74
	Heparin	3/72 (4.2)	1/72 (1.4)	1/72 (1.4)
Simonneau et al[189] (1993)	Enoxaparin	0/67	0/67	3/67 (4.5)
	Heparin	0/67	0/67	2/67 (3.0)
Lindmarker et al[188] (1994)	Dalteparin	5/101 (5.0)	1/101	2/101 (2.0)
	Heparin	3/103 (2.9)	0/103	3/103 (2.9)
Simonneau et al[194] (1997)	Tinzaparin	5/304 (1.6)	3/304 (1.0)	12/304 (3.9)
	Heparin	6/308 (1.90)	5/308 (1.6)	14/308 (4.5)
Decousus et al[190] (1998)	Enoxaparin	10/195 (5.1)	7/195 (3.6)	10/195 (5.1)
	Heparin	12/205 (5.0)	8/205 (3.9)	15/205 (7.3)

TABLE 140-9. PREDOMINANTLY OUTPATIENT TREATMENT OF PROXIMAL DEEP VEIN THROMBOSIS WITH LOW-MOLECULAR-WEIGHT HEPARIN VERSUS INPATIENT TREATMENT WITH INTRAVENOUS HEPARIN

STUDY	TREATMENT	RECURRENT DVT No. (%)	MAJOR BLEEDING No. (%)
Levine et al[191] (1996)	Enoxaparin versus heparin	13/247 (5.3) 17/253 (6.7)	5/247 (2.0) 3/253 (1.2)
Koopman et al[192] (1996)	Nadroparin versus heparin	14/202 (6.9) 17/198 (8.6)	1/202 (0.5) 4/198 (2.0)
Columbus Study[193] (1997)	Reviparin versus heparin	27/510 (5.3) 24/511 (4.9)	16/510 (3.1) 12/511 (2.3)

DVT = deep venous thrombosis.

drug administration.[200] During the first few days of warfarin therapy, the prothrombin time (PT) reflects mainly the depression of factor VII, which has a half-life of 5 to 7 hours. Equilibrium levels of factors II, IX, and X are not reached until about 1 week after the initiation of therapy. The use of small initial daily doses (e.g., 5.0 to 10 mg) is the preferred approach for initiating warfarin treatment.

The dose-response relationship to warfarin therapy varies widely among individuals and, therefore, the dose must be carefully monitored to prevent overdosing or underdosing. A number of drugs interact with warfarin. Critical appraisal of the literature reporting such interactions indicates that the evidence substantiating many of the claims is limited.[201] Nonetheless, patients must be warned against taking any new drugs without the knowledge of their attending physician.

Laboratory Monitoring and Therapeutic Range

The laboratory test most commonly used to measure the effects of warfarin is the one-stage PT test. The PT is sensitive to reduced activity of factors II, VII, and X but is insensitive to reduced activity of factor IX. Confusion about the appropriate therapeutic range has occurred because the different tissue thromboplastins used for measuring the PT vary considerably in sensitivity to the vitamin K–dependent clotting factors and in response to warfarin.[202]

Rabbit brain thromboplastin, which was widely used in North America, is less sensitive than standardized human brain thromboplastin, which has been widely used in the United Kingdom and other parts of Europe. A PT ratio of 15:20 using rabbit brain thromboplastin (i.e., the traditional therapeutic range in North America) is equivalent to a ratio of 4.0:6.0 using human brain thromboplastin.[202] Conversely, a twofold to threefold increase in the PT using standardized human brain thromboplastin is equivalent to a 1.25- to 1.5-fold increase in the PT using rabbit brain thromboplastin.

To promote the standardization of the PT for monitoring oral anticoagulant therapy, the World Health Organization (WHO) developed an international reference thromboplastin from human brain tissue and recommended that the PT ratio be expressed as the International Normalized Ratio. The INR is the PT ratio obtained by testing a given sample using the WHO reference thromboplastin. For practical clinical purposes, the INR for a given plasma sample is equivalent to the PT ratio obtained using a standardized

human brain thromboplastin known as the *Manchester comparative reagent*, which has been widely used in the United Kingdom.

Warfarin is administered in an initial dosage of 5.0 to 10 mg/day for the first 2 days. The daily dose is then adjusted according to the INR. Heparin therapy is discontinued on the fourth or fifth day following initiation of warfarin therapy, provided the INR is prolonged into the recommended therapeutic range (INR, 2.0 to 3.0).[198] Because some individuals are either fast or slow metabolizers of the drug, the selection of the correct dosage of warfarin must be individualized. Therefore, frequent INR determinations are required initially to establish therapeutic anticoagulation.

Once the anticoagulant effect and patient's warfarin dose requirements are stable, the INR should be monitored at regular intervals throughout the course of warfarin therapy for venous thromboembolism. If there are factors that may produce an unpredictable response to warfarin (e.g., concomitant drug therapy), the INR should be monitored frequently to minimize the risk of complications due to poor anticoagulant control.[198] Several warfarin nomograms and computer software programs are now available to assist caregivers in the control of warfarin therapy.

LONG-TERM TREATMENT

Patients with established venous thrombosis or pulmonary embolism require long-term anticoagulant therapy to prevent recurrent disease. Warfarin therapy is highly effective and is preferred in most patients.[198, 202] Adjusted-dose subcutaneous heparin is the treatment of choice when long-term oral anticoagulants are contraindicated, as in pregnancy. Adjusted-dose subcutaneous heparin, or unmonitored LMW heparin has been used for long-term treatment when oral anticoagulant therapy proves to be very difficult to control.[203] In patients with proximal vein thrombosis, long-term therapy with warfarin reduces the frequency of objectively documented recurrent venous thromboembolism from 47% to 2%.[127] The use of a less intense warfarin regimen (INR, 2.0 to 3.0) markedly reduces the risk of bleeding, from 20% to 4%, without loss of effectiveness in comparison with more intense warfarin.[202]

With the improved safety of oral anticoagulant therapy using a less intense warfarin regimen, there has been renewed interest in evaluating the long-term treatment of thrombotic disorders. In clinical trials in patients with atrial fibrillation, oral anticoagulant treatment has been given safely with a low risk of major bleeding complications (1% to 2% per year).[204] In trials such as these, the safety of oral anticoagulant treatment depends heavily on the maintenance of a narrow therapeutic INR range. These and other studies have emphasized the importance of maintaining careful control of oral anticoagulant therapy, particularly with the use of anticoagulant management clinics if oral anticoagulants are going to be used for extended periods of time.

Data from clinical trials have documented an unacceptably high incidence of recurrent venous thromboembolism, including fatal pulmonary embolism, during the long-term clinical course of patients with proximal DVT who are treated according to the current practice with intravenous heparin for several days, followed by oral anticoagulant treatment for 3 to 6 months.[113, 205–209] Three groups of patients who have a particularly poor prognosis have been identified[210, 211]:

- Patients with idiopathic, recurrent venous thromboembolism
- Patients who are carriers of genetic mutations that predispose to venous thromboembolism, such as factor V Leiden mutation
- Patients with cancer

Duration of Oral Anticoagulants After a First Episode of Deep Vein Thrombosis

It has been recommended that all patients with a first episode of venous thromboembolism receive warfarin therapy for 3 to 6 months. Attempts to decrease the treatment to 4 weeks[212, 213] or 6 weeks[208] resulted in higher rates of recurrent thromboembolism in comparison with either 12 or 26 weeks of treatment (11% to 18% recurrent thromboembolism in the following 1 to 2 years). Most of the recurrent thromboembolic events occurred in the 6 to 8 weeks immediately after anticoagulant treatment was stopped, and the incidence was higher in patients with continuing risk factors, such as cancer and immobilization.[208, 213] Treatment with oral anticoagulants for 6 months reduced the incidence of recurrent thromboembolic events, but there was a cumulative incidence of recurrent events at 2 years (11%) and an ongoing risk of recurrent thromboembolism of approximately 5% to 6% per year.[208]

In patients with a first episode of idiopathic venous thromboembolism treated with intravenous heparin followed by warfarin for 3 months, continuation of warfarin for 24 months led to a significant reduction in the incidence of recurrent venous thromboembolism when compared with placebo.[214] The continued risk of recurrent thromboembolism even with 6 months' treatment after a first episode of deep vein thrombosis has encouraged the development of clinical trials evaluating the effectiveness of long-term anticoagulant treatment beyond 6 months.

Duration of Oral Anticoagulant Treatment in Patients with Recurrent Deep Vein Thrombosis

In a multicenter clinical trial, Schulman and colleagues randomized patients with a first recurrent episode of venous thromboembolism to receive oral anticoagulants either for 6 months or continued indefinitely, with a targeted INR of 2.0 to 2.85.[209] The analysis was reported at 4 years. In the patients receiving anticoagulants for 6 months, recurrent thromboembolism occurred in 20.7%, compared with 2.6% of patients receiving the indefinite treatment ($p <$ .001). However, the rates of major bleeding were 2.7% in the 6-months group, compared with 8.6% in the indefinite group. In the indefinite group, two of the major hemorrhages were fatal; in the 6-months group, there were no fatal hemorrhages. This study showed that extending the duration of oral anticoagulants for approximately 4 years resulted in a significant decrease in the incidence of recurrent venous thromboembolism but with a higher incidence of major bleeding. Without a mortality difference, the risk of hemorrhage versus the benefit of decreased recurrent thromboembolism with the use of extended warfarin treatment remains uncertain and will require further clinical trials.

For patients experiencing a first episode of venous thromboembolism, long-term anticoagulant therapy should be continued for at least 3 to 6 months using oral anticoagulants to prolong the prothrombin time to an INR of 2.0 to 3.0.[127] For patients with recurrent venous thromboembolism or a continuing risk factor, such as immobilization, heart failure, or cancer, anticoagulants should be continued for a longer period of time and possibly indefinitely, particularly for those patients with more than one recurrent episode of thrombosis.[127]

Adverse Effects

The major side effect of oral anticoagulant therapy is bleeding.[215] Bleeding during well-controlled oral anticoagulant therapy is usually due to surgery or other forms of trauma, or to local lesions such as peptic ulcer or carcinoma.[215] Spontaneous bleeding may occur if warfarin sodium is given in an excessive dose, resulting in marked prolongation of the INR; this bleeding may be severe and even life-threatening. The risk of bleeding can be substantially reduced by adjustment of the warfarin dose to achieve a less intense anticoagulant effect than has traditionally been used in North America (INR, 2.0 to 3.0; prothrombin time, 1.25 to 1.5 times control value obtained using a rabbit brain thromboplastin, such as Simplastin or Dade-C).[202]

Nonhemorrhagic side effects of oral anticoagulant differ according to whether coumarin derivatives (e.g., warfarin sodium) or indanediones are administered. Such side effects are uncommon with coumarin anticoagulants, and the coumarins are therefore the oral anticoagulants of choice.

Coumarin-induced skin necrosis is a rare but serious complication that requires immediate cessation of oral anticoagulant therapy.[216, 217] It usually occurs between 3 and 10 days after therapy has commenced, is commoner in women, and most often involves areas of abundant subcutaneous tissues, such as the abdomen, buttocks, thighs, and breast. The mechanism of coumarin-induced skin necrosis, which is associated with microvascular thrombosis, is uncertain but it appears to be related, at least in some patients, to depression of protein C level. Patients with congenital deficiencies of protein C may be particularly prone to the development of coumarin skin necrosis.

Management of Patients Who Require Surgical Intervention During Long-term Oral Anticoagulant Therapy

Physicians are commonly confronted with the problem of managing oral anticoagulants in individuals who require temporary interruption of treatment for surgery or other invasive procedures.[218–223] In the absence of data from randomized clinical trials, recommendations can be made based only on cohort studies, retrospective reviews, and expert opinions. The most common conditions requiring long-term anticoagulant therapy are atrial fibrillation, mechanical or prosthetic heart valve replacement, and venous thromboembolism.[224, 225] For each of these conditions, the risk of arterial or venous thromboembolism when anticoagulants have been discontinued must be weighed against the risk of bleeding if intravenous heparin is applied before or after the surgical procedure, or if oral anticoagulant therapy is continued at the therapeutic level.

The possible choices based on the risk/benefit assessment in the individual patient include[224]:

1. Discontinuing warfarin for 3 to 5 days before the procedure to allow the INR to return to normal and then restarting therapy shortly after surgery.

2. Lowering the warfarin dose to maintain an INR in the lower or subtherapeutic range during the surgical procedure.

3. Discontinuing warfarin and treating the patient in-hospital with intravenous heparin before and after the surgical procedure, until warfarin therapy can be reinstituted. LMW heparin is now being used in some of the circumstances.

In a recent review that attempted to estimate the risk-benefit for the temporary discontinuation of oral anticoagulants and temporary use of heparin in patients with different conditions requiring oral anticoagulation, further revised recommendations were made.[224] Until further randomized clinical trials are carried out in these patients, no firm recommendations can be made, but the preceding guidelines have proved useful in clinical practice.

Antidote to Oral Anticoagulant Agents

The antidote to the vitamin K antagonists is vitamin K_1. If an excessive increase of the INR occurs, the treatment depends on the degree of the increase and whether or not the patient is bleeding. If the increase is mild and the patient is not bleeding, no specific treatment is necessary other than reduction in the warfarin dose. The INR can be expected to decrease during the next 24 hours with this approach. With a more marked increase of the INR in patients who are not bleeding, treatment with small doses of vitamin K_1, given either orally or by subcutaneous injection (1.0 to 2.0 mg), might be considered. With very marked increase of the INR, particularly in a patient who is either actively bleeding or at risk of bleeding, the coagulation defect should be corrected.

Reported side effects of vitamin K include flushing, dizziness, tachycardia, hypotension, dyspnea, and sweating.[198] Intravenous administration of vitamin K_1 should be performed with caution to avoid inducing an anaphylactoid reaction. The risk of anaphylactoid reaction can be reduced by slow administration of vitamin K_1. In most patients, intravenous administration of vitamin K_1 produces a demonstrable effect on the INR within 6 to 8 hours and corrects the increased INR within 12 to 24 hours. Because the half-life of vitamin K_1 is less than that of warfarin sodium, a repeated course of vitamin K_1 may be necessary. If bleeding is very severe and life-threatening, vitamin K therapy can be supplemented with concentrations of factors II, VII, IX, and X.

Upper Extremity Deep Vein Thrombosis

The treatment of upper extremity DVT is the same as for proximal venous thrombosis (i.e., heparin or LMW heparin plus warfarin for at least 3 months).[25] Patients with recent-onset upper extremity DVT have been treated with thrombolytic agents, but there is no evidence from clinical trials that this decreases long-term sequelae. The rare patient with thoracic outlet obstruction may benefit from surgery (see Chapter 85).

Recurrent Venous Thrombosis

The diagnosis of recurrent DVT is problematic, particularly if previous investigations are not available.[205, 226] Abnormalities persist on ultrasound studies for more than 12 months in the majority of patients, and the impedance plethysmography test remains abnormal at 3 months in approximately 30% of patients.[226] If these tests have reverted to negative and become positive with a symptomatic recurrence or if a new defect is detected in the same leg or the contralateral leg, the diagnosis is quite evident.[205] A new intraluminal filling defect on repeated venography is diagnostic. There is hope that the D-dimer assay may be of use in the exclusion of recurrent venous thrombosis, but this has not been adequately tested.[226] The finding of a new defect on ventilation perfusion lung scanning is helpful in making the diagnosis of pulmonary embolism. Otherwise, at present, if it is not possible to make a firm diagnosis of recurrent venous thromboembolism by objective tests, clinical judgment must be used.

Superficial Thrombophlebitis

In the absence of associated DVT, the treatment of superficial thrombophlebitis is usually confined to symptomatic relief with analgesia and rest of the affected limb. The exception is the patient with superficial thrombophlebitis involving a large segment of the long saphenous vein, particularly when it occurs above the knee. Chapter 143 discusses in detail current controversies and management, but it is our opinion that these patients should be treated with heparin or LMW heparin with or without oral anticoagulant therapy or superficial venous ligation. The presence of associated DVT requires the usual treatment with heparin or LMW heparin along with warfarin, for at least 3 months.

SUMMARY

Over the past 20 years, a large number of Level I clinical trials have been carried out on the prevention and medical management of acute DVT. Patterns of practice have changed dramatically in response to these studies. In this chapter, we have concentrated on the results of Level 1 clinical trials, but at the same time we have identified areas where further research is required. Many of the remaining questions should be answered in the near future based on the large number of Level I clinical trials currently being undertaken.

REFERENCES

1. Bertina RM, Koeleman BP, Koster T, et al: Mutation in blood coagulation factor V associated with resistance to activated protein C. Nature 369:64–67, 1994.
2. Dahlbäck B: Physiological anticoagulation: Resistance to activated protein C and venous thromboembolism. J Clin Invest 94:923–927, 1994.
3. Ridker PM, Miletich JP, Stampfer MJ, et al: Factor V Leiden and risks of recurrent idiopathic venous thromboembolism. Circulation 92:2800–2802, 1995.
4. Franco RF, Araujo AG, Guerreiro JF, et al: Analysis of the 677 C-T mutation of the methylenetetrahydrofolate reductase gene in different ethnic groups. Thromb Haemost 79:119–121, 1998.
5. D'Angelo, Selhub J: Homocysteine and thrombotic disease. Blood 90:1–11, 1997.
6. Simioni P, Prandoni P, Burlina A, et al: Hyperhomocysteinemia and deep vein thrombosis. Thromb Haemost 76(6):883–885, 1996.
7. Poort SR, Rosendaal FR, Reitsma PH, Bertina RM: A common genetic variation in the 3'-untranslated region of the prothrombin gene is associated with elevated plasma prothrombin levels and an increase in venous thrombosis. Blood 88:3698–3703, 1996.
8. Price DT, Ridker PM: Factor V Leiden mutation and the risks for thromboembolic disease: A clinical perspective. Ann Intern Med 127:895–903, 1997.
9. Lane DA, Mannucci PM, Bauer KA, et al: Inherited thrombophilia: Part 1. Thromb Haemost 76(5):651–662, 1996.
10. Hellgren M, Svensson PJ, Dahlbäck B: Resistance to activated protein C as a basis for venous thromboembolism associated with pregnancy and oral contraceptives. Am J Obstet Gynecol 173:210–213, 1995.
11. Koeleman BP, Reitsma PH, Allaart CF, Bertina RM: Activated protein C resistance as an additional risk factor for thrombosis in protein C–deficient families. Blood 84:103–105, 1994.
12. Middledrop S, Henkens CMA, Koopman MMW, et al: The incidence of venous thromboembolism in family members of patients with factor V Leiden mutation and venous thrombosis. Ann Intern Med 128:15–20, 1998.
13. Pepe G, Richards O, Vanegas OC, et al: Prevalence of factor V Leiden mutation in non-European populations. Thromb Haemost 77(2):329–331, 1997.
14. Hillarp A, Zöller B, Svensson P, Dahlbäck B: The 20210 A allele of the prothrombin gene is a common risk factor among Swedish outpatients with verified deep venous thrombosis. Thromb Haemost 78:990–992, 1997.
15. Hull RD, Hirsh J, Carter CJ, et al: Diagnostic efficacy of impedance plethysmography for clinically suspected deep vein thrombosis: A randomized trial. Ann Intern Med 102:21–28, 1985.
16. Huisman MV, Buller HE, ten Cate JW, et al: Serial impedance plethysmography for suspected deep venous thrombosis in outpatients: The Amsterdam General Practitioner Study. N Engl J Med 314:823–828, 1986.
17. Kakkar VV, Flanc C, Howe CT, et al: Natural history of postoperative deep vein thrombosis. Lancet 2:230–233, 1969.
18. Lagerstedt CI, Fagher BO, Olsson CG, et al: Need for long-term anticoagulant treatment in symptomatic calf vein thrombosis. Lancet 2:515–518, 1985.
19. Lohr JM, James KV, Deshmukh RM, Hasselfeld KA: Calf vein thrombi are not a benign finding. Am J Surg 170:86–90, 1995.
20. Moser KM, Le Moine JR: Is embolic risk conditioned by location of deep venous thrombosis? Ann Intern Med 94:439–444, 1981.
21. Sevitt S, Gallagher N: Venous thrombosis and pulmonary embolism: A clinicopathological study in injured and burned patients. Br J Surg 48:475–489, 1961.
22. Mavor GE, Galloway JMD: The iliofemoral venous segment as a source of pulmonary emboli. Lancet 1:871–874, 1967.
23. Hull RD, Hirsh J, Carter CJ, et al: Diagnostic value of ventilation-perfusion lung scanning in patients with suspected pulmonary embolism. Chest 88:819–828, 1985.
24. A collaborative study by the PIOPED investigators: Value of the ventilation/perfusion scan in acute pulmonary embolism: Results of the Prospective Investigation of Pulmonary Embolism Diagnosis (PIOPED). JAMA 263:2753–2769, 1990.
25. Prandoni P, Polistena P, Bernardi E, et al: Upper-extremity deep vein thrombosis. Arch Intern Med 157:57–62, 1997.
26. Martinelli I, Cattaneo M, Panzeri D, et al: Risk factors for deep venous thrombosis of the upper extremities. Ann Intern Med 126:707–711, 1997.
27. Bounameaux H, Reber-Wasem MA: Superficial thrombophlebitis and deep vein thrombosis. Arch Intern Med 157:1822–1824, 1997.
28. McLachlin J, Richard T, Paterson JC: An evaluation of clinical signs in the diagnosis of venous thrombosis. Arch Surg 85:738–742, 1962.
29. Kakkar VV, Adams PC: Preventive and therapeutic approach to venous thromboembolism: Can death from pulmonary embolism be prevented? J Am Coll Cardiol 8:146B–158B, 1986.
30. Skinner DB, Salzman EW: Anticoagulant prophylaxis in surgical patients. Surg Gynecol Obstet 125:741–746, 1967.
31. Shephard RM, White HA, Shirkey AL: Anticoagulant prophylaxis of thromboembolism in post-surgical patients. Am J Surg 112:698–702, 1966.
32. Coventry MB, Nolan DR, Beckenbaugh RD: "Delayed" prophylactic anticoagulation: A study of results and complications in 2,012 total hip arthoplasties. J Bone Joint Surg (Am) 55:1487–1492, 1973.
33. Eskeland G, Solheim K, Skhorten F: Anticoagulant prophylaxis, thromboembolism and mortality in elderly patients with hip fracture: A controlled clinical trial. Acta Chir Scand 131:16–29, 1986.
34. Murray DW, Britton AR, Bulstrode CJK: Thromboprophylaxis and death after total hip replacement. J Bone Joint Surg 78(6) 863–870, 1996.
35. Campling EA, Devlin HB, Hoile RW, Lunn JN: The report of the National Confidential Enquiry into Perioperative Deaths (NCEPOD) 1991/1992, London.
36. Salzman EW, Davies GC: Prophylaxis of venous thromboembolism: Analysis of cost-effectiveness. Ann Surg 191:207–218, 1980.
37. Hull R, Hirsh J, Sackett DL, et al: Cost-effectiveness of primary and secondary prevention of fatal pulmonary embolism in high risk surgical patients. Can Med Assoc J 127:990–995, 1982.
38. Oster G, Tuden RL, Colditz GA: A cost-effectiveness analysis of prophylaxis against deep vein thrombosis in major orthopedic surgery. JAMA 257:203–208, 1987.
39. Bergqvist D, Matzsch T, Jendteg S, et al: The cost-effectiveness of prevention of post-operative thromboembolism. Acta Chir Scand (Suppl) 556:36–41, 1990.
40. Hauch O, Khattar SC, Jorensen LN: Cost-benefit analysis of prophylaxis against deep vein thrombosis in major orthopaedic surgery. JAMA 257:203–208, 1987.
41. Sharnoff JG, Deblassio G: Prevention of fatal postoperative thromboembolism by heparin prophylaxis. Lancet 2:1006–1007, 1970.
42. Kearon C, Hirsh J: Starting prophylaxis for venous thromboembolism postoperatively. Arch Intern Med 155:366–372, 1995.
43. Bergqvist D, Benoni G, Bjorell O, et al: Low molecular weight heparin (enoxaparin) as prophylaxis against venous thromboembolism after total hip replacement. N Engl J Med 335(10):696–700, 1996.
44. Planes A, Vochelle N, Darmon JY, et al: Risk of deep-venous thrombosis after hospital discharge in patients having undergone total hip replacement: Double-blind randomized comparison of Enoxaparin versus placebo. Lancet 348:224–228, 1996.
45. Dahl OE, Andreassen G, Aspelin T, et al: Prolonged thromboprophylaxis following hip replacement surgery—results of a double-blind prospective, randomized, placebo-controlled study with dalteparin (Fragmin). Thromb Haemost 77(1):26–31, 1997.
46. Robinson KS, Anderson DR, Gross M, et al: Ultrasonographic screening before hospital discharge for deep venous thrombosis after arthroplasty: The post-arthroplasty screening study: A randomized controlled trial. Ann Intern Med 127:439–445, 1997.
47. Ricotta S, Iorio A, Parise P, et al: Post discharge, clinically overt venous thromboembolism in orthopaedic surgery patients with negative venography: An overview analysis. Thromb Haemost 76(6):887–892, 1996.

48. Vandermeulen EP, Van Aken H, Vermylen J: Anticoagulants and spinal-epidural anesthesia. Anesth Analg 79:1165–1177, 1994.
49. Bergqvist D, Lindblad B, Matzsch T: Risk of combining low molecular weight heparin for thromboprophylaxis and epidural or spinal anesthesia. Semin Thromb Hemost 19 (Suppl 1):147–151, 1993.
50. Dahlgren N, Tornebrandt K: Neurological complications after anaesthesia; A follow-up of 18,000 spinal and epidural anesthetics performed over three years. Acta Anaesthesiol Scand 39:872–880, 1995.
51. Horlocker TT, Heit JA: Low molecular weight heparin: Biochemistry, pharmacology, perioperative prophylaxis regimens, and guidelines for regional anesthetic management. Anesth Analg 85:874–885, 1997.
52. Clagett GP, Anderson FA, Heit J, et al: Prevention of venous thromboembolism. Chest 108(4):312S–334S, 1995.
53. Nicolaides AN, Bergqvist D, Hull RD, et al: Prevention of venous thromboembolism: International consensus statement. Int Angiol 16:3–38, 1997.
54. Cook DJ, Guyatt GH, Laupacis A, et al: Rules of evidence and clinical recommendations on the use of antithrombotic agents. Chest 108(4):227S–230S, 1995.
55. Collins R, Scrimgeour A, Yusef S, et al: Reduction in fatal pulmonary embolism and venous thrombosis by perioperative administration of subcutaneous heparin. N Engl J Med 318:1162–1173, 1988.
56. International Multicentre Trial: Prevention of fatal postoperative pulmonary embolism by low doses of heparin. Lancet 2:45–64, 1975.
57. Leyvraz PF, Bachmann F, Hoek J, et al: Prevention of deep vein thrombosis after hip replacement: Randomized comparison between unfractionated heparin and low molecular weight heparin. BMJ 303:543–548, 1991.
58. Kakkar V V, Cohen AT, Edmonson RA, et al: Low molecular weight versus standard heparin for prevention of venous thromboembolism after major abdominal surgery. Lancet 341:259–265, 1993.
59. Kakkar V V, Boeckl O, Boneau B, et al: Efficacy and safety of a low molecular weight heparin and standard unfractionated heparin for prophylaxis of postoperative venous thromboembolism: European multicenter trial. World J Surg 21:2–9, 1997.
60. Bergqvist D, Matzsch T, Brumark U, et al: Low molecular weight heparin given the evening before surgery compared with conventional low dose heparin in prevention of thrombosis. Br J Surg 75:888–891, 1988.
61. Caen JP: A randomized double-blind study between a low molecular weight heparin Kabi 2154 and standard heparin in the prevention of deep vein thrombosis in general surgery: A French multicentre trial. Thromb Haemost 59:216–220, 1988.
62. Bergqvist D, Burmark US, Flordal PA, et al: Low molecular weight heparin started before surgery as prophylaxis against deep vein thrombosis: 2500 versus 5000 X_{al} units in 2070 patients. Br J Surg 82:496–501, 1995.
63. Nurmohamed MT, Verhaeghe R, Haas S, et al: A comparative trial of a low molecular weight heparin (enoxaparin) versus standard heparin for the prophylaxis of postoperative deep vein thrombosis in general surgery. Am J Surg 169:567–571, 1995.
64. ENOXACAN Study Group: Efficacy and safety of enoxaparin versus unfractionated heparin for prevention of deep vein thrombosis in elective cancer surgery: A double-blind randomized multicentre trial with venographic assessment. Br J Surg 84:1099–1103, 1997.
65. The Danish Enoxaparin Study Group: Low molecular weight heparin (enoxaparin) vs. dextran 70. Arch Intern Med 151:1621–1624, 1991.
66. Levine MN, Hirsh J, Gent M, et al: Prevention of deep vein thrombosis after elective hip surgery: A randomized trial comparing low molecular weight heparin with standard unfractionated heparin. Ann Intern Med 114(7):545–551, 1991.
67. Eriksson BI, Kälebo P, Anthmyr BA, et al: Prevention of deep vein thrombosis and pulmonary embolism after total hip replacement. J Bone Joint Surg (Am) 73-A(4):484–493, 1991.
68. Planes A, Vochelle N, Fagola M, et al: Prevention of deep vein thrombosis after total hip replacement: The effect of low molecular weight heparin with spinal and general anaesthesia. J Bone Joint Surg (Br) 73-B:418–423, 1991.
69. Colwell CW, Spiro TE, Trowbridge AA, et al: Use of enoxaparin, a low molecular weight heparin, and unfractionated heparin for the prevention of deep venous thrombosis after elective hip replacement. J Bone Joint Surg 76-A(1):3–14, 1994.
70. Hull RD, Raskob GE, Pineo GF, et al: A comparison of subcutaneous low molecular weight heparin with warfarin sodium for prophylaxis against deep vein thrombosis after hip or knee implantation. N Engl J Med 329:1370–1376, 1993.
71. Hamulyak K, Lensing AWA, van der Meer J, et al: Subcutaneous low molecular weight heparin or oral anticoagulants for the prevention of deep vein thrombosis in elective hip and knee replacement? Thromb Haemost 74(6):1428–1431, 1995.
72. Francis CW, Pellegrini RV, et al: Prevention of deep vein thrombosis after total hip arthroplasty. J Bone Joint Surg 79-A(9):1365–1372, 1997.
73. Leclerc JR, Geerts WH, Desjardins L, et al: Prevention of deep vein thrombosis after major knee surgery: A randomized, double-blind trial comparing a low molecular weight heparin fragment (enoxaparin) to placebo. Thromb Haemost 67(4):417–423, 1992.
74. Leclerc JR, Geerts WH, Desjardins L, et al: Prevention of venous thromboembolism after knee arthroplasty: A randomized, double-blind trial comparing enoxaparin with warfarin. Ann Intern Med 124:619, 1996.
75. Heit JA, Berkowitz SD, Bona R, et al: Efficacy and safety of low molecular weight heparin (ardeparin sodium) compared to warfarin for the prevention of venous thromboembolism after total knee replacement surgery: A double blind, dose ranging study. Thromb Haemost 77(1):32–38, 1997.
76. Leizorovicz A, Haugh MC, Chapuis FR, et al: Low molecular weight heparin in prevention of perioperative thrombosis. BMJ 305:913–920. 1992.
77. Nurmohamed MT, Rosendaal FR, Buller HR, et al: Low molecular weight heparin in the prophylaxis of venous thrombosis: A meta-analysis. Lancet 340:152–156, 1992.
78. Koch A, Bouges S, Ziegler S, et al: Low molecular weight heparin and unfractionated heparin in thrombosis prophylaxis after major surgical intervention: Update of previous meta-analyses. Bri J Surg 84:750–759, 1997.
79. Palmer AJ, Koppenhagen K, Kirchhof B, et al: Efficacy and safety of low molecular weight heparin, unfractionated heparin and warfarin for thromboembolism prophylaxis in orthopaedic surgery: A meta-analysis of randomised clinical trials. Haemostasis 27:75–84, 1996.
80. O'Brien BJ, Anderson DR, Goeree R: Cost-effectiveness of enoxaparin versus warfarin prophylaxis against deep vein thrombosis after total hip replacement. Can Med Assoc J 150(7):1083–1089, 1994.
81. Menzin J, Colditz GA, Regan MM, et al: Cost-effectiveness of enoxaparin vs. low-dose warfarin in the prevention of deep vein thrombosis after total hip replacement surgery. Arch Intern Med 155:757–764, 1995.
82. Hull RD, Raskob GE, Pineo GF, et al: Warfarin prophylaxis after knee or hip surgery was more cost-effective than tinzaparin in the United States but not in Canada. Arch Intern Med 157:298–303, 1997.
83. Geerts WH, Jay RM, Code KI, et al: A comparison of low dose heparin with low molecular weight heparin as prophylaxis against venous thromboembolism after major trauma. N Engl J Med 335(10):701–707, 1996.
84. Harenberg J, Roebruck P, Heene DL, on behalf of the Heparin Study in Internal Medicine Group: Subcutaneous low molecular weight heparin versus standard heparin and the prevention of thromboembolism in medical inpatients. Haemostasis 26:127–139, 1996.
85. Bergmann JF, Neuhart E: A multicenter randomized double-blind study of enoxaparin compared with unfractionated heparin in the prevention of venous thromboembolic disease in elderly inpatients bedridden for an acute medical illness. Thromb Haemost 7(4):529–534, 1996.
86. Gallus A, Cade J, Ockelford P, et al: Orgaran (Org 10172) or heparin for preventing venous thromboembolism after elective surgery for malignant disease? A double-blind, randomized multicentre comparison. Thromb Haemost 70:562–567, 1993.
87. Bergqvist D, Kettunen K, Fredin H, et al: Thromboprophylaxis in hip fracture patients: A prospective randomized comparative study between ORG 10172 and dextran. Surgery 109:617–622, 1991.
88. Gerhart TN, Yett HS, Robertson LK, et al: Low molecular weight heparinoid compared with warfarin for prophylaxis of deep vein thrombosis in patients who are operated on for fracture of the hip: A prospective, randomized trial. J Bone Joint Surg 73-A(4):494–502, 1991.
89. Hoek J, Nurmohamed MT, ten Cate H, et al: Prevention of deep vein thrombosis following total hip replacement by a low molecular weight heparinoid. Thromb Haemost (Suppl) 62:1637, 1989.

90. Francis CW, Pellegrini VD, Marder VJ, et al: Comparison of warfarin and external pneumatic compression in prevention of venous thrombosis after total hip replacement. JAMA 267(21):2911–2915, 1992.

91. Paiement GD, Wessinger SJ, Waltman WC, et al: Low dose warfarin versus external pneumatic compression. Ann Intern Med 112:423–428, 1990.

92. Francis CW, Pellegrini VD Jr, Leibert KM: Comparison of two warfarin regimens in the prevention of venous thrombosis following total knee replacement. Thromb Haemost 5(75):706–716, 1996.

93. Power PJ, Gent M, Jay R, et al: A randomized trial of less intense postoperative warfarin or aspirin therapy in the prevention of venous thromboembolism after surgery for fractured hip. Arch Intern Med 149:771–774, 1989.

94. Poller L, McKernan A, Thomson JM, et al: Fixed minidose warfarin: A new approach to prophylaxis against venous thrombosis after major surgery. BMJ 285:1309–1312, 1988.

95. Bern MM, Lokich JJ, Wallach SR, et al: Very low doses of warfarin can prevent thrombosis in central venous catheters. Ann Intern Med 112:423–428, 1990.

96. Dale C, Gallus A, Wycherley A, et al: Prevention of venous thrombosis with minidose warfarin after joint replacement. Br Med J 303:224, 1991.

97. Robert VC, Sabri S, Beely AH, et al: The effect of intermittently applied external pressure on the hemodynamics of the lower limb in man. Br J Surg 59:233–236, 1972.

98. Ramos R, Salem BI, Pawlikowski MP, et al: The efficacy of pneumatic compression stockings in the prevention of pulmonary embolism after cardiac surgery. Chest 109(1):82–85, 1996.

99. Turpie AGG, Gallus A, Beattie WS, et al: Prevention of venous thrombosis in patients with intracranial disease by intermittent pneumatic compression of the calf. Neurology 27:435–438, 1977.

100. Turpie AGG, Delmore T, Hirsh J, et al: Prevention of venous thrombosis by intermittent sequential calf compression in patients with intracranial disease. Thromb Res 16:611–616, 1979.

101. Skillman JJ, Collins RR, Coe NP, et al: Prevention of deep vein thrombosis in neurosurgical patients: A controlled, randomized trial of external pneumatic compression boots. Surgery 83:354–358, 1978.

102. Hull RD, Raskob G, Gent M, et al: Effectiveness of intermittent pneumatic leg compression for preventing deep vein thrombosis after total hip replacement. JAMA 263:2313–2317, 1990.

103. Hull RD, Delmore TJ, Hirsh J, et al: Effectiveness of intermittent pulsatile elastic stockings for the prevention of calf and thigh vein thrombosis in patients undergoing elective knee surgery. Thromb Res 16:37–45, 1979.

104. McKenna R, Galante J, Bachmann F, et al: Prevention of venous thromboembolism after total knee replacement by high-dose aspirin or intermittent calf and thigh compression. Br Med J 1:514–517, 1980.

105. Meyerowitz BR, Nelson R: Measurement of the velocity of blood in lower limb veins with and without compression surgery. Surgery 56:481–486, 1964.

106. Sigel B, Edelstein AL, Felix WR: Compression of the deep venous system of the lower leg during inactive recumbency. Arch Surg 106:38–43, 1973.

107. Wells PS, Lensing AWA, Hirsh J: Graduated compression stockings in the prevention of postoperative venous thromboembolism: A meta-analysis. Arch Intern Med 154:67–72, 1994.

108. Eriksson BI, Ekman S, Kalebo P, et al: Prevention of deep vein thrombosis after total hip replacement: Direct thrombin inhibition with recombinant hirudin, CGP 39393. Lancet 347:635–639, 1996.

109. Eriksson BI, Goteborg SE, Lindbratt S, et al: Prevention of thromboembolism with use of recombinant hirudin. J Bone Joint Surg 79-A(3):326–333, 1997.

110. Antiplatelet Trialists' Collaboration: Collaborative overview of randomized trials of antiplatelet therapy: III. Reduction in venous thrombosis and pulmonary embolism by antiplatelet prophylaxis among surgical and medical patients. BMJ 308:235–246, 1994.

111. Ginsberg JS, Hirsh J: Use of antithrombotic agents during pregnancy. Chest 100(4):305S–311S, 1995.

112. Brandjes DPM, Buller HR, Hejiboer H, et al: Randomised trial of effect of compression stockings in patients with symptomatic proximal vein thrombosis. Lancet 349:759–762, 1997.

113. Franzeck UK, Schaich I, Jager KA, et al: Prospective 12-year follow-up study of clinical and haemodynamic sequelae after deep vein thrombosis in low risk patients (Zurich study). Circulation 93:74–79, 1996.

114. Lane DA: Heparin binding and neutralizing protein. In Lane DA, Lindahl U (eds): Heparin: Chemical and Biological Properties, Clinical Applications. London, Edward Arnold, pp 363–391.

115. Lindahl U, Backstrom G, Hook M, et al: Structure of the antithrombin-binding site of heparin. Proc Natl Acad Sci U S A 76:3198–3102, 1979.

116. Lindahl U, Thunberg L, Backstrom G, et al: Extension and structural variability of the antithrombin-binding sequence in heparin. J Biol Chem 259:12368–12376, 1984.

117. Rosenberg RD, Lam L: Correlation between structure and function of heparin. Proc Natl Acad Sci 76:1218–1222, 1979.

118. Casu B, Oreste P, Torri G, et al: The structure of heparin oligosaccharide fragments with high anti-(factor X_a) activity containing the minimal antithrombin III–binding sequence. Biochem J 197:599–609, 1981.

119. Weitz JI, Hudoba M, Massel D, et al: Clot-bound thrombin is protected from inhibition by heparin–antithrombin III but is susceptible to inactivation by antithrombin III–independent inhibitors. J Clin Invest 86:385–391, 1990.

120. Salzman EW, Rosenberg RD, Smith MH, et al: Effect of heparin and heparin fractions on platelet aggregation. J Clin Invest 65:64–73, 1980.

121. Rollefsen DM, Majerus DW, Blank MK: Heparin cofactor II: Purification and properties of a heparin-dependent inhibitor of thrombin in human plasma. J Biol Chem 257(5):2162–2169, 1982.

122. Hoppensteadt D, Walenga JM, Fasanella A, et al: TFPI antigen levels in normal human volunteers after intravenous and subcutaneous administration of unfractionated heparin and low molecular weight heparin. Thromb Res 77(2):175–185, 1995.

123. Barzu T, Molho P, Tobelem G, et al: Binding of heparin and low molecular weight heparin fragments to human vascular endothelial cells in culture. Nouv Rev Fr Haematol 26:243–247, 1984.

124. Blajchman MA, Young E, Ofosu FA: Effects of unfractionated heparin, dermatan sulfate and low molecular weight heparin on vessel wall permeability in rabbits. Ann N Y Acad Sci 556:245–254, 1989.

125. Gallus A, Jackaman J, Tillett J, et al: Safety and efficacy of warfarin started early after submassive venous thrombosis or pulmonary embolism. Lancet ii:1293–1296, 1986.

126. Hull RD, Raskob GE, Rosenbloom D, et al: Heparin for 5 days as compared with 10 days in the initial treatment of proximal venous thrombosis. N Engl J Med 322:1260–1264, 1990.

127. Hyers TN, Hull RD, Weg JG: Antithrombotic therapy for venous thromboembolic disease. Chest 108(4):335S–351S, 1995.

128. Hull RD, Raskob GE, Rosenbloom D, et al: Optimal therapeutic level of heparin therapy in patients with venous thrombosis. Arch Intern Med 152:1589–1595, 1992.

129. Hull RD, Raskob GE, Brant RF, et al: Relation between the time to achieve the lower limit of the APTT therapeutic range and recurrent venous thromboembolism during heparin treatment for deep vein thrombosis. Arch Intern Med 157:2562–2568, 1997.

130. Hull RD, Raskob GE, Brant RF, et al: The importance of initial heparin treatment on long-term clinical outcomes of antithrombotic therapy. Arch Intern Med 157:2317–2321, 1997.

131. Brill-Edwards P, Ginsberg S, Johnston M, et al: Establishing a therapeutic range for heparin therapy. Ann Intern Med 119:104–109, 1993.

132. Campbell N, Hull RD, Brant R, et al: Aging and heparin-related bleeding. Arch Intern Med 156:857–860, 1996.

133. White RH, Zhou H, Woo L, Mungall D: Effect of weight, sex, age, clinical diagnosis and thromboplastin reagent on steady-state intravenous heparin requirements. Arch Intern Med 157:2468–2472, 1997.

134. Juergens CP, Semsarian C, Keech AC, et al: Hemorrhagic complications of intravenous heparin use. Am J Cardiol 80:150–153, 1997.

135. Fennerty A, Thomas P, Backhouse G, et al: Audit of control of heparin treatment. Br Med J 290:27–28, 1985.

136. Wheeler AP, Jaquiss RD, Newman JH: Physician practices in the treatment of pulmonary embolism and deep venous thrombosis. Arch Intern Med 148:1321–1325, 1988.

137. Cruickshank MK, Levine MN, Hirsh J, et al: A standard nomogram for the management of heparin therapy. Arch Intern Med 151:333–337, 1991.

138. Raschke RA, Reilly BM, Guidry JR, et al: The weight-based heparin-

dosing nomogram compared with a "standard care" nomogram. Ann Intern Med 119:874–881, 1993.

139. Raschke R, Gollihare B, Peirce JC: The effectiveness of implementing one weight-based heparin nonogram as a practice guideline. Arch Intern Med 156:1645–1649, 1996.

140. Hirsh J, Raschke R, Warkentin TE, et al: Heparin: Mechanism of action, pharmacokinetics, dosing consideration, monitoring, efficacy and safety. Chest 108(4):258S–275S, 1995.

141. Kelton JG: Heparin-induced thrombocytopenia. Haemostasis 16:173–186, 1986.

142. Warkentin TE, Elavathil LJ, Hayward CPM, et al: The pathogenesis of venous limb gangrene associated with heparin-induced thrombocytopenia. Ann Intern Med 127:804–812, 1997.

143. Boshkov LK, Warkentin TE, Hayward CPM, et al: Heparin-induced thrombocytopenia and thrombosis: Clinical and laboratory studies. Br J Haematol 84:322–328, 1993.

144. Arepally G, Reynolds C, Tomaski A, et al: Comparison of PF4/heparin ELISA assay with the (^{14}C) serotonin release assay in the diagnosis of heparin-induced thrombocytopenia. Am J Clin Pathol 104(6):648–654, 1995.

145. Greinacher A, Michel I, Kiefel V, et al: A rapid and sensitive test for diagnosis of heparin-associated thrombocytopenia. Thromb Haemost 66:734–736, 1991.

146. Warkentin TE, Chong BH, Greinacher A: Heparin-induced thrombocytopenia: Towards consensus. Thromb Haemost 79:1–7, 1998.

147. Magnani HN: Heparin-induced thrombocytopenia (HIT): An overview of 230 patients treated with orgaran (Org 10172). Thromb Haesmost 70:554–561, 1993.

148. Greinacher A, Volpel H, Porzsch B: Recombinant hirudin in the treatment of patients with heparin-induced thrombocytopenia (HIT) (Abstract). Blood 88:281a, 1996.

149. Matsuo T, Kario K, Chikahira Y, et al: Treatment of heparin-induced thrombocytopenia by use of argatroban, a synthetic thrombin inhibitor. Br J Haematol 82:627–629, 1992.

150. Demers C, Ginsberg JS, Brill-Edwards P, et al: Rapid anticoagulation using ancrod for heparin-induced thrombocytopenia. Blood 78:2194–2197, 1991.

151. Weitz JI: Low molecular weight heparins. N Engl J Med 337:688–698, 1997.

152. Hirsh J, Levine MN: Low molecular weight heparin. Blood 79:1–17, 1992.

153. Fareed J, Hoppensteadt D, Jeske W, et al: The available low molecular weight heparin preparations are not the same. Thromb Haemost 3 (Suppl 1):S38–S52, 1997.

154. Bara L, Samama MM: Pharmacokinetics of low molecular weight heparin. Acta Chir Scand 545:65–72, 1988.

155. Briant L, Caranobe C, Saivin S, et al: Unfractionated heparin and CY216: Pharmacokinetics and bioavailabilities of the anti–factor X$_a$ and II$_a$: Effects of intravenous and subcutaneous injection in rabbits. Thromb Haemost 61:348–353, 1989.

156. Anderson L-O, Barrowcliffe TW, Holmer E, et al: Molecular weight dependency of the heparin-potentiated inhibition of thrombin and activated factor X: Effect of heparin neutralization in plasma. Thromb Res 115:531–538, 1979.

157. Fareed J, Walenga JM, Racanelli A, et al: Validity of the newly established low molecular weight heparin standard in cross referencing low molecular weight heparins. Haemostasis 3(Suppl):33–47, 1988.

158. Barrowcliffe TW, Curtis AD, Johnson EA, et al: An international standard for low molecular weight heparin. Thromb Haemost 60:1–7, 1988.

159. Holmer E, Soderberg K, Bergqvist D, et al: Heparin and its low molecular weight derivatives: Anticoagulant and antithrombotic properties. Haemostasis 16(Suppl 2):1–7, 1986.

160. Carter CJ, Kelton JG, Hirsh J, et al: The relationship between the hemorrhagic and antithrombotic properties of low molecular weight heparins and heparin. Blood 59:1239–1245, 1982.

161. Cade JF, Buchanan MR, Boneu B, et al: A comparison of the anti-thrombotic and haemorrhagic effects of low molecular weight heparin fractions: The influence of the method of preparation. Thromb Res 35:613–625, 1985.

162. Andriuoli G, Mastacchi R, Barnti M, et al: Comparison of the antithrombotic and hemorrhagic effects of heparin and a new low molecular weight heparin in the rat. Haemostasis 15:324–330, 1985.

163. Lensing AW, Prins MH, Davidson BL, et al: Treatment of deep

164. Monreal M, Lafoz E, Salvador R, et al: Adverse effects of three different forms of heparin therapy: Thrombocytopenia, increased transaminases, and hyperkalaemia. Eur J Clin Pharmacol 37:415–418, 1989.

165. Monreal M, Vinas L, Monreal L, et al: Heparin-related osteoporosis in rats: A comparative study between unfractionated heparin and a low molecular weight heparin. Haemostasis 20:204–207, 1990.

166. Matzsch T, Bergqvist D, Hedner U, et al: Effects of low molecular weight heparin and unfragmented heparin on induction of osteoporosis in rats. Thromb Haemost 63:505–509, 1990.

167. Shaughnessy SG, Young E, Deschamps P, Hirsh J: The effects of low molecular weight and standard heparin on calcium loss from fetal rat calvaria. Blood 86:1368–1373, 1995.

168. Warkentin TE, Levine MN, Hirsh J, et al: Heparin-induced thrombocytopenia in patients treated with low molecular weight heparin or unfractionated heparin. N Engl J Med 332(20):1330–1335, 1995.

169. Forestier F, Daffos F, Capella-Pavlovsky M: Low molecular weight heparin (PH 10169) does not cross the placenta during the second trimester of pregnancy: Study by direct fetal blood sampling under ultrasound. Thromb Res 34:557–560, 1984.

170. Omri A, Delaloye FJ, Andersen H, et al: Low molecular weight heparin Novo (LHN-1) does not cross the placenta during the second trimester of pregnancy. Thromb Haemost 61:55–56, 1989.

171. Andrew M, Cade J, Buchanan MR, et al: Low molecular weight heparin does not cross the placenta (Abstract). Thromb Haemost 50:225, 1983.

172. Melissari E, Parker CJ, Wilson NV, et al: Use of low molecular weight heparin in pregnancy. Thromb Haemost 68:652–656, 1992.

173. Sturridge F, de Swiet M, Letsky E: The use of low molecular weight heparin for thromboprophylaxis in pregnancy. Br J Obstet Gynaecol 101:69–71, 1994.

174. Wahlberg TB, Kher A: Low molecular weight heparin as thromboprophylaxis in pregnancy: A retrospective analysis from 14 European clinics. Haemostasis, 24:55–56, 1994.

175. Hunt BJ, Doughty H-A, Majumdar G, et al: Thromboprophylaxis with low molecular weight heparin (Fragmin) in high-risk pregnancies. Thromb Haemost 77(1):39–43, 1997.

176. Dalitzk M, Pauzner R, Langevitz P, et al: Low molecular weight heparin during pregnancy and delivery: Preliminary experience with 41 pregnancies. Obstet Gynecol 87:380–383, 1996.

177. Boneu B, Caranobe C, Cadroy Y, et al: Pharmacokinetic studies of standard unfractionated heparin, and low molecular weight heparins in the rabbit. Semin Thromb Hemost 14:18–27, 1988.

178. Boneu B, Buchanan MR, Cade JF, et al: Effects of heparin, its low molecular weight fractions and other glycosaminoglycans on thrombus growth in vivo. Thromb Res 40:81–89, 1985.

179. Bratt G, Tornebohm E, Granqvist S, et al: A comparison between low molecular weight heparin (KAEI 2165) and standard heparin in the intravenous treatment of deep venous thrombosis. Thromb Haemost 54:813–817, 1985.

180. Holm HA, Ly B, Handeland GF, et al: Subcutaneous heparin treatment of deep venous thrombosis: A comparison of unfractionated and low molecular weight heparin. Haemostasis 16:30–37, 1986.

181. Albada J, Nieuwenhuis HK, Sixma JJ: Treatment of acute venous thromboembolism with low molecular weight heparin (Fragmin): Results of a double-blind randomized study. Circulation 80:935–940, 1989.

182. Bratt G, Aberg W, Johansson M, et al: Two daily subcutaneous injections of Fragmin as compared with intravenous standard heparin in the treatment of deep venous thrombosis (DVT). Thromb Haemost 64:506–510, 1990.

183. Harenberg J, Huck K, Bratsch H, et al: Therapeutic application of subcutaneous low molecular weight heparin in acute venous thrombosis. Haemostasis 20 (Suppl 1):205–219, 1990.

184. Siegbahn A, Y-Hassan S, Boberg J, et al: Subcutaneous treatment of deep venous thrombosis with low molecular weight heparin: A dose finding study with LMWH-Novo. Thromb Res 55:267–278, 1989.

185. Hull RD, Raskob GE, Pineo GF, et al: Subcutaneous low molecular weight heparin compared with continuous intravenous heparin in the treatment of proximal vein thrombosis. N Engl J Med 326:975–938, 1992.

186. Prandoni P, Lensing AW, Buller HR, et al: Comparison of subcutaneous low molecular weight heparin with intravenous standard heparin in proximal deep vein thrombosis. Lancet 339:441–445, 1992.

venous thrombosis with low molecular weight heparins. Arch Int Med 155:601–607, 1995.

187. Lopaciuk S, Meissner AJ, Filipecki S, et al: Subcutaneous low molecular weight heparin versus subcutaneous unfractionated heparin in the treatment of deep vein thrombosis: A Polish muticentre trial. Thromb Haemost 68:14–18, 1992.

188. Lindmarker P, Holmstrom M, Granqvist S, et al: Comparison of once-daily subcutaneous Fragmin with continuous intravenous unfractionated heparin in the treatment of deep venous thrombosis. Thromb Haemost 72:186–190, 1994.

189. Simonneau G, Charbonnier B, Decousus H, et al: Subcutaneous low molecular weight heparin compared with continuous intravenous unfractionated heparin in the treatment of proximal deep vein thrombosis. Arch Intern Med 153:1541–1546, 1993.

190. Decousus H, Leizorovicz A, Parent F, et al: A clinical trial of vena caval filters in the prevention of pulmonary embolism in patients with proximal deep vein thrombosis. N Engl J Med 338:409–415, 1998.

191. Levine M, Gent M, Hirsh J, et al: A comparison of low molecular weight heparin administered primarily at home with unfractionated heparin administered in the hospital for proximal deep vein thrombosis. N Engl J Med 334:677–681, 1996.

192. Koopman MMW, Prandoni P, Piovella F, et al: Treatment of venous thrombosis with intravenous unfractionated heparin administered in the hospital as compared with subcutaneous low molecular weight heparin administered at home. N Engl J Med 334:682–687, 1996.

193. The Columbus Investigators: Low molecular weight heparin in the treatment of patients with venous thromboembolism. N Engl J Med 337:657–662, 1997.

194. Simonneau G, Sors H, Charbonnier B, et al: A comparison of low molecular weight heparin with unfractionated heparin for acute pulmonary embolism. N Engl J Med 337:663–669, 1997.

195. Hull RD, Raskob GE, Rosenbloom D, et al: Treatment of proximal vein thrombosis with subcutaneous low molecular weight heparin vs. intravenous heparin: An economic perspective. Arch Intern Med 157:289–294, 1997.

196. Van den Belt AGM, Bossuyt PMM, Prins MH, et al: Replacing inpatient care by outpatient care in the treatment of deep vein thrombosis: An economic evaluation. Thromb Haemost 79:259–263, 1998.

197. Freedman MD: Oral anticoagulants: Pharmacodynamics, clinical indications and adverse effects. J Clin Pharmacol 32:196–209, 1992.

198. Hirsh J, Dalen JE, Deykin D, et al: Oral anticoagulants; Mechanism of action, clinical effectiveness and optimal therapeutic range. Chest 108(4):231S–246S, 1995.

199. Clouse LH, Comp PC: The regulation of haemostasis: The protein C system. N Engl J Med 314:1298–1304, 1986.

200. O'Reilly RA, Aggeler PM: Studies on coumarin anticoagulant drugs: Initiation of warfarin therapy without a loading dose. Circulation 38:169–177, 1968.

201. Wells PS, Holbrook AM, Crowther R, Hirsh J: Warfarin and its drug/food interactions; A critical appraisal of the literature. Ann Intern Med 121:676–683, 1994.

202. Hull RD, Hirsh J, Jay RM, et al: Different intensities of oral anticoagulant therapy in the treatment of proximal vein thrombosis. N Engl J Med 307:1676–1681, 1982.

203. Hull RD, Delmore T, Carter C, et al: Adjusted subcutaneous heparin versus warfarin sodium in the long-term treatment of venous thrombosis. N Engl J Med 306:189–194, 1982.

204. Laupacis A, Albers G, Dalen J, et al: Antithrombotic therapy in atrial fibrillation. Chest 108:352S–359S, 1995.

205. Hull RD, Carter CJ, Jay RM, et al: The diagnosis of acute, recurrent deep vein thrombosis: A diagnostic challenge. Circulation 67:901–906, 1983.

206. Prandoni P, Lensing AWA, Cogo A, et al: The long-term clinical course of acute deep venous thrombosis. Ann Intern Med 125:1–7, 1996.

207. Beyth RJ, Cohen AM, Landefeld CS: Long-term outcomes of deep vein thrombosis. Arch Intern Med 155:1031–1037, 1995.

208. Schulman S, Rhedin AS, Lindmarker P, et al: A comparison of six weeks with six months of oral anticoagulation therapy after a first episode of venous thromboembolism. N Engl J Med 332:1661–1665, 1995.

209. Schulman S, Granqvist S, Holmstrom M, et al: The duration of oral anticoagulant therapy after a second episode of venous thromboembolism. N Engl J Med 336:393–398, 1997.

210. Prandoni P, Lensing A, Buller H, et al: Deep vein thrombosis and the incidence of subsequent symptomatic cancer. N Engl J Med 327:1128–1133, 1992.

211. Simioni P, Prandoni P, Lensing AWA, et al: The risk of recurrent venous thromboembolism in patients with Arg^{506}–Gin mutation in the gene for factor V (factor V Leiden). N Engl J Med 336:339–403, 1997.

212. Research Committee of the British Thoracic Society: Optimum duration of anticoagulation for deep vein thrombosis and pulmonary embolism. Lancet 340:873–876, 1992.

213. Levine MN, Hirsh J, Gent M, et al: Optimal duration of oral anticoagulant therapy: A randomized trial comparing four weeks with three months of warfarin in patients with proximal deep vein thrombosis. Thromb Haemost 74:606–611, 1995.

214. Kearon C for the LAFIT Investigators: Two years of warfarin vs. placebo following three months of anticoagulation for a first episode of idiopathic venous thromboembolism (VTE) (Abstract). Thromb Haemost 77:767, 1997.

215. Levine MN, Raskob GE, Hirsh J: Hemorrhagic complications of long-term anticoagulant therapy. Chest 95(Suppl 2):26S, 1989.

216. Grimaudo V, Gueissaz F, Hauert J, et al: Necrosis of skin induced by coumarin in a patient deficient in protein S. Br Med J 298:233, 1989.

217. Becker CG: Oral anticoagulant therapy and skin necrosis: Speculation on pathogenesis. Adv Exp Med Biol 214:217, 1987.

218. Rustad H, Myhre E: Surgery during anticoagulant treatment. Acta Med Scand 173:115–119, 1963.

219. McIntyre H: Management during dental surgery of patients on anticoagulants. Lancet 2:99–100, 1966.

220. Tinker JH, Tarhan S: Discontinuing anticoagulant therapy in surgical patients with cardiac valve prostheses. JAMA 239:738–739, 1978.

221. Katholi RE, Nolan SP, McGuire LB: The management of anticoagulation during non-cardiac operations in patients with prosthetic heart valves. Am Heart J 96:163–165, 1978.

222. Bodnar AG, Hutter AM: Anticoagulation in valvular heart disease preoperatively and postoperatively. Cardiovasc Clin 14:247–264, 1984.

223. Eckman MH, Beshansky JR, Duranad-Zaleski I, et al: Anticoagulation for non-cardiac procedures in patients with prosthetic heart valves. JAMA 263:1513–1521, 1990.

224. Kearon C, Hirsh J: Management of anticoagulation before and after elective surgery. N Engl J Med 336(21):1506–1511, 1997.

225. Stein PD, Alpert JS, Copeland JG, et al: Antithrombotic therapy in patients with mechanical and biological prosthetic heart valves. Chest 108(4):371S–379S, 1995.

226. Huisman MV, Beaumont-Koopman MAW: The diagnosis of recurrent deep vein thrombosis. In Hall RD, Raskob GE, Pineo GF: Venous Thromboembolism: An Evidence-Based Atlas. Armonk, NY, Futura Publishing Company, 1996.

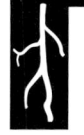

C H A P T E R 1 4 1

Interventional Treatments for Iliofemoral Venous Thrombosis

Robert Rutherford, M.D., Bo Eklof, M.D., and
Mark Mewissen, M.D.

This chapter discusses the role of early removal of thrombus, by thrombectomy or thrombolysis, in the management of iliofemoral venous thrombosis. The rationale and the preference for such interventions over conservative management with anticoagulant therapy are presented. We also recommend indications and guidelines for appropriate case selection and review results of the thrombectomy and thrombolysis. Finally, an algorithm for selective use of these interventions in the treatment of iliofemoral venous thrombosis is offered.

PREVALENT VIEWS REGARDING MANAGEMENT

Most clinicians recognize that the majority of cases of chronic venous insufficiency (CVI) of the lower extremities are post-thrombotic in origin. Although the tremendous toll attributable to the late sequelae of deep venous thrombosis (DVT) is well documented, there appears to be widespread apathy among many, particularly primary care physicians, regarding the use of thrombolysis or thrombectomy to prevent or mitigate these sequelae in iliofemoral venous thrombosis (IFVT), in spite of encouraging results reported in the literature.

This is attributable, in part, to a primary focus on the initial treatment, i.e., preventing pulmonary embolism and the propagation or recurrence of thrombosis, and to a lack of experience with or attention to the late sequelae. There is apparently also a lack of appreciation of the different natural history of IFVT compared with more distal DVT, a lack of understanding of the different pathophysiologic changes that occur following DVT, and the relative contribution of these changes to the pathogenesis and severity of the post-thrombotic syndrome. Traditional thinking is that the thrombosed segments eventually recanalize but their valve function is destroyed; therefore, reflux in these segments leads to high venous pressures under gravitational stress, thereby causing the post-thrombotic sequelae.

Along with this simplistic view, it is thought that these interventions have little chance of preventing late reflux in the involved segments. However this is an oversimplification and represents only part of the pathophysiology and pathogenesis of the late post-thrombotic sequelae. In this chapter, the authors not only demonstrate that early and complete thrombus removal can preserve valve function in the involved segment but also present an important addi-

tional perspective, namely, that obstruction also plays a significant role in pathogenesis, both early and late, particularly after IFVT. This not only affects the involved venous segment but also causes incompetence in segments distal to this obstruction.

Pathogenesis of Post-thrombotic Sequelae

Outcome after DVT can be categorized into four subgroups: those with neither detectable obstruction nor valvular insufficiency, those with obstruction alone, those with valvular insufficiency alone, and those with both outflow obstruction and distal valvular insufficiency. Noninvasive testing[1] suggests that less than 20% of those with documented DVT do not have either significant obstruction or reflux. These are presumably patients with short segmental venous involvement in whom residual obstruction or valvular insufficiency is limited to the involved segment, with no global changes in venous function detectable by noninvasive testing. Estimates of those with significant residual obstruction after lower extremity DVT are close to 10% with the CVI in most of the remainder being attributed to valvular reflux. The combination of reflux and obstruction is often overlooked.

The overall outcome of DVT in terms of disturbed venous pathophysiology depends to a large degree on the location of the thrombosed segments and the extent of involvement (i.e. single or multiple segments). The location relates to the likelihood of recanalization of the thrombosed segment, which, in the lower extremity, decreases as one moves proximally. Venographic studies, which were commonly performed in the 1950s and 1960s, showed that close to 95% of popliteal or tibial thromboses recanalize completely,[2] and at least 50% of superficial femoral venous thromboses recanalize.[3] In contrast, the minority of iliofemoral thromboses (>20%) completely recanalize and form a normal, unobstructed lumen.[4]

However, if one takes a closer look at thromboses involving the iliofemoral venous segment, it becomes apparent that only 20% completely recanalize spontaneously and another 60% recanalize partly or at least develop adequate collaterals, testing negative for obstruction on noninvasive studies (e.g., impedance plethysmography). Thus, in reality, only about 20% remain significantly occluded or have collaterals so poor that detectable and symptomatic venous outflow obstruction results. Nevertheless, a significant degree of obstruction persists for 3 to 6 months in most patients with IFVT.

It has also been pointed out that, if the distal venous valves (and particularly those in the popliteal segment) remain competent, the post-thrombotic sequelae are relatively modest and controllable by conservative measures.[5] What is not well appreciated is that persisting proximal obstruction, even if it is ultimately relieved by partial recanalization or collateral development, can lead to progressive breakdown of distal valves, resulting in reflux.

The severity of post-thrombotic sequelae correlates with the level of *ambulatory venous pressure* (AVP), as shown by Nicolaides and coworkers.[6] It is impressive how steadily the frequency of ulceration climbs with increasing levels of ambulatory pressure. This suggests that anything that significantly reduces AVP will reduce the severity of the post-thrombotic sequelae, and vice versa. Nicolaides and coworkers have also shown that the highest levels of AVP are found in patients with both obstruction and reflux.[7] These two observations underscore a major point to be made in regard to the disturbed pathophysiology associated with IFVT and the pathogenesis of post-thrombotic sequelae. Obstruction alone is rarely sufficient to cause venous claudication; it mostly causes increased swelling with activity. Valvular insufficiency alone causes most of the "stasis sequelae" (i.e., brawny edema, subcutaneous fibrosis, pigmentation, and ulceration), but these can be managed, in the compliant patient, with elastic stockings and elevation. However, those with both obstruction *and* valvular insufficiency have severe post-thrombotic sequelae, so severe that management is difficult even in a compliant patient.

Possibly of greater importance is the lack of appreciation of the changes that occur with time after major DVT of the lower extremity. While accepting that obstruction is present early on, most clinicians focus on valve insufficiency of the recanalized segments as the only cause of the late post-thrombotic sequelae. However, proximal obstruction, if unrelieved for any significant period of time, can lead to secondary valvular incompetence in distal segments, segments that were not involved in the original thrombotic process.

Patients with IFVT are usually advised to elevate their legs and wear elastic stockings initially. They are also frequently advised to progressively increase ambulation and the time spent in the upright position during the rehabilitation period. This advice typically is given in the early weeks soon after hospital discharge. At this early time, patients rarely complain of much swelling or pain, since they have been spending most of their time off their feet with only limited periods of activity; however, most of them still have residual obstruction at this time. In considering the impact of advising ambulation and being upright, one should appreciate the differences in extremity blood flow between the resting state, or one of very limited activity, and the state of full activity and periods of moderate exercise. At rest, the venous collaterals that have formed may enable venous outflow to occur at reasonable venous pressures, but with ambulation, the exercising muscles demand significant additional arterial inflow, so that overall extremity flow may increase severalfold. As a direct corollary to this, venous outflow must increase proportionately, and, whereas the existing collaterals may have been able to handle resting flow rates at moderate venous pressures, the increased flow

rates associated with exercise cannot be accommodated readily, so the venous pressure distal to the point of obstruction increases dramatically.

The effect of persisting obstruction, particularly in the patients who are trying to rehabilitate by steadily increasing their levels of activity, is to create frequent periods of severe venous hypertension associated with dilation of the distal venous segments. Ultimately, these repeated periods of engorgement and dilation of the distal veins cause progressive stretching and incompetence of the valves, so that valvular incompetence develops with time in previously uninvolved distal segments.

What is the evidence that this actually occurs? The best studies on this are the result of a program of ongoing duplex scan surveillance of patients with DVT being carried on by Strandness and associates. In a series of articles, Strandness and coworkers showed that 20% to 50% of initially uninvolved distal veins become incompetent by 2 years.[8] They also demonstrated that the combination of reflux and obstruction, as opposed to either alone, correlated with the severity of symptoms and was present in 55% of symptomatic patients[9] and that 25% of all venous segments developed reflux in time, of which 32% were not involved previously with thrombosis.[10] Finally, in a study of the posterior tibial veins located below a popliteal segment involved with thrombosis, 55% of the distal veins became incompetent if the segment remained obstructed, compared with 7.5% of those below a popliteal vein that recanalized.[11]

These changes in the distal veins occur early enough that they cannot be blamed on proximal valvular reflux, although this also comes into play with time. Thus, it appears that the early relief of obstruction (by thrombectomy or thrombolysis) should prevent more extensive post-thrombotic sequelae if only by protecting the distal veins against progressive valvular incompetence. This point has not been well recognized, not only in terms of basic pathogenesis but also in judging the results of thrombectomy and thrombolysis, in which critics have largely ignored the restoration of proximal patency while focusing on the presence or absence of valve reflux. This topic will be discussed further, as we look at the results of these two methods of thrombus removal.

ILIOFEMORAL VENOUS THROMBECTOMY

Historical Background

During the 1940s, surgical interruption of veins, often combined with local thrombectomy, was the prevailing method for prophylaxis and treatment of DVT from the superficial femoral vein proximally, the main goal being the prevention of a pulmonary embolus (PE). Anticoagulation therapy was slowly being accepted at that time. The modern era of thrombectomy (TE) in the United States started with Mahorner's description of a "new management for thrombosis of deep veins of extremities," presented in 1954, in which he advocated TE followed by restoration of vein lumen rather than ligation, plus regional heparinization.[12] He presented 6 patients, 5 of whom had an excellent result, with rapid disappearance of leg swelling, very little late morbidity, and minimum leg edema. There was no PE prior or subsequent to surgery. In a subsequent paper in 1957, he and associates reported 16 patients on whom TE was performed in 14 legs and two arms, with excellent results in 12, good in two, and poor in 2 patients.[13] Mahorner's report created a wave of enthusiasm for TE that rolled over the United States from the South (Table 141–1). Postoperative mortality was high (9%) but the mortality from fatal PE was low, and the clinical results were good in more than 75%, if the history of the DVT was short (less than 10 days).

The enthusiastic wave created by Mahorner was given major impetus by Haller and Abrams in 1963, who reported on 45 patients with IFVT who underwent TE.[16] In 34 patients with short histories of DVT (less than 10 days), flow was successfully restored in 31 (91%). At follow-up after an average of 18 months, 26 of these 31 patients (84%) had normal legs, and venography in 13 patients showed normal patency of the deep venous system in 11 (85%).

Enthusiasm was dramatically dampened by Lansing and Davis in 1968 with their 5-year follow-up of Haller and Abrams' patients.[14] Of the 34 patients who had had thrombectomy within 10 days of DVT, only 17 patients (50%) were interviewed. Sixteen patients were found to have swelling of the leg requiring elastic stockings, and one had an ulcer. Ascending venography in the supine position in 15 patients showed patent veins, but the involved area of the deep venous system was found to be incompetent in all cases, and there were no functioning valves. Unfortunately, Lansing and Davis used ascending phlebography in the supine position, a technique that does not assess valve competency reliably and often does not give good visualization of the iliac segment. The apparent excellent patency was ignored and the (flawed) assessment of venous valve function was stressed. In discussing this paper, Haller stated that he was never consulted about the follow-up report and during a recent visit to Louisville, he had studied 17 patients in whom total removal of the thrombus had been possible, and none had residual edema. Despite the expression of support for TE at this and subsequent surgical meetings, the impact of Lansing and Davis' published report was striking, and only a few series of TE for IFVT were later reported by American investigators. All, however, showed very good clinical results, with success rates above 75% (Table 141–2).

One other report that also had a negative impact on TE for IFVT was Karp and Wylie's brief report of 10 patients, among whom eight had reocclusion of the femoral vein before discharge.[23] Unfortunately, few realized that these were all patients in whom TE was performed for extensive IFVT with phlegmasia cerulea dolens, in which rethrombosis using the techniques of the day was quite high. However, TE continued to be performed, and improved technically, in centers in Europe and elsewhere in the world, where the impact of the American literature was small. It is this modern experience with TE upon which current recommendations are made. The results will be presented later, after a discussion of management and technique.

Diagnosis and Preoperative Management

The clinical picture of acute IFVT is typical, with sudden swelling and pain of the whole leg, which usually is pale in color (phlegmasia alba dolens), seldom bluish (phlegmasia cerulea dolens), and rarely progressing into venous gangrene. Duplex scanning confirms the presence of the thrombus in the leg with high accuracy, but a femoral venogram from the opposite side is required to determine the upper limit of the thrombus, for if the inferior vena

TABLE 141–1. ILIOFEMORAL VENOUS THROMBECTOMY IN THE UNITED STATES BEFORE LANSING AND DAVIS (1968)

STUDY (YEAR)	NO. OF PATIENTS	PERIOPERATIVE MORTALITY No. (%)	NO. OF FPEs	POSTOPERATIVE VENOGRAPHY (%)	CLINICAL SUCCESS (%)
Mahorner et al[13] (1957)	14	1 (7)	0	39	85
DeWeese et al[15] (1960)	11	3 (27)	1	—	75
Haller and Abrams[16] (1963)	34*	3 (9)	0	58	84
	11†	3 (27)	2	50	13
DeWeese[17] (1964)	29	4 (14)	1	64	80
Bradham and Buxton[18] (1964)	16	3 (19)	1	62	100
Kaiser et al[19] (1965)	48	9 (19)	0	—	82
Hafner et al[20] (1965)	49‡	1 (2)	1	—	86
Smith[21] (1965)	18	1 (6)	1	24	82
Fogarty et al[22] (1966)	31	0 (0)	0	55	89
Karp and Wylie[23] (1966)	10	— —	—	80	—
Britt[24] (1966)	16	0 (0)	0	—	42
Wilson and Britt[25] (1967)	36	1 (3)	1	31	39
TOTAL	323	29 (9)	8	—	71

From Eklof B, Kistner RL: Is there a role for thrombectomy in iliofemoral venous thrombosis? Semin Vasc Surg 9:34–45, 1996.
*Symptoms for less than 10 days.
†Symptoms 14–21 days.
‡With venous interruption in 41 cases.
FPE = fatal pulmonary embolism.

TABLE 141–2. ILIOFEMORAL VENOUS THROMBECTOMY IN THE UNITED STATES AFTER LANSING AND DAVIS (1968)

STUDY (YEAR)	NO. OF PATIENTS	PERIOPERATIVE MORTALITY No. (%)		FPE	POSTOP VENOGRAPHY (%)	CLINICAL SUCCESS (%)
Harris and Brown[26] (1968)	17	0	0	0	100	88
Mahorner[27] (1969)	93	6	6	1	+	83
Barner et al[28] (1969)	70	12	17	1	29	76
Edwards et al[29] (1970)	58	1	2	0	+	80
Stephens[30] (1976)	16	0	0	0	—	75
Kistner and Sparkuhl[31] (1979)	77	0	0	0	74	86

From Eklof B, Kistner RL: Is there a role for thrombectomy in iliofemoral venous thrombosis? Semin Vasc Surg 9:34–45, 1996.
FPE = fatal pulmonary embolism.

cava (IVC) is affected, surgery is more complex. Ventilation-perfusion radionuclide lung scan is routinely performed before surgery as baseline information. When the diagnosis is established, heparin infusion is started. Two units of blood are ordered for routine femoral TE, 6 units if a caval approach is contemplated. The cell-saver autotransfusion device is used during the latter procedure. Prophylactic antibiotics are given to reduce the incidence of wound infection in the groin.

Surgical Technique

Surgery is performed with the patient under general intubation anesthesia with positive end-expiratory pressure (PEEP) of 10 cm of water, added during manipulation of the thrombus to prevent intraoperative PE. The involved leg and the abdomen are prepared. A longitudinal incision is made in the groin to expose the long saphenous vein, which is followed to its confluence with the common femoral vein (CFV), which is dissected up to the inguinal ligament. The superficial femoral artery 3 to 4 cm below the femoral bifurcation is prepared for construction of the arteriovenous fistula (AVF). Further dissection depends upon the etiology of the IFVT.

A longitudinal venotomy is made in the CFV, and a venous Fogarty TE catheter is passed through the thrombus into the IVC. The balloon is inflated, and repeated passes with the Fogarty catheter are made until no more thrombotic material is extracted. With the balloon inflated in the common iliac vein, a suction catheter is introduced to the level of the internal iliac vein to evacuate thrombi from this vein. Back-flow is not a reliable sign of clearance, since a proximal valve in the external iliac vein may be present in 25% of cases, preventing retrograde flow in a cleared vein. In contrast, back-flow can be excellent from the internal iliac vein and its tributaries despite a remaining occlusion of the common iliac vein. Therefore, an intraoperative completion venogram is mandatory. An alternative is the use of an angioscope, which enables removal of residual thrombus material under direct vision.

The distal thrombus in the leg is normally removed by manual massage of the elevated leg, starting at the foot. The Fogarty catheter can sometimes be advanced gently in retrograde fashion, but this usually is needed only in extensive or late thrombus. If iliac patency is established but the

thrombus in the femoral vein is too old to remove, then we prefer ligation of the superficial femoral vein.

In a 13-year follow-up after superficial femoral vein (SFV) ligation, Masuda and associates found excellent clinical and physiologic results without post-thrombotic syndrome.[32] If normal flow in the SFV cannot be reestablished, we recommend extending the incision distally enough to evacuate thrombus fully from the deep femoral branches, using a smaller Fogarty catheter. The SFV is then ligated. The venotomy is closed with continuous suture, and an AVF is created using the adjacent saphenous vein, anastomosing it end-to-side to the superficial femoral artery. An intraoperative venogram is performed through a catheter inserted in a branch of the AVF. After a satisfactory completion venogram, the wound is closed. If iliac vein compression is demonstrated, which can occur in about 50% of cases of left-sided IFVT, we recommend intraoperative angioplasty and stenting (see Chapter 151).

If phlegmasia cerulea dolens or venous gangrene is present, we start the operation with fasciotomy of the calf compartments to release the pressure and immediately improve the circulation. If there is extension of the thrombus into the IVC, it is approached transperitoneally through a right subcostal incision. The IVC is exposed by reflecting the ascending colon and duodenum medially. Depending on the venographic findings relative to the top of the thrombus, the IVC is controlled, usually just below the renal veins. The IVC is opened and the thrombus is removed by massage, especially of the iliac venous system. If the iliofemoral segment is also involved, the operation is continued in the groin as just described. When laparotomy is contraindicated in poor-risk patients, a caval filter of the Greenfield type can be introduced before the TE is carried out from below, to protect against fatal PE.

Heparin is continued at least 5 days postoperatively, and warfarin is started on the first postoperative day and continued for 6 months. The patient starts walking the day after the operation, wearing a compression stocking. The patient is usually readmitted after 6 weeks for closure of the fistula. One of the authors (R.B.R.) does not employ a fistula in early operations on young patients with phlegmasia alba dolens, but its *overall* benefit has been well demonstrated.

Loeprecht and colleagues, in an experimental study, showed 80% rethrombosis without AVF compared with none in dogs with AVF.[33] Vollmar and Hutschenreiter confirmed the advantage of the temporary AVF, showing 82% patency of the iliac vein in 93 patients with AVF versus 54% in 26 patients without an AVF.[34] The technical difficulties associated with fistula closure have been obviated by percutaneous techniques.[35] The approach is made through the contralateral groin, and, before the fistula is closed by coil or balloon, an angiogram is performed to demonstrate iliac patency without residual outflow stenosis, which, if encountered, is stented at that time.

Results of Surgical Treatment

Mortality

One of the reasons that surgeons abandoned TE in the 1960s was the high mortality (9%; see Table 141–1). Surgery still bears a risk but, with modern perioperative care, the results are much better. In a series of over 200 patients of one of the authors (B.E.), only two died: one in acute respiratory failure due to chronic pulmonary fibrosis (with no fresh PE seen at autopsy); the other had cirrhosis of the liver and died in multiorgan failure on the 32nd postoperative day following intra-abdominal hemorrhage and severe shock due to postoperative overanticoagulation.

Pulmonary Embolism

In the same author's experience (B.E.), there have been no cases of fatal perioperative PE. To avoid this problem, it is important to have a preoperative venogram to exclude extension of the thrombus into the IVC (which modifies the technique), and to apply PEEP during proximal thrombectomy in other cases. In a prospective randomized study in Sweden, positive perfusion scans were found on admission in 45% of all patients, with additional defects seen after 1 and 4 weeks in 11% and 12% of the conservatively treated group, respectively, and in the thrombectomized group in 20% and 0%, respectively.[36] Mavor and colleagues demonstrated that incomplete clearance of the thrombus in the iliac vein increased the incidence of rethrombosis and PE.[37] In the Swedish series no additional perfusion defects developed after the first postoperative week following TE with AVF. Since the AVF effectively prevented rethrombosis, it can be assumed that the fistula was one reason for the low incidence of postoperative PE.

Rethrombosis

In the prospective randomized study from Sweden using an AVF, early rethrombosis of the iliac vein occurred in 13%.[38] This low rate of early rethrombosis using a temporary AVF is corroborated by a collected series of 555 patients (Table 141–3) showing 12% rethrombosis. Important factors in avoiding this complication are:

1. Avoid operation if the symptoms of iliac obstruction were present more than 7 days.
2. Use of the Fogarty catheter to clear the external and common iliac vein, confirmed by intraoperative venography or venoscopy, and special attention to establish flow from the internal iliac vein.
3. Direct caval approach when the IVC is involved.
4. Use of a temporary AVF.

TABLE 141–3. THROMBECTOMY WITH TEMPORARY ARTERIOVENOUS FISTULA: EARLY ILIAC VEIN PATENCY

STUDY (YEAR)	NO. OF PATIENTS	PATENT ILIAC VEIN (%)
Delin et al[39] (1982)	13	85
Plate et al[38] (1984)	31	87
Piquet et al[40] (1985)	92	80
Einarsson et al[41] (1986)	51	88
Juhan et al[42] (1987)	42	93
Vollmar and Hutschenreiter[34] (1989)	93	82
Kniemeyer et al[43] (1990)	185	96
Negien et al[44] (1991)	48	89
TOTAL	555	88

From Eklof B, Kistner RL: Is there a role for thrombectomy in iliofemoral venous thrombosis? Semin Vasc Surg 9:34–45, 1996.

5. Early ambulation wearing compression stockings.
6. Carefully monitored postoperative anticoagulation.

Other Complications

Postoperative bleeding with hematoma formation in the groin is not uncommon, despite drainage of the wound, as full anticoagulation with heparin is continued for 5 days after operation. To avoid compression of the vein with risk of thrombosis and infection, major hematomas should be evacuated. Venous gangrene is very rare and in most cases is associated with underlying malignancy. With liberal indications for fasciotomy in phlegmasia cerulea dolens, it can be prevented. Groin infection is common unless prophylactic antibiotics are used. Lymph leak may occur, but it usually stops after 2 to 3 weeks.

Late Outcome

There are few reports on long-term results after TE with AVF. In eight clinical series totaling 521 patients *with more than 2 years' follow-up* "clinical success" is achieved in 62% (Table 141–4). There are five series totaling 247 patients in which iliac vein patency was assessed *after more than 2 years' follow-up,* showing 82% patency (range, 77% to 88%) (Table 141–5). There are five studies reporting on distal (femoropopliteal) valvular competence *after more than 2 years' follow-up,* totaling 259 patients and showing 60% competence (range, 36% to 84%) (Table 141–6).

The best longitudinal data come from the prospective, randomized study from Sweden.[36, 48, 56] After 6 months, there was a highly significant difference in the number of asymptomatic patients, with 42% in the surgical group versus 7% in the conservatively treated group. At 5 years, 37% of the operated patients were asymptomatic, compared with 18% in the conservative group. At 10 years, 54% in the surgical group were basically asymptomatic (class 0-2 CEAP classification) compared with 23% in the conservative group (not statistically significant, n.s.s.). Iliac vein patency at 6 months was 76% in the surgical group compared with 35% in the conservative group, demonstrated by venography. This significant difference was maintained after 5 and 10 years with 77% and 77% patency in the surgical group versus 30% and 47% in the conservative

TABLE 141–4. THROMBECTOMY WITH TEMPORARY ARTERIOVENOUS FISTULA: CLINICAL RESULTS

STUDY (YEAR)	NO. OF PATIENTS	FOLLOW-UP (mo)	CLINICAL SUCCESS (%)
Poilleux et al[45] (1975)	27	—	78
Plate et al[38] (1984)	31	6	42
Piquet et al[40] (1985)	82	51	51
Einarsson et al[41] (1986)	55	10	75
Juhan et al[42] (1987)	36	12–48	93
Gänger et al[46] (1989)	17	91	88
Winter et al[47] (1989)	100	12	64
Kniemeyer et al[43] (1990)	147	43	51
Plate et al[48] (1990)	19	60	37
Rasmussen et al[49] (1990)	25	20	68
Loeprecht et al[50] (1991)	112	36	59
Neglén et al[44] (1991)	37	24	83
Törngren et al[51] (1991)	63	66	43
Juhan et al[52] (1997)*	44	60	82
Juhan et al[52] (1997)*	16	120	81

From Eklof B, Kistner RL: Is there a role for thrombectomy in iliofemoral venous thrombosis? Semin Vasc Surg 9:34–45, 1996.
*Data updated by author.

group, respectively. Femoropopliteal valvular competence at 6 months was 52% in the surgical group compared with 26% in the conservatively treated group, using descending venography with Valsalva, a significant difference. After 5 years, the patients who underwent TE had significantly lower ambulatory venous pressures, improved venous emptying as shown by plethysmography, and a better calf pump function with less reflux, as measured by foot volumetry.

Combining the results of all functional tests, 36% of the surgical patients had normal venous function compared with 11% of the conservatively treated group (n.s.s.). At 10 years, by means of duplex scanning, popliteal reflux

TABLE 141–5. THROMBECTOMY WITH TEMPORARY ARTERIOVENOUS FISTULA: "LONG-TERM" ILIAC VEIN PATENCY

STUDY (YEAR)	NO. OF PATIENTS	FOLLOW-UP (mo)	PATENT ILIAC VEIN (%)
Plate et al[38] (1984)	31	6	76
Piquet et al[40] (1985)	57	39	80
Einarsson et al[41] (1986)	58	10	61
Vollmar[53] (1986)	93	53	82
Juhan et al[42] (1987)	36	12–48	93
Törngren et al[54] (1988)	54	19	54
Plate et al[48] (1990)	19	60	77
Rasmussen et al[49] (1990)	24	20	75
Neglén et al[44] (1991)	34	24	88
Juhan et al[52] (1997)*	44	60	84
Juhan et al[52] (1997)*	16	120	80

From Eklof B, Kistner RL: Is there a role for thrombectomy in iliofemoral venous thrombosis? Semin Vasc Surg 9:34–45, 1996.
*Data updated by author.

TABLE 141–6. THROMBECTOMY WITH TEMPORARY ARTERIOVENOUS FISTULA: "LONG-TERM" COMPETENCE OF THE FEMOROPOPLITEAL VEIN

STUDY (YEAR)	NO. OF PATIENTS	FOLLOW-UP (mo)	COMPETENCE (%)
Plate et al[38] (1984)	31	6	52
Einarsson et al[41] (1986)	53	10	42
Gänger et al[46] (1989)	17	91	82
Kniemeyer et al[43] (1990)	147	43	44
Plate et al[48] (1990)	14	60	36
Neglén et al[44] (1991)	37	24	56
Kniemeyer et al[55] (1992)	37	55	84
Juhan et al[52] (1997)*	44	60	84
Juhan et al[52] (1997)*	16	120	56

Used with permission from Eklof B, Kistner RL: Is there a role for thrombectomy in iliofemoral venous thrombosis? Semin Vasc Surg 9:34–45, 1996.
*Data updated by author.

was found in 32% in the surgical group compared with 67% in the conservative group. Six patients who had a successful TE without obstruction of the iliac vein at the time of surgery were still available for follow-up at 10 years. All were asymptomatic, with patent iliac veins, and 50% had competent popliteal veins.[56] From these data, it seems clear that successful TE confers long-term benefit.

THROMBOLYSIS

Historical Background

As with TE, after a wave of initial enthusiasm and some proof of efficacy, thrombolysis was discredited by a single well-publicized report of its failure to prevent venous valvular insufficiency. Kakkar and associates reported no significant difference in the presence or absence of reflux, as judged by foot volumetry, between those treated with systemic streptokinase and those managed with heparin and warfarin alone.[57] This one negative report by an authority in the field of anticoagulation seems to have carried the day, in spite of contemporary analyses by Arneson and colleagues[58] and Elliott and colleagues[59] of careful clinical follow-up of DVT treated by systemic streptokinase, in which there was clearly less leg edema and, in the latter report, less ulceration.

It was shown ultimately, as summarized in Comerota's review of 13 comparative clinical trials, that systemic lytic therapy achieves far superior results than anticoagulant therapy alone.[60] Systemic thrombolysis achieved, on average, only about 50% patency. Protection of the distal valves by successful lysis is an important issue. Jeffery and co-workers, in a 5-year follow-up of those subjected to systemic streptokinase, showed that those who achieved complete lysis had only a 9% incidence of popliteal reflux, whereas those with incomplete lysis had a 77% incidence of popliteal reflux.[61] Thus, when thrombolysis was successful it appeared to confer long-term functional and clinical benefit. Nevertheless, with only a 50% patency rate to offset the risks of systemic lytic therapy, it is not surprising that clinicians did not embrace this therapy. Safer and more complete lysis was needed.

It was inevitable that the catheter-directed techniques that were developed to deal with native artery and graft thromboses would be applied to proximal venous thrombosis. After sporadic reports with small numbers of cases, a sizeable series—27 treated limbs in 21 patients—was reported by Semba and Dake in 1994.[62] They achieved 72% complete and 20% significant partial lysis in the 93% of cases in which successful access was achieved, usually via the internal jugular vein. Thus complete lysis was achieved in two thirds of all patients, a remarkable achievement considering that 26% were "chronic" (between 2 weeks and 1 year). In the latter cases, and 50% of the total, residual iliac vein narrowing was found and stented. Seventeen of 21 patients were followed for a mean of 13.5 months, with an 88% primary and 94% secondary patency rate. There was a 12% rethrombosis rate within 1 year.

This experience stimulated the development of a multicenter venous registry to see whether these results could be duplicated nationwide. The trial recently closed after enrollment of almost 500 patients. The results have not yet been published but have been presented at several meetings, the last in 1997.[63] The major findings are summarized here.

Complete data with follow-up of at least 6 months were collected on nearly 300 patients, 70% of whom had IFVT. Access was obtained most commonly through the popliteal vein, followed by contralateral femoral and internal jugular veins, with less than 10% having pedal infusions. Lysis was monitored venographically every 12 hours, continuing until complete lysis was achieved or no further lysis was seen for 12 hours. Treatment duration averaged more than 48 hours, with close to 7 million units of urokinase administered in those with direct intraclot delivery. One third of the patients received adjunctive stenting for residual narrowing, but this was close to 40% in the IFVT group and close to half of those with left-sided involvement. Lysis was graded as I, less than 50%; II, more than 50%; and III, 100%. Grades II and III lysis showed similar outcomes and were achieved in over 80% of cases. Together, they are termed "significant" lysis in the following discussion. Complete lysis was achieved in close to one third of patients.

Because there were no strict exclusions in this trial, the location of the thrombus, site of access, duration of symptoms before therapy, and history of previous DVT varied independently, and analysis of *pure* subgroups suffers from reduced numbers of patients. Nevertheless, the data indicate a favorable outcome for the type of patients discussed in this chapter. The preliminary data indicate better results for IFVT versus femoropopliteal thrombosis, for acute (less than 10 days) versus subacute or chronic thrombosis, and for first episode versus repeated DVT. Results were inferior with pedal infusion.

The use of popliteal vein access using ultrasound guidance became increasingly favored during the course of the study. If one focuses on the results of direct infusions for acute, first episode IFVT, which is the focus of this chapter, *complete* lysis was seen almost twice as often (about 60%), with continued patency in close to 90% of these at 6 months. Seventy per cent of those with *significant* lysis were still patent beyond 6 months. Reflux at 6 months' follow-up, including the involved segments, was less than 30% in those with complete lysis, about 45% in those with greater than 50% lysis, but over 60% in those with less than 50% initial lysis, again showing the greater protective effect of complete thrombus removal. There were only two deaths in the entire study (0.4%), one from intracranial hemorrhage and one in one of the six patients who suffered a PE (1.2%). Longer follow-up, including of those who still had incomplete data at 6 months, should provide more definitive recommendations based on careful subgroup analysis and functional evaluation.

Current Technique

The ipsilateral popliteal venous approach is preferred by the author (M.M.) because it is often difficult to penetrate an occluded SFV from either superior approach (i.e., the internal jugular vein or the contralateral common femoral vein), due to venous valves that may prevent safe catheter and guide wire manipulations. The popliteal vein should be accessed under ultrasound guidance with a small-gauge echogenic needle to avoid inadvertent puncture of the popliteal artery. A 5 French (Fr.) short sheath is then introduced, through which all subsequent catheters can be introduced and exchanged.

Following baseline venography obtained via a catheter introduced through the popliteal sheath, the occluded venous segment is crossed with a straight-tip 5 Fr. catheter and a 0.035-inch curved-tip glide wire. Venography is then repeated to confirm transluminal passage of the catheter, which is then exchanged for a 5 Fr. coaxial infusion system, consisting of a proximal multi-sidehole catheter and a distal infusion wire. It is crucial to position the infusion system directly into the thrombus, to maximize plasminogen activation throughout the site of obstruction.

Urokinase therapy is initiated at 150,000 to 200,000 U per hr, evenly split between the infusing ports. In practice, a total dose of 200,000 U per hr of urokinase is rarely exceeded regardless of the thrombus burden. Intravenous heparin is concomitantly administered via the popliteal sheath at a rate of 500 to 1000 U per hr following a 5000-U bolus of heparin. Patients are monitored in the ICU or in a "step-down" unit, similar to those receiving thrombolytic treatment for acute PE or an arterial occlusion.

Because the duration of therapy may be in excess of 48 hours, it is not practical (or necessary) to assess the progress of lysis very frequently. Follow-up venograms every 12 hours are sufficient, and are used primarily to reposition the infusion devices in or close to the remaining thrombis. Gentle thrombus maceration with a 6-mm balloon angioplasty catheter may be helpful, particularly in the superficial femoral vein, where focal narrowings, probably representing sites of organized thrombus, are at times encountered. Ordinarily, unless a complication dictates otherwise, lytic therapy is continued until complete lysis is achieved or until no discernible progress is demonstrated during the previous 12 hours compared with the prior venogram. Since the degree of thrombolysis has been shown in the Venous Registry to be a strong predictor of continued patency, it is important that complete lysis be achieved if possible. Residual narrowing in the iliac vein after lysis is treated with stenting. Although the long-term benefits of this admittedly have not yet been demonstrated, leaving the narrowing untreated appears to be associated with a significant risk of early rethrombosis.

Suggested Management

Preliminary data from the Venous Registry, following on the experience of Semba and Dake,[62] suggest that, in selected cases, catheter-directed thrombolysis produces results comparable with modern thrombectomy, but with less associated morbidity. Thus it would seem, from the literature presented, that *early* thrombus removal regardless of the technique employed, can reduce late post-thrombotic sequelae significantly. The remaining questions, then, are (1) which patients with IFVT deserve intervention, and (2) which intervention should be chosen?

Indications for Intervention

Obviously, major interventions such as thrombectomy or catheter-directed thrombolysis *cannot* ordinarily be justified in chronically ill, bedridden, high-risk, or aged patients, or those with serious intercurrent disease and limited longevity. In such patients, early thrombus removal can be justified only for limb threat, that is, *cases of phlegmasia cerulea dolens with signs of impending venous gangrene or compartment syndrome,* although early removal of the thrombus will likely reduce acute morbidity in other cases with such extensive thrombosis. However, in active, *healthy* patients with acute iliofemoral venous thrombosis with phlegmasia alba dolens, the results of catheter-directed thrombolysis or thrombectomy would appear to justify those interventions on the grounds of significantly reducing, if not completely avoiding, post-thrombotic sequelae. These are the patients whose remaining life is most likely to be significantly affected by post-thrombotic sequelae and these are also the patients who can more readily tolerate these interventions.

Choice of Method of Thrombus Removal

In applying these two methods of thrombus removal to carefully selected IFVT patients, at either extreme of the disease spectrum for either acute morbidity with limb salvage or avoidance of significant late post-thrombotic sequelae, the question of which technique to choose still remains, because TE and catheter-directed thrombolysis vie for essentially the same patients and produce similar success rates. A treatment algorithm is suggested for this (Fig. 141–1) with the following explanation.

Assuming that one has appropriate grounds for intervention based on the preceding discussion, the next question to ask is whether or not there are contraindications to lytic therapy. IFVT not uncommonly occurs after trauma, after surgery, or around the time of delivery. These and other standard contraindications, e.g., brain tumor and recent GI bleeding, as outlined in Chapter 28, must first be considered.

There are other preliminary considerations. If the patient is a *prohibitive* operative risk, thrombolysis should be chosen, although the risk of TE is higher from uncompensated blood loss than from the anesthetic. Conversely, if there is an urgent need for thrombus removal, as in cases with massive IFVT and phlegmasia cerulea dolens progressing toward venous gangrene or compartment compression syndrome, TE would be chosen, since catheter-directed thrombolysis often takes 48 hours to complete. Also, because of the time and expense of thrombolytic therapy, one might prefer to treat very early cases of phlegmasia alba dolens in healthy young patients by TE without an AVF. But, with these few exceptions, catheter-directed thrombolysis is the initial choice, as the gentler and less morbid means of thrombus removal, and one that can be successfully applied after longer delays than can TE (e.g., optimal limits of 10 days versus 5 days, respectively). If access cannot be obtained or if lysis does not proceed satisfactorily or lead to adequate clearance, usually it is appropriate to cross over

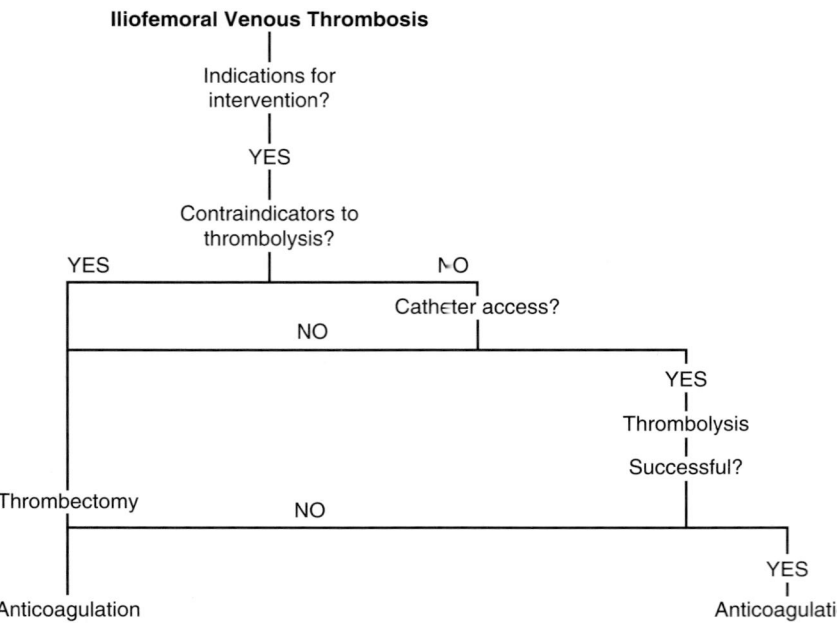

Iliofemoral Venous Thrombosis

Indications for intervention?

YES

Contraindicators to thrombolysis?

YES   NO

Catheter access?

NO

YES

Thrombolysis

Successful?

Thrombectomy   NO

YES

Anticoagulation   Anticoagulation

FIGURE 141–1. An algorithm summarizing the application of either thrombectomy or catheter-directed thrombolysis to selected patients with iliofemoral venous thrombosis, as discussed in the text.

to TE, since a valid indication to intervene has already been determined. Obviously then, both methods of thrombus removal should be applied for individual considerations rather than pursuing a blind preference for one or the other.

Finally, even though this may seem to some to represent an aggressive approach to IFVT, it is recommended *only* in carefully selected patients. Anticoagulant therapy will still be used in the majority of patients because of such other overriding considerations as advanced age, serious intercurrent disease, sedentary lifestyle, limited extent of thrombosis (in those with phlegmasia alba dolens), and lack of threat of venous gangrene or compartment compression (in those with phlegmasia cerulea dolens), or, unfortunately, when there are excessive delays in presentation or referral. This still leaves a significant number of patients who can benefit from intervention, or conversely who would unnecessarily suffer serious sequelae if treated by the prevailing conservative therapy with anticoagulant therapy. It is particularly important to establish these selective indications for these interventions now because, if the new approach of treating DVT on an ambulatory basis using low-molecular-weight heparin is widely adopted, the patients who might benefit may not be considered for admission or evaluated for these interventions.

REFERENCES

1. Lindner DJ, Edwards JM, Phinney ES, et al: Long-term hemodynamic and clinical sequelae of lower extremity deep vein thrombosis. J Vasc Surg 4:436, 1986.
2. Arenander E: Varicosity and ulceration of the lower limb: A clinical follow-up study of 247 patients examined phlebographically. Acta Chir Scand 12:135, 1957.
3. Thomas ML, McAllister V: The radiological progression of deep venous thrombosis. Radiology 99:37, 1971.
4. Mavor GE, Galloway JMD: Iliofemoral venous thrombosis: Pathological considerations and surgical management. Br J Surg 56:45, 1969.
5. Schull KC, Nicolaides AN, Fernandes é Fernandes J, et al: Significance of popliteal reflux in relation to ambulatory venous pressure. Arch Surg 114:1304, 1979.
6. Nicolaides AN, Hussein MK, Szendro G, et al: The relation of venous ulceration with ambulatory venous pressure measurements. J Vasc Surg 17:414, 1993.
7. Nicolaides AN, Sumner DS (eds): Investigation of Patients with Deep Vein Thrombosis and Chronic Venous Insufficiency. Los Angeles, Med-Orion Publishing Co, 1991.
8. Markel A, Manzo R, Bergelin R, Strandness DE: Valvular reflux after deep vein thrombosis: Incidence and time of occurrence. J Vasc Surg 15:377, 1992.
9. Johnson BF, Manzo RA, Bergelin RO, Strandness DE Jr.: Relationship between changes in the deep venous system and the development of the post-thrombotic syndrome after an acute episode of lower limb deep venous thrombosis: A one- to six-year follow-up. J Vasc Surg 21:307, 1995.
10. Caps MT, Meissner MH, Bengelin RO, Strandness DE Jr: Venous valvular reflux in veins not involved at the time of acute deep venous thrombosis. Presented at the American Venous Forum, Fort Lauderdale, Fla, February 23, 1995.
11. Strandness DE Jr: Descending venous incompetence in uninvolved segments after acute DVT (Abstract). Personal communication.
12. Mahorner H: New management for thrombosis of deep veins of extremities. Am Surg 20:487–498, 1954.
13. Mahorner H, Castleberry JW, Coleman WO: Attempts to restore function in major veins which are the site of massive thrombosis. Ann Surg 146:510–522, 1957.
14. Lansing AM, Davis WM: Five-year follow-up study of iliofemoral venous thrombectomy. Ann Surg 168:620–628, 1968.
15. DeWeese JA, Jones TI, Lyon J, Dale WA: Evaluation of thrombectomy

16. Haller JAJ, Abrams BL: Use of thrombectomy in the treatment of acute iliofemoral venous thrombosis in forty-five patients. Ann Surg 158:561–569, 1963.
17. DeWeese JA: Thrombectomy for acute iliofemoral venous thrombosis. J Cardiovasc Surg 5:703–712, 1964.
18. Bradham RR, Buxton JT: Thrombectomy for acute iliofemoral venous thrombosis. Surg Gynecol Obstet 119:1271–1275, 1964.
19. Kaiser GC, Murray RC, Willman VL, Hanlon CR: Iliofemoral thrombectomy for venous occlusion. Arch Surg 90:574–577, 1965.
20. Hafner CD, Cranley JJ, Krause RJ, Strasser ES: Venous thrombectomy: Current status. Ann Surg 161:411, 1965.
21. Smith GW: Therapy of iliofemoral venous thrombosis. Surg Gynecol Obstet 121:1298–1302, 1965.
22. Fogarty TJ, Dennis D, Krippaehne WW: Surgical management of iliofemoral venous thrombosis. Am J Surg 112:211–217, 1966.
23. Karp RB, Wylie EJ: Recurrent thrombosis after iliofemoral venous thrombectomy. Surg Forum 17:147–149, 1966.
24. Britt LG: Iliofemoral veno-occlusive disease: Results with thrombectomy in 16 cases. Am Surg 32:103–106, 1966.
25. Wilson H. Britt LG: Surgical treatment of iliofemoral thrombosis. Ann Surg 165:355–859, 1967.
26. Harris EJ, Brown WH: Patency of the thrombectomy for iliofemoral thrombosis. Ann Surg 167:91, 1968.
27. Mahorner H: Results of surgical operations for venous thrombosis. Surg Gynecol Obstet 129:66–70, 1969.
28. Barner HB, Willman VL, Kaiser GC, Hanlon CR: Thrombectomy for iliofemoral venous thrombosis. JAMA 28:2442, 1969.
29. Edwards WH, Sawyers JL, Foster JH: Iliofemoral venous thrombosis: Reappraisal of thrombectomy. Ann Surg 171:961–970, 1970.
30. Stephens GGL: Current opinion on iliofemoral venous thrombectomy. Am Surg 42:108–115, 1976.
31. Kistner RL, Sparkuhl MD: Surgery in acute and chronic venous disease. Surgery 85:31–43, 1979.
32. Masuda EM, Kistner RL, Ferris EB: Long-term effects of superficial femoral vein ligation: Thirteen-year follow-up. J Vasc Surg 16:741–749, 1992.
33. Loeprecht H, Vollmar J, Heyes H, et al: Beeinflussung des Spontanverlaufs der Phlebothrombose und ihrer operativen Behandlungsergebnisse durch Anderung der Hamodynamik. Vasa 5:135–141, 1976.
34. Vollmar JF, Hutschenreiter S: Surgical treatment of acute thromboembolic disease: The role of vascular endoscopy. In Veith FJ (ed): Current Critical Problems in Vascular Surgery. St. Louis, Quality Medical Publishing, 1989, pp 154–160.
35. Endrys J, Eklof B, Neglén P, et al: Percutaneous balloon occlusion of surgical arteriovenous fistulae following venous thrombectomy. Cardiovasc Intervent Radiol 12:226–229, 1989.
36. Plate G, Ohlin P, Eklof B: Pulmonary embolism in acute iliofemoral venous thrombosis. Br J Surg 72:912, 1985.
37. Mavor GE, Galloway JMD: The iliofemoral venous segment as a source of pulmonary emboli. Lancet 1(7495)871–874, 1967.
38. Plate G. Einarsson E, Ohlin P, et al: Thrombectomy with temporary arteriovenous fistula: The treatment of choice in acute iliofemoral venous thrombosis. J Vasc Surg 1(7495):871–874, 1967.
39. Delin A, Swedenborg J, Hellgren M, et al: Thrombectomy and arteriovenous fistula for iliofemoral venous thrombosis in fertile women. Surg Gynecol Obstet 154:69–73, 1982.
40. Piquet P. Tournigand P, Josso B, Mercier C: Traitement chirurgical des thromboses ilio-caves: exigences et resultats. In Kieffer E (ed): Chirurgie de la Veine Cave Inferieure et de Ses Branches. Paris, Expansion Scientifique Francaise, 1985, pp 210–216.
41. Einarsson E, Albrechtsson U, Eklof B: Thrombectomy and temporary AV-fistula in iliofemoral vein thrombosis: Technical considerations and early results. Int Angiol 5:65–72, 1986.
42. Juhan C, Cornillon B, Tobiana F, et al: Patency after iliofemoral and iliocaval venous thrombectomy. Ann Vasc Surg 1:529–533, 1987.
43. Kniemeyer HW, Merckle R, Stuhmeier K, Sandmann W: Chirurgische Therapie der akuten und embolisierenden tiefen Beinvenenthrombose—Indikation, technisches Prinzip, Ergebnisse. Klin Wochenschr 68:1208–1216, 1990.
44. Neglén P, al-Hassan HK, Endrys J, Nazzal MM, et al: Iliofemoral venous thrombectomy followed by percutaneous closure of the temporary arteriovenous fistula. Surgery 110:493–499, 1991.
45. Poilleux J, Chermet J, Bigot JM, Deliere T: Les thromboses veineuses iliofemorales recentes. Ann Chir 29:713–718, 1975.
46. Ganger KH, Nachbur BH, Ris HB, Zurbrugg H: Surgical thrombec-

tomy versus conservative treatment for deep venous thrombosis: Functional comparison of long-term results. Eur J Vasc Surg 3:529–538, 1989.

47. Winter C, Weber H, Loeprecht H: Surgical treatment of iliofemoral vein thrombosis; Technical aspects: Possible secondary interventions. Int Angiol 8:188–193, 1989.

48. Plate G, Akesson H, Einarsson E, et al: Long-term results of venous thrombectomy combined with a temporary arterio-venous fistula. Eur J Vasc Surg 4:483–489, 1990.

49. Rasmussen A, Mogensen K, Nissen FH, et al: Acute iliofemoral venous thrombosis: Twenty-six cases treated with thrombectomy, temporary arteriovenous fistula and anti-coagulants. Ugeskr Laeger 152:2928–2930, 1990.

50. Loeprecht H, Weber H, Krawielitzky B: Indikationen zur Gefasschirurgischen Behandlung der Iliofemoralvenenthrombose. In Maurer PC, Doorler J, v. Sommoggy S (eds): Gefasschirurgie im Fortschritt: Neuentwicklungen, Kontroversen, Grenzen, Perspektiven. Stuttgart, Georg Thieme Verlag., 1991, pp 180–185.

51. Törngren S, Bremme K, Hjertberg R, Swedenborg J: Late results of the thrombectomy for iliofemoral iliothrombosis. Phlebology 6:249–254, 1991.

52. Juhan CM, Alimi YS, Barthelemy TJ, et al: Late results of iliofemoral venous thrombectomy. J Vasc Surg 25:417–422, 1997.

53. Vollmar JF: Advances in reconstructive venous surgery. Int Angiol 5:117–129, 1986.

54. Törngren S, Swedenborg J: Thrombectomy and temporary arteriovenous fistula for ilio-femoral venous thrombosis. Int Angiol 7:14–18, 1988.

55. Kniemeyer HW, Sandmann W, Schwindt C, et al: Thrombectomy with AV fistula—the better alternative to prevent recurrent pulmonary embolism. Presented at the 4th Annual Meeting of the American Venous Forum, Coronado, Calif, February 26–28, 1992.

56. Plate G, Eklof B, Norgren L, et al: Venous thrombectomy for iliofemoral vein thrombosis: 10-year results of a prospective randomized study. Eur J Endo Vasc Surg 14:367–374, 1997.

57. Kakkar VV, Lawrence D: Hemodynamic and clinical assessment after therapy for acute deep vein thrombosis: A prospective study. Am J Surg 150:28, 1985.

58. Arnesen H, Hoiseth A, Ly B: Streptokinase or heparin in the treatment of deep vein thrombosis: Follow-up results of a prospective study. Acta Med Scand 211:65, 1982.

59. Elliot MS, Immelman EJ, Jeffery P, et al: A comparative randomized trial of heparin versus streptokinase in the treatment of acute proximal venous thrombosis: An interim report of a prospective trial. Br J Surg 66:838, 1979.

60. Comerota AJ: Venous thromboembolism. In Rutherford RB (ed): Vascular Surgery, 4th ed. Philadelphia, WB Saunders, 1995, p 1785.

61. Jeffery P, Immelman E, Amoore J: Treatment of deep vein thrombosis with heparin or streptokinase: Long-term venous function assessment. (Abstract No. S20.3). In Proceedings of the Second International Vascular Symposium, London, 1986.

62. Semba CP, Dake MD: Iliofemoral deep venous thrombosis: Agressive therapy with catheter-directed thrombolysis. Radiology 191:487, 1994.

63. Mewissen MW: Data presented at the Venous Registry Investigators Meeting, San Diego, September 13, 1997.

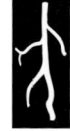

CHAPTER 142
Caval Interruption Procedures

Lazar J. Greenfield, M.D.

HISTORICAL PERSPECTIVE

John Hunter performed the first femoral vein ligation for thrombophlebitis in 1784. However, not until 1893 did Bottini report successful ligation of the inferior vena cava to prevent pulmonary embolism (PE). In the United States, venous ligation was also the earliest surgical technique used. Bilateral common femoral vein ligation was undertaken first as suggested by Homans, but an unacceptable incidence of recurrent PE and lower extremity venous stasis sequelae led to abandonment of the procedure. Ligation of the infrarenal inferior vena cava provided theoretical control of the final common path to the pulmonary circulation for most emboli and was performed commonly until the late 1960s. However, high postoperative mortality, recurrent PE, and adverse lower extremity sequelae were unacceptable outcomes.

Nasbeth and associates[34] and Amador and coworkers[2] found mortality rates after inferior vena caval ligation of 19% and 39%, respectively; rates were highest in patients

with underlying cardiac disease (41% and 19%). Among patients who had normal cardiac function and who were classified as good preoperative risks, an operative mortality rate of 4% was still observed; cited causes included recurrent PE arising at the site of caval ligation and phlegmasia cerulea dolens. In follow-up studies, Ferris and colleagues found recurrent PE in three of 20 patients within 2 months after vena caval ligation.[12] Although thrombus can form above the ligation, large ovarian and ascending lumbar venous collaterals were the probable conduits for emboli from lower extremity sources because acute thrombi were present below the ligation site in 40% to 50% of cases. Lower extremity sequelae in the series of Nasbeth and associates included leg edema (40%), development of new varicose veins (20%), stasis pigmentation (18%), leg discomfort (14%), disabling venous claudication (14%), and ulceration (6%).[34]

More recent data have also suggested an underappreciation of cardiac output limitation after vena caval ligation in patients without preexisting heart disease. Miller and Staats' exercise and gas exchange study of such patients found significant impairment of cardiac output secondary to inadequate venous return.[32]

Against this background, the first techniques to provide filtration of emboli without vena caval occlusion evolved. For more than a decade, vena caval suture, staple plication, and externally applied clip devices were used to provide a limited orifice flow through the inferior vena cava.[1, 27, 43] These techniques added the morbidity of general anesthesia and laparotomy. Although inferior vena caval clips are still being applied at the time of surgery in some instances, it is the author's opinion that there is considerably less morbidity if an intracaval filter is placed preoperatively. Despite promising early patency data, high rates of caval occlusion with external devices were noted after a relatively short follow-up.[3, 8, 10]

The development of transvenous approaches under local anesthesia was the next logical step. The earliest transvenous approaches demonstrated the ease of access to the vena cava under local anesthesia and fluoroscopy. Although various devices were developed, the Mobin-Uddin umbrella became the most popular because it could be readily positioned below the renal veins. However, it was found to have a high rate of subsequent vena caval thrombosis and was associated with additional complications of proximal thrombus formation and occasional migration into the pulmonary artery.[6] It was withdrawn from the market, and a new generation of devices was developed to facilitate placement, reliable capture of thromboemboli, and long-term caval patency.

INDICATIONS FOR VENA CAVAL FILTER PLACEMENT

Currently accepted indications for inferior vena caval filter insertion include:

1. Documented deep venous thrombosis (DVT) or PE with a recognized contraindication to anticoagulation.
2. Recurrent PE despite adequate anticoagulation.
3. Bleeding complications requiring that anticoagulation therapy for DVT or PE be discontinued.
4. After pulmonary embolectomy.
5. Failure of another form of caval interruption, demonstrated by recurrent thromboembolism (Table 142–1).

Case-selective or relative indications include:

1. The presence of iliofemoral thrombosis with a 5-cm or longer free-floating tail.
2. Septic PE.
3. Chronic PE in a patient with cor pulmonale.
4. A high-risk patient (e.g., one who has significant cardiopulmonary disease, occlusion of more than 50% of the pulmonary bed, or both) who would not tolerate any recurrent thromboembolism.

As long-term favorable experience with the Greenfield vena caval filter has accumulated, there have been suggestions to liberalize further the indications for filter insertion. Two new uses for vena caval filters have been suggested:

1. As a method of pure prophylaxis, they have been placed in patients who have sustained massive trauma and

TABLE 142–1. INDICATIONS FOR INSERTION OF A VENA CAVAL FILTER

Absolute Indications

Deep venous thrombosis or documented thromboembolism in a patient who has a contraindication to anticoagulation
Recurrent thromboembolism despite adequate anticoagulation
Complications of anticoagulation that have forced therapy to be discontinued
Immediately after pulmonary embolectomy
Failure of another form of caval interruption, demonstrated by recurrent thromboembolism

Relative Indications

A large free-floating iliofemoral thrombus demonstrated on venography in a high-risk patient
A propagating iliofemoral thrombus despite adequate anticoagulation
Chronic pulmonary embolism in a patient with pulmonary hypertension and cor pulmonale
A patient who has occlusion of more than 50 per cent of the pulmonary vascular bed and would not tolerate any additional thrombus
Presence of recurrent septic embolism

remain at high risk of thromboembolism but do not actually have the disease.[26, 37, 40]

2. Some physicians such as Cohen and colleagues,[7] Lossef and Barth,[28] and Rosen and colleagues[41] advocate the use of filters in patients with malignancy who are at risk or who have thromboembolism.

Each of these indications remains unproved in randomized studies, but in smaller series they have proven efficacy. Recommendations have included routine use of the filter for DVT instead of anticoagulation, in high-risk general surgical patients, in older patients, or in pregnant women with DVT or PE[7, 13] instead of anticoagulation. Additional studies are required to determine whether the risk of anticoagulation outweighs the risk of filter placement alone. At present, the author continues to recommend the use of appropriate anticoagulation to control the underlying thrombotic disorder in patients who are eligible for anticoagulant therapy.

STAINLESS STEEL GREENFIELD FILTER

The current benchmark for performance of transvenous vena caval filters is the stainless steel Greenfield filter, for which 20 years of long-term follow-up is available.[19] The Greenfield filter was developed to maintain caval patency after trapping emboli and to preserve prograde caval flow, avoiding stasis and facilitating lysis of the trapped emboli (Fig. 142–1). The cone-shaped filter is 4.6 cm long from apex to base. The base is formed by the filter's six legs, which provide for caval fixation by means of small, recurved hooks at their distal ends. The spacing between the legs is 2 mm at the apex of the cone and a maximum of 5 to 6 mm at the base when the device is expanded, depending on inferior vena cava size. The spacing between limbs is such that the filter effectively traps most emboli 3 mm or greater in diameter.[44]

The conical geometry allows progressive central filling while maintaining circumferential blood flow, thus avoiding

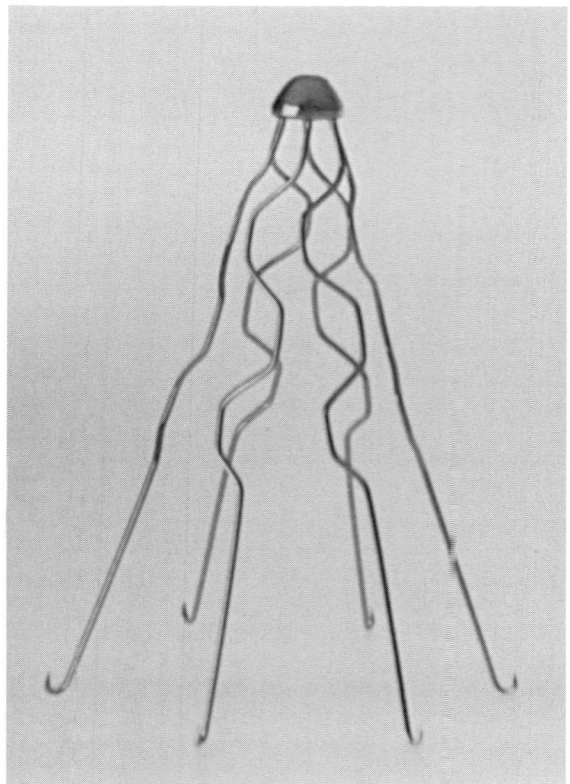

FIGURE 142–1. Original stainless steel Greenfield filter introduced in 1972 for mechanical protection against pulmonary thromboembolism.

progressive venous thrombosis, caval obstruction, and venous hypertension. When thrombus fills the filter to 70% of its depth, only 49% of the cross-sectional area is blocked. Experience has shown that no distal venous pressure increase occurs until 80% of the filter is filled with clot, at which point more than 64% of the cross-sectional area is blocked (Fig. 142–2). These design features result in superior patency rates and a minimal incidence of stasis sequelae. In addition, an unexpected result of flow preservation was the evidence of progressive lysis of the trapped thrombus over time.

The stainless steel Greenfield filter had a 4% rate of recurrent embolism over a 12-year period of observation in 469 patients, and a long-term filter patency rate of 98%.[20] Similar results have been obtained in other follow-up series, with long-term patency rates in excess of 95%.[6, 14] Our 20-year experience demonstrated the same low rate of recurrent PE and high rate of caval patency as seen in the earlier reports.[21] This reinforces the durability of findings with this device. This high level of patency has allowed placement of the Greenfield filter above the level of the renal veins when needed because of thrombus at that level or in pregnant women to avoid contact between the gravid uterus and the filter. The results with suprarenal filter placement are quite comparable, with a 100% patency rate in the 22 patients studied long term of the series of 69 filters placed at this level since 1976.[17]

The patency rate of the Greenfield filter is not dependent on prolonged anticoagulation, and the termination of anticoagulant therapy is dictated by the patient's underlying

thrombotic disorder. The few associated complications include misplacement due to premature discharge or inaccurate fluoroscopic control of the carrier, rare limb penetration of the cava, and filter limb fracture. Although it is possible to retrieve a misplaced device, misplacements into the renal, hepatic, or iliac veins have not caused functional problems. The only functional consequence of venous misplacement may be inadequate filtration of vena caval flow.

Because of its reliable preservation of caval patency, the filter has adapted well to a variety of unusual clinical problems, such as the rare need for superior vena caval placement. The filter has also been a useful adjunct in the successful management of septic thrombophlebitis. This is possible because preserved prograde venous flow through the filter permits in vivo sterilization of any infected thrombus within it by parenteral antibiotic treatment.[35]

Technical Considerations for Filter Insertion

The procedure should be performed under optimal fluoroscopy. This can be achieved in the operating room with a C-arm fluoroscope in most circumstances, or in the radiology suite, where better imaging can be obtained, e.g., for the obese patient. A preoperative venacavogram should be obtained and be available for review at the time of insertion. In some cases, it may be desirable to place the filter using intravascular ultrasound in order to image the vena cava, determine its true diameter, and locate the renal and other tributary veins. Examples of patient situations that might make this useful include severely unstable patients who cannot be moved from the intensive care unit, pregnant patients who are at risk from radiation, and those with a contraindication to contrast medium.

The Greenfield filters are designed for either surgical or percutaneous placement. Although the majority of filters

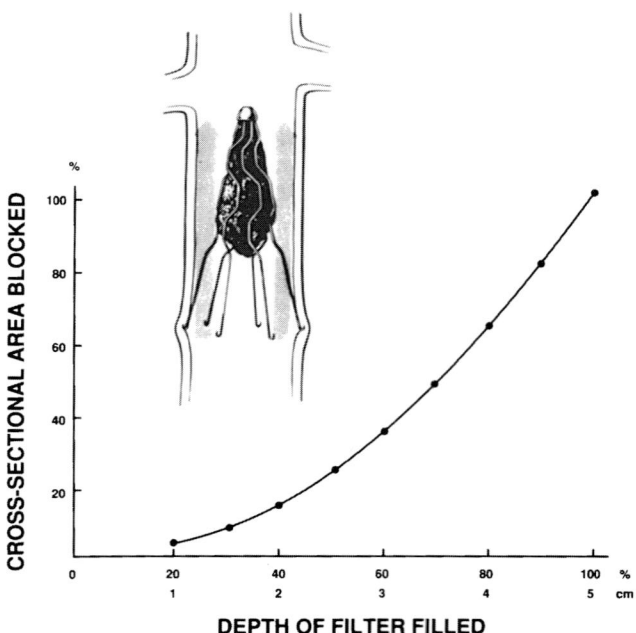

FIGURE 142–2. Relationship between the volume of thrombus trapped within the filter and the percentage of cross section occluded.

sold now are the percutaneous type, a number of the 24 Fr. design continue to be placed. Regardless of the method of delivery, it is important to assure the security of the device prior to delivery. This is achieved by the over-the-wire technique with the 24 Fr. design and the protective sheath used with titanium. The newest percutaneous filter also uses a sheath and an over-the-wire system to prevent misplacement. In the majority of cases, the ideal site is the L2 or L3 level; however, the suprarenal inferior vena cava and superior vena cava may be indicated in some situations.

The radiographic diameter of the vena cava should be measured, with correction for magnification, which can be as much as 25% to 30%. Very large vena cavas (> 30 mm in diameter) may be found in patients with right-sided heart failure. In these patients, it is safer to introduce separate filters into each iliac vein. Fortunately, the vena cava is narrower in the anteroposterior diameter than it is in the transverse diameter, which provides an additional measure of security for fixation.

Unlike the original stainless steel filter, the percutaneous devices are preloaded in the carrier system. An intravascular sheath is inserted, then the carrier system is advanced through the sheath until it is seen to exit at the desired level for placement. Use of the standard stainless steel carrier follows a similar path over the guide wire to the level of L2 to L3. At this point, the stylet is unlocked, and the carrier is gradually retracted until the filter springs open at the appropriate level in the vena cava. The introducer system and the guide wire should then be withdrawn, with no further attempts being made to manipulate the filter. Any delay in positioning can be associated with thrombus formation inside the carrier; therefore, heparinized saline should be used to flush the system through the attached Luer-Lok connection either periodically or continuously. Contrast medium can also be injected, if necessary, to verify the filter's position as well as its proximity to any thrombus that might be in the inferior vena cava.

Thrombus within the vena cava should not be allowed to contact the filter, because this can lead to propagation of thrombus through the filter and above the level of mechanical protection. If thrombus does extend to the level of the renal veins or if the distal inferior vena cava is thrombosed, the filter should be placed at the level of T12, above the renal veins. After removal of the carrier system and the guide wire, a follow-up abdominal radiograph is obtained to confirm the position of the filter. Often a discrepancy is noted between the fluoroscopic impression of the level of the filter and the filter level indicated by the abdominal radiograph; this difference is due to slight parallax of the fluoroscopic image.

PERCUTANEOUS FILTER DEVICES

Percutaneous insertion of devices designed to provide effective filtration of thromboemboli in the vena cava offers a number of potential advantages for the patient, including reduced discomfort, insertion time, and procedural cost because of the use of the radiology suite rather than the operating room.[24] Insertion is made possible by use of the Seldinger technique, which allows the percutaneous insertion of progressively larger dilators and a sheath over a polytetrafluoroethylene (Teflon)-coated guide wire. A newer technique is use of single-wall needles to limit the risk of puncturing the femoral artery during the attempt to enter the vein. Ultrasound guidance has also been used when the internal jugular vein has been the selected site for placement. Enlarging the skin incision permits tract expansion either by a balloon or dilators to allow the insertion of a larger sheath.

Percutaneously inserted caval devices are customarily placed through the right femoral vein, but they may also be inserted through the neck by way of the jugular vein. The latter route is less desirable because of the risk of air embolism. Although the left femoral approach is more challenging due to more difficult anatomy, it has also been used as an access site. With introduction of the flexible delivery system for the percutaneous stainless steel filter, the left femoral vein has been used with greater ease and success

Initial efforts at percutaneous introduction of the standard 24 Fr. carrier system of the stainless steel Greenfield filter required a very large sheath (28 Fr.) and prolonged compression of the insertion site; this resulted in a 30% to 40% incidence of insertion site venous thrombosis.[25] This complication led to the enthusiastic proliferation of many innovative devices that could be inserted percutaneously using smaller-diameter delivery systems (Fig. 142–3) in an effort to retain the advantage of percutaneous insertion while minimizing the incidence of insertion site venous thrombosis. Despite the insertion of large numbers of these alternative filter devices (Fig. 142–4), it has been difficult to obtain accurate follow-up information in order to compare their effectiveness (Table 142–2).

Bird's Nest Filter

In 1984, Roehm and coworkers reported the use of a percutaneously placed intracaval device that consisted of four stainless steel wires preshaped into a crisscrossing array of nonmatching bends.[38] Placement of such a complex array was intended to provide multiple barriers to thromboemboli. Each of these wires is 25 cm long, is 0.18 mm

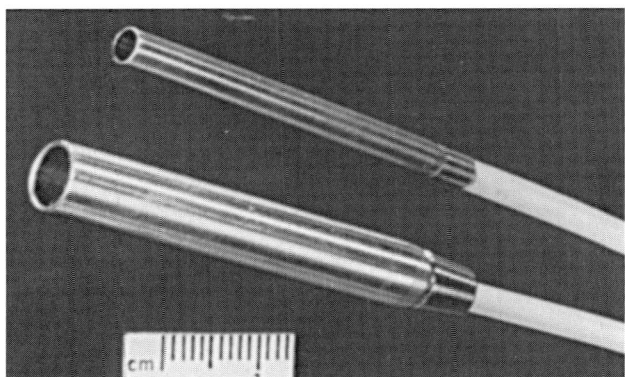

FIGURE 142–3. Comparison of the carriers used for the available models of the Greenfield filter: the 12 French (Fr.) carrier for the modified-hook titanium Greenfield filter (*top*) and the 24 Fr. carrier for the stainless steel Greenfield filter (*bottom*).

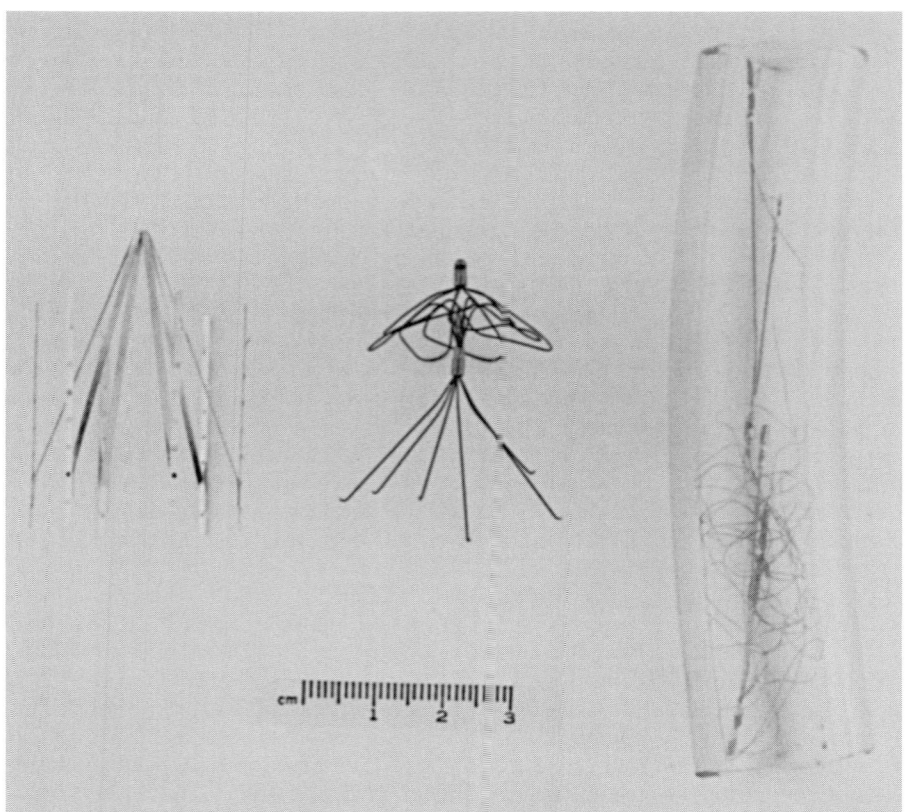

FIGURE 142–4. Commercially available vena caval filter devices: the Vena Tech filter (*left*), the Simon Nitinol filter (*center*), and the bird's nest filter (*right*).

in diameter, and ends in a strut that is connected to a fixation hook. One strut is Z-shaped, so that a pusher wire can be attached.

As initially described, the device was preloaded into an 8 Fr. (Teflon) catheter. Problems with proximal migration of this model led to redesign of the struts in 1986, with a stiffer, 0 46-mm wire used in an attempt to improve fixation. This modification required a concomitant increase in diameter of the catheter system to 12 Fr. During placement of this modified device, the pusher is used to set the first group of hooks into the caval wall; the wires are then extruded with the goal of closely packing the formed loops into a 7-cm-long segment of infrarenal vena cava (see Fig. 142–4). Finally, the second group of hooks is pushed into the caval wall. The pusher is then disengaged by being unscrewed from the filter, and the catheter is withdrawn.

Purported but unproved advantages of this device include:

1. The ability to trap smaller emboli by virtue of the tighter meshing of wires.

2. Avoidance of the need for intraluminal centering with this configuration.

3. The ability to accommodate to vena cavas as large in diameter as 40 mm.

4. The possibility that wires may be able to occlude nearby collaterals.

5. The lack of radially oriented struts, which limits the tendency toward caval wall penetration.

A series of 481 patients was reported on in 1988.[39] Only 37 patients with the filter in place 6 months or longer had

been studied by venacavography or ultrasonography, so long-term data are limited. Of these patients, 7 (19%) had an occluded vena cava. Three patients underwent pulmonary angiography for suspicion of recurrent embolism, which was confirmed in one case (3%). As indicated previously, the original model showed a troublesome tendency to migrate proximally, despite what appeared to be adequate placement. This problem was encountered in five patients and resulted in the death of one, who 10 days after placement was found to have the filter embedded within a massive pulmonary embolus. In a later series of 32 patients in whom the modified strut version was used, three instances of proximal migration were encountered.[31] Two of these occurred within 24 hours of placement and could be corrected by angiographic manipulation. The third instance was not detected until 6 months after insertion, at which point the filter was not able to be repositioned from the right side of the heart, where it had become embedded.

Nitinol Filter

Nitinol is a nickel-titanium alloy that can be drawn into a straight wire. Although pliable when cooled, it rapidly is transformed into a previously imprinted rigid shape on warming to body temperature. Although a filter composed of this alloy was initially described in 1977, the preliminary results of a multicenter clinical trial were not available until 1989.[42]

The filter design makes use of a 28-mm dome of eight overlapping loops, below which six diverging legs form a cone (see Fig. 142–4). Each leg has end-hooks designed to

TABLE 142–2. COMPARISON OF INFERIOR VENA CAVAL FILTERS

PARAMETER	GREENFIELD STAINLESS STEEL	GREENFIELD TITANIUM	VENA TECH	BIRD'S NEST	SIMON NITINOL
Evaluation	Registry (1988)	Clinical trial (1991)	Clinical trial (1990)	Clinical trial (1988)	Clinical trial (1990)
Duration	12 yr	30 days	1 yr	6 mo	6 mo
Number	469	186 (123 at follow-up)	97 (77 at follow-up)	568 (440 at 6 mo)	224 (102 at follow-up)
Recurrent pulmonary embolism	4%	3%	2%	2.7% (33%–67% in subset with objective follow-up)	4% based on those who had follow-up
Caval patency	98%	100%	92%	97%	81%
Filter patency	98%	Not reported	63% without thrombus	81%	Not reported
Insertion site deep venous thrombosis	41% (percutaneous)	8.7%	23%	Few reported clinically	11%
Migration	35% >3 mm	11% >9 mm	14% >10 mm	9% with original model	1.2% of those with follow-up
Penetration	Not reported	1%	Not reported	Not reported	0.6% of those with follow-up
Misplacement	4%	0.5%	Not reported	Not reported	Not reported
Incomplete opening	Not seen	2%	6%	Not reported	Not reported
Means of follow-up	Physical examination, inferior vena cava scan, x-ray study, noninvasive vascular examination	Physical examination, x-ray study, computed tomography, noninvasive vascular examination	Objective data vary by site (cavagram, computed tomography, duplex scanning, x-ray study)	Phone interview, objective data are random and only available for 40 of 440	Clinical, x-ray, laboratory tests

engage the caval wall. Insertion requires that iced normal saline be continuously infused through a 9 Fr. delivery system. During placement, the cooled filter wire is rapidly advanced by the feeder pump and discharged from the storage catheter. Purportedly, the filter then instantly reshapes itself into its predetermined configuration and locks into place.

Of the 103 placements recorded in the initial multicenter trial, detailed information is available on 44. During a limited follow-up period, two patients sustained recurrent PE (5%). In one individual, thrombus propagating above the filter was seen on venacavography. There were seven cases of confirmed vena caval occlusion, and in two cases occlusion was suspected on the basis of clinical findings, resulting in an overall caval occlusion rate of 18%. Five patients (11%) had stasis sequelae. Insertion site thrombosis was seen in five of 18 patients (28%) studied with ultrasonography. Proximal migration was noted in one instance.

A subsequent report on the use of this device in 224 patients indicated that of the 102 individuals followed up and the 65 in whom 6-month follow-up evaluations had been completed, 4 patients experienced recurrent embolism (4%) and one died (1%). In addition, there were 20 documented caval occlusions (20%).[11] A smaller series of 20 patients had follow-up in 16 patients for an average of 14 months. Caval penetration was seen in five patients (31%), caval thrombosis was seen in four patients (25%), filter migration into the pulmonary artery was found in one patient, and filter leg fracture was noted in two patients.[30]

Vena Tech Filter

The Vena Tech filter, introduced in 1986, is a stamped, cone-shaped filter made of Phynox, a material with properties similar to the alloy Elgiloy, which is used in temporary cardiac pacing wires. The filter cone consists of six angled radial prongs, each of which is connected to a hooked stabilizing strut; this array is designed to center and immobilize the device within the vena cava (see Fig. 142–4). It is generally inserted via a right internal jugular approach by means of a 12 Fr. catheter system that is positioned over a guide wire. After the filter is pushed through the entire length of the insertion catheter, it is released by quick withdrawal of the catheter.

The initial reported experience was from France, where the design was introduced as the "LGM" filter.[36] In a series of 100 patients, the indication for filter placement was thromboembolism in 77%, prophylaxis in iliocaval thrombosis in 13%, and contraindication to anticoagulation in 9%. As a result, most patients remained on anticoagulation after filter placement. In 100 attempted percutaneous insertions via the jugular route, 98 filters were discharged and 82 were positioned correctly. Eight filters had a 15-degree or greater tilt, five did not open completely, and three additional filters had both conditions, resulting in a 16% incidence of malposition. The investigators commented that many of these instances were early in their experience and might have been operator dependent. Recurrent PE was seen in two patients (2%), both of whom had incompletely opened filters. One-year follow-up demonstrated 7 caval occlusions (8%). Twenty-nine per cent of patients had

lower extremity edema despite the use of support stockings. Migration of the device both proximally to the renal veins (4%) and distally to the iliac veins (9%) was observed.

Another small series reported a 2.5% incidence of recurrent embolism and an occlusion rate of 8%.[29] There was a 13% rate of either tilting or incomplete opening and a similar rate of distal migration. A more recent experience with this filter showed an occlusion rate of 22%.[33] Breakage of stabilizer struts has also been reported in individual cases.[4] Long-term studies of this device by Crochet and associates have demonstrated that there has been a 37% incidence of filter occlusion with this device over time,[9] and laboratory studies in sheep demonstrated a strong association between length of placement and increased amounts of hyperplastic tissue that could be seen as early as 8 weeks following placement.

Titanium Greenfield Filter

A recent development is the modified-hook titanium Greenfield filter, which is inserted using a 12 Fr. introducer through a 14 Fr. sheath. Its conical shape is similar to that of the stainless steel Greenfield filter, but it is 8 mm wider at the base and 0.5 cm taller (Fig. 142–5). Studies have demonstrated that titanium remains as inert as stainless steel in the tissues, and there is no evidence of any additional thrombogenicity.

The mechanical properties of the titanium Greenfield filter have been tested extensively, and it shows remarkable resistance to flexion fatigue and induced corrosion.[23] Be-

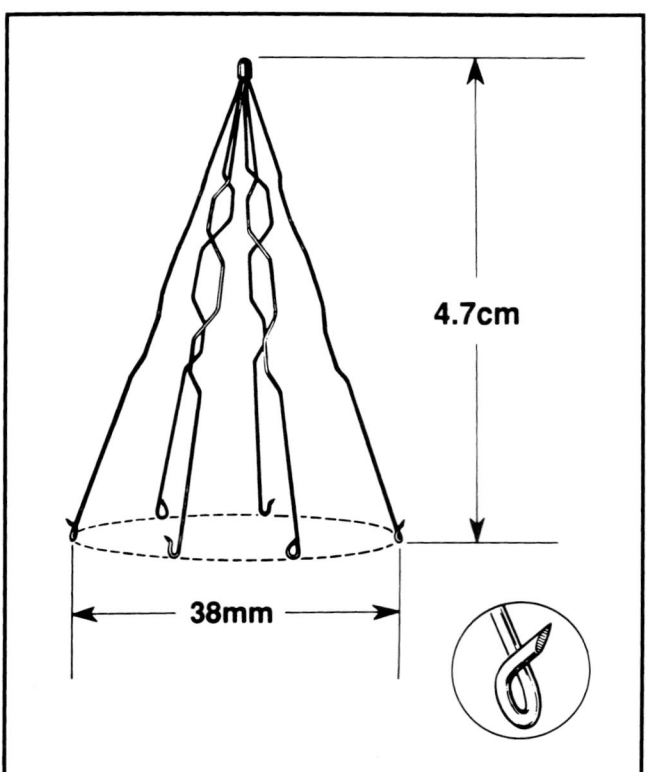

FIGURE 142–5. Modified-hook titanium Greenfield filter. The recurved hooks are set at an angle of 80 degrees for stabilization without full penetration of the vena cava.

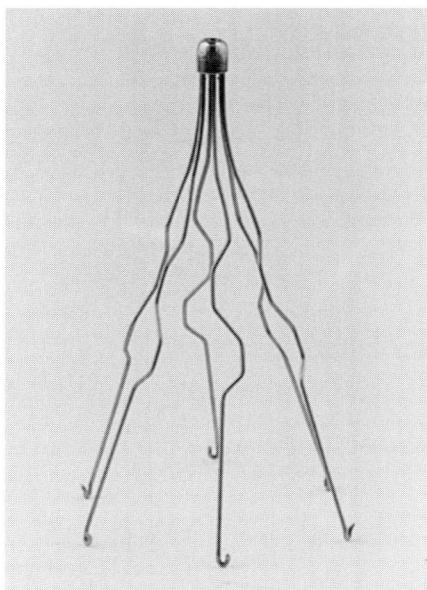

FIGURE 142–6. The percutaneous stainless steel filter has an improved fixation system with two of the four recurved hooks directed in a downward direction to oppose distal migration.

cause this filter is sufficiently elastic to allow it to be folded into the 12 Fr. carrier, modification of the original hook design was necessary to improve filter stabilization in the vena cava against upward and downward vectors of force (see Fig. 142–5). This modified-hook design has reduced the incidence of filter migration and caval penetration found with the hook design of the original titanium filter.[15, 18]

This filter can be inserted through either the jugular or the femoral vein, but usually the femoral vein is preferred for ease of entry. The titanium Greenfield filter can also be inserted at the time of laparotomy, either through a pursestring suture in the vena cava or through a small venous tributary. Under these circumstances, fluoroscopy is not required because the proper position of the carrier can be established by palpation, and the filter can be discharged at the appropriate level.

The delivery system differs from that of the stainless steel version in that a guide wire is not used for axial stabilization of the filter during insertion. This may result in tilting of the filter and occasional asymmetry of the legs if the sheath-carrier is displaced against the wall of the vena cava; however, subsequent alignment of the legs of the filter has been seen on most follow-up radiographs.

The 12 Fr. stainless steel filter is an alternative device for percutaneous placement. Clinical trials have demonstrated it to be comparable to the 24 Fr. and titanium filters with respect to efficacy (95%) and patency (95%).[5] It allows for over-the-wire delivery and a flexible carrier system to facilitate safe delivery. It is the tallest of the Greenfield devices at 4.9 cm, with a resting base diameter of 3.2 cm that lies between the titanium Greenfield filter (3.8 cm) and the original (3.0 cm). To facilitate secure fixation within the vena cava, two of the six hooks are angled distally (Fig. 142–6). The device is manufactured from the same No. 316 stainless steel as the original stainless Greenfield filter, but the wires exit from the apex at a 0- versus 17-degree angle, which facilitates delivery via a 12 Fr. system (Figure 142–7, all three filters).

Filter Insertion Technique

With local anesthesia, a 4-mm stab incision is made over the right femoral vein, which is entered with a thin-walled needle that allows passage of a 0.035-inch guide wire (Fig. 142–8). The guide wire is passed into the upper reaches of the inferior vena cava, after which the dilator-sheath system is introduced and passed into the inferior vena cava (Fig. 142–9). The dilator is withdrawn, and the preloaded carrier is passed under fluoroscopic control through the sheath to the desired level of filter placement (Fig. 142–10). If resistance is encountered at the level of the common iliac vein as it angles out of the pelvis, the sheath and carrier should be advanced together, which will usually facilitate passage.

Once the carrier has been seen to exit from the sheath, the base of the sheath is secured to the carrier and the filter tip is positioned at the desired level of introduction (Fig. 142–11). As a unit, the carrier catheter and sheath are retracted to release the filter. The carrier and sheath are then withdrawn, and gentle pressure is applied to the

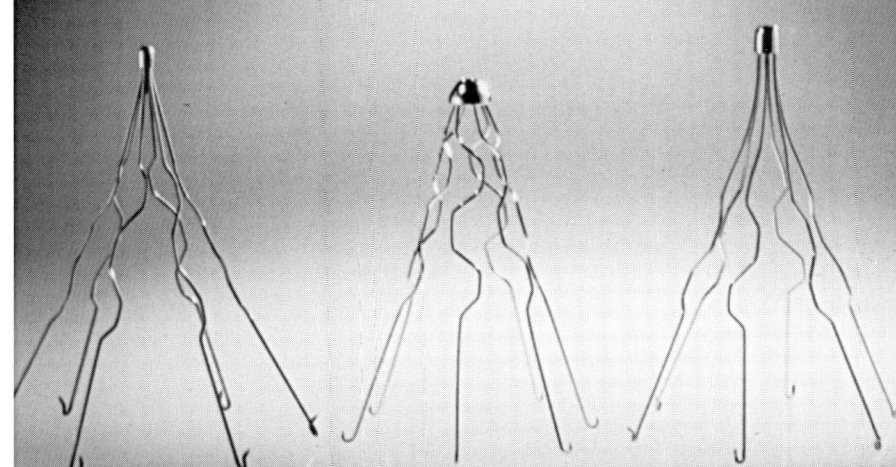

FIGURE 142–7. The three marketed Greenfield filters share a similar conical shape, which has demonstrated long-term protection from pulmonary embolism while maintaining caval patency in more than 95% of cases.

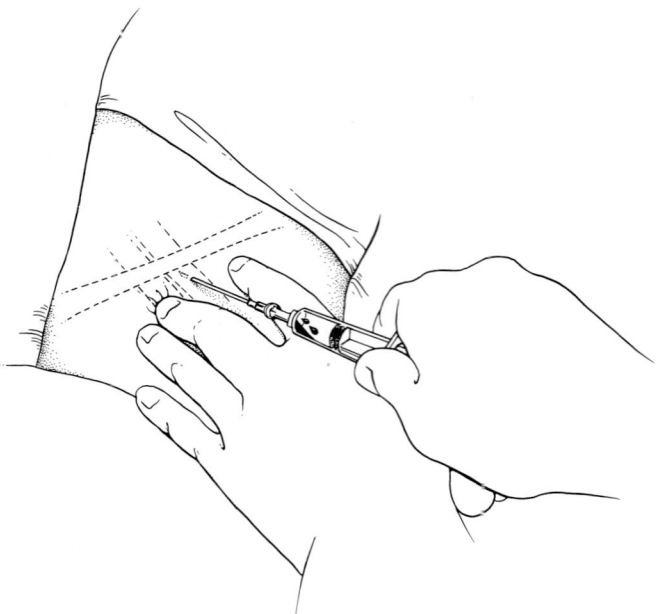

FIGURE 142–8. Percutaneous needle insertion into the common femoral vein is shown medial to the femoral artery, which is palpated with the middle finger. (Reprinted with permission from Greenfield LJ: Percutaneous placement of the Greenfield filter. *In* Vanoer Salm TJ, Cutler BS, Wheeler HB [eds]: Atlas of Bedside Procedures, 2nd ed. Boston, Little, Brown & Co, 1988, pp 107–110.)

insertion site. An additional advantage to the use of the sheath-carrier is that premature discharge of the filter would be into the sheath rather than into the patient. The filter is preloaded into the carrier system, obviating concern about crossed limbs.

Clinical Experience

Experience with the modified-hook titanium Greenfield filter has accrued since the device was approved by the Food and Drug Administration in 1991. The initial prospective multicenter trial showed that filter insertion was successful in 181 of 186 patients (97%); placement of the remainder was precluded only by unfavorable anatomy.[16] All but two of the insertions were performed percutaneously. At the time of insertion, incomplete opening was seen in 2%, but this was readily corrected by guide wire manipulation in each case. Leg asymmetry was seen in 5%, but there was no association between this asymmetry and either recurrent embolism or penetration of the wall of the vena cava. Filter apex perforation of the vena cava at the time of insertion occurred in one patient after introduction from the left groin, and there was misplacement of one filter into a lumbar vein in another. No clinical sequelae were seen in either patient, although a second filter was inserted into each patient. The only symptomatic complication noted in the series was a hematoma at the insertion site in one patient.

Initial follow-up data, obtained from all participating institutions at 30 days, showed minimal filter movement in 11%; there was no significant proximal migration. Computed tomographic scans were obtained when the diameter of the base of the filter was seen to have enlarged more

than 5 mm. There was evidence of penetration of the wall of the vena cava in only one case (0.8%), with no clinical sequelae.

A second clinical study of the titanium Greenfield filter extended the follow-up period to at least 12 months. The late patency rate was 99%, and recurrent PE was seen in 3.7% of the 176 who were enrolled.[22] Although it is too soon to report on long-term findings for the percutaneous stainless steel Greenfield filter, reports for 9 patients observed for 1 year indicated similar outcomes.[5]

Temporary Filters

Interest in a vena caval filter that could be removed in whole or part has been expressed by some orthopedic and trauma surgeons. The rationale is that there is a very limited period of risk in these cases, and surgeons do not want to

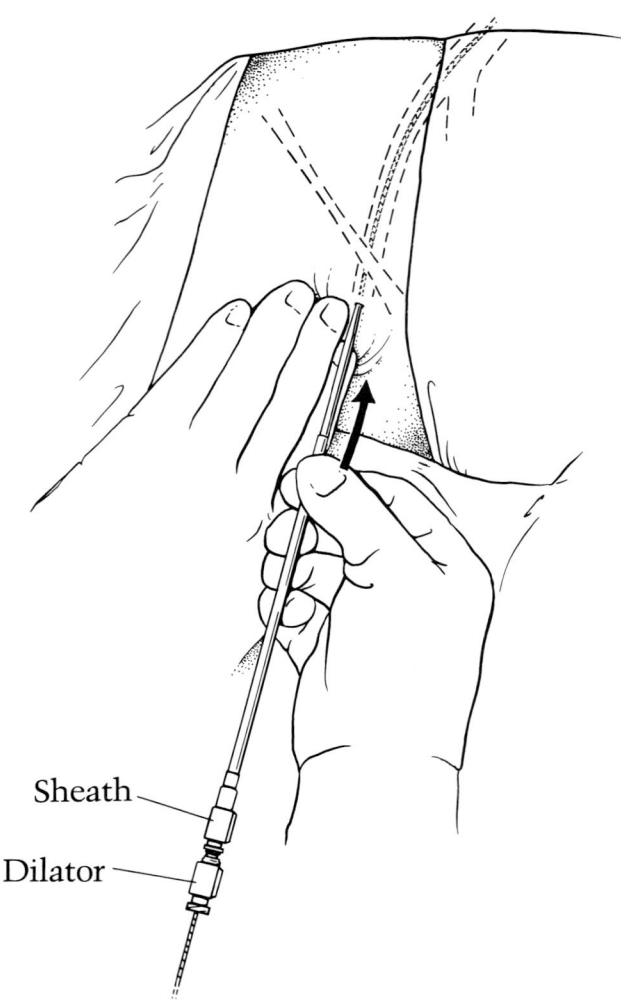

FIGURE 142–9. The dilator with attached sheath is passed under fluoroscopy over the guide wire to the desired level of discharge of the filter. The dilator and guide wire are then withdrawn, leaving the sheath in place. The sheath should then be flushed with heparinized saline. Digital control of the sheath orifice is necessary to minimize blood loss. (Reprinted with permission from Greenfield LJ: Percutaneous placement of the Greenfield filter. *In* Vanoer Salm TJ, Cutler BS, Wheeler HB [eds]: Atlas of Bedside Procedures, 2nd ed. Boston, Little, Brown & Co, 1988, pp 107–110.)

leave a permanent device in a young person with years of life ahead of him or her. It has also been suggested that a temporary device might also be used during administration of lytic therapy or thromboembolectomy.

Although superficially appealing, further consideration of these indications raises unanswered questions: (1) how to determine the period during which the patient is at risk, and (2) how to remove safely a filter that has trapped a large embolus without dislodging it, resulting in PE? In addition, the device may need to be replaced if sepsis developed, and the patient must return to the radiology suite for removal of the device. Each of these factors would increase the cost of the procedures.

SUMMARY

There is considerable ingenuity in the numerous devices now available for clinical use as vena caval filters. The

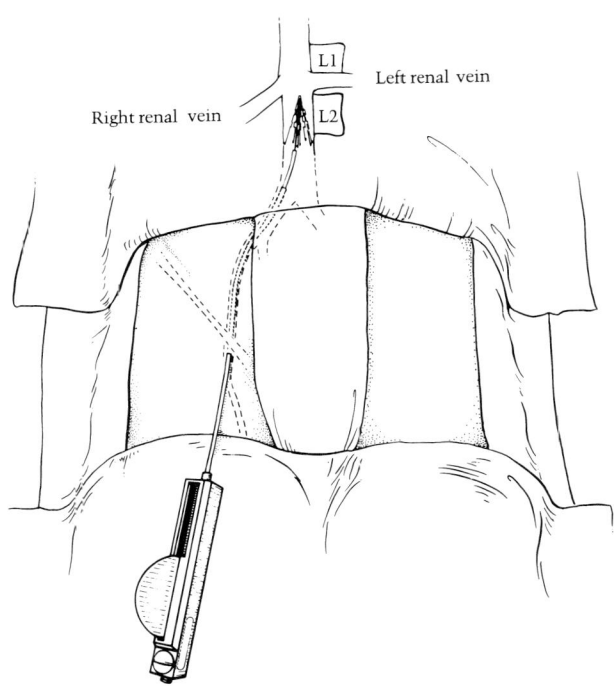

FIGURE 142–11. The carrier tip should be positioned under fluoroscopy at the level of L2–L3. The locking mechanism on the control handle is released by moving the control tab with the thumb to the left. The control tab is then pulled backward to uncover the filter, which will be discharged within the vena cava. Once the filter has been discharged, no attempt should be made to alter its position. (Reprinted with permission from Greenfield LJ: Percutaneous placement of the Greenfield filter. *In* Vanoer Salm TJ, Cutler BS, Wheeler HB [eds]: Atlas of Bedside Procedures, 2nd ed. Boston. Little, Brown & Co, 1988, pp 107–110.)

primary objective, to provide a safe and effective device for permanent implantation, should lead to continued evolution of materials and design. The standard for comparison, however, should remain the stainless steel Greenfield filter, with data available since its introduction in 1972. It seems clear that advances in percutaneous techniques will make percutaneous placement the obvious choice for the future, but the long-term safety and efficacy of the conical design of the Greenfield filter suggest that a new design may not be needed.

In the overall management of the patient with thrombotic disease, it is imperative to understand that any filtration device plays only a limited role, and it is incumbent on the physician who treats the patient to assume the responsibility for the ongoing management and long-term follow-up of the underlying disorder.

REFERENCES

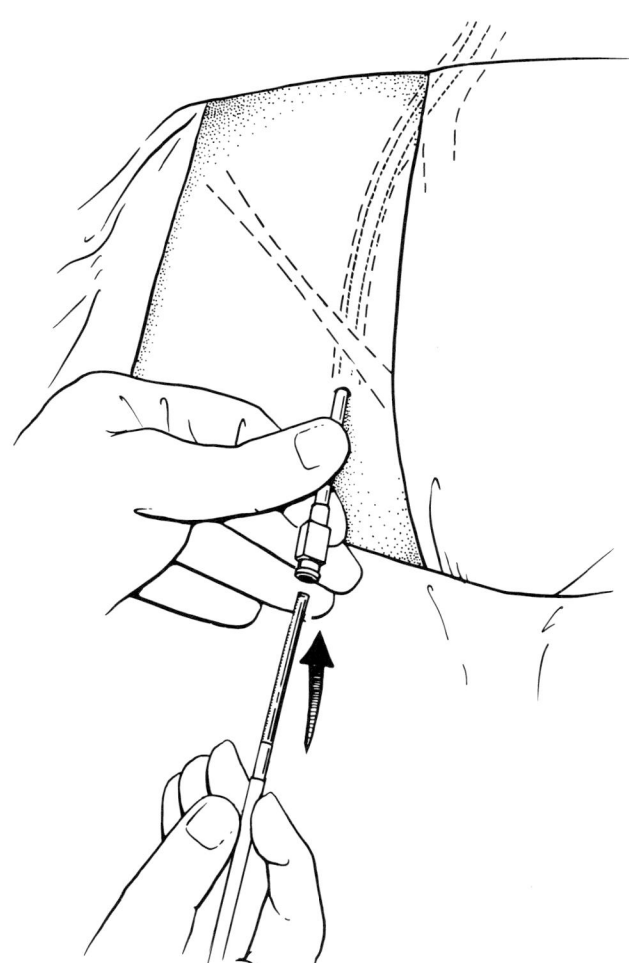

FIGURE 142–10. The filter carrier is introduced into the sheath, and if difficulty is encountered in exiting from the pelvis, both carrier and sheath should be advanced together. The carrier should be advanced through the sheath until the sheath hub contacts the control handle to prevent release of the filter into the sheath. (Reprinted with permission from Greenfield LJ: Percutaneous placement of the Greenfield filter. *In* Vanoer Salm TJ, Cutler BS, Wheeler HB [eds]: Atlas of Bedside Procedures, 2nd ed. Boston, Little, Brown & Co, 1988, pp 107–110.)

1. Adams JT, DeWeese JA: Partial interruption of the inferior vena cava with a new plastic clip. Surg Gynecol Obstet 123:1087, 1966.
2. Amador E, Ting KL, Crane C: Ligation of inferior vena cava for thromboembolism. JAMA 206:1758–1760, 1968.
3. Askew AR, Gardner AMN: Long-term follow-up of partial caval occlusion by clip. Am J Surg 140:441–443; 1980.
4. Awh M, Taylor F, Lu CT: Spontaneous fracture of a Vena-Tech inferior vena caval filter. AJR Am J Roentgenol 157:177–178, 1991.
5. Cho KJ, Greenfield LJ, Proctor MC, et al: Evaluation of a new

percutaneous stainless steel Greenfield filter. J Vasc Interv Radiol 8:181–187, 1997.

6. Cimochowski GE, Evans RH, Zarins CK: Greenfield filter versus Mobin-Uddin umbrella: The continuing quest for the ideal method of vena caval interruption. J Thorac Cardiovasc Surg 79:358, 1980.
7. Cohen J, Tenenbaum M, Citron M: Greenfield filter as primary therapy for deep venous thrombosis and/or pulmonary embolism in patients with cancer. Surgery 109:12–15, 1991.
8. Couch NP, Baldwin SS, Crane C: Mortality and morbidity rates after inferior vena caval clipping. Surgery 77:106–112, 1975.
9. Crochet DP, Stora O, Ferry D, et al: Vena Tech-LGM filter: Long-term results of a prospective study. Radiology 188:857–850, 1993.
10. DeMeester T, Rutherford RB, Blazek JV, et al: Plication of the inferior vena cava for thromboembolism. Surgery 62(1):56–65, 1967.
11. Dorfman GS: Percutaneous inferior vena caval filters. Radiology 174:987–992, 1990.
12. Ferris EJ, Vittimberga FJ, Byrne JJ, et al: The inferior vena cava after ligation and plication: A study of collateral routes. Radiology 89:1–10, 1967.
13. Fink JA, Jones BT: The Greenfield filter as the primary means of therapy in venous thromboembolic disease. Surg Gynecol Obstet 172:253–256, 1991.
14. Gomez GA, Cutler BS, Wheeler HB: Transvenous interruption of the inferior vena cava. Surgery 93:612, 1983.
15. Greenfield LJ, Cho KJ, Pais O, et al: Preliminary clinical experience with the titanium Greenfield vena caval filter. Arch Surg 124:657–659, 1989.
16. Greenfield LJ, Cho KJ, Proctor MC, et al: Results of a multicenter study of the modified-hook titanium Greenfield filter. J Vasc Surg 14:253–257, 1991.
17. Greenfield LJ, Cho KJ, Proctor MC, et al: Late results of suprarenal Greenfield vena cava filter placement. Arch Surg 127:969–973, 1992.
18. Greenfield LJ, Cho KJ, Tauscher J: Evolution of hook design for fixation of the titanium Greenfield filter. J Vasc Surg 12:345–353, 1990.
19. Greenfield LJ, McCurdy JR, Brown PP, et al: A new intracaval filter permitting continued flow and resolution of emboli. Surgery 73:599–606, 1973.
20. Greenfield LJ, Michna BA: Twelve-year clinical experience with the Greenfield vena caval filter. Surgery 104:706–712, 1988.
21. Greenfield LJ, Proctor MC: Twenty-year clinical experience with the Greenfield filter. Cardiovas Surg 3:199–205, 1995.
22. Greenfield LJ, Proctor MC, Cho KJ, et al: Extended evaluation of the titanium Greenfield vena caval filter. J Vasc Surg 20:458–465, 1994.
23. Greenfield LJ, Savin M: Comparison of titanium and stainless steel Greenfield vena caval filters. Surgery 106:820–828, 1989.
24. Hye R, Mitchell A, Dory C, et al: Analysis of the transition to percutaneous placement of Greenfield filters. Arch Surg 125:1550–1553, 1990.

25. Kantor A, Glanz S, Gordon DH, et al: Percutaneous insertion of the Kimray-Greenfield filter: Incidence of femoral vein thrombosis. Am J Roentgenol 149:1065–1066, 1987.
26. Khansarinia S, Dennis JW, Veldenz HC, et al: Prophylactic Greenfield filter placement in selected high-risk trauma patients. J Vasc Surg 22:231–236, 1995.
27. Lindenauer SM: Prophylactic staple plication of the inferior vena cava. Arch Surg 107:669–675, 1973.
28. Lossef SV, Barth K: Outcome of patients with advanced neoplastic disease receiving vena caval filters. J Vasc Interv Radiol 6:273–277, 1995.
29. Maquin P, Fajadet P, Railhac N: LGM and Gunther: Two complementary vena cava filters. Radiology 173:476, 1989.
30. McCowan T, Ferris E, Carver DK, et al: Complications of the nitinol vena caval filter. J Vasc Interv Radiol 3:401–408, 1992.
31. McCowan TC, Ferris EJ, Keifsteck JE: Retrieval of dislodged Bird's Nest inferior vena cava filter: Progress report. J Interv Radiol 3:179, 1988.
32. Miller TD, Staats BA: Impaired exercise tolerance after inferior vena caval interruption. Chest 93:776–780, 1988.
33. Millward S, Peterson R, Rasuli P, et al: LGM (Vena Tech) vena cava filter: Clinical experience in 64 patients. J Vasc Interv Radiol 2:429–433, 1991.
34. Nasbeth DC, Moran JM: Reassessment of the role of inferior vena cava ligation in thromboembolism. N Engl J Med 273:1250–1253, 1965.
35. Peyton JWR, Hylemon MB, Greenfield LJ, et al: Comparison of Greenfield filter and vena caval ligation for experimental septic thromboembolism. Surgery 93:533–537, 1983.
36. Ricco JB, Crochet DP, Sebilotte P, et al: Percutaneous transvenous caval interruption with "LGM" filter. Ann Vasc Surg 2:242–247, 1988.
37. Rodriguez JL, Lopez JM, Proctor MC, et al: Early placement of prophylactic vena caval filters in injured patients at high risk for a pulmonary embolism. J Trauma 40:797–804, 1996.
38. Roehm J, Gianturco C, Barth M, et al: Percutaneous transcatheter filter for the inferior vena cava: A new device for treatment of patients with pulmonary embolism. Radiology 150:255–257, 1984.
39. Roehm J, Johnsrude I, Barth M, et al: The Bird's Nest inferior vena cava filter: Progress report. Radiology 168:745–749, 1988.
40. Rogers FB, Shackford SR, Wilson J, et al: Prophylactic vena cava filter insertion in severely injured trauma patients: Indications and preliminary results. J Trauma 35:637–642, 1993.
41. Rosen M, Porter DH, Kim D: Reassessment of vena caval filter use in patients with cancer. J Vasc Interv Radiol 5:501–506, 1994.
42. Simon M, Athanasoulis C, Kim D, et al: Simon nitinol inferior vena cava filter: Initial clinical experience. Radiology 172:99–103, 1989.
43. Spencer F: Plication of the vena cava for pulmonary embolism. Surgery 62:388–392, 1967.
44. Verstraete M: Thrombolytic treatment. BMJ 311:582–583, 1995.

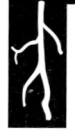

C H A P T E R 1 4 3

Superficial Thrombophlebitis: Diagnosis and Management

Ralph G. DePalma, M.D., and
George Johnson, Jr., M.D.

The seriousness of thrombosis involving the superficial venous system has been underestimated in the past. Although at times superficial thrombophlebitis causes significant discomfort, it generally has been considered to be benign and self-limiting. However, some authors now report that superficial thrombophlebitis can progress to deep venous thrombosis in as high as 11% of cases.[9] Superficial venous thrombosis can be caused by trauma such as catheter insertion, direct intimal injury and infection, and stasis in varices, or it can relate to abnormalities in blood coagulation. Here superficial thrombophlebitis may signal the presence of abnormalities in antithrombin III and protein C or S.[21]

A relationship between oral contraceptives[14, 23] and pregnancy[11] and superficial thrombophlebitis has been demonstrated in women, particularly individuals with abnormal activated protein C. An association with certain malignancies has long been noted, and procoagulant factors have been identified in acute lymphocytic leukemia[3] and cholangiocarcinoma.[20] Each factor can be seen to represent the components of *Virchow's triad*: intimal injury, stasis, and changes in blood coagulation.

CATEGORIES

Traumatic Thrombophlebitis

Superficial venous thrombosis can occur after direct injury, usually of an extremity. It presents as a tender cord along the course of a vein, juxtaposing the area of trauma. Ecchymosis is often present, indicating extravasation of blood associated with the injury. Thrombophlebitis at the site of an intravenous infusion is usually the result of irritating drugs or hypertonic solutions and, less commonly, intimal injury caused by the catheter. This presentation is seen in hospitalized patients or in ambulatory individuals using or receiving drugs. Redness, pain, and tenderness sometimes signal its development while the infusion is in progress. Thrombosis remains as a cord or lump for days or weeks after cessation of intravenous therapy.

Thrombophlebitis in Varicose Veins

Superficial thrombophlebitis frequently occurs in varicose veins. On occasion, the process extends the length of the saphenous vein or, more frequently, remains confined segmentally or involves cluster varicosities away from the saphenous vein. Thrombosis sometimes follows trauma to a varix, but the process more often appears without antecedent cause, possibly due to stasis. Thrombophlebitis presents as a tender, hard nodule surrounded by a zone of erythema in a previously noted varicose vein. Rarely, bleeding occurs if an inflammatory reaction extends through the vein wall and skin at the ankle. Localized thrombosis and woody induration often surround venous stasis ulcers, owing to round cell inflammation and cytokine elaboration.

Thrombophlebitis and Infection

DeTakats in 1932 speculated that dormant infection in varicose veins was a factor in the development of thrombophlebitis, which might be exacerbated after operations, injection treatments, trauma, or exposure to radiation therapy.[13] Altemeier and colleagues suggested that the presence of l-forms and other atypical bacterial forms in the blood play an etiologic role in thrombophlebitis.[1] However, septic phlebitis caused by intravenous cannulation is a special case; this is a serious, potentially lethal complication.

Aerobic and anaerobic as well as mixed infections occur.[5] Aerobic organisms include *Staphylococcus aureus*, *Pseudomonas*, and *Klebsiella*; anaerobic bacteria include *Peptostreptococcus*, *Propionibacterium*, *Bacteroides fragilis*, *Prevotella*, and *Fusobacterium*. In children and neonates as well as in elderly people, septicemia might present in one third of patients. Most patients exhibit localizing signs, but a search with a high index of suspicion should be made of intravenous sites in older people and infants with an unexplained fever. Treatment includes discontinuing cannulation, prompt excision of suppurating veins, and an appropriate systemic antibiotic regimen.[10]

Migratory Thrombophlebitis

Migratory thrombophlebitis, according to Glasser,[15] was first described by Jadioux in 1845 as an entity characterized by repeated thrombosis of superficial veins at varying sites, commonly involving the lower extremity. The association with carcinoma was first reported by Trousseau in 1856. Sproul emphasized that migratory thrombophlebitis was particularly prevalent with carcinoma of the tail of the pancreas.[27] Migratory phlebitis occurs in diseases associated with vasculitis, such as polyarteritis nodosa (periarteritis nodosa) and Buerger's disease. Buerger noted phlebitis in eight of 19 patients,[7] and it has been reported in 43% of 255 patients followed for extended periods.[26] Upper extremity involvement occurs in Buerger's disease. Inflammatory lesions mimicking migratory phlebitis include erythema nodosum, erythema induratum, and Behçet's disease.[16, 17]

Mondor's Disease: Thrombophlebitis of Superficial Veins of the Breast

Mondor's disease is rare. Superficial thrombophlebitis involves the veins at the anterolateral aspect of the upper portion of the breast or in the region extending from the lower portion of the breast across the submammary fold toward the costal margin and the epigastrium. Characteristically, a tender, cord-like structure can be demonstrated by tensing the skin, as by elevating the arm. As with other cases of thrombophlebitis, a search for malignancy may be indicated. Mondor's disease has occurred after breast surgery, with use of oral contraceptives, with hereditary protein C deficiency, and in the presence of anticardiolipin antibodies.[28]

Unusual Forms

Thrombophlebitis can involve the dorsal penile vein; this entity is sometimes called penile Mondor's disease. Main etiologic factors include prolonged excessive sexual intercourse, hernia operations, and, as with other forms of superficial thrombophlebitis, deep venous involvement.[24] Ultrasound diagnosis has been suggested[20] and is useful to rule out deep involvement. Therapy includes nonsteroidal anti-inflammatory drugs (NSAIDs) as well as dorsal penile vein resection for patients not responding to medical therapy.

Another unusual form of superficial thrombophlebitis has been described in the palmar digital veins in women, with vein involvement over the proximal interphalangeal joints.[18] In five women, no history of trauma was elicited and no underlying cause was noted. Four of the five were treated with excision, which confirmed the diagnosis.

DIAGNOSIS

Diagnosis of superficial thrombophlebitis is usually obvious. The patient complains of a painful, cord-like structure along the course of the affected vein. A perivenous inflammatory reaction frequently gives rise to redness along the course of the vein. Duplex scanning documents the thrombus in the superficial vein, yielding critical information about extension into the deep venous system.

Lutter and associates reported that 12% of 186 patients with superficial thrombophlebitis of the great saphenous vein above the knee had extension into the deep venous system.[19] More recently, Bounameaux and Reber-Wassem[5] described associations with deep vein thrombosis, with reported frequencies of 12% to 44%. In their data base, 31 cases, or 5.6%, with a confidence interval of 3.8% to 7.9%, had associated deep vein thrombosis. During a 3-month follow-up thromboembolic events were detected in 1.7%.

Although the association with deep vein thrombosis might be considered modest, this remains a risk, particularly when superficial involvement is detected in an immobilized patient. Phlebography is not needed to confirm the diagnosis; in fact, this procedure makes the process worse. Rarely, phlebography is useful in excluding the diagnosis of proximal deep involvement; here computed tomographic scanning of the caval segments can be used effectively.

TREATMENT

The treatment of superficial venous thrombosis depends on its etiology, extent, and severity of symptoms. Duplex scanning gives an accurate appraisal of the extent of disease, permitting more rational therapy. For the superficial, localized, mildly tender area of thrombophlebitis involving a varicose vein, treatment with a NSAID, such as aspirin, and the use of elastic support usually suffice. Patients are encouraged to continue their usual daily activities.[12] With localized varicosities or when symptoms persist, phlebectomy of the involved segment can speed recovery.

More extensive thrombophlebitis, as indicated by severe pain, redness, and diffuse involvement, has been treated traditionally by bed rest, with elevation of the extremity and application of massive warm, wet compresses. The latter measure seems to be more effective using a large, bulky dressing, including a blanket and plastic sheeting, followed by an aquathermal pad. The immobilization may be as beneficial as the moist heat in some cases. Long-leg heavy-gauge elastic stockings or elastic (Ace) bandages are indicated when the patient becomes ambulatory. Antibiotics are usually not needed unless an ulcer or lymphangitis accompanies the process.

In the past, excision of the vein was recommended as early definitive therapy for ascending phlebitis.[24] However, this approach has been questioned and will be further considered. Operative treatment is not indicated in a massive inflammatory response as described.

Certain anti-inflammatory drugs are of benefit. Salicylates, indomethacin, and ibuprofen have all been reported to be effective. The salicylates, ibuprofen, and dipyridamole have been recommended as antithrombotic agents, but their effectiveness has not been documented in this setting. Because thrombophlebitis is primarily due to inflammation and fibrin clot, antithrombotic or anti–platelet-aggregating agents would seem to have little value. Anticoagulants are indicated when the process extends to or approximates the deep venous system; these sites are usually at the saphenofemoral junction or at the popliteal vein.

Although past wisdom suggested saphenectomy or saphenofemoral junction ligation, particularly when the process extended into the thigh, a 1995 report[2] describes nonoperative treatment of 20 patients with saphenofemoral junctional thrombophlebitis. Significantly, 40% of these patients already had concurrent deep involvement, indicating a perceived need for full heparin anticoagulation in a hospital setting, followed by warfarin for 6 months. In another report,[4] superficial saphenous thrombophlebitis extended into the common femoral vein in 8.6% of cases, among which 10% embolized to the lungs. These authors also recommended standard anticoagulation. The availability of low-molecular-weight heparin might make a difference in the long-term approach to this problem.

In contrast, particularly when serial duplex scanning reveals ascending superficial thrombophlebitis, the authors have selectively followed traditional advice,[16] approaching the saphenofemoral junction in a young, active individual or immediately post partum with good outcomes. One can meticulously expose the saphenofemoral junction, ligate it, or even remove encroaching thrombus from the deep system. It is crucial not to cause embolization by securing atraumatic control of the saphenofemoral junction early. External stripping of the involved long saphenous segment completes the procedure and may speed recovery The need for this intervention is admittedly rare. In other instances (e.g., for elderly or immobilized patients), standard anticoagulation is also a safe alternative.

More data using low-molecular-weight heparin and case-selected prospective studies are needed to address rational management alternatives in individual cases. In the interim, neither intelligent case selection for operative intervention nor anticoagulation can be criticized. As mentioned previously, suppurative thrombophlebitis due to a catheter or cannula insertion clearly demands immediate aggressive surgical treatment, including excision of the involved vein, leaving the wound open, and using appropriate systemic antibiotic therapy based on culture results.

PROGNOSIS AND LONG-TERM MANAGEMENT

The prognosis of patients with superficial thrombophlebitis depends on etiology, extent of involvement, and extension into the deep venous system. Deep extension is not ubiquitous but occurs in certain cases with varying frequencies. Because of this, serial duplex surveillance appears advisable in all cases. If the process persists or recurs, a search for coagulation abnormalities, including protein C, protein S, antithrombin III, and activated protein C resistance, is indicated. Such screening, although costly, is important in young women when superficial thrombophlebitis occurs while they are receiving oral contraception. A final caution exists in vascular laboratory reporting of "superficial" femoral vein thrombophlebitis,[8] which, in actuality, is deep venous involvement. Whereas such confusion is unlikely among surgeons, the primary care community might be misled into believing that a relatively benign prognosis exists.

REFERENCES

1. Altemeier WA, Hill EO, Fullen WD: Acute recurrent thromboembolic disease: A new concept of etiology. Ann Surg 170:547, 1969.
2. Ascer E, Lorenson E, Pollina RM, et al: Preliminary results of a non-operative approach to saphenofemoral junctional thrombophlebitis. J Vasc Surg 22:616, 1995.
3. Bilgrami S, Greenberg BR, Weinstein RE, et al: Recurrent venous thrombosis as the presenting manifestation of acute lymphocytic leukemia. Med J Pediatr Oncol 24:40, 1995.
4. Blumenberg RM, Barton E, Gelfand, ML et al: Occult deep venous thrombosis complicating superficial thrombophlebitis. J Vasc Surg 27.338, 1998.
5. Boumameaux H, Reber-Wassem MA: Superficial deep vein thrombosis: A controversial association. Arch Intern Med 157:1822, 1997.
6. Brook I, Frazier EH: Aerobic and anaerobic microbiology of superficial suppurative thrombophlebitis. Arch Surg 131:95, 1996.
7. Buerger L: The veins in thromboangiitis obliterans: With particular reference to arteriovenous anastomosis as a cure for the condition. JAMA 52:1319, 1909.
8. Bundens WP, Bergan JJ, Halasz NA, et al: The superficial femoral vein. A potentially lethal misnomer. JAMA 274:1296, 1995.
9. Chengelis D, Berdick PJ, Glover JL, et al: Progression of superficial venous thrombosis to deep vein thrombosis. J Vasc Surg 24:745, 1996.
10. Cho KH, Kim YG, Yang SG, et al: Inflammatory nodules of the lower legs: A clinical and histological analysis of 234 cases. J Dermatol 24:522, 1997.
11. Cook G, Walker ID, McCall F, et al: Familial thrombophilia and activated protein C resistance: Thrombotic risk in pregnancy. Br J Haematol 87:873, 1994.
12. Cranley JJ: Thrombophlebitis in obstetrics and gynecology. In Rakel RE (ed): Conn's Current Therapy. Philadelphia, WB Saunders, 1984.
13. DeTakats G: "Resting infection" in varicose veins: Its diagnosis and treatment. Am J Med Sci 184:57, 1932.
14. Girolami A, Simioni P, Girolami B, et al: Homozygous patients with APC resistance may remain paucisymptomatic or asymptomatic during oral contraception. Blood Coagul Fibrinolysis 7:590, 1996.
15. Glasser ST: Principles of Peripheral Vascular Surgery. Philadelphia, FA Davis, 1959.
16. James RV, Lohr JM, Deshmukh RM, Cranely JJ: Venous thrombotic complications of pregnancy. Cardiovasc Surg 4:777, 1996.
17. Kahn EA, Correa AS, Baker CJ: Suppurative thrombophlebitis in children: A ten-year experience. Pediatr Infect Dis J 16:63, 1997.
18. Lanzetta M, Morrison WA: Spontaneous thrombosis of palmar digital veins. J Hand Surg 21:410, 1996.
19. Lutter KS, Kerr TM, Roedersheimer LR, et al: Superficial thrombophlebitis diagnosed by duplex scanning. Surgery 110:42, 1991.
20. Martins EP, Flemming RA, Garrido MC, et al: Thrombophlebitis, dysplasia, and cholangiocarcinoma in primary sclerosing cholangitis. Gastroenterology 107:537, 1994.
21. Pabinger I, Schneider B: Thrombotic risk in hereditary antithrombin III, protein C, and protein S deficiency. Arterioscler Thromb Vasc Biol 16:742, 1996.
22. Sagdic R, Ozer ZG, Saba D, et al: Venous lesions in Behçet's disease. Eur J Vasc Endovasc Surg 11:537, 1996.
23. Samama MM, Simon D, Horellou MH, et al: Diagnosis and clinical characteristics of inherited activated protein C resistance. Haemostasis 26(Supp 4):325, 1996.
24. Sasso F, Gulino G, Bsar M, et al: Penile Mondor's disease, an underestimated pathology. Br J Urol 77:729, 1996.
25. Shapiro RJ: Superficial dorsal penile vein thrombosis (penile Mondor's phlebitis): Ultrasound diagnosis. J Clin Ultrasound 24:272, 1996.
26. Shionoya S: Buerger's Disease: Pathology, Diagnosis and Treatment. Nagoya, Japan, University of Nagoya Press, 1990.
27. Sproul EE: Carcinoma and venous thrombosis: Frequency of association of carcinoma in body or tail of pancreas with multiple venous thrombosis. Am J Cancer 34:566, 1938.
28. Wester JP, Kuenen BC, Menwissen OJ: Mondor's disease as the first thrombotic event in hereditary protein C deficiency and anticardiolipin antibodies. Neth J Med 50:85; 1997.

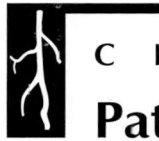

C H A P T E R   1 4 4

Pathophysiology of Chronic Venous Insufficiency

Gregory L. Moneta, M.D., Mark R. Nehler, M.D., and John M. Porter, M.D.

EPIDEMIOLOGY AND SOCIETAL IMPACT

A number of risk factors are associated with venous disease. The risk factors for varicose veins include prolonged standing,[1] heredity,[2] history of phlebitis,[3] female sex,[2, 3] and parity.[4] Age-adjusted multivariate analysis, however, suggests that a history of phlebitis, female sex and a family history of varicose veins are the most important risk factors for superficial varicosities.[3]

Risk factors for venous ulceration differ from those for varicose veins. Conditions associated with venous ulcers include increased age, obesity, hypertension diabetes, congestive heart failure, renal insufficiency, rheumatoid arthritis, male sex, low socioeconomic class, lower extremity trauma, and a history of venous thrombosis.[5–10] Many of these conditions are associated with older age. Indeed, the prevalence of venous disease increases progressively with age. The median age for patients with venous ulcers has been reported as high as 70 and 77 years.[6, 7] The overall incidence of venous ulcers in patients older than 45 years of age is estimated at 3.5 per thousand per year.[11] Age-adjusted multivariate analysis suggests that in addition to age the principal risk factors for venous ulceration are male sex, obesity, and a history of deep venous thrombosis (DVT) and serious lower extremity trauma.[3]

Chronic venous insufficiency (CVI) is both prevalent and costly to individuals and society at large. About 27% of the American adult population has some form of detectable lower extremity venous abnormality, primarily varicose veins or telangiectasias.[1] The incidence of CVI in the adult population, based on American and European studies, is between 0.5 and 3.0%.[12–14] European data indicate that up to 1.5% of European adults will suffer a venous stasis ulcer at some point in their lives.[15] Afflicted patients have a severely impaired quality of life. Nearly 70% experience some type of negative emotional impact, including feelings of anger, depression, isolation, and diminished self-image.[16] Eighty per cent experience a decrease in mobility.[16]

Although the symptoms of CVI such as edema and leg fatigue, discomfort, and heaviness are troublesome, the skin changes and their ulcerative sequelae are the most significant. Many epidemiologic studies have documented the societal impact of venous ulceration. A postal survey in Edinburgh, Scotland, by the National Health Service identified 1477 patients within this community of 1 million people who were receiving treatment for lower extremity ulceration.[17] From the 1477 identified patients, a representative sample of 600 patients, with a total of 827 ulcerated lower extremities, was examined in detail. Seventy-six per cent of the ulcerated limbs in this sample were classified as venous in origin. Of all the ulcerated limbs, 67% had a recurrent ulcer at the time of the survey and 35% of ulcerated limbs had four or more recurrences. Two hundred seventy patients (45%) had lower extremity ulceration for more than 10 years.

Baker and associates[18] studied 259 patients with chronic ulceration of 286 lower extremities. On the basis of a shortened venous recovery time, 57% of the ulcerated limbs were identified as having ulcerations secondary to CVI. Of all patients, 75% had a history of recurrent ulceration and 28% had a history of 10 or more episodes of ulceration. Thirty-four per cent had lower extremity ulceration for more than 10 years.

Of venous ulcer patients, 42% note moderate to severe limitation of their leisure activities. Forty per cent of employed persons with leg ulcers experience earning capacity limited by the presence of the ulcer. Five per cent lose their jobs secondary to lower extremity ulceration.[19] Up to 2 million workdays are lost each year in the United States secondary to venous ulceration.[20] Annual health care costs for venous ulceration are estimated at 290 million pounds in the United Kingdom, 14.7 billion francs in France, 420 million deutsche marks in Germany, 1,638 billion liras in Italy, 17,240 pesetas in Spain, and $1 billion in the United States.[21]

PATHOPHYSIOLOGY: THE MACROCIRCULATION

The term *macrocirculation* refers to the deep, superficial, and communicating veins of the lower extremity. Signs and symptoms of secondary CVI result from venous obstruction, venous reflux, calf muscle pump dysfunction, or combinations of these factors. In most cases, however, reflux is thought to serve as the principal cause of the development of the signs and symptoms of CVI. Venous insufficiency is usually described as "primary" or "secondary." *Primary valvular incompetence* is the diagnosis when no obvious underlying etiologic mechanism of valvular dysfunction can be identified. Most cases of apparently isolated superficial venous insufficiency are considered examples of primary venous insufficiency. Such cases may develop from a loss of elasticity of the vein wall.[22] Patients with primary varicose veins have venous elasticity that is significantly lower than that of controls,[23] and loss of elasticity precedes valvular incompetence in patients identified as having primary venous insufficiency.[24]

Valvular incompetence is described as *secondary* when there is an obvious antecedent event, most frequently a DVT, that may have led to destruction or dysfunction, or both, of the venous valves. Most information on the natural history and pathophysiology of CVI derives from patients with presumed secondary CVI.

Abnormal Venous Functions

Because *valvular reflux* is present in almost all cases of moderate to severe CVI, most techniques in the evaluation of CVI focus on identification and quantification of venous reflux. An understanding of the techniques of investigation of CVI is crucial to an understanding of its pathophysiology. These techniques are detailed in Chapters 11 and 145.

Evaluation of the macrocirculation in CVI first used invasive measurements of *ambulatory venous pressure* (AVP) and *venous recovery time* (VRT) as indicators of valvular dysfunction. AVP has been and continues to be the simplest and most direct measure of venous hypertension. AVP measurements clearly implicate the presence of venous hypertension as being strongly associated with CVI. Patients with an AVP of below 40 mmHg have a minimal incidence of venous ulceration compared with an 80% incidence of venous ulceration in patients with an AVP of greater than 80 mmHg.[25]

AVP does not, however, completely characterize the function of the lower extremity venous system. AVP correlates poorly with clinical outcome after deep venous reconstructive procedures and with symptoms of CVI.[26] A review of AVPs in 207 limbs found that 25 of 52 limbs (48%) classified as having severe ambulatory venous hypertension (a less than 25% decrease in venous pressure with exercise) were only mildly symptomatic or asymptomatic.[27] In addition, AVP measurements are a measure of the overall function of the lower extremity venous system. They cannot distinguish the combined effects of reflux and obstruction, evaluate the role of the calf muscle pump itself, or localize sites of reflux.

Air plethysmography (see Chapters 11 and 145) has been reintroduced into the study of venous physiology.[28, 29] The air plethysmograph theoretically permits evaluation of venous reflux (venous filling index [VFI]), calf muscle pump function (ejection fraction [EF]), and overall lower extremity venous function (residual volume fraction [RVF]). Abnormalities in RVF, which correlates with ambulatory venous pressure, may reflect inadequate calf muscle pump action (decreased EF), the presence of valvular reflux (increased VFI), or combinations of both. This type of information may allow more precise preoperative stratification of patients being considered for deep venous reconstructions or superficial vein ablative procedures. Patients with increased VFIs and normal EFs would theoretically appear to be appropriate candidates for antireflux procedures, whereas those with normal VFIs and diminished EFs would be unlikely to benefit from antireflux surgery.

Air plethysmography has been used as a method of evaluating calf muscle function in patients with CVI. Poor calf muscle pump function, as measured by air plethysmography, has also been shown to independently influence the severity of CVI when corrected for the magnitude and location of lower extremity venous reflux.[30] The technique has been used to document the effects of ankle range of motion on calf muscle pump function in patients with CVI. Ankle range of motion correlated with air plethysmography measurements of EF and RVF and indicated that ankle range of motion and calf muscle function impairment are correlated with a deterioration in the clinical severity of CVI.[31]

Distribution of Venous Reflux

Duplex scanning is now also employed for noninvasive detection and quantification of venous reflux at specific anatomic sites (see Chapter 145). With the patient upright and non–weight bearing, pneumatic cuffs are deflated at different limb levels and reflux velocities are measured with the duplex scanner (Fig. 144–1). Reproducible times to valve closure, venous diameters, peak reflux velocities, and calculated volume flow at peak reflux (VFPR) can be determined at specific locations in both the deep and the superficial venous systems. Ninety-five per cent of normal valves close within 0.5 second of cuff deflation.[32] A high incidence of lipodermatosclerosis has been demonstrated in patients with a cumulative VFPR in the greater saphenous, lesser saphenous, and popliteal venous segments that is greater than 10 ml/sec.[33]

The location of venous reflux also appears to be important in the pathophysiology of CVI. Whereas proximal deep venous reflux has been felt to be of primary importance in the development of venous ulcers, work from a number of centers now indicates that reflux in the popliteal and infrapopliteal veins is more important than more proximal reflux to the development of skin changes and ulcers associated with advanced CVI.[34–36] In addition, venous ulceration can occur with superficial incompetence alone, without accompanying detectable deep venous or communicating vein insufficiency.[37, 38]

Hanrahan and coworkers[35] used duplex scanning to examine the superficial and deep venous systems in 95 ulcerated limbs in 78 patients. Twenty-six of the patients (33%) had a history of DVT. Thirty-four limbs (36%) had incompetence of the popliteal vein. The tibial veins were not evaluated, and 16 of the ulcerated limbs (17%) had only isolated superficial venous incompetence. Depending on the series, 0% to 17% of patients with venous ulceration appear to have reflux limited to the superficial system alone.[34–38]

Moore and associates[36] used duplex scanning to examine the superficial and deep venous segments for sites of valvular reflux in 122 patients with CVI of various degrees of severity. Ninety-three of the 174 symptomatic limbs (53%) had a history of prior DVT. In addition, although 162 of the symptomatic limbs (93%) had evidence of valvular incompetence by duplex examination, so did 41 of the asymptomatic limbs (59%). Ten per cent of limbs with ulceration had isolated superficial venous insufficiency. Reflux in the distal (popliteal-tibial) deep venous system correlated most closely with clinical disease severity.

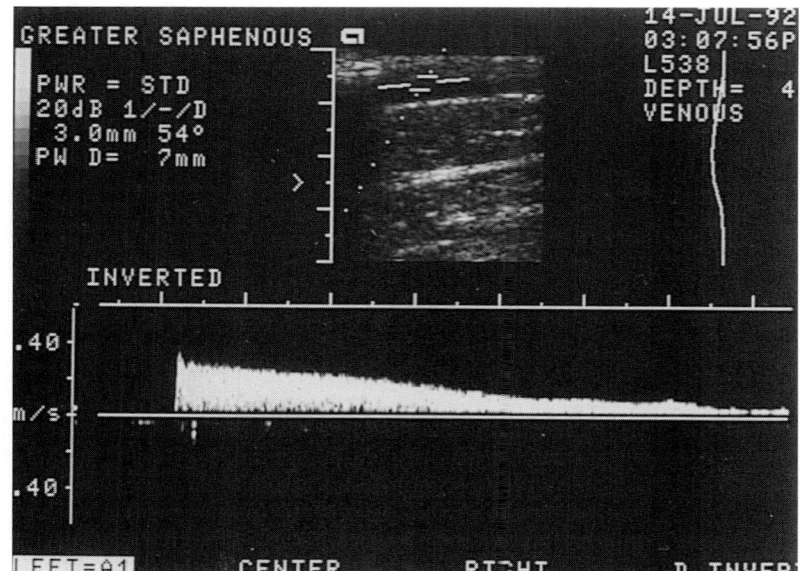

FIGURE 144–1. Immediately after deflation of a leg blood pressure cuff, duplex scanning demonstrates extensive reflux in the greater saphenous vein.

An additional study of 98 consecutive patients (196 limbs) who had CVI of various degrees of clinical severity used phlebography and duplex scanning to evaluate the superficial and deep venous systems.[34] There was a history of DVT in only 13 limbs (7%). Insufficiency of the posterior tibial veins was associated with more severe clinical disease. Valvular insufficiency was demonstrated in multiple asymptomatic limbs. There was, however, no history of venous ulceration in any of the 38 limbs with isolated superficial venous insufficiency.

Perforator Vein Incompetence

Incompetent communicating veins may also be present in patients with a competent deep system.[39] Although communicating veins have long been thought by some to be important in the development of venous ulceration, there has been little proof other than "guilt by association." Data derived from duplex examination of communicating veins in the region of a venous ulcer do, however, indicate communicating vein incompetence in the region of the venous ulcer in up to 86% of ulcers.[40] Communicating vein incompetence may also contribute to ulcer recurrence after vein-stripping procedures.[41]

Therapeutic Considerations of Venous Dysfunction

Duplex scanning offers the potential of tailoring specific venous procedures to the individual patient on the basis of the site and the severity of valvular reflux. For example, a patient with significant venous insufficiency and a combined calculated VFPR of 12 ml/sec, 8 ml/sec of which is present in the superficial veins, may be adequately treated by obliteration of the superficial veins with either sclerotherapy or surgery. Similarly, a patient with a VFPR of 20 ml/sec in the popliteal vein would be unlikely to benefit from a superficial venous procedure alone and is perhaps better treated with deep venous reconstruction or nonoperative therapy.

Patients with communicating vein incompetence in the region of a venous ulcer may be best treated by interruption of incompetent communicating veins. Alternatively, because there is no convincing evidence that communicating vein interruption reverses the skin changes of CVI or decreases the long-term recurrence of venous ulceration, the best candidates for communicating vein interruption may be patients with incompetent communicating veins and early lipodermatosclerosis prior to the onset of venous ulceration. Such scenarios, although attractive, have yet to be subjected to evaluation by appropriate clinical trial.

Natural History of Acute Deep Venous Thrombosis

Several studies have followed up patients with documented DVT to determine the frequency of development of CVI symptoms, the location of valvular dysfunction, and the severity of disease in relationship to the extent and location of the initial thrombosis. In one study, 61 patients (65 limbs) with DVT documented by either contrast or isotope phlebography were followed up at 6-month intervals for 1 to 144 months (mean, 39 months).[42] Patients were evaluated for clinical symptoms or signs of CVI. Photoplethysmographic venous refill times were also determined. Continuous wave venous Doppler examinations were used to demonstrate sites of venous obstruction, venous reflux, or both. No attempt was made to determine recanalization of the originally occluded segments by Doppler examination because of the difficulty in separating venous collaterals from a recanalized segment. Strain-gauge plethysmography was employed to evaluate venous outflow. Forty-one patients (66%) had symptoms of pain, swelling, or both during follow-up. Lipodermatosclerotic skin changes developed in 19 limbs at or during follow-up, and ulcers developed in three of these.

Doppler examination revealed that 39 limbs had deep veins distal to the most proximal site of the previously documented DVT that were either involved in the original occlusion or had developed reflux. Of these limbs with

Doppler-determined distal deep venous abnormalities, 77% were in patients with symptoms of pain, swelling, or both. Eighty-nine per cent of the limbs with lipodermatosclerotic skin changes and all of the limbs with venous ulceration had valvular incompetence or occlusion *distal* to the site of the previous DVT. Venous recovery times were shorter in patients with symptoms than in those who were asymptomatic. No differences were found in maximal venous outflow between symptomatic and asymptomatic patients.

Another series used photoplethysmographically determined VRT and AVPs, in addition to Doppler examination of deep and superficial venous segments, to evaluate 47 patients (54 limbs) with phlebographically determined DVT at 5 and 10 years of follow-up.[43] Seventy-nine per cent of patients were symptomatic, but venous ulceration developed in only two patients. Abnormal venous hemodynamics developed in 83% of patients. Symptoms correlated with the extent of the initial thrombus, and eight of 10 asymptomatic patients had DVT limited to the calf. However, only three of the 10 asymptomatic patients had normal venous hemodynamics.

A third study examined 21 heparin-treated patients with DVT who had duplex scanning at 7, 30, 90, 180, and 270 days after diagnosis of DVT.[44] Evidence of recanalization of the thrombosed venous segments was present in 44% of patients at 7 days, in 94% of patients at 30 days, and in all patients by 90 days after the diagnosis of DVT. The degree of venous segmental occlusion at each observation time was also determined as a percentage of the segments occluded at initial presentation. The percentage of segmental occlusion fell from 93% at 7 days to 14% at 90 to 270 days. Fifty-three per cent of patients underwent recanalization of all occluded segments by 90 days. In three patients, thrombus propagation occurred within the first 7 days and in four patients within 30 and 180 days while they were receiving apparently therapeutic levels of anticoagulation. Valvular incompetence was determined as a percentage of all patent venous segments. At 30 days after the DVT diagnosis, 8% of patent venous segments were incompetent. This figure rose to 25% by 180 days, then remained stable. There was great variability in the development of valvular incompetence, and eight patients had no evidence of valvular incompetence at the end of the 270-day study period.

This important study demonstrates that venous recanalization following DVT generally occurs early, whereas valvular incompetence appears later. It also appears that veins not involved with thrombosis also can become incompetent.[45] Incorporation of venous valves in the thrombotic process therefore may not be the only cause of venous reflux following DVT. In addition, the appearance and localization of valvular insufficiency following DVT in an individual patient appear unpredictable and may relate to the interval between thrombus formation and recanalization.

Conclusion

A large percentage of patients with deep venous insufficiency do not have a known history of DVT. Although deep venous insufficiency is important in the development of CVI,[46] it is not an absolute prerequisite for venous ulcer-

ation, and even lesser saphenous vein insufficiency may result in a venous ulcer.[47] In many patients, subclinical DVT may be cause of deep vein reflux because only an estimated 40% to 50% of above-knee deep vein thrombi and 5% of isolated calf vein thrombi are symptomatic.[48, 49]

It is thus likely that asymptomatic DVT is important in the etiology of CVI, especially since distal valvular incompetence appears most important in the development of clinical symptoms[32, 35, 40] and distal leg vein thrombi are much more likely to be clinically asymptomatic than proximal thrombi. The observation that the development of reflux in individual venous segments does not precisely correlate with the prior location of venous thrombus or the time course of recanalization after known DVT suggests that the mechanisms of the development of valvular incompetence are undoubtedly more complex than simple valvular destruction by organizing thrombi. Valvular incompetence, in some instances, may arise secondary to venous distention resulting from proximal obstruction. Prolonged distention of distal venous segments may result in permanent valvular incompetence after several months of unrelenting distention.[50]

CELLULAR AND MICROCIRCULATORY CONSIDERATIONS

The end-organ in CVI is the skin and subcutaneous tissue. Advanced CVI is characterized by functional and morphologic abnormalities of the cutaneous capillaries and lymphatics. Several theories have been proposed to explain the abnormalities of the cutaneous microcirculation in patients with lipodermatosclerosis or venous stasis ulceration and to link these abnormalities with reflux in the deep venous system, the superficial venous system, or both. Without doubt, the transmission of high venous pressures from the superficial or deep venous systems to the venous end of the cutaneous microcirculation is crucial to the initiation of microcirculatory damage. The end result of microcirculatory abnormalities in CVI is a combination of the disruption of nutrient delivery to the skin and the release of toxic metabolites or enzymes that result in tissue destruction.

Venous Endothelium

Microcirculatory capillary endothelial cells are morphologically and functionally altered in CVI. The endothelial cells have increased pinocytic vesicles, a more irregular surface, and a widening of the interendothelial space from a normal of 15 nm up to 180 nm, all suggesting low-grade endothelial injury.[51–53] Increased production of the inflammatory mediators intracellular adhesion molecule (ICAM) and interleukin-1 has also been demonstrated in the capillary endothelial cells in patients with CVI.[53, 54] A pro-inflammatory response is also suggested by lymphocyte and monocyte infiltration in the skin of patients with CVI. These mononuclear cells, normally required for wound healing, have diminished function in CVI.[55]

The etiology of diminished mononuclear cell function in the skin of CVI patients is unclear but suggests diminished capacity for cellular proliferation in CVI, perhaps explaining, in part, the difficulty of healing a venous ulcer. Other investigators have also noted that dermal fibroblasts have a decreased response to cytokines and growth factors associated with normal wound healing.[56]

Arteriovenous Shunting

The oldest microcirculatory theory of venous ulceration comes from gross observations at the time of vein stripping. "Arterial" bleeding as well as pulsations within varicose veins at the time of operation led to the proposal that small arteriovenous fistulae were a cause of CVI. It was postulated that microarteriovenous fistulae transmitted arterial pressure to the veins, leading to increased vascular permeability. This in turn induced abnormalities in the skin and subcutaneous capillaries that adversely affected tissue nutrition. The potential existence of such fistulae is supported by measurements of relatively high oxygen saturations in blood from varicose veins.[57] In addition, skin temperature is higher in limbs with varicose veins than in control limbs.[58] Finally, several radiologic studies have suggested an abnormally early venous phase during arteriography in patients with varicose veins.[59, 60]

Despite these historical studies, no recent data support the existence of microcirculatory arteriovenous fistulae in patients with CVI. Conversely, radiolabeled albumin has been used to measure the percentage of total shunt volume referable to the lower extremities. No difference has been found between patients with varicose veins and controls.[61] Arteriovenous fistula is no longer widely accepted as the primary mechanism of the cutaneous alterations associated with CVI. The presence of such fistulae has never been demonstrated with ultrastructure studies.

Capillary Circulation

Initial histologic studies of the perimalleolar skin and subcutaneous tissues in patients with CVI revealed an apparent increase in capillary number.[62] More recently, with the advent of videomicroscopy, these same capillary beds can be examined in vivo. Videomicroscopic studies reveal tortuous perimalleolar capillaries in patients with CVI. The absolute number, however, is similar to that in normal skin. The discrepancy between standard histologic studies and videomicroscopic examination may be a sectioning artifact in preparing the histologic specimens. In vivo microscopy studies also reveal areas of capillary microthrombosis in lipodermatosclerotic skin[63] and reductions in capillary numbers in areas of prior ulceration (atrophie blanche).[64] These data suggest that actual destruction of the cutaneous nutrient circulation may contribute to venous ulceration and recurrence.

Lymphatic Circulation

Videomicroscopic results of cutaneous lymphatics are also abnormal in patients with CVI. (FITC)–dextran is a dye that can be injected into the subdermal space and observed with videomicroscopic techniques.[65] The dye fills the cutaneous lymphatic network and renders the cutaneous lymphatics visible as an interlacing network. Anatomic lymphatic abnormalities are not present in skin without trophic

changes but are easily observed in areas of induration and hyperpigmentation. In areas of damaged skin, the number of visible collecting channels is decreased and the lymphatic network is disrupted.[64]

The Fibrin Cuff Theory

Studies of the skin microcirculation in CVI indicate that diffusion abnormalities may be important in the development of lipodermatosclerosis. Burnand and associates[66] used implanted Guyton capsules[67] in the subcutaneous tissue to sample the interstitial fluid of canine hindlimbs in an animal model of venous hypertension. Radiolabeled sodium, albumin, and fibrinogen (selected for their increasing molecular weights) were injected intravenously. After circulation and diffusion times were allowed for, the contents of the Guyton capsules were aspirated and the radiolabeled substrates were assayed. Of the three molecules, fibrinogen was the only one found at higher concentrations within the interstitium of venous hypertensive limbs than within control limbs, suggesting a diffusion abnormality in CVI that increases large molecule capillary permeability.

Additional evidence of a diffusion abnormality in CVI is suggested by capillary videomicroscopy. Diffusion patterns of sodium fluorescein in patients with CVI and control subjects have been examined with appropriate filters, video techniques, and densitometric analysis of light intensity.[68–70] Compared with those of controls, the cutaneous capillaries of patients with CVI developed much larger fluorescing pericapillary cuffs ("halos") after intravenous injection of sodium fluorescein, suggesting increased transcapillary diffusion in these patients (see Fig. 144–2). These halos likely represent pericapillary edema. When they are punctured with appropriate microsurgical techniques, the halos decrease dramatically in size.[64]

The major theory of venous ulcer pathogenesis that depends in large part on capillary diffusion abnormalities is the so-called fibrin cuff theory.[71] It is postulated that semiocclusive pericapillary fibrin cuffs result from leakage of fibrinogen into the interstitium. These cuffs then act as a barrier to oxygen and nutrient diffusion to interstitial tissues and cutaneous skin cells. These cuffs, however, are more complex than originally thought.[72] They appear to be composed not solely of fibrin but of a number of extracellular matrix proteins that can serve as potent chemoattractants and leukocyte and platelet activators and conceivably may serve as the basis for the chronic inflammatory response in CVI noted previously.

Less fibrinolytic activity has been observed within vein walls of patients with varicose veins than within controls.[73] Lotti and associates[74] demonstrated less plasma fibrinolytic activity in patients with CVI and lipodermatosclerosis than in controls. In addition, studies in canine models of limb venous hypertension have documented increased pericapillary fibrin deposition and increased lymphatic concentration of fibrinogen.[75] Skin biopsy specimens from patients with CVI and lipodermatosclerosis have demonstrated pericapillary fibrin deposition.[76] The presence of fibrin cuffs in CVI thus appears well documented. The importance of these cuffs in producing tissue hypoxia is more controversial. Investigators thus far have been unable to conclusively

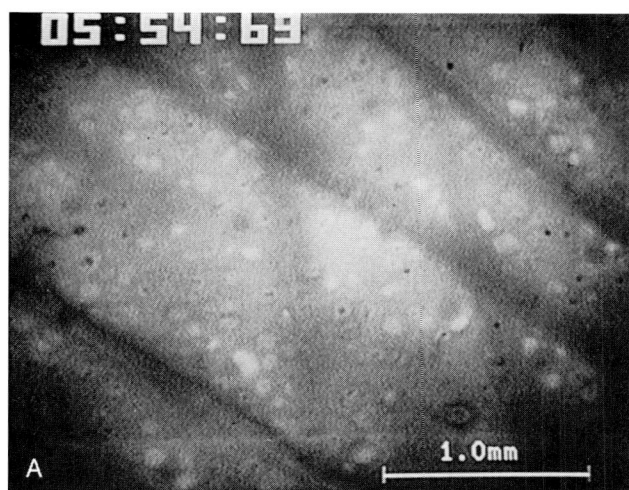

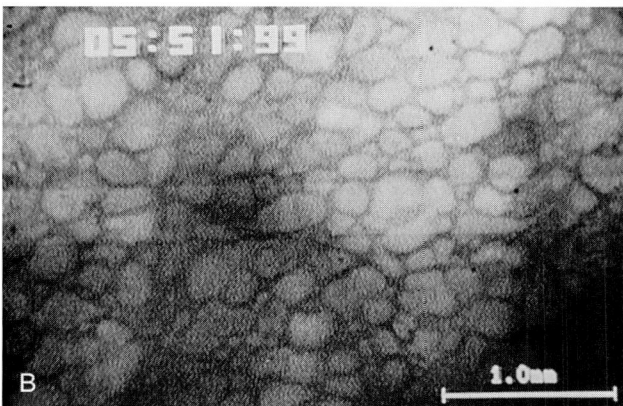

FIGURE 144-2. *A,* Normal capillary video microscopy findings after intravenous fluorescein injection. Note the uniform small pericapillary "halos" containing the fluorescein tracer. *B,* Abnormal capillary video microscopy findings after intravenous fluorescein injection in a patient with chronic venous insufficiency and lipodermatosclerosis. Note the irregular-sized large pericapillary halos containing the fluorescein tracer. (From Nehler MN, Moneta GL, Porter JM: The lower extremity venous system: II. The pathophysiology of chronic venous insufficiency. Perspect Vasc Surg 5:89, 1992.)

demonstrate hypoxia of the perimalleolar tissues in patients with CVI.

Tissue Hypoxia

Biochemical markers of ischemia have been reported in patients with CVI. Magnetic resonance spectroscopy of radiolabeled phosphate (phosphorus 31) from gastrocnemius muscle biopsy specimens was used to evaluate levels of creatine phosphate, adenosine triphosphate (ATP), adenosine diphosphate (ADP), and inorganic phosphate as a measure of muscle energy stores in seven patients with symptomatic CVI.[77] All specimens demonstrated flattened spectral waveforms in the high-energy phosphate region, with increased spectral peaks in the low-energy phosphate region. Evidence of muscle atrophy was noted in each specimen on histologic sectioning. Despite the small sample size, these data are at least suggestive of a potential biochemical defect in cellular oxidative metabolism of the limb in patients with CVI.

Radioactively labeled oxygen (oxygen-15), a short-lived photon-emitting isotope, has been used during positron emission tomography (PET) to investigate oxygen levels in limbs of patients with CVI. Patterns of photon emission are mapped, permitting calculations of the original molecular distribution within the tissue. Eleven patients with venous stasis ulceration and five patients with lipodermatosclerosis underwent lower extremity PET.[78] Regional blood flow was markedly *increased* in areas of venous ulceration, with reduced oxygen extraction at the same sites. This suggests an oxygen diffusion defect with resultant tissue hypoxia, although the study does not exclude the possibility of a defect in tissue oxygen delivery.

Multiple reports have described transcutaneous oxygen measurements of the lower extremity in various conditions. Transcutaneous partial pressure oxygen ($tcPo_2$) is measured during heat-induced local hyperemia. Unfortunately, the techniques of obtaining perimalleolar $tcPo_2$ measurements in patients with CVI have not been consistent. By convention, $tcPo_2$ measurements are made with the probe heated to 43°C. Under these conditions, the $tcPo_2$ in the perimalleolar skin of CVI patients with venous ulcers is lower than normal.[79-81] However, when measurements of $tcPo_2$ are made with the unheated electrode, $tcPo_2$ is higher in limbs with CVI and venous ulcers than in controls.[82] There is no widely accepted explanation for these seemingly disparate findings. Perhaps low oxygen tensions detected with the heated sensor represent a deficiency in microvascular regulation that may act to prevent effective capillary recruitment and nutrient delivery in lipodermatosclerotic skin. There is some precedent for this reasoning because attenuated skin blood flow responses to hyperemia have also been demonstrated in patients with diabetes mellitus.[83]

A measure of local cutaneous blood flow can be obtained with laser Doppler flowmetry.[84] The scattering of laser light across skin capillary beds is measured using the Doppler principle. A baseline laser Doppler flux tracing is generated, and any deviations above or below the baseline are considered a measure of increased or decreased net cutaneous blood flow in the area examined by the probe. Flux depends on both the velocity and concentration of red cells moving within the area sampled by the laser Doppler probe.

Patients with CVI have higher levels of resting laser Doppler flux in perimalleolar skin than do normal controls.[85] This appears to be due to higher concentrations of red blood cells in the area sampled by the probe.[86] Interestingly, both leg elevation and external compression—treatment modalities associated with healing of venous ulcers—result in increases in microcirculatory flow velocities in patients with CVI.[87, 88]

Cheatle and associates[89] used laser Doppler flowmetry to examine skin blood flow in the limbs of 17 controls and 17 patients with CVI and lipodermatosclerosis. With the use of inflatable cuffs of varying pressures, periods of arterial and venous occlusion were produced. Patients with CVI and lipodermatosclerosis showed no hyperemic response after 3 minutes of arterial occlusion, whereas areas of normal skin in the same patients demonstrated attenuated hyperemia. Control limbs also demonstrated attenuated hyperemia after 30 minutes of venous occlusion, possibly indicating that the changes in vascular regulation seen in patients with CVI can be reproduced in normals with periods of induced venous hypertension. These findings may partially explain the results of tcPo$_2$ measurements. Perhaps patients with CVI have resting hyperemia, compared with controls, and are unable to recruit additional capillaries in response to stimuli that provoke a normal hyperemic response.

Local Neural Control

There is also evidence of abnormal activation of local neural control mechanisms within the subcutaneous microcirculation in CVI. A local sympathetic axonal reflex, the venoarteriolar reflex, results in microvascular vasoconstriction in response to venous pressures above 25 mmHg.[90] Normally, this reflex is abolished by activation of the calf muscle pump and reduction in venous pressure.

In addition, axonal nociceptive C-fibers appear to be abnormal in CVI. These fibers are responsible both for transmitting pain sensation to the central nervous system, thereby preventing repetitive trauma to areas of injury, and for stimulating the release of vasodilator neuropeptides that act as growth factors for epidermal cells and fibroblasts.[91] Laser Doppler flowmetry was used to study C-fibers in 15 older patients with venous ulcers.[92] Vasodilatation was measured by determining changes in skin blood flow in response to either electrical stimulation or chemical stimulation with topical acetylcholine or nitroprusside and was compared in patients with CVI and controls. Patients with CVI demonstrated an attenuated electrically stimulated (neurogenic) vasodilatory response when compared with controls. There were no detectable differences in response to local stimulation by acetylcholine and nitroprusside between patients with CVI and controls.

Because baseline foot skin blood flow was not significantly different between the two groups, it appears that the components of the cutaneous vasodilatory response mediated by nociceptive C-fiber input are dysfunctional in patients with severe CVI. This may contribute to venous ulceration by making the patient less sensitive to local trauma and diminishing vasodilator neuropeptides that could act as growth factors to stimulate healing after injury.

The Theory of White Blood Cell Trapping

The most recent theory of venous ulceration to attract widespread interest suggests that white blood cell trapping within the skin microcirculation is important in venous ulceration. The proposed mechanism is that white blood cells become trapped in the microcirculation of patients with CVI, leading to microvascular congestion and thrombosis. The trapped white blood cells migrate into the interstitium and release lysosomal enzymes, resulting in tissue destruction. It was originally observed that venous blood from dependent limbs of normal subjects had proportionately lower white blood cell counts than did venous blood from the same limbs in the supine position.[93] Approximately 20% of white blood cells, predominantly monocytes, are lost in lower extremity venous effluent after 40 minutes of dependency, suggesting that limb dependency results in microcirculatory white blood cell trapping or

leakage into the interstitium. Additional work suggests that venous hypertension results in upregulation and expression of leukocyte adhesion molecules. These permit adherence of leukocytes to the capillary endothelial cells, the first step in trapping the white blood cells within the cutaneous microcirculation of CVI patients.[94]

Patients with CVI have confirmed lower numbers of white blood cells in femoral venous samples after 30 minutes of lower limb dependency than in control limbs.[95, 96] As noted previously, Bollinger and Leu,[63] using capillary microscopy, also described capillary microthrombosis in the perimalleolar skin of patients with CVI that may be secondary to sludging of white blood cells in the cutaneous microcirculation.

Work by Scott and associates[97] is compatible with these data. These workers used capillary microscopy to examine the perimalleolar skin in 10 patients with CVI, both with patients supine and after 30 minutes of limb dependency. In addition, femoral vein blood was obtained at the time of microscopy examination. After the dependent interval, there were fewer visible capillary loops on videomicroscopy in nine of the 10 patients. Loss of visible capillary loops correlated with decreases in femoral vein white blood cell counts. Other investigators have also demonstrated that lipodermatosclerotic skin biopsy specimens taken from patients with CVI and a history of ulceration reveal significantly more white blood cells per cubic millimeter than do biopsy specimens from controls (217 versus 6.2 cells/mm^3),[97] presumably because of increased trapping of white blood cells within the microcirculation and the resultant migration into the interstitium.

SUMMARY

No single proposed mechanism adequately explains all the observed changes within the macrocirculation or microcirculation of patients with CVI. Venous hypertensive effects are clearly much more complex than previously realized. It appears, however, that venous hypertension transmitted to the cutaneous microcirculation results in a set of interrelated cellular, microangiopathic, and functional abnormalities that together result in the end-point of lipodermatosclerosis and venous ulceration. Improving the treatment of CVI will depend on increased detailed understanding of these complex relationships.

REFERENCES

1. Brand FN, Dannenberg AL, Abbott RD, Kannel WB: The epidemiology of varicose veins: The Framingham study. Am J Prev Med 4:96, 1988.
2. Jamieson WG: State of the art of venous investigation and treatment. Can J Surg 36:119, 1993.
3. Scott TE, La Morte WW, Gorin DR, et al: Risk factors for chronic venous insufficiency: A dual case-control study. J Vasc Surg 22:622, 1995.
4. Criado E, Johnson G Jr: Venous disease. Current Problems 28:339, 1991.
5. Nelzen O, Bergqvist D, Lindhagen A: Leg ulcer etiology: A cross-sectional population study. J Vasc Surg 14:557, 1991.
6. Baker SR, Stacey MC, Jopp-McKay AG, et al: Ulcers. Br J Surg 78:864, 1991.

7. Cornwall JV, Dore CJ, Lewis JD: Leg ulcers: Epidemiology and aetiology. Br J Surg 73:693, 1986.

8. Callum M, Ruckley CV, Harper DR, et al: Chronic ulceration of the leg: Extent of the problem and provision of care. Br Med J 29:1855, 1985.

9. Miller WL: Chronic venous insufficiency. Cardiovasc Clin 22:67, 1992.

10. Ruckley CV, Dale JJ, Callum MJ, et al: Causes of chronic leg ulcer. Lancet 2:615, 1982.

11. Lees TA, Lambert D: Prevalence of lower limb ulcers in an urban health district. Br J Surg 79:1032, 1992.

12. Coon WW, Willis PW, Keller JB: Venous thromboembolism and other venous disease in the Tecumseh community health study. Circulation 48:839, 1973.

13. Margolis DJ, Cohen JH: Management of chronic venous leg ulcers: A literature guided approach. Clin Dermatol 12:19, 1994.

14. Biland L, Widmer LK: Varicose veins (VV) and chronic venous insufficiency (CVI): Medical and socio-economic aspects, Basle study. Acta Chir Scand Suppl 544:9, 1988.

15. Madar G, Widmer LK, Zemp E, Maggs M: Varicose veins and chronic venous insufficiency—a disorder or disease? A critical epidemiological review. Vasa 15:126, 1986.

16. Phillips T, Stanton B, Provan A, et al: A study of the impact of leg ulcers on quality of life: Financial, social, and psychologic implications. J Am Acad Dermatol 31:49, 1994.

17. Callam MJ, Harper DR, Dale JJ, Ruckley CV: Chronic ulcer of the leg: Clinical history. Br Med J 294:1389, 1987.

18. Baker SR, Stacey MC, Jopp-Mckay AG, et al: Epidemiology of chronic venous ulcers. Br J Surg 78:864, 1991.

19. Callam MJ, Harper DR, Dale JJ, Ruckley CV: Chronic leg ulceration: Socioeconomic aspects. Scott Med J 33:358, 1988.

20. Browse NL, Burnand KG, Thomas ML: Diseases of the Veins: Pathology, Diagnosis and Treatment. London, Hodder and Stoughton, 1988.

21. Abenhaim L, Kurx X, and VEINES Study Collaborators: The VEINES Study: An international cohort study on chronic venous disorders of the leg. Angiology 48:59, 1997.

22. Clarke GH: Venous elasticity. Doctoral Thesis, University of London, London 1989.

23. Clarke H, Smith SR, Vasdekis SN, et al: Role of venous elasticity in the development of varicose veins. Br J Surg 76:577, 1989.

24. Clarke GH, Vasdekis SN, Hobbs JT, Nicolaides AN: Venous wall function in the pathogenesis of varicose veins. Surgery 111:402, 1992.

25. Nicolaides AN, Zukowski AJ: The value of dynamic pressure measurements. World J Surg 10:919, 1986.

26. Raju S, Fredericks R: Valve reconstruction procedures for nonobstructive venous insufficiency: Rationale, techniques, and results in 107 procedures with two- to eight-year follow-up. J Vasc Surg 7:301, 1988.

27. Randhawa GK, Dhillon JS, Kistner RL, Ferries EB: Assessment of chronic venous insufficiency using dynamic venous pressure studies. Am J Surg 148:203, 1984.

28. Christopoulos D, Nicolaides AN, Cook A, et al: Pathogenesis of venous ulceration in relation to the calf muscle pump function. Surgery 106:829, 1989.

29. Christopoulos DG, Nicolaides AN, Szendro G, et al: Air plethysmography and the effect of elastic compression on venous hemodynamics of the leg. J Vasc Surg 3:49, 1986.

30. Araki CT, Back TL, Padberg FT, et al: The significance of calf muscle pump function in venous ulceration. J Vasc Surg 20:872, 1994.

31. Back TL, Padberg FT, Araki CT, et al: Limited range of motion is a significant factor in venous ulceration. J Vasc Surg 22:519, 1995.

32. van Bemmelen PS, Bedford G, Beach K, Strandness DE: Quantitative segmental evaluation of venous valvular reflux with duplex ultrasound scanning. J Vasc Surg 10:425, 1989.

33. Vasdekis SN, Clarke GH, Nicolaides AN: Quantification of venous reflux by means of duplex scanning. J Vasc Surg 10:670, 1989.

34. Rosfors S, Lamke LO, Nordstrom E, Bygdeman S: Severity and location of venous valvular insufficiency: The importance of distal valve function. Acta Chir Scand 156:689, 1990.

35. Hanrahan LM, Araki CT, Rodriguez AA, et al: Distribution of valvular incompetence in patients with venous stasis ulceration. J Vasc Surg 13:805, 1991.

36. Moore DJ, Himmel PD, Sumner DS: Distribution of venous valvular incompetence in patients with the postphlebitic syndrome. J Vasc Surg 3:49, 1986.

37. Sethia KK, Darke SG: Long saphenous incompetence as a cause of venous ulceration. Br J Surg 71:754, 1984

38. Hoare MC, Nicolaides AN, Miles CR, et al: The role of primary varicose veins in venous ulceration. Surgery 92:450, 1982.

39. Burnand KG, O'Donnell TF, Thomas ML, Browse NL: The relative importance of incompetent communicating veins in the production of varicose veins and venous ulcers. Surgery 82:9, 1977.

40. Labropoulos N, Giannoukas AD, Nicolaides AN, et al: New insights into the pathophysiologic condition of venous ulceration with color-flow duplex imaging: Implications for treatment? J Vasc Surg 22:45, 1995.

41. Linton RR, Hardy IB: Postthrombotic syndrome of the lower extremity: Treatment by interruption of the superficial femoral vein and ligation and stripping of the long and short saphenous veins. Surgery 24:452, 1948.

42. Strandness DE, Langlois Y, Cramer M, et al: Long-term sequelae of acute venous thrombosis. JAMA 250:1289, 1983.

43. Lindner DJ, Edwards JM, Phinney ES, et al: Long-term hemodynamic and clinical sequelae of lower extremity deep vein thrombosis. J Vasc Surg 4:436, 1986.

44. Killewich LA, Bedford GR, Beach KW, Strandness DE: Spontaneous lysis of deep venous thrombi: Rate and outcome. J Vasc Surg 9:89, 1989.

45. Caps MT, Manzo RA, Bergelin RO, et al: Venous valvular reflux in veins not involved at the time of acute deep venous thrombosis. J Vasc Surg 22:524, 1995.

46. Welch HJ, Young CM, Semegran AB, et al: Duplex assessment of venous reflux and chronic venous insufficiency. The significance of deep venous reflux. J Vasc Surg 24:755, 1996.

47. Bass A, Chayen D, Weinmann EE, et al: Lateral venous ulcer and short saphenous vein insufficiency. J Vasc Surg 25:654, 1997.

48. Oster G, Tuden RL, Colditz GA: A cost-effective analysis of prophylaxis against deep-vein thrombosis in major orthopedic surgery. JAMA 257:203, 1987.

49. Lagerstedt CI, Fagher BO, Olsson CG, et al: Need for long-term anticoagulant treatment in symptomatic calf-vein thrombosis. Lancet 2:515, 1985.

50. van Bemmelen PS: Venous Valvular Incompetence: An Experimental Study in the Rat. Alblasserdam, The Netherlands, Offsetdrukkerij Kanters BV, 1984.

51. Leu HJ: Morphology of chronic venous insufficiency: Light and electron microscopic examinations. Vasa 20:330, 1991.

52. Wenner A, Leu HJ, Spycher M, et al: Ultrastructural changes of capillaries in chronic venous insufficiency. Exp Cell Biol 48:1, 1980.

53. Coleridge Smith PD: The role of white cell trapping in the pathogenesis of venous ulceration. Phlebol Dig 4:4, 1992.

54. Veraart JCJM, Verhaegh MEJM, Neumann HAM, et al: Adhesion molecule expression in venous leg ulcers. Vasa 2:243, 1993.

55. Pappas PJ, Teehan EP, Fallek SR, et al: Diminished mononuclear cell function is associated with chronic venous insufficiency. J Vasc Surg 22:580, 1995.

56. Hasan A, Murata H, Falabella A, et al: Dermal fibroblasts from venous ulcers are unresponsive to the action of transforming growth factor-3. J Dermatol Sci 16:59, 1997.

57. Blalock A: Oxygen content of blood in patients with varices. Arch Surg 19:898, 1929.

58. Haeger KH, Bergman L: Skin temperature of normal and varicose legs and some reflections on the aetiology of varicose veins. Angiology 14:473, 1963.

59. Piulachs P, Vidal-Barraquer E: Pathogenic study of varicose veins. Angiology 4:59, 1953.

60. Haimovich H: Abnormal arteriovenous shunts associated with chronic venous insufficiency. J Cardiovasc Surg 17:473, 1976.

61. Lindemayer W, Lofferer O, Mostbeck A, Partsch H: Arteriovenous shunts in primary varicosis? A critical essay. Vasc Surg 6:9, 1972.

62. Burnand KG, Whimster I, Clemenson G, et al: The relationship between the number of capillaries in the skin of the venous ulcer-bearing area of the lower leg and the fall in foot vein pressure during exercise. Br J Surg 68:297, 1981.

63. Bollinger A, Leu AJ: Evidence for microvascular thrombosis obtained by intravital fluorescence videomicroscopy. Vasa 20:252, 1991.

64. Leu AJ, Leu H-J, Franzeck UK, et al: Microvascular changes in chronic venous insufficiency: A review. Cardiovasc Surg 3:237, 1995.

65. Bollinger A, Jager K, Sgier F, et al: Fluorescence microlymphography. Circulation 64:1195, 1981.

66. Burnand KG, Clemenson G, Whimster I, et al: The effect of sustained venous hypertension on the skin capillaries of the canine hind limb. Br J Surg 69:41, 1982.

67. Guyton AC: Interstitial fluid pressure: II. Pressure-volume curves of interstitial space. Circ Res 16:452, 1965.

68. Hasselbach P, Vollenweider U, Moneta G, Bollinger A: Microangiopathy in severe chronic venous insufficiency evaluated by fluorescence video-microscopy. Phlebology 1:159, 1986.

69. Bollinger A, Jager K, Geser A, et al: Transcapillary and interstitial diffusion of Na-fluorescein in chronic venous insufficiency with white atrophy. Int J Microcirc Clin Exp 1:5, 1982.

70. Fagrell E: Local microcirculation in chronic venous incompetence and leg ulcers. Vasc Surg 13:217, 1979.

71. Burnand KG, Whimster I, Naidoo A, Browse NL: Pericapillary fibrin in the ulcer-bearing skin of the leg: The cause of lipodermatosclerosis and venous ulceration. Br Med J 285:1071, 1982.

72. Herrick SE, Sloan P, Mcgurk M, et al: Sequential changes in histologic pattern and extracellular matrix deposition during the healing of chronic venous ulcers. Am J Pathol 141:1085, 1992.

73. Wolf JH, Morland M, Browse NL: The fibrinolytic activity of varicose veins. Br J Surg 66:185, 1979.

74. Lotti T, Chimenti M, Bianchini G, et al: Cutaneous and plasmatic fibrinolytic activity in the subject of stasis dermatitis. Ital Gen Rev Dermatol 20:9, 1983.

75. Leach RD, Browse NL: Effect of venous hypertension on canine hind limb lymph. Br J Surg 72:275, 1985.

76. Vanscheidt W, Laaf H, Wokalck H, et al: Pericapillary fibrin cuff: A histologic sign of venous ulceration. J Cutan Patho 17:266, 1990.

77. Taheri SA, Pollack L, Loomis R: P-31-NMR studies of muscle in patients with venous insufficiency. Int Angiol 6:95, 1987.

78. Hopkins NF, Spinks TJ, Rhodes CG, et al: Positron emission tomography in venous ulceration and liposclerosis: Study of regional tissue function. Br Med J 286:333, 1983.

79. Clyne CA, Ramsden WH, Chant AD, Webster JH: Oxygen tension on the skin of the gaiter area of limbs with venous disease. Br J Surg 72:644, 1985.

80. Mani R, White JE, Barrett DF, Weaver PW: Tissue oxygenation, venous ulcers and fibrin cuffs. J R Soc Med 82:345, 1989.

81. Franzeck UK, Bollinger A, Huch R, Huch A: Transcutaneous oxygen tension and capillary morphology characteristics and density in patients with chronic venous incompetence. Circulation 70:806, 1984.

82. Dodd HJ, Gaylarde PM, Sarkany I: Skin oxygen tension in venous insufficiency of the lower leg. J R Soc Med 78:373 1985.

83. Rayman G, Williams SA, Spencer PD, et al: Impaired microvascular response to minor skin trauma in type 1 diabetes. Br Med J 292:1295, 1986.

84. Tenland T: On laser Doppler flowmetry: Methods and microvascular applications. Linkoping Studies in Science and Technology Dissertations. 1982, p 83.

85. Partsch H: Hyperaemic hypoxia in venous ulceration. Br J Dermatol 110:249, 1984.

86. Sindrup JH, Avnstorp C, Steenfos HH, et al: Transcutaneous Po2 and laser Doppler blood flow measurements in 40 patients with venous leg ulcers. Acta Derm Venereol 67:160, 1987.

87. Abu-Own A, Scurr JH, Coleridge Smith PD: Effect of leg elevation on the skin microcirculation in chronic venous insufficiency. J Vasc Surg 20:705, 1994.

88. Abu-Own A, Shami SK, Chittendon SJ, et al: Microangiopathy of the skin and the effect of leg compression in patients with chronic venous insufficiency. J Vasc Surg 19:1074, 1994.

89. Cheatle TR, Coleridge Smith PD, Scurr JH: Skin microcirculatory responses in chronic venous insufficiency: The effect of short term venous hypertension. Vasa 20:63, 1991.

90. Henriksen O: Local sympathetic reflex mechanism in regulation of blood flow in human subcutaneous adipose tissue. Acta Physiol Scand Suppl 450:7, 1977.

91. Dalsgaard CJ, Haltgardh-Nilsson A, Haegerstrand A, Nilsson J: Neuropeptides as growth factors: Possible role in human diseases. Regul Pept 25:1, 1989.

92. Ardron ME, Helme RD, McKernan S: Microvascular skin responses in elderly people with varicose leg ulcers. Age Ageing 20:124, 1991.

93. Moyses C, Cederholm-Williams SA, Michel CC: Haemoconcentration and accumulation of white cells in the feet during venous stasis. Int J Microcirc Clin Exp 5:311, 1987.

94. Thomas PR, Nash GB, Dormandy JA: White cell accumulation in dependent legs of patients with venous hypertension: A possible mechanism for trophic changes in the skin. Br Med J 290:1693, 1988.

95. Thomas PR, Nash GB, Dormandy JA: Increased white cell trapping in the dependent legs of patients with chronic venous insufficiency. J Mal Vasc 15:35, 1990.

96. Saharay M, Shields DA, Porter JB, el al: Leukocyte activity in the microcirculation of the leg in patients with chronic venous disease. J Vasc Surg 25:265, 1997.

97. Scott HJ, Coleridge Smith PD, Scurr JH: Histologic study of white blood cells and their association with lipodermatosclerosis and venous ulceration. Br J Surg 78:210, 1991.

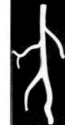

CHAPTER 1 4 5

A Practical Approach to the Diagnosis and Classification of Chronic Venous Disease

Robert L. Kistner, M.D., and Elna M. Masuda, M.D.

While the field of chronic venous disease has undergone important changes in diagnostic techniques and in treatment modalities over the past 25 years, standardization in diagnosis has not yet been achieved. The criteria that define a proper diagnosis are that it be (1) accurate in identifying the pathologic problem and (2) definitive in ruling out conditions that are not present. To be practical, it should be appropriate to the patient's clinical setting and it should achieve accuracy within that setting by including tests needed to identify the problem and avoiding those that have no value. The purpose of this chapter is to examine the diagnostic evaluation of the patient with chronic venous disease and how it can achieve the goals set forth earlier. The technical details of the different diagnostic tests are discussed in Chapters 11 and 13.

Treatment modalities for chronic venous disease today

vary from simple external support of the extremity to complex venous reconstructions for both reflux and obstructive problems. The variety of treatment options increases the importance of accurate, thorough diagnosis, which is necessary not only to select an appropriate treatment for a given patient but also to be able to compare results of different therapies. For instance, the currently important subject of perforator vein surgery requires accurate diagnosis to determine the relative efficacy of ligation of incompetent perforating veins, when the deep system is competent or when it is incompetent.[1, 2] It is essential to know the cause of the disease (primary or secondary), its distribution in the affected extremity, and its pathophysiologic mechanism (reflux or obstruction) because these data guide in the treatment and in analysis of results.

When the only treatment option that will be considered is external support, we have only to identify that the problem is due to venous disease, rather than to some other cause. This can be accomplished with the history and physical examination findings, supplemented by the hand-held, continuous wave Doppler or photoplethysmography, all studies that can be performed entirely in the office. These data are frequently sufficient to identify the venous system as the basis of the problem but do not identify the causes, mechanisms, or the segmental locations that are involved. This limited evaluation is appropriate for incapacitated patients or those with a limited life expectancy, for whom the future development of progressive venous insufficiency is of no importance.

In most patients, it is necessary to determine the specific cause, anatomic distribution, and pathophysiologic mechanisms, which requires that testing progress from the office into the vascular laboratory. When endovascular intervention or reconstructive venous surgery is planned, more invasive evaluation including contrast-enhanced venography, is needed. With increasing complexity of the treatment methods, the need for accurate and thorough evaluation of the entire venous tree requires every bit as much detail as does arterial diagnosis before surgical revascularization.

Figure 145–1 shows varicose veins, skin discoloration, and ulceration in a limb. The possible underlying conditions that might have produced this state are multiple and include:

1. Varicose veins due to primary disease of the greater saphenous vein.

2. Varicose veins (as in No. 1) plus perforator incompetence of the thigh or calf, or of both.

3. Varicose veins (as in No. 1) plus perforator incompetence (as in No. 2) plus deep vein reflux due to primary valvular incompetence.

4. Varicose veins plus perforator incompetence plus post-thrombotic reflux or obstruction, or both, in the deep veins.

5. Varicose veins plus perforator incompetence and post-thrombotic changes in the lower extremity plus post-thrombotic occlusion of the iliac veins.

If surgical treatment is planned for the patient in Figure 145–1, it is clear that definitive testing would be necessary. Since the office diagnosis is inadequate to differentiate between the possible causes, the diagnostic process must involve vascular laboratory tests, the most useful of which

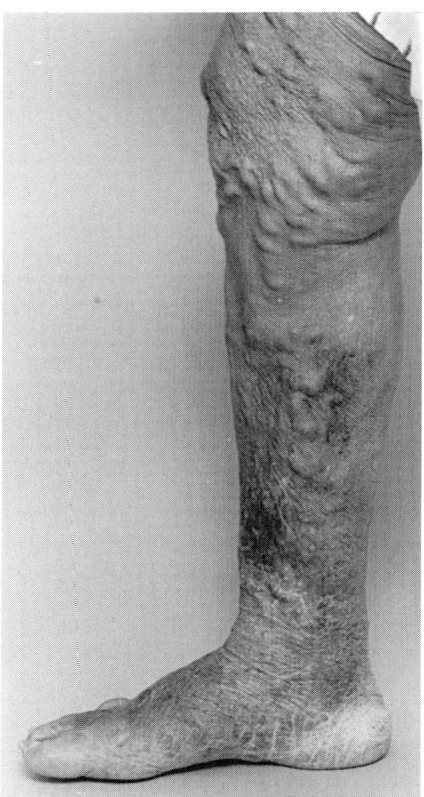

FIGURE 145–1. This photograph shows a typical "post-thrombotic" leg, but the disease may have many other causes. This illustrates the need for accurate CEAP (i.e., class, etiology, anatomical distribution, pathomechanism) classification of chronic venous disease.

is the duplex ultrasound scan. Duplex ultrasonography identifies sites of reflux and obstruction and localizes the process to the venous segments that are involved. To quantify the extent of reflux or of obstruction, plethysmography by one of several techniques (air, strain-gauge, or photoplethysmography) can provide additional data. In obstructive states, venous pressure studies are used to estimate the physiologic importance of venous occlusion. With more complicated problems, the differentiation of primary from secondary disease is aided by ascending and descending venography. For the best map of the veins in the extremity, ascending venography is the "gold standard" and is very helpful in planning surgical procedures. Descending venography is required to identify the location of valve sites.

Computed tomography (CT) is performed in patients with proximal venous occlusion to exclude pelvic lesions (tumor, retroperitoneal fibrosis). Magnetic resonance imaging has been used with increasing frequency to identify primary or secondary venous tumors and vascular malformations associated with acute or chronic venous disease.

CEAP CLASSIFICATION

In consideration of the diagnostic needs of patients with chronic venous disease, an international group of experts met in 1994 under the auspices of the American Venous

TABLE 145–1. CLINICAL CLASSIFICATION OF CHRONIC VENOUS DISEASE*

Class 0: No visible or palpable signs of venous disease
Class 1: Telangiectases or reticular veins
Class 2: Varicose veins
Class 3: Edema
Class 4: Skin changes ascribed to venous disease (e.g., pigmentation, venous eczema, lipodermatosclerosis)
Class 5: Skin changes, as defined above, with healed ulceration
Class 6: Skin changes, as defined above, with active ulceration

Modified from The Consensus Group: Classification and grading of chronic venous disease in the lower limbs. A consensus statement. Vasc Surg 30:5–11, 1996.
*The presence or absence of symptoms such as pain or aching, as contrasted to the signs listed above, which are enumerated as classes 1 through 6, is denoted by a (asymptomatic) or s (symptomatic), to modify the class description.

Forum and devised the CEAP classification. [2] This classification was designed to define the clinical class (C) and the etiology (E) of the problem, its anatomic (A) distribution in the veins of the extremity; and its pathologic mechanism (P) of development (reflux or obstruction, or both; Tables 145–1 through 145–5). According to signs of chronic venous disease, patients are assigned to one of seven clinical classes (C_{0-6}):

- No signs of venous disease (C_0)
- Telangiectasias and spider veins (C_1)
- Varicose veins (C_2)
- Edema due to venous disease (C_3)
- Skin changes and lipodermatosclerosis (C_4)
- Healed ulcers (C_5)
- Active (C_6) venous ulcers

The document also provides a severity rating scale (Table 145–6) and a disability scale (Table 145–7) for affected patients.

At first glance, the CEAP method may seem too complex for routine use, but with practice it becomes a familiar process, well organized and worth the effort. To make this classification practical, the diagnostic methods need to be adapted to the severity of the problem being addressed. With a simple problem such as telangiectasia or straightforward varicose veins, the definitive diagnosis can frequently be made quickly in the office after the history and physical examination, supplemented with the hand-held Doppler examination if needed (level I diagnosis) In most patients, level II diagnostic tests are needed in the vascular laboratory and, as discussed earlier, candidates for interventions require level III investigations with contrast venography (Table 145–8). These levels of testing represent increasing complexity, expense, and risk. While they add certainty

TABLE 145–2. ETIOLOGIC CLASSIFICATION

Congenital	(E_c)
Primary	(E_p), undetermined cause
Secondary	(E_s), known cause
Post-thrombotic	
Post-traumatic	
Other	

Modified from The Consensus Group: Classification and grading of chronic venous disease in the lower limbs. A consensus statement. Vasc Surg 30:5–11, 1996.

TABLE 145–3. ANATOMIC CLASSIFICATION

Superficial	(A_s)
Perforator	(A_p)
Deep	(A_d)

Modified from The Consensus Group: Classification and grading of chronic venous disease in the lower limbs. A consensus statement. Vasc Surg 30:5–11, 1996.

to the diagnosis, they must be justified by the need for accuracy.

INITIAL OFFICE VISIT

At the first visit, the diagnosis begins with identification of the clinical problem, followed by determination of the patient's health status and occupation and way of life. The effect of the venous problem on the patient's life should be identified and used to determine how to proceed with the workup (Table 145–9). The impact of the problem could be categorized as follows:

- *Cosmetic only*—may include spiders, varicose veins, swelling, or pigmentation pain or disability of any sort
- *Annoyance*—includes mild aching and swelling that is not severe enough to alter the way of life or the activity level but still adequate to prompt an office visit and a desire for treatment
- *Lifestyle limitation*—may be mild (e.g., the need to wear stockings) or severe (e.g., the need to change occupation or other accustomed aspects of daily life)

Painful, extensive ulceration may lead to significant disability.

TABLE 145–4. EIGHTEEN ANATOMIC SEGMENTS

	NO.	SEGMENT
Superficial Veins (A_s)		Telangiectases/reticular veins
	1	Greater (long) saphenous
	2	Above knee
	3	Below knee
	4	Lesser (short) saphenous
	5	Nonsaphenous
Deep Veins (A_d):		
	6	Inferior vena cava
		Iliac
	7	Common
	8	Internal
	9	External
	10	Pelvic/gonadal, broad ligament, other
		Femoral
	11	Common
	12	Deep
	13	Superficial
	14	Popliteal
	15	Crural: anterior tibial, posterior tibial, peroneal (all paired)
	16	Muscular: gastrocnemius, soleus, other
Perforating Veins (A_p)		
	17	Thigh
	18	Calf

Modified from The Consensus Group: Classification and grading of chronic venous disease in the lower limbs. A consensus statement. Vasc Surg 30:5–11, 1996.

TABLE 145–5. PATHOPHYSIOLOGIC CLASSIFICATION*

Reflux	(P_R)
Obstruction	(P_O)
Reflux and obstruction	$(P_{R,O})$

Modified from The Consensus Group: Classification and grading of chronic venous disease in the lower limbs. A consensus statement. Vasc Surg 30:5–11, 1996.

*The elements of reflux and obstruction may be reported by using the anatomic segments in Table 145–3 to accurately define the extent of the process, segment by segment. Alternatively, obstruction can be simplified by using familiar segmental regions of occlusion, namely caval, iliac, femoral, popliteal, and crural (respectively designated P_{O-CAV}, P_{O-I}, P_{O-F}, P_{O-P}, P_{O-C}).

Along with this estimation of the impact of the clinical status on the patient's lifestyle, the initial visit includes the physical examination and a continuous-wave hand-held Doppler examination, and from these data the outline of an appropriate diagnostic workup is tailored to the individual.

DIAGNOSIS

Testing

Diagnostic testing varies with the clinical setting. After the office examination, testing usually begins in the vascular laboratory with the duplex scan, which is the single most useful test of chronic venous disease.

Plethysmography and venous pressure testing may be added to quantitate the extent of reflux or obstruction. These tests often raise new questions about the type or distribution of disease or its potential for repair, and these questions prompt venography.

Ascending venography is the best method of producing a map of the extremity veins and of distinguishing primary from secondary disease. Distorted veins, excessive collaterals, and intraluminal defects are pathognomonic for post-thrombotic disease, and their absence suggests primary valvular incompetence. Although the presence of reflux is established by duplex scanning, the distinction between primary and secondary causes of reflux is not adequately made by duplex scan in many cases. *Ascending* venography is helpful for differentiating primary from secondary disease, and *descending* venography is needed to show the sites and the competence of individual valves. Perforator vein incompetence and size can be determined by duplex study

TABLE 145–6. CLINICAL SEVERITY*

Pain	0 = none; 1 = moderate, not requiring analgesics
	2 = severe, requiring analgesics
Edema	0 = none; 1 = mild/moderate; 2 = severe
Venous claudication	0 = none; 1 = mild/moderate; 2 = severe
Pigmentation	0 = none; 1 = localized; 2 = extensive
Lipodermatosclerosis	0 = none; 1 = localized; 2 = extensive
Ulcer size (largest)	0 = none; 1 = <2 cm diameter; 2 = >2 cm
Ulcer duration	0 = none; 1 = <3 mo; 2 = >3 mo
Ulcer recurrence	0 = none; 1 = once; 2 = more than once
Ulcer number	0 = none; 1 = single; 2 = multiple

Modified from The Consensus Group: Classification and grading of chronic venous disease in the lower limbs. A consensus statement. Vasc Surg 30:5–11, 1996.

*This schema can be simplified to denote severity of symptom/sign; thus 0 = absent; 1 = mild, moderate (localized, single); 2 = severe (extensive, multiple).

TABLE 145–7. DISABILITY SCORE

0	Asymptomatic
1	Symptomatic, can function without support device
2	Can work 8-hour day *only* with support device
3	Unable to work even with support device

Modified from The Consensus Group: Classification and grading of chronic venous disease in the lower limbs. A consensus statement. Vasc Surg 30:5–11, 1996.

and checked with ascending venography if the venography is performed in a manner tailored to show perforators.

Classification

Diagnostic evaluation of patients is discussed according to the clinical classes of the CEAP classification. Examples of the acronyms of different conditions written in CEAP terms are presented at the end of the chapter.

Class 1: Telangiectasias or Reticular Veins

Telangiectasias and spider veins are frequent cosmetic problems that do not interfere with the patient's occupation or way of life, although there are exceptions. The examination generally can be done in the office. It consists of history, physical examination, and continuous wave, hand-held, Doppler scanning to search for occult reflux in the saphenous and deep veins. When reflux is found, further duplex scanning is usually justified.

Class 2: Varicose Veins

Evaluation of varicose veins requires a search for valvular incompetence in both the greater and lesser saphenous veins, the perforating veins, and the deep veins. This is first done with the hand-held Doppler device in the office. As the veins are examined, the Doppler imager traces the greater saphenous vein up the thigh, checking for Valsalva-induced reflux. Finger occlusion of the proximal saphenous vein can determine whether all of the reflux is coming from the saphenofemoral junction or whether perforator or pelvic veins contribute to the reflux. The saphenopopliteal junction is checked in a somewhat similar fashion, and the deep veins are checked for reflux or obstructive disease. This testing is done with the patient positioned semi-erect or standing. When saphenous reflux is found, effective, long-term therapy requires control of the reflux by high ligation, usually with stripping; when saphenous reflux is

TABLE 145–8. TESTING FOR VARIOUS LEVELS OF CHRONIC VENOUS DISEASE

Level 1 *Office visit diagnosis*
   History and physical examination, continuous wave Doppler ultrasonography

Level 2 *Vascular laboratory diagnosis*
   Duplex scan, plethysmography (air, strain-gauge or photoplethysmography), venous pressure measurements

Level 3 *Invasive radiologic testing*
   Ascending venography, descending venography, iliocavography, varicography

TABLE 145–9. STEPS IN DIAGNOSIS OF CHRONIC VENOUS DISEASE

1. Determine the nature of the problem.
2. Determine the severity of the problem.
3. Perform diagnostic testing.
4. Determine CEAP classification.
5. Weigh treatment alternatives.

CEAP = clinical class, etiology, anatomic distribution, and pathologic mechanism.

absent, sclerotherapy of the varices or local phlebectomy is definitive treatment.

Etiology

Varicose veins are most frequently classified as *primary* venous disease (see Table 145–2). *Secondary* varicosities include post-thrombotic lesions and varicose veins due to an arteriovenous fistula or nonthrombotic proximal venous occlusion. Patients with congenital malformations have persistent varicose embryonic superficial veins. Although pure post-thrombotic disease in the saphenous vein is possible, in most cases, superficial thrombophlebitis develops on a background of primary disease when a segment of the dilated vein becomes thrombosed.

Anatomy (see Tables 145–3 and 145–4)

The sources of venous reflux can be estimated by Doppler imaging, but duplex scanning is needed to identify the actual sites of reflux (deep, superficial, perforator).

Pathophysiology (see Table 145–5)

In primary disease, the pathophysiologic problem is limited to reflux. Obstruction in superficial veins occurs as a result of previous episodes of thrombophlebitis or surgical interruption.

Testing Methods

When saphenous vein reflux is found by Doppler examination and the patient is a surgical candidate, a duplex scan is used to define the saphenous anatomy and search for other sites of reflux, such as incompetent perforator veins. In patients with primary varicosity, plethysmography provides information on venous function, but venous pressure measurements and venography are reserved for suspected deep venous occlusion or other unusual congenital or acquired venous problems.

Class 3: Edema

A discussion of the full differential diagnosis of edema transcends this chapter, but attention to the venous causes of edema is appropriate. The history taking and physical examination are more complex than for class 1 or 2 disease because both local and systemic causes of edema need to be considered. Unilateral edema is the main sign that directs attention to the veins and lymphatics of the extremity.

For class 3 problems, the CEAP system requires definition of etiology, anatomic divisions, and pathophysiologic involvement in the segments to be complete. Primary reflux or post-thrombotic obstruction or reflux, or both, may be present. Reflux in the superficial, perforator, or deep veins, or in any combination of these may cause edema. Some

cases are due to pure reflux, others to obstruction, and many to a combination.

Etiology

Edema may be due to primary, secondary, or congenital causes, and at least duplex scanning in the vascular laboratory is necessary to make the distinction. For patients who give a history of thrombophlebitis, it is important to determine how the diagnosis was established in the first place and to check the duplex findings for clues to earlier thrombophlebitis. Some clues are distorted deep veins that have intraluminal defects, segments of occlusion or stenosis, collateral vessels, and thickening of the walls of the veins with loss of wall compliance. Sometimes it is possible to differentiate between primary and secondary disease until venography is done.

Anatomy

Persons with chronic venous disease require duplex scanning to rule out deep—and proximal and distal—sites of reflux or obstruction that might cause edema. Various venography techniques may be helpful, including radionuclide venography for the iliofemoral and caval anatomy and contrast venography for definitive preoperative study. Neither venous pressure nor plethysmography is of much help in defining the anatomy.

Pathophysiology

Distinguishing reflux from obstruction is important in the study of edema, and is frequently accomplished by duplex scanning. With primary disease there is only reflux, but with post-thrombotic or congenital disease there may be both reflux and obstruction, and it can be difficult to determine which is physiologically dominant. Plethysmography is very useful for differentiating reflux from obstruction. In general, for estimating reflux, it is quite sensitive, whereas for estimating obstruction it is not very sensitive.

When obstruction plays a significant role, venous pressure measurements are useful for demonstrating sustained venous hypertension at the pedal, femoral, or popliteal level. The determination of pedal venous pressure and femoral venous pressure has been widely practiced and studied,[6] whereas the arm-foot measurement has been advocated by Raju.[9]

Testing Methods

Edema can be a simple annoyance or a debilitating condition that causes people to change their occupation. The sophistication of the evaluation will be tailored to the potential treatment. For instance, if external support and lifestyle accommodation will be the prescription regardless of the findings, there is little to be gained by doing any tests beyond the office examination or a duplex scan. When the problem is more severe, and especially when it affects the patient's occupation or lifestyle, definitive study begins with duplex scanning and proceeds through the other vascular laboratory and venographic steps until the explanation is found. If definitive surgery is an option, a full venous evaluation in the vascular laboratory and by venography may be worthwhile.

Class 4: Skin Changes
Class 5: Healed Ulcer
Class 6: Active Ulcer

With the appearance of skin changes due to chronic venous disease comes advanced-stage disease. Skin changes cover a wide range: stasis discoloration due to pigmentation from diapedesis of red blood cells; thickening of dermal and subdermal tissues that progresses to sclerosis of these tissues; and, ultimately, the ulcerative state. Lipodermatosclerosis is often complicated by inflammation of these tissues that contributes to the local problem. From physiologic testing it has become clear that there is no discernible difference between the severity of the venous dysfunctions associated with, respectively, advanced skin changes and ulcerations.[13] The following comments that apply to class 4 disease apply also to classes 5 and 6.

Diagnosis of class 4, 5, or 6 disease requires a thorough history to search for prior deep venous thrombosis, problems with swelling or varicose veins (to indicate long-standing primary venous disease), or earlier trauma that might have caused bleeding in the leg but left dark discoloration that is not at all related to venous disease.[4] The physical examination should differentiate thickening and sclerosis of the leg from simple discoloration and should identify sites of lipodermatosclerosis. Tenderness over subcutaneous fascial defects may reveal perforator veins that are incompetent. The Doppler examination in the office seeks deep, perforator and superficial reflux or obstruction, and sites of perforator reflux. Ulcers, active or healed, may indicate perforators that are incompetent in those sites.

Etiology

Skin changes may be due to primary, secondary, or congenital causes. The evaluation for a cause begins with the duplex scan. Special attention to the perforators is warranted when searching for the cause of skin discoloration or lipodermatosclerosis, because perforators are frequently involved and may be due to either primary or secondary disease. Because of the difficulty of identifying all of the tibial veins, especially when they are distorted by disease, venography is often more reliable than duplex scanning in establishing the etiology.

Anatomy

Duplex scan is always needed to achieve a definitive study of the anatomic abnormalities that give rise to skin changes, and venography is often needed to add certainty to the diagnosis established by Duplex scanning. Although the venous Doppler examination and palpation of the leg for perforators are useful tests in skilled hands, they are not definitive studies of sites and causes of venous disease.

Pathophysiology

Although the assignment of reflux or obstruction to the anatomic segments of the leg is done largely by duplex scanning, venography is frequently necessary for confirmation. Knowledge is only now evolving about which segments and divisions of the leg veins need to be involved to give rise to advanced chronic skin changes. It is becoming clear that involvement of multiple divisions (superficial, perforator, deep) and segments are more conducive to advanced changes in the skin than are isolated changes in any one site.[3, 5] Skin changes require careful evaluation, because many cases of dark, discolored skin and thickening of the skin are due to trauma or hematoma rather than to chronic venous disease.

Testing Methods

Vascular laboratory testing by duplex scan determine:

- Primary reflux or post-thrombotic disease
- The sites of the reflux and obstructions in the deep, perforator, and superficial veins
- Whether the patient is a candidate for repair of one or more of these problems

When disease is limited to the saphenous and perforator veins, duplex scanning is often the definitive test. Additional evaluation by plethysmography, venous pressure measurement, and venography should be done selectively for those who might be candidates for surgical intervention. Plethysmography is helpful for many reasons. One of these is that any obstruction on plethysmography is strong evidence of post-thrombotic disease.

While duplex scan usually distinguishes between primary and post-thrombotic disease, there are exceptions, and for such cases venography is needed to tell the difference. In some cases, even ascending venography findings are inconclusive. Then, descending venography is needed to identify the sites and leakage pattern of refluxing primary valves, in preparation for surgical repair.

WRITING THE CEAP ACRONYM

The CEAP classification can be expressed as an acronym that summarizes the result of the diagnostic evaluation of chronic venous disease. The composition of the acronym for routine clinical use is determined by noting each of the clinical classes present in a given case (e.g., C2, C3, C4). This is followed by the subscript for symptomatic (s) or asymptomatic (a) patients; the indication for etiology, Ep (primary) or Es (secondary); and by the anatomic divisions involved As,p,o (superficial, perforator, deep). Finally, the pathophysiologic mechanism of reflux (Pr) or obstruction (Po) is assigned to the segments involved by disease (see Tables 145–1 through 145–5).

The CEAP classification in class 1 disease is simple. It denotes only the class number and any symptoms by using the modifiers (s) for symptomatic and (a) for asymptomatic. The acronym *C1 (a) or C1 (s)* is a definitive CEAP for class 1.

An example of the diagnostic acronym for varicose veins with swelling, skin discoloration, and active ulcer due to varicosity of the greater saphenous vein, perforator reflux in the calf, and primary reflux in the superficial femoral and popliteal veins is as follows:

CEAP: C2,3,4,6 (s)—Ep–As,p,d—Pr2.3,13,14,18.

C2,3,4,6 reflects the presence of varicose veins (2) with edema (3) and skin changes (4) and an active ulcer (6). *Ep* reflects that the cause is primary. *As,p,d* describes involve-

				RIGHT	LEFT
CLINICAL	No visible sign of venous disease		0		
	Telangiectases or reticular		1		
	Varicose veins		2		
	Edema		3		
	Skin changes		4		
	Skin changes + healed ulcer		5		
	Skin changes + active ulcer		6		
	ASYMPTOMATIC		A		
	SYMPTOMATIC		S		

				RIGHT	LEFT
ETIOLOGIC	Congenital (at birth or later)		C		
	Primary (undetermined cause)		P		
	Secondary (PTS, Other)		S		

					RIGHT	LEFT
ANATOMIC	SUPERFICIAL	T&RV	S	1		
		GSV Above knee		2		
		GSV Below knee		3		
		LSV		4		
		Non Saphenous		5		
	DEEP	Inf vena cava	D	6		
		Common Iliac		7		
		Internal Iliac		8		
		External Iliac		9		
		Pelvic, Gonadal, Broad lig, other		10		
		Common Femoral		11		
		Deep Femoral		12		
		Superficial Femoral		13		
		Popliteal		14		
		Crural (ant tib, post tib, peroneal)		15		
		Muscular, gastrocnemial, soleal		16		
	PERFORATING VEINS	Thigh	P	17		
		Calf		18		

			RIGHT	LEFT
PATHOPHYSIOLOGY	Reflux	R		
	Obstruction	O		
	Both	RO		

CEAP Classification:

RIGHT	LEFT

A

FIGURE 145–2. *See legend on opposite page*

CLINICAL SCORE			RIGHT	LEFT
PAIN	None	0		
	Moderate, no analgesics	1		
	Severe, analgesics required	2		
EDEMA	None	0		
	Mild, Moderate	1		
	Severe	2		
V CLAUDICATION	None	0		
	Mild, Moderate	1		
	Severe	2		
PIGMENTATION	None	0		
	Localized	1		
	Extensive	2		
LIPODERMATOSCLEROSIS	None	0		
	Localized	1		
	Extensive	2		
ULCER, SIZE	None	0		
	<2 cm diam	1		
	>2 cm diam	2		
ULCER, DURATION	None	0		
	<3 Months	1		
	>3 Months	2		
ULCER, RECURRENCE	None	0		
	Once	1		
	More than once	2		
ULCER NUMBER	None	0		
	Single	1		
	Multiple	2		
TOTAL CLIN SCORE				
ANATOMIC SCORE	(Number of segments 1-13)			

			RIGHT	LEFT
DISABILITY SCORE	Asymptomatic	0		
	Symptomatic, works without support	1		
	8 h/day only W/support	2		
	Unable to work	3		

Severity (CAD) Score:

(C#A#D#=Total Score)

RIGHT	LEFT

B

FIGURE 145–2. This worksheet is a convenient way to record the CEAP (i.e., class, etiology, anatomical distribution pathomechanisms) classification (A) and the scoring of clinical severity (B). CAD = clinicoanatomic disability; s = superficial; D = deep, P = perforating; V = vein; t = telangiectasis; R = reticular; LSV = lesser saphenous vein; GSV = greater saphenous vein. (Courtesy of J. Jerome Guex, M.D., and Michel Perrin, M.D., by personal communication.)

ment of the superficial (s), perforator (p), and deep (d) veins. Pr2,3,13,14,18 describes reflux in the greater saphenous vein of the thigh (2) and calf (3), and in the superficial femoral (13) and popliteal (14) veins of the deep system, and in the perforator veins of the calf (18).

For class 3, 4, 5, or 6 disease, the following acronyms can be used: C 3 or 4 or 5 or 6 (a) or (s)—E ɔ or s—As,p, and/or d—Pr or o, followed by description of the anatomic segments (see Table 145–4).

The CEAP classification can be used for longitudinal study of the individual case by adding a date to indicate the day it was determined. At a future time, after an interval treatment, or after a change in the patient's condition, a new CEAP determination can be made and compared with the patient's original status.

A useful method of estimating the reliability of the CEAP determination is to indicate the levels and methods of testing used to arrive at the CEAP (Table 145–8). For instance, the clinical class can be accurately determined by the office visit, but to be reliable, the etiology, pathophysiology, and anatomic distribution require more sophisticated testing in the vascular laboratory. In advanced cases when questions are left unanswered by the vascular laboratory studies, ascending and descending venography add confirmation and clarity. This is especially useful for differentiating between primary and secondary reflux (as the duplex scan can be misleading) and for identifying venous valves and estimating their functional integrity.

SEVERITY SCORING

A useful adjunct was developed at the creation of the CEAP classification when the committee devised a scoring system for venous problems (see Table 145–7). Its purpose is to indicate the severity of the condition at a given point in time so that it can be used to study outcome by repeating the severity scoring at intervals, such as after treatment, or after a given time interval. The method devised by Guex and Perrin in France is a handy way to make this estimation when the patient is seen in the office for evaluation and follow-up (Fig. 145–2).

DISABILITY SCORING

The CEAP classification contains a simple disability rating scale (see Table 144–7) that demonstrates the overall effect on the patient of the venous problem. In this scale, the categories are related to the patient's ability to perform accustomed activities and to whether external compression is needed to achieve an "active" rating.

DISCUSSION

Physicians have been slow to recognize that diagnosis of chronic venous disease carries the same requirements that diagnosis in arterial disease imposes. The idea that an examiner can tell what is wrong with the veins inside the extremity just by looking at external signs is manifestly erroneous, just as it is not possible to identify arterial lesions by looking at an ischemic foot. In each case, it is necessary to visualize the vessels and to determine pressures and flow channels—and, in this way, the cause of the problem and the site where physiologic processes are altered.

It is curious to speculate why disease in the veins has not been carefully identified in the past. The answer probably lies in the nature of venous disease, which is bothersome and at times serious but rarely threatens limb or life. This is a major difference from arterial disease, which has such serious sequelae. The second reason is the reluctance through the years to perform definitive venography for chronic venous disease because it is painful, expensive, and has some risk of complications. There has grown a mystique that venous disease is somehow not understandable because of variations in anatomy and because of the great capacity for collateralization and compensation found in the veins.

Now is the time to change these concepts, because the noninvasive ultrasound technology has opened up the veins to inspection in situ, and ways have been developed to surgically treat most reflux and many occlusive problems. In ulcer disease, which is regarded as the most serious manifestation of chronic venous disease, thorough investigation of the veins has shown that at least 70% of such lesions can be treated surgically with good and long-lasting results. This is because 30% to 50% of venous ulcers are due to primary reflux disease localized to the superficial and perforator veins, and most of these can be successfully treated by conventional surgery. For an additional 30% of ulcers, primary deep vein disease can be surgically repaired with a 75% chance of long-term success (extending beyond 8 to 15 years).[7, 8, 10, 11] Vein transplantation and transposition are useful in selected cases of post-thrombotic reflux, and cross-pubic bypass is successful for as many as 75% of iliac vein occlusions. These cases will be discovered—and treated—only when the diagnostic approach to chronic venous disease becomes objective and thorough. The CEAP approach is a big step in that direction.

Some say that definitive diagnosis of chronic venous disease is too complicated to be practical. This statement is true for physicians who limit their treatment to bandaging and prescriptions of salves, antibiotics, rest, and lifestyle alterations. For those who desire to forge ahead to specific treatment of the problems of chronic venous disease, the disease processes can now be catalogued in an orderly, scientific manner by thorough diagnosis and classification.

REFERENCES

1. Burnand K, O'Donnell T, Lea MT, Browse NL: Relationship between post-phlebitic changes in deep veins and results of surgical treatment of venous ulcers. Lancet I:936–938, 1976.
2. Gl*oviczki P, Bergan JJ, Menawat SS, et al: Safety, feasibility, and early efficacy of subfascial endoscopic perforator surgery (SEPS): A preliminary report from the North American Registry. J Vasc Surg 25:94–105, 1997.
3. Hanrahan LM, Araki CT, Rodrigues AA, et al: Distribution of valvular incompetence in patients with venous stasis ulceration. J Vasc Surg 13:805–811, 1991.

4. Kistner RL: Definitive diagnosis and definitive treatment in chronic venous disease: A concept whose time has come. J Vasc Surg 24:703–710, 1996.
5. Labropoulos N, Giannoukas AD, Nicolaides AN, et al: New insights into the pathophysiologic condition of venous ulceration with color-flow duplex imaging: Implications of treatment. J Vasc Surg 22:45–50, 1995.
6. Labropoulis N, Leon M, Geroulakos G, et al: Venous hemodynamic abnormalities in patients with leg ulceration. Am J Surg 169:572–574, 1995.
7. Lurie F: Results of deep-vein reconstruction. Vasc Surg 31:275–276, 1997.
8. Masuda E, Kistner RL: Long-term results of venous valve reconstruction: A 14- to 21-year follow-up. J Vasc Surg 19:391–403, 1994.
9. Raju S: New approaches to the diagnosis and treatment of venous obstruction. J Vasc Surg 4:42–54, 1986.
10. Raju S, Fredericks RK, Neglen PN, Bass JD: Durability of venous valve reconstruction techniques for "primary" and postthrombotic reflux. J Vasc Surg 23:357–367, 1996.
11. Sottiurai VS: Results of deep-vein reconstruction. Vasc Surg 31:276–278, 1997.
12. The Consensus Group: Classification and grading of chronic venous disease in the lower limb: A consensus statement. Vasc Surg 30:5–11, 1996.
13. Welch HJ, Faliakou EC, McLaughlin RL, et al: Comparison of descending phlebography with quantitative photoplethysmography, air plethysmography, and duplex quantitative valve closure time in assessing deep venous reflux. J Vasc Surg 16:913–919, 1992.

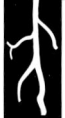

CHAPTER 146
Nonoperative Treatment of Chronic Venous Insufficiency

Gregory L. Moneta, M.D., and John M. Porter, M.D.

Nonoperative therapy has been the basic treatment for chronic venous insufficiency (CVI) and venous ulceration for decades. Elevation of the lower extremities that includes the feet above the thighs when one is sitting and above the heart when one is supine is nearly universally accepted as effective treatment for venous ulceration. It is, however, impractical for most patients, especially employed persons, as anything but a short-term solution to a refractory or enlarging ulcer. The goals of nonoperative therapy for venous ulceration are to promote healing of existing ulcers and prevent recurrence while allowing the patient to maintain a normal ambulatory status. Nonoperative therapy is highly effective in controlling symptoms of CVI and promoting healing of venous ulcers. Healing, however, can be prolonged and in some cases painful. Recurrence of venous ulceration after healing remains a significant problem.

COMPRESSION THERAPY

Compression therapy remains the primary treatment for CVI despite progress in both ablative[1] and reconstructive[2, 3] venous surgery. The actual mechanism by which compression therapy obviates the adverse effects of venous hypertension on the skin and subcutaneous tissues remains unknown. Many studies, however, have focused on the possible venous hemodynamic effects of compression therapy. Some investigators using either invasive or noninvasive techniques have shown no change in ambulatory venous pressure (AVP) or venous recovery time (VRT) with compression therapy.[4–6] Others have reported statistically significant improvements in AVP and VRT with compression therapy.[7–12] Even in reports suggesting improved hemodynamics with compression, detected changes are often small and AVP measurements are rarely normalized.

Another possible explanation for the benefits of compression therapy is a direct effect on subcutaneous interstitial pressures. Increased interstitial pressure counteracts transcapillary Starling's forces and promotes fluid resorption and resolution of edema with improved diffusion of nutrients to the skin and subcutaneous tissues. Several studies have examined the skin microcirculation in limbs with CVI after the resolution of edema following compression therapy. Skin capillary density, as determined by videomicroscopy (see Chapter 144), predictably increases after edema reduction.[13] Several authors have demonstrated an increase in skin transcutaneous oxygen pressure ($tcPo_2$) after edema reduction,[14, 15] with others unable to demonstrate a significant change in skin $tcPo_2$ after edema removal by pneumatic compression.[16]

Elastic Compression Stockings

Jobst invented gradient ambulatory compression therapy in the 1950s after personally suffering for years from venous ulceration.[17] He observed that his leg symptoms were alleviated when he stood upright in a swimming pool. He therefore designed the first ambulatory gradient compression hosiery to mimic hydrostatic forces exerted by water in a swimming pool (Fig. 146–1). Forty years later, the use of ambulatory compression hosiery remains the primary

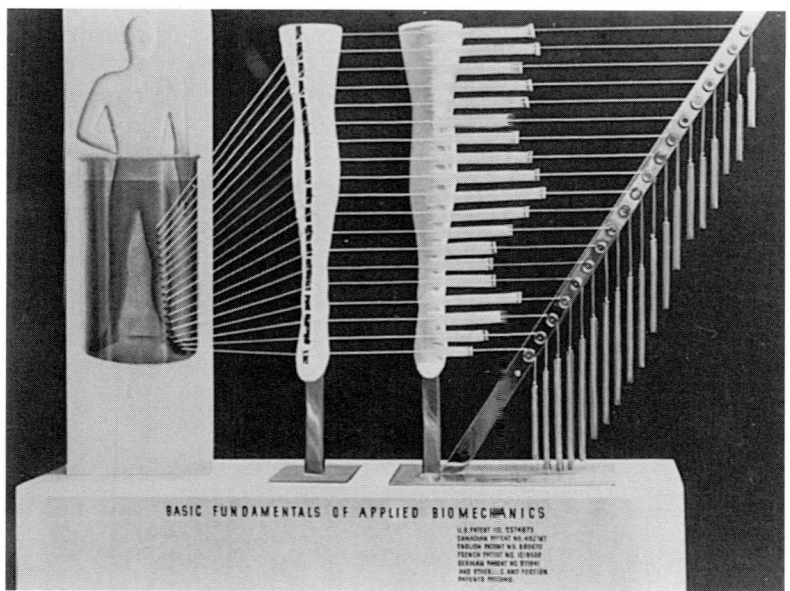

FIGURE 146–1. Model demonstrating the effect of hydrostatic pressure on the lower extremity in a water tank and its relationship to gradient compression hosiery. The pressure obtained by each is represented by the weights of various sizes, with the largest located at the ankle. (From Bergan JJ: Conrad Jobst and the development of pressure gradient therapy for venous disease. In Bergan JJ, Yao JS [eds]: Surgery of the Veins. Orlando, Fla, Grune & Stratton, 1985, pp 529–540.)

treatment of CVI. Manufacturers provide elastic compression stockings of various strengths, compositions, and lengths.

Many reports demonstrate benefit of compression stockings in the treatment of CVI and venous ulceration.[18–20] At the authors' institution, venous ulceration is treated primarily with local wound care and elastic compression therapy.[21] Patients with venous ulcers are first assessed for the presence of infection and the extent of lower extremity edema. When necessary, a period of bed rest of 5 to 7 days is prescribed to help resolve the edema. Cellulitis is treated with short-term intravenous or oral antibiotics in conjunction with local wound care (dry gauze dressings changed every 12 hours). When the edema or cellulitis has resolved, patients are fitted with below-knee 30- to 40-mmHg elastic compression stockings. Two pairs are prescribed to permit laundering on alternate days. Patients are instructed to wear the stockings at all times while they are ambulatory and to remove them on going to bed.

Wound care throughout the course of compression therapy consists of a simple daily washing of the ulcer with soap and water. Topical corticosteroids may be applied to surrounding areas of significant stasis dermatitis, but they are not applied to the ulcer itself. Other topical agents are avoided. The ulcer is covered with a dry gauze dressing held in place by the compression stocking. Once the ulcer has healed, the patient is instructed to continue ambulatory compression therapy.

One hundred thirteen patients were treated over 15 years (from 1975 to 1990). Of these patients, 102 (90%) were compliant with stocking use, and 105 (93%) experienced complete ulcer healing, with a mean healing time of 5.3 months. Seventy-three patients had long-term follow-up (mean, 30 months), and 58 (79%) adhered to the recommendation of perpetual ambulatory compression therapy. The total ulcer recurrence in patients who were compliant with long-term therapy was 16%. Recurrence was 100% in patients who were noncompliant with long-term therapy. Recurrence was not related to previous ulceration, previous venous surgery, or arterial insufficiency.[21]

Erickson and colleagues[22] also examined the effects of failure to comply with the use of elastic stockings following healing of a venous ulcer. Follow-up of 91 patients with healed venous ulcers revealed that 56% recurred at a median of 10.4 months following initial healing. Age, sex, diabetes, ankle-brachial index (ABI), toe pressure, evidence of DVT by duplex ultrasound, original ulcer location, area, quantity, depths, or photoplethysmography (PPG)-derived VRTs were not associated with recurrence. Total recurrence was, however, higher in patients who were not compliant with the use of elastic stockings after healing (60%) versus those who were compliant with the use of stockings after healing (37%).[22]

Several problems have been recognized with compression therapy for venous ulcers. The most noteworthy is poor patient compliance.[23] Often patients have hypersensitive skin in the lipodermatosclerotic area adjacent to the ulcer or at the site of a previously healed ulcer. These patients can be initially intolerant of the sensation of compression. Frequently, the stockings can be worn only for brief periods during the initial phase of therapy. When beginning therapy, patients should be instructed to wear elastic compression stockings for only as long as tolerable (perhaps only 10 to 15 minutes at first) and to increase gradually the time they wear them. Occasionally, patients may initially need to be fitted with a lesser degree of compression (20 to 30 mmHg).

Many weak, elderly, or arthritic patients have difficulty applying elastic stockings. In a study of 166 patients with leg ulcers, presumably predominantly venous ulcers, attempts were made to treat with elastic stockings. The patients were mostly women (69%) and elderly (mean age, 72 years). Fifteen per cent were incapable of applying stockings and 26% could put them on only with great difficulty.[24] Both silk "booties" and commercially available devices that assist in the application of the stockings can be useful for such patients. With open-toed stockings, an inner silk sleeve is placed over the patient's toes and forefoot to allow the stocking material to slide smoothly during application. The sleeve is removed through the toe opening after the stockings are on. Another device allows the patient to load the stocking onto a wire frame. The patient then simply steps into the stocking and pulls the device upward along the leg, applying the stocking (Fig. 146–2). These techniques, coupled with the use of home health services as needed and extensive counseling of the patient and family concerning the importance of compression therapy, are helpful in improving patient compliance.

An additional concern with elastic compression therapy is the possibility of exacerbating concomitant arterial insufficiency. One study noted that 49 of 154 general surgeons (32%) had experience with a patient who had worsening of clinical leg ulceration after compression therapy.[25] Twelve cases resulted in amputation. Callam and associates[26] analyzed 600 patients with 827 ulcerated limbs and found an ABI of less than 0.9 in 176 limbs (21%). They concluded that arterial disease represented a serious risk for patients with leg ulcers and recommended against compression therapy in patients with evidence of arterial insufficiency.

The rare patient with a venous ulcer and significant arterial insufficiency, therefore, should be considered for arterial reconstruction if the ulcer fails to improve with elastic compression therapy. However, arterial reconstructions are necessary in very few patients. Patients with critical leg ischemia (ABI < 0.4) should undergo arterial reconstruction as part of the initial management of the venous ulcer.

Paste Gauze (Unna) Boots

The paste gauze compression dressing was developed by the German dermatologist Unna in 1896.[27] The current dressing (Dome paste) contains calamine, zinc oxide, glycerin, sorbitol, gelatin, and magnesium aluminum silicate and is popularly called the *Unna boot*. This dressing is designed to provide both compression and topical therapy. The Unna boot consists of a three-layer dressing. It is preferentially applied by trained medical personnel. The Dome paste rolled gauze bandage is first applied with graded compression from the forefoot to just below the knee. The next layer consists of a 4-inch-wide continuous gauze dressing. An elastic wrap with graded compression constitutes the outer layer. The bandage becomes stiff after drying. The relatively unyielding nature of the Unna boot may aid in preventing edema formation. Bandages are generally changed weekly.

The Unna boot has the advantage of requiring minimal patient compliance because the dressing is usually applied and removed by a health care professional. Disadvantages include the inability to monitor the ulcer between dressing changes, the need for health care personnel to apply the bandage, the relative discomfort of the bulky dressing, and the operator-dependent nature of the compression achieved after wrapping.[28] Contact dermatitis may occur secondary to the paraben preservative and may require boot removal.

The Unna boot has been compared with other treatments. A randomized, prospective trial of 21 patients with venous ulcers compared Unna boot therapy with mild compression stocking therapy (24 mmHg at the ankle). Although 70% of the total number of ulcers healed in both groups, the average time for healing in the Unna boot group was 7.3 weeks but 18.4 weeks in the compression stocking group.[29] The authors qualify this finding by noting that the average healing time for the compression stocking

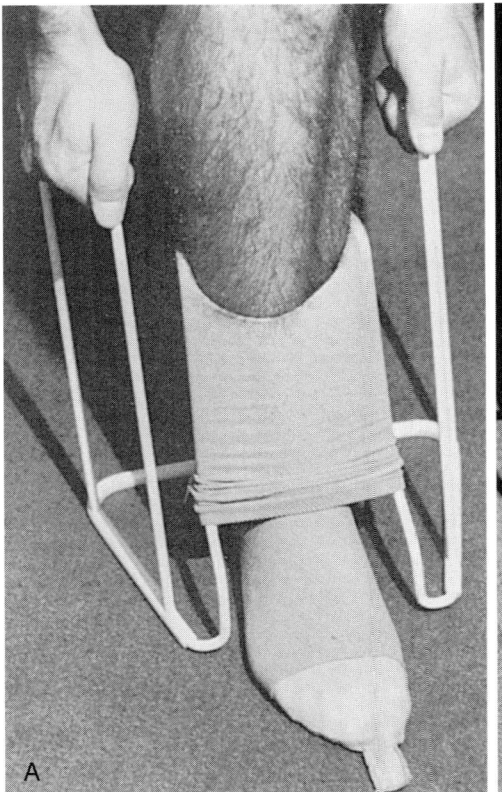
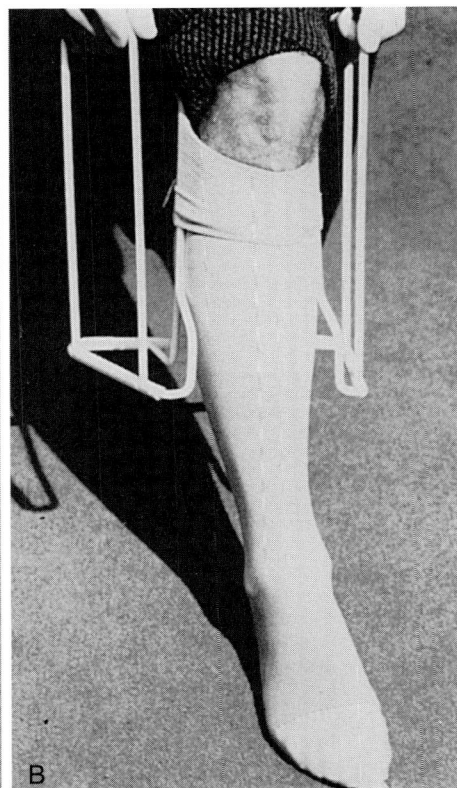

FIGURE 146–2. *A* and *B*, Compression stocking being sequentially fitted onto the leg with the Butler device. (*A* and *B*, From Mayberry JC, Moneta GL, Taylor LM, Porter JM: Nonoperative treatment of venous stasis ulcer. *In* Bergan JJ, Yao JS [eds]: Venous Disorders. Philadelphia, WB Saunders, 1991, pp 381–395.)

group was 11.8 weeks after the exclusion of a single patient in the stocking group who took 78 weeks to heal extensive calf ulcerations. Stronger compression therapy was not used in this study.

An additional randomized study of 26 patients who had CVI and venous ulcers compared Unna boots with polyurethane foam dressings and elastic compression wraps.[30] After 12 months, patients in the Unna boot group had faster healing rates and greater overall wound healing. More than 50% of the patients in the polyurethane dressing group withdrew before completion of the study.

Unna boots were also compared with hydrocolloid dressings (DuoDerm) in a 6-month trial treating 87 venous ulcers in 84 patients.[31] Seventy per cent of the ulcers treated with Unna boots healed; only 38% of those treated with the hydrocolloid dressings alone healed. A more recent study compared Unna boots with hydrocolloid dressings and elastic compression bandages and found no statistical difference in healing rates after 12 weeks.[32]

Other Forms of Elastic Compression

Additional forms of elastic compression include simple elastic wraps and multilayered wrapped dressings. Although achieving and maintaining appropriate pressure gradients with elastic wraps of any sort is highly operator- and technique-dependent, satisfactory dressings can be applied. Ankle pressures achieved with a multilayer wrap of orthopedic wool, crepe bandages, and elastic cohesive wraps (Coban) decrease only 10% after 1 week.[33] A four-layer dressing used to treat 126 consecutive patients (148 ulcerated limbs) whose ulcers had previously been refractory to treatment with simple elastic wraps resulted in complete healing of 74% of the ulcers at 12 weeks. In general,

however, the results obtained with elastic wraps in the healing of venous ulceration have been inferior to those achieved with compression stockings or Unna boots.[34–37] The combination of inferior reesults, coupled with the inconvenience and applicator dependency of elastic wraps, makes them suboptimal for the treatment of most patients with venous ulcers.

A new legging orthosis (Circ-Aid) is available (Fig. 146–3).[38] It consists of multiple pliable, rigid, adjustable compression bands that wrap around the leg from the ankle to the knee and are held in place with Velcro tape. The device offers the rigid compression of the Unna boot with increased ease of application. Because of the adjustable nature of the bands, it can be tailored to the individual as limb edema resolves. Anecdotally, the orthosis appears to be efficient in promoting resolution of edema, especially in patients who may be unable or unwilling to wear compression hosiery. Clinical trials of this device are ongoing. One preliminary study suggests the Circ-Aid orthosis may be superior to elastic stockings in preventing limb swelling in patients with advanced CVI.[39]

Adjunctive Compression Devices

External pneumatic compression devices serve as adjunctive measures in the treatment of lower extremity edema, venous ulceration, or both. They may be particularly applicable to patients with massive edema or morbid obesity. Commercially available devices apply either intermittent compression of uniform strength or intermittent sequential gradient compression. Relative contraindications to external pneumatic compression are arterial insufficiency and uncontrolled congestive heart failure.

Pneumatic compression devices that provide sequential

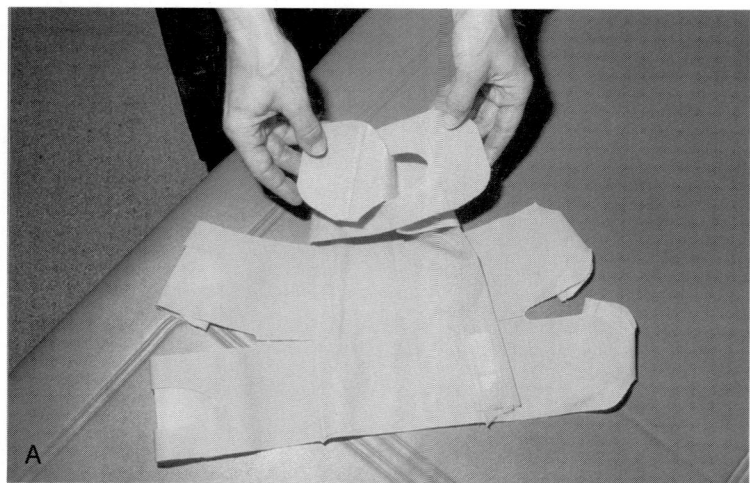

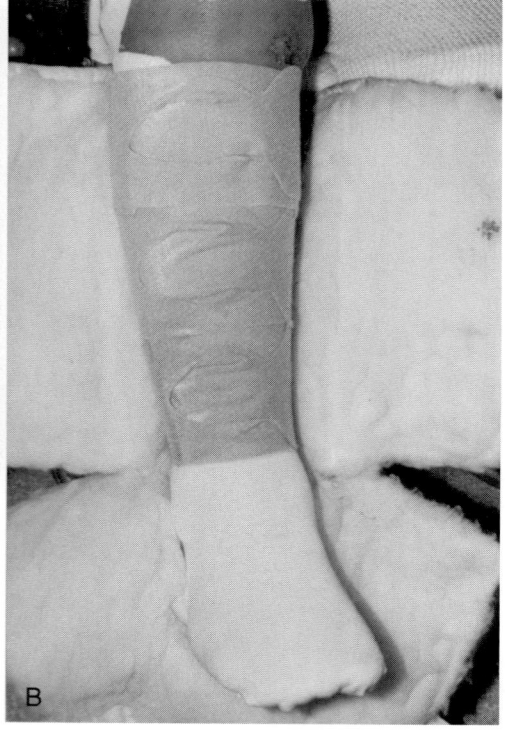

FIGURE 146–3. The Circ-Aid legging orthosis provides rigid, adjustable compression. The device appears particularly useful in patients with very large or unusually shaped legs. *A* illustrates the interlocking Velcro straps that provide adjustable compression. *B* shows the device in place.

gradient *intermittent pneumatic compression* (IPC) have received the most attention. They have gained widespread use in the prevention of deep venous thrombosis (DVT) in nonambulatory hospitalized patients. Several reports have also described the use of these devices to treat venous ulcers. The results suggest improvement in ulcer healing with the use of pneumatic compression but must be qualified by the fact that patients undergoing IPC therapy may also elevate their legs longer each day than "nonpumped" patients.

One group treated eight patients who had phlebographically documented CVI and stasis ulcers present from 1 month to 5 years with IPC for 45-minute sessions 5 days a week, for a total of 2 weeks.[40] IPC was then continued twice a week until the ulcer healed. Between treatments with IPC, the limbs were bandaged in elastic compression wraps and the ulcers were dressed with wet-to-dry dressings. All ulcers healed (mean time, 5 weeks). The authors compared this result with a mean healing time of 13 weeks in their previous patients who had treatment with elastic compression bandages alone. They concluded that the addition of IPC therapy led to a superior rate of ulcer healing.

A randomized study of 45 patients who had duplex-confirmed CVI and venous ulcers of at least 12 weeks' duration compared treatment consisting of IPC and 30- to 40-mmHg ambulatory compression stockings with the use of compression stockings alone.[41] The study continued until the ulcers had healed or until 3 months had elapsed. Only 1 of 24 patients treated with stockings alone had ulcer healing, and 10 of 21 patients in the IPC group had healing. The use of adjunctive intermittent compression has not, however, gained widespread acceptance. This is despite the results of the few available studies indicating it may be useful in the treatment of venous ulcers, especially those refractory to ambulatory compression therapy alone.

PHARMACOLOGIC THERAPY

Diuretics have little role in the treatment of chronic venous insufficiency. They can be used occasionally for short periods in patients with severe edema, but they must be used cautiously. Injudicious application, particularly in older patients without chronic intravascular volume overload, can lead to hypovolemia and associated metabolic complications.

There are multiple other drug therapies to treat lipodermatosclerosis and venous ulceration. These agents are relatively unknown in the United States. They have been primarily studied in Europe, where they are widely consumed. In a 1993 German study, 11% of persons 15 years and older consumed medication dispensed for venous disease during the previous 12 months.[42]

Zinc

Several investigators have noted that patients with CVI and venous ulceration may have depressed levels of serum zinc.[43, 44] Greaves and Skillen[45] subsequently reported complete ulcer healing after 4 months of oral zinc therapy and compression bandage use in 13 of 18 patients with low serum zinc levels and previously refractory venous ulceration of more than 2 years' duration.

A double-blind trial of 27 patients with venous ulceration and various serum zinc levels compared the combination of zinc therapy and compression bandage use with the use of compression bandages alone.[46] Additional zinc was found to be beneficial only if pretreatment zinc levels were low. A double-blind trial of 38 patients with venous ulceration and unknown zinc levels compared zinc therapy and compression bandage use with bandage use alone. Zinc did not increase ulcer healing.[47] Two additional studies of oral zinc therapy in patients with venous ulcers also showed no benefit of oral zinc therapy.[48, 49]

Fibrinolytic Agents

In general, the use of fibrinolytic agents in the treatment of CVI has been disappointing.

Stanozolol

Stanozolol is an androgenic steroid with significant fibrinolytic activity. Browse and associates[50] originally reported encouraging results in 14 patients with CVI and lipodermatosclerosis who were treated for 3 months with stanozolol. All patients had subjective and objective improvement (based on lipodermatosclerotic area). Serum parameters of fibrinolytic activity improved. However, a placebo-controlled crossover study of 23 patients with CVI and long-standing lipodermatosclerosis refractory to stocking therapy demonstrated no difference between stanozolol and stockings versus stockings alone with respect to the area of lipodermatosclerosis.[51] Skin biopsy specimens did not show a reduction in tissue fibrin with the steroid treatment. Leg volumes demonstrated increased fluid retention with use of the drug. Other studies have also been unable to demonstrate major benefits in patients with CVI after anabolic steroid treatment.[52, 53]

Oxpentifylline

Oxpentifylline is a cytokine antagonist with some profibrinolytic activity. The results of one small study suggest that it may be effective in ulcer healing.[54] The drug has significant side effects, however, including edema, vomiting, dyspepsia, diarrhea, and depression, that make it unattractive for widespread use.

Phlebotrophic Agents
Hydroxyrutosides

Hydroxyrutosides are a class of flavonoid drug derived from plant glycosides. Initial studies demonstrated a reduction in capillary permeability after thermal injury.[55] Studies of hydroxyrutosides in the treatment of patients with CVI without ulceration have suggested marginal subjective symptomatic improvement in CVI-associated pain, night cramps, and restless legs. The hydroxyrutosides also appear to be slightly more effective than placebo in controlling lower extremity edema as measured by ankle circumference.[56–58] They have not been demonstrated to promote healing of venous ulcers.[59]

Calcium Dobesilate

Calcium 2,5-dihydroxybenzenesulfonate (calcium dobesilate) increases lymphatic flow and macrophage-mediated proteolysis. The net effect is a reduction in edema.[60–62] This agent has not been extensively evaluated in the treatment of CVI. Subjective improvements in the symptoms of CVI have been demonstrated in female patients with clinically "mild" CVI.[63]

Troxerutin

Troxerutin (trihydroxy-ethylutoside) is another flavonoid derived semisynthetically from *Sophora japonica*. It appears to have an antierythrocyte aggregation effect that may improve capillary dynamics in patients with mild degrees of CVI.[64] Its effect on healing of venous ulceration is unknown.

Hemorrheologic Agents

Pentoxifylline

Pentoxifylline is a well-known hemorrheologic agent that has been used in the treatment of venous ulceration. In addition to its hemorrheologic effects, it reduces white blood cell adhesiveness, inhibits cytokine-mediated neutrophil activation, and reduces the release of superoxide free radicals produced in neutrophil degranulation.[65] In one double-blind, placebo-controlled study of 59 patients with venous ulceration, 87% of patients receiving the study drug had improvement in their venous ulcers, compared with 45% of the placebo group.[66] A multicenter trial of 80 patients with venous ulceration demonstrated a significant reduction in ulcer size after 6 months in the patients treated with pentoxifylline and compression stockings compared with those treated with compression therapy alone. Sixty per cent of the patients receiving pentoxifylline demonstrated ulcer healing compared with 29% of the controls.

Aspirin

An increased rate of venous ulcer healing has been reported with the use of 300 mg/day of enteric coated aspirin.[67] The mechanism of aspirin benefit in healing of venous ulcers is unknown. It is speculated that aspirin may promote ulcer healing by decreasing associated inflammation or inhibiting platelet function.[68]

Free Radical Scavengers

Free radical scavengers have been evaluated in the treatment of CVI. One hundred thirty-three patients who had CVI and venous ulcers were divided into three groups. Patients in the first two groups were treated with compression stocking therapy and either allopurinol or dimethyl sulfoxide as topical free radical scavenger agents.[69] Patients in the third group were treated with compression therapy alone and served as controls. At 12 weeks, patients given topical free radical scavengers had improved rates of ulcer healing. Average ulcer areas at 12 weeks were 0.2 to 0.3 cm^2 in the treatment groups compared with 1.3 cm^2 in controls.

Prostaglandins

Prostaglandin E

Prostaglandin E_1 (FGE$_1$) has multiple microcirculatory effects. It reduces white blood cell activation, inhibits platelet aggregation, and decreases small vessel vasodilation.[70] This drug, which must be administered intravenously, has been used in the treatment of venous ulcers. In a trial of PGE$_1$ treatment of venous ulceration, 44 patients were treated with compression bandages and either placebo or PGE$_1$.[71] Patients receiving PGE$_1$ showed significant improvement in edema and ulcer healing. Forty per cent of the patients in the PGE$_1$-treated group had ulcer healing compared with only 9% in the control group.

Prostaglandin F

Horse-chestnut seed extract stimulates release of prostaglandins from the PGF series. PGFs mediate vasoconstriction. A randomized clinical trial has found horse-chestnut seed extract to be superior to placebo and equivalent to compression stockings in reducing leg edema.[72] At least in the short term (<12 months), adverse effects appear minimal.

Topical Therapies

Antibiotics

Topical antibiotics have been advocated as a treatment of venous ulceration for years. However, without evidence of local infection, wound bacteriology appears to have little impact on healing.[73] The application of antiseptic agents is counterproductive to wound healing. Commercially available concentrations of povidone-iodine, acetic acid, hydrogen peroxide, and sodium hypochlorite are 100% cytotoxic to cultured fibroblasts.[74]

Iodine

Cadexomer iodine (Iodosorb) is an iodine-containing hydrophilic starch powder employed as a topical dressing for venous ulcers. It absorbs wound exudate and releases iodine as a bactericidal agent. Sixty-one patients with venous ulcers were treated with either Iodosorb or a standard topical antibiotic dressing.[35] Patients treated with the Iodosorb dressing demonstrated superior healing. A trial comparing Iodosorb with another hydrophilic powder containing propylene glycol (Scherisorb) in 95 patients with venous ulcers resulted in healing of 29% of ulcers by 10 weeks.[34] There was no difference in healing rates between the two groups.

Iodosorb was also compared with dextranomer powder (Debrisan) in the treatment of 27 patients with venous ulcers.[75] All limbs were also treated with elastic compression bandages. After 8 weeks, the ulcers healed in 64% of the Iodosorb group and in 50% of the Debrisan group.

Finally, a multicenter randomized trial compared Iodosorb treatment with saline dressing treatment in 93 patients whose venous ulcers had been present at least 3 months.[76] All limbs were also treated with elastic compression bandages. At 6 weeks, the mean ulcer size in the Iodosorb group had decreased 34% compared with 5% in the saline group.

Ketanserin

Ketanserin, a serotonin-2 antagonist, is reported to increase fibroblast collagen synthesis. A double-blind study of 23 patients with venous ulcers compared the use of topical 2% ketanserin and compression bandages with bandage use alone.[77] Wound improvement was demonstrated in 91% of the ketanserin-treated group in contrast to 50% of controls.

Amnion

Several agents have been evaluated in attempts to promote ingrowth of granulation tissue in venous ulcer beds. Five days of treatment using human amnion as a topical occlusive dressing in combination with bed rest was reported in an uncontrolled trial of 15 patients.[78] Amnion-treated ulcer beds had improved ingrowth of granulation tissue. The patients reported almost immediate pain relief with the application of the amnion dressings.

Occlusive Dressings

Hydrocolloid occlusive dressings (DuoDerm) maintain a moist wound environment, are often comfortable for the patient, and may promote more rapid epithelialization of granulating wounds.[79] A randomized trial of 55 patients with venous ulcers compared elastic compression bandages with either hydrocolloid occlusive dressings or gauze bandages for efficiency in ulcer healing. No difference in healing rate was found. In addition, occlusive hydrocolloid dressings may be associated with up to a 25% infectious complication rate.[31] Although occlusive dressings may be more comfortable for the patient, they may not produce more rapid healing and may lead to an increased number of local infectious complications.

Growth Factors and Cytokines

There is considerable interest in the use of topically applied growth factors and cytokines in the treatment of chronic nonhealing wounds. To date, however, no large-scale clinical trials demonstrate safety or efficacy of these substances in the treatment of venous ulcers. Preliminary studies, however, have demonstrated efficacy in healing a series of chronic wounds of mixed etiology.[80] Clearly, these agents should be the focus of continued investigation.

SKIN SUBSTITUTES

Advances in biotechnology have led to the development of human skin substitutes. The intent is to promote permanent closure of open wounds, including venous ulcers. These products vary from simple acellular skin substitutes to complete living bioengineered bilayered human skin equivalents with allogenic epidermal and dermal layers. The mechanism of action in promoting wound healing is uncertain. Living products may possibly serve as a delivery vehicle for various growth factors and cytokines important in wound healing.

Apligraf is a bioengineered product consisting of a keratinocyte-containing epidermis and a dermal layer of fibroblasts in a collagen matrix separated by a basement membrane (Fig. 146–4).[81] Both keratinocytes and fibroblasts are derived from neonatal foreskin. The epidermal and dermal layers are both mitotically active and secrete collagen and other matrix elements. In a randomized clinical trial of Apligraf versus multilayered compression therapy, Apligraf was effective in inducing healing of venous ulcers. Large ulcers (>6 cm) and long-standing ulcers (>12 months) showed the greatest benefit with the Apligraf skin substitute.[82]

SUMMARY

When all of the data on the nonoperative treatment of CVI are analyzed, compression therapy continues to offer the best combination of simplicity and efficacy. Compression therapy provides symptomatic relief, promotes ulcer healing, and aids in preventing ulcer recurrence. It continues to be the standard of nonoperative therapy for CVI against which all other therapies for venous ulcer and CVI should

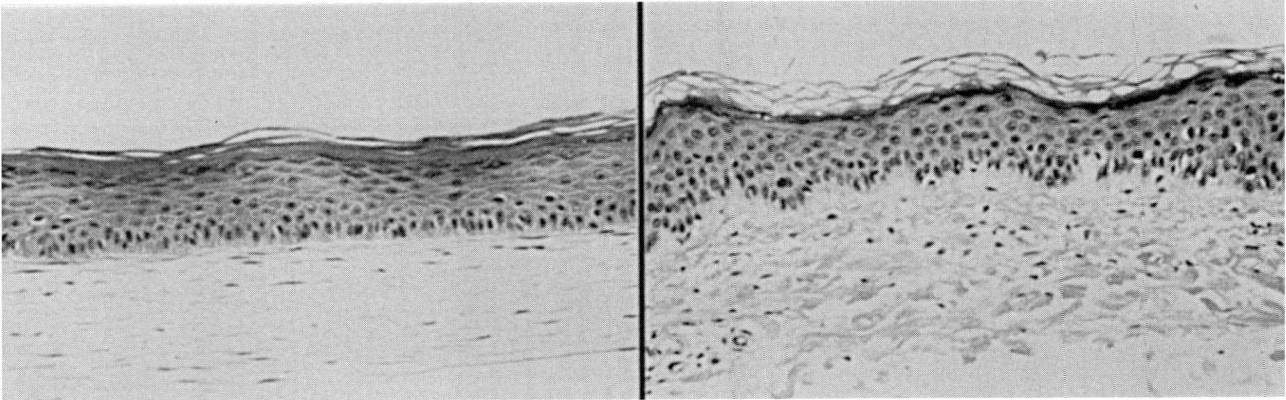

FIGURE 146–4. Histologic photographs of the bioengineered skin substitute Apligraf (*left*) and normal human skin (*right*). The bioengineered product appears very similar to normal human skin. It produces numerous growth factors, and both dermal and epidermal layers are mitotically active.

be compared. New therapies for venous ulceration, both operative and nonoperative, should have as their goal more rapid promotion of healing with less pain and decreased late recurrence than is currently achieved with optimal application of compression therapy.

REFERENCES

1. Cikrit DF, Nichols WK, Silver D: Surgical management of refractory venous stasis ulceration. J Vasc Surg 7:473, 1988.
2. Bergan JJ, Yao JST, Flinn WR, McCarthy WJ: Surgical treatment of venous obstruction and insufficiency. J Vasc Surg 3:174, 1986.
3. Raju S, Fredericks R: Valve reconstruction procedures for nonobstructive venous insufficiency: Rationale, techniques, and results in 107 procedures with two- to eight-year follow-up. J Vasc Surg 7:301, 1988.
4. Mayberry JC, Moneta GL, DeFrang RD, Porter JM: The influence of elastic compression stockings on deep venous hemodynamics. J Vasc Surg 13:91, 1991.
5. O'Donnell TF, Rosenthal DA, Callow AD, Ledig FL: The effect of elastic compression on venous hemodynamics in postphlebitic limbs. JAMA 242:2766, 1979.
6. Husni EA, Ximenes JOC, Goyette EM: Elastic support of the lower limbs in hospital patients: A critical study. JAMA 214:1456, 1970.
7. Noyes LD, Rice JC, Kerstein MD: Hemodynamic assessment of high-compression hosiery in chronic venous disease. Surgery 102:813, 1987.
8. Somerville JJF, Brow GO, Byrne PJ, et al: The effect of elastic stockings on superficial venous pressures in patients with venous insufficiency. Br J Surg 61:979, 1974.
9. Norris CS, Turley G, Barnes RW: Noninvasive quantification of ambulatory venous hemodynamics during elastic compressive therapy. Angiology 35:560, 1984.
10. Christopoulos DG, Nicolaides AN, Szendro G, et al: Air-plethysmography and the effect of elastic compression on venous hemodynamics of the leg. J Vasc Surg 5:148, 1987.
11. Jones NA, Webb PJ, Rees RI, Kakkar VV: A physiological study of elastic compression stockings in venous disorders of the leg. Br J Surg 67:569, 1980.
12. Horner J, Fernandes JF, Nicolaides AN: Value of graduated compression stockings in deep venous insufficiency. Br Med J 75:820, 1980.
13. Mahler F, Chen D: Intravital microscopy for evaluation of chronic venous incompetence. Int J Microcirc Clin Exp 106(Suppl):1, 1990.
14. Neumann HA: Possibilities and limitations of transcutaneous oxygen tension: Measurements in chronic venous insufficiency. Int J Microcirc Clin Exp 105(Suppl):1, 1990.
15. Kolari PJ, Pekanmaki K: Effects of intermittent compression treatment on skin perfusion and oxygenation in lower legs with venous ulcers. Vasa 16:312, 1987.
16. Nemeth AJ, Falanga V, Alstadt SA, Eaglstein WH: Ulcerated edematous limbs: Effect of edema removal on transcutaneous oxygen measurements. J Am Acad Dermatol 120:191, 1989.
17. Bergan JJ: Conrad Jobst and the development of pressure gradient therapy for venous disease. In Bergan JJ, Yao JS (eds): Surgery of the Veins. Orlando, Fla, Grune & Stratton, 1985, pp 529–540.
18. Wright AD: The treatment of indolent ulcer of the leg. Lancet 1:457, 1931.
19. Anning ST: Leg ulcers: The results of treatment. Angiology 7:505, 1956.
20. Kitahama A, Elliot LF, Kerstein MD, Menendez CJ: Leg ulcer: Conservative management or surgical treatment? JAMA 247:197, 1982.
21. Mayberry JC, Moneta GL, Taylor LM, Porter JM: Fifteen-year results of ambulatory compression therapy for chronic venous ulcers. Surgery 109:575, 1991.
22. Erickson CA, Lanza DJ, Karp DL, et al: Healing of venous ulcers in an ambulatory care program: The roles of chronic venous insufficiency and patient compliance. J Vasc Surg 22:629, 1995.
23. Chant AD, Davies LJ, Pike JM, Sparks MJ: Support stockings in practical management of varicose veins. Phlebology 4:167, 1989.
24. Franks PJ, Oldroyd MI, Dickson D, et al: Risk factors for leg ulcer recurrence: A randomized trial of two types of compression stockings. Age Ageing 24:490, 1995.
25. Callam MJ, Ruckley CV, Dale JJ, Harper DR: Hazards of compression treatment of the leg: An estimate from Scottish surgeons. Br Med J 295:1382, 1987.
26. Callam MJ, Harper DR, Dale JJ, Ruckley CV: Arterial disease in chronic leg ulceration: An underestimated hazard? Lothian and Forth Valley leg ulcer study. Br Med J 294:929, 1987.
27. Unna PG: Ueber Paraplaste, eine neue Form medikamentoser Pflaster. Wien Med Wochenschr 43:1854, 1896.
28. Elder DM, Greer BE: Venous disease: How to heal and prevent chronic leg ulcers. Geriatrics 50:30, 1995.
29. Hendricks WM, Swallow RT: Management of stasis leg ulcers with Unna's boots versus elastic support stockings. J Am Acad Dermatol 12:90, 1985.
30. Rubin JR, Alexander J, Plecha EJ, Marman C: Unna's boots vs. polyurethane foam dressings for the treatment of venous ulceration. Arch Surg 125:489, 1990.
31. Kitka MJ, Schuler JJ, Meyer JP, et al: A prospective, randomized trial of Unna's boots versus hydroactive dressing in the treatment of venous stasis ulcers. J Vasc Surg 7:478, 1988.
32. Cordts PR, Hanrahan LM, Rodriguez AA, et al: A prospective, randomized trial of Unna's boot versus DuoDERM CGF hydroactive dressing plus compression in the management of venous leg ulcers. J Vasc Surg 15:480, 1992.
33. Blair SD, Wright DD, Backhouse LM, et al: Sustained compression and healing of chronic venous ulcers. Br Med J 297:1159, 1988.
34. Stewart AJ, Leaper DJ: Treatment of chronic leg ulcers in the community: A comparative trial of Scherisorb and Iodosorb. Phlebology 2:115, 1987.
35. Ormiston MC, Seymour MT, Venn GE, et al: Controlled trial of Iodosorb in chronic venous ulcers. Br Med J 291:308, 1985.
36. Ryan TJ, Biven HF, Murphy JJ, et al: The use of a new occlusive dressing in the management of venous stasis ulceration. In Ryan TJ (ed): An Environment for Healing: The Role of Occlusion. London, Royal Society of Medicine, 1984, pp 99–103.
37. Eriksson G: Comparative study of hydrocolloid dressing and double layer bandage in treatment of venous stasis ulceration. In Ryan TJ (ed): An Environment for Healing: The Role of Occlusion. London, Royal Society of Medicine, 1984, pp 111–113.
38. Vernick SH, Shapiro D, Shaw FD: Legging orthosis for venous and lymphatic insufficiency. Arch Phys Med Rehabil 68:459, 1987.
39. Spence RK, Cahall E: Inelastic versus elastic leg compression in chronic venous insufficiency: A comparison of limb size and venous hemodynamics. J Vasc Surg 24:783, 1996.
40. Pekanmaki K, Kolari PJ, Kiistala U: Intermittent pneumatic compression treatment for post-thrombotic leg ulcers. Clin Exp Dermatol 12:350, 1987.
41. Coleridge Smith P, Sarin S, Hasty J, Scurr JH: Sequential gradient pneumatic compression enhances venous ulcer healing: A randomized trial. Surgery 108:871, 1990.
42. Uber A: The socioeconomic profile of patients treated by phlebotropic drugs in Germany. Angiology 48:595, 1997.
43. Greaves MW, Boyde TR: Plasma zinc concentrations in patients with psoriasis, other dermatoses, and venous leg ulceration. Lancet 2:1019, 1967.
44. Withers AF, Baker H, Musa M, Dormandy TL: Plasma zinc in psoriasis. Lancet 2:278, 1968.
45. Greaves MW, Skillen AW: Effects of long-continued ingestion of zinc sulphate in patients with venous leg ulceration. Lancet 2:889, 1970.
46. Hallbook T, Lanner E: Serum-zinc and healing of venous leg ulcers. Lancet 2:780, 1972.
47. Greaves MW, Ive FA: Double blind trial of zinc sulphate in the treatment of chronic venous ulceration. Br J Dermatol 87:632, 1972.
48. Myers MB, Cherry G: Zinc and the healing of chronic ulcers. Am J Surg 120:77, 1970.
49. Phillips A, Davidson M, Greaves MW: Venous leg ulceration: Evaluation of zinc treatment, serum zinc and rate of healing. Clin Exp Dermatol 2:395, 1977.
50. Browse NL, Jarrett PE, Morland M, Burnand K: Treatment of lipodermatosclerosis of the leg by fibrinolytic enhancement: A preliminary report. Br Med J 2:434, 1977.
51. Burnand K, Lemenson G, Morland M, et al: Venous lipodermatosclerosis: Treatment by fibrinolytic enhancement and elastic compression. Br Med J 280:7, 1980.
52. McMullin GM, Watkin GT, Coleridge Smith PD, Scurr JH: The efficacy of fibrinolytic enhancement with stanozolol in the treatment of venous insufficiency. Aust NZ J Surg 61:306, 1991.

53. Layer GT, Stacey MC, Burnand KG: Stanozolol and the treatment of venous ulceration: An interim report. Phlebology 1:197, 1986.

54. Colgan M, Dormandy JA, Jones PW, et al: Oxpentifylline treatment of venous ulcers of the leg. BMJ 300:972, 1990.

55. Arturson G: Effects of 0-(B-hydroxyethyl)-rutosides (HR) on the increased microvascular permeability in experimental skin burns. Acta Chir Scand 138:111, 1972.

56. Balmer A, Limoni C: A double-blind placebo-controlled trial of venorutin on the symptoms and signs of chronic venous insufficiency. Vasa 9:76, 1980.

57. Pulvertaft TB: Paroven in the treatment of chronic venous insufficiency. Practitioner 223:838, 1979.

58. Pulvertaft TB: General practice treatment of symptoms of venous insufficiency with oxyrutins: Results of a 660 patient multicenter study in the UK. Vasa 12:373, 1983.

59. Mann RJ: A double-blind trial of oral 0: B-hydroxy-ethyl rutosides for stasis leg ulcers. Br J Clin Pract 35:79, 1981.

60. Casley-Smith JR, Casley-Smith JR: The effects of calcium dobesilate on acute lymphedema (with and without macrophages) and on burn edema. Lymphology 18:37, 1985.

61. Casley-Smith JR: The effect of variations in tissue protein concentration and tissue hydrostatic pressure on fluid and protein uptake by the initial lymphatics, and the action of calcium dobesilate. Microcirc Endothelium Lymphatics 2:385, 1985.

62. Casley-Smith JR: A double-blind trial of calcium dobesilate in chronic venous insufficiency. Angiology 39:853, 1988.

63. Hachen HJ, Lorenz P: Double-blind clinical and plethysmographic study of calcium dobesilate in patients with peripheral microvascular disorders. Angiology 33:480, 1982.

64. Boissean MR, Taccoen A, Garrean C, et al: Fibrinolysis and hemorrheology in chronic venous insufficiency: A double blind study of troxerutin efficiency. J Cardiovasc Surg 36:369, 1995.

65. Sullivan GW, Carper HT, Novick WJ, Mandell GL: Inhibition of the inflammatory action of interleukin-1 and tumor necrosis factor-α on neutrophil function by pentoxifylline. Infect Immun 56:1722, 1988.

66. Weitgasser H: The use of pentoxifylline (Trental 400) in the treatment of leg ulcers: The results of a double blind trial. Pharmatherapeutica 3(Suppl 1):143, 1983.

67. Layton AM, Ibbotson SH, Davies JA, et al: The effect of oral aspirin in the treatment of chronic venous leg ulcers. Lancet 344:164, 1994.

68. Ibbotsen SH, Layton AM, Davies JA, et al: The effect of aspirin on haemostatic activity in the treatment of chronic venous leg ulceration. Br J Dermatol 132: 422, 1995.

69. Salim AS: The role of oxygen-derived free radicals in the management of venous (varicose) ulceration: A new approach. World J Surg 15:264, 1991.

70. Sinzinger H, Virgolini I, Fitscha P: Pathomechanisms of atherosclerosis beneficially affected by prostaglandin E₁ (PGE₁): An update. Vasa 28(Suppl):6, 1989.

71. Rudofsky G: Intravenous prostaglandin E in the treatment of venous ulcers: A double-blind, placebo controlled trial. Vasa 28(Suppl):39, 1989.

72. Diehm C, Trampisch HJ, Lange S, et al: Comparison of leg compression stockings and oral horse-chestnut seed extract in patients with chronic venous insufficiency. Lancet 347:292, 1996.

73. Gilchrist B, Reed C: The bacteriology of chronic venous ulcers treated with occlusive hydrocolloid dressings. Br J Dermatol 121:337, 1989.

74. Lineaweaver W, Howard R, Souey D, et al: Topical antimicrobial toxicity. Arch Surg 120:267, 1985.

75. Tarvainen K: Cadexomer iodine (Iodosorb) compared with dextranomer (Debrisan) in the treatment of chronic leg ulcers. Acta Chir Scand Suppl 544:57, 1988.

76. Hillstrom L: Iodosorb compared to standard treatment in chronic venous leg ulcers: A multicenter study. Acta Chir Scand Suppl 544:53, 1988.

77. Roelens P: Double-blind placebo-controlled study with topical 2% ketanserin ointment in the treatment of venous ulcers. Dermatologica 178:98, 1989.

78. Bennett JP, Matthews R, Faulk WP: Treatment of chronic ulceration of the legs with human amnion. Lancet 1:1153, 1980.

79. Alvarez OM, Mertz PM, Eaglstein WH: The effect of occlusive dressings on collagen synthesis and re-epithelialization in superficial wounds. J Surg Res 35:142, 1983.

80. Ganio C, Tenewitz FE, Wilson RC, et al: The treatment of chronic nonhealing wounds using autologous platelet-derived growth factors. J Foot Ankle Surg 32:263, 1993.

81. Wilkins LM, Watson SR, Prosky SJ, et al: Development of a bilayered living skin construct for clinical applications. Biotechnol Bioeng 43:747, 1994.

82. Falanga V, Margolis D, Alvarez O, et al: Rapid healing of venous ulcers and lack of clinical rejection with an allogenic cultured human skin equivalent. Arch Dermatol 134:283, 1998.

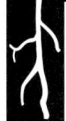

C H A P T E R   1 4 7

Varicose Veins: Treatment by Surgery and Sclerotherapy

John J. Bergan, M.D., F.A.C.S.

The care of venous stasis in all of its manifestations is the responsibility of surgeons in general and of vascular surgeons in particular. With varicose veins, such care is directed toward ablation of diseased vessels. Ablation is achieved by removing them surgically or by obliterating them with sclerotherapy. Large varicose clusters, axial veins (greater and lesser saphenous veins) that show gross reflux, and varicosities above the knee are best treated by removal.[1] Other vessels, especially telangiectasias, may be subjected to sclerotherapy.

RELEVANT ANATOMY

The gross anatomy of the venous system is well known to surgeons.[2] Valve-containing deep veins transport venous blood by means of muscular contraction. Less physiologically important superficial veins also contain valves that direct their flow upward, and these veins connect with the deep system by means of perforating veins that penetrate the deep fascia of the lower extremities. Check valves in the perforating veins protect the poorly supported venules superficial to the tela aponeurotica from compartmental exercise pressure.

Less surgically appreciated is the reticular subdermal venous network, which also contains valves (Fig. 147–1). Because it is the most superficially located vein network of the lower extremities, this plexus is the most poorly supported and is the source of the earliest subcutaneous varicosities.[3]

Superficial to this network in the dermis, postcapillary venules run horizontally, range in size from 12 to 35 μm, and empty into collecting venules twice as large in the mid-dermis.[2, 3] One-way valves are found in venules at the dermis-adipose junction and also in areas of anastomosis of small to large venules. Larger venules also contain valves not necessarily associated with junctional points. Free edges of valves are always directed away from the smaller vessels and toward the larger ones. These valves serve to direct blood flow toward the deeper venous system. The valve structure in these small venules is identical to that found in larger deep veins, consisting of valve sinuses, cusps, and aggeres in relation to vein walls.

Of greatest concern to the physician treating venous problems in the lower extremity is the greater saphenous vein. The term *saphenous* is derived from the Greek word for "visible."[4] The saphenous vein (1) originates on the dorsum of the foot in the dorsal venous arch, (2) passes anterior to the medial malleolus, (3) progresses through the medial calf across the posteromedial aspect of the popliteal space, (4) ascends in the medial thigh, and (5) terminates in the femoral vein (Fig. 147–2).

The anatomy of the greater saphenous vein is relatively constant. It is well appreciated that this vein lies on the deep fascia of the leg and thigh. Less well recognized, however, is that it lies below or deep to the superficial fascia. Even contemporary descriptions of the anatomy of the veins of the lower extremity do not make this distinction.[5] Yet this fact is important to knowledge of the development of varicosities.

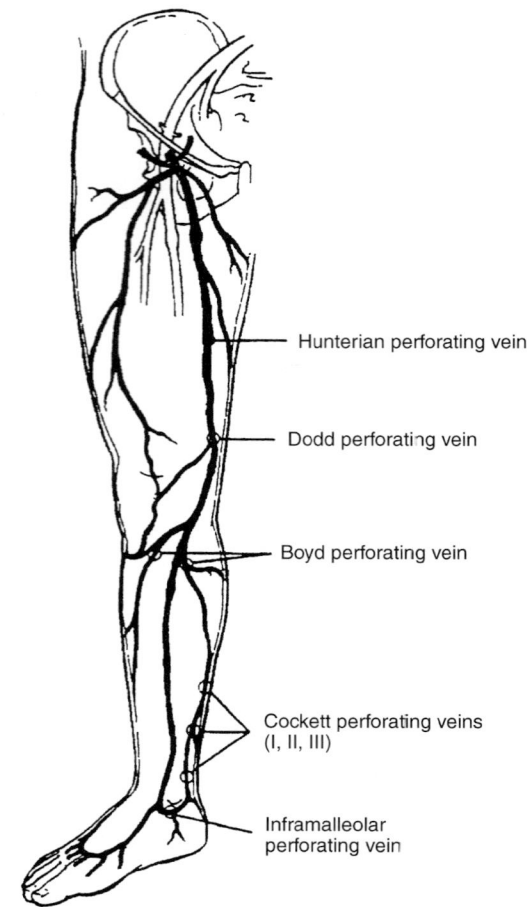

FIGURE 147–2. The location of the most important perforating veins associated with the greater saphenous system is shown. The Cockett and inframalleolar perforating veins are actually separate from the greater saphenous system. The Boyd perforating vein is constantly present, but it may drain the saphenous vein or its tributaries. Perforating veins in the distal third of the thigh are referred to as "Dodd perforators," whereas those in the middle third of the thigh are referred to as "Hunterian perforators."

In varicose venous anatomy, the important tributaries to the greater saphenous vein extending upward from below are:

1. The posterior arch vein, which receives the three Cockett's perforating veins.

2. The anterior tributary vein to the saphenous system, which lies below the patella and collects blood from the anterior and lateral surface of the leg.

3. The posterior tributary vein, which also empties into the greater saphenous vein in the upper anteromedial calf.

Other tributaries that may terminate high in the saphenous system near the groin are the posteromedial thigh vein and the anteromedial thigh vein. Either of these veins may become the site of varicose clusters.

Less common in primary varicosities and more important in recurrent varicose veins after surgery are other tributaries to the greater saphenous vein where it terminates in the fossa ovalis. They are the superficial external pudendal vein, the superior epigastric vein, and the superficial circumflex iliac vein.

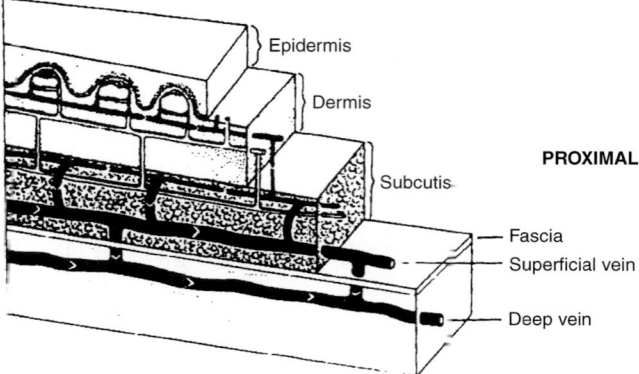

FIGURE 147–1. Dermal postcapillary venular network. Valves within these tiny vessels all direct blood flow deeper into large collecting veins. Failure of check valve function allows high-pressure venous blood to flow into unsupported dermal vessels, thus producing telangiectatic blemishes.

Posteriorly, the most important of the axial veins is the lesser saphenous vein (Fig. 147–3).[4] This vein originates on the lateral aspect of the foot in the dorsal venous arch and ascends virtually in the midline of the calf. Unlike the greater saphenous vein, the lesser saphenous vein may penetrate the deep fascia at any point from the middle third of the calf upward. This fact explains the segmental rather than total nature of reflux found in the lesser saphenous vein.

Important tributaries to the saphenous vein are inconstant but may include the posteromedial tributary vein. Superiorly, this tributary may be associated with a lateral thigh vein called the anterolateral superficial thigh vein. Another important and commonly encountered vein is the ascending superficial vein, which leaves the popliteal space and progresses proximally to join the saphenous vein medially at a point high in the thigh. This vessel is the vein of Giacomini.

The importance of knowing the regular features of the gross anatomy of the superficial veins of the lower extremity is that one of these systems may be the site of growth of clusters of varicosities. Such clusters can be referred to by the name of the normal vein in that location. All named

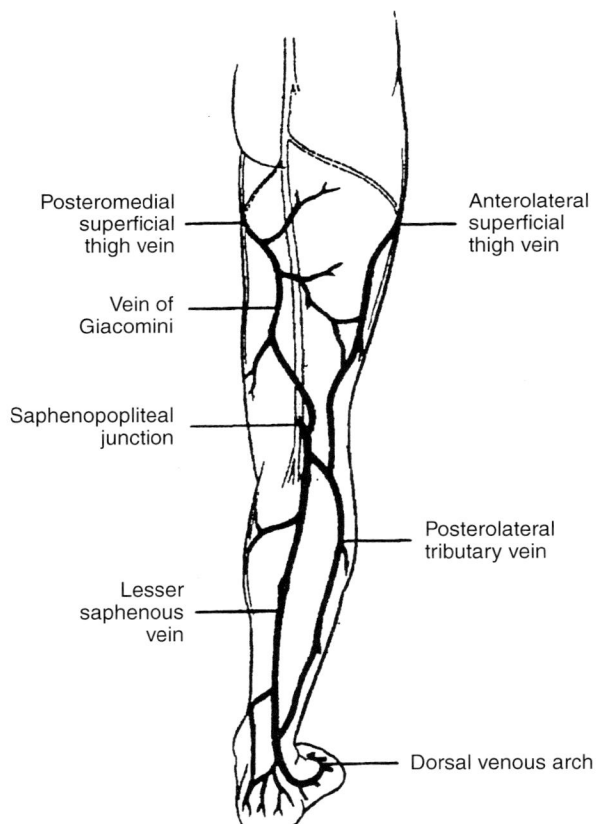

FIGURE 147–3. The lesser saphenous vein dominates the posterolateral superficial venous drainage and originates in the dorsal venous arch. At the posterolateral ankle, it is intimately associated with the sural nerve. Note the important posterolateral tributary vein and the posterior thigh vein, which ascend and connect the lesser saphenous venous system with the greater saphenous system. The anterolateral superficial thigh vein and the posterolateral tributary vein can be very important in congenital venous anomalies, such as Klippel-Trenaunay syndrome.

tributaries to the greater and lesser saphenous system lie superficial to the membranous fascia and are relatively unsupported in comparison with the greater and lesser saphenous veins and the deep veins of the muscular compartments.

IMPORTANT PERFORATING VEINS

Veins that connect the superficial venous system to the deep venous system and penetrate the fascia are properly called *perforating veins* (see Fig. 147–2). In the past, they were called "communicating veins." Any one of these veins, or any combination of them, may be the source of the hydrodynamic forces of venous hypertension that produce superficial varicosities. It is the abnormally high pulses of hydrodynamic pressure transmitted through incompetent perforating vein valves that affect relatively unsupported superficial veins. Such pulses of increased fluid force originate to some extent from increased abdominal pressure but to a greater extent from increased compartmental pressure during muscular contraction.

The best-recognized connections between the superficial venous system and the deep venous system are the saphenofemoral and saphenopopliteal junctions. Incompetence of the check valves at their termination has been suggested as the cause of distal varicosities from gravitational reflux. This reverse flow is said to dilate more distal veins in a progressive fashion. Such reflux is neither always present nor the cause of highest hydrodynamic pressure. Gravitational reflux is referred to as *hydrostatic pressure*.

Because it is frequently the site of the first varicose veins or the first reticular veins that become varicose, Boyd's perforating vein in the anteromedial calf now receives great attention from physicians who treat venous problems.[6] Experience with duplex ultrasound scanning reveals that venous incompetence at this level may be isolated and may be the first reflux to appear. Such incompetence may be asymptomatic. However, when the incompetence is symptomatic, it produces aching pain, fatigue, and even a throbbing discomfort. These symptoms can be relieved by firm local pressure. In some patients, the next perforator system to become incompetent is the distal thigh perforating vein.

The frequency of varicosities in this location is documented in a graph by Cotton[7] that tabulates the number of varices in limbs in the monumental and informative study he performed in 1957. It was Cotton who pointed out that the "most extreme degree of tortuosity is exhibited by small tributaries which are found close to, and draining into, communicating [perforating] veins." In the figures illustrating Cotton's thesis, one can see the normal deep veins and the abnormal perforating veins *receiving* blood from "intensely tortuous veins which are seen to be varicose tributaries entering the communicating (perforating) veins."[7]

HYDRODYNAMIC PRESSURE

Reversing this observation, we can visualize pulses of compartmental exercise pressure being delivered to unsupported superficial veins through incompetent perforators. Once we realize that intracompartmental pressure can be transmitted through incompetent check valves of perforating veins to unsupported tributaries to these veins, it is easy to see how the hydrostatic forces of gravitational reflux are additive to the hydrodynamic forces of muscular contraction. These very high pressures approach 150 to 300 mmHg as they are generated within the muscular compartments. When transmitted outward, they produce localized blowouts or varicosities.

Progressing proximally from Boyd's perforating vein are the perforating veins in the distal third of the thigh. These veins, named for Harold Dodd, may be found in any location along the saphenous pathway in the distal third of the thigh.

The third important series of perforating veins, named for John Hunter, are found in the mid-thigh. Tung and colleagues[8] have surveyed phlebograms to study the anatomy of mid-thigh perforating veins. They found that 61% of limbs had one or more of these veins in the middle third of the thigh. In addition, they noted that 27% of the limbs had a perforating vein in the lower third of the thigh. Only 11% of the 100 phlebograms showed no evidence of perforating veins.

A concurrent study from St. Mary's Hospital in London found that the incompetent thigh perforating veins may occur anywhere in the thigh from the upper edge of the patella to a few centimeters below the saphenofemoral junction; 71% were found in the middle third of the thigh, and 20% of the limbs had more than one perforating vein.[9] All of the incompetent thigh perforating veins communicated directly with the long saphenous vein. It is interesting to note that five patients who underwent complete saphenous vein stripping also had connections of thigh perforating veins with residual saphenous vein trunks. This observation emphasizes the need for removal of the entire refluxing saphenous vein in the thigh.

In the leg, the principal communicating veins have been named for Frank Cockett. Many surgeons incorrectly assume that the perforating veins on the medial aspect of the ankle and calf connect the deep system to the greater saphenous vein. These perforating veins actually connect the posterior tibial deep venous system with the posterior arch vein (vein of Michelangelo). Posterior tibial veins are frequently paired, and phlebography may show their connection through perforating veins to the superficial system and the posterior arch vein.[10] Cockett has described the medial communicating veins as if they were relatively constant in location, but they are not. The location is commonly given as the distance from the sole of the foot. Figures given from the heel pad are 6, 12, and 18 cm from this point (see Fig. 147–2). Other important perforating veins in the distal part of the extremity include the inframalleolar perforating vein. Frequently, this is the site of a painful ulceration. A flare of intradermal telangiectasias below this perforating vein is called a *corona phlebectatica*.

Perforating veins on the posterior aspect of the lower extremity are much less well known. However, several are encountered frequently and are found to be the site of varicose clusters. Among these are the lateral thigh perforating vein, which may be located in the middle third of the thigh on its lateral aspect, and the lateral leg perforating

vein, also invariably located in the middle or proximal third of the calf on its lateral aspect.

PATTERNS OF VARICOSITIES

Recognizing the normal anatomy and the most common perforating vein sources of varicosities makes identification of patterns of varicosities relatively easy (Table 147–1). As noted earlier, varicosities arising from the location of Boyd's perforating vein may be the first to appear and may occur in the absence of varicose veins elsewhere in the lower extremity. Such varicosities may consist of the anterior tributary vein varicose cluster or, more commonly, a posterior varicose cluster. The first manifestations may be pain, aching, and heaviness. Relief may be obtained by applying local pressure under an elastic stocking and then by performing local excision of the cluster of varicosities and its perforating vein. Whether sclerotherapy for this pattern of varicosities will give long-term benefit is undetermined, but the best method of treatment is phlebectomy.

Of some importance is the relationship of the saphenous nerve to Boyd's perforating veins and its varicose clusters. In a study of this relationship, the most common vein-nerve pattern was found to be the saphenous vein and saphenous nerve that meet a few centimeters below the knee.[11] Below this point, the vein and the nerve were inseparable as far as the medial malleolus. This pattern was noted in 41 of 60 limbs studied. The next most common pattern, seen in 10 limbs, was the nerve joining the saphenous vein a few centimeters more proximally. Thus, in 50 of 60 limbs, nerve injury could be a problem in limbs in which the saphenous vein is exposed below Boyd's perforating vein.

Another isolated pattern of varicosities arises from the anteromedial tributary to the saphenofemoral junction. These veins may form prominent rope-like varicosities across the anterior surface of the thigh, coursing laterally and descending on the lateral aspect of the thigh. They may cross the popliteal space and arborize distally on the calf.

Other prominent varicose cluster patterns originate from the perforating veins of Hunter at the mid-thigh and of Dodd in the distal thigh and are sometimes isolated clusters of varicosities. Usually, they occur in association with greater saphenous vein reflux. In fact, recognition that these clusters of varicosities are markers of saphenous vein reflux alerts the interested physician to study the saphenofemoral junction. The probable cause of greater saphenous insufficiency when varicose clusters of the mid-thigh or distal

TABLE 147–1. PATTERNS OF VARICOSITIES

LOCATION OF VARICES	PERFORATOR
Medial thigh, mid-third	Hunterian
Medial thigh, distal third	Dodd's
Medial leg, upper third	Boyd's
Ankle, posteromedial	Cockett's
Ankle, anteromedial	Sherman's
Posterolateral knee crease	Unnamed

thigh are present can then be confirmed by Doppler evaluation.

In a study intended to classify the clinical appearance of uncomplicated varicose veins, Goren and Yellin[12] found that 71% of the limbs of patients studied demonstrated typical saphenous vein varicosities. Of the 164 limbs, 147 demonstrated greater saphenous vein incompetence, whereas only 17 limbs showed lesser saphenous vein incompetence. Only 22% of limbs did not show saphenous vein incompetence; these showed isolated perforating vein incompetence.

The necessity of reconciling preservation of the saphenous vein for subsequent arterial surgery with the need for varicose vein surgery is considerably aided by the recognition that greater saphenous vein incompetence may not be present in some limbs with gross varicosities. In such instances (22% of the limbs in the study by Goren and Yellin[12]), the greater saphenous vein can be spared yet the operation can be done properly to remove symptomatic varicosities. Doppler evaluation with confirmation by duplex scanning aids considerably in the planning of such surgical interventions. However, one should also understand that in more than 75% of limbs, the greater saphenous vein may have to be sacrificed.

VARICOSE VEINS AND TELANGIECTASIAS

Varicose veins, telangiectatic blemishes, and dilated, tortuous, flat, blue-green reticular veins are not normal physical findings. They are evidence of venous dysfunction. The visible physical findings, more often than not, cause symptoms of aching pain, leg fatigue, and a poorly described discomfort that makes the individual harboring this venous dysfunction wish to elevate the legs to a more comfortable position. Ultimately, the target of venous dysfunction is the skin. With long-standing venous dysfunction, the skin darkens as a result of hemosiderin deposition; if an inflammatory process is triggered, the subcutaneous tissues harden, and minor breaks in the epidermis are slow to heal, producing white, depressed scars.

The aching pain, which is the most common symptom, is related to pressure of the dilated vessels on a dense network of somatic nerve fibers that is present in subcutaneous tissues adjacent to affected veins. The magnitude of symptoms is not related to the length or diameter of the malfunctioning vein.[13] Patients with telangiectasias, for the most part, have symptoms identical to those of patients with protuberant, saccular varicosities.[14] It is these symptoms that drive the patient to a physician, who more likely than not dismisses the symptoms and their cause as unimportant.[15] Nevertheless, in best medical practice, the patient's complaint is acknowledged, and after appropriate diagnosis, treatment is instituted.

Indications for therapeutic intervention are listed in Table 147–2. Physicians might recognize that treatment is indicated when the patient has had superficial thrombophlebitis in varicose clusters or has experienced external bleeding from high-pressure venous blebs. Certainly, treatment such as elastic support would be offered for advanced

TABLE 147–2. VARICOSE VEINS: INDICATIONS FOR INTERVENTION

General appearance	External bleeding
Aching pain	Ankle hyperpigmentation
Leg heaviness	Lipodermatosclerosis
Easy leg fatigue	Atrophie blanche
Superficial thrombophlebitis	Venous ulcer

changes of chronic venous insufficiency. The much more common symptoms, such as aching pain, leg fatigue, and leg heaviness, and the appearance of the leg, however, are likely to be dismissed. Nevertheless, they should be acknowledged and cared for.

Specific findings on physical examination that lead to surgical intervention rather than sclerotherapy are the findings of axial vein reflux in the greater saphenous vein or, perhaps, the lesser saphenous vein. Experience teaches that sclerotherapy of varicosities in the presence of saphenous vein reflux will fail.[16] Furthermore, large varices lend themselves to surgical removal rather than sclerotherapy, and the trend worldwide is toward ambulatory phlebectomy rather than sclerotherapy for such varicose clusters.[17] H.A.M. Neumann, a dermatologist, has emphasized this issue, recommended that one should "always operate: insufficient saphenous junctions, major insufficiency of long saphenous vein ... and big insufficient (incompetent) perforating veins."[18] Others have found that surgery is indicated even when saphenofemoral junction incompetence is not present.[19]

When such phlebectomies are carried out, patient satisfaction is virtually unanimous.[20] At present, such surgery can be carried out as day-case surgery, with no additional workload being given to the primary care physician.[21]

Extensive availability of duplex ultrasound technology has revealed another reason for operating on varicose veins—deep venous function is improved by superficial venous surgery.[22] Increased dilatation of the deep venous system has been noted to accompany superficial venous reflux and was described in a phlebographic study by Fischer and Siebrecht[23] as early as 1970. They observed that greater dilatation of deep veins was seen in the absence of post-thrombotic manifestations.

Such deep venous dysfunction has been thought to be the most important complication of superficial axial vein incompetence.[24] Although observations of deep venous dilatation and elongation were made in phlebographic studies in preoperative patients, such studies were not carried out uniformly in postoperative patients. When duplex ultrasound technology is applied to the study of postoperative patients, ablation of preoperative deep vein reflux has been an almost uniform finding.[22, 25, 26] This important finding provides a strong argument for treatment of varicose veins with the best method possible, which is ambulatory phlebectomy.

SURGICAL TREATMENT

Objectives

When surgery is decided upon, the surgeon must keep three goals in mind in planning the treatment[27]:

- Permanent removal of the varicosities with the source of venous hypertension
- As cosmetic a result as possible
- Minimum number of complications

The source of venous hypertension as described previously is gravitational reflux (hydrostatic) or compartmental pressure developed during muscular contraction through perforator outflow (hydrodynamic). Therefore, removal of gravitational reflux by means of axial vein removal and detachment of hydrodynamic forces by superficial varicosity excision has been found to accomplish both objectives.[28] Experience in treating recurrent varicose veins has revealed that an inadequate procedure at the saphenofemoral junction is a principal finding.[29, 30] An equally important cause of recurrent varicosities is failure of the primary procedure to remove the offending varicosities completely.

The Plan

The planned operation for a given patient must be completely individualized. As indicated previously, Doppler evaluation and duplex scanning have shown that in 70% of limbs selected for surgery, typical saphenofemoral junction reflux is present. In such limbs, the saphenous vein at the femoral junction must be operated on. However, atypical varicosities without saphenofemoral junction reflux do occur in some 20% of limbs. In other limbs atypical reflux points cause their varicosities.[12] Clearly, no standard operation fits every patient perfectly.

The techniques of saphenous surgery are well described in standard surgical texts.[29, 31] Their outpatient variations have come into vogue.[32, 33] This means that older methods requiring inpatient care, general anesthesia, long operating time, radical avulsion of varicose veins, and stripping of varicose veins to the ankle can be largely abandoned.[27] The operation of removal of the saphenous vein is now done by groin-to-knee downward stripping of the varicose vein.[34, 35] Techniques to decrease hematoma after downward stripping include irrigation and adrenaline-gauze packing of the saphenectomy tunnel.[12, 28, 36] Tourniquets should be used during saphenous vein stripping for huge varicosities.[37, 38]

Options

Options available for surgical treatment of varicose veins are:

- Ankle-to-groin saphenous vein stripping (with stab avulsion)
- Segmental saphenous vein stripping (with stab avulsion)
- Saphenous vein ligation: high, low, or both
- Saphenous vein ligation and sclerotherapy
- Saphenous vein ligation and stab avulsion of varices
- Stab avulsion of varices without saphenous vein stripping (phlebectomy)

Objectives of surgical treatment should be (1) ablation of the hydrostatic forces of axial and saphenous vein reflux and (2) removal of the hydrodynamic forces of perforating vein reflux. These maneuvers should be combined with extraction of the varicose vein clusters in as cosmetic a fashion as possible.

Saphenous Vein Ligation

Ligation of the saphenous vein at the saphenofemoral junction has been practiced widely in the belief that it would control gravitational reflux while preserving the vein for subsequent arterial bypass. It is true that the saphenous vein is largely preserved after proximal ligation.[39] Reflux continues, however, and hydrostatic forces are not controlled.[40]

Before the accurate delineation of the sites of origin of varicosities, ankle-to-groin stripping of the saphenous vein was considered the standard operation that should be performed in every operated case. Turn-of-the-century publications had conveyed the belief that reflux was uniformly distributed over the entire length of the saphenous vein.[41–43] This belief led to excessively radical saphenous vein stripping and the desire of surgeons to perform proximal saphenous vein ligation without saphenous vein stripping.

The objective of excision of the saphenous vein is to remove its gravitational reflux and detach its perforator vein tributaries in the thigh. Therefore, it has been found unnecessary to remove the below-knee portion. Perforating veins of the medial thigh are largely a part of the saphenous system; in the lower leg, however, this is not the case. Below the knee, important perforating veins are part of the posterior arch circulation. A further argument against routine removal of the saphenous vein below the knee is the discovery of saphenous nerve injury associated with the operation. Such injury has occurred in the upper third of the leg as well as adjacent to the ankle incision.[44]

Recurrent varicose veins are more common after saphenous vein ligation than after stripping.[45] Recurrent varicose veins are also more common after saphenous vein ligation and sclerotherapy than after stripping and sclerotherapy.[28] A prospective randomized trial comparing proximal saphenous vein ligation and stab avulsion of varices with stripping of the thigh portion of the saphenous vein and stab avulsion of varices has found superior results for the latter procedure.[46]

Studies of recurrent varicose veins have found preservation of the patency of the saphenous vein and continued reflux in the saphenous vein to be the most common element in the recurrence.[9, 47, 48] In patients presenting for surgical relief of recurrent varicosities, Stonebridge and colleagues[47] found that two thirds required removal of the saphenous vein as part of the second procedure. For all of these reasons, simple proximal saphenous vein ligation should be done only in very special cases.

Surgical Procedure

As indicated previously, knowledge of the pathophysiologic hydrodynamics, relevant venous anatomy, and results of the various surgical procedures allows precise prescription of the proper surgical procedure for each patient and each limb to be benefited by surgical intervention. In surgical practice, because greater saphenous vein reflux is found in two thirds of patients,[12] groin-to-knee stripping is part of the operation chosen (Fig. 147–4).

In nearly all patients, this procedure is supplemented with stab avulsion of clusters of varicosities. In one third of patients, the saphenofemoral junction is found to be

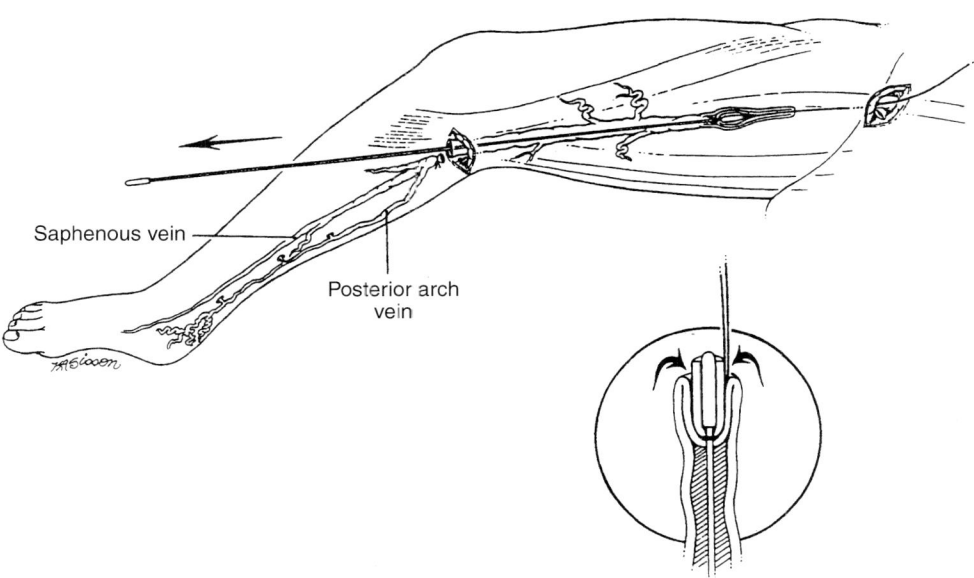

FIGURE 147–4. Removal of the thigh portion of the saphenous vein is the mainstay in surgical treatment of primary venous insufficiency. The endoluminal device, commonly a disposable plastic stripper, can be introduced from above downward, the vein ligated around the stripper proximally. As distal traction is applied, the vein is then inverted into itself and removed distally in the region of the knee. This minimizes tissue trauma but accomplishes the desired result of detaching the superficial venous system from perforating veins that are transmitting intercompartmental pressure to unsupported subcutaneous venous networks.

Saphenous vein

Posterior arch vein

competent and therefore can be left intact. However, stab avulsion of clusters of varicosities derived from reflux from the Hunter or Dodd perforating veins may be necessary. This maneuver may remove segments of the greater saphenous vein. Finally, approximately 15% of patients are found to have lesser saphenous vein incompetence, and the operation in such patients must include careful removal of some or all of that structure.

Greater Saphenous Vein Stripping

In principle, incisions at the groin, ankle, and knee are transverse and are placed within skin lines. For incisions made elsewhere, experience has revealed that best cosmetic results are obtained with vertical incisions throughout the leg and thigh, which also allow preservation of lymphatics. Transverse incisions are used only in knee creases. Oblique incisions in skin lines are appropriate over the patella. Preoperative marking must be accurate so as to outline the extent of varicose clusters, clinical points of control of varices, and clinically identified locations of perforating veins.

In the groin, an oblique variation of the transverse incision is appropriate. This incision should be placed either in or 1 cm above the visible skin crease. It should not be made below the inguinal skin crease. This placement allows accurate and direct identification of the junction. Anatomy of the named tributaries is infinitely variable; the general appearance, however, is shown in Figure 147–2.

In order not to leave a network of interanastomosing inguinal tributaries behind, the surgeon should make a special effort to draw into the groin incision each of the saphenous tributaries. Traction should be put on them until their primary or even secondary tributaries can be controlled. The importance of this maneuver is underscored by Ruckley's description of the residual inguinal network as an important cause of varicose recurrence.[47]

A major cause of discomfort and occasional permanent skin pigmentation is blood extravasated subcutaneously

during and after saphenous vein stripping. This can be minimized by:

- Use of a hemostatic tourniquet
- Leg elevation prior to and during the actual stripping
- Internal packing of the stripper tract with the use of 5-cm-wide roller gauze soaked in lidocaine 0.5% with added epinephrine

The disposable plastic Codman vein stripper can be introduced from above downward, because Doppler evaluation and duplex scanning will have confirmed saphenous junction incompetence. Angioscopic examination of the saphenous vein has revealed remarkably few valves in those saphenous vein that have come to surgery.[49] Valves that have been observed to be present have been monocuspid, deformed, or even perforated. The reasons for these deformities have not been elucidated but could include leukocyte trapping and activation in valve cusps.[50] Because the valves consist of only collagen and epithelium,[51] elaboration of collagenase by activated leukocytes could explain all of the valve damage that has been observed.

The vein stripper, introduced from above, can be exposed distally with a short transverse incision in the knee skin crease at the medial edge of the popliteal space. This is one of the three places where the saphenous vein is anatomically constant; it is helpful for this location to be marked preoperatively while the patient is standing. The skin incision in this location is cosmetically acceptable.

If the stripper passes relatively unobstructed to the ankle, it can be exposed there with an exceedingly small skin incision placed in a carefully chosen skin line. Passage of the stripper from above downward to the ankle has proved absence of functioning valves, and stripping of the vein from above downward is unlikely to cause nerve damage (see Fig. 147–3). At the ankle, the vein should be very cleanly dissected to free it from surrounding nerve fibers before the actual stripping is done.

Stripping of the saphenous vein has been shown to produce profound distal venous hypertension. This effect can be seen in virtually every such operation. Therefore, if considerable stab avulsion is to be performed. it is best for the surgeon to perform this procedure before the actual downward stripping. The stab avulsion, performed with the use of the Varady dissector, Müller hooks or other such devices, successfully detaches perforating veins from their tributary varicose clusters. Dissection of each perforator at fascial level is neither necessary nor cosmetically acceptable. Neither is it necessary to ligate or clip retained vein ends after stab avulsion. The elevated leg, trauma-induced venospasm, and direct pressure will ensure adequate hemostasis.

Techniques of phlebectomy have been markedly refined by experienced workers in Europe.[52] The size of the incision depends on the size of the varicose vein the thickness of the vein wall, and the vein's adherence to perivenous tissues. Incisions are 1 to 2 mm in length. They are oriented vertically except in areas where skin lines are obviously horizontal. The varicosity is exteriorized by hook or forcep technique, divided, and then avulsed as far as is possible. Subsequent incisions are made as widely spaced as possible. Following avulsion of the varicosity, skin edges can be approximated with tape or with a single absorbable suture.

Surgery of the Lesser Saphenous Vein

Surgery of the lesser saphenous vein is very little like surgery of the greater saphenous vein. There is one similarity; the anatomy of the saphenopopliteal junction is just as irregular as that of the saphenofemoral junction. Indications for surgery of the lesser saphenous vein are similar to those for surgery of the greater saphenous vein; that is, reflux in the lesser saphenous vein accompanied by symptomatic varices tributary to that system.

Although earlier surgeons described a normal low or high termination of the saphenous vein in the popliteal fossa, this area has been more carefully defined by duplex scanning. Now it is known that a very low termination below the knee joint occurs in only 2% of cases. In 42% of cases, the termination is within 5 cm of the knee joint crease and is the saphenous vein's only termination. However, the lesser saphenous vein may continue up into the thigh and terminate elsewhere. For example, it terminates in the vein of Giacomini in about 12% of cases, in half of which there is also a standard saphenopopliteal junction. The lesser saphenous vein may terminate higher, in a femoropopliteal vein or posterior subcutaneous thigh vein. In nearly half of these cases, the femoropopliteal vein enters a thigh perforating vein or, more rarely, splits into two or more branches that may reach the gluteal area. One third of these cases also demonstrate a standard saphenopopliteal junction.[52]

Because of the variability of the anatomy and the limited nature of lesser saphenous vein reflux, it is essential that examination with a continuous-wave, hand-held Doppler instrument be supplemented by duplex scanning. The objectives of duplex scanning are to confirm lesser saphenous vein reflux and to identify the termination of the lesser saphenous vein. The termination can be marked on the skin if the examination is performed immediately preoperatively; more often, however, because the duplex examination is remote in time from the operative procedure, the

distance from the heel pad to the termination of the saphenous vein is carefully measured and recorded in the duplex scanning report. In a patient who has not undergone duplex scanning, it may be possible to locate the termination of the lesser saphenous vein by careful examination with a continuous-wave, hand-held Doppler instrument; that is, assessing location of reflux and the proximal extent of reflux will locate the lesser saphenous vein termination.

Hobbs[53] recommends on-table lesser saphenous varicography. Many of his observations were made before the days of duplex scanning. To perform on-table saphenous vein varicography, the surgeon does the following:

1. Cannulates a varicose cluster on the posterior aspect of the calf.
2. Places the leg in a lateral position with the x-ray film below the knee joint.
3. Marks skin creases in the popliteal spaces with steel hypodermic needles.
4. Exposes the film during injection of 20 ml of contrast solution.

Further differences between the lesser saphenous vein and the greater saphenous vein include the fact that in the posterior leg, the lesser saphenous vein has segmental reflux in most cases. van Bemmelen and associates[54] found that the proximal part of the vein was incompetent in 36% of cases and the mid-calf portion was incompetent in 31%. In more than half of the affected lesser saphenous veins, the incompetence was limited to only one segment; in the distal half of the leg, the lesser saphenous vein was normal in 26% of cases. The importance of this finding derives from the fact that the sural nerve is vulnerable to injury in the retromalleolar space on the lateral aspect of the ankle.

The surgical procedure is performed with the patient prone and the popliteal space relaxed by knee flexion. The incision is made over the termination of the lesser saphenous vein and centered on the junction between the middle and lateral thirds of the popliteal space. It can be made 5 cm long to expose the deep fascia. This structure can be further relaxed by more knee flexion. The incision in the deep fascia can be made parallel to the skin incision or longitudinally to achieve more exposure. The sural nerve should be identified and preserved. Frequently, the lesser saphenous vein or tributaries to it encircles one or more of these nerve structures. When the encircling veins are varicose, the dissection may be tricky indeed.

Division of the tributaries, and especially the proximal tributary to the vein of Giacomini, mobilizes the lesser saphenous vein termination. The vein can be divided and suture-ligated near its termination in the popliteal vein. Distally, stripping can be carried out with the disposable plastic Codman vein stripper or, better, with the Oesch stripper. Because there are no equivalents to the Hunter or Dodd perforating vein in the posterior calf, the stripping can be limited to the proximal lesser saphenous vein to above mid-calf in most cases. Goren and Yellin[55] have provided a concise description of this technique.

After ligation, my colleagues and I have followed the original Oesch technique, which dictates that after the saphenous vein is divided, the stainless steel stripper is passed with its angled tip in a downward direction. The stripper usually passes only to the varicose cluster in the posterior calf. There, the angled tip of the stripper can be palpated through the skin, and skin pressure allows the stripper to perforate the vein wall and become subcutaneous. A 3-mm stab incision exposes the tip of the stripper, and the actual vein, which has been penetrated, is not visualized. A strong, nonabsorbable suture is tied to the end of the stainless steel stripper, and this suture in turn is fixed to the end of the vein so that it can be inverted into itself as the stripper is removed distally.

Once the inverted vein appears in the distal incision, it can be grasped directly with the hemostat, and traction can be placed on the vein as close to the skin as possible to avoid tearing the relatively fragile lesser saphenous vein. Gastrocnemius veins should be searched for in the proximal incision, because their persistence may contribute to recurrent varicosities in the posterior calf.

SCLEROTHERAPY

Although many credit Pravaz with the invention of the syringe in 1851, it was actually Rynd who developed this radical advance in 1845.[56] Case reports of sclerotherapy appear throughout the latter half of the 19th century.[57] A variety of caustics were used, including carbolic acid. Profound inflammation and suppuration followed such treatments in the pre-Listerian era. All early agents were thrombogenic. After investigations showing that quinine obliterated small vessels by intimal damage, the focus of sclerotherapy changed.[58] This change led directly to the use of hypertonic saline in 1924 and sodium morrhuate in 1930.[59]

Credit should be given to Biegeleisen[60] for the invention of microsclerotherapy after 1930. The technique languished somewhat until after 1970, although in some centers, treatment of varicosities of all sizes continued throughout this time.[61, 62]

Indications for the use of sclerotherapy are listed in Table 147–3. Sclerotherapy is the only modality effective in the ablation of telangiectatic blemishes. It can also erase reticular veins and varicosities, particularly those less than 4 mm

TABLE 147–3. INDICATIONS FOR SCLEROTHERAPY

Optimal Indications

Telangiectasias
Reticular varicosities and reticular veins
Isolated varicosities*
Below-knee varicosities*
Recurrent varicosities*

Less Than Optimal Indications

Symptomatic reflux
Aged or infirm patient
Patients who are not surgical candidates

Questionable Indications

Greater saphenous vein reflux
Lesser saphenous vein reflux
Large varicosities

Contraindication

Allergy to the sclerosant*

*In the absence of gross saphenous vein reflux.

in diameter. Below the knee, where effective compression is most efficient, sclerosants can ablate larger varicosities and small clusters of varices not associated with gross saphenous vein reflux. Furthermore, sclerotherapy is useful in obliterating residual varicosities after surgical treatment and varicosities that appear at times remote from surgery after saphenous vein reflux has been totally corrected.

Many individuals, especially nonsurgeons, use sclerotherapy for nearly all varicosities. Some even believe that axial vein reflux through saphenous veins can be halted effectively by sclerosants.[3] Furthermore, sclerotherapy is used by some for thigh varicosities of nonsaphenous origin and even for large varices associated with principal named perforating veins. As mentioned in Table 147–3, these are not ideal indications. It is the use of sclerotherapy in suboptimal situations that has contributed to its inferior reputation.

In general, sclerotherapy finds its greatest utility in the smallest incompetent vessels. These, then, may be telangiectasias or small varices below the knee. Proximal venous reflux and venous hypertension must be corrected first.[63–68] Under less than ideal circumstances, sclerotherapy also finds a distinct usefulness in palliation, for the aged or infirm patient. In addition, in situations that violate these guidelines, sclerotherapeutic ablation of symptomatic varicosities can temporarily prove to be gratifyingly beneficial.

When telangiectasias are treated by sclerotherapy, the process is termed *microsclerotherapy*.[69] When sclerotherapy is used to obliterate larger veins, it is referred to as *macrosclerotherapy*.

Sclerotherapeutic Agents

Drugs available for sclerotherapy may cause thrombosis, fibrosis, or both. Excessive thrombosis is undesirable and may lead to excessive perivascular inflammation and recanalization of the vessel. More desirable endothelial damage may be provoked by a number of mechanisms, including:

• Changes in the surface tension of the plasma membrane
• Modification of the physical or chemical environment of the endothelial cell
• Alteration in intravascular pH or osmolality

For effective microsclerotherapy, the endothelial damage must produce vascular necrosis in a significant portion of the vascular wall.[62]

Agents that change the surface tension of the plasma membrane are *detergents*. They include sodium morrhuate, sodium tetradecyl sulfate, and polidocanol. Their action produces endothelial damage through interference with cell surface lipids.[70]

Hypertonic solutions, including hypertonic saline, hypertonic dextrose, and sodium salicylate, cause dehydration of endothelial cells through osmosis. Possibly, fibrin deposition with thrombus formation occurs through modification of the electrostatic charge on the endothelial cells.[71]

Chemical irritants, such as chromated glycerin and polyiodinated iodine, act directly on the endothelial cells to produce endosclerosis. After endothelial damage occurs, fibrin is deposited in the sclerosed vessels. Platelets adhere to the underlying elastin, collagen, or basement membrane.[72]

TABLE 147–4. RELATIVE STRENGTHS OF
SCLEROSING SOLUTIONS

Category 1: Strongest

Sodium tetradecyl sulfate, 1.5–3.0%
Polidocanol, 3–5%
Polyiodinated iodine, 3–12%

Category 2: Strong

Sodium tetradecyl sulfate, 0.5–1.0%
Polidocanol, 1–2%
Polyiodinated iodine, 2%
Sodium morrhuate, 5%

Category 3: Moderate

Sodium tetradecyl sulfate, 0.25%
Polidocanol, 0.75%
Polyiodinated iodine, 1%
Hypertonic saline, 23.4%
Sodium morrhuate, 2.5%

Category 4: Weak

Sodium tetradecyl sulfate, 0.1%
Polidocanol, 0.25–0.50%
Chromated glycerin, 50%
Polyiodinated iodine, 0.1%
Hypertonic saline, 11.7%
Sodium morrhuate, 1%

Table 147–4 ranks sclerosing agents according to strength. The strongest solutions are used in the largest veins, including the saphenopopliteal and saphenofemoral junctions, selective perforating veins, and larger varicose clusters. At the other end of the scale are the weakest solutions, which are used for telangiectasias and other vessels smaller than 0.4 mm in diameter. Weak solutions are useful for vessels of up to 2 mm in diameter, and strong solutions for vessels of 3 to 5 mm in diameter.

The only two sclerosant solutions approved by the U.S. Food and Drug Administration (FDA) and listed in the *Physician's Desk Reference* are detergents. The oldest, sodium morrhuate, is a mixture of sodium salts of saturated and unsaturated fatty acids present in cod liver oil. This agent experienced early popularity in the 1930s. This enthusiasm was dampened by reports of anaphylactic reactions.

The other agent, sodium tetradecyl sulfate, was widely utilized after 1950[73] and was advocated for use in dilute solution for the treatment of telangiectasias after 1978.[74] Although it is widely used, this agent does produce epidermal necrosis when infiltrated in concentrations greater than 0.2%. Allergic reactions have been reported, and post-sclerotherapy hyperpigmentation is commonly seen. Curiously, the manufacturer recommends an intravenous test injection as a precaution against anaphylaxis.

Not approved by the FDA at present but undergoing Phase 2 trials in anticipation of approval is the most widely used sclerotherapeutic agent, polidocanol. It was synthesized and introduced as a local and topical anesthetic agent that clearly differed from the class of anesthetic agents that were "-caine" compounds. Polidocanol is a urethane whose optimum anesthetic effect occurs at a concentration of 3%. Because intravascular and intradermal instillations of this agent produced sclerosis of small-diameter blood vessels, polidocanol was withdrawn as an anesthetic agent and proposed as a sclerosing agent after 1967. An optimal concentration for treating telangiectasias is 0.5%, whereas

varicose veins may be treated with a 1% or greater concentration.[75]

Treatment of Telangiectatic Blemishes (Microsclerotherapy)

Telangiectatic blemishes may be thought of as extremely small varicose veins. Therefore, principles of treatment remain the same. The source of venous hypertension that has produced the elongation, tortuosity, and dilatation of the vessel must be controlled if treatment is to be effective. Telangiectasias may receive their pulse of venous hypertension directly through minute incompetent perforating veins.[66] This may be identifiable through careful Doppler examination; more often, the offending perforating vein is not specifically identified. Treatment of the telangiectatic blemish in such a situation may fail simply because the sclerosant solution does not reach the feeding vein in a concentration sufficient to obliterate it.

Telangiectasias may receive their pulse of venous hypertension from the subdermal reticular network (Fig. 147–5). These are seen as thin-walled, blue, superficial, dilated veins that are eventually tributaries to the main superficial venous system. Doppler studies have shown that free reflux occurs in such a network in association with telangiectasias. The reflux may proceed upward against the flow of gravity.[80] The reticular network may receive venous hypertension by gravitational effects, from incompetent perforators, or from a hydrostatic or hydrodynamic cause as described earlier in this chapter.

Knowledge of anatomy and pathophysiology dictates that the treatment of telangiectasias begin with the source of venous hypertension. When the source can be identified as a reticular dilated vein, the sclerosant solution may be seen to enter the telangiectasia directly from the feeding vein. The reverse may be true; injecting telangiectasias may allow the observer to watch the sclerosant solution enter a feeding vein from the site of injection. If it is impossible to identify the source of the venous hypertension, telangiectasias

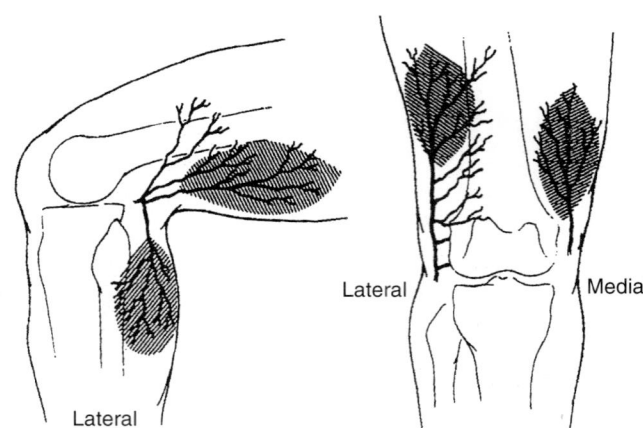

FIGURE 147–5. Common locations of telangiectatic blemishes on the medial distal thigh and the proximal leg both laterally and medially. Such telangiectatic blemishes may be connected to reticular feeding veins, which can be identified and sclerosed. Commonly, these feeding veins are connected to the deep venous circulation and transmit hydrodynamic forces to the dermal venules.

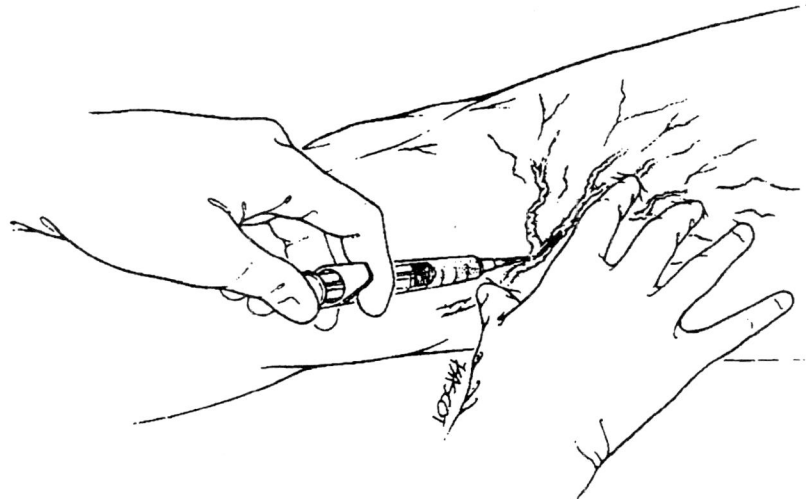

FIGURE 147–6. Placement of the needle in a feeding vein to treat the reticular varicosity found in association with a large telangiectatic blemish. Note the stretching of the skin, the penetration of the reticular varicosity with the needle, and the deft management of the plunger to clear blood from the entire blemish during injection.

should be treated beginning at the point at which the branches converge. The actual injection method varies somewhat among authorities.[70, 81, 82]

The patient is in a horizontal position, either prone or supine. The skin is cleansed with alcohol to remove excess keratin and allow better visualization of the target vessel. Thirty-gauge needles are used, and they are bent to 10 to 20 degrees. The bevel of the needle may be placed either down or up, but the needle should be parallel to the skin surface. Small syringes, either 1 or 3 ml in volume, are most convenient. The skin adjacent to the blemish must be stretched, and the firmly supported needle and syringe are then moved so that the needle pierces the skin and vein while pressure on the plunger ejects the sclerosant solution (Fig. 147–6).

Magnification and good light may allow the operator to recognize the appearance of the needle within the lumen of the target vessel. Pressure on the plunger allows the operator to see the development of a wheal if there is extravasation or a clearing of the telangiectatic web if intravascular injection is achieved. Some operators favor preceding injection of the sclerosant with a bolus (0.05 ml) of air. This allows the operator to check the position of the needle and may cause a greater spread of the sclerosant solution.[83]

Injections should be performed very slowly, and the amount of sclerosant should be limited to 0.1 or 0.2 ml per injection site. Injection over 10 to 15 seconds is optimal. If a precise intravascular injection with rapid clearing of the telangiectasias is achieved, the operator must control his or her enthusiasm and must sharply limit the amount of sclerosant given in any one particular site.

Minimizing the volume, pressure, and duration of the injection minimizes pain, risk of extravasation, and skin infarction. If persistent blanching of the skin to a waxy white color is seen or if a larger amount of sclerosant is inadvertently given in a single site, the area should be flushed thoroughly with hypodermic normal saline. This maneuver will dilute areas of extravasation and help to relieve vessel spasm. Vessels being treated that are larger than 0.5 mm and those that protrude above the skin surface should be compressed immediately, and compression should be maintained without interruption. Cotton balls,

gauze, or foam rubber can be taped over the site with hypoallergenic tape in preparation for the eventual compression bandage or stocking.

After all telangiectatic blemishes and reticular varicosities have been injected and the injection session has been completed, elastic compression can be applied over the entire treated area. Again, practice varies, with some operators using compression with elastic bandages and others with elastic stockings. Furthermore, the duration of compression varies among authorities. Some use no compression, some limit compression to 18 hours, and some advise compression for as long as 2 weeks. It is generally agreed that protuberant telangiectasias or telangiectasias associated with large reticular veins should be treated with compression for 72 hours or more. Nonprotuberant telangiectasias require no compression. Patients are encouraged to walk and not to restrict their activities. The number of treatment sessions depends on the level of success of each session. It is common, however, for the patient to require three or four sessions, and the interval between injection sessions is usually 2 to 4 weeks.

The treatment of reticular varicosities and feeding veins is slightly different from the treatment of telangiectasias. The patient is in a horizontal position. A No. 30 needle is optimal and can be inserted directly into the flat, blue-green reticular vein. The operator will feel resistance at the skin level and also at the vein wall. After the vein has been pierced, the plunger may be pulled back, and a flash of blood will be seen in the transparent syringe hub. This is possible even with a No. 30 needle. The volume injected should be maintained at less than 0.5 ml, and, as in treatment of varicosities, multiple puncture sites aid in successful obliteration of the reticular varicosity.

Solutions used in treating reticular veins and telangiectatic blemishes must be dilute. The use of 0.1% or 0.2% sodium tetradecyl sulfate or its equivalent is satisfactory. If 11.7% or 23.4% hypertonic saline is used, an air block test of the injection site is advocated, because this solution is caustic enough to cause cutaneous damage during extravasation. Once polidocanol is approved by the FDA,[84] 0.5% polidocanol solution may be used in treating reticular veins and telangiectatic blemishes.[76]

Treatment of Varicose Veins (Macrosclerotherapy)

Intervention in patients with varicose veins is indicated for relief of symptoms that include aching pain, limb tiredness or heaviness after prolonged standing or sitting, and an exacerbation of symptoms at the termination of a menstrual cycle and on the first day of a menstrual period. The unsightly appearance of varicose veins and telangiectasias is important to patients and is an indication for treatment. Protuberant, saccular, bulging varicosities; the discoloration of dilated veins of telangiectasias; and the purple stain of the corona phlebectatica at the ankle all bring patients to the physician.

If greater or lesser saphenous vein reflux is excessive, as determined by Doppler examination, it should be corrected surgically before sclerotherapy. However, palliation can be achieved for 2 to 4 years in the presence of axial vein reflux even though recurrence of varices may be expected. For example, in an older patient who experiences external bleeding from varicose blebs, uncorrected axial vein reflux does not affect local sclerotherapy to obliterate the blebs and prevent further bleeding episodes. Similarly, if recurrent thrombophlebitis in varicosities has occurred, the varicosities themselves can be obliterated by sclerotherapy even without control of the proximal venous hypertension.

Contraindications to sclerotherapy include:

- Presence of arterial occlusive disease
- Patient immobility
- Presence of uncontrolled malignant tumor
- Hypersensitivity to the drug
- Acute thrombophlebitis
- Huge varicosities with large communications to deep veins

In addition to the clinical examination to determine the sites of varicosities and the origin of their venous hypertension, examination with a continuous wave, hand-held Doppler instrument is essential. This measure may be supplemented in particular cases with duplex scanning. Other assessments of venous function, such as impedance plethysmography, photoplethysmography, and venous pressure tests, are indirect and are not essential. Invasive phlebography is also not required. Classic tests, including the Perthes and Trendelenburg tests, have been replaced by the Doppler examination.

The objective of sclerotherapy is to produce endothelial damage and subsequent fibrosis of the entire vein wall without recanalization. Therefore, the ideal sclerosant solution would produce endothelial destruction with a minimum of thrombus formation. Unfortunately, FDA-approved agents are detergents, which are thrombogenic. Hypertonic saline is also used for sclerotherapy, although it is approved by the FDA for use only as an abortifacient. It does produce rapid endothelial damage. Hypertonic saline is available in a concentration of 23.4% and has been used extensively at this strength. Its single appeal is its total lack of allergenicity. However, it is common practice to add heparin, procaine, or lidocaine to hypertonic saline; additives, of course, offset the appeal of hypoallergenicity. Hypertonic saline at a concentration of 11.7% is equal to 23.4% in effect.[76]

Treatment of varicose veins 3 to 8 mm in diameter requires 0.5% to 1.0% sodium tetradecyl sulfate or its equivalent. Such large varicosities necessitate a stronger solution than telangiectasias do.

Because of the commonplace nature of varicosities and the very large number of people who treat them, a variety of techniques have developed. In principle, small-caliber (No. 25) butterfly needles are placed in varicosities while the patient is standing with the veins distended. The needles are attached to capped plastic extension tubing. A proximal tourniquet is neither necessary nor desirable. The multiple needles are placed either within a cluster of varicosities or in linear continuity in varices. An attempt to identify and to inject into a source of reflux aids in achieving long-term success.

The needles are held in place with tape until all have been inserted. Then the patient is asked to lie down, and the leg is elevated so that the veins will be empty. Duplex scanning verification of superficial venous collapse with the leg elevated to 45 degrees is useful.[77]

While injection of 0.5 to 1.0 ml of solution proceeds, there should not be any pain, irritation, or burning sensation. The presence of any of these symptoms indicates extravasation rather than intravascular injection. Extravasation demands cessation of injection.

At each injection site, after the needle has been withdrawn, a pressure pad of gauze, cotton, dental roll, or foam rubber is applied and taped in place with hypoallergenic tape. Elastic bandages may be used, wrapped from the toes proximally as they are gently stretched. The wrap is carried to 3 inches above the most proximal injection site. An elastic stocking may be fitted over the elastic bandage for additional compression or may be used instead of the elastic bandage.

The duration of compression varies with the individual preferences of the operator. For varicosities of 3 to 8 mm in diameter, a constant compression for 3 to 7 days is advised. A large school of French phlebologists practice minimal or no compression, but the influential work of Fegan mandates 6 weeks of constant compression. The controversy over the use of compression continues. Histologic studies suggest that 12 days of fibroblastic healing is required for obliteration of moderate-sized varicosities.[62, 78, 79]

Nearly all workers in this field advise that the patient should walk around the clinic for 30 minutes after the procedure. This measure allows symptoms and signs of an allergic reaction to appear and be treated. The comfort of the elastic compression can be evaluated, and the deep venous circulation can be stimulated to be flushed of any sclerosant that has entered from the superficial injection.

Side Effects of Sclerotherapy

The fear of adverse sequelae of sclerotherapy keeps many physicians and surgeons from including this treatment modality in their therapeutic armamentarium. However, the incidence of complications is exceedingly low.[70, 82] Undesirable sequelae include[85]:

- Anaphylaxis
- Allergic reactions
- Thrombophlebitis

- Cutaneous necrosis
- Pigmentation
- Neoangiogenesis

Anaphylaxis is an immunoglobulin E–mediated, mast cell–activated reaction that occurs within minutes of reexposure to an antigen.[85] Other classes of immunoglobulin may contribute to the reaction. Risk of anaphylaxis increases with repeated exposure to a given antigen, a fact that applies directly to repetitive episodes of sclerotherapy. Mast cell concentrations are high in the skin. Mediators derived from mast cells, including histamine, can produce clinical anaphylactic manifestations. These may range in severity from mild pruritus and urticaria to shock and death. Manifestations that should alert the physician to serious problems are itching, flushing, erythema, and developing angioedema. Mucous membranes of the eyes, nose, and mouth are frequently involved, and this involvement may precede upper airway obstruction caused by edema of the larynx. This, in turn, is heralded by respiratory stridor. Unrelated to respiratory obstruction is hypotensive shock, which is thought to be due to peripheral vasodilatation and increased vascular permeability.[86]

Rapid treatment of anaphylaxis is crucial. Therefore, the equipment necessary for resuscitation must be present and must be used aggressively. Epinephrine is the drug of choice for the treatment of systemic reactions, because it (1) counteracts vasodilatation and bronchoconstriction and (2) inhibits further release of mediators from mast cells. Antihistamines and corticosteroids are not the drugs of choice in initial treatment, but both may be administered after epinephrine. Endotracheal intubation, oxygen, and intravenous therapy may be necessary, and patients with serious reactions should be admitted directly to the hospital.

Sodium morrhuate has been implicated as the most common cause of anaphylaxis among the sclerosing agents. However, nearly all of the reactions reported occurred before 1950. Goldman,[70] who reviewed the medical literature regarding anaphylaxis and sodium tetradecyl sulfate, found only 47 cases of nonfatal allergic reactions in a review of 14,404 patients. The product manufacturer has reported only two fatalities associated with the use of sodium tetradecyl sulfate, neither of which was from an anaphylactic reaction.

Polidocanol has the lowest incidence of allergic reactions, including anaphylaxis. Furthermore, patients allergic to sodium tetradecyl sulfate have been successfully treated with polidocanol. A single case of fatal anaphylactic shock has been reported with the use of polidocanol.

Alone, hypertonic saline shows no evidence of inducing an allergic reaction or of having a toxic effect. However, additives such as lidocaine or heparin may, in and of themselves, induce allergic reactions.

Thrombophlebitis and its sequelae were commonly reported before the use of compression after sclerotherapy. The actual incidence of superficial thrombophlebitis is difficult to ascertain but it ranges around 1% to 3%. Duffy[81] estimated that it occurred in 0.5% of his patients.

Deep venous thromboembolic events are obviated by post-sclerotherapy exercise that flushes the deep veins. There are scattered reports of pulmonary embolization following sclerotherapy.

Although serious reactions such as anaphylaxis, allergy, and thromboembolic events may be uncontrollable, the less severe complications of sclerotherapy can be diminished in frequency by attention to the details of injection. Skin ulceration and cutaneous necrosis may result from extravasation of solution. More commonly, they are due to arterial occlusion caused by sclerosant reaching a terminal arteriole. Other causes are reactive vasospasm from a too great volume of injection or excessive cutaneous pressure. Complications of extravasation are minimized by the use of extremely dilute solution, especially in the treatment of telangiectatic blemishes. Dilute 0.1% and even 0.2% sodium tetradecyl sulfate may extravasate without complication. The same is true of 0.5% polidocanol. However, extravasation of hypertonic saline into the skin may result in cutaneous necrosis if the solution remains undiluted. Intra-arterial infiltration of sclerosant is avoided through strict adherence to the practice of injecting small quantities into each site.

Hyperpigmentation is common after sclerotherapy for veins and telangiectatic blemishes. It may occur in up to 30% of patients but is most common in patients treated with sodium tetradecyl sulfate and hypertonic saline. It is seen least in patients treated with polidocanol and is uncommon after the use of chromated glycerin. Neither of the latter two sclerosants had been approved by the FDA at the time of this writing.

Pigmentation, which is hemosiderin, derives from extravasation of red blood cells, which may appear in the dermis through either diapedesis or fracture of vessel walls. The following measures may reduce the incidence of post-sclerotherapy pigmentation:

- Using weaker concentrations of solution
- Limiting the magnitude of intravascular pressure produced during injection
- Removing the post-sclerotherapy coagula that may appear in protuberant telangiectasias, reticular veins, or varicosities

Removal of such coagula can be achieved by incising the skin with a No. 21 or No. 18 needle to allow expulsion of the entrapped blood through pressure. During expression of the coagula, all must be evacuated in order to avoid tattooing of the dermis with further extravasation of red blood cells. Post-sclerotherapy hyperpigmentation largely disappears over a prolonged period, and it has been estimated that 90% is gone after 12 months.

Treatment of hyperpigmentation is unsuccessful. Bleaching agents affect only melanin, not hemosiderin. Exfoliants carry the risk of scarring and hypopigmentation. Topical retinoic acid has produced a varied response. Successful chelation of the iron with ethylenediaminetetraacetic acid ointment has been reported but is unconfirmed.

The new appearance of red telangiectasias in a site of prior sclerotherapy has been termed *telangiectatic matting* or *neoangiogenesis*. Although such matting may result from simple blockage of a crucial efferent vessel, it is usually thought to be a complex process in which new vessels actually grow in response to endothelial growth factors, mast cell products, or platelet-derived growth factors. Estrogen has been implicated as playing a role in the development of such neovascularization.

Prevention of neoangiogenesis is best achieved through (1) the use of dilute concentrations of sclerosant solution, (2) injection under low pressure, and (3) use of only 0.1 to 0.2 ml of injectate per injection site. Treatment is relatively ineffective, but the process usually resolves over a short period (3 to 6 months). Pulsed-dye laser therapy for neoangiogenesis has been successful but is expensive.

SUMMARY

Manifestations of telangiectasias, reticular varicosities, and varicose veins can be looked upon as elongated and dilated veins with incompetent valves. They are stretched by hydrodynamic and hydrostatic forces and pressures on somatic nerves to cause definitive symptoms. Though regarded as cosmetic nuisances, in fact they generally cause some symptoms, which occasionally are severe.

Treatment can be accomplished by removing the malfunctioning vessels. Surgical removal is best for vessels larger than 2 to 3 mm and sclerotherapy suffices for vessels smaller than 2 mm.

REFERENCES

1. Bergan JJ: Surgery versus sclerotherapy in treatment of varicose veins. In Veith FJ (ed): Current Critical Problems in Vascular Surgery. St. Louis, Quality Medical Publishing, 1989.
2. Bergan JJ: Common anatomic patterns of varicose veins. In Bergan JJ, Goldman MP (eds): Varicose Veins and Telangiectasias: Diagnosis and Management. St. Louis, Quality Medical Publishing, 1993.
3. Braverman IM: Ultrastructure and organization of the cutaneous microvasculature in normal and pathologic states. J Invest Dermatol 93:28, 1989.
4. Goldman MP, Fronek A: Anatomy and pathophysiology of varicose veins. J Dermatol Surg Oncol 15:138–145, 1989.
5. Nehler MR, Moneta GL: The lower extremity venous system: Anatomy and normal physiology. Perspect Vasc Surg 4:104–116, 1991.
6. Boyd AM: Treatment of varicose veins. Proc Roy Soc Med 41:633–639, 1948.
7. Cotton LT. Varicose veins: Gross anatomy and development. Br J Surg 48:589–598, 1961.
8. Tung KT, Chan O, Lea Thomas M: The incidence and sites of medial thigh communicating veins: A phlebologic study. Clin Radiol 41:339–340, 1990.
9. Papadakis K, Christodoulou C, Christopoulos D, et al: Number and anatomic distribution of incompetent thigh perforating veins. Br J Surg 76:581–584, 1988.
10. O'Donnell TF Jr: Surgical treatment of incompetent communicating veins. In Bergan JJ, Kistner RL (eds): Atlas of Venous Surgery. Philadelphia, WB Saunders, 1992.
11. Holme JB, Holme K, Sorensen LS: The anatomic relationship between the long saphenous vein and the saphenous nerve. Acta Chir Scand 154:631–633, 1988.
12. Goren G, Yellin AE: Primary varicose veins: Topographic and hemodynamic correlations. J Cardiovasc Surg 31:672–677, 1990.
13. Goldman MP, Weiss RA, Bergan JJ: Diagnosis and treatment of varicose veins: A Review. J Am Acad Dermatol 31:393–414, 1994.
14. Weiss RA, Weiss MA: Resolution of pain associated with varicose and telangiectatic leg veins after compression sclerotherapy. J Dermatol Surg Oncol 16:333–336, 1990.
15. Weiss RA, Weiss MA, Goldman MP: Negative physician perception of sclerotherapy for venous disorders: Results of a survey and a review of a 7-year positive American experience with modern sclerotherapy. South Med J 11:1101–1106, 1992.
16. Bergan JJ: Surgical management of primary and recurrent varicose veins. In Gloviczki P, Yao JST (eds): Handbook of Venous Disorders. Andover, England, Chapman & Hall, 1996.
17. Weiss RA, Weiss MA: Ambulatory phlebectomy compared to sclerotherapy for varicose and telangiectatic veins: Indications and complications. Adv Dermatol 11:3–16, 1996.
18. Neumann HAM: Ambulant minisurgical phlebectomy. J Dermatol Surg Oncol 18:53–54, 1992.
19. Abu-Own A, Scurr JH, Coleridge Smith PD: Saphenous vein reflux without incompetence at the saphenofemoral junction. Br J Surg 81:1452–1454, 1994.
20. Baker DM, Turnbull NB, Pearson JCG, Makin GS: How successful is varicose vein surgery? A patient outcome study following varicose vein surgery using the SF-36 health assessment questionnaire. Eur J Vasc Endovasc Surg 9:299–304, 1995.
21. Ramesh S, Umeh HN, Galland RB: Day-case varicose vein operations: Patient suitability and satisfaction. Phlebology 10:103–105, 1995.
22. Walsh JC, Bergan JJ, Beeman S, Comer TP: Femoral venous reflux is abolished by greater saphenous stripping. Ann Vasc Surg 8:566–570, 1994.
23. Fischer H, Siebrecht H: Das kaliber der tiefen unterschenkelvenen bei der primaren varicose und beim postthrombotischen syndrome (Eine phlebographische Studie). Der Hautarzt 5:205–211, 1970.
24. Hach-Wunderle V: Die sekundare popliteal und femoral venen insuffizienz. Phlebology 21:52–58, 1992.
25. Sales CM: Correction of lower extremity deep venous incompetence by ablation of superficial reflux. Ann Vasc Surg 10:186–189, 1996.
26. Ballard J: unpublished data.
27. Bergan JJ: Surgical procedures for varicose veins: Axial stripping and stab avulsion. In Bergan JJ, Kistner RL (eds): Atlas of Venous Surgery. Philadelphia, WB Saunders, 1992.
28. Neglen P: Treatment of varicosities of saphenous origin: Comparison of ligation, selective excision, and sclerotherapy. In Bergan JJ, Goldman MP (eds): Varicose Veins and Telangiectasias: Diagnosis and Treatment. St. Louis, Quality Medical Publishing, 1993.
29. Ruckley CV: Surgical Management of Venous Disease. London, Wolfe Medical Publications, 1988.
30. Labropoulos N, Touloupakis E, Giannoukas AD, et al: Recurrent varicose veins: Investigation of the pattern and extent of reflux with color-flow duplex scanning. Surgery 119:406–410, 1996.
31. Lumley JSP: Color Atlas of Vascular Surgery. Baltimore, Williams & Wilkins, 1986.
32. Greenhalgh RM: Vascular Surgical Techniques. Philadelphia, WB Saunders, 1989.
33. Bishop CCR, Jarrett PEM: Outpatient varicose vein surgery under local anaesthesia. Br J Surg 73:821–822, 1986.
34. Samuels PB: Technique of varicose vein surgery. Am J Surg 142:239–244, 1981.
35. Conrad P: Groin-to-knee downward stripping of long saphenous vein. Phlebology 7:20–22, 1992.
36. Furuya T, Tada Y, Sato O: A new technique for reducing subcutaneous hemorrhage after stripping of the great saphenous vein (Letter). J Vasc Surg 3:493–494, 1992.
37. Corbett R, Jayakumar JN: Clean-up varicose vein surgery—use a tourniquet. Ann R Coll Surg Engl 71:57–58, 1989.
38. Thompson JF, Royle GT, Farrands PA, et al: Varicose vein surgery using a pneumatic tourniquet: Reduced blood loss and improved cosmesis. Ann R Coll Surg Engl 72:119–122, 1990.
39. Rutherford RB, Sawyer JD, Jones DN: The fate of residual saphenous vein after partial removal or ligation. J Vasc Surg 12:422–428, 1990.
40. McMullin GM, Coleridge Smith PD, Scurr JH: Objective assessment of high ligation without stripping the long saphenous vein. Br J Surg 78:1139–1142, 1991.
41. Mayo CH: Treatment of varicose veins. Surg Gynecol Obstet 2:385–388, 1906.
42. Babcock WW: A new operation for extirpation of varicose veins. N Y Med J 86:1553–1557, 1907.
43. Keller WL: A new method for extirpating the internal saphenous and similar veins in varicose conditions: A preliminary report. N Y Med J 82:385–389, 1905.
44. Bergan JJ: Surgery of the Veins of the Lower Extremity. Philadelphia, WB Saunders, 1985.
45. Munn SR, Morton JB, MacBeth WAAG, McLeish AR: To strip or not to strip the long saphenous vein? A varicose veins trial. Br J Surg 68:426–428, 1981.
46. Sarin S, Scurr JH, Coleridge Smith PD: Assessment of stripping the long saphenous vein in temperature treatment of primary varicose veins. Br J Surg 79:889–893, 1992.

47. Stonebridge PA, Chalmers N, Beggs I, et al: Recurrent varicose veins: A varicographic analysis leading to a new practical classification. Br J Surg 82:60–62, 1995.
48. Darke SG: The morphology of recurrent varicose veins. Eur J Vasc Surg 6:512–517, 1992.
49. Gradman WS, Segalowitz J, Grundfest W: Venoscopy in varicose vein surgery: Initial experience. Phlebology 8:145–150, 1993.
50. Ono T, Bergan JJ, Schmid-Schönbein GW, Takase S: Monocyte infiltration into venous valves. J Vasc Surg 27:158–166, 1998.
51. Butterworth DM, Rose SS, Clark P, et al: Light microscopy, immunohistochemistry, and electron microscopy of the valves of the lower limb veins and jugular veins. Phlebology 7:1–3, 1992.
52. Ricci S, Georgiev M, Goldman MP: Ambulatory Phlebectomy. St. Louis, CV Mosby, 1995.
53. Hobbs JT: Perioperative venography to ensure accurate saphenopopliteal vein ligation. Br Med J 280:1578, 1980.
54. van Bemmelen PS, Bedford G, Beach K, Strandness DE Jr: Quantitative segmental evaluation of venous valvular reflux with ultrasound scanning. J Vasc Surg 10:425–431, 1989.
55. Goren G, Yellin AE: Invaginated axial saphenectomy by a semirigid stripper: Perforate-invaginate stripping. J Vasc Surg 20:970–977, 1994.
56. Garrison FH: Introduction to the History of Medicine. Philadelphia, WB Saunders, 1929.
57. Bergan JJ: History of surgery of the somatic veins. In Bergan JJ, Kistner RL (eds): Atlas of Venous Surgery. Philadelphia, WB Saunders, 1992.
58. Genevrier M: Du traitement des varices par les injections coagulantes concentrées de sels de quinine. Soc Med Mil Fr 15:169, 1921.
59. Rogers L, Winchester AH: Intravenous sclerosing injections. Br Med J 2:120, 1930.
60. Biegeleisen HI: Telangiectasias associated with varicose veins. JAMA 102:2092, 1934.
61. Foley WT: The eradication of venous blemishes. Cutis 15:665, 1975.
62. Fegan WG: Varicose Veins: Compression Sclerotherapy. Dublin, Wm Heinemann Medical Books, 1967.
63. Miani A, Rubertsi U: Collecting venules. Minerva Cardioangiol 41:541, 1958.
64. Wokalek H, Vanscheidt W, Martan K, Leder O: Morphology and localization of sunburst varicosities: An electron microscopic study. J Dermatol Surg Oncol 15:149, 1989.
65. deFaria JL, Morales I: Histopathology of the telangiectasia associated with varicose veins. Dermatologica 127:321, 1963.
66. Bohler-Sommeregger K, Karnel F, Schuller-Petrovic SS, Sautler R: Do telangiectasias communicate with the deep venous system? J Dermatol Surg Oncol 18:403, 1992.
67. Wells HS, Youman JB, Miller DG: Tissue pressure (intracutaneous, subcutaneous, and intramuscular) as related to venous pressure, capillary filtration, and other factors. J Clin Invest 17:489, 1938.
68. Cockett HFB, Jones BE: The ankle blow-out syndrome: A new approach to the varicose ulcer problem. Lancet 1:17, 1953.
69. Green D: Compression sclerotherapy: Techniques. Dermatol Clin 7:137, 1989.
70. Goldman MP: Sclerotherapy. St. Louis, Mosby–Year Book, 1991.
71. Imhoff E, Stemmer R: Classification and mechanism of action of sclerosing agents. Soc Fr Phlebol 22:143, 1969.
72. Lindemayer H, Santler R: The fibrinolytic activity of the vein wall. Phlebologie 30:151, 1977.
73. Reiner L: The activity of anionic surface active compounds on producing vascular obliteration. Proc Soc Exp Biol Med 62:49, 1946.
74. Tretbar LL: Spider angiomata: Treatment with sclerosant injections. J Kansas Med Soc 79:198, 1978.
75. Carlin MC, Ratz JL: Treatment of telangiectasias: Comparison of sclerosing agents. J Dermatol Surg Oncol 13:1181, 1987.
76. Sadick NS: Sclerotherapy of varicose and telangiectatic leg veins: Minimal sclerosant concentration of hypertonic saline and its relationship to vessel diameter. J Dermatol Surg Oncol 17:65, 1991.
77. Foley DP, Forrestal MD: A comparative evaluation of the empty vein utilizing duplex ultrasonography. In Raymond-Martimbeau P, Prescott R, Zummo M (eds): Phlébologie. Montrouge, France, John Libbey Eurotext, 1992.
78. Vin F: Principe, technique, et résultats du traitement rapide des saphènes internes incontinentes par scléro-herapie. In Raymond-Martimbeau P, Prescott R, Zummo M (eds) Phlébologie. Montrouge, France, John Libbey Eurotext, 1992.
79. Sigg K: The treatment of varicosities and accompanying complications. Angiology 3:355, 1952.
80. Tretbar LL: The origin of reflux in incompetent blue reticular/telangiectatic veins. In Davy A, Stemmer R (eds): Phlébologie 89. Montrouge, France, John Libbey Eurotext, 1989.
81. Duffy DM: Small-vessel sclerotherapy: An overview. Adv Dermatol 3:221, 1988.
82. Goldman MP: Sclerotherapy of superficial venules and telangiectasias of the lower extremities. Dermatol Clin 5:369, 1987.
83. Bodian EL: Techniques of sclerotherapy for sunburst venous blemishes. J Dermatol Surg Oncol 11:696, 1985.
84. Goldman MP: Polidocanol (aethoxysclerol) for sclerotherapy of superficial venules and telangiectasias. J Dermatol Surg Oncol 15:204, 1989.
85. Bochner BS, Lichtenstein LM: Anaphylaxis. N Engl J Med 324:1785, 1991.
86. Bergan JJ, Goldman MP: Complications of sclerotherapy. In Bernhard VM, Towne JB (eds): Complications of Vascular Surgery. St. Louis, CV Mosby, 1991.

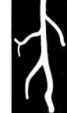

C H A P T E R 1 4 8
Management of Perforator Vein Incompetence

Peter Gloviczki, M.D., and Jeffrey M. Rhodes, M.D.

Incompetent perforating veins were observed in patients with venous ulceration by John Gay as early as the 1860s,[1] but surgical interruption of these veins to prevent ulceration was not suggested until 1938, by Linton.[2] Linton attributed a key role to perforator vein incompetence in the pathomechanism of venous ulcerations, an idea embraced later by Cockett,[3, 4] Dodd,[5] and several other investigators.[6–18] Linton's original operative technique, which used a long skin incision, has been largely abandoned because of frequent wound complications and need for prolonged

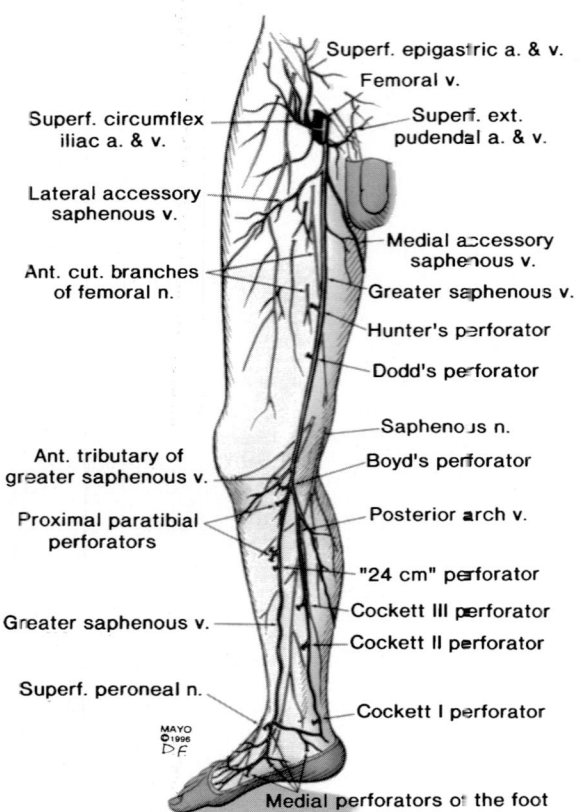

FIGURE 148–1. Anatomy of medial superficial and perforating veins of the leg. (From Mozes G, Gloviczki P, Menawat SS, et al: Surgical anatomy for endoscopic subfascial division of perforating veins. J Vasc Surg 24:800–808, 1996.)

hospitalization. Attempts to interrupt perforators with less invasive surgical techniques included the use of shorter skin incisions[3–10] and blind avulsion of the perforators with a shearing instrument.[19] Subfascial endoscopic perforator vein surgery (SEPS) has rapidly developed as an effective, minimally invasive technique to interrupt perforating veins.[11, 15–18, 20–26]

In this chapter we review the surgical anatomy of the perforating veins and discuss available evidence that supports the role of perforators in chronic venous disease. We describe surgical indications and preoperative evaluation of the patients and present the currently used open and endoscopic surgical techniques for interruption of perforators. Finally, we review data in the literature on efficacy of perforator vein interruption.

SURGICAL ANATOMY OF PERFORATOR VEINS

Perforator veins connect the superficial to the deep venous system either directly to the main axial veins (direct perforators) or indirectly to muscular tributaries or soleal venous sinuses (indirect perforators). The term *communicating veins* is reserved now for veins that interconnect portions of the same system. Although flow through perforators of the

foot is usually from deep to superficial,[27] in normal limbs unidirectional flow from the greater and lesser saphenous systems toward the deep veins in calf and thigh perforators is ensured by venous valves.

In the mid and distal calf, the most important direct medial perforators do not originate directly from the greater saphenous vein (Fig. 148–1). This observation may be the most important aspect of the anatomy of leg veins because stripping of the greater saphenous vein does not affect flow through incompetent medial calf perforators in most patients. The Cockett perforators connect the posterior arch vein (Leonardo's vein) to the paired posterior tibial veins. In some patients the posterior arch veins are not well developed, and other posterior tributaries of the greater saphenous vein are connected through perforators to the deep system.

Three groups of Cockett perforators have been identified. The *Cockett I* perforator is located just behind the medial malleolus, the *Cockett II* veins are located at 7 to 9 cm proximally from the lower border of the medial malleolus, and the *Cockett III* perforators are at 10 to 12 cm (Fig. 148–2).[28] These veins are usually at 2 to 4 cm posterior from the medial edge of the tibia (Linton's line or "lane").[29–31] The more proximal paratibial perforating veins of the calf connect the greater saphenous or its tributaries to the posterior tibial or popliteal veins. These perforators are found 1 to 2 cm medially from the medial border of the tibia.

In their studies, Mozes and coworkers found three groups of paratibial perforators at 18 to 22 cm, 23 to 27 cm, and 28 to 32 cm from the medial malleolus, respectively (Fig. 148–3; see also Fig. 148–1).[28] The 18- to 22-cm group corresponds to the "24-cm" perforator described by Sherman, who used the sole of the foot as his point of reference.[31] The most proximal calf perforator just distal to the knee (Boyd's perforator) connects the greater saphenous

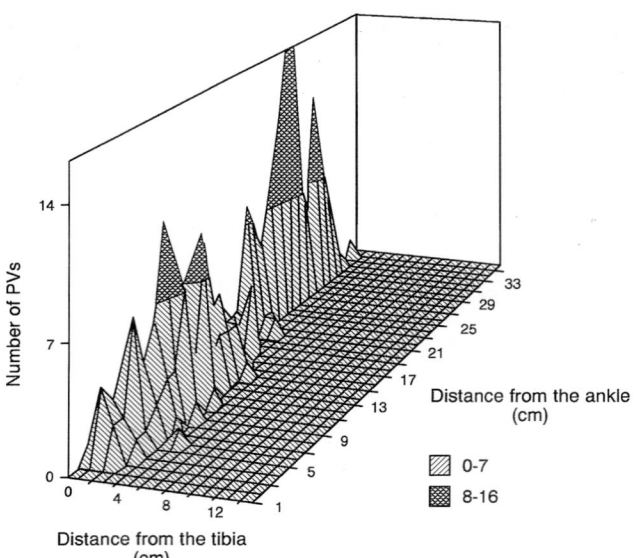

FIGURE 148–2. Number and location of 287 medial direct perforating veins (PVs) in 40 legs. (From Mozes G, Gloviczki P, Menawat SS, et al: Surgical anatomy for endoscopic subfascial division of perforating veins. J Vasc Surg 24:800–808, 1996.)

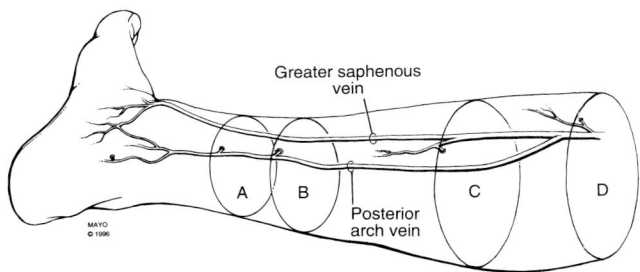

FIGURE 148–3. Superficial and perforating veins in the medial side of the leg. The cross sections shown in Figure 148–4 are indicated (*A–D*). (From Mozes G, Gloviczki P, Menawat SS, et al: Surgical anatomy for endoscopic subfascial division of perforating veins. J Vasc Surg 24:800–808, 1996.)

vein to the popliteal vein.[28] Although during anatomic dissections an average of 14 medial direct and indirect perforators per limb can be identified, in most patients with chronic venous insufficiency (CVI) only three to five larger, clinically significant incompetent perforators are found.[16]

Certain anatomic considerations specific to the endoscopic interruption of medial calf perforators must be mentioned. In cadaver dissections, Mozes and coworkers noted that only 63% of all medial perforators were directly acces-

sible from the posterior superficial compartment (Fig. 148–4).[28] This is an important observation because major incompetent perforators can be missed during surgery if additional dissection of planes through the endoscope is not performed. Two areas should be explored. One is the posterior deep compartment, and the other is the intermuscular septum in Linton's lane, which can be a duplication of the deep fascia. The paratibial and the Cockett veins can be found under the fascia of the deep posterior compartment, while the Cockett veins can be located also within the intermuscular septum.

A deceiving anatomic variation of the Cockett II perforator can be a division with a posterior branch directing toward the soleus muscle. Although this posterior division is easily visible when it penetrates the posterior superficial compartment, the more important anterior division is hidden by the intermuscular septum or by the deep posterior fascia, and it may be missed (Fig. 148–5). Sixteen per cent of Cockett III and 68% of Cockett II perforators are hidden by a septum or fascia that needs to be divided during endoscopic surgery; otherwise, major perforators will be left behind.[28]

In the calf, anterior and lateral perforators are also found, and in patients with lateral ulceration these veins are clinically significant. The anterior perforators connect tributaries of the greater and lesser saphenous veins directly to the anterior tibial veins. The lateral perforating veins consist of

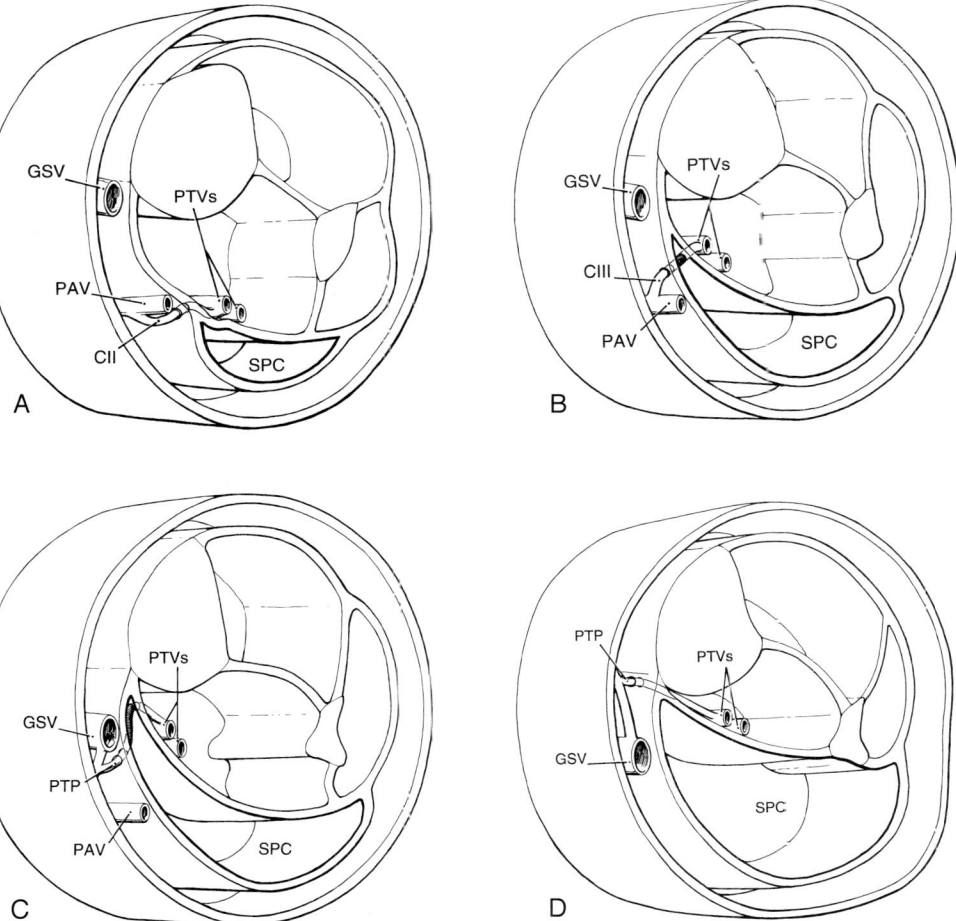

FIGURE 148–4. Compartments and medial veins of the leg. Cross sections are at the levels of Cockett II (*A*), Cockett III (*B*), "24-cm" (*C*), and more proximal paratibial (*D*) perforating veins. GSV = greater saphenous vein, PAV = posterior arch vein, PTVs = posterior tibial veins, SPC = superficial posterior compartment, CII = Cockett II, CIII = Cockett III, PTP = paratibial perforator. (From Mozes G, Gloviczki P, Menawat SS, et al: Surgical anatomy for endoscopic subfascial division of perforating veins. J Vasc Surg 24:800–808, 1996.)

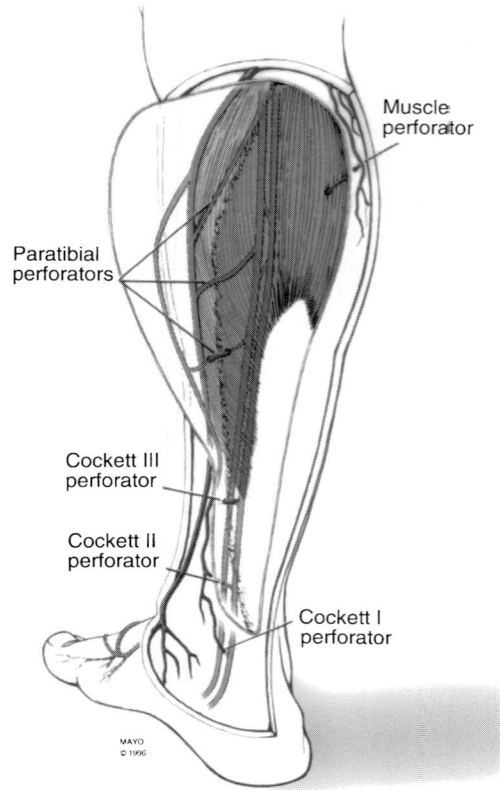

FIGURE 148–5. Relationship of the superficial, perforating, and deep veins to the fascia of the superficial posterior compartment. Note that Cockett III and the lowest proximal paratibial perforator ("24-cm perforator") are readily accessible from the subfascial space. (From Mozes G, Gloviczki P, Kadar A, Carmichael SW: Surgical anatomy of perforating veins. In Gloviczki P, Bergan JJ [eds]: Atlas of Endoscopic Perforator Vein Surgery. London, Springer-Verlag, 1998, pp 17–28.)

both direct and indirect perforators. In the distal calf, the lesser saphenous vein is connected by direct perforators to the peroneal veins (Bassi's perforator). The indirect perforators connect tributaries of the lesser saphenous vein to either the muscular venous sinuses or the gastrocnemius or soleus veins before the deep axial system is entered. The largest indirect muscular perforators are referred to as the *soleus* and *gastrocnemius points* (Fig. 148–6).

As the greater saphenous vein continues cephalad through the thigh, there are two additional groups of perforators (Fig. 148–7). The *Dodd perforator* and the *Hunterian* perforator connect the greater saphenous to the proximal popliteal or the superficial femoral veins (see Fig. 148–1). Because a well-developed double saphenous system is present in at least 8% of the patients, removal of one saphenous vein does not always guarantee interruption of these perforator veins.

HEMODYNAMIC SIGNIFICANCE OF PERFORATING VEINS

Chapter 144 covers the pathophysiology of CVI, but data on the hemodynamic significance of the perforator veins are briefly addressed here. Although the pathophysiology of CVI at the cellular level remains controversial, most authors agree that venous hypertension in the erect position and during ambulation is the most important factor responsible for the development of skin changes and venous ulcerations. Reflux of venous blood due to primary or post-thrombotic valvular incompetence, in addition to calf pump failure, is the most frequent cause of CVI. Linton attributed a key role to ambulatory venous hypertension,[32] as did Cockett, who coined the term "ankle blowout syndrome" to differentiate perforator incompetence from the usually more benign isolated saphenous incompetence.[3, 4]

Indeed, perforator vein incompetence can raise pressures in the supramalleolar network well above 100 mmHg during calf muscle construction, a phenomenon best described by Negus and Friedgood using the analogy of a "broken bellows."[9] Experiments of Bjordal confirmed a net outward flow of 60/ml/min through incompetent perforating veins.[33] The importance of incompetent perforators is also supported by the observation that skin changes and venous ulcers almost always develop in the gaiter area of the leg (the area between the distal edge of the soleus muscle and the ankle), where large incompetent medial perforating veins are located.

Although severe isolated incompetence of the superficial system may also lead to high ambulatory pressures and to the development of ulcers, evidence is increasing that the majority of patients with venous ulcers have multisystem (superficial, deep, and perforator) incompetence, involving at least two of the three venous systems.[26, 35–38] In the recent report of the North American Subfascial Endoscopic Perforator Surgery (NASEPS) registry, only 28% of the patients with advanced CVI were free of deep venous reflux or obstruction.[25] In a much-quoted series from a Middlesex hospital, 53% of 79 limbs with venous ulcers had a competent deep system.[39] All these patients had saphenous incompetence, but incompetence of perforating veins in this study was not addressed.

The large prevalence of perforator incompetence in ulcer patients is emphasized even in those studies that favor operation on the incompetent superficial system only.[40] At Boston University, 95 limbs with venous ulcerations were studied with duplex scanning; isolated superficial incompetence was found in 17% only, and 63% had perforator incompetence.[38] Similarly, a 60% incidence of perforator incompetence in ulcer patients was demonstrated by duplex scanning by Lees and Lambert[41] and a 56% incidence by Labrapoulos and associates.[36] In several surgical series, incompetent perforators were noted to be more prevalent.[9, 10, 16]

Although few argue today that incompetent perforators occur in at least two thirds of the patients with venous ulcerations, the contribution of perforating vein incompetence to the hemodynamic derangement in limbs with CVI remains a topic of debate.[42, 43] Because functional studies cannot reliably differentiate perforator from deep vein incompetence in most patients, the task of documenting hemodynamic problems related directly to perforator incompetence, even if it is confirmed with duplex scanning, remains difficult. The question will be difficult to answer because isolated perforator vein incompetence in CVI is rare[36] and because incompetent perforators with outward flow have been observed in normal limbs as well; in one study 21% of normal limbs had outward flow in perforating veins.[44]

In a study using Doppler ultrasonography and ambula-

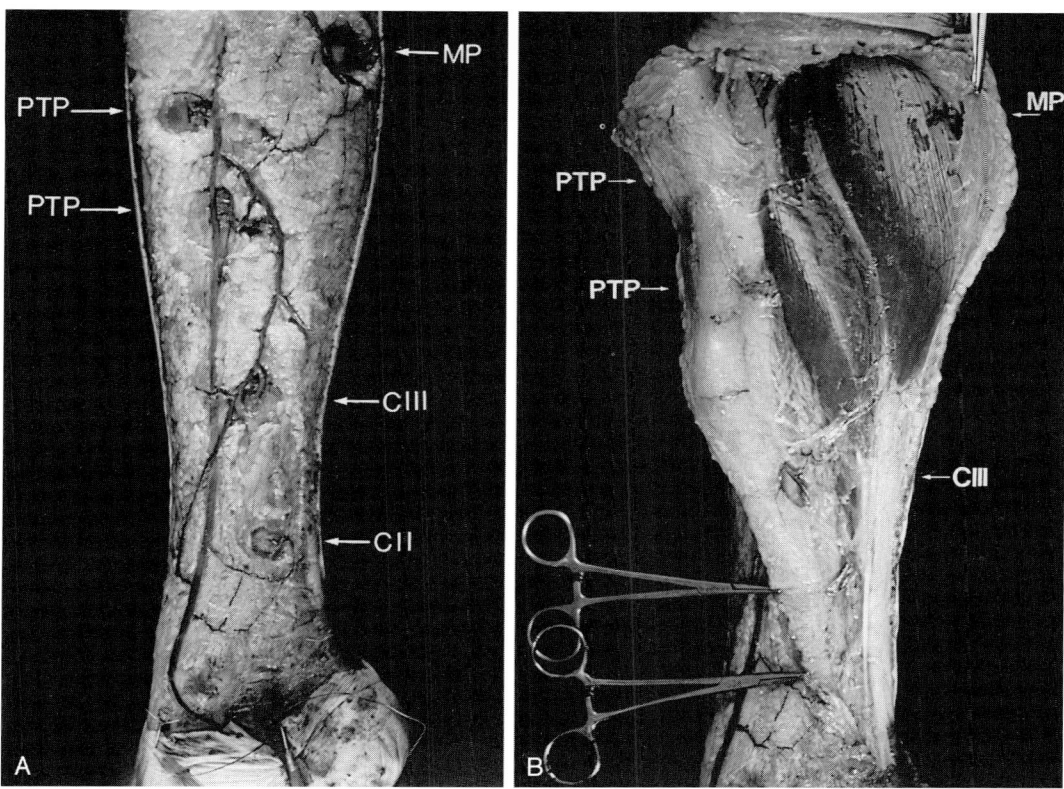

FIGURE 148–6. Corrosion cast of leg veins. *A,* Skin and a portion of subcutaneous fat were removed. *B,* Fascia has been incised and rolled anteriorly to expose the superficial posterior compartment. Note that only the lower paratibial perforator and Cockett III perforators are now accessible in the superficial posterior compartment. MP = muscle perforator, PTP = paratibial perforator, CII = Cockett II, CIII = Cockett III. (From Mozes G, Gloviczki P, Menawat SS, et al: Surgical anatomy for endoscopic subfascial division of perforating veins. J Vasc Surg 24:800–808, 1996.)

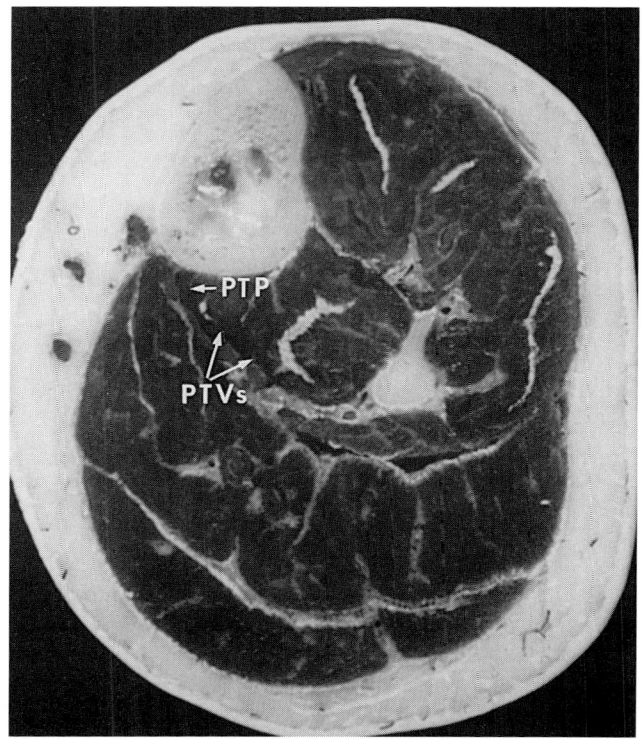

FIGURE 148–7. Cross section of the upper third of the leg. Note a paratibial perforating vein (PTP) passing between the periosteum of the tibia and the fascia of the superficial posterior compartment. Veins were filled with blue latex. PTVs = posterior tibial veins. (From Mozes G, Gloviczki P, Menawat SS, et al: A Surgical anatomy for endoscopic subfascial division of perforating veins. J Vasc Surg 24:800–808, 1996.)

tory venous pressure measurements to assess functional significance of incompetent perforating veins, however, Zukowski and Nicolaides found that 70% of incompetent perforators were of moderate or major hemodynamic significance.[45] More importantly, hemodynamic deterioration caused by incompetent perforators correlated with the severity of CVI. A correlation between the number and size of incompetent perforating veins, as detected by duplex, and the severity of CVI was also demonstrated by Labrapoulos and coworkers.[37] In patients with advanced disease more incompetent perforators were found, and their diameters were also larger. This study is significant because, contrary to previously published data,[44] it failed to confirm perforator incompetence in 106 normal volunteers.

Data have been accumulating from hemodynamic studies performed after surgical interruption of incompetent perforating veins. These are discussed later in this chapter.

INDICATIONS FOR PERFORATOR INTERRUPTION

The presence of incompetent perforators in patients with advanced CVI (clinical classes 4 to 6) is an indication for surgical treatment in a fit patient. While most authors performing open perforator ligation prefer to operate only in patients with healed ulcerations, a clean, granulating open ulcer is not a contraindication for a SEPS procedure. Contraindications include associated chronic arterial occlusive disease, infected ulcer, morbid obesity, and a nonambulatory or high-risk patient. Diabetes, renal failure, or ulcers in patients with rheumatoid arthritis or scleroderma are relative contraindications. Patients with previous perforator interruption or those with extensive skin changes, circumferential large ulcers, or large legs may not be suitable for SEPS. Those with lateral ulcerations, if appropriate, should be managed by open interruption of lateral or posterior perforators.

PREOPERATIVE EVALUATION

Chapter 145 discusses in general the evaluation of patients with CVI. Potential candidates with an indication for perforator interruption, as listed earlier, should undergo imaging studies to document superficial, deep, and perforator incompetence to confirm the clinical suspicion and to guide the operative intervention. Before perforator interruption, we favor duplex scanning (Fig. 148–8) to phlebography (Fig. 148–9) and reserve contrast studies for patients with underlying occlusive disease or for those who are candidates for deep venous reconstruction. In our practice, all candidates for SEPS, which has become our preferred technique, undergo duplex ultrasonography of the deep, superficial, and perforator systems to document location of reflux and presence of venous obstruction.[46]

Perforator mapping, a time-consuming test, is done only the day before surgery because the sites of incompetent perforators are marked on the skin of the patient with a nonerasable marker. The patient is on a tilted examining table in a near upright non–weight-bearing position for the affected extremity. Perforator incompetence is defined as outward flow of more than 0.3 second (or 0.5 second by some authors) during the relaxation phase after release of manual compression (see Fig. 148–8). Although duplex scanning misses smaller perforator veins, it has 100% specificity and the highest sensitivity of all diagnostic tests to predict the sites of incompetent perforating veins (Table 148–1).

In addition to duplex scanning, strain-gauge or air plethysmography may be performed before and after surgery. This technique can quantitate the degree of incompetence before surgery and then assess the hemodynamic results of the surgical intervention.[14, 26]

SURGICAL TECHNIQUES

Open Technique of Perforator Interruption

Linton's radical operation of subfascial ligation, which included long medial, anterolateral, and posterolateral calf

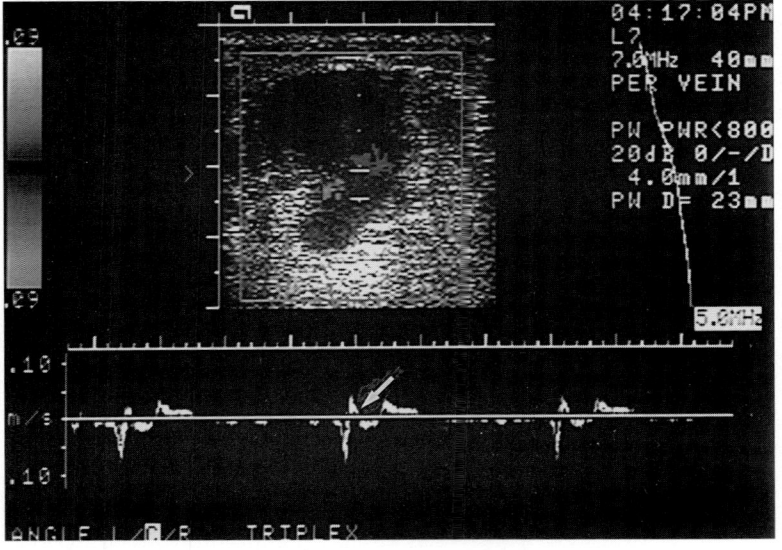

FIGURE 148–8. Color Doppler and spectral tracing of an enlarged incompetent perforating vein. Spectral analysis demonstrates bidirectional flow (*arrow*). (From Gloviczki P, Lewis BD, Lindsey JR, McKusick MA: Preoperative evaluation of chronic venous insufficiency with Duplex scanning and venography. *In* Gloviczki P, Bergan JJ [eds]: Atlas of Endoscopic Perforator Vein Surgery. London, Springer-Verlag, 1998, pp 81–91.)

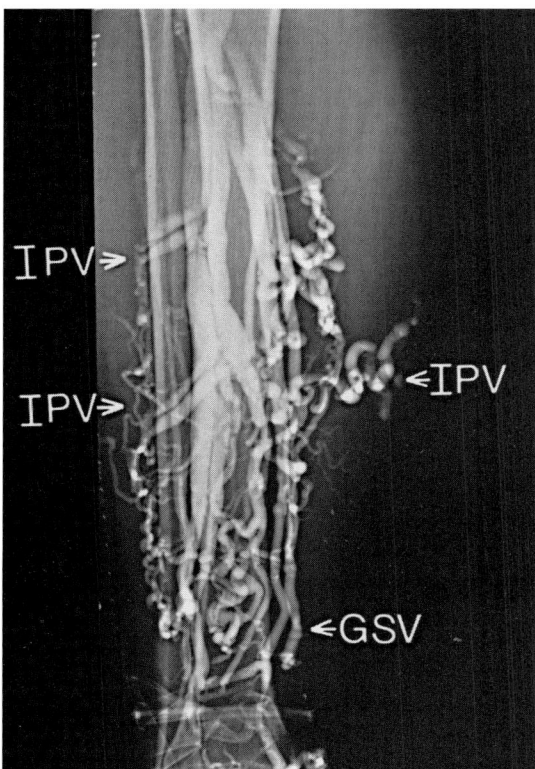

FIGURE 148–9. Ascending venogram in anteroposterior projection of the right calf of a 41-year-old female with nonhealing venous ulcer due to primary valvular incompetence. Note medial and lateral incompetent perforators (IPV) filling the superficial system with contrast. GSV = greater saphenous vein. (From Gloviczki P, Lewis BD, Lindsey JR, McKusick MA: Preoperative evaluation of chronic venous insufficiency with Duplex scanning and venography. In Gloviczki P, Bergan JJ (eds): Atlas of Endoscopic Perforator Vein Surgery. London, Springer-Verlag, 1998, pp 81–91.)

incisions, was soon abandoned because of its association with wound complications.[2] In a report published in 1953, Linton advocated only a long medial incision from the ankle to the knee to interrupt all medial and posterior perforating veins.[32] His operative technique also included stripping of the greater and lesser saphenous veins and excision of a portion of the deep fascia. (His suggestion to interrupt axial reflux by ligation of the superficial femoral vein is of historical interest only.) Wound complications caused by the incision made in the lipodermatosclerotic skin were, however, still frequent and hospitalization of the patients prolonged.

Several other authors have proposed further changes in

TABLE 148–1. DIAGNOSTIC TESTS TO PREDICT THE SITES OF INCOMPETENT PERFORATING VEINS

TEST	SENSITIVITY (%)	SPECIFICITY (%)
Physical examination[29]	60	0
Continuous wave Doppler ultrasonography[29]	62	4
Ascending phlebography[29]	60	50
Duplex scanning[18]	79	100

the open procedure to limit wound complications. These suggestions include the use of shorter medial incisions and a more posteriorly placed stocking seam type of incision. Cockett advocated ligation of the perforating veins above the deep fascia,[3, 4] a technique distinctly different from that of Linton. DePalma achieved good results using multiple, parallel bipedicled flaps placed along skin lines to access and ligate the perforating veins above or below the fascia (Figs. 148–10 and 148–11).[7] The operation was combined with saphenous stripping, ulcer excision, and skin grafting.

To decrease wound complications, a technique to ablate incompetent perforating veins from sites remote from diseased skin was first reported by Edwards in 1976.[19] Edwards designed a device, called the *phlebotome,* which is inserted through a medial incision just distal to the knee, deep to the fascia, and advanced to the level of the medial malleolus (Fig. 148–11). Resistance is felt as perforators are engaged and subsequently disrupted with the leading edge. Other authors have subsequently reported successful application of this device, passed either in the subfascial or extrafascial plane.[47]

Interruption of perforators through stab wounds and hook avulsion is another possibility, and accuracy of this blind technique will improve if duplex scanning is used for mapping. Another proposed technique was to place sutures around the perforators without a skin incision being made. Sclerotherapy to occlude perforating veins is described in Chapter 147.

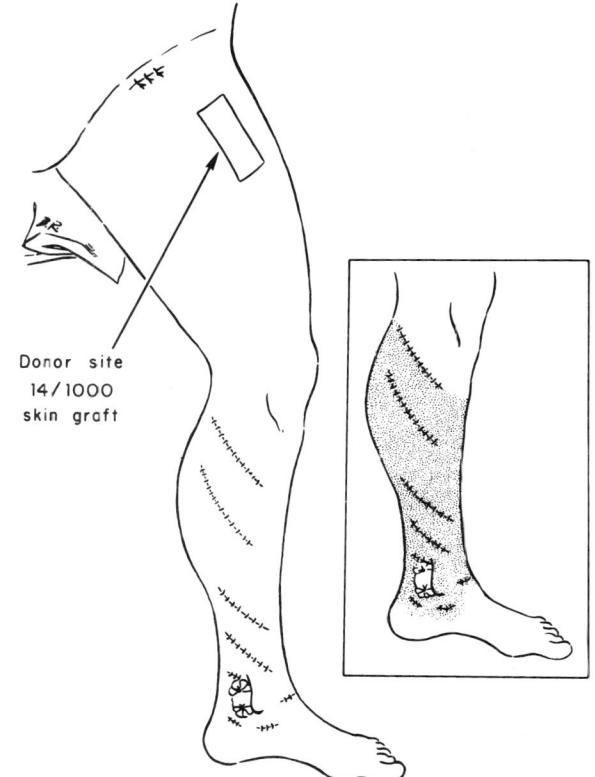

FIGURE 148–10. Linton operation modified by DePalma. Note the extent of the area that is dissected (shaded area in *inset*). Also note the submalleolar skin line incisions. (From DePalma RG: Surgical therapy for venous stasis surgery. Surgery 76:910–917, 1975.)

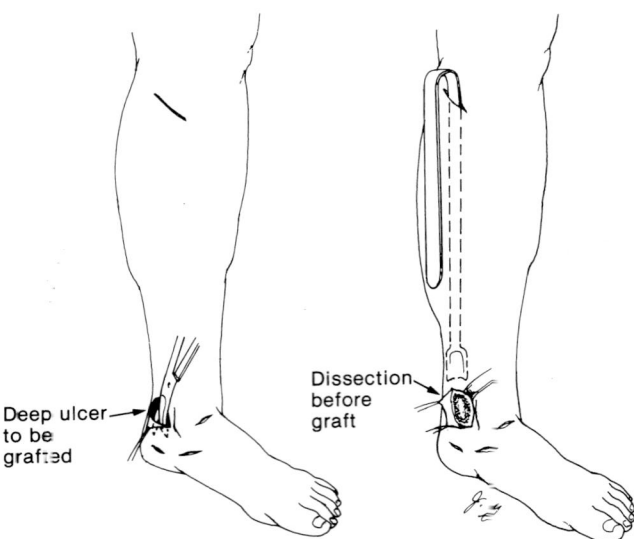

FIGURE 148–11. Excision and dissection of a deep ulcer prior to extrafascial shearing operation. The submalleolar incisions allow division of the retromalleolar perforator. (From DePalma RG: Surgical therapy for venous stasis surgery. Surgery 76:910–917, 1975.)

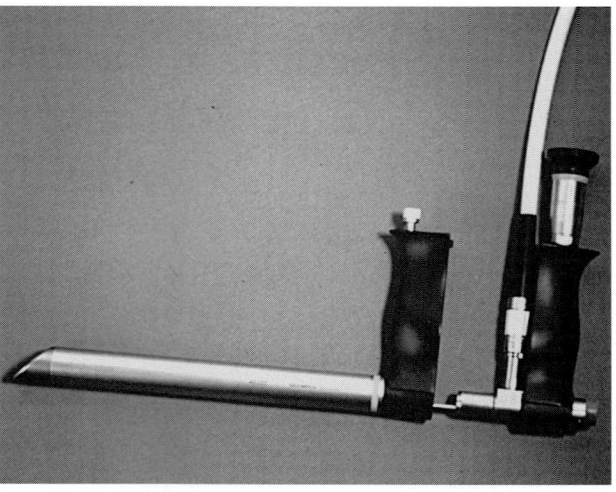

FIGURE 148–12. Olympus endoscope for the subfascial perforating vein interruption. The scope can be used with or without carbon dioxide insufflation. It has an 85-angle field of view, and the outer sheath is either 16 or 22 mm in diameter. The working channel is 6 × 8.5 mm, with a working length of 20 cm. (From Bergan JJ, Ballard JL, Sparks S: Subfascial endoscopic perforator surgery: The open technique. *In* Gloviczki P, Bergan JJ [eds]: Atlas of Endoscopic Perforator Vein Surgery. London, Springer-Verlag, 1998, 141–149.)

Techniques of Subfascial Endoscopic Perforator Surgery

Initial experience with endoscopic ablation of perforating veins, achieved through a scope placed subfascially at a site distant to the skin changes and ulceration, was reported by Hauer in 1985.[20] Since its introduction, two main techniques for SEPS have emerged. The first, based on the original work of Hauer[20] and Fischer and associates[11, 48, 49] and further developed by Bergan and coworkers,[15, 50] Pierik and coworkers,[17, 18] and Wittens,[51] uses a single scope to both view and work in the channel (Fig. 148–12). Perforating veins are either electrocauterized or clipped and divided. Until recently, instrumentation for this technique has not allowed carbon dioxide insufflation into the subfascial plane.

The second technique, involving instrumentation from laparoscopic surgery, was initiated by O'Donnell[13] and developed by our group at the Mayo Clinic[23] and by Conrad in Australia.[22] We also use a thigh tourniquet that is inflated to 300 mmHg after the limb is exsanguinated by an Esmarque bandage (Fig. 148–13). Two 10-mm-diameter endoscopic ports are then placed 6 to 10 cm from each other proximal from the diseased skin in the calf (Fig. 148–14). We prefer using a 10-mm video camera because smaller, 5- or 2-mm scopes have inferior image quality. Carbon dioxide is insufflated into the subfascial space, and pressure is maintained around 30 mmHg to improve access to the perforators (Fig. 148–15). Using laparoscopic scissors inserted through the second port, we sharply divide the remaining loose connective tissue between the calf muscles and the superficial fascia.

The subfascial space is widely explored from the medial border of the tibia to the posterior midline and down to the level of the ankle. All perforators encountered are interrupted. Perforators less than 2 mm are divided with the harmonic scalpel, and all others are divided sharply

between clips (Figs. 148–16 through 148–18). As discussed previously, we perform paratibial fasciotomy by incising the fascia of the posterior deep compartment close to the tibia to avoid any injury to the posterior tibial vessels and the tibial nerve. Paratibial and Cockett perforators can frequently be found under the fascia. The Cockett II and Cockett III perforators, when located in an intermuscular septum, are dissected and divided between clips. The medial insertion of the soleus muscle to the tibia may also have to be exposed to visualize proximal paratibial perforators.

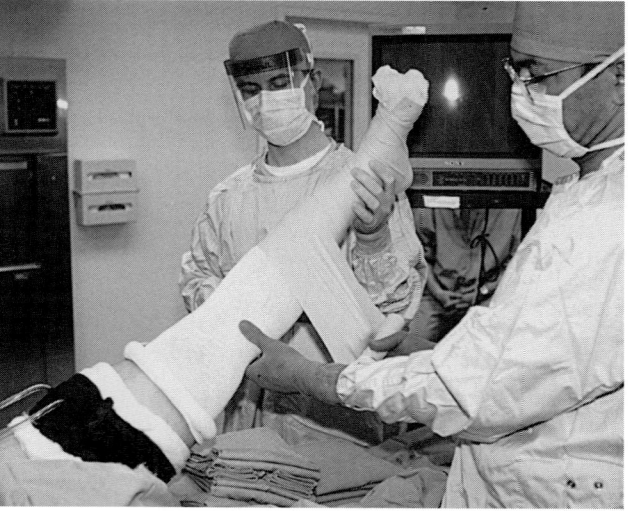

FIGURE 148–13. Endoscopic perforator division is performed in a bloodless field. A pneumatic tourniquet is placed on the thigh, and the extremity is exsanguinated with an Esmarque bandage. (From Gloviczki P, Canton LG, Cambria RA, Rhee RY: Subfascial endoscopic perforator vein surgery with gas insufflation. *In* Gloviczki P, Bergan JJ [eds]: Atlas of Endoscopic Perforator Vein Surgery. London, Springer-Verlag, 1998, pp 125–138.)

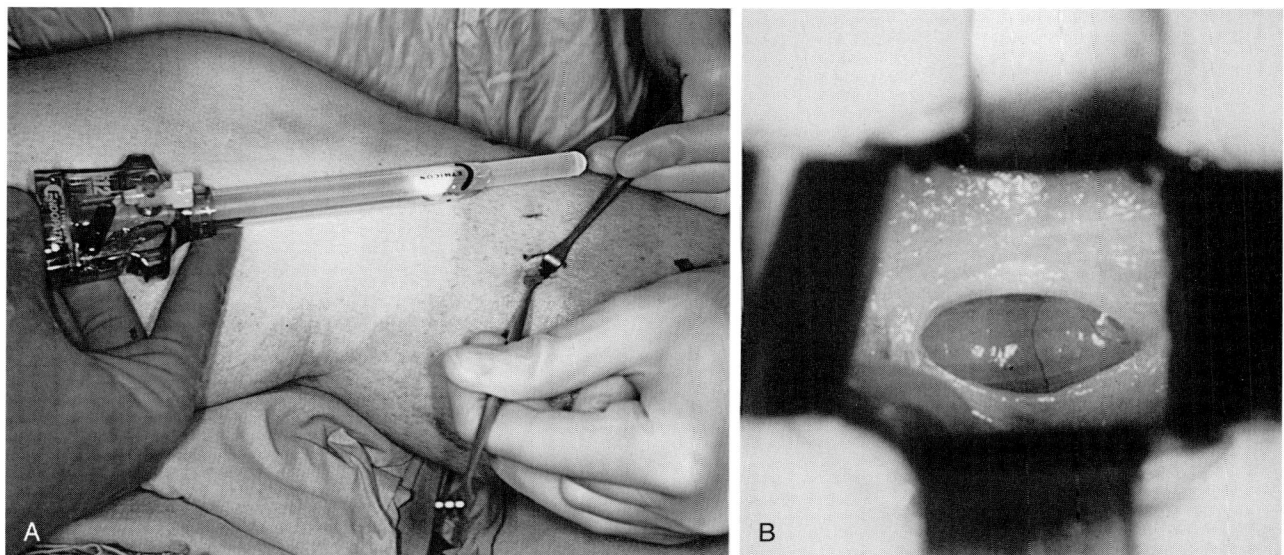

FIGURE 148–14. *A,* A 10-mm laparoscopic port is placed into the subfascial space with the help of a blunt obturator. *B,* Incision of the fascia of the superficial posterior compartment. Note the small skin incision to allow an air seal around the port. (From Gloviczki P, Cambria RA, Rhee RY, et al: Surgical technique and preliminary results with endoscopic subfascial division of perforating veins. J Vasc Surg 23:517–523, 1996.)

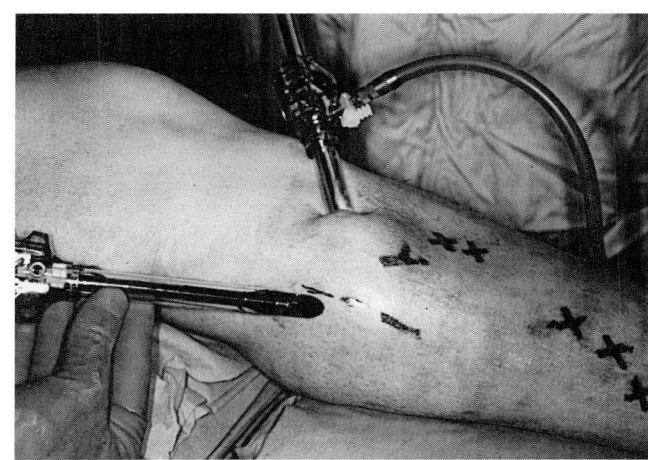

FIGURE 148–15. Carbon dioxide is insufflated through the first port, which is used for the video camera. Placement of a second 10-mm port is performed under video control. Incompetent perforators were marked with an X preoperatively with duplex scanning. (From Gloviczki P, Cambria RA, Rhee RY, et al: Surgical technique and preliminary results with endoscopic subfascial division of perforating veins. J Vasc Surg 23:517–523, 1996.)

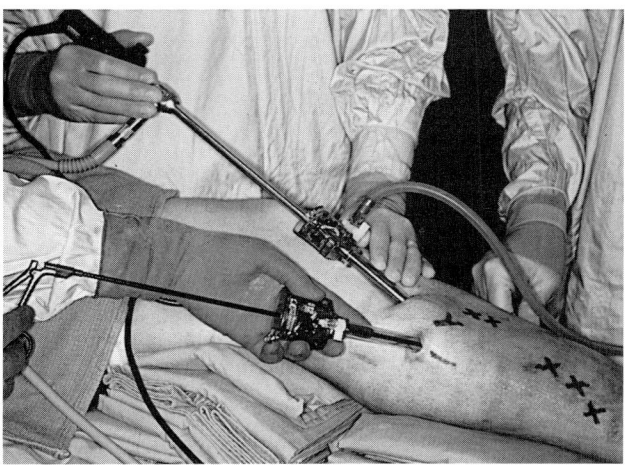

FIGURE 148–16. Clipping and division of perforators is performed with laparoscopic instruments placed through the second port; the first port is used for video control. (From Gloviczki P, Cambria RA, Rhee RY, et al: Surgical technique and preliminary results with endoscopic subfascial division of perforating veins. J Vasc Surg 23:517–523, 1996.)

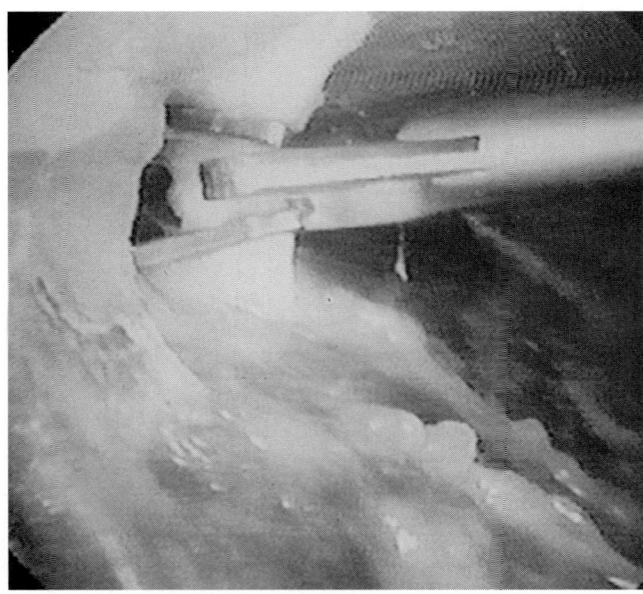

FIGURE 148–17. Division of the perforator with endoscopic scissors after placement of vascular clips. (From Gloviczki P, Cambria RA, Rhee RY, et al: Surgical technique and preliminary results with endoscopic subfascial division of perforating veins. J Vasc Surg 23:517–523, 1996.)

One can approach the more proximal perforators by rotating the ports cephalad and continuing the dissection up to the level of the knee. Even though the addition of a paratibial fasciotomy can aid in distal exposure, retromalleolar Cockett I perforators cannot usually be reached endoscopically. An incompetent Cockett I perforator, identified by preoperative duplex scanning, may require a separate small incision over it to gain direct exposure (Figs. 148–19 and 148–20).

At the completion of the endoscopic portion of the procedure, the instruments and ports are removed, the carbon dioxide is manually expressed from the limb, and the tourniquet is deflated. If concomitant superficial reflux is present, high ligation and stripping of the incompetent portion of the greater saphenous vein (usually from groin to below the knee) is performed. Stab avulsion of varicosities is also performed, and lesser saphenous reflux, if present, is corrected by ligation or stripping. Wounds are closed with subcutaneous and subcuticular absorbable sutures, and the limb is wrapped with an elastic bandage. Leg

elevation is maintained postoperatively, and after 3 hours ambulation is permitted. This is an outpatient procedure, and the patients are discharged the same day or the next morning after overnight observation.

Progress in technology has resulted in continuous improvements in instrumentation, video equipment, endoscopes (see Fig. 148–12), and dissecting devices. Fogarty's balloon dissecting device should be mentioned because it has been used with increasing frequency to widen the subfascial space and to facilitate access after port placement (Figs. 148–21 and 148–22).[52]

RESULTS OF SURGICAL TREATMENT

Clinical Results of Perforator Interruption

Clinical benefit attributed directly to interruption of incompetent perforating veins has been difficult to assess because concomitant ablation of saphenous reflux has frequently

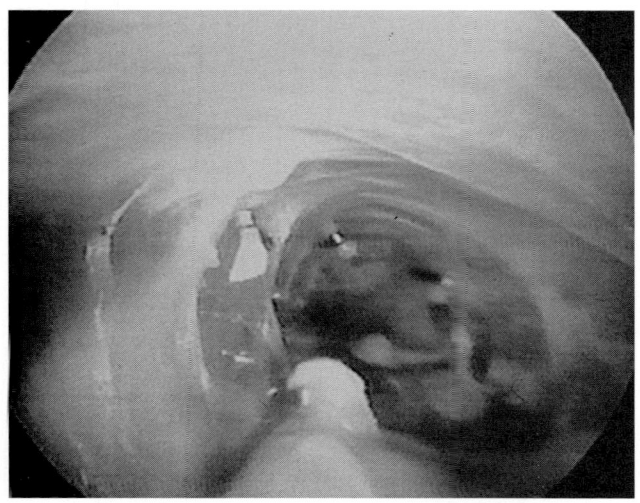

FIGURE 148–18. Full view of the superficial posterior compartment after clipping and division of the medial perforating veins. (From Gloviczki P, Cambria RA, Rhee RY, et al: Surgical technique and preliminary results with endoscopic subfascial division of perforating veins. J Vasc Surg 23:517–523, 1996.)

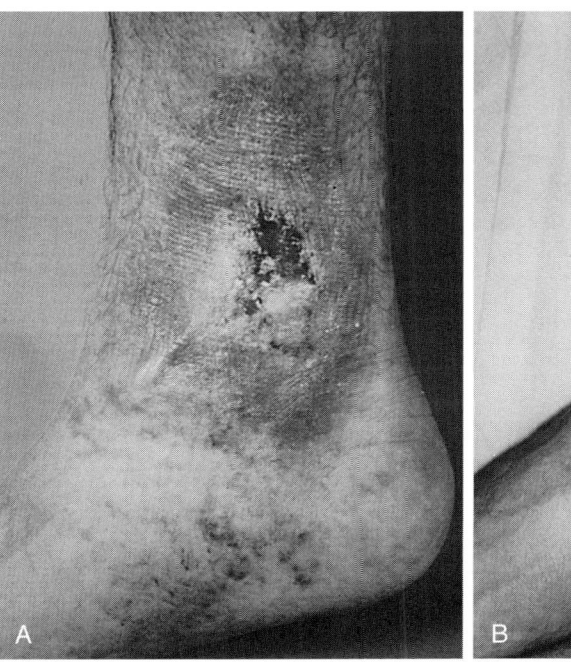
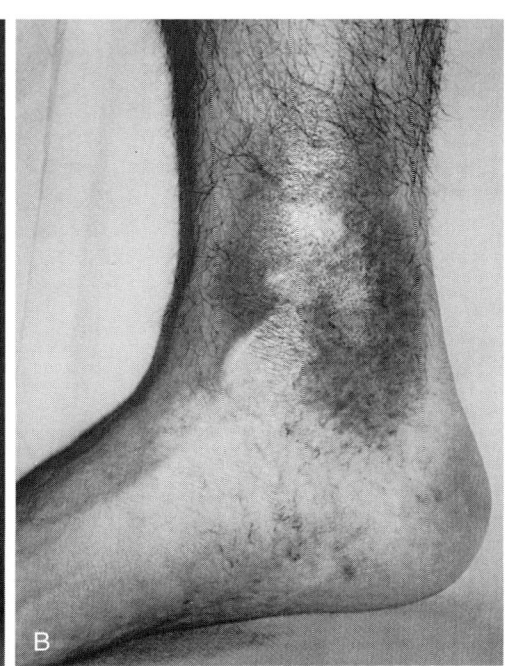

FIGURE 148–19. *A,* Thirty-six-year-old male with post-thrombotic ulcer of the right ankle before endoscopic division of six medial perforating veins. *B,* Same leg 10 months later with healed ulcer. (From Gloviczki P, Canton LG, Cambria RA, Rhee RY: Subfascial endoscopic perforator vein surgery with gas insufflation. *In* Gloviczki P, Bergan JJ [eds]: Atlas of Endoscopic Perforator Vein Surgery. London, Springer-Verlag, 1998, pp 125–138.)

been performed. In addition, in many studies the follow-up of a large number of patients was insufficient to predict ulcer recurrence. Because level 1 evidence of the effectiveness of perforator ligation (or of any surgical treatment) over nonoperative management is currently not available, postoperative results should be compared with results of larger series of nonoperative management (Table 148–2), as detailed in Chapter 146.[53–56]

In their classic papers, Linton[2, 32] and Cockett[3, 4] reported

benefits from open perforator ligation, and these benefits were later supported by data from several other investigators.[5–10, 54–57] In nine large series,[6, 9, 10, 17, 57–62] ulcer recurrence rates ranged from 0% to 55%, and they averaged 22% (Table 148–3). In one study that included 108 limbs with venous ulcers, 84% were free of ulcerations up to 6 years after perforator vein ligation.[53]

Wound complications after open procedures were significant in most series; they ranged from 12% to 53% and

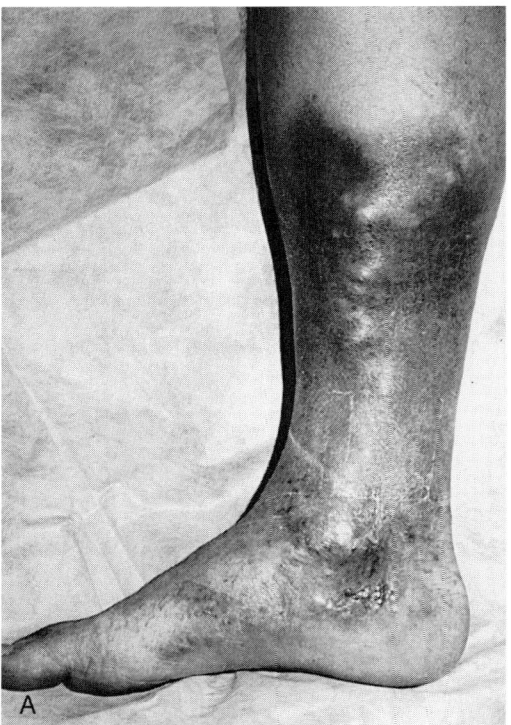
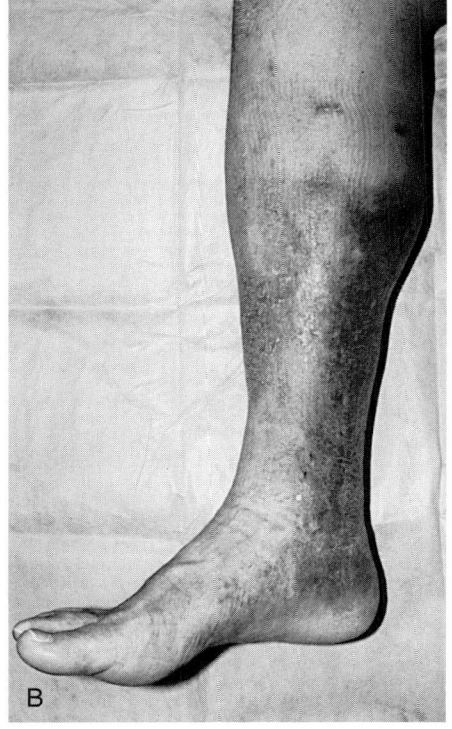

FIGURE 148–20. *A,* Right leg of a 64-year-old male who has a 2-year history of ulcer and severe post-thrombotic syndrome. *B,* Postoperative picture at 6 weeks shows healed ulcer and incisions following subfascial endoscopic perforator vein surgery, stripping, and avulsion of varicose veins. Three years later the patient is asymptomatic, does not use elastic stockings, and has had no ulcer recurrence. (From Gloviczki P, Canton LG, Cambria RA, Rhee RY: Subfascial endoscopic perforator vein surgery with gas insufflation. *In* Gloviczki P, Bergan JJ [eds]: Atlas of Endoscopic Perforator Vein Surgery. London, Springer-Verlag, 1998, pp 125–138, with permission.)

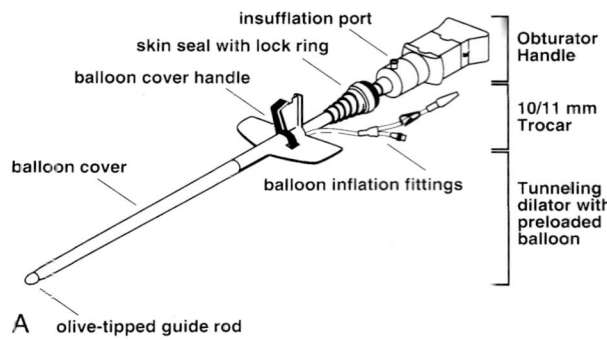

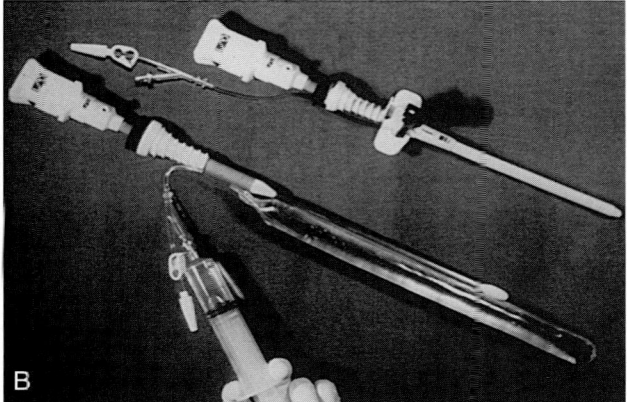

FIGURE 148–21. *A,* Components of balloon dissector (General Surgical Innovations, Palo Alto, Calif.) for creation of a large subfascial working space. An integral 10-mm endoscopic port is included. *B,* The balloon dissector device before *(top)* and after *(bottom)* balloon cover removal. Note the degree of radial and distal balloon expansion that occurs when fully inflated with saline solution. (From Allen RC, Tawes RL, Wetter A, Fogarty T: Endoscopic perforator vein surgery: Creation of a subfascial space. *In* Gloviczki P, Bergan JJ [eds]: Atlas of Endoscopic Perforator Vein Surgery. London, Springer-Verlag, 1998, pp 153–162.)

averaged 24% (see Table 148–3). Controversy over the efficacy of the operation emerged when Burnand and co-workers reported a 55% recurrence rate in their patients, with 100% recurrence in a subset of 23 patients with post-thrombotic syndrome.[60] The ulcer recurrence rate in the same study in patients without post-thrombotic damage of the deep veins, however, was only 6%.

One of the few prospective randomized studies in venous surgery investigated the rates of wound complications after open perforator ligation and after SEPS.[1] Thirty-nine patients were randomized, and wound complications were found to have occurred in 53% in the open group versus 0% in the SEPS group. During a mean follow-up of 21 months, no ulcer recurrence was noted in either group of patients.

Considerable experience with SEPS has accumulated in several medical centers (Table 148–4), and results from the Mayo Clinic of 57 consecutive SEPS procedures in 48 patients were recently presented.[26] Forty-one limbs had concomitant ablation of saphenous reflux. The minor wound complication rate was 5%, and one patient had an early recurrent deep venous thrombosis. Twenty-two limbs had active ulcers, and all healed within a median of 36

days after surgery. A recurrent or new ulcer developed in 9% of all patients but in 12% of those with preoperative class 5 and class 6 disease during follow-up that extended to 52 months and averaged 17 months. Post-thrombotic deep vein obstruction was associated with both delayed healing and ulcer recurrence.

The relative safety of SEPS was also confirmed in the NASEPS registry, in which a 6% wound complication rate was reported, with one deep venous thrombosis at 2 months after surgery. Mid-term (24-month) results of 146 patients followed up in the registry revealed that cumulative ulcer healing at 1 year was 88%, with a median time to healing of 54 days (Fig. 148–23). Cumulative ulcer recurrence at 1 year was 16%, and at 2 years was 28% (standard error < 10%) (Fig. 148–24). Post-thrombotic limbs had a higher 2-year cumulative recurrence rate (46%) than those with primary valvular incompetence (20%) (*p* < .05) (Fig. 148–25). Twenty-eight (23%) of the 122 patients who had active or healed ulcer (class 5 or 6) before surgery had active ulcer at last follow-up. These recurrence rates are high but still compare favorably with results of nonoperative management (Table 148–5).

Hemodynamic Results of Perforator Interruption

Alterations in venous hemodynamics have been measured with a variety of noninvasive techniques, most frequently by foot volumetry, photo-gauge, strain-gauge, or air plethysmography complemented by bidirectional Doppler studies, or, more recently, by duplex scanning. Similar to the debate over clinical effectiveness, there is ongoing controversy about hemodynamic improvement that can be attributed to perforator interruption. Because perforator

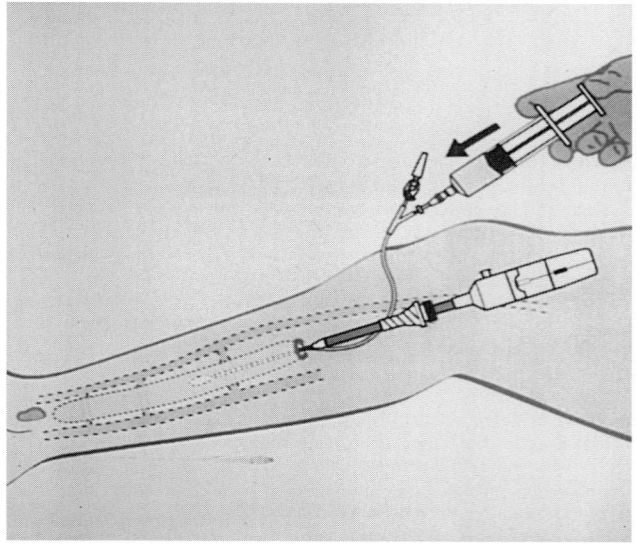

FIGURE 148–22. Balloon inflation is performed with 200 to 300 ml of saline. The balloon expands both radially and distally with minimal trauma to surrounding tissue, thus creating a large bloodless working space. (From Allen RC, Tawes RL, Wetter A, Fogarty T: Endoscopic perforator vein surgery: Creation of a subfascial space. *In* Gloviczki P, Bergan JJ [eds]: Atlas of Endoscopic Perforator Vein Surgery. London, Springer-Verlag, 1998, pp 153–162.)

TABLE 148–2. RESULTS OF NONOPERATIVE MANAGEMENT FOR ADVANCED CHRONIC VENOUS DISEASE

AUTHOR AND YEAR	NO. OF LIMBS TREATED	NO. OF LIMBS WITH ULCER*	TREATMENT	ULCER HEALING NO. (%)	ULCER RECURRENCE† NO. (%)	MEAN FOLLOW-UP (MO.)
Anning,[54] 1956	100	100	Stockings	100 (100)	59 (59)	64
Negus,[53] 1985	25	0	Stockings	—‡	17 (67)	—
Mayberry et al,[55] 1991	113	113	Stockings	105 (93)	24 (33)	30
Erickson et al,[56] 1995	99	99	Stocking/Una's boot	91 (92)	51 (56)	—
Total No. of limbs (%)	337 (100)	312 (93)		296/312 (95)	151/289 (52)	—

*Only class 6 (active ulcer) patients are included.
†Percentage accounts for patients lost to follow-up.
‡Only class 5 (healed ulcer) patients were admitted in this study.

TABLE 148–3. RESULTS OF OPEN PERFORATOR INTERRUPTION FOR THE TREATMENT OF ADVANCED CHRONIC VENOUS DISEASE

AUTHOR AND YEAR	NO. OF LIMBS TREATED	NO. OF LIMBS WITH ULCER*	WOUND COMPLICATIONS NO. (%)	ULCER HEALING NO. (%)	ULCER RECURRENCE† NO. (%)	MEAN FOLLOW-UP (YEARS)
Silver et al,[6] 1971	31	19	4 (14)	—	— (10)	1–15
Thurston et al,[57] 1973	102	0	12 (12)	—‡	11 (13)	3.3
Bowen,[58] 1975	71	8	31 (44)	—	24 (34)	4.5
Bergan et al,[50] 1976	41	0	—	—‡	24 (55)	—
Negus and Friedgood,[9] 1983	108	108	24 (22)	91 (84)	16 (15)	3.7
Wilkinson and Maclaren,[59] 1986	108	0	26 (24)	—‡	3 (7)	6
Cikrit et al,[10] 1988	32	30	6 (19)	30 (100)	5 (19)	4
Bradbury et al,[14] 1993	53	0	—	—‡	14 (26)	5
Pierik et al,[17] 1997	19	19	10 (53)	17 (90)	0 (0)	1.8
Total No. of limbs (%)	565 (100)	184 (33)	113/468 (24)	138/157 (88)	97/443 (22)	—

*Only class 6 (active ulcer) patients are included.
†Recurrence calculated for class 5 and 6 limbs only, where data available and percentage accounts for patients lost to follow-up.
‡Only class 5 (healed ulcer) patients were admitted in this study.

TABLE 148–4. RESULTS OF SUBFASCIAL ENDOSCOPIC PERFORATOR VEIN SURGERY FOR TREATMENT OF ADVANCED CHRONIC VENOUS DISEASE

AUTHOR AND YEAR	NO. OF LIMBS TREATED	NO. OF LIMBS WITH ULCER*	CONCOMITANT SAPHENOUS ABLATION NO. (%)	WOUND COMPLICATIONS NO. (%)	ULCER HEALING NO. (%)	ULCER RECURRENCE† NO. (%)	MEAN FOLLOW-UP (MO.)
Jugenheimer and Junginger,[21] 1992	103	17	97 (94)	3 (3)	16 (94)	0 (0)	27
Pierik et al,[63] 1995	40	16	4 (10)	3 (8)	16 (100)	1 (2.5)	46
Bergan,[15] 1996	31	15	31 (100)	3 (10)	15 (100)	(C)	—
Wolters et al,[64] 1996	27	27	0 (0)	2 (7)	26 (96)	2 (8)	12–24
Padberg et al,[65] 1996	11	0	11 (100)	—	—‡	0 (C)	16
Pierik et al,[17] 1997	20	20	14 (70)	0 (0)	17 (85)	0 (C)	21
Rhodes et al,[26] 1998	57	22	41 (72)	3 (5)	22 (100)	5 (12)	17
Gloviczki et al,[24] 1998	146	101	86 (59)	9 (6)	85 (84)	26 (21)	24
Total No. of limbs (%)	435 (100)	218 (50)	284/435 (65)	23/424 (5)	197/218 (90)	34/303 (11)	—

*Only class 6 (active ulcer) patients are included.
†Recurrence calculated for class 5 and 6 limbs only, where data available and percentage accounts for patients lost to follow-up.
‡Only class 5 (healed ulcer) patients were admitted in this study.

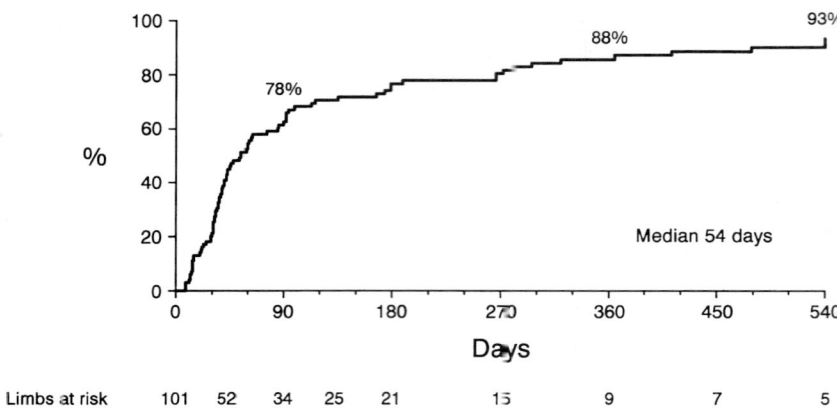

Limbs at risk   101   52   34   25   21   15   9   7   5

FIGURE 148–23. Cumulative ulcer healing in 101 patients after subfascial endoscopic perforator vein surgery. The 90-day, 1-year, and 1.5-year healing rates are indicated. The standard error is less than 10% at all time points. (From Gloviczki P, Bergan JJ, Rhodes JM, et al: North American Study Group: Mid-term results of endoscopic perforator vein interruption for chronic venous insufficiency: Lessons learned from the North American Subfascial Endoscopic Perforator Surgery (NASEPS) registry. J Vasc Surg 29:489–499, 1999.)

FIGURE 148–24. Cumulative ulcer recurrence in 106 patients after subfascial endoscopic perforator vein surgery (SEPS). The 1-, 2-, and 3-year recurrence rates are indicated. All class 5 limbs at the time of SEPS and class 6 limbs that subsequently healed are included. The start point (day 0) for time to recurrence in class 6 patients was the date of initial ulcer healing. The standard error is less than 10% at all time points. (From Gloviczki P, Bergan JJ, Rhodes JM, et al: North American Study Group: Mid-term results of endoscopic perforator vein interruption for chronic venous insufficiency: Lessons learned from the North American Subfascial Endoscopic Perforator Surgery (NASEPS) registry. J Vasc Surg 29:489–499, 1999.)

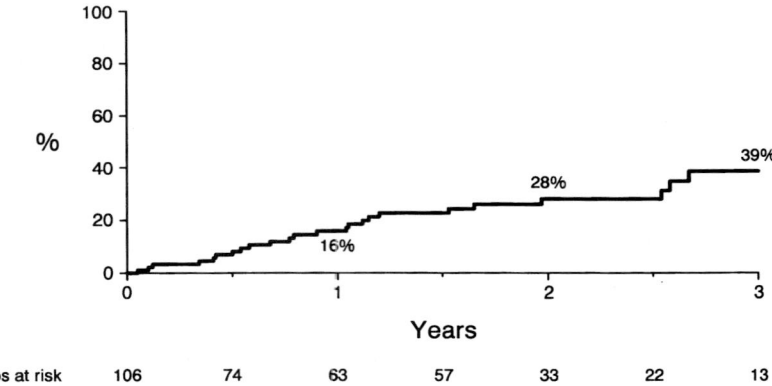

Limbs at risk   106   74   63   57   33   22   13

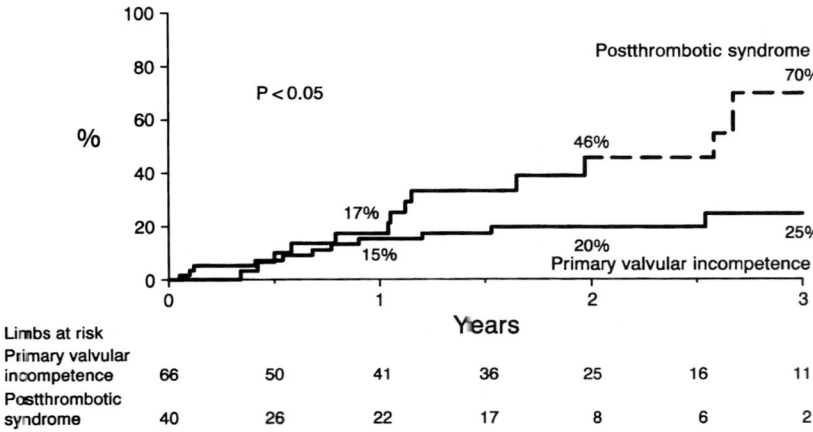

Limbs at risk
Primary valvular
incompetence   66   50   41   36   25   16   11
Postthrombotic
syndrome   40   26   22   17   8   6   2

FIGURE 148–25. Ulcer recurrence based on cause of chronic venous insufficiency. Limbs were separated into primary valvular incompetence (n = 66) and post-thrombotic syndrome (n = 40). The 1-, 2-, and 3-year recurrence rates are indicated. The *dashed line* represents a standard error of greater than 10%. Primary valvular incompetence versus post-thrombotic syndrome, *p* < .05. (From Gloviczki P, Bergan JJ, Rhodes JM, et al: North American Study Group: Mid-term results of endoscopic perforator vein interruption for chronic venous insufficiency: Lessons learned from the North American Subfascial Endoscopic Perforator Surgery (NASEPS) registry. J Vasc Surg 29:489–499, 1999.)

TABLE 148–5. STUDIES REPORTING LIFE-TABLE ANALYSIS FOR TREATMENT OF ADVANCED CHRONIC VENOUS DISEASE TREATMENTS

AUTHOR AND YEAR	TREATMENT	NO. OF LIMBS TREATED	LIMBS WITH ULCER* (NO.)	ULCER HEALING (%)	ULCER RECURRENCE†
Mayberry, 1991[55]	Compression therapy	113	113	93	29% 5 yr, compliant patients 100% 3 yr, noncompliant
Erickson, 1995[56]	Compression therapy	99	99	92	41% 2 yr, compliant patients 71% 2 yr, noncompliant
Johnson, 1985[61]	Open perforator ablation	47	0	—‡	22% at 1 yr 51% at 5 yr
Robison, 1992[62]	Open perforator ± saphenous stripping	18	18	89	37% at 3 yr
Rhodes, 1998[26]	SEPS ± saphenous stripping	57	22	100	18% at 2 yr 30% at 3 yr
Gloviczki, 1998[24]	SEPS ± saphenous stripping	146	101	84	28% at 2 yr 39% at 3 yr

*Only class 6 (active ulcer) patients are included.
†Recurrence calculated for class 5 and 6 limbs only, where data available.
‡Class 5 (healed ulcer) at time of entry.
SEPS = subfascial endoscopic perforator vein surgery.

incompetence is frequently treated together with ablation of superficial reflux, postoperative hemodynamic measurements reflect results of a combined operation.

In a classic study, however, using ambulatory venous pressure measurements, Schanzer and Pierce[8] documented significant hemodynamic improvements after isolated perforator interruption in 22 patients. Improvement in both calf muscle pump function and venous incompetence could be demonstrated and hemodynamic improvement correlated with clinical results. Twenty patients in this series remained free of ulcer recurrence during a mean follow-up period of 15 months.[8] These results were confirmed in a 1992 air plethysmographic study by Padberg and colleagues.[65] These authors also observed significant hemodynamic improvements, with no ulcer recurrence up to 2 years after perforator ligation with concomitant correction of superficial reflux.

These results contrast with those of Akesson and associates, who measured hemodynamic changes with ambulatory venous pressure (AVP) measurements before and after saphenous stripping at a first operation and perforator interruption at a second operation.[66] A significant reduction in AVP was seen after saphenous stripping, but the improvement in mean AVP did not reach significance after perforator interruption. In this study, however, AVP did not correlate with clinical outcome.

Using foot volumetry, Stacey and coworkers demonstrated that perforator vein ligation with ablation of saphenous reflux improved calf muscle pump function in limbs with primary valvular incompetence, although the relative expelled volume did not return to normal.[67] No hemodynamic benefit was found in post-thrombotic limbs.

In the Mayo Clinic series, Rhodes and colleagues used strain-guage plethysmography to quantitate calf muscle pump function and venous incompetence before and after SEPS (Fig. 148–26).[25] The authors observed significant improvement in both calf muscle pump function and venous incompetence in 31 limbs studied within 6 months after SEPS. Twenty-four of the 31 limbs underwent saphenous stripping in addition to SEPS. Normalization of venous incompetence occurred in up to 50% of limbs stud-

ied, and this improvement was associated with a favorable clinical outcome. Although limbs undergoing SEPS alone had significant clinical benefits, the hemodynamic improvements did not reach statistical significance. This is likely related to both the small number of patients and the predominance of post-thrombotic syndrome in this subgroup. Post-thrombotic limbs had both poorer clinical and hemodynamic improvements after perforator interruption.

Bradbury and coworkers used foot volumetry and duplex scanning to assess hemodynamic improvement after saphenous and perforator ligation in 43 patients with recurrent ulcers.[14] At a median follow-up of 66 months, 34 patients had no ulcer recurrence, and in these patients both expulsion fraction and half-refilling time had improved significantly after surgery, as measured with foot volumetry and tourniquet occlusion of the superficial veins.

Studies of Zukowski and Nicolaides indicate that only 70% of patients with venous ulcers have incompetent perforators of moderate or major significance.[45] As suggested

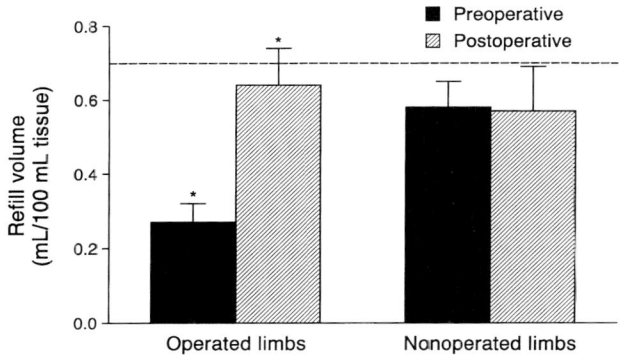

FIGURE 148–26. Calf muscle pump function (refill volume) measured in 28 limbs before and after subfascial endoscopic perforator vein surgery and in 18 contralateral nonoperated limbs. Asterisk indicates $p < .01$; dashed line indicates normal refill volume ≥ 0.7 ml/100 ml tissue. (From Rhodes JM, Gloviczki P, Canton LG, et al: Endoscopic perforator vein division with ablation of superficial reflux improves venous hemodynamics. J Vasc Surg 28:839–847, 1998.)

by the authors, variable hemodynamic improvement observed after perforator interruption may be explained by the fact that perforators with no or minor hemodynamic effects were treated. Further research for the best preoperative test with which to determine the hemodynamic effects of incompetent perforators and to help select patients for perforator interruption is clearly justified.

SUMMARY

Perforator incompetence, caused by primary valvular incompetence or by previous deep venous thrombosis, contributes to ambulatory venous hypertension and to the development of chronic venous disease. Incompetent perforators occur in at least two thirds of patients with venous ulceration and are found together with superficial or deep venous incompetence in most patients. Although the exact role and contribution of perforators to the development of ulcers is under debate, poor results with nonoperative management to prevent ulcer recurrence justify surgical attempts of perforator ligation, in addition to ablation of superficial reflux.

The endoscopic technique of perforator interruption produces significantly less wound complications than the open technique. Interruption of incompetent perforators with ablation of the superficial reflux, if present, is effective and durable to decrease symptoms of CVI and rapidly heal ulcers. Ulcer recurrence after correction of perforator and superficial reflux in patients with post-thrombotic syndrome is much higher than in patients with primary valvular incompetence. Prospective randomized studies are needed to define the exact benefit of interruption of incompetent perforators in patients with advanced chronic venous disease.

REFERENCES

1. Gay J: Lettsomian Lectures 1867. Varicose Disease of the Lower Extremities. London, Churchill, 1868.
2. Linton RR: The communicating veins of the lower leg and the operative technique for their ligation. Ann Surg 107:582–593, 1938.
3. Cockett FB, Jones BD: The ankle blow-out syndrome: A new approach to the varicose ulcer problem. Lancet i:17–23, 1953.
4. Cockett FB: The pathology and treatment of venous ulcers of the leg. Br J Surg 44:260–278, 1956.
5. Dodd H, Cockett FR: The management of venous ulcers. In The Pathology and Surgery of the Vein of the Lower Limbs. New York, Churchill Livingstone, 269–296, 1976.
6. Silver D, Gleysteen JJ, Rhodes GR: Surgical treatment of the refractory postphlebitic ulcer. Arch Surg 103:554–560, 1971.
7. De Palma RG: Surgical therapy for venous stasis: Results of a modified Linton operation. Am J Surg 137:810–813, 1979
8. Schanzer H, Pierce EC: A rational approach to surgery of the chronic venous stasis syndrome. Ann Surg 195:25–29, 1982.
9. Negus D, Friedgood A: The effective management of venous ulceration. Br J Surg 70:623–627, 1983.
10. Cikrit DF, Nichols WK, Silver D: Surgical management of refractory venous stasis ulceration. J Vasc Surg 7:473–478, 1988.
11. Fischer R: Surgical treatment of varicose veins: Endoscopic treatment of incompetent Cockett veins. Phlebologie 1040–1041, 1989.
12. Raju S, Fredricks R: Venous obstruction: An analysis of one hundred thirty-seven cases with hemodynamic, venographic, and clinical correlations. J Vasc Surg 14:305–313, 1991.
13. O'Donnell TF: Surgical treatment of incompetent communicating veins. In Bergan JJ, Kistner RL (eds): Atlas of Venous Surgery. Philadelphia, WB Saunders, 1992, pp 111–124.
14. Bradbury AW, Stonebridge PA, Callam MJ, et al: Foot volumetry and duplex ultrasonography after saphenous and subfascial perforating vein ligation for recurrent venous ulceration. Br J Surg 80:845–848, 1993.
15. Bergan JJ, Murray J, Greason K: Subfascial endoscopic perforator vein surgery: A preliminary report. Ann Vasc Surg 10:211–219, 1996.
16. Gloviczki P, Bergan JJ, Menawat SS, et al: Safety, feasibility, and early efficacy of subfascial endoscopic perforator surgery: A preliminary report from the North American Registry. J Vasc Surg 25:94–105, 1997.
17. Pierik EGJM, van Urk H, Hop WCJ, Witten CHA: Endoscopic versus open subfascial division of incompetent perforating veins in the treatment of venous leg ulceration: A randomized trial. J Vasc Surg 26:1049–1054, 1997.
18. Pierik EGJM, Toonder IM, van Urk H, Wittens CHA: Validation of duplex ultrasonography in detecting competent and incompetent perforating veins in patients with venous ulceration of the lower leg. J Vasc Surg 26:49–52, 1997.
19. Edwards JM: Shearing operation for incompetent perforating vein. Br J Surg 63:885–886, 1976.
20. Hauer G: The endoscopic subfascial division of the perforating veins: Preliminary report. Vasa 14:59–61, 1985.
21. Jugenheimer M, Junginger T: Endoscopic subfascial sectioning of incompetent perforating veins in treatment of primary varicosities. World J Surg 16:971–975, 1992.
22. Conrad P: Endoscopic exploration of the subfascial space of the lower leg with perforator vein interruption using laparoscopic equipment: A preliminary report. Phlebology 9:154–157, 1994.
23. Gloviczki P, Cambria RA, Rhee RY, et al: Surgical technique and preliminary results of endoscopic subfascial division of perforating veins. J Vasc Surg 23:517–523, 1996.
24. Gloviczki P, Bergan JJ, Rhodes JM, et al, North American Study Group: Mid-term results of endoscopic perforator vein interruption for chronic venous insufficiency: Lessons learned from the North American Subfascial Endoscopic Perforator Surgery (NASEPS) registry. J Vasc Surg 29:489–499, 1999.
25. Rhodes JM, Gloviczki P, Canton LG, et al: Endoscopic perforator vein division with ablation of superficial reflux improves venous hemodynamics. J Vasc Surg 28:839–847, 1998.
26. Rhodes JM, Gloviczki P, Canton LG, et al: Factors affecting clinical outcome following endoscopic perforator vein ablation. Am J Surg 176:162–167, 1998.
27. Lofgren EP, Myers TT, Lofgren KA: The venous valves of the foot and ankle. Surg Gynecol Obstet 127:289–290, 1968.
28. Mozes G, Gloviczki P, Menawat SS, et al: Surgical anatomy for endoscopic subfascial division of perforating veins. J Vasc Surg 24:800–808, 1996.
29. O'Donnell TF, Burnand KG, Clemenson G, et al: Doppler examination vs clinical and phlebographic detection of the location of incompetent perforating veins. Arch Surg 112:31–35, 1977.
30. Negus D (ed): Leg Ulcers: A Practical Approach to Management, 2nd ed. Oxford, Butterworth-Heinemann, Ltd, 1995, pp 3–10, 30–41.
31. Sherman RS: Varicose veins: Further findings based on anatomic and surgical dissections. Ann Surg 130:218–232, 1949.
32. Linton RR: The post-thrombotic ulceration of the lower extremity: Its etiology and surgical treatment. Ann Surg 138:415–432, 1953.
33. Bjordal RI: Circulation patterns in incompetent perforating veins of the calf in venous dysfunction. In May R, Partsch J, Staubesand J (eds): Perforating Veins. Baltimore, Urban & Schwarzenberg, 1981, pp 77–88.
34. Sethia KK, Darke SG: Long saphenous incompetence as a cause of venous ulceration. Br J Surg 71:754–755, 1984.
35. van Rij AM, Solomon C, Christie R: Anatomic and physiologic characteristics of venous ulceration. J Vasc Surg 20:759–764, 1994.
36. Labropoulos N, Leon M, Geroulakos G, et al: Venous hemodynamic abnormalities in patients with leg ulcerations. Am J Surg 169:572–574, 1995.
37. Labropoulos N, Mansour MA, Kong SE, Gloviczki P, Baker WH: New insights into perforator vein incompetence. J Vasc Indovascular Surg (in press).
38. Hanrahan LM, Araki CT, Rodriguez AA, et al: Distribution of valvular incompetence in patients with venous stasis ulceration. J Vasc Surg 13:805–812, 1991.
39. Shami SK, Sarin S, Cheatle TR, et al: Venous ulcers and the superficial system. J Vasc Surg 17:487–490, 1993.

40. Darke SG, Penfold C: Venous ulceration and saphenous ligation. Eur J Vasc Surg 6:4–9, 1992.
41. Lees TA, Lambert D: Patterns of venous reflux in limbs with skin changes associated with chronic venous insufficiency. Br J Surg 80:725–728, 1993.
42. Coleridge Smith P: Calf perforating veins—time for an objective appraisal (Editorial)? Phlebology 11:135–136, 1996.
43. Gloviczki P: Endoscopic perforator vein surgery: Does it work (Editorial)? Vasc Surg 32:303–305, 1998.
44. Sarin S, Scurr JH, Coleridge-Smith PD: Medial calf perforators in venous disease: The significance of outward flow. J Vasc Surg 16:40–46, 1992.
45. Zukowski AJ, Nicolaides AN, Szendro G, et al: Haemodynamic significance of incompetent calf perforating veins. Br J Surg 78:625–629, 1991.
46. Gloviczki P, Lewis BD, Lindsey JR, McKusick MA: Preoperative evaluation of chronic venous insufficiency with duplex scanning and venography. In Gloviczki P, Bergan JJ (eds): Atlas of Endoscopic Perforator Vein Surgery. London, Springer-Verlag, 1998, pp 81–91.
47. De Palma RG: Linton's operation and modification of the open techniques. In Gloviczki P, Bergan JJ (eds): Atlas of Endoscopic Perforator Vein Surgery. London, Springer-Verlag, 1998, pp 107–113.
48. Fischer R, Sattler G, Vanderpuye R: The current status of endoscopic treatment of perforators [in French]. Phlebologie 46:701–707, 1993.
49. Fischer R, Schwahn-Schreiber C, Sattler G: Conclusions of a consensus conference on subfascial endoscopy of perforating veins in the medial lower leg. Vasc Surg 32:339–347, 1998.
50. Bergan JJ, Ballard JL, Sparks S: Subfascial endoscopic perforator surgery: The open technique. In Gloviczki P, Bergan JJ (eds): Atlas of Endoscopic Perforator Vein Surgery. London, Springer-Verlag, 1998, pp 141–149.
51. Wittens CHA: Comparison of open Linton operation with subfascial endoscopic perforator vein surgery. In Gloviczki P, Bergan JJ (eds): Atlas of Endoscopic Perforator Vein Surgery. London, Springer-Verlag, 1998, pp 177–185.
52. Allen RC, Tawes RL, Wetter A, Fogarty TJ: Endoscopic perforator vein surgery: Creation of a subfascial space. In Gloviczki P, Bergan JJ (eds): Atlas of Endoscopic Perforator Vein Surgery. London, Springer-Verlag, 1998, pp 153–162.
53. Negus D: Prevention and treatment of venous ulceration. Ann R Coll Surg Engl 67:144–148, 1985.
54. Anning ST: Leg ulcers: The results of treatment. Angiology 7:505–516, 1956.
55. Mayberry JC, Moneta GL, Taylor LM Jr, Porter JM: Fifteen-year results of ambulatory compression therapy for chronic venous ulcers. Surgery 109:575–581, 1991.
56. Erickson CA, Lanza DJ, Karp DL, et al: Healing of venous ulcers in an ambulatory care program: The role of chronic venous insufficiency and patient compliance. J Vasc Surg 22:629–636, 1995.
57. Thurston OG, Williams HTG: Chronic venous insufficiency of the lower extremity. Arch Surg 106:537–539, 1973.
58. Bowen FH: Subfascial ligation of the perforating leg veins to treat post-thrombophlebitic syndrome. Am Surg 148–151, 1975.
59. Wilkinson GE, Maclaren IF: Long term review of procedures for venous perforator insufficiency. Surg Gynecol Obstet 163:117–120, 1986.
60. Burnand K, et al: Relation between postphlebitic changes in the deep veins and results of surgical treatment of venous ulcers. Lancet 1:936–938, 1976.
61. Johnson WC, et al: Venous stasis ulceration: Effectiveness of subfascial ligation. Arch Surg 120:797–800, 1985.
62. Robison JG, Elliott BM, Kaplan AJ: Limitations of subfascial ligation for refractory chronic venous stasis ulceration. Ann Vasc Surg 6:9–14, 1992.
63. Pierik EGJM, Wittens CHA, van Urk H: Subfascial endoscopic ligation in the treatment of incompetent perforator veins. Eur J Vasc Endovasc Surg 5:38–41, 1995.
64. Wolters U, Schmitz-Rixen T, Erasmi H, et al: Endoscopic dissection of incompetent perforating veins in the treatment of chronic venous leg ulcers. Vasc Surg 30:481–487, 1996.
65. Padberg FT, Pappas PJ, Araki CT, et al: Hemodynamic and clinical improvement after superficial vein ablation in primary combined venous insufficiency with ulceration. J Vasc Surg 24:711–718, 1996.
66. Akesson H, Brudin L, Cwikiel W, et al: Does the correction of insufficient superficial and perforating veins improve venous function in patients with deep venous insufficiency? Phlebology 5:113–123, 1990.
67. Stacey MC, Burnand KG, Layer GT, Pattison M: Calf pump function in patients with healed venous ulcers is not improved by surgery to the communicating veins or by elastic stockings. Br J Surg 75:436–439, 1988.

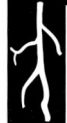

C H A P T E R   1 4 9
Surgical Treatment of Deep Venous Valvular Incompetence

Seshadri Raju, M.D.

Chronic venous insufficiency is a significant cause of disability in the workplace. Surveys have indicated that 4% of the work force in the industrialized world may be affected.[22] The incidence in the population overall is estimated to be approximately 2%. The direct and indirect costs of treating it are staggering.

ETIOLOGY AND PATHOPHYSIOLOGY

Chronic venous insufficiency can result from congenital, "primary," or post-thrombotic causes of valvular reflux (Fig.

149–1; see Chapter 145). Congenital causes of reflux include valve aplasia and dysplasias, such as avalvular duplication conduits that circumvent valve structures, and a wide variety of valvular malformations that predispose to poor valve function and reflux (Fig. 149–2). *Conduit dysplasias* occur more frequently than valve abnormalities (5% and 1% incidence, respectively). *Klippel-Trenaunay syndrome* is often associated with venous valve aplasia and dysplasias.

Primary valve reflux, once considered a rare entity, is now recognized as a common cause of chronic venous insufficiency.[26] In the author's medical center, it currently

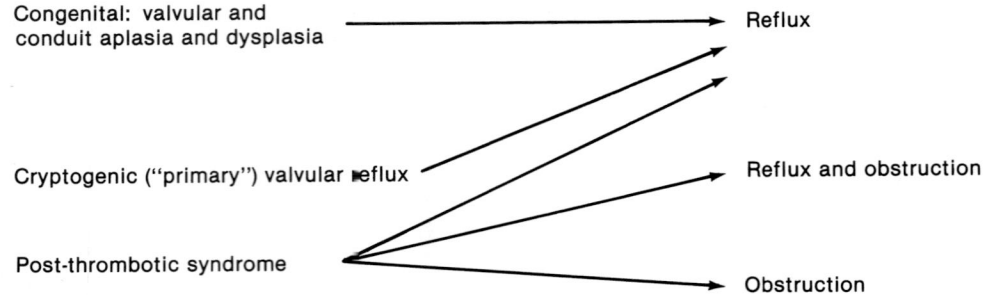

FIGURE 149–1. Etiologic mechanisms of chronic venous insufficiency.

occurs in about 30% of patients. With primary valve reflux, the valve leaflets appear normal in texture but are redundant and have a tendency to evert. This results in poor coaptation of the leaflets, which permits reflux (Fig. 149–3). Because thrombotic changes in and around the valve cusps usually are not evident in affected persons, it is assumed that the defect arises from a developmental mechanism. The precise structural defect and its cause, however, have not been determined.

Primary valve reflux may result in *deep venous thrombosis* from reflux stasis.[27] Patients often present with primary reflux in the femoral area and distal thrombosis in the calf veins. Recurrent bouts of deep venous thrombosis in these patients may be relieved by correction of the proximal valve reflux.

Deep venous thrombosis remains the most common cause of advanced chronic venous insufficiency. It accounts for about 65% of cases (including proximal "primary" reflux with distal thrombosis) in the author's hospital practice. The precise incidence and evolution of chronic venous insufficiency after deep venous thrombosis are not known, because few long-term longitudinal studies have been undertaken in the context of modern anticoagulant therapy. In a study that extended as long as 4 years after the appearance of deep venous thrombosis, approximately 25%

of the patients studied were already severely symptomatic from postphlebitic syndrome.[18] Because the development of clinical manifestations of post-thrombotic venous insufficiency is a slow and insidious process, with a predilection for recurrent thrombosis, in many patients the full impact of the disease may not be apparent until 15 to 20 years after the initial episode. The valve structure may be completely destroyed by thrombosis and recanalization (see Fig. 149–3); or less extensive damage—ranging from thickening of valve cusps, to shortening and fibrosis of the leaflets, perforations, or adhesion to another leaflet or a sinus wall—may be evident. Curiously, the valve structure is preserved intact in some cases and the reflux is attributed to relative redundancy produced by contraction and foreshortening of the wall around the valve cusps (Fig. 149–4).

Serial duplex examination of post-thrombotic extremities has revealed delayed onset of new reflux in venous segments *proximal* to the earlier thrombosis.[18] Reflux resulting from a post-thrombotic cause is often associated with residual venous obstruction from the thrombotic process. Post-thrombotic abnormalities of the calf venous pump mechanism, such as reduced venous capacitance and poor wall compliance (Fig. 149–5), compound the refluxive and obstructive pathophysiologic mechanisms to produce the full-blown post-phlebitic syndrome. Collaterals that develop in

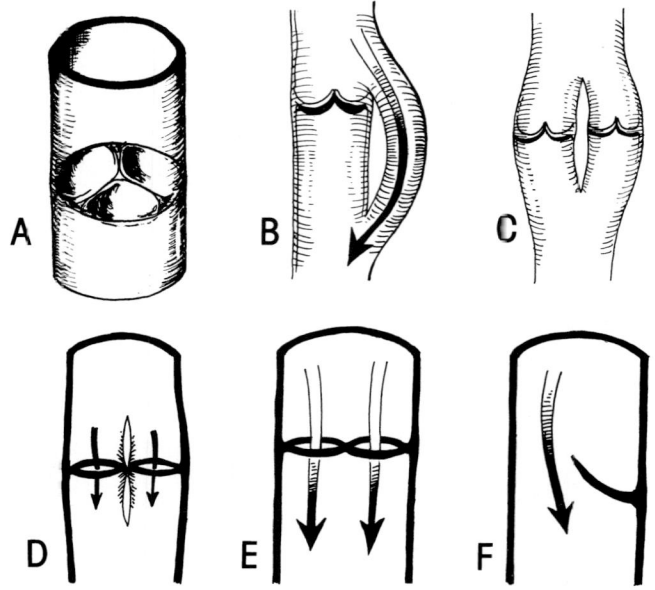

FIGURE 149–2. Congenital anomalies of the venous conduit and the valve structure. These are frequently associated with venous reflux. A, Tricuspid valve. B, Avalvular duplication conduit. C, Duplication conduit with refluxive valves. D, Duplication of the valve with an intervening septum. E, Duplication of the valve without a septum. F, Refluxive monocuspid valve.

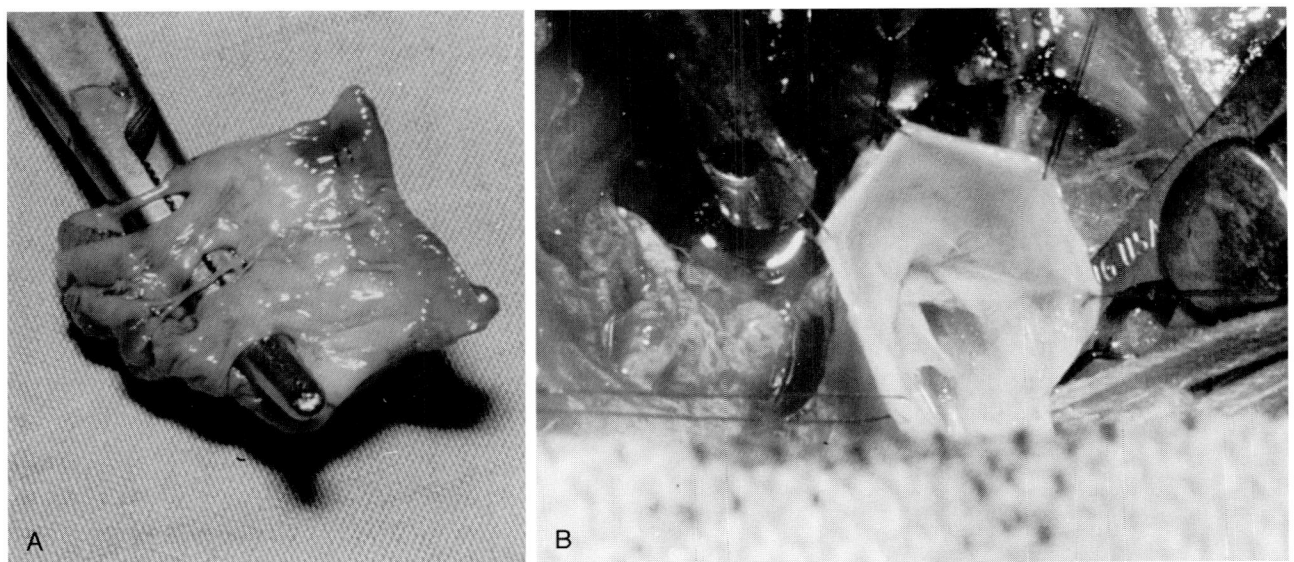

FIGURE 149–3. *A*, Post-thrombotic valve with destruction of the valve structure. *B*, "Primary" valve reflux with everting valve cusps.

the post-thrombotic limb are an important source of (often massive) reflux in the affected extremity. Collateral connections that develop between the profunda femoris and popliteal veins in the presence of femoral vein thrombosis often persist even after the thrombus has become fully recanalized. The rapidity with which this collateral pathway develops after thrombosis of the superficial femoral vein is remarkable and may have an embryonic origin.[34] The profunda femoris vein may undergo compensatory enlargement (axial transformation) when superficial femoral outflow is compromised by post-thrombotic changes. Profunda femoris vein reflux usually results from dilatation of the vein in this situation and is frequently associated with venous stasis ulceration of the limb (Fig. 149–6).[34] In these

cases, the axially transformed profunda femoris vein attains the caliber of the superficial femoral vein, and its course in the limb is so smooth that it is often mistaken for the native superficial femoral vein.

HEMODYNAMIC CHANGES

Hemodynamic abnormalities are discussed in Chapter 144, but a few important points should be mentioned to clarify

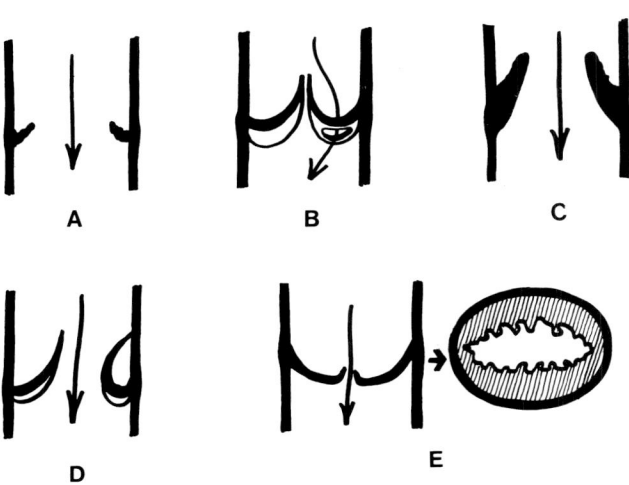

FIGURE 149–4. Pathology of post-thrombotic valve reflux. The degree of valve damage is variable. *A*, Destroyed valve cusp. *B*, Perforated cusp. *C*, "Frozen" and thickened valve cusp. *D*, Adherent valve cusp with some thickening. *E*, Redundant refluxive valve is indistinguishable from "primary valve reflux." (From Raju S: Pathophysiology of venous thrombosis. *In* Ernst CB, Stanley JC [eds]: Current Therapy in Vascular Surgery, 3rd ed. St. Louis, Mosby–Year Book, 1995, p 878.)

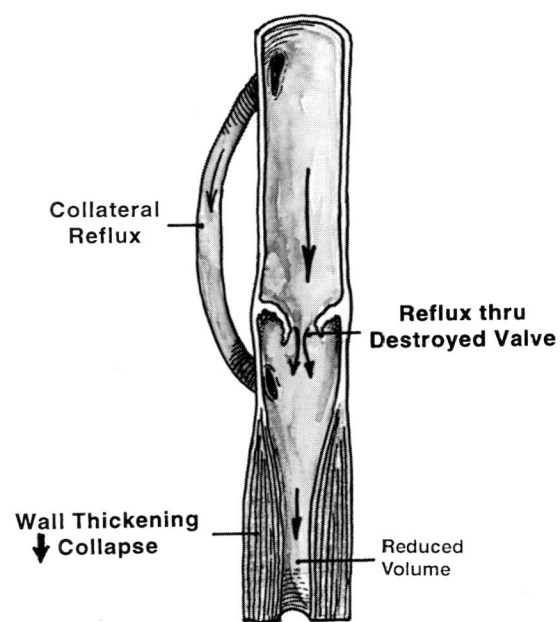

FIGURE 149–5. Pathophysiology of post-thrombotic syndrome: Reflux through the post-thrombotic valve and through collaterals is compounded by post-thrombotic abnormalities of the calf venous pump. Reduced venous capacitance and post-thrombotic compliance changes decrease the efficiency of the calf venous pump and produce ambulatory venous hypertension.

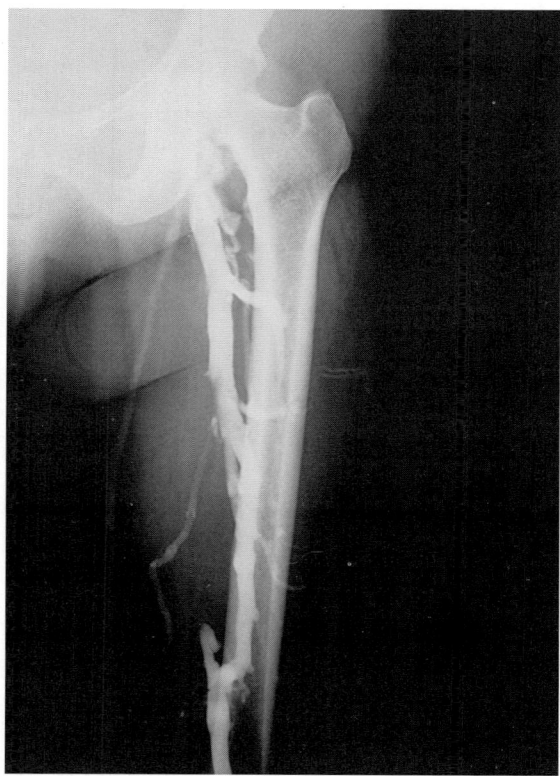

FIGURE 149–6. Axial transformation of the profunda femoris vein. Note the remnant of the thrombosed superficial femoral vein in the distal thigh. (From Raju S, Fountain T, Neglén P, et al: Axial transformation of the profunda femoris vein. J Vasc Surg 27:651–659, 1998.)

the rationales of valve repair. Reflux is clearly associated with stasis ulceration (Fig. 149–7). The resulting ambulatory venous hypertension can be shown to correlate with the incidence of stasis ulceration (Table 149–1).[23] However,

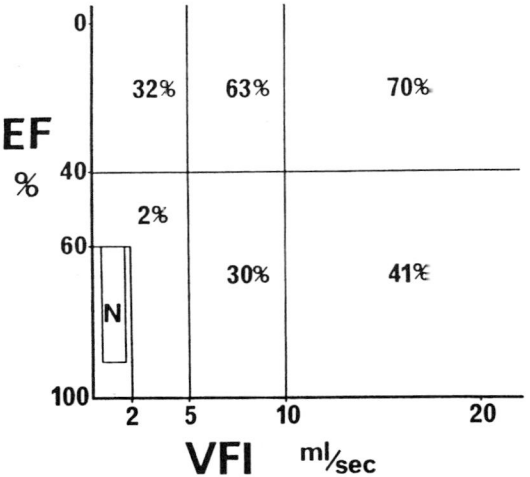

FIGURE 149–7. Incidence of leg ulceration in relation to the venous filling index (VFI) and the ejection fraction (EF) of the calf muscle pump as measured by air plethysmography in 175 limbs with venous problems. Normal range (N) for these parameters is indicated by inset. (From Nicolaides AN, Sumner DS: Investigation of Patients with Deep Vein Thrombosis and Chronic Venous Insufficiency. Los Angeles, Med-Orion Publishing, 1991, p 49.)

TABLE 149–1. INCIDENCE OF LEG ULCERATION (ACTIVE OR HEALED) IN RELATION TO AMBULATORY VENOUS PRESSURE (P) IN 251 LIMBS

NO. OF LIMBS	PRESSURE (mmHg)	ULCERATION (%)
34	<30	0
44	31–40	12
51	41–50	22
45	51–60	38
34	61–70	57
28	71–80	68
15	>80	73

From Nicolaides AN, Sumner DS (eds): Ambulatory venous pressure measurements. In Investigation of Patients with Deep Vein Thrombosis and Chronic Venous Insufficiency. Los Angeles, Med-Orion Publishing, 1991, p 50.

approximately 25% of patients with reflux and stasis ulceration have ambulatory venous pressures that are considered to be in the normal range.[35] Thus, the precise interrelation between venous reflux, ambulatory venous hypertension, and the genesis of stasis ulceration is not fully understood.

There is increasing appreciation that the volume of reflux is more important than its location (i.e., in the superficial or the deep system).[23] Stasis ulceration can develop in patients who have massive reflux that is largely confined to the superficial system.[1] More frequently, however, patients with stasis-induced skin changes demonstrate multivalvular, multisystem reflux.[27] Deep system reflux, alone or in association with superficial reflux, is commonly identified in this patient population (Table 149–2).[20] Symptom expression also correlates with increasing incidence of deep valvular and perforator reflux (Table 149–3).[21] The common association between deep venous reflux and stasis-related lesions is probably related to the large volume of reflux required to overwhelm the compensatory mechanisms of the calf venous pump.[38] Primary valve reflux is often global, affecting both the superficial and the deep systems. In post-thrombotic syndrome, deep venous reflux is predominant after an earlier episode of deep venous thrombosis. Thus, the high incidence of deep venous reflux in stasis ulceration should not be surprising, in view of the propensity of the major etiologic mechanisms to affect the deep system, either alone or in combination with superficial venous insufficiency.

When both obstruction and reflux are present, reflux is thought to be more important in the genesis of stasis skin changes.[36, 40] Patients with deep venous obstruction present

TABLE 149–2. INCIDENCE OF SUPERFICIAL AND DEEP VEIN REFLUX IN 485 DESCENDING VENOGRAMS

REFLUX SITE	INCIDENCE (%)
Saphenous vein only	2
Superficial femoral vein only	19
Deep femoral vein only	12
Superficial and deep femoral veins	51
Saphenous vein with superficial femoral vein, deep femoral vein, or both	16

From Morano JU, Raju S: Chronic venous insufficiency: Assessment with descending venography. Radiology 174:441–444, 1990.

TABLE 149–3. FREQUENCY OF SUPERFICIAL AND PERFORATOR INCOMPETENCE, DEEP VEIN REFLUX, AND HEMODYNAMIC TESTS IN 56 LOWER LIMBS ACCORDING TO CLINICAL SEVERITY STAGING

CLINICAL SEVERITY CLASS	NO. OF LIMBS	AMBULATORY VENOUS PRESSURE (% DROP)*	VENOUS FILLING TIME (SEC)	SUPERFICIAL INCOMPETENCE† (%)	PERFORATOR INCOMPETENCE‡ (%)	DEEP VEIN REFLUX§ (%)
0	15	58 ± 7	39 ± 21	20	20	20
1	19	57 ± 5	33 ± 16	58	69	26
2	8	49 ± 12	16 ± 12	63	88	63
3	14	41 ± 11	9 ± 7	71	100	86

From Neglén P, Raju S: A comparison between descending phlebography and duplex Doppler investigation in the evaluation of reflux in chronic venous insufficiency: A challenge to phlebography as the "gold standard." J Vasc Surg 1992;16:687.
*Class 0 + class 1 is significantly different from class 2 + class 3 for ambulatory venous pressure ($p < .001$) and venous filling time ($p < .001$).
†Established by ultrasonography.
‡Established on ascending venography.
§Established on descending venography.

primarily with swelling and pain; stasis changes in the gaiter area develop with recanalization of the thrombosed vein and the onset of reflux. A transition from obstructive symptoms in the early years to refluxive venous stasis in the later years may be observed on long-term follow-up of deep venous thrombosis.

CLINICAL PRESENTATION

The clinical presentation of chronic venous insufficiency can vary from mild to severe,[26] depending on the extent of underlying disease. In advanced cases, the triad of pain, swelling, and stasis skin changes is present in various combinations and intensities of these components. For reasons not known, one or more of this triad is entirely absent in some patients even when they have advanced hemodynamic and pathologic changes. In patients with varicosities in the lower leg, sometimes punctate skin necrosis develops over distended varices that can lead to impressive hemorrhage when the patient is in the erect position. This should not be confused with the classic stasis ulcer that is associated with extensive areas of lipodermatosclerosis and skin changes around the stasis ulcer itself (Fig. 149–8).

PREOPERATIVE EVALUATION

In this author's practice, before valve reconstruction is undertaken, investigation of patients who present with symptoms of chronic venous insufficiency has these objectives:

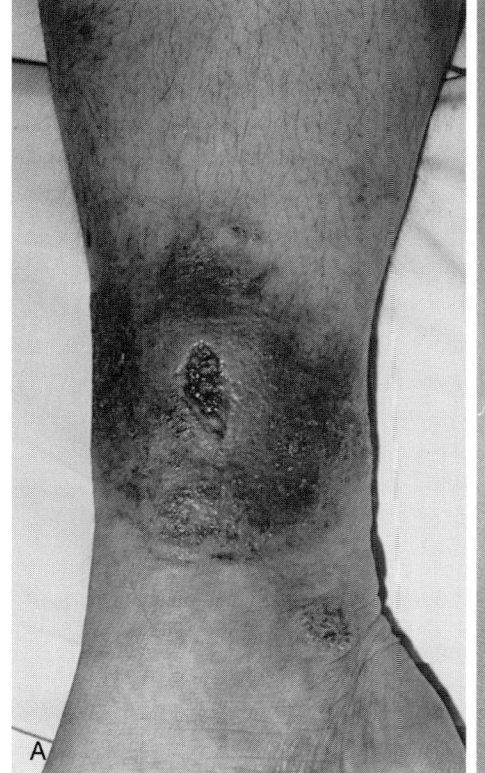
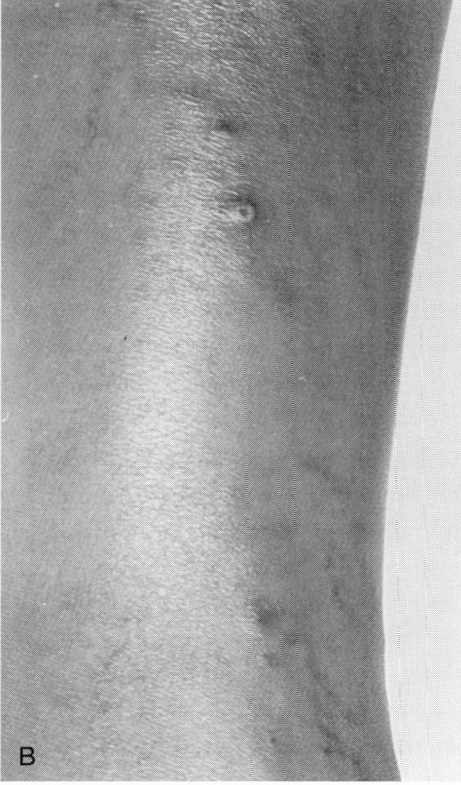

FIGURE 149–8. *A,* Typical stasis ulcer with necrosis and surrounding areas of lipodermatosclerosis. This lesion should not be confused with the punctate pressure ulcers (*B*) sometimes seen over prominent varicosities. *B,* Pinpoint ulcers can bleed profusely when the patient is in the erect position. Note the absence of skin changes around the punctate "varicose" ulcer.

1. Confirmation of the diagnosis of reflux and assessment of its degree and extent.

2. Detection of any associated obstruction and determination of its severity and location.

3. Identification of a possible cause (e.g., primary or post-thrombotic reflux).

4. Evaluation of the status of the lymphatics when swelling is a presenting symptom.

A detailed discussion of evaluation can be found in Chapter 145.

It is generally impossible to differentiate chronic venous obstruction from reflux on the basis of clinical presentation alone. Similarly, primary valvular reflux cannot be differentiated with certainty from the post-thrombotic type on the basis of history and physical findings. Patients who report previous episodes of "phlebitis" may have normal venographic findings. Conversely, extensive post-thrombotic changes may be evident on venography, even when there is no clinical history of deep venous thrombosis. All patients with evidence of earlier episodes of thrombosis should undergo screening for hypercoagulability syndromes. This information is essential for determining the necessary intensity and duration of postoperative anticoagulation. Older patients with thrombosis should be investigated for occult malignancies. Patients with large stasis ulcers are often deficient in nutrients essential to wound healing. These deficits should be corrected before surgery.

Duplex Scanning

In most laboratories, duplex Doppler ultrasonography has superseded other modalities for screening patients suspected to have chronic venous insufficiency. The presence, extent, and location of reflux can be assessed noninvasively with this technique.[20, 21] In most laboratories however, the sensitivity of duplex scanning in detecting reflux is in the range of only 75%.[20] It is therefore recommended that additional independent techniques, such as air plethysmography or ambulatory venous pressure measurement, be incorporated in the investigative protocol,[20] because they provide global measurements of reflux and yield important additional information about the efficiency of the calf venous pump mechanism. The presence and degree of hemodynamic obstruction cannot be reliably assessed with the duplex technique. The arm-foot venous pressure differential[28] provides this information.

Phlebography

Patients in whom reconstructive valve surgery is contemplated should undergo additional phlebographic examination, including ascending and descending venography. These studies supply anatomic information essential for surgical exploration. *Ascending venography* provides information on the patency of axial channels, perforator incompetence, evidence of previous deep venous thrombosis, postphlebitic changes, sites of obstruction, and abnormal collateral vessels.

Descending phlebography[19] is used to identify and measure the extent of reflux. It yields information on the location of refluxing valve stations and provides details of valve anatomy. Uncomplicated primary valve reflux is usually easily distinguished from advanced post-thrombotic reflux by descending venography. Surgical experience, however, indicates that a large group of patients have indeterminate venographic features, so that the precise cause cannot be established preoperatively from the venographic appearance alone.

Although several grading systems have been devised to assess reflux on descending phlebography, their correlations with hemodynamic parameters of reflux are inconsistent.[37] Findings of descending phlebography may be false-negative for reflux in the presence of proximal venous obstruction.[19, 20] Conversely, patients who are asymptomatic or only mildly symptomatic may demonstrate impressive reflux on descending phlebography.[19] A decision to operate, therefore, should not be based on phlebographic findings alone; this test, however, is most useful in guiding surgical exploration once the decision to operate has been made on other grounds.

Nucleotide Lymphoscintigraphy

Nucleotide lymphoscintigraphy should be used to investigate chronic leg swelling. The origin of the swelling may be purely venous, purely lymphatic, or a combination of the two. A surprisingly large percentage of patients with chronic venous insufficiency (25%) have associated lymphatic abnormalities.[17, 38]

DIFFERENTIAL DIAGNOSIS

A wide variety of nonvenous conditions, such as periarteritis nodosa, acanthosis, restless leg syndrome, idiopathic calf cramps, lymphedema, Marjolin's ulcer, fungus infections, vasculitis of various types, and acrocyanosis, mimic some features of venous insufficiency. These conditions are often observed in patients with demonstrable venous insufficiency because it is so prevalent. Careful identification of the true cause of the symptoms is therefore essential. Atypical ulcers and skin lesions should always undergo biopsy.

INDICATIONS FOR SURGERY

Surgery may be considered when conservative therapy has failed to relieve severe stasis symptoms when complications, such as recurrent cellulitis and recurrent deep venous thrombosis during conservative therapy, occur. Finally, certain ancillary factors—relatively young age, desire for speedy rehabilitation to return to work or pursue an active lifestyle, inability to conform to a strict regimen of conservative measures among others—may be relative indications.

Noncompliance in use of support stockings is quite common.[34] The reasons include poor fit (or "binding") by the compression stockings, with a sensation of cutting off the circulation; warm climate; onset of contact dermatitis; and cosmetic or lifestyle considerations. Patients with arthritis and other disabling conditions of the extremities may not be able to keep their legs elevated or to apply tight-fitting stockings. Elderly patients who live alone or in minimal-assistance settings may not have the economic or personnel resources to comply with daily compression therapy. Surgical correction, applied to carefully selected patients, can provide substantial improvement in quality of life for this challenging group of patients. For the most part, surgery should be reserved for patients who present with class 4 or higher[25] skin changes that do not respond to conservative therapy or those, who cannot tolerate conservative therapy. After failure of conservative therapy, patients who present primarily with painful swelling or pain alone may be considered for surgery if hemodynamically massive reflux can be demonstrated.

Although considerable alleviation of leg swelling may be obtained frequently with valve reconstruction surgery, complete resolution is less common. Painless swelling without skin changes is therefore a relative contraindication for surgery. Because they are constantly in pain, patients with disabling venous insufficiency often exhibit personality alterations. Many have an exaggerated pain syndrome: they feel pain that is out of proportion to the extent of their disease. Other extraneous factors, such as a desire for disability or workers' compensation payments, may also color the clinical presentation with exaggerated symptoms. Treatment of this group of patients poses a difficult challenge, because successful surgical correction of reflux may not relieve symptoms. Considerable clinical judgment is required in selecting patients from this group for surgery.

SURGICAL TECHNIQUE

Surgical correction is directed toward the valve stations that were identified to be refluxive on the preoperative evaluation. The uppermost superficial femoral valve, which nearly always lies below the takeoff point of the deep femoral vein, is most frequently repaired. With post-thrombotic disease, the axially transformed profunda femoris vein may function as an important reflux channel[34] and may be reconstructed. Less commonly, valve reconstruction procedures are undertaken at sites farther distal, such as the distal superficial femoral vein in the adductor canal,[40, 42] the popliteal vein, and the posterior tibial vein.

Single valve repairs for "primary" reflux have yielded excellent results—about 60% ulcer-free actuarial survival at 5 years; however, about 20% of ulcers recur early or never heal after the procedure.[40] Early onset of reflux at the repaired valve site accounts for many of these treatment failures. Roughly half are intraoperative failures (i.e., failure to create a totally competent valve at surgery) and the other half are due to early failure of the repaired valve from unknown causes.[40, 42] In light of these findings, an argument could be made for routine repair of a second valve whenever feasible, in the hope of reducing the rates of early failures and recurrences. The second superficial femoral valve is an excellent candidate for such backup repair. Although its location is more variable than that of the first valve, it is frequently accessible through the groin incision.

Techniques of valve reconstruction in post-thrombotic syndrome are currently evolving. Because of the presence of tributary and collateral reflux in this syndrome, reconstruction of multiple valves at various levels would appear

to be a logical move.[30, 42] Several reconstruction techniques are available to accommodate differences in valve lesions, valve location, and other variables (e.g., speed of execution)

Technique of Valve Reconstruction

Exposure and Identification of Valve Station

The first and second superficial femoral valves are approached through an oblique groin incision. The profunda femoris vein can be exposed through the same incision by dividing the fascia that attaches to the sartorius muscle and retracting it laterally. A 2- to 3-inch segment of profunda femoris vein located in the fibrofatty tissue deep to the superficial femoral vein can be exposed in this fashion.

For repair of either vessel, the adjoining segment of common femoral vein must be exposed. The valve station to be repaired and 2 to 3 cm of vein distally should be cleared of branches to test the valve for competence by the strip test.[27, 38] Parallel collateral branches that circumvent valve structures are common and should be identified and divided.

At this stage of the operation, surgical manipulation and the resulting venoconstriction may have rendered a refluxive valve competent. A prosthetic sleeve in situ technique of reconstruction (see later) may be appropriate in such cases. When the valve is still refluxive, valve attachment lines should be exposed in their entirety by careful adventitial dissection (Fig. 149–9).[42] This is an essential first step in most valve reconstruction techniques. Absence of valve attachment lines despite adequate adventitial dissection denotes post-thrombotic dissolution; no more time should be wasted in a futile search for the nonexistent valve cusps through a venotomy. The surgeon should proceed forthwith with an axillary vein transfer. When valve attachment lines are present and have been clearly exposed, they provide

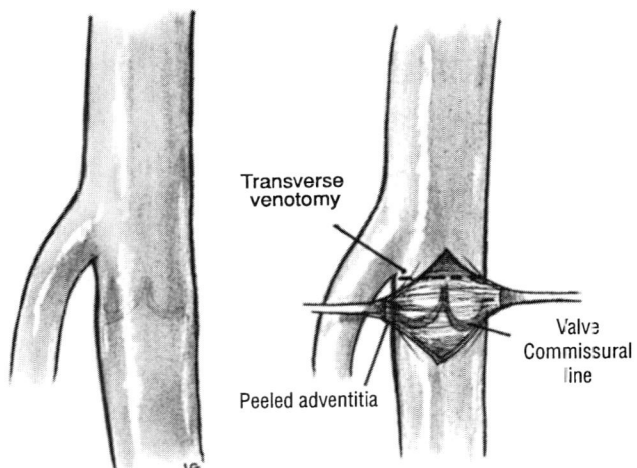

FIGURE 149–9. Exposure of valve attachment lines by adventitial dissection is an important initial step in most valve reconstruction techniques. Careful peeling/excision of the adventitial covering with loop magnification will expose portions of the valve attachment lines, which then should be followed to expose the lines in their entirety. (From Raju S, Hardy JD: Technical options in venous valve reconstruction. J Vasc Surg 173:301–307, 1997.)

the necessary landmarks for placement of the venotomy for internal valvuloplasty and for precise placement of sutures in external and transcommissural techniques.

Alternative Sites for Valve Reconstruction

The mid-superficial femoral vein is exposed through a mid-thigh incision entering the subsartorius tunnel medial to this muscle. More distal parts of the vein can be approached at the adductor hiatus by taking down the adductor tendon.[4] A distal femoral valve is present here in about 60% of cases. The author prefers a medial approach to the tibiopopliteal trunk. Wide exposure and the necessary length of the vein for valve repair are easily obtained by taking down the medial head of the gastrocnemius muscle at its attachment. This maneuver is particularly useful in obese patients and when duplex ultrasonography of the popliteal vein shows it to be compressed when the gastrocnemius is contracted[16]; reattachment of the muscle is not necessary after valve repair. Choice of an alternative site for valve repair is particularly useful in valve reconstructions when the initial repair fails after a while. Reentry through cicatrix from the original incision should be avoided when possible.

Internal Valvuloplasty

The valve may be approached either through a longitudinal incision extending between valve cusp attachments (Kist-

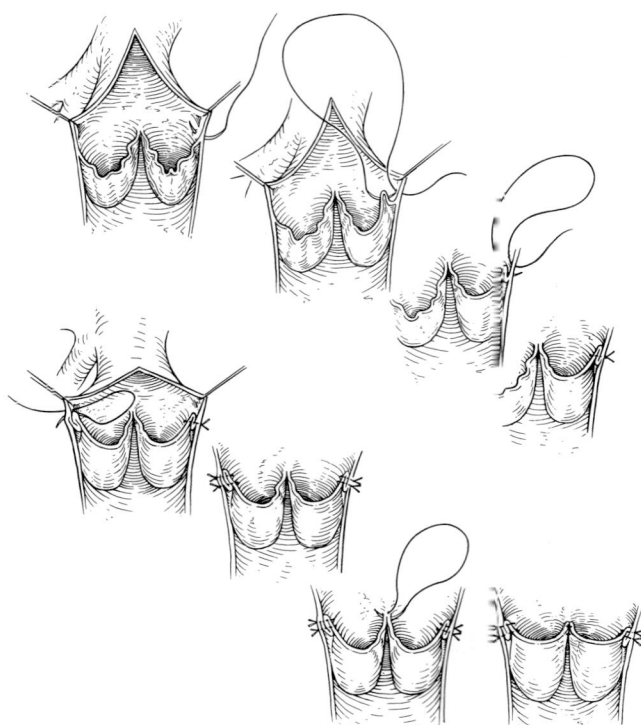

FIGURE 149–10. Internal valvuloplasty technique (Kistner's). The valve cusps are approached via a longitudinal venotomy made through the anterior commissure. *Note:* Plication sutures have been placed at each commissure to eliminate cusp redundancy. (From Bergan JJ, Kistner RL, [eds]: Atlas of Venous Surgery. Philadelphia, WB Saunders, 1992, p 128.)

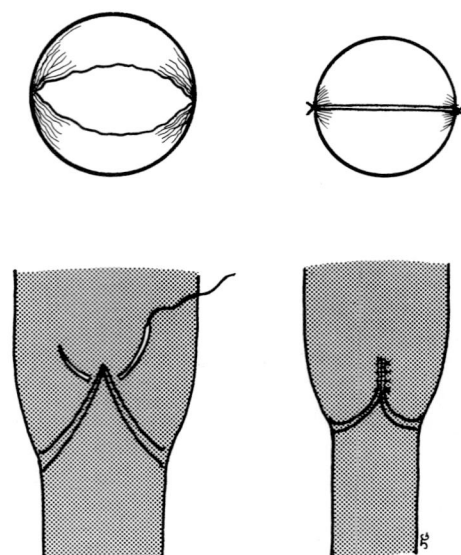

FIGURE 149–11. Transcommissural "repair" utilizes transluminal sutures to close the commissural valve angle while simultaneously tightening the valve cusp. Use of the angioscope is optional. This type of repair is preferred over external valvuloplasty, which closes the valve angle by transmural sutures *without* tightening the valve cusps. (From Raju S, Hardy JD: Technical options in venous valve reconstruction. J Vasc Surg 173:301–307, 1997.)

ner's incision[9]; Fig. 149–10) or through a supravalvular transverse (Raju's)[38] or **T** (Sottiurai's)[43] incision. Fine sutures of 7–0 polypropylene are used to gather up the redundant valve cusp edges at each commissure.

External and Transcommissural Techniques

An external technique for repairing the valve without a venotomy has been described.[11] The valve attachment lines are brought together by transmural partial-thickness sutures placed near each commissure. The technique is less precise and more prone to failure than internal valvuloplasty, but it has the advantages of being more expeditious and of being applicable to small-caliber veins. The transcommissural technique of valve reconstruction is similar to the external technique except that the sutures are transluminal, traversing the valve cusps near their attachments to the wall (Fig. 149–11). As the sutures are tied, the valve attachment lines are coapted, as in external valvuloplasty; but, in addition, the cusps are tightened, a measure that might possibly produce superior outcomes. As yet, long-term data to confirm this expectation are not available.

Angioscopic Techniques

Gloviczki[7] and Hoshino[8] have described valve reconstruction techniques performed with angioscopic control. The transcommisural technique is derived from the suture technique originally described by Gloviczki as part of the angioscopic method. Although considerable dexterity is required, use of the angioscope ensures precise placement of sutures across the valve cusps Valve tightening can be progressively monitored as each suture is placed, to achieve

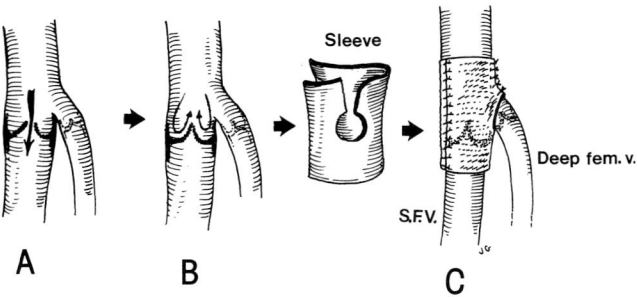

FIGURE 149–12. Prosthetic sleeve in situ. A refluxive superficial femoral valve (A) becomes competent with surgical manipulation and venoconstriction (B). A prosthetic sleeve is fitted around the slightly contracted valve ring to maintain competency (C). The sleeve may be fashioned around the profunda-femoral junction as shown. Superficial femoral vein (SFV).

an optimal result without compromising the lumen. Angioscopic irrigation after completion of the repair aids in visual testing of the competence of the valve.

Prosthetic Sleeve in Situ

A refluxive vein valve sometimes becomes competent with venoconstriction caused by surgical manipulation (Fig. 149–12).[38] An appropriate-sized polyester (Dacron) or ringed polytetrafluoroethylene (PTFE) sleeve can be placed around the valve in the slightly contracted position to maintain competency. The technique is quick to perform, avoids venotomy, and is applicable to small-caliber veins. An adjustable silicone sleeve designed on this principle is commercially available.[15] Too aggressive tightening of the device, in a misguided attempt to render an overtly refluxive valve competent, may cause iatrogenic venous obstruction.

Axillary Vein Transfer

When the valve cannot be repaired by one of the techniques discussed earlier or when it has been completely destroyed by earlier thrombosis, axillary vein valve transfer may be considered.[29, 31, 32, 46] A competent valve-bearing segment of axillary vein is excised and transferred to the superficial femoral vein below the inguinal ligament or to one of the alternative sites.

A seemingly simple procedure, axillary vein transfer in fact demands exacting technique to achieve a competent result (Fig. 149–13). Interrupted sutures are used to allow expansion of the suture line when the patient assumes erect posture. The axillary vein is ligated without repair; significant obstructive sequelae have not been observed (mild episodic symptoms in 2% of the patients). The transferred axillary vein segment should be wrapped with a prosthetic sleeve to avoid late dilatation, which may occur from a compliance mismatch between the transferred venous segment and the native vein in the lower limb (Fig. 149–14). About 40% of axillary vein valves are incompetent in situ.[38, 42] A competent valve can usually be located, however, farther proximal or distal in the axillary vein segment. Failing this, bench repair of the incompetent axillary valve can be carried out to render the graft competent before it is transferred.

Bench repair utilizing the external valvuloplasty technique has been largely unsuccessful but the transcommissural technique appears to work very well for this purpose.[42] Sottiurai has successfully used the internal valvuloplasty technique for bench repairs.[43]

Several of the previously described techniques can be combined to perform multiple-valve reconstruction (Fig. 149–15).

Other Antireflux Procedures

A variety of less commonly used techniques, including venoplastic procedures,[42] Kistner's segment transfer,[10, 12] valve reconstruction de novo,[42] and others,[2] are available for use in special circumstances. The large repertoire of techniques should allow successful reconstruction in most cases, despite variations in anatomy and in lesions.

FIGURE 149–13. Technique of axillary vein transfer. The valve should be inserted under optimal tension without torsion. The shallow axillary valves are susceptible to malcoaptation and reflux due to technical deficiencies such as torsion or excessive or inadequate tension (inset). (From Raju S, Hardy JD: Technical options in venous valve reconstruction. J Vasc Surg 173:301–307, 1997.)

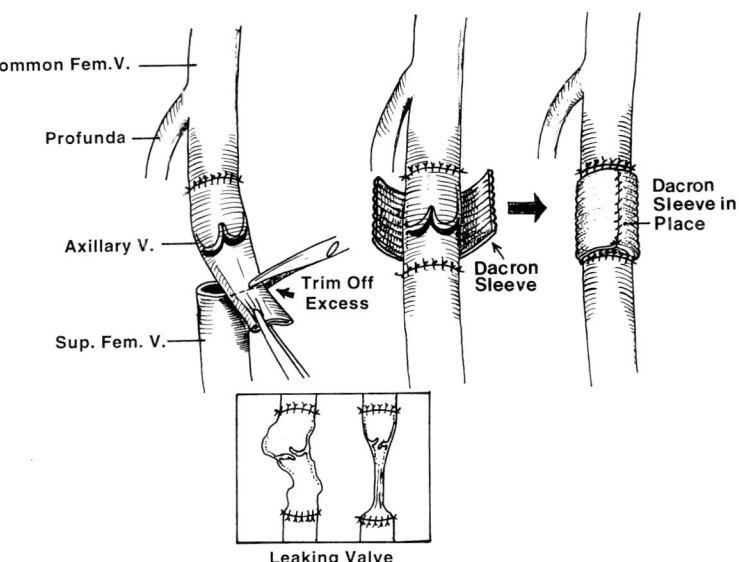

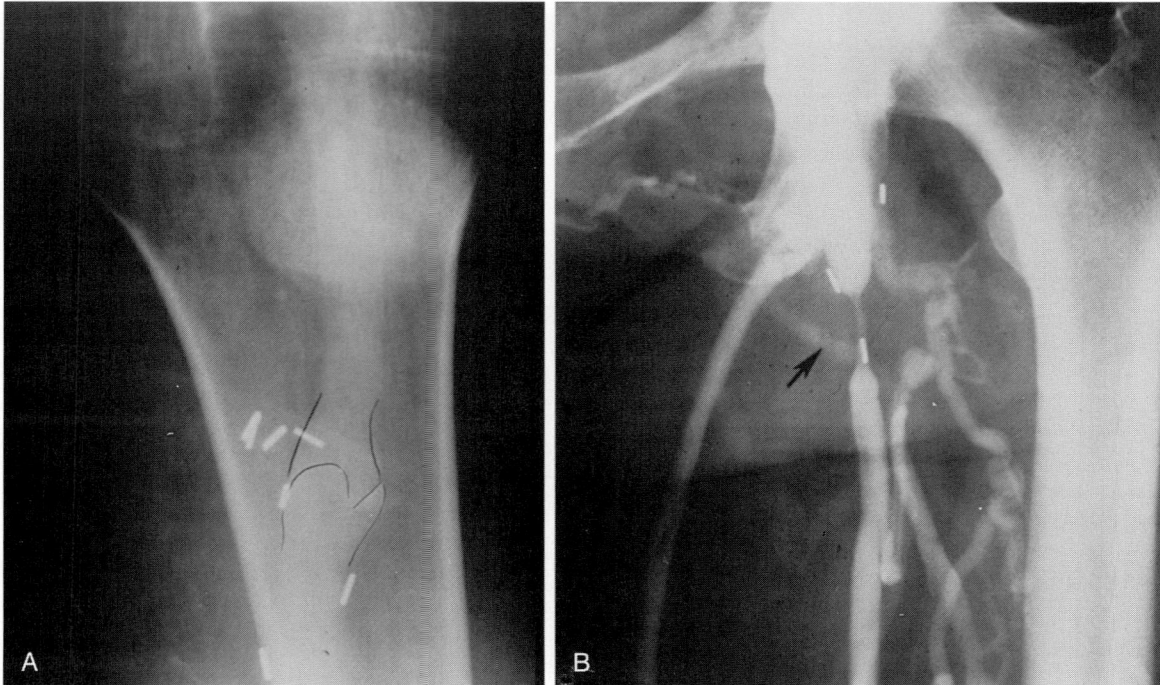

FIGURE 149–14. Late failure of transferred axillary vein valve. *A,* Recurrent reflux through a transferred axillary vein valve that was not fitted with a prosthetic sleeve. *B,* Less commonly, the transferred valvular segment may become stenotic *(arrow)* after functioning satisfactorily for a number of years.

Choice of Technique

Internal valvuloplasty is a proven technique with an established track record. It is clearly the preferred technique when single-valve repair for "primary" reflux is contemplated. Prosthetic sleeve in situ, when used very selectively as described earlier, produces equally good results.[40] Unlike the internal technique, it is rapid, does not require venotomy, and is applicable to small-caliber veins. Because of

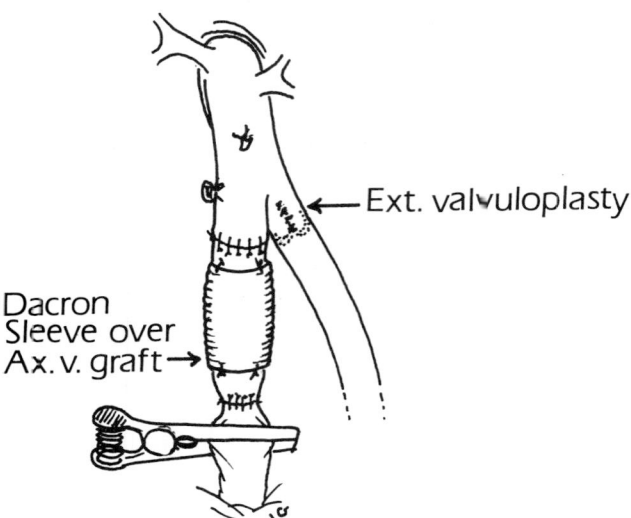

FIGURE 149–15. Different techniques can be combined to perform multiple venous valve reconstructions. An axillary vein (Ax. v.) transfer with a prosthetic sleeve to reconstruct the superficial femoral vein and an external (Ext) valvuloplasty of the profunda femoris venous valve are shown.

the aforementioned limitations, the internal technique is not readily suitable for simultaneous multiple valve reconstructions or for small-caliber veins. For such cases, this author prefers the transcommissural technique. The angioscopic technique and other special-use procedures will find favor according to individual preferences and specific circumstances.

Axillary vein transfer remains the mainstay for valves destroyed beyond direct repair. Bench repair techniques, as described earlier, have greatly extended its availability. Earlier fears that axillary vein transfer might yield clinical results inferior to those of direct valvuloplasty[38] have not been borne out.[32, 40] Nevertheless, duplex follow-up data indicate that axillary vein valves are more likely to fail than repairs by direct valvuloplasty.[40] Furthermore, axillary vein transfer is a more extensive and more complex procedure and should not be used as an "easy" substitute for a direct valve repair technique except when that is not feasible.

TABLE 149–4. COMPLICATIONS IN 550 VALVE REPAIRS IN 347 PATIENTS[42]

COMPLICATION	PREVALENCE (%)
Postoperative deep vein thrombosis (3 mo)	3.5
Thrombosis of valve repair	0.7
Pulmonary embolus	0.3*
Hematoma/seroma	5
Deep wound infections	2
Prosthetic sleeve infections	2

From Raju S, Hardy JD: Technical options in venous valve reconstruction. Am J Surg 173:301, 1997.
*Successfully resolved with thrombolysis.

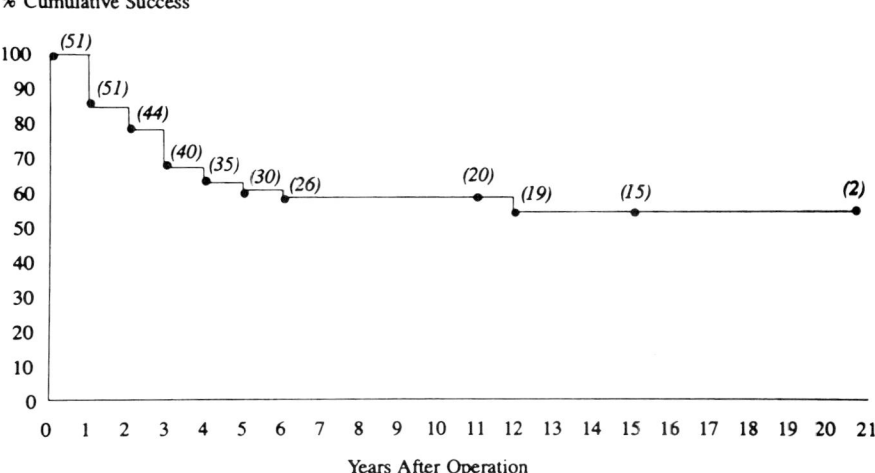

FIGURE 149–16. Cumulative clinical success rates for class 0 or 1 result after venous valve reconstruction for all limbs. Numbers in parentheses represent total limbs at risk for each time interval. (From Masuda EM, Kistner RL: Long-term results of venous valve reconstruction: A four- to twenty-one-year follow-up. J Vasc Surg 19:391–403, 1994.)

Ancillary Procedures

Saphenous vein stripping and modified perforator interruption[5] can be performed simultaneously with valve reconstruction to abolish reflux in these segments.[9, 42] In some post-thrombotic cases, the saphenous vein and the perforators may appear on ascending venography to provide a collateral pathway around an obstruction in the deep vein. These collateral venous segments are dilated and refluxive as well. Traditional teaching forbids interruption of these secondary varicosities. This admonition notwithstanding, in this situation saphenectomy[33] and perforator interruption[36] are clinically helpful; reflux is reduced without compromising outflow.

Collateral reflux may be abolished by dividing persistent collateral connections, for instance the profunda femoris–popliteal connection. This should be performed only when the superficial femoral vein has become satisfactorily recanalized lest outflow obstruction result.[30] In the presence of axial transformation of the patent profunda femoris vein, a severely damaged post-thrombotic superficial femoral vein may be ligated instead of undertaking valve reconstruction.[34]

PERIOPERATIVE MANAGEMENT

Heparin (2000 to 10,000 units) is given intraoperatively, the amount depending on the technique of valve repair and the coagulation status of the patient. For techniques that do not require venotomy or prolonged clamping of the vein (e.g., transcommissural repair), the smaller dose of heparin may suffice. Heparin is not "reversed" at the end of the procedure. Dalteparin sodium is administered, 2500 units subcutaneously twice daily, starting in the recovery room and continuing postoperatively for 5 to 7 days. Oral warfarin sodium is started on the first postoperative day and titrated to International Normalized Ratio (INR) 2.0 to 2.5 for 6 weeks, and later to 1.7 to 2.0. Patients at increased risk for recurrent thrombosis should use an anticoagulant indefinitely. Others discontinue anticoagulation after 4 months.

For long-term anticoagulation, the author prefers a low-dose warfarin regimen (1 mg/day). This regimen has been useful in other patients at high risk for thrombosis.[24] A pneumatic cuff or another compression device should be used in the postoperative period to reduce swelling. Prophylactic antibiotics are used routinely during the first 48 to 72 hours after surgery.

POSTOPERATIVE COMPLICATIONS

Valve reconstruction is associated with low risk of morbidity (Table 149–4). Wound complications can be minimized by routine use of closed drainage and meticulous surgical technique. It is noteworthy that wound infections, including prosthetic sleeve infections, have been rare, even

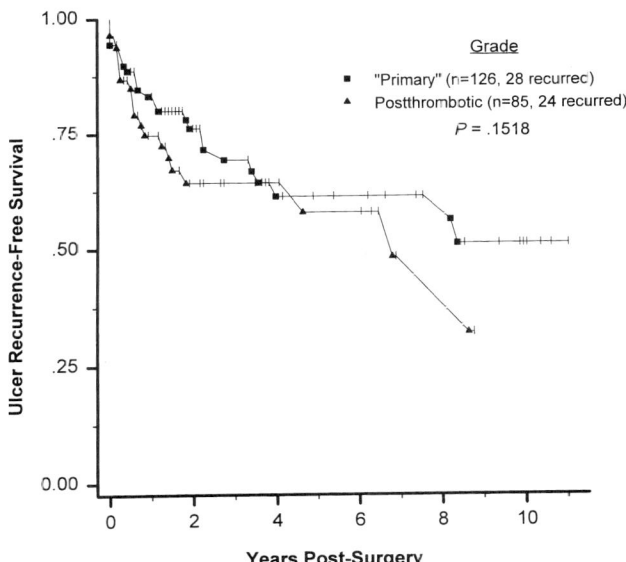

FIGURE 149–17. Actuarial ulcer-free survival in primary and post-thrombotic reflux. (From Raju S, Fredericks RK, Neglén PN, et al: Durability of venous valve reconstruction techniques for "primary" and postthrombotic reflux. J Vasc Surg 23:357–367, 1996.)

TABLE 149–5. WORLDWIDE EXPERIENCE WITH VALVE RECONSTRUCTION

INVESTIGATOR	NO. OF CASES	ULCER HEALING (%)	FOLLOW-UP (YR)
Eriksson	19	85	7
Kistner	51	60*	10
Perrin	11	91	2
O'Donnell	15	79	4
Raju	126	63*	7
Sottiurai	21	80	6

*Actuarial data.

though 31% of patients had an open stasis ulcer at the time of surgery.

RESULTS

Primary Valve Reflux

Valve reconstruction procedures produce satisfactory long-term results.[14] The results of internal valvuloplasty have been durable: few recurrences are reported after the first 3 or 4 years after surgery (Fig. 149–16). Similar results have now been reported for a wide variety of techniques from multiple centers worldwide (Table 149–5).[3, 4, 6, 8, 40, 45, 47] Most patients whose valve reconstruction successfully heals stasis ulceration and relieves other stasis symptoms stop using support stockings.[38, 40]

Post-thrombotic Reflux

Experience with valve reconstruction in post-thrombotic syndrome is not yet extensive. In our own center, results similar to those for "primary" reflux have been obtained (Fig. 149–17).[32, 40] Others' experiences have been mixed.[14]

Hemodynamic Improvement

Significant improvements in ambulatory venous pressure,[13, 40] air plethysmography findings,[3] and other reflux parameters[38] have been documented after venous valve reconstruction. As a rule, however, ambulatory venous pressure does not completely normalize. Determinants of ambulatory venous pressure are complex and are related in part to the nonlinear volume-pressure relationship that obtains in collapsible tubes.[39, 41] A reduction in the volume of reflux is therefore reflected in improvement of ambulatory venous pressure in a variable manner. Venous stasis ulceration is frequently, but not invariably,[35] associated with ambulatory venous hypertension. The precise pathophysiologic relationship between ambulatory venous hypertension and venous stasis ulceration is poorly understood and remains to be precisely defined.

REFERENCES

1. Bjordal RI: Pressure patterns in the saphenous system in patients with venous leg ulcers. Acta Chir Scand 137:495, 1971.
2. Burkhart HM, Fath SW, Dalsing MC, et al: Experimental repair of venous valvular insufficiency using a cryopreserved venous valve allograft aided by a distal arteriovenous fistula. J Vasc Surg 26:817, 1997.
3. Bry JD, Muto PA, O'Donnell TF, et al: The clinical and hemodynamic results after axillary-to-popliteal vein valve transplantation. J Vasc Surg 21:110, 1995.
4. Cheatle TR, Perrin M: Venous valve repair: Early results in fifty-two cases. J Vasc Surg 19:404, 1994.
5. DePalma RG: Surgical therapy for venous stasis: Results of a modified Linton operation. Am J Surg 137:810, 1979.
6. Eriksson I, Almgren B: Influence of the profunda femoris vein on venous hemodynamics of the limb: Experience from thirty-one deep vein valve reconstructions. J Vasc Surg 4:390, 1986.
7. Gloviczki P, Merrell SW, Bower TC: Femoral vein valve repair under direct vision without venotomy: A modified technique use of angioscopy. J Vasc Surg 14:645, 1991.
8. Hoshino S, Satakawa H, Iwaya F, et al: External valvuloplasty under preoperative angioscopic control. Phlebologie 46:521, 1993.
9. Kistner RL: Surgical repair of the incompetent femoral vein valve. Arch Surg 114:1304, 1979.
10. Kistner RL: Transposition techniques. In Bergan JJ, Kistner RL (eds): Atlas of Venous Surgery. Philadelphia, WB Saunders, 1992, pp 153–155.
11. Kistner R: Surgical technique of external venous valve repair. Proc Straub Pacific Health Found 55:15, 1990.
12. Kistner RL: Reflux disease: Valvuloplasty/transposition/valve transplant. Proc Straub Pacific Health Found 57:37, 1993.
13. Kistner RL, Eklof B, Masuda EM: Deep venous valve reconstruction. Cardiovasc Surg 3:129, 1995.
14. Masuda EM, Kistner RL: Long-term results of venous valve reconstruction: A four- to twenty-one-year follow-up. J Vasc Surg 19:391, 1994.
15. Lane RJ: Repair of incompetent venous valves: A new technique. Presentation: Meeting of the Australian and New Zealand Society of Phlebology. Sydney, Australia, May 4, 1991.
16. Leon M, Volteas N, Labropoulos N, et al: Popliteal vein entrapment in the normal population. Eur J Vasc Surg 6:623, 1992.
17. LePage PA, Villavicencio JL, Gomez ER, et al: The valvular anatomy of the iliac system and its clinical applications. J Vasc Surg 14:678, 1991.
18. Markel A, Manzo RA, Bergelin RO, Strandness DE Jr: Valvular reflux following deep vein thrombosis: Incidence and time of occurrence. J Vasc Surg 15:377, 1992.
19. Morano JU, Raju S: Chronic venous insufficiency: Assessment with descending venography. Radiology 174:441, 1990.
20. Neglén P, Raju S: A comparison between descending phlebography and duplex Doppler investigation in the evaluation of reflux in chronic venous insufficiency: A challenge to phlebography as the "gold standard." J Vasc Surg 16:687, 1992.
21. Neglén P, Raju S: A rational approach to detect significant reflux using duplex Doppler scan and air plethysmography. J Vasc Surg 17:590, 1993.
22. Nicolaides AN: The investigation of chronic venous disorders of the lower limb: A consensus statement. J Vasc Surg 29:1050–1064, 1999.
23. Nicolaides AN, Summer DS (eds): Investigation of Patients with Deep Vein Thrombosis and Chronic Venous Insufficiency. Los Angeles, Med-Orion Publishing, 1991.
24. Poller L, McKernan A, Thomson JM, et al: Fixed minidose warfarin: A new approach to prophylaxis against venous thrombosis after major surgery. Br Med J 295:1309, 1987.
25. Porter JM, Rutherford RB, Clagett GP, et al: Reporting standards in venous disease. J Vasc Surg 8:172, 1988.
26. Raju S: Venous insufficiency of the lower limb and stasis ulceration: Changing concepts and management. Ann Surg 197:688, 1983.
27. Raju S: Valve reconstruction procedures for chronic venous insufficiency. Semin Vasc Surg 1:101, 1988.
28. Raju S: New approaches to the diagnosis and treatment of venous obstruction. J Vasc Surg 4:42, 1986.
29. Raju S: Axillary vein transfer for postphlebitic syndrome. In Bergan JJ, Kistner RL (eds): Atlas of Venous Surgery. Philadelphia, WB Saunders, 1992, pp 147–152.
30. Raju S: Multiple-valve reconstruction for venous insufficiency: Indications, optimal technique, and results. In Veith FJ (ed): Current Critical Problems in Vascular Surgery, 4th ed. St. Louis, Quality Medical Publishing, 1992, pp 122–125.
31. Raju S: Discussion in Johnson ND, Queral LA, Flinn WR, et al: Late

objective assessment of venous valve surgery. Arch Surg 116:1461, 1981.
32. Raju S, Doolittle J, Neglén P: Axillary vein transfer in trabeculated postphlebitic veins. J Vasc Surg (in press).
33. Raju S, Easterwood L, Fountain T, et al: Saphenectomy in the presence of chronic venous obstruction. Surgery 123:637–644, 1998.
34. Raju S, Fountain T, Neglén P, et al: Axial transformation of the profunda femoris vein. J Vasc Surg 27:651, 1998.
35. Raju S, Fredericks R: Hemodynamic basis of stasis ulceration: A hypothesis. J Vasc Surg 13:491, 1991.
36. Raju S, Fredericks R: Venous obstruction: An analysis of 137 cases with hemodynamic, venographic and clinical correlations. J Vasc Surg 14:305, 1991.
37. Raju S, Fredericks R: Evaluation of methods for detecting venous reflux: Perspectives in venous insufficiency with descending venography. Arch Surg 125:1463, 1990.
38. Raju S, Fredericks R: Valve reconstruction procedures for non-obstructive venous insufficiency: Rationale, techniques, and results in 107 procedures with 2–8-year follow-up. J Vasc Surg 7:301, 1988.
39. Raju S, Fredericks R, Lishman P, et al: Observations on the calf venous pump mechanism: Determinants of post-exercise pressure. J Vasc Surg 17:459, 1993.
40. Raju S, Fredericks RK, Neglén PN, et al: Durability of venous valve reconstruction techniques for "primary" and postthrombotic reflux. J Vasc Surg 23:357, 1996.
41. Raju S, Green AB, Fredericks RK, et al: Tube collapse and valve closure in ambulatory venous pressure regulation: Studies with a mechanical model. J Endovasc Surg 5:42, 1998.
42. Raju S, Hardy JD: Technical options in venous valve reconstruction. Am J Surg 173:301, 1997.
43. Sottiurai VS: Supravalvular incision for valve repair in primary valvular insufficiency. In Bergan JJ, Kistner RL (eds): Atlas of Venous Surgery. Philadelphia, WB Saunders, 1992, pp 137–138.
44. Sottiurai VS: Surgical correction of recurrent venous ulcer. J Cardiovasc Surg 32:104, 1991.
45. Sun JM, Zhang PH: Venous valve transplant in the treatment of incompetent deep veins of the lower extremities. Chung Hua Wai Ko Tsa Chih 23:752, 1985.
46. Taheri SA, Lazar L, Elias S, et al: Surgical treatment of postphlebitic syndrome with vein valve transplant. Am J Surg 144:221, 1982.
47. Zhang PH, Sun JM Shang HZ: Treatment of primary valvular incompetence of the deep veins of the leg with repair of femoral vein valves. Chung Hua Wai Ko Tsa Chih 23:137, 1985.

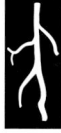

CHAPTER 150
Surgical Treatment of Chronic Deep Venous Obstruction

Peter Gloviczki, M.D., and Jae-Sung Cho, M.D.

Valvular incompetence is the most common cause of chronic venous insufficiency (CVI) of the lower extremities; deep venous obstruction is responsible for signs and symptoms of venous congestion in less than 10% of patients.[1] Although the first successful venous reconstruction in a patient was reported more than 40 years ago by Warren and Thayer,[2] results of surgical treatment for venous obstructions have been less than satisfactory for many years. Only in the last two decades have improvements in diagnosis, patient selection and surgical technique and the availability of better graft materials resulted in more frequent successful implantation of venous bypasses in patients.[3] Current results of venous bypasses are, however, still inferior to those obtained with arterial reconstructions.

In this chapter, we discuss indications, patient selection, and preoperative evaluation for surgical treatment of popliteal, femoral, iliac, and inferior vena caval venous obstructions. We examine causes of graft failure in the venous system and list advantages of different adjuncts used currently to improve patency of venous grafts.

Finally, we describe techniques of venous bypasses used for femoropopliteal, iliac, and inferior vena caval occlusions and present available data on long-term results. See Chapter 151 for techniques and results of endovascular treatment of large vein obstruction, and Chapter 152 for vena caval reconstruction in treatment of malignant tumors. For details on venous reconstruction after trauma, see Chapter 59.

ETIOLOGY

Deep venous thrombosis is the most common cause of venous obstructions. In symptomatic patients, recanalization of the thrombosed veins is incomplete and collateral circulation is inadequate. Venous occlusion may also develop because of trauma or irradiation or as a result of external compression of deep veins by:

- Retroperitoneal fibrosis[4]
- Benign or malignant, primary or metastatic tumors[5–7]
- Cysts
- Aneurysms
- Abnormally inserted muscle (popliteal vein entrapment)[8]
- Fibrous bands or ligaments (soleal arch syndrome,[9] femoral vein compression by the inguinal ligament[10])

Compression of the left common iliac vein by the overriding right common iliac artery (May-Thurner or Cockett syndrome) (Fig. 150–1) is a frequently overlooked cause of left iliofemoral venous thrombosis.[11–14] May and Thurner

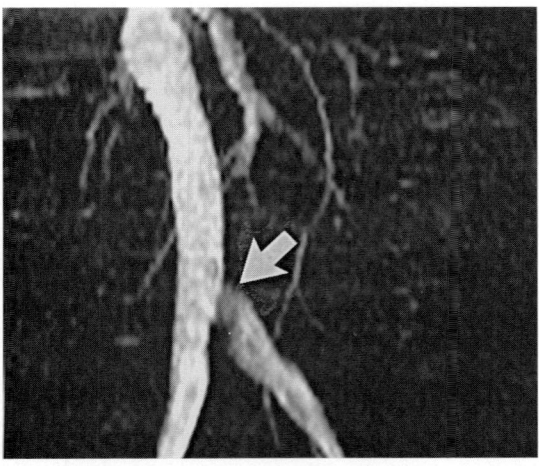

FIGURE 150–1. Magnetic resonance venography of the iliocaval bifurcation. *Arrow* indicates compression of the left common iliac vein by the overriding right common iliac artery (May-Thurner syndrome).

observed secondary changes, such as an intraluminal web or "spur," in the proximal left common iliac vein in 20% of 430 autopsies. Congenital anomalies, such as membranous occlusion of the suprahepatic inferior vena cava (IVC) with or without associated thrombosis of hepatic veins (*Budd-Chiari syndrome*),[15] aplasia, and hypoplasia of the iliofemoral veins (Fig. 150–2) as in *Klippel-Trenaunay syndrome*,[16, 17] can also cause CVI.

PREOPERATIVE EVALUATION

Preoperative evaluation of the patient should reveal the etiology and functional significance of deep venous ob-

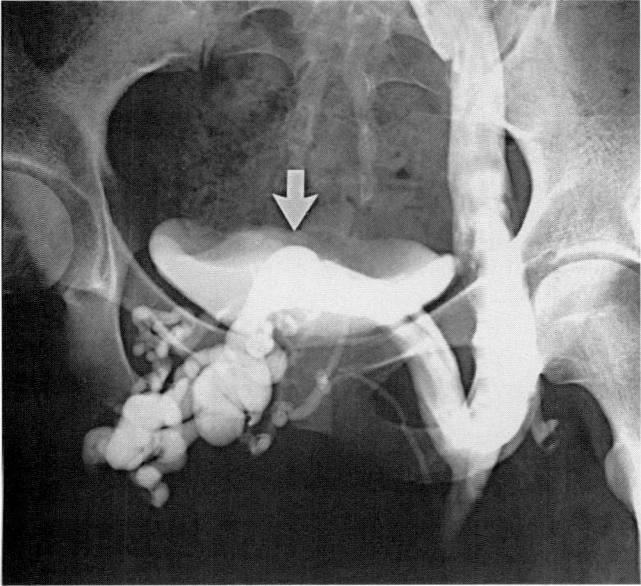

FIGURE 150–2. Venogram of agenesis of the right iliac vein in a 22-year-old woman. A huge suprapubic venous collateral (*arrow*) drains the entire right lower extremity. (From Gloviczki P, Stanson AW, et al: Klippel-Trenaunay syndrome: The risks and benefits of vascular interventions. Surgery 110:469–479, 199.)

struction and the extent and severity of associated venous incompetence. In at least two thirds of patients with venous outflow obstruction, however, distal reflux due to valvular incompetence contributes greatly to development of CVI.[18] For details of the clinical and diagnostic evaluation of the patients with CVI, see Chapter 145. Specific aspects of the evaluation of patients with suspected deep venous occlusion are emphasized here.

History and Physical Examination

History and physical examination, complemented by examination with a hand-held Doppler instrument, should reveal signs and symptoms typical of venous congestion. Patients with venous occlusion have swelling and experience exercise-induced pain in the thigh muscles, referred to as *venous claudication*. This pain is described as a "bursting" pain in the thigh and sometimes in the calf that occurs after exercise and is relieved by rest but more effectively by elevation of the legs.

Signs of CVI, such as edema, varicose veins, skin changes, lipodermatosclerosis, eczema, and ulceration, should be noted. Distended varicose veins are present even in the supine patient with CVI, and suprapubic and abdominal wall collaterals develop in patients with pelvic occlusion. Bleeding from high-pressure varicosities is not infrequent. The swollen leg has a cyanotic hue, and bilateral swelling indicates bilateral iliofemoral or vena caval occlusion or systemic disease. In some patients, venous congestion results in hyperhidrosis and significant fluid loss through the skin. Associated chronic high-output or low-output lymphedema (see Chapter 155) may also develop.

The patient's evaluation should identify risk factors of deep vein thrombosis (DVT), including:

- Previous deep venous thrombosis
- Pulmonary embolism
- Family history of venous thrombosis
- Obesity
- Decreased activity level
- Recent pregnancy
- Malignancy
- Hormonal treatment
- Hypercoagulability
- Recent trauma
- Surgical history

Associated chronic arterial occlusive disease as well as congenital venous malformation manifesting as limb hypertrophy, port-wine stains, and lateral atypical varicose veins (Klippel-Trenaunay syndrome), and the presence of a thrill or bruit indicating arteriovenous fistula (*Parkes-Weber syndrome*) should be excluded. Patients with membranous occlusion of the vena cava frequently have evidence of hepatic failure and portal hypertension as well.[15]

A simple technique to test femoropopliteal venous occlusion in the office is the *Perthes test*. A tourniquet is placed on the proximal calf, and the patient is asked to walk. Exercise results in rapid emptying of superficial vein through patent perforators into a patent deep system. Distention of superficial veins distal to the tourniquet following ambulation indicates deep venous occlusion. Examination with a hand-held Doppler instrument also yields evidence for deep venous occlusion, but the diagnosis should be established by more accurate means, primarily duplex ultrasonographic scanning. A complete evaluation to establish the clinical class of venous disease is necessary.

Noninvasive Venous Evaluation

Although duplex scanning and plethysmography are the tests needed to establish deep venous occlusion and to determine the extent of valvular incompetence and calf muscle pump failure, it is equally important to exclude any abdominal or pelvic disease (tumor, cyst, retroperitoneal fibrosis) with computed tomography (CT) or magnetic resonance imaging (MRI). Outflow plethysmography is useful to confirm functional venous outflow obstruction and to document improvement following treatment.

Ambulatory venous pressure measurements suggest venous hypertension, and measurements of foot-arm pressure differences, as described by Raju,[19] quantitate venous hypertension. A resting arm-foot pressure differential greater than 4 mmHg is considered evidence of significant obstruction. For purposes of testing, exercise consists of 10 dorsiflexions of the ankles or 20 isometric contractions of the calf muscle. In potential candidates for proximal venous reconstruction, femoral and central venous pressure measurements are required to document the severity of proximal iliac or iliocaval obstruction. Either a pressure difference of at least 5 mmHg between the femoral and the central pressures in the supine patient or a two-fold increase in femoral vein pressure after exercise indicates hemodynamically significant proximal stenosis or occlusion.[20–24]

Contrast Phlebography

In patients being considered for venous reconstruction, detailed contrast phlebography is performed. In our practice, we use both ascending and descending phlebography to evaluate obstruction and any associated valvular incompetence.[22, 23] Iliocavography and abdominal venacavography through a brachial approach may also be necessary in some patients to visualize the vena cava proximal to the occlusion. The femoral access is useful not only for descending phlebography and iliocavography but also for measuring femoral venous pressures. Magnetic resonance phlebography (see Fig. 150–1) is a promising new technique that may further decrease the number of contrast radiographic examinations in the future.

Contrast phlebography is covered in Chapter 17.

FACTORS AFFECTING GRAFT PATENCY

Grafts placed in the venous system undergo thrombosis more frequently than those implanted for arterial reconstruction. This difference is attributed to several factors. Flow in venous grafts in general is lower than in arterial grafts placed at the same location, primarily because of the collateral venous circulation that developed to compensate for the chronic obstruction. Distal venous obstruction and incompetence further decrease inflow to the graft, contrib-

uting to potential failure.[18, 23] Pressure in the venous system is low, and grafts can collapse under increased abdominal pressure or in tightly confined spaces, such as the area under the inguinal ligament and the retrohepatic space, or when tunneled through the diaphragm. Many patients with previous deep venous thrombosis lack circulating anticoagulants, such as protein C, protein S, and antithrombin III, and thus have greater thrombogenicity. The thrombogenic surface of the prosthetic graft also increases the risk of graft failure.

VENOUS GRAFTS AND ADJUNCTS TO IMPROVE PATENCY

As a result of extensive laboratory efforts made in the past decades,[25–37] patency of grafts implanted in the venous circulation has considerably improved. The availability of large-diameter autologous and prosthetic grafts, the use of adjuncts such as a distal arteriovenous fistula, rigid external support of the grafts, perioperative and postoperative anticoagulation, the use of perioperative intermittent-compression pumps, and postoperative surveillance with duplex scanning all have contributed to better patency and improved clinical outcome.

Venous Graft Materials

Autologous grafts in the infrainguinal location have the best chance of long-term success. The greater saphenous vein, because of its low thrombogenicity, and its suitability in size and length in most patients, is the best choice, when available. As a spiral or panel graft, it can be used for large vein reconstruction as well, although in our experience, these grafts do not perform as well for iliocaval reconstructions as they do for superior vena caval replacement (see Chapter 153).[22, 23] The contralateral superficial femoral vein and the arm veins, especially the basilic-brachial-axillary vein, are other potential sources of autogenous grafts, as are the external and, occasionally, even the internal jugular veins. Harvesting contralateral deep veins in patients with a history of DVT, however, may be the source of significant added morbidity.

Experiments with cryopreserved femoral vein grafts have been promising,[38] and a first-phase clinical trial has been completed. Data at this point are insufficient, however, to support recommendation of this graft for routine clinical use.

Of the available prosthetic materials, the expanded polytetrafluoroethylene (ePTFE) graft has been used most frequently for large vein replacement.[4–7, 21–25, 39–46] Because of a large diameter, sufficient length, immediate availability, and the external ring or spiral support associated with relatively low thrombogenicity, ePTFE grafts are currently the best choice for prosthetic replacement of large veins.

Arteriovenous Fistula

Multiple experiments have confirmed that a distal arteriovenous fistula, first suggested by Kunlin and Kunlin[30] in 1953, improves patency of grafts placed in the venous system.[25, 28, 33, 34] An arteriovenous fistula increases flow and decreases platelet and fibrin deposition in prosthetic grafts (Fig. 150–3).[33] Prosthetic grafts have significantly higher thrombotic threshold velocity than autologous grafts and require higher flow to maintain patency.

Disadvantages of an arteriovenous fistula include the longer operating time needed to create the fistula and the inconvenience of additional procedures to close the fistula at a later date by means of either endovascular techniques (embolization) or a cutdown. A potential side effect is an elevated cardiac output, caused by high fistula flow; the latter can also defeat the purpose of the operation by increasing venous pressure at the groin and causing venous outflow obstruction. Experimental work in our laboratory revealed that to avoid deleterious effect on venous outflow from the leg, the optimal ratio between the diameters of the fistula and the graft should not exceed 0 3.[47] Elevated intraoperative pressure in the femoral vein after placement of a fistula should be taken as a warning sign, and the fistula diameter should be decreased through banding of the conduit.

The configuration and location of the fistula have been the subjects of much controversy. A large side branch of the greater saphenous vein or the saphenous vein itself can be used to perform one anastomosis only. Most recently, we have placed the venous end of the arteriovenous fistula right onto the hood of the venous graft at the distal anastomosis, using either a 4-mm vein as a free graft (saphenous vein or a large tributary) or a 4-mm PTFE graft. The advantage of a vein or a polyester (Dacron) fistula is that flow can be calibrated with an electromagnetic flowmeter, and large flows (>300 ml/min) can be avoided.

The arterial anastomosis is usually made to the superficial femoral artery. We place a small polymeric silicone (Silastic) sheet around the fistula to prevent healing and to facilitate dissection of the fistula during a second procedure to occlude it. A 2-0 polypropylene suture is also tied loosely around the fistula, and its end is positioned in the subcutaneous tissue, close to the incision, for later identification; intraoperative duplex scanning facilitates identification of the fistula. Percutaneous closure of the fistula with transcatheter embolization is also an option.

At present, for all prosthetic grafts anastomosed to the femoral vein and all longer (>10 cm) iliocaval grafts implanted at our institution, a femoral arteriovenous fistula is added to maintain patency (Fig. 150–4). The fistula is left open for at least 6 months after the operation, but patients without any side effects benefit from long-term fistula flow to prolong patency.

Thrombosis Prophylaxis

Intravenous heparin, in a dose of 5000 units, is given before cross-clamping, and anticoagulation is maintained during and after the procedure in most patients. We administer low-dose heparin (500 to 800 U/hour) locally through a small polyethylene catheter in the perioperative period (Fig. 150–5), until complete systemic heparinization is achieved through an increase in the dose, as demonstrated by an increase in activated partial thromboplastin time to twice normal by 48 hours after surgery. The catheter is then removed, heparinization is continued intravenously through an arm vein or central line, and the patient begins oral anticoagulation therapy with warfarin.

An intermittent pneumatic compression pump, leg elevation, elastic bandages, and early ambulation are also used in the perioperative period to improve the success of venous reconstruction.[48] The patient is fitted with 30 to 40 mmHg graduated-compression elastic stockings before discharge. Warfarin is continued in patients with autogenous grafts for at least 3 months; in most patients with prosthetic grafts or with an underlying coagulation abnormality, however, oral anticoagulation is maintained indefinitely.

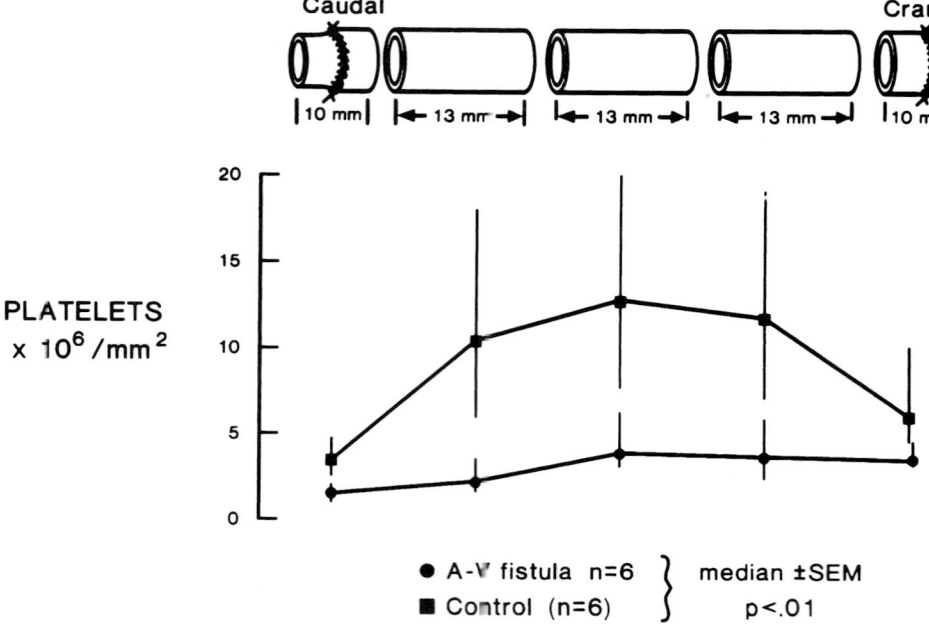

FIGURE 150–3. Platelet deposition on polytetrafluoroethylene vena caval grafts in dogs with and without arteriovenous fistula 3 hours after perfusion. (From Gloviczki P, Hollier LH, Dewanjee MJ, et al: Experimental replacement of the inferior vena cava: Factors affecting patency. Surgery; 95:657–666, 1984.)

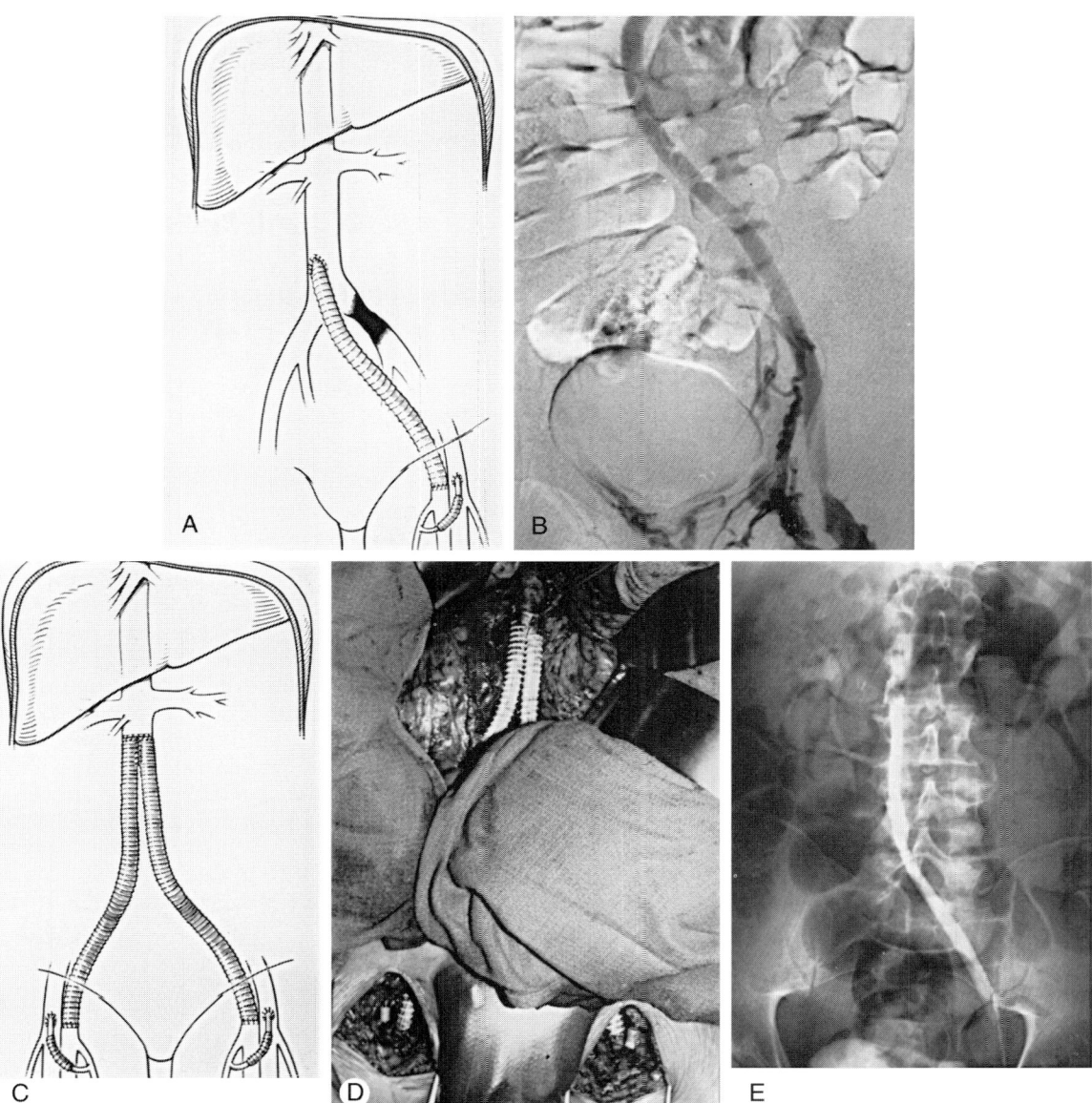

FIGURE 150–4. *A,* Illustration of a left femorocaval polytetrafluoroethylene (ePTFE) graft with a femoral arteriovenous fistula. *B,* Postoperative venogram shows patent graft. Narrowing at the site of the femoral anastomosis is an artifact caused by inflow from the arteriovenous fistula. *C* and *D,* Artist's conception and intraoperative photograph of a bifemorocaval PTFE graft with bilateral femoral arteriovenous fistula. *E,* Left femoral venogram at 6 months confirmed a patent graft. (From Gloviczki P, Pairolero PC, Cherry KJ, Hallett JW: Reconstruction of the vena cava and of its primary tributaries: A preliminary report. J Vasc Surg 11:373-381, 1990.)

Graft Surveillance

Intraoperative duplex scanning is now performed in most patients to ensure patency, good flow, and lack of thrombus deposition. Direct pressure measurements are made before wound closure in every patient with and without graft flow to document the hemodynamic benefit. In venous or polyester conduits, fistula flow can be measured and calibrated with an electromagnetic flowmeter. If flow is higher than 300 ml/min, banding of the fistula should be considered.

On the first postoperative day, we perform contrast phlebography through the catheter, which is positioned at the distal anastomosis of the graft (see Fig. 150–5). Any stenosis or thrombosis detected at this time is revised during a reoperation. Postoperatively, the grafts are observed with duplex scanning at 3 and at 6 months and then twice yearly afterward. Outflow plethysmography is also performed to document improvement. In symptomatic patients, however, contrast phlebography is usually performed to exclude graft stenosis.

INDICATIONS FOR SURGICAL TREATMENT

Failure of conservative management of symptomatic venous obstruction is a potential indication for endovascular or surgical treatment. The severity of venous stenosis, the

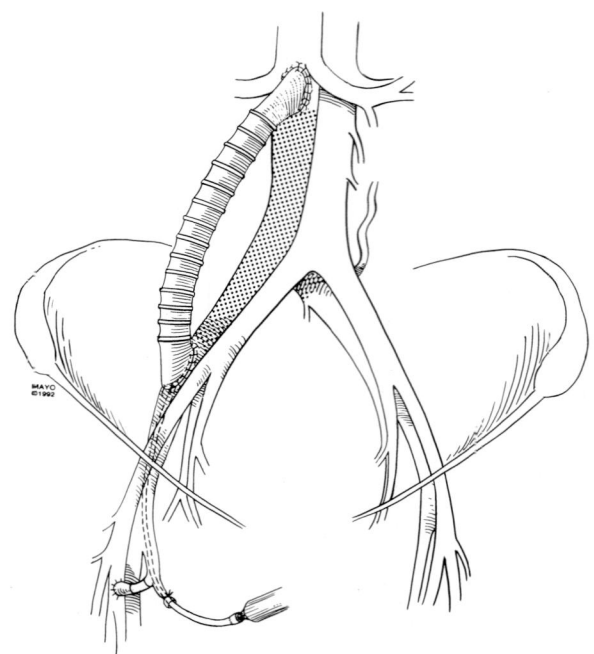

FIGURE 150–5. Illustration of a right iliac vein inferior vena caval externally supported polytetrafluoroethylene graft. Note the arteriovenous fistula at the right groin and a 20-gauge catheter, which is introduced through a tributary of the saphenous vein for perioperative heparin infusion. (From Gloviczki P, Pairolero PC, Toomey BJ, et al: Reconstruction of large veins for nonmalignant venous occlusive disease. J Vasc Surg 16:750–761, 1992. With permission of Mayo Foundation.)

location and length of venous occlusion, the age of the thrombus, the nature of any external compression (e.g., tumor, retroperitoneal fibrosis), any underlying malignant disease, and the risks of a surgical intervention all play a role in determining whether to continue nonoperative management or to attempt endovascular or direct surgical intervention. In recent years, short segmental stenosis of the proximal common iliac vein (*May-Thurner syndrome*) or of the retrohepatic vena cava has been treated more frequently with angioplasty and stenting. In our experience, however, multiple stent placements for long, chronic occlusions in the venous system seldom have had lasting results. In such cases, if the patients are low-risk surgical candidates, bypass is a better alternative.

Admittedly, a few series of successful stent placements for chronic venous disease with short-term follow-up have been published (see Chapter 151). Indications and results in patients with malignant tumors who undergo venous reconstructions are reviewed in Chapter 152.

SURGICAL PROCEDURES

Saphenopopliteal Bypass

First advocated by Warren and Thayer[2] in 1954 and reintroduced by Husni[49] and May[50] in the 1970s, saphenopopliteal bypass (*May-Husni operation*) has been designed for patients with occlusion of the superficial femoral or proximal popliteal veins.

Technique

In the original operation, the ipsilateral saphenous vein is used for conduit. A single distal anastomosis is performed, usually end-to-side, between the mobilized and divided saphenous vein and the distal popliteal vein, with standard atraumatic vascular surgical techniques and fine, 6-0 or 7-0 monofilament, nonabsorbable running sutures. A temporary arteriovenous fistula can be constructed at the ankle between the posterior tibial artery and one of the paired posterior tibial veins or even with the saphenous vein at the ankle, in an end-to-side fashion.[42, 51] An alternative to the traditional technique of saphenous vein transposition is a popliteofemoral or popliteosaphenous bypass (Figs. 150–6 and 150–7) with a free graft that uses either the ipsilateral or contralateral saphenous vein or an arm vein.

Results

The original May-Husni transposition is rarely performed now, and popliteofemoral bypasses are also uncommon. For nine reported series comprising 218 operated patients, functional improvement was reported in 77% of cases.[42, 51–58] In an earlier review of 59 operations, Smith and Trimble[59] reported clinical success in 76% of patients. With the exception of one series,[57] cumulative patency rates have not been reported. Crude patency rates at variable follow-up intervals ranged from 5% to 100%, but only four of the

TABLE 150–1. RESULTS OF SAPHENOPOPLITEAL BYPASS

FIRST AUTHOR	YEAR	NO. OF LIMBS	FOLLOW-UP (YEARS)	POSTOPERATIVE IMAGING (%)	PATENCY RATE (%)	CLINICAL IMPROVEMENT (%)
Frileux[52]	1972	22	1–3	32	71	N/A
Dale[53]	1979	6	N/A	83	50	50
Husni[54]	1983	27	1–11	N/A	63	76
Gruss[51]	1985	12	5–10	N/A	75	42
Dale[55]	1985	14	N/A	N/A	60	
O'Donnell[56]	1987	6	>3	100	100	100
AbuRahma[57]	1991	19	5.5	100	56 (7-year cumulative)	58
Danza[58]	1991	8	N/A	N/A	N/A	75
Gruss[42]	1991	14	Up to 19	N/A	78	50

N/A = not available.

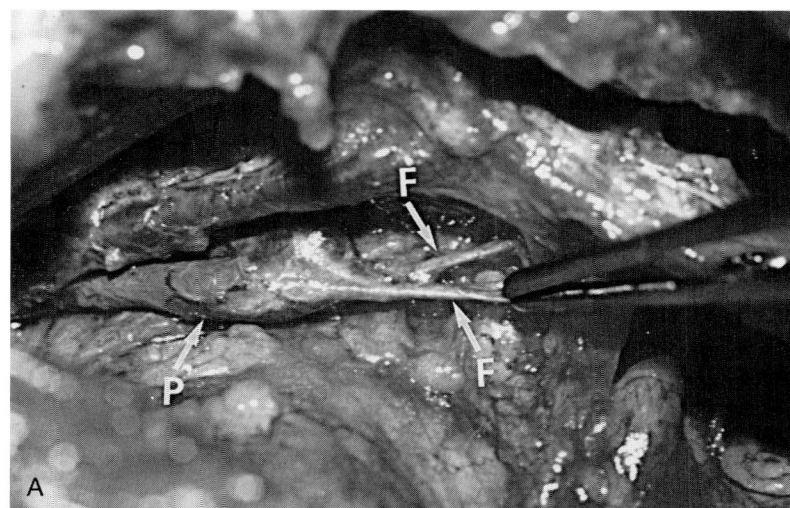

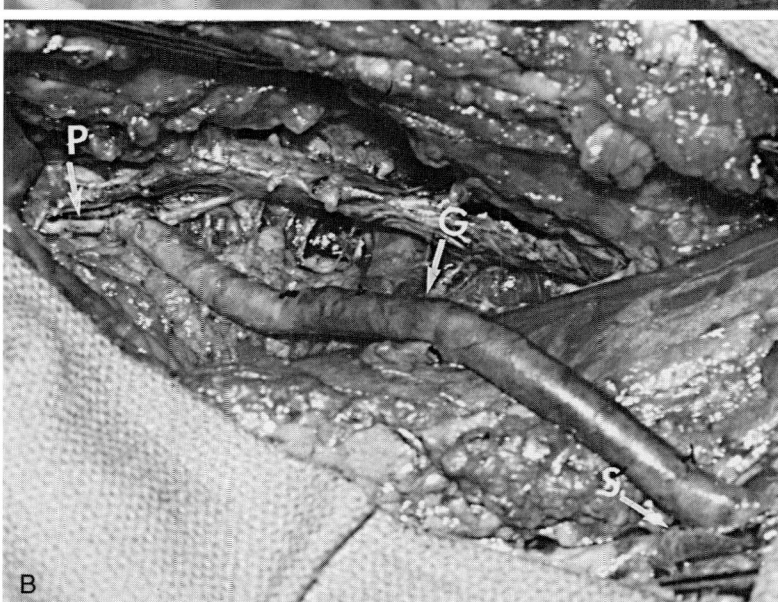

FIGURE 150–6. *A*, Klippel-Trenaunay syndrome with atresia of the right superficial femoral vein in a 20-year-old patients. P = popliteal vein; F = fibrous bands replacing the superficial femoral vein. *B*, Intraoperative photograph of the contralateral saphenous vein graft interposed between the patient's popliteal and proximal greater saphenous vein. P = popliteal vein; G = vein graft. S = greater saphenous vein. (From Gloviczki P, Stanson AW, Stickler GB, et al: Klippel-Trenaunay syndrome: The risks and benefits of vascular interventions. Surgery 110:469–479, 1991.)

nine studies reported on late imaging of the grafts to ascertain patency (Table 150–1).[42, 51–58]

Cross-Pubic Venous Bypass

Initially described 40 years ago by Palma and colleagues[60] in Uruguay and popularized by Dale[55, 61, 62] in the United States, the *Palma-Dale procedure* has remained a useful technique for venous reconstruction in patients with proximal outflow obstruction (Fig. 150–8). This operation, which was designed for patients with chronic unilateral iliac vein obstruction of any etiology, requires a normal contralateral iliofemoral venous system to ensure venous drainage. Results have been better in the presence of intact inflow, when the affected limb has no infrainguinal obstruction or deep venous incompetence.

We favor this operation especially in young women who present with residual chronic iliac vein occlusion following acute left iliofemoral venous thrombosis that developed as a result of May-Thurner syndrome.

Technique

For the original operation, the contralateral saphenous vein is used. Preoperative imaging of the potential graft conduit with phlebography or duplex scanning is recommended, because varicose saphenous veins or veins smaller than 4 mm in diameter have poor chance of long-term success.

Endoscopic harvesting of a 25- to 30-cm segment of the contralateral saphenous vein ensures excellent cosmetic result; otherwise, the vein can be dissected through two or three small skin incisions.

After ligation and division of all tributaries, the graft is gently distended (Fig. 150–9) with heparinized papaverine solution and is tunneled to the contralateral groin in a suprapubic, subcutaneous position. Dissection of the femoral vein on the affected side should be minimal; usually, just the anterior and lateral vein wall is freed up for proximal and distal clamps or for a side-biting clamp to occlude the femoral artery for the anastomosis. Excision of intraluminal fibrous bands following venotomy may be needed. The anastomosis between the saphenous and femoral veins

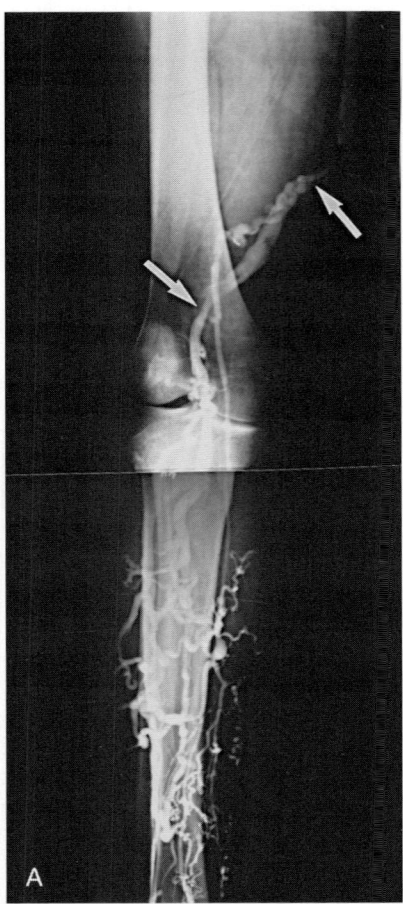

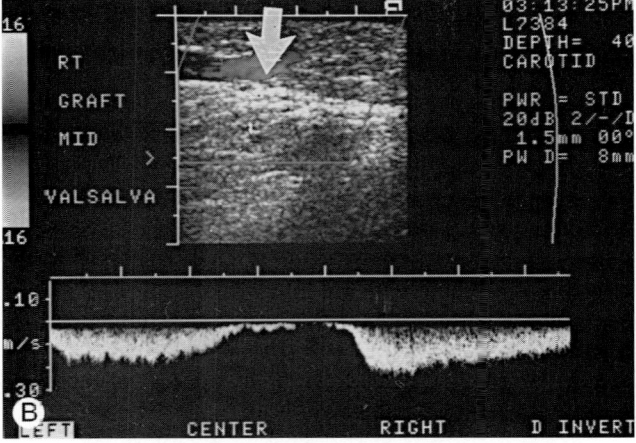

FIGURE 150–7. *A,* Venogram performed 5 months after popliteal saphenous vein interposition graft. *Arrow* indicates proximal and distal anastomoses of the patent graft. Note absence of the right superficial femoral vein. *B,* Duplex scan of the patent saphenous vein graft. *Arrow* indicates flow and Valsalva maneuver confirming competence of the valve in the vein graft. The vein has been patent and competent at 8 years, 6 months. (From Gloviczki P, Stanson AW, Stickler GB, et al: Klippel-Trenaunay syndrome: The risks and benefits of vascular interventions. Surgery 110:469–479, 1991.)

is performed in an end-to-side fashion with standard atraumatic vascular surgical technique. If the vein is small, interrupted 5-0 or 6-0 sutures are preferred to permit later dilatation of the vein and to avoid "pursestringing" of the

venous anastomosis. A small catheter can be placed through a tributary of the ipsilateral saphenous vein for immediate low-dose heparinization and postoperative phlebography (Fig. 150–10). A temporary arteriovenous fistula can also be placed to improve flow and to aid early patency.

If the traditional transposition results in significant kinking of the saphenous vein at the contralateral groin, free vein grafting should be considered. For autologous graft material, the contralateral or even the ipsilateral saphenous vein (with lysis of any competent valve) or an arm vein can be used.

Kistner[63] reported another ingenious idea for an autologous suprapubic graft. Through a retroperitoneal approach, the ipsilateral iliac vein is mobilized to the site of the occlusion. The internal iliac vein is ligated and divided to provide adequate length for the conduit. The common iliac vein is then divided and used for suprapubic subcutaneous transposition, with a single anastomosis performed between the iliac and the contralateral femoral veins.

When suitable autologous conduit is not available, an 8-mm, externally supported ePTFE graft is the best alternative.[64]

Results

Analysis of results of 412 operations published in nine series revealed clinical improvement in 63% to 89% of patients (Table 150–2).[21, 24, 42, 53, 54, 57, 60, 62, 65] Reported patency rates ranged between 70% and 85%, but follow-up periods were variable and objective graft assessment with imaging in all patients was rarely performed. The largest series, of 85 crossover venous bypasses, was reported by

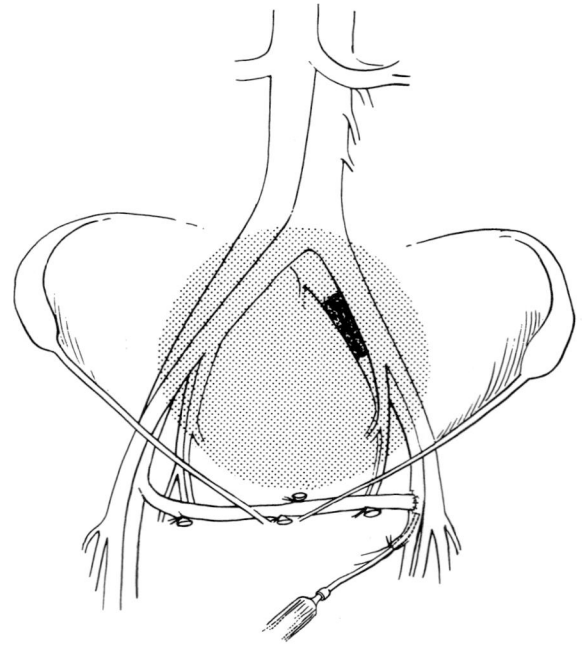

FIGURE 150–8. Left to right femorofemoral venous bypass (Palma procedure) for left common iliac vein obstruction. A small polyethylene catheter can be placed through a side branch of the greater saphenous vein for immediate perioperative heparinization to improve chances of patency. An arteriovenous fistula with saphenous vein is usually not necessary. (From Rhee RY, Gloviczki P, Luthra HS et al: Iliocaval complications of retroperitoneal fibrosis. Am J Surg 168:179–183, 1994.)

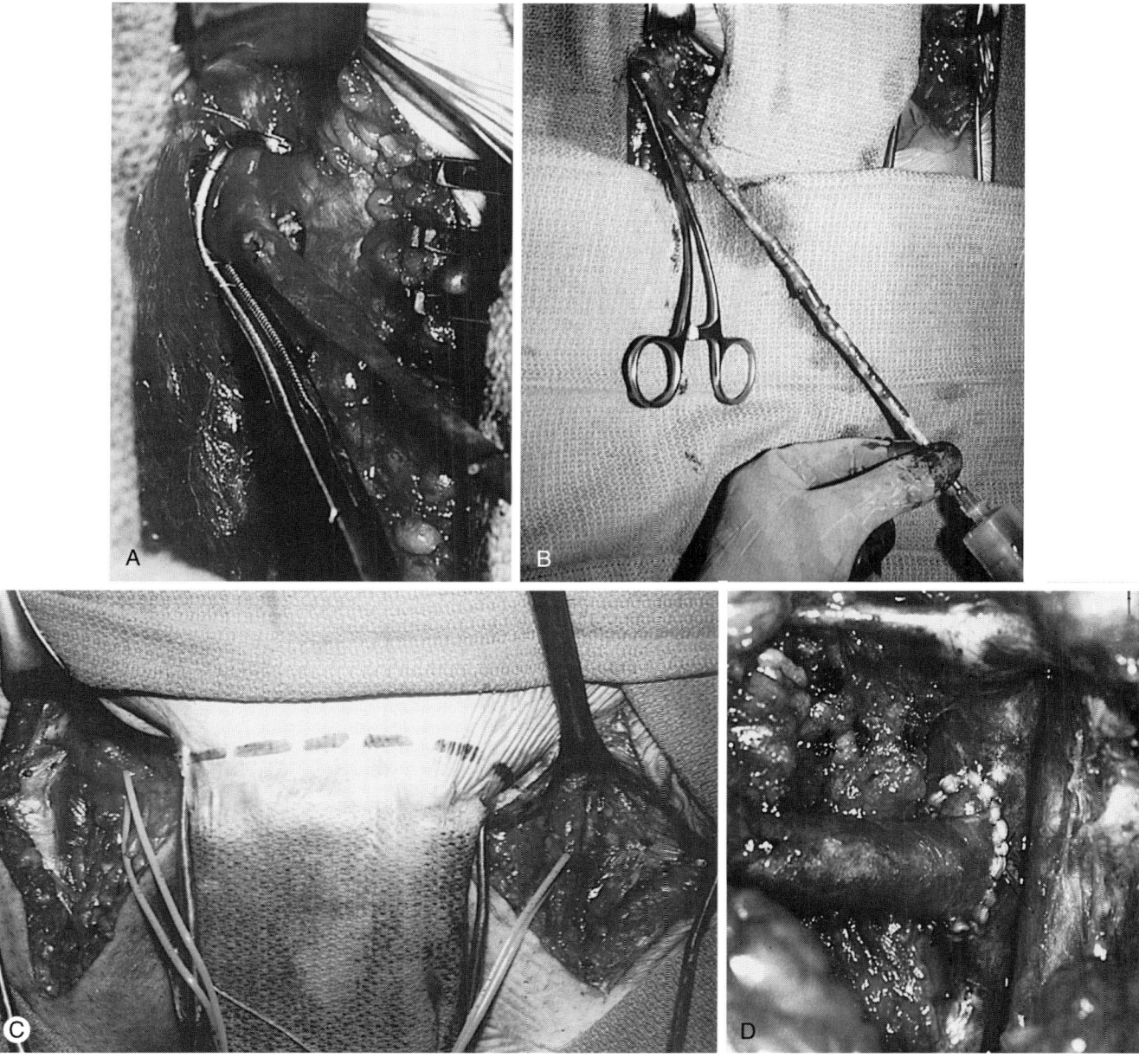

FIGURE 150–9. *A,* The contralateral saphenous vein is dissected, and a vascular clamp is placed on the common femoral vein. *B,* The vein is distended with papaverine solution. *C* and *D,* The saphenous vein is tunneled to the left groin and anastomosed end-to-side to the common femoral vein.

TABLE 150–2. RESULTS OF FEMORO-FEMORAL CROSSOVER BYPASS

FIRST AUTHOR	YEAR	NO. OF LIMBS	FOLLOW-UP (YEARS)	POSTOPERATIVE IMAGING (%)	PATENCY RATE (%)	CLINICAL IMPROVEMENT (%)	GRAFT MATERIAL
Palma[60]	1960	8	Up to 3	13	N/A	88	Vein
Dale[53]	1979	48	Up to 12	N/A	N/A	77	Vein
May[21]	1981	66	N/A	N/A	73	N/A	Vein
Dale[62]	1983	56	N/A	N/A	N/A	80	Veins
Husni[54]	1983	85	0.5–15	N/A	70	74	Vein (n = 83); PTFE (n = 2)
Halliday[65]	1985	47	Up to 18	72	75 (5-year cumulative)	89	Vein
Danza[58]	1991	27	N/A	N/A	N/A	81	Vein
AbuRahma[57]	1991	24	5.5	100	75 (7-year cumulative)	63	Vein
Gruss[24, 42]	1997	19	N/A	N/A	71	82 overall	Vein
		32	N/A	N/A	85		PTFE

N/A = not available.

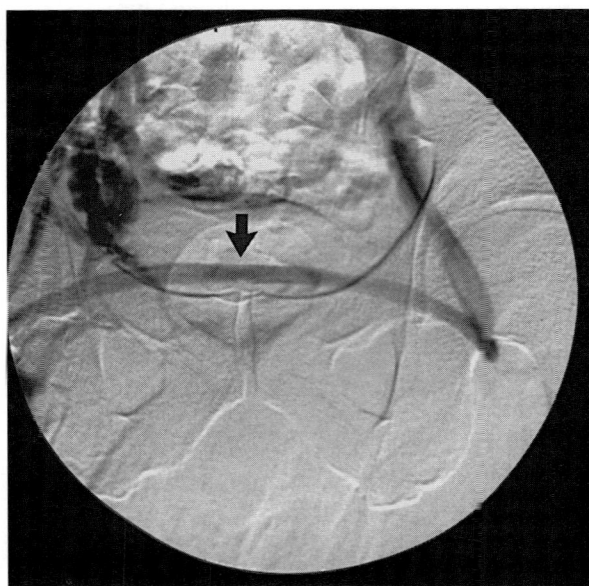

FIGURE 150–10. Postoperative venogram of a right to left femorofemoral crossover vein graft (*arrow*) (Palma procedure).

Husni.[54] At last follow-up visits, ranging from 6 months to 15 years after operation, 47 of 67 grafts were patent. Results in this study were better when a temporary distal arteriovenous fistula was used. Patency of grafts implanted for extrinsic compression of the iliac vein without distal disease was 100%, compared with 67% in patients with post-thrombotic syndrome.

In a review of 50 consecutive operations performed in 47 patients, Halliday and associates[65] reported a cumulative patency rate of 75% at 5 years confirmed by phlebography. Clinical improvement in this series was seen in 89% of patients. The cumulative patency rate in another series of 24 patients was 75% at 7 years, but the standard error in these calculations was high because of the low number of patients studied.

Danza and colleagues[58] noted better results with use of the saphenous vein as a free graft than with saphenous transposition. Gruss[24] and Gruss and Hiemer[42] reported good results for ePTFE grafts. Although the length of follow-up was not mentioned, long-term patency was noted in 22 of 26 grafts. On the basis of these results and that of others,[64] Gruss recommends using externally supported ePTFE grafts with arteriovenous fistula for all cross-femoral venous bypasses.[24]

Plethysmographic evidence of outflow obstruction was an independent predictor of clinical outcome in the report by AbuRahma and coworkers.[57] Eighty-eight per cent of their patients undergoing the Palma procedure who had abnormal preoperative maximum venous outflow showed significant clinical improvement, whereas 86% of those with normal preoperative maximum venous outflow had no improvement after operation.

Prosthetic Femorocaval, Iliocaval, or Inferior Vena Caval Bypass

Anatomic in-line iliac or iliocaval reconstruction can be performed for (1) unilateral disease when autologous conduit for suprapubic graft is not available or (2) bilateral iliac, iliocaval, or inferior vena caval occlusion. Extensive venous thrombosis, not infrequently following previous placement of a vena caval clip, tumors, and retroperitoneal fibrosis not responding to nonoperative therapy are potential indications. Failure of previous endovascular attempts and occlusion after placement of multiple stents have also been indications for bypass.

Technique

The femoral vessels (for the arteriovenous fistula or for the site of the distal anastomosis) are exposed at the groin through a vertical incision. The iliac vein or the distal segment of the IVC is exposed through a right oblique flank incision through the retroperitoneal approach. The vena cava at the level of the renal veins is best exposed through a midline or a right subcostal incision (see Fig. 150–4D). The ascending colon is mobilized medially, and the vena cava is exposed retroperitoneally. The infrarenal IVC is reconstructed with a 16- to 20-mm graft, the iliocaval segment usually with a 14-mm graft, and the femorovenacaval segment with a 10- or 12-mm PTFE graft. The arteriovenous fistula is constructed first in patients who undergo a long iliocaval bypass (see Fig. 150–5).

Short iliocaval bypass with significant pressure gradient can be performed without an arteriovenous fistula, as discussed previously. Reconstruction of the vena cava with a straight PTFE graft, if the inflow is good, is also usually performed without an additional arteriovenous fistula. In

TABLE 150–3. RESULTS OF FEMOROCAVAL/ILIOCAVAL BYPASS

FIRST AUTHOR	YEAR	NO. OF LIMBS	FOLLOW-UP (MONTHS)	IMAGING (%)	PATENCY RATE (%)	CLINICAL IMPROVEMENT (%)	GRAFT MATERIAL
Gloviczki[23]	1992	12	1–60	100	58	67	11 PTFE; 1 Dacron
Husfeldt[68]	1981	4	4–30	100	100	100	PTFE
Dale[41]	1984	3	1–30	100	100	100	PTFE
Alimi[40]	1997	8	mean: 19.5	100	88	88	PTFE
Sottiurai[67]	1998	45	11–139	100†	93*	89‡	PTFE

*Includes six femoroiliac, 26 femorofemoral, eight femorocaval, and five femorofemorocaval grafts.
†Postoperative duplex scan, followed by annual air plethysmography and selective venography.
‡An additional eight patients (18%) experienced recurrent ulcers during follow-up.
PTFE = polytetrafluoroethylene.

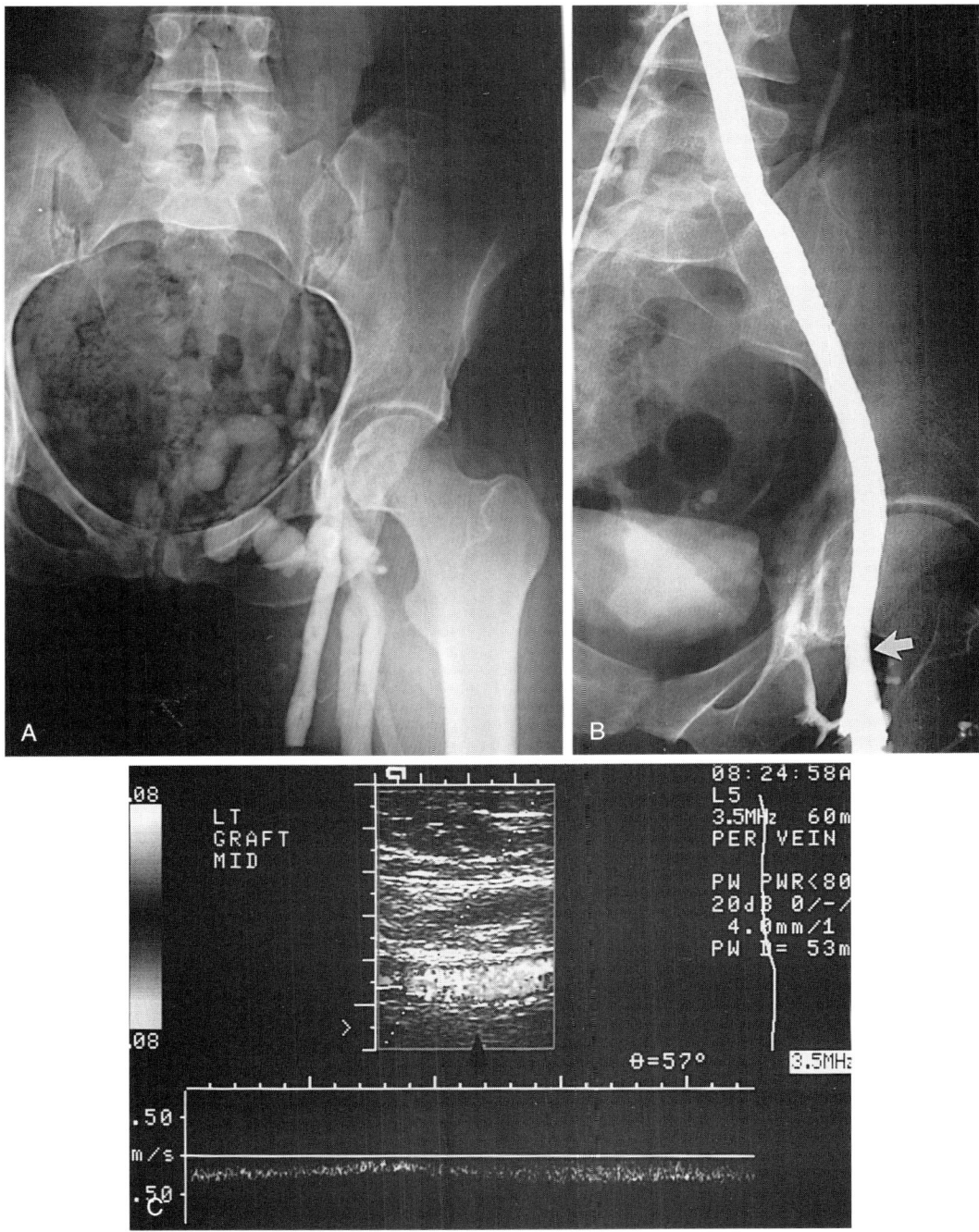

FIGURE 150-11. *A,* Preoperative venogram of left iliac vein thrombosis in a 36-year-old female patient. *B,* Venogram 1.6 years after implantation confirms widely patent 10 mm polytetrafluoroethylene graft. *Arrow* indicates site of the end-to-end femoral anastomosis. *C,* This patient is free of symptoms 10 years after the operation with duplex evidence (*arrow*) of graft patency.

patients who undergo femorocaval bypass, we perform the proximal and distal anastomoses of the bypass first and then place the arteriovenous fistula before opening up the circulation through the graft. As discussed previously, we usually use a tributary of the greater saphenous vein. The operation is performed with the patient in full anticoagulation with intravenous heparin, and at the end of the operation, as mentioned, a small polyethylene catheter is placed to the level of the distal anastomosis to infuse low-dose heparin (500 U/hour).

Results

Experience with femorocaval or iliovenacaval bypass is limited, and only a few series are available (Table 150-3). We reported on 12 such bypasses with a follow-up that extended up to 5 years after operation.[23] Seven grafts were patent at last follow-up, and six of the seven patients remained free of symptoms (Figs. 150-11 to 150-14). Improvement in the seventh patient was also documented.

Alimi and colleagues[40] reported results of eight iliac vein

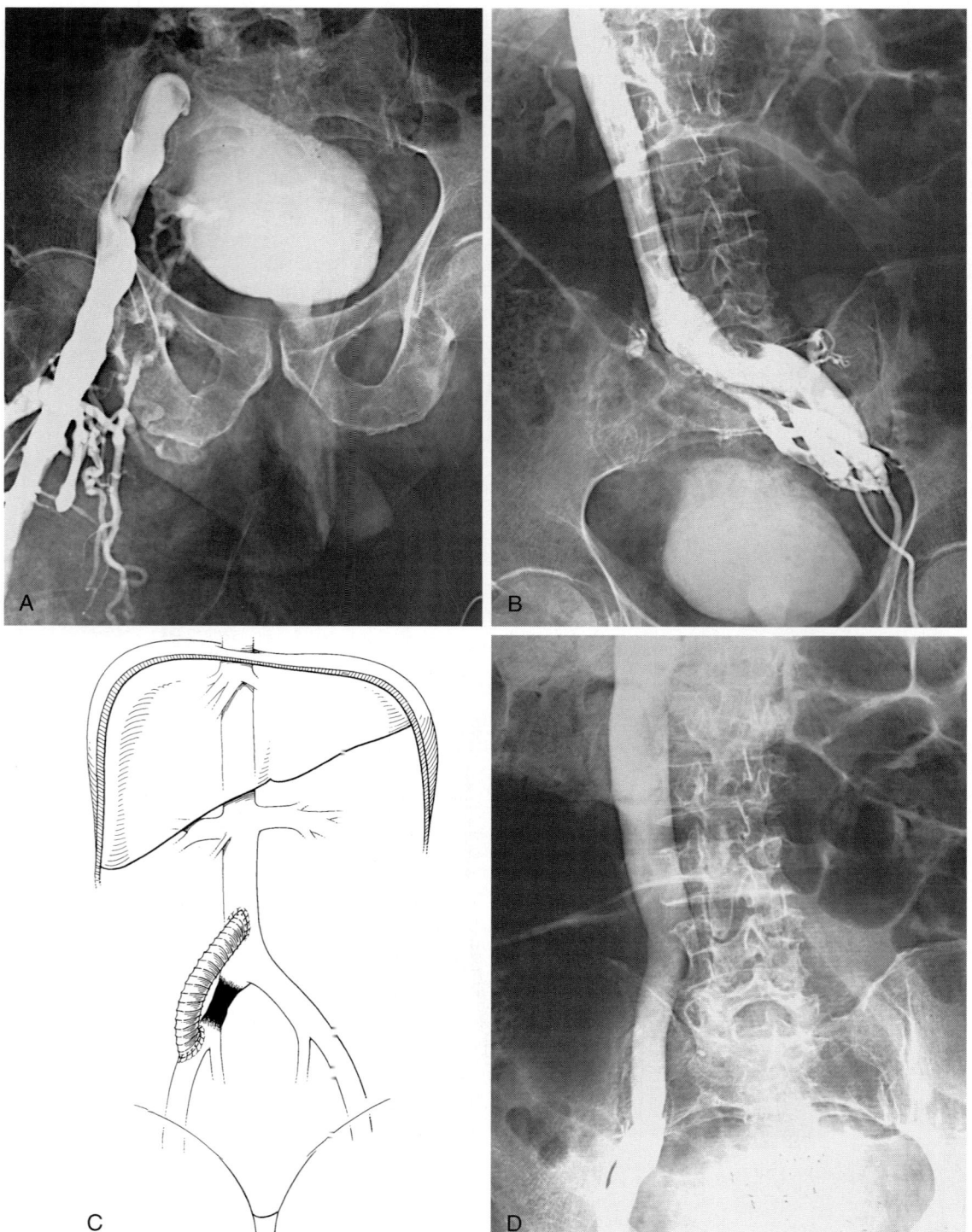

FIGURE 150–12. *A,* Preoperative venogram confirms occlusion of the right common iliac vein with a remarkable lack of collateral circulation. *B,* Left iliocavogram confirms normal anatomy. *C,* Illustration of a right external iliac inferior vena cava ringed polytetrafluoroethylene graft. *D,* Patent graft on venogram 3 months later.

reconstructions with femorocaval or iliocaval bypasses for both acute and chronic obstructions. In the four patients who had chronic obstruction, three grafts were patent at last follow-up. Eklof and associates[66] observed only one occlusion in five grafts followed for 14 to 22 months after operation, in which bypass was combined with venous

thrombectomy for acute deep venous thrombosis. Dale and associates[41] implanted the first iliovenacaval bifurcated PTFE graft in 1984, and our group reported on placement of a bifemorocaval bypass with bilateral arteriovenous fistulae in 1988.[22]

The largest experience with PTFE reconstruction of large

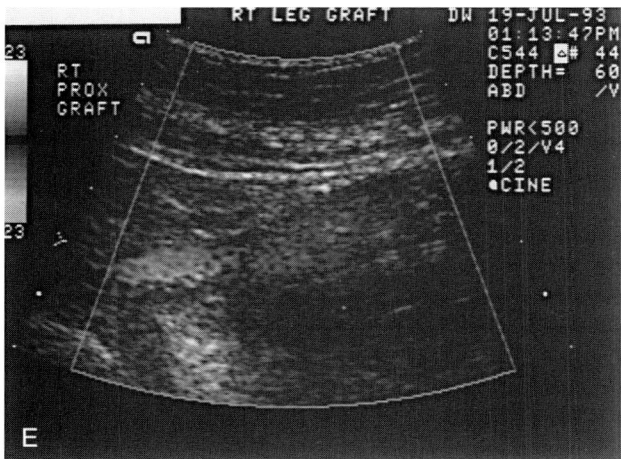

FIGURE 150–12 *Continued* E, Duplex scan documented graft patency at 4 years, 8 months after surgery.

veins was presented by Sottiurai and coworkers.[67] Fifty-two of 56 grafts (93%), including 13 femorovenacaval grafts and 26 femorofemoral grafts, which were used for a variety of central vein reconstructions, were reported to be patent at 1 year after implantation. Arteriovenous fistula in this study was constructed with a saphenous vein between the adjacent artery and the graft. The site of the fistula was at 2 cm proximal to the distal heel of the graft, where an ovoid 4 × 10 mm defect was cut in the graft wall to standardize flow through the fistula. Dale did not favor the use of an arteriovenous fistula with PTFE grafts[41, 53]; like Sottiurai and coworkers,[67] however, we believe that all femorocaval or longer iliocaval grafts require the benefit of a distal arteriovenous fistula to maintain patency. Our policy now is to keep the fistula patent as long as possible.[47]

Iliac Vein Decompression

Compression of the left iliac vein between the right common iliac artery (see Fig. 150–1) and the fifth lumbar vertebra was described first by McMurrich[69] in 1908 and later in much more detail in a large autopsy study by May and Thurner, who also recognized the clinical implications of the iliac "spurs" leading to acute deep vein thrombosis.[11, 70] Cockett and associates[12] coined the term "iliac vein compression syndrome" in 1965 and called attention to the obstructive symptoms in affected patients, who are often seen without clinical signs of previous deep venous thrombosis. *May-Thurner (Cockett) syndrome* is observed more frequently in females between the second and fourth decades of life.[4, 12–14] Left leg swelling, venous claudication, pain, and chronic stasis skin changes, including rare ulceration, may develop.

An acute complication is left iliofemoral deep venous thrombosis. Although a literature review[64] found fewer than 100 reported cases, the true incidence of this condition, leading to left iliofemoral venous thrombosis, is most likely higher. Some surgeons suggest repair of any lesion discovered,[72] but we advocate reconstruction only for symptomatic patients, including those who already had an episode of acute deep venous thrombosis due to this condition. Endovascular techniques with stenting (see Chapter 151) should be considered as an alternative, although late results for such treatment are not available.

Technique

In patients with chronic obstructive symptoms (swelling, venous claudication), our first choice has been to decompress the venous system with a Palma-Dale procedure. In patients with stenosis or short iliac occlusion, direct explora-

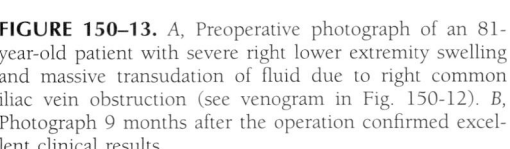

FIGURE 150–13. *A,* Preoperative photograph of an 81-year-old patient with severe right lower extremity swelling and massive transudation of fluid due to right common iliac vein obstruction (see venogram in Fig. 150-12). *B,* Photograph 9 months after the operation confirmed excellent clinical results.

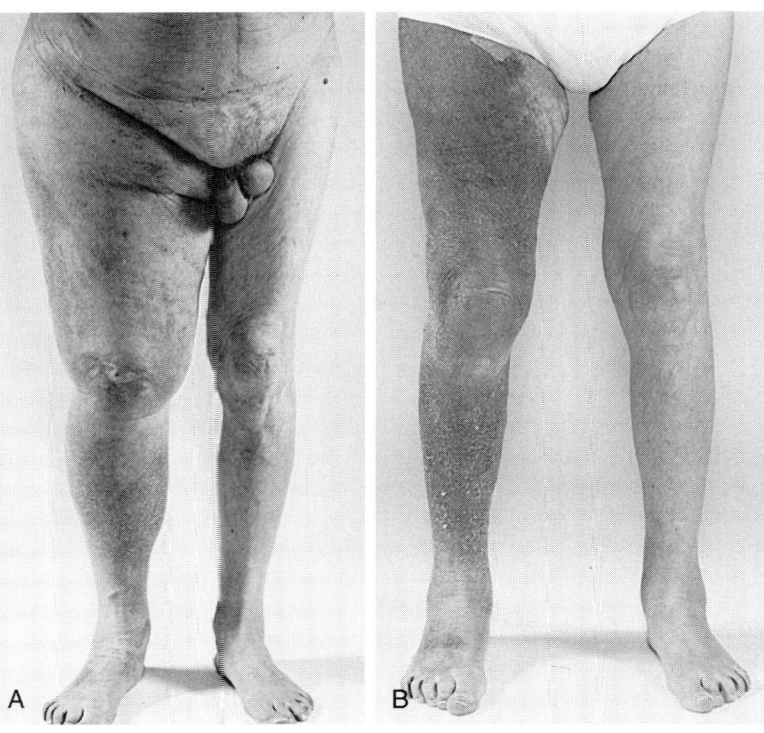

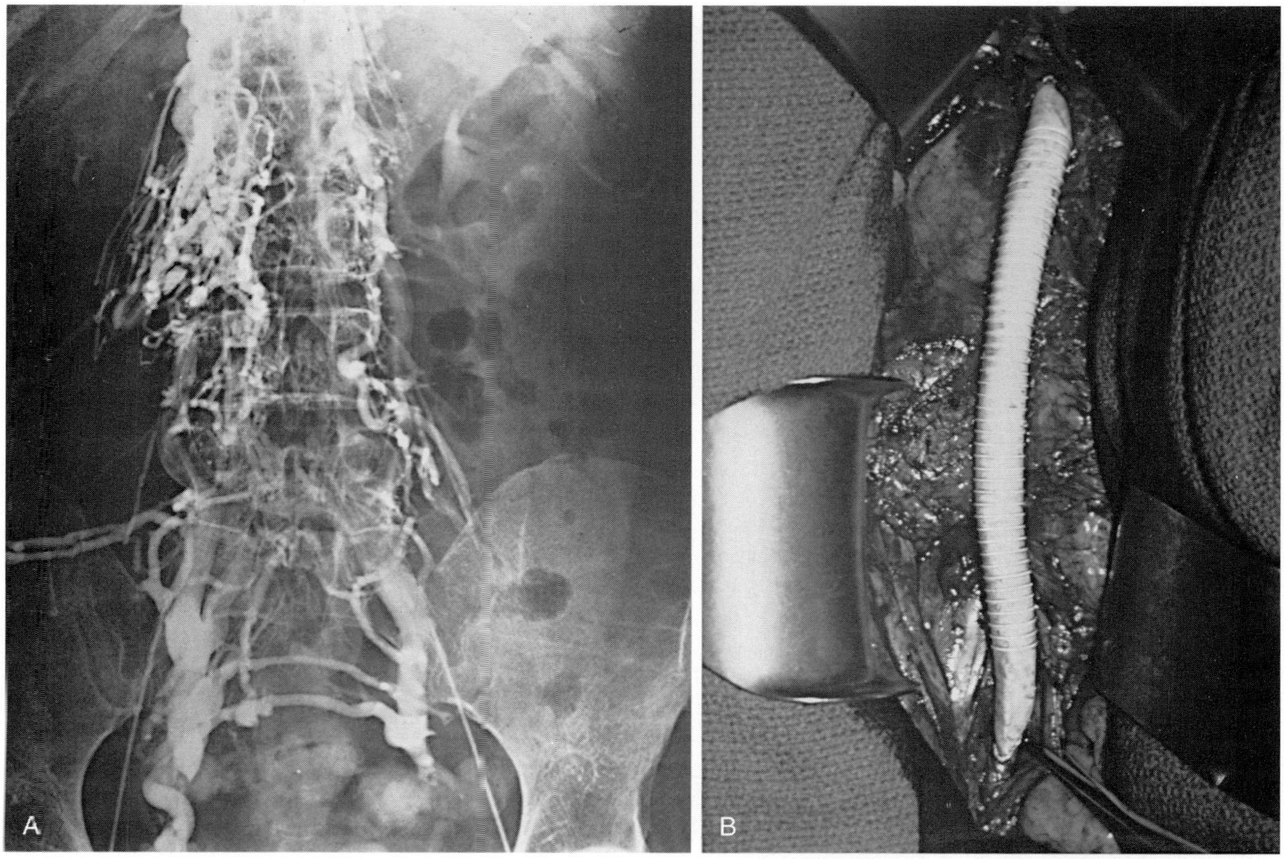

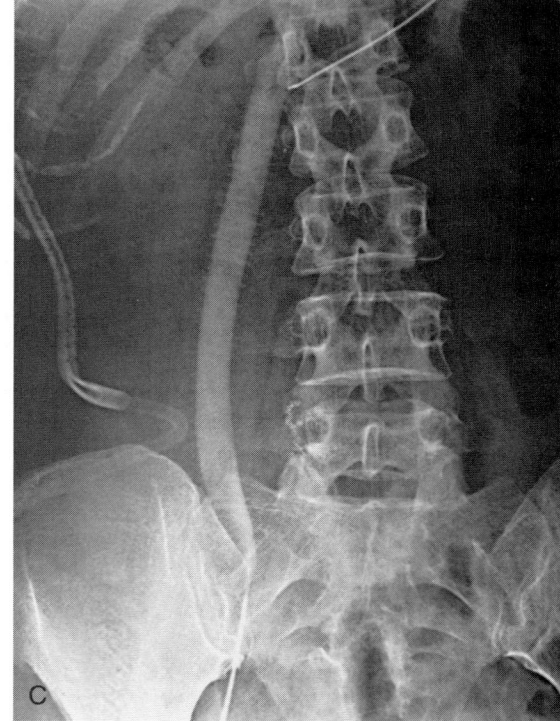

FIGURE 150–14. *A* and *B*, Extensive iliocaval obstruction in a 47-year-old patient treated with right iliocaval bypass with a right saphenous vein common femoral artery arteriovenous fistula. *C*, Postoperative venogram shows patent graft. The graft was patent at 3 years, 4 months after surgery.

tion of the vena caval bifurcation has been recommended, with the use of a variety of techniques to release the iliac venous obstruction. The iliac vein is fully mobilized, and any external compressing band is transected. Excision of any intraluminal web and vein or PTFE patch angioplasty may have to be performed; other surgeons recommend transposition of the iliac artery behind the iliac vein.[6, 71–73] Cormier[73] suggested transposition of the right common iliac into the left internal iliac artery to decompress the left common iliac vein.

Results

Lalka[64] analyzed results of iliac vein decompression operations in detail, although lack of larger series in the literature and the use of a multitude of techniques make evaluation of these procedures difficult. It is likely that failed attempts at repair were not reported. In their review, Akers and colleagues[71] found that of 80 reported patients undergoing iliac vein decompression, 65 (85%) had significant improvement postoperatively.

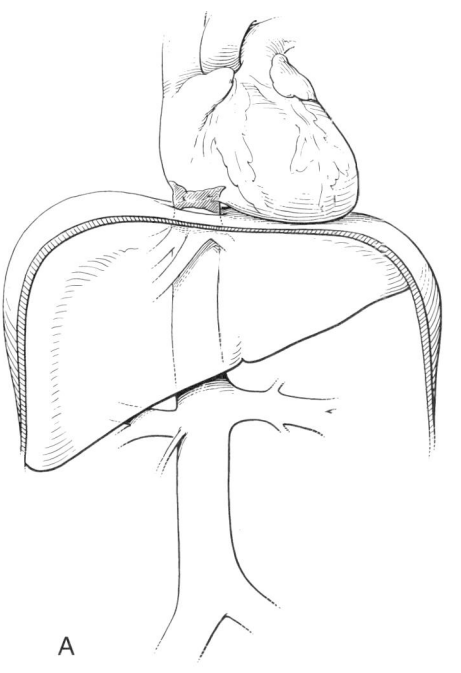

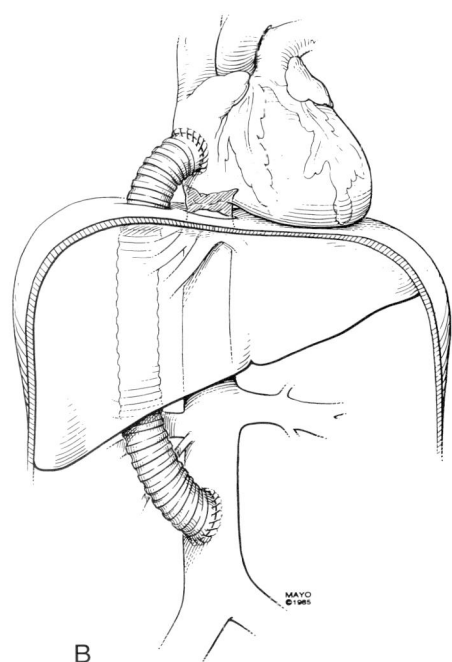

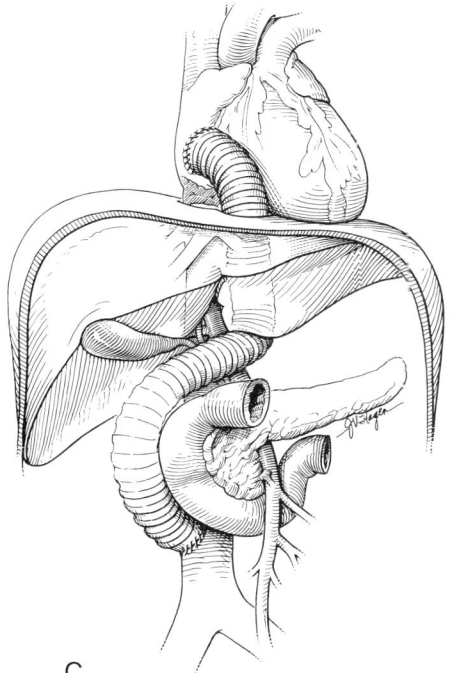

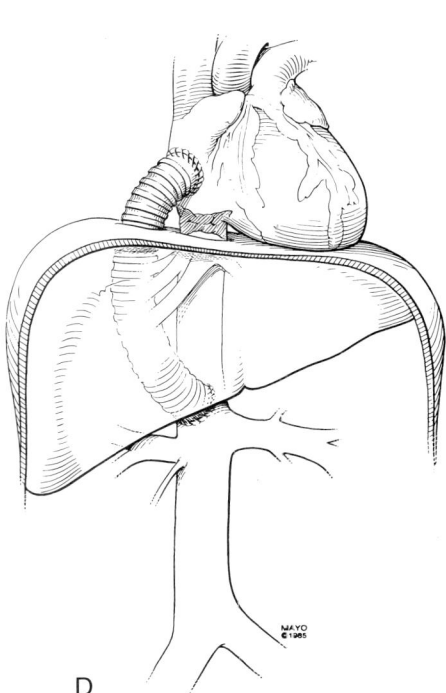

FIGURE 150–15. Different configurations of cavoatrial bypass performed for membranous occlusion (A) of the inferior vena cava. Reinforced polytetrafluoroethylene graft can originate from the infrarenal (B) or suprarenal (D), inferior vena cava and routed behind the right lobe of the liver. Another potential position of the graft is behind the left lobe of the liver (C). (With permission of Mayo Foundation.)

Suprarenal Inferior Vena Caval Reconstruction

The most common reason to reconstruct the suprarenal IVC for benign disease is membranous occlusion of the IVC, which is frequently associated with occlusion of the hepatic veins (Budd-Chiari syndrome), subsequent portal hypertension, and liver failure. Occlusion of the suprahepatic IVC usually does not cause significant congestion of lower extremity veins, although leg edema and venous claudication may still develop in affected patients. Although attempts to reconstruct the IVC with autologous grafts using spiral vein graft or superficial femoral vein have been reported, most surgeons agree that externally supported PTFE graft is the best option for vena caval or cavoatrial bypass. If percutaneous transluminal balloon angioplasty, stenting, or transatrial dilatation of the membranous occlusion has not been successful, and portosystemic shunting is not required, venacavoatrial bypass is an effective technique to decompress the IVC.

Technique

The retrohepatic segment of the vena cava and the right atrium are exposed through a right anterolateral thoracotomy, with extension of the incision across the costal arch so that the peritoneal cavity is entered through the diaphragm.[39] The liver is retracted anteriorly, and the paravertebral gutter is exposed together with the suprarenal segment of the IVC. The pericardium is opened anterior to the right phrenic nerve, and the right atrium is isolated. The IVC is cross-clamped with a partial-occlusion clamp above the renal vein, and a 16- or 18-mm, externally supported PTFE graft is sutured end-to-side to the IVC with running 5-0 or 6-0 Prolene sutures. The graft is then passed parallel to the IVC up to the right atrium or the suprahepatic IVC. The central anastomosis is performed after placement of a partial-occlusion clamp on the vena cava or the right atrium. Before completion of the anastomosis, air is carefully flushed from the graft to avoid air embolization.

An anterior approach was suggested by Kieffer and associates,[45] who performed segmental replacement of the suprahepatic IVC by a short ringed PTFE graft (Fig. 150–15). Tunneling of a long cavoatrial graft in front of the liver or under the left lobe was also reported.

Results

Wang and colleagues[15] reported on 100 patients with Budd-Chiari syndrome, 12 of whom underwent cavoatrial bypasses. Clinical improvement with patent graft was noted in 10 patients at a median follow-up period of 1.5 years after surgery. In their experience, Kieffer and associates[45] observed only one occlusion in grafts placed for membranous occlusion of the vena cava. In another series, Victor and colleagues[74] reported patent grafts at 21 months to 6 years after the operation in five patients.

Three cavoatrial grafts placed for nonmalignant disease were reported by our group: The patient with the PTFE graft was asymptomatic at 10 years, the long Dacron graft

became occluded at 3 years, and the spiral vein graft underwent occlusion within 1 year. Chapter 152 details the reconstruction of the vena cava for malignant disease, including the need for partial bypass.

SUMMARY

The number of operations performed for chronic venous occlusion is still small. Because the experience of vascular surgeons with venous reconstruction is limited, caution in patient selection is most important. Indications for such operations should be obvious, and occlusion, not valvular incompetence, must be the main cause of advanced, symptomatic CVI in surgical candidates for reconstruction.

Utmost attention to technical details during the operation, selection of an appropriate graft, careful preoperative thrombosis prophylaxis, and close follow-up are mandatory. Progress in endovascular surgery will require careful analysis of results to determine appropriate procedures for patients with chronic venous occlusion. More experience is clearly needed, but current results indicate that venous reconstructive surgery for chronic occlusion has become an effective tool in the treatment of carefully selected patients with advanced chronic venous disease.

REFERENCES

1. Raju S: Venous insufficiency of the lower limb and stasis ulceration: Changing concepts and management. Ann Surg 197:688, 1983.
2. Warren R, Thayer TR: Transplantation of the saphenous vein for postphlebitic stasis. Surgery 35:867, 1954.
3. Bergan JJ, Yao JS, Flinn WR, McCarthy WJ: Surgical treatment of venous obstruction and insufficiency (Review). J Vasc Surg 3:174, 1986.
4. Rhee RY, Gloviczki P, Luthra HS, et al: Iliocaval complications of retroperitoneal fibrosis. Am J Surg 168:179, 1994.
5. Dzsinich C, Gloviczki P, van Heerden JA, et al: Primary venous leiomyosarcoma: A rare but lethal disease. J Vasc Surg 15:595, 1992.
6. Bower TC, Nagorney DM, Toomey BJ, et al: Vena cava replacement for malignant disease: Is there a role? Ann Vasc Surg 7:51, 1993.
7. Bower TC: Primary and secondary tumors of the inferior vena cava. In Gloviczki P, Yao JST (eds): Handbook of Venous Disorders: Guidelines of the American Venous Forum. London, Chapman & Hall, 1996, pp 529–550.
8. Rich NM, Hughes CW: Popliteal artery and vein entrapment. Am J Surg 113:696, 1967.
9. Servelle M, Babilliot J: Syndrome du soléaire. Phlebologie 21:399, 1968.
10. Gullmo A: The strain obstruction syndrome of the femoral vein. Acta Radiol 47:119, 1957.
11. May R, Thurner J: Ein Gefäßsporn in der Vena iliaca communis sinistra als Ursache der ubegend linksseitigen Beckenvenenthrombosen. Ztsch Kreislaufforschung 45:912, 1956.
12. Cockett FB, Thomas ML: The iliac compression syndrome. Br J Surg 52:816, 1965.
13. David M, Striffling V, Brenot R, et al: Syndrome de Cockett acquis: À propos de trois cas opérés dont deux forés inhabituelles. Ann Chir 35:93, 1981.
14. Steinberg JB, Jacocks MA: May-Thurner syndrome: A previously unreported variant. Ann Vasc Surg 7:577, 1993.
15. Wang Z, Zhu Y, Wang S, et al: Recognition and management of Budd-Chiari syndrome: Report of one hundred cases. J Vasc Surg 10:149, 1989.
16. Gloviczki P, Stanson AW, Stickler GB, et al: Klippel-Trenaunay syn-

drome: The risks and benefits of vascular interventions. Surgery 110:469, 1991.

17. Jacob AG, Driscoll DJ, Shaughnessy WJ, et al: Klippel-Trenaunay syndrome: Spectrum and management. Mayo Clin Proc 73:28, 1998.

18. Schanzer H, Skladany M: Complex venous reconstruction for chronic iliofemoral vein obstruction. Cardiovasc Surg 4:837, 1996.

19. Raju S: New approaches to the diagnosis and treatment of venous obstruction. J Vasc Surg 4:42, 1986.

20. Negus D, Cockett FB: Femoral vein pressures in post-phlebitic iliac vein obstruction. Br J Surg 54:522, 1967.

21. May R: The Palma operation with Gottlob's endothelium preserving suture. In May R, Weber J (eds): Pelvic and Abdominal Veins: Progress in Diagnostics and Therapy. Amsterdam, Excerpta Medica. 1981, pp 192–197.

22. Gloviczki P, Pairolero PC, Cherry KJ, Hallett JW: Reconstruction of the vena cava and of its primary tributaries: A preliminary report. J Vasc Surg 11:373, 1990.

23. Gloviczki P, Pairolero PC, Toomey BJ, et al: Reconstruction of large veins for nonmalignant venous occlusive disease. J Vasc Surg 16:750, 1992.

24. Gruss JD: Venous bypass for chronic venous insufficiency. In Bergan JJ, Yao JST (eds): Venous Disorders. Philadelphia, WB Saunders, 1991, pp 316–330.

25. Yamaguchi A, Eguchi S, Iwasaki T, Asano K: The influence of arteriovenous fistulae on the patency of synthetic inferior vena caval grafts. J Cardiovasc Surg 9:99, 1968.

26. Soyer T, Lempinen M, Cooper P, et al: A new venous prosthesis. Surgery 72:864, 1972.

27. Chiu CJ, Terzis J, Mac Rae ML: Replacement of superior vena cava with the spiral composite vein graft. Ann Thorac Surg 17:555, 1974.

28. Wilson SE, Jabour A, Stone RT, Stanley TM: Patency of biologic prosthetic inferior vena cava grafts with distal limb fistula. Arch Surg 113:1174, 1978.

29. Hobson RW 2nd, Wright CB: Peripheral side to side arteriovenous fistula. Am J Surg 126:411, 1978.

30. Kunlin K, Kunlin A: Experimental venous surgery. In May R (ed): Surgery of the Veins of the Leg and Pelvis. Philadelphia, WB Saunders, 1979, pp 37–75.

31. Hutschenreiter S, Vollmar J, Loeprecht H, et al: Reconstructive interventions of the venous system: Clinical evaluation of late results using functional and vascular anatomic criteria. Chirurgica 50:555, 1979.

32. Fiore AC, Brown JW, Cromartie RS, et al: Prosthetic replacement for the thoracic vena cava. J Thorac Surg 84:560, 1982.

33. Gloviczki P, Hollier LH, Dewanjee MK, et al: Experimental replacement of the inferior vena cava: Factors affecting patency. Surgery 95:657, 1984.

34. Plate G, Hollier LH, Gloviczki P, et al: Overcoming failure of venous vascular prostheses. Surg 96:503, 1984.

35. Chan EL, Bardin JA, Bernstein EF: Inferior vena cava bypass: Experimental evaluation of externally supported grafts and initial clinical application. J Vasc Surg 95:657, 1984.

36. Robison RJ, Peigh PS, Fiore AC, et al: Venous prostheses: Improved patency with external stents. J Surg Res 36:306, 1984.

37. Koveker GB, Burkel WE, Graham LM, et al: Endothelial cell seeding of expanded polytetrafluoroethylene vena cava conduits: Effects of luminal production of prostacyclin, platelet adherence, and fibrinogen accumulation. J Vasc Surg 7:600, 1988.

38. Burkhart HM, Fath SW, Dalsing MC, et al: Experimental repair of venous valvular insufficiency using a cryopreserved venous valve allograft aided by a distal arteriovenous fistula. J Vasc Surg 26:817, 1997.

39. Gloviczki P, Pairolero PC: Venous reconstruction for obstruction and valvular incompetence. Perspect Vasc Surg 1:75, 1988.

40. Alimi YS, DiMauro P, Fabre D, Juhan C: Iliac vein reconstructions to treat acute and chronic venous occlusive disease. J Vasc Surg 25:673, 1997.

41. Dale WA, Harris J, Terry RB: Polytetrafluoroethylene reconstruction of the inferior vena cava. Surgery 95:625, 1984.

42. Gruss JD, Hiemer W: Bypass procedures for venous obstruction: Palma and May-Husmi bypasses, Raju perforator bypass, prosthetic bypasses, and primary and adjunctive arteriovenous fistulae. In Raju S, Villavicencio JL (eds): Surgical Management of Venous Disease. Baltimore, Williams & Wilkins, 1997, pp 289–305.

43. Gloviczki P, Berens E: Vena cava syndrome. In Raju S, Villavicencio JL

(eds): Surgical Management of Venous Disease. Baltimore, Williams & Wilkins, 1997, 397–420.

44. Gloviczki P, Pairolero PC: Prosthetic replacement of large veins. In Bergan JJ, Kistner RL (eds): Atlas of Venous Surgery. Philadelphia, WB Saunders, 1992, pp 191–214.

45. Kieffer E, Bahnini A, Koskas F: Nonthrombotic disease of the inferior vena cava: Surgical management of 24 patients. In Bergan JJ, Yao JST (eds): Venous Disorders. Philadelphia, WB Saunders, 1991, pp 501–516.

46. Lalka SG: Venous bypass graft for chronic venous occlusive disease. In Gloviczki P, Yao JST (eds): Handbook of Venous Disorders. London, Chapman & Hall, 1996, pp 446–470.

47. Menawat SS, Gloviczki P, Mozes G, et al: Effect of a femoral arteriovenous fistula on lower extremity venous hemodynamics after femorocaval reconstruction. J Vasc Surg 24:793, 1996.

48. Hobson RW 2nd, Lee BC, Lynch TG, et al: Use of intermittent pneumatic compression of the calf in femoral venous reconstruction. Surg Gynecol Obstet 159:284, 1984.

49. Husni EA: Clinical experience with femoropopliteal venous reconstruction. In Bergan JJ, Yao JST (eds): Venous Problems. Chicago, Year Book Medical Publishers, 1978, pp 485–491.

50. May R: Der Femoralisbypass beim Postthrombotischen Zustandsbild. Vasa 1:267, 1972.

51. Gruss JD: The saphenopopliteal bypass for chronic venous insufficiency (May-Husni operation). In Bergan JJ, Yao JST (eds): Surgery of the Veins. Orlando, Fla, Grune & Stratton, 1985, pp 255–265.

52. Frileux C, Pillot-Bienayme P, Gillot C: Bypass of segmental obliterations of ilio-femoral venous axis by transposition of saphenous vein. J Cardiovasc Surg 13:409, 1972.

53. Dale WA: Reconstructive venous surgery. Arch Surg 114:1312, 1979.

54. Husni EA: Reconstruction of veins: The need for objectivity. J Cardiovasc Surg 24:525, 1983.

55. Dale WA: Peripheral venous reconstruction. In Dale WA (ed): Management of Vascular Surgical Problems. New York, McGraw-Hill, 1985, pp 493–521.

56. O'Donnell TF, Mackey WC, Shepard AD, Callow AD: Clinical, hemodynamic and anatomic follow-up of direct venous reconstruction. Arch Surg 122:474, 1987.

57. AbuRahma AF, Robinson PA, Boland JP: Clinical hemodynamic and anatomic predictors of long-term outcome of lower extremity venous bypasses. J Vasc Surg 14:635, 1991.

58. Danza R, Navarro T, Baldizan J: Reconstructive surgery in chronic venous obstruction of the lower limbs. J Cardiovasc Surg 32:98, 1991.

59. Smith DE, Trimble C: Surgical management of obstructive venous disease of the lower extremity. In Rutherford RB (ed): Vascular Surgery. Philadelphia, WB Saunders, 1977, pp 1247–1268.

60. Palma EC, Esperon R: Vein transplants and grafts in the surgical treatment of the postphlebitic syndrome. J Cardiovasc Surg 1:94, 1960.

61. Dale WA, Harris J: Cross-over vein grafts for iliac and femoral venous occlusion. J Cardiovasc Surg 10:458, 1969.

62. Dale WA: Crossover vein grafts for iliac and femoral venous occlusion. Resident Staff Physician March:58, 1983.

63. Kistner RL: Autogenous iliofemoral bypass. In Bergan JJ, Kistner RL (eds): Atlas of Venous Surgery. Philadelphia, WB Saunders, 1992, pp 187–190.

64. Lalka SG: Management of chronic obstructive venous disease of the lower extremity. In Rutherford RB (ed): Vascular Surgery. Philadelphia, WB Saunders, 1995, pp1862–1882.

65. Halliday P, Harris J, May J: Femoro-femoral crossover grafts (Palma operation): A long-term follow-up study. In Bergan JJ, Yao JST (eds): Surgery of the Veins. Orlando, Fla, Grune & Stratton, 1985, pp 241–254.

66. Eklof B, Broome A, Einarsson E: Venous reconstruction in acute iliac vein obstruction using PTFE grafts. In May R, Weber J (eds): Pelvic and Abdominal Veins. Amsterdam, Excerpta Medica, 1981, pp 259–264.

67. Sottiurai VS, Gonzales J, Cooper M, et al: A new concept of arteriovenous fistula in venous bypass requiring no fistula interruption: Surgical technique and long-term results. Ann Vasc Surg (in press).

68. Husfeldt KJ: Venous replacement with Gore-Tex prosthesis: Experimental and first clinical results. In May R, Weber J (eds): Pelvic and Abdominal Veins: Progress in Diagnostics and Therapy. Amsterdam, Excerpta Medica, 1981, pp 249–253.

69. McMurrich JP: The occurrence of congenital adhesions in the common iliac veins and their relation to thrombosis of the femoral and iliac veins. Am J Med Sci 135:342, 1908.
70. May R, Thurner S: The cause of the predominantly sinistral occurrence of thrombosis of the pelvic veins. Angiology 8:419, 1957.
71. Akers DL Jr, Creado B, Hewitt RL: Iliac vein compression syndrome: Case report and review of the literature. J Vasc Surg 35:477, 1996.
72. Taheri SA, Williams J, Powell S, et al: Iliocaval compression syndrome. Am J Surg 154:169, 1987.
73. Cormier JM: Transposition de l'artère iliaque primitive sur l'hypogastrique controlatérale. Nouv Presse Med 9:2015, 1980.
74. Victor S, Jayanthi V, Kandasamy I, et al: Retrohepatic cavoatrial bypass for coarctation of inferior vena cava with a polytetrafluoroethylene graft. J Thorac Cardiovasc Surg 91:99, 1986.

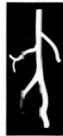

CHAPTER 151
Endovascular Treatment of Chronic Occlusions of Large Veins

Robert P. Liddell, M.S., and Michael D. Dake, M.D.

Chronic occlusions of the superior vena cava (SVC) and inferior vena cava (IVC) form a heterogeneous group of vascular lesions, of various causes, and prognosis.[1-4] As outlined in the preceding chapters, there have been a number of modern developments in the medical and surgical management of venous disease. Simultaneous advances in radiographic imaging and catheter-based interventional procedures now offer clinicians safe, less invasive, and effective treatment alternatives to traditional therapy for these diseases. The purpose of this chapter is to outline recent advances in the fields of thrombolysis, percutaneous transluminal angioplasty (PTA), and endoluminal stenting, focusing on their applications in the treatment of chronic large vein occlusions.

Traditionally, the treatments of choice for vena caval obstruction included external-beam radiation, chemotherapy, systemic anticoagulation, and systemic thrombolytic therapy. Success rates for these procedures have generally been disappointing.[5-7] Also, a number of different operative approaches have been presented in the surgical literature. Surgical bypass, an invasive approach, has usually been reserved for relief of symptoms caused by diseases other than neoplastic ones.[7-10] In many series, short-term patency rates for surgical bypass have have been better than those for medical management alone[6, 11]; however, symptoms of caval obstruction recur in a large proportion of patients.[8, 12]

The goal of endovascular interventions is to provide a safe, noninvasive approach to the management of acute and chronic venous occlusions. Endovascular techniques have been used for palliation of symptoms of venous obstruction associated with malignant neoplasm for a number of years.[13, 14] Recently, however, primary venous angioplasty and stenting have been performed with increasing frequency for benign venous occlusive disease, and in institutions where caval occlusions are treated principally with surgical bypass, endovascular techniques have been used to salvage failing vena cava grafts.[15, 16]

INDICATIONS FOR INTERVENTION

Endovascular interventions are indicated for patients whose symptoms have not resolved after either a standard course of anticoagulation or surgical bypass and who have persistent symptoms consistent with chronic SVC or IVC occlusion. The decision to exclude a patient from endovascular intervention is based primarily on contraindications to anticoagulation or fibrinolytic therapy.

The treatment of caval occlusions secondary to benign processes remains a serious challenge for endoluminal therapies, as patients often outlive their repairs. In patients with a known malignancy, the clinician must weigh the patient's quality of life against the potential complications of the procedure. The patient must understand that the endovascular procedure will not treat the underlying malignancy and is merely palliative.

INTERVENTIONAL STRATEGIES

The four primary strategies for endovascular interventions in the SVC and IVC systems are venography, thrombolysis, angioplasty, and endoluminal stenting or stent-grafting. For both chronic SVC and IVC occlusions, a combination of these techniques is used to restore and maintain good drainage into the right atrium. The interventions listed earlier can be performed entirely in the angiographic suite under sterile conditions.

Superior Vena Cava

Occlusion of the superior vena cava and of associated central veins of the thorax can produce a wide range of clinical findings which, collectively, are referred to as supe-

rior vena cava syndrome. SVC syndrome (see Chapter 153) consists of facial, periorbital, neck, and bilateral upper extremity edema, dilated superficial veins over the anterior and lateral chest wall, dysphagia, dyspnea, and cognitive dysfunction secondary to cerebral venous hypertension. Rarely is SVC syndrome alone a life-threatening emergency; however, the quality of life for many of these patients is poor owing to limited use of their arms, inability to lie flat (due to venous congestion), and severe facial edema.[1, 2]

The clinical syndrome is caused by compression or complete obstruction of the SVC plus altered venous return from the head, neck, and upper extremities. The severity of the SVC syndrome depends on how fast occlusion develops and the associated pattern of collateral vessels. The more acute the occlusion and the more limited the development of collateral vessels, the more severe are the symptoms. SVC syndrome has both benign and malignant causes (Table 151–1). Before the advent of antibiotic therapy, a large percentage of cases of SVC syndrome were caused by pathogens. Today, malignant disease accounts for 85% to 97% of all cases, but, as the number of central venous catheters placed for long-term access continues to rise, non-neoplastic causes will increase proportionetely.[2]

Patients suffering from SVC syndrome should undergo complete diagnostic evaluation to rule out malignancy, including a detailed history and physical examination, chest radiography, and thoracic computed tomography (CT). Chest radiographs reveal malignant intrathoracic processes in 85% of patients with SVC syndrome. Two-thirds of these lesions are situated in the right upper lobe near the SVC, and a right-sided pleural effusion is present in about a quarter of patients.[3, 4] Venography is not usually part of the initial evaluation but typically is reserved for patients who will undergo some form of endovascular intervention. In our experience, patients who have recently been found to have radiosensitive tumors are usually treated immediately with radiation, chemotherapy, or both. Prompt therapy with these modalities often relieves the symptoms of SVC syndrome. Consequently, patients do not usually require endovascular intervention acutely. Patients with a malignancy who have been treated with radiation, chemotherapy, or surgery can present several months later with SVC syndrome secondary to radiation-induced fibrosis of central veins.

Venography and Catheterization of Superior Vena Cava Occlusion

Venography is still considered the "gold standard" for diagnosis and localization of occlusive disease in the SVC. With the patient lying supine or semi-recumbent, and to the

TABLE 151–1. ETIOLOGY OF SUPERIOR VENA CAVAL OBSTRUCTION

Benign	Malignant
Central venous catheters	Bronchogenic carcinoma
Radiation fibrosis	Mediastinal tumors
Mediastinal fibrosis	Lymphoma
Pacemaker leads	Thyroid carcinoma
Dialysis fistula–related stenosis	Metastatic disease
Substernal thyroid goiter	

extent it is clinically tolerated, bilateral access is obtained through both the right and left basilic veins. When there is an SVC occlusion with extension of acute thrombus into both brachiocephalic veins, each subclavian vein must be traversed with catheters and wires advanced into the SVC and right atrium. To gain access to a chronically occluded SVC involved by fibrosis the right femoral or right internal jugular approach may be necessary to provide for a better mechanical advantage. If the patient has a dialysis fistula, access may be gained through direct puncture of the fistula. Once venipuncture has been performed, simultaneous bilateral upper extremity venography is performed to document the extent and degree of stenosis or occlusion (Fig. 151–1).

In patients with upper extremity edema, venipuncture of the basilic vein may prove very difficult. Standard tourniquet techniques are often unsuccessful, since the basilic vein lies well below the the skin surface. One technique involves cannulating a small hand vein and performing venography to map the basilic vein in the antecubital region with an arm tourniquet in place. The contrast medium–infiltrated basilic vein is then punctured under direct fluoroscopic guidance. A second popular method involves ultrasound-guided needle puncture of the basilic vein using a 5- or 7-MHz transducer with an arm tourniquet in place.

Once vascular access has been achieved in both arms, the basilic venipuncture sites are converted to 5 French (Fr.) or 6 Fr. angiographic side-arm sheaths. Attempts are then made to pass a 5. Fr. angiographic catheter with a simple curve (Berenstein Glidecatheter, Boston Scientific, Watertown, Mass.) and a 0.035-inch steerable hydrophilic guide wire (Glidewire, Boston Scientific) through the occluded vein segment. For more organized fibrotic occlusions, extra stiffness may be needed to avoid buckling of the catheter when it encounters resistance. In this situation, we would convert to a coaxial system consisting of a 7 or 8 Fr. braided coronary guiding catheter fitted with a Touhy-Borst adapter to allow placement of the 5 Fr. catheter and guide wire. The guiding catheter provides a better mechanical advantage and reduces the tendency of the 5 Fr. catheter to recoil. Once the lesion has been successfully traversed, pressure measurements can be recorded to inform future therapy.

Catheter-Directed Venous Thrombolytic Therapy

Catheter-directed thrombolytic therapy in the setting of SVC syndrome was first described in a 1974 report of a patient whose acute thrombosis was caused by a pacemaker lead.[17] Since then, a number of studies have documented the efficacy and safety of central venous thrombolysis, with and without supplemental PTA and endoluminal stenting.[15, 18–22] The goal of catheter-directed thrombolysis in the acute setting is clear: to "lyse" the fresh thrombus, relieve the venous congestion, and restore venous return to the right atrium. Adjunctive PTA or stent placement should then be considered to treat the underlying lesion. In a chronically occluded SVC that is impenetrable by standard guide wire and catheter techniques, catheter-directed thrombolysis often serves to soften or partially recanalize the thrombus, to eventually allow a guide wire to cross the lesion. Once the

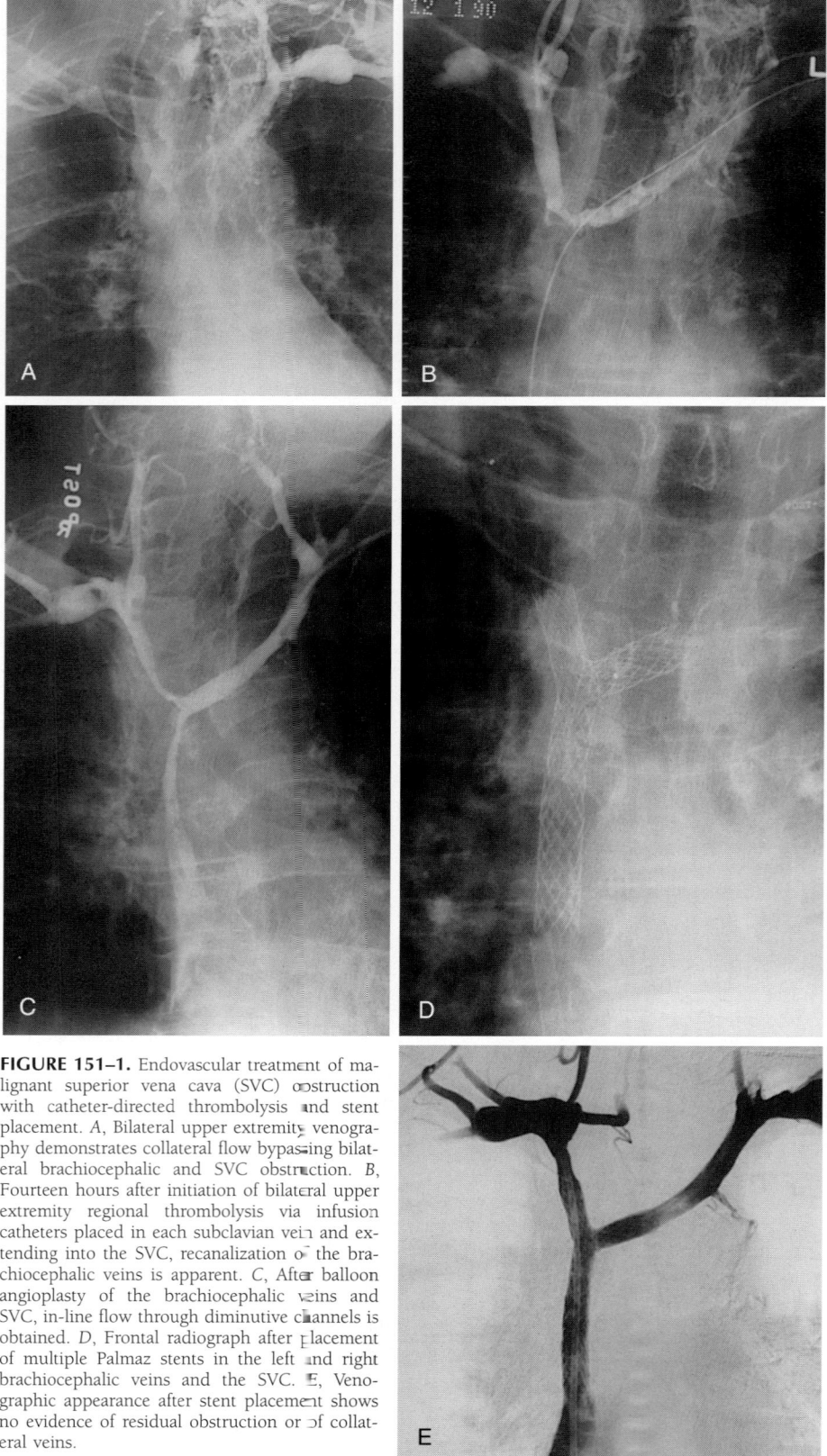

FIGURE 151–1. Endovascular treatment of malignant superior vena cava (SVC) obstruction with catheter-directed thrombolysis and stent placement. *A,* Bilateral upper extremity venography demonstrates collateral flow bypassing bilateral brachiocephalic and SVC obstruction. *B,* Fourteen hours after initiation of bilateral upper extremity regional thrombolysis via infusion catheters placed in each subclavian vein and extending into the SVC, recanalization of the brachiocephalic veins is apparent. *C,* After balloon angioplasty of the brachiocephalic veins and SVC, in-line flow through diminutive channels is obtained. *D,* Frontal radiograph after placement of multiple Palmaz stents in the left and right brachiocephalic veins and the SVC. *E,* Venographic appearance after stent placement shows no evidence of residual obstruction or of collateral veins.

guide wire has safely traversed the obstruction, again, PTA and stenting can dilate the occluded segment. Although many patients derive substantial benefit from thrombolysis alone, only a minority enjoy complete relief of symptoms.[15]

Locally delivered catheter-directed thrombolytic therapy has a number of distinct advantages over systemic lytic therapy for treatment of chronic occlusions. Catheter-directed thrombolysis ensures that the thrombolytic agent is delivered directly to the site of occlusion, in higher concentration and to a larger surface area of the thrombus, than a systemic peripheral can deliver. This more efficient delivery technique may be particularly benificial for patients with large clot burdens involving long venous segments and may be particularly important in terms of limiting the length of the vein that requires endoluminal stenting. In contrast, a systemically administered thrombolytic agent is directed away from occluded venous segments by collateral channels and, consequently, is less efficient and more likely to produce complications.[23] Finally, catheter-directed thrombolysis generally requires a smaller total dose of thrombolytic agent and takes less time as compared with systemic thrombolysis.[23, 24]

Two major thrombolytic delivery systems are currently available: the coaxial multicomponent system and the multiple side-hole single-catheter system. The coaxial system is the simplest to use and is easy to manage. With this system, the occlusion is first crossed with an 0.035-inch Glidewire and a 5 Fr. angiographic catheter, as described earlier. Once the end-hole catheter is safely through the occluded segment of vein, the Glidewire is exchanged for a specially designed 0.035-inch thrombolytic guide wire. The thrombolytic guide wires are designed to "weep" or drip urokinase (1) through an end hole (Sos wire; USCI, Billerica, Mass.; Cragg wire; Medi-Iech) or (2) along the distal few centimeters of the wire (Katzen infusion wire; Medi-Tech). The thrombolytic infusion wire is advanced out through the end of the 5-Fr. catheter and then secured using a Touhy-Borst adapter. From the basilic approach, the catheter is gently pulled back to the leading edge of the thrombus and the guide wire is placed approximately two thirds of the way into the thrombosed arterial segment.

The multiple side-hole catheter system consists of either a 5 Fr. catheter (Mewissen catheter, Medi-Tech, or Pulse Spray catheter, AngioDynamics, Queensbury, N.Y.) or a multilumen catheter (EDM catheter, Mallinckrodt). An occlusion wire prevents the urokinase from leaking out through the end hole and instead forces it through a number of side holes in the multiple side-hole catheter. The multilumen catheter has two ports. One drips urokinase through the guide wire end hole, and the other infuses four separate lumina that feed multiple side holes. The 4.8 Fr. multilumen catheter allows simultaneous infusion of heparin through the sidearm of a 5 Fr. angiographic sheath.

The safety and efficacy of urokinase (Abbokinase; Abbott Laboratories, Chicago) when used in both arterial and venous systems, has been reported.[24-26] Urokinase is available in 250,000 IU vials and requires reconstitution with using 10 ml of sterile water. The maximum recommended dose of urokinase is 4,400 IU/kg/hr. For catheter-directed thrombolysis, urokinase doses range from 150,000 to 200,00 IU/hr.

A tumor-induced hypercoagulable state is not uncommon in patients undergoing palliative SVC reconstruction who have underlying malignant disease.[27] Once the urokinase infusion is started, a bolus of 5000 units of heparin is given an infused initially at 1000 units/hr. Subsequently, they take antiplatelet prophylaxis, including 325 mg of aspirin daily, for at least 6 months. In an effort to reduce the length of hospital stay during the transition from intravenous anticoagulation with heparin to oral warfarin, a loading dose of 10 mg of warfarin is administered on the first 2 days of the endovascular procedure. Subsequently, daily doses are titrated and International Normalized Ratio (INR) levels are followed on an outpatient basis with the target INR between 2.0 and 3.0.

Thrombolysis in most cases of chronic disease is performed for 24 to 48 hours, and follow-up venography daily. The thrombolytic infusion is discontinued before the 48-hour, point if follow-up venography demonstrates no residual thrombus, if a complication related to regional thrombolysis occurs, or if the fibrinogen level falls below 100 mg/dl (1.0 g/L). During a regional urokinase infusion, both partial thromboplastin time (PTT) and fibrinogen level are checked every 6 hours. PTT is maintained between 60 and 90 seconds, and fibrinogen levels are kept above 100 mg/dl. Fibrinogen levels below 100 mg/dl indicate a systemic fibrinolytic state and are associated with increased the risk of hemorrhagic complications. Thrombolytic therapy is contraindicated for patients who have bleeding disorders or metastatic cancer that involves brain or spinal cord, those who have had a hemorrhagic stroke, and pregnant women.

Venous Angioplasty and Stenting

The role of PTA in the treatment of chronic central venous stenoses and occlusions has changed dramatically as endoluminal stenting has come into widespread use. Early studies reported encouraging technical results, owing but to the extensive recoil of diseased veins, PTA without stent placement has generally proved ineffective.[28-33] PTA is now principally used to recanalize occluded veins before stenting. Endoluminal stenting, unlike PTA alone, prevents elastic recoil and has greatly increased the long-term patency of venous endovascular therapy (see Fig. 151–1).[15, 34, 35]

In the SVC, the advisability of stent placement depends on (1) whether disease in the vein is focal or diffuse; (2) whether the cause of the obstruction is benign or malignant; (3) the venous anatomy; and (4) the personal preference of the clinician. In general, "long-segment venous disease" and lesions that include the brachiocephalic veins tend not to respond well to balloon dilation alone and almost inevitably require stenting. Patients with SVC occlusion secondary to cancer tend to experience dramatic and rapid relief of symptoms (e.g., facial edema, dyspnea, cognitive function, upper limb swelling) after stent placement, results that can significantly improve their quality of life.[36, 37] Patients with benign disease, on the other hand, may require close monitoring and subsequent interventions, since they often survive long after their primary endovascular procedure. Secondary patency rates reported in this patient population have ranged between 25% and 85%.[15, 22]

Reports of large clinical series document recent experience with three endoluminal stents used for central venous reconstruction: the Palmaz stent (Johnson & Johnson Interventional Systems), the Wallstent (Schneider), and the Gianturco Z-stent (Cook). Because all three have their advantages and disadvantages, the choice of which one to use is very subjective and inevitably based on the individual patient's clinical condition and venous anatomy and on the interventionalist's experience and biases.

The Palmaz stent has been described in a number of studies as being effective in treating vena caval and central venous stenoses.[15, 38, 39] Palmaz stents are balloon-expandable, rigid, stainless steel cylinders. The Principal advantages of the Palmaz design are its superior hoop strength, accuracy of placement, and limited foreshortening (Fig. 151-2). The main disadvantage is its susceptibility to plastic deformation from extrinsic compression by surrounding structures, including tumors.[40] Palmaz stents come in a variety of lengths, ranging from 10 to 78 mm, and some can be dilated to 17 mm. In the SVC these stents are usually deployed from the right femoral vein with a very long sheath (9 or 10 Fr.).

Earlier reports of the Wallstent applied to treatment of SVC obstruction cited mixed results.[40, 41] The Wallstent is a longitudinally flexible, self-expanding, metal stent. The principal advantages of Wallstents are their relatively low delivery profile, their flexibility, and the capability they afford of treating longer lesions with a single stent unit. For diameters smaller than 14 mm, the stent is mounted on a 7 or 8 Fr. delivery catheter. The catheter makes it easy to introduce from the basilic vein, and, because of its flexibility, it passes more easily through the curved innominate and subclavian veins. It is available in lengths up to 90 mm and in diameters of 5 to 24 mm, features that make it appropriate for treating long segments of diseased vein. In addition, the fine-braid pattern of the stent and its large metallic surface area limit the size of the interstices, a feature that may prevent tumor ingrowth. The Wallstent is designed to foreshorten as it is deployed the lumen of the vessel. Consequently, in certain anatomic areas, precise placement is difficult. In response to this limitation, the manufacturer recently designed a deployment system that allows the operator to safely reconstrain and then reposition the stent before it is finally deployed. Other arguable disadvantages of the Wallstent are its relatively low radial force, which is more apparent in larger-diameter stents, and its relatively large total metallic surface area as compared with other stents', features that make it relatively thrombogenic in the low–flow velocity venous system.

The Gianturco Z-stent was the first commercially available stent to be used by a number of centers to treat SVC syndrome.[12, 42, 43] Since the early reports, a large-volume of data have documented the safety and efficacy of the device.[13, 14, 37, 44, 45] It is a relatively rigid, self-expanding stent. Among its advantages, the Z-stent comes in a wide variety of diameters (8 to 40 mm), possesses good hoop strength, and does not foreshorten during deployment. In addition, its small surface area, large interstices, and low thrombogenicity allow it to be placed across feeding veins. The small surface area and open design of the Z-stent, however, may allow tumor infiltration. The constrained stent is delivered into the appropriate delivery sheath by a blunt-tipped mandrel that is used as a pusher to advance the device to the target. The stent is deployed by fixing the pusher and withdrawing the sheath. Accurate deployment of this particular stent is not difficult; however, as it is currently designed, it cannot be repositioned.

Our experience suggests that stenting of short segmental occlusions offers better and longer-lasting relief of symptoms than extensive stenting of diffuse disease. We prefer to use Wallstents for the treatment of brachiocephalic vein stenosis and use Palmaz stents in the SVC. *Acute* complications of stent deployment in the venous system (i.e., those that develop within 30 days) include stent migration, extrinsic compression, and thrombosis.[46–51] Long-term complications are related principally to stent patency and to development of intimal hyperplasia, thrombus deposition, and progression of the underlying pathophysiologic process.[52]

Stent migration can result from incomplete expansion of the stent or improper positioning. Most migration complications occur at the junction of the SVC with the right atrium, a point where there is an abrupt increase in transverse diameter and where stents that are not seated high enough in the SVC may develop emboli. The dislodged stent may become entangled in the trabecula of the right ventricle, damage the tricuspid valve, or embolize to the pulmonary arteries. Stents that remain in the right ventricle or pulmonary artery for any length of time may eventually become covered with fibrous tissue and endothelialized and, so, impossible to remove percutaneously.[48, 49] In light of this fact, and depending on the patient's clinical condition, an immediate decision must be made to either leave the stent or retrieve it and deploy it in the intended site or in a "safe" area such as the infrarenal IVC or the common iliac vein. Balloons, baskets, loop snares, and a variety of endovascular techniques have been used successfully to retrieve migrated stents.[53, 54]

Balloon-expandable stents such as the Palmaz are susceptible to plastic deformation when external, two-point compression is applied. This phenomenon has been observed in the subclavian vein, where stents may be subjected to compression by external forces applied to the vein as it runs over the first rib, typically from the scalenus and subclavius muscles.[50, 51] Theoretically, both self-expanding and balloon-expandable stents may be compressed by tumor that encases the SVC, a sequela that results in either stenosis or occlusion of the SVC with the development of SVC syndrome. If the problem is caught early enough, redilation or restenting of these lesions often produces very good secondary patency.

Stent in the venous system carry the risk for thrombosis because of the foreign body surface area and the low flow velocity of venous blood. After stent placement, patients continue treatment with intravenous heparin while they are "transitioning" warfarin therapy. Anticoagulant therapy is adjusted to maintain an INR of 2.0 to 2.5. Patients with an underlying malignancy receive oral anticoagulation as long as this is clinically feasible. For patients with benign disease, anticoagulation is discontinued at 6-month follow-up if clinical patency has been maintained.[15, 46]

Stent-Grafts

The use of stent-grafts for the treatment of aneurysmal disease is well documented.[55] There are, however, case

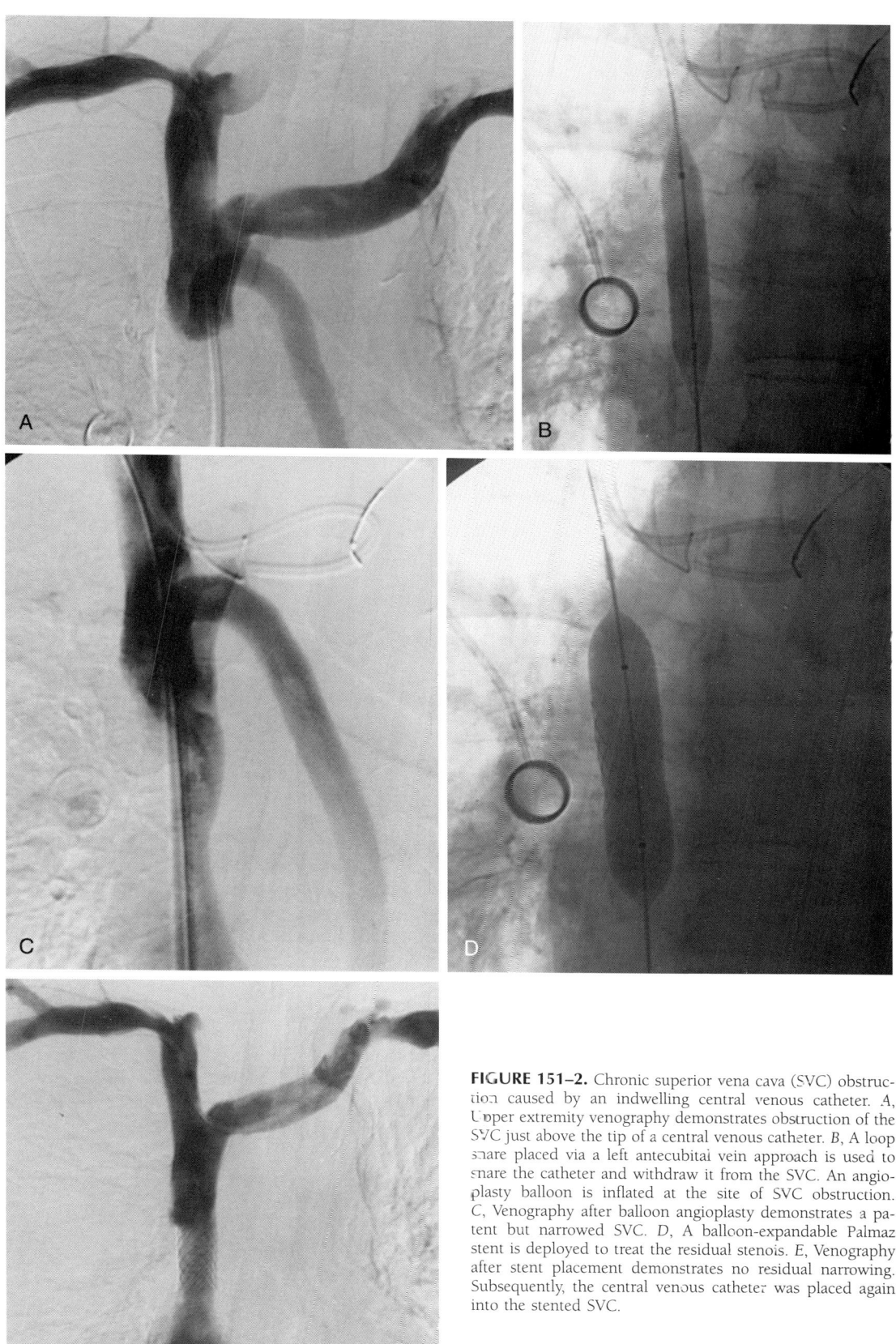

FIGURE 151–2. Chronic superior vena cava (SVC) obstruction caused by an indwelling central venous catheter. A, Upper extremity venography demonstrates obstruction of the SVC just above the tip of a central venous catheter. B, A loop snare placed via a left antecubital vein approach is used to snare the catheter and withdraw it from the SVC. An angioplasty balloon is inflated at the site of SVC obstruction. C, Venography after balloon angioplasty demonstrates a patent but narrowed SVC. D, A balloon-expandable Palmaz stent is deployed to treat the residual stenois. E, Venography after stent placement demonstrates no residual narrowing. Subsequently, the central venous catheter was placed again into the stented SVC.

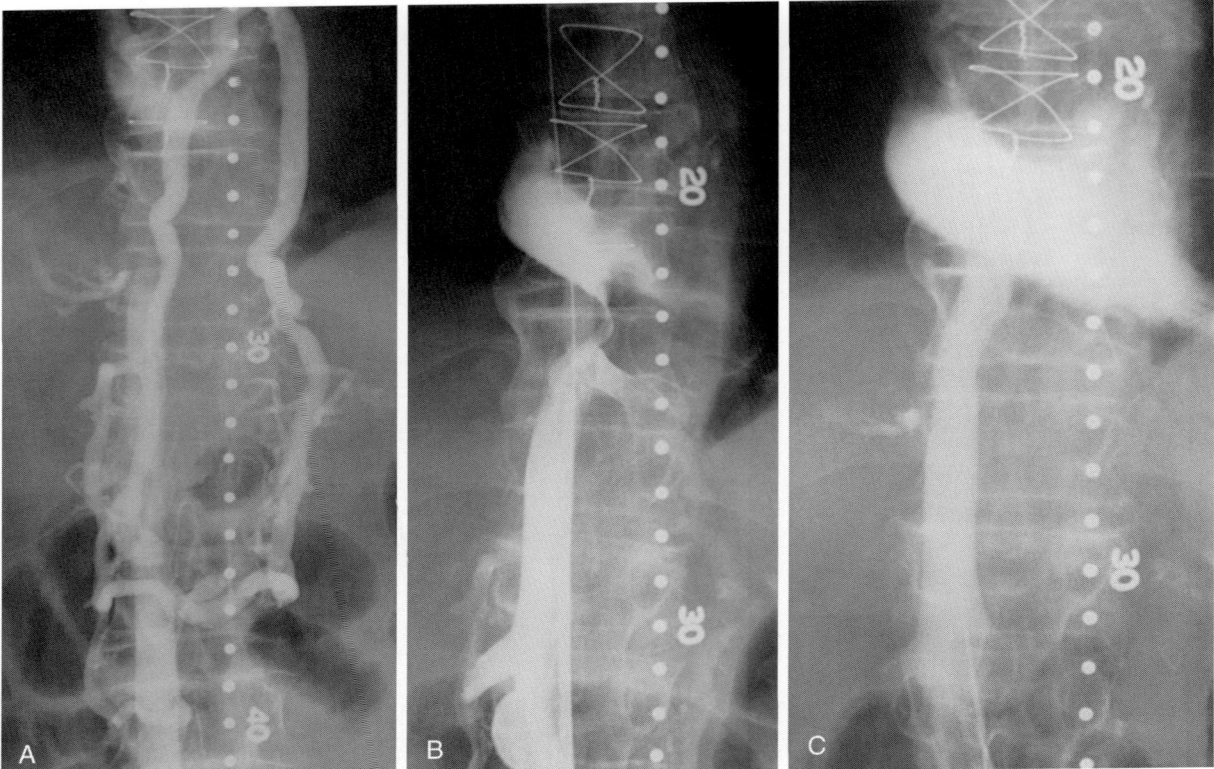

FIGURE 151–3. Focal chronic obstruction of the intrahepatic inferior vena cava (IVC). *A*, Inferior venacavogram demonstrates obstruction of the IVC with abundant collateral opacification. *B*, After balloon angioplasty, residual stenosis of the intrahepatic IVC is evident. *C*, No residual narrowing is noted after placement of two Palmaz stents at the site of IVC obstruction.

reports of similar devices being used in the venous system and in transjugular intrahepatic portosystemic shunt (TIPS) revisions.[56, 57] There has been only one case report of stent-graft placement in the SVC. It describes the use of Z-stents covered with nonporous polyester graft material (Meadox Medicals, Oakland, N.J.). In this particular case, the stent-graft was placed to treat a previously stented malignant obstruction that had been reoccluded by tumor ingrowth. After a course of aggressive thrombolysis, a residual filling defect was noted on the cavogram. The filling defect was considered to represent invading tumor or thrombus in the

lumen of the previously stented SVC. The rationale for using such a device is that the graft material covering the stent acts as a barrier to further ingrowth of tumor and development of thrombus. Follow-up was limited because the patient died only 19 days after the procedure owing to the effects of the underlying malignancy. In contrast to stent-grafts placed in the arterial system to exclude aneurysms, the current role of endoluminal stent grafting in the venous system appears palliative, not yet a definitive, first-line therapy.

Although experience with stent-grafting in the venous system is very limited, there are a number of potential complications. The most important one may be related to stent-graft misplacement. Because graft material covers the stent, the interventionalist must be careful not to place the device across important feeding veins. This could exacerbate symptoms, particularly in chronic cases when a rich network of collaterals has formed. Thrombosis of the stent-graft is another possible complication. There may be a predisposition to thrombosis when the diameter of the stent-graft has been oversized or it has not fully expanded, because in the low-pressure venous system any redundancy in graft material may serve as a nidus for thrombus formation.

Unlike placement in the arterial system, Stent-grafts placed in the venous system do not require introduction through a surgical venotom; percutaneous access is still feasible for delivery systems up to 24 Fr. in most patients.

TABLE 151–2. ETIOLOGY OF INFERIOR VENA CAVAL OBSTRUCTION

Benign
    Membranous occlusion
    Hypercoagulability disorders
    Inferior vena caval interruption
        Post-transplant surgery
        Inferior vena caval filter thrombosis
    Dialysis fistula–related stenosis
    Retroperitoneal fibrosis
    Inflammation
    Trauma
    Infection
Malignant
    Hepatocellular carcinoma
    Renal cell carcinoma
    Lymphoma

Inferior Vena Cava

Chronic occlusions of the IVC are a heterogeneous group of lesions of varied causes and unpredictable prognoses (Table 151–2).[58, 59] IVC occlusion may be associated with a wide range of clinical manifestations, including bilateral lower extremity pain and edema, thoracoabdominal varicosities, massive ascites, back pain, umbilical herniation, venous ulceration, and even disrupted liver and kidney function if the intrahepatic vena cava or renal veins are involved.[5, 58–60] Medical management alone has not been successful in treating chronic IVC occlusions, whereas surgery has been reserved for the most severe cases. (Chapter 153 details the results of surgical treatment of IVC occlusion.[7, 9, 10, 61, 63]) Initial patency rates, reported for PTA were very good.[64, 65] Long-term patency rates however, were disappointing, and repeat angioplasty was necessary in many cases.[66–68] The further development of endovascular stents has greatly improved endovascular patency rates and reduced the need for repeated PTA.[44, 69–73]

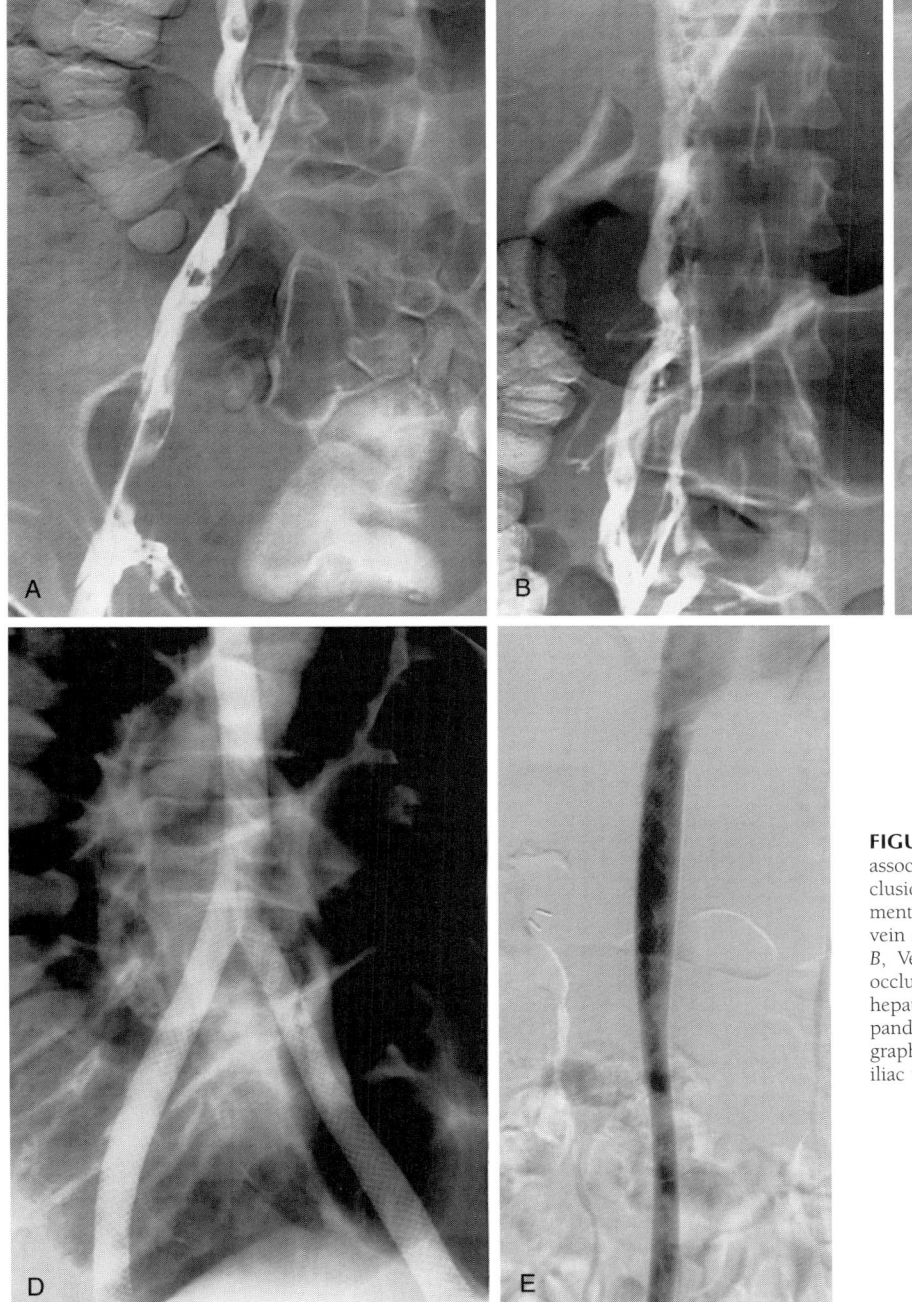

FIGURE 151–4. Acute iliac deep vein thrombosis associated with chronic inferior vena cava (IVC) occlusion. Endovascular treatment by Wallstent placement. *A,* Pelvic venogram demonstrates right iliac vein obstruction with abundant collateral formation. *B,* Venographic appearance of the abdomen shows occlusion of the IVC from its bifurcation to its intrahepatic segment. *C,* Deployment of 24-mm, self-expanding Wallstent within the IVC. *D* and *E,* Venographic appearance after Wallstent placement in the iliac vein and IVC.

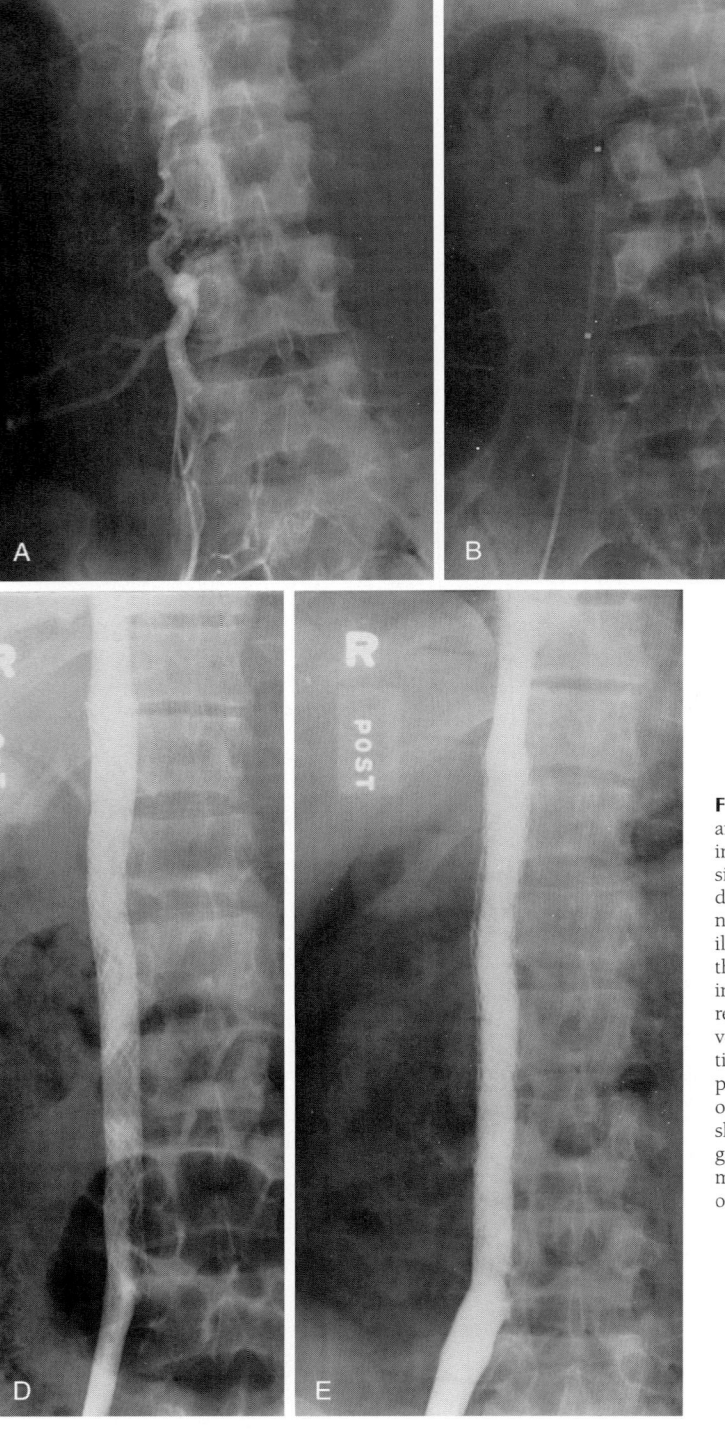

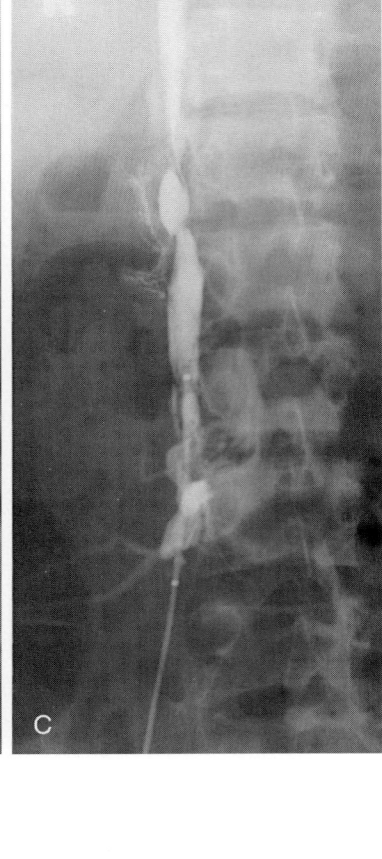

FIGURE 151–5. Catheter-directed thrombolysis and stent placement for recanalization of an inferior vena cava (IVC) obstruction. The occlusion was associated with multiple femoral hemodialysis catheters and was first documented venographically 4 years before this study. *A,* Right iliac venogram shows obstruction of the IVC at the level of its bifurcation. *B,* Multiple-sidehole infusion cathether placed within the IVC for regional thrombolysis with urokinase. *C,* Inferior venacavogram performed 12 hours after initiation of catheter-directed thrombolysis shows partial recanalization of the IVC. *D,* Appearance of IVC after placement of multiple Palmaz stents shows no residual stenosis. *E,* Follow-up cavogram 3 years after stent placement demonstrates mild intimal hypertrophy lining the stents without significant narrowing of the IVC.

Membranous and discrete segmental occlusions are the most frequent benign occlusive diseases of the suprahepatic and intrahepatic IVC (Fig. 151–3).[58] Focal segmental occlusion of the IVC is thought to be an advanced form of membranous obstruction.[61] Both forms can be associated with thrombosis of the hepatic veins (Budd-Chiari syndrome) and may cause liver failure, portal hypertension, bilateral leg swelling, and, rarely, venous claudication. Iliocaval venous thrombosis after IVC interruption is the most common benign cause of infrarenal IVC occlusion (Fig. 151–4).[58] These patients are more likely than those with suprahepatic and intrahepatic IVC occlusions to develop lower limb swelling and deep venous thrombosis (DVT).

Venography and Catheterization of Inferior Vena Caval Occlusion

As described earlier, all patients with IVC occlusion are studied venographically. Percutaneous venous access is initially obtained through either the common femoral or jugular veins. Transfemoral or transjugular cavograms are used to demonstrate the location, length, and severity of occlusive lesions. Both access routes allow measurement of pressure gradients across stenoses and evaluation of the results after PTA stent deployment.

In cases of acute obstruction, it may be easy to traverse the occlusion by passing a catheter and guide wire system from a single access site. As an access site, however, the femoral vein may prove difficult to puncture in patients who have lower extremity edema or an iliofemoral occlusion. It may be necessary to place the patient in the prone position and make the venipuncture into the popliteal vein.

Once venous access has been achieved from the common femoral, jugular, or popliteal approach, the venipuncture site is converted to a hemostatic angiographic sheath. Initial attempts should be made at passing a 5 Fr. angiographic catheter with a simple pre-formed curve and a 0.035-inch steerable hydrophilic guide wire through the occluded venous segment. Chronically occluded vena caval and iliocaval segments may require conversion to a coaxial system of catheters to provide better mechanical advantage. This may entail the use of a coronary guiding catheter to support the 5 Fr. angiographic catheter and wire.

Catheter-Directed Venous Thrombolytic Therapy

Thrombolytic therapy alone is effective in a very small percentage of patients.[74, 75] When combined with PTA and stent placement, however, local thrombolytic therapy contributes to successful recanalization (Fig. 151–5).[76] As in the SVC, catheter-directed thrombolytic infusions create a channel through acute thrombus and soften chronic thrombus. In accordance with the protocol described for SVC occlusions, a single infusion system is placed in the thrombus to deliver urokinase for 12 to 48 hours. If the occlusion includes the iliofemoral system bilaterally, two infusion systems should be introduced to treat each lower extremity.

Venous Angioplasty and Stenting

The first reported attempt at balloon dilation of an occluded IVC in 1974 used a Fogarty balloon catheter.[77] It was not until almost 10 years later that Gruntzig-type balloons were used in IVC occlusions, and initial results were encouraging.[64, 65] Successful recanalization and dilations were achieved by simultaneous inflation of four balloons in the obstructed IVC segment. Recent developments in catheter design now allow production of balloons with a diameter large enough to treat the entire IVC (12 to 24 mm). Like the results of PTA for venous disease in the SVC, long-term patency rates of PTA alone in the IVC have been disappointing.[71]

The role of stents in IVC occlusions is to prevent the elastic recoil typically seen after PTA. The three stents most used are the Palmaz stent, the Wallstent, and the Gianturco Z-stent. All three stents can be placed via either a transfemoral or a transjugular approach with good results.

A review of the literature reveals that Gianturco Z-stents are the ones most often used for IVC occlusions. This may be due to the stent's small surface area and robust radial force, especially if the stent is oversized. Results have been particularly encouraging in the treatment of Budd-Chiari and anastamotic stenosis after liver transplantation.[78, 79] Use of Wallstents has also been reported for treating chronic occlusions due to long-term indwelling femoral hemodialysis catheters.[80] Also, Palmaz stents have been used to a limited degree in treating IVC occlusion.[81] Their relatively short lengths preclude easy and effective treatment of long-segment venous occlusions.

Stent-Grafts

The use of stent-grafts has not been reported in the IVC, perhaps because of lower incidence of invading tumors as compared with the SVC.

BIBLIOGRAPHY

1. Escalante CP: Causes and management of superior vena cava syndrome. Oncology 7:61, 1993.
2. Abner A: Approach to the patient who presents with superior vena cava obstruction. Chest 103:394S, 1993.
3. Lochridge SK, Knibbe WP, Doty DB: Obstruction of superior vena cava. Surgery 85:14, 1979.
4. Adar R, Rosenthal T, Mozes M: Venal caval obstruction in 76 patients. Angiology 25:433, 1974.
5. Davenport D, Ferree C, Blake D: Radiation therapy in the treatment of superior vena cava obstruction. Cancer 42:2600, 1966.
6. Levitt SH, Jona TK, Kilpatrick SJ, Bogardus CR: Treatment of malignant superior vena cava syndrome. Semin Oncol 5:123, 1978.
7. Gloviczki P, Pairolero P, Toomey B, et al: Reconstruction of large veins for nonmalignant venous disease. J Vasc Surg 16:750, 1992.
8. Doty DB: Bypass of superior vena cava: Six years experience with spiral vein graft for the obstruction of superior vena cava due to benign or malignant disease. J Thorac Cardiovasc Surg 83:326, 1982.
9. McCarthy PM, vonHeerden JA, Adson MA, et al: Budd-Chiari syndrome: Medical and surgical management of thirty patients. Arch Surg 120:657, 1985.
10. Iwashi K: Surgical correction of the inferior vena cava obstruction with Budd-Chiari syndrome. Nippon Geka Hokan 50:559, 1981.
11. Sarkar R, Eilber FR, Gelabert HA, et al: Prosthetic replacement of the inferior vena cava for malignancy. J Vasc Surg 28:75, 1998.
12. Rosch J, Bedell JE, Putman J, et al: Gianturco expandable wire stents in the treatment of superior vena cava syndrome recurring after maximum-tolerance radiation. Cancer 60:1243, 1987.
13. Shah R, Sabanthan S, Lowe RA, et al: Stenting in malignant obstruction of the superior vena cava. J Thorac Cardiovasc Surg 112:335, 1996.

14. Irving J, Dondelinger R, Reid J, et al: Gianturco self-expanding stents: Clinical experience in the vena cava and large veins. Cardiovasc Intervent Radiol 15:328, 1992.

15. Kee ST, Kinoshita L, Razavi, et al: Superior vena cava syndrome: Treatment with catheter-directed thrombolysis and endovascular stent placement. Radiology 206:187, 1998.

16. Alimi YS, Gloviczki P, Vrtiska T, et al: Reconstruction of the superior vena cava: Benefits of postoperative surveillance and secondary endovascular techniques. J Vasc Surg 27:287, 1998.

17. Williams DR, Demos NJ: Thrombosis of superior vena cava caused by pacemaker wire and managed with streptokinase. J Thorac Cardiovasc Surg 68:134, 1974.

18. Mico G, Robles I, Catalan M, et al: Superior vena cava syndrome caused by pacemaker cable, treated with streptokinase. Rev Clin Esp 177:358, 1985.

19. Montgomery J, D'Souza V, Dyer R, et al: Non-surgical treatment of superior vena cava: Management of upper extremity central venous obstruction using interventional radiology. Ann Vasc Surg 12:202, 1998.

20. Blackburn T, Dunn M: Pacemaker-induced superior vena cava syndrome: Consideration of management. Am Heart J 116:893, 1988.

21. Crow MT, Davies CH, Gaines PA: Percutaneous management of superior vena cava occlusions. Cardiovasc Intervent Radiol 18:367, 1995.

22. Kalman PG, Lindsay TF, Clarke K, et al: Management of upper extremity central venous obstruction using interventional radiology. Ann Vasc Surg 12:202, 1998.

23. Becker GJ, Holden RW, Rabe FE, et al: Low-dose fibrinolytic therapy: Results and new concepts. Radiology 149:769, 1983.

24. van Breda A, Katzen BT, Deutsch AS: Urokinase versus streptokinase in local thrombolysis. Radiology 165:109, 1987.

25. McNamara TO, Fischer JR: Thrombolysis of arterial and graft occlusions: Improved results using high-dose urokinase. Am J Roentgenol 144:769, 1985.

26. Becker GJ, Rabe FE, Richmond BD, et al: Low-dose fibrinolytic therapy: Results and new concepts. Radiology 148:663, 1983.

27. Naschitz JE, Yeshurun D, Lev LM: Thromboembolism in cancer: Changing trends. Cancer 71:1384, 1993.

28. Sherry C, Diamond N, Meyers T, et al: Successful treatment of superior vena cava syndrome by venous angioplasty. Am J Roentgenol 147:834, 1986.

29. Ingram TL, Reid SH, Tisnade J, et al: Percutaneous transluminal angioplasty of brachiocephalic vein stenoses in patients with dialysis shunts. Radiology 166:45, 1988.

30. Walpole H, Lovett K, Chaung V, et al: Superior vena cava syndrome treated by percutaneous balloon angioplasty. Am Heart J 115:1303, 1988.

31. Davidson C, Newman G, Sheikh K, et al: Mechanisms of angioplasty in hemodialysis fistula stenoses evaluated by intravascular ultrasound. Kidney Int 40:91, 1991.

32. Wisselink W, Maoney SR, Becker MD, et al: Comparison of operative reconstruction and percutaneous balloon dilation central venous obstruction. Am J Surg 166:200, 1993.

33. Kovalik E, Newman G, Suhocki P, et al: Correction of central venous stenoses: Use of angioplasty and vascular Wallstents. Kidney Int 45:1117, 1994.

34. Gaines PA, Belli AM, Anderson PB, et al: Superior vena caval obstruction managed by the Gianturco Z-stent. Clin Radiol 49:202, 1994.

35. Oudkerk M, Kuijpers TJ, Schmitz PI, et al: Self-expanding metal stents for palliative treatment of superior vena caval syndrome. Cardiovasc Intervent Radiol 19:146, 1996.

36. Dyet JF, Nicholson AA, Cook AM: The use of the Wallstent endovascular prosthesis in the treatment of malignant obstruction of the superior vena cava. Clin Radiol 48:381 1993.

37. Oudkerk, Kuijpers TJ, Schmitz PI, et al: Self-expanding metal stents for palliative treatment of superior vena cava syndrome. Cardiovasc Intervent Radiol 19:146, 1996.

38. Palmaz J: Balloon expandable intravascular stent. AJR Am J Roentgenol 150:1263, 1988.

39. Solomam N, Holey M, Jarmolowski L: Intravascular stents in the management of superior vena cava syndrome. Cathet Cardiovasc Diagn 23:245, 1991.

40. Antonucci F, Salmonowitz C, Stuckmann G, et al: Placement of venous stents: Clinical experience with a self-expanding prosthesis. Radiology 183:493, 1992.

41. Watkinson AF, Hansell DM: Expandable Wallstent for the treatment of obstruction of the superior vena cava. Thorax 48:915, 1993.

42. Charnsangavej C, Carrusco CH, Wallace S, et al: Stenosis of the vena cava: Preliminary assessment of treatment with expandable metallic stents. Radiology 161:295, 1986.

43. Putman JS, Uchida BT, Antonovic R, et al: Superior vena cava syndrome associated with massive thrombosis: Treatment with expandable wire stents. 167:727, 1988.

44. Gaines PA, Belli AM, Anderson PB, et al: Superior vena caval obstruction managed by the Gianturco Z stent. Clin Radiol 49:202, 1994.

45. Kazushi K, Sonomura T, Mitouzane K, et al: Self-expandable metallic stent therapy for superior vena cava syndrome: Clinical observations. Radiology 189:531, 1993.

46. Rosch J, Petersen BD, Lakin PC: Venous stents: Indications, techniques, results. In Perler BA, Becker GJ (eds): Vascular Intervention: A Clinical Approach. New York, Thieme, 1998, p 706.

47. Carrasco CH, Charnsangavej C, Wright K, et al: Use of self-expanding stents in stenoses of the superior vena cava. J Vasc Interv Radiol 3:409, 1992.

48. Entwisle KG, Watkinson AF, Reidy J: Case report: Migration and shortening of a self-expanding metallic stent complicating the treatment of malignant superior vena cava stenosis. Clin Radiol 51:593, 1996.

49. Gray RJ, Dolmatch BL, Horton KM, et al: Migration of Palmaz stents following deployment for venous stenoses related to hemodialysis access. J Vasc Interv Radiol 5:117, 1994.

50. Bjarnason H, Hunter DW, Crain MR, et al: Collapse of a Palmaz stent in the subclavian vein. AJR Am J Roentgenol 160:1123, 1993.

51. Prischl FC, Weber T, Lenglinger F, et al: Conservative management of late Palmaz stent embolization to the pulmonary artery—a complication after PTA with stent implantation of a fistula-draining right subclavian vein stenosis. Nephrol Dial Transplant 12:119, 1997.

52. Nishibe MK, Ohkashiw MH, Takahashi OH, et al: Gianturco stents for the venous system: A detailed pathological study. Surg Today 28:396, 1998.

53. Rhee JS, Slonim SM, Dake MD, et al: Retrieval of intravascular stents. Radiology 205:431, 1997.

54. Cekirge S, Foster R, Weiss JP, et al: Percutaneous removal of an embolized Wallstent during a transjugular intrahepatic portosystemic shunt procedure. J Vasc Interv Radiol 4:559, 1993.

55. Dake MD, Miller C, Semba CP, et al: Transluminal placement of endovascular stent-grafts for the treatment of descending thoracic aortic aneurysms. N Engl J Med 331:1729, 1994.

56. Chin DH, Peterson BD, Timmermans H, et al: Stent-graft in the management of superior vena cava syndrome. Cardiovasc Intervent Radiol 19:302, 1996.

57. Saxon RR, Timmermans HA, Uchida BT, et al: Stent-grafts for revision of TIPS stenoses and occlusions: A clinical pilot study. J Vasc Interv Radiol 8:539, 1997.

58. Harris R: The etiology of inferior vena caval obstruction and compression. Crit Rev Clin Radiol Nucl Med 8:57, 1976.

59. Missal ME, Robinson JA, Tatum RW: Inferior vena cava obstruction: Clinical manifestation, diagnostic methods, and related problems. Ann Intern Med 62:133, 1965.

60. Sonin AH, Mazer MJ, Powers TA: Obstruction of the inferior vena cava: A multiple-modality demonstration of causes, manifestations, and collateral pathways. RadioGraphics 12:309, 1992.

61. Hirooka M, Kimura C: Membranous obstruction of the hepatic portion of the inferior vena cava. Arch Surg 100:656, 1970.

62. Kimura C, Matsuda S, Koie H, et al: Membranous obstruction of the hepatic portion of the inferior vena cava: Clinical study of nine cases. Surgery 72:551, 1972.

63. Wilson SE, Jabour H, Stone R, et al: Patency of biological and prosthetic inferior vena cava grafts with distal limb fistula. Arch Surg 113:1174, 1992.

64. Yamada R, Sato M, Kawabata M, et al: Segmental obstruction of the hepatic inferior vena cava treated by transluminal angioplasty. Radiology 49:91, 1983.

65. Jeans WD, Bourne JT, Read AE: Treatment of hepatic vein and inferior vena caval obstruction by balloon dilatation. Br J Radiol 56:687, 1983.

66. Lois JF, Hartzman S, Mcglade CT, et al: Budd-Chiari syndrome: Treatment with percutaneous transhepatic recanalization and dilation. Radiology 170:791, 1989.

67. Martin LG, Henderson JM, Millikan WJ Jr, et al: Angioplasty for long-term treatment of patients with Budd-Chiari syndrome. AJR Am J Roentgenol 154:1007, 1990.

68. Sato M, Yamada R, Tsuji K, et al: Percutaneous transluminal angio-

plasty in segmental obstruction of the hepatic inferior vena cava: Long-term results. Cardiovasc Intervent Radiol 13:189, 1990.

69. Gilliams A, Dick R, Platts A, et al: Dilation of the inferior vena cava using an expandable metal stent in Budd-Chiari syndrome. J Hepatol 13:149, 1991.

70. Carrasco C, Charnsangavej C, Wright K, et al: Use of the Gianturco self-expanding stent in stenosis of the superior and inferior venae cavae. J Vasc Interv Radiol 3:409, 1992.

71. Venbrux AC, Mitchell SE, Savader SJ, et al: Long-term results with the use of metallic stents in the inferior vena cava for treatment of Budd-Chiari syndrome. J Vasc Interv Radiol 5:411, 1994.

72. Park JH, Chung JW, Han JK, et al: Interventional management of benign obstruction of the hepatic inferior vena cava. J Vasc Interv Radiol 5:403, 1994.

73. Simo G, Echenagusia A, Camunez F, et al: Stenosis of the inferior vena cava after liver transplantation: Treatment with Gianturco expandable metallic stents. Cardiovasc Intervent Radiol 18:212, 1995.

74. Maddrey WC: Hepatic vein thrombosis (Budd-Chiari syndrome). Hepatology 4(Suppl):44s, 1984.

75. Frank JW, Kamath PS, Stanson AW: Budd-Chiari syndrome: Early

76. Ishiguchi T, Fukatsu H, Itoh S, et al: Budd-Chiari syndrome with long segmental inferior vena cava obstruction: Treatment with thrombolysis, angioplasty, and intravascular stents. J Vasc Interv Radiol 3:421, 1992.

77. Eguchi S, Takeuchi Y, Asano K: Successful balloon membranotomy for obstruction of the hepatic portion of the inferior vena cava. Surgery 76:837, 1974.

78. Berger H, Hilbert T, Zunlke K, et al: Balloon dilatation and stent placement of suprahepatic caval anastamotic stenosis following liver transplantation. Cardiovasc Intervent Radiol 16:384, 1993.

79. Baijil SS, Roy S, Phadke RV, et al: Management of isiopathic Budd-Chiari syndrome with primary stent placement: Early results. J Vasc Interv Radiol 7:545, 1995.

80. Chang TC, Zaleski GX, Lin BHJ, et al: Treatment of inferior vena cava obstruction in hemodialysis patients using Wallstents: Early and intermediate results. AJR Am J Roentgenol 171:125, 1998.

81. Elson JD, Becker GJ, Wholey MH, et al: Vena caval and central venous stenoses: Management with Palmaz balloon-expandable intraluminal stents. J Vasc Interv Radiol 2:215, 1991.

intervention with angioplasty and thrombolytic therapy. Mayo Clin Proc 69:877, 1994.

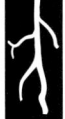

CHAPTER 152

Diagnosis and Management of Tumors of the Inferior Vena Cava

Thomas C. Bower, M.D., and Anthony Stanson, M.D.

Tumors of the inferior vena cava (IVC) are rare and often malignant.[1-4] The management of these patients is difficult for several reasons:

1. Both primary and secondary tumors cause symptoms at a late stage, and this delays diagnosis and worsens patient prognosis.

2. Adjuvant therapy has resulted in little reduction in tumor burden or palliation of symptoms.

3. Surgical resection and caval replacement is a major operation with high risk and unknown long-term benefit to the patient.

Because surgical resection, with or without venous reconstruction, remains the only hope for cure or control of symptoms for many of these patients, surgeons have become more aggressive in their operative approach. Improvements in surgical techniques, anesthesia support, postoperative critical care, and the development and successful use of externally supported synthetic grafts to replace large veins for benign disease (see Chapter 150) have resulted in a number of case reports and small clinical series documenting successful resection of the tumor and replacement of all segments of the IVC.[4-26]

This chapter reviews the types of IVC tumors, their clinical presentation, the current methods of diagnosis, and

surgical treatment. A variety of terms have been used to describe the different segments of the IVC. We divide the IVC into three segments, as described by Kieffer and coworkers[12]:

The *suprahepatic* IVC is the segment between the hepatic veins in the right atrium.

The *suprarenal* IVC is the segment between the renal and hepatic veins. The retrohepatic portion of the suprarenal IVC lies behind the liver. The infrahepatic portion is between the inferior edge of the liver and the renal vein confluence.

The *infrarenal* segment extends from the confluence of the common iliac veins to the renal veins (Fig. 152–1) (see Color Plate).

TUMOR TYPES

Primary tumors originate from within the wall of the IVC, while secondary tumors surround, compress, or invade the vein (Table 152–1) The most common primary vascular tumor is *leiomyosarcoma*, which arises from the smooth muscle cell of the vessel wall.[27] Vascular leiomyosarcomas are rare, with only one case noted by Hallock and associates in more than 34,000 autopsies.[28] These tumors involve

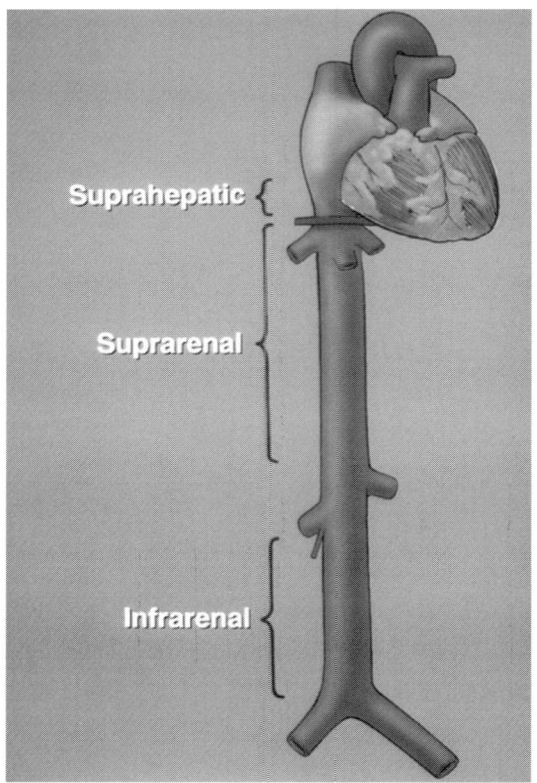

FIGURE 152–1. Segments of the inferior vena cava. See Color Plate.

veins more commonly than arteries and represent fewer than 2% of all leiomyosarcomas.[27]

Perl first described a *primary venous leiomyosarcoma* (PVL) from an autopsy case in 1871[29]; since that time, only a few hundred cases have been reported.[3, 4] PVL arises from the IVC more often than from other central or peripheral

TABLE 152–1. TUMORS OF THE INFERIOR VENA CAVA
(IVC)

Primary
　IVC leiomyosarcoma
Secondary
　Retroperitoneal soft tissue tumors
　　Liposarcoma
　　Leiomyosarcoma
　　Malignant fibrous histiocytoma
　Hepatic tumors
　　Cholangiocarcinoma
　　Hepatocellular carcinoma
　　Metastatic (e.g. colorectal)
　Pancreaticoduodenal cancers
Secondary Tumors That May Have Tumor Thrombus
　Renal cell carcinoma
　Pheochromocytoma
　Adrenocortical carcinoma
　Sarcomas of uterine origin
　　Leiomyomatosis
　　Endometrial stromal cell
　Germ cell tumors
　　Embryonal
　　Teratocarcinoma

veins. The IVC was involved in 33 of 68 cases reported in one review of vascular sarcomas in 1973,[30] and in a more recent review, Dzsinich and coauthors found 60% of the 210 reported cases of PVL to arise from the IVC.[4] Primary caval tumors may arise from any segment of the vena cava. In a review of 144 cases by Mingoli and colleagues, three fourths of the tumors arose from the suprarenal (42%) and infrarenal (34%) segments, and one fourth involved the suprahepatic segment (Fig. 152–2).[3] The true prevalence of PVL is unknown because the slow growth of these tumors delays their detection. Among all types of retroperitoneal sarcomas, approximately 6% of cases are classified as primary venous leiomyosarcomas.[31]

These tumors are usually polypoid or nodular in pathologic appearance. They are firmly attached to the vessel of origin and exhibit less intratumor hemorrhage and necrosis than other retroperitoneal sarcomas do (Fig. 152–3).[4, 27, 31] The most common growth pattern is intraluminal, but the tumor can extend through the adventitial surface of the vein wall and invade adjacent structures because the vein wall is thin.[31] This characteristic makes them difficult to differentiate from other retroperitoneal sarcomas. Such extraluminal growth may occur early in the course of the disease, which would account for the presence of distant metastases in almost half of patients at the time of diagnosis.[3, 4, 27, 32] Metastases to the lung, liver, kidney, bone, pleura or chest wall occur hematogenously or by lymphatic spread.[4, 27, 32] If the lesion remains untreated, survival is measured in months, with the patient dying of complications from locoregional growth or metastatic disease. Min-

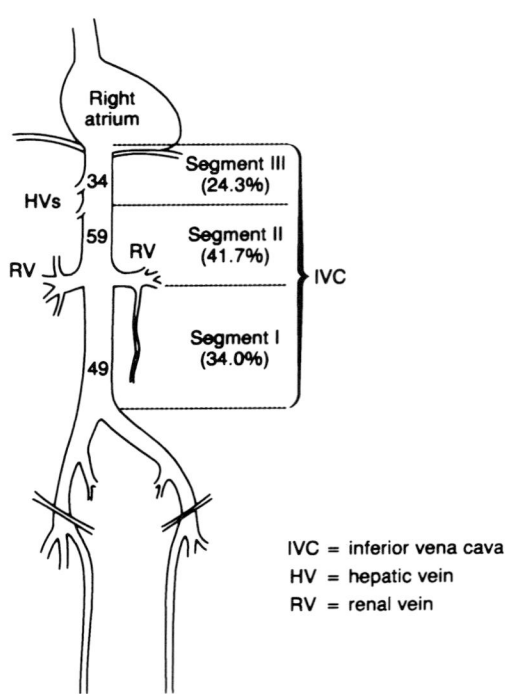

FIGURE 152–2. Distribution of primary inferior vena cava leiomyosarcomas. (Data based on a review by Mingoli A, Feldhaus RJ, Cavallaro A, Stipa S: Leiomyosarcoma of the inferior vena cava. *In* Bergan JJ, Yao ST [eds]: Surgery of the Veins. New York, Grune & Stratton, 1985, pp 423–443. By permission of Mayo Foundation.)

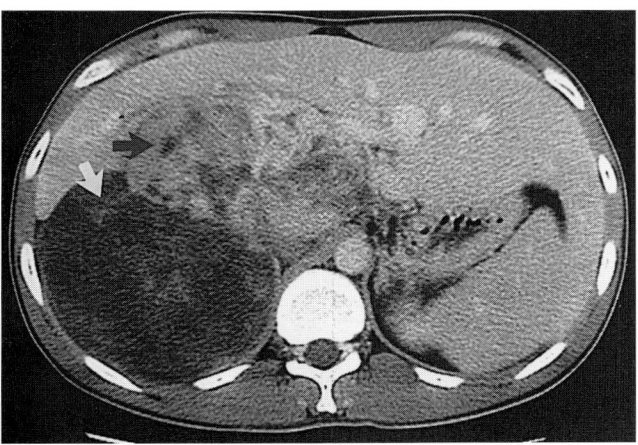

FIGURE 152–3. CT scan of a large retroperitoneal leiomyosarcoma involving the organs of the right upper quadrant, including the liver and retrohepatic vena cava. Note the necrotic areas within the tumor (*arrow*). (From Bower TC: Primary and secondary tumors of the inferior vena cava. *In* Gloviczki P, Yao JST [eds]: Handbook of Venous Disorders: London, Chapman & Hall, 1996, pp 529–550.

goli and associates reported a mean survival of 3 months for untreated patients in their series.[3]

Microscopically, grading of the malignancy can be difficult and extensive sampling of the tumor is necessary. Of the criteria used to determine malignancy in leiomyosarcomas, such as size, degree of cellularity, presence of necrosis within the tumor, cellular atypia, and mitotic activity, the most important determinant of malignancy is mitotic activity.[27, 33]

Secondary malignancies affecting the vena cava include the following categories (see Table 152–1):

- Primary or metastatic cancer of the liver
- Duodenal, pancreatic, intestinal, adrenal or renal malignancy
- Retroperitoneal sarcomas, such as liposarcoma, malignant fibrous histiocytoma, and leiomyosarcoma

These cancers invade the wall of the vena cava and obstruct its lumen by extrinsic compression, invasion of the caval wall, or intraluminal growth of tumor thrombus (Fig. 152–4).

Similar to PVL, retroperitoneal sarcomas can invade or obstruct any segment of the IVC and they are the most common cause of malignant obstruction of the infrarenal segment.[1] They are usually covered by a pseudocapsule and often displace, but do not invade, adjacent structures. Retroperitoneal leiomyosarcomas originate from smooth muscle tissue either from the wall of retroperitoneal veins or from wolffian remnants[31] and behave similarly to PVL. When these tumors invade beyond their pseudocapsule and become adherent to the vena cava, they can be indistinguishable pathologically from primary tumors of the IVC that have grown outside the lumen. In addition to intraluminal growth with PVL, two growth patterns are predominant with retroperitoneal sarcomas. In two thirds of cases, these sarcomas grow extrinsic to the major arteries and veins. A combination of extraluminal and intraluminal growth from invasion of the vena cava is seen in as many as one third

of cases and is the second most common growth pattern (see Fig. 152–4).[31, 33]

Cancers of the solid organs or the intestines invade or obstruct the segment of the IVC in anatomic proximity to the site of origin of the neoplasm. Primary hepatic malignancies, such as hepatocellular carcinoma, cholangiocarcinoma, mixed tumors, and metastatic lesions, involve the retrohepatic suprarenal vena cava up to and including the hepatic veins.[1] Duodenal, pancreatic, and large renal or adrenal malignancies may obstruct the suprarenal vena cava at or above the level of the renal veins. Unlike sarcomas, these cancers have no pseudocapsule; when they involve the vena cava, they adhere to adjacent structures and often obliterate normal tissue planes around the IVC.

Some cancers (e.g., renal cell carcinoma, adrenocortical carcinoma, pheochromocytoma, sarcomas of uterine origin, and germ cell tumors, such as embryonal cell carcinoma and teratocarcinoma) exhibit an unusual growth pattern and extend themselves as tumor thrombus within the lumen of the IVC toward the heart (Fig. 152–5) (see Color Plate).[34–57]

The most common malignancy with intracaval tumor thrombus is renal cell carcinoma, also the most common cancer involving the IVC in patients undergoing surgical resection.[34–37, 57] Tumor thrombus is found in the renal veins in 15% to 20% of cases and in the IVC in 4 to 15%.[44, 46, 57]

Tumor thrombus is usually associated with large renal cell carcinomas and reflects a large local tumor burden.[36, 44, 48] Kallman and colleagues, in review of preoperative radiologic studies on 431 patients subjected to radical nephrectomy for renal cell carcinoma between 1985 and 1989, found the size of the carcinoma to be predictive for the detection of tumor thrombus. No patient with a carcinoma smaller than 4.5 cm in diameter had intracaval extension of thrombus.[58] Additionally, tumor thrombus occurs more often from carcinomas involving the right kidney.[44, 48, 58] Neves and Zincke, in a review of 54 patients treated by radical nephrectomy and caval tumor thrombectomy, found the right kidney involvement by tumor in 41 patients and left kidney involvement in only 13.[36] Classification of the extent of vena cava tumor thrombus is helpful for surgeons planning operative intervention. A variety of classification schemes have been reported, and most are based on the extent of thrombus either above or below the level of the diaphragm and whether the thrombus involves the right heart chambers (Fig. 152–6) (see Color Plate).[35, 36, 44, 53, 57]

In approximately 50% of patients with renal cell carcinoma and tumor thrombus, the thrombus extends into the IVC near the renal vein confluence (level I). In almost 40% of the cases, thrombus extends into the infrahepatic portion of the suprarenal IVC (level II) or into the retrohepatic (intrahepatic) segment to the level of the hepatic veins (level III). Extension of tumor thrombus into the right heart (level IV) occurs in approximately 10% of cases (see Fig. 152–6).[36, 44, 57]

In a study by Neves and Zincke, 10 patients had thrombus at level I; 29, at level II; 14, at level III; and one, at level IV.[36] Similarly, in a contemporary series of 37 patients undergoing radical nephrectomy and tumor thrombectomy reported by Nesbitt and colleagues, nine patients had a

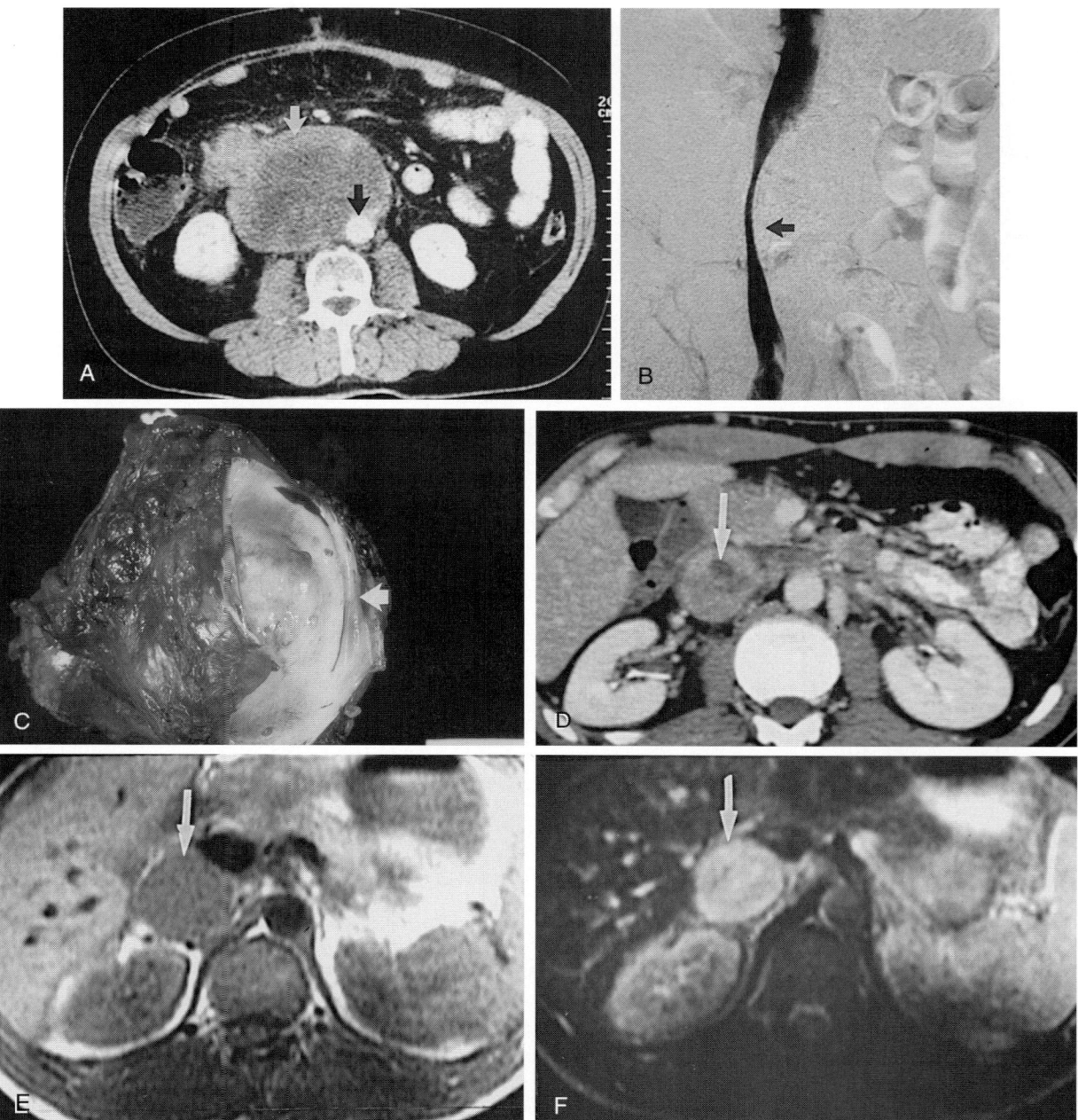

FIGURE 152–4. Patterns of growth in tumors of the inferior vena cava (IVC). *A,* CT scan of the abdomen showing a large retroperitoneal tumor which surrounds the IVC and obliterates its lumen *(white arrow).* The tumor also abuts the abdominal aorta *(dark arrow). B,* Venacavogram shows compression and bowing of the IVC. (From Phillips M, Bower T, Orszulak TO, Hartmann L: Intracardiac extension of an intracaval sarcoma of endometrial origin. Ann Thorac Surg 59:742–744, 1995.) *C,* Pathology specimen from the same patient after resection showing invasion of the lumen of the IVC *(arrow). D,* Venacavogram showing the typical filling defect seen with tumors confined to the lumen of the IVC *(arrow). D,* From Bower TC: Primary and secondary tumors of the inferior vena cava. *In* Gloviczki P, Yao JST [eds]: Handbook of Venous Disorders: London, Chapman & Hall, 1996, pp 529–550.

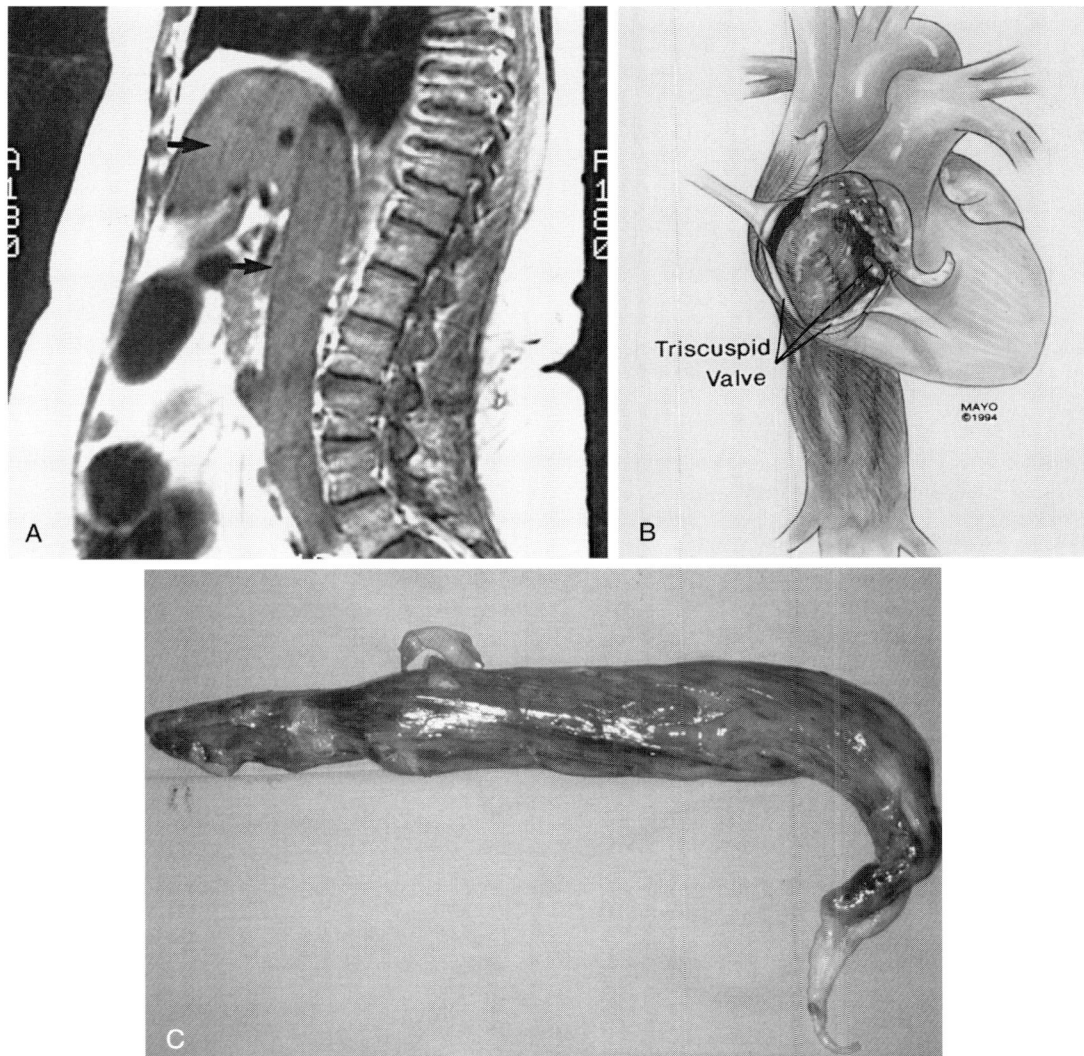

FIGURE 152–5. Intracaval tumor thrombus extending into the right heart chambers shown on MRI (A) and depicted schematically (B). Pathologic specimen (C) revealed endometrial stromal cell sarcoma. See Color Plate for C. (A, From Bower TC: Primary and secondary tumors of the inferior vena cava. *In* Gloviczki P, Yao JST [eds]: Handbook of Venous Disorders: London, Chapman & Hall, 1996, pp 529–550.)

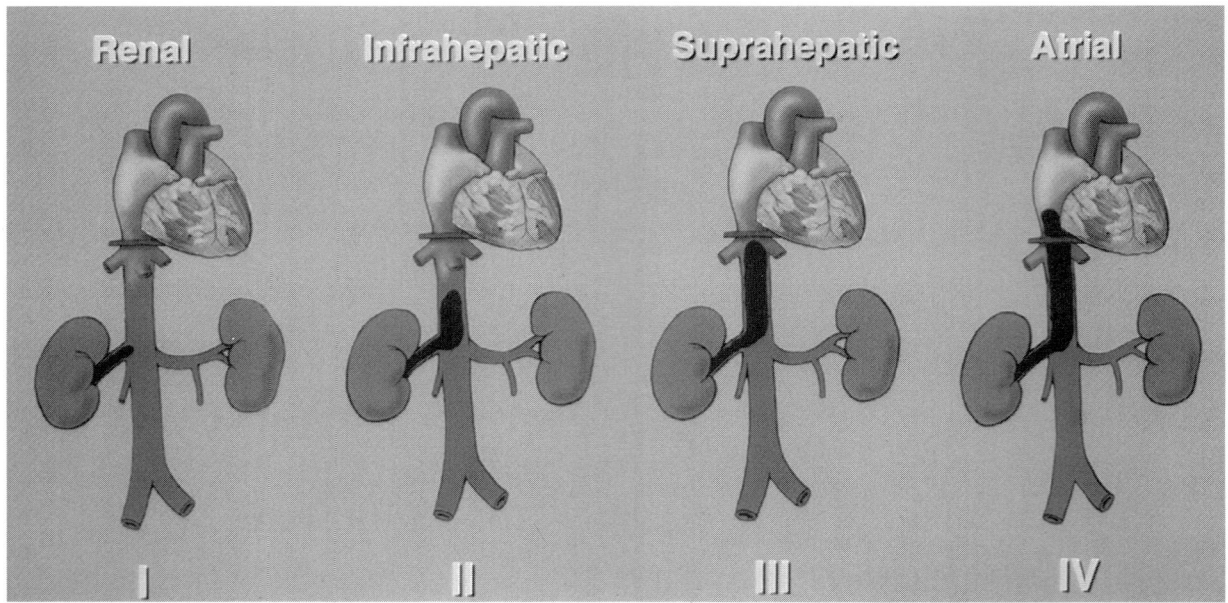

FIGURE 152–6. Classification of level of inferior vena caval thrombus associated with renal cell carcinoma. See Color Plate. (From Montie, JE: Inferior vena cava tumor thrombus. *In* Montie JE, Purtes JE, Bukowski RM [eds]: Clinical Management of Renal Cell Cancer. St. Louis, Mosby–Year Book, 1990.)

level I thrombus; seven, level II; and 19, level III; of these, three patients had extension of the thrombus above the hepatic veins but not into the right heart. Only two patients had a tumor thrombus in the right atrium.[57]

Cancers that secondarily involve the IVC also carry a poor prognosis. Like patients with primary IVC tumors, these patients often have extensive locoregional spread or distant metastases at the time of diagnosis. Because patients with secondary caval malignancies are older than those with primary tumors, they often have other associated medical co-morbidities and may be more debilitated from their disease at presentation. Survival from most secondary cancers is usually less than 1 year without treatment.[1]

CLINICAL PRESENTATION

Primary leiomyosarcoma of the vena cava is much more prevalent in women than men compared with venous leiomyosarcomas of the extremities, which occurs equally in men and women.[3, 4, 27] Nine of 13 patients with PVL reported by Dzsinich and coworkers had involvement of the vena cava, and only one of these patients was male.[4] In a review of the world's literature on IVC leiomyosarcoma through 1989 by Mingoli and colleagues, 118 of 144 patients (81.9%) were women.[3] Mean age of the patients in this series was 54.4 ± 13.6 years, but there was a wide age range from 15 to 83 years. These tumors have been reported in infants, and we have previously operated on an 88-year-old woman with an IVC leiomyosarcoma.[1]

Clinical presentation of patients with primary caval tumors is related to symptoms or signs from metastatic disease or from obstruction of the vena cava. Rarely, these tumors are detected at an early stage as incidental findings during evaluation of nonspecific symptoms, such as back or abdominal pain. Only four of 144 patients with PVL

reviewed by Mingoli's group were asymptomatic at diagnosis.[3] All other patients had multiple symptoms or signs when first seen. Abdominal pain was present in 95 patients (66.0%); an abdominal mass in 69 (47.9%); and lower limb edema in 56 (38.9%). Budd-Chiari syndrome occurred in 32 patients (22.2%); loss of weight, in 44 (30.6%); and nonspecific symptoms, such fever, weakness, anorexia, nausea, vomiting, nocturnal sweating, and dyspnea, in fewer than 15%.[3] Consumption coagulopathy and abnormalities of red blood cells have also been noted.[27]

Secondary tumors of the IVC, such as retroperitoneal sarcomas and germ cell tumors, occur over a wide age range, whereas most patients with renal cell carcinoma and primary hepatic, pancreatic, or intestinal cancers are detected in the fifth, sixth or seventh decades of life.[34–35, 57, 59]

Most patients with secondary IVC malignancies present with symptoms and signs related to the cancer. Invasion or obstruction of the IVC in some of these patients may cause few clinical sequelae and is discovered only on imaging studies.[1, 36, 44] In other cases, the segment of the vena cava affected by the tumor and the degree of venous outflow obstruction from adjacent organs determines the presenting symptoms or signs (Table 152–2). Tumor or thrombus that involves the right side of the heart may cause cardiac arrhythmias, syncope, pulmonary embolism, pulmonary hypertension, and even right-sided heart failure. Hepatic venous outflow obstruction results in Budd-Chiari syndrome with hepatomegaly, jaundice, massive ascites, or liver failure. Occlusion of the suprarenal IVC between the renal and hepatic veins rarely occurs, and only a few patients with involvement of this caval segment have venous or renal insufficiency.

More commonly, cancers that invade the retrohepatic IVC cause right upper quadrant or epigastric pain, biliary tract symptoms, nausea, vomiting, or tenderness on abdominal examination. Caval obstruction at the level of the renal veins may result in renal insufficiency or nephrotic syndrome, but frank renal failure is unusual because the renal, gonadal, and lumborenal branches of the left renal vein usually allow for venous decompression of the kidney. Patients with tumors of the infrarenal IVC present with abdominal pain or a palpable mass; neurologic symptoms and pain caused by growth of the tumor into the vertebral bodies, the lumbosacral plexus, the nerve roots, or the psoas muscle; or edema of the lower extremities because of inadequate collateral venous drainage of the obstructed IVC. In patients with slow, progressive IVC obstruction, dilated abdominal wall veins may develop but lower extremity venous thrombosis is a rare presentation. Deep venous thrombosis is more often seen as the initial presentation in patients with primary tumors of the iliac or peripheral veins.[1-5, 12, 13, 27, 31, 36, 60]

EVALUATION

We prefer a multidisciplinary approach to evaluation and treatment. Specialists in medical and surgical oncology, vascular, general, hepatobiliary, urologic, or cardiothoracic surgery help to direct the work-up and choose the type of imaging studies to determine resectability of the cancer.

The goals in the evaluation are to:

- Determine the type of tumor
- Define the local extent of the malignancy and the presence of metastatic disease
- Assess the degree of caval obstruction and the adequacy of collateral venous drainage
- Identify the presence and extent of intraluminal tumor thrombus

If the lesion appears to be locally resectable and if there is no evidence of metastases, the patient's medical risk for operation is assessed. A thorough cardiopulmonary evaluation is essential, as most of our postoperative morbidity has been related to heart or lung problems. Additonally, we have found an assessment of the patient's physical activity to be helpful for risk assessment. We use the criteria outlined by the Eastern Cooperative Oncology Group (ECOG) to further stratify risk and to help judge the impact of the operation on the quality of life after tumor resection.[1, 61]

A variety of radiologic imaging studies are performed in patients with suspected intra-abdominal and retroperitoneal malignancies. Initially, many patients have chest and abdominal roentgenograms. Multiple lung lesions and mediastinal or hilar adenopathy is consistent with pulmonary and lymph node metastases. In most patients, abdominal roentgenograms are not diagnostic, but in some sarcomas,

calcification is seen within a retroperitoneal mass.[4] For patients with renal cell carcinomas or retroperitoneal sarcomas who present with urologic symptoms, distortion or displacement of the kidney, ureter, or renal calyces is discovered on excretory urography or a filling void is present on the nephrogram.[31]

The four most useful modalities for visualizing the cancer and the IVC are[1, 36, 44, 53]:

- Ultrasonography
- Computed tomography (CT)
- Magnetic resonance imaging (MRI)
- Venacavography

Often a combination of studies is needed to determine surgical resectability and to plan vena cava reconstruction.

Ultrasonography provides visualization of the entire IVC, including the retrohepatic segment; however, distortion of the major venous structures by tumor and the presence of bowel gas impair evaluation of the vena cava and are the major limitations with this technique. Nevertheless, when adequate imaging of the vena cava is achieved, ultrasonography is as sensitive as MRI and venacavography for defining patency of the vena cava and the presence and extent of intraluminal tumor thrombus.[58]

CT and *MRI* are perhaps the two most common tests used in the evaluation of patients with IVC tumors.[62] CT and MRI scans of the chest and abdomen not only define the local extent of the cancer and the level of venous involvement but also help to delineate regional or distant metastases.[1, 44, 58, 62] In some cases, the location and appearance of the tumor on these studies allow diagnosis of the type of tumor (see Fig. 152-4).[62] Both techniques detect primary intracaval tumors and cancers with tumor thrombus. In early stages, a primary IVC tumor appears as a localized mass or filling defect within the IVC. Filling defects and distention of the IVC are also seen in patients with secondary cancers that have intraluminal caval thrombus. Differentiation of tumor thrombus from bland thrombus on a single study may be difficult in the absence of an adjacent mass, but enlargement and distention of the vena cava on serial examinations suggest the presence of a caval tumor. Such changes in the caliber of the IVC may be seen in patients with unusual endometrial tumors.[56]

MRI has evolved into one of the most versatile techniques for evaluation because it allows imaging of the tumor and vena cava in axial, coronal, and sagittal planes. MRI is especially useful for patients with renal cell carcinoma and intracaval tumor thrombus.[62] Enlargement of one renal vein, compared to the other in a patient with renal cell carcinoma, suggests the presence of tumor thrombus. However, an enlarged vein that quickly tapers is a more

TABLE 152-2. CLINICAL PRESENTATIONS RELATED TO LEVEL OF INFERIOR VENA CAVA OBSTRUCTION

LEVEL	POSSIBLE SYMPTOMS AND SIGNS
1. Suprahepatic	Cardiac arrhythmias, syncope, pulmonary embolism
2. Suprarenal	
a. Retrohepatic with hepatic vein involvement	Budd-Chiari syndrome, ascites
b. Retrohepatic between hepatic and renal veins	Nonspecific abdominal pain, biliary symptoms, nausea
c. At renal vein confluence	Renal insufficiency, nephrotic syndrome
3. Infrarenal	Pain, dilated veins on abdominal wall, palpable mass, lower extremity edema

specific finding. Kallman and associates believe the optimal MRI technique for detecting tumor thrombus is a combination of axial and sagittal T-weighted and SE pulse sequences with axial single breath-hold gradient echo images.[58] In their experience, this imaging technique has proved almost 100% sensitive for detecting intracaval tumor thrombus associated with renal cell cancers; this rate is similar to that for venacavography. MRI is more sensitive but not as specific as CT in these situations. False-positive results with MRI are usually caused by flow artifacts.[58] Additionally, both CT and MRI are useful for postoperative cancer surveillance and for monitoring graft patency when venous reconstruction is performed.[1, 4, 5]

Venography has long been the "gold standard" for the evaluation of patients with suspected peripheral or central venous obstruction. Venacavography aids the planning of surgical resection and IVC reconstruction because it defines the location and extent of vena cava involvement by the cancer and the presence and extent of intracaval tumor thrombus. If the IVC is occluded on antegrade images, retrograde cavography via the internal jugular vein is used to assess the proximal extent of caval occlusion in relation to the renal and hepatic veins.[12] As software and instrumentation improve, venography will likely be supplanted by ultrasonography, CT, and MRI.

Preoperative fine needle aspiration or true-cut needle biopsy with CT or ultrasound guidance is sometimes used when the histologic diagnosis will affect treatment.[62] Transvenous biopsy has also been used for diagnosis when intracaval tumor cannot be differentiated from bland thrombus. Except for patients with germ cell cancer, most primary and secondary malignancies of the vena cava do not respond well to radiation or chemotherapy; thus, preoperative tissue sampling has little role in treatment.[1, 4, 44] Additionally, the amount of material obtained by biopsy may be inadequate to provide pathologic diagnosis. This is especially true for patients with PVL or other retroperitoneal sarcomas for whom adequate tissue sampling is needed to determine whether the tumor is benign or malignant.

TREATMENT

In past years, surgical procedures were rarely performed for patients with primary and secondary tumors of the vena cava because of the advanced stage of the malignancy at the time of diagnosis, the overall poor prognosis from the tumor, the higher operative risk related to the extent of surgical resection and caval replacement, and the debilitated state of many of the patients. Patients with diffuse metastatic disease, severe cardiopulmonary dysfunction, major medical comorbidity or inanition are not candidates for surgical resection. More recently, improvements in preoperative imaging studies for staging, surgical technique, intraoperative anesthetic management, and postoperative critical care, and the success of prosthetic and autogenous grafts to replace major veins have provided the impetus for a more aggressive surgical approach in small selected groups of patients. Patients with localized tumors, a good performance status, and few associated medical co-morbidities are now considered candidates for operation.[1, 12, 13]

Surgical Approach

Operative treatment depends on the following:

- Type of cancer
- Extent of the cancer
- The segment of vena cava involved by the tumor or thrombus
- Degree of caval obstruction and venous collaterals

The choice of incision depends on the patient's body habitus, the need for major liver resection, the segment of IVC to be reconstructed, and the possible need for cardiopulmonary bypass (Fig. 152–7). A midline abdominal incision is useful for tumors involving the infrarenal vena cava extending to the confluence of the renal veins. A right thoracoabdominal incision through the eighth or ninth interspace or a bilateral subcostal or midline abdominal incision combined with median sternotomy is useful in selected patients with cancers affecting the suprarenal or suprahepatic IVC.[5, 12, 13, 37, 46] These latter approaches allow complete mobilization of the liver, control and reconstruction of the suprahepatic and suprarenal vena cava, and removal of the tumor under direct vision. Patients with tumor thrombus extending into the right heart may require cardiopulmonary bypass, and a combination of a median sternotomy with either a midline or subcostal abdominal incision may be used for similar reasons.[1, 12, 37, 46]

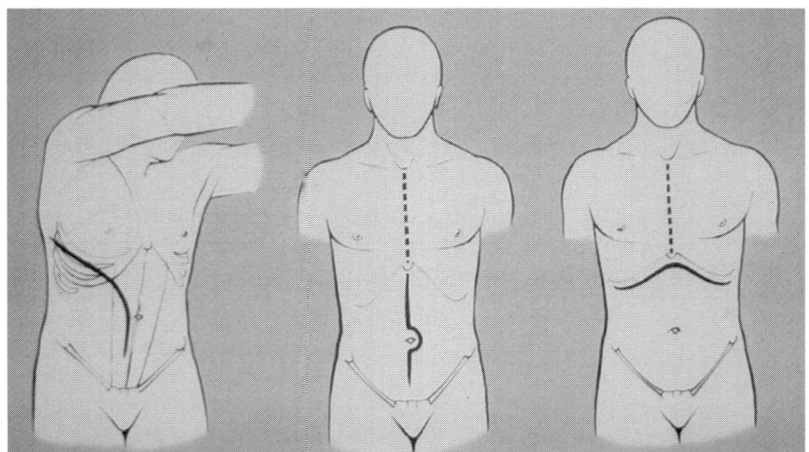

FIGURE 152–7. Various incisions used to approach the inferior vena cava.

Inferior Vena Cava Resection Without Replacement

Resection of the infrarenal vena cava without replacement is usually well tolerated in patients with IVC occlusion who have no lower extremity edema but do have well-developed venous collaterals.[3, 32, 60, 63] Resection of the suprarenal vena cava without venous replacement has been reported but carries more risk of renal dysfunction and lower extremity edema compared with resection of the infrarenal segment.[13, 26] When the suprarenal IVC is occluded, blood is rerouted via collateral lumbar, epigastric, renal, adrenal, gonadal, and paravertebral pathways which may adequately decompress the kidneys and lower extremities in some patients.[64]

The ability to predict preoperatively which patients will tolerate suprarenal IVC ligation without complications is difficult. Of six patients who had suprarenal IVC resection reported by Huguet and colleagues, two did not undergo venous replacement.[13] One of these patients had no postoperative renal dysfunction or lower extremity edema because the IVC was chronically occluded and collateral veins were well developed. The other patient experienced caval thrombosis and moderate lower extremity venous insufficiency as a result of rapid, progressive obstruction of the IVC preoperatively, which did not allow for the development of venous collaterals. During follow-up, visible abdominal wall collateral veins developed as venous insufficiency improved.[13]

Failure to reconstruct either the suprarenal IVC or the renal veins may lead to transient or permanent renal dysfunction in as many as 50% of patients.[65] This complication is more likely to occur in patients who have had previous right nephrectomy or those who require concomitant right nephrectomy and left renal vein ligation.[13] Adequate venous drainage from the left kidney is critical in preventing postoperative renal failure in these situations. Postoperative acute renal failure occurred in one of two patients, reported by Huguet and coworkers, who had undergone resection of the suprarenal IVC and ligation of the left renal vein. In another patient, intraoperative anuria occurred but was reversed after reimplantation of the left renal vein onto the caval graft.[13]

Careful monitoring of urine output intraoperatively and measurement of renal vein pressures help guide the need for reconstruction of the renal veins. Anuria, marked slowing of urine output after caval resection, or renal vein pressures exceeding 40 mmHg with test clamping, indicates the need for renal vein reconstruction or reimplantation.[13, 47] On the basis of their experience, Huguet and associates now advise reconstruction of the suprarenal IVC for the majority of patients.[13] Our preference has been to replace this segment as well, and others share this opinion.[5, 12]

Renal Cell Carcinoma with Inferior Vena Cava Tumor Thrombus

The most common operative procedure performed on the vena cava is removal of intracaval tumor thrombus in patients with renal cell carcinoma. Usually, this tumor thrombus is removed en bloc with the cancer by open thrombectomy.[34–55, 57] Resection of large renal cell cancers with tumor and thrombus extending behind the liver is

difficult. In these cases, Nesbitt and colleagues suggest nephrectomy first, with ligation and amputation of the renal vein rather than complete en bloc resection, to better facilitate access to and exposure of the vena cava.[57] In patients with large cancers, renal artery embolization 24 to 72 hours preoperatively may be used to reduce tumor vascularity and to contract the tumor thrombus.[52, 57] Patients with tumor thrombi extending to or above the hepatic veins and those with intra-atrial tumor thrombi require complete mobilization of the liver to allow access to the retrohepatic segment of the IVC. In these instances, intraoperative transesophageal echocardiography is a useful adjunct to define the proximal extent of the thrombus to determine the need for cardiopulmonary bypass.[57]

If only a small tongue of tumor is found to protrude into the atrium as discovered on intraoperative exploration or echocardiography, Nesbitt[57] and Skinner[38] and their colleagues prefer to gently palpate the tumor at the cavoatrial junction and to manipulate it into the suprahepatic IVC. A vascular cross-clamp can then be safely applied across the IVC below the cavoatrial junction, avoiding the need for cardiopulmonary bypass. The surgeon must perform this maneuver carefully in order to prevent tumor embolization. Hepatic vascular exclusion, which isolates the retrohepatic IVC by cross-clamping both the inflow of blood to the liver (Pringle maneuver) and the IVC above and below the level of the tumor thrombus, is a useful technique to facilitate tumor removal in an essentially bloodless field.[66–68] Complete tumor thrombectomy and a technically precise IVC closure serve to minimize the risk of pulmonary embolization or caval thrombosis with reestablishment of blood flow.[36, 57]

Primary closure of the suprarenal IVC at the renal vein confluence can be safely done in most patients because of the large size of the IVC at this level; however, if primary closure causes significant narrowing of the IVC or if a cuff of vena cava requires resection because of adherent tumor, a synthetic or venous patch should be used to close the cavotomy. Partial resection of the wall of the IVC with patch angioplasty is useful technique for reconstruction of the IVC at all levels and is preferable to segmental caval replacement because it is safer and simpler to perform.[1, 12]

Large tumor thrombus extending into the right heart chambers should be removed with cardiopulmonary bypass.[57] Concomitant deep hypothermia, with or without or circulatory arrest, may be necessary in some patients. This latter technique has been safely performed but it is probably not necessary in every case. The risk of coagulopathy and organ dysfunction with hypothermia and circulatory arrest must weighed against the advantage this technique provides for removal of the tumor.[34–39, 41–44, 57] These operative principles apply to other cancers with IVC tumor extension as well.[56]

Inferior Vena Cava Replacement

We believe that the IVC at any level should be replaced if it is only partially obstructed and if most of its circumference requires resection for tumor clearance.[1, 5] Our preference has been to use an externally supported expanded polytetrafluoroethylene (ePTFE) graft to replace the IVC (Fig. 152–8). Numerous case reports and clinical series docu-

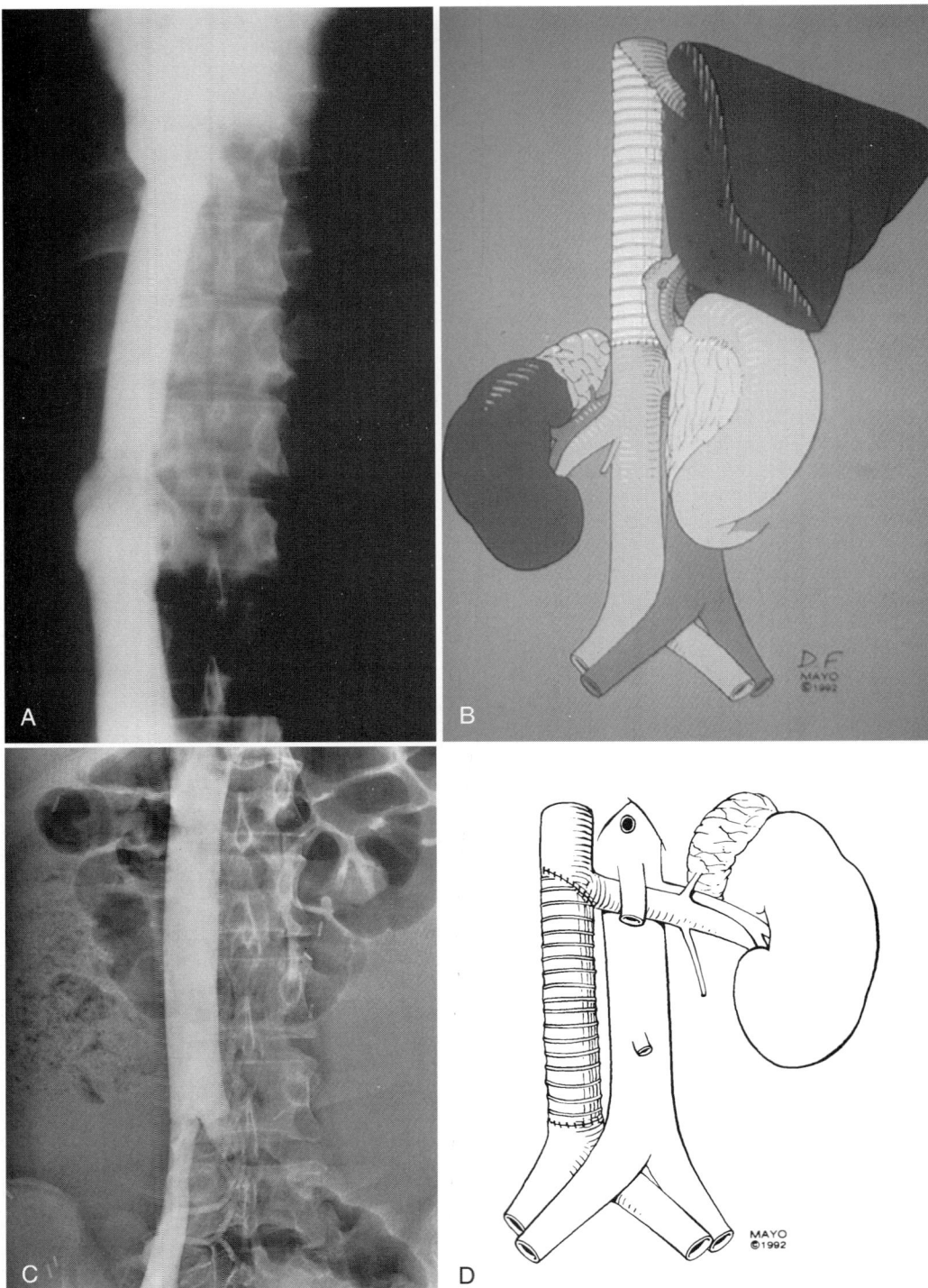

FIGURE 152–8. Postoperative cavograms and accompanying diagrams demonstrating patency of expanded polytetrafluoroethylene grafts used to replace the retrohepatic vena cava after liver resection (*A* and *B*) and the infrarenal vena cava after tumor removal (*C* and *D*). See Color Plate for *B*. (*A, B,* and *D,* From Bower TC, Nagorney DM, Toomey BJ, et al: Vena cava replacement for malignant disease: Is there a role? Ann Vasc Surg 7:51–62, 1993, with permission).

ment the successful use of large-diameter synthetic grafts for vena cava replacement for either benign or malignant disease.[1, 4–26] Synthetic grafts are advantageous because they are readily available and are easily matched to the size of the IVC with regard to its diameter and length.[1, 12] These prostheses have a theoretic advantage of resisting the positive intra-abdominal pressure and compression from the viscera and are preferable, in our opinion, to the use of spiral saphenous vein or superficial femoral vein grafts in this location.[1, 5, 12, 13]

Replacement of the Retrohepatic Suprarenal Vena Cava in Conjunction with Major Liver Resection

Successful resection of primary and secondary tumors involving the suprarenal vena cava in conjunction with major liver resection has been reported by many authors.[5, 7–9, 12–14] Hepatic vascular exclusion, selective use of venovenous bypass to maintain hemodynamics, and isolation of the fixed portion of the supradiaphragmatic extrapericardial IVC as a location for the upper cross-clamp are all important adjuncts for minimizing operative risks.[5, 12, 13]

Our approach and surgical technique are illustrated in Figure 152–8. A bilateral subcostal abdominal incision or a right thoracoabdominal incision through the eighth or ninth interspace with radial incision of the diaphragm is used to expose the suprahepatic vena cava. Careful abdominal exploration is performed to exclude metastatic disease. Bimanual palpation of the liver and intraoperative ultrasonography are used to define the presence of additional liver nodules, which may preclude resection. Ultrasonography provides accurate visualization of tumor proximity to the major vascular structures.

Control of the major vascular structures to the liver and the IVC above and below the level of the tumor is performed early in the operation. In most cases, early ligation of the appropriate hepatic artery, vein, and portal vein branches demarcates the area to be resected and minimizes blood loss during the hepatic resection. However, to avoid injury to this vessel, no attempt is made to isolate the hepatic veins draining the liver segment to be preserved. Hepatic resection is performed using the CUSA ultrasonic dissector (Valley Lab, Boulder, Col.) device to further minimize blood loss. A few patients with liver parenchymal disease may require hepatic vascular exclusion to control blood loss during the hepatic resection.

Just before the en bloc tumor resection is completed, a test clamp of the suprahepatic vena cava is performed to determine the hemodynamic effects. If intravenous volume loading does not maintain systolic blood pressures at 100 mmHg or more, venovenous bypass is instituted via a cannula is inserted into the infrarenal IVC (14 to 20 Fr.) at the level of the gonadal vein and a cannula is placed into the right jugular vein (8.5 Fr.). A magnetically coupled mechanical pump model 520D (Bio-Medicus, Eden Prairie, Minn.) is used to recirculate the blood. Blood flow rates are modified to maintain the systolic blood pressure at 100 mmHg or above and to maintain the central venous pressure at 12 mmHg or higher. In our experience, patients over age 50 years and those with preoperative cardiopulmonary dysfunction are most likely to require venovenous

bypass.[5] A low-dose of intravenous heparin (usually 1000 to 2500 units) is given prior to caval clamping, depending on the amount of blood lost during the liver resection.

Hepatic vascular exclusion is used to complete the tumor and retrohepatic caval resection and the upper IVC reconstruction (Fig. 152–9) The upper caval anastomosis, performed first, often incorporates the remaining hepatic vein. The inflow occlusion clamp to the liver is released, keeping the suprahepatic caval clamp in place to flush acid metabolites from the liver. The suprahepatic clamp is then moved and placed across the graft and blood flow is restored through the liver. The length of time required to complete tumor resection and perform the upper caval anastomosis is usually less than 30 to 60 minutes and well within the tolerable limits of warm ischemia to the liver.[5, 13, 66–68] Liver ischemia exceeding 1 hour has also been reported with few long-term sequelae.[13]

The lower caval anastomosis is then performed. With the patient's head lowered and the lungs inflated to 30 torr, back-bleeding and forebleeding are allowed to avoid air embolism. The anastomosis is completed, and blood flow is established through the graft. Intraoperative duplex ultrasonography is used to assess graft patency in patients who require replacement of more than one caval segment (long grafts) or who need left renal vein reimplantation. The remaining segment of liver is fixed to its ligamentous attachments to avoid torsion or occlusion of the hepatic venous outflow tract, and the graft is covered with omentum to minimize the possibility of secondary infection from bile leak from the cut liver surface.

A transient elevation in liver function studies is common, usually peaking within the first 2 to 3 days after operation and then returning to normal.[5, 13] Most patients undergoing concomitant major liver resection remain anticoagulated for 24 to 48 hours. Lower extremity pneumatic compression devices and subcutaneous heparin are used to augment venous blood flow and to minimize the risk of vein thrombosis until the patients are ambulatory. Patients are discharged from the hospital on warfarin to maintain the International Normalized Ratio between 2.0 and 3.0.[5] Because of the rapid blood flow in the suprarenal IVC, we along with others believe that the risk of graft thrombosis is low.[5, 12, 13] Thus, these patients are now maintained only on antiplatelet therapy with aspirin.

OUTCOMES

Perioperative Mortality and Morbidity

Replacement of the IVC for malignancy has been safely accomplished at several centers, but only a few authors report experiences with more than one or two patients.[1, 4–19] Kieffer and associates reported two postoperative deaths among 18 patients surgically treated for primary or secondary tumors of the IVC.[12] One death was caused by massive acute gastrointestinal hemorrhage in a patient in whom a duodenal fistula developed after resection of a large leiomyosarcoma; the other death occurred from hepatic failure in a patient who had undergone a palliative mesoatrial bypass because of Budd-Chiari syndrome related to caval extension of a large renal cell carcinoma.

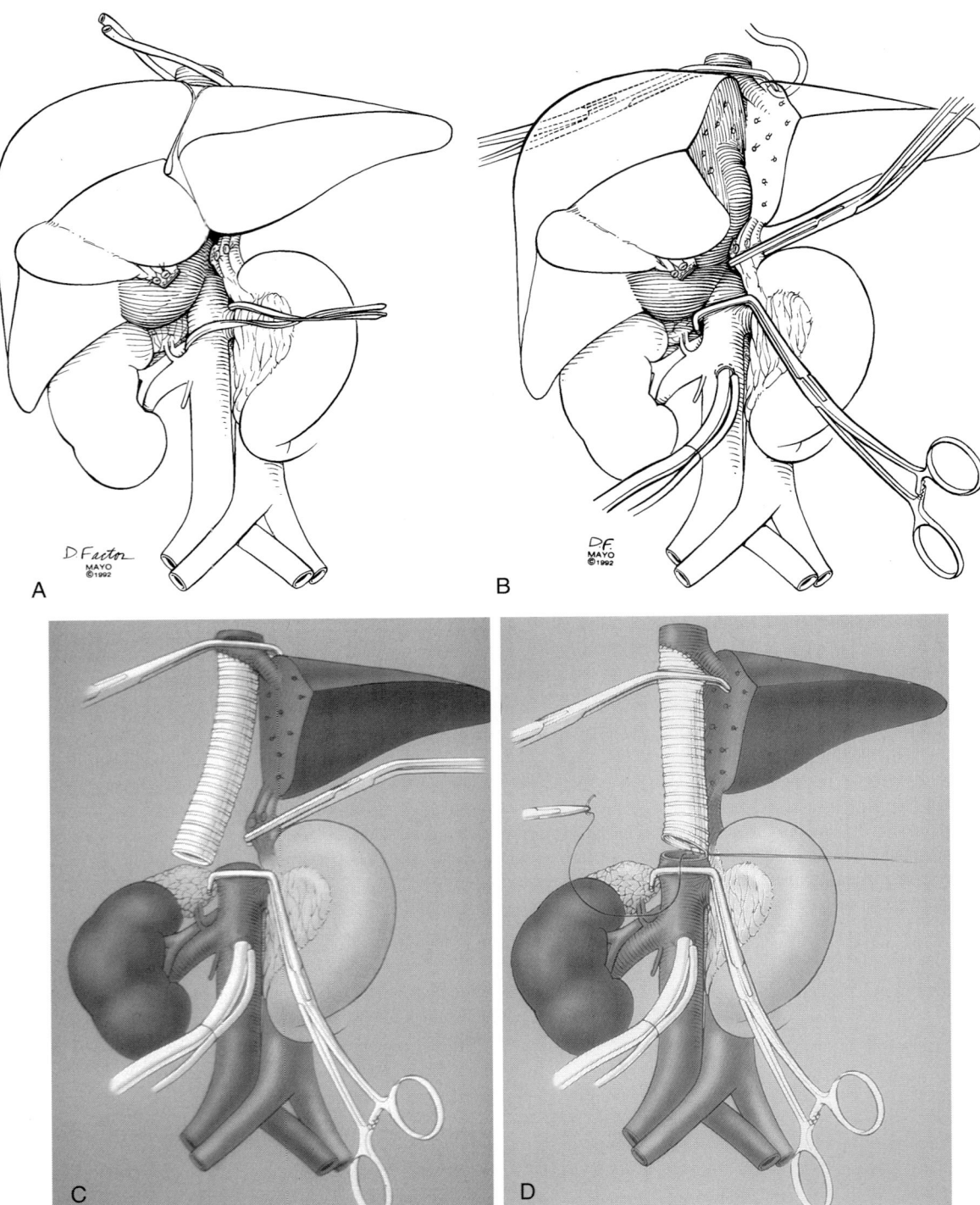

FIGURE 152–9. Operative technique for replacement of the retrohepatic inferior vena cava (IVC) in conjunction with major liver resection. *A*, Isolation of the IVC above and below the level of the tumor as well as isolation and division of the hepatic artery and portal vein branch performed first if the lesion is found to be resectable. *B*, Hepatic vascular exclusion is utilized to complete resection of the liver, tumor, and retrohepatic IVC. If necessary a venovenous bypass via a canula can be used. *C*, The upper caval anastomosis is performed first. *D*, The suprahepatic caval clamp is then placed across the graft after acid metabolites have been flushed from the liver. The lower caval anastomosis is completed. See Color Plate for *C* and *D*. (*B*, From Bower TC, Nagorney DM, Toomey BJ, et al. Vena cava replacement for malignant disease: Is there a role? Ann Surg 7:51–62, 1993, with permission).

In the study by Huguet and associates, one patient died of renal failure among four patients who had undergone graft replacement of the suprarenal vena cava.[13] A study from the Mayo Clinic reported no operative deaths among 11 patients undergoing replacement of the superior or IVC for malignant disease.[5]

The major perioperative morbidity rate must be acceptable and should not result in a significant change of quality of life if these extensive operations are to have a role. With eight patients undergoing IVC graft replacement at the Mayo Clinic, bleeding requiring reoperation, myocardial infarction, and late wound infection occurred in one patient each. No patient experienced renal failure, liver failure, or graft infection.[5] In the Huguet study, one patient had a biliary leak and another had a subphrenic abscess, which was percutaneously drained; however, graft infection did not occur in either patient during follow-up.[13]

Operative mortality rates for patients undergoing radical nephrectomy and IVC tumor thrombectomy have ranged between 2.7% and 13% (Table 152–3).[35–40, 45, 53, 57] The addition of cardiopulmonary bypass or hypothermic circulatory arrest in most series has not significantly increased operative mortality, which ranges from 4.7% to 11%.[37, 39, 41–43] Cardiopulmonary problems are the primary cause of perioperative death, but the risk of these problems continues to decrease.

In a study by Neves and Zincke, five of 54 patients died (9.3% mortality), four of pulmonary emboli and one of myocardial infarction.[36] In the series reported by Nesbitt and coauthors in 1997, one of 37 patients died of myocardial infarction (2.7% mortality).[57] Preoperative cardiac evaluation has been recommended for patients older than 65 years of age or for those with a history of coronary artery disease.[57] The most common postoperative complications are myocardial ischemia, pulmonary complications (e.g., prolonged ventilation, pneumonitis, pulmonary embolism), atrial arrhythmias, renal insufficiency, and bleeding. Major morbidity is as high as 10% to 31%.[36, 53, 57] Pulmonary emboli have been a major cause of postoperative morbidity and mortality.[36, 44]

Therefore, clipping of the vena cava or placement of an IVC filter to avoid embolization is recommended for patients with occlusion or with nonocclusive bland thrombus in the infrarenal IVC.[36, 44, 57] The use of cardiopulmonary bypass or hypothermic circulatory arrest increases the overall blood loss and the length of operation and carries a greater risk of perioperative coagulopathy compared with operations performed without bypass.[37–39, 41–43, 45, 46, 57]

Graft Patency

Early and late patency for short, large-diameter, intra-abdominal prosthetic grafts is good, regardless of which segment of the vena cava is replaced or whether the graft is used for benign or malignant disease (see Fig. 152–8).[5, 12, 13, 20, 22, 23] Huguet and associates reported no graft occlusion among three survivors with prosthetic replacement of the suprarenal IVC, and these patients demonstrated good functional results.[13] None of the eight IVC grafts thrombosed in the Mayo Clinic series.[5]

Because prosthetic grafts tend to form a thick pseudointima, it is important to use grafts with a large diameter (≥ 16 mm) and to keep the length as short as possible to minimize the risk of graft thrombosis.[69] The use of an adjunctive arteriovenous fistula to improve graft patency is controversial. Kieffer and colleagues use a centrally placed fistula if graft flow needs to be enhanced[12]; others place the fistula at the femoral vein level.[70] We rarely place femoral arteriovenous fistulae in patients with infrarenal IVC reconstructions, and consider it only in patients who need a long (>15 cm), small-diameter (<14 mm) graft. An arteriovenous fistula is not needed for reconstruction of the suprarenal or suprahepatic vena cava because of the rapid blood flow at this level.[1, 5, 8, 12, 13]

Survival and Quality of Life

The most important outcome in patients who undergo venous replacement for malignancy is not necessarily the long-term patency of the graft but, rather, the impact on survival, control of local recurrence, and the quality of life afforded by aggressive surgical management. At present, complete resection of the tumor provides the best chance of patient survival and the lowest risk of local or regional recurrent disease regardless of tumor type.

Survival in patients with PVL depends on whether tumor-free margins can be achieved with resection. Dzsinich and coworkers reported the median survival after initial operation in patients with PVL at all sites to be 3.5 years (range, 6 months to 17 years).[4] Survival was not affected by tumor size, location of the lesion, grade of the malignancy, or use of adjuvant therapy. These findings are inter-

TABLE 152–3. OPERATIVE MORTALITY AND FIVE-YEAR CUMULATIVE SURVIVAL OF PATIENTS WITH RENAL CELL CARCINOMAS AND INFERIOR VENA CAVA TUMOR THROMBECTOMY

STUDY	NO. OF PATIENTS	OPERATIVE MORTALITY (%)	SURVIVAL, %, NO METASTASES	SURVIVAL, %, WITH METASTASES (LYMPH NODE OR DISTANT)
Neves and Zincke, 1987[36]	54	9.3	68	12.5
Skinner et al, 1989[38]	53	13	40	0
Libertino et al, 1990[35]	71	NA	72	16
Montie et al, 1991[39]	68	7.4	30	25 (2 year)
Hatcher et al, 1991[43]	44	6.8	42	13
Swierzewski et al, 1994[40]	100	NA	64	19.6
Nesbitt et al, 1997[57]	37	2.7	45	24.6

NA = not available.

esting because the primary determinant of survival in most patients with retroperitoneal leiomyosarcomas is usually the grade of the tumor.

Survival of patients with primary IVC leiomyosarcoma, reported by Mingoli's group, averaged 3 months in patients not having an operation, 21 months in patients undergoing palliative resection, and 36.8 months in patients undergoing radical resection. In that series, a 5-year survival of 28% was achieved with curative resection.[3]

In another study, Mingoli and associates analyzed data of 120 patients from the International Registry of IVC leiomyosarcomas to determine the influence of limited versus extensive resection on tumor recurrence and patient survival.[60] In one group, 53 patients underwent limited resection of the IVC wall with primary or patch closure. In the other group, 67 patients underwent extensive IVC resection. Seventeen patients in this group underwent IVC reconstructions with prosthetic (n = 14) or autogenous vein grafts (n = 3). Three early deaths occurred, and 39 patients (33%) died of recurrent disease at a mean of 40 ± 3 months postoperatively. Of 53 survivors available for long-term follow-up, 36 were alive with no evidence of disease at a mean of 63 ± 13 months postoperatively, and 17 patients were alive with recurrent disease at a mean of 68 ± 9 months. Overall, 57% of the patients developed recurrent disease within 3 years after operation. Of six patients with local recurrence in the vena cava, three had undergone partial resection and three had extensive IVC resection. Multivariate analysis showed no significant difference in survival or disease recurrence between the group with limited wall resection of the IVC compared to the group with segmental IVC resection. Survival rates between these groups were 55% and 37% at 5 years and 42% and 23% at 10 years, respectively.[50]

Nonetheless, resection with tumor-free margins remains the primary goal for patients undergoing operative intervention for sarcomas in any location.[60, 71, 72] Although adjuvant therapy with radiation and other mitotic chemotherapeutic agents is usually given to patients postoperatively, there has been no clear beneficial effect of these modalities on prolongation of survival or on the prevention of local or regional recurrence.[33] Survival in untreated patients with secondary malignancies affecting the IVC is usually measured in months, not years.

The limited data available suggest that length of survival may be improved with tumor resection and IVC replacement. In an initial report from the Mayo Clinic, five of eight patients who underwent IVC replacement because of malignant disease experienced tumor recurrence either in regional or distant sites but not in the bed of resection. Local control of these tumors and palliation of symptoms were excellent.[5]

In Kieffer's experience of 16 patients, seven late deaths occurred after tumor dissemination, and two of nine survivors had pulmonary metastases. Of five survivors in the series by Huguet's group, one patient was alive 16 months postoperatively but had recurrent renal cell carcinoma; the other four patients died at 4, 6, 37, and 42 months after operation.[13]

Patients with renal cell carcinoma and caval tumor thrombus have very good (50%) 5-year survival rates after aggressive surgical treatment.[44] Survival as high as 68%

may be possible in patients with no distant or regional metastases.[36] The primary determinants of survival are (1) the presence of diffuse metastases, (2) lymph node involvement, and (3) completeness of tumor resection.[35, 36, 38, 39, 43, 50, 57] Tumor thrombus as an independent factor probably does not affect patient survival.[37, 38, 43, 51, 57]

Patients with diffuse metastases have 1-year survival rates ranging from 10% to 68% and 5-year survival rates of only 0% to 8%.[39, 44] Patients with metastatic disease have a higher chance (2.76 times) of dying than do patients without metastatic disease.[39] The data of Nesbitt and coauthors suggested a reduced survival of patients with distant metastases only if there also were positive lymph nodes at the time of resection and tumor thrombectomy. Some of their patients with distant metastases and negative nodes had improved survival with resection, but those patients who benefited could not be predicted.[57] Palliation of symptoms or local control of the cancer can be achieved with radical resection in selected patients with metastatic disease.[57] These findings suggest that tumor biology and behavior may differ between patients and tumor growth and spread may be indolent and unpredictable.

Lymph node involvement also reduces survival. Although the Skinner and Montie groups found no effect on survival in patients with lymph node metastases, most other clinical series document a worse prognosis in the presence of positive lymph nodes.[35, 36, 38, 39, 57] Five-year survival rates of 50% to 68% have been achieved for patients with complete tumor resection and absent lymph node metastases compared to 5-year survival rates less than 17% for patients with positive nodes.[35, 36, 39, 43, 57]

Another factor that worsens survival is incomplete tumor resection. Only a handful of patients survive 5 years if they are left with residual cancer.[36, 38, 43, 57]

Finally, the presence of tumor thrombus in the IVC does not appear to affect survival. Nesbitt and associates found no significant difference in survival based on the level of tumor thrombus even though there was a trend for improved 2-year survival in patients with tumor thrombus at the renal vein confluence (78%) in contrast to patients with thrombus in the infrahepatic (57%) and retrohepatic (58%) IVC segments.[57] Similar findings have been noted by other authors.[37, 43, 51] However, there may be a trend toward poorer survival in patients with tumor thrombus in the right heart than in patients with thrombus at lower levels of the IVC.[38, 39, 41, 54]

Postoperative quality of life is an important issue that must be addressed if IVC replacement for malignancy is to be efficacious. However, this issue is difficult to assess objectively with the currently available tools. Although few clinical series report performance status (physical limitations) of patients after resection, we are impressed by the fact that with careful preoperative selection, most patients have no or minimal restriction in physical activity postoperatively. In our initial review, 82% of patients who underwent vena cava replacement for malignant disease had a good or excellent performance status, and this trend has continued.[5] Even patients with regional or distant recurrent disease can maintain a good performance status months after resection.[5, 12, 13, 57, 60] Although the benefits of aggressive surgical management of patients with renal cell carcinoma and vena cava tumor thrombus, and with localized primary IVC leiomyosarcomas appear certain, similar benefits for patients with other secondary malignancies involving the IVC are not proven.

SUMMARY

Primary and secondary malignancies that involve the IVC are rare, are usually at advanced stages at the time of diagnosis, and carry a poor prognosis if left untreated. Until cancers can be detected at earlier stages and effective preoperative and postoperative adjuvant therapies can be developed, surgical resection remains the only chance for cure or control of symptoms. Careful patient selection, thorough preoperative evaluation and staging, and a coordinated effort between the oncologist and surgical subspecialist to plan therapy are the keys to a successful outcome.

Patients with no evidence of metastatic disease, few medical co-morbidities and good performance status should be considered candidates for surgical resection with or without venous replacement. If vena cava reconstruction is necessary, it can be performed safely with few graft-related complications. More experience and longer observation of patients are needed to determine the optimal therapy.

REFERENCES

1. Bower TC: Primary and secondary tumors of the inferior vena cava. In Gloviczki P, Yao JST (eds): Handbook of Venous Disorders. London, Chapman & Hall, 1996, pp 529–550.
2. Kieffer E, Berrod JL, Chomette G: Primary tumors of the inferior vena cava. In Bergann JJ, Yao JST (eds): Surgery of the Veins. New York, Grune & Stratton, 1985, pp 423–443.
3. Mingoli A, Feldhaus RJ, Cavallaro A, Stipa S: Leiomyosarcoma of the inferior vena cava: Analysis and search of world literature on 141 patients and report of three new cases. J Vasc Surg 14:688–699, 1991.
4. Dzsinich C, Gloviczki P, van Heerden JA, et al: Primary venous leiomyosarcoma: A rare but lethal disease. J Vasc Surg 15:595–603, 1992.
5. Bower TC, Nagorney DM, Toomey BJ, et al: Vena cava replacement for malignant disease: Is there a role? Ann Vasc Surg 7:51–62, 1993.
6. Starzl TE, Koep LJ, Weil R, et al: Right trisegmentectomy for hepatic neoplasms. Surg Gynecol Obstet 150:208–214, 1980.
7. Kumada K, Shimahara Y, Fujui K, et al: Extended right hepatic lobectomy: Combined resection of inferior vena cava and its reconstruction by ePTFE graft. Acta Chir Scand 154:481–483, 1988.
8. Iwatsuki S, Todo S, Starzl TE: Right trisegmentectomy with a synthetic vena cava graft. Arch Surg 123:1021–1022, 1988.
9. Miller CM, Schwartz ME, Nishizaki T: Combined hepatic and vena caval resection with autogenous caval graft replacement. Arch Surg 126:106–108, 1991.
10. Risher WH, Arensman RM, Oschsner JL, Hollier LH: Retrohepatic vena cava reconstruction with polytetrafluoroethylene graft. J Vasc Surg 12:367–370, 1990.
11. Yamaoka Y, Ozawa K, Kumada K, et al: Total vascular exclusion for hepatic resection in cirrhotic patients: Application of venovenous bypass. Arch Surg 127:276–280, 1992.
12. Kieffer E, Bahnini A, Koskas F: Nonthrombotic disease of the inferior vena cava: Surgical management of 24 patients. In Bergan JJ, Yao JST (eds): Venous Disorders. Philadelphia, WB Saunders, 1991, pp 501–516.
13. Huguet C, Ferri M, Gavelli A: Resection of the suprarenal inferior vena cava: The role of prosthetic replacement. Arch Surg 130:793–797, 1995.
14. Yagyu T, Shimizu R, Nishida M, et al: Reconstruction of the hepatic vein to the prosthetic inferior vena cava in right extended hemihepatectomy with ex situ procedure. Surgery 115:700–744, 1994.
15. Okada Y, Kumada K, Habuchi T, et al: Total replacement of the suprarenal inferior vena cava with an expanded polytetrafluoroethylene tube graft in 2 patients with tumor thrombi from renal cell carcinoma. J Urol 141:111–114, 1989.
16. Kraybill WG, Callery MP, Heiken JP, Fley MW: Radical resection of tumors of the inferior vena cava with vascular reconstruction and kidney autotransplantation. Surgery 121:31–36, 1997.
17. Yanaga K, Okadome K, Ito H, et al: Graft replacement of pararenal inferior vena cava for leiomyosarcoma with the use of venous bypass. Surgery 113:109–112, 1993.
18. Habib NA, Michaeil NE, Boyle T, Bean A: Resection of the inferior vena cava during hepatectomy for liver tumours. Br J Surg 81:1023–1024, 1994.
19. Silva MB, Silva HC, Sandager GP, et al: Prosthetic replacement of the inferior vena cava after resection of pheochromocytoma. J Vasc Surg 19:169–173, 1994.
20. Dale WA, Harris J. Terry RB: Polytetrafluoroethylene reconstruction of the inferior vena cava Surgery 95:625–630, 1984.
21. Katz NM, Spence LJ, Wallace RB: Reconstruction of the inferior vena cava with a polytetrafluoroethylene tube graft after resection for hypernephroma of the right kidney. J Thorac Cardiovasc Surg 87:791–797, 1984.
22. Gloviczki P, Pairolero PC, Cherry KJ, et al: Reconstruction of the vena cava and of its primary tributaries: A preliminary report. J Vasc Surg 11:373–381, 1990.
23. Gloviczki P, Pairolero PC, Toomey BJ, et al: Reconstruction of large veins for nonmalignant venous occlusive disease. J Vasc Surg 16:750–761, 1992.
24. Victor S, Jayanthi V, Kandasamy I, et al: Retrohepatic cavoatrial bypass for coarctation of inferior vena cava with a polytetrafluoroethylene graft. J Thorac Cardiovasc 39:485–491, 1985.
25. Chan EL, Bardine JA, Bernstein EF: Inferior vena cava bypass: Experimental evaluation of externally supported grafts and initial clinical application. J Vasc Surg 1:675–680, 1984.
26. Duckett JW, Lifland JH, Peters PC: Resection of the inferior vena cava for adjacent malignant diseases. Surg Gynecol Obstet 136:711–716, 1973.
27. Enzinger FM, Weiss SW: Soft Tissue Tumors, 3rd ed. In Gay SM (ed): St. Louis, Mosby–Year Book, 1995, pp 505–510.
28. Hallock P, Watson CJ, Berman L: Primary tumor of inferior vena cava with clinical features suggestive of Chari's disease. Arch Intern Med 66:50, 1940.
29. Perl L: Ein fall von sarkom der vena cava inferior. Virchow's Arch [A] 53:378–383, 1971.
30. Kevorkian J, Cento DP: Leimyosarcoma of large arteries and veins. Surgery 73:390–400, 1973.
31. Hartman DS, Hayes WS, Choyke PL, Tibbetts GP: Leiomyosarcoma of the retroperitoneum and inferior vena cava: Radiologic-pathologic correlation RadioGraphics 12:1203–1220, 1992.
32. Burke AP, Virmani R: Sarcomas of the great vessels. Cancer 71:761–73, 1993.
33. Chang AE, Sondak VK: Clinical evaluation and treatment of soft tissue tumors. In Gay SM (ed): Soft Tissue Tumors, 3rd ed. St. Louis, Mosby–Year Book, 1995, pp 17–38.
34. Concepcion RS, Koch MO, McDougal WS, et al: Management of primary nonrenal parenchymal malignancies with vena caval thrombus. J Urol 145:243–247, 1991.
35. Libertino JA, Burke WE, Zinman L: Long-term results of 71 patients with renal cell carcinoma with venous, vena caval, and atrial extension (Abstract). J Urol 143:294A, 1990.
36. Neves RJ, Zincke H: Surgical treatment of renal cancer with vena cava extension. Br J Urol 59:390–395, 1987.
37. Novick AC, Kaye MC, Cosgrove DM, et al: Experience with cardiopulmonary bypass and deep hypothermic circulatory arrest in the management of retroperitoneal tumors with large vena caval thrombi. Ann Surg 212:472–477, 1990.
38. Skinner DG, Pritchett TR, Lieskovsky G, et al: Vena caval involvement by renal cell carcinoma. Ann Surg 210:387–394, 1989.
39. Montie JE, El Ammar R, Pontes JE, et al: Renal cell carcinoma with inferior vena cava tumor thrombi. Surg Gynecol Obstet 173:107–115, 1991.
40. Swierzewski DJ, Swierzewski JA: Radical nephrectomy in patients with renal cell carcinoma with venous, vena caval, and atrial extension. Am J Surg 168:205–209, 1994.
41. Marshall FF, Dietrick DD, Baumgartner WA, et al: Surgical manage-

ment of renal cell carcinoma with intracaval neoplastic extension of the hepatic veins. J Urol 139:1165–1172, 1988.

42. Shahain DM, Libertino JA, Zinman LN, et al: Resection of cavoatrial renal cell carcinoma employing total circulatory arrest. Arch Surg 125:727–732, 1990.

43. Hatcher PA, Anderson EE, Paulson DF, et al: Surgical management and prognosis of renal cell carcinoma invading the vena cava. J Urol 145:20–24, 1991.

44. Couillard DR, White RWD: Surgery of renal cell carcinoma. Urol Clin North Am 20:263–275, 1993.

45. Klein EA, Kaye MC, Novick AC: Management of renal cell carcinoma with vena caval thrombi via cardiopulmonary bypass and deep hypothermic circulatory arrest. Urol Oncol 18:445–447, 1991.

46. Stewart JA, Carey JA, McDougal WS, et al: Cavoatrial tumor thrombectomy using cardiopulmonary bypass without circulatory arrest. Ann Thorac Surg 51:717–722, 1991.

47. Clayman RV, Gonzalez R, Fraley EE: Renal cell cancer invading the inferior vena cava: Clinical review and anatomic approach. J Urol 123:157–163, 1980.

48. Gancharenko V, Gerlock JA Jr, Kadir S, et al: Incidence and distribution of venous extension in 70 hypernephromas. Am J Roentgenol 133:263, 1979.

49. Glazer AA, Novick AC: Long-term follow-up after surgical treatment for renal cell carcinoma extending into the right atrium. J Urol 155:448–450, 1996.

50. Tongaonkar HB, Dandekar NP, Dalal AV, et al: Renal cell carcinoma extending to the renal vein and inferior vena cava: Results of surgical treatment and prognostic factors. J Surg Oncol 59:94–100, 1995.

51. Cherrie RJ, Goldman DG, Lindner, A, et al: Prognostic implications of vena caval extension of renal cell carcinoma. J Urol 128:910–912, 1982.

52. Swanson DA, Wallace S, Johnson DE: The role of embolization and nephrectomy in the treatment of metastatic renal carcinoma. J Urol Surg 7:719–730, 1980.

53. Suggs WD, Smith RB, Dodson TF, et al: Renal cell carcinoma with inferior vena caval involvement. J Vasc Surg 14:43–48, 1991.

54. Sosa RE, Muecke EC, Vaugn ED, et al: Renal cell carcinoma extending into the inferior vena cava: The prognostic significance of the level of the vena caval involvement. J Urol 132:1097–1100, 1984.

55. Langenburg SE, Blackbourne LH, Sperling JW, et al: Management of renal tumors involving the inferior vena cava. J Vasc Surg 20:385–388, 1994.

56. Phillips M, Bower T, Orszulak TO, Hartmann L: Intracardiac extension of an intracaval sarcoma of endometrial origin. Ann Thorac Surg 59:742–744, 1995.

57. Nesbitt JC, Soltero ER, Dinney CPN, et al: Surgical management of renal cell carcinoma with inferior vena cava tumor thrombus. Ann Thorac Surg 63:1592–1600, 1997.

58. Kallman DA, King BF, Hattery RR, et al: Renal vein and inferior vena cava tumor thrombus in renal cell carcinoma: CT, US, MRI and venacavography. J Comput Assist Tomogr 16:240–247, 1992.

59. Nagorney DM, vanHeerden JA, Ilstrup DM, et al: Primary hepatic malignancy: Surgical management and determinants of survival. Surgery 106:740–749, 1989.

60. Mingoli A, Sapienza P, Cavallaro A, et al: The effect of extent of caval resection in the treatment of inferior vena cava leiomyosarcoma. Anticancer Res 17:3877–3882, 1997.

61. American Joint Commission on Cancer: General rules for staging cancer. In Beahrs OH, Henson DE, Hutter RVP, et al (eds): Manual for Staging of Cancer, 3rd ed. Philadelphia: JB Lippincott, 1988, p 9.

62. Stanson AW, Breen JF: Computed tomography and magnetic resonance imaging. In Gloviczki P, Yao JST (eds): Handbook of Venous Disorders: Guidelines of the American Venous Forum, pp 529–550.

63. Spitz A, Wilson TG, Kawachi MH, et al: Vena caval resection for bulky metastatic germ cell tumors: An 18-year experience. J Urol 158:1813–1818, 1997.

64. Perhoniemi V, Salmenkivi K, Vorne M: Venous haemodynamics in the legs after ligation of the inferior vena cava. Acta Chir Scand 152:23–27, 1986.

65. McCullough DL, Gittes RF: Ligation of the renal in the solitary kidney: Effects on renal function. J Urol Surg 113:295–299, 1975.

66. Delva E, Camus Y, Norlinger B, et al: Vascular occlusions for liver resections: Operative management and tolerance to hepatic ischemia: 142 cases. Ann Surg 209:211–218, 1989.

67. Bismuth H, Castaing D, Garden OJ: Major hepatic resection under total vascular exclusion. Ann Surg 210:13–19, 1989.

68. Huguet C, Gavelli A, Addario Chieco P, et al: Liver ischemia for hepatic resection: Where is the limit? Surgery 111:251–259, 1992.

69. Gloviczki P, Hollier LH, Dewanjee MK, et al: Experimental replacement of the inferior vena cava: Factors affecting patency. Surgery 95:657–666, 1984.

70. Wilson SE, Jabour A, Stone RT, et al: Patency of biologic and prosthetic inferior vena cava grafts with distal limb fistula. Arch Surg 113:1174–1179, 1978.

71. McGrath PC, Neifeld JP, Lawrence W Jr, et al: Improved survival following complete excision of retroperitoneal sarcomas. Ann Surg 200:200–204, 1984.

72. Singer S, Corson JM, Demetri GD, et al: Prognostic factors predictive of survival for truncal and retroperitoneal soft-tissue sarcoma. Ann Surg 221:185–195, 1995.

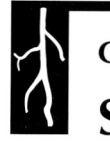

C H A P T E R   1 5 3

Surgical Treatment of Superior Vena Cava Syndrome

Peter Gloviczki, M.D., and Terri J. Vrtiska, M.D.

Few areas of venous surgery provide more satisfying experience for both the patient and the vascular surgeon than reconstruction for superior vena cava (SVC) syndrome. Relief from severe, frequently incapacitating symptoms of chronic venous congestion of the head and neck is almost instantaneous, and benefit following reconstruction is generally long lasting.

In this chapter, we review the etiology, clinical presentation, and diagnostic evaluation of SVC syndrome. Because endovascular treatment is reviewed in Chapter 151, we focus on surgical management of SVC and innominate vein occlusions.

ETIOLOGY

Metastatic pulmonary or mediastinal malignancy is the most frequent cause of SVC syndrome. In a collected series of 1986 patients with SVC syndrome, 85% had metastatic pulmonary or mediastinal malignant disease.[1] The primary tumor most often causing obstruction of central veins by metastases in the mediastinum is adenocarcinoma of the lung. Mediastinal malignancies leading to SVC syndrome include medullary or follicular carcinoma of the thyroid, mediastinal lymphoma, thymoma, teratoma, angiosarcoma, and synovial cell carcinoma.[1-5] Mediastinal fibrosis and granulomatous fungal disease, such as histoplasmosis, have been the most frequent benign causes of SVC and innominate vein obstruction.[6-10] However, SVC syndrome caused by indwelling central venous catheters and pacemaker lines has increased in the 1980s and 1990s.[6, 7, 9, 11-16] Previous radiotherapy to the mediastinum and retrosternal goiter can also cause SVC syndrome. The risk of venous thrombosis is increased in patients with deficiencies in circulating natural anticoagulants, such as antithrombin III, protein S, and protein C.

CLINICAL PRESENTATION

Signs and symptoms of venous congestion of the head, neck, and upper extremities are determined by the duration and extent of the venous occlusive disease and by the amount of collateral venous circulation that develops. Patients with SVC syndrome present with a feeling of fullness in the head and neck that is more severe when the patient bends over or lies flat in bed. The severity of the disease can be graded easily by the number of pillows needed by the patient for comfortable sleeping. Venous hypertension may cause headache, dizziness, visual symptoms, or even blackout spells. Patients may complain of mental confusion, dyspnea, orthopnea, or cough. Swelling of the face, neck, and eyelids is characteristic (Fig. 153-1). Ecchymosis and dilated jugular veins accompany cyanosis and the development of chest wall collateral veins. Although symptoms are usually localized to the head and neck, mild to moderate upper extremity swelling may also develop (Table 153-1). Additional signs or symptoms of malignant SVC syndrome include hemoptysis, hoarseness, weight loss, or palpable cervical tumor or lymph nodes. Patients with lymphoma may also present with fever and night sweats.

DIAGNOSTIC EVALUATION

The diagnosis of SVC obstruction is usually suggested from a detailed clinical history and physical examination. The clinical diagnosis may be confirmed by a variety of tools, including plain film radiographs, ultrasonography, radionuclide imaging, computed tomography (CT), venography, and magnetic resonance imaging (MRI). The appropriate diagnostic study for an individual patient includes not only the demonstration of the underlying cause but also the site and extent of obstruction as well as the routes of collateral venous circulation.

Radiography

Plain film radiographs of the chest are readily available and are often abnormal in patients with SVC obstruction. Findings most commonly include mediastinal widening, pleural effusion, right hilar mass, and upper lobe collapse; however, a normal radiograph of the chest does not preclude the diagnosis of SVC obstruction. Occasionally, dilated collateral veins may be visible, especially enlargement of the azygos vein or superior intercostal vein (aortic nipple) draining the hemiazygos system.

Ultrasonography

Ultrasound evaluation is an effective, noninvasive screening technique in the patient with suspected SVC obstruction. The subclavian veins are accessible to sonographic evaluation and can provide indirect evidence of SVC patency or obstruction. Patent subclavian veins demonstrate respiratory flow variation that is due to changes in intrathoracic

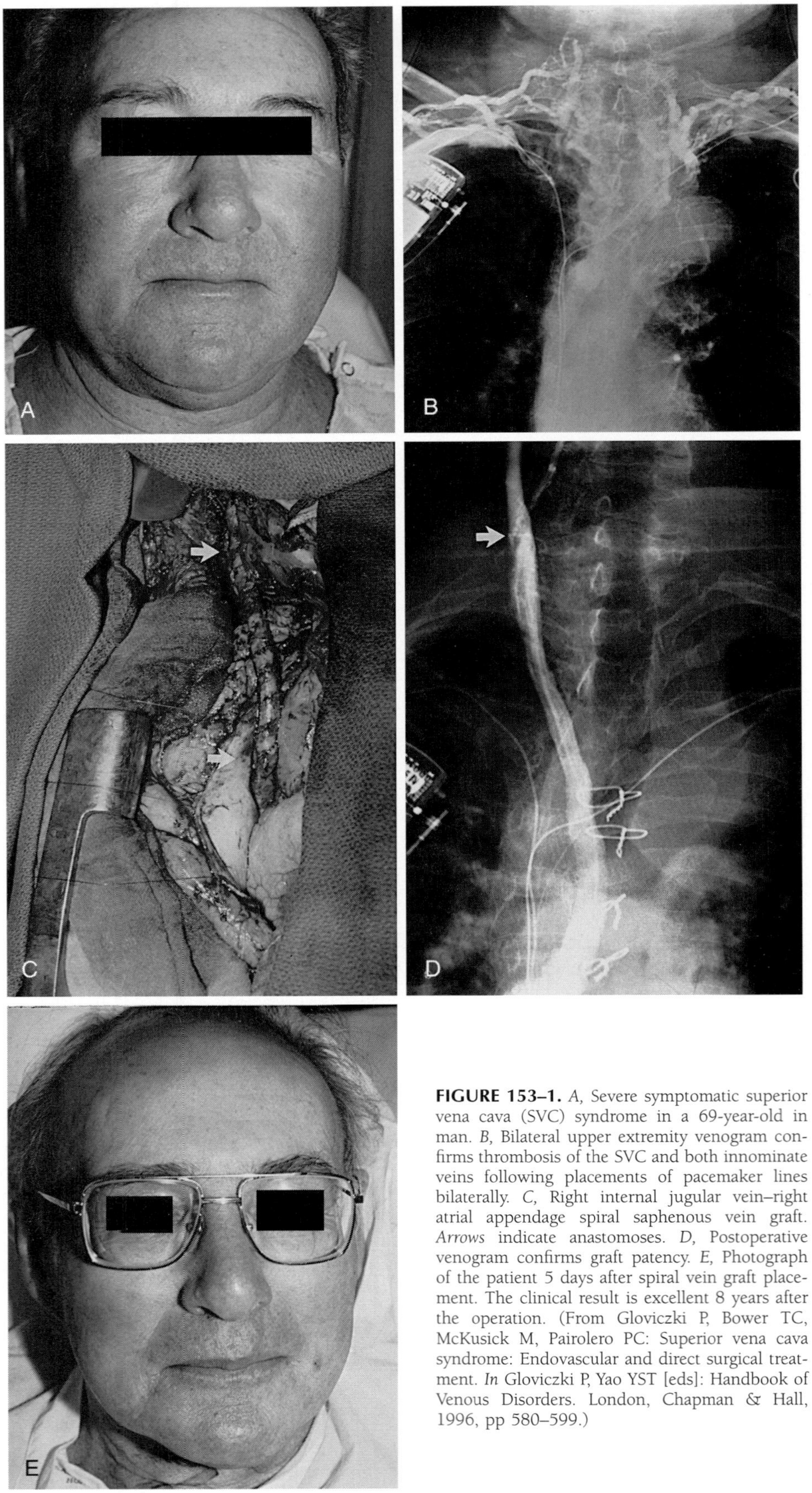

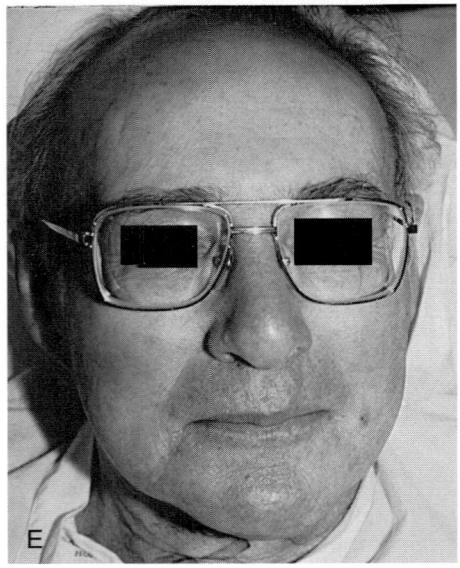

FIGURE 153–1. *A,* Severe symptomatic superior vena cava (SVC) syndrome in a 69-year-old in man. *B,* Bilateral upper extremity venogram confirms thrombosis of the SVC and both innominate veins following placements of pacemaker lines bilaterally. *C,* Right internal jugular vein–right atrial appendage spiral saphenous vein graft. *Arrows* indicate anastomoses. *D,* Postoperative venogram confirms graft patency. *E,* Photograph of the patient 5 days after spiral vein graft placement. The clinical result is excellent 8 years after the operation. (From Gloviczki P, Bower TC, McKusick M, Pairolero PC: Superior vena cava syndrome: Endovascular and direct surgical treatment. *In* Gloviczki P, Yao YST [eds]: Handbook of Venous Disorders. London, Chapman & Hall, 1996, pp 580–599.)

TABLE 153–1. SIGNS AND SYMPTOMS OF SUPERIOR VENA CAVA SYNDROME IN 19 PATIENTS WITH BENIGN DISEASE

	NO. OF PATIENTS	%
Signs		
Head and neck swelling	19	100
Large chest wall venous collaterals	17	89
Arm swelling	11	58
Facial cyanosis	8	42
Symptoms		
Feeling of fullness in head or neck	14	74
Dyspnea on exertion or orthopnea	12	63
Headaches	7	37
Visual problems, painful eyes	5	26
Cough	6	32

From Alimi YS, Gloviczki P, Vrtiska TJ, et al: Reconstruction of the superior vena cava: The benefits of postoperative surveillance and secondary endovascular interventions. J Vasc Surg 27:298–299, 1998.

pressures. The diameter and blood flow through the patent subclavian veins quickly change in response to respiratory maneuvers such as a sudden sniff maneuver or a Valsalva maneuver. Occasionally, collateral vessels may be detected within the chest wall or in the area of the subclavian veins. The advantage of ultrasound is the absence of exposure to ionizing radiation and no requirement for the administration of iodinated contrast material. In addition, patency of the internal jugular veins must be confirmed in candidates for surgical reconstruction. Since upper extremity venography is usually unable to visualize the internal jugular veins, ultrasound remains an important preoperative diagnostic test in these patients. The disadvantage of ultrasound includes not only the lack of direct visualization of the SVC but also the inability to determine the extent of an obstructing lesion.

Radionuclide Imaging

Radionuclide venography has been used in the diagnosis of SVC syndrome. A technetium 99m pertechnetate scan (^{99m}Tc), performed with bilateral simultaneous injection of the radionuclide tracer into the arm veins, has been used not only to demonstrate the presence of SVC obstruction and associated collateral pathways but also to provide functional aspects of the SVC obstruction using time-density curves. An advantage is the potential usefulness as a follow-up examination in determining therapeutic response. The disadvantage of radionuclide venography is the lower-resolution anatomic detail and the inability to determine the cause of the SVC obstruction.

Computed Tomography

The diagnosis of the SVC obstruction can be made by CT of the chest. Multiple authors have demonstrated CT findings in the diagnosis of SVC obstruction. These findings include nonopacification or decreased opacification of the central veins of the chest with increased opacification of collateral venous routes. These collateral pathways include the (1) azygos-hemiazygos pathway, (2) internal mammary pathway, (3) lateral thoracic-thoracoepigastric pathway, and

(4) vertebral pathway. A second, less common abnormal CT finding is an intense focal enhancement in the medial segment of the left lobe of the liver that is due to collateral circulation.

CT imaging accurately depicts the location and extent of the obstruction and distinguishes various types of benign and malignant mediastinal disease. The extent of venous collateral formation is also well demonstrated. Disadvantages include the requirement for intravenous contrast material, which may be contraindicated in patients with a history of allergic reaction or renal failure.

Venography

Venography has been considered the standard for accurate depiction of central venous obstruction, and it is used as an anatomic road map prior to reconstructive surgery. Venography also depicts the presence and direction of venous collateral flow. Stanford and Doty[17] described four venographic patterns of SVC syndrome, each having a different venous collateral network depending on the site and extent of SVC obstruction (Fig. 153–2 and Table 153–2). *Type I* is partial and *type II* is complete or near complete SVC obstruction, both with antegrade azygos flow. *Type III* patients with 90% to 100% obstruction have reversed azygos blood flow (Fig. 153–3A), whereas *type IV* patients have extensive mediastinal venous occlusion with venous return occurring through the inferior vena cava (see Fig. 153–1B).

The disadvantage of contrast venography is its invasiveness and the requirement of contrast material administration. Catheter-directed venography is also limited by the site of contrast administration. Only veins and collateral pathways between the injection site and right atrium are visualized.

Magnetic Resonance Imaging

MRI may provide a new standard for venographic imaging in the future, especially with the ability to acquire veno-

TABLE 153–2. VENOGRAPHIC CLASSIFICATION OF 19 PATIENTS WHO UNDERWENT RECONSTRUCTION FOR BENIGN SUPERIOR VENA CAVA (SVC) SYNDROME

TYPE*		NO. OF PATIENTS	%
I.	Stenosis (up to 90%) of the SVC with patency and antegrade flow of the azygos–right atrial pathway	3	16
II.	>90% stenosis or occlusion of the SVC with patency and antegrade flow in the azygos–right atrial path	3	16
III.	>90% stenosis or occlusion of the SVC with reversal of azygos blood flow	6	32
IV.	Occlusion of the SVC and one or more of the major caval tributaries, including the azygos systems	7	37
	Total	19	100

From Alimi YS, Gloviczki P, Vrtiska TJ, et al: Reconstruction of the superior vena cava: The benefits of postoperative surveillance and secondary endovascular interventions. J Vasc Surg 27:298–299, 1998.
*Classification of Stanford and Doty.[17]

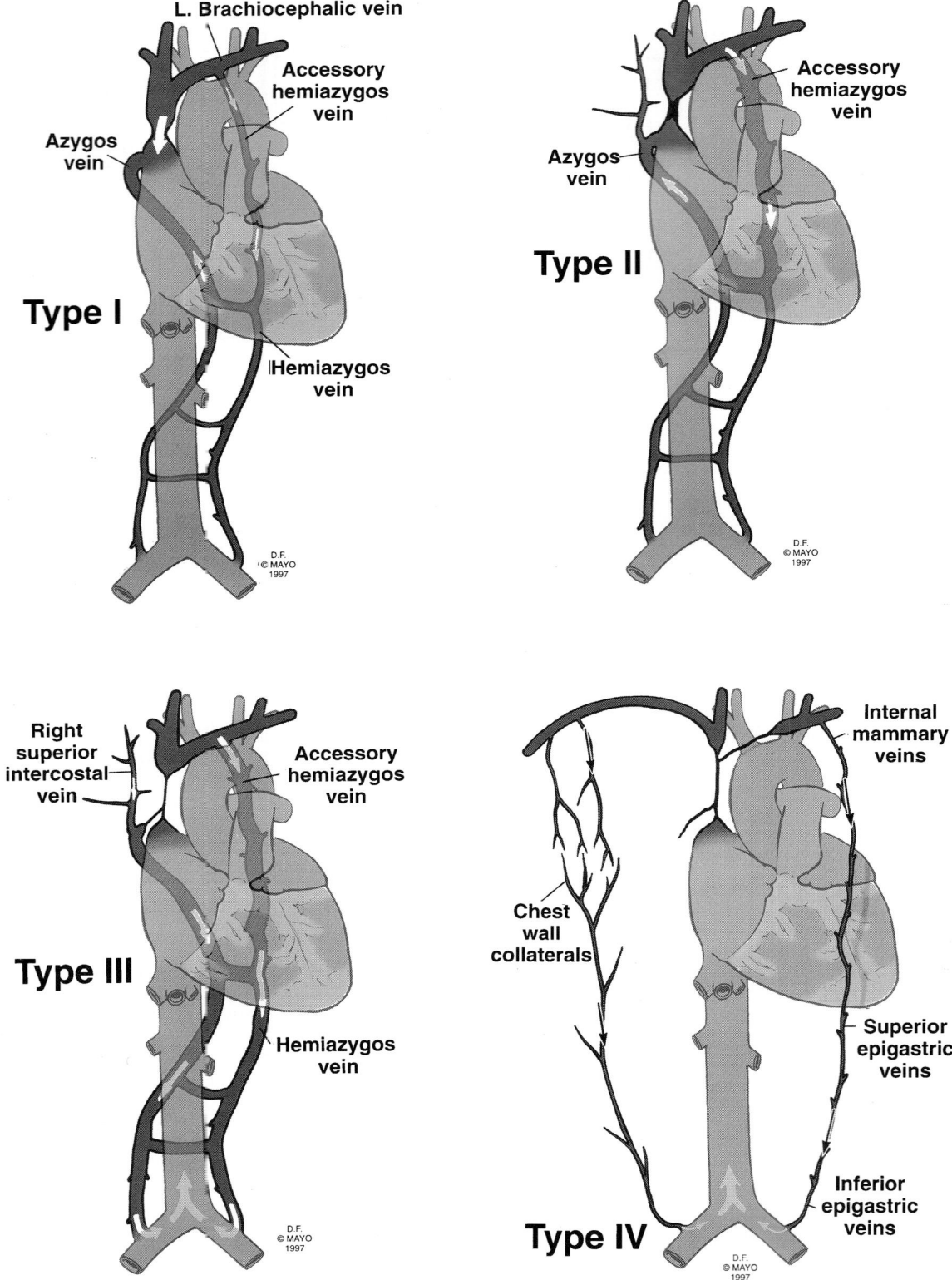

FIGURE 153–2. Venographic classification of superior vena cava (SVC) syndrome according to Stanford and Doty.[17] *A, Type I,* High-grade SVC stenosis with normal direction of blood flow, but still normal direction of blood flow through the SVC and azygos veins. Increased collateral circulation through hemiazygos and accessory hemiazygos veins. *B, Type II,* Greater than 90% stenosis or occlusion of the SVC, but patent azygos vein with normal direction of blood flow. *C, Type III,* Occlusion of the SVC with retrograde flow in both the azygos and hemiazygos veins. *D, Type IV,* Extensive occlusion of the SVC and innominate and azygos veins with chest wall and epigastric venous collaterals. (From Alimi YS, Gloviczki P, Vrtiska TJ, et al: Reconstruction of the superior vena cava: The benefits of postoperative surveillance and secondary endovascular interventions. J Vasc Surg 27:298–99, 1998.)

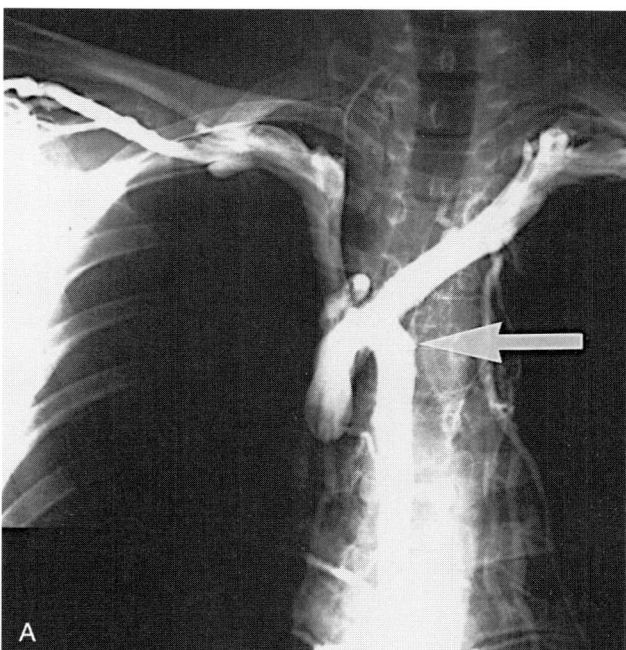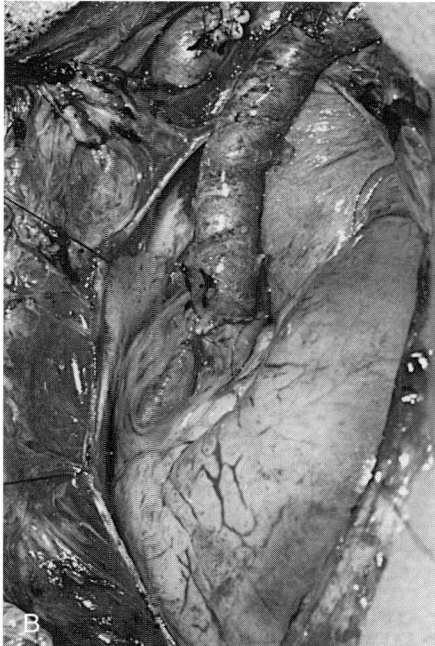

FIGURE 153–3. *A,* Bilateral upper extremity venogram documents obstruction of the superior vena cava and retrograde flow through the azygos vein (*arrow*). *B,* Left innominate vein—right atrial appendage spiral vein graft. (From Gloviczki P, Pairolero PC, Cherry KJ, Hallett JW: Reconstruction of the vena cava and of its primary tributaries: A preliminary report. J Vasc Surg 11:373–381, 1990.)

graphic images during the peak phase of gadolinium enhancement. The advantages of MRI include the ability to demonstrate anatomic structures in multiple planes and to delineate the central venous chest veins and collateral vessels. MRI is a relatively noninvasive modality and does not require the administration of iodinated contrast material. The disadvantage is its contraindication in patients with pacemakers and aneurysm clips.

CONSERVATIVE THERAPY

Conservative measures are used first in every patient to relieve symptoms of venous congestion and to decrease progression of venous thrombosis. These measures include elevation of the head during the night on pillows, modifications of daily activities by avoiding bending over, and avoidance of wearing constricting garments or a tight collar. Patients frequently need diuretic agents to decrease, at least temporarily, excessive edema of the neck and head.

Patients with acute SVC syndrome, caused by malignant disease, are generally treated with intravenous or low-molecular-weight heparin, followed by warfarin, to prevent recurrence and to protect the venous collateral circulation. Thrombolytic treatment is considered in most patients with benign acute SVC syndrome, whereas those with metastatic malignant disease are candidates for treatment by endovascular stents, with or without thrombolytic treatment (see Chapter 151).

Symptoms of SVC syndrome caused by mediastinal malignancy frequently improve after irradiation or chemotherapy.[4, 5] Chen and associates[4] treated 42 patients with malignant SVC syndrome using external beam radiotherapy or chemotherapy. Symptoms resolved in 80% of the patients within 4 weeks following radiotherapy.

SURGICAL TREATMENT

Indications

Patients with SVC syndrome can have severe, frequently incapacitating symptoms, which cannot be alleviated fully by conservative measure. *Endovascular* or *surgical* treatment in these patients should be considered. Those with extensive chronic venous thrombosis (type III or IV) and those with less extensive disease (type I or II) who have not benefited from endovascular attempts or who have elected not to have endovascular treatment are candidates for surgical reconstruction. Studies of endovascular treatment of nonmalignant SVC syndrome are limited to case reports and small series with short follow-up.[18–28] Indications for surgical treatment, however, are better defined, because experience dates back many years and long-term results are good. We have performed caval reconstruction for obstruction caused by mediastinal fibrosis, central venous catheters, pacemaker electrodes, or ventriculoatrial shunt or in patients with antithrombin III deficiency or idiopathic venous thrombosis.[7, 9, 29] The indications for reconstruction of the SVC in patients with benign disease were similar in the reports by Doty[6] and Moore and Hollier.[30]

Surgical reconstruction of the SVC also has been performed in patients with different types and stages of malignant disease.[31–40] However, endovascular techniques in such patients should always be considered unless the tumor is resectable and median sternotomy is contemplated. We believe that most patients with a malignant tumor should

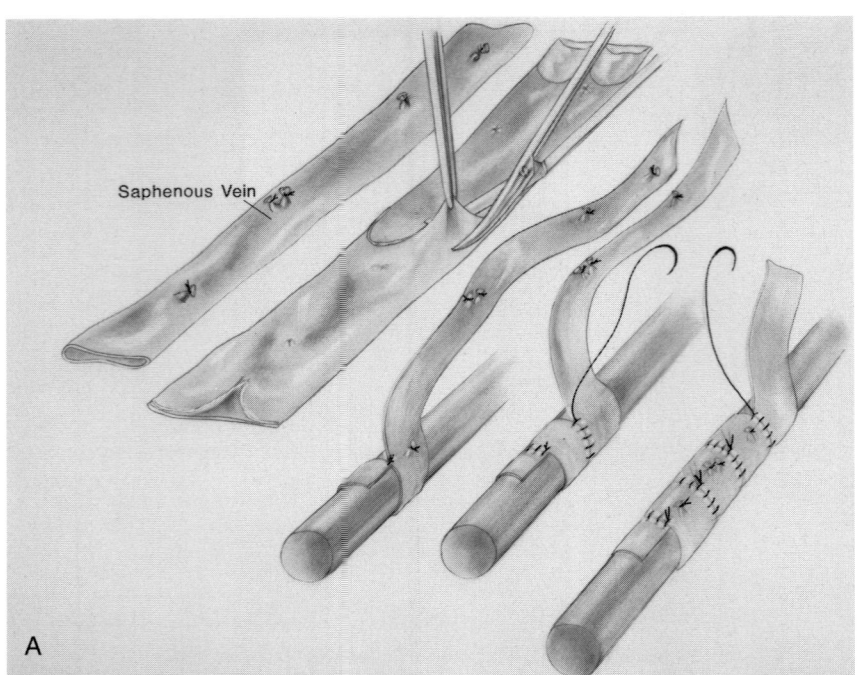

Saphenous Vein

A

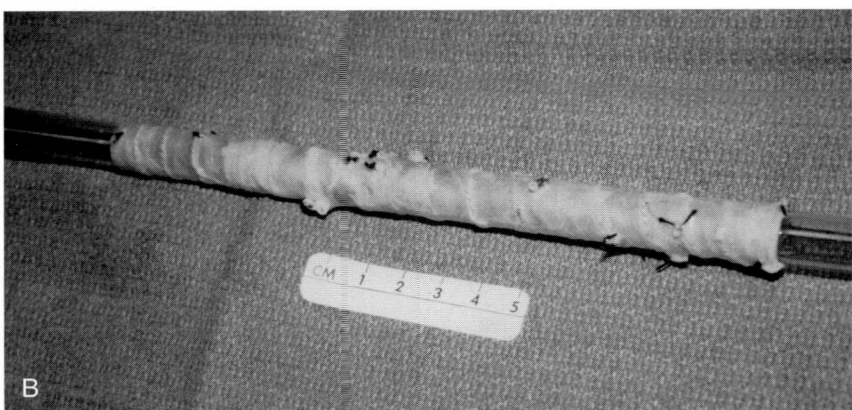

B

FIGURE 153–4. *A,* Technique for a spiral saphenous vein graft. The saphenous vein is opened longitudinally, valves are excised, the vein is wrapped around an argyle chest tube, and the vein edges are approximated with sutures. *B,* A 15-cm long spiral saphenous vein graft ready for implantation. *C,* Technique of left internal jugular—right atrial spiral vein graft implantation. (From Gloviczki PG, Pairolero PC: Venous reconstruction for obstruction and valvular incompetence. *In* J Goldstone [ed]: Perspectives in Vascular Surgery. St. Louis, Quality Medical Publishing, Inc., 1988, pp 75–93.)

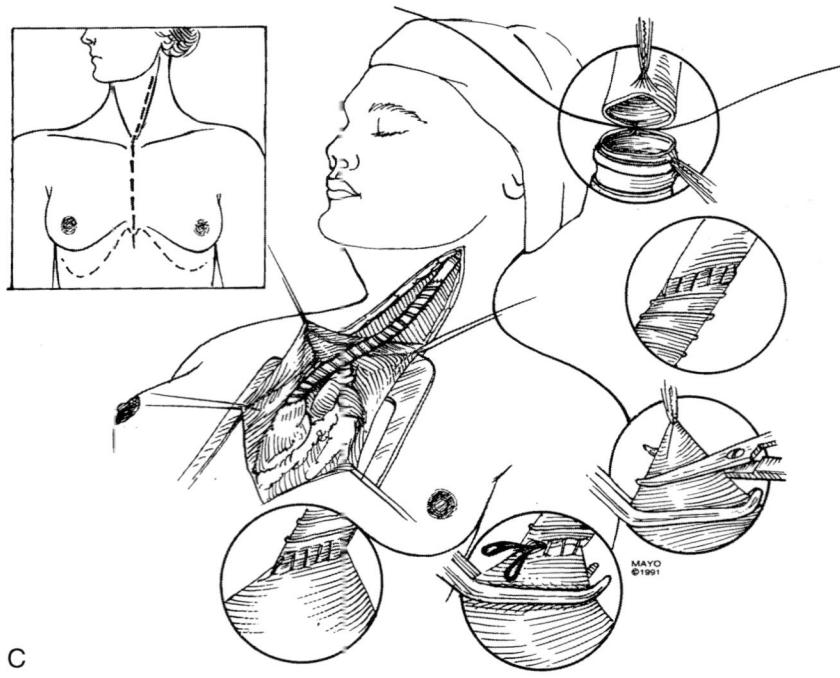

C

undergo reconstruction through median sternotomy only if their life expectancy is greater than 1 year. Extra-anatomic subcutaneous bypass between the jugular vein and the femoral vein using a composite saphenous vein graft is an alternative if symptoms are severe and endovascular techniques fail or are not possible.[38, 39]

Graft Materials

Grafting of large veins has been difficult, because large-diameter autologous vein graft is not available. The *greater saphenous vein* is usually not suitable because of poor size mismatch. The *superficial femoral vein* has been used with success[41, 42] is often and excellent in size and length.[41, 42] If the patient has underlying thrombotic abnormalities, however, removal of a deep leg vein may result in at least moderate lower extremity venous problems.

Spiral Saphenous Vein Graft

Spiral saphenous vein graft is autologous tissue with low thrombogenicity. Although its length is limited by the available saphenous vein segment, its diameter can be easily matched to that of the internal jugular or innominate vein (see Figs. 153–1 and 153–3). Disadvantages include the additional incision and the time (60 to 90 minutes) needed to prepare the graft. Described in experiments first by Chiu and colleagues,[43] this graft was implanted first in patients by Doty.[44] Our technique of preparing the spiral graft is illustrated in Figure 153–4.[19, 20]

The saphenous vein is removed, distended with papaverine-saline solution, and opened longitudinally. We excise the valves and wrap the saphenous vein around a 32 or 36 French (Fr.) polyethylene chest tube. To prepare the spiral vein graft, we suture the edges of the vein with running 6–0 or 7–0 monofilament nonabsorbable sutures. Harvesting vein from the groin to the knee results in a spiral saphenous vein graft approximately 10 cm long.

Expanded Polytetrafluoroethylene Graft

Of the available prosthetic materials, externally supported expanded polytetrafluoroethylene (ePTFE) graft (Fig. 153–5) is used almost exclusively for large vein reconstruction.[45] Short, large-diameter (10 to 14 mm) grafts have excellent long-term patency because flow through the innominate vein usually exceeds 1000 ml/min. If the peripheral anastomosis is performed with the subclavian vein, venous inflow is significantly less and the addition of an arteriovenous fistula is usually required in the arm to ensure graft patency. If an internal jugular-atrial appendage bypass is necessary, we prefer to use a spiral saphenous vein graft if available. An additional arteriovenous fistula with direct flow into the graft has not been performed for jugular grafts. Prosthetic graft is our choice in patients with a tight mediastinum and usually for all patients with malignancy, because external compression of recurrent tumor has a greater chance to occlude a vein graft.

Iliocaval Allograft

Iliocaval allograft can be considered in rare cases when immunosuppressive treatment is indicated for protection of

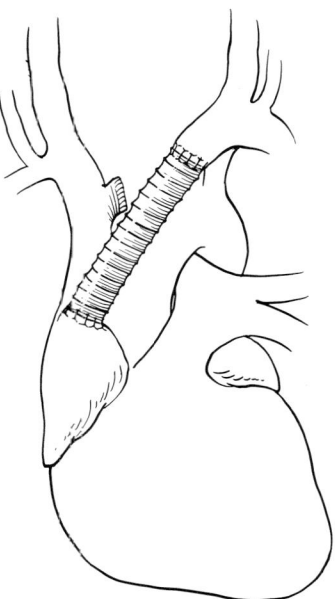

FIGURE 153–5. Left innominate vein–right atrial bypass using externally supported expanded polytetrafluoroethylene (ePTFE) graft.

a transplanted organ (Fig. 153–6).[46] Cryopreserved femoral vein grafts are potential alternatives, as are grafts prepared from autogenous or bovine pericardium.[47]

Surgical Technique

The operation is performed through median sternotomy. If the internal jugular vein is used for inflow, the mid-line incision is extended obliquely to the neck along the anterior border of the sternocleidomastoid muscle on the appropriate side. The mediastinum is exposed, and biopsy of the mediastinal mass or resection of the tumor is performed before caval reconstruction.

Once biopsy or tumor resection is done, the pericardial sac is opened to expose the right atrial appendage, which is used most frequently for the central anastomosis. A side-biting Satinsky clamp is placed on the right atrial appendage, which is opened longitudinally. Some trabecular muscle is excised, and the end-to-side anastomosis with the vein graft is performed with running 5–0 monofilament suture (see Fig. 153–4C). If it is not involved in the fibrosing process, a patent SVC central to the occlusion can also be used for this purpose. The peripheral anastomosis of the graft is performed with the internal jugular or innominate vein in an end-to-side or, preferably, an end-to-end fashion.

Although we have performed bifurcated spiral vein grafts (Fig. 153–7) or bifurcated prosthetic grafts in a few patients, a single straight graft from the internal jugular or innominate vein (see Figs. 153–1 and 153–3) is our current operation for SVC reconstruction. Because collateral circulation in the head and neck is almost always adequate, unilateral reconstruction is sufficient to relieve symptoms in most patients. When only a small portion of the venous wall is invaded by the tumor, resection and caval patch angioplasty using prosthetic or autogenous material, such as saphenous vein or pericardium, are also a viable option.

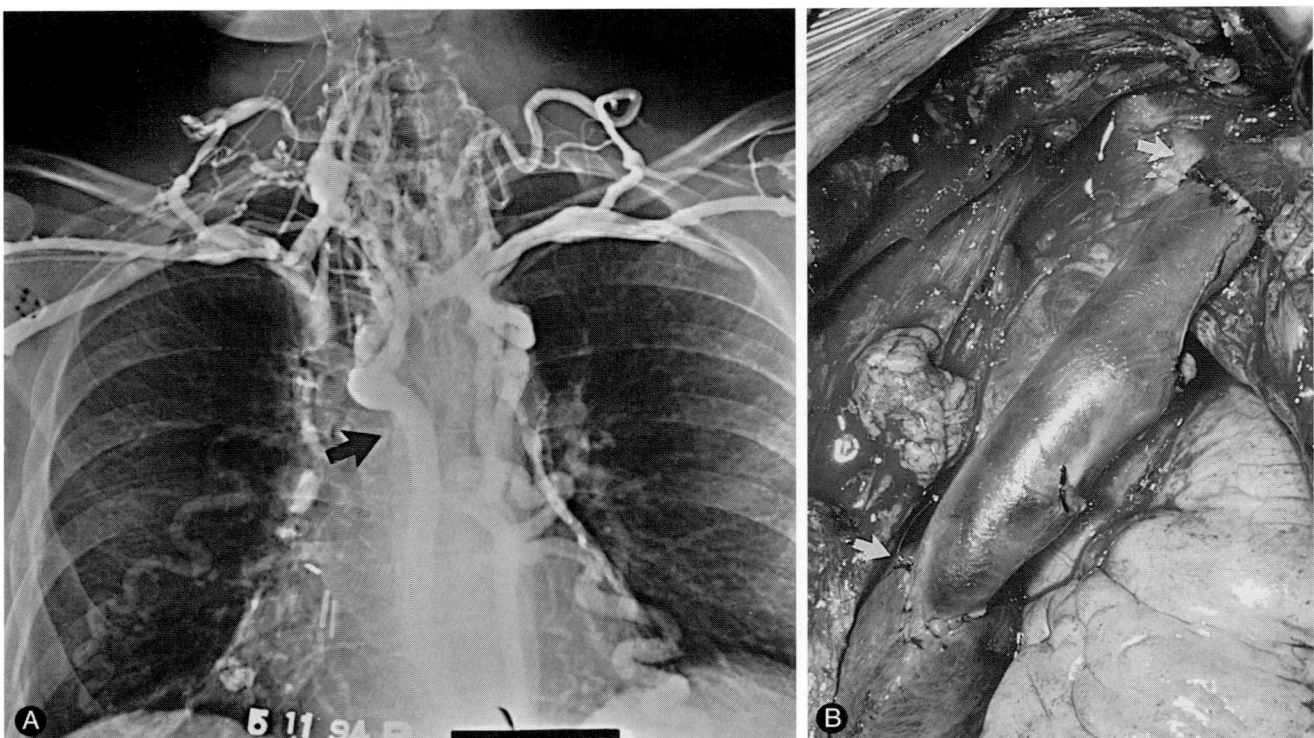

FIGURE 153–6. *A,* Venography in a 41-year-old woman with mediastinal fibrosis and liver failure, demonstrating type III superior vena cava (SVC) occlusion with retrograde flow in the azygos vein *(arrow). B,* Left innominate vein–right atrial appendage bypass was performed concomitant to orthotopic liver transplantation, using an iliocaval allograft. *Arrows* indicate the anastomoses. The graft is patent and the patient is asymptomatic from SVC syndrome 3 years after surgery. (From Rhee Y, Gloviczki P, Steers JL, et al: Superior vena cava reconstruction using an iliocaval allograft. Vasc Surg 30:77–83, 1996.)

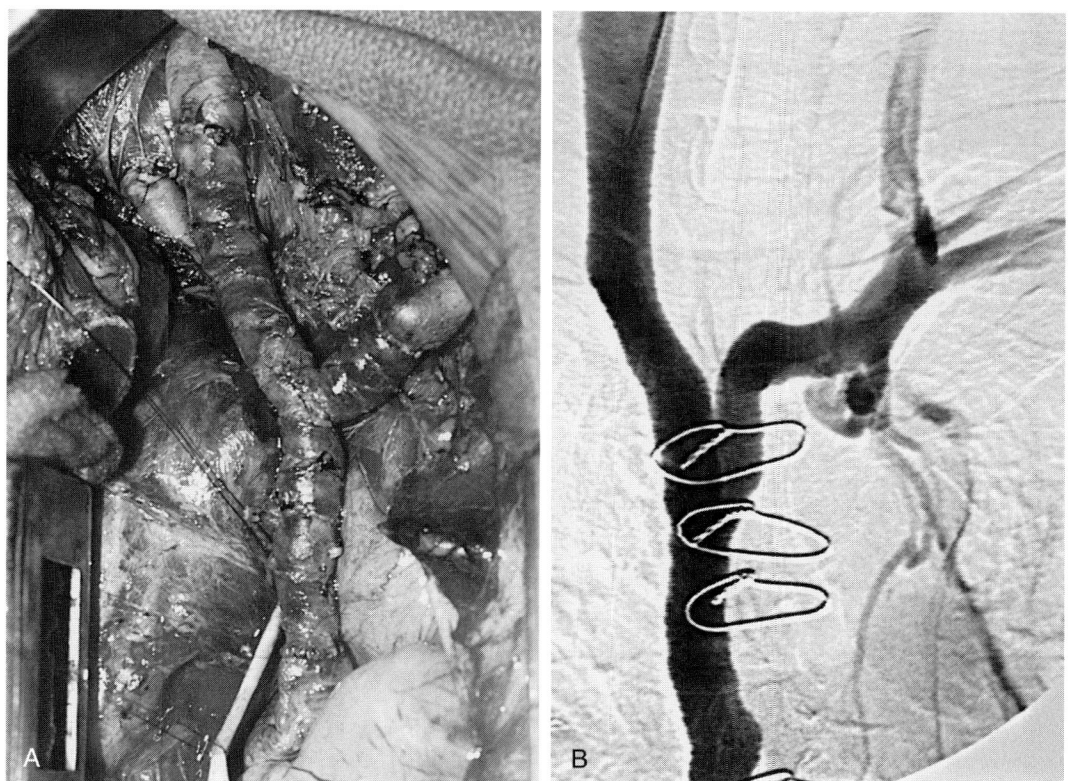

FIGURE 153-7. *A,* Bifurcated spiral saphenous vein graft in a 43-year-old woman. *B,* Venogram at 37 months reveals patent limbs of the bifurcated graft. (From Alimi YS, Gloviczki P, Vrtiska TJ, et al: Reconstruction of the superior vena cava: The benefits of postoperative surveillance and secondary endovascular interventions. J Vasc Surg 27:298–299, 1998.)

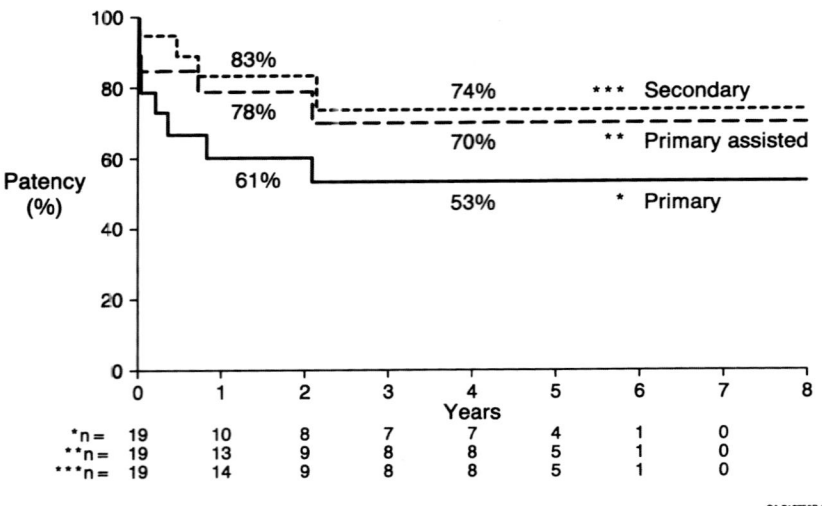

FIGURE 153–8. Cumulative patency rates of 19 bypass grafts used for superior vena cava reconstruction. (From Alimi YS, Gloviczki P, Vrtiska TJ, et al: Reconstruction of the superior vena cava: The benefits of postoperative surveillance and secondary endovascular interventions. J Vasc Surg 27:298–299, 1998.)

Postoperative anticoagulation is started 24 to 48 hours later with heparin, and the patient is discharged on an oral anticoagulation regimen. Patients with a spiral or femoral vein graft who have no underlying coagulation abnormality are maintained on warfarin (Coumadin) for 3 months only. Those with underlying coagulation disorders and most patients with ePTFE grafts continue lifelong anticoagulation therapy.

Results

We recently reported on the long-term results in 19 patients who underwent SVC reconstruction because of obstruction caused by nonmalignant disease.[9] Fourteen received spiral vein graft, four had externally supported ePTFE graft implanted, and one patient received an iliocaval allograft (see Fig. 153–6).

No early deaths or pulmonary thromboembolism occurred. Three patients had early reoperation for graft thrombosis and one for high-grade early restenosis. Three of these four grafts could be salvaged, for a discharge patency of 95%. During a mean follow-up of 49.5 months, high-grade stenosis of the graft developed in four additional patients, and one or several secondary endovascular interventions were required.

Primary and secondary patency rates of all the grafts at 5 years were 53% and 74%, respectively (Fig. 153–8). Of the different graft types, straight spiral vein grafts performed the best, with 90% patency at 5 years, 11 of the 12 grafts patent at last follow-up, and good to excellent clinical results (Fig. 153–9). Endovascular procedures (angioplasty, with or without stent) saved two of three spiral vein grafts with postoperative stenosis (Fig. 153–10).

Doty[6] reported on long-term patency in nine patients who underwent spiral vein grafting for SVC syndrome caused by benign disease. Seven of nine grafts remained patent during follow-up, which extended from 1 to 15 years, and all but one of the patients became asymptomatic.

However, increasing success with superficial femoral vein as an arterial conduit has resurrected this autologous graft for large vein reconstructions as well.[41, 42] Recent reports on good early results indicate that autologous femoropop-

liteal vein when available, shows promise for replacement of large central veins.[42] Still, the morbidity of harvesting a deep vein in patients with thrombotic potentials and venous thrombosis elsewhere in the body is not well known. One of our two patients who underwent SVC reconstruction using the femoral vein has mild but persistent leg swelling and venous claudication.

Results with ePTFE grafts implanted into the mediastinum in several series showed excellent patency. We reported on five patients who underwent SVC reconstruction using ePTFE grafts.[9, 32] Patency beyond 1 year, however, was documented only in three grafts. However, Dartevelle and coworkers[31] reported excellent results with ePTFE grafts, with 20 of 22 grafts patent at a mean of 23 months after surgery. None of the 10 PTFE grafts that Moore and Hollier[30] implanted failed at a mean follow-up of 30 months. In eight patients, however, an additional arteriovenous fistula at the arm was used to maintain patency.

Magnan and associates[33] reported on 10 patients, nine with malignant tumor, who underwent SVC reconstruction using ePTFE grafts. Although early mortality was high, with only two survivals during the follow-up period, no patients

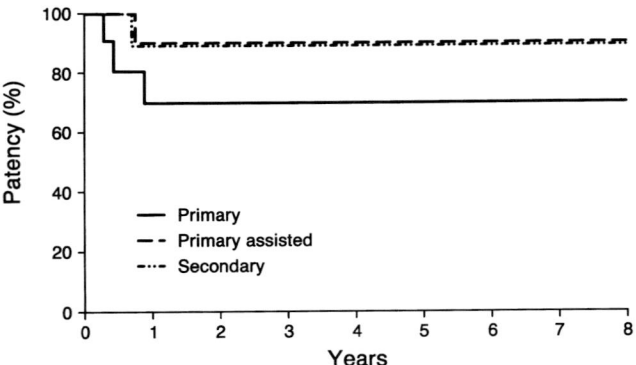

FIGURE 153–9. Cumulative patency rates of 12 straight spiral saphenous vein grafts used for superior vena cava reconstruction. (From Alimi YS, Gloviczki P, Vrtiska TJ, et al: Reconstruction of the superior vena cava: The benefits of postoperative surveillance and secondary endovascular interventions. J Vasc Surg 27:298–299, 1998.)

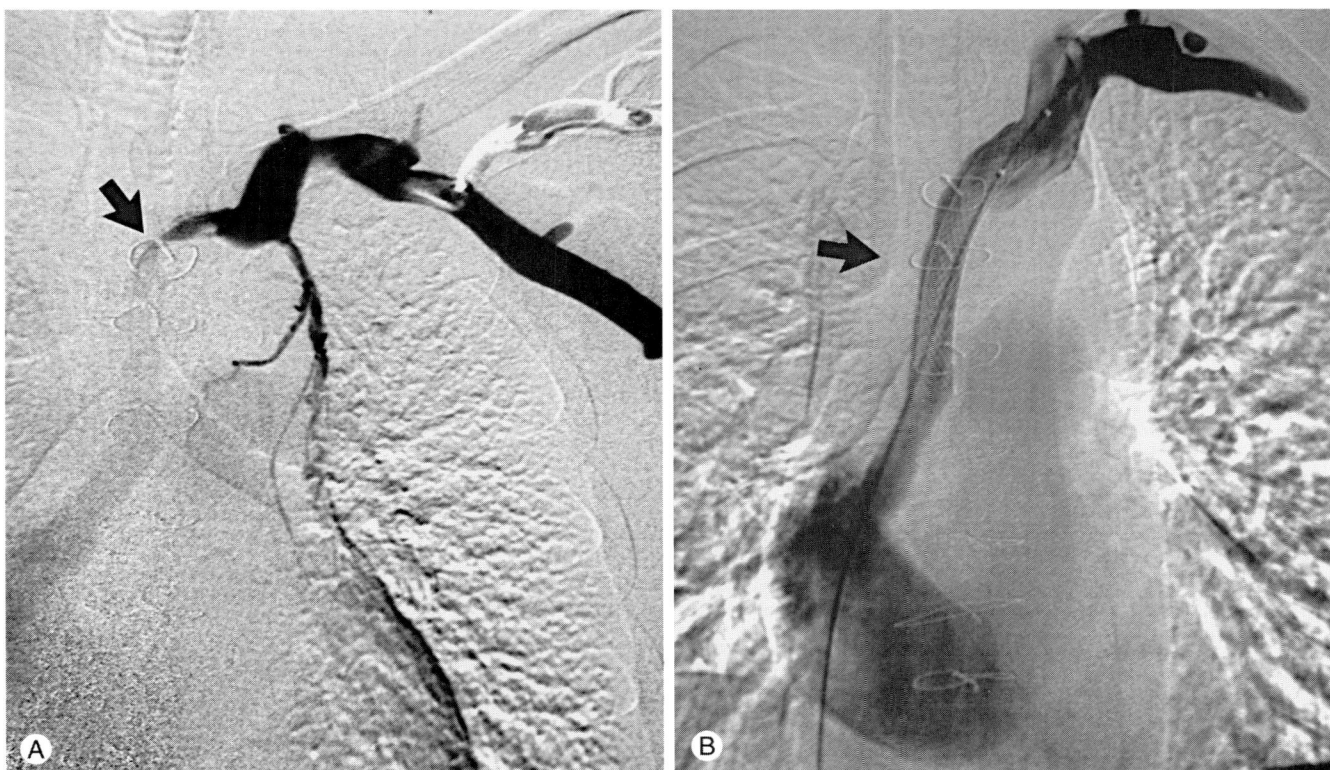

FIGURE 153–10. *A,* Venogram 10 months after placement of a left innominate vein–right atrial appendage spiral vein graft reveals severe stenosis at the proximal anastomosis (*arrow*). *B,* Successful reconstruction with placement of a WallStent. (From Alimi YS, Gloviczki P, Vrtiska TJ, et al: Reconstruction of the superior vena cava: The benefits of postoperative surveillance and secondary endovascular interventions. J Vasc Surg 27:298–299, 1998.)

experienced recurrent symptoms of SVC syndrome. Reviewing multiple series from the literature, we found that patency of ePTFE grafts at 2 years was approximately 70%.[7, 9, 30–37] Thrombosis occurs more frequently in patients in whom the distal anastomosis is performed with the internal jugular or the subclavian veins, and results appear much better in patients with innominate or SVC interposition grafts. Although spiral vein graft continues to be our first choice for SVC replacement, short, large-diameter ePTFE graft is an excellent alternative.

Postoperative follow-up is important, but unfortunately duplex scan provides only indirect evidence of patency of an intrathoracic graft. Therefore, contrast or magnetic resonance venography is used, and it is performed before discharge and once at 3 to 6 months after surgery. In our experience, most graft stenoses presented within 1 year after implantation. Endovascular therapy is most useful as an adjunctive measure to correct graft stenosis and to improve long-term graft patency.[9]

SUMMARY

Surgical treatment of SVC syndrome is effective and provides long-term relief in patients with nonmalignant disease. Spiral saphenous vein graft and femoral vein are the best autologous conduits, whereas externally supported ePTFE is the least thrombogenic prosthetic graft for SVC reconstruction. As experience with endovascular techniques increases, it is likely that surgical treatment will be reserved

for patients who do not improve after less invasive techniques or for those who are not candidates for endovascular management. If excision of malignant mediastinal tumor is possible, concomitant venous reconstruction can be performed. Otherwise, endovascular techniques should be attempted first for palliation in patients with metastatic malignant disease. Endovascular techniques are also helpful adjuncts to prolong the patency of grafts implanted for SVC replacement.

REFERENCES

1. Ahmann FR: A reassessment of the clinical implications of the superior vena cava syndrome. J Clin Oncol 4:961–969, 1984.
2. Parish JM, Marschke RF, Dines DE, Lee RE: Etiologic considerations in superior vena cava syndrome. Mayo Clinic Proc 56:407–413, 1981.
3. Sculier JP, Feld R: Superior vena cava obstruction syndrome: Recommendations for management. Cancer Treat Rev 12:209–218, 1985.
4. Chen JC, Bongard F, Klein SR: A contemporary perspective on superior vena cava syndrome. Am J Surg 160:207–211, 1990.
5. Yellin A, Rosen A, Reichert N, Lieberman Y: Superior vena cava syndrome: The myth—the facts. Am Rev Respir Dis 141:1114–1118, 1990.
6. Doty DB: Bypass of superior vena cava: Fifteen years' experience with spiral vein for obstruction of superior vena cava caused by benign disease. J Thorac Cardiovasc Surg 99:889–896, 1990.
7. Gloviczki P, Pairolero PC, Toomey BJ, et al: Reconstruction of large veins for nonmalignant venous occlusive disease. J Vasc Surg 16:750–761, 1992.
8. Gupta DK, Mathur AS: Cervical and mediastinal fibrosis presenting with superior vena cava syndrome. Indian Heart J 31:302–304, 1979.
9. Alimi YS, Gloviczki P, Vrtiska TJ, et al: Reconstruction of the superior

vena cava: Benefits of postoperative surveillance and secondary endovascular interventions. J Vasc Surg 27:287–299, 1998.

10. Dodds GA, Harrisson JK, O'Laughlin MP, et al: Relief of superior vena cava syndrome due to fibrosing mediastinitis using the Palmaz stent. Chest 106:315, 1994.

11. Spittell PC, Vliestra RE, Hayes DL, Higano ST: Venous obstruction due to permanent transvenous pacemaker electrodes: Treatment with percutaneous transluminal balloon venoplasty. PACE 13:271–274, 1990.

12. Grace AA, Sutters M, Schofield PM: Balloon dilatation of pacemaker induced stenosis of the superior vena cava. Br Heart J 65:225–226, 1991.

13. Sunder SK, Ekong EA, Silvalingam K, Kumar A: Superior vena cava thrombosis due to pacing electrodes: Successful treatment with combined thrombolysis and angioplasty. Am Heart J 123:790–792, 1992.

14. Lindsay HSJ, Chennells PM, Perrins EJ: Successful treatment by balloon venoplasty and stent insertion of obstruction of the superior vena cava by an endocardial pacemaker lead. Br Heart J 71:363–365, 1994.

15. Frances CM, Starkey IR, Errington ML, Gillepsie IN: Venous stenting as treatment for pacemaker-induced superior vena cava syndrome. Am Heart J 129:836–837, 1995.

16. Kastner RJ, Fisher WG, Blacky AR, Bacon ME: Pacemaker-induced superior vena cava syndrome with successful treatment by balloon venoplasty. Am J Cardiol 77:789–790, 1996.

17. Stanford W, Doty DB: The role of venography and surgery in the management of patients with superior vena cava obstruction. Ann Thorac Surg 41:158–163, 1986.

18. Dake MD, Semba CP, Enstrom RJ, et al: Percutaneous treatment of venous occlusive disease (Abstract). J Vasc Interv Radiol 4:42, 1993.

19. Kishi K, Sonomura T, Mitsunaze K, et al: Self-expandable metallic stent therapy for superior vena cava syndrome: Clinical observations. Radiology 189:531–535, 1993.

20. Furui S, Sawada S, Kuramoto K, et al: Gianturco stent placement in malignant caval obstruction: Analysis of factors for predicting the outcome. Radiology 195:147–152, 1995.

21. Rosch J, Uchida BT, Hall LD, et al: Gianturco-Rosch expandable Z-stents in the treatment of superior vena cava syndrome. Cardiovasc Intervent Radiol 15:319–327, 1992.

22. Charnsangavej C, Carrasco CH, Wallace S, et al: Stenosis of the vena cava: Preliminary assessment of treatment with expandable metallic stents. Radiology 161:295–298, 1986.

23. Sherry CS, Diamond NG, Meyers TP, Martin RL: Successful treatment of superior vena cava syndrome by venous angioplasty. AJR 147:834–835, 1986.

24. Putnam JS, Uchida BT, Antonovic R, Rösch J: Superior vena cava syndrome associated with massive thrombosis: Treatment with expandable wire stents. Radiology 167:727–728, 1988.

25. Walpole HT, Lovett KE, Chuang VP, et al: Superior vena cava syndrome treated by percutaneous transluminal balloon angioplasty. Am Heart J 115:1303–1304, 1988.

26. Solomon N, Wholey MH, Jarmolowski CR: Intravascular stents in the management of superior vena cava syndrome. Cathet Cardiovasc Diagn 23:245–252, 1991.

27. Chatelain P, Meier B, Friedli B: Stenting of superior vena cava and inferior vena cava for symptomatic narrowing after repeated atrial surgery for D-transposition of the great vessels. Br Heart J 66:466–468, 1991.

28. Dondelinger RF, Trotteur G: Expandable stents in the venous system.

Abstracts of the International Symposium, Leuven, Belgium, December 14, 1996.

29. Gloviczki P, Pairolero PC, Cherry KJ, Hallett JW: Reconstruction of the vena cava and of its primary tributaries: A preliminary report. J Vasc Surg 11:373–381, 1990.

30. Moore WM Jr, Hollier LH: Reconstruction of the superior vena cava and central veins. In Bergan JJ, Yao JST (eds): Venous Disorders. Philadelphia, WB Saunders, 1991, pp 517–527.

31. Dartevelle PG, Chapelier AR, Pastorino U, et al: Long-term follow-up after prosthetic replacement of the superior vena cava combined with resection of mediastinal-pulmonary malignant tumors. J Thorac Cardiovasc Surg 102:259–265, 1991.

32. Bower TC, Nagorney DM, Toomey BJ, et al: Vena cava replacement for malignant disease: Is there a role? Ann Vasc Surg 7:51–62, 1993.

33. Magnan PE, Thomas P, Giudicelli R, et al: Surgical reconstruction of the superior vena cava. Cardiovasc Surg 2:598–604, 1994.

34. Bergeron P, Reggi M, Jausseran J, et al: Our experience in superior vena cava surgery [in French]. Ann Chir: Chir Thorac Cardiovasc 39:485–491, 1985.

35. Herreros J, Glock Y, Fuente Adl, et al: The superior vena cava compression syndrome: Our experience of twenty six cases [in French]. Ann Chir: Chir Thorac Cardiovasc 39:495–500, 1985.

36. Ricci C, Benedetti VF, Colini GF, et al: Reconstruction of the superior vena cava: 15 years' experience using various types of prosthetic material. Ann Chir 39:492–495, 1985.

37. Masuda H, Ogata T, Kikuche K, et al: Total replacement of superior vena cava because of invasive thymoma: Seven years' survival. J Thorac Cardiovasc Surg 95:1083–1085, 1988.

38. Vincze K, Kulka F, Csorba L: Saphenous-jugular bypass as palliative therapy of superior vena cava syndrome caused by bronchial carcinoma. J Thorac Cardiovasc Surg 83:272–277, 1982.

39. Graham A, Anikin V, Curry R, McGuigan J: Subcutaneous jugulofemoral bypass: A simple surgical option for palliation of superior vena cava obstruction. J Cardiovasc Surg 36:615–617, 1995.

40. Gloviczki P, Bower TC, McKusick M, Pairolero PC: Superior vena cava syndrome: Endovascular and direct surgical treatment. In Gloviczki P, Yao JST (eds): Handbook of Venous Disorders. London, Chapman, & Hall, 1996, pp. 580–599.

41. Marshall WG Jr, Kouchoukos NT: Management of recurrent superior vena caval syndrome with an externally supported femoral vein bypass graft. Ann Thorac Surg 46:239–241, 1988.

42. Hagino RT, Bengtson TD, Fosdick DA, et al: Venous reconstruction using the superficial femoral-popliteal vein. J Vasc Surg 26:829–837, 1997.

43. Chiu CJ, Terzis J, Mac Rae ML: Replacement of superior vena cava with the spiral composite vein graft. Ann Thorac Surg 17:555–560, 1974.

44. Doty DB: Bypass of superior vena cava: Six years' experience with spiral vein graft for obstruction of superior vena cava due to benign and malignant disease. J Thorac Cardiovasc Surg 83:326–338, 1982.

45. Gloviczki P, Pairolero PC: Prosthetic replacement of large veins. In Bergan JJ, Kistner RL (eds): Atlas of Venous Surgery. Philadelphia, WB Saunders, 1992, pp 191–214.

46. Rhee RY, Gloviczki P, Steers JL, et al: Superior vena cava reconstruction using an iliocaval allograft. Vasc Surg 30:77–83, 1996.

47. Zembala M, Kustrzycki A, Ostapczuk S, et al: Pericardial tube for obstruction of superior vena cava by malignant teratoma. J Thorac Cardiovasc Surg 91:469–471, 1986.

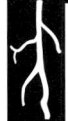

C H A P T E R   1 5 4

Lymphedema: An Overview

Peter Gloviczki, M.D.

I think I have proved, that the lymphatic vessels are the absorbing vessels . . .; that they are the same as the lacteals; and that . . . with the thoracic duct, constitute one great and general system, dispersed through the whole body for absorption.

William Hunter, 1784

When the transport capacity of the lymphatic system is reduced by obstruction or abnormal development of the lymph vessels or lymph nodes, protein-rich interstitial fluid accumulates and lymphedema develops. Chronic limb swelling due to lymphedema is not only a marked cosmetic deformity; in most patients, it is also a disabling and distressing condition. Complications can be severe and include bacterial and fungal infections, chronic inflammation, wasting, immunodeficiency, and occasionally malignancy. Lymphedema, long a neglected field in medicine, has received considerable attention in recent years owing to progress in ultrastructural and physiologic investigations and to improvements in diagnosis and management of the disease. This new information and experience with lymphedema is based on a substantial knowledge of the lymphatic system that has been accumulating for centuries.

HISTORICAL BACKGROUND

Lymph vessels and nodes were mentioned in early times by Hippocrates (460–377 B.C.), who described "white blood" and "glands, that everyone has in the armpit,"[1] by Aristotle (384–322 B.C.), who wrote about "nerves . . . which contain colorless liquids,"[2] and by Erasistratus (310–250 B.C.) of the Alexandrian School of Medicine, who recognized the lacteals as "arteries on the mesentery of sucking pigs full of milk."[3] It was not until the Renaissance, however, that further progress was made in this field. Eustachius, dissecting a horse in 1563, was the first to observe the thoracic duct, but he did not recognize its significance and named it the *vena alba thoracis*.[4]

The discovery of the lymphatic system is attributed to Gasparo Asellius, Professor of Anatomy and Surgery at Pavia, Italy. On July 23, 1622, during a vivisection, he observed the mesenteric lymphatics in a well-fed dog.[5] Asellius named the lymphatics the *vasa lactea* and recognized their function of absorbing chyle from the intestines. He assumed, however, that the mesenteric lymphatics transported lymph to the liver. It was Jean Pecquet, in 1651, who described the exact route of mesenteric lymphatic drainage to the "receptaculum chyli" and from there into the thoracic duct.[6] In subsequent years, Bartholin and Rudbeck clarified other details of the lymphatic circulation and the anatomy of the thoracic duct (Fig. 154–1).[7, 8] The term *lymphatic* was first used by Bartholin. The valvular structure in the lymph vessels was demonstrated by Ruysch[9] in 1665 and later in 1692 by Anton Nuck, who injected mercury into the lymph vessels for his anatomic studies.[10]

The gross anatomy of the lymphatic system was remarkably well documented by the great anatomists of the 18th century. Cruikshank, a student of William Hunter, published *The Anatomy of the Absorbing Vessels of the Human Body* in 1786.[11] His work, however, was surpassed by the atlas of Paolo Mascagni, who published exceptionally detailed and clear illustrations of the entire lymphatic system (Figs. 154–2 to 154–4).[12] It was not until 100 years later that our knowledge of the anatomy of the lymphatic system was further broadened by the works of Sappey[13] and then by those of Ranvier.[14]

The lymphatics as an integrated system responsible for absorption were recognized at the end of the 18th century by William Hunter, his brother John, and two of his stu-

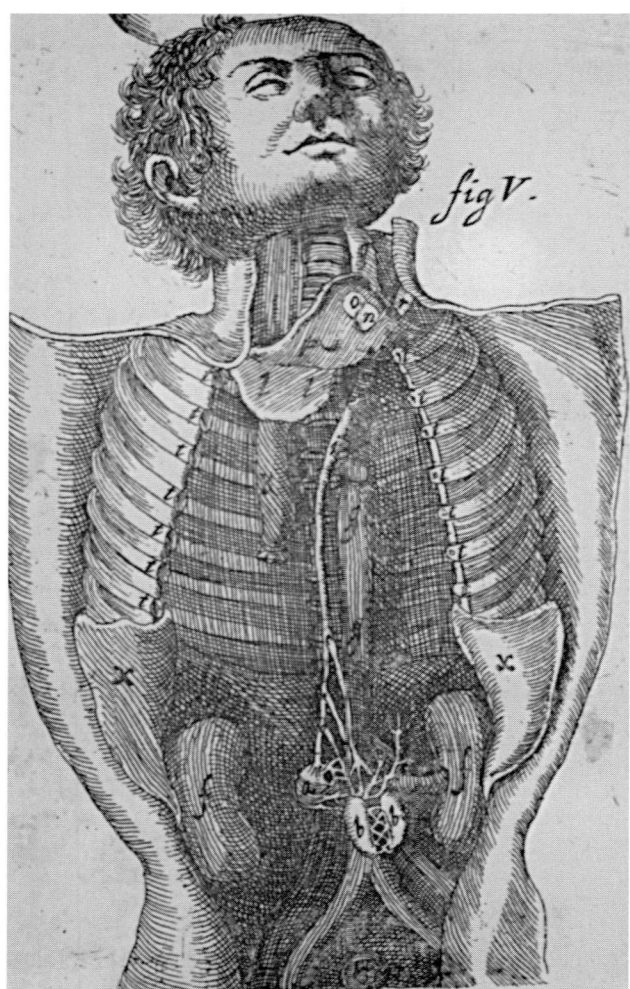

FIGURE 154–1. The receptaculum chyli and the thoracic duct in humans. (From Bartholin T: Vasa Lymphatica. Hafniae, Petrus Hakius, 1653.)

Földi, and Szabó.[23] With the introduction of a clinically practical technique of contrast lymphangiography in the early 1950s, Kinmonth gave a special impetus toward clinical research of the lymphatic system and focused much-needed attention on the diagnosis and management of chronic lymphedema.[24]

LYMPHEDEMA: AN ENIGMA?

Lymphedema, a disease known for centuries, has been considered by many clinicians to be one of the enigmas of medicine.[25] The reasons are legion. Lymphedema is caused by a fault in a system that is hardly visible. It frequently occurs years after the initial insult to the lymph vessels and lymph nodes following a long period of apparent well-being and normal functioning. It is difficult, and frequently frustrating, to treat and almost impossible to cure.

dents, Hewson and Cruikshank.[15] However, their theory that the lymphatic system was the only absorbing system of the body was rightly criticized, even by their peers.

Although Hunter thought that the lymphatics were closed tubes, Hewson suggested that they had physiologic orifices and acted as "capillary tubes" that were "capable of absorbing the chyle and the lymph."[16] The "open mouth" theory—that the lymphatics had completely open distal ends—was advocated by von Kölliker[17] and later by von Recklinghausen, who also discovered the endothelial lining of the lymphatics.[18]

As Drinker stated,[19] however, "The modern history of lymph formation and lymph movement began with Starling." At the turn of the 20th century, Starling confirmed the relationship between the hydrostatic pressure in the blood capillaries and the oncotic pressure of the plasma proteins.[20] His work was a continuation of the theory of Ludwig, who suggested that lymph was formed by filtration of the blood through the walls of the capillaries.[21] Drinker and his colleagues at Harvard University deserve the credit for explaining the absorption of proteins from the intercellular space via the lymphatic system.[22] Further details of lymphatic physiology were elaborated later by members of the Hungarian school of lymphology, headed by Rusznyák,

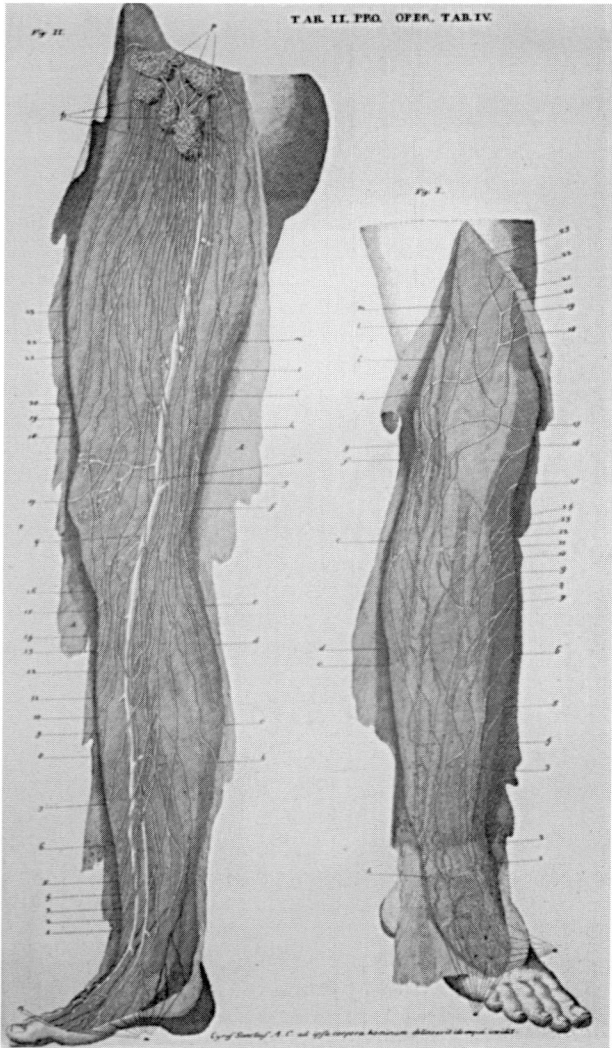

FIGURE 154–2. The lymphatic system of the lower extremity according to Mascagni. (From Mascagni P: Vasorum Lymphaticorum Corporis Humani Historia et Ichnographia. Vol 138. Senis, P Carli, 1787.)

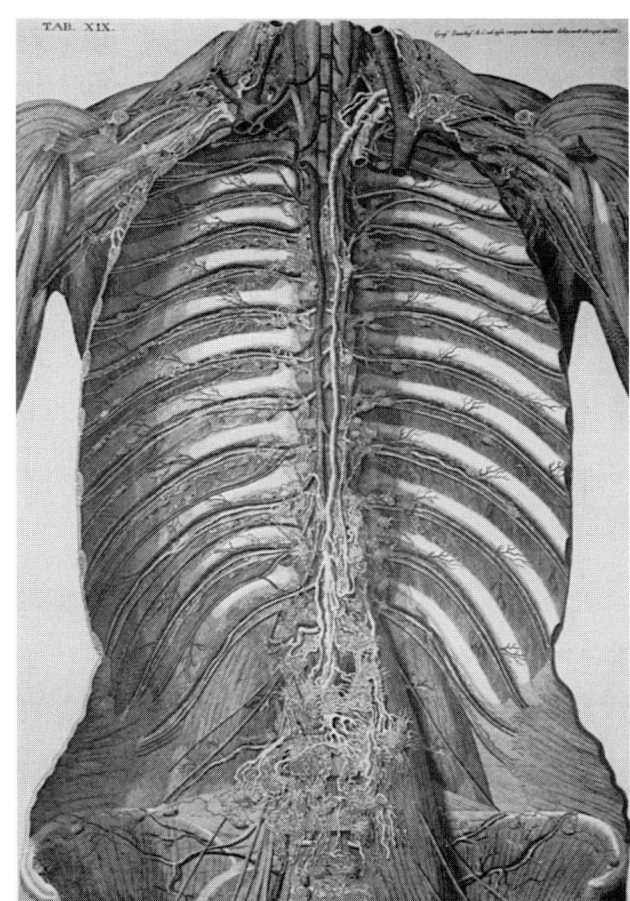

FIGURE 154–3. Anatomy of the thoracic duct, as illustrated by Mascagni. (From Mascagni P: Vasorum Lymphaticorum Corporis Humani Historia et Ichnographia. Vol 138. Senis, P Carli, 1787.)

Lymphatic Physiology

Nonetheless, our understanding of lymphatic physiology has markedly improved in recent years. Chapter 155 provides new perspectives on the three-dimensional anatomy of the blood capillary–interstitial lymph interface and on the formation and propulsion of lymph. The spontaneous intrinsic contractility of the lymph vessels is recognized now as the pivotal mechanism by which lymph is propelled under normal conditions.

In regard to new theories of the pathophysiology of lymphedema, it must be emphasized that the lymphatic system is not comparable to the venous system. They are not two identical, unidirectional canalicular systems that are responsible for the return of excess interstitial fluid to the bloodstream and the heart. The major difference is that the *venous system* is filled with a liquid column, which responds immediately to changes in pressure or resistance. The *lymphatic system,* however, is not fully primed. Only if there is long-standing stasis does the lymph column fill the lymphatic channels completely. Only under these conditions are factors other than intrinsic contractility, such as muscle contractions and external massage, important in the forward propulsion of lymphatic flow.

Progress in angiogenesis research has been extended to the lymphatic system, and Chapter 155 includes an update on lymphangiogenesis and its critical role in abnormalities

of the lymphatic circulation. In the future, genetic manipulation of "lymphangiogenesis genes" may have the potential to stimulate formation of new lymph vessels and enhance abnormal lymphatic transport.

Diagnosis

In most patients with limb swelling, the diagnosis of lymphedema is based on the history and physical findings. Once a systemic cause of edema has excluded, one should keep in mind that chronic venous insufficiency is more often a local cause of limb swelling than is lymphedema. Secondary lymphedema, on the other hand, is more common than primary lymphedema.[26] Lymphoscintigraphy has become the study of choice for confirming that edema is lymphatic in origin (see Chapter 156).[27] It is still essential to perform computed tomography in most adult patients suspected to have lymphedema to exclude underlying ma-

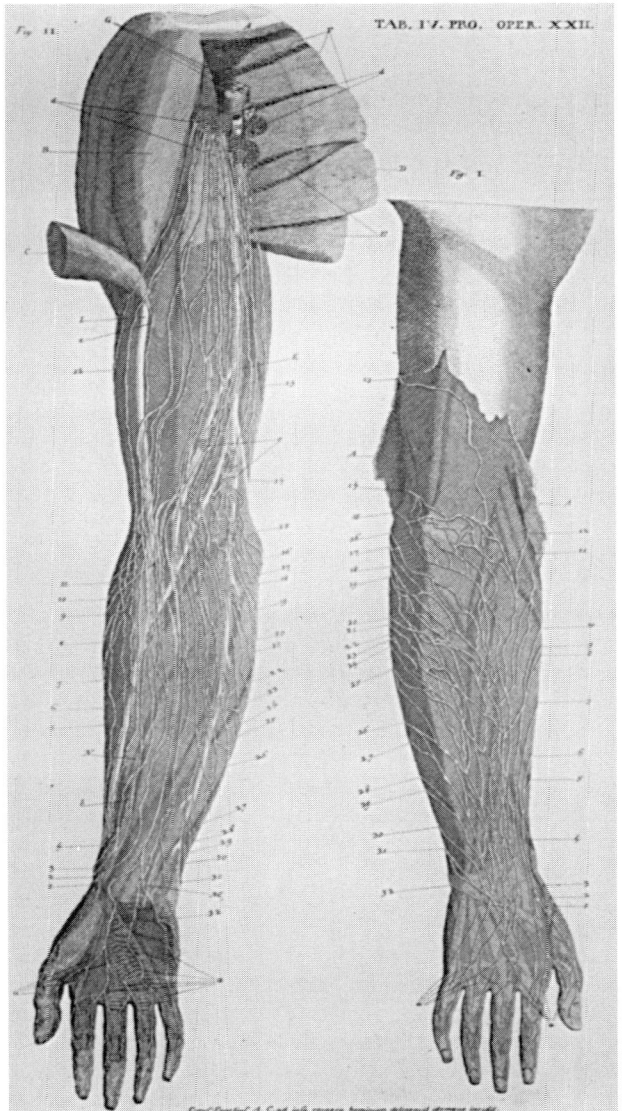

FIGURE 154–4. Anatomy of the lymphatic system of the upper extremity by Mascagni. (From Mascagni P: Vasorum Lymphaticorum Corporis Humani Historia et Ichnographia. Vol 138. Senis, P Carli, 1787.)

lignancy. Magnetic resonance imaging is being used with increasing frequency to image the anatomy of lymph nodes, and it has the potential to become the most useful complement to lymphoscintigraphy.

Although direct contrast lymphangiography still provides the finest details of lymphatic anatomy,[24, 28] it is an invasive study that has potential side effects, and its use has been markedly restricted in patients with lymphedema. In our practice, contrast lymphangiography is reserved for the preoperative evaluation of patients with lymphangiectasia and for selected patients who are candidates for direct operations on the lymph vessels or the thoracic duct.

Prevention

Prevention of primary lymphedema is not possible at present. The incidence of secondary lymphedema, however, can be reduced by preventive measures. Filariasis, which affects almost 100 million people worldwide, was eradicated from Europe and North America by public health measures and control of mosquito breeding.[29] The introduction of similar measures in Third World countries, in addition to prophylactic antifilarial medications and immediate treatment of infected persons, can decrease a worldwide epidemic.

An important form of secondary lymphedema in developed countries is still postmastectomy lymphedema. In well-documented studies, Kissin and colleagues[30] noted that extensive axillary lymphadenectomy, axillary radiotherapy, and nodal involvement with disease are the most important independent risk factors for lymphedema. Although treatment of malignancy should not be compromised, excision of lymphatic tissue for either diagnostic or therapeutic purposes should be restricted to a minimum. The prevention of infectious complications is equally important in patients who have undergone lymph node dissection or who already have lymphedema. It is achieved by observing meticulous personal hygiene measures, avoiding skin injury, and controlling fungal infections.

Treatment

The mainstays of treatment of lymphedema continue to be conservative measures, including (1) leg elevation, (2) elastic or rigid compression, (3) manual physical decongestion, and (4) intermittent pneumatic compression.

Leg elevation continues to be the simplest way of reducing lymphedema, although it requires hospitalization, bed rest, and elevation of the extremity in an edema sling for several days. Elastic and nonelastic external compression of the limb remains the most important conservative measure to control lymphedema.

Manual physical decongestive therapy has been popularized in Europe by Földi and colleagues,[31] and this effective physical therapy regimen (see Chapter 157) has gained acceptance in the United States. Gamble and colleagues describe the complex physical therapy program practiced at the Mayo Clinic Lymphedema Center, which includes limb elevation, therapeutic exercises, standardized techniques of manual lymph drainage massage, and complex multilayer low-stretch wrapping.

Intermittent pneumatic compression is a widely used conservative treatment for lymphedema. Data from a prospective study of Pappas and O'Donnell support its long-term effectiveness.[32] Their protocol included 2 to 3 days' hospitalization with daily treatment with a sequential, high-pressure, intermittent pneumatic compression pump. The edema status was then maintained with two-way stretch elastic compression stockings. Limb girth reduction was maintained in 90% of patients, and excellent results were recorded in 53% at a mean follow-up interval of 25 months.

Excisional debulking operations are recommended by Miller[33] for patients who have significant functional impairment due to excessive lymphedema (see Chapter 158). In the late stage of the disease, when irreversible skin and subcutaneous changes have occurred, this may be the only way to decrease the volume of the extremity. Among the different excisional operations, the staged subcutaneous excision beneath flaps has provided the most satisfying results.[33, 34]

Reconstruction of the obstructed lymphatic circulation has been attempted with direct operations on the lymph vessels (lymphovenous anastomoses, lymphatic grafting)[35–37] or operations designed to promote the formation of new lympholymphatic anastomoses (omental transposition,[38] mesenteric bridge operation,[39] lymph node transplantation[40]). Substantial controversy has attended these procedures. Although the long-term patency and function of lymphovenous anastomoses and lymphatic grafting still have not been proved, well-documented studies from two centers have claimed long-term improvement after microsurgical lymphatic reconstructions.[36, 37]

A variation of lymphatic grafting was reported by Campisi, who treated 64 patients with upper or lower extremity lymphedema by creating a lymphatic-venous-lymphatic anastomosis with autologous interposition graft.[41] When an isolated vein segment is used, the anastomosis is not exposed to intraluminal blood and theoretically is better protected from thrombotic occulusion. Clinical evaluation and volumetric assessment confirmed marked or moderate improvement in 90% of the patients 5 years after surgery. Unfortunately, graft patency was not studied in these patients. As an editorial writer observed in 1991, however, the lack of prospective clinical trials and the imperfect nature of current treatment modalities continue to generate disagreement about what constitutes optimal management of chronic lymphedema.[42]

SUMMARY

The problems that we have to face in dealing with lymphatic diseases are still substantial. Lymphedema, however, should no longer be considered an enigma of medicine. The authors writing on lymphedema in this new volume of *Vascular Surgery* sincerely hope that the information presented here will stimulate further basic and clinical research and much-needed prospective clinical trials of this difficult and long-neglected problem. This section assigned to the management of lymphedema is a testimony to the indisputable progress that has been made in the past decades in the field of lymphatic diseases.

REFERENCES

1. Kanter MA: The lymphatic system: An historical perspective. Plast Reconstr Surg 79:131, 1987.
2. Bartels P: Das Lymphgefässsystem. Jena, G Fischer, 1909, p 2.
3. Wolfe JHN: The pathophysiology of lymphedema. *In* Rutherford RB (ed): Vascular Surgery, 3rd ed. Philadelphia, WB Saunders, 1989, pp 1648–1656.
4. Eustachi B: Opuscula Anatomica. Venetiis, V Luchinus, 1564, p 301.
5. Asellius G: De Lactibus sive Lacteis Venis Quarto Vasorum Mesaraicorum Genere Novo Inuento. Mediolani, JB Biddellium, 1627.
6. Pecquet J: Experimenta Nova Anatomica, Quibus Incognitum Lactenus Chyli Receptaculum, et ab eo per Thoracem in Ramos Usque Subclavio Vasa Lactea Deteguntur. Paris, Cramoisy, 1651.
7. Bartholin T: Vasa Lymphatica. Hafniae, Petrus Hakius, 1653.
8. Rudbeck O: Novo Exercitatio Anatomica, Exhibens Ductus Hepaticos, Aquoso et Vasa Glandularum Serosa. Arosiae, kexud. e. Lauringerus 1653 [English translation in Bull Hist Med 11:304, 1942.]
9. Ruysch F: Dilucidatio Valvularium in Vasis Lymphaticis, et Lacteis. Hagaecomitiae, Harmani Gael, 1665.
10. Nuck A: Adenographia Curiosa et Uteri Foeminei Anatome Nova. Lugduni Batavorum, Jordanum Luchtmans, 1692.
11. Cruikshank WC: The Anatomy of the Absorbing Vessels of the Human Body. London, G Nicol, 1786.
12. Mascagni P: Vasorum Lymphaticorum Corporis Humani Historia et Ichnographia, Vol. 138. Senis, Pazzini Carli, 1787, p. 27.
13. Sappey PC: Anatomie, Physiologie, Pathologie des Vaisseaux Lymphatiques, Considérés chez l'Homme et chez les Vertebrés. Paris, Delahaye et Lecrossier, 1874.
14. Ranvier L: Morphologie et developpment des vaisseaux lymphatiques chez mammiferes. Arch d'Anat Microscopique 1:69, 1897.
15. Hunter W: Hunter's Lectures of Anatomy. Amsterdam, Elsevier, 1972.
16. Hewson W: The Lymphatic System in the Human Subject, and in Other Animals. London, J Johnson, 1774.
17. von Kölliker A: Handbuch der Gewebelehre des Menschen. Leipzig, W. Engelmann, 1855.
18. von Recklinghausen F: Die Lymphgefässe und ihre Beziehungen zum Bindegewebe. Berlin, Hirschwald, 1862.
19. Drinker CK: The Lymphatic System: Its Part in Regulating Composition and Volume of Tissue Fluid. Stanford, Calif. Stanford University Press, 1942.
20. Starling EH: On the absorption of fluids from the connective tissue spaces. J Physiol (Lond) 19:312, 1896.
21. Ludwig CFW: Lehrbuch der Physiologie des Menschen, 2nd ed. Leipzig, 1858–1861, p 562.
22. Yoffey JM, Courtice FC: Lymphatics, Lymph and the Lymphomyeloid Complex. New York, Academic Press, 1970.
23. Rusznyák I, Földi M, Szabö G: Lymphatics and Lymph Circulation. New York, Pergamon Press, 1960.
24. Kinmonth JB: The Lymphatics: Surgery, Lymphography and Diseases of the Chyle and Lymph Systems. London, Edward Arnold, 1982.
25. Olszewski W: The enigma of lymphedema—search for answers. Lymphology 24:100, 1991.
26. Browse NL: The diagnosis and management of primary lymphedema. J Vasc Surg 3:181, 1986.
27. Gloviczki P, Calcagno D, Schirger A, et al: Non-invasive evaluation of the swollen extremity: Experiences with 190 lymphoscintigraphic examinations. J Vasc Surg 9:683, 1989.
28. Clouse ME, Wallace S: Lymphatic Imaging. Lymphography, Computed Tomography, and Scintigraphy, 2nd ed. Baltimore, Williams & Wilkins, 1985.
29. Reynolds WD, Sy FS: Eradication of filariasis in South Carolina: A historical perspective. J SC Med Assoc 85:331, 1989.
30. Kissin MW, della Rovere GQ, Easton D, Westbury G: Risk of lymphoedema following the treatment of breast cancer. Br J Surg 73:580, 1986.
31. Földi E, Földi M, Clodius L: The lymphedema chaos: A lancet. Ann Plast Surg 22:505, 1989.
32. Pappas CJ, O'Donnell TF Jr: Long-term results of compression treatment for lymphedema. J Vasc Surg 16:555, 1992.
33. Miller AJ: The history of the lymphatics of the heart. *In* Miller AJ (ed): Lymphatics of the Heart. New York, Raven Press, 1982, pp 1–43.
34. Pflug JJ, Schirger A: Chronic peripheral lymphedema. *In* Clement DL, Shepherd JT (eds): Vascular Diseases in the Limbs: Mechanisms and Principles of Treatment. St. Louis, Mosby–Year Book, 1993, pp 221–238.
35. Gloviczki P, Fisher J, Hollier LH, et al: Microsurgical lymphovenous anastomosis for treatment of lymphedema: A critical review. J Vasc Surg 7:647, 1988.
36. O'Brien BMC, Mellow CG, Khazanchi RK, et al: Long-term results after microlymphatico-venous anastomoses for the treatment of obstructive lymphedema. Plast Reconstr Surg 85:562, 1990.
37. Baumeister RG, Siuda S: Treatment of lymphedemas by microsurgical lymphatic grafting: What is proved? Plast Reconstr Surg 85:64, 1990.
38. Goldsmith HS: Long-term evaluation of omental transposition for chronic lymphedema. Ann Surg 180:847, 1974.
39. Hurst PA, Stewart G. Kinmonth JB, Browse NL: Long-term results of the enteromesenteric bridge operation in the treatment of primary lymphoedema. Br J Surg 72:272, 1985.
40. Trevidic P, Cormier JM: Free axillary lymph node transfer. *In* Cluzan RV (ed): Progress in Lymphology XIII. Amsterdam, Elsevier, 1992, pp 415–420.
41. Campisi C, Tosatti E, Casaccia M, et al: Lymphatic microsurgery. Minerva Chir 41:469, 1986.
42. Witte CL, Witte, MH: The enigma of lymphedema—a search for answers. Lymphology 24:100, 1991.

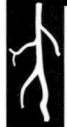

Circulatory Dynamics and Pathophysiology of the Lymphatic System

Charles L. Witte, M.D., and Marlys H. Witte, M.D.

> Any proteid which leaves these vessels . . . is lost for the time to the vascular system. . . . it must be collected by lymphatics and restored to the vascular system by way of the thoracic or right lymphatic duct.
>
> *Starling, 1897*

In a narrow sense, the lymph circulation is a unidirectional vascular system that merely transports surplus tissue fluid back to the bloodstream. In a broader sense, however, this network stabilizes the mobile intercellular liquid and extracellular matrix microenvironment to ensure parenchymal cellular integrity and function. In its entirety, the lymphatic system is composed of vascular conduits, lymphoid organs (including the lymph nodes, spleen, Peyer's patches, thymus, and nasopharyngeal tonsils), and cellular elements (such as lymphocytes and macrophages that circulate in the liquid lymph). These migrating cells cross the blood-capillary barrier along with a multitude of immunoglobulins, polypeptides, plasma protein complexes, and cytokines and enter lymphatics to return to the bloodstream.

Whereas body water circulates very rapidly as a plasma suspension of red blood cells in the blood vascular compartment, it percolates slowly outside the bloodstream as a tissue fluid–lymph suspension of lymphocytes through lymph vessels and lymph nodes. As a specialized subcompartment of the extracellular space, therefore, the lymphatic system completes a closed loop for the circulation by returning liquid, macromolecules, and other blood elements that "escape," or "leak," from blood capillaries (Fig. 155–1). Disruption of this blood-lymph loop promotes tissue swelling and is responsible for a variety of syndromes characterized by scarring, wasting, immunodeficiency, and dysangiogenesis.

TOPOGRAPHY

Macroscopic Anatomy

The discovery early in the 17th century of chylous mesenteric lacteals in a well-fed dog by Gasparo Aselli set off a flurry of anatomic dissections in England and continental Europe that established the nearly ubiquitous presence of lymphatics throughout the body and their important role in

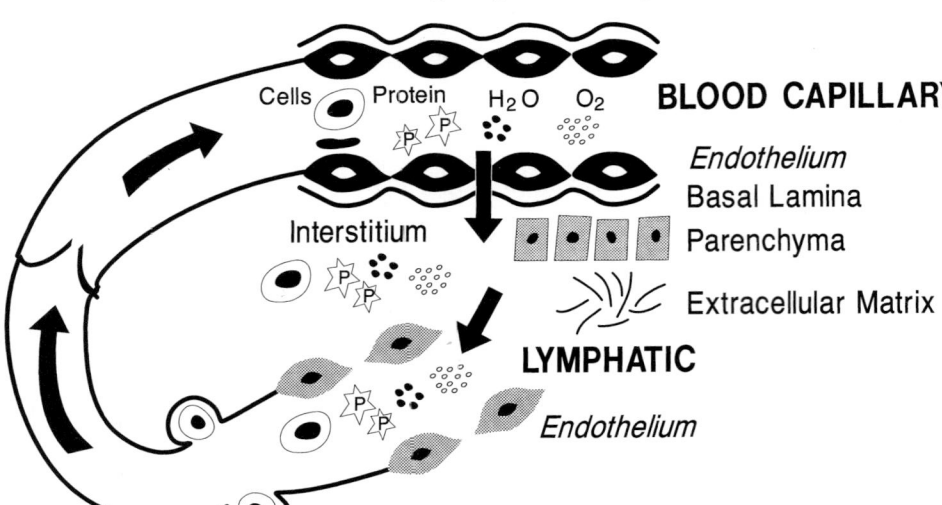

FIGURE 155–1. The closed liquid circulation of the body. In the bloodstream, water flows rapidly, as a plasma suspension of red blood cells; outside the bloodstream, it flows slowly, as a tissue fluid–lymph suspension of lymphocytes through lymphatics and lymph nodes. Small and large molecules, including plasma proteins (P), cells, and respiratory gases cross the blood capillary-endothelial barrier to nourish the parenchyma and then return in the lymph stream.

the absorption of nutrients.[1] These lymphatic "absorbents" accompany venous trunks everywhere except in the central nervous system and in the cortical bony skeleton.

In general, lymph from the lower torso and viscera enters the bloodstream via the thoracic duct at the left subclavian–jugular venous junction. Lymphatics from the head and neck and the upper extremities enter the central veins either independently or via a common supraclavicular cistern. Numerous interconnections exist in this rich vascular network, and subvariant anatomic pathways are plentiful. For example, the bulk of cardiac and pulmonary lymph as well as the intraperitoneal fluid, which drains through fenestrae of the diaphragm into substernal mediastinal collectors, unites as a common trunk to empty into the great veins in the right neck. Intestinal lymph transports cholesterol and fat-soluble vitamins, such as A, K, D, and long-chain triglycerides as chylomicra after oral ingestion. Unlike intestinal blood, which flows directly into the liver (via the portal vein), intestinal lacteals course retroperitoneally to the aortic hiatus to form, with other visceral and retroperitoneal lymphatics, the multichannel cisterna chyli and the thoracic duct. The bulk of the lymph formed in the liver flows retrograde, or countercurrent to the portal blood flow, and enters intestinal lymph collectors just before the origin of the thoracic duct. Only a small amount of hepatic lymph drains antegrade along the major hepatic veins to the anterior mediastinum and the right lymph duct.

Although these topographic variants influence the development and progression of peripheral (lymph)edema only indirectly, these features are nonetheless essential for a broad understanding of edema syndromes, including those accompanied by visceral lymphatic abnormalities, celomic effusions, and chylous reflux. Technically, the brain and retina do not have a lymphatic apparatus, but they possess analogous circulations, such as the aqueous humor–canal of Schlemm in the anterior chamber of the eye or the cerebrospinal fluid–subarachnoid villi connections (pacchionian bodies). Glial elements and non–endothelium-lined intracerebral perivascular (Virchow-Robin) spaces probably also transport interstitial fluid to nearby intracranial venous sinuses. Extensive interruption of cervical lymphatic trunks (e.g., after bilateral radical neck dissection), therefore, causes prominent facial suffusion and a transient neurologic syndrome resembling pseudotumor cerebri,[2] whereas an infusion of crystalloid solution directly into the canine cisterna magna causes elevation of intracranial pressure and increases lymph flow from draining neck lymphatics.[3, 4] Although abundant lymphatic pathways thus are available to return surplus tissue fluid to the bloodstream, homeostasis of the internal environment still depends on an intact interstitial-lymph fluid circulatory system (see Fig. 155–1).

Microscopic Anatomy

As an afferent vascular system, the lymphatics originate in the interstitium as specialized capillaries, although in certain organs (such as the liver) they seem to emanate from nonendothelialized precapillary channels (e.g., the spaces of Disse).[5] Lymphatic capillaries are remarkably porous and readily permit entry of even large macromolecules (>1000 kd). In this respect, they resemble the uniquely "leaky" fenestrated sinusoidal blood capillaries of the liver but are distinctively different from most other blood capillaries, which are relatively impervious to macromolecules, even those the size of albumin (MW = 69 kd).[6]

Under light microscopy without pre–paraffin-embedded tracer or intravascular latex injection, it is difficult to distinguish between blood and lymph vessels, although the latter are usually thin-walled and tortuous, have wider, more irregular lumina and are largely devoid of red blood cells. Many staining features have been proposed to differentiate between blood and lymph microvasculature, such as the endothelial marker factor VIII: vWF (von Willebrand's factor). Although staining characteristics vary in both normal tissue and that involved by disease, and at different sites (perhaps because of endothelial cell de-differentiation), in general, lymphatic staining resembles, but is less intense than, its blood vessel counterpart; that is, the staining differences, if any, are more quantitative than qualitative.[7–9]

Ultrastructurally, lymph capillaries display both "open" and "closed" (or so-called tight) endothelial junctions, often with prominent convolutions.[8] Depending on the extent of tissue "activity," these capillaries can dramatically adjust their shape and lumen size. Unlike blood capillaries, a basal lamina (basement membrane) is tenuous or lacking altogether in lymph capillaries.[10, 11] Moreover, complex elastic fibrils, termed *anchoring filaments,* tether the outer portions of the endothelium to a fibrous gel matrix in the interstitium.[12, 13] These filaments allow the lymph microvessels to open wide in response to sudden increases in tissue fluid load and pressure, in contrast to the simultaneous collapse of adjacent blood capillaries (Fig. 155–2).

Just beyond the lymph capillaries are the terminal lymphatics. In contrast to more proximal and larger lymph collectors and trunks, these are devoid of smooth muscle, although the endothelial lining is rich in the contractile protein actin.[7] Intraluminal bicuspid valves are also prominent features, and they serve to partition the lymphatic vessels into discrete contractile segments termed *lymphangions.*[14] These specialized microscopic features of the lymphatic network support the function of this delicate apparatus, that of absorbing and transporting lymph node elements and the large protein moieties, cells, and foreign agents of the bloodstream (e.g., viruses, bacterial) that have gained access to the interstitial space (Fig. 155–3).

PHYSIOLOGY

General Principles

Because it is a fine adjuster of the tissue microenvironment, the lymphatic system is neglected in most treatises on vascular diseases. Yet this delicate system, very inconspicuous during life and collapsed after death, participates in (1) maintenance of the liquid, protein, and osmotic equilibrium around cells; (2) absorption and distribution of nutrients, disposal of wastes, and (3) exchange of oxygen and carbon dioxide in the local *milieu interieur.*

Two thirds of the human body is water, and most of it is contained in the cells. It is the remainder existing outside the cells, however, that continuously circulates. In a series of epochal experiments conducted nearly a century ago,

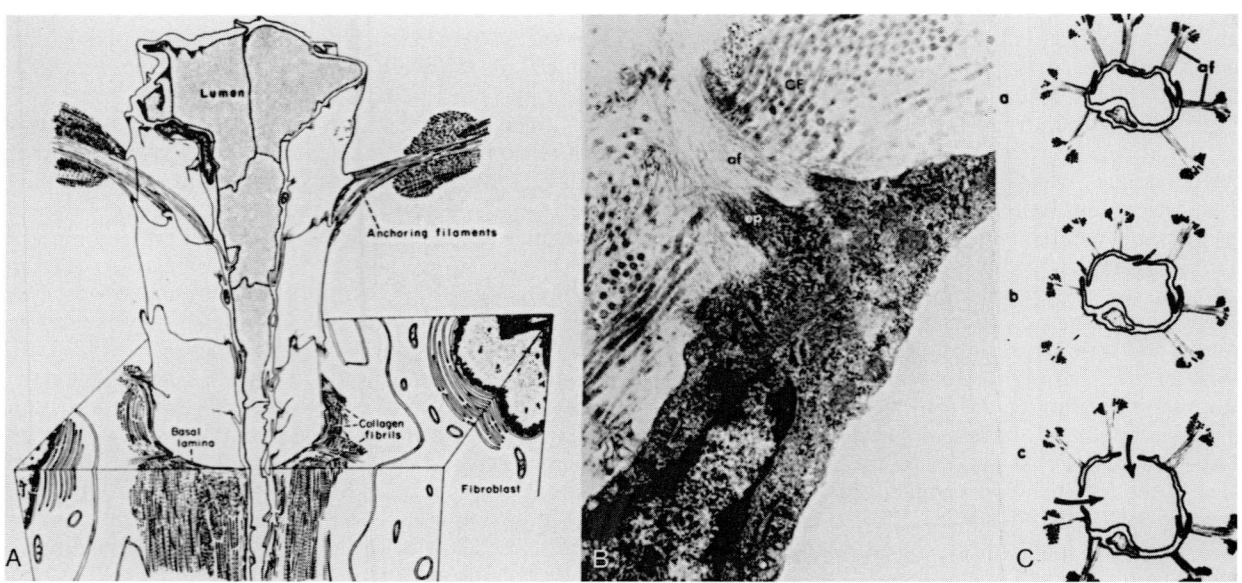

FIGURE 155–2. *A,* Three-dimensional diagram of a lymphatic capillary reconstructed from collated electron micrographs. The lymphatic anchoring filaments originate from the abluminal surface of the endothelial cells and extend into adjacent collagen bundles, forming a firm connection between the lymphatic capillary wall and the surrounding interstitium. *B,* Transmission electron micrograph demonstrating anchoring filaments (af) that derive from the lymphatic endothelium (ep) and join nearby collagen bundles (CF). *C,* Response of lymphatic capillaries to an increase in interstitial fluid volume. As the tissue matrix expands, the tension on the anchoring filaments (af) rises, and the lymph capillaries open widely to allow more rapid entry of liquid and solute (a-c). In contrast to the stretching of the lymph capillaries, a rise in matrix pressure collapses the blood capillaries, restricting further plasma filtration. (*A-C,* From Leak LV, Burke JF: Ultrastructural studies on the lymphatic anchoring filaments. Reproduced from Cell Biol 30:129–149, 1968, by copyright permission of the Rockefeller University Press; and Leak LV: Electron microscopic observation on lymphatic capillaries and the structural components of the connective tissue–lymph interface. Microvasc Res 2:361, 1970.)

the English physiologist Ernest Starling outlined the pivotal factors that regulate the partition of extracellular fluid.[15, 16]

The distribution of fluid between the blood vascular compartment and tissues and the net flux of plasma escaping from the bloodstream depends principally on the transcapillary balance of hydrostatic and protein osmotic pressure gradients as modified by the character (i.e., the hydraulic conductance) of the filtering microvascular surface (Fig. 155–4). Normally, a small surplus of tissue fluid forms continuously (net capillary filtration), which enters the lymphatics and returns to the venous system.

In contrast to blood, which flows in a "circular" pattern at the rate of several liters per minute, lymph flows in one direction only and, at rest, amounts to only 2 to 2.5 L/day. This limited volume is the result of a slight hydrodynamic imbalance that favors fluid, salt, and macromolecular movement from plasma into tissue spaces. Although blood capillary beds vary in hydraulic conductance, disturbances in the transcapillary hydrostatic and protein osmotic pressure gradients (Starling forces) tend to promote edema fluid that is low in protein content (<1.0 gm/dl), whereas impedance to lymph flow (lymph stasis) promotes protein-rich lymph-edema fluid content (>1.5 gm/dl).

Unlike blood flow, which is propelled by a powerful and highly specialized muscular pump, the heart, lymph is propelled predominantly by spontaneous intrinsic segmental contractions of larger (and probably also small) lymph trunks (Fig. 155–5),[17–19] and, to a lesser extent, by extrinsic "haphazard forces" such as breathing, sighing, yawning, muscle squeezing (e.g., alimentary peristalsis), and transmitted arterial pulsations.[19, 20] The contractions of lymphatic segments between intraluminal valves (i.e., the

lymphangions) are very responsive to lymph volume. Thus, an increase in lymph formation is accompanied by more frequent and more powerful lymphangion contractions (Fig. 155–6), a lymphodynamic response that resembles Starling's other major physiologic principle, "the Law of the Heart."[14, 21]

Lymphatic truncal contraction, like venous and arterial vasomotion, is mediated by sympathomimetic agents (both alpha- and beta- adrenergic agonists),[22, 23] by-products of arachidonic acid metabolism (thromboxanes and prostaglandins),[24–27] and neurogenic stimuli (Fig. 155–7).[28, 29] Oddly, in different regions of the body, lymphatic trunks seem to exhibit different sensitivities to vasoactive and neurogenic stimulants.[23, 30, 31] Although the importance of truncal vasomotion as mediated by tunica smooth muscle is well established, it remains unclear whether terminal lymphatics or lymphatic capillaries also are capable of vasomotion or are simply passive channels. In some ways, this controversy parallels the prolonged dispute about whether blood capillary endothelial cells are capable of vasoactivity, a question now clearly resolved in the affirmative. Because lymphatic endothelium, like blood endothelium, is rich in actin[7] (a principal contractile protein), it is reasonable to assume that lymphatic microvessels also exhibit vasomotion.

In addition to their central immune function, lymph nodes are potential sites of impedance to lymph flow. Unlike frogs, which lack lymph nodes but possess four or more strategically placed "lymph hearts," which propel large quantities of peripheral lymph back to the bloodstream,[32, 33] mammals possess immunoreactive lymph nodes, which, when swollen, fibrotic, or atrophic, may

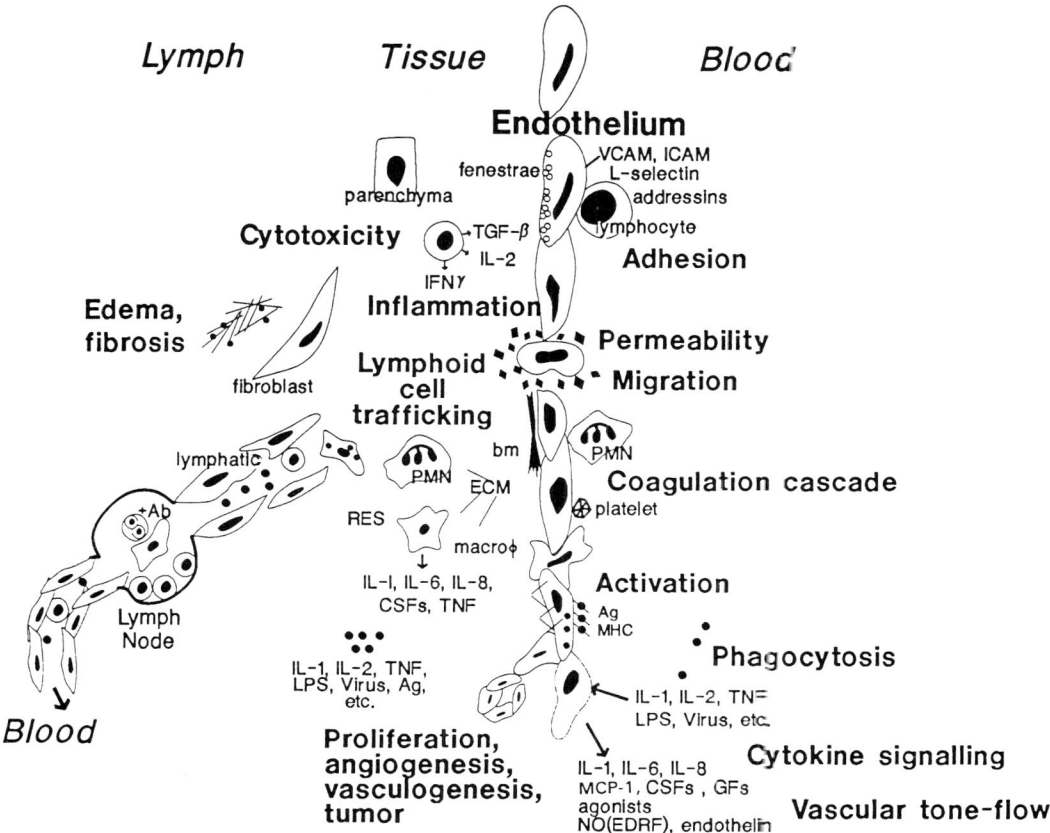

FIGURE 155–3. Schematic illustration depicting the postulated role of endothelial processes in microcirculatory events bearing on angiogenesis in the blood-lymph loop. These include macromolecular and liquid permeability, vasoreponsiveness, leukocyte adhesion and transmigration, coagulation cascade, particulate phagocytosis, antigen presentation and cytokine activation, lymphoid cell trafficking, and proliferative events leading to growth of new vessel or tumor. Although scarcely studied, processes corresponding to those implicated at the blood–vascular endothelial surface probably also occur at the lymphatic-endothelial interface. The relative anatomic and dynamic relationships among blood and lymph vascular endothelium, parenchymal and extravascular connective tissues, and transmigrating leukocytes are shown. Ag = antigen; bm = basement membrane; CSFs = colony-stimulating factors; ECM = extracellular matrix; EDRF = endothelium-derived relaxing factor; GFs = growth factors; ICAM = intercellular adhesion molecule; IFN = interferon; IL = interleukin; LPS = lipopolysaccharide; macroϕ = macrophage; MCP-1 = monocyte chemoattractant protein 1; MHC = major histocompatibility complex; NO (EDRF) = nitric oxide (endothelium derived relaxing factor; PMN = polymorphonuclear leukocyte; RES = reticuloendothelial system; TGF = transforming growth factor; TNF = tumor necrosis factor; VCAM = vascular cell adhesion molecule; ● = exogenous particulates; ■ = macromolecules; drops represent fluid (plasma, interstitial, or lymph).

$$\Delta \text{IFV} = \int K_f \left[(P_c - P_t) - \sigma(\pi_p - \pi_t) \right] - \int Q_L$$

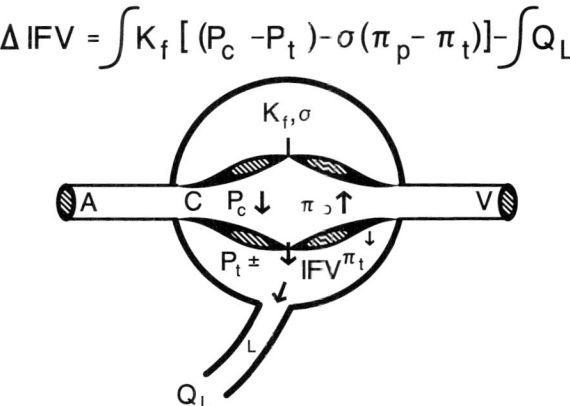

FIGURE 155–4. Schematic diagram of the primary forces regulating fluid flux into the interstitium and the importance of lymph flow in maintaining steady-state interstitial fluid volume and, hence, a stable partition of extracellular fluid between the bloodstream and the interstitium.

Normal: $\Delta \text{IFV} = 0$

A = arteriole $\quad$ P_c = capillary pressure $\quad$ K_f = filtration coefficient
V = venule $\quad$ P_t = tissue pressure $\quad$ σ = solute coefficient
C = capillary $\quad$ π_p = plasma oncotic pressure $\quad$ IFV = interstitial fluid volume
L = lymph $\quad$ π_t = tissue oncotic pressure $\quad$ Q_L = lymph flow

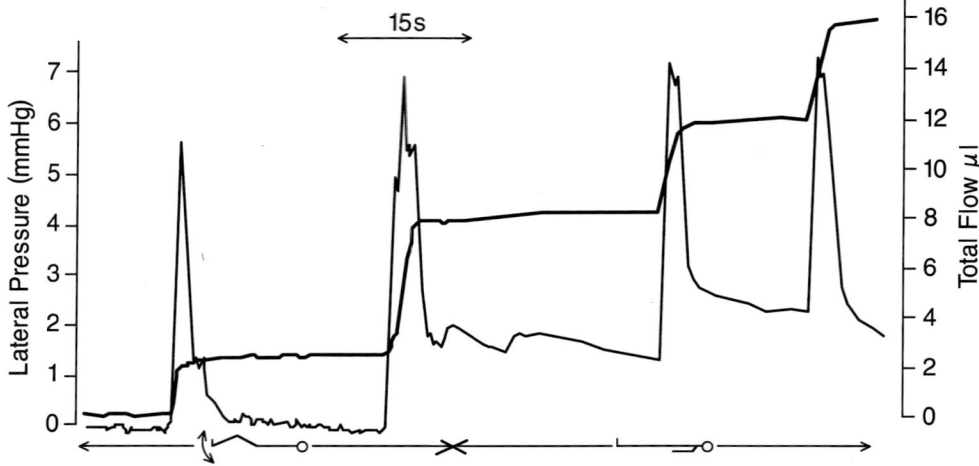

FIGURE 155–5. Lateral pressure (*curve with sharp peaks*) and cumulative lymph flow (*stepwise rising curve*) in a subcutaneous leg lymphatic of a healthy man lying supine (1) during movement of the foot and (2) at rest. Note that lymph flow occurs only during rhythmic contraction of the lymphatic collector and, specifically, not by voluntary contraction of calf muscles. s = seconds. (From Olszewski WL, Engeset A: Intrinsic contractility of prenodal lymph vessels and lymph flow in the human leg. Am J Physiol 239:H775, 1980.)

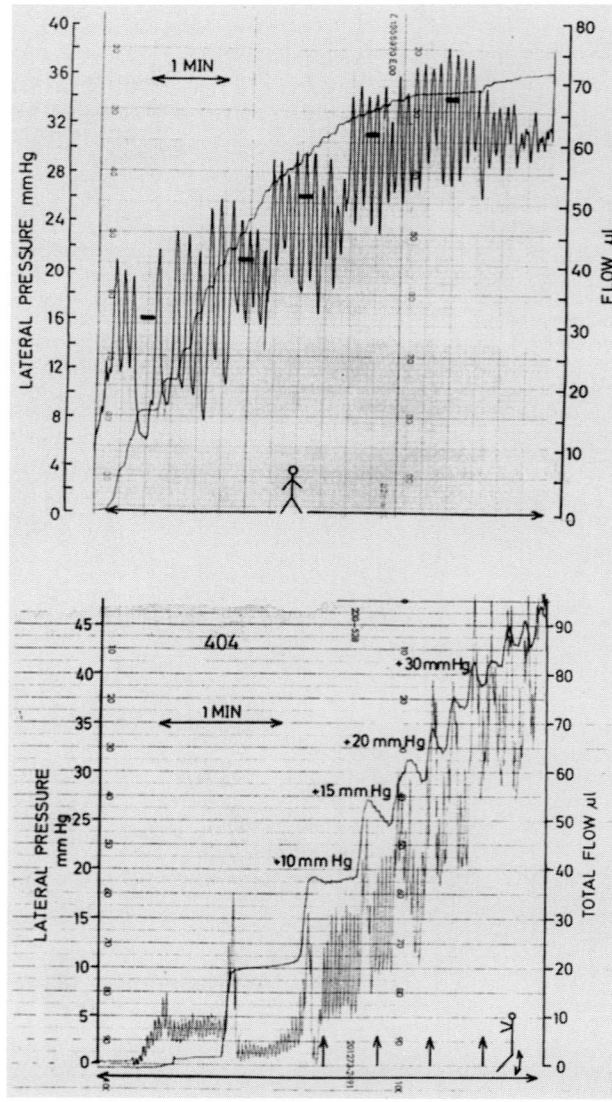

FIGURE 155–6. A human leg lymphatic has been cannulated retrograde, and the external tip of the cannula has been progressively raised, gradually increasing hydrostatic pressure above the level of the cannulated lymphatic. While the subject is upright (*upper tracing*), sequential increases in outflow resistance cause an increase in lymphatic pulse frequency with subsequent decreases in pulse amplitude, lymph flow (*stepwise ascending curve*), and stroke volume. When the intralymphatic pressure reaches 34 mmHg, lymph flow ceases despite a high pulsation rate. The lower tracing was made while the subject walked on tiptoes and rising outflow pressure induced more frequent lymphatic pulsations. Note, again, that calf muscle contraction with up-and-down foot motion is not associated with greater lymph propulsion. At higher pressures, each flow wave is followed by sporadic retrograde flow (reflux), which probably relates to intraluminal valve incompetence in the distending lymph vessel. (From Olszewski WL: Lymph pressure and flow in limbs. *In* Lymph Stasis: Pathophysiology, Diagnosis, and Treatment. Boca Raton, Fla, CRC Press, 1991, pp 136–137.)

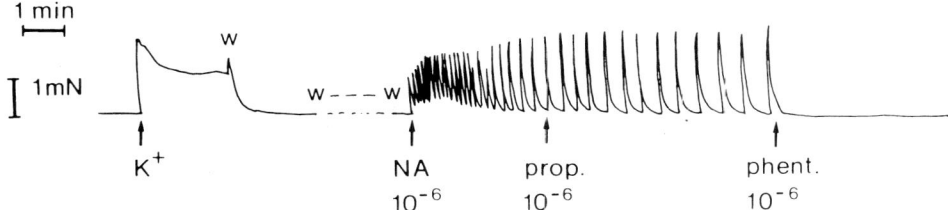

FIGURE 155–7. Tracing taken from a human lower leg lymphatic segment. Noradrenaline (NA) 10^{-6}M induces phasic lymphatic contractions that are not affected by the beta-blocker propranolol (prop) 10^{-6}M but are abolished by phentolamine (phent) 10^{-6}M. K$^+$ indicates previous potassium–induced (124 mM) contraction, and W indicates washout with fresh Krebs buffer solution. (From Sjöberg T, Steen S: Contractile properties of lymphatics from the human lower leg. Lymphology 24:16, 1991.)

initiate or perpetuate lymph stasis.[34, 35] Perhaps the intrinsic contraction of mammalian lymphatic trunks represents a phylogenetic vestige of amphibian lymph heart activity (see Flow-Pressure Dynamics).

Flow-Pressure Dynamics

Although lymphatics, like veins, are thin-walled, flexible conduits that return liquid to the heart, the flow-pressure

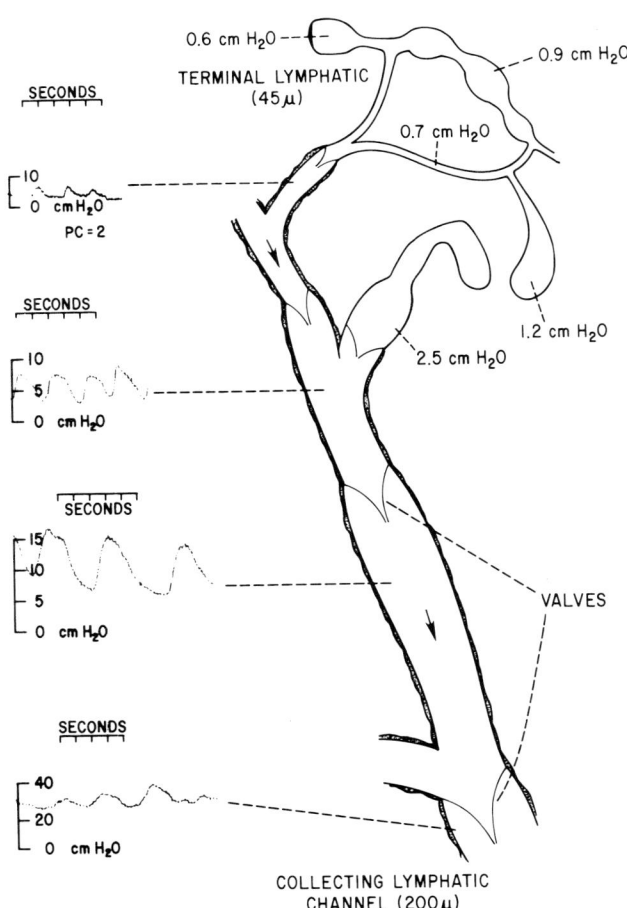

FIGURE 155–8. Composite drawing of terminal lymphatic network reconstructed from several mesenteric preparations in the rat demonstrated a gradual rise in intralymphatic pressure from 0.6 cm H_2O in the terminal lymphatics to 30 cmH$_2$O in the larger collecting duct. Note also the rhythmic pressure pulsations in the collecting trunks. (From Zweifach BW, Prather JW: Micromanipulation of pressure in terminal lymphatics in the mesentery. Am J Physiol 228: 1326, 1975.)

relationships in the venous and lymphatic systems are quite different. The energy to drive blood in the venous system derives primarily from the thrust of the heart. The cardiac propulsive boost maintains a pressure head through the arteries and blood capillaries into the veins that is sufficient to overcome venous vascular resistance. In the presence of competent venous valves, muscle contractions such as those produced by walking and running, supplement cardiac action in facilitating return of blood to the heart.

Lymph vessels in tissues, however, are not directly contiguous with the blood vessels, and most of the energy for lymph propulsion emanates from the intrinsic lymphatic truncal wall contractions (propulsor lymphaticum).[17–23] Like amphibian lymph heart tissue (cor lymphaticum), mammalian lymphatic smooth muscle beats rhythmically and, in the presence of a well-developed intraluminal valve system, facilitates lymph transport (Fig. 155–8).[36] In a sense, the lymphatics function as micropumps that respond to fluid challenges with increases in both rate and stroke volume.[14, 24] Ordinarily, resistance to flow in the lymphatic vessels is relatively high, as compared with the resistance in the venous system,[37] but the pumping capacity of the lymphatics is able to overcome this impedance by generating intraluminal pressures of 30 to 50 mmHg (see Fig. 155–6) and sometimes pressures that even equal or exceed arterial pressure.[17, 37, 38] This formidable lymphatic ejection force is modulated not only by filling pressure but also by temperature, sympathomimetics, neurogenic stimuli, circulating hormones, and locally released paracrine and autocrine cytokine secretions.[39]

It is often (mistakenly) thought that lymph return, like venous return, is directly enhanced by truncal compression from skeletal muscle and other adjacent structures. Whereas muscle contraction and external massage clearly accelerate lymph return in the presence of edema,[38] under normal conditions, peripheral lymph flow is regulated primarily by spontaneous contraction of the lymphatics themselves.[38, 39] In peripheral lymphatics (unlike peripheral veins), the column of liquid is incomplete. Accordingly, with normal intralymphatic pressure, external compression is ineffective for propelling lymph onward (Fig. 155–9), although it may increase the frequency and amplitude of lymphatic contractions. Lymphatics, therefore, in contrast to veins, are not sufficiently "primed."[40] During lymphatic obstruction and persistent lymph stasis, hydrostatic pressure in the draining tissue watersheds and lymphatics rises as intrinsic truncal contractions fail to expel lymph completely. In this circumstance, unlike the normal situation, the fluid column in the lymphatics becomes continuous,

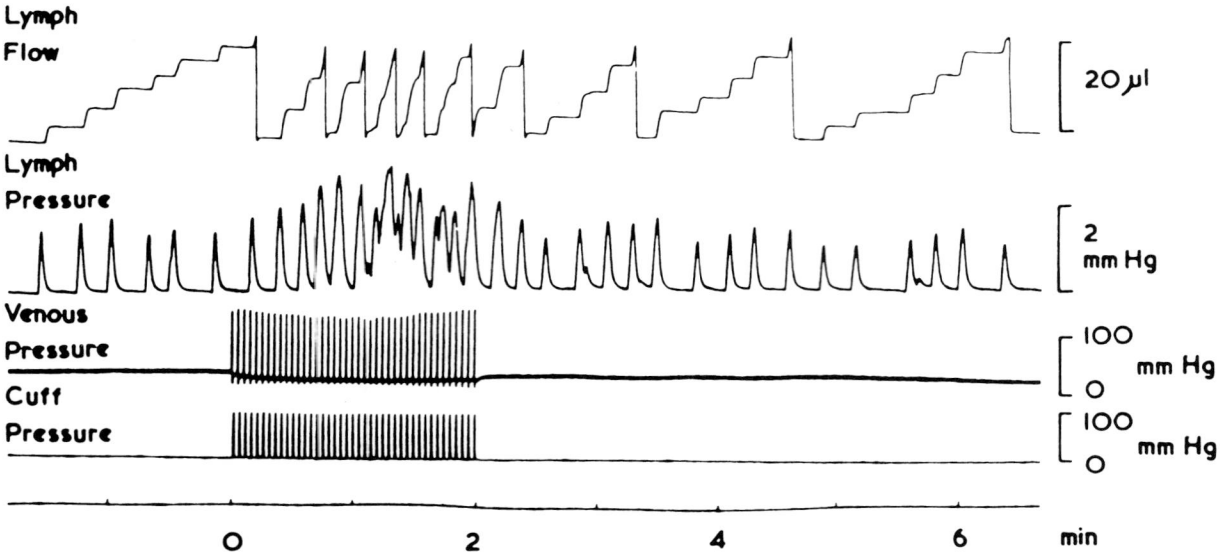

FIGURE 155–9. Effect of intermittent external pneumatic compression of the sheep foot on peripheral lymph flow, lymph outflow pressure, and venous pressure. Note that before external compression the lymphatic contracts spontaneously, and each contraction extrudes a small quantity of lymph, which appears as a step increment in the flow record. In the 2-minute period during which the foot cuff is intermittently inflated, each compression causes a synchronous pressure rise in peripheral venous pressure but not in lymph pressure. The frequency and amplitude of spontaneous lymphatic contractions increase, however, and this increase is associated with a concomitant rise in lymph flow. (From Pippard C, Roddie IC: Comparison of fluid transport systems in lymphatics and veins. Lymphology 20:224, 1987.)

and skeletal muscle or forceful external compression then becomes an effective pumping mechanism that aids lymph transport.[38, 40]

Results of studies of the effects of gravity on peripheral lymphatic and venous pressure conform to these findings. Whereas assuming an erect position sharply raises distal venous pressure, peripheral intralymphatic pressure is not affected, although lymphatic truncal pulsation increases in both frequency and amplitude.[40] This arrangement favors the removal of tissue fluid by the lymphatics during dependency because, unlike the veins, the lymphatics operate at much lower hydrostatic pressures. Once the lymphatics become obstructed, truncal contractions quicken at first; however, the intraluminal valves then gradually give way. As the lymphatic fluid column becomes continuous, this mechanical advantage is lost and chronic lymphedema supervenes (Table 155–1).

PATHOPHYSIOLOGY

Overview

Because both congenital absence and radical excision of regional lymph nodes (and thus lymphatics) are associated with edema, it seems reasonable to conclude that lymphedema is simply the end result of insufficient lymphatic drainage. Nevertheless, peripheral lymphedema has proved difficult to simulate in experimental animals and to treat.

Initial experimental attempts to simulate the clinical condition using lymphatic sclerosis and radical excision were notoriously unsuccessful and revealed a remarkable capacity of obstructed lymphatics to regenerate and "bridge the gap" or bypass the induced blockage with spontaneous opening of auxiliary lymphatic-venous shunts.[41, 42] Although transient swelling was common, these compensa-

TABLE 155–1. CIRCULATORY DYNAMICS OF VASCULAR CONDUITS

FEATURE	LYMPHATIC	VEIN	ARTERY
Primary propulsive unit	Lymphangion*	Heart	Heart
Secondary propulsive force	Haphazard†	Skeletal muscle	Vasomotion
Distal (upright) pressure (mmHg)	2–3	90–100	20
Central pressure (mmHg)	6–10	0–2	100
Flow rate	Very low	High	High
Vascular resistance	Relatively high	Very low	High
Intraluminal valves	Innumerable	Several	None
Impediment to flow	Lymph nodes	None	None
Conduit fluid column	Incomplete	Complete	Complete
Conduit failure	Edema (>1.5 gm/dl)	Edema (<1.0 gm/dl)	Claudication
	Brawny induration	Skin pigmentation	Rest pain
	Acanthosis	"Stasis" ulceration	Tissue necrosis

*A contractile segment of lymph vessel between two lymphatic valves.
†Breathing, sighing, yawning, peristalsis, transmitted arterial pulsation. Skeletal muscle contraction also increases the amplitude and frequency of lymph vessel contractions and squeezes interstitial fluid into initial lymphatics (i.e., lymph capillaries).

tory mechanisms were thought to circumvent the development of permanent edema solely from obstruction to lymphatic drainage. The general failure of early lymph stasis experiments to reproduce unremitting peripheral edema reinforced a long-held theory that overt or subclinical bacterial infection (lymphangitis) was indispensable to the evolution of chronic lymphedema.[43] By disrupting microvascular integrity and promoting lymphatic obliteration, recurring infection was thought to exaggerate tissue scarring and, eventually, to cause unremitting lymphedema. This widely held belief was consistent with the commonly observed delayed onset and unpredictability of arm and leg edema after radical mastectomies and groin dissections, respectively, and the grotesque deformities of tropical lymphedema (so-called elephantiasis) associated with filariasis (*Wuchereria bancrofti* and *Brugia malayi*).

Although understanding is still incomplete, it is nonetheless now clear that nonpitting, brawny extremity edema can arise from lymph stasis alone and the associated unremitting accumulation of protein-rich fluid in the extracellular matrix. With repeated intralymphatic injections of silica particles, Drinker and colleagues[44] first succeeded in simulating chronic lymphedema in dogs by inducing extensive lymphatic sclerosis. Subsequently, Danese,[45] Olszewski,[35] and Clodius and Altorfer[46] and their associates established that refractory lymphedema could result solely from the mechanical interruption of peripheral lymphatics. An experimental model of circumferential lymphatic transection revealed that tissue swelling was prompt at first (acute lymphedema), disappeared by 4 to 6 weeks, and remained absent for months to years (latent lymphedema) but later reappeared and persisted (chronic lymphedema).

A similar sequence of events occurs in experimental (B. malayi) filariasis.[47] During the latent phase, when edema is not visible, conventional oil lymphography corroborates ongoing lymphatic destruction.[35] Progressive truncal tortuosity and dilatation give way to massive lymphangiectasis, valvular incompetence, and retrograde flow (dermal backflow). Serial microscopy discloses mononuclear cell infiltration, intramural destruction of lymphatic collectors, and collagen deposition throughout the soft tissues. Eventually, the lymph trunks lose their distinctive smooth muscle and endothelial lining, and the boundary lines between lymph collectors and the surrounding matrix progressively blur.[35, 46]

These studies definitively demonstrate that extensive impairment of lymph drainage is sufficient, by itself, to cause chronic lymphedema (Fig. 155–10). The key observation is the long interval between the disruption of the lymph trunks and the development of refractory edema, which helps to explain the inconstancy and unpredictability of limb swelling after radical operations for treatment of cancer and other disorders of lymphatic transport. As with deep venous occlusive disease, which is associated with valve destruction, venous stasis, and, eventually, overt edema (post-thrombophlebitic syndrome) with characteristic trophic skin changes (hyperpigmentation and ulceration), the absence or obliteration of the lymphatics is associated with lymphatic valve incompetence, lymph stasis, and, eventually, intractable edema (postlymphangitic syndrome), with its characteristic trophic skin changes

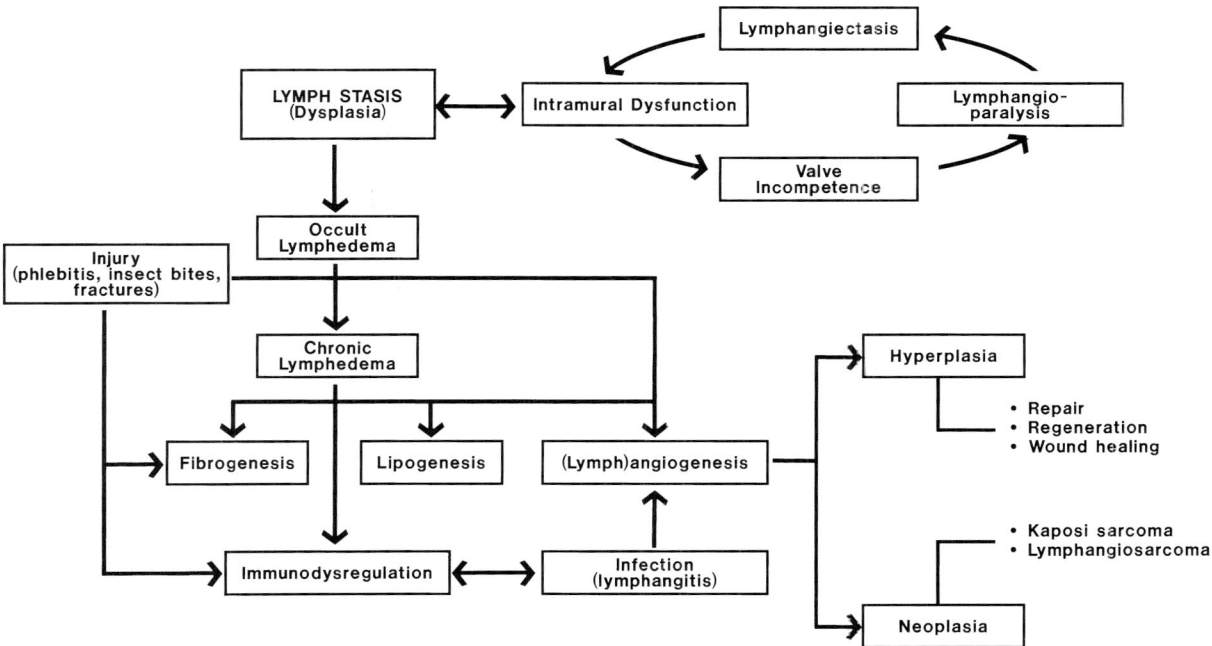

FIGURE 155–10. Flow chart illustrates the pathogenesis of peripheral lymphedema and some of its sequelae. According to this scheme, congenitally deficient or obstructed lymphatics promote lymph stasis, which is accompanied by deranged truncal contractility, progressive valve incompetence, destruction of contractile elements (lymphangioparalysis), and gradual ectasia of lymphatic collectors. After a variable period (occult lymphedema), sometimes aggravated by environmental trauma, a series of events is set into motion that culminates in chronic lymphedema. This clinical state is characterized not only by progressive swelling but also by deposition of fat and scar tissue, immunodysregulation, a propensity for cellulitis, and microvascular proliferation. These processes, on the one hand, are essential for repair and regeneration, but on the other hand they may result in bizarre and poorly understood new vascular growths.

(thickened toe skin folds, or Stemmer's sign, warty overgrowth, and brawny induration).[48]

Infection

Recurrent cellulitis is a devastating sequela of peripheral lymphedema. Erysipelas resulting from beta-hemolytic streptococcal infection is most common, but a variety of microorganisms may cause fulminant soft tissue infection.[49] To a certain extent, vulnerability to superimposed infection exists whenever tissue fluid stagnates. Thus, pyelonephritis with urinary retention, cholangitis with common duct stones, and spontaneous bacterial peritonitis with "cirrhotic" ascites are vivid examples of this phenomenon. Yet lymphedema (in contrast to edema states arising from imbalances in transcapillary hydrodynamic forces) is so prone to recurring lymphangitis that, at one time, it was mistaken as the *since qua non* of lymphedema (see earlier discussion).

The reasons for the extraordinary susceptibility of an extremity involved with lymphedema to secondary bacterial infection remain perplexing. Studies of canine-induced and human filarial lymphedema implicate defective complement activation and immunodysregulation.[35] Alternative hypotheses include the depopulation of regional lymph nodes and replacement by fat and scar tissue[34] and deficient protease activity of extravascular macrophages.[50] It remains unclear, however, whether these immune-mediated perturbations are systemic, strictly regional, or even peculiar to lymphedema. Nevertheless, the onset of overt lymphedema is often precipitated by sudden infection or injury in an extremity already exhibiting defective lymphatic function. Moreover, episodes of thrombophlebitis and trauma, including bone fractures and multiple insect bites, are associated with "lymphangitis" and exacerbation of peripheral

lymphedema. Walking barefoot particularly in Third World countries where proper hygiene is often unavailable predisposes to overt or occult cellulitis and local foot infections that aggravate filaria-induced lymphedema and exaggerate exuberant skin verrucae and dermal scarring. Thus, in an extremity where lymphatic drainage is already marginal, even minor trauma and infection may initiate a protracted and pernicious cycle that, in extreme cases, culminates in a deformity resembling an elephantine limb and that, on rare occasions, leads to a very aggressive vascular malignancy (see Fig. 155–10 and earlier discussion).

Fibrosis

Like the sequela of superimposed infection, the complication of progressive interstitial fibrosis also sets apart lymphedema from other edematous states. Whereas the pathogenetic sequence linking scarring to lymphedema is still ill defined, it has long been recognized that conditions associated with edema fluid of high protein content (such as that of lymphedema) are characterized by fibrous proliferation.

Altered cytokine production, perturbed immunoreactivity, accumulation of abnormal plasma protein moieties, including growth factors in the extracellular matrix, proliferation of mast cells with release of vasomediators such as histamine,[51, 52] and activation of a complement cascade with "fixation" to immune complexes, may exert, singly or in toto, both microvascular and chemotactic effects that facilitate tissue infiltration of chronic inflammatory cells (e.g., lymphocytes and macrophages).[53] As fibrin-and cell-binding circulating fibronectins accumulate in the stagnant edema fluid, they act as the scaffolding and support glue for the migration of fibroblasts and the laying down of collagen.[54] In addition, lymph stasis and the build-up of plasma proteins trapped in the interstitium overwhelm in-

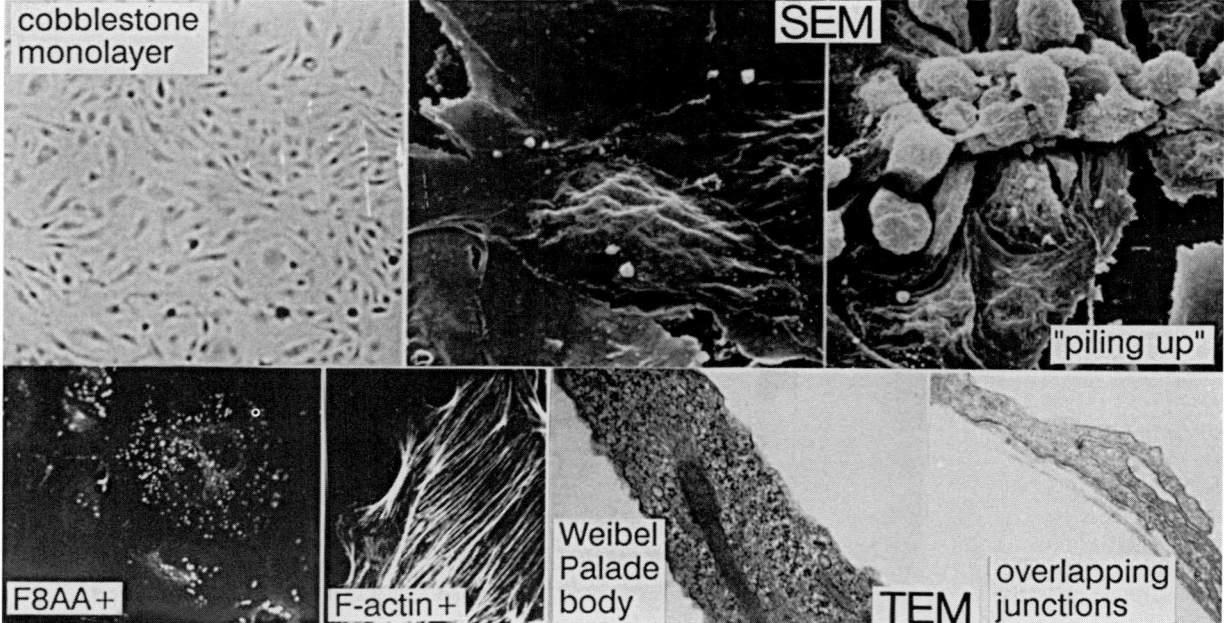

FIGURE 155–11. Lymphatic endothelial cell line derived from a retroperitoneal lymphangioma. Note the cobblestone morphology and on scanning electron microscopy (SEM) the polygonal cells in some areas that are "piling up," the positive stain for von Willebrand (vWf) factor 8 and F-actin, and, on transmission electron microscopy (TEM), the presence of Weibel-Palade bodies and typical lymphatic overlapping cell junctions. (From Way L, et al: Lymphatic endothelial cell line (CH3) from a recurrent retroperitoneal lymphangioma. In Vitro 23:647, 1987).

trinsic neutrophil and macrophage proteases and provoke diffuse scarring.[55]

Intensive neoangiogenesis associated with enhanced migration of endothelial cells further aggravates these matrix derangements. Ironically, these same processes are also critical to the repair of wounds, in which scar formation is also the final common outcome.

Neoplasia

A rare, but nonetheless revealing, sequela of long-standing peripheral lymphedema is (lymph)angiosarcoma. This aggressive vascular tumor was once thought to arise only after radical mastectomy and irradiation for local control of breast cancer (Stewart-Treves syndrome).[56, 57] Now, however, lymphangiosarcoma has been documented in association with other secondary lymphedemas, and even in congenital, or primary, lymphedema.[58] Because the preexisting swelling has usually persisted for many years and may occur in either primary or secondary lymphedema and in the absence of radiotherapy, the lymphedema process itself has been thought to be the principal cause.

More recently, Kaposi's sarcoma, a vascular tumor akin to Stewart-Treves syndrome and allied closely with acquired immunodeficiency syndrome (AIDS), has been linked to an origin from lymphatic endothelium.[59–62] Perhaps immunodysregulation, particularly in the antigen-presenting afferent loop (i.e., dysregulated lymphangiogenesis and hemangiogenesis), underlies a wide range of bizarre vasoproliferative and lymphologic syndromes, including hemolymphangioma, Klippel-Trenaunay syndrome, angiofollicular hyperplasia (epithelioid hemangioma), lymphangioleiomyomatosis, and lymphangitic metastatic carcinomatosis (see Fig. 155–10).

Lymphangiogenesis

In contrast to uncontrolled new growth (lymphangiosarcoma), programmed proliferation of lymphatic endothelium with tube formation (lymphangiogenesis) is critical to a host of physiologic and pathologic processes. During the past several decades, since the phenomenon of angiogenesis was first reproduced in endothelial cell– and mixed vascular tissue cultures,[63, 64] considerable attention has been directed to furthering understanding of this process, although largely in the context of blood vessel growth or "hemangiogenesis."[65] The "lymphatic" counterpart (i.e., lymphangiogenesis) has received only scant attention, even though

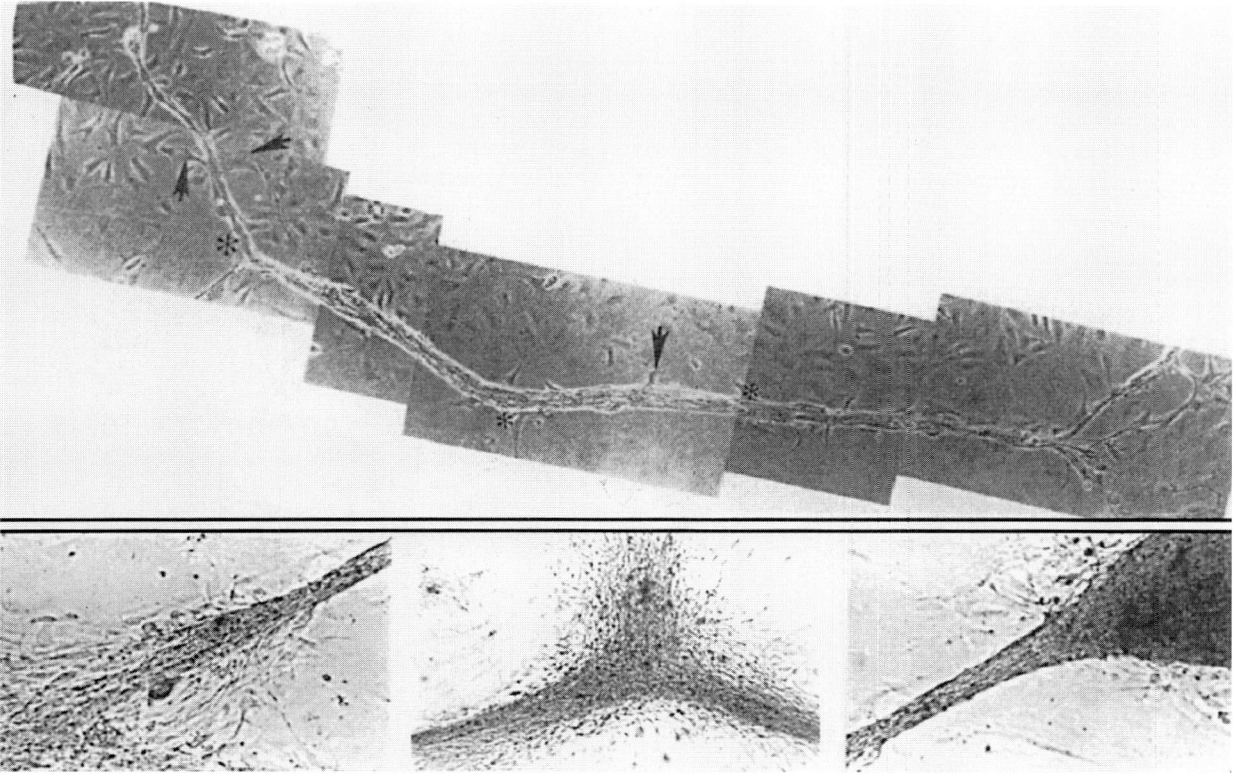

FIGURE 155–12. Lymphangiogenesis in vitro.

Top, At 1 to 3 days after treatment of lymphatic endothelial cells in tissue culture with collagen type 1. Adjacent cells (*arrows*) continue to migrate and adhere to tubular points with an increase in their dimension and length. Adhesion of cells (*asterisk*) at various points along the length of the tubular structures is accompanied by branching and the subsequent formation of elaborate capillary-like networks in the culture dishes. This lymphatic capillary tube that formed in vitro was derived from bovine lymphatic endothelialcells (×155). (From Leak LV, Jones M: Lymphatic endothelium isolation, characterization and long-term culture. Anat Rec 236:641, 1993.)

Bottom, Spontaneous lymphangiogenesis in cell culture derived from a lymphatic ductal malformation (lymphangioma). Note loose clusters of lymphatic endothelial cells sprouting into branches (*left*), which are more prominent (*middle*) and evolve into a sheet-like aggregate with intense lymphatic-like sprouting branches (*right*).

(From Witte CL, Witte MH: Lymphatics and blood vessels, lymphangiogenesis and hemangiogenesis: From cell biology to clinical medicine. Lymphology 20:257, 1987.)

lymphatic (re)generation is essential to health and disorders of lymph flow are common, often disfiguring, and sometimes life- and limb-threatening.[65]

After experimental hindlimb circumferential skin incision, new lymphatics traverse the integumentary gap as early as postoperative day 4. By the 8th day, lymphatic continuity is restored anatomically (delineated by distribution of intradermal India ink particles) and physiologically (transient peripheral edema remits).[41, 66] Bellman and Odén meticulously documented by Thorotrast microlymphangiography the time course and extent of newly formed lymphatics in circumferential wounds in the rabbit ear, including lymphatic bridging through newly formed scar.[67, 68] As lymphatics increased in caliber, intraluminal valves and sinuous dilatations appeared. Subsequent studies have documented restoration of distinctive ultrastructural features in newly regenerated lymphatic vessels, including the characteristic overlapping junctional complexes and Weibel-Palade bodies (storage depots for vWf-XIII; see later).[69–71]

In now classic studies, Clark and Clark documented the extension of lymphatic capillaries by outgrowth from preexisting lymph vessels in rabbit ear transparent chambers.[72] Later, Pullinger and Florey emphasized that, despite the similar appearance of the three types of vascular endothelium, lymphatics consistently connected to lymphatics, veins to veins, and arteries to arteries, without intermingling.[73] Like the more than 1 trillion blood vascular endothelial cells that normally are dormant,[74, 75] lymphatic endothelial cell turnover is also minuscule.[76] With injury, however, incorporation of tritiated thymidine into proliferating lymphatic endothelium increases sharply.[76] Moreover, fetal lymphatics show "greater labeling" than do neonatal and adult lymphatics, whereas visceral lymphatic endothelium proliferates more rapidly than that of peripheral lymphatics.[77]

Lymphatic endothelium was first isolated in vitro from bovine mesenteric lymphatics[78] and later that year (1984) from a patient with a large cervicomediastinal lymphangioma.[79] Lymphatic endothelial cells have now also been isolated, passed in culture, and studied (from canine and human thoracic duct and ovine, rat, and ferret lymphatic collectors) by techniques similar to those used for blood large vessel and microvessel isolations. Lymphatic endothelium grown in monolayer and on microcarrier beads exhibits the cobblestone morphology and typical endothelial structural features and staining characteristics (Fig. 155–11).[80]

Lymphangiogenesis in vitro was also first demonstrated more than a decade ago, when formation of tubes and cyst-like structures was induced, spontaneously or after addition of collagen matrix, in tissue culture.[65, 79] Later, lymphatic explant proliferation with lymphatic sprouting was detected (Fig. 155–12).[81, 82] Growing evidence suggests that lymphangiogenesis is under genetic control. For example, one or more genes expressed by nonactivated portions of the inactivated X chromosome or from the Y chromosome are likely involved in the development of lymphatics, and one or more deficiencies of these genes or their products are responsible for Turner's syndrome (XO ovarian dysgenesis), a disorder that exhibits a variety of lymphatic and other cardiovascular anomalies. Other chromosomal aneuploidy disorders, such as trisomy 21 (Down's syndrome), also occasionally present with strangulating fetal cystic hygroma, lymphedema, and intestinal lymphangiectasia.[83]

A spectrum of other hereditary lymphedema-angiodysplasia syndromes (often of autosomal-dominant inheri-

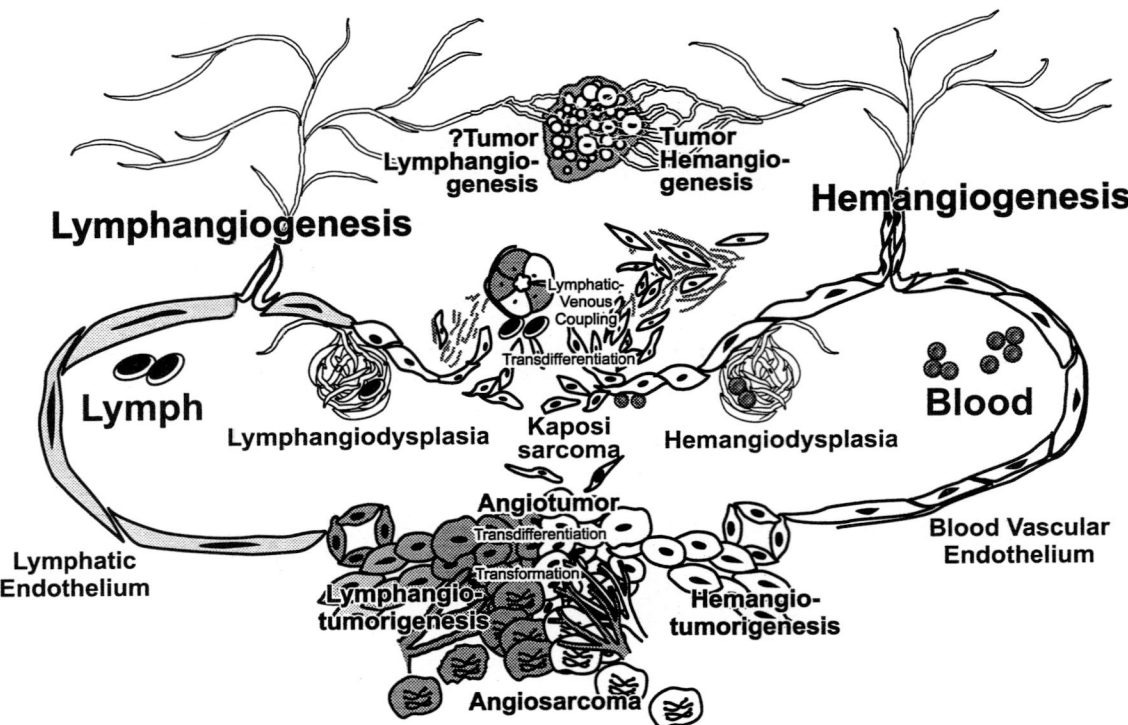

FIGURE 155–13. Schematic representation of physiological and pathological processes involving growth of lymphatic vessels (lymphangiogenesis) analogous to and accompanied by hemangiogenesis. Among these entities are tumor-associated angiogenesis, angiodysplasias, Kaposi's sarcoma, and angiotumorigenesis, including angiosarcoma.

tance) also provide clues to potential sites of "lymphangio-genesis genes."[83, 84] Most notable is *Milroy's disease,* a familial disorder characterized by progressive lymphedema present at birth or appearing in early childhood as a consequence of lymphatic truncal hypoplasia. Whereas the underlying mechanisms governing lymphangiogenesis are ill understood, a variety of stimulatory (e.g., vascular endothelial growth factor-C or VEGF-2) and inhibitory factors modulate the growth, development, and (dys)function of the lymphatic network, in common with or distinct from the blood vasculature.[85] These angiomodulatory agents are very likely crucial to understanding clinical conditions as diverse as cystic hygroma, Klippel-Trenaunay syndrome, (lymph)-angiosarcoma, elephantine overgrowth, and a broad constellation of peripheral and visceral disorders characterized by swelling, scarring, immunodysregulation, and malnutrition (Fig. 155–13).

Chylous Reflux

Abnormal retrograde transport of intestinal lymph is responsible for chylous disorders. Because cholesterol and long-chain triglycerides, in the form of chylomicra, are absorbed only by the lymphatic system, dysfunction (in the form of disruption, compression, obstruction, or fistulization) of mesenteric lacteals, the cisterna chyli, and the thoracic duct is directly linked to chylothorax, chylous ascites, and chyluria. In some patients with high-grade blockage of intestinal lymph flow, dilatation of the peripheral lymphatics gradually develops, and, with progressive valvular incompetence, lactescent lymph refluxes into the soft tissues of the pelvis, scrotum, and lower extremities (chylous vesicles and edema; Fig. 155–14).

SUMMARY

Disturbances in microcirculatory perfusion and exchange of liquid, macromolecules, and cells across intact and abnormal microvessels and deranged lymph kinetics are, individually and together, associated with disorders of tissue swelling. Low-output failure of the lymph circulation manifested as peripheral lymphedema typically is indolent for many years before lymphatic insufficiency and tissue swelling accelerate and become persistent. Nonetheless, impedance of lymph flow is by itself sufficient to explain at least mild to moderate lymphedema.

Chronic lymphedema is characterized by trapping of fluid, extravasated plasma proteins, and other macromolecules in the skin and subcutaneous tissues. It is typical to find impaired immune cell trafficking (lymphocytes, Langerhans cells, monocytes), abnormal transport of autologous and foreign antigens, probably intact hydrodynamic (Starling) transcapillary forces,[86] and an increased propensity to superimposed infection. Additional characteristics include progressive obliteration of lymphatics (lymphangiopathy "die-back" or lymphangitis), defective lymphangion contractility, mononuclear cell infiltrate (chronic interstitial inflammation), epidermal cell–fibroblast proliferation, collagen deposition, altered immunoreactivity, and vasoactive mediator imbalance with increased production of local cy-

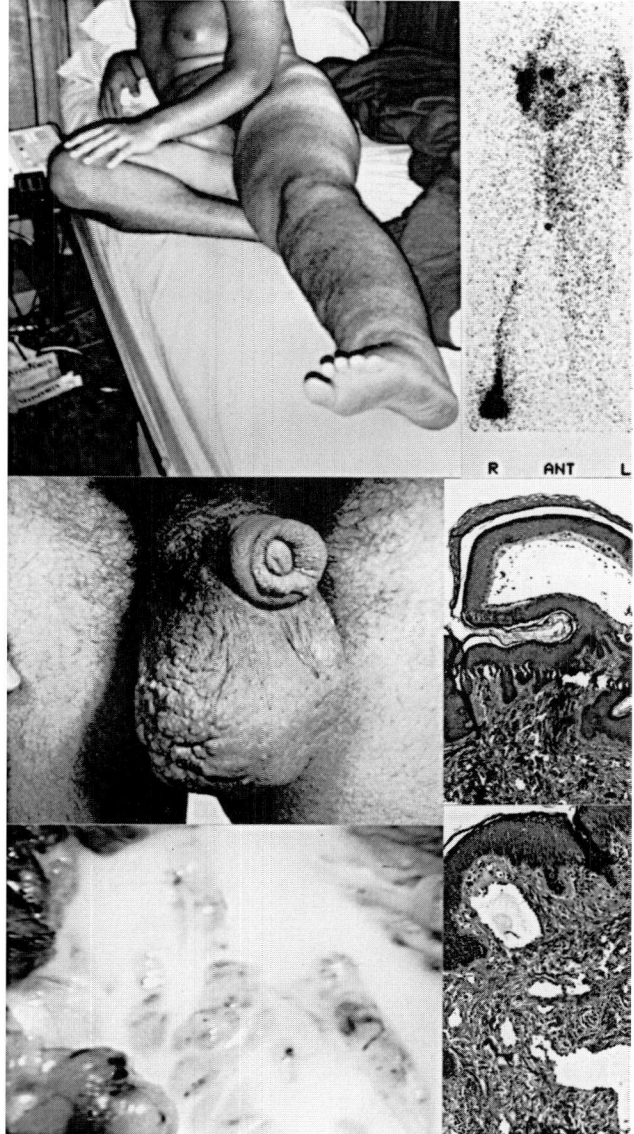

FIGURE 155–14. Chylous reflux syndrome in a 16-year-old male, characterized by left leg, penile, and scrotal lymphedema with multiple small chyle-containing vesicles. Lymphoscintigraphy (*upper right*) showed that tracer (technetium 99m [^{99m}Tc] human serum albumin) injected intradermally into the right foot crossed to the left side and flows retrograde to outline dermal lymphatics in the contralateral leg. During a scrotal debulking operation, chylous lymph flooded the operative field (*lower left*), and light microscopy of the excised skin showed large endothelium-lined channels (*center and lower right*) that are consistent with ectatic dermal lymphatics.

tokines and growth factors, including autocrine and paracrine hormones.

In contrast to the blood circulation, where flow depends principally on the propulsive force of the myocardium, lymph propulsion depends predominantly on intrinsic truncal contraction, a mechanism that is a phylogenetic remnant of amphibian lymph heart function. Whereas venous plasma flows rapidly (2.5 to 3 L/min) against low vascular resistance, lymph "plasma" flows slowly (1.0 ml/min) against high vascular resistance. On occasion, impaired transport of intestinal lymph may be associated with reflux and accumulation or leakage of intestinal chyle into swollen legs. In extreme circumstances, these factors, operating together, may be responsible for the grotesque deformities known as *elephantiasis*.

Transdifferentiation and transformation of endothelium and other vascular accessory cells associated with lymph stasis may also be pivotal factors in a wide range of dysplastic and neoplastic vascular disorders, including Stewart-Treves syndrome, AIDS-associated Kaposi's sarcoma, and lymphangitic metastatic carcinomatosis. These phenomena have their origin in controlled and uncontrolled lymphangiogenesis and apparently are regulated at specific sites in the genome, the manipulation of which may offer new avenues of therapy for both primary and secondary lymphedema and related angiodysplasia syndromes.

REFERENCES

1. Rusznyák I, Földi M, Szabo G: History of the discovery of lymphatics and lymph circulation. In Lymphatics and Lymph Circulation, 2nd ed. Oxford, Pergamon Press, 1967, pp 15–24.
2. Földi M: Lymphogenous encephalopathy. In Diseases of Lymphatics and Lymph Circulation. Springfield, Ill, Charles C Thomas, 1969, pp 91–117.
3. Bradbury MWB, Westrop RJ: Factors influencing exit of substances from cerebrospinal fluid into deep cervical lymph of the rabbit. J Physiol 339:519, 1983.
4. Leeds SE, Kong AK, Wise BL: Alternative pathways for drainage of cerebrospinal fluid in the canine brain. Lymphology 22:144, 1989.
5. Casley-Smith JR: Lymph and lymphatics. In Kaley G, Altura BM (eds): Microcirculation, Vol. 1. Baltimore, University Park Press, 1977, pp 423–502.
6. Leak LV: Physiology of the lymphatic system. In Abramson DI, Dobrin PB (eds): Blood Vessels and Lymphatics in Organ Systems. Orlando, Fla, Academic Press, 1984, pp 134–164.
7. Way D, Hendrix M, Witte MH, et al: Lymphatic endothelial cell line (CH3) from a recurrent retroperitoneal lymphangioma. In Vitro 23:647, 1987.
8. Gnepp DR, Chandler W: Tissue culture of human and canine thoracic duct endothelium. In Vitro 21:200, 1985.
9. Johnston MG, Walker MA: Lymphatic endothelial and smooth-muscle cells in tissue culture. In Vitro 20 566, 1984.
10. Casley-Smith JR: The lymphatic system. In Földi M, Casley-Smith JR (eds): Lymphangiology. Stuttgart, FK Schattauer-Verlag, 1983, pp 89–164.
11. Leak LV, Burke JF: Fine structure of the lymphatic capillary and the adjoining connective tissue area. Am J Anat 118:785, 1966.
12. Leak LV, Burke JF: Ultrastructural studies on the lymphatic anchoring filaments. J Cell Biol 36:129, 1968.
13. Leak LV: Electron microscopic observation on lymphatic capillaries and the structural components of the connective tissue–lymph interface. Microvasc Res 2:361, 1970.
14. Mislin H: The lymphangion. In Földi M, Casley-Smith JR (eds): Lymphangiology. Stuttgart, FK Schattauer-Verlag, 1983, pp 165–175.
15. Starling EH: Physiologic factors involved in the causation of dropsy. Lancet 1:1267, 1896.
16. Starling EH: The fluids of the body. In: The Herter Lectures. Chicago, WT Keener, 1909, p 81.
17. Hall JG, Morris B, Woolley G: Intrinsic rhythmic propulsion of lymph in the unanaesthetised sheep. J Physiol (Lond) 180:336, 1965.
18. Mawhinney HJD, Roddie IC: Spontaneous activity in isolated bovine mesenteric lymphatics. J Physiol 229:339, 1973.
19. Olszewski WL, Engeset A: Intrinsic contractility of prenodal lymph vessels and lymph flow in the human leg. Am J Physiol 239:H775, 1980.
20. Gnepp DR: Lymphatics. In Staub NC, Taylor AE (eds): Edema. New York, Raven Press, 1984, pp 263–298.
21. McHale NG, Roddie IC: The effect of transmural pressure on pumping activity in isolated bovine lymphatic vessels. J Physiol 261:255, 1976.
22. McHale NG, Roddie IC: The effect of intravenous adrenaline and noradrenaline infusion on peripheral lymph flow in the sheep. J Physiol 341:517, 1983.
23. Johnston MG: The intrinsic lymph pump: Progress and problems. Lymphology 22:116, 1989.
24. Sinzinger H, Kaliman J, Mannheimer E: Regulation of human lymph contractility by prostaglandins and thromboxane. Lymphology 17:43, 1984.
25. Johnston MG, Gordon JL: Regulation of lymphatic contractility by arachidonate metabolites. Nature 293:294, 1981.
26. Johnston MG, Feuer C: Suppression of lymphatic vessel contractility with inhibitors of arachidonic acid metabolism. J Pharmacol Exp Ther 226:603, 1983.
27. Ohhashi T, Kawai Y, Azuma T: The response of lymphatic smooth muscles to vasoactive substances. Pflügers Arch 375:183, 1978.
28. McHale NG, Roddie IC, Thornbury K: Nervous modulation of spontaneous contractions in bovine mesenteric lymphatics. J Physiol 309:461, 1980.
29. McGeown JG, McHale NG, Thornbury K: Popliteal efferent lymph flow response to stimulation of the sympathetic chain in the sheep. J Physiol 387:55P, 1987.
30. Sjöberg T, Alm P, Andersson KE, et al: Contractile response in isolated human groin lymphatics. Lymphology 20:152, 1987.
31. Sjöberg T, Steen S: Contractile properties of lymphatics from the human lower leg. Lymphology 24:16, 1991.
32. Swemer RL, Foglia VG: Fatal loss of plasma volume after lymph heart destruction in toads. Proc Soc Exp Biol Med 53:14, 1943.
33. Conklin R: The formation and circulation of lymph in the frog: I. The rate of lymph production. Am J Physiol 95:79, 1930.
34. Kinmonth JB, Wolfe JH: Fibrosis in the lymph nodes in primary lymphedema. Ann R Coll Surg 62:344, 1980.
35. Olszewski W: On the pathomechanism of development of post surgical lymphedema. Lymphology 6:35, 1973.
36. Zweifach BW, Prather JW: Micromanipulation of pressure in terminal lymphatics in the mesentery. Am J Physiol 228:1326, 1975.
37. Pippard C, Roddie IC: Resistance in the sheep's lymphatic system. Lymphology 20:230, 1987.
38. Olszewski WL: Lymph pressure and flow in limbs. In Lymph Stasis: Pathophysiology, Diagnosis and Treatment. Boca Raton, Fla, CRC Press, 1991, pp 109–156.
39. McHale NG: Influence of autonomic nerves on lymph flow. In Olszewski WL (ed): Lymph Stasis: Pathophysiology, Diagnosis and Treatment, Boca Raton, Fla, CRC Press, 1991, pp 85–107.
40. Pippard C, Roddie IC: Comparison of fluid transport systems in lymphatics and veins. Lymphology 20:224, 1987.
41. Reichert FL: The regeneration of the lymphatics. Arch Surg 13:871, 1926.
42. Blalock A, Robinson CS, Cunningham RS, Gray ME: Experimental studies on lymphatic blockade. Arch Surg 34:1049, 1937.
43. Halsted WS: The swelling of the arm after operations for cancer of the breast. Elephantiasis chirurgica—its cause and prevention. Johns Hopkins Hosp Bull 32:309, 1921.
44. Drinker CK, Field MJ, Homans J: The experimental production of edema and elephantiasis as a result of lymphatic obstruction. Am J Physiol 108:509, 1934.
45. Danese CA, Georgalas-Bertakis M, Morales LE: A model of chronic postsurgical lymphedema in dogs' limbs. Surgery 64:814, 1968.
46. Clodius L, Altorfer J: Experimental chronic lymphostasis of extremities. Folia Angiol 25:137, 1977.
47. Case T, Leis B, Witte M, et al: Vascular abnormalities in experimental and human lymphatic filariasis. Lymphology 24:174, 1991.
48. Földi M: Lymphoedema. In Földi M, Casley-Smith JR (eds): Lymphangiology. Stuttgart, FK Schattauer-Verlag, 1983, pp 668–670.
49. Edwards EA: Recurrent febrile episodes and lymphedema. JAMA 184:102, 1963.
50. Casley-Smith JR, Casley-Smith JR: High-Protein Oedemas and the Benzopyrones. Sydney, JB Lippincott, 1986, pp 126–152.
51. Ehrich WE, Seifter J, Alburn HE, Begamy AJ: Heparin and heparinocytes in elephantiasis scroti. Proc Soc Exp Biol Med 70:183, 1949.
52. Dumont AE, Fazzini E, Jamal S: Metachromatic cells in filarial lymphoedema. Lancet 2:1021, 1983.
53. Gaffney RM, Casley-Smith JR: Lymphedema without lymphostasis: Excess proteins as the cause of chronic inflammation. In: Weissleder H, Bartos V, Clodius L, Malek P (eds): Progress in Lymphology. Proceedings of the VII International Congress. Prague, Avicenum, 1981, pp 213–216.
54. Poslethwaite AE, Keski-Oja J, Balian G, Kang AH: Induction of fibroblast chemotaxis by fibronectin. J Exp Med 153:494, 1981.
55. Földi M: Insufficiency of lymph flow. In Földi M, Casley-Smith JR (eds): Lymphangiology. Stuttgart, FK Schattauer-Verlag, 1983, p 195.

56. Stewart FW, Treves N: Lymphangiosarcoma in post mastectomy lymphedema: A report of six cases in elephantiasis chirurgica. Cancer 1:64, 1948.
57. Unruh H, Robertson DI, Karasewich E: Post-mastectomy lymphangiosarcoma. Can J Surg 22:586, 1979.
58. Woodward AH, Ivins JC, Sorle EH: Lymphangiosarcoma arising in chronic lymphedematous extremities. Cancer 30:562, 1972.
59. Dorfman RF: Kaposi's sarcoma: Evidence supporting its origin from the lymphatic system. Lymphology 21:45, 1988.
60. Witte MH, Stuntz M, Witte CL: Kaposi's sarcoma: A lymphologic perspective. Int J Dermatol 28:561, 1989.
61. Witte MH, Fiala M, McNeill GC, et al: Lymphangioscintigraphy in AIDS-associated Kaposi sarcoma. AJK Am J Roentgenol 155:311, 1990.
62. Beckstead JH, Wood GS, Fletcher V: Evidence for the origin of Kaposi's sarcoma from lymphatic endothelium. Am J Pathol 119:294, 1985.
63. Folkman J, Haudenschild C: Angiogenesis in vitro. Nature 288:551, 1980.
64. Folkman J: Clinical applications of research on angiogenesis. N Engl J Med 26:1757, 1995.
65. Witte MH, Witte CL: Lymphatics and blood vessels, lymphangiogenesis and hemangiogenesis: From cell biology to clinical medicine. Lymphology 20:171, 1987.
66. Casley-Smith JR: The regenerative capacity of the lymphvascular system. In Földi M, Casley-Smith JR (eds): Lymphangiology. Stuttgart, FK Schattauer-Verlag, 1983, p 276.
67. Bellman S, Odén B: Regeneration of surgically divided lymph vessels: An experimental study on the rabbit's ear. Acta Chir Scand 116:99, 1958–1959.
68. Odén B: A microlymphangiographic study of experimental wounds healing by second intention. Acta Chir Scand 120:100, 1960.
69. Magari S, Asano S: Regeneration of the deep cervical lymphatics—light and electron microscopic observations. Lymphology 11:57, 1978.
70. Magari S: Comparison of fine structure of lymphatics and blood vessels in normal conditions and during embryonic development and regeneration. Lymphology 20:189, 1987.
71. Leak L: Interaction of the peritoneal cavity to intraperitoneal stimulation: A peritoneal nodal system to monitor cellular and extracellular events in the formation of granulation tissue. Am J Anat 173:171, 1985.
72. Clark ER, Clark EL: Observations on the new growth of lymphatic vessels as seen in transparent chambers introduced into the rabbit's ear. Am J Anat 51:49, 1932.
73. Pullinger DB, Florey HW: Proliferation of lymphatics in inflammation. J Pathol Bacteriol 45:157, 1937.
74. Jaffe EA: Cell biology of endothelial cells. Hum Pathol 18:234, 1987.
75. Denekamp J: Angiogenesis, neovascular proliferation and vascular pathophysiology as targets for cancer therapy. Br J Radiol 66:181, 1993.
76. Junghans BM, Collin HB: Limbal lymphangiogenesis after corneal injury: An autoradiographic study. Current Eye Res 8:91, 1989.
77. Travella W, Dugan MC: Endothelial interactions. In Nishi M, Uchino S, Yabuki S (eds): Progress in Lymphology XII. Amsterdam, Elsevier Scientific, 1990, p 269.
78. Johnston M, Walker M: Lymphatic endothelial and smooth muscle cells in tissue culture. In Vitro 20:566, 1984.
79. Bowman C, Witte MH, Witte CL, et al: Cystic hygroma reconsidered: Hamartoma or neoplasm? Primary culture of an endothelial cell line from a massive cervicomediastinal cystic hygroma with bony lymphangiomatosis. Lymphology 17:15, 1984.
80. Way D, Hendrix M, Witte M, et al: Lymphatic endothelial cell line (CH3) from a recurrent retroperitoneal lymphangioma. In Vitro 23:647, 1987.
81. Leak LV, Jones M: Lymphatic endothelium: Isolation, characterization and long-term culture. Anat Rec 236:641, 1993.
82. Nicosia RF: Angiogenesis and the formation of lymphatic-like channels in cultures of thoracic duct. In Vitro Cell Develop Biol 23:167, 1987.
83. Witte MH, Way DL, Witte CL, Bernas M: Lymphangiogenesis: Mechanisms, significance and clinical implications. In Goldberg IV, Rosen EM (eds): Regulation of Angiogenesis. Basel, Birkhäuser Verlag, 1997, p 65.
84. Greenlee R, Hoyme H, Witte M, et al: Developmental disorders of the lymphatic system. Lymphology 26:156, 1993.
85. Witte MH, Witte CL: Control of lymphangiogenesis. In Jiménez Cossío JA, Farrajota A, Samaniego E, et al (eds): Progress in Lymphology XVI. Lymphology 31(Suppl):37, 1998.
86. Kirk RM: Capillary filtration rates in normal and lymphedematous legs. Clin Sci 27:363, 1964.

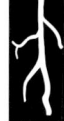

CHAPTER 156

Clinical Diagnosis and Evaluation of Lymphedema

Peter Gloviczki, M.D., and
Heinz W. Wahner, M.D., F.A.C.P.

Chronic lymphedema is a progressive, usually painless swelling of the extremity that results from a decreased transport capacity of the lymphatic system. Lymphedema may be caused by developmental abnormalities of the lymph vessels, such as aplasia, hypoplasia, or hyperplasia with valvular incompetence,[1, 2] or it may be the result of congenital or acquired obstruction of the lymph vessels and lymph nodes.[3–6] The diagnosis of lymphedema is suspected in most patients after the history is obtained and the physical examination performed. The goal of further evaluation is to confirm the cause and determine the type and site of lymphatic obstruction. It is equally important, however, to diagnose any underlying malignancy and to exclude other systemic or local causes of limb swelling such as venous disease or congenital vascular malformation.

In this chapter, the current classifications of lymphedema are presented and the clinical presentation of patients with this disease is reviewed. The methods of noninvasive evaluation are discussed, and the technique and interpretation of lymphoscintigraphy, which has become the test of choice to confirm or exclude lymphatic disease, are presented in detail. The role of contrast lymphangiography in the diagnosis of lymphatic disorders is delineated. Finally, the differential diagnosis of lymphedema is discussed, and a diagnostic protocol for the evaluation of patients with a swollen extremity is suggested.

CLINICAL CLASSIFICATIONS

Standard clinical classifications distinguish lymphedemas based on etiology (primary versus secondary), genetics (familial versus sporadic), and time of onset of the edema (congenital, praecox, tarda) (Table 156–1).[1, 2, 7] Although these systems are useful for categorizing all lymphedemas, they do not address the clinical severity of the disease and are usually not relevant to therapy. More recent classifications focus on the clinical stage of lymphedema[8] or emphasize the underlying anatomic abnormality of the lymphatic system in an attempt to plan therapy.[3, 4, 9]

Primary Lymphedema

The most accepted etiologic classification divides lymphedemas into two major groups, *primary* and *secondary* lymphedemas. These terms were suggested in 1934 by Allen, from the Mayo Clinic, who evaluated 300 patients with lymphedema of the extremities.[7] He further divided the primary or idiopathic group into *congenital* and *praecox* types (Fig. 156–1). The congenital included patients who developed edema before 1 year of age. Kinmonth later added another group to the primary lymphedemas comprising those who develop the disease after 35 years of age (lymphedema *tarda*).[2]

Although it has been assumed that all primary or idiopathic lymphedemas have an underlying developmental abnormality in the lymphatic system (i.e., aplasia, hypoplasia, or hyperplasia of the lymph vessels), fibrotic occlusion of lymph vessels and lymph nodes has been described in primary lymphedema by Kinmonth[10] and Wolfe.[11] Studies by Browse suggest that the most likely cause of primary lymphedema praecox in many patients is acquired fibrotic

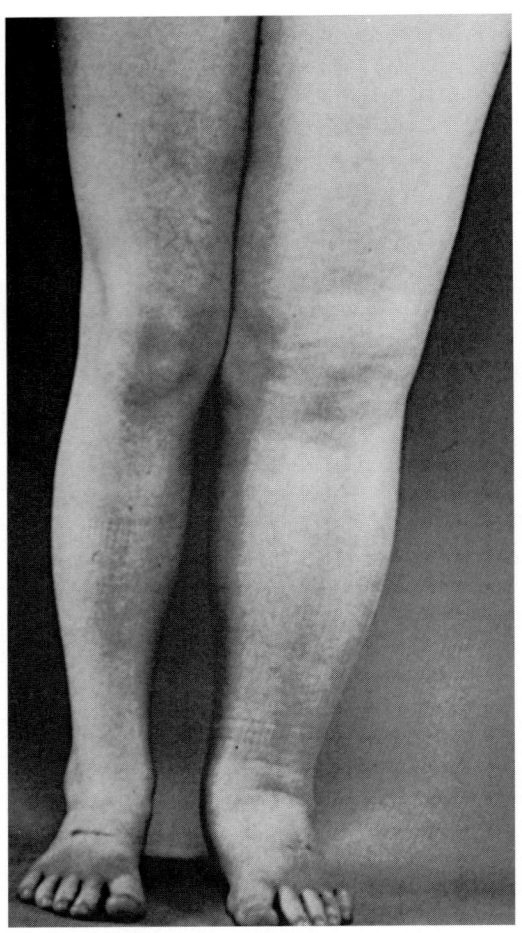

FIGURE 156–1. Primary lymphedema praecox of both lower extremities, more significantly of the left. Leg swelling in this patient, a 9-year-old boy, was first noted at age 4 years.

obliteration of the lymph vessels and the lymph-conducting elements of the lymph nodes.[3, 4, 9]

Primary lymphedema is fortunately rare. Based on data collected by the Rochester Group Study,[12] it affects 1.15 per 100,000 persons younger than 20 years of age. It occurs more frequently in girls, and the incidence peaks between the ages of 12 and 16 years. Of 125 patients with primary lymphedema treated at the Mayo Clinic, 97 (78%) were females and 28 (22%) were males, yielding a female:male ratio of 3.5:1.0.[13] The ratio of unilateral to bilateral lymphedema was 3:1.

Congenital lymphedema occurred more frequently in males than in females. In these patients, the edema was usually bilateral and involved the entire lower extremity. In contrast, the typical patient with lymphedema praecox was female and had unilateral involvement, with swelling usually extending up to the knee only.[13]

Familial Lymphedema

The familial form of primary lymphedema was first described in 1865 by Letessier,[14] and additional cases were later published by Nonne[15] and Milroy.[16, 17] The report of Milroy in 1892 described lower limb lymphedema that

---

TABLE 156–1. ETIOLOGIC CLASSIFICATION OF LYMPHEDEMA

I. Primary lymphedema
   A. Congenital (onset before 1 year of age)
      1. Nonfamilial
      2. Familial (Milroy's disease)
   B. Praecox (onset 1 to 35 years of age)
      1. Nonfamilial
      2. Familial (Meige's disease)
   C. Tarda (onset after 35 years of age)
II. Secondary lymphedema
   A. Filariasis
   B. Lymph node excision ± radiation
   C. Tumor invasion
   D. Infection
   E. Trauma
   F. Other

was observed in 22 members of the same family over six generations.[16] In all except two patients, the edema was present at birth. The term *Milroy's disease* should be reserved for patients with familial lymphedema that is present at birth or is noted soon thereafter. A familial form of lymphedema that becomes manifest only during puberty was later described by Meige.[18] The term *Meige's disease*, therefore, refers to the familial form of lymphedema praecox.

In a collected series of 291 patients with primary lymphedema, 42 (14%) had a family history of lymphedema. Fourteen patients (5%) had congenital lymphedema, the onset of which was noted before 1 year of age, and 28 (9%) had lymphedema praecox.[13] In the Mayo Clinic series, 10 of 125 patients (8%) had a positive family history of lymphedema.

Functional Classification of Primary Lymphedemas

The functional classification of primary lymphedema by Browse is based on the underlying lymphatic anatomy as determined by lymphangiography.[3, 4] This classification describes three different anatomic abnormalities, which are associated with different clinical presentations. More importantly, however, the classification is treatment oriented and selects appropriate groups that may respond to medical or surgical treatment.

Based on the underlying anatomic abnormality of the lymphatic system, Browse subdivided primary lymphedemas into three groups (Table 156–2):

1. Distal obliteration.
2. Proximal obliteration.
3. Congenital hyperplasia.

Distal obliteration occurs in 80% of patients and affects predominantly females. The swelling is frequently bilateral.[4, 9] Lymphangiography demonstrates absent or a diminished number of superficial leg lymphatics in these patients. This group was also described by Kinmonth and Wolfe as having aplasia or hypoplasia.[2, 10] The course of the disease is usually benign, progression is slow, and the edema is usually responsive to conservative compression treatment.

Ten percent of patients with primary lymphedema have proximal occlusion in the aortoiliac or inguinal lymph nodes.[9] This disease is frequently unilateral and involves the entire lower extremity, affecting both males and females.

This form of lymphedema frequently develops rapidly, and progression is usual. The edema responds poorly to conservative management. Distal dilatation with proximal occlusion, however, may be suitable for mesenteric bridge operation or for microvascular lymph vessel reconstruction (see Chapter 159).

Hyperplasia and incompetence of the lymph vessels are observed in the remaining 10% of patients. Most of these patients have bilateral lymphedema, and males are more frequently affected than females.[11] One subgroup of these patients has megalymphatics, and, because of concomitant involvement of the mesenteric lymphatics, reflux of chyle frequently results. The leg edema is unilateral in most of these patients.[10, 11] Protein-losing enteropathy, chyluria, chylous drainage through the vagina, and chylorrhea from small vesicles in the labia majora, scrotum, or lower extremities may also develop (Fig. 156–2).[19–21] The leg edema responds well to elevation, but recurs rapidly with ambulation. These patients are candidates for surgical treatment consisting of ligation and excision of the incompetent retroperitoneal lymphatics (see Chapter 159).

Although this functional classification is helpful in selecting patients for further management, the overlap in the first two groups may be quite significant. In addition, without contrast lymphangiography, separation of the groups is not always possible.

Secondary Lymphedema

Secondary acquired lymphedema results from a well-defined disease process that causes obstruction or injury to the lymphatic system. The most frequent cause of secondary lymphedema in the world is parasitic infestation by filariasis.[22, 23] In North America and Europe, the most frequent cause of secondary lymphedema is surgical excision and irradiation of the axillary or inguinal lymph nodes as part of the treatment of an underlying malignancy, most frequently cancer of the breast (Fig. 156–3),[24–29] cervical cancer,[30] soft tissue tumors (Fig. 156–4), or malignant melanoma of the leg.[31] Other causes of secondary lymphedema are tumors invading the lymph vessels and nodes,[32] bacterial and fungal infections, lymphoproliferative diseases, and trauma.[33]

Less frequent causes of secondary lymphedema are contact dermatitis, tuberculosis, rheumatoid arthritis, and infection after a snake or insect bite. Factitious edema induced by application of a tourniquet on the arm or leg or

TABLE 156–2. FUNCTIONAL CLASSIFICATION OF PRIMARY LYMPHEDEMA

	DISTAL OBLITERATION (80%)	PROXIMAL OBLITERATION (10%)	HYPERPLASIA* (10%)
Gender	Female	Male or female	Male or female
Onset			
Time	Puberty	Any age	Congenital
Location	Ankle; bilateral	Whole leg, thigh; unilateral	Whole leg; unilateral or bilateral
Progression	Slow	Rapid	Progressive
Family history	Frequently positive	None	Frequently positive

Adapted from Browse NL: The diagnosis and management of primary lymphedema. J Vasc Surg 3:181, 1986.
*With or without reflux of chyle.

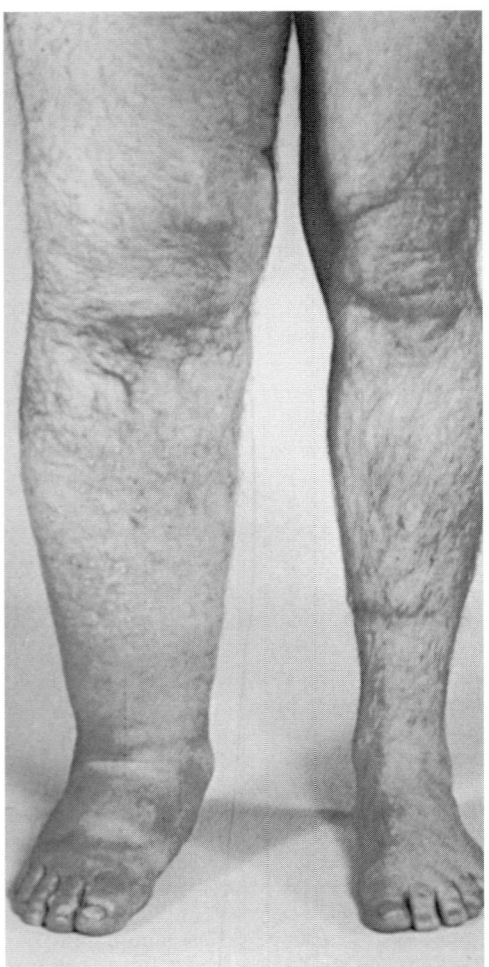

FIGURE 156–2. Primary lymphedema of the right leg caused by hyperplasia of the lymphatics and valvular incompetence. Note skin vesicles at mid-calf containing milky fluid because of reflux of chyle.

by maintenance of the limb in an immobile or dependent state should also be considered in some patients.[34]

Filariasis

Lymphatic filariasis is caused by the developing and adult forms of three parasites: *Wuchereria bancrofti, Brugia malayi,* and *B. timori.* Of the estimated 90.2 million people in the world who are infected, more than 90% have bancroftian filariasis.[23] The disease is most frequent in subtropical and tropical countries, such as China, India, and Indonesia. It is transmitted by different types of mosquitos, and transmission is closely related to poor urban sanitation.[35]

Perilymphatic inflammation, fibrosis, and sclerosis of the lymph nodes are caused by the indwelling adult worms. Lymph node fibrosis, reactive hyperplasia, and dilation of the lymphatic collecting channels are caused by the worm products, by physical injury to the valves and vessel walls caused by the live worms, and by the immune response of the host.[36] Eosinophilia is found in the peripheral blood smear, and microfilaria can be demonstrated in peripheral nocturnal blood, in the centrifuged urine sediment, or in the lymphatic fluid.[37] Filarial lymphedema rapidly develops

into grossly incapacitating elephantiasis that is extremely difficult to treat.

Lymph Node Excision and Irradiation

Postmastectomy lymphedema is the most distressing and unpleasant complication following operation for breast cancer. During past decades, when radical mastectomy was routinely performed, clinically significant lymphedema was reported to occur in 6% to 60% of patients.[24] Axillary vein obstruction and episodes of lymphangitis contributed significantly to the further development of edema (see Fig. 156–3). With the introduction of more conservative breast cancer operations, the incidence of postmastectomy lymphedema markedly decreased. The reported incidence of arm lymphedema after modified radical mastectomy is 15.4%[25]; after local excision and total axillary lymphadenectomy it is 2.1% to 3.1%[26, 27]; and after wide local excision and radiotherapy it is 2.3%.[28] Few studies, however, have objectively documented the degree of limb swelling in these patients.

Kissin and colleagues studied the development of lymphedema in 200 patients following different breast cancer operations.[29] Chronic lymphedema, with an increase of over 200 ml in the volume of the extremity, developed in 25.5% of the patients. Independent risk factors contributing to lymphedema included extensive axillary lymphadenectomy ($p < .05$), axillary radiotherapy ($p < .001$), and pathologic nodal status ($p < .10$). Extensive axillary lymph

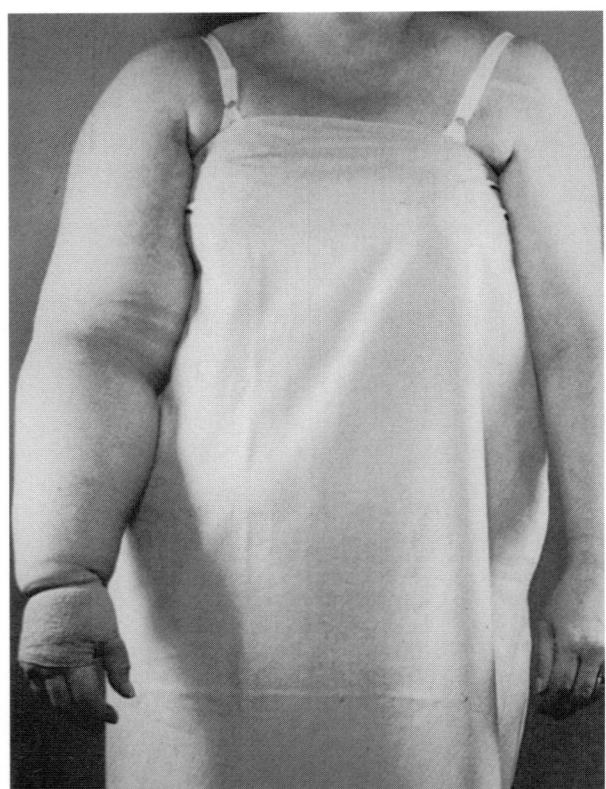

FIGURE 156–3. Right arm lymphedema after modified radical mastectomy and radiation treatment. The edema was aggravated by obstruction of the right axillary vein.

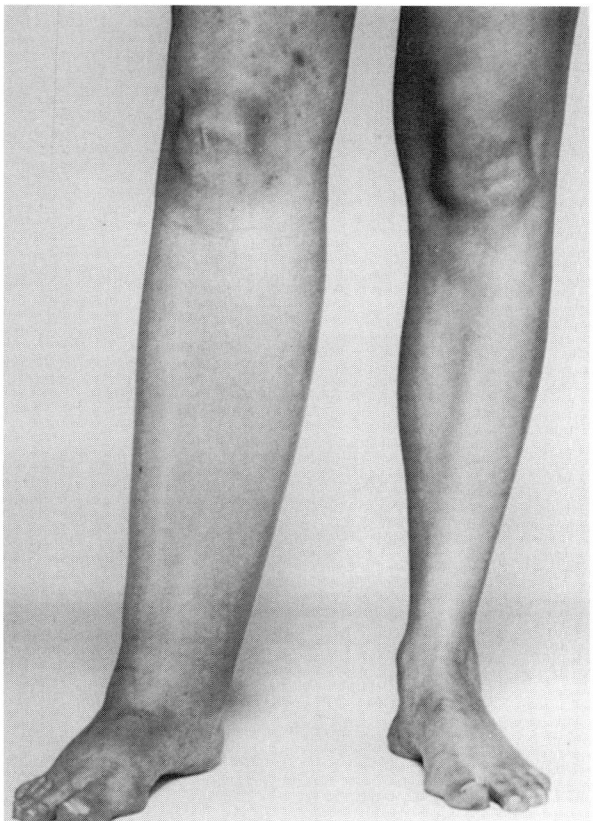

FIGURE 156–4. Secondary lymphedema of the right leg in a 29-year-old woman after excision of Ewing's sarcoma of the thigh and irradiation.

node dissection followed by radiotherapy resulted in the highest incidence, with 38.3% of the patients developing lymphedema.[29]

In a series of 91 patients who underwent regional lymphadenectomy for invasive primary melanoma, chronic lymphedema developed in 80% of those followed for more than 5 years.[31] Most swelling occurred in the thigh. In a series of 402 patients from Norway who underwent radical hysterectomy and pelvic lymphadenectomy for cervical cancer, severe lymphedema occurred in 5%[30] and mild to moderate lymphedema developed in 23.4%[30] All patients with severe lymphedema had adjuvant preoperative and postoperative radiation treatments.

Tumor Invasion

Lymphedema may be the first manifestation of a malignant tumor infiltrating the regional lymph nodes. In a series of 650 patients with lymphedema, De Roo found 60 in whom limb swelling developed as the first clinical marker of a malignant process.[32] The most frequent tumor was metastatic ovarian carcinoma, followed by carcinoma of the uterus with inguinal metastases and lymphosarcoma. All these patients were 28 years old or older, and in two thirds of the patients limb edema started in the *proximal* region of the extremity. In our experience, the most frequent tumor causing secondary lymphedema is carcinoma of the prostate in men and malignant lymphoma in women.[33]

Infection

Obstructive lymphangitis, caused most frequently by beta-hemolytic streptococci or, rarely, staphylococci, not only is a severe complication of an already existing lymphedema but also is itself an important cause of secondary lymphedema. Swelling may develop after an episode of cellulitis caused by an insect bite, trauma, excoriation, or fungal infection. It is possible that many patients who present with inflammatory lymphedema already have an impairment of lymphatic transport due to lymphatic hypoplasia or primary fibrotic occlusion of the lymph vessels or lymph nodes.

Clinical Staging of Lymphedema

Because none of the classic classification schemes addresses the clinical stage of the disease, the Working Group of the 10th International Congress of Lymphology in 1985 suggested staging chronic lymphedemas regardless of etiology. A latent, subclinical stage and three clinical grades were established as suggested by Brunner.[8] Each grade was subclassified as mild, moderate, and severe.

In the latent phase excess fluid accumulates, and fibrosis occurs around the lymphatics, but no edema is apparent clinically. In *Grade I,* edema pits on pressure and is reduced largely or completely by elevation; there is no clinical evidence of fibrosis. *Grade II* edema does not pit on pressure and is not reduced by elevation. Moderate to severe fibrosis is evident on clinical examination. *Grade III* edema is irreversible and develops from repeated inflammatory attacks, fibrosis, and sclerosis of the skin and subcutaneous tissue. This is the stage of lymphostatic elephantiasis.

The advantage of this classification is that it permits evaluation of the effectiveness of a treatment and comparison of different treatment modalities. A drawback, however, is that appropriate staging in some cases may be difficult without performing a biopsy of the subcutaneous tissue.

CLINICAL PRESENTATION OF LYMPHEDEMA

History

A careful history of the disease frequently reveals the cause of the swelling and suggests the diagnosis of lymphedema. A family history that is positive for leg swelling may indicate familial lymphedema. The development of painless leg swelling in a female in her teens without any identifiable cause strongly suggests *primary* (idiopathic) lymphedema. A history of diarrhea and weight loss is a clue to mesenteric lymphangiectasia, whereas intermittent drainage of milky fluid from skin vesicles in these patients indicates reflux of chyle. In patients with *secondary* lymphedema, a cause of limb swelling is evident in the history, such as previous lymph node dissection, irradiation, tumor, trauma, or infection. In patients who have traveled in tropical countries, filariasis is suspected. Although the cause of primary lymphedema is different from that of secondary lymphedema, the clinical presentation and characteristic physical findings of the diseases are frequently similar.

Signs and Symptoms

Edema

Patients with chronic lymphedema usually present with slowly progressive, painless swelling of the limb. The edema is partially pitting early in the course of the disease but is usually nonpitting in chronic lymphedema owing to the secondary fibrotic changes in the skin and subcutaneous tissue.

The distribution of swelling in lymphedema is characteristic. It starts distally in the extremity in most patients and involves the perimalleolar area, with disappearance of the contours of the ankle in advanced cases (tree trunk or elephantine configuration). The dorsum of the forefoot is usually involved, resulting in the typical appearance of a "buffalo hump" (Fig. 156–5). Squaring of the toes (Stemmer's sign) is also a characteristic feature and results from the high protein content of the excess tissue fluid (Fig. 156–6).

Skin Changes

In the early stage of lymphedema, the skin usually has a pinkish-red color and a mildly elevated temperature due to the increased vascularity. In long-standing lymphedema, however, the skin becomes thick and shows areas of hyperkeratosis, lichenification, and development of a "peau d'orange." The term *pigskin* reflects the reactive changes of the dermis and epidermis in response to the chronic inflammation caused by lymphatic stasis.[38] Recurrent chronic eczematous dermatitis or excoriation of the skin may occur, but frank ulcerations are rare. Unlike the situation in venous stasis, the skin maintains a higher degree of hydration and elasticity for a long time in lymphedema, and ischemic changes due to high skin tension and disruption of the circulation to the skin and subcutaneous tissue are rare.[39]

Additional skin changes in chronic lymph stasis, primarily in patients with hyperplasia of the lymphatics and valvular incompetence, include verrucae or small vesicles, which frequently drain clear lymph (lymphorrhea). In patients with lymphangiectasia and reflux of the chyle, drainage from the vesicles is milky in appearance (chylorrhea) (see Fig. 156–2).

Primary lymphedema may be associated with yellow

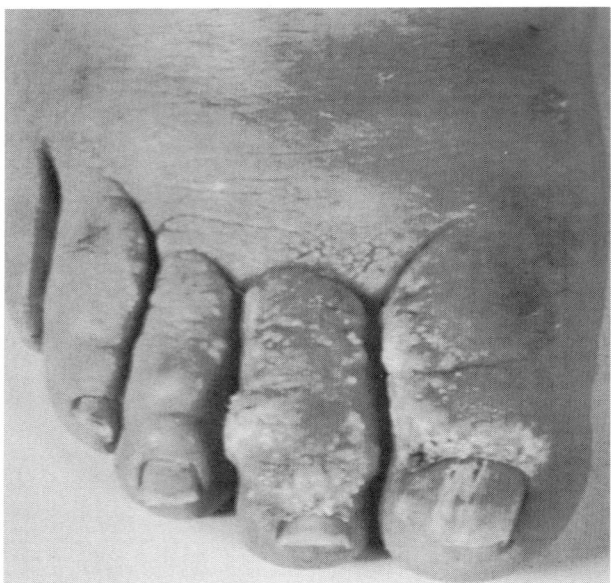

FIGURE 156–6. Squaring of the toes, small verrucae of the skin, and onychomycosis in a patient with primary lymphedema praecox. (From Gloviczki P, Schirger A: Lymphedema. *In* Spittell JA Jr (ed): Clinical Medicine. Philadelphia, Harper & Row, 1985, pp 1–10.)

discoloration of the nails.[40–42] In the yellow nail syndrome, pleural effusion is also present. The pale yellow color of the nails is most likely caused by impaired lymphatic drainage. Severe clubbing, transverse ridging, friability of the nail, and a decreased rate of nail growth are also observed.[41, 42]

Pain

Although some aching or heaviness of the limb is a frequent complaint, significant pain is rare. If the patient with lymphedema complains of marked pain, infection or neuritic pain in the area of scar tissue or radiation treatment should be suspected. Other possible causes of leg swelling, such as venous edema or reflex sympathetic dystrophy, should also be considered (see later section on differential diagnosis).

Complications

Infection

The lymphedematous limb is highly sensitive to fungal infections, such as dermatophytosis and onychomycosis (see Fig. 156–6). Fungal infections in the interdigital spaces are also sites of entry for bacteria, most frequently beta-hemolytic streptococci, which may cause cellulitis or lymphangitis in the affected limb. Cellulitis may present with high fever and chills, and the skin of the affected extremity is red and tender. Repeated episodes of cellulitis aggravate lymphedema.

Malnutrition and Immunodeficiency

Lymphangiectasia with protein-losing enteropathy or chylous ascites or chylothorax may result in severe loss of proteins, long-chain triglycerides, cholesterol, and calcium.[19, 20] As discussed in Chapter 155, losses of lympho-

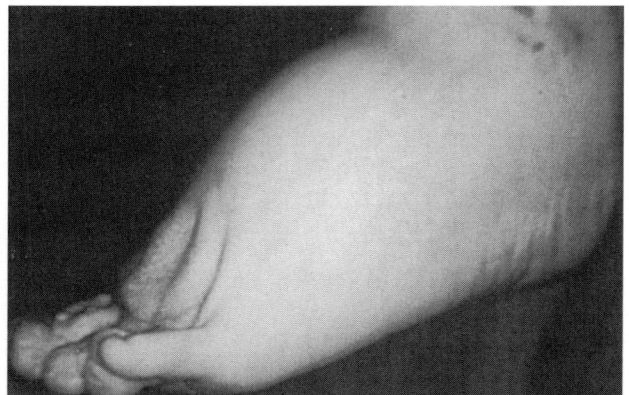

FIGURE 156–5. Lymphedema of the forefoot showing the typical "buffalo hump."

cytes, different immunoglobulins, polypeptides, and cytokines result in a state of immunodeficiency that decreases the ability of these patients to resist infections or malignancy.

Malignancy

Nonhealing "bruises," the development of multiple rounded, purple-red nodules with persistent ulcerations, should alert the physician to the possibility of malignancy.[43-45] Lymphangiosarcoma after long-standing secondary lymphedema, originally described by Stewart and Treves,[43] is a rare malignant disease that frequently results in loss of a limb or even the life of the patient.

NONINVASIVE EVALUATION

The most frequent noninvasive imaging modalities used to evaluate patients with lymphatic diseases include lymphoscintigraphy, computed tomography (CT), and magnetic resonance imaging (MRI).

Lymphoscintigraphy

Interstitially injected colloids labeled with a radioactive tracer were used as long ago as 1953, when Sherman and Ter-Pergossian injected radioactive gold (^{198}Au) into the parametrium to produce lymph node necrosis in an attempt to treat metastatic cancer.[46] The first application of plasma protein labeled with radioactive iodine (^{131}I) for diagnostic evaluation of the lymphatic system in lymphedema was reported by Taylor and associates in 1957.[47] Because of advances in imaging techniques, the introduction of a better radioactive label (technetium 99), and selection of the optimal size of the labeled particles, the technique of diagnostic lymphoscintigraphy has improved continuously during the last two decades.[48-56]

At this time, lymphoscintigraphy with radiocolloids is used principally for evaluation of the swollen extremity. For detection of lymph node metastases, radiolabeled monoclonal antibodies are being used with increasing frequency.

Radiopharmaceuticals

The biokinetic behavior of interstitially applied colloid particles depends on their surface charge and particle size. Particles with small diameters are absorbed into capillaries, whereas those in the 10-nm range (antimony trisulfide [Sb_2S_3]) are absorbed into the lymphatic system. The time needed for activity to appear in the regional lymph nodes has been variably defined according to the physical characteristics of the imaging agent. For example, small particles such as technetium Tc 99m (^{99m}Tc) human serum albumin may appear in the pelvic nodes within 10 minutes,[55] whereas relatively large agents including rhenium and Sb_2S_3 colloid should arrive within 30 minutes[51] or 1 hour,[54] respectively. In our experience, which now includes studies in over 500 limbs, ^{99m}Tc-Sb_2S_3 has been used for lymphoscintigraphy with satisfactory results.[54, 57, 58] Others have reported similar success with the use of technetium-labeled human serum albumin.[52, 53, 55, 59]

Technique

Lymphoscintigraphy is performed with the patient comfortably positioned supine on the imaging table. The feet are attached to a foot ergometer, and the patient is instructed in the proper use of the device. For lymphoscintigraphy of the upper extremity, we employ a plastic squeezable ball the size of a tennis ball that is compressed on command.

After proper positioning and instruction, a subcutaneous injection of 11 MBq (350 to 450 μCi) of ^{99m}Tc-Sb_2S_3 colloid is made into the web space between the second and the third toes (or fingers) bilaterally. The number of particles in the injected solution (0.1 to 0.2 ml) ranges from 10^9 to 10^{13}. The tracer dose is prepared previously in tuberculin syringes (one for each side), and the injection is made with a 27-gauge needle. The injection is associated with an often very intense stinging sensation lasting for 5 to 10 seconds. Absorption of Sb_2S_3 is rapid, and up to 30% of the injected tracer is absorbed by 3 hours. In the United States, this radiopharmaceutical is regulated as an investigational drug by the U.S. Food and Drug Administration.

Immediately after the injection, a gamma camera with a large field of view is positioned to include the groin region in the upper field of view. An all-purpose collimator is used, and a 20% window is placed symmetrically around the 140-keV photopeak of the ^{99m}Tc isotope.

Dynamic anterior images (made every 5 minutes during the first hour, for a total of 12 frames in 1 hour) of the groin are obtained during the first hour (Fig. 156–7). The patient is requested to exercise with the foot ergometer for 5 minutes initially and then 1 minute out of every 5 minutes for the rest of the hour. The same exercise schedule with the squeeze ball is used for the upper extremity. Measured exercise is important to obtain reproducible appearance times in the groin.

At the end of the first hour the patient is scanned with a dual-headed gamma camera (Siemens) for a total body image. Imaging time is about 20 minutes. Similar total body images are obtained at 3 hours (Fig. 156–8) and, for selected patients, at 6 and 24 hours. The patient is encouraged to ambulate in the times between the total body images. Like others, we have experimented with multiple injection sites (two or more sites on each side) or used an injection site behind the lateral malleolus to obtain access to the deep lymphatic system. We have not been convinced, however, that any advantage results from these modifications of the standard technique.

Reading a Lymphoscintigram

At the end of the study, the following information is available to the reviewer for diagnostic interpretation:

1. *Evidence of proper injection.* No uptake is seen in the liver initially, and only faint activity is present at 1 hour. Early liver uptake without activity in the abdominal nodes and channels suggests intravenous tracer injection.

2. *Appearance time of activity in regional lymph nodes (groin or axilla) after tracer injection.* Normal transit time is between 15 and 60 minutes. Less than 15 minutes indicates rapid transport, and more than 60 minutes suggests delayed lymphatic transport (see Fig. 156–7).

3. *The absence or presence and the pattern of lymph channels in the leg; the number, size, and symmetry of tracer activity in*

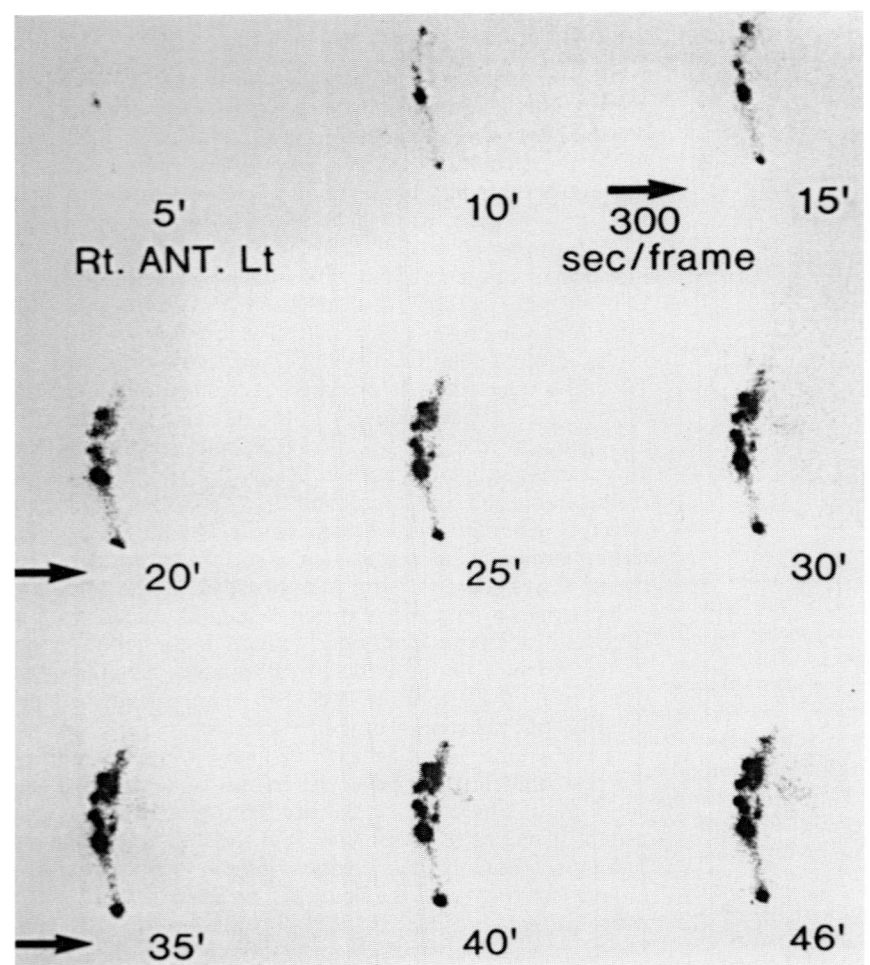

FIGURE 156–7. Lymphoscintigraphic images of the groin taken every 5 minutes after injection of the colloid into both feet. Normal lymphatic transport and image pattern of the inguinal nodes on the right, and no visualization of the lymphatics of the left. This 30-year-old woman had primary lymphedema of the left leg.

the groin lymph nodes. For the upper extremity, similar observations are made for the axilla and arms.

4. *The pattern of lymph nodes and channels in the pelvis and abdomen and activity in the liver.* For the arm, the uptake pattern in axillary lymph nodes is observed.

The data are recorded in a standardized report format, which helps to create reproducible reports when many physicians review these tracings. Such a report form is shown in Table 156–3 and is an adaptation of a form proposed by Kleinhans and colleagues for the estimation of a transport index.[60]

Uptake of the tracer by lymph nodes is not always predictable even in normal patients. Thus, when interpreting a lymphoscintigram, a detailed evaluation for the number of lymph nodes present in the groin is not possible. Nevertheless, abnormal patterns for nodes can be defined, such as (1) no lymph node uptake, (2) marked asymmetry, and (3) mild asymmetry.

The Normal Lymphoscintigram

After the tracer injection, visible activity gradually ascends the anteromedial aspect of the leg. The injection site, because of the relatively large tracer dose given, does not show details, and no information about lymph distribution in the feet is obtainable. Several lymph channels may be

identified in the calf. In the thigh, however, the lymph vessels run close to each other; separate activity in each larger channel is seldom seen on lymphoscintigrams (see Fig. 156–8).

With standardized exercise, as mentioned before, tracer activity should be seen clearly in the inguinal lymph nodes by 60 minutes (range, 15 to 60 minutes). A faint hepatic uptake, activity in the bladder, and faint traces in the para-abdominal nodes are visible at 1 hour. Three-hour images show intense uptake in the liver, symmetric and good uptake in the lymph nodes of the groin, pelvis, and abdomen, and occasionally a tracer focus in the left supraclavicular area at the site of the distal thoracic duct.

Scintigraphic Findings in Lymphedema

Abnormal lymphoscintigrams may show (1) an abnormally slow removal or no removal of the tracer from the injection site (Figs. 156–9 and 156–10); (2) the presence of collaterals or a cutaneous pattern (dermal back-flow) in the extremities (Figs. 156–11 and 156–12A); (3) reduced, faint, or no uptake in the lymph nodes of the groin, the aortoiliac nodes, and the axillary nodes; and (4) abnormal tracer accumulation suggestive of extravasation, lymphocele, or lymphangiectasia (Fig. 156–13A).

Primary and secondary lymphedema are associated with similar abnormalities on lymphoscintigraphy. These include

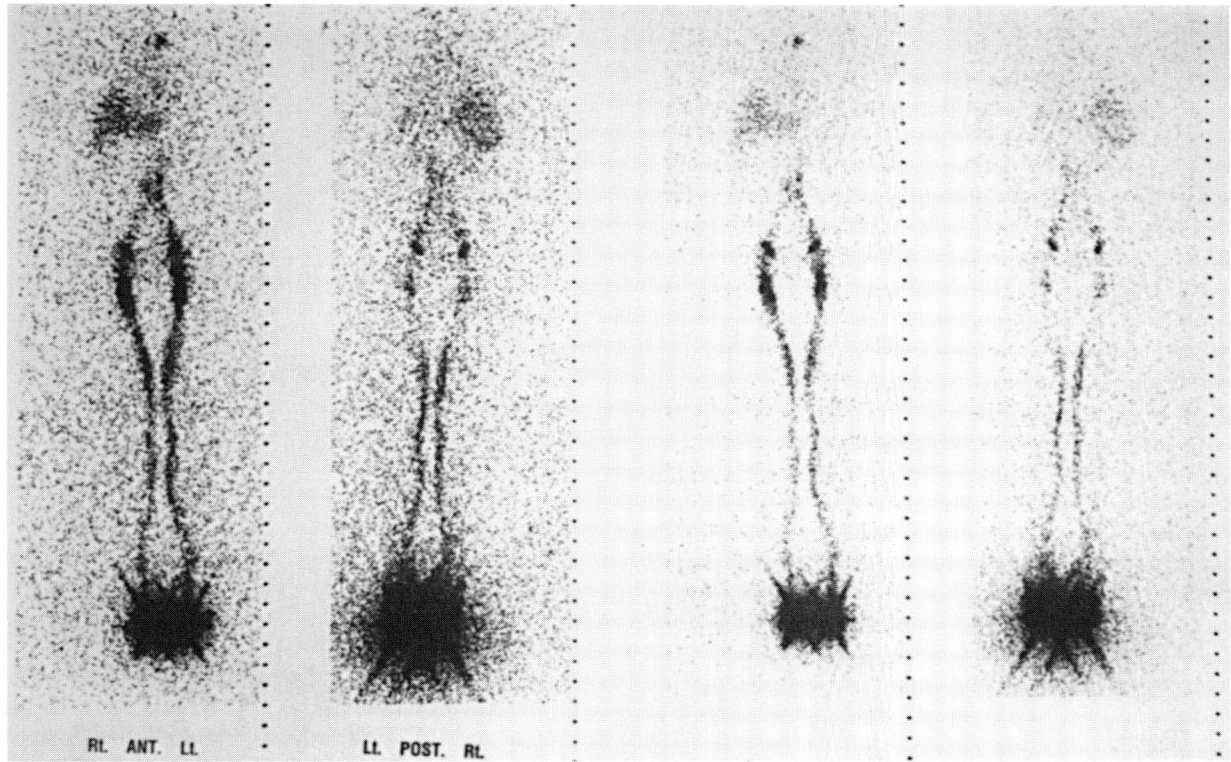

FIGURE 156–8. Image display from total body scan with dual-headed gamma camera. Anterior and posterior images are displayed in two intensity settings. *Left,* Anterior and posterior images of a normal lymphoscintigram. *Right,* Higher-intensity settings in the same patient. Large area of high activity and scatter is seen at the feet where the injection was made. The single well-outlined band in each leg represents the main lymphatic channels. Lymph nodes in the groin, pelvic and para-aortic nodes, liver, and an area at the site of the upper thoracic duct are visualized.

TABLE 156–3. EVALUATION FORM FOR CALCULATION OF LYMPHATIC TRANSPORT INDEX

Patient's Initials _____

Clinic Number _____   Date _____

LYMPHOSCINTIGRAPHY
DATA EVALUATION
☐ Arms   ☐ Legs

IMAGE	1 HR		3 HR		6 HR		24 HR	
	R	L	R	L	R	L	R	L
Lymph transport kinetics: 0 = no delay, 1 = rapid, 3 = low-grade delay, 5 = extreme delay, 9 = no transport								
Distribution pattern: 0 = normal, 2 = focal abnormal tracer, 3 = partial dermal, 5 = diffuse dermal, 9 = no transport								
Lymph node appearance time: Minutes								
Assessment of lymph nodes: 0 = clearly seen, 3 = faint, 5 = hardly seen, 9 = no visualization								
Assessment of lymph vessels: 0 = clearly seen, 3 = faint, 5 = hardly seen, 9 = no visualization								
Abnormal sites of tracer accumulation (describe)								

Adapted from Kleinhans E, Baumeister RGH, Hahn D, et al: Evaluation of transport kinetics in lymphoscintigraphy: Follow-up study in patients with transplanted lymphatic vessels. Eur J Nucl Med 10:349, 1985. Courtesy of Springer-Verlag.

a delay in transport from the injection site (Fig. 156–14), dermal back-flow, the presence of large collaterals, occasionally extravasated activity, fewer visualized lymph nodes, and "crossover" filling of contralateral inguinal (or axillary) lymph nodes as a sign of collateral pathways.[54, 57, 58] In primary lymphedema, it may be possible to distinguish aplasia from hypoplasia if imaging is performed early in the evolution of the disease. In aplasia, there is usually little or no (1) removal of tracer from the injection site, (2) tracer in regional lymph nodes on 1- and 3-hour images, (3) dermal back-flow, and (4) visualized lymph channels. In hypoplasia, these scintigraphic features may be variably present. Regardless of etiology, lymphatic vessels of normal caliber are not seen in patients with long-standing lymphedema.[55]

Qualitative interpretation of images has resulted in excellent sensitivity (92%) and specificity (100%) for the diagnosis of lymphedema.[57] Quantitative lymphoscintigraphy with measurement of lymphatic clearance may improve detection of early disease,[55] but the results obtained in our studies have been equivocal.[54, 57] Neither the image pattern nor the quantitative parameters can reliably distinguish primary from secondary lymphedema.[54, 57, 58]

Scintigraphic Findings in Lymphangiectasia

Dilated on lymph channels with only mild or no delay in lymph transport are frequently seen on lymphoscinti-

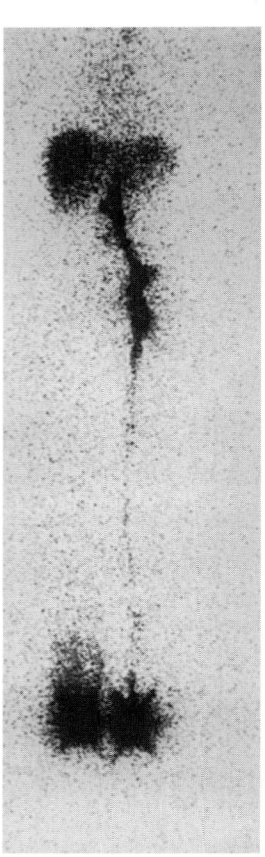

FIGURE 156–10. Lymphoscintigram of a 65-year-old woman with primary lymphedema tarda of the right lower extremity. There is minimal dermal back-flow above the right ankle 3 hours after injection, and no lymph vessels or lymph nodes are visualized. Normal pattern in left leg.

graphic images. Injection of the colloid into the unaffected lower extremity may reflux into the affected lymphedematous leg because of lymphatic valvular incompetence. Similar reflux of the colloid may be seen in the dilated mesenteric lymphatics (see Fig. 156–13A) or in the retroperitoneum, perineum, or scrotum (Fig. 156–15). Ruptured lymphatics cause extravasation of the colloid into the abdominal cavity or the chest of patients with chylous ascites or chylothorax. The images are generally not helpful, however, in determining the exact site of the lymphatic leak.

Computed Tomography

The greatest value of CT in the evaluation of patients with a swollen leg is to exclude any obstructing mass that may result in decreased transport capacity of the lymphatic system. For patients with lymphedema, CT confirms the presence of coarse, nonenhancing, tubular reticular structures in the subcutaneous tissue.[61–63] This honeycomb appearance in the subcutaneous tissue is caused either by lymphatic channels or by free fluid accumulating in tissue planes. However, CT is not able to distinguish subcutaneous fat from tissue fluid. In our experience, this test is not sensitive enough to define the cause of lower extremity swelling.

Magnetic Resonance Imaging

Because of continuous improvements in technology, MRI has become the most important noninvasive imaging test

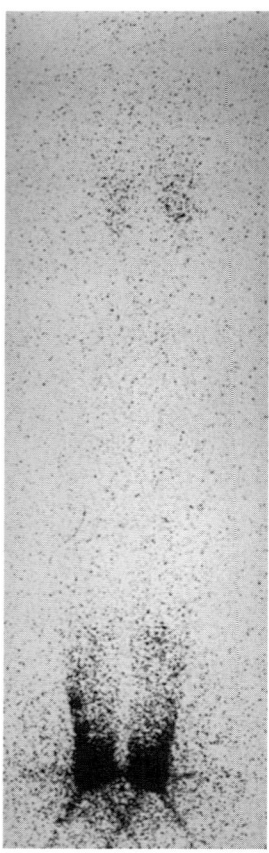

FIGURE 156–9. Lymphoscintigram of a 25-year-old woman with congenital familial lymphedema of both lower extremities, Note absence of lymph vessels and lymph nodes at 6 hours, with only minimal dermal back-flow visible in the distal calves. This patient also had recurrent familial cholestasis due to absence of intrahepatic bile ducts (Aagenaes syndrome).

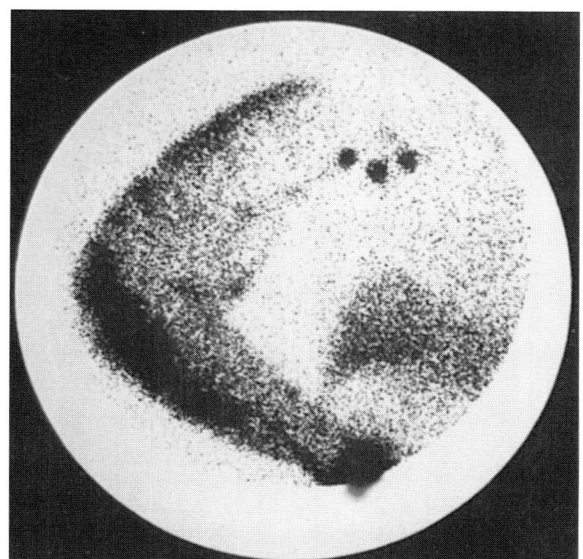

FIGURE 156–11. Lymphoscintigram of the right arm of a 51-year-old woman with postmastectomy lymphedema. Note extensive dermal backflow resulting from lymphatic obstruction. Three groups of axillary nodes are still visualized.

for the diagnosis of congenital vascular malformations and the identification of soft tissue tumors. The value of MRI in the diagnosis of the swollen leg, however, has not been evaluated until recently. Duewell and colleagues found MRI scanning useful in differentiating the three major forms of limb swelling: lipedema, chronic venous edema, and

lymphedema.[64] Lipedema was characterized by an increased amount of subcutaneous fat without increased vascularity or signal changes suggesting excess fluid. The ratio of the superficial to the deep compartment was found to be increased. In lymphedema and venous edema, however, there was no change in the superficial-to-deep compartment ratio. Like findings observed on CT, a honeycomb pattern was seen in the subcutaneous tissues of patients with lymphedema.[64]

MRI is particularly useful in complementing findings observed on lymphoscintigraphy.[65, 66] MRI is helpful for delineating nodal anatomy in addition to imaging soft tissue changes and the larger lymphatic trunks and nodes in different tissue planes (Fig. 156–16). MRI is also suitable for imaging lymphatic trunks and nodes proximal to the site of lymphatic obstruction, which cannot be visualized by lymphoscintigraphy. Experience that is accumulating with the use of supermagnetic agents (e.g., iron oxide) appears promising for delineation of the lymphatic truncal-nodal anatomy in greater detail.[67]

LYMPHANGIOGRAPHY

Visual Lymphangiography (Dye Test)

Hudack and McMaster were the first, in 1933, to use subcutaneous injection of vital dyes to visualize the superficial lymphatics of the thigh and the forearm.[63] Subcutaneous injection of patent blue V or isosulfan blue (Lymphazurin) dye in the first or second interdigital space of the foot results in fast, selective uptake of the large-molecular-

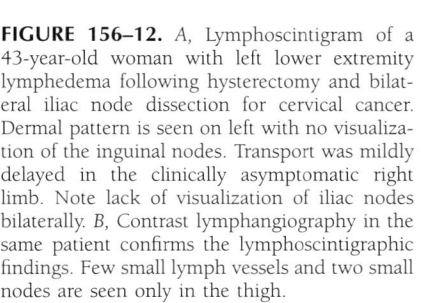

FIGURE 156–12. *A,* Lymphoscintigram of a 43-year-old woman with left lower extremity lymphedema following hysterectomy and bilateral iliac node dissection for cervical cancer. Dermal pattern is seen on left with no visualization of the inguinal nodes. Transport was mildly delayed in the clinically asymptomatic right limb. Note lack of visualization of iliac nodes bilaterally. *B,* Contrast lymphangiography in the same patient confirms the lymphoscintigraphic findings. Few small lymph vessels and two small nodes are seen only in the thigh.

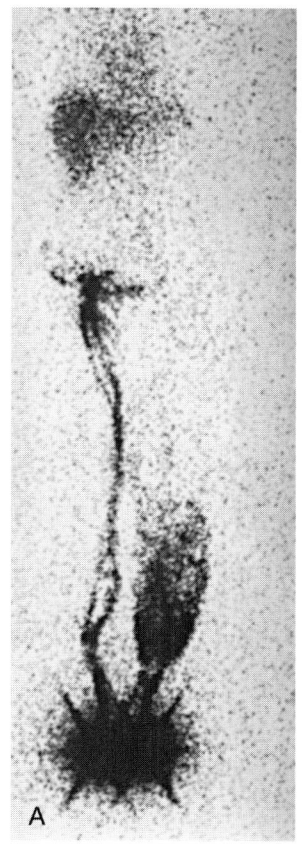

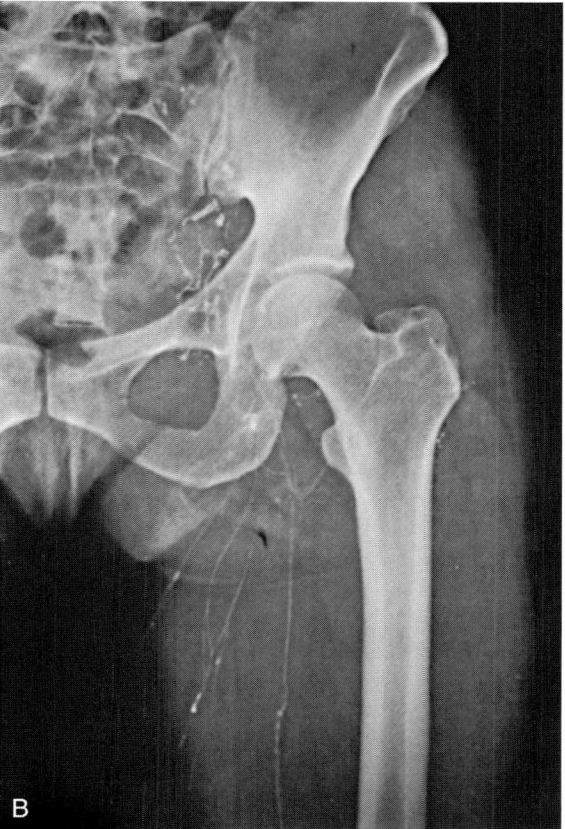

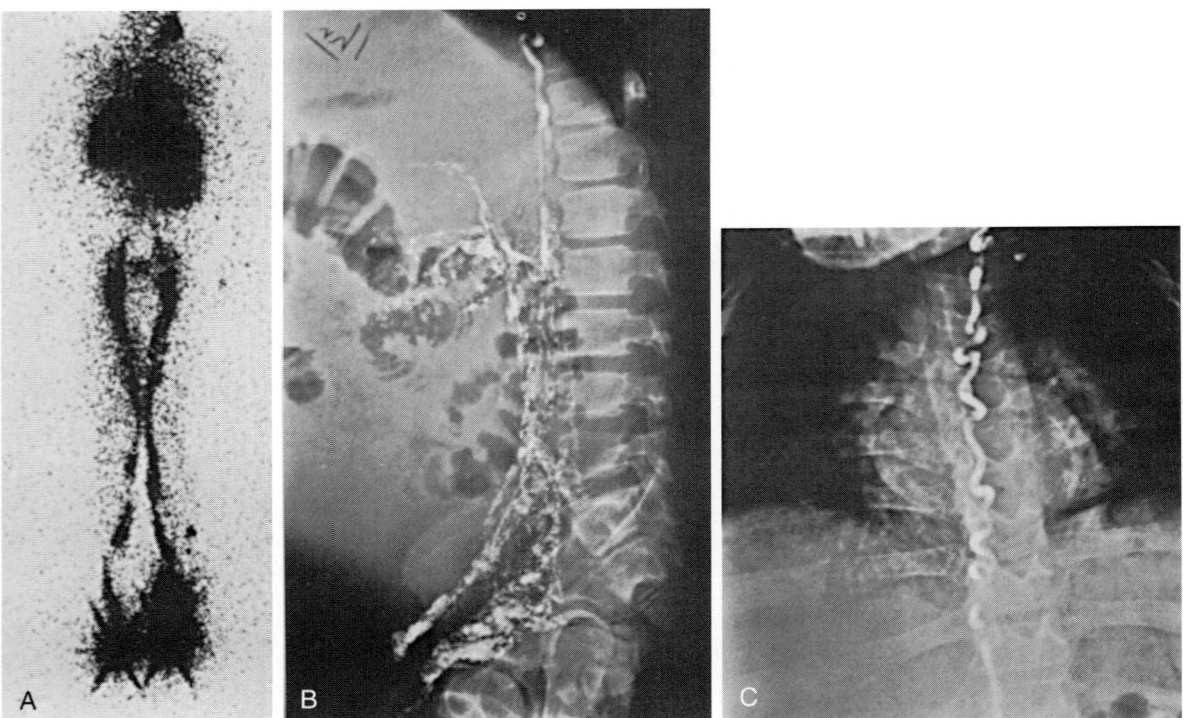

FIGURE 156–13. *A,* Lymphoscintigram of an 18-year-old man with lymphangiectasia, protein-losing enteropathy, and chylous ascites. Note large leg lymphatics and reflux of colloid into the mesenteric lymph vessels, filling almost the entire abdominal cavity. *B,* Lymphangiogram of the same patient reveals reflux of dye into the dilated mesenteric lymphatics. *C,* Note extremely dilated and tortuous but patent thoracic duct.

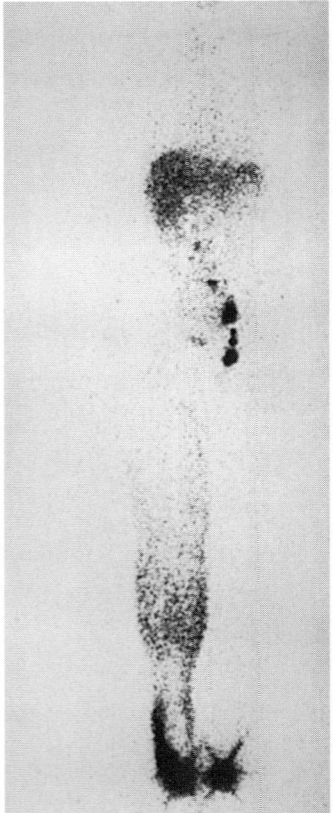

FIGURE 156–14. Lymphoscintigram of a 47-years-old woman with primary lymphedema tarda of the right lower extremity. Note markedly delayed transport with dermal pattern in the right leg. The right inguinal or iliac nodes were not visualized.

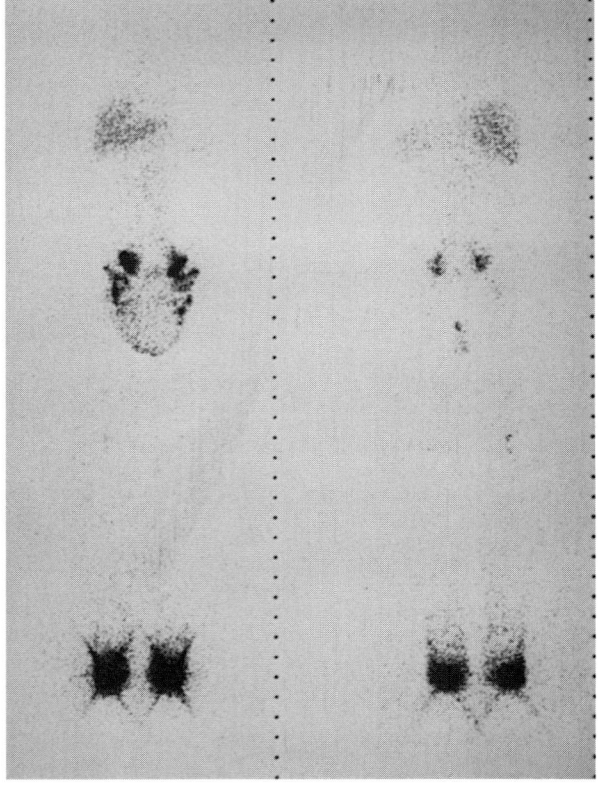

FIGURE 156–15. Bilateral leg scintigraphy with anterior (*left*) and posterior (*right*) views in a 24-year-old man outlines the swollen scrotum in the 6-hour image. Reflux of the colloid resulted from dilatation and valvular incompetence of the lymphatics.

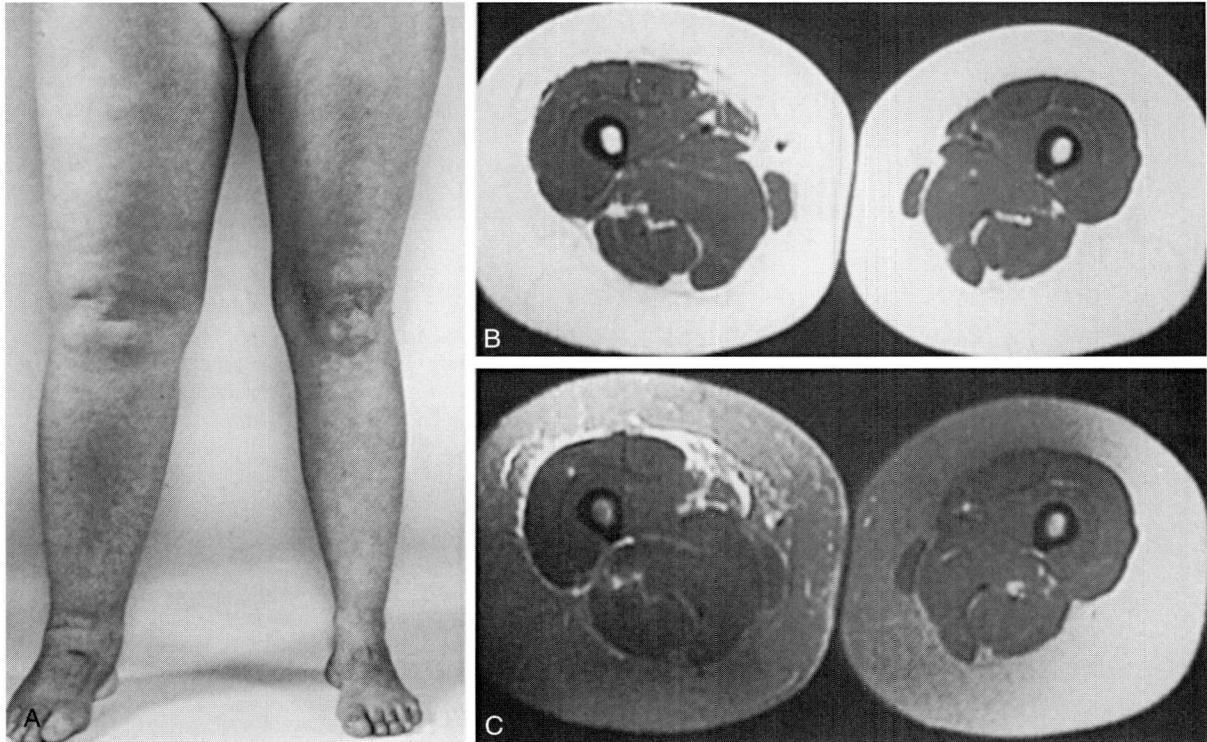

FIGURE 156–16. *A,* Secondary lymphedema of the right lower extremity, in a 36-year-old woman, *B,* MRI of the legs reveals enlargement of the subcutaneous tissues and the deep compartment on the right with considerable stranding within the subcutaneous tissues, predominantly anteriorly and medially. *C,* T2-weighted image reveals the region of soft tissue stranding that is now of high signal intensity in the deep layers of the subcutaneous tissue.

weight dye into the lymphatic system. With normal lymphatic circulation, the dye is transported to the inguinal lymph nodes 5 to 10 minutes after injection. In patients with lymphatic stasis in the superficial lymph collectors, dermal back-flow is observed soon after injection (Fig. 156–17). If positive, the test is reliable to diagnose lymphatic stasis, but failure to demonstrate dermal back-flow may also indicate extensive lymphatic obstruction, hypoplasia, or aplasia.

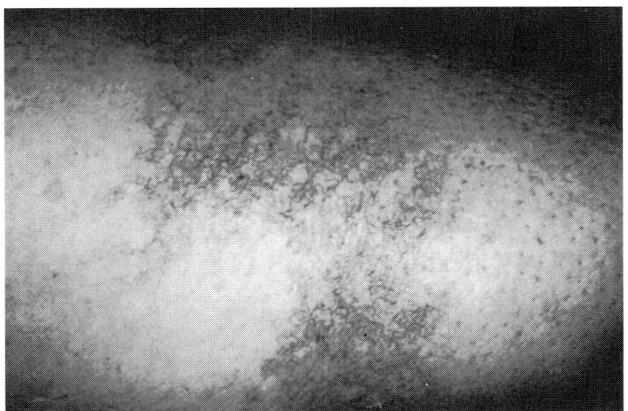

FIGURE 156–17. Visual lymphangiography in secondary lymphedema. Lymphazurine dye injected into the first interdigital space of the foot delineates the dermal lymphatics at the mid-calf owing to obstruction in the proximal main lymphatic vessels.

Direct Contrast Lymphangiography

Contrast lymphangiography was first performed by Servelle in 1943,[69] but the current technique of subcutaneous injection of a vital dye to identify the foot lymphatics for cannulation and direct injection of the contrast material was developed by Kinmonth.[70] Lymphangiography with lipid-soluble contrast material provided a major stimulus to the investigation of the lymphatic system in patients with both lymphedema and malignancy. Since the availability of CT and MRI, the utility of lymphangiography in the clinical staging of malignancies has significantly diminished. With the availability of isotope lymphoscintigraphy. the use of contrast lymphangiography for patients with lymphedema has also significantly decreased.

Technique of Pedal Lymphangiography

Contrast lymphangiography is performed under local anesthesia using a 1% lidocaine (Xylocaine) solution. A small transverse incision is made in the mid-dorsum of the foot after 1 ml of isosulfan blue (Lymphazurin) dye has been injected subcutaneously into the first and second interdigital spaces. Because the dye injection itself is uncomfortable and painful, we mix the dye with equal amounts of 1% lidocaine solution.

The lymph vessels are dissected under loupe magnification, and a 30-gauge needle attached to a polyethylene tube is inserted into the lymph vessels. A constant infusion of lipid-soluble contrast material (ethiodized oil) is started at

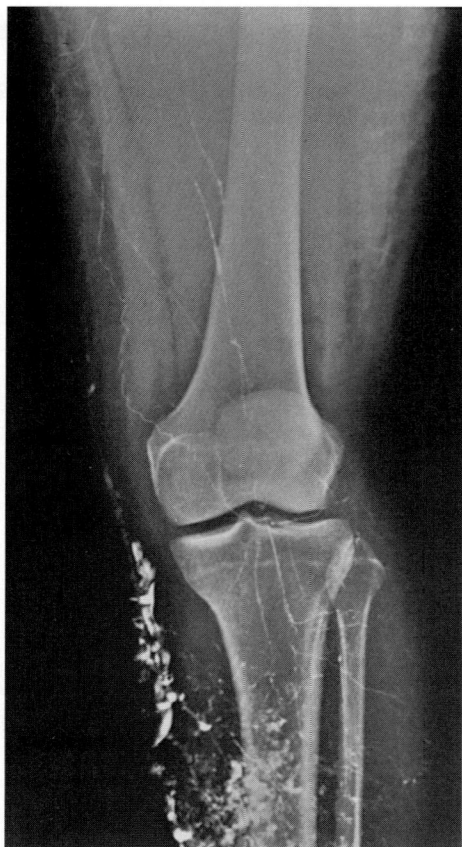

FIGURE 156–18. Extensive occlusion of most lymph vessels in the thigh with extravasation of the dye distal to the knee after contrast lymphangiography in a patient with secondary lymphedema.

a rate of 1 ml in 8 minutes, as suggested by Wolfe.[71] A maximum of 7 ml is injected into each limb, making a total infusion that does not exceed 14 ml. If the injection is made too fast, the dye will extravasate through the wall of the lymph vessels, and interpretation of the images will be difficult (Fig. 156–18). If the amount of extravasation is significant, the rate of infusion should be decreased. At the end of the procedure the needle is removed, and the incision is closed meticulously with interrupted 5-0 nylon vertical mattress sutures.

Serial films are taken of the lower extremities, groin, pelvis, lumbar area, and upper abdomen and chest during the injection. Additional films are taken several hours after injection and 24 hours later. The oily contrast material may remain in the lymph nodes for several months after injection.

Arm Lymphangiography

Lymphangiography of the upper extremity is now rarely performed. The technique is similar to that used for pedal lymphangiography, except that a small lymphatic on the dorsum of the hand is cannulated. The amount of contrast should be limited to 4 to 5 ml of ethiodized oil (Ethiodol).[71]

Interpretation of Lymphangiograms

Injection of a dorsal pedal lymph vessel fills the superficial medial lymphatic vessels and most of the inguinal lymph nodes. Five to 15 lymph vessels are seen in normal patients at the medial aspect of the thigh (Fig. 156–19), with valves frequently visualized every 5 to 10 mm. Lateral lymphatics and deep lymphatics are not visible on normal lymphangiograms but may be seen in patients with lymphatic obstruction (Fig. 156–20). The deep lymph vessels are frequently paired and follow the main blood vessels of the extremity. The normal lymphatic nodes have a ground-glass appearance. Normally the iliac lymph vessels and lymph nodes fill within 30 to 45 minutes after the injection is started. The thoracic duct may only show up on images several hours after the injection (see Fig. 156–13C).

Most patients with primary lymphedema have an obstruction of some or most of the lymph vessels and lymph-conducting elements of the lymph nodes. As mentioned previously, distal obliteration of the lymph vessels in the leg is much more frequent than proximal, pelvic lymphatic obstruction. With pelvic obstruction the inguinal and iliac lymph nodes are few or absent, but the leg lymphatics are patent and are frequently distended and tortuous (Fig. 156–21). Back-flow of the contrast into dilated dermal lymphatics is observed. The lymphangiographic findings in proximal obliteration are similar to those seen in secondary lymphedema. With time, however, fibrotic occlusion of the dilated distal lymph vessels frequently occurs. This retrograde occlusion of the lymph vessels (die-back) was observed in patients with both secondary and primary lymphedemas.[72]

Patients with lymphangiectasia frequently need larger amounts of contrast to image the dilated, incompetent lymphatics. The number of pelvic lymph nodes may be diminished. Contrast material may reflux into the mesenteric lymphatics (see Fig. 156–13B). The thoracic duct in some of the patients is occluded or absent, whereas in others it is dilated and tortuous (see Fig. 156–13C).

Complications

Contrast lymphangiography is an invasive and lengthy procedure that is frequently uncomfortable for the patient. Obstructive lymphangitis and progression of lymphedema after lymphangiography have also been noted.[73] Symptomatic pulmonary embolization due to the oily contrast material may complicate lymphangiography. This problem may be caused by using excessive amounts of contrast, or it may be the result of embolization through spontaneous lymphovenous anastomoses. In patients who have had previous pulmonary irradiation, cerebral embolization through pulmonary arteriovenous fistulae may also occur.[71] The use of ethiodized oil (Ethiodol) is contraindicated in patients who are allergic to iodine.

Indications for Direct Contrast Lymphangiography

Contrast lymphangiography is a test that is now rarely and only selectively used for the diagnosis of lymphedema. It is indicated for some patients who are candidates for microvascular lymphatic reconstruction. It is also useful in the preoperative evaluation of patients with lymphangiectasia and reflux of chyle (see Chapter 146). Although the diagnosis of lymphangiectasia can be made with lymphoscintigraphy, the extent and location of the dilated lymphat-

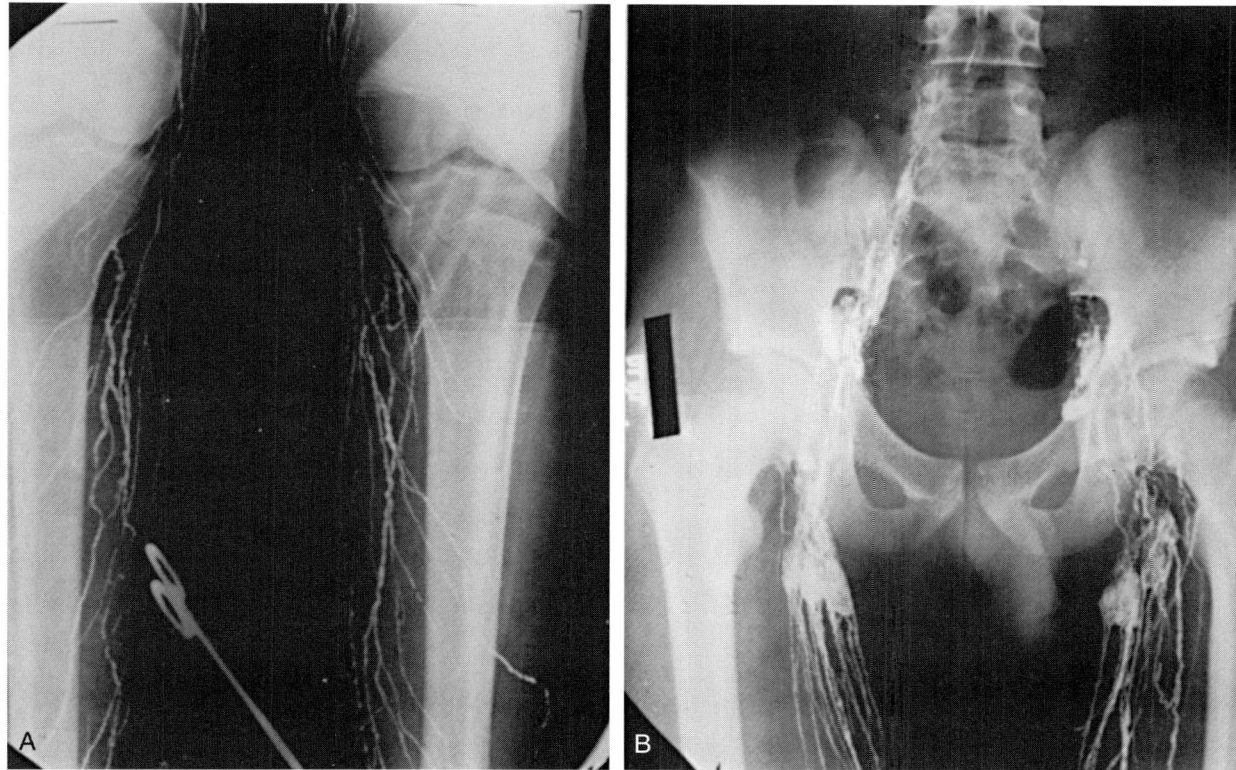

FIGURE 156–19. *A* and *B,* Normal bipedal lymphangiogram with only mild dilatation and tortuosity of the lymph vessels of the calf. Note the presence of 10 to 15 superficial lymphatic collectors in the thighs.

ics are best delineated by contrast lymphangiography. Lymphangiography remains the best test for imaging the thoracic duct and for identifying the exact location of some pelvic, abdominal, and thoracic lymphatic fistulae.

Indirect Contrast Lymphangiography

Because of the difficulties encountered with direct cannulation of the lymphatics and the use of oily contrast material, increasing research has focused in recent years on indirect lymphangiography. This is performed with subepidermal infusion of a water-soluble contrast material (iotasul, iopamidol).[74] The dermal lymphatics and in some patients the distal lymph collectors can be imaged with this technique. In primary lymphedema, absence, hypoplasia, or hyperplasia of the dermal lymphatics can be demonstrated with indirect lymphangiography. In secondary lymphedema, hyperplasia of the initial lymphatics is the most frequent finding. Although indirect lymphangiography is helpful for diagnosing lymphatic stasis and for imaging the fine initial lymph vessels, the limitations of the current technique are still important: larger lymphatic collectors or nodes distant to the site of the injection are not visualized.[75]

DIFFERENTIAL DIAGNOSIS OF LYMPHEDEMA

During the evaluation of patients with chronic limb swelling, a systemic cause of the disease should be excluded first. Underlying cardiac diseases such as congestive heart failure, chronic constrictive pericarditis, and severe tricuspid regurgitation are the most frequent systemic causes leading to pitting or bilateral leg swelling. Hepatic or renal failure, hypoproteinemia, malnutrition, and endocrine disorders (myxedema) are other possible causes of leg swelling. Allergic reactions, hereditary angioedema, and idiopathic cyclic edema are rare systemic causes that should be considered. Chronic use of diuretics may lead to generalized swelling, which most frequently affects the extremities and the face. Other drugs that may cause swelling include steroids, some of the antihypertensive drugs, and anti-inflammatory agents (Table 156–4).

Remember that, among the local or regional causes of limb swelling, chronic venous insufficiency is much more common than lymphedema. In some patients with chronic iliac or iliocaval obstruction massive swelling of the entire extremity can develop (Fig. 156–22A). The usual causes of proximal venous occlusion are deep venous thrombosis or external compression of the vein by tumor or retroperitoneal fibrosis. Although lymphedema is usually painless, venous hypertension results in marked pain and cramps after prolonged standing or at the end of the day. Patients with proximal venous obstruction may complain of typical claudication, which presents with throbbing pain in the thigh or calf after walking. The pain resolves with rest, although elevation of the extremity provides the fastest relief. The presence of varicosity, pigmentation, induration, or venous ulcers makes the diagnosis of venous insufficiency easier. Chronic inflammation in the subcutaneous tissue due to venous stasis may result in destruction of the collecting lymph channels, and a mixed venous-lymphatic edema develops in these patients.

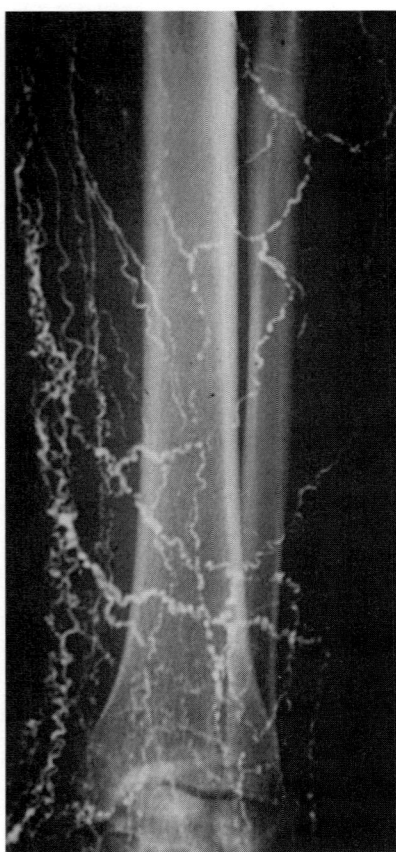

FIGURE 156–20. Dilated tortuous lymph vessels with valvular insufficiency and filling of lateral lymph vessels in a patient with lymphedema praecox. (From Gloviczki P, Schirger A: Lymphedema. *In* Spittell JA Jr (ed) Clinical Medicine. Philadelphia, Harper & Row, 1985, pp 1–10.)

Patients with congenital vascular malformations frequently have a larger extremity that may be difficult to distinguish from lymphedema (Fig. 156–22*B*). An increase in the length of the affected extremity, the presence of atypical lateral varicosity, and port-wine stain with underlying developmental abnormality of the deep venous system is characteristic of Klippel-Trenaunay syndrome.[76] Although hypertrophy of the soft tissues and bones is caused by an abnormality in mesenchymal development, congenital lymphedema may also be present in these patients. In patients with high-shunt, high-flow arteriovenous malformations the extremity is larger and is also frequently longer.[77] A bruit and thrill are present, the superficial veins are dilated and frequently pulsatile, and the distal arterial pulses may be diminished.

Lipedema is characterized by deposition of a large amount of fatty tissue in the subcutaneous layers. Most of these patients have morbid obesity, although some, mostly females, have fat deposition primarily localized to the lower half of the body. Evaluation of the lymphatic system with lymphoscintigraphy or lymphangiography shows essentially normal findings.

Trauma and subsequent reflex sympathetic dystrophy may result in painful swelling of the extremity. Because of disuse, a varying degree of osteoporosis can be observed, and increased sympathetic activity occurs in the limb of these patients. The swelling is usually the result of a "high-

output" lymphatic failure, and increased lymphatic transport on lymphoscintigraphy may be demonstrated (Fig. 156–23*A* and *B*). Baker's cyst, soft tissue tumor, hematoma, and inflammation such as tenosynovitis or arthritis are additional local causes of limb swelling that should be considered in the differential diagnosis of lymphedema.

DIAGNOSTIC PROTOCOL FOR EVALUATION OF CHRONIC EDEMA

Clinical examination of the patient frequently reveals the correct cause of limb swelling. Initial laboratory examinations should include routine blood tests to look for signs of renal or hepatic failure, eosinophilia, or hypoproteinemia. Urinalysis may indicate proteinuria. Once a systemic cause of edema is excluded, the local or regional cause should be confirmed (Fig. 156–24).

CT has become a routine test in our practice for most adult patients with leg swelling to exclude underlying malignancy. Noninvasive venous studies, such as Doppler examination or strain-gauge plethysmography, are frequently sufficient to diagnose venous disease. In some patients, however, duplex scanning is necessary to exclude obstruction of the deep veins. MRI provides the most accurate information in patients with clinical signs of congenital vascular malformation, soft tissue tumor, or retroperitoneal fibrosis.

Lymphoscintigraphy is now the test of choice for the confirmation of lymphedema, and a normal lymphoscintigraphic examination essentially excludes the diagnosis of lymphedema. Patients with chronic venous insufficiency may have abnormal results on lymphoscintigraphic examination with delayed transport because of mixed, lymphatic, and venous edema. Direct contrast lymphangiography should be performed selectively and should not be included routinely in the evaluation of patients with chronic limb swelling.

TABLE 156–4. DIFFERENTIAL DIAGNOSIS OF CHRONIC LEG SWELLING

SYSTEMIC CAUSES	LOCAL OR REGIONAL CAUSES
Cardiac failure	Chronic venous insufficiency
Hepatic failure	Lymphedema
Renal failure	Lipedema
Hypoproteinemia	Congenital vascular malformation
Hyperthyroidism (myxedema)	Arteriovenous fistula
Allergic disorders	Trauma
Idiopathic cyclic edema	Snake or insect bite
Hereditary angioedema	Infection, inflammation
	Hematoma
Drugs	Dependency
	Rheumatoid arthritis
Antihypertensives	Postrevascularization edema
Methyldopa	Soft tissue tumor
Nifedipine	Hemihypertrophy
Hydralazine	
Hormones	
Estrogen	
Progesterone	
Anti-inflammatory drugs	
Phenylbutazone	
Monoamine oxidase inhibitors	

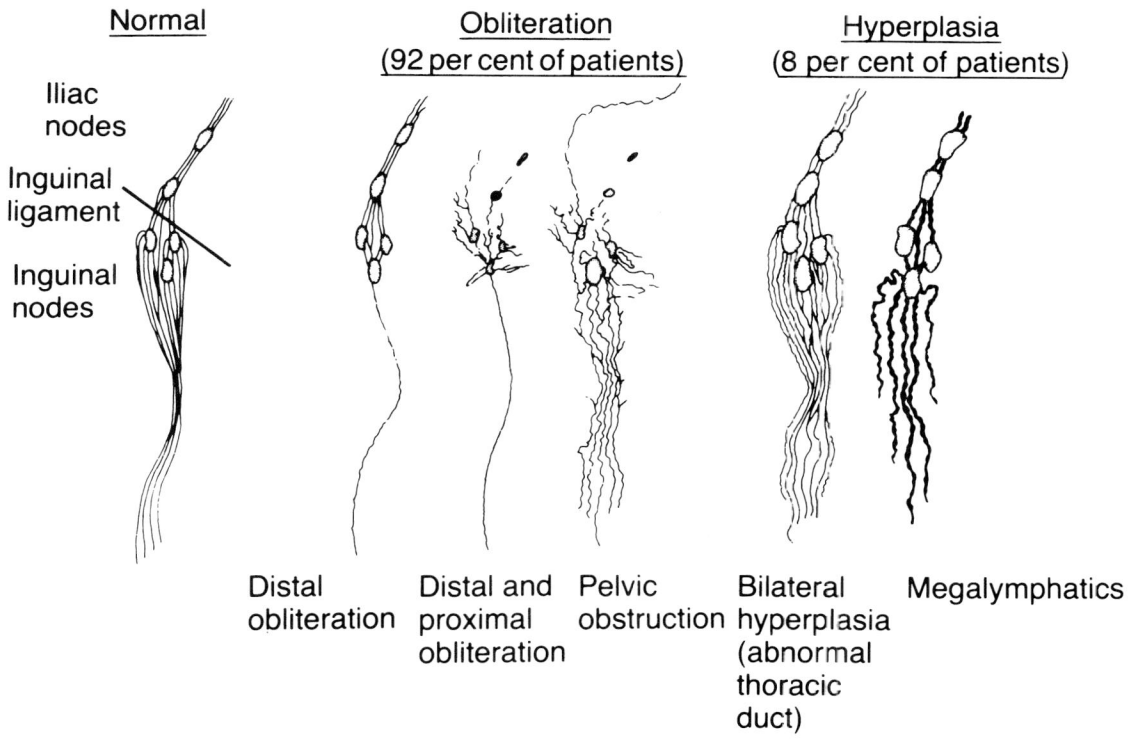

FIGURE 156–21. Lymphangiographic patterns in normal patient and in patients with different types of primary lymphedema.

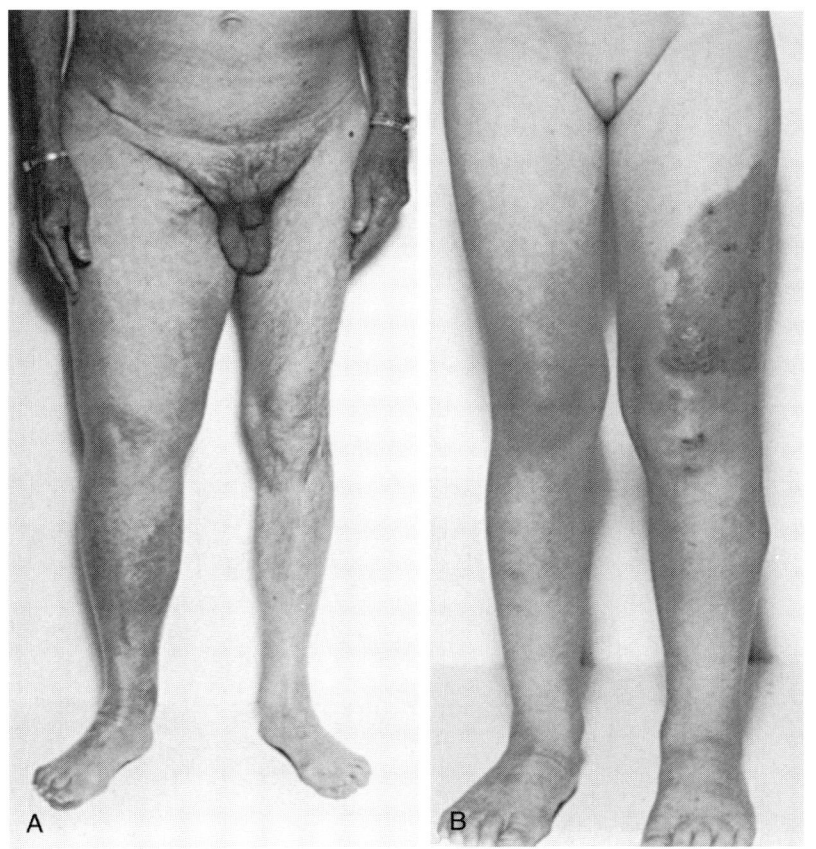

FIGURE 156–22. Venous disease in the differential diagnosis of limb edema. *A*, Right leg swelling due to venous insufficiency, caused by chronic iliofemoral venous thrombosis. *B*, Left leg edema associated with congenital vascular malformation (Klippel-Trenaunay syndrome).

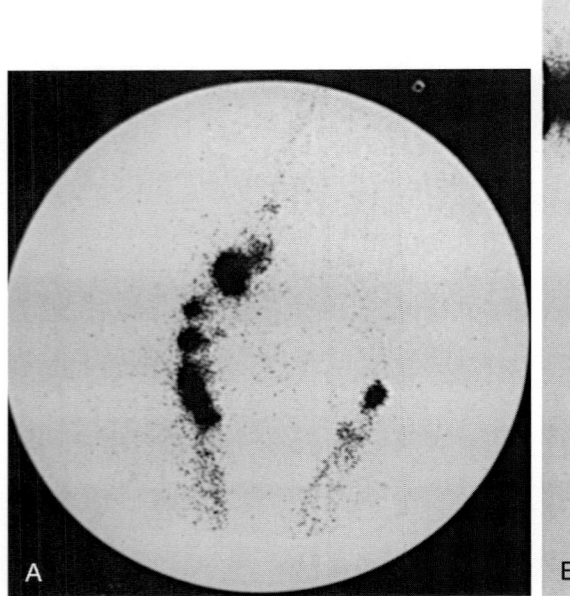
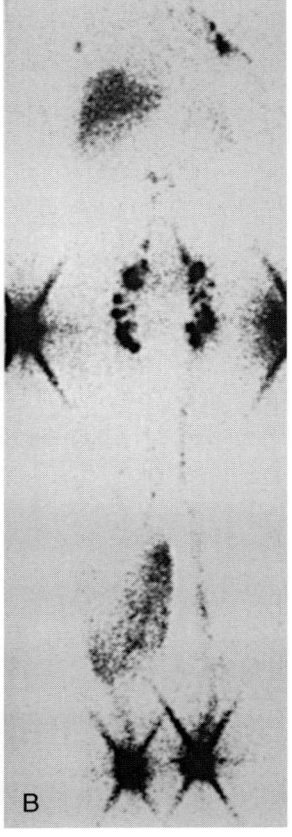

FIGURE 156–23. Lymphoscintigraphy in "high-output" lymphatic failure due to reflex sympathetic dystrophy of the right leg. *A,* Fast lymphatic transport in the affected right leg compared with the normal left leg on the image taken of the inguinal nodes 20 minutes after injection. *B,* Total body image taken at 3 hours shows dermal pattern on the right but no evidence of proximal lymphatic obstruction.

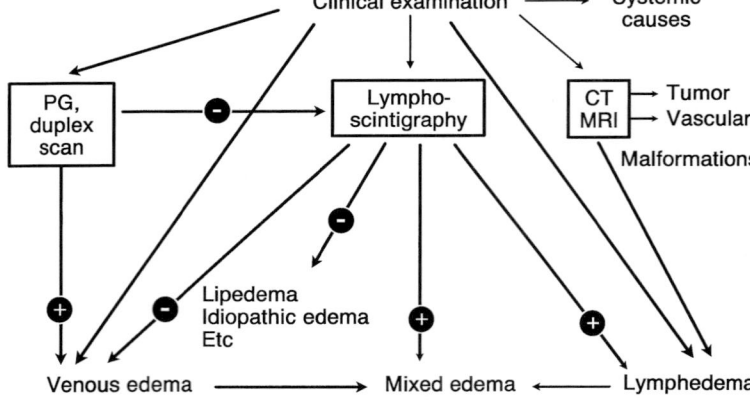

FIGURE 156–24. Diagnostic protocol for patients with chronic limb swelling. PG = plethysmography.

REFERENCES

1. Kinmonth JB, Taylor GW, Tracy GD, et al: Primary lymphoedema: Clinical and lymphangiographic studies of a series of 107 patients in which the lower limbs were affected. Br J Surg 45:1, 1957.
2. Kinmonth JB: The lymphoedemas. General considerations. In Kinmonth JB (ed): The Lymphatics: Surgery, Lymphography and Diseases of the Chyle and Lymph Systems. London, Edward Arnold, 1982, pp 83–104.
3. Browse NL, Stewart G: Lymphoedema: Pathophysiology and classification. J Cardiovasc Surg 26:91, 1985.
4. Browse NL: The diagnosis and management of primary lymphedema. J Vasc Surg 3:181, 1986.
5. Gloviczki P, Schirger A: Lymphedema. In Spittell JA Jr (ed): Clinical Medicine. Philadelphia, Harper & Row, 1985, pp 1–10.
6. O'Donnell TF, Howrigan P: Diagnosis and management of lymphedema. In Bell PRF, Jamieson CW, Ruckley CV (eds): Surgical Management of Vascular Disease. Philadelphia, WB Saunders, 1992, pp 1305–1327.
7. Allen EV: Lymphedema of the extremities: Classification, etiology and differential diagnosis: A study of three hundred cases. Arch Inter Med 54:606, 1934.
8. Casley-Smith JR, Földi M, Ryan TJ, et al: Lymphedema: Summary of the 10th International Congress of Lymphology Working Group Discussions and Recommendations, Adelaide, Australia, August 10–17, 1985. Lymphology 18:175, 1985.
9. Browse NL: Primary lymphedema. In Ernst C, Stanley J (eds): Current Therapy in Vascular Surgery. Philadelphia, BC Decker, 1987, pp 454–457.
10. Kinmonth JB, Wolfe JH: Fibrosis in the lymph nodes in primary lymphoedema: Histological and clinical studies in 74 patients with lower-limb oedema. Ann R Coll Surg Engl 62:344, 1980.
11. Wolfe JHN: The prognosis and possible cause of severe primary lymphoedema. Ann R Coll Surg Engl 66:251, 1984.
12. Kurland LT, Molgaard CA: The patient record in epidemiology. Sci Am 245:54, 1981.
13. Smeltzer DM, Stickler GB, Schirger A: Primary lymphedema in children and adolescents: A follow-up study and review. Pediatrics 76:206, 1985.
14. Letessier EE: Cited by Schroeder E, Helweg-Larsen HF: Chronic hereditary lymphedemia (Nonne-Milroy-Meige disease). Acta Med Scand 137:198, 1950.
15. Nonne M: Vier Fälle von Elephantiasis congenita hereditaria. Arch Pathol Anat Physiol 125:189, 1891.
16. Milroy WF: An undescribed variety of hereditary edema. NY Med J 56:505, 1892.
17. Milroy WF: Chronic hereditary edema: Milroy's disease. JAMA 91:1172, 1928.
18. Meige H: Dystrophie oedemateuse hereditaire. Presse Med 2:341, 1898.
19. Servelle M: Congenital malformation of the lymphatics of the small intestine. J Cardiovasc Surg 32:159, 1991.
20. Kinmonth JB, Cox SJ: Protein-losing enteropathy in lymphoedema: Surgical investigation and treatment. J Cardiovasc Surg 16:111, 1975.
21. Gloviczki P, Soltesz L, Solti F, et al: The surgical treatment of lymphedema caused by chylous reflux. In Bartos V, Davidson JW (eds): Advances in Lymphology. Proceedings of the 8th International Congress of Lymphology, Montreal, 1981. Prague, Czechoslovak Medical Press, 1982, pp 502–507.
22. Lymphatic filariasis—tropical medicine's origin will not go away. Lancet 1:1409, 1987.
23. Mak JW: Epidemiology of lymphatic filariasis. Ciba Found Symp 127:5, 1987.
24. Lobb AW, Harkins HN: Postmastectomy swelling of the arm with note on effect of segmental resection of axillary vein at time of radical mastectomy. West J Surg 57:550, 1949.
25. Leis HP: Selective moderate surgical approach for potentially curable breast cancer. In Gallagher HS, Leis HP, Snyderman RK, Urban JA (eds): The Breast. St. Louis, CV Mosby, 1978, pp 232–247.
26. Hayward JL, Winter PJ, Tong D, et al: A new approach to the conservative treatment of early breast cancer. Surgery 95:270, 1984.
27. Veronesi U, Saccozzi R, Del Vecchio M, et al: Comparing radical mastectomy with quadrantectomy, axillary dissection, and radiotherapy in patients with small cancers of the breast. N Engl J Med 305:6, 1981.
28. Osborne MP, Ormiston N, Harmer CL, et al: Breast conservation in the treatment of early breast cancer. A 20-year follow-up. Cancer 53:349, 1984.
29. Kissin MW, della Rovere GQ, Easton D, Westbury G: Risk of lymphoedema following the treatment of breast cancer. Br J Surg 73:580, 1986.
30. Martimbeau PW, Kjorstad KE, Kolstad P: Stage IB carcinoma of the cervix, the Norwegian Radium Hospital, 1968–1970: Results of treatment and major complications. I. Lymphedema. Am J Obstet Gynecol 133:389, 1978.
31. Papachristou D, Fortner JG: Comparison of lymphedema following incontinuity and discontinuity groin dissection. Ann Surg 185:13, 1977.
32. De Roo T: Analysis of lymphoedema as first symptom of a neoplasm in a series of 650 patients with limb involvement. Radiol Clin (Basel) 45:236, 1976.
33. Smith RD, Spittell JA Jr, Schirger A: Secondary lymphedema of the leg: Its characteristics and diagnostic implications. JAMA 185:80, 1963.
34. Földi M: Classification of lymphedema and elephantiasis. 12th International WHO/TDR/FIL Conference on Lymphatic Pathology and Immunopathology in Filariasis, Thanjavur, India, November 18–22, 1985. Lymphology 18:159, 1985.
35. Chernin E: The disappearance of bancroftian filariasis from Charleston, South Carolina. Am J Trop Med Hyg 37:111, 1987.
36. Case T, Leis B, Witte M, et al: Vascular abnormalities in experimental and human lymphatic filariasis. Lymphology 24:174, 1991.
37. Dandapat MC, Mohapatro SK, Dash DM: Management of chronic manifestations of filariasis. J Indian Med Assoc 84:210, 1986.
38. Schirger A: Lymphedema. In Spittell JA Jr (ed): Cardiovascular Clinics. Philadelphia, FA Davis, 1983, pp 293–305.
39. Chant ADB: Hypothesis: Why venous oedema causes ulcers and lymphoedema does not. Eur J Vasc Surg 6:427, 1992.
40. Samman PD, White WF: The "yellow nail" syndrome. Br J Dermatol 76:153, 1964.
41. Taylor JS, Young JR: The swollen limb: Cutaneous clues to diagnosis and treatment. Cutis 21:553, 1978.
42. Fields CL, Roy TM, Ossorio MA, Mercer PJ: Yellow nail syndrome: A perspective. J Ky Med Assoc 89:563, 1991.
43. Stewart FW, Treves N: Lymphangiosarcoma in postmastectomy lymphedema: A report of six cases in elephantiasis chirurgica. Cancer 1:64, 1948.
44. Alessi E, Sala F, Berti E: Angiosarcomas in lymphedematous limbs. Am J Dermatopathol 8:371, 1986.
45. Muller R, Hajdu SI, Brennan MF: Lymphangiosarcoma associated with chronic filarial lymphedema. Cancer 59:179, 1987.
46. Sherman AI, Ter-Pergossian M: Lymph node concentration of radioactive colloidal gold following interstitial injection. Cancer 6:1238, 1953.
47. Taylor GW, Kinmonth JB, Rollinson E, et al: Lymphatic circulation studied with radioactive plasma protein. Br Med J 1:133, 1957.
48. Ege GN: Internal mammary lymphoscintigraphy—the rationale, technique, interpretation, and clinical application. Radiology 118:101, 1976.
49. Jackson FI, Bowen P, Lentle BC: Scintilymphangiography with 99mTc-antimony sulfide colloid in hereditary lymphedema (Nonne-Milroy disease). Clin Nucl Med 3:296, 1978.
50. Sty JR, Starshak RJ: Atlas of pediatric radionuclide lymphography. Clin Nucl Med 7:428, 1982.
51. Stewart G, Gaunt JI, Croft DN, Browse NL: Isotope lymphography: A new method of investigating the role of the lymphatics in chronic limb oedema. Br J Surg 72:906, 1985.
52. Nawaz K, Hamad MM, Sadek S, et al: Dynamic lymph flow imaging in lymphedema: Normal and abnormal patterns. Clin Nucl Med 11:653, 1986.
53. Ohtake E, Matsui K: Lymphoscintigraphy in patients with lymphedema: A new approach using intradermal injections of technetium-99m human serum albumin. Clin Nucl Med 11:474, 1986.
54. Vaqueiro M, Gloviczki P, Fisher J, et al: Lymphoscintigraphy in lymphedema: An aid to microsurgery. J Nucl Med 27:1125, 1986.
55. Weissleder H, Weissleder R: Lymphedema: Evaluation of qualitative and quantitative lymphoscintigraphy in 238 patients. Radiology 167:729, 1988.
56. Collins PS, Villavicencio JL, Abreu SH, et al: Abnormalities of lym-

phatic drainage in lower extremities: A lymphoscintigraphic study. J Vasc Surg 9:145, 1989.

57. Gloviczki P, Calcagno D, Schirger A, et al: Noninvasive evaluation of the swollen extremity: Experiences with 190 lymphoscintigraphic examinations. J Vasc Surg 9:683, 1989.

58. Cambria RA, Gloviczki P, Naessens JM, Wahner HW: Noninvasive evaluation of the lymphatic system with lymphoscintigraphy: A prospective, semiquantitative analysis in 386 extremities. J Vasc Surg 18:773, 1993.

59. McNeill GC, Witte MH, Witte CL, et al: Whole-body lymphangioscintigraphy: Preferred method for initial assessment of the peripheral lymphatic system. Radiology 172:495, 1989.

60. Kleinhans E, Baumeister RGH, Hahn D, et al: Evaluation of transport kinetics in lymphoscintigraphy: Follow-up study in patients with transplanted lymphatic vessels. Eur J Nucl Med 10:349, 1985.

61. Gamba JL, Silverman PM, Ling D, et al: Primary lower extremity lymphedema: CT diagnosis. Radiology 149:218, 1983.

62. Hadjus NS, Carr DH, Banks L, Pflug JJ: The role of CT in the diagnosis of primary lymphedema of the lower limb. Am J Roentgenol 144:361, 1985.

63. Göltner E, Gass P, Haas JP, Schneider P: The importance of volumetry, lymphoscintigraphy and computer tomography in the diagnosis of brachial edema after mastectomy. Lymphology 21:134, 1988.

64. Duewell S, Hagspiel KD, Zuber J, et al: Swollen lower extremity: Role of MR imaging. Radiology 184:227, 1992.

65. Weissleder R, Thrall JH: The lymphatic system: Diagnostic imaging studies. Radiology 172:315, 1989.

66. Case TC, Witte CL, Witte MH, et al: Magnetic resonance imaging in human lymphedema: Comparison with lymphangioscintigraphy. J Magn Reson Imag 10:549, 1992.

67. Weissleder R, Elizondo G, Wittenburg J, et al: Ultrasmall superparamagnetic iron oxide: An intravenous contrast agent for assessing lymph nodes with MR imaging. Radiology 175:494, 1990.

68. Kanter MA: The lymphatic system: An historical perspective. Plast Reconstr Surg 79:131, 1987.

69. Servelle M: La lymphographie moyen d'étude de la physiopathologie des grosses jambes. Rev Chir 82:251, 1944.

70. Kinmonth JB: Lymphangiography in man: A method of outlining lymphatic trunks at operation. Clin Sci 11:13, 1952.

71. Wolfe JHN: Diagnosis and classification of lymphedema. In Rutherford RB (ed): Vascular Surgery, 3rd ed. Philadelphia, WB Saunders, 1989, pp 1656–1667.

72. Fyfe NCM, Wolfe JHN, Kinmonth JB: "Die-back" in primary lymphedema—lymphographic and clinical correlations. Lymphology 15:66, 1982.

73. O'Brien BMcC, Mellow CG, Khazanchi RK, et al: Long-term results after microlymphatico-venous anastomoses for the treatment of obstructive lymphedema. Plast Reconstr Surg 85:562, 1990.

74. Partsch H, Urbanek A, Wenzel-Hora B: The dermal lymphatics in lymphoedema visualized by indirect lymphography. Br J Dermatol 110:431, 1984.

75. Gloviczki P: Invited commentary. In Gan JL, Chang TS, Fu DK, et al: Indirect lymphography with Isovist-300 in various forms of lymphedema. Eur J Plast Surg 14:109, 1991.

76. Gloviczki P, Stanson AW, Stickler GB, et al: Klippel-Trenaunay syndrome: The risks and benefits of vascular interventions. Surgery 110:469, 1991.

77. Gloviczki P, Hollier LH: Arteriovenous fistulas. In Haimovici H (ed): Vascular Surgery: Principles and Techniques, 3rd ed. Norwalk, CT, Appleton & Lange, 1989, pp 698–716.

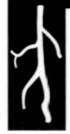

CHAPTER 1 5 7

Nonoperative Management of Chronic Lymphedema

Gail L. Gamble, M. D., Thom W. Rooke, M. D., and Peter Gloviczki, M. D.

Persons who suffer from chronic lymphedema seek dramatic and prompt resolution of their disabling symptoms. Although, at present, cure is not possible, most patients benefit from some mode of long-term nonoperative management. Patient expectations, prevention measures, treatment options, and available resources are all key components in the development of successful strategies for managing lymphedema. Overall, conservative care of lymphedema can focus on three major areas: (1) public health and education measures to prevent or limit progression of edema; (2) pharmacologic therapy to treat infection, which is frequently a cause (but also a sequela) of lymphedema, and (3) physical therapeutic measures to mechanically reduce edema and maintain reduction. Because the psychosocial impact of lymphedema is also significant, as it affects the patient's self-image and perceived quality of life,[1, 2] these areas should considered by the physician and addressed in a comprehensive conservative management program.

PREVENTIVE MEASURES

It is generally easier to prevent lymphedema than to treat it. Although by definition, *primary* lymphedema occurs in the absence of any known precipitating factors, many possible causes of *secondary* lymphedema can be avoided or minimized by taking appropriate measures.

Filarial Disease

Worldwide, the most common cause of lymphedema is infection, and this type of lymphedema is prevalent in

TABLE 157–1. PROPHYLACTIC SKIN MANAGEMENT

Skin hygiene
    Daily washing
    Moisturizer (not alcohol-based)
    Air drying
Clothing
    Cotton against skin, avoid synthetics
    Loose fit
Avoidance of trauma
    Protective clothing for work outdoors
    Avoid cuts, scrapes, puncture wounds
    Avoid sunburn
Control fungal infections
    Topical antifungal agents
    Oral medication if necessary

regions where climate enhances its development and public health efforts are compromised. In regions where filarial disease is prevalent, the likelihood of infection can be reduced by taking simple precautions aimed at avoiding transmission of the parasites (*Wuchereria bancrofti, Brugia malayi*) by mosquito bites. Public health measures are control of mosquito breeding,[3, 4] use of protective clothing and mosquito netting, and, in some cases, prophylactic antifilarial medications. Prompt therapy with diethylcarbamazine (DEC) or ivermectin should be instituted when filarial infections are discovered.[5–8] Population-wide treatments using combination therapy of ivermectin and DEC or albendazole (a newer broad-spectrum antihelminth drug) have been advocated.[9–11]

Malignancy

In industrialized nations, lymphedema is most often identified after surgical or radiation therapy for breast, pelvic, or prostate cancer. The incidence and severity of lymphedema may be minimized if the extent of axillary or inguinal lymph node dissections was limited,[12–14] although the invasiveness of the operation depends on the size, type, and location of the lesion. Sentinel node biopsy, rather than extensive lymph node dissection, will decrease the risk for lymphedema secondary to certain tumor resections.[15–18] Early patient education after surgical excision or tumor irradiation is important, since skin precautions, limb elevation, and appropriate exercise reduce the incidence of lymphedema.

TABLE 157–2. PROPHYLACTIC ANTIBIOTIC REGIMEN

NO. OF EPISODES OF CELLULITIS	PROPHYLAXIS
Cellulitis × 1	Oral Penicillin-VK, 250–500 q.i.d. × 7–10 days, or an equivalent
Cellulitis × 1	Keep antibiotic prescription at home; take immediately at onset of symptoms
Cellulitis >4×/yr	Prophylaxis with antibiotics 1 week/month (combined with rigorous edema control)
Refractory cellulitis	Daily oral antibiotics using PEN VK; then use cephalosporin, rotating monthly to avoid development of resistance

Infection

Recurrent clinical or subclinical infections contribute to lymph vessel destruction and to the development of lymphedema. In addition, a lymphedematous limb is extremely susceptible to bacterial invasion, which would further compromise the already impaired lymphatic system. Practical precautions are necessary to prevent infection in extremeties involved by lymphedema (Table 157–1).

Attention to daily skin hygiene of the limbs is imperative, yet it is often difficult for patients because of inadequate bathing facilities or morbid obesity, and they may need assistance. The limbs should be washed regularly with soap and water, and, while still moist, lubricated with an alcohol-free emollient cream that traps moisture, minimizing the risk of skin fissures. Patients with a history of trichophytosis should use topical antifungal medication routinely. Clotrimazole cream (1%) or miconazole nitrate lotion or cream (2%) is sufficient for most patients, although long-term systemic griseofulvin treatment (250 to 1000 mg daily) may be required in refractory cases.

Prompt administration of appropriate antibiotic therapy in patients with lymphangitis is essential.[19] The pathogen is usually a penicillin-sensitive group A streptococcus. *Staphylococcus* species and other organisms are less common ones. At the first sign of cellulitis, treatment should be started with oral penicillin VK, 250 or 500 mg four times daily (Table 157–2). High-dose intravenous penicillin infusion, hospitalization, and bed rest with leg elevation may be needed for some patients with fulminant lymphangitis (erysipelas). Erythromycin or a first-generation cephalosporin is a reasonable alternative for those who cannot take penicillin. Antibiotic therapy should be continued for 7 to 10 days or until all signs and symptoms of infection have clearly resolved. There is no consensus on optimal treatment of recurrent cellulitis in lymphedema (see Table 157–2). When spontaneous episodes occur more often than four to six times a year, a regular prophylactic program—penicillin VK (or an equivalent), 250 mg four times daily for 7 days of each month—should be considered. An alternative regimen is penicillin G benzathine 1.2 million IU units given intramuscularly once a month. For some patients, even this program may not be sufficient to prevent recurrent infections, and they may need daily antibiotic prophylaxis. If they can tolerate it, two, or even three,

TABLE 157–3. EDEMA PREVENTIVE MEASURES

Limb elevation
    Above heart
    Periodic daily elevation
    Elevated bed positioning (pillows or wedge to elevate leg)
Exercise
    Daily exercise to increase lymph flow in limb
    Avoid rough, repetitive, resistive exercise
Dietary
    Well-balanced meals, *including protein*
    Low sodium
    Minimal or no alcohol intake
    Weight management
Pressure avoidance
    Blood pressure cuff not to be applied to affected limb
    No tight jewelry or clothing
    No purse, backpack, other source of shoulder pressure

different antibiotics can be given in monthly rotations. Recently, sodium selenite, in combination with physical therapy, was found to significantly decrease recurrences of cellulitis and to minimize the need for maintenance antibiotic therapy.[20] This treatment requires further study.

Other Measures

Prolonged elevation of an involved limb can help to reduce edema, especially in the early stages of the disease (Table 157–3). Exercise, particularly walking and isometric exercise, promote lymph flow.[21, 22] Dietary restrictions have been advocated, and one recent study suggested that lowering triglyceride values has some effect.[23] Morbid obesity compounds lymphedema, and weight reduction enhances effects of other measures for edema reduction. When offering "do's and don'ts," medical myths must be separated from sound medical advice, especially in such "unregulated" areas as nutritional supplements. These issues require rigorous investigational study.

A well-informed patient has the best chance of avoiding complications. Patient education materials are available through patient advocacy groups such as the National Lymphedema Network in the USA, and much is also available on the Internet. Very few often recommended prophylactic measures, however, are grounded in research. Some observations (e.g., the beneficial effect of lowered airplane cabin pressure) deserve further investigation.[24]

PHARMACOLOGIC THERAPY

Pharmacologic agents to enhance lymph transport have had a limited role in the treatment of lymphedema.

Diuretics

Diuretics are included in the treatment programs of some authors[25] but not others.[26] Regular treatment with diuretics is not appropriate for patients with chronic lymphedema. Their effect is temporary, and secondary hemoconcentration is a serious possible side effect.[27] In some circumstances, however, short-term diuretic therapy may be helpful. In patients hospitalized for edema reduction (and treated with strict bed rest, elevation of the extremity, and physical therapy), the response to acute treatment can be maximized by administering 40 to 80 mg of furosemide daily. For women whose periodic exacerbations of edema correspond to the menstrual cycle, short-term use of diuretics may be helpful. Finally, patients in the terminal phase of a malignant disease who have painful swelling of the extremity, may need diuretics to alleviate symptoms.

Benzopyrones

Benzopyrones are thought to decrease lymphedema by stimulating tissue macrophages and thus altering the (macrophage-dependent) balance between protein deposition and lysis.[28–30] As a result of increased macrophage activity, the intercellular protein concentration is reduced, which promotes tissue softening and remodeling. In a random-

ized, double-blind study, 31 patients with postmastectomy lymphedema of the arm and 21 patients with leg lymphedema received 400 mg 5, 6-benzo-(alpha)-pyrone or placebo for 6 months.[30] Limb measurements showed that the drug reduced the volume the arms from 46% to 26% above normal ($p < .001$) and the volume of the legs from 25% to 17% above normal ($p < .001$). The limb tissue softened, skin temperatures dropped, and the episodes of infection diminished. The authors concluded that 5,6-benzo-(alpha)-pyrone produced slow but safe reduction of lymphedema.

In a more recent study, 140 women were followed after breast cancer treatment in a prospective randomized crossover study comparing the effects of a benzopyrone, coumarin, with placebo.[31] The patients received coumarin, 400 mg daily, or placebo for 6 months and then the opposite treatment for 6 months. Measurements included calculated arm volumes (from serial circumference measures) and monthly patient self-report questionnaires. At the end of the study, upper extremity volumes and patient reports showed no difference. The average arm volumes increased 40 ml after placebo and 50 ml after coumarin. There were also reports of increases in liver enzymes in 6% of patients. Because of potential hepatotoxicity, coumarin has been withdrawn from the market in several countries, and it has not been approved for use in the United States.

Another benzopyrone, without known hepatotoxicity, has received increased attention. A purified, micronized, flavonoid fraction (PMFF), has been shown to increase lymphatic transport.[32] A randomized double-blind study was undertaken 48 patients with post-mastectomy upper extremity edema received placebo, and 46 others received the compound. Although several measurement parameters failed to show statistically significant differences, a subgroup of 24 patients with more severe lymphedema showed a statistically significant reduction in limb circumference.[32] Further studies will be necessary to determine if this agent will, indeed, play a major role in lymphedema management.

In another effort to control edema, intralymphatic steroid injections have been used to decrease fibrotic occlusion in lymph nodes and improve lymphatic transport. In a pilot study of 20 patients with primary lymphedema, eight showed improvement as long as 9 months after treatment.[33] The effectiveness of steroid treatment, however, remains unproved. Investigators in Japan have attempted to treat secondary lymphedema by injecting autologous lymphocytes into the main artery of the affected limb.[34] Although five of seven patients showed short-term improvement, further evidence in support of this treatment is lacking. The beneficial effect of oral amitriptyline, reported to reduce postmastectomy lymphedema,[35] also awaits further confirmation.

MECHANICAL REDUCTION OR LIMB SWELLING

Reducing the size of the limb is the primary goal of therapy for lymphedema. Early in the course of the disease, when the tissues are still soft and pitting, it may be possible to restore the limb to its original size and volume. After fibrosis has developed in the subcutaneous regions, the brawny tissues typically do not normalize completely after treatment, and some residual subcutaneous thickening and swelling may have to be accepted. A comprehensive therapy approach should include a standardized measure of changes in limb size to gauge response to treatment. Changes in limb size can be followed subjectively or by objective measures, including (1) circumferential measurements obtained at prescribed levels and (2) volumetric assessments using water-displacement or other techniques. Newer methods using computed tomography[36] and bioelectrical impedance analysis[37] techniques have been reported; however, these techniques are not yet ready for routine clinical use.

Reduction of edema can be accomplished by a variety of techniques, discussed next, which may be employed individually or in combinations, to best fit a given patient's needs.

Elevation

Elevation is a simple and effective way of reducing lymphedema.[38] The patient is positioned comfortably, and the limb is elevated as tolerated, usually 45 degrees or more. A variety of arm boards and lymphedema slings[25] (Fig. 157–1) have been developed for this purpose. With continuous bed rest, gravity usually produces maximal reduction within 2 to 5 days. This method of acute treatment of lymphedema has been used in the authors' institution for decades, with excellent results, and it is still used for refractory cases with severe cellulitis (Fig. 157–2).

If hospitalization is utilized for strict elevation, an appropriate compression garment must be provided for maintenance before the patient is discharged; otherwise, any reduction will be lost. Today, inpatient treatment is less often an option, and patients often find elevation therapy outside the hospital impractical and ineffective. The authors' outpatient limb reduction program still incorporates overnight

and regular daily periods of limb elevation. O'Donnell and Howrigan[39] have suggested that 4- to 6-inch blocks be placed under the legs of the bed to provide adequate overnight elevation for patients with lower extremity edema. In our institution, we often use the wedge for limb elevation (Fig. 157–3).

Complex Physical Therapy

A comprehensive program of elevation, therapeutic exercise, manual massage techniques, and compression wrapping has been advocated for decades.[21] In more recent years, a combined approach based on the complex program popularized in Europe by Földi and coworkers[26] and advocated by the Casley-Smiths in Australia[40] has been used more. The success of these treatments has been documented in the literature worldwide, including in the United States.[41–46] The program involves four discrete components with two phases (Table 157–4) and is a resource-intensive treatment that requires large investments of therapist's and patient's time.

Massage

Therapists must be specially trained to perform standardized techniques of manual lymph drainage massage and complex multilayered wrapping, and few recognized training programs are available. Thus, this treatment, although successful, currently is offered only in more specialized treatment centers.

The massage is light and superficial (in contrast to deeper decongestive massage). An attempt is made to move the fluid via superficial lymphatics from a drainage basin that is obstructed to an area that has an open drainage system. It is also believed that the massage techniques loosen subcutaneous fibrosis. Manual lymph drainage is performed in steps. The trunk is divided into quadrants, and treatment

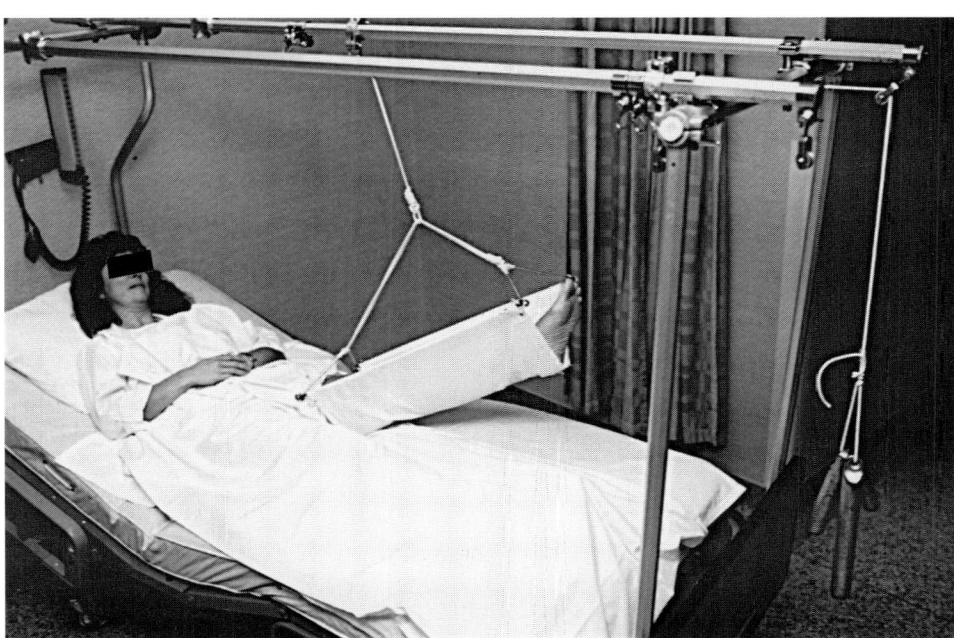

FIGURE 157–1. The lymphedema sling is used to elevate the patient's leg during bed rest, typically 45 degrees or more.

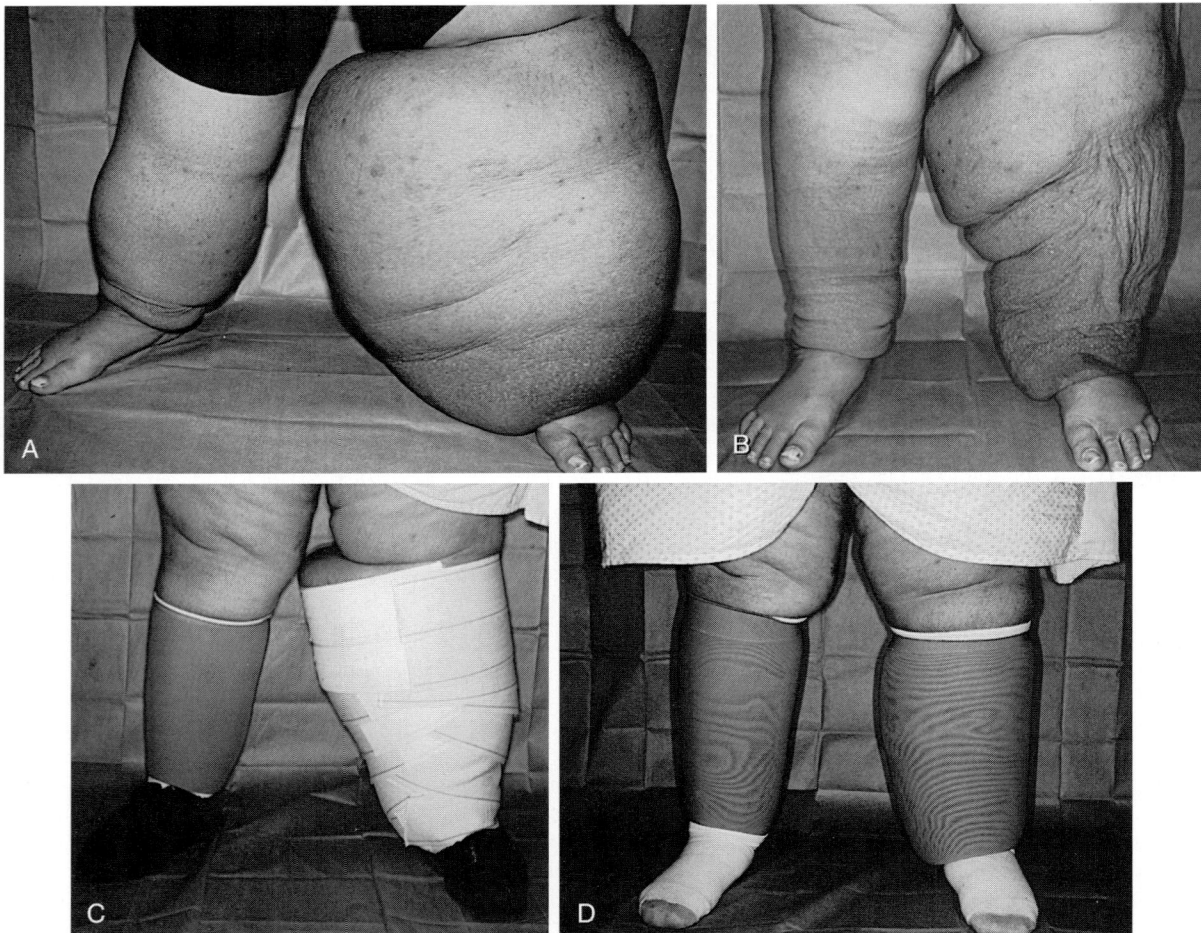

FIGURE 157–2. Severe primary lymphedema of the lower extremities in a 36-year-old man. *A,* Limbs on presentation. *B,* The legs after 2 weeks of continuous leg elevation, elastic wrapping, and pneumatic compression treatment. Much of the residual deformity distal to the knee is fatty deposition. *C,* The legs after application of bilateral custom-made elastic stockings and a nonelastic wrapping to reinforce the stocking on the left. *D,* The legs 1 month after initiation of therapy.

is initiated by massaging the quadrant *contralateral* to the affected limb.

In theory, the massage stimulates lymph flow and helps to drain cutaneous lymph from the "normal" skin, preparing it to receive lymph fluid from the adjacent, involved area. Massage is performed next over the trunk adjacent to the affected limb. Fluid is pushed out. Some of it drains directly into the veins or deep lymphatics, and some of it crosses through the superficial anastomotic lymph vessels into the freshly drained contralateral quadrant. The operator repeats the process in stages along the length of the limb, moving slowly from proximal-to distal but massaging each small segment in a distal-to-proximal direction (Figs. 157–4 and 157–5).

Wrapping

The wrapping techniques are quite complex and use low-stretch wrap instead of the more traditional high-stretch elastic bandages (Fig. 157–6). The high-stretch wraps provide high pressures when the limb is resting but yield when the limb moves, and they do not assist the muscle pump action as vigorously as the low-stretch wrap, which is

comfortable at rest but with movement provides unyielding resistance to augment the muscle pump action. Frequently, foam padding is used to enhance the pressure provided with the low-stretch wrap techniques (Fig. 157–7). During the active, intensive treatment time, the low-stretch wraps are worn 24 hours a day except when the patient is receiving massage. In the maintenance phase, a compression garment (discussed later) is worn during the day and the patient is instructed to do simple self-massage techniques but to use the wrap at night.

TABLE 157–4. DECONGESTIVE LYMPHATIC THERAPY

Intensive therapy (phase I)
    Manual lymph drainage massage
    Multilayered low-stretch wrapping
    Exercise techniques
    Skin care and elevation principles
Maintenance therapy (phase II)
    Daily wear of pressure garment
    Nightly wrapping
    Self-massage
    Exercise and skin care

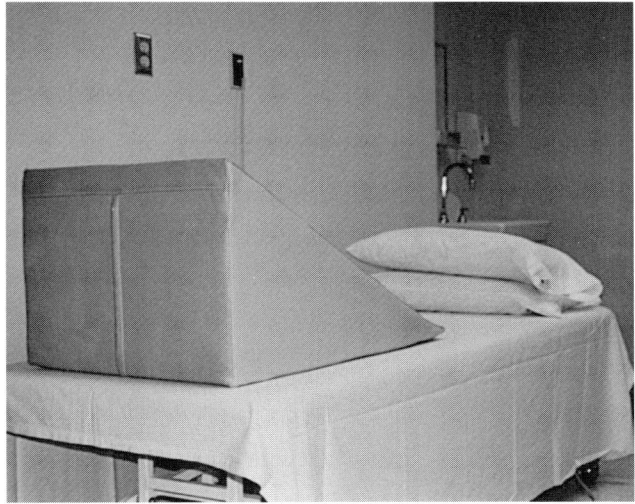

FIGURE 157–3. (Lymph wedge). The wedge can be used at several angles and provides a portable, firm support for elevation.

In our program, we use low-stretch wrapping techniques and manual massage, with pumps (occasionally) or alone, depending on the patient's condition, often with good results. Prospective studies should be conducted to assess the relative efficacy of each component of massage and wrapping, as the multiweek treatment regimen of decongestive therapy hardly fits Americans' lifestyles and finances.

Exercise

Appropriate exercise regimens are an integral part of this lymphedema management program in both the intensive and maintance phases and should be individualized to the patient to maximize gravity assist and muscle pump action in achieving reduction. Meticulous skin care and patient education are also part of the program. We have in our

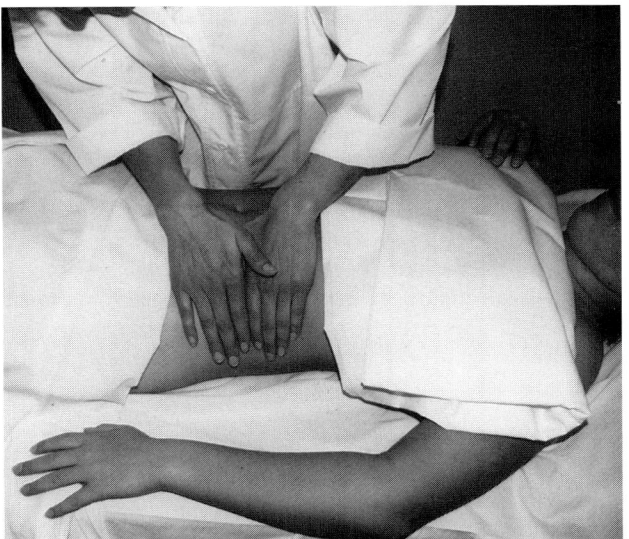

FIGURE 157–4. Manual lymph drainage massage of the trunk involves light movements first in truncal areas to stimulate and open proximal lymph channels.

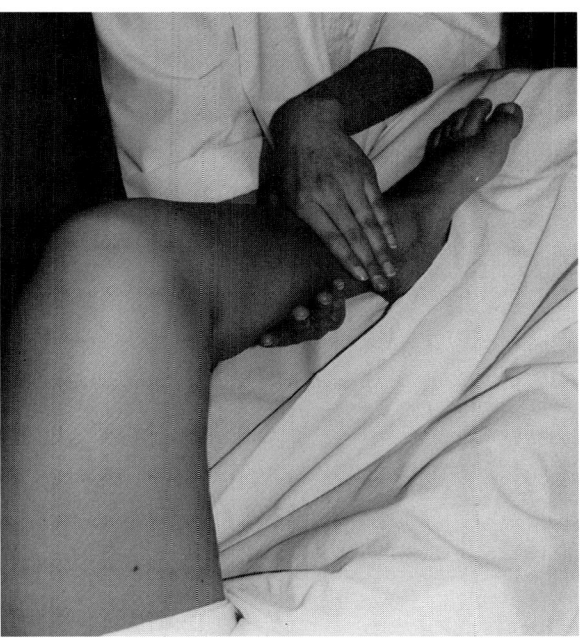

FIGURE 157–5. Manual lymph drainage of the limb is performed with distal to proximal hand movements over short segments, which are treated sequentially, beginning with proximal portion of the limb.

institution experienced remarkable success with it, not only with moderately effected limbs but specifically with advanced, refractory lymphedema. Although it is hoped that this regimen will eventually become the standard of care for all treatment centers,[46] this more complex approach is not appropriate for each patient. There can be extenuating factors, such as co-morbidity, focal tumor recurrence, impaired cognitive status, and poor social supports, obstacles that would preclude the use of the program, which requires long-term patient self-management at home.

Compression Pumping

An alternative, and more traditional, method for achieving limb reduction uses intermittent pneumatic compression. Pneumatic pumping has for decades been the traditional physical therapeutic intervention in the United States. The affected limb is placed in a pneumatic cuff, or sleeve, which is alternately inflated and deflated, the pressure gradient thus created forces lymph fluid out of the affected limb and back into the trunk. These devices are quite diverse and may utilize either a single uniform-pressure sleeve or a sleeve built with a series of overlapping chambers within that can be inflated sequentially.[47–56] The direction of sequential inflation has always been distal to proximal. A theoretical disadvantage of the single-chamber device is that high pressure is exerted both proximally and distally that can potentially force fluid farther distal in the extremity. Because of the longer duration of the pressure cycle, it may also be uncomfortable for the patient.

In a controlled study, Richmand and associates[49] failed to achieve an acute response in 30% of patients treated with a single-chamber pump. These authors also found that the proximal portion of the limb responded poorly to the unicell device. The data of Zanolla and colleagues,[50]

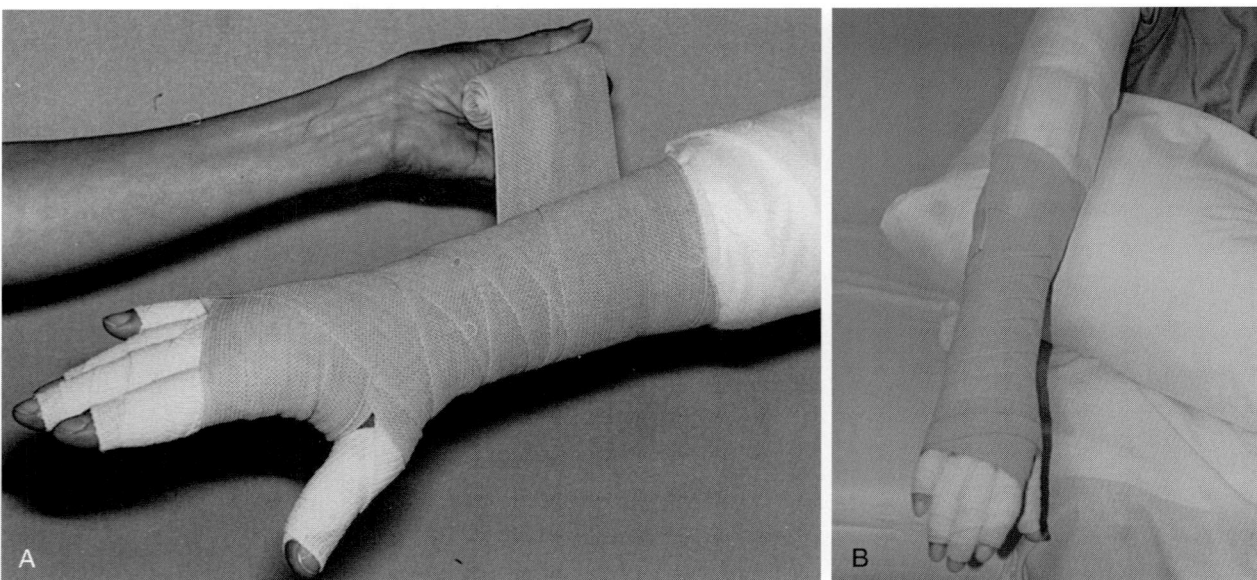

FIGURE 157–6. *A* and *B,* The multilayered wrap technique allows maximal pressures without causing the patient discomfort.

however, support the effectiveness of the single-chamber device in the treatment of postmastectomy lymphedema. In their study, the acute treatment period of 1 week included 6-hour treatments daily, using a 90-mmHg cuff pressure with a ratio of 1:3 for compression and decompression. A 21% reduction in limb circumference was achieved in 20 patients and was maintained at 3 months.

With the sequential pneumatic compression device developed by Zelikovski and colleagues,[48, 51] the chambers are inflated in a distal-to-proximal direction, producing a dynamic pressure gradient and "milking" the limb (Fig. 157–8). Pressures of 100 mmHg or more are typically tolerated with these devices owing to the short duration of each inflation cycle (typically 20 seconds to 1 to 2 minutes). Treatment sessions may last from 1 hour to as

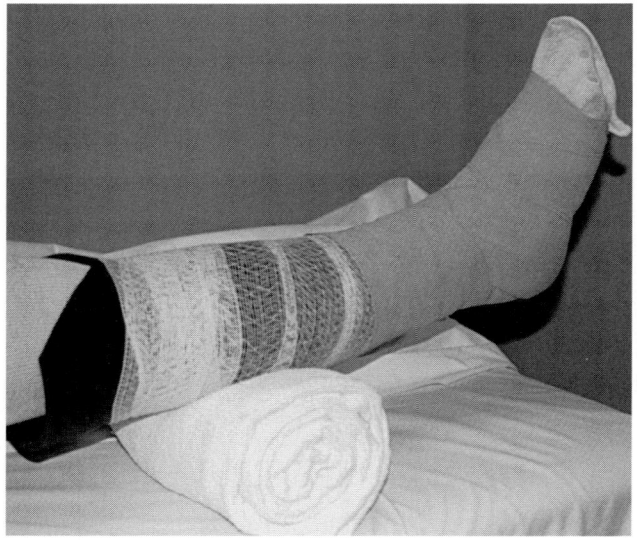

FIGURE 157–7. Complex wrapping of the leg with foam. The use of foam pads allows for extra pressure to help contour focal, hardened areas.

long as 8 to 10 hours, depending on the magnitude and refractoriness of the edema. In recent years, many therapy programs have achieved successful reduction with much lower pressures, and in our program the standard pressure is approximately 50 mmHg.

In another prospective nonrandomized clinical study, Pappas and O'Donnell[52] confirmed the long-term effectiveness of compression for lymphedema. Their protocol included 2 to 3 days hospitalization and daily 6- to 8-hour treatment sessions with sequential high-pressure intermittent pneumatic compression using the Lymphapress device (Camp International, Jackson, Mich.). The reduction was maintained by custom-made two-way stretch elastic compression stockings. Some patients continue to use the Lymphapress at home. Limb girth measurements for 49 patients were obtained at nine levels serially during a follow-up period that averaged 25 months. This protocol resulted in long-term maintenance of limb girth reduction in 90%, and the improvement remained excellent at late follow-up in 26 of 49 patients: absolute reductions in calf and ankle girths of were 5.37 ± 1.01 cm and 4.63 ± 0.88 cm, respectively, as compared with pretreatment dimensions. The most important factor affecting outcome was the degree of subcutaneous fibrosis. More than 80% of patients whose response to the treatment was poor had had lymphedema for more than 10 years. These data also confirm that conservative pneumatic compression treatment should be started early, before a chronic inflammatory reaction develops and fibrosis in the subcutaneous tissues is irreversible.

Other multicellular intermittent pneumatic compression devices include the three-celled Hemoflow II unit (Camp International) and the three-celled Wright linear pump (Wright-Linear Pump, Imperial, Pa.). Klein and coworkers[53] used the Wright linear pump in 78 extremities of 73 patients with lymphedema. Acute treatment included 48 hours of hospitalization with bed rest and leg elevation and pump treatment sessions lasting up to 8 hours. After ther-

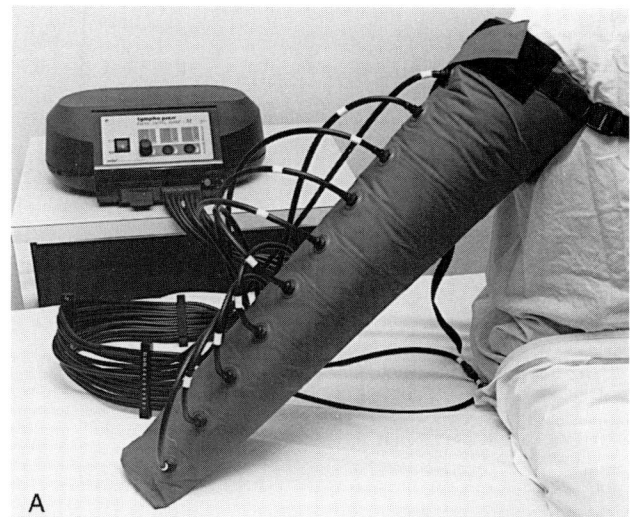

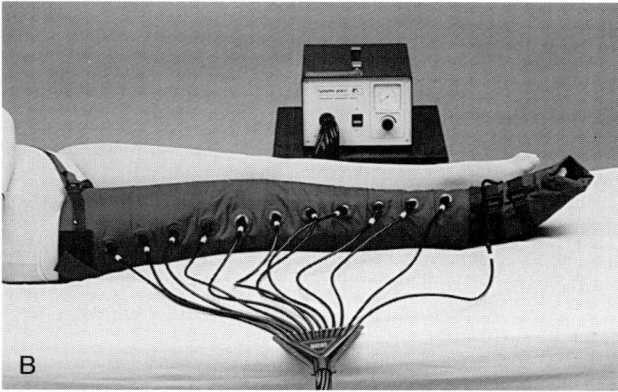

FIGURE 157–8. Sequential pneumatic pump used for intermittent compression treatment of upper (A) or lower (B) extremity lymphedema. (A and B, Courtesy of Camp International, Inc., Jackson, Mich.)

apy, 90% of the patients showed reductions in limb circumference at the ankle or the mid-calf ranging from 1.6 to 2.1 cm. The results of long-term maintenance of the reduced volume in this study were not reported. In comparing the three different multichamber devices in a small group of pediatric patients with congenital lymphedema, McLeod and colleagues[54] found that the Lymphapress was superior to the Hemoflow II and the Wright linear pump.

In a recent study, Bergan[55] randomized 35 patients with lymphedema to a 2-hour long treatment session with one of three types of compression pumps: (1) a unicompartmental pump using 50 mmHg pressure, (2) a three-compartment pump with segmental pressures of 50 mmHg in each cell, or (3) a multicompartmental gradient pressure pump with 10 cells ranging in pressures from 80 mmHg distally to 30 mmHg proximally. Mean percentage volume change was +0.4% in the first group, +7.3% in the second, and −31.6% in the third. The authors concluded that multicompartment sequential compression achieves the best reduction of limb volume after a single treatment for chronic lymphedema.

Although pneumatic compression therapy is helpful in the management of lymphedema, there is other evidence of limited utility.[56] Which type of compression may be best

is still in question, as is which pressures are most useful.[57] Controversy persists about whether pneumatic compression or complex physiotherapy involving compression bandaging and manual lymph drainage massage is the better first-line treatment. These issues clearly need to be studied in an organized fashion.

Most recently, a randomized study compared manual lymph drainage (Vodder) massage techniques with a sequential pneumatic compression pump (40 to 60 mmHg). Patients were followed for a relatively short time, 2 weeks. At the end of treatment time, both methods had decreased arm volume and the difference was not statistically significant.[58] Ultimately, the appropriate treatment regimen, whether manual lymph drainage therapy or intermittent pneumatic compression, needs to fit the needs of the patient to maximize compliance. If the patient is motivated and compliant, any treatment has a better chance of success.

Heat

Heat therapy as a means of reducing lymphedema has been practiced in the Orient, and elsewhere, for centuries. Heating the limb presumably mobilizes fluid and softens the tissues; tight wrappings are applied between treatments to reduce and maintain the limb's size. In a study from China of 1045 patients with lymphedema, 68% achieved an effective reduction in the volume of the extremity with heat therapy and reported subsequent decreases in the frequency of lymphangitis episodes.[59] Traditional methods have used ovens heated to 80° to 90°C, but newer methods involving microwave heating have been reported to be successful in descriptive studies.[60–62] No controlled comparative study is available, however, to prove the effectiveness of this treatment.

Recently, a study of low-level laser therapy with 2-year follow-up reported effective control of "post–radical mastectomy edema" in seven of 10 patients.[63] Theoretically, heat should increase lymph production, and the mechanism whereby volume is reduced remains obscure. More investigations are clearly needed.

MAINTENANCE OF LIMB SIZE

The pressure garment is the eventual maintenance component of nearly any lymphedema management program. Although intermittent outpatient therapy with manual lymphatic drainage, pneumatic compression, elevation, or another method can help to reduce the size of the swollen limb, external support—elastic or nonelastic—is necessary to maintain the reduction.

Graduated Elastic Support

Strict daily use of properly fitting, appropriately graduated, elastic compression garments remains the key to maintaining limb size for most patients.[64] Support garments come in a variety of sizes, compression strengths, and materials, and the combination of these features must be tailored to the needs and dimensions of the individual.[65]

Although many swollen limbs can be fitted with over-the-counter prefabricated garments, those with significant swelling or an unusual shape may need custom-made stockings to obtain the best fit. It is better to use a mechanical aid to don the stocking (rubber gloves, metal frame) than to sacrifice needed pressure.

Compression

Stockings are classified according to the amount of compression they deliver at the ankle, and the compression they produce may be "graduated" or "nongraduated." Graduated stockings are made to provide the greatest compression in the distal portion of the limb and progressively less pressure approaching the trunk. Over-the-counter "support stockings" usually provide 7 to 15 mmHg of compression and are not graduated. "Antiembolism stockings," such as TED hose, provide 15 to 20 mmHg of compression and tend to be graduated. "Therapeutic" elastic stockings designed for chronic venous insufficiency or lymphedema, come in a variety of compression strengths (20 to 30, 30 to 40, 40 to 50, and 50 to 60 mmHg) and lengths. Limbs with lymphedema generally require at least 40 to 50 mmHg of compression at the ankle to control the swelling; however, for hospitalized patients with arthritis, arterial occlusive disease, or another problem that may limit the use of high-compression stockings, stockings with pressures of 30 to 40 mmHg may be tried. Low-compression (<30 mmHg) or nongraduated stockings usually provide little, if any, control of even mild lymphedema.

Length

Stocking length is frequently an issue for patients with lymphedema (Fig. 157–9). As a rule, stockings should be long enough to cover the edematous portion of the limb, but patient preference and physical limitations must be taken into account. If a stocking that, from the physician's viewpoint, is less than optimal is more acceptable to the patient, that stocking is probably the better long-term choice, as compliance may well be enhanced. This is especially true for male patients, whose compliance tends to be better with below-knee stockings than with above-knee or full-length ones.

Materials and Brands

Stockings come in a variety of knits and materials; most are composed of some combination of latex, spandex, nylon, cotton, and silk.[36] Differences in construction, sizing, and materials can significantly affect the "feel" and function of various brands and styles for a given patient. Unfortunately, predicting which patient will do best with a particular stocking is almost impossible. For this reason, a patient may need to try a variety of brands and styles to find the one that works best for him. Like O'Donnell and Howrigan,[39] the authors prefer two-way stretch elastic stockings, although no controlled study has proved the superiority of any of the available stockings (e.g., Sigvaris, Jobst, Camp, Medi-Strumpf, Bell Horn, Juzo, Venosan). It should be noted that with repeated washing all brands exhibit fatigue

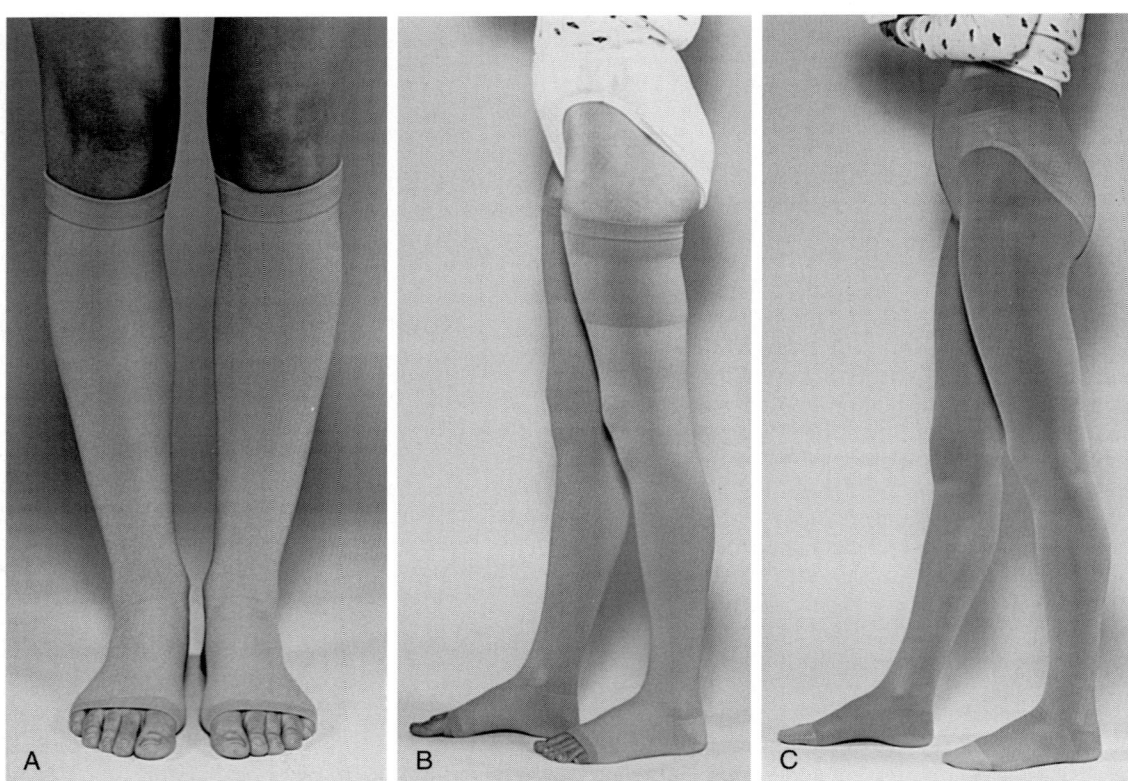

FIGURE 157–9. Different types of high-compression graduated elastic stockings for patients with lower extremity lymphedema: below-knee (A), thigh-high (B), and pantyhose lengths (C).

and that garments should be replaced several times each year.

Nonelastic Support

Although nonelastic support devices were once widely used to control limb swelling, they have been largely replaced by modern elastic stockings. Commercial devices employing the principle of nonelastic support have been reintroduced for the control of lymphedema and are being received with patient enthusiasm. The Circ Aid (Shaw Therapeutics, Rumson, N.J.) uses Velcro fastenings to readjust a series of nonelastic support bands around the leg and ankle. Whether this approach is superior, or comparable, to conventional elastic support hose remains to be determined. We had patients who were pleased with the Circ Aid device and achieved excellent reduction of the limb. As adjuncts to a compression garment, nonelastic supports have been worn over the garment, especially during periods of exercise or prolonged dependency.

Another form of nonelastic support, the Reid sleeve, which has multiple air cell chambers custom-inflated but then left static and applied to the limb (with wide Velcro bands), has been reported to help to control edema.[66] We find it helpful to patients who are unable by themselves to manage a program of complex wrapping (Fig. 157–10).

OTHER TREATMENT CONSIDERATIONS

Psychological and Functional Impairment, Economic Issues

The psychological and functional impairments of lymphedema should not be underestimated. Smeltzer and associates[1] examined the psychologic impact of lymphedema. Their findings suggest that related emotional problems are

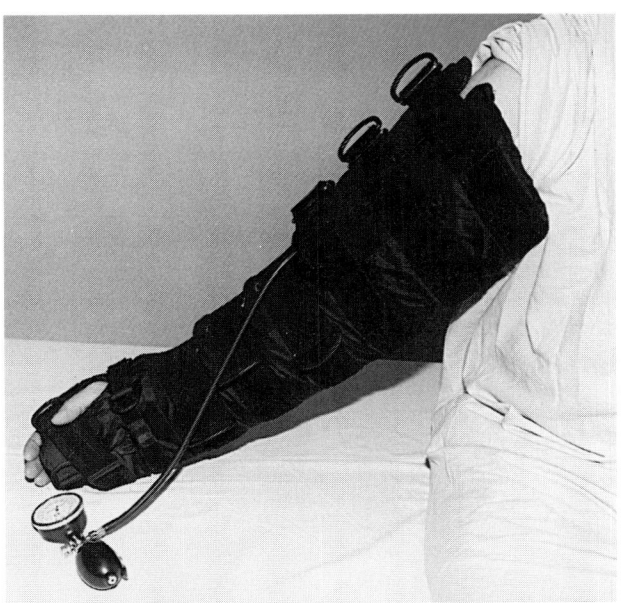

FIGURE 157–10. The Reid sleeve is easy to put on yet provides "custom" low-stretch resistance.

not uncommon and are often neglected by physicians. The need to address the psychological aspects of long-term disfigurement, especially in adolescents, cannot be overemphasized. Also discussed in this study is the functional impact of lymphedema on lifestyle. Twelve per cent of patients reported that because of the edema they were limited to desk jobs or ones that allowed frequent sitting. Employees' impressions that job promotion was withheld because of the edema have also been reported. Some patients limit their participation in exercise or sports because of an uncomfortable or heavy sensation in the affected limb.

Very frustrating for the patient is the fact that some insurance companies deem the edema to be only a cosmetic problem and deny payment for both treatment and garments. This misperception often necessitates repeated communications between insurance companies and physicians to justify well-deserved treatment for the patient.

Malignancy

Late-onset malignancies are potentially devastating, and fortunately rare, complications of long-standing lymphedema. In most series, they develop in no more than 1% of patients with lymphedema.[1, 67] The most common ones are angiosarcomas[58] and lymphangiosarcomas,[69, 70] which are thought to represent, respectively, neoplastic transformations of blood vessels and of lymphatics.

Histologically and clinically, it is difficult to distinguish these two sarcomas, and, for most purposes, they can be considered identical. The association between angiosarcoma (or lymphangiosarcoma) and lymphedema is commonly called the *Stewart-Treves syndrome*.[69] Sarcomas can develop in patients with long-standing lymphedema of any cause—primary lymphedema[71] or lymphedema secondary to filariasis,[72] hysterectomy,[73] trauma,[73] or mastectomy.[74] Other malignancies, including Hodgkin's and non-Hodgkin's lymphoma,[75] Kaposi's sarcoma,[76] squamous cell carcinoma,[77, 78] and malignant melanoma,[79] have been reported in association with chronic lymphedema. Limbs with edema must therefore be inspected frequently to permit early detection and appropriate treatment of tumors.

SUMMARY

Conservative, nonsurgical management continues to be the mainstay of treatment for lymphedema. Preventive measures include immediate medical treatment for bacterial infections affecting the limbs or for parasitic infections known to cause filariasis. No effective drug therapy to decrease chronic lymphedema is now available in the United States, although studies of several agents continue. Long-term use of diuretics has not been shown to be helpful and is not recommended. Mechanical reduction of lymphedema can best be achieved with elevation or with a program of decongestive lymphatic therapy (including manual lymphatic drainage) or intermittent pneumatic compression. Patients generally prefer sequential pneumatic cells, and they are more useful than the single-chamber compression pump. Maintaining the volume reduction is an integral part of any program and can be achieved in most patients with regular use of high-compression elastic stockings and/or continued wrapping most frequently using low-stretch elastic bandages.

The psychological aspects of the disease should be recognized and addressed to help patients cope with their functional impairment and cosmetic deformity. Regular medical follow-up is necessary to ensure compliance and to recognize immediately any malignant disease of late onset. Lymphedema remains a disabling medical condition that requires knowledgeable physicians so that they may intervene and serve as advocates for patients.

REFERENCES

1. Smeltzer D, Stickler GB, Schirger A: Primary lymphedema in children and adolescents: A follow-up study and review. Pediatrics 76:206, 1985.
2. Mirolo BR, et al: Psychosocial benefits of post mastectomy lymphedema therapy. Cancer Nursing 18:197, 1995.
3. Chernin E: The disappearance of bancroftian filariasis from Charleston, South Carolina. Am J Trop Med Hyg 37:111, 1987.
4. Mak JW: Epidemiology of lymphatic filariasis. Ciba Found Symp 127:5, 1987.
5. Ottesen EA: Description, mechanisms and control of reactions to treatment in the human filariases. Ciba Found Symp 127:265, 1987.
6. Subrahmanyam D: Antifilarials and their mode of action. Ciba Found Symp 127:246, 1987.
7. Dandapat MC, Mohapatro SK, Dash D: Management of chronic manifestations of filariasis. J Indian Med Assoc 84:210, 1986.
8. Meyerowitsch DW, Simonsen PE: Long-term effect of mass diethylcarbamazine chemotherapy on bancroftian filariasis: Results at four years after start of treatment. Trans R Soc Trop Med Hyg 92:98, 1998.
9. Meyerowitsch DW, Simonsen PE: Long-term effect of mass diethylcarbamazine chemotherapy on bancroftian filariasis: Results at four years after start of treatment. Trans R Soc Trop Med Hyg 92:98, 1998.
10. Ismail MM: Efficacy of single dose combinations of albendazole, ivermectin and diethylcarbamazine for the treatment of bancroftian filariasis. Trans R Soc Trop Med 92:94, 1998.
11. Ottesen EA, Duke BO: Strategies and tools for the control/elimination of lymphatic filariasis. Bull WHO 75(6):491–503, 1997.
12. Kissin MW, Querci-della-Rovere G, Easton D, et al: Risk of lymphoedema following the treatment of breast cancer. Br J Surg 73:580, 1986.
13. Markby R, Baldwin E, Kerr P: Incidence of lymphoedema in women with breast cancer. Prof Nurse 6:502, 1991.
14. Schunemann H, Willich N: Secondary lymphedema of the arm following primary therapy of breast carcinoma. Zentralbl Chir 116:220–225, 1992.
15. Giuliano AE, Kirgan DM, Guenther JM, et al: Lymphatic mapping and sentinel lymphadenectomy for breast cancer. Ann Surg 220(3):391–398, 1994.
16. Giuliano AE, Jones RC, Brennan M, et al: Sentinel lymphadenectomy in breast cancer. J Clin Oncol 15(6):2345–2350, 1997.
17. Albertini JJ, Lyman GH, Cox C, et al: Lymphatic mapping and sentinel node biopsy in the patient with breast cancer. JAMA 276(22):1818–1822, 1996.
18. Veronesi U, Paganelli G, Galimberti V, et al: Sentinel-node biopsy to avoid axillary dissection in breast cancer with clinically negative lymph nodes. Lancet 349:1864–1867, 1997.
19. Babb RR: Prophylaxis of recurrent lymphangitis complicating lymphedema. JAMA 195:871, 1966.
20. Kasseroller R: Sodium selenite as prophylaxis of erysipelas in secondary lymphedema. Anticancer Res 18:227–2230, 1998.
21. Stillwell GK, Redford JWB: Physical treatment of postmastectomy lymphedema. Mayo Clin Proc 33:1, 1958.
22. Thiadens SRJ, Rooke TW, Cooke JP: Lymphedema. In Cooke JP, Frohlich ED (eds): Current Management of Hypertensive and Vascular Diseases. St. Louis, Mosby–Year Book, 1992, pp 314–319.
23. Soria P, Cuesta A: Dietary treatment of lymphedema by restriction of long-chain triglycerides. Angiology 45:703–707, 1994.
24. Casley-Smith JR: Lymphedema initiated by aircraft flights. Aviat Space Environ Med 67:52–56, 1996.
25. Schirger A: Lymphedema. Cardiovasc Clin 13:293, 1983.
26. Földi E, Földi M, Weissleder H: Conservative treatment of lymphoedema of the limbs. Angiology 36:171, 1985.
27. Tiedjen KV, Kluken N: The lymphostatic edema? The therapeutic effect of diuretic treatment compared with physiological and physical methods in an isotope study. Presented at the 13th World Congress of the International Union of Angiology, Rochester, Minn, 1983.
28. Casley-Smith JR, Casley-Smith JR: The pathophysiology of lymphedema and the action of benzopyrones in reducing it. Lymphology 21:190, 1988.
29. Piller NB: Macrophage and tissue changes in the developmental phases of secondary lymphoedema and during conservative therapy with benzopyrone. Arch Histol Cytol Suppl 53:209, 1990.
30. Casley-Smith JR, Morgan RG, Piller NB: Treatment of lymphedema of the arms and legs with 5, 6-benzo-(alpha)-pyrone. N Engl J Med 329:1158, 1993.
31. Loprinzi C, Kugler J, Sloan JA, et al: Lack of effect of coumarin in women with postmastectomy lymphedema. N Engl J Med 340:346–350, 1999.
32. Pecking AP, Fevrier B, et al: Efficacy of Daflon 500 mg in the treatment of lymphedema (secondary to conventional therapy of breast cancer). Angiology 48:93–98, 1997.
33. Fyfe NC, Rutt DL, Edwards JM, et al: Intralymphatic steroid therapy for lymphoedema: Preliminary studies. Lymphology 15:23, 1982.
34. Katoh I, Harada K, Tsuda Y, et al: Intraarterial lymphocytes injection for treatment of lymphedema. Jpn J Surg 14:331–334, 1984.
35. Winstone DJ: Amitriptyline and lymphoedema. Med J Aust 2:119, 1982.
36. Collins CD, Mortimer PS: Computed tomography in the assessment of response to limb compression in unilateral lymphoedema. Clin Radiol 50:541–544, 1995.
37. Cornish BH, Bunce IH: Bioelectrical impedance for monitoring the efficacy of lymphoedema treatment programmes. Breast Cancer Res Treat 38:169–176, 1996.
38. Swedborg I, Norrefalk JR: Lymphoedema post-mastectomy: Is elevation alone an effective treatment? Scand J Rehabil Med 25:79–82, 1993.
39. O'Donnell TF, Howrigan P: Diagnosis and management of lymphoedema. In Bell PRF, Jamieson CW, Ruckley CV (eds): Surgical Management of Vascular Disease. Philadelphia, WB Saunders, 1992, pp 1305–1327.
40. Casley-Smith JR, Casley-Smith JR, Mason MR: Complex physical therapy for lymphoedema in Australia. Phlebology 6:21, 1991.
41. Boris M, Weindorf S: Lymphedema reduction by noninvasive complex lymphedema therapy. Oncology 8:95–106; Discussion 109–110, 1994.
42. Boris M, Weindorf S: Persistence of lymphedema reduction after noninvasive complex lymphedema therapy. Oncology 11:99–109; Discussion 110, 1997.
43. Ko DS, Lerner R, Lkose G: Effective treatment of lymphedema of the extremities. Arch Surg 133:452–458, 1998.
44. Daane S, Poltoratszy P, Rockwell WB: Postmastectomy lymphedema management: Evolution of the complex decongestive therapy technique. Ann Plast Surg 40:128–134, 1998.
45. Murthy G, Ballard RE, Breit GA, et al: Intramuscular pressures beneath elastic and inelastic leggings. Ann Vasc Surg 8:543–548, 1994.
46. Witte MH, Witte CL, Bernas M: ISL Consensus Document revisited: Suggested modifications (summarized from discussions at the 16th ICL, Madrid, Spain, September 1997, and the Interim ISL Executive Committee meeting). Lymphology, 31(3):138–140, 1998.
47. Thiadens SRJ: Advances in the management of lymphedema. In Goldstone J (ed): Perspectives in Vascular Surgery. St. Louis, Quality Medical Publishing, 1990, pp 125–141.
48. Zelikovski A, Deutsch A, Reiss R: The sequential pneumatic compression device in surgery for lymphedema of the limbs. J Cardiovasc Surg 24:122, 1983.
49. Richmand DM, O'Donnell TF Jr, Zelikovski A: Sequential pneumatic compression for lymphedema: A controlled trial. Arch Surg 120:1116, 1985.
50. Zanolla R, Monzeglio C, Balzarini A, et al: Evaluation of the results of three different methods of postmastectomy lymphedema treatment. J Surg Oncol 26:210, 1984.
51. Zelikovski A, Melamed I, Kott I, et al: The "Lymphapress": A new pneumatic device for the treatment of lymphedema: Clinical trials and results. Folia Angiol 28:165, 1980.
52. Pappas CJ, O'Donnell TF: Long-term results of compression treatment for lymphedema. J Vasc Surg 16:555, 1992.
53. Klein MJ, Alexander MA, Wright JM, et al: Treatment of adult lower

extremity lymphedema with the Wright linear pump: Statistical analysis of a clinical trial. Arch Phys Med Rehabil 69:202, 1988.

54. McLeod A, Brooks D, Hale J, et al: A clinical report on the use of three external pneumatic compression devices in the management of lymphedema in a paediatric population. Physiother Can 43:28, 1991.

55. Bergan JJ, Sparks S, Angle N: Lymphedema: A comparison of compression pumps in the treatment of lymphedema, Vasc Surg 32:455–462, 1998.

56. Dini D, Del Mastrol L, et al: The role of pneumatic compression in the treatment of postmastectomy lymphedema: A randomized phase III study. Ann Oncol 9:187–190, 1998.

57. Palmar A, Macchiaverna J, Braun A, et al: Compression therapy of limb edema using hydrostatic pressure of mercury. Angiology 42:533, 1991.

58. Johansson K, Lie E, Ekdahl C, Lindfeldt J: A randomized study comparing manual lymph drainage with sequential pneumatic compression for treatment of postoperative arm lymphedema. Lymphology 31:56–64, 1998.

59. Ti-sheng Z, Wen-yi H, Liang-yu H, et al: Heat and bandage treatment for chronic lymphedema of extremities: Report of 1,045 patients. Chin Med J 97:567, 1984.

60. Gloviczki P: Treatment of secondary lymphedema. In Ernst CB, Stanley JC (eds): Current Therapy in Vascular Surgery, 2nd ed. Philadelphia, BC Decker, 1991, pp 1030–1036.

61. Gan JL, Li SL: Microwave heating in the management of postmastectomy upper limb lymphedema. Ann Plast Surg 36:576–581, 1996.

62. Chang TS, Gan JL, Fu KD: The use of 5, 6 benzo-(alpha)-pyrone (coumarin) and heating by microwaves in the treatment of chronic lymphedema of the legs. Lymphology 29:106–111, 1996.

63. Piller NB, Thelander A: Treatment of chronic postmastectomy lymphedema with low level laser therapy: A 2.5 year follow-up. Lymphology 31:74–86, 1998.

64. Pierson S, Pierson D, Swallow R, et al: Efficacy of graded elastic compression in the lower leg. JAMA 249:242, 1983.

65. Johnson G Jr: Role of elastic support in treatment of the chronically swollen limb. In Bergan JJ, Yao JST (eds): Venous Disorders. Philadelphia, WB Saunders, 1991, pp 372–378.

66. Szuba A, Cooke JP, Rockson SG: A novel therapy for lymphedema complicated by lymphorrhea. Vasc Med 1:247–250, 1996.

67. Servelle M: Surgical treatment of lymphedema: A report of 652 cases. Surgery 101:485, 1987.

68. Schmitz-Rixen, Horsch S, Arnold G, Peters PE: Angiosarcoma in primary lymphedema of the lower extremity—Stewart-Treves syndrome. Lymphology 17:50, 1984.

69. Merli GJ: Lymphedema. Clin Podiatry 1:363, 1984.

70. Witte MH, Witte CL: Lymphangiogenesis and lymphologic syndromes. Lymphology 19:21, 1986.

71. Kobayashi MR, Miller TA: Lymphedema. Clin Plast Surg 14:303, 1987.

72. Muller R, Hajdu SI, Brennan MF: Lymphangiosarcoma associated with chronic filarial lymphedema. Cancer 1:179, 1987.

73. Alessi E, Sala F, Berti E: Angiosarcomas in lymphedematous limbs. Am J Dermatopathol 8:371, 1986.

74. Benda JA, Al-Jurf AS, Benson AB 3d: Angiosarcoma of the breast following segmental mastectomy complicated by lymphedema. Am J Clin Pathol 87:651, 1987.

75. Tatnall FM, Mann BS: Non-Hodgkin's lymphoma of the skin associated with chronic limb lymphoedema. Br J Dermatol 113:751, 1985.

76. Ruocco V, Astarita C, Guerrera V, et al: Kaposi's sarcoma on a lymphedematous immunocompromised limb. Int J Dermatol 23:56, 1984.

77. Shelly WB, Wood MG: Transformation of the common wart into squamous cell carcinoma in a patient with primary lymphedema. Cancer 1:820, 1981.

78. Epstein JI, Mendelsohn G: Squamous carcinoma of the foot arising in association with long-standing verrucous hyperplasia in a patient with congenital lymphedema. Cancer 1:943, 1984.

79. Bartal AH, Pinsky CM: Malignant melanoma appearing in a postmastectomy lymphedematous arm: A novel association of double primary tumors. J Surg Oncol 30:16, 1985.

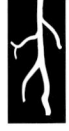

C H A P T E R   1   5   8

Excisional Operations for Chronic Lymphedema

Dominic F. Heffel, M.D.,
and Timothy A. Miller, M.D.

Conservative therapy is the mainstay of treatment for lymphedema, and most patients can be adequately managed without surgical intervention. For the few (10%) patients who ultimately require surgical treatment,[2, 5] the likelihood of benefit and satisfaction depends, in large part, on the indication for surgery. Functional impairment caused by inability to control the size of the extremity is clearly the best indication for surgery. Those who experience recurrent lymphangitis are also likely to benefit from surgical treatment. The aim of surgical therapy is to reduce extremity size, improve limb function, and decrease the frequency of infections.

The frustration encountered in the surgical management of lymphedema is reflected in the numerous techniques offered to patients during the past 80 years. A review of the surgical literature suggests less of an evolution of techniques and more of a trial-and-error approach. Long-term follow-up studies are few, and, objective or quantitative data are usually absent. Qualitative terms such as *satisfactory, good,* and *excellent* pepper the literature but preclude comparison of one technique with another. Sometimes one surgeon's *good* is another's *satisfactory.*

Volumetric measurements of the involved extremity before and after surgery are probably the ideal objective method to quantify changes in extremity volume. These data, for one reason or another, are often absent in surgical reports. Photographic logs documenting extremity status over time provide important objective follow-up data. To reflect the success of therapy accurately, volumetric and photographic evaluation should be standardized and completed after the patient has carried out a normal day of activity, not after the patient has been recumbent for 8 to 12 hours. In many reports, it is unclear when the photographs were taken, and sometimes close examinations of the photographs suggest that the extremity was decompressed prior to photography.

Lymphoscintigraphy may also serve a role in presurgical and postsurgical evaluations. This nuclear medicine study, however, also suffers from deficiencies. To date, there is no consensus on what constitutes a normal lymphoscintigraphic finding. Furthermore, the lymphoscintigraphic protocol varies according to the institution, possibly precluding inter-institution comparisons.

Typically, during a lymphoscintigraphic study a unilaterally enlarged extremity is compared with what *appears* to be a normal contralateral extremity. A curve depicting radiolabeled tracer clearance is then generated, and a qualitative statement, such as "delayed clearance," is made. Because no normal value is currently available, lymphoscintigraphy is useful but limited. The practice of comparing the enlarged extremity with the normal-appearing contralateral extremity seems itself open to scientific criticism. In simple terms, with no known normal clearance value, how is one certain whether the "normal" extremity is normal?

After a review of the literature, it becomes difficult to unequivocally state that one procedure is superior to another, because the data are not standardized from one clinic or institution to another. Moreover, long-term follow-up studies are few. The lymphedema literature is replete with clinician and surgeon bias toward a particular procedure, and active debate continues as to the best surgical approach to lymphedema. Clearly, some conclusions may be based on the complications with and difficulty of performing a given procedure, but to state that microsurgery, for example, is superior to a debulking procedure would be *premature*. The data are not conclusive. This being the case, the most logical approach is to utilize a procedure that has minimal operator dependence, useful long-term follow-up data, and a low incidence of short-term and long-term complications.

This chapter reviews the best available surgical option for palliation of a lymphedematous extremity. Regardless of etiology, long-term follow-up studies demonstrate that, with one probable exception, only one operation for the lymphedematous extremity provides lasting improvement: *staged subcutaneous tissue excision*. The exception may be procedures that bypass isolated lymphatic obstructions. The various microsurgical approaches have shown early promise, but extensive data are not available. For primarily historical reasons, a brief description of the *Thompson* and *Charles procedures* is provided. Although these last two procedures do reduce extremity size, the staged subcutaneous excision is simpler to execute than both and is cosmetically superior to the Charles procedure.

Operations for lymphedema can be divided into two major groups: (1) *physiologic* and (2) *excisional*. Using physiologic procedures, one attempts to reconstruct lymphatic drainage either by bypassing a segmental lymphatic ob-

struction or by establishing communication between a lymphatic-rich flap and the edematous limb. Excisional procedures involve removal of varying amounts of the involved skin and subcutaneous tissue, thereby reducing extremity size.

As shown in Figure 158–1 reductions in extremity circumference can have significant effects on extremity volume and, therefore, extremity weight. Reductions in extremity weight of only 3 to 4 pounds can significantly decrease a patient's sense of fatigue. Some procedures, such as Thompson's buried dermal flap, are combinations of physiologic and excisional procedures.[16]

Excisional procedures continue to be the mainstay of surgical treatment for chronic whole-limb edema with poor distal lymphatic function. All patients must understand that surgery is palliative and that a cosmetically perfect result is unattainable. At present, no surgical procedure can be offered as a cure.

STAGED SUBCUTANEOUS EXCISION BENEATH FLAPS

Staged subcutaneous excision beneath flaps was first described by Sistrunk[14] in 1918 and was later modified and

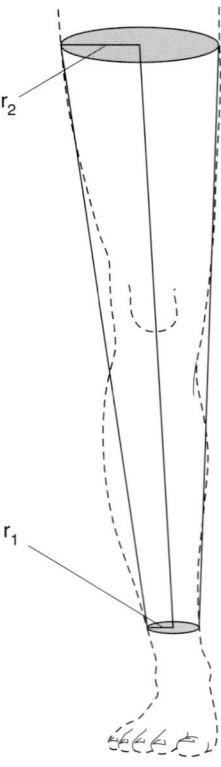

FIGURE 158–1. A method used to estimate extremity volume. The volume varies with the square of the radius:

$$\text{volume} = (\text{length})(\pi/3)(r_1^2 + r_1 r_2 + r_2^2)$$

A 10% increase in the measured circumferences of the extremity can result in a 20% increase in volume. Likewise, a decrease in the circumference of the extremity (i.e., debulking) can result in a substantial decrease in volume and weight. Each liter of fluid gained or lost results in a weight increase or decrease, respectively, of 2.2 pounds.

popularized by Homans.[7] This technique provides the most reasonable surgical approach. It offers reliable improvement while minimizing the likelihood of unfavorable postoperative complications. Relative to microsurgical procedures, the technique is operator independent and probably less expensive.

Improvement is directly related to the amount of skin and subcutaneous tissue removed. As shown in Figure 158–1, small changes in extremity circumference greatly affect extremity volume and weight. The surgical procedure is offered to patients as a means of managing lymphedema, not as a cure.[11] The surgeon removes subcutaneous tissue and skin to an extent that preserves primary closure. To maintain extremity contour, the closure should be snug.[4, 11, 12] The surgical approach is described next.

Preoperative Care

Absolute bed rest with extremity elevation is begun 3 days before surgery. This step can begin at home. When possible, sequential pneumatic pumps are used to facilitate fluid loss. After bed rest and extremity elevation, a patient with lower extremity lymphedema usually loses 4 to 10 pounds of fluid. The rate of edema resolution depends on the duration of the condition and the amount of subcutaneous fibrosis that exists. Edema resolution results in skin laxity, allowing greater amounts of tissue excision. The patient is admitted 1 to 2 days preoperatively. Other than a single preoperative prophylactic dose, antibiotics are not used.

Operation on the Lower Extremity

Surgical Technique

The procedure is usually performed in two stages. The medial excision is performed first, because more tissue can be excised (Fig. 158–2). The lateral excision is performed 3 months later. A third stage can be performed if needed.

Medial Incision

A pneumatic tourniquet is placed as proximally as possible, and the extremity is exsanguinated. A medial incision is made at the level of the ankle, beginning 1 cm posterior to the medial malleolus and extending proximally into the thigh. Flaps approximately 1.5 cm thick are elevated anteriorly and posteriorly to the mid-sagittal plane in the calf, with less extensive dissection in the knee and ankle. All subcutaneous tissue beneath the flaps is removed, with care taken to preserve the sural nerve. The deep fascia of the calf is incised over the tibia and resected. The fascia about the knee and ankle is spared in order to preserve joint integrity. Redundant skin is then resected. It is not unusual to remove a 4- to 10-cm width of skin. The tourniquet is deflated, and hemostasis is obtained.

A suction catheter is placed in the dependent portion of the posterior flap and is left in place for 5 days. Interrupted 4-0 nylon is employed for skin closure. When the area around the knee and ankle is sutured, portions of the deep fascia are included in the suture to fix the skin and ensure contour. No subcutaneous or dermal sutures are placed.

Lateral Incision

The lateral excision is performed 3 months after the first stage. The incision can extend superiorly as needed. The sensory branches of the peroneal nerve should be identified and preserved.

Postoperative Care

The extremity is immobilized with a posterior splint. The patient is kept at absolute bed rest for 9 days with the extremity elevated. Sutures are usually removed on the eighth day and replaced with tape immobilization. The patient is measured for an elastic compression stocking, and dependency of the leg is begun on the ninth day, but only with the leg tightly wrapped with elastic bandages. This procedure is continued for 3 weeks postoperatively.

During the first month, the protective wrapping and pressure are important for preventing seroma formation and optimizing healing and contouring. Ambulation is started on the 11th postoperative day, but only with the leg tightly wrapped. Postoperatively, elastic stockings must be used on a regular basis.

Operation On the Arm

Surgical Technique

A medial incision is made from the distal ulna across the medial epicondyle of the humerus to the posterior medial upper arm (Fig. 158–3). Flaps approximately 1 cm thick are elevated to the mid-sagittal aspect of the forearm, and the dissection is tapered distally and proximally. The edematous subcutaneous tissue is removed, but the deep fascia is spared. The ulnar nerve is identified in the region of the medial epicondyle and preserved. The redundant skin is excised. The tourniquet is deflated, and hemostasis is obtained. (If necessary, the tourniquet can be removed, the area prepared, and the operation continued into the axilla.) A suction catheter is placed, and the skin is closed with 4-0 nylon suture. No subcutaneous or dermal sutures are placed.

Postoperative Care

The arm is immobilized and elevated for 5 days. In many instances, the suction catheter can be removed after the third day. Otherwise, postoperative management is similar to that described for the leg.

Results

There is a clear relationship between reduction of leg volume and improvement of leg function. The degree to which patients complied with medical management had a favorable influence on long-term outcome. In no patients was there complete elimination of edema, even when extremity volume was greatly reduced. Prolonged standing worsened the inevitable recurrence of edema, and this fact complicated postoperative evaluation.

One of the chapter authors (T.A.M.) has performed staged subcutaneous tissue and skin excision on more than

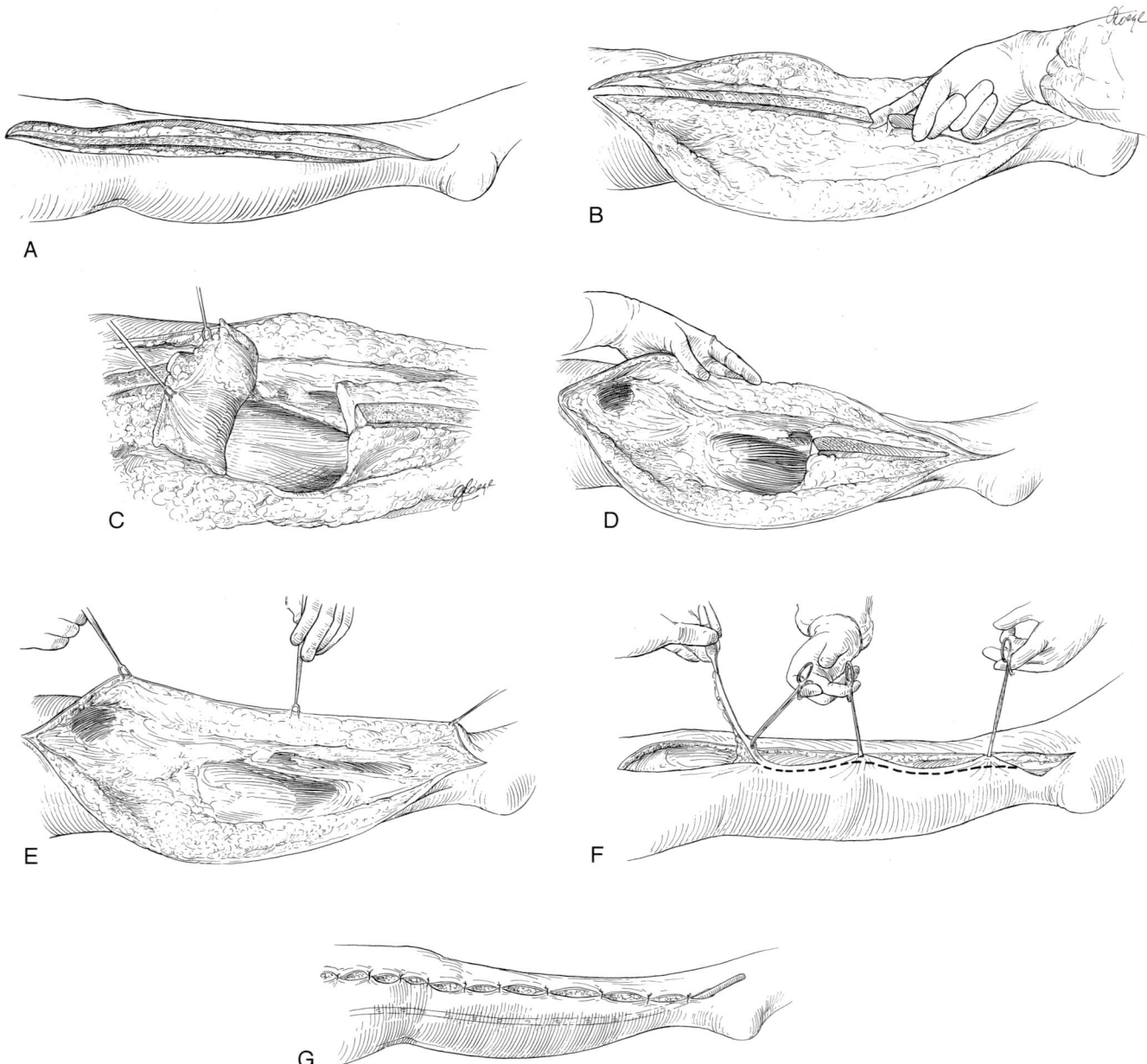

FIGURE 158–2. The staged subcutaneous tissue and skin excision procedure in the lower extremity. *A,* An incision is made posterior to the medial malleolus and extends into the thigh. *B,* Flaps approximately 1.5 cm thick are elevated anteriorly and posteriorly. *C–E,* The deep fascia of the calf is incised over the tibia and resected; the fascia about the knee and ankle is spared. The sural nerve should be identified and preserved. *F,* Redundant skin is resected. *G,* A suction catheter is placed in the dependent portion of the posterior flap, and the skin is closed with 4-0 nylon. When areas about the knee and ankle are sutured, portions of the deep fascia are included in the suture to fix the skin and ensure contour.

100 patients. Recently, a long-term follow-up study was conducted. Thirty-eight patients (six male, 32 female) with lower extremity lymphedema were observed for an average of 14 years (3 to 27 years). Surgical results were documented by various methods: physical examination, volume displacement, serial photography, lymphoscintigraphy, and patient survey. Of all the methods available for the evaluation of surgical therapy, photographs provided a simple and accurate means by which improvement could be studied and documented. A representative photograph depicting long-term maintenance of form is shown in Figure 158–4.

Thirty of the 38 patients experienced a significant reduction in extremity size, improved contour, and a reduction in or elimination of the incidence of cellulitis. No differences in the long-term results were seen with acquired, in contrast to congenital, lymphedema. Two patients were essentially unchanged on short-term follow-up. Five patients experienced continuing enlargement in the leg after surgery. In one patient, postoperative improvement occurred during the first 2 years. Swelling recurred, however, as significant weight gain occurred. Men did not experience as much improvement as women did.

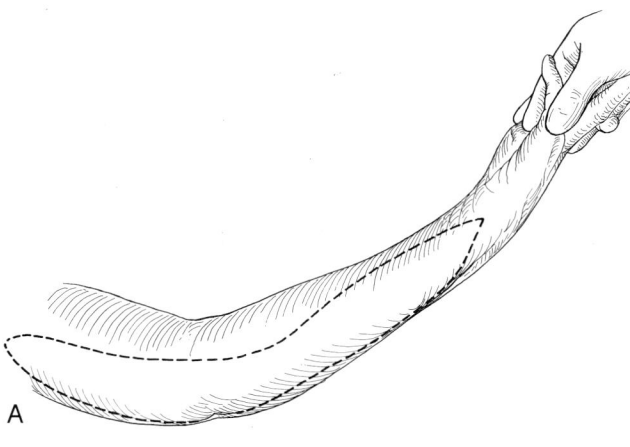

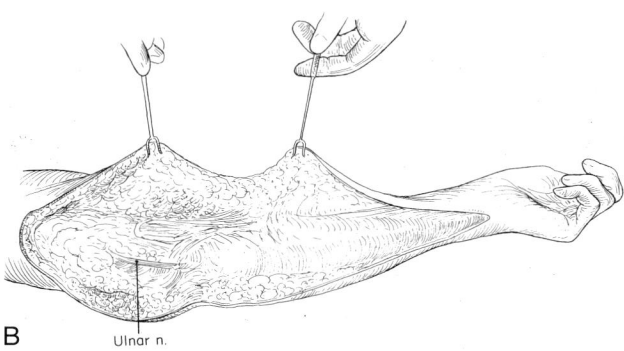

FIGURE 158–3. The staged subcutaneous tissue and skin excision procedure in the upper extremity is analogous to the same procedure in the lower extremity. *A,* A medial elliptical incision is made from the distal ulna across the medial epicondyle of the humerus to the posterior medial upper arm. An ellipse of skin is excised so that the scar occurs on the mid-medial aspect of the arm. *B,* The ulnar nerve is identified in the region of the medial epicondyle and preserved. The edematous subcutaneous tissue is removed; the deep fascia is spared. Closure is performed in a fashion similar to that in the lower extremity.

Skin and subcutaneous excision has not been effective for upper extremity lymphedema. In 1984, the results of 14 patients managed over 11 years were reported.[12] Although extremity volume was reduced by 250 to 1200 ml in 10 patients, four patients noted hand swelling postoperatively. In four other patients, arm swelling continued to progress despite an initial reduction postoperatively. The reason for the difference in postoperative results between the upper and lower extremity is unclear. Staged subcutaneous tissue and skin excision should not be performed on patients with average postmastectomy lymphedema. Fortunately, for these patients, some authors employing a microsurgical approach have noted a reduction in hand swelling after reconstruction.[13] However, it would be premature to conclude that one operation is indicated in the upper extremity and another in the lower extremity.

Except for partial wound separation in one patient and three instances of ischemic flap necrosis (which healed by secondary intention), there were no significant postoperative complications. Although many patients experienced

decreased sensation at the incision site, this has not been a source of complaint. None of these patients had inadvertent nerve injury, and no alteration in hand or foot sensation occurred.

TOTAL SUBCUTANEOUS EXCISION (CHARLES' PROCEDURE)

Surgical Technique

Charles described a surgical technique for the treatment of scrotal edema in 1901. The adaptation of this technique for treatment of lower extremity lymphedema led to the eponym the "Charles procedure." This operation is the most extensive of the excisional procedures.[3]

In the lower extremity, all of the skin and subcutaneous tissue is excised from the tibial tuberosity to the malleoli. Tissues overlying the tibial tuberosity, malleoli, and tendons of the calcaneus are not removed. Although some surgeons resect the deep fascia in its entirety,[15] others remove only heavily fibrosed segments.[8] The excision of the tissue is tapered at the proximal and distal margins of the resection to prevent a step deformity.

The defect is closed with a split-thickness or full-thickness skin graft from the resected specimen, or a split-thickness skin graft can be used from an uninvolved donor site. Coverage with a *split-thickness* skin graft is technically easier and gives a satisfactory initial appearance. However, these grafts are injured easily, ulcerate frequently, scar extensively, and a severe hyperkeratotic weeping dermatitis may develop. Hyperpigmentation of the grafted segment is also common. Coverage with a single *full-thickness* skin graft is technically more demanding but produces a better cosmetic result and a more durable graft site. Nevertheless, regions of graft breakdown and substantial scar formation can also occur with full-thickness grafts.

A complete description of the operative procedure has been provided by Hocpes.[8] We think that this operation leads to a cosmetic result that is often worse than the initial presentation.

BURIED DERMIS FLAP (THOMPSON'S PROCEDURE)

In Thompson's procedure, a portion of the lymphedematous subcutaneous tissue is resected beneath flaps, a flap edge is de-epithelialized, and the resulting "dermis flap" is buried in the underlying muscle compartment. Thompson's operation has three theoretical advantages:

1. The buried dermis permits the formation of lymphatic connections between the subdermal lymphatic plexus of the flap and the deep lymphatics of the muscle compartment.

2. Muscle contractions increase the lymphatic flow rate through the subdermal plexus.

3. The buried flap provides a physical barrier against deep fascia regeneration.[17]

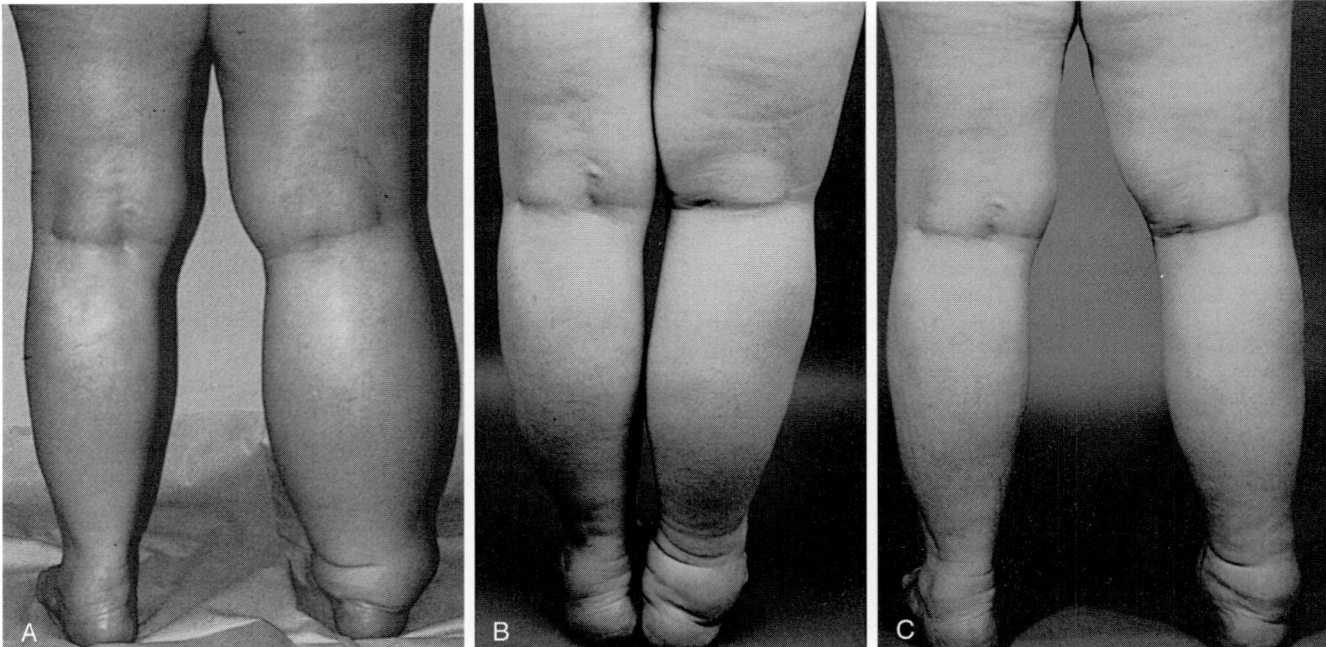

FIGURE 158–4. Photographs documenting long-term changes. *A*, A preoperative view of a lymphedematous right lower extremity. *B*, Postoperative view of the same right lower extremity 3 years after a staged subcutaneous tissue and skin excision. Note the reduction in leg volume. *C*, Postoperative view of the same right lower extremity 8 years after a staged subcutaneous tissue and skin excision. In the postoperative views, note the return of symmetry and the maintenance of contour.

The operation is both excisional and physiologic in approach.[16]

Surgical Technique

In the lower limbs, the initial operation is usually performed on the lateral aspect of the involved extremity. If additional volume reduction is desired, the procedure is repeated on the medial aspect of the limb 3 months after the first operation. The surgical incision is placed at the junction of the anterior and middle thirds of the lateral thigh and leg but curves posteriorly at the knee to traverse its mid-lateral aspect. Anterior and posterior flaps 1 to 2 cm in thickness are elevated to the mid-sagittal line. The subcutaneous tissue and the underlying fascia are excised to expose the muscle compartments. Some subcutaneous tissue is retained over the proximal fibula, and the common peroneal nerve is carefully preserved.

A 4- to 5-cm wide split-thickness skin graft is harvested from the edge of the posterior flap. The entire epidermis must be removed; burial of the dermal flap with retained epidermal islands will lead to formation of draining sinus tracts at the suture line. The dermal flap is sutured to the lateral wall of the femoral canal in the thigh and to the intramuscular space between the tibialis anterior and the extensor hallucis longus muscles in the leg. A drain is placed beneath each flap, and the anterior flap is closed over the dermal flap in a "vest over pant" fashion with mattress sutures.

Depending on the extent of disease, this procedure may be limited to the leg and distal thigh or extended onto the proximal thigh and foot. A similar operation is available for the medial aspect of the lower limb and for both lateral and medial aspects of the upper extremity.[17–19]

Operative success is attributed to the formation of lymphatic connections between the flap and the muscle compartment, and radioactive iodine–tagged human serum albumin (RIHSA) clearance studies have demonstrated postoperative improvement in the rate of lymphatic isotope clearance.[1, 6, 18] Postoperative lymphangiography, however, has failed to demonstrate any lymphatic anastomosis.[3] Moreover, subcutaneous excision alone has been shown to increase the rate of RIHSA clearance.[9, 10] It may be the excisional component of the operation that actually produces most of the postoperative improvement.

SUMMARY

The best indication for an excisional surgical procedure is functional impairment of the limb due to excessive lymphedema refractory to medical management. During the excisional procedures, a varying amount of skin and subcutaneous tissue is removed from the extremity. The Charles' operation, which includes circumferential resection of all skin and subcutaneous tissue with split-thickness or full-thickness skin coverage, should be reserved for those few patients who have extreme lymphedema with severe skin changes. The benefit of Thompson's buried dermis flap operation is most likely related to the amount of subcutaneous tissue excised. The best cosmetic and functional result is achieved with the staged subcutaneous excision underneath flaps. Although these procedures decrease the volume of the extremity and improve function, they cannot cure lymphedema.

REFERENCES

1. Amar R, Rosello R, Meline F, Bureau H: L'utilisation de la serum albumine humaine marquee a l'iode-131 pour l'exploration des lymphoedemes chirurgicaux des membres. Etude preliminaire. Ann Chir Plast 21:49, 1976.
2. Barsotti J, Gaisne E: Surgical treatment of lymphedema. J Mal Vasc 15:163, 1990.
3. Charles RH: Elephantiasis scroti. In Latham A (ed): A System of Treatment. Vol 3. London, Churchill, 1912.
4. Fonkalsrud EW, Coulson WF: Management of congenital lymphedema in infants and children. Ann Surg 177:280, 1973.
5. Gloviczki P: Treatment of secondary lymphedema. In Ernst CB, Stanley JC (eds): Current Therapy in Vascular Surgery, 2nd ed. Philadelphia, BC Decker, 1991.
6. Harvey RF: The use of[131] I-labeled human serum albumin in the assessment of improved lymph flow following buried dermis flap operation in cases of post-mastectomy lymphedema of the arm. Br J Radiol 42:260, 1969.
7. Homans J: The treatment of elephantiasis of the legs: Preliminary report. N Engl J Med 215:1099, 1936.
8. Hoopes JE: Lymphedema of the extremity. In Cameron JL (ed): Current Surgical Therapy. Vol 3. Philadelphia, BC Decker, 1989, p 630.
9. Kinmonth JB: Primary lymphoedema of the lower limb: Response to discussion. Proc R Soc Med 58:1031, 1965.
10. Miller T, Harper J, Longmire WP: The management of lymphedema by staged subcutaneous excision. Surg Gynecol Obstet 136:586, 1973.
11. Miller TA: Surgical management of lymphedema of the extremity. Plast Reconstr Surg 56:633, 1975.
12. Miller TA: Surgical approach to lymphedema of the arm after mastectomy. Am J Surg 148:152, 1984.
13. O'Brien BM, Mellow CG, Khazanchi RK, et al: Long-term results after microlymphaticovenous anastomoses for the treatment of obstructive lymphedema. Plast Reconstr Surg 85(4):562, 1990.
14. Sistrunk WE: Further experiences with the Kondoleon operation for elephantiasis. JAMA 71:800, 1918.
15. Taylor GW: Surgical management of primary lymphedema. Proc R Soc Med 58:1024, 1965.
16. Thompson N, Wee JTK: Twenty years' experience of the buried dermis flap operation in the treatment of chronic lymphedema of the extremities. Chir Plast (Berl) 5:147, 1980.
17. Thompson N: Surgical treatment of chronic lymphedema of the lower limb. With preliminary report of new operation. Br Med J 2:1566, 1962.
18. Thompson N: Surgical treatment of primary and secondary lymphedema of the extremities by lymphatic transposition. Proc R Soc Med 58:1026, 1965.
19. Thompson N: The surgical treatment of chronic lymphedema of the extremities. Surg Clin North Am 47:445, 1967.

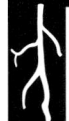

CHAPTER 159
Lymphatic Reconstructions

Peter Gloviczki, M.D., and
Audra A. Noel, M.D.

The many different operations that have been proposed to improve lymphatic transport are testimony to the frustration that surgeons have experienced in treating chronic lymphedema. *Direct* operations on the lymphatics to reconstruct obstructed pathways include lymphovenous anastomoses[1–12] and lymphatic grafting.[13, 14] *Indirect* lymphatic reconstructions designed to improve lymphatic drainage include the use of an omental flap,[15, 16] the mesenteric bridge operation,[17, 18] and autotransplantation of lymphatic tissue as a free flap.[19] These procedures are based on the ability of the lymphatic system to form spontaneous lympholymphatic anastomoses to improve collateral lymphatic drainage to the mesentery or to regions of the body where lymphatic drainage is normal.

Although some of these operations have been performed for several decades, none of them has proven long-term effectiveness and their use continues to be controversial. Because cure of lymphedema at present is not possible and clinical improvement after each of the operations has been reported by at least one experienced surgical team, a review

of these procedures is still warranted. Although the main goal of this chapter is to update current attempts at lymphatic reconstructions and discuss operations for chylous disorders, no less important is the authors' intent to stimulate further clinical research in this difficult field.

DIRECT LYMPHATIC RECONSTRUCTIONS

Lymphovenous Anastomoses

Surgical lymphovenous anastomoses intended to bypass the obstructed lymphatic system in patients with chronic lymphedema have been performed in the last three decades.[1–12] The rationale for the operation is based on the observation that in patients with chronic lymphedema contrast lymphangiography occasionally demonstrates spontaneous lymphovenous anastomoses.[19] These spontaneous channels are considered compensatory mechanisms of the

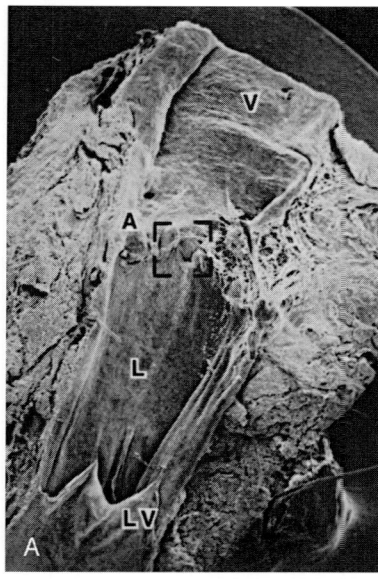
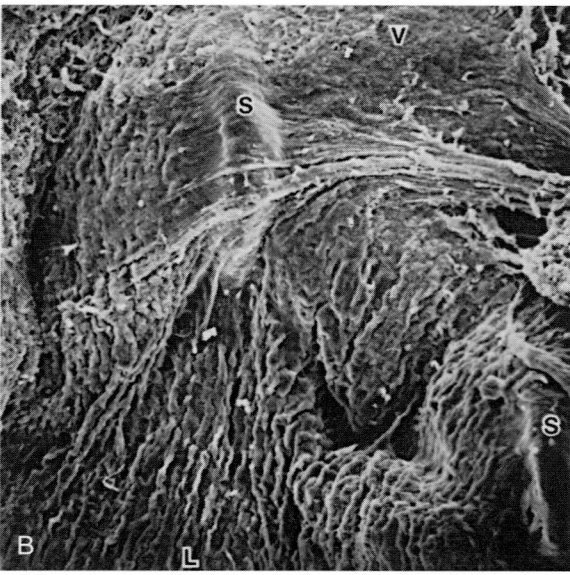

FIGURE 159–1. *A* and *B,* Scanning electron micrographs of patent lymphovenous anastomosis 4 weeks after operation in a dog. Endothelial cells cover suture line. A = anastomosis, L = lymph vessel, LV = lymphatic valve, S = suture, V = vein. (*A,* Original magnification, ×10; *B,* original magnification, ×200.) (*A* and *B,* From Gloviczki P, Hollier LH, Nora FE, Kaye MP: The natural history of microsurgical lymphovenous anastomoses: An experimental study. J Vasc Surg 4:148, 1986.)

body to decrease the lymphatic hypertension that occurs early in the course of the disease.

Nielubowicz and Olszewski suggested anastomosing the inguinal lymph nodes to the femoral or greater saphenous vein.[21] Although improvement in patients with lymph node–vein anastomoses has been reported,[3, 21, 22] enthusiasm for this operation faded because early occlusion due to thrombosis and fibrosis over the cut surface of the node is likely.[22]

The development of microvascular surgery and the availability of fine instruments and suture materials enabled microsurgeons to develop techniques to anastomose blood vessels less than 2 mm in diameter with excellent patency. Successful direct anastomoses between lymph vessels and veins were reported in experiments as early as 1962 by Jacobson[24] and soon after by Laine and Howard.[25] Subsequent experiments from several groups documented a 50% to 70% patency rate several months after surgery.[26–29] The authors' group performed end-to-end anastomoses between normal femoral lymph vessels and a tributary of the femoral vein in dogs and noted a 50% patency rate up to 8 months after the operation.[30] The anastomoses were done with 11-0 monofilament nonabsorbable interrupted sutures with the help of an operating microscope with high-power magnification. Cinelymphangiography and scanning electron microscopy were used to document patency (Figs. 159–1 and 159–2). Most anastomoses that occluded were performed at the beginning of the experiments, suggesting the importance of technical expertise in performing these operations. However, Puckett and colleagues failed to confirm the patency of lymphovenous anastomoses 3 weeks after surgery in an experimental model of chronic lymphedema.[30]

Attempts to improve patency of lymphovenous anastomoses include the use of polytetrafluoroethylene (Teflon) stents.[31] In experiments, lymph vessels were anastomosed with adjacent veins in rabbits with 1.5-mm internal stents. Patency rate at 1 week was 71% compared with 38% in the sutured, nonstented anastomoses. All lymphovenous anastomoses, however, were occluded at 4 weeks. Initial good patency rates indicate that stenting is feasible, but refinement of such techniques is required.

Indications

Patients with secondary lymphedema of recent onset without previous episodes of cellulitis or lymphangitis are potential candidates for surgical treatment unless they can be managed easily with conservative measures. In the late

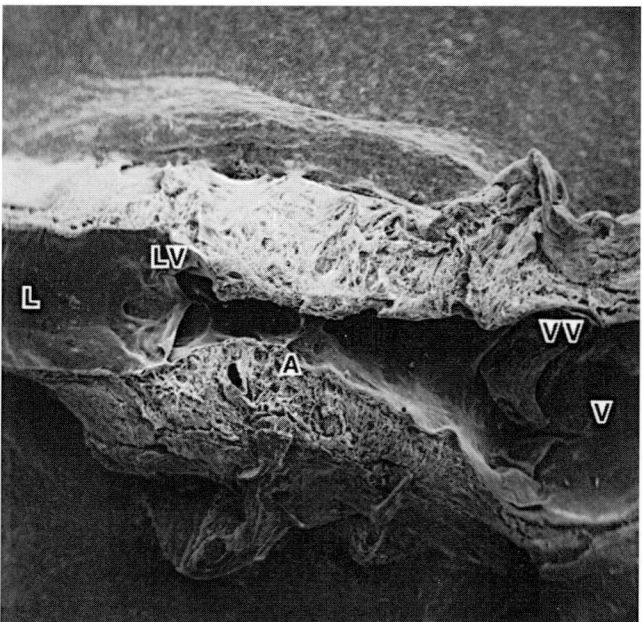

FIGURE 159–2. Scanning electron micrograph of a patent lymphovenous anastomosis 3 months after operation in a dog. A = anastomosis, L = lymph vessel, LV = lymphatic valve, V = vein; VV = venous valve. (Original magnification, ×10). (From Gloviczki P, Hollier LH, Nora FE, Kaye MP: The natural history of microsurgical lymphovenous anastomoses: An experimental study. J Vasc Surg 4:148, 1986.)

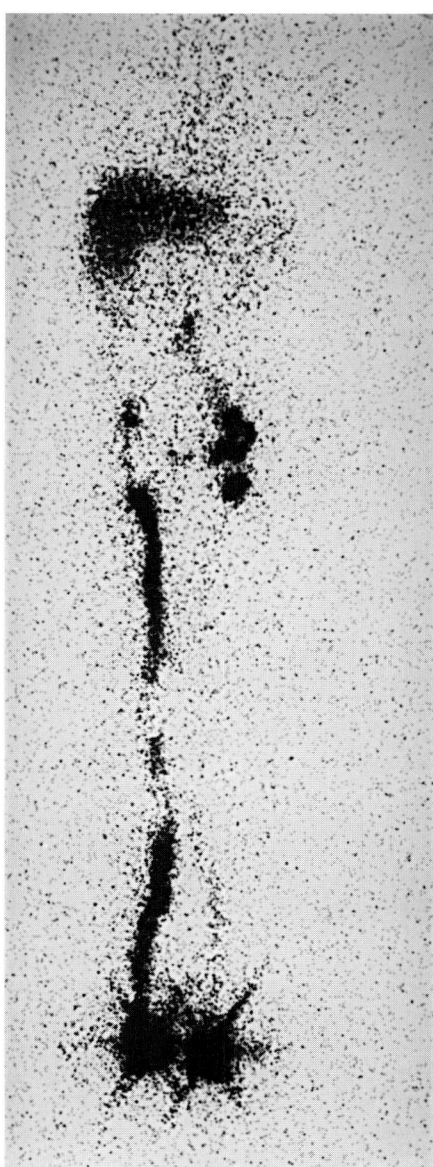

FIGURE 159–3. Bilateral lower extremity lymphoscintigram in a patient with right lower extremity lymphedema secondary to obstruction of the right iliac nodes. Note dilated lymph vessels in the right thigh distal to the obstruction suitable for direct lymphatic reconstruction.

dates, it confirms the presence of dilated infrainguinal lymph vessels with proximal pelvic lymphatic obstruction (Fig. 159–3). Although it does not differentiate between primary and secondary lymphedema, and even though it is primarily a functional and not an anatomic study, semiquantitative lymphoscintigraphy with 99m-technetium antimony trisulfide colloid can identify reliably the pattern of lymphatic transport.[32] In selected patients, however, direct contrast lymphangiography can be performed to show the fine details of the lymphatic circulation.

Other preoperative tests include noninvasive venous studies and duplex scanning of the deep veins. Computed tomography (CT) is used in most patients to exclude any underlying mass or malignant tumor. Once surgery has been decided on, the patients are hospitalized for 28 to 48 hours to elevate the extremity in a lymphedema sling and to allow use of intermittent compression treatment with a pump to decrease the volume of the extremity.

Surgical Technique

Because the operation lasts many hours, general anesthesia is preferred. For lower extremity lymphedema, a transverse incision at the mid-thigh or a longitudinal incision close to the saphenofemoral junction is performed to allow dissection of the lymphatics of the superficial medial bundle (Fig. 159–4). The greater saphenous vein and any tributaries are also dissected. An attempt is made to visualize the lymph vessels by injecting subcutaneously 5 ml of isosulfan blue (Lymphazurin) dye; half of this amount is directed toward the first interdigital space and half toward the area 10 to 15 cm distal to the site of incision. Because of lymphatic obstruction, however, lymph flow even in patent lymphatics may be minimal, and the dye usually is not visible during dissection. With experience, the whitish fluid-filled lymphatics, frequently with vascularized adventitia, can be distinguished from small subcutaneous nerves or fibrotic bands.

If contrast lymphangiography is performed within 24 hours of the operation, the contrast-filled lymphatics are easily identifiable and can be located during the operation with an image intensifier and a C-arm (Fig. 159–5A). Contrast lymphangiography in some patients helps to avoid many hours of unsuccessful searching for patent lymphatics in the groin. Once the lymphatic vessels and the veins are isolated, a standard microsurgical technique is used to perform an end-to-end anastomosis, using six to eight interrupted 11-0 monofilament sutures (Fig. 159–5B–D). The operation is performed with a Zeiss operating microscope with ×4 to ×40 magnification.

For arm lymphedema, the lymphatics are dissected either through a transverse incision at the wrist or in the mid-cubital fossa or through a longitudinal incision at the medial aspect of the arm, a few centimeters proximal to the elbow. The lymphatics of the superficial medial lymphatic bundle usually are used for anastomoses (Fig. 159–6), which are performed with the mid-cubital, basilic, or brachial veins or their tributaries in an end-to-side or end-to-end fashion.

Postoperatively, the limb is wrapped with elastic bandage

stage of lymphedema, fibrosis and valvular incompetence of the main lymph vessels develop, the intrinsic contractility of the vessel wall is lost, and interstitial pressure decreases owing to secondary changes in the subcutaneous tissue (see Chapter 155). The chances of success with lymphovenous anastomoses in such limbs are clearly diminished. Because venous hypertension impedes forward flow through the anastomoses, patients with chronic venous insufficiency are not candidates for this operation.

Preoperative Evaluation

Isotope lymphoscintigraphy usually is sufficient for preoperative imaging of the lymphatic system. In ideal candi-

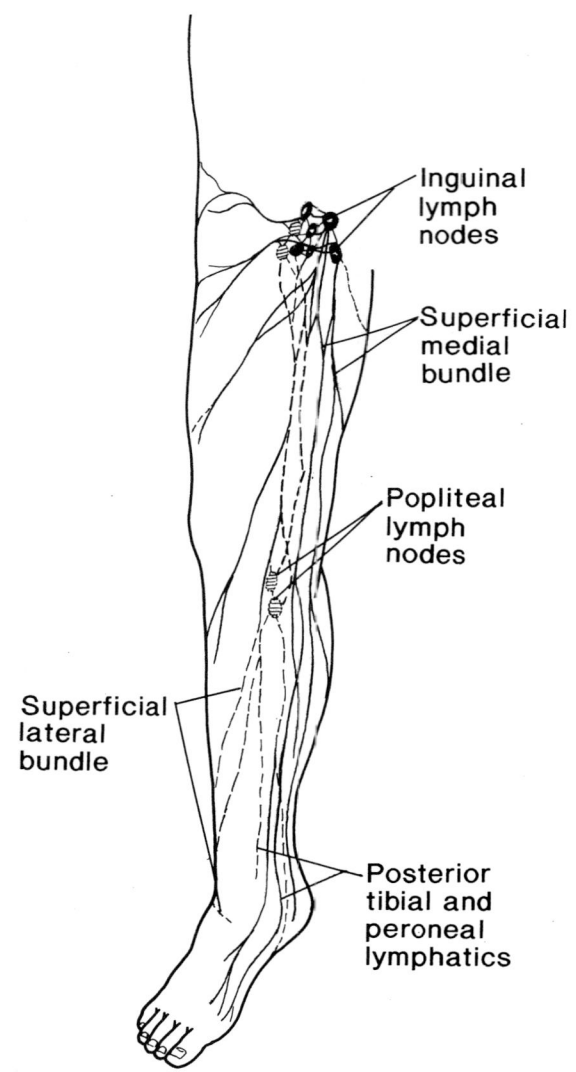

FIGURE 159–4. The lymphatic system of the lower extremity. (By permission of Mayo Foundation.)

Inguinal lymph nodes

Superficial medial bundle

Popliteal lymph nodes

Superficial lateral bundle

Posterior tibial and peroneal lymphatics

and elevated at 30 degrees with two pillows for the arm or, for the lower extremity, elevation of the foot of the bed.

Results

Objective evaluation of the long-term effectiveness of lymphovenous anastomoses in patients has been difficult (Table 159–1). Decrease in circumference or volume of the extremity, patient satisfaction, decrease in episodes of cellulitis, and improvement in lymphatic clearance as measured by lymphoscintigraphy have been used as the criteria of success. In a review of 14 patients who underwent lymphovenous anastomosis at the authors' institution, however, only five limbs remained improved at a mean follow-up time of 46 months after surgery.[10] Improvement was observed in four of seven patients with secondary lymphedema but in only one of eight patients with primary lymphedema. Improvement in lymphatic clearance from the injection site was the only indirect sign of patency of

the shunts. Therefore, the authors' group was not able to provide objective evidence of late patency of the lymphovenous anastomoses in these patients.

The largest experience with lymphovenous shunts was reported in Australia. O'Brien and colleagues published a well-documented report with long-term follow-up studies of 90 patients who underwent lymphovenous anastomoses for chronic lymphedema.[12] Although a significant number of patients underwent additional excisional operations, improvement was documented even in patients who underwent only lymphovenous anastomoses. Of the patients who underwent lymphovenous anastomosis only, 73% had subjective improvement and 42% had objective long-term improvement. Seventy-four percent of all patients discontinued the use of elastic stockings. Because direct contrast lymphangiography has occasionally resulted in progression of lymphedema due to chemical lymphangitis or accumulation of the contrast material in the lymph nodes due to poor lymphatic transport, this test was not used to document late patency of the anastomoses. Therefore, objective evidence that the improvement in these patients was due to patent and functioning lymphovenous anastomoses is still lacking.

Lymphatic Grafting

Baumeister and colleagues introduced lymphatic grafting for upper extremity and unilateral lower extremity secondary lymphedema.[13, 33–38] Because lymph is devoid of platelets and coagulates less than blood, the chances of patency in successful lympholymphatic anastomoses appear to be better than those in lymphovenous anastomoses. Also, an elevated venous pressure, which may interrupt flow intermittently through lymphovenous anastomoses, is not a factor in this procedure. In their experiments, Baumeister and colleagues achieved 100% short- to medium-term patency of lymphatic interposition grafts.[33] Indisputably, this operation requires special microsurgical expertise.

A variation of lymphatic grafting was reported by Campisi and coworkers, who treated 64 patients with upper and lower extremity lymphedema by creating a lymphatic-venous-lymphatic anastomosis with autologous interposition vein graft.[14] Experimental data from lymphatic-vessel-to-isolated-vein anastomoses in the dog suggests improved patency rates.[39] With an isolated vein segment, the anastomosis is not exposed to intraluminal blood and theoretically is protected from thrombotic occlusion. The isolated vein-lymphatic graft technique represents the increasing efforts at improving patency of lymphatic reconstructions.

Preoperative Evaluation

Preoperative evaluation is similar to that needed for patients who undergo lymphovenous anastomoses. It is important to image the donor leg lymphatics with lymphoscintigraphy because a normal lymphatic system is a prerequisite for the use of lymph vessels from the leg for grafting. In the experience of Baumeister and coworkers, which now amounts to 95 patients, postoperative leg swelling occurred in only one limb due to post-thrombotic venous disease.[37] Patients with bilateral leg edema are not candidates for this procedure.

TABLE 159–1. CLINICAL RESULTS OF MICROSURGICAL LYMPHATIC RECONSTRUCTIONS

STUDY	NO. OF PATIENTS	EXTREMITY Upper	Lower	TYPE OF OPERATION	FOLLOW-UP (MO)	RESULTS: EXCELLENT OR GOOD (%)
Krylov et al,[4] 1982	50	+		LVA	?	30
Nieuborg,[5] 1982	47	+		LVA	6–12	68
Gong-Kang et al,[6] 1985	91		+	LVA	24*	79
Zhu et al,[9] 1987	48		+	LVA	6–52	33
	185		+	LVA	6–52	73
Gloviczki et al,[10] 1988	6	+		LVA	} 36.6*	50
	8		+	LVA		25
O'Brien et al,[12] 1990	46	+		LVA		54
	30		+	LVA	} 51*	83
	6†	+		LVA		33
	8†		+	LVA		50
Baumeister and Siuda,[13] 1990	36	+		LG	>12	33
	12		+	LG	>24	8
Campisi et al,[14] 1995	5	+		LVL	>60	} 90.5
	59		+	LVL		

*Mean.
†Lymphovenous anastomosis plus excisional procedure.
LVA = lymphovenous anastomoses; LG = lymphatic grafting; LVL = lymphatic-venous-lymphatic graft with autologous vein.

Surgical Technique

The operation on the lower extremity is very similar to a suprapubic saphenous vein graft, as performed by Palma for unilateral iliac vein obstruction (see Chapter 150). As in lymphovenous anastomoses, the superficial thigh lymphatics in the edematous limb are dissected first through a longitudinal incision made just distal to the saphenofemoral junction. Five milliliters of isosulfan blue (Lymphazurin) dye is injected subcutaneously into the first interdigital space of the normal foot, and the thigh lymphatics are exposed through a 25- to 30-cm incision along the greater saphenous vein with loupe magnification (Fig. 159–7). Two or three lymphatics are selected for grafting. They are transected distally after double ligation and tunneled subcutaneously above the pubis to the contralateral side, where end-to-end lympholymphatic anastomoses are performed under the operating microscope with 11-0 or 12-0 interrupted sutures (Fig. 159–8).

For postmastectomy lymphedema, the two or three lymphatics from the leg are harvested and used as free interposition grafts. They are placed in a subcutaneous tunnel from the upper medial arm to the neck and then sutured end to end first to the superficial medial bundle lymphatics in the arm and then to the descending neck lymphatics in the supraclavicular fossa. Postoperative care for these patients is similar to that given to patients with lymphovenous anastomoses.

In patients treated with peripheral lymphatic-venous-lymphatic anastomoses, autologous vein is harvested from the volar aspect of the forearm for upper extremity procedures, or the ipsilateral greater or lesser saphenous veins are used for lower extremity lymphedema. The lymph vessels proximal and distal to the lymphatic occlusion are anastomosed to the vein graft with a telescoping anastomosis with 8-0 or 9-0 nylon suture (Fig. 159–9). This technique allows the invagination of several lymphatic afferent vessels into the vein graft. As stated above, isosulfan blue can be used to delineate lymphatics as well as to confirm patency of the anastomosis intraoperatively.[14]

Results

In a report evaluating 55 patients undergoing this operation with a follow-up of more than 3 years, Baumeister and associates documented a decrease in the volume of the extremity in 80% of the patients.[13] Volume measurements were diminished significantly in 36 patients with arm lymphedema, and 16 patients were improved clinically for more than 2 years after surgery. Significant improvement was documented in eight of 12 patients with lower extremity lymphedema more than 1 year after suprapubic grafting.

Thirty patients were studied by lymphoscintigraphy. With a semi-quantitative assessment and a lymphatic transport index, some improvement in lymphatic clearance could be demonstrated in all patients. Although several grafts were imaged by lymphoscintigraphy, the patency rate of the implanted lymphatic grafts was not reported.

Since their initial report, Baumeister and coworkers have treated 127 limbs in 122 patients with microsurgical lymphatic grafting (79 with arm edema, 48 with lower extremity edema).[38] Most patients with arm edema experienced a decrease in volume measurements. In addition, the authors documented the use of both lymphoscintigraphy and indirect lymphography with non-ionic water-soluble contrast injection to demonstrate patent grafts; however, graft patency was not recorded. Significant experience with this operation has not been gained by other surgical teams. In two of the patients operated on by the authors' group with this technique, lymphoscintigraphy suggested graft patency (Fig. 159–10). This result, however, was associated with significant early reduction of the swelling in only one patient, in whom edema recurred at 2 years despite an apparently patent and functioning graft.

The 64 patients operated on by Campisi and coworkers who underwent lymphatic-venous-lymphatic grafts were studied for 5 years. Marked improvement in edema occurred in 40 (62.5%) patients, moderate improvement in 18 (28%), and mild edema regression in six (9.5%).[14] Unfortunately, graft patency was not studied in these patients. Clinical evaluation and mean volumetric assessment

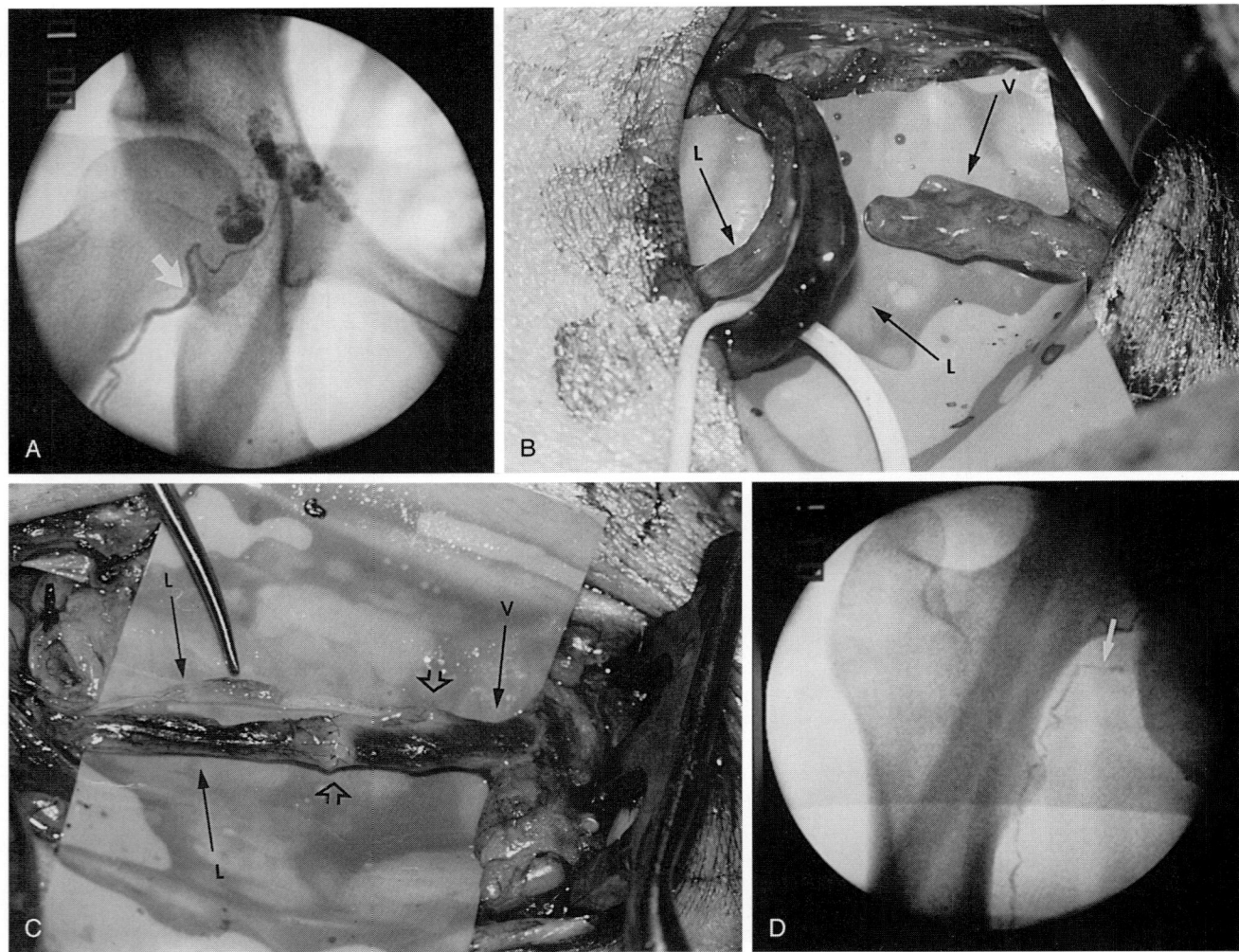

FIGURE 159–5. *A,* Localization of groin lymphatics before lymphovenous anastomosis operation. The patient underwent contrast lymphangiography 24 hours before operation. *Arrow* indicates the lymphatics selected for anastomosis. *B,* Two dilated lymphatics (L) and a tributary of the saphenous vein with a small side branch (V) were dissected for end-to-end lymphovenous anastomosis. *C,* End-to-end lymphovenous anastomosis completed between two lymph channels (L) and the bifurcated vein (V). *Open arrows* indicate the sites of the anastomoses. *D, Arrow* indicates patent lymphovenous anastomosis in the same patient. (*B* and *C,* From Gloviczki P: Treatment of secondary lymphedema—medical and surgical. *In* Ernst CB, Stanley JC [eds]: Current Therapy in Vascular Surgery, 2nd ed. Philadelphia, BC Decker, 1991, pp 1030–1036.)

of edema, however, suggest long-term improvement in most patients.

Conclusions

Meticulous microsurgical technique, fine instruments, and high-power magnification with the operating microscope enable microsurgeons to perform anastomoses between lymph vessels or between a lymph vessel and a vein with good immediate success. Although long-term improvement in patients has been reported, these results remain to be confirmed by different surgical teams and then compared with results obtained in patients treated by conservative measures. Because lymph coagulates significantly less than blood, lympholymphatic anastomoses with lymphatic grafts or venous interposition grafts into the lymphatic system have a potential advantage over lymphovenous anastomoses, in which thrombosis on the venous side may occur.

The long-term patency and function of these anastomoses in patients, however, are still unknown. More important, the main questions remain unanswered:

- Does restoring the patency of two or three lymph channels result in restoration of normal lymphatic transport?
- Does lymphovenous anastomosis or lymphatic grafting reverse changes that have already occurred in the distal lymphatic circulation, the subcutaneous tissue, or the skin of patients with chronic lymphedema?
- Is clinical improvement superior to those results obtained with current nonsurgical techniques?

Until these important questions are answered, patients should be made aware of the unproven benefit of this type of treatment.

INDIRECT LYMPHATIC RECONSTRUCTIONS

Mesenteric Bridge Operation

Patients with fibrotic occlusion or surgical excision of the iliac nodes may be candidates for the mesenteric bridge

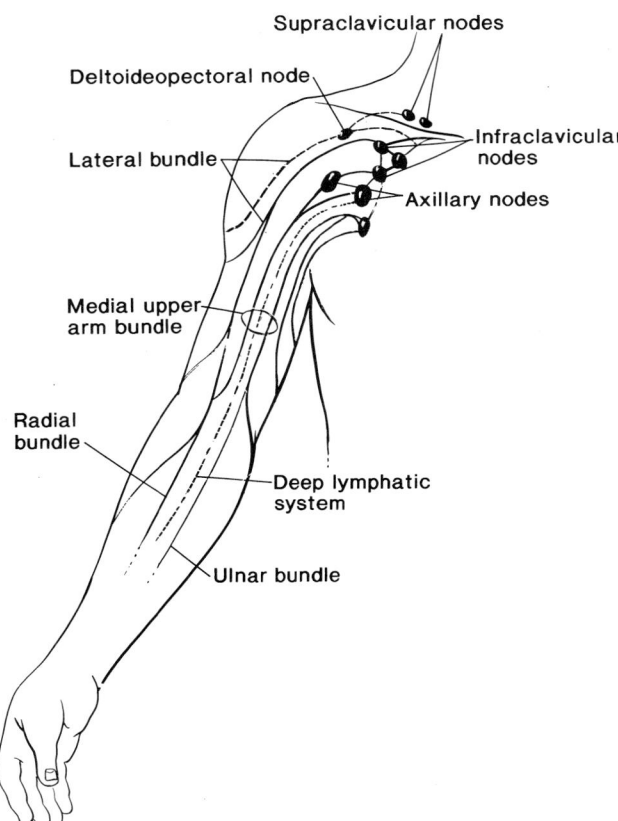

FIGURE 159–6. The lymphatic system of the upper extremity. (By permission of Mayo Foundation.)

operation. Designed by Kinmonth and colleagues, this procedure includes isolation of a segment of the ileum without division or ligation of its blood supply or lymphatic circulation (Fig. 159–11).[17] The ileum is opened longitudinally, its mucosa is removed, and the bowel wall is sewn over the transected distal iliac or inguinal nodes. The continuity of the small bowel is reestablished by end-to-end ileostomy.

Hurst and colleagues reported the late results in eight patients who underwent enteromesenteric bridge operation for ilioinguinal lymph node obliteration.[18] Significant reduction in the volume of the swollen extremity and a decrease in discomfort was noted in five of the eight patients at a follow-up that extended more than 5 years. Lymphangiographic evidence of communications between the inguinal nodes and the mesenteric lymphatic circulation was obtained in five patients. Five of eight patients also had normal lymphatic clearance with lymphoscintigraphy 5 years after the operation, as reported later by Browse.[40] Unfortunately, patients with proximal lymphatic obstruction and intact inguinal or external iliac lymph nodes are rare. As Wolfe emphasized, the lymphatic obstruction for this procedure must be quite proximal for the pedicle to reach beyond it without tension.[41] In addition, patients who have obstruction proximal to the mesenteric vessels and those with hyperplasia are not candidates for this operation.

Omental Flap

Goldsmith and associates suggested the use of an omental flap to improve lymphatic drainage of the swollen limb through spontaneous lympholymphatic anastomoses, which supposedly develop between patent lymphatics in the limb and the lymphatics of the greater omentum.[15] Using patent blue dye injected into the leg, they documented passage of the dye to the omentum 1 month after surgery. In the experiments of Danese and associates, however, contrast lymphangiography failed to demonstrate similar communications 3 months after surgery.[42] At exploration, the pedicles were found to have developed a fibrous capsule around them that prevented any communication between the leg lymphatics and the omentum.

In a follow-up study that extended up to 7 years and included 22 patients, Goldsmith admitted that poor results occurred in one third of his patients.[16] More importantly, he reported significant complications in eight patients, including wound infection, bowel obstruction, pulmonary embolization, and hernia. For these reasons, this operation has largely been abandoned as a treatment option for lymphedema.

In the more recent experiments of O'Brien and associates, however, canine lymphedema was successfully decreased

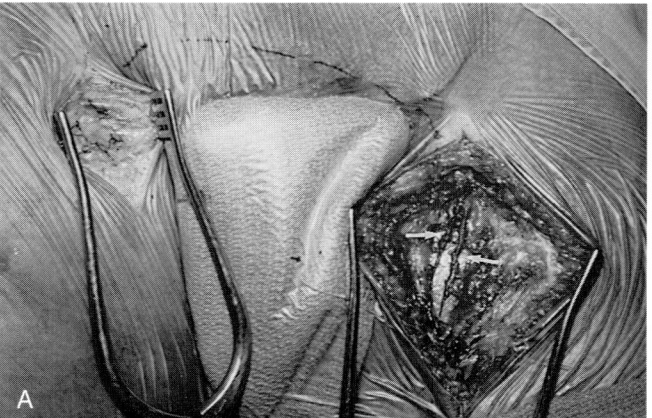
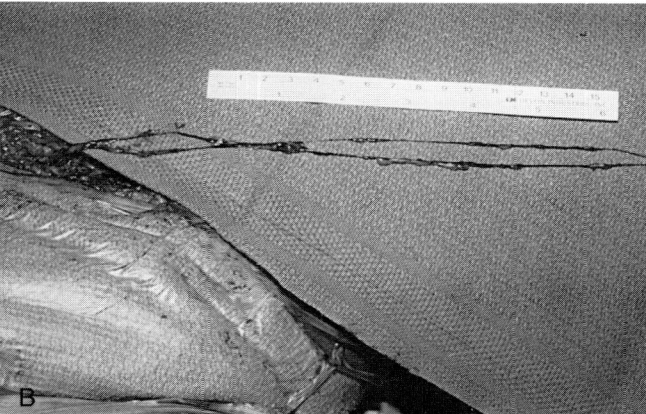

FIGURE 159–7. A, Exposure of lymph vessels for suprapubic transposition. Note two major lymph vessels of the left thigh that will be used for grafting (arrows). B, Two lymphatic grafts divided at the distal thigh are prepared for lymphatic grafting. (By permission of Mayo Foundation.)

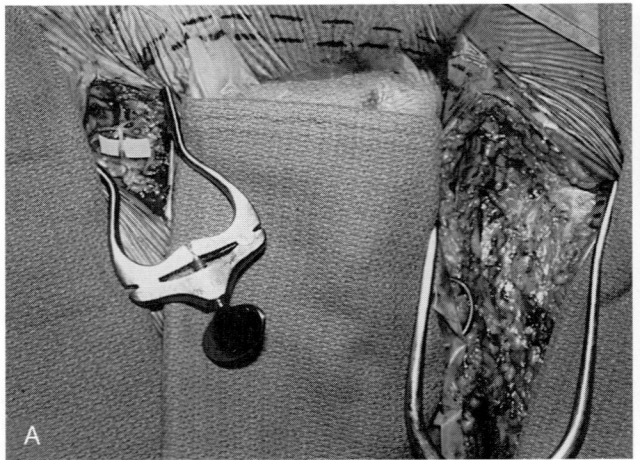
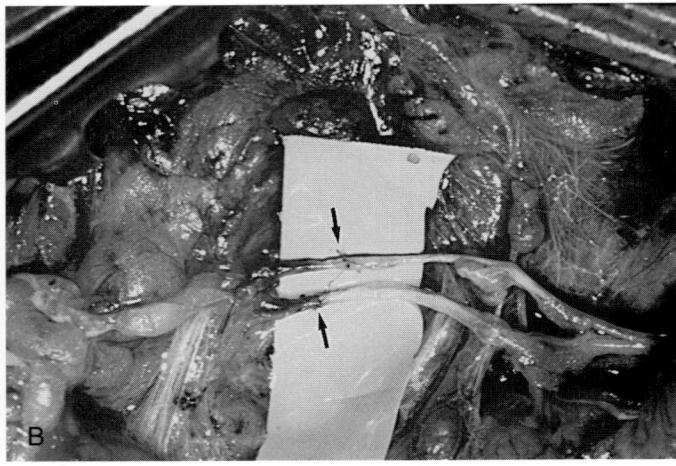

FIGURE 159–8. A, Completed suprapubic lymph graft with two lympholymphatic anastomoses at right groin. Dashed line indicates position of suprapubic lymphatic grafts. B, Magnified photograph of two end-to-end lympholymphatic anastomoses (arrows) performed with 11 = 0 interrupted monofilament sutures. (By permission of Mayo Foundation.)

by the use of a vascularized free omental flap.[43, 44] Blue dye injected into the leg 6 months after surgery could be identified in the dilated lymphatics of the omentum implanted to bridge the lymphatic defect in the lower extremity in dogs. Although whether the omentum can provide adequate lymphatic drainage continues to be controversial, the easy availability of the omentum as a vascularized flap and at least some success in experiments warrant continuation of further research.

Autotransplantation of Free Lymphatic Flap

Trevidic and Cormier performed autotransplantation of a free axillary lymph node flap from the contralateral axillary fossa to the side of the lymphedematous arm in patients with postmastectomy lymphedema.[19] The inferior axillary nodes were removed with a vascularized flap composed of

a portion of the latissimus dorsi muscle with a segment of skin. The blood supply to the flap consisted of the subscapular artery and vein. This lymphatic tissue flap was then transplanted into the supraclavicular fossa, where anastomoses were created with the subclavian artery and vein. The authors reported results in 19 patients who underwent axillary lymph node transplantation. The graft failed in one patient. Improvement was documented in 75% of patients, and direct contrast lymphography demonstrated the development of new lympholymphatic anastomoses in some patients. Lymphoscintigraphy showed improved lymphatic transport in 75% of the patients. Further experience and longer follow-up periods with this operation are needed to assess its efficacy.

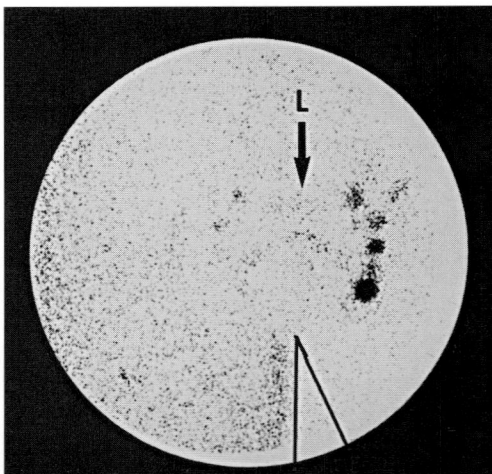

FIGURE 159–10. Lymphoscintigram 3 months after suprapubic lymphatic grafting for secondary lymphedema of the right lower extremity. Labeled colloid was injected into the right foot only. Arrow indicates suprapubic graft. Note intense filling of the left inguinal nodes. Preoperative lymphoscintigram in this patient showed no activity at the groin. L = lymphatic graft. (From Gloviczki P: Treatment of secondary lymphedema—medical and surgical. In Ernst CB, Stanley JC [eds]: Current Therapy in Vascular Surgery, 2nd ed. Philadelphia, BC Decker, 1991, pp 1030–1036.)

FIGURE 159–9. Techniques of lymphatic reconstructions according to Campisi with interposition vein graft (A) or lymphovenous anastomosis (B). C, Technique of invagination of multiple lymphatics into interposition vein graft (lymphatic-venous-lymphatic anastomoses). (By permission of Mayo Foundation.)

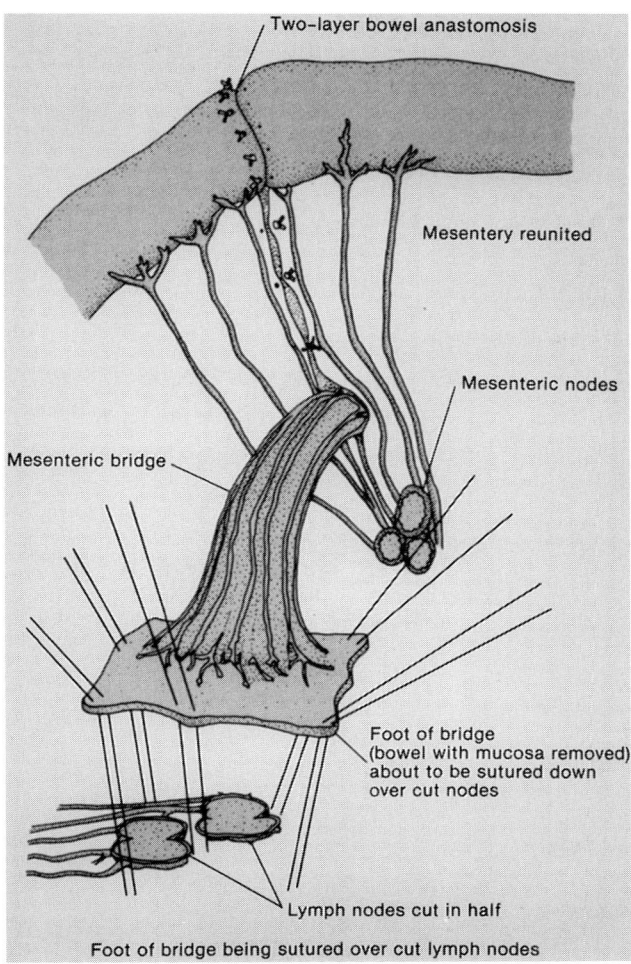

Two-layer bowel anastomosis

Mesentery reunited

Mesenteric nodes

Mesenteric bridge

Foot of bridge
(bowel with mucosa removed)
about to be sutured down
over cut nodes

Lymph nodes cut in half

Foot of bridge being sutured over cut lymph nodes

FIGURE 159–11. Technique of mesenteric bridge operation.

Conclusions

Because of the paucity of lymphatics in the omentum and the reported complications with omental flaps, the authors do not recommend omentoplasty for the treatment of lymphedema. The complexity of the mesenteric bridge operation, its possible complications, and the small number of suitable patients limit acceptance of this procedure as well. The most promising operation among indirect reconstructions of the lymphatic drainage remains autotransplantation of a free vascularized lymphatic flap. The rich lymphatic tissue in the axillary flap provides the best opportunity for the spontaneous development of lympholymphatic anastomoses. Further research with this operation, therefore, is clearly warranted.

OPERATIONS FOR PRIMARY CHYLOUS DISORDERS

Chylous disorders are characterized by an accumulation of chyle in abnormal areas of the body. Chylous ascites, chylothorax, or chylocutaneous fistula may be caused by malignant tumors, most frequently lymphoma, or by

trauma to the mesenteric lymphatics or the thoracic duct, which may also occur during vascular surgical procedures as discussed in detail in Chapter 40.

Primary chylous disorders are usually caused by congenital lymphangiectasia or megalymphatics, which in some patients are associated with obstruction of the thoracic duct. In patients with lymphangiectasia and lymphatic valvular incompetence, chyle may reflux into the lower extremities, the perineum, or the genitalia.[45–49] Depending on the site of the dilated lymphatics and the site of the chylous leak, these patients may also have protein-losing enteropathy, chylous ascites, chylothorax, chylopericardium, or reflux of chyle into the lungs and tracheobronchial tree.[45–51] Medical treatment is aimed at decreasing production of chyle by means of a medium-chain triglyceride diet or occasionally by parenteral nutrition (see Chapter 156). Repletion of proteins and calcium lost with chyle is as important as the need to strengthen the defense mechanism of the body because lymphocytes and important immunoglobulins are also wasted in these patients. Only surgical treatment can provide long-term improvement and occasionally cure by ligation of the incompetent retroperitoneal lymph vessels and oversewing of the site of the lymphatic leak. In some patients, attempts to reconstruct the obstructed thoracic duct by creation of thoracic duct–azygos vein anastomoses have also been reported.

Chylous Reflux Into the Lower Extremity or Genitalia

Although many patients with lymphangiectasia and reflux of chyle have lower extremity lymphedema that is unilateral in most cases, the main discomfort for the patients is intermittent or continuous discharge of chyle from cutaneous vesicles in the lower extremity or in the genitalia. The first five patients known to have suffered from this rare condition were described in 1949 by Servelle and Deysson.[52]

Preoperative evaluation of patients with chylous reflux into the lower extremity or genitalia should include lymphoscintigraphy (Fig. 159–12A).[53] Contrast lymphangiography, however, is the definitive test to confirm the diagnosis and to localize the dilated retroperitoneal lymphatics and, frequently, also the site of the lymphatic leak. Radical excision and ligation of the incompetent retroperitoneal lymph vessels is the only effective technique for controlling reflux of the chyle and its drainage through skin vesicles in the perineum, labia, scrotum, or lower extremity. The authors' group uses the technique of Servelle and performs the entire reflux operation in two stages through flank incisions using the retroperitoneal approach.[46] Four hours before the procedure, the patient ingests 60 gm of butter and drinks 8 ounces of whipping cream. The fatty meal allows ready visualization of the retroperitoneal lymphatics during exploration (Fig. 159–12B–D). Ligation of the lymph vessels should be done with the utmost care to avoid tearing or avulsing the lymphatics, resulting in residual leaks or rupture. In recent years, sclerotherapy of the dilated lymphatics has been added to ligation to increase efficacy of the operation. Tetracycline solution, 500 to 1000 mg diluted in 20 ml of normal saline, is injected directly

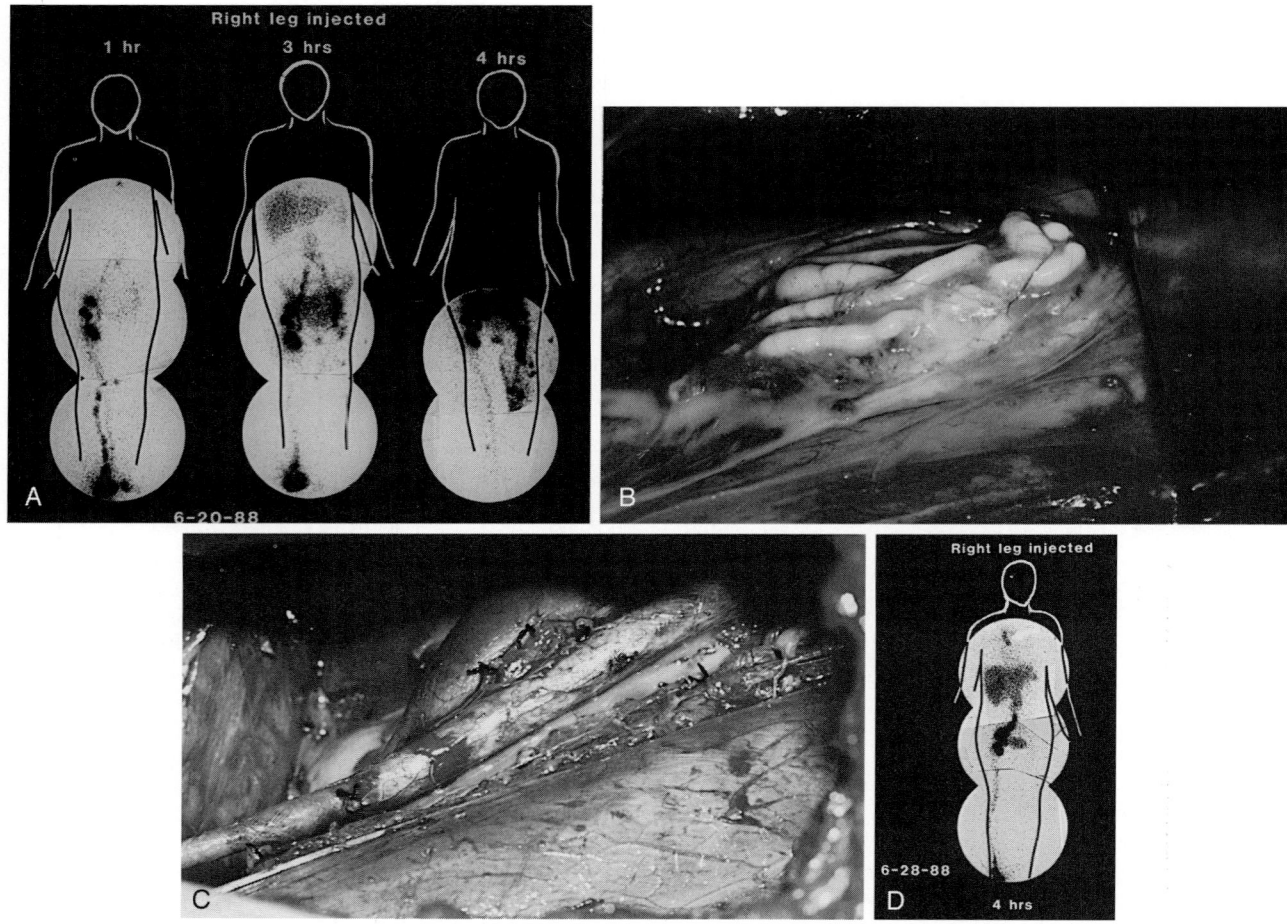

FIGURE 159–12. *A*, Right lower extremity lymphoscintigram in a 16-year-old female with lymphangiectasia and severe reflux into the genitalia and left lower extremity. Injection of the isotope into the right foot reveals reflux into the pelvis at 3 hours and into the left lower extremity at 4 hours. *B*, Intraoperative photograph reveals dilated incompetent retroperitoneal lymphatics in the left iliac fossa containing chyle. *C*, Radical excision and ligation of the lymph vessels were performed. In addition, two lymphovenous anastomoses were also performed between two dilated lymphatics and two lumbar veins. *D*, Postoperative lymphoscintigram performed in a similar fashion reveals no evidence of reflux at 4 hours. The patient has no significant reflux 4 years after surgery. (*A–D*, From Gloviczki P, et al: Noninvasive evaluation of the swollen extremity: Experiences with 190 lymphoscintigraphic examinations. J Vasc Surg 9:683, 1989.)

into the dilated retroperitoneal lymph vessels to provoke obstructive lymphangitis.

As reported by Molitch and associates, percutaneous computed tomography (CT)-guided or magnetic resonance imaging (MRI)-guided cannulation of these dilated lymphatics may also be possible, and sclerotherapy to decrease reflux can be performed repeatedly, if necessary.[54] Lymphovenous anastomoses with the dilated lymphatics can also be performed. Reflux of blood into the dilated and incompetent lymphatics, however, can occur. A competent valve on the venous side completely avoids reflux and increases the chance of successful lymphatic drainage.[50, 55]

Results

The largest group of patients studied was reported by Servelle, who operated on 55 patients with chylous reflux into the lower extremity or genitalia and reported durable benefit in most patients.[46] In a series of 19 patients who underwent ligation of the retroperitoneal lymphatics for chylous reflux to the limbs and genitalia by Kinmonth, permanent cure was achieved in five patients and alleviation of symptoms, frequently after several operations, in 12 patients.[45] No improvement or failure was noted in only two cases.

Chylous Ascites

Chylous ascites usually results from intraperitoneal rupture of the mesenteric or retroperitoneal lymphatics or from exudation of the chyle into the peritoneal cavity.[49] Evaluation of such patients should include CT or magnetic resonance imaging (MRI) to exclude abdominal malignancy. The diagnosis of lymphangiectasia is confirmed by bipedal contrast lymphangiography. Paracentesis is both diagnostic and therapeutic. If conservative measures fail and ascites returns, abdominal exploration should be performed after a fatty meal as described previously. If chylous ascites is due to primary lymphangiectasia, abdominal exploration may reveal ruptured lymphatics, which can be oversewn. In some patients, large chylous cysts develop, which should be excised (Fig. 159–13). If the condition is associated with protein-losing enteropathy and the disease is localized to a segment of the small bowel, the bowel segment should be resected.

The outcome of the operation usually is good if a well-defined abdominal fistula is found. If the mesenteric lymphatic trunks are fibrosed, aplastic, or hypoplastic and exudation of the chyle is the main source of the ascites, however, the prognosis is poor and recurrence is frequent. In these patients, an attempt to control the ascites using a LeVeen's peritoneal-venous shunt should be made. Results with peritoneal-venous shunts have been mixed. It is noteworthy that in the experience of Browse and coworkers with nine peritoneal-venous shunts, all became occluded within 3 to 6 months after insertion.[49]

Chylothorax

As with chylous ascites, the most frequent cause of chylothorax is trauma or malignant disease.[45] Primary lymphatic disorders that cause chylothorax include lymphangiectasia

with or without thoracic duct obstruction. However, chylothorax may also result from chylous ascites passing through the diaphragm. In these patients, the chylothorax is cured when the chylous ascites is controlled. Preoperative lymphangiography in these patients should be performed because it may localize the site of the chylous fistula or document occlusion of the thoracic duct (Fig. 159–14).

Thoracentesis usually is not effective in curing the disease, and chyle that leaks from the thoracic duct or one of the large intercostal, mediastinal, or diaphragmatic collaterals reaccumulates. Injection of tetracycline is frequently ineffective because it is diluted by the leaking chyle. The best treatment for chylothorax is surgical pleurodesis with excision of the parietal pleura and prolonged pleural suction.[52] During thoracotomy, which is performed after a fatty meal, a careful search for the leaking lymphatics should be undertaken, and the site of the leak should be oversewn.

Thoracic Duct Reconstruction

If occlusion of the cervical or upper thoracic duct (Fig. 159–15) is the cause of lymphangiectasia and reflux of chyle into the pleural or peritoneal cavity, thoracic duct–azygos vein anastomosis can be attempted to reconstruct the duct and to improve lymphatic transport. Preoperative imaging of the duct with contrast pedal lymphangiography is important because if occlusion of the entire duct is present it precludes anastomoses.

The operation is performed through a right posterolateral thoracotomy, and the anastomosis between the lower thoracic duct and the azygos vein is performed in an end-to-end fashion with 8-0 or 10-0 nonabsorbable interrupted sutures and magnification with a loupes or operating microscope. Only a few patients undergoing this operation have been reported.[45, 53] Both patients operated on by the authors' group had good immediate patency, and excellent flow of chyle was observed through the anastomosis intraoperatively (Fig. 159–16). Although none had postoperative contrast lymphangiography, the recurrent chylothorax that was the main indication for the procedure ultimately resolved in both. Browse reported two successes in three patients who underwent thoracic duct reconstruction.[53] Kinmonth performed this procedure in two patients, however, and concluded that the anastomosis alone is not effective for decompressing the thoracic duct; ligation of the abnormal mediastinal lymphatics and oversewing of the sites of the lymphatic leak are also necessary.[45]

SUMMARY

Primary chylous disorders are fortunately rare. The underlying abnormality usually is congenital lymphangiectasia and fibrotic occlusion or atresia of the thoracic duct. Surgical treatment is frequently the only effective way to control chylous reflux or leak, and ligation of the incompetent retroperitoneal lymphatics and oversewing of the ruptured lymphatics can produce long-term improvement or even cure in many patients. In selected symptomatic patients with obstruction of the thoracic duct, a thoracic duct–azygos vein anastomosis may be considered as a surgical option.

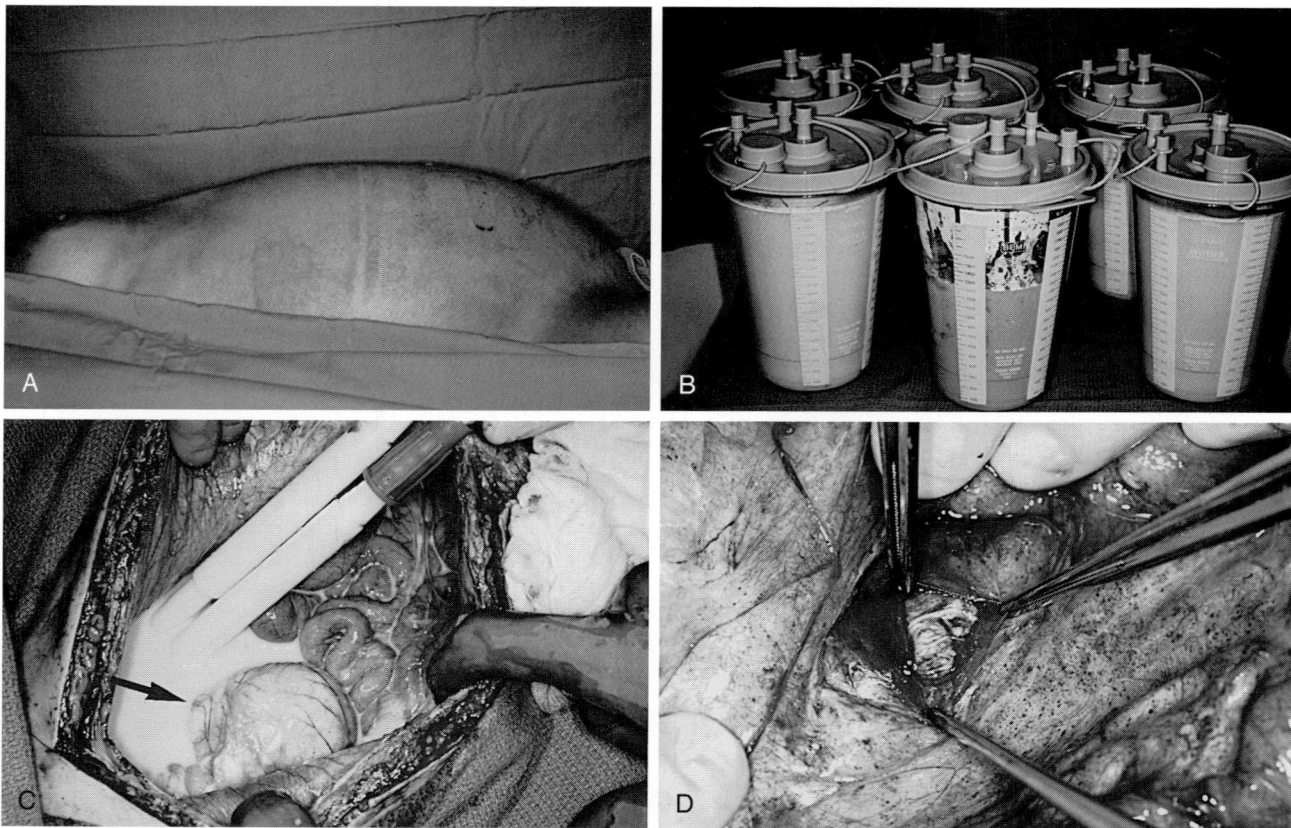

FIGURE 159–13. *A*, Preoperative photograph of an 18-year-old female with lymphangiectasia and recurrent chylous ascites. *B*, During the operation, 12 L of chyle was aspirated from the abdomen. *C*, The chylous ascites was caused by ruptured lymphatic and leaking large mesenteric lymphatic cysts (*arrow*). *D*, The dilated retroperitoneal lymphatics containing chyle were ligated and excised. The patient has an excellent clinical result 8 months after the operation.

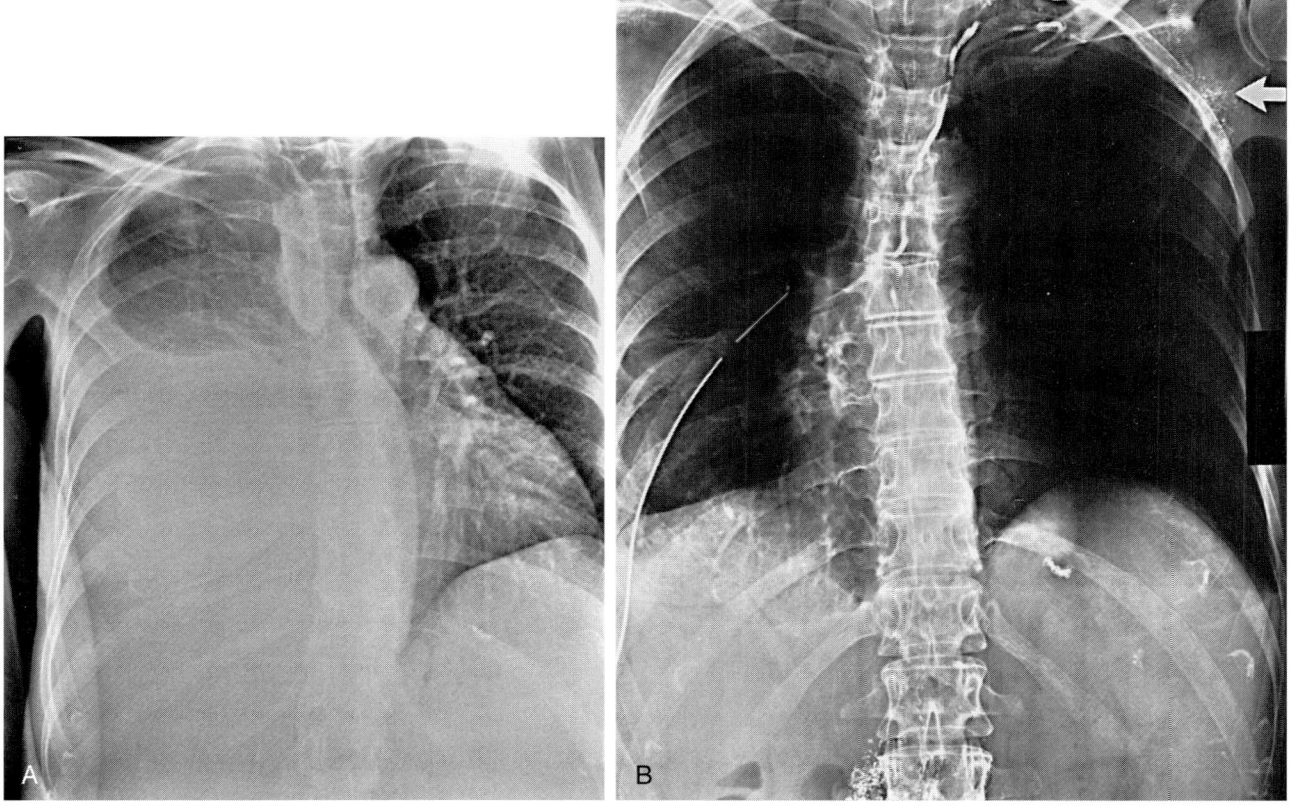

FIGURE 159–14. *A*, Right chylothorax in a 63-year-old woman. *B*, Bipedal lymphangiography confirmed thoracic duct obstruction at the base of the neck. Note contrast in the supraclavicular and left axillary lymphatics (*arrows*).

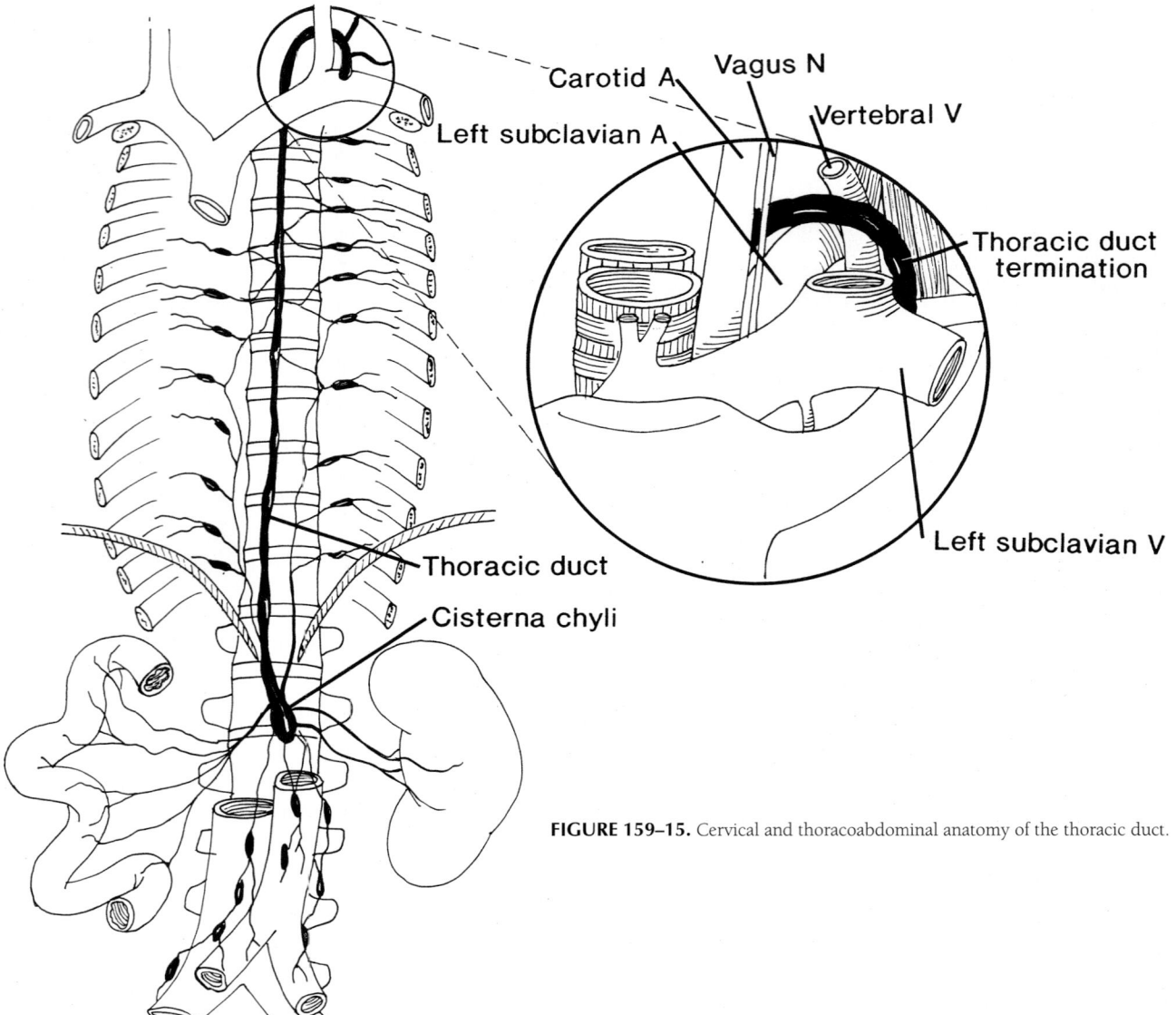

Carotid A.

Vagus N

Left subclavian A

Vertebral V

Thoracic duct termination

Thoracic duct

Cisterna chyli

Left subclavian V

FIGURE 159–15. Cervical and thoracoabdominal anatomy of the thoracic duct.

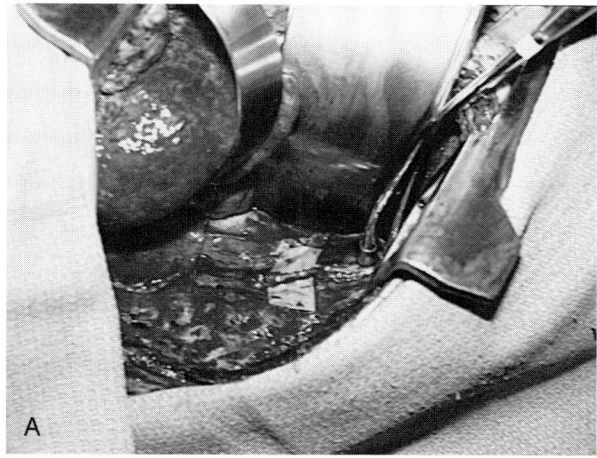
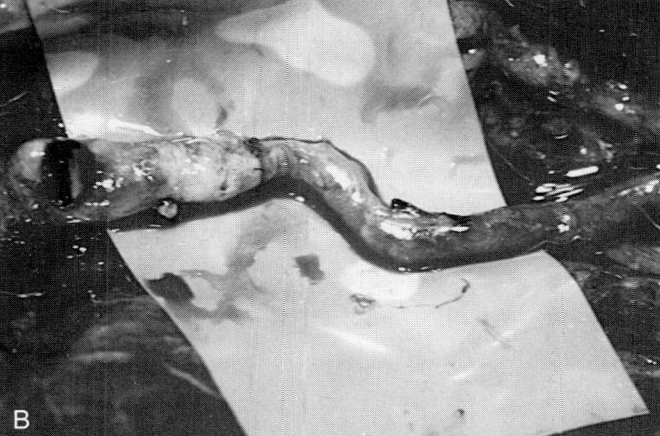
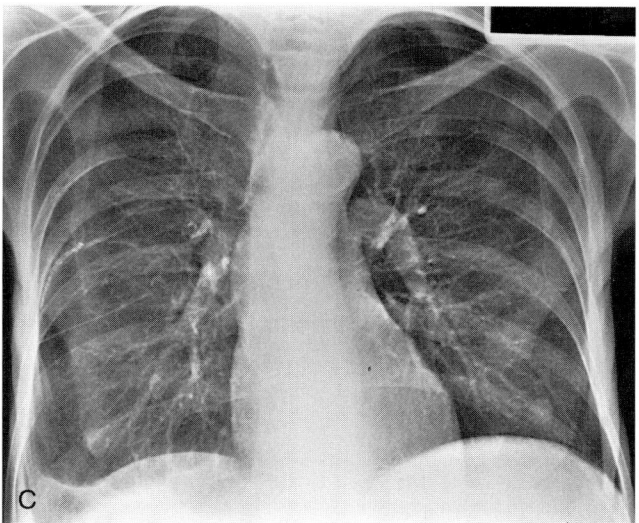

FIGURE 159–16. *A* and *B*, Thoracic duct–azygos vein anastomosis performed through a right posterolateral thoracotomy in an end-to-end fashion with interrupted 8-0 polypropylene (Prolene) sutures. *C*, Chest roentgenogram 2 years later confirms absence of chylothorax.

REFERENCES

1. O'Brien BMC, Shafiroff BB: Microlymphaticovenous and resectional surgery in obstructive lymphedema. World J Surg 3:3, 1979.
2. Huang GK, Ru-Qi H, Zong-Zhao L, et al: Microlymphaticovenous anastomosis for treating lymphedema of the extremities and external genitalia. J Microsurg 3:32, 1981.
3. Jamal S: Lymphovenous anastomosis in filarial lymphedema. Lymphology 14:64, 1981.
4. Krylov V, Milanov N, Abalmasov K: Microlymphatic surgery of secondary lymphoedema of the upper limb. Ann Chir Gynaecol 71:77, 1982.
5. Nieuborg L: The Role of Lymphaticovenous Anastomoses in the Treatment of Postmastectomy Oedema. Alblasserdam, The Netherlands, Offsetdrukkerij Kanters BV, 1982.
6. Gong-Kang H, Ru-Qi H, Zong-Zhao L, et al: Microlymphaticovenous anastomosis in the treatment of lower limb obstructive lymphedema: Analysis of 91 cases. Plast Reconstr Surg 76:671, 1985.
7. Ingianni G, Holzmann T: Clinical experience with lymphovenous anastomosis for secondary lymphedema. Handchirurgie 17:43, 1985.
8. Campisi C, Tosatti E, Casaccia M, et al: Lymphatic microsurgery. Minerva Chir 41:469, 1986.
9. Zhu JK, Yu GZ, Liu JX, et al: Recent advances in microlymphatic surgery in China. Clin Orthop 215:32, 1987.
10. Gloviczki P, Fisher J, Hollier LH, et al: Microsurgical lymphovenous anastomosis for treatment of lymphedema: A critical review. J Vasc Surg 7:647, 1988.
11. Ipsen T, Pless J, Fredericksen PB: Experience with microlymphatico-
venous anastomoses for congenital and acquired lymphoedema. Scand J Plast Reconstr Surg 22:233, 1988.
12. O'Brien BM, Mellow CG, Khazanchi RK, et al: Long-term results after microlymphaticovenous anastomoses for the treatment of obstructive lymphedema. Plast Reconstr Surg 85:562, 1990.
13. Baumeister RG, Siuda S: Treatment of lymphedemas by microsurgical lymphatic grafting: What is proved? Plast Reconstr Surg 85:64, 1990.
14. Campisi C, Boccardo F, Tacchella M: Reconstructive microsurgery of lymph vessels: The personal method of lymphatic-venous-lymphatic (LVL) interpositioned grafted shunt. Microsurgery 16:161, 1995.
15. Goldsmith HS, De Los Santos R, Beattie EJ: Relief of chronic lymphoedema by omental transposition. JAMA 203:19, 1968.
16. Goldsmith HS: Long term evaluation of omental transposition for chronic lymphedema. Ann Surg 180:847, 1974.
17. Kinmonth JB, Hurst PAE, Edwards JM, Rutt DL: Relief of lymph obstruction by use of a bridge of mesentery and ileum. Br J Surg 65:829, 1978.
18. Hurst PA, Stewart G, Kinmonth JB, Browse NL: Long-term results of the enteromesenteric bridge operation in the treatment of primary lymphoedema. Br J Surg 72:272, 1985.
19. Trevidic P, Cormier JM: Free axillary lymph node transfer. In Cluzan RV (ed): Progress in Lymphology. Vol 13. Amsterdam, Elsevier Science Publishers, 1992, pp 415–420.
20. Edwards JM, Kinmonth JB: Lymphovenous shunts in man. Br Med J 4:579, 1969.
21. Nielubowicz J, Olszewski W: Surgical lymphaticovenous shunts in patients with secondary lymphoedema. Br J Surg 55:440, 1968.
22. Olszewski W, Clodius L, Földi M: The enigma of lymphedema—a search for answers. Lymphology 24:100, 1991.
23. Calderon G, Roberts B, Johnson LL: Experimental approach to the

surgical creation of lymphatic-venous communications. Surgery 61:122, 1967.

24. Jacobson JH: Discussion. Arch Surg 84:9, 1962.

25. Laine JB, Howard JM: Experimental lymphatico-venous anastomosis. Surg Forum 14:111, 1963.

26. Yamada Y: The studies on lymphatic venous anastomosis in lymphedema. Nagoya J Med Sci 32:1, 1969.

27. Gilbert A, O'Brien BM, Vorrath JW, Sykes PJ: Lymphaticovenous anastomosis by microvascular technique. Br J Plast Surg 29:355, 1976.

28. Gloviczki P, LeFloch P, Hidden G: Anastomoses lymphaticoveineuses experimentales. J Chir (Paris) 116:437, 1979.

29. Gloviczki P, Hollier LH, Nora FE, Kaye MP: The natural history of microsurgical lymphovenous anastomoses: An experimental study. J Vasc Surg 4:148, 1986.

30. Puckett CL, Jacobs GR, Hurvitz JS, Silver D: Evaluation of lymphovenous anastomoses in obstructive lymphedema. Plast Reconstr Surg 66:116, 1980.

31. Shaper NJ, Rutt DR, Browse NL: Use of Teflon stents for lymphovenous anastomosis. Br J Surg 79:633, 1992.

32. Cambria RA, Gloviczki P, Naessens JM, Wahner HW: Noninvasive evaluation of the lymphatic system with lymphoscintigraphy: A prospective, semiquantitative analysis in 386 extremities. J Vasc Surg 18:773, 1993.

33. Baumeister RG, Seifert J, Wiebecke B: Homologous and autologous experimental lymph vessel transplantation—initial experience. Int J Microsurg 3:19, 1981.

34. Baumeister RG, Seifert J: Microsurgical lymph vessel transplantation for the treatment of lymphedema: Experimental and first clinical experiences. Lymphology 14:90, 1981.

35. Baumeister RG, Siuda S, Bohmert H, Moser E: A microsurgical method for reconstruction of interrupted lymphatic pathways: Autologous lymph-vessel transplantation for treatment of lymphedemas. Scand J Plast Reconstr Surg 20:141, 1986.

36. Kleinhans E, Baumeister RGH, Hahn D, et al: Evaluation of transport kinetics in lymphoscintigraphy: Follow-up study in patients with transplanted lymphatic vessels. Eur J Nucl Med 10:349, 1985.

37. Baumeister RGH, Frick A, Hofmann T: 10 years experience with autogenous microsurgical lymph vessel transplantation. Eur J Lymphol 6:62, 1991.

38. Baumeister RGH, Fink U, Tatsch K, Frick A: Microsurgical lymphatic grafting: First demonstration of patent grafts by indirect lymphography and long term follow-up studies. Lymphology (Suppl) 27:787, 1994.

39. Kinjo O, Kusara A: Lymphatic vessel-to-isolated-vein anastomosis for secondary lymphedema in a canine model. Surg Today 25:633, 1995.

40. Browse NL: The diagnosis and management of primary lymphedema. J Vasc Surg 3:181, 1986.

41. Wolfe JHN: Treatment of lymphedema. In Rutherford RB (ed): Vascular Surgery, 3rd ed. Philadelphia, WB Saunders, 1989, pp 1668–1678.

42. Danese CA, Papioannou AN, Morales LE, Mitsuda S: Surgical approaches to lymphatic blocks. Surgery 64:821, 1968.

43. O'Brien BM, Hickey MJ, Dvir E, et al: Microsurgical transfer of greater omentum in the treatment of canine lymphoedema. Br J Plast Surg 43:440, 1990.

44. Knight KR, Hurley JV, Hickey MJ, et al: Combined coumarin and omental transfer treatment for canine proximal obstructive lymphoedema. Int J Exp Pathol 72:533, 1991.

45. Kinmonth JB: Chylous diseases and syndromes, including references to tropical elephantiasis. In Kinmonth JB (ed): The Lymphatics: Surgery, Lymphography and Diseases of the Chyle and Lymph Systems, 2nd ed. London, Edward Arnold, 1982, pp 221–268.

46. Servelle M: Surgical treatment of lymphedema: A report on 652 cases. Surgery 101:485, 1987.

47. Servelle M: Congenital malformation of the lymphatics of the small intestine. J Cardiovasc Surg 32:159, 1991.

48. Kinmonth JB, Cox SJ: Protein losing enteropathy in lymphedema Surgical investigation and treatment. J Cardiovasc Surg 16:111, 1975.

49. Browse NL, Wilson NM, Russo F, et al: Aetiology and treatment of chylous ascites. Br J Surg 79:1145, 1992.

50. Gloviczki P, Soltesz L, Solti F, et al: The surgical treatment of lymphedema caused by chylous reflux. In Bartos V, Davidson JW (eds): Advances in Lymphology. Proceedings of the 8th International Congress of Lymphology, Montreal, 1981. Prague, Czechoslovak Medical Press, 1982, pp 502–507.

51. Sanders JS, Rosenow EC III, Piehler JM, et al: Chyloptysis (chylous sputum) due to thoracic lymphangiectasia with successful surgical correction. Arch Intern Med 148:1465, 1988.

52. Servelle M, Deysson H: Reflux du chyle dans les lymphatiques jambiers. Arch Mal Coeur 12:1181, 1949.

53. Browse NL: The surgery of lymphedema. In Veith FJ (ed): Current Critical Problems in Vascular Surgery. St. Louis, Quality Medical Publishing, 1989, pp 408–409.

54. Molitch HI, Unger EC, Witte CL, vanSonnenberg E: Percutaneous sclerotherapy of lymphangiomas. Radiology 194:343, 1995.

55. Gloviczki P, Calcagno D, Schirger A, et al: Noninvasive evaluation of the swollen extremity: Experiences with 190 lymphoscintigraphic examinations. J Vasc Surg 9:683, 1989.

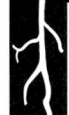

C H A P T E R   1 6 0

Overview of Extremity Amputations

William C. Krupski, M.D.

Although improved limb salvage rates for patients with peripheral vascular disease have improved substantially, amputation may be the only practical treatment for a limb severely affected by trauma, infection, tumor, or the end stages of ischemia. Unfortunately, vascular surgeons have traditionally viewed amputations as manifestations of failure—failure to comprehend or control the disease process, failure of the referring physician or patient to seek help in a timely fashion, or failure of the vascular surgeon to perform successful revascularization. This negative bias should be condemned because it may contribute to the poor results reported in many series of major limb amputations in contrast to the advances made in arterial reconstructions. Instead, amputation surgery should be considered an important *reconstructive* surgical technique in the total management of patients with limb-threatening disorders of the extremities.

Currently, most patients with peripheral vascular occlusive disease have had a previous bypass graft, some other arterial reconstruction such as profundaplasty or thromboendarterectomy, or a percutaneous endovascular procedure such as transluminal angioplasty or atherectomy that was either unsuccessful or failed after a variable length of time. Although there has been recent interest in therapeutic angiogenesis by direct injection of vascular endothelial growth factor (VEGF), this experimental treatment for patients with profound ischemia after failed arterial reconstructions or for those with unreconstructable vascular disease is far from clinical application.[37] For these patients and for those who present with extensive tissue necrosis or infection, amputation may be preferable to increasingly complex reoperative vascular reconstructions, which carry attendant risks of morbidity and death. The decision to amputate limbs rather than to attempt revascularization must be individualized and is often complicated and difficult. Importantly, the patient must actively participate in making this judgment.

The immediate aims of amputation are (1) removal of diseased tissue; (2) relief of pain; (3) primary healing of the amputation at the level chosen; and (4) construction of a stump and provision of a prosthesis that will permit useful function. The purpose of this overview is to provide historical perspective and background and to introduce the detailed chapters that follow.

HISTORICAL PERSPECTIVE

The history of amputation surgery is long and colorful (Table 160–1). In neolithic times and in pre-Columbian America (as well as in some parts of the world today) it was a religious ritual or a form of punishment.[8, 19] In the Babylonian era, the hands of the surgeon whose treatment caused blindness or death were amputated.[3] Hammurabi (King of Babylon in 1792–1750 B.C.) dictated that if a surgeon caused blindness, serious injury, or death in a free man, the surgeon's hands were cut off, whereas he was required only to replace a slave who died under his care.

Hippocrates (c. 460–370 B.C.) first reported extremity amputation as treatment for disease in patients with gangrene after vascular occlusion.[2] He advised amputation through devitalized tissue to avoid the greater risk of hemorrhage when cutting through living tissue. The Roman aristocrat and historian Aulus Cornelius Celsus (c. A.D. 25–50), often mistaken for a physician because of his meticulous treatises on medical subjects, elucidated important principles of amputation surgery. He proposed amputation through viable tissue, use of a rasp to smooth bone, and use of hemostatic ligatures.[42] In the latter part of the first century, Archigenes of Apamea, who lived under the rule of Emperor Trajan, advocated identification and ligation of blood vessels *before* completing an amputation.[31] Only if hemorrhage persisted did he resort to cautery with hot irons or boiling water.

The introduction of gunpowder in 1338 resulted in an unprecedented number of severe battle wounds requiring amputation.[3] Much of modern surgery was developed from lessons learned from war. Thus, it is not surprising that a

TABLE 160–1. SOME IMPORTANT EVENTS IN AMPUTATION SURGERY

ERA	NOTABLE INDIVIDUALS	DATES	EVENTS
Babylonian	Hammurabi	1792–1750 B.C.	Amputation as punishment
Greek	Hippocrates	c. 460–370 B.C.	First medical amputation
Roman	Celsus	c. A.D. 25–50	Amputation through viable tissue, hemostatic ligatures
Middle Ages	Hans von Gerssdorf	1485–1545	Opium for amputation, postoperative pressure dressings
Renaissance	Ambroise Paré	1510–1590	Abandoned scalding oil and reintroduced ligatures for hemostasis; designed prostheses; attention to rehabilitation
The "Enlightenment"	John Hunter	1728–1793	Surgeon-scientist, opposed primary amputation
Napoleonic wars	Dominique Jean Larrey	1766–1842	Expeditious evacuations of wounded; advocated primary amputation, débridement and healing by secondary intention
U.S. Civil War	Samuel D. Gross	1861–1865	Advised amputation of compound fractures, ignored asepsis
Franco-Prussian War	Joseph Lister	1827–1912	Successful treatment of compound fractures with carbolic acid dressings
World War I	Alexis Carrel	1914–1918	Abandonment of prophylactic amputation of compound fractures; developed Carrel-Dakin solution
World War II	Michael DeBakey	1939–1945	Blood banks, antibiotics; below-knee amputation more common than above-knee amputation
Korean conflict	"MASH" units	1950–1953	Sharp fall in amputation rate because of arterial injury repair
Vietnam War	Norman Rich	1965–1975	Improved vascular techniques; rapid evacuation
Post-Vietnam	Ernest Burgess	1975–present	Replantation, improved prostheses and rehabilitation

From Krupski WC, Bass A: Amputations for traumatic vascular injury. In Bongard FS, Wilson SE, Perry MO (eds): Vascular Injuries in Surgical Practice. San Mateo, Calif, Appleton & Lange, 1991, pp 313–325.

German military surgeon, Hans von Gerssdorf, became a preeminent amputation surgeon, performing over 200 amputations for gangrene or erysipelas.[61] His two major contributions to amputation surgery were the administration of opium prior to the operation and the use of a pressure bandage fashioned from an ox bladder to reduce postoperative bleeding.

Ambroise Paré (1510–1590), the distinguished father of French surgery, ranks as one of the Renaissance's most acclaimed surgeons whose contributions to amputation surgery are legendary. His accomplishments include (1) discontinuation of application of scalding oil for hemostasis, (2) reintroduction of hemostatic ligatures, (3) classification of amputation as a reconstructive procedure, (4) suggestion that amputation be performed through viable tissue, (5) description of phantom limb pain, (6) selection of amputation levels based on later prosthetic use, and (7) design of several upper and lower extremity prostheses.[20] Delivering advice that is equally befitting today, Paré wrote, "You say that tying up the blood vessels after amputation is a new method, and should therefore not be used. That is a bad argument for a doctor."[22]

Celsus had written about circular amputation incisions in the 11th century. This technique remained standard for 1600 years, until Verdusi (1696), Ravaton (1749), and Vermale (1765) advocated longitudinal incisions for the purpose of creating flaps for improved coverage of bone.[31, 42, 56] During this era, surgeons debated the proper timing of amputation for traumatic injuries. Some advocated primary amputation on the battlefield to prevent the fatal complications attendant from compound fractures and gangrene. Opponents argued that it was preferable to allow patients to recover from the initial trauma before imposing another injury.[3] Ironically, the brilliant London surgeon John Hunter (1728–1793), renowned for his contributions to our understanding of the physiology of collateral circulation and repair of peripheral arterial aneurysms, was an ardent pro-

ponent of delayed amputation; his recommendations strongly influenced surgical practice in his day.[26]

At the age of 22 years, Pierre Joseph Desault (1744–1795) was already chief surgeon at the Hotel Dieu hospital in Paris. Although he became well known for private lectures, he later abandoned this teaching method in favor of bedside teaching. He spent much of his career observing wound healing and introduced the term débridement for treatment of traumatic wounds. Desault's most famous student, Dominique Jean Larrey (1766–1842), became Napolean's chief surgeon. Larrey accompanied Napolean's troops in 400 skirmishes, 60 major battles, and 25 campaigns.[17] In Borodino on the road to Moscow, during the first great battle of the Russian campaign, Larrey performed 200 amputations in 24 hours—averaging one amputation every 7 minutes![3] On the Russian front, he learned to pack the amputation stump in ice and snow to decrease pain. Larrey contributed greatly to amputation and trauma surgery. He recognized the importance of prompt treatment after injury and developed the ambulance volante ("flying ambulance") corps of the French army to expedite evacuation of the wounded, who otherwise often remained unattended on the battlefield for days waiting for the fighting to end.[34] Larrey was also the first to perform amputation at the hip. He advocated (1) extensive wound débridement, (2) removal of all foreign bodies, (3) delayed amputation only in severely infected wounds, (4) closure of traumatic wounds by secondary intention, (5) immobilization of extremities to promote healing, and (6) therapeutic wound débridement with maggots.[3, 22] Remarkably, these achievements preceded the development of anesthesia or asepsis.

When ether and chloroform were introduced in 1846 and 1847, respectively, the need for excessive haste in performing amputations disappeared. On one occasion, the endeavor to complete the procedure with extraordinary speed resulted in amputation of not only the patient's extremity but also both his testicles and two fingers of an assistant![56] Robert Liston (1794–1847) routinely performed amputations in less than 30 seconds, holding the knife in his mouth.[3]

The catastrophic suffering in the American Civil War motivated interest in amputation surgery among American surgeons. Samuel D. Gross, the acclaimed Civil War surgeon and educator, published a treatise on amputations in 1862 that echoed the tenets proposed 50 years earlier by Larrey. Nevertheless, more limbs were lost by American soldiers in the Civil War than in any other military conflict, despite continuing development of more destructive weapons. Confederate soldiers suffered an estimated 25,000 major amputations, while in the Union army about 21,000 major amputations were performed.[3, 44] The mortality for major amputations approached 80% because of the staggeringly high incidence of postoperative wound infection.[30]

In 1865, Joseph Lister (1827–1912) reported successful treatment of 11 patients with compound fractures using occlusive dressings soaked in carbolic acid.[35] The surgical community was subsequently divided between those who advocated "laudable pus" and those who favored aseptic technique. Surprisingly, Samuel D. Gross was a severe critic of Professor Lister. The Franco-Prussian war was instrumental in settling the issue when it became apparent that wounded Prussians, who were treated by the Listerian method, fared far better than the French, who were not.[11]

Half a million men required amputations in World War I, including over 4000 Americans.[3, 41] Higher muzzle velocities and more powerful explosives produced more extensive injuries than in previous conflicts. Anaerobic bacteria from heavily fertilized European soil were responsible for the 28% mortality from gas gangrene, which occurred in 5% of wounds.[23] Nevertheless, several advances in amputation surgery arose from the lessons learned in World War I, including delayed primary closure of contaminated wounds after serial dressing changes with antiseptic solution, repudiation of prophylactic amputations in all compound fractures, and development of orthopedic external fixation splints.

The availability of antibiotics and blood transfusions transformed trauma surgery dramatically in World War II. Nonetheless, amputation rates after major extremity injury actually *increased* from 2% in World War 1 to 5% in World War II because of the damage caused by even more powerful weapons. Nearly 16,000 Americans underwent major amputations. There was improvement in treatment of compound fractures and preservation of the knee joint, thus resulting in better long-term rehabilitation. The ratio of above-knee to below-knee amputation in World War I was 2.5:1, falling to 1:1 in World War II.[44] Moreover, mortality from wound infections decreased from 8% in World War I to 4.5% in World War II.[50]

Mortality related to wounds continued to decrease in the Korean conflict to 2.5%.[44] Amputations were necessary in only 13% of severely injured extremities because of improvements in rapid evacuation of the wounded and refinements in repair of vascular injuries. Similar rates were reported in the Vietnam war.[47, 57] The vascular registry developed by Dr. Norman Rich in the Vietnam war has been instrumental in improving outcome after civilian arterial trauma.

During the past three decades, the lessons learned from traumatic amputations were applied to amputations performed for nontraumatic causes. In the mid-1960s, Burgess and associates introduced important advances in amputation techniques, leading to increased acceptance of prostheses and less psychological trauma postoperatively.[9, 10] The concept of immediate fitting of prostheses after amputation, proposed in 1958 by Berlemont in France,[6] was expanded by the group at the San Francisco Veterans Administration Medical Center in the 1970s.[43] During the 1990s, most achievements in amputation surgery involved lower limb vascular reconstruction, prosthetic materials and design, and rehabilitation methods. Improvements in these areas have resulted in an increased number of useful extremities.

SCOPE OF THE PROBLEM

As the average age of the population has risen, the incidence of peripheral vascular disease and diabetes mellitus has increased. More than 90% of the 60,000 amputations performed in the United States each year are for ischemic or infective gangrene.[23] Similar statistics have been reported in Great Britain.[40] Most lower extremity amputations are performed for vascular and infectious complications of diabetes mellitus, and 15% to 35% of diabetic amputees will lose a second leg within 5 years.[24, 46, 53, 60] da Silva, for the Audit Committee of the Vascular Surgical Society of Great Britain and Ireland, recently reported the management and outcome of critical limb ischemia in diabetic patients from a national survey.[16] The limb salvage rate and mortality rate were 60% and 15%, respectively, in diabetic patients and 73% and 12%, respectively, in nondiabetic patients who presented with critical limb ischemia. Other indications for lower extremity amputation include nondiabetic infection with ischemia, ischemia without infection, chronic osteomyelitis, trauma, and miscellaneous causes. The evaluation and preparation of patients for amputation with respect to these different presentations are discussed in Chapter 161.

A recently published list of the 20 most commonly performed major procedures in general surgery based on the 1987 National Hospital Survey conspicuously omits extremity amputation, even though the number performed nationally would place it nearly in the top 10 operations.[59] This suggests that many amputations are performed by orthopedic surgeons and emphasizes the importance of exchanging information between specialists in the various disciplines. Moreover, few general surgery training programs offer extensive experience in the technical performance of amputation or, of equal importance, in postoperative rehabilitation or use of prostheses.[15] It is therefore prudent for surgeons with experience in these areas to work closely with orthopedic colleagues, rehabilitation specialists, and local prosthetists to develop a comprehensive program in amputation surgery.[12, 49]

Economic expenditures for amputations are substantial. In the United Kingdom, £33 million are spent per year on prostheses alone.[40] At the end of the 1970s, Malone and coworkers estimated that by applying a team approach to the treatment of potential amputees, the U.S. Veterans Administration could save $80 million over a 5-year period.[39] The actual expense of amputation varies widely, depending on the locale, year and success rate (i.e., primary healing). For example, in a comparison of the costs of revascularization versus amputation, Gupta and the group from New York City reported in 1982 that an uncomplicated amputation amounted to $27,225 ± $2,896.[21] Mackey and colleagues in 1986 analyzed the extended costs of revascularization versus amputation, including the costs of secondary complications, and reported a value of $40,563 ± $4,729.[36] In 1992, Cheshire found that the cost of primary amputation in the United Kingdom averaged £20,416.[13] Some of the reasons for these discrepancies are discussed in Chapter 166.

LEVEL OF AMPUTATION

Amputation should be performed at the level at which healing is most likely to be complete but which will also permit the most efficient use of the limb after rehabilitation. In the upper extremity, circulatory impairment rarely constitutes an indication for amputation. In the lower extremities, in which vascular insufficiency is much more likely, the circulatory status at different levels may be determined by measurement of the peripheral pulses and the capillary refill time and by noting the presence of rubor, the condition of the skin, and the presence of ischemic atrophy. At present, no single measurement of blood flow can reliably predict the best level of healing. The best predictions are based on clinical assessment by an experienced surgeon, assisted by one of several techniques for determining amputation level. In patients with distinct lines of demarcation and in those with tumors, the amount of tissue that must be removed is more obvious.

Maximum limb length should be preserved to maintain ambulation as near normal as possible with the least energy expenditure. The increased energy expenditure and metabolic consequences of extremity amputation are frequently underappreciated.[45] For example, compared with normal walking, energy expenditure is increased 10% to 40% for a unilateral below-knee amputation, 50% to 57% for a unilateral above-knee amputation, and 60% for crutch walking.[58] Consequently, whereas 70% of below-knee amputees attain bipedal gait, only 10% to 30% of above-knee amputees eventually walk again.[4, 48, 51]

Ancillary tests to assist in determination of optimal amputation level include segmental Doppler systolic pressure measurements, fluorescein dye measurements, laser-Doppler velocimetry, photoelectric skin perfusion pressure, isotope measurement of skin perfusion pressure, isotope measurement of skin blood flow, measurement of skin temperature, and measurement of transcutaneous oxygen tension. These techniques are elaborated in detail in Chapter 162. Specific lower extremity amputations are also discussed.

COMPLICATIONS OF AMPUTATION

Chapter 163 covers complications of amputation in depth. Adverse outcomes are unfortunately common despite refinements in *preoperative* assessment, *intraoperative* management, and *postoperative* care. The authors discuss complications in relation to these periods of time. In addition, late complications may affect the ability of amputees to use prostheses effectively. These unfavorable consequences include stump congestion, bulbous stump, excessive residual soft tissue, callosities and cysts, neuropathy and phantom limb, bone spurs, osteoporosis, bone overgrowth, adherent scar, loss of the contralateral limb, and requirement for revision of stumps.

THE TEAM APPROACH

Dramatic improvement in the rehabilitation of amputees has been achieved after institution of a team approach. In addition to the surgeon, the ideal group of individuals charged with caring for patients requiring amputation includes a physiatrist, rehabilitation nurse, physical therapist, occupational therapist, recreation or vocational therapist, prosthetist, medical social worker, and psychologist/counselor. Such a team enhances patient care immensely. Expectations for the amputee should be well defined and evaluated on a regular basis. The benefits of a team approach were established by Malone and colleagues, who compared the team approach with historical controls.[38] The results are summarized in Table 160–2. Chapter 164 presents the case for a comprehensive approach for the rehabilitation of amputees. The importance of patient education and a team approach cannot be overemphasized.[7]

UPPER EXTREMITY AMPUTATIONS

Upper extremity amputations comprise 15% to 20% of all amputations. Almost 8000 new upper extremity amputations are performed each year in the United States.[5] Ten per cent of these amputees have involvement of the other upper extremity. In contrast to lower extremity amputees, most upper extremity amputations are performed for trauma. Other indications, in order of decreasing frequency, are tumor, congenital anomalies, vascular disease, infections, and iatrogenic causes (e.g., extravasation of caustic chemicals or vasopressor therapy).

Reestablishment of a functional limb depends on preoperative counseling and explanation of realistic expectations, meticulous surgical technique, attention to the principles of prosthetic fitting and rehabilitation, and recognition and treatment of the psychological trauma imposed by loss of all or part of the upper limb.[32] The features of upper extremity amputation are reviewed in Chapter 165.

AMPUTATION VERSUS REVASCULARIZATION

The final chapter in Section XXI, Chapter 166, extensively reviews the arguments for and against amputation as opposed to revascularization for patients with end-stage peripheral vascular disease. Those in favor of primary amputation cite the large numbers of patients subjected to

TABLE 160–2. TEAM VERSUS NONTEAM APPROACH TO REHABILITATION

	HEALING (%)	HOSPITAL DAYS	REHABILITATION DAYS	REHABILITATION RATE (%)
Team approach	97	38	31	100
Nonteam approach	63	68	128	69

Adapted from Malone JM, Moore W, Leal JM, Childers SJ: Rehabilitation for lower extremity amputation. Arch Surg 116:93, 1981. Copyright 1981, American Medical Association.

revascularization who ultimately require a major amputation, the level of which may be adversely affected by a failed bypass.[29, 52] Multiple reoperations increase morbidity and mortality rates. Furthermore, rehabilitation of amputees has become increasingly successful.

Proponents of revascularization note that limb salvage rates generally surpass bypass graft patency rates by 15% to 20%.[4, 55] They point out that patients with severely ischemic extremities have a limited life expectancy, and a "palliative" revascularization is advantageous so that the patient can maintain as normal a lifestyle as possible for the remainder of life. However, a recent report from the Oregon Health Sciences University examined the functional outcome after infrainguinal bypass for limb salvage in a group of 513 patients. Of 29 nonambulatory patients (preoperatively), only 6 became ambulatory postoperatively. At 5 years, the overall survival rate was 48%.[1]

In a similar outcome study from Europe, Holdsworth and McCollum analyzed resource implications of treating end-stage limb ischemia.[25] There were 228 patients treated by revascularization with 275 severely ischemic limbs. Although the limb salvage rate was a respectable 65% at 4 years, for reconstructive vascular surgery, excluding amputation and rehabilitation, there were 383 hospital admissions covering 7343 days. Only 64% of patients were treated in a single admission, and the median hospital stay for a first admission was 16 days.

The prudence of attempting lower limb revascularization in patients with end-stage renal disease (ESRD) is a particularly controversial topic. Johnson and associates reviewed 53 patients with ESRD undergoing arterial reconstructions.[28] The 30-day operative mortality rate was 10%, and the 2-year survival rate was 38%. The cumulative limb salvage rate was only 57% at 2 years. In the group of patients who required amputations (22 patients), 59% were performed despite a patent bypass. The authors concluded that primary amputation should be considered for ESRD patients with foot gangrene. Similar findings have been reported by others.[18, 27]

Young amputees do not necessarily fare better than older ones. Valentine and colleagues recently reported that fewer than half of individuals requiring ischemic limb amputations before age 50 years ever achieve ambulation.[54] By 4 years postoperatively, about 40% of these patients had died, the same percentage as in a population of atherosclerotic amputees between ages 60 and 75 years.

The controversy concerning amputation versus revascularization arises from many factors, including differences in patient populations, different institutional philosophies, variable technical abilities of surgeons, different levels of expertise in support services (e.g., radiology versus rehabili-

tation medicine), and a lack of objective preoperative criteria on which to base the decision of when to attempt revascularization or primary amputation. Chapter 166 presents a comprehensive update of this problem. A analysis of fiscal considerations is also presented.

REFERENCES

1. Abou-Zamzam AM Jr, Lee RW, Moneta GL, et al: Functional outcome after infrainguinal bypass for limb salvage. J Vasc Surg 25:287, 1997.
2. Adams F: The Genuine Works of Hippocrates. Translated from Greek with preliminary discourse and annotations. New York, Williams, Wood, 1891.
3. Aldea PA, Shaw WW: The evolution of the surgical management of severe lower extremity trauma. Clin Plast Surg 13:549, 1986.
4. Bartlett ST, Olinde AJ, Flinn WR, et al: The reoperative potential of infrainguinal bypass: Long-term limb and patient survival. J Vasc Surg 5:170, 1987.
5. Beasley RW: General considerations in managing upper limb amputations. Orthop Clin North Am 12:743, 1981.
6. Berlemont M: Notre expérience de l'appareillage précoce des amputées du membre inférieur aux établissements Helios Marius de Berck. Ann Med Phys 4:4, 1961.
7. Boulton AJ: Why bother educating the multi-disciplinary team and the patient—the example of prevention of lower extremity amputation in diabetes. Pat Educ Counselling 26:183, 1995.
8. Brothwell D, Moller-Christensen V: Medico-historical aspects of a very early case of mutilation. Dan Med Bull 10:21, 1963.
9. Burgess EM: Amputation surgery and postoperative care. In Banerjee SN (ed): Rehabilitation Management of Amputees. Baltimore, Williams & Wilkins, 1982, pp 163–180.
10. Burgess EM, Romano RJ, Zettl JH, Schrock RD Jr: Amputation of the leg for peripheral vascular insufficiency. J Bone Joint Surg 53:874, 1971.
11. Cartwright RR: The Development of Modern Surgery. New York, Thomas Crowell, 1968.
12. Chang BB, Jacobs RL, Darling RC III, et al: Foot amputations. Surg Clin North Am 75:773, 1995.
13. Cheshire NJ, Wolfe JH, Noone MA, et al: The economics of femorocrural reconstruction for critical leg ischemia with and without saphenous vein. J Vasc Surg 15:167, 1992.
14. Couch NP, David JK, Tilney NL, Crane C: Natural history of the leg amputee. Am J Surg 133:469, 1977.
15. Cutson TM, Bongiorni DR: Rehabilitation of the older lower limb amputee: A brief review. J Am Geriatr Soc 44:1388, 1996.
16. da Silva AF, for the Audit Committee of the Vascular Surgical Society of Great Britain and Ireland: The management and outcome of critical limb ischaemia in diabetic patients: Results of a national survey. Diabet Med 13:726, 1996.
17. Dibble JH: DJ Larrey, a surgeon of the revolution, consulate and empire. Med Hist 3 100, 1959.
18. Edwards JM, Taylor LM, Porter JM: Limb salvage in end-stage renal disease. Arch Surg 123:1164, 1988.
19. Friedmann LW: Amputation in pre-Columbian America. Arch Phys Med Rehabil 54:323, 1973.
20. Garrison FH: An Introduction to the History of Medicine, 4th ed. Philadelphia, WB Saunders, 1929.
21. Gupta SK, Veith FJ, Samson RH, et al: Cost analysis of operations for infrainguinal arteriosclerosis. Circulation 66(Suppl 2):11-9, 1982.

22. Haeger K: The Illustrated History of Surgery. New York, Bell Publishing, 1988.
23. Hardaway RM: Vietnam wound analysis. J Trauma 18:635, 1978.
24. High RM, McDowell DE, Savin RA: A critical review of amputation in vascular patients. J Vasc Surg 1:653, 1984.
25. Holdsworth RJ, McCollum PT: Results and resource implications of treating end-stage limb ischaemia. Eur J Endovasc Surg 13:164, 1997.
26. Hunter JA: Treatise on the Blood, Inflammation and Gunshot Wounds. Philadelphia, Thomas Bradford, 1796.
27. Isiklar MH, Kulbaski M, MacDonald MJ, Lumsden AB: Infrainguinal bypass in end-stage renal disease: When is it justified? Semin Vasc Surg 10:42, 1997.
28. Johnson BL, Glickman MH, Bandyk DF, et al: Failure of foot salvage in patients with end-stage renal disease after surgical revascularization. J Vasc Surg 22:280, 1995.
29. Kazmers M, Satiani B, Evans WE: Amputation level following unsuccessful distal limb salvage operations. Surgery 87:683, 1980.
30. Keen WW: The contrast between the surgery of the Civil War and that of the present war. N Y Med J 101:817, 1915.
31. Kirk NT: The development of amputation. Bull Med Lib Assoc 32:132, 1944.
32. Kneisl JS: Function after amputation, arthrodesis, or arthroplasty for tumors about the shoulder. J South Orthop Assoc 4:228, 1995.
33. Krupski WC, Skinner HB, Effeney DJ: Amputation. In Way LW (ed): Current Surgical Diagnosis and Treatment, San Mateo, Calif, Appleton & Lange, 1988, pp 704–714.
34. Larrey DJ: Memoires de Chirurgie Militaire et Campagnes. Paris, J Smith, 1812–1817.
35. Lister J: On a method of treating compound fractures, abscesses, etc., with observations of the conditions of suppuration. Lancet 1:326, 1867.
36. Mackey WC, McCollough JL, Conlon TP, et al: The costs of surgery for limb-threatening ischemia. Surgery 99:26, 1986.
37. Majesky MW: A little VEGF goes a long way: Therapeutic angiogenesis by direct injection of vascular endothelial growth factor–encoding plasmid DNA. Circulation 94:3062, 1996.
38. Malone JM, Moore W, Leal JM, Childers SJ: Rehabilitation for lower extremity amputation. Arch Surg 116:93, 1981.
39. Malone JM, Moore WS, Goldstone J, Malone SJ: Therapeutic and economic impact of a modern amputation program. Ann Surg 189:798, 1979.
40. McColl I: Review of Artificial Limb and Appliance Centre Services. Department of Health and Human Services Report. London, Her Majesty's Stationery Office, 1986.
41. The Medical Department of the United States Army in the World War. Vol 13, Part I—General Surgery, Orthopedic Surgery, Neurosurgery. Washington DC, U.S. Government Printing Office, 1927.
42. Mettler CC: History of Medicine. Philadelphia, Blakiston, 1947.
43. Moore WS, Hall AP, Lim RC: Below-the-knee amputation for ischemic gangrene: Comparative results of conventional operation and immediate postoperative fitting. AM J Surg 124:127, 1972.
44. Office of the Surgeon General, United States Army: Orthopedic Surgery in the Zone of the Interior: Surgery in World War II. Washington, DC, Medical Department, 1970.
45. Pinzur MS: The metabolic cost of lower extremity amputation. Clin Podiatr Med Surg 14:599, 1997.
46. Powell TW, Burnham SJ, Johnson G Jr: Second leg ischemia: Lower extremity bypass versus amputation in patients with contralateral lower extremity amputation. Am Surg 11:577, 1984.
47. Rich NM, Braugh JH, Hughes CW, et al: Acute arterial injuries in Vietnam: 1000 cases. J Trauma 10:359, 1970.
48. Roon AJ, Moore WS, Goldstone J: Below-knee amputation: A modern approach. Am J Surg 134:153, 1977.
49. Sanders LJ: Transmetatarsal and midfoot amputations. Clin Podiatr Med Surg 14:741, 1997.
50. Simeone FA: Studies of trauma and shock in man: William S. Stone's role in the military effort. J Trauma 24:181, 1984.
51. Steinberg FU, Sunwoo I, Roettger RF: Prosthetic rehabilitation of geriatric amputee patients: A follow-up study. Arch Phys Med Rehabil 66:742, 1985.
52. Stoney RJ: Ultimate salvage for the patient with limb-threatening ischemia: Realistic goals and surgical considerations. Am J Surg 136:228, 1978.
53. Stuck RM, Sage R, Pinxur, Osterman H: Amputations in the diabetic foot. Clin Podiatr Med Surg 12:141, 1995.
54. Valentine RJ, Myers SI, Inman MH, et al: Late outcome of amputees with premature atherosclerosis. Surgery 119:487, 1997.
55. Veith FJ, Gupta SK, Samson RH, et al: Progress in limb salvage by reconstructive arterial surgery combined with new or improved adjunctive procedures. Ann Surg 194:386, 1981.
56. Wagensteen OH, Smith J, Wagensteen SD, et al: Some highlights in the history of amputation reflecting lessons in wound healing. Bull Hist Med 41:97, 1967.
57. Walter Reed Army Medical Center: Battle Casualties in Korea. Vol 3. The Battle Wound: Clinical Experiences. Washington, DC, Army Medical Service Graduate School, 1955.
58. Waters RL, Perry J, Antonelli D, et al: Energy cost of walking amputees: The influence of level of amputation. J Bone Joint Surg 58:42, 1976.
59. Wheeler HB: Myth and reality in general surgery. Bull Am Coll Surg 78:21, 1993.
60. Whitehouse FW, Jurgensen C, Block MA: The later life of the diabetic amputee: Another look at fate of the second leg. Diabetes 17:520, 1968.
61. Zimmerman LM, Veith I: Great Ideas in the History of Surgery. New York, Dover, 1967.

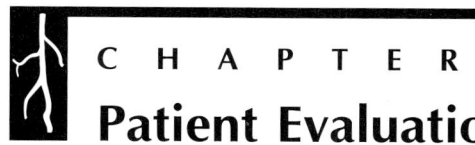

C H A P T E R   1 6 1

Patient Evaluation and Preparation for Amputation

Kenneth E. McIntyre, Jr., M.D., and Scott S. Berman, M.D.

Amputation of the lower extremity is often regarded as "the final chapter" for patients who have chronic lower extremity occlusive disease. Moreover, leg amputation exposes the limits of modern limb salvage techniques for treatment of lower extremity ischemia. Despite technical advances in lower extremity revascularization, the number of amputations performed annually has not decreased. This finding should come as no surprise because amputations are more prevalent in older patients and the mean age of the population continues to increase.[1-3] In addition to circulatory impairment of the lower extremities, older patients may also have coexisting diseases that influence outcomes after amputations.[4] Therefore, a thorough preoperative evaluation must be performed to minimize the significant morbidity and mortality associated with lower extremity amputation.[5] Loss of a limb is also associated with acute depression, which should be anticipated and treated to optimize postoperative rehabilitation.[6, 7]

This chapter reviews the epidemiology of amputation and the evaluation of concurrent diseases that influence perioperative outcome and rehabilitation. A treatment algorithm is presented to identify important preoperative conditions that contribute to postoperative morbidity.

Nontraumatic amputations are most often a consequence of acute ischemia, chronic ischemia, or diabetes with infectious gangrene.[8, 9] The preoperative evaluation of patients with these conditions is important because the specific underlying condition that has necessitated amputation may contribute to unique perioperative problems.[10]

AMPUTATION FOR ACUTE ISCHEMIA

Acute ischemia requiring lower extremity amputation results from either arterial thrombosis or embolism. More than 20 years ago, Blaisdell and coworkers documented the morbid outcome of acute lower extremity ischemia after thromboembolism.[11] Today, despite the widespread use of the Fogarty thrombectomy catheter,[12] arterial bypass,[13] and catheter-directed thrombolytic infusions,[14, 15] the limb loss rate after acute ischemia remains between 9% and 30% and mortality rates are up to 18%.[13-16]

It is often difficult to distinguish thrombosis from embolism as the cause of acute lower extremity ischemia. Typically, patients with embolism tend to be older, and they usually have a cardiac embolic source. Arterial embolism may occur as a consequence of arrhythmia (e.g., atrial fibrillation), acute myocardial infarction, valvular heart dis-

ease, or ventricular aneurysm. Less commonly, embolism is from a more proximal arterial source.[17, 18] In contrast, in situ thrombosis often occurs in patients with a history of lower extremity vascular occlusive disease, including symptoms of claudication, ischemic rest pain, earlier interventional or vascular reconstructive procedures, or even previous amputation.

In most cases, careful history and physical examination reveal the cause of acute lower extremity ischemia. In patients with unilateral lower extremity ischemia secondary to embolism, pulses in the contralateral leg are often normal. An irregularly irregular pulse readily identifies atrial fibrillation. A precordial murmur may indicate valvular heart disease. In patients with thrombosis, pulses in the contralateral extremity may be diminished or absent. In addition, the contralateral extremity may exhibit other important signs, such as absence of hair over the toes and dorsum of the foot, thickening of the toenails, atrophy of the subcutaneous tissue, pallor with foot elevation, and rubor with dependency. Even after a thorough history and physical examination. however, the precise cause of tissue ischemia may remain elusive. Additional tests are then required.

Transthoracic echocardiography is less sensitive than transesophageal echocardiography (TEE) for examination of the left atrium as a source for embolism, although it is used more often.[19] Although actual thrombi may not be visualized, ventricular wall motion abnormalities and stagnant flow in the left atrium, findings that often predispose to thrombus formation, can readily be identified.[19] In addition, TEE offers the advantage of viewing the thoracic aorta, a potential source of atheroembolism.[20] Even if a cardiac embolic source is not identified, anticoagulation with intravenous heparin should be instituted immediately. This therapy prevents additional embolic episodes that may result in stroke, myocardial infarction, or renal failure. Systemic heparinization also further reduces lower extremity ischemia by limiting propagation of thrombus.[11, 21, 22]

Before and after an episode of acute thromboembolism, myocardial infarction is an important risk factor that contributes to the prognosis for both patient and extremity.[18] A resting electrocardiogram and myocardial enzyme determinations are obtained to rule out acute myocardial infarction, which may both precipitate limb ischemia and complicate its management. Myocardial infarction as a cause of acute thromboembolism is important to recognize not only during embolectomy but also before a definitive amputation. Congestive heart failure also greatly increases the risk to life and limb.[18, 23] Aggressive treatment of ventricular dysfunction and anticoagulation therapy may help to reduce the high risk of operation and recurrent thromboembolism. Chapters 2 and 40 offer more detailed information on these topics.

When acute ischemia develops from thrombosis in the presence of preexisting disease, the diagnosis should generally be confirmed by arteriography. Arteriography helps to determine the operative strategy when reconstruction is deemed feasible. When adequate healing of a below-knee amputation is in doubt (see Chapter 162), arteriography may identify a proximal arterial stenosis or occlusion that might be amenable to either surgical reconstruction or angioplasty. In addition to defining the level of obstruction, arteriography also offers an opportunity to deliver intra-arterial thrombolytic agents.[14, 16] Arteriography, however, necessarily delays operative treatment, and time is a crucial factor for limb salvage.

AMPUTATION FOR CHRONIC ISCHEMIA

Even with modern arterial reconstructive techniques, chronic ischemia still accounts for nearly 20,000 amputations each year.[5] Patients are not considered candidates for primary amputation unless a significant part of the weight-bearing surface of the foot is affected with gangrene or necrosis. For elderly patients who do not walk, are mentally incompetent, have flexion contractures secondary to immobility or arthritis, have a concurrent terminal illness, or have no reconstructable calf or foot vessels, primary amputation is appropriate, however.[24]

Prevention of significant perioperative complications and reduction of mortality have traditionally been cited as justification for evaluating and treating patients with ischemic heart disease before they undergo vascular surgery.[25] However, more recent reports question the benefit of preoperative cardiac evaluations before elective vascular procedures.[26, 27] Nonetheless, patients who require amputation as a consequence of chronic ischemia commonly have advanced atherosclerosis of the coronary arteries and require special consideration.[28] In diabetic patients silent (asymptomatic) myocardial infarction is particularly common. Therefore, the absence of ischemic heart disease, by history alone, may be unreliable. For patients with a recent history of myocardial infarction, congestive heart failure, unstable angina pectoris, or significant mitral or aortic valvular disease, further cardiac evaluation is often advisable before the amputation (see Chapter 40).[24]

The standard technique for the diagnosis of ischemic heart disease is the exercise treadmill stress test, which has been validated as both specific and sensitive for ischemic heart disease.[29, 30] Unfortunately, to be considered valid, the exercise stress test requires the patient to walk at a rate that elevates the heart rate to a target value.[31] Therefore, it is not useful for patients with claudication, ischemic rest pain, or a gangrenous foot, or for those whose contralateral extremity has been amputated.

An alternative to the exercise stress test is arm exercise ergometry, which monitors the electrocardiogram, heart rate, and blood pressure during a standard exercise protocol that uses an arm crank ergometer.[31, 32] This test is a safe and effective alternative for the detection of coronary artery disease in patients who cannot walk vigorously, although direct concordance with coronary arteriographic findings has not been confirmed. Of note, ergometry has a role in determining safe exercise levels and may be a predictor of successful prosthetic use for patients in rehabilitation after amputation.[31, 32]

A test that has commonly been used to evaluate patients for suspected ischemic heart disease is dipyridamole thallium scintigraphy (DTS). Initially, there was much enthusiasm, because it was believed to predict which patients are at greatest risk for perioperative cardiac events.[33] Unfortunately, more recent work has documented the inability of DTS to accurately identify persons at risk for cardiac events.[34, 35] When amputation is necessary, it is prudent to proceed with that procedure without an extensive preoperative cardiac evaluation unless there is a history of recent myocardial infarction, unstable angina, congestive heart failure, or significant valvular heart disease.

In patients with chronic ischemia, amputation generally is performed as an elective procedure. In addition to adequate preoperative evaluation and treatment of co-morbid conditions, the elective nature of amputation in these patients allows for initiation of preoperative physical training and psychologic counseling, encouraging better adaptation to amputation and rehabilitation. Bradway and colleagues have described four stages of adaptation to amputation: (1) preoperative, (2) immediate postoperative, (3) in-hospital, and (4) at-home rehabilitation.[6] All amputees must work through these adaptive stages.

Ideally, a multidisciplinary team of surgeon, prosthetist, physical therapist, occupational therapist, social worker, and psychologist or psychiatrist can begin working with the patient in the preoperative period to optimize rehabilitation potential. Successful application of this team approach, with special attention to the psychologic needs of the amputee, can enhance rehabilitation and avoid the need for long-term psychiatric care.[6]

AMPUTATION FOR INFECTIOUS GANGRENE

Infectious gangrene requiring amputation usually occurs in patients who have diabetes mellitus. When superficial foot infections progress to deep closed-space infections that jeopardize the foot, blood glucose becomes difficult to control. Ketoacidosis develops, and patients become relatively "insulin-resistant" and metabolically unstable. Dehydration caused by osmotic diuresis and hyperosmolarity contributes to worsening of ischemia of the extremity as well as in other vascular beds. Urgent, aggressive foot débridement is necessary to document the extent of infection, to provide adequate drainage of necrotic and purulent tissue, and to obtain adequate culture material from deep tissues.[36]

The foot is not salvageable when the infection has destroyed the plantar architecture and a functional weight-bearing surface is absent after radical débridement. When necrosis with active purulence is present and the foot is considered unsalvageable after thorough inspection in the operating room, an ankle *guillotine* operation, rather than a definitive one-stage amputation, should be performed.[37–39] Supramalleolar guillotine amputation is an easy method of alleviating gangrenous foot infections that have destroyed the architecture of the foot. In addition, because the wound is left open, lymphatics contaminated with bacteria are allowed to drain, thus arresting ascending infection. Immediately after guillotine amputation, blood glucose levels become easier to manage and ketoacidosis resolves quickly, so that metabolic and hemodynamic stabilization are promoted. Before the definitive below-knee amputation is performed, generally 5 to 7 days after guillotine amputation, a more complete elective preoperative evaluation is conducted.

Several authors have shown that preparatory guillotine amputation in patients with infectious gangrene is associated with a lower incidence of complications than one-stage definitive amputation.[37–39] In addition, no significant difference in operative mortality rates is associated with one-stage and two-stage amputations.[37–39]

Infectious gangrene in patients with diabetes is generally polymicrobial and adjunctive treatment with parenteral broad-spectrum antibiotics is needed.[36, 38, 40, 41] Specimens for culture, obtained by either ulcer curettage or deep tissue biopsy, are more accurate for defining the offending organisms than culture of material collect by superficial wound swabbing.[36, 41] Even when the microbiology laboratory fails to grow anaerobic organisms in culture, the characteristic putrid odor emanating from the foot suggests their presence.

Once the grossly infected and nonviable tissue has been removed by débridement or guillotine amputation, the wound must be closely observed before a definitive amputation is performed at a more proximal level. After the

infection is under control and sepsis has resolved, antibiotics may be discontinued. Before the definitive below-knee amputation, however, antibiotics should be given perioperatively to provide coverage for organisms cultured during the initial débridement or guillotine amputation.[38] This practice may help to reduce the risk of subsequent infection in the "definitive amputation" stump.

SUMMARY

Lower extremity amputations are necessary as a consequence of acute and chronic leg ischemia as well as overwhelming infection, which occurs principally in patients with diabetes mellitus. Although the indications for amputation differ, several common denominators must be considered carefully before operation.

The surgeon must endeavor to perform amputations below the knee, because rehabilitation potential is enhanced by preserving the knee joint owing to the significantly lower energy expenditure required to walk with a below-knee prosthesis as compared with an above-knee device.[42] Even though no test currently available reliably predicts postamputation healing,[43] the surgeon must be reasonably confident that the blood supply is adequate to support skin healing at the proposed level of amputation. If the status of skin perfusion is in question, arteriography may be useful for identifying a proximal arterial lesion that is ame-

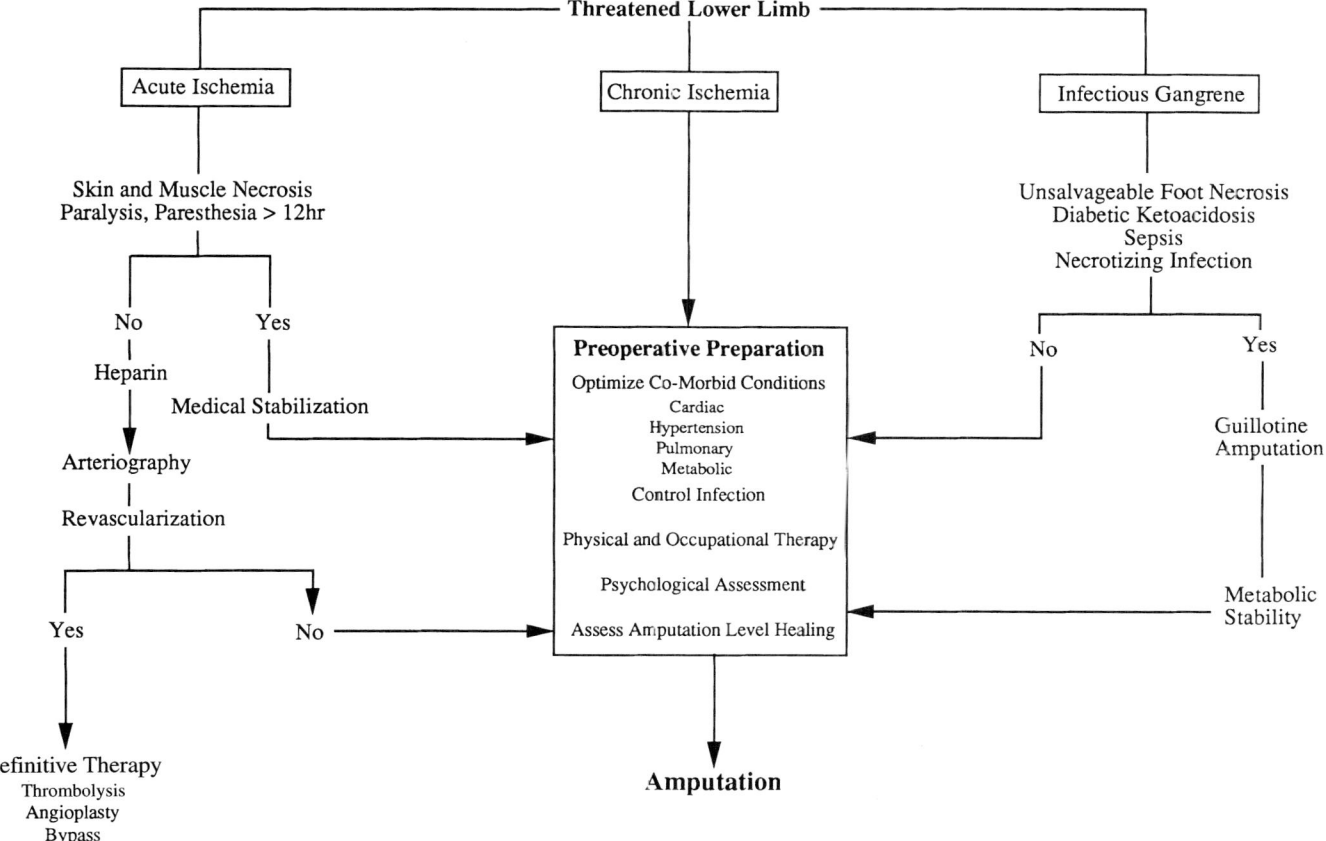

FIGURE 161–1. Algorithm for preoperative evaluation of amputation patients.

nable to surgical or interventional repair. Often, a procedure such as iliac angioplasty provides sufficient increase in perfusion to the ischemic extremity to ensure healing at the below-knee level.

The cause of tissue ischemia should also be considered. If acute tissue ischemia is a consequence of embolism, further ischemia may develop in the lower extremity or other target organs. Infection must be eradicated before definitive amputation is undertaken. By performing a supramalleolar guillotine amputation in patients who have an unsalvageable foot and ascended infection or gangrene, the surgeon can successfully extirpate the infection. It is often necessary to perform this procedure emergently to achieve metabolic and hemodynamic stability in a diabetic patient with sepsis.

Finally, myocardial ischemia is a major contributor to the high perioperative mortality rate associated with nontraumatic lower extremity amputation. Therefore, it is necessary to evaluate cardiac function in patients with a pertinent history to identify those at greatest risk for perioperative myocardial ischemia. An algorithm for the preoperative evaluation and management of the candidate for amputation is depicted in Figure 161–1.

REFERENCES

1. Veith FJ, Gupta SK, Wengerter KR, et al: Changing arteriosclerotic disease patterns and management strategies in lower-limb–threatening ischemia. Ann Surg 212:402, 1990.
2. Taylor LM Jr, Hamre D, Dalman RL, et al: Limb salvage vs. amputation for critical ischemia: The role of vascular surgery. Arch Surg 126:1251, 1991.
3. Kald A, Carlsson R, Nilsson E: Major amputation in a defined population: Incidence, mortality and results of treatment. Br J Surg 76:308, 1989.
4. Roth EJ, Wiesner SL, Green D, et al: Dysvascular amputee rehabilitation: The role of continuous noninvasive cardiovascular monitoring during physical therapy. Am J Phys Med Rehabil 69:16, 1990.
5. Malone JM: Complications of lower extremity amputation. In Moore WS, Malone JM (eds): Lower Extremity Amputation. Philadelphia, WB Saunders, 1989.
6. Bradway JK, Malone JM, Racy J, et al: Psychological adaptation to amputation: An overview. Orthot Prosthet 38:46, 1984.
7. Steinberg FU, Sunwoo IS, Roettger RF: Prosthetic rehabilitation of geriatric amputee patients: A follow-up study. Arch Phys Med Rehabil 66:742, 1985.
8. Bild DE, Selby JV, Sinnock P, et al: Lower-extremity amputation in people with diabetes: Epidemiology and prevention. Diabetes Care 12:24, 1989.
9. Gregory-Dean A: Amputations: Statistics and trends. Ann R Coll Surg Engl 73:137, 1991.
10. Thomas JH, Steers JL, Keushkerian SM, et al: A comparison of diabetics and nondiabetics with threatened limb loss. Am J Surg 156:481, 1988.
11. Blaisdell FW, Steele M, Allen RE: Management of acute lower extremity arterial ischemia due to embolism and thrombosis. Surgery 84:822, 1978.
12. Fogarty TJ, Cranley JJ, Krause RJ, et al: A method of extraction of arterial emboli and thrombi. Surg Gynecol Obstet 116:241, 1963.
13. Yeager RA, Moneta GL, Taylor LM Jr, et al: Surgical management of severe acute lower extremity ischemia. J Vasc Surg 15:385, 1992.
14. Ouriel K, Shortell CK, DeWeese JA, et al: A comparison of thrombolytic therapy with operative revascularization in the initial treatment of acute peripheral arterial ischemia. J Vasc Surg 19:1021, 1994.
15. Ouriel K, Veith FJ, Sasahara AA: Thrombolysis or peripheral arterial surgery: Phase I results. J Vasc Surg 23:64, 1996.
16. Jivegård L, Holm J, Shersten T: The outcome in arterial thrombosis misdiagnosed as arterial embolism. Acta Chir Scand 152:251, 1986.
17. Machleder HI, Takiff H, Lois JF, et al: Aortic mural thrombus: An occult source of arterial thromboembolism. J Vasc Surg 4:473, 1986.
18. Ljungman C, Adami HO, Bergqvist D, et al: Risk factors for early lower limb loss after embolectomy for acute arterial occlusion: A population-based case-control study. Br J Surg 78:1482, 1991.
19. Rubin BG, Barzilai B, Allen BT, et al: Detection of the source of arterial emboli by transesophageal echocardiography: A case report. J Vasc Surg 15:573, 1992.
20. Hoffmann T, Kasper W, Meinertz T, et al: Echocardiographic evaluation of patients with clinically suspected arterial emboli. Lancet 336:1421, 1990.
21. Clagett GP, Graor RA, Salzman EW: Antithrombotic therapy in peripheral arterial occlusive disease. Chest 102:517S, 1992.
22. Elliott JP, Hageman JH, Szilagyi E, et al: Arterial embolization; Problems of source, multiplicity, recurrence, and delayed treatment. Surgery 88:833, 1980.
23. Ouriel K, Green RM, DeWeese JA, et al: Outpatient echocardiography as a predictor of perioperative cardiac morbidity after peripheral vascular surgical procedures. J Vasc Surg 22:671, 1995.
24. Harris KA, van Schie L, Carroll SE, et al: Rehabilitation potential of elderly patients with major amputations. J Cardiovasc Surg 32:463, 1991.
25. Brewster DC, Edwards JD: Cardiopulmonary complications related to vascular surgery. In Bernhard VM, Towne JB (eds): Complications in Vascular Surgery. St. Louis, Quality Medical Publishing, 1991.
26. Mason JJ, Owens DK, Harris RA, et al: The role of coronary angiography and coronary revascularization before noncardiac vascular surgery. JAMA 273:1919, 1995.
27. Taylor LM Jr, Yeager RA, Moneta GL, et al: The incidence of perioperative myocardial infarction in general vascular surgery. J Vasc Surg 15:52, 1991.
28. Kallero KS, Bergqvist D, Cederholm C, et al: Arteriosclerosis in popliteal artery trifurcation as a predictor for myocardial infarction after arterial reconstructive operation. Surg Gynecol Obstet 159:133, 1984.
29. McCabe CJ, Reidy NC, Abbott WM, et al: The value of electrocardiogram monitoring during treadmill testing for peripheral vascular disease. Surgery 89:183, 1981.
30. Cutler B: Prevention of cardiac complications in peripheral vascular surgery. Surg Clin North Am 66:281, 1986.
31. Priebe M, Davidoff G, Lampman RM: Exercise testing and training in patients with peripheral vascular disease and lower extremity amputation. West J Med 154:598, 1991.
32. Finestone HM, Lampman RM, Davidoff GN, et al: Arm ergometry exercise testing in patients with dysvascular amputations. Arch Phys Med Rehabil 72:15, 1991.
33. Eagle KA, Singer DE, Brewster DC, et al: Dipyridamole-thallium scanning in patients undergoing vascular surgery. JAMA 257:2185, 1987.
34. Baron VF, Mundler O, Vertrand M, et al: Dipyridamole-thallium scintigraphy and gated radionuclide angiography to assess cardiac risk before abdominal aortic surgery. N Engl J Med 330:663, 1994.
35. Mangano DT, London MJ, Tubau JF, et al: Dipyridamole thallium scintigraphy as a preoperative screening test: A re-examination of its predictive potential. Circulation 84:493, 1991.
36. McIntyre KE: Control of infection in the diabetic foot: The role of microbiology, immunopathology, antibiotics, and guillotine amputation. J Vasc Surg 5:787, 1987.
37. McIntyre KE, Bailey SA, Malone JM, et al: Guillotine amputation in the treatment of nonsalvageable lower-extremity infections. Arch Surg 119:450, 1984.
38. Fisher DF, Clagett GP, Fry RE, et al: One-stage versus two-stage amputation for wet gangrene of the lower extremity: A randomized study. J Vasc Surg 8:428, 1988.
39. Desai Y, Robbs JV, Keenan JP: Staged below-knee amputations for septic peripheral lesions due to ischemia. Br J Surg 73:392, 1986.
40. Erstad BL, McIntyre KE Jr: Prospective, randomized comparison of ampicillin/sulbactam and cefoxitin for diabetic foot infections. Vasc Surg 31:419, 1997.
41. Borrero E, Rossini M Jr: Bacteriology of 100 consecutive diabetic foot infections and in vitro susceptibility to ampicillin/sulbactam versus cefoxitin. Angiology 43:357, 1992.
42. Huang CT, Jackson JR, Moore NB, et al: Amputation: Energy cost of ambulation. Arch Phys Med Rehabil 60:18, 1979.
43. Malone JM, Ballard JL: Complications of lower extremity amputation. In Bernhard VM, Towne JB (eds): Complications in Vascular Surgery. St. Louis, Quality Medical Publishing, 1991.

Lower Extremity Amputation Levels: Indications, Determining the Appropriate Level, Technique, and Prognosis

Joseph R. Durham, M. D.

Virtually every surgeon is presented with the unfortunate patient who has painful, dying, or infected tissue coupled with unreconstructable lower extremity arterial anatomy. Additionally, there are cases of established gangrene of an extremity when even a patent vascular reconstruction would not salvage the limb. In such cases, the surgeon must accept multiple challenges, specifically:

1. Providing an amputation that will remove the painful, infected, or dead part of the limb.
2. Performing the amputation at a level that has an excellent potential for healing.
3. Selecting a level of amputation that will provide the best opportunity for successful rehabilitation.
4. Creating an amputation stump that will function in harmony with a prosthetic device.
5. Caring for the patient beyond the immediate postoperative period through the various stages of rehabilitation.

A thorough knowledge of the physiology of the underlying pathologic process, coupled with experience with amputation and rehabilitation techniques, is essential to achieving these goals.

In all cases, an experienced surgeon should be involved in the planning and execution of any amputation of an ischemic limb. These operations should not be delegated to novice surgeons, although this often happens. A recent British study has confirmed this notion that amputations by "junior level" surgeons have a higher incidence of stump-related complications and subsequently, decreased likelihood of successful ambulation with a prosthesis.[170] Any amputation for infection or ischemia should be regarded as a potential new beginning for that patient. As Moore concluded,

> A properly performed amputation cannot only be life-saving to the patient, but may often be a better therapeutic alternative than an ill-conceived, valiant, but often futile attempt at vascular reconstruction that is doomed to fail for lack of adequate recipient vessels to accommodate a distal extremity bypass.[111]

The qualities essential for the successful amputation surgeon include objectivity, dedication, compassion, and technical expertise.

INDICATIONS

General indications for amputation of an ischemic lower extremity (Table 162–1) include:

1. Severe acute ischemia caused by unreconstructible arterial disease.
2. Irreversible tissue compromise secondary to acute and prolonged ischemia.
3. Unreconstructible chronic ischemia producing rest pain, gangrene, nonhealing skin lesions, osteomyelitis, or infection refractory to systemic antibiotics and aggressive local would care measures.
4. Overwhelming foot sepsis in patients with diabetes mellitus.

SELECTION OF LEVEL

Accurate selection of amputation level is of crucial importance not only for minimal morbidity and mortality results but also because it affects rehabilitation potential. A proximal, mid-thigh amputation may deprive a patient of the opportunity for subsequent rehabilitation and ambulation, even if the amputation wound heals well. Conversely, if the amputation site is too distal, inadequate blood supply may lead to wound dehiscence or infection, thereby requiring subsequent operative revisions to achieve healing. This latter approach is demoralizing to the patient, may result in increased morbidity and mortality, and may culminate in rehabilitation failure. Even so, more below-knee amputations should be performed than those at an above-knee level.

The ultimate objective of amputation level selection is to identify the most distal site at which an amputation will heal reliably. The proposed amputation must accomplish removal of all infected, painful, or necrotic tissue and still yield a stump that may be readily fitted with an effective

TABLE 162–1. INDICATIONS FOR LOWER EXTREMITY AMPUTATION

	OCCURRENCE (%)
Complications of diabetes mellitus	60–80
Nondiabetic infection with ischemia	15–25
Ischemia without infection	5–10
Chronic osteomyelitis	3–5
Trauma	2–5
Miscellaneous	5–10

From Malone JM: Lower extremity amputations. In Moore WS (ed): Vascular Surgery: A Comprehensive Review, 4th ed. Philadelphia: WB Saunders, 1993, p 810.

prosthesis. Objective determination of the adequacy of blood supply at the proposed amputation site is a challenge for amputation surgeons. Rehabilitation potential hinges on this determination, because ambulation requires a *10% to 40%* increase in energy expenditure for a unilateral below-knee prosthesis compared with a *50% to 70%* with a unilateral above-knee prosthesis.[45, 51, 168] Consequently, successful rehabilitation is achieved after about *70%* of all below-knee amputations but after only *10% to 30%* of all above-knee amputations.[18, 29, 43, 100, 108, 139, 154]

Historically, virtually all amputations for ischemic disease were performed at above-knee level, and this level is still typically selected in some areas of the world. Although the rehabilitation rate for empirical above-knee amputation does approach a 100%, the average rehabilitation potential (<30%) is unacceptable.

Many methods have been proposed for selecting optimal amputation levels objectively. Unfortunately, none is foolproof. The value of any objective test lies in its *sensitivity*, in this case its ability to predict accurately whether local cutaneous blood flow is adequate to produce successful wound healing. The *specificity* of such a test is defined as its ability to detect truly inadequate local blood flow that would cause healing failure of the amputation stump at a given level. No method of preamputation level selection to assess local blood flow should be too specific, unless its sensitivity is also great, because, although it may produce a 100% healing rate, it may also result in unnecessarily high levels of amputation.

The following methods have been utilized for preoperative selection of amputation levels in "dysvascular" limbs:

- Clinical judgment
- Doppler systolic segmental blood pressure measurements
- Fluorescein dye measurements
- Laser Doppler velocimetry
- Laser Doppler measurement of skin perfusion pressure
- Photoelectric skin perfusion pressures
- Isotope measurement of skin perfusion pressures
- Isotope skin blood flow measurements
- Skin temperature measurements
- Transcutaneous oxygen measurements (tcPO_2)
- Transcutaneous carbon dioxide measurements (tcPCO_2)

The goal of each technique is to produce a numerical value above which all amputations will heal and below which none will. Such an infallible technique does not currently exist. Many of these techniques are useful guides, however. Newer modalities such as magnetic resonance blood flowmetry are in the early stages of development and await clinical trials.[30]

Clinical Judgment and Empirical Amputation Level Selection

Empirical selection of the amputation site results in successful healing of roughly 80% of below-knee amputations and 90% of above-knee amputations.[21, 82, 94, 137] The results are even worse below the ankle, for empirical selection of this level results in a *healing* rate of only 40%.[149]

Most physical examination findings are not helpful in improving the empirical healing rates just noted. Although the presence of pulses immediately above the proposed site of amputation is a good positive prognostic indicator, the absence of such a pulse does not necessarily lead to failure of wound healing.[38, 66, 84] Similarly, subjective assessment of skin temperature, correlation with arteriographic findings, and skin edge bleeding at the time of operation may lead to erroneous assumptions and suboptimal level selections. The only consistently liable physical findings are dependent ischemic rubor and gangrene at the level of amputation. These signs indicate severe ischemia; amputation through ruborous or gangrenous skin invariably fails and should not be attempted. Unfortunately, the *absence* of dependent rubor does not ensure successful healing and cannot be used as the sole indicator in selection of amputation level.

The value of an *experienced* clinical opinion cannot be overemphasized because objective tests are not infallible.[167] If clinical judgment contradicts laboratory values, more proximal amputation should not be chosen based on vascular laboratory results alone. Amputation at a lower level is especially desirable for young, motivated patients, even if the findings of objective studies are marginal. For older, sicker patients with limited rehabilitation potential, a higher level may be more appropriate.[171, 174]

Segmental Doppler Systolic Blood Pressure Measurements

Initial attempts at objective determination of the potential for amputation wound healing employed measurement of segmental Doppler systolic blood pressures, as outlined in Chapters 9 and 10. Although this method can inform the decision for above-knee or below-knee amputation,[13, 126] it is markedly less reliable for ankle, foot, and forefoot amputations.[49, 50, 109, 169, 172] Some of the problems with this technique stem from the falsely elevated pressures that often result from calcification of the arterial wall, especially in the tibial arteries of diabetic patients. Adjunctive pulse volume recordings[22, 49, 50, 130] and infrared photoplethysmographic determinations of toe blood pressures[7, 11, 66, 164] help to alleviate this shortcoming. The poor predictive value should be no surprise, because these techniques do not measure arterial perfusion of the *skin* at that level. Although these Doppler-derived segmental blood pressure measurements are inexpensive, noninvasive, and easy to obtain, their major shortcoming lies in their relative inability to predict which amputations will not heal. It is generally agreed that absence of *all* Doppler flow at the popliteal artery indicates that a distal amputation will not heal. Bone and Pomajzl[11] have shown that, in diabetic patients, toe blood pressures are much more useful than ankle-brachial indices, absolute pressures of less than 30 mmHg being indicative of poor healing. The digital arteries have less tendency to be affected by medial wall calcification.

Fluorescein Dye Measurements

A technique utilizing ultraviolet Wood's light fluorescence in conjunction with new fiberoptic and microcomputer technology to quantitate skin blood flow based on the measurement of local skin fluorescence was reported by Bongard and colleagues in 1984.[12] After intravenous injection of fluorescein dye, the skin at the proposed site of amputation is viewed with a fiberoptic fluorometer, which gives a digital numerical readout that is proportional to the volume of skin blood flow at that site. This technique appears to be applicable and reliable at all levels of amputation.

Compared with segmental Doppler systolic pressures, skin fluorescence testing helps the surgeon to select a more distal level of amputation that has a high probability of healing.[105] Initial reports not only demonstrated an optimal reference point between healing and nonhealing amputations but also led to the definition of a dye fluorescence *index* that could achieve 93% accuracy for amputation level selection.[149] Whereas this test appears to be readily reproducible and is minimally invasive, it has not gained widespread popularity because of its unreliability in the presence of active cellulitis or inflammation, which commonly accompany gangrene or impending tissue loss.

Laser Doppler Velocimetry

The working principle of the laser Doppler velocimeter is derived from the fact that a laser light beam incident upon tissue is scattered by the static structures (skin) and by the moving components (red blood cells). According to the Doppler effect, light beams back-scattered by the moving red cells undergo a frequency shift that is proportional to their velocity. Beams scattered in the static tissue remain unshifted in frequency. These return signals are guided from the skin surface onto the probe's photodetector, extracted, and processed to produce a numerical value that is proportional to the flow in the microcirculation. This flow calculation depends not only on the average velocity of the red blood cells but also on the density of red blood cells per measured volume. The advantage of using light as the tissue "probe" is the limited depth of penetration (1 mm), which avoids any interference from blood flow in the deeper major blood vessels, which would compromise accurate assay of the local microvascular flow in the skin (Fig. 162–1).

Resting measurements of cutaneous blood flow by the

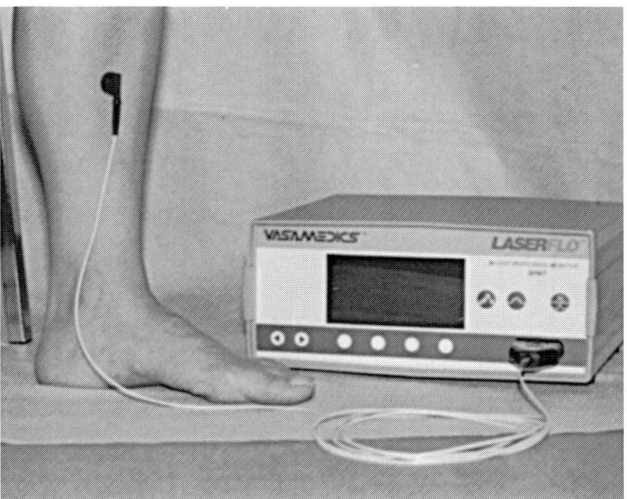

FIGURE 162–1. Laser Doppler velocimetry device with skin surface probe in place, connected to the monitor. This technique is noninvasive, reproducible, and portable. (Courtesy of Vasamedics, Inc., St. Paul, Minn.)

laser Doppler principle in dysvascular limbs are in the same general range as similar measurements in limbs that have no significant arterial disease; however, when the skin beneath the laser probe is heated to 44°C for 10 minutes, patients with significant arterial disease demonstrate markedly diminished hyperemic responses compared with normovascular control subjects.[58, 61, 104] Such local skin heating may make the laser Doppler technique more accurate as a potential preoperative assay for predicting amputation healing. Laser Doppler measurement sites are employed at these levels:

- *Toe amputation:* on the dorsal surface of the foot at the metatarsal head of the involved digit
- *Forefoot amputation:* midway between the first metatarsal head and the medial malleolus
- *Below-knee:* 10 cm distal to the tibial tuberosity and 10 cm proximal to the patella

All perfusion measurements are performed with the patient supine.[2] Reliability has been enhanced by combining the results obtained by laser Doppler velocimetry with those derived from transcutaneous assay of local skin oxygen tension (see later).[78]

Laser Doppler Measurement of Skin Perfusion Pressure

Skin perfusion pressure is defined as the amount of external pressure required to arrest microcirculatory blood flow. Newer techniques allow this determination by application of external pressure and by the return of microcirculatory flow, as detected by laser Doppler velocimetry, by photoelectric assay, or by photoplethysmographic techniques.[103] When a transparent plastic bladder is used to apply pressure, the laser Doppler and photoplethysmographic parameters can be obtained readily and noninvasively.[20] Preheating the skin to 45°C may increase accuracy.[2]

These noninvasive bedside techniques are readily available and not unduly expensive; moreover, they measure pressure in the microcirculatory bed at the skin level and should circumvent the inaccuracies inherent in segmental Doppler studies that may yield spurious information due to medial wall calcification of the tibial or digital arteries.

Photoelectric Skin Perfusion Pressure

Skin perfusion pressure may be measured by isotope washout techniques (see later), but these studies are time-consuming and invasive and require expensive, sophisticated equipment. Photoelectric measurement of skin perfusion pressure is a less invasive and simpler means of determining skin blood flow.[62–68, 121, 156] The equipment consists of a photodetector, which is placed on the patient's skin and connected to a plethysmograph. External pressure to a suprasystolic level is then applied over the photodetector with a blood pressure cuff. As the pressure is gradually reduced at a constant rate, the plethysmographic tracing changes direction when capillary inflow begins. The skin perfusion pressure is defined as the minimum external pressure that prevents reddening of the skin after it has been blanched; this numerical value (empressed in millimeters of mercury [mmHg]) is the point at which the plethysmographic tracing changes direction and capillary inflow begins.[156]

To avoid the difficulties inherent in interpreting the tracings from patients with diminished lower extremity systolic blood pressures, a standardized reading technique has been developed so that the systolic pressure is measured directly by a strain-gauge technique at the same level of the extremity where the photoelectric tracing is being obtained.[156] Although proponents of this technique conclude that it can replace isotope washout assays in many cases, the isotope techniques, if available, should be the method of choice when technically satisfactory photoelectric tracings cannot be made or when the systolic blood pressures cannot be accurately measured.[121]

Isotope Measurement of Skin Perfusion Pressure

Estimation of local tissue perfusion pressure by isotope washout was originally described by Nilsen[119] and Holstein[68] and their associates using xenon 133 in muscle and skin. Holstein began with the radioisotope clearance method originally described for assay of muscle perfusion and modified it for use in skin perfusion pressure measurement, defining the skin perfusion pressure as the amount of external counterpressure necessary to stop the clearance of the intradermally injected isotope.[62]

Because xenon 133 can be trapped within the subcutaneous fat, and because medical-grade xenon 133 is no longer commercially available, other isotopes have been proposed for this assay, such as sodium iodine 131, iodine 131 antipyrine, and technetium 99m pertechnetate. Several subsequent studies have verified the utility of Holstein's method.[62-65, 67, 114, 115] Although these reports do suggest a correlation between isotope-derived skin perfusion pressure and successful amputation wound healing, until recently there was no threshold skin perfusion pressure value above which all amputations would heal and below which none would heal. Data on skin perfusion pressure from the Netherlands (using a modified ^{123}I-iodoantipyrine technique) has demonstrated excellent amputation wound healing predictive values. The threshold value was 20 mmHg. Reliable healing occurred when skin perfusion pressure values were over 20 mmHg, and poor healing when they were less than 20 mmHg ($p < .001$; positive predictive value 89%; negative predictive value 99%).[38]

Isotope Measurement of Skin Blood Flow

Skin blood flow can be determined by using an intradermal injection of xenon 133 gas that has been dissolved in saline solution[34, 100, 112] or an intracutaneous injection of iodine 125 iodoantipyrine[169]; the subsequent rate of isotope clearance from the point of injection is measured with a gamma camera interfaced to a minicomputer. Dual-point testing with a separation of 1 cm is done to eliminate injection error. As described by Malone and associates,[98, 99] the monoexponential washout rate of the intradermal xenon 133 during the first 6 minutes after injection is used to calculate the rate of skin blood flow in milliliters per minute per 100 gm of tissue.

One of the major drawbacks to the universal application of xenon 133 skin blood flow measurements for preoperative selection of amputation level has been the difficulty in reproducing results from one center to another. In addition, the technique is invasive and expensive; sophisticated nuclear scanning devices along with computing equipment and software are required. Nonetheless, in experienced hands, primary healing of amputation wounds has been accurately predicted from the toe (83% success) to the below-knee level (93% success), on up to the above-knee level (100% success).[36, 99] These results were obtained by using the discriminant value of blood flow of 2.4 to 2.6 ml/min per 100 gm of tissue; blood flow above this level was associated with successful healing of amputations. Harris and associates,[54] however, have suggested that these recommendations of the lowest flow consistent with healing have been set too high, because they observed clinical success in 94% of below-knee amputations when the local skin blood flow value was only 1.0 ml/min per 100 gm of tissue. A modification of this technique utilizes *epicutaneous*, rather than *intradermal*, injection of xenon 133, with excellent results.[86]

Measurement of Skin Temperature

Although clinical assessment of skin temperature by physical examination is not a sound basis for selecting the amputation level,[66] studies have suggested that *objective* skin temperature measurement may yield valid data for preoperative selection of amputation level.[152] This technique has been particularly valuable in discriminating between below-knee and above-knee levels (with 90% accuracy[167]) and has been correlated with isotopically derived measurements of skin blood flow.[152] Thus, thermographic mapping appeared to hold some promise for objective preoperative amputation level selection, especially because the examinations are easy to perform and may be tailored to provide a contoured isothermic map of the limb, which might be useful in designing the amputation flaps. No recent work in this area has been pursued, however, since other techniques seem more readily applicable.

Measurement of Transcutaneous Oxygen Tension

Use of a miniaturized, heated Clark electrode to measure the oxygen tension at the surface of the skin was reported simultaneously in 1972 by Huch and Eberhard and their respective associates.[39, 69] These reports led to widespread clinical application of this technique in the setting of neonatal critical care monitoring because the $tcPO_2$ values so derived were found to correlate strongly with more invasive arterial blood PO_2 values. Unfortunately, results were not reproducible in adult populations.

At normal room temperature, the PO_2 on the surface of adult skin approaches zero.[42] Therefore, the clinically relevant measurements of $tcPO_2$ rely on the maximal dilatation of the local vasculature in the upper dermis, an effect produced by local heating of the skin surface via heating the Clark electrode to 43° to 45°C. The theoretical basis of transcutaneous blood gas measurement has been presented in elegant detail by Lubbers.[96]

Several groups have reported encouraging work in the

evaluation of dysvascular patients using the modified Clark-type heated oxygen electrode.[17, 46, 56, 74, 79, 87, 102, 104, 116, 131, 133, 153] All of these studies have suggested that the $tcPO_2$ measurements can predict the *healing* of a specific amputation level with a high degree of accuracy; however, their ability to predict accurately the *failure* to heal is not as reliable.[171] Additionally, the failure of healing of an amputation wound may often be due to numerous perioperative factors, so that a preoperative test of any nature should not be expected to always predict the outcome with complete certainty.[131] Decreased $tcPO_2$ levels correlate with increased probability of failure to heal; however, even a $tcPO_2$ level of zero does not *invariably* lead to failure of amputation wound healing.

The discrepancy between $tcPO_2$ and actual skin blood flow measurements at low (<10 mmHg) $tcPO_2$ levels has been addressed in several studies that provide a partial explanation for why some amputations heal at low $tcPO_2$ levels that usually indicate failure.[104] Matsen and associates[104] reported that there is a nonlinear relationship between $tcPO_2$ and local cutaneous blood flow; they demonstrated that $tcPO_2$ readings of 0 were obtained in the presence of significant local cutaneous blood flow (arteriovenous gradients of 13 to 34 mmHg). Measurements of $tcPO_2$ depend on the ratio of arterial to venous gradients and vascular resistance. Heating the skin under the electrode minimizes local vascular resistance and tends to make the $tcPO_2$ measurements more parallel with the local cutaneous blood flow. Spence and associates[153] have suggested that the $tcPO_2$ values are not directly related to *actual* tissue PO_2 and thus may not represent the true local oxygen availability, because oxygen extraction and utilization are significantly altered in ischemic tissue. They concluded, however, that $tcPO_2$ may be closely related to the actual arterial perfusion pressure, especially in ischemic areas, since ischemic tissue is maximally vasodilated.

Other modifications to improve accuracy include $tcPO_2$ measurements while the patient is breathing supplemental oxygen[56, 113, 116, 145] and measurements following intravenous infusion of naftidrofuryl, which increases cellular metabolism.[116] Ito and associates[74] have mapped out transcutaneous "isobars" on the lower limb based on circumferential $tcPO_2$ measurements; this technique should allow the objective preoperative modification of skin flap design to achieve maximal healing potential and to avoid any "islands of ischemia" described by Rhodes and Cogan.[132] Transcutaneous oxygen recovery half-time after temporarily induced limb ischemia has provided increased discrimination for objective evaluation of room air $tcPO_2$ values.[87] Harward[56] and Oishi[120] and their groups evaluated the accuracy of $tcPO_2$ measurements while patients were breathing room air and again while they were breathing supplemental oxygen; this technique increased the accuracy of amputation level selection at all levels.

Finally, investigators at the Mayo Clinic defined the pressure for successful healing of amputations as $tcPO_2$ of more than 40 mmHg and that for failure of healing as less than 20 mmHg. In an attempt to enhance the predictability of the intervening "gray zone" of $tcPO_2$ between 20 and 40 mmHg, repeat $tcPO_2$ measurements were obtained during elevation of the lower limbs to 30 degrees for 3 minutes. Decreases in $tcPO_2$ of *more than* 15 mmHg were predictive

of amputation healing failure, whereas decreases of *less than* 15 mmHg were usually associated with successful wound healing.[1] It appears that $tcPO_2$ levels greater that 30 to 40 mmHg are associated with a good likelihood of healing in most instances.[1, 5, 15]

Measurement of Transcutaneous Carbon Dioxide Tension

Some transcutaneous gas monitors now have a combination sensor electrode that allows simultaneous monitoring of $tcPCO_2$ in addition to the $tcPO_2$. Less experience is available on assay of $tcPCO_2$, and exact correlations among the $tcPCO_2$, skin blood flow, and subsequent amputation healing have not yet been defined. Thus, the door is open for future studies to determine whether the addition of $tcPCO_2$ to the preoperative evaluation may assist in the selection of the optimal level of amputation.

Conclusion

Transcutaneous measurement of gases is a useful preoperative test to assist in selecting the most distal amputation site that will heal successfully. Yet, using $tcPO_2$ and $tcPCO_2$ values for such decisions requires a few caveats.

First, different manufacturers of transcutaneous gas monitors often give different absolute numerical values for discriminatory purposes, and this fact makes comparisons of findings very difficult from one institution to another. One possible solution to this problem is to use an indexed value using the limb $tcPO_2$ or the limb $tcPCO_2$ results as the numerator with a reference chest wall reading of $tcPO_2$ or $tcPCO_2$ as the denominator, as described by Hauser and Shoemaker.[57]

A second problem inherent in the interpretation of $tcPO_2$/$tcPCO_2$ results is that excellent positive predictive values (approaching 100%) are produced, whereas the negative predictive value is only 50%.[36] This can lead to an increased number of amputations at a higher level. Perhaps these problems will be resolved as additional studies are completed.[102]

Finally, cellulitis and edema often result in inaccurate transcutaneous gas levels, and each of these situations should be controlled before any definitive operative decisions are made.[5]

AMPUTATION LEVELS: INDICATIONS, OBJECTIVE LEVEL SELECTION, TECHNIQUES, AND PROGNOSIS

General Principles

Preoperative evaluation and preparation of the patient decrease perioperative morbidity and mortality rates. Important ancillary factors that should improve the healing and recovery rates include optimization of cardiorespiratory status, renal function, nutritional status,[34] and diabetes management. Preoperative hemodilution may also be helpful.[3, 47, 77] Preoperative, prophylactic, intravenous antibiotic coverage[70, 136, 151] in conjunction with control or eradication of any existing septic focus can also improve outcomes. Control of the infected portion of the ischemic limb may be accomplished with systemic intravenous antibiotics, local drainage and débridement, cryoamputation,[53, 71] or open guillotine amputation.[33, 106] Most often, a combination of these modalities is required.

Surprisingly, the presence of diabetes mellitus has no significant impact on successful primary healing of major lower extremity amputations.[60, 72, 97–99] In fact, diabetic patients generally do better with management at an early stage. Typically, patients who have had the worst profiles have been young, white, male nondiabetic smokers with coronary artery disease.[35, 82, 155] More recent studies underscore the multifactoral complexity of vascular disease that necessitates amputation. In a group of diabetic patients, African Americans had a higher mortality rate after lower extremity amputation than did non-Hispanic whites. Hispanics with heart failure and stroke had the most significant associated adverse factors.[91] The Danish Amputation Register also focused on diabetic amputees and found higher mortality rates for women and younger patients. The mortality rate was eight times greater for diabetic amputees than for diabetic person who had not had an amputation.[40]

Precise surgical technique is essential to achieving optimal healing of amputations performed for complications of ischemia. The surgeon should strive to preserve the longest stump that will reliably heal; at times, achieving this requires performing a vascular reconstructive procedure before the planned amputation that will allow healing at a lower level, resulting in better potential for rehabilitation. Because some amputations do follow revascularization operations,[134] atypical skin flaps are often preferable to amputation at a more proximal site; these flaps may be mapped out preoperatively using the objective tests outlined in the preceding section.

Bones must be transected at a comfortable distance above the skin flaps. Appropriate beveling of angulated bone remnants and bony prominences should be done carefully to create smooth contours. The periosteum should not be stripped away excessively, lest bony overgrowth or sequestrum formation develop.

Small nerves should be divided sharply while firm but not excessive traction is applied to the nerve trunk. This allows retraction of the nerve remnant above the level of bone division, placing any subsequent neuroma well above points of pressure. Excessive traction on the nerve during division may lead to unnecessary neuralgia and stump pain. The blood supply to large nerves, such as the sciatic nerve, should be suture ligated proximally before being transected because the vasa nervorum may cause substantial bleeding if not controlled.

Muscles may be divided sharply or with electrocautery. In either instance, hemostasis must be precise; mass ligature incorporating large clumps of tissue is unacceptable. The use of a proximal tourniquet is contraindicated during amputation of an ischemic limb. Myodesis procedures, too, should usually be avoided.

Hemostasis is essential to ensuring optimal healing; a hematoma may elevate tenuous skin flaps or may result in infection. *Careful* use of electrocautery allows pinpoint control of bleeding sites. Indiscriminate use of electrocautery should be avoided to prevent damage to surrounding soft tissues. The use of bone wax should be discouraged because it acts as a foreign body.

If absolute hemostasis is not possible, judicious use of closed-system suction drains is indicated to prevent hematoma formation. Such drains should be removed within 24 to 48 hours. Before closure of the wound, as hemostasis is being achieved, the wound should be thoroughly irrigated to remove clots and debris. Many surgeons use an antibiotic solution (e.g., bacitracin-kanamycin) for irrigation, although convincing data that show that "local" antibiotics are beneficial have not been published. Similarly, such an antibiotic solution may be used throughout the operation to prevent desiccation of the tissues and to keep bacterial counts down.

The surgeon must close the skin of an amputation stump atraumatically using precise suture placement without using skin forceps. Perfect coaptation of the skin edges will be rewarded with faster and successful primary healing. In addition to monofilament sutures, metal staples or tape strips are efficient and effective alternative means of closing the skin when atraumatic techniques with minimal use of tissue forceps are employed.

Lower limb amputation after an unsuccessful vascular reconstruction attempt may be complicated when the bypass conduit is a prosthetic material. Rubin and associates[141] documented that removal of the thrombosed graft in the presence of an infected wound or removal of an infected graft at the time of major limb amputation decreased the incidence of amputation wound complications and subsequent graft remnant infections. In another study, Rubin's group also provided evidence to support removal of the *entire* failed prosthetic graft at the time of amputation, even when there is no evidence of wound or graft infection at that time.[142] Firm recommendation for adding this potentially extensive procedure to an amputation awaits confirmation in other centers.

Lower extremity amputations may also follow previous orthopedic procedures, sometimes from long ago. Metallic prostheses used for fracture fixation or joint reconstruction must be anticipated by a thorough history and physical examination. Unsuspected orthopedic hardware can create unnecessary difficulties or complications, most often during above-knee amputations. Survey radiographs can define the nature of a metallic implant in a patient with "suspicious" surgical scars. In this manner, the amputation operation can be tailored to avoid the prosthesis; if necessary, a plan for orderly transection or removal of the device with special equipment and personnel can be formulated preoperatively.[80]

With the exception of amputations of the digits or single ray amputations, immediate postoperative application of a precisely fitted rigid dressing produces the most prompt and successful healing and rehabilitation of all amputations through or distal to the knee joint. The use of an immediately fitted rigid postoperative dressing need not always be combined with an immediate postoperative prosthesis. A rigid postoperative amputation stump dressing is not a panacea and it requires an intimate knowledge of the technique; misapplication can lead to serious wound problems. Some authors are quick to point out the disadvantages of such a rigid dressing protocol in the immediate postoperative period[28] and report better postoperative courses when soft compression dressings are employed. Such reports are dated, however, and reflect lack of experience with rigid postoperative dressings. Findings are contrary to those of larger studies that emphasize a *team approach* that involves the surgeon, the prosthetist, and the physiatrist.[97]

Early postoperative mobilization and perioperative use of a pneumatic compression device on the contralateral limb addresses the significant problem of lower extremity deep venous thrombosis in the amputee. Yeager and colleagues documented a 12.5% incidence of deep venous thrombosis during the perioperative period after lower extremity amputation. Patients with a history of chronic venous disease or another amputation were at highest risk.[175] While prophylactic anticoagulation is not routinely warranted, an aggressive investigative approach with duplex venous ultrasound should be employed in the presence of unexpected limb edema or prolonged recumbency.

Toe Amputation

Indications

Amputation of a toe is the most common amputation of the lower limb. "Dry" gangrene is best treated by allowing autoamputation; epithelialization proceeds beneath the dead portion of the gangrenous, but uninfected, digit. This approach should be selected only for reliable, conscientious patients whose clinical course can be closely monitored. The presence of dry gangrene also permits preamputation vascular reconstruction, if warranted. If the gangrenous process is "wet," an active infectious process is under way that may be progressive, and prompt surgical removal of all dead, infected tissue is mandatory. Antibiotics are a useful adjunct but are not to be used *alone* when the infection involves the entire toe or when osteomyelitis is present; instead, prompt digital amputation with concurrent antibiotic administration enhances recovery and rehabilitation.[83]

Indications for toe amputation include gangrene, infection, osteomyelitis, and neuropathic ulceration that is confined to the middle or distal phalanx. Amputation of a painful but uninfected ischemic toe may also be indicated.

Contraindications

Specific contraindications to amputation at the toe level include:

1. Dependent rubor of the toes.
2. Cellulitis proximal to the site of proposed toe amputation.
3. Forefoot or plantar space infection.
4. Infection or osteomyelitis involving the metatarsophalangeal joint or the metatarsal head.
5. Inadequate blood supply.

Prediction of Healing

The various methods of preoperative evaluation of the arterial circulation for amputation at the toe level are outlined in Table 162–2. Clinical findings still play a most important role in predicting the success of toe amputation.[93] Although empirical selection at this level yields a

TABLE 162–2. PREOPERATIVE LEVEL SELECTION: TOE AMPUTATION

SELECTION CRITERION	SUCCESSFUL HEALING, PRIMARY AND SECONDARY/TOTAL (%)	REFERENCE
Empirical	86/115 (75)	127
Presence of pedal pulses	357/365 (98)	150
Doppler toe pressure > 30 mmHg	47/60 (78)	68
Doppler ankle pressure > 35 mmHg	44/46 (96)	163
Photoplethysmographic digit or TMA pressure > 20 mmHg	20/20 (100)	146
Xenon 133 skin blood flow > 2.6 ml/100 gm tissue/min	5/6 (83)	98

TMA = transmetatarsal.

disappointing healing rate of 75% in the absence of foot pulses, the presence of palpable pedal pulses is associated with a 98% healing rate. When pedal pulses are not palpable, determination of the digit (or forefoot) systolic blood pressure via photoplethysmography is the best available predictor of healing. Furthermore, experience with photoplethysmographically derived toe or transmetatarsal pressures indicates that a systolic digital pressure greater than 40 mmHg used as the index for successful healing is a reliable prognostic parameter.

Surgical Technique

Amputation of a single toe should never be performed by disarticulation through a phalangeal joint because this leads to exposure of the avascular cartilage of the proximal joint capsule. Instead, the surgeon transects the proximal phalanx, leaving a small button of bone to protect the metatarsal head. Skin flaps may be of any design (e.g., fish-mouth, plantar-based, dorsally based, or side-to-side), but the most commonly used incision is circular (Fig. 162–2). Any flaps

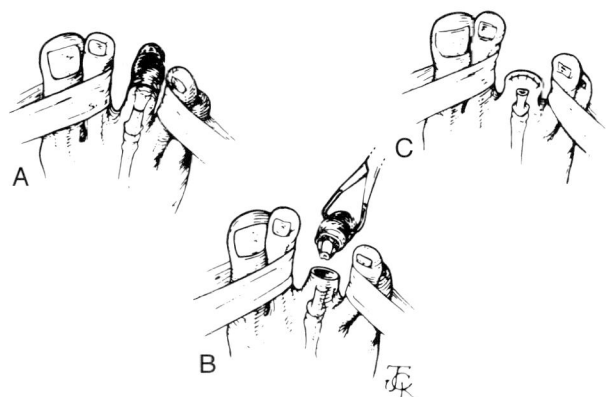

FIGURE 162–2. A, While the adjacent toes are retracted medially and laterally, a circular incision proximal to the proximal interphalangeal joint is made. B, Dissection exposes the proximal phalanx, which is divided. C, The circular incision is then closed in a transverse direction with interrupted, carefully placed, coapting sutures.

must be tailored to allow tension-free closure over the phalangeal stump.

A circular skin incision minimizes the length of the resultant wound and should help to reduce the risk of skin edge devascularization that may occur with any type of skin flap. The incision is then carried down to the phalanx, which is divided. The bony remnant may be smoothed carefully with a rasp. Any tendinous structures must be sharply excised while they are held on gentle traction. Electrocautery should be used sparingly, if at all. Irrigation fluid is used to cleanse the wound thoroughly. Meticulous hemostasis and careful, atraumatic, edge-to-edge skin closure will be rewarded with enhanced wound healing. Minimally reactive monofilament suture material is used because often these sutures must remain in place for long periods (4 to 6 weeks) to ensure complete wound healing. In the presence of an active infectious process, the amputation wound should be left open for healing by secondary intention.

Advantages and Disadvantages

The principal advantages of simple toe amputation are the minimal amount of tissue removed and the minimal impact on rehabilitation. Total resection of the great toe, or of *all* the toes of a given foot, however, may lead to minor imbalance during ambulation. Preservation of the metatarsal fat pads affords relatively normal weight-bearing mechanics. The main disadvantage of a simple toe amputation is the risk of stump breakdown due to ischemia or intervening infection.

Prosthetic Requirements and Rehabilitation Potential

No prosthesis is necessary after toe amputation. The potential for rehabilitation should be 100%. Amputation of all the toes of one foot causes minor gait disturbances at a slow pace and becomes more troublesome at a fast pace because of the loss of "pushoff"; squatting and tiptoeing are difficult or impossible. Consequently, a shoe filler is helpful for very active patients. Continued close follow-up care is essential because almost 75% of these patients may require a more proximal amputation within 3½ years after the toe amputation.[95]

Ray Amputation
Indications

Localized gangrene or infection adjacent to the metatarsophalangeal crease or involving the metatarsal head precludes a simple toe amputation. In such cases, extending the amputation to excise the metatarsal head accomplishes removal of all necrotic, infected, and compromised tissue and leaves adequate viable skin for successful wound closure without tension.

Contraindications

Dependent rubor, cellulitis, infection, or gangrene proximal to the metatarsophalangeal crease are specific contraindica-

tions to performance of a ray amputation; osteomyelitis of a metatarsal shaft is also a contraindication. Some cases of cellulitis that preclude immediate safe performance of a ray amputation may be initially treated with appropriate intravenous antibiotics as a first-line measure, followed by the ray amputation if the cellulitis subsides.

Involvement of three or more toes is a relative contraindication; a transmetatarsal amputation would be more suitable in this case. Ray amputation of the great toe may also be considered a relative contraindication *in active patients,* because removal of the first metatarsal head leads to unstable weight bearing, difficulty with ambulation, and late skin ulceration of the plantar surface. A ray amputation of the great toe is a worthwhile procedure in patients whose activity levels were already limited.

Finally, caution has been advised in the performance of a ray amputation in an insensitive, dysvascular foot because these problems are associated with a high failure rate owing to the subsequent development of a "transfer lesion." This lesion is an ulceration resulting from abnormal weight bearing due to the transfer of pressure points after removal of a metatarsal head. When this type of ulceration develops in the ray amputee with an insensate foot, the amputation level must be revised, often to the below-knee level.[48]

Prediction of Healing

The same objective preoperative parameters used for predicting the outcome of simple toe amputations are applicable to evaluating the potential success of a ray amputation (see Table 162–2).

Surgical Technique

A racquet-type incision is started with a vertical component (the "handle" of the racquet) on the dorsum of the foot to expose the metatarsal head (Fig. 162–3). This incision is then carried distally, bifurcating medially and laterally to encircle the toe. The two bifurcated limbs of the incision

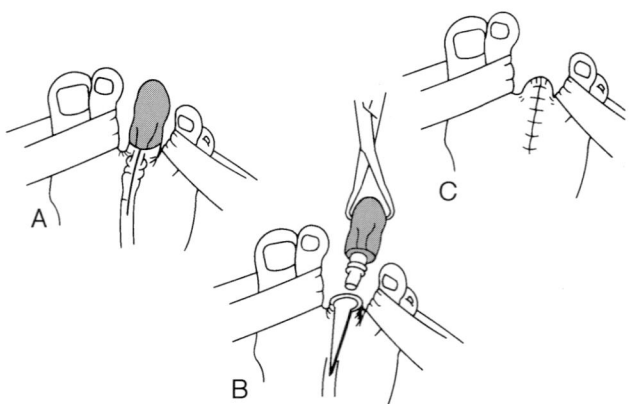

FIGURE 162–3. Artist's rendition of the steps involved in a single-ray amputation of the foot. *A,* The incision is designed to expose the distal metatarsal phalangeal region. *B,* The distal metatarsal is divided far enough proximally to permit closure without tension. *C,* Following excision of the specimen, including the intact metatarsal phalangeal joint, the dorsal portion of the incision is closed in its original direction, and the circular portion of the plantar incision is closed transversely.

are then joined on the plantar aspect of the foot to create a circle at the base of the toe (the "head" of the racquet). As the incision is taken down to the level of the bone, care must be exercised to avoid injuring the digital arteries that course along the metatarsal shaft. Additional caution is employed to avoid entry into the deep tendon or joint spaces of the adjacent digits.

The distal metatarsal shaft is divided at its neck with a 45-degree plantar bevel that minimizes the risk of plantar ulceration from a sharp plantar bony prominence pressure point. Structures attached to the detached metatarsal head are divided sharply, and the intact specimen (consisting of the toe, the metatarsophalangeal joint, and the metatarsal head) may then be removed in continuity.

All tendon remnants are sharply excised as far proximally as possible. Hemostasis is achieved with careful, conservative use of electrocautery or fine monofilament sutures. The space created by removal of the metatarsal head is irrigated thoroughly with an antibiotic solution before skin closure. Monofilament sutures that incorporate the deep tissues are placed to coapt the skin edges exactly, or the wound may be closed in layers. A *closed* drain should be utilized only if excellent hemostasis cannot be achieved, and it should be removed within 24 hours. If the metatarsal head is infected or if there is extensive distal infection, the wound may be left open, packed, and allowed to heal by delayed primary closure or by secondary intention. A soft compression dressing helps to avoid tension on the suture line and to minimize the potential dead space in the bed of the metatarsal head.

Advantages and Disadvantages

The advantages of a ray amputation are minimal tissue loss and no subsequent limitations on activity. Drawbacks include the risks of nonhealing, chronic osteomyelitis of the metatarsal shaft remnant, and hematoma or infection in the deep tissue space. Certainly, these risks are minimized with proper patient selection and exacting surgical technique. Ray amputation of the great toe may make ambulation difficult, and late plantar skin breakdown may occur because of the loss of the balance and pushoff provided by the first metatarsal head and the great toe.

Prosthetic Requirements and Rehabilitation Potential

Although no prosthetic device is required for rehabilitation after ray amputation, a specially constructed orthotic shoe definitely improves balance and minimizes skin trauma for very active patients. Rehabilitation potential is 100%.

Transmetatarsal Amputation
Indications

Gangrene or infection confined to several toes or involving only the great toe is the ideal indication for transmetatarsal amputation. This procedure may also be used if the disease process extends only a short way past the metatarsophalangeal crease, provided that the plantar skin is healthy.

Contraindications

Specific contraindications to amputation at this level include:

- Dependent rubor, cellulitis, lymphangitis, and osteomyelitis at the mid-foot
- Deep forefoot (plantar space) infection
- Gangrene or ischemia of the plantar skin of the foot

Open transmetatarsal amputation may be used successfully in the presence of infection if the forefoot infectious process does not extend proximally beyond the level of the metatarsal heads and if no significant ischemia exists.[37]

Prediction of Healing

The most accurate objective techniques for preoperative determination of successful healing at the transmetatarsal level are fiberoptic fluorometry, xenon 133 (or iodine 125 iodoantipyrine) skin blood flow assay, and transcutaneous oxygen and carbon dioxide measurements (Table 162–3). Doppler ankle systolic blood pressure measurements are useful as a second-line technique when the other tests are not available; however, the Doppler-derived pressures suffer from lack of sensitivity, and the absolute ankle systolic pressure required to predict healing success reliably is at least 60 to 70 mmHg. If the objective tests listed earlier are not available, photoplethysmographic toe pressures offer the most reliable guide to successful transmetatarsal amputation healing, especially in diabetic patients, whose amputations with photoplethysmographically derived toe pressures less than 38 mmHg invariably failed to heal.[164] Unfortunately, this does not seem to hold true for persons who do not have diabetes; for them, no obvious relationship between toe pressures and healing outcomes was noted. Studying nondiabetic patients, Vitti and coworkers documented some successful wound healing, even at toe pressure values of 10 mmHg or less.[164]

Finally, pulsatile pulse volume recordings at the transmetatarsal level with normal amplitude and contour are a reliable guide to successful wound healing.

Surgical Technique

Excellent descriptions of the technique of transmetatarsal amputation have been published by McKittrick[107] and Effeney[41] and their colleagues. The skin incision is designed to utilize a total plantar flap and virtually no dorsal skin flap component. A slightly curved dorsal incision is carried from one side of the foot to the other, just distal to the anticipated line of bone transection at the middle portion of the metatarsal shafts. The incision extends to the base of the toes medially and laterally in the mid-plane axis of the foot and then across the plantar surface at the metatarsophalangeal crease (Fig. 162–4). Once the skin incision has been sharply defined, the dorsal component is carried down to the metatarsal shafts, which are transected 5 to 10 mm proximal to the line of the dorsal skin incision with a power oscillating saw with a small blade. The bony ends are carefully smoothed with a rasp if necessary.

The plantar tissues of the distal forefoot are sharply excised from the metatarsal shafts. Tendons are sharply

TABLE 162–3. PREOPERATIVE LEVEL SELECTION: FOOT AND FOREFOOT AMPUTATION

SELECTION CRITERION		SUCCESSFUL HEALING, PRIMARY AND SECONDARY/TOTAL (%)	REFERENCE
Empirical		11/24 (46)	127
		36/50 (72)	169
Doppler ankle pressure	<40 mmHg	5/9 (56)	109, 169
	>40 mmHg	20/60 (33)	10
	40–60 mmHg	4/5 (80)	169
	>50 mmHg	14/21 (66)	68
	>60 mmHg	68/91 (75)	109, 169
	>70 mmHg	70/93 (75)	4, 118, 146
Doppler toe pressure	>30 mmHg	4/5 (80)	68
Doppler ankle-brachial pressure index	>0.45 (nondiabetic)	58/60 (97)	125
	>0.50 (diabetic)		
Photoplethysmographic toe pressure	>55 mmHg	14/14 (100)	11
	>45 < 55 mmHg	2/8 (25)	11
	<45 mmHg	0/8 (0)	11
	<38 mmHG (diabetic)	0/21 (0)	164
Fiberoptic fluorometry (dye fluorescence index > 44)		18/20 (90)	149
Laser Doppler velocimetry		2/6 (33)	61
Iodine 125 iodopyrine skin blood flow > 8 ml/100 gm tissue/min		18/18 (100)	169
Xenon 133 skin blood flow > 2.6 ml/100 gm tissue/min		23/25 (92)	36
Transcutaneous $P_{O_2} > 10$ mm (or a >10 mm increase on $FI_{O_2} = 1.0$)		6/8 (75)	56
Transcutaneous $P_{O_2} > 28$ mmHg		3/3 (100)	36
Transcutaneous $P_{CO_2} < 40$ mmHg		3/3 (100)	36

transected under tension and are allowed to retract into the depths of the foot. The plantar skin flap is then tailored and thinned sharply to achieve a natural fit when it is rotated dorsally for closure. The avascular volar plates are sharply excised, as is any redundant muscle or fat. Meticulous hemostasis is essential; precise electrocautery is preferable to bone wax. Thorough irrigation with an antibiotic solution precedes closure of the deep tissues with a layer of absorbable interrupted sutures.

Finally, the surgeon performs a tension-free skin closure using monofilament sutures in a vertical mattress technique. If there is tension along the suture line at this point, the surgeon revises the closure by shortening the metatarsal shafts enough to allow absolutely tension-free closure.

The completed stump is then dressed with sterile bandages and protected by a well-padded short-leg plaster cast. Such a rigid dressing helps to control edema and to prevent trauma to the vulnerable transmetatarsal stump. Weight bearing on the amputated limb is not allowed for at least 7 to 10 days, at which time a cast change routine is initiated. Sutures are usually left intact for at least 3 to 4 weeks.

Once the transmetatarsal amputation wound has completely healed, a very durable stump results. Stumps thought to be at high risk for subsequent infection or wound breakdown may be left open (Fig. 162–5A). Rapid wound closure and rehabilitation may be accomplished by placement of a partial-thickness skin graft on the open transmetatarsal stump when it is clean and covered by granulation tissue. Any ischemic or infectious process must be corrected if this approach is to be successful. With time, wound contracture can lead to complete closure of the skin defect created by the open transmetatarsal amputation without the need for a potentially vulnerable partial-thickness skin graft (Fig. 162–5B).[37]

Advantages and Disadvantages

The main advantage of a well-healed transmetatarsal amputation is its excellent function and minimal, if any, disability. It avoids the equinus and equinovalgus deformities that may occur with the more proximal mid-foot amputations of Lisfranc, Chopart, and Pirogoff.[161] These three proximal foot amputations are not often indicated in dysvascular limbs, but they are sometimes successful if performed appropriately.[22, 23]

The main disadvantage is the risk of nonhealing due to ischemia, infection, trauma, or hematoma, which would necessitate a subsequent revision to a higher level. When the appropriate objective preoperative tests to predict healing potential are used, these risks are minimized.

An open transmetatarsal amputation is a safe surgical option that is preferable to a mid-foot or below-knee amputation for the treatment of severe forefoot infection or gangrene even if the distal plantar skin flap is nonviable.[37] Transmetatarsal amputation in patients with peripheral neuropathy carries risk of subsequent mal perforans ulceration than does amputation in patients with a normally sensate foot.[107] Adjunctive revascularization enhances the rate of successful healing in marginally ischemic limbs.[110]

Prosthetic Requirements and Rehabilitation Potential

No specific prosthesis is necessary for adequate ambulation after transmetatarsal amputation, but a shoe modification that incorporates a steel shank in the sole allows normal toe pushoff and prevents excessive dorsiflexion. The steel spring shank reproduces the action of the longitudinal arch of the foot during ambulation. A custom-molded foam pad, lamb's wool, or a toe block is used to fill the toe portion

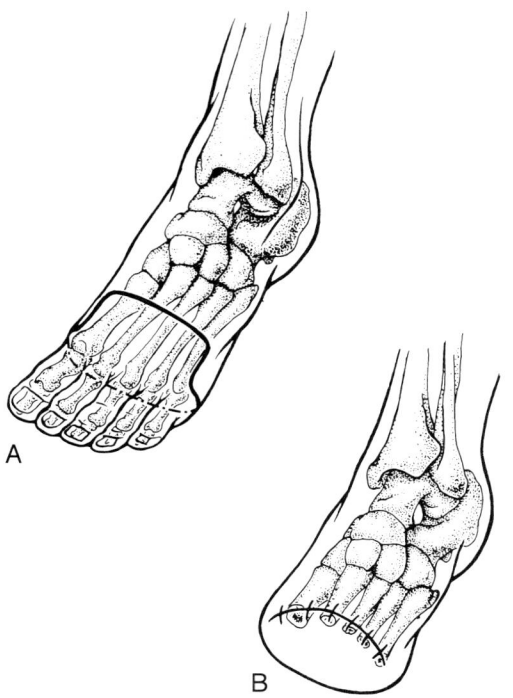

FIGURE 162–4. Illustration of the steps in a transmetatarsal amputation of the forefoot. *A,* The skin incision is placed to provide a total posterior flap while allowing excision of the forefoot with division through all five metatarsals in the mid-metatarsal region. *B,* After excision of the forefoot, the plantar flap is thinned to remove capsule and tendinous material, and a meticulous closure of the plantar and anterior skin is performed.

of the shoe to prevent shoe buckling. A second footwear option is a custom-molded shoe that utilizes a roller-shaped sole to provide the toe pushoff motion during ambulation.[100] There are no limitations on rehabilitation after transmetatarsal amputation, provided suitable footwear is furnished. Proper construction and fit help to prevent subsequent problems with neuropathy-associated ulceration and stump breakdown.

Mid-foot Amputations

Indications

When the gangrenous or infectious process precludes amputation at the transmetatarsal level, a more proximal amputation through the mid-portion of the foot may be considered if ischemia is absent or correctable.[22, 23, 27, 52, 135] Although technically demanding operations, the amputation of Lisfranc and Chopart can produce more functional stumps than an ankle-level or below-knee amputations (Fig. 162–6). If ischemia is present, every effort should be made to provide the most direct revascularization to the foot.

Contraindications

Mid-foot amputations are doomed to fail if significant ischemia is present (see later). Neuropathy in the foot is a *relative* contraindication, as postoperative neuropathic ulcerations may result from abnormal weight bearing on the foot remnant.

Prediction of Healing

Toe pressures and transmetatarsal pulse volume recordings are usually not attainable in these patients owing to tissue loss at these levels. Since these amputations are based on plantar flap coverage, $tcPo_2$ values are not often helpful because of the thick plantar skin. The most reliable predictor of adequate healing is a "believable" Doppler-derived systolic ankle pressure of at least 30 mmHg. These amputations are doomed to fail if the ankle pressure is less than 30 mmHg[23, 24] or if plantar tissue loss is extensive or involves the heel pad. If there is any question of ischemia or unreliability of the noninvasive perfusion parameters, prompt angiography and aggressive attempts at revascularization will enhance amputation wound healing results.

Surgical Technique

The *Lisfranc amputation* is a disarticulation of the mid-foot between the tarsal and metatarsal bones, whereas *Chopart*

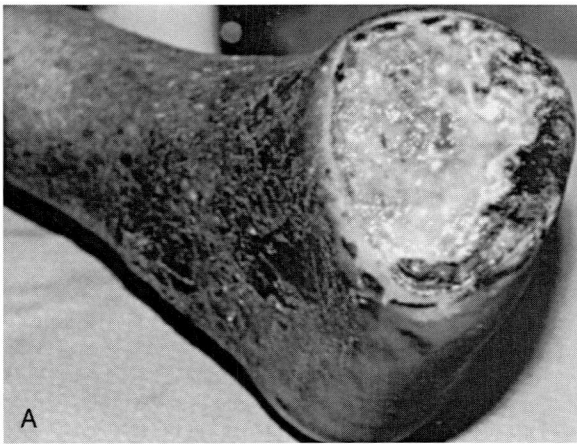
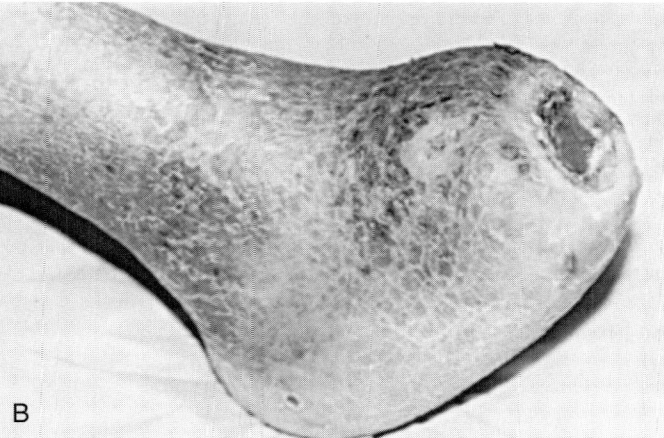

FIGURE 162–5. *A,* Open transmetatarsal amputation stump resulting from resection of all gangrenous and infected tissue in a patient with an advanced diabetic forefoot infection. *B,* Same patient 9 months later with almost complete wound closure owing to wound contraction. This patient was fully ambulatory.

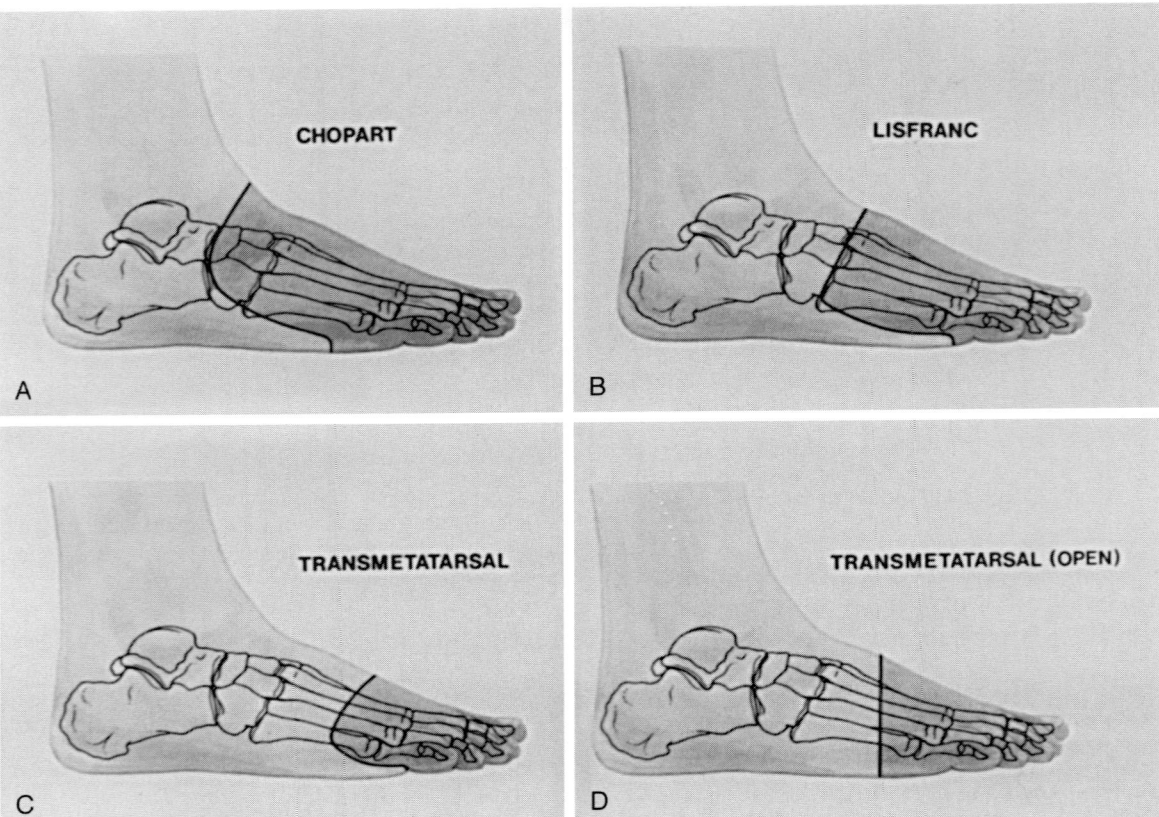

FIGURE 162–6. A–D, The various skin flaps required for closure of mid-foot and forefoot amputations. (From Durham JR, McCoy DM, Sawchuk AP, et al: Open transmetatarsal amputation in the treatment of severe foot infections. Am J Surg 158:128, 1989.)

amputation is disarticulation of the talonavicular and calcaneocuboid joints. Details of surgical technique are similar to those for the more conventional transmetatarsal amputation. Typical skin flaps are shown in Figure 162–6, but the flaps, which are usually based on medial or lateral pedicles, are often not truly symmetric owing to preexisting tissue loss.

A common complication of the Chopart amputation is an equinovarus foot deformity that results from unopposed tendon traction. An important modification of the standard Chopart technique involves severance of the heel cord just above its insertion to the calcaneus. This simple maneuver "lengthens" the heel cord and allows the foot to remain in neutral position, thereby minimizing postoperative development of equinus that would otherwise result from the unopposed pull of the gastrocnemius muscle.[22, 23] Excellent comprehensive reviews of these unconventional mid-foot amputations have been presented by Chang and Pinzur and their associates.[22, 23, 125]

A closed suction drain may be required to manage oozing from cancellous bone surfaces. A soft, bulky dressing without elastic compression is applied. Sutures are typically left intact for 4 to 6 weeks. Full weight bearing is not allowed until the amputation stump has completely healed, usually at 6 to 8 weeks.

Advantages and Disadvantages

A successful Lisfranc amputation often allows relatively normal ambulation with only minor, inexpensive orthotic devices placed in a regular shoe. The main disadvantage is the unpredictable healing process of this amputation. In addition, disruption of the insertion of the peroneus brevis muscle onto the base of the fifth metatarsal head can result in a varus foot deformity; fortunately, it can usually be overcome by appropriate physical therapy. Modification of Chopart's amputation with division of the heel cord minimizes the risk for development of a steep equinus foot deformity, which can result in stump ulceration or abnormal gait.

Adequate ambulation over considerable distances is possible with the clam-shell prosthesis (described later). Short trips in the home, for example to the bathroom, are possible without the prosthesis. Either of these two mid-foot amputations is far preferable to an ankle-level disarticulation or a below-knee amputation. Expert surgical technique and adequate arterial perfusion are imperative to achieving satisfactory results.

Prosthetic Requirements and Rehabilitation Potential

A successfully healed Lisfranc amputation requires only the minor alterations in footwear that are typically employed for a transmetatarsal amputation. A foam filler placed in the toe of a regular shoe is all that is necessary for walking in most instances; however, some patients may require a high-topped shoe or a special ankle-foot orthosis. Not surprisingly, rehabilitation success is quite good. The more proximal nature of Chopart's amputation leaves a much smaller walking platform that must be protected with a specially fitted polypropylene clam-shell prosthesis. This particular prosthesis allows ambulation with a regular oxford shoe and minimizes the up-and-down pumping action that can lead to skin breakdown with this proximal mid-foot amputation.[22]

Once the stump has healed completely, short trips around the house can be made without the prosthesis. Proper prosthetic fitting and diligent follow-up are essential. Aggressive physical therapy minimizes the chances of equinus or varus deformities that can develop with these more proximal mid-foot amputations.

The Ankle-Level Amputations of Syme and Pirogoff

Indications

Indications for an ankle-level amputation are generally the same as those for a transmetatarsal or mid-foot amputation, except that the *Syme* and *Pirogoff* amputations do not require healthy plantar skin distally. The ideal indication for a Syme or a Pirogoff amputation is a distal forefoot or toe infection that involves the plantar skin and thereby precludes a mid-foot or hindfoot amputation. In this situation, an ankle-level amputation is indicated, as long as prognostic tests suggest there is a reasonable chance of successful healing. Healing of these amputations depends on good blood supply to the skin flap via the posterior tibial artery. Thus, this amputation is rarely indicated or appropriate for truly ischemic limbs.

Contraindications

Any abnormality of the heel or heel pad is a contraindication to the *Syme* or *Pirogoff* amputation: (1) gangrene or infection involving the heel; (2) an open lesion of the heel or ankle; or (3) dependent rubor, cellulitis, or lymphangitis of the heel. Pedal neuropathy in a diabetic patient that involves the heel is an absolute contraindication to amputation at this level because the absence of sensation invariably leads eventually to stump breakdown and failure. Moreover, the presence of diabetes mellitus should be a relative contraindication to the Syme amputation because of the risk of subsequent development of distal neuropathy and ulceration of the stump, even after initial success. Malone has reported eventual long-term failure of Syme's amputation in 17 of 32 diabetic patients (53%) who initially enjoyed successful postoperative healing and rehabilitation.[101]

Prediction of Healing

The same objective parameters used preoperatively to predict the healing of foot and forefoot amputations are useful in patients being considered for the Syme amputation (see Table 162–3). Calcification of the tibial arteries with false elevation of ankle-level blood pressure should be a concern. Again, pulsatile pulse volume recordings with relatively normal amplitude and contour are a good prognostic parameter.

Surgical Technique

From a technical standpoint, the ankle-level amputations of Syme and Pirogoff are indisputably among the most demanding and least forgiving lower extremity amputations. Although the Pirogoff amputation helps to preserve limb length, it is rarely performed (see other excellent descriptions of surgical technique.[22, 23, 117]). The Syme amputation is described in detail later. Exacting attention to surgical details is crucial to its success, because the skin flap is easily devascularized and the heel pad can migrate posteriorly if it is not properly affixed to the tibia and fibula. The two-stage *Wagner's modification* is superior to the classic one-stage Syme's amputation[55] in patients with ischemia of the lower extremity. The two-stage procedure also yields a less bulbous, cosmetically more acceptable, more easily fitted stump than does the one-stage technique. Wagner has described both techniques in elegant detail.[166]

The skin incision is planned to create a single long posterior flap that incorporates the heel pad; the incision for the two-stage technique is begun 1 to 1.5 cm farther distal than that for the classic Syme amputation to allow for the additional volume of the retained malleoli. The dorsal incision extends across the ankle from the tip of the medial malleolus to the tip of the lateral malleolus (Fig. 162–7). The plantar incision begins at a 90-degree angle from the dorsal incision and courses around the plantar aspect of the foot distal to the heel pad, cutting all layers to the bone. The dorsal incision is then carried through the subcutaneous tissues to the bone without dissection in the tissue planes.

The tendons are sharply transected under tension and are allowed to retract. The anterior tibial artery is ligated. The capsule of the tibiotalar joint is entered across the

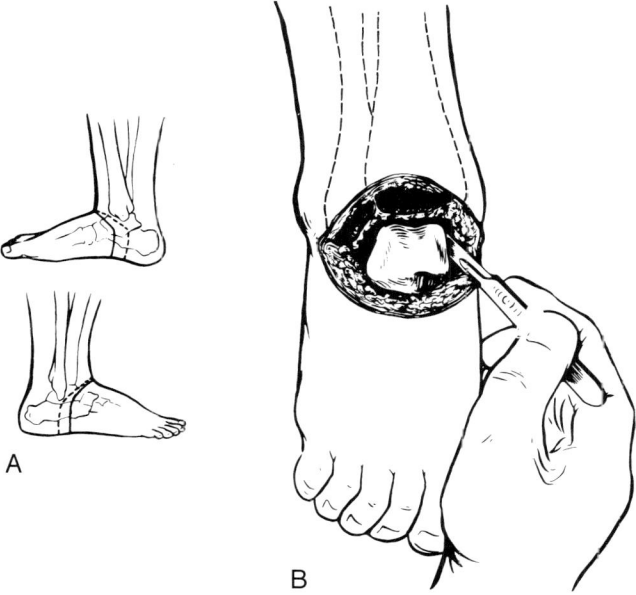

FIGURE 162–7. *A*, Incision for two-stage technique is 1 to 1.5 cm more distal than classic Syme's amputation to allow for volume of malleoli. *B*, Collateral ligaments are divided side to side to allow talus to dislocate distally. (From Wagner FW Jr: The Syme amputation. *In* American Academy of Orthopaedic Surgeons: Atlas of Limb Prosthetics: Surgical and Prosthetic Principles. St. Louis, CV Mosby, 1981.)

dorsum of the talar neck. After the posterior tibialis tendon is divided, the foot is forced into plantar flexion to provide increased exposure of the tibiotalar joint. The mediolateral collateral ligaments are then divided, a maneuver that allows the talus to be dislocated. Great caution must be exercised during dissection along the medial malleolus to avoid damaging the posterior tibial artery, which provides the only blood supply to the heel pad flap.

The peroneus brevis and tertius tendons are transected. Beginning on its superolateral surface, the calcaneus is sharply dissected from the heel pad. At this point, direct inspection of the posterior tibial vascular bundle permits transection *distal* to its branching into the medial and lateral plantar branches. Continued dissection distally allows medial retraction of the vascular bundle and medial dissection of the calcaneus. Transection of the Achilles tendon at its insertion on the calcaneus is performed with great care because, at this point, the tendon is virtually subcutaneous. Penetration, or "buttonholing," of the skin at this step may lead to failure of wound healing (Fig. 162–8). Excision of the forefoot is completed by subperiosteal dissection of the calcaneus and division of the plantar aponeurosis.

Hemostasis is achieved, and thorough irrigation of the wound is performed. A closed suction drainage tube is introduced through a separate small incision and is placed within the joint cavity. The heel pad is rotated anteriorly and placed against the malleoli and plafond; its length is tailored precisely to enable tension-free closure. The deep fascia over the anterior tibia and the remnants of the collateral ligaments are sutured to the deep fascia of the

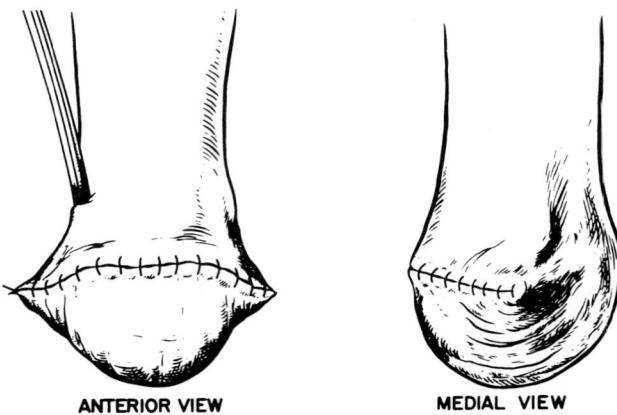

ANTERIOR VIEW   **MEDIAL VIEW**

FIGURE 162–9. No attempt is made to tailor dog ears at closure of first stage. Further posterior dissection narrows base of flap and jeopardizes its circulation. (From Wagner FW Jr: The Syme amputation. *In* American Academy of Orthopaedic Surgeons: Atlas of Limb Prosthetics: Surgical and Prosthetic Principles. St. Louis, CV Mosby, 1981.)

plantar flap. A single layer of monofilament interrupted vertical mattress sutures is used to complete the atraumatic skin closure.

Either a soft compression dressing or a rigid plaster cast is used as the postoperative dressing; most authors prefer a short-leg plaster cast, which helps to maintain correct alignment of the heel pad and to avoid trauma to the stump. Caution must be exercised with the use of a rigid dressing to avoid injury to the medial and lateral skin flaps, or "dog-ears" (Fig. 162–9).

In most cases, adequate healing occurs at about 6 weeks, and the second—and definitive—stage of the amputation may be performed at this time. Two elliptical incisions are made over the malleoli to remove the dog-ears (Fig. 162–10). The amount of tissue removed must be equal to the volume of each malleolus. Sharp dissection is carried down to the bone, with care taken not to damage the posterior tibial vascular bundle along the posteromedial aspect. Close dissection around the medial malleolus protects these vessels.

After periosteal resection, the malleoli are removed flush with the joint surface; the tibial articular cartilage is not

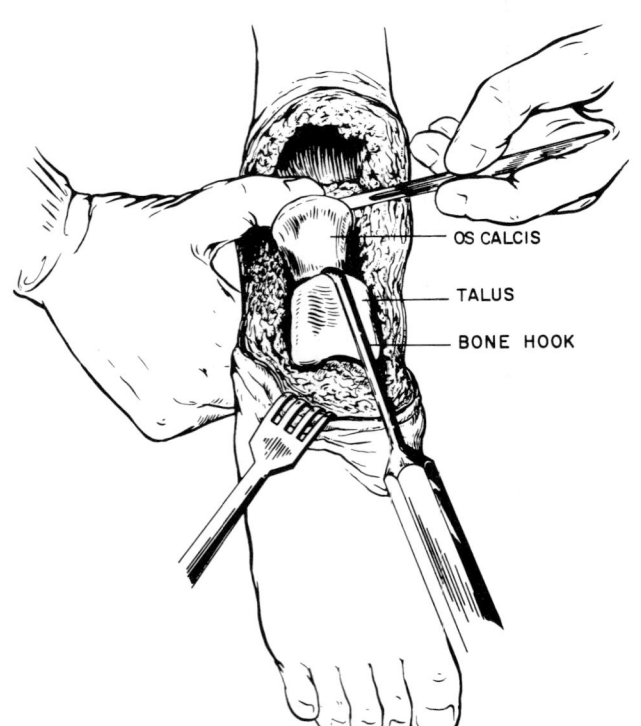

OS CALCIS

TALUS

BONE HOOK

FIGURE 162–8. The surgeon must take care not to buttonhole skin when dividing the Achilles tendon, which is almost subcutaneous at this point. (From Wagner FW Jr: The Syme amputation. *In* American Academy of Orthopaedic Surgeons: Atlas of Limb Prosthetics: Surgical and Prosthetic Principles. St. Louis, CV Mosby, 1981.)

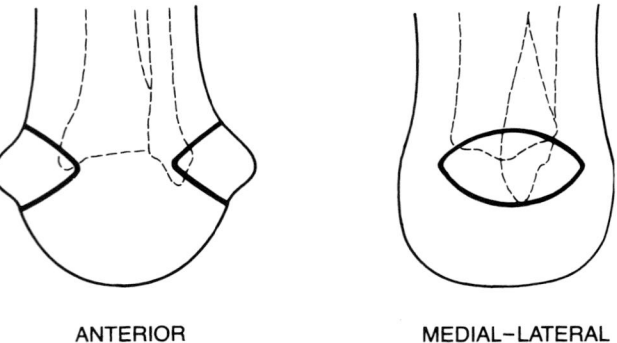

ANTERIOR   **MEDIAL–LATERAL**

FIGURE 162–10. Second-stage Syme's amputation. Elliptical incision removes tissue equal in volume to bone removed. (From Wagner FW Jr: The Syme amputation. *In* American Academy of Orthopaedic Surgeons: Atlas of Limb Prosthetics: Surgical and Prosthetic Principles. St. Louis, CV Mosby, 1981.)

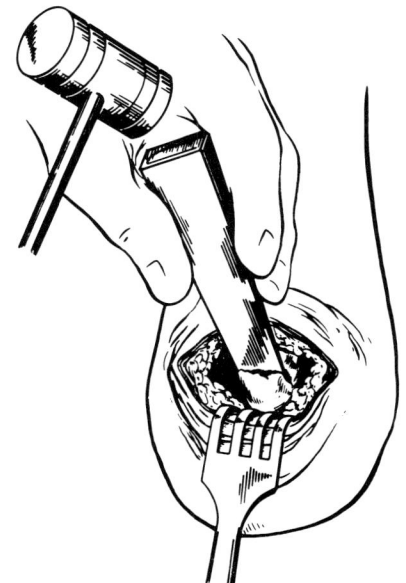

FIGURE 162–11. Second-stage Syme's amputation. Malleoli are removed flush with joint surface. Central cartilage is not disturbed. (From Wagner FW Jr: The Syme amputation. *In* American Academy of Orthopaedic Surgeons: Atlas of Limb Prosthetics: Surgical and Prosthetic Principles. St. Louis, CV Mosby, 1981.)

disturbed (Fig. 162–11). The distal tibia and fibula are then exposed in a subperiosteal plane to a point 3 to 6 cm above the ankle joint; the tibial and fibular flares are removed with an osteotome and smoothed with a rongeur. This step results in a relatively square stump that subsequently simplifies prosthetic fitting (Fig. 162–12). When the wounds are closed, the heel pad must be anchored to bone. If the heel pad is loose after the removal of the malleoli, it must be secured to the tibia and fibula through drill holes. The skin is then closed with monofilament sutures, and a soft compression dressing or a rigid cast dressing is applied to maintain proper heel pad alignment.[100, 124, 166] Rehabilitation is initiated with a 3-week period of non–weight-bearing followed by 3 to 4 weeks in a short-leg walking cast.

Advantages and Disadvantages

The advantage of a well-healed Syme or Pirogoff amputation is that rehabilitation is usually successful because the associated increases in energy consumption are minor, compared with those of normal bipedal ambulation.[168] For daily use, a below-knee patellar-tendon–bearing (PTB) prosthesis

is used. The stump is not durable enough to allow long periods of unprotected weight bearing, but no prosthesis is required for short walks inside the home, such as a trip to the bathroom at night.

The disadvantages of amputation at the ankle level all stem from wound healing complications; hematoma formation and secondary infection are all too common. Failure of healing at this level invariably leads to reamputation at the below-knee level. Another problem with the Syme amputation in diabetic patients is that progressive neuropathy later may create problems in the Syme amputation stump.

Prosthetic Requirements and Rehabilitation Potential

Typically, ankle-level amputees require a patellar-tendon–bearing prosthesis consisting of a plastic foot and a lightweight plastic shell that incorporates the lower leg and stump. Ambulation around the home or for short distances may also be achieved with a simple strap-on cap slipper with a built-up heel. Since ambulatory energy consumption is, at most, 10% greater than for a non-amputee, no significant disability should be expected in the Syme or Pirogoff amputee who has a well-healed stump and a well-fitted prosthesis. Most people with ankle-level amputations resume normal daily and work activities.

Below-Knee Amputation

Indications

Amputation below the knee joint is indicated in patients who have gangrene, infection, "unreconstructible" rest pain, or nonhealing ulcerations of the foot that preclude a more distal amputation. A below-knee amputation should be considered as a first choice over a Syme amputation for diabetic patients, as outlined earlier. Below-knee amputation is indicated as the definitive procedure after an initial staged open-ankle guillotine amputation for the treatment of unsalvageable lower limb infections.[33, 106]

Contraindications

Any patient with a fixed flexion contracture of the knee of 15 degrees or more should not undergo below-knee amputation because fitting a prosthesis is impossible and the stump is vulnerable to decubitus ulceration in bedridden patients. Such knee flexion contractures are most common among stroke victims, demented patients, and those with severe, chronic rest pain who have adopted the fetal

FIGURE 162–12. Second-stage Syme's amputation. Removal of malleoli and distal flare through lateral and medial incisions. (From Wagner FW Jr: The Syme amputation. *In* American Academy of Orthopaedic Surgeons: Atlas of Limb Prosthetics: Surgical and Prosthetic Principles. St. Louis, CV Mosby, 1981.)

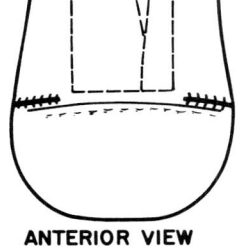

ANTERIOR VIEW

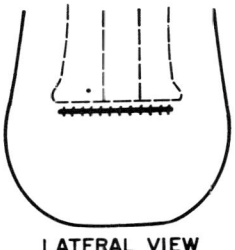

LATERAL VIEW

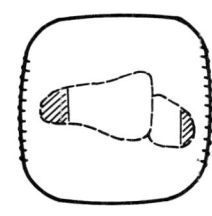

END VIEW

position in response to the pain. Patients who are totally bedridden with no chance for ambulation should rarely undergo a below-knee amputation because the risk of non-healing is not warranted in this population. Instead, a through-knee disarticulation or a long above-knee amputation provides substantial limb leverage for mobility in bed but does not risk stump decubitus ulceration or breakdown should a knee flexion contracture develop.

A gangrenous or infectious process that extends close to the tibial tuberosity or that involves the proposed skin flap consistently results in failure of a primarily closed amputation at the below-knee level, as does amputation through ruborous, cellulitic, or gangrenous skin. One technique that may allow salvage of the knee joint in infected cases is an *open-ankle guillotine amputation* with concurrent administration of sensitivity-directed antibiotics. This approach may allow regression of the cellulitis to a point distal to the proposed skin flap margins, thus permitting safe performance of a below-knee amputation later. Moreover, a patient who has been cured of systemic sepsis is more physiologically stable and a much better operative risk.[33, 106]

On occasion, especially in limbs involved by trauma or gangrene due to hypotension and vasopressors, a sharp delineation between healthy skin and nonviable skin appears; this line of demarcation may prevent the creation of standard musculocutaneous flaps for primary closure of an amputation. In carefully selected patients, an *open* below-knee amputation may be performed. Retraction of the wound edges is minimized by gentle traction applied with skin hooks or even "old-fashioned" Buck's skin traction.

Closure of the wound is subsequently accomplished by using partial-thickness skin grafts (Fig. 162–13). Because contemporary below-knee prostheses place the weight burden on the patellar tendon and the femoral condyles, rather than on the end of the stump, the skin graft covering the stump is not compromised.

A final contraindication to below-knee amputation is a definite, inadequate blood flow, as discovered by preoperative objective tests. These objective measurements are especially important when clinical examination of the patient indicates questionable healing potential.

Age alone is not a contraindication to amputation below the knee. Impressive success may be achieved in the geriatric amputees who were ambulatory before a below-knee amputation.[19, 29, 84, 154]

Prediction of Healing

Because the below-knee amputation is the highest-level amputation for which rehabilitation potential is still good (and above which rehabilitation attempts are poor), every patient has a *reasonable* chance of healing a below-knee amputation should be offered this procedure. However, a below-knee amputation in a patient who has little chance of successful healing will compound the morbidity and mortality that accompany wound breakdown, possible sepsis, and an overall setback in rehabilitation. The methods of choosing below-knee or above-knee amputation are listed in Table 162–4.

The available tests for preoperative evaluation for below-

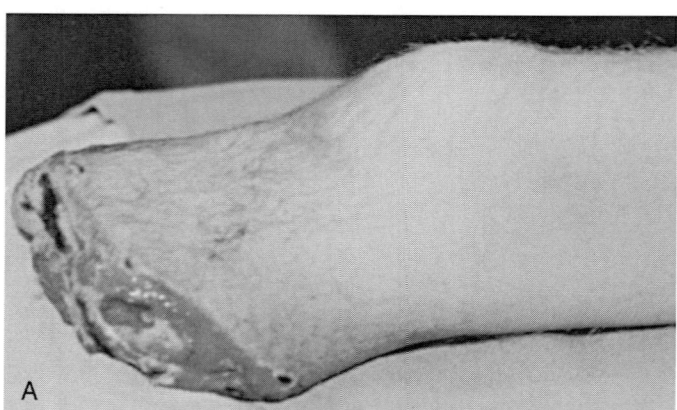
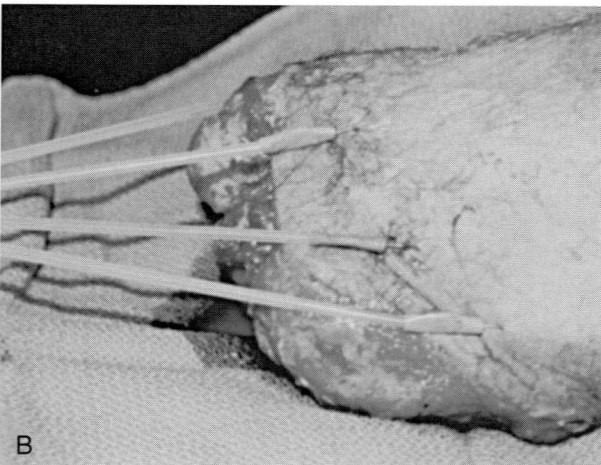
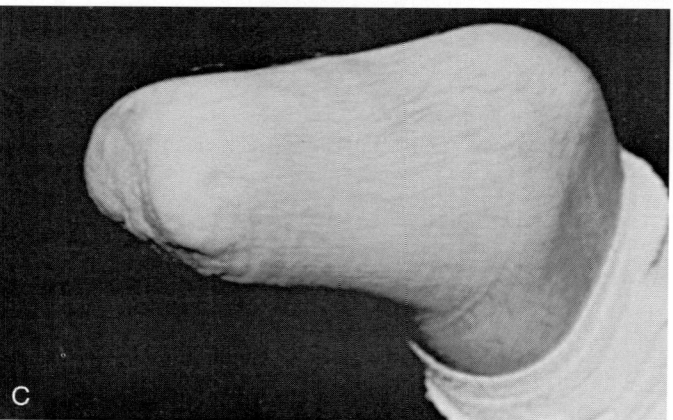

FIGURE 162–13. Series of photographs depicting the course of an open below-knee amputation performed for gangrene following disseminated intravascular coagulation due to systemic *Legionella* sepsis in a young carpenter. *A,* Proximal open below-knee amputation just proximal to eventual sharp line of demarcation between healthy skin and gangrenous tissue. *B,* Traction applied to skin wound edges by hooks placed under gentle traction (5 pounds). *C,* Result at 6 weeks following partial-thickness skin graft. The patient then underwent successful rehabilitation on bilateral below-knee prostheses.

TABLE 162–4. PREOPERATIVE LEVEL SELECTION: BELOW-KNEE AMPUTATION

SELECTION CRITERION		SUCCESSFUL HEALING, PRIMARY AND SECONDARY/TOTAL (%)	REFERENCE
Empirical		794/974 (82)	21, 82, 94, 127, 137
Doppler ankle pressure	<30 mmHg	66/70 (94)	118, 130
Doppler calf pressure	>50 mmHg	36/36 (100)	173
	>68 mmHg	96/97 (99)	6, 118
Doppler thigh pressure	>100 mmHg	31/31 (100)	92
	>80 mmHg	104/113 (92)	7, 150, 173
Fluorescein dye		24/30 (80)	105
Fiberoptic fluorometry (dye fluorescence index > 44)		12/12 (100)	149
Laser Doppler velocimetry		33/34 (97)	61, 88
Skin perfusion pressure			
Pertechnetate 99m		24/26 (92)	64
Iodine 131 or 125 antipyrine > 30 mm		60/62 (97)	66
Photoelectric skin perfusion pressure > 20 mm		60/71 (85)	121, 156
Xenon 133 skin blood flow			
Epicutaneous > 0.9 ml/100 gm tissue/min		14/15 (93)	24, 86
Intradermal > 2.4 ml/100 gm tissue/min		83/89 (93)	36, 59, 98, 148
Intradermal > 1.0 ml/100 gm tissue/min		11/12 (92)	54
Transcutaneous $P_{O_2} = 0$		0/3 (0)	17
>10 mmHg (or >10 mmHg increase on $FI_{O_2} = 1.0$)		76/80 (95)	46, 56
>10 but <40 mmHg		5/7 (71)	36
>20 mmHg		25/26 (96)	26
>35 mmHg		51/51 (100)	17, 36, 79, 131
Transcutaneous P_{O_2} index > 0.59		17/17 (100)	79
Transcutaneous P_{CO_2} < 40 mmHg		7/8 (88)	36

knee amputation include fiberoptic fluorometry, laser Doppler velocimetry, photoelectric and radioisotope measurements of skin perfusion pressure, xenon 133 skin blood flow, and transcutaneous assay of oxygen and carbon dioxide. As shown in Table 162–4, these methods are fairly comparable in accuracy. Which test is utilized will depend on available equipment and facilities. Multisensor transcutaneous oximetric mapping of the anterior and posterior skin of the leg, particularly when values are compared with skin tcP_{O_2} at a reference site, is an accurate method of predicting successful wound healing of the below-knee amputation.[89] If none of these testing modalities is available, careful interpretation of Doppler segmental systolic arterial blood pressures is a useful second-line technique.[13] When implemented properly, any of the objective tests increases successful healing rates compared with the 80% rate that can be expected from nothing more than *empirical* selection of below-knee amputation.

Surgical Technique

The design of the skin flaps for closure of the below-knee amputation depends on the distribution of gangrenous or infected tissues, the presence of surgical scars, and documented "islands of ischemia."[132] One of four basic skin flap designs are utilized in most of below-knee amputations in the dysvascular patient:

1. A long, posterior myocutaneous flap based on the underlying gastrocnemius and soleus muscles.
2. Anterior and posterior flaps of equal length (*fish-mouth flaps*).
3. Medial and lateral myocutaneous flaps of equal length created via sagittal incisions (*skew flaps*).
4. A medially based myocutaneous flap.

Because open wounds or surgical incisions may be present at the time of amputation, however, an ingeniously designed atypical skin flap is preferable to amputation at a more proximal level.

The long posterior flap technique is used most often, owing to theoretical considerations related to the marginal blood supply to the ischemic leg. The theory holds that the blood supply to the posterior gastrocnemius–soleus muscle group is usually better than that to the anterior compartment of the leg.[32, 162] Accordingly, the equal-length anterior and posterior flap technique should be associated with higher failure rates. Recent findings challenge this contention, however, and report excellent healing rates with the equal-length anterior and posterior flap technique[44] and sagittal incisions to create medial and lateral myocutaneous flaps of equal length.[76, 122, 158] Holloway and Burgess[59] reported a series of long posterior flap closures that were studied with the xenon 133 clearance skin blood flow method. They found that postoperative blood flow in the posterior flap was actually less than that in the undissected anterior skin flap, as did Johnson and coworkers.[76]

Theoretical concerns notwithstanding, most surgeons report excellent results with the posterior myocutaneous flap method. The equally based sagittal incision flap method is useful in patients with infection, ischemia, or necrosis involving the boundaries of a proposed posterior flap. With both techniques, it is imperative that all collateral vessels and vessels between the skin and the underlying muscle be preserved by avoiding dissection along tissue planes. The creation of a myocutaneous flap preserves these essential blood vessels. One isolated study has reported that plugging the medullary canal of the tibial stump with cortex of the removed bone led to a 67% increase in blood flow to the amputation stump muscles,[123] but these results have not been reproduced in other centers.

Because the long posterior myocutaneous flap technique is used most and is the basis for comparison with other techniques, its construction is outlined here. If gangrenous or ischemic skin changes do not allow safe construction of the classic posterior myocutaneous flap, alternative flap designs may be used to avoid amputation above the knee. The Kendrick below-knee amputation method employs a slightly shorter posterior myocutaneous flap.[81] The medially based myocutaneous flap[75] and the sagittal incision method for creating equal-length medial and lateral myocutaneous flaps[122] are discussed elsewhere.

For the routine below-knee amputation, the level of tibial transection is generally 10 to 12 cm below the tibial tuberosity, or approximately one hand breadth including the thumb. When indicated by local disease processes, this length may be shortened. The *absolute minimum* length of bone for a functional below-knee amputation starts just below the tibial tuberosity, because the insertion of the patellar tendon *must* be preserved for knee extension. The skin incision should be placed about 1 cm distal to the planned level of tibial transection. Preincision measurement and outlining of the skin flaps are described by Sanders and Augspurger (Fig. 162–14).[144]

The skin incision is begun on the anterior surface of the leg and is carried down to the tibia. It then follows the marked outline laterally and medially before turning distally, initially penetrating only the skin and superficial fascia. The muscles of the anterior compartment are divided, and the anterior tibial neurovascular bundle is identified, suture ligated proximally, and divided. After circumferential scoring of the periosteum of the tibia, a periosteal elevator is used to mobilize the periosteum to a point just proximal to the site of planned bone division. The tibia is divided in a steep bevel to avoid pressure on the overlying skin, and the fibula is transected at a point 1 to 2 cm proximal to the tibial stump.

Once the bony structures have been divided, the posterior tibial and common peroneal neurovascular bundles are identified; the arteries, veins, and nerves are suture ligated and divided. The posterior flap is created next, leaving the gastrocnemius and soleus muscles as the base of the myocutaneous flap. The posterior muscle mass may require additional tailoring to form a flap that can readily be rotated anteriorly to close it to the anterior skin over the tibia. This beveling of the muscle flap must remove enough muscle so that the end of the stump is not bulbous but not so much that the tibia will have inadequate soft tissue coverage. The distal tibia is then beveled at a 45- to 60-degree angle, and all bone surfaces are smoothed with a rasp (Fig. 162–15).

Complete hemostasis is essential and is followed by thorough irrigation with an antibiotic solution. A drain is not usually needed for amputation of an ischemic limb, but if one is required, it should be a closed suction drain, because Penrose-type drains may disrupt the wound.[77]

The posterior muscle flap is then rotated anteriorly, and

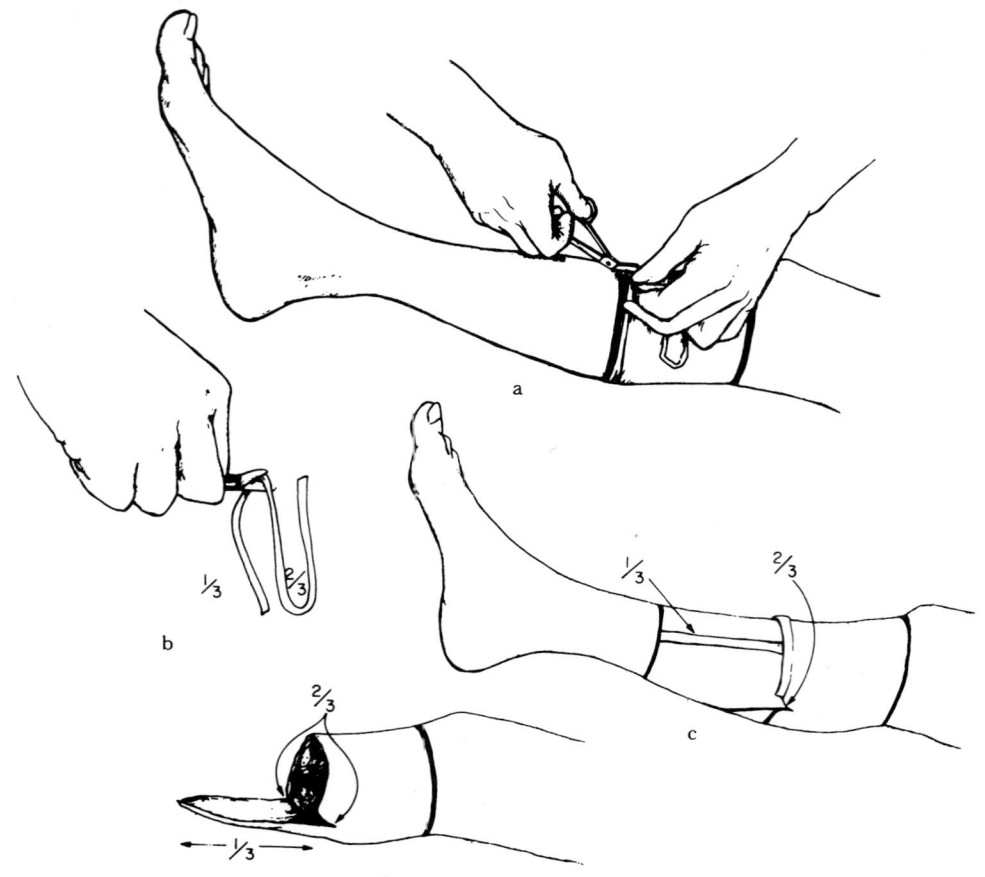

FIGURE 162–14. Technique for measuring the length of skin flaps in below-knee amputations. *a,* Umbilical tape or string is used to measure the circumference of the leg at the point of bone transection. *b,* Tape is divided in one-third and two-third lengths. *c,* The one-third piece measures the length of the posterior flap. The two-thirds piece measures the length of the anterior incision. Dog ears at each corner are avoided by cutting a curved triangle of skin from the anterior flap. *d,* The completed amputation before closure. (From Sanders RJ, Augspurger R: Skin flap measurement for below-knee amputation. Surg Gynecol Obstet 145:740, 1977. By permission of Surgery, Gynecology & Obstetrics.)

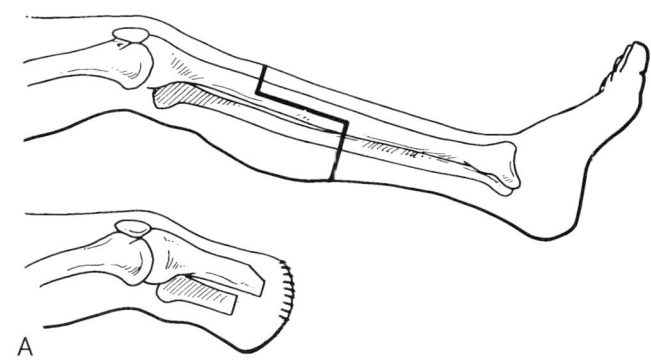

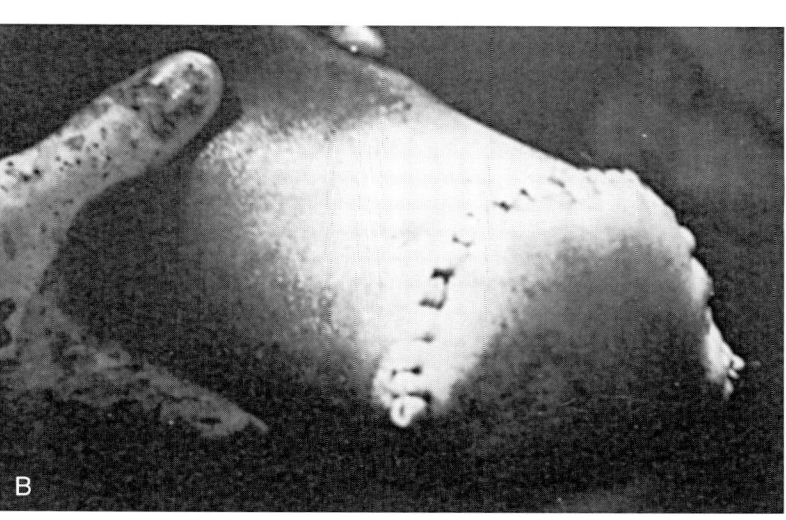

FIGURE 162–15. *A,* The standard posterior flap below-knee amputation. Notice the beveled tibia and the proximal shortening of the fibula compared with the tibia. *B,* An intraoperative photograph showing a below-knee amputation. Notice the skin coaptation with interrupted sutures and the minimal dog ears. (From Malone JM, Goldstone J: Lower extremity amputation. *In* Moore WS, [ed]: Vascular Surgery: A Comprehensive Review, 2nd ed. Orlando, Fla, Grune & Stratton, 1986, p 1165.)

the muscle fascia of the posterior flap is sewn to the anterior fascia with interrupted absorbable sutures. The skin edges are approximated atraumatically and precisely using interrupted vertical mattress sutures of monofilament, metal staples, or subcuticular sutures with sterile tapes for skin closure.

A rigid postoperative dressing that incorporates the knee is ideal, regardless of whether immediate postoperative application of a prosthesis is planned. A rigid dressing helps to minimize edema, promote healing, protect the vulnerable stump in the immediate postoperative period, and prevent development of a flexion contracture. In the hands of a well-coordinated team of surgeons, prosthetists, and physiatrists, immediate postoperative rigid dressings set the standard for optimal initiation of rehabilitation of the below-knee amputee.[97]

For surgeons who are not thoroughly familiar with the application of rigid dressings, using soft compression dressings is safer. An alternative method of managing the below-knee amputation stump in the immediate postoperative period is an *air splint.* Reports on the air splint claim that it helps to achieve the primary goals of decreased wound edema, decreased pain, earlier mobilization, and better primary healing.[147] An even more sophisticated device, the *controlled-environment unit,* has been developed in Edinburgh. This unit not only offers adjustable air pressure but also provides a flow of warmed, bacteriologically filtered

air.[143] Although the limb and amputation stump are fully visible at all times with this device, the theoretical advantages are offset, to some degree, by the practical drawbacks of immobility and noise.

Advantages and Disadvantages

The main advantages of the below-knee amputation are its durability after successful healing and its excellent potential for prosthetic ambulation. Disadvantages include the need for a relatively expensive prosthesis and the increased energy expenditure required for prosthetic ambulation.

Prosthetic Requirements and Rehabilitation Potential

Some form of below-knee prosthesis is required to achieve energy-efficient ambulation after below-knee amputation. Advances have been achieved in the design of lightweight, energy-storing prostheses (see Chapter 164).

Crutch walking without a prosthesis is a very inefficient form of ambulation for below-knee amputees, since it uses considerably more energy than independent ambulation with a unilateral below-knee prosthesis.[168] Although ambulation with a well-fitted below-knee prosthesis increases the relative energy cost by 10% to 40% as compared with walking on two intact limbs, amputees modify their walking speed to keep the heart rate, respiratory quotient, and relative energy costs within normal limits.[168] These calculations of energy expenditure were determined using conventional below-knee prostheses; newer lightweight prostheses should reduce energy expenditure even more. It should be no surprise that successful independent prosthetic ambulation can be achieved by 70% to 100% below-knee amputees, regardless of age, provided that they were ambulatory before the amputation.[43, 100, 139, 154] Even *bilateral* below-knee amputees have reasonably good rehabilitation potential. Some 33% to 71% of them who are young and in good mental and physical condition achieve successful ambulation.[29, 43, 154, 159, 165]

The amputation team must maintain a consistent follow-up protocol for below-knee amputees because there is substantial risk of arterial compromise of the *contralateral* limb as well as significant risk of death during the ensuing years. Couch and associates[29] demonstrated 49% survival at 3 years and 31% 5 years after unilateral amputation (below-knee or above-knee), rates similar to the 50% 3-year survival reported by Bodily and Burgess.[9] Standard life-table analysis also demonstrated that within 2 years of amputation, 50% of the *surviving* amputees required a contralateral amputation.[9]

Powell and colleagues have concluded that "an independent, aggressive approach for evaluation and surgical revascularization should not be overlooked for the ischemic, remaining lower extremity in the dysvascular unilateral amputee."[128]

Knee Disarticulation

Indications

Disarticulation of the knee *(through-knee amputation)* may be indicated for the occasional patient who has gangrene, infection, or cellulitis that precludes the creation of the flaps necessary for closure of a below-knee amputation. A patient with an uncorrectable flexion contracture of the knee but adequate blood supply to heal a below-knee amputation may also require knee disarticulation. A bedridden, debilitated patient with no hope for ambulatory rehabilitation may be spared subsequent contracture of a below-knee amputation stump by undergoing primary through-knee amputation; the resultant stump provides a long lever arm for better mobility and balance in bed.[176] Although it is most appropriate for young, healthy patients whose amputation is performed for trauma or tumor, the knee disarticulation has some limited utility in patients with ischemia-related tissue loss.

Contraindications

Objective preoperative findings of blood flow that is inadequate to heal a below-knee amputation should be considered a contraindication to knee disarticulation. Except for patients with one of the specific contraindications to below-knee amputation described earlier, knee disarticulation that sacrifices the knee joint should not be preferred over below-knee amputation. Obvious ischemia, ulceration, gangrene, or infection involving the knee joint or its surrounding tissues contraindicates knee disarticulation.

Finally, this amputation is contraindicated for patients with a fixed hip flexion deformity of more than a few degrees because the contracture would prohibit appropriate kinetic function of the intrinsic knee mechanism of the prosthesis. In this situation, a long above-knee amputation is preferable.

Prediction of Healing

Because disarticulation of the knee involves the creation of substantial skin flaps to enable tension-free closure of the wound (especially if the femoral condyles are not remodeled), the same preoperative objective parameters applied for below-knee amputation should be used to determine the adequacy of blood supply at this level (see Table 162–4).

Surgical Technique

Two techniques have been described for disarticulation of the knee for an ischemic lower limb. The two main variations involve (1) management of the femoral condyles and (2) skin flap design. Transection of the femoral condyles requires more dissection but affords easier and safer skin flap closure. Further, this remodeled stump accepts a prosthesis more readily. Alternatively, transection of the condyles is not indicated for patients who are not expected to pursue a rehabilitation program aimed at prosthesis-assisted ambulation. When the condyles are left intact, the articular cartilage remains, and prolonged suction drainage of the amputation wound is essential to prevent accumulation of joint fluid beneath the skin flaps.

Three basic skin flap designs are used for closure of the knee disarticulation (Fig. 162–16):

- The classic long anterior flap[8]
- Equal-length anterior and posterior flaps[16]
- Equal-length medial and lateral flaps, via sagittal incisions[85, 138]

The sagittal incision technique, which produces short medial and lateral flaps and the equal-length anterior and posterior flaps provide more reliable healing in ischemic limbs than the technique using the long anterior flap design.[161]

Operation may be performed with the patient prone or supine. The hip joint is hyperextended by placing a "bump" beneath the thigh to provide ready access to the anterior or posterior aspect of the leg and thigh. The knee is flexed. A marking pen is used to outline the exact skin flap design before an incision is made. Great care must be taken to create flaps that will allow absolutely tension-free skin closure.

The initial steps of the procedure involve dissection anteriorly down to the insertion of the patellar tendon on the tibia, where the tendon is divided. Deep medial dissection reveals the four inner hamstring muscle tendons, which are divided and allowed to retract. The deep fascia is retracted as a unit along with the skin and tendon flap. Dissection along the lateral side of the knee reveals the biceps femoris muscle tendon and the iliotibial band, both of which are divided distally. The knee joint is then entered

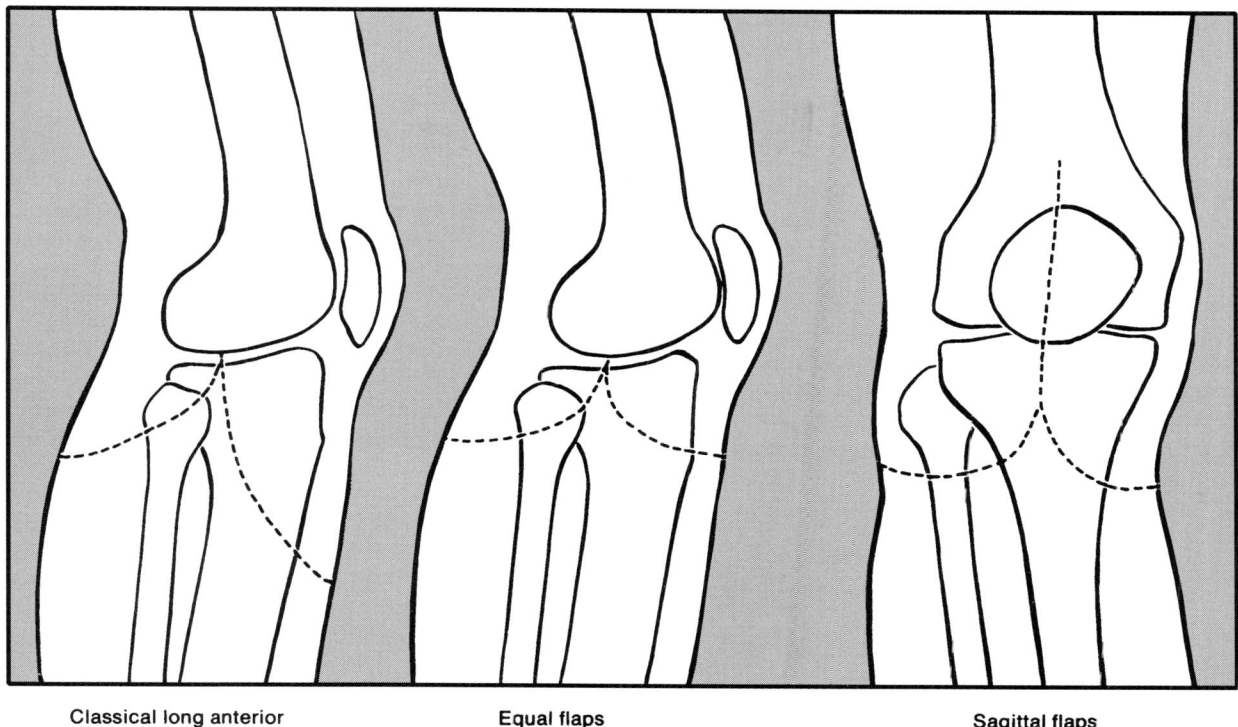

Classical long anterior   **Equal flaps**   **Sagittal flaps**

FIGURE 162–16. Skin incisions available for knee disarticulation. These may be modified further, depending on availability of suitable skin for development of flaps. (From Burgess EM: Disarticulation of the knee: A modified technique. Arch Surg 112:1250–1255, 1977. Copyright 1977, American Medical Association.)

from the front, and as the knee is flexed, the cruciate ligaments are cut at their tibial insertions.

The posterior structures are transected after individual control and suture ligation of the contents of the popliteal neurovascular bundle has been completed. The popliteal artery should be ligated distal to the origin of its superior geniculate branches. The tibial and peroneal nerves are transected sharply and allowed to retract. The patella is removed in a subperiosteal plane; the fascial defect thus created in the patellar tendon is closed with interrupted sutures.

The femoral condyles are transected transversely 1.5 cm above the knee joint (Fig. 162–17). Any sharp distal femoral margins are carefully remodeled with smooth contours. Remaining articular cartilage on the femur and any remaining synovium need not be removed. Next, the patellar tendon is pulled well down into the intracondylar notch under moderate tension and is sewn to the stump of the cruciate ligaments. In similar fashion, the tendons of the semitendinous and biceps femoris muscles are pulled into the notch, tailored, and sewn to the stump of the patellar tendon and cruciate ligaments; this provides muscle stability. After thorough irrigation and meticulous hemostasis are established, the superficial fascia is closed with interrupted absorbable sutures. The skin is then closed atraumatically. A closed suction drain is optional. Immediate application of a rigid dressing is recommended, even if an immediate postoperative prosthesis is not employed.[16, 99, 100]

Advantages and Disadvantages

The advantages of the through-knee amputation include (1) excellent and durable end weight–bearing capacity, (2)

retention of a long and powerful muscle-stabilized femoral lever arm, (3) improved stump proprioception, and (4) potential for excellent control of the prosthesis. Even for a bedridden, debilitated patient, the long lever arm allows greater mobility than an above-knee stump, and there is no risk of decubitus ulceration of a below-knee stump that becomes fixed in flexion.[176]

The main disadvantages of amputation at this level are the loss of the knee joint, which increases ambulatory energy expenditure (compared with a below-knee amputation), and the fact that the requisite long skin flaps are prone to wound healing problems in most ischemic limbs that require amputation at this level.

Prosthetic Requirements and Rehabilitation Potential

Improved prosthetic designs with lightweight polycentric hydraulic knee joints and endoskeletal systems now offer excellent rehabilitation results for knee disarticulation patients and overcome many of the problems of knee axis misalignment. To approach the efficiency of a below-knee amputee's gait, the knee disarticulation prosthesis must have an effective joint mechanism. With the proper prosthetic design, the rehabilitation potential of through-knee amputees should rival that of below-knee amputees.

Above-Knee Amputation
Indications

Indications for amputation of the lower limb at the above-knee level are usually related to advanced ischemia that

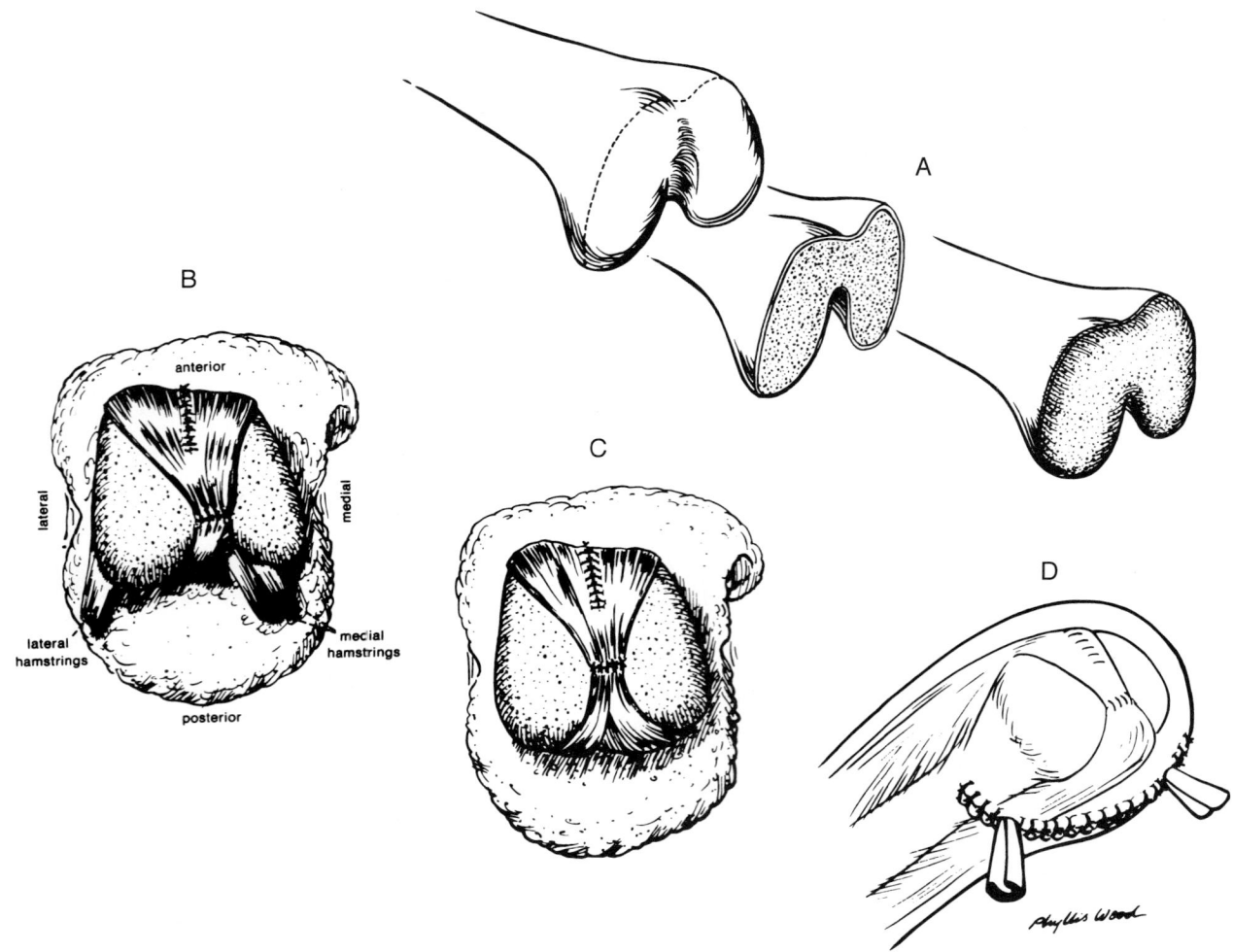

FIGURE 162–17. *A,* Weight-bearing surface of femoral condyles illustrating bone preparation: transverse cut 1.5 cm above condylar ends and femoral margins contoured. *B,* Muscle stabilization with patellar tendon sewn to cruciate ligaments. Biceps tendon and medial hamstrings are also sutured in intracondylar notch. One or more medial hamstrings may be stabilized. Site of patellar removal and repair is shown. *C,* Surgical closure of aponeurosis: hamstrings sutured through femoral notch to patellar tendon and cruciate ligaments. *D,* Closed wound over drainage using classic long anterior skin flap. (From Burgess EM: Disarticulation of the knee: A modified technique. Arch Surg 112:1250–1255, 1977. Copyright 1977, American Medical Association.)

precludes reliable chances of healing at a level farther distal. Rubor, infection, and open ischemic lesions at the level of the knee joint are all contraindications to below-knee amputation and thus are indications for above-knee amputation. A disabled patient who is not expected to walk again is another "indication" for above-knee amputation because disuse of a below-knee amputation in a bedridden patient may lead to a decubitus ulcer on the bottom of the stump. Similarly, a fixed flexion contracture of the knee is another indication for above-knee, rather than below-knee, amputation.

Contraindications

The most common contraindication to amputation at the above-knee level is an infection or gangrene that extends to the proposed level of amputation. A relative contraindication may be preoperative objective documentation of inadequate local blood flow to ensure successful healing at that level. Bunt cites three specific relative contraindications

to above-knee amputations *unless* there is definite *objective* evidence that the local blood flow will sustain a viable stump[14]:

1. Acute thrombosis of a combined inflow and outflow revascularization attempt.

2. Superficial femoral artery occlusion associated with an occluded or highly stenotic profunda femoris artery.

3. Absence of a femoral pulse coupled with no detectable pulse volume recordings at the level of the proximal thigh.

Preamputation revascularization to correct any of these situations enhances amputation wound healing.[14, 90]

Prediction of Healing

Many surgeons assume that virtually all above-knee amputations will heal. Unfortunately, this is not true; about 2% to 10% of such amputations fail to heal.[100] Because this failure rate is relatively low, one may question the need for objective preoperative assay of blood flow in this patient group; however, the consequences of a failed above-knee amputation can be disastrous, even fatal. Thus, appropriate selection of candidates for preamputation revascularization procedures may avert such untoward sequelae in the severely ischemic thigh. Moreover, occasionally after a revascularization procedure, an even farther distal amputation heals at the below-knee or through-knee level.

Scientific studies reaffirm the notion that *empirical* selection of patients for amputation at the above-knee level will be associated with successful healing in 91%.[82, 127] Proper use of preoperative testing methods, however, should allow appropriate patient selection, resulting in successful healing of above-knee amputations at a rate approaching 100% (Table 162–5). The particular tests any surgeon uses of course depend on local availability.

Surgical Technique

There are three general levels for amputation of the lower extremity above the knee (Fig. 162–18). Owing to the loss of the knee joint, the length of the residual femur is crucial because it functions as the lever arm during prosthetic ambulation. In general, the longer the femoral shaft is, the less energy is required for prosthetic ambulation and the more likely it is that the patient will successfully ambulate with a prosthesis. Moreover, a longer femoral shaft remnant provides a mechanical advantage for easier transfers and better balance for prolonged sitting. Amputation at a higher level, when forced by infection, gangrene, or ischemia, reduces the chances of successful prosthetic ambulation because of the mechanical disadvantage of the shorter femoral shaft. Modification of the Gritti-Stokes knee disarticulation with femur transection at the supracondylar level produces the longest above-knee amputation stump.[176]

Two basic incision designs are applicable to above-knee amputation:

1. The *circular incision* is planned 2 to 3 cm below the level of proposed femur transection (Fig. 162–19).
2. A *fish-mouth incision* defines anterior and posterior skin flaps of equal length.

The proximal extent of the incisions lies at the level of femur division, and the length of each flap is designed to be at least half the anteroposterior diameter of the thigh at

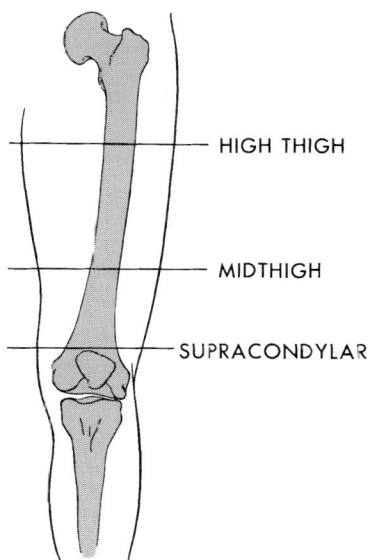

FIGURE 162–18. Potential levels of bone division of the femur. The three common levels are a supracondylar above-knee amputation, a mid-thigh amputation, and a high-thigh amputation.

the level of bone transection. With either flap design, the incision is carried through the skin, subcutaneous tissue, and fascia.

Retraction of the skin and fascia superiorly allows division of the thigh muscles farther proximal. The femoral arteries and veins are identified in the subsartorial canal and are individually controlled and suture ligated. All remaining muscles of the anterior, medial, and lateral portions of the thigh are transected; this allows their proximal retraction to expose the femur. Some surgeons use a long amputation knife to divide muscle groups in one swift incision, thereby avoiding creation of multiple tissue planes.

At the site of planned bone transection, the periosteum is scored circumferentially and is elevated superiorly, allowing transection of the femur well above the skin incision. The sciatic nerve is isolated; ligation and division are performed with gentle traction on the nerve so that the proximal nerve remnant will retract well into the depths of the thigh

TABLE 162–5. PREOPERATIVE LEVEL SELECTION: ABOVE-KNEE AMPUTATION

SELECTION CRITERION	SUCCESSFUL HEALING, PRIMARY AND SECONDARY/TOTAL (%)	REFERENCE
Empirical	390/430 (91)	82, 116
Fiberoptic fluorometry (dye fluorescence index > 44)	6/7 (86)	149
Laser Doppler velocimetry	6/6 (100)	61
Photoelectric skin perfusion pressure > 21 mm	19/19 (100)	121
Skin perfusion pressure (Iodine 131 or 125 antipyrine)	44/48 (92)	65, 67
Xenon 133 skin blood flow intradermal > 2.6 ml/100 gm tissue/min	20/20 (100)	36, 98, 148
Transcutaneous P_{O_2}		
>10 mmHg (or >10 mmHg increase on $F_{IO_2} = 1.0$)	15/23 (65)	56
>20 mmHg	12/12 (100)	26
>23 mmHg	2/2 (100)	36
>35 mmHg	21/24 (88)	36, 131
Transcutaneous P_{CO_2} < 38 mmHg	5/5 (100)	36

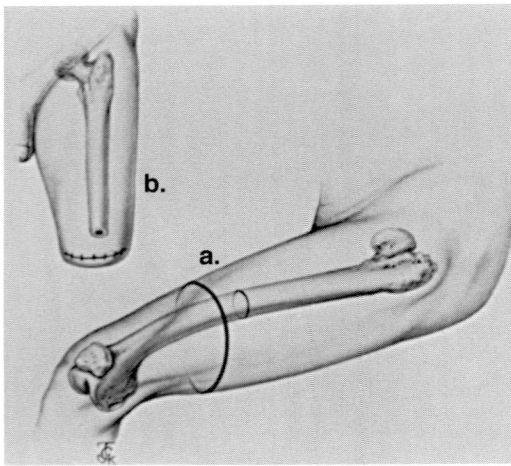

FIGURE 162–19. *a,* A circular incision is placed well distal to the point of proposed bone division. *b,* Each successive deeper tissue layer is circularly divided at a more proximal level to create a conical effect. The transverse closure of the fascia and skin following removal of the specimen is shown here.

muscle mass. Now the posterior musculature of the thigh may be divided.

The roughened edges of the femoral stump are smoothed with a rasp, with special attention given to the anterolateral aspect, which must be flattened to prevent subsequent point pressure on the overlying soft tissues. Thorough irrigation with an antibiotic solution removes all bone fragments and tissue debris. Hemostasis is achieved; no bone wax should be used. The skin edges are then coapted manually to ensure that the skin closure will be tension-free. If there appears to be too much tension or if the soft tissue coverage appears inadequate, the femur may be shortened at this time to allow optimal closure of the soft tissues.

Once the adequacy of femoral coverage is ensured, the wound is closed in layers. No myodesis procedures are utilized in the amputation of ischemic limbs. Perfect skin closure is performed atraumatically with interrupted vertical monofilament mattress sutures. Only in cases of severe proximal gangrene or extensive infection should the amputation wound be left open. As in any major amputation, any thrombosed prosthetic bypass graft should generally be removed at the time of amputation to decrease the risk of wound healing complications and to prevent the subsequent infection of retained graft material.[141, 142]

A rigid dressing is not as advantageous for amputations above the knee and, in fact, is often cumbersome. Consequently, a soft compression dressing is utilized. The dressing is suspended with an elastic bandage or with a modified waist suspension belt to maintain its proper position.[129] Provision of a temporary prosthesis is often delayed until the wound has healed well, usually around 2 to 4 weeks after the operation.

Advantages and Disadvantages

The main advantage of above-knee amputation is the exceptionally high incidence of successful primary healing.

The principal disadvantage is the lower rate of successful rehabilitation as compared with more distal amputations.

Prosthetic Requirements and Rehabilitation Potential

The absolute minimum prosthetic requirement for above-knee amputees is a wheelchair or a set of walking crutches; however, either is a poor alternative to independent ambulation with a prosthetic limb. Newer designs of prosthetic devices for above-knee amputees incorporate strong, ultralightweight materials, endoskeletal design, sophisticated joints, and even energy storage capability. All of these features combine to increase the rehabilitation rate for above-knee amputees, especially in the geriatric population.[73]

Rehabilitation potential after above-knee amputation of an ischemic limb depends on several variables, including the patient's nutritional and physical status, concurrent diseases, stump length, motivation, and rehabilitation training. Compared with normal bipedal ambulation, the relative energy cost for above-knee prosthetic ambulation is increased 50% to 70%. Whereas *below-knee* amputees are able to modify their walking speed to maintain relatively normal energy costs, dysvascular *above-knee* amputees are less able to do this; thus, greater oxygen consumption, increased heart rate, and a significantly increased respiratory quotient are the results.[168] Crutch walking without a prosthesis imposes similar energy demands on above-knee amputees, in contrast to all other amputee groups, who use *less energy* walking with a prosthesis.[168]

Because of the dramatically increased energy requirements for ambulation after unilateral above-knee amputation, the rate of successful rehabilitation ranges from 36% to 76%.[29, 100] Age alone need not be considered the major determinant of success or failure, because rehabilitation failure is more often a result of concurrent medical disease or mental deterioration.[154]

Patients who have a single above-knee amputation who survive 2 years are at significant risk (up to 50%) for problems that require amputation of the contralateral limb.[9, 84] Ambulatory rehabilitation of bilateral amputees who have one above-knee amputation succeeds in only 10% to 24% of cases,[43, 100, 165] whereas for those with bilateral above-knee amputations it approaches zero. Thus, the goal of the dysvascular bilateral amputee with at least one above-knee amputation is wheelchair mobility, which requires only a 9% increase in relative energy costs over normal ambulation.[51]

Long-term survivors of unilateral above-knee amputation must be observed closely to detect quickly any imminent ischemic or infectious problems in the intact limb. Such follow-up makes possible an aggressive approach to revascularization to overt a second, contralateral, amputation.

Hip Disarticulation

Indications

Typical indications for hip joint disarticulation are malignant bone tumors of the femur below the lesser trochanter and malignant soft tissue tumors of the middle or lower thigh.[157] Less frequent indications are extensive trauma, uncontrolled infections, extensive gangrene, and compromise of healing of a high above-knee amputation by infection or ischemia.[140, 160] Objective preoperative evidence of inadequate local blood flow to heal a high-level above-knee amputation may constitute an indication for hip disarticulation if revascularization of the thigh is not feasible.

Contraindications

Contraindications include tumor, infection, or gangrene that involves the skin flaps or musculature at the proposed level of amputation. Hip disarticulation performed for ischemic complications of above-knee amputation may be hazardous unless proximal vascular reconstruction is carried out before the disarticulation.[90]

Prediction of Healing

Owing to the fortunate fact that hip disarticulations are not often performed for ischemic complications, no data are available on objective preoperative determinations of wound healing potential. Consequently, observation of the contraindications outlined previously ensures the best results that currently are possible. As an adjunct, transcutaneous mapping of oxygen and carbon dioxide levels may help to guide the surgeon in designing skin flaps in much the same manner as it does for more distal amputations.

Surgical Technique

An excellent detailed narrative with complete illustrations of the surgical technique for hip disarticulation has been published by Sugarbaker and Chretien.[157] A summary of their technique follows (Figs. 162–20 and 162–21).

The patient is in a posterolateral position. In the first phase of the procedure, the surgeon stands anterior to the

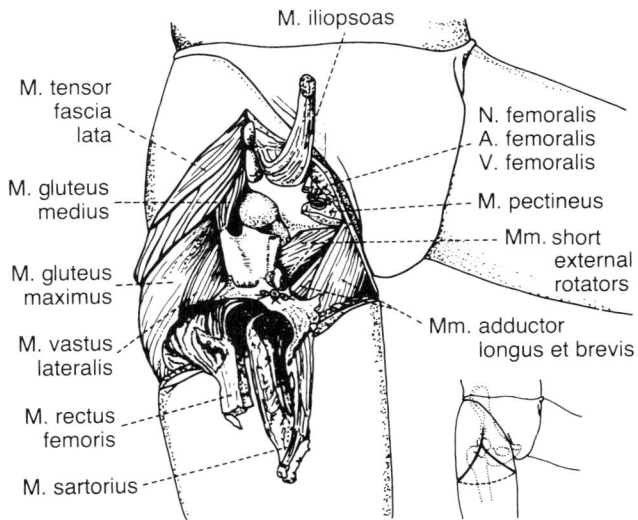

FIGURE 162–20. Stage of anatomic disarticulation following ligation of the femoral vessels and nerves and detachment of the sartorius, rectus femoris, pectineal, and iliopsoas muscles. The inset shows the line of the incision. (From Boyd HB: Anatomic dislocation of the hip. Surg Gynecol Obstet 84:346, 1947. By permission of Surgery, Gynecology & Obstetrics.)

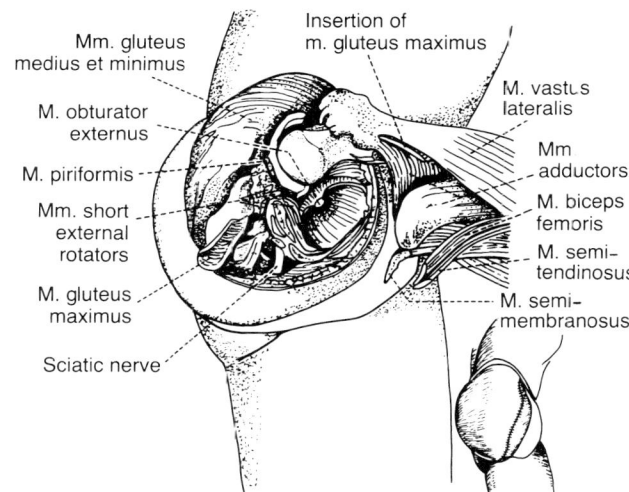

FIGURE 162–21. Stage of the anatomic disarticulation following separation of the gluteal muscles from their insertions, division of the sciatic nerve, severance of the short rotators, and detachment of the hamstring muscles from the ischial tuberosity. The inset shows the stump after closure of the wound. (From Boyd HB: Anatomic dislocation of the hip. Surg Gynecol Obstet 84:347, 1947. By permission of Surgery, Gynecology & Obstetrics.)

patient. After incision of the skin and division of the femoral vessels and nerve, muscles of the anterior thigh are transected off the pelvic bone, from lateral to medial, starting with the sartorius and finishing with the adductor magnus. Muscles are divided at their origin except for the iliopsoas and obturator externus, which are divided at their insertion on the lesser trochanter of the femur. The quadratus femoris muscle is identified and preserved: the flexor muscles are then transected at their site of origin from the ischial tuberosity.

During the next phase, the surgeon is posterior to the patient. The pelvis is rotated from the posterolateral to the anterolateral position. After the skin incision is completed, the gluteal fascia, tensor fascia latae, and the gluteus maximus muscles are divided and dissected free of their posterior attachments to expose the muscles inserting by way of a common tendon onto the greater trochanter. These muscles are transected at their insertion on the bone. The posterior aspect of the joint capsule is then exposed and transected.

Finally, the sciatic nerve is divided and allowed to retract beneath the piriformis muscle. To close the wound, the preserved muscles surgeon approximates over the joint capsule and secures the gluteal fascia to the inguinal ligament over suction drains. The skin is closed with interrupted sutures.

Advantages and Disadvantages

The only true advantage of hip disarticulation for ischemic problems is that it may result in a well-healed amputation wound that will allow a prosthesis to be fitted when above-knee amputation has failed or is contraindicated. Also, disarticulation of the hip may be life-saving for a patient with sepsis. The disadvantage of this amputation is its low incidence of successful ambulatory rehabilitation in the dysvascular patient population.

Prosthetic Requirement and Rehabilitation Potential

Although a number of prostheses are available for hip disarticulation patients, most employ a "Canadian-type" pelvic bucket of endoskeletal of construction to minimize its weight. Very few utilize sophisticated knee joints, ankle joints, or "moving" feet. Compared with normal bipedal ambulation, ambulation with the hip disarticulation prosthesis uses 150% to 250% more energy. Because of this massive energy requirement, successful ambulatory rehabilitation after hip disarticulation is very uncommon (<10% for dysvascular patients[100]); thus, prescription of a prosthesis for this level of amputation is done very selectively.

REFERENCES

1. Bacharach JM, Rooke TW, Osmundson PJ, Gloviczki P: Predictive value of transcutaneous oxygen pressure and amputation success by use of supine and elevation measurements. J Vasc Surg 15:558, 1992.
2. Back TL, Padberg FT, Thompson, Hobson RW II: Probability of successful wound outcome determined by laser Doppler measurements using a heated probe (LDHP). J Vasc Tech 18:67, 1994.
3. Bailey MJ, Johnston CLW, Yates CJP, et al: Preoperative haemoglobin as predictor of outcome of diabetic amputations. Lancet 28:168, 1979.
4. Baker WH, Barnes RW: Minor forefoot amputation in patients with low ankle pressure. Am J Surg 133:331, 1977.
5. Ballard JL, Eke CC, Bunt TJ, Killeen JD. A prospective evaluation of transcutaneous oxygen measurements in the management of diabetic foot problems. J Vasc Surg 22:485, 1995.
6. Barnes RW, Shanik GD, Slaymaker EE: An index of healing in below-knee amputation: Leg blood pressure by Doppler ultrasound. Surgery 79:13, 1976.
7. Barnes RW, Thornhill B, Nix L, et al: Prediction of amputation wound healing: Roles of Doppler ultrasound and digit photoplethysmography. Arch Surg 116:80, 1981.
8. Batch JW, Spittler AW, McFadden JG: Advantages of the knee disarticulation over amputations through the thigh. J Bone Joint Surg 36A:921, 1954.
9. Bodily KC, Burgess EM: Contralateral limb and patient survival after leg amputation. Am J Surg 146:280, 1983.
10. Boeckstyns MEH, Jensen CM: Amputation of the forefoot: Predictive value of signs and clinical physiological tests. Acta Orthop Scand 55:224, 1984.
11. Bone GE, Pomajzl MJ: Toe blood pressure by photoplethysmography: An index of healing in forefoot amputations. Surgery 89:569, 1981.
12. Bongard FS, Upton RA, Elings VB, et al: Digital cutaneous fluorometry: Correlation between blood flow and fluorescence. J Vasc Surg 1:635, 1984.
13. Borozan PG, Schuler JJ, Flanigan DP: The accuracy of segmental Doppler pressures in predicting healing of below-knee amputation in diabetic patients. Unpublished data presented at the Association of Veterans Administration Surgeons Meeting, Los Angeles, May 9–12, 1984.
14. Bunt TJ: Gangrene of the immediate postoperative above-knee amputation stump: Role of emergency revascularization in preventing death. J Vasc Surg 2:874, 1985.
15. Bunt TJ: TcPO2 as an accurate predictor of therapy in limb salvage. Ann Vasc Surg 10:224, 1996.
16. Burgess EM: Disarticulation of the knee: A modified technique. Arch Surg 112:1250, 1977.
17. Burgess EM, Matsen FA, Wyss CR, et al: Segmental transcutaneous measurements of PO_2 in patients requiring below the knee amputation for peripheral vascular insufficiency. J Bone Joint Surg 64A:378, 1982.
18. Campbell WB, St. Johnston JA, Kernick VFM, Rutter EA: Lower limb amputation: Striking the balance. Ann R Coll Surg Engl 76:201, 1994.
19. Castronuovo JJ, Deane LM, Deterling RA, et al: Below-knee amputation: Is the effort to preserve the knee joint justified? Arch Surg 115:1184, 1980.
20. Castronuovo JJ: Diagnosis of critical limb ischemia with skin perfusion pressure measurements. J Vasc Tech 21:175, 1997.
21. Cederberg PA, Pritchard DJ, Joyce JW: Doppler-determined segmental pressures and wound-healing in amputations for vascular disease. J Bone Joint Surg 65A:363, 1983.
22. Chang BB, Bock DEM, Jacobs RL, et al: Increased limb salvage by the use of unconventional foot amputations. J Vasc Surg 19:341, 1994.
23. Chang BB, Jacobs RL, Darling RC III, et al: Foot amputations. Surg Clin North Am 75:773, 1995.
24. Cheng EY: Lower extremity amputation level: Selection using noninvasive hemodynamic methods of evaluation. Arch Phys Med Rehabil 63:475, 1982.
25. Chleboun JO, Martins R, Rao S: Laser Doppler velocimetry and platelet-derived growth factor as prognostic indicators for the healing of ulcers and ischaemic lesions of the lower limb. Cardiovasc Surg 3:285, 1995.
26. Christensen KS, Klarke M: Transcutaneous oxygen measurement in peripheral occlusive disease: An indicator of wound healing in leg amputation. J Bone Joint Surg 68B:423, 1986.
27. Christie J, Clowes CB, Lamb DW: Amputations through the middle part of the foot. J Bone Joint Surg 62B:473, 1980.
28. Cohen SI, Goldman LD, Salzman EW, et al: The deleterious effect of immediate postoperative prosthesis in below-knee amputation for ischemic disease. Surgery 76:992, 1974.
29. Couch NP, David JK, Tilney NL, et al: Natural history of the leg amputee. Am J Surg 133:469, 1977.
30. Cunha SXS, Beebe HC: Magnetic resonance blood flowmetry: A review. J Vasc Tech 18:141, 1994.
31. Daly MJ, Henry RE: Quantitative measurement of skin perfusion with xenon-133. J Nucl Med 21:156, 1980.
32. Dellon AL, Morgan RF: Myodermal flap closure of below the knee amputation. Surg Gynecol Obstet 153:383, 1981.
33. Desai Y, Robbs JV, Keenan JP: Staged below knee amputations for septic peripheral lesions due to ischaemia. Br J Surg 73:392, 1986.
34. Dickhaut SC, Delee JC, Page CP: Nutritional status: Importance in predicting wound healing after amputation. J Bone Joint Surg 66A:71, 1984.
35. Dormandy J, Belcher G, Broos P, et al: Prospective study of 713 below-knee amputations for ischaemia and the effect of a prostacyclin analogue on healing. Br J Surg 81:33, 1994.
36. Durham JR, Anderson GG, Malone JM: Methods of preoperative selection of amputation level. In Flanigan DP (ed): Perioperative Assessment in Vascular Surgery. New York, Marcel Dekker, 1987, pp 61–82.
37. Durham JR, McCoy DM, Sawchuk AP, et al: Open transmetatarsal amputation in the treatment of severe foot infections. Am J Surg 158:127, 1989.
38. Dwars BJ, van den Broek TAA, Rauwerda JA, Bakker FC: Criteria for reliable selection of the lowest level of amputation in peripheral vascular disease. J Vasc Surg 15:536, 1992.
39. Eberhard P, Mindt W, Hammacher K: Percutane Messung der Sauerstatpartaldrukes: Methodick and Anwendungen. Stuttgart, Proc Medizin-Technik, May 16, 1972.
40. Ebskov IB: Relative mortality in lower limb amputees with diabetes mellitus. Prosthet Orthot Int 20:147, 1996.
41. Effeney DJ, Lim RC, Schechter WP: Transmetatarsal amputation. Arch Surg 112:1366, 1977.
42. Evans NTS, Naylor PFD: The oxygen tension gradient across human epidermis. Respir Physiol 3:38, 1967.
43. Evans WE, Hayes JP, Vermilion BD: Rehabilitation of the bilateral amputee. J Vasc Surg 5:589, 1987.
44. Fearon J, Campbell DR, Hoar CS, et al: Improved results with diabetic below-knee amputations. Arch Surg 120:777, 1985.
45. Fisher SV, Gullickson G Jr: Energy cost of ambulation in health and disability: A literature review. Arch Phys Med Rehabil 59:124, 1978.
46. Franzeck UK, Talke P, Bernstein EF, et al: Transcutaneous PO_2 measurement in health and peripheral arterial occlusive disease. Surgery 91:156, 1982.
47. Gatti JE, LaRossa D, Neff SR, et al: Altered skin flap survival and fluorescein kinetics with hemodilution. Surgery 92:200, 1982.
48. Gianfortune P, Pulla RJ, Sage R: Ray resections in the insensitive or dysvascular foot: A critical review. J Foot Surg 24:103, 1985.

49. Gibbons GW, Wheelock FC Jr, Hoar CS Jr, et al: Predicting success of forefoot amputations in diabetics by noninvasive testing. Arch Surg 114:1034, 1979.

50. Gibbons GW, Wheelock FC Jr, Siembrieda C, et al: Noninvasive prediction of amputation level in diabetic patients. Arch Surg 114:1253, 1979.

51. Gonzalez EG, Corcoran PJ, Reyes RL: Energy expenditure in below-knee amputees: Correlation with stump length. Arch Phys Med Rehabil 55:111, 1974.

52. Hamit HF: The Boyd-Syme forefoot amputation technique. Contemp Orthop 23:321, 1991.

53. Harbrecht PJ, Netheny H, Ahmad W, Fry DE: A technic for freezing an extremity in preparation for amputation. Am J Surg 135:859, 1978.

54. Harris JP, McLaughlin AF, Quinn RJ, et al: Skin blood flow measurement with xenon-133 to predict healing of lower extremity amputations. Aust N Z J Surg 56:413, 1986.

55. Harris RI: Syme's amputation: The technical details essential for success. J Bone Joint Surg 38B:614, 1956.

56. Harward TRS, Volny J, Golbranson F, et al: Oxygen inhalation–induced transcutaneous Po₂ changes as a predictor of amputation level. J Vasc Surg 2:220, 1985.

57. Hauser CJ, Shoemaker WC: Use of a transcutaneous Po₂ regional perfusion index to quantify tissue perfusion in peripheral vascular disease. Ann Surg 197:337, 1983.

58. Holloway GA Jr, Watkins BW: Laser Doppler measurement of cutaneous blood flow. J Invest Dermatol 69:300, 1977.

59. Holloway GA Jr, Burgess EM: Cutaneous blood flow and its relation to healing of below-knee amputation. Surg Gynecol Obstet 146:750, 1978.

60. Holloway GA Jr: Cutaneous blood flow responses to injection trauma measured by laser Doppler velocimetry. J Invest Dermatol 74:1, 1980.

61. Holloway GA Jr, Burgess EM: Preliminary experiences with laser Doppler velocimetry for the determination of amputation levels. Prosthet Orthot Int 7:63, 1983.

62. Holstein P: Distal blood pressure as a guide in choice of amputation level. Scand J Clin Lab Invest 31(Suppl 128):245, 1973.

63. Holstein P, Lund P, Larsen B, Schomacker T: Skin perfusion pressure measured as the external pressure required to stop isotope washout: Methodological considerations and normal values on the legs. Scand J Clin Lab Invest 30:649, 1977.

64. Holstein P, Lassen NA: Assessment of safe level of amputation by measurement of skin blood pressure. In Rutherford RB (ed): Vascular Surgery. Philadelphia, WB Saunders, 1977, pp 105–111.

65. Holstein P, Sager P, Lassen NA: Wound healing in below knee amputations in relation to skin perfusion pressure. Acta Orthop Scand 40:49, 1979.

66. Holstein P: Level selection in leg amputation for arterial occlusive disease: A comparison of clinical evaluation and skin perfusion pressure. Acta Orthop Scand 53:821, 1982.

67. Holstein P, Trap-Jensen J, Bagger H, Larsen B: Skin perfusion pressure measured by isotope washout in legs with arterial occlusive disease. Clin Physiol 3:313, 1983.

68. Holstein P: The distal blood pressure predicts healing of amputations on the feet. Acta Orthop Scand 55:227, 1984.

69. Huch A, Huch R, Mentzer K, et al: Eine schnelle, behitze problachenelektrode zur Kontinuier lichen Uberwach und des Po₂ bemenschen: A Elektrodenaut bau und eigen Schaften. Stuttgart, Proc Medizin-Technik, May 16, 1972.

70. Huizinga WFJ, Robbs JV, Kritzinger NA: Prevention of wound sepsis in amputations by peri-operative antibiotic cover with an amoxycillin–clavulanic acid combination. South Afr Med J 63(15):71, 1983.

71. Hunsaker RH, Schwartz JA, Keagy BA, et al: Dry ice cryoamputation: A twelve year experience. J Vasc Surg 2(6):812, 1985.

72. Huston CC, Bivins BA, Ernst CB, Griffen WO Jr: Morbid implications of above-knee amputations: Report of a series and review of the literature. Arch Surg 115:165, 1980.

73. Isakov E, Susak Z, Becker E: Energy expenditure and cardiac response in above-knee amputees while using prostheses with open and locked knee mechanisms. Scand J Rehabil Med Suppl 12:108, 1985.

74. Ito K, Ohgi S, Mori T, et al: Determination of amputation level in ischemic legs by means of transcutaneous oxygen pressure measurement. Int Surg 69:59, 1984.

75. Jain AS, Stewart CPU, Turner MS: Transtibial amputation using a medially based flap. J R Coll Surg Edinb 40:263, 1995.

76. Johnson WC, Watkins MT, Hamilton J, Baldwin D: Transcutaneous partial oxygen pressure changes following skew flap and Burgess-type below-knee amputations. Arch Surg 132:261, 1997.

77. Kacy SS, Wolma FJ, Flye MW: Factors affecting the results of below-knee amputation in patients with and without diabetes. Surg Gynecol Obstet 155:513, 1982.

78. Karanfilian RG, Lynch TG, Zirul VT, et al: The value of laser Doppler velocimetry and transcutaneous oxygen tension determination in predicting healing of ischemic forefoot ulcerations and amputations in diabetic and nondiabetic patients. J Vasc Surg 4:511, 1986.

79. Katsamouris A, Brewster DC, Megerman J, et al: Transcutaneous oxygen tension in selection of amputation level. Am J Surg 147:510, 1984.

80. Kaufman JL, Glockner F, Chang BB, et al: Impact of the presence of orthopedic hardware on technical performance of major amputations. Ann Vasc Surg 4:356, 1990.

81. Kaufman JL: Alternative methods for below-knee amputation: Reappraisal of the Kendrick procedure. J Am Coll Surg 181:511, 1995.

82. Keagy BA, Schwartz JA, Kotb M, et al: Lower extremity amputations: The control series. J Vasc Surg 4:321, 1986.

83. Kerstein MD, Welter W, Gahtan V, Roberts AB: Toe amputation in the diabetic patient. Surgery 122:546, 1997.

84. Kihn RB, Warren R, Beebe GW: The "geriatric" amputee. Ann Surg 176:305, 1972.

85. Kjolbye J: The surgery of through-knee amputation. In Murdock G (ed): Prosthetic and Orthotic Practice. London, Edward Arnold, 1970, pp 255–257.

86. Kostuik JP, Wood D, Hornby R, et al: Measurement of skin blood flow in peripheral vascular disease by the epicutaneous application of xenon-133. J Bone Joint Surg 58A:833, 1976.

87. Kram HB, Appel PL, White RA, et al: Assessment of peripheral vascular disease by postocclusive transcutaneous oxygen recovery time. J Vasc Surg 1:628, 1984.

88. Kram HB, Appel PL, Shoemaker WC: Prediction of below-knee amputation wound healing using noninvasive laser Doppler velocimetry. Am J Surg 158:29, 1989.

89. Kram HB, Appel PL, Shoemaker WC: Multisensor transcutaneous oximetric mapping to predict below-knee amputation wound healing: Use of critical Po₂. J Vasc Surg 9:796, 1989.

90. Kwaan JHM, Connolly JE: Fatal sequelae of the ischemic amputation stump: A surgical challenge. Am J Surg 138:49, 1979.

91. Lavery LA, van Houtum AH, Armstrong DG, et al: Mortality following lower extremity amputation in minorities with diabetes mellitus. Diabetes Res Clin Pract 37:41, 1997.

92. Lepantalo MJA, Haajanen J, Linfors O, et al: Predictive value of preoperative segmental blood pressure measurements in below-knee amputations. Acta Chir Scand 148:581, 1982.

93. Light JT Jr, Rice JC, Kerstein MD: Sequelae of limited amputation. Surgery 103:294, 1988.

94. Lim RC Sr, Blaisdell FW, Hall AD, et al: Below-knee amputation for ischemic gangrene. Surg Gynecol Obstet 125:493, 1967.

95. Little JM, Stephen MS, Zylstra PL: Amputation of the toes for vascular disease: Fate of the affected leg. Lancet 2:1318, 1976.

96. Lubbers DW: Theoretical basis of the transcutaneous blood gas measurements. Crit Care Med 9:721, 1981.

97. Malone JM, Moore WS, Goldstone J, Malone SJ: Therapeutic and economic impact of a modern amputation program. Ann Surg 189:798, 1979.

98. Malone JM, Leal JM, Moore WS, et al: The "gold standard" for amputation level selection: Xenon-133 clearance. J Surg Res 30:449, 1981.

99. Malone JM, Goldstone J: Lower extremity amputation. In Moore WS (ed): Vascular Surgery: A Comprehensive Review. New York, Grune & Stratton, 1984, pp 909–974.

100. Malone JM, Goldstone J: Lower extremity amputation. In Moore WS (ed): Vascular Surgery: A Comprehensive Review, 2nd ed. Orlando, Fla, Grune & Stratton, 1986, pp 1139–1209.

101. Malone JM: Unpublished data, personal communication, 1987.

102. Malone JM, Anderson GG, Lalka SG, et al: Prospective comparison of noninvasive techniques for amputation level selection. Am J Surg 154:179, 1987.

103. Malvezzi L, Castronuovo JJ, Swayne LC, et al: The correlation between three methods of skin perfusion pressure measurement: Ra-

dionuclide washout, laser Doppler flow, and photophlethysmography. J Vasc Surg 15:823, 1992.

104. Matsen FA, Wyss CR, Robertson CL, et al: The relationship of transcutaneous Po₂ and laser Doppler measurements in a human model of local arterial insufficiency. Surg Gynecol Obstet 159:418, 1984.

105. McFarland DC, Lawrence PF: Skin fluorescence: A method to predict amputation site healing. J Surg Res 32:410, 1982.

106. McIntyre KE Jr, Bailey SA, Malone JM, et al: Guillotine amputation in the treatment of nonsalvageable lower-extremity infections. Arch Surg 119:450, 1984.

107. McKittrick LS, McKittrick JB, Risby TS: Transmetatarsal amputation for infection or gangrene in patients with diabetes mellitus. Ann Surg 130:826, 1949.

108. McWhinnie DL, Gordon AC, Collin J, et al: Rehabilitation outcome 5 years after 100 lower-limb amputations. Br J Surg 81:1596, 1994.

109. Mehta K, Hobson RW II, Jamil Z, et al: Fallibility of Doppler ankle pressure in predicting healing of transmetatarsal amputation. J Surg Res 28:466, 1980.

110. Miller N, Dardik H, Wolodinger F, et al: Transmetatarsal amputation: The role of adjunctive revascularization. J Vasc Surg 13:705, 1991.

111. Moore WS: Introduction to amputation symposium. Arch Surg 116:79, 1981.

112. Moore WS, Henry RE, Malone JM, et al: Prospective use of xenon-133 clearance for amputation level selection. Arch Surg 116:86, 1981.

113. Moosa HH, Makaroun MS, Peitzman AB, et al: TcPo₂ values in limb ischemia: Effects of blood flow and arterial oxygen tension. J Surg Res 40:482, 1986.

114. Munck O, Anderson AM: Decomposition of iodine labelled antipyrine. Scand J Lab Invest 19:256, 1967.

115. Munck O, Anderson AM, Binder C: Clearance of 4-iodo-antipyrine-125-I after subcutaneous injection in various regions. Scand J Lab Invest 99(Suppl):39, 1967.

116. Mustapha NM, Jain SK, Dudley P, Redhead RG: The effect of oxygen inhalation and intravenous naftidrofuryl on the transcutaneous partial oxygen pressure in ischemic lower limbs. Prosthet Orthot Int 8:135, 1984.

117. Nakhgevary KB, Rhoads JE Jr: Ankle-level amputation. Surgery 95:549, 1984.

118. Nicholas GG, Myers JL, Demuth WE: The role of vascular laboratory criteria in the selection of patients for lower extremity amputation. Ann Surg 195:469, 1982.

119. Nilsen R, Dahn I, Lassen NA, Wastling GA: On the estimation of local effective perfusion pressure in patients with obliterative arterial disease by means of external compression over a xenon-133 depot. Scand J Clin Lab Invest 99(Suppl):29, 1967.

120. Oishi CS, Fronek A, Golbranson FL: The role of non-invasive vascular studies in determining levels of amputation. J Bone Joint Surg 70A:1520, 1988.

121. Ovesen J, Stockel M: Measurement of skin perfusion pressure by photoelectric technique: An aid to amputation level selection in arteriosclerotic disease. Prosthet Orthot Int 8:39, 1984.

122. Persson BM: Sagittal incision for below-knee amputation in ischaemic gangrene. J Bone Joint Surg 56B:110, 1974.

123. Pilegard HK, Madsen MR, Hansen-Leth C, et al: Muscle blood flow after amputation: Increased flow with medullary plugging. Acta Orthop Scand 56:500, 1985.

124. Pinzur MS, Jordan C, Rana NA: Syme's two stage amputation in diabetic dysvascular disease. Ill Med J 160:23, 1981.

125. Pinzur M, Kaminsky M, Sage R, et al: Amputations at the middle level of the foot. J Bone Joint Surg 68A:1061, 1986.

126. Pollack SB, Ernst CB: Use of Doppler pressure measurements in predicting success in amputation of the leg. Am J Surg 139:303, 1980.

127. Porter JM, Baur GM, Taylor LM Jr: Lower extremity amputations for ischemia. Arch Surg 116:89, 1981.

128. Powell TW, Burnham SJ, Johnson G Jr: Second leg ischemia: Lower extremity bypass versus amputation in patients with contralateral lower extremity amputation. Am Surg 50:577, 1984.

129. Puddifoot PC, Weaver PC, Marshall SA: A method of supportive bandaging for amputation stumps. Br J Surg 60:729, 1973.

130. Raines JK, Darling RC, Buth J, et al: Vascular laboratory criteria for the management of peripheral vascular disease of the lower extremities. Surgery 79:21, 1976.

131. Ratliff DA, Clyne CAC, Chant ADB, et al: Prediction of amputation wound healing: The role of transcutaneous Po₂ assessment. Br J Surg 71:219, 1984.

132. Rhodes GR, Cogan F: "Islands of ischemia": Transcutaneous PtcO₂ documentation of pedal malperfusion following lower limb revascularization. Am Surg 51:407, 1985.

133. Rhodes GR: Uses of transcutaneous oxygen monitoring in the management of below-knee amputations and skin envelope injuries (SKI). Am Surg 51:701, 1985.

134. Rhodes GR, King TA: Delayed skin oxygenation following distal tibial revascularization (DTR): Implications for wound healing in late amputations. Am Surg 52:519, 1986.

135. Roach JJ, Deutsch A, McFarlane DS: Resurrection of the amputations of Lisfranc and Chopart for diabetic gangrene. Arch Surg 122:931, 1987.

136. Robbs JV, Kritzinger NA, Mogotlane KA, et al: Antibiotic prophylaxis in amputations (débridement) with or without arterial reconstructions for septic ischaemic lower limb lesions. South Afr J Surg 19(3):181, 1981.

137. Robbs JV, Ray R: Clinical predictors of below-knee stump healing following amputation for ischaemia. South Afr J Surg 20(4):305, 1982.

138. Robinson K: Amputation in vascular disease. Ann R Coll Surg Engl 62:87, 1980.

139. Roon AJ, Moore WS, Goldstone J: Below-knee amputation: A modern approach. Am J Surg 134:153, 1977.

140. Rosental JJ: Discussion in Kwaan JHM, Connolly JE: Fatal sequelae of ischemic amputation stump: A surgical challenge. Am J Surg 138:52, 1979.

141. Rubin JR, Yao JST, Thompson RG, et al: Management of infection of major amputation stumps after failed femorodistal grafts. Surgery 98(4):810, 1985.

142. Rubin JR, Marmen C, Rhodes RS: Management of failed prosthetic grafts at the time of major lower extremity amputation. J Vasc Surg 7:673, 1988.

143. Ruckley CV, Rae A, Prescott RJ: Controlled environment unit in the care of the below-knee amputation stump. Br J Surg 73:11, 1986.

144. Sanders RJ, Augspurger R: Skin flap measurement for below-knee amputation. Surg Gynecol Obstet 145:740, 1977.

145. Scheffler A, Rieger H: A comparative analysis of transcutaneous oximetry (TcPo₂) during oxygen inhalation and leg dependency in severe peripheral arterial occlusive disease. J Vasc Surg 16:218, 1992.

146. Schwartz JA, Schuler JJ, O'Connor RJA, et al: Predictive value of distal perfusion pressure in the healing of amputation of the digits and the forefoot. Surg Gynecol Obstet 154:865, 1982.

147. Sher MH, Liebman P: The air splint: A method of managing below-knee amputations. J Cardiovasc Surg 23:407, 1982.

148. Silberstein EB, Thomas S, Cline J, et al: Predictive value of intracutaneous xenon clearance for healing of amputation and cutaneous ulcer sites. Radiology 147:227, 1983.

149. Silverman DG, Rubin SM, Reilly CA, et al: Fluorometric prediction of successful amputation level in the ischemic limb. J Rehabil Res Dev 22:29, 1985.

150. Sizer JS, Wheelock FC: Digital amputations in diabetic patients. Surgery 72:980, 1972.

151. Sonne-Holm S, Boeckstyns M, Menck H, et al: Prophylactic antibiotics in amputation of the lower extremity for ischemia. J Bone Joint Surg 67A(5):800, 1985.

152. Spence VA, Walker WF: The relationship between temperature isotherms and skin blood flow in the ischemic limb. J Surg Res 36:278, 1984.

153. Spence VA, McCollum PT, Walker WF, et al: Assessment of tissue viability in relation to the selection of amputation level. Prosthet Orthot Int 8:67, 1984.

154. Steinberg FU, Sunwoo I, Roettger RF: Prosthetic rehabilitation of geriatric amputee patients: A follow-up study. Arch Phys Med Rehabil 66:742, 1985.

155. Stewart CPU: The influence of smoking on the level of lower limb amputation. Prosthet Orthot Int 11:113, 1987.

156. Stockel M, Ovesen J, Brochner-Mortensen J, et al: Standardized photoelectric technique as routine method for selection of amputation level. Acta Orthop Scand 53:875, 1982.

157. Sugarbaker PH, Chretien PB: A surgical technique for hip disarticulation. Surgery 90:546, 1981.

158. Termansen NB: Below-knee amputation for ischaemic gangrene:

Prospective, randomized comparison of a transverse and a sagittal operative technique. Acta Orthop Scand 48:311, 1977.

159. Thornhill HL, Jones GD, Brodzka W, et al: Bilateral below-knee amputations: Experience with 80 patients. Arch Phys Med Rehabil 67:159, 1986.

160. Tooms RE, Hampton FL: Hip disarticulation and hemipelvectomy amputation. In American Academy of Orthopaedic Surgeons: Atlas of Limb Prosthetics, Surgical and Prosthetic Principles. St. Louis, CV Mosby, 1981, p 403.

161. Tooms RE: Amputations of lower extremity. In Crenshaw AH (ed): Campbell's Operative Orthopaedics, 8th ed. Vol. 2. St. Louis, Mosby–Year Book, 1992, pp 689–702.

162. Towne JD, Condon RE: Lower extremity amputations for ischemic disease. Adv Surg 13:199, 1979.

163. Verta MJ, Gross WS, Van Bellan B, et al: Forefoot perfusion pressure and minor amputation surgery. Surgery 80:729, 1976.

164. Vitti MJ, Robinson DV, Hauer-Jensen M, et al: Wound healing in forefoot amputations: The predictive value of toe pressure. Ann Vasc Surg 8:99, 1994.

165. Volpicelli LJ, Chambers RB, Wagner FW: Ambulation levels of bilateral lower extremity amputees. J Bone Joint Surg 65A:599, 1983.

166. Wagner FW: The Syme amputation. In American Academy of Orthopaedic Surgeons: Atlas of Limb Prosthetics: Surgical and Prosthetic Principles. St. Louis, CV Mosby, 1981, pp 326–340.

167. Wagner WH, Keagy BA, Kotb MM, et al: Noninvasive determination

168. Waters RL, Perry J, Antonelli D, et al: Energy cost of walking amputees: The influence of level of amputation. J Bone Joint Surg 58A:42, 1976.

169. Welch GH, Leiberman DP, Pollock JG, et al: Failure of Doppler ankle pressure to predict healing of conservative forefoot amputations. Br J Surg 72:888, 1985.

170. White SA, Thompson MM, Zickerman AM, et al: Lower limb amputation and grade of surgeon. Br J Surg 84:509, 1997.

171. Wutschert R, Bounameaux H: Determinations of amputation level in ischemic limbs: Reappraisal of the measurement of $TcPO_2$. Diabetes Care 20:1315, 1997.

172. Wyss CR, Robertson C, Love SJ, et al: Relationship between transcutaneous oxygen tension, ankle blood pressure, and clinical outcome of vascular surgery in diabetic and non-diabetic patients. Surgery 101:56, 1987.

173. Yao JST, Bergan JJ: Application of ultrasound to arterial and venous diagnosis. Surg Clin North Am 54(1):23, 1974.

174. Yao JST: Choice of amputation level. J Vasc Surg 8:544, 1988.

175. Yeager RA, Moneta GL, Edwards JM, et al: Deep vein thrombosis associated with lower extremity amputation. J Vasc Surg 22:612, 1995.

176. Yusuf SW, Baker DM, Wenham PW, et al: Role of Gritti-Stokes amputation in peripheral vascular disease. Ann R Coll Surg 79:102, 1997.

of healing of major lower extremity amputation: The continued role of clinical judgment. J Vasc Surg 8:703, 1988.

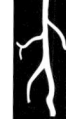

C H A P T E R   1 6 3
Complications of Amputation

Frank A. Gottschalk, M.D., F.R.C.S.Ed., F.C.S.(S.A.)Orth., and Daniel F. Fisher, Jr., M.D.

Despite improved techniques in amputation surgery, patients frequently develop one of the various complications related to the procedure itself or to the postoperative rehabilitation. The patient's ability to deal with these complications is often affected by his or her overall preoperative condition and ultimate desire to walk again. Multiple minor complications can be just as devastating as a single major complication.

This chapter is divided into *preoperative, intraoperative,* and *postoperative* complications. In reality, this division oversimplifies the situation because many of these problems are integrally interrelated and frequently coexist. Any treatment directed at a specific complication should take into account the overall status of the patient, the potential for recovery, and the likelihood of ultimate ambulation.

PREOPERATIVE CONSIDERATIONS TO AVOID COMPLICATIONS

Patients about to undergo amputation may have several preexisting medical conditions that can markedly affect the approach to surgery.

Cardiovascular Status

Many older patients undergoing amputation for vascular insufficiency have compromised cardiac function (see Chapters 2, 40, and 161). Detailed attention by a team of physicians, including an internist or cardiologist, should be directed at improving the patient's cardiac status to minimize cardiac complications. In extreme cases of congestive heart failure, Swan-Ganz catheterization may be required to monitor the patient's cardiac output and manage inotropic support. Occasionally, in severely ill patients with septic extremities, a "medical" (i.e., packing the extremity in ice) or guillotine amputation may afford time to improve the patient's hemodynamics.[10, 16, 22, 26, 33, 38, 58, 98] A definitive amputation can later be performed under optimal conditions.

Respiratory Status

In general, most lower extremity amputations can be performed adequately under spinal or epidural anesthesia, which avoids having to extubate a patient who may have severely compromised pulmonary reserve. However, spinal anesthesia may produce hypotension unless the patient's preoperative volume status is satisfactory. Central venous pressure or Swan-Ganz catheter monitoring in conjunction with the judicious administration of fluids and systemic vasodilators or vasopressors may help correct volume deficits and avoid hypotension at the onset of spinal or general anesthesia.

Preoperative Activity Level

Before any amputation is performed, the surgeon should evaluate critically the patient's rehabilitation potential. This may require consultation with physicians specializing in rehabilitation medicine.[27, 61, 67, 93] Inactive and bedridden patients, such as those with preexisting stroke or dementia who are not candidates for ambulation, may develop flexion contractures and stump breakdown if transtibial amputations are performed, ultimately requiring revision to the transfemoral level. The authors generally perform transfemoral amputations in patients with no rehabilitation potential to avoid the development of knee flexion contractures and subsequent stump complications.[62]

Joint Deformities

Preexisting joint problems, such as severe knee or hip flexion contractures, may compromise the potential for walking. In these circumstances, the authors usually perform transfemoral amputations to ensure healing, with less emphasis on femur length. Severe arthritis in the knee joint is a relative contraindication to a transtibial amputation. Failed total knee replacement associated with an ischemic limb necessitates a transfemoral amputation, or, in some instances, a knee disarticulation.

Previous Orthopedic Surgery

Before any patient is taken to the operating room for amputation surgery, the surgeon should question the patient about any previous orthopedic operations and examine the extremity for scars indicative of an orthopedic procedure. Prior hip or femur surgery may involve the placement of an implant, *which cannot be cut with standard saws*. If there is a question about the type of orthopedic implant at the site of the proposed bone transection, standard bone radiographs, which should include the joint above and below, are helpful in planning the amputation. It is often advisable to remove an intramedullary nail through a separate hip incision before performing bone transection for a transfemoral amputation. Long-stemmed hip implants may require transection with special saws. Stemmed total knee replacements may produce similar problems[83] (Fig. 163-1).

Osteomyelitis

Bone infections unresponsive to intensive antibiotic and surgical therapy require amputation at a level *above* the infection. If circulatory status is adequate, osteomyelitis in the digit generally responds to a ray amputation. Osteomyelitis in the tibia or fibula requires a knee disarticulation, and osteomyelitis of the knee or femur requires a transfemoral amputation. If an amputation is performed in close proximity to a site of osteomyelitis, a specimen of bone at

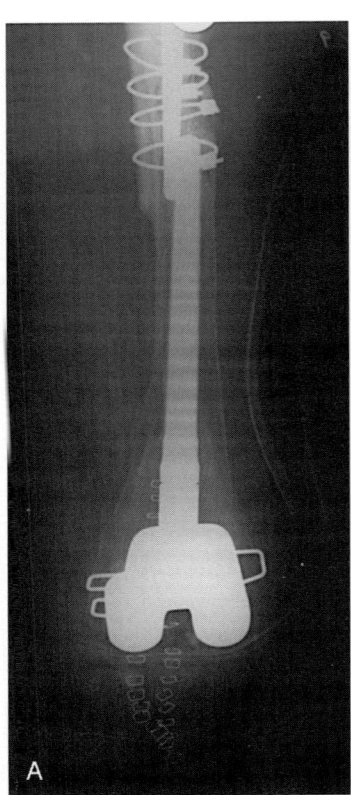
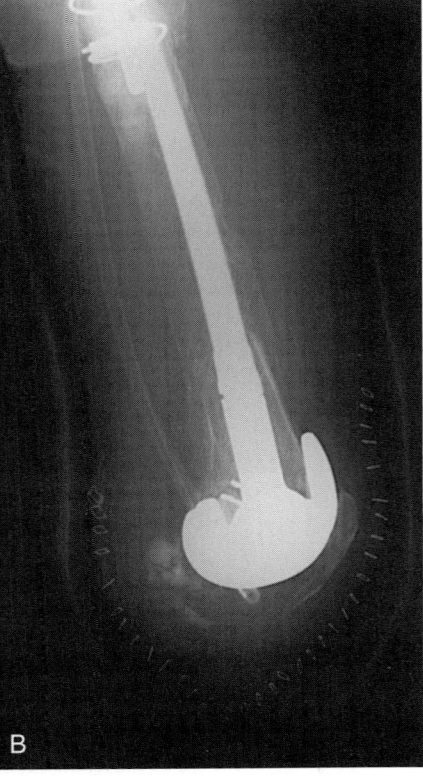

FIGURE 163-1. *A* and *B.* Knee disarticulation through total knee replacement in patient with unreconstructable vascular disease. Stemmed femoral component abutting against a femoral hip replacement component.

the amputation margin should be sent to the bacteriology laboratory for culture and sensitivity studies.

Soft Tissue Infections

Diabetic patients with insensitive feet are particularly prone to severe forefoot ulceration and infection. Medical management of such patients should include broad-spectrum antibiotics that cover aerobic and anaerobic organisms and an assessment of local arterial circulation.[50, 81, 97] If septicemia ensues, an open guillotine ankle amputation can be expeditiously performed for rapid relief of sepsis and associated lymphangitis that may accompany the foot infection.[10, 16, 22, 26, 33, 38, 58] Revision to a formal transtibial amputation is accomplished after resolution of any cellulitis or lymphangitis in the residual extremity.

Neurotrophic Ulcers

Patients with peripheral neuropathies from any cause are extremely prone to develop plantar ulcers, which may not be secondary to arterial ischemia per se.[14, 40] If treated early, these ulcers can be healed with a combination of pressure distribution, shoe modification, and patient education. If a toe or forefoot amputation becomes necessary, recurrent ulceration at a later date frequently occurs unless the amputation is performed above the level of insensitivity. Likewise, a transmetatarsal or Syme's amputation in these patients with diminished sensation may also be unsuccessful on a long-term basis.[20, 59, 95]

Diabetes or Renal Failure

The combination of these two metabolic problems leads to poor wound healing, especially of the skin. Some authors have suggested that a primary amputation is the operation of choice in all dialysis-dependent diabetics with gangrene of the foot because the healing potential of these patients is so poor, regardless of the patency of a bypass graft.[72, 73] Because of the risk of wound edge necrosis in these patients, the surgeon should pay the utmost attention to gentle handling of tissues and precise skin closure.[18, 19, 45, 92]

Traumatic or Crush Injuries

A combination of massive bone, nerve, muscle, and skin trauma occasionally dictates that an emergency amputation must be performed, and this is one setting in which an intraoperative tourniquet can be used. If the lower leg is involved, a knee disarticulation may lead to a very functional amputation level.[12] If the knee is involved, a transfemoral amputation may be the only reasonable choice. Usually, the level of amputation is dictated by the location and severity of injury.[79]

Absent Femoral Pulse

Approximately 10% of all patients undergoing a transfemoral amputation do not have a palpable femoral pulse. These patients are at high risk for necrosis of the stump, even if the amputation is performed at the mid-thigh level. Revascularization to the femoral artery level should be

considered in these cases. If wound edge gangrene occurs or is persistent, excruciating stump pain develops and the hip disarticulation may be unavoidable if revascularization of the profunda femoris artery cannot be accomplished. If hip disarticulation is performed before infection develops in the transfemoral amputation incision, the patient has an 80% chance of healing the disarticulation.[11, 47, 94]

Deep Venous Thrombosis

A severe case of deep venous thrombosis may result in secondary arterial compromise of the leg (phlegmasia cerulea dolens).[7, 99] If anticoagulation, directed thrombolytic therapy, lower leg fasciotomy, and possibly venous thrombectomy do not improve circulatory status, the lower leg may develop gangrene. Most of these rare patients require a transfemoral amputation. Necrosis of skin flaps may occur because of venous hypertension in the residual limb. Distal compression with an elastic bandage may help to reduce the residual edema.

Postphlebitic Syndrome

Rarely, patients require amputation for refractory venous stasis ulcers alone, and others undergo amputation for a combination of arterial and venous insufficiency. Patients with hyperpigmentation of the lower leg are particularly prone to develop posterior skin flap ulceration after a transtibial amputation that otherwise has enough arterial circulation to heal. If a transtibial amputation is chosen in this setting, immediate stump compression with some type of rigid plaster dressing or elastic bandage is mandatory until well after the stump has healed (up to 6 weeks). Thereafter, a support stocking is recommended whenever the patient is ambulatory.

Smoking

Cigarette smoking is a major risk factor for atherosclerosis. A Danish study found that the risk of stump infection and reamputation was twice as high in smokers as in nonsmokers. By measuring digital blood flow, platelet aggregation, hematocrit, and fibrinogen levels of patients who smoke, it was concluded that patients should stop smoking for at least a week to reduce the acute effects of nicotine on cutaneous and subcutaneous vasoconstriction.[51]

Blue Toe Syndrome

Distal microembolization can occur from any embolizing lesion located more proximally in the arterial tree. If the patient is an operative candidate, the embolizing lesion should be corrected to prevent recurrent embolization to the remaining limb, regardless of whether a distal amputation is necessary.[23] Progressive embolization can lead to necrosis of a healed stump, or, depending on the location of the embolic source, it can threaten the contralateral extremity. In the classic case of blue toe syndrome associated with normal pedal pulses, a distal toe disarticulation or a formal ray amputation usually cures gangrene in the forefoot. In more severe cases in which pedal pulses may not be present (such as those associated with embolization of large amounts of debris from aortic, femoral, or popliteal aneurysms), a transtibial or higher amputation may be necessary.

Impending Gangrene, Unreconstructible Vessels

Patients in this category usually have ischemic rest pain with or without open foot lesions. Arteriography demonstrates that vessels are diseased to serve as target arteries. Nevertheless, in 80% to 85% of these patients, a carefully performed transtibial amputation will heal unless a more compelling reason to perform a transfemoral amputation exists.[13, 36] Overall, amputation healing can be raised to over 90% if a transfemoral amputation is offered to those patients who do not have an audible popliteal artery Doppler signal.[3]

Previous Incisions

If possible, old scars should be excised or used to create amputation flaps, to prevent the chance of skin necrosis between old and new incisions. This becomes an issue more often in patients who have failed vascular procedures in the lower leg and who are thought to be candidates for a transtibial amputation. Although most authorities believe that transtibial amputations are best performed using long posterior and shorter anterior flaps, other flaps can be used in selected circumstances to prevent "skin island" necrosis. A skew flap provides good closure and has healing rates similar to those of long posterior flaps. Equal sagittal flaps may also provide satisfactory healing.[21, 34, 77]

Failed Bypass

In an effort to prevent amputation, it is always reasonable to consider distal reconstruction initially unless the extremity is unsalvageable. However, there is an unresolved controversy in the literature about whether a failed distal bypass will compromise healing at the transtibial amputation level (see Chapter 166).[15, 19, 21, 32, 43, 92] If the bypass fails and amputation becomes necessary, it still may be feasible and desirable to attempt a transtibial amputation. Amputation success will most likely depend on whether the thrombus extends into the host vessels beyond the distal graft in patients in whom bypasses end *above* the proposed level of amputation.

In general, the longer the time interval between the presumed graft thrombosis and amputation, the greater the chance of transtibial amputation healing. In such cases, the surgeon should plan the operation to start initially with a transtibial amputation, and if bleeding is totally inadequate, he or she can proceed with a transfemoral amputation. The experience of the authors has demonstrated that transtibial amputation healing frequently occurs after bypass surgery (Fig. 163–2).

Unsalvageable Foot, Patent Bypass

Since the advent of in situ bypass grafting, the authors have seen patients with distal foot lesions that have not healed despite a patent bypass.[57] The surgeon reluctantly

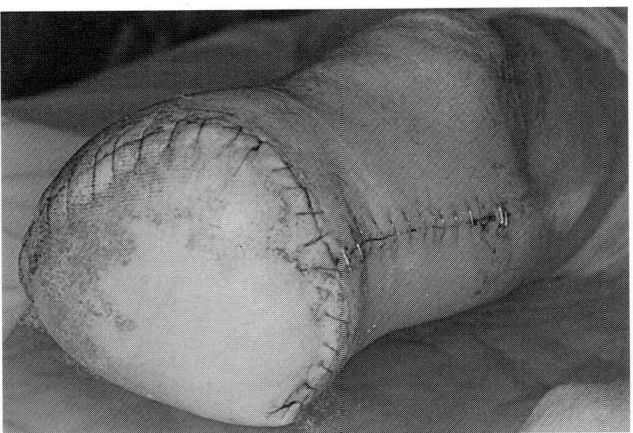

FIGURE 163–2. Healing of transtibial amputation and incision for bypass surgery.

may have to perform an amputation in this situation but may have concern that a transtibial amputation will result in acute graft thrombosis that might severely jeopardize stump healing.[92] In an effort to preserve the knee joint, the authors have had reasonable success in performing transtibial amputations in this circumstance. If possible, the posterior flap should be created as long as possible to avoid graft ligation. An alternative to standard transtibial amputation is to use the patent bypass as a source of arterial inflow for a microvascular free myocutaneous flap.

INTRAOPERATIVE PROBLEMS

Cardiovascular Collapse with Induction of Anesthesia

Cardiac collapse is a complication that usually occurs in patients who have deficient intravascular volume to compensate for the vasodilatory effects of spinal or general anesthetics. If this occurs, it is generally better to postpone the amputation until the patient's hemodynamic instability can be elucidated and treated appropriately. If the patient's hypotension is thought to be secondary to sepsis from a foot infection, an expeditious open guillotine amputation can be performed in less than 5 minutes.[16, 22, 58] This can significantly improve the patient's hemodynamic status in a matter of hours.

One other cause of cardiovascular collapse can be anaphylaxis secondary to antibiotics, usually cephalosporins. Although the cross-allergenicity between the penicillin and cephalosporin family of drugs is thought to be less than 5% to 10%, the authors have seen three cases of anaphylaxis after cephalosporins were administered. Profound hypotension necessitated an epinephrine drip and cancellation of surgery for several days. If the patient gives a strong history of a life-threatening reaction to penicillin or cephalosporins, or both, these antibiotics should be avoided. Ideally, antibiotics should be chosen on the basis of culture results, and nonallergenic alternative agents are usually available.

Stump Failure Secondary to Technical Problems

A variety of problems may severely affect prosthetic utilization but may not cause pain or threaten stump viability. These include (1) an excessively long fibula or inadequate beveling of the tibia in transtibial amputations; (2) an excessively long femur in transfemoral amputations; (3) an excessive muscle or soft tissue mass in the end of the stump, which may cause pistoning in a prosthesis; and (4) skin separation after suture removal. In most stumps with an adequate blood supply, these problems can be improved or cured by local remedial surgery without shortening the residual limb and jeopardizing the overall amputation level.[31] If the bone must be resected, the residual bone should be kept as long as feasible. Bulky soft tissue or muscle masses always interfere with optimal prosthetic fitting, which is facilitated by revision to a tapered, cylindrical stump. In some instances, the stump remodels itself with wrapping, as do the small dog-ears of a posterior flap.

Failed Prosthetic Bypass

Many extremities come to amputation after a failed above-knee or below-knee prosthetic bypass. Although some reports suggest that all such bypasses should be completely removed at the time of amputation, the authors take a modified approach.[75, 76] If the bypass is infected, it is removed as the first stage of a two-stage procedure. If possible, the amputation is delayed until the infection is eradicated. If the bypass is not infected, the graft is left in place and is resected as high as possible during the amputation in a single, one-stage procedure.

Inadequate Bleeding in Skin and Muscle

Patients with ruborous lower extremities at the mid-calf level, previously failed distal bypasses, or absent Doppler popliteal or femoral pulse are poor candidates for healing at the transtibial amputation level. For these patients, the entire lower leg should be prepared for surgery. If the skin incision does not bleed or if the muscle does not react when stimulated with electrocautery, the surgeon should abort plans for a transtibial amputation.[4, 6] The next best level for predictable healing is the transfemoral level, because knee disarticulations have unpredictable healing in very ischemic extremities.[39, 44, 62, 69]

Inadequate Posterior Skin Flap

In optimal circumstances, the authors transect the tibia at least 9 cm or more distal to the tibial tubercle in transtibial amputations to allow maximal transtibial stump length.[35, 80] In amputations with equal flaps, the length of the posterior skin flap should always be at least as long as the anterior skin flap, and in patients who have a large lower leg, the posterior flap should be longer (12 to 14 cm). Redundant posterior skin can always be trimmed and discarded. If the posterior flap is cut too short, the tibia should be cut shorter to determine whether the posterior flap can then be closed. This may require removal of more muscle in the posterior flap. If the flap still cannot be closed, the tibia

can be shortened more but the residual stump function will be compromised severely. Nevertheless, a short transtibial stump is better than a transfemoral stump.

Excessive Muscle in Posterior Flap

The posterior flap should be carefully fashioned to prevent a bulky, noncylindrical stump. If this flap contains too much gastrocnemius and soleus muscle, preventing a snug fit of the flap over the end of the tibia, prosthetic fitting may be quite difficult. Ideally, the soft tissue in the posterior flap should be a direct extension of the tibia.[2, 55] Soft tissue redundancy at the end of the stump serves no useful purpose and complicates prosthetic fitting and wearing. Excessive muscle and soft tissue should be excised during the amputation procedure to prevent the need for later revision.

Inadequate Beveling of the Tibia

The tibia must be beveled (45 to 60 degrees) so that there is no residual sharp point on this bone. Beveling can be done with a variety of saws, but the authors have found that pneumatic saws are especially useful for this purpose. A file can also be useful to smooth sharp edges.

Use of Foreign Material

Any material that can cause a foreign body reaction should be avoided. This includes the use of bone wax to stop bone marrow bleeding and the use of multifilament sutures such as silk. The authors routinely use polyglycolic acid (Dexon), polyglactin (Vicryl), or Polydioxanone (PDS) sutures for fascial closure.

Avoiding Excessive Tissue Destruction

Some authors have strong opinions regarding the use of the electrocautery in performing amputations through ischemic muscle. These authors prefer muscle transection with a scalpel. Other authors routinely use a cautery and feel that it may reduce blood loss and prevent the need for an intraoperative drain. Regardless of the surgeon's opinion, ischemic tissue should be handled with care to try to prevent any focal necrosis that might condemn the stump to failure.

Stump Hematoma

Often there is a slow ooze of blood after the posterior flap is fashioned despite an inability to find a focal bleeding point. The use of drains is controversial. The authors never hesitate to drain any stump that has persistent oozing. Our drains of choice are either a Hemovac or Jackson-Pratt closed-suction drain. These drains can be removed in 24 to 48 hours in almost all circumstances except knee disarticulations, which may require prolonged drainage for up to 7 days to evacuate synovial fluid. Postoperative stump hematomas, which can become secondarily infected, should almost always be avoidable with selective drainage.[58, 74]

Redundant Edges (Dog-Ears)

Ideally, the extent of the anterior skin incision in transtibial amputations should be equal to that of the posterior skin, as previously discussed. This is rarely the case because the posterior skin flap is usually longer. This can be partially avoided by extending the anterior skin incision farther posteriorly on the medial and lateral aspects of the flap. Most small dog-ears remodel spontaneously. Unless the dog-ears are extremely large, they should not be excised because injudicious excision can jeopardize the blood supply to the remaining flap (Fig. 163–3). With the use of long posterior flaps, "dog-ears" can be minimized by rounding the corners of the flap.

Wound Edge Necrosis

The surgeon should always try to avoid wound edge necrosis because it may cause the demise of an otherwise perfect amputation (Fig. 163–4). It is best to avoid picking up the skin with instruments. Delicate skin forceps should be used, if needed, to pick up the subcutaneous tissue, not the skin. Plastic surgery skin hooks may be useful. Sutures should gently approximate the skin, which should not be excessively tight. Because fascial sutures are placed so close to the wound edge, subcutaneous sutures are generally not necessary. Usually, good skin approximation can be achieved with simple sutures placed close to the wound edge. Occasionally, vertical mattress sutures may be required to achieve good skin coaptation. Although skin staples are an expedient method of closing the skin, the authors feel that, in general, skin closure is better performed with sutures.

Residual Stump Problems

The immediate postoperative dressing for transtibial amputees should prevent swelling and external trauma, should prevent knee flexion contracture, and should feel comfortable. All of these objectives can be accomplished easily with a rigid plaster dressing that is correctly applied.[63] If the surgeon has no experience in applying this device, the stump should be wrapped snugly in an elastic bandage and

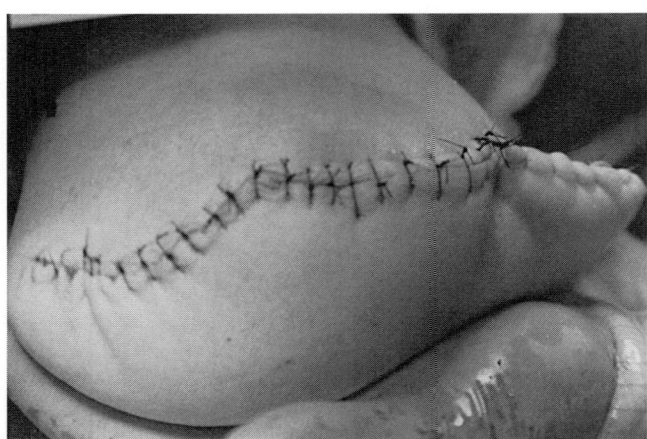

FIGURE 163–3. Redundant edges as a result of inadequate fashioning of flaps.

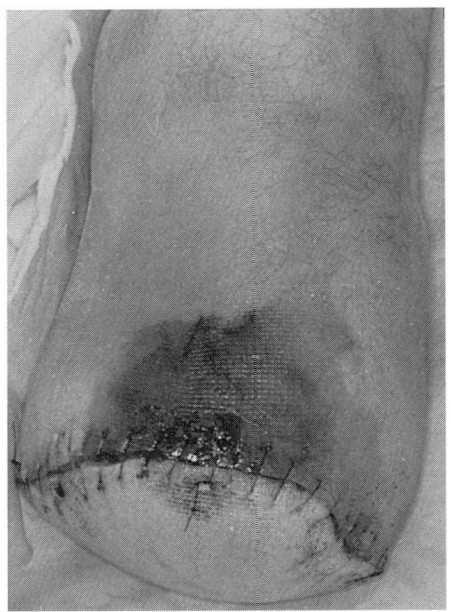

FIGURE 163–4. Wound edge necrosis with incipient gangrene of anterior flap.

the knee can be held in full extension with a knee immobilizer or a posterior plaster splint. If the splint is used, the surgeon should take care to avoid a skin plaster burn by placing an adequate amount of cotton wrapping between the skin and the plaster. In addition, tape should not be applied directly to ischemic skin to avoid a severe "tape burn" when it is removed.

POSTOPERATIVE COMPLICATIONS

General Considerations
Death

As a result of improvements in preoperative and intraoperative management, mortality should be 6% or less for transtibial amputations and about 11% to 12% for transfemoral amputations.[8, 78] The higher mortality for transfemoral amputations reflects the fact that these patients, in general, are older and have more extensive atherosclerosis. Death is most commonly caused by ischemic heart disease and stroke. Despite a successful operation, older amputees are still at significant risk for death. By using life-table survival curves, Bodily and Burgess showed that 50% of all elderly lower extremity amputees died within 36 months of the initial amputation.[8, 12]

Prevention of Stump Infection

Patients undergoing amputation (non-infection indications) should receive prophylactic perioperative antibiotic coverage for staphylococcal organisms primarily.[46, 60] Most surgeons today use cephalosporins for this purpose. Patients undergoing amputation performed for wet gangrene or other infectious indications should receive coverage with culture-specific antibiotics if culture results are available. If not, broad-spectrum coverage should include antibiotics active against gram-positive, gram-negative, and anaerobic organisms.

Stump Trauma

Stump trauma is a potentially avoidable complication that occurs with alarming frequency. Some patients forget that the leg has been amputated and may even try to "walk" on the stump. Rigid plaster dressings or knee immobilizers can help prevent the complications of stump trauma.[5, 63] If a hematoma develops and the stump remains viable, expectant therapy is indicated. If the stump is forced open by the trauma itself or opens spontaneously to decompress the hematoma, reamputation to a higher level will almost certainly be necessary (Fig. 163–5).

Swelling

All stumps swell, especially transtibial amputation stumps. Excessive swelling may prolong significantly the interval between amputation and prosthetic fitting. Rigid plaster dressings should be rapidly reapplied to transtibial stumps to prevent swelling between changes. If swelling continues to be a problem, careful compressive wrapping with an elastic bandage usually results in an eventual loss of edema.

Deep Vein Thrombosis

Deep venous thrombosis (DVT) occurs after 5% to 40% of amputation operations.[42, 99] The diagnosis should be considered whenever the surgeon observes that a stump has suddenly become more swollen. In addition, the *contralateral* leg is also at risk; hence, prophylaxis against DVT (e.g., a sequential compression stocking or low-dose subcutaneous heparin) should be strongly considered. DVT usually occurs about 3 to 7 days after amputation. Documenta-

tion by the standard venogram may be impossible, but a Doppler examination of the femoral venous system is usually diagnostic.

If DVT is strongly suspected or identified, therapeutic doses of heparin can be instituted with little fear of bleeding into the amputation site, especially if the stump is immobilized in a plaster cast or knee immobilizer. Stump swelling may be a significant problem and may mandate removal of a plaster dressing. Excessive swelling may tend to pull skin edges apart, jeopardizing stump viability. If anticoagulation therapy is contraindicated, a Greenfield inferior vena caval filter can be placed to prevent the development of pulmonary embolism.

Decubitus Heel Ulcers

Bedridden patients are extremely susceptible to the development of heel ulcers on the contralateral foot. The ulcer can quickly cause necrosis of all the thin subcutaneous tissue covering the calcaneus, eventually leading to an amputation of this limb.[8] Foam heel protectors should be applied to the contralateral limb of all patients to avoid this preventable complication. Frequent changes in position are mandatory. Occasionally, the authors apply a total contact cast to this contralateral leg to distribute the weight of the leg over the entire surface area of the cast.

Decubitus Sacral Ulcers

Decubitus sacral ulcers frequently develop in nonambulatory patients. Special mattresses and frequent turning are invaluable in preventing this calamity. Occasionally, radical surgery is necessary to cure these pressure problems by removal of the underlying bone.[48, 66, 90, 91, 94]

Overall Nutrition

Optimal wound healing and ambulation training require good nutrition. In patients with inadequate caloric intake, temporary tube feedings may be indicated. However, if tube feeding is necessary for longer than 2 to 3 weeks, it is extremely unlikely that the patient will be a candidate for rehabilitation. Because of the expense and complications involved with intravenous hyperalimentation, it has little applicability to most amputees.

Upper Body Strength

It should be remembered that ambulation training for lower limb amputations requires upper body strength, especially in the arms. While patients are recuperating from the amputation itself, it is important to start early upper body rehabilitation to maintain the patient's upper body strength.

Bone Erosion

Transtibial amputation bone erosion typically occurs because the tibia was inadequately beveled. If this complication occurs and revision becomes necessary, the surgeon should use an elliptical incision that encompasses the old incision and the area of bone erosion through the skin. The tibia should be shortened 1 to 2 cm and beveled correctly.

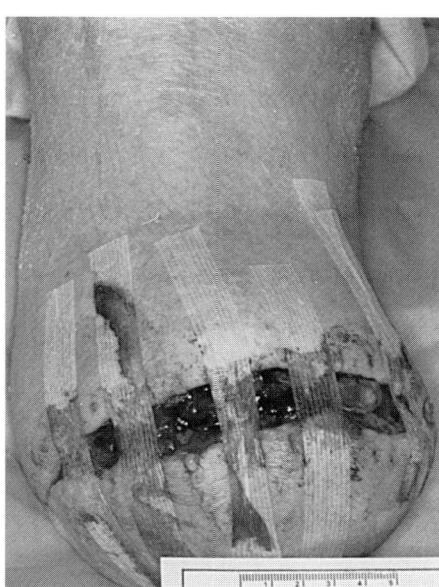

FIGURE 163–5. Stump gaping after minor trauma. Taping of wound is not correct, and additional surgery is required.

If the stump is also bulbous, the posterior flap can be modified appropriately.

Transfemoral amputation bone erosion typically occurs because the femur was left too long. Because the hip flexors are stronger than the hip extensors, the femur tends to erode through the anterior aspect of the skin incision (Fig. 163–6). The authors have generally reamputated the entire transfemoral stump, making sure that the femur is adequately short. If the patient is expected to ambulate, the femur should be left as long as is consistent with adequate wound closure.

Early or Late Ischemic Stump Ulceration

When stump ulceration occurs, revision to a higher level of amputation may be the only feasible option.[47] Occasionally, lower extremity vascular reconstruction to save an ischemic amputation stump is technically possible. Most transtibial amputation failures heal at the transfemoral level, and most transfemoral failures heal at a very high transfemoral level. Rarely, hip disarticulation is necessary in very ischemic limbs that have totally occluded the common femoral and profunda femoris arteries.[9, 91, 94] The authors have a small experience with dismal results upon trying to salvage failing stumps with a variety of revascularization procedures, although others have reported limited success with these procedures.[11]

Early Complications

Localized Problems

The most common complications seen in the early postoperative period (first 3 to 4 weeks) are infection, gangrene, and poor wound healing (Fig. 163–7). Frequently, these are directly related to an inappropriately low level of amputation and are further compounded by the patient's poor medical and nutritional condition. Despite the current trend to amputate at as low a level as possible, in some instances this may result in unnecessary complications that delay patient rehabilitation. Once a local problem is identi-

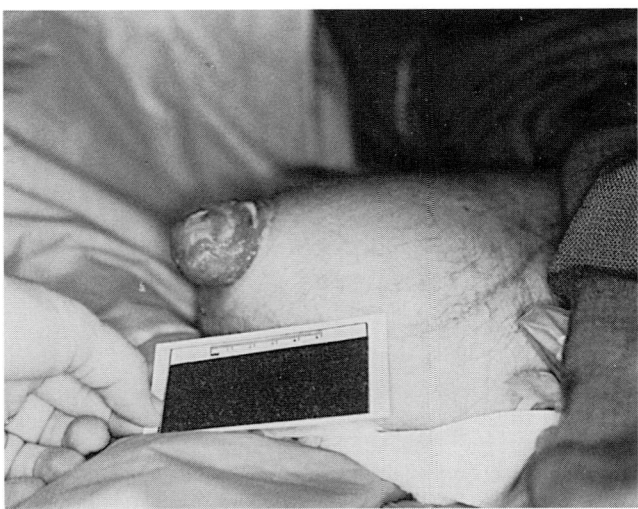

FIGURE 163–6. Erosion of distal femur through anterior aspect of skin.

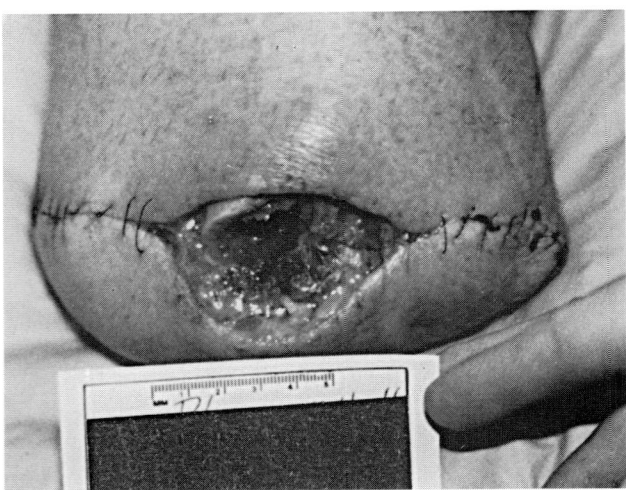

FIGURE 163–7. Wound breakdown and infection of soft tissue. Note sharp end of tibia as a result of inadequate beveling.

fied, the surgeon must decide whether revision surgery or local débridement is required. This decision should be made expeditiously to encourage early rehabilitation.

EARLY EXCESSIVE PAIN. Most amputations, regardless of level, result in a tolerable amount of pain in 4 to 7 days. Stumps that seem to be causing excessive amounts of pain after this time may have underlying ischemic muscle or frank muscle necrosis. Such extremities almost always require reamputation at a higher level for pain relief and healing.[47]

Infection

The incidence of stump infection is directly related to the indication for the amputation and ranges from 12% to 28%.[50, 53, 54, 58] In patients with a preexisting infection, antibiotic therapy, together with a guillotine amputation or wide drainage of the infection prior to the definitive amputation, is usually effective in reducing the incidence of this complication.[16, 58] An ankle guillotine amputation prior to definitive transtibial amputation for a septic foot has been shown to significantly decrease the rate of stump infection from 22% for a one-stage procedure to 3% for a two-stage operation.[10, 16, 22, 26, 33, 38, 58]

The authors recommend treating patients who have preoperative infections with broad-spectrum antibiotics that provide aerobic and anaerobic coverage. In a 1988 article, the combination of gentamicin and clindamycin was very effective in reducing postoperative infections in diabetic patients, in whom the incidence of mixed anaerobic infections may be as high as 60%.[22] However, many non-nephrotoxic broad-spectrum antibiotics provide good coverage without the risks of renal inefficiency from aminoglycosides.

An established infection in a stump must be adequately drained with a widely opened incision. This almost always requires later revision to a higher-level amputation. The seriousness of the complication is emphasized by the fact that in the elderly patient, conversion from a transtibial to a transfemoral amputation is often the difference between successful ambulation and not walking.

Prevention of stump hematoma is very important because there is a high correlation between hematoma formation and the development of infection. Hemostasis in flaps must be meticulous. The authors recommend placing closed suction drains for all amputations in which there is any significant oozing from the tissues.

Wound Healing

Failure of a wound to heal may be due to (1) inadequate blood supply at the level selected for amputation, (2) rough or traumatic intraoperative handling of marginally vascularized tissue, (3) a stump hematoma with or without secondary infection (Fig. 163–8), or (4) metabolic factors (e.g., malnutrition, immunosuppression). The incidence of nonhealing after major lower extremity amputation ranges from 3% to 28%.[4, 6, 53, 54, 74] An overall healing rate of 80% to 85% for transtibial amputations and 85% to 90% for transfemoral amputations should generally be expected.[13]

The authors' experience with forefoot and Syme's amputations in the dysvascular patient is not as good as that quoted in the literature.[25, 68] It has been disappointing how few patients heal a transmetatarsal or Syme's amputation, especially those patients with diabetes mellitus who do not have a palpable pedal pulse prior to amputation.[25] Appropriate vascular reconstruction may help lower the level of amputation by improving the local blood supply.

Failure of an amputation stump to heal may be related to any of the four categories previously listed. With respect to nutrition, several investigators have shown that if the lymphocyte count is less than 1500/mm^3 or if the serum albumin is less than 3.5 gm/dl, wound healing may be severely compromised.[17] This may occur in both diabetic and nondiabetic patients. Although nutritional status cannot be immediately corrected, awareness of the patient's debilitated state allows provision for prolonged wound healing and delayed fitting of a prosthesis.

Other factors that have been shown to adversely affect healing of transtibial amputations include (1) absence of a popliteal pulse, (2) presence of central cardiovascular disease, and (3) absence of intraoperative skin flap bleeding.[52]

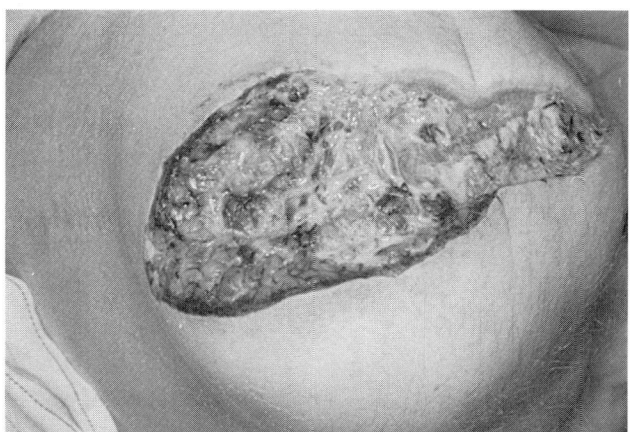

FIGURE 163–8. Failure of wound to heal, with necrotic tissue in base. Revision to higher level is necessary

Poor surgical technique resulting in inadequate skin flaps that have an excessive tension may contribute to wound breakdown in the early postoperative period. Excessive postoperative swelling may further aggravate an already compromised skin flap. Prevention and reduction of the swelling can best be controlled by either a rigid dressing or a pneumatic sleeve applied to the stump. Previous venous congestion in a limb, which may involve part of the skin flap, is also a contributing factor to postoperative stump congestion and wound breakdown.

Knowledge of the vascularity of the flap is important for preventing potential wound-healing problems. Studies of the blood supply of various types of flaps have helped in planning surgery for transtibial amputations.[37] The local blood supply is an important factor in healing, and the integrity of the skin-fascia interface is essential in closing the defect. Local treatment for unsuccessful transtibial amputations may be possible in some cases of wound breakdown. Necrotic tissue is excised, and some bone shortening may be necessary. Placement of a gentamicin collagen sponge within the wound may potentially reduce local infection, and the sponge is absorbed without the need for additional surgery.[89]

Flexion Contractures

Flexion contractures of the hip or knee joint are not uncommon after major lower limb amputation. The contractures tend to occur early in the postoperative phase in ambulatory and nonambulatory patients if the patient is not adequately monitored.[53, 54, 63] Pillows should not be placed under the thigh or the knee, and patients should be encouraged to avoid positions that keep the joints flexed. The rigid dressing for transtibial amputations will prevent flexion contractures at the knee by keeping the knee straight.

The role of the therapist in the early postoperative phase is extremely important in preventing these deformities. The presence of joint contractures compromises the fitting of a prosthesis and, therefore, the patient's ability to walk. It is generally accepted that a flexion contracture of *10 degrees* or more at the hip and *15 degrees* or more at the knee cannot be satisfactorily fitted with a prosthesis and limits the patient's ability to walk.

Muscle Stabilization

Inadequate and insufficient muscle stabilization at the time of surgery may result in a stump that is too flabby or that contains too much bony prominence. Another effect of the poor stabilization is poor stump control and unopposed muscle action of the opposing muscle group. This is frequently seen in transfemoral amputations, in which the femur may be pulled into abduction because of inadequate anchoring of the adductor group of muscles (Fig. 163–9). The eventual outcome is tenting of the skin on the lateral side of the thigh, with callus formation. Although the frequency of this problem has not been rigorously studied, it does affect the fitting of a prosthesis.[28]

The biomechanics of transfemoral amputations emphasizes the importance of the adductor magnus as a stabilizer of the femur. A muscle-preserving transfemoral amputation

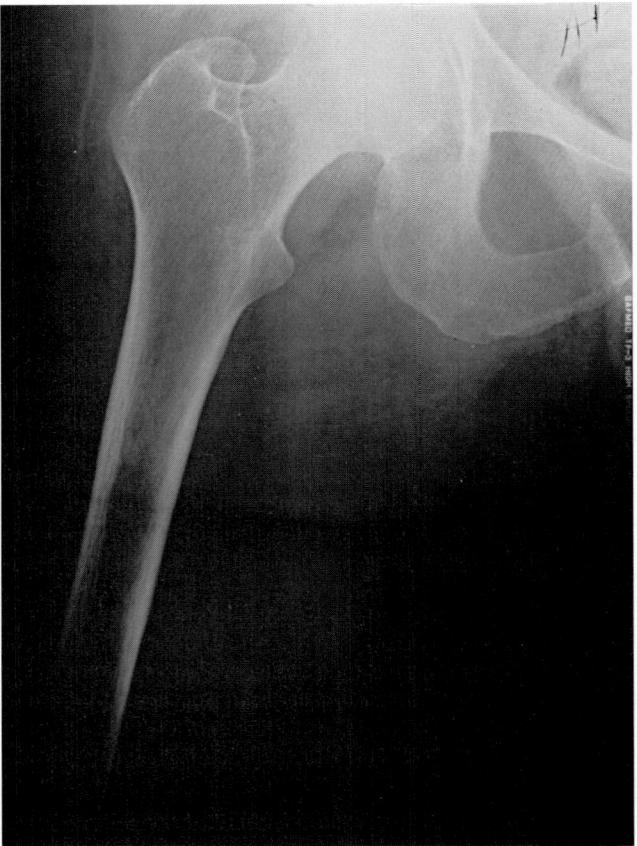

FIGURE 163–9. Residual femur in fixed abduction. (From Gottschalk F, Kourosh S, Stills M, et al: Does socket configuration influence the position of the femur in above knee amputation? J Prosthetics Orthotics 2:97, 1989.)

that keeps the adductor magnus intact minimizes the abduction deformity that frequently occurs. Loss of the distal third of the adductor magnus attachment results in a 70% loss of the effective moment arm of the muscle, which then leads to the abducted femur in standard transfemoral amputations.[30] Preservation of the adductor magnus and use of muscle myodesis to hold the residual femur adducted prevent some of the fitting problems and gait abnormalities associated with transfemoral amputation[29] (Fig. 163–10). In transtibial amputations, anchoring the gastrocnemius tendon to the periosteum of the anterior tibia helps reduce the posterior muscle sag and popliteal fossa discomfort associated with wearing a prosthesis.

Pain

Phantom limb *sensation* is a painless limb image that is experienced by most amputees. It is a feeling that the limb is still present, and it varies in intensity. Phantom limb *pain,* however, is poorly localized and may be burning, cramping, aching, or stabbing.[1] Melzack[56] noted that phantom limb pain had four major properties:

1. It lasted long after healing of the injured tissue.
2. It had trigger zones that could spread to healthy areas.
3. It developed in patients who had experienced pain

for a prolonged period before amputation and resembled in quality and location the pain present before amputation.

4. It could be abolished by temporary increases or decreases in somatic input.

A study of 59 patients who had hemipelvectomy or hip disarticulation showed that phantom limb *sensation* occurred in all patients and that 14 of 16 patients who had preamputation pain experienced postoperative phantom limb *pain.* In eight of nine patients with no preamputation pain, postoperative phantom limb pain subsequently developed.[96]

Various reports in the literature cite the incidence of disabling stump pain and phantom limb pain after major lower extremity amputation as between 5% and 30%.[1, 65, 84–87] Sherman and associates reported that 85% of patients responding to a survey had significant stump pain.[84–87] This high incidence of postoperative pain was attributed to the fact that most studies have not closely surveyed for its presence. A prospective study documented that the presence of preamputation pain significantly increased the incidence of stump pain and phantom pain; in 42% of patients, the phantom pain closely resembled the pain experienced at the time of amputation.[64]

Phantom limb pain is very difficult to treat; treatment modalities include medications, local injections, and surgery. No single or combined therapy has been shown to have consistent success. It has been described that patients with phantom pain often have a personality disorder and exhibit psychologic aberrations. This seems to occur more frequently in younger patients who have undergone ampu-

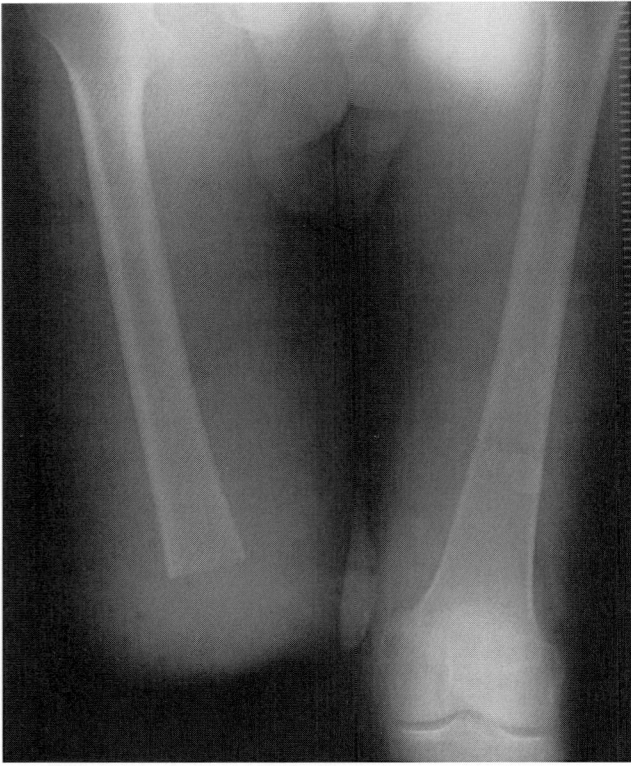

FIGURE 163–10. Residual femur in adduction following muscle-preserving adductor myodesis.

tations for trauma. Severe pain is less common in older patients undergoing amputation for vascular disease.

Amputations occurring as a result of trauma may develop a local agonizing burning pain associated with trophic changes in the remaining part of the limb. This burning pain, originally called causalgia, is now considered to be part of the syndrome of reflex sympathetic dystrophy.[82] The skin of the involved limb becomes mottled, cool, and shiny, and the bones become osteopenic. Early sympathetic anesthetic blocks or surgical sympathectomy may abort the process, but no individual modality is invariably successful.

The experience of Malone and others showed that an aggressive amputation rehabilitation program reduced the incidence of disabling pain after major lower extremity amputations to less than 5%, especially when the amputation was performed for ischemic rest pain or gangrene.[53, 54, 71, 74] This was attributed to the rapidity and success of rehabilitation as well as postoperative rigid dressings.

Late Complications

Various types of late complications may occur in the stump, related to poor fitting of the proshesis and the patient's general condition.

Stump Congestion

Incorrectly fitting sockets may predispose the stump to edema because of pressure distribution that disturbs the circulation. This edema is unrelated to the surgical trauma and usually is due to mechanical factors of poor prosthetic fit and obesity. A commonly seen problem is *verrucous hyperplasia,* which results in a wart-like appearance of the entire distal stump (Fig. 163–11).[49] The etiology is thought to be related to lymphatic and venous congestion from a poor-fitting prosthesis. This condition is best treated by a better-fitting prosthesis with total contact distally to support the stump rather than surgical revision of the amputation.

Bulbous Stump

The persistence of a bulbous end to the stump after the early maturation phase may complicate the fitting of a prosthesis and lead to uneven pressure distribution and skin breakdown. Resection of excessive residual soft tissue may be required to produce a more cylindrically shaped stump. This applies to both transtibial and transfemoral amputations. The most common cause of bulbous stumps is insufficient excision of muscle during flap closure.

Excessive Residual Soft Tissue

An excessively flabby stump resulting from redundant soft tissue severely compromises an adequate prosthetic fit so that the prosthesis cannot be satisfactorily suspended. Pressure points may develop where the soft tissue is compressed in the prosthesis (Fig. 163–12).

Thigh muscle atrophy following transtibial and transfemoral amputation interferes with the patient's ability to control the prosthesis efficiently during daily activities.[41] The shorter the stump, the more pronounced the atrophy and

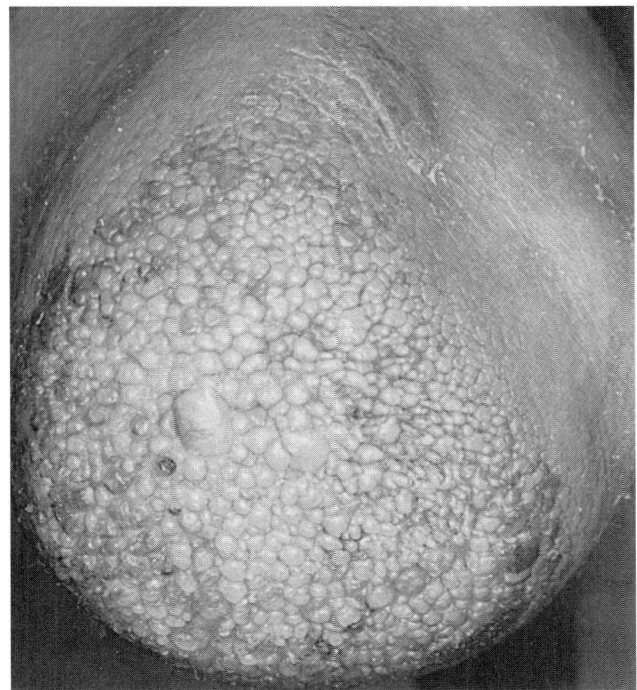

FIGURE 163–11. Verrucous hyperplasia of distal stump due to poor-fitting prosthesis.

loss of thigh muscle strength. Therapy aimed at strengthening thigh musculature will improve standing balance and quality of gait.

Calluses and Cysts

The development of calluses around the knee or the groin area may occur in long-term prosthetic users and is associated with areas of increased weight bearing in a prosthesis, particularly over bony prominences. Occasionally, these areas may break down or become painful. Calluses commonly occur at the end of the stump when insufficient soft tissue has been left over the tibial tuberosity and the ischium.

Other frequently occurring problems related to long-term prosthetic use are inspissated hair follicles and epidermoid cysts. Both are caused by mechanical pressure and are seen in hairy limbs, especially behind the knee and in the groin.[49] If realignment of the prosthesis or adjustment of the socket does not relieve the problem, surgical drainage or excision is indicated. However, recurrence of the cysts at the same site or in close proximity is not uncommon.

Neuroma

Neuroma formation cannot be uniformly prevented; it is a manifestation of a natural healing phenomenon. If the neuroma forms in an area that is subjected to pressure or is not well buried in the deep muscle tissue, the patient experiences a deep, aching pain that may be unresponsive to conservative treatment.[24] The best way to ensure that a neuroma is least likely to cause a problem is to gently cut the nerve deep in muscle tissue so that the nerve does not

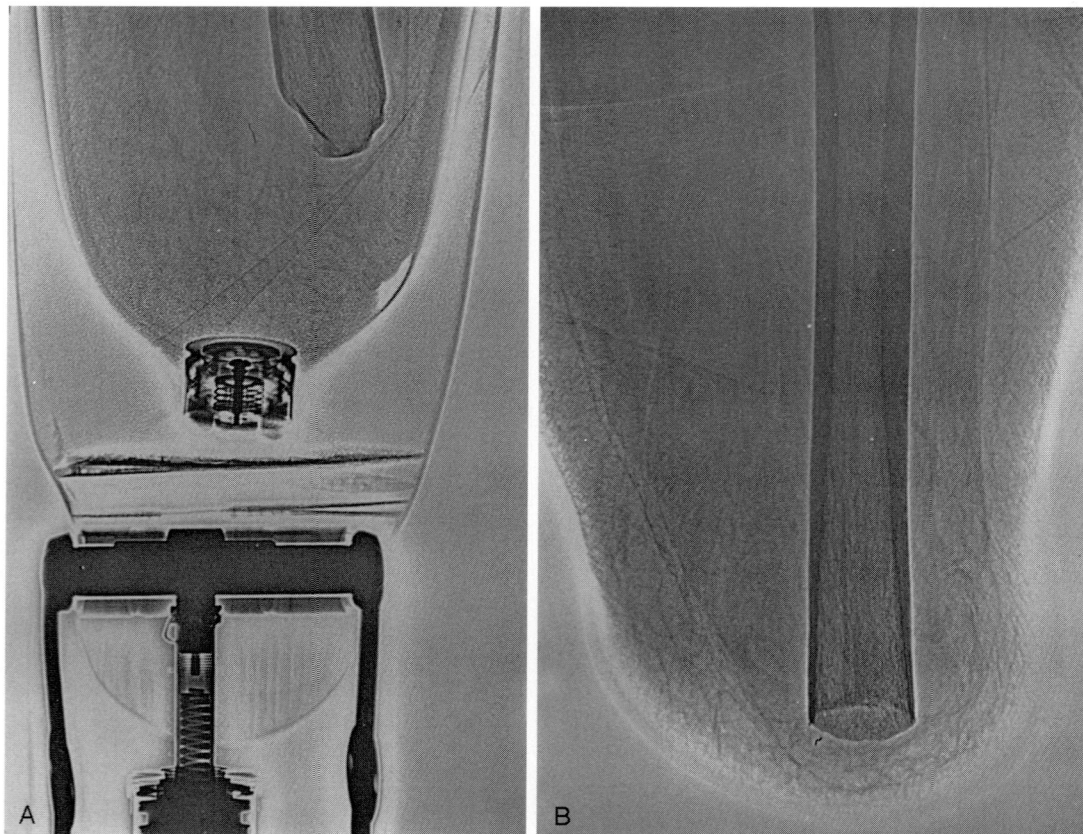

FIGURE 163–12. *A,* Xerogram of excessive residual soft tissue squeezed into prosthetic socket. *B,* Postoperative xerogram showing excision of redundant soft tissue.

lie adjacent to the sharp edge of the transected bone. Even gentle traction on a major nerve can result in a traction neuropathy, suggesting that any traction on a nerve should be avoided. If central vessels in the nerve bleed, they should be *individually* ligated. The authors prefer not to use an electrocautery for nerve transection to prevent excessive trauma to the nerve. A heavy ligature will not prevent neuroma formation and may irritate that portion of the nerve to which it is applied.

It is generally agreed that a neuroma buried in scar or located in a vulnerable position may impair the amputee severely. Rigid dressings in the early postoperative phase reduce symptoms from neuromas and phantom pain.[53, 54, 63]

Bone Spurs

Although bone callus does not form around the transected bone, it is not unusual for bone spurs to form at some point on the circumference, probably related to periosteal stripping. If the spur is in a location near the subcutaneous border, it may lead to a pressure point.

Osteoporosis

Osteoporosis develops in the residual bone in the stump in long-standing amputees because of disuse (Fig. 163–13). The bone is not stressed during activities because it is shielded by the prosthesis. Osteoporosis is usually asymptomatic, but it causes the bone to be prone to fracture.

Patients are susceptible to fractures when they wear a prosthesis. The long lever arm provided by the prosthesis and its weight, in conjunction with a fall, may fracture one of the bones in the residual extremity (Fig. 163–14).

Bone Overgrowth

Amputations through the long bones in children are uncommon and are usually a result of major trauma. Bone overgrowth has been noted in the femur, tibia, and humerus, which does not occur in congenital amputations of these bones. The cause of the overgrowth relative to the soft tissues is unknown, but it is proposed that children are at risk for this complication because of the periosteum's contribution to bone growth and the lack of stimulation for growth of the soft tissues.[88] Overgrowth does not occur in disarticulations. Surgical maneuvers to prevent this overgrowth include capping the transected end of the bone with cartilage.

Adherent Scar

Adherent skin and scar tissue, which is subjected to weight-bearing stresses, may break down and become infected. Judicious placement of surgical incisions is important to prevent these soft tissues from becoming adherent to the underlying bone as the wounds heal.

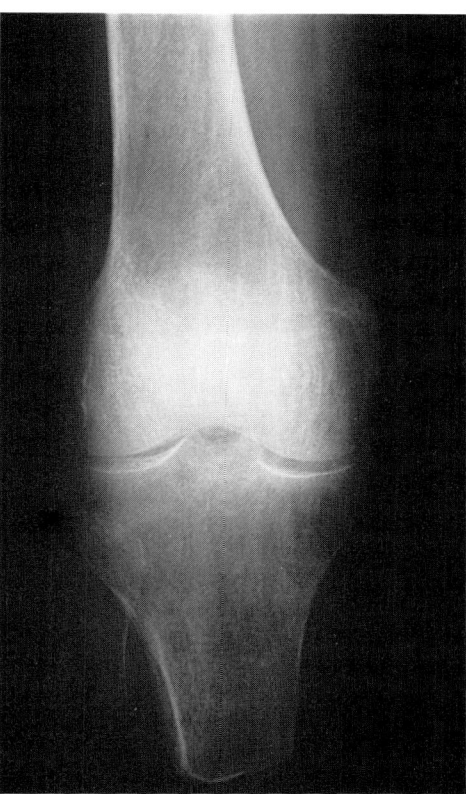

FIGURE 163–13. Osteoporosis of remaining tibia. Note loss of cortical thickness and trabeculae.

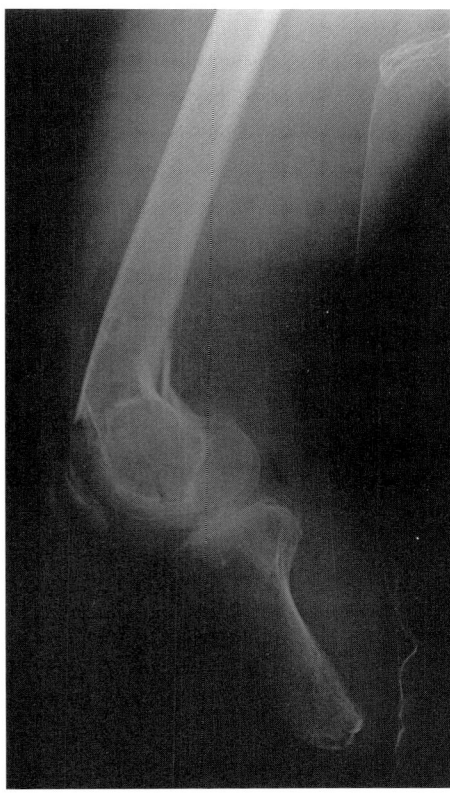

FIGURE 163–14. Supracondylar fracture of the femur on the side of a transtibial amputation.

Opposite Limb

The patient's other limb may be prone to vascular complications. In addition, contractures and skin breakdown may occur if care is not appropriate and if the patient is bedridden. The risk of contralateral amputation is very high in the diabetic or dysvascular patient, and precautions should be taken to prevent complications that might lead to amputation of the contralateral limb. It is reported that contralateral limb amputation may be as high as 40% within a mean time interval of 17.2 months.[8]

Revision Surgery

Because of increasing longevity, more stumps requiring surgical treatment are presenting. However, the need for revision is related to the level of amputation, adequate prosthetic fitting, and well-supervised postoperative follow-up and care. In long-term prosthetic users with chronic stump problems, revision may be the only means of resolving the problematic stump.

REFERENCES

1. Abramson AS. Feibel A: The phantom phenomenon: Its use and disuse. Bull N Y Acad Med 57:99, 1981.
2. Abrahamson MA, Skinner HD, Effeney DJ, et al: Prescription options for the below-knee amputee. Orthopedics 8:210, 1985.
3. Barnes RW, Thornbill B, Nix L, et al: Prediction of amputation wound healing: Roles of Doppler ultrasound and digit photoplethysmography. Arch Surg 116:80, 1981.
4. Baur GM, Porter JM, Axthelm S, et al: Lower extremity amputation for ischemia. Am Surg 44:472, 1978.
5. Behar TA, Burnham SJ, Johnson G: Major stump trauma following transtibial amputation: Outcome and recommendations for therapy. J Cardiovasc Surg 32:753, 1991.
6. Berardi RS, Keonin Y: Amputations in peripheral vascular occlusive disease. Am J Surg 135:231, 1978.
7. Bernstein EF: Operative management of acute venous thromboembolism. In Rutherford RB (ed): Vascular Surgery, 2nd ed. Philadelphia, WB Saunders, 1984, pp 1367–1384.
8. Bodily RC, Burgess EM: Contralateral limb and patient survival after leg amputations. Am J Surg 146:280, 1983.
9. Boyd HB: Anatomic disarticulation of the hip. Surg Gynecol Obstet 84:346, 1947.
10. Bunt TJ: Physiologic amputation for acute pedal sepsis. Am Surg 56(9):530, 1990.
11. Bunt TJ: Gangrene of the immediate postoperative transfemoral amputation stump: Role of emergency revascularization in preventing death. J Vasc Surg 2:874, 1985.
12. Burgess EM: Disarticulation of the knee. Arch Surg 112:1250, 1977.
13. Burgess EM, Matsen FA, Wyss CR, et al: Segmental transcutaneous measurements of Po₂ in patients requiring below the knee amputation for peripheral vascular insufficiency. J Bone Joint Surg 64A:378, 1982.
14. Ctercteko GC, Dhanendran M, Hutton WC, et al: Vertical forces acting on the feet of diabetic patients with neuropathic ulceration. Br J Surg 68:608, 1981.
15. Dardik H, Kahn M, Dardik I, et al: Influence of failed vascular bypass procedures on conversion of transtibial to transfemoral amputation levels. Surgery 91:64, 1982.
16. Desai Y, Robbs JV, Keenan JP: Staged transtibial amputations for septic peripheral lesions due to ischemia. Br J Surg 73:392, 1986.
17. Dickhaut SC, DeLee JC, Page CP: Nutritional status: Importance in predicting wound-healing after amputation. J Bone Joint Surg 66A:71, 1984.
18. Dossa CD, Shepard AD, Amos AM, et al: Results of lower extremity amputations in patients with end-stage renal disease. J Vasc Surg 20:14, 1994.
19. Edwards JM, Taylor LM, Porter JM: Limb salvage in end-stage renal

20. Effeney DJ, Lim RC, Schecter WP: Transmetatarsal amputation. Arch Surg 112:1366, 1977.
21. Evans WE, Hayes JP, Vermillion BD: Effect of a failed distal reconstruction on the level of amputation. Am J Surg 160:217, 1990.
22. Fisher DF, Clagett GP, Fry RE, et al: One-stage vs. two-stage amputation for wet gangrene of the lower extremity: A randomized study. J Vasc Surg 8:428, 1988.
23. Fisher DF Jr, Clagett GP, Brigham RA, et al: Dilemmas in dealing with the blue toe syndrome: Aortic versus peripheral source. Am J Surg 148:836, 1984.
24. Fisher GT, Boswick JA: Neuroma formation following digital amputations. J Trauma 23:136, 1983.
25. Francis H, Roberts JR, Clagett GP, et al: The Syme amputation: Success in elderly diabetic patients with palpable ankle pulses. J Vasc Surg 12:237, 1990.
26. Garrison AF, Jelenko C III, Brahn G, et al: The MCG boot: A device which facilitates physiologic amputation. Am Surg 39:637, 1973.
27. Gonzales EG, Corcoran PJ, Reyes RL: Energy expenditure in transtibial amputees: Correlation with stump length. Arch Phys Med Rehabil 55:111, 1974.
28. Gottschalk F, Kourosh S, Stills M, et al: Does socket configuration influence the position of the femur in transfemoral amputation? J Prosthet Orthot 2:97, 1989.
29. Gottschalk F: Transfemoral amputation. In Bowker J, Michael J (eds): Atlas of Limb Prosthetics, 2nd ed. St. Louis, Mosby–Year Book, 1992.
30. Gottschalk F, Stills M: The biomechanics of trans-femoral amputation. Prosthet Orthot Int 18:12, 1994.
31. Hadden W, Marks R, Murdock G, Stewart C: Wedge resection of amputation stumps: A valuable salvage procedure. J Bone Joint Surg 69B:306, 1987.
32. Haimovici H: Failed grafts and level of amputation. J Vasc Surg 2:271, 1985.
33. Harbrecht PJ, Nethery H, Ahmad W, et al: A technique for freezing an extremity in preparation for amputation. Am J Surg 135:859, 1978.
34. Harrison JD, Southworth S, Callum KG: Experience with the "skew flap" transtibial amputation. Br J Surg 74:930, 1987.
35. Hicks L, McClelland RN: Transtibial amputations for vascular insufficiency. Am Surg 46:239, 1980.
36. Holloway GA Jr, Burgess EM: Cutaneous blood flow and its relation to healing of transtibial amputation. Surg Gynecol Obstet 146:750, 1978.
37. Humzah MD, Gilbert PM: Fasciocutaneous blood supply in transtibial amputation. J Bone Joint Surg 79B:441, 1997.
38. Hunsaker RH, Schwartz JA, et al: Dry ice cryoamputation: A twelve-year experience. J Vasc Surg 2:312, 1985.
39. Huston CC, Bivins BA, Ernst CB, et al: Morbid implications of transfemoral amputations: Report of a series and review of the literature. Arch Surg 115:165, 1980.
40. American Academy of Orthopaedic Surgeons: Instructional Course Lectures, XXVIII. St. Louis, CV Mosby, 1979, pp 118–165.
41. Isakov E, Burger H, Gregoric M, et al: Stump length as related to atrophy and strength of the thigh muscles in transtibial amputees. Prosthet Orthot Int 20:96, 1996.
42. Johnson G Jr: Superficial venous thrombosis. In Rutherford RB (ed): Vascular Surgery, 4th ed. Philadelphia, WB Saunders, 1995.
43. Kazmers M, Satiani B, Evans WE: Amputation level following unsuccessful distal limb salvage operations. Surgery 87:683, 1980.
44. Kihn RB, Warren R, Beebe GW: The "geriatric" amputee. Ann Surg 176:305, 1972.
45. Knighton DR, Fylling CP, Fiegel VD, Cerra F: Amputation prevention in an independently reviewed at-risk diabetic population using a comprehensive wound care protocol. Am J Surg 160:466, 1990.
46. Krebs B: The use of antibiotic prophylaxis in amputations of the lower extremity. Acta Orthop Scand 56:179, 1985.
47. Kwaan JHM, Connolly JE: Fatal sequelae of the ischemic amputation stump: A surgical challenge. Am J Surg 138:49, 1979.
48. Lawton RL, DePinto V: Bilateral hip disarticulation in paraplegics with decubitus ulcers. Arch Surg 122:1040, 1987.
49. Levy SW: Skin Problems of the Amputee. St. Louis, Warren H. Green, 1983, p 153.
50. LeFrock JL, Joseph WS: Lower extremity infections in diabetics. Infect Surg 5:135, 1986.
51. Lind J, Kramhoft M, Bodtker S: The influence of smoking on compli-

cations after primary amputation of the lower extremity. Clin Orthop 267:211, 1991.
52. Low CK, Chew W, Howe T, et al: Factors affecting healing of below knee amputation. Singapore Med J 37:392, 1996.
53. Malone JM, Moore WS, Leal JM, Childers SJ: Rehabilitation for lower extremity amputation. Arch Surg 116:93, 1981.
54. Malone JM, Moore WS, Goldstone J, et al: Therapeutic and economic impact of a modern amputation program. Ann Surg 189:798, 1979.
55. Medhat MA: Rehabilitation of vascular amputee. Orthop Rev 12:51, 1983.
56. Melzack R: Phantom limb implications for treatment of pathological pain. Anesthesiology 35:401, 1971.
57. Memsic L, Busuttil RW, Machleder H, et al: Interval gangrene occurring after successful lower extremity revascularization. Arch Surg 122:1060, 1987.
58. McIntyre KE Jr, Bailey SA, Malone JM, et al: Guillotine amputation in the treatment of nonsalvageable lower-extremity infections. Arch Surg 119:450, 1984.
59. McKittrick LS, McKittrick JB, Risley TS: Transmetatarsal amputation for infection or gangrene in patients with diabetes mellitus. Ann Surg 130:826, 1949.
60. Moller BN, Krebs B: Antibiotic prophylaxis in lower limb amputation. Acta Orthop Scand 56:327, 1985.
61. Mooney V: Innovations in care of the amputee. Tex Med 75:43, 1979.
62. Mooney V: Transfemoral amputations. In American Academy of Orthopaedic Surgeons: Atlas of Limb Prosthetics: Surgical and Prosthetic Principles. St. Louis, CV Mosby, 1981, pp 378–382.
63. Mooney V, Harvey JP Jr, McBride E, et al: Comparison of postoperative stump management: Plaster vs. soft dressings. J Bone Joint Surg 53A:241, 1971.
64. Nikolajsen L, Ilkjaer S, Kronerk J, et al: The influence of preamputation pain on post-amputation stump and phantom pain. Pain 72:393, 1997.
65. Parkes CM: Factors determining persistence of phantom pain in the amputee. J Psychosomat Res 17:97, 1973.
66. Pearlman NW, McShane RH, Jochimsen PR, Shirazi SS: Hemicorpectomy for intractable decubitus ulcers. Arch Surg 111:1139, 1976.
67. Perry J, Waters RL: Physiological variances in lower limb amputees. In American Academy of Orthopaedic Surgeons: Atlas of Limb Prosthetics: Surgical and Prosthetic Principles. St. Louis, CV Mosby, 1981, pp 410–416.
68. Pinzur M, Kaminsky M, Sage R, et al: Amputations at the middle level of the foot: A retrospective and prospective review. J Bone Joint Surg 68A:1061, 1986.
69. Pinzur MS, Smith DG, Daluga DJ, Osterman H: Selection of patients for through-the-knee amputation. J Bone Joint Surg 79A:746, 1988.
70. Porter JM, Baur GM, Taylor LM Jr: Lower extremity amputation for ischemia. Arch Surg 116:89, 1981.
71. Potts JR, Wendelken JR, Elkins RC, et al: Lower extremity amputations: Review of 110 cases. Am J Surg 138:924, 1979.
72. Robicsek F: Vascular surgery: Possible adverse effect on extent of subsequent lower limb amputation. South Med J 85:1190, 1992.
73. Robicsek F: Regarding impact of arterial surgery and balloon angioplasty on amputation: A population-based study of 1155 procedures between 1973 and 1992. J Vasc Surg 26:353, 1997.
74. Roon AJ, Moore WS, Goldstone J: Transtibial amputation: A modern approach. Am J Surg 134:153, 1977.
75. Rubin JR, Yao JST, Thompson RG, et al: Management of infection of major amputation stumps after failed femorodistal grafts. Surgery 98:810, 1985.
76. Rubin JR, Marmen C, Rhodes RS: Management of failed prosthetic grafts at the time of major lower extremity amputation. J Vasc Surg 7:673, 1988.
77. Ruckley CV, Stonebridge PA, Prescott RJ: Skew flap vs. long posterior flap in transtibial amputations: Multicenter trial. J Vasc Surg 13:423, 1991.
78. Rush DS, Huston CC, Bivins BA, et al: Operative and late mortality rates of transfemoral and transtibial amputations. Am Surg 47:36, 1981.
79. Russell WL, Sailors DM, Whittle TB, et al: Limb salvage versus traumatic amputation: A decision based on a seven-part predictive index. Ann Surg 213:473, 1991.
80. Sanders RJ, Augspurger R: Skin flap measurement for transtibial amputation. Surg Gynecol Obstet 145:741, 1977.
81. Sapico FL, Whitte JL, Canawati HN, et al: The infected foot of the

diabetic patient: Quantitative microbiology and analysis of clinical features. Rev Infect Dis 6:S171, 1984.

82. Schnell MD, Bunch WM: Management of pain in the amputee. In American Academy of Orthopaedic Surgeons: Atlas of Limb Prosthesis: Surgical and Prosthetic Principles. St. Louis, CV Mosby, 1981, pp 464–472.

83. Schwartz ME, Harrington EB, Harrington M, et al: Transfemoral amutation in patients with prior hip surgery: A caveat. J Vasc Surg 11:480, 1990.

84. Sherman RA: Published treatment of phantom pain. Am J Phys Med 59:232, 1980.

85. Sherman RA, Sherman CJ, Gall NG: A survey of current phantom limb pain treatment in the United States. Pain 8:85, 1980.

86. Sherman RA, Sherman CJ, Parker L: Chronic phantom and stump pain among American veterans: Results of a survey. Pain 18:83, 1984.

87. Sherman RA, Tippens JK: Suggested guidelines for treatment of phantom limb pain. Orthopaedics 5:1595, 1982.

88. Speer DP: The pathogenesis of amputation stump overgrowth. Clin Orthop 159:294, 1981.

89. Spruit M, Bosman CHR: Revision of failed transtibial amputation. Eur J Surg 160:267, 1994.

90. Strinden WD, Mixter RC, Dibbell DG: Internal hemipelvectomy as a treatment for end-stage pressure sores. Ann Plast Surg 22:529, 1989.

91. Sugarbaker PH, Cretien PB: A surgical technique for hip disarticulation. Surgery 90:546, 1981.

92. Taylor LM, Hamre D, Dalman RL, Porter JM: Limb salvage vs. amputation for critical ischemia: The role of vascular surgery. Arch Surg 126:1251, 1991.

93. Traugh GH, Corcoran PJ, Reyes RL: Energy expenditure of ambulation in patients with transfemoral amputations. Arch Phys Med Rehabil 56:67, 1975.

94. Unruh T, Fisher DF, Unruh TA, et al: Hip disarticulation: An 11-year experience. Arch Surg 125:791, 1990.

95. Wagner FW Jr: The Syme amputation. In American Academy of Orthopaedic Surgeons: Atlas of Limb Prosthetics: Surgical and Prosthetic Principles. St. Louis, CV Mosby, 1981, pp 326–340.

96. Wall R, Novotny JP, MacNamara T: Does preamputation pain influence phantom limb pain in cancer patients? South Med J 78:34, 1985.

97. Wheat IJ, Allen SD, Henry M, et al: Diabetic foot infections. Arch Intern Med 146:1935, 1986.

98. Winburn G, Wood M, Hawkins M, et al: Current role of cryoamputation. Am J Surg 162:647, 1991.

99. Yeager RA, Moneter GL, Edwards JM, et al: Deep vein thrombosis associated with lower extremity amputation. J Vasc Surg 22:612, 1995.

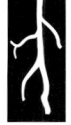

CHAPTER 164
Rehabilitation of the Person with an Amputation

Robert H. Meier III, M.D.

PHILOSOPHY OF THE AMPUTATING SURGEON

Amputation surgery must be viewed as a means of providing patients with improved function that requires the removal of nonviable tissue, alleviation of pain, extirpation of dysfunctional tissue, and construction of a limb that can be fitted with a prosthesis if the patient is a prosthetic candidate. Neither the surgeon nor the patient should view the amputation as a failure of therapy but, instead, should approach the operation as the prelude to more comfort and improved function—with or without a prosthesis.

The level of amputation largely determines the prognosis for the functional outcome. In most cases, the longer the residual limb, the better the function. Three levels may not follow this rule: (1) a hindfoot amputation, (2) a long transtibial amputation (distal to the taper of the gastrocnemius–soleus muscle belly), and (3) a long transfemoral amputation (distal to the junction of the middle and distal thirds of the femur).

A brief discussion of upper extremity amputation is found at the end of the chapter.

PHASES OF REHABILITATION

For purposes of rehabilitation staging and planning, the phases of amputee management are divided into nine phases (Table 164–1):

1. Preoperative.
2. Amputation with surgical reconstruction.
3. Acute postoperative.
4. Preprosthetic.
5. Prosthetic prescription and fabrication.
6. Prosthetic training.
7. Community reintegration.
8. Vocational rehabilitation.
9. Functional follow-up.

Staging the rehabilitation program assists in the development of a system of rehabilitation care that can be customized for differing institutional settings and rehabilitation team structures. Utilizing a conceptual framework permits each team member to develop particular responsibilities in the assessment and treatment plan for the amputee. In addition, this framework assists the team in developing goals and timelines for accomplishing each phase. Staging should also provide more continuity of care and helps develop outcome measures to assess the benefits of amputee rehabilitation.

Preoperative Phase

Functional outcome of amputation is optimal when the patient is in the most favorable cardiovascular condition

TABLE 164-1. PHASES OF AMPUTEE REHABILITATION

PHASE	HALLMARKS
1. Preoperative	Assessment of body condition, patient education; discussion of surgical level, postoperative prosthetic plans
2. Amputation with surgical reconstruction	Length, myoplastic closure, soft tissue coverage, nerve handling, rigid dressing
3. Acute postoperative	Wound healing, pain control, proximal body motion, emotional support
4. Preprosthetic	Shaping and shrinking of amputation stump, improvement of muscle strength, restoration of patient as locus of control
5. Prosthetic prescription and fabrication	Team consensus on prosthetic prescription, experienced limb prosthetic fabrication
6. Prosthetic training	Increased wearing of prosthesis and mobility skills
7. Community reintegration	Resumption of roles in family and community activities; regaining of emotional equilibrium and healthy coping strategies; pursuit of recreational activities
8. Vocational rehabilitation	Assessment and planning of vocational activities for future; possible need for further education, training, or job modification
9. Functional follow-up	Lifelong prosthetic, functional, medical, and emotional support; regular assessment of functional level and prosthetic problem solving

and has been mobile before the amputation. At minimum, the potential amputee should avoid being wheelchair-bound and should ambulate with a walker or crutches, at least for short distances. Strengthening the hip extensor and abductor muscles as well as the knee extensors hastens postamputation rehabilitation. Additionally, this is an appropriate time for the rehabilitation team to discuss phantom limb sensation, phantom pain, and residual limb pain with the patient. The staging of the rehabilitation plan, the potential for prosthetic use, and the approximate timetable for the rehabilitation program should be detailed. Discussion of the emotional adaptive process is also important during the preoperative phase. It is essential to prevent flexion contractures of the hip or knee joints of the affected limb and the other leg. Any hip or knee contracture of more than 5 to 10 degrees from full extension substantially increases the difficulty of using the prosthesis and augments the energy expenditure it requires.

Amputation with Surgical Reconstruction

This topic has been covered elsewhere in this text, but it cannot be stated strongly enough that careful reconstruction of the amputated limb at the time of surgery is the *sine qua non* for optimal functional outcomes. The techniques that seem to determine successful prosthetic fit and comfort are related to (1) identification of a level of tissue viability that will heal primarily, (2) formation of a cylindrical residual limb (Fig. 164–1), (3) myoplastic closure for prevention of movement of the residual bone in the soft tissues (see Chapter 163), (4) beveling of the ends of the residual bones, (5) control of postoperative edema with immediate postoperative rigid dressings, and (6) burying of the ends of major peripheral nerves.

Acute Postoperative Phase

After the amputation, the residual limb is best placed in an immediate postoperative rigid dressing to diminish postoperative edema, enhance wound healing, and decrease pain. Various postoperative rigid dressing protocols have been proposed and are part of a comprehensive, coordinated

amputee management system.[1, 2] If a soft dressing is applied at the conclusion of the surgery, no attempt should be made to use elastic compression to shrink the stump or to decrease the edema until the wound shows evidence of primary healing (at least 3 weeks on average).

An alternative to the soft dressing that can provide im-

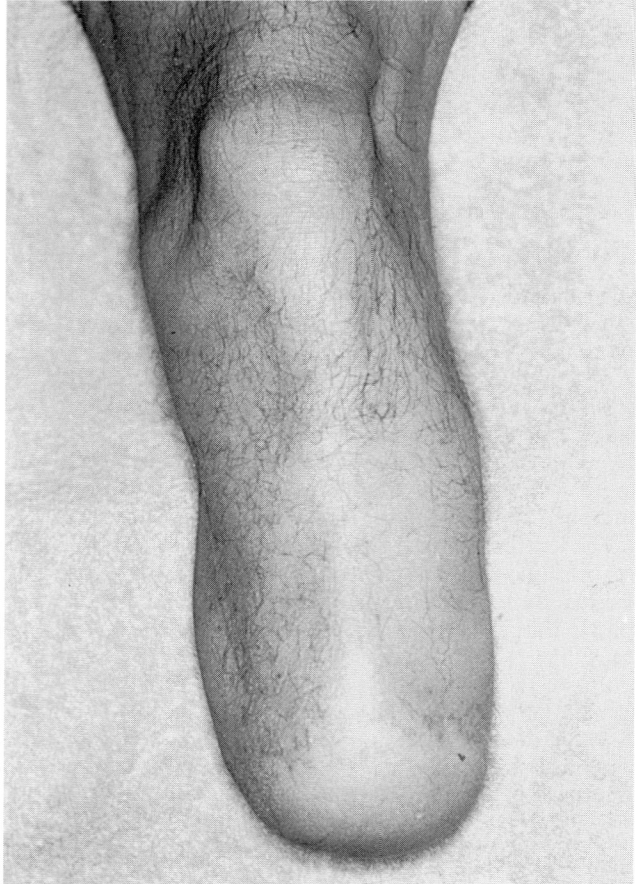

FIGURE 164–1. Transtibial amputation residual limb demonstrating the preferred cylindrical shape of the soft tissues below the knee.

portant protection to the fresh incision is the removable rigid dressing.[3] It can be applied shortly after the patient has undergone the amputation. This cap protects the stump from trauma and should be changed as edema decreases or when the rigid dressing becomes loose.

If a rigid dressing is not employed postoperatively, a long posterior splint should be affixed behind the knee to hold it in extension. In addition, an elevating leg rest for wheelchair mobility assists in keeping the knee in full extension. The patient should lie prone for prolonged periods to assist in maintaining full extension of the hip. Limiting the time the patient spends in the sitting position diminishes the development of hip flexion tightness.

After skin sutures or staples have been removed, a more aggressive program of residual limb shaping and shrinking can begin. Suture removal marks the beginning of the preprosthetic phase if the patient has the potential for using a prosthesis. The important components of rehabilitation during this period consist of controlling pain, promoting wound healing, and increasing upper limb, trunk, and remaining limb muscle strength. During this acute postoperative phase, the emphasis should be put on the remaining body parts that will substitute for the part that has been amputated. These activities enhance mobility before use of a prosthesis is desirable or practical. This is an ideal time for the patient to adjust to the new appearance of the body and to learn functional skills without using a prosthesis.

The debate about the use of rigid, semi-rigid, or soft dressings after amputation continues in the United States; a consensus conference on amputation surgical techniques was held at Strathclyde, Scotland, in 1990.[4] Whether rigid dressings or some other dressings are employed, a center-specific protocol for amputee care should be developed. Members of the team caring for amputees should understand their roles in effecting the goals of rehabilitation.[5]

In addition to the surgeon, an ideal rehabilitation team consists of a physiatrist, rehabilitation nurse, physical therapist, occupational therapist, psychologist, medical social worker, recreational therapist, vocational rehabilitationist, prosthetist, case manager, and pastoral counselor. These team members can evaluate the individual amputee and design a plan with functional goals that can be measured objectively at regular intervals. This team should be able to predict accurately the patient's expected function at varying intervals from the time of the amputation. It should provide a complete array of services to facilitate the patient's return to optimal function in the most timely and cost-effective manner. Amputation rehabilitation has progressed beyond the point at which the patient with a healed amputation was sent to the prosthetist with a generic prosthetic prescription in hand. If the patient's quality of life is to reach its zenith, he or she should be carefully guided through each phase of amputee rehabilitation with input from this team of health professionals.

Nail and preventive foot care for the remaining limb should be established early because this limb will always be subjected to more weight-bearing force than when the individual had two feet on which to bear weight during ambulation. The health care team should inspect the shoes customarily worn and ensure that the patient acquires properly fitted shoes if needed. In order to prevent plantar pressure problems from developing in the remaining foot

of the dysvascular amputee, an accommodative insole may be needed to more evenly distribute pressures over the plantar surface.

Preprosthetic Phase

Once the wound has developed adequate tensile strength, the stump must undergo a process of shaping and shrinking. A rigid dressing, changed weekly, or an Unna paste dressing can be employed. Elastic compression with a shrinker garment or elastic rolled bandages can be used.[6] If elastic rolled bandages are used, they must be applied in a figure-of-eight fashion (Figs. 164–2 and 164–3). The elastic bandages are anchored by incorporating the next proximal joint, and bandages should be rewrapped every 4 hours. When they are removed, they should not remain off for more than 15 minutes so that extracellular fluid does not reaccumulate. Usually, 2 weeks of shaping and shrinking should produce enough residual limb change to allow creation of a cast for the initial prosthetic socket.

During this phase, increasing the strength of the residual and opposite limb muscles is of paramount importance. The remaining muscles must compensate for those lost in the amputation. Knee stability is enhanced not just by the quadriceps muscle but, more importantly, by the hip extensors, including the gluteus maximus muscle and the hamstrings (Fig. 164–4).[7] These muscles are essential for knee stability during prosthetic stance. The hip abductor mechanism, generated by the gluteus medius, gluteus minimus, and tensor fasciae latae muscles, is of prime importance for pelvic stability during the stance phase of prosthetic gait (Fig. 164–5). Trunk and upper limb strengthening is also essential. This is also a time to improve cardiovascular fitness and endurance with the use of aerobic training, unless they are contraindicated.

Psychosocial issues are very important during the preprosthetic period.[8] All rehabilitation team members play important roles in the patient's psychosocial adaptation to limb loss. A psychologist or social worker knowledgeable about the process of adapting to limb loss and change in body image is essential for optimal rehabilitation. Often these aspects of rehabilitation, not simply the provision of the optimal prosthesis, are the basis of a successful outcome. Psychologic counseling helps the amputee adapt to altered body image and function, with or without a prosthesis. Team members responsible for psychosocial issues should actively interact with the amputee throughout all phases of the rehabilitation program.

The preprosthetic phase of rehabilitation is concluded when the patient is ready for prosthetic fitting. This period usually lasts from 6 to 10 weeks from the date of surgery for a dysvascular limb and often is shorter for the primarily healed limb lost to trauma. In general, the patient should first be fitted with a preparatory (temporary) prosthesis, which should be used for several weeks to months. These preparatory prostheses are best made from thermoplastic materials rather than from plaster by an experienced prosthetist. A definitive prosthesis of plastic laminate should be fabricated after the soft tissues have responded to the pressure of weight bearing during use of the preparatory prosthesis. The process of stump shaping occurs over several months to several years. In most cases, however, the resid-

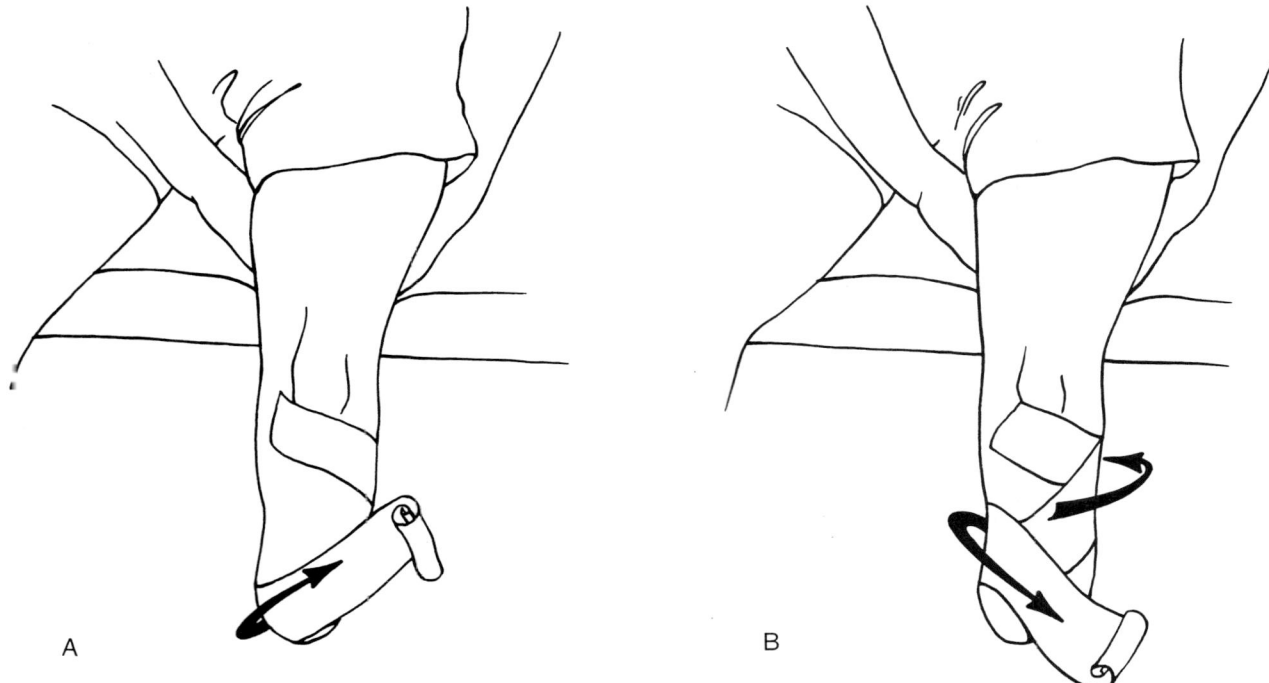

FIGURE 164–2. Elastic wrap procedure for transtibial amputation. *A,* Make all turns on the diagonal. Never use horizontal turns because they tend to constrict circulation. *B,* Do not encircle the end of the residual limb with one turn because this tends to cause skin creases in the scar. Alternatively, cover the inside and outside of the end in successive turns.

ual limb tissues stabilize within the first 12 months. Less frequent prosthetic adjustments are required after this initial period.

Prosthetic Prescription and Fabrication

Prosthetic fabrication should be a brief phase beginning with the decision whether the amputee is a candidate for a prosthesis. If a decision is made to proceed with a prosthesis, the team, together with the amputee and the family, should discuss the prosthetic options. If the amputee can stand independently and walk for short distances on one leg using a walker or crutches, he or she is a potential prosthetic candidate. Even if the prosthesis is to be used only for transferring from a wheelchair to another surface, provision of a prosthesis may be warranted. Only rarely should a leg prosthesis be prescribed for purely cosmetic reasons.

Whenever possible, prosthesis component options should be tried before the final prosthetic prescription is developed. This flexibility requires a willing prosthetist and third-party payer. Third-party sponsorship for the prosthesis should be obtained as quickly as possible. Most prosthetists should be able to fabricate any type of leg prosthesis with n 2 weeks of casting of the prosthesis.

It is important to discuss with the patient the length of time that is expected for fabrication of the prosthesis. In addition, the amputee must be educated about the steps in fabrication and the approximate number of visits to the prosthetist's laboratory that will likely be required before the prosthesis is ready to wear and prosthetic training can begin.

Prosthetic Training

Prosthetic training begins with the delivery of the prosthesis from the prosthetic laboratory, ideally within 3 to 8 weeks of the amputation surgery. Training should occur under the guidance of an experienced physician, therapist, and prosthetist, all of whom understand the biomechanics and principles of prosthetic use.[9–11] The decision whether to use an inpatient or outpatient setting for prosthetic training depends on many factors. In most instances, a patient with a unilateral transtibial or transfemoral amputation can be trained as an outpatient. The transfemoral amputee with significant cardiopulmonary compromise or multiple medical problems, however, probably needs initial inpatient training. Some patients with bilateral leg amputation may also require inpatient gait training.

Short periods of wearing the prosthesis and instruction in donning and doffing it should be the initial focus. Walking while wearing the prosthesis, although a very exciting prospect for the amputee, is often inappropriate early in training because the proximal leg muscles have not yet been properly strengthened or do not have the endurance to provide adequate knee, hip, or pelvic stability. Periods of standing supported by parallel bars with weight shifting should be attempted initially. Good hip and knee stability must be attained prior to advancing to the next stage—walking with a gait aid.

Whenever possible, the amputee should be discouraged from using a wheelchair and should be encouraged to walk with a walker and then to walk using crutches or a cane. Use of a walker never permits a normal gait pattern and frequently limits the environment in which the prosthesis can be used. Use of the prosthesis in the home should be

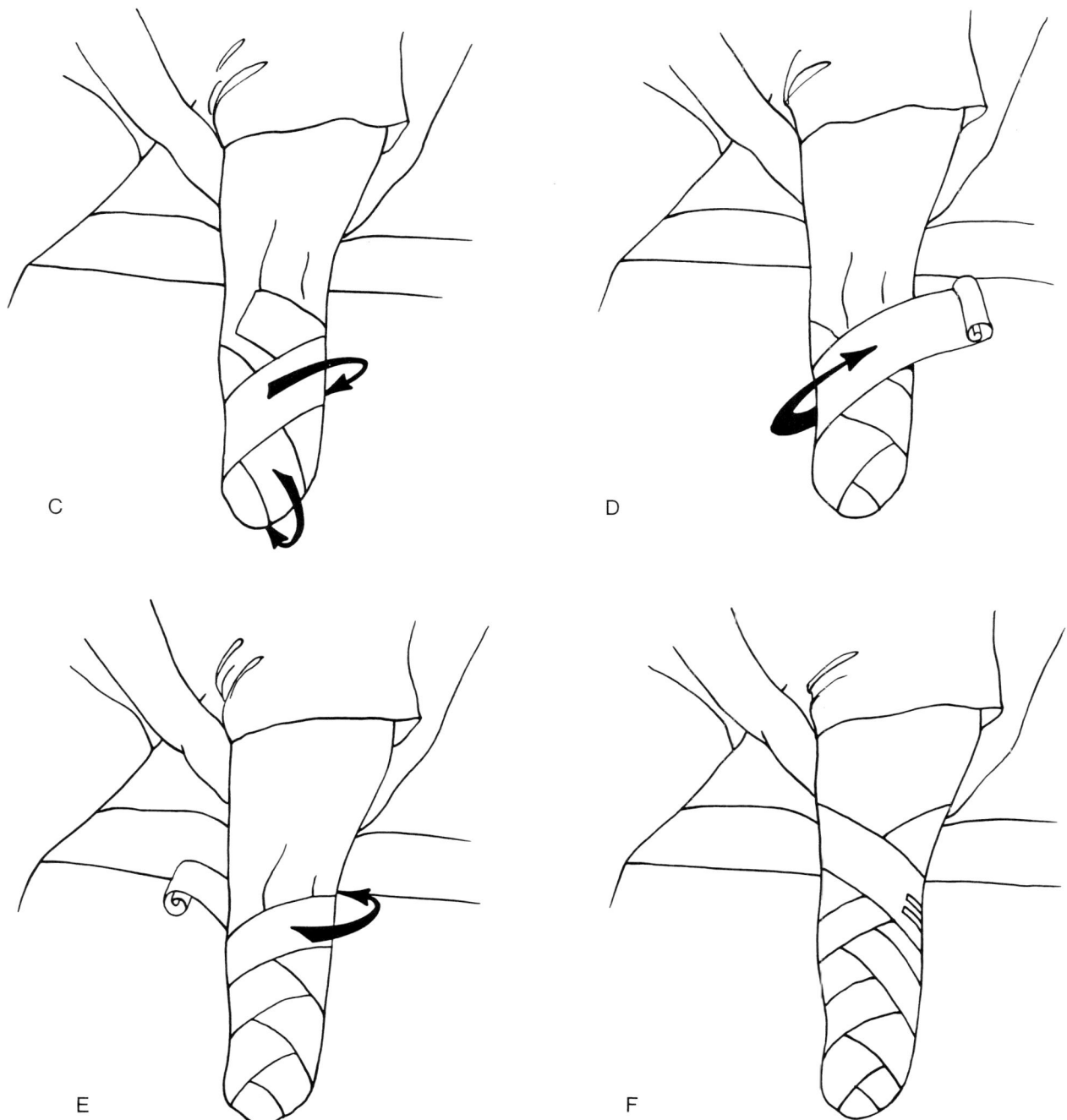

FIGURE 164–2 *Continued C*, Continue making diagonal turns, exerting firm pressure over the distal end of the residual limb. *D*, Bandage pressure should become lighter as you continue to wrap proximally. *E*, Extend the wrap above the knee. There should be at least one turn above the kneecap. *F*, Return to below the knee. If bandage remains, finish the bandage with diagonal turns *over the end* of the residual limb. Anchor the bandage with tape. Do not use safety pins. Rewrap the residual limb every 3 to 4 hours, or more often if necessary. (From Karacoloff LA, Hammersley CS, Schneider FJ: Lower Extremity Amputation: A Guide to Functional Outcomes in Physical Therapy Management, 2nd ed. Gaithersburg, Md, Aspen Publishers, 1992, pp 16–17. © 1992, Aspen Publishers.)

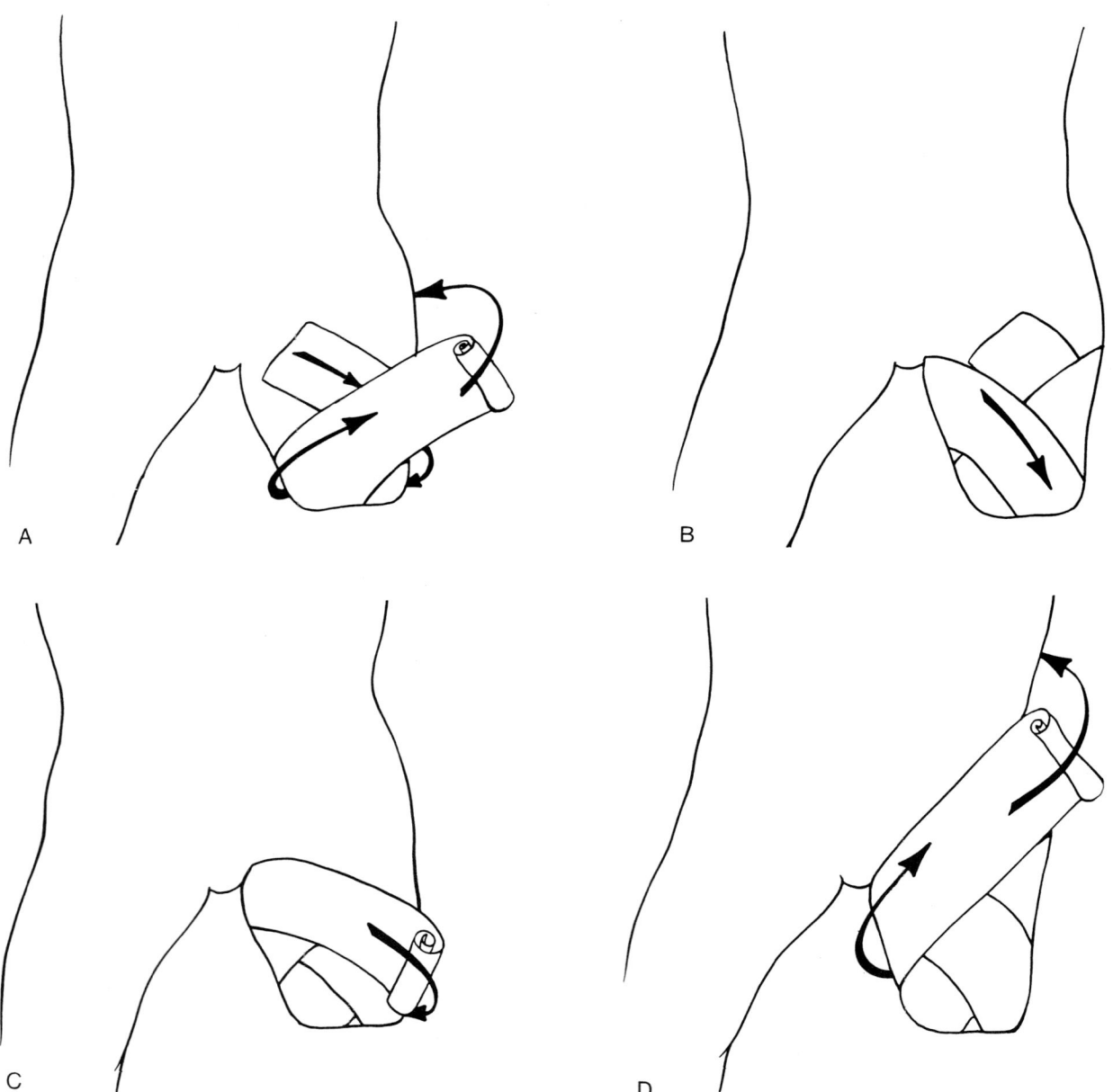

FIGURE 164–3. Elastic wrap procedure for transfemoral amputation. *A*, Start with the bandage in the groin area. Roll toward the outside, then behind and around the residual limb, covering the medial thigh. Keep the bandage smooth. Avoid wrinkles because they may cause skin irritations. *B*, Roll around the posterior residual limb. Continue down and around the lateral half of the distal end. *C*, Continue making diagonal turns around the residual limb until all skin is covered with at least two layers of bandage and firm pressure is obtained over the end. Avoid encircling the end with one turn because this tends to cause skin creases in the scar. Never use circular turns because this constricts circulation. Pressure should be greatest at the end, becoming lighter as you wrap toward the hip. Include all soft tissue on the medial thigh at the groin. *D*, Begin the hip spica as shown here. Place the bandage as high as possible on the medial thigh, and then cross it over the hip joint.

observed by the training therapist, and training on curbs, ramps, and stairs should be offered to maximize mobility. Most older persons have a fear of falling. Training in falling techniques and arising from a fall help to minimize the dangers and fear associated with falling. Exploration of the use of the prosthesis for driving, recreation, and vocational needs should also be part of this phase.

The amputee's perception of the prosthesis, its meaning to the quality of life, the effort needed to use it, and how closely it simulates the lost leg should be assessed. Often the artificial limb does not meet the fantasized expectations

of the amputee in regard to what a prosthesis should look like, what function it provides, and how it feels to walk with it compared with normal walking before the amputation.

This training phase is completed when the amputee achieves full use of the prosthesis.

Community Reintegration

Reentering society with an altered body image and a change in function is often an emotionally stressful time for an

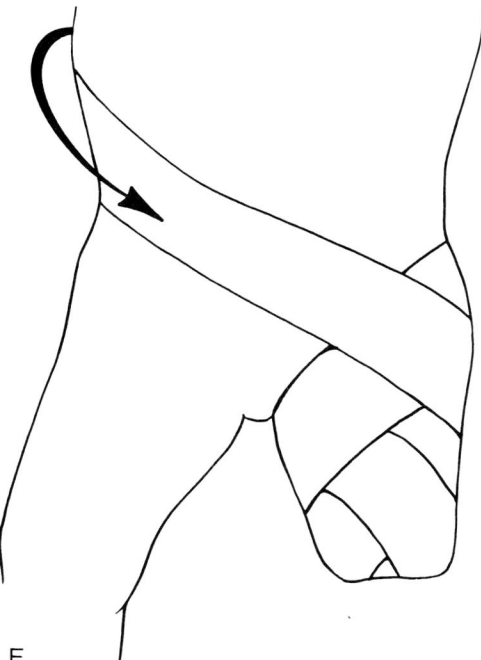

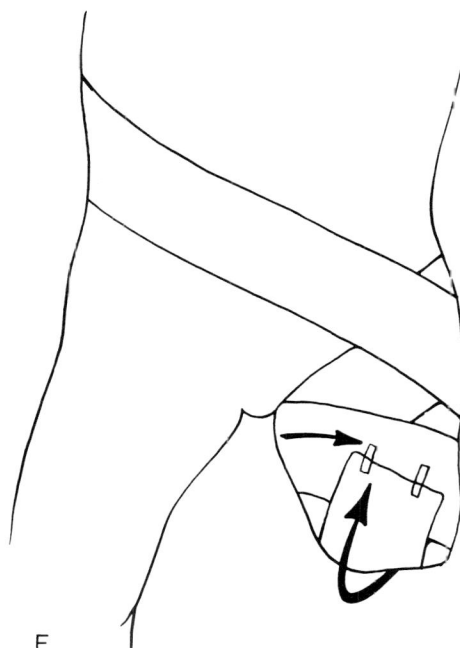

FIGURE 164–3 *Continued E*, Carry the bandage behind and around the pelvis, crossing just below the waist on the sound side. Returning to the amputated side, cross over the hip joint again. *F*, Finish the bandage by making diagonal turns around the end of the residual limb. Anchor the bandage with tape. Do not use safety pins. The bandage should not cause pain. If it does, remove it and rewrap. Rewrap the residual limb every 3 to 4 hours or more often if necessary. (From Karacoloff LA, Hammersley CS, and Schneider, FJ: Lower Extremity Amputation: A Guide to Functional Outcomes in Physical Therapy Management, 2nd ed. Gaithersburg, Md, Aspen Publishers, 1992, pp 17–18. © 1992, Aspen Publishers.)

amputee. Identification of a meaningful support structure in the community is one of the most important roles of the rehabilitation team. Often this is a time in an older amputee's life when changes in support systems are overwhelming. Spouse and friends are dying, living settings are changing, vocational life is winding down or has stopped, and the amputee may have fewer activities to enjoy and anticipate. Whenever possible, previous community supports need to be enlisted. On occasion, however, an extended care facility may provide the best environment in which the leg amputee can enhance prosthetic skills and proficiency in activities of daily living before returning to previous living conditions.

All aspects of a person's life should be addressed during this phase. The person's function in society, although changed, should be made as meaningful and satisfying as possible. This integrative model draws on all persons and resources in the community: spouse, family, merchants, employer, senior citizens' center, clergy, social workers, health professionals, municipal government, and the federal government working in concert to assist in restoring these persons to their rightful place in society. This phase of rehabilitation continues to influence the amputee for the remainder of his or her life.

Vocational Rehabilitation

Unfortunately, the vocational rehabilitation phase is often overlooked for the geriatric amputee. More and more today, individuals older than age 65 years find that continuing to work is an important part of their mature years. Despite

the loss of a limb, their dreams and plans should not be discouraged. They may still retain significant potential for full-time or part-time employment. A careful discussion of the patient's vocational plans should be included in the rehabilitation plan. Vocational services should be provided for the older amputee who has questions about future vocational options. In such cases, an understanding of the amputee's maximal prosthetic functional skills should help in proper vocational rehabilitation planning. For the younger person with a traumatic amputation, this is an essential part of amputee rehabilitation.

Functional Follow-up

Careful patient follow-up remains the single most important phase of amputee rehabilitation after hospital discharge. It is during this lifelong phase that attention to functional outcome, with or without a prosthesis, determines the quality of life achieved by the amputee.[12] Emphasis should not be placed on the prosthesis but, instead, on the ultimate functional capability of the amputee. The patient's emotional well-being and role in the family and community are continually assessed and are enhanced whenever possible by the rehabilitation team.

Follow-up visits to the physiatrist should be as frequent as visits to the internist or vascular surgeon. Any prosthetic fitting problem should receive prompt attention, and any decrease in the level of function should be investigated for its cause. Often, correction of the problem requires more than just a visit to the prosthetist, and the matter should be discussed with the rehabilitation team.

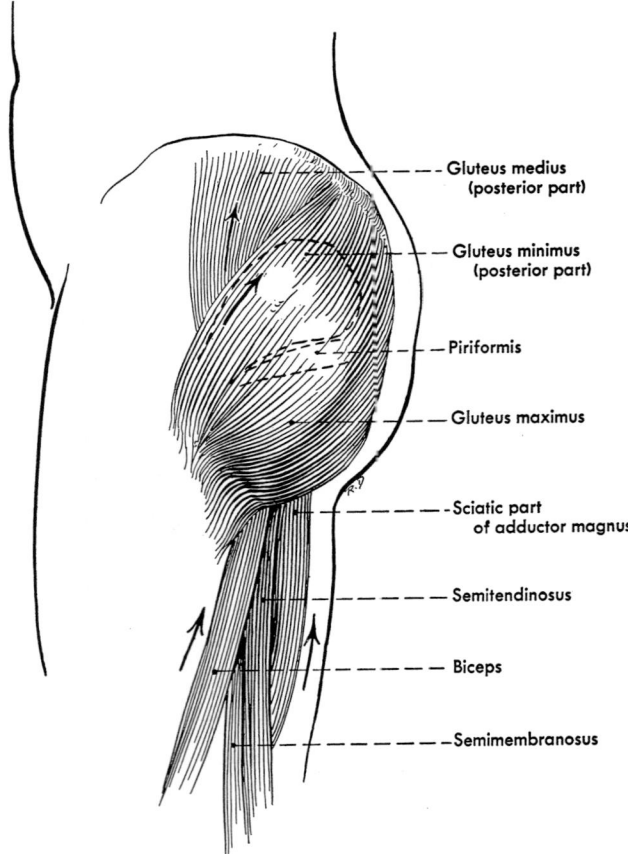

FIGURE 164–4. Extensor muscles of the thigh. (From Jenkins DB: Movements of the thigh and leg. *In* Hollinsheads Functional Anatomy of the Limbs and Back, 6th ed. Philadelphia, WB Saunders, 1991, p 272.)

Only with a comprehensive array of amputation rehabilitation services can the wide variety of amputee issues be dealt with thoroughly and in a coordinated fashion. This highly structured system provides health care to the amputee in the most efficient and cost-effective manner. Such a system produces the best functional outcome and quality of life after amputation.

PROSTHETIC COMPONENT OPTIONS AND PRESCRIPTION

The options for prosthetic restoration, in terms of socket design, interface materials, suspension designs, and components, have burgeoned in the past decade. It is not the author's intent to provide information on each of the new components available, but rather to give examples of contemporary prosthetic prescription and design for the common levels of lower extremity amputation. Also, prosthetic prescription practices are often regionally determined, and what seems to work well on the East Coast of the United States may not be what is in vogue on the West Coast.

Few data exist, however, to support the superiority of the new technology over that developed in the 1950s. Certainly, the cost-effectiveness of these more expensive designs has not been established. Nevertheless, subjective patient feedback does affirm that the newer designs provide better comfort and function.

Partial Foot

Usually, the portion of the foot missing is replaced with a molded toe filler approximately the size of the other foot. The toe filler is usually attached to an insole that slips into a Blucher shoe or athletic-type shoe that laces to hold the residual foot and insole with minimal shear at the skin-insole interface.[13] To achieve improved rollover and simulation of toe push-off, a rocker bar built into the shoe sole and a long steel or carbon graphite shank approximate a more anatomic gait.

In patients with hindfoot amputations, the prosthetic foot restoration can be attached to a molded plastic shell that crosses the ankle and extends up the lower leg (Fig. 164–6). This design provides functional ankle and hindfoot control and a larger surface over which to distribute the pressures.

Syme's Amputation

Two basic prosthetic designs are generally used for patients with Syme's amputation: (1) a windowed plastic shell and (2) an expandable inner lining. Both of these systems have outer walls of plastic laminated material that extend up to the knee region and may provide some patellar tendon weight bearing rather than allow loading of all the weight directly onto the end of the Syme heel pad. The windowed plastic shell permits the bulbous end of the residual limb to pass through the window into the end of the socket. The window is closed and held in place, providing a

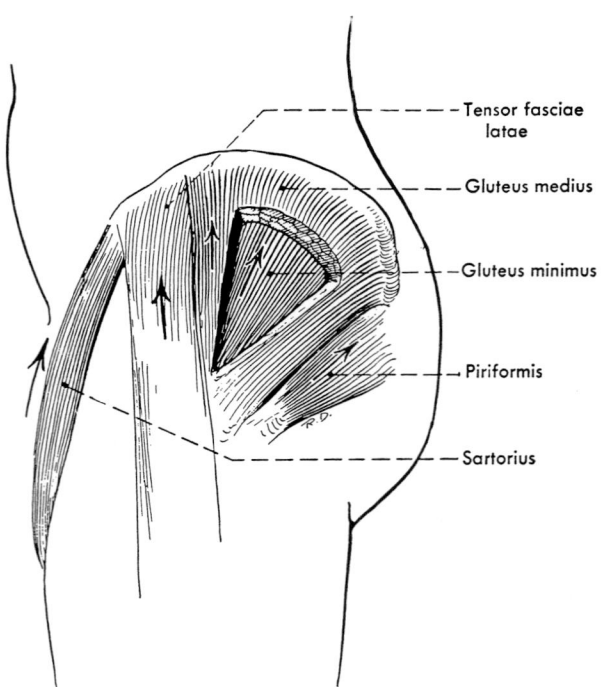

FIGURE 164–5. Abductor muscles of the thigh. (From Jenkins DB: Movements of the thigh and leg. *In* Hollinshead's Functional Anatomy of the Limbs and Back, 6th ed. Philadelphia, WB Saunders, 1991, p 273.)

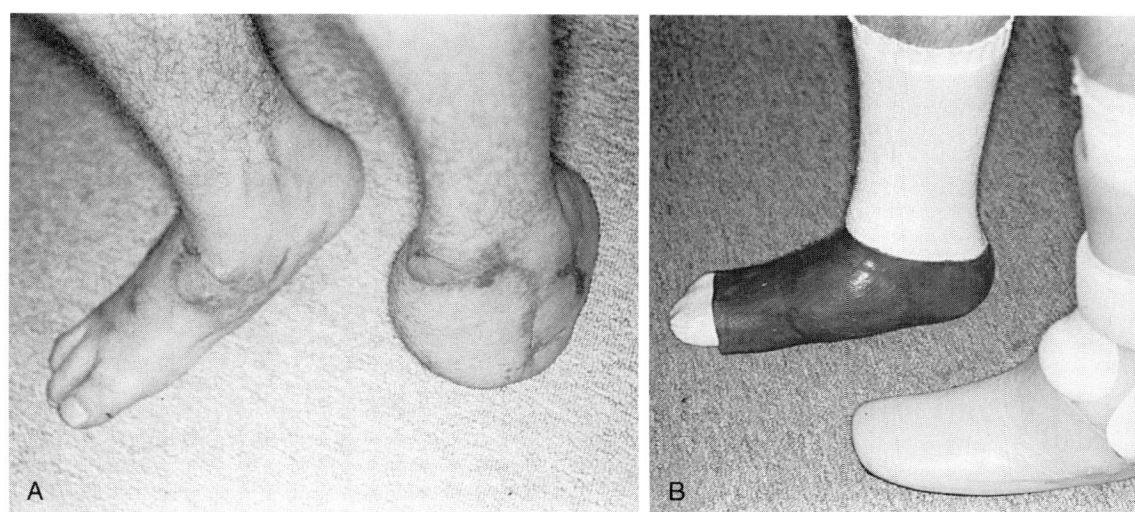

FIGURE 164–6 *A*, Left Lisfranc amputation. *B*, Bivalved hindfoot prosthesis extends above the ankle to stabilize the residual hindfoot in the prosthesis while one is wearing a shoe.

means of self-suspension. In the alternative suspension, the residual limb is placed through an inner distensible lining. The lining closes over the bulbous end, and the prosthesis is self-suspended. Although fewer prosthetic feet are available for this level of amputation, some do provide dynamically responsive features.

Transtibial Amputation

The traditional design developed for transtibial amputation became popular in the 1950s and has proved to be very durable. This design, the patellar-tendon-bearing (PTB) prosthesis, places weight-bearing pressures in pressure-tolerant areas while relieving pressure in pressure-intolerant areas.[14] In the past, this prosthesis was held in place with a supracondylar cuff and had a solid ankle cushion heel (SACH) foot attached. This remains a durable option, but newer systems have been designed.

Most commonly, an inner lining of cushioning material is placed on the residual limb and inserted into the plastic laminate socket. Today, an increasingly more popular way of suspending the socket makes use of an elasticized sleeve that fits around the outside of the prosthesis and is unrolled up onto the knee and thigh (Fig. 164–7). This sleeve does not appear to have an adverse effect on circulation to the skin or distal leg.

Another popular new system, referred to as the silicone suction socket,[35] uses a silicone or gel sleeve placed against the below-knee skin and then unrolled over the knee with a knurled pin that locks into the end of the prosthetic socket (Fig. 164–8). This is a self-suspending design that works much like a finger-trap.[15] Several gel or silicone sleeves have become available, each differing in material, thickness, durability, and color.

There are many prosthetic foot and ankle design options. Michael[16] and Esquenazi and Torres[17] have categorized them in a systematic way (Table 164–2). The dynamically responsive designs include the Seattle Lightfoot, the Flex-Foot, and the Carbon Copy (Fig. 164–9). A new design, called the Cirrus Foot, is a dynamically responsive foot in

which the responsiveness can be readily adjusted for the individual amputee (Fig. 164–10). These designs restore more normal foot and ankle dynamics and permit a greater amount of physical activity. Some designs also significantly

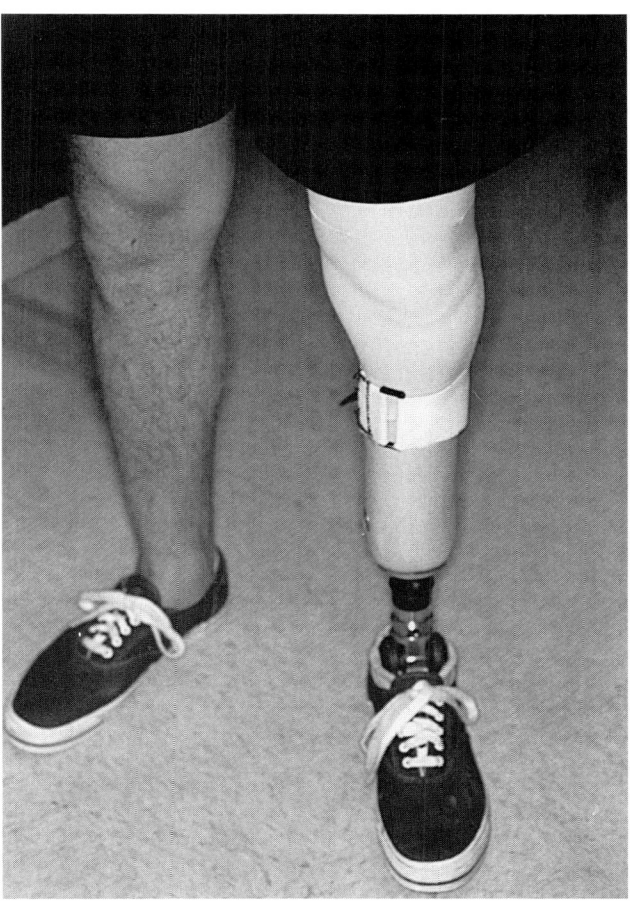

FIGURE 164–7. Transtibial below-knee (BK) amputee with patellar-tendon-bearing prosthesis utilizing elastic sleeve suspension.

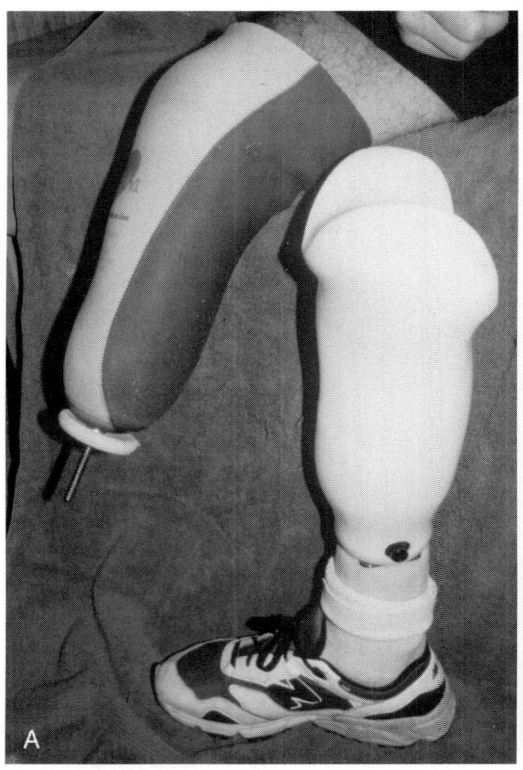
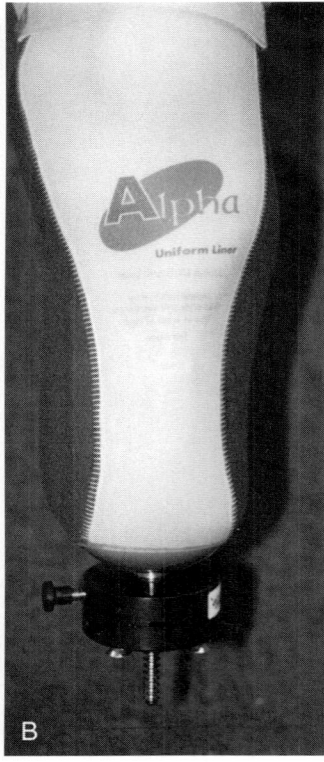

FIGURE 164–8. Components of Triple S system. *A,* Silicone suction socket (3S) suspension system for a patellar-tendon-bearing prosthesis. Gel sleeve is placed over the soft tissues of the residual limb. *B,* Distal pin locks into the distal end of the prosthetic socket.

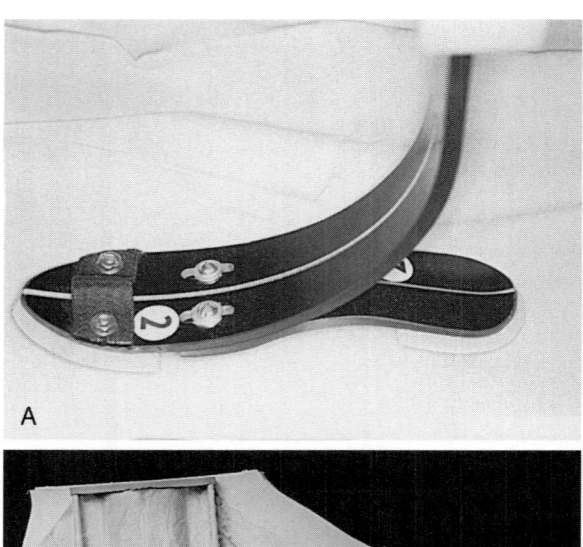
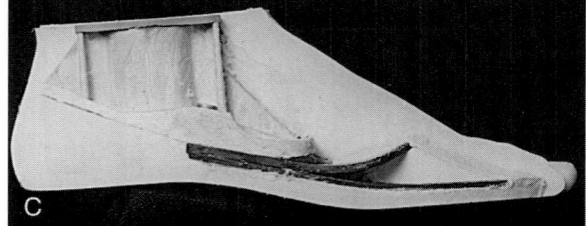
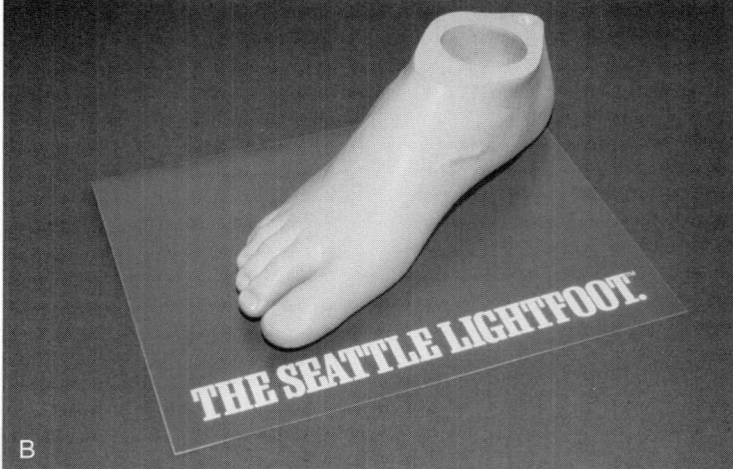

FIGURE 164–9. Dynamically responsive (energy-storing) feet. *A,* Modular III Flex-Foot. (Courtesy of Flex-Foot, Inc., Laguna Hills, Calif.) *B,* Seattle Lightfoot. (Courtesy of Model and Instrument Development Corp., Seattle.) *C,* Carbon Copy II. (Courtesy of The Ohio Willow Wood Co., Mount Sterling, Ohio.)

TABLE 164-2. RECOMMENDED FOOT-ANKLE SYSTEMS ACCORDING TO LEVEL OF AMPUTATION AND LEVEL OF ACTIVITY

	WEIGHT (gm)	BELOW-KNEE SEDENTARY	ABOVE-KNEE SEDENTARY	SYME'S SEDENTARY	BILATERAL SEDENTARY	BELOW-KNEE ACTIVE	ABOVE-KNEE ACTIVE	SYME'S ACTIVE	BILATERAL ACTIVE
Carbon Copy II	495	2	1	2	1	3	3	2	2
Carbon Copy III	900	2	NA	NA	0	3	NA	NA	3
Dynamic	550	1	1	NA	1	1	2	NA	1
Flex-Foot	900	0	0	NA	1	3	3	NA	2
Flex-Walk	550	1	1	NA	1	3	1	NA	3
Flex Syme's	900	NA	NA	1	NA	NA	NA	3	NA
Graph-Lite	600	1	2	NA	1	2	2	NA	2
Greissinger	850	1	1	NA	1	1	2	NA	1
Endolite with ankle	800	0	0	NA	1	1	2	NA	1
Multiflex	540	3	3	NA	3	2	2	NA	2
Quantum	540	2	2	2	2	1	1	1	1
RAX	425	2	1	NA	2	1	1	NA	1
Sabolich	500	0	0	NA	0	3	3	NA	2
S.A.F.E. I & II	750	1	1	2	1	2	1	3	2
Seattle Lightfoot with ankle	715	1	1	NA	1	2	1	NA	2
Seattle Lightfoot	470	3	3	2*	2	2	1	1*	2
Spring-Lite	900	0	0	NA	0	3	3	NA	2
STEN	685	1	0	NA	0	1	0	NA	1

From Esquenazi A, Torres MM: Prosthetic feet and ankle mechanisms. Phys Med Rehabil Clin North Am 2:299, 1991.
*To be used without ankle.
Key: 0, Not recommended; 1, good; 2, very good; 3, excellent.
NA, Not available.

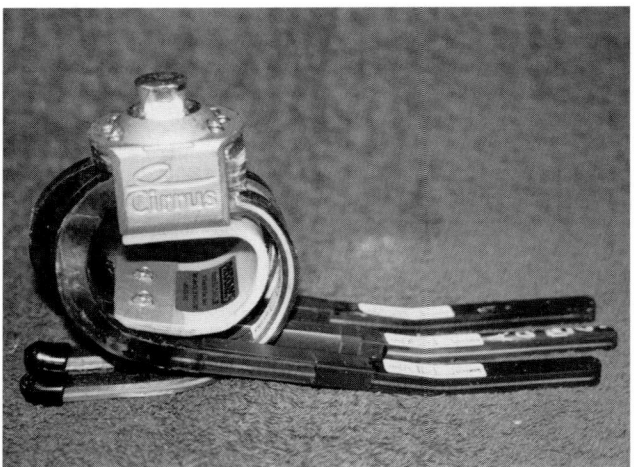

FIGURE 164–10. Cirrus Foot. A dynamically responsive foot with carbon graphite springs that can be interchanged provides more or less responsiveness, depending on the individual amputee's needs.

decrease the weight of the total prosthesis and therefore change the location of the center of mass of the prosthesis, which may cause less skin friction and decrease stump-socket interface forces.

Multiaxial foot designs, such as the Genesis Foot (Fig. 164–11), have become more commonplace as the weight has decreased and the durability of the foot design has increased. Often the amputee appreciates the more natural feel of the articulating ankle. In addition, the improved ability to achieve footflat position easily using an articulated ankle enhances knee stability during the early part of prosthetic stance. In addition, the resistance to dorsiflexion and

plantarflexion (i.e., stiffness) can be adjusted to produce the most desirable gait. These designs also improve the amputee's ability to walk on uneven terrain.

Socket design has been modified to place windows or cutouts in the pressure-sensitive areas, permitting tissue expansion into these windowed areas. Such a design is seen in the Icelandic–Swedish–New York University (ISNY) socket (Fig. 164–12).[18]

Knee Disarticulation

Knee disarticulation has become a more popular level of amputation because it provides an end weight-bearing surface for prosthetic use and a longer lever arm for prosthetic function.[37] A significant disadvantage for some knee disarticulation amputees is the wide appearance of the distal end of the thigh socket when a prosthesis is worn. This cosmetic appearance may not be acceptable to persons with slim thighs. The prosthetic prescription for this amputation level may provide a socket window that closes over the femoral condyle protrusions and is therefore self-suspending. Another form of suspension uses suction with an ischium-containing, narrow mediolateral socket. With the advent of the polycentric knee, knee components can be fitted close to the end of the thigh socket, and the cosmetic appearance of the prosthetic knee has been improved. The distal shin portion should usually be of endoskeletal components. A dynamically responsive foot completes this prescription.

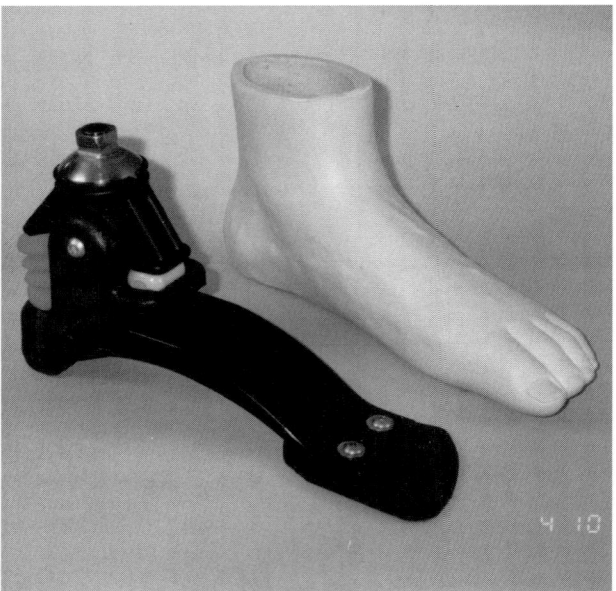

FIGURE 164–11. Genesis Foot. A multiaxial foot that provides more anatomic movement in both the medial-lateral and dorsiflexion-plantarflexion directions. The bumpers can be changed to provide more or less resistance to dorsiflexion and plantarflexion providing the best gait characteristics. This type of foot is especially accommodating on uneven terrain.

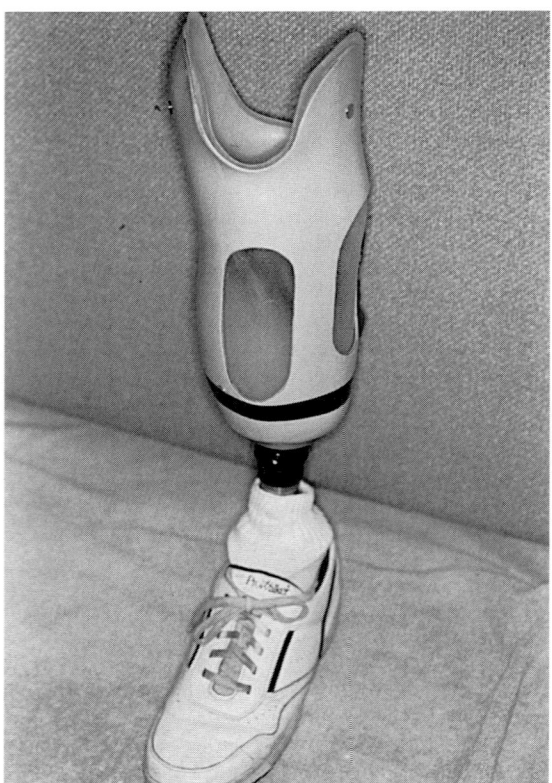

FIGURE 164–12. Patellar-tendon-bearing prosthesis of endoskeletal design showing the cut-out windows in the plastic laminate socket that are present in an Icelandic–Swedish–New York University design.

Transfemoral Amputation

Perhaps one of the most significant changes in prosthetic design for transfemoral amputees in the past few years has been the move away from quadrilateral above-knee sockets to the ischium-containing narrow mediolateral socket.[19, 20] This design, with its variety of fabrication methods, is meant to lock onto the pelvis by encompassing the ischial tuberosity and the inferior pubic ramus. The proximal brim of the socket extends higher on the residual limb and contains the lateral and posterior gluteal muscle masses (Fig. 164–13). This feature permits better stabilization of the superincumbent body over the prosthesis.

This socket design is also frequently fabricated with an ISNY design utilizing suction suspension (Fig. 164–14). In this device, a thermoplastic, vacuum-molded inner socket is formed from polypropylene or polyethylene. This socket can be applied without the traditional pull sock; instead, a skin lotion or gel is applied to the skin, and the residual limb is slipped into the suction socket with minimal effort. A total elastic suspension (TES) belt, which is flexible and encircles the waist, can be used for supplemental suspension (Fig. 164–15).

Positioning the femur in the socket has become a point of controversy, but it is generally agreed that the femur should be kept in as normal anatomic adduction as possible.[21] This femoral alignment permits better hip abductor muscle mechanics, which enhance pelvic stability and allow more normal gait. Gottschalk[22] has discussed the surgical handling of the adductor muscles during transfemoral amputation (see Chapter 163).

Most geriatric amputees prefer a lighter-weight prosthesis. The weight of the finished prosthesis can be decreased with use of an endoskeletal design. The supporting skeletal structure is fabricated from aluminum, titanium, or carbon-graphite pylons and couplings (Fig. 164–16). In addition, some of the dynamically responsive feet and newer knee units can help to decrease the total prosthetic weight so that a current above-knee prosthesis should weigh between 6 and 8 pounds.

Michael[38] has suggested a paradigm for selecting the most appropriate knee unit (Table 164–3). He separates the many knee units available today into five functional categories:

- Constant friction
- Stance control
- Polycentric (Fig. 164–17)
- Manual locking
- Fluid controlled

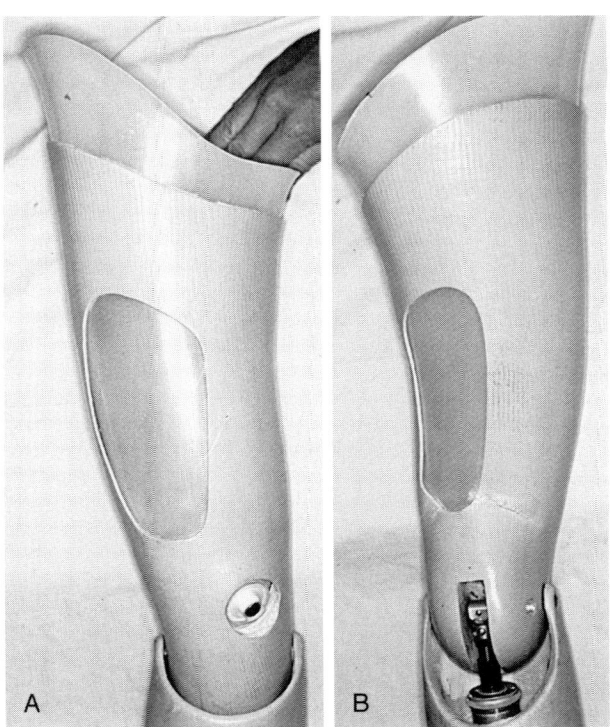

FIGURE 164–14. *A,* Anterior view. Transfemoral prosthesis with an Icelandic–Swedish–New York University socket design and suction suspension. *B,* Posterior view.

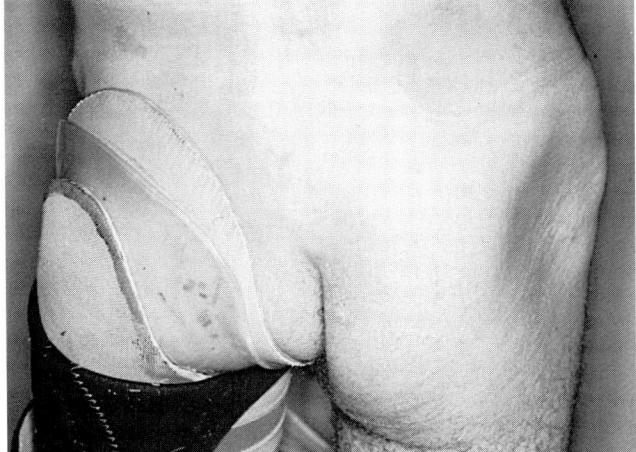

FIGURE 164–13. Posterior aspect of a transfemoral amputee with an ischial containment socket. The socket includes portions of the gluteus medius and maximus muscles.

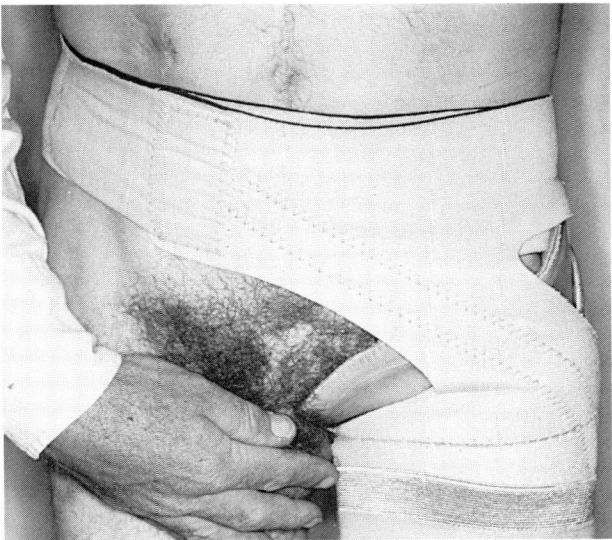

FIGURE 164–15. Total elastic suspension (TES) system for suspension of a transfemoral prosthesis.

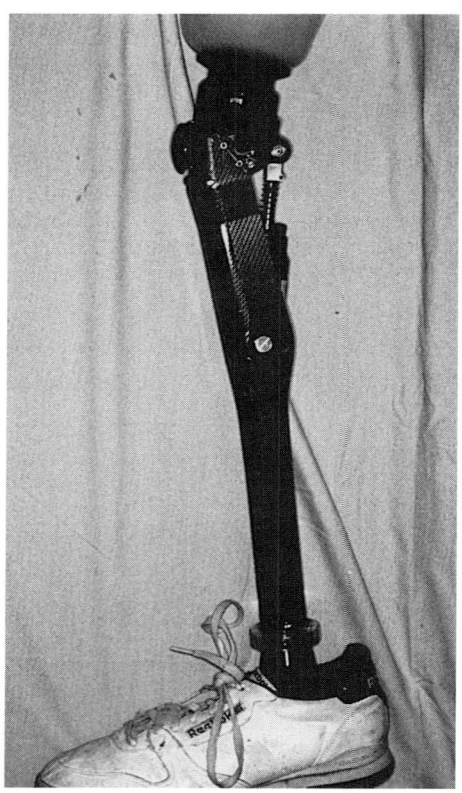

FIGURE 164–16. Endoskeletal (Endolite) device is made of carbon graphite material to decrease the final weight of the prosthesis.

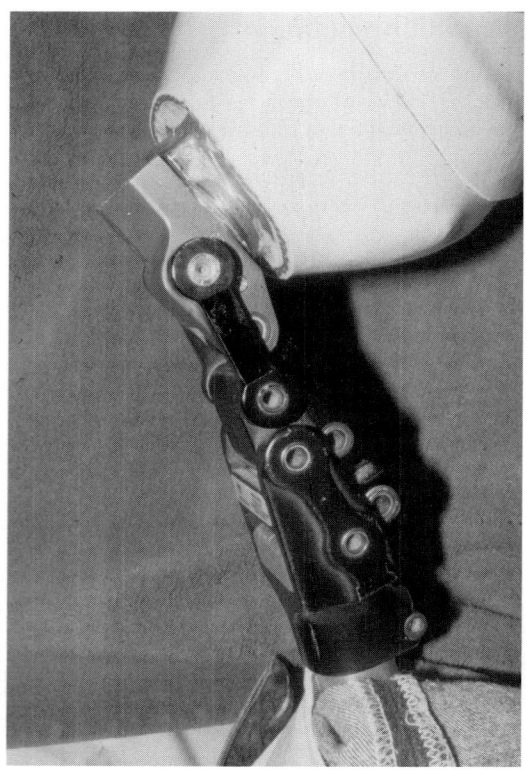

FIGURE 164–17. Polycentric knee mechanism (Total Knee) with multibar linkages characterized by multiple centers of knee rotation as the knee flexes. This knee offers excellent stance stability and ease of swing phase flexion.

Safety knee (stance controlled) units are often prescribed for geriatric patients to provide a friction brake for added knee stability in the extended position. Hydraulic knee mechanisms (fluid control) can also be used in prostheses for the active dysvascular patient to achieve a more cosmetic gait when velocity of walking is changed. Locking knee units should be avoided, as a rule. If the amputee cannot control a knee mechanism that is not locked, he or she will generally not have much functional use of the prosthesis. Rather than providing a locked knee prosthesis, the rehabilitation team should emphasize improvement of

TABLE 164–3. CLASSIFICATION OF PROSTHETIC KNEE MECHANISMS

FUNCTIONAL CLASS	GENERAL INDICATIONS	ADVANTAGES	DISADVANTAGES
Constant friction CF ("Single axis")	Single speed walking on level surfaces, provided hip control is good	Inexpensive Reliable	Low stability Fixed cadence
Stance control SC ("Safety")	Geriatric Short RL General debility Uneven surfaces	Improved knee stability	Slightly increased weight, cost, maintenance Must unload fully to flex
Polycentric PC ("Four Bar")	Same as stance control Knee disarticulation	Excellent knee stability Cosmesis for disarticulations, very long RL	Greater weight, cost, maintenance
Manual locking ML ("Lock")	Knee of last resort	Ultimate knee stability	Abnormal gait Awkward sitting
Fluid controlled FC ("Pneumatic" = light duty) ("Hydraulic" = heavy duty)	Active walkers	Variable cadence Smoothest gait Sophisticated stability (Mauch SNS only)	Greatest weight, cost, maintenance

Reproduced in part from Michael JW: Prosthetic knee mechanisms. Phys Med Rehabil State Art Rev 8:147, 1994. Courtesy of Hanley & Belfus, Philadelphia.
RL = residual limb; SNS = Swing-N-Stance.

the strength and the endurance of the hip extensor muscles, including the gluteus maximus and the residual hamstring muscles. Prosthetic training then focuses on prosthetic knee stability during stance on the prosthesis. A rotator unit that permits rotation of the prosthetic socket on the distal components should also be considered for patients who play golf or participate in other outdoor activities requiring rotational movement.

Hip Disarticulation

Geriatric dysvascular amputees can rarely tolerate the high energy expenditure required to use a prosthesis for hip disarticulation. Certainly, if a prosthesis is considered, an endoskeletal design is preferable. The lightest components must be employed to minimize the total weight of the final design.

ENERGY EXPENDITURE WITH PROSTHETIC AMBULATION

Several investigators have discussed the energy costs of prosthetic use and have compared these costs in younger, traumatically injured amputees with those in the older, dysvascular amputee population (Table 164–4).[23, 24] From these studies, it is apparent that every effort should be made to salvage the knee joint, because it may make the difference between an amputee who successfully walks with a prosthesis and one who is wheelchair-bound. The transtibial amputee walking with a prosthesis requires 25% to 40% more energy than normal walking. In contrast, the above-knee amputee walking with a prosthesis requires 65% to 100% more energy expenditure than normal. Wheelchair use on level surfaces requires an energy expenditure 8% greater than normal. Thus, many dysvascular amputees with cardiopulmonary disease are unable to sustain the increased energy demands of ambulating with a prosthesis. Instead, they choose to be sedentary and to get around with a wheelchair. A slower speed of ambulation with a prosthesis puts less demand on cardiopulmonary

reserves. Nonetheless, even amputees with limited cardiopulmonary function benefit from prosthetic restoration for transfers and short distance ambulation, especially for toilet and hygiene activities.

FUNCTIONAL OUTCOMES FOR THE PERSON WITH A LEG AMPUTATION

In today's health care environment, increased emphasis is placed on comparing the benefits and cost of health care measures. Rehabilitation professionals have begun to assess carefully the outcomes achieved for a number of specific disabilities. No uniform, nationally applied measures have been developed as yet for the lower limb amputee, with or without prosthetic restoration. Granger and Hamilton[39] have developed the Functional Independence Measure (FIM). However, this rating system is most appropriately applied to individuals with central nervous system disabilities. Other published amputee outcome scoring systems do not provide uniform measurements and usually do not assess the psychosocial outcomes.

Moore and colleagues[40] have reported that in transtibial amputees of all ages, two thirds achieved functional prosthetic ambulation even though 48% had coronary artery disease. There was no statistically significant relationship between sex, diabetes mellitus, pulmonary disease, or musculoskeletal disease and prosthetic ambulation in the 157 major lower extremity amputees in this study. Only 46% of the patients with transfemoral amputation were successful in prosthetic ambulation. Only one fifth of 27 patients with bilateral lower extremity amputation were ambulatory.

Walker and associates,[41] in the United Kingdom, reported that 71% of transtibial amputees responding to a questionnaire could regularly walk from about one quarter of a mile to more than a mile.[41] Surprisingly, 84% of transfemoral amputees could walk with their prostheses for this same distance. In this study, 42% of respondents with transtibial amputations and 15.4% of those with transfemoral amputations ceased all sporting activity after their amputations.

TABLE 164–4. ENERGY EXPENDITURE: UNILATERAL AMPUTEES

AMPUTEES	SPEED (m/min)	O₂ RATE (ml/kg · min)	O₂ COST (ml/kg · m)	PULSE (beats/min)
Vascular				
TF	36	10.8	0.28	126
TT	45	9.4	0.20	105
AD	54	9.2	0.17	108
Surgical				
TP	40	11.5	0.29	97
HD	47	11.1	0.24	99
Traumatic				
TF	52	10.3	0.20	111
KD	61	13.4	0.23	109
TT	71	12.4	0.16	106

From Waters RL: The energy expenditure of amputee gait. In Bowker JH, Michael JW (eds): Atlas of Limb Prosthetics: Surgical, Prosthetic, & Rehabilitation Principles, 2nd ed. St. Louis, Mosby–Year Book, 1992, p 385; data from Nowroozi F, Salvanelli ML, Gerber LH: Energy expenditure in hip disarticulation and hemipelvectomy amputees. Arch Phys Med Rehabil 64:300–303, 1983; and Waters RL, Perry J, Antonelli D, et al: The energy cost of walking of amputees—influence of level of amputation. J Bone Joint Surg 58A:42–46, 1976.

TF = transfemoral; TT, transtibial; AD = ankle disarticulation; TP = transpelvic; HD = hip disarticulation; KD = knee disarticulation.

Smith and coworkers[42] reported the SF-36 Health Status Profile on 20 traumatic transtibial amputees with a mean age of 36 years. The 36-Item Short Form (SF-36) scores were significantly decreased in the categories of physical function and role limitations due to physical health problems and pain. However, there were no significant differences from published normal age-matched scores in the areas of role limitations due to emotional problems, social function, mental health, energy versus fatigue, and health perception.

Volpicelli and Evans and their colleagues[43, 44] have evaluated the function of bilateral lower limb amputees. They found that successful ambulation is more likely if both amputations are at the transtibial level (80%) than if one amputation is transtibial and the other transfemoral (24%). Few patients with bilateral transfemoral amputations (5%) achieve ambulatory status.

Tables 164–5 and 164–6 are empirical "checklists" of ideal functional outcomes for unilateral transtibial and transfemoral prostheses, respectively. These checklists can be used by the rehabilitation team and prosthetic training therapist to set goals for transtibial and transfemoral amputees. If an amputee does not achieve a specific function on the checklist, the team should decide whether it is a realistic rehabilitation target for the patient or whether co-morbid factors prohibit its achievement.

Outcome studies for the person with an amputation must consider more than the functional use of the prosthesis. They must also assess emotional well-being and quality of life.[46]

Additional prospective national multicenter outcome studies for the lower limb amputee must be undertaken if we are to learn the most efficient way to deliver health care to the person who undergoes an amputation. Moreover, to better determine the cost-effectiveness of the variety of prosthetic designs and rehabilitation programs, we must have standardized outcome parameters for the amputee. These studies will be essential for scientific comparison of the costs of amputation and limb salvage (see Chapter 166).

TABLE 164–5. FUNCTIONAL OUTCOMES FOR TRANSTIBIAL PROSTHETIC USE

1. Ambulates with prosthesis on level and uneven surfaces, stairs, ramps, and curbs
2. Ambulates with minimal or no gait aids
3. Independent with dressing
4. Independent in donning and doffing prosthesis
5. Independent in stump wrapping or applying a shrinker
6. Able to drive
7. Can participate in shopping activities
8. Has returned to previous work, with or without modifications
9. Can stand for up to 2 continuous hours
10. Can sit for up to 2 continuous hours
11. Can arise from the kneeling position
12. Comfortable with falling techniques and can arise from the floor
13. Can hunt, fish, run, bicycle (if part of previous lifestyle)
14. Knows how to purchase properly fitting footwear for the remaining foot
15. Knows proper skin and nail care for remaining foot
16. Can safely perform aerobic conditioning program
17. Climbs stairs foot over foot

From Leonard JA, Meier RH: Upper and lower extremity prosthetics. *In* Delisa JA, Gans BM (eds): Rehabilitation Medicine: Principles and Practice, 3rd ed. Philadelphia, Lippincott-Raven, 1998, p 692.

TABLE 164–6. FUNCTIONAL OUTCOMES FOR TRANSFEMORAL PROSTHETIC USE

1. Ambulates with prosthesis on level and uneven surfaces, stairs, ramps, and curbs
2. Ambulates with minimal or no gait aids
3. Independent with dressing
4. Independent in donning and doffing prosthesis
5. Independent in stump wrapping or applying a shrinker
6. Able to drive
7. Can participate in shopping activities
8. Has returned to previous work, with or without modifications
9. Can stand for up to 2 continuous hours
10. Can sit for up to 2 continuous hours
11. Can arise from the kneeling position
12. Comfortable with falling techniques and can arise from the floor
13. Can hunt, fish, run, bicycle (if part of previous lifestyle)
14. Knows how to purchase properly fitting footwear for the remaining foot
15. Knows proper skin and nail care for remaining foot
16. Can safely perform aerobic conditioning program
17. Stairs are generally climbed one at a time
18. Can run (if amputee desires, has adequate cardiopulmonary reserve and residual limb length)
19. Uses no more than a cane for ambulation

From Leonard JA, Meier RH: Upper and lower extremity prosthetics. *In* Delisa JA, Gans BM (eds): Rehabilitation Medicine: Principles and Practice, 3rd ed. Philadelphia, Lippincott-Raven Publishers, 1998, p 692.

The younger traumatic amputee is often differentiated from the more elderly dysvascular amputee in functional studies. To some extent, this is an example of ageism in our society. Whereas the older amputee may have more comorbid factors that can influence prosthetic use, it should not be assumed that such a patient will be unsuccessful. Studies in the geriatric population have shown that appropriate muscle training can produce improved strength and endurance.[47, 48] Geriatric amputees should routinely participate in an exercise program that increases both muscle strength and aerobic conditioning. If they are unable to tolerate this type of program, the likelihood of successful prosthetic use is low.

In a study of 116 lower extremity amputees older than 65 years of age, Steinberg and colleagues[49] found that 98% of subjects fitted with transtibial prostheses used their prostheses for meaningful function. Of those fitted with transfemoral prostheses, 64% had achieved meaningful function. Age alone was not a major determining factor in the failure or success of prosthetic rehabilitation; rather, failures were related to concurrent medical illnesses or mental deterioration. Leonard[50] reported that prosthetic success in some geriatric individuals may be limited to the use of the prosthesis for activities such as transferring. Esquenazi[51] and Andrews[52] have provided excellent reviews of the issues encountered with the geriatric leg amputee.

Partial Foot Amputation

With a prosthetic toe filler, most partial foot or transmetatarsal amputees should be able to ambulate around the living quarters on both level surfaces and stairs. They can also negotiate uneven terrain, curbs, and ramps. They may have a shortened stride from the affected foot onto the normal foot and have difficulty jogging and participating in some sports-related activities.

Syme's Amputation

With good prosthetic restoration, persons with Syme's amputation should be quite functional in most if not all activities in which they participated prior to the amputation. They may be able to do even *more* than they could before the amputation if the dysvascular leg prevented them from actively walking and functioning on two legs.

Transtibial Amputation

With 10 to 18 cm of leg remaining below the medial tibial plateau, adequate soft tissue, and a well-placed scar, the transtibial amputee should be very functional in almost any desired activity that is tolerated by the heart, lungs, other leg, and muscles. The amputee should be encouraged to lead a very active and "normal" life (see Table 164–5).

Knee Disarticulation

The long femoral lever arm provided by knee disarticulation permits excellent powering of the prosthesis but does require more energy than that needed for a prosthesis with amputation at the transtibial level or below. If the patient has good cardiopulmonary reserve and the other leg is strong, he or she should be functional on all surfaces and can enjoy many recreational opportunities.

Transfemoral Amputation

Functional expectations after transfemoral amputation vary according to residual limb length and the cardiopulmonary condition of the amputee. With a mid-thigh or longer residual femoral lever arm and a well-fitted prosthesis, the amputee should be able to perform all ambulatory activities, including negotiation of stairs, ramps, curbs, and uneven terrain (see Table 164–6). Athletic endeavors of all types may be possible, such as running, golf, baseball, hunting, and fishing.

With a shorter residual limb or significant cardiopulmonary compromise, however, even ambulation on a level surface may be compromised. Transfer activities and short distance ambulation may be all that are possible. The use of a walker, crutches, or cane may also be important adjuncts for safe ambulation. The combination of a prosthesis and a wheelchair may provide the most functional combination for household and community activities.

Hip Disarticulation

Prosthetic restoration for hip disarticulation is best accomplished in the younger, previously active person who has no significant cardiopulmonary problems. Even the most physically fit person may find the energy expenditure and discomfort of wearing the prosthesis excessive. Many such amputees find that walking with crutches or using a wheelchair may be preferable to the slow gait achieved with a hip disarticulation prosthesis.

Bilateral Amputations

Various combinations of bilateral leg amputations permit different functional abilities. Loss of portions of both feet shortens the stride length but generally does not limit activities other than running. Bilateral Syme's amputations present minimal functional limitation. Walking with bilateral transtibial prostheses increases the energy expenditure needed to more than 40% above normal but yields good functional results. As previously mentioned, however, a combination of transtibial and transfemoral amputations is severely limiting for older amputees (Table 164–7). Bilateral transfemoral amputations are catastrophic for successful function. Even a healthy young amputee finds this combination excessively difficult to utilize for walking. For almost all bilateral transfemoral amputees, the wheelchair becomes the most practical method of achieving mobility.

Activities

Recreational activities should be explored for every person who undergoes an amputation.[25] After satisfactory prosthetic restoration, the patient can resume many preamputation leisure activities, including swimming, golf, tennis, dancing, hunting, fishing, and running.

Another area of functional concern is the amputee's ability to drive an automobile. Driving should be possible for below-knee and above-knee amputees without a major alteration of the automobile, although it is always advisable for the vehicle to have an automatic transmission. Driver evaluation and driver training, when indicated, may be necessary. When the remaining foot is the left one, a left-footed accelerator can be useful.

A total body conditioning program should be initiated to enhance cardiopulmonary function and endurance. A variety of exercise equipment can be utilized, but the author has found the Versaclimber to be especially adaptable to the lower limb amputee (Fig. 164–18).

GAIT TRAINING WITH A LEG PROSTHESIS

The requirements for fulfilling functional prosthetic expectations include a rigorous preprosthetic training program to prepare the entire body for the increased energy expenditure imposed by use of the prosthesis.[9–11] The elements of such a program are:

1. Strengthening of the upper body and trunk.
2. Strengthening of the remaining lower extremity.
3. Stretching of any lower extremity joint that does not have full range of motion.
4. Specific programs aimed at increasing the strength and endurance of the hip extensors and abductors bilaterally.
5. Increasing the strength of the remaining knee extensors.
6. Cardiovascular conditioning (usually requiring upper arm ergometry).

Once these preprosthetic goals have been achieved, the prosthesis is fabricated and early prosthetic gait training is initiated. Certain therapeutic guidelines must be followed, including careful attention to the details of gait to decrease energy requirements and enhance function. Gait training should emphasize:

TABLE 164–7. ENERGY EXPENDITURE IN BILATERAL AMPUTEES

AMPUTEES	SPEED (m/min)	O₂ RATE (ml/kg · min)	O₂ COST (ml/kg · m)	PULSE (beats/min)
Traumatic				
TT/TT*	67	13.6	0.20	112
TF/TF*	54	17.6	0.33	104
Vascular				
AD/AD*	62	12.8	0.21	99
TT/TT*	40	11.6	0.31	113
Stubbies†	46	9.9	0.22	86

From Waters RL: The energy expenditure of amputee gait. *In* Bowker JH, Michael JW (eds): Atlas of Limb Prosthetics: Surgical, Prosthetic, and Rehabilitation Principles, 2nd ed. St. Louis, Mosby–Year Book, 1992, p 386.

*Data from Waters RL, Perry J, Chambers R: Energy expenditure of amputee gait. *In* Moore WS, Malone JM (eds): Lower Extremity Amputation. Philadelphia, WB Saunders CO, 1989, pp 250–260.

†Data from Wainapel SF, March H, Steve L: Stubby prostheses: An alternative to conventional prosthetic devices. Arch Phys Med Rehabil 66:264–266, 1985.

TT = transtibial; TF = transfemoral; AD = ankle disarticulation.

1. Equal stride length.
2. Active hip extension to provide knee stability, especially at heel strike.
3. Encouraging a pattern of heel strike to footflat rather than one that initiates stance with a footflat position.
4. Stance phase training to load the prosthetic toe during pushoff.
5. Discouragement of significant lateral trunk bending (Fig. 164–19).
6. Balance training.
7. Withdrawal of the wheelchair and gait aids at the appropriate time to enhance reliance on and use of the prosthesis.

Unfortunately, we are experiencing a shortage of thera-

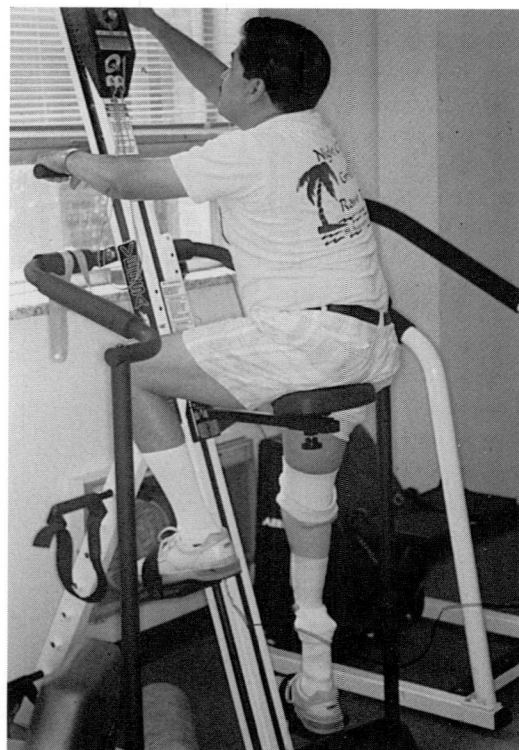

FIGURE 164–18. Versaclimber equipment can be used for cardiopulmonary conditioning for the transtibial or transfemoral amputee.

pists who are educated in training techniques to maximize the functions of contemporary prosthetics. There is also a decrease in the quantity of therapy that will be sponsored by third-party payers for prosthetic training. These two limitations in access to the quality and quantity of prosthetic training may lead to a national decrease in prosthetic function after lower extremity prosthetic restoration.

VOCATIONAL FUNCTION

Loss of a limb does not necessarily signal the end of a productive vocational life. Most below-knee amputees can return to their previous employment. A transfemoral amputee who has a job requiring prolonged standing, walking on uneven surfaces, or climbing ladders may need to consider alternative employment. Such a person may also benefit from vocational rehabilitation if the preamputation job is not feasible. It is often useful for the therapist to visit the worksite and make suggestions for worksite modifications to enhance the amputee's safety and function.

PREVENTIVE CARE OF THE REMAINING LIMB

Every effort must be made to protect the remaining foot and leg from the need for amputation. Perhaps the single most important preventive measure is the use of proper footwear. The author normally recommends careful fitting of appropriately sized shoes, which provide even pressure distribution over the plantar aspect of the foot. Shock-absorbing systems should be used through the addition of insoles that conform to the plantar contours. An alternative is the use of athletic-type shoes that have an air or gel cushion built into the forefoot and the heel. When significant edema is present, the use of compressive stockings providing 30 to 40 mmHg of pressure is helpful. The patient should be instructed in the proper care of calluses and toenails.

EMOTIONAL ADAPTATION TO LIMB LOSS

The process of emotional adaptation to an amputation is an individual one that follows a variable course.[27] Many

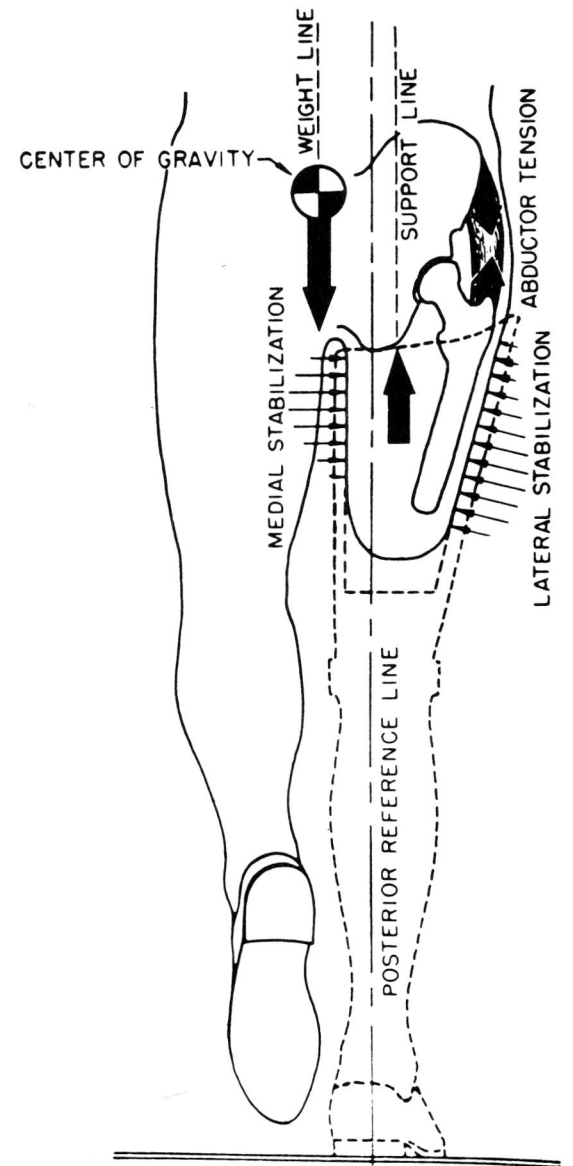

FIGURE 164–19. Use of hip abductors for lateral stabilization of the pelvis can be achieved only by providing adequate lateral support to the femur. (From Radcliff CW: Biomechanics of prosthetic use. Artif Limbs 2:38, 1955. Courtesy of the National Academy of Sciences, Washington, DC.)

persons experience a period of grieving as for the death of a close family member. This emotional process can be supported through open discussion of the amputee's feelings of body loss, the presence of pain, anxiety, concern about the loss of control, uncertainty about the future, and frustration with the condition that caused the change in body image. Any rehabilitation team member may lend an ear and support, but it is desirable for team members experienced in psychosocial services to be available to counsel the patient and the family; ideally, these members are a psychologist, a social worker, and a pastoral counselor.

Emotional adaptation to amputation may proceed at varying rates. This is a time for amputees to be open about

their feelings and concerns with the members of both their immediate support system and the rehabilitation team. Acknowledgment of feelings of loss, anxiety, and depression is often helpful in dealing with this difficult event. The adaptive process and the way in which the emotional needs of the amputee are met are among the most important aspects of amputee rehabilitation. The rehabilitation team should enhance the amputee's sense of empowerment.[53]

COMPLICATIONS OF WEARING A PROSTHESIS

Many complications of prosthesis use are related to the presence of excessive pressure at the stump-socket interface that produces redness, blistering, and ulceration. Shear forces resulting from pistoning of the residual limb against the wall of the socket frequently cause these skin problems. Common areas of skin trauma are near the fibular head, at the anterior distal tibia (kick point), at the proximal medial and lateral tibial flares, and at points of scar that meet normal soft tissue. In addition, hair follicles become plugged, and as they build up bacteria folliculitis develops.[28] This process may progress to involve the pilosebaceous apparatus, forming an infected sebaceous cyst. The skin of the residual limb may become sensitive to the materials used in the prosthesis or the substances used to clean the socket.

Superficial infections usually respond to administration of antibiotics, whereas an infected sebaceous cyst requires incision, drainage, and excision. For allergic dermatitis, use of the prosthesis should be discontinued and topical steroids applied. Painful redness, blisters, or ulcerations also require discontinuation of prosthesis use until the proper adjustments can be made by the prosthetist. On occasion, the addition or removal of stump socks can help to alleviate the excessive pressure. Changes in size and shape of the residual limb can also cause frequent fitting problems. These changes require the addition or deletion of stump socks or modifications in the prosthetic socket.

PAIN IN THE AMPUTEE

Phantom limb sensation, phantom limb pain, and residual limb pain must be differentiated to be understood by the amputee and to determine the best modalities for treatment.

Phantom Limb Sensation

Phantom limb sensation occurs in almost everyone with an acquired amputation and does not usually require treatment. It is usually no more than a minor annoyance and on occasion may be useful during the phase of prosthetic training. It is felt most strongly in the immediate postoperative period and normally decreases in intensity but may continue throughout life.

Phantom Limb Pain

Phantom limb pain begins in the acute postamputation period, generally subsides, and is seldom a long-term problem. In a few amputees, however, phantom limb pain results in a chronic pain syndrome that may be refractory to treatment. Such pain may alter lifestyle and become the focus of the patient's existence.

Treatment methods are numerous and have produced inconsistent success.[29, 30] During the immediate postoperative period, it is essential that the new amputee be pain-free for a period of 72 to 96 hours to decrease the potential for development of problematic phantom pain. The use of narcotics, synthetic narcotics, or other addictive substances is contraindicated after the immediate postoperative phase. Other modalities commonly used to diminish this pain are (1) transcutaneous electrical nerve stimulation (TENS), (2) percussion, (3) vibration, (4) massage, (5) acupuncture, (6) biofeedback, (7) hypnosis, and (8) relaxation techniques. Regional neurologic blockade has had some success, especially if sympathetic nervous tone appears to be a significant part of the pain; injection near or into a neuroma is useful. More invasive procedures for pain control are sympathectomy, neuroma excision, dorsal root entry zone rhizotomy, epidural spinal cord stimulation, and sensory thalamic stimulation.[54]

Medications currently available to diminish phantom limb pain are (1) analgesics, (2) neuroleptics, (3) anticonvulsants, (4) tricyclic antidepressants, (5) beta-blockers, (6) sodium channel blockers, and (7) baclofen. These medications should be tried in an orderly fashion; for problematic phantom limb pain, they should be used in the maximally tolerated doses. Combination therapy is often necessary for optimal pain relief.

Residual Limb Pain

Residual limb pain is defined as pain in the remaining part of the limb that does not descend into the "phantom." This pain may be caused by neuroma formation or physical changes in the residual limb. A common cause is the pressure caused by an ill-fitting prosthesis, and prosthetic modification often alleviates this type of pain. If the pain seems to be related to a neuroma, local infiltration with anesthesia with or without steroids may improve it. Local resection of the neuroma or relocation of the terminal end of the nerve deeper into the residual limb may improve the symptoms.

BONE LENGTHENING AND SOFT TISSUE COVERAGE

Very short transtibial and transfemoral residual limbs should now be considered for lengthening techniques that use a free bone graft or an Ilizarov procedure. These reconstructive operations can add significant length, providing a longer lever arm to power the prosthesis. Inadequate soft tissue coverage or significant scarring can be removed and replaced with a full-thickness skin graft or a myocutaneous flap.[31] The provision of scar-free skin and full-thickness subcutaneous tissues can greatly improve prosthetic function. Occasionally, these procedures should be considered before prosthetic fitting is attempted.

UPPER LIMB AMPUTATION AND PROSTHETIC REHABILITATION

The tragedy of arm amputation occurs most commonly in the formative and productive years of a young man's life.[32, 33] The loss of this particular body part often results from a work-related injury and usually robs the victim of his dominant hand and arm. Postoperatively, such a patient should also be fitted with an immediate rigid dressing to control edema and pain. Within 30 days of the amputation, the patient should be fitted for and trained to use a preparatory prosthesis that will help him or her incorporate the prosthesis as a functional assist to the remaining limb. This "window of opportunity" for successful wear and function of a prosthesis has been studied by Malone and colleagues.[34] It appears that the upper limb amputee becomes "one-handed" after this time and has increasing difficulty in incorporating the prosthesis successfully into daily activities.

In the United States, three types of prosthetic systems are used to replace the upper limb:

- Cosmetic system
- Body-powered prosthesis
- Externally powered prosthesis

The first system is primarily a cosmetic one that is passive in nature and has no moving parts. The materials composing such prostheses are fairly life-like but are not particularly durable. They do provide some assistive function but cannot actively grasp and release, and they do not provide any sensory feedback. They are the lightest in weight of all the upper limb prostheses and provide the most acceptable facsimile of the usual body appearance.

The most commonly prescribed upper limb system is a *body-powered prosthesis* that is controlled through straps, harnesses, and cables, which capture residual body movement to actively power the moving parts of the artificial arm. These moving parts are most frequently the terminal device and the elbow for use with the transhumeral or more proximal amputation levels. The body-powered terminal devices used most commonly are voluntary opening hooks or hands; a few voluntary closing devices are also available. The voluntary opening devices are limited in their pinch force by the number of rubber bands or the spring mechanism built into the hand. The amputee opens such a terminal device by pulling on a cable using the force provided by residual scapular abduction and humeral flexion. Voluntary closing devices also operate through a cable control and can generate more closing pinch force but are heavier.

The voluntary opening hand is heavier than the voluntary opening hook but does appear more natural. Because of its bulk, however, it covers more of the visual sight lines than the hook does. Proficient wearers of body-powered prostheses find that the harnessing and cable control systems actually give the user some sensory feedback, which is useful in sensing where the terminal device is located and how much pinch force has been applied to an object that has been grasped.

The third system, an *externally powered prosthesis*, is available in two types: myoelectric and switch control. Except in some unusual, patient-specific circumstances, the myoelectric design is more widely applied. Myoelectric prostheses take advantage of human-generated electrical signals normally transmitted to the residual limb muscles from the nervous system. These signals are picked up from the surface of the skin through contact electrodes placed inside the prosthetic socket. They are amplified and fed into motors that drive the movable prosthetic fingers and may also move a rotating wrist unit or an electric elbow. These designs diminish the amount of harnessing and cable strapping necessary to operate the body-powered design. This decrease in strapping often makes the prosthesis more comfortable, but the motors and electrical components add weight. Another advantage of this prosthesis is provided by the electric motors, which supply greater grip force than body-powered methods. A disadvantage of these designs is that they are significantly more expensive than their body-powered counterparts.

Despite the advantages and disadvantages of these prosthetic options, fewer than half of unilateral amputees wear and use an arm prosthesis for most of the day. If the patients are fitted within 30 days of the amputation or if they are rehabilitated in a comprehensive medical center treating upper limb amputees, these results may improve. Successful use of an upper limb prosthesis is related to how amputees perceives their future and how they interpret the role of the prosthesis in that future.

The emotional well-being of the amputee should always be the primary focus of the rehabilitation team's effort because the amputee's future may or may not include a prosthesis. Even if the person who has lost an arm becomes a successful prosthetic user, will society permit such an amputee to return to a productive and fulfilling vocation? Vocational rehabilitation professionals often have a poor understanding of the functional abilities of a one-handed person or of someone who uses an artificial arm. There is a societal "Captain Hook" stigma for anyone who wears a terminal device that looks different from a human hand. American society has difficulty recognizing that individuals have significant contributions to make if they appear different. It is to be hoped that the Americans with Disabilities Act[35] will help the public begin to recognize the fallacy of these beliefs and behaviors.

For the best prosthetic functional outcomes and the most cost-effective care, upper limb amputees should be treated in a comprehensive rehabilitative center with experience in upper limb amputee care. Such centers provide multidisciplinary rehabilitation for many arm amputees each year.

REFERENCES

1. Burgess EM, Romano RL, Zettl JH: The Management of Lower Extremity Amputations. Bulletin TR 10-6. Washington, DC, U.S. Government Printing Office, 1969.
2. Malone JM, Moore WS, Goldstone J, Malone SJ: Therapeutic and economic impact of a modern amputation program. Ann Surg 189:789, 1979.
3. Wu Y, Krick H: Removable rigid dressing for below-knee amputees. Clin Prosthet Orthot 11:33, 1987.
4. Murdoch G, Jacobs NA, Wilson AB (eds): Papers Presented at the ISPO Consensus Conference on Amputation Surgery, University of Strathclyde, Scotland, October 15–17, 1990.
5. King JC, Titus MD: Prescriptions, referrals, and the rehabilitation team. In DeLisa JA (ed): Rehabilitation Medicine: Principles and Practice. Philadelphia, JB Lippincott, 1993.
6. Banerjee SN (ed): Rehabilitation Management of Amputees. Baltimore, Williams & Wilkins, 1982.
7. Anderson MH, Bray JJ, Hennessy CA: Prosthetic Principle: Above-Knee Amputations. Springfield, Ill, Charles C Thomas, 1960.
8. Dise-Lewis J: In Atkins DJ, Meier RH (eds): Psychological adaptations to limb loss. In Comprehensive Management of the Upper Limb Amputee. New York, Springer-Verlag, 1989.
9. Gailey RS, McKenzie A: Prosthetic Gait Training Program for Lower Extremity Amputees. Miami, Fla, University of Miami School of Medicine, Department of Orthopaedics and Rehabilitation, Division of Physical Therapy, 1989.
10. Karacoloff L, Hammersley CS, Schneider FJ: Lower Extremity Amputation: A Guide to Functional Outcomes in Physical Therapy Management, 2nd ed. Gaithersburg, Md, Aspen Publishing, 1992.
11. Mensch G, Ellis P: Physical Therapy Management of Lower Extremity Amputation. Rockville, Md, Aspen Publishing, 1986.
12. Fuhrer MJ (ed): Rehabilitation Outcomes: Analysis and Measurement. Baltimore, Paul Brookes, 1987.
13. Wu KK: Foot Orthoses. Baltimore, Williams & Wilkins, 1990.
14. Radcliffe CW, Foort J: The Patellar-Tendon-Bearing Below-Knee Prosthesis. Berkeley, Calif, Biomechanics Laboratory, University of California Berkeley, 1961.
15. Kapp S, Cummings D: Transtibial amputation: Prosthetic management. In Bowker JH, Michael JW (eds): Atlas of Limb Prosthetics: Surgical, Prosthetic, and Rehabilitation Principles, 2nd ed. St. Louis, Mosby–Year Book, 1992.
16. Michael J: Energy-storing feet: Clinical comparison. Clin Prosthet Orthot 11:154, 1987.
17. Esquenazi A, Torres MM: Prosthetic feet and ankle mechanisms. Phys Med Rehabil Clin North Am 2:299, 1991.
18. Fishman S, Berger N, Krebs D: The ISNY (Icelandic–Swedish–New York University) flexible above-knee socket. Phys Ther 65:742, 1985.
19. Michael JW: Current concepts in above-knee socket design. Instr Course Lect 39:373, 1990.
20. Staros A, Rubin G: Prescription considerations in modern above-knee prosthetics. Phys Med Rehabil Clin North Am 2:311, 1991.
21. Long I: Normal shape–normal alignment (NSNA) above-knee prosthesis. Clin Prosthet Orthot 9:9, 1985.
22. Gottschalk F: Transfemoral amputation—surgical procedures. In Bowker JH, Michael JW (eds): Atlas of Limb Prosthetics: Surgical, Prosthetic, and Rehabilitation Principles, 2nd ed. St. Louis, Mosby–Year Book, 1992.
23. Gonzalez EG, Corcoran PJ, Reyes RL: Energy expenditure in below-knee amputees: Correlation with stump length. Arch Phys Med Rehabil 55:111, 1974.
24. Waters RL, Perry J, Antonelli D, et al: The energy cost of walking of amputees: Influence of level of amputation. J Bone Joint Surg (Am) 58:42, 1976.
25. Kegel B: Adaptations for sports and recreation. In Bowker JH, Michael JW (eds): Atlas of Limb Prosthetics: Surgical, Prosthetic, and Rehabilitation Principles, 2nd ed. St. Louis, Mosby–Year Book, 1992.
26. Slocumb DB: Atlas of Amputations. St. Louis, CV Mosby, 1949.
27. Kohl SJ: The process of psychological adaptation to traumatic limb loss. In Krueger DW (ed): Emotional Rehabilitation of Physical Trauma and Disability. New York, SP Medical and Scientific Books, 1984.
28. Levy SW: Skin Problems of the Amputee. St. Louis, Warren H Green, 1983.
29. Sherman R: Stump and phantom limb pain. Neurol Clin 7:249, 1989.
30. Davis R: Phantom sensation, phantom pain and stump pain. Arch Phys Med Rehabil 74:79, 1993.
31. Shenaq SM, Krouskop T, Stal S, Spira M: Salvage of amputation stumps by secondary reconstruction utilizing microsurgical free-tissue transfer. Plast Reconstr Surg 79:861, 1987.
32. Atkins DJ, Meier RH (eds): Comprehensive Management of the Upper-Limb Amputee. New York, Springer-Verlag, 1989.
33. Leonard JA, Meier RH: Upper and lower extremity prosthetics. In DeLisa JA (ed): Rehabilitation Medicine: Principles and Practices. Philadelphia, JB Lippincott, 1993.
34. Malone JM, Fleming LL, Leal JM, et al: Immediate, early and late postsurgical management of the upper extremity amputation. J Rehabil Res Dev 21:33, 1984.
35. Anmuth CJ, Kamen L: Small business concerns regarding compliance with the Americans with Disabilities Act. Arch Phys Med Rehabil 73:978, 1992.

36. Fillauer CE, Pritham CH, Fillauer KD: Evolution and development of the Silicone Suction Socket (3S) for below knee prostheses. J Prosthet Orthot 1:92, 1989.
37. Pinzur MS, Smith DG, Daluga DJ, Osterman H: Selection of patients for through the knee amputation. J Bone Joint Surg 70A:746, 1988.
38. Michael JW: Prosthetic knee mechanisms. Phys Med Rehab State Art Rev (Hanley & Belfus) 8:147, 1994.
39. Granger CV, Hamilton BB: The uniform data system for medical rehabilitation report of first admission for 1991. Am J Phys Med Rehabil 72:33, 1993.
40. Moore TJ, Barron J, Hutchinson F, et al: Prosthetic usage following major lower extremity amputation. Clin Orthop 238:219, 1989.
41. Walker CRC, Ingram RR, Hullin MG, McCreath SW: Lower limb amputation following injury: A survey of long-term functional outcome. Injury 25:387, 1994.
42. Smith DG, Horn P, Malchow D, et al: Prosthetic history, prosthetic changes and functional outcome of isolated, traumatic below-knee amputee. J Trauma 38:44, 1995.
43. Volpicelli LJ, Chambers RB, Wagner FW: Ambulation levels of bilateral lower-extremity amputees. J Bone Joint Surg 65A: 599, 1983.
44. Evans WE, Hayes JP, Vermilion BD: Rehabilitation of the bilateral amputee. J Vasc Surg 5:589, 1987.
45. Leonard, JA, Meier RH: Upper and lower extremity prosthetics. In Delisa JA, Gans BM (eds): Rehabilitation Medicine: Principles and Practice, 3rd ed. Philadelphia, Lippincott-Raven, 1998.
46. Granger CV: The emerging science of functional assessment: Our tool for outcomes analysis. Arch Phys Med Rehabil 79:235, 1998.
47. Posner JD, Gorman KM, Windsor-Landsberg L, et al: Low to moderate intensity endurance training in healthy older adults: Physiological responses after four months. J Am Geriatr Soc 40:1, 1992.
48. Pyka G, Linderberger E, Charette S, Marcus R: Muscle strength and fiber adaptations to a year-long resistance training program in elderly men and women. J Gerontol 49:M22, 1994.
49. Steinberg FU, Sunwoo I, Roettger RF: Prosthetic rehabilitation of geriatric amputee patients: A follow-up study. Arch Phys Med Rehabil 66:742, 1985.
50. Leonard JA: The elderly amputee. In Felsenthal G, Garrison SJ, Steinberg FU (eds): Rehabilitation of the Aging and Elderly Patient. Baltimore, Williams & Wilkins, 1994.
51. Esquenazi A: Geriatric amputee rehabilitation. Clin Geriatr Med 4:731, 1993.
52. Andrews KL: Rehabilitation in limb deficiency. The geriatric amputee. Arch Phys Med Rehabil 77:S-14, 1996.
53. Meier RH, Purtilo R: Ethical issues and the patient-provider relationship. Am J Phys Med Rehabil 73:365, 1994.
54. Saris SC, Iacono RP, Nashold BS: Dorsal root entry zone lesions for post-amputation pain. J Neurosurg 62:72, 1985.

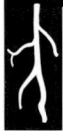

CHAPTER 165

Upper Extremity Amputation

Michael J. V. Gordon, M.D., F.A.C.S., and
Lawrence L. Ketch, M.D., F.A.C.S., F.A.A.P.

Primary atherosclerotic vascular disease of the upper extremity, in contrast to the familiar lower extremity disease process, is distinctly uncommon. To be sure, those diseases that lead to ischemia in the lower extremities can also produce complications in the upper extremity, but much less frequently. In a study comparing diabetic and nondiabetic patients using duplex Doppler examination, arterial disease in the upper extremity occurred in 2.3% of diabetic patients versus 0% in nondiabetic patients; arterial disease in the lower extremity occurred in 31.8% of diabetic patients versus 18.4% in nondiabetic patients.[1]

Other disorders also cause vascular compromise in the upper extremity. Vasospastic disorders (including vibration syndromes), Buerger's disease (thromboangiitis obliterans), thoracic outlet syndrome, arterial steal syndromes in patients on hemodialysis with arteriovenous fistulas, and arterial malformations are well-recognized entities leading to upper extremity symptoms. However, trauma is the most common etiology for upper extremity vascular compromise. Of traumatic injuries, most are associated with direct mechanical trauma, but some are related to secondary factors such as embolization from misplaced drug injection, blunt trauma leading to occlusive disease, and surgical and radiation damage after treatment for breast cancer.[2] When possible, treatment is directed at correction of the underlying pathology (such as cessation of smoking in Buerger's disease). Occasionally, upper extremity ischemia responds to sympathectomy for vasospastic diseases, bypasses for occlusive disease, or thrombolytic therapy.

Unfortunately, many of these diseases affecting the upper extremity share a common final pathway leading to some form of amputation. If the process is diffuse, without clear anatomic definition to the location of the vascular obstruction (such as in the vasospastic diseases or in severe diabetes mellitus), the principle of conservatism and conservation of parts is vital, because aggressive surgical procedures may aggravate the ischemic process. In the cases in which the vascular obstruction is more clearly defined, the same principles as used in traumatic amputations are invoked to provide the best functional result for the patient.

Upper extremity amputations comprise 15% to 20% of all amputations. In contrast to lower extremity amputees, individuals requiring amputations of the upper extremity are younger, with a mean age ranging from 20 to 40 years. Psychologic, emotional, and financial considerations play an even greater role in upper than in lower extremity amputations. The majority of upper extremities are lost to trauma (90%), with tumors, congenital anomalies, vascular insufficiency, infections, and iatrogenic causes (e.g., cardiac catheterization mishaps, extravasation of vasopressors) accounting for the remainder. It has been estimated that there currently are 75,000 upper extremity amputees in the United States, with 7800 new amputations each year.

GENERAL CONSIDERATIONS

Three primary issues are be considered in the assessment of patients requiring an upper extremity amputation. First, a thorough evaluation of the injury, tumor, or ischemia is required to determine the best surgical procedure. Only through extensive experience can one estimate the degree of functional recovery possible at the time of an injury. Nevertheless, such information is important in determining optimal surgical strategy for the patient.

Second, evaluation of "extrinsic" factors, including the patient's age, gender, handedness, general medical condition, other associated injuries, occupation, and hobbies, is necessary. These features determine the suitability of the patient for initial repair, secondary operations, and extended rehabilitation; thus, they guide the surgeon in recommending replantation, definitive amputation, or alternative complex reconstructive options.

Third, the most difficult assessment involves evaluation of the patient's "intrinsic" factors. These include the patient's own self-image and desires for the final functional and cosmetic result. Consideration must be given to the patient's social and cultural background. In some cultural settings, even a minor cosmetic deformity is more debilitating than *any* functional impairment.

After the overall patient evaluation, a decision must be made about immediate care. Often this involves a determination about whether replantation is either surgically possible or functionally desirable. If replantation has been eliminated as a possibility, closure of the wound must be considered. The timing of wound closure is critical and depends on several factors. In cases of traumatic injury, the nature of the wound (the contamination of the offending agent) and the amount of time elapsed since the injury dictate whether immediate closure is possible. It is best to adhere to general surgical principles of wound management. Although it is technically possible to close upper extremity traumatic amputation sites immediately most of the time, delayed closure is reasonable if conditions warrant.

A much more difficult problem is the selection of the type of closure to perform. This decision depends on the level of amputation and is discussed in detail in subsequent sections with respect to each amputation level. General considerations in this regard are determined by the principles of the reconstructive ladder. This approach dictates that one begin with the simplest closure and progress to more complex closure patterns as required by lack of simpler methods or by functional (or esthetic) considerations. In practical terms, one considers direct closure first, and then skin grafting, local flaps, distant flaps, and finally free-flap coverage. Before dealing with these issues in detail, one must pay attention to how the different anatomic structures are handled. In general, one usually considers bone, cartilage, tendons, muscles, nerves, vessels, and cutaneous coverage.

Length

Although preservation of length is a fundamental principle of amputation surgery, length does not always correlate directly with function, depending on the type of prosthetic application contemplated. In certain cases, it may be wise to sacrifice length in favor of better prosthetic fit. Such decisions are almost never possible in emergency situations, and ideally it is desirable to consult with an experienced prosthetist or rehabilitation specialist in these matters.

Bone

Whatever length is ultimately chosen for the amputation, the bony prominences must be optimally contoured. Lack of attention to the bony prominences or irregularities in contour leads to aesthetic abnormalities and difficulties with prosthetic fit. This results from inadequate débridement of traumatized and displaced bony fragments, improper initial contouring of the bone, or failure to identify bone-producing periosteum, which must also be contoured. Visual identification of the periosteum is easiest at the time of the initial injury, and achievement of a natural contour of the bone is greatly assisted by palpating the end of the bone through the skin prior to closure. This is even more important in amputations through joints, where natural anatomic flares of the bone produce aesthetically unnatural contours and interfere with prosthetic fitting.

Vessels

After proper débridement of the bony structures, the vessels are identified and ligated or coagulated, depending on their size and location.

Tendons

The hand represents a very delicate balance between extensor and flexor forces. It is extremely difficult to duplicate the balance of these forces through *myodesic* methods (i.e., suturing of tendons or muscles to bones) or *myoplastic* techniques (i.e., suturing of tendons or muscles to tendons or muscles of the opposite functional group, for example, suturing an extensor tendon directly to a flexor tendon over a bony amputation site). In general, then, such techniques are not used distally in the fingers and hand because they often *add* to the functional deficit. However, they do have value more proximally, where the balance is not as critical and reeducation and adaptation are easier.

Nerves

Prevention of neuroma is the major and most difficult problem in upper extremity amputation. As in all of medicine, the existence of many methods of treatment usually indicates that none of them is exceptionally good. Such is the case with neuromas. Distal ligation, proximal ligation, coagulation, chemical ablation of the end, simple division, traction and division, nerve repair to other divided nerves, and immediate burial of the transected nerve end have all been attempted with varying degrees of success. The desire to eliminate painful focal sensation must be balanced against the secondary loss of sensibility induced by many of these techniques.

One must accept the fact that a divided nerve always attempts to regenerate and, in so doing, produces a neuroma of variable clinical significance. Thus, in reality the goal is not to prevent the formation of a neuroma altogether but to prevent the patient from experiencing pain or dysesthesias from the neuroma that will predictably develop. In general, locating the divided, free nerve end as far from external stimuli as possible and placing it in a healthy, nonscarred bed of tissue are the best preventive measures. In addition, early postoperative therapy (desensitization or sensory reeducation) is an extremely important determinant of the patient's ability to tolerate the dysesthesias that result from an amputation.

Soft Tissue Coverage

Historically, the matter of soft tissue coverage has been indistinguishable from the issue of length. Previously, if soft tissue coverage was not adequate, one merely shortened the extremity until closure could be achieved. The concept of grafts and flaps has dramatically changed this approach. Skin grafts are applicable when the underlying bed is acceptable, but one must be sensitive to the ultimate functional needs of the amputation site; in some cases, skin grafts may not be durable enough.

Local flaps (see Fingertip Amputation next) abound, but their applicability, owing to the anatomy at more proximal amputation sites, is limited. *Pedicled* flaps (regional or distal) have a long, productive history in hand surgery; however, these have been increasingly replaced by free tissue transfers. This change is based on (1) better matching of the tissue transferred (in terms of thickness and ultimate functional performance), (2) avoidance of additional surgery (whether for division or thinning of the flap), and (3) lack of the joint limitations that result from the immobility that is necessary until the pedicled flap is divided.

SPECIFIC AMPUTATIONS

Fingertip Amputation

Distal digital amputations are extremely common. The most frequent mechanism causing such injuries is a crushing blow, such as from a closing door. Although many people arrive in the emergency department with the tips of the finger available for reattachment, this injury is usually too distal for microsurgical reattachment. Many surgeons have attempted composite reattachment (i.e., reattachment without specific revascularization) with generally poor results. At present, such composite grafts are not indicated except in younger children (<2 years of age), in whom there is an increased chance of graft survival.[3] The reason for failure of these composite grafts is twofold:

1. The amount of tissue is generally more that can survive the ischemia until new circulation develops.

2. The zone of injury is greater than the area of amputation (i.e., the tip is usually damaged and thus is not capable of surviving as a composite graft).

Closure of the amputation site is then the problem. If the proximal portion of the distal phalanx is not severely injured so that the insertions of the flexor digitorum profundus and extensor tendons are intact, preservation of that portion of bone is indicated for functional length. If these areas are involved beyond repair, disarticulation through the distal interphalangeal joint is indicated. The overriding issues are the status of the nail and what type of coverage can be provided. Generally, the amputation occurs through a portion of the nailbed. If enough proximal nailbed (~50%) is present to provide a functional nail, the bed should be repaired under optical magnification with absorbable 6-0 or 7-0 sutures.

The distal phalanx is usually rongeured back so that the end of the bone is not exposed. If the final cutaneous defect is then less than 1 cm², simply allowing the wound to close by secondary intention is acceptable. Other wound closures have been attempted, including every conceivable type of local or regional flap. However, given the fact that the flap closures are frequently insensate (and take no less time to heal), the ultimate functional recovery appears to be better after secondary healing because the resulting scar contracture diminishes the size of the sensory defect.

If the cutaneous defect is greater than 1 cm², the amount of time needed for closure and the ultimate functional result no longer warrant healing by secondary intention. If there is no exposed bone, a skin graft is possible. The temptation is to use the amputated part as a donor source for the skin graft. This should be avoided because the amputated portion has been traumatized, and therefore the overall success of these skin grafts is less than might be expected. Nevertheless, one advantage of such grafts is that they may serve as temporary biologic dressings even if they do not survive.

Nontraumatized skin graft donor sites that may be considered are:

1. The ulnar border of the palm (within the operative field and a good color match).

2. The forearm (the medial portion of the forearm or the elbow crease, although hypertrophic scarring can lead to some cosmetic deformity).

3. The groin (a well-hidden donor area, although the color match is not good and some unwanted hair may also be transferred).

As previously mentioned, many alternative flaps are often useful for cutaneous defects of the fingertip; some of the more common local flaps include:

- The Kutler flap,[4] a lateral V-Y flap for closure of a central tip defect
- The Atasoy flap,[5] a palmar V-Y flap
- The palmar flap,[6] based on both digital neurovascular bundles in which the entire soft tissue coverage of the digit above the tendon sheath is elevated and advanced to cover the tip of the finger
- Radius-based or ulna-based local flaps, which preserve the cutaneous innervation on the appropriate digital nerve,[7] with skin grafting of the donor site as necessary.

In addition to these local flaps, numerous *regional* flaps can be used, such as (1) dorsal skin cross-finger flaps, (2) palmar skin cross-finger flaps, and (3) thenar flaps. Although it is sometimes necessary to use these regional pedicled flaps, they carry significant additional morbidity by creating joint stiffness because of the obligatory period of immobility needed for attachment of the flap. Even in young people who have had good physical therapy, this can cause a long-term problem.

In addition, a rare patient may require distant pedicled flaps for coverage. Many such flaps have been described, including abdominal flaps, infraclavicular flaps, supraclavicular flaps, cross-arm flaps, and cross-hand flaps. Again, secondary morbidity resulting from immobility is usually higher than warranted, and simpler techniques are preferable. Free tissue transfer is almost never indicated for these injuries except in the case of thumbtip amputations (discussed later).

Digital Amputations

Digital amputations are classified by level. Amputations that leave more than half the proximal phalanx may be functional for the patient. These amputations, then, represent variations of fingertip amputations. First, the bone is rongeured back a short distance to allow soft tissue coverage. Tendons that have been separated from their bony insertions by the amputation are placed on traction, divided, and allowed to retract into the palm. Digital nerves are a potentially more difficult problem. It is preferable to divide them under mild traction and allow them to retract beneath healthy vascularized tissue. Excessive traction may denervate the new tip of the digit. No traction leaves the cut nerve adjacent to the amputation site, allowing postinjury trauma and producing significant pain. The associated soft tissue defect is managed in the same manner as a fingertip amputation.

Amputation proximal to the mid-portion of the proximal phalanx typically is not a functional amputation. If enough digit remains, it may be possible for patients to wear a cosmetic prosthesis that may allow some functional restoration; however, most patients find the remaining digit a nuisance (Fig. 165–1). Each time they reach into their pocket or a purse for a small object, the object falls through the opening left in the hand by the remaining short digit, which cannot flex adequately to close the space. As a result, these patients frequently choose to undergo a secondary ray amputation. Regardless of the certainty of this dénouement, ray amputation should *not* be offered to the patient at the time of the initial wound closure. Elective deletion of the remaining portion of the digit is a decision each patient should come to by experience.

Ray amputation often provides a far more cosmetically acceptable hand; in most cases, the appearance of a three-fingered hand with normal border contours is so natural that it goes unnoticed. Nevertheless, the operation is not without its own set of risks. First, the procedure narrows the palm by approximately 20% to 25%. This reduces the hand's ability to stabilize objects. Second, the operation is a more extensive procedure, producing more proximal postoperative pain, edema, and stiffness than were produced by the injury to the digit. However, in the final analysis, ray amputation is very functional and cosmetically appealing, and there are few dissatisfied patients.

Thumb Amputations

Constituting 40% of the function of the hand, the thumb deserves special attention in any amputation involving the hand. Clearly, the major emphasis is on reattachment of the thumb. However, the desire for reattachment has led some surgeons to attempt replantation in circumstances that would otherwise be considered contraindications (e.g., severe avulsion injuries). Although thumb replantation has not been universally accepted, it has produced encouraging results even after avulsion injuries.[8] Nonreplantable amputations at the level of the interphalangeal joint are quite functional, and most patients do not request or require additional reconstruction. More proximal thumb amputations may be reconstructed by pollicization, osteoplasty, bone-lengthening techniques, or toe-to-thumb transfer (great toe, second toe, or toe wrap-around).

The issues of closure of the amputation site are basically the same as those already discussed with respect to digital amputations, except that there must be greater emphasis on retention of length. Local flaps, such as the neurovascular island flap from the dorsum of the index finger, may be useful in these injuries.[9]

Hand-Wrist Amputations

Whatever can be salvaged from a hand amputation *should* be salvaged. A short palm hand may seem dysfunctional, but as an assist hand it may be preferable to a prosthesis in some individuals. All patients should be allowed to function with such a partial hand to determine whether they would prefer to have a more proximal amputation, with subsequent fitting of a standard prosthesis. The advantage of the short palm is that it retains some valuable wrist flexion-extension (particularly if the remaining portion has good sensibility). If the injured extremity is the dominant one and the patient wants to rehabilitate the extremity to an independently functional unit, he or she will probably benefit from wrist disarticulation and fitting with a hook prosthesis (Fig. 165–2).

If it is decided to proceed with a wrist disarticulation, the radial and ulnar styloid processes are trimmed but not completely resected after removal of the proximal carpal row. This allows more secure fitting of the prosthesis and good transmission of pronation and supination capability without causing wear by the bony prominences.

The radial, ulnar, and median nerves can present difficulties. The ulnar and median nerves are frequently avulsed at a more proximal level with these traumatic amputations; if they are apparent in the wound, they can be severed with mild traction and allowed to retract. Retraction of the ends usually positions the nerves away from contact with a prosthesis. The sensory branch of the radial nerve, however, is quite superficial throughout its course in the forearm (covered only by the brachioradialis muscle). Neuromas from this nerve are not uncommon, and division of the nerve in the proximal forearm may be considered at the time of the initial amputation. Sensibility of the forearm skin is not directly determined by these nerves but instead is controlled by brachial cutaneous nerves. These can cause

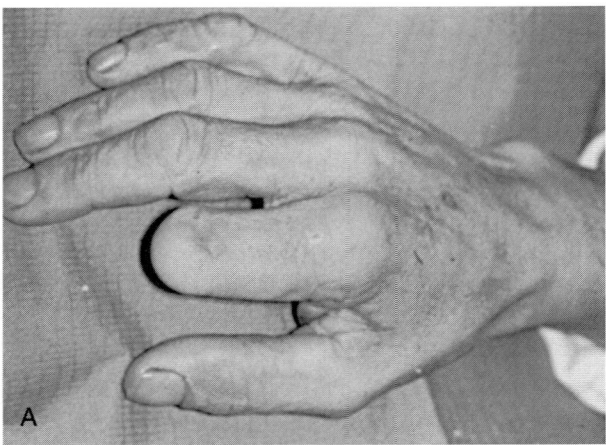

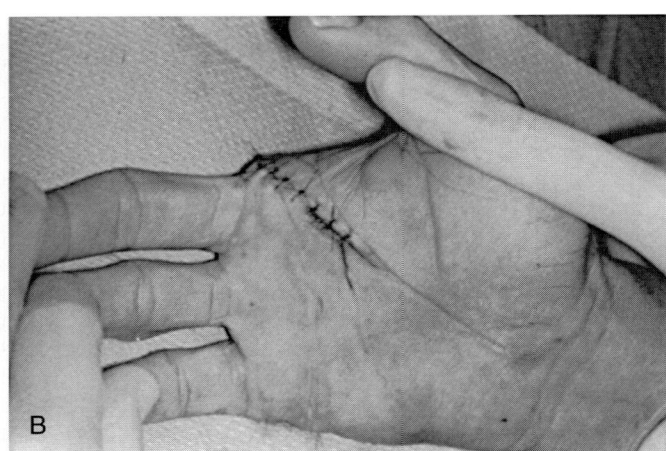

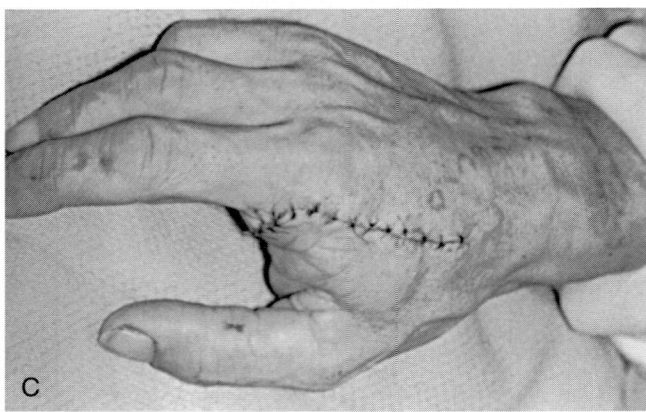

FIGURE 165–1. *A–C,* The patient is a 30-year-old man who lost his index finger at the proximal interphalangeal joint. He does not use the index remnant, bypassing it to use his long digit. He requested elective ray resection because of a feeling that the index remnant was "getting in the way" and creating an unsightly appearance.

similar difficulties to the superficial branch of the radial nerve. In contrast, it is preferable not to divide these nerves far proximally because sensibility of the forearm skin will be sacrificed.

The wrist is the most distal level of amputation at which tenodesis may be safely considered. Suturing of the flexor and extensor tendons over the amputation stump may provide some extra soft tissue padding at the amputation site as well as maintaining some forearm muscle mass.

A difficult problem that is sometimes encountered is whether the patient is best rehabilitated with a hook prosthesis or a myoelectric hand. The myoelectric prosthesis adds length to the amputation site and is more cosmetically positioned with removal of several additional centimeters of distal forearm (Fig. 165–3). The amputee usually cannot make such decisions near the time of the initial injury. Proximal revision of these amputations may be done at any time in the future, and no bridges should be burned until the patient has had ample time to evaluate the consequences of his or her decision.

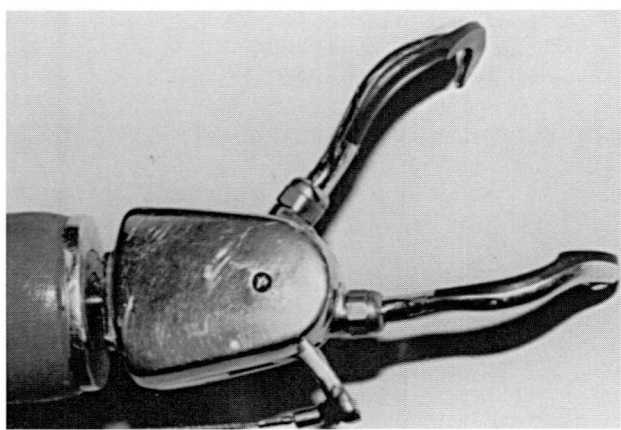

FIGURE 165–2. Example of a voluntary-closing terminal device. Internal springs provide opening power.

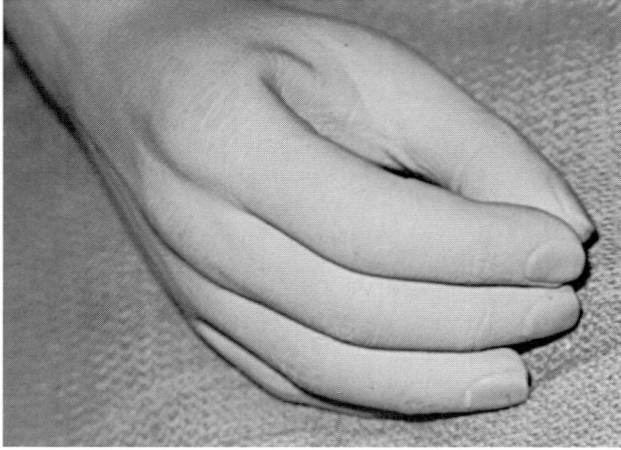

FIGURE 165–3. An Otto Bock myoelectric hand with standard rubber glove.

Forearm Amputations

There are two considerations in forearm amputation. First, as much length as possible should be preserved to maintain maximal pronation and supination. The more proximal the amputation, the less movement arm remains for rotation, and, if far enough proximal, the muscles that create pronation and supination are lost. This principle is illustrated graphically in Figure 165–4.

Second, the patient's ability to wear a prosthesis is a major issue. Preservation of the elbow joint is critical, and a prosthesis must fit well without interfering with the motion of the joint. So important is the elbow that the use of free-flap soft tissue coverage to preserve length or even distraction osteogenesis is a viable consideration in the case of very short below-elbow amputations. With the exception of these very special cases, however, heroic efforts at preserving length are not indicated.

Heeding these caveats, the surgeon can trim the bony tissues adequately to permit soft tissue closure. Flexor and extensor tendons (or muscles more proximally) should be sutured to each other over the ends of the amputation site. Nerves (radial, median, ulnar, and superficial cutaneous nerves) are either transposed to deeper layers or placed on traction and divided (allowing them to retract into deeper, more protected, and healthier tissue).

Reconstruction of the amputation is generally accomplished by means of a fitted prosthesis. As described by Tubiana,[10] however, bilateral upper extremity amputations can be functionally improved by using the Krukenberg procedure, in which a sensate pincer is created between the radius and the ulna (Fig. 165–5). Although the cosmetic result is far from desirable, the functional improvement is great, and the procedure should be given serious consideration in those rare instances of bilateral injuries in blind individuals or when prosthetic reconstruction is not practical.[11]

Elbow Disarticulation and Upper Arm Amputations

Surgical recommendations for specific amputations still depend on the type of prosthetic fitting that can be expected.

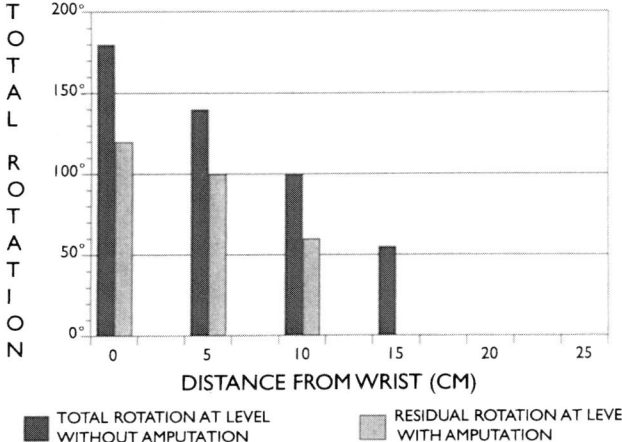

FIGURE 165–4. Residual forearm rotation after amputation.

Although improvements in upper extremity prostheses continue, the rate of improvement and the funds available for research are limited. Many of the systems that have been used are expensive, and the funding of the prosthetic fitting is a substantial financial issue (e.g., the Utah elbow with terminal device can run from $39,000 to $50,000).

Compared with the forearm, which has two bones with a functional noncircular cross section and thin soft tissue coverage that allows transmission of rotational forces (pronation and supination), the upper arm has a single bone with a relatively circular cross section and less rotational stability because of its thicker soft tissue. Thus, there has been considerable emphasis on retention of the full length of the humerus to take advantage of the flare of the condyles as a method of achieving better prosthetic fit (prevention of rotation of the prosthesis) and preserving some rotational movement of the upper arm. In so doing, however, the upper arm will appear longer than the normal arm in order to accommodate an internal elbow joint. It is possible to fit the patient with an external elbow joint, but these joints are substantially less durable.

Another approach to this problem involves the construction of an artificial asymmetry by means of angulation osteotomy.[12] Although this method has gained popularity in Europe, it is not routinely practiced in the United States because of the obvious cosmetic deformity induced in the proximal remaining stump.

Surgical considerations with above-elbow amputations are essentially the same as those in forearm amputations with respect to the treatment of bone, muscles, tendons, nerves, and skin. Wood and Cooney have reported that replantation should be considered even in these high amputations.[13] Although functional recovery of the hand may not be expected, it may be possible to convert an obvious above-elbow amputation to a below-elbow amputation, which is far more functional.

The shorter the remaining stump, the more difficult the prosthetic fit and the less functional the prosthesis will be. As a result, several new techniques have been developed to facilitate this type of reconstruction. The use of free flaps can provide additional soft tissue and bone length for a short upper arm amputation. Functional restoration of the glenohumeral joint may be accomplished with a free fibular transfer. The proximal humerus can be completely replaced with the fibula and its proximal joint with reattachment of the muscular insertions.[14, 15] Particularly in patients with malignant tumors, limbs that would otherwise have to be sacrificed can now be salvaged. Fibular flaps can also be used in conjunction with soft tissue coverage from a latissimus dorsi flap (pedicled or free) to provide an acceptable length of upper arm for fitting a prosthesis.

One final technique used to achieve adequate bony length is distraction osteogenesis.[16] Although this technique was developed in the 1960s by Ilizarov, it has become widely used worldwide only in the 1990s. Initial reports of this method of treatment have been encouraging.

As indicated previously, every effort should be made to avoid high amputations. Even when the amputation will be a functional shoulder disarticulation (amputation proximal to the insertions of the deltoid and pectoralis major),

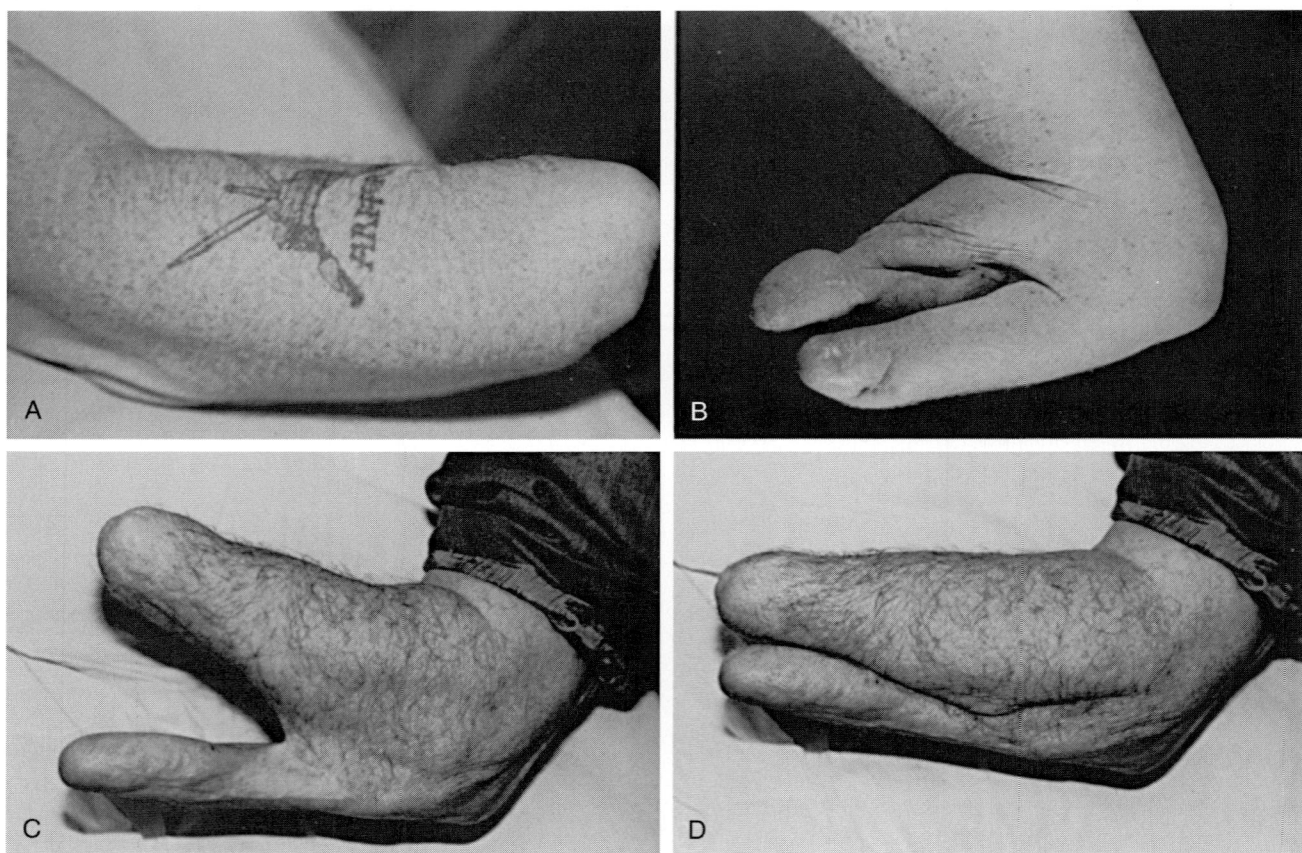

FIGURE 165–5. A–D, In the bilateral blind amputee, use of any standard prosthesis is impossible because of the absence of visual feedback or proprioception in the prosthesis. Under such circumstances, separation of the radius and ulna with Krukenberg's procedure can provide a proprioceptive "feeling" extremity capable of simple grasp-release.

the maximal proximal length of humerus should be salvaged for either prosthetic fitting or reconstruction.

Shoulder Disarticulation and Forequarter Amputations

The shoulder disarticulation and forequarter amputation are the most complex and difficult procedures from a prosthetic and functional standpoint. Considerations are (1) loss of potential motor units as drivers of the prosthetic device, and (2) difficulty of fitting the prosthesis to contour. The shoulder disarticulation (after rounding off the bony prominences that may cause wear) leaves a contour adequate to provide a snug fit for the prosthesis. In addition, scapular function is retained and can be used (with some difficulty) as a motor unit for the prosthetic device. The forequarter amputation (which is done almost exclusively for malignant processes), however, offers little hope for functional restoration of the limb.

The surgical techniques for these amputations are well described in the literature. The anterior approach, described by Berger,[17] and the posterior approach, described by Littlewood,[18] differ only in the exposure of the vascular structures hidden behind the clavicle. Both approaches are well accepted. The same principle that were described previously apply in terms of removing the bony promi-

nences, treating the nerves and muscles, and providing adequate soft tissue coverage.

Postoperative Management

Aside from routine postoperative care, several other issues deserve mention. Immediate application of postoperative prostheses has been advocated to decrease edema and facilitate earlier rehabilitation. The poor vascularity and problems in wound healing inherent in lower extremity amputations are rarely encountered in the upper extremity.

A major issue frequently overlooked in the amputee is the psychologic disturbance created first by the amputation itself and then by the subsequent impact on the patient's life. The hand and upper extremity are so intricately involved in daily existence that the complete or partial loss of either demands psychologic readjustment in *all* cases. This principle applies as much to children as to adults. In many cases, a young man or woman may make light of the psychologic issues and insist that there are no problems. Although as surgeons we welcome quick adjustment to disability and anticipate the patient moving ahead with the rest of his or her life, it is necessary for the amputee to experience a grieving process similar to that encountered with the death of a close relative. In detailing some of the principles learned in the treatment of hand injuries during World War II, Cleveland pointed out that ". . . the hand is more important than the eye, and is next in importance to the brain itself . . . ."[19] Grunert and colleagues studied the physiologic issues involved in upper extremity amputation and confirmed their importance.[20]

REFERENCES

1. Mackaay AJ, Beks PJ, Dur AH, et al: The distribution of peripheral vascular disease in a Dutch Caucasian population: Comparison of type II diabetic and non-diabetic subjects. Eur J Vasc Endovasc Surg 9:170–175, 1995.
2. Taylor PJ, Cooper GG, Sarkar TK: Upper-limb arterial disease in women treated for breast cancer. Br J Surg 82:1089, 1995.
3. Rosslein R, Simmen BR: Finger tip amputations in children. Handchir Mikrochir Plast Chir 23:312–317, 1991.
4. Kutler W: New method for fingertip amputation. JAMA 133:39, 1947.
5. Atasoy E, Ioakimidis E, Kasdan M, et al: Reconstruction of the amputated fingertip with a triangular volar flap. J Bone Joint Surg 52(A): 921, 1970.
6. Snow JW: The use of a volar flap for repair of fingertip amputations: A preliminary report. Plast Reconstr Surg 52:299, 1973.
7. Venkataswami R, Subramanian N. Oblique triangular flap: A new method of repair for oblique amputations of the fingertip and thumb. Plast Reconstr Surg 66:296–300, 1980.
8. Bowen CV, Beveridge J, Milliken RG, Johnston GH. Rotating shaft avulsion amputations of the thumb. J Hand Surg [Am] 16:117–121, 1991.
9. Leupin P, Weil J, Buchler U: The dorsal middle phalangeal finger flap: Mid-term results of 43 cases. J Hand Surg [Br] 22:362–371, 1997.
10. Tubiana R: Krukenberg's operation. Orthop Clin North Am 12:819–826, 1981.
11. Gu YD, Zhang LY, Zheng YL: Introduction of a modified Krukenberg operation. Plast Reconstr Surg 97:222–226, 1996.
12. Neusel E, Traub M, Blasius K, Marquardt E. Results of humeral stump angulation osteotomy. Arch Orthop Trauma Surg 116:263–265, 1997.
13. Wood MB, Cooley WF 3d: Above elbow limb replantation: Functional results. J Hand Surg [Am] 11:682–687, 1986.
14. Huckstep RL, Sherry E: Replacement of the proximal humerus in primary bone tumours. Aust N Z J Surg 66:97–100, 1996.
15. Yajima H, Tamai S, Ono H, Kizaki K: Vascularized bone grafts to the upper extremities; Plast Reconstr Surg 101:727–735; discussion, 736–737.
16. Ilizarov GA: The principles of the Ilizarov method. Bull Hosp Joint Dis 56:49–33, 1997.
17. Berger P: L'amputation du Membre Superieur dans la Contiguite du Tronc (Amputation Interscapulo-Thoracic). Paris, G Masson, 1887.
18. Littlewood H: Amputations at the shoulder and at the hip. Br Med J 1:381, 1922.
19. Cleveland M: Hand injuries in the European theater of operations. In Surgery in World War II: Hand Surgery, Washington, DC, Office of the Surgeon General, Department of the Army, 1955.
20. Grunert BK, Matloub HS, Sanger JR, Yousif NJ: Treatment of post-traumatic stress disorder after work-related hand trauma. J Hand Surg [Am] 15:511–515, 1990.

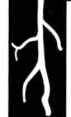

CHAPTER   1 6 6
Revascularization Versus Amputation

James M. Malone, M.D., F.A.C.S.

The selection of arterial revascularization versus amputation for a given patient presenting with advanced ischemia is a clinical decision that frequently challenges the surgical judgment of all vascular surgeons. The development of ever more sophisticated and innovative distal arterial reconstructive procedures, noninvasive or percutaneous reconstructive procedures, and a team approach for microsurgery and free flaps complicates the question of when to perform a primary amputation rather than use arterial reconstructive techniques.

Even when it is technically possible to perform revascularization in some clinical situations, a better approach for the patient might be primary amputation. Commonly asked questions are or should be, "How many reoperations should be performed for attempted revascularization?" and "When should enough be enough?"

Past publications have focused on independent and multiple variables to consider when one is choosing between amputation and arterial reconstruction: patient age, life expectancy, operative mortality and morbidity, presence of diabetes with and without foot sepsis, functional status of the patient and the involved limb, risk of graft failure or the presence of previous graft failures, presence of graft sepsis, poor graft runoff, lack of a suitable autogenous vein, and, more recently, cost-effectiveness. We must also pay attention to race and gender, in addition to diabetes mellitus, because there is an increased incidence of amputation in African Americans and Hispanics, compared with whites.[1–3] Also, data are emerging to suggest that patients with end-stage renal disease may best be treated with a primary amputation despite our technical ability to perform advanced reconstructive procedures.[4] Almost all vascular surgeons are familiar with these variables and their individual and multiple impacts on a specific patient. However, opinions vary from surgeon to surgeon about which procedures should be performed on any given patient.

Part of the disparity in approaches can be attributed to variability and conflicting data within the reported literature. Not all study groups are comparable, not all studies are prospective, and not all studies are controlled for important variables such as race, gender, fasting blood glucose, and careful classification of coexisting diseases. In addition, although we try to assess the variables independently, the spectrum of disease (i.e., severity index) within each variable may not be comparable, thereby giving rise to conflicting reports from what appear to be similar studies. This chapter examines variables that are included in the framework for deciding the optimal management of a patient who presents with limb-threatening ischemia.

OVERVIEW

The answer to the conundrum: amputation or revascularization is perhaps as much philosophic as it is scientific. Few data in the literature compare the experience and training of the surgeon and the degree of sophistication of either the revascularization team or the amputation team. Most important, long-term comparable data are nonexistent. The data are complex, surgeons have multiple and variable backgrounds, and in the absence of objective, comparable criteria, it is impossible to identify unequivocally which patients would benefit from revascularization and which would best be served by early amputation and rehabilitation. Traditionally, vascular surgeons analyzed their results based upon graft patency, complication rates, and long-term outcomes. Changes within contemporary American medicine now require analysis of quality of life, cost-effectiveness, and cost of extended care for those patients who are not returned to ambulatory status.

Before examining "comparative" data, it is important to distinguish between amputation versus revascularization for patients with acute ischemia, and amputation versus revascularization for patients with progressive chronic ischemia.

ACUTE ISCHEMIA

The choice of amputation for the management of acute ischemia in a patient whose arterial tree is considered unreconstructable or in a patient who presents late in the course of acute ischemia, such that arterial reconstruction may be contraindicated, is a decision-making process that will tax the judgment of even the most experienced surgeon. In addition, urgent or emergency amputation is usually associated with the greatest morbidity and mortality within the entire field of amputation surgery. The degree of urgency for amputation in the presence of acute arterial ischemia is governed by multiple factors that include, but are not limited to:

- Extent of extremity ischemia
- Duration of ischemia
- Changes in neurosensory function
- Presence of signs of systemic toxicity from products of muscle necrosis or bacteremia
- Degree of diabetic control in those patients who are afflicted with diabetes mellitus

If the affected ischemic area is small and there are no supervening signs of systemic toxicity, amputation can and should be postponed as long as possible to allow maximal

development of collateral circulation. Adequate drainage of any purulence, débridement of dead or infected tissue, systemic heparin, low-molecular-weight dextran, or the use of fibrinolytic agents may all be valuable adjuncts to maintain or increase blood flow through marginally ischemic tissues during the period of observation when collateral channels are enlarging. However, the presence of severe pain, extensive muscle necrosis, or systemic toxicity may require emergency amputation, with less preoperative patient preparation. Systemic toxicity, especially due to a necrotizing infection, necessitates emergency amputation. For patients with significant comorbid medical conditions or systemic toxicity, cryologic or physiologic amputation extends time for patient preparation for operation and decreases mortality.[5–7]

Several features are helpful in the decision-making process. The location of nonviable skin is important in determining the extent of the amputation. Areas of hyposensitivity, although possibly due to a diabetic neuropathy, also may indicate severe skin ischemia that precludes healing. The presence of significant calf muscle swelling or muscle rigidity is an ominous sign suggestive of myonecrosis and most probably requires major limb amputation. As discussed, the presence of systemic toxicity or significant changes in neurologic examination are indications for proceeding with immediate amputation, or at least physiologic amputation. In addition, myoglobinuria or cardiovascular instability often require an immediate amputation.

When observation is selected, prophylaxis against renal damage from precipitation of myoglobin pigment should include diuresis in a range of 70 to 100 ml/hr by the administration of intravenous fluids and osmotic diuretics such as mannitol. The urine pH should be maintained alkaline, because myoglobin precipitates in the renal tubules when the pH is less than 7.0. Finally, infection in an ischemic extremity is an ominous complication that may mandate immediate major limb amputation. As long as there is continual improvement in the collateral blood supply to an acutely ischemic extremity, there are no signs of systemic or renal toxicity, and neurologic function is stable or improving, then observation should be continued. Failure to see those changes or improvements requires reevaluation for urgent revascularization or amputation.

Evaluation for potential revascularization in a patient with a clear-cut demarcation of a nonviable area of the lower limb after a period of observation is not likely to be beneficial; however, marginal viability of a significant amount of tissue above an area that is believed to be nonviable warrants evaluation for vascular reconstruction to preserve limb length.[8]

PROGRESSIVE CHRONIC ISCHEMIA

The patient with progressive chronic ischemia usually presents for amputation with one or more of the following problems: rest pain, nonhealing skin lesion or ulceration, gangrene, or gangrene with superimposed infection. Gangrene complicated by infection is a special problem that is not addressed in this chapter; however, this condition almost always requires emergency amputation and appropriate medical support, including intravenous antibiotics and prophylaxis for renal failure.

From the patient's perspective, ischemic rest pain is probably one of the more compelling indications for amputation; however, this symptom usually justifies evaluation for revascularization if the patient is an appropriate candidate. In absence of systemic toxicity or supervening infection, and if the ischemic rest pain can be controlled with medication such as heparin and analgesics, the patient can be observed and carefully evaluated. Another manifestation of chronic ischemia is ischemic skin ulceration or nonhealing skin lesions. In the absence of systemic sepsis, emergency treatment is not necessary and the patient almost always can be evaluated for revascularization. Even in patients who present with frank tissue loss, provided that tissue loss is small and there are no signs of systemic toxicity, there is sufficient time to evaluate the patient for revascularization. Preoperative evaluation of such patients should also include attention to all associated medical diseases. Almost all patients with chronic limb ischemia should be considered for vascular reconstruction for limb salvage prior to amputation. Revascularization should always be attempted unless contraindicated by the patient's medical condition or anatomic constraints.

LIMB REVASCULARIZATION: THE JUSTIFICATION

Proponents of limb revascularization, even to the level of the foot and ankle, base their assertion on the following:

1. Limb salvage rates are usually 10% to 20% higher than graft patency rates.
2. Most patients die of other causes but are still ambulatory with a salvaged limb.
3. Mortality rates are actually higher for primary amputation than they are for revascularization.

In addition, those authorities challenge the concept that a failed revascularization may cause a higher level of amputation and cite low morbidity and mortality rates even for secondary vascular reconstruction. In a study by Panayiotopoulos and colleagues, primary amputation was associated with an in-hospital mortality rate of 18% in contrast to 10% for revascularization; however, 3-year survival rates were comparable.[9]

Whether increased rates of revascularization reduce the number of amputations is controversial. Mattes and associates suggested that the reduction in major amputations was secondary to a decrease in the incidence of peripheral arterial occlusive disease, rather than increased vascular reconstructive operations.[10] In a 12-year population-based study from Findland, Luther and associates noted that amputation rates as a measure of the efficiency of an arterial reconstruction policy should be employed only on a population basis.[11] Those authors reported that data from a referral center are skewed. In contrast, Karlstrom and colleagues reported that increased vascular intervention led to improved limb salvage rates and reduced amputation rates.[12] It is interesting that most of the reduction in amputation rates in that study were in the primary amputation group. That report stressed the importance of identifying good responders to revascularization because the choice of initial treatment influenced limb salvage but not overall survival.[12] The Westcoast Vascular Study Group from Sweden did not demonstrate that the amputation rates were decreased by increased revascularization rates, and suggested that patients undergoing vascular reconstruction versus amputation represented different population groups.[13]

Perhaps the most compelling study comparing amputation and revascularization rates was that published by Hallett and colleagues, which was a population-based investigation between 1973 and 1992.[14] Revascularization procedures increased in the first decade of the study, but reached a plateau after 1985. Angioplasty rates initially lagged behind surgery and then significantly surpassed surgery and did not plateau. The authors noted that all minor amputation rates remained unchanged for the duration of the study. More importantly, the authors noted that there was an approximate 50% reduction in the incidence of major limb amputations, and they concluded that increased vascular surgery and balloon angioplasty have coincided with a significant reduction in major limb amputation rates over the past 10 years.[14]

PRIMARY AMPUTATION: THE JUSTIFICATION

Advocates of primary amputation base their arguments on the following: (1) shortened patient hospitalization, (2) lower overall patient morbidity, (3) identical survival rates, (4) increased morbidity associated with failed revascularization, (5) the possibility of higher levels of amputation after a failed bypass, and (6) the excessive cost of a revascularization plus amputation compared with a primary amputation. In selected patient populations, proponents of primary amputation have been able to demonstrate acceptable operative mortality, especially in medically compromised patients.

In centers specializing in amputation and rehabilitation, excellent rates of postoperative ambulation and rehabilitation have been reported.[15] It is important to emphasize, however, that studies from amputation referral centers probably do not reflect amputee care in the average community hospital. In addition, the variables of surgical training and experience are probably just as great as the variables of the patient populations being studied. Vascular surgeons accustomed to performing reconstructive procedures at distal levels and who perform a high volume of these operations have a solid foundation from which to recommend revascularization over primary amputation for almost all patients. In contrast, vascular surgeons who practice in large amputation referral centers, who have excellent results with patient rehabilitation after amputation and who also have the ability to perform distal revascularizations, base their recommendations for revascularization versus primary amputation on specific patient disease. The experience of the vascular/amputation surgeon is crucial (and underappreciated) in the decision-making process. Table 166–1 outlines the basic considerations that constitute the algorithm for primary amputation rather than vascular reconstruction.

The decision for primary amputation versus vascular reconstruction is a balance of relative risk, cost, and quality of life. The bias of the author, like that of most other

TABLE 166–1. INDICATIONS FOR PRIMARY AMPUTATION

Absolute

Psychosocial	Patient is nonambulatory, has no transfer capability, has ipsilateral limb contractures, or has limited cognitive ability
	Patient has ipsilateral paralysis or insensate limb
	Patient has limited mobility, and an amputation is not expected to worsen mobility
Anatomic	No reconstructible vessels
	Uncontrolled pedal sepsis in a native limb or in a limb after reconstruction with a patent or occluded graft
	Progressive gangrene beyond mid-forefoot

Relative

Anatomic	Large hindfoot ulcer with no donor vessel available for free flap
Situational	Patient has an expected survival of less than 1 year
	Patient's co-morbidities push risk of death after revascularization to an excessive level
	Life-threatening hemorrhage or sepsis
	Patient has been evaluated by a surgeon skilled in distal bypass who has excluded reconstruction as an option
Less important	Only synthetic conduit is available
	No trained surgeon is available (patient must be transferred)

vascular surgeons, is that the basic mission of vascular surgery is to salvage tissue, whether cerebral, visceral, or lower extremity. The decision favoring revascularization versus amputation then becomes a matter of comparing risk to the patient; expected outcome; and, in today's managed-care market, the direct and indirect costs to the system or the patient.

COMPARATIVE MORBIDITY AND MORTALITY

Comparison of operative mortality and morbidity for revascularization versus amputation is not as straightforward as it might seem because of differences in data reporting. Conclusions deduced from five major studies are listed in Table 166–2, and the following discussion provides a detailed analysis of the data.

In 1985, Gregg reported an experience of 18 surgeons at several community hospitals over a 4-year period,[16] including both suprainguinal and infrainguinal arterial reconstructions. There were 289 procedures in 275 patients, including 62 aortic reconstructions, 69 extra-anatomic bypasses, and 150 infrainguinal bypasses. Predictably, there was a difference in mortality based on age. The mortality was 15% for 101 patients over 70 years of age and 3% for 188 patients under the age of 70 years. In addition, the mortality rate for amputations (16%) and revascularization (17%) were comparable in the over-70 age group.[16] The mortality rate for 80 primary amputations compared with 49 amputations done after failed revascularization was not different (17% versus 12%), but these patient groups were not comparable. Significantly, the percentage of transfemo-

ral amputations rose from 16% for those under age 55 years to 50% for those over age 55 years.

Gregg analyzed his data using risk factors and divided his results into two patient groups: high risk and low risk. The preoperative risk factors included angina, prior myocardial infarction, atrial fibrillation, hypertension, cardiac decompensation, pacemaker, chronic obstructive pulmonary disease, and stroke with residual neurologic findings. A 100% mortality was reported by Gregg if four risk factors were present. Eighteen per cent of the high-risk patients died, and 18% required subsequent amputation. Only 7 high-risk patients were ambulatory 1 year after surgery. In marked contrast, the mortality rate in 110 low-risk patients was 4%, and 13% required eventual amputation.[16]

On the basis of an institutional policy of preferential revascularization, Hobson and colleagues reported a 5-year revascularization experience in 1985.[17] Three hundred seventy-five patients underwent revascularization (64% femoropopliteal; 37% femorotibial). The operative mortality and rate was 3%, the long-term survival rate was 58%. In contrast, 172 patients underwent primary transtibial amputations with a 13% operative mortality and a 57% long-term survival. The similar survival between patients undergoing revascularization versus primary amputation has been reported by other authors.[18] In the Hobson series, of those patients who underwent primary amputation, 64% were successfully rehabilitated but 23% required revision to transfemoral amputation.[17] Of note, Hobson's data did not suggest the need for revision to a higher level of amputation in those patients with failure of a prior revascularization versus those with successful revascularization (23% versus 19%).[17]

Criticisms of the Hobson study include an unacceptably high mortality rate for amputation compared with other series[18]; no explanation of the reasons for the high amputation and mortality rates; and indefinite indications for primary amputation (the amputation portion of the series includes 92 secondary amputations). By comparison, Bunt and Malone reported an amputation mortality rate of 1.5% in patients, regardless of age.[18] In the Bunt study, however, all patients with pedal sepsis were treated with physiologic amputation.[6, 7]

Outcomes in 362 patients over a 25-year period in an institution that favored primary amputation for patients with significant medical problems was reported by Ouriel and colleagues in 1988.[19] Two hundred four patients underwent revascularization (56% femoropopliteal; 44% femorodistal) for specific limb salvage indications, whereas 158 patients underwent primary transtibial amputation for what would appear to be equivalent limb salvage indications. Revascularization failures, trauma, infection, and nonreconstructible limbs were specifically excluded. The populations in the two groups were comparable.[19] In addition, patient risk was assessed by both Dripps anesthesia and Goldman Cardiopulmonary Risk Protocols.

The patients were divided into three categories according to risk analysis: low (A), moderate (B), and high (C). In the revascularization group, Ouriel and associates reported lower mortality, shorter hospital stays, and higher rates of postoperative ambulation. There was a statistically signifi-

TABLE 166–2. COMPARATIVE MORBIDITY AND MORTALITY FOR REVASCULARIZATION VERSUS PRIMARY AMPUTATION

AUTHOR (YEAR)	PROCEDURE	NO. OF PATIENTS	MORTALITY (%)	LONG-TERM SURVIVAL (%)
Hobson et al[17] (1985)	Revascularization	375	3	58 at 5 yr
	Amputation	172	13	57 at 5 yr
			($p < .01$)	
Ouriel et al[19] (1988)	Revascularization	204	2.9	
	Amputation	158	7.6	
			($p < .05$)	
Schina et al[20] (1992)	Revascularization	211	2	
	Amputation	122	4	
			(NSS)	
Bunt and Malone[18] (1994)	Age < 70 yr	183	2.2	
	Revascularization	212	1.5	
	Amputation		(NSS)	
	Age > 70 yr	119	8.0	84 at 1 yr
	Revascularization	253	1.5	50 at 1 yr
	Amputation		($p < .01$)	
Panayiotopoulos et al[9] (1997)	Revascularization	109		62 at 3 yr
	Amputation	43		39 at 3 yr
				(NSS)

NSS = Not statistically significant.

cant difference in the mortality rate for revascularization compared with primary amputation (2.9% versus 7.6%; $p < .05$).[19] Nearly all deaths in both groups occurred in Class C patients. Length of hospital stay for revascularization patients compared with that for primary amputation patients was 10 ± 1 days versus 19 ± 2 days for the A group, and 14 ± 2.1 days versus 31 ± 3 days for the C group ($p < .05$). Although an increased rate of ambulation for those undergoing revascularization (87%) versus those undergoing primary amputation (63%; $p < .01$) was reported, it is difficult to interpret these data because that institution has not reported amputation rehabilitation data at a center of excellence and compared their amputation data with other published reports.[15, 18]

Based upon literature reviews and our own results, we have reported that conventional rehabilitation techniques achieve an average rate of rehabilitation of 64%, whereas accelerated rehabilitation with immediate postoperative prostheses results in success rates as high as 100% in the short term, with over 90% sustained successful rehabilitation at 5 years.[15] With such findings, it is difficult to interpret the report by Ouriel and colleagues with respect to differences in ambulatory status of amputees versus patients undergoing revascularization. Ouriel and colleagues concluded that their conservative approach, in which amputation was offered preferentially to patients deemed medically compromised, was not supported by their data, because revascularization was performed with a lower mortality rate and better rates of postoperative ambulation than primary amputation. However, the amputation group had significantly more Class C patients ($p < .01$) and fewer A patients ($p < .05$).[19]

In 1991, our group analyzed the effect of an aggressive policy of limb salvage, reserving amputation for psychosocial considerations (see Table 166–1) or operatively determined inability to perform revascularization.[18] The amputation cohort was further subdivided into operations urgently performed for pedal sepsis versus those done electively.

The latter amputee group more closely approximates the clinical profile of patients who undergo revascularization. The independent effective age on mortality and morbidity was also analyzed.

Three hundred sixty-two primary revascularizations and 465 primary amputations were performed; 62% of the operations were performed in patients over 70 years of age. The mortality rate for revascularization versus amputation in the under-70 group was not statistically different (2.2% versus 1.5%). In the over-70 group, however, the mortality rate for revascularization was significantly higher than that for elective amputation (8% versus 1.5%; $p < .01$). The operative mortality rate of urgent amputations was 22%, ranging from 66% (12/18) for emergency amputation, to 25% (3/12) for guillotine amputation for pedal sepsis, to 8% (6/69) for definitive operative amputation after physiologic amputation ($p < .01$).[18] The improved 1-year survival for the over-70 age group for revascularization (84%) versus amputations (50%) may be inaccurate because there was no mortality correction for diabetes mellitus. We have shown in previous reports that the expected survival for amputees without diabetes is approximately normal, whereas the expected mortality rate after amputation for patients with diabetes is excessively high (71% at 5 years).[15]

In 1992, Schina and coworkers reported 266 patients treated over a 7-year period.[20] Two hundred eleven patients underwent 295 infrainguinal limb salvage operations and 122 underwent major lower extremity amputations (23 transmetatarsal, 70 transtibial, and 29 transfemoral). Amputations were performed in unreconstructible patients and in 39 patients with failed revascularizations. There was no overall difference in mortality between revascularization and amputation (2% versus 4%; not significant).[20] This report is interesting because the authors compared all *morbidity*, defined as all perioperative complications. The complication rate was 48% for primary revascularization, 35% for secondary revascularization ($p < .05$ compared with primary revascularization) and 37% for amputation ($p <$

.05 compared with primary revascularization). The most common complications were cardiac-, wound-, or graft-related. There was a significantly greater incidence of cardiac complication after primary revascularization ($p <$ .05).[20]

In 1997, Panayiotopoulos and associates reported a prospective analysis of 109 consecutive patients undergoing femorocrural-pedal bypass for critical lower limb ischemia in a singular vascular unit.[9] In addition, 43 amputations for unreconstructable distal disease were also analyzed. The outcomes included mortality, amputation, rehabilitation, and knee salvage rates. Primary amputees had a higher hospital mortality (18% versus 10%) but similar 3-year survival rates when compared with secondary amputees (30% versus 37%; not significant). Although patients with successful revascularization had higher survival rates at 3 years than amputees (62% versus 39%), this difference was not statistically significant. Factors associated with knee salvage in patients undergoing revascularization were the condition of inflow, patency of the profunda femoris artery, and graft material. Previous attempts at revascularization had a statistically significant deleterious effect on knee loss in those patients with unsuccessful reconstruction, but the authors nevertheless concluded that failure of a distal graft did not affect the final amputation level.[9]

DATA ANALYSIS SUMMARY

The preceding discussion emphasizes the difficulty in comparing primary revascularization and primary amputation. First, data on morbidity and mortality of revascularization versus amputation are based on different indications for amputation. There are significant differences in the clinical indications for amputation, and most series do not differentiate those patients presenting with acute foot sepsis requiring urgent amputation and those patients who undergo elective amputation. In many cases, elective revascularization is being compared with combined elective *and* emergency amputation.

Second, age is not addressed in most series. We have noted the effect of increasing age on mortality for both revascularization and amputation,[18] and our data are consistent with larger community studies, such as the Cleveland Metropolitan Registry data,[21] which demonstrated a linear effect of increasing age on operative mortality in vascular operations. The mortality rate for distal revascularization increased from 2.2% for patients under 75 years of age to 6.7% for patients over 75 years of age ($p <$ .01). Similarly, the amputation mortality increased from 9.8% to 14.7% ($p <$ .01) for patients younger than 75 years of age compared with those older than 75 years of age.

Gregg reported similar results from his reported community experience, in which the operative mortality rate increased from 3.5% to 15% for those under 70 versus those over 70 years of age.[16] Smaller single institutions may have different mortality rates. In 1986, Scher and colleagues, reported a mortality rate of only 6% in 168 patients over 80 years of age who had limb salvage procedures.[22] Friedman and associates reported a series of 50 patients over 80 years of age with 3.1% mortality,[23] and Edwards and associates described a 3.5% mortality in patients over 80 years

of age who underwent infrainguinal operations.[24] Owing to the reporting variability previously discussed, it is difficult to compare the smaller series with the larger series.

Third, it is the combination of the elderly patient with sepsis or urgent indications for amputation that predisposes the patient to excessive mortality when such patients are subjected to emergency amputation. Liberal use of physiologic amputation produced an overall mortality rate of 2.7% in 262 transfemoral amputations and 0.5% in 213 transtibial amputations in our series.[18] Physiologic amputation delays anesthesia and operative risks to an elective time frame, allowing control of sepsis and metabolic and hemodynamic stabilization.[6, 7, 18] Unfortunately, most of the other studies listed in Table 166–2 did not make use of physiologic amputation for elderly septic patients, so it is difficult to compare the authors' data with those reported by others.

COST-BENEFIT COMPARISON

The choice of operative procedure—revascularization versus primary amputation—cannot ethically be based on economic factors alone; however, the increasing importance of economic costs does force us to take a careful look at the cost-benefit ratios. Cost-comparison data are shown in Table 166–3.

A frequently quoted report by Gupta and colleagues in 1982 analyzed costs for revascularization versus primary amputation in their institution, where a policy of limb salvage was evaluated in 313 patients over a 3-year period.[25] Two hundred eighty-nine patients underwent either femoropopliteal (166) or femorodistal (123) bypasses, whereas only 24 patients underwent primary amputation. The choice of amputation was based on unreconstructible vascular disease, advanced gangrene, or psychosocial reasons. The two groups are not comparable based on operative indications and sample size, although Gupta and associates considered the groups to be similar, except for a higher incidence of foot necrosis in the amputation group. Costs included all hospital, physician, and rehabilitation charges. The costs and length of stay of revascularization versus the costs and length of stay of amputation are shown in Table 166–3. More important than the comparison of costs of amputation versus revascularization was the recognition that *unsuccessful* revascularization substantially increased costs and length of stay.[25]

The Gupta report is consistent with a study reported by Perler in 1994.[26] In the latter study, the costs for revascularization and primary amputation were similar when the costs of a prosthesis and rehabilitative therapy were included in the calculations for amputation.[26] Perler correctly points out that a flaw in analysis in many studies is that many patients with primary amputation do not ambulate, and therefore long-term institutionalization costs should be included in a cost analysis.

The present authors believe that amputation in patients who do not ambulate is not comparable to either amputation in patients who do ambulate or revascularization in other patients. Perler reported a significant increase in the costs of revascularization when the attempted revascularization failed ($28,374 versus $56,809).[26] Perler wrote, "The

TABLE 166–3. COMPARATIVE COSTS OF REVASCULARIZATION VERSUS AMPUTATION

AUTHOR (YEAR)	NO. OF PATIENTS	SURGERY	COST	HOSPITAL STAY (DAYS)
Gupta et al[25] (1982)	289	Revascularization	$26,194 ± 876	50 ± 2.3
	24	Amputation	$27,225 ± 2.896	60 ± 2.3
		Failure to amputate	$42,107 ± 486	78
Mackey et al[27] (1986)	78	Revascularization	$40,769 ± 3,726	67 ± 6
		Average	$28,374	
		Simple	$56,809	
	28	Amputation (average)	$40,563 ± 4,729	85 ± 10
Raviola et al[28] (1988)	94	Revascularization		15.4
		Simple	$20,300	
		Complex	$42,200	
	53	Amputation		18.4
		Simple	$20,400	
		Complex	$40,600	
Cheshire et al[29] (1992)	130	Revascularization		
		Simple	$6,898	
		Complex (PTFE)	$20,416	
		Complex (autogenous)	$15,024	
		Amputation	$21,726	
Perler[26] (1994)		Revascularization (secondary)	$28,344	
			$56,809	
Luther et al[11] (1996)		PTA	$11,353–22,482	
		Failed revascularization	$50,935	
		Failed	$15,059–16,033	
			$25,515	

PTA = percutaneous transluminal angioplasty; PTFE = polytetrafluoroethylene.

key to minimizing health care costs in this population is careful patient selection for initial revascularization, with aggressive long-term surveillance to ensure graft patency and limb viability." We would agree with that conclusion but add that fair comparisons for cost of amputation must emanate from centers of excellence with accelerated rehabilitation programs and that patients who are not candidates for ambulation after surgery cannot fairly be compared with patients undergoing revascularization.

Another cost-benefit analysis was published by Mackey and colleagues in 1986, which included the extended costs of revascularization versus amputation (i.e., long-term secondary complications as well as initial hospital costs).[27] As shown in Table 166–3, the cost for revascularization was $40,769 ± $3,726, compared with the cost of amputation of $40,563 ± $4,729. These costs did not include physician fees; inclusion of surgeon charges would most likely increase the cost of revascularization compared with amputation. The revascularization group had 2.4 ± 0.2 hospitalizations, with an average hospital stay of 67 ± 6 days; patients undergoing amputation had 2.2 ± 0.3 hospitalizations, with an average hospital stay of 85 ± 10 days. A successful initial revascularization procedure cost approximately half that of a failed revascularization. When patient groups were analyzed for indications of limb salvage, patients presenting with tissue loss incurred greater costs than those with rest pain alone.[27] An amputation done for tissue loss costs more than revascularization, but an amputation done for rest pain costs less than revascularization for the same indication.[27]

In 1988, Raviola and associates reported costs of amputations.[28] The data included hospital costs and professional fees. Rehabilitation costs averaged $6,400 per patient, because all services were performed on an outpatient basis. In this series, the average cost for 53 primary transtibial amputations was $20,400 (18.4 hospital days), which increased to $40,600 if complications occurred.[28] The average cost for 94 femoropopliteal bypass grafts was $20,300 (15.4 hospital days), which increased to $28,700 if the grafts were successfully revised, and $42,200 if the graft failure led to amputation.[28] This is a noteworthy report because it came from a center of excellence in amputation surgery.

In 1992, Cheshire and colleagues evaluated primary and secondary expenses for revascularization versus amputation and compared the variable of autogenous versus polytetrafluoroethylene (PTFE) grafts.[29] One hundred thirty patients who presented with limb salvage indications over a 5-year period underwent femorodistal reconstruction (41 with PTFE grafts and 89 autologous saphenous vein grafts), and the costs of these procedures were compared with the costs of primary amputation. Operative mortality was less than 1% for revascularization procedures but over 10% for the amputation group. Survival was 80% at a mean follow-up of 20 months for both groups. The significantly increased mortality rate for amputation is controversial in the Cheshire study and, unfortunately, its impact on cost was not analyzed. The mean cost of a revascularization procedure was $6,898 for both PTFE and autologous grafts, which increased to $7,074 for revisional surgery.[29] When revision costs are included, the *total* cost for autologous vein grafts was $15,024 and $20,416 for PTFE grafts. The costs for primary amputation were $21,726. It is unclear why the base revascularization costs ($6,898) are so low, approximately one third to one fourth of what others have reported. Cheshire and associates summarized their data as follows: revascularization was 44% less expensive than amputation for autologous vein grafts and 6% less expensive for synthetic grafts.[29] In addition, they reported that only one third of amputees achieved ambulatory status, as opposed to 80% of revascularization patients. Again, this is a surprisingly low rate of ambulation.[15]

Cost analysis data are equally as difficult to compare as morbidity and mortality data, for many of the same reasons discussed previously. Cost analysis becomes even more confusing if the variable of percutaneous transluminal angioplasty (PTA) is introduced. Luther and colleagues compared costs between PTA and femoropopliteal bypass for patients with chronic limb ischemia due to femoropopliteal disease.[11] As shown in Table 166–3, PTA was less expensive than revascularization. The cost of both PTA and revascularization increased with revisions, whereas with failure of treatment the cost of PTA more than doubled the cost of a failed revascularization.[11]

The costs of prostheses are not well examined in the literature. Transtibial prostheses range in price from several thousand to over $10,000. Clearly, prosthetic costs can have a significant impact on cost comparison data. Unpublished data from our group, based upon our experience with an aggressive accelerated rehabilitation program in Phoenix, which utilizes extensive outpatient occupational therapy and functional but conservatively priced prostheses, demonstrate that patients undergoing primary transtibial amputations can be treated for a total cost of approximately $25,000. Ambulation success rates are in excess of 90% at 1 and 3 years. Unfortunately, comparison of our own revascularization versus primary amputation data is flawed because of the same variables discussed previously.[18] At a county hospital in metropolitan Phoenix, we determined that the cost (surgeon, prosthetist, hospital, rehabilitation, and prosthesis) of primary amputation was lower ($42,000 versus $47,000) and successful postamputation rehabilitation was higher (95% versus 60%) in those patients treated with immediate postoperative prostheses[30] compared with conventional rehabilitation techniques.

In general, we might conclude the following:

1. An amputation done without prescribing a lower limb prosthesis is less costly than one that involves a prosthesis and rehabilitation cost.

2. An amputation done for relief of rest pain is less costly than that done for tissue loss (encouraging performance of earlier amputation before patients deteriorate).

3. Complications of either revascularization or amputation substantially increase costs.

4. The impact of new or endovascular procedures on the cost comparisons between revascularizations and primary amputations are unknown at present.

5. The surgeons' skill and judgment and the institution's experience with amputation rehabilitation will greatly influence comparative costs and cannot be easily accounted for in cost comparison studies.

It is fair to say that a well-done revascularization that results in limb salvage and ambulation probably costs less than primary amputation. In addition, it is established that operative complications from revascularization produce costs that are far higher than primary amputation. However,

the total cost of primary amputation must include the postoperative ambulatory status of the patient, the cost of rehabilitation, and the cost of a prosthesis. Although, cost data cannot singularly be used to justify a surgical approach, we should strive to lower the costs of the chosen approach in every patient.

RISK OF HIGHER-LEVEL AMPUTATION

Predictably, some studies support contrary positions: (1) failure of primary revascularization leads to a higher level of amputation, decreased rehabilitation, and increased overall morbidity from the combined operative procedures; and (2) revascularization saves many patients from amputation and does not raise amputation levels if bypasses fail. Advocates for both sides of this controversy admit that patients in whom poorly planned or poorly executed operations of either type are performed sustain amputations at a higher level than expected. Again, it is difficult to assess the merits of either position because of many uncontrolled variables in studies supporting one side or the other.

Stoney set the stage for discussion with his eloquent publication in 1978, in which he noted that in four series of revascularizations, half of all failures led to higher levels of amputation.[31] He suggested that the surgeon recognize his or her obligation to provide the operation most likely to benefit the patient, not the surgeon. In 1982, Dardik and colleagues reported that femoropopliteal grafts failed more often than femorotibial grafts and that the graft failures resulted in an unanticipated higher level of amputation.[32] However, other authors have reported little difference in the healing rates of primary transtibial amputation versus one performed after failure of revascularization, with healing rates ranging from 75% to 85%.

Reports from more recent literature further confuse the picture. As previously discussed, Hallett and associates reported that increased vascular reconstructive surgery and balloon angioplasty rates have coincided with a significant reduction in major amputation rates.[14] In 1997, Karlstrom and Bergqvist reported that increased vascular intervention produced improved limb salvage rates and decreased amputation rates.[12] They also suggested that it was important for ethical and economic reasons to identify the appropriate patient for revascularization because the choice of operation influenced limb salvage but not survival.

In 1980, Kazmers and colleagues designed a prospective study to asses the outcome of 40 limbs amputated after failed bypass and compared the *actual* level of amputation with that *predicted* by Doppler pressure measurements performed prior to revascularization.[37] A Doppler popliteal arterial pressure of 60 mmHg predicted an 87% healing rate, based upon published literature. It is important to point out, however, that Lim and colleagues reported in 1967 that transtibial amputations done in "all comers" without preselection resulted in a combined primary and secondary rate of healing of 85%,[33] challenging the utility of Doppler pressures. In the Kazmers study, 33 of the 40 amputated limbs had a popliteal arterial pressure of 60 mmHg or higher; 52% of transtibial amputations healed in these patients. Four of 7 patients with pressure of less than

60 mmHg also healed. The authors concluded that the observed decrease in healing rate from a theoretical 87% to 52% was related to the failed bypass.[37] Moreover, a healing rate of 52%, compared with Lim's reported 85% with no testing, probably does represent a real decrease in limb salvage rates due to failed bypass. However, such comparisons of noncontrolled series from different centers and different authors are problematic. In addition, the Kazmers study included 7 patients who had tibial explorations without revascularizations and 7 patients who underwent primary transfemoral amputations.

In 1990, Evans and associates compared 210 amputations after failed revascularization procedures with 551 primary amputations; 319 primary amputations were performed, with a 6.6% perioperative mortality and a 92% healing rate.[39] Ninety-two per cent of the patients with a popliteal pressure of 60 mmHg or more healed, but 56% of those with popliteal pressures of less than 60 mmHg also healed. The inability of absolute popliteal arterial pressure to predict accurately transtibial amputation healing has been reported by others.[15] After a failed bypass, there was a 3% mortality and a 77% rate of primary healing in 147 transtibial amputations ($p < .01$). Of those 147 patients, 61% with popliteal arterial pressures of 60 mmHg or more healed primarily, whereas 64% of those patients with pressures of 60 mmHg or less healed primarily.[39] A 77% healing rate for transtibial amputation in limbs with a failed bypass, compared with the 92% ($p < .01$) healing rate for primary amputations performed at the same institution, is an important observation.

Sethia and associates concluded that injudicious attempts at bypass raised the level of amputation; of note, healing problems were almost as common after transfemoral amputations as transtibial amputations,[40] thereby raising questions about patient selection or operative technique. Epstein and colleagues reported a significantly higher proportion of transfemoral amputations after 32 failed revascularizations, compared with 43 primary amputations. They also reported that the transtibial amputation primary healing rate was 85%, but that only 64% of secondary amputations healed.[41]

At this point, we can conclude the following:

1. Although revascularization salvages limbs, there does not appear to be a difference in survival rates between those patients undergoing revascularization compared with those patients undergoing primary amputation.

2. Injudicious revascularization or multiple attempts at revascularization probably lead to higher levels of amputation.

3. Secondary amputations are equivalent in those patients undergoing revascularization with synthetic grafts and autologous grafts.

4. The controversy over raised amputation level after failed revascularization remains unanswered.

5. Distal revascularizations should have the incisions planned so that graft failure does not lead to a compromised amputation.

SPECIAL CONSIDERATIONS

Calcific Vessels

Patients with diabetes mellitus commonly have arterial medial calcinosis. In some patients, rigid pipe-like casts of the trifurcation vessels or the pedal vessels are visible on plain radiograph. The success of distal bypass is increasingly dependent on technical perfection the lower the anastomosis is placed in the arterial tree. Calcific vessels make arteriotomy difficult. The intima and the walls tend to fragment. Suturing is difficult, and the application of excessive force, or "pushing the needle through the wall," may result in arterial laceration or injury. Because of these technical issues, some surgeons consider heavily calcified vessels to be a contraindication to revascularization. However, calcific vessels can serve as targets for successful bypasses if the surgeon uses perseverance and patience. Employment of temporary tourniquet occlusion rather than standard clamps, use of special tempered steel needles, and the application of the fracture-crush technique described in 1986 by Ascer and associates facilitates construction of these anastomoses.[42] That report documented 75% patency of grafts to severely calcified vessels at 30 days, and 47% at 3 years. Those patency rates are not significantly different for anastomosis to less severely calcified vessels.[42, 43]

Poor Outflow

As illogical as it seems, patency rates for bypass grafts to isolated popliteal arteries (segments) are equivalent to those for revascularization procedures to nonisolated popliteal arteries.[44] In addition, Ascer and associates reported excellent results with bypass grafts to plantar arteries, a procedure they define as an extended approach to limb salvage.[43] The excellent results reported by Ascer and associates underscore the precision in surgical technique required when one is "pushing the limits" of revascularization. The published data, therefore, suggest that there is little reason to prohibit revascularization based on outflow alone; however, superb surgical technique is important if one expects to achieve excellent patency rates.

Synthetic Versus Autogenous Grafts

When synthetic grafts rather than autogenous veins are used as conduits, all published series on lower extremity revascularization report a decreased patency for below-knee bypasses, and especially for femorodistal bypasses.

The key question is, Should a distal reconstruction be attempted if an autogenous conduit is inadequate or unavailable? Multiple reports suggest that successful long-term limb salvage can be achieved using cephalic vein bypass grafts.[45–47] Dardik and colleagues have described using a distal arteriovenous fistula as a potential adjunct to increase patency rates with human umbilical vein.[48] Newer small series suggest that use of "Taylor" patches for synthetic PTFE grafts in distal revascularization increases patency and improves limb salvage. It remains to be seen in carefully controlled large prospective studies whether these new techniques truly improve limb salvage.

The absence of an autogenous vein should seldom represent an indication for primary amputation. Failure of an autogenous vein bypass with no suitable autologous vein, thereby requiring a secondary or tertiary reconstruction with a synthetic conduit, is a soft indication for primary amputation. However, several revascularization failures of synthetic grafts (not mere revisions to achieve extended patency) mandate amputation rather than another recon-struction with prosthetic material that would in all proba-bility fail.

Nontechnical Considerations

It is increasingly common for patients with a prior amputa-tion to present with a threatened contralateral limb.[49] The decision regarding revascularization of the remaining leg should be made using the same clinical and psychosocial indications used in patients without an amputation. The ability to walk with or without a prosthesis and the ability to transfer are important considerations for continued self-sufficiency.

It is important to remember that the rate of contralateral limb loss in diabetic patients who have undergone one major limb amputation is 15% to 33% over 5 years.[15] In all probability, however, a diabetic amputee is more likely to die of cardiac complications prior to contralateral limb loss.[15] Because of the risk of contralateral limb loss, espe-cially in diabetic patients, careful attention should be paid to the contralateral limb after revascularization or amputa-tion. It is extremely important to instruct diabetic patients about foot care, diet, insulin, blood glucose testing, and physician follow-up, because amputation in diabetic pa-tients can be postponed or avoided with good foot care, control of fasting blood glucose levels, control of hyperten-sion, and maintenance of normal hemoglobin A_{1C}.

Large Foot Ulcers

Large ulcers, particularly those involving the heel and the calcaneus, have been thought to represent a contraindica-tion to successful revascularization. Limb salvage can be achieved with distal revascularization combined with mi-crovascular transfer of free flaps.[50] Whether or not it is safe to use a distal bypass graft as a source of donor inflow for a free flap is as yet unresolved. However, a combination of a distal bypass with a microvascular free flap represents a heroic measure to limb salvage and such combined proce-dures substantially increase costs. To date, cost analysis of such a combined approach has not been done. Neverthe-less, a large forefoot or heel ulcer is neither a contraindica-tion for distal revascularization nor a major indication for primary amputation: A complicating factor for patients with large foot ulcers is osteomyelitis or low-grade pedal sepsis, which increases the morbidity and mortality for either revascularization or primary amputation.[51]

End-Stage Renal Disease

End-stage renal disease (ESRD) requiring dialysis, especially in the presence of diabetes mellitus, has been uniformly associated with decreased limb salvage after revasculariza-tion.[52, 53] In contrast, ESRD in diabetic patients does not seem to influence the mortality or rehabilitation rates for patients undergoing primary transtibial amputation in cen-ters of amputation excellence.[15] Edwards and associates suggest that primary amputation should be performed in patients presenting with profound limb ischemia and ESRD.[52] A more recent study by Simsir and group reported that more liberal use of primary amputation for patients

with ESRD with critical leg ischemia may be indicated.[4] Patients undergoing amputation and revascularization were similar in age, cause, duration of renal failure, and the presence of coronary artery disease. The operative mortality rate in the revascularization patients compared with the amputation patients was 13% versus 20%, and 71% of the deaths were caused by sepsis. Limb salvage at 1 year was 67%, and 1-year survival in both the primary amputation and revascularization groups was 72%.[4] In 1990, Harring-ton and associates analyzed 39 patients (59 limbs) with ESRD who underwent limb salvage procedures.[53] Primary patency was 77% at 1 year and operative mortality was 7.7%, but 3-year survival was only 39%. The poor survival is not surprising for patients with diabetes mellitus.[15] Of the patients who were alive at 3 years in the Harrington study, 84% had a salvaged limb.[53]

REVISION VERSUS REOPERATION FOR FAILED GRAFT

In analyzing revascularization and primary amputation, we must distinguish reoperation for revision of a *failing* graft from reoperation for a *failed* graft. Many failing grafts can be successfully revised to achieve secondary patencies not dissimilar to those of primary grafts. In general, the mor-bidity and mortality for revision of failing grafts is quite low, and revision of a failing graft is clearly superior to primary amputation. However, reoperation for a failed graft starts to beg the question, "When is enough, enough?" In the authors' experience, two attempts at lower extremity revascularization (not including graft revision) are reason-able, four attempts are probably unreasonable, and it is unclear whether or not a third attempt is justified. The decision-making process must be individualized for each patient according to (1) medical condition, (2) expected limb salvage potential, (3) technical and anatomic consider-ations, and (4) the surgeon's experience and skills.

GRAFT INFECTION

Some authors have suggested that primary amputation is the preferable solution for infection in a lower extremity bypass graft.[54] More recent reports have suggested that limb salvage in the face of graft infection is not only possible but reasonably probable.[55, 56] Although graft infection does not mandate amputation, careful analysis of each patient is required. Overly aggressive attempts at limb salvage with lower extremity graft infection will increase patient mortal-ity, but careful, well-planned attempts at lower extremity salvage with prosthetic graft infection are appropriate in selected patients. Of note, Rubin and associates reported that amputation complications in patients with prior lower extremity graft infections are substantially higher than in uninfected patients.[57]

PATIENT EDUCATION

Although the focus of this chapter is to provide information on which to base the decision for primary amputation versus revascularization, perhaps our efforts should concentrate on patient education. As previously mentioned, lower extremity amputation in diabetic patients can be postponed or avoided. In 1989, our group reported a prospective randomized series showing that a diabetic educational program could lower the incidence of major limb amputation threefold ($p < .025$).[58] This original study had 1 year's follow-up. We have recently completed a 10-year review of those same study patients and have found that the rates of major limb amputation were 5% in the education group and 15% in the noneducation group ($p < .044$).

SUMMARY

The controversy over primary amputation versus revascularization remains unresolved. As extensively discussed, data analysis is confounded by lack of prospective randomized studies, inability to compare one series with another, differences in technique and judgment of different surgeons, and wide disparity in results among centers specializing in lower limb revascularization and centers specializing in accelerated rehabilitation after amputation. Thus, there is no single recommendation for an individual patient other than careful, thoughtful consideration by the surgeon.

In addition, although economic data should not be used to justify one surgical procedure against another, patient morbidity and mortality and economic costs are variables that weigh into the ultimate decision to perform primary amputation versus revascularization for limb salvage. For most vascular surgeons and patients, limb salvage is the primary goal that usually can be achieved at acceptable morbidity, mortality, and monetary costs. The final deciding factor may very well be the results of rehabilitation following amputation and the durability of amputation compared with the durability of revascularization.

REFERENCES

1. Laverly LA, vanHoutum WH, Armstrong DG, et al: Mortality following lower extremity amputation in minorities with diabetes mellitus. Diabetes Res Clin Pract 37(1):41–47, 1997.
2. Guadagnoli E, Ayanian JZ, Gibbons G, et al: The influence of race on the use of surgical procedures for treatment of peripheral vascular disease of the lower extremities. Arch Surg 130(4):381–386, 1995.
3. Laverly LA, Ashry HR, vanHoutum W, et al: Variation in the incidence and proportion of diabetes-related amputations in minorities. Diabetes Care 19(1):48–52, 1996.
4. Simsir SA, Cabellon A, Kohlman-Trigoboff D, et al: Factors influencing limb salvage and survival after amputation and revascularization in patients with end-stage renal disease. Am J Surg 170(2):113–117, 1995.
5. Brinker MR, Timberlake GA, Goff JM, et al: Below-knee physiologic cryoanesthesia in the critically ill patient. J Vasc Surg 7:433–438, 1988.
6. Bunt TJ: Physiologic amputation for acute pedal sepsis. Am Surg 56(9):520, 1990.
7. Bunt TJ, Manship LR, Bynol RP, Haynes JL: Lower extremity amputation: A low mortality operation. Am Surg 50(11):581, 1984.
8. Johansen K, Burgess EM, Zorn R, et al: Improvement of amputation level by lower extremity revascularization. Surg Gynecol Obstet 153:707–709, 1981.
9. Panayiotopoulos YP, Reidy JF, Taylor PR: The concept of knee salvage: Why does a failed femorocrural/pedal arterial bypass not affect the amputation level? Eur J Vasc Endovasc Surg 13(5):477–485, 1997.
10. Mattes E, Norman PE, Jamrozik K: Falling incidence of amputation for peripheral occlusive arterial disease in Western Australia between 1980–1992. Eur J Vasc Endovasc Surg 13(1):14–22, 1997.
11. Luther M, Lepantalo M, Alback A, et al: Amputation rates as a measure of vascular surgical results. Br J Surg 83(2):241–244, 1996.
12. Karlstrom L, Bergqvist D: Effects of vascular surgery on amputation rates and mortality. Eur J Vasc Endovasc Surg 14(4):273–283, 1997.
13. The Westcoast Vascular Surgeons (WVS) Study Group: Variations of rates of vascular surgical procedures for chronic critical limb ischaemia and lower limb amputation rates in western Swedish counties. Eur J Vasc Endovasc Surg 14(4):310–314, 1997.
14. Hallett JW Jr, Byrne J, Gayari MM, et al: Impact of arterial surgery and balloon angioplasty on amputation: A population-based study of 1155 procedures between 1973 and 1992. J Vasc Surg 25(1):29–38, 1997.
15. Malone JM: Lower extremity amputation. In Moore WS: Vascular Surgery: A Comprehensive Review, 5th ed. Philadelphia, WB Saunders, 1998.
16. Gregg RO: Bypass or amputation? Concomitant review of bypass arterial grafting and major amputations. Am J Surg 149(3):397, 1985.
17. Hobson RW, Lynch TG, Zafor J, et al: Results of revascularization and amputation in severe lower extremity ischemia: A five-year experience. J Vasc Surg 2(1):174, 1985.
18. Bunt TJ, Malone JM: Revascularization or amputation in the over 70 year old. Am Surg 60(5):349–352, 1994.
19. Ouriel K, Fiore WM, Geary JE: Limb-threatening ischemia in the medically compromised patient: Amputation or revascularization? Surgery 104(4):667, 1988.
20. Schina MJ Jr, Atnip RG, Healy DA, Thiele BL: The relative risk of limb revascularization and amputation in the modern era. J Vasc Surg Cardiovasc Surg 2:754, 1994.
21. Plecha FR, Bertin VS, Plecha EJ, et al: The early results of vascular surgery in patients 75 years of age and older: Analysis of 3,259 cases. J Vasc Surg 2:769, 1985.
22. Scher LA, Veith FJ, Ascer E, et al: Limb salvage in octogenarians and nonagenarians. Surgery 99(2):160, 1986.
23. Friedman SG, Kerner BA, Friedman MS, Moccio CG: Limb salvage in elderly patients: Is aggressive surgical therapy warranted? J Cardiovasc Surg 30(5):848, 1989.
24. Edwards WH, Mueherin JL Jr, Rogers DM: Vascular reconstruction in the octogenarian. South Med J 75:648, 1982.
25. Gupta SK, Veith FJ, Samson RH, et al: Cost analysis of operations for infrainguinal arteriosclerosis (Abstract). Circulation 66(Suppl 2):II-9, 1982.
26. Perler BA: Vascular disease in the elderly patient. Surg Clin North Am 74(1):200–216, 1994.
27. Mackey WC, McCullough JL, Conlon TP, et al: The costs of surgery for limb-threatening ischemia. Surgery 99(1):26, 1986.
28. Raviola CA, Nichter LA, Baker JD: Cost of treating advanced leg ischemia: Bypass graft vs. primary amputation. Arch Surg 123(8):495, 1988.
29. Cheshire NJW, Wolfe SHN, Nocne MA, et al: The economics of femorocrural reconstruction for critical leg ischemia with and without autologous vein. J Vasc Surg 15(1):170, 1992.
30. Pippinich L, Malone JM: Cost effectiveness of lower extremity immediate postoperative prosthesis. Presented at the Pan-Pacific Prosthetic Conference, Hawaii, 1996.
31. Stoney RJ: Ultimate salvage for the patient with limb-threatening ischemia. Am J Surg 136:228, 1978.
32. Dardik H, Hahn M, Dardik I, et al: Influence of failed vascular bypass procedures on conversion of below knee to above-knee amputation levels. Surgery 91:64, 1982.
33. Samson RH, Gupta SK, Scher LA, Veith FJ: Level of amputation after failure of limb salvage procedures. Surg Gynecol Obstet 154(1):56, 1982.
34. Burgess EM, Marsden FW: Major lower extremity amputations following arterial reconstruction. Arch Surg 108:655, 1976.
35. Schlenker JD, Wolkoff JS: Major amputations after femoropopliteal bypass procedures. Am J Surg 129:495, 1975.
36. Kihn RB, Warren R, Beebe GW: The geriatric amputee. Ann Surg 176:305, 1972.
37. Kazmers M, Satiani B, Evans WE: Amputation level following unsuccessful distal limb salvage operations. Surgery 87(6):683, 1980.
38. Lim RC Jr, Blaisdell FW, Hall AD, et al: Below-knee amputation for ischemic gangrene. Surg Gynecol Obstet 125:493–501, 1967.
39. Evans WE, Hayes JP, Vermilion BD: Effect of a failed distal reconstruction on the level of amputation. Am J Surg 160(8):217, 1990.

40. Sethia KK, Berry AR, Morrison JD, et al: Changing pattern of lower limb amputation for vascular disease. Br J Surg 73(9):701, 1986.

41. Epstein SB, Worth MH, El Ferzli G: Level of amputation following failed vascular reconstruction for lower limb ischemia. Curr Surg May-June:185, 1989.

42. Ascer E, Veith FJ, Flores SAW: Infrapopliteal bypasses to heavily calcified rock-like arteries: Management and results. Am J Surg 152(8):220, 1986.

43. Ascer E, Veith FJ, Gupta SK: Bypass to plantar arteries: An extended approach to limb salvage. J Vasc Surg 8(4):434, 1988.

44. Mannick JA, Jackson BT, Coffman JD: Success of bypass vein grafts in patients with isolated popliteal artery segments. Surgery 61:17–35, 1967.

45. Harris RW, Andros G, Dulana LB, et al: Successful long-term limb salvage using cephalic vein bypass grafts. Ann Surg 200:785–794, 1984.

46. Londrew GL, Bosher LP, Brown PW, et al: Infrainguinal reconstruction with arm vein, lesser saphenous vein, and remnants of greater saphenous vein: A report of 257 cases. J Vasc Surg 20:451–457, 1994.

47. Sesto ME, Sullivan TM, Hertzer NR, et al: Cepahlic vein grafts for lower extremity revascularization. J Vasc Surg 15:543–549, 1992.

48. Dardik H, Berry SM, Dardik A, et al: Infrapopliteal prosthetic graft patency by use of distal adjunctive arteriovenous fistula. J Vasc Surg 3(5):685, 1991.

49. Powell TW, Burnham SJ, Johnson G Jr: Second leg ischemia: Lower extremity bypass vs. amputation in patients with contralateral lower extremity amputation. Am Surg 50(11):577, 1984.

50. Greenwald LL, Comefota A, Mitra A, et al: Free vascularized tissue transfer for limb salvage in peripheral vascular disease. Ann Vasc Surg 4(3):244, 1990.

51. Rubin JR, Pitluk HC, Graham LM: Do operative results justify tibial artery reconstruction in the presence of pedal sepsis? Am J Surg 156:144, 1988.

52. Edwards JM, Taylor LM, Porter JM: Limb salvage in end-stage renal disease (ESRD): Comparison of modern results in patients with and without ESRD. Arch Surg 123(9):1164, 1988.

53. Harrington EB, Harrington ME, Schnazer H, et al: End-stage renal disease: Is infrainguinal limb revascularization justified? J Vasc Surg 12(6):691, 1990.

54. Kitka MJ, Goodson SF, Bishara RA, et al: Mortality and limb loss with infected infrainguinal bypass grafts. J Vasc Surg 5:566, 1987.

55. Baytes BT, Mesh CL, McGee GS, et al: Lung-threatening ischemia complicated by perigeniculate infection. J Surg Res 54:163, 1993.

56. Bunt TJ: Vascular graft infections: A personal experience. J Cardiovasc Surg 1:489, 1993.

57. Rubin JR, Yao JST, Thompson RG, et al: Management of infection of major amputation stumps after failed femorodistal grafts. Surgery 98(4):810, 1985.

58. Malone JM, Synder J, Anderson G, et al: Prevention of amputation by diabetic education. Am J Surg 158:520–524, 1989.

INDEX

Note: Page numbers in *italics* refer to illustrations; page numbers followed by t refer to tables.

i